Nursing Care Plan

Guidelines

CONGRATULATIONS

You now have access to Mosby's "Get Connected" Bonus Package!

Here's what's included to help you "Get Connected"

sign on at:

http://www.harcourthealth.com/MERLIN/Wong/maternal/

A website just for you as you learn maternity and pediatric nursing with the 2nd edition of **Maternal Child Nursing Care**

what you will receive:

Whether you're a student, an instructor, or a clinician, you'll find information just for you. Things like:

- Special Features
- Links to Related Products
- Author Information... and more

plus:

LIFT HERE

PASSCODE INSIDE

If passcode sticker is removed, this textbook cannot be returned to Mosby, Inc.

Mosby WebLinks

An exciting program that allows you to directly access hundreds of active websites keyed specifically to the content of this book. The WebLinks are continually updated, with new ones added as they develop. **Peel the top layer only from the sticker on this page and register with the listed passcode.**

MERLIN

Mosby's Electronic Resource Links & Information Network

Mosby
A Harcourt Health Sciences Company

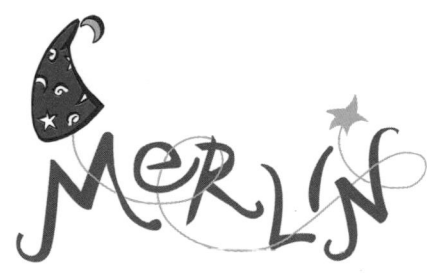

Maternal Child Nursing Care

2nd EDITION

Maternal Child Nursing Care

DONNA L. WONG, PhD, RN, PNP, CPN, FAAN

Adjunct Associate Professor, University of Oklahoma College of Medicine—Tulsa;
Adjunct Professor, University of Oklahoma College of Nursing;
Adjunct Professor/Consultant
Oral Roberts University Anna Vaughn School of Nursing Tulsa, Oklahoma;
Consultant, Children's Hospital at Saint Francis, Tulsa, Oklahoma;
Consultant, Texas Children's Hospital, Houston, Texas

SHANNON E. PERRY, PhD, RN, CNS, FAAN

Professor, School of Nursing
Coordinator, Child and Adolescent Development Program
Marion Wright Edelman Institute
San Francisco State University
San Francisco, California

MARILYN J. HOCKENBERRY, PhD, RN-CS, PNP, FAAN

Professor, Department of Pediatrics
Baylor College of Medicine;
Director of Nurse Practitioners, Texas Children's Cancer Center
Texas Children's Hospital, Houston, Texas

Associate Editor

DEITRA LEONARD LOWDERMILK, PhD, RNC, FAAN

Clinical Professor, School of Nursing
University of North Carolina at Chapel Hill
Chapel Hill, North Carolina

Mosby

A Harcourt Health Sciences Company

St. Louis London Philadelphia Sydney Toronto

Mosby
A Harcourt Health Sciences Company

Vice President, Publishing Director: Sally Schrefer
Senior Editors: Michael S. Ledbetter *and* Loren S. Wilson
Senior Developmental Editors: Laurie K. Muench *and* Michele D. Hayden
Project Manager: Deborah Vogel
Production Editor: Ed Alderman
Book Designer: Teresa Breckwoldt

SECOND EDITION

NOTICE:
Pharmacology is an ever-changing field. Standard safety precautions must be followed, but as new research and clinical experience broaden our knowledge, changes in treatment and drug therapy may become necessary or appropriate. Readers are advised to check the most current product information provided by the manufacturer of each drug to be administered to verify the recommended dose, the method and duration of administration, and contraindications. It is the responsibility of the treating appropriately licensed health care provider, relying on experience and knowledge of the patient, to determine dosages and the best treatment for each individual patient. Neither the publisher nor the editor assumes any liability for any injury and/or damage to persons or property arising from this publication.

Mosby, Inc.
A Harcourt Health Sciences Company
11830 Westline Industrial Drive
St. Louis, MO 63146

Printed in the United States of America

Library of Congress Cataloging-in-Publication Data

Wong, Donna L., 1948-
Maternal child nursing care / Donna L. Wong, Shannon E. Perry, Marilyn Hockenberry; associate editor, Deitra Leonard Lowdermilk.—2nd ed.
p. ; cm.
Includes bibliographical references and index.
ISBN 0-323-01399-6 (alk. paper)
1. Maternity nursing. 2. Pediatric nursing. I. Perry, Shannon E. II. Hockenberry, Marilyn J. III. Lowermilk, Deitra Leonard.
[DNLM: 1. Maternal-Child Nursing—methods. 2. Pediatric Nursing—methods. WY 157.3 W872m 2001
RG951 .W87 2001
610.73′62—dc21

2001030745

01 02 03 04 05 GW/KPT 9 8 7 6 5 4 3 2 1

Preface

This second edition of *Maternal Child Nursing Care* combines essential information on maternity and pediatric nursing into one text. The text focuses on the care of women during their reproductive years and on children from newborn through adolescence. Issues and concerns of childbearing women and the health care of children are the primary concentrations. The promotion of wellness and the management of common women's health problems and child development are also addressed.

Maternal Child Nursing Care was developed to provide students with the knowledge and skills they need to become competent, critical thinkers, and to attain the sensitivity needed to become caring nurses. This second edition has been revised and refined in response to comments and suggestions from educators, clinicians, and students. It includes the most accurate, current, and clinically relevant information available. As we move further into the 21st Century, this second edition of *Maternal Child Nursing Care* is designed to address the changing needs of women and children during their childbearing and developing years.

Many exciting changes will be evident throughout the book; they demonstrate the different dimensions of health care for women and children. However, we have retained the underlying philosophy of the previous edition: we believe that pregnancy and childbirth, and the developmental changes in a woman's life, are natural processes; we believe that the promotion of normal childhood growth and development is an essential nursing function. Our goal continues to be to help students understand and recognize these normal processes before asking them to identify any complications and to comprehend their implications for care.

The goal of nursing education is to prepare today's student to meet the challenges of tomorrow. This preparation must extend beyond the mastery of facts and skills. Nurses must be able to combine competence with caring and critical thinking. They must address both the physiologic and the psychosocial needs of patients. Above all, they must look beyond the condition and see women and children as individuals with distinctive needs but living in the context of the family.

APPROACH

Professional nursing practice continues to evolve and adapt to society's changing health priorities. The rapidly changing health care delivery system offers new opportunities for nurses to alter the practice of maternity and pediatric nursing and to improve the way care is given. Consumers of maternity and pediatric care vary in age, ethnicity, culture, language, social status, marital status, and sexual orientation. They seek care from obstetricians, gynecologists, pediatricians, family practice physicians, nurse midwives, nurse practitioners, and other health care providers in a variety of health care settings, including the home.

Nursing education must reflect these changes. Clinical education must be planned to offer students a variety of health care experiences in settings that include hospitals and birth centers, homes, clinics, private physicians' offices, shelters for the homeless or for women and children in need of protection, and other community-based settings. The changing needs of nursing students must also be addressed. Today's nursing students are challenged to learn more than ever before—and often in less time than their predecessors.

Care Management has been used as an organizing framework for discussion in the nursing care chapters. This approach demonstrates how nursing must collaborate with other health care disciplines to provide the most comprehensive care possible to women and children. Assessments, nursing diagnoses, expected outcomes, nursing implementation, and evaluation of care are highlighted throughout the chapters. Nursing care plans reinforce the problem-solving approach to patient care. In chapters that focus on complications of childbearing, reproductive conditions, and childhood illnesses, medical interventions are presented first and followed by nursing care management.

Health care today emphasizes *wellness.* This focus is an integral part of our philosophy. The developmental changes that a woman experiences throughout her life are considered to be natural and normal. Understanding normal growth and development of the child is essential to our philosophy of care. The goal of promoting wellness is achieved through imparting knowledge of the body and its normal functions, and developing awareness of conditions that require medical intervention. The unit on reproductive concerns has been expanded to emphasize the wellness aspect of care. This unit has been placed before the units on pregnancy because many of the aspects of assessment and care can be applied to later chapters. We present normal aspects of the childbearing cycle before discussing potential complications.

The pediatric section of the book is organized by first emphasizing health promotion and wellness of the child from infancy through adolescence. This is presented from a developmental context with the family as the focus of care. The care of healthy children who experience common health problems is presented within these chapters. The remaining chapters present the more serious health problems experienced by children and adolescents that are not specific to a particular age group.

Patient education is an essential component of nursing care of women and children. The chapter on women's health promotion and screening emphasizes teaching for self-care to promote wellness and to encourage preventive care. A new chapter on transition to parenthood focuses on teaching for new mothers and infants at home. Special boxes highlight home care throughout the text. Family focus boxes incorporate family considerations important to care of women and children. Issues concerning grandparents, siblings, and different family constellations are addressed. In the pediatric chapters, these boxes focus on the special learning needs of families caring for their child.

To implement *preventive care,* nurses must be able to recognize signs and symptoms of emergent problems. Throughout the discussion of assessment and care, we alert the nurse to signs of potential problems and provide information boxes that highlight warning signs and emergency situations.

Chapter 2 includes a discussion of cultural implications and focuses on specific customs related to childbearing and women's health. This chapter also stresses the importance of assessing both the nurse's and the patient's cultural beliefs. Cultural implications are integrated throughout the text to emphasize the wide range of ethnic diversity and its affect on the health of women and children. Boxes throughout the text highlight cultural aspects of care. Two new chapters on care in the community and home have been added to prepare the student to provide care for women and children in a variety of settings.

Nurses confront ethical and legal challenges daily. Nurses need to develop a reflective stance that assesses new technologies and policies in light of their potential to influence human well-being. Legal tips are integrated throughout the maternity section to emphasize these issues as they relate to the care of women and children.

FEATURES

This second edition features a contemporary design with logical, easy-to-follow headings and attractive four-color design that highlights important content and increases visual appeal. Hundreds of color photographs and drawings throughout the text illustrate important concepts and techniques to further enhance comprehension.

To help students learn essential information quickly and efficiently, we have included numerous features that prioritize, condense, simplify, and emphasize important aspects of nursing care. In addition, the text encourages students to *think critically.* The organizing framework, *Care Management,* is used consistently to discuss nursing care. The five steps of the *Nursing Process* are incorporated into this framework. *Nursing Care Plans* are included to help students apply the nursing process in the clinical setting. The *Nursing Care Plans* use NANDA-approved nursing diagnoses, describe expected outcomes, and provide rationales for interventions. *Care Paths, Protocols,* and *Procedures* are included in the maternity chapters to provide students with examples of various approaches to the implementation of care.

SPECIAL FEATURES

- **Learning Objectives** focus students' attention on the important content to be mastered.
- **Home Care** boxes emphasize guidelines for the patient to practice self-care and provide information to help students transfer learning from the hospital to the home setting.
- **Cultural Considerations** boxes describe beliefs and practices about pregnancy, childbirth, parenting, and women's health concerns.
- **Family Focus** boxes highlight the needs or concerns of families that should be addressed when family-centered care is provided.
- **Patient Teaching** boxes assist students to help patients and families become involved in their own care with optimal outcomes.
- **Nursing Care Plans** are provided for all commonly encountered situations and disorders. NANDA-accepted nursing diagnoses are included in the care plans. Rationales are added to nursing interventions for which the rationale might not be immediately evident to students.
- **Critical Thinking** boxes encourage students to consider real-life clinical situations and make appropriate clinical judgments.
- **Nurse Alerts** call the reader's attention to critical information that could lead to deteriorating or emergency situations.
- **Emergency** boxes alert students to the signs and symptoms of various emergency situations and provide interventions for immediate implementation.
- **Atraumatic Care** boxes emphasize the importance of providing competent care while minimizing undue physical and psychologic distress for the child and family.
- **Research findings** summarized in the Cochrane Pregnancy and Childbirth Database are included in chapters that address pregnancy and childbirth. Findings that confirm effective practices or that identify practices with unknown, ineffective, or harmful effects are identified by the ■ icon in the margin.
- During assessment, the nurse must be alert for **Signs of Potential Complications;** these are included as boxes in chapters that cover uncomplicated pregnancy and childbirth.
- **Legal Tips** are integrated throughout to provide students with relevant information to deal with important legal areas in the context of maternity nursing.
- **Key Points,** located at the end of each chapter, help the reader summarize major points, make connections, and synthesize information.
- A highly detailed, cross-referenced **index** allows readers to quickly access needed information.

TEACHING/LEARNING PACKAGE

1. **Study Guide**—Includes reviews of key concepts and content and critical thinking questions.
2. **Instructor's Electronic Resource**—Includes chapter outlines with teaching strategies, case studies with community-based applications, updated test bank questions, and an Electronic Image Collection with over 500 full-color images from the text.
3. **Whaley & Wong's Pediatric Nursing Video Series**—Set of six individual videotapes narrated by Donna Wong. Topics include Pediatric Assessment, Growth and Development, Medications and Injections, Family-Centered Care, Pain Assessment and Management, and Communicating with Children and Families.

ACKNOWLEDGMENTS

Thanks to Irene Bobak for starting a tradition of excellence. Thanks also to Jane McAteer for developing nursing care plans and to Karen Piotrowski for writing the Instructor's Resource Manual and Study Guide. I would also like to thank the following photographers: Michael S. Clement, MD, Mesa, AZ; Marjorie Pyle, RNC, Lifecircle, Costa Mesa, CA; Gregory Vogel, Bloomington, IL; and Kathy Allen, Newport News, VA. Special words of gratitude are extended to Michael Ledbetter for his encouragement and assistance. I would expecially like to thank Laurie Muench for her encouraging words, her attention to myriad details, and her excellent follow-up of all my quesitons and concerns. Her support was crucial for the completion of this project.

Shannon E. Perry

Very special thanks go to all the individuals at Harcourt Health Sciences who were committed to making this book the best it could be. Special gratitude goes to Shelly Hayden and Loren Wilson for their exceptional devotion to pediatric nursing; their high standards do not go unnoticed.

I wish to also thank my son, Andrew, for teaching me the most about caring for children.

Marilyn J. Hockenberry

The authors wish to express their gratitude to Patrick Barrera, Contributing Editor to the book, for his commitment to excellence. His work on this book has provided its readers with the most current and accurate information available to nurses caring for mothers and their children. We are grateful for his attention to detail and devotion to nursing education.

The authors would also like to acknowledge the following individuals for contributions to the seventh edition of *Maternity & Women's Health Care* and the sixth edition of *Wong's Essentials of Pediatric Nursing:*

Kathryn Rhodes Alden, MSN, RN, IBCLC; Kari Anderson, RN, MSN, EdD; Debbie Fraser Askin, MN, RNC; Jean A. Bachman, DSN; Kitty Cashion, RN, C, MSN; Jane G. Conner, MSN, WHCNP, RNC; Gayle Tart Davis, BSN, MSN, EdD, CPNP; Lienne D. Edwards, RN, PhD; Anne H. Fishel, PhD, RN, CS; Catherine Ingram Fogel, RNC (WHNP), PhD, FAAN; Margaret Comerford Freda, RN, EdD, CHES, FAAN; Cynthia Garrett, RNC, BSN, MSN; S. Kim Genovese, RNC, MSN, CARN, MSA; Bette B. Hammond, RN, BSN, MSN; Betty G. Harris, RN, PhD; Mildred G. Harvey, BSN, MSN, RNC; Sharon E. Lock, PhD, RN, FNP; Jane McAteer, RN, BSN, MN; Esther Megerman, MA, PhD; Margaret Shandor Miles, RN, MSN, PhD, FAAN; Mary Courtney Moore, RN, RD, PhD; Amy A. Nichols, RN, PCNS, EdD; Karen A. Piotrowski, RNC, MSN; Judith H. Poole, PhD, RNC, FACCE; Barbara C. Rynerson, RN, MS, CS; Rebecca Burdette Saunders, RNC, PhD; Barbara Peterson Sinclair, MN, RNC, OGNP, FAAN; Linda H. Snell, DNS; Susan M. Tucker, MSN, RN, PHN, CNAA; Wendy Wetzel, RN, MSN, FNP, HNC; Rhea P. Williams, RN, MN, PhD; Jan Lamarche Zdanuk, RNC, MSN, CNS, CFNP. Elizabeth Ahmann, ScD, RN; Chris L. Algren, EdD, MSN, RN; Rose A. Urdiales Baker, MSN, RN, CS; Sarah J. Bottomley, MN, RN, CPNP; Christine A. Brosnan, DrPH, RNC; Jean Park Brown, MS, RNC; Melody Brown, MS, RN, CPON; Rosalind Bryant, MN, RN-CS, PNP; Helen Currier, CNN, RN; Martha R. Curry, MS, RNC, CPNP; Carolyn V. Daigneau, MS, RN-CS, PNP; Jennifer A. Disabato, MS, RN, CPNP; Pam DiVito-Thomas, MS, RN; Kim D. Evans, MSN, RN, CPNP, ACRN; Kristi M. Kana, BSN, RN; Nancy E. Kline, PhD, RN, CPNP; Linda M. Kollar, MSN, RN; Christine Golazeski Leyden, MSN, RN, A-CCC; Rosemary Liguori, PhD, ARNP, CPNP; Mary Mondozzi, MSN, RN, CS; Barbara Montagnino, MS, RN, CNS; Dottie Needham, MSN, CPNP, APRN; Patricia O'Brien, MSN, RN-CS, PNP; Amy N. Romanczuk, MSN, RN, CNS; Tamara E. Scott, MSN, RN, CPNP, CPON; Rebecca Stroud, MSN, RN, CPNP; C. Nolan Thomas, DMin, MDiv, MS, NCC; Margaret R. Ugalde, DrPH, RN-CS, PNP; Lisa M. Vallino, BSN, RN; Donna P. Williams, MS, RN, FNP.

Contents

PART I
Maternity Nursing

UNIT 1
INTRODUCTION TO MATERNITY NURSING

UNIT 2
REPRODUCTIVE YEARS

PART II
Pediatric Nursing

UNIT 7
CHILDREN, THEIR FAMILIES, AND THE NURSE

UNIT 8
ASSESSMENT OF THE CHILD AND FAMILY

APPENDIXES

CHAPTER 1

Contemporary Maternity Nursing

http://www.harcourthealth.com/MERLIN/Wong/maternal/

Learning Objectives

On completion of this chapter the reader will be able to:

- Describe the scope of maternity nursing.
- Evaluate contemporary issues and trends in maternity nursing.
- Describe sociopolitical issues affecting the care of women and infants.
- Compare selected biostatistical data among races.
- Examine social concerns in maternity nursing.
- Give examples of standards of practice in the delivery of nursing care.
- Debate ethical issues in perinatal nursing.
- Examine the *Healthy People 2010* goals related to maternal and infant care.

Maternity nursing focuses on the care of childbearing women and their families through all stages of pregnancy and childbirth, as well as the first 4 weeks after birth. Throughout the prenatal period, nurses, nurse practitioners, and nurse-midwives provide care for women in clinics and physicians' offices and teach classes to help families prepare for childbirth. Nurses care for childbearing families during labor and birth in hospitals; in birthing centers; and, less often, in the home. Nurses with special training may provide intensive care to high risk neonates in special care units and to high risk mothers in antepartum units, in critical care obstetric units, or in the home. Maternity nurses teach about pregnancy; the process of labor, birth, and recovery; and parenting skills. Nurses provide continuity of care throughout the childbearing cycle.

There exists in the United States serious problems related to the health and health care of mothers and infants. One-sixth of all Americans, or 44.3 million people, have no health insurance (Sheridan-Gonzalez, 2000). A lack of access to prepregnancy and pregnancy-related care for all women, as well as the lack of reproductive health services for adolescents, are major concerns. Sexually transmitted infections including AIDS (acquired immunodeficiency syndrome) continue to adversely affect reproduction.

Racial and ethnic diversity is increasing within North America. It is estimated that within 40 years, 50% of the population will be European-American, 22% will be African-American, 18% will be Hispanic, and 10% will be Asian-American (Gary, Sigsby, and Campbell, 1998).

There is significant disparity in health outcomes among people of various racial and ethnic groups. In addition, people may have lifestyles, health needs, and health care preferences related to their ethnic or cultural backgrounds. They may have dietary preferences and health practices that are not understood by caregivers. To meet the health care needs of a culturally diverse society, it is essential that the nursing workforce reflect the diversity of its patient population.

The focus of the first part of this book is maternity nursing. Chapter 1 presents a general overview of issues and trends related to the health and health care of women and infants during the maternity cycle. The second part, which begins with Chapter 29, addresses the issues and trends related to the health care of children.

CONTEMPORARY ISSUES AND TRENDS

Changing Childbirth Practices

Changing Health Care Delivery Structure. Changes in the health care market are influencing the way health care providers can care for their patients. The number of professional nurses in hospitals has declined, and unlicensed assistive personnel and multiskilled workers have been substituted. The role of the nurse is evolving from primary caregiver to the leader of an interdisciplinary care team. Advanced practice roles are increasing as nurses assume more responsibility for care of patients.

Integrative Health Care. Integrative health care encompasses complementary and alternative therapies in combination with conventional Western modalities of treatment. Many popular alternative healing modalities offer human-centered care based on philosophies that recognize the value of the patient's input and honor the individual's beliefs, values, and desires. The focus of these modalities is on the whole person, not just on a disease complex. Patients often find that alternative modalities are more consistent with their own belief systems and also allow for more patient autonomy in health care decisions (Astin, 1998).

Increasing numbers of American adults are seeking alternative and complementary health care. It is estimated that more than 629 million such visits were made in 1997, an increase of 47% over previous numbers of visits. This volume exceeds visits paid to primary health care providers. Approximately 45% of the general population uses complementary therapies (King, Pettigrew and Reed, 1999). Annual expenditures related to alternative therapies are estimated at $27 billion, approximately half of which is out-of-pocket expense not covered by medical insurance (Eisenberg et al, 1998; Eisenberg, Kessler, and Forster, 1993).

Eisenberg and colleagues (1993) reported that approximately 60 million Americans used an alternative medical therapy in 1990. They also found that the number of visits to providers of alternative medicine in that period exceeded the number of visits to U.S. primary care physicians, and that over 70% of users of alternative therapy did not tell their physician.

Changing Maternity Care. Maternity care has evolved in response to consumer demands. Women can choose either a physician or a nurse-midwife as their primary care provider. In 1997, physicians attended 92% and nurse-midwives attended 7% of all births (Curtin and Park, 1999). Hospital births accounted for 99% of births. Of the out-of-hospital births, 64% were in the home, 28% in free-standing birth centers, and 2% in clinics or doctor's offices (Curtin and Park, 1999). Women who choose nurse-midwives as their primary providers actively participate in childbirth decisions and receive fewer interventions such as epidural analgesia for labor (Callister, 1995).

Women can give birth in a hospital labor room (rather than a delivery room), in a birthing room, in a free-standing birthing center, or at home. Women may stay in the same room for the entire birth experience (i.e., labor, delivery, recovery, and postpartum) and one nurse may care for both mother and baby (couplet or mother-baby care). Lactation consultants are available to assist mothers with breastfeeding.

The method of analgesia and the positions for labor and birth vary, depending on the condition and choice of the mother and the preferences of the providers. No longer are laboring mothers and their support people separated. With family-centered care, fathers, partners, grandparents, siblings, and friends may be present for labor and birth. Fathers or partners may be present for cesarean births. Doulas—trained and experienced female labor attendants—provide a continuous, one-on-one, caring presence throughout the labor and birth. Newborn infants remain with the mother and are encouraged to breastfeed immediately after birth. Parents participate in the care of their infants in nurseries and neonatal intensive care units (NICUs).

Discharge of a mother and baby within 24 to 48 hours of birth is a common practice and has created a growing need for follow-up or home care. In some settings, discharge may occur as early as 6 hours after birth. Legislation has been enacted to ensure that mothers and babies are permitted to stay in the hospital at least 48 hours after vaginal birth and 96 hours after cesarean birth. There is a need for focused and efficient teaching to enable the parents and infant to make a safe transition from hospital to home. Nurses may use follow-up telephone calls or home visits to assist families needing information and reassurance.

Neonatal security in the hospital setting is receiving increasing attention. A number of cases of "baby-napping" and of sending parents home with the wrong baby have been reported. Security systems are being placed in nurseries, and nurses are required to wear photo identification.

Changing Views of Women. Women must be viewed holistically and in the context in which they live. Their physical, mental, and social needs must be considered because these areas are interdependent and influence health and illness. Even the language health care professionals use to describe women and their problems needs to be examined (Freda, 1995). For example, practitioners may describe a woman as having an "incompetent cervix," as "failing to progress," or as having an "arrest" of labor. They may describe a fetus as having intrauterine growth "retardation," or providers may "allow" women a "trial" of labor. Practitioners instead should use phrases such as "the woman who has recurrent premature dilation of the cervix" or "the fetus whose intrauterine growth has been restricted" (Freda, 1995). There is a movement to refer to spontaneous pregnancy loss as a "miscarriage" instead of the more politically charged "abortion."

CRITICAL THINKING

POLICIES ON BREASTFEEDING

Call five major companies located in your vicinity that employ or are frequented by large numbers of women to identify whether they have policies related to breastfeeding or resources to enable continued breastfeeding. These companies can include industries, department stores, grocery stores, and others.

- **How many of the companies have a policy related to breastfeeding? What does the policy cover? Does the company know the benefits of breastfeeding? Is the company aware of the benefits to the employer in relation to a decrease in absenteeism for infant illness in breastfeeding mothers?**
- **Can a breastfeeding mother bring her nursing infant to work? Can a woman breastfeed in a public area of the company? Is lactation consultation available?**
- **Does the company have a place for a breastfeeding mother to pump and store milk? Does the company provide a breast pump? Are women allowed to take breaks to pump?**
- **Does the human resources department keep track of absenteeism related to pregnancy and lactation? Have they noticed a decrease in absenteeism as a result of less infant illness in breastfeeding mothers in contrast to bottle-feeding mothers?**
- **What conclusions can you draw from your survey of companies? What public policy initiatives are necessary to promote breastfeeding in your community?**

Violence is a major factor affecting pregnant women. This includes battering (which may increase during pregnancy), rape or other sexual assaults, and attacks with various weapons. It is estimated that 8% of pregnant women are battered. Violence is associated with complications of pregnancy such as bleeding.

Cases of perinatally acquired immunodeficiency syndrome (AIDS) peaked in 1992; the rate of AIDS among infants declined from 8.9 per 100,000 births in 1992 to 2.8 per 100,000 births in 1996. Of mothers who tested positive for HIV before giving birth, 91% received zidovudine. This contributed to the decrease in infants infected with the virus (Lindegren et al, 1999).

Healthy People 2010 Goals

Healthy People 2010 is the nation's agenda for improving health. It has two overarching goals: to increase the quality and years of healthy life; and to eliminate health disparities. Within *Healthy People 2010,* there are 467 objectives to improve health that are organized into 28 specific focus areas including one related to maternal, infant, and child health (Box 1-1). Current information about the goals of *Healthy People 2010* is available on the Internet at: www.health.gov/healthypeople.

Trends in Fertility and Birthrate

Fertility trends and birthrates reflect women's needs for health care. Box 1-2 defines biostatistical terminology useful in analyzing maternity health care. In 1998 the fertility rate (i.e., the number of births to women of childbearing age [15 to 44 years]), was 65.6 live births per 1000 women (Guyer et al, 1999). This is a 1% increase from the 65.0 rate in 1997. The highest birthrates (number of births per 1000 women) were for women between ages 20 and 29, but the birthrate for women in their 40s (7.3 per 1000) has nearly doubled since 1983 (Guyer et al, 1999). Almost one third of all births in the United States in 1997 were to unmarried women, with much variation in proportion among racial groups (African-American 69.0%, Hispanic 41.6%, and Caucasian 21.9%) (Guyer et al, 1999). Births to unmarried women are often related to less favorable outcomes because there are typically a large number of teenagers in the unmarried group (78.8% in 1998) (Guyer et al, 1999).

BOX 1-1

Healthy People 2010, Focus Area 16, Maternal, Infant, and Child Health

Goal: Improve the health and well-being of women, infants, children, and families

Fetal, infant, and child deaths
Maternal death and illness
Prenatal care
Obstetrical care
Risk factors
Developmental disabilities and neural tube defects
Prenatal substance exposure
Breastfeeding, newborn screening, and service systems

From US Department of Health and Human Services: *Healthy People 2010* (conference edition, in two volumes), Washington, DC, 2000, USDHHS.

Incidence of Low Birth Weight

Babies born weighing less than 2500 g are classified as low birth weight (LBW), and their risks for morbidity and mortality increase. In 1998 the incidence of LBW was 7.8%, and the incidence of very low birth weight (VLBW) was 1.45% (Guyer et al, 1999). There is racial disparity in the incidence of LBW. African-American babies are more than twice as likely as Caucasian babies to be LBW and to die within the first year of life. By race, the incidence of LBW for African-American births was 13%; for Hispanic births, 6.4%; and for Caucasian births, 6.6%. Cigarette smoking is associated with LBW, prematurity, and intrauterine growth restriction. In 1997, 13.2% of pregnant women smoked, a proportion that has declined by one third since 1989 (Guyer et al, 1999).

The proportion of preterm infants (i.e., those born before 38 weeks of gestation) was 17.4% for African-American births and 9.8% for Caucasian births (Guyer et al, 1999). The number of multiple births increased to 27.4 per 1000 in 1996, with most of the increase attributed to the use of fertility drugs (Guyer et al, 1999).

Infant Mortality in the United States

A common indicator of the adequacy of prenatal care and the health of a nation as a whole is the infant mortality rate (i.e., deaths per 1000 live births). The preliminary infant mortality rate for 1998 was 7.2, a rate that matches the lowest ever recorded in the United States (Guyer et al, 1999). The infant mortality rate continues to be higher for African-American babies (14.1 per 1000) than for Caucasian babies (6.0 per 1000). Limited maternal education, young maternal age, unmarried status, poverty, and lack of prenatal care appear to be associated with higher infant mortality rates. Poor nutrition, smoking and alcohol use, and maternal conditions such as poor health or hypertension are also important contributors to infant mortality.

BOX 1-2

Maternal-Infant Biostatistical Terminology

Abortus—An embryo or fetus that is removed or expelled from the uterus at 20 weeks' gestation or less, weighs 500 g or less, or measures 25 cm or less.

Birthrate—Number of live births in 1 year per 1000 population.

Fertility rate—Number of births per 1000 women between the ages of 15 and 44 years (inclusive), calculated on a yearly basis.

Infant mortality rate—Number of deaths of infants under 1 year of age per 1000 live births.

Maternal mortality rate—Number of maternal deaths from births and complications of pregnancy, childbirth, and puerperium (the first 42 days after termination of the pregnancy) per 100,000 live births.

Neonatal mortality rate—Number of deaths of infants under 28 days of age per 1000 live births.

Perinatal mortality rate—Number of stillbirths and the number of neonatal deaths per 1000 live births.

Stillbirth—An infant who, at birth, demonstrates no signs of life, such as breathing, heartbeat, or voluntary muscle movements.

A shift from the current emphasis on high-technology medical interventions to a focus on improving access to preventive care for low-income families is necessary.

International Trends in Infant Mortality

The infant mortality rate of Canada ranks sixteenth and that of the United States ranks twenty-third when compared with other industrialized nations (Guyer et al, 1999). One reason for this is the high rate of LBW infants in the United States compared with other countries.

Maternal Mortality Trends

In 1996, the annual mortality rate (number of maternal deaths per 100,000 live births) was 7.5 in the United States. There are significant racial differences in the rates: African-American women have a maternal mortality rate four times higher than that of Caucasian women. Maternal mortality was 20.3 per 100,000 for African-American women, in contrast with 5 per 100,000 for Caucasian women (CDC, 1998). The predominant causes of these deaths are hemorrhage, infection, pregnancy-induced hypertension, and ectopic pregnancy. The *Healthy People 2010* goal of 3.3 maternal deaths per 100,000 poses a significant challenge.

The Trend Toward Earlier Prenatal Care

First trimester care increased for the ninth consecutive year to 82.8% in 1998. The percent of women seeking early care varied among racial groups: Caucasians 87.9%, African-Americans 73.3%, and Hispanics 74.3% (Guyer et al, 1999). Early prenatal care enables health care providers to detect and manage conditions that affect pregnancy. Education about health-promoting behaviors can occur.

The Trend Toward High-Technology Care

Advances in scientific knowledge and the large number of high risk pregnancies have contributed to a health care system that emphasizes high-technology care. Maternity care has branched out to preconception counseling, more and better scientific techniques to monitor the mother and fetus, more definitive tests for hypoxia and acidosis, and neonatal intensive care units. Robotic aids may become common (Buus-Frank, 1999). Telemedicine, which uses electronic means to gather information and communicate, permits specialists including nurses to provide health care and consultation when distance separates them from those needing care. Strides are being made in identifying genetic codes, and genetic engineering is taking place. In general, high-technology care has flourished while "health" care has been relatively neglected. These technologic advances have also contributed to higher health care costs. Nurses must use caution and prospective planning and assess the effect of the emerging technology (Buus-Frank, 1999).

CRITICAL THINKING

REPRODUCTIVE HEALTH

Examine a daily newspaper for 7 days. Identify articles reporting topics related to maternity or reproductive health.

- **How many articles did you identify? What are the topics? Are they local or national issues?**
- **Who is the reporter, that is, health reporter, local or national columnist, male or female?**
- **What is the "slant" of the articles? Are the reports favorable to women and reproductive health? Does the tenor of the articles limit reproductive freedom or infringe on women's rights?**
- **What conclusions can you draw related to the treatment of women's issue and reproductive health in your community?**

Home Health Care

A shift in settings, from acute care institutions to the home, has taken place. Even high risk childbearing women may now be cared for in the home. Technology previously available only in the hospital is now found in the home. This has affected the organizational structure of care, the skills required to provide such care, and the cost to consumers. Home health care also has a community focus. Nurses are involved in caring for women and infants in homeless shelters, in caring for adolescents in schools, and in promoting health at community sites. Nursing education curricula are increasingly community based.

Escalation of High Risk Pregnancies

The number of high risk pregnancies has increased, which means that a greater number of women are at risk for poor pregnancy outcomes. Escalating drug use (ranging from 11% to 27% of pregnant women, depending on geographic location) has contributed to higher incidences of prematurity, LBW, congenital defects, learning disabilities, and withdrawal symptoms in infants. Alcohol use in pregnancy has been associated with miscarriages (spontaneous abortions), mental retardation, LBW, and fetal alcohol syndrome.

The two most common reported maternal medical risk factors are hypertension associated with pregnancy and diabetes (Guyer et al, 1999). The multiple birthrate is increasing, with the birthrate of higher-order multiple (triplet, quadruplet, and greater) jumping 16% from 1996 to 1997 (Guyer et al, 1999). Multiple births now account for nearly 3% of all births (Guyer et al, 1999). The cesarean birthrate increased to 21.2% in 1998, with primary cesareans rising to 14.9% and vaginal births after cesarean dropping 4% to 26.3 per 100 (Guyer et al, 1999). About 3.6% of the births of babies born vaginally are assisted with forceps and 7.8% with vacuum extraction. Electronic fetal monitoring was used in 83% of women in labor; 64% of mothers had an ultrasound during pregnancy; and 18% of labors were induced and 17% were stimulated (Curtin and Park, 1999).

Trends and the Issue of High Costs

Health care is one of the fastest growing sectors of the U.S. economy. Even though the United States spends proportionately more on health care than any of the other 190 countries that make up the World Health Organization, it ranks thirty-seventh in quality (Rubin, 2000). A shift in demographics, an increased emphasis on high-cost technology, and the liability costs of a litigious society contribute to the high cost of care. Most researchers agree that the costs of caring for the increased number of LBW infants in NICUs contributes significantly to the overall health care costs.

Midwifery care has helped contain some health care costs, but not all insurance carriers reimburse nurse-practitioners and clinical nurse-specialists as direct care providers, a situation that continues to be a problem.

Early discharge programs are also used to reduce costs. The American Academy of Pediatrics has published minimum criteria for early discharge of a newborn (American Academy of Pediatrics Committee on Fetus and Newborn, 1995).

Problems with Access to Care

The proportion of women in 1998 who began prenatal care in the first trimester was 82.8%, the highest level ever reported. Only 3.9% of pregnant women delayed care until the third trimester or had no care (Guyer et al, 1999).

Barriers to access need to be removed so that pregnancy outcomes can be improved. The most significant barrier to access is the inability to pay. Lack of transportation and dependent child care are other barriers. In addition to a lack of insurance and high costs, there is a lack of providers for women with low incomes because many physicians refuse to take Medicaid patients or take only a few such patients. This presents a problem because a significant proportion of births are to mothers who receive Medicaid.

TRENDS IN NURSING PRACTICE

The increasing complexity of care for maternity patients has contributed to specialization of nurses working with these patients. This specialized knowledge is being gained through experience, advanced degrees, and certification programs. Nurses in advanced practice (e.g., nurse practitioners and nurse-midwives) may provide primary care throughout a woman's life, including the pregnancy cycle. In some settings, the clinical nurse specialist and nurse practitioner roles are blended and nurses delivery high quality, comprehensive, and cost-effective care in a variety of settings (Sperhac and Strodtbeck, 1997). Lactation consultants provide services in the postpartum unit or on an outpatient basis.

Nursing Interventions Classification

When the National Institutes of Medicine proposed that patient records be computerized by the year 2000, the need for a common language to describe the contributions of nurses to patient care became evident (Eganhouse, McCloskey, and Bulachek, 1996). A comprehensive standardized language that describes the interventions performed by generalist or specialist nurses is included in the Nursing Interventions Classification (NIC). Interventions commonly used by maternal-child nurses include those in Box 1-3.

BOX 1-3

Childbearing Care Interventions

LEVEL 1 DOMAIN: FAMILY
Care that supports the family unit

LEVEL 2 CLASS: CHILDBEARING CARE
Interventions to assist in understanding and coping with the psychologic and physiologic changes during the childbearing period

LEVEL 3: INTERVENTIONS
Amnioinfusion
Anticipatory guidance
Attachment promotion
Birthing
Bleeding reduction: antepartum uterus
Bleeding reduction: postpartum uterus
Bottle-feeding
Breastfeeding assistance
Cesarean-section care
Childbirth preparation
Electronic fetal monitoring: antepartum
Electronic fetal monitoring: intrapartum
Environmental management: attachment process
Family integrity promotion: childbearing family
Family planning: contraception
Family planning: infertility
Family planning: unplanned pregnancy
Genetic counseling
Grief work facilitation: perinatal death
High risk pregnancy care
Infant care
Intrapartal care
Kangaroo care
Labor induction
Labor suppression
Lactation counseling
Lactation suppression
Newborn care
Newborn monitoring
Nonnutritive sucking
Parent education: childbearing family
Phototherapy: neonate
Postpartal care
Preconception counseling
Pregnancy termination care
Prenatal care
Reproductive technology management
Resuscitation: fetus
Resuscitation: neonate
Risk identification: childbearing family
Surveillance: late pregnancy
Teaching: infant care
Tube care: umbilical line
Ultrasonography: limited obstetric

From Iowa Intervention Project: 2000. *Nursing interventions classification (NIC)*, ed 3, St Louis, 2000, Mosby.

Outcomes Orientation

Outcomes of care (i.e., the effectiveness of interventions and quality of care) are receiving increased emphasis. Outcomes-oriented care measures effectiveness of care against benchmarks or standards based on results achieved by others. It is a measure of the value of nursing using quality indicators such as cost, length of stay, and patient satisfaction (Oermann and Huber, 1999). Nurses commonly conduct studies of patient satisfaction.

Best Practices as the Goal of Care

A program or service that has been recognized for excellence is considered to be a best practice. A best practice must provide a better or a new way to achieve goals (Lewis, 1998) and be sound from operational, clinical, and financial perspectives (Fitzgerald, 1998). To determine best practices, information is collected from similar institutions. Staff members then identify solutions that have been successful in addressing specific needs and select one that incorporates the best resolutions of the problem and that fits the agency's own population and mission characteristics. The agency continually compares its performance against the best in the industry and the best of a specific function.

Clinical Benchmarking

Clinical benchmarking is a process used to compare one's own performance against the performance of the best in an area of service (Fitzgerald, 1998). Benchmarking supports and promotes continuous quality improvement, and assists the organization to remain competitive within the health care market. The Best Practices Network uses collaborative benchmarking, which involves sharing strategies and outcomes and leads to the development of new best practices (Reclaiming benchmarking, 1999/2000). The Best Practices Network can be accessed on the Internet at http://best4health.org.

Perinatal nurses can use standards set by such organizations as the Association of Women's Health, Obstetric, and Neonatal Nurses (AWHONN); the National Association of Neonatal Nurses (NANN); the American College of Obstetricians and Gynecologists; and the American Academy of Pediatrics. Areas of practice routinely monitored in perinatal nursing include hospital length of stay, maternal mortality, infant mortality, cesarean birthrate, hysterectomy rate, epidural rate, and episiotomy rate.

A Global Perspective

Advances in medicine and nursing have resulted in increased knowledge and understanding in the care of mothers and infants and reduced perinatal morbidity and mortality. However, these advances have primarily affected the industrialized nations (Vidyasagar and Edelman, 1997). As the world becomes smaller through improved travel and communication technologies, nurses and other health care providers are gaining a global perspective and taking part in activities that improve the health and health care of people worldwide. Nurses participate in medical outreach by providing obstetric, surgical, ophthalmologic, orthopedic, or other services; by attending international meetings; by conducting research; and by providing international consultation. International student and faculty exchanges take place (Fig. 1-1), and more articles about health care in other countries are being published in nursing journals. Several schools of nursing in the United States are World Health Organization Collaborating Centers.

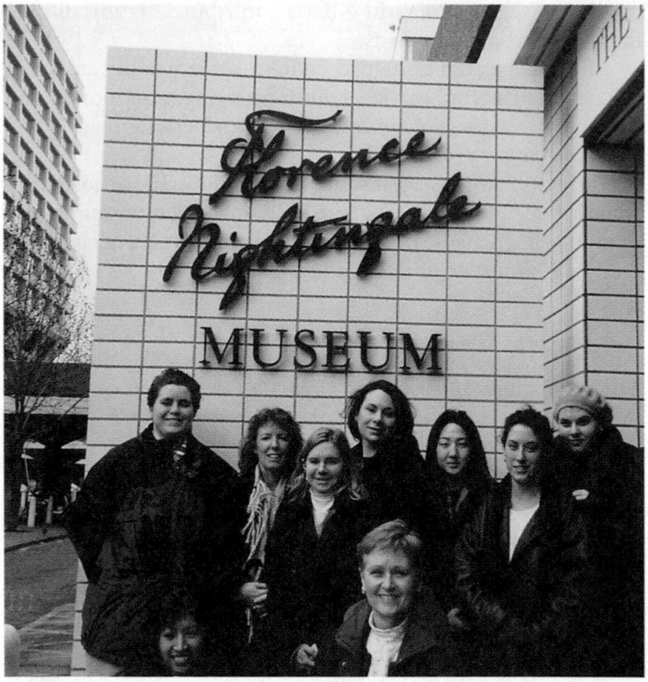

FIG. 1-1 • Nursing students visit a museum as part of an international community service learning experience. (Courtesy Shannon Perry, San Jose, CA.)

STANDARDS OF PRACTICE AND LEGAL ISSUES IN DELIVERY OF CARE

Nursing standards of practice in perinatal and women's health nursing have been described by several organizations. These include the American Nurses Association (ANA), which publishes standards for maternal-child health nursing; AWHONN, which publishes standards of practice and education; and the National Association of Neonatal Nurses (NANN), which publishes standards of practice for neonatal nurses. These standards reflect current knowledge and represent levels of practice agreed upon by leaders in the specialty (AWHONN, 1998) (Box 1-4). Because nursing practice, society, and health care systems are dynamic rather than static, standards change over time.

In addition to these more formalized standards, agencies often have their own policy-and-procedure books that outline standards to be followed in that setting. In determining legal negligence, the care given is compared with the standards of care. If the standard was not met, and the result was harm to the patient, negligence occurred. The number of legal suits in the perinatal area has typically been high. As a consequence, malpractice insurance rates are high for physicians, nurse-midwives, and nurses in labor and delivery.

LEGAL TIP • Standard of care When you are uncertain about how to perform a procedure, consult the agency procedure book and follow the printed guidelines. These guidelines are the standard of care for that agency.

BOX 1-4

Standards of Care for Women and Newborns

STANDARDS THAT DEFINE THE NURSE'S RESPONSIBILITY TO THE PATIENT

Assessment
Collection of health data of the woman or newborn

Diagnosis
Analysis of data to determine nursing diagnosis

Outcome Identification
Identification of expected outcomes that are individualized

Planning
Development of a plan of care

Implementation
Performance of interventions for the plan of care

Evaluation
Evaluation of the effectiveness of interventions in relation to expected outcomes

STANDARDS OF PROFESSIONAL PERFORMANCE THAT DELINEATE ROLES AND BEHAVIORS FOR WHICH THE PROFESSIONAL NURSE IS ACCOUNTABLE

Quality of Care
Systemic evaluation of nursing practice

Peformance Appraisal
Self-evaluation in relation to professional practice standards and other regulations

Education
Participation in ongoing educational activities to maintain knowledge for practice

Collegiality
Contribution to the development of peers, students, and others

Ethics
Use of Code for Nurses to guide practice

Collaboration
Involvement of patient, significant others, and other health care providers in the provision of patient care

Research
Use of research findings in practice

Resource Utilization
Consideration of factors related to safety, effectiveness, and costs in planning and delivering patient care

Practice Environment
Contribution to the environment of care delivery

Accountability
Legal and professional responsibility for practice

Source: Association of Women's Health, Obstetric, and Neonatal Nurses (AWHONN): *Standards and guidelines for professional nursing practice in the case of women and newborns,* ed 5, Washington, DC, 1998, AWHONN.

ETHICAL ISSUES IN PERINATAL NURSING

Ethical concerns and debates have multiplied with increasing use of technology and with scientific advances. For example, with reproductive technology, pregnancy is now possible in women who thought they would never bear children, including some who are menopausal or postmenopausal. Should scarce resources be devoted to achieving pregnancies in older women? Is giving birth to a child at an older age worth the risks involved? Should third-party payers assume the costs of reproductive technology? Potential patients, nurses, physicians, ethicists, and lawmakers must discuss and debate these questions. With induced ovulation and in vitro fertilization, multiple pregnancies occur, and multifetal pregnancy reduction (selectively terminating one or more fetuses) may be considered. Innovations such as intrauterine fetal surgery, fetoscopy, therapeutic insemination, genetic engineering, surrogate childbearing, surgery for infertility, "test tube" babies, fetal research, and treatment of VLBW infants have resulted in questions about informed consent and allocation of resources. The introduction of long-acting contraceptives has created moral choices and policy dilemmas for health care providers and legislators. For example, should some women (such as substance abusers, women with low incomes, or women who are HIV positive) be required to take the contraceptives (Moskowitz, Jennings, and Callahan, 1995)? With the potential for great good that can come from fetal tissue transplantation, what research is ethical? What are the rights of the embryo (Sams, 1997)? Discussion and debate about these issues will occur for many years. Nurses and patients, as well as scientists, physicians, attorneys, and members of the clergy, must be involved in these discussions.

RESEARCH INTO PRACTICE

Evidence-Based Practice

There is increasing emphasis on providing practice based on evidence gained through research and clinical trials. Although not all practice can be evidence-based, practitioners must use the best available information on which to base their interventions. The first consensus initiative of the Coalition for Improving Maternity Services is the Mother Friendly Childbirth Initiative (1997). This is an evidence-based model that focuses on prevention and wellness as alternatives to costly programs of screening, diagnosis, and treatment. AWHONN's *Standards and Guidelines for Professional Nursing Practice in the Care of Women and Newborns* (AWHONN, 1998) includes an evidence-based approach to practice.

The incorporation of research findings into practice is essential to develop a science-based practice. AWHONN has completed four research-based practice projects: Transition of an Infant from an Incubator to an Open Crib, Management of Second-Stage Labor, Urinary Continence in Women, and Neonatal Skin Care. These projects were multistate, and staff nurses were involved in their implementation and in data collection. Additional projects are on pelvic pain and comfort management and on nursing management of preterm labor. AWHONN is also creating new practice guidelines to incorporate evidence-based practices for second-stage labor management, continence for women, breastfeeding support, assessment of midlife women, and intrapartum-perioperative-perianesthesia care. Using such guidelines and published reports, nurses can develop protocols and procedures based on published research and incorporate an evidence base into their practice. AWHONN research priorities through 2001 include the above topics as well as family violence, fetal surveillance, genetics, infertility, and early parenting.

Cochrane Pregnancy and Childbirth Database

The Cochrane Pregnancy and Childbirth Database was first planned in 1976 with a small grant from the World Health Organization to Dr. Iain Chalmers and colleagues at Oxford, England. In 1993 the Cochrane Collaboration was formed, and the Oxford Database of Perinatal Trials became known as the Cochrane Pregnancy and Childbirth Database. The Cochrane Collaboration oversees up-to-date, systematic reviews of randomized controlled trials of health care and disseminates these reviews. The premise of the project is that these types of studies provide the most reliable evidence about the effects of care.

The evidence from these studies should encourage practitioners to implement useful measures and to abandon those measures that are useless or harmless. Studies are ranked in six categories:

1. Beneficial forms of care
2. Forms of care that are likely to be beneficial
3. Forms of care with a trade-off between beneficial and adverse effects
4. Forms of care with unknown effectiveness
5. Forms of care that are unlikely to be beneficial
6. Forms of care that are likely to be ineffective or harmful

Practices that have been reviewed by the collaboration will be identified with a ■■ throughout the maternity portion of the text.

Key Points

- Maternity nursing focuses on women and their infants and families during the childbearing cycle.
- Nurses caring for women can play an active role in shaping health care systems to be responsive to the needs of contemporary women.
- Childbirth practices have changed to become more family-focused and to allow alternatives in care.
- Home care is a cost-effective alternative locus of care.
- The United States ranks twenty-third among industrialized nations in infant mortality.
- Ethical concerns have multiplied with increasing use of technology and scientific advances.
- *Healthy People 2010* provides goals for maternal and infant health.

References

American Academy of Pediatrics Committee on Fetus and Newborn: Hospital stay for healthy term newborns, *Pediatrics* 96(4 pt. 1):788-790, 1995.

Association of Women's Health, Obstetric, and Neonatal Nurses (AWHONN): *Standards and guidelines for professional nursing practice in the care of women and newborns,* ed 5, Washington, DC, 1998, AWHONN.

Astin J: Why patients use alternative medicine, *JAMA* 278: 1548-1553, 1998.

Buus-Frank M: Nurse versus machine: slaves or masters of technology? *J Obstet Gynecol Neonatal Nurs* 28(5):433-441, 1999.

Callister L: Beliefs and perceptions of childbearing women choosing different primary health care providers, *Clin Nurs Res* 4(2):168-180, 1995.

Centers for Disease Control and Prevention: Maternal mortality—United States, 1982-1996, *MMWR* 47:705-707, 1998.

Curtin S, Park M: Trends in the attendant, place, and timing of births, and in the use of obstetric interventions: United States, 1989-97, *National Vital Statistics Reports* 47(27):1-16, 1999.

Eganhouse D, McCloskey J, Bulachek G: How NIC describes MCH nursing, *MCN Am J Matern Child Nurs* 21(5):247-252, 1996.

Eisenberg D et al: Trends in alternative medicine use in the United States, 1970-1997, *JAMA* 280:1569-1575, 1998.

Eisenberg D, Kessler R, Forster C: Unconventional medicine in the United States, *N Engl J Med* 328(4):246-252, 1993.

Fitzgerald K: Clinical benchmarking: implications for perinatal nursing, *J Perinat Neonatal Nurs* 12(1):23-30, 1998.

Freda M: Arrest, trial, and failure, *J Obstet Gynecol Neonatal Nurs* 24(5):393-394, 1995.

Gary F, Sigsby L, Campbell D: Preparing for the 21st century: diversity in nursing education, research, and practice, *J Prof Nurs* 14(5):272-279, 1998.

Guyer B et al: Annual summary of vital statistics—1998, *Pediatrics* 104(6):1229-1246, 1999.

King M, Pettigrew A, Reed F: Complementary, alternative, integrative: have nurses kept pace with their patients? *Medsurg Nurs* 8(4):249-256, 1999.

Lewis J: Best practices: ideas that work, *AORN J* 68(3):444-446, 1998.

Lindegren M et al: Trends in perinatal transmission of HIV/AIDS in the United States, *JAMA* 282(6):531-538, 1999.

The Mother Friendly Childbirth Initiative: The first consensus initiative of the coalition for improving maternity services, *J Nurs Midwifery* 42(1):59-63, 1997.

Moskowitz E, Jennings B, Callahan D: Long-acting contraceptives: ethical guidance for policymakers and health care providers, *Hastings Center Rep* 25(1):S1-S8, 1995.

Oermann M, Huber D: Patient outcomes: a measure of nursing's value, *AJN* 99(9):40-48, 1999.

Reclaiming benchmarking for clinicians, *AWHONN Lifelines* 3(6):41, 1999/2000.

Rubin R: U.S. ranks 37th in health care, *USA Today* June 21, 2000, p. 1.

Sams L: Ethical dilemmas in maternal-fetal research, *MCN Am J Matern Child Nurs* 22:67-71, 1997.

Sheridan-Gonzalez J: It's not my patient , *AJN* 100(1):13, 2000.

Sperhac A, Strodtbeck F: Advanced practice nursing: new opportunities for blended roles, *MCN Am J Matern Child Nurs* 22:287-293, 1997.

U.S. Department of Health and Human Services: *Healthy People 2010* (conference edition in two volumes), Washington, DC, 2000, USDHHS.

Vidyasagar D, Edelman A: Perinatology/neonatology: a global perspective, *J Perinatol* 17:1-2, 1997.

CHAPTER

2

The Family and Culture

http://www.harcourthealth.com/MERLIN/Wong/maternal/

Learning Objectives

On completion of this chapter the reader will be able to:

- Identify key factors in determining the quality of family health.
- Differentiate between various family forms.
- Explain family functions that contribute to the well-being of its members and society.
- Explain family dynamics and how the components of family dynamics contribute to accomplishing family functions.
- Compare three theoretic approaches (i.e., family systems theory, family developmental theory, and family stress theory) for working with childbearing families.
- Relate the impact of culture on childbearing families.

The family is one of society's most important institutions. It represents a primary social group that influences and is influenced by other people and institutions. The family assumes major responsibility for the introduction and socialization of children. It transmits its fundamental cultural background to its members. Despite modern stresses and strains, the family, through its structure and function, forms a social network that acts as a potent support system for its members. The current emphasis in working with families is on wellness and empowerment for families to achieve control over their lives. Language reflects our views when we refer to the family as patient, client, or partner (Mohr, 2000).

DEFINING THE FAMILY

Families are defined in many ways. Definitions of the family usually involve explaining family *structure, functions, composition,* and *affectional ties.* These definitions include a variety of family forms such as the nuclear family, the extended family, the binuclear family, and the reconstituted family.

Family Structure

The family structure or family composition consists of individuals, each with a socially recognized status and position, who interact with one another on a regular, recurrent basis in socially sanctioned ways. When members are gained or lost through events (e.g., marriage, divorce, birth, death, abandonment, or incarceration), the family composition is altered and roles must be redefined or redistributed. Children may belong to several different family groups during their lifetimes.

Nuclear Family. The nuclear family consists of parents and their dependent children (natural or adopted) who live in a common household (Fig. 2-1). The family lives apart from either the husband's or wife's family of origin and is usually economically independent.

This is the reproductive unit in which the marital tie (legally or otherwise sanctioned) is the chief binding force. A strongly functional nuclear family is the prototype of human relationships and the basic unit from which more complex family forms are derived.

Extended Family. The extended family includes the nuclear family and other people related by blood. Called kin, these people include grandparents, aunts, uncles, and cousins (Fig. 2-2) (Friedman, 1998). Through its kinship network, the extended family provides role models and support to all members.

In the extended family, childrearing is often a shared responsibility. Relatives are present and available to help young parents with household chores and child care activities. The daily lives of the children are organized around the needs and requirements of the family, with assigned tasks and obligations.

Single-Parent Family. The single-parent family may result from the loss of spouse by death, divorce, separation, or desertion; from the out-of-wedlock birth of a child; or from the adoption of a child. Almost half of all children in the United States either currently live with a single parent or have lived with one in the past.

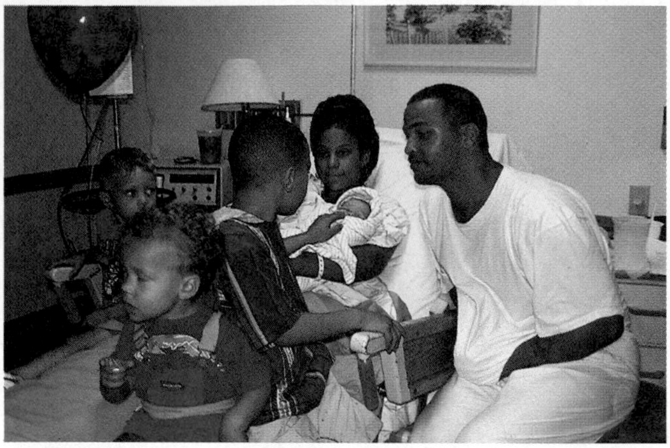

FIG. 2-1 • Nuclear family. (Courtesy Marjorie Pyle, RNC, Lifecircle, Costa Mesa, CA.)

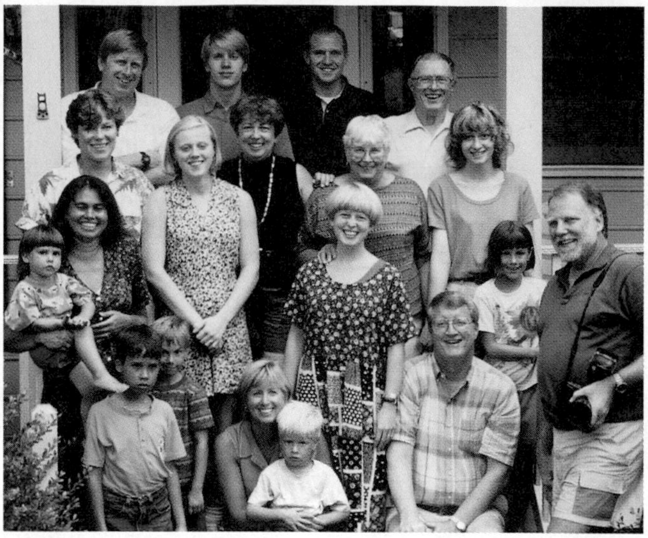

FIG. 2-2 • Extended family. (Courtesy Kathy Allen, Newport News, VA.)

It is becoming increasingly common in divorce settlements for fathers to be awarded custody of dependent children. A significant number of single-parent families result from a single mother who wants to have a child but does not choose to have a husband. Also, unmarried mothers often choose to keep and raise their children rather than place them for adoption or marry.

The single-parent family tends to be vulnerable both economically and socially. Many single-mother households are poor, and many of the most disadvantaged children live with mothers who were never married. For other adults, the single-parent family is a chosen lifestyle that provides a free and open system for development of parents and children.

Binuclear Family. Binuclear family refers to the family after divorce, in which the child is a member of both maternal and paternal nuclear households. The degree of cooperation between parents varies among these families. In joint custody, the court assigns divorcing parents equal rights to and responsibilities for the minor child or children. These alternate family forms are efforts on the part of those concerned to view divorce as a process of reorganization and redefinition of a family rather than as a family dissolution.

Reconstituted Family. The reconstituted family (also called a blended, combined, or remarried family) includes stepparents and stepchildren. Separation, divorce, and remarriage are commonplace in the United States, where approximately 50% of marriages end in divorce. Divorce and remarriage may occur at any time in the family life cycle and affect family function differently depending on when in the cycle they occur. Whatever the timing, effort is required to constitute and stabilize the new family groups. Through creativity and flexibility, satisfying rituals for the new family can be established.

Homosexual (Lesbian and Gay) Family. A same-sex, homosexual, or gay/lesbian family is one in which there is a common-law tie between two persons of the same sex who have children. It is estimated that 6 to 14 million children reside in gay or lesbian households. Although most children in gay/lesbian households are biologic offspring from a former legal marriage, there are other means by which homosexual adults acquire children. For example, they may be foster or adoptive parents. Lesbian mothers may conceive through artificial insemination. A gay male couple may become parents through use of a surrogate mother or by adoption. Because this family form is more common than most people may realize, it is important for the nurse to understand that gay/lesbian families are simply different from heterosexual families, not necessarily better or worse.

Family Functions

Although family functions have evolved and adapted over time in response to social and economic changes (Friedman, 1998), the family progresses through its life cycle (Table 2-1) and continues to carry out certain functions for the well-being of family members and the wider society.

Friedman (1998) describes the family functions as the affective, socialization, reproductive, economic, and health care functions. The affective function is one of the most vital and focuses on meeting family members' needs for affection and understanding. The socialization function refers to the learning experiences provided within the family to teach children their culture and how to function and assume adult social roles. This is a lifelong process. The reproductive function ensures family continuity over the generations and the survival of society. Economic functions involve the family's provision and allocation of sufficient resources. Health care functions are met by the provision of such physical necessities as food, clothing, shelter, and health care.

Some functions are emphasized more in one phase of a family's life cycle; others are continuous for the family's survival and progress. Many functions previously performed almost exclusively by one gender (e.g., child care and financial

TABLE 2-1
Stages of the Family Life Cycle

Stage of Family Life Cycle	Emotional Process of Transition: Key Principles	Second-Order Changes in Family Status Required to Proceed Developmentally
Leaving home: single young adults	Accepting emotional and financial responsibility for self	Differentiation of self in relation to family of origin Development of intimate peer relationships Establishment of self through work and financial independence
Joining of families through marriage: new couple	Commitment to new system	Formation of marital system Realignment of relationships with extended families and friends to include spouse
Families with young children	Accepting new members into system	Adjusting marital system to make space for child(ren) Joining in childrearing, financial, and household tasks Realignment of relationships with extended family to include parenting and grandparenting roles
Families with adolescents	Increasing flexibility of family boundaries to include children's independence and grandparents' frailties	Shifting of parent-child relationships to permit adolescent to move in and out of system Refocus on midlife marital and career issues Beginning shift toward joint caring for older generation
Launching children and moving on	Accepting multitude of exits from and entries into the family system	Renegotiation of marital system as a dyad Development of adult-to-adult relationships between grown children and their parents Realignment of relationships to include in-laws and grandchildren Dealing with disabilities and death of parents (grandparents)
Families in later life	Accepting shifting of generational roles	Maintaining own and/or couple functioning and interests in face of physiologic decline; exploration of new familial and social role options Support for a more central role of middle generation Making room in the system for wisdom and experience of elderly members; supporting older generation without overfunctioning for them Dealing with loss of spouse, siblings, and other peers and preparation for own death; life review and integration

From Carter B, McGoldrick M: *The expanded family life cycle: individual, family, and social perspectives*, ed 3, Needham Heights, MA, 1999, Allyn & Bacon.

support) are today shared between genders. Although goals for socialization and childrearing practices differ from culture to culture, in most societies the family appears to have three major objectives in relation to children: caregiving, nurturing, and training.

Family Dynamics

Families work cooperatively to accomplish family functions. Through family dynamics (interactions and communication), family members assume appropriate social roles. Social roles in the family are learned in pairs (e.g., mother-father, parent-child, and brother-sister). Role pairing enables social interactions to take place in an orderly, predictable manner; the roles are said to be complementary. Some families maintain a traditional pairing of roles, whereas other families change behavior patterns to suit a change in family lifestyle. Rather than mother-father, brother-sister, the roles may be mother-daughter, mother-son. Negotiation brings these pair roles into a new alignment. Negotiation is essential to maintain family equilibrium.

Each family sets up boundaries between itself and society. People are conscious of the difference between "family members" and "outsiders," or people without kinship status. Some families isolate themselves from the outside community; others have a wide community network to help in times of stress. Although boundaries exist for every family, family members set up channels through which they interact with society. These channels also ensure that the family receives its share of social resources.

Ideally, the family uses its resources to provide a safe, intimate environment for the biopsychosocial development of the family members. The family provides for the nurturing of the newborn and the gradual socialization of the growing child. Children form their earliest and closest relationships with their parents or parenting persons; these affiliations continue throughout a lifetime. For better or worse, parent-child relationships influence self-worth and the ability to form later relationships. The family also influences the child's perceptions of the outside world. The family provides the growing child with an identity that possesses both a past and a sense of the future. Cultural values and rituals are passed from one generation to the next through the family (Friedman, 1998).

Through everyday interactions, the family develops and uses its own patterns of verbal and nonverbal communication. These patterns give insight into the emotional exchange within a family and act as reliable indicators of interpersonal functioning. Family members not only react to the communication or actions of other family members, but also interpret and define them.

Over time the family develops protocols for problem solving, particularly regarding important decisions such as having a baby, buying a house, or sending children to college. The criteria used in making decisions are based on family values and attitudes about the appropriateness of the behavior and the moral, social, political, and economic events of society. The power to make critical decisions is given to a family member through tradition or negotiation. This power is not always stated. Power reflects the family's concepts of male or female dominance and cultural practices, social customs, and community norms. As a result, family members attain certain statuses or hierarchies. They play out these statuses by assuming various roles. Most families have a member who "takes charge" or "is supportive" or "can't be expected to do anything."

Family Theories

A family theory can be used to describe families and how the family unit responds to events both within and outside the family. Each family theory makes certain assumptions about the family and has inherent strengths and limitations. Most nurses use a combination of theories in their work with families. A brief discussion of three family theories (i.e., systems, developmental, and stress theories) and their implications for maternal-child nursing is presented here.

Family Systems Theory. Family systems theory is derived from general system theory, a science of "wholeness" that is characterized by interaction among the components of the system and between the system and the environment. Wright and Leahy (2000) list the following as key characteristics of family systems theory:

- A family system is part of a larger suprasystem and comprises many subsystems.
- The family as a whole is greater than the sum of its individual members.
- A change in one family member affects all family members.
- The family is able to create a balance between change and stability.
- Family members' behaviors are best understood from a view of circular rather than linear causality; that is, an individual's behavior affects and is affected by the behavior of others.

The family systems theory encourages nurses to view individual family members as part of a larger family system influenced by and influencing others. Application of these concepts can guide assessment and interventions for the family. For example, the childbearing family interacts as a system with many elements in the environmental suprasystem, including the health care community. The extent to which this suprasystem influences the family in matters such as prenatal care, childbirth education, and infant care depends on the family's boundary permeability. A relatively closed family may want instructions only from others within the family, whereas a relatively open family may be more receptive to instruction from health care providers.

Family Developmental Theory. Family developmental theory focuses on the family as it moves across time. Family members pass through phases of growth from dependence to active independence to interdependence. The family's structure and function also varies over time. Taken together, the stages that follow constitute the family life cycle (Carter and McGoldrick, 1988):

- Leaving home: single young adults
- Joining of families through marriage: the new couple
- Families with young children
- Families with adolescents
- Launching children and moving on
- Families in later life

The developmental perspective provides many useful insights into family functioning. Family members—as a group and as individuals—engage in developmental tasks simultaneously. Disharmony results when the developmental task of the family does not correspond with that of the person. For example, the adolescent father may be grappling with the need to break from his own family ties while also trying to establish monetary and other support for his new family. Or the toddler who is learning socially acceptable behaviors may revert to infantile behavior when introduced to a new sibling. The developmental approach presents a realistic, constantly evolving concept of family. Using this knowledge the nurse can help the family develop appropriate coping mechanisms (Nursing Care Plan).

Family Stress Theory. Family stress theory is concerned with the ways families react to stressful events. Boss (1988) believes that family stress must be studied within the internal and external contexts in which the family is living. The internal context involves elements that a family can change or control, such as family structure (e.g., boundaries and roles), psychologic defenses (e.g., perception of the event), and philosophic values and beliefs. The external context consists of the time and place in which a particular family finds itself. A family has no control over these elements, which include the culture of the larger society, the time in history during which the events happen to the family, the economic state of society, maturity of the individuals involved, success of the family in coping with stressors, and genetic inheritance.

Nurses working with childbearing families may find the family stress theory particularly useful because of its realistic and practical approach. Birth is one of the expected developmental (maturational) stressor events. Although a birth is expected and normal, its occurrence causes family dynamics to shift, thus having the potential to change a family's stress level. Families experience increased stress at each transition point.

Nurses can be instrumental in assisting families to change their stress levels by helping them exercise control of internal context factors. For example, if a family's perception of a stressful event is based on incorrect or incomplete information, the nurse intervenes through educational strategies. Nurses can explain various dimensions of the external context. For example,

Nursing Care Plan INCORPORATING THE INFANT INTO THE FAMILY

NURSING DIAGNOSIS Family coping, potential for growth related to adaptation of family to new infant

EXPECTED OUTCOME Family members will verbalize that individual as well as family goals are met during a smooth transition of new family member into the home.

Nursing Interventions/*Rationales*

Assess type and amount of support available to family on a daily basis during the postpartal period *to facilitate adaptation of the family to situation of a new member.*

Encourage family to use past successful coping mechanisms *to enhance ability to cope with new situation and promote self-esteem.*

Encourage mother to use family and other support or services to carry out daily household tasks *to permit her to focus on herself and infant.*

Suggest that woman take time to rest when infant sleeps *to conserve energy for healing and limit responsibility to herself and infant.*

Give suggestions regarding potential roles of siblings and grandparents, taking into account developmental stages and availability of grandparents *to include all family members in creative ways and facilitate goals of all family members.*

Assess family structure and relationships, including culture *to evaluate if longer period of adjustment may be expected.*

Teach family about sensory needs and capabilities of infant *to motivate family to meet infant's needs and set realistic expectations for infant's capabilities.*

Refer to parent support group or community agencies, as needed *to facilitate and validate ongoing positive adjustment of family to new family member.*

NURSING DIAGNOSIS Role performance, altered, related to developmental challenge of addition of new family member

EXPECTED OUTCOME Each family member will verbalize realistic expectations regarding his or her role in the family and formulate a plan to incorporate role into overall family goals.

Nursing Interventions/*Rationales*

Assess family structure, roles, and each member's perception of his or her role in the family *to evaluate the impact of the new member on the structure and roles of the family as perceived by the members.*

Evaluate individual's perception of goals and new roles during this transition *to promote early intervention and correct any misinterpretation.*

Encourage discussion of family members' thoughts and feelings regarding this transition *to promote open communication and trust.*

Provide positive reinforcement for family members' actions that promote a positive environment for the infant *to increase self-esteem and provide encouragement.*

Refer to community support groups *to provide group reinforcement and further assistance.*

Give information about sibling and grandparent classes and support groups as available *to promote empowerment and self-esteem for significant others in the family.*

explaining normal infant growth and development (maturation) may reduce the stress of parenting.

KEY FACTORS IN FAMILY HEALTH

Family dynamics, family socioeconomics, and family response to stress and culture are important in determining the quality of family health. For example, family dynamics (see previous discussion) encompass the coordination of intrafamilial roles, distribution of power within the family, and the decision-making process. Family dynamics also affect the use of health services.

Family socioeconomic characteristics influence the family's ability to access and use health care services. Socioeconomic factors govern expectations, obligations, and rewards, all of which affect the use of health services. In addition, the family acts as the primary economic unit in which incomes may be pooled, expenditure decisions made jointly, and services rendered internally.

Friedman (1998) considers a family's social class as the prime molder of its lifestyle. Socioeconomic factors and cultural background influence family values and practices, family behavior patterns, socialization, and world experiences. The interplay among stress, perception, and resources affects the level of support afforded family members. The family's response to stress influences its members' physiologic and psychologic well-being. Cultural responses to childbearing and use of related health care services play a central role in family health.

Cultural Factors Related to Family Health

Cultural Context of the Family. The family process within its cultural context is a central concern in nursing, especially when the nurse is providing care to the childbearing family. A critical life experience, such as childbearing, is often bound by traditional beliefs and practices. A culture's beliefs and practices regarding childbearing are embedded in its economic, religious, kinship, and political structures. All cultures have behavioral norms and expectations for each stage of the perinatal cycle. These norms and expectations relate to each culture's view of how people stay healthy and prevent illness. To practice with cultural competence, nurses must focus on the way people of different cultures perceive life events and the health care system. Patients have the right to expect that their physiologic and psychologic health care needs will be met and that their cultural beliefs will be respected.

Many subcultures may be found within each culture. Subculture refers to a group that retains its own characteristics while existing within a larger cultural system. A subculture may be an ethnic group or a group organized in another way. In the United States there are many ethnic subcultures (e.g., African-Americans, Asian-Americans, and Hispanics) as well as subcultures within these groups. Nurses should remember that the Caucasian population in the United States also has diverse and multiple subcultures. Although recent literature in the area of ethnicity and health has focused on people of color, little has been written about Caucasian ethnic communities (e.g., Italian-Americans, Polish-Americans, and German-Americans) (Spector, 1996). In issues of health, illness, and major life transitions, greater differences than have generally been acknowledged may exist among Caucasian groups.

Each subculture holds rich and complex traditions, including health practices, that have proved effective over time. These traditions vary from group to group. In a multicultural society, many groups can influence these traditions and practices. As cultural groups come in contact with each other, acculturation and assimilation may occur.

Acculturation refers to changes that occur in one or both groups when people from different cultures come in contact with one another. People may retain some of their own culture while adopting some cultural practices of the dominant society. This familiarization among cultural groups results in much overt behavioral similarity, especially in mannerisms, styles, and practices. Dress, language patterns, food choices, and health practices especially show differences among cultural groups within a society. In the United States, acculturation is generally thought to take three generations. The adult grandchild of the immigrant is usually fully Americanized (Spector, 1996). An example of acculturation is the adoption of ethnic food practices in the United States.

Assimilation, on the other hand, occurs when a cultural group loses its identity and becomes a part of the dominant culture. According to Friedman (1998), "assimilation denotes the more complete and one-way process of one culture being absorbed into the other." Assimilation is the process by which groups "melt" into the mainstream, thus accounting for the notion of a "melting pot." This phenomenon has been said to occur in the United States. However Spector (1996) asserts that in the United States, the melting pot, with its dream of a common culture "has proved to be a myth and has faded; it is now time to identify the mosaic phenomenon and both accept and appreciate the differences among people."

A wide range of cultural diversity exists within society. The health care provider striving to provide culturally appropriate health care must assess the beliefs and practices of patients. Nurses must be aware of factors that may prevent some health care practitioners from delivering optimum care. Understanding the concepts of ethnocentrism and cultural relativism may be helpful to nurses caring for families in a multicultural society.

Ethnocentrism refers to "the view that one's culture's way of doing things is the right and natural way" (Galanti, 1997). Essentially, ethnocentrism supports the notion that "my group is the best." Although the United States is a culturally diverse nation, the prevailing practice of health care is based on beliefs and practices held by members of the dominant culture, primarily Caucasians of European descent. This practice is based on the biomedical model that represents pregnancy and childbirth as phenomena with inherent risk, most appropriately managed through specific knowledge and technology. When encountering behavior in women unfamiliar with this model, the nurse may become frustrated and impatient. The nurse may label the behavior inappropriate and believe that it conflicts with "good" health practices. If the Western health care system provides the nurse's only standard for judgment, the behavior of the nurse is ethnocentric.

Cultural relativism is the opposite of ethnocentrism. It involves learning about and applying the standards of another person's culture to activities within that culture. To be culturally relativistic, the nurse recognizes that people from different cultural backgrounds comprehend the same objects and situa-

Critical Thinking

CULTURE AND VIEWS OF HEALTH

In a prenatal clinic, interview families from at least two different cultural backgrounds.

- **What do they believe will keep them healthy in pregnancy?**
- **What are the roles of men and women in childbirth? Who should be present at birth?**
- **What is the role of technology in the childbirth process?**
- **Are there restrictions on activity and diet in the postpartum period?**
- **What is the preferred method of infant feeding? How soon after birth should breastfeeding begin?**
- **Are there special foods that should be eaten during pregnancy or after childbirth?**
- **What will keep the baby healthy after birth?**

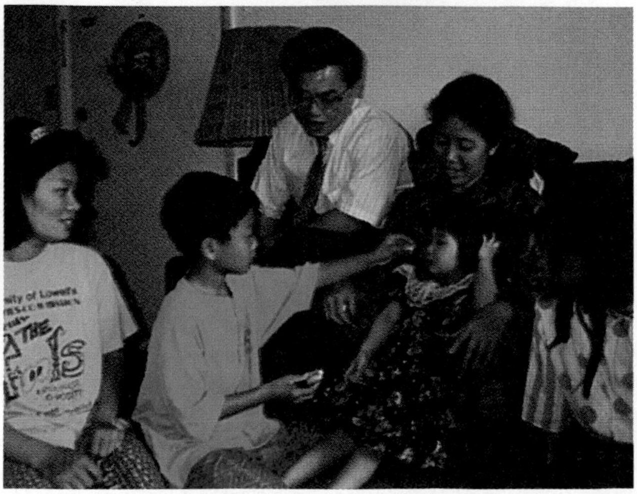

FIG. 2-3 • Southeast Asian families may be large and closely spaced. They are often a closely knit group. (From Dickason E, Silverman B, Kaplan J: *Maternal-infant nursing care,* ed 3, St Louis, 1998, Mosby.)

tions differently; that is, that culture determines a person's viewpoint.

Cultural relativism does not require nurses to accept the beliefs and values of another culture; rather, nurses recognize that the behavior of others may be based on a system of logic different from their own. Cultural relativism affirms the uniqueness and value of every culture.

Childbearing Beliefs and Practices. Nurses working with childbearing families in the United States and Canada care for families from different cultures and ethnic groups (Fig. 2-3). To provide culturally competent care, the nurse should be aware of the cultural beliefs and practices important to individual families. Countless beliefs and practices stem from a religious or ethnic origin and may be observed by families with differing cultural backgrounds.

A nurse should consider the products of culture—including communication, space, time, and family roles—when working with childbearing families. Communication often creates the most difficult problem for nurses working with patients from another cultural group. Communication includes understanding not only the individual's language, varied dialect, and style, but also volume of speech and the meaning of touch and gestures. When the patient and/or family do not speak the same language as the nurse, a translator can be used to address the family's health care needs in a culturally competent manner. When working with a translator, the nurse respects the family by addressing questions to them and not the translator (Box 2-1).

Personal space needs and feelings of territoriality develop in a cultural context. Although personal space varies from person to person and with the situation, dimensions of comfort zones differ from culture to culture. Actions such as touching, placing the patient in proximity to others, taking away personal possessions, and making decisions for the patient can decrease personal security and heighten anxiety. On the other hand, respecting the need for distance allows the patient to maintain control over personal space and support personal autonomy, thereby increasing the sense of security. For example, Chinese-Americans are traditionally a noncontact group, and some members of this group may consider closeness, increased eye contact, and touch offensive or impolite. Misunderstandings can be reduced by providing explanations when performing tasks that require close contact. Nurses often use touch, espe-

Box 2-1

Working with a Translator

STEP 1: BEFORE THE INTERVIEW

A. Outline your statements and questions. List the key pieces of information you want/need to know.
B. Learn something about the culture so that you can converse informally with the translator.

STEP 2: MEETING WITH THE TRANSLATOR

A. Introduce yourself to the translator and converse informally. This is the time to find out how well he or she speaks English. No matter how proficient or what age the translator is, be respectful. Some ways to show respect are to ask a cultural question to acknowledge that you can learn from the translator, or you could learn one word or phrase from the translator.
B. Emphasize that you do want the patient to ask questions because some cultures consider this inappropriate behavior.
C. Make sure the translator is comfortable with the technical terms you need to use. If not, take some time to explain them.

STEP 3: DURING THE INTERVIEW

A. Ask your questions and explain your statements (see Step 1).
B. Make sure that the translator understands which parts of the interview are most important. You usually have limited time with the translator, and you want to have adequate time at the end for patient questions.
C. Try to get a "feel" for how much is "getting through." No matter what the language is, if in relating information to the patient the translator uses far fewer or far more words than you do, "something else" is going on.
D. Stop every now and then and ask the translator, "How is it going?" You may not get a totally accurate answer, but you will have emphasized to the translator your strong desire to focus on the task at hand, if there are language problems: (1) speak *slowly;* (2) use gestures (e.g., fingers to count or point to body parts); and (3) use pictures.
E. Ask the translator to elicit questions. This may be difficult, but it is worth the effort.
F. Identify cultural issues that may conflict with your requests or instructions.
G. Use the translator to help problem solve or at least give insight into possibilities for solutions.

STEP 4: AFTER THE INTERVIEW

A. Speak to the translator and try to get an idea of what went well and what could be improved. This will help you to be more effective with this or another translator.
B. Make notes on what you learned for your future reference or to help a colleague.

Remember:

Your interview is a *collaboration* between you and the translator. *Listen* as well as speak.

Notes:

1. The translator may be a child, grandchild, or sibling of the patient. Be sensitive to the fact that the child is playing an adult role.
2. Be sensitive to cultural and situational differences (e.g., an interview with someone from urban Germany will likely be different from an interview with someone from a transitional refugee camp).
3. Younger females telling older males what to do may be a problem for both a female nurse and a female translator. This is not the time to pioneer new gender relations. Be aware that in some cultures it is difficult for a woman to talk about some topics with a husband or a father present.

Courtesy Elizabeth Whalley, PhD, San Francisco State University.

cially in areas such as labor and delivery. The acceptance and effectiveness of these approaches must be considered in a cultural context.

Nurses must also understand time as it pertains to culture. People in cultural groups may be oriented to the past, present, or future. People who focus on the past strive to maintain tradition and have little motivation for formulating future goals. Some individuals who focus on the present neither save for the future nor appreciate the past; these individuals may not adhere to strict, time-structured schedules. Individuals oriented to the future use the present to achieve future goals.

The time orientation of the childbearing family may affect nursing care. For example, bringing the infant to the clinic for follow-up examinations at a specific time may be difficult for the family that focuses on the present. On the other hand, a family with a future-oriented sense of time, in which events are planned, may be much more likely to return for scheduled visits. Despite differences in time orientation, each family may be equally concerned for the well-being of its newborn.

Family roles involve the expectations and behaviors associated with a member's position in the family (e.g., mother, father, or grandparent). Social class and cultural norms also affect these roles; distinct roles for men and women may be stressed. For example, culture may influence whether a man actively participates in pregnancy and childbirth. In turn, the way that health care practitioners manage a family's care molds its experience in and perception of the Western health care system. Maternity care practitioners expect fathers to be involved, but this role expectation may conflict with that of Mexican-Americans and Arab-Americans, who usually view the birthing experience as a female affair (Cultural Considerations box).

Cultural Considerations

QUESTIONS TO OBTAIN CULTURAL EXPECTATIONS ABOUT CHILDBEARING

1. **What do you and your family think you should do to remain healthy during pregnancy?**
2. **What are the things you can do or cannot do to improve your health and the health of your baby?**
3. **Who do you want with you during your labor?**
4. **What actions are important for you and your family to do after the baby's birth?**
5. **What do you and your family expect from the nurse(s) caring for you?**
6. **How will family members participate in your pregnancy, childbirth, and parenting?**

Critical Thinking

FAMILY GENOGRAM

Interview members of a family. Prepare a genogram based on the information you obtained. How many variations in family composition are present in this family? Are there indications of any genetic disorders in the genogram? How could you use this information to provide care to the family? Discuss the genogram with the family and provide them with a copy. What was their response to the genogram?

The nurse needs to be familiar with each woman as an individual and validate her cultural beliefs. The nurse supports and nurtures the beliefs that promote physical or emotional adaptation to childbearing. However, if certain beliefs might be harmful, the nurse should carefully explore them with the woman and use them in the reeducation and modification process.

Table 2-2 provides examples of some cultural beliefs and practices surrounding childbearing. Most of these cultural beliefs and customs reflect the traditional culture and are not practiced by all members of the cultural group in the United States and Canada. Variables such as degree of acculturation, educational and income levels, and amount of contact with the older generations influence the extent to which these customs are practiced. Women from these cultural and ethnic groups may adhere to some, all, or none of the practices listed.

Family-centered care is "based on mutually beneficial partnerships among childbearing women, infants, family members, and health care providers" (Gordon and Johnson, 1999). In planning the care of a family or individual family member, the nurse may find it useful to view the family as being at a developmental phase in the life cycle, as facing stressful life events, or as operating as a system. A family assessment tool such as the one outlined by Friedman (1998) can be used as a guide for assessing the aspects of family discussed in this chapter, including family development, family structure, family functions, and family stress and coping. A family genogram (Fig. 2-4) provides valuable information about a family and can be placed in the nursing care plan for easy access by care providers.

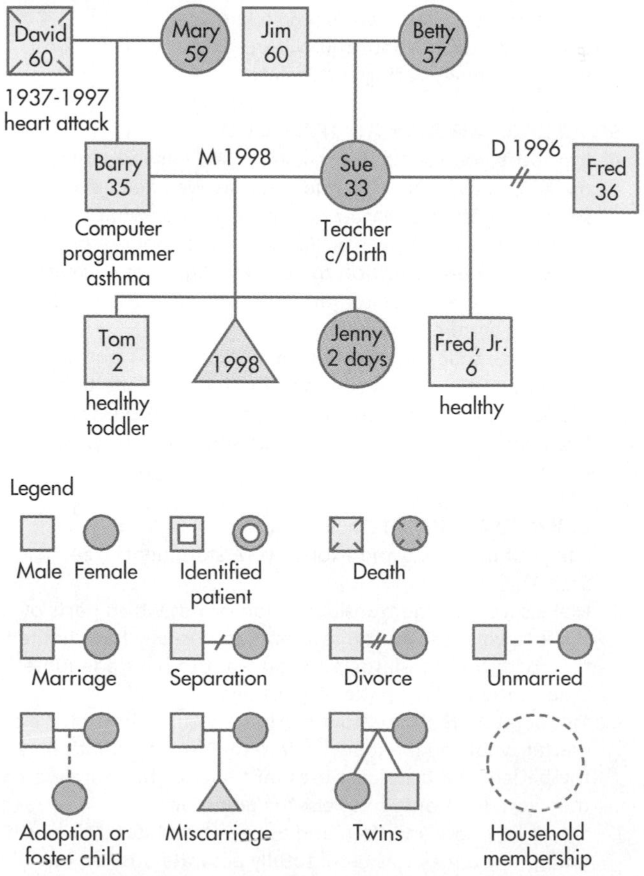

FIG. 2-4 • Example of a family genogram.

TABLE 2-2

Traditional* Cultural Beliefs and Practices: Childbearing and Parenting

Pregnancy	Childbirth	Parenting
HISPANIC (Based primarily on knowledge of Mexican-Americans; members of the Hispanic community have their origins in Spain, Cuba, Central and South America, Mexico, Puerto Rico, and other Spanish-speaking countries.)		
Pregnancy Pregnancy desired soon after marriage Late prenatal care Expectant mother influenced strongly by mother or mother-in-law Cool air in motion considered dangerous during pregnancy Unsatisfied food cravings thought to cause a birthmark Some pica observed in the eating of ashes or dirt (not common) Milk avoided because it causes large babies and difficult births Many predictions about sex of baby May be unacceptable and frightening to have pelvic examination by male health care provider Use of herbs to treat common complaints of pregnancy Drinking chamomile tea thought to ensure effective labor	**Labor** Use of "partera" or lay midwife preferred in some places; may prefer presence of mother rather than husband After birth of baby, mother's legs brought together to prevent air from entering uterus Loud behavior in labor **Postpartum** Diet may be restricted after birth; for first 2 days only boiled milk and toasted tortillas permitted (special foods to restore warmth to body) Bed rest for 3 days after birth Keep warm Delay bathing Mother's head and feet protected from cold air; bathing permitted after 14 days Mother often cared for by her own mother 40-day restriction on sexual intercourse	**Newborn** Breastfeeding begun after third day; colostrum may be considered "filthy" or "spoiled" Olive oil or castor oil given to stimulate passage of meconium Male infant not circumcised Female infant's ears pierced Belly band used to prevent umbilical hernia Religious medal worn by mother during pregnancy; placed around infant's neck Infant protected from "evil eye" Various remedies used to treat "Mal ojo" (evil eye) and fallen fontanel (depressed fontanel)
AFRICAN-AMERICAN (Members of the African-American community, many of whom are descendants of slaves, have different origins. Today a number of Black Americans have emigrated from Africa, the West Indian Islands, the Dominican Republic, Haiti, and Jamaica.)		
Pregnancy Acceptance of pregnancy depends on economic status Pregnancy thought to be state of "wellness," which is often the reason for delay in seeking prenatal care, especially by lower-income African-Americans "Old wives' tales" include having a picture taken during pregnancy will cause stillbirth and reaching up will cause cord to strangle baby Craving for certain foods, including chicken, greens, clay, starch, and dirt Pregnancy may be viewed by African-American men as a sign of their virility Self-treatment for various discomforts of pregnancy, including constipation, nausea, vomiting, headache, and heartburn	**Labor** Use of "Granny midwife" in certain parts of United States Varied emotional responses: some cry out, some display stoic behavior to avoid calling attention to selves Patient may arrive at hospital in far-advanced labor Emotional support often provided by other women, especially own mother **Postpartum** Vaginal bleeding seen as sign of sickness; tub baths and shampooing of hair prohibited Sassafras tea thought to have healing power Eating liver thought to cause heavier vaginal bleeding because of its high "blood" content	**Newborn** Feeding very important: "Good" baby thought to eat well Early introduction of solid foods May breastfeed or bottle-feed; breastfeeding may be considered embarrassing Parents fearful of spoiling baby Commonly call baby by nicknames May use excessive clothing to keep baby warm Belly band used to prevent umbilical hernia Abundant use of oil on baby's scalp and skin Strong feeling of family, community, and religion

Data from Amaro H: Women in the Mexican-American community: religion, culture, and reproductive attitudes and experiences, *J Comm Psych* 16(1):6-19, 1994; Bar-Yam N: Learning about culture: a guide for birth practitioners, *Int J Childbirth Educ* 9(2):8-10, 1994; Galanti, G: *Caring for patients from different cultures: case studies from American hospitals,* ed 2, Philadelphia, 1997, University of Pennsylvania Press; Geissler E: *Pocket guide to cultural assessment,* St Louis, 1994, Mosby; Mattson S: Culturally sensitive prenatal care for Southeastern Asians, *J Obstet Gynecol Neonatal Nurs* 24(4):335-341, 1995; Spector R: *Cultural diversity in health and illness,* ed 5, Upper Saddle River, NJ, 2000, Prentice Hall Health; and Williams R: Issues in women's health care. In Johnson B, editor: *Psychiatric mental health nursing: adaptation and growth.* Philadelphia, 1989, JB Lippincott.

NOTE: Most of these cultural beliefs and customs reflect the traditional culture and are not universally practiced. These lists are not intended to stereotype patients but rather to serve as guidelines while discussing meaningful cultural beliefs with a patient and her family. Examples of other cultural beliefs and practices are found throughout this text.

*Variations in some beliefs and practices exist within subcultures of each group.

Continued

TABLE 2-2—cont'd

Traditional* Cultural Beliefs and Practices: Childbearing and Parenting

Pregnancy	Childbirth	Parenting
ASIAN-AMERICANS (Typically refers to groups from China, Korea, the Philippines, Japan, Southeast Asia [particularly Thailand], Indochina, and Vietnam)		
Pregnancy Pregnancy considered time when mother "has happiness in her body" Pregnancy seen as natural process Strong preference for female health care provider Belief in theory of hot and cold May omit soy sauce in diet to prevent dark-skinned baby Prefer soup made with ginseng root as general strength tonic Milk usually excluded from diet because it causes stomach distress Inactivity or sleeping late may cause difficult delivery	**Labor** Mother admitted by other women, especially her own mother Father does not actively participate Labor in silence Cesarean birth not welcome **Postpartum** Must protect self from yin (cold forces) for 30 days Ambulation limited Shower and bathing prohibited Warm room Chinese mother avoids fruits and vegetables Diet: Warm fluids Some patients are vegetarians Korean mother served seaweed soup with rice Chinese diet high in hot foods	**Newborn** Concept of family important and valued Father is head of household; wife plays a subordinate role Birth of boy preferred May delay naming child Some groups (e.g., Vietnamese) believe colostrum is dirty; therefore they may delay breastfeeding until milk comes in
EUROPEAN-AMERICAN (Members of the European-American [Caucasian] community have their origins in countries such as Ireland, Great Britain, Germany, Italy, and France.)		
Pregnancy Pregnancy viewed as a condition that requires medical attention to ensure health Emphasis on early prenatal care Variety of childbirth education programs available and participation encouraged Technology driven Emphasis on nutritional science Involvement of the father valued Written source of information valued	**Labor** Birth is a public concern Technology dominated Birthing process in institutional setting valued Involvement of father expected Physician seen as head of team **Postpartum** Emphasis or focus on early bonding Medical interventions for dealing with discomfort Early ambulation and activity emphasized Self-care valued	**Newborn** Increased popularity of breastfeeding Breastfeeding begins as soon as possible after childbirth **Parenting** Motherhood and transition to parenting seen as stressful time Nuclear family valued, although single parenting and other forms of parenting more acceptable than in the past Women often deal with multiple roles Early return to prenatal activities

Data from Amaro H: Women in the Mexican-American community: religion, culture, and reproductive attitudes and experiences, *J Comm Psych* 16(1):6-19, 1994; Bar-Yam N: Learning about culture: a guide for birth practitioners, *Int J Childbirth Educ* 9(2):8-10, 1994; Galanti, G: *Caring for patients from different cultures: case studies from American hospitals,* ed 2, Philadelphia, 1997, University of Pennsylvania Press; Geissler E: *Pocket guide to cultural assessment,* St Louis, 1994, Mosby; Mattson S: Culturally sensitive prenatal care for Southeastern Asians, *J Obstet Gynecol Neonatal Nurs* 24(4):335-341, 1995; Spector R: *Cultural diversity in health and illness,* ed 5, Upper Saddle River, NJ, 2000, Prentice Hall Health; and Williams R: Issues in women's health care. In Johnson B, editor: *Psychiatric mental health nursing: adaptation and growth.* Philadelphia, 1989, JB Lippincott.

NOTE: Most of these cultural beliefs and customs reflect the traditional culture and are not universally practiced. These lists are not intended to stereotype patients but rather to serve as guidelines while discussing meaningful cultural beliefs with a patient and her family. Examples of other cultural beliefs and practices are found throughout this text.

*Variations in some beliefs and practices exist within subcultures of each group.

TABLE 2-2—cont'd

Traditional* Cultural Beliefs and Practices: Childbearing and Parenting

Pregnancy	Childbirth	Parenting
NATIVE AMERICAN (Many different tribes exist within the Native American culture; viewpoints vary according to tribal customs and beliefs.)		
Pregnancy Pregnancy considered as a normal, natural process Late prenatal care Avoid heavy lifting Herb teas encouraged	**Labor** Prefers female attendant, although husband, mother, or father may assist with birth Birth may be attended by whole family Herbs may be used to promote uterine activity Birth may occur in squatting position **Postpartum** Herb teas to stop bleeding	**Newborn** Infant not fed colostrum Use of herbs to increase flow of milk Use of cradle boards for infant Babies not handled often

Key Points

- There are a variety of family forms in contemporary American society.
- The family is a social network that acts as an important support system for its members.
- Ideally, the family provides a safe, intimate environment for the biopsychosocial development of its members.
- Family systems, developmental, and stress theories provide nurses with useful guides to understand family function.
- Family socioeconomics, response to stress, and culture are key factors influencing family health.
- The reproductive beliefs and practices of a culture are embedded in its economic, religious, kinship, and political structures.

References

Amaro H: Women in the Mexican-American community: religion, culture, and reproductive attitudes and experiences, *J Comm Psych* 16(1):6-19, 1994.

Bar-Yam N: Learning about culture: a guide for birth practitioners, *Int J Childbirth Educ* 9(2):8-10, 1994.

Boss P: *Family stress management,* Newbury Park, CA, 1988, Sage.

Carter B, McGoldrick M, editors: *The changing family life cycle: a framework for family therapy,* ed 2, Needham Heights, MA, 1988, Allyn & Bacon.

Dickason E, Silverman B, Kaplan J: *Maternal-infant nursing care,* ed 3, St Louis, 1998, Mosby.

Friedman M: *Family nursing theory and assessment,* ed 4, New York, 1998, Appleton & Lange.

Galanti G: *Caring for patients from different cultures: case studies from American hospitals,* ed 2, Philadelphia, 1997, University of Pennsylvania Press.

Geissler E: *Pocket guide to cultural assessment,* St Louis, 1994, Mosby.

Gordin P, Johnson B: Technology and family-centered perinatal care: conflict or synergy? *J Obstet Gynecol Neonatal Nurs* 28(4):401-408, 1999.

Mattson S: Culturally sensitive prenatal care for Southeastern Asians, *J Obstet Gynecol Neonatal Nurs* 24(4):335-341, 1995.

Mohr W: Partnering with families, *J of Psychosocial Nurs* 38(1):15-22, 2000.

Spector R: *Cultural diversity in health and illness,* ed 5, Upper Saddle River, NJ, 2000, Prentice Hall Health.

Williams R: Issues in women's health care. In Johnson B, editor: *Psychiatric mental health nursing: adaptation and growth.* Philadelphia, 1989, JB Lippincott.

Wright L, Leahey M: *Nurses and families: a guide to family assessment and intervention,* ed 3, Philadelphia, 2000, F.A. Davis.

CHAPTER

3

Community and Home Care

http://www.harcourthealth.com/MERLIN/Wong/maternal/

Learning Objectives

On completion of this chapter the reader will be able to:

- Compare community-based health care and community health (population or aggregate focused) care.
- Select appropriate methods of community assessment for specific situations.
- List health indicators of community health status and their relevance to perinatal health care.
- Discuss perinatal concerns and related nursing interventions for selected vulnerable populations: homeless, migrant laborers, and refugees.
- List the potential advantages and disadvantages of home visits.
- Identify and define common perinatal conditions amenable to home care.
- Discuss safety and infection control principles as they apply to the care of patients in their homes.
- Describe the nurse's role in perinatal home care.

Most health care for women occurs outside the acute care setting. The movement to reduce health care costs has shortened hospitalization time and led to an increase of home- and community-based options for the provision of care (Henry, 1997). The U.S. national health objectives in *Healthy People 2010* focus attention on the unequal distribution of disease and disability and the need to reach out to vulnerable populations not being adequately served by the current health system. Hospital-based nurses are increasingly involved in follow-up of patients and families after discharge (Fowler et al, 1997). Chapter 2 contains an overview of family and cultural theory and assessment. In this chapter the larger system of which the family is a part—the community—is discussed. Methods of community assessment and the special perinatal health needs of vulnerable aggregates in the population are identified. Included are guidelines and issues related to the provision of home care for patients across the perinatal continuum.

ASSESSING LEVELS OF COMMUNITY WELLNESS

Definitions of Community

There are many definitions of community, but most share three characteristics: people, place, and interaction or function. This discussion is limited to geographically based communities. The people are the residents of the community; place refers to geographic dimensions; function refers to the activities of the community that meet the needs of the residents (Shuster and Goeppinger, 1996). Fig. 3-1 shows the core of the community surrounded by the multiple systems that serve to meet its collective needs. The people who reside there make up the core of the community. Significant characteristics include the demographics of the population and the residents' values, beliefs, and culture. Economics, education, public safety, environmental factors, and availability of health and social services all have significant impact on community health and well-being. The broken lines between the segments emphasize the interaction and interdependence among the subsystems of the community (Anderson and McFarlane, 1996).

Methods of Community Assessment

The organization and focus of perinatal care at the community level must be responsive to the unique characteristics of the populations and their special needs.

Multiple sources of data about communities are available. A nurse who is providing family-focused home care may be primarily interested in becoming familiar with the neighborhoods and resources with which his or her patients interact. A community health agency must conduct a comprehensive needs assessment in order to plan and evaluate health services for the community as a whole. Methods of data collection include windshield surveys, participant observation, interviews, focus groups, analysis of existing data, and surveys.

Using one's senses while traveling through a community is the essence of the windshield (or walking) survey (Table 3-1).

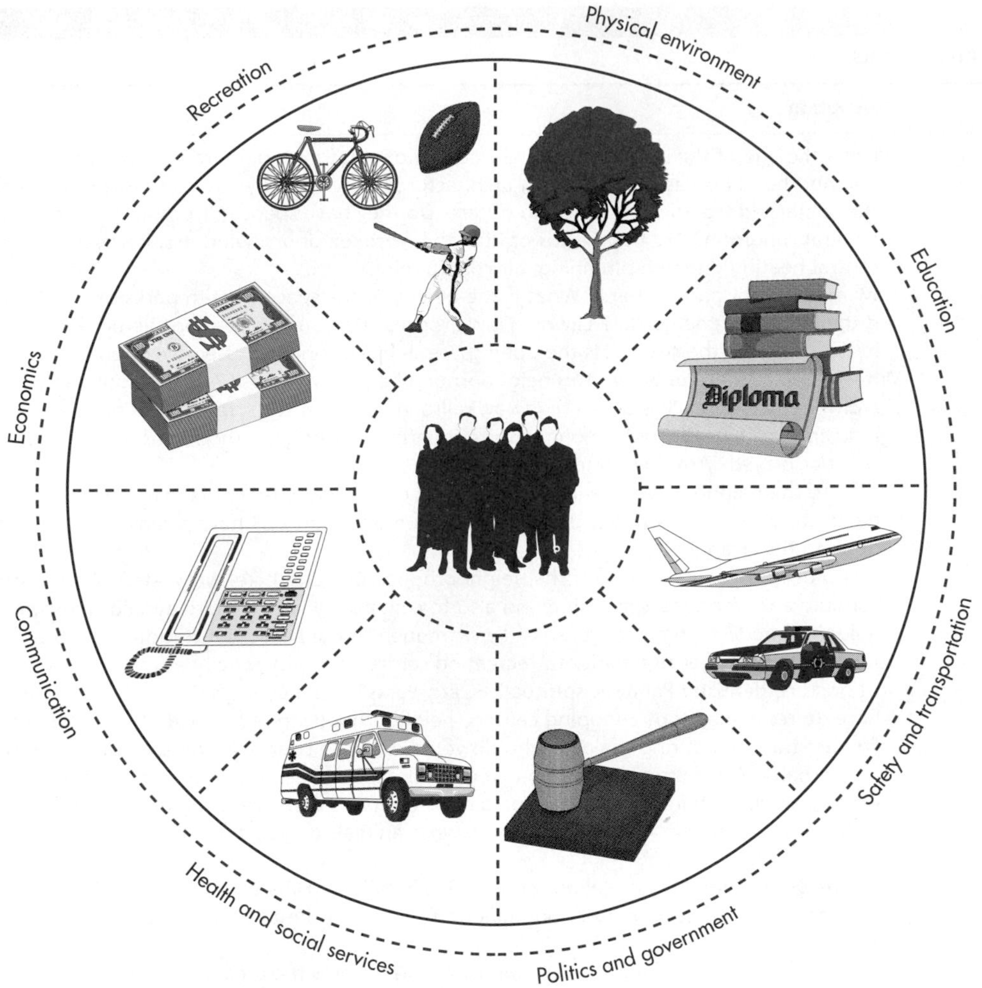

FIG. 3-1 • The community assessment wheel, the assessment segment of the community-as-partner model. (From Anderson E, McFarlane J: *Community as partner: theory and practice in nursing,* ed 2, Philadelphia, 1996, JB Lippincott.)

By using skills of observation during a trip through a community, a nurse can obtain significant information about its sociocultural characteristics and the environment, housing, transportation, and local community agencies. By using participant observation, in which nurses are part of the situation they wish to learn about, it is possible to more fully understand the people and processes involved and to validate perceptions and inferences.

Every 10 years the U.S. government conducts a national census. Census data offer a broad range of information that is extremely helpful to nurses and other health care providers who wish to become familiar with a community. These data include population size; age, sex, and ethnic distribution; socioeconomic status; educational level; employment; and housing characteristics. Data on socioeconomic status and environmental stressors have been used to identify women at risk for delivery of a low-birth-weight (LBW) infant. Based on this information, outreach activities can be appropriately targeted (O'Campo et al, 1997).

Vital Statistics and Other Sources of Health Data. Official records of births and deaths are reported annually for the preceding year by city, county, and state health departments. In addition to the number of births and deaths, certificates include the types of births, and any complications, as well as the causes of deaths. The National Center for Health Statistics publishes annual National Health Survey data that describe health trends on a national sample. Many state and local governments report health and planning agency data that assist the nurse in assessing the community. Voluntary agencies may conduct needs assessments: for example, the March of Dimes Birth Defects Foundation has supported perinatal needs assessments in many communities across the United States.

Interviews with selected individuals in positions of leadership (key informants) allow input from many different perspectives. Persons such as health care providers or administrators, religious leaders, government officials, representatives of voluntary health organizations, service clubs, and cultural

TABLE 3-1
Windshield Survey Components

Element	Description
Housing and zoning	What is the age of the houses, their architecture, of what materials are they constructed? Are all the neighborhood houses similar in age, architecture? How would you characterize the differences? Are they detached from or connected to others? Do they have space in front and behind? What is their general condition? Are there signs of disrepair—broken doors, windows, leaks, locks missing? Is there central heating, modern plumbing, air conditioning?
Open space	How much open space is there? What is the quality of the space—green parks or rubble-filled lots? What is the lot size of the houses? Lawns? Flower boxes? Do you see trees on the pavements, a green island in the center of the streets? Is the open space public or private? Used by whom?
Boundaries	What signs are there of where this neighborhood begins and ends? Are the boundaries natural—a river, a different terrain? Physical—a highway, railroad? Economic—difference, in real estate or presence of industrial, commercial units along with residential? The neighborhood has an identity, a name? Do you see it displayed? Are there unofficial names?
"Commons"	What are the neighborhood hangouts? For what groups, at what hours (e.g., schoolyard, candy store, bar, restaurant, park, 24-hour drugstore)? Does the "commons" have a sense of "territoriality" or is it open to the stranger?
Transportation	How do people get in and out of the neighborhood? Car, bus, bike, walk, etc.? Are the streets and roads conducive to good transportation and also to community life? Is there a major highway near the neighborhood? Whom does it serve? How frequent is public transportation available?
Service centers	Do you see social agencies, patients, recreation centers, signs of activity at the schools? Are there offices of doctors, dentists? Palmists, spiritualists, etc. Parks? Are they in use?
Stores	Where do residents shop? Shopping centers, neighborhood stores? How do they travel to shop?
Street people	If you are traveling during the day, who do you see on the street? An occasional housewife, a mother with a baby? Do you see anyone you would not expect? Teenagers, unemployed males? Can you spot a welfare worker, an insurance collector, a door-to-door salesman? Is the dress of those you see representative or unexpected? Along with people, what animals do you see? Stray cats, dogs, pedigreed pets, "watchdogs"?
Signs of decay	Is this neighborhood on the way up or down? Is it "alive"? How would you decide? Trash, abandoned cars, political posters, neighborhood meeting posters, real estate signs, abandoned houses, mixed-zoning usage?
Race	Are the residents Caucasian, African-American, Asian,* or is the area integrated?
Ethnicity	Are there indices of ethnicity—food stores, churches, private schools, information in a language other than English?
Religion	Of what religion are the residents? Do you see evidence of heterogeneity or homogeneity? What denomination are the churches? Do you see evidence of their use other than on Sunday mornings?
Health and morbidity	Do you see evidence of acute or of chronic diseases or conditions? Of accidents, communicable diseases, alcoholism, drug addiction, mental illness, etc.? How far is it to the nearest hospital? Clinic?
Politics	Do you see any political campaign posters? Is there a headquarters present? Do you see any evidence of a predominant party affiliation?
Media	Do you see outdoor TV antennas? What magazines, newspapers do residents read? Do you see *Forward Times, Hampton Post, Enquirer, Readers' Digest* in the stores? What media seem most important to the residents? Radio? TV?

Source: Anderson E, McFarlane J: *Community as partner: application of the nursing process,* Philadelphia, 1996, Lippincott.
*Added by author.

groups can provide an "insider's" viewpoint not available in published documents. Similarly, focus groups can be conducted with potential patients or collaborators to discuss needs and services important to the community. Formal surveys, either by mail, telephone, or face-to-face, are expensive and time consuming but can be sources of information not available from secondary sources. Knowledge of support groups, educational programs, and social service agencies allows the nurse to make appropriate referrals for perinatal patients. Information about community resources may be obtained from many of the sources listed previously, as well as the local United Way organization, telephone directory, or community services directory.

HEALTH AND WELLNESS IN THE COMMUNITY

Community Health Status Indicators

The data collected about communities can be compared with state or national standards to assess the well-being of the population as a whole and answer questions such as the following: Do most women begin prenatal care in the first trimester? What are the fetal and infant mortality rates?

Box 3-1 displays a set of community health status indicators developed by a committee of experts from many community health-related organizations. Infant mortality, because it is affected by the preconceptional health and prenatal and intra-

Box 3-1

Consensus Set of Indicators* for Assessing Community Health Status

INDICATORS OF HEALTH STATUS OUTCOME

1. Race/ethnicity-specific infant mortality, as measured by the rate (per 1000 live births) of deaths among infants younger than 1 year of age

Death rates (per 100,000 population)† for

2. Motor vehicle crashes
3. Work-related injury
4. Suicide
5. Lung cancer
6. Breast cancer
7. Cardiovascular disease
8. Homicide
9. All causes

Reported incidence (per 100,000 population) of

10. Acquired immunodeficiency syndrome
11. Measles
12. Tuberculosis
13. Primary and secondary syphilis

INDICATORS OF RISK FACTORS

14. Incidence of LBW, as measured by percentage of total number of liveborn infants weighing less than 2500 g at birth
15. Births to adolescents (females age 10 to 17 years) as a percentage of total live births
16. Prenatal care, as measured by percentage of mothers delivering live infants who did not receive prenatal care during first trimester
17. Childhood poverty, as measured by the proportion of children younger than 15 years of age living in families at or below the poverty level
18. Proportion of persons living in counties exceeding U.S. Environmental Protection Agency standards for air quality during previous year

From U.S. Department of Health and Human Services: Consensus set of indicators for assessing community health status, *MMWR* 40(27):449, 1991.
*Position or number of the indicator does not imply priority.
†Age-adjusted to the 1940 standard population.

partal care of the mother, as well as living conditions for the infant after birth, is a statistic widely used to compare the health status of different populations. Three of the five indicators of risk (i.e., incidence of low birth rate, adolescent pregnancy, and early prenatal care) refer to maternal-infant health. Poverty and a high percentage of young children in a community are strongly associated with significant community health needs (Zyzanski, Williams, and Flocke, 1996).

Healthy People 2010 has set national goals for maternal-child health. One of the overall goals is to reduce disparities in health between groups within the U.S. population. Infant mortality in the African-American population remains twice that of the nation as a whole in spite of efforts to address this concern. The rate of pregnancy in young adolescents is still higher than the targeted goal. Reported child abuse and neglect continue to increase. These and many other health problems require intervention at the community level in addition to assisting individuals to improve their personal health behaviors.

Critical Thinking

HEALTH NEEDS OF VULNERABLE POPULATIONS

Read your local newspaper and identify articles describing health needs of vulnerable populations in your community. Consult the yellow pages of the telephone book. Are there agencies in your area that specifically deal with meeting those needs? If you encountered a patient with one of the needs, to whom would you refer her?

Population- or Aggregate-Focused Care

Levels of Prevention. Population-focused health care uses a framework of levels of prevention:

- Primary prevention includes efforts made before the development of illness to promote general health and well-being. It also includes the use of specific protections, such as immunizations or approved infant car seats.
- Secondary prevention involves early detection of health problems so that treatment can begin before significant disability occurs. This includes various methods of health screening, such as prenatal care.
- Tertiary prevention is the treatment and rehabilitation of persons who have developed disease. Because most women are healthy during pregnancy, maternal-newborn nursing emphasizes primary and secondary prevention activities regardless of where care is provided. However, in general, the ill, hospitalized patient is the focus of tertiary prevention. This would include women with severe preeclampsia or other high risk condition.

High Risk Aggregates or Vulnerable Populations

Definition of Vulnerability. Vulnerable populations are groups at higher risk of developing physical, mental, or social health problems or who are more likely to have worse outcomes from these health problems than the population as a whole (Aday, 1997; Sebastian, 1996).

Many special population groups are more vulnerable to reproductive health risks. These include pregnant adolescents, substance abusers, violence-prone families, the mentally ill, people with sexually transmitted or other communicable diseases, and those with malnutrition. These groups are often served by community health nurses.

The Homeless. The term homeless, as defined by the U.S. Department of Housing and Urban Development, includes people who are homeless (e.g., living on the streets or in shelters) and those who are at risk of being homeless (e.g., those sharing housing and people who are transients). Each year an estimated 2.5 to 3 million people lack access to a conventional dwelling. Families are the fastest growing segment of this population. Families with children account for 33% to 43% of the homeless. Young, single women head 53% of homeless families. Many of these women have a history of physical or sexual abuse as children and have also abused alcohol or drugs (American Academy of Pediatrics, 1996; Stanhope and Lancaster, 1996). It is estimated that as many as 2 million homeless adolescents may be living on the streets of major cities. Many engage in "survival sex," exchanging sexual favors for food, clothing, and shelter, making them vulnerable to sexually transmitted infections and unintended pregnancies. They seldom appear at agencies serving the adult homeless population (Rew, 1996).

Many homeless women are covered by Medicaid and may go to private offices and hospitals for care. Distrust of the system may lead them to try to hide their status, making it difficult to do follow-up. Nurses working with homeless women and families agree that treating patients with dignity and respect is basic to establishing a therapeutic relationship. Case management is recommended to coordinate the various agencies and disciplines that may be involved in meeting the multiple needs of these families.

Migrants. An estimated 3 to 5 million people in America are classified as migrant farm workers; 16% of these are women (Maternal Child Health Bureau, 1997). Migrant laborers are those who must establish temporary residence in various areas on a seasonal basis in order to obtain employment. Most live in temporary housing for at least 6 months out of the year; others move continuously throughout the year. Ethnic groups among migrants include African-Americans, European-Americans, Hispanics, Haitians, and some Southeast Asians. Those in the western and central states are predominantly Mexican; the population in the east, traveling north from Florida, is more varied (Lambert, 1995; Rodriguez, 1996).

Migrant laborers and their families face many problems, including financial instability, child labor, poor housing, lack of education, language and cultural barriers, and limited access to health and social services (Clemen-Stone, Eigsti, and McGuire, 1998). The average life expectancy for migrant laborers is 49 years (as compared with 75 years for the population as a whole). Substance abuse and domestic violence are significant problems.

Higher rates of miscarriage, inadequate prenatal care, and infant mortality are reported in this population. There is concern about the reproductive effects of exposure to toxic chemicals. Less consistent use of contraception and increased rates of sexually transmitted infections, including human immunodeficiency virus (HIV), and inflammatory conditions of the cervix, vagina, and vulva are reported (Lambert, 1995). Migrants are more likely to initiate prenatal care later and to have inadequate pregnancy weight gain. The infant mortality rate is 2.5 times the national average (Sandhaus, 1998).

Although a system of 100 federally funded Migrant Health Centers has been established in the United States and Puerto Rico, these facilities see less than 15% of the 3 to 5 million farm workers, and the gap is not closed by the various voluntary agencies that also serve this community. Lack of trust (e.g., reluctance to share personal problems with a stranger or an undocumented person's fear of being reported to the Immigration and Naturalization Services) prevents many migrants from obtaining care.

Providing culturally competent care to a multiethnic population is a challenge for health care workers (Jones and Schenk, 1996; Lambert, 1995). (See Chapter 2 for a discussion of cultural competence.) One approach that has been successful is the use of lay camp aides to assist in outreach and health education. Among Hispanic women the use of camp volunteers (known as *romotoras*) who assist families in obtaining prenatal, postpartum, and infant care and meeting other health needs, has been effective. This partnership with the community provides a link between the formal health care system and traditional practices (Rodriguez, 1996). Guidance and information about other resources is available to health care providers through the National Migrant Resource Program and the Migrant Clinicians Network.

Refugees and Immigrants. One of every 140 people in the United States is of refugee origin (U.S. Committee on Refugees, 1995). The surge in refugee immigration began with Southeast Asians after the Vietnam War and continued with those from Ethiopia, Cuba, Bosnia and Eastern Europe, and the Kurds from Iraq. Other countries whose emigrants are not always officially recognized as refugees include Haiti, China, and uncounted numbers from Central America. Refugees are automatically eligible for permanent resident status and additional services and support. Problems of women refugees include being raped while in transit or in refugee camps and having no previous experience with prenatal care and family planning.

The World Health Organization recommends that reproductive health programs for refugee women include a minimum package of care related to issues of family planning; maternal mortality; unwanted pregnancy; sexually transmitted infections, including HIV and acquired immunodeficiency syndrome (AIDS); and physical and sexual violence. If they have lost children during the exodus from their country, women may want to rebuild their families soon after resettlement (Djeddah, 1995). Bicultural professionals and trained community workers from the refugee group have successfully reached women and families who were reluctant to interact with the health system of the new country (Lipson and Omidian, 1997). When refugee and other immigrant women are hospitalized, a cultural liaison who can interpret not only language but also differing cultural expectations is invaluable. Understanding reproductive health needs through the eyes of refugee communities is an essential step toward providing appropriate and culturally sensitive services and information (Djeddah, 1995; Gany and Bocanegra, 1996). Many immigrants who have strong ties to traditional medical practices from their homeland also respect Western or scientific practices. This pluralistic view allows them to combine both modalities without conflict (Kang, Kahler, and Tesar, 1998; Rodriguez, 1996).

Critical Thinking

HEALTH NEEDS OF A MIGRANT WORKER

The agency receives a referral for a home visit to a 16-year-old Spanish-speaking mother who is a migrant worker. She has a 2-week-old infant and is expected to return to the fields to work.

- **What should be taken into consideration by the nursing supervisor in assigning a nurse to this home visit?**
- **What additional information would the nurse need to develop a plan of care?**
- **What health teaching is likely to be needed?**
- **Describe the environmental assessment that would be appropriate.**
- **Identify community resources that are available to this mother.**

HOME CARE ACROSS THE PERINATAL CONTINUUM OF CARE

A continuum of care is defined as a range of clinical services provided for an individual or group that reflects care given during a single hospitalization or care for multiple conditions over a lifetime. Home care is one delivery component available along the perinatal continuum of care (Fig. 3-2). This continuum begins with family planning and continues with preconception care, prenatal care, intrapartum care, postpartum care, newborn care, interconceptional care, and infant care until the infant is 1 year old. Independent self-care, ambulatory care, home care, low risk hospitalization, or specialized intensive care may be appropriate at different points along this continuum.

Communication to Bridge the Continuum

As maternity care continues to consist of frequent and brief contacts with health care providers throughout the prenatal and postpartum periods, nurses must develop innovative nursing delivery methods as well as innovative ways to communicate that care is provided. Some hospitals have provided cross-training for hospital-based nurses to make postpartum home visits (Fowler et al, 1997; Pignatello et al, 1998). Another approach is the development of outpatient centers for postpartum follow-up, staffed by nurses from the maternity unit (Blystad-Keppler, 1995).

Telephonic Nursing Care. Telephonic nursing care—through services such as warm lines, nurse advice lines, and telephonic nursing assessments—is emerging as a valuable way to manage health care problems and bridge the gaps among acute, outpatient, and home care services. This type of nursing care occurs by telephone and is very interactive and responsive to the immediate questions consumers have about particular health care needs. Warm lines are telephone lines that are offered as a community service to provide new parents with support, encouragement, and basic parenting education. Nurse advice lines, or toll-free nurse consultation services, provide answers to medical questions, guide callers through urgent health care situations, suggest treatment options, and provide health education (Bleich, 1998). Telephonic nursing assessments are commonly used after a postpartum home care visit to reassess a woman's knowledge about the signs and symptoms of adequate hydration in breastfeeding; or, after initiating home phototherapy, to assess the caregiver's knowledge regarding problems with equipment.

Guidelines for Nursing Practice

Although the home care industry continues to grow rapidly, perinatal home care nursing practice is still emerging. The role of the perinatal home care nurse, and the ways this role differs from other health care providers, is still being molded by clinical practice and regulatory and accreditation organizations.

The Association of Women's Health, Obstetric, and Neonatal Nurses (AWHONN) (1998) defined home care as:

> . . . the provision of technical, psychological, and other therapeutic support in the patient's home rather than in an institution. The scope of nursing care delivered in the home setting is necessarily limited to practices deemed safe and appropriate to be carried out in an environment that is physically separated from a health care institution and its resources. . . . Nursing practice at home is consistent with federal and state regulations . . . that direct home care practice. The nurse demonstrates practice competence through formalized orientation and ongoing clinical education and performance evaluation in the respective home care agency. Standards for practice from key specialty organizations such as AWHONN, the American College of Obstetricians and Gynecologists (ACOG), the American Academy of Pediatrics, and the Intravenous Nursing Society (INS) provide the basis for clinical protocols and pathways and organizational programs in home care practice. The Joint Commission on Accreditation of Healthcare Organizations (JCAHO) provides criteria for home care operations.

AWHONN (1994) developed standards of practice and identified essential knowledge and skills to provide safe perinatal home care. Health care agencies and individuals can use these to assess the nurse's skills and learning needs.

A wide range of professional health care services and health products can be delivered or used in the home. The primary difference between health care in a hospital and home care is the absence of the continuous presence of professional health care providers in a patient's home. Most home health care is given as intermittent care with the professional staff visiting in the patient's home or providing care on site for fewer than 4 hours at a time. The home health care agency maintains on-call professional staff to assist home care patients who have questions about their care and for emergencies such as equipment failure.

Perinatal Services

Home care perinatal services may be provided by hospital-based programs, by independent proprietary (for profit) or nonprofit home care agencies, or by official or tax-supported agencies. Home visits have both advantages and disadvantages. The mother is able to maintain bed rest (if indicated), and vulnerable neonates are not exposed to the weather or external sources of infection. The nurse can observe and interact with family members in their most natural and secure environment. Adequacy of resources and safety factors can be assessed. Teaching can be tailored to the actual home conditions and other

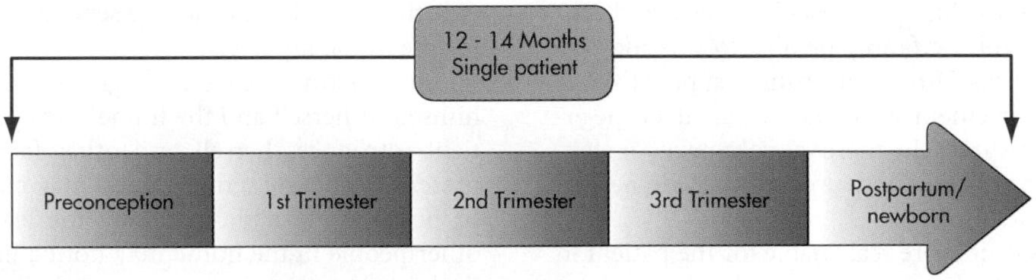

FIG. 3-2 • Perinatal continuum of care.

family members can be included. Antepartal home care that prolongs gestation and reduces neonatal intensive care hospitalization is cost-effective. Even home infusion services at a cost of $225 to $325 per day provide a substantial saving over an average hospitalization ($1500 per day) (Monical, 1998).

Although a home visit is less expensive than a day's hospitalization, a 60- to 90-minute visit requires 2.5 to 3 hours of nursing time, including travel and documentation. It is more cost-effective to see patients in an office setting because professional time is not spent in travel. The availability of nurses with expertise in maternity care may be limited, and concerns about the nurse's physical safety may limit visits in some communities.

Visits for outreach and health promotion are an integral part of community (or public) health nursing. Until recently, private insurers did not reimburse for health promotion visits. Managed care organizations now recognize that anticipatory guidance is cost-effective, but home visit programs are still targeted to specific high risk populations such as young adolescents or women at risk for preterm labor.

Home care agencies are subject to regulation by governmental and professional organizations. They provide interdisciplinary services including social work, nutrition, and occupational and physical therapy. Their caseloads are increasingly made up of patients who require high-technologic care such as infusions or home monitoring. Preconception care and low risk antepartum care can usually be provided more efficiently in office settings, and are not currently reimbursable. High risk antepartum care is often provided by home care agencies. Women with hyperemesis gravidarum, who require parenteral nutrition, may be treated at home. Conditions requiring bed rest, such as preterm labor and hypertension, are common indications for home care.

Postpartum home care is a growing area of perinatal services. Some insurers reimburse for at least one visit to families after early discharge or in the presence of high risk factors. Home phototherapy is used for treatment of neonatal hyperbilirubinemia and to avoid separation of mother and infant. Many other neonates who require long-term high-technology care are also managed with home care. Consumer demand and the education of insurers by case managers are increasing the availability of home care options (Malnory, 1997; Women's Health Center Management, 1997).

Patient Selection and Referral. The office- or hospital-based nurse is often the key person in making effective referrals to home care. When considering a referral to home care, the following factors must be evaluated:

- Health status of mother and fetus or infant: Is the condition serious enough to warrant home care, and is it stable enough for intermittent observation to be sufficient?
- Availability of professionals to provide the needed services within the patient's community.
- Family resources, including psychosocial, social, and economic resources: Will the family be able to provide care between nursing visits? Are relationships supportive? Is third-party reimbursement available or can it be negotiated with the insurer? Is there a voluntary or tax-supported community agency that could provide needed care without payment?
- Cost-effectiveness: Is it more reasonable for the patient to receive these services at home or to go to a local outpatient facility to receive them?

Community referrals should not be limited to women with physiologic complications of pregnancy that require medical treatment. Patients at risk (e.g., young adolescents, families with history of abuse, members of vulnerable population groups, and developmentally disabled individuals) may need follow-up care at home. In consultation with the social worker, the hospital-based nurse should become familiar with local agencies that accept such referrals.

Admission to Home Care. Once the patient is admitted to the agency, the determination of staffing is addressed by nursing management. Patient assignments are generally determined according to diagnosis, geographic location, potential length of service, and skill level of the home care nurse. An agency may have a number of nurses with various clinical backgrounds and certifications. Clinical nurse specialists are assuming leadership roles in many perinatal home care agencies.

Preparing for the Home Visit. The home care nurse reviews available clinical data, demographic information, and the completed plan of care form; then consults with the home care pharmacist or other health care team members who have previously contacted the woman to determine the goals of the visit. At this point the nurse uses the medical diagnosis and stage on the perinatal continuum as a starting point to organize the woman's care. The nurse reviews agency policies and procedures, professional literature about the diagnosis, and community resources as part of the previsit preparation work (Box 3-2).

Before going on a home visit, the nurse contacts the woman to make necessary arrangements. Contact by telephone has several goals besides establishing a convenient date and time for the visit and obtaining directions to the home. It is essential to set the stage for the first home care visit. The nurse identifies himself or herself by name, title, and agency; then explains who referred the woman to the agency and the purpose of the home care visits. The nurse briefly explains what will occur during the visit and approximately how long the visit will last. The patient should be asked to restrain any pets during the visit. Last, the nurse asks about health supplies that may be needed for the woman's care. Medications and specialized equipment are collected in preparation for the visit.

CARE MANAGEMENT

First Home Care Visit

Making the first home care visit can be stressful for the nurse and the patient. The home care nurse is faced with an unknown environment controlled by the woman and her family. The woman and her family also experience feelings of the unknown, such as anxiety about the way the nurse will treat them, or what the nurse will do during the visit. The challenge for the home care nurse is to establish a nurse-patient relationship and provide the prescribed home care services within the time provided for the initial home visit.

Introductions generally begin the visit; the nurse identifies himself or herself and the home care agency (Fig. 3-3). The patient introduces herself and other family members who are present. Sometimes, the woman may feel uncertain of her role or be uncomfortable in taking the lead in introductions, so other people in the home may not be introduced to the nurse. In these situations the nurse can politely ask about other people in the home and their relationship to the woman.

Box 3-2

Protocol for Perinatal Home Visits

PREVISIT INTERVENTIONS

1. Contact family to arrange details for home visit.
   a. Identify self, credentials, and agency role.
   b. Review purpose of home visit follow-up.
   c. Schedule convenient time for visit.
   d. Confirm address and route to family home.
2. Review and clarify appropriate data.
   a. All available assessment data for mother and fetus or infant (i.e., referral forms, hospital discharge summaries, family identified learning needs).
   b. Review records of any previous nursing contacts.
   c. Contact other professional caregivers as necessary to clarify data (i.e., obstetrician, nurse-midwife, pediatrician, referring nurse).
3. Identify community resources and teaching materials appropriate to meet needs already identified.
4. Plan the visit, and prepare bag with equipment, supplies, and materials necessary for assessments of mother and fetus or infant, actual care anticipated, and teaching.

IN-HOME INTERVENTIONS: ESTABLISHING A RELATIONSHIP

1. Reintroduce self and establish purpose of visit for mother, infant, and family; offer family opportunity to clarify their expectations of contact.
2. Spend brief time socially interacting with family to become acquainted and establish trusting relationship.

IN-HOME INTERVENTIONS: WORKING WITH FAMILY

1. Conduct systematic assessment of mother and fetus or newborn to determine physiologic adjustment and any existing complications.
2. Throughout visit, collect data to assess the emotional adjustment of individual family members to pregnancy or birth and lifestyle changes. Note evidence of family-newborn bonding and sibling rivalry; note relationships among mother, father, children, and grandparents.
3. Determine adequacy of support system.
   a. To what extent does someone help with cooking, cleaning, and other home management tasks?
   b. To what extent is help being provided in caring for the newborn and any other children?
   c. Are support persons encouraging the new mother to care for herself and get adequate rest?
   d. Who is providing helpful information? Emotional support?
4. Throughout the visit, observe home environment for adequacy of resources:
   a. Space: privacy, safe play of children, sleeping.
   b. Overall cleanliness and state of repair.
   c. Number of steps pregnant woman/new mother must climb.
   d. Adequacy of cooking arrangements.
   e. Adequacy of refrigeration and other food storage areas.
   f. Adequacy of bathing, toilet, and laundry facilities.
   g. Arrangements in home for newborn: sleeping, bathing, formula preparation (if needed), layette items, and diapers.
5. Throughout the visit, observe home environment for overall state of repair and existence of safety hazards:
   a. Storage of medications, household cleaners, and other substances hazardous to children.
   b. Presence of peeling paint on furniture, walls, or pipes.
   c. Factors that contribute to falls, such as dim lighting, broken steps, scatter rugs.
   d. Presence of vermin.
   e. Use of crib or playpen that fails to meet safety guidelines.
   f. Existence of emergency plan in case of fire; fire alarm or extinguisher.
6. Provide care to mother, newborn, or both as prescribed by their respective primary care provider or in accord with agency protocol.
7. Provide teaching on basis of previously identified needs.
8. Refer family to appropriate community agencies or resources, such as warm lines and support groups.
9. Ascertain that woman knows potential problems to watch for and whom to call if they occur.
10. Ensure that used disposable items have been handled appropriately and that reusable items are cleaned and repacked appropriately in the nurse's bag.

IN-HOME INTERVENTIONS: ENDING THE VISIT

1. Summarize the activities and main points of the visit.
2. Clarify future expectations, including schedule of next visit.
3. Review teaching plan and provide major points in writing.
4. Provide information about reaching the nurse or agency if needed before the next scheduled visit.

POSTVISIT INTERVENTIONS

1. Document the visit thoroughly, using the necessary agency forms to serve as a legal record of the visit and to allow third-party reimbursement, as possible.
2. Initiate the plan of care on which the next encounter with the woman/family will be based.
3. Communicate appropriately (by telephone, letter, progress notes, or referral form) with primary care provider, other health professionals, or referral agencies on behalf of woman/family.

Before performing any services, the home care nurse must obtain written agreement and consent for the home health care services. This consent-for-care serves two major purposes: (1) agreement for care; and (2) authorization to release medical information. Many third-party payers require written documentation of the services provided. Therefore the agency obtains authorization from the woman to give information to her physician and any individual or company involved in payment for the services. Agencies that bill third-party payers for the rendered services will include agreement language for assignment of benefits and financial remuneration. By agreeing to assign insurance benefits to the agency, the woman allows her insurance company to pay the home health care agency directly.

All patients have the right to actively participate in their home care plan of care. These patient rights and responsibilities should begin the discussion about the nurse-patient roles during this initial visit.

Assessment and Nursing Diagnoses

The primary goals of the assessment phase are to develop a trusting relationship and collect data by various methods to obtain a comprehensive patient profile. It may not be feasible or appropriate to collect in-depth information about all areas of assessment during the first visit (Clemen-Stone, Eigsti, and McGuire, 1998). However, in many instances the nurse may be limited to one visit and must obtain information pertinent to the current situation in that hour.

The establishment of a trusting relationship begins with the previsit telephone call. An interview style that reflects sensitivity; a nonjudgmental, accepting attitude; and respect for the woman's rights facilitates the development of that trusting relationship. A skillful interviewer avoids barriers to communication such as false reassurance, advice giving, excessive talking, and the showing of approval or disapproval (Clemen-Stone, Eigsti, and McGuire, 1998). This nurse-patient relationship continues to develop over the course of home visits.

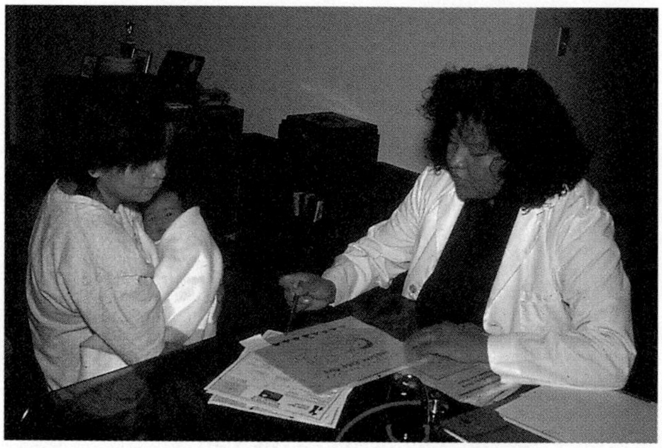

FIG. 3-3 • Home care nurse visiting with woman and her infant. (Courtesy Michael S. Clement, MD, Mesa, AZ.)

The nurse is a guest in the woman's home and should show respect for her and her belongings. Some adaptation of the home visit schedule may need to occur if there are numerous distractions during a visit, such as caring for the needs of small children. The nurse may need to ask to have the volume of the television lowered, or suggest moving to another room where it is more quiet and private.

The major areas of the assessment are demographics, medical history, general health history, medication history, sociocultural assessment, home and community environment, and physical assessment. Some of this information can be obtained from patient records sent to the home care agency at the time of referral or from the previsit interview. These data will be used to develop the nursing care plan and to complete the plan of care, which is required for many licensed home health care agencies. Two areas requiring further discussion are the social assessment and the home environment assessment.

Social assessment includes information regarding the number and roles of each household member, which family members or individuals have taken on the role of caregiver, and the woman's social support network. Identifying the roles of each member is helpful in developing the nursing care plan (Box 3-3).

Physical assessment of the home environment is an essential part of the home care assessment. The major areas of this assessment include physical features of the home, access to the home, sanitary conditions, the presence of utilities (e.g., telephone and electricity), safety features, and access to transportation and emergency support. Some of this information can be collected during an interview. However, a physical inspection of the areas of the home essential to care is critical in developing an accurate nursing care plan. Before any physical inspection,

Box 3-3

Psychosocial Assessment

LANGUAGE
Identify the primary language spoken in the home
Assess whether there are any language barriers to receiving support

COMMUNITY RESOURCES/ACCESS TO CARE
Identify primary and secondary means of transportation
Identify community agencies family currently uses for health care and support
Assess cultural and psychosocial barriers to receiving care

SOCIAL SUPPORT
Determine the people living with the pregnant woman
Identify who assists with household chores
Identify who assists with child care/parenting activities
Identify who the pregnant woman turns to for problems or during a crisis

INTERPERSONAL RELATIONSHIP
Identify the way decisions are made in the family
Identify the family's perception of the need for home care
Identify roles of adults in caring for family members

CAREGIVER
Identify the primary caregiver for home care treatments
Identify other caregivers and their roles
Assess the caregiver's knowledge of treatments and care process
Identify potential strain from the caregiver role
Identify the level of satisfaction with the caregiver role

STRESS AND COPING
Identify what the woman perceives as life-style changes and their impact on her and her family
Identify the changes she and her family have made to adjust to her health condition and home health care treatments

the home care nurse should ask the patient or caregiver for permission and assistance in identifying areas in the home that will be involved in caregiving activities. During the physical inspection, care should be taken to avoid moving personal belongings that are not affected by the care.

Each specific plan of care has a different emphasis in the home environment. For example, women on infusion therapy for hyperemesis gravidarum need to store medications and infusion supplies in a safe place out of reach of small children in the home. The home care nurse should incorporate the agency policies and procedures for the storage and handling of infusion supplies into the walk-through inspection. During the walk-through, the home care nurse looks for supply storage areas that are dry, clean, and where the temperature can be maintained. The home care nurse should include an inspection of the work areas (e.g., countertops, tabletops, sinks, and trash areas) that the woman or caregiver may use for mixing medications, changing infusion tubing, handling supplies, or disposing of used equipment and supplies.

Patients using electronic home health care equipment such as phototherapy equipment or infusion pumps require physical inspection of the electrical outlets, electrical cords, and extension cords that will be used. Homes with faulty electrical wiring may place the patient at risk for being involved in an electrical fire; such wiring may require inspection and repair by a professional electrician before electronic devices are used. Findings from the assessment are incorporated into the plan of care. Nursing diagnoses are derived from the data collected at the first home visit (Nursing Care Plan).

Plan of Care and Interventions

Development of the nursing care plan is based on the individual health care needs of the woman. The care plan describes the nursing diagnoses and the interventions needed to meet the woman's health care needs. The frequency of skilled nursing visits may vary with the individual plan of care, nursing care plan, and the reimbursement criteria established by third-party payers.

Home care nurses working in HCFA-regulated home health care agencies use a plan of care that uses patient demographics, the health care provider's orders, home care goals, and the level of functioning as a basis for nursing care plans. This document is initiated at the time of referral to the home care agency and must be updated every 60 days or as specified by state regulations.

Nurse safety and infection control are two important aspects specific to home care.

Safety Issues for the Home Care Nurse. The nurse should be fully aware of the environment in the home and in the neighborhood in which the home care is being provided. Unlike hospitals, in which the environment is more predictable and controlled, conditions in the patient's neighborhood and home are less certain. Home care nurses should take necessary safety precautions and avoid dangerous areas.

Agencies that serve patients in high-crime areas may conduct a violence-potential assessment by telephone before the visit, and enlist the patient's cooperation in minimizing risk (Hunter, 1997). Others have hired full-time security personnel to accompany nurses on their visits. Personal strategies recommended for nurses visiting families with a history of violence or substance abuse include the following: (1) self-awareness; (2) environmental assessment; (3) using listening and observation skills with patients to be aware of behavioral changes indicating aggression or lack of impulse control; (4) advance planning to deal with aggressive behavior (e.g., allowing personal space and taking a nonaggressive stance); (5) making visits in pairs; and (6) having access to a cellular phone at all times.

Personal Safety. The home care nurse must be aware of personal safety behaviors before going on a home visit. Dress should be casual but professional in appearance and include a name-identification tag. Jewelry should be eliminated or limited. Valuable personal items, such as an expensive purse or coat, should not be worn on a visit. Carrying an extra set of car keys in the nursing home care bag will save time and frustration if the nurse becomes locked out of the automobile. Automobile keys, held between the fingers with sharp ends outward, can be used as a weapon if necessary. The same common-sense behaviors and precautions that guide a person's behavior when alone in any setting should be followed by home care nurses.

The agency should have a copy of the nurse's home care itinerary, including contact telephone numbers (if the patient does

Nursing Care Plan COMMUNITY AND HOME CARE

NURSING DIAGNOSIS Family coping, potential for growth, related to family growth and development in new community

EXPECTED OUTCOME Family will identify at least three community groups that can serve as appropriate resources for an expectant family with small children.

Nursing Interventions/*Rationales*

Assess family structure and availability of significant others, friends, or family members to assist family with new baby and siblings *to provide database for further interventions.*

Encourage family to enlist assistance of individuals who are available to help family at birth of new baby *to provide physical and emotional support.*

Using therapeutic communication, assist the family to assess coping strategies used in the past for new situations *to provide clarification and promote empowerment of family in new situations.*

Suggest strategies to find resources available in the community *to assist family during pregnancy, with new baby, and small siblings.*

Give information regarding community workshops, classes, or support groups *to promote networking, community bonding, and support.*

not have a telephone) and information on the nurse's car (i.e., make, model, color, and license plate number). Many home care nurses carry agency-provided pagers or cellular telephones. This allows the agency to contact the nurse throughout the day with information on patient updates, changes in orders or services, schedule changes, and new patients who require an initial visit. The telephone is also useful to notify patients when the nurse is delayed.

The automobile used for the home care visits, whether a personal vehicle or an agency-owned, should have regular preventive maintenance, adequate fuel, and road safety items stored in the trunk. Items to carry in the vehicle include change for telephone calls and tolls, maps, emergency telephone numbers, a flashlight, a first aid kit, flares, a blanket, and equipment for inclement weather.

All valuable items should be stored out of sight before leaving the office. While driving to the patient's home, the home care nurse should assess the neighborhood for safety, especially if unfamiliar with the area. The nurse should park in a safe place, visible from the street and the patient's home and away from alleys or other hiding places, and lock the car. While walking to the patient's home, nurses should not walk near groups of strangers hanging out in doorways or alleys, enter vacant buildings, or enter a yard that has an unrestrained dog. The home or building should not be entered if the nurse has any safety concerns. All home care agencies should have policies in place for such situations (Occupational Safety and Health Administration, 1996).

Patient's Home. Once inside the woman's home, the nurse may encounter unsafe situations such as the presence of weapons, abusive behavior, or health hazards. Each potentially hazardous situation must be dealt with according to agency policies and procedures. If abuse or neglect is reasonably suspected, the home care nurse should follow home care agency and state and federal regulations for reporting and documenting the situation. Nurses should maintain their own safety first and act accordingly throughout the visit.

Infection Control. The nurse carries the supplies and equipment necessary to provide nursing care to the woman. Home care bags should contain infection control supplies such as personal protection equipment; disposable nonsterile, sterile, and utility gloves; disinfectants; disposable cardiopulmonary resuscitation (CPR) masks, gowns, shoe covers, and caps; leakproof and puncture-resistant specimen containers; a sharps container; dry hand disinfectants; and leakproof barriers. Proper infection control techniques should be used in stocking, storing, handling, and transporting this bag. When a procedure is to be performed, the nurse should set up a "clean" area for necessary supplies. A "dirty" area with a trash bag is designated for the collection of soiled equipment and supplies. Hands are washed before the supplies and equipment needed for the visit are removed from the bag and placed in the clean area.

The importance of infection control does not diminish when nursing care is provided in the patient's home rather than in a hospital. Patients are not likely to become infected because of their home environment, but the nurse may become exposed to a communicable disease. Standard Precautions should be used whenever a treatment is performed.

Handwashing remains the single most important infection control procedure. Hands should be washed before and after each patient contact. Wearing gloves does not eliminate the necessity for handwashing. If running water or clean facilities are unavailable, the hands can be cleaned with a self-drying antiseptic solution.

Using gloves reduces the incidence of exposure to bloodborne pathogens. Gloves should be selected according to the nursing activity to be performed. Nonsterile latex or vinyl gloves should be worn with each procedure that has the potential for contact with bodily substances (e.g., performing venipunctures, heel sticks on a newborn, and perineal care). Sterile gloves should be worn with clinical procedures that require sterile technique, such as insertion of peripherally inserted central lines and certain dressing changes. General-purpose utility gloves should be used for housekeeping activities such as cleaning equipment or spills. After one use, nonsterile and sterile gloves should be discarded in a leak-resistant waste receptacle. Utility gloves may be disinfected and reused.

Disposable personal protection equipment should be removed after each use and discarded in a plastic trash container. Safety glasses or goggles can be cleaned with soap and water after each use.

Whenever specimens are collected, Standard Precautions should be used. Any specimen of bodily fluids should be placed in a leakproof bag and secured in a puncture-proof container. The outside of the container is washed off (if it was soiled) before transporting. Specimens should be labeled with the woman's name and additional identifying information according to the home health care agency or laboratory policies. If specimens are being transported, they should be placed in a container on a flat surface in the vehicle. An insulated container may be used to keep specimens cool in transit.

Sharps containers—puncture-proof and leakproof containers labeled with a biohazard sign on the outside—should be used to collect needles and other sharp objects. The home care nurse covers information about storage and handling as part of the patient teaching process. Patients are instructed to fill containers only two-thirds to three-fourths full to prevent spillage of contents. When the container reaches its maximum capacity, it should be returned to the home health care agency and a new one left in its place.

The patient should be instructed regarding the proper disposal of medical waste in the home. Medical waste such as urine and secretions can be discarded through the sewer or septic system. Contaminated dressings and disposable supplies should be placed in a leakproof plastic bag and securely fastened for disposal at the patient's home. Agency policies and procedures and local waste-management ordinances should be consulted before the patient is instructed.

Nursing Considerations

In home care the woman or family members are responsible for administration of medications in the absence of the nurse. A careful medication history should be obtained to see if the patient is taking her medications correctly and understands the desired action and potential side effects. Sometimes, when orders are changed, women continue to take both the old and new prescriptions; this can lead to dangerous overdoses or medication interactions. The nurse ensures that there is an adequate supply of medications and a safe place for their proper storage to prevent deterioration or accidental ingestion by children or pets. The nurse inquires about any other medications that the woman might be taking concurrently. Over-the-counter drugs or herbal supplements may not be considered medications by the woman; if so, such information will not be provided unless it is specifically asked for.

High-technology home care involves many diagnostic and therapeutic procedures. A focused physical assessment is always part of the visit. Nurses involved in perinatal home care must be skilled in prenatal, postpartal, and newborn assessment. Many women require additional diagnostic tests. The nurse may need to collect blood or other specimens. Portable fetal monitoring or even ultrasound equipment can be used in the home for fetal assessment. Home infusion for women with hyperemesis gravidarum often replaces hospitalization. Women with preterm labor may receive parenteral tocolytic therapy. Phototherapy or apnea monitors for newborns can be provided in the home. Family members may need to be taught how to monitor equipment and prevent accidental damage between nurse visits.

Medical emergencies may occur during or between the nurse's visits to the home. Prior planning and education can reduce the risk of problems. All parents of newborns should know infant CPR. There should be immediate telephone access to call for emergency medical assistance. Women and their families should be taught to recognize danger signs related to their condition. For example, women at risk for preterm labor should learn to palpate the uterus and recognize contractions in the absence of pain; women with diabetes must learn the signs of hypoglycemia and what to do if it occurs; and women with preeclampsia must know the danger signs that indicate their condition is worsening and that they must notify the health care provider immediately.

Patient and family education in home care includes information about the specific high risk condition or conditions involved, implications for pregnancy outcome, and measures for self-monitoring. Verbal explanations should be supplemented with clearly written instructions. General information to promote well-being, such as nutrition and common discomforts of pregnancy, should also be included. The need for preparation for childbirth can be addressed with books or videos and supplemented by individual teaching at home. The woman with a high risk pregnancy may have a problem coping with bed rest or other limitation of activity. The nurse can share strategies that others have used, help with time management, and provide information about support services. Teaching about infant care or the special needs of the preterm infant may be appropriate during the prenatal period.

Clear documentation of assessments, problems identified, treatments and interventions performed, and the patient's responses is essential. Third-party payers base reimbursement on the nurse's written record of providing skilled nursing care and assessments that support the woman's continuing need for those services. The nurse must promptly inform the health care provider by telephone or facsimile of any significant changes.

The home care nurse reassesses the patient's condition and response to the interventions during every home visit, then revises the nursing diagnoses and care plan as needed. Nursing documentation should reflect an objective description of the nursing assessment data collected at each visit. Statements such as "no change" or "same as last visit" do not accurately reflect the monitoring of the patient condition that occurred during the skilled nursing visit. Once the home care outcomes are achieved, and the patient is discharged from the home care agency, documentation should include information about the patient's status at the time of discharge, progress toward attaining health care goals, and plans for follow-up care.

Key Points

- Community-oriented practice is targeted to the community, the population group in which healthful change is sought.
- Assessing community health requires gathering and interpreting data.
- Methods of collecting data useful to the nurse working in the community include windshield surveys, analysis of existing data, informant interviews, and participant observation.
- The health care system is giving increasing attention to health promotion and disease prevention for populations and aggregates.
- Vulnerable populations are groups at higher risk for developing physical, mental, or social health problems.
- Perinatal home care is a unique nursing practice that incorporates knowledge from community health nursing, acute care nursing, family therapy, health promotion, and patient education.
- Perinatal home care can be provided for women and infants throughout the perinatal period, beginning before conception and ending in the postpartum period.
- Perinatal home care nurses should incorporate personal safety and infection control practices into the nursing care plan.

References

Aday L: Vulnerable populations: a community-oriented perspective, Part 1, *Fam Comm Health* 19(4):1-16, 1997.

American Academy of Pediatrics, Committee on Community Health Services: Health needs of homeless children and families, *Pediatrics* 98(4 pt 1):789-791, 1996.

Anderson E, McFarlane J: *Community as partner: theory and practice in nursing,* ed 2, Philadelphia, 1996, JB Lippincott.

Association of Women's Health, Obstetric, and Neonatal Nurses (AWHONN): *Didactic content and clinical skills verification for professional nurse providers of perinatal home care,* Washington, DC, 1994, AWHONN.

Association of Women's Health, Obstetric, and Neonatal Nurses (AWHONN): *Standards and guidelines for professional nursing practice in the care of women and newborns,* ed 5, Washington, DC, 1998, AWHONN.

Bleich M: Growth strategies to optimize the functions of telephonic nursing call centers, *Nurs Econ* 4(6):215-218, 1998.

Blystad-Keppler A: Postpartum care center: follow-up care in a hospital-based clinic, *J Obstet Gynecol Neonatal Nurs* 24(1):17-21, 1995.

Clemen-Stone S, Eigsti D, McGuire S: *Comprehensive community health nursing: family, aggregate, and community practice,* ed 4, St Louis, 1998, Mosby.

Djeddah C: Refugee families, *World Health* 48(6):10-11, 1995.

Fowler B et al: Cross-training to develop a home visit program: a rural experience, *Mother Baby Journal* 2(2):30-38, 1997.

Gany F, Bocanegra H: Maternal-child immigrant health training: changing knowledge and attitudes to improve health care delivery, *Patient Educ Couns* 27:23-31, 1996.

Henry J: Community nursing centers: models of nurse managed care, *J Obstet Gynecol Neonatal Nurs* 26(2):224-228, 1997.

Hunter E: Violence prevention in the home health setting, *Home Healthc Nurse* 15(6):403-409, 1997.

Jones K, Schenk C: MIgrant health issues. In Stanhope M, Lancaster J, editors: *Community health nursing: promoting the health of aggregates, families, and individuals,* ed 4, St Louis, 1996, Mosby.

Kang D, Kahler L, Tesar C: Cultural aspects of caring for refugees, *Am Fam Physician* 57:1245-1246, 1249-1250, 1253-1254, 1998.

Lambert M: Migrant and seasonal farm worker women, *J Obstet Gynecol Neonatal Nurs* 24(3):65-68, 1995.

Lipson J, Omidian P: Afghan refugee issues in the U.S. social environment, *West J Nurs Res* 19(1):10-126, 1997.

Malnory M: Mother-infant home care drives quality in a managed care environment: the quality challenge in managed care, *J Nurs Care Qual* 4(11):3-26, 1997.

Maternal Child Health Bureau: Pregnancy-related behaviors among migrant farm workers—four states, 1989-1993, *MMWR* 46(13):283, 1997.

Monical W: Managing high risk pregnancies at home, *Home Health Cons* 5:28-31, 1998.

O'Campo P et al: Neighborhood risk factors for low birthweight in Baltimore: a multilevel analysis, *Am J Public Health* 87(7):1113-1118, 1997.

Occupational Safety and Health Administration: *Guidelines for preventing workplace violence for health care and social service workers* (OSHA 3148-1996), Washington, DC, 1996, United States Department of Labor (Internet: http://www.osha.gov/oshapubs/workplace/).

Pignatello C et al: Expanding the role of the pediatric nurse from inpatient to community health, *Nurs Adm Q* 4:48-53, 1998.

Rew L: Health risks of homeless adolescents: implications for holistic nursing, *J Holist Nurs* 14(4):348-359, 1996.

Rodriguez R: Promoting healthy partnerships with migrant farm workers: Colorado. In Anderson E, McFarlane J: *Community as partner: theory and practice in nursing,* ed 2, Philadelphia, 1996, JB Lippincott.

Sandhaus S: Migrant health: a harvest of poverty, *Am J Nurs* 98:52, 54, 1998.

Sebastian J: Vulnerability and vulnerable populations: an introduction. In Stanhope M, Lancaster J, editors: *Community health nursing: promoting the health of aggregates, families, and individuals,* ed 4, St Louis, 1996, Mosby.

Shuster G, Goeppinger J: Community as client: using the nursing process to promote health. In Stanhope M, Lancaster J, editors: *Community health nursing: promoting the health of aggregates, families, and individuals,* ed 4, St Louis, 1996, Mosby.

Stanhope M, Lancaster J: *Community health nursing: promoting the health of aggregates, families, and individuals,* ed 4, St Louis, 1996, Mosby.

U.S. Committee on Refugees: *World refugee survey,* Washington, DC, 1995, Immigration and Refugee Services of America.

Women's Health Center Management: Making insurers want to pay for home care, *Women's Health Care Management* 5(1):2, 1997.

Zyzanski S, Williams R, Flocke S: Selection of key community descriptors for community-oriented primary care, *Family Practice* 13(3):280-288, 1996.

CHAPTER 4

Health Promotion and Prevention

http://www.harcourthealth.com/MERLIN/Wong/maternal/

Learning Objectives

On completion of this chapter the reader will be able to:

- Identify reasons for women to enter the health care delivery system.
- Explain conditions and characteristics that increase health risks for women during their childbearing years.
- Review programs of anticipatory guidance that promote health and prevention.
- Suggest community resources to combat violence against women.
- Explain the cycle of violence and its use in assessment and intervention for battered women.
- Discuss the incidence of battering in pregnant women.

In addition to regular health care needs, women have unique and special health circumstances related to their reproductive capacity. As a result, many women initially enter the health care system because of some reproductive system–related situation such as pregnancy, irregular menses, a desire for contraception, or an episodic illness such as a vaginal infection. It is important that health care providers recognize the importance of health promotion and preventive health maintenance and provide these services as part of lifelong care for women.

PRECONCEPTION COUNSELING

Preconception health promotion provides women and their partners with information needed to make decisions about their reproductive future. Preconception counseling guides couples on how to avoid unintended pregnancies. It also stresses risk management, and identifies healthy behaviors that promote the well-being of the woman and her potential fetus. Some couples simply want information pertaining to normal physiology or the timing of coitus to achieve pregnancy; others want to have their myths or beliefs confirmed or dispelled.

Activities that promote healthy mothers and babies must be initiated before the period of critical fetal organ development, which is between 17 and 56 days after fertilization. By the end of the eighth week after conception—and certainly by the end of the first trimester—any major structural anomalies in the fetus are already present. Because many women do not realize that they are pregnant, and do not seek prenatal care until well into the first trimester, the rapidly growing fetus may be exposed to many types of intrauterine environmental hazards during this most vulnerable developmental phase. Thus preconception health care should occur well in advance of an actual pregnancy.

Every woman of childbearing age should be viewed as a potential mother. Identifying and treating risk factors and providing anticipatory guidance with emphasis on healthy lifestyles may therefore be the key to improving the health of the next generation. The components of preconception care (i.e., health promotion, risk assessment, and interventions) are outlined in Box 4-1.

Preconception care is especially important for women who have had a problem with a previous pregnancy (e.g., miscarriage or preterm birth). Although causes are not always identifiable, in many cases problems can be identified and treated and do not recur in subsequent pregnancies. Preconception care is also important to minimize fetal malformations. For example, research has consistently shown that offspring of women who have type 1 diabetes mellitus have significantly more congenital anomalies than do children of mothers without diabetes. Furthermore, it has been shown that the rate of malformation is greatly reduced when the insulin-dependent diabetic woman has excellent blood glucose control when she becomes pregnant and maintains euglycemia (normal blood sugar) throughout the period of organ development in the fetus. Therefore education and glucose control must begin before conception for the woman and her fetus to benefit from this knowledge (Casele and Laifer, 1998).

BOX 4-1

Components of Preconception Care

HEALTH PROMOTION: GENERAL TEACHING

Nutrition
- Healthy diet, including folic acid
- Optimum weight

Exercise and rest

Avoidance of substance abuse (tobacco, alcohol, "recreational" drugs)

Use of safer sex practices

Attending to family and social needs

RISK FACTOR ASSESSMENT

Medical history
- Immune status (e.g., rubella, hepatitis B)
- Family history (e.g., genetic disorders)
- Illnesses (e.g., infections)
- Current use of medication (prescription, nonprescription)

Reproductive history
- Contraceptive
- Obstetric

Psychosocial history
- Spouse/partner and family situation, including domestic violence
- Availability of family or other support systems
- Readiness for pregnancy (e.g., age, life goals, stress)

Financial resources

Environmental (home, workplace) conditions
- Safety hazards
- Toxic chemicals
- Radiation

INTERVENTIONS

Anticipatory guidance/teaching

Treatment of medical conditions and results
- Medications
- Cessation/reduction in substance use/abuse
- Immunizations (e.g., rubella, tuberculosis, hepatitis)

Nutrition, diet, and weight management

Exercise

Referral for genetic counseling

Referral to and use of
- Family planning services
- Family and social needs management

The same concept is true for folic acid as a means to prevent neural tube defects such as spina bifida and anencephaly in the offspring. All women of reproductive age are urged to take a daily vitamin or to eat fortified cereal daily to obtain the 400 μg of supplemental folic acid necessary to protect an actual or potential fetus (Burke, 1999).

Many examples illustrate effects of maternal age or illnesses; conditions that produce anomalies in the fetus (teratogenic agents), such as drugs, viruses, and chemicals; genetically inherited diseases; or other conditions that might be harmful to the woman should a pregnancy occur. In many instances, counseling can allow for behavior modification before damage is done, or the woman can make an informed decision about her willingness to accept potential hazards.

BOX 4-2

Contraceptive Health Promotion

Child spacing and quality maternity care improve perinatal outcomes and health in general of mother and children.

Achieving desired family size enables a better sharing of all resources with attendant increases in education, health care, and other positive societal parameters.

Contraceptives themselves may positively affect future health. For example, use of condoms may prevent acquisition of HIV infection; combined OCs may provide some protection against later development of cancer of ovary and endometrium; barrier methods decrease transmission of STIs, which can develop into pelvic inflammatory disease with resultant infertility or sterility and thus affect future childbearing capacity.

PREGNANCY

A woman's entry into health care is often associated with pregnancy, either for diagnosis or for actual care. Early entry into prenatal care allows for identification of the woman at risk for complications and initiation of measures to prevent problems or treat them if they arise. Extensive discussion of pregnancy is found in Unit 3.

WELL-WOMAN CARE

Many women first enter the health care delivery system for a Papanicolaou (Pap) smear or for contraception. Visits to the nurse may be their only contact with the system unless they become ill. Some women postpone examination until a specific need arises, such as pregnancy, infertility, pain, abnormal bleeding, or vaginal discharge. Fertility control and infertility are addressed in Chapter 7. Health promotion concepts related to contraception are listed in Box 4-2.

Conditions and Characteristics that Increase Health Risks in the Childbearing Years

Maintaining optimum health is a goal for all women. Essential components of health maintenance are the identification of unrecognized problems and potential risks and the education and health promotion needed to reduce them. This is especially important for a woman in her childbearing years because conditions that increase her health risks concern not only her well-being but also may be associated with negative outcomes for both mother and baby in the event of a pregnancy. Prenatal care is the prime example of prevention that is practiced after conception. However, prevention and health maintenance are needed before conception because many of the mother's risks can be identified and eliminated, or at least modified. An overview follows of the conditions and circumstances that increase health risks in the childbearing years.

Demographics

Age

Adolescents. As a female progresses through developmental ages and stages, she is faced with conditions that are age-related. All teens undergo progressive growth of sexual characteristics. They also undertake the developmental tasks of adolescence such as establishing identity, developing sexual preference, emancipating from family, and establishing career goals. Some of these situations can produce great stress for the adolescent, and the health care provider should treat her very carefully. Female teenagers who enter the health care system usually do so for screening (Pap smears start at age 18 or when sexually active) or because of a problem such as episodic illness or accidents. Gynecologic problems are often associated with menses (either bleeding irregularities or dysmenorrhea), vaginitis or leukorrhea, sexually transmitted infection (STI), contraception, or pregnancy.

Most young women begin having sex in the mid to late teens; for those who do not, the likelihood of having intercourse increases steadily with age. A sexually active teen who does not use contraception has a 90% chance of pregnancy within 1 year (Alan Guttmacher Institute, 1998).

Teenage Pregnancy. Pregnancy in the teenager who is 16 years of age or younger often introduces additional stress on an already stressful developmental period. The emotional level of such teens is commonly characterized by impulsiveness and self-centered behavior, and they often place primary importance on the beliefs and actions of their peers. In attempts to establish a personal and independent identity, many teens do not realize the consequences of their behavior; their thinking processes do not include planning for the future (Muscari, 1998).

Unless very young, teens are sufficiently mature to physically support the pregnancy, but they may not adhere to many areas of prenatal instruction, especially nutrition and continuing care. Children of teen mothers may be at risk for abuse or neglect because of the teen's inadequate knowledge of growth, development, and parenting. Implementation of specialized adolescent programs in schools, communities, and health care systems is demonstrating continued success in lowering the birth rate in teens as evidenced by an overall 15% decline in teenage pregnancy between 1991 and 1997 (National Center for Health Statistics, 1998).

Young and Middle Adulthood. Because women aged 20 to 40 years have a need for contraception, pelvic and breast screening, and pregnancy care, they may prefer to use their gynecologic or obstetric provider as their primary care provider. During these years the woman may be "juggling" family, home, and career responsibilities with resulting increases in stress-related conditions. Health maintenance includes not only pelvic and breast screening but also promotion of a healthy lifestyle: that is, good nutrition, regular exercise, no smoking, moderate or no alcohol consumption, sufficient rest, stress reduction, and referral for medical conditions and other specific problems. Common conditions in well-woman care include vaginitis, urinary tract infections, menstrual variations, obesity, sexual and relationship issues, and pregnancy.

Parenthood After Age 35. The woman aged more than 35 years does not have a different physical response to a pregnancy per se, but has had health status changes as a result of time and the aging process. These changes may be responsible for age-related pregnancy conditions. For example, a woman with type 2 diabetes may not have had expression of her diabetes at age 22 years but may have full-blown disease at age 38 years. Other chronic or debilitating diseases or conditions increase in severity with time and these, in turn, may predispose to increased risks during pregnancy. Of significance to women in this age group is the risk for certain genetic anomalies (e.g., Down syndrome), and the opportunity for genetic counseling should be available to all (see Chapter 8).

Women of later reproductive age are often experiencing change and reordering personal priorities. In general, the goals of education, career, marriage, and family have been achieved, and now the woman has increased time and opportunity for new interests and activities. Conversely, divorce rates are high at this age, and children leaving home may produce an "empty nest syndrome" that results in levels of depression. Chronic diseases also become more apparent. Most problems for the well woman are associated with perimenopause (e.g., bleeding irregularities and vasomotor symptoms). Health maintenance screening continues to be of importance because some conditions such as breast disease or ovarian cancer occur more often during this stage.

Social/Cultural. Differences exist among people from different socioeconomic levels and ethnic groups with respect to risk for illness and distribution of disease and death. Some diseases are more common among people of selected ethnicity; for example, sickle cell anemia in African-Americans, Tay-Sachs disease in Ashkenazi Jews, adult lactase deficiency in Chinese, β-thalassemia in Mediterranean peoples, and cystic fibrosis in northern Europeans. Cultural and religious influences also increase health risks because the woman and her family may have life and societal values and a view of health and illness that dictate practices different from those expected in the Judeo-Christian Western model. These may include food taboos or frequencies, methods of hygiene, effects of climate, care-seeking behaviors, willingness to undergo screening and diagnostic procedures, and value conflicts. Culturally induced belief in magic can cause illness and death (Murray and Zentner, 1997).

Socioeconomic contrasts result in major health differences, as exemplified in birth outcomes. The rates of perinatal and maternal deaths, preterm births, and low-birth-weight babies are considerably higher in disadvantaged populations (National Center for Health Statistics, 1998). Social consequences for poor women as single parents are great because many mothers with few skills are caught in the bind of insufficient income to afford child care. These families generate fewer and fewer resources and increase their risks for health problems. Multiple roles for women in general produce overload, conflict, and stress, resulting in higher risks for psychosocial health care (Cox, 1997).

Health Behaviors

Smoking. Cigarette smoking is a major preventable cause of death and illness. Smoking is linked to cardiovascular heart disease, various types of cancers (especially lung and cervical), chronic lung disease, and negative pregnancy outcomes. Tobacco contains nicotine, which is an addictive substance that creates physical and psychologic dependence. Tobacco smoke contains known carcinogens. The average cigarette smoker shortens his or her life by 6 to 8 years. The incidence of smoking among persons 18 years of age and over remains stable at 25.5%. However, the age of smoking initiation has been dropping over the last 10 years, and girls as young as age 12 or 13 are currently starting to smoke (Pohl and Caplan, 1998). Among adolescents and young adults, more women than men smoke, with non-Hispanic white women significantly more likely to be frequent smokers than either Hispanic or African-American women (Grimes, 1998). Smoking in persons over age 25 ranges from 12% for college graduates to 38% for those with less than a high school education.

Cigarette smoking impairs fertility in both women and men, may reduce the age for menopause, and increases the risk for osteoporosis after menopause. Passive or secondhand smoke (environmental tobacco smoke [ETS]) contains similar hazards and presents additional problems for the smoker, as well as harm for the nonsmoker. The American College of Obstetricians and Gynecologists (ACOG) (1997) reports widespread exposure to ETS, with 9 of 10 nonsmoking Americans showing blood levels of a chemical metabolized from nicotine.

Approximately one third of women who become pregnant are smokers at the time of conception (ACOG, 1997). Smoking in pregnancy is known to cause a decrease in placental perfusion and is one cause of low birth weight in infants (ACOG, 1997). The harmful effects of smoking are numerous because the oxygen-carrying capacity of hemoglobin is decreased when carbon monoxide passes through the placenta. Furthermore, nicotine causes vasoconstriction, and smokers generally have a nutrient-poor diet. Finally, smoking interferes with the body's ability to process essential vitamins and minerals, resulting in calcium loss from the bones, a decreased intestinal synthesis of vitamin B_{12}, and increased usage of vitamin C. The woman who smokes during pregnancy is at risk for a variety of complications (Box 4-3).

Substance Use and Abuse. The use of illicit drugs and the inappropriate use of prescription drugs continue to increase; the problem is found in all ages, races, ethnic groups, and socioeconomic strata. When abused, psychoactive (mind-altering) drugs can disturb relationships, cause psychologic and physical dependency, and create serious health problems. Such substances interfere with the brain's neurotransmitters and normal chemistry; this in turn affects an individual's moods. They particularly affect the part of the brain that produces euphoria, pleasure, or pain release and, as a result, lead easily to abuse. Risk increases with the strength, amount, frequency, and route of administration.

Addiction to substances is seen as a biopsychosocial disease with several factors adding to risk. These factors include biogenetic predisposition, lack of resilience to stressful life experiences, and poor social support (Jessup, 1997). Women are less likely than men to abuse drugs, but the rate in women is increasing significantly. Substance-abusing pregnant women create severe problems for themselves and their offspring, including interference with optimal growth and development and addiction. In many instances, the use of substances is identified through screening programs in prenatal clinics and obstetric units (Li et al, 1999).

Alcohol. Women aged 35 to 49 years have the highest rates of chronic alcoholism, but women aged 21 to 34 years have the highest rates of specific alcohol-related problems (Jessup, 1997). About one third of alcoholics are women, and many relate onset of their drinking problem to stressful events. Women who are problem drinkers are often depressed, have more motor vehicle injuries, and have a higher incidence of attempted suicide than do women in the general population. Also, they are at particular risk for alcohol-related liver damage. Early case finding and early treatment are important in alcoholism for both the ill individual and for family members.

Alcohol abuse during pregnancy is the leading cause of mental retardation in the United States (Lewis and Woods, 1994). In addition, alcohol abuse during pregnancy has been associated with fetal growth restriction, altered facies, and developmental problems. For this reason, abstinence from alcohol consumption during pregnancy is recommended (Cefalo and Moos, 1995).

Illicit Drugs

Cocaine. Cocaine is a powerful central nervous system stimulant that is addictive because of the tremendous sense of pleasure that it creates. It can be snorted, smoked, or injected. Crack or rock cocaine is a form of the drug that is exceedingly potent and even more highly addictive. (Some say that an individual is "hooked" after the first use or, at the least, after two or three "hits.") After ingestion of cocaine, an intensely pleasurable high results that is followed by an uncomfortable low; this increases the urge to repeat the drug.

Cocaine affects all of the major body systems. Among other complications, it produces cardiovascular stress that can lead to heart attack or stroke, liver disease, central nervous system stimulation that can cause seizures, and even perforation of the nasal septum. Users are often poorly nourished and commonly have STIs. If the user is pregnant, there is an increased incidence of miscarriage, preterm labor, small-for-gestational-age babies, abruption of placenta, and stillbirth. Anomalies have been reported (Fox, 1994).

Heroin. Heroin is an opiate that is usually injected but can also be smoked or snorted. It produces euphoria, relaxation, relief from pain, and "nodding out" (i.e., apathy, detachment from reality, impaired judgment, and drowsiness). Signs and symptoms are constricted pupils, nausea, constipation, slurred speech, and respiratory depression (Stuart and Sundeen, 1998). Users are at increased risk for human immunodeficiency virus (HIV) and hepatitis B, C, and D, primarily because of sharing needles that contain contaminated blood. Perinatal effects in-

BOX 4-3

Maternal Complications of Pregnancy Associated with Smoking

- Ectopic pregnancy
- Miscarriage (especially after in vitro fertilization)
- Premature rupture of membranes
- Preterm birth
- Placenta previa
- Abruptio placentae
- Chorioamnionitis

Source: American College of Obstetricians and Gynecologists: *Smoking and women's health,* (ACOG Technical Bulletin no. 240), Washington, DC, 1997, ACOG.

clude interference with fetal growth, premature rupture of membranes, preterm labor, and prematurity. Newborns can be born addicted to heroin and may need to undergo a withdrawal process.

Marijuana. Marijuana is a substance derived from the cannabis plant. It is usually rolled into cigarettes and smoked. It may also be mixed into food and eaten. It produces an intoxicating and sensory-distorting high. Marijuana smoke has the same characteristics as tobacco smoke and, for this reason, has similar dangers. It also readily crosses the placenta and has the effect of increasing carbon monoxide levels in the mother's blood, reducing the oxygen supply to the fetus.

Other Illicit Drugs. A number of other street drugs pose risk to users. A few are derived from organic materials, but more and more are synthetically produced in laboratories. Variations of stimulants (e.g., "speed," "meth," and "ice") produce signs and symptoms similar to cocaine, although fewer maternal and fetal complications have been attributed to them. Sedatives such as "downers," "yellow jackets," or "red devils" are used to come off of "highs." Hallucinogens alter perception and body function. PCP ("angel dust") and LSD produce vivid changes in sensation, often with agitation, euphoria, paranoia, and a tendency toward antisocial behavior. Their use may lead to flashbacks, chronic psychosis, and violent behavior. Hallucinogens taken during pregnancy may have negative neurobehavioral effects on the newborn.

Prescription Medications

Psychotherapeutic Medications. Stimulants, sleeping pills, tranquilizers, and pain relievers are used by an estimated 2% of American women (Epps and Stewart, 1995). Such medications can bring relief from undesirable conditions such as insomnia, anxiety, and pain; but because the medications have mind-altering capacity, misuse can produce psychologic and physical dependency in the same manner as illicit drugs. Risk-to-benefit ratios should be considered when such medications are used for more than a very short period of time. When taken during pregnancy, all of these categories of drugs have some effect on the fetus and must be very carefully monitored.

Stimulants. These medications increase energy and reduce appetite. In the past they were occasionally used for weight loss, but because of their tendency to create dependence they are no longer sanctioned for this purpose. They may be prescribed for narcolepsy or attention deficit disorder.

Sleeping Pills. Barbiturates and hypnotics are used to relieve insomnia; but with long-term use, tolerance develops and larger amounts are needed for the same effect. Larger amounts of the medications can result in poor concentration, mood swings, anxiety, and depression. Again, dependency occurs. Withdrawal symptoms can include emotional distress, anxiety, headache, gastrointestinal disturbances, and restlessness.

Narcotics. The use of opiate narcotics is of great benefit in many circumstances because they act on the brain and nervous system to decrease sensitivity to pain and to produce a sense of well-being. However, they are highly addictive over time and can produce severe physical and mental symptoms when withdrawn.

Tranquilizers. Tranquilizers provide short-term relief from anxiety and stress caused by unexpected emotional conflict or trauma. Their effect is similar to that of alcohol; low doses produce relaxation and buoyancy, and higher doses produce intoxication. Tranquilizers are not appropriate for long-term therapy. Withdrawal effects are similar to those of sleeping pills, but less severe.

Psychotropic Medications. Depression is the most common mental health problem in women. Everyone has a case of the "blues" periodically, but true depression impairs the ability to live a normal life and involves symptoms of pervasive sadness, isolation, fatigue, changes in eating and sleeping patterns, and general negativity. Severely depressed people are at risk for suicide. Typical medications used to treat depression are tricyclic antidepressants (e.g., imipramine [Tofranil] and amitriptyline [Elavil]); monoamine oxidase (MAO) inhibitors (e.g., phenelzine [Nardil]); selective serotonin reuptake inhibitors (SSRIs) (e.g., fluoxetine [Prozac] or sertraline [Zoloft]); and lithium. Tricyclic antidepressants relieve symptoms of depression without the artificial mood enhancement seen with stimulants.

Caffeine. Caffeine is found in society's most popular drinks: coffee, tea, and soft drinks. It is a stimulant that can affect mood and interrupt body functions by producing anxiety and sleep interruptions. Heart arrhythmias may be made worse by caffeine, and there can be interactions with certain medications such as lithium. Birth defects have not been related to caffeine consumption; however, high intake has been related to a slight decrease in birth weight. The U.S. Food and Drug Administration recommends that pregnant women eliminate or limit their consumption of caffeine to less than 300 mg per day (3 cups of coffee or cola).

Nutrition. Good nutrition is essential to good health. A well-balanced diet helps prevent illness and also is used to treat certain health problems. Conversely, poor eating habits, eating disorders, and obesity are linked to disease and discomfort.

Overt disease caused by a lack of certain nutrients is rarely seen in the United States. However, insufficient amounts or imbalances of nutrients do pose problems for individuals and families. Overweight or underweight status, listlessness, fatigue, frequent colds and other minor infections, constipation, dull hair and nails, and dental caries are examples of problems that could be nutritionally related and indicate the need for further nutritional assessment. Poor nutrition, especially related to obesity and high fat and cholesterol intake, may lead to more serious conditions and is said to contribute to 6 of the 10 leading causes of death in the United States: heart disease, cancer, stroke and hypertension, arteriosclerosis, cirrhosis of the liver, and diabetes (Lean et al, 1999).

To maintain good nutrition, women should be counseled to include recommended servings from the major food categories of the Food Guide Pyramid (see Fig. 12-4). Complex carbohydrates, including grains, breads, fruits, and vegetables, should make up 45% to 60% of daily intake. Moderate amounts of proteins, sugars, and salt should be ingested, and diets should be low in total fat (i.e., no more than 30% of total calories), saturated fat (i.e., no more than 10%), and cholesterol (under 300 mg per day). Recommended servings from the food groups also provide for adequate vitamins, minerals, iron, and fiber. Fluid intake is not included in the Food Guide Pyramid, but individuals should be encouraged to drink at least four to six glasses of water every day in addition to other fluids such as juices. Coffee, tea, soft drinks, and alcoholic beverages should be used in moderation if used at all.

The diet can be assessed using a standard assessment form—a 24-hour recall is adequate and quick—and then food likes and

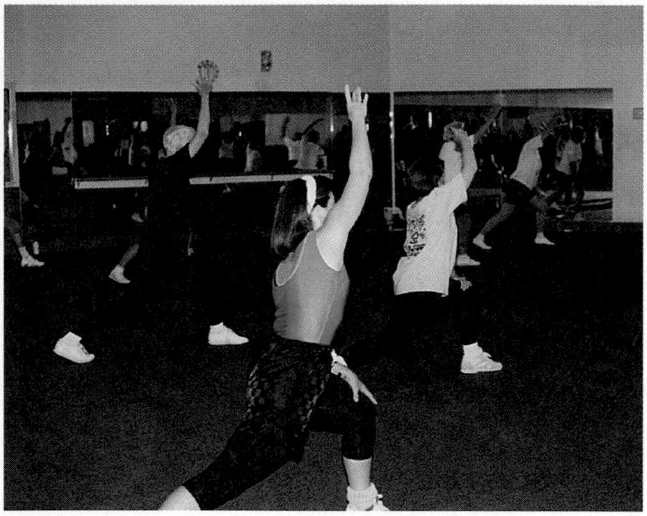

FIG. 4-1 • Weight-bearing exercise may delay bone loss and increase bone mass. (Courtesy Jonas McCoy, Raleigh, NC.)

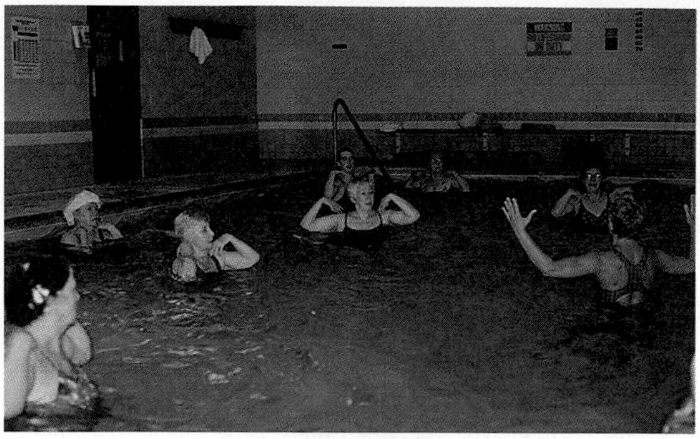

FIG. 4-2 • Water aerobics improves cardiovascular function. (Courtesy Jonas McCoy, Raleigh, NC.)

dislikes, including cultural variations and typical food portions and dietary habits, should be discussed and incorporated into counseling. The nurse should actively involve the woman in evaluating her intake, using a standard food group guide, and should suggest modifications in the diet where needed. Many women have a fair knowledge of food groups and their importance for various nutrients; with guidance they can critique their own intake and suggest changes to improve nutrition. Many women, especially if they are obese or know they are not eating as they should, are sensitive about diet. Unless the motivation to change food habits is intrinsic, efforts to change the diet will fail.

Although many people are aware of the association between high fat and cholesterol and disease, they may not know the major sources of saturated fat and may need help in changing eating patterns established during childhood. Fiber-rich foods can be substituted for foods high in fat; these foods delay digestion and absorption and increase the feeling of satiety.

Most women do not recognize the importance of calcium to health, and have diets insufficient in calcium. The ideal daily calcium intake is not known, but it is agreed that most women, especially adolescents, should increase their intake. Women under age 50 need 1000 mg of calcium per day, and postmenopausal women over age 50 need 1500 mg per day. Pregnant and lactating women also need 1500 mg per day. If calcium supplementation is necessary, calcium carbonate, which contains more elemental calcium than other preparations, is preferable.

Physical Fitness and Exercise. Exercise contributes to good health by lowering risks for a variety of conditions that are influenced by obesity and a sedentary lifestyle. It is effective in the prevention of cardiovascular disease and in the management of chronic conditions such as hypertension, arthritis, diabetes, respiratory disorders, and osteoporosis. Exercise also contributes to stress reduction and weight maintenance. Women report that engaging in regular exercise improves their body image and self-esteem and acts as a mood enhancer. Aerobic exercise produces cardiovascular involvement because increasing amounts of oxygen are delivered to working muscles. Anaerobic exercise, such as weight training, improves individual muscle mass without stress on the cardiovascular system. Because women are concerned about both cardiovascular and bone health, weight-bearing aerobic exercises such as walking, running, racket sports, and dancing are preferred. However, excessive or strenuous exercise can lead to hormonal imbalances, resulting in amenorrhea and its consequences. Physical injury is also a potential risk.

Physical activity and exercise counseling for persons of all ages should be undertaken at schools, worksites, and primary care settings. It is characterized as integrating short bouts of exercise into daily living (Pender, 1996). Specific recommendations include 20 to 30 minutes of moderate activity at least three times per week. Few Americans exercise this often, and physical inactivity increases with age, especially during adolescence and early adulthood. Even small increases in activity can be beneficial. The nurse should stress the importance of daily exercise throughout life for weight management and health promotion, suggesting exercises that are enjoyable to the individual (Figs. 4-1 and 4-2).

During pregnancy, an ongoing exercise regimen can be continued but should be decreased in intensity and duration. Sedentary women should obtain medical clearance to initiate exercise during pregnancy, and should begin with low-intensity and low-impact workouts.

Kegel Exercises. Kegel exercises, or pelvic muscle exercises, were developed to strengthen the supportive pelvic floor muscles to control or reduce involuntary urine loss. These exercises are also beneficial during pregnancy and postpartum. They strengthen the muscles of the pelvic floor, providing support for the pelvic organs, and control of the muscles surrounding the vagina and urethra.

The Association of Women's Health, Obstetric, and Neonatal Nurses conducted a research utilization project focused on continence for women (Sampselle et al, 1997). The Patient Teaching box describes Kegel exercise teaching strategies that were compiled by nurse researchers involved in the project.

Stress. The modern woman faces increasing levels of stress and, as a result, is prone to a variety of stress-induced com-

Patient Teaching

KEGEL EXERCISES

Description and Rationale

Kegel exercise, or pelvic muscle exercise, is a technique used to strengthen the muscles that support the pelvic floor. This exercise involves regularly tightening (contracting) and relaxing the muscles that support the bladder and urethra. By strengthening these pelvic muscles, a woman can prevent or reduce accidental urine loss.

Technique

The woman needs to learn how to target the muscles for training and how to contract them correctly. One suggestion for teaching is to have the woman pretend she is trying to prevent the passage of intestinal gas. Have her use this tightening motion on the muscles around her vagina and the upper pelvis. She should feel these muscles drawing inward and upward. Other suggested techniques are to have the woman pretend she is trying to stop the flow of urine in midstream or to have her think about how her vagina is able to contract around and move up the length of the penis during intercourse.

The woman should avoid straining or bearing-down motions while performing the exercise. She should be taught how bearing down feels by having her take a breath, hold it, and push down with her abdominal muscles as though she were trying to have a bowel movement. Then the woman can be taught how to avoid straining down by exhaling gently and keeping her mouth open each time she contracts her pelvic muscles.

Specific Instructions

1. Each contraction should be as intense as possible without contracting the abdomen, thighs, or buttocks.
2. Contractions should be held for at least 10 seconds. The woman may have to start with as little as 2 seconds per contraction until her muscles get stronger.
3. The woman should rest for 10 seconds or more between contractions so that the muscles have time to recover and each contraction can be as strong as the woman can make it.
4. The woman should feel the pulling up and over the three muscle layers so that the contraction reaches the highest level of her pelvis.

Other Suggestions for Implementation

1. At first the woman should set aside about 15 minutes a day to do the Kegel exercises.
2. The woman may want to put up reminders, such as notes on her bathroom mirror, her refrigerator, her TV, or a calendar, to do the exercises.
3. Guidelines for practicing Kegel exercises suggest performing between 30 and 80 contractions a day; however, positive results can be achieved with only 30 a day.
4. The best position for learning how to do Kegel exercises is to lie supine with the knees bent. Another position to use is on the hands and knees. Once the woman learns the proper technique, she can perform the exercises in other positions such as standing or sitting.

Source: Breeding D: You don't have to live with incontinence, *Female Patient* 53:29, 1996; Sampselle C, Miller J: Pelvic muscle exercise: effective patient teaching, *Female Patient* 21:29, 1996; and Sampselle C et al: Continence for women: evidence-based practice, *J Obstet Gynecol Neonatal Nurs* 26(4):375-385, 1997.

plaints and illnesses. Stress often occurs because of multiple roles which conflict (e.g., coping with job and financial responsibilities versus parenting and home). To add to this burden, women are socialized to be caretakers, which is emotionally draining by itself. They also may find themselves in positions of minimal power without control over their everyday environments (Epps and Stewart, 1995). Some stress is normal and, in fact, contributes to positive outcomes. Many women thrive in busy surroundings. However, excessive or high levels of ongoing stress trigger physical reactions such as rapid heart rate, elevated blood pressure, slowed digestion, release of additional neurotransmitters and hormones, muscle tenseness, and weakened immune system.

Consequently, constant stress can contribute to clinical illnesses such as flare-ups of arthritis or asthma, frequent colds or infections, gastrointestinal upsets, cardiovascular problems, and infertility. Box 4-4 lists physical symptoms that may be related to chronic or extreme stress. Psychologic symptoms such as anxiety, irritability, eating disorders, depression, insomnia, and substance abuse have also been associated with stress.

Stress Management. Because it is neither possible nor desirable to avoid all stress, women must learn how to manage stress. The nurse should assess each woman for signs of stress, using therapeutic communication skills to determine risk factors and the woman's ability to function.

Some women must be referred for counseling or other mental health therapy. Women are twice as likely as men to suffer from depression, anxiety, or panic attacks (Japenga, 1998). Nurses must be alert to the symptoms of serious mental disorders, such as depression and anxiety, and make referrals to mental health practitioners when necessary. Women experiencing major life changes, such as separation and divorce, bereavement, serious illness, and unemployment, also need special attention.

For many women the nurse is able to provide comfort, reassurance, and advice concerning helping resources such as support groups. Many centers offer support groups to help women prevent or manage stress. The nurse can help women become more aware of the relationship between good nutrition, rest, re-

BOX 4-4

Physical Symptoms of Stress

- Headache
- Dizziness or feeling faint
- Muscle tension
- Backache
- Grinding of teeth
- Skin rash or hives
- Sweaty palms
- Indigestion
- Nausea, vomiting
- Diarrhea
- Constipation
- Loss of appetite
- Shortness of breath
- Pounding heart
- Nonradiating chest pain
- Frequent colds

Modified from Epps R, Stewart S: *The women's complete healthbook,* New York, 1995, The Philip Lief Group, Inc.

laxation, exercise, and diversion and the ability to deal with stress. In the case of role overload, it is important to determine what needs immediate attention and what can wait. Practical advice includes regular breaks, taking time for friends, developing interests outside of work or the home, setting realistic goals, and learning self-acceptance. Discussing how women can maintain meaningful relationships is important. Social support and good coping skills can improve a woman's self-esteem and give her a sense of mastery. Anticipatory guidance for developmental or expected situational crises can help her plan strategies for dealing with potentially stressful events. Role-playing, relaxation techniques, biofeedback, meditation, desensitization, imagery, assertiveness training, yoga, diet, exercise, and weight control are all techniques nurses can include in their repertoire of helping skills.

Sexual Practices. Potential risks related to sexual activity include undesired pregnancy and STIs.

The risks are particularly high for adolescents and young adults, who are engaging in sexual intercourse at earlier and earlier ages. Adolescents report many reasons for wanting to be sexually active; among these are peer pressure, to love and be loved, experimentation, to enhance self-esteem, and to have fun (Murray and Zentner, 1997). However, many teens do not have the decision-making or values-clarification skills needed to take this important step. They may also lack knowledge about contraception and STIs. Many do not believe that pregnancy or getting an STI will happen to them. Pregnancy raises further issues: continuing the pregnancy versus abortion, adoption versus childrearing, continuing with education and career goals versus quitting school and accepting jobs that require little skill.

Although some STIs can be cured with antibiotics, many can cause significant problems. Possible sequelae include infertility, ectopic pregnancy, neonatal morbidity and mortality, genital cancers, acquired immunodeficiency syndrome, and even death (Hatcher et al, 1998). Sexually transmitted infections are increasing rapidly and are in epidemic proportion. Choice of contraception has an impact on the risk of contracting an STI. Natural family planning, hormones, and intrauterine devices offer no protection. Diaphragms offer some cervical protection. Condoms combined with a spermicide offer the most protection. No method of contraception offers complete protection. (See Chapter 6 for a discussion of STIs and Chapter 7 for a discussion of contraception.)

Safer Sexual Practices. Prevention of STIs is predicated on the reduction of high risk behaviors by educating toward a behavioral change. Behaviors of concern include multiple and casual sexual partners and unsafe sexual practices. Specific self-care measures for safer sex are listed in Box 4-5. The abuse of alcohol and drugs is also a high risk behavior resulting in impaired judgment and thoughtless acts. Behavioral changes must come from within, and therefore the nurse must provide sufficient information for the individual or group to "buy into" the need for change.

Education for STIs includes the following: (1) verbal desensitizing (e.g., talking about sex and sexual practices); (2) offering specific information (e.g., the signs and symptoms of diseases, their complications, and how to prevent disease); (3) endorsing use of condoms (although not 100% effective, condoms are the best form of protection and should be used each and every time unless abstinence or mutual monogamy is ensured); (4) providing behavioral scripts (e.g., suggest ways to handle sexual situations before they actually occur); and (5) providing referrals for screening (even in the absence of symptoms), additional information, or treatment (see Chapter 6).

In addition to the prevention of STIs, women of childbearing years need information and behavioral considerations regarding contraception and family planning (see Chapter 7). Education is a powerful tool in health promotion and prevention of STIs and pregnancy. However, it works best when delivered in a way that takes into account the language, culture, and lifestyle of the intended listener.

BOX 4-5

"Safer" Sex

"Safer" sex is possible only if there is no oral, genital, or rectal exchange of body fluids.

Correct use of condoms, although greatly reducing risk, is not exclusively protective.

Use of spermicides may offer additional protection.

Select sexual partners with extreme care.

Ask partner about history of STIs.

Medical Conditions

Most women of reproductive age are relatively healthy. However, certain medical conditions present during pregnancy can have deleterious effects on both mother and fetus. Of particular concern are risks from all forms of diabetes, urinary tract disorders, thyroid disease, hypertensive disorders of pregnancy, cardiac disease, and seizure disorders. Effects on the fetus vary and include intrauterine growth restriction, macrosomia, anemia, prematurity, immaturity, and stillbirth. Effects on the mother can also be severe. Refer to Chapters 13 and 14 for information on specific conditions.

Gynecologic Conditions Affecting Pregnancy. Gynecologic conditions that may contribute negatively to pregnancy include the following:

- Pelvic inflammatory disease (PID) can cause stricture or occlusion of uterine (fallopian) tubes and result in infertility or ectopic pregnancy.
- Endometriosis occurs when endometrial tissue grows outside of the uterus; it responds to hormonal influences and causes scarring and adhesions in the tubes.

Community Focus

CULTURE SENSITIVE HEALTH MESSAGES

General health messages have limited usefulness in certain communities. A participatory, culture-sensitive approach directed to specific subcultures of a community is likely to be more effective. Identification of unmet needs of a target group and training lay women from those subcultures to take health education messages, in the appropirate language, back to the target group has demonstrated effectiveness. This approach may also break down barriers between the community and professionals.

Data from: Hampton K: Communicating health messages to marginalized communities—a culture sensitive approach, *Int J Health Promot Educ* 38(2):40-46, 2000.

- Some STIs can be vertically transmitted to the fetus (e.g., HIV and syphilis) or cause damage during the birth process (e.g., Chlamydia, *Neisseria gonorrhoeae,* herpes simplex virus [HSV], or group B streptococci).
- Fibroids, benign fibrous growths from the uterine muscle that are under the influence of estrogen, can press on the lining of the uterus, causing infertility. Occasionally they impinge on the space needed by the growing fetus and require surgical removal and cesarean birth.
- Uterine deformities (e.g., bicornuate uterus) can cause miscarriage, preterm labor, and fetal growth problems.
- Vaginal infection caused by Trichomonas, Candida, or bacterial vaginosis can result in uncomfortable vaginal discharge and be confused with normal leukorrhea. Candida has a propensity for the glycogen-laden vaginal epithelium found during pregnancy, and reinfections can occur.
- Reproductive or breast cancer treatments (i.e., radiation, surgery, and chemotherapy) can cause fetal anomalies, miscarriage, and preterm labor.

Risks for Gynecologic Cancers. Women are at risk for cancer. Risk factors differ, depending on the type of cancer.

Cervical Cancer. Risks for cervical cancer include the following:

- **Early age of first sexual intercourse**—This introduces foreign bodies to the young teen's rapidly changing cells at the junction of columnar tissue from the endometrium and squamous tissue from the vagina.
- **Cigarette smoking**—Organic residues from tobacco are preferentially deposited in the cervix.
- **Human papillomavirus (HPV) infection**—A few particular strains of HPV, such as types 16, 18, 45, and 56, are associated with cervical cancer.
- **Multiple sexual partners**—This exposes the cervix to many microorganisms.

In the United States, African-American women have the highest rate of cervical cancer, followed by Hispanic women. Abnormal spotting or vaginal bleeding is the primary symptom (American Cancer Society, 1999).

Endometrial Cancer. The most common malignancy of the reproductive system is endometrial cancer. Estrogen-related exposures such as nulliparity, unopposed estrogen therapy, infertility, and early or late menopause are the most significant risk factors. Other risk factors include obesity, hypertension, diabetes, gallbladder disease, and family history of breast or ovarian cancer. Use of birth control pills and pregnancy appear to provide some protection against endometrial cancer. It occurs most commonly in Caucasian women and after menopause. Abnormal uterine bleeding is the cardinal sign (ACS, 1997).

Ovarian Cancer. Ovarian cancer is the most malignant of all gynecologic cancers, accounting for the most deaths from these cancers. Risk factors include family history of ovarian or breast cancer and having no children or having them late in life. Native American women have the highest rates of ovarian cancer in the United States. There are usually no early warning symptoms (ACS, 1997).

Other Gynecologic Cancers. Cancers of the vulva, vagina, and uterine tubes account for less than 6% of all female reproductive cancers. Cancer of the vulva and vagina have been linked to HPV and HSV. The cause of uterine tube cancer is unknown. These cancers occur most often in postmenopausal women. Lesions are often the first sign of vulvar cancer. Women with vaginal or uterine tube cancer may be asymptomatic or have vaginal bleeding (DiSaia and Creasman, 1997).

Environmental and Workplace Hazards

Environmental hazards in the home, workplace, and community can contribute to poor health at all ages. Categories and examples of health-damaging hazards include the following: (1) pathogenic agents (e.g., viruses, bacteria, fungi, and parasites); (2) natural and synthetic chemicals (e.g., natural toxins from animals, insects, and plants; consumer and industrial products such as pesticides and hydrocarbon gases; medical and diagnostic devices; tobacco; fuels; and drug and alcohol abuse); (3) radiation (e.g., radon, heat waves, and sound waves); (4) food substances (e.g., added components that are not necessary for nutrition); and (5) physical objects (e.g., moving vehicles, machinery, weapons, water, and building materials) (Pender, 1996).

Environmental hazards can affect fertility, fetal development, live birth, and the child's future mental and physical development. Children are at special risk for poisoning from lead found in paint and soil. Everyone is at risk from air pollutants such as tobacco smoke, carbon monoxide, smog, suspended particles (e.g., dust, ash, and asbestos), and cleaning solvents; noise pollution; pesticides; chemical additives; and poor preparation of food. Workers also face safety and health risks caused by ergonomically poor workstations and stress. The lists could go on and on. It is important that risk assessments continue to be in effect to identify and understand environmental public health problems.

Violence Against Women

Violence against women is a major health care problem in the United States, affecting 2 to 4 million women each year and costing millions of dollars in annual medical costs. Women of all racial, ethnic, educational, religious, and socioeconomic backgrounds are affected. Pregnancy is often a time when violence begins or escalates. The magnitude of the problem is far greater than statistics indicate because violent crimes against women are the most underreported. This is a result of fear, lack of understanding, and the stigma surrounding violent situations (Stringham, 1999).

Community Focus

VIOLENCE AGAINST WOMEN AND REPRODUCTIVE HEALTH CARE

The majority of women in the United States seek reproductive health services each year. This provides an opportunity for identifying women at risk of or who are experiencing violence from an intimate partner. National professional associations have endorsed screening for violence; however, not all settings provide this screening. Appropriate, sensitive, and effective care must be increased for women who are at risk for or affected by intimate partner violence.

Data from: Parsons L, Goodwin M, Petersen R: Violence against women and reproductive health: toward defining a role for reproductive health care, *Matern Child Health J* 4(2):135-140, 2000.

Maternity and women's health nurses, by the very nature of their practice, are in a unique position to conduct case finding, provide sensitive care to women experiencing abusive situations, engage in prevention activities, and influence health care and public policy toward decreasing the violence.

Battered Women. *Wife battering, spouse abuse,* and *domestic* or *family violence* are all terms applied to a pattern of assaultive and coercive behaviors that includes physical, sexual, and psychologic attacks, as well as economic coercion inflicted by a male partner in a marriage or in another heterosexual, significant, intimate relationship. The terms *domestic violence* and *spouse abuse* connote that abuse can occur by either partner against the other and do not acknowledge that women are the victims of abuse at a rate much greater than that for men victims.

Relationship violence rarely consists of a single episode, but is a pattern that may start with intimidation or threats and progress to more aggressive physical and sexual acts resulting in injury to the woman. Common elements of battering are economic deprivation, sexual abuse, intimidation, isolation, and stalking and terrorizing victims and their children.

Characteristics of Women in Battering Relationships. Every segment of society is represented among abused women. Race, religion, social background, age, and educational level do not differentiate women at risk. Poor and uneducated women tend to be disproportionately represented because they end up in emergency departments, are financially more dependent, have fewer resources and support systems, and have fewer problem-solving skills.

Battered women may believe they are to blame for their situations because they are "not good enough" for their partner. The woman blames herself for bringing on the violent behavior in her relationship because she believes she needs to "try harder" to please the abuser. In many cases there is a traumatic bonding with the man that hinges on loyalty, fear, terror, and learned helplessness. Many women have low self-esteem and may have histories of domestic violence in their families of origin. They fear societal rejection if they discuss their problem openly.

Cycle of Violence: The Dynamics of Battering. Battering is neither random nor constant; rather, it occurs in repeated cycles. A three-phase cyclic pattern to the battering behavior includes a period of *increasing tension* leading to the *battery,* which is then followed by a period of *calm and remorse* in which the male partner displays kind, loving behavior and pleas for forgiveness. This "honeymoon" phase lasts until stress or other factors cause conflict and tension to mount again toward another episode of battering. Over time, the tension and battering phases last longer and the calm phase becomes shorter until there is no honeymoon phase (Walker, 1984).

Battery During Pregnancy. Between 40% and 60% of pregnant women admit being battered during pregnancy (McFarlane et al 1999; Parker and McFarlane, 1991); battering in teenage pregnancies ranges from 26% to 28% (Parker, McFarlane, and Soeken, 1994).

Battery during pregnancy results in a higher rate of miscarriages, preterm, low-birth-weight, and stillborn infants; and maternal complications of low weight gain, infections, and anemia. In addition, the woman may smoke or use alcohol or other drugs as means of coping (Curry, 1998).

During pregnancy, the nurse should assess for abuse at each prenatal visit and on admission to labor. Pregnancy is a time of initial or increased battering episodes in violent relationships for a number of reasons: (1) the stresses of pregnancy may strain the relationship beyond the couple's ability to cope;

Nursing Care Plan: THE BATTERED WOMAN

NURSING DIAGNOSIS Risk for self-directed violence related to history of battering by partner as evidenced by physical injuries

EXPECTED OUTCOME Patient will identify factors leading to cycle of violence and develop plan for future safety.

Nursing Interventions/*Rationales*

Using therapeutic communication, provide opportunity to verbalize feelings in a nonthreatening atmosphere *to obtain clarification and give emotional support.*

Assess on an ongoing basis for cues indicative of battering *to provide baseline and database for further interventions and referrals.*

Provide information on options available to battered woman (i.e., shelters, legal assistance) *to assist in developing a future plan for safety for herself and her children.*

Refer to social services and support groups *to coordinate options, give further information, and share common experiences.*

NURSING DIAGNOSIS Risk for situational low self-esteem related to repeated cycle of domestic violence

EXPECTED OUTCOME Patient will verbalize a positive self-assessment.

Nursing Interventions/*Rationales*

Using therapeutic communication, encourage expression of feelings *to clarify and correct any misconceptions regarding the cycle of violence.*

Encourage questions and provide information regarding domestic violence *to alleviate possible feelings of guilt and low self-esteem, which may be enhanced by the situation.*

Refer to support groups or other victims of domestic violence *to assist with resolution of feelings and clarify perception of situation.*

Provide written information regarding domestic violence, shelters, support groups, and legal implications *to assist patient to have reference material at a later date and provide control over the situation.*

(2) the man may be jealous of the fetus; (3) the man may be angry at the unborn child or the woman; and (4) the beating may be the man's conscious or subconscious attempt to end the pregnancy. After birth the mother may be so physically and emotionally drained that she may have difficulty bonding with her infant. She may be at risk of becoming an abusive mother whether or not she remains in the abusive relationship.

The target body parts of pregnant women change during abusive episodes; physical blows are directed to the head, breasts, abdomen, and genitalia. Sexual assault is common (McFarlane, 1993). The battered pregnant woman should be treated as a high risk obstetric patient because she is prone to anxiety, depression, alcohol and drug use, and inadequate and late prenatal care (Campbell et al, 1992; Curry, 1998).

If the pregnant woman remains with her partner, she is at additional risk for repeated physical and psychologic trauma. If battering begins in pregnancy, it is likely to continue after the birth. This information is vital to share with the woman and other nurses involved in her care.

Plan of Care and Interventions. Establishing a therapeutic relationship and skillful interviewing will help women disclose and describe their abuse. Language is important when talking with women. For example, using the term *victim* connotes powerlessness and hopelessness (Ryan and King, 1998); a more empowering term is *survivor.*

The nurse can help the woman formulate a plan: What referrals (e.g., shelters, agencies, and legal aid) can help her? Where can she go if she needs to leave immediately? What necessary documents and personal items should be packed so that they can easily be accessed? The woman must be told that help is available and that she does not deserve to be abused. The nurse's goal is to empower the woman. The woman needs to gain a feeling of control over her life, set her own goals, and make her own decisions (Nursing Care Plan).

Rape. Rape is an act of violence, not a sexual act. Rape is a legal term and not a medical entity. In its strictest sense, rape is the penile penetration of the female sex organ or labia without the female's consent. Sexual assault, a term used interchangeably with rape, is also an act of force and has a much broader definition to include unwanted or uncomfortable touches, kisses, hugs, petting, intercourse, or other sexual acts. States may also use different legal definitions of rape.

Hymenal penetration or ejaculation does not have to occur to qualify as rape. The key feature to establish rape is lack of consent: threat or coercion implies the lack of consent. The court must prove absence of consent; thus the term alleged rape or alleged sexual assault is used in medical records.

Many people (perhaps even the victim of the rape) will believe that the woman "invited" the rape through either seductive dress or behavior. The fact is that no one deserves to be forced into any sexual behavior.

The types of rape are reported as date or acquaintance rape, marital rape, gang rape, stranger rape, and psychic rape. Acquaintance rape is sexual assault by persons who know one another (e.g., a classmate, neighbor, family member, or a date) and occurs when the trust of that relationship is violated and one person is forced by another into sexual activity (Stuart and Sundeen, 1998). Date and acquaintance rape occur most often to women between 15 and 19 years of age.

Marital rape occurs partly because men may believe it is their right to engage in sex whenever they desire, regardless of the partner's desire or condition. It commonly occurs along with physical abuse of the woman.

Gang rape occurs when one woman is raped by more than one man. In stranger rape, an unknown attacker actively seeks a woman who is vulnerable. This is the type of rape most feared by women (Aguilera, 1994).

Psychic rape occurs when one's personal dignity and self-respect are assaulted (Stuart and Sundeen, 1998). Sexual harassment, although not classified as rape, is another form of using power and control tactics to victimize women sexually, particularly in the workplace. The anticipatory fear of rape, the trauma experienced during an attack, and the terror that persists after the attack are all damaging to women's lives.

Female Genital Mutilation. Female genital mutilation is practiced in more than 45 countries, with the majority of these countries being in Africa. These procedures involve the intentional removal of all or part of the external female genitalia (Affara, 2000). As emigrants from those counties arrive in North America, nurses in the United States and Canada will see patients who have had such procedures performed. Complications of female genital mutilation include infection, hemorrhage, and urinary complications, as well as higher maternal and infant morbidity and mortality during labor (Affara, 2000).

ANTICIPATORY GUIDANCE FOR HEALTH PROMOTION AND PREVENTION

Over the last several decades, women have made tremendous strides in education, careers, policy making, and overall participation in today's complex society. There have been costs for these advances, and although women are living longer, they may not be living better. As a result, the health care system needs to pay greater attention to the health consequences for women. In addition, women must be active participants in their own health promotion and illness prevention. Pender (1996) de-

Critical Thinking

COMMUNITY RESOURCES FOR RAPE SURVIVORS

Investigate resources in your community for victims of rape. Do local hospitals have rape counselors? What educational efforts have the police made? Are there telephone hotlines for advice and referral? How would a victim of rape learn of these resources? Prepare a list of community resources appropriate for distribution in the community.

Critical Thinking

ANTICIPATORY GUIDANCE FOR HEALTH PROMOTION

Prepare a consultation plan for a 35-year-old, divorced, nulliparous woman needing general anticipatory guidance for health promotion and prevention.

- **Ascertain her opinion regarding her health status.**
- **Identify need for counseling regarding nutrition, exercise, stress management, and safer sexual practices.**
- **Suggest recommendations for screening based on information obtained.**

scribes health promotion as the motivation to increase well-being and actualize health potential. Prevention is the desire to avoid illness, to detect it early, or to maintain optimal functioning when illness is present.

Nurses have a major opportunity and responsibility to help women understand risk factors and to motivate them to adopt healthy lifestyles that prevent disease. Lifestyle factors that affect health—and that the woman has some control over—include diet; tobacco, alcohol, and substance use; exercise; sunlight exposure; stress management; and sexual practices. Other influences, such as genetic and environmental factors, may be beyond the woman's control, although some opportunities for prevention exist (e.g., through environmental legislative activism or genetic counseling services).

Knowledge alone is not enough to bring about healthy behaviors. The woman must be convinced that she has some control over her life and that healthy life habits, including periodic health examinations, are a sound investment. She must believe in the efficacy of prevention, early detection, and therapy, and in her ability to perform self-care practices such as breast self-examination. Many people believe that they have little control over their health, or they become so immobilized by fear and anxiety in the face of life-threatening illnesses, such as cancer, that they delay seeking treatment. The nurse must explore the reality of each woman's perceptions about health behaviors and individualize teaching if it is to be effective.

Substance Use Cessation

All women at all ages will receive substantial and immediate benefits from smoking cessation. This is not easy, however, and most people will attempt to stop several times before they accomplish their goal. Many are never able to do so.

New approaches are needed to increase cessation among smokers and to discourage smoking among young women, especially in adolescence and during pregnancy. Health care providers can have an impact on smoking behavior and should attempt to motivate smokers to stop (Box 4-6). Raising questions about social consequences (e.g., stained teeth and foul-smelling breath and clothes) is sometimes effective with young people.

Those who wish to stop smoking can be referred to a smoking cessation program in which individualized methods can be implemented. At the very least, individuals should be guided to self-help materials available from the March of Dimes Birth Defects Foundation, the American Lung Association, and the American Cancer Society. During pregnancy, women seem to be highly motivated to stop or at least to limit smoking to 10 or fewer cigarettes a day. Insult to the fetus can be reduced or even avoided if this is done by the end of the first trimester.

Alcohol and other drugs exact a staggering toll on society, not only in terms of personal health, but also in their association with poverty and homelessness, family disorganization, violence, crime, motor vehicle injuries, reduced productivity, and economic costs. The abuse of alcohol and other drugs increases the risk of victimization and date rape and of acquiring HIV through shared needles or sexual contact. Alcohol use and drug use are the leading preventable causes of birth defects.

A national awareness of the seriousness of problems associated with substance abuse has led to raising the legal drinking age to 21 in all states and to tighter controls on advertising. Stronger regulation of advertising and tougher laws and law enforcement for alcohol- and drug-related offenses are being implemented. There is still much that must be done to increase the accessibility to care for low-income people, minorities, and young people. Women—especially pregnant women and the mothers of young children—have special needs that must be addressed.

All primary care providers should screen for alcohol and other drug use problems, with an understanding of the obvious problems in relying on self-reporting of these behaviors. The use of over-the-counter drugs by women should also be explored. Counseling women who appear to be drinking excessively or using drugs may include strategies to increase self-esteem and teaching new coping skills to resist and maintain resistance to alcohol abuse and drug use. Appropriate referrals

BOX 4-6

Interventions for Smoking Cessation: The Four *A*'s

ASK

What was her age when she started smoking? How many cigarettes does she smoke a day? When was her last cigarette? Has she tried to quit? Does she want to quit?

ASSESS

What are her reasons for not being able to quit before, or what made her start again? Does she have anyone who can help her? Does anyone else smoke at home? Does she have friends or family who have quit successfully?

ADVISE

Give her information about the effects of smoking on pregnancy and her fetus, on her own future health, and on the members of her household.

ASSIST

Provide support; give self-help materials. Encourage her to set a quit date. Refer to a smoking cessation program or provide information about nicotine replacement products (not recommended during pregnancy) if she is interested. Teach and encourage use of stress reduction activities. Provide for follow-up with a phone call, letter, or clinic visit.

Source: American College of Obstetricians and Gynecologists: *Smoking and women's health,* (ACOG Technical Bulletin No. 240), Washington, DC, 1997, ACOG.

BOX 4-7

National Groups Offering Help for Chemical Dependency

Alcoholics Anonymous (for individuals who are alcohol dependent) 1-212-686-1100*
- Al-Anon (for families of alcoholics)
- Al-Ateen (for teenager children of alcoholics)

COCAINE Hotline 1-800-COCAINE

National Alcohol and Drug Abuse Hotline 1-800-252-6465

Narcotics Anonymous (for drug abusers) 1-888-336-4066*

*Also check your telephone book for local listing.

should be made, with the health care provider arranging the contact and then following up to ensure that appointments are kept. General referral to sources of support should also be provided. National groups that provide information and support for those who are chemically dependent are listed in Box 4-7. Many of these organizations have local branches or contacts that are listed in the telephone book.

Anticipatory guidance includes teaching about the health and safety risks of alcohol and mind-altering substances; and discouraging drug experimentation among preteen and high school students, because the use of drugs at an early age tends to predict greater involvement later.

Health Screening Schedule

Periodic health screening includes history, physical examination, education, counseling, and selected diagnostic and laboratory tests. This regimen provides the basis for overall health promotion, prevention of illness, early diagnosis of problems, and referral for appropriate management. Such screening should be customized according to a woman's age and risk factors. In most instances it is completed in health care offices, clinics, or hospitals; however, portions of the screening are now being carried out at events such as community health fairs. An overview of health screening recommendations for women over 18 years of age is provided in Table 4-1. Consistent with infor-

TABLE 4-1

Health Screening Recommendations for Women 18+ Years of Age

Intervention	Recommendation*
PHYSICAL EXAMINATION	
Blood pressure	Every visit, but at least every 2 years
Height and weight	
Pelvic examination	
Breast examination	
Self-examination	Initiated/taught at time of first pelvic examination; done monthly at end of menses.
Clinical breast examination†	Every 1 to 3 years starting at age 30 years; annually over age 40 years
High risk	Annually over age 18 with history of premenopausal breast cancer in first-degree relative
Risk groups	At least annually:
Skin examination	Family history of skin cancer or increased exposure to sunlight
Oral cavity examination	Mouth lesion or exposure to tobacco or excessive alcohol
LABORATORY/DIAGNOSTIC TESTS	
Blood cholesterol†	Every 5 years
High risk	More often per clinical judgment with potential for cardiac or lipid abnormalities
Papanicolaou smear†	Initially at age 18 years or when sexually active; after three normal consecutive annual examinations, Pap can be per risk, based on discussion with health care provider‖
Mammography‡	Annually over age 50 years† Annually over age 40 years§,‖
Fecal occult blood test	Annually over age 50 years‖
Sigmoidoscopy	Every 5 years after age 50 years‖
Colonoscopy	Every 10 years over age 50 years‖
Risk groups	
Fasting blood sugar	Annually with family history of diabetes, gestational diabetes, or woman who is significantly obese
Hearing	Annually with exposure to excessive noise
STI screen	As needed with multiple sexual partners
Tuberculin skin test	Annually with exposure to persons with tuberculosis or in risk categories for close contact with the disease
Endometrial biopsy	At menopause for women at risk for endometrial cancer‖
IMMUNIZATIONS	
Tetanus-diphtheria	Booster is given every 10 years after primary series
Measles, mumps, rubella	Once if born after 1956 and no evidence of immunity
Hepatitis B	Primary series of three for all who are in risk categories
Influenza	Annually after age 65 years or in risk categories, such as chronic diseases, immunosuppression, renal dysfunction

Source: United States Preventive Services Task Force: *Guide to clinical preventive services,* ed 2, Baltimore, 1996, Williams & Wilkins.
*Unless otherwise noted, the recommended intervention should be performed routinely every 1 to 3 years.
†United States Preventive Services Task Force (1996).
‡Note: There is no consensus regarding mammograms for women between ages 40 and 49, thus various recommendations are listed. Women are urged to discuss circumstances with their health care providers.
§American College of Obstetricians and Gynecologists (1997a).
‖American Cancer Society (1999).

mation provided earlier in this chapter, it is important for the nurse to continually educate and counsel on diet, exercise, cessation of smoking, alcohol moderation, help for drug abuse, and stress management.

Health Risk Prevention

Often, simple safety factors are forgotten or perceived not to be important; yet injuries continue to have a major impact on the health status of all age groups. Awareness of hazards and implementation of safety guidelines will reduce risks. The nurse should regularly reinforce the following commonsense concepts that will protect the individual:

- Wear seat belts at all times in a moving vehicle.
- Wear safety helmets when riding a motorcycle or bicycle.
- Follow driving rules of the road.
- Have working smoke alarms in place throughout the home and workplace.
- Avoid secondhand smoke.
- Reduce noise pollution or safeguard against hearing loss.
- Protect skin from ultraviolet light via sunscreen and clothing.
- Handle and store firearms appropriately.
- Practice water safety.

Taking necessary precautions and avoiding dangerous situations are imperative.

Health Protection

Nurses can make a difference in stopping violence against women and in preventing further injury. Educating women that abuse is a violation of their rights and facilitating their access to protective and legal services constitutes a first step. Encouraging health care institutions to implement appropriate domestic violence screening programs is also of great value (Gantt and Bickford, 1999). Other measures that may help women avoid falling into abusive relationships are promoting assertiveness and self-defense courses; suggesting support and self-help groups that encourage positive self-regard, confidence, and empowerment; and recommending educational and skills development classes that will enhance independence (or at least the ability to take care of oneself).

Many national and local organizations provide information and assistance for women in abusive situations. Nurses and victims may find these resources helpful. Box 4-8 lists national resources and hotlines. All nurses who work in women's health care should become familiar with local services and legal options.

BOX 4-8

Resources for Violence Against Women

Center for Women Policy Studies
2000 P St. NW, Suite 508
Washington, DC 20036
(202) 872-1770
(Publications and current federal legislation information)

National Child Abuse Hotline
(800) 422-4453

National Coalition Against Domestic Violence
(202) 544-7358
National Domestic Violence/Abuse Hotline: (800) 799-SAFE
(Many states have local coalitions against domestic violence.)

National Coalition Against Sexual Assault
912 North 2nd St.
Harrisburg, PA 17102
(717) 232-6771

National Organization for Women (NOW) Legal Defense and Education Fund
99 Hudson St.
New York, NY 10013-2871
(212) 925-6635

National Resource Center for Domestic Violence
1-800-537-2238

The National Center on Women and Family Law
799 Broadway, Room 402
New York, NY 10003
(212) 674-8200
(Legal information)

Key Points

- Culture, religion, socioeconomic status, personal circumstances, the uniqueness of the individual, and the stage of development influence a person's recognition of need for care and the response to the health care system and therapy.
- Preconception counseling allows identification and possible remediation of potentially harmful personal and social conditions, medical and psychologic conditions, environmental conditions, and barriers to care before pregnancy occurs.
- Conditions that increase a woman's health risks also increase risks for her offspring.
- Health promotion and prevention assists women to actualize health potential by increasing motivation, providing information, and suggesting how to access specific resources.
- Violence against women is a major social and health care problem in the United States; domestic violence includes physical, sexual, emotional, psychologic, and economic abuse.
- Battering affects all races; all socioeconomic, educational, and religious groups; and many pregnant women.

References

Affara F: Correspondence from abroad. When tradition maims, *Am J Nurs* 100(8):52-57, 58-59, 60, 2000.

Aguilera D: *Crisis intervention: theory and methodology,* ed 7, St Louis, 1994, Mosby.

Alan Guttmacher Institute: *Risks and realities of early childbearing,* New York, 1998, The Institute.

American Cancer Society: *Cancer facts and figures 1997,* New York, 1997, American Cancer Society.

American Cancer Society: *Cancer facts and figures 1999,* New York, 1999, American Cancer Society.

American College of Obstetricians and Gynecologists: *Smoking and women's health (ACOG Tech Bull No. 240),* Washington, DC, 1997, ACOG.

Burke B: *Preventing neural tube birth defects: a prevention model and resource guide,* Atlanta, 1999, Centers for Disease Control and Prevention.

Campbell et al: Correlates of battering during pregnancy, *Res Nurs Health* 15:219-226, 1992.

Casele H, Laifer S: Factors influencing preconception control of glycemia in diabetic women, *Arch Intern Med* 158(12): 1321-1324, 1998.

Cefalo R, Moos M: *Preconceptional health care,* St Louis, 1995, Mosby.

Cox R: Family health care delivery for 21st century, *J Obstet Gynecol Neonatal Nurs* 26(1):109, 1997.

Curry M: The interrelationships between abuse, substance use, and psychosocial stress during pregnancy, *J Obstet Gynecol Neonatal Nurs* 27(6):692-699, 1998.

DiSaia P, Creasman W: *Clinical gynecologic oncology,* ed 5, St Louis, 1997, Mosby.

Epps R, Stewart S: *The women's complete healthbook,* New York, 1995, The Philip Lief Group, Inc.

Fox C: Cocaine use in pregnancy, *J Am Board Fam Pract* 7(3):225-228, 1994.

Gantt L, Bickford A: Screening for domestic violence, *AWHONN Lifelines* 3(2):36-42, 1999.

Grimes D, editor: Helping patients stop smoking: a new treatment option, *Contraceptive Report* 9(3):12, 1998.

Hatcher R et al: *Contraceptive technology,* ed 17, New York, 1998, Irvington.

Japenga A: Depression: are men hiding? *USA Weekend,* Jan. 2, 1998, p. 20.

Jessup M: Addiction in women: prevalence, profiles, and meaning, *J Obstet Gynecol Neonatal Nurs* 26(4):449-458, 1997.

Lean M et al: Impairment of health and quality of life using new U.S. federal guidelines for identification of obesity, *Arch Intern Med* 159(8):837-843, 1999.

Lewis D, Woods S: Fetal alcohol syndrome, *Am Fam Physician* 50(5):1025, 1994.

Li C et al: Implementation of substance use screening in prenatal clinics, *S D J Med* 52(2):59-64, 1999.

McFarlane J: Abuse during pregnancy: the horror and the hope, *AWHONN Clin Issues Perinat Women's Health Nurse* 4(30):350-362, 1993.

McFarlane J et al: Severity of abuse before and during pregnancy for African-American, Hispanic, and Anglo women, *J Nurse Midwifery* 44(2):139-144, 1999.

Murray R, Zentner J: *Health assessment promotion strategies through the life span,* ed 6, Stamford, CT, 1997, Appleton & Lange.

Muscari M: Rebels with a cause, *Am J Nurs* 98(12):26-30, 1998.

National Center for Health Statistics: *Health, United States, 1998,* Atlanta, 1998, Centers for Disease Control and Prevention.

Parker B, McFarlane J: Identifying and helping battered pregnant women, *MCN Am J Matern Child Nurs* 16:161-164, 1991.

Parker B, McFarlane J, Soeken K: Abuse during pregnancy: effects on maternal complications and birth weight in adult and teenage women, *Obstet Gynecol* 84(3):323-328, 1994.

Pender N: *Health promotion in nursing practice,* ed 3, Stamford, CT, 1996, Appleton & Lange.

Pohl J, Caplan D: Smoking cessation: using group intervention methods to treat low-income women, *Nurs Pract* 23(12):13, 17-18, 20, 1998.

Ryan J, King M: Scanning for violence, *AWHONN Lifelines* 2(3):36-41, 1998.

Sampselle C et al: Continence for women: evidence-based practice, *J Obstet Gynecol Neonatal Nurs* 26(4):375-385, 1997.

Stuart G, Sundeen S: *Principles and practices of psychiatric nursing,* ed 6, St Louis, 1998, Mosby.

Stringham P: Domestic violence, *Prim Care* 26(2):373-384, 1999.

Walker L: *The battered woman syndrome,* ed 6, New York, 1984, Springer.

CHAPTER

5

Health Assessment

http://www.harcourthealth.com/MERLIN/Wong/maternal/

Learning Objectives

On completion of this chapter the reader will be able to:

- Identify the structures and functions of the female reproductive system.
- Summarize the menstrual cycle in relation to hormonal, ovarian, and endometrial response.
- Identify the four phases of the sexual response cycle.
- Discuss how assessment and physical examination can be adapted for women with special needs.
- Identify indications of abuse, appropriate screening, and referral to community agencies.
- Define components of taking a woman's history and performing a physical examination.
- Identify the correct procedure for assisting with and collecting Papanicolaou smear specimens.
- Review patient teaching of breast self-examination.

The purpose of this chapter is to review female anatomy and physiology, the menstrual cycle, and gynecologic health assessment.

FEMALE REPRODUCTIVE SYSTEM

The female reproductive system consists of external structures (visible from the pubis to the perineum) and internal structures (located in the pelvic cavity). The external and internal female reproductive structures develop and mature in response to estrogen and progesterone. This process starts in fetal life and continues through puberty and the childbearing years. Reproductive structures atrophy with age or in response to a decrease in ovarian hormone production. A complex nerve and blood supply supports the functions of these structures. The appearance of the external genitalia varies greatly among women. Heredity, age, race, and the number of children a woman has borne influence the size, shape, and color of her external organs.

External Structures

The external genital organs, or vulva, include all structures visible externally from the pubis to the perineum: the mons pubis, labia majora, labia minora, clitoris, vestibular glands, vaginal vestibule, vaginal orifice, and urethral opening. The external genital organs are illustrated in Fig. 5-1.

The mons pubis is a fatty pad that lies over the anterior surface of the symphysis pubis. In the postpubertal female, the mons is covered with coarse, curly hair. The labia majora are two rounded folds of fatty tissue covered with skin that extend downward and backward from the mons pubis. The labia are highly vascular structures that develop hair on the outer surfaces after puberty. They protect the inner vulvar structures. The labia minora are two flat, reddish folds of tissue visible when the labia majora are separated. There are no hair follicles on the labia minora, but many sebaceous follicles and a few sweat glands are present. The interior of the labia minora is composed of connective tissue and smooth muscle, and is supplied with extremely sensitive nerve endings. Anteriorly, the labia minora fuse to form the prepuce (i.e., the hoodlike covering of the clitoris) and the frenulum (i.e., the fold of tissue under the clitoris). The labia minora join to form a thin, flat tissue called the fourchette underneath the vaginal opening at midline. The clitoris is located underneath the prepuce. It is a small structure composed of erectile tissue with numerous sensory nerve endings. During sexual arousal the clitoris increases in size.

The vaginal vestibule is an almond-shaped area enclosed by the labia minora that contains openings to the urethra, Skene's glands, vagina, and Bartholin glands. The urethra is not a reproductive organ but is discussed here because of its location. It usually is found about 2.5 cm below the clitoris. Skene's glands are located on each side of the urethra and produce mucus, which aids in lubrication of the vagina. The vaginal opening is in the lower portion of the vestibule and varies in shape and size. The hymen, a connective tissue membrane that surrounds the vaginal opening, can be perforated during strenuous exercise, insertion of tampons, masturbation, and vaginal intercourse. Bartholin's glands lie under the constrictor muscles of

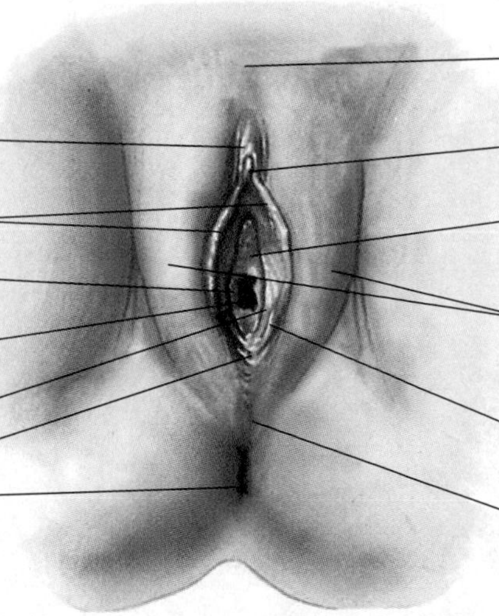

FIG. 5-1 • External female genitalia.

the vagina and are located posteriorly on the sides of the vaginal opening, although the ductal openings are usually not visible. During sexual arousal the glands secrete a clear mucus to lubricate the vaginal introitus.

The area between the fourchette and the anus is the perineum, a skin-covered muscular area that covers the pelvic structures. The perineum forms the base of the perineal body, a wedge-shaped mass that serves as an anchor for the muscles, fascia, and ligaments of the pelvis. The muscles and ligaments form a sling that supports the pelvic organs.

Internal Structures

The internal structures include the vagina, uterus, uterine tubes, and ovaries.

The vagina is a fibromuscular, collapsible, tubular structure that lies between the bladder and rectum and extends from the vulva to the uterus. During the reproductive years the mucosal lining is arranged in transverse folds called rugae. These rugae allow the vagina to expand during childbirth. When estrogen deprivation occurs after childbirth, during lactation, and at menopause, it causes dryness and thinness of the vaginal walls and causes the rugae to become smooth. The vagina, particularly the lower segment, has few sensory nerve endings. Vaginal secretions are slightly acidic (pH 4 to 5) so that the vagina's susceptibility to infections is reduced. The vagina serves as a passageway for menstrual flow, as a female organ of copulation, and as a part of the birth canal for vaginal childbirth. The uterine cervix projects into a blind vault at the upper end of the vagina. There are anterior, posterior, and lateral pockets called fornices (singular: fornix) that surround the cervix. The internal pelvic organs can be palpated through the thin walls of these fornices.

The uterus is a muscular organ shaped like an upside-down pear that sits midline in the pelvic cavity, between the bladder and rectum and above the vagina. Four pairs of ligaments (i.e., the cardinal, uterosacral, round, and broad) support the uterus. Single anterior and posterior ligaments also support the uterus. The cul-de-sac of Douglas is a deep pouch or recess posterior to the cervix formed by the posterior ligament.

The uterus is divided into two major parts, an upper triangular portion called the corpus and a lower cylindrical portion called the cervix (Fig. 5-2). The fundus is the dome-shaped top of the uterus and is the site at which the uterine tubes enter the uterus. The isthmus, or lower uterine segment, is a short, constricted portion that separates the corpus from the cervix.

The uterus serves for reception, implantation, retention, and nutrition of the fertilized ovum and later the fetus during pregnancy and expulsion of the fetus during childbirth. It also is responsible for cyclic menstruation.

The uterine wall comprises three layers: the endometrium, the myometrium, and part of the peritoneum. The endometrium is a highly vascular lining that is itself made up of three layers, the outer two of which are shed during menstruation. The myometrium is made up of layers of smooth muscles that extend in three different directions (i.e., longitudinal, transverse, and oblique) (Fig. 5-3). Longitudinal fibers of the outer myometrial layer are found mostly in the fundus, and this arrangement assists in expelling the fetus during birth. The middle layer contains fibers from all three directions, forming a figure-eight pattern encircling large blood vessels. This arrangement assists in ligating blood vessels after childbirth and controls blood loss. Most of the circular fibers of the inner myometrial layer are around the site where the uterine tubes enter the uterus and around the internal cervical os (opening). These fibers help keep the cervix closed during pregnancy and prevent menstrual blood from flowing back into the uterine tubes during menstruation.

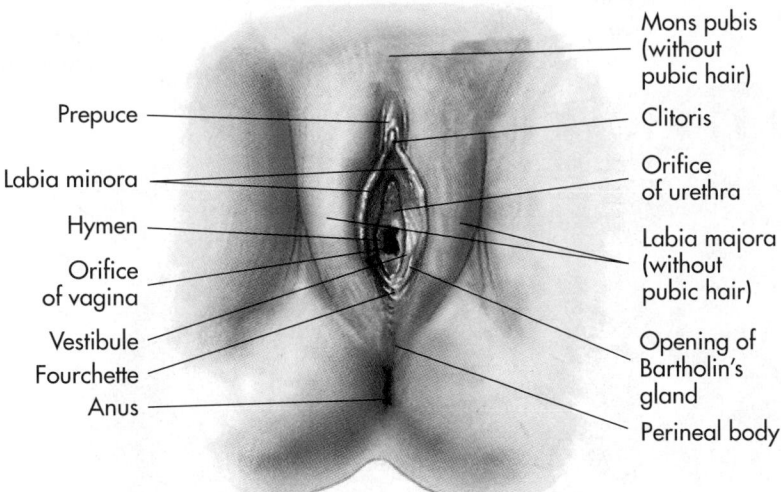

The cervix is made up mostly of fibrous connective tissues and elastic tissue, making it possible for the cervix to stretch during vaginal childbirth. The opening between the uterine cavity and the canal that connects the uterine cavity to the vagina (endocervical canal) is the internal os. The narrowed opening between the endocervix and the vagina is the external os, a small circular opening in women who have never been pregnant. The

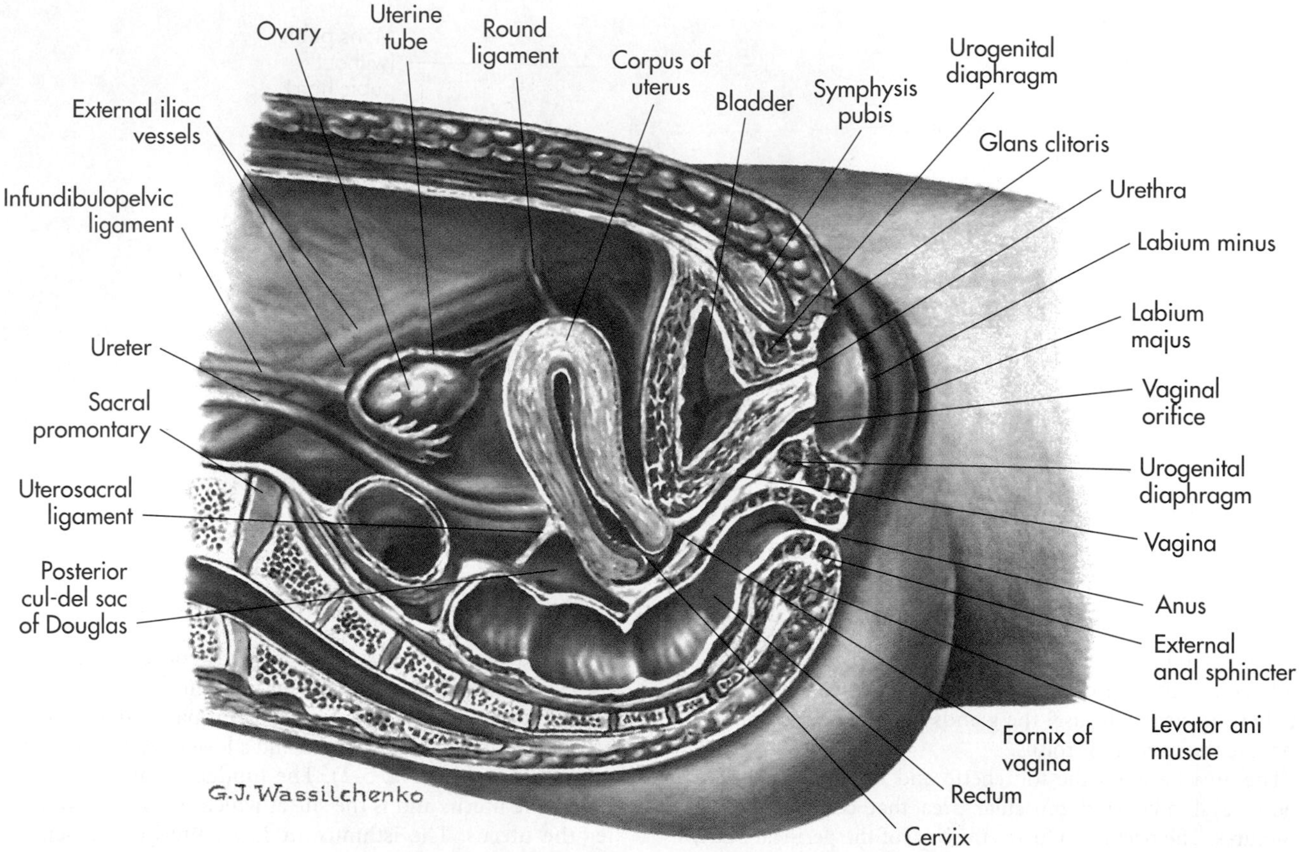

FIG. 5-2 • Midsagittal view of female pelvic organs with woman lying supine.

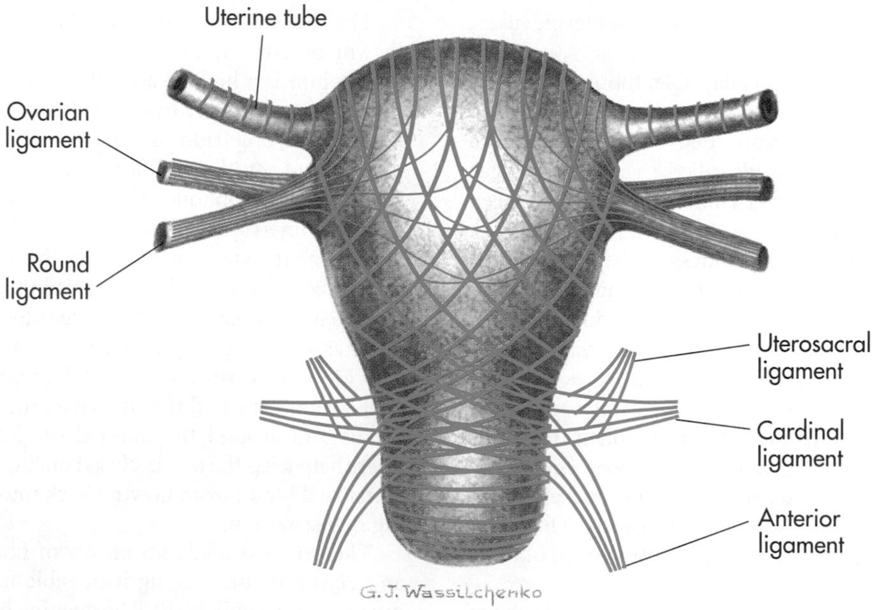

FIG. 5-3 • Schematic arrangement of directions of muscle fibers. Note that uterine muscle fibers are continuous with supportive ligaments of uterus.

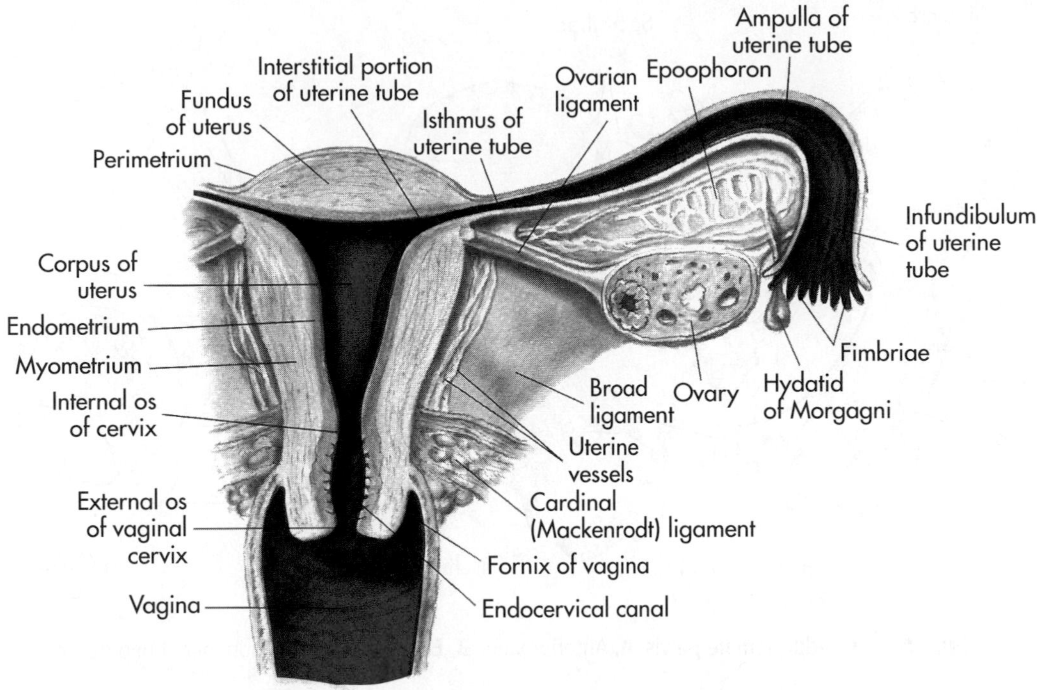

FIG. 5-4 • Cross section of uterus, adnexa, and upper vagina.

cervix feels firm (like the end of a nose) with a dimple in the center that marks the external os.

The outer cervix is covered with a layer of squamous epithelium. The mucosa of the cervical canal is covered with columnar epithelium and contains numerous glands that secrete mucus in response to ovarian hormones. The squamocolumnar junction, where the two types of cells meet, is usually located just inside the cervical os. This junction is the most common site for neoplastic changes, and cells from this site are scraped for the Papanicolaou test.

The uterine tubes (fallopian tubes) attach to the uterine fundus and are supported by the broad ligaments. These tubes range from 8 to 14 cm in length and are divided into four sections: the interstitial portion, closest to the uterus; the isthmus and the ampulla, the two middle portions; and the infundibulum, closest to the ovary (Fig. 5-4). The uterine tubes provide a passage between the ovaries and the uterus for the ovum. The end of the tubes are fimbriated (fringed) and pull the ovum into the tube. The ovum is pulled along the tubes to the uterus by rhythmic contractions of muscles and by the current produced by the movement of the cilia that line the tubes. Fertilization by sperm usually takes place in the outer third of one of the tubes.

The ovaries are almond-shaped organs located on each side of the uterus below and behind the uterine tubes. During the reproductive years, they are approximately 3 cm long, 2 cm wide, and 1 cm thick; they diminish in size after menopause. Before menarche, each ovary has a smooth surface; after menarche they become nodular because of repeated ruptures of follicles at ovulation. The ovaries serve two functions: ovulation and hormone production. Ovulation is the release of a mature ovum from the ovary at intervals (usually monthly). Estrogen, progesterone, and androgen are the hormones produced by the ovaries.

The Bony Pelvis

The bony pelvis serves three primary purposes: protection of the pelvic structures, accommodation of the growing fetus during pregnancy, and anchorage of the pelvic support structures. The pelvis comprises four bones: the two innominate (hip) bones (consisting of ilium, ischium, and pubis); the sacrum; and the coccyx (Fig. 5-5). Cartilage and ligaments form the symphysis pubis, sacrococcygeal, and two sacroiliac joints that separate the pelvic bones.

The pelvis is divided into two parts: the false pelvis and the true pelvis (Fig. 5-6). The false pelvis is the upper portion above the pelvic brim or inlet. The true pelvis is the lower curved bony canal, which includes the inlet, the cavity, and the outlet through which the fetus passes during vaginal birth. The upper portion of the outlet is at the level of the ischial spines, and the lower portion is at the level of the ischial tuberosities and the pubic arch. Variations in the size and shape of the pelvis are usually due to age and race. Pelvic ossification is complete at about 20 years of age.

Breasts

The breasts are paired mammary glands located between the second and sixth ribs (Fig. 5-7). About two thirds of the breast overlies the pectoralis major muscle, between the sternum and midaxillary line, with an extension to the axilla referred to as the tail of Spence. The lower one third of the breast overlies the serratus anterior muscle. The breasts are attached to the muscles by connective tissue or fascia.

The breasts of the healthy, mature woman are approximately equal in size and shape, but often are not absolutely symmetric. The size and shape vary with the woman's age, heredity, and nutrition. However, the contour should be smooth with no retrac-

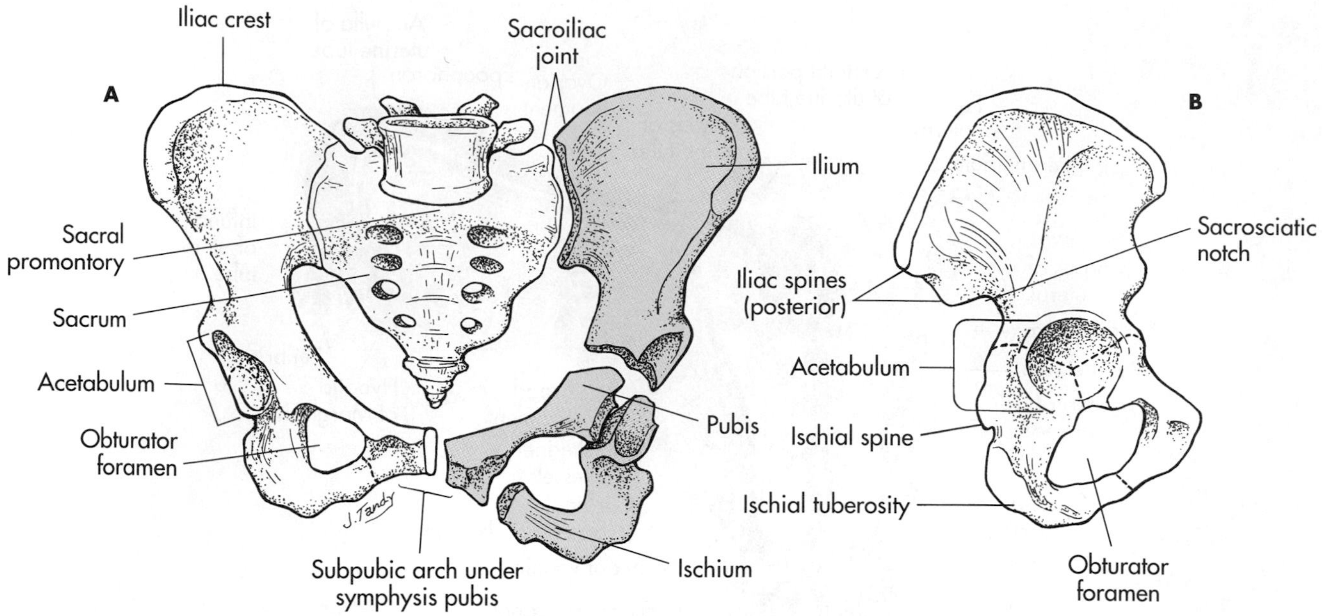

FIG. 5-5 • Adult female pelvis. **A,** Anterior view. **B,** External view of innominate bone (fused).

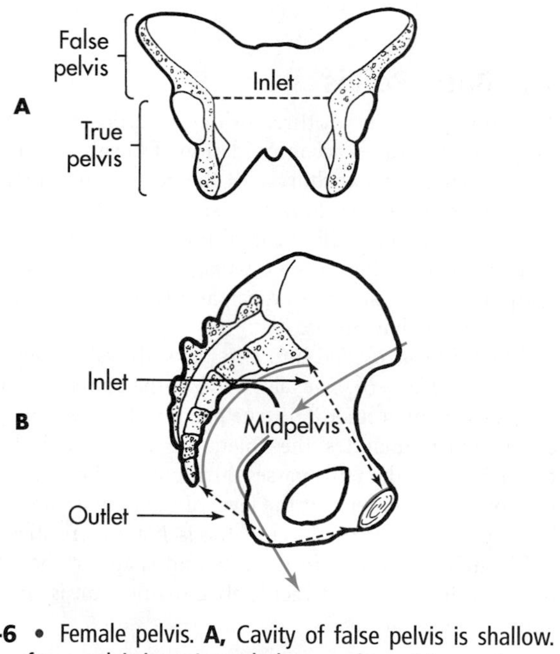

FIG. 5-6 • Female pelvis. **A,** Cavity of false pelvis is shallow. **B,** Cavity of true pelvis is an irregularly curved canal (*arrows*).

tions, dimpling, or masses. Estrogen stimulates growth of the breast by inducing fat deposition, development of stromal tissue (i.e., increase in its amount and elasticity), and growth of the extensive ductile system. Estrogen also increases the vascularity of breast tissue.

When ovulation begins in puberty, progesterone levels increase. This causes maturation of mammary gland tissue, specifically the lobules and acinar structures. During adolescence, fat deposition and growth of fibrous tissue contribute to the increase in the glands' size. Full development of the breasts is not achieved until after the end of the first pregnancy or in the early period of lactation.

Each mammary gland is made of 15 to 20 lobes, which are divided into lobules. Lobules are clusters of acini. An acinus is a saclike terminal part of a compound gland emptying through a narrow lumen or duct. In discussions of mammary glands, acinus (the correct anatomic term) is often used interchangeably with the term alveolus. The acini are lined with epithelial cells that secrete colostrum and milk. Just below the epithelium is the myoepithelium, which contracts to expel milk from the acini. The ducts from the clusters of acini that form the lobules merge to form larger ducts draining the lobes. Ducts from the lobes converge in a single nipple (mammary papilla) surrounded by an areola. Just as the ducts converge, they dilate to form common lactiferous sinuses, which are also called ampullae. The lactiferous sinuses serve as milk reservoirs. Many tiny lactiferous ducts drain the ampullae and exit in the nipple.

The glandular structures and ducts are surrounded by protective fatty tissue and are separated and supported by fibrous suspensory Cooper's ligaments. Cooper's ligaments provide support to the mammary glands while permitting their mobility on the chest wall (see Fig. 5-7). The nipple is usually round, slightly elevated, and projects slightly upward and laterally. It contains 15 to 20 openings from lactiferous ducts. The nipple is surrounded by fibromuscular tissue and covered by wrinkled skin. Except during pregnancy and lactation, there is normally no discharge from the nipple.

The nipple and surrounding areola are usually more deeply pigmented than the skin of the breast. The rough appearance of the areola is caused by sebaceous glands (i.e., Montgomery tubercles) directly beneath the skin. These glands secrete a fatty substance thought to lubricate the nipple. Smooth muscle fibers in the areola contract to stiffen the nipple to make it easier for the breastfeeding infant to grasp.

The vascular supply to the mammary gland is abundant. In the nonpregnant state the skin does not have an obvious vascu-

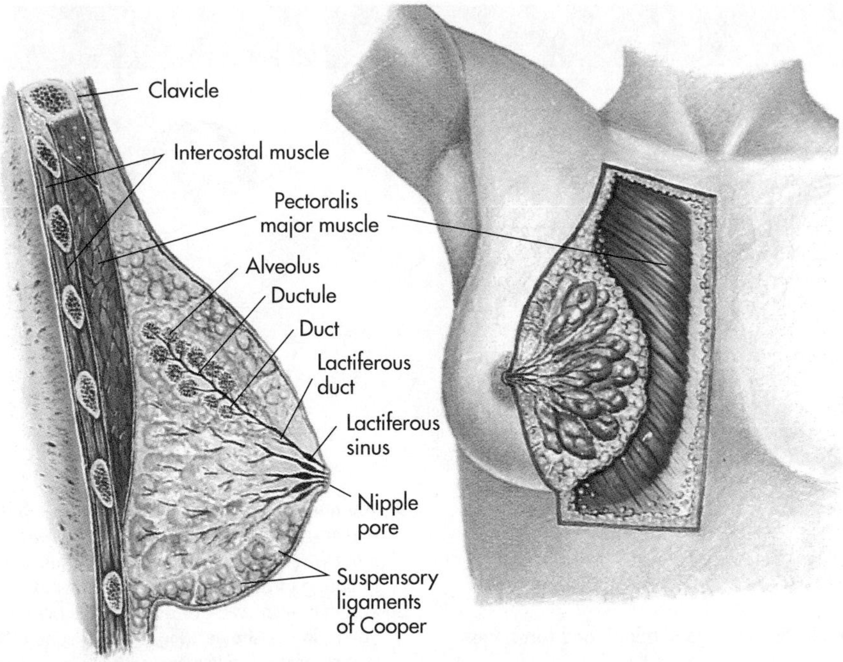

FIG. 5-7 • Anatomy of the breast, showing position and major structures. (From Seidel H et al: *Mosby's guide to physical examination,* ed 4, St Louis, 1999, Mosby.)

lar pattern. The normal skin is smooth without tightness or shininess. The skin covering the breasts contains an extensive superficial lymphatic network that serves the entire chest wall and is continuous with the superficial lymphatics of the neck and abdomen. The lymphatics form a rich network in the deeper portions of the breasts. The primary deep lymphatic pathway drains laterally toward the axillae.

Besides their function of lactation, breasts function as organs for sexual arousal in the mature adult.

The breasts change in size and nodularity in response to cyclic ovarian changes throughout reproductive life. Increasing levels of both estrogen and progesterone in the 3 to 4 days before menstruation increase vascularity of the breasts, induce growth of the ducts and acini, and promote water retention. The epithelial cells lining the ducts proliferate in number, the ducts dilate, and the lobules distend. The acini become enlarged and secretory, and lipid (fat) is deposited within their epithelial cell linings. As a result, breast swelling, tenderness, and discomfort are common symptoms just before the onset of menstruation. After menstruation, cellular proliferation begins to regress, acini begin to decrease in size, and retained water is lost. After breasts have undergone changes numerous times in response to the ovarian cycle, the proliferation and involution (regression) are not uniform throughout the breast. In time, after repeated hormonal stimulation, small persistent areas of nodulations may develop. This normal physiologic change must be remembered when breast tissue is examined. Nodules may develop just before and during menstruation, when the breast is most active. The physiologic alterations in breast size and activity reach their minimum level about 5 to 7 days after menstruation stops. Therefore breast self-examination (BSE), which is the systematic palpation of breasts to detect signs of breast cancer or other changes, is best carried out during this phase of the menstrual cycle (Guidelines box).

MENSTRUATION

Menarche and Puberty

Although young girls secrete small, rather constant amounts of estrogen, a marked increase occurs between 8 and 11 years of age. The term menarche denotes first menstruation. Puberty is a broader term that denotes the entire transitional stage between childhood and sexual maturity. Increasing amounts and variations in gonadotropin and estrogen secretion develop into a cyclic pattern at least a year before menarche. In North America this occurs in most girls about 13 years of age.

Initially periods are irregular, unpredictable, painless, and anovulatory. After 1 or more years, a hypothalamic-pituitary rhythm develops, and the ovary produces adequate cyclic estrogen to make a mature ova. Ovulatory periods tend to be regular, monitored by progesterone.

Although pregnancy can occur in exceptional cases of true precocious puberty, most pregnancies in young girls occur after the normally timed menarche. All girls would benefit from knowing pregnancy can occur at any time after the onset of menses.

Menstrual Cycle

Menstruation is the periodic uterine bleeding that begins approximately 14 days after ovulation. It is controlled by a feedback system of three cycles: endometrial, hypothalamic-pituitary, and ovarian. The average length of a menstrual cycle is 28 days, but variations are normal. The first day of bleeding is desig-

Guidelines

BREAST SELF-EXAMINATION

1. The best time to do breast self-examination is after your period, when breasts are not tender or swollen. If you do not have regular periods or sometimes skip a month, do it on the same day every month.
2. Lie down and put a pillow under your right shoulder. Place your right arm behind your head (Fig. 1).
3. Use the finger pads of your three middle fingers on your left hand to feel for lumps or thickening. Your finger pads are the top third of each finger.
4. Press firmly enough to know how your breast feels. If you're not sure how hard to press, ask your health care provider, or try to copy the way your health care provider uses the finger pads during a breast examination. Learn what your breast feels like most of the time. A firm ridge in the lower curve of each breast is normal.
5. Move around the breast in a set way. you can choose either circles (Fig. 2, *A*), vertical lines (Fig. 2, *B*), or wedges (Fig. 2, *C*). Do it the same way every time. It will help you to make sure that you've gone over the entire breast area and to remember how your breast feels.
6. Gently compress the nipple between your thumb and forefinger and look for discharge.
7. Now examine your left breast using the finger pads of your right hand.
8. If you find any changes, see your health care provider right away.

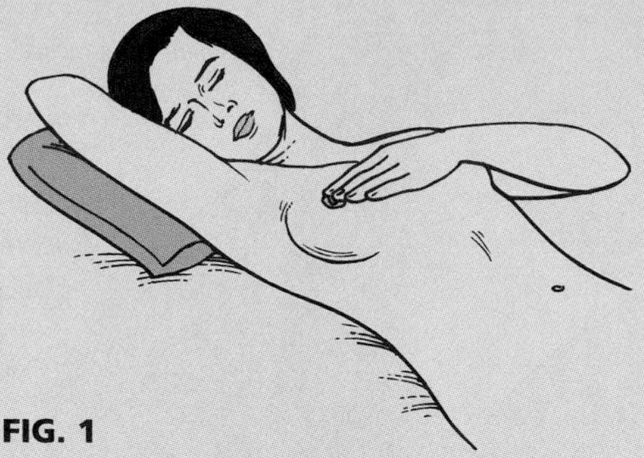

FIG. 1

9. You may want to check your breasts while standing in front of a mirror right after you do your breast self-examination each month. See if there are any changes in the way your breasts look: dimpling of the skin, changes in the nipple, or redness or swelling.
10. You may also want to do an extra breast self-examination while you're in the shower (Fig. 3). Your soapy hands will glide over the wet skin, making it easy to check how your breasts feel.
11. It is important to check the area between the breast and the underarm and the underarm itself. Also examine the area above the breast to the collarbone and to the shoulder.

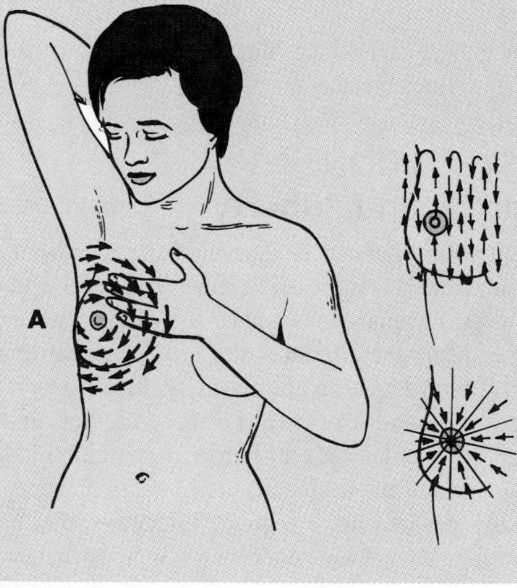

FIG. 2

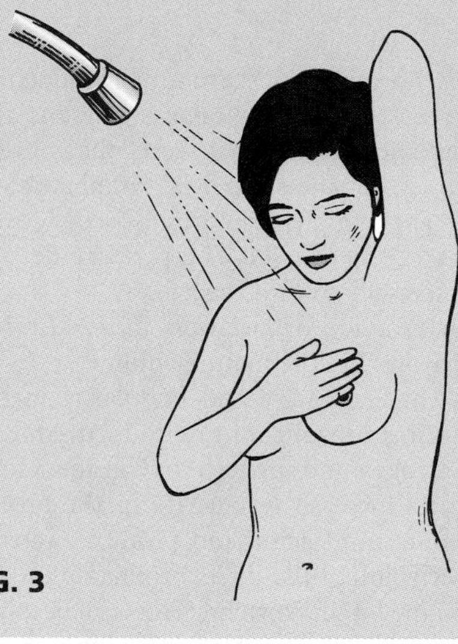

FIG. 3

nated as day 1 of the menstrual cycle, or menses (Fig. 5-8). The average duration of menstrual flow is 5 days (with a range of 3 to 6 days) and the average blood loss is 50 ml (with a range of 20 to 80 ml), but these vary greatly.

For about 50% of women, menstrual blood does not appear to clot. The menstrual blood clots within the uterus, but the clot usually liquefies before being discharged. Uterine discharge includes mucus and epithelial cells in addition to blood.

The menstrual cycle is a complex interplay of events that occur simultaneously in the endometrium, hypothalamus and pituitary glands, and ovaries. The menstrual cycle prepares the uterus for pregnancy. When pregnancy does not occur, menstruation follows. A woman's age, physical and emotional status, and environment influence the regularity of her menstrual cycles.

Endometrial Cycle. The four phases of the endometrial cycle are (1) the menstrual phase, (2) the proliferative phase, (3) the secretory phase, and (4) the ischemic phase (see Fig. 5-8). During the menstrual phase, shedding of the functional two thirds of the endometrium (the compact and spongy layers) is initiated by periodic vasoconstriction in the upper layers of the endometrium. The basal layer is always retained, and regeneration begins near the end of the cycle from cells derived from the remaining glandular remnants or stromal cells in the basalis.

The proliferative phase is a period of rapid growth lasting from about the fifth day to the time of ovulation. The endome-

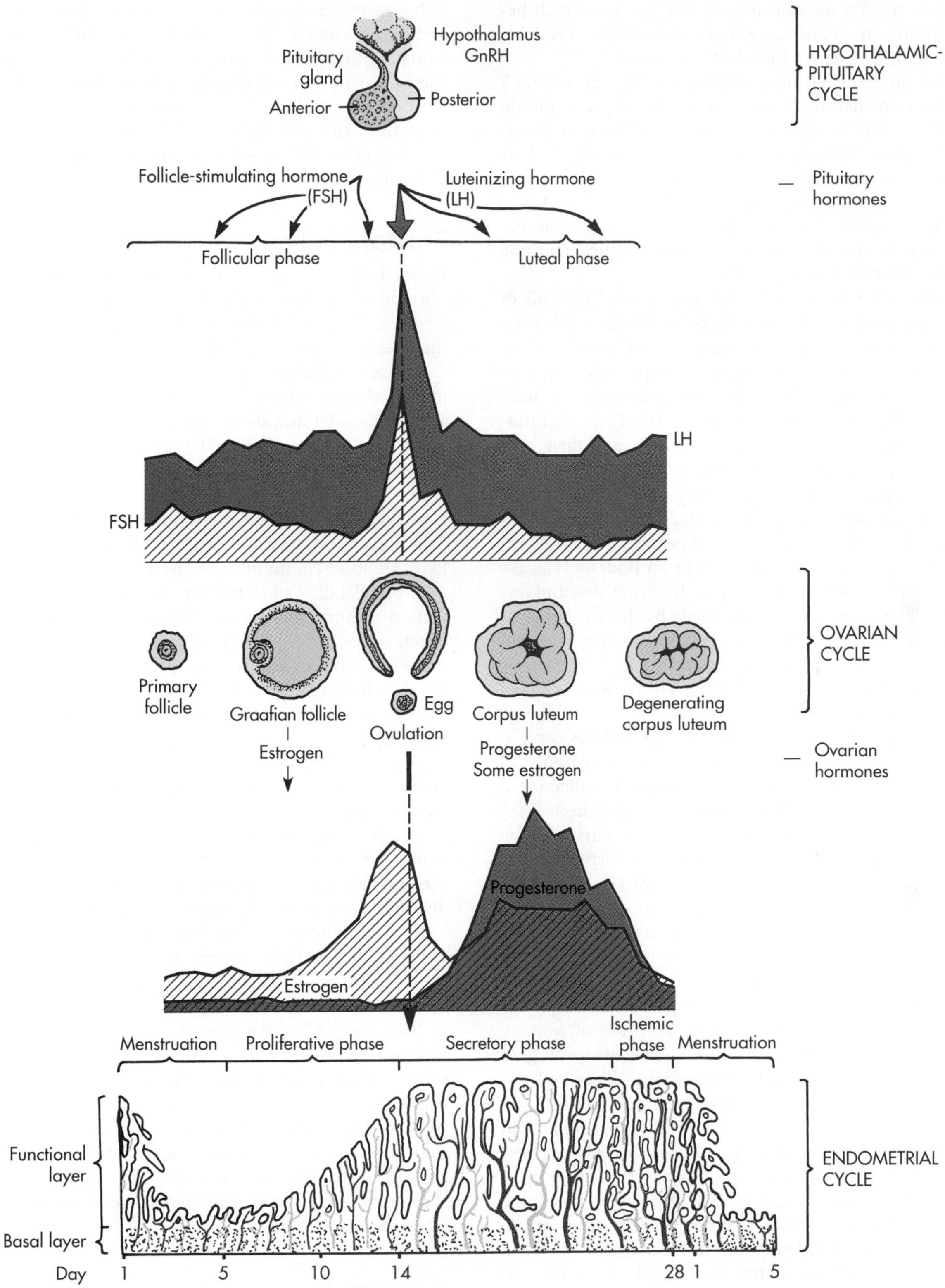

FIG. 5-8 • Menstrual cycle: hypothalamic-pituitary, ovarian, and endometrial.

trial surface is completely restored in approximately 4 days, or slightly before bleeding ceases. From this point on an eightfold to tenfold thickening occurs, with a leveling off of growth at ovulation. The proliferative phase depends on estrogen stimulation derived from ovarian follicles.

The secretory phase extends from the day of ovulation to about 3 days before the next menstrual period. After ovulation, larger amounts of progesterone are produced. An edematous, vascular, functional endometrium is now apparent.

At the end of the secretory phase the fully matured secretory endometrium reaches the thickness of heavy, soft velvet. It becomes luxuriant with blood and glandular secretions, a suitable protective and nutritive bed for a fertilized ovum.

Implantation of the fertilized ovum generally occurs about 7 to 10 days after ovulation. If fertilization and implantation do not occur, the corpus luteum, which secretes estrogen and progesterone, regresses. With the rapid fall in progesterone and estrogen levels, the spiral arteries go into spasm. During the ischemic phase, the blood supply to the functional endometrium is blocked and necrosis develops. The functional layer separates from the basal layer, and menstrual bleeding begins, marking day 1 of the next cycle (see Fig. 5-8).

Hypothalamic-Pituitary Cycle. Toward the end of the normal menstrual cycle, blood levels of estrogen and progesterone fall. Low blood levels of these ovarian hormones stimulate the hypothalamus to secrete gonadotropin-releasing hormone (GnRH). In turn, GnRH stimulates anterior pituitary secretion of follicle-stimulating hormone (FSH). FSH stimulates development of ovarian graafian follicles and their production of estrogen. Estrogen levels begin to fall, and hypothalamic GnRH triggers the anterior pituitary release of luteinizing hormone (LH). A marked surge of LH and a smaller peak of estrogen (day 12; see Fig. 5-8) precede the expulsion of the ovum from the graafian follicle by about 24 to 36 hours. LH peaks about the day 13 or 14 of a 28-day cycle. If fertilization and implantation of the ovum have not occurred by this time, regression of the corpus luteum follows. Levels of progesterone and estrogen decline, menstruation occurs, and the hypothalamus is once again stimulated to secrete GnRH. This process is called the hypothalamic-pituitary cycle.

Ovarian Cycle. The primitive graafian follicles contain immature oocytes (primordial ova). Before ovulation, from 1 to 30 follicles begin to mature in each ovary under the influence of FSH and estrogen. The preovulatory surge of LH affects a selected follicle. The oocyte matures, ovulation occurs, and the empty follicle begins its transformation into the corpus luteum. This follicular phase (preovulatory phase) (see Fig. 5-8) of the ovarian cycle varies in length from woman to woman. Almost all variations in ovarian cycle length are the result of variations in the length of the follicular phase. On rare occasions (i.e., 1 in 100 menstrual cycles) more than one follicle is selected, and more than one oocyte matures and undergoes ovulation.

After ovulation, estrogen levels drop. For 90% of women, only a small amount of withdrawal bleeding occurs and it goes unnoticed. In 10% of women, there is sufficient bleeding for it to be visible, resulting in what is termed midcycle bleeding.

The luteal phase begins immediately after ovulation and ends with the start of menstruation. This postovulatory phase of the ovarian cycle usually requires 14 days (with a range of 13 to 15 days). The corpus luteum reaches its peak of functional activity 8 days after ovulation, secreting the steroids estrogen and progesterone. Coincident with this time of peak luteal functioning, the fertilized ovum is implanted in the endometrium. If no implantation occurs, the corpus luteum regresses and steroid levels drop. Two weeks after ovulation, if fertilization and implantation do not occur, the functional layer of the uterine endometrium is shed through menstruation.

Other Cyclic Changes. When the hypothalamic-pituitary-ovarian axis functions properly, other tissues undergo predictable responses. Before ovulation the woman's basal body temperature (BBT) is often below 37° C; after ovulation, with rising progesterone levels, her BBT rises. Changes in the cervix and cervical mucus follow a generally predictable pattern. Preovulatory and postovulatory mucus is viscous (thick) so that sperm penetration is discouraged. At the time of ovulation, cervical mucus is thin and clear. It looks, feels, and stretches like egg white. This stretchable quality is termed *spinnbarkheit.* At the time of ovulation, some women experience localized lower abdominal pain called *mittelschmerz.*

Prostaglandins

Prostaglandins (PGs) are oxygenated fatty acids classified as hormones. The different kinds of PGs are distinguished by letters (e.g., PGE and PGF), numbers (e.g., PGE_2), and letters of the Greek alphabet (e.g., $PGF_{2\alpha}$).

PGs are produced in most organs of the body, including the uterus. Menstrual blood is a potent prostaglandin source. PGs are metabolized quickly by most tissues. They are biologically active in minute amounts in the cardiovascular, gastrointestinal, respiratory, urogenital, and nervous systems. They also exert a marked effect on metabolism, particularly on glycolysis. Prostaglandins play an important role in many physiologic, pathologic, and pharmacologic reactions. $PGF_{2\alpha}$, PGE_4, and PGE_2 are most commonly used in reproductive medicine.

Prostaglandins affect smooth muscle contractility and modulation of hormonal activity. Indirect evidence supports PGs' effects on ovulation, fertility, changes in the cervix and cervical mucus that affect receptivity to sperm, tubal and uterine motility, sloughing of endometrium (menstruation), onset of miscarriage and induced abortion, and onset of labor (term and preterm).

After exerting their biologic actions, newly synthesized PGs are rapidly metabolized by tissues in such organs as the lungs, kidneys, and liver.

PGs may play a key role in ovulation. If PG levels do not rise along with the surge of LH, the ovum remains trapped within the graafian follicle. After ovulation, PGs may influence production of estrogen and progesterone by the corpus luteum.

The introduction of PGs into the vagina or into the uterine cavity (from ejaculated semen) increases the motility of uterine musculature, which may assist the transport of sperm through the uterus and into the oviduct.

PGs produced by the woman cause regression of the corpus luteum; regression of the endometrium; and sloughing of the endometrium, resulting in menstruation. PGs increase myometrial response to oxytocic stimulation, enhance uterine contractions, and cause cervical dilation. They may be a factor in the initiation of labor, the maintenance of labor, or both. They may also be involved in the following pathologic states: dysmenorrhea, hypertensive states, preeclampsia/eclampsia, and anaphylactic shock.

Climacteric

The climacteric is a transitional phase during which ovarian function and hormone production decline. This phase spans the years from the onset of premenopausal ovarian decline to the postmenopausal time when symptoms stop. Menopause (from the Latin *mensis,* month, and Greek *pauses,* to cease) refers only to the last menstrual period. Unlike menarche, however, menopause can only be dated with certainty 1 year after menstruation ceases. The average age at natural menopause is 51.4 years, with an age range of 35 to 60 years.

SEXUAL RESPONSE

The hypothalamus and anterior pituitary glands in females regulate the production of FSH and LH. The target tissue for these hormones is the ovary, which produces ova and secretes estrogen and progesterone. A feedback mechanism—between hormone secretion from the ovaries, the hypothalamus, and the anterior pituitary—aids in the control of sex cell production and steroid sex hormone secretion.

Physiologic Response to Sexual Stimulation

Although the first outward appearance of maturing sexual development occurs at an earlier age in females, both females and males achieve physical maturity at approximately 17 years of age; however, individual development varies greatly. Anatomic and reproductive differences notwithstanding, women and men are more alike than different in their physiologic response to sexual excitement and orgasm. For example, the glans clitoris and the glans penis are embryonic homologues. Not only is there little difference between female and male sexual response, but the physical response is essentially the same whether stimulated by coitus, fantasy, or masturbation. According to Masters (1992), physiologic sexual response can be analyzed in terms of two processes: vasocongestion and myotonia.

Sexual stimulation results in circumvaginal blood vessels (lubrication in the female), causing engorgement and distention of the genitalia. Venous congestion is localized primarily in the genitalia, but it also occurs to a lesser degree in the breasts and in other parts of the body. Arousal is characterized by myotonia (i.e., increased muscular tension), resulting in voluntary and involuntary rhythmic contractions. Examples of sexually stimulated myotonia are pelvic thrusting, facial grimacing, and spasms of the hands and feet (carpopedal spasms).

The sexual response cycle is divided into four phases: excitement phase, plateau phase, orgasmic phase, and resolution phase. The four phases occur progressively with no sharp dividing line between any two phases. Specific body changes take place in sequence. The time, intensity, and duration for cyclic completion also vary for individuals and situations. Table 5-1 compares male and female body changes during each of the four phases of the sexual response cycle.

TABLE 5-1
Four Phases of Sexual Response

Reactions Common to Both Sexes	Female Reactions	Male Reactions
EXCITEMENT PHASE		
Heart rate and blood pressure increase. Nipples become erect. Myotonia begins.	Clitoris increases in diameter and swells. External genitals become congested and darken. Vagina lubrication occurs; upper two thirds of vagina lengthen and extend. Cervix and uterus pull upward. Breast size increases.	Erection of the penis begins; penis increases in length and diameter. Scrotal skin becomes congested and thickens. Testes begin to increase in size and elevate toward the body.
PLATEAU PHASE		
Heart rate and blood pressure continue to increase. Respirations increase. Myotonia becomes pronounced; grimacing occurs.	Clitoral head retracts under the clitoral hood. Lower one third of vagina becomes engorged. Skin color changes occur—red flush may be observed across breasts, abdomen, or other surfaces.	Head of penis may enlarge slightly. Scrotum continues to grow tense and thicken. Testes continue to elevate and enlarge. Preorgasmic emission of 2 or 3 drops of fluid appears on the head of the penis.
ORGASMIC PHASE		
Heart rate, blood pressure, and respirations increase to maximum levels. Involuntary muscle spasms occur. External rectal sphincter contracts.	Strong rhythmic contractions are felt in the clitoris, vagina, and uterus. Sensations of warmth spread through the pelvic area.	Testes elevate to maximum level. Point of "inevitability" occurs just before ejaculation and an awareness of fluid in the urethra. Rhythmic contractions occur in the penis. Ejaculation of semen occurs.
RESOLUTION PHASE		
Heart rate, blood pressure, and respirations return to normal. Nipple erection subsides. Myotonia subsides.	Engorgement in external genitalia and vagina resolves. Uterus descends to normal position. Cervix dips into seminal pool. Breast size decreases. Skin flush disappears.	Fifty percent of erection is lost immediately with ejaculation; penis gradually returns to normal size. Testes and scrotum return to normal size. Refractory period (time needed for erection to occur again) varies according to age and general physical condition.

HEALTH ASSESSMENT

Current women's health trends have expanded beyond a reproductive focus to include a holistic approach to health care across the life span. Women's health assessment and screening focuses on a systems evaluation that begins with a careful history and physical examination. During the assessment and evaluation, the responsibility for self-care, health promotion, and enhancement of wellness is emphasized.

A nurse often takes the history, orders diagnostic tests, interprets test results, makes referrals, coordinates care, and directs attention to problems requiring medical intervention. Advanced practice nurses who have specialized in women's health (e.g., nurse practitioners, clinical nurse specialists, and nurse midwives) perform complete physical assessments including gynecologic examinations.

Nursing care should be delivered with an awareness of cultural diversity while respecting the unique qualities of each woman. Nurses must acknowledge their own values, beliefs, and communication styles in order to understand what they contribute to cross-cultural communication (Lipson, Dibble, and Minarik, 1996).

Interview

The interview should be conducted in a private, comfortable, and relaxed setting (Fig. 5-9). The woman is addressed by her title and name (e.g., Mrs. Martinez) and the nurse introduces herself or himself using name and title. It is important to phrase questions in a sensitive and nonjudgmental manner and to assure the woman of strict confidentiality. Body language should match oral communication. For many women, fear, anxiety, and modesty make the examination a dreaded and stressful experience. Many women are uninformed, misguided by myths, or afraid they will appear ignorant by asking questions about sexual or reproductive functioning. The woman is assured that no question is irrelevant. The history begins with an open-ended question such as, "What brings you into the office/clinic/hospital today?" and is furthered by other questions such as "Anything else?" and "Tell me about it." Additional ways to encourage women to share information include the following:

- **Facilitation**—Using a word or posture that communicates interest, such as leaning forward, making eye contact, or saying "Mm-hmmm" or "Go on."
- **Reflection**—Repeating a word or phrase that a woman has used.
- **Clarification**—Asking the woman what is meant by a stated word or phrase.
- **Empathic responses**—Acknowledging the feelings of a woman by statements such as "That must have been frightening."
- **Confrontation**—Identifying something about the woman's behavior or feelings not expressed verbally or apparently inconsistent with her history.
- **Interpretation**—Putting into words what you infer about the woman's feelings or about the meaning of her symptoms, events, or other matters.

Direct questions may be necessary to get specific details. This should be worded in language that is understandable to the woman and expressed neutrally so that the woman will not be led into a specific response. The nurse asks about one item at a time and proceeds from the general to the specific (Seidel et al, 1999).

Biographic Information. The woman's name, age, marital status, race, ethnicity, address, phone numbers, occupation, and date of visit are recorded. A subjective judgment about the reliability of the person giving the history (e.g., the woman, parent, spouse, or other historian) is recorded.

Cultural and Communication Variations. Recognition of signs and symptoms of disease, and the decision of when to seek treatment, are influenced by cultural perceptions. Culture evolves over time and is a system of symbols that are learned, shared, and passed on through generations of a social group. It is essential that a nurse have respect for cultural diversity and the rich and unique qualities of individuals and trust that the woman is the expert on her life, culture, and experiences. The nurse communicates in an even-toned and nonjudgmental manner, keeping a calm facial expression and recognizing that modifications may be necessary for the physical examination. In some cultures it may be considered inappropriate for the woman to completely disrobe for the physical examination. In many cultures, a woman examiner is preferred.

Women with Special Needs. Women with emotional or physical disorders have special needs. Women who have vision, hearing, emotional, or physical disabilities should be involved in the assessment and physical examination to the full

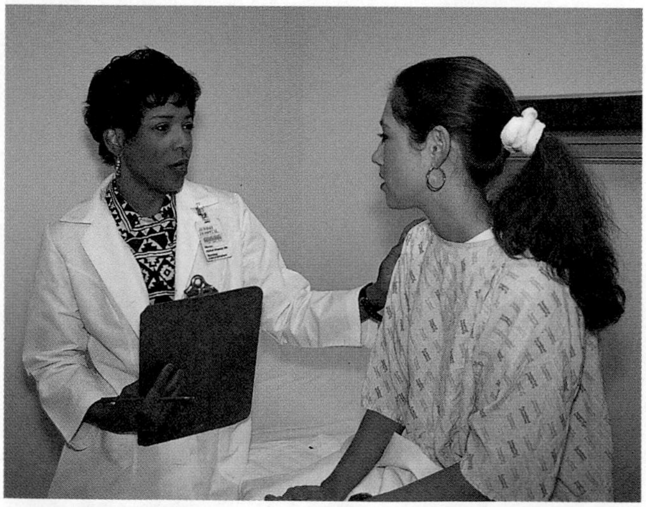

FIG. 5-9 • Nurse interviews patient as part of annual physical examination. (From Potter PA, Perry AG: *Basic nursing: a critical thinking approach,* ed 4, St Louis, 1997, Mosby.)

> *Critical Thinking*
>
> **TEACHING BREAST SELF-EXAMINATION**
>
> **You are assigned to teach breast self-examination (BSE) at a clinic for non-English-speaking women from Vietnam. The clinic provides you with an aide who is bilingual.**
>
> - **Compare the immigrant women's perceptions and beliefs about health and BSE to your own.**
> - **Analyze how these factors may affect the health-seeking behaviors of these women.**
> - **How would you incorporate this knowledge into your teaching plan?**

extent of their abilities. The nurse should communicate openly and directly and with sensitivity. It is often helpful to learn about the disability directly from the woman while maintaining eye contact. Family and significant others should be relied on only when absolutely necessary. The assessment and physical examination can be adapted to each woman's individual needs.

Communication with a woman who is hearing impaired can be accomplished without difficulty. Many of these women read lips, write, or both; the interviewer who speaks and enunciates each word slowly and in full view may be easily understood. If a woman is not comfortable with lipreading, she may use an interpreter. In this case, it is important to continue to address the woman directly, avoiding the temptation to speak directly with the interpreter. The visually impaired woman needs to be oriented to the examination room and may have her guide dog with her. As with all patients, the visually impaired woman needs a full explanation of what the examination entails before proceeding. Before touching her, the nurse explains, "Now I am going to take your blood pressure. I am going to place the cuff on your right arm." To reduce her anxiety, the woman can be asked if she would like to touch each of the items that will be used in the examination.

Many physically disabled women cannot comfortably lie in the lithotomy position for the pelvic examination. Several alternative positions may be used, including a lateral (side-lying) position, a V-shaped position, a diamond-shaped position, and an M-shaped position (Fig. 5-10). The woman can be asked what has worked best for her previously. If she has never had a pelvic examination, or has never had a comfortable pelvic examination, the nurse proceeds slowly by showing her a picture of various positions and asking her which one she prefers. The nurse's support and reassurance can help the woman to relax, which will make the examination go more smoothly. The woman is informed that she is in charge, and if the examination must stop for any reason, it can be rescheduled at a later date.

Abused Women. Nurses should screen all women entering the health care system for potential abuse. Abuse is a life-threatening public health problem that affects millions of women and their children. Help for the woman may depend on the sensitivity with which the nurse screens for abuse, the discovery of abuse, and subsequent intervention. The nurse must be familiar with the laws governing abuse in the state in which she or he practices and inform the patient of these laws before eliciting this information. Awareness of the law can ensure the woman's confidentiality and trust.

Critical Thinking

CARING FOR A WOMAN WITH A PHYSICAL DISABILITY

A woman with severe scoliosis who uses a wheelchair arrives at the clinic for a physical examination and Pap smear.

- **What modifications in your usual assessment procedure are needed?**
- **Does the clinic have obstacles that would prevent patients with disabilities from receiving appropriate care?**
- **What needs to be changed? What can you do to bring about change?**

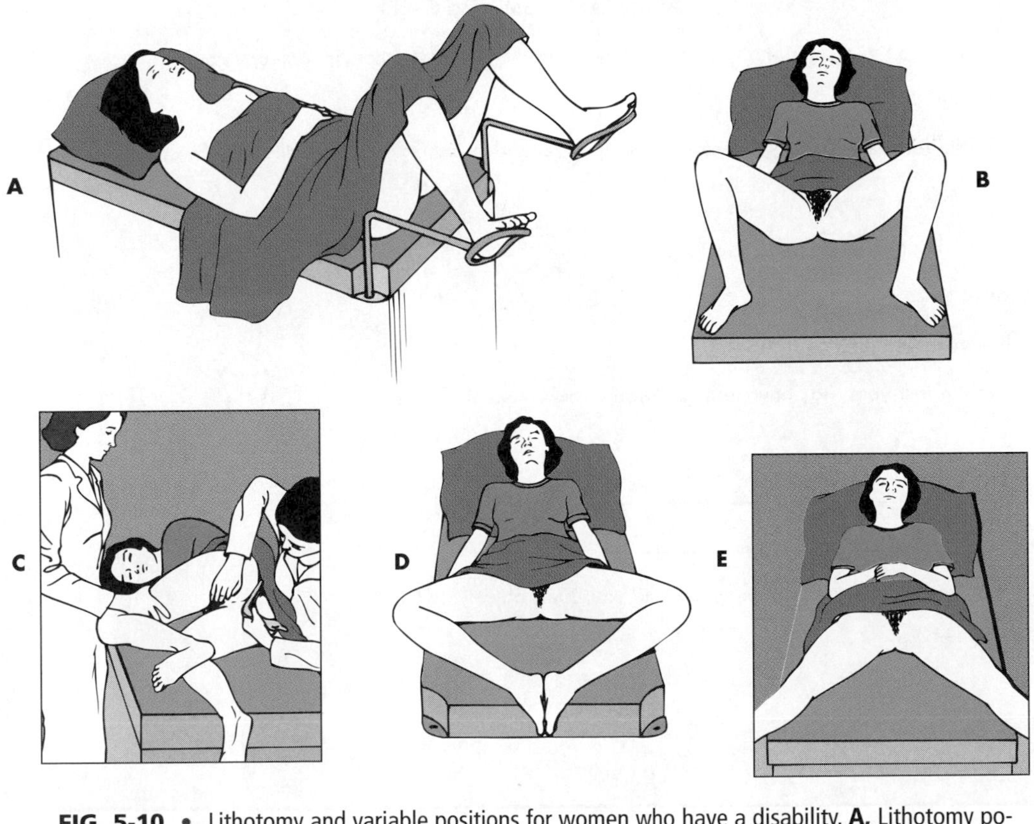

FIG. 5-10 • Lithotomy and variable positions for women who have a disability. **A,** Lithotomy position. **B,** M-shaped position. **C,** Side-lying position. **D,** Diamond-shaped position. **E,** V-shaped position.

LEGAL TIP • Mandatory Reporting of Domestic Violence. Forty states and the District of Columbia have laws that mandate health care providers report any situation in which a woman has an injury that may have been caused by a deadly weapon. Some states also require reports when there is a reason to believe the woman's injury may have resulted from an illegal act or an act of violence. Only six states have mandatory reporting laws specific to domestic violence or adult abuse.

Pocket cards listing emergency numbers (e.g., abuse counseling, legal protection, and emergency shelter) may be obtained from local police departments, women's' shelters, or emergency departments. It is helpful to have these on hand when screening is done. An abuse assessment screen (Fig. 5-11) can be used as part of the interview or written history (Poirier, 1997). Reports show an increase in identification of victims of domestic violence when screening takes place at each visit. If a male partner is present, he should be asked to leave the room because the woman may not disclose experiences of abuse in his presence, or he may try to answer questions for her to protect himself. The same procedure would apply for partners of lesbians or the adult children of older women.

Fear, guilt, and embarrassment may keep many women from giving information about family violence. Clues in the history and evidence of injuries on physical examination should give a high index of suspicion (Box 5-1). The areas most commonly injured in women are the head, neck, chest, abdomen, breasts, and upper extremities. Other signs are burns and bruises in patterns resembling hands, belts, cords, or other weapons; and multiple traumatic injuries. Attention should be given to women who repeatedly seek treatment for somatic complaints such as headaches, insomnia, choking sensations, hyperventilation, gastrointestinal symptoms, and pain in the chest, back, or pelvis.

If a woman discloses battering, this disclosure is acknowledged and affirmed as behavior that is unacceptable. The

Box 5-1

Indicators of Possible Abuse

1. Change in appointment pattern, either increased appointments with somatic, vague complaints or frequently missed appointments.
2. Self-directed abuse, depression, attempted suicide
3. Severe anxiety, insomnia, or violent nightmares
4. Alcohol or drug abuse; overuse or abuse of prescription medications
5. Bruises

Data from Edge V, Miller M: *Women's health care,* St Louis, 1994, Mosby.

ABUSE ASSESSMENT SCREEN

1. Have you ever been emotionally or physically abused by your partner or someone important to you?

YES ☐ NO ☐

2. Within the last year, have you been hit, slapped, kicked, or otherwise physically hurt by someone?

YES ☐ NO ☐

If YES, by whom ____________________

Number of times ____________________

Mark the area of injury on body map.

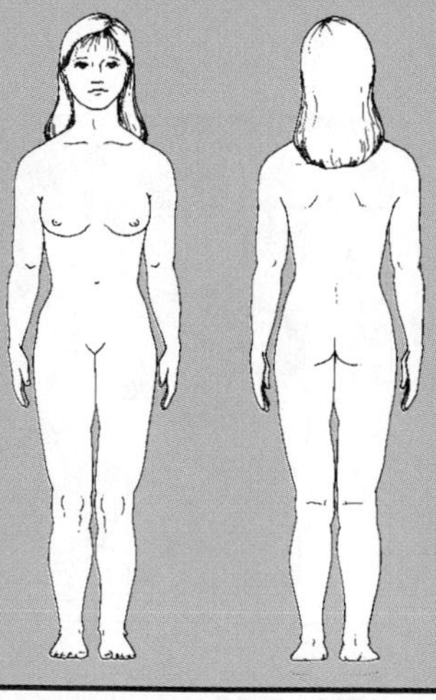

3. Within the last year, has anyone forced you to have sexual activities?

YES ☐ NO ☐

If YES, by whom ____________________

Number of times ____________________

4. Are you afraid of your partner or anyone you listed above?

YES ☐ NO ☐

FIG. 5-11 • Abuse assessment screen. (Modified from the Nursing Research Consortium on Violence and Abuse, 1991.)

woman is told that she is at risk for recurrence. She also needs to know that battering is a common problem, because she may think that she is alone in experiencing violence perpetrated by a family member or loved one. She needs to be informed about the cycle of violence (see Chapter 4). She must be told that help is available and that she does not deserve to be abused.

Because the nurse's goal is to empower the woman, it is vital for the nurse to communicate two messages: (1) the nurse is deeply concerned for her welfare, and (2) the woman does not deserve to be abused (U.S. Department of Health and Human Services, 1997). Each nurse can plan care that points out the woman's strengths and raises her self-esteem.

Adolescents (Ages 13 to 19 Years). A maturing young woman should be asked the same questions included in any history. Particular attention should be paid to hints about risky behaviors, eating disorders, and depression. Sexual activity is addressed after rapport has been established; it is best to talk to a teen with the parent (or partner or friend) out of the room. Questions should be asked with sensitivity and in a gentle and nonjudgmental manner (Seidel et al, 1999).

Injury prevention should be a part of the counseling at routine health examinations, with special attention to seat belts, helmets, firearms, recreational hazards, and sports involvement. The use of drugs and alcohol and the nonuse of seat belts contribute to motor vehicle injuries, which account for the greatest proportion of accidental deaths in women (Fogel and Woods, 1995). Contraceptive options, including the use of condoms, should be addressed during visits. As she progresses rapidly through emotional and physical change, the teen is egocentric. Her feelings of invulnerability may lead to misconceptions such as the belief that unprotected sexual intercourse will not lead to pregnancy (Youngkin and Davis, 1994).

History

A medical history usually includes information elicited in the following areas:

1. Chief complaint(s): A verbatim response to the question "What problem or symptom brought you here today?" If a lengthy list is recited, it may be necessary to tell the woman that her two complaints with the highest priority will be addressed today. Then in order to give all of her problems the full attention they deserve, a follow-up appointment in 1 to 2 weeks will be scheduled.
2. History of present illness: A chronologic narrative that includes onset of the problem, the setting in which it developed, its manifestations, and any treatments received. The woman's state of health before the onset of the present problem is determined. If the problem is long standing, the reason for seeking attention at this time is elicited. The principal symptoms should be described as to location, quality, quantity or severity, timing (e.g., onset, duration, and frequency), setting, factors that aggravate or relieve, and associated manifestations.
3. Past medical history: Determine general state of health:
   - **Infectious diseases**—measles, mumps, rubella, whooping cough, chickenpox, rheumatic fever, scarlet fever, diphtheria, polio, tuberculosis (TB), hepatitis
   - **Chronic disease and system disorders**—arthritis, cancer, diabetes, heart, lung, kidney, seizures, thyroid, stroke, ulcers
   - **Injuries, accidents, illnesses, disabilities, hospitalizations, blood transfusions**—note if the injury occurred on the job (workers' compensation) or if potential litigation is being considered
4. Present health status: Includes current information on these topics:
   - **Allergies**—medications, previous transfusion reactions, and environmental allergies
   - **Immunizations**—diphtheria; pertussis; tetanus; polio; measles, mumps, rubella (MMR); hepatitis B; varicella; influenza; pneumococcal vaccine; last TB skin test
   - **Screening tests**—Papanicolaou smear, mammogram, stool for occult blood, sigmoidoscopy/colonoscopy, chest x-ray, hematocrit, hemoglobin, rubella titer, urinalysis, cholesterol test; blood type/Rh; last eye examination; last dental examination
   - **Environmental/chemical hazards**—exposure in home, school, work, and leisure setting; exposure to extreme heat/cold, noise; industrial toxins such as asbestos or lead; pesticides; diethylstilbestrol (DES); radiation; cat feces; and cigarette smoke
   - **Use of safety measures**—seat belts, bicycle helmets, athletic protective devices, and designated driver
   - **Exercise and leisure activities**
   - **Sleep patterns**—length and quality
   - **Sexuality**—sexually active? With men, women, or both? Are condoms used?
   - **Diet**—including beverages (24-hour dietary recall)
   - **Oral hygiene**—brush teeth three times daily; floss daily
   - **Medications**—name, dose, frequency, duration, reason for taking, and compliance with dosage instructions; home remedies, over-the-counter drugs, vitamin and mineral or herbal supplements used over a 24-hour period
   - **Nicotine, alcohol, or recreational drugs**—type, amount, frequency, duration, and reactions
   - **Caffeine**—coffee, tea, cola, or chocolate intake
5. Past surgical history: Type, date, reason, outcome, and any complications should be noted.
6. Family history: Information about age and health of family members (e.g., age, health/death of parents, siblings, spouse,

Community Focus

PREVALENCE OF MENTAL DISORDERS AMONG OBSTETRIC-GYNECOLOGIC PATIENTS

Limited assessment for mental disorders occurs among obstetric and gynecologic patients, who are usually viewed as younger, healthy women. Patients in seven obstetric-gynecologic outpatient clinics being cared for by 63 clinicians were assessed. Assessment parameters included psychosocial stressors, functional status measures, days on disability, use of health care, diagnoses by mental health professionals, PRIME-MD questionnaire diagnoses, and treatment or referral recommendations.

Mental disorders were present in 20% of these 3000 women, but diagnosis rarely led to therapeutic intervention. Since the prevalence of mental disorders is significant in the obstetric-gynecologic population, nurses working with these women must be alert for signs of mental disorders and perform appropriate screening and referral when necessary. Good listening skills, and support for women who are stressed are important.

Data from: Spitzer R et al: Validity and utility of the PRIME-MD Patient Health Questionnaire in assessment of 3000 obstetric-gynecologic patients: the PRIME-MD Patient Health Questionnaire Obstetrics-Gynecology Study, *Am J Obstet Gynecol* 183(3):759-769, 2000.

and children) may be presented in a narrative or as a genogram (see Fig. 2-5). Check for history of disorders such as diabetes; heart disease; hypertension; stroke; respiratory, renal, or thyroid problems; cancer; bleeding disorders; hepatitis; allergies; asthma; arthritis; TB; epilepsy; mental illness; and human immunodeficiency virus (HIV).

7. Social history: Note birthplace, education, employment, marital status, living accommodations, children, persons at home, and hobbies. Does she enjoy what she is doing?
   - **Screen for abuse**—Has she ever been hit, kicked, slapped, or forced to have sex against her wishes? Is she verbally or emotionally abused? Is there a history of childhood sexual abuse? If yes, has she received counseling or does she need referral (Seng and Petersen, 1995)?
8. Review of systems: It is probable that not all questions in each system will be included every time a history is taken. But some questions regarding each system should be included in every history. The essential areas to be explored are listed in the following head-to-toe sequence. If a woman gives a positive response to a question about an essential area, more detailed questions should be asked:
   - **General**—weight change, fatigue, weakness, fever, chills, night sweats
   - **Skin**—skin, hair and nail changes, itching, bruising, bleeding, rashes, sores, lumps, moles
   - **Lymph nodes**—enlargement, inflammation, pain, suppuration (pus), drainage
   - **Head, eyes, ears, nose, and throat**—
     - **Head**—trauma, vertigo (dizziness), convulsive disorder, syncope (fainting), headache location, frequency, pain type, nausea/vomiting, visual symptoms
     - **Eyes**—glasses, contact lenses, blurriness, tearing, itching, photophobia, diplopia, inflammation, trauma, cataracts, glaucoma, acute visual loss
     - **Ears**—hearing loss, tinnitus (ringing), vertigo, discharge, pain, fullness, recurrent infections, mastoiditis
     - **Nose/sinuses**—trauma, rhinitis, nasal discharge, epistaxis, obstruction, sneezing, itching, allergy, smelling impairment
     - **Mouth/throat/neck**—hoarseness, voice changes, soreness, ulcers, bleeding gums, goiter, swelling, enlarged nodes
   - **Breasts**—masses, pain, lumps, dimpling, nipple discharge, fibrocystic changes or implants, BSE
   - **Respiratory**—shortness of breath, wheezing, cough, sputum, hemoptysis, pneumonia, pleurisy, asthma, bronchitis, emphysema, TB, last chest x-ray
   - **Cardiac**—hypertension, rheumatic fever, murmurs, angina, palpitations, dyspnea, tachycardia, orthopnea, edema, chest pain, cough, cyanosis, cold extremities, ascites, intermittent claudication (leg pain), phlebitis, skin color changes
   - **Gastrointestinal**—appetite, nausea, vomiting, indigestion, dysphagia, abdominal pain, ulcers, hematochezia (bleeding with stools), melena (black, tarry stools), bowel habit changes, diarrhea, constipation, bowel movement frequency, food intolerance, hemorrhoids, jaundice or hepatitis, sigmoidoscopy, colonoscopy, barium enema, ultrasound
   - **Genitourinary**—frequency, hesitancy, urgency, polyuria, dysuria, hematuria, nocturia, incontinence, stones, infection, or urethral discharge; dysmenorrhea, intermenstrual bleeding, dyspareunia, discharge, sores, itching, sexually transmitted infections, gravidity, parity, problems in pregnancy, contraception, menopause, hot flashes or sweats (may be included here or as part of endocrine)
   - **Vascular**—leg edema, claudication, varicose veins, thromboses, emboli
   - **Endocrine**—heat/cold intolerance, dry skin, excessive sweating, polyuria, polydipsia, polyphagia, thyroid problems, diabetes, secondary sex characteristic changes, age at menarche, length/flow of menses, last menstrual period (LMP), age at menopause, libido, sexual concerns
   - **Hematologic**—anemia, easy bruising, bleeding, petechiae, purpura, transfusions
   - **Musculoskeletal**—muscle weakness, pain, joint stiffness, scoliosis, lordosis, kyphosis, range-of-motion instability, redness, swelling, arthritis, gout
   - **Neurologic**—loss of sensation, numbness, tingling, tremors, weakness, vertigo, paralysis, fainting, twitching, blackouts, seizures, convulsions, loss of consciousness or memory
   - **Psychiatric**—moodiness, depression, anxiety, obsessions, delusions, illusions or hallucinations
   - **Functional assessment**—should be done on women with disabilities and women age 70 years and over

Physical Examination

In preparation for the physical examination, the woman is instructed to undress and given a gown to wear during the examination. She is usually given the opportunity to undress privately.

Objective data are recorded by system or location. A general statement of overall health status is a good way to start. Findings are described in detail.

- **General appearance**—age, race, sex, state of health, posture, height, weight, development, dress, hygiene, affect, alertness, orientation, cooperativeness, communication skills
- **Vital signs**—temperature, pulse, respiration, blood pressure
- **Skin**—color; integrity; texture; hydration; temperature; edema; excessive perspiration; unusual odor; presence and description of lesions; hair texture and distribution; nail configuration; color, texture, condition, presence of nail clubbing
- **Head**—size, shape, trauma, masses, scars, rashes or scaling; facial symmetry; presence of edema or puffiness
- **Eyes**—pupil size, shape, reactivity, conjunctival injection, scleral icterus, fundal papilledema, hemorrhage, lids, extraocular movements, visual fields and acuity
- **Ears**—shape and symmetry, tenderness, discharge, external canal, and tympanic membranes; hearing—Weber should be midline (loudness of sound equal in both ears) and Rinne negative (no conductive or sensorineural hearing loss); should be able to hear whisper at 3 feet
- **Nose**—symmetry, tenderness, discharge, mucosa, turbinate inflammation, frontal or maxillary sinus tenderness; discrimination of odors
- **Mouth and throat**—hygiene, condition of teeth, dentures, appearance of lips, tongue, buccal and oral mucosa, erythema, edema, exudate, tonsillar enlargement, palate, uvula, gag reflex, ulcers
- **Neck**—mobility, masses, range of motion, trachea deviation, thyroid size, carotid bruits
- **Lymphatic**—cervical, intraclavicular, axillary, trochlear, or inguinal adenopathy; size, shape, tenderness, consistency

- **Breasts**—skin changes, dimpling, symmetry, scars, tenderness, discharge or masses; characteristics of nipples and areolae
- **Heart**—rate, rhythm, murmurs, rubs, gallops, clicks, heaves, or precordial movements
- **Peripheral vascular**—jugular vein distention, bruits, edema, swelling, vein distention, Homans sign, or tenderness of extremities
- **Lungs**—chest symmetry with respirations, wheezes, crackles, rhonchi, vocal fremitus, whispered pectoriloquy, percussion, and diaphragmatic excursion; breath sounds equal and clear bilaterally
- **Abdomen**—shape, scars, bowel sounds, consistency, tenderness, rebound, masses, guarding, organomegaly, liver span, percussion (tympany, shifting, dullness), costovertebral angle tenderness
- **Extremities**—edema, ulceration, tenderness, varicosities, erythema, tremor, or deformity
- **Genitourinary**—external genitalia, perineum, vaginal mucosa, cervix, inflammation, tenderness, discharge, bleeding, ulcers, nodules, masses, internal vaginal support, bimanual, and rectovaginal; palpation of cervix, uterus, adnexa
- **Rectal**—sphincter tone, masses, hemorrhoids, rectal wall contour, tenderness; stool for occult blood
- **Musculoskeletal**—posture, symmetry of muscle mass, muscle atrophy, weakness, appearance of joints, tenderness or crepitus, joint range of motion, instability, redness, swelling, spine deviation
- **Neurologic**—mental status, orientation, memory, mood, speech clarity and comprehension, cranial nerves II to XII, sensation, strength, deep tendon and superficial reflexes, gait, balance, and coordination with rapid alternating motions

Pelvic Examination. Many women fear the gynecologic portion of the physical examination. The nurse can be instrumental in allaying these fears by providing information and assisting the woman to express her feelings to the examiner.

The woman is assisted into the lithotomy position (see Fig. 5-10, *A*) for the pelvic examination. When in the lithotomy position, the woman's hips and knees are flexed with buttocks at the edge of the table and feet are supported by heel or knee stirrups.

Some women prefer to keep their shoes or socks on, especially if the stirrups are not padded. Many women express feelings of vulnerability and strangeness when in the lithotomy position. During the procedure the nurse assists the woman with relaxation techniques. One method of helping the woman relax is to have her place her hands on her chest at about the level of the diaphragm, breathe deeply and slowly (in through her nose and out through her O-shaped mouth), concentrate on the rhythm of breathing, and relax all body muscles with each exhalation (Barkauskas et al, 1998). This breathing technique is particularly helpful for the adolescent and for the woman whose introitus may be especially tight or for whom the experience is new or may provoke tension. Some women relax when they are encouraged to become involved with the examination (e.g., with a mirror placed so that they can view the area being examined). This type of participation helps with health teaching as well. Distraction (e.g., placement of interesting pictures on the ceiling over the head of the table) is another technique that can be used effectively.

Many women find it distressing to attempt to converse in the lithotomy position. Most women appreciate an explanation of the procedure as it unfolds, as well as coaching for the type of sensations they may expect. Generally, however, women prefer not to have to respond to questions until they are again upright and at eye level with the examiner. Questioning during the procedure, especially if they cannot see their questioner's eyes, may make women tense.

A teen's first speculum examination is the most important. This is because she will develop perceptions that will remain with her for future examinations. What the examination entails should be discussed with the teen while she is dressed. Models or illustrations can be used to show exactly what will happen. All of the necessary equipment should be assembled so that there are no interruptions. Pediatric specula that are 1 to 1.5 cm wide can be inserted with minimal discomfort. If the teen is sexually active, a small adult speculum may be used.

External Inspection. The examiner sits at the foot of the table for the inspection of the external genitalia and for the speculum examination. To facilitate open communication, and to help the woman relax, the woman's head is raised on a pillow and the drape is arranged so that eye-to-eye contact can be maintained. In good lighting, external genitalia are inspected for sexual maturity, clitoris, labia, and perineum. After childbirth or other trauma there may be healed scars.

External Palpation. The examiner proceeds with the examination using palpation and inspection. The examiner wears gloves for this portion of the assessment. Before touching the woman, the examiner explains what is going to be done and what the woman should expect to feel (e.g., pressure). The examiner may touch the woman in a less sensitive area such as the inner thigh to alert her that the genital examination is beginning. This gesture may put the woman more at ease. The labia are spread apart to expose the structures in the vestibule: urinary meatus, Skene's glands, vaginal orifice, and Bartholin's glands (Fig. 5-12). To assess the Skene's glands, the examiner inserts one finger into the vagina and "milks" the area of the urethra. Any exudate from the urethra or the Skene's glands is cultured. Masses and erythema of either structure are assessed further. Ordinarily the openings to the Skene's glands are not visible; prominent openings may be seen if the glands are in-

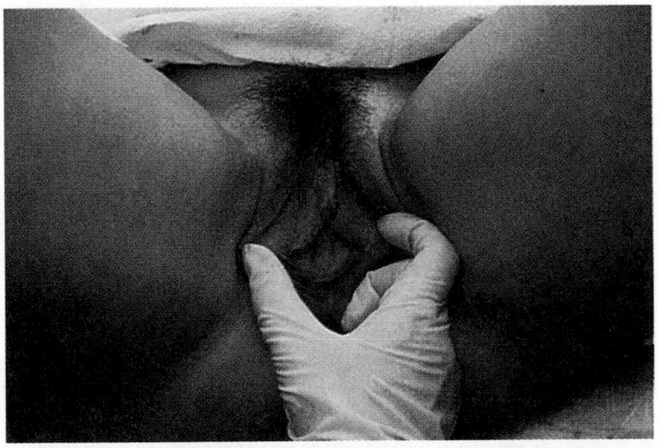

FIG. 5-12 • External examination. Separation of the labia. (From Edge V, Miller M: *Women's health care,* St Louis, 1994, Mosby.)

fected (e.g., with gonorrhea). During the examination, the examiner keeps in mind the data from the review of systems, such as history of burning on urination.

The vaginal orifice is examined. Hymenal tags are normal findings. With one finger still in the vagina, the examiner repositions the index finger near the posterior part of the orifice. With the thumb outside the posterior part of the labia majora, the examiner compresses the area of Bartholin's glands located at the 8 o'clock and 4 o'clock positions and looks for swelling, discharge, and pain.

The support of the anterior and posterior vaginal wall is assessed. The examiner spreads the labia with the index and middle finger and asks the woman to strain down. Any bulge from the anterior wall (i.e., urethrocele or cystocele) or posterior wall (i.e., rectocele) is noted and compared with the history, such as constipation or difficulty starting the stream of urine.

The perineum (i.e., the area between the vagina and anus) is assessed for scars from old lacerations or episiotomies, thinning, fistulas, masses, lesions, and inflammation. The anus is assessed for hemorrhoids, hemorrhoidal tags, and integrity of the anal sphincter. The anal area is also assessed for lesions, masses, abscesses, and tumors. If there is a history of sexually transmitted disease, the examiner may want to obtain a culture specimen from the anal canal at this time. Throughout the genital

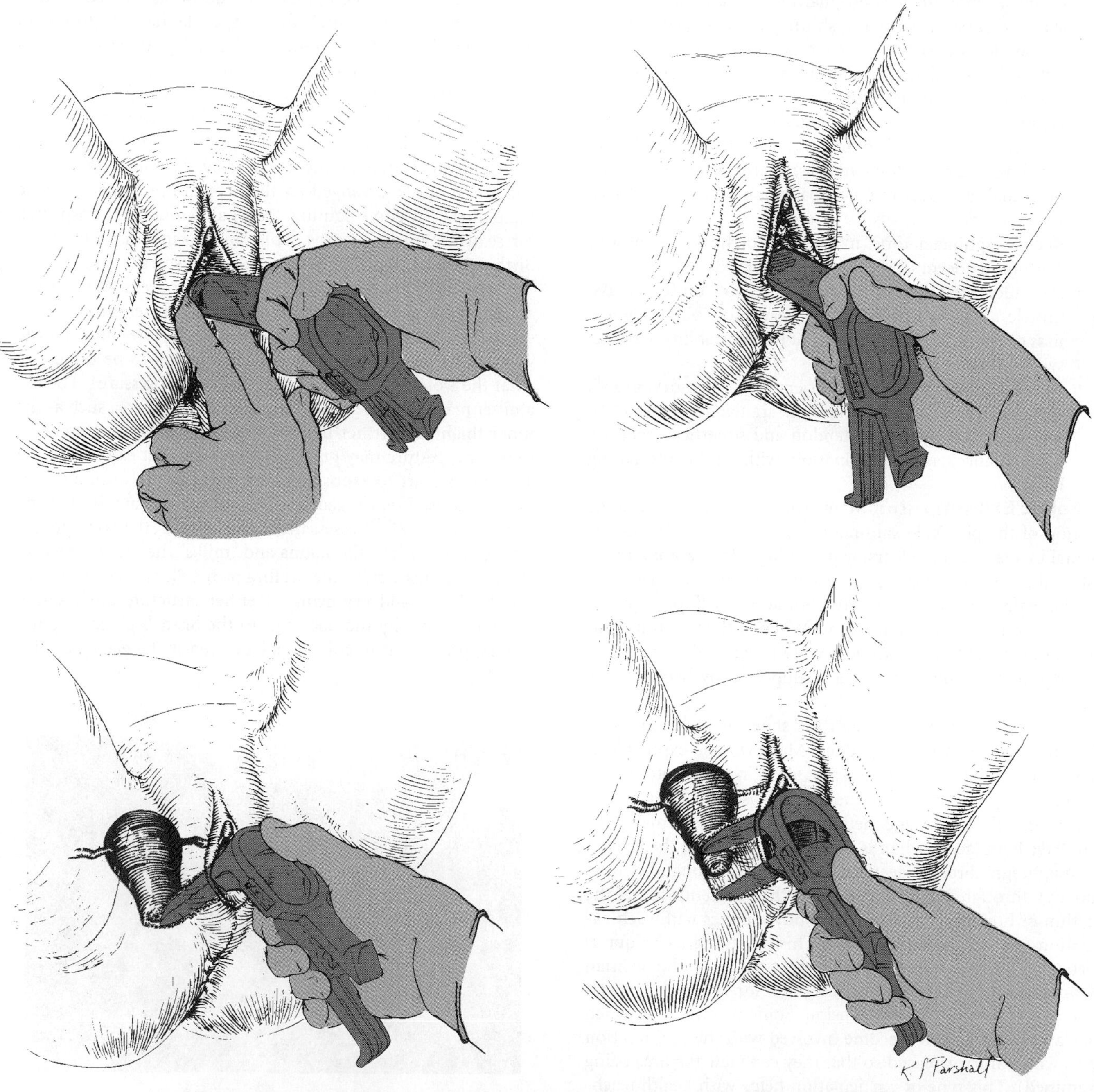

FIG. 5-13 • Insertion of speculum for vaginal examination. **A,** Opening of the introitus. **B,** Oblique insertion of the speculum. **C,** Final insertion of the speculum. **D,** Opening of the speculum blades. (From Barkauskas V et al: *Health and physical assessment,* ed 2, St Louis, 1998, Mosby.)

examination, the examiner notes any odor, which may indicate infection or poor hygiene.

Vulvar Self-Examination. The pelvic examination provides a good opportunity for the practitioner to emphasize the need for regular vulvar self-examination (VSE) and to teach this procedure. Because there has been a dramatic increase in cancerous and precancerous conditions of the vulva in recent years, a VSE should be an integral part of preventive health care for all women who are sexually active or 18 years of age or older. VSE should be performed monthly between menses or more often if there are symptoms or a history of serious vulvar disease. Most lesions, including malignancy, condyloma acuminatum (wartlike growth), and Bartholin cysts, can be seen or palpated and are easily treated if diagnosed early.

The examination can be performed by the practitioner and woman together using a mirror. A simple diagram of the anatomy of the vulva can be given to the woman, with instructions to perform the examination herself that evening to reinforce what she has learned. She does the examination in a sitting position with adequate lighting, holding a mirror in one hand and using the other hand to expose the tissues surrounding the vaginal introitus. She then systematically examines the mons pubis, clitoris, urethra, labia majora, perineum, and perianal area and palpates the vulva, noting any changes in appearance or abnormalities (e.g., ulcers, lumps, warts, and changes in pigmentation).

Internal Examination. A vaginal speculum consists of two blades and a handle. Speculums come in a variety of types and styles. A vaginal speculum is used to view the vaginal vault and cervix (Box 5-2). The speculum is gently placed into the vagina and inserted to the back of the vaginal vault. The blades are opened to reveal the cervix and are locked into the open position. The cervix is inspected for position and appearance of the os (e.g., color, lesions, bleeding, and discharge) (Fig. 5-13). Cervical findings not within normal limits include ulcerations, masses, inflammation, and excessive protrusion into the vaginal vault. Anomalies, such as a cockscomb (a protrusion over the cervix that looks like a rooster's comb), a hooded or collared cervix (seen in DES daughters), or polyps, are noted.

Collection of specimens. The collection of specimens for cytologic examination is an important part of the gynecologic examination. Examination of specimens collected during the pelvic examination can diagnose infections such as *Candida albicans, Trichomonas vaginalis,* bacterial vaginosis, b-hemolytic streptococci, *Neisseria gonorrhoeae, Chlamydia trachomatis,* and herpes simplex virus. Once the diagnoses have been made, treatment can be instituted.

Papanicolaou Smear. Carcinogenic conditions, whether potential or actual, can be determined by a Papanicolaou (Pap) smear, an examination of cells from the cervix collected during the pelvic examination (Box 5-3, Fig. 5-14).

Box 5-2

Procedure: Assisting with Pelvic Examination (Fig. 5-13)

Wash hands. Assemble equipment.

Ask woman to empty her bladder before the examination (obtain clean-catch urine specimen as needed).

Assist with relaxation techniques. Have the woman place her hands on her chest at about the level of the diaphragm, breathe deeply and slowly (in through her nose and out through her O-shaped mouth), concentrate on the rhythm of breathing, and relax all body muscles with each exhalation (Barkauskas et al., 1998).

Encourage the woman to become involved with the examination if she shows interest. For example, a mirror can be placed so that she can see the area being examined.

Assess for and treat signs of problems such as supine hypotension.

Warm the speculum in warm water if a prewarmed one is not available.

Instruct the woman to bear down when the speculum is being inserted.

Apply gloves and assist the examiner with collection of specimens for cytologic examination, such as a Pap test. After handling specimens, remove gloves and wash hands.

Lubricate the examiner's fingers with water or water-soluble lubricant before bimanual examination.

Assist the woman at completion of the examination to a sitting position.

Provide tissues to wipe lubricant from perineum.

Provide privacy for the woman while she is dressing.

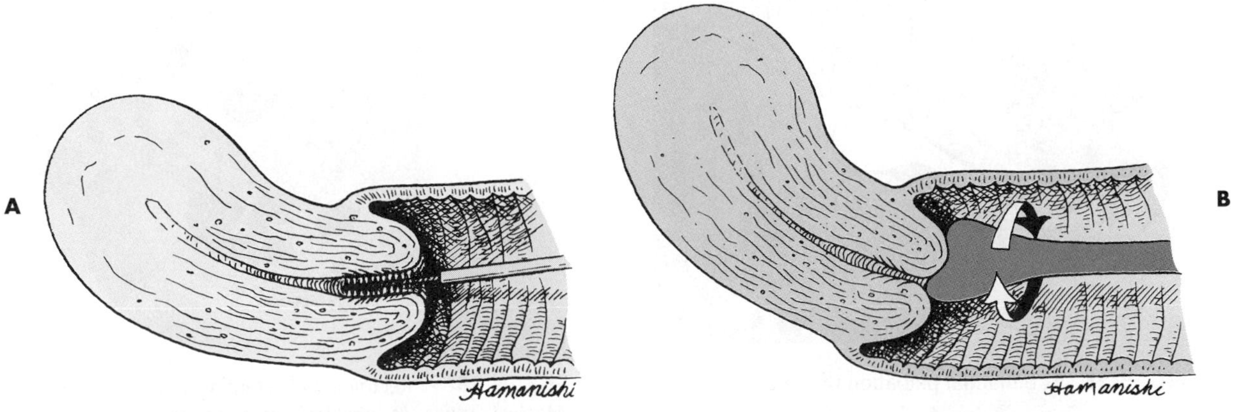

FIG. 5-14 • Pap smear. **A,** Collecting cells from the endocervix using a cytobrush. **B,** Obtaining cells from the transformation zone using a wooden spatula. (From Mishell D et al: *Comprehensive gynecology,* ed 3, St Louis, 1997, Mosby.)

Box 5-3
Procedure: Papanicolaou Smear

In preparation, make sure the woman has not douched, used vaginal medications, or had sexual intercourse for at least 24 hours before the procedure. Reschedule the test if the woman is menstruating.

The woman is assisted into a lithotomy position. A speculum is inserted into the vagina.

Explain to the woman the purpose of the test and what sensations she will feel as the specimen is obtained (e.g., pressure but not pain).

The cytologic specimen is obtained before any digital examination of the vagina is made or endocervical bacteriologic specimens are taken with cotton swabbing of the cervix.

The Pap smear is obtained by using an endocervical sampling device (Cytobrush, Cervex-Brush, papette, or broom) (see Fig. 5-14). If the two-sample method of obtaining cells is used, the cytobrush is inserted into the canal and rotated 90 to 180 degrees, followed by a gentle smear of the entire transformation zone using a spatula. Broom devices are inserted and rotated 360 degrees five times. They obtain endocervical and ectocervical samples at the same time. If the patient has had a hysterectomy, the vaginal cuff is sampled. Areas that appear abnormal on visualization will require colposcopy and biopsy. If using a one-slide technique, the spatula sample is smeared first. This is followed by applying the cytobrush sample (rolling the brush in the opposite direction from which it was obtained), which is less subject to drying artifact, and then the slide is sprayed with preservative within 5 seconds.

The ThinPrep Pap Test is an improved method of preserving cells that reduces blood, mucus, and inflammation. The Pap specimen is obtained in the manner described above, and the collection device (brush, spatula, or broom) is simply rinsed in a vial of preserving solution that is provided by the lab. The sealed vial with solution is sent off to the appropriate lab. A special processing device filters the contents, and a thin layer of cervical cells is deposited on a slide, which is then examined microscopically. Initial reports state that specimen adequacy is improved by 50% and detection of low-grade and more severe lesions is improved by 65%.

Label the slides with the woman's name and site. Include on the form to accompany the slides the woman's name, age, LMP, parity, and chief complaint or reason for taking the cytologic specimens.

Send specimens to the pathology laboratory promptly for staining, evaluation, and a written report, with special reference to abnormal elements, including cancer cells.

Advise the woman that repeat smears may be necessary if the specimen is not adequate.

Instruct the woman concerning routine checkups for cervical and vaginal cancer. The American Cancer Society advises that women over 18 years of age and those under 18 who are sexually active have the test yearly. After three or more consecutive normal menses, less frequent screening may be performed based on risk.

Record the examination date on the woman's record.

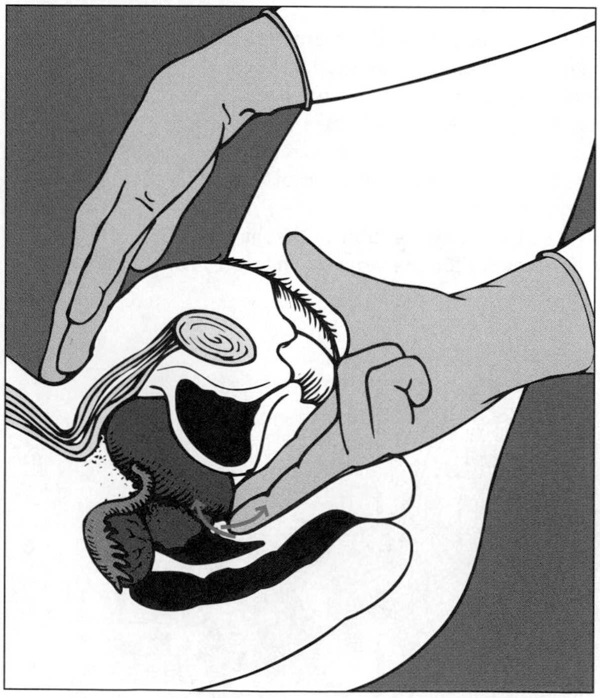

FIG. 5-15 • Bimanual palpation of the uterus.

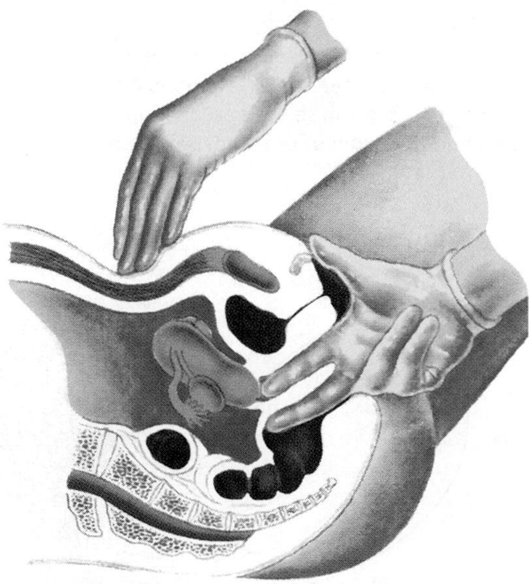

FIG. 5-16 • Rectovaginal examination. (From Seidel H et al: *Mosby's guide to physical examination,* ed 4, St Louis, 1999, Mosby.)

Vaginal Examination. After the specimens are obtained, the vagina is viewed when the speculum is rotated. The speculum blades are unlocked and partially closed. As the speculum is withdrawn, it is rotated and the vaginal walls are inspected for color, lesions, rugae, fistulas, and bulging.

Bimanual Palpation. The examiner stands for this part of the examination. A small amount of lubricant is placed on the first and second fingers of the gloved hand for the internal examination. To avoid tissue trauma and contamination, the thumb is abducted and the ring and little fingers are flexed into the palm (Fig. 5-15).

The vagina is palpated for distensibility, lesions, and tenderness. The cervix is examined for position, shape, consistency, motility, and lesions. The fornix around the cervix is palpated.

The other hand is placed on the abdomen halfway between the umbilicus and symphysis pubis and exerts pressure downward toward the pelvic hand. Upward pressure from the pelvic hand traps reproductive structures for assessment by palpation. The uterus is assessed for position, size, shape, consistency, regularity, motility, masses, and tenderness.

With the abdominal hand moving to the right lower quadrant and the fingers of the pelvic hand in the right lateral fornix, the adnexa is assessed for position, size, tenderness, and masses. The examination is repeated on the woman's left side.

Just before the intravaginal fingers are withdrawn, the woman is asked to tighten her vagina around the fingers as much as she can. If the muscle response is weak, the woman is assessed for her knowledge about Kegel exercises.

Rectovaginal Palpation. To prevent contamination of the rectum from organisms in the vagina (such as *Neisseria gonorrhoeae*), it is necessary to change gloves, add fresh lubricant, and then reinsert the index finger into the vagina and the middle finger into the rectum (Fig. 5-16). Insertion is facilitated if the woman strains down. The maneuvers of the abdominovaginal examination are repeated. The rectovaginal examination permits assessment of the rectovaginal septum, the posterior surface of the uterus, and the region behind the cervix and the adnexa. The vaginal finger is removed and folded into the palm, leaving the middle finger free to rotate 360 degrees. The rectum is palpated for rectal tenderness and masses.

After the rectal examination, the woman is assisted into a sitting position, given tissues or wipes to cleanse herself, and privacy to dress. The examiner returns after the woman is dressed to discuss findings and the plan of care.

Laboratory and Diagnostic Procedures

The following laboratory and diagnostic procedures are ordered at the discretion of the clinician, considering the patient and family history: hemoglobin, fasting glucose, total cholesterol, lipid profile, urinalysis, syphilis serology (VDRL or RPR), screening tests for sexually transmitted infections, Pap smear, mammogram, tuberculosis screening, hearing, visual acuity, electrocardiogram, chest x-ray, pulmonary function, fecal occult blood, flexible sigmoidoscopy, and bone mineral density (DEXA scan). Tests for HIV, hepatitis B, and drug screening may be offered with informed consent in high risk populations (see Table 4-1).

Key Points

- Normal feedback regulation of the menstrual cycle depends on an intact hypothalamic-pituitary-gonadal mechanism.
- The female's reproductive tract structures and breasts respond predictably to changing levels of sex steroids across her life span.
- The myometrium of the uterus is uniquely designed to expel the fetus and promote hemostasis after birth.
- Health promotion and prevention assist women to actualize health potential by increasing motivation, providing information, and suggesting how to access specific resources.
- Periodic health screening, including history, physical examination, and diagnostic and laboratory tests, provides the basis for overall health promotion, prevention of illness, early diagnosis of problems, and referral for management.
- Monthly breast self-examination, routine screening mammography, and yearly breast examinations by practitioners are recommended for early detection of breast cancer.

References

Barkauskas V et al: *Health and physical assessment,* ed 2, St Louis, 1998, Mosby.

Fogel C, Woods N: *Women's health care. A comprehensive handbook,* Thousand Oaks, CA, 1995, Sage.

Lipson J, Dibble S, Minarik P: *Culture and nursing care: a pocket guide.* San Francisco, 1996, UCSF Nursing Press.

Masters W: *Human sexuality,* ed 4, New York, 1992, HarperCollins.

Poirier L: The importance of screening for domestic violence in all women, *Nurse Pract* 22(5):105-122, 1997.

Seidel H et al: *Mosby's guide to physical examination,* ed 4, St Louis, 1999, Mosby.

Seng J, Petersen B: Incorporating routine screening for history of childhood sexual abuse in well-women and maternity care, *J Nurse Midwifery* 40(1):26-30, 1995.

U.S. Department of Health and Human Services, Public Health Service: *Clinician's handbook of preventive services,* Washington, DC, 1997, U.S. Government Printing Office.

Youngkin E, Davis M: *Women's health. A primary care clinical guide,* Norwalk, CT, 1994, Appleton & Lange.

CHAPTER

6

Common Health Problems

http://www.harcourthealth.com/MERLIN/Wong/maternal/

Learning Objectives

On completion of this chapter the reader will be able to:

- Develop a nursing care plan for the woman with primary dysmenorrhea.
- Outline patient teaching about premenstrual syndrome.
- Relate the pathophysiology of endometriosis to associated symptoms.
- Evaluate the use of alternative therapies for menstrual disorders.
- Describe prevention and treatment of sexually transmitted infections in women.
- Summarize the care of women with selected viral infections (i.e., HIV and hepatitis B).
- Differentiate signs, symptoms, and management of selected vaginal infections.
- Discuss the pathophysiology and emotional effects of selected benign breast conditions and malignant neoplasms of the breasts found in women.

At some point in her lifetime the average woman is likely to have some concerns related to her menstrual and gynecologic health and will experience bleeding, pain, or discharge or infections associated with her reproductive organs or functions. This chapter provides information on common menstrual problems, sexually transmitted infections, and selected other infections that can affect reproductive functions; and benign breast conditions. Breast cancer is also included as the most common reproductive cancer occurring in women.

MENSTRUAL PROBLEMS

Normal menstrual patterns are averages based on observations and reports from large groups of healthy women. Although no woman's cycle is exactly the same length every month, the typical month-to-month variation in an individual's cycle is usually plus or minus 2 days; greater but still normal variations are commonly noted.

Women typically have menstrual cycles for about 40 years. Once a cyclic, predictable pattern of monthly bleeding is established, women may worry about any deviation from that pattern or from what they have been told is normal for all menstruating women. A sign such as amenorrhea or excess menstrual bleeding can be a source of severe distress and concern for a woman.

Amenorrhea

Amenorrhea, or the absence or cessation of menstrual flow, is a clinical symptom of a variety of disorders. Generally, the following circumstances should be evaluated: (1) the absence of both menarche and secondary sexual characteristics by age 14 years; (2) the absence of menses by age 16, regardless of normal growth and development (primary amenorrhea); or (3) a 6-month cessation of menses after a period of menstruation (secondary amenorrhea) (Fogel, 1997).

Amenorrhea is most commonly the result of pregnancy. Although amenorrhea is not a disease, it is often a sign of disease. It may occur from any defect or interruption in the hypothalamic-pituitary-ovarian-uterine axis. It may also result from anatomic abnormalities; other endocrine disorders, such as hypothyroidism or hyperthyroidism; chronic diseases such as type 1 diabetes; medications, such as phenytoin (Dilantin); eating disorders; strenuous exercise; emotional stress; and oral contraceptive use.

Assessment of amenorrhea begins with a thorough history and physical examination. An important initial step is to be sure that the woman is not pregnant. Specific components of the assessment process depend on a patient's age (e.g., adolescent, young adult, or perimenopausal) and whether she has previously menstruated.

Hypogonadotropic Amenorrhea. Hypogonadotropic amenorrhea reflects a problem in the central hypothalamic-pituitary axis. In rare instances, a pituitary lesion or the genetic inability to produce follicle-stimulating hormone (FSH) and luteinizing hormone (LH) is at fault. Hypogonadotropic amenorrhea often results from hypothalamic suppression as a result of two principal influences: stress (e.g., in the home, school, or workplace) or a body fat-to-lean ratio that is inappropriate for an individual woman, especially during a normal growth period. Research has demonstrated a biologic basis for the relation of stress to physiologic processes. Women who are more than

20% underweight for height, or who have experienced rapid weight loss, may report amenorrhea as may women with eating disorders such as anorexia nervosa or bulimia. Amenorrhea is one of the classic signs of anorexia nervosa, and the interrelation of disordered eating, amenorrhea, and premature osteoporosis has been described as the female athlete triad (Birch and George, 1999; West, 1998). A loss of calcium from the bone, comparable to that seen in postmenopausal women, may occur with this type of amenorrhea.

Exercise-associated amenorrhea can occur in women undergoing vigorous physical and athletic training (Birch and George, 1999; Castiglia, 1996) and is thought to be associated with many factors, including body composition (e.g., height, weight, and percentage of body fat); type, intensity, and frequency of exercise; nutritional status; and presence of emotional or physical stressors (McGee, 1997).

Management. When amenorrhea is due to hypothalamic disturbances, the nurse is the ideal health professional to assist women because many of the causes (e.g., stress and weight loss for nonorganic reasons) are potentially reversible. Counseling and education are primary nursing interventions and appropriate nursing roles. Together the nurse and woman plan ways to do the following: correct weight loss, decrease or discontinue medications known to affect menstruation, deal more effectively with psychologic stress, and eliminate substance abuse. Deep-breathing exercises and relaxation techniques are simple yet effective stress-reduction measures. Referral for biofeedback or massage therapy also may be useful. In some instances, referrals for psychotherapy may be indicated.

If a woman's exercise program is thought to contribute to her amenorrhea, she may be encouraged to decrease the intensity or duration of her training or to gain 2% to 3% in body weight. This may be difficult for the person committed to a strenuous exercise regimen. Many young female athletes may not understand that low bone density or osteoporosis is related to stress fractures. The nurse and woman should investigate other factors that may be contributing to the amenorrhea and develop plans for altering lifestyle and decreasing stress.

If amenorrhea continues after a woman has decreased her exercise level or gained weight and altered her lifestyle, hormonal therapy may be indicated to prevent additional problems. Estrogen therapy is used in exercise-associated amenorrhea (Castiglia, 1996). Oral contraceptive pills (OCPs) and calcium are commonly used to treat extremely low levels of estrogen and to prevent osteoporosis. A daily calcium intake of 1200 to 1500 mg, accomplished by drinking 3 glasses of skim milk or by taking a calcium supplement, is recommended for women experiencing amenorrhea associated with the female athlete triad (West, 1998). OCPs have the additional advantage of providing pregnancy protection in sexually active women.

Dysmenorrhea

Dysmenorrhea, or painful menstruation, is one of the most common gynecologic problems in women of all ages. Most adolescents experience dysmenorrhea in the first 3 years after menarche. Between 50% and 80% of women report some level of discomfort associated with menses, and 10% to 18% report severe dysmenorrhea (Fankenauser, 1996; Fogel, 1995b). The amount of disruption caused in women's lives, however, is difficult to determine. It has been estimated that up to 10% of women who experience dysmenorrhea have pain severe enough to interfere with their functioning for 1 to 3 days a month (Fankenauser, 1996). Menstrual problems, including dysmenorrhea, are more common in women who smoke (Parazzini et al, 1994). Dysmenorrhea improves in most women after a full-term pregnancy (Speroff, Glass and Kase, 1999). Symptoms usually begin with menstruation, although some women experience discomfort several hours before onset of flow, and symptoms may last several hours or several days. The range and severity of symptoms differ from woman to woman and from cycle to cycle in the same woman.

Primary Dysmenorrhea. Primary dysmenorrhea, a condition associated with ovulatory cycles, is due to myometrium contractions induced by prostaglandins in the second half of the menstrual cycle. During the luteal phase and subsequent menstrual flow, prostaglandin $F2_{\alpha}$ ($PGF2_{\alpha}$) is secreted. The uterine muscle of both normal and dysmenorrheic women is sensitive to prostaglandins; however, the amount of prostaglandin produced is the major differentiating factor (Speroff, Glass, and Kase, 1999). Excessive release of $PGF2_{\alpha}$ increases the amplitude and frequency of uterine contractions and causes vasospasm of the uterine arterioles, resulting in ischemia and cyclic lower abdominal cramps. Systemic responses to $PGF2_{\alpha}$ include backache, weakness, sweating, gastrointestinal symptoms (e.g., anorexia, nausea, vomiting, and diarrhea), and central nervous system symptoms (e.g., dizziness, syncope, headache, and poor concentration). Pain begins at the onset of menstrual flow and lasts from 8 to 48 hours.

Though not normal, primary dysmenorrhea is not a pathologic condition but a physiologic alteration in some women. Anovulatory bleeding, common in the first few months or years after menarche, is painless. Primary dysmenorrhea usually appears within 6 to 12 months after menarche when ovulation is established. Because both estrogen and progesterone are necessary for primary dysmenorrhea to occur, it is experienced only with ovulatory cycles. This problem is most commonly experienced by women in their late teens and early 20s; the incidence declines with age. Psychogenic factors may influence symptoms, but symptoms are definitely related to ovulation and do not occur when ovulation is suppressed.

Management. Management of primary dysmenorrhea depends on the severity of the problem and the individual woman's response to various treatments. Important components of nursing care are information and support of the woman's feelings of positive sexuality and self-worth. Nurses can correct myths and misinformation about menstruation and dysmenorrhea by providing facts about what is normal.

Often more than one alternative for alleviating menstrual discomfort and dysmenorrhea can be offered. Women can decide which options work best for them. Heat (e.g., a heating pad or hot bath) minimizes cramping by increasing vasodilation and muscle relaxation and by minimizing uterine ischemia. Massaging the lower back can reduce pain by relaxing paravertebral muscles and by increasing pelvic blood supply. Soft rhythmic rubbing of the abdomen (i.e., effleurage) may be useful because it provides distraction and an alternative focal point. Biofeedback, progressive relaxation, hatha yoga, and meditation also have been used successfully to decrease menstrual discomfort.

Exercise helps relieve menstrual discomfort through the following: increased vasodilation and subsequent decreased ischemia; release of endogenous opiates, specifically beta-endorphins; suppression of prostaglandins; and shunting of blood flow away from the viscera, resulting in less pelvic congestion. Specific exercises that nurses can suggest to their patients include pelvic rock and the heels-over-the-head yoga position.

In addition to maintaining good nutrition at all times, specific dietary changes may be helpful. Decreased salt and refined sugar intake in the 7 to 10 days before expected menses may reduce fluid retention. Natural diuretics such as asparagus, cranberry juice, peaches, parsley, and watermelon may help reduce edema and related discomforts. Decreasing red meat intake and switching to a low-fat diet may also help minimize dysmenorrheal symptoms.

Medications used to treat primary dysmenorrhea include prostaglandin synthesis inhibitors, primarily nonsteroidal anti-inflammatory drugs (NSAIDs) (Apgar, 1997) (Table 6-1). NSAIDs are effective if begun 2 to 3 days before menses or with the first sign of bleeding (Speroff, Glass, and Kase, 1999). All NSAIDs have potential gastrointestinal side effects (e.g., nausea, vomiting, and indigestion). All women taking NSAIDs should be warned to report dark-colored stools because this may be an indication of gastrointestinal bleeding. Women with a history of aspirin sensitivity or allergy should avoid all NSAIDs. Often if one NSAID is ineffective, a different one will be effective. Approximately 80% of dysmenorrheic women obtain relief with prostaglandin inhibitors. If the second drug is unsuccessful after a 6-month trial, OCPs may be used.

The benefits of OCP use are attributed to decreased prostaglandin synthesis associated with an atrophic decidualized endometrium (Speroff, Glass, and Kase, 1999). No single OCP has been shown to be superior to another for the relief of primary dysmenorrhea. Although generally prescribed on a 21-day cycle of hormones, followed by 7 hormone-free days, OCPs can be used continuously in an attempt to produce amenorrhea if women have severe dysmenorrhea during withdrawal bleeding (Lipscomb and Ling, 1997). OCPs combine contraception with a positive effect on dysmenorrhea, menstrual flow, and menstrual irregularities. Since OCPs have side effects, women may not wish to use them for dysmenorrhea. (See Chapter 7 for a complete discussion of oral contraceptives.)

Over-the-counter (OTC) preparations that are indicated for primary dysmenorrhea contain the same active ingredients (e.g., ibuprofen or naproxen sodium) as prescription preparations. However, the labeled recommended dose may be subtherapeutic. Preparations containing acetaminophen are even less effective because acetaminophen does not have the antiprostaglandin properties of NSAIDs.

Secondary Dysmenorrhea. Secondary dysmenorrhea is menstrual pain that develops later in life than primary dysmenorrhea, typically after age 25. It is associated with pelvic pathology such as adenomyosis, endometriosis, pelvic inflammatory disease, endometrial polyps, submucous or interstitial myomas (fibroids), or the use of an intrauterine device (IUD). Pain often begins a few days before menses, but it can be present at ovulation and continue through the first days of menses or start after menstrual flow has begun. In contrast to primary dysmenorrhea, the pain of secondary dysmenorrhea is often characterized by dull, lower abdominal aching that radiates to the back or thighs. Often women experience feelings of bloating or pelvic fullness. In addition to a physical examination with a careful pelvic examination, diagnosis may be assisted by ultrasound, dilation and curettage (D&C), endometrial biopsy, or la-

TABLE 6-1

Medications Used to Treat Dysmenorrhea: NSAIDs

Drug	Side Effects*	Comments	Contraindications
Aspirin†	Gastrointenstinal irritation; tinnitus with excess dose	Not as potent a prostaglandin synthesis inhibitor as NSAIDs Do not take with NSAIDs	Hemophilia, hemorrhagic states, bleeding ulcers
Fenoprofen (Nalfon)†	Diarrhea, abdominal distention, nausea and vomiting, dyspepsia, constipation	For mild-to-moderate pain Take with meals Avoid alcohol	See aspirin
Ibuprofen (Motrin, Advil, Nuprin)	Nausea, dyspepsia, rash, pruritus	Most commonly used Take with meals Do not take with aspirin Avoid alcohol Side effects more likely	See aspirin
Mefenamic acid (Ponstel)	Diarrhea, nausea, abdominal distention	Very potent and effective prostaglandin synthesis inhibitor Antagonizes already formed prostaglandins Increased incidence of adverse GI side effects	See aspirin
Naproxen sodium (Anaprox, Aleve)	Nausea, abdominal distress, dyspepsia, rash, pruritus	See ibuprofen	See aspirin

Adapted from Fogel C: Common symptoms. In Fogel C, Woods N, editors: *Women's health care,* Thousand Oaks, Calif, 1995, Sage; Facts and Comparisons: *Loose-leaf drug information service,* St Louis, 1995, Facts and Comparisons.

*Risk with all NSAIDs is gastrointestinal ulceration, possible bleeding, and prolonged bleeding time. Incidence of side effects is dose related. Reported incidence 3% to 9%.

†Unlabeled indications for use in treating dysmenorrhea.

paroscopy. Treatment is directed toward removal of the underlying pathology. Many of the measures described for pain relief of primary dysmenorrhea are also helpful for women with secondary dysmenorrhea.

Premenstrual Syndrome

PMS is the appearance of one or more of a large number (more than 100) of physical and psychologic symptoms, beginning in the luteal phase of the menstrual cycle, occurring to such a degree that lifestyle or work is affected, and followed by a symptom-free period. Approximately 40% of women report problems related to their menstrual cycle, and 2% to 10% report a degree of impact on work or lifestyle (Speroff, Glass, and Kase, 1999). All age groups are affected, with women in their 20s and 30s most often reporting symptoms. The existence, diagnosis, and etiology of PMS are hotly and widely debated. Readers are encouraged to explore current feminist, medical, and social science literature for more information about PMS.

Symptoms of PMS include fluid retention (e.g., abdominal bloating, pelvic fullness, edema of the lower extremities, breast tenderness, and weight gain); behavioral or emotional changes (e.g., depression, crying spells, irritability, panic attacks, and impaired ability to concentrate); premenstrual cravings (e.g., for sweets, salt, increased appetite, and food binges); and headache, fatigue, and backache. In contrast, some women experience a heightened sense of creativity and increased mental and physical energy. A diagnosis of PMS is made only if the following criteria are met:

- Symptoms occur in the luteal phase and resolve within a few days of onset of menses.
- A symptom-free period occurs in the follicular phase.
- Symptoms are recurrent.

The cause of PMS is unknown (Box 6-1). It has been theorized that PMS has a significant psychologic component or may be due to cultural beliefs that lead to the menstrual cycle being associated with a variety of negative reactions. Speroff, Glass, and Kase (1999) suggest that PMS has a basic psychophysiologic origin tied to the menstrual cycle, primarily biologic but with a psychologic overlay. Furthermore, it can be a learned response or a response triggered in vulnerable individuals by normal neuroendocrine and hormonal changes.

Box 6-1

Possible Causes of Premenstrual Syndrome

Low progesterone levels
High estrogen levels
Falling estrogen levels
Changes in estrogen-progesterone levels
Increased aldosterone activity
Increased renin-angiotensin activity
Increased adrenal activity
Endogenous endorphin withdrawal
Subclinical hypoglycemia
Central changes in catecholamines
Response to prostaglandins
Vitamin deficiencies (vitamin B_6)
Excess prolactin secretion

Management. There is little agreement on management. A careful, detailed history and daily log of symptoms and mood fluctuations spanning several cycles may give direction to a plan of management. Any changes that assist a woman with PMS to exert control over her life have a positive impact. For this reason, lifestyle changes are often effective in the treatment of PMS.

Diet and exercise changes are a useful way to begin and provide symptom relief for some women. Nurses can suggest that patients not smoke and limit their consumption of refined sugar (to less than 5 tbsp/day), salt (to less than 3 g/day), red meat (less than 3 oz/day), alcohol (less than 1 oz/day), and caffeinated beverages. Patients can be encouraged to include whole grains, legumes, seeds, nuts, vegetables, fruits, and vegetable oils in their diet. The use of natural diuretics (see the section on dysmenorrhea management earlier in this chapter) may help reduce fluid retention. Nutritional supplements may assist in symptom relief. Calcium (at least 1200 mg/day), magnesium, and vitamin E have been shown to be moderately effective in relieving symptoms, to have few side effects, and to be safe. Natural hormones may be effective (Borkin, 1999).

Daily supplements of evening primrose oil are thought to relieve breast symptoms with minimal side effects. Women who exercise regularly seem to have less premenstrual anxiety than nonathletic women. It is thought that aerobic exercise increases beta-endorphin levels to offset symptoms of depression and to elevate mood. Patients should exercise for at least 30 minutes four times per week. A monthly program that varies in intensity and type of exercise according to PMS symptoms is best.

Counseling, in the form of support groups or individual or couple counseling, may be helpful (Taylor, 1999). Stress-reduction techniques may also assist with symptom management (Baker, 1998).

If these strategies do not provide significant symptom relief in 1 to 2 months, medication often is begun. Medications often used in the treatment of PMS include diuretics, prostaglandin inhibitors (NSAIDs), progesterone, and OCPs. Selective serotonin reuptake inhibitors (SSRIs) (e.g., fluoxetine [Prozac] and clomipramine [Anafranil]) are often used for PMS with a resultant decrease in emotional symptoms, especially depression

Community Focus

PREMENSTRUAL SYNDROME EXPERIENCES

The experiences of women in the United States who have been diagnosed with premenstrual syndrome (PMS) are a cause for concern. Women may seek help for a number of years before diagnosis is given; they may seek help from several physicians before satisfactory help is received; physicians are not thought to be adequately prepared to treat women with PMS; a minority of physicians use a symptom chart for diagnosis (the only current way to diagnose PMS); only 26% of physicians surveyed offered a helpful treatment. Diagnosis occurred in most instances after a suggestion from the woman. Vitamins, diet modifications, and exercise were the most common treatments. Nurses working in settings where women are cared for are in prime positions to do case-finding, provide education and referrals, and raise awareness of other health care providers to PMS, its diagnosis and treatment.

Data from: Kraemer G, Kraemer R: Premenstrual syndrome: diagnosis and treatment experiences, *J Womens Health* 7(7):893-907, 1998.

Nursing Care Plan PREMENSTRUAL SYNDROME

NURSING DIAGNOSIS Pain related to cyclic breast changes as evidenced by patient report

EXPECTED OUTCOME Patient will report a decrease in the intensity of pain or discomfort following interventions.

Nursing Interventions/*Rationales*

Assess timing and intensity of pain or discomfort *to validate relationship to cyclic changes.*

Administer hormonal medications or diuretics if prescribed *to minimize breast tenderness.*

Suggest that patient wear a supportive bra *to minimize breast tenderness.*

NURSING DIAGNOSIS Situational low self-esteem related to cyclic hormonal changes as evidenced by patient verbal report

EXPECTED OUTCOME Patient will report increased number of feelings of self-worth.

Nursing Interventions/*Rationales*

Provide therapeutic communication *to validate patient feelings of depression and mood swings.*

Encourage patient to limit caffeine and eat small, frequent meals *to lessen irritability aggravated by caffeine and hypoglycemia.*

Refer patient to support groups *to encourage the sharing of experiences, feelings, and self-help tips.*

NURSING DIAGNOSIS Fluid volume excess related to cyclic hormonal influences as evidenced by weight gain before start of menstrual period

EXPECTED OUTCOME Patient will report no significant changes in body weight before start of menstrual period.

Nursing Interventions/*Rationales*

Encourage patient to limit intake of salt- and sodium-containing foods *to decrease fluid retention.*

Administer diuretics as prescribed *to facilitate fluid excretion.*

(Baker, 1998; Chandraiah, 1996). Melfenamic acid (e.g., 250 mg daily during the luteal phase of the menstrual cycle) may relieve or resolve many symptoms—specifically fatigue, headaches, general aches and pains, and mood swings (Chuong, Pearsall-Otey, and Rosenfeld, 1995). Bromocriptine (e.g., 5 mg daily at night on days 10 to 26 of the cycle) helps reduce breast tenderness and swelling (Nursing Care Plan).

Endometriosis

Endometriosis is characterized by the presence and growth of endometrial tissue outside of the uterus. The tissue may be implanted on the ovaries, cul-de-sac, uterine ligaments, rectovaginal septum, sigmoid colon, pelvic peritoneum, cervix, and inguinal area (Fig. 6-1). Endometrial lesions may be found in the vagina and surgical scars, as well as on the vulva, perineum, bladder, and sites far from the pelvic area such as the thoracic cavity, gallbladder, and heart. A chocolate cyst is a cystic area of endometriosis in the ovary. The dark coloring of the contents of the cyst is caused by old blood.

Endometrial tissue contains glands and stoma and responds to cyclic hormonal stimulation in the same way that the uterine endometrium does but often out of phase with it. The endometrial tissue grows during the proliferative and secretory phases of the cycle. During or immediately after menstruation, the tissue bleeds, resulting in an inflammatory response with subsequent fibrosis and adhesions to adjacent organs.

The overall incidence of endometriosis is about 10% in reproductive-age women, 25% to 35% in infertile women, and 28% in women with chronic pelvic pain (Corwin, 1997; Speroff, Glass, and Kase, 1999; Wellbery, 1999). Each year endometriosis affects between 1.7 million and 5.6 million American women and accounts for about 49,000 hysterectomies (Ryan and Taylor, 1997). Although the condition usually develops in the third or fourth decade of life, endometriosis has been found in adolescents with disabling pelvic pain or abnormal vaginal bleeding. Endometriosis may worsen with repeated cycles, or it may remain asymptomatic and undiagnosed, eventually disappearing after menopause. The condition appears equally in Caucasian and African-American women and slightly more in Asian women. It occurs across all socioeconomic levels (Sangi-Haghpeykar and Poindexter, 1995). There appears to be a familial tendency to develop endometriosis (Hadfield et al, 1997).

One of the most widely accepted, long-debated theories about the cause of endometriosis is transtubal migration, or retrograde menstruation. According to this theory, endometrial tissue is regurgitated or mechanically transported from the uterus during menstruation to the uterine (fallopian) tubes and into the peritoneal cavity, where it implants on the ovaries and other organs. Retrograde menstruation has been documented in a number of surgical studies and is estimated to occur in 96% of menstruating women (Corwin, 1997). For most women, endometrial tissue outside the uterus is destroyed before it can implant or seed in the peritoneal cavity or elsewhere. An explanation for why only 10% to 15% of women develop endometriosis may lie in differences in the functioning of an individual's immune system. It may also reflect differences in genetic makeup or environmental challenges (Speroff, Glass, and Kase, 1999).

Symptoms, from nonexistent to incapacitating, vary among women. Severity of symptoms can change over time and may not reflect the extent of the disease. The major symptoms of endometriosis are dysmenorrhea and deep pelvic dyspareunia

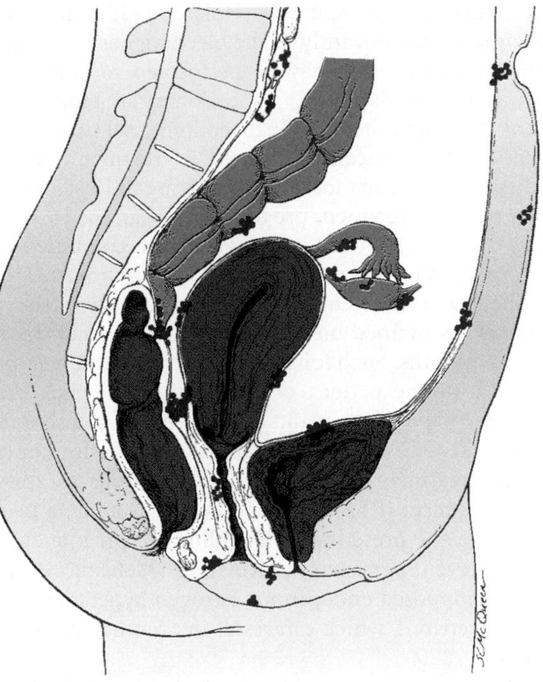

FIG. 6-1 • Common sites of endometriosis. (From Mishell D et al: *Comprehensive gynecology,* ed 3, St Louis, 1997, Mosby.)

(painful intercourse). Women also experience chronic noncyclic pelvic pain, pelvic heaviness, or pain radiating into the thighs. Many women report bowel symptoms such as diarrhea, pain with defecation, and constipation secondary to avoiding defecation because of the pain. Less common symptoms include abnormal bleeding (e.g., hypermenorrhea, menorrhagia, or premenstrual staining) and pain during exercise as a result of adhesions.

Management. Treatment is based on the severity of symptoms and the goals of the woman or couple. Women without pain who do not want to become pregnant need no treatment. In women with mild pain who may desire a future pregnancy, treatment may be limited to use of NSAIDs during menstruation (see earlier discussion of these medications).

Suppression of endogenous estrogen production and subsequent endometrial lesion growth is the cornerstone of management of the disease. Two main classes of medications are currently used to suppress endogenous estrogen levels: gonadotropin-releasing hormone (GnRH) agonists and androgen derivatives. GnRH agonist therapy (e.g., with leuprolide [Lupron] or nafarelin [Synarel]) acts by suppressing pituitary gonadotropin secretion. FSH and LH stimulation to the ovary declines markedly, and ovarian function decreases significantly. A medically induced menopause develops, resulting in anovulation and amenorrhea. Shrinkage of already established endometrial tissue, significant pain relief, and an interruption in further lesion development follow. The hypoestrogenism results in hot flashes in almost all women. Trabecular bone loss is common, although most loss is reversible within 12 to 18 months after the medication is stopped. Both leuprolide (e.g., 3.75 mg intramuscular injection given once a month) or nafarelin (e.g., 200 mg administered twice daily by nasal spray) are effective and well tolerated. Both medications reduce endometrial lesions and pelvic pain associated with endometriosis and have posttreatment pregnancy rates similar to that of danazol therapy (Speroff, Glass, and Kase, 1999). Common side effects of these drugs are those of natural menopause—hot flashes and vaginal dryness. Occasionally women report headaches and muscle aches. Treatment is usually limited to 6 months to minimize bone loss. Although unlikely, it is possible for a woman to become pregnant on a GnRH agonist. Because the potential teratogenicity of this drug is unclear, women should use a barrier contraceptive during treatment.

Critical Thinking

RESPONSES OF A WOMAN TO ENDOMETRIOSIS

Interview a woman with endometriosis to determine her responses to the condition.

- **What are her perceptions about how others view her condition?**
- **Examine how her response compare with theoretic responses, as well as your own perceptions.**
- **What therapies has she used to treat her condition? How effective were the therapies?**
- **Formulate realistic expected outcomes using the data from the interview.**

Danazol (Danocrine), a mildly androgenic synthetic steroid, suppresses FSH and LH secretion, thus producing anovulation and hypogonadotropism with resulting decreased secretion of estrogen and progesterone and regression of endometrial tissue. Danazol can produce side effects that can cause a woman to discontinue the drug. Side effects include masculinizing traits in the woman (e.g., weight gain, edema, decreased breast size, oily skin, hirsutism, and deepening of the voice), all of which often disappear when treatment is discontinued (Salek et al, 2000). Other side effects include amenorrhea, hot flashes, vaginal dryness, insomnia, and decreased libido. Migraine headaches, dizziness, fatigue, and depression are also reported. Danazol treatment has been reported to adversely affect lipids, with a decrease in high-density lipoprotein (HDL) levels and an increase in low-density lipoprotein (LDL) levels. Danazol should never be prescribed when pregnancy is suspected, and contraception should be used with it because ovulation may not be suppressed. Danazol can produce pseudohermaphroditism in female fetuses. The medication is contraindicated in women with liver disease and should be used with caution in women with cardiac and renal disease.

Women who have severe pain and who can postpone pregnancy may be treated with oral contraceptives that have a low estrogen-to-progestin ratio to shrink endometrial tissue. Often the daily dosage has to be increased to 2 or 3 pills to maintain amenorrhea. Side effects such as nausea, edema, and breakthrough bleeding often lead women to discontinue this therapy. When therapy is stopped, patients often experience high rates of recurrence of pain and other symptoms. Most recently, mifepristone (RU-486) has been used to treat endometriosis successfully (Kettel et al, 1998).

Surgical intervention is often needed for severe, acute, or incapacitating symptoms. Decisions regarding the extent and type of surgery are influenced by a woman's age, desire for children, and location of the disease. For women who do not want to preserve their ability to have children, the only definite cure is total abdominal hysterectomy with bilateral salpingo-oophorectomy (TAH with BSO). In women who are in their childbearing years and who want children, and in whom the disease does not prevent it, reproductive capacity should be retained through careful removal by surgery or laser therapy of all endometrial tissue possible with retention of ovarian function (Garner, 1995).

Regardless of the type of treatment (short of TAH with BSO), endometriosis recurs in approximately 40% of women. Thus for many women endometriosis is a chronic disease with conditions such as chronic pain and infertility. Counseling and education are critical components of nursing care for women with endometriosis. Women need an honest discussion of treatment options, with potential risks and benefits of each option reviewed. Because pelvic pain is a subjective, personal experience that can be frightening, support is important. Sexual dysfunction resulting from dyspareunia is common and may necessitate referral for counseling. Support groups for women with endometriosis may be found in some locations. Resolve, an organization for infertile couples, may also be helpful. The nursing care discussed in the section on dysmenorrhea is appropriate for managing chronic pelvic pain and dysmenorrhea experienced by the woman with endometriosis.

Dysfunctional Uterine Bleeding

Dysfunctional uterine bleeding (DUB) refers to a wide variety of menstrual irregularities, but most often it is associated with excessive bleeding of some type (e.g., flow that is too frequent, too heavy, too prolonged, or irregular). Box 6-2 lists possible causes of dysfunctional uterine bleeding. A diagnosis of DUB is made only after all other causes of abnormal menstrual bleeding have been ruled out (Rosenfeld, 1996).

When uterine bleeding is severe, and a woman's hemoglobin level is less than 8 g/100 ml (i.e., a hematocrit of 23% or 24%), the woman may be hospitalized and given conjugated estrogens (e.g., Premarin) intravenously (Hillard, 1999) until bleeding stops or slows significantly. If the bleeding has not stopped in 12 to 24 6ours, D&C may be performed to control severe bleeding and hemorrhage. An endometrial biopsy may be done at the same time to evaluate endometrial tissue or to rule out endometrial cancer. Following this treatment, oral conjugated estrogen is given for 21 days. During the last 7 to 10 days of this estrogen regimen, progesterone (e.g., medroxyprogesterone [Provera]) is added. Alternatively, a combined OCP is given for 21 days after intravenous therapy (Starr, Lommel, and Shanon, 1995). Once the acute phase has passed, the woman is maintained on cyclic, low-dose oral contraceptives for 3 to 6 months. Such long-term treatment will help prevent recurrence of the pattern of dysfunctional uterine bleeding and hemorrhage. If she wants contraception, she should continue to take OCPs. If the woman has no need for contraception, the treatment may be stopped in order to assess her bleeding pattern. If her menses does not resume, a progestin regimen may be prescribed after ruling out pregnancy. This is done to prevent persistent anovulation (Mehring, 1997) with chronic unopposed endogenous estrogen hyperstimulation of the endometrium, which can result in eventual atypical tissue changes.

If the recurrent, heavy bleeding is not controlled by hormonal therapy or D&C, ablation of the endometrium through laser treatment may be performed. Nursing roles include informing patients of their options, counseling and education as indicated, and referring to the appropriate specialists and health care services.

Care Management

➤ Assessment

In addition to taking a careful menstrual, obstetric, sexual, and contraceptive history, the nurse should explore the woman's perceptions of her condition, cultural or ethnic influences, ex-

Box 6-2

Possible Causes of Dysfunctional Uterine Bleeding

ANOVULATION
Hypothalamic dysfunction
Polycystic ovary syndrome

PREGNANCY-RELATED CONDITIONS
Threatened or spontaneous abortion
Retained products of conception after elective abortion
Ectopic pregnancy

LOWER REPRODUCTIVE TRACT INFECTIONS
Chlamydial cervicitis
Pelvic inflammatory disease

NEOPLASMS
Endometrial hyperplasia
Cancer of cervix and endometrium
Endometrial polyps
Hormonally active tumors (rare)
Leiomyomata
Vaginal tumors (rare)

TRAUMA
Genital injury (accidental, coital trauma, sexual abuse)
Foreign body
Primary coagulation disorders

SYSTEMIC DISEASES
Diabetes mellitus
Thyroid dysfunction (hypothyroidism, hyperthyroidism)
Severe organ disease (renal or liver failure)

IATROGENIC CAUSES
Exogenous hormone use (oral contraceptives, menopausal hormone therapy)
Medications with estrogenic activity
Herbal preparation (ginseng)

Sources: Hillard P: Diagnosing and controlling abnormal uterine bleeding, *Contemporary Adolescent Gynecology* 4(1):4-11, 1999; Speroff L, Glass R, Kase N: *Clinical gynecologic endocrinology and infertility,* ed 6, Baltimore, 1999, Lippincott/Williams & Wilkins.

periences with other caregivers, lifestyle, and patterns of coping. The amount of pain or bleeding experienced and its effect on daily activities should be evaluated. Home remedies and prescriptions to relieve discomfort are noted. A symptom diary, in which the woman records emotions, behaviors, physical symptoms, diet, and exercise and rest patterns, is a useful diagnostic tool.

➤ Nursing Diagnoses

Nursing diagnoses for women experiencing menstrual disorders may include the following:

- Risk for ineffective individual or family coping related to:
  - —Insufficient knowledge of the cause of the disorder
  - —Emotional and physiologic effects of the disorder
- Knowledge deficit related to:
  - —Self-care
  - —Available therapy for the disorder
- Risk for body image disturbance related to:
  - —Menstrual disorder
  - —Sexual dysfunction

➤ Expected Outcomes

The expected outcomes for the woman with a menstrual disorder are that she will do the following:

- Verbalize her understanding of reproductive anatomy, etiology of her disorder, medication regimen, and diary use.
- Develop personal goals that benefit her emotionally and physically.
- Choose appropriate therapeutic measures for her menstrual problems.
- Adapt successfully to the condition if cure is not possible.

➤ Plan of Care and Implementation

During the history and diagnostic workup, the clinician's concern for and acceptance of the woman's symptoms as valid is in itself therapeutic. Data from the daily diary about emotional status, subjective feelings, and physical state are correlated with physiologic changes. If the woman has a partner, both the woman and her partner should keep separate diaries that include how each perceives the other's responses day by day. Through the diaries, feelings are vented, problems are identified and clarified, insights occur, and possible solutions begin to develop. The clinician facilitates insights and suggests therapeutic options. The woman (or couple) then makes choices considered best for her (or them).

Nurses should discuss the options available to women with menstrual disorders. Women must understand basic information about anatomy and physiology, pathophysiology, psychologic impact, and treatment for the condition, including alternative therapies. Support groups are an important resource. Nurses can use a local women's center or clinic to bring together women who want to learn more about their condition and support each other.

➤ Evaluation

The nurse can be assured that care has been effective when the woman reports improvement in the quality of her life, skill in self-care, and a positive self-concept and body image.

> *Critical Thinking*
>
> **ALTERNATIVE THERAPIES FOR MENSTRUAL PROBLEMS**
>
> **Review the literature for studies determining effectiveness of alternative therapies for menstrual problems. In a clinical conference, discuss therapies that have been shown to be beneficial, are likely to be beneficial, have unknown effects, or have effects that are likely not to be beneficial or may be harmful. Discuss how nurses can use this information in their clinical practice.**

INFECTIONS

Infections of the reproductive tract can occur throughout a woman's life and are often the cause of significant morbidity and mortality. The direct economic costs of these infections can be substantial and the indirect cost equally overwhelming. Some consequences of maternal infection (e.g., infertility) last a lifetime. The emotional costs may include damaged relationships and lowered self-esteem.

Sexually Transmitted Infections (STIs)

Sexually transmitted infections (STIs), or sexually transmitted diseases (STDs), are infections or infectious disease syndromes primarily transmitted by close, intimate contact (Box 6-3). These terms, used interchangeably in this text, have replaced the older designation, venereal disease, which primarily described gonorrhea and syphilis. STIs include more than 25 infectious organisms that are transmitted through sexual activity and the dozens of clinical syndromes that they cause (Institute of Medicine, 1997). The U.S. Surgeon General has targeted STIs as a priority for prevention and control efforts. Still, STIs are among the most common health problems in the United States (Institute of Medicine, 1997). The Centers for Disease Control and

> Box 6-3
>
> **Sexually Transmitted Infections**
>
> **BACTERIA**
> Chlamydia
> Gonorrhea
> Syphilis
> Chancroid
> Lymphogranuloma venereum
> Genital mycoplasmas
> Group B streptococci
>
> **VIRUSES**
> Human immunodeficiency virus
> Herpes simplex virus, types 1 and 2
> Cytomegalovirus
> Viral hepatitis A and B
> Human papillomavirus
>
> **PROTOZOA**
> Trichomoniasis
>
> **PARASITES**
> Pediculosis (may or may not be sexually transmitted)
> Scabies (may or may not be sexually transmitted)

Prevention (CDC) estimates that more than 12 million Americans are infected with STIs every year (Centers for Disease Control and Prevention, Division of STD/HIV Prevention, 1995). The most common STIs in women are chlamydia, human papillomavirus, gonorrhea, herpes simplex virus type 2, syphilis, and human immunodeficiency virus (HIV) infection. These are discussed in this chapter. Neonatal effects of STIs are discussed in Chapter 28.

Prevention of STIs. Preventing infection (primary prevention) is the most effective way of reducing the adverse consequences of STIs for women and for society. With the advent of serious and potentially lethal STIs that are either not readily cured or incurable, primary prevention becomes critical. Prompt diagnosis and treatment of current infections (secondary prevention) can prevent personal complications and transmission to others.

Preventing the spread of STIs requires that women at risk for transmitting or acquiring infections avoid risky behaviors. A critical first step is for the nurse to include questions about a woman's sexual history, sexual risk behaviors, and drug-related risky behaviors as a part of her assessment (Box 6-4). When risk factors or risky behaviors are identified, the nurse has an opportunity to provide prevention counseling. Effective techniques in providing prevention counseling include using open-ended questions, using understandable language, and reassuring the woman that treatment will be provided regardless of consideration such as ability to pay, language spoken, or lifestyle (Centers for Disease Control and Prevention, 1998a). Prevention messages should include descriptions of specific actions to be taken to avoid acquiring or transmitting STIs (e.g., refrain from sexual activity if you have STI-related symptoms) and should be tailored to the individual woman with attention given to her specific risk factors (Guidelines box).

To be motivated to take preventive actions, a woman must believe that catching a disease will be serious for her and that she is at risk for infection. Most individuals tend to underestimate their personal risk of infection in a given situation. Thus many women may not perceive themselves as being at risk for contracting an STI, and telling them that they need to carry condoms may not be well received. Though levels of awareness of STIs are generally high, widespread misconceptions or specific gaps in knowledge also exist. Therefore nurses have a responsibility to ensure that their patients have accurate, complete knowledge about transmission and symptoms of STIs and the behaviors that place them at risk for contracting infections. Risk-free options include complete abstinence from sexual activities that transmit semen, blood, or other body fluids; or that allow for skin-to-skin contact (Hatcher et al, 1998). Involvement in a mutually monogamous relationship with an uninfected partner also eliminates risk of contracting STIs.

Safer Sex Practices. An essential component of primary prevention is counseling women regarding safer sex practices, including knowledge of her partner, reduction of number of partners, low risk sex, and avoiding the exchange of body fluids.

Box 6-4

Assessing STI/HIV Risk Behaviors

Answer these questions for all the times in your life from 1977* to now.

SEXUAL RISK

Are you sexually active now?
If no, have you had sex in the past?
Ever had an oral, vaginal, or anal sexual experience with another person?
With how many different people? 1? 2 or 3? 4 to 10? More than 10?
Have your partners been men, women, both?
Ever thought that a sex partner put you at risk for AIDS/STI (IV drug user, bisexual)?
Ever had an STI (herpes, gonorrhea, genital warts, chlamydia)?
Ever had sex against your will?
What do you do to protect yourself from AIDS/STIs?
Do you use male condoms? Female condoms? Other barriers?

DRUG USE-RELATED RISK

Ever injected drugs using shared equipment, including street drugs, steroids?
Ever had sex with a person who uses and shares?
Ever had sex while stoned, high, or drunk, so that you can't remember the details?
Ever exchanged sex for drugs, money, shelter?

BLOOD-RELATED RISKS

Ever had a blood transfusion?
Ever had sex with a person who had a blood transfusion?
Ever had sex with a person with hemophilia?
Ever received donor semen, egg, transplanted organ or tissue?
Ever shared equipment for tattoo, body piercing?

OTHER

Ever had a test for HIV?
Ever worried about AIDS and would like to talk with someone about it?

Adapted from Hatcher R et al: *Contraceptive technology* ed 17, New York, 1998, Ardent Media, Inc.
*Relates to risk of HIV–infection not known to exist in humans until this time.

Guidelines

PREVENTION OF GENITAL TRACT INFECTIONS IN WOMEN

- **Practice genital hygiene.**
- **Choose underwear or hosiery with a cotton crotch.**
- **Avoid tight-fitting clothing (especially tight jeans).**
- **Select cloth car seat covers instead of vinyl.**
- **Limit the time spent in damp exercise clothes (especially swimsuits, leotards, and tights).**
- **Limit exposure to bath salts or bubble bath.**
- **Avoid colored or scented toilet tissue.**
- **If sensitive, discontinue use of feminine hygiene deodorant sprays.**
- **Use condoms.**
- **Void before and after intercourse.**
- **Decrease dietary sugar.**
- **Drink yeast-active milk and eat yogurt (with lactobacilli).**
- **Do not douche.**

No aspect of prevention is more important than knowing one's partner. Reducing the number of partners and avoiding partners who have had many previous sexual partners decreases a woman's chances of contracting an STI. Women should be taught low risk sexual practices as well as which sexual practices to avoid. Sexual fantasizing is safe, as are caressing, hugging, body rubbing, and massage. Mutual masturbation is low risk as long as there is no contact with a partner's semen or vaginal secretions. All sexual activities are safe when both partners are monogamous, trustworthy, and known (by testing) to be free of disease.

The physical barrier promoted for the prevention of sexual transmission of HIV and other STIs is the male condom. Explicit instructions for how to apply a male condom are included in Box 7-9.

The female condom—a lubricated polyurethane sheath with a ring on each end that is inserted into the vagina—is also an effective mechanical barrier to virus, including HIV (Centers for Disease Control and Prevention, 1998a). Furthermore, clinical studies have documented its effectiveness in providing protection from recurrent trichomoniasis. Whether condoms lubricated with spermicide are more effective than other lubricated condoms in protecting against STIs (including HIV) has not been established, nor has it been determined that condoms used with vaginal spermicides are more effective in preventing STI (including HIV) transmission than those used without spermicide (Centers for Disease Control and Prevention, 1998a). Nurses should stress that the consistent use of condoms for every act of sexual intimacy where there is the possibility of transmission of disease is essential.

Women should be counseled to watch out for situations that make it hard to talk about and practice safer sex. These include romantic times when condoms are not available and when alcohol or drugs make it impossible to make wise decisions about safer sex.

Sexually Transmitted Bacterial Infections

Chlamydia. *Chlamydia trachomatis* is the most common and fastest-spreading STI in American women, with an estimated 2.6 million new cases each year (Institute of Medicine, 1997). These infections are often silent and highly destructive; their sequelae and complications can be very serious. In women, chlamydial infections are difficult to diagnose; the symptoms, if present, are nonspecific, and culturing the organism is expensive.

Early identification of *C. trachomatis* is important because untreated infection often leads to acute salpingitis or pelvic inflammatory disease. Pelvic inflammatory disease is the most serious complication of chlamydial infections, and past chlamydial infections are associated with an increased risk of ectopic pregnancy and tubal factor infertility. Furthermore, chlamydial infection of the cervix causes an inflammation that results in microscopic cervical ulcerations, and thus may increase the risk of acquiring HIV infection.

Sexually active women younger than age 20 years are two to three times as likely to become infected with chlamydia as women between 20 and 29 years. Women over age 30 years have the lowest rate of infection. Risky behaviors, including multiple partners and nonuse of barrier methods of birth control, increase a woman's risk of chlamydial infection. Lower socioeconomic status may be a risk factor, especially with respect to treatment-seeking behaviors.

Screening and Diagnosis. In addition to obtaining information about the presence of risk factors, the nurse should inquire about the presence of any symptoms. The CDC (1998a) strongly urges screening of asymptomatic, high risk women in whom infection would otherwise go undetected; that is, sexually active adolescents, women between ages 20 and 34 years, women who do not use barrier contraceptives, and women with new or multiple partners. In addition, whenever possible, all women with two or more of the risk factors for chlamydia should have cervical cultures. All pregnant women should have cervical cultures for chlamydia at the first prenatal visit. Reculturing late in the third trimester (e.g., at 36 weeks) should be carried out if the woman was previously positive or if she is less than age 25 years or has a new sex partner or multiple sex partners.

Although usually asymptomatic, some women with chlamydia may experience spotting or postcoital bleeding, mucoid or purulent cervical discharge, or dysuria. Bleeding results from inflammation and erosion of the cervical columnar epithelium. Women taking oral contraceptives may experience breakthrough bleeding.

Diagnosis of chlamydia is by culture, a method that is expensive, requires special transport and storage, and takes up to 10 days for results. Special culture media and proper handling of specimens are important, so the nurse should always know what is required in the individual practice site.

Management. CDC recommendations for the treatment of urethral, cervical, and rectal chlamydial infections are doxycycline (100 mg orally twice a day for 7 days) or azithromycin (1 g orally in a single dose) (CDC, 1998a). Azithromycin is often prescribed when compliance may be a problem because only one dose is needed; however, expense is a concern with this medication. If the woman is pregnant, erythromycin (500 mg orally four times a day for 7 days) or amoxicillin (500 mg orally three times a day for 7 days) is used. Women who have a chlamydial infection and are also infected with HIV should be treated with the same regimen as those who are not infected with HIV.

Because chlamydia is often asymptomatic, the woman should be cautioned to take all medication prescribed. All exposed sexual partners should be treated. Women treated with doxycycline or azithromycin do not need to be retested unless symptoms continue. Women treated with erythromycin may be retested 3 weeks after completing the medication, although the validity of this practice has not been established (Centers for Disease Control and Prevention, 1998a).

Gonorrhea. Gonorrhea is probably the oldest communicable disease in the United States. An estimated 800,000 American men and women contract gonorrhea each year. The incidence of drug-resistant cases of gonorrhea, in particular penicillinase-producing *Neisseria gonorrhoeae* (PPNG), is rising dramatically in the United States.

Gonorrhea is caused by the aerobic, gram-negative diplococci *Neisseria gonorrhoeae.* The principal means of transmission is genital-to-genital contact during sexual activity; however, it is also spread by oral-genital and anal-genital contact. There is also evidence that infection may spread in females from vagina to rectum. Although the organism has been recovered from inanimate objects artificially inoculated with the bacteria, there is no evidence that natural transmission occurs this way (Schaffer, 1998).

The majority of those contracting gonorrhea are under 20 years of age; adolescent females have the highest rates of infection, and the incidence is higher in African-American adolescents than in Hispanic or Caucasian teens (Bonny and Biro, 1998). The reported incidence of gonococcal disease is higher in minority groups; many of the apparent differences in infection rates can be explained by the disproportionate representation of African-Americans among the nation's poor and among inner city dwellers. Rates of gonorrhea are higher in urban areas than in rural areas, with even higher rates in the inner city. Sex workers and their partners, intravenous drug users, and crack cocaine users are considered high risk groups. Other risk factors include early onset of sexual activity and multiple sexual partners.

Women are often asymptomatic, with one third of infections in adolescent women going unnoticed. When symptoms are present, they are often less specific than the symptoms in men. They may have a purulent endocervical discharge, but discharge is usually minimal or absent. Menstrual irregularities may be the presenting symptom, or women may complain of pain (e.g., chronic or acute severe pelvic or lower abdominal pain or longer, more painful menses). Infrequently, dysuria, vague abdominal pain, or low backache prompts a woman to seek care. Gonococcal rectal infection may occur in women following anal intercourse. Rectal gonorrhea may be completely asymptomatic or, conversely, cause severe symptoms with profuse purulent anal discharge, rectal pain, and blood in the stool. Rectal itching, fullness, pressure, and pain are also common symptoms, as is diarrhea. A diffuse vaginitis with vulvitis is the most common form of gonococcal infection in prepubertal girls. There may be few signs of infection; or vaginal discharge, dysuria, and swollen, reddened labia may be present.

Gonococcal infections in pregnancy potentially affect both mother and infant. Women with cervical gonorrhea may develop salpingitis in the first trimester. Perinatal complications of gonococcal infection include premature rupture of membranes, preterm birth, chorioamnionitis, neonatal sepsis, intrauterine growth restriction, and maternal postpartum sepsis. Amniotic infection syndrome—manifested by placental, fetal, and umbilical cord inflammation following premature rupture of the membranes—may result from gonorrheal infection during pregnancy. Gonorrhea also can be transmitted to the newborn by direct contact with gonococcal organisms in the cervix during birth and result in ophthalmia neonatorum.

Screening and Diagnosis. Because gonococcal infections in women often are asymptomatic, the CDC (1998a) recommends screening all women at risk for gonorrhea. All pregnant women should be screened at the first prenatal visit, and infected women and those identified with risky behaviors rescreened at 36 weeks of gestation. Cultures should be obtained from the endocervix, rectum, and, when indicated, from the pharynx. Because coinfection is common, any woman suspected of having gonorrhea should have a chlamydial culture and serologic test for syphilis unless one has been done within the past 2 months.

Management. Management of gonorrhea is straightforward, and with appropriate antibiotic therapy, the cure is usually rapid. Single-dose efficacy is a major consideration in selecting an antibiotic regimen for women with gonorrhea. Another important consideration is the high proportion (45%) of women with coexisting chlamydial infections. The treatment of choice for uncomplicated urethral, endocervical, and rectal infections in pregnant and nonpregnant women is ceftriaxone (125 mg IM once). The CDC (1998a) suggests concomitant treatment for chlamydia because coinfection is common. All women with both gonorrhea and syphilis should also be treated for syphilis according to CDC guidelines (see discussion of syphilis in this chapter).

Gonorrhea is highly communicable. Recent (i.e., within 30 days) sexual partners should be examined, cultured, and treated with appropriate regimens. Most treatment failures result from reinfection. The patient needs to be informed of this, as well as of the consequences of reinfection in terms of chronicity, complications, and potential infertility. Women are counseled to use condoms. All patients with gonorrhea should be offered confidential counseling and testing for HIV infection.

LEGAL TIP • Gonorrhea Gonorrhea is a reportable communicable disease. Health care providers are legally responsible for reporting all cases of gonorrhea to health authorities (usually the local health department in the patient's county of residence). Women should be informed that the case will be reported, told why, and informed of the possibility of being contacted by a health department epidemiologist.

Treatment failure following combined ceftriaxone/doxycycline therapy is rare; therefore follow-up culture (test of cure) is not essential. A more cost-effective approach is reexamination with a culture 1 to 2 months after treatment. This approach will detect both treatment failures and reinfections. Patients should be counseled to return if symptoms persist after treatment.

Syphilis. Syphilis, one of the earliest described sexually transmitted diseases, is caused by *Treponema pallidum,* a motile spirochete. Transmission is thought to be by entry in the subcutaneous tissue through microscopic abrasions that can occur during sexual intercourse. The disease can also be transmitted through kissing, biting, or oral-genital sex. Transplacental transmission may occur at any time during pregnancy; the degree of risk is related to the quantity of spirochetes in the maternal bloodstream.

There are an estimated 120,000 new cases of syphilis in the United States each year. Rates are highest among young adult African-Americans in urban areas and in southern states (Centers for Disease Control and Prevention, 1998b). Much of the rise in cases seen since 1990 is directly attributable to use of illicit drugs (particularly crack cocaine) and to the exchange of sex for drugs and money.

Syphilis is a complex disease that can lead to serious systemic disease and even death if untreated. Infection manifests itself in distinct stages with different symptoms and clinical manifestations. Primary syphilis is characterized by a primary lesion, the chancre, that appears 5 to 90 days after infection. This lesion often begins as a painless papule at the site of inoculation and then erodes to form a nontender, shallow, indurated, clean ulcer several millimeters to centimeters in size (Fig. 6-2). Secondary syphilis occurs 6 weeks to 6 months after the appearance of the chancre. It is characterized by a widespread, symmetric, maculopapular rash on the palms and soles; and generalized lymphadenopathy. The infected individual also may experience fever, headache, and malaise.

Condylomata lata (broad, painless, pink-gray, wartlike infectious lesions) may develop on the vulva, perineum, or anus. If the woman is untreated, she enters a latent phase that is asymptomatic for the majority of individuals. Left untreated, about one third of these women will develop tertiary syphilis. Neurologic, cardiovascular, musculoskeletal, or multiorgan system complications can develop in the third stage.

Screening and Diagnosis. All women who are diagnosed with another STI or with HIV should be screened for syphilis. All pregnant women should be screened for syphilis at the first prenatal visit and again in the late third trimester. Diagnosis is dependent on microscopic examination of primary and secondary lesion tissue and serology during latency and late infection. Any test for antibodies may not be reactive in the presence of active infection because it takes time for the body's immune system to develop antibodies to any antigens. Two types of serologic tests are used: nontreponemal and treponemal. Nontreponemal antibody tests such as the VDRL (Venereal Disease Research Laboratories) or RPR (rapid plasma reagin) are used as screening tests. False-positive results are not unusual, particularly when conditions such as acute infection, autoimmune disorders, malignancy, pregnancy, and drug addiction exist and after immunization or vaccination. The treponemal tests—fluorescent treponemal antibody absorbed (FTA-ABS) and microhemagglutination assays for antibody to *T. pallidum* (MHA-TP)—are used to confirm positive results. Test results in patients with early primary or incubating syphilis may be negative. Seroconversion usually takes place 6 to 8 weeks after exposure, so testing should be repeated in 1 to 2 months when a suspicious genital lesion exists. Positive treponemal antibody tests stay positive for life regardless of treatment or disease activity (Centers for Disease Control and Prevention, 1998a).

Tests for concomitant STIs (e.g., wet preps and cultures) should be performed, and HIV testing should be offered if indicated.

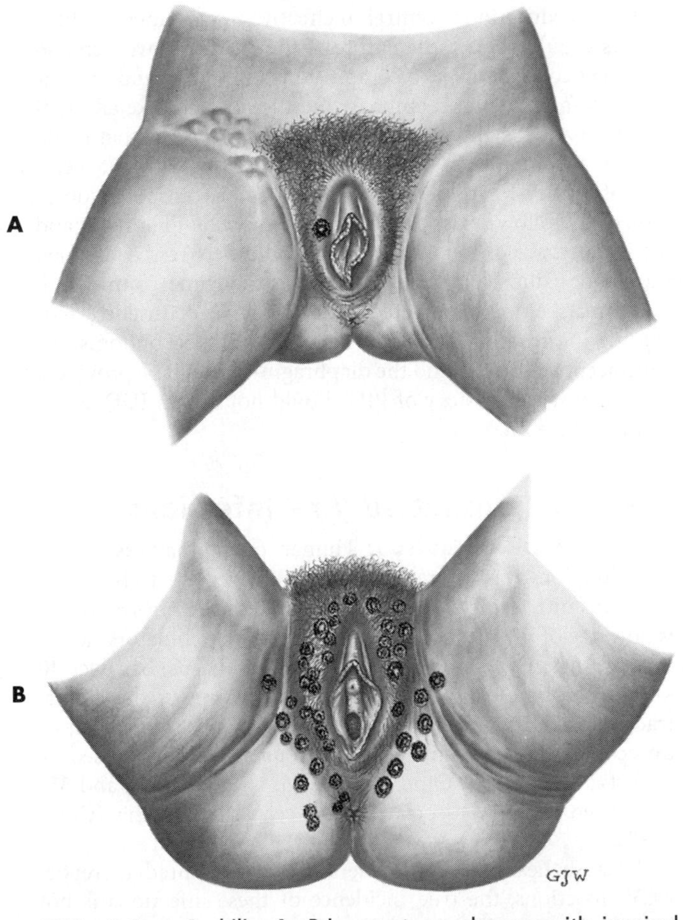

FIG. 6-2 • Syphilis. **A,** Primary stage: chancre with inguinal adenopathy. **B,** Secondary stage: condyloma lata.

Management. Penicillin is the preferred drug for treating patients with syphilis. It is the only proven therapy that has been widely used for patients with neurosyphilis, congenital syphilis, or syphilis during pregnancy. Intramuscular penicillin G benzathine (as 2.4 million units IM once) is used to treat primary, secondary, and early latent syphilis. Women with syphilis of greater than 1 year's duration (i.e., in late latent or tertiary stages) require weekly treatment of 2.4 million units of penicillin G benzathine for 3 weeks. Although doxycycline, tetracycline, and erythromycin are alternative treatments for penicillin-allergic patients, both tetracycline and doxycycline are contraindicated in pregnancy, and erythromycin is unlikely to cure a fetal infection. Therefore pregnant women should, if necessary, receive skin testing and be treated with penicillin, or be desensitized (Centers for Disease Control and Prevention, 1998a).

NURSE ALERT • Patients treated for syphilis may experience a Jarisch-Herxheimer reaction. This is an acute febrile reaction often accompanied by headache, myalgias, and arthralgias that develops within the first 24 hours of treatment. Women treated in the second half of pregnancy are at risk for preterm labor and birth if treatment precipitates this reaction. They should be advised to contact their health care provider if they notice any change in fetal movement or if they have any contractions.

Monthly follow-up is mandatory so that retreatment may be given if needed. The nurse should emphasize the necessity of long-term serologic testing even in the absence of symptoms. The woman should be advised to practice sexual abstinence until treatment is completed, all evidence of primary and secondary syphilis is gone, and serologic evidence of a cure is demonstrated. Women should be told to notify all partners who may have been exposed. They should be informed that the disease is reportable. Preventive measures should be discussed.

Pelvic Inflammatory Disease. Pelvic inflammatory disease (PID) is an infectious process that most commonly involves the uterine (fallopian) tubes (salpingitis), uterus (endometritis), and, more rarely, the ovaries and peritoneal surfaces. Multiple organisms have been found to cause PID, and most cases are associated with more than one organism. In the past the most common causative agent was thought to be *N. gonorrhoeae;* however, *C. trachomatis* is now estimated to cause one half of all cases of PID. In addition to gonorrhea and chlamydia, a wide variety of anaerobic and aerobic bacteria cause PID.

Most PID results from the ascending spread of microorganisms from the vagina and endocervix to the upper genital tract.

This spread most commonly happens at the end of or just after menses following reception of an infectious agent. During the menstrual period, several factors facilitate the development of an infection: the cervical os is slightly open, the cervical mucus barrier is absent, and menstrual blood is an excellent medium for growth. PID also may develop following an abortion, pelvic surgery, or childbirth.

Each year more than 1 million women in the United States have an episode of symptomatic PID (Institute of Medicine, 1997). Risk factors for acquiring PID are those associated with the risk of contracting an STI, including young age, multiple partners, high rate of new partners, and a history of STIs. Women who use IUDs may be at increased risk for PID if they have more than one sexual partner or if the partner has other sexual partners because they are at higher risk for acquiring an STI (Hatcher et al, 1998). Most of this risk occurs in the first months after IUD insertion. PID tends to recur, with nearly 1 in 5 patients experiencing recurrent PID (Bonny and Biro, 1998).

Women who have had PID are at increased risk for ectopic pregnancy, infertility, and chronic pelvic pain. Other problems associated with PID include dyspareunia, pyosalpinx (pus in the uterine tubes), tubo-ovarian abscess, and pelvic adhesions.

The symptoms of PID vary depending on whether the infection is acute, subacute, or chronic; however, pain is common to all clinical presentations. It may be dull, cramping, and intermittent (subacute); or severe, persistent, and incapacitating (acute). The woman with acute PID also may complain of intermenstrual bleeding. Physical examination reveals adnexal tenderness, with or without rebound, and exquisite tenderness with cervical movement (Chandelier sign). Pelvic tenderness is usually bilateral. There may or may not be a palpable adnexal swelling or thickening. A urethral or cervical discharge, often purulent in nature, may be present. A fever of 39° C or above is characteristic. Significant laboratory data include an elevated white blood cell count and markedly elevated erythrocyte sedimentation rate. Fever and peritonitis are more characteristic of gonococcal PID than of PID caused by other organisms that are more likely to be "silent." Because PID caused by chlamydia is more commonly asymptomatic, it more often results in tubal obstruction from delayed diagnosis or inadequate treatment.

Screening and Diagnosis. A careful history is necessary to distinguish between PID and other conditions that cause abdominal pain, such as an ectopic pregnancy or appendicitis. A menstrual history is useful in establishing the relationship of onset of pain to menses and in identifying any variations from normal in the cycle. Other relevant history includes recent pelvic surgery, birth, abortion, or dilation of the cervix; purulent vaginal discharge; irregular bleeding; and a longer, heavier menstrual period. A sexual history will assist in identifying possible increased risk for STI exposure. Symptoms of an STI in a woman's partner(s) also should be noted.

Vital signs are obtained and a complete physical examination performed. CDC routine criteria for diagnosing PID include oral temperature greater than 38.3° C, abnormal cervical or vaginal discharge, elevated erythrocyte sedimentation rate, and laboratory documentation of cervical infection with *N. gonorrhoeae* or *C. trachomatis.* Physical findings of lower abdominal tenderness, bilateral adnexal tenderness, and cervical motion tenderness are important in making a clinical diagnosis of PID. Essential laboratory data are a complete blood count with differential and cervical cultures for gonorrhea and chlamydia.

Management. Perhaps the most important nursing intervention is prevention. Primary prevention is education to avoid acquisition of sexually transmitted infections, whereas secondary prevention involves preventing a lower genital tract infection from ascending to the upper genital tract. Instructing women in self-protective behaviors such as practicing safer sex and using barrier methods is critical. Women using hormonal contraception or an IUD and those who have chosen tubal ligation must be reminded to use a condom with intercourse when indicated. Also important is the detection of asymptomatic gonorrheal and chlamydial infections through routine screening of women who practice risky behaviors or have specific risk factors such as age. Partner notification when an STI is diagnosed is essential to prevent reinfection.

Although treatment regimens vary with the infecting organism, generally a broad-spectrum antibiotic is used. Several antimicrobial regimens have proved to be effective, and no single therapeutic regimen of choice exists. The woman with acute PID should be on bed rest in a semi-Fowler's position. Comfort measures include analgesics for pain and all other nursing measures applicable to a patient confined to bed. Few pelvic examinations should be done during the acute phase of the disease. During the recovery phase, the woman should restrict her activity and make every effort to get adequate rest and a nutritionally sound diet. Follow-up laboratory work after treatment should include endocervical cultures for a test of cure.

Health education is central to effective management of PID. Nurses should explain the nature of the disease to women and should encourage them to comply with all therapy and prevention recommendations, emphasizing the need to take all medication, even if symptoms disappear. Any problems that could prevent a woman from completing a course of treatment (i.e., a lack of money for prescriptions or a lack of transportation to return for follow-up appointments) should be identified, and the importance of follow-up visits should be stressed. Women should be counseled to refrain from sexual intercourse until their treatment is completed. Contraceptive counseling—including information on barrier methods such as condoms, the contraceptive sponge, and the diaphragm—should be provided. A woman with a history of PID should not use an IUD as her contraceptive method.

Sexually Transmitted Viral Infections

Human Papillomavirus. Human papillomavirus (HPV) infection, previously named genital or venereal warts, is a sexually transmitted infection that was first described in 25 AD and is now one of the most common STIs seen in ambulatory health care settings. HPV, a double-stranded DNA virus, has over 40 known serotypes; more than 20 types can infect the genital tract. Most HPV infections are asymptomatic, subclinical, or unrecognized. The visible genital lesions are usually caused by HPV types 6 and 11. Other types (e.g., 16, 18, 31, 33, and 35) have been strongly associated with cervical dysplasia (CDC, 1998a).

Because health care providers are not required to report HPV infections, the true incidence of these infections is not known. An estimated 24 million Americans are infected with HPV, and as many as 1 million new infections occur yearly

(CDC, 1998a). In addition to the general risk factors for STIs noted earlier, cigarette smoking and use of oral contraceptives for more than 5 years have been found to be risk factors for HPV.

In women, HPV lesions (also called condylomata acuminata) are most commonly seen in the posterior part of the introitus; however, lesions also are found on the buttocks, vulva, vagina, anus, and cervix (Fig. 6-3). Typically the lesions are small (i.e., 2 to 3 mm in diameter and 10 to 15 mm in height), soft, papillary swellings occurring singly or in clusters on the genital and anal-rectal region. Infections of long duration may appear as a cauliflower-like mass. In moist areas such as the vaginal introitus, the lesions may appear to have multiple, fine, fingerlike projections. Vaginal lesions are often multiple. Flat-topped papules, 1 to 4 mm in diameter, are seen most often on the cervix. Often these lesions are visualized only under magnification. Warts are usually flesh colored or slightly darker on Caucasian women; black on African-American women; and brownish on Asian women. Usually painless, the lesions may also be uncomfortable, particularly when very large, inflamed, or ulcerated. Chronic vaginal discharge, pruritus, or dyspareunia can occur.

HPV infections are thought to be more common in pregnant than in nonpregnant women, with an increase in incidence from the first trimester to the third. Furthermore, a significant proportion of preexisting HPV lesions enlarge greatly during pregnancy, a proliferation presumably resulting from the relative state of immunosuppression present during pregnancy. Lesions may become so large during pregnancy that they affect urination, defecation, mobility, and fetal descent, although birth by cesarean is rarely necessary (American College of Obstetricians and Gynecologists, 1994). Initial observation of large growths can be misleading, suggesting that the entire vagina is involved. However, all of the growth may derive from one stalk, and in such cases it may be possible to push the large mass to the side, allowing the baby to pass through. HPV infection may be acquired by the neonate during birth; the incidence of such transmission is unknown.

Screening and Diagnosis. A woman with HPV lesions may complain of symptoms such as a profuse, irritating vaginal discharge, itching, dyspareunia, or postcoital bleeding. She also may report "bumps" on her vulva or labia. History of a known exposure is important; however, because of the potentially long latency period and the possibility of subclinical infections in men, the lack of a history of known exposure cannot be used to exclude a diagnosis of HPV infection.

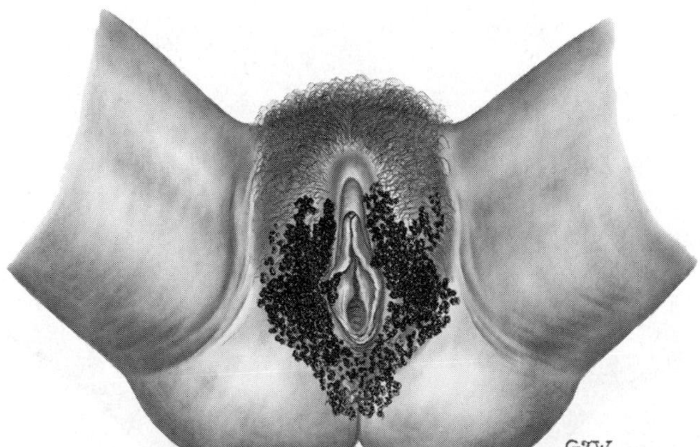

FIG. 6-3 • HPV infection. Condyloma acuminata.

Physical inspection of the vulva, perineum, anus, vagina, and cervix is essential whenever HPV lesions are suspected or seen in one area. Because speculum examination of the vagina may block some lesions, it is important to rotate the speculum blades until all areas are visualized. When lesions are visible, the characteristic appearance previously described is considered diagnostic. However, in many instances, cervical lesions are not visible, and some vaginal or vulvar lesions also may be unobservable to the naked eye. Because of the potential spread of vulvar or vaginal lesions to the anus, gloves should be changed between vaginal and rectal examinations.

Diagnosis is made by colposcopy and direct visualization of the growths or by biopsy. Cervical examination with a Papanicolaou (Pap) smear is imperative for women who either have vulvar HPV or who have partners with HPV. Pap smears of the cervical transformation zone are used as a screening technique; however, because of false-negative results, a negative Pap smear does not indicate absence of disease. The severity of any cervical lesion reported on a Pap smear is best determined by colposcopy and biopsy. Vinegar solution may be used to highlight early or flat cervical lesions; however, it is important to note that a positive reaction may also be obtained with any inflammatory reaction, after sexual intercourse, and with vaginal trauma.

HPV lesions must be differentiated from molluscum contagiosum and condylomata lata. Molluscum contagiosum lesions are half-domed, smooth, flesh-colored to pearly white papules with depressed centers. Condylomata lata are a form of secondary syphilis and generally are flatter and wider than genital warts. A serologic test for syphilis would confirm the diagnosis of secondary syphilis.

Management. Treatment of genital warts is often difficult and should be guided by preference of the woman, available resources, and experience of the health care provider. No therapy has been shown to eradicate HPV. The goal of treatment therefore is removal of warts and relief of signs and symptoms, not the eradication of HPV (Centers for Disease Control and Prevention, 1998a). Often the patient must make multiple office visits; commonly, many different treatment modalities will be used. Eradication of the virus is not considered conclusive even after there is no visible evidence of wart tissue because of the high incidence of recurrence. Imiquimod, podophyllin, and podofilox are common treatments, but should not be used during pregnancy. Because the lesions can proliferate and become friable during pregnancy, many experts recommend their removal using cryotherapy or various surgical techniques (CDC, 1998a).

Women who are experiencing discomfort associated with genital warts may find that bathing with an oatmeal solution and drying the area with cool air from a hair dryer will provide some relief. Keeping the area clean and dry will also decrease the growth of the warts. Cotton underwear and loose-fitting clothes that decrease friction and irritation also may lessen discomfort. Women should be advised to maintain a healthy lifestyle to aid the immune system; and be counseled regarding diet, rest, stress reduction, and exercise.

Patient counseling should address how the virus is transmitted, that no immunity is conferred with infection, and that reacquisition of the infection is likely with repeated contact. Women need to know that partners should be checked even if they are asymptomatic. Because HPV is highly contagious, the majority of women's partners will be infected and should be treated. All sexually active women with multiple partners or a history of HPV should be encouraged to use latex condoms and a vaginal spermicide for intercourse to decrease acquisition or transmission of condylomata.

Instructions for all medications and treatments must be detailed. Women should be informed before treatment of the possibility of posttreatment pain associated with specific therapies. The importance of thorough treatment of concurrent vaginitis or STI should be emphasized. The link between cervical cancer and HPV infections and the need for close follow-up should be discussed.

Annual health examinations are recommended to assess disease recurrence and screening for cervical cancer. Biannual Pap smears should be done for the first 2 years after treatment and annually thereafter on women who have been treated for HPV infections (National Institutes of Health, 1996). When the cervix is treated, a Pap smear should be done in 4 to 6 months; after two negative Pap smears at 6-month intervals, an annual Pap smear can be performed (Centers for Disease Control and Prevention, 1998a). Women should understand the advisability of treatment before becoming pregnant.

Women with HPV infection may radically alter their sexual practices both from fear of transmission to and from a partner and from genital discomfort associated with treatment, which may have a negative impact on their sexual relationships. Unless the partner accepts and understands the necessary precautions, it may be difficult for the woman to follow the treatment regimen. The nurse can offer to discuss feelings that the woman may have. When indicated, joint counseling can be suggested.

Herpes Simplex Virus. Unknown until the middle of the twentieth century, herpes simplex virus (HSV) infection is now widespread in the United States, especially in women. HSV infection results in painful, recurrent genital ulcers. It is caused by two different antigen subtypes of herpes simplex virus: herpes simplex virus type 1 (HSV-1) and herpes simplex virus type 2 (HSV-2). HSV-2 is usually transmitted sexually; HSV-1 is usually transmitted nonsexually. Although HSV-1 is more commonly associated with gingivostomatitis and oral labial ulcers (fever blisters) and HSV-2 with genital lesions, both types are not exclusively associated with the respective sites.

Although HSV infection is not a reportable disease, it is estimated that at least 45 million Americans are infected with genital herpes (Centers for Disease Control and Prevention, 1998a) and that 200,000 to 500,000 persons contract an initial (or primary) infection each year. Recurrent HSV infections are much more common (Hatcher et al, 1998). Estimates suggest that at least 1 in every 4 women will become infected in her lifetime (Institute of Medicine, 1997).

An initial HSV genital infection is characterized by multiple painful lesions, fever, chills, malaise, and severe dysuria, and may last 2 to 3 weeks. Women generally have a more severe clinical course than do men. Women with primary genital herpes have many lesions that progress from macules to papules; then to form vesicles, pustules, and ulcers that crust and heal without scarring (Fig. 6-4). These ulcers are extremely tender, and primary infections may be bilateral. Women also may have itching, inguinal tenderness, and lymphadenopathy. Severe vulvar edema may develop, and women may have difficulty sitting. HSV cervicitis also is common with initial HSV-2 infections. The cervix may appear normal or be friable, reddened, ulcerated, or necrotic. A heavy, watery to purulent vaginal discharge is common. Extragenital lesions may be present because of autoinoculation. Urinary retention and dysuria may occur secondary to autonomic involvement of the sacral nerve root.

Women experiencing recurrent episodes of HSV infections commonly have only local symptoms that are usually less severe than those associated with the initial infection. Systemic symptoms are usually absent, although the characteristic prodromal genital tingling is common. Recurrent lesions are unilateral, are less severe, and usually last 5 to 7 days. Lesions begin as vesicles and progress rapidly to ulcers. Few women with recurrent disease have cervicitis.

During pregnancy, maternal infection with HSV-2 can have adverse effects on both the mother and fetus. Viremia occurs during the primary infection, and congenital infection is possible, though rare. Primary infections during the first trimester have been associated with increased miscarriage rates. The most severe complication of HSV infection is neonatal herpes, a potentially fatal or severely disabling disease occurring at a rate of 1 in 2000 to 1 in 10,000 live births. Most mothers of infants who contract neonatal herpes lack a history of clinically evident genital herpes. Risk of neonatal infection is highest among women with primary herpes infection who are near term; risk is low among women with recurrent herpes (Centers for Disease Control and Prevention, 1998a). There is a 60% infant mortality rate associated with infants who contract HSV infection, and about 50% of those who survive suffer serious neurologic damage (Corder-Mabe, 1998).

An association between cervical cancer and HSV-2 has been observed. It is theorized that genital herpes is a marker for high risk sexual behaviors that could transmit other STIs, including HPV (DiSaia and Creasman, 1997).

Screening and Diagnosis. A diagnosis of herpes is facilitated by a careful history; exposure to an infected person is important, although infection from an asymptomatic individual is possible. A history of viral symptoms such as malaise, headache, fever, or myalgia is suggestive. Local symptoms such as vulvar pain, dysuria, itching or burning at the site of infection, and painful genital lesions that heal spontaneously are also highly suggestive of HSV infections. The nurse should ask about prior history of a primary infection, prodromal symptoms, vaginal

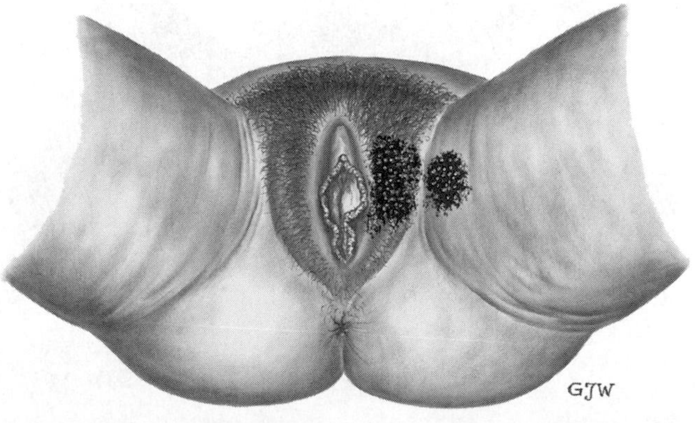

FIG. 6-4 • Herpes genitalis.

discharge, and dyspareunia. Pregnant women should be asked whether they or their partner(s) have had genital lesions.

During the physical examination, the nurse should assess for inguinal and generalized lymphadenopathy and elevated temperature. The entire vulvar, perineal, vaginal, and cervical areas should be carefully inspected for vesicles or ulcerated or crusted areas. A speculum examination may be very difficult for the woman because of the extreme tenderness often associated with herpes infections. Any suspicious or recurrent lesions found during pregnancy should be cultured to document HSV. Although a diagnosis of herpes infection may be suspected from the history and physical, it is confirmed by laboratory studies. A viral culture is obtained by swabbing exudate during the vesicular stage of the disease. Preliminary results are available in 48 hours, with final results in 1 to 2 weeks (Youngkin, 1995). In primary HSV infection, viral shedding is prolonged and HSV is more easily isolated.

Management. Genital herpes is a chronic and recurring disease for which there is no known cure. Management is directed toward specific treatment during primary and recurrent infections, prevention, self-help measures, and psychologic support.

Systemic antiviral medications partially control the symptoms and signs of HSV infections when used for the primary or recurrent episodes or when used as daily suppressive therapy. However, these medications do not eradicate the infection, nor do they alter subsequent risk, frequency, or recurrences after the medication is stopped. Three antiviral medications provide clinical benefit: acyclovir, valacyclovir, and famciclovir. Safety and efficacy have been clearly shown in persons taking acyclovir daily for up to 3 years. The safety of acyclovir, valacyclovir, and famciclovir therapy during pregnancy has not been established; however, the first clinical episode of genital herpes during pregnancy may be treated with oral acyclovir. In the presence of life-threatening maternal HSV infection, acyclovir IV is indicated (Centers for Disease Control and Prevention, 1998a). Continued investigation is needed of HSV therapy with these medications during pregnancy.

Cleaning lesions twice a day with saline will help prevent secondary infection. Bacterial infection must be treated with appropriate antibiotics. Measures that may increase comfort for women when lesions are active include warm sitz baths with baking soda; keeping lesions dry by using cool air from a hair dryer or by patting dry with a soft towel; wearing cotton underwear and loose clothing; using drying aids such as hydrogen peroxide, Burow's solution, or oatmeal baths; applying cool, wet, black tea bags to lesions; and applying compresses with an infusion of cloves or peppermint oil and clove oil to lesions.

Oral analgesics such as aspirin or ibuprofen may be used to relieve pain and systemic symptoms associated with initial infections. Because the mucous membranes affected by herpes are extremely sensitive, any topical agents should be used with caution. Nonantiviral ointments, especially those containing cortisone, should be avoided. A thin layer of lidocaine ointment or an antiseptic spray may be applied to decrease discomfort, especially if walking is difficult.

A diet rich in vitamin C, B-complex vitamins, zinc, and calcium is thought to help prevent recurrences. Daily use of kelp powder (2 capsules) and sunflower seed oil (1 tbsp) has been recommended to decrease recurrences (Ammer, 1989). The amino acid L-lysine has been used in doses of 750 to 1000 mg daily while lesions are active and doses of 500 mg during asymptomatic periods. It is thought that L-lysine has an inhibitory effect on the multiplication of the herpes simplex virus.

Counseling and education are critical components of the nursing care of women with herpes infections. Information regarding the etiology, signs and symptoms, transmission, and treatment should be provided. The nurse should explain that each woman is unique in her response to herpes and emphasize the variability of symptoms. Women should be helped to understand when viral shedding and thus transmission to a partner is most likely, and that they should refrain from sexual contact from the onset of prodrome until complete healing of lesions. Some authorities recommend consistent use of condoms for all persons with genital herpes. Condoms may not prevent transmission, particularly male-to-female transmission; however, this does not mean that the partners should avoid all intimacy. Women can be encouraged to maintain close contact with their partners while avoiding contact with lesions. Women should be taught how to look for herpetic lesions using a mirror and good light source and a wet cloth or finger covered with a finger cot to rub lightly over the labia. The nurse should ensure that women understand that when lesions are active, sharing intimate articles (e.g., washcloths or wet towels) that come into contact with the lesions should be avoided. Plain soap and water is all that is needed to clean hands that have come in contact with herpetic lesions; isolation is not necessary or appropriate.

The role of precipitating factors in the reactivation of the latent virus and recurrent episodes should be discussed. Stress, menstruation, trauma, febrile illnesses, chronic illness, and ultraviolet light have all been found to trigger genital herpes. Women may wish to keep a diary to identify stressors that seem to be associated with recurrent herpes attacks so that they can then avoid these stressors when possible. The role of exercise in reducing stress can be discussed. Referral for stress reduction therapy, yoga, or meditation classes may be indicated. Avoiding excessive heat and sun and hot baths and using a lubricant during sexual intercourse to reduce friction may also be helpful. Women in their childbearing years should be counseled regarding the risk of herpes infection during pregnancy. They should be instructed to use condoms if there is any risk of contracting an STI from a sexual partner. If they are using acyclovir therapy, they should be counseled to use contraception because of the potential teratogenicity of acyclovir. Women who are breastfeeding should not use acyclovir.

Because neonatal HSV infection is such a devastating disease, prevention is critical. Current recommendations include carefully examining and questioning all women about symptoms at onset of labor (Eisenstat, 1995). Diagnosis of genital herpes in any pregnant woman with active, visible lesions should be confirmed with culture. If visible lesions are not present at onset of labor, vaginal birth is acceptable. Cesarean birth, within 4 hours after labor begins or after membranes rupture, is recommended if visible lesions are present. Infants who are delivered through an infected vagina should be carefully observed and cultured. Some experts recommend presumptive treatment of infants who were exposed to HSV during birth. Because HSV infection may be associated with cervical dysplasia, women must be encouraged to have yearly Pap smears and gynecologic examinations.

The emotional impact of contracting herpes is considerable. No cure is available, and most women experience recurrences. At diagnosis many emotions may surface—helplessness, anger, denial, guilt, anxiety, shame, or inadequacy. Women need the opportunity to discuss their feelings and help in learning to live with the disease. A woman can be encouraged to think of herself as someone who is healthy and merely inconvenienced from time to time. Herpes can affect a woman's sexuality, her sexual practices, and her current and future relationships. She may need help in discussing her HSV status with her partner or with future partners.

Viral Hepatitis. Five different viruses (i.e., hepatitis viruses A, B, C, D, and E) account for almost all cases of viral hepatitis in humans. Hepatitis viruses A, B, and C are discussed in this section. Hepatitis D and E viruses, common among users of intravenous drugs and recipients of multiple blood transfusions, are not included in this discussion.

Hepatitis A. Hepatitis A virus (HAV) infection is acquired primarily through a fecal-oral route by ingestion of contaminated food, particularly milk, shellfish, or polluted water, or person-to-person contact. Women living in the western United States, Native Americans, Alaskan Natives, and children and employees in day care centers are at high risk (Centers for Disease Control and Prevention, 1996a).

HAV infection is characterized by flu-like symptoms with malaise, fatigue, anorexia, nausea, pruritus, fever, and upper right quadrant pain. Serologic testing to detect the IgM antibody is done to confirm acute infections. The IgM antibody is detectable 5 to 10 days after exposure and can remain positive for up to 6 months. Because HAV infection is self-limited and does not result in chronic infection or chronic liver disease, treatment is usually supportive. Women who become dehydrated from nausea and vomiting, or who have fulminating hepatitis A, may need to be hospitalized. Medications that might cause liver damage or that are metabolized in the liver should be used with caution. No specific diet or activity restrictions are necessary. Immune globulin (gamma globulin) or immune-specific globulin is indicated for any pregnant woman exposed to HAV to provide passive immunity through injected antibodies. All household contacts of the woman should also receive gamma globulin.

Hepatitis B. Hepatitis B virus (HBV) infection is a sexually transmitted disease and is the virus most threatening to the fetus and neonate (Corrarino, 1998). It is caused by a large DNA virus and is associated with three antigens and their antibodies: hepatitis B surface antigen (HBsAG), HBV antigen (HBeAG), HBV core antigen (HBcAG), antibody to HBsAG (anti-HBs), antibody to HBeAG (anti-HBe), and antibody to HBcAG (anti-HBc). Screening for active or chronic disease or disease immunity is based on testing for these antigens and their antibodies.

Factors considered to place a woman at risk for HBV are those associated with STI risk in general: history of multiple sexual partners, multiple STIs, and intravenous drug use; and behaviors that are associated with blood contact (e.g., work or treatment in a dialysis unit, history of multiple blood transfusions, public safety workers exposed to blood in the workplace, and health care workers). Although HBV can be transmitted via blood transfusion, the incidence of such infections has decreased significantly since testing of blood for HBsAG became a routine procedure. Drug abusers who share needles are at risk, as are health care workers exposed to blood and needle sticks. In addition, women of Asian, Pacific Islander (e.g., Polynesian, Micronesian, and Melanesian), or Alaskan Eskimo descent and of Haitian or sub-Saharan Africa birth are considered to be at risk.

HBV infection is transmitted parenterally and through intimate contact. It is 50 to 100 times more contagious than HIV. The hepatitis B carrier state affects 5% of the world's population, with higher percentages found in tropical areas and Southeast Asia. Hepatitis B surface antigen has been found in blood, saliva, sweat, tears, vaginal secretions, and semen. Perinatal transmission does occur; however, the fetus is not at risk until it comes in contact with contaminated blood during birth. Infants born to mothers who are highly infectious (i.e., positive for both HBsAG and HBeAG) have a 70% to 90% chance of acquiring perinatal hepatitis B infection. Approximately 85% to 90% of infected infants will become chronic carriers. HBV has also been transmitted by artificial insemination.

HBV infection is a disease of the liver and is often a silent infection. In the adult, the course of the infection can be fulminating and the outcome fatal. Symptoms of HBV infection are similar to those of hepatitis A: arthralgias, arthritis, lassitude, anorexia, nausea, vomiting, headache, fever, and mild abdominal pain. Later the woman may have clay-colored stools, dark urine, increased abdominal pain, and jaundice. Between 5% and 10% of individuals with HBV have persistence of HBsAg and become chronic hepatitis B carriers. Twenty-five percent of chronic carriers die from primary hepatocellular carcinoma or cirrhosis of the liver.

Screening and Diagnosis. All women at high risk for contracting HBV should be screened on a regular basis. Since screening only individuals at high risk may not identify up to 50% of HBsAg-positive women, current CDC guidelines recommend screening for the presence of HBsAg on all women at the first prenatal visit and repeated later in pregnancy for women with high risk behaviors (Centers for Disease Control and Prevention, 1998a).

Testing for HBV is complex. Patients with acute hepatitis B generally have detectable serum HBsAG levels in the late incubation phase of the disease, 2 to 5 weeks before symptoms appear. Anti-HBs with a negative HBsAG test signals immunity. Anti-HBs with a positive antigen denotes a chronic carrier state; during this time, the disease can be transmitted. During the recovery phase, the patient may continue to be infectious even though HBsAG cannot be detected. This is called the "window phase" and is identified by anti-HBc in the absence of anti-HBs. Women should be prepared for repeat testing because HBV screening tests may also be used to monitor the progression of the disease.

Components of the history to be obtained when hepatitis B is suspected include inquiry about the symptoms of the disease and risk factors outlined earlier. Physical examination includes inspection of the skin for rashes, inspection of the skin and conjunctiva for jaundice, and palpation of the liver for enlargement and tenderness. Weight loss, fever, and general debilitation should be noted. If the HBsAG is positive, further laboratory studies may be ordered (e.g., anti-HBe, anti-HBc, serum glutamic-oxaloacetic transaminase [SGOT], alkaline phosphatase, and liver panel). If the HBsAG is negative in early pregnancy and the woman could be in the window phase, or if high risk behaviors continue during pregnancy, a repeat HBsAG should be ordered in the third trimester.

Management. There is no specific treatment for hepatitis B. Recovery is usually spontaneous in 3 to 16 weeks. Usually pregnancies complicated by acute viral hepatitis are managed on an outpatient basis. Women should be advised to increase bed rest; eat a high-protein, low-fat diet; and increase their fluid intake. They should avoid medications metabolized in the liver, drugs, and alcohol. Women with a definite exposure to HBV should be given hepatitis B immune globulin and should begin the hepatitis B vaccine series within 14 days of the most recent contact to prevent infection (CDC, 1998a). Vaccination during pregnancy is not thought to pose risks to the fetus.

All nonimmune women at high or moderate risk of hepatitis should be informed of the existence of hepatitis B vaccine. Vaccination is recommended for all individuals who have had multiple sex partners within the past 6 months (Centers for Disease Control and Prevention, 1998a). In addition, intravenous drug users, residents of correctional or long-term care facilities, persons seeking care for an STI, prostitutes, women whose partners are intravenous drug users or bisexual, and women whose occupation exposes them to high risk should be vaccinated. The vaccine is given in a series of three (some authorities recommend four) doses over a 6-month period with the first two doses given at least 1 month apart. The vaccine is given in the deltoid muscle (CDC, 1998a).

Patient education includes explaining the meaning of hepatitis B infection, including transmission, state of infectivity, and sequelae. The nurse should also explain the need for immunoprophylaxis for household members and sexual contacts. To decrease transmission of the virus, women with hepatitis B or who test positive for HBV should be advised to maintain a high level of personal hygiene (e.g., wash hands after using the toilet; carefully dispose of tampons, pads, and bandages in plastic bags; do not share razor blades, toothbrushes, needles, or manicure implements; have male partner use a condom if unvaccinated and without hepatitis; avoid sharing saliva through kissing, or through sharing of silverware or dishes; and wipe up blood spills immediately with soap and water). They should inform all health care providers of their carrier state. Breastfeeding is not contraindicated if the infant receives prophylaxis at birth and is currently on the immunization schedule.

Hepatitis C. Hepatitis C virus (HCV) infection has become an important health problem as increasing numbers of persons acquire the disease. Fourteen percent of the United States population is infected with HCV (Hunt, Carson, and Sharara, 1997). Because up to 70% of patients with HCV infection progress to chronic hepatitis, hepatitis C represents nearly 50% of chronic viral hepatitis. Risk factors for pregnant women include women with STIs such as hepatitis B and HIV, multiple sexual partners, history of blood transfusions, and history of intravenous drug use. Hepatitis C is readily transmitted through exposure to blood. It is transmitted much less efficiently by means of semen, saliva, and urine.

Most patients with hepatitis C are asymptomatic or have general flu-like symptoms similar to hepatitis A. About 10% have fatigue, nausea, and anorexia (Hunt, Carson, and Sharara, 1997). HCV infection is confirmed by the presence of anti-C antibody during laboratory testing. Testing for hepatitis C is not done widely (Freitag-Koontz, 1996); however, screening of high risk patients is recommended (Hunt, Carson, and Sharara, 1997).

Interferon alfa-2b is the main therapy for HCV infection, although effectiveness of this treatment varies. Currently there is no vaccine for use with hepatitis C. Transmission of HCV through breastfeeding has not been reported.

Human Immunodeficiency Virus. Although HIV has been thought of as a disease primarily related to homosexual behavior, heterosexual transmission is now the most common means of transmission in women. Furthermore, women are now the fastest-growing population of individuals with HIV infection and acquired immunodeficiency syndrome (AIDS) (Wortley and Flemming, 1997). In 1993, AIDS became the fourth leading cause of death in the United States in women ages 25 to 44 years. In many larger cities on the East Coast it is the leading cause of death (Cotton and Watts, 1997).

Transmission of HIV, a retrovirus, occurs primarily through exchange of body fluids (e.g., semen, blood, or vaginal secretions). Severe depression of the cellular immune system associated with HIV infection characterizes AIDS. Although behaviors that place women at risk have been well documented, all women should be assessed for the possibility of HIV exposure. Until recently HIV infection has commonly been reported at a later disease stage in women; however, this is changing with revised CDC definitions of AIDS. For both men and women, the most commonly reported opportunistic diseases are *Pneumocystis carinii* pneumonia (PCP), candida esophagitis, and wasting syndrome. Other viral infections such as HSV and cytomegalovirus infections seem to be more prevalent in women than men (Wildschut, Weiner, and Peters, 1996). PID may be more severe in HIV-infected women, and rates of HPV and cervical dysplasia may be higher. The clinical course of HPV infection in women with HIV infection is accelerated, and recurrence is more frequent.

Once HIV enters the body, seroconversion to HIV positivity usually occurs within 6 to 12 weeks. Although HIV seroconversion may be totally asymptomatic, it usually is accompanied by a viremic, influenza-like response. Symptoms include fever, headache, night sweats, malaise, generalized lymphadenopathy, myalgias, nausea, diarrhea, weight loss, sore throat, and rash.

Laboratory studies may reveal leukopenia, thrombocytopenia, anemia, and an elevated erythrocyte sedimentation rate. HIV has a strong affinity for surface-marker proteins on T lymphocytes. This affinity leads to significant T-cell destruction. Both clinical and epidemiologic studies have shown that declining CD4 levels are strongly associated with increased incidence of AIDS-related diseases and death in many different groups of HIV-infected persons (Cotton and Watts, 1997).

Screening and Diagnosis. Screening, teaching, and counseling regarding HIV risk factors, indications for being tested, and testing are major roles for nurses caring for women today. A number of behaviors that place women at risk for HIV infection have been identified. These include intravenous drug use, high risk sexual partners, multiple sex partners, and a previous history of multiple STIs. HIV infection is usually diagnosed by using HIV-1 antibody tests. Antibody testing is done first with a sensitive screening test such as the enzyme immunoassay. Reactive screening tests must be confirmed by an additional test, such as the Western blot or an immunofluorescence assay. If a positive antibody test is confirmed by a supplemental test, it means that a woman is infected with HIV and is capable of infecting others. HIV antibodies are detectable in at least 95% of patients within 6 months after infection. Although a negative antibody test usually indicates that a person is not infected, antibody tests cannot exclude infection that occurred less than 6 months before the test. Because HIV antibody crosses the placenta, its presence in children less than 18 months of age is not diagnostic of HIV infection (Centers for Disease Control and Prevention, 1998a).

CDC guidelines recommend offering HIV testing to all women whose behavior places them at risk for HIV infection (Centers for Disease Control and Prevention, 1998a). It may be useful to allow women to self-select for HIV testing. On entry to the health care system a woman can be handed written information about the risk factors for the AIDS virus and asked to inform the nurse if she believes she is at risk. She should be told that she does not have to say why she may be at risk, only that she thinks she might be.

Counseling for HIV Testing. Counseling before and after HIV testing is standard nursing practice today. It is a nursing responsibility to assess a woman's understanding of the information such a test would provide and to be sure the patient thoroughly understands the emotional, legal, and medical implications of a positive or negative test before she is ready to take an HIV test. One's life is profoundly altered by knowledge of HIV seropositivity. A unique stigma is associated with HIV infection that can have a profound impact on the quality of life of those infected. This stigma extends to those who are asymptomatic but seropositive.

Pregnancy is not encouraged for women who are HIV positive. Preconception counseling is recommended; contraceptive counseling should be offered to HIV-positive women who do not desire pregnancy. HIV-infected women should be informed specifically about the risks for perinatal infection. Current evidence indicates that 15% to 25% of infants born to untreated HIV-infected women are infected with HIV; the virus also can be transmitted through breastfeeding (Centers for Disease Control and Prevention, 1998a).

All pregnant women should be offered HIV testing as early in pregnancy as possible (Centers for Disease Control and Prevention, 1995). This recommendation is essential because of the available treatments that can reduce the likelihood of perinatal transmission and maintain the health of the woman. HIV-infected women should be specifically informed about the risks for perinatal transmission. Insufficient information is available regarding the safety of zidovudine or any other antiretroviral drugs during early pregnancy; however, zidovudine is indicated for the prevention of maternal-fetal HIV transmission. Zidovudine reduces transmission risk to 8% if given in late pregnancy, during labor, and to infants for the first 6 weeks of life (Centers for Disease Control and Prevention, 1994). Therefore zidovudine treatment should be offered to all HIV-positive pregnant women. Current protocol includes oral zidovudine at 14 to 34 weeks of gestation, intravenous zidovudine during labor, and zidovudine syrup to the neonate after birth (Centers for Disease Control and Prevention, 1998a). Elective cesarean birth has been found to decrease perinatal transmission of HIV (Elective caesarean-section, 1999; Towers et al, 1998). HIV-infected women should be advised not to breastfeed their infants because the virus is transmitted through breast milk.

Given the strong social stigma attached to HIV infection, nurses must consider confidentiality and documentation before providing counseling and offering HIV testing to patients.

LEGAL TIP • HIV Testing If test results are placed in the woman's chart—the appropriate place for all health information—they are available to all who have access to the chart. The woman must be informed of this before testing. Informed consent must be obtained before an HIV test is performed. In some states written consent is mandated. All pretest and posttest counseling should be documented.

There is generally a 1- to 3-week waiting period after testing for HIV, and this can be a very anxious time for the woman. It is helpful if the nurse informs her that this time period between blood drawing and test results is routine. Test results, whatever they are, must always be communicated in person, and women should be informed in advance that this is the procedure. Whenever possible, the person who provided the pretest counseling should also tell the woman her test results. Some women, when informed of negative results, may escalate risk behaviors because they equate negativity with immunity. Others may believe that negative means "bad" and positive means "good." The woman's reaction to a negative test should be explored by asking, "How do you feel?" HIV-negative result counseling sessions are another opportunity to provide education. Emphasis can be placed on ways in which a woman can remain HIV free. She should be reminded that if she has been exposed to HIV in the past 6 months she should be retested, and that she should have ongoing testing if she continues high risk behaviors.

As the number of HIV-infected women escalates, prevention, education, and counseling activities must be directed toward all women. It is very difficult to keep abreast of the ever-changing picture of AIDS. Important sources of information include the following: National AIDS Hot-line, 1-800-342-2437 (English), 1-800-344-7432 (Spanish), 1-800-243-7889 (hearing-impaired); and the National AIDS Information Clearing House, P.O. Box 6003, Rockville, MD 20850, 1-800-458-5231.

Management. During the initial contact with an HIV-infected woman, the nurse should establish what the woman knows about HIV infection. The nurse should ensure that the woman is being cared for by a medical practitioner or a facility with expertise in caring for persons with HIV infections, including AIDS. Psychologic referral also may be indicated. Resources such as counseling for death and dying, suicide prevention, financial assistance, and legal advocacy may be appropriate. All women who are drug users should be referred to a substance abuse program. A major focus of counseling is prevention of transmission of HIV to partners.

Nurses counseling seropositive women who wish to receive contraceptive information may recommend oral contraceptives and latex condoms, Norplant implants and latex condoms, or tubal sterilization or vasectomy and latex condoms. The IUD is not an ideal choice for the HIV-infected woman, but it is not totally contraindicated (Johnstone, 1997). Insertion in a woman who is immunocompromised should be avoided. Spermicides, female condoms, or abstinence can be offered to women whose partners refuse to use condoms. In a study of female sex workers, nonoxynol-9 did not protect against infection with HIV and may have increased the transmission rate; the CDC is currently revising its prevention guidelines (Gayle, 2000).

No cure is available for HIV infection at this time. Rare and unusual diseases are characteristic of HIV infection. Opportunistic infections and concurrent diseases should be managed vigorously with treatment specific to the infection or disease.

Discussion of the medical care of HIV-positive women and women with AIDS is beyond the scope of this chapter. The reader is referred to the Centers for Disease Control and Prevention, AIDS hotlines, and Internet websites for current information and recommendations.

Group B Streptococcus. Group B streptococcus (GBS) may be considered a normal vaginal flora in a woman who is not pregnant, and is present in 10% to 30% of healthy pregnant women. GBS infection has been suggested as a factor in preterm labor, chorioamnionitis, urinary tract infections during pregnancy, and postpartum infections (Gibbs and Sweet, 1999). Furthermore, GBS infections are an important factor in perinatal and neonatal morbidity and mortality, usually resulting from vertical transmission from the birth canal of the infected mother to the infant during birth (Lieu et al, 1998; Smaill, 2000).

Risk factors for neonatal GBS infection include positive prenatal culture for GBS in the current pregnancy; previous preterm birth of less than 37 weeks of gestation; premature rupture of membranes for longer than 18 hours; intrapartum maternal fever higher than 38° C; and a positive history for early-onset neonatal GBS.

Identification of GBS status during pregnancy is difficult because duration of carrier status is variable. Prenatal screening before the last few weeks of pregnancy may not identify a woman who is a carrier at onset of labor. Current recommendations are to screen all pregnant women for GBS infection at 36 to 37 weeks of gestation. Cultures should be obtained from the anorectal and vaginal areas and not the cervix. To decrease the risk of neonatal GBS infection, it is recommended that all women who develop risk factors for GBS during the antepartum and intrapartum period should be treated during labor (Centers for Disease Control and Prevention, 1996b). In addition, all women who test positive for GBS during the 36- to 37-week screening, or who go into labor before 37 weeks, should be treated. The recommended treatment is penicillin G 5 million units IV loading dose and then 2.5 million units IV every 4 hours during labor. Ampicillin 2 g loading dose IV followed by 1 g IV every 4 hours is an alternative therapy (Home Care box).

Home Care

SEXUALLY TRANSMITTED INFECTIONS

- Take your medication as directed.
- Use comfort measures for symptom relief as suggested by your health care provider.
- Keep your appointment for repeat cultures or checkups after your treatment to make sure your infection is cured.
- Inform your sexual partner(s) to be tested and treated, if necessary.
- Abstain from sexual intercourse until your treatment is completed or for as long as you are advised by your health care provider.
- Use safer sex practices when sexual intercourse is resumed.
- Call your health care provider immediately if you notice bumps, sores, rashes, or discharges.
- Keep all future appointments with your health care provider, even if things appear normal.

Vaginal Infections

Vaginal discharge and itching of the vulva and vagina are among the most common reasons a woman seeks help from a health care provider. Indeed, more women complain of vaginal discharge than any other gynecologic symptom. Vaginal discharge resulting from infection must be distinguished from normal secretions. Normal vaginal secretions (or leukorrhea) are clear to cloudy in appearance. The discharge may turn yellow after drying; is slightly slimy; is nonirritating; and has a mild, inoffensive odor. Normal vaginal secretions are acidic, with a pH range of 3.8 to 4.2. The amount of leukorrhea present differs with phases of the menstrual cycle, with greater amounts occurring at ovulation and just before menses. Leukorrhea is also increased during pregnancy. Normal vaginal secretions contain lactobacilli and epithelial cells. Women who have adequate endogenous or exogenous estrogen will have vaginal secretions.

Abnormal vaginal discharge (or vaginitis) is related to infection by a microorganism. The most common vaginal infections are bacterial vaginosis, candidiasis, and trichomoniasis. Inflammation of the vulva and vagina (or vulvovaginitis) may be caused by vaginal infection; copious amounts of leukorrhea, which can cause maceration of tissues; and chemical irritants, allergens, and foreign bodies, which may produce inflammatory reactions.

Bacterial Vaginosis. Bacterial vaginosis (BV), formerly called nonspecific vaginitis, Haemophilus vaginitis, or Gardnerella, is the most common type of vaginitis today (Plourd, 1997). BV is associated with preterm labor and birth; treatment with antibiotics does not prevent preterm birth in the genera obstetric population (Carey et al, 2000) but does reduce the rate of preterm birth in women with a history of previous preterm birth (Brocklehurst, Hannah, and McDonald, 2000). The exact etiology of BV is unknown. It is a syndrome in which normal H_2O_2 producing lactobacilli are replaced with high concentrations of anaerobic bacteria (e.g., Gardnerella and Mobiluncus). With the proliferation of anaerobes, the level of vaginal amines is raised and the normal acidic pH of the vagina is altered. Epithelial cells slough and numerous bacteria attach to their surfaces (clue cells). When the amines are volatilized, the characteristic odor of BV occurs.

Most, but not all, women with BV complain of a characteristic "fishy odor." The odor may be noticed by the woman or her partner after heterosexual intercourse because semen releases the vaginal amines. When present, the BV discharge is usually profuse; thin; and white, gray, or milky in appearance. Some women also may experience mild irritation or pruritus.

Screening and Diagnosis. A careful history may help distinguish BV from other vaginal infections if the woman is symptomatic. Reports of fishy odor and increased thin vaginal discharge are most significant, and report of increased odor after intercourse is also suggestive of BV. Women with previous occurrence of similar symptoms, diagnosis, and treatment should be queried, because women with BV often have been treated incorrectly because of misdiagnosis.

Microscopic examination of vaginal secretions is always done (Table 6-2). Both normal saline and 10% potassium hydroxide smears should be made. The presence of clue cells confirmed by wet smear is highly diagnostic because the phenomenon is specific to BV. Vaginal secretions should be tested for pH and amine odor. Nitrazine paper is sensitive enough to detect a

TABLE 6-2
Wet Smear Tests for Vaginal Infections

Infection	Test	Positive Findings
Trichomoniasis	Saline wet smear (vaginal secretions mixed with normal saline on a glass slide)	Presence of many white blood cell protozoa
Candidiasis	Potassium hydroxide (KOH) prep (vaginal secretions mixed with KOH on a glass slide)	Presence of hyphae and pseudohyphae (buds and branches of yeast cells)
Bacterial vaginosis	Normal saline smear Whiff test (vaginal secretions mixed with KOH)	Presence of clue cells (vaginal epithelial cells coated with bacteria) Release of fishy odor

pH of 4.5 or greater. The fishy odor of BV will be released when KOH is added to vaginal secretions on the lip of the withdrawn speculum.

Management. Treatment of bacterial vaginosis with oral metronidazole (Flagyl) is most effective (Centers for Disease Control and Prevention, 1998a). Metronidazole is an antiprotozoal and antibacterial agent. In the past metronidazole was contraindicated in the first trimester of pregnancy; however, because of the increased risk of preterm birth, current CDC guidelines recommend treatment of all high risk asymptomatic pregnant women, as well as all symptomatic pregnant women (CDC, 1998a). The medication is contraindicated if the woman is breastfeeding because high concentrations have been found in infants. If it is necessary to prescribe metronidazole for the lactating woman, she can suspend breastfeeding temporarily and resume it 48 to 72 hours after taking the last dose. Metronidazole is contraindicated in patients with blood dyscrasia or central nervous system disease because in rare cases it may affect the hematopoietic or central nervous system.

The many side effects of metronidazole include a sharp, unpleasant metallic taste in the mouth; furry tongue; central nervous system reactions; and urinary tract disturbances. When oral metronidazole is taken, the patient is advised not to drink alcoholic beverages because they produce severe side effects of abdominal distress, nausea, vomiting, and headache. Gastrointestinal symptoms are common whether alcohol is consumed or not. Treatment of sexual partners is not recommended because sexual transmission of BV has not been proven (CDC, 1998a).

Candidiasis. Vulvovaginal candidiasis, or yeast infection, is the second most common type of vaginal infection in the United States. Although vaginal candidiasis infections are common in healthy women, those seen in women with HIV infection are often more severe and persistent. Genital candidiasis lesions may be painful, coalescing ulcerations necessitating continuous, prophylactic therapy.

The most common organism is *Candida albicans;* it is estimated that 80% to 95% of the yeast infections in women are caused by this organism. However, in the past 10 years, the incidence of non–*C. albicans* infections has risen steadily. Women with chronic or recurrent infections often are infected with a higher percentage of non–*C. albicans* species than are women who are experiencing their first infection or who have few recurrences.

Numerous factors have been identified as predisposing a woman to yeast infections. These include antibiotic therapy, particularly broad-spectrum antibiotics such as ampicillin, tetracycline, cephalosporins, and metronidazole; diabetes, especially when uncontrolled; pregnancy; obesity; diets high in refined sugars or artificial sweeteners; use of corticosteroids and exogenous hormones; and immunosuppressed states. Clinical observations and research have suggested that tight-fitting clothing and underwear or pantyhose made of nonabsorbent materials create an environment in which a vaginal fungus can grow.

The most common symptom of yeast infection is vulvar and possibly vaginal pruritus. The itching may be mild or intense, may interfere with rest and activities, and may occur during or after intercourse. Some women report a feeling of dryness; others may experience painful urination as the urine flows over the vulva. The latter usually occurs in women who have excoriations resulting from scratching. Most often the discharge is thick, white, lumpy, and cottage cheese–like. The discharge may be found in patches on the vaginal walls, cervix, and labia. Commonly the vulva is red and swollen, as are the labial folds, vagina, and cervix. Although there is no odor characteristic of yeast infections, sometimes a yeasty or musty smell occurs.

Screening and Diagnosis. In addition to a careful history of the woman's symptoms and their onset and course, the history is a valuable screening tool for identifying predisposing risk factors. Physical examination should include a thorough inspection of the vulva and vagina. A speculum examination is always done. Commonly saline and KOH wet smear and vaginal pH are obtained. Vaginal pH is normal with a yeast infection; if the pH is greater than 4.5, trichomoniasis or BV should be suspected. The characteristic pseudohyphae (i.e., bud or branching of a fungus) may be seen on a wet smear done with normal saline; however, these may be confused with other cells and artifacts.

Management. A number of antifungal preparations are available for the treatment of *C. albicans.* In 1990 many of these medications (e.g., Monistat and Gyne-Lotrimin) were made available as over-the-counter agents. The first time a woman suspects that she may have a yeast infection, she should see a health care provider for confirmation of the diagnosis and treatment recommendation. If she experiences another infection, she may wish to purchase an OTC preparation and self-treat. If she elects to do this, she should always be counseled to seek care for numerous recurrent or chronic yeast infections. If vaginal discharge is extremely thick and copious, vaginal debridement with a cotton swab followed by application of vaginal medication may be useful.

Women who have extensive irritation, swelling, and discomfort of the labia and vulva may find sitz baths helpful in decreasing inflammation and increasing comfort. Adding Aveeno powder to the bath may also increase the woman's comfort. Not wearing underpants to bed may help decrease symptoms and prevent recurrences. Completing the full course of treatment as prescribed is essential to removing the pathogen, and women are instructed to continue medication even during menstruation. They should be counseled not to use tampons during menses because the medication will be absorbed by the tampon. If possible, intercourse is avoided during treatment; if this is not feasible, the woman's partner should use a condom to prevent introduction of more organisms. Suggested measures to prevent genital tract infections are outlined in the Guidelines box on page 76.

Trichomoniasis. Trichomonas vaginalis is almost always a sexually transmitted infection. It is also a common cause of vaginal infection (up to 25% of all vaginitis) and discharge and thus is discussed in this section.

Trichomoniasis is caused by *Trichomonas vaginalis,* an anaerobic, one-celled protozoan with characteristic flagella. Although trichomoniasis may be asymptomatic, commonly women experience yellowish to greenish, frothy, mucopurulent, copious, and malodorous discharge. Inflammation of the vulva, vagina, or both may be present, and the woman may complain of irritation and pruritus. Dysuria and dyspareunia are often present. Typically, the discharge worsens during and after menstruation. Often the cervix and vaginal walls demonstrate the characteristic "strawberry spots" or tiny petechiae, and the cervix may bleed on contact. In severe infections, the vaginal walls, cervix, and occasionally the vulva may be acutely inflamed.

Screening and Diagnosis. In addition to obtaining a history of current symptoms, a careful sexual history should be obtained. Any history of similar symptoms in the past and any treatments used should be noted. The nurse should determine whether the patient's partner(s) were treated, and if she has had subsequent sexual relations with new partners.

A speculum examination is always done, even though it may be very uncomfortable for the woman; relaxation techniques and breathing exercises may help the woman with the procedure. Any of the classic signs may or may not be present on physical examination. The typical one-celled flagellate trichomonads are easily distinguished on a normal saline wet prep. Trichomoniasis also may be identified on Pap smears. Because trichomoniasis is an STI, once diagnosis is confirmed, appropriate laboratory studies for other STIs should be carried out.

Management. The recommended treatment is metronidazole, 2 g orally in a single dose (Centers for Disease Control and Prevention, 1998a). Although the male partner is usually asymptomatic, it is recommended that he receive treatment also, because he often harbors the trichomonads in the urethra or prostate. It is important that nurses discuss the importance of partner treatment with patients because it is likely that the infection will recur if partners are not treated.

Women with trichomoniasis need to understand the sexual transmission of this disease. The patient must know that the organism may be present without symptoms being present, perhaps for several months, and that it is not possible to determine when she became infected. Women should be informed of the necessity for treating all sexual partners and helped with ways to raise the issue with their partners.

Infection Control

Infection control measures are essential to protect care providers and to prevent nosocomial infection of patients, regardless of the infectious agent. The risk for occupational transmission varies with the disease. Even when the risk is low, as with HIV, the existence of any risk warrants reasonable precautions. Precautions against airborne disease transmission are available in all health care agencies. Standard Precautions (precautions to use in care of all persons for infection control) and additional precautions for labor and birth settings are listed in Box 6-5.

PROBLEMS OF THE BREAST

Fibrocystic Changes

Approximately 50% of women experience a breast problem at some point in their adult life. The most common benign breast problem is fibrocystic change. Fibrocystic change is not a disease, as previously believed, but a condition found in varying degrees in healthy women's breasts. Fibrocystic change is characterized by lumpiness, with or without tenderness, and usually occurs with changes in the menstrual cycle (Link, 1993).

Approximately 70% of fibrocystic changes are nonproliferative lesions without atypia (i.e., benign growing cells) and the rest are proliferative lesions with atypical hyperplasia. The risk of breast cancer is increased when atypical hyperplasia is present (Edge and Miller, 1994). When fibrocystic breast changes are present in a woman with a family history of breast cancer, the relative risk of breast cancer is increased (Powell and Stelling, 1994).

Etiology. No known etiologic agent is responsible for benign breast disease, although an imbalance of estrogen and progesterone may be responsible. One theory is that estrogen excess and progesterone deficiency in the luteal phase of the menstrual cycle may cause changes in breast tissue. Risk factors are associated with benign breast disease, including nulliparity, low parity, later menopause, and estrogen therapy (Powell and Stelling, 1994).

Clinical Manifestations and Diagnosis. The usual clinical presentation of fibrocystic change is lumpiness in both breasts. However, single simple cysts may also occur. Symptoms usually develop about 1 week before menstruation begins and subside about 1 week after menstruation ends. When symptoms do occur, they include dull, heavy pain and a sense of fullness and tenderness that increases premenstrually (McCool, Stone-Condry, and Bradford, 1998). The woman with fibrocystic change may form cysts that manifest as painful enlarging lumps in her breasts. Cysts are common in premenopausal women who are not receiving estrogen therapy. The cysts are soft on palpation, well differentiated, and movable. Deeper cysts, especially aggregations of cysts, are indistinguishable by palpation from carcinomas, which are malignant growths that infiltrate surrounding tissue.

A first step in the workup of a breast lump is ultrasonography to determine if it is fluid filled or solid. Fluid-filled cysts are aspirated, and the woman is followed on a routine basis for development of other cysts. If the lump is solid, mammography is obtained if the woman is more than 50 years of age. A fine-needle aspirate (FNA) is then performed, regardless of the woman's age, to determine the nature of the lump. In some cases, a core biopsy may need to follow FNA to harvest adequate amounts of tissue for pathologic examination (Link, 1993).

Management. Treatment for fibrocystic change is usually conservative and follows a two-pronged approach. Diet changes and vitamin supplements constitute the first therapy. Although still controversial, some advocate eliminating dimethylxanthines such as caffeine and theophylline. Patients are encouraged to stop consuming coffee, cola, tea, and chocolate, and discontinue certain respiratory drugs to decrease the premenstrual tenderness associated with fibrocystic changes (Love and Lindsey, 1995). Researchers have found no association among cigarette smoking, alcohol consumption, and fibrocystic changes (Powell and Stelling, 1994), although some women do report relief of symptoms by avoiding alcohol and not smoking.

Women also report decreased symptoms with measures such as taking vitamin E supplements and decreasing sodium intake or taking mild diuretics shortly before menses. Other pain relief measures include taking analgesics or nonsteroidal antiinflammatory drugs (NSAIDs) such as ibuprofen, wearing a supportive bra, and applying heat to the breasts. Some women report relief while taking oral contraceptives, but others report worsening of symptoms (Love and Lindsey, 1995).

Women may need to try several approaches for a number of months before improvement is noted. The recommended therapies are based on mostly anecdotal evidence; scientific validation of treatment strategies is lacking.

Box 6-5

Standard Precautions

Medical history and examination cannot reliably identify all persons infected with HIV or other blood-borne pathogens. Standard Precautions should therefore be used consistently in the care of all persons. These precautions apply to blood, body fluids, and all secretions and excretions, except sweat, nonintact skin, and mucous membranes. Standard Precautions are recommended to reduce the risk of transmission of microorganisms from known and unknown sources of infection (Centers for Disease Control and Hospital Infection Control Practices Advisory Committee, 1996).

1. Handwashing is recommended promptly and thoroughly between patient contacts. Hands and other skin surfaces should be washed immediately and thoroughly if contaminated with blood or other body fluids. Hands should be washed immediately after gloves are removed.
2. In addition to handwashing, all health care workers should routinely use appropriate barrier precautions to prevent skin and mucous membrane exposure when contact with blood or other body fluids of any person is anticipated. *Latex gloves* should be worn for touching blood and body fluids, mucous membranes, or nonintact skin of all persons; for handling items or surfaces soiled with blood or body fluids; and for performing venipuncture and other vascular access procedures. Gloves should be changed after contact with each patient. *Masks and protective eyewear* or face shields should be worn during procedures that are likely to generate droplets of blood or other body fluids to prevent exposure of mucous membranes of the mouth, nose, and eyes. *Gown or aprons* should be worn during procedures that are likely to generate splashes of blood or other body fluids.

   Leg coverings, boots, or shoe covers also can be worn to provide protection against splashes and may be recommended for certain procedures such as surgery.
3. All health care workers should take precautions to prevent injuries caused by needles, scalpels, and other sharp instruments or devices during procedures; when cleaning used instruments; during disposal of used needles; and when handling sharp instruments after procedures. *To prevent needle-stick injuries,* needles should not be recapped, purposely bent or broken by hand, removed from disposable syringes, or otherwise manipulated by hand. After they are used, disposable syringes and needles, scalpel blades, and other sharp items should be immediately placed in a puncture-resistant container for disposal; puncture-resistant containers should be located as close as is practical to the use area.
4. Although saliva has not been implicated in HIV transmission, to minimize the need for emergency mouth-to-mouth resuscitation, mouthpieces, resuscitation bags, or other ventilation devices should be available for use in areas in which the need for resuscitation is predictable.
5. Health care workers who have exudative lesions or weeping dermatitis should refrain from all direct patient care and from handling patient care equipment until the condition resolves.

PRECAUTIONS FOR INVASIVE PROCEDURES

An invasive procedure is surgical entry into tissues, cavities, or organs; or repair of major traumatic injuries (1) in an operating or birthing room, emergency department, or out-of-hospital setting, including both physicians' and dentists' offices; and (2) a vaginal or cesarean birth or other invasive obstetric procedure during which bleeding may occur. Standard Precautions, combined with the following precautions, should serve as minimum precautions for all such invasive procedures:

1. All health care workers who participate in invasive procedures must routinely use appropriate barrier precautions to prevent skin and mucous membrane contact with blood and other body fluids of all patients. Gloves and surgical masks must be worn for all invasive procedures. Protective eyewear or face shields should be worn for procedures that commonly result in the generation of droplets, splashing of blood or other body fluids, or the generation of bone chips. Gowns or aprons made of materials that provide an effective barrier should be worn during invasive procedures that are likely to result in the splashing of blood or other body fluids. All health care workers who perform or assist in vaginal or cesarean births should wear gloves and gowns when handling the placenta or the infant until blood and amniotic fluid have been removed from the infant's skin. Gloves should be worn during infant eye prophylaxis, care of the umbilical cord, circumcision site, parenteral procedures, diaper changes, contact with colostrum, and postpartum assessments.
2. If a glove is torn or a needle stick or other injury occurs, the glove should be removed and a new glove used as promptly as patient safety permits; the needle or instrument involved in the incident also should be removed from the sterile field.
3. Any needle stick or other injury should be reported and appropriate treatment obtained as specified by the health care facility.

Surgical removal of nodules is attempted only in selected cases. In the presence of multiple nodules, the surgical approach involves multiple incisions and tissue manipulation and may not prevent the development of more nodules.

Fibroadenomas

The next most common benign condition of the breast is fibroadenoma. Fibroadenomas occur in women from puberty through menopause. Masses are solid, encapsulated, nontender, and most often found in the upper outer quadrant of the breast.

The cause of fibroadenomas is unknown. Fibroadenomas are characterized by discrete, usually solitary lumps less than 3 cm in diameter (Link, 1993). Occasionally the woman with a fibroadenoma will experience tenderness in the tumor during the menstrual cycle (Stelling and Powell, 1994). Fibroadenomas increase in size during pregnancy and decrease in size as the woman ages. However, generally fibroadenomas do not increase in size in response to the menstrual cycle (in contrast to fibrocystic cysts). The mass tends to remain the same size or increase in size slowly over time (McCool, Stone-Condry, and Bradford, 1998).

Diagnosis is made by a review of the history and physical examination. Mammography, ultrasonography, or magnetic resonance imaging (MRI) may be used to determine the type of lesion. FNA may be used to determine the underlying disorder. Surgical excision may be necessary if the lump is suspicious or if the symptoms are severe. Fibroadenomas do not respond to either dietary changes or hormonal therapy. Periodic observation of masses by professional physical examination or mammography may be all that is necessary for those masses not needing surgical intervention.

Lipomas

A lipoma is a tumor, composed of fat, that is soft and has discrete borders. The cause of lipoma is unknown. Lipomas are often found in women over 45 years of age, usually located on the chest wall and breast. They are characterized as palpable soft masses that are mobile and nontender. Mammography can be used to make a diagnosis; biopsy usually is not needed. Lipomas can be surgically excised if removal is desired (Stelling and Powell, 1994).

Nipple Discharge

Nipple discharge is a common occurrence that concerns many women. Although most nipple discharge is physiologic, each woman who has discharge must be evaluated carefully because a small percentage will be found to have a serious endocrine disorder or malignancy. Bilateral, serous discharge expressed during nipple stimulation can be considered a normal finding. Patient education and reassurance are indicated (Jardines, 1996).

Another form of breast discharge not related to malignancy is galactorrhea. Galactorrhea manifests as a bilaterally spontaneous, milky, sticky discharge. It is a normal finding in pregnancy. It can also occur as the result of elevated prolactin levels. Increased prolactin levels may occur as a result of a thyroid disorder, pituitary tumor, or chest wall surgery or trauma. A complete medication history is essential. Oral contraceptives and neuroleptic drugs are known to precipitate galactorrhea in some women. Diagnostic tests that may be indicated included prolactin levels, microscopic analysis of the discharge, a thyroid profile, a pregnancy test, and a mammogram (Hawkins, Roberto-Nichols, and Stanley-Haney, 1997).

Mammary Duct Ectasia

Mammary duct ectasia is an inflammation of the ducts behind the nipple. The cause of mammary duct ectasia is unknown, although chronic inflammation and dilation of the lactiferous ducts has been suggested. It occurs most often in perimenopausal women and is characterized by a nipple discharge that is thick; sticky; and white, brown, green, or purple. Often the patient will experience a burning pain, itching, or a palpable mass behind the nipple.

The workup includes a mammogram and aspiration and culture of fluid. Generally treatment is symptomatic and consists of encouraging good breast hygiene and avoidance of breast stimulation (Nettles-Carlson, 1995). Development of an infection in the inflamed area requires antibiotic therapy, and incision and drainage is necessary if an abscess develops. Treatment also may include a local excision of the affected duct(s) if the woman has no future plans to breastfeed.

Table 6-3 compares common manifestations of benign breast masses.

TABLE 6-3
Comparison of Common Manifestations of Benign Breast Masses

Fibrocystic Changes	Fibroadenoma	Lipoma	Mammary Duct Ectasia
Multiple lumps	Single lump	Single lump	Mass behind nipple
Nodular	Well delineated	Well delineated	Not well delineated
Palpable	Palpable	Palpable	Palpable
Movable	Movable	Movable	Nonmobile
Round, smooth	Round, lobular	Round, lobular	Irregular
Firm or soft	Firm	Soft	Firm
Tenderness influenced by menstrual cycle	Usually asymptomatic	Nontender	Painful, burning itching
Bilateral	Unilateral	Unilateral	Unilateral
May or may not have nipple discharge	No nipple discharge	No nipple discharge	Thick, sticky nipple discharge

Care Management

Assessment should include a careful history and physical examination. The history should focus on risk factors for breast diseases, events related to the breast mass, and health maintenance practices. Risk factors for breast cancer are discussed later in this chapter. Information related to the breast mass should include how, when, and by whom the mass was discovered. The interval between discovery and seeking care is crucial. The answers to these questions can give clues about breast self-examination (BSE) practice and access to care. The nurse should document the following patient information: pain, whether symptoms increase with menses, dietary habits, smoking habits, use of oral contraceptives, regular BSE, and the examination technique used. The patient's emotional status, including her stress level, fears, and concerns, and her ability to cope should also be assessed.

Physical examination may include assessment of the breasts for symmetry, masses (including size, number, consistency, and mobility), and nipple discharge.

Nursing actions might include the following:

- Demonstrate correct BSE technique.
- Discuss the intervals for and facets of breast screening, including professional examination and mammography.
- Provide written educational materials.
- Encourage the verbalization of fears and concerns about treatment and prognosis.
- Provide specific information regarding the woman's condition and treatment, including dietary changes, drug therapy, comfort measures, stress management, and surgery.
- Describe pain-relieving strategies in detail, and collaborate with the primary health care provider to ensure effective pain control.

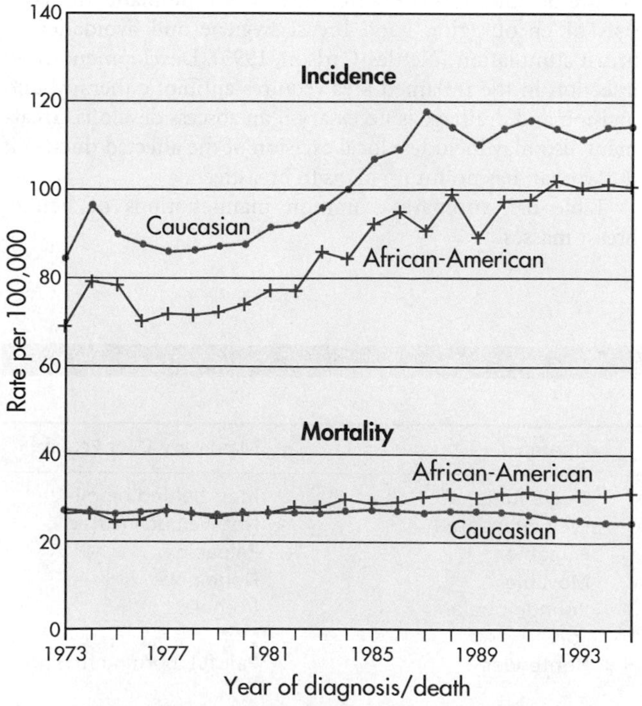

FIG. 6-5 • Breast cancer incidence and mortality rates—Caucasian females vs. African-American females. (Courtesy National Cancer Institute, Washington, DC.)

- Encourage discussion of feelings about body image.
- Refer to a support group or stress management resource if needed to cope with long-term consequences of benign breast conditions.

Malignant Conditions of the Breast

The United States has one of the highest rates of breast carcinoma in the world. One in eight American women will develop breast cancer in her lifetime. The incidence of breast cancer rose about 4% per year beginning in 1980 and leveled off in the 1990s to about 110 cases per 100,000 women. The rising incidence may be related to better detections of early-stage breast cancer. The incidence of breast cancer is higher in Caucasian women than in African-American women, but the mortality rate for African-American women with breast cancer is higher (Fig. 6-5). Even though African-American women practice BSE and obtain clinical breast examinations and mammograms by a professional with a frequency the same as or greater than that of Caucasian women, more African-American women are initially diagnosed with a later stage of breast cancer (Douglass et al, 1995; National Cancer Institute, 1999).

Etiology. Although the exact cause of breast cancer continues to elude investigators, certain factors that increase a women's risk for developing a malignancy have been identified. The factors are listed in Box 6-6.

The most important predictor of risk for breast cancer is age; a woman's risk of breast cancer increases as her age increases. Most of the other risk factors involve the effects of the menstrual-reproductive cycle (probably the effect of estrogen or progesterone) on the development of breast cancer. Fewer menstrual cycles and early childbearing appear to have a protective effect (McCool, Stone-Condry, and Bradford, 1998). Another important variable appears to be related to diet, weight, and exercise. Maintaining normal weight, eating a diet rich in fruits and vegetables and low in fat, and regular exercise seem to exert a protective effect against the development of breast cancer

Box 6-6

Risk Factors for Breast Cancer*

- Age
- Previous history of breast cancer
- Family history of breast cancer, especially a mother or sister (particularly significant if premenopausally)
- Previous history of ovarian, endometrial, colon, or thyroid cancer
- Early menarche (before age 12 years)
- Late menopause (after age 55 years)
- Nulliparity or first pregnancy after age 30 years
- Use of estrogen replacement therapy
- Daily alcohol use
- Obesity after menopause
- Previous history of benign breast disease with epithelial hyperplasia
- Race (Caucasian women have highest incidence)
- High socioeconomic status
- Sedentary lifestyle

*Risk factors are cumulative—the more risk factors present, the greater the likelihood of breast cancer occurring.

(Henderson, 1995; Nicholson, 1996; Stoll, 1996). Many risk factors are additive. However, risk factors help identify fewer than 30% of women who will eventually develop breast cancer. Women at increased risk should be screened more frequently (McCool, Stone-Condry, and Bradford, 1998).

Although most breast cancers are not related to genetic factors, the identification of the BRCA1 and BRCA2 genes has demonstrated the role of heredity and genetic mutations in this disease. Only about 5% of all breast cancers are attributed to heredity, but it is believed that a higher percentage of women with breast cancer before age 40 have abnormalities in the BRCA1 and BRCA2 genes (Daudt, Alberg, and Helzlsouer, 1996).

The ability to test for BRCA1 and BRCA2 has generated heated ethical debate within the health care community. Testing is expensive and often not covered by insurance. The questions of who should be tested and who should pay for it have not been adequately addressed. What to do when a positive result is discovered is not universally agreed upon. Debate also centers around how often screening should be performed; whether prophylactic mastectomies should be recommended; and whether there would be employment discrimination if this information is contained in a woman's medical record. Women requesting testing must be fully informed of the possible risks and benefits of testing before consenting to the procedure (Burke et al, 1997).

There has been much discussion about possible links between breast cancer and hormonal therapy. Although studies are conflicting, a number of researchers believe there may be an increased risk of breast cancer associated with the use of estrogen therapies (Helzlsouer and Couzi, 1995). The safest course of action for women with a history of breast cancer is to avoid estrogen and progesterone replacement therapy (Isaacs and Swain, 1994).

Clinical Manifestations and Diagnosis. It is estimated that 90% of all breast lumps are detected by the woman. Of this 90%, only 20% to 25% are malignant. More than half of all lumps are discovered in the upper outer quadrant of the breast (Fig. 6-6). The most common initial symptom is a lump or thickening of the breast. The lump may feel hard and fixed or soft and spongy. It may have well-defined or irregular borders. It may be fixed to the skin, thereby causing dimpling to occur. A unilateral nipple discharge that is spontaneous (i.e., without nipple stimulation) and bloody or clear also may be present.

Early detection and diagnosis reduces the mortality rate because the cancer is found when it is smaller, lesions are more localized, and there tends to be a lower percentage of positive nodes. Regular BSE, the use of clinical examination by a qualified health care provider, and screening mammography may aid in the early detection of breast cancers.

When a suspicious finding on mammogram is noted, or when a lump is detected, diagnosis is confirmed by FNA or by a needle localization biopsy. The latter procedure requires the collaborative efforts of both the radiologist and the surgeon and may take place in two different environments (i.e., radiology and surgery). Patients need specific information regarding procedures, duration, and outcomes.

Many studies support the theory that breast cancer is a systemic disease; micrometastasis could be present at the initial presentation with or without nodal involvement (Fiorica, 1997). However, nodal involvement and tumor size are the most significant prognostic criteria for long term survival. Women with estrogen receptor (ER) tumors respond better to therapy and have higher survival rates.

Management. Medical management of breast cancer includes surgery, breast reconstruction, radiation therapy, adjuvant hormone therapy, and chemotherapy.

Surgery. The most commonly recommended surgical approaches are lumpectomy and modified radical mastectomy (Fig. 6-7). Lumpectomy (also called tylectomy, partial mastectomy, or segmental mastectomy) involves the removal of the breast tumor, a small amount of surrounding tissue, and a sampling of axillary lymph nodes, leaving the pectoralis major muscle intact. Modified radical mastectomy is the removal of the entire breast and a sample of lymph nodes, sparing the pectoral muscles. The woman's selection of option should be based on an informed choice; a decision board was developed to provide information on the benefits and risks of various options (Whelan et al, 1999).

Women who have these surgeries experience cosmetic changes. Change in shape (because of lumpectomy) or loss of a breast results in a change in body image, which can cause significant alterations in perceptions of femininity and sexual image and interest (Fiorica, 1997; Kraus, 1999).

Breast Reconstruction. The goals of surgical breast reconstruction are achievement of symmetry and preservation of body image. Autologous flap reconstruction involves the use of the woman's own tissue to create a breast. The three types of autologous flaps are the latissimus dorsi flap, the transverse rectus abdominis myocutaneous (TRAM) flap, and the inferior gluteus free flap. After the reconstruction is done, postoperative care specific to these procedures focuses on monitoring the skin flap for signs of decreased capillary refill, hematoma, infection, and necrosis. The breast may also be reconstructed using saline-

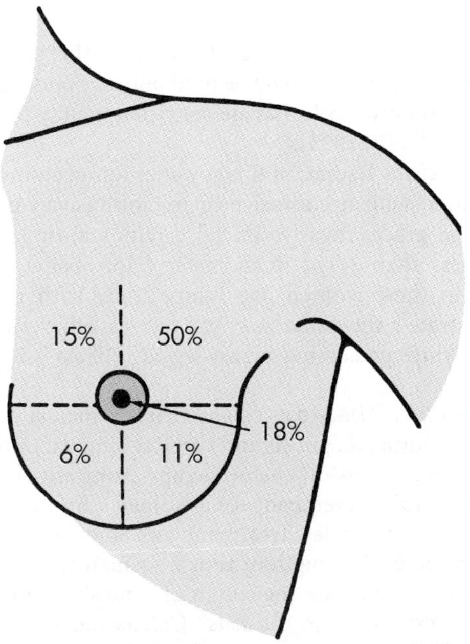

FIG. 6-6 • Relative location of malignant lesions of the breast. (Modified from DiSaia, P, Creasman W: *Clinical gynecologic oncology,* ed 5, St Louis, 1997, Mosby.)

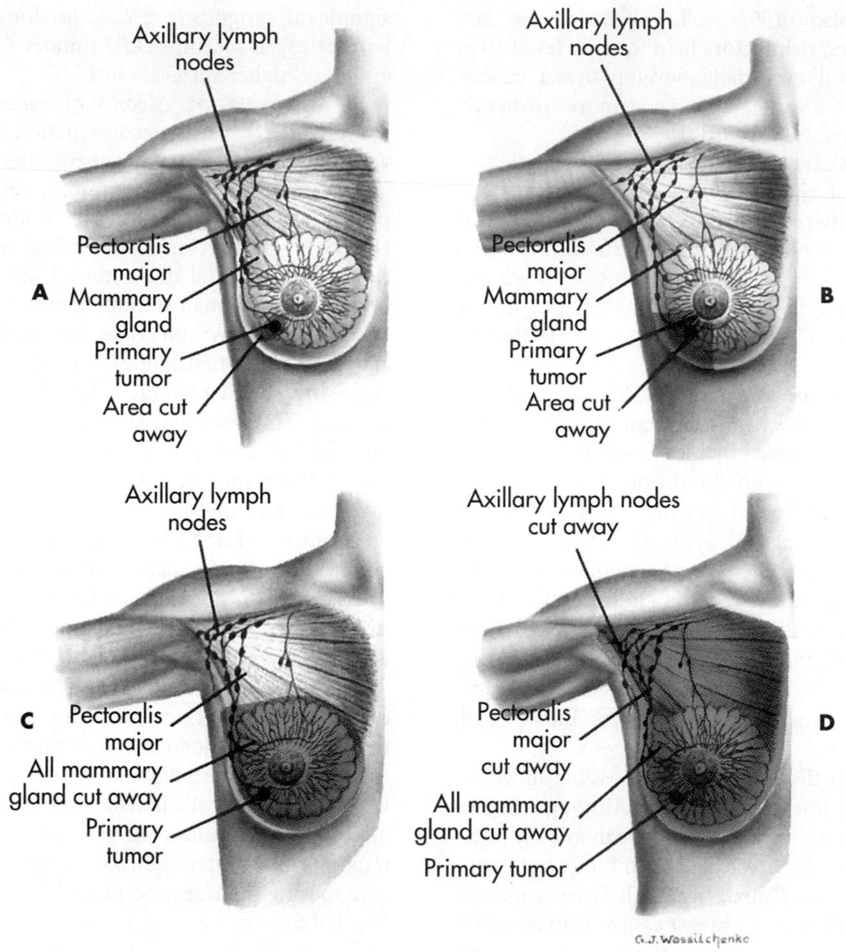

FIG. 6-7 • Surgical alternatives for breast cancer. **A,** Lumpectomy (tylectomy). **B,** Quadrectomy (segmental resection). **C,** Total (simple) mastectomy. **D,** Radical mastectomy.

filled tissue expanders. The safety of silicone breast implants has been questioned. They may be used only in Food and Drug Administration protocols that are restricted mainly to reconstruction (Logothetis, 1995).

Radiation. Radiation therapy after lumpectomy is reserved for women with noninvasive or microinvasive cancer; or any histologic grade, invasive ductal carcinoma, or lobular carcinoma less than 1 cm in diameter (Hortobagyi and Buzdar, 1995). In these women, the lumpectomy with radiation has demonstrated the same survival rate as other surgical techniques while preserving breast tissue (DiSaia and Creasman, 1997).

Adjuvant Therapy. Chemotherapy that is administered soon after initial diagnosis and surgical removal of the tumor is referred to as adjuvant chemotherapy. Adjuvant chemotherapy is most useful in premenopausal women who have breast cancer with positive nodes. Treatment with adjuvant chemotherapy often increases the length of time a woman with breast cancer lives and may increase the length of time she is free of disease (Early Breast Cancer Trialists' Collaborative Group, 1992; Hacker, 1998). Adjuvant chemotherapy may be given alone or with hormonal therapy.

Tamoxifen is an oral antiestrogen medication that mimics progesterone and estrogen. Tamoxifen attaches to the hormone receptors on cancer cells and prevents natural hormones from attaching to the receptors (McKeon, 1997). When tamoxifen fits into the receptors, the cell is unable to grow. Adjuvant hormonal therapy using tamoxifen, recommended for all women over 50 years of age, improves disease-free survival and in some cases length of survival.

Chemotherapy drugs are most effective when used in combination. Chemotherapy drugs include Cytoxan, methotrexate, 5-fluorouracil, cyclophosphamide, doxorubicin, and epirubicin. These chemotherapy drugs can cause leukopenia, neutropenia, thrombocytopenia, anemia, gastrointestinal side effects (e.g., nausea, vomiting, anorexia, and mucositis), and partial or full hair loss.

Care Management. Preoperatively, women need to be assessed for psychologic preparation and specific teaching needs. A visit from a woman who has had a similar experience may be beneficial preoperatively, as well as postoperatively.

Postoperative nursing care focuses on recovery. Precautions should be taken to avoid measuring the blood pressure, giving injections, or taking blood from the arm on the affected side. The woman may have drainage tubes from the incision site that will need to be assessed and drained. Incisional care may include dressing changes. If postoperative arm exercises are appropriate, these may be initiated during the early postoperative

Home Care

AFTER A MASTECTOMY

Wash hands well before and after touching incision area or drains.

Empty surgical drains twice a day and as needed, recording the date, time, drain site (if more than one drain is present), and amount of drainage in milliliters in a diary you will take to each surgical checkup until your drains are removed. (Before discharge, you may receive a graduated container for emptying drains and measuring drainage.)

Avoid driving, lifting more than 10 pounds, or reaching above your head until given permission by surgeon.

Take medications for pain as soon as pain begins.

Perform arm exercises as directed.

Call physician if inflammation of incision or swelling of the incision or the arm occurs.

Avoid tight clothing, tight jewelry, and other causes of decreased circulation in the affected arm.

Until drains are removed, wear loose-fitting underwear (camisole or half-slip) and clothes, pinning surgical drains inside of clothing. (You will be taught how to do this safely.)

After drains are removed and surgical sites are healing and still tender, wear a mastectomy bra or camisole with a cotton-filled, muslin temporary prosthesis. Temporary prostheses of this type are often available from Reach to Recovery.

Avoid depilatory creams, strong deodorants, and shaving of affected chest area, axilla, and arm.

Sponge bathe until drains are removed.

Return to the surgeon's office for incision check, drain inspection, and possible drain removal as directed.

Contact Reach to Recovery for assistance obtaining external prosthesis and lingerie when dressings, drains, and staples are removed and wound is healing and nontender.

Contact insurance company for information about coverage of prosthesis and wig if needed. Obtain prescriptions for prosthesis and wig to submit with receipts of purchase for these items to the insurance company. If insurance does not pay for these items, contact hospital or agency social worker or local American Cancer Society for assistance.

Continue with monthly BSE of unaffected side and affected surgical site and axilla.

Encourage mother, sisters, and daughters (if applicable) to learn and practice monthly BSE and to have annual professional breast examinations and mammography (if appropriate).

Keep follow-up visits for professional examination, mammography, and testing to detect recurrent breast cancer.

Expect decreased sensation and tingling at incision sites and in the affected arm for weeks to months after surgery.

Resume sexual activities as desired.

period. The woman is given self-care instructions and usually discharged to home after 24 hours or more, depending on the type of procedure done (Home Care box). Arm exercises are encouraged at least four times daily (Guidelines box). A referral for home nursing care may be made if the woman needs assistance caring for her incision. A referral to the American Cancer Society's Reach to Recovery program will result in a visit by a breast cancer survivor who has been trained in how to offer information. The resources offered may include such things as a list of sources for prostheses and lingerie.

Concerns about appearance after breast surgery may affect the woman's self-concept. Before surgery, the woman and her partner need information about what the woman's postoperative appearance will be like. Both the woman and her partner need to be able to discuss feelings and concerns about accepting the changes. Information about community resources and support groups such as Reach to Recovery may be beneficial. Invaluable resources are the National Comprehensive Cancer Network (NCCN) and the American Cancer Society, which provide specific, up-to-date recommendations on breast cancer treatments on the Internet.

Care of the woman with breast cancer is effective if the woman verbalizes satisfaction with the decision-making process

Guidelines

POSTMASTECTOMY ARM EXERCISES

Exercise: Climbing the Wall

1. Stand facing wall with toes close to wall.
2. Bend elbows and place palms of hands against wall at shoulder level.
3. Move both hands parallel to each other up the wall as far as possible until incisional pull or pain occurs.
4. Move both hands down to starting position.
5. Goal is complete extension with elbow straight.
6. Perform activities that use the same action: reaching top shelves, hanging out clothes, washing windows, hanging curtains, setting hair.

Exercise: Arm Swinging

1. Bend forward from waist, permitting both arms to relax and hang naturally.
2. Swing arms together left to right (motion comes from shoulder).
3. Swing arms in circles parallel to floor, clockwise and counterclockwise.
4. Straighten up slowly.

Exercise: Rope Pull

1. Attach a rope over a shower rod or hook.
2. Grasp each end of rope, alternately pulling on each end, raising arm on affected side to a point of incisional pull or pain.
3. Shorten rope over time until arm on affected side is raised almost directly overhead.

Exercise: Elbow Spread

1. Clasp hands behind neck.
2. Raise elbows to chin level, holding head erect; move slowly and rest when incisional pull or pain occurs.
3. Gradually spread elbows apart; rest when pull or pain occurs.

From American Cancer Society: *Reach to recovery,* New York, The Society.

Critical Thinking

CHOICES REGARDING RECONSTRUCTIVE SURGERY AFTER MASTECTOMY

Interview a woman who selected reconstructive surgery after mastectomy to treat breast cancer and one who did not select such surgery.

- What were their reasons for their decisions?
- What influence did their partner have on their decision?
- Did their age affect their treatment decision?

What social and community support did they receive to deal with their diagnosis and treatment? How will this information assist you in caring for patients having mastectomy, with or without reconstructive surgery?

Nursing Care Plan THE WOMAN WITH BREAST CANCER

NURSING DIAGNOSIS Pain related to surgical incision and surgical drains as evidenced by patient verbalizations

EXPECTED OUTCOME Patient will report minimal intensity and decreased number of painful episodes.

Nursing Interventions/*Rationales*

Utilize pain scale to assess for type and intensity of pain *to provide accurate database.*

Administer analgesics as ordered *to decrease perception of pain.*

Reposition patient with affected arm elevated *to promote comfort and lymphatic channel return.*

NURSING DIAGNOSIS Risk for infection related to disruption of skin integrity and removal of lymph nodes

EXPECTED OUTCOME Patient will experience no clinical manifestations of infection.

Nursing Interventions/*Rationales*

Assess for clinical manifestations of infection at the incision and drain sites that may include redness, swelling, localized heat, fever, increasing pain, and foul-smelling drainage *to facilitate prompt treatment.*

Demonstrate the procedure for emptying and recording the amount of drainage from the Jackson-Pratt drain(s) *to provide information to the surgeon as to the appropriate removal time of drains. Drains are usually removed when 24 hours of drainage does not exceed 30 ml of fluid.*

Explain the need to avoid trauma or irritation to the affected arm *to reinforce to the patient that alterations in sensation and removal of some lymph nodes may affect ability to sense irritation and prevent infection.*

Reinforce to patient the need to protect arm from injury and to avoid venipunctures or blood pressures to be taken on the affected arm *to avoid trauma and infection, since decreased sensation may be present as well as decreased lymphatic return.*

Explain the importance of reporting any clinical manifestations of infection to the caregiver as soon as possible *to provide identification and treatment of problem.*

NURSING DIAGNOSIS Body-image disturbance related to loss of all or part of a breast as evidenced by patient statements

EXPECTED OUTCOME Patient will maintain a positive body image.

Nursing Interventions/*Rationales*

Provide opportunity through therapeutic communication to express feelings about body image changes *to clarify and validate feelings.*

Provide information about breast prostheses and other cosmetic devices *to assist in maintaining an intact body image.*

Encourage woman to speak to physician about the possibility of breast reconstructive surgery *to provide additional resources for body image enhancement.*

Refer to support groups *to facilitate verbalization of feelings with women who have similar concerns.*

about treatment options and if she gets appropriate support from significant others through all stages of treatment and recovery (Nursing Care Plan).

Key Points

- Menstrual disorders diminish the quality of life for affected women and their families.
- Premenstrual syndrome (PMS) is a disorder that begins in the luteal phase of the menstrual cycle and ends with the onset of menses.
- Endometriosis is characterized by secondary amenorrhea, dyspareunia, abnormal uterine bleeding, and infertility.
- Alternative therapies are beneficial in relieving some discomforts associated with menstrual disorders.
- Safer sex practices are key STI prevention strategies.
- STIs are responsible for substantial mortality and morbidity, great personal suffering, and heavy economic burden in the United States.
- Pregnancy confers no immunity against infection; both mother and fetus must be considered when a pregnant woman contracts an infection.
- Blood and body fluid precautions should be used consistently for everyone all the time.
- Approximately 50% of women experience a breast problem at some point in their adult life; the risk of an American woman developing breast cancer is 1 in 8.
- Monthly BSE, yearly clinical breast examinations by a health care provider, and routine screening mammograms are recommended for early detection of breast cancer.
- Treatment for breast cancer includes surgery, radiation, and chemotherapy.

References

American College of Obstetricians and Gynecologists: *Genital human papillomavirus infections (ACOG Tech Bull No. 194),* Washington, DC, 1994, ACOG.

Ammer C: *The new A-to-Z of woman's health: a concise encyclopedia,* New York, 1989, Facts on File, Inc.

Apgar B: Dysmenorrhea and dysfunctional bleeding, *Prim Care* 24(1):161-178, 1997.

Baker S: Menstruation and related problems and concerns. In Youngkin E, Davis M, editors: *Women's health,* Stamford, CT, 1998, Appleton & Lange.

Birch K, George K: Overtraining the female athlete, *J Bodywork Movement Ther* 3(1):24-29, 1999.

Bonny A, Biro F: Recognizing and treating STDs in adolescent girls, *Contemp Pediatr* 15(3):123,125 passim, 1998.

Borkin M: Avoiding problems with progesterone, *Altern Med* (31):38-42, 44, 47-48 passim, 1999.

Brocklehurst P, Hannah M, McDonald H: Interventions for treating bacterial vaginosis in pregnancy, *Cochrane Database Syst Rev* 2000 (2):CD000262.

Burke W et al: Recommendations for follow-up care of individuals with an inherited predisposition to cancer: BRCA1 and BRCA2, *JAMA* 277(12):997-1003, 1997.

Carey J et al: Metronidazole to prevent preterm delivery in pregnant women with asymptomatic bacterial vaginosis. National Institute of Child Health and Human Development Network of Maternal-Fetal Medicine Units, *N Engl J Med* 342(8):534-540, 2000.

Castiglia P: Amenorrhea, *J Pediatr Health Care* 10(5):226-227, 1996.

Centers for Disease Control and Prevention: Recommendations of the U.S. Public Health Service Task Force on the use of zidovudine to reduce perinatal transmission of human immunodeficiency virus, *MMWR* 43(RR-11), on-line issue, 1994.

Centers for Disease Control and Prevention: Recommendations of the U.S. Public Health Service Task Force for human immunodeficiency virus counseling and voluntary testing for pregnant women, *MMWR* 44(RR-7):1-12, 1995.

Centers for Disease Control and Prevention: Prevention of hepatitis A through active or passive immunization: recommendations of the advisory committee on immunization practice, *MMWR* 45(RR-15):1-30, 1996a.

Centers for Disease Control and Prevention: Prevention of perinatal group B streptococcal disease: a public health perspective, *MMWR* 45(RR-7):1-24, 1996b.

Centers for Disease Control and Prevention: 1998 guidelines for treatment of sexually transmitted diseases, *MMWR* 47(RR-1):1-117, 1998a.

Centers for Disease Control and Prevention: Primary and secondary syphilis—United States, 1997, *MMWR* 47(24): 493-497, 1998b.

Centers for Disease Control and Prevention, Division of STD/HIV Prevention: *Annual report 1994,* U.S. Department of Health and Human Services, Atlanta, 1995, CDC.

Centers for Disease Control and Prevention and Hospital Infection Control Practices Advisory Committee: Special recommendations: guidelines for isolation precautions in hospitals. Part II. Recommendations for isolation precautions in hospitals, *Am J Infect Control* 24(1):24-52, 1996.

Chandraiah S: Premenstrual syndrome. In Blackwell R, editor: *Women's medicine,* Cambridge, MA, 1996, Blackwell Science.

Chuong C, Pearsall-Otey L, Rosenfeld B: A practical guide to relieving PMS, *Contemp Nurse Pract* 1(3):31-34, 36-37, 1995.

Corder-Mabe J: Complications of pregnancy. In Youngkin E, Davis M, editors: *Women's health care: a clinical guide,* ed 2, Stamford, CT, 1998, Appleton & Lange.

Corrarino J: Perinatal hepatitis B: update and recommendations, *MCN Am J Matern Child Nurs* 23(5):246-253, 1998.

Corwin E: Endometriosis: pathology, diagnosis and treatment, *Nurs Pract* 22(10):35-36, 38, 40-42, 45, 48, 50-51, 1997.

Cotton D, Watts D: *The medical management of AIDS in women,* New York, 1997, Willey-Liss.

Daudt A, Alberg A, Helzlsouer K: Epidemiology, prevention, and early detection of breast cancer, *Curr Opin Oncol* 8:455-461, 1996.

DiSaia P, Creasman W: *Clinical gynecologic oncology,* ed 5, St Louis, 1997, Mosby.

Douglass M et al: Breast cancer early detection: differences between African-American and white women's health beliefs and detection practices, *Oncol Nurs Forum* 22(5):835-837, 1995.

Early Breast Cancer Trialists' Collaborative Group: Systemic treatment of early breast cancer by hormonal, cytotoxic or immune therapy: 133 randomized trials involving 31,000 recurrences and 24,000 deaths among 75,000 women, *Lancet* 339:1-15, 71-85, 1992.

Edge V, Miller M: *Women's health care,* St Louis, 1994, Mosby.

Eisenstat S: Infectious exposure and immunization during pregnancy. In Carlson K et al, editors: *Primary care of women,* St Louis, 1995, Mosby.

Elective caesarean-section versus vaginal delivery in prevention of vertical HIV-1 transmission: a randomized clinical trial. The European Mode of Delivery Collaboration, *Lancet* 353(9158):1035-1039, 1999.

Fankenauser M: Treatment of dysmenorrhea and premenstrual syndrome, *J Am Pharmaceutical Association* NS36(8): 503-513, 1996.

Fiorica J: Breast cancer. In Leppert P, Howard F, editors: *Primary care for women,* Philadelphia, 1997, Lippincott-Raven.

Fogel C: Common symptoms. In Fogel C, Woods N, editors: *Women's health care,* Thousand Oaks, CA, 1995b, Sage.

Fogel C: Endocrine causes of amenorrhea, *Primary Care Practice* 1(5):507-518, 1997.

Freitag-Koontz M: Prevention of hepatitis B and C transmission during pregnancy and the first year of life, *J Perinat Neonatal Nurs* 10:40-55, 1996.

Garner C: Infertility. In Fogel C, Woods N, editors: *Women's health care,* Thousand Oaks, CA, 1995, Sage.

Gayle H: *Dear Colleague.* Letter from U.S. Department of Health and Human Services, Public Health Service, Centers for Disease Control, August 4, 2000. Retrieved from http://www.cdc.gov/hiv/pubs/mmwr/mmwr11aug00.htm.

Gibbs R, Sweet R: Maternal and fetal infectious diseases. In Creasy R, Resnik R, editors: *Maternal-fetal medicine,* ed 4, Philadelphia, 1999, WB Saunders.

Hacker N: Breast disease: a gynecologic perspective. In Hacker N, Moore J, editors: *Essentials of obstetrics and gynecology,* ed 3, Philadelphia, 1998, WB Saunders.

Hadfield R et al: Endometriosis in monozygotic twins, *Fertil Steril* 68:941-942, 1997.

Hatcher R et al: *Contraceptive technology,* ed 17, New York, 1998, Ardent Media, Inc.

Hawkins J, Roberto-Nichols D, Stanley-Haney J: *Protocols for nurse practitioners in gynecologic settings,* ed 6, New York, 1997, Tiresias Press.

Helzlsouer K, Couzi R: Hormones and breast cancer, *Cancer* 76(10 Suppl):2059-2062, 1995.

Henderson M: Nutritional aspects of breast cancer, *Cancer* 76(10 Suppl):2053-2058, 1995.

Hillard P: Diagnosing and controlling abnormal uterine bleeding, *Contemporary Adolescent Gynecology* 4(1):4-11, 1999.

Hortobagyi G, Buzdar A: Current status of adjuvant systemic therapy for primary breast cancer: progress and controversy, *CA Cancer J Clin* 45(4):199-226, 1995.

Hunt C, Carson K, Sharara A: Hepatitis C in pregnancy, *Obstet Gynecol* 89(5, pt 2):883-890, 1997.

Institute of Medicine, Committee on Prevention and Control of Sexually Transmitted Diseases: *The hidden epidemic: confronting sexually transmitted diseases,* Washington, DC, 1997, National Academy of Sciences.

Isaacs C, Swain S: Hormone replacement therapy in women with a history of breast cancer, *Hematol Oncol Clin North Am* 8(1):179-195, 1994.

Jardines L: Management of nipple discharge, *American Surgeon* 62:119-122, 1996.

Johnstone F: Contraception for the HIV-infected woman, *J Int Assoc Phys AIDS Care* October 1997:10-15.

Kettel L et al: Preliminary report on the treatment of endometriosis with low-dose mifepristone (RU 486), *Am J Obstet Gynecol* 178: 1151-1156, 1998.

Kraus P: Body image, decision making, and breast cancer treatment, *Cancer Nurs* 22(6):421-429, 1999.

Lieu T et al: Neonatal group B streptococcal infection in a managed care population, *Obstet Gynecol* 92(1):21-27, 1998.

Link J: Benign breast disease, *Nurse Pract Forum* 4(2):96-99, 1993.

Lipscomb G, Ling F: Chronic pelvic pain and dysmenorrhea. In Scott S, McNeeley S, editors: *Gynecology for the primary care provider,* Philadelphia, 1997, WB Saunders.

Logothetis M: Women's reports of breast implant problems and silicone-related illness, *J Obstet Gynecol Neonatal Nurs* 24(7):609-616, 1995.

Love S, Lindsey K: *Dr. Susan Love's breast book,* ed 2, Indianapolis, IN, 1995, Addison-Wesley.

McCool W, Stone-Condry, M, Bradford H: Breast health care: a review, *J Nurse Midwifery* 43(6):406-430, 1998.

McGee G: Secondary amenorrhea leading to osteoporosis: incidence and prevention, *Nurs Pract* 22(5):38, 41-45, 1997.

McKeon V: The breast cancer prevention trial: evaluating tamoxifen's efficacy in preventing breast cancer, *J Obstet Gynecol Neonatal Nurs* 26(1):79-90, 1997.

Mehring P: Dysfunctional uterine bleeding, *Adv Nurse Pract* 5(1):26, 1997.

National Cancer Institute: *Breast cancer information.* Available on-line at: http://www.cancertrials.NCI.NIH.gov. Accessed March 15, 1999.

National Institutes of Health: *Consensus development conference statement on cervical cancer,* April 1-3, Bethesda, MD, 1996, National Institutes of Health.

Nettles-Carlson B: Problems of the breast. In Fogel C, Woods N, editors: *Women's health care,* Thousand Oaks, CA, 1995, Sage.

Nicholson A: Diet and the prevention and treatment of breast cancer, *Alternative Therapies* 2(6):32-38, 1996.

Parazzini F et al: Cigarette smoking, alcohol consumption, and risk of primary dysmenorrhea, *Epidemiology* 5(4):469-472, 1994.

Plourd D: Practical guide to diagnosing and treating vaginitis, *Medscape Women's Health* 2(1):1-13, 1997.

Powell D, Stelling C: *The diagnosis and detection of breast disease,* St Louis, 1994, Mosby.

Rosenfeld R: Treatment of menorrhagia due to dysfunctional uterine bleeding, *Am Fam Physician* 53(1):166-172, 1996.

Ryan I, Taylor R: Endometriosis and infertility: new concepts, *Obstet Gynecol Surv* 52(6):365-371, 1997.

Sangi-Haghpeykar H, Poindexter A: Epidemiology of endometriosis among parous women, *Obstet Gynecol* 85(6): 983-992, 1995.

Schaffer S: Vaginitis and sexually transmitted diseases. In Youngkin E, Davis M, editors: *Women's health: a primary care clinical guide,* ed 2, Stamford, CT, 1998, Appleton & Lange.

Salek et al: Danazol for pelvic pain associated with endometriosis, *The Cochrane Library* (Oxford) issue 1, 2000.

Smaill F: Intrapartum antibiotics for Group B streptococcal colonization, *The Cochrane Library* (Oxford) 2000 issue 1(6p), 2000.

Speroff L, Glass R, Kase N: *Clinical gynecologic endocrinology and infertility,* ed 6, Baltimore, 1999, Lippincott/Williams & Wilkins.

Starr W, Lommel L, Shanon M: *Women's primary health care: protocols for practice,* Washington, DC, 1995, American Nurses Publishing.

Stelling C, Powell D: Circumscribed breast masses. In Powell D, Stelling C, editors: *The diagnosis and detection of breast disease,* St Louis, 1994, Mosby.

Stoll B: Diet and exercise regimens to improve breast carcinoma prognosis, *Cancer* 78(12):2465-2469, 1996.

Taylor D: Effectiveness of professional-peer group treatment: symptom management for women with PMS, *Res Nurs Health* 22(6):496-511, 1999.

Towers CV et al: A "bloodless cesarean section" and perinatal transmission of the human immunodeficiency virus, *Am J Obstet Gynecol* 179(3 Pt 1):708-714, 1998.

Wellbery C: Diagnosis and treatment of endometriosis, *Am Fam Physician* 60(6):1753-1762, 1767-1768, 1999.

West R: The female athlete. The triad of disordered eating, amenorrhea, and osteoporosis, *Sports Med* 26(2):63-71, 1998.

Whelan T et al: Mastectomy or lumpectomy? Helping women make informed choices, *J Clin Oncol* 17(6):1727-1735, 1999.

Wildschut H, Weiner C, Peters T: *When to screen in obstetrics and gynecology,* Philadelphia, 1996, WB Saunders.

Wortley P, Flemming P: AIDS in women in the United States: recent trends, *JAMA* 278(11):911-916, 1997.

Youngkin E: Sexually transmitted diseases: current and emerging trends, *J Obstet Gynecol Neonatal Nurs* 24(8):743-758, 1995.

CHAPTER 7

Infertility, Contraception, and Abortion

http://www.harcourthealth.com/MERLIN/Wong/maternal/

Learning Objectives

On completion of this chapter the reader will be able to:

- List common causes of infertility.
- Discuss the psychologic impact of infertility.
- List common diagnoses and treatments for infertility.
- Compare reproductive alternatives for couples experiencing infertility.
- State the advantages and disadvantages of methods of contraception.
- Explain common nursing interventions that facilitate contraceptive use.
- Describe the techniques used for medical and surgical interruption of pregnancy.
- Recognize ethical, legal, cultural, and religious considerations of infertility, contraception, and elective abortion.

This chapter addresses infertility, associated tests, and common therapies; contraception; and abortion. Available alternatives and psychosocial implications are discussed.

INFERTILITY

Incidence

Infertility is a serious medical concern that affects quality of life and is a problem for 10% to 15% of reproductive-age couples (American Society for Reproductive Medicine, 1999; Hatcher et al, 1998). Infertility implies subfertility, a prolonged time to conceive, as opposed to sterility, or the inability to conceive. A fertile couple has approximately a 25% chance of conception in each ovulatory cycle. Primary infertility applies to a woman who has never been pregnant; secondary infertility applies to a woman who has been pregnant in the past.

The prevalence of infertility is relatively stable among the overall population; in the individual, it increases with the age of the woman. An estimated 1 of every 12 women in the United States is involuntarily childless (Seibel, 1997). Infertility among all childless women older than 35 years is thought to be 21%. Probable causes include the trend toward delaying pregnancy until later in life, when fertility decreases naturally and the incidence of diseases such as endometriosis and ovulatory dysfunction is increased.

The diagnosis and treatment of infertility requires considerable physical, emotional, and financial investment over an extended period. Men and women often perceive infertility differently, with women having more stress from tests and treatments, placing greater importance on having children, being more accepting of indicated treatments, and wanting children more than men (Stephen and Chandra, 1998).

Factors Associated with Infertility

Many factors, in both the male and female, contribute to normal fertility. A normally developed reproductive tract in both the male and female partner is essential. Normal functioning of an intact hypothalamic-pituitary-gonadal axis supports gametogenesis (the formation of sperm and ova). Timing of intercourse is critical: infertility may be caused by something as simple as poor timing or inadequate frequency of intercourse. Although sperm remain viable in the female's reproductive tract for 48 hours or more, probably only a few retain fertilization potential for more than 24 hours. Ova remain viable for about 24 hours, but the optimum time for fertilization may be no more than 1 to 2 hours (Cunningham et al, 1997). Implantation of the blastocyst must occur within 7 to 10 days in a hormone-prepared endometrium. The conceptus must develop normally, reach viability, and be born in good condition for extrauterine life.

An alteration in one or more of these structures, functions, or processes results in some degree of impaired fertility. In general, a female factor such as ovulatory dysfunction or pelvic factors is responsible for infertility in 50% of infertile couples (American Society for Reproductive Medicine, 1999). A male factor (e.g., sperm and semen abnormalities) is responsible for infertility in about 35% of couples. Unexplained factors and unusual problems account for 10% and 5% of infertility, respectively (Mishell et al, 1997; Session et al, 1998). Box 7-1 lists factors affecting female fertility; Box 7-2 lists factors affecting male fertility.

Critical Thinking

INFERTILITY WORKUP

Jane and Andrew are in their early 30s. They have been trying to achieve pregnancy for the 10 years of their marriage. They have come for an infertility workup. What are the psychosocial issues that such a couple is facing? What are likely pressures they are experiencing? Is an infertility workup and in vitro or other assisted reproductive technologies covered by insurance in the state in which you reside? What are myths you have heard about how to achieve pregnancy?

Box 7-1

Factors Affecting Female Fertility

CONGENITAL OR DEVELOPMENTAL FACTORS
Abnormal external genitals
Absence of internal reproductive structures

OVARIAN FACTORS
Anovulation-primary
  Pituitary or hypothalamic hormone disorder
  Adrenal gland disorder
    Congenital adrenal hyperplasia
Anovulation-secondary
  Disruption of hypothalamic-pituitary-ovarian axis
Amenorrhea after discontinuing OCP
Early menopause
Increased prolactin levels

TUBAL/PERITONEAL FACTORS
Tubal motility reduced
Absence of fimbriated end of tube
Absence of a tube
Inflammation within the tube
Tubal adhesions

UTERINE FACTORS
Developmental anomalies
Endometrial and myometrial tumors
Asherman's syndrome (uterine adhesions or scar tissue)

Care Management

➤ Assessment

The nurse assists in the assessment by obtaining data relevant to fertility through interview and physical examination. The database needs to include information to identify whether infertility is primary or secondary. Religious, cultural, and ethnic data are noted because these may place restrictions on tests and treatments.

Some of the data needed to investigate impaired fertility are of a sensitive, personal nature. Obtaining these data may be viewed as an invasion of privacy. The tests and examinations are occasionally painful and intrusive and can take the romance out of lovemaking. A high level of motivation is needed to endure the investigation.

Because multiple factors involving both partners are common, the investigation of impaired fertility is conducted systematically and simultaneously for both male and female partners. Both partners must be interested in the solution to the problem. The medical investigation requires time (e.g., 3 to 4 months) and considerable financial expense. It also causes

Box 7-2

Factors Affecting Male Fertility

STRUCTURAL OR HORMONAL DISORDERS
Undescended testes
Hypospadias
Varicocele
Low testosterone levels
Testicular damage caused by mumps

OTHER FACTORS
Endocrine disorders
Genetic disorders
Psychologic disorders
Sexually transmitted infections
Exposure to workplace hazards such as radiation or toxic substances
Exposure of scrotum to high temperatures

SUBSTANCE ABUSE
Changes in sperm
  Smoking, heroin, marijuana, amyl nitrate, butyl nitrate, ethyl chloride, methaqualone
Monoamine oxidase
Decrease in sperm
  Hypopituitarism
  Debilitating or chronic disease
  Trauma
  Gonadotropic inadequacy

OBSTRUCTIVE LESIONS OF THE EPIDIDYMIS AND VAS DEFERENS

NUTRITIONAL DEFICIENCIES
Decrease in libido
  Heroin, methadone, SSRIs, and barbiturates
Impotence
  Alcohol
  Antihypertensive medications

emotional distress and strain on the couple's interpersonal relationship. Couples should be cautioned that everything can be normal and conception may still not occur; and conversely, that poor test results do not mean a pregnancy will not occur.

Assessment of Female Infertility. Investigation of impaired fertility begins for the woman with a complete history and physical examination. The history explores the duration of infertility and past obstetric events and contains a detailed sexual history. Medical and surgical conditions are evaluated. Exposure to reproductive hazards in the home (e.g., mutagens such as plastic-vinyl chlorides, teratogens such as alcohol, and emotional stresses) and workplace are explored.

A complete general physical examination is followed by a specific assessment of the reproductive tract. The endocrine system is evaluated for abnormalities. Inadequate development of secondary sex characteristics (e.g., inappropriate distribution of body fat and hair) may point to problems with the hypothalamic-pituitary-ovarian axis or genetic aberrations (e.g., polycystic ovarian syndrome or Turner's syndrome).

A woman may have an abnormal uterus and tubes (Fig. 7-1) as a result of in utero exposure to diethylstilbestrol (DES). A history of infection of the genitourinary system is noted. Bimanual examination of internal organs may reveal a lack of mobility of the uterus or abnormal contours of the uterus and adnexa. Laboratory data, including routine urine and blood tests, are assembled.

Diagnosis. The basic infertility survey of the female involves evaluation of the cervix, uterus, tubes, and peritoneum; assessment of immunologic compatibility; and evaluation of psychogenic factors (Angard, 1999; Morell, 1997) (Table 7-1).

TABLE 7-1
Tests for Impaired Fertility

Test/Examination	Timing (Menstrual Cycle Days)	Rationales
Hysterosalpingogram (installation of radioopaque dye in uterus) (Fig. 7-2)	7-10	Late follicular, early proliferative phase; will not disrupt a fertilized ovum; may open uterine tubes before time of ovulation; detect uterine and/or tubal abnormalities
Postcoital test	1-2 days before ovulation	Ovulatory late proliferative phase; look for normal motile sperm in cervical mucus
Sperm immobilization antigen-antibody reaction	Variable, ovulation	Immunologic test to determine sperm and cervical mucus interaction
Assessment of cervical mucus	Variable, ovulation	Cervical mucus should have low viscosity, high spinnbarkeit
Ultrasound diagnosis of follicular collapse	Ovulation	Collapsed follicle is seen after ovulation
Serum assay of plasma progesterone	20-25	Midluteal midsecretory phase; check adequacy of corpus luteal production of progesterone
Hormone analysis	Variable	Determine blood levels of prolactin, FSH, LH, and thyroid hormone
Basal body temperature	Chart entire cycle	Elevation occurs in response to progesterone; documents ovulation
Endometrial biopsy	21-27	Late luteal, late secretory phase; check endometrial response to progesterone and adequacy of luteal phase
Sperm penetration assay	After 2 days but no more than 1 week of abstinence	Evaluation of ability of sperm to penetrate an egg
Laparascopy (Fig. 7-3)	7-12	Detect adhesions, endometriosis, fibroids, etc.; done early in menstrual cycle to prevent disruption of fertilized ovum
Ultrasound	Variable	Abdominal or vaginal ultrasound to detect various pelvic conditions (abnormalities, development of follicles, confirm intrauterine vs. ectopic pregnancy)

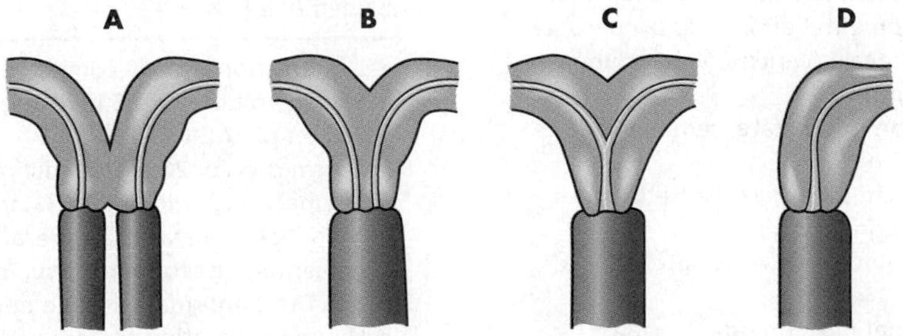

FIG. 7-1 • Abnormal uterus. **A,** Complete bicornuate uterus with vagina divided by a septum. **B,** Complete bicornuate uterus with normal vagina. **C,** Partial bicornuate uterus with normal vagina. **D,** Unicornuate uterus.

Test findings that are favorable to fertility are summarized in Box 7-3.

Assessment of Male Infertility. The systematic investigation of infertility in the male patient begins with a thorough history and physical examination. Assessment of the male patient starts with noninvasive tests.

Semen analysis. The basic test for male infertility is the semen analysis. A complete semen analysis, study of the effects of cervical mucus on sperm forward motility and survival, and evaluation of the sperm's ability to penetrate an ovum provide basic information. Sperm counts vary from day to day and are dependent on emotional and physical status and sexual activity. Therefore a single analysis may be inconclusive (Hargreave and Ghosh, 1998). Usually several specimens taken at monthly intervals are evaluated (Trantham, 1996).

Semen is collected by ejaculation into a clean container or a plastic sheath that does not contain a spermicidal agent (Speroff, Glass, and Kase, 1994). The specimen is usually collected by masturbation following 2 to 5 days of abstinence from ejaculation. The semen is taken to the laboratory in a sealed container within 2 hours of ejaculation. Exposure to excessive heat or cold is avoided. Normal values for semen characteristics are given in Box 7-4.

Hormone analyses are done for testosterone, gonadotropin, follicle-stimulating hormone (FSH) and luteinizing hormone (LH). The sperm penetration assay may be used to evaluate the ability of sperm to penetrate an egg. Because human oocytes are not readily available, hamster eggs are used as a substitute to evaluate sperm penetration abilities (no actual fertilization occurs) (Hargreave and Ghosh, 1998). Testicular biopsy may be warranted.

Assessment of the Couple

Postcoital Test. The postcoital test (PCT), also called the Sims-Huhner test, is one method used to test for adequacy of coital technique, cervical mucus, sperm, and degree of sperm penetration through cervical mucus. The test is performed within several hours after ejaculation of semen into the vagina. A specimen of cervical mucus is obtained from the cervical os and examined under a microscope. The quality of mucus and the number of forward moving sperm are noted. A PCT with good mucus and motile sperm is associated with fertility (Hargreave and Ghosh, 1998).

Intercourse is synchronized with the expected time of ovulation (as determined from evaluation of basal body temperature [BBT], cervical mucus changes, and usual length of menstrual cycle or use of LH detection kit to determine LH surge). Intercourse is performed only in the absence of vaginal infection. Couples may experience some difficulty abstaining from intercourse for 2 to 4 days before expected ovulation, and then having intercourse with ejaculation on schedule. Sex on demand may strain the couple's interpersonal relationship. A problem may arise if the expected day of ovulation occurs when facilities or the physician is unavailable (such as over a weekend or holiday).

Box 7-3

Summary of Findings Favorable to Fertility

1. Follicular development, ovulation, and luteal development are supportive of pregnancy:
   a. BBT (presumptive evidence of ovulatory cycles) is biphasis, with temperature elevation that persists for 12 to 14 days before menstruation
   b. Cervical mucus characteristics change appropriately during phases of menstrual cycle
   c. Laparoscopic visualization of pelvic organs verifies follicular and luteal development
2. The luteal phase is supportive of pregnancy:
   a. Levels of plasma progesterone are adequate
   b. Findings from endometrial biopsy samples are consistent with day of cycle
3. Cervical factors are receptive to sperm during expected time of ovulation:
   a. Cervical os is open
   b. Cervical mucus is clear, watery, abundant, and slippery and demonstrates good spinnbarkeit and arborization (fern pattern)
   c. Cervical examination reveals no lesions or infections
   d. Postcoital test findings are satisfactory (adequate number of live, motile, normal sperm present in cervical mucus)
   e. No immunity to sperm demonstrated
4. The uterus and uterine tubes are supportive of pregnancy:
   a. Uterine and tubal patency are documented by
      (1) Spillage of dye into peritoneal cavity
      (2) Outlines of uterine and tubal cavities of adequate size and shape, with no abnormalities
   b. Laparoscopic examination verifies normal development of internal genitals and absence of adhesions, infections, endometriosis, and other lesions
5. The male partner's reproductive structures are normal:
   a. No evidence of developmental anomalies of penis, testicular atrophy, or varicocele (varicose vein on the spermatic vein in the groin)
   b. No evidence of infection in prostate, seminal vesicles, and urethra
   c. Testes are more than 4 cm in largest diameter
6. Semen is supportive of pregnancy:
   a. Sperm (number per milliliter) are adequate in ejaculate
   b. Most sperm show normal morphology
   c. Most sperm are motile, forward moving
   d. No autoimmunity exists
   e. Seminal fluid is normal

Box 7-4

Semen Analysis

- Liquefaction usually complete within 10 to 20 minutes
- Semen volume 2 to 5 ml (range 1 to 7 ml)
- Semen pH 7.2 to 7.8
- Sperm density 20 to 200 million cells/ml
- Normal morphology, ≥60% normal oval
- Motility (important consideration in sperm evaluation), percentage of forward-moving sperm estimated with respect to abnormally motile and nonmotile sperm ≥50%
- Ovum penetration test (may be done if further evaluation necessary)

NOTE: These values are not absolute, only relative to final evaluation of the couple as a single reproductive unit.

➤ Nursing Diagnoses

Examples of nursing diagnoses related to impaired fertility include the following:

- Body image or self-esteem disturbance related to:
  —Impaired fertility.
- Decisional conflict related to:
  —Therapies for impaired fertility.
  —Alternatives to therapy (e.g., childfree living or adoption).
- Altered patterns of sexuality related to:
  —Loss of libido secondary to medically imposed restrictions.
- Risk for social isolation related to:
  —Impaired fertility, its investigation, and management.

➤ Expected Outcomes

The expected outcomes are phrased in patient-centered terms and may include that the couple will do the following:

- Verbalize understanding of the anatomy and physiology of the reproductive system.
- Verbalize understanding of treatment for any abnormalities identified through various tests and examinations and be able to make an informed decision about treatment.
- Resolve guilt feelings and not need to focus blame.
- Conceive or, failing to conceive, decide on an alternative acceptable to both of them (e.g., childfree living or adoption).

➤ Plan of Care and Implementation

Psychosocial. Within the United States, feelings connected to impaired fertility are numerous and complex. Infertility is recognized as a major life stressor that can affect self-esteem; relations with the spouse, family, and friends; and careers. Couples often need assistance in separating their concepts of personal success and failure from success and failure related to treatment for infertility. The woman or couple facing infertility may exhibit grieving behaviors usually associated with other types of loss. Recognizing the significance of infertility as a loss, and resolving these feelings, is crucial to putting infertility into perspective, even if treatment is successful (Boxer, 1996).

Their psychologic responses to the diagnosis of infertility may tax a couple's capacity for physical and sexual closeness. The prescriptions and proscriptions for achieving conception may add tension to a couple's sexual functioning. Couples may report decreased desire for intercourse, orgasmic dysfunction, or midcycle erectile disorders.

To be able to deal comfortably with a couple's sexuality, nurses must be comfortable with their own sexuality so that they can better help couples understand why the private act of lovemaking needs to be shared with health care professionals. Nurses need up-to-date factual knowledge about human sexual practices, and must be able to accept the preferences and activities of others without being judgmental. They must be skilled in interviewing and in therapeutic use of self, sensitive to the nonverbal cues of others, and knowledgeable regarding each couple's sociocultural and religious tenets (Johnson, 1996).

The support systems of the couple with impaired fertility need to be explored. This exploration should include data about persons available to assist, their relationship to the couple, their ages, their availability, and the cultural or religious support that is available.

If the couple conceives, the concerns and problems of the previously infertile couple may not be over. Many couples are overjoyed with the pregnancy; however, some are not. Some couples rearrange their lives, sense of self, and personal goals within their acceptance of their infertile state. The couple may feel that those who worked with them to identify and treat impaired fertility expect them to be happy with the pregnancy. The couple may be shocked to find that they themselves feel resentment because the pregnancy, once a cherished dream, now necessitates another change in goals, aspirations, and identities. The normal ambivalence toward pregnancy may be perceived as reneging on the original choice to become parents. The couple might choose to abort the pregnancy at this time. Other couples worry about miscarriage. If the couple wishes to continue with the pregnancy, they will need the care other expectant couples need.

If the couple does not conceive, they are assessed regarding their desire to be referred for help with adoption, therapeutic intrauterine insemination, other reproductive alternatives, or choosing a childfree state. The couple may find helpful a list of agencies, support groups, and other resources in their community (Box 7-5).

Nonmedical Therapies. Simple changes in lifestyle may be effective in the treatment of subfertile men. Only water-soluble lubricants should be used during intercourse because many commonly used lubricants contain spermicides or have spermicidal properties. High scrotal temperatures may be caused by daily hot tub baths or saunas that keep the testes at temperatures too high for efficient spermatogenesis. Wearing boxer shorts may be recommended.

Treatment is available for women who have immunologic reactions to sperm. The use of condoms during genital intercourse for 6 to 12 months will reduce female antibody production in most women who have elevated antisperm antibody titers. After the serum reaction subsides, condoms are used at all times except at the expected time of ovulation. Approximately

Box 7-5

Fertility Resources

1. RESOLVE, 1310 Broadway, Somerville, MA 02144, (617) 623-0744
   www.resolve.org
   Counseling, referral, and support for infertile individuals and couples; education and assistance for professionals.
2. American Society for Reproductive Medicine, 1209 Montgomery Hwy., Birmingham, AL 35216
   (205) 978-5000
   www.asrm.org
   Consumer literature is available.
3. International Council on Infertility Information Dissemination, (703) 379-9178
   www.inciid.ord
   Clearinghouse for infertility information.
4. The American College of Obstetricians and Gynecologists (ACOG), 409 12 St., SW, Washington, DC 20024-2188
   (202) 638-5577
   www.acog.org
   Ask for a full list of brochures and publications available for consumers.
5. www.ihr.com
   Infertility organization for consumers.

one third of couples with this problem conceive by following this course of action.

Medical Therapies. Pharmacologic therapy is often an expensive but important component of care for female infertility. Ovulatory stimulants may be warranted to induce ovulation. Clomiphene (Clomid, Serophene), an oral preparation, stimulates the ovarian follicle. It is used to treat anovulation caused by hypothalamic suppression when the hypothalamic-pituitary-ovarian axis is intact. Multifetal pregnancy rates are less than 10%, with most being twin gestations. Bromocriptine (Parlodel), a synthetic ergot alkaloid that inhibits the release of prolactin, is used to treat anovulation caused by elevated levels of prolactin. Thyroid stimulating hormone (Synthroid) is indicated if the woman has hypothyroidism.

Human menopausal gonadotropin (Pergonal) or pure FSH (Metrodin) is used when clomiphene fails to induce ovulation or when pregnancy has not been achieved in 6 to 12 ovulatory cycles. These medications are extremely potent and require daily monitoring with ovarian ultrasonography and monitoring of estradiol levels to prevent hyperstimulation (Angard, 1999). The incidence of multiple pregnancy with the use of these medications is greater than 25%. When ovulation is caused either by hypothalamic-pituitary dysfunction or failure, or failure to respond to clomiphene, gonadotropin-releasing hormone (GnRH) may be used.

Hormone replacement therapy may be indicated. The woman who has low estrogen levels is a candidate for conjugated estrogens and medroxyprogesterone. A hypoestrogenic condition may result from a high stress level or from a decreased percentage of body fat as a result of an eating disorder (e.g., anorexia nervosa) or excessive exercise. Hydroxyprogesterone supplementation with vaginal suppositories or intramuscular injection is used to treat luteal phase defects. In the presence of adrenal hyperplasia, prednisone, a glucocorticoid, is taken orally. Treatment of endometriosis may include danazol, progesterones, combined oral contraceptives, or gonadotropin-releasing hormone agonists (Session et al, 1998; Speroff, Glass, and Kase, 1994). Infections are treated with appropriate antimicrobial formulations.

Medications may be indicated for male infertility. Problems with the thyroid or adrenal glands are corrected with appropriate medications. Clomiphene may be given for idiopathic subfertility, although its effectiveness in enhancing fertility rates has been poorly documented. Infections are identified and treated with antimicrobials.

Surgical Treatment. A number of surgical procedures can be used for problems causing female infertility. Ovarian tumors must be excised. Whenever possible, functional ovarian tissue is left intact. Scar tissue adhesions caused by chronic infections may cover much or all of the ovary. These adhesions usually necessitate surgery to free and expose the ovary so that ovulation can occur.

Hysterosalpingography is useful for identification of tubal obstruction and also for the release of blockage (Fig. 7-2). During laparoscopy, delicate adhesions may be divided and removed and endometrial implants may be destroyed by electrocoagulation or laser (Fig. 7-3). Laparotomy and even microsurgery may be required to do extensive repair of the damaged tube. Prognosis is dependent on the degree to which tubal patency and function can be restored.

A woman with a relatively small uterus may become pregnant, but the uterus may then be incapable of accommodating the enlarging fetus and a miscarriage results. In such cases recurrent or habitual (three or more) miscarriages often occur. No medical therapy has been effective for the enlargement of an abnormally small uterus. Observation suggests that women who do become pregnant, but who miscarry, often abort at a later time with each successive pregnancy. After two or three pregnancy losses, they may finally give birth to a viable infant. Apparently, actual growth of the uterus occurs with each pregnancy. Reconstructive surgery (e.g., the unification operation for bicornuate uterus) often improves a woman's ability to conceive and carry the fetus to term.

Surgical removal of tumors or fibroids involving the endometrium or uterus often improves the woman's chance of

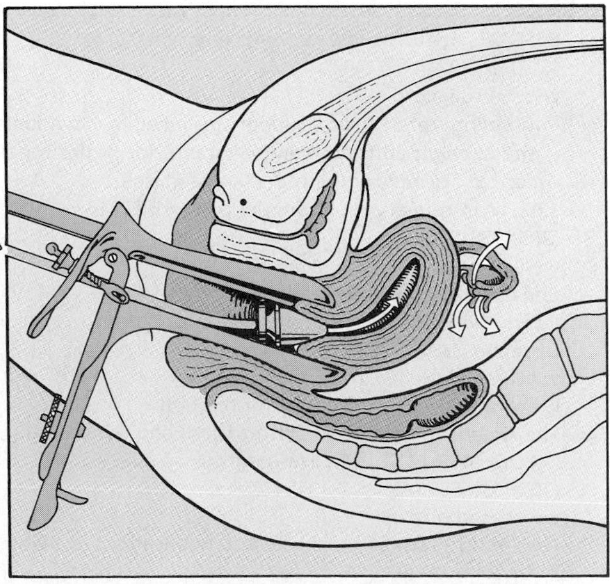

FIG. 7-2 • Hysterosalpingography. Note contrast medium flows through intrauterine cannula and out through the uterine tubes.

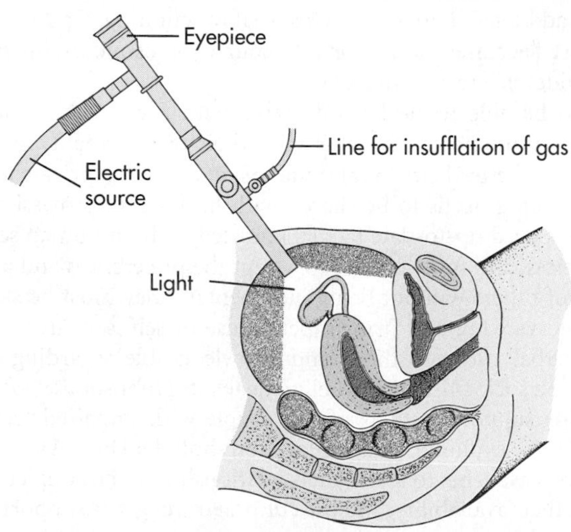

FIG. 7-3 • Laparoscopy.

conceiving and maintaining the pregnancy to viability. Surgical treatment of uterine tumors or maldevelopment that results in successful pregnancy usually requires birth by cesarean surgery near term gestation. The uterus may rupture as a result of weakness in the area of surgical healing.

Chronic inflammation and infection can be eliminated by radial chemocautery (destruction of tissue with chemicals) or thermocautery (destruction of tissue with heat, usually electrical) of the cervix; cryosurgery (destruction of tissue by application of extreme cold, usually liquid nitrogen); or conization (excision of a cone-shaped piece of tissue from the endocervix). When the cervix has been deeply cauterized or frozen, or when extensive conization has been performed, extreme limitation of mucous production by the cervix may result. The absence of a mucous bridge from the vagina to the uterus may therefore make sperm migration difficult or impossible. Therapeutic intrauterine insemination may be necessary to carry the sperm directly through the internal os of the cervix.

Surgical procedures may also be used for problems causing male infertility. Surgical repair of varicocele has been relatively successful in increasing sperm count but not fertility rates. A varicocele on the left side is found in a substantial number of subfertile men.

Microsurgery to reanastomose (restore tubal continuity) the sperm ducts can result in pregnancy rates greater than 50% (Speroff, Glass, and Kase, 1994). The rate of success decreases as the time since the procedure increases.

Reproductive Alternatives

There have been remarkable developments in reproductive medicine. Assisted reproductive therapies (ARTs) are creating ethical and legal dilemmas. The lack of information, or misleading information about success rates and the risks and benefits of treatment alternatives, prevents couples from making informed decisions. Some of the ARTs for treatment of infertility include in vitro fertilization-embryo transfer (IVF-ET), gamete intrafallopian transfer (GIFT) (Fig. 7-4), zygote intrafallopian transfer (ZIFT), ovum transfer (oocyte donation), embryo adoption, embryo hosting, and surrogate parenting. Table 7-2 describes these procedures and the possible indications for ARTs. Other options include intracytoplasmic sperm injection, assisted hatching, therapeutic donor insemination (TDI), adoption, and surrogate mothering.

LEGAL TIP • Cryopreservation of Human Embryos
Couples who have excess embryos frozen for later transfer must be fully informed before consenting to the procedure, to make decisions regarding the disposal of embryos in the event of death, divorce, or the decision that the couple no longer wants the embryos at a later time.

Complications. Other than the established risks associated with laparoscopy and general anesthesia, few risks are associated with IVF-ET, GIFT, and ZIFT. The more common transvaginal needle aspiration requires only local or intravenous analgesia. Congenital anomalies occur no more frequently than among naturally conceived embryos. Ectopic pregnancies do occur more often, however, and these carry a significant maternal risk. There is no increase in maternal or perinatal complications with TDI; the same incidences of anomalies (about 5%) and obstetric complications (between 5% and 10%) that accompany natural insemination (i.e., through sexual intercourse) also apply to TDI.

Preimplantation Genetic Diagnosis. Preimplantation genetic diagnosis (PGD) is a form of early genetic testing designed to eliminate embryos with serious genetic diseases before implantation through one of the ARTs. There are over 20 centers around the world where PGD is being used clinically. By avoiding implantation of defective embryos, future termination of pregnancy for genetic reasons is eliminated (Fasouliotis and Schenker, 1999; Harper and Wells, 1999). Jones and Krysa (1998) suggest comfort care interventions to enable families at risk to use available technologies. Experts caution that use of

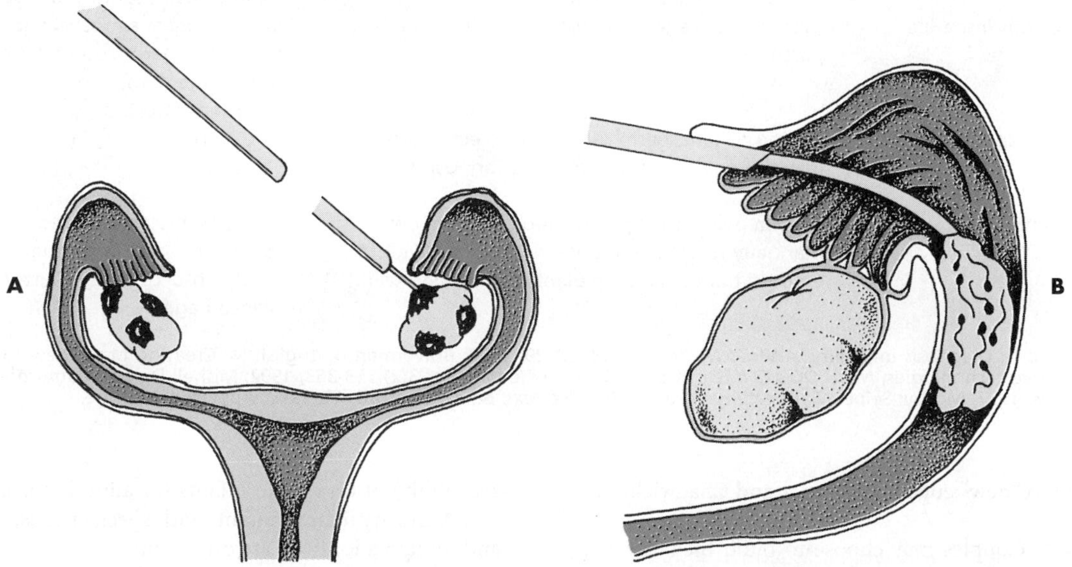

FIG. 7-4 • GIFT. **A,** Through laparoscopy, a ripe follicle is located and fluid containing the egg is removed. **B,** The sperm and egg are placed separately in the uterine tube, where fertilization occurs.

TABLE 7-2
Assisted Reproductive Therapies (ARTs)

Procedure	Definition	Indications
In vitro fertilization-embryo transfer (IVF-ET)	A woman's eggs are collected from her ovaries, fertilized in the laboratory with sperm, and transferred to her uterus after normal embryo development has occurred.	Tubal disease or blockage; severe male infertility; endometriosis; unexplained infertility; cervical factor; immunologic infertility
Gamete intrafallopian transfer (GIFT)	Oocytes are retrieved from the ovary, placed in a catheter with washed motile sperm, and immediately transferred into the fimbriated end of the uterine tube. Fertilization occurs in the uterine tube.	Same as for IVF-ET, *except* there must be normal tubal anatomy, patency, and absence of previous tubal disease in at least one uterine tube
IVF-ET and GIFT with donor sperm	This process is the same as described above except in cases where the husband's fertility is severely compromised and donor sperm can be used; if donor sperm are used, the wife must have indications for IVF and GIFT.	Severe male infertility; azoospermia; indications for IVF-ET or GIFT
Zygote intrafallopian transfer (ZIFT)	This process is similar to IVF-ET; after in vitro fertilization the ova are placed in one uterine tube during the zygote stage.	Same as for GIFT
Donor oocyte	Eggs are donated by an IVF procedure, and the donated eggs are inseminated. The embryos are transferred into the recipient's uterus, which is hormonally prepared with estrogen/progesterone therapy.	Early menopause; surgical removal of ovaries; congenitally absent ovaries; autosomal or sex-linked disorders; lack of fertilization in repeated IVF attempts because of subtle oocyte abnormalities or defects in oocyte/spermatozoa interaction
Donor embryo (embryo adoption)	A donated embryo is transferred to the uterus of an infertile woman at the appropriate time (normal or induced) of the menstrual cycle.	Infertility not resolved by less aggressive forms of therapy; absence of ovaries; male partner is azoospermic or is severely compromised
Gestational carrier (embryo host); surrogate mother	A couple undertakes an IVF cycle and the embryo(s) is transferred to another woman's uterus (the carrier) who has contracted with the couple to carry the baby to term. The carrier has no genetic investment in the child. Surrogate motherhood is a process by which a woman is inseminated with semen from the infertile woman's partner and then carries the baby until birth.	Congenital absence or surgical removal of uterus; a reproductively impaired uterus, myomas, uterine adhesions, or other congenital abnormalities; a medical condition that might be life-threatening during pregnancy, such as diabetes, immunologic problems, or severe heart, kidney, or liver disease
Therapeutic donor insemination (TDI)	Donor sperm are used to inseminate the female partner.	Male partner is azoospermic or has a very low sperm count; couple has a genetic defect; male partner has antisperm antibodies
Intracytoplasmic sperm injection	Selection of one sperm cell that is injected directly into the egg to achieve fertilization. Used with IVF.	Same as TDI
Assisted hatching	The zona pellucida is penetrated chemically or manually to create an opening for the dividing embryo to hatch and implant into uterine wall.	Recurrent miscarriages; to improve implantation rate in women with previously unsuccessful IVF attempts; advanced age

Data from Angard N: Diagnosis infertility, *AWHONN Lifelines* 3(3):22–29, 1999; Braverman A, English M: Creating brave new families with advanced reproductive technologies, *NAACOG's Clin Issu Perinat Womens Health Nurs* 3(2):353-363, 1992; Mishell D et al: *Comprehensive gynecology,* ed 3, St Louis, 1997, Mosby; Seibel M: *Infertility: a comprehensive text,* ed 2, Stamford, CT, 1997, Appleton & Lange.

PGD may lead to "new" eugenics (Draper and Chadwick, 1999; King, 1999).

Adoption. Couples may choose to build their family by adopting children who are not their own biologically. However, with increased availability of birth control and abortion, and an increase in single mothers who choose to keep their babies, the availability of Caucasian infants for adoption is extremely limited. Minority infants, infants with special needs, older children, and foreign adoptions are other options.

Couples who seek to adopt a child have decided that being a parent of a child is more important than the actual process of birthing the child. The birth process is a very small aspect of

Nursing Care Plan THE COUPLE EXPERIENCING INFERTILITY

NURSING DIAGNOSIS Knowledge deficit related to lack of understanding of the reproductive process with regard to conception as evidenced by patient questions

EXPECTED OUTCOME Patient and partner will verbalize understanding of the components of the reproductive process, common problems leading to infertility, usual infertility testing, and the importance of completing testing in a timely manner.

Nursing Interventions/*Rationales*

Assess woman's current level of understanding of the factors promoting conception *to identify gaps or misconceptions in knowledge base.*

Provide information in a supportive manner regarding factors promoting conception including common factors leading to infertility of either partner *to raise couples' awareness and promote trust in caregiver.*

Identify and describe the basic infertility tests and the rationale for precise scheduling *to enhance completion of the diagnostic phase of the infertility workup.*

NURSING DIAGNOSIS Risk for ineffective individual/family coping related to inability to conceive as evidenced by patient and partner statements

EXPECTED OUTCOME Patient and partner will identify situational stressors and positive coping methods to deal with testing and unknown outcomes.

Nursing Interventions/*Rationales*

Provide opportunities through therapeutic communication to discuss feelings and concerns *to identify common feelings and perceived stressors.*

Evaluate couple's support system, including support of each other during this process *to identify any barriers to effective coping.*

Identify support groups and refer as needed *to enhance coping by sharing experiences with other couples experiencing similar problems.*

having a baby and becoming a parent. The question to be answered by couples who want to adopt is, "Do you want to have a baby, or do you want to become parents?"

Surrogate Mothers. Surrogate motherhood can be achieved by two methods. The first is to have the surrogate mother inseminated with semen from the infertile woman's partner and carry the baby until the birth. The baby is then formally adopted by the infertile couple. The second, less common method is to retrieve an ovum from the infertile woman, fertilize it with her partner's sperm, and place it into the uterus of a surrogate, who becomes a gestational carrier. These newer interventions raise considerable legal and ethical issues that require extensive counseling of couples and the women who choose to become pregnant.

➤ Evaluation

Evaluation of the effectiveness of care of the couple experiencing impaired fertility is based on the previously stated outcomes (Nursing Care Plan).

CONTRACEPTION

Contraception is the voluntary prevention of pregnancy. In 1995, more than 90% of women in the United States at risk for pregnancy used a method of contraception. Despite the large numbers of men and women who use contraception, almost half of the 6.3 million pregnancies in the United States every year are unintended (Henshaw, 1998). Those who use contraception may be at risk for pregnancy if their choice of contraceptive method is not perfect or is used incorrectly.

Care Management

A multidisciplinary approach may assist a woman in choosing and correctly using an appropriate contraceptive method. Nurses, nurse-midwives, nurse practitioners, and other advanced practice nurses and physicians can assist a woman in making decisions about contraception that will satisfy the woman's personal, social, cultural, and interpersonal needs.

➤ Assessment

A history (including menstrual, contraceptive, and obstetric), physical examination (including pelvic examination), and laboratory tests are usually completed. The woman's knowledge about contraception and her sexual partner's commitment to any particular method are determined. Data are required about the frequency of coitus, number of sexual partners, level of contraceptive involvement, and her or her partner's objections to any methods. The woman's level of comfort and willingness to touch her genitals and cervical mucus are assessed. Myths are identified, and religious and cultural factors are determined. The woman's verbal and nonverbal responses to hearing about the various available methods are carefully noted. An individual's reproductive life plan must be considered.

Informed consent is a vital component in the education of the woman concerning contraception or sterilization. The nurse has the responsibility of documenting information provided and the understanding of that information by the woman.

➤ Nursing Diagnoses

Examples of nursing diagnoses regarding contraception include:

- Risk for decisional conflict related to:
  —Contraceptive alternatives

- Risk for infection related to:
  —Being sexually active
  —Use of contraceptive method
  —Broken skin or mucous membrane secondary to surgery, IUD insertion, and hormonal implant
- Spiritual distress related to:
  —Discrepancy between religious or cultural beliefs and choice of contraception

➤ Expected Outcomes

The expected outcomes are stated in patient-centered terms and may include that the woman or couple will:

- Verbalize understanding about contraceptive methods.
- State comfort and satisfaction with the method chosen.
- Use the contraceptive method correctly and consistently.
- Experience no adverse sequelae as a result of the chosen method of contraception.

➤ Plan of Care and Implementation

Unbiased patient teaching is fundamental to initiating and maintaining any form of contraception. The nurse counters myths with facts, clarifies misinformation, and fills in gaps of knowledge. The ideal contraceptive should be safe, easily available, economical, acceptable, simple to use, and promptly reversible. Although no method may ever achieve all these objectives, impressive progress has been made.

Contraceptive failure rate refers to the percentage of contraceptive users expected to experience an accidental pregnancy during the first year even when they use a method consistently and correctly. Contraceptive effectiveness varies from couple to couple and depends on both the properties of the method and the characteristics of the user (Guest, 1998). Failure rates decrease over time, either because a user gains experience with and uses a method more appropriately or because the less effective users stop using the method.

Safety of a method depends on the patient's medical history, tobacco use (associated with abnormal and decreased number of sperm and chromosome damage), and age. Barrier methods offer some protection from STIs, and oral contraceptives may lower the incidence of ovarian and endometrial cancer but increase the risk of thromboembolic problems (Box 7-6).

Critical Thinking

CONTRACEPTION FOR ADOLESCENTS

Alicia is a 15-year-old Chinese female who comes to the Family Planning Clinic seeking contraception. She has recently become sexually active and is concerned that her mother will find out. What are the issues facing sexually active adolescents? How does her culture affect her use of contraception? Can a 15 year old give informed consent for contraception? Give advantages and disadvantages to a 15-year-old female of various types of contraceptives.

Box 7-6
Signs of Potential Complications with Oral Contraceptives

Before oral contraceptives are prescribed and periodically throughout hormone therapy, the woman is alerted to stop taking the pill and to report any of the following symptoms to the health care provider immediately. The word *aches* helps in retention of this list:

A—Abdominal pain: may indicate a problem with the liver or gallbladder
C—Chest pain or shortness of breath: may indicate possible clot problem within lungs or heart
H—Headaches (sudden or persistent): may be caused by cardiovascular accident or hypertension
E—Eye problems: may indicate vascular accident or hypertension
S—Severe leg pain: may indicate a thromboembolic process

Methods of Contraception

The following discussion of contraceptive methods provides the nurse with information needed for patient teaching. After implementing the appropriate teaching for contraceptive use, the nurse supervises return demonstrations and practice to assess patient understanding. The woman is given written instructions and phone numbers for questions. If the woman has difficulty understanding written instructions, she (and her partner, if available) is offered graphic material and a phone number to call as necessary or is offered an opportunity to return for further instruction.

Coitus Interruptus (Withdrawal). Coitus interruptus involves the man withdrawing his penis from the woman's vagina before he ejaculates. Although coitus interruptus has been criticized as being an ineffective method of contraception, it is a good choice for couples who do not have another contraceptive available (Kowal, 1998). Effectiveness is similar to barrier methods and depends on the man's ability to withdraw his penis before ejaculation. The percentage of women who will experience an unintended pregnancy within the first year of typical use (failure rate) of withdrawal is about 19% (Kowal, 1998). Coitus interruptus does not protect against STIs or human immunodeficiency virus (HIV) infection.

Periodic Abstinence. Periodic abstinence, or natural family planning (NFP), provides contraception by using methods that rely on avoidance of intercourse during fertile days. It is the only method of contraception acceptable to the Roman Catholic

Community Focus

EDUCATION FOR CONTRACEPTIVE USE

Education on contraceptive use in the postpartum period is a common component of discharge planning in many countries, with wide variation among health care delivery systems. Education at this time assumes women's receptiveness to information about contraception, and that education or receptiveness to such information will be less at a later period. Clinical trials have not demonstrated the effectiveness of education in the immediate postpartum period. When assessing effectiveness of contraceptive education, attendance at family planning clinics, cessation of breastfeeding, knowledge about contraception, unplanned pregnancies, and satisfaction with care should be included as factors affecting or measuring effectiveness. The content, timing, and organization of contraceptive education offered in the postpartum period needs to be addressed. Nurses provide discharge planning after childbirth; they commonly staff family planning clinics and provide contraceptive information; evaluation of the effectiveness of their efforts must be implemented and results used to make appropriate changes.

Data from: Hiller J, Griffith E: Education for contraceptive use by women after childbirth (Cochrane Review), *The Cochrane Library,* Issue 3, 2000, Oxford: Update Software.

Church. Fertility awareness is the combination of charting signs and symptoms of the menstrual cycle with the use of abstinence or other contraceptive methods during fertile periods. Signs and symptoms most commonly used are menstrual bleeding, cervical mucus, and BBT (Jennings, Lamprecht, and Kowal, 1998).

The human ovum can be fertilized no later than 16 to 24 hours after ovulation. Motile sperm have been recovered from the uterus and the oviducts as long as 60 hours after coitus. However, their ability to fertilize the ovum probably lasts no longer than 24 to 48 hours. Pregnancy is unlikely to occur if a couple abstains from intercourse for 4 days before and for 3 or 4 days after ovulation (fertile period). However, Wilcox, Weinberg, and Baird (1995) found that pregnancy occurred only in couples who had intercourse within the 6 days before and including the day of ovulation.

Unprotected intercourse on the other days of the cycle (safe period) should not result in pregnancy. However, the exact time of ovulation cannot be predicted accurately, and couples may find it difficult to abstain from sexual intercourse for several days before and after ovulation. Women with irregular menstrual periods have the greatest risk of failure with this form of contraception. The typical failure rate for all fertility awareness methods is 25% during the first year of use (Jennings, Lamprecht, and Kowal, 1998).

Calendar Rhythm Method. Practice of the calendar rhythm method (also known as the rhythm method or menstrual cycle charting) is based on the number of days in each cycle counting from the first day of menses (Jennings, Lamprecht, and Kowal, 1998). The fertile period is determined after accurately recording the lengths of menstrual cycles for 6 months. The beginning of the fertile period is estimated by subtracting 18 days from the length of the shortest cycle. The end of the fertile period is determined by subtracting 11 days from the length of the longest cycle. If the shortest cycle is 24 days and the longest is 30 days, application of the formula is as follows:

SHORTEST CYCLE (24) − 18 = 6th day

LONGEST CYCLE (30) − 11 = 19th day

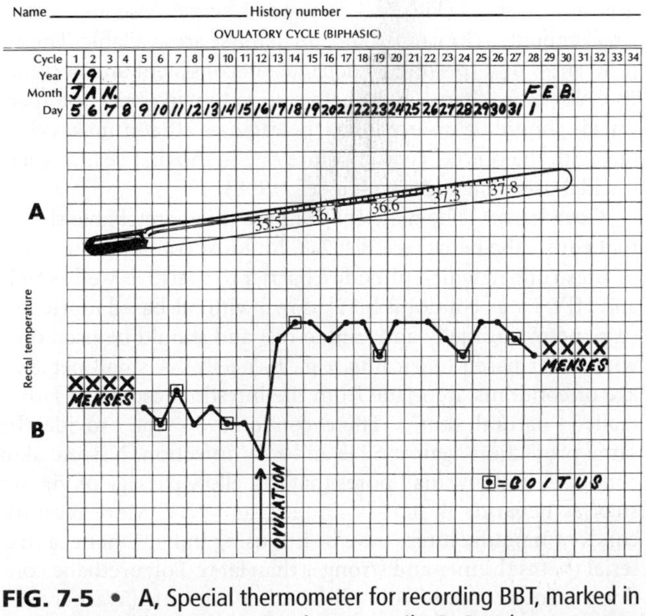

FIG. 7-5 • **A,** Special thermometer for recording BBT, marked in tenths to enable person to read more easily. **B,** Basal temperature record shows drop and sharp rise at time of ovulation. Biphasic curve indicates ovulatory cycle.

To avoid conception the couple would abstain during the fertile period—days 6 through 19.

If the woman has very regular cycles of 28 days each, the formula indicates the fertile days to be as follows:

SHORTEST CYCLE (28) − 18 = 10th day

LONGEST CYCLE (28) − 11 = 17th day

To avoid conception, the couple abstains from day 10 through 17 because ovulation occurs on day 14 + 2 days.

A major drawback of the calendar method is that one is trying to predict future events with past data. The unpredictability of the menstrual cycle is also not taken into consideration. The calendar rhythm method is most useful as an adjunct to the BBT or cervical mucus method.

Basal Body Temperature. The BBT is the lowest body temperature of a healthy person, taken immediately after waking and before getting out of bed. The BBT usually varies from 36.2° to 36.3° C during menses and for approximately 5 to 7 days afterward (Fig. 7-5).

About the time of ovulation a slight drop in temperature (approximately 0.05° C) may be seen by some women, but others see no drop at all. After ovulation, in concert with the increasing progesterone levels of the early luteal phase of the cycle, the BBT rises slightly (approximately 0.2° to 0.4° C). The temperature remains on an elevated plateau until 2 to 4 days before menstruation. Then it drops to the low levels recorded during the previous cycle unless pregnancy has occurred, and the temperature remains elevated.

If ovulation fails to occur, the pattern of lower body temperature continues throughout the cycle. Infection, fatigue, less than 3 hours of sleep per night, awakening late, and anxiety may cause temperature fluctuations and alter the expected pattern. If a new BBT thermometer is purchased, this fact is noted on the chart because the readings may vary slightly. Jet lag, alcohol taken the evening before, or sleeping in a heated waterbed must also be noted on the chart because these affect the BBT.

The drop and subsequent rise in temperature are referred to as the thermal shift. When the entire month's temperatures are recorded on a graph, the pattern described is more apparent. It is more difficult to perceive day-to-day variations without the entire picture (Guidelines box). Therefore the BBT alone is not a reliable method to predict ovulation. To determine if a rise in temperature is indeed the thermal shift, the woman must be

Guidelines

BASAL BODY TEMPERATURE

Discuss BBT with the woman.

Show woman a diagram depicting the phases of the menstrual cycle.

Discuss the hormones in the woman's body that are responsible for her menstrual cycle and ovulation. Leave time for questions.

Show the woman a sample BBT graph (see Fig. 7-6) and the biphasic line seen in ovulatory cycles.

Show the woman the BBT thermometer and how it is calibrated.

Provide a demonstration.

Encourage woman to demonstrate taking and reading the thermometer and graphing the temperature while the nurse watches.

Encourage the woman to start a log to keep track of any other activity that might interfere with her true BBT.

Guidelines

CERVICAL MUCUS CHARACTERISTICS

Setting the Stage

Show charts of menstrual cycle along with changes in the cervical mucus.
Have woman practice with raw egg white.
Supply her with a BBT log and graph if she does not already have one.
Explain that the assessment of cervical mucus characteristics is best when mucus is not mixed with semen, contraceptive jellies or foams, or discharge from infections.

Content Related to Cervical Mucus

Explain to woman (couple) how cervical mucus changes throughout the menstrual cycle.
Right before ovulation, the watery, thin, clear mucus becomes more abundant and thick. It feels like a lubricant and can be stretched 5+ cm between the thumb and forefinger, this is called **spinnbarkeit**. This characteristic indicates the period of maximum fertility. Sperm deposited in this type of mucus can survive until ovulation occurs.

Assessment Technique

Stress that good handwashing is imperative to begin and end all self-assessment.
Start observation from last day of menstrual flow.
Assess cervical mucus several times a day for several cycles. Mucus can be obtained from vaginal introitus; no need to reach into vagina to cervix.
Record findings on the same record on which her BBT is entered.

aware of other signs of approaching ovulation while she continues to assess the BBT (see the discussion that follows on using the symptothermal method for other indicators of ovulation).

Most counselors advise the couple who wish to prevent conception to avoid unprotected intercourse from the last day of the menses until after 3 days of elevated temperature (Jennings, Lamprecht, and Kowal, 1998).

Cervical Mucus Method. The cervical mucus method (also called the Billings method and the Creighton model ovulation method) requires that the woman recognize and interpret the cyclic changes in amount and consistency that characterize her own unique pattern of cervical mucus changes. The cervical mucus that accompanies ovulation is necessary for viability and motility of sperm. To ensure an accurate assessment of changes, the cervical mucus should be free from semen, contraceptive gels or foams, and blood or discharge from vaginal infections for at least one full cycle. Other factors that create difficulty in identifying mucus changes include douches and vaginal deodorants; being in the sexually aroused state (which thins the mucus); and taking medications such as antihistamines, which dry up the mucus.

Some women may find this method unacceptable if they are uncomfortable touching their genitals. Whether or not a woman wants to use this method for contraception, it is to her advantage to learn to recognize mucus characteristics at ovulation (Guidelines box).

Symptothermal Method. The symptothermal method combines the BBT and cervical mucus methods with awareness of secondary, cycle phase–related symptoms. The woman gains fertility awareness as she learns the psychologic and physiologic symptoms that mark the phases of her cycle. Secondary symptoms include increased libido, midcycle spotting, mittelschmerz, pelvic fullness or tenderness, and vulvar fullness.

The woman is taught to palpate the cervix to assess for changes indicating ovulation: the os dilates slightly, the cervix softens and rises in the vagina, and cervical mucus is copious and slippery. The woman notes days on which coitus, changes in routine, illness, and so on have occurred (Fig. 7-6). Calendar calculations and cervical mucus changes are used to estimate the onset of the fertile period; changes in cervical mucus or the BBT are used to estimate its end.

Predictor Test for Ovulation. All the methods previously discussed are indicative of ovulation but do not prove the occurrence and exact timing of ovulation. The predictor test for ovulation is a major assist to the periodic abstinence methods for women who want to plan the time of their pregnancies and for those women who are trying to conceive. The predictor test for ovulation detects the sudden surge of LH that occurs approximately 12 to 24 hours before ovulation. Unlike BBT, the test is not affected by illness, emotional upset, or physical activity. Available for home use, a test kit contains sufficient material for several days' testing during each cycle. A positive response indicating an LH surge is noted by a color change that is easy to read. Directions for use of this home test kit vary with the manufacturer.

Barrier Methods. Barrier contraceptives have gained in popularity not only as a contraceptive method but also as protection against the spread of STIs. Chemical barriers such as nonoxynol-9 have been shown to reduce slightly the risk of infection with gonorrhea and chlamydia (Cates and Raymond, 1998; Heath and Sulik, 1997), but to increase the transmission of HIV (Gayle, 2000). Male and female condoms provide a mechanical barrier to STIs (Stewart F, 1998).

Spermicides. A vaginal spermicide is a physical barrier to sperm penetration that also has a chemical action on sperm. Nonoxynol-9 is the most commonly used spermicidal chemical in the United States. Intravaginal spermicides are marketed as aerosol foams, foaming tablets, suppositories, creams, films, gels, and sponges (Fig. 7-7). Preloaded, single-dose applicators small enough to be carried in a small purse are available. The effectiveness of a spermicide depends on consistent and accurate use. Not more than 1 hour before sexual intercourse, the spermicide should be inserted into the vagina so that it makes contact with the cervix. Typical failure rate in the first year of spermicidal use alone is 26% (Trussell, 1998).

Condoms. The male condom is a thin, stretchable sheath that covers the penis (see Fig. 7-8, *B*). Most condoms are made of latex rubber, which provide a barrier to sperm as well as STIs and HIV. Latex condoms break down with oil-based lubricants (e.g., petroleum jelly and suntan oil) and should be used only with water-based lubricants (e.g., K-Y jelly). A small percentage of condoms are made from the intestinal cecum of lambs (called "natural skin"). These condoms do not provide the same protection against STIs and HIV infection. Natural skin condoms contain small pores that can allow passage of viruses such as hepatitis B, herpes simplex, and HIV. More recently, condom manufacturers have begun using polyurethane, a material that is thinner and stronger than latex. Polyurethane condoms can be used with oil-based lubricants (Warner and Hatcher, 1998). Studies are being conducted to determine the effectiveness of polyurethane condoms in protecting against STIs and HIV.

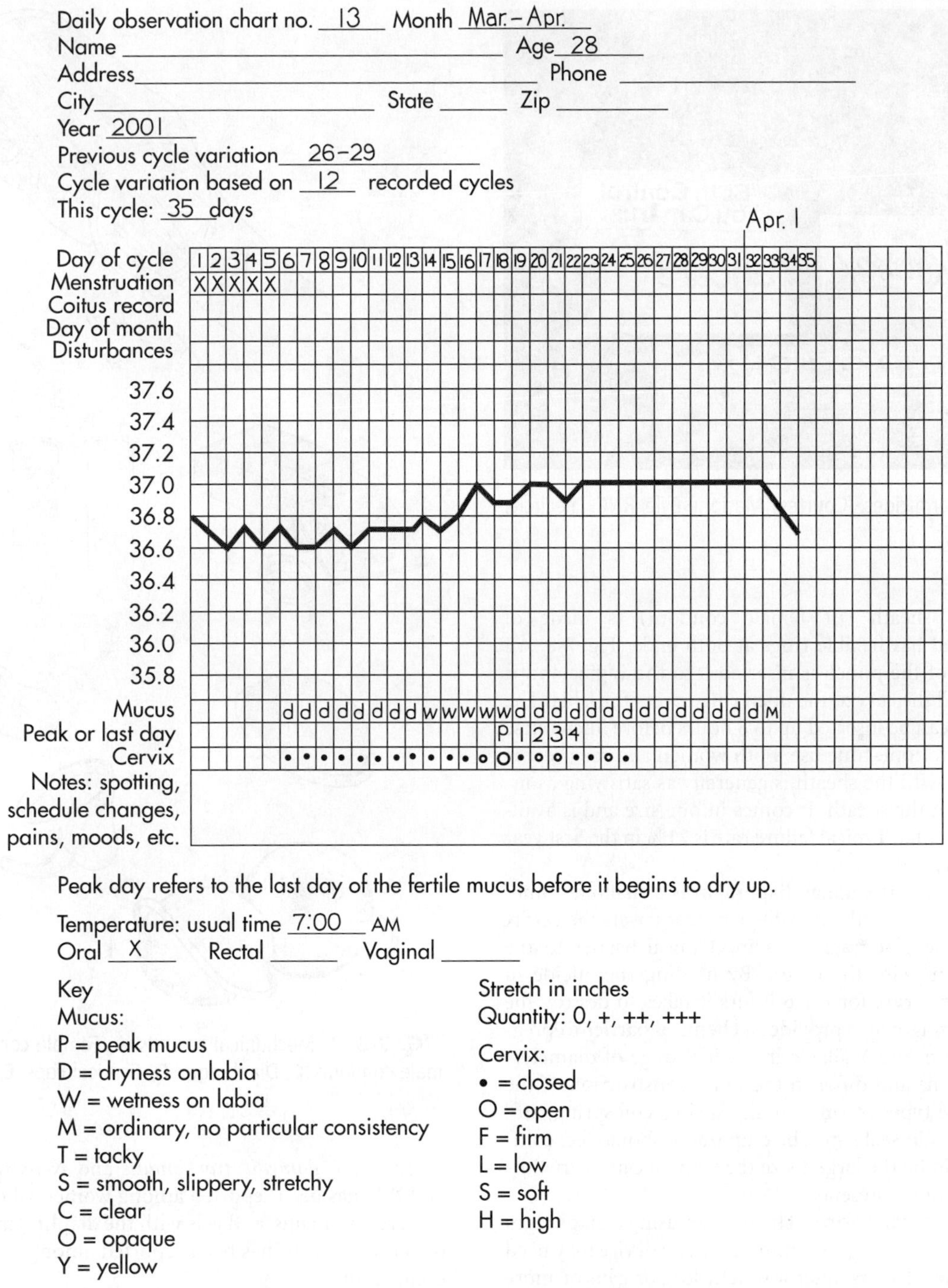

FIG. 7-6 • Example of completed symptothermal chart.

NURSE ALERT • **All patients should be questioned about the potential for latex allergy. Latex condom use is contraindicated for patients with latex sensitivity.**

A functional difference in condom shape is the presence or absence of a sperm reservoir tip. To enhance vaginal stimulation, some condoms are contoured and rippled or have ribbed or roughened surfaces. Thinner construction increases heat transmission and sensitivity; a variety of colors increases their acceptability and attractiveness (Warner and Hatcher, 1998). A wet jelly or dry powder lubricates some condoms. Spermicide is added to the interior or exterior surfaces of some condoms. Typical failure rate for the first year of use of the male condom is 14% (Warner and Hatcher, 1998).

NURSE ALERT • **It is a false assumption that everyone knows how to use condoms. To prevent unintended pregnancy and the spread of STIs, it is essential that condoms be used correctly. Proper instructions in use must be provided. The sheath is applied over the erect penis before insertion and before the loss of preejaculatory drops of semen (Box 7-7).**

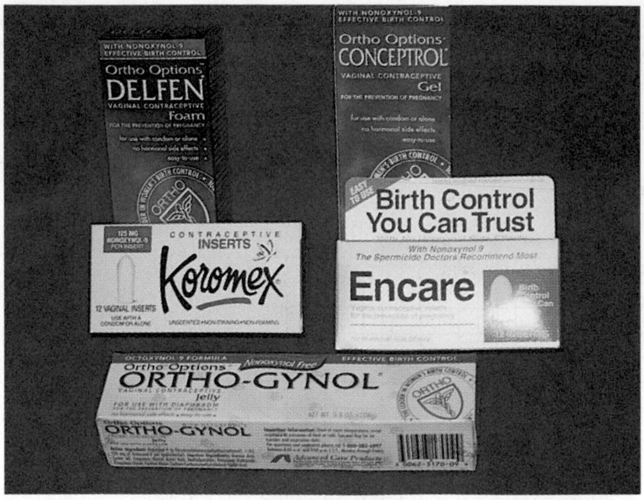

FIG. 7-7 • Spermicides. (Courtesy Marjorie Pyle, RNC, Lifecircle, Costa Mesa, CA.)

The vaginal sheath (or female condom) is made of polyurethane and has flexible rings at both ends (Fig. 7-8, *A*). The closed end of the pouch is inserted into the vagina and is anchored around the cervix; the open ring covers the labia. The female condom can be inserted up to 8 hours before intercourse and is intended for one-time use. Both women and men report that intercourse with the sheath is generally as satisfying as intercourse without the sheath. It comes in one size and is available over-the-counter. Typical failure rate is 21% in the first year of use (Stewart F, 1998).

Diaphragm. The vaginal diaphragm is a shallow, dome-shaped, rubber device with a flexible rim that covers the cervix (Fig. 7-8, *C*). The diaphragm is a mechanical barrier to the meeting of sperm with the ovum. By holding spermicide in place against the cervix for the 6 hours it takes to destroy the sperm, the diaphragm also provides a chemical barrier to pregnancy. Diaphragms are available in a wide range of diameters (i.e., 50 to 95 mm) and differ in the inner construction of the circular rim. The types of rims are flat spring, coil spring, arcing spring, and wide-seal rim. The diaphragm should feel comfortable. It should be the largest size the woman can wear without being aware of its presence.

Nursing Considerations. The woman using a diaphragm needs an annual gynecologic examination. The device may need to be refitted after 2 years, after a weight loss or gain of more than 22 kg, or after a term birth or a second-trimester miscarriage (Stewart F, 1998). Because there are various types of diaphragms on the market, the package insert is used for teaching the woman how to use and care for the diaphragm (Home Care box).

Except for occasional allergic responses to the diaphragm or spermicide, there are no side effects from a well-fitted device. To increase spontaneity, the diaphragm can be inserted as long as 6 hours before intercourse; but spermicide must be added each time intercourse is repeated. It must be left in place for at least 6 hours after the last intercourse. The woman who engages in intercourse infrequently may choose this barrier method. The spermicide offers additional lubrication if it is needed. A decreased incidence of vaginitis, cervicitis (including cervicitis caused by *Chlamydia trachomatis* and *Neisseria gonorrhoeae*), and PID has been reported among women who use contraceptive creams, foams, and gels with the diaphragm. A reduced risk of cervical cancer has been reported among women who use a diaphragm.

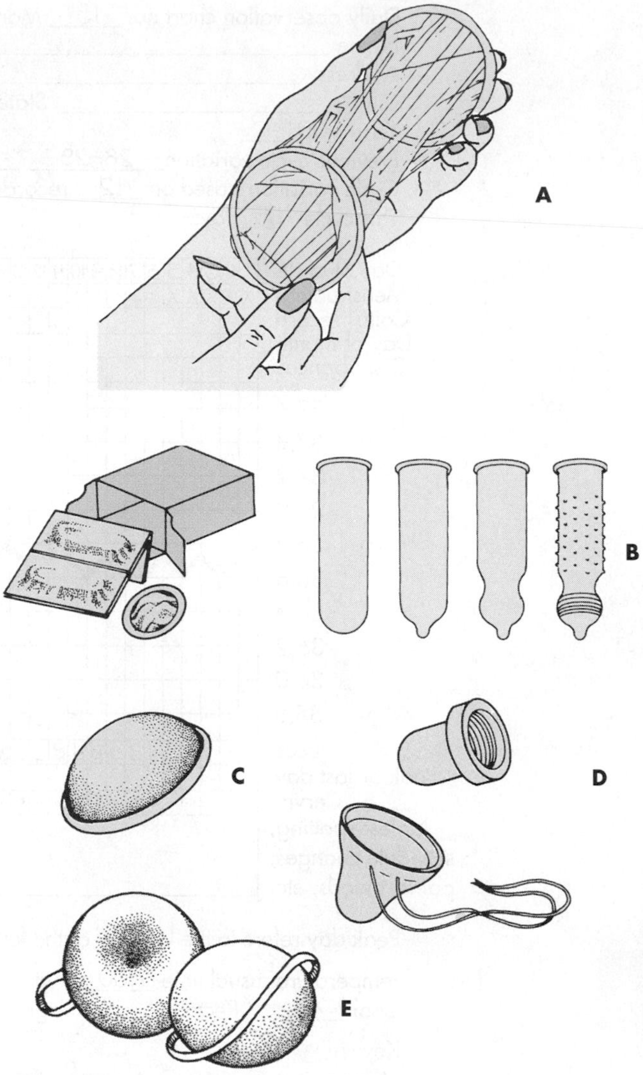

FIG. 7-8 • Mechanical barriers. **A,** Female condom. **B,** Types of male condoms. **C,** Diaphragm. **D,** Cervical caps. **E,** Sponge.

Disadvantages of using a diaphragm include the reluctance of some women to insert and remove the device. A cold diaphragm and a cold gel temporarily reduce vaginal response to sexual stimulation if insertion of the diaphragm occurs immediately before intercourse. Some women or couples object to the messiness of the spermicide. These annoyances of diaphragm use, along with failure to insert the device once foreplay has begun, are the most common reasons for failures of this method. Side effects may include irritation of tissues related to contact with spermicides. Urethritis and recurrent cystitis, caused by upward pressure of the diaphragm rim against the urethra, may be increased. Diaphragms are contraindicated for women with pelvic relaxation (uterine prolapse) or a large cystocele. Women with a latex allergy should not use latex diaphragms.

Box 7-7
Male Condoms

MECHANISM OF ACTION
Sheath is applied over the erect penis before insertion or before loss of preejaculatory drops of semen. Used correctly, condoms prevent sperm from entering the cervix. Spermicide-coated condoms cause ejaculated sperm to be immobilized rapidly, thus increasing contraceptive effectiveness.

FAILURE RATE
Typical users, 14%
Correct and consistent users, 3%

ADVANTAGES
Safe
No side effects
Readily available
Premalignant changes in cervix can be prevented or ameliorated in women whose partners use condoms
Method of male nonsurgical contraception

DISADVANTAGES
Must interrupt lovemaking to apply sheath.
Sensation may be altered.
If used improperly, spillage of sperm can result in pregnancy.
Occasionally, condoms may tear during intercourse.

STI PROTECTION
If a condom is used throughout the act of intercourse and there is no unprotected contact with female genitals, a latex rubber condom, which is impermeable to viruses, can act as a protective measure against STIs. The addition of a spermicide increases protection against transmission of STIs, including HIV.

NURSING CONSIDERATIONS
Teach man to do the following:
- Use a new condom (check expiration date) for each act of sexual intercourse or other acts between partners that involve contact with the penis.

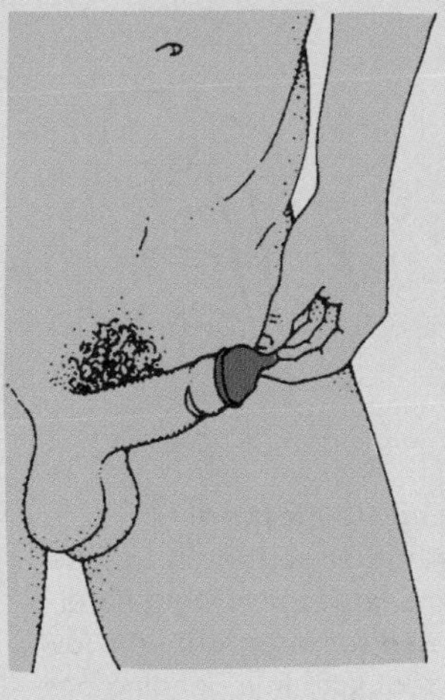
Fig. A

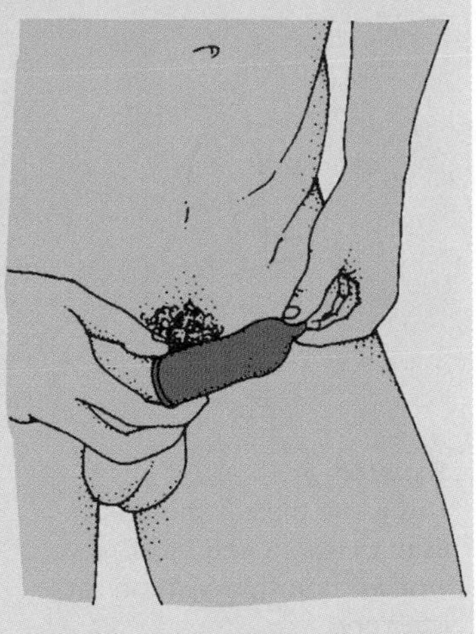
Fig. B

- Place condom after penis is erect and before intimate contact.
- Place condom on head of penis (Fig. A) and unroll it all the way to the base (Fig. B).
- Leave an empty space at the tip (Fig. A); remove any air remaining in the tip by gently pressing air out toward the base of the penis.
- If a lubricant is desired, use water-based products such as K-Y Jelly. Do not use petroleum-based products because they can cause the condom to break.
- After ejaculation, carefully withdraw the still-erect penis from the vagina, holding onto condom rim; remove and discard the condom.
- Store unused condoms in a cool, dry place.
- Do not use condoms that are sticky, brittle, or obviously damaged.

Toxic shock syndrome (TSS), although reported in very small numbers, can occur in association with the use of the contraceptive diaphragm (Stewart F, 1998). Measures to reduce the risk for TSS include handwashing before insertion and removal, prompt removal 6 to 8 hours after intercourse, not using the diaphragm during menses, and learning and watching for danger signs of TSS.

NURSE ALERT • The nurse should be alert for signs of TSS in women who use a diaphragm or cervical cap as a contraceptive method. The most common signs include sudden onset of a fever greater than 38.4° C, hypotension (systolic BP less than 90 mm Hg or orthostatic dizziness), and a rash.

Cervical Cap. The cervical cap has a 22 to 31 mm soft natural rubber dome with a firm but pliable rim (see Fig. 7-8, *D*). It fits snugly around the base of the cervix close to the junction of the cervix and vaginal fornices. The device is available in four sizes. It is recommended that the cap remain in place no less than 8 hours and not more than 48 hours. It is left in place at least 6 hours after the last act of intercourse. The seal provides a physical barrier to sperm; spermicide inside the cap adds a chemical barrier.

The extended period of wear is an added convenience for women who previously used the diaphragm. Instructions for the actual insertion and use of the cervical cap closely resemble the instructions for use of the contraceptive diaphragm. Some of the differences are that the cervical cap can be inserted hours before sexual intercourse without a later need for additional spermicide, the cervical cap requires less spermicide than the diaphragm when initially inserted, and no additional spermicide is required for repeated acts of intercourse.

Women who are not good candidates for wearing the cervical cap include those with abnormal Pap test results, those who cannot be fitted properly with the existing cap sizes or who find the insertion and removal of the device too difficult, those with

Home Care

USE AND CARE OF THE DIAPHRAGM
Positions for Insertion of Diaphragm

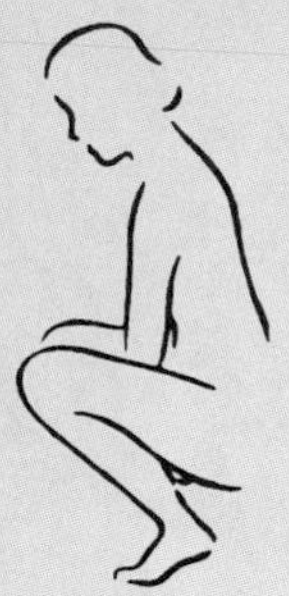

Squatting
This is the most commonly used position, and most women find this position satisfactory.

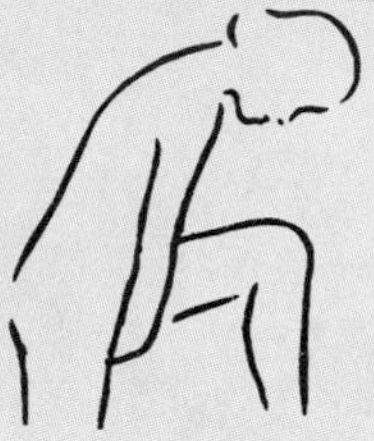

Leg Up Method
Another position is to raise the left foot (if right hand is used for insertion) on a low stool, and in a bending position the diaphragm is inserted.

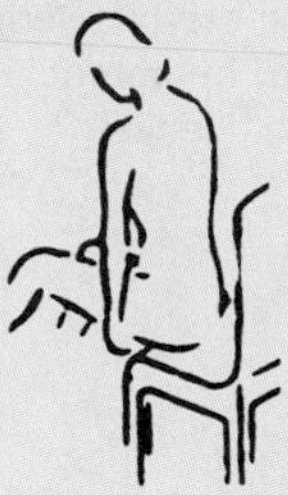

Chair Method
Another practical method for diaphragm insertion is for you to sit far forward on the edge of a chair.

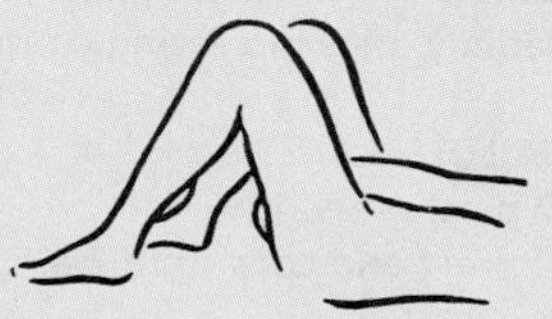

Reclining
You may prefer to insert the diaphragm while in a semi-reclining position in bed.

Inspection of Diaphragm
Your diaphragm must be inspected carefully before each use. The best way to do this is:

Hold the diaphragm up to a light source. Carefully stretch the diaphragm at the area of the rim, on all sides, to make sure there are no holes. Remember, it is possible to puncture the diaphragm with sharp fingernails.

Another way to check for pinholes is to carefully fill the diaphragm with water. If there is any problem, it will be seen immediately.

If your diaphragm is puckered, especially near the rim, this could mean thin spots.

The diaphragm should not be used if you see any of the above; consult your health care provider.

Preparation of Diaphragm
Rinse off cornstarch. Your diaphragm must always be used with a spermicidal lubricant to be effective. Pregnancy cannot be prevented effectively by the diaphragm alone.

Always empty your bladder before inserting the diaphragm. Place about 2 teaspoonfuls of contraceptive jelly or contraceptive cream on the side of the diaphragm that will rest against the cervix (or whichever way you have been instructed). Spread it around to coat the surface and the rim. This aids in insertion and offers a more complete seal. Many women also spread some jelly or cream on the other side of the diaphragm (see Fig. A).

Insertion of Diaphragm
The diaphragm can be inserted as long as 6 hours before intercourse. Hold the diaphragm between your thumb and fingers. The dome can either be up or down, as directed by your health care provider. Place your index finger on the outer rim of the compressed diaphragm (see Fig. B). Use the fingers of the other hand to spread the labia (lips of the vagina). This will assist in guiding the diaphragm into place.

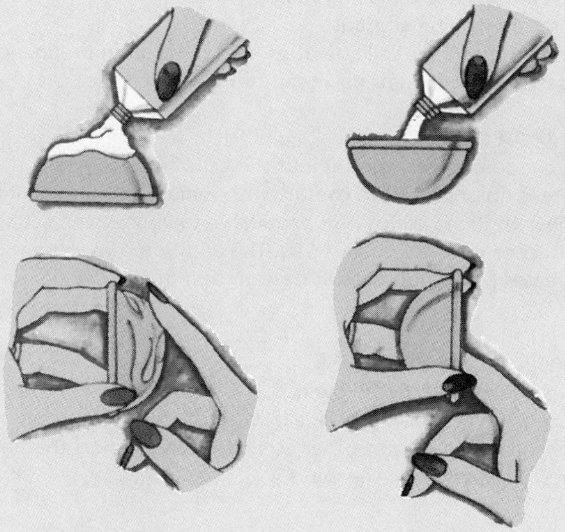

Fig. A

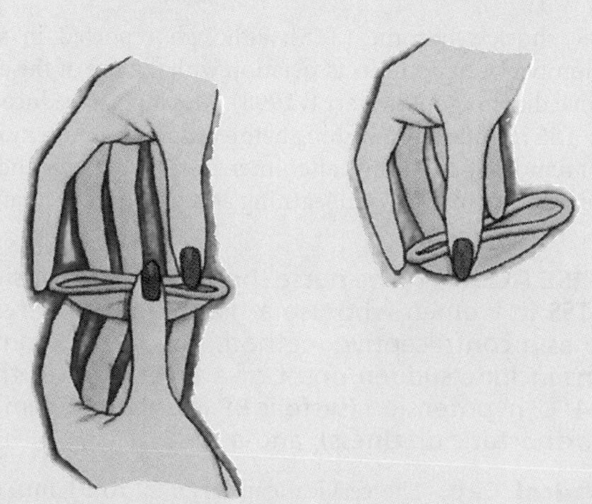

Fig. B

Home Care

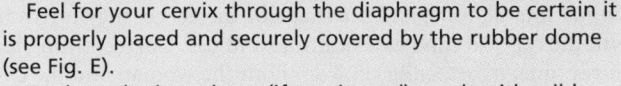

USE AND CARE OF THE DIAPHRAGM—cont'd

Insertion of Diaphragm

Insert the diaphragm into the vagina. Direct it inward and downward as far as it will go to the space behind and below the cervix (see Fig. C).

Tuck the front of the rim of the diaphragm behind the pelvic bone so that the rubber hugs the front wall of the vagina (see Fig. D).

Feel for your cervix through the diaphragm to be certain it is properly placed and securely covered by the rubber dome (see Fig. E).

To clean the introducer (if one is used), wash with mild soap and warm water and rinse and dry thoroughly.

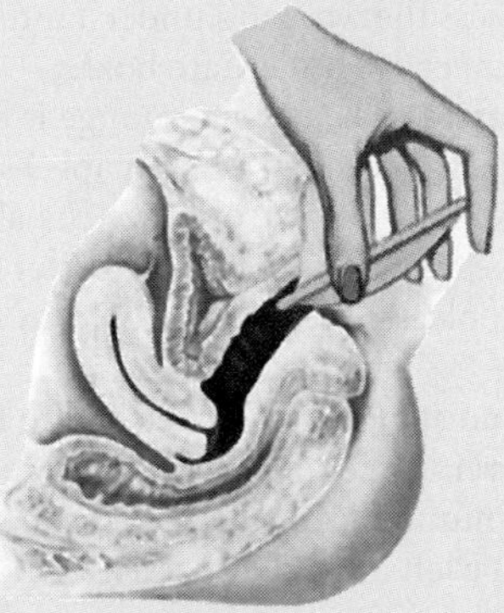

Fig. C

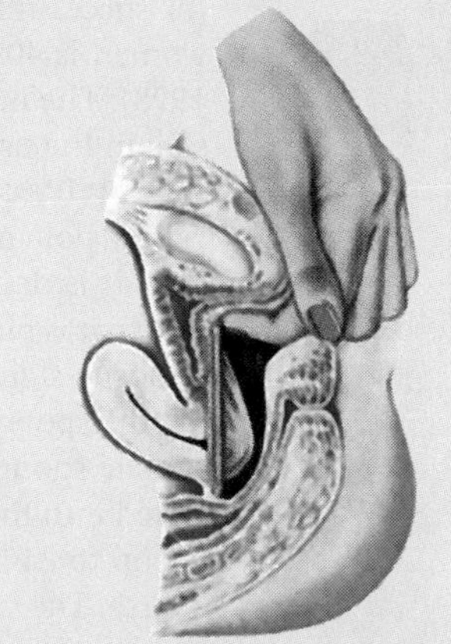

Fig. D

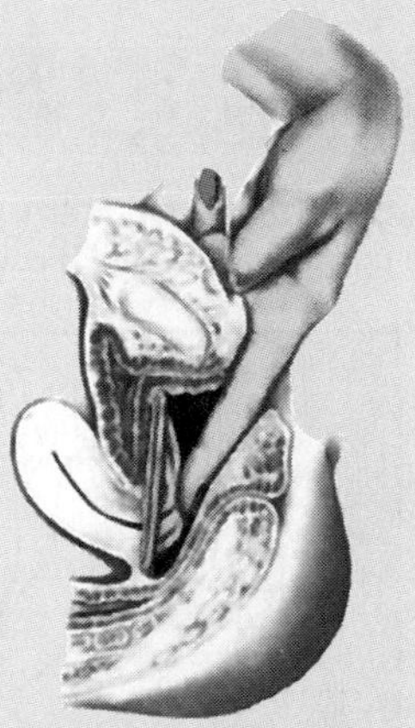

Fig. E

General Information

Regardless of the time of the month, this method of contraception must be used each and every time intercourse takes place. Your diaphragm must be left in place for at least 6 hours after the last intercourse. If you remove your diaphragm before the 6-hour period, your chance of becoming pregnant could be greatly increased.

Removal of Diaphragm

The only proper way to remove the diaphragm is to insert your forefinger up and over the top side of the diaphragm, and slightly to the side.

Next, turn the palm of your hand downward and backward, hooking the forefinger firmly on top of the inside of the upper rim of the diaphragm, *breaking the suction* (Fig. F).

Pull the diaphragm down and out. This avoids the possibility of tearing the diaphragm with the fingernails. The diaphragm *should not* be removed by trying to catch the rim from *below* the dome.

Care of Diaphragm

When using a vaginal diaphragm, avoid using products that may contain petroleum, such as certain body lubricants, vaginal lubricants, or vaginitis preparations. These products can weaken the rubber.

A little care means longer wear for your diaphragm. After each use the diaphragm should be washed in warm water and mild soap. Do not use detergent soaps, cold cream soaps, deodorant soaps, and soaps containing petroleum because they can weaken the rubber.

After washing, the diaphragm should be dried thoroughly. All water and moisture should be removed with your towel. The diaphragm should then be dusted with *cornstarch.* Scented talc, body powder, baby powder, and the like should not be used because they can weaken the rubber.

The diaphragm should then be placed back in the plastic case for storage. It should not be stored near a radiator or heat source or exposed to light for an extended period.

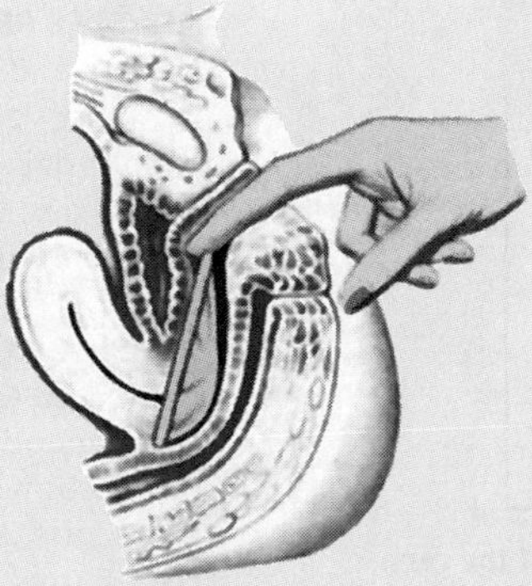

Fig. F

a history of TSS or with vaginal or cervical infections, and those who experience allergic responses to the cap or to spermicide.

Nursing Considerations. The angle of the uterus, the vaginal muscle tone, and the shape of the cervix may interfere with the cervical cap's ease of fitting and use. Correct fitting requires time, effort, and skill from both the woman and the clinician. The woman must check the position of the cap before and after each act of intercourse. Current research has not found an association between cervical cap use and Pap smear abnormalities.

Although no link has been discovered between TSS and the use of the cervical cap, such an association remains possible. The package insert recommends that another form of birth control be used during menstrual bleeding and for at least 6 weeks postpartum. The cap should be checked for proper fit after any gynecologic surgery or birth and after major weight loss or gain. Otherwise, the size should be checked at least once a year.

Strong patient motivation is the most important criterion for successful cap use. Failure rate with typical use for parous women is 40% and for nulliparous women is 20% (Stewart F, 1998). The nurse should assess the woman's understanding and skill in the use of the cervical cap (Home Care box).

Contraceptive Sponge. The vaginal sponge is a small, round, polyurethane sponge that contains nonoxynol-9 spermicide. It is designed to fit over the cervix (one size fits all). The side that is placed next to the cervix is concave for better fit. The opposite side has a woven polyester loop to be used in removing the sponge.

The sponge should be moistened with water before it is inserted into the vagina to cover the cervix. It provides protection for up to 24 hours and for numerous instances of sexual intercourse. The sponge should be left in place for at least 6 hours af-

Home Care

USE AND CARE OF THE CERVICAL CAP

Push cap up into vagina until it covers cervix.

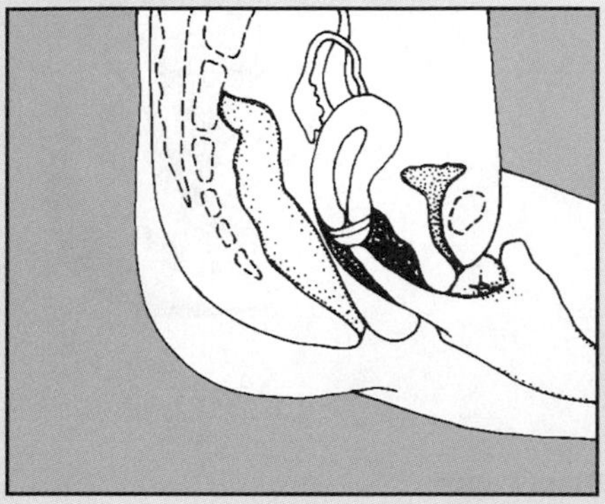

Press rim against cervix to create a seal.

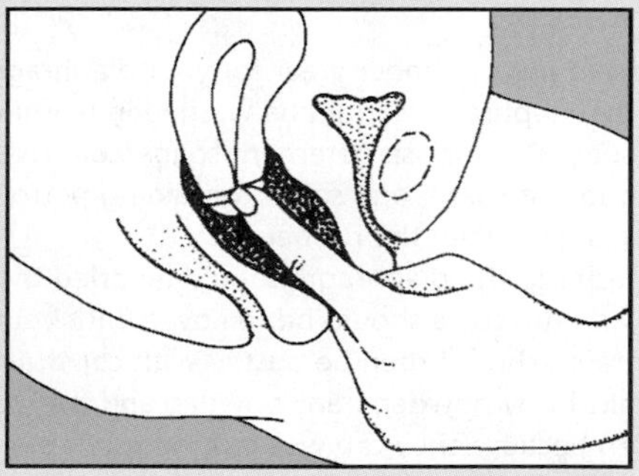

To remove: Push rim toward right or left hip to loosen from cervix and then remove.

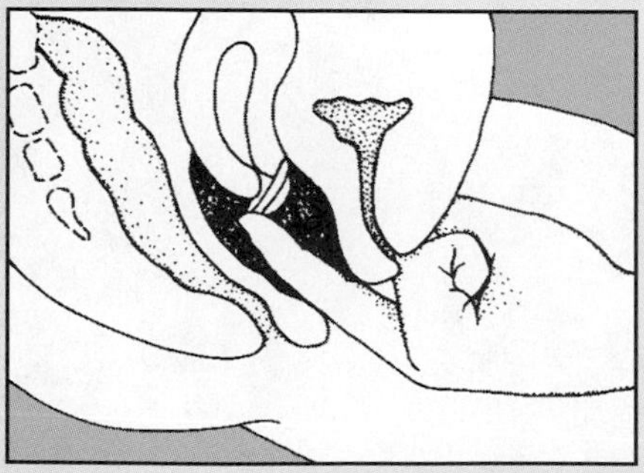

The woman can assume a number of positions to insert the cervical cap. See the four positions shown for inserting the diaphragm on p. 114.

Box 7-8

Combined Estrogen-Progestin Oral Contraceptives

ACTION

Suppresses action of the hypothalamus and anterior pituitary leading to inappropriate secretion of FSH and LH; ovarian follicles do not mature; ovulation is inhibited. Causes endometrium to slough when hormones are removed (withdrawal bleeding).

INDICATION

Prevention of pregnancy.

DOSAGE AND ROUTE

1 tablet orally daily until the pack is finished. If 28-day pack, start next pack the next day. If 21-day pack, wait 7 day start again. Doses of estrogen and progesterone vary by brand and are prescribed according to woman's response. Lowest possible effective dose is used.

ADVERSE REACTIONS

Nausea and vomiting, dizziness, edema, leg cramps, increase in breast size, breast tenderness, chloasma, visual changes, weight gain, decreased libido, hypertension, vascular headaches, bleeding irregularities, depression, headaches, change in glucose tolerance.

NURSING CONSIDERATIONS

Combined OCPs should be taken at same time every day to maintain adequate hormone levels. Effectiveness of OCPs decreases when taking phenytoin sodium, carbamazepine, primidone, topirimate, grieseofulvin, and rifampin. Use a backup method of contraception when taking broad-spectrum antibiotics for the duration of the antibiotic plus 7 days.

ter the last act of sexual intercourse. Longer wearing time (i.e., greater than 24 to 30 hours) is not recommended because the woman may be at risk for TSS (Stewart F, 1998).

Hormonal Methods. Over 30 different hormonal contraceptive formulations are available in the United States today. Because of the wide variety of preparations available, the woman and nurse must read the package insert for information about specific products prescribed. Formulations include combined estrogen-progestin steroidal medications or progestin-only agents. The formulations are administered orally, subdermally, or by implantation. Box 7-8 lists combined estrogen-progestin medications.

There are many different preparations of oral hormonal contraceptives. Because of the wide variations, each woman must be clear about the unique dosage regimen for the preparation prescribed for her and follow directions on the package insert. Directions for care after missing one or two tablets also vary (Fig. 7-9). Signs of potential complications associated with the use of oral contraceptives must be reviewed with the woman (Box 7-9). Oral contraceptives do not protect a woman against STIs. A barrier method such as condoms and spermicide should also be used if this kind of protection is desired.

Progestin-Only Contraception. Progestin-only methods impair fertility by inhibiting ovulation, thickening and decreasing the amount of cervical mucus, and thinning the endometrium (Hatcher, 1998).

Oral progestins (minipill). Progestin-only pills are less effective than combined OCPs. Failure rate for typical users is 5% in the first year of use (Hatcher, 1998). Effectiveness is increased if minipills are taken correctly. Because minipills contain such a low dose of progestin, the minipill must be taken at the same time every day. Users often complain of irregular bleeding.

Injectable progestins. Medroxyprogesterone (DMPA, Depo-Provera) 150 mg is given intramuscularly in the deltoid or gluteus maximus. Injections should be administered every 12 weeks (Hatcher, 1998).

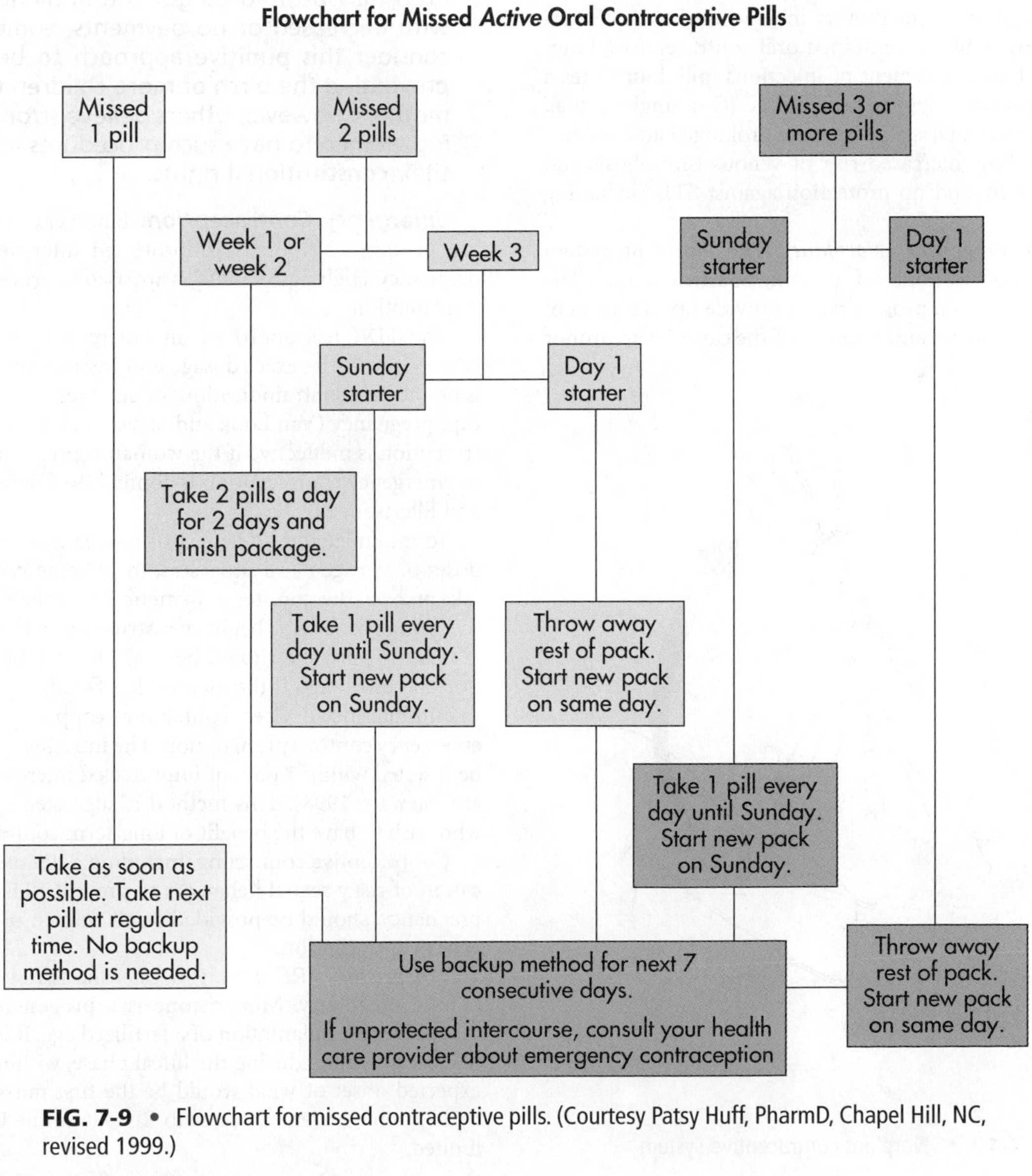

FIG. 7-9 • Flowchart for missed contraceptive pills. (Courtesy Patsy Huff, PharmD, Chapel Hill, NC, revised 1999.)

Box 7-9

Signs of Potential Complications with IUDs

Signs of potential complications related to IUDs can be remembered in this manner:

P—Period late, abnormal spotting or bleeding
A—Abdominal pain, pain with intercourse
I—Infection exposure, abnormal vaginal discharge
N—Not feeling well, fever, or chills
S—String missing, shorter or longer

Hatcher R et al: *Contraceptive technology (1994-1996),* ed 16, New York, 1994, Irvington Publishers.

NURSE ALERT • When administering an intramuscular injection of progestin (e.g., Depo-Provera), the site should not be massaged after the injection because this action can hasten the absorption and shorten the period of effectiveness.

The advantages of Depo-Provera include a contraceptive effectiveness comparable to combined oral contraceptives, long-lasting effects, the requirement of injections only four times a year, and lactation not likely to be impaired (Cunningham et al, 1997; Hatcher, 1998). Disadvantages are prolonged amenorrhea or uterine bleeding, increased risk of venous thrombosis and thromboembolism, and no protection against STIs (including HIV).

Implantable Progestins (Norplant). The Norplant system consists of six flexible, nonbiodegradable Silastic capsules. The Silastic capsules contain progestin and provide up to 5 years of contraception. Insertion and removal of the capsules are minor surgical procedures involving a local anesthetic, a small incision, and no sutures. The capsules are placed subdermally in the inner aspect of the upper arm (Fig. 7-10). The progestin prevents some, but not all, ovulatory cycles and thickens cervical mucus. The effectiveness is greater than 99% over 5 years. Other advantages include reversibility and long-term continuous contraception that is not coitus related.

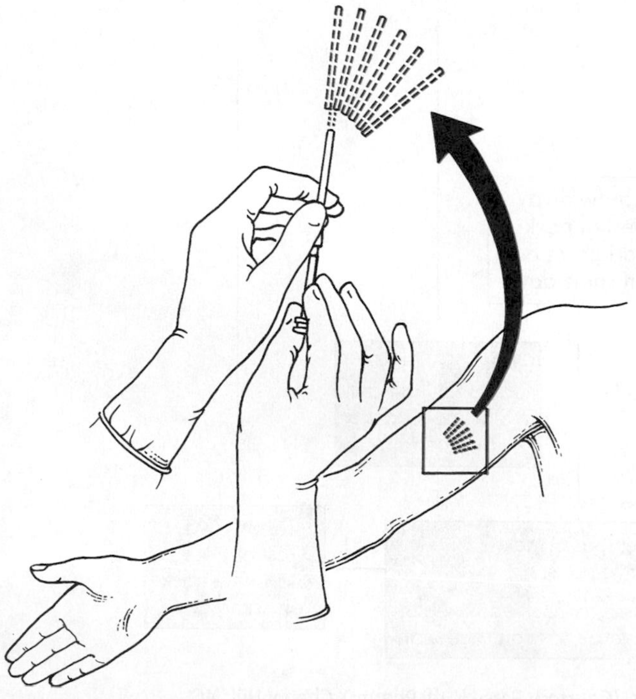

FIG. 7-10 • Norplant contraceptive system

Irregular menstrual bleeding is the most common side effect. Less common side effects include headaches, nervousness, nausea, skin changes, and vertigo. No STI protection is provided with the Norplant method; condoms should be used if protection is desired. The Food and Drug Administration has approved Norplant 2, which uses two Silastic capsules (Hatcher, 1998).

NURSE ALERT • The nurse may be confronted with an ethical dilemma concerning enforced contraception for a patient. There have been some judicial rulings for women convicted of child abuse to either obtain a Norplant device or face a jail term. Other women receiving public assistance for children may be told to get the implant or be faced with decreased or no payments. Some nurses may consider this punitive approach to be effective in preventing the birth of more children to unsuitable mothers; however, others believe strongly that forcing women to have such procedures interferes with their constitutional rights.

Emergency Contraception. Emergency contraception is used within 72 hours of unprotected intercourse to prevent pregnancy. High doses of OCPs are used to prevent ovulation or implantation.

The FDA has approved an emergency contraception kit (Preven) with the exact dosage and instructions for use. There is no medical contraindication for emergency contraception except pregnancy (Van Look and Stewart, 1998). Emergency contraception is ineffective if the woman is pregnant. Effectiveness of emergency contraception is about 75% (Trussell, Rodriguez, and Ellertson, 1998).

To minimize the side effect of nausea that occurs with high doses of estrogen and progestin, the woman can be advised to take an over-the-counter antiemetic 1 hour before each dose. If the woman does not begin menstruation within 21 days after taking the pills, she should be evaluated for pregnancy. Abortion can be offered if the method has failed.

Intrauterine devices containing copper provide another emergency contraception option. The intrauterine device should be inserted within 7 days of unprotected intercourse (Van Look and Stewart, 1998). This method is suggested only for women who wish to have the benefit of long-term contraception.

Contraceptive counseling, including a discussion of modification of risky sexual behaviors to prevent STIs and unwanted pregnancy, should be provided to all women requesting emergency contraception.

Mifepristone (RU 486). Progesterone is essential for maintaining pregnancy. Mifepristone is a progesterone antagonist that prevents implantation of a fertilized egg. It is most effective in early gestation, during the luteal phase, within 10 days of the expected onset of what would be the first missed period after conception. Currently, access to RU 486 in the United States is limited.

Intrauterine Devices. An intrauterine device (IUD) is a small T-shaped device inserted into the uterine cavity. Medicated IUDs are loaded with either copper or a progestational agent (Fig. 7-11). These chemically active substances are released continuously (copper-bearing devices for up to 10 years and progesterone devices for 1 year). IUDs are impregnated with barium sulfate for radiopacity. Evidence strongly supports a true contraceptive effect in preventing fertilization (Mishell, 1998). The copper-bearing IUD damages sperm in transit to the uterine tubes and few sperm reach the ovum, thus preventing fertilization.

The progesterone-bearing IUD causes progestin-related effects on cervical mucus and endometrial maturation. Because the effect is local, there is no disruption of the woman's ovulatory pattern. Copper-bearing IUDs have a lower failure rate than progesterone-releasing IUDs. The typical failure rate of the IUD ranges from 0.1% to 2.0% (Stewart G, 1998).

The IUD offers constant contraception without the need to remember to take pills each day or engage in other manipulation before or between coital acts. If pregnancy can be excluded, an IUD can be placed at any time during the menstrual cycle. An IUD may be inserted immediately after childbirth or abortion.

The absence of interference with hormonal regulation of menstrual cycles makes the IUD more appropriate than hormonal contraception for heavy smokers, women over age 35 years, women who have hypertension, or those with a history of vascular disease or familial diabetes. Contraceptive effects are reversible. When pregnancy is desired, the IUD may be removed by the health care provider.

The progesterone IUD offers two important noncontraceptive progesterone-related advantages: less blood loss during menstruation and decreased primary dysmenorrhea. The average blood loss is increased for the copper IUD. This blood loss may be clinically significant in undernourished individuals.

The IUD is contraindicated for women with a history of PID, known or suspected pregnancy, undiagnosed genital bleeding, suspected genital malignancy, or a distorted intrauterine cavity.

Disadvantages of IUD use include the risk of PID, especially within 3 months of insertion; and risk of bacterial vaginosis, uterine perforation, and infection at time of insertion. The IUD offers no protection against STIs. The IUD is not recommended for teenagers, but primarily is recommended for women who have had at least one child and who are involved in a stable, monogamous relationship.

Nursing Considerations. The woman must check for the presence of the IUD thread after menstruation and at the time of ovulation, as well as before coitus, to rule out expulsion of the device. If pregnancy occurs with the IUD in place, the IUD should be removed immediately, if possible. Retention of the IUD during pregnancy increases the risk of septic miscarriage and ectopic pregnancy (Stewart G, 1998). Some women allergic to copper develop a rash, necessitating removal of the copper-bearing IUD.

Sterilization. Sterilization refers to surgical procedures intended to render the person infertile. Most procedures involve the occlusion of the passageways for the ova and sperm (Fig. 7-12, *A*). For the female, the oviducts (uterine tubes) are occluded; for the male, the sperm ducts (vas deferens) are occluded. Only surgical removal of the ovaries (oophorectomy) or uterus (hysterectomy) or both will result in absolute sterility for the woman. All other operations have a small but definite failure rate; that is, pregnancy may result.

Female Sterilization. Female sterilization may be performed immediately after giving birth (within 24 to 48 hours), concomitantly with abortion, or as an interval procedure (dur-

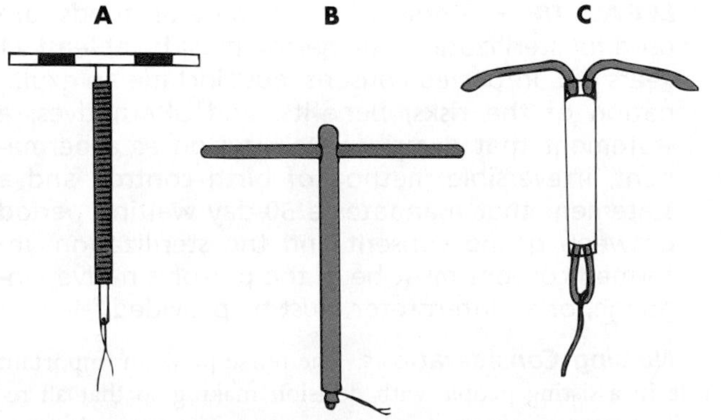

FIG. 7-11 • Intrauterine devices. **A,** Copper T380A. **B,** Progesterone T. **C,** Levonorgestrel-releasing IUD.

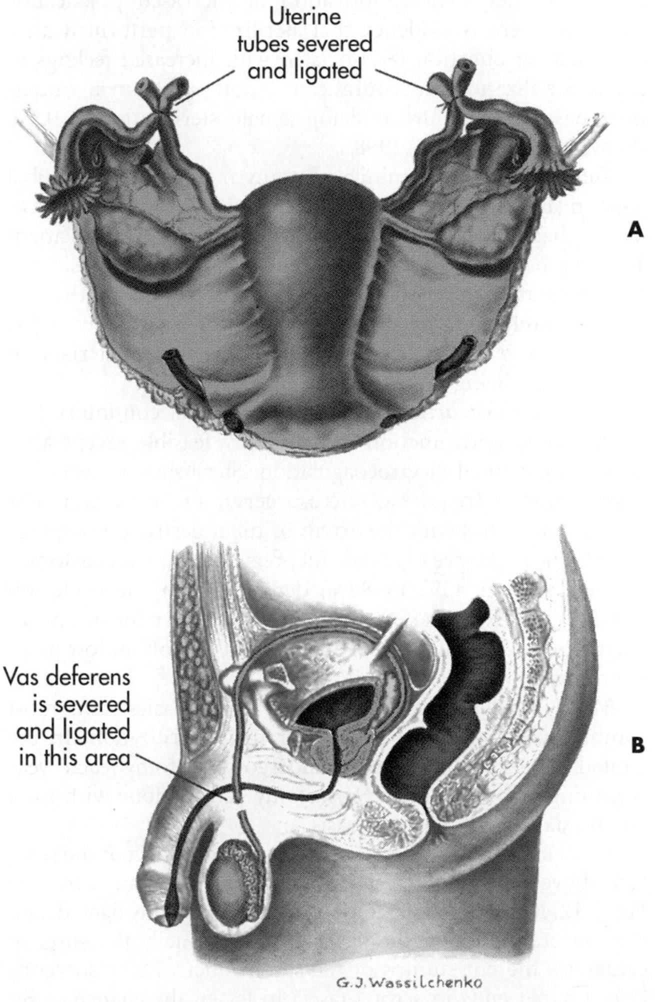

FIG. 7-12 • Sterilization. **A,** Uterine tubes ligated and severed (tubal ligation). **B,** Sperm duct ligated and severed (vasectomy).

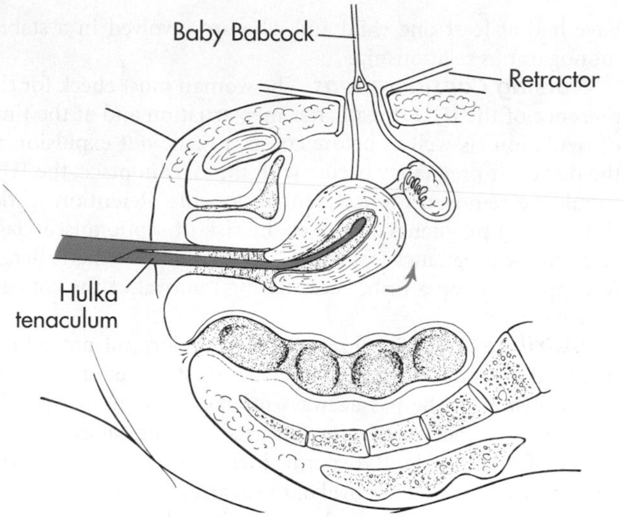

FIG. 7-13 • Use of minilaparotomy to gain access to uterine tubes for occlusion procedures. Tenaculum is used to lift uterus upward *(arrow)* toward incision.

ing any phase of the menstrual cycle). Most sterilization procedures are performed immediately after a pregnancy, probably because of heightened motivation or increased practicality. However, there is evidence that sterilization performed after childbirth or abortion is associated with increased feelings of regret. Sterilization procedures can be done safely on an outpatient basis. The failure rate for female sterilization is 0.5% (Stewart and Carignan, 1998).

Tubal Occlusion. A minilaparotomy may be used for tubal ligation (Fig. 7-13), tubal electrocoagulation, or for the application of bands or clips (e.g., Hulka, Filshe, and Wolf) (Patient Teaching box). Electrocoagulation and ligation are considered to be permanent methods. Use of the bands or clips has the theoretic advantage of possible removal and return of tubal patency. Transcervical approaches to inject occlusive material into the tubes are being investigated (Reifsnider, 1997).

Tubal Reconstruction. Restoration of tubal continuity (reanastomosis) and function is technically feasible except after laparoscopic tubal electrocoagulation. Sterilization reversal is costly, difficult (requiring microsurgery), and uncertain. The success rate varies with the extent of tubal destruction and removal. The incidence of successful pregnancy after reanastomosis ranges from 43% to 88%, depending on the occlusion method. The loss of a segment of tube necessary for sperm capacitation and fertilization is probably the reason for low pregnancy rates.

Male Sterilization. Vasectomy is the easiest and most commonly employed operation for male sterilization. In the United States, 500,000 men undergo vasectomy each year (Cunningham et al, 1997). Vasectomy can be done with local anesthesia on an outpatient basis.

Small incisions are made into the anterior aspect of the scrotum above and lateral to each testis over the spermatic cord (see Fig. 7-12, *B*). Each vas deferens is identified, doubly ligated, and then severed between the ligatures. Occasionally the surgeon cauterizes the cut stumps of the sperm ducts. Many surgeons bury the cut ends in scrotal fascia to lessen the chance of reunion. Then the skin incisions are closed. Usually one suture is used for closure of each skin incision and a dressing is applied.

Patient Teaching

WHAT TO EXPECT AFTER TUBAL LIGATION

You should expect no change in hormones and their influence.
Your menstrual period will be approximately the same as before the sterilization.
You may feel pain of ovulation.
The ovum disintegrates within the abdominal cavity.
It is highly unlikely that you will get pregnant.
You should not experience a change in sexual functioning; in fact, you may enjoy sexual relations more because you will not be concerned about getting pregnant.
Sterilization offers no protection against STIs; therefore you may need to use condoms.

Endocrine production of testosterone continues so that secondary sex characteristics are not affected. Complications after bilateral vasectomy are uncommon and usually not serious. They include bleeding (usually external), suture reaction, and reaction to the anesthetic agent. Men occasionally may develop a hematoma, infection, or epididymitis. Less common are painful granulomas from accumulation of sperm. The failure rate for male sterilization is 15% (Stewart and Carignan, 1998).

Tubal Reconstruction. Microsurgery to reanastomose and restore tubal continuity of the sperm ducts can be accomplished successfully (i.e., sperm in the ejaculate) in 98% of cases; however, the fertility rate is much lower (16% to 79%) (Stewart and Carignan, 1998). The rate of success decreases as the time since the procedure increases. The vasectomy may result in permanent changes in the testes that leave men unable to father children. The changes are those ordinarily seen only in the elderly (e.g., interstitial fibrosis [scar tissue between the seminiferous tubules]). Some men develop antibodies against their own sperm (autoimmunization).

Laws and Regulations. All states have strict regulations for informed consent. Many states permit voluntary sterilization of any mature, rational woman without reference to her marital or pregnancy status. Although the partner's consent is not required by law, the woman is encouraged to discuss the situation with the partner, and health care providers may request the partner's consent. Sterilization of minors or mentally incompetent individuals is restricted by most states and often requires the approval of a board of eugenicists or other court-appointed individuals.

LEGAL TIP • Sterilization If federal funds are used for sterilization, the person must be at least 21 years old. Informed consent must include an explanation of the risks, benefits, and alternatives; a statement that describes sterilization as a permanent, irreversible method of birth control; and a statement that mandates a 30-day waiting period between giving consent and the sterilization. Informed consent must be in the person's native language, or an interpreter must be provided.

Nursing Considerations. The nurse plays an important role in assisting people with decision making so that all requirements for informed consent are met. The nurse also provides information about alternatives to sterilization, such as contraception.

Nursing Care Plan SEXUAL ACTIVITY AND CONTRACEPTION

NURSING DIAGNOSIS **Decisional conflict related to contraceptive alternatives**

EXPECTED OUTCOME Patient and partner will verbalize understanding of different methods of contraception and will choose the method best suited for their needs.

Nursing Interventions/*Rationales*

Provide information regarding reliability, use, indications, contraindications, and side effects of different methods of contraception *to facilitate the decision-making process.*

Utilize privacy and therapeutic communication during discussion of sexual activity and methods of contraception *to provide clarification of information and patient trust of caregiver.*

NURSING DIAGNOSIS **Risk for infection related to ongoing sexual activity as evidenced by patient history**

EXPECTED OUTCOME Patient and her partner will remain free of sexually transmitted infections.

Nursing Interventions/*Rationales*

Provide information regarding safer sex practices, use of spermicides and barrier methods *to raise patient awareness of methods to prevent infection.*

Information must be given about what is entailed in the various procedures, how much discomfort or pain can be expected, and what type of care is needed. Many individuals fear sterilization procedures because of the imagined effect on their sexual life. They need reassurance concerning the hormonal and psychologic basis for sexual function, and that uterine tube occlusion or vasectomy has no biologic sequelae in terms of sexual adequacy (Stewart and Carignan, 1998).

Preoperative care includes health assessment, which includes a psychologic assessment, physical examination, and laboratory tests. Postoperative care depends on the procedure performed, for example, laparoscopy or laparotomy for tubal occlusion, or vasectomy. General care includes recovery after anesthesia, vital signs, fluid-electrolyte balance (e.g., intake and output and laboratory values), prevention of or early identification and treatment of infection or hemorrhage, control of discomfort, and assessment of emotional response to the procedure and recovery.

Discharge planning depends on the type of procedure performed. In general, the patient is given written instructions about observing for and reporting symptoms and signs of complications, the type of recovery to be expected, and the date and time for a follow-up appointment.

➤ Evaluation

The nurse can be reasonably assured that care was effective when the patient-centered expected outcomes have been achieved (Nursing Care Plan).

ABORTION

Induced abortion is the purposeful interruption of a pregnancy before 20 weeks gestation. (Miscarriage is discussed in Chapter 14.) If the abortion is performed at the woman's request, the term elective abortion is usually used; if performed for reasons of maternal or fetal health or disease, the term therapeutic abortion usually applies. Many factors contribute to a woman's decision to have an abortion. Indications include (1) preservation of the life or health of the mother, (2) genetic disorders of the fetus, (3) rape or incest, and (4) the pregnant woman's request. The control of birth, dealing as it does with human sexuality and the question of life and death, is one of the most emotional components of health care and has been the most controversial social issue in the last half of the twentieth century (Soriano, 1998). Abortion as a surgical alternative to contraception is regulated in most countries (World Health Organization, 1995). Regulations exist to protect the mother from the complications of abortion.

> ### Critical Thinking
> **TERMINATION OF PREGNANCY**
>
> **Tricia is a 24-year-old single woman, engaged to be married, whose contraceptive failed. She is 6 weeks pregnant and is seeking termination of the pregnancy. What procedure is most likely to be chosen at this gestation? What are the risks associated with the procedure? Should her fiancé be involved in the decision to terminate the pregnancy? What are your feelings about terminating this pregnancy? Would you feel differently if Tricia were pregnant as a result of rape or incest? Would you feel differently if the fetus has congenital anomalies incompatible with life?**

The majority of women having abortions are Caucasian, younger than 24 years old, and unmarried (Centers for Disease Control and Prevention, 1996). Only one fourth of abortions are obtained by married women (Wallach and Zacur, 1995). Sixty percent of women having abortions say they used a contraceptive, but it failed. The U.S. Supreme Court set aside previous antiabortion laws in January 1973, holding that first trimester abortion is permissible inasmuch as the mortality rate from interruption of early gestation is less than the mortality rate after normal term delivery; 90% of abortions are performed at this point in pregnancy (Wallach and Zacur, 1995). Second trimester abortion was left to the discretion of the individual states (Cates and Ellertson, 1998). Hospitals maintained by Roman Catholics, and others maintained by strict fundamentalists, forbid abortion (and often sterilization) despite legal challenges.

LEGAL TIP • Induced Abortion It is important for nurses to know the laws regarding abortion in their state of practice before they offer abortion counseling or nursing care to a woman choosing an abortion. Many states enforce a mandatory delay or state-directed counseling before a woman may legally obtain an abortion.

The woman facing an abortion is pregnant and will exhibit the emotional responses shared by all pregnant women, including the possibility of postbirth depression. Nurses often struggle with the same values and moral convictions as those of the pregnant woman. The conflicts and doubts of the nurse can be nonverbally communicated to women who are already anxious and overly sensitive. Health care professionals need assistance to identify and come to terms with their own feelings. It is not uncommon for confusion to arise when beliefs are challenged by the reality of care.

NURSE ALERT • Nurses whose religious or moral beliefs do not support abortion have the right to refuse such an assignment. Reassignment is usually an option so that the abortion patient receives needed care.

First Trimester Abortion

Methods for performing early elective abortion include vacuum aspiration; and medical methods (e.g., mifepristone with prostaglandin, and methotrexate with misoprostol).

Vacuum aspiration abortion is the most common procedure, with about 97% of all procedures being performed by suction curettage. Very early abortions (e.g., menstrual extraction and endometrial aspiration) can be done without cervical dilation or anesthesia with a small, flexible, plastic cannula. The insertion of a small laminaria tent (i.e., a cone of dried seaweed that swells as it absorbs moisture and dilates the cervix) retained by a vaginal tampon for 4 to 24 hours will atraumatically dilate the cervix two or three times its original diameter. This usually facilitates the purposeful interruption of a first trimester pregnancy greater than 8 weeks of gestation (Wallach and Zacur, 1995). On removal of the laminaria tent, the insertion of an adequate-sized aspiration cannula (8.5 to 10.5 mm) is almost always possible. Prostaglandin gel may also be used to soften the cervix (Cunningham et al, 1997).

Aspiration abortion may be performed in a physician's office, clinic, or hospital. The suction procedure for performing an early elective abortion (ideal time is 8 to 12 weeks after the last menstrual period) usually requires less than 5 minutes. During the procedure, the woman is kept informed about what to expect next (e.g., menstrual-like cramping and sounds of the suction machine) and her vital signs are assessed. The aspirated uterine contents must be carefully inspected to ascertain whether all fetal parts and adequate placental tissue have been evacuated. After the abortion the woman rests on the table until she is ready to stand. She then remains in the recovery area or waiting room for 1 to 3 hours for detection of excessive cramping or bleeding. She may be discharged alone or in the company of a relative or friend, depending on the anesthetic used. If the procedure is done in the physician's office, preoperative sedation is usually not given, and local anesthesia is usually used.

Bleeding after the operation is normally about the equivalent of a heavy menstrual period, and cramps are rarely severe. Excessive vaginal bleeding and infection, such as endometritis or salpingitis, are the most common complications of induced abortion. Retained products of conception are the primary cause of vaginal bleeding. Evacuation of the uterus, uterine massage, and administration of oxytocin or methylergonovine (Methergine) may be necessary (Cates and Ellertson, 1998; World Health Organization, 1995). Prophylactic antibiotics have been shown to decrease the risk of infection and should be considered (Grimes, 1995).

Nursing Considerations. Postabortal instructions differ among health care providers (e.g., tampons should not be used for at least 3 days or should be avoided for up to 3 weeks, and resumption of sexual intercourse may be permitted within 1 week or discouraged for 3 weeks). The woman may shower daily. Instruction is given to watch for excessive bleeding (i.e., more than one large pad per hour for 4 hours), cramps, or fever, and to avoid douches of any type. The woman may expect her menstrual period to resume 4 to 6 weeks after the day of the procedure. The nurse offers information about the birth control method the woman prefers, if this has not been done during the counseling interview that usually precedes the decision to have an abortion. The woman must be strongly encouraged to return for her follow-up visit so that complications can be detected and an acceptable contraceptive method prescribed. A pregnancy test may also be performed to determine if the pregnancy has been successfully terminated.

Other First Trimester Abortions

Methotrexate. Methotrexate can be given intramuscularly followed by vaginal placement of misoprostol (prostaglandin analog). Oral methotrexate followed by vaginal misoprostol also has been shown to be effective with few side effects (Carbonell et al, 1998). If abortion does not occur by the next day, misoprostol is repeated (Creinin et al, 1996).

Mifepristone. Mifepristone (RU 486) can be taken up to 5 weeks after conception. The effectiveness of mifepristone is inversely related to gestational age as determined by b-human chorionic gonadotropin levels and the duration of amenorrhea (Creinin et al, 1996). However, it is considered to be an effective and safe method for termination of early pregnancy.

Uterine bleeding begins within 4 days of administration of the first dose. Usually a period of painless heavy bleeding is reported. Termination of pregnancy occurs for most women. When mifepristone is combined with administration of a prostaglandin agent 36 to 48 hours later, the rate of abortion increases.

Supporters of this method believe that even with known disadvantages, mifepristone offers a reasonable alternative to surgical abortion, which carries the risk of anesthesia, surgical complications, and infertility (Cates and Ellertson, 1998). Others have taken a strong stand against the use of mifepristone. In the United States it is still not readily available for terminating pregnancy.

Second Trimester Abortion

Second trimester abortion is associated with an increase of complications and higher costs. Dilation and evacuation, induction of uterine contractions, and major operations are the methods used.

Dilation and Evacuation. Dilation and evacuation (D&E) can be performed at up to 20 weeks of gestation (Cates and Ellertson, 1998). It is the predominant method of abortion used beyond the first trimester (Wallach and Zacur, 1995). The cervix requires more dilation because the products of conception are larger. Often laminaria are inserted several hours or several days before the procedure. Nursing care includes monitoring vital signs, providing emotional support, administering analgesics, and postoperative monitoring. Disadvantages of D&E may be long-term harmful effects on the cervix.

Prostaglandins. The most common technique for medical termination in the second trimester is the administration of prostaglandins. Prostaglandins can be administered in suppository form, as a gel, or by intrauterine injection. Unpleasant side effects (e.g., nausea, vomiting, and diarrhea) usually occur. Repeated doses may be needed for expulsion of the products of conception.

Complications After Abortion

The most common complications after abortion include infection, retained products of conception or intrauterine blood clots, continuing pregnancy, cervical or uterine trauma, and excessive bleeding (Cates and Ellertson, 1998; Wallach and Zacur, 1995). Preoperative antibiotic prophylaxis has been effective in reducing the risk of infection. Women are advised to report fever, pelvic pain, and excessive bleeding. Prophylactic chlamydia and gonorrhea treatment and the use of an oral ergonovine postoperatively may reduce the incidence of infection and retained products of conception.

Nursing Considerations. The woman considering an abortion will need help to explore the meaning of the various alternatives and consequences to herself and her significant others. It is often difficult for a woman to express her true feelings (e.g., what abortion means to her now and in the future and what support or regret her friends and peers may demonstrate). A calm, matter-of-fact approach on the part of the nurse can be helpful. Clarifying, restating, and reflecting statements; open-ended questions; and feedback are communication techniques that can be used to maintain a realistic focus on the situation and bring the woman's problems into the open. Once a decision has been made, the woman must be assured of continued support. Information must be given about what various procedures entail, how much discomfort or pain can be expected, and what type of care is needed. If family or friends cannot be involved, scheduling time for nursing personnel to give the necessary support is an essential component of the care plan.

➤ Evaluation

The nurse can be reasonably sure that care was effective when the expected outcomes have been met.

Key Points

- Infertility is the inability to conceive and to carry a child to term gestation at a time the couple has chosen to do so.
- Infertility affects between 10% to 15% of otherwise healthy adults. Infertility increases in women older than 35 years.
- In the United States, about 50% of infertility is related to female causes; 35% is related to male causes; and 10% to 15% of the causes are unexplained.
- Common etiologic factors of infertility include decreased sperm production, ovulation disorders, tubal occlusion, and endometriosis.
- Reproductive alternatives for family building include IVF-ET, GIFT, ZIFT, oocyte donation, embryo donation, TDI, surrogate motherhood, and adoption.
- A variety of contraceptive methods with various effectiveness rates, advantages, and disadvantages are available.
- Women and their partners should choose the contraceptive method(s) best suited to them.
- Effective contraceptives are available through both prescription and nonprescription sources.
- Proper concurrent use of spermicides and latex condoms provides protection against STIs.
- Tubal ligations and vasectomies are permanent sterilization methods used by increasing numbers of women and men.
- Induced abortion performed in the first trimester is safer and less complex than an abortion performed in the second trimester.
- The most common complications of induced abortion include infection, retained products of conception, and excessive vaginal bleeding.

References

American Society for Reproductive Medicine: *Results of joint SART/ASRM, CDC, and RESOLVE 1996 assisted reproductive technology success rate report,* 1999. Accessed on-line at www.asrm.com.

Angard N: Diagnosis infertility, *AWHONN Lifelines* 3(3):22-29, 1999.

Boxer A: Images of infertility, *Nurse Pract Forum* 7(2):60-63, 1996.

Carbonell J et al: Oral methotrexate and vaginal misoprostol for early abortion, *Contraception* 57(2):83-88, 1998.

Cates W, Ellertson C: Abortion. In Hatcher R et al, editors: *Contraceptive technology,* ed 17, New York, 1998, Ardent Media.

Cates W, Raymond E: Vaginal spermicides. In Hatcher R et al, editors: *Contraceptive technology,* ed 17, New York, 1998, Ardent Media.

Centers for Disease Control and Prevention: CDC surveillance summaries (abortion surveillance—United States, 1991), *MMWR* 45(SS-3):1-43, 1996.

Creinin M et al: Methotrexate and misoprostol for early abortion: a multicenter trial. I. Safety and efficacy, *Contraception* 53(6):321-327, 1996.

Cunningham F et al: *Williams' obstetrics,* ed 20, Stamford, CT, 1997, Appleton & Lange.

Draper H, Chadwick R: Beware! Preimplantation genetic diagnosis may solve some old problems but it also raises new ones, *J Med Ethics* 25:114-120, 1999.

Fasouliotis S, Schenker J: Social aspects in assisted reproduction, *Human Reproduction Update* 5(1):26-39, 1999.

Gayle H: Dear Colleague, Centers for Disease Control and Prevention, 2000; available online at http://www.cdc.gov/hiv/pubs/mmwr/mmwr11aug00.htm.

Grimes D: Sequelae of abortion. In Baird D, Grimes D, Van Look P, editors: *Modern methods of inducing abortion,* London, 1995, Blackwell Scientific.

Guest F: Education and counseling. In Hatcher R et al, editors: *Contraceptive technology,* ed 7, New York, 1998, Ardent Media.

Hargreave T, Ghosh C: Male fertility disorder, *Endocrinol Metab Clin North Am* 27(4):765-782, 1998.

Harper J, Wells D: Recent advances and future developments in PGD, *Prenat Diagn* 19(13):1193-1199, 1999.

Hatcher R: Depo-Provera, Norplant, and progestin-only pills (minipills). In Hatcher R et al, editors: *Contraceptive technology,* ed 17, New York, 1998, Ardent Media.

Hatcher R et al: *Contraceptive technology,* ed 17, New York, 1998, Ardent Media.

Heath C, Sulik S: Contraception and preconception counseling, *Women's Health* 24(10):123-133, 1997.

Henshaw S: Unintended pregnancy in the United States, *Fam Plann Perspect* 30:24-29, 46, 1998.

Jennings V, Lamprecht V, Kowal D: Fertility awareness methods. In Hatcher R et al, editors: *Contraceptive technology,* ed 17, New York, 1998, Ardent Media.

Johnson C: Regaining self-esteem: strategies and interventions for the infertile woman, *J Obstet Gynecol Neonatal Nurs* 25(4):291-295, 1996.

Jones S, Krysa L: Comfort care interventions in a preimplantation genetic testing program, *Holist Nurs Pract* 12(3):20-29, 1998.

King D: Preimplantation genetic diagnosis and the 'new' genetics, *J Med Ethics* 25:176-182, 1999.

Kowal D: Coitus interruptus (withdrawal). In Hatcher R et al, editors: *Contraceptive technology,* ed 17, New York, 1998, Ardent Media.

Mishell D: Intrauterine devices: mechanisms of action, safety, and efficacy, *Contraception* 58(suppl 3):45S-53S, 1998.

Mishell D et al: *Comprehensive gynecology,* ed 3, St Louis, 1997, Mosby.

Morell V: Basic infertility assessment, *Prim Care* 24(1):195-204, 1997.

Reifsnider E: On the horizon: new options for contraception, *J Obstet Gynecol Neonatal Nurs* 26(1):91-100, 1997.

Seibel M: *Infertility: a comprehensive text,* ed 2, Stamford, CT, 1997, Appleton & Lange.

Session D et al: Recent advances in infertility treatment, *Minnesota Medicine* 81(10):27-32, 1998.

Soriano C: Abortion: new common ground, *USA Weekend,* January 9-11, 1998.

Speroff L, Glass H, Kase G: *Clinical gynecologic endocrinology and infertility,* ed 5, Baltimore, 1994, Williams & Wilkins.

Stephen E, Chandra A: Updated projections of infertility in the United States, 1995-2025, *Fertil Steril* 70(1):30-34, 1998.

Stewart F: Vaginal barriers. In Hatcher R et al, editors: *Contraceptive technology,* ed 17, New York, 1998, Ardent Media.

Stewart G: Intrauterine devices (IUDs). In Hatcher R et al, editors: *Contraceptive technology,* ed 17, New York, 1998, Ardent Media.

Stewart G, Carignan C: Female and male sterilization. In Hatcher R et al, editors: *Contraceptive technology,* ed 17, New York, 1998, Ardent Media.

Trantham P: The infertile couple, *Am Fam Physician* 54(3):1001-1010, 1996.

Trussell J: Contraceptive efficacy. In Hatcher R et al, editors: *Contraceptive technology,* ed 17, New York, 1998, Ardent Media.

Trussell J, Rodriguez G, Ellertson C: New estimates of the effectiveness of the Yuzpe regimen of emergency contraception, *Contraception* 57(6):363-369, 1998.

Van Look P, Stewart F: Emergency contraception. In Hatcher R et al, editors: *Contraceptive technology,* ed 17, New York, 1998, Ardent Media.

Wallach E, Zacur H: *Reproductive medicine and surgery,* St Louis, 1995, Mosby.

Warner D, Hatcher R: Male condoms. In Hatcher R et al, editors: *Contraceptive technology,* ed 17, New York, 1998, Ardent Media.

Wilcox A, Weinberg C, Baird D: Timing of sexual intercourse in relation to ovulation. Effects on the probability of conception, survival of the pregnancy, and sex of the baby, *N Engl J Med* 333:1517-1521, 1995.

World Health Organization: *Complications of abortion,* Geneva, 1995, World Health Organization.

CHAPTER

8 Genetics, Conception, and Fetal Development

http://www.harcourthealth.com/MERLIN/Wong/maternal/

Learning Objectives

On completion of this chapter the reader will be able to:

- Explain basic principles of genetics.
- Describe the Human Genome Project.
- Describe the nurse's role in genetics.
- Examine ethical dimensions of genetic screening.
- Summarize the process of fertilization.
- Describe the development, structure, and functions of the placenta.
- Describe the composition and functions of the amniotic fluid.
- Identify three organs or tissues arising from each of the three primary germ layers.
- Summarize the significant changes in growth and development of the embryo and fetus.
- Identify the potential effects of teratogens during vulnerable periods of embryonic and fetal development.

This chapter presents a brief discussion of genetics and the role of the nurse in genetics. It also provides an overview of the process of fertilization and of the development of the normal embryo and fetus.

GENETICS

Genetic causes of disease have assumed increasing importance as the incidence of communicable diseases has decreased. For most genetic conditions, therapeutic or preventive measures do not exist or are very limited. Consequently, the most useful means of reducing the incidence of these disorders is by preventing their transmission. It is standard practice to assess all pregnant women for heritable disorders to identify potential problems (Creasy and Resnik, 1999). The incidence of chromosomal aberrations is estimated to be 0.5% to 0.6% in newborns. Approximately 50% of miscarriages and 5% to 7% of stillbirths and perinatal deaths are caused by chromosomal abnormalities (Lashley, 1998).

Genetic disease affects people of all ages, from all socioeconomic levels, and from all racial and ethnic backgrounds. Genetic disease affects not only individuals, but also families, communities, and society. Advances in genetic testing and genetically based treatments have altered the care provided to affected individuals. Improvements in diagnostic capability have resulted in earlier diagnosis and enabled individuals who previously would have died in childhood to survive into adulthood (Lashley, 1998). The genetic aberrations that lead to disease are present at birth but may not be manifested for many years, or possibly, not at all.

Some disorders appear more often in ethnic groups (Creasy and Resnik, 1999). Examples include Tay-Sachs disease in Ashkenazi Jews; β-thalassemia in Italians and Greeks; sickle cell anemia in African-Americans; α-thalassemia in Southeast Asians and North Africans; lactase deficiency in adult Chinese and Thailanders; cleft lip and palate and Oguchi disease in Japanese; ear anomalies in Navajo Indians; clubfoot in Polynesians; phenylketonuria in Irish, Scots, Scandinavians, Icelanders, and Polish; cystic fibrosis in Scots and English; Niemann-Pick disease, Type D, in Nova Scotia Acadians; and tyrosinemia in French-Canadians from the Lac St. Jean–Chicoutimi region of Quebec (Fanaroff and Martin, 1997; Lashley, 1998).

Relevance of Genetics to Nursing

Genetic disorders span every clinical practice specialty and site including school, clinic, office, hospital, mental health agency, and community health settings. Because the potential impact on families and the community is significant (Box 8-1) genetics must be integrated into nursing education and practice (Lashley, 1998). A genetic paradigm must be embraced; that is, genetic information, technology, and testing must be incorporated in health care services (Anderson et al, 2000). Skills needed by nurses include the ability to interview, to take a history over three generations, to recognize risk for genetic disorders, to refer for evaluation and counseling, and to explain and interpret the purpose and results of genetic tests (Lashley, 1998).

Although diagnosis and treatment of genetic disorders requires medical skills, nurses with advanced preparation are assuming important roles in counseling people about genetically transmitted or genetically influenced conditions. Nurses are usually the ones who provide follow-up care and maintain contact with the patients. Community health nurses can identify groups within populations that are high risk for illness, as well as provide care to individuals, families, and groups (Williams, 1998). They are a vital link in follow-up for newborns who may need newborn screening. The International Society of Nurses in Genetics (ISONG) has developed a Statement on the Scope and Standards of Genetics Clinical Nursing Practice (Anderson et al, 2000).

Referral to appropriate agencies is an essential part of the follow-up management. Many organizations and foundations (e.g., the Cystic Fibrosis Foundation and the Muscular Dystrophy Association) help provide services and equipment for affected children. There are also numerous parent groups in which the family can share experiences and derive mutual support from other families with similar problems.

Probably the most important of all nursing functions is providing emotional support to the family during all aspects of the counseling process. Feelings that are generated under the real or imagined threat posed by a genetic disorder are as varied as the people being counseled (McGowan, 1999). Responses may include a variety of stress reactions such as apathy, denial, anger, hostility, fear, embarrassment, grief, and loss of self-esteem.

Box 8-1

Potential Impact of Genetic Disease on Family and Community

- Financial cost to family
- Decrease in planned family size
- Loss of geographic mobility
- Decreased opportunities for siblings
- Loss of family integrity
- Loss of career opportunities and job flexibility
- Social isolation
- Lifestyle alterations
- Reduction in contributions to their community by families
- Disruption of husband-wife or partner relationship
- Threatened family self-concept
- Coping with intolerant public attitudes
- Psychologic effects
- Stresses and uncertainty of treatment
- Physical health problems
- Loss of dreams and aspirations
- Cost to society of institutionalization or home or community care
- Cost to society because of additional problems and needs of other family members
- Cost of long-term care
- Housing and living arrangement changes

From Lashley F: *Clinical genetics in nursing practice,* ed 2, New York, 1998, Springer.

Genetics Counseling Services

The most efficient counseling services are associated with the larger universities and major medical centers. This is also where support services are available (e.g., biochemistry and cytology laboratories), usually from a group of specialists under the leadership of a physician trained in medical genetics. Health professionals should become familiar with people who provide genetic counseling and the places that offer counseling services in their area of practice. Box 8-2 contains information on genetics resources.

Box 8-2

Genetics Resources on the World Wide Web

SITES FOR HEALTH PROFESSIONALS

The National Center for Human Genome Research
http://www.nhgri.nih.gov

Online Mendelian Inheritance in Man (OMIM)
http://www.ncbi.nlm.nih.gov/Omim

Understanding Gene Testing
http://www.gene.com/ae/AE/AEPC/NIH/index.html

Visible Embryo
http://visembryo.ucsf.edu

Webget
http://med.upenn.edu/bioethic/webget

Gene Tests
http://www.hslib.washington.edu/helix

MEDLINE: PubMed and Internet Grateful Med
http://www.nlm.nih.gov/databases/freemedl.html

International Society of Nurses in Genetics (ISONG)
http://www.nursing.creighton.edu/isong

The National Society of Genetic Counselors
http://members.aol.com/nsgcweb/nsgchome.htm

SITES FOR PARENTS AND FAMILIES

The Alliance of Genetic Support Groups
http://www.geneticalliance.org

A Family Guide to Cystic Fibrosis Genetic Testing
http://www.phd.msu.edu/cf/fam.html

National Marfan Foundation
http://www.marfan.org

Ask NOAH About: Pregnancy
http://www.noah.cuny.edu/pregnancy/pregnancy.html

Neurofibromatosis
http://www.nf.org/

National Down Syndrome Society
http://www.ndss.org

The National Fragile X Foundation
http://www.nfxf.org

Osteogenesis Imperfecta Foundation
http://www.oif.org

A World of Genetics Societies
http://faseb.org/genetics/mainmenu.htm

Data from Hetterberg C, Trangenstein P: Genetics and the World Wide Web: an introduction, *Neonat Netw* 18(4):9-13, 1999.

Ethical Considerations

Researchers have proposed using fetal neurologic, liver, and pancreatic tissues to treat adults with Parkinson disease, metabolic disorders, or head and spinal cord injury. The use of fetal tissue in research was banned for several years, but the ban was lifted in 1993.

Most genetic testing is offered prenatally in order to identify genetic disorders in fetuses (White, 1999). When an affected fetus is identified, termination of the pregnancy is an option. Other requests for genetic testing occur; for sex selection or for late onset disorders. An ethic of social responsibility should guide genetic counselors in their interactions with patients (White, 1999) while recognizing that people make their choices by integrating personal values and beliefs with their new knowledge of genetic risk and medical treatments (Anderson, 1998).

Other ethical issues relate to autonomy, privacy, and confidentiality. Should genetic testing be done when there is no treatment available for the disease? When is it appropriate to warn family members at risk for inherited diseases? When should presymptomatic testing be done? Some who might benefit from genetic testing choose not to have it, fearing discrimination based on the risk of a genetic disorder. Several states have prohibitions against insurance discrimination; other states are expected to follow their lead (O'Connor, 1998). Until guidelines for genetic testing are created, caution should be exercised. The benefits of testing should be weighed carefully against the potential for harm (O'Connor, 1998).

Preimplantation genetic diagnosis (PGD) is available in a limited number of centers. In this procedure, embryos are tested prior to implantation by in vitro fertilization (IVF) (Jones and Krysa, 1998). PGD has the potential to eliminate specific disorders in pregnancies conceived by IVF.

The Human Genome Project

The Human Genome Project began in 1990 as an international effort to map and sequence the genetic makeup of humans; it is funded by the National Institutes of Health (NIH) and the Department of Energy. There are 22 Human Genome Project research centers in the United States (Rice, 1998). It was expected that by 2005, the entire human genome (i.e., the copy of the genetic material in humans) would be mapped and that all of the 5 billion nucleic acid base pairs and 100,000 genes would be identified. However, initial sequencing of the human genome was completed in June 2000, well ahead of schedule. The map will facilitate study of hereditary diseases and will provide the potential for making changes at the gene level to treat or prevent hereditary diseases. Mapping is significant because there are more than 7000 single-gene disorders known (Munro, 1999).

An integral part of the Human Genome Project is the Ethical, Legal, and Social Implications (ELSI) program. This program addresses the potential that genetic information may be used to discriminate against individuals or for eugenic purposes. Continued awareness of and vigilance against such misuse of information is the collective responsibility of health care providers, ethicists, and society.

> *Community Focus*
>
> **USE OF GENETIC MATERIALS AND INFORMATION**
>
> **Rapid technologic advances have created complex questions for which there are no easy answers. Mapping of the human genome and other advances occurred before adequate debate on legal, ethical, social, and clinical issues by professionals and the public had taken place. Currently there are inadequate laws to protect the interests of stakeholders: donors, researchers, and insurers. There is no agreement on what encompasses "proper use" of such information. Continued discussion and debate must occur among ethicists, health professionals, representatives of the legal profession, and the public.**
>
> Data from: Giarelli E, Jacobs L: Issues related to the use of genetic material and information, *Oncol Nurs Forum* 27(3):459-467, 2000.

Management of Genetic Disorders

At this time, no cures exist for genetic disorders, although remedies can be implemented to prevent or reduce the harmful effects of a few disorders. Structural defects can sometimes be modified to produce normal or near-normal function. Surgical therapy is employed for congenital heart defects and cosmetic defects such as cleft lip. Advances in fetal surgery are occurring. Other conditions are treated with product replacement (e.g., thyroid for hereditary cretinism), diet modification (e.g., low phenylalanine diet for phenylketonuria), and corrective devices for missing limbs. Research is being conducted on methods to influence or change genes directly by placing substitute DNA in the cells of those with a genetic mutation, thereby preventing or curing the disease process or relieving symptoms.

The possibility exists that understanding embryonic stem cells (primitive cells that can develop into all types of body tissue, including muscles, nerves, and bones) will lead to new medical discoveries. The successful cloning of sheep, cattle, mice, and pigs; the production of rhesus monkeys through nuclear transfer of embryonic cells; and the isolation of stem cells constitute breakthroughs in technology. They also raise other ethical questions. On August 25, 2000, the NIH published guidelines for research using human stem cells (National Institutes of Health, 2000). The nurse involved in genetics must keep abreast of new developments and be prepared to discuss ethical implications with patients and other health care providers.

Estimation of Risk. The risks of recurrence of a genetic disorder are determined by the mode of inheritance. The risk of recurrence for disorders caused by a factor that segregates during cell division (i.e., genes and chromosomes) can be estimated with a high degree of accuracy by application of mendelian principles. In a dominant disorder the risk is 50%, or 1 in 2, that a subsequent offspring will be affected; an autosomal recessive disease carries a one-in-four risk of recurrence; and an X-linked disorder is related to the child's sex, as described in the section related to X-linked inheritance. Translocation chromosomes have a high risk of recurrence.

Disorders in which a subsequent pregnancy would carry no more risk than there is for pregnancy alone (estimated at 1 in 30) include those resulting from isolated incidences not likely to be present in another pregnancy. These disorders include maternal infections (e.g., rubella and toxoplasmosis), maternal ingestion of drugs, most chromosomal abnormalities, and a disorder determined to be the result of a fresh mutation.

Interpretation of Risk. Counselors explain the risk estimates to patients without making recommendations or decisions and without allowing their own biases to interfere. The counselor provides appropriate information about the nature of the disorder, the extent of the risks in the specific case, the probable consequences, and (if appropriate) alternative options available; however, the final decision to become pregnant or to continue a pregnancy must be left to the family. An important nursing role is reinforcing the information the families are given and continuing to interpret this information on their level of understanding.

The most important concept that must be emphasized to families is that *each pregnancy is an independent event.* For example, in monogenic disorders, in which the risk factor is 1 in 4 that the child will be affected, the risk remains the same no matter how many affected children are already in the family. Families may make the erroneous assumption that the presence of one affected child ensures that the next three will be free of the disorder. However, "chance has no memory." The risk is 1 in 4 for each pregnancy. On the other hand, in a family with a child who has a disorder with multifactorial causes, the risk increases with each subsequent child born with the disorder.

GENES AND CHROMOSOMES

The hereditary material carried in the nucleus of each somatic (body) cell determines an individual's physical characteristics. This material, called deoxyribonucleic acid (DNA), forms threadlike strands known as chromosomes. Each chromosome is composed of many smaller segments of DNA referred to as genes. Genes or combinations of genes contain "coded" information that determines an individual's unique characteristics. The code consists of the specific linear order of the molecules that combine to form the strands of DNA.

All normal human somatic cells contain 46 chromosomes arranged as 23 pairs of homologous (matched) chromosomes; one chromosome of each pair is inherited from each parent. There are 22 pairs of autosomes, which control most traits in the body; and one pair of sex chromosomes, which determines sex and some other traits. The large female chromosome is called the X; the tiny male chromosome is the Y. When one X and one Y chromosomes are present, the embryo develops as a male. When two X chromosomes are present, the embryo develops as a female.

Because each gene occupies a specific chromosome location, and because chromosomes are inherited as homologous pairs, each person has two genes for every trait. In other words, if an autosome has a gene for hair color, its partner also has a gene for hair color—in the same location on the chromosome. Although both genes code for hair color, however, they may not code for the same hair color. Different genes coding for different variations of the same trait are called alleles. An individual with two copies of the same allele for a given trait is said to be homozygous for that trait; with two different alleles, the person is heterozygous for the trait.

Some genes are dominant, and their characteristics are expressed even if another allele is present on the other chromosome. Other genes are recessive, and their characteristics are expressed only if they are carried by both homologous chromosomes. When an egg and a sperm unite, the combination of alleles becomes that individual's entire genetic makeup, or genotype. This includes all the genes that the person carries and that can be passed to offspring. The genotype determines the person's physical appearance, or phenotype, but this is affected by the dominant or recessive nature of the allele.

The pictorial analysis of the number, form, and size of an individual's chromosomes is known as a karyotype. A karyotype can be obtained from a blood sample that has been treated and stained to make the replicating chromosomes visible under a mi-

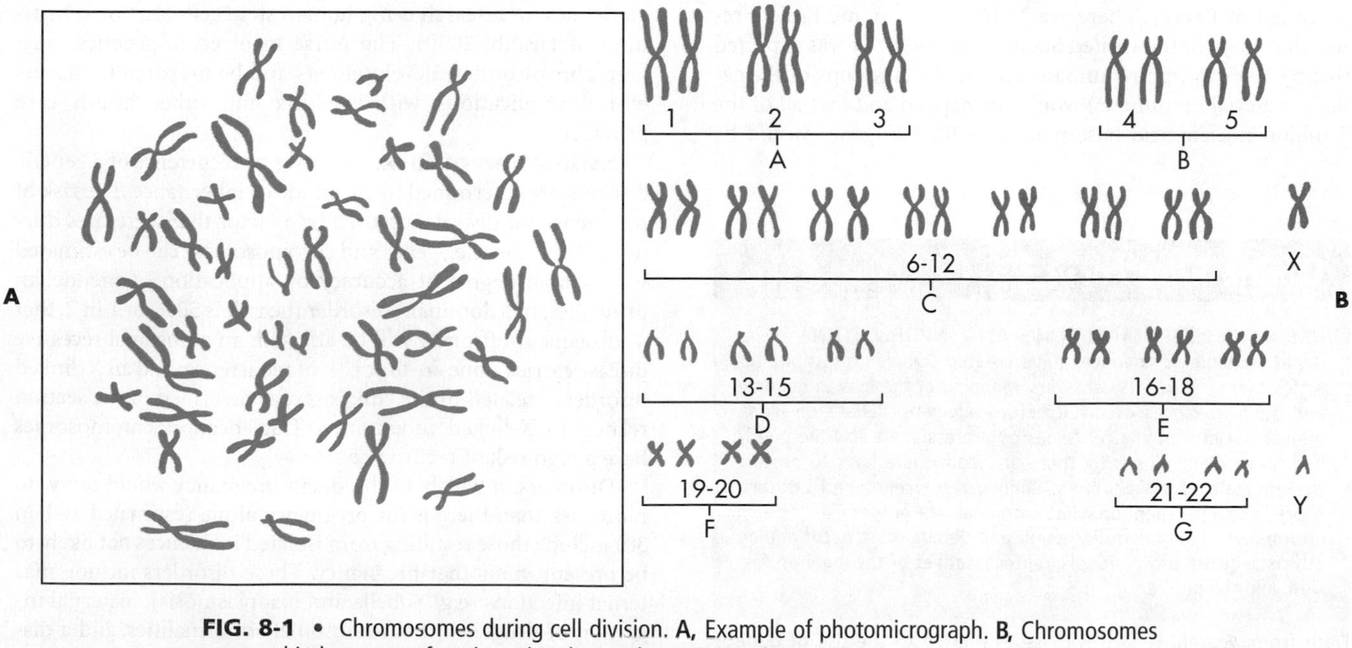

FIG. 8-1 • Chromosomes during cell division. **A,** Example of photomicrograph. **B,** Chromosomes arranged in karyotype; female and male sex-determining chromosomes.

croscope. The photographed chromosomes are cut out and arranged in a specific numeric order according to their length and shape. Fig. 8-1 illustrates the chromosomes in a body cell and a karyotype. Karyotypes can be used to determine the sex of a child and the presence of any gross chromosomal abnormalities.

Chromosomal Abnormalities

Errors resulting in chromosomal abnormalities can occur in mitosis or meiosis. These occur in either the autosomes or the sex chromosomes. Even without the presence of obvious structural malformations, small deviations in chromosomes can cause problems in fetal development.

Autosomal Abnormalities. Autosomal abnormalities involve differences in the number or structure of chromosomes resulting from unequal distribution of the genetic material during gamete formation.

Abnormalities of Chromosome Number. An abnormality of chromosome number, or aneuploidy, is most often caused by nondisjunction. Nondisjunction occurs during meiosis when a pair of chromosomes fails to separate, and one resulting cell contains both chromosomes while the other contains none. The product of the union of a normal gamete with a gamete containing an extra chromosome is a trisomy. The resulting individual has 47 chromosomes in each cell.

The most common trisomal abnormality is Down syndrome, or trisomy 21 (see Fig. 42-5 and discussion in Chapter 42). Other autosomal trisomies that have been identified are trisomy 18 (Edwards syndrome) and trisomy 13 (Patau syndrome). Both conditions have a very poor prognosis, and most affected children die from cardiac or respiratory complications within 6 months of birth.

The product of the union of a normal gamete (ovum or sperm) with a gamete that is missing a chromosome is a monosomy. This individual would have only 45 chromosomes in each cell. The lack of an autosomal chromosome always results in death of the embryo.

Nondisjunction can also occur during mitosis. If this occurs early in development, when cell lines are forming, the individual has a mixture of cells, some with a normal number of chromosomes and others either missing a chromosome or containing an extra chromosome. This condition is known as mosaicism.

Abnormalities of Chromosome Structure. Abnormalities of chromosome structure involve chromosome breakage, usually resulting from one of two events: (1) translocation, and (2) additions and/or deletions. Translocation occurs when genetic material is transferred from one chromosome to another, different chromosome. Thus instead of two normal pairs of chromosomes, the individual has one normal chromosome of each pair and a third chromosome that is a fusion of the other two chromosomes. As long as all genetic material is retained in the cell, the individual is unaffected but is a carrier of a balanced translocation.

If a gamete receives the two normal chromosomes or the fused chromosome, the resulting offspring will be clinically normal. If the gamete receives one of the two normal chromosomes and the fused version, the resulting offspring will have an extra copy of one of the chromosomes. This condition is called an unbalanced translocation and often has serious clinical effects.

Whenever a portion of a chromosome is deleted from one chromosome and added to another, the gamete produced may have either extra copies of genes or too few copies. The clinical effects produced may be mild or severe depending on the amount of genetic material involved.

Sex Chromosome Abnormalities. Several sex chromosome abnormalities have been identified that are caused by nondisjunction during gametogenesis in either parent. The most common deviation in females is Turner's syndrome, or monosomy X (having only one X chromosome); the affected female exhibits juvenile external genitalia with undeveloped ovaries. She is usually short in stature with webbing of the neck. Intelligence may be impaired. Most affected embryos miscarry spontaneously.

The most common deviation in males is Klinefelter's syndrome, or trisomy of the sex chromosomes XXY (an extra X chromosome). The affected male has poorly developed secondary sexual characteristics and small testes. He is infertile, usually tall, and effeminate. Males who are mosaic for Klinefelter's syndrome may be fertile. Subnormal intelligence is usually present.

Patterns of Genetic Transmission

Heritable characteristics are those that can be passed on to offspring. The patterns by which genetic material is transmitted to the next generation are affected by the number of genes involved in the expression of the trait. Many phenotypic characteristics result from two or more genes on different chromosomes acting together (referred to as multifactorial inheritance); others are controlled by a single gene (unifactorial inheritance).

Defects at the gene level cannot be determined by conventional laboratory methods such as karyotyping. Instead, genetic counselors predict the probability of the presence of an abnormal gene from the known occurrence of the trait in the individual's family and the known patterns by which the trait is inherited.

Multifactorial Inheritance. Most common congenital malformations, such as cleft lip and palate and neural tube defects, result from multifactorial inheritance, a combination of genetic and environmental factors. Each malformation may range from mild to severe, depending on the number of genes for the defect present or the amount of environmental influence. Multifactorial disorders tend to occur in families. Some malformations occur more often in one sex than the other.

Unifactorial Inheritance. If a single gene controls a particular trait, disorder, or defect, its pattern of inheritance is referred to as unifactorial mendelian or single-gene inheritance. The number of unifactorial abnormalities far exceeds the number of chromosomal abnormalities. This is understandable, considering that 50,000 to 100,000 genes in the haploid number (23) of chromosomes are passed on to an offspring from each parent.

Unifactorial or single-gene disorders follow the inheritance patterns of dominance, segregation, and independent assortment described by Mendel and include autosomal dominant, autosomal recessive, and X-linked dominant and recessive modes of inheritance (Fig. 8-2).

Autosomal dominant inheritance. Autosomal dominant inheritance disorders are those in which the abnormal gene for the trait is expressed even when the other member of the pair is normal. The abnormal gene may appear as a result of a mutation, a spontaneous and permanent change in the normal gene structure. In this case the disorder occurs for the first time in the family. Usually an affected individual comes from multiple generations having the disorder (Fig. 8-2, *B* and *C*). Males and females are equally affected.

Examples of common autosomal dominantly inherited disorders are Marfan syndrome (a disorder of connective tissue resulting in skeletal, ocular, and cardiovascular abnormalities), achondroplasia (dwarfism), polydactyly (extra digits), Huntington disease, and polycystic kidney disease.

Nursing Care Plan THE FAMILY WITH A NEONATE WITH FRAGILE X SYNDROME

NURSING DIAGNOSIS Risk for altered family processes related to birth of a neonate with an inherited disorder

EXPECTED OUTCOME The couple will verbalize accurate information about fragile X disorder including implications for future pregnancies.

Nursing Interventions/*Rationales*

Assess knowledge base of couple regarding the clinical signs and symptoms of fragile X syndrome and inheritance patterns *to correct any misconceptions and establish basis for teaching plan.*

Provide information throughout the genetics evaluation regarding risk status and clinical signs and symptoms of fragile X syndrome *to give couple a realistic picture of neonate's defects and assist with decision making for future pregnancies.*

Use therapeutic communication during discussions with the couple *to provide opportunity for expression of concern.*

Refer to support groups, social services, or counseling *to assist with family cohesive actions and decision making.*

Refer to child development specialist *to provide family with realistic expectations regarding cognitive and behavioral differences of child with fragile X syndrome.*

NURSING DIAGNOSIS Situational low self-esteem related to diagnosis of inherited disorder as evidenced by parents' statements of guilt and shame

EXPECTED OUTCOME The parents will express an increased number of positive statements regarding the birth of a neonate with fragile X syndrome.

Nursing Interventions/*Rationales*

Assist parents to list strengths and coping strategies which have been helpful in past situations *to use appropriate strategies during this situational crisis.*

Encourage expression of feelings using therapeutic communication *to provide clarification and emotional support.*

Clarify and provide information regarding fragile X syndrome *to decrease feelings of guilt and gradually increase feelings of positive self-esteem.*

Refer for further counseling as needed *to provide more in-depth and ongoing support.*

NURSING DIAGNOSIS Risk for altered parenting related to birth of neonate with fragile X syndrome

Nursing Interventions/*Rationales*

Assist parents to see and describe normal aspects of infant *to promote bonding.*

Encourage and assist with breastfeeding if that is parent's choice of feeding method *to facilitate closeness with infant and provide benefits of breastmilk.*

Assure parents that information regarding the neonate will remain confidential *to assist the parents to maintain some situational control and allow for time to work through their feelings.*

Discuss and role play with parents ways of informing family and friends of infant's diagnosis and prognosis *to promote positive aspects of infant and decrease potential isolation from social interactions.*

Provide anticipatory guidance about what to expect as infant develops *to assist family to be prepared for behavior problems or mental deficits.*

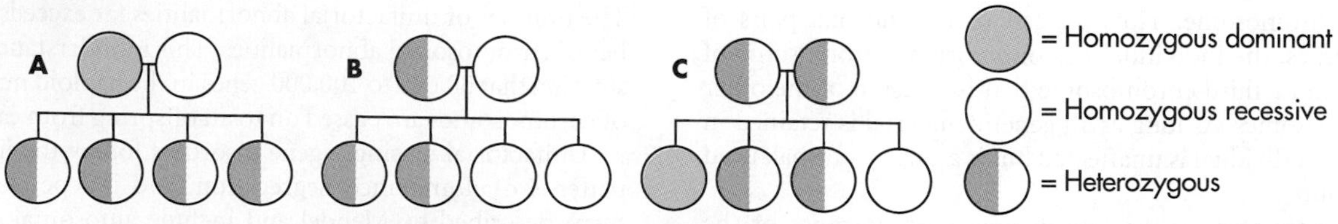

FIG. 8-2 • Possible offspring in three types of matings. **A,** Homozygous-dominant parent and homozygous-recessive parent. Children all heterozygous, displaying dominant trait. **B,** Heterozygous parent and homozygous-recessive parent. Children 50% heterozygous, displaying dominant trait; 50% homozygous, displaying recessive trait. **C,** Both parents heterozygous. Children 25% homozygous, displaying dominant trait; 25% homozygous, displaying recessive trait; 50% heterozygous, displaying dominant trait.

Autosomal Recessive Inheritance. Autosomal recessive inheritance disorders are those in which both genes of a pair must be abnormal for the disorder to be expressed. Heterozygous individuals have only one abnormal gene and are unaffected clinically because their normal gene overshadows the abnormal gene. They are known as carriers of the recessive trait. For the trait to be expressed, two carriers must each contribute the abnormal gene to the offspring (Fig. 8-2, *C*). Males and females are equally affected. Most inborn errors of metabolism, such as phenylketonuria, galactosemia, maple syrup urine disease, Tay-Sachs disease, sickle cell anemia, and cystic fibrosis, are autosomal recessive inherited disorders.

X-Linked Dominant Inheritance. X-linked dominant inheritance disorders occur in males and heterozygous females. Because the females also have a normal gene, the effects are less severe than in affected males. Affected males transmit the abnormal gene only to their daughters on the X chromosome. Fragile-X syndrome is an example of an X-linked dominant inherited disorder (Nursing Care Plan). (See discussion in Chapter 42.)

X-Linked Recessive Inheritance. Abnormal genes for X-linked recessive inheritance disorders are carried on the X chromosome. Females may be heterozygous or homozygous for traits carried on the X chromosome because they have two X chromosomes. Males are hemizygous because they have only one X chromosome carrying genes, with no alleles on the Y chromosome. Therefore X-linked recessive disorders are most often manifested in the male with the abnormal gene on his single X chromosome. Hemophilia, color blindness, and Duchenne muscular dystrophy are all X-linked recessive disorders.

Inborn Errors of Metabolism. Disorders of protein, fat, or carbohydrate metabolism that reflect absent or defective enzymes generally follow a recessive pattern of inheritance. Enzymes, the actions of which are genetically determined, are essential for all the physical and chemical processes that sustain body systems. Defective enzyme action interrupts the normal series of chemical reactions from the affected point onward. The result may be an accumulation of a damaging product such as phenylalanine or the absence of a necessary product such as thyroxin or melanin. (See Table 25-2 for screening tests for inborn errors of metabolism.)

Phenylketonuria (PKU) is an uncommon disorder caused by autosomal recessive genes. A deficiency in the liver enzyme phenylalanine hydroxylase results in failure to metabolize the amino acid phenylalanine, allowing its metabolites to accumulate in the blood. The incidence of this disorder is 1 in every 10,000 to 20,000 births. Screening for PKU is routinely performed on all infants in the newborn nursery through a blood test.

Tay-Sachs disease, inherited as an autosomal recessive trait, results from a deficiency in hexosaminidase. It occurs primarily in Jewish families. Infants appear normal until 4 to 6 months of age, then the clinical symptoms appear: apathy and regression in motor and social development, and decreased vision. Death occurs between ages 3 and 4 years of age. No known treatment exists.

Cystic fibrosis (mucoviscidosis or fibrocystic disease of the pancreas) is inherited as an autosomal recessive trait and is characterized by generalized involvement of exocrine glands. Clinical features are related to the altered viscosity of mucus-secreting glands throughout the body. Overall incidence is 1 per every 2000 births. Advances in diagnosis and treatment have improved the prognosis; many affected individuals live to adulthood. Some affected women have borne children, but men generally are sterile.

Meconium ileus occurs in about 10% of newborns with cystic fibrosis. Although an initial stool may be passed from the rectum with none thereafter, usually no meconium is passed during the first 24 to 48 hours. The abdomen becomes increasingly distended, and eventually the newborn requires a laparotomy for diagnosis and treatment of the condition. (See discussion in Chapter 46.)

Nongenetic Factors Influencing Development

Not all congenital disorders are inherited. Congenital means that the condition was present at birth. Some congenital malformations may be the result of teratogens, that is, environmental substances or exposures that result in functional or structural disability. In contrast to other forms of developmental disabilities, disabilities caused by teratogens are, in theory, totally preventable. Known human teratogens are drugs and chemicals, infections, exposure to radiation (Scialli, 1997), and certain maternal conditions such as diabetes and PKU (Box 8-3). A teratogen has the greatest effect on the organs and parts of an embryo during its periods of rapid differentiation. This occurs during the embryonic period, specifically from days 15 to 60. During the first 2 weeks of development, teratogens either have no effect on the embryo or have effects so severe that they cause

Box 8-3

Etiology of Human Malformations

ENVIRONMENTAL

Maternal Conditions

Alcoholism, diabetes, endocrinopathies, phenylketonuria, smoking, nutritional problems

Infectious Agents

Rubella, toxoplasmosis, syphilis, herpes simplex, cytomegalic inclusion disease, varicella, Venezuelan equine encephalitis

Mechanical Problems (Deformations)

Amniotic band constrictions, umbilical cord constraint, disparity in uterine size and uterine contents

Chemicals, Drugs, Radiation, Hyperthermia

GENETIC

Single Gene Disorders

Chromosomal Abnormalities

UNKNOWN

Polygenic/Multifactorial (Gene-Environment Interactions)

"Spontaneous" errors of development

Other Unknowns

Modified from Fanaroff A, Martin R: *Neonatal-perinatal medicine: diseases of the fetus and infant,* St Louis, 1997, Mosby.

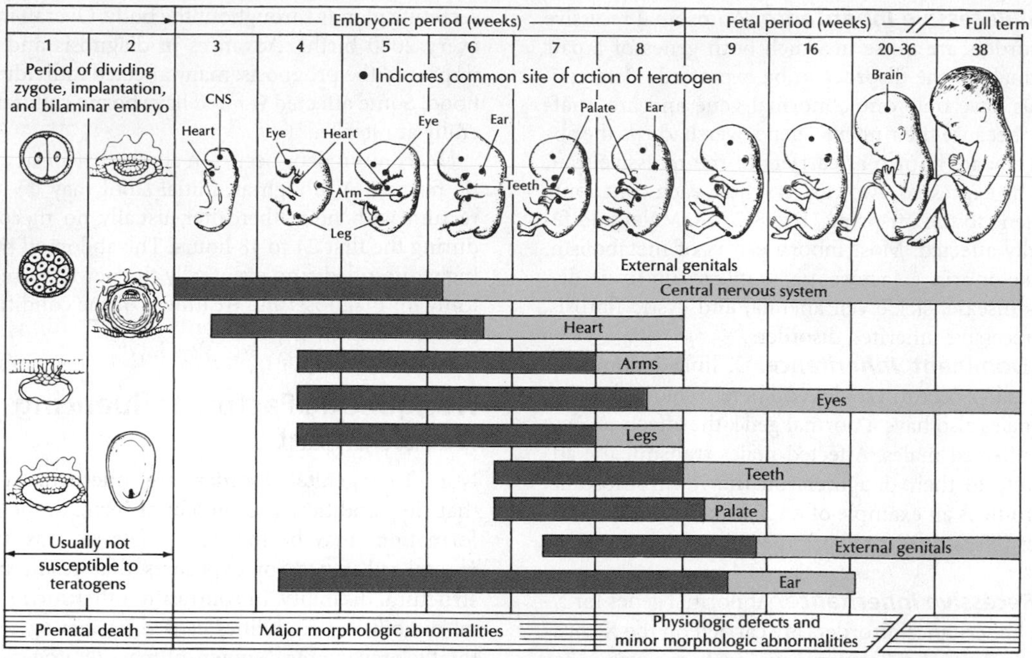

FIG. 8-3 • Sensitive, or critical, periods in human development. Dark color denotes highly sensitive periods; light color indicates stages that are less sensitive to teratogens. (From Moore K, Persaud T: *Before we are born: basic embryology and birth defects,* ed 5, Philadelphia, 1998, Saunders.)

Critical Thinking

WEB RESOURCES ON GENETICS

Select two web addresses for resources on genetics for parents from the list provided in this chapter. Access the sites.

- **Compare and contrast the appearance, the readability, and the information contained in the sites.**
- **To whom would you recommend these sites?**
- **Is the information contained culturally relevant?**
- **What information would parents need?**
- **How could you as a nurse use this information?**

miscarriage. Brain growth and development continue during the fetal period, and teratogens can severely affect mental development throughout gestation (Fig. 8-3).

In addition to genetic makeup and the influence of teratogens, the adequacy of maternal nutrition influences development. The embryo and fetus must obtain the nutrients they need from the mother's diet; they cannot tap the maternal reserves. Malnutrition during pregnancy produces low-birth-weight (LBW) newborns who are susceptible to infection. Malnutrition also affects brain development during the latter half of gestation and may result in learning disabilities in the child.

The field of behavioral genetics is engaged in discovering links between genetics and environment in explaining normal and deviant behavior (Sherman et al, 1997). This represents a movement away from the belief that human behavior is almost completely the result of influences of the environment. For example, memory and intelligence, activity level, sociability, and shyness all have some degree of genetic influence (Sherman et al, 1997).

CONCEPTION

Cell Division

Cells are reproduced by two different methods: mitosis and meiosis. In mitosis, the body cells replicate to yield two cells with the same genetic makeup as the parent cell. First the cell makes a copy of its DNA; then it divides, with each daughter cell receiving one copy of the genetic material. The purpose of mitotic division is growth and development or cell replacement.

Meiosis produces gametes (eggs and sperm). Each homologous pair of chromosomes contains one chromosome received from the mother and one from the father; thus meiosis results in cells that contain one of each of the 23 pairs of chromosomes. Because these germ cells contain 23 single chromosomes, half of the genetic material of a normal somatic cell, they are called haploid. When the female gamete (egg or ovum) and the male gamete (spermatozoon) unite to form the zygote, the diploid number of human chromosomes (46, or 23 pairs) is restored.

The process of DNA replication and cell division in meiosis allows different alleles for genes to be distributed at random by each parent and then rearranged on the paired chromosomes. The chromosomes then separate and proceed to different gametes. Because the two parents have genotypes derived from four different grandparents, many combinations of genes on each chromosome are possible. This random mixing of alleles accounts for the variation of traits seen in the offspring of the same two parents.

Gametogenesis

When a male reaches puberty, his testes begin the process of spermatogenesis. The cells that undergo meiosis in the male are

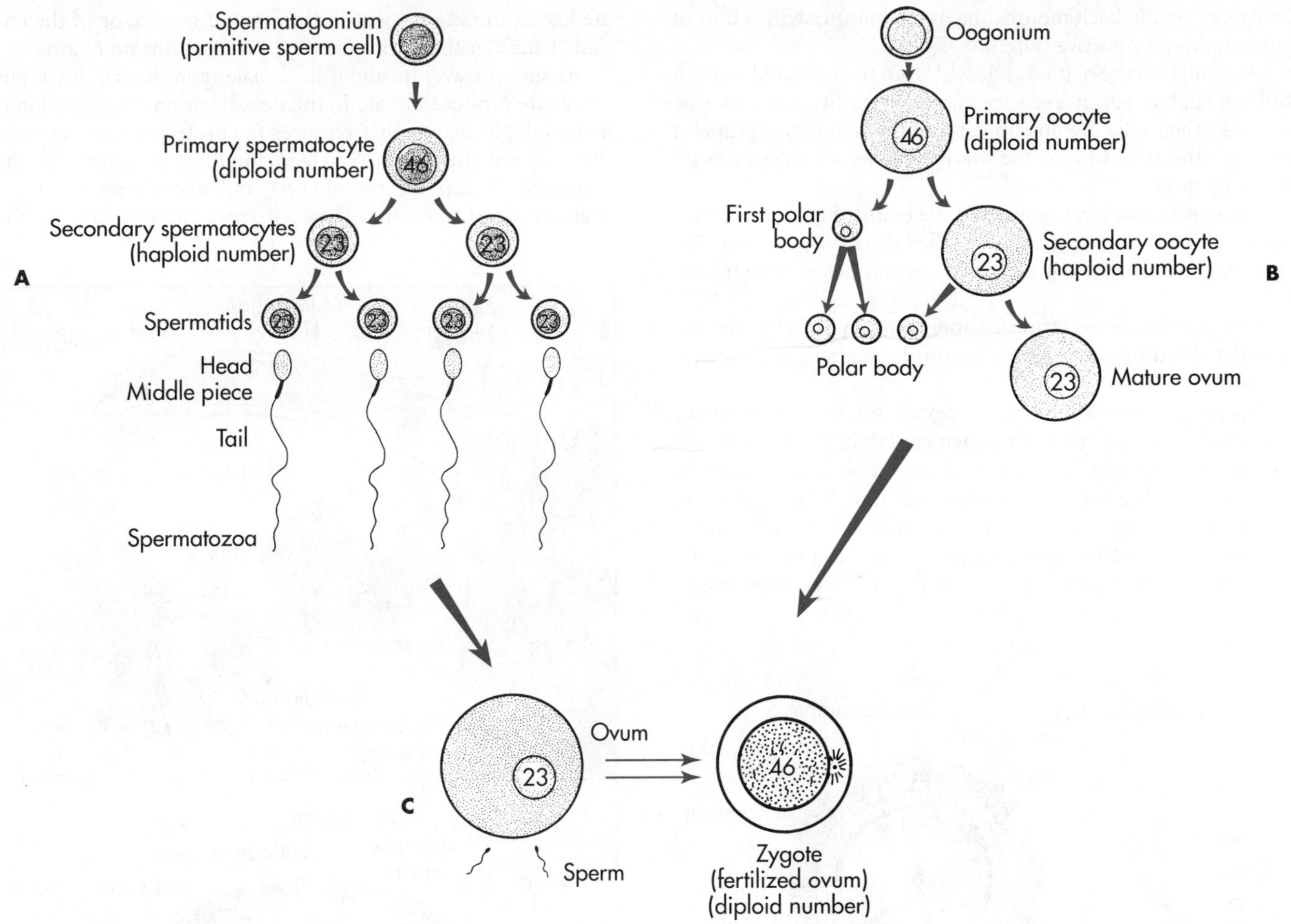

FIG. 8-4 • Spermatogenesis. **A,** Gametogenesis in the male produces four mature gametes, the sperm. **B,** Oogenesis. Gametogenesis in the female produces one mature ovum and three polar bodies. Note relative difference in overall size between ovum and sperm. **C,** Fertilization results in the single-cell zygote and restoration of the diploid number of chromosomes.

called spermatocytes. The primary spermatocyte, which undergoes the first meiotic division, contains the diploid number of chromosomes. The cell has already copied its DNA before division, so four alleles for each gene are present. Because the copies are bound together (i.e., one allele plus its copy on each chromosome), the cell is still considered diploid.

During the first meiotic division, two haploid secondary spermatocytes are formed, each containing 22 autosomes and one sex chromosome; one contains the X chromosome (plus its copy) and the other the Y chromosome (plus its copy). During the second meiotic division the male produces two gametes with an X chromosome and two gametes with a Y chromosome, all of which will develop into viable sperm (Fig. 8-4, *A*).

Oogenesis, the process of egg (ovum) formation, begins during fetal life of the female. All the cells that may undergo meiosis in a woman's lifetime are contained in her ovaries at birth. The majority of the estimated 2 million primary oocytes (the cells that undergo the first meiotic division) degenerate spontaneously. Only 400 to 500 ova will mature during the approximately 35 years of a woman's reproductive life. The primary oocytes begin the first meiotic division (i.e., they replicate their DNA) during fetal life, but remain suspended at this stage until puberty (Fig. 8-4, *B*). Then, usually monthly, one primary oocyte matures and completes the first meiotic division, yielding two unequal cells: the secondary oocyte and a small polar body. Both contain 22 autosomes and one X sex chromosome.

At ovulation the second meiotic division begins. However, the ovum does not complete the second meiotic division unless fertilization occurs. At fertilization, a second polar body and the zygote (the united egg and sperm) are produced (Fig. 8-4, *C*). The three polar bodies degenerate. If fertilization does not occur, the ovum also degenerates.

Conception

Conception, defined as the union of a single egg and sperm, marks the beginning of a pregnancy. Conception does not occur in isolation; a series of events surround it. These events include gamete (egg and sperm) formation, ovulation (release of the egg), union of the gametes (which results in an embryo), and implantation in the uterus.

Ovum. Meiosis is the process by which germ cells divide and decrease their chromosomal number by half. In the female this meiotic process occurs in the ovarian follicles and produces an egg, or ovum. Each month, one ovum matures with a host of surrounding supportive cells.

At ovulation the ovum is released from the ruptured ovarian follicle. High estrogen levels increase the motility of the uterine tubes so their cilia are able to capture the ovum and propel it through the tube toward the uterine cavity. An ovum cannot move by itself.

Two protective layers surround the ovum (Fig. 8-5). The inner layer is a thick, acellular layer called the zona pellucida. The outer layer, called the corona radiata, is composed of elongated cells.

Ova are considered fertile for about 24 hours after ovulation. If unfertilized by a sperm, the ovum degenerates and is reabsorbed.

Sperm. Ejaculation during sexual intercourse normally propels almost a teaspoon of semen containing as many as 200 to 500 million sperm into the vagina. The sperm swim by means of the flagellar movement of their tails. Some sperm can reach the site of fertilization within 5 minutes, but average transit time is 4 to 6 hours. Sperm remain viable within the woman's reproductive system for an average of 2 to 3 days. Most sperm are lost in the vagina, within the cervical mucus, or in the endometrium; or they enter the tube that contains no ovum.

As sperm travel through the female reproductive tract, enzymes are produced to aid in their capacitation. Capacitation is a physiologic change that removes the protective coating from the heads of the sperm. Small perforations then form in the acrosome (a cap on the sperm) and allow enzymes (e.g., hyaluronidase) to escape. These enzymes are necessary for the

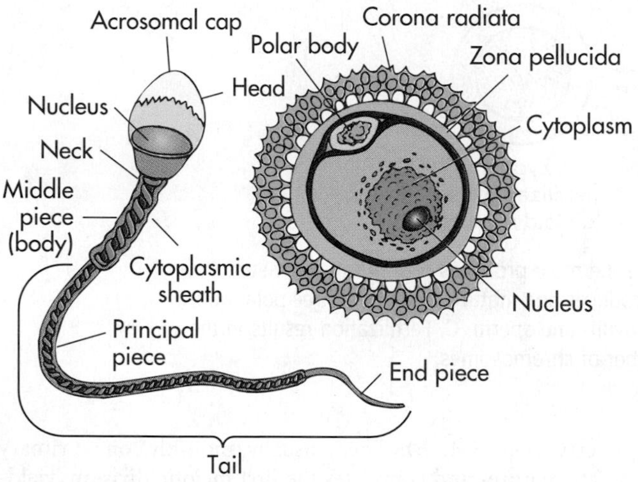

FIG. 8-5 • Sperm and ovum.

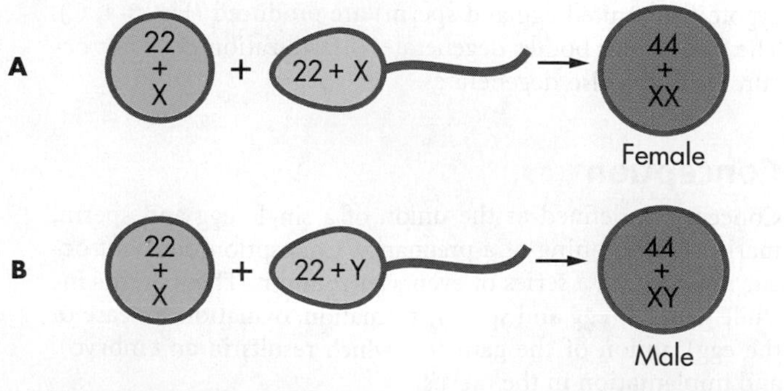

FIG. 8-6 • Fertilization. **A,** Ovum fertilized by X-bearing sperm to form female zygote. **B,** Ovum fertilized by Y-bearing sperm to form male zygote.

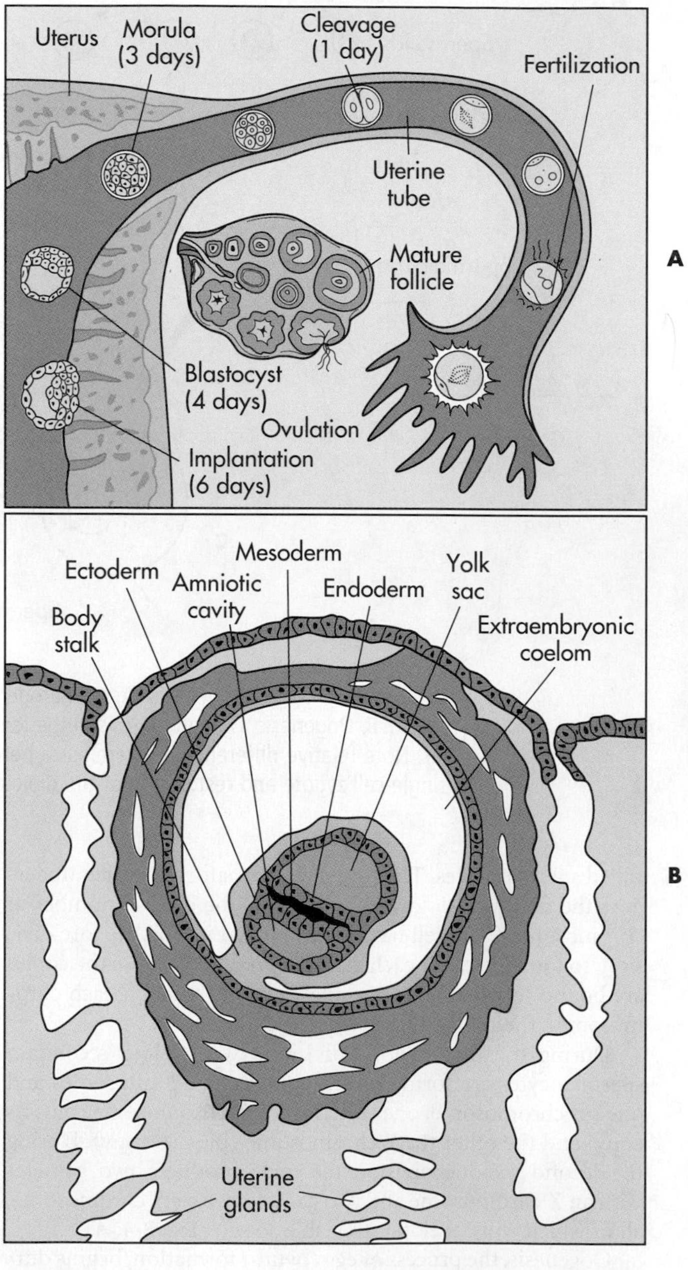

FIG. 8-7 • **A,** First weeks of human development. Follicular development in ovary, ovulation, fertilization and transport of early embryo down uterine tube and into uterus, where implantation occurs. **B,** Blastocyst embedded in endometrium. Germ layers forming. (A, from Carlson B: *Human embryology and developmental biology,* St Louis, 1994, Mosby; B, adapted from Langley L et al: *Dynamic human anatomy and physiology,* ed 5, New York, 1980, McGraw-Hill.)

sperm to penetrate the protective layers of the ovum before fertilization.

Fertilization

Fertilization takes place in the ampulla (the outer third) of the uterine tube. When a sperm successfully penetrates the membrane surrounding the ovum, both sperm and ovum are enclosed within the membrane, and the membrane becomes impenetrable to other sperm; this is termed the zona reaction. The second meiotic division of the oocyte is then completed, and the ovum nucleus becomes the female pronucleus. The head of the sperm enlarges to become the male pronucleus, and the tail degenerates. The nuclei fuse and the chromosomes combine, restoring the diploid number (46) (Fig. 8-6). Conception, the formation of the zygote (the first cell of the new individual), has been achieved.

Mitotic cellular replication, called cleavage, begins as the zygote travels the length of the uterine tube into the uterus. This voyage takes 3 to 4 days. Because the fertilized egg divides rapidly with no increase in size, successively smaller cells, called blastomeres, are formed with each division. A 16-cell morula, a solid ball of cells, is produced within 3 days, and is still surrounded by the protective zona pellucida (Fig. 8-7, *A*). Further development occurs as the morula floats freely within the uterus. Fluid passes through the zona pellucida into the intercellular spaces between the blastomeres, separating them into two parts; the trophoblast (which gives rise to the placenta), and the embryoblast (which gives rise to the embryo). A cavity forms within the cell mass as the spaces come together, forming a structure called the blastocyst cavity. When the cavity becomes recognizable, the whole structure of the developing embryo is known as the blastocyst. The outer layer of cells surrounding the cavity is the trophoblast.

Implantation

The zona pellucida degenerates, and the trophoblast attaches itself to the uterine endometrium, usually in the anterior or posterior fundal region. Between 6 and 10 days after conception, the trophoblast secretes enzymes that enable it to burrow into the endometrium until the entire blastocyst is covered. This is known as implantation. Endometrial blood vessels erode, and some women experience slight implantation bleeding (slight spotting and bleeding during the time of the first missed menstrual period). Chorionic villi, or fingerlike projections, develop out of the trophoblast and extend into the blood-filled spaces of the endometrium. These villi are vascular processes that obtain oxygen and nutrients from the maternal bloodstream and dispose of carbon dioxide and waste products into the maternal blood.

After implantation, the endometrium is called the decidua. The portion directly under the blastocyst, where the chorionic villi tap the maternal blood vessels, is the decidua basalis. The portion covering the blastocyst is the decidua capsularis, and the portion lining the rest of the uterus is the decidua vera (Fig. 8-8).

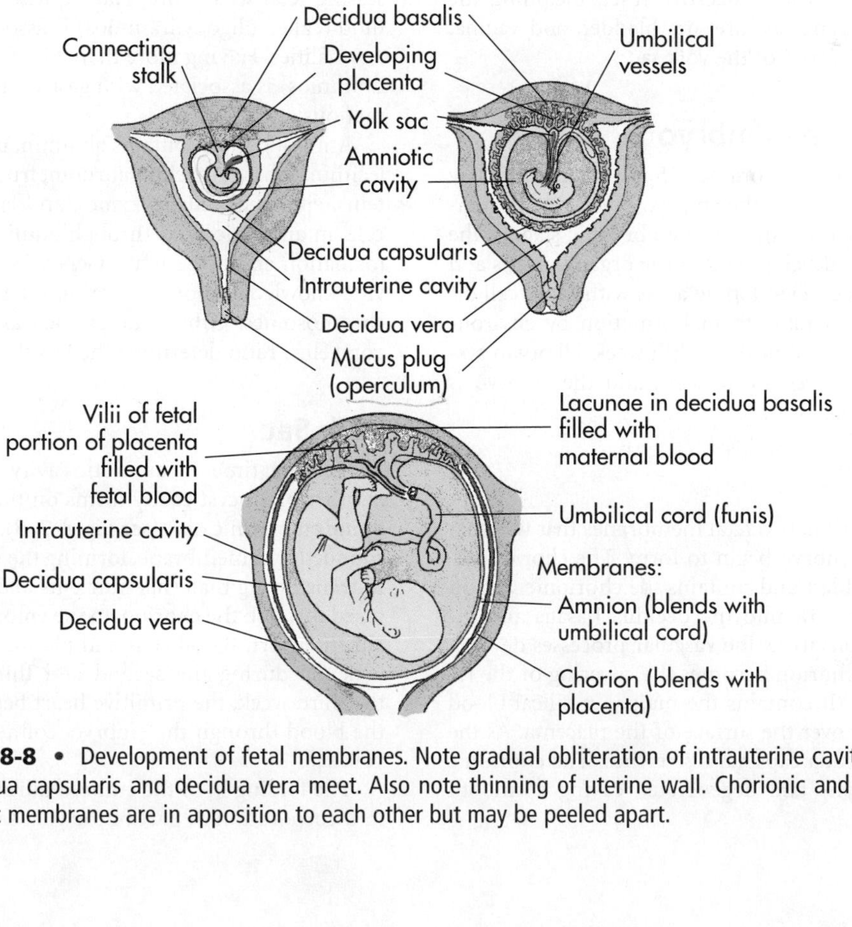

FIG. 8-8 • Development of fetal membranes. Note gradual obliteration of intrauterine cavity as decidua capsularis and decidua vera meet. Also note thinning of uterine wall. Chorionic and amnionic membranes are in apposition to each other but may be peeled apart.

THE EMBRYO AND FETUS

Pregnancy lasts approximately 10 lunar months (9 calendar months, 40 weeks, or 280 days). Length of pregnancy is computed from the first day of the last menstrual period (LMP) until the day of birth. However, conception occurs approximately 2 weeks after the first day of the LMP. Thus the postconception age of the fetus is 2 weeks less, for a total of 266 days or 38 weeks. Postconception age is used in the discussion of fetal development.

Intrauterine development is divided into three stages: ovum or preembryonic, embryo, and fetus (see Fig. 8-3). The stage of the ovum lasts from conception until day 14. This period covers cellular replication, blastocyst formation, initial development of the embryonic membranes, and establishment of the primary germ layers.

Primary Germ Layers

During the third week after conception the embryonic disk differentiates into three primary germ layers: the ectoderm, mesoderm, and endoderm or entoderm (see Fig. 8-7, *B*). All tissues and organs of the embryo develop from these three layers.

The ectoderm, or upper layer of the embryonic disk, gives rise to the epidermis, glands, nails and hair, the central and peripheral nervous systems, lens of the eye, tooth enamel, and the floor of the amniotic cavity.

The mesoderm, or middle layer, develops into the bones and teeth, muscles (skeletal, smooth, and cardiac), dermis and connective tissue, cardiovascular system and spleen, and urogenital system.

The endoderm, or lower layer, gives rise to the epithelium lining the respiratory tract and digestive tract, including the oropharynx, liver and pancreas, urethra, bladder, and vagina. The endoderm forms the roof of the yolk sac.

Development of the Embryo

The stage of the embryo lasts from day 15 until approximately 8 weeks after conception, when the embryo measures approximately 3 cm from crown to rump. The embryonic stage is the most critical time in the development of the organ systems and the main external features. Developing areas with rapid cell division are the most vulnerable to malformation by environmental teratogens. At the end of the eighth week, all organ systems and external structures are present, and the embryo is unmistakably human (Fig. 8-3).

Membranes

At the time of implantation, two fetal membranes that will surround the developing embryo begin to form. The chorion develops from the trophoblast and contains the chorionic villi on its surface. The villi burrow into the decidua basalis and increase in size and complexity as the vascular processes develop into the placenta. The chorion becomes the covering of the fetal side of the placenta. It contains the major umbilical blood vessels that branch out over the surface of the placenta. As the embryo grows, the decidua capsularis stretches. The chorionic villi on this side atrophy and degenerate, leaving a smooth chorionic membrane.

The inner cell membrane, the amnion, develops from the interior cells of the blastocyst. The cavity that develops between this inner cell mass and the outer layer of cells (trophoblast) is the amniotic cavity (see Fig. 8-7, *B*). As it grows larger, the amnion forms on the side opposite to the developing blastocyst (see Fig. 8-7, *B*, and Fig. 8-8). The developing embryo draws the amnion around itself to form a fluid-filled sac. The amnion becomes the covering of the umbilical cord and covers the chorion on the fetal surface of the placenta. As the embryo grows larger, the amnion enlarges to accommodate the embryo/fetus and the surrounding amniotic fluid. The amnion eventually comes in contact with the chorion surrounding the fetus.

Amniotic Fluid

At first the amniotic cavity derives its fluid by diffusion from the maternal blood. The amount of fluid increases weekly, and 800 to 1200 ml of transparent liquid are normally present at term. The volume of amniotic fluid changes constantly. The fetus swallows fluid, and fluid flows into and out of the fetal lungs. The fetus urinates into the fluid, greatly increasing its volume.

The amniotic fluid serves many functions for the embryo/fetus. Amniotic fluid helps maintain a constant body temperature. It serves as a source of oral fluid and as a repository for waste. It cushions the fetus from trauma by blunting and dispersing outside forces. It allows freedom of movement for musculoskeletal development. The fluid keeps the embryo from tangling with the membranes, facilitating symmetric growth of the fetus. If the embryo does intersect with the membranes, amputations of extremities or other deformities can occur from constricting amniotic bands.

The volume of amniotic fluid is an important factor in assessing fetal well-being. Having less than 300 ml of amniotic fluid (called oligohydramnios) is associated with fetal renal abnormalities. Having more than 2 L of amniotic fluid (called hydramnios) is associated with gastrointestinal and other malformations.

Amniotic fluid contains albumin, urea, uric acid, creatinine, lecithin, sphingomyelin, bilirubin, fructose, fat, leukocytes, proteins, epithelial cells, enzymes, and lanugo hair. Study of fetal cells in amniotic fluid through amniocentesis yields much information about the fetus. Genetic studies (karyotyping) provide knowledge about the sex and the number and structure of chromosomes. Other studies such as the L/S (lecithin/sphingomyelin) ratio determine the health or maturity of the fetus.

Yolk Sac

At the same time the amniotic cavity and amnion are forming, another blastocyst cavity forms on the other side of the developing embryonic disk (see Fig. 8-7, *B*). This cavity becomes surrounded by a membrane, forming the yolk sac. The yolk sac aids in transferring maternal nutrients and oxygen, which have diffused through the chorion, to the embryo. Blood vessels form to aid transport. Blood cells and plasma are manufactured in the yolk sac during the second and third weeks. At the end of the third week, the primitive heart begins to beat and circulate the blood through the embryo, connecting stalk, chorion, and yolk sac.

The folding in of the embryo during the fourth week results in incorporation of part of the yolk sac into the embryo's body as the primitive digestive system. Primordial germ cells arise in the yolk sac and move into the embryo. The shrinking remains of the yolk sac degenerate (see Fig. 8-7, *B*), and by the fifth or sixth week, the remnant has separated from the embryo.

Umbilical Cord

By day 14 after conception the embryonic disk, amniotic sac, and yolk sac are attached to the chorionic villi by the connecting stalk. During the third week the blood vessels develop to supply the embryo with maternal nutrients and oxygen. During the fifth week, after the embryo has curved inward on itself from both ends (bringing the connecting stalk to the ventral side of the embryo), the connecting stalk becomes compressed from both sides by the amnion and forms the narrower umbilical cord (see Fig. 8-8). Two arteries carry blood to the chorionic villi from the embryo, and one vein returns blood to the embryo. One percent of umbilical cords contain only two vessels: one artery and one vein. This occurrence is sometimes associated with congenital malformations.

The cord rapidly increases in length. At term the cord is 2 cm in diameter and ranges from 30 to 90 cm in length (with an average of 55 cm). It twists spirally on itself and loops around the embryo/fetus. A true knot is rare, but false knots occur as folds or kinks in the cord and may jeopardize circulation to the fetus. Connective tissue called Wharton's jelly prevents compression of the blood vessels and ensures continued nourishment of the embryo/fetus. Compression can occur if the cord lies between the fetal head and the pelvis or if it is twisted around the fetal body. When the cord is wrapped around the fetal neck, it is called a nuchal cord.

Because the placenta develops from the chorionic villi, the umbilical cord is usually located centrally. A peripheral location is less common and is known as a battledore placenta. The blood vessels are arrayed out from the center to all parts of the placenta.

Placenta

Structure. The placenta begins to form at implantation. During the third week after conception the trophoblast cells of the chorionic villi continue to invade the decidua basalis. As the uterine capillaries are tapped, the endometrial spiral arteries fill with maternal blood. The chorionic villi grow into the spaces with two layers of cells: the outer syncytium and the inner cytotrophoblast. A third layer develops into anchoring septa, dividing the projecting decidua into separate areas called cotyledons. In each of the 15 to 20 cotyledons, the chorionic villi branch out, and a complex system of fetal blood vessels forms. Each cotyledon is a functional unit. The whole structure is the placenta (Fig. 8-9).

The maternal-placental-embryonic circulation is in place by day 17, when the embryonic heart starts beating. By the end of the third week, embryonic blood is circulating between the embryo and the chorionic villi. In the intervillous spaces, maternal blood supplies oxygen and nutrients to the embryonic capillaries in the villi (Fig. 8-10). Waste products and carbon dioxide diffuse into the maternal blood.

The placenta functions as a means of metabolic exchange. Exchange is minimal at this time because the two cell layers of the villous membrane are too thick. Permeability increases as

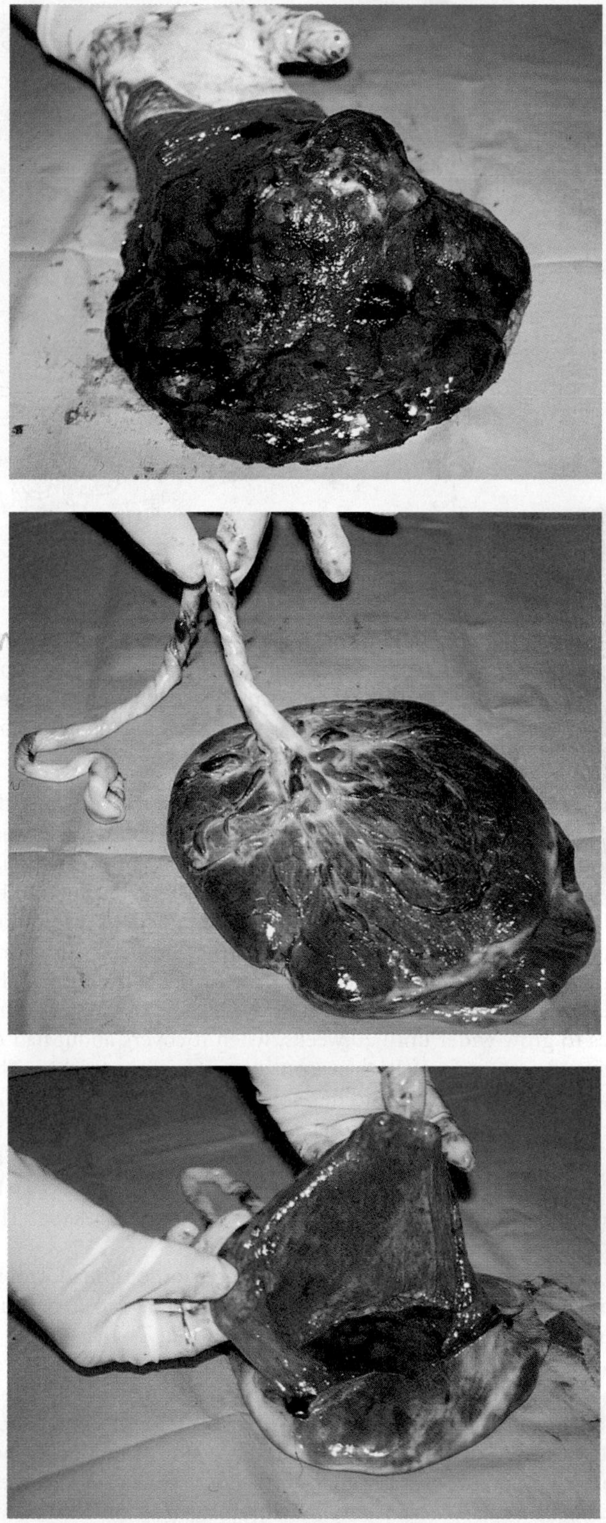

A

B

C

FIG. 8-9 • Full-term placenta. **A,** Maternal (or uterine) surface, showing cotyledons and grooves. **B,** Fetal (or amniotic) surface, showing blood vessels running under amnion and converging to form umbilical vessels at attachment of umbilical cord. **C,** Amnion and smooth chorion are arranged to show that they are (1) fused and (2) continuous with margins of placenta. (Courtesy Marjorie Pyle, RNC, Lifecircle, Costa Mesa, CA.)

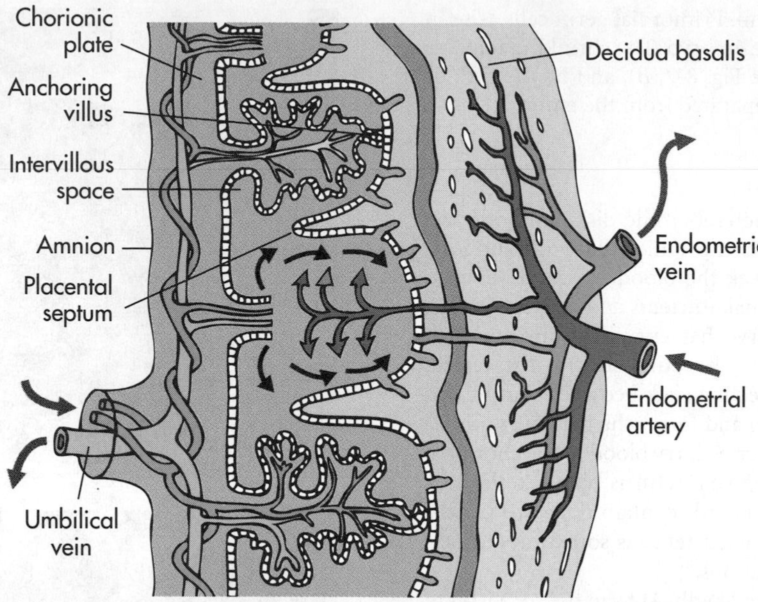

FIG. 8-10 • Schematic drawing of placenta illustrating how it supplies oxygen and nutrition to embryo and removes its waste products. Deoxygenated blood leaves fetus through the umbilical arteries and enters placenta, where it is oxygenated. Oxygenated blood leaves placenta through the umbilical vein, which enters the fetus via the umbilical cord.

the cytotrophoblast thins and disappears; by the fifth month, only the single layer of syncytium is left between the maternal blood and the fetal capillaries. The syncytium is the functional layer of the placenta. By the eighth week, genetic testing may be done on a sample of chorionic villi obtained by aspiration biopsy; however, limb defects have been associated with chorionic villi sampling done before 10 weeks. The structure of the placenta is complete by the twelfth week. The placenta continues to grow wider until 20 weeks, when it covers about half of the uterine surface. It then continues to grow thicker. The branching villi continue to develop within the body of the placenta, increasing the functional surface area.

Functions. One of the early functions of the placenta is as an endocrine gland that produces four hormones necessary to maintain the pregnancy and support the embryo/fetus. The hormones are produced in the syncytium.

The protein hormone human chorionic gonadotropin (hCG) can be detected in the maternal serum by 8 to 10 days after conception, or shortly after implantation. This hormone is the basis for pregnancy tests. The hCG preserves the function of the ovarian corpus luteum, ensuring a continued supply of estrogen and progesterone needed to maintain the pregnancy. Miscarriage occurs if the corpus luteum stops functioning before the placenta can produce sufficient estrogen and progesterone. The hCG reaches its maximum level at 50 to 70 days, then begins to decrease.

The other protein hormone produced by the placenta is human chorionic somatomammotropin (hCS) or human placental lactogen (hPL). This substance is similar to a growth hormone and stimulates maternal metabolism to supply needed nutrients for fetal growth. This hormone increases the resistance to insulin, facilitates glucose transport across the placental membranc, and stimulates breast development to prepare for lactation.

The placenta eventually produces more of the steroid hormone progesterone than the corpus luteum does during the first few months of pregnancy. Progesterone maintains the endometrium, decreases the contractility of the uterus, and stimulates development of breast alveoli and maternal metabolism.

By 7 weeks after fertilization, the placenta is producing most of the maternal estrogens, which are steroid hormones. The major estrogen secreted by the placenta is estriol, while the ovaries produce mostly estradiol. Measuring estriol levels is a clinical assay for placental functioning. Estrogen stimulates uterine growth and uteroplacental blood flow. It causes a proliferation of the breast glandular tissue and stimulates myometrial contractility. Placental estrogen production increases greatly toward the end of pregnancy. One theory for the cause of the onset of labor is the decrease in circulating levels of progesterone and the increased levels of estrogen.

The metabolic functions of the placenta are respiration, nutrition, excretion, and storage. Oxygen diffuses from the maternal blood across the placental membrane into the fetal blood, and carbon dioxide diffuses in the opposite direction. In this way the placenta functions as a lung for the fetus.

Carbohydrates, proteins, calcium, and iron are stored in the placenta for ready access to meet fetal needs. Water, inorganic salts, carbohydrates, proteins, fats, and vitamins pass from the maternal blood supply across the placental membrane into the fetal blood, supplying nutrition. Water and most electrolytes with a molecular weight less than 500 readily diffuse through the membrane. Hydrostatic and osmotic pressures aid in the flow of water and some solutions. Facilitated and active transport assists in the transfer of glucose, amino acids, calcium, iron, and substances with higher molecular weights. Amino acids and calcium are transported against the concentration gradient between the maternal blood and fetal blood.

The fetal concentration of glucose is lower than the glucose level in the maternal blood because of its rapid metabolism by the fetus. This fetal requirement demands larger concentrations of glucose than simple diffusion can provide. Therefore, maternal glucose moves into the fetal circulation by active transport.

Pinocytosis is a mechanism used for transferring large molecules (e.g., albumin and gamma globulins) across the placental membrane. This mechanism conveys the maternal immunoglobulins that provide early passive immunity to the fetus.

Metabolic waste products of the fetus cross the placental membrane from the fetal blood into the maternal blood. The maternal kidneys then excrete them. Many viruses can cross the placental membrane and infect the fetus. Some bacteria and protozoa first infect the placenta and then infect the fetus. Drugs can also cross the placental membrane and may harm the fetus. Caffeine, alcohol, nicotine, carbon monoxide and the other toxic substances in cigarette smoke, and prescription and recreational drugs (e.g., marijuana and cocaine) readily cross the placenta.

Although no direct link exists between the fetal blood in the vessels of the chorionic villi and the maternal blood in the intervillous spaces, only one cell layer separates them. Breaks occasionally occur in the placental membrane. Fetal erythrocytes then leak into the maternal circulation, and the mother may develop antibodies to the fetal red blood cells. This is often how the Rh-negative mother becomes sensitized to the erythrocytes of her Rh-positive fetus (see the discussion of isoimmunization in Chapter 28).

Though the placenta and fetus are living tissue transplants, they are not destroyed by the host mother (Cunningham, MacDonald, and Gant, 1997). Either the placental hormones suppress the immunologic response, or the tissue evokes no response.

Placental function depends on the maternal blood pressure supplying the circulation. Maternal arterial blood, under pressure in the small uterine spiral arteries, spurts into the intervillous spaces (see Fig. 8-10). As long as rich arterial blood continues to be supplied, pressure is exerted on the blood already in the intervillous spaces, pushing it toward drainage by the low-pressure uterine veins. At term gestation, 10% of the maternal cardiac output goes to the uterus.

If there is interference with the circulation to the placenta, the placenta cannot supply the embryo/fetus. Vasoconstriction, such as that caused by hypertension or cocaine use, diminishes uterine blood flow. Decreased maternal blood pressure or cardiac output also diminishes uterine blood flow.

When a woman lies on her back with the pressure of the uterus compressing the vena cava, blood return to the right atrium is diminished (see the discussion of supine hypotension in Chapter 11). Excessive maternal exercise that diverts blood to the muscles away from the uterus compromises placental circulation. Optimum circulation is achieved when the woman is lying at rest on her side. Decreased uterine circulation may lead to intrauterine growth restriction of the fetus and infants who are small for gestational age.

Braxton Hicks contractions seem to enhance the movement of blood through the intervillous spaces, aiding placental circulation. However, prolonged contractions or too-short intervals between contractions during labor can reduce the blood flow to the placenta.

Fetal Maturation

The fetal stage lasts from 9 weeks (when the embryo becomes recognizable as a human being) until the pregnancy ends. Changes during the fetal period are not as dramatic, since refinement of structure and function is taking place. The fetus is less vulnerable to teratogens, except those that affect central nervous system functioning.

Viability refers to the capability of the fetus to survive outside the uterus. In the past the earliest age at which fetal survival could be expected was 28 weeks after conception. With modern technology and advances in maternal and neonatal care, viability is now possible at 20 weeks after conception (22 weeks since LMP; fetal weight of 500 g or more). The limitations on survival outside the uterus are based on central nervous system function and oxygenation capability of the lungs.

Respiratory System. The respiratory system begins development during embryonic life and continues through fetal life and into childhood. The development of the respiratory tract begins in week 4 and continues through week 17 with formation of the trachea, bronchi, and lung buds. Between 16 and 24 weeks the bronchi and terminal bronchioles enlarge, and vascular structures and primitive alveoli are formed. Between 24 weeks and term birth, more alveoli form. Specialized alveolar cells, Type I and Type II cells, secrete pulmonary surfactants to line the interior of the alveoli. After 32 weeks, sufficient surfactant is present in developed alveoli to provide infants with a good chance of survival.

Pulmonary Surfactants. The detection of the presence of pulmonary surfactants (surface-active phospholipids) in amniotic fluid has been used to determine the degree of fetal lung maturity, or the ability of the lungs to function after birth. Lecithin (L) is the most critical alveolar surfactant required for postnatal lung expansion. It increases in amount after the twenty-fourth week. Another pulmonary phospholipid, sphingomyelin (S), remains constant in amount. Thus the measure of lecithin in relation to sphingomyelin, or the L/S ratio, is used to determine fetal lung maturity. When the L/S ratio reaches 2:1, the infant's lungs are considered to be mature. This occurs at approximately 35 weeks of gestation (Creasy and Resnik, 1999).

Certain maternal conditions that cause decreased maternal placental blood flow accelerate lung maturity. This apparently is caused by the resulting fetal hypoxia, which stresses the fetus and increases the blood levels of corticosteroids that accelerate alveolar and surfactant development. Conditions such as maternal hypertension, placental dysfunction, infection, or corticosteroid use accelerate fetal lung maturity.

Conditions such as gestational diabetes and chronic glomerulonephritis can retard fetal lung maturity. The use of intrabronchial synthetic surfactant in the treatment of respiratory distress syndrome in the newborn has greatly improved the chances of survival for preterm infants.

Fetal respiratory movements have been seen on ultrasound as early as the eleventh week. These fetal respiratory movements may aid in development of the chest wall muscles and regulate lung fluid volume. The fetal lungs produce fluid that expands the air spaces in the lungs. The fluid drains into the amniotic fluid or is swallowed by the fetus.

Before birth, secretion of lung fluid decreases. The normal birth process squeezes out approximately one third of the fluid. Infants of cesarean births do not benefit from this squeezing process; thus they may have more respiratory difficulty at birth. The fluid remaining in the lungs at birth is usually reabsorbed into the infant's bloodstream within 2 hours of birth.

Fetal Circulatory System. The cardiovascular system is the first organ system to function in the developing human. Blood vessel and blood cell formation begins in the third week and supplies the embryo with oxygen and nutrients from the mother. By the end of the third week the tubular heart begins to beat, and the primitive cardiovascular system links the embryo, connecting stalk, chorion, and yolk sac. During the fourth and fifth weeks the heart develops into a four-chambered organ. By the end of the embryonic stage the heart is developmentally complete.

The fetal lungs do not function for respiratory gas exchange, so a special circulatory pathway, the ductus arteriosus, bypasses the lungs. Oxygen-rich blood from the placenta flows rapidly through the umbilical vein into the fetal abdomen (Fig. 8-11). When the umbilical vein reaches the liver, it divides into two branches. One branch circulates some oxygenated blood through the liver. Most of the blood passes through the ductus venosus into the inferior vena cava. There it mixes with the deoxygenated blood from the fetal legs and abdomen on its way to the right atrium. Most of this blood passes straight through the right atrium and through the foramen ovale, an opening into the left atrium. There it mixes with the small amount of deoxygenated blood returning from the fetal lungs through the pulmonary veins.

The blood flows into the left ventricle and is squeezed out into the aorta, where the arteries supplying the heart, head, neck, and arms receive most of the oxygen-rich blood. This pattern of supplying the highest levels of oxygen and nutrients to the head, neck, and arms enhances the cephalocaudal (head-to-rump) development of the embryo/fetus.

Deoxygenated blood returning from the head and arms enters the right atrium through the superior vena cava. This blood

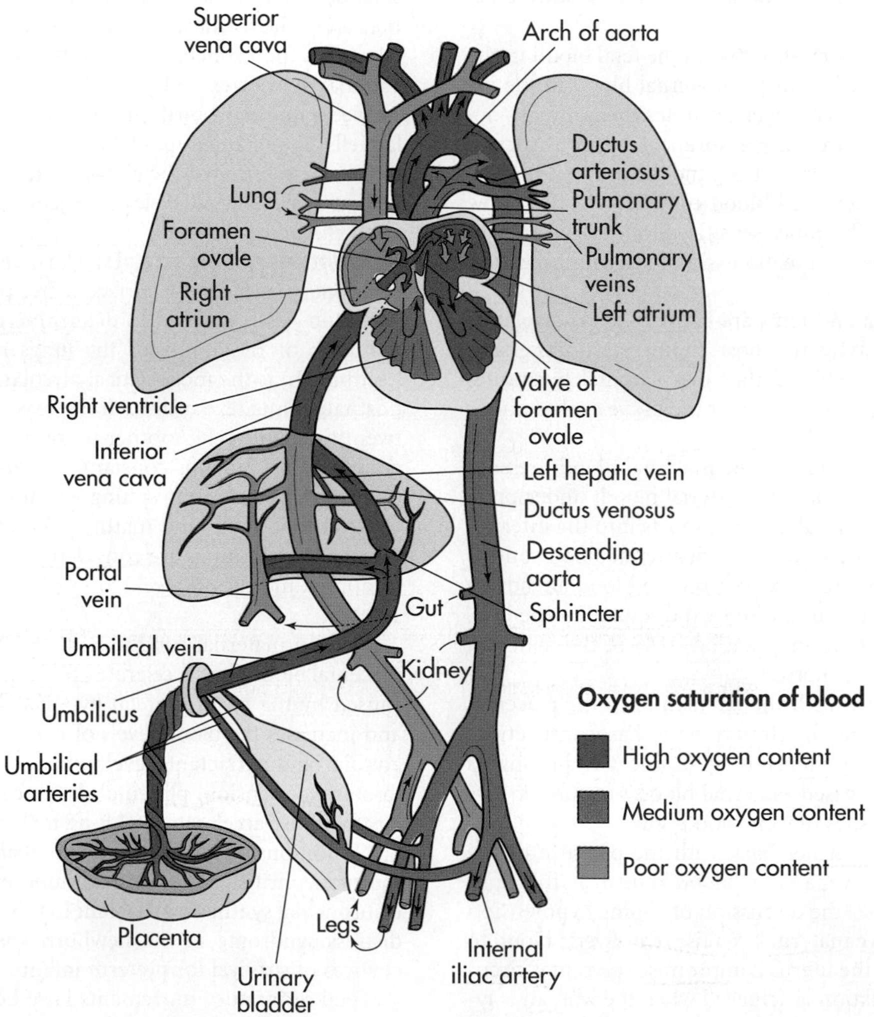

FIG. 8-11 • Schematic illustration of the fetal circulation. The colors indicate the oxygen saturation of the blood, and the arrows show the course of the blood from the placenta to the heart. The organs are not drawn to scale. Observe that three shunts permit most of the blood to bypass the liver and lungs: (1) ductus venosus, (2) foramen ovale, and (3) ductus arteriosus. The poorly oxygenated blood returns to the placenta for oxygen and nutrients through the umbilical arteries. (From Moore K, Persaud T: *Before we are born: essentials of embryology and birth defects,* ed 5, Philadelphia, 1998, WB Saunders.)

is directed downward into the right ventricle, where it is squeezed into the pulmonary artery. A small amount of blood circulates through the resistant lung tissue, but the majority follows the path with less resistance through the ductus arteriosus into the aorta, distal to the point of exit of the arteries supplying the head and arms with oxygenated blood. The oxygen-poor blood flows through the abdominal aorta into the internal iliac arteries, where the umbilical arteries direct most of it back through the umbilical cord to the placenta. There the blood gives up its wastes and carbon dioxide in exchange for nutrients and oxygen. The blood remaining in the iliac arteries flows through the fetal abdomen and legs, ultimately returning through the inferior vena cava to the heart.

Hematopoietic System. Hematopoiesis, or the formation of blood, occurs in the yolk sac (see Fig. 8-7, *B*) beginning in the third week. Hematopoietic stem cells seed the fetal liver during the fifth week, and hematopoiesis begins there during the sixth week. This accounts for the relatively large size of the liver between the seventh and ninth weeks. Stem cells seed the fetal bone marrow, spleen and thymus, and lymph nodes between weeks 8 and 11.

The antigenic factors that determine blood type are present in the erythrocytes soon after the sixth week. For this reason the Rh-negative woman is at risk for isoimmunization in any pregnancy that lasts longer than 6 weeks after fertilization.

Hepatic System. The liver and biliary tract develop from the foregut during the fourth week of gestation. Hematopoiesis begins during the sixth week and requires that the liver be large. The embryonic liver is prominent, occupying most of the abdominal cavity. Bile, a constituent of meconium, begins to form in the twelfth week.

Glycogen is stored in the fetal liver beginning at week 9 or 10. At term, glycogen stores are twice those of the adult. Glycogen is the major source of energy for the fetus and for the neonate stressed by in utero hypoxia, extrauterine loss of the maternal glucose supply, the work of breathing, or cold stress. Iron is also stored in the fetal liver. If maternal intake is sufficient, the fetus can store enough iron to last for 5 months after birth.

During fetal life the liver does not have to conjugate bilirubin for excretion because the unconjugated bilirubin is cleared by the placenta. Therefore the glucuronyl transferase enzyme needed for conjugation is present in the fetal liver in amounts less than those required after birth. This predisposes the neonate to hyperbilirubinemia.

Coagulation factors II, VII, IX, and X cannot be synthesized in the fetal liver because of the lack of vitamin K synthesis in the sterile fetal gut. This coagulation deficiency persists after birth for several days and is the rationale for the prophylactic administration of vitamin K to the newborn.

Gastrointestinal System. During the fourth week the shape of the embryo changes from being almost straight to a C shape as both ends fold in toward the ventral surface. A portion of the yolk sac is incorporated into the body from head to tail as the primitive gut (digestive system).

The foregut produces the pharynx, part of the lower respiratory tract, esophagus, stomach, the first half of the duodenum, liver, pancreas, and the gallbladder. These structures evolve during the fifth and sixth weeks. Malformations that can occur in these areas include esophageal atresia, hypertrophic pyloric stenosis, duodenal stenosis or atresia, and biliary atresia.

The midgut becomes the distal half of the duodenum, the jejunum and ileum, the cecum and appendix, and the proximal half of the colon. The midgut loop projects into the umbilical cord between weeks 5 and 10. A malformation (or omphalocele) results if the midgut fails to return to the abdominal cavity, causing the intestines to protrude from the umbilicus. Meckel's diverticulum is the most common malformation of the midgut. It occurs when a remnant of the yolk stalk that has failed to degenerate attaches to the ileum, leaving a blind sac.

The hindgut develops into the distal half of the colon, the rectum and parts of the anal canal, urinary bladder, and urethra. Anorectal malformations are the most common abnormalities of the digestive system.

The fetus swallows amniotic fluid beginning in the fifth month. Gastric emptying and intestinal peristalsis occur. Fetal nutrition and elimination needs are taken care of by the placenta. As the fetus nears term, fetal waste products accumulate in the intestines as dark green to black, tarry meconium. Normally this substance is passed through the rectum within 48 hours of birth. Sometimes with a breech presentation or fetal hypoxia, meconium is passed in utero into the amniotic fluid. The failure to pass meconium after birth may indicate atresia somewhere in the digestive tract; an imperforate anus; or meconium ileus, in which a firm meconium plug blocks passage (seen in infants with cystic fibrosis).

The metabolic rate of the fetus is relatively low, but the infant has great growth and development needs. Beginning in week 9 the fetus synthesizes glycogen for storage in the liver. Between 26 and 30 weeks the fetus begins to lay down stores of brown fat in preparation for extrauterine cold stress. Thermoregulation in the neonate requires increased metabolism and adequate oxygenation.

The gastrointestinal system is mature by 36 weeks. Digestive enzymes (except pancreatic amylase and lipase) are present in sufficient quantity to facilitate digestion. The neonate cannot digest starches or fats efficiently. Little saliva is produced.

Renal System. The kidneys form during the fifth week and begin to function approximately 4 weeks later. Urine is excreted into the amniotic fluid and forms a major part of the amniotic fluid volume. Oligohydramnios is indicative of renal dysfunction. Because the placenta acts as the organ of excretion and maintains fetal water and electrolyte balance, the fetus does not need functioning kidneys while in utero. At birth, however, the kidneys are required immediately for excretory and acid-base regulatory functions.

A fetal renal malformation can be diagnosed in utero. Corrective or palliative fetal surgery may treat the malformation successfully, or plans can be made for treatment immediately after birth (Jona, 1998).

At term the fetus has fully developed kidneys. However, the glomerular filtration rate (GFR) is low, and the kidneys lack the ability to concentrate urine. This makes the newborn more susceptible to both overhydration and dehydration.

Most newborns void within 24 hours of birth. With the loss of the swallowed amniotic fluid and the metabolism of nutrients provided by the placenta, voidings for the first days of life are scant until fluid intake increases.

Neurologic System. The nervous system originates from the ectoderm during the third week after fertilization. The open neural tube forms during the fourth week. It initially closes at what will be the junction of the brain and spinal cord, leaving both ends open. The embryo folds in on itself lengthwise at this time, forming a head fold in the neural tube at this junction. The cranial end of the neural tube closes, then the caudal end closes. During week 5, different growth rates cause more flexures in the neural tube, delineating three brain areas: the forebrain, midbrain, and hindbrain.

The forebrain develops into the eyes (cranial nerve II) and cerebral hemispheres. The development of all areas of the cerebral cortex continues throughout fetal life and into childhood. The olfactory system (cranial nerve I) and thalamus also develop from the forebrain. Cranial nerves III and IV (oculomotor and trochlear) form from the midbrain. The hindbrain forms the medulla, pons, cerebellum, and the remainder of the cranial nerves. Brain waves can be recorded on an electroencephalogram by week 8.

The spinal cord develops from the long end of the neural tube. Another ectodermal structure, the neural crest, develops into the peripheral nervous system. By the eighth week, nerve fibers traverse throughout the body. By week 11 or 12 the fetus makes respiratory movements, moves all extremities, and changes position in utero. The fetus can suck his or her thumb, swim in the amniotic fluid pool, turn somersaults, and sometimes ties a knot in the umbilical cord. Sometime between 16 and 20 weeks, when the movements are strong enough to be perceived by the mother as "the baby moving," quickening has occurred. The perception of movement occurs earlier in the multipara than in the primipara. The mother also becomes aware of the sleeping and waking cycles of the fetus.

Sensory Awareness. Purposeful movements of the fetus have been demonstrated in response to a firm touch transmitted through the mother's abdomen. Invasive procedures to be done on a fetus require anesthesia.

Fetuses respond to sound by 24 weeks. Different types of music evoke different movements. The fetus can be soothed by the sound of the mother's voice. Acoustic stimulation can be used to evoke a fetal heart rate (FHR) response. The fetus becomes accustomed to noises heard repeatedly. Hearing is fully developed at birth.

The fetus is able to distinguish taste. By the fifth month, when the fetus is swallowing amniotic fluid, a sweetener added to the fluid causes the fetus to swallow faster. The fetus also reacts to temperature changes. A cold solution placed into the amniotic fluid can cause fetal hiccups.

The fetus can see. Eyes have both rods and cones in the retina by the seventh month. A bright light shone on the mother's abdomen in late pregnancy causes abrupt fetal movements. During sleep time, rapid eye movements (REMs) have been observed similar to those occurring in children and adults while dreaming (Cole, 1997).

At term the fetal brain is approximately one-fourth the size of an adult brain. Neurologic development continues. Stressors on the fetus and neonate (e.g., chronic poor nutrition or hypoxia, drugs, environmental toxins, trauma, or disease) cause damage to the central nervous system long after the vulnerable embryonic time for malformations in other organ systems. Neurologic insult can result in cerebral palsy, neuromuscular impairment, mental retardation, and learning disabilities.

Endocrine System. The thyroid gland develops along with structures in the head and neck during the third and fourth weeks. The secretion of thyroxine begins during the eighth week. Maternal thyroxine does not readily cross the placenta; therefore the fetus that does not produce thyroid hormones will be born with congenital hypothyroidism. If untreated, hypothyroidism can result in severe mental retardation. Screening for hypothyroidism is typically included in the testing when screening for PKU after birth.

The adrenal cortex is formed during the sixth week and produces hormones by the eighth or ninth week. As term approaches, the fetus produces more cortisol. This is believed to aid in initiation of labor by decreasing the maternal progesterone and stimulating production of prostaglandins.

The pancreas forms from the foregut during the fifth through eighth weeks. The islets of Langerhans develop during the twelfth week. Insulin is produced by the twentieth week. In infants of mothers with uncontrolled diabetes, maternal hyperglycemia produces fetal hyperglycemia, stimulating hyperinsulinemia and islet cell hyperplasia. This results in a macrosomatic (large-sized) fetus. The hyperinsulinemia also blocks lung maturation, placing the neonate at risk for respiratory distress and hypoglycemia when the maternal glucose source is lost at delivery. Control of the maternal glucose level before and during pregnancy minimizes problems for the fetus and infant.

Reproductive System. Sex differentiation begins in the embryo during the seventh week. Distinguishing characteristics appear around the ninth week and are fully differentiated by the twelfth week. When a Y chromosome is present, testes are formed. By the end of the embryonic period, testosterone is being secreted and causes formation of the male genitalia. By week 28 the testes begin descending into the scrotum. After birth, low levels of testosterone continue to be secreted until the pubertal surge.

The female, with two X chromosomes, forms ovaries and female external genitalia. By the sixteenth week, oogenesis has been established. At birth the ovaries contain the female's lifetime supply of ova. Most female hormone production is delayed until puberty. However, the fetal endometrium responds to maternal hormones, and withdrawal bleeding or vaginal discharge (pseudomenstruation) may occur at birth when these hormones are lost. The high level of maternal estrogen also stimulates mammary engorgement and secretion of fluid ("witch's milk") in newborn infants of both sexes.

Musculoskeletal System. Bones and muscles develop from the mesoderm by the fourth week of embryonic development. At that time the cardiac muscle is already beating. The mesoderm next to the neural tube forms the vertebral column and ribs. The parts of the vertebral column grow toward each other to enclose the developing spinal cord. Ossification, or bone formation, begins. If there is a defect in the bony fusion, spina bifida may occur. A large defect affecting several vertebrae

Critical Thinking

FETAL DEVELOPMENT

You are asked to speak about fetal development to a group of pregnant adolescent girls.

- **What would be the purpose of such a presentation?**
- **How would the materials you prepare differ from those you would prepare for women in their 20s and 30s?**
- **How much information about teratogens would you include?**
- **What implications does this information have for the daily lives of these young women?**

may allow the membranes and spinal cord to pouch out from the back, producing neurologic deficits and skeletal deformity.

The flat bones of the skull develop during the embryonic period, and ossification continues throughout childhood. At birth, connective tissue sutures exist where the bones of the skull meet. The areas where more than two bones meet (called fontanels) are especially prominent. The sutures and fontanels allow the bones of the skull to mold, or move during birth, enabling the head to pass through the birth canal.

The bones of the shoulders, arms, hips, and legs appear in the sixth week as a continuous skeleton with no joints. Differentiation occurs, producing separate bones and joints. Ossification will continue through childhood to allow growth. Beginning in the seventh week, muscles contract spontaneously. Arm and leg movements are visible on ultrasound, although the mother does not perceive them until sometime between 16 and 20 weeks.

Integumentary System. The epidermis begins as a single layer of cells derived from the ectoderm at 4 weeks. By the seventh week, there are two layers of cells. The cells of the superficial layer are sloughed and become mixed with the sebaceous gland secretions to form the white, cheesy vernix caseosa, the material that protects the skin of the fetus. The vernix is thick at 24 weeks but becomes scant by term.

The basal layer of the epidermis is the germinal layer, which replaces lost cells. Until 17 weeks the skin is thin and wrinkled, with blood vessels visible underneath. The skin thickens, and all layers are present at term. After 32 weeks, as subcutaneous fat is deposited under the dermis, the skin becomes less wrinkled and red in appearance.

By 16 weeks the epidermal ridges are present on the palms of the hands, the fingers, the bottom of the feet, and the toes. These handprints and footprints are unique to that infant.

Hairs form from hair bulbs in the epidermis that project into the dermis. Cells in the hair bulb keratinize to form the hair shaft. As the cells at the base of the hair shaft proliferate, the hair grows to the surface of the epithelium. Very fine hairs, called lanugo, appear first at 12 weeks on the eyebrows and upper lip. By 20 weeks they cover the entire body. At this time the eyelashes, eyebrows, and scalp hair are beginning to grow. By 28 weeks the scalp hair is longer than the lanugo, which thins and may disappear by term gestation.

Fingernails and toenails develop from thickened epidermis at the tips of the digits beginning during the tenth week. They grow slowly. Fingernails usually reach the fingertips by 32 weeks, and toenails reach toetips by 36 weeks.

Immunologic System. During the third trimester, albumin and globulin are present in the fetus. The only immunoglobulin that crosses the placenta, IgG, provides passive acquired immunity to specific bacterial toxins. The fetus produces IgM immunoglobulins by the end of the first trimester. These are produced in response to blood group antigens, gram-negative enteric organisms, and some viruses. IgA immunoglobulins are not produced by the fetus; however colostrum, the precursor to breast milk, contains large amounts of IgA and can provide passive immunity to the neonate who is breastfed.

The normal term neonate can fight infection, but not as effectively as an older child. The preterm infant is at much greater risk for infection.

Table 8-1 summarizes embryonic and fetal development.

Multifetal Pregnancy

Twins. When two mature ova are produced in one ovarian cycle, both have the potential to be fertilized by separate sperm. This results in two zygotes, or dizygotic twins (Fig. 8-12). There are always two amnions, two chorions, and two placentas that may be fused together. These dizygotic or fraternal twins may be the same sex or different sexes and are genetically no more alike than siblings born at different times. Dizygotic twinning occurs in families, is more common among African-American women than Caucasian women, and is least common among Asian-American women. Dizygotic twinning increases in frequency with maternal age up to 35 years, with parity, and with the use of fertility drugs.

Identical or monozygotic twins develop from one fertilized ovum, which then divides (Fig. 8-13). They are the same sex and have the same genotype. If division occurs soon after fertilization, two embryos, two amnions, two chorions, and two placentas that may be fused will develop. Most often, division occurs between 4 and 8 days after fertilization, and there are two embryos, two amnions, one chorion, and one placenta. Rarely, division occurs after the eighth day following fertilization. In this case there are two embryos within a common amnion and a common chorion with one placenta. This often causes circulatory problems because the umbilical cords may tangle together, and one or both fetuses may die. If division occurs very late, cleavage may not be complete, and conjoined or "Siamese" twins could result. Monozygotic twinning occurs in approximately 1 of 250 births (Cunningham, MacDonald, and Gant, 1997). There is no association with race, heredity, maternal age, or parity. Fertility drugs increase the incidence of monozygotic twinning.

Other Multifetal Pregnancies. The occurrence of multifetal pregnancies with three or more fetuses has increased

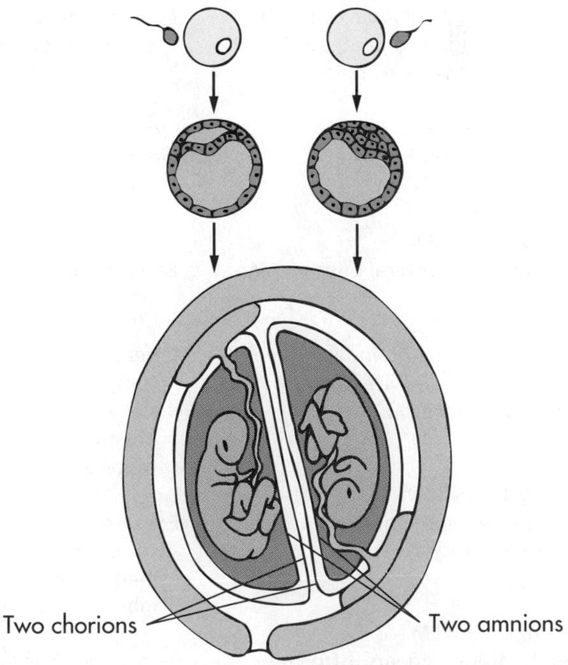

FIG. 8-12 • Formation of dizygotic twins. There is fertilization of two ova, two implantations, two placentas, two chorions, and two amnions.

TABLE 8-1

Milestones in Human Development Before Birth Since Last Menstrual Period (LMP)

4 Weeks	8 Weeks	12 Weeks
EXTERNAL APPEARANCE		
Body flexed, C shaped; arm and leg buds present; head at right angles to body	Body fairly well formed; nose flat, eyes far apart; digits well formed; head elevating; tail almost disappeared; eyes, ears, nose, and mouth recognizable	Nails appearing; resembles a human; head erect but disproportionately large; skin pink, delicate
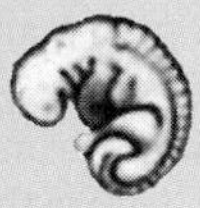	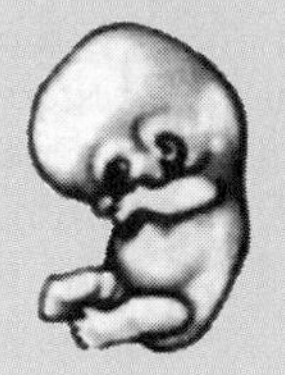	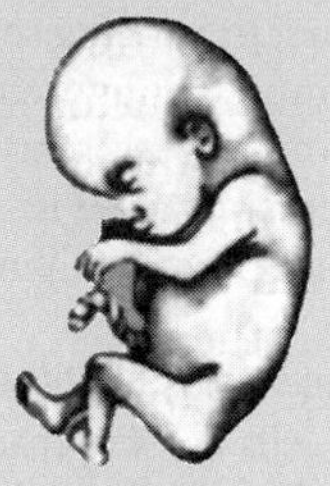
CROWN-TO-RUMP MEASUREMENT; WEIGHT		
0.4 to 0.5 cm; 0.4 g	2.5 to 3 cm; 2 g	6 to 9 cm; 19 g
GASTROINTESTINAL SYSTEM		
Stomach at midline and fusiform; conspicuous liver; esophagus short; intestine a short tube	Intestinal villi developing; small intestines coil within umbilical cord; palatal folds present; liver very large	Bile secreted; palatal fushion complete; intestines have withdrawn from cord and assume characteristic positions
MUSCULOSKELETAL SYSTEM		
All somites present	First indication of ossification—occiput, mandible, and humerus; fetus capable of some movement; definitive muscles of trunk, limbs, and head well represented	Some bones well outlined, ossification spreading; upper cervical to lower sacral arches and bodies ossify; smooth muscle layers indicated in hollow viscera
CIRCULATORY SYSTEM		
Heart develops, double chambers visible, begins to beat; aortic arch and major veins completed	Main blood vessels assume final plan; enucleated red cells predominate in blood	Blood forming in marrow
RESPIRATORY SYSTEM		
Primary lung buds appear	Pleural and pericardial cavities forming; branching bronchioles; nostrils closed by epithelial plugs	Lungs acquire definite shape; vocal cords appear
RENAL SYSTEM		
Rudimentary ureteral buds appear	Earliest secretory tubules differentiating; bladder-urethra separates from rectum	Kidney able to secrete urine; bladder expands as a sac
NERVOUS SYSTEM		
Well-marked midbrain flexure; no hindbrain or cervical flexures; neural groove closed	Cerebral cortex begins to acquire typical cells; differentiation of cerebral cortex, meninges, ventricular foramina, cerebrospinal fluid circulation; spinal cord extends entire length of spine	Brain structural configuration almost complete; cord shows cervical and lumbar enlargements; fourth ventricle foramina are developed; sucking present
SENSORY ORGANS		
Eye and ear appearing as optic vessel and otocyst	Primordial choroid plexuses develops; ventricles large relative to cortex; development progressing; eyes converging rapidly; internal ear developing	Earliest taste buds indicated; characteristic organization of eye attained
GENITAL SYSTEM		
Genital ridge appears (fifth week)	Testes and ovaries distinguishable; external genitalia sexless but begin to differentiate	Sex recognizable; internal and external sex organs specific

Modified from Wong D: *Whaley & Wong's nursing care of infants and children,* St Louis, 1979, Mosby.

TABLE 8-1
Milestones in Human Development Before Birth Since Last Menstrual Period (LMP)—cont'd

16 Weeks	20 Weeks	24 Weeks
EXTERNAL APPEARANCE		
Head still dominant; face looks human; eyes, ears, and nose approach typical appearance on gross examination; arm/leg ratio proportionate; scalp hair appears	Vernix caseosa appears; lanugo appears; legs lengthen considerably; sebaceous glands appear	Body lean but fairly well proportioned; skin red and wrinkled; vernix caseosa present; sweat glands forming
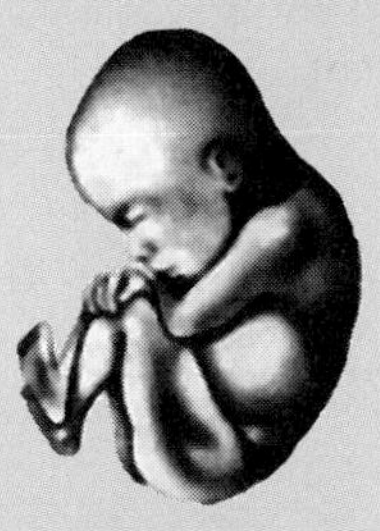	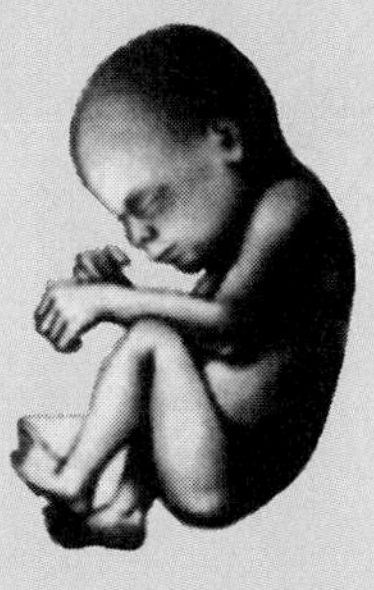	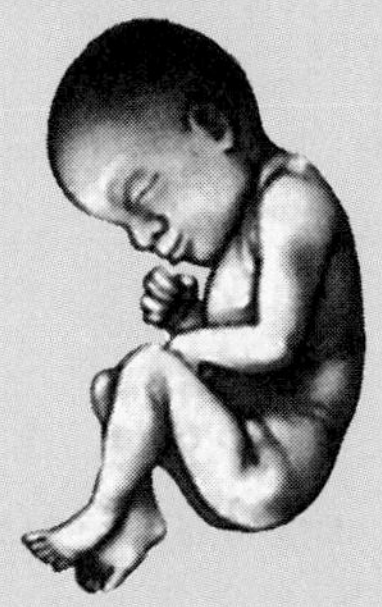
CROWN-TO-RUMP MEASUREMENT; WEIGHT		
11.5 to 13.5 cm; 100 g	16 to 18.5 cm; 300 g	23 cm; 600 g
GASTROINTESTINAL SYSTEM		
Meconium in bowel; some enzyme secretion; anus open	Enamel and dentine depositing; ascending colon recognizable	
MUSCULOSKELETAL SYSTEM		
Most bones distinctly indicated throughout body; joint cavities appear; muscular movements can be detected	Sternum ossifies; fetal movements strong enough for mother to feel	
CIRCULATORY SYSTEM		
Heart muscle well developed; blood formation active in spleen		Blood formation increases in bone marrow and decreases in liver
RESPIRATORY SYSTEM		
Elastic fibers appears in lungs; terminal and respiratory bronchioles appear	Nostrils reopen; primitive respiratory-like movements begin	Alveolar ducts and sacs present; lecithin begins to appear in amniotic fluid (weeks 26 to 27)
RENAL SYSTEM		
Kidney in position; attains typical shape and plan		
NERVOUS SYSTEM		
Cerebral lobes delineated; cerebellum assumes some prominance	Brain grossly formed; cord myelination begins; spinal cord ends at level of first sacral vertebra (S-1)	Cerebral cortex layered typically; neuronal proliferation in cerebral cortex ends
SENSORY ORGANS		
General sense organs differentiated	Nose and ears ossify	Can hear
GENITAL SYSTEM		
Testes in position for descent into scrotum: vagina open		Testes at inguinal ring in descent to scrotum

Continued

TABLE 8-1
Milestones in Human Development Before Birth Since Last Menstrual Period (LMP)—cont'd

28 Weeks	30-31 Weeks	36 and 40 Weeks
EXTERNAL APPEARANCE		
Lean body, less wrinkled and red; nails appear	Subcutaneous fat beginning to collect; more rounded appearance; skin pink and smooth; has assumed birth position 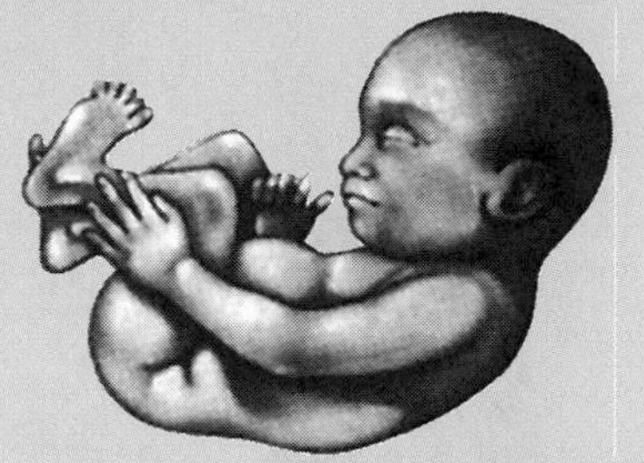	**36 Weeks** Skin pink, body rounded; general lanugo disappearing; body usually plump **40 Weeks** Skin smooth and pink; scant vernix caseosa; moderate to profuse hair; lanugo on shoulders and upper body only; nasal and alar cartilage apparent
CROWN-TO-RUMP MEASUREMENT; WEIGHT		
27 cm; 1100 g	31 cm; 1800 to 2100 g	**36 Weeks** 35 cm; 2200 to 2900 g **40 Weeks** 40 cm: 3200+ g
MUSCULOSKELETAL SYSTEM		
Astragalus (talus, ankle bone) ossifies; weak, fleeting movements, minimum tone	Middle fourth phalanxes ossify; permanent teeth primordia seen; can turn head to side	**36 Weeks** Distal femoral ossification centers present; sustained, definite movements; fair tone; can turn and elevate head **40 Weeks** Active, sustained movement; good tone; may lift head
RESPIRATORY SYSTEM		
Lecithin forming on alveolar surfaces	L/S ratio = 1.2:1	**36 Weeks** L/S ratio ≥ 2:1 **40 Weeks** Pulmonary branching only two-thirds complete
RENAL SYSTEM		
		36 Weeks Formation of new nephrons ceases
NERVOUS SYSTEM		
Appearance of cerebral fissures, convolutions rapidly appearing; indefinite sleep-wake cycle; cry weak or absent; weak suck reflex		**36 Weeks** End of spinal cord at level of third lumbar vertebra (L-3); definite sleep-wake cycle **40 Weeks** Myelination of brain begins; patterned sleep-wake cycle with alert periods; cries when hungry or uncomfortable; strong suck reflex
SENSORY ORGANS		
Eyelids reopen; retinal layers completed, light receptive; pupils capable of reacting to light	Sense of taste present; aware of sounds outside mother's body	
GENITAL SYSTEM		
	Testes descending to scrotum	**40 Weeks** Testes in scrotum; labia majora well developed

Modified from Wong D: *Whaley & Wong's nursing care of infants and children,* St Louis, 1979, Mosby.

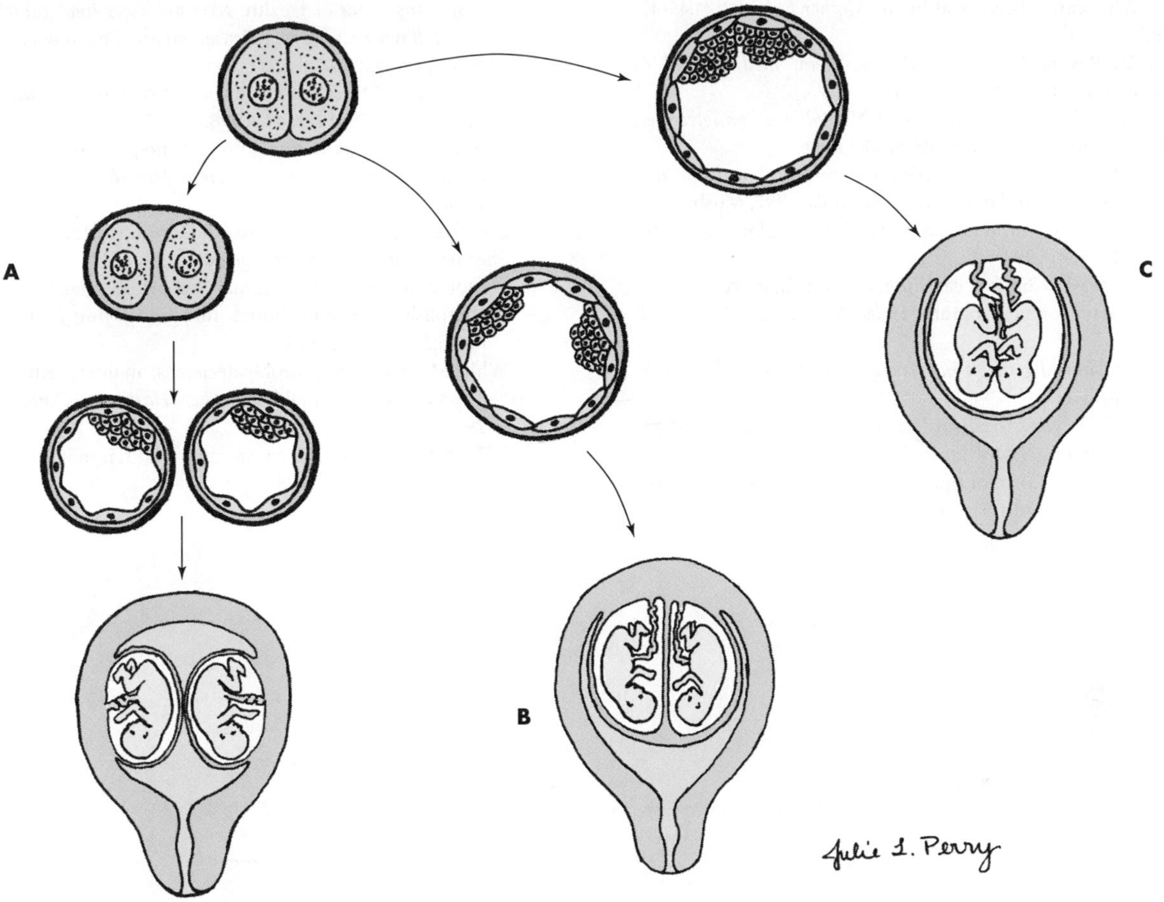

FIG. 8-13 • Formation of monozygotic twins. **A,** One fertilization: blastomeres separate, resulting in two implantations, two placentas, and two sets of membranes. **B,** One blastomere with two inner cell masses, one fused placenta, one chorion, and separate amnions. **C,** One blastomere with incomplete separation of cell mass resulting in conjoined twins.

with the use of fertility drugs and in vitro fertilization. Triplets occur in about 1 of 7600 pregnancies. They can occur from the division of one zygote into two, with one of the two dividing again, producing identical triplets. Triplets can also be produced from two zygotes, one dividing into a set of identical twins and the second zygote a single fraternal sibling; or from three zygotes. Quadruplets, quintuplets, sextuplets, and so on, have similar possible derivations.

Key Points

- Genetic disease affects people of all ages, from all socioeconomic levels, and from all racial and ethnic backgrounds.
- Genetic disorders span every clinical practice specialty.
- Nurses with advanced preparation are assuming important roles in genetic counseling.
- Genes are the basic units of heredity responsible for all human characteristics. They comprise 23 pairs of chromosomes: 22 pairs of autosomes and one pair of sex chromosomes.
- Genetic disorders follow mendelian inheritance patterns of dominance, segregation, and independent assortment of normal genetic transmission.
- Multifactorial inheritance includes both genetic and environmental contributions.
- Human gestation is approximately 280 days after the LMP or 266 days after conception.
- Fertilization occurs in the uterine tube within 24 hours of ovulation. The zygote undergoes mitotic divisions, creating a 16-cell morula.
- Critical periods occur in human development during which the embryo/fetus is vulnerable to environmental teratogens.

References

Anderson G: Storytelling: a holistic foundation for genetic nursing, *Holist Nurs Pract* 12(3):64-76, 1998.

Anderson G et al: Preparing the nursing profession for participation in a genetic paradigm in health care, *Nurs Outlook* 48(1):23-27, 2000.

Cole J: What can babies see at birth? *Mother Baby J* 2(4):45-47, 1997.

Creasy R, Resnik J, editors: *Maternal-fetal medicine,* ed 4, Philadelphia, 1999, WB Saunders.

Cunningham F, MacDonald P, Gant N: *Williams' obstetrics,* ed 20, Stamford, CT, 1997, Appleton & Lange.

Fanaroff A, Martin R, editors: *Neonatal-perinatal medicine: diseases of the fetus and infant,* ed 6, St Louis, 1997, Mosby.

Jona J: Advances in fetal surgery, *Pediatr Clin North Am* 45(3):599-604, 1998.

Jones S, Krysa L: Comfort care interventions in a preimplantation genetic testing program, *Holist Nurs Pract* 12(3):20-29, 1998.

Lashley F: *Clinical genetics in nursing practice,* ed 2, New York, 1998, Springer.

McGowan R: Beyond the disorder: one parent's reflection on genetic counseling, *J Med Ethics* 25(2):195-199, 1999.

Munro C: Implications for nursing of the Human Genome Project, *Neonat Netw* 18(3):7-12, 1999.

National Institutes of Health: *NIH publishes final guidelines for stem cell research,* News Release, retrieved from www.nih.gov/news/pr/aug2000.

O'Connor D: Ethical issues in the age of genetics, *Patient Care* 32(18):137-149, 142-144, 1998.

Rice E: The Human Genome Project and gene therapy: a genetic counselor's perspective, *J Perinat Neonat Nurs* 12(3):16-25, 1998.

Scialli A: Toxicology, *Contemp OB GYN* 42(5):15, 1997.

Sherman S et al: Behavioral genetics '97: ASHG Statement. Recent developments in human behavioral genetics: past accomplishments and future directions, *Am J Hum Genet* 60(6):1265-1275, 1997.

White M: Making responsible decisions: an interpretive ethic for genetic decision-making, *The Hastings Center Report* 29(1):14-21, 1999.

Williams J: Genetics and community health nursing, *Holist Nurs Pract* 12(3):30-37, 1998.

CHAPTER

9

puerperium

Assessment for Risk Factors

http://www.harcourthealth.com/MERLIN/Wong/maternal/

Learning Objectives

On completion of this chapter the reader will be able to:

- Explore the scope of high risk pregnancy.
- Examine risk factors identified through history, physical examination, and diagnostic techniques.
- Describe diagnostic techniques and implications of findings.
- Describe the nursing role in antepartal risk assessment.

Approximately 500,000 of the 4 million births that occur in the United States each year are categorized as high risk because of maternal or fetal complications. Perinatal outcome depends on the early recognition and management of problems. Identification of the risks, together with appropriate and timely intervention, can prevent morbidity and mortality among mothers and infants.

With the changing demographics in the United States, more women and families can be identified as at risk because of factors other than biophysical criteria. Among those at risk are homeless, single, and uninsured pregnant women, who are unlikely to be able to access prenatal care early or at all. Psychosocial factors that involve maternal behaviors and adverse lifestyles have a negative effect on the health of the mother and fetus (Fogel and Lewallen, 1995).

Care of these high risk patients requires the unified efforts of medical and nursing personnel. The high risk patient and the factors associated with a diagnosis of high risk are discussed in this chapter; diagnostic techniques used to monitor the maternal-fetal unit are also described.

DEFINITION AND SCOPE OF THE PROBLEM

A high risk pregnancy is one in which the life or health of the mother or infant is jeopardized by a disorder coincidental with or unique to pregnancy. For the mother, the high risk status arbitrarily extends through the puerperium (30 days after childbirth). Postbirth maternal complications usually are resolved within a month of birth, but perinatal morbidity may continue for months or years.

Maternal Health Problems

The leading causes of maternal death attributable to pregnancy differ throughout the world. In general, three major causes have persisted for the last 40 years: hypertensive disorders, infection, and hemorrhage.

From 1982 to 1996 the maternal death rate in the United States remained approximately the same at 7.5 per 100,000 live births. Maternal mortality continues to be higher among women of color: 20.3 per 100,000 for African-American women, compared with 5 per 100,000 for Caucasian women (Centers for Disease Control and Prevention, 1998). Factors strongly related to maternal death include age (increased if less than 20 years or greater than 35 years), lack of prenatal care, low educational attainment, single status, and non-Caucasian (Koonin et al, 1997).

Although the overall number of maternal deaths is small, maternal mortality remains a significant problem because a high proportion of these deaths are preventable, mainly through improving the access to and use of prenatal care services. Nurses can be instrumental in educating the public about the importance of obtaining early and regular care during pregnancy. Reaching the *Healthy People 2010* goal of 3.3 maternal deaths per 100,000 poses a significant challenge.

Fetal and Neonatal Health Problems

The leading causes of death in the neonatal period are congenital anomalies, disorders relating to short gestation and low birth weight (LBW), respiratory distress syndrome, and the effects of maternal complications. Increased rates of survival during the neonatal period have resulted largely from the improvement in high-quality prenatal care and the improvement in perinatal services, including technologic advances in neonatal intensive care and obstetrics.

To achieve significant decline of the infant mortality rate and to eliminate racial and ethnic differences in pregnancy outcomes, a national, state, and local commitment to these goals is necessary. Reducing infant mortality requires the removal of financial, educational, sociocultural, and logistic barriers to care so that pregnant women can seek and receive health services.

dystocia [io] abruptio placenta

Box 9-1

Categories of High Risk Factors

BIOPHYSICAL

1. **Genetic**—may interfere with normal fetal/neonatal development, result in congenital anomalies, and/or create difficulties for the mother. Includes defective genes, transmittable inherited disorders, chromosome anomalies, multiple pregnancy, large fetal size, and ABO incompatibility.
2. **Nutritional status**—one of the most important determinants of pregnancy outcome. Fetal growth and development cannot progress normally without adequate nutrition. Includes very young age; three pregnancies in the past 2 years; tobacco, alcohol, or drug use; inadequate intake because of chronic illness or food fads; inadequate or excessive weight gain; and hematocrit less than 33%.
3. **Medical and obstetric**—medical complications of current and past pregnancies, obstetric-related illnesses, and pregnancy losses. See Box 9-2.

PSYCHOSOCIAL

1. **Smoking**—strong, consistent, causal relationship between maternal smoking and reduced birth weight has been established. Risks include LBW infants, especially with increased age; higher neonatal mortality rates; increased miscarriages; and increased incidence of premature rupture of membranes. Risks aggravated by low socioeconomic status, poor nutritional status, and concurrent use of alcohol.
2. **Caffeine**—not been shown to cause birth defects in humans. High intake (3 or more cups of coffee/day) has been related to a slight decrease in birth weight.
3. **Alcohol**—although exact effects of use in pregnancy have not been quantified and mode of action is largely unexplained, alcohol exerts adverse effects on the fetus, resulting in fetal alcohol syndrome (FAS) and fetal alcohol effects (FAEs), learning disabilities, and hyperactivity.
4. **Drugs**—may adversely affect a developing fetus through several mechanisms: they can be teratogenic, cause metabolic disturbances, produce chemical effects, or cause depression and/or alteration of central nervous system function. Includes medications prescribed by health care provider or bought over the counter as well as commonly abused drugs such as heroin, cocaine, and marijuana.
5. **Psychologic status**—childbearing triggers profound and complex physiologic, psychologic, and social changes, with evidence to suggest a relationship between emotional distress and birth complications. Includes specific intrapsychic disturbances and addictive lifestyles; history of child or spouse abuse; inadequate support systems; family disruption or dissolution; maternal role changes/conflicts; noncompliance with cultural norms; unsafe cultural, ethnic, or religious practices; and situational crises.

SOCIODEMOGRAPHIC

1. **Low income**—poverty underlies many other risk factors and leads to inadequate financial resources for food and prenatal care, poor general health, and increased risk of medical complications of pregnancy; adverse environmental influences more prevalent.
2. **Lack of prenatal care**—major factor in placing woman at risk since opportunity is lost for early diagnosis and treatment of complications. May be caused by financial barriers or lack of access to care; depersonalization of the system resulting in long waits, routine visits, variability in health care personnel, and unpleasant physical surroundings; lack of understanding of need for early and continued care or cultural beliefs that do not support the need; and fear of health care providers and the system.
3. **Age**—women at both ends of the childbearing years have a higher incidence of poor outcomes; age may not be a risk factor in all patients. Both physiologic and psychologic risks should be evaluated.

   Adolescents: more complications are seen in the very young (younger than 15 years old) who have a 60% higher mortality rate than those over age 20. Complications include anemia, pregnancy-induced hypertension (PIH), prolonged labor, contracted pelvis, and cephalopelvic disproportion. Long-term social implications of early motherhood are lower educational-attainment, lower income, increased dependence on government support programs, higher divorce rates, and higher parity.

   Mature mothers: risks do not arise from age alone, but are affected by other factors, such as number and spacing of previous pregnancies; genetic disposition of the parents; and medical history, lifestyle, nutrition, and prenatal care. Increased likelihood of chronic diseases that adversely affect pregnancy outcomes; more invasive medical management of older women's pregnancies and labors, with resulting complications; and demographic characteristics put an older woman at risk. Medical conditions more likely to be experienced by mature women include hypertension and PIH, diabetes, extended labor, cesarean birth, placenta previa, abruptio placentae, and mortality. Her fetus is at greater risk for both LBW and macrosomia, chromosomal abnormalities, congenital malformations, and neonatal mortality.
4. **Parity**—number of previous pregnancies is a risk factor associated with age. Includes all first pregnancies and first pregnancy at either end of the childbearing age continuum; incidence of PIH and dystocia is higher with a first birth.
5. **Marital status**—mortality and morbidity rates are higher for nonmarried women. Includes greater risk for PIH and inadequate prenatal care; more often occur in lower age-groups.
6. **Residence**—availability and prenatal care quality varies greatly with geographic region. Women in metropolitan areas have more prenatal visits than those in rural areas; those in rural areas have higher incidence of maternal mortality and have fewer opportunities for specialized care. Health care in an inner city may be of poorer quality than in a more affluent section, and those women are usually poorer and begin childbearing earlier and continue longer.
7. **Ethnicity**—although ethnicity alone is not a major risk, race is an indicator of other sociodemographic factors. Non-Caucasian women are more than 4 times as likely as Caucasian women to die of pregnancy-related causes; infant mortality rates among African-Americans are more than twice as high as those among Caucasians: African-American babies have the highest rates of prematurity and LBW.

ENVIRONMENTAL

Various environmental substances can effect fertility and fetal development, the chance of a live birth, and the child's subsequent mental and physical development. Environmental influences include infections, radiation, chemicals such as pesticides, therapeutic drugs, illicit drugs, industrial pollutants, cigarette smoke, stress, and diet. Paternal exposure to mutagenic agents in the workplace has been associated with increased risk of miscarriage.

Perinatal services must be modified to meet contemporary health care needs (Dooley, Freels, and Turnock, 1997).

Regionalization of Health Care Services

Mortality decreases when high risk status is identified and when intensive care is applied. Follow-up studies have shown that serious residual handicaps (both physical and mental) of surviving infants have been dramatically reduced when such identification and intervention exist.

It is neither feasible nor reasonable for each hospital to develop and maintain the full spectrum of services required for high risk perinatal patients. As a consequence, there emerged regionalization of health care (i.e., facilities within a geographic region organized to provide different levels of care).

In ambulatory settings, providers must distinguish themselves by the level of care they provide. *Basic care* is provided by obstetricians, family physicians, certified nurse midwives, and other advanced practice clinicians approved by local governance. Routine risk-oriented prenatal care, education, and support are included. Providers offering *specialty* care are obstetricians who must provide fetal diagnostic testing and management of obstetric and medical complications in addition to basic care. *Subspecialty care* is provided by maternal-fetal medicine specialists and includes the aforementioned as well as genetic testing, advanced fetal therapies, and management of severe maternal and fetal complications (American Academy of Pediatrics/American College of Obstetricians and Gynecologists [AAP/ACOG], 1997).

In hospital settings, perinatal services are also designated as basic, specialty, or subspecialty. Criteria for basic perinatal services include care of all patients admitted to the service, with an established triage system for high risk patients who should be transferred to a higher level of care; ability to perform a cesarean birth within 30 minutes of a decision to do so; availability of blood and blood products; availability of radiology, anesthesia, and laboratory services on a 24-hour basis; presence of nursery and postpartum care; resuscitation and stabilization of all neonates born in hospital; availability of transport for all sick neonates; family visitation; and data collection and retrieval (AAP/ACOG, 1997).

Specialty hospital care includes the above requirements in addition to care of high risk mothers and fetuses, stabilization of ill neonates before transfer, and care of preterm infants with a birth weight of 1500 g or more. Preterm labor or impending births of 32 weeks of gestation or less should be transferred for subspecialty care. Other criteria for subspecialty care include comprehensive prenatal services, research and educational support, and use of high risk technologies. Collaboration among providers to meet the patient's needs is key in reducing perinatal morbidity and mortality (AAP/ACOG, 1997).

Assessment for Risk Factors

In the past, risk factors were viewed only from the medical model; thus only medical, obstetric, or physiologic risk factors were considered to place the patient at risk. Today a more comprehensive approach to high risk pregnancy is used, and the factors associated with high risk childbearing are grouped into broad categories based on threats to health and pregnancy outcome. Categories of risk include biophysical, psychosocial, sociodemographic, and environmental (Fogel and Lewallen, 1995) (Box 9-1). *Biophysical* risks include factors that originate within the mother or fetus and affect the development or functioning of either or both. *Psychosocial* risks are comprised of maternal behaviors and adverse lifestyles that have a negative effect on the health of the mother and/or fetus. These risks may include emotional distress and disturbed interpersonal relationships, inadequate social support, and unsafe cultural practices. Box 9-2 lists assessment factors for an antepartum cultural assessment. *Sociodemographic* risks arise from the mother and her family and place the mother and fetus at risk. *Environmental* risks include hazards of the workplace and the woman's general environment.

Box 9-2

Antepartum Cultural Assessment

All cultures recognize pregnancy as a special transitional period and have particular customs and beliefs that dictate behavior during this time. In the antepartum period the nurse should assess the following:

- Beliefs of whether pregnancy is a state of illness or health
- Behavioral expectations of the mother and of the health care provider
- Dietary prescriptions or restrictions and of the health care provider
- Dietary prescriptions or restrictions (e.g., hot/cold balance theory, pica)
- Activity restrictions or prescriptions (e.g., use of massage)
- Availability of advice (e.g., from whom and at what time advice will be sought and when prenatal care will begin [if at all])
- Considerations of modesty

Risk factors are interrelated and cumulative in their effects. Box 9-3 lists pregnancy problems and risk factors. Box 9-4 outlines risk factors of the postpartum woman and the neonate. The development of a comprehensive database for pregnancy risk assessment will help generate appropriate nursing diagnoses.

ANTEPARTUM TESTING/BIOPHYSICAL ASSESSMENT

The major expected outcome of antepartum testing is the detection of potential fetal compromise. Ideally the technique used will identify fetal compromise before intrauterine asphyxia of the fetus so that the health care provider can take measures to prevent or minimize adverse perinatal outcomes. No single test can provide this information. Assessment tests should be selected based on their effectiveness and the results must be interpreted in light of the complete clinical picture. The most reliable evidence for effectiveness is provided by randomized controlled trials. Nurses can be informed about the most recent research on fetal assessment by using the Cochrane Pregnancy and Childbirth Database. Table 9-1 lists evidence for recommending care for fetal assessment screening based on this database.

Box 9-3

Specific Pregnancy Problems and Related Risk Factors

PRETERM LABOR

Age less than 16 or more than 35 years
Low socioeconomic status
Maternal weight below 50 kg
Poor nutrition
Previous preterm birth
Incompetent cervix
Uterine anomalies
Smoking
Drug addiction and alcohol abuse
Pyelonephritis, pneumonia
Multiple gestation
Anemia
Abnormal fetal presentation
Preterm rupture of membranes
Placental abnormalities
Infection
Abdominal surgery in current pregnancy
History of cervical surgery

POLYHYDRAMNIOS

Diabetes mellitus
Multiple gestation
Fetal congenital anomalies
Isoimmunization (Rh or ABO)
Nonimmune hydrops
Abnormal fetal presentation

INTRAUTERINE GROWTH RESTRICTION (IUGR)

Multiple gestation
Poor nutrition
Maternal cyanotic heart disease
Prior pregnancy with IUGR
Maternal collagen diseases
Chronic hypertension
Pregnancy-induced hypertension
Recurrent antepartum hemorrhage
Smoking
Maternal diabetes with vascular problems
Fetal infections
Fetal cardiovascular anomalies
Drug addiction and alcohol abuse
Fetal congenital anomalies
Hemoglobinopathies

OLIGOHYDRAMNIOS

Renal agenesis (Potter's syndrome)
Prolonged rupture of membranes
IUGR
Intrauterine fetal death

POSTTERM PREGNANCY

Anencephaly
Placental sulfatase deficiency
Perinatal hypoxia, acidosis
Placental insufficiency

CHROMOSOMAL ABNORMALITIES

Maternal age 35 years or more
Balanced translocation (maternal and paternal)

Data from DeCherney A, Pernoll M, editors: *Current obstetric and gynecologic diagnosis and treatment,* ed 8, Norwalk, CT, 1994, Appleton & Lange.

Box 9-4

Factors that Place the Postpartum Woman and Neonate at High Risk

MOTHER

Hemorrhage
Infection
Abnormal vital signs
Traumatic labor of birth
Psychosocial factors

INFANT (FOR ADMISSION TO NICU)

High Risk Category

Infants continuing or developing signs of RDS or other respiratory distress
Asphyxiated infants (Apgar scores less than 6 at 5 minutes); resuscitation required at birth
Preterm infants; dysmature infants
Infants with cyanosis or suspected cardiovascular disease; persistent cyanosis
Infants with major congenital malformations requiring surgery; chromosomal anomalies
Infants with convulsions, sepsis, hemorrhagic diathesis, or shock
Meconium aspiration syndrome
CNS depression for longer than 24 hours
Hypoglycemia
Hypocalcemia
Hyperbilirubinemia

Moderate Risk Category

Dysmaturity
Prematurity (weight between 2000 and 2500 g)
Apgar score less than 5 at 1 minute
Feeding problems
Multifetal birth
Transient tachypnea
Hypomagnesemia or hypermagnesemia
Hypoparathyroidism
Failure to gain weight
Jitteriness or hyperactivity
Cardiac anomalies not requiring immediate catheterization
Heart murmur
Anemia
CNS depression for less than 24 hours

CNS, Central nervous system; *NICU,* neonatal intensive care unit; *RDS,* respiratory distress syndrome.

TABLE 9-1

Fetal Assessment Screening: Recommendations for Care

Fetal Assessment Test	Recommendation/Conclusion
Doppler ultrasound use in pregnancy at high risk for fetal compromise	Beneficial effects
Ultrasound use to estimate gestational age in first and early second trimesters Ultrasound use to confirm multiple pregnancy Ultrasound use for placental location in placenta previa Early second trimester amniocentesis for identification of chromosomal abnormalities Transabdominal instead of transvaginal chorionic villus sampling (CVS)	Effects likely to be beneficial
Formal systems of risk scoring Routine use of early ultrasound CVS versus amniocentesis for diagnosing chromosomal abnormalities Serum alpha fetoprotein screening for neural tube defects Routine fetal movement counts to improve perinatal outcome	There is a trade-off between beneficial and adverse effects
Placental grading by ultrasound to improve perinatal outcome Biophysical profile for fetal surveillance	Unknown effectiveness
Routine use of ultrasound for fetal anthropometry (body measurements) in late pregnancy Use of Doppler ultrasound in all pregnancies Measurement of placental hormones (estriol)	Unlikely to be beneficial
Nipple stimulation test to improve perinatal outcome Nonstress test to improve perinatal outcome Contraction stress test to improve perinatal outcome	Likely to be ineffective or harmful

Source: Enkin M, et al: Effective care in pregnancy and childbirth, *Birth 22*(2):101-110, 1995.

Daily Fetal Movement Count

Assessment of fetal activity by the mother is a simple yet valuable method for monitoring the condition of the fetus. The daily fetal movement count (DFMC) is simple to understand, is noninvasive, can be done at home, and does not interfere with most daily routines. The presence of fetal movements is generally a reassuring sign of fetal health.

Several protocols are used for counting. Except for noting a very low number of daily fetal movements (FMs) or a trend toward decreased motion, the clinical value of the absolute number of FMs has not been established. The only exception is if FMs cease entirely for 12 hours (the fetal alarm signal). Generally, a count of fewer than three FMs within 1 hour warrants further evaluation by nonstress or contraction stress testing, biophysical profile (BPP), or a combination of these. Patients should be taught the significance of fetal movements, the procedure to use for counting, and how to record findings on a daily fetal movement record (see Guidelines box on p. 417).

NURSE ALERT • In assessing fetal movements, it is important to remember that they are usually not present during the fetal sleep cycle; they may be temporarily reduced if the woman is taking depressant medication, drinking alcohol, or smoking a cigarette. They do not usually decrease as the woman nears term.

Ultrasonography

Diagnostic ultrasonography is an important technique in antepartum fetal surveillance. Ultrasound can be done abdominally or transvaginally during pregnancy. Both methods produce a three-dimensional view from which a pictorial image is obtained. Abdominal ultrasonography is more useful after the first trimester when the pregnant uterus becomes an abdominal organ. For the procedure the woman is usually required to have a full bladder (to push the uterus up) to get a better image of the fetus. Transmission gel or paste is applied to the abdomen before a transducer is moved over the skin to enhance transmission and reception of the sound waves.

Transvaginal ultrasonography, in which the probe is inserted into the vagina, allows pelvic anatomy to be evaluated in greater detail and allows intrauterine pregnancy to be diagnosed earlier (Cunningham et al, 1997). A transvaginal ultrasound examination is well tolerated by most patients because it alleviates the need for a full bladder. It is especially useful in obese patients whose thick abdominal layers cannot be penetrated adequately by an abdominal approach. Transvaginal ultrasonography is used in the first trimester to detect ectopic pregnancies, monitor the developing embryo, help identify abnormalities, and help establish gestational age. In some instances it may be used as an adjunct to abdominal scanning to evaluate preterm labor in second- and third-trimester pregnancies (Guzman et al, 1998).

For an abdominal ultrasound the woman is positioned comfortably with small pillows under her head and knees. The display panel should be positioned so that the woman and her partner can observe the images on the screen if they desire. A transvaginal ultrasound may be performed either with the woman in a lithotomy position or with her pelvis elevated by towels, cushions, or a folded pillow. This pelvic tilt is optimal to image the pelvic structures. A protective cover such as a condom, the finger of a clean rubber surgical glove, or a special cover provided by the manufacturer is used to cover the probe. The probe is lubricated with a water-soluble gel and placed in the vagina either by the examiner or by the woman herself. During the examination the position of the probe or the tilt of the examining table may be changed to view the complete pelvis. The procedure is not physically painful, although the woman will feel pressure as the probe is moved.

Indications for Use. Major indications for the use of obstetric sonography vary by trimester. During the first trimester, ultrasound examination is performed to obtain information on the following: (1) number, size, and location of gestational sacs; (2) presence or absence of fetal cardiac and body movements; (3) presence or absence of uterine abnormalities (e.g., bicornuate uterus and fibroids) or adnexal masses (e.g., ovarian cysts and ectopic pregnancy); (4) pregnancy dating (i.e., crown-rump length); and (5) presence and location of an intrauterine contraceptive device.

During the second and third trimesters, information on the following is sought: (1) fetal viability, number, position, gestational age, growth pattern, and anomalies; (2) amniotic fluid volume; (3) placental location and maturity; (4) uterine fibroids and anomalies; (5) adnexal masses; and (6) cervical length.

Ultrasonography can lead to earlier diagnosis, allowing therapy to be instituted early in pregnancy. This decreases the severity and duration of morbidity, both physical and emotional, for the family.

Fetal Heart Activity. Fetal heart activity can be demonstrated as early as 6 to 7 weeks by real-time echo scanners and at 10 to 12 weeks by Doppler mode. By 9 to 10 weeks, gestational trophoblastic disease can be diagnosed. Fetal death can be confirmed by lack of heart motion, the presence of fetal scalp edema, and maceration and overlap of the cranial bones.

Gestational Age. Gestational dating by ultrasonography is indicated for conditions such as the following: (1) uncertain dates for the last normal menstrual period, (2) recent discontinuation of oral contraceptives, (3) bleeding episode during the first trimester, (4) uterine size that does not agree with dates, and (5) other high risk conditions.

During the first 18 to 20 weeks of gestation, ultrasonography provides an accurate assessment of gestational age because most normal fetuses grow at the same rate. With increased fetal age, the accuracy of gestational age estimates using ultrasound also increases because more variables are measured. Four methods of fetal age estimation are used: (1) determination of gestational sac dimensions (at about 8 weeks), (2) measurement of crown-rump length (between 7 and 14 weeks), (3) measurement of the biparietal diameter (BPD) (after 12 weeks), and (4) measurement of femur length (after 12 weeks). Fetal BPD at 36 weeks should be approximately 8.7 cm. Term pregnancy and fetal maturity can be diagnosed with some confidence if the biparietal measurement by ultrasound is greater than 9.8 cm (Figs. 9-1 and 9-2, Table 9-2), especially when this is combined with appropriate femur length measurement.

In later gestations the accuracy of fetal age determination is enhanced by serial measurements. Two and preferably three composite measurements are recommended, at least 2 weeks apart, and these are plotted against standard fetal growth

TABLE 9-2
Correlation of Fetal Weight and BPD

BPD (cm)	Estimated Fetal Weight
8.2	2290 g
8.5	2500 g
8.8	2730 g
9.4	3180 g
10.0	3630 g
10.6	4070 g

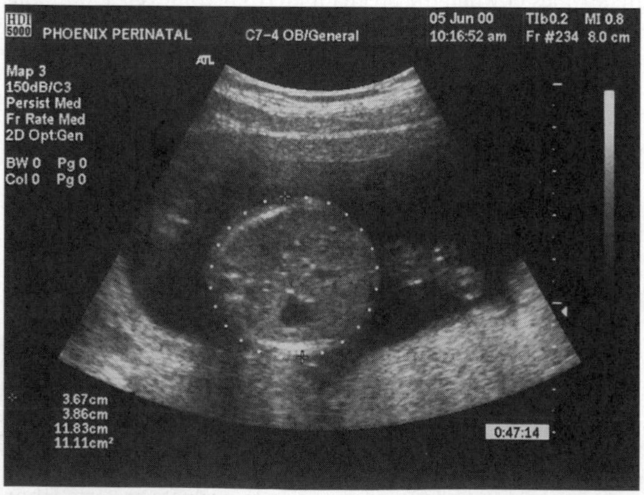

FIG. 9-1 • Biparietal cephalometry by ultrasound. (Courtesy Michael S. Clement, MD, Mesa, AZ.)

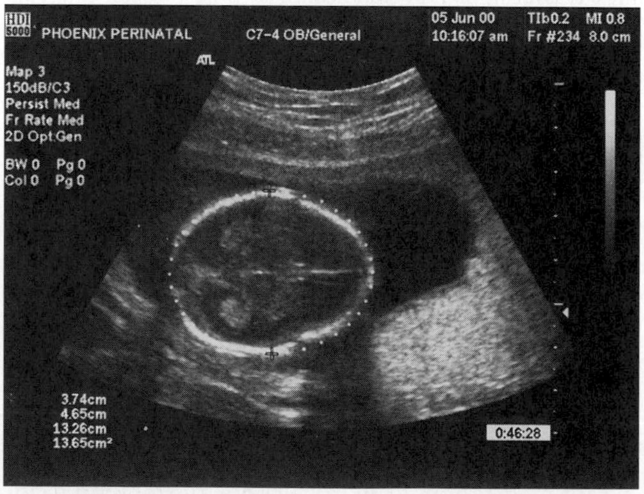

FIG. 9-2 • Head circumference. (Courtesy Michael S. Clement, MD, Mesa, AZ.)

curves. This method, when applied between 24 and 32 weeks of gestation, yields an estimation error of 10 days more or less than the actual age (Manning, 1999a).

Fetal Growth. Fetal growth is a result of interaction between intrinsic growth potential and the environmental factors that may enhance or inhibit that growth. Conditions that indicate the need for ultrasound assessment of fetal growth include: (1) poor maternal weight gain or pattern of weight gain, (2) previous intrauterine growth restriction (IUGR), (3) chronic infections, (4) ingestion of drugs (e.g., tobacco, alcohol, over-the-counter, and street drugs), (5) maternal diabetes mellitus, (6) hypertension, (7) multifetal pregnancy, and (8) other medical or surgical complications.

Serial evaluations of BPD and limb length can differentiate between size discrepancy resulting from inaccurate dates and true IUGR. IUGR may be symmetric (i.e., the fetus is small in all parameters) or asymmetric (i.e., head and body growth vary). Symmetric IUGR implies a chronic or long-standing insult and may be caused by low genetic growth potential, intrauterine infection, maternal undernutrition, heavy smoking, or chromosomal aberration. Asymmetric growth reflects an acute or late-occurring deprivation such as placental insufficiency resulting from hypertension, renal disease, or cardiovascular disease.

Macrosomic infants (those weighing 4000 g or more) are at increased risk for trauma during birth. Fetal macrosomia associated with maternal glucose intolerance carries an increased risk of intrauterine death.

Adjunct to Amniocentesis, Percutaneous Umbilical Blood Sampling, and Chorionic Villus Sampling. The safety of amniocentesis is increased when the physician knows the exact position of the fetus, placenta, and pockets of amniotic fluid. Ultrasound scanning has reduced the risks previously associated with amniocentesis, such as fetomaternal hemorrhage from a pierced placenta. Percutaneous umbilical blood sampling (PUBS) and chorionic villus sampling (CVS) are also guided by ultrasound to identify accurately the cord and chorion frondosum.

Fetal Anatomy. Depending on the gestational age, the following structures may be identified: head (including ventricles and blood vessels), neck, spine, heart, stomach, small bowel, liver, kidneys, bladder, limbs, and umbilical cord. Ultrasonography permits the confirmation of normal anatomy (Fig. 9-3) or the detection of major fetal malformations. The presence of an anomaly may influence the birth location (e.g., delivery room instead of a labor-delivery-recovery room or a subspecialty center versus a basic care center) and the method of birth to optimize neonatal outcomes. The number of fetuses and their presentation also may be assessed by ultrasonography, allowing plans to be made for therapy and mode of birth.

Placental Position and Function. The pattern of uterine and placental growth and the fullness of the maternal bladder influence the apparent location of the placenta as viewed by ultrasound. By 14 to 16 weeks the placenta can be clearly defined, but its relationship to the internal cervical os can sometimes be altered dramatically by changing the degree of fullness of the maternal bladder. In approximately 15% to 20% of all pregnancies in which ultrasound scanning is performed in the second trimester, the placenta seems to be overlying the os, but at term the incidence of placenta previa is only 0.5%. Thus the diagnosis of placenta previa can seldom be confirmed before 27 weeks, primarily because of the elongation of the lower uterine segment as pregnancy advances.

Another use of ultrasound is the grading of placental maturation. Calcium deposits are of significance in postterm pregnancies because as they increase, the available surface area that can be adequately bathed by maternal blood decreases. At exactly what point this results in fetal wastage and hypoxia cannot be pinpointed precisely; however, effects usually are observable by 42 weeks and progress thereafter (Gilbert and Harmon, 1998).

Fetal Well-Being. Physiologic measurements that can be performed with fetal ultrasound scanning include amniotic fluid volume, vascular waveforms from the fetal circulation, heart motion, fetal breathing movements, fetal urine production, and fetal limb and head movements. Assessment of these parameters, singly or in combination, yields a fairly reliable picture of fetal well-being. The significance of these findings is discussed in the following sections.

Amniotic Fluid Volume. Abnormalities of amniotic fluid volume (AFV), whether excessive or diminished, are often associated with fetal disorders. Subjective criteria for the assessment of oligohydramnios (decreased fluid) include the absence of fluid pockets in the uterine cavity and the impression of crowding of fetal small parts (arms and legs). An objective criterion of decreased AFV is met when the largest pocket of fluid measured in two perpendicular planes is less than 2 cm. In the case of polyhydramnios (increased fluid), the criteria include multiple large pockets of fluid greater than 12 cm in the vertical axis, the impression of a floating fetus, and free movement of fetal limbs (Manning, 1999a). The total AFV can be evaluated by a method in which the depths (in centimeters) of amniotic fluid in all four quadrants surrounding the maternal umbilicus are totaled, resulting in an amniotic fluid index (AFI). An AFI is normal if the summed value is more than 80 mm and less than 180 mm (Manning, 1999a).

Oligohydramnios is associated with congenital anomalies (such as renal agenesis), IUGR, and fetal distress in labor. Polyhydramnios is associated with neural tube defects, obstruction of the fetal gastrointestinal tract, multiple fetuses, and fetal hydrops.

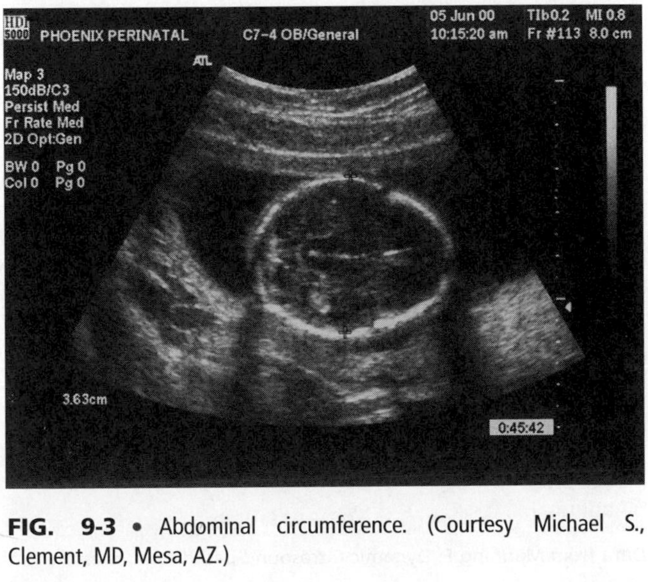

FIG. 9-3 • Abdominal circumference. (Courtesy Michael S., Clement, MD, Mesa, AZ.)

Doppler Blood Flow Analysis. One of the major advances in perinatal medicine is the ability to study blood flow noninvasively in the fetus and placenta. Doppler ultrasound is a useful adjunct in the management of pregnancies at risk because of hypertension, IUGR, diabetes mellitus, multiple fetuses, or preterm labor (Miller, 1998). The velocity of the RBCs can be determined by measuring the change in the frequency in the sound wave reflected off them.

Velocity waveforms from umbilical and uterine arteries, reported in systolic/diastolic (S/D) ratios, can be first detected at 15 weeks of pregnancy. Because of progressive decline in resistance in both the umbilical and the uterine arteries, this ratio decreases as pregnancy advances. Most fetuses achieve an S/D ratio of 3 or less by 30 weeks (Fig. 9-4). Persistent elevation of S/D ratios after 30 weeks is associated with IUGR, usually resulting from uteroplacental insufficiency (UPI). Abnormal velocity study results are also seen in postterm pregnancies with a poorly perfused placenta, with certain chromosomal abnormalities (i.e., trisomy 13 and 18), and with lupus erythematosus in the mother. Exposure to nicotine from maternal smoking also increases the S/D ratio.

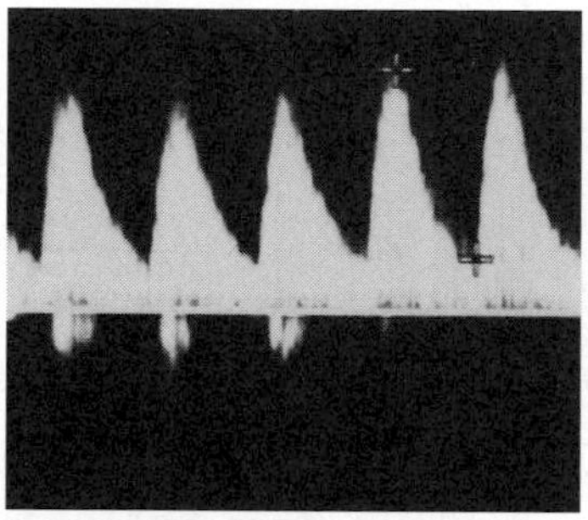

FIG. 9-4 • Umbilical artery velocity waveform in a 17-week fetus with S/D ratio of 4.4, which is normal for this stage. (Courtesy Michael S. Clement, MD, Mesa, AZ.)

Biophysical Profile. Real-time ultrasound permits detailed assessment of the physical and physiologic characteristics of the developing fetus to such an extent that it is possible to examine the fetus in detail and to catalog normal and abnormal biophysical responses to stimuli. The biophysical profile (BPP) is a noninvasive dynamic assessment of a fetus and its environment, employing ultrasonography and external fetal monitoring.

BPP scoring is a method of fetal risk surveillance based on the assessment of acute and chronic markers of fetal disease. The BPP includes fetal breathing movements, fetal movements, fetal tone, fetal heart rate patterns by means of a nonstress test (NST), and AFV. The procedure may be considered as a physical examination of the fetus, including determination of vital signs. The fetus responds to central hypoxia by alterations in movement, muscle tone, breathing, and heart rate patterns. The presence of normal fetal biophysical activities shows that the central nervous system is fully functional and that therefore the fetus is not hypoxemic (Manning, 1999b). BPP variables and scoring are detailed in Table 9-3.

The BPP is an accurate indicator of impending fetal death. Fetal acidosis can be diagnosed early with a nonreactive NST and absent fetal breathing movements. When an abnormal score and oligohydramnios are encountered, labor induction is warranted (Manning, 1995). Fetal infection in women whose membranes rupture prematurely (at less than 37 weeks' gestation) can be diagnosed early. The change in biophysical activities precedes the clinical signs of infection and indicates the necessity for immediate birth. When BPP score is normal and the risk of fetal death low, intervention is indicated only for obstetric or maternal factors.

TABLE 9-3
Biophysical Profile

Variables	Normal (Score = 2)	Abnormal (Score = 0)
Fetal breathing movements	One or more episodes in 30 min, each lasting ≥30 sec	Episodes absent or no episode ≥30 sec in 30 min
Gross body movements	Three or more discrete body or limb movements in 30 min (episodes of active continuous movement being considered as a single movement)	Less than three episodes of body or limb movements in 30 min
Fetal tone	One or more episodes of active extension with return to flexion of fetal limb(s) or trunk, opening and closing of hand being considered normal tone	Slow extension with return to flexion, movement of limb in full extension, or fetal movement absent
Reactive fetal heart rate	Two or more episodes of acceleration (≥15 beats/min) in 20 min, each lasting ≥15 sec and associated with fetal movement	Less than two episodes of acceleration or acceleration of <15 beats/min in 20 min
Qualitative amniotic fluid volume	One or more pockets of fluid measuring ≥1 cm in two perpendicular planes	Pockets absent or pocket <1 cm in two perpendicular planes
SCORE		
Normal	8-10 (if Amniotic Fluid Index is adequate)	
Equivocal	6	
Abnormal	<4	

Data from Manning F: Dynamic ultrasound-based fetal assessment: the fetal biophysical profile score, *Clin Obstet Gynecol* 38(1):26-44, 1995.

Safety of Diagnostic Ultrasonography. In the 30 years that diagnostic ultrasonography has been used, no conclusive evidence of any harmful effects on humans has emerged. Although the possibility of unidentified biologic effects exists, the benefits to the patient of prudent use of diagnostic ultrasonography appear to outweigh any possible risk (Anthony, 1996).

Magnetic Resonance Imaging

Magnetic resonance imaging (MRI) is a noninvasive tool that can be used for obstetric and gynecologic diagnosis.

MRI can evaluate the following: (1) fetal structure (e.g., central nervous system, thorax, abdomen, genitourinary tract, and musculoskeletal system), and overall growth; (2) placenta (e.g., position, density, and presence of gestational trophoblastic disease); (3) amniotic fluid quantity; (4) maternal structures (e.g., uterus, cervix, adnexa, and pelvis); (5) biochemical status (e.g., pH and adenosine triphosphate content) of tissues and organs; and (6) soft tissue, metabolic, or functional malformations.

The woman is placed on a table in a supine position and slid into the bore of the main magnet that is similar in appearance to a CT scanner. Depending on the reason for the study, the entire procedure may take 20 to 60 minutes, during which time the woman must be perfectly still except for short respites. Because of the long time needed to produce magnetic resonance images, it is likely that the fetus will move and obscure anatomic details. The only way to ensure that the fetus will not move is to administer a sedative to the mother, but this approach should be reserved for selected cases in which visualization of fetal detail is critical.

MRI has little effect on the fetus; concerns that the fetal heart rate or fetal movement would decrease have not been supported (Poutamo et al, 1998).

BIOCHEMICAL ASSESSMENT

Biochemical assessment involves the study of biologic components such as genes or exfoliated cells and chemical components such as the lecithin/sphingomyelin (L/S) ratio and bilirubin levels (Table 9-4). Procedures used to obtain the specimens needed for study include amniocentesis, percutaneous umbilical blood sampling, chorionic villus sampling, and maternal assays.

Amniocentesis

Amniocentesis is performed to obtain amniotic fluid, which contains fetal cells. Under direct ultrasonic visualization, a needle is inserted transabdominally into the uterus, amniotic fluid is withdrawn into a syringe, and various amniotic fluid assessments are performed. Amniocentesis is possible after week 14 of pregnancy, when the uterus becomes an abdominal organ and sufficient amniotic fluid is available for testing (Table 9-4, Fig. 9-5). Indications for the procedure include prenatal diagnosis of genetic disorders or congenital anomalies (neural tube defects in particular), assessment of pulmonary maturity, and diagnosis of fetal hemolytic disease.

Complications in the mother and fetus occur in less than 1% of the cases and include the following:

Maternal—Hemorrhage, fetomaternal hemorrhage with possible maternal Rh isoimmunization, infection, labor, abruptio placentae, inadvertent damage to the intestines or bladder, amniotic fluid embolism. Because of the possibility of fetomaternal hemorrhage, it is standard practice to administer immune globulin D (RhoGAM) to the woman who is Rh negative after an amniocentesis.

Fetal—Death, hemorrhage, infection (amnionitis), direct injury from the needle, miscarriage or preterm labor, and leakage of amniotic fluid.

TABLE 9-4
Summary of Biochemical Monitoring Techniques

Test	Possible Findings	Clinical Significance
MATERNAL BLOOD		
Coombs test	Titer of 1:8 and rising	Significant Rh incompatibility
AFP	See below	See below
AMNIOTIC FLUID ANALYSIS		
Color	Meconium	Possible hypoxia or asphyxia
Lung profile		
L/S ratio	>2	Fetal lung maturity
Phosphatidylglycerol	Present	
Creatinine	>2 mg/dl	Gestational age >36 weeks
Bilirubin (ΔOD 450/nm)	<0.015	Gestational age >36 weeks, normal pregnancy
	High levels	Fetal hemolytic disease in Rh isoimmunized pregnancies
Lipid cells	>10%	Gestational age >35 weeks
AFP	High levels after 15-week gestation	Open neural tube or other defect
Osmolality	Decline after 20-week gestation	Advancing nonspecific gestational age
Genetic disorders	Dependent on cultured cells for karyotype and enzymatic activity	Counseling possibly required
Sex-linked		
Chromosomal		
Metabolic		

Many of the complications have been minimized or eliminated by performing the procedure under ultrasound guidance.

Genetic Problems. Prenatal assessment of genetic disorders is indicated for women over age 35 years, for those with a previous child with a chromosomal abnormality, and those with a family history of chromosomal anomalies. Inherited errors of metabolism and other disorders for which marker genes are known may also be detected.

Cells are cultured for karyotyping of chromosomes (see Chapter 8). The incidence of fetal chromosomal aberrations increases with age of the mother. Fetal cells can be assessed for sex chromatin; sex determination is important if a sex-linked disorder is suspected.

Alpha-fetoprotein (AFP) levels are assessed as a follow-up for elevated levels of maternal serum AFP. High AFP levels in the amniotic fluid occur in the presence of an open neural tube defect such as spina bifida or anencephaly, or with an open abdominal wall defect such as omphalocele. AFP levels also may be elevated in a normal multifetal pregnancy and with intestinal atresia, presumably caused by lack of fetal swallowing. Concurrent ultrasound examination is recommended in these patients.

Fetal Maturity. Accurate assessment of fetal maturity is possible through examination of amniotic fluid or its exfoliated cellular contents (Box 9-5). Table 9-4 includes laboratory studies that are used to demonstrate term pregnancy and fetal maturity.

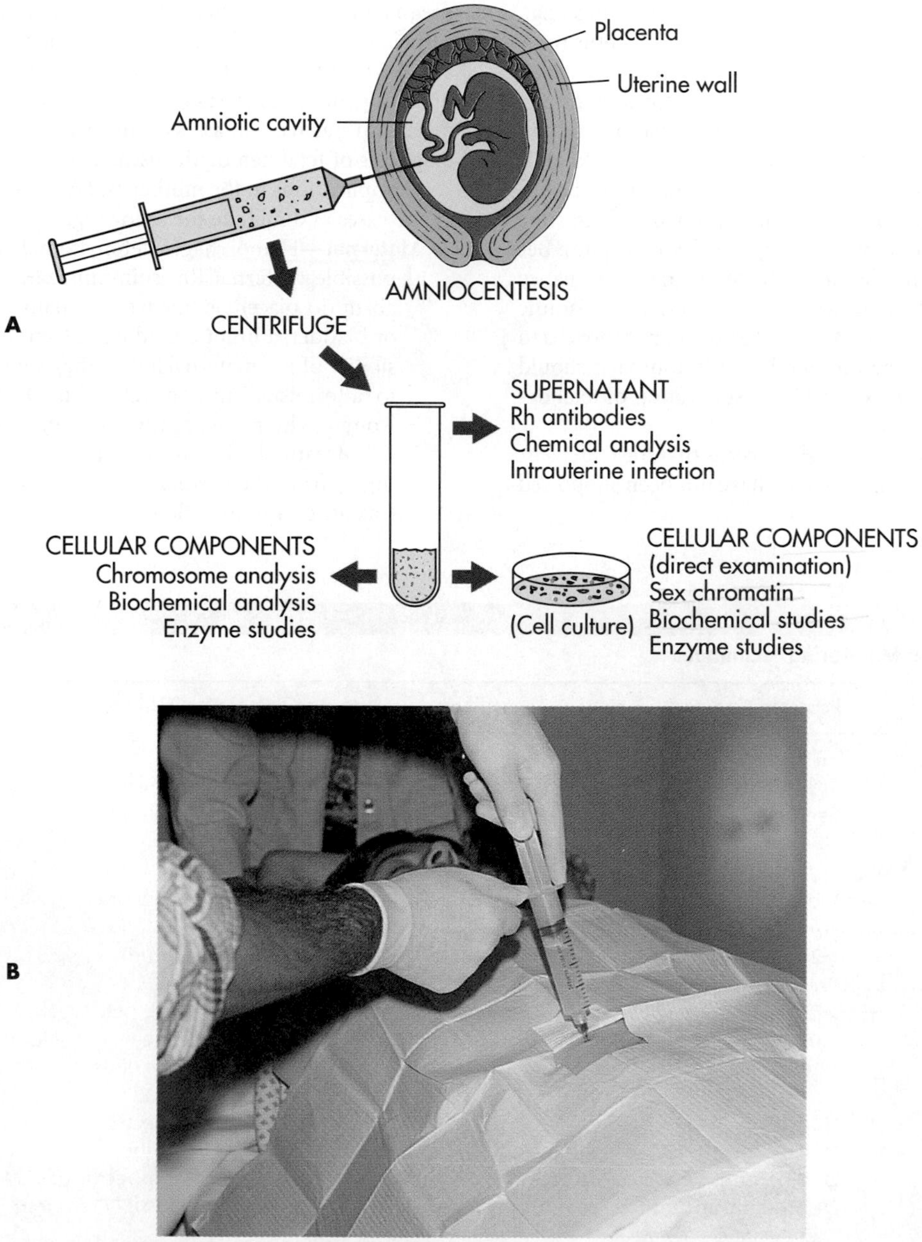

FIG. 9-5 • **A,** Amniocentesis and laboratory use of amniotic fluid aspirant. **B,** Transabdominal amniocentesis. (B, courtesy Marjorie Pyle, RNC, Lifecircle, Costa Mesa, CA.)

Fetal Hemolytic Disease. Amniocentesis is used to identify and follow-up fetal hemolytic disease in cases of isoimmunization. The procedure is usually not done until the mother's serum antibody titer reaches 1:8 and is rising. Currently, percutaneous umbilical blood sampling is the procedure of choice to evaluate and treat fetal hemolytic disease (Box 9-6).

Meconium. The presence of meconium in the amniotic fluid is usually determined by visual inspection of the sample. The significance of meconium in the amniotic fluid varies depending on when it is found.

Antenatal Period. Meconium in the amniotic fluid before early labor begins is not usually associated with an adverse fetal outcome. The finding may be the result of an acute and subsequently corrected fetal stress, chronic ongoing stress, or simply the physiologic passage of meconium. Because some association has been found between meconium in amniotic fluid in the third trimester and hypertensive conditions and postmaturity, the fetus should undergo further antepartum evaluation if the birth is not imminent (Glantz and Woods, 1999).

Intrapartal Period. Intrapartal meconium-stained amniotic fluid is an indication for more careful evaluation by electronic fetal monitoring (EFM) and perhaps fetal scalp blood sampling. The presence of meconium, however, should not be the sole indicator for intervention.

Three possible reasons exist for the passage of meconium during the intrapartal period: (1) it is a normal physiologic function that occurs with maturity (meconium passage is uncommon before weeks 23 to 24, but there is an increased incidence after 38 weeks); (2) it is the result of hypoxia-induced peristalsis and sphincter relaxation; and (3) it may be a sequela to umbilical cord compression–induced vagal stimulation in mature fetuses. Thick, fresh meconium passed for the first time in late labor, associated with nonremediable severe variable or late FHR decelerations, is an ominous sign.

NURSE ALERT • The birth team should be ready to suction the nasopharynx of the neonate at time of the birth, ideally before the first breath is taken. Suctioning at this time is effective in reducing the incidence and severity of meconium aspiration in the neonate.

Percutaneous Umbilical Blood Sampling

Direct access to the fetal circulation during the second and third trimesters is possible through percutaneous umbilical blood sampling (PUBS), or cordocentesis. PUBS is the most widely used method for fetal blood sampling and transfusion. PUBS involves the insertion of a needle directly into the fetal umbilical vessel under ultrasound guidance. Ideally, the umbilical cord is punctured 1 to 2 cm from its placental insertion (Fig. 9-6). At this point the cord is well anchored and will not move, and the risk of maternal blood contamination (from the placenta) is slight. Generally, 1 to 4 ml of blood is removed during the puncture and immediately tested by the Kleihauer-Betke procedure to ensure that it is fetal blood. Indications for use of PUBS include prenatal diagnosis of inherited blood disorders, karyotyping of malformed fetuses, detection of fetal infection, determination of the acid-base status of fetuses with IUGR, and assessment and treatment of isoimmunization and thrombocytopenia in pregnant women (Harmon, 1999). Complications that can occur include leaking of blood from the puncture site, cord laceration, thromboembolism, preterm labor, premature rupture of membranes, and infection.

Box 9-5

Shake Test for the Presence of Phospholipids

A quick means of determining an approximate L/S ratio is the shake test, foam test, or bubble stability test. Serial dilutions of fresh amniotic fluid are mixed with ethanol and shaken. After 15 minutes, the amount of bubbles present at different dilutions indicates the presence of surfactant.

Box 9-6

Apt Test for Differentiation of Maternal and Fetal Blood

The Apt test is used to differentiate maternal and fetal blood when vaginal bleeding occurs during pregnancy or labor. It may be performed quickly by the following method: Add 0.5 ml bloody fluid to 4.5 ml distilled water and shake. Add 1 ml 0.25N sodium hydroxide. Fetal and cord blood remains pink for 1 to 2 minutes. Maternal blood turns brown in 30 seconds. A Kleihauer-Betke procedure can be done in the laboratory to confirm the presence of fetal blood.

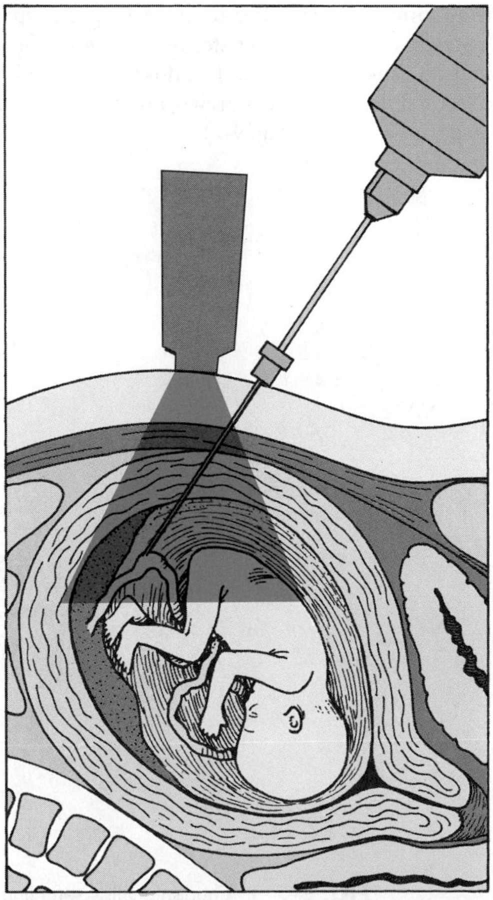

FIG. 9-6 • Technique for PUBS guided by ultrasound.

In fetuses at risk for isoimmune hemolytic anemia, PUBS permits precise identification of fetal blood type and RBC count and may prevent further intervention. If the fetus is positive for the presence of maternal antibodies, a direct blood test can confirm the degree of anemia resulting from hemolysis. Intrauterine transfusion of severely anemic fetuses can be done 4 to 5 weeks earlier than through the intraperitoneal route.

Follow-up includes continuous FHR monitoring for several minutes to 1 hour and a repeat ultrasound examination 1 hour later to ensure that no bleeding or hematoma formation has occurred.

Chorionic Villus Sampling

The combined advantages of earlier diagnosis and rapid results have made chorionic villus sampling a popular technique for genetic studies, although some risks to the fetus exist. The procedure is performed between 10 and 12 weeks of gestation and involves the removal of a small tissue specimen from the fetal portion of the placenta. Because chorionic villi originate in the zygote, that tissue reflects the genetic makeup of the fetus.

CVS can be accomplished either transcervically or transabdominally. In transcervical sampling, a sterile catheter is introduced into the cervix under continuous ultrasonographic guidance and a small portion of the chorionic villi is aspirated with a syringe. The aspiration cannula and obturator must be placed at a suitable site, and rupture of the amniotic sac must be avoided.

If the abdominal approach is used, an 18-gauge spinal needle with stylet is inserted under sterile conditions through the abdominal wall into the chorion frondosum under ultrasound guidance. The stylet is then withdrawn, and the chorionic tissue is aspirated into a syringe (Fig. 9-7).

Complications of the procedure include vaginal spotting or bleeding immediately afterward; miscarriage (0.3%), rupture of membranes (0.1%), and chorioamnionitis (0.5%). Because of the possibility of fetomaternal hemorrhage, women who are Rh negative should receive RhoGAM to avoid isoimmunization (Gilbert and Harmon, 1998). An increased risk of limb anomalies has been noted when CVS is done before 10 weeks of gestation (Box 9-7).

Indications for CVS are similar to those for amniocentesis. About 90% of the procedures are performed because of advanced maternal age (i.e., over age 35) (Scioscia, 1999). Other indications include biochemical and molecular assays for infections or metabolic disorders.

Maternal Assays

Alpha-fetoprotein. AFP is produced by the fetal liver and is detectable in increasing quantities in the serum of pregnant women from 14 to 34 weeks. Maternal serum AFP (MSAFP) is used in pregnancy as a screening tool for neural tube defects (NTDs) and is usually done between 15 and 22 weeks gestation. Through MSAFP, approximately 80% to 85% of all open NTDs

> Box 9-7
> **Fetal Rights**
>
> Amniocentesis, PUBS, and CVS are prenatal tests used for diagnosing fetal defects in pregnancy. They are invasive and carry risks to the mother and fetus. A consideration of abortion is linked to the performance of these tests because there is no treatment for genetically affected fetuses. Thus the issue of fetal rights is a key ethical concern in prenatal testing for fetal defects.

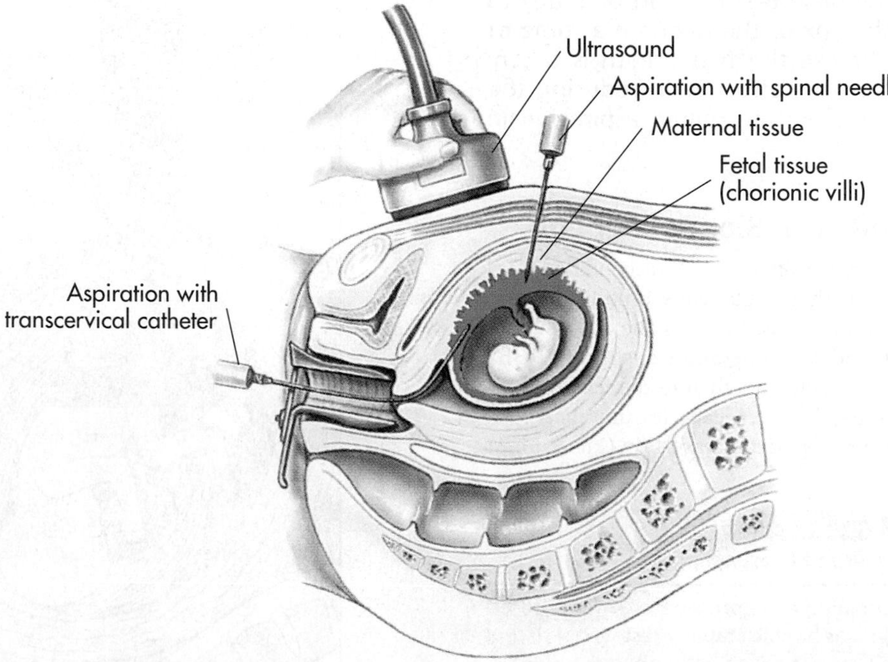

FIG. 9-7 • Chorionic villus sampling (abdominal and transcervical methods). (Courtesy Medical and Scientific Illustration, Crozet, VA.)

can be detected early in pregnancy. If findings are abnormal, follow-up procedures include genetic counseling for families with a history of NTD, repeat AFP, ultrasound examination, and possibly amniocentesis.

Down syndrome—and probably other autosomal trisomies—is associated with lower-than-normal levels of MSAFP and amniotic fluid AFP. The triple-marker test is also performed at 16 to 18 weeks of gestation and uses the levels of three markers, MSAFP, unconjugated estriol, and human chorionic gonadotropin (hCG), in combination with maternal age to calculate a new risk. If a fetus has Down syndrome, the MSAFP and unconjugated estriol levels are low and the hCG level is elevated. With the two additional screening tests, approximately 60% of fetuses with Down syndrome can be identified (Ross and Elias, 1997).

As with MSAFP, these tests are screening procedures only and are not diagnostic. A definitive examination of amniotic fluid for AFP and chromosomal analysis, combined with ultrasound visualization of the fetus, is necessary for diagnosis.

Coombs Test. The Coombs test for Rh incompatibility is discussed in Chapter 28. If the maternal titer for Rh antibodies is greater than 1:8, amniocentesis for bilirubin in amniotic fluid or PUBS is indicated to determine the severity of fetal anemia from hemolysis. The Coombs test can also detect other antibodies that may place the fetus at risk for incompatibility with maternal antigens.

ASSESSMENT USING ELECTRONIC FETAL MONITORING

Indications

Assessment during the first and second trimesters is directed primarily at the diagnosis of fetal anomalies. The goal of third-trimester testing is to determine whether the intrauterine environment continues to be supportive to the fetus. The testing often is used to determine the timing of childbirth for patients at risk for uteroplacental insufficiency (i.e., the gradual decline in the delivery of needed substances to the fetus). Gradual loss of placental function results first in inadequate nutrient delivery to the fetus, then leads to IUGR. Subsequently, respiratory function is compromised, resulting in fetal hypoxia. Indications for both the NST (or fetal activity determination [FAD]) and the contraction stress test (CST) are listed in Box 9-8.

No clinical contraindications exist for the NST, but results may be inconclusive if gestation is 26 weeks or less. Absolute contraindications for the CST are rupture of membranes, previous classic incision for cesarean birth, preterm labor, placenta previa, and abruptio placentae. Multifetal pregnancy, previous preterm labor, hydramnios, more than 36 weeks' gestation, and incompetent cervix are relative contraindications for CST. As a rule, reactive patterns with the NST or negative results with the CST are associated with favorable outcomes.

Box 9-8

Indications for the Nonstress Test and the Contraction Stress Test

- Maternal diabetes mellitus
- Chronic hypertension
- Hypertensive disorders in pregnancy
- IUGR
- Sickle cell disease
- Maternal cyanotic heart disease
- Postmaturity
- History of previous stillbirth
- Decreased fetal movement
- Isoimmunization
- Meconium-stained amniotic fluid at third-trimester amniocentesis
- Hyperthyroidism
- Collagen disease
- Older pregnant woman
- Chronic renal disease

Fetal Responses to Hypoxia and Asphyxia

Hypoxia or asphyxia elicits a number of responses in the fetus. There is a redistribution of blood flow to certain vital organs. This series of responses (redistribution of blood flow favoring vital organs, decreased total oxygen consumption, and anaerobic glycolysis) is a temporary mechanism that enables the fetus to survive up to 30 minutes of limited oxygen supply without decompensation of vital organs. However, during more severe asphyxia or sustained hypoxemia, these compensatory responses are no longer maintained, and a decrease in the cardiac output, arterial blood pressure, and blood flow to the brain and heart occurs (Parer, 1999), with characteristic FHR patterns reflecting these changes.

Variability

Considerable evidence supports the clinical belief that FHR variability represents an intact nervous pathway through the cerebral cortex, midbrain, vagus nerve, and cardiac conduction system. Thus the integrity of this pathway is intact in the presence of normal FHR variability. With 98% accuracy in predicting fetal well-being, the presence of normal FHR variability is a reassuring indicator. Input from various areas of the brain decreases after cerebral asphyxia, leading to a decrease in variability after failure of the fetal hemodynamic compensatory mechanisms to maintain cerebral oxygenation (Parer, 1999).

Nonstress Test (Fetal Activity Determination)

The NST is the most widely applied technique for antepartum evaluation of the fetus. The basis for the NST, or FAD, is that the normal fetus produces characteristic FHR patterns in response to fetal movements (FM). In the healthy fetus with an intact central nervous system, 90% of gross fetal body movements are associated with FHR accelerations. This response can be blunted by hypoxia, acidosis, drugs (e.g., analgesics, barbiturates, and beta blockers), fetal sleep, and some congenital anomalies (Tucker, 2000).

NST can be performed easily in an outpatient setting because it is noninvasive. It also is relatively inexpensive and has no known contraindications. Disadvantages center around the high rate of false-positive results for nonreactivity as a result of fetal sleep cycles, medications, and fetal immaturity. The test is slightly less sensitive in detecting fetal compromise than are the CST or BPP.

Procedure. The woman is seated in a reclining chair (or in semi-Fowler's position) to avoid supine hypotension. The FHR is recorded by Doppler transducer, and a tocotransducer is applied to detect uterine contractions or FMs. The strip chart is observed for signs of fetal activity and a concurrent acceleration of FHR. If evidence of FM is not apparent on the strip, the woman may be asked to depress a button on a hand-held event marker connected to the monitor when she feels FM. The FM is then noted on the strip. Because almost all accelerations are accompanied by FM, the movements need not be recorded with accelerations for the test to be considered reactive. The test usually takes 20 to 30 minutes, but it may take longer if the fetus needs to be awakened from a sleep state.

It is common that a woman is asked to drink orange juice or be given glucose to raise her blood sugar and thereby stimulate fetal movements; there is no research evidence that this practice is effective (McCarthy and Narrigan, 1995). Other methods that have been used to stimulate fetal activity (e.g., manipulating the woman's abdomen or using a transvaginal light) have not been effective either. Only acoustic stimulation has had some impact (Marden et al, 1997).

Interpretation. Generally accepted criteria for a reactive tracing are as follows:

- Two or more accelerations of 15 beats/min lasting for 15 seconds over a 20-minute period
- Normal baseline rate
- Long-term variability amplitude of 10 or more beats/min

If the test does not meet the criteria after 40 minutes, it is considered nonreactive (Fig. 9-8, Table 9-5), in which case further assessments are needed with a CST or BPP. The current recommendation is that NST be performed twice weekly (after 28 weeks of gestation) with patients who are diabetic or at risk for fetal death.

Fetal Acoustic Stimulation

The acoustic stimulation test is another method of testing antepartum FHR response. The test takes approximately 15 minutes to complete, with the fetus monitored for 5 to 10 minutes before stimulation to obtain a baseline FHR. The sound source (usually a laryngeal stimulator) is then activated for 3 seconds on the maternal abdomen over the fetal head. Monitoring con-

TABLE 9-5
Interpretation of the Nonstress Test

Result	Interpretation	Clinical Significance
Reactive	Two or more accelerations of FHR of 15 beats/min lasting 15 seconds or more, associated with each FM in a 20-minute period	As long as twice-weekly NSTs remain reactive, most high-risk pregnancies are allowed to continue.
Nonreactive	Any tracing with either no FHR accelerations or accelerations <15 beats/min or lasting <15 seconds throughout any FM during testing period	Further indirect monitoring may be attempted with abdominal fetal electrocardiography (ECG) in an effort to clarify FHR pattern and quantitative variability; external monitoring should continue, and a CST or BPP should be done.
Unsatisfactory	Quality of FHR recording not adequate for interpretation	Test is repeated in 24 hours or a CST is done, depending on the clinical situation.

BPP, Biophysical profile; *CST,* contraction stress test; *FHR,* fetal heart rate; *NST,* nonstress test.

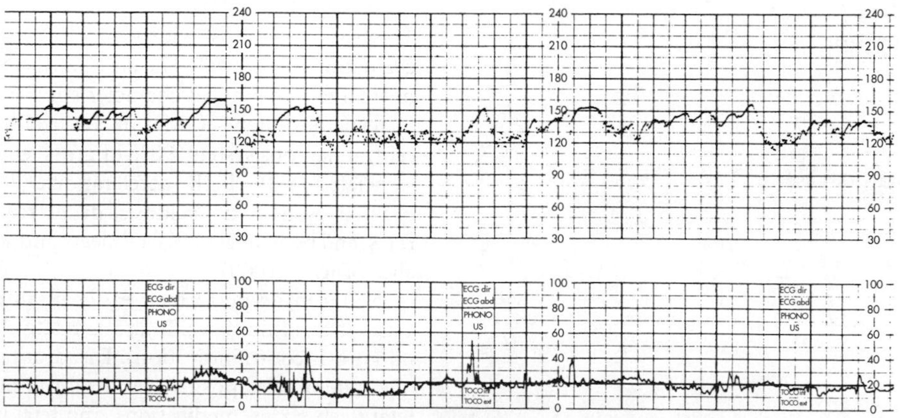

FIG. 9-8 • Reactive NST. FHR accelerations with fetal movement. (From Tucker S: *Pocket guide to fetal monitoring and assessment,* ed 4, St Louis, 2000, Mosby.)

tinues for another 5 minutes, after which the monitor tracing is assessed. A test is considered reactive if there is an immediate and sustained increase in long-term variability and heart rate accelerations. The test may be repeated at 1-minute intervals up to three times when there is no response. Further evaluation is needed with BPP or CST if the pattern is still nonreactive.

Contraction Stress Test

The CST was one of the first electronic methods to be developed for assessment of fetal well-being. It was devised as a graded stress test of the fetus, and its purpose was to identify the fetus in jeopardy who was stable at rest but showed evidence of compromise with stress. Uterine contractions decrease uterine blood flow and placental perfusion. If this decrease is sufficient to produce hypoxia in the fetus, a deceleration in FHR results, beginning at the peak of the contraction and persisting after its conclusion (late deceleration).

NURSE ALERT • In a healthy fetoplacental unit, uterine contractions usually do not produce late decelerations; when there is underlying uteroplacental insufficiency, contractions will produce late decelerations.

The CST provides a warning of fetal compromise earlier than the NST and with fewer false-positive tests. In addition to the contraindications described earlier, CST is more time-consuming and expensive than an NST. It also is an invasive procedure if exogenous oxytocin stimulation is required.

Critical Thinking

ACOUSTIC STIMULATION TEST

Yu Mei approaches the antepartum testing center for an acoustic stimulation test. She does not speak English and is by herself and appears anxious. How would you explain the procedure and its rationale to her? What is the significance of a positive or a negative test? If the test is negative, what additional tests might be ordered?

Procedure. The woman is placed in semi-Fowler's position or sits in a reclining chair. She is monitored indirectly, and the strip is observed for 10 minutes for baseline rate, long-term variability, and the possible occurrence of spontaneous contractions. Two methods of CST are the nipple-stimulated contraction test and the oxytocin-stimulated contraction test.

Nipple-Stimulated Contraction Test. After the procedure is explained to the woman, warm, moist washcloths are applied to both breasts for several minutes. The woman is then asked to massage one nipple for 10 minutes. Massaging the nipples causes a release of oxytocin from the posterior pituitary. An alternative approach is for her to massage the nipple for 2 minutes, rest for 2 minutes, and continue for four cycles of massage and rest. If unilateral stimulation does not achieve adequate contractions (three occurring within a 10-minute window), unilateral continuous stimulation should be tried (if the intermittent approach was used), followed by bilateral stimulation for 10 minutes. When adequate contractions are achieved or hyperstimulation occurs, stimulation should be stopped. If the stimulation and rest cycle method is used, it can be performed indefinitely until considered unsuccessful (Devoe, 1995).

Oxytocin-Stimulated Contraction Test. If the nipple stimulation is not successful, an exogenous oxytocin-stimulated CST should be performed. An intravenous (IV) infusion is begun with a scalp needle. The oxytocin is diluted in an IV solution (usually 10 units to 1000 ml fluid) and infused through a piggyback port into the tubing of the main IV device. An infusion pump is used to ensure accurate dosage. The oxytocin infusion usually is begun at 0.5 mU/min and increased by 0.5 mU/min at 15- to 30-minute intervals until three uterine contractions of good quality are observed within a 10-minute period. The typical rate of oxytocin infusion used to elicit uterine contractions is 4 to 5 mU/min; rarely is more than 8 mU/min required. The oxytocin infusion rate should probably not be increased to more than 20 mU/min; each case should be assessed individually (Devoe, 1995).

Interpretation. If no late decelerations are observed with the contractions, the findings are considered to be negative (Fig. 9-9). Repetitive late decelerations, occurring with most contractions, render the test results positive (Fig. 9-10, Table 9-6).

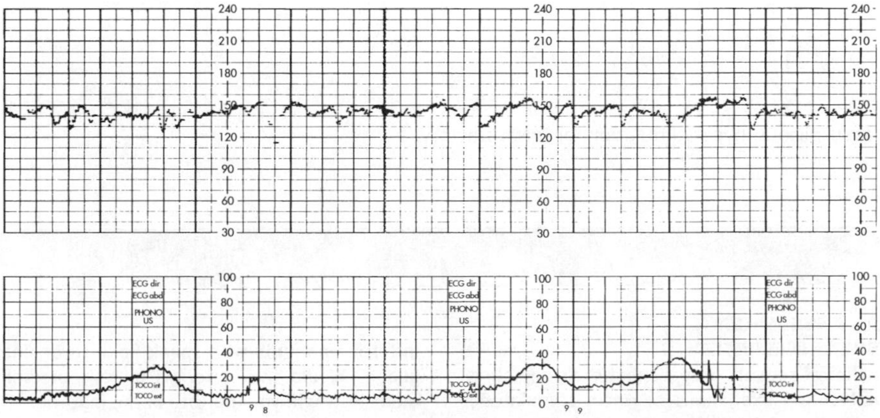

FIG. 9-9 • Negative CST. (From Tucker S: *Pocket guide to fetal monitoring and assessment,* ed 4, St Louis, 2000, Mosby.)

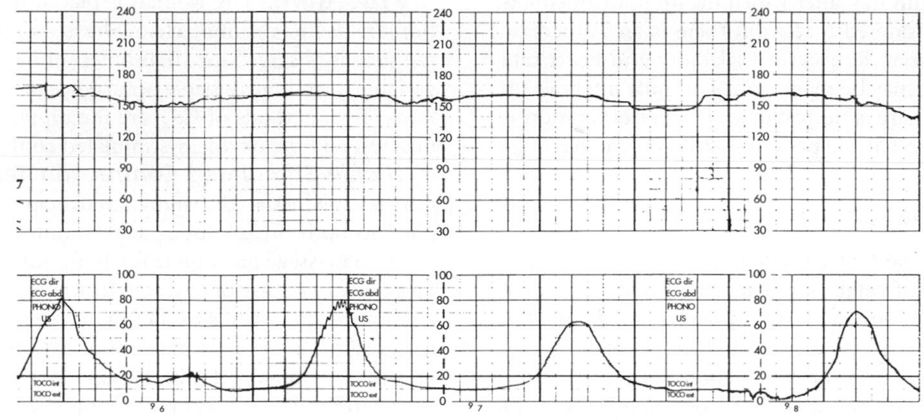

FIG. 9-10 • Positive CST, compromised fetus. (From Tucker S: *Pocket guide to fetal monitoring and assessment,* ed 4, St Louis, 2000, Mosby.)

TABLE 9-6
Interpretation of the Contraction Stress Test

Interpretation	Clinical Significance
NEGATIVE	
No late decelerations, with minimum of three uterine contractions lasting 40 to 60 sec within 10-min period (see Fig. 9-9)	Reassurance that the fetus is likely to survive labor should it occur within 1 week; more frequent testing may be indicated by clinical situation
POSITIVE	
Persistent and consistent late decelerations occurring with more than half of contractions (Fig. 9-10).	Management lies between use of other tools of fetal assessment such as BPP and termination of pregnancy; a positive test result indicates that fetus is at increased risk for perinatal morbidity and mortality; physician may perform expeditious vaginal birth after successful induction or may proceed directly to cesarean birth; decision to intervene is determined by fetal monitoring and presence of FHR reactivity
SUSPICIOUS	
Late decelerations occurring in less than half of uterine contractions once adequate contraction pattern established	NST and CST should be repeated within 24 hr; if interpretable data cannot be achieved, other methods of fetal assessment must be used*
HYPERSTIMULATION	
Late decelerations occurring with excessive uterine activity (contractions more often than every 2 min or lasting longer than 90 sec) or persistent increase in uterine tone	
UNSATISFACTORY	
Inadequate uterine contraction pattern or tracing too poor to interpret	

*Applies to results noted as suspicious, hyperstimulation, or unsatisfactory.

Critical Thinking

EDUCATION ON FETAL ASSESSMENT FOR NON–ENGLISH-SPEAKING PATIENTS

With classmates in your clinical section, prepare materials depicting NST, CST (nipple stimulated and exogenous oxytocin stimulated), and acoustic stimulation tests in pictorial form. Would the materials differ for patients who speak Spanish or Chinese or any other language? Would the materials be suitable for patients who do not read? How will you indicate in the materials that the patient can ask questions?

After interpretation of the FHR pattern, the oxytocin infusion is discontinued, and the maintenance IV solution infused until the uterine activity has returned to the prestimulation level. If the CST is negative, the IV device is removed and the fetal monitor disconnected. If the CST is positive, continued monitoring and further evaluation of fetal well-being are indicated.

NURSING ROLE IN ANTENATAL ASSESSMENT FOR RISK

The nurse's role is that of educator and support person when the woman is undergoing examinations such as ultrasonography, MRI, CVS, PUBS, and amniocentesis. In some instances the nurse may assist the physician with the procedure. In many antenatal settings, nurses perform NSTs, CSTs, BPPs, and basic ultrasounds; conduct an initial assessment; and begin necessary interventions for nonreassuring patterns. These nursing actions are accomplished after additional education and training, under guidance of established protocols, and in collaboration with physicians (Treanor, 1998). Patient teaching, which is an integral component of this role, involves preparing the patient for the procedure, interpreting the findings, and providing psychosocial support when needed.

All women who undergo antenatal assessments are at risk for real and potential problems and may be anxious. With rare exceptions, the tests are ordered because of suspected fetal compromise or deterioration of a maternal condition, or both. In the third trimester, pregnant women are most concerned about protecting themselves and their fetuses and consider themselves most vulnerable to outside influences. The label of high risk will increase this sense of vulnerability.

Most patients have incomplete knowledge related to the procedure, the implications of findings, or the need for further evaluation or counseling. Perinatal nurses can provide the required education, and by keeping the patients well informed, can also promote a positive parental self-image in these high risk individuals.

Community Focus

SUPPORT FOR AT-RISK PREGNANT WOMEN

Researchers have consistently found a relationship between social disadvantage and low-birth-weight babies. Multiple trials of providing social support to women believed to be at risk for giving birth to low-birth-weight babies have been conducted. Nurses, social workers, and midwives—as well as trained lay persons—have provided support. The assistance provided was emotional support such as counseling, sympathetic listening, reassurance, and education or advice at home or in the clinic. In addition, transportation to the clinic or assistance with care of children in the home has been provided. While such programs have demonstrated improved short term psychosocial outcomes, medical outcomes have not improved. Preterm births still pose a significant problem in the care of pregnant women and their families. Efforts to reduce the incidence of preterm births must continue.

Hodnett E: Support during pregnancy for women at increased risk of low birthweight babies, *(Cochrane Review),* The Cochrane Library, Issue 3, 2000. Oxford: Update Software.

Key Points

- A high risk pregnancy is one in which the life or well-being of the mother or infant is jeopardized by a biophysical or psychosocial disorder coincidental with or unique to pregnancy.
- The pregnancy, fetus, or neonate can be placed at risk by biophysical, sociodemographic, psychosocial, and environmental factors.
- Psychosocial perinatal warning indicators include characteristics of the parents, the child, their support systems, and family circumstances.
- Maternal and perinatal mortality rates for Caucasians are considerably lower than for other ethnic groups in the United States.
- Mortality rate decreases when risks are identified early and intensive care is applied.
- Biophysical assessment techniques include fetal movement counts, ultrasonography, and MRI.
- Biochemical monitoring techniques include amniocentesis, PUBS, CVS, and MSAFP.
- Reactive NSTs and negative CSTs suggest fetal well-being.
- Most assessment tests have some degree of risk for the mother and fetus, and usually cause some anxiety for the woman and her family.

References

American Academy of Pediatrics/American College of Obstetricians and Gynecologists (AAP/ACOG): *Guidelines for perinatal care,* ed 4, Elk Grove, IL, 1997, AAP/ACOG.

Anthony A: Biologic effects and safety. In DuBose T, editor: *Fetal sonography,* Philadelphia, 1996, WB Saunders.

Centers for Disease Control and Prevention: Maternal mortality—United States, 1982-1996, *MMWR* 47:705-707, 1998.

Cunningham F et al: *Williams obstetrics,* ed 20, Stamford, CT, 1997, Appleton & Lange.

Devoe L: Nonstress and contraction stress testing. In Sciarra J, editor: *Gynecology and obstetrics vol 3: maternal and fetal medicine,* Philadelphia, 1995, JB Lippincott.

Dooley S, Freels S, Turnock B: Quality assessment of perinatal regionalization by multivariate analysis: Illlinois, 1991-1993, *Obstet Gynecol* 89(2):193-198, 1997.

Fogel C, Lewallen L: High risk childbearing. In Fogel C, Woods N, editors: *Women's health care: a comprehensive handbook,* Thousand Oaks, CA, 1995, Sage.

Gilbert E, Harmon J: *Manual of high risk pregnancy and delivery,* ed 2, St Louis, 1998, Mosby.

Glantz J, Woods J: Significance of amniotic fluid meconium. In Creasy R, Resnik R, editors: *Maternal-fetal medicine,* ed 4, Philadelphia, 1999, WB Saunders.

Guzman E et al: Longitudinal assessment of endocervical canal length between 15 and 24 weeks' gestation in women at risk for pregnancy loss or preterm birth, *Obstet Gynecol* 92:31-37, 1998.

Harmon C: Percutaneous fetal blood sampling. In Creasy R, Resnik R, editors: *Maternal-fetal medicine,* ed 4, Philadelphia, 1999, WB Saunders.

Koonin L et al: Pregnancy-related mortality surveillance—United States, 1987-1990, *MMWR* 46:17-36, 1997.

Manning F: Dynamic ultrasound-based fetal assessment: the fetal biophysical profile score, *Clin Obstet Gynecol* 38(1):26-44, 1995.

Manning F: General principles and applications of ultrasound. In Creasy R, Resnik R, editors: *Maternal-fetal medicine,* ed 4, Philadelphia, 1999a, WB Saunders.

Manning F: Fetal assessment by evaluation of biophysical variables: fetal biophysical profile score. In Creasy R, Resnik R, editors: *Maternal-fetal medicine,* ed 4, Philadelphia, 1999b, WB Saunders.

Marden D et al: A randomized controlled trial of a new fetal acoustic stimulation test for fetal well-being, *Am J Obstet Gynecol* 176(6):1386-1388, 1997.

McCarthy K, Narrigan D: Is there scientific support for the use of juice to facilitate the nonstress test? *J Obstet Gynecol Neonatal Nurs* 24(4):303-306, 1995.

Miller D: Antepartum testing, *Clin Obstet Gynecol* 41(3): 647-653, 1998.

Parer J: Fetal heart rate. In Creasy R, Resnik R, editors: *Maternal-fetal medicine,* ed 4, Philadelphia, 1999, WB Saunders.

Poutamo J et al: MRI does not change fetal cardiotocographic parameters, *Prenat Diagn* 18:1149-1154, 1998.

Ross H, Elias S: Maternal serum screening for fetal genetic disorders, *Obstet Gynecol Clin North Am* 24(1):33-47, 1997.

Scioscia A: Prenatal genetic diagnosis. In Creasy R, Resnik R, editors: *Maternal-fetal medicine,* ed 4, Philadelphia, 1999, WB Saunders.

Treanor C: Exploring nurses' roles in limited ultrasound, *AWHONN Lifelines* 2:13-14, 1998.

Tucker S: *Pocket guide to fetal monitoring and assessment,* ed 4, St Louis, 2000, Mosby.

CHAPTER 10

Anatomy and Physiology of Pregnancy

http://www.harcourthealth.com/MERLIN/Wong/maternal/

Learning Objectives

On completion of this chapter the reader will be able to:

- Explain the expected maternal anatomic and physiologic adaptation to pregnancy.
- Differentiate among presumptive, probable, and positive signs of pregnancy.
- Identify maternal hormones produced during pregnancy, their target organs, and their major effects on pregnancy.
- Compare the characteristics of the abdomen, vulva, and cervix of the nullipara and multipara.
- Determine gravidity and parity using the five- and four-digit systems.
- Describe the various types of pregnancy tests.

The goal of maternity care is a healthy pregnancy with a physically safe and emotionally satisfying outcome for mother, infant, and family. Consistent health supervision and surveillance are of utmost importance. Many maternal adaptations are unfamiliar to pregnant women and their families. Helping the pregnant woman recognize the relationship between her physical status and the plan for her care assists her in making decisions and encourages her to participate in her own care.

GRAVIDITY AND PARITY

An understanding of the following terms used to describe pregnancy and the pregnant woman is essential to the study of maternity care:

- **Gravida**—A woman who is pregnant
- **Gravidity**—Pregnancy
- **Multigravida**—A woman who has had two or more pregnancies
- **Multipara**—A woman who has completed two or more pregnancies to the stage of fetal viability
- **Nulligravida**—A woman who has never been pregnant
- **Nullipara**—A woman who has not completed a pregnancy with a fetus or fetuses who have reached the stage of viability
- **Parity**—The number of pregnancies in which the fetus or fetuses have reached viability, not the number of fetuses (e.g., twins) born. Whether the fetus is born alive or is stillborn (i.e., showing no signs of life at birth) after viability is reached does not affect parity.
- **Postdate or postterm**—Pregnancy that goes beyond 42 weeks of gestation
- **Preterm**—Born after 20 weeks of gestation but before completion of 37 weeks of gestation
- **Primigravida**—A woman who is pregnant for the first time
- **Primipara**—A woman who has completed one pregnancy with a fetus or fetuses who have reached the stage of fetal viability
- **Term**—Born between the beginning of week 38 of gestation and the end of week 42 of gestation
- **Viability**—Capacity to live outside the uterus, occurring about 22 to 24 weeks since last menstrual period or when weight of fetus is greater than 500 g

Gravidity and parity information is obtained during history-taking interviews and may be recorded in several ways in patient records. A two-digit system uses abbreviations that stand for gravity and parity. For example, the abbreviation "I/O" means that a woman is pregnant for the first time (primigravida) and has not carried a pregnancy to viability (nullipara).

Another abbreviation commonly employed in maternity centers is more detailed. It consists of five digits with hyphens for separation. The first digit represents the total number of pregnancies, including the present one (gravidity); the second digit represents the total number of full-term births; the third indicates the number of preterm births; the fourth identifies the number of abortions (miscarriage or elective termination of pregnancy before viability); and the fifth is the number of children currently living. The acronym GTPAL may be helpful in remembering this numeric abbreviation. For example, if a woman pregnant only once with twins gives birth at the thirty-fifth week and the babies survive, the abbreviation that represents this information is "1-0-1-0-2." During her next pregnancy the abbreviation is "2-0-1-0-2." Table 10-1 provides additional examples.

Others prefer a four-digit system. The first digit of the five-digit system, which signifies gravidity, is dropped.

PREGNANCY TESTS

Early detection of pregnancy allows for early initiation of care. Human chorionic gonadotropin (hCG) is the biologic marker on which pregnancy tests are based. Production of hCG begins as early as the day of implantation and can be detected in the blood as early as 6 days after conception, or about 20 days since the last menstrual period (LMP), and in urine about 26 days after conception (Cunningham et al, 1997). The level of hCG rises until it peaks at about 60 to 70 days of pregnancy and then begins to decline. The lowest level is reached between 100 to 130 days of pregnancy and remains constant until birth (Varney, 1997).

Serum and urine pregnancy tests are performed in clinics, offices, women's health centers, and laboratory settings. Both serum tests and urine tests provide accurate results. A 7 to 10 ml sample of venous blood is collected for serum testing. Most urine tests require a first-voided morning urine specimen because it contains levels of hCG approximately the same as those in serum. Random urine samples usually have lower levels. Urine tests are less expensive and provide more immediate results than serum tests (Hatcher et al, 1998).

Many different tests are available, but they all depend on recognition of hCG or a beta subunit of hCG. The wide variety of tests precludes discussion of each; however, the nurse should read the manufacturer's directions for the test to be used.

Enzyme-linked immunosorbent assays (ELISA) testing is the most popular testing procedure for pregnancy. It uses a specific monoclonal antibody (anti-hCG) with enzymes that bond with hCG in urine. Depending on the specific test, levels of hCG as low as 5 to 50 mIU/ml can be detected as early as 4 days after implantation (Hatcher et al, 1998). As an office or home procedure, it requires minimal time and offers results in 5 minutes. A positive test is indicated by a simple color change reaction.

ELISA technology is the basis for most over-the-counter home pregnancy tests. With these one-step tests, the woman usually applies urine to a strip and reads the results. The test kit comes with directions for collection of the specimen, the testing procedure, and reading of results. Most manufacturers of the kits provide a toll-free telephone number to call if users have concerns and questions about test procedures or results. The most common error in performing home pregnancy tests is doing the test too early in pregnancy (Hatcher et al, 1998).

Interpreting the results of pregnancy tests requires some judgment. The type of pregnancy test and its degree of sensitivity (i.e., the ability to detect low levels of a substance) and specificity (i.e., the ability to discern the absence of a substance) have to be considered in conjunction with the woman's history. This includes the date of the last normal menstrual period (LNMP), her usual cycle length, and results of previous pregnancy tests. It is important to know if the woman abuses substances, and also what medications she is taking. This is because medications such as anticonvulsants and tranquilizers can cause false-positive results whereas diuretics and promethazine can cause false-negative results (Pagana and Pagana, 2000). Improper collection of the specimen, hormone-producing tumors, and laboratory errors may also be responsible for inaccurate results.

Critical Thinking

OTC PREGNANCY HOME TEST KITS

In a pharmacy in your neighborhood, how many different types of OTC pregnancy home test kits are available? Read the labels on three different types of OTC pregnancy home test kits. Do the kits provide for more than one test? Are the directions printed in more than one language? After reading the directions, do you have questions about how to perform the test or how to interpret the results? If so, what does that say about the likelihood that the tests will be used correctly?

TABLE 10-1
Gravidity and Parity Using Five-Digit (GTPAL) and Two-Digit Systems

	Five-Digit System					Two-Digit System
Condition	Pregnancies (Gravidity, G)	Term Birth (T)	Preterm Birth (P)	Abortions (A)	Living Children (L)	Gravidity/ Parity
Kathy is pregnant for the first time.	1	0	0	0	0	I/O
She carries the pregnancy to term, and the neonate survives.	1	1	0	0	1	I/I
She is pregnant again.	2	1	0	0	1	II/I
Her second pregnancy ends in abortion.	2	1	0	1	1	II/I
During her third pregnancy, she gives birth to preterm twins.	3	1	1	1	3	III/II

When there is any question, further evaluation or retesting may be appropriate.

ADAPTATIONS TO PREGNANCY

Maternal physiologic adaptations are attributed to the hormones of pregnancy and to mechanical pressures arising from the enlarging uterus and other tissues. These adaptations protect the woman's normal physiologic functioning, meet the metabolic demands that pregnancy imposes on her body, and provide a nurturing environment for fetal development and growth. Although pregnancy is a normal phenomenon, problems can occur. The nurse needs a foundation in normal maternal physiology to provide optimal nursing care.

Signs of Pregnancy

Some physiologic adaptations are recognized as the signs and symptoms of pregnancy. Three commonly used categories of these signs and symptoms are: (1) presumptive, those changes felt by the woman (e.g., amenorrhea, fatigue, and breast changes); (2) probable, those changes observed by an examiner (e.g., Hegar's sign, ballottement, and pregnancy tests); and (3) positive, those signs attributed only to the presence of the fetus (e.g., hearing fetal heart tones, visualizing the fetus, and palpating fetal movements). Table 10-2 summarizes these signs of pregnancy in relation to when they might occur and gives other possible causes for their occurrence.

Reproductive System and Breasts

Uterus

Changes in Size, Shape, and Position. High levels of estrogen and progesterone stimulate phenomenal uterine growth in the first trimester. Early uterine enlargement results from increased vascularity and dilation of blood vessels, hyperplasia (i.e., production of new muscle fibers and fibroelastic tissue) and hypertrophy (i.e., enlargement of preexisting muscle fibers and fibroelastic tissue), and development of the decidua. By 7 weeks gestation the uterus is the size of a large hen's egg; by 10 weeks it is the size of an orange (twice its nonpregnant size); and by 12 weeks of gestation, it is the size of a grapefruit. After the third month, uterine enlargement is primarily the result of mechanical pressure of the growing fetus (Varney, 1997).

As the uterus enlarges, it also changes in weight, shape, and position. At conception the uterus is shaped like an upside-down pear. During the second trimester, as the muscular walls strengthen and become more elastic, the uterus becomes spherical or globular. Later, as the fetus lengthens, the uterus becomes larger and more ovoid and rises out of the pelvis into the abdominal cavity.

The pregnancy may "show" after the fourteenth week, although this depends to some degree on the woman's height and weight. Abdominal enlargement may be less apparent in the nullipara with good abdominal muscle tone (Fig. 10-1). Posture also influences the type and degree of abdominal enlargement that occurs. In normal pregnancies the uterus enlarges at a predictable rate. Uterine enlargement is determined by measuring

TABLE 10-2
Signs of Pregnancy

Time of Occurrence (Gestational Age)	Sign	Other Possible Causes
	PRESUMPTIVE	
3-4 weeks	Breast changes	Premenstrual changes, oral contraceptives
4 weeks	Amenorrhea	Stress, vigorous exercise, early menopause, endocrine problems, malnutrition
4-14 weeks	Nausea, vomiting	Gastrointestinal virus, food poisoning
6-12 weeks	Urinary frequency	Infection, pelvic tumors
12 weeks	Fatigue	Stress, illness
16-20 weeks	Quickening	Gas, peristalsis
	PROBABLE	
5 weeks	Goodell's sign	Pelvic congestion
6-8 weeks	Chadwick's sign	Pelvic congestion
6-12 weeks	Hegar's sign	Pelvic congestion
4-12 weeks	Positive pregnancy test (serum)	Hydatidiform mole, choriocarcinoma
6-12 weeks	Positive pregnancy test (urine)	Pelvic infection, tumors
16 weeks	Braxton Hicks contractions	Myomas, other tumors
16-28 weeks	Ballottement	Tumors, cervical polyps
	POSITIVE	
5-6 weeks	Visualization of fetus by ultrasound, X-ray films	No other causes
6 weeks	Fetal heart tones (FHTs) by ultrasound	
10-17 weeks	FHTs by Doppler	
17-19 weeks	FHTs by stethoscope	
19-22 weeks	Fetal movements palpated	
Late pregnancy	Visible	

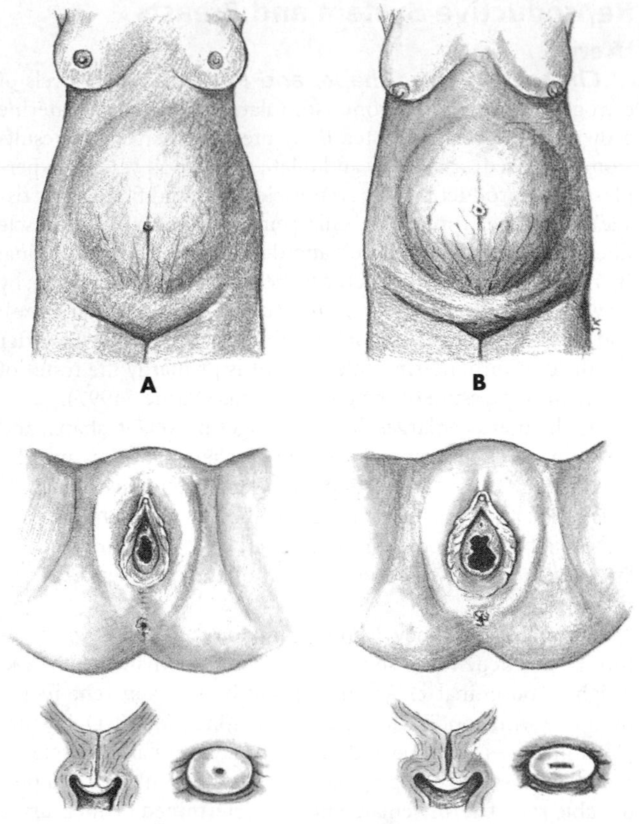

FIG. 10-1 • Comparison of abdomen, vulva, and cervix in **A,** nullipara, and **B,** multipara, at the same stage of pregnancy,

fundal height. This measurement is commonly used to estimate the duration of pregnancy. However, variation in the position of the fundus or the fetus, variations in the amount of amniotic fluid present, the presence of more than one fetus, maternal obesity, and variation in examiner technique can reduce the accuracy of this estimation of the duration of pregnancy.

As the uterus grows and fills the pelvic cavity, it is elevated out of the pelvic area. It may be palpated above the symphysis pubis some time between the twelfth and fourteenth weeks of pregnancy (see Fig. 10-2). The uterus rises gradually to the level of the umbilicus at 22 to 24 weeks gestation, and nearly reaches the xiphoid process at term. Between weeks 38 and 40, fundal height decreases as the fetus begins to descend and engage in the pelvis (lightening). Generally, lightening occurs in the nullipara about 2 weeks before the onset of labor and at the start of labor in the multipara.

Generally the uterus rotates to the right as it elevates, probably because of the presence of the rectosigmoid colon on the left side. However, the extensive hypertrophy (enlargement) of the round ligaments keeps the uterus in the midline. Eventually the growing uterus touches the anterior abdominal wall and displaces the intestines to either side of the abdomen (Fig. 10-2). When a pregnant woman stands, most of her uterus rests against the anterior abdominal wall and contributes to altering her center of gravity.

During the early weeks of pregnancy an increase in uterine blood flow and lymph causes pelvic congestion and edema. As a result, the uterus, cervix, and isthmus soften perceptibly and progressively, and the cervix takes on a bluish color (i.e., Chadwick's sign, a probable sign of pregnancy) (Creasy and Resnik, 1999).

At approximately 6 weeks gestation, softening and compressibility of the lower uterine segment (uterine isthmus) occurs (Hegar's sign). This results in exaggerated uterine anteflexion during the first 3 months of pregnancy (Fig. 10-3). In this position the uterine fundus presses on the urinary bladder, causing the woman to experience urinary frequency.

Changes in Contractility. Soon after the fourth month of pregnancy, uterine contractions can be felt through the abdominal wall. These contractions are referred to as Braxton Hicks contractions, a probable sign of pregnancy. Braxton Hicks contractions are irregular, painless contractions that occur intermittently throughout pregnancy. These contractions facilitate uterine blood flow through the intervillous spaces of the placenta and promote oxygen delivery to the fetus. Although Braxton Hicks contractions are not painful, some women do complain that they are annoying. After the twenty-eighth week, these contractions become more definite, but they usually cease with walking or exercise. Braxton Hicks contraction can be mistaken for true labor; however, they do not increase in intensity or duration or cause cervical dilation. Because the woman cannot distinguish between Braxton Hicks contractions and preterm labor, childbirth educators should either not teach about Braxton Hicks contractions or should emphasize signs of preterm labor and when to call the primary health care provider.

Uteroplacental Blood Flow. Placental perfusion depends on the maternal blood flow to the uterus. Blood flow increases rapidly as the uterus increases in size. Although uterine blood flow increases twentyfold, the fetoplacental unit grows even more rapidly. Consequently, more oxygen is extracted from the uterine blood during the latter part of pregnancy (Cunningham et al, 1997). In a normal term pregnancy, one sixth of the total maternal blood volume is within the uterine vascular system. Three factors known to decrease uterine blood flow are low mean maternal arterial pressure, contractions of the uterus, and maternal position. Estrogen stimulation may increase uterine blood flow.

Using an ultrasound device or a fetal stethoscope, the health care provider may hear the uterine souffle or bruit, a rushing or blowing sound of maternal blood flowing through uterine arteries to the placenta that is synchronous with the maternal pulse. The funic souffle, which is synchronous with the fetal heart rate and is caused by fetal blood coursing through the umbilical cord, may also be heard as well as the actual heartbeat of the fetus.

Cervical Changes. In a normal, unscarred cervix, a softening of the cervical tip may be observed about the beginning of the sixth week. This probable sign of pregnancy, Goodell's sign, is brought about by increased vascularity, slight hypertrophy, and hyperplasia (increase in number of cells). The muscle and its collagen-rich connective tissue become loose, edematous, highly elastic, and increased in volume. The glands near the external os proliferate beneath the stratified squamous epithelium, giving the cervix the velvety consistency characteristic of pregnancy. Friability is increased; that is, the cervix bleeds easily when scraped or touched. Increased friability is the cause of the few drops of blood seen after coitus with deep penetration or after vaginal examination. These few drops are usually within normal limits.

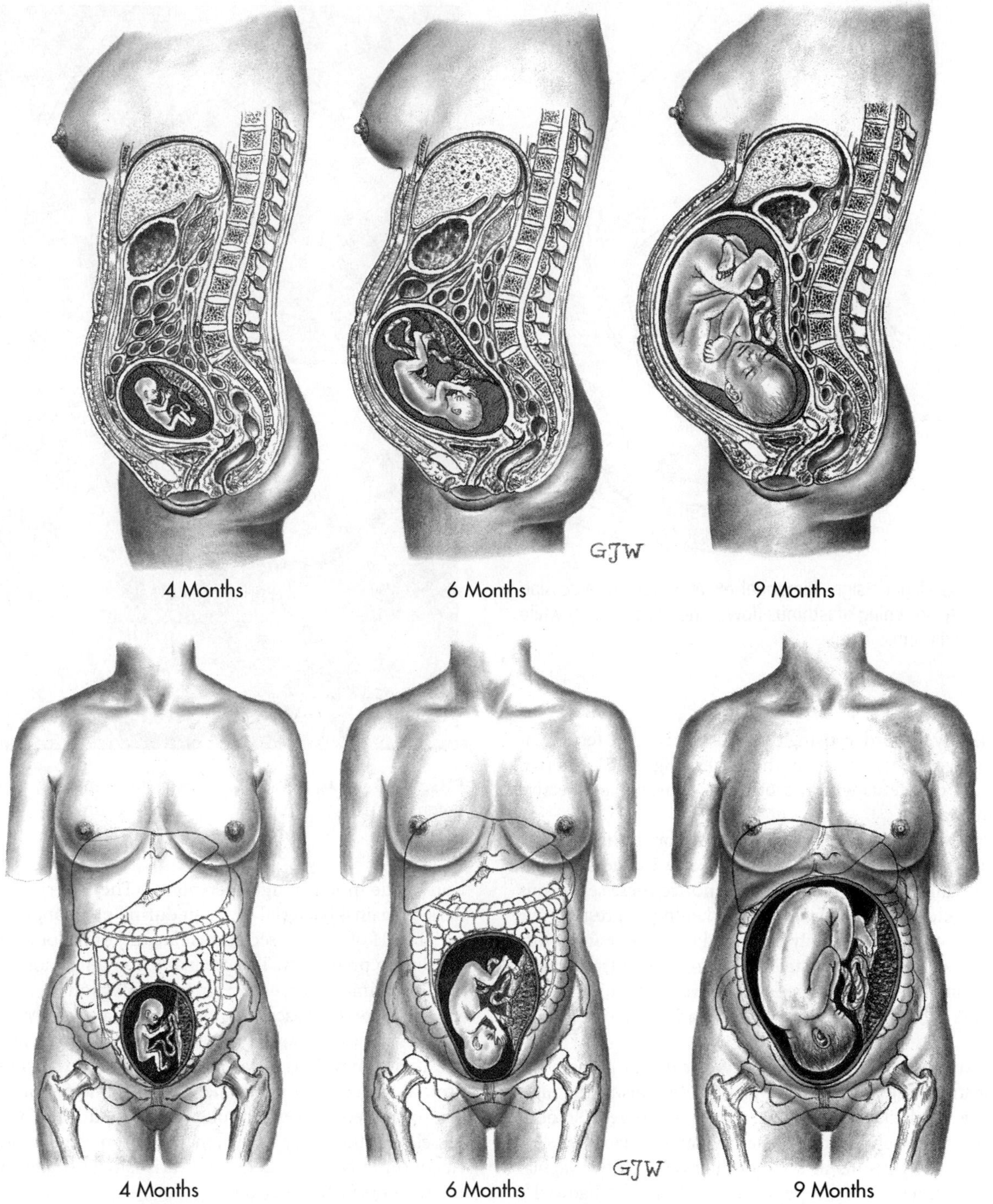

FIG. 10-2 • Displacement of internal abdominal structures and diaphragm by the enlarging uterus at 4, 6, and 9 months gestation.

Pregnancy can also cause the squamocolumnar junction (the site for obtaining cells for cervical cancer screening) to be located away from the cervix. Because of these changes, evaluation of abnormal Papanicolaou tests during pregnancy can be complicated. However, a careful assessment of all pregnant women is important because about 3% of all cervical cancers are diagnosed during pregnancy (Creasy and Resnik, 1999).

The cervix of the nullipara is rounded. Lacerations of the cervix almost always occur during the birth process. With or without lacerations, after childbirth the cervix becomes more oval in the horizontal plane, and the external os appears as a transverse slit (Fig. 10-4).

Changes Related to the Presence of the Fetus. Passive movement of the unengaged fetus is called ballottement and can be identified generally between the sixteenth and eighteenth week. Ballottement is a technique of palpating a floating structure by bouncing it gently and feeling it rebound. To palpate the fetus, the examiner places a finger within the vagina

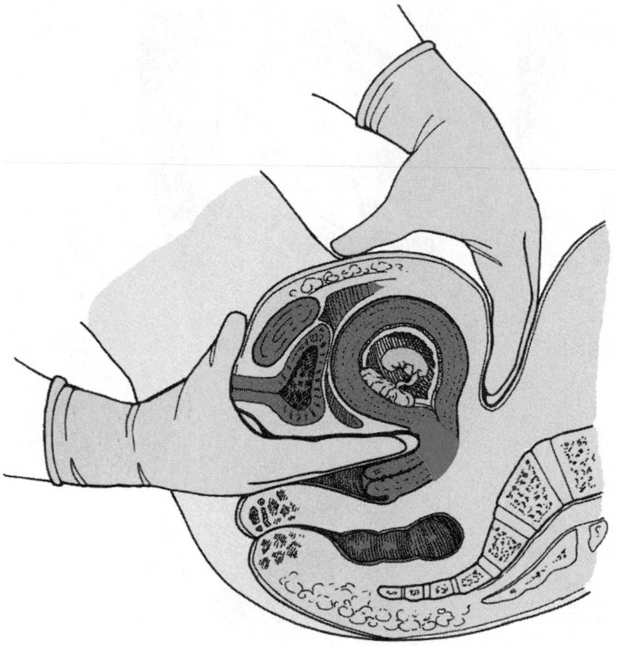

FIG. 10-3 • Hegar's sign. Bimanual examination for assessing compressibility, softening of isthmus (lower uterine segment) while the cervix is still firm.

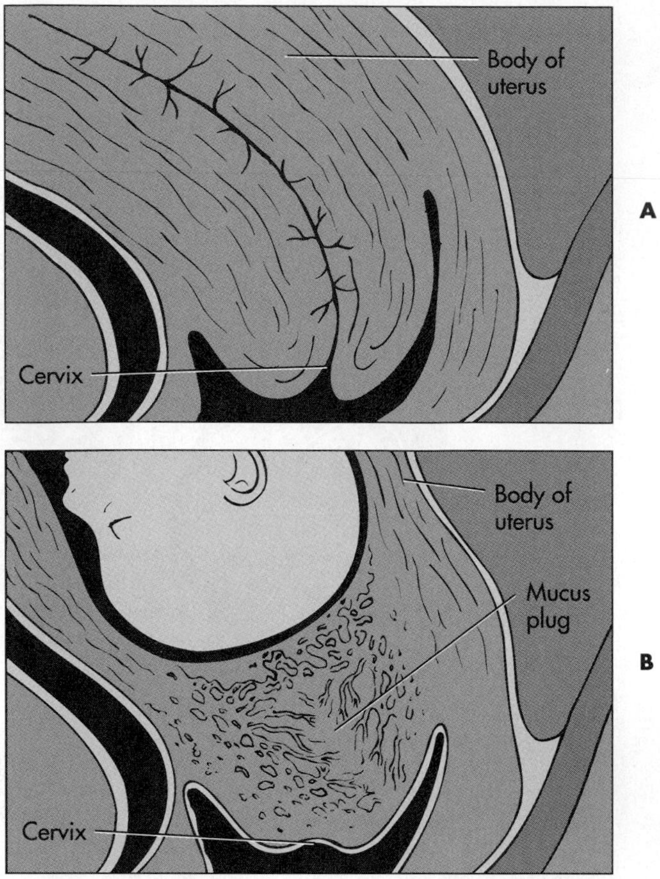

FIG. 10-4 • **A,** Cervix in nonpregnant woman. **B,** Cervix during pregnancy.

and taps gently upward, causing the fetus to rise. The fetus then sinks, and a gentle tap is felt on the finger (Fig. 10-5). Internal ballottement of a fetus within a uterus is a probable objective sign of pregnancy.

The first recognition of fetal movements, or "feeling life," by the multiparous woman may occur as early as the sixteenth week. The nulliparous woman may not notice these sensations until the eighteenth week or later. Quickening, a presumptive sign of pregnancy, is commonly described as a flutter and is difficult to distinguish from peristalsis. Fetal movements gradually increase in intensity and frequency. The week in which quickening occurs provides a tentative clue in dating the duration of gestation.

Vagina and Vulva. Pregnancy hormones prepare the vagina for stretching during labor and birth by causing the vaginal mucosa to thicken, connective tissue to loosen, smooth muscle to hypertrophy, and the vaginal vault to lengthen. Increased vascularity results in a violet-blue color of the vaginal mucosa and cervix. The deepened color, termed Chadwick's sign, may be evident as early as the sixth week but is easily noted by the eighth week of pregnancy.

Leukorrhea is a white or slightly gray mucoid discharge with a faint musty odor. This copious mucoid fluid occurs in response to cervical stimulation by estrogen and progesterone. The fluid is whitish because of the presence of many exfoliated vaginal epithelial cells caused by normal pregnancy hyperplasia. This vaginal discharge is never pruritic or blood stained. Because of the progesterone effect, ferning usually does not occur in the dried cervical mucus smear, as it would in a smear of amniotic fluid. Instead, a beaded or cellular crystallizing pattern formed in the dried mucus is seen (Cunningham et al, 1997). The mucus fills the endocervical canal, resulting in the formation of the mucus plug (operculum). The operculum acts as a barrier against bacterial invasion during pregnancy.

The pH of vaginal secretions ranges from about 4.0 to about 6.5 during pregnancy. The pregnant woman is more vulnerable to vaginal infections, especially yeast infections.

The increased vascularity of the vagina and other pelvic viscera results in a marked increase in sensitivity. The increased sensitivity may lead to a high degree of sexual interest and arousal, especially during the second trimester of pregnancy. The increased congestion, plus the relaxed walls of the blood vessels and the heavy uterus, may result in edema and varicosities of the vulva. The edema and varicosities usually resolve during the postpartum period.

External structures of the perineum are enlarged during pregnancy because of an increase in vasculature, hypertrophy of the perineal body, and deposition of fat. The labia majora of nullipara approximate and obscure the vaginal introitus; those of the parous woman separate and gape after childbirth and perineal or vaginal injury (see Fig. 10-1).

Breasts. Fullness, heightened sensitivity, tingling, and heaviness of the breasts begin as early as the sixth week of gestation in response to increased levels of estrogen and progesterone. These changes are considered presumptive signs of pregnancy because other factors can cause them to occur. Breast sensitivity varies from mild tingling to sharp pain. Nipples and areolae become more pigmented; secondary pinkish areolae de-

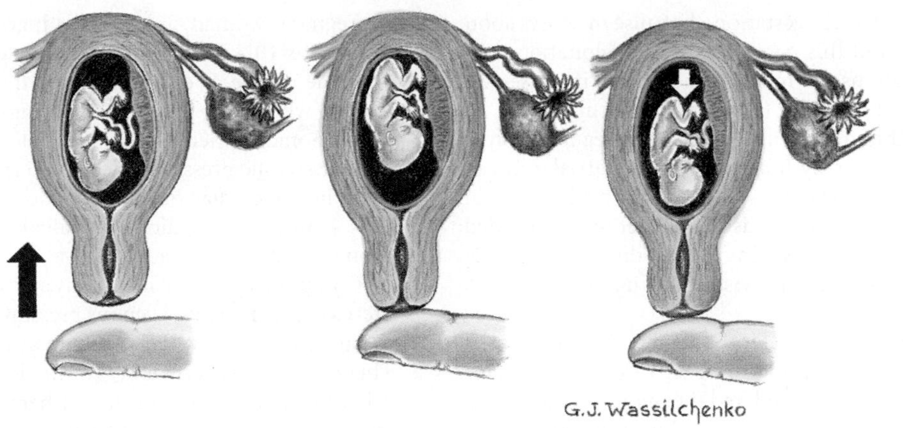

FIG. 10-5 • Internal ballottement (18 weeks).

velop, extending beyond the primary areolae; and nipples become more erectile. Hypertrophy of the sebaceous (oil) glands embedded in the primary areolae, called Montgomery tubercles, may be seen around the nipples. These sebaceous glands may have a protective role in that they keep the nipples lubricated for breastfeeding. Suppleness of the nipples is jeopardized if the protective oils are washed off with soap.

The richer blood supply causes the vessels beneath the skin to dilate. Once barely noticeable, the blood vessels become visible, often appearing in an intertwining blue network beneath the surface of the skin. Venous congestion in the breasts is more obvious in the primigravida. Striae gravidarum may appear at the outer aspects of the breasts.

During the second and third trimesters, growth of the mammary glands accounts for the progressive breast enlargement. The high levels of luteal and placental hormones in pregnancy promote proliferation of the lactiferous ducts and lobule-alveolar tissue; thus palpation of the breasts reveals a generalized, coarse nodularity. Glandular tissue displaces connective tissue, and as a result the tissue becomes softer and looser.

Although development of the mammary glands is functionally complete by midpregnancy, lactation is inhibited until a drop in estrogen level occurs after birth. A thin, clear, viscous secretory material (precolostrum) can be found in the acini cells by the third month of gestation. Colostrum, the creamy, white-to-yellowish-to-orange premilk fluid, may be expressed from the nipples as early as 16 weeks of gestation (Lawrence, 1999). See Chapter 26 for discussion of lactation.

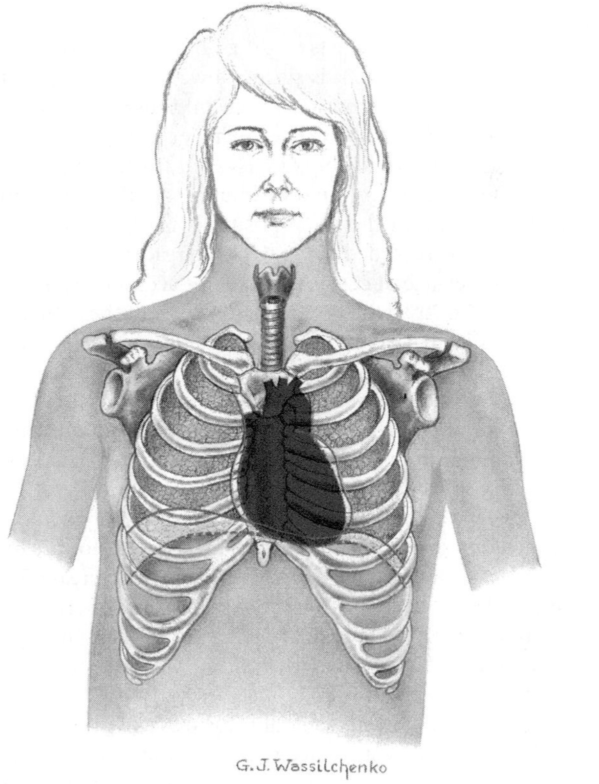

FIG. 10-6 • Changes in position of heart, lungs, and thoracic cage in pregnancy. *Broken line,* nonpregnant state; *solid line,* change that occurs in pregnancy.

General Body Systems

Cardiovascular System. Maternal adjustments to pregnancy involve extensive anatomic and physiologic changes in the cardiovascular system. Cardiovascular adaptations protect the woman's normal physiologic functioning, meet the metabolic demands pregnancy imposes on her body, and provide for fetal developmental and growth needs.

Slight cardiac hypertrophy (enlargement) is probably secondary to increased blood volume and cardiac output. The heart returns to its normal size after childbirth. As the diaphragm is displaced upward by the enlarging uterus, the heart is elevated upward and rotated forward to the left (Fig. 10-6). The apical impulse, a point of maximum intensity (PMI), is shifted upward and laterally about 1 to 1.5 cm. The degree of shift depends on the duration of pregnancy and the size and position of the uterus.

The changes in heart size and position, and increases in blood volume and cardiac output, contribute to auscultatory changes common in pregnancy. There is more audible splitting of S_1 and S_2, and S_3 may be readily heard after 20 weeks of gestation. Additionally, systolic and diastolic murmurs may be heard over the pulmonic area. These changes are transient and disappear shortly after the woman gives birth (Cunningham et al, 1997).

Between 14 and 20 weeks gestation, the pulse increases about 10 to 15 beats/min and this persists to term. Palpitations may occur. In twin gestations the maternal heart rate increases significantly in the third trimester (Cunningham et al, 1997).

The cardiac rhythm may be disturbed. The pregnant woman may experience sinus arrhythmia, premature atrial contractions, and premature ventricular systole. In the healthy woman with no underlying heart disease, no therapy is needed; however, women with preexisting heart disease will need close medical and obstetric supervision during pregnancy (see Chapter 13).

Blood Pressure. Arterial blood pressure (brachial artery) varies with age, activity level, and presence of health problems. Additional factors must be considered during pregnancy. These factors include maternal anxiety, maternal position, and type of blood pressure apparatus.

Maternal anxiety can elevate readings. If an elevated reading is found, the woman is given time to rest, and the reading is repeated.

Maternal position affects readings. Brachial blood pressure is highest when the woman is sitting; lowest when she is lying in the lateral recumbent position; and intermediate when she is supine, except for some women who experience hypotensive syndrome (see the following discussion). Therefore at each prenatal visit the reading should be obtained in the same arm and with the woman in the same position. The position and arm used should be recorded along with the reading.

The proper size of cuff is essential for accurate readings. The cuff should be 20% wider than the diameter of the patient's arm (i.e., about 12 to 14 cm for average-sized individuals and 18 to 20 cm for obese persons). A cuff that is too small yields a falsely high reading; a cuff that is too large yields a falsely low reading. Caution should be used when comparing auscultatory and oscillatory blood pressure readings because discrepancies can occur (Green and Froman, 1996).

In the first trimester, blood pressure usually remains at the prepregnancy level. During the second trimester of pregnancy, both systolic pressure and diastolic pressure decrease 5 to 10 mm Hg. This decrease is probably the result of peripheral vasodilation caused by hormonal changes during pregnancy. During the third trimester, maternal blood pressure should return to first trimester levels.

Calculating the mean arterial pressure (MAP) (mean of the blood pressure in the arterial circulation) increases the diagnostic value of the findings. Normal MAP readings in the nonpregnant woman are 86.4 mm Hg $\pm$ 7.5 mm Hg. MAP readings for a pregnant woman are slightly higher (Creasy and Resnik, 1999). Box 10-1 illustrates one way to calculate a MAP.

Box 10-1

Calculation of Mean Arterial Pressure

Blood pressure: 106/70

$$\text{Formula: } \frac{\text{Systolic} + 2(\text{Diastolic})}{3}$$

$$\frac{106 + 2\,(70)}{3}$$

$$\frac{106 + 140}{3}$$

246/3 = 82 mm Hg

Some degree of compression of the vena cava occurs in all women who lie on their backs during the second half of pregnancy. Some women experience a fall of more than 30 mm Hg in their systolic pressure. After 4 to 5 minutes a reflex bradycardia is noted, cardiac output is reduced by half, and the woman feels faint. This condition is called supine hypotensive syndrome (Cunningham et al, 1997).

Compression of the iliac veins and inferior vena cava by the uterus causes increased venous pressure and reduced blood flow in the legs, except when the woman is in the lateral position. These alterations contribute to the dependent edema, varicose veins in the legs and vulva, and hemorrhoids experienced by women in the latter part of term pregnancy (Fig. 10-7).

Blood Volume and Composition. The degree of blood volume expansion varies considerably. Blood volume increases by approximately 1500 ml, or 40% to 50% above nonpregnancy levels (Cunningham et al, 1997). This increase consists of 1000 ml of plasma plus 450 ml of red blood cells (RBCs). The increase in volume starts at weeks 10 to 12, peaks at weeks 32 to 34, and decreases slightly at week 40. The volume in a multiple gestation increases above that for a single pregnancy (Creasy and Resnik, 1999). Increased blood volume is a protective mechanism. It is essential for meeting the blood needs of the hypertrophied vascular system of the enlarged uterus, for adequately hydrating fetal and maternal tissues when the woman assumes an erect or supine position, and for providing a fluid reserve to compensate for blood loss during birth and the puerperium. Peripheral vasodilation maintains a normal blood pressure despite the increased blood volume in pregnancy.

During pregnancy there is an accelerated production of RBCs (the normal RBC count is 4.2 to 5.4 million/mm^3). The

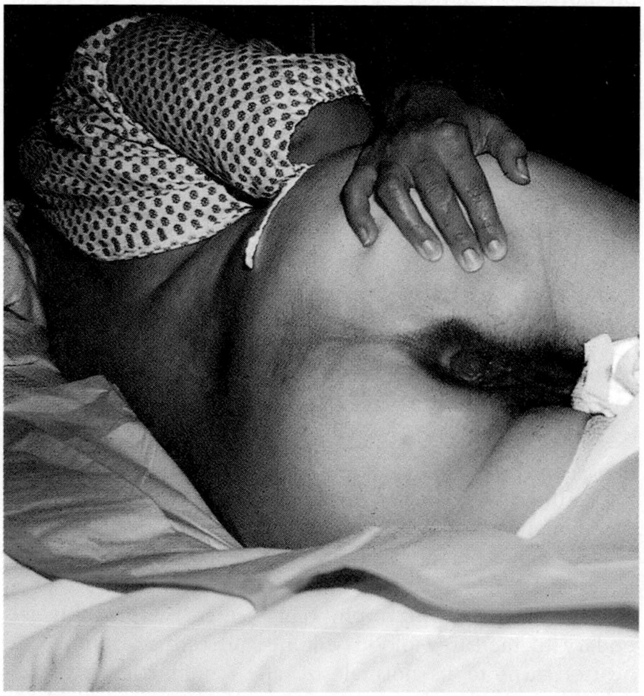

FIG. 10-7 • Hemorrhoids. (Courtesy Marjorie Pyle, RNC, Lifecircle, Costa Mesa, CA.)

percentage of this increase depends on the amount of iron available, but the RBC mass increases by about 17% (Creasy and Resnik, 1999).

Because the plasma increase is greater than the increase in RBC production, there is a decrease in normal hemoglobin values (to 12 to 16 g/dl blood) and hematocrit values (to 37% to 47%). This state of hemodilution is referred to as physiologic anemia. The decrease is more noticeable during the second trimester, when rapid expansion of blood volume occurs faster than RBC production. If the hemoglobin value drops to 10 g/dl or less, or if the hematocrit drops to 35% or less, the woman is considered anemic.

The total white blood cell (WBC) count increases during the second trimester and peaks during the third trimester. This increase is primarily in the granulocytes; the lymphocyte count stays about the same throughout pregnancy.

Cardiac Output. Cardiac output has increased 30% to 50% by week 32 of pregnancy; this declines to about a 20% increase at 40 weeks gestation. This elevated cardiac output is largely a result of increased stroke volume and heart rate and occurs in response to increased tissue demands for oxygen (Creasy and Resnik, 1999).

Cardiac output in late pregnancy is appreciably higher when the woman is in the lateral recumbent position than when she is supine. In the supine position the large, heavy uterus often impedes venous return to the heart and affects blood pressure. Cardiac output increases with any exertion, such as labor and birth. Box 10-2 summarizes cardiovascular changes in pregnancy.

Circulation and Coagulation Times. The circulation time decreases slightly by week 32. It returns to near normal at term. There is a greater tendency for blood to coagulate (clot) during pregnancy because of increases in various clotting factors (i.e., factors VII, VIII, IX, X, and fibrinogen). This, combined with the fact that fibrinolytic activity (the splitting up or dissolving of a clot) is depressed during pregnancy and the postpartum period, provides a protective function to decrease the chance of bleeding but also makes the woman more vulnerable to thrombosis, especially after cesarean birth.

Respiratory System. Structural and ventilatory adaptations occur during pregnancy to provide for both maternal and fetal needs. Maternal oxygen requirements increase in response to the acceleration in metabolic rate and the need to add to the tissue mass in the uterus and breasts. In addition, the fetus requires oxygen and a way to eliminate carbon dioxide.

Elevated levels of estrogen cause the ligaments of the rib cage to relax, permitting increased chest expansion (see Fig. 10-6). The transverse diameter of the thoracic cage increases by about 2 cm and the circumference by 6 cm (Cunningham et al, 1997). The costal angle increases and the lower rib cage appears to flare out. The chest may not return to its prepregnant state after birth (Seidel et al, 1999).

The diaphragm is displaced by as much as 4 cm during pregnancy. With advancing pregnancy, chest breathing replaces abdominal breathing, and descent of the diaphragm with inspiration becomes less possible. Thoracic breathing is primarily accomplished by the diaphragm rather than by the costal muscles.

The upper respiratory tract becomes more vascular in response to elevated levels of estrogen. As the capillaries become engorged, edema and hyperemia develop within the nose, pharynx, larynx, trachea, and bronchi. This congestion within the tissues of the respiratory tract gives rise to several conditions commonly seen during pregnancy, including nasal and sinus stuffiness, epistaxis (nosebleed), changes in the voice, and marked inflammatory response to even a mild upper respiratory infection.

Increased vascularity of the upper respiratory tract also can cause the tympanic membranes and eustachian tubes to swell, giving rise to symptoms of impaired hearing, earaches, or a sense of fullness in the ears.

Pulmonary Function. The pregnant woman breathes deeper, increasing her tidal volume (i.e., the volume of gas moved into or out of the respiratory tract with each breath). The respiratory rate remains unchanged or is only slightly increased (by about two breaths per minute). The expiratory reserve volume and residual volume decrease progressively during pregnancy. The inspiratory capacity increases slightly, whereas the vital capacity remains unchanged. The total lung capacity decreases slightly. These changes are related to the elevation of the diaphragm and chest wall changes (Creasy and Resnik, 1999). Box 10-3 lists respiratory changes in pregnancy.

During pregnancy, changes in the respiratory center result in a lowered threshold for carbon dioxide. Progesterone and estrogen are presumed to be responsible for the increased sensitivity of the respiratory center to carbon dioxide. In addition, pregnant women experience increased awareness of the need to breathe; some may complain of dyspnea at rest.

Although pulmonary function is not impaired by pregnancy, diseases of the respiratory tract may be more serious during this time (Cunningham et al, 1997). One important factor responsible for this may be the increase in oxygen requirements.

Box 10-2

Cardiovascular Changes in Pregnancy

Heart rate	Increases 10-15 beats/min
Blood pressure	Remains at prepregnancy levels in first trimester Slight decrease in second trimester Returns to prepregnancy levels in third trimester
Blood volume	Increased by 1500 ml or 40%-50% above prepregnancy level
Red blood cell mass	Increases 17%
Hemoglobin	Decreases
Hematocrit	Decreases
White blood cell count	Increases in second and third trimester
Cardiac output	Increases 30%-50%

Box 10-3

Respiratory Changes in Pregnancy

Respiratory rate	Unchanged or slightly increased
Tidal volume	Increased 30%-40%
Vital capacity	Unchanged
Inspiratory capacity	Increased
Expiratory volume	Decreased
Total lung capacity	Unchanged to slightly decreased
Oxygen consumption	Increased 15%-20%

Basal Metabolic Rate. The basal metabolic rate (BMR) varies considerably in women at the beginning and during pregnancy; it usually increases 15% to 20% by term (Worthington-Roberts and Williams, 1997). The BMR returns to nonpregnant levels by 5 to 6 days postpartum. The elevation in BMR reflects increased oxygen demands of the uterine-placental-fetal unit and greater oxygen consumption because of increased maternal cardiac work (Chamberlain and Pipkin, 1998). Peripheral vasodilation and acceleration of sweat gland activity help dissipate the excess heat resulting from the increased BMR during pregnancy. Pregnant women may experience heat intolerance. Lassitude and fatigability after only slight exertion are experienced by many women in early pregnancy. These feelings, along with a greater need for sleep, may persist and may be caused in part by the increased metabolic activity.

Acid-Base Balance. Progesterone may be responsible for increasing the sensitivity of the respiratory center receptors, so that tidal volume is increased and Pco_2 falls, the base excess (HCO_3, or bicarbonate) falls, and pH rises slightly. These alterations in acid-base balance indicate that pregnancy is a state of respiratory alkalosis compensated by mild metabolic acidosis (Chamberlain and Pipkin, 1998). These changes also facilitate the transport of CO_2 from the fetus and O_2 release from the mother to the fetus. Box 10-4 lists acid-base values during pregnancy.

Renal System. The kidneys are responsible for maintaining electrolyte and acid-base balance, regulating extracellular fluid volume, excreting waste products, and conserving essential nutrients.

Anatomic Changes. Changes in renal structure result from hormonal activity (i.e., estrogen and progesterone), pressure from an enlarging uterus, and an increase in blood volume. As early as the tenth week of pregnancy, the renal pelves and the ureters dilate. Dilation of the ureters is more pronounced above the pelvic brim, in part because they are compressed between the uterus and the pelvic brim. In most women the ureters below the pelvic brim are of normal size. The smooth-muscle walls of the ureters undergo hyperplasia and hypertrophy and muscle tone relaxation. The ureters elongate, become tortuous, and form single or double curves. In the latter part of pregnancy the renal pelvis and ureter dilate more on the right side than on the left because the heavy uterus is displaced to the right by the sigmoid colon.

Because of these changes, a larger volume of urine is held in the pelves and ureters, and urine flow rate is slowed. Urinary stasis or stagnation has several consequences, including the following:

- There is a lag between the time urine is formed and when it reaches the bladder. Therefore clearance test results may reflect substances contained in glomerular filtrate several hours before.
- Stagnated urine is an excellent medium for the growth of microorganisms. In addition, the urine of pregnant women contains greater amounts of nutrients, including glucose, that increase the pH (i.e., make the urine more alkaline). Pregnant women are therefore more susceptible to urinary tract infection.

Bladder irritability, nocturia, and urinary frequency and urgency (without dysuria) are commonly reported in early pregnancy. These bladder symptoms may return near term, especially after lightening occurs. Urinary frequency results initially from increased bladder sensitivity and later from compression of the bladder. In the second trimester the bladder is pulled up out of the true pelvis into the abdomen. The urethra lengthens to 7.5 cm as the bladder is displaced upward. The pelvic congestion that occurs in pregnancy is reflected in hyperemia of the bladder and urethra. This increased vascularity causes the bladder mucosa to be traumatized and bleed easily. Bladder tone may decrease, which increases the bladder capacity to 1500 ml. At the same time, the bladder is compressed by the enlarging uterus, resulting in the urge to void even if the bladder contains only a small amount of urine.

Functional Changes. In normal pregnancy, renal function is altered considerably. Glomerular filtration rate (GFR) and renal plasma flow (RPF) increase early in pregnancy (Cunningham et al, 1997). These changes are caused by pregnancy hormones, an increase in blood volume, the woman's posture, physical activity, and nutritional intake. The woman's kidneys must manage the increased metabolic and circulatory demands of the maternal body and also the excretion of fetal waste products.

Renal function is most efficient when the woman lies in the lateral recumbent position and least efficient when the woman assumes a supine position. A side-lying position increases renal perfusion, which increases urine output and decreases edema. When the pregnant woman is lying supine, the heavy uterus compresses the vena cava and the aorta, and cardiac output decreases. As a result, blood flow to the brain and heart is continued at the expense of other organs, including the kidneys and uterus.

Fluid and Electrolyte Balance. Selective renal tubular reabsorption maintains sodium and water balance regardless of changes in dietary intake and losses through sweat, vomitus, or diarrhea. From 500 to 900 mEq of sodium is normally retained during pregnancy to meet fetal needs. To prevent excessive sodium depletion, the maternal kidneys undergo a significant adaptation by increasing tubular reabsorption. Because of the need for increased maternal intravascular and extracellular fluid volume, additional sodium is needed to expand fluid volume and to maintain an isotonic state. As efficient as the renal system is, it can be overstressed by excessive dietary sodium intake or restriction or by use of diuretics. Severe hypovolemia and reduced placental perfusion are two consequences of using diuretics during pregnancy.

The capacity of the kidneys to excrete water is more efficient during the early weeks than later in pregnancy. As a result, some women feel thirsty in early pregnancy because of the greater amount of water loss. The pooling of fluid in the legs in the latter part of pregnancy decreases renal blood flow and GFR. This pooling is sometimes referred to as physiologic or dependent

Box 10-4

Acid-Base Values in Arterial Blood of Pregnant Women

Po_2	104-108 mm Hg (increased)
Pco_2	27-32 mm Hg (decreased)
Sodium bicarbonate (HCO_3)	18-31 mEq/L (decreased)
Blood pH	7.40-7.45 (slightly increased—more alkaline)

From Gabbe S, Niebyl J, Simpson J: *Obstetrics: normal and problem pregnancies,* ed 3, New York, 1996, Churchill Livingstone.

edema, and requires no treatment. The normal diuretic response to the water load is triggered when the woman lies down, preferably on her side, and the pooled fluid reenters general circulation.

Normally the kidney reabsorbs almost all the glucose and other nutrients from the plasma filtrate. In pregnant women, however, tubular reabsorption of glucose is impaired so that glucosuria occurs at varying times and to varying degrees. Although glucosuria may be found in normal pregnancies (1+ levels may be seen with increased anxiety states), the possibility of diabetes mellitus and gestational diabetes must be kept in mind.

Proteinuria does not usually occur in normal pregnancy except during labor or after birth (Cunningham et al, 1997). However, the increased amounts of amino acids that need to be filtered may exceed the capacity of the renal tubules to absorb them, and small amounts of protein may be lost in the urine. Values of trace to 1+ protein (by dipstick assessment), or less than 300 mg/24 hr, are acceptable during pregnancy. However, a pregnant woman with hypertension and proteinuria must be carefully evaluated because she may be at greater risk for an adverse pregnancy outcome. Box 10-5 lists renal changes during pregnancy.

Integumentary System. Alterations in hormonal balance and mechanical stretching are responsible for several changes in the integumentary system during pregnancy. General changes include increases in skin thickness and subdermal fat, hyperpigmentation, increased hair and nail growth, accelerated sweat and sebaceous gland activity, and increased circulation and vasomotor activity. Cutaneous elastic tissues are more fragile, resulting in striae gravidarum (or "stretch marks"). Cutaneous allergic responses are enhanced.

Hyperpigmentation is stimulated by the anterior pituitary hormone melanotropin, which is increased during pregnancy. Darkening of the nipples, areolae, axillae, and vulva occurs about the sixteenth week of gestation. Facial melasma (also called chloasma or mask of pregnancy) is a blotchy, brownish hyperpigmentation of the skin over the cheeks, nose, and forehead, especially in dark-complected pregnant women. Chloasma appears in 50% to 70% of pregnant women, beginning after the sixteenth week and increasing gradually until term. The sun intensifies this pigmentation in susceptible women. Chloasma caused by normal pregnancy usually fades after delivery.

The linea nigra (Fig. 10-8) is a pigmented line extending from the symphysis pubis to the top of the fundus in the midline. This line is known as the linea alba before hormone-induced pigmentation. In primigravidas the extension of the linea nigra, beginning in the third month, keeps pace with the rising height of the fundus; in multigravidas the entire line often appears earlier than the third month. Not all pregnant women develop lineae nigra.

Striae gravidarum (Fig. 10-9) appear over the lower abdomen in 50% to 90% of pregnant women during the second half of pregnancy. These may be caused by the action of adrenocorticosteroids. Striae reflect separation within the underlying connective (collagen) tissue of the skin. These slightly depressed streaks tend to occur over areas of maximum stretch (i.e., the abdomen, thighs, and breasts). The stretching sometimes causes a sensation that resembles itching. The tendency to develop striae may be familial. After birth they usually fade, although they never disappear completely. Color of striae varies depending on the pregnant woman's skin color. The striae appear pinkish on a woman with light skin and are lighter than the surrounding skin in dark-skinned women. In the multipara, in addition to the striae of the present pregnancy, glistening silvery lines (in light-skinned women) or purplish lines (in dark-skinned women) are commonly seen. These represent the scars of striae from previous pregnancies.

Box 10-5
Renal Changes in Pregnancy

Bladder capacity	Increased
Glomerular filtration rate (GFR)	Increased 30%-50%
Renal plasma flow (RPF)	Increased 30%
Blood urea nitrogen (BUN)	Decreased
Creatinine	Decreased
Glucose (in urine)	Present in 20% of pregnant women

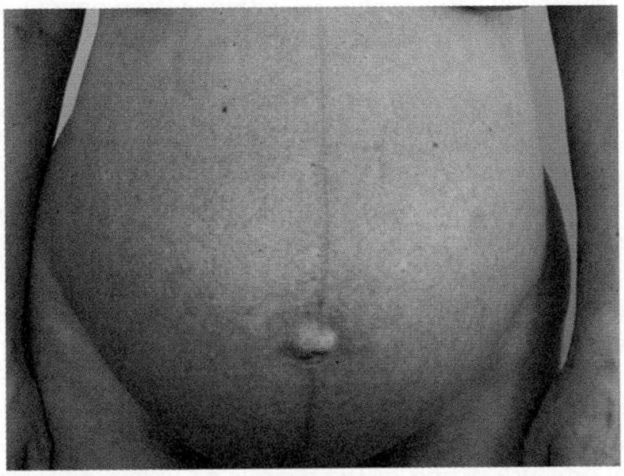

FIG. 10-8 • Linea nigra. (From Seidel H et al: *Mosby's guide to physical examination,* ed 4, St Louis, 1999, Mosby.)

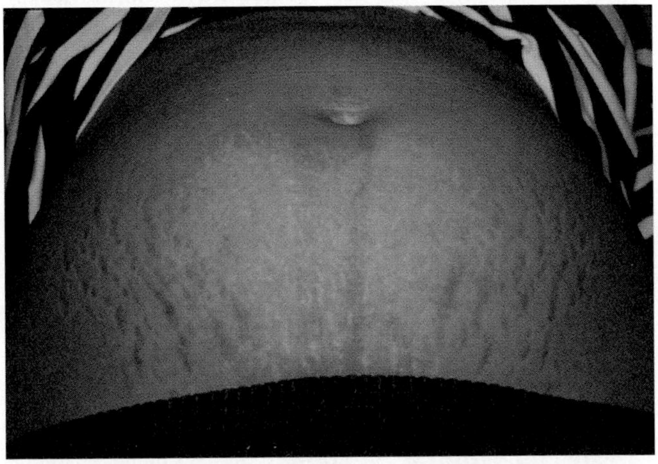

FIG. 10-9 • Striae gravidarum, or "stretch marks." (Courtesy Michael S. Clement, MD, Mesa, AZ.)

Critical Thinking

AWARENESS OF PHYSIOLOGIC CHANGES OF PREGNANCY

Interview two pregnant women, one who is pregnant with her first baby and one who is pregnant for the second or third time. Select five physiologic changes of pregnancy (e.g., ptyalism, striae gravidarum, morning sickness, heart rate, relaxation of smooth muscle leading to heartburn or constipation). Have the women been aware of these changes? When in their pregnancy did they occur? Has their health care provider informed them of changes to expect during pregnancy? What "old wives' tales" have they heard in relation to those changes? What patient teaching is appropriate for these women? Share these findings in your clinical group and compare them with the findings of your classmates.

Box 10-6

Ethnic Considerations for Skin Assessment During Pregnancy

Integumentary system changes vary greatly among women of different racial backgrounds. For example, vascular spiders and palmar erythema are seen more often in Caucasian women than in African-American women. Areolar pigmentation varies by race: African-American women have the darkest areolae, Caucasian women have the lightest, and Asian women and Native American women have intermediate pigmentation. When performing physical assessments, the color of the woman's skin should be noted along with any changes that may be attributed to pregnancy.

Angiomas are commonly referred to as vascular spiders. These tiny, star-shaped or branched, slightly raised, and pulsating end-arterioles are usually found on the neck, thorax, face, and arms. They occur as a result of elevated levels of circulating estrogens. The spiders are bluish in color and do not blanch with pressure. Vascular spiders appear during the second to fifth month of pregnancy in 65% of Caucasian women and 10% of African-American women. The spiders usually disappear after birth.

Pinkish red, diffusely mottled or well-defined blotches are seen over the palmar surfaces of the hands in about 60% of Caucasian women and 35% of African-American women during pregnancy (Cunningham et al, 1997). These color changes, called palmar erythema, are related primarily to increased estrogen levels. Box 10-6 lists ethnic considerations for skin assessment during pregnancy.

Pruritus is a relatively common dermatologic symptom in pregnancy, with cholestasis of pregnancy being the most common cause of pruritic rash. The goal of management is to relieve the itching. Topical steroids are the usual treatment, although systemic steroids may be needed. The problem usually resolves in the postpartum period.

Gum hypertrophy may occur. An epulis (gingival granuloma gravidarum) is a red, raised nodule on the gums that bleeds easily. This lesion may develop around the third month and usually continues to enlarge as pregnancy progresses. It is usually controlled by avoiding trauma to the gums (e.g., using a soft toothbrush). An epulis usually regresses spontaneously after birth.

Nail growth may be accelerated. Some women may notice thinning and softening of the nails. Oily skin and acne vulgaris may occur during pregnancy. For other women the skin clears and looks radiant. Hirsutism, the excessive growth of hair or growth of hair in unusual places, is commonly reported. An increase in fine hair growth may occur but tends to disappear after pregnancy. However, growth of coarse or bristly hair does not usually disappear after pregnancy.

Increased blood supply to the skin leads to increased perspiration. Women feel hotter during pregnancy, possibly related to a progesterone-induced increase in body temperature and the increased BMR.

Musculoskeletal System. The gradually changing body and increasing weight of the pregnant woman usually cause noticeable alterations in her posture (Fig. 10-10) and in the way she walks. The great abdominal distention gives the pelvis a forward tilt, decreased abdominal muscle tone, and increased weight bearing. The woman's center of gravity shifts forward, requiring a realignment of the spinal curvatures. An increase in the normal lumbosacral curve (lordosis) develops, and a compensatory curvature in the cervicodorsal region (i.e., exaggerated anterior flexion of the head) develops to help her maintain balance. Aching, numbness, and weakness of the upper extremities may result. Large breasts and a stoop-shouldered stance will further accentuate the lumbar and dorsal curves. Walking is more difficult, and the waddling gait of the pregnant woman, called "the proud walk of pregnancy" by Shakespeare, is well known. The ligamentous and muscular structures of the middle and lower spine may be severely stressed. These and related changes often cause musculoskeletal discomfort.

The young, well-muscled woman may tolerate these changes without complaint. However, older women or those with a back disorder or a faulty sense of balance may have a considerable amount of back pain during and just after pregnancy.

Slight relaxation and increased mobility of the pelvic joints is normal during pregnancy. This is secondary to the exaggerated elasticity and softening of connective and collagen tissue caused by increased circulating steroid sex hormones, especially estrogen. Relaxin, an ovarian hormone, assists in this relaxation and softening. These adaptations permit enlargement of pelvic dimensions to facilitate labor and birth. The degree of relaxation varies, but considerable separation of the symphysis pubis and the instability of the sacroiliac joints may cause pain and difficulty in walking. Obesity or multifetal pregnancy tend to increase the pelvic instability. Peripheral joint laxity also increases as pregnancy progresses, but the cause is not known (Schauberger et al, 1996).

The muscles of the abdominal wall stretch and ultimately lose some tone. During the third trimester the rectus abdominis muscles may separate (Fig. 10-11), allowing abdominal contents to protrude at the midline. The umbilicus flattens or protrudes. After birth the muscles gradually regain tone. However, separation of the muscles (diastasis recti abdominis) may persist.

Neurologic System. Little is known regarding specific alterations in function of the neurologic system during pregnancy, aside from hypothalamic-pituitary neurohormonal changes. Specific physiologic alterations resulting from preg-

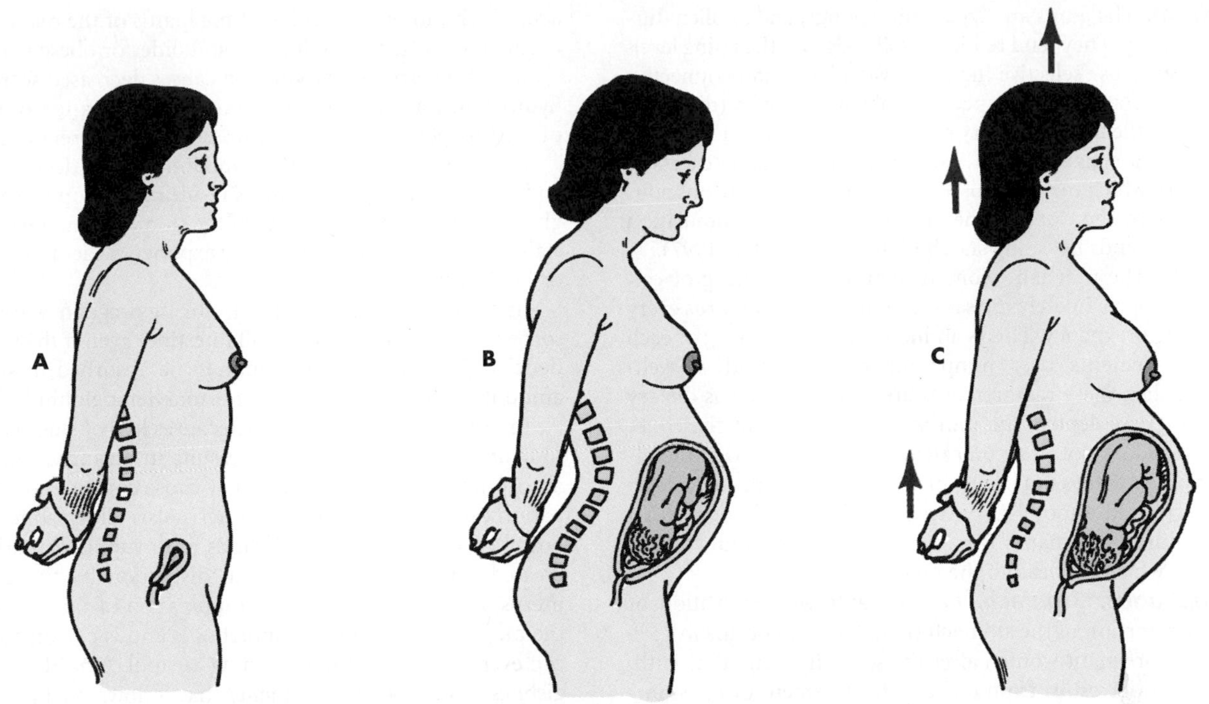

FIG. 10-10 • Postural changes during pregnancy. **A,** Nonpregnant. **B,** Incorrect posture. **C,** Correct posture.

nancy may cause the following neurologic or neuromuscular symptoms:

- Compression of pelvic nerves or vascular stasis caused by enlargement of the uterus may result in sensory changes in the legs.
- Dorsolumbar lordosis may cause pain because of traction on nerves or compression of nerve roots.
- Edema involving the peripheral nerves may result in carpal tunnel syndrome during the last trimester. The edema compresses the median nerve beneath the carpal ligament of the wrist. The syndrome is characterized by paresthesia (i.e., an abnormal sensation such as burning or tingling caused by a disorder of the sensory nervous system) and pain in the hand, radiating to the elbow. The dominant hand is usually affected most, although as many as 80% of women report symptoms in both hands. Symptoms usually regress after pregnancy. Some patients may require surgical treatment (Cunningham et al, 1997).
- Acroesthesia (numbness and tingling of the hands) is caused by the stoop-shouldered stance (Fig. 10-10, *B*) assumed by some women during pregnancy. The condition is associated with traction on segments of the brachial plexus.
- Tension headache is common when anxiety or uncertainty complicates gestation. However, vision problems such as refractive errors, sinusitis, or migraine may also be responsible for headaches.
- "Lightheadedness," faintness, and even syncope (fainting) are common during early pregnancy. Vasomotor instability, postural hypotension, or hypoglycemia may be responsible.
- Hypocalcemia may cause neuromuscular problems such as muscle cramps or tetany.

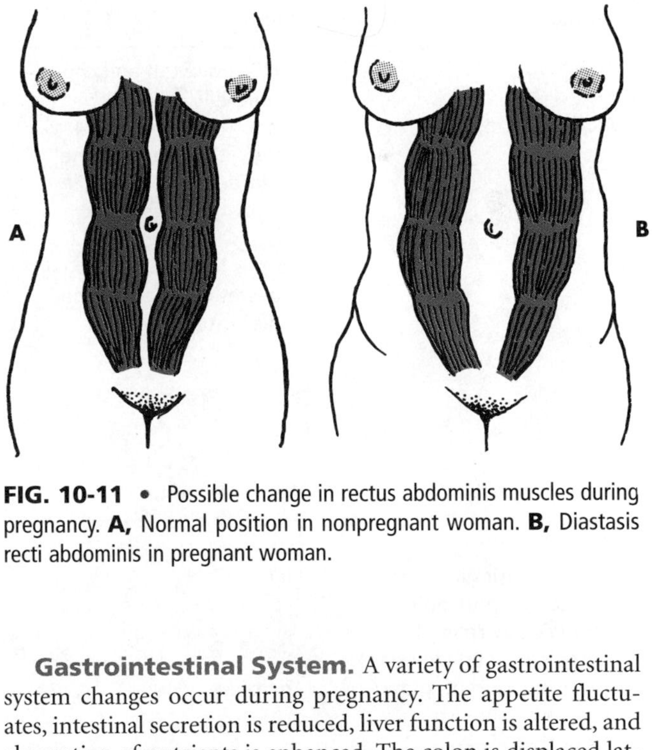

FIG. 10-11 • Possible change in rectus abdominis muscles during pregnancy. **A,** Normal position in nonpregnant woman. **B,** Diastasis recti abdominis in pregnant woman.

Gastrointestinal System. A variety of gastrointestinal system changes occur during pregnancy. The appetite fluctuates, intestinal secretion is reduced, liver function is altered, and absorption of nutrients is enhanced. The colon is displaced laterally upward and posteriorly. Peristaltic activity (motility) decreases. As a result, bowel sounds are diminished and constipation, nausea, and vomiting are common. Blood flow to the pelvis increases, as does venous pressure, contributing to hemorrhoid formation in later pregnancy. (For further discussion of nutrition in pregnancy, see Chapter 12.)

Mouth. The gums are hyperemic, spongy, and swollen during pregnancy. They tend to bleed easily because the rising levels of estrogen cause selective increased vascularity and connective tissue proliferation (a nonspecific gingivitis). Epulis (discussed earlier with the integumentary system) may develop at the gumline. Some pregnant women complain of ptyalism (excessive salivation), which may be caused by the decrease in unconscious swallowing by the woman when nauseated or from stimulation of salivary glands by eating starch (Cunningham et al, 1997).

Teeth. The pregnant woman requires about 1.2 g of calcium and approximately the same amount of phosphorus every day during pregnancy. This is an increase of about 0.4 g of each of these elements over nonpregnant needs. With a well-balanced diet, these requirements are satisfied. Serious dietary deficiency may deplete the mother's bony stores of these elements, but does not draw on calcium in her teeth. Demineralization of teeth does not occur during pregnancy; the old adage, "for every child a tooth" is untrue. Gingivitis and poor dental hygiene during pregnancy (or anytime) may contribute to dental caries, which can lead to the loss of a tooth.

Esophagus, Stomach, and Intestines. Herniation of the upper portion of the stomach (hiatal hernia) occurs in 15% to 20% of pregnant women after the seventh or eighth month. This condition results from upward displacement of the stomach, which causes a widening of the hiatus of the diaphragm. It occurs more often in multiparas and older or obese women.

Increased estrogen production causes decreased secretion of hydrochloric acid. Therefore peptic ulcer formation or flare-up of existing peptic ulcers is uncommon during pregnancy.

Increased progesterone production causes decreased tone and motility of smooth muscles resulting in esophageal regurgitation, slower emptying time of the stomach, and reverse peristalsis. As a result, the woman may experience "acid indigestion" or heartburn (pyrosis).

In response to increased needs during pregnancy, iron is absorbed more readily in the small intestine. Even if the woman is deficient in iron, it will continue to be absorbed in sufficient amounts for the fetus to have a normal hemoglobin level.

Increased progesterone (which causes loss of smooth muscle tone and decreased peristalsis) results in an increase in water absorption from the colon and may cause constipation. Constipation can also result from hypoperistalsis (sluggishness of the bowel), food choices, lack of fluids, iron supplementation, decreased activity level, abdominal distention by the pregnant uterus, and displacement and compression of the intestines. If the pregnant woman has hemorrhoids and is constipated, they can evert or bleed during straining at stool. A mild ileus (sluggishness and lack of movement) that follows birth, as well as

TABLE 10-3

Hormones and Effects of Changes During Pregnancy

Hormone	Source	Effects of Changes During Pregnancy
hCG	Fertilized ovum and chorionic villi	Maintains corpus luteum's production of estrogen and progesterone until placenta takes over the function
Progesterone	Corpus luteum until 14 wks gestation, then by the placenta	Suppresses secretion of FSH and LH by the anterior pituitary; maintains pregnancy by relaxing smooth muscles decreasing uterine contractility; causes fat to deposit in subcutaneous tissues over the maternal abdomen, back, and upper thighs; decreases mother's ability to use insulin
Estrogen	Corpus luteum until 14 wks gestation, then by the placenta	Suppresses secretion of FSH and LH by the anterior pituitary; causes fat to deposit in subcutaneous tissues over the maternal abdomen, back, and upper thighs; promotes enlargement of genitals, uterus, and breasts; increased vascularity; relaxes pelvic ligaments and joints, interferes with folic acid metabolism, increases the level of total body proteins, promotes retention of sodium and water; decreases secretion of hydrochloric acid and pepsin; decreases mother's ability to use insulin
Serum prolactin	Anterior pituitary	Responsible for initial lactation
Oxytocin	Posterior pituitary	Stimulates uterine contractions; stimulates the let-down or milk-ejection reflex
Human chorionic somatomammotropin (previously called human placental lactogen)	Placenta	Acts as a growth hormone; contributes to breast development; decreases maternal metabolism of glucose; increases the amount of fatty acids for metabolic needs
Thyroxine-binding globulin, thyroxine, triiodothyronine	Thyroid	Causes moderate enlargement of the thyroid gland but woman remains euthyroid; possibly play role in early neural development of the fetus
Parathyroid	Parathyroid	Controls calcium and magnesium metabolism
Insulin	Pancreas	Decreases production of insulin to protect fetus and its need for glucose
Cortisol	Adrenal glands	Stimulates production of insulin; increases peripheral resistance to insulin
Aldosterone	Adrenal glands	Stimulates reabsorption of excess sodium from the renal tubules

postbirth fluid loss and perineal discomfort, contribute to continuing constipation.

Gallbladder and Liver. The gallbladder is often distended because of its decreased muscle tone during pregnancy. Increased emptying time and thickening of bile caused by prolonged retention are typical changes. These features, together with slight hypercholesterolemia from increased progesterone levels, may account for the development of gallstones during pregnancy.

Hepatic function is difficult to appraise during pregnancy. However, only minor changes in liver function develop. Occasionally, intrahepatic cholestasis (i.e., retention and accumulation of bile in the liver caused by factors within the liver) occurs late in pregnancy in response to placental steroids. It may result in pruritus gravidarum (severe itching) with or without jaundice. These distressing symptoms subside soon after birth.

Abdominal Discomfort. Intraabdominal alterations that can cause discomfort include pelvic heaviness or pressure, round ligament tension, flatulence, distention and bowel cramping, and uterine contractions. In addition to displacement of intestines, pressure from the expanding uterus causes an increase in venous pressure in the pelvic organs. Although most abdominal discomfort is a consequence of normal maternal alterations, the health care provider must be constantly alert to the possibility of disorders such as bowel obstruction or an inflammatory process.

Appendicitis may be difficult to diagnose in pregnancy because the appendix is displaced upward and laterally, high and to the right, away from McBurney's point (Fig. 10-12).

Endocrine System

During pregnancy, there are profound endocrine changes. These are essential for maintaining the pregnancy, for stimulating normal fetal growth, and for postpartum recovery. Hormones, their sources, and their effects on the pregnancy are presented in Table 10-3.

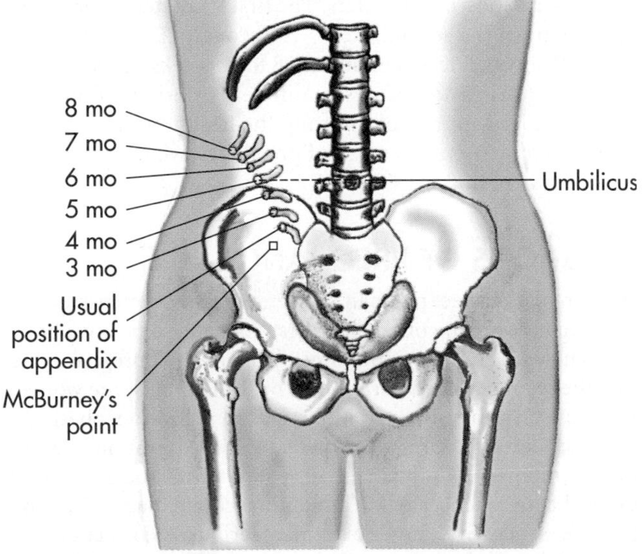

FIG. 10-12 • Change in position of appendix in pregnancy. Note McBurney's point.

Key Points

- Adaptations to pregnancy protect the woman's normal physiologic functioning, meet the metabolic demands that pregnancy imposes, and provide for fetal developmental and growth needs.
- Maternal adaptations are attributed to the hormones of pregnancy and to mechanical pressures arising from the enlarging uterus and other tissues.
- The ability to recognize the beta subunit of hCG through monoclonal antibody technology has revolutionized endocrine tests for pregnancy.
- Presumptive, probable, and positive signs of pregnancy aid in the diagnosis of pregnancy; only positive signs (i.e., identification of a fetal heart tone, verification of fetal movements, and visualization of the fetus) can establish the diagnosis of pregnancy.
- The rise in pH of the pregnant woman's vaginal secretions makes her more vulnerable to vaginal infections.
- Increased vascularity and sensitivity of the vagina and other pelvic viscera may lead to a high degree of sexual interest and arousal.
- Some adaptations to pregnancy result in discomforts such as fatigue, urinary frequency, nausea, constipation, and breast sensitivity.
- Balance and coordination are affected by changes in joints and in the woman's center of gravity as pregnancy progresses.

References

Chamberlain G, Pipkin F, editors: *Clinical physiology in obstetrics,* ed 3, Oxford, 1998, Blackwell Scientific.

Creasy R, Resnik R: *Maternal-fetal medicine,* ed 4, Philadelphia, 1999, WB Saunders.

Cunningham F et al: *Williams obstetrics,* ed 20, Stamford, CT, 1997, Appleton & Lange.

Green L, Froman R: Blood pressure measurement during pregnancy: auscultating versus oscillatory methods, *J Obstet Gynecol Neonatal Nurs* 25(2):155-159, 1996.

Hatcher R et al: *Contraceptive technology,* ed 17, New York, 1998, Ardent Media.

Lawrence R: *Breastfeeding: a guide for the medical profession,* ed 4, St Louis, 1999, Mosby.

Pagana K, Pagana T: Mosby's *diagnostic and laboratory test reference,* ed 5, St Louis, 2000, Mosby.

Schauberger C et al: Obstetrics: peripheral joint laxity increases in pregnancy but does not correlate with serum relaxin levels, *Am J Obstet Gynecol* 174(2):667-671, 1996.

Seidel H et al: *Mosby's guide to physical examination,* ed 3, St Louis, 1999, Mosby.

Varney H: *Varney's midwifery,* ed 3, Sudbury, MA, 1997, Jones & Bartlett.

Worthington-Roberts B, Williams S: *Nutrition in pregnancy and lactation,* ed 6, St Louis, 1997, Mosby.

CHAPTER

11 Nursing Care During Pregnancy

http://www.harcourthealth.com/MERLIN/Wong/maternal/

Learning Objectives

On completion of this chapter the reader will be able to:

- Describe the processes of confirming pregnancy and estimating the date of birth.
- Summarize the physical, psychosocial, and behavioral changes that usually occur as the mother and other family members adapt to pregnancy.
- Discuss the benefits of prenatal care and problems of accessibility for some women.
- Outline the patterns of health care provided to assess maternal and fetal health status at the initial and at follow-up visits during pregnancy.
- Discuss education needed by pregnant women to understand physical discomforts related to pregnancy and to recognize the signs and symptoms of potential complications.
- Explain the impact of culture, age, parity, and number of fetuses on the response of the family to the pregnancy and on the prenatal care provided.
- Identify the purposes of childbirth education.
- Compare the advantages and disadvantages of choosing different care providers.

The prenatal period is a time of physical and psychologic preparation for birth and parenthood. Becoming a parent represents one of the maturational milestones of adult life, and as such it is a time of intense learning for parents and those close to them. The prenatal period provides a unique opportunity for nurses and other members of the health care team to influence family health. During this period, essentially healthy women seek regular care and guidance. The nurse's health promotion interventions can affect the well-being of the woman, her unborn child, and the rest of her family for many years.

Regular prenatal visits, ideally beginning soon after the first missed menstrual period, offer opportunities to ensure the health of the expectant mother and her infant. Prenatal health care permits diagnosis and treatment of preexisting maternal disorders and those that may develop during the pregnancy. Care is designed to monitor the growth and development of the fetus and to identify abnormalities that may interfere with the course of normal labor. The woman and her family can seek support to reduce stress and to learn parenting skills.

Pregnancy lasts 9 calendar months. However, health care providers use the concept of lunar months, which last 28 days (or 4 weeks) to describe the duration of pregnancy or gestational age. Thus normal pregnancy lasts about 10 lunar months; that is, 40 weeks, or 280 days. Pregnancy is divided into three 3-month periods, or trimesters. The first trimester covers weeks 1 through 13; the second, weeks 14 through 26; and the third, weeks 27 through term gestation (38 to 40 weeks). Prenatal care during each trimester focuses on different priorities of care. The focus of this chapter is on meeting the health needs of the expectant family over the course of pregnancy, which is known as the prenatal period.

DIAGNOSIS OF PREGNANCY

Women may suspect pregnancy when they miss a menstrual period. Many women come to the first visit after a positive home pregnancy test. However, the clinical diagnosis of pregnancy before the second missed period may be difficult in some women. Factors such as physical variations, lack of relaxation, obesity, or tumors, may confound even the experienced examiner. Accuracy is important, however, because emotional, social, medical, or legal consequences related to an inaccurate diagnosis, either positive or negative, can be extremely serious. A correct date for the first day of the last (normal) menstrual period (LMP), the date of intercourse, or the basal body temperature (BBT) record may be of great value in the accurate diagnosis of pregnancy.

Signs and Symptoms

Great variability is possible in the subjective and objective symptoms of pregnancy. Therefore the diagnosis of pregnancy may be uncertain for a time. The diagnosis of pregnancy is based on signs and symptoms that are reported during history taking or found during physical examination. These signs and symptoms are classified as presumptive, probable, and positive (see Table 10-2).

Estimating Date of Birth

When pregnancy is confirmed, the woman's first question usually concerns the time she will give birth. This date has traditionally been called the estimated date of confinement (EDC); however, to promote a more positive perception of both pregnancy and birth, the term estimated date of birth (EDB) is usually used. Because the exact date of conception is usually unknown, several formulas have been suggested for calculating the EDB. None of these guides is infallible, but Nägele's rule is reasonably accurate and is the method usually used.

Nägele's rule is as follows: After determining the first day of the LMP, subtract 3 months, add 7 days and 1 year; or alternatively, add 7 days to the LMP and count forward 9 months. For example, if the first day of the LMP was July 10, 2001, the EDB is April 17, 2002.

Nägele's rule assumes that the woman has a 28-day menstrual cycle and that the pregnancy occurred on the fourteenth day of the cycle. An adjustment is in order if the cycle is longer or shorter than 28 days. Only about 4% to 10% of pregnant women give birth spontaneously on the EDB as determined by Nägele's rule; most give birth in a period extending from 7 days before to 7 days after the EDB.

> *Family Focus*
>
> **CONCERNS ABOUT THE FETUS**
>
> **Parental concern for the health of the child seems to vary during the course of pregnancy. The first concern appears in the first trimester and relates to the possibility of spontaneous abortion. Many women delay telling others about the pregnancy until this time passes. As the child becomes more of a reality, with movement and an audible heartbeat and through ultrasound examination, parental anxiety focuses on possible defects in the child.**

> *Family Focus*
>
> **PREGNANCY AND THE FAMILY**
>
> **Family adaptation to pregnancy takes place within a cultural environment that is influenced by societal trends. Scholars in the United States and Canada have carried out much of their investigation of family dynamics in pregnancy by studying Caucasian, middle-class families; the findings may not apply to families who do not fit the traditional American model. Terms such as spouse, husband, and wife, for example, are used consistently in family literature but may not fit the configuration of a given family. The nurse can adapt various terms, if appropriate, to avoid offense to the family and embarrassment to the nurse.**

ADAPTATION TO PREGNANCY

Pregnancy affects all family members, and each family member must adapt to the pregnancy and interpret its meaning in light of his or her own needs.

Maternal Adaptation

Women of all ages use the months of pregnancy to adapt to the maternal role. Early in pregnancy nothing seems to be happening, and much time is spent sleeping. With the perception of fetal movement in the second trimester, the woman turns her attention inward to her pregnancy.

Pregnancy is a maturational milestone and requires mastery of certain developmental tasks: accepting the pregnancy, identifying with the role of mother, reordering the relationships between herself and her mother and between herself and her partner, establishing a relationship with the unborn child, and preparing for the birth experience (Lederman, 1996). The partner's emotional support is an important factor in the successful accomplishment of these developmental tasks. Single women with limited support may have difficulty making this adaptation.

Accepting the Pregnancy. The first step in adapting to the maternal role is accepting the idea of pregnancy and assimilating the pregnant state into the woman's way of life. Mercer (1995) described this process as cognitive restructuring and credited Reva Rubin (1984) as the nurse theorist who pioneered our understanding of maternal role attainment.

Initially, many women are dismayed at finding themselves pregnant. Eventual acceptance of pregnancy parallels the growing acceptance of the reality of a child. Nonacceptance of the pregnancy should not be equated with rejection of the child. A woman may dislike being pregnant but feel love for the child to be born. Women who are happy and pleased about their pregnancy have high self-esteem and tend to be confident about outcomes for themselves, their babies, and other family members.

Many pregnant women are surprised to experience emotional lability, that is, rapid and unpredictable changes in mood. Increased irritability, explosions of tears and anger, and feelings of great joy and cheerfulness alternate, apparently with little or no provocation.

Most women experience ambivalent feelings during pregnancy. Ambivalence, or having conflicting feelings at the same time, is considered a normal response in people preparing for a new role. Even women who are pleased to be pregnant may experience feelings of hostility toward the pregnancy or the unborn child from time to time. Intense feelings of ambivalence that persist through the third trimester may indicate an unresolved conflict with the motherhood role (Mercer, 1995). After the birth of a healthy child, memories of these ambivalent feelings usually are dismissed. If the child is born with a defect, a woman may look back at the times when she did not want the pregnancy and feel intense guilt; she may believe that her ambivalence caused the birth defect. She will need reassurance that her feelings were not responsible for the problem.

Identifying with the Mother Role. The process of identifying with the mother role begins early in each woman's life at the time she is being mothered as a child. Practice roles, such as playing with dolls, baby-sitting, and taking care of siblings, may increase her understanding of what being a mother entails.

Many women have always wanted a baby; they like children, and look forward to motherhood. Their high motivation to become a parent promotes acceptance of pregnancy and eventual prenatal and parental adaptation. Other women apparently have not considered in any detail what motherhood means to them. During pregnancy, conflicts such as not wanting the pregnancy and career-related decisions need to be resolved.

Reordering Personal Relationships. Close relationships held by the pregnant woman undergo change as she prepares emotionally for the new role of mother. As family members learn their new roles, periods of tension and conflict may occur. Promoting effective communication patterns between the expectant mother and her own mother and between the expectant mother and her partner are common nursing interventions provided during the prenatal visits.

Family Focus

MATERNAL ADAPTATION

Adaptation to the maternal role involves a complex social and cognitive learning process. Pregnancy functions as a rite of passage and indicates that maturity has been reached. Reva Rubin began studying maternal role adaptation in the 1960s. She described the *developmental tasks* of pregnancy as accepting the pregnancy, identifying the role of mother, reordering the relationships between her mother and herself and between herself and her partner, establishing a relationship with the unborn child, and preparing for the birth experience.

The partner's emotional support is an important factor in the successful accomplishment of these developmental tasks. Women prepared to accept a pregnancy seek medical validation early. When pregnancy is confirmed, a woman's emotional responses may range from delight to shock, disbelief, and despair. A general state of well-being predominates, but emotional liability is common. These rapid mood changes include increased irritability, explosions of tears and anger, and feelings of great joy and cheerfulness. Such changes are often attributed to hormonal changes.

Rubin described changes in pregnancy as follows. The subjective experience of time and space changes during pregnancy; early in pregnancy, nothing seems to be happening, and the woman spends much time sleeping. With quickening (feelings of fetal movement) in the second trimester, there is a reduction of time and space, both geographic and social, as the woman turns her attention inward to her pregnancy. She examines or fosters relationships with her mother and other women who have been or are pregnant. With the third trimester, there is a slower pace and a sense that time is running out as the woman's activities are curtailed. A mother's reaction to her daughter's pregnancy signifies her acceptance of the grandchild and of her daughter. If the mother is supportive, the daughter has an opportunity to discuss pregnancy and labor and her feelings of joy or ambivalence with a knowledgeable and accepting woman.

Women express two major needs within the partner relationship during pregnancy: feeling loved and valued, and having the child accepted by the partner. The addition of a child changes forever the nature of the bond between partners. The partner can be a stabilizing influence, a good listener to expressions of doubts and fears, and a source of physical and emotional reassurance. The partner can also feel jealous of the unborn baby. Lesbian and unpartnered women have received little attention in the literature. Some suggest that a woman partner may be better able to understand and meet more effectively the needs of her partner for nurturing. An unpartnered woman may seek out her mother or other women friends to meet her dependence needs.

Data from Mercer R: *Becoming a mother,* New York, 1995, Springer.

The woman's relationship with her mother is significant in adapting to pregnancy and motherhood. Important components in the pregnant woman's relationship with her mother are the mother's availability (past and present), her reactions to the daughter's pregnancy, respect for her daughter's autonomy, and the willingness to reminisce (Mercer, 1995).

The mother's reaction to the daughter's pregnancy signifies her acceptance of the grandchild and of her daughter. If the mother is supportive, the daughter has an opportunity to discuss pregnancy and labor and her feelings of joy or ambivalence with a knowledgeable and accepting woman (Fig. 11-1). Reminiscing about the pregnant woman's early childhood and sharing the grandmother-to-be's account of her childbirth experience help the daughter anticipate and prepare for labor and birth.

Although the woman's relationship with her mother is significant in considering her adaptation in pregnancy, the most important person to the pregnant woman is usually the father of her child. A woman who is nurtured by her partner during pregnancy has fewer emotional and physical symptoms, fewer labor and childbirth complications, and an easier postpartum adjustment.

The marital or committed relationship is not static but evolves over time. The addition of a child changes forever the nature of the bond between partners. Partners who trust and support each other are able to share mutual-dependency needs (Mercer, 1995).

As pregnancy progresses, changes in body shape, body image, and levels of discomfort influence both partners' desire for sexual expression. During the first trimester the woman's sexual desire may decrease, especially if she experiences breast tenderness, nausea, fatigue, or sleepiness. As she progresses into the second trimester, her sense of well-being, combined with the in-

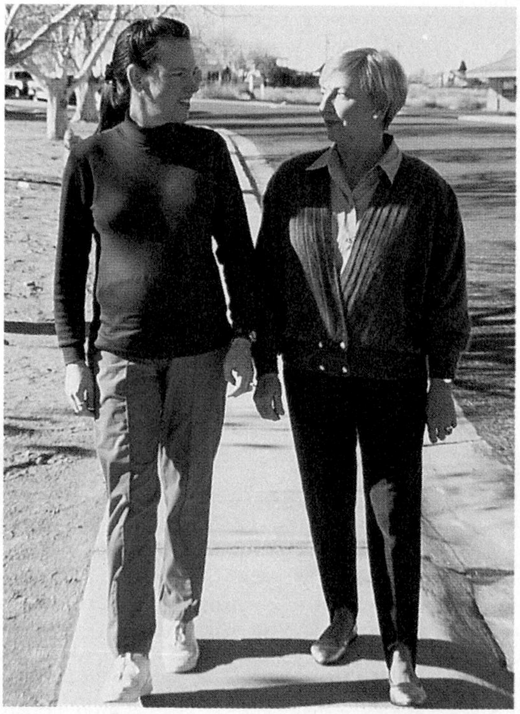

FIG. 11-1 • A pregnant woman and her mother enjoy a walk together. (Courtesy Michael S. Clement, MD, Mesa, AZ.)

creased pelvic congestion that occurs at this time, may increase her desire for sexual release. In the third trimester, somatic complaints and physical bulkiness may increase her physical discomfort and diminish her interest in sex.

Establishing a Relationship with the Fetus. Emotional attachment to the child begins during the prenatal period as women use fantasizing and daydreaming to prepare themselves for motherhood (Rubin, 1975). They think of themselves as mothers and imagine maternal qualities they would like to possess. Expectant parents desire to be warm, loving, and close to their child. The mother-child relationship progresses through pregnancy as a developmental process. Three phases in the developmental pattern become apparent.

In phase 1 the woman accepts the biologic fact of pregnancy. She needs to be able to state, "I am pregnant." In phase 2 the woman accepts the growing fetus as distinct from herself and as a person to nurture. She can now say, "I am going to have a baby." During phase 3, the woman prepares realistically for the birth and parenting of the child. She expresses the thought, "I am going to be a mother" and defines the nature and characteristics of the child. She may, for example, speculate about the child's sex and personality traits based on patterns of fetal activity.

Family Focus

MATERNAL-PATERNAL-FETAL RELATIONSHIP

Emotional attachment to the child begins during the prenatal period. Parents fantasize and daydream to prepare for parenthood. Early in pregnancy the woman accepts the biologic fact of pregnancy and incorporates the idea of a child into her body and self-image. When the fetus is viewed on ultrasound, it becomes more real. During the second trimester there is growing awareness of the child as a separate being. When she accepts the reality of the child, the woman becomes more introspective. She seems to withdraw and to concentrate her interest on the unborn child. Her partner may feel left out, and other children in the family become more demanding in efforts to redirect the mother's attention to themselves.

The *fantasy child* may have familial characteristics and superior abilities; its appearance may be that of a 3- or 4-month-old infant. Both parents and siblings believe the unborn child responds in an individualized, personal manner. Some families become involved by picking the child's name and anticipating the child's sex if it is not already known. Some families select the child's name as early as the first month of pregnancy. Family tradition, religious customs, and continuation of one's own name or names of relatives and friends are important in the selection process. Family members may interact a great deal with the unborn child by trying to listen, talk to, and play with the fetus; and stroking or kissing the mother's abdomen, especially when the fetus moves.

Nurses must continue to seek to understand and foster attitudes and behaviors that promote early attachment and reduce the risk of negative long-term effects such as child neglect and abuse. More research relating psychologic variables to prenatal attachment and maternal-paternal-fetal interaction with maternal-paternal-child interaction is needed, including research with lesbian couples and unpartnered women. Tools to measure maternal-fetal attachment are the Maternal-Fetal Attachment Scale (MFAS)* and the Prenatal Attachment Inventory (PAI).†

*Cranley M: Development of a tool for the measurement of maternal attachment during pregnancy, *Nurs Res* 30:28, 1981.

†Müller M: Development of the prenatal attachment inventory, *West J Nurs Res* 15:199, 1993.

Preparing for Childbirth. Many women actively prepare for birth. They read books, view films, attend parenting classes, and talk to other women (Lederman, 1996). They seek the best caregiver possible for advice, monitoring, and caring.

Anxiety can arise from concern about safe passage for herself and her child during the birth process (Mercer, 1995; Rubin, 1975). These feelings persist despite statistical evidence about the safe outcome of pregnancy for mothers and their infants. Many women fear the pain of childbirth or mutilation because they do not understand anatomy and the birth process. Education by the nurse can alleviate many of these fears.

Toward the end of the third trimester breathing is difficult and fetal movements become vigorous enough to disturb the mother's sleep. Backaches, frequency and urgency of urination, constipation, and varicose veins can become troublesome. The bulkiness and awkwardness of her body interfere with the woman's ability to care for other children, perform routine work-related duties, and assume a comfortable position for sleep and rest. A strong desire to see the end of pregnancy, to be over and done with it, makes women at this stage ready to move on to childbirth.

Paternal Adaptation

The father's beliefs and feelings about the ideal mother and father and his cultural expectation of appropriate behavior during pregnancy affect his response to his partner's need for him. For most men, pregnancy can be a time of preparation for the parental role with intense learning.

Accepting the Pregnancy. In older societies, the man enacted the ritual couvades; that is, he behaved in specific ways

Family Focus

PATERNAL ADAPTATION

A man's emotional responses to becoming a father, his concerns, and his informational needs change during the course of pregnancy. Three styles of involvement provide examples of different ways men can experience pregnancy (May, 1980, 1982). Men may be involved in pregnancy as an observer, that is, avoiding direct involvement in activities such as parent education classes and decisions about breastfeeding. Others are more expressive and display a strong emotional response to pregnancy and a desire to be a full partner in the project; some expectant fathers even experience the couvade syndrome and have pregnancy-like symptoms such as nausea and other gastrointestinal complaints, fatigue, and other physical discomforts. Other fathers adopt the instrumental style, seeing tasks they can perform in their role as manager of the pregnancy. They feel responsible for the outcome of pregnancy and are protective and supportive of their wives.

The father's beliefs and feelings about the ideal mother and father and his cultural expectation of appropriate behavior during pregnancy affect his response to his partner's need for him. One man may engage in nurturing behavior; another may feel lonely and alienated as the woman becomes physically and emotionally engrossed in the unborn child. The man may seek comfort and understanding outside the home, or become interested in a new hobby or involved with his work. Some men view pregnancy as a proof of their masculinity and their dominant role. To others, pregnancy has no meaning in terms of responsibility to either mother or child. For most men, however, pregnancy is a time of preparation for the parental role, of fantasy, of great pleasure, and of intense learning.

and respected taboos associated with pregnancy and giving birth. In this way the man's new status was recognized and endorsed. His behavior acknowledged his psychosocial and biologic relationship to the mother and child. In Western societies, the participation of fathers in childbirth has risen dramatically over the past 25 years, and the father in the role of labor coach is common.

Identifying with the Father Role. Each father brings to pregnancy attitudes that affect the way in which he adjusts to the pregnancy and parental role. Some men are highly motivated to nurture and love a child. They may be excited and pleased about the anticipated role of father. Others may be more detached or even hostile to the idea of fatherhood.

Reordering Personal Relationships. The partner's main role in pregnancy is to nurture and respond to the pregnant woman's feelings of vulnerability. Some aspects of a partner's behavior indicate rivalry. Direct rivalry with the fetus may be evident, especially during sexual activity. Men may protest that fetal movements prevent sexual gratification, or that the fetus is watching them during sexual activity.

The woman's increased introspection may cause her partner to feel uneasy as she becomes preoccupied with thoughts of the child and of motherhood, with her growing dependence on her physician or midwife, and with her reevaluation of the couple's relationship.

Establishing a Relationship with the Fetus. The father-child attachment can be as strong as the mother-child relationship, and fathers can be as competent as mothers in nurturing their infants. The father-child attachment begins in pregnancy. A father may rub or kiss the maternal abdomen, try to listen to the fetus, or play with the fetus as he notes fetal movement.

Men prepare for fatherhood in many of the same ways that women prepare for motherhood—by reading, fantasizing, and daydreaming about the baby. As the birth day approaches, fa-

Box 11-1

Tips for Sibling Preparation

PRENATAL

1. Adjust the timing and content of information about an anticipated infant to the age and understanding of the older child.
2. Take your child on a prenatal visit. Let the child listen to the fetal heartbeat and feel the baby move.
3. Involve the child in preparations for the baby, such as helping decorate the baby's room.
4. Move the child to a bed (if still sleeping in a crib) at least 2 months before the baby is due.
5. Read books, show videos, or take child to sibling preparation classes, including a hospital tour.
6. Answer your child's questions about the coming birth, what babies are like, and any other questions.
7. Take your child to the homes of friends who have babies so that the child has realistic expectations of what babies are like.

DURING THE HOSPITAL STAY

1. Have someone bring the child to the hospital to visit you and the baby (unless you plan to have the child attend the birth).
2. Don't force interactions between the child and the baby. Often the child will be more interested in seeing you and being reassured of your love.
3. Help the child explore the infant by showing how and where to touch the baby.
4. Give the child a gift (from you or from you, the father, and the baby).

GOING HOME

1. Leave the child at home with a relative or babysitter.
2. Have someone else carry the baby from the car so that you can hug the child first.

ADJUSTMENT AFTER THE BABY IS HOME

1. Arrange for a special time with the child alone with each parent.
2. Don't exclude the child during infant feeding times. The child can sit with you and the baby and feed a doll or drink juice or milk with you or sit quietly with a game.
3. Prepare small gifts for the child so that when the baby gets gifts, the sibling won't feel left out. The child can also help open the baby gifts.
4. Praise the child for acting age appropriately (so that being a baby does not seem better than being older).

Family Focus

SIBLING ADAPTATION TO PREGNANCY AND BIRTH

Sibling responses to pregnancy vary with age and dependency needs. The 1-year-old infant seems largely unaware of the process, but the 2-year-old child notices the change in the mother's appearance and may comment, "Mommy's fat." The 2-year-old child's need for sameness in the environment makes the child aware of any change. Toddlers may exhibit more clinging behavior and revert to dependent behaviors in toilet training or eating.

By age 3 or 4 years, children like to be told the story of their own beginning and accept its being compared to the present pregnancy. They like to listen to heartbeats and feel the baby moving in utero (Fig. 11-2). Sometimes they worry about how the baby is being fed and what it wears.

School-age children take a more clinical interest in their mother's pregnancy. They may want to know in more detail, "How did the baby get in there?" and "How will it get out?" Children in this age-group notice pregnant women in stores, churches, and schools and sometimes seem shy if they need to approach a pregnant woman directly. On the whole they look forward to the new baby, see themselves as "mothers" or "fathers," and enjoy buying baby supplies and readying a place for the baby. Because they still think in concrete terms and base judgments on the here and now, they respond positively to their mother's current good health.

Early and middle adolescents preoccupied with the establishment of their own sexual identity may have difficulty accepting the overwhelming evidence of the sexual activity of their parents. They reason that if they are too young for such activity, certainly their parents are too old. They seem to take on a critical parental role and may ask, "What will people think?" or "How can you let yourself get so fat?" Many pregnant women with teenage children confess that their teenagers are the most difficult factor in their current pregnancy.

Late adolescents do not appear to be unduly disturbed. They realize that they soon will be gone from home. Parents usually report they are comforting and act more like other adults than children.

thers have more questions about fetal and newborn behaviors. Some fathers are shocked or amazed at how small the clothes and furniture for the baby are.

Preparing for Childbirth. The father's major concerns are getting the mother to a medical facility in time for the birth and not appearing ignorant. He may fantasize about different situations and plan what he will do in response to them; he may rehearse taking various routes to the hospital, timing each route at different times of the day. The father may have fears concerning safe passage of his partner and the mutilation or death of his partner or child. With the exception of childbirth preparation classes, a father has few opportunities to learn ways to be an involved and active partner in this rite of passage into parenthood.

Sibling Adaptation

Sharing the spotlight with a new brother or sister may be the first major crisis for a child. The older child often experiences a sense of loss or feels jealous at being "replaced" by the new baby. Some of the factors that influence the child's response are age, the parents' attitudes, the father's role, the length of separation from the mother, the hospital's visitation policy, and how the child has been prepared for the change.

The mother with other children must devote time and energy to reorganizing her relationships with these children. She needs to prepare siblings for the birth of the baby (Box 11-1; also see Fig. 11-3) and begin the process of role transition in the family by including the children in the pregnancy and being sympathetic to older children's protests at losing their places in the family hierarchy. No child willingly gives up a familiar position.

Classes to prepare children for the birth of a new brother or sister are available in many communities (Fig. 11-3).

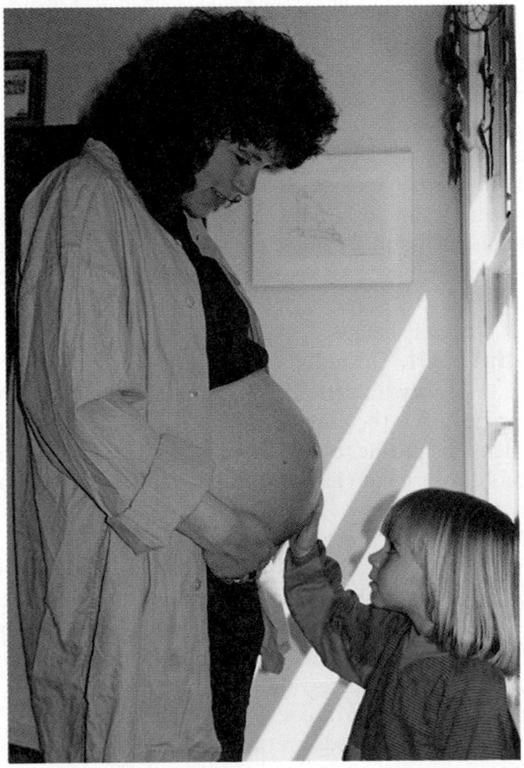

FIG. 11-2 • A sibling feels the movement of a fetus. (Courtesy Kim Molloy, Knoxville, IA.)

CARE MANAGEMENT

The purpose of prenatal care is to identify existing risk factors and other deviations from normal so that pregnancy outcomes may be enhanced (Beischer, MacKay, and Colditz, 1997). Major emphasis is placed on preventive aspects of care, primarily to motivate the pregnant woman to practice optimal self-care and to report unusual changes early so that problems can be minimized or prevented. In providing holistic care, nurses also provide information and guidance about the psychosocial impact of pregnancy on the woman and members of her family. The goals of prenatal nursing care, therefore, are not only to foster a safe birth for the infant and mother but also to promote satisfaction of the mother and family with the pregnancy and birth experience.

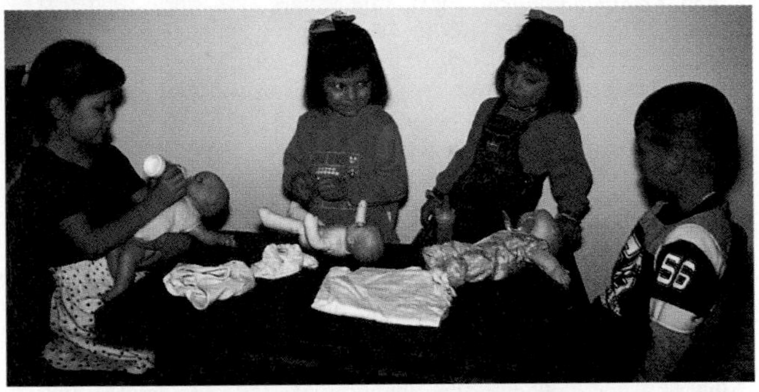

FIG. 11-3 • A sibling class of preschoolers learns infant care using dolls. (Courtesy Michael S. Clement, MD, Mesa, AZ.)

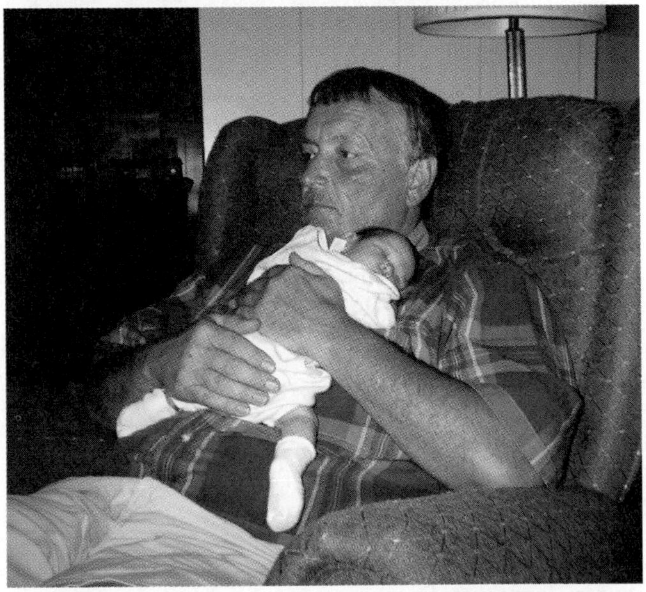

FIG. 11-4 • A grandfather relaxes with his granddaughter. (Courtesy Gregory Vogel, Bloomington, IL.)

Family Focus

GRANDPARENT ADAPTATION TO PREGNANCY AND BIRTH

Every pregnancy affects all family relationships. For expectant grandparents, a first pregnancy in a child is undeniable evidence that they are growing older. Many think of a grandparent as old, white haired, and becoming feeble of mind and body; however, some people face grandparenthood while still in their 30s or 40s. A mother-to-be announcing her pregnancy to her mother may be greeted by a negative response that indicates she is not ready to be a grandmother. Both daughter and mother may be startled and hurt by the response.

Some expectant grandparents not only are nonsupportive but also use subtle means to decrease the self-esteem of the young parents-to-be. Mothers may talk about their terrible pregnancies; fathers may discuss the endless cost of rearing children; and mothers-in-law may complain that their sons are neglecting them because their concern is now directed toward the pregnant daughters-in-law.

However, most grandparents are delighted with the prospect of a new baby in the family. It reawakens their feelings of their own youth, the excitement of giving birth, and their delight in the behavior of the parents-to-be when they were infants. They set up a memory store of their child's first smiles, first words, and first steps that can be used later for "claiming" the newborn as a member of the family. Their and the parents' satisfaction comes with the realization that continuity between past and present is guaranteed.

The grandparent is the historian who transmits the family history, a resource person who shares knowledge based on experience, a role model, and a support person. The grandparent's presence and support can strengthen family systems by widening the circle of support and nurturance (Fig. 11-4). Other sources of information cannot replace the unique contribution that grandparents make.

Many women report that their pregnancies bridged the final gap between them and their own mothers. The estrangement that began in adolescence disappears as the now-pregnant daughter experiences joys, concerns, and anxieties similar to those her mother felt before her.

Expectant grandparenthood can be a maturational milestone for the parent of an expectant parent. To be truly family oriented, maternity care must include the grandparent in implementing the nursing process with childbearing families. A class for grandparents is one method of incorporating the grandparents into the family system and of encouraging communication between the generations.

Prenatal care is sought routinely by women of middle or high socioeconomic status. However, women living in poverty or who lack health insurance may not be able to use public medical services or gain access to private care. Likewise, immigrant women from cultures in which prenatal care is not emphasized may not know to seek routine prenatal care. Birth outcomes in these populations are thus less positive, with higher rates of maternal and fetal or newborn complications. In particular, problems with low birth weight (less than 2500 g) and infant mortality have been associated with inadequate prenatal care.

Barriers to obtaining health care during pregnancy include inadequate numbers of health care providers, distance from health care facilities, lack of transportation, fragmentation of services, inadequate finances, and personal attitudes. The availability and accessibility of prenatal care may be improved by the increasing use of advanced practice nurses in collaborative practice with physicians (Mvula and Miller, 1998) or midwives

Critical Thinking

LATE ENTRY INTO PRENATAL CARE

Angelina, G5 P4, is seen in the clinic for her first prenatal visit when she is 8 months pregnant. She explained that she did not come sooner because pregnancy is normal, she is not sick, she has had other babies with no problems, and there was no need to bother a doctor. How would you approach this situation? What needs might Angelina have that she does not recognize? What assessments are necessary? Identify at least three priorities for the care of Angelina.

Family Focus

FAMILY AND THE INITIAL INTERVIEW

Often the woman is accompanied by a family member or members at her initial assessment. The nurse builds a relationship with these people as part of the social context of the patient. They also are helpful in recalling and validating information related to the patient's health. With the patient's permission, those accompanying her can be included in the initial prenatal interview. Observations and information about the woman's family are part of the interview. For example, if the woman is accompanied by small children, the nurse can inquire about her plans for child care during the forthcoming labor and birth.

(Oakley et al, 1996). The effectiveness of a regular schedule of home visiting by nurses during pregnancy also has been validated (Chestnut, 1998). Prenatal care is ideally a multidisciplinary activity in which nurses work with physicians or midwives, nutritionists, social workers, and others. Collaboration among these individuals is necessary to provide holistic care.

➤ Assessment

Once the presence of pregnancy has been confirmed and the woman's desire to continue the pregnancy has been validated, prenatal care is begun. The assessment process begins at the initial prenatal visit and is continued throughout the pregnancy. Assessment techniques include the interview, physical examination, and laboratory tests. Because the initial visit and follow-up visits are distinctly different in content and process, they are described separately below.

Initial Visit. The initial evaluation includes a comprehensive health history that emphasizes the current pregnancy, previous pregnancies, the family, a psychosocial profile, a physical assessment, diagnostic testing, and an overall risk assessment. A prenatal history form (Fig. 11-5) is the best way to document information obtained.

Interview. The therapeutic relationship between the nurse and the woman is established during the initial assessment interview. It is a time for planned, purposeful communication that focuses on specific content. The data collected are of two types: the woman's subjective appraisal of her health status; and the nurse's objective observations of the woman's affect, posture, body language, skin color, and other physical and emotional signs. Special needs are noted at this time (e.g., wheelchair access, assistance in getting on and off the examining table, and cognitive deficits) (Fig. 11-6)

Reason for Seeking Care. Although pregnant women are scheduled for "routine" prenatal visits, they often come to the

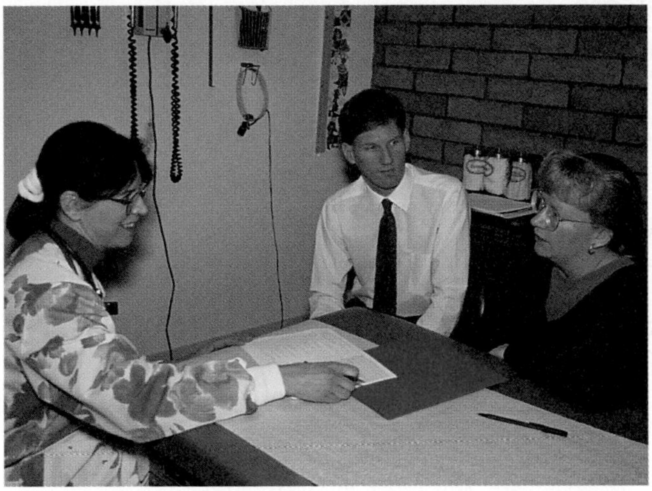

FIG. 11-6 • Prenatal interview.

health care provider seeking information or reassurance about a particular concern. When the woman is asked a broad, open-ended question such as "How have you been feeling?" she may reveal problems that could otherwise be overlooked. The woman's chief concerns should be recorded in her own words to alert other personnel to the priority of needs identified by her. A typical desire at the initial visit is for information about what is normal in the course of pregnancy.

Current Pregnancy. The presumptive signs of pregnancy may be of great concern to the woman. A review of symptoms she is experiencing and how she is coping with them helps establish a database to develop a plan of care. Some early teaching may be provided at this time.

Obstetric/Gynecologic History. Data are gathered on the woman's age at menarche, menstrual history, contraceptive history, the nature of any infertility or gynecologic conditions, history of any STIs, her sexual history, and a detailed history of all her pregnancies (including the present pregnancy) and their outcomes. The date of the last Papanicolaou test and the result are noted. The date of her LMP is obtained to establish the EDB.

Medical History. The medical history includes those medical or surgical conditions that may affect the pregnancy or that may be affected by the pregnancy. For example, a pregnant woman who has diabetes or epilepsy requires special care. Because most women are anxious during the initial interview, the nurse's reference to cues such as a Medic-Alert bracelet can prompt the woman to explain allergies, chronic diseases, or medications being taken (e.g., cortisone, insulin, or anticonvulsants).

The nature of previous surgical procedures should also be described. If a woman has had uterine surgery or extensive repair of the pelvic floor, a cesarean birth may be necessary; appendectomy rules out appendicitis as a cause of right lower quadrant pain; and spinal surgery may contraindicate the use of spinal or epidural anesthesia. Any injury involving the pelvis is noted.

Many women who have chronic or handicapping conditions forget to mention them during the initial assessment because they have adapted to them. Special shoes or a limp may indicate the existence of a pelvic structural defect, an important consideration in pregnant women. The nurse who observes these special characteristics and sensitively inquires about them can obtain individualized data that will provide the basis for a comprehensive nursing care plan. Observations are a vital component of the interview process because they prompt the nurse and the woman to focus on the specific needs of the woman and her family.

Nutritional History. The nutritional status of a pregnant woman has a direct effect on the growth and development of the fetus. A dietary assessment can reveal special diet practices, food allergies, eating behaviors, and other factors related to nutritional status. Usually, pregnant women are motivated to learn about good nutrition and respond well to nutritional advice generated by this assessment.

History of Drug Use. A woman's past and present use of legal drugs (e.g., over the counter [OTC] and prescription drugs, caffeine, alcohol, and nicotine) and illegal drugs (e.g., marijuana, cocaine, and heroin) needs to be assessed because many substances cross the placenta and may harm the developing fetus. Periodic urine toxicology screening tests are often recommended during pregnancy for women who have a history of illegal drug use.

Nurses may have ethical concerns if pregnant women are not informed of the possibility of random urine testing for presence of drugs. They may also be concerned about the unborn child and whether the mother has a duty not to harm him or her.

Family History. The family history provides information about the woman's immediate family, including parents, siblings, and children. These data help identify familial or genetic disorders or conditions that could affect the present health status of the woman or her fetus.

Social and Experiential History. Situational factors such as the family's ethnic and cultural background and socioeconomic status are assessed while the history is obtained.

The following information may be obtained over several encounters. The woman's perception of this pregnancy is explored by asking her questions about the following: Is this pregnancy wanted or not, planned or not? Is the woman/couple pleased or displeased, accepting or nonaccepting? What problems related to finances, career, or living accommodations may arise as a result of the pregnancy? The family support system is determined by asking her such questions about the following: What primary support is available to her? Are changes needed to promote adequate support? What are the existing relationships among mother, father/partner, siblings, and in-laws? What preparations are being made for her care and that of dependent family members during labor and for the care of the infant after birth? Is financial, educational, or other support needed from the community?

What are the woman's ideas about childbearing, her expectations of the infant's behavior, and her outlook on life and the female role? Other areas to question include the following: What does the woman think it will be like to have a baby in the home? How is her life going to change by having a baby? What plans will having a baby interrupt? In interviews throughout the pregnancy, the nurse should remain alert for the appearance of potential parenting problems such as depression, lack of family support, and inadequate living conditions. The nurse needs to assess the woman's attitude toward health care, particularly during childbearing; her expectations of health care providers; and her view of the relationship between herself and the nurse.

Coping mechanisms and patterns of interacting are identified. Early in the pregnancy the nurse should determine the woman's knowledge of pregnancy, maternal changes, fetal growth, self-care, and care of the newborn, including feeding. It is important to ask about attitudes toward unmedicated or medicated childbirth and about her knowledge of the availability of parenting skills classes. Before planning for nursing care, the nurse needs information about the woman's decision-

PRENATAL RECORD

Name	Religion	Date
Address		Telephone
Occupation	Business address	Business telephone
Husband's/father's name	Business address	Business telephone
Husband's/father's occupation	Referred by	

Age	Gravida	Para	Term	Premature	Abortions	Living

LMP	PMP	Quickening	EDD

Significant history

Significant findings

Date													
Wt. ( )													
BP													
Edema													
Ht. of fundus													
Position													
FH													
Urine	Sug / Pro												
Gestation													
Movement													
Initials													
RTC													

Blood group	Rh	STS	Hgb. HCT.	Pap	HBsAg
Rubella	Glucola	Alpha feto protein	GC	HIV	
PPD	Chest x-ray	Vitamin supplement	Breast/bottle	Anesthesia preference	Pediatrician

Problem list

☐ Family planning information

FIG. 11-5 • A sample prenatal history form.

Name:

Present Pregnancy

Nausea:	Vomiting:	Other symptoms of pregnancy:	
Bleeding:	Cramping:	Pain:	Edema:
Pregnancy test	Date		

Previous Pregnancies

No.	Date delivered	Feeding	Sex	Wt.	Wks. preg.	Condition		Duration of labor	Type of delivery	Remarks
						Birth	Now			
1										
2										
3										
4										
5										
6										

Past History

Menstruation onset	Frequency	Duration	Flow	Pain
Usual childhood illnesses	Rheumatic fever	Heart disease	Pulmonary disease	
Convulsions	Venereal disease	Allergies	Blood transfusion	
Injuries	Operations	Urinary disease		
Alcohol	Smoking	Drugs	Medication	

Family History

Mother	Father	Siblings	Other
Diabetes		Twins	

Physical Examination

General	Ht.	BP	Eyes	Fundi
Ears	Mouth	Teeth	Throat	Thyroid
Chest	Breasts	Nipples	Heart	Lungs
Abdomen	Extremities			

Ext. genitalia		Perineum	
Vagina		Cervix	
Uterus			
Adnexa			
BI cm	DC cm	Arch	
Sacrum		Spines	
Post. sagittal	SS ligaments	Coccyx	

Signature

FIG. 11-5—cont'd • A sample prenatal history form.

making abilities and living habits (e.g., exercise, sleep, diet, diversional interests, personal hygiene, and clothing). Common stressors during childbearing include the baby's welfare, the labor and birth process, the behaviors of the newborn, the relationship with the baby's father, changes in body image, physical symptoms, and changes in family dynamics.

Attitudes concerning the range of acceptable sexual behaviors during pregnancy are explored. Questions such as the following could be asked: What has your family (partner, friends) told you about sex during pregnancy? The woman's sexual self-concept is given emphasis by asking questions such as: How do you feel about the changes in your appearance? How does your partner feel about your body now? How do you feel about wearing maternity clothes?

History of Physical Abuse. All women should be assessed for a history or risk of physical abuse, particularly since the likelihood of abuse increases during pregnancy. Although visual cues from the woman's appearance or behavior may suggest the possibility, abuse may be missed if questioning is limited to those who fit the supposed profile of the battered woman. Identification of abuse and an immediate clinical intervention that includes information about safety can result in behavior that may prevent future abuse and increase the safety and well-being of the woman and her infant (McFarlane et al, 1998).

Review of Systems. During this portion of the interview, the woman is asked to identify and describe preexisting or concurrent problems with any of the body systems, and her mental status is assessed. The woman is questioned about physical symptoms she has experienced, such as shortness of breath or pain. Pregnancy affects and is affected by all body systems; therefore information on the present status of body systems is important in planning care. For each sign or symptom described, the following additional data should be obtained: body location, quality, quantity, chronology, aggravating or alleviating factors, and associated manifestations (e.g., onset, character, and course) (Seidel et al, 1999).

Physical Examination. The initial physical examination provides the baseline for assessing subsequent changes. The examiner should determine the woman's needs for basic information regarding reproductive anatomy and provide this information, along with a demonstration of the equipment that may be used during the examination and an explanation of the procedure itself. The interaction requires an unhurried, sensitive, and gentle approach with a matter-of-fact attitude.

The physical examination begins with assessment of vital signs including blood pressure, height, and weight. The bladder should be empty before pelvic examination. This may provide the opportunity to collect a urine specimen to test for protein, glucose, leukocytes, or for other tests.

Each examiner develops a routine for proceeding with the physical examination; most choose the head-to-toe progression. Heart and breath sounds are evaluated and extremities examined. The skin is assessed for changes in pigmentation, rashes, and edema. Distribution, amount, and quality of body hair is of particular importance because the findings reflect nutritional status, endocrine function, and attention to hygiene. The thyroid

TABLE 11-1
Laboratory Tests in Prenatal Period

Laboratory Test	Purpose
Hemoglobin/hematocrit/WBC, differential	Detects anemia/detects infection
Hemoglobin electrophoresis	Identifies women with hemoglobinopathies (e.g., sickle cell anemia, thalassemia)
Blood type, Rh, and irregular antibody	Identifies those fetuses at risk for developing erythroblastosis fetalis or hyperbilirubinemia in neonatal period
Rubella titer	Determines immunity to rubella
Tuberculin skin testing; chest film after 20 weeks' gestation in women with reactive tuberculin tests	Screens for exposure to tuberculosis
Urinalysis, including microscopic examination of urinary sediment; pH, specific gravity, color, glucose, albumin, protein, RBCs, WBCs, casts, acetone; hCG	Identifies women with unsuspected diabetes mellitus, renal disease, hypertensive disease of pregnancy; infection; occult hematuria
Urine culture	Identifies women with asymptomatic bacteriuria
Renal function tests: BUN, creatinine, electrolytes, creatinine clearance, total protein excretion	Evaluates level of possible renal compromise in women with a history of diabetes, hypertension, or renal disease
Pap test	Screens for cervical intraepithelial neoplasia, herpes simplex type 2, and HPV
Vaginal or rectal smear for *Neisseria gonorrhoeae, Chlamydia,* HPV, GBS	Screens high risk population for asymptomatic infection. GBS done at 35-37 weeks
RPR/VDRL/FTA-ABS	Identifies women with untreated syphilis
HIV* antibody, hepatitis B surface antigen, toxoplasmosis	Screens for infection
1-hr glucose tolerance	Screens for gestational diabetes; done at initial visit for women with risk factors; done at 28 weeks for all pregnant women
3-hr glucose tolerance	Screens for diabetes in women with elevated glucose level after 1-hr test; must have two elevated readings for diagnosis
Cardiac evaluation: ECG, chest x-ray film, and echocardiogram	Evaluates cardiac function in women with a history of hypertension or cardiac disease

BUN, Blood urea nitrogen; *ECG,* electrocardiogram; *FTA-ABS,* fluorescent treponemal antibody absorption test; *GBS,* group B streptococcus; *hCG,* human chorionic gonadotropin; *HIV,* human immunodeficiency virus; *HPV,* human papillomavirus; *RPR,* rapid plasma reagin.
*With patient permission.

gland is assessed carefully, as are the breasts and abdomen. The height of the fundus is noted if the first examination occurs after the first trimester of pregnancy. The typical basic examination is usually completed without much discomfort for the healthy woman. During the examination, the examiner needs to remain alert to the woman's cues that give direction to the remainder of the assessment and that indicate imminent untoward response such as supine hypotension. See Chapter 5 for a detailed description of the physical examination.

Whenever a pelvic examination is performed, the tone of the pelvic musculature and the woman's knowledge of Kegel exercises are assessed. Particular attention is paid to the size of the uterus because this is an indication of the timing of gestation. The nurse present during the examination can coach the woman at this time in breathing and relaxation techniques as needed. Onc vaginal examination during pregnancy is recommended, but another is usually not done unless medically indicated (Bergsjo and Villar, 1997).

Laboratory Tests. The laboratory data yielded from laboratory examination of specimens add important information concerning the symptoms of pregnancy and the health status (Table 11-1). Both nursing and medical diagnoses stem from such information.

Specimens are collected at the initial visit so any abnormal findings can be treated. Tine or purified protein derivative (PPD) tuberculin tests are administered to assess for exposure to tuberculosis. Testing for antibody to the human immunodeficiency virus (HIV) is strongly recommended for all pregnant women (Box 11-2).

The finding of risk factors during pregnancy may indicate the need to repeat some tests at other times. For example, exposure to tuberculosis or an STI would necessitate repeat testing. STIs are common in pregnancy and may have negative effects on mother and fetus. Careful assessment and screening is essential (Jackson and Soper, 1997).

Follow-Up Visits. Monthly visits are scheduled routinely during the first and second trimesters, although additional appointments may be made as the need arises. During the third trimester, however, the possibility for complications increases, and closer monitoring is warranted. Starting with week 28, visits are scheduled every 2 weeks until week 36, and then every week until birth, unless the health care provider individualizes the schedule. Individual needs and risks of the pregnant woman may warrant visits more or less often. The pattern of interviewing the woman first and then assessing physical changes and performing laboratory tests is maintained.

Interview. Follow-up visits are less intensive than the initial prenatal visit. At each of these follow-up visits, the woman is asked to summarize relevant events that have occurred since the previous visit. She is asked about her general emotional and physiologic well-being, complaints or problems, and about any questions she may have. Personal and family needs are also identified and explored.

Emotional changes are common during pregnancy, and therefore it is reasonable for the nurse to ask whether the woman has experienced any mood swings, reactions to changes in her body image, bad dreams, or worries. Positive feelings (her own and that of her family) are also noted and recorded.

How the woman is progressing through the developmental tasks of pregnancy is also assessed. By the beginning of the second trimester, most women have accepted the biologic fact of pregnancy. Usually by the fifth month, a pregnant woman experiences a growing awareness of the child as a separate being, distinct from herself; she can say "I am going to have a baby." With quickening, she turns her attention inward (becomes introspective) to her pregnancy and toward her relationships with others (e.g., her mother and partner).

During the third trimester, current family situations and their effects on the mother are assessed, for example, the response of siblings and grandparents to the pregnancy and the coming child. The nurse needs to assess the parents' understanding of the following: the warning signs of emergencies, such as bleeding and abdominal pain; the signs of preterm and term labor; the labor process and anxieties about labor; fetal development; and methods to assess fetal well-being. The nurse should ascertain whether the woman is planning to attend childbirth preparation classes, and what she knows about the control of discomfort during labor.

A review of the woman's physical systems is appropriate at each visit, and any suspicious signs or symptoms are assessed in depth. Discomforts reflecting adaptations to pregnancy are identified.

Physical Examination. Reevaluation is a constant aspect of a pregnant woman's care. At each visit, pulse and respirations

Box 11-2

HIV Screening

Pregnant women are ethically obligated to seek reasonable care during pregnancy and to avoid causing harm to the fetus. Maternity nurses should be advocates for the fetus, but not at the expense of the pregnant woman.

Mandatory HIV screening involves ethical issues related to privacy invasion, discrimination, social stigma, and reproductive risks to the pregnant woman. Incidence of perinatal transmission from an HIV-positive mother to her fetus ranges from 25% to 35%. Methods of preventing maternal-fetal transmission are not available. However, zidovudine decreases perinatal transmission with no adverse effect*. Until there is a change in technology that alters the diagnosis or treatment of the fetus, testing of the pregnant woman should be voluntary, although some professional groups now advocate mandatory testing. Health care providers have an obligation to make sure the pregnant woman is well informed about HIV symptoms, testing, and methods of decreasing maternal-fetal transmission.

*Culnane M et al: Lack of long-term effects of in utero exposure to zidovudine among uninfected children born to HIV-infected women, *JAMA* 281:151-157, 1999.

Emergency

SUPINE HYPOTENSION

Signs/Symptoms

Pallor
Dizziness, faintness, breathlessness
Tachycardia
Nausea
Clammy (damp, cool) skin; sweating

Interventions

Position woman on her side until her signs/symptoms subside and vital signs stabilize within normal limits.

are measured. BP is taken at every visit using the same arm and with the woman seated. Her weight is measured and the appropriateness of the weight gain is evaluated. Urine may be checked by dipstick. The presence and degree of edema are noted. At each visit, after emptying the bladder, the fundal height is measured. While the woman lies on her back, the nurse should be alert for the occurrence of supine hypotension (Emergency box). When a woman is lying in this position, the weight of the abdominal contents may compress the vena cava and aorta, causing a drop in BP and a feeling of faintness.

Careful interpretation of BP is important in the risk factor analysis of all pregnant women. BP is evaluated on the basis of absolute values and the length of gestation and is interpreted in the light of modifying factors (Box 11-3).

An absolute systolic BP of 140 mm Hg or more and a diastolic BP of 90 mm Hg or more suggests the presence of hypertension (Helewa et al, 1997). A rise in systolic BP of 30 mm Hg or more than the baseline pressure, or rise in the diastolic BP of 15 mm Hg more than the baseline pressure, is also a significant finding regardless of the absolute values. An increase of 20 mm Hg or more in the mean arterial pressure (MAP) is also an indicator of hypertension (Gilbert and Harmon, 1998).

The pregnant woman is monitored continuously for a range of signs and symptoms that indicate potential complications in addition to hypertension. For example, persistent and excessive vomiting and ketonuria may indicate the development of hyperemesis gravidarum. Uterine cramping and vaginal bleeding are signs of threatened miscarriage. Chills and fever are symptoms of infection. Discharge from the vagina may be amniotic fluid or associated with infection (Box 11-4).

Fetal Assessment. Toward the end of the first trimester, before the uterus is an abdominal organ, the fetal heart tones (FHTs) can be heard with an ultrasound fetoscope or an ultrasound stethoscope. To hear the FHTs the instrument is placed in the midline, just above the symphysis pubis, and firm pressure is applied. The woman and her family should be offered the op-

Box 11-3

Protocol for Blood Pressure Measurement

1. Measure blood pressure with the woman seated (ambulatory) or in a 30-degree tilt on her left side.
2. After positioning, allow the woman at least 5 minutes of quiet rest before blood pressure measurement, to encourage relaxation.
3. Use the right arm for blood pressure measurement.
4. Hold the arm in a roughly horizontal position at heart level.
5. Use the proper-sized cuff (cuff should cover approximately 80% of the upper arm).
6. Maintain a slow, steady deflation rate.
7. Take the average of two readings at least 6 hours apart to minimize recorded blood pressure variations across time.
8. Use Korotkoff phase V (disappearance of sound) for recording the diastolic value (some sources recommend recording both phase IV [the muffled sound] and phase V).
9. Use accurate equipment.
10. If interchanging manual and electronic devices, use caution in interpreting different blood pressure values.

Box 11-4

Signs of Potential Complications During the First, Second, and Third Trimesters

FIRST TRIMESTER

Signs/Symptoms	Possible Causes
Severe vomiting	Hyperemesis gravidarum
Chills, fever	Infection
Burning on urination	Infection
Diarrhea	Infection
Abdominal cramping; vaginal bleeding	Miscarriage, ectopic pregnancy

SECOND AND THIRD TRIMESTERS

Signs/Symptoms	Possible Causes
Persistent, severe vomiting	Hyperemesis gravidarum, hypertension, pregnancy-induced hypertension (PIH)
Sudden discharge of fluid from vagina before 37 weeks	Premature rupture of membranes (PROM)
Vaginal bleeding, severe abdominal pain	Miscarriage, placenta previa, abruptio placentae
Chills, fever, burning on urination, diarrhea	Infection
Severe backache or flank pain	Kidney infection or stones; preterm labor
Change in fetal movements: absence of fetal movements after quickening, any unusual change in pattern or amount	Fetal jeopardy or intrauterine fetal death
Uterine contractions; pressure; cramping before 37 weeks	Preterm labor
Visual disturbances: blurring, double vision, or spots	Hypertensive conditions, PIH
Swelling of face or fingers and over sacrum	Hypertensive conditions, PIH
Headaches: severe, frequent, or continuous	Hypertensive conditions, PIH
Muscular irritability or convulsions	Hypertensive conditions, PIH
Epigastric or abdominal pain (perceived as severe stomachache)	Hypertensive conditions, PIH, abruptio placentae
Glycosuria, positive glucose tolerance test reaction	Gestational diabetes mellitus
Sudden weight gain 2+ kg/wk	PIH

portunity to listen to the FHTs. The health status of the fetus is assessed at each visit for the remainder of the pregnancy.

Fundal Height. During the second trimester, the uterus becomes an abdominal organ. The fundal height, or measurement of the height of the uterus above the symphysis pubis, is used as one indicator of fetal growth. The measurement also provides a gross estimate of the duration of pregnancy. During the second and third trimesters (weeks 18 to 30), the height of the fundus in centimeters is approximately the same as the number of weeks gestation, if the woman's bladder is empty at the time of measurement (Cunningham et al, 1997). In addition, measurement of fundal height may aid in the identification of high risk factors. A stable or decreased fundal height may indicate the presence of intrauterine growth restriction (IUGR); an excessive increase could indicate the presence of multifetal gestation or hydramnios.

A paper tape measure or a pelvimeter may be used to measure fundal height. To increase the reliability of the measurement, the same person could examine the pregnant woman at each of her prenatal visits; often this is not possible. Ideally a protocol should be established for the setting in which the measurement technique is explicitly set forth, and the woman's position on the examining table, the measuring device, and method of measurement used are specified. Fig. 11-7 presents two methods of measuring fundal height.

Gestational Age. In an uncomplicated pregnancy, fetal gestational age is estimated after the duration of pregnancy and the EDB are determined. Fetal gestational age is determined from the menstrual history, contraceptive history, and pregnancy test results, and the following findings obtained from the clinical evaluation:

- First uterine size estimate: date, size
- FH first heard: date, Doppler stethoscope, fetoscope
- Date of quickening
- Current fundal height, estimated fetal weight (EFW)
- Current week of gestation by history of LMP and/or ultrasound
- Ultrasound: date, week of gestation, biparietal diameter (BPD)
- Reliability of dates

Quickening ("feeling life") refers to the mother's first perception of fetal movement. It usually occurs between weeks 16 and 20 of gestation and is initially experienced as a fluttering sensation.

Routine use of ultrasound examination (also called a sonogram) in early pregnancy has been recommended (Crowley, 1998), and many health care providers have this equipment available in the office. This procedure may be used to establish the duration of pregnancy if the woman cannot give a precise date for her LMP or if the size of the uterus does not conform to the EDB as calculated by Nägele's rule. Ultrasound also provides information about the well-being of the fetus; however, the routine use of ultrasound has not been found to substantively improve fetal outcome (Neilson, 1998).

Health Status. The assessment of fetal health status includes consideration of fetal movement, the fetal heart rate and rhythm, and abnormal maternal or fetal symptoms.

The mother is instructed to note the extent and timing of fetal movements and to report immediately if the pattern changes or if movement ceases. Regular movement has been found to be a reliable indicator of fetal health. The FHR is checked on routine visits once it has been heard (Fig. 11-8). Early in the second trimester the heartbeat may be heard with the Doppler stethoscope (Fig. 11-8, *B*). Before the fetus can be palpated by Leopold's maneuvers (see Fig. 18-5), the scope is moved around the abdomen until the heartbeat is heard. Each nurse develops a set pattern for searching the abdomen for the heartbeat: for example, starting in the midline about 2 to 3 cm above the symphysis, followed by the left lower quadrant, and so on. The FHR is counted, and the quality and rhythm are noted. Later in the second trimester the FHR can be determined with the fetoscope or Pinard's stethoscope (Fig. 11-8, *A* and *C*). A normal rate and rhythm are other good indicators of fetal health. Once the heartbeat is noted, its absence is cause for immediate investigation.

Intensive investigation of fetal health status is initiated if any maternal or fetal complications arise (e.g., maternal hypertension, IUGR, premature rupture of membranes [PROM], irregular or absent FHR, absence of fetal movements after quickening). Careful, precise, and concise recording of patient responses and laboratory results contributes to the continuous supervision vital to ensuring the well-being of the mother and fetus.

Laboratory Tests. The number of routine laboratory tests done during pregnancy is limited. A clean-catch urine specimen is used to test for levels of glucose, protein, and nitrites and leukocytes at each follow-up visit. Urine specimens for culture and sensitivity, as well as blood samples, are obtained only if signs and symptoms warrant. A hematocrit determination is done at each visit in some offices. A blood specimen is obtained at 16 weeks to determine the alpha-fetoprotein (AFP) level.

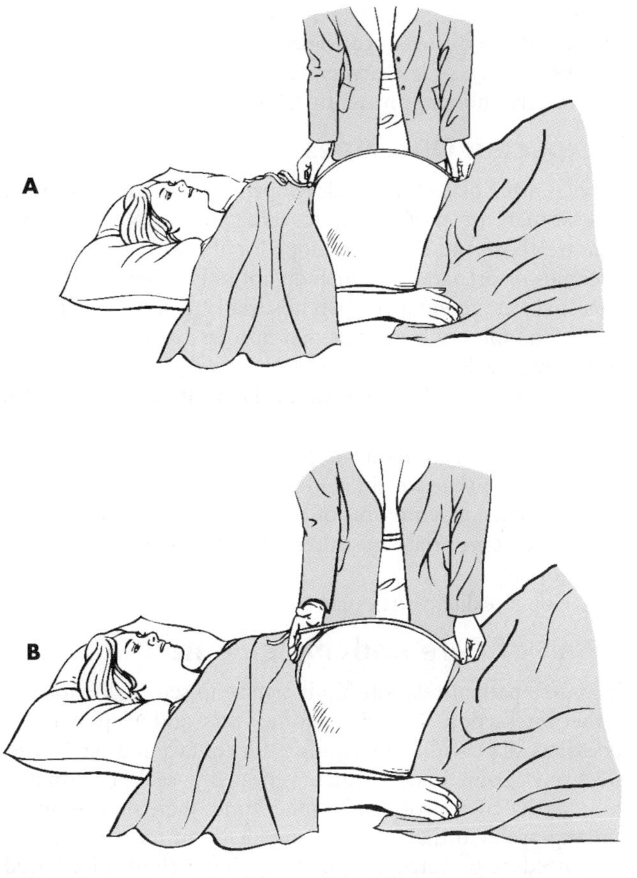

FIG. 11-7 • Measurement of fundal height from symphysis that **A,** includes the upper curve of the fundus and **B,** does not include the upper curve of the fundus. Note position of hands and measuring tape.

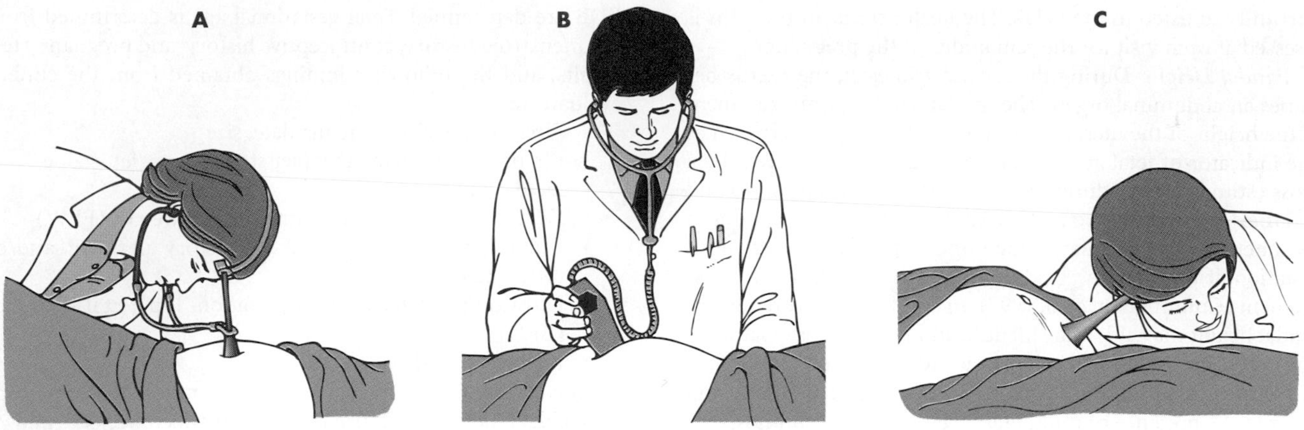

FIG. 11-8 • Detecting fetal heartbeat. **A,** Fetoscope (18 to 20 weeks). **B,** Doppler ultrasound stethoscope (12 weeks). **C,** Pinard's stethoscope. NOTE: Hands should not touch stethoscope while nurse is listening.

The multiple marker test, or triple screen test, is used to detect Down syndrome. Done between 16 and 18 weeks of gestation, it measures maternal serum alpha-fetoprotein (MSAFP), hCG, and unconjugated estriol. Adjusted values are combined to yield the risk for Down syndrome. Low levels may be associated with Down syndrome and other chromosomal abnormalities (Cunningham et al, 1997).

The following blood tests are repeated as necessary: RPR/VDRL test for syphilis; complete blood count with hematocrit, hemoglobin, and differential values; antibody screen (Kell, Duffy, rubella, toxoplasmosis, anti-Rh, HIV); sickle cell; and level of folacin when indicated. If not done earlier in pregnancy, a glucose screen for women over age 25 is performed. Glucose challenge is usually done between 24 and 28 weeks. Cervical and vaginal smears are repeated as necessary to examine for chlamydia organisms, gonorrhea, and herpes simplex virus types 1 and 2. Group B streptococcus (GBS) testing is done between 35 and 37 weeks of gestation; cultures collected earlier will not accurately predict GBS status at time of birth.

Other Tests. Other diagnostic tests are available to assess the health status of both the pregnant woman and the fetus. Ultrasonography, for example, may be performed to determine the status of the pregnancy and to confirm gestational age of the fetus. Amniocentesis, a procedure used to obtain amniotic fluid for analysis, may be needed to evaluate the fetus for genetic disorders or gestational maturity. These and other tests used to determine health risks for the mother and infant are described in Chapters 9 and 17.

➤ Nursing Diagnoses

The diagnoses that follow are examples of the nursing diagnoses that may be appropriate in the prenatal period:

- Anxiety related to:
  —Physical discomforts of pregnancy
  —Ambivalent and labile emotions
  —Changes in family dynamics
  —Fetal well-being
  —Ability to manage anticipated labor
- Altered family processes related to:
  —Changing roles and responsibilities
  —Inadequate understanding of physical and emotional changes in pregnancy
  —Increased concern about labor
- Altered health maintenance related to knowledge deficit regarding self-care measures for:
  —Posture and body mechanics
  —Rest and relaxation
  —Personal hygiene
  —Activity and exercise
  —Safety
- Sleep pattern disturbance related to:
  —Discomforts of late pregnancy
  —Anxiety about approaching labor

➤ Expected Outcomes

Individualized plans that are developed mutually with the pregnant woman are more likely to result in desirable outcomes than are those the nurse develops for the woman. Measured outcomes of prenatal care include not only physical outcomes but also developmental and psychosocial outcomes. The following are examples of outcomes that may be expected. The pregnant woman will:

- Indicate decreased anxiety about the health of her fetus and herself.
- Describe improved family dynamics.
- Show appropriate weight gain patterns.
- Report signs or symptoms of complications.
- Describe appropriate measures taken to relieve physical discomforts.
- Develop a realistic birth plan.

➤ Plan of Care and Implementation

The nurse-patient relationship is critical in setting the tone for further interaction. The clinic, home visits, and telephone conversations all provide opportunities for contact and can be used effectively. Sometimes women repeatedly seek information about a particular problem. At other times there may be an underlying problem that the woman is hesitant to bring up. The nurse needs to be perceptive in identifying such unvoiced needs and can help the woman by asking for a patient-generated solution and a subsequent report of its effectiveness.

Care Paths. Because of the large number of health care professionals involved in care of the expectant mother, unintentional gaps or overlaps in care may occur. To better coordinate prenatal care services for childbearing families, care paths are used to improve consistency of care and reduce costs (Simon, Heaps, and Chodroff, 1997). Care paths may also contribute to improved satisfaction of families with the prenatal care provided (Fig. 11-9).

Education for Self-Care. Health maintenance is an important aspect of prenatal care. Patient participation in the care ensures prompt reporting of untoward responses to pregnancy. Patient assumption of responsibility for health maintenance is assisted by a readiness to learn and by the nurse's understanding of maternal adaptations to the growth of the unborn child. Nurses provide women with the information necessary for adherence to health care guidelines.

The expectant mother needs information about many topics. The nurse who is observant, listens, and knows typical concerns of expectant parents can anticipate what questions will be asked and can also prompt mothers and their partners to discuss what is on their minds. Printed literature can be given to supplement the individualized teaching the nurse provides, and women often avidly read books and pamphlets related to their own experience. When nurses read the literature before they distribute it, they have an opportunity to point out areas that may not correspond with local health care practices. Patients who receive conflicting advice or instruction are likely to grow increasingly frustrated with members of the health care team and the care provided. Several topics that may cause concern in pregnant women are discussed in the following sections.

Nutrition. Proper nutrition is important in the maintenance of maternal health during pregnancy and in the provision of adequate nutrients for embryonic and fetal development. The nourishment the fetus receives from its mother influences health in later life (Campbell-Brown and Hytten, 1998). Assessing a woman's nutritional status and providing information on nutrition are part of the nurse's responsibilities in providing prenatal care. In some settings a registered dietitian conducts classes for pregnant women on the topics of nutritional status and nutrition during pregnancy or interviews them to assess their knowledge of these topics. Nurses can refer women to a registered dietitian if a need is revealed during the nursing assessment. (For detailed information concerning maternal and fetal nutritional needs and related nursing care, see Chapter 12.)

Personal Hygiene. During pregnancy, the sebaceous (sweat) glands are highly active because of hormonal influences, and women often perspire freely. They may be reassured that the increase is normal and that their previous patterns of perspiration will return after the postpartum period. Washing the body regularly is basic to good personal hygiene. Baths and warm showers can be therapeutic because they relax tense, tired muscles; help counter insomnia; and make the pregnant woman feel fresh. Tub bathing is permitted even in late pregnancy because little water enters the vagina unless under pressure. However, later in pregnancy, when the woman's center of gravity lowers, she is at risk for falling. Tub bathing is contraindicated after rupture of the membranes.

Prevention of Urinary Tract Infection. Because of dramatic changes that occur in the renal system during pregnancy, urinary tract infections are common, but they may be asymptomatic. Women should be instructed to inform their health care provider if blood or pain occurs with urination. These infections pose a risk to the mother and fetus; thus, the prevention or early treatment of these infections is essential (Polivka, Nickel, and Wilkins, 1997).

The nurse can assess the woman's understanding and use of good handwashing techniques before and after urinating and whether she knows to wipe from front to back. Soft, absorbent toilet tissue (preferably white and unscented) should be used; harsh, scented, or printed toilet paper may cause irritation. Bubble bath or other bath oils should be avoided because these may be irritating to the urethra. Women should wear underpants and panty hose with a cotton crotch and avoid wearing tight-fitting slacks or jeans for long periods; anything that allows a buildup of heat and moisture in the genital area may foster the growth of bacteria.

Some women do not consume enough fluid and food. After ascertaining the woman's food preferences, the nurse should advise the woman to drink 2 to 3 liters (8 to 12 glasses) of liquid a day to maintain an adequate fluid intake that ensures frequent urination. Pregnant women should not limit fluids in an effort to reduce the frequency of urination. Women need to know that if urine looks dark (concentrated), they need to increase their fluid intake. The consumption of yogurt and acidophilus milk may also help prevent urinary tract and vaginal infections.

The nurse should review healthy urination practices with the woman. Women should be told not to ignore the urge to urinate because holding urine lengthens the time bacteria are in the bladder and allows them to multiply. Women should plan ahead when faced with situations that may normally require them to delay urination (e.g., a long car ride). They should always urinate before going to bed at night. Bacteria also can be introduced during intercourse. Women are therefore advised to urinate before and after intercourse and then drink a large glass of water to promote additional urination.

Kegel Exercises. Kegel exercises (exercises for the pelvic floor) strengthen the muscles around the reproductive organs and improve muscle tone. Many women are not aware of the muscles of the pelvic floor until it is pointed out that these are the muscles used during urination and sexual intercourse and can be consciously controlled. The pelvic floor muscles encircle the outlet through which the baby must pass; it is important that they be exercised because a toned muscle can stretch and contract readily at birth. Practice of pelvic muscle exercise during pregnancy also results in fewer complaints of urinary incontinence in late pregnancy and postpartum (Sampselle et al, 1998). (See Patient Teaching box, p. 39.)

Preparation for Breastfeeding the Newborn. Pregnant women are usually eager to discuss their plans for feeding the newborn. Breast milk is the food of choice, in part because breastfeeding is associated with a decreased incidence in perinatal morbidity and mortality. The American Academy of Pediatrics recommends breastfeeding for at least 1 year. However, a deep-seated aversion to breastfeeding by the mother or partner; the mother's need for certain medications; and certain medical complications, such as active tuberculosis, newly diagnosed breast cancer, and hepatitis C, are contraindications to breastfeeding (Lawrence, 1999). Hepatitis B antigen has not been shown to be transmitted through breast milk; it is recommended as an added precaution, however, that infants born to hepatitis B antigen–positive women receive the hepatitis B vaccine and the hepatitis B immune globulin (HBIG) immediately after birth. Nursing is discouraged in women who are HIV positive because of the risk of HIV transmission.

A woman's decision about the method of infant feeding is made before pregnancy (Skinner et al, 1997), thus it is essential to educate women of childbearing age about the benefits of

Prenatal Care Pathway

PRENATAL EDUCATION CLINICAL PATHWAY

INITIAL VISIT AND ORIENTATION ________ SOCIAL SERVICE ________ DIETITIAN:

I. EARLY PREGNANCY (WEEKS 1-20) (initial and date after education given)

Fetal growth and development ________
Maternal changes ________
Lifestyle: exercise/stress/nutrition ________
  Drugs, OTC, tobacco, alcohol ________
  STIs ________
Psycho/social adjustments: ________
  FOB involved/accepts ________
  Baby for adoption ________

Testing: Labs ________ Ultrasound ________
Possible complications: ________
  a. Threatened miscarriage ________
  b. Diabetes ________
  c. ____________ ________
Introduction to breastfeeding ________
Acceptance ________
  and childbirth preparation ________
Dietary follow-up ________

II. MIDPREGNANCY (WEEKS 21-27) (initial and date after education given)

Fetal growth and development ________
Maternal changes ________
Daily fetal movement ________
Possible complications: ________
  a. Preterm labor prevention ________
  b. PIH symptoms ________
  c. ____________ ________

Breast or bottle-feeding ________
Birth plan initiated ________
Childbirth preparation ____________________
____
Dietary follow-up ________

III. LATE PREGNANCY (WEEKS 28-40) (initial and date after education given)

Fetal growth and development ________
Fetal evaluation: ________
Daily movement ________ NSTs ________
Kick counts ________ BPPs ________
Maternal changes ________
Possible complications:
  a. Preterm labor prevention ________
  b. PIH symptoms ________
  c. ____________ ________
Breastfeeding preparation:
  Nipple assessment ________
Dietary follow-up ________

Childbirth preparation:
  S/S of labor; labor process ________
  Pain management: natural childbirth, ________
    meds, epidural
  Cesarean; VBAC ________
  Birth plan complete ________
  Review hospital policies ________
Parenting preparation:
Pediatrician ________ Childcare ________
Siblings ________ Immunizations ________
Car seat/safety ________
Postpartum:
  P.P. care/checkup ________
  Emotional changes ________
  B.C. options ________
  Safe sex/STIs ________

Signature: ____________________ ____________________ ____________________

FIG. 11-9 • Prenatal care pathway.

breastfeeding. The woman and her partner are encouraged to decide what method of feeding is suitable for them; however, the benefits of breastfeeding should be emphasized. Once the couple has been given information about the advantages and disadvantages of bottle-feeding and breastfeeding, they can make an informed choice. Health care providers support these decisions and provide any needed assistance.

The pinch test is done to determine whether the nipple is everted or inverted (Fig. 11-10). To perform the pinch test, the woman places her thumb and forefinger on her areola and presses inward gently. This action will cause her nipple either to stand erect or to invert. Most nipples will stand erect.

Exercises to break the adhesions that cause the nipple to invert do not work and may in fact cause uterine contractions (Lawrence, 1999). The use of breast shells by women with flat or inverted nipples is recommended (Fig. 11-11). Breast shells work by exerting a continuous, gentle pressure around the areola that pushes the nipple through a central opening in the inner shield. Breast shells should be worn for 1 to 2 hours daily during the last trimester of pregnancy. They should be worn for gradually increasing lengths of time (Lawrence, 1999). Breast stimulation is contraindicated in women at risk for preterm labor.

The woman is taught to cleanse the nipples with warm water to prevent blocking of the ducts with dried colostrum. Soap, ointments, alcohol, and tinctures should not be applied because they remove protective oils that keep nipples supple. The use of these substances may cause the nipple to crack during early lactation (Lawrence, 1999).

The woman who plans to breastfeed should purchase a nursing bra that will accommodate her increased breast size during the last few months of pregnancy and during lactation. If her breasts are very heavy, or if the woman feels uncomfortable with the weight unsupported, the bra can be worn day and night.

Dental Health. Dental care during pregnancy is especially important because nausea during pregnancy may lead to poor oral hygiene and allow dental caries to develop. However, no physiologic alteration during gestation can cause dental caries. Because calcium and phosphorus in the teeth are fixed in enamel, the old adage "for every child a tooth" is not true.

There is no scientific evidence indicating that filling teeth or even dental extraction using local or nitrous oxide/oxygen anesthesia causes miscarriage or premature labor. Antibacterial therapy should be considered for sepsis, however, especially in pregnant women who have had rheumatic heart disease or nephritis. Emergency dental surgery is not contraindicated during pregnancy; however, the risks and benefits of surgery need to be explained to the mother.

Physical Activity. Physical activity promotes a feeling of well-being in the pregnant woman. It improves circulation, promotes relaxation and rest, and counteracts boredom (as it does in the nonpregnant woman). Detailed exercise tips for pregnancy are presented in the Home Care box.

Exercises that help relieve the low back pain that often arises during the second trimester because of the increased weight of the fetus are demonstrated in Fig. 11-12.

A

B

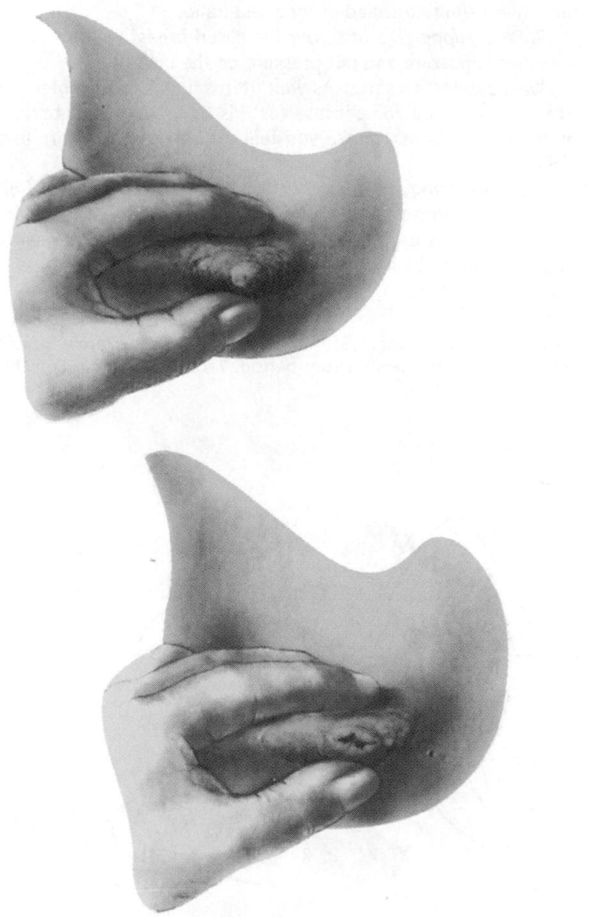

FIG. 11-10 • Pinch test. **A,** Normal nipple everts with gentle pressure. **B,** Inverted nipple inverts with gentle pressure. (Modified from Lawrence R: *Breastfeeding: a guide for the medical profession,* ed 5, St Louis, 1999, Mosby.)

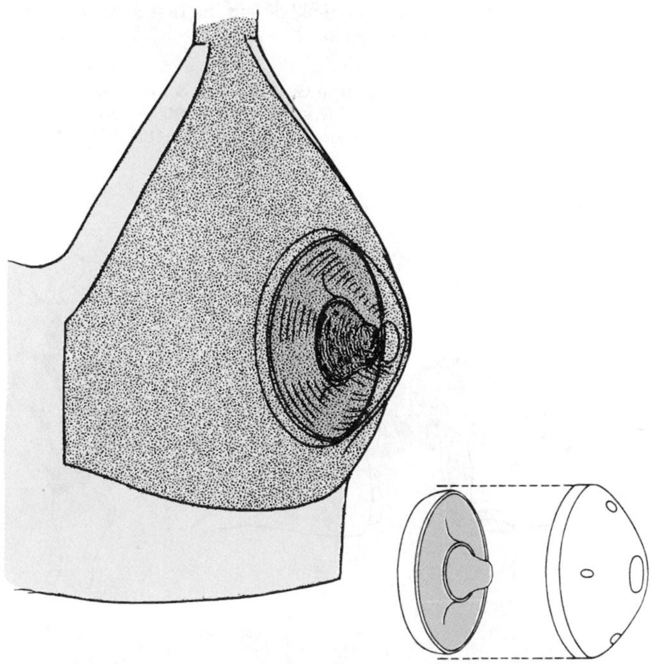

FIG. 11-11 • Breast shell in place inside bra to evert nipple. (Modified from Lawrence R: *Breastfeeding: a guide for the medical profession,* ed 5, St Louis, 1999, Mosby.)

Home Care

EXERCISE TIPS FOR PREGNANT WOMEN

Consult your health care provider when you know or suspect you are pregnant. Discuss your medical and obstetric history, your current exercise regimen, and the exercises you would like to continue throughout pregnancy.

Seek help in determining an exercise routine that is well within your limit of tolerance, especially if you have not been exercising regularly.

Consider decreasing weight-bearing exercises (jogging, running) and concentrating on non–weight-bearing activities such as swimming, cycling, or stretching. If you are a runner, starting in your seventh month, you may wish to walk instead.

Avoid risky activities such as surfing, mountain climbing, skydiving, and racquetball because such activities that require precise balance and coordination may be dangerous. Avoid activities that require holding your breath and bearing down (Valsalva's maneuver). Jerky, bouncy motions also should be avoided.

Exercise regularly at least three times a week, as long as you are healthy, to improve muscle tone and increase or maintain your stamina. If you do exercises sporadically, this may put undue strain on your muscles. Limit activity to shorter intervals. Exercise for 10 to 15 minutes, rest for 2 to 3 minutes, then exercise for another 10 to 15 minutes.

Decrease your exercise level as your pregnancy progresses. The normal alterations of advancing pregnancy, such as decreased cardiac reserve and increased respiratory effort, may produce physiologic stress if you exercise strenuously for a long time.

Take your pulse every 10 to 15 minutes while you are exercising. If it is more than 140 beats/min, slow down until it returns to a maximum of 90 beats/min. You should be able to converse easily while exercising. If you cannot, you need to slow down.

Avoid becoming overheated for extended periods of time. It is best not to exercise for more than 35 minutes, especially in hot, humid weather. As your body temperature rises, the heat is transmitted to your fetus. Prolonged or repeated elevation of fetal temperature may result in birth defects, especially during the first 3 months. Your temperature should not exceed 38° C.

Avoid the use of hot tubs and saunas.

Warm-up and stretching exercises prepare your joints for more strenuous exercise and lessen the likelihood of strain or injury to your joints. After the fourth month of gestation you should not perform exercises flat on your back.

A cool-down period of mild activity involving your legs after an exercise period will help bring your respiration, heart, and metabolic rates back to normal and prevent the pooling of blood in the exercised muscles.

Rest for 10 minutes after exercising, lying on your side. As the uterus grows, it puts pressure on a major vein in your abdomen, which carries blood to your heart. Lying on your side removes the pressure and promotes return circulation from your extremities and muscles to your heart, thereby increasing blood flow to your placenta and fetus. You should rise gradually from the floor to prevent dizziness or fainting (orthostatic hypotension).

Drink two or three 8 oz glasses of water after you exercise to replace the body fluids lost through perspiration. While exercising, drink water whenever you feel the need.

Increase your caloric intake to replace the calories burned during exercise and provide the extra energy needs of pregnancy. (Pregnancy alone requires an additional 300 kcal/day.) Choose such high-protein foods as fish, milk, cheese, eggs, or meat.

Take your time. This is not the time to be competitive or train for activities requiring speed or long endurance.

Wear a supportive bra. Your increased breast weight may cause changes in posture and put pressure on the ulnar nerve.

Wear supportive shoes. As your uterus grows, your center of gravity shifts and you compensate for this by arching your back. These natural changes may make you feel off balance and more likely to fall.

Stop exercising immediately if you experience shortness of breath, dizziness, numbness, tingling, pain of any kind, more than four uterine contractions per hour, decreased fetal activity, or vaginal bleeding, and consult your health care provider.

Modified from Artal R, Subak-Sharpe G: *Pregnancy & exercise,* New York, 1992, Delacorte Press; Fishbein E, Phillips M: How safe is exercise during pregnancy? *J Obstet Gynecol Neonatal Nurs* 19(1):45, 1990; ACOG: Exercise during pregnancy and the postpartum period, *Technical Bulletin* Feb:189, 1994; Pivarnik J: Maternal exercise in pregnancy, *Sports Med* 18:215, 1994.

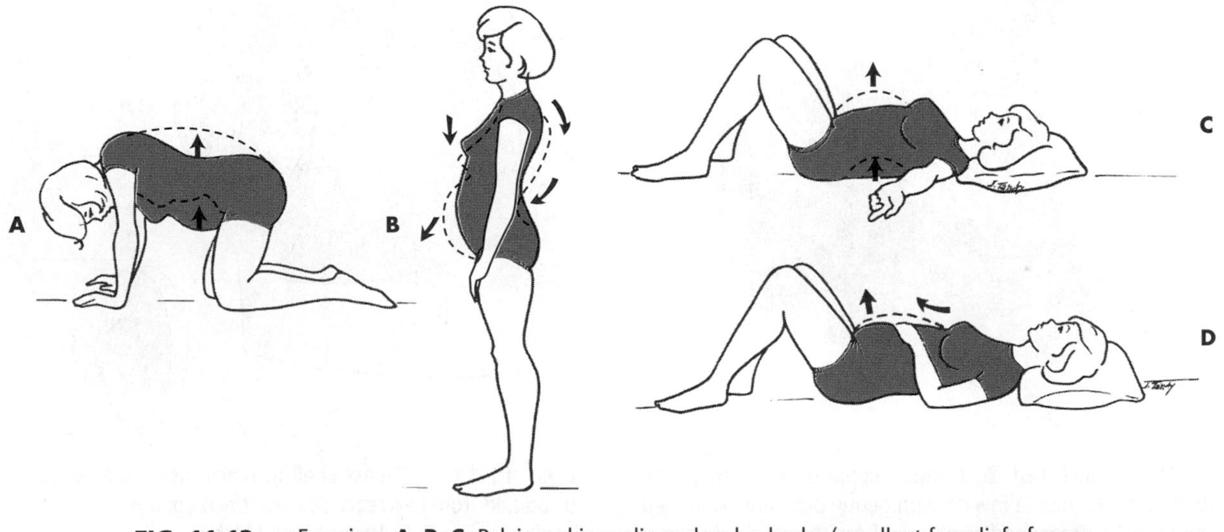

FIG. 11-12 • Exercises. **A, B, C,** Pelvic rocking relieves low backache (excellent for relief of menstrual cramps as well). **D,** Abdominal breathing aids relaxation and lifts abdominal wall off uterus.

Posture and Body Mechanics. Many maternal adaptations predispose the woman to suffering backache and incurring possible injury. The pregnant woman's center of gravity changes, pelvic joints soften and relax, and stress is placed on abdominal musculature as pregnancy progresses. Poor posture and body mechanics contribute to the discomfort and potential for injury. To minimize these problems, women can acquire a kinesthetic sense for good body posture (Fig. 11-13). The activities described in the Home Care box can also promote greater physical comfort.

Community Focus

AEROBIC EXERCISE DURING PREGNANCY

Maternal exercise affects the fetus. Increases in fetal heart rate following brief periods of maternal exercise have been documented. Regular exercise is recommended for pregnant women to maintain physical fitness. Aerobic exercise has documented beneficial effects on maternal fitness with no major benefits or risks identified for the fetus. Prenatal education programs and community centers could provide a major service to pregnant women by appropriate exercise counseling or by initiating exercise classes for women in various states of pregnancy. Posters and pamphlets could be made available as part of the education efforts.

Data from: Kramer M: Regular aerobic exercise during pregnancy (Cochrane Review), *The Cochrane Library,* Issue 3, 2000. Oxford: Update Software.

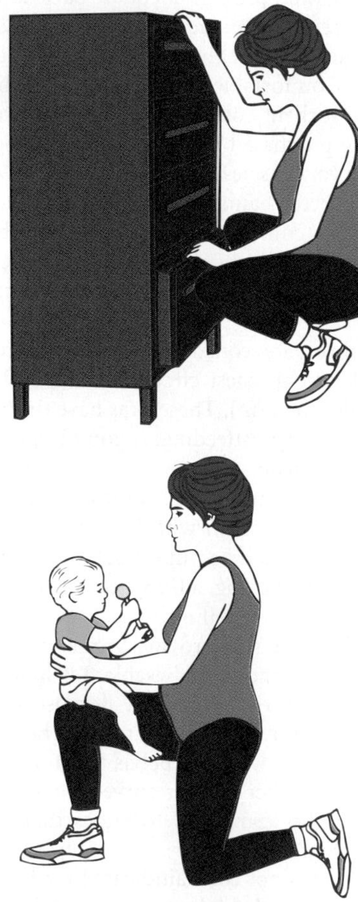

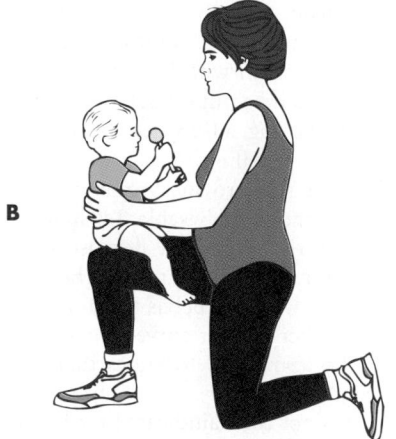

FIG. 11-13 • Correct body mechanics. **A,** Squatting. **B,** Lifting.

Rest and Relaxation. The pregnant woman is encouraged to plan regular rest periods, particularly as pregnancy advances. The side-lying position is recommended to promote uterine perfusion and fetoplacental oxygenation by eliminating pressure on the ascending vena cava and descending aorta, which can lead to supine hypotension. The mother should also be shown the way to rise slowly from a side-lying position to prevent strain on the back and to minimize the orthostatic hypotension caused by changes in position common in the latter part of pregnancy. To stretch and rest back muscles at home or at work, the nurse can suggest the woman do the following exercises:

- Stand behind a chair. Support and balance yourself using the back of the chair (Fig. 11-14). Squat for 30 seconds; stand for 15 seconds. Repeat six times, in several sets per day, as needed.
- While sitting in a chair, lower your head to your knees for 30 seconds. Raise your head up. Repeat six times, several times per day, as needed.

Conscious relaxation is the process of releasing tension from the mind and body through deliberate effort and practice. The ability to relax consciously and intentionally can be beneficial for the following reasons:

- It can relieve the normal discomforts related to pregnancy.
- It can reduce stress and therefore diminish pain perception during the childbearing cycle.

Home Care

POSTURE AND BODY MECHANICS

To Prevent or Relieve Backache

Do pelvic tilt:

- Pelvic tilt (rock) on hands and knees (see Fig. 11-12, *A*) and while sitting in straight-back chair.
- Pelvic tilt (rock) in standing position against a wall, or lying on floor (see Fig. 11-12, *B* and *C*).
- Perform abdominal muscle contractions during pelvic tilt while standing, lying, or sitting to help strengthen rectus abdominis muscle (see Fig. 11-12, *D*).
- Use good body mechanics.
- Use leg muscles to reach objects on or near floor. Bend at the knees, not the back. Knees are bent to lower body to squatting position. Feet are kept 12 to 18 inches apart to provide a solid base to maintain balance (Fig. 11-13, *A*).
- Lift with the legs. To lift heavy object (e.g., young child), one foot is placed slightly in front of the other and kept flat as woman lowers herself onto one knee. She lifts the weight holding it close to her body and never higher than the chest. To stand up or sit down, one leg is placed slightly behind the other as she raises or lowers herself (Fig. 11-13, *B*).

To Restrict the Lumbar Curve

For prolonged standing (e.g., ironing or because of employment), place one foot on low footstool or box; change positions often.

Move car seat forward so that knees are bent and higher than hips. If needed, use a small pillow to support low back area.

Sit in chairs low enough to allow both feet to be placed on floor, preferably with knees higher than hips.

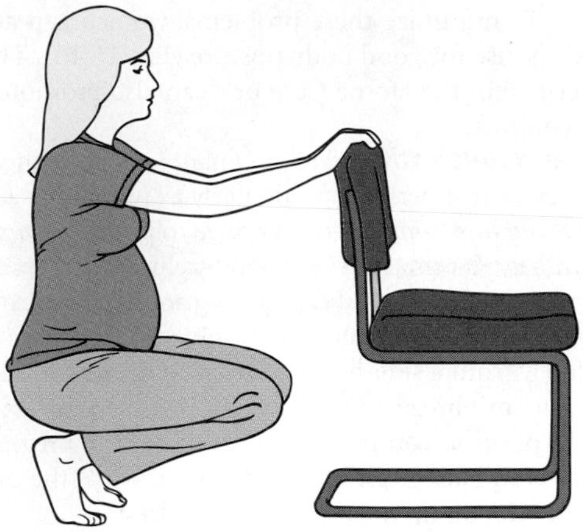

FIG. 11-14 • Squatting for muscle relaxation and strengthening and for keeping leg and hip joints flexible.

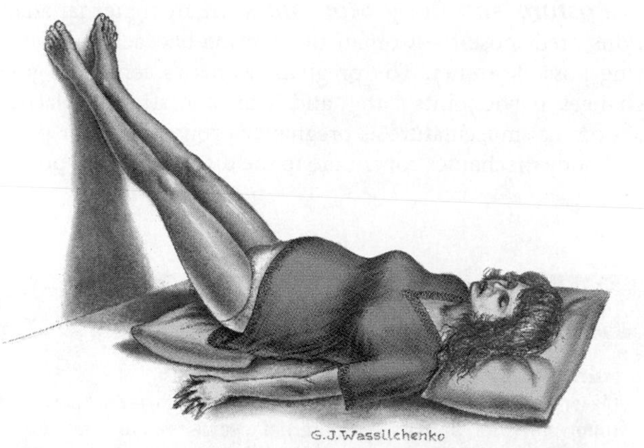

FIG. 11-15 • Position for resting legs and for reducing edema and varicosities. Encourage the woman with vulvar varicosities to include a pillow under her hips.

Box 11-5

Conscious Relaxation Tips

Preparation: Loosen clothing, assume a comfortable sitting or side-lying position with all parts of body well supported with pillows. The use of soothing music is optional.

Beginning: Allow self to feel warm and comfortable. Inhale and exhale slowly, and imagine peaceful relaxation coming over each part of the body, starting with the neck and working down to the toes. People who learn conscious relaxation often speak of feeling relaxed even if some discomfort is present.

Maintenance: Use imagery (fantasy or daydream) to maintain the state of relaxation. Using *active imagery,* imagine yourself moving or doing some activity and experiencing its sensations. Using *passive imagery,* imagine yourself watching a scene, such as a lovely sunset.

Awakening: Return to the wakeful state gradually. Slowly begin to take in stimuli from the surrounding environment.

Further retention and development of the skill: Practice regularly for some periods each day, for example, at the same hour for 10 to 15 minutes each day, to feel refreshed, revitalized, and invigorated.

- It can heighten self-awareness and trust in one's own ability to control responses and functions.
- It can help the woman cope with stress in everyday life situations, whether she is pregnant or not.

The techniques for conscious relaxation are numerous and varied. The guidelines given in Box 11-5 can be used by anyone.

Employment. Employment of pregnant women usually has no adverse effects on pregnancy outcomes. Job discrimination that is based solely on pregnancy is illegal. However, some job environments pose potential risk to the fetus (e.g., dry cleaning plants, chemical laboratories, and parking garages).

Activities that require a good sense of balance should be discouraged, especially during the last half of pregnancy. Commonly, excessive fatigue is the deciding factor in the termination of employment. Women in sedentary jobs need to walk around at intervals and should neither sit nor stand in one position for long periods. This will counter the sluggish circulation in the legs, which can cause varices and thrombophlebitis to develop. Women should also avoid crossing their legs at the knees because this also fosters such conditions. Standing for long periods also increases the risk of preterm labor. The pregnant woman's chair should provide adequate back support. Use of a footstool can prevent pressure on veins, relieve strain on varicosities, and minimize swelling of feet.

Clothing. Comfortable, loose clothing is best. Washable fabrics (e.g., absorbent cottons) are often preferred. Maternity clothes may be purchased new or found in good condition at thrift shops or garage sales because they rarely wear out. Tight bras and belts, stretch pants, garters, tight-top knee socks, panty girdles, and other constrictive clothing should be avoided because tight clothing over the perineum encourages vaginitis and miliaria (heat rash), and impaired circulation in the legs can cause varices.

Maternity bras are constructed to accommodate the increased breast weight, chest circumference, and size of breast tail tissue (under the arm). These bras have drop-flaps over the nipples to facilitate breastfeeding. A good bra can help prevent neckache and backache.

Elastic hose give considerable comfort and promote greater venous emptying in women with large varicose veins. Ideally, support stockings should be put on before the woman gets out of bed in the morning. Fig. 11-15 demonstrates a position to rest the legs and reduce swelling.

Comfortable shoes that provide firm support and promote good posture and balance are advisable. Tall high heels and platform shoes are not recommended because of the woman's changed center of gravity, which can cause her to lose her balance. In addition, the woman's pelvis tilts forward in the third trimester, increasing her lumbar curve. The resulting leg aches and cramps will be aggravated by shoes that do not provide good support (Fig. 11-16).

Travel. Travel is not contraindicated for low-risk pregnant women, but those with high risk pregnancies are advised to avoid long distance travel after fetal viability has been reached so as to avert the economic and psychologic consequences of

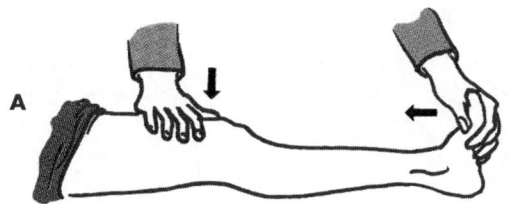

FIG. 11-16 • Relief of muscle spasm (leg cramps). **A,** Another person dorsiflexes foot with knee extended. **B,** Woman stands and leans forward, thereby dorsiflexing foot of affected leg.

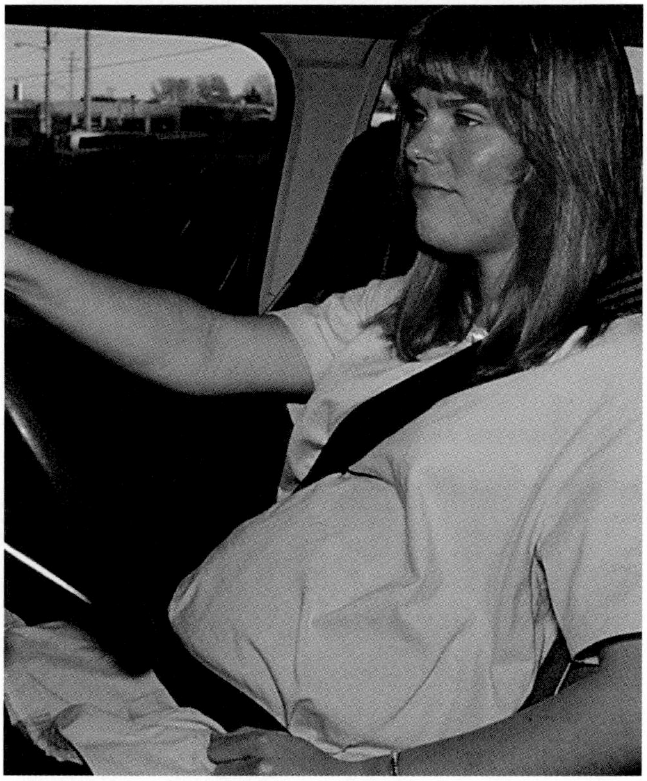

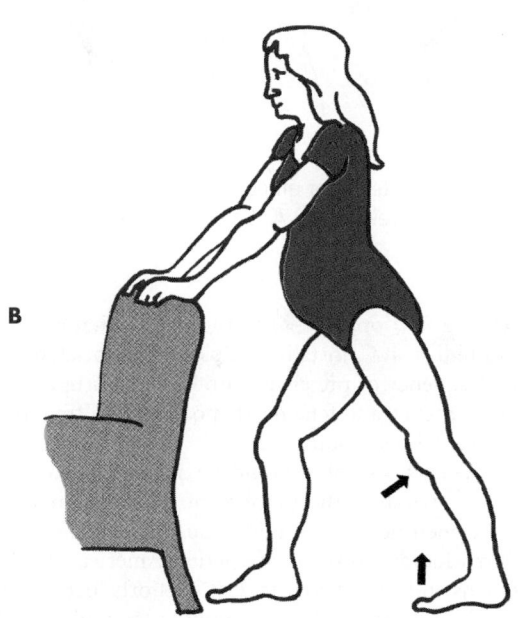

FIG. 11-17 • Proper use of seat belt and headrest. (Courtesy Michael S. Clement, MD, Mesa, AZ.)

giving birth to a preterm infant far from home. Travel to areas where medical care is poor, water is untreated, and malaria is prevalent should be avoided if possible. Women who contemplate foreign travel should be aware that many health insurance carriers do not cover birth in a foreign setting or even hospitalization for preterm labor.

Pregnant women who travel for long distances should schedule periods of activity and rest. While sitting the woman can practice deep breathing, foot circling, and alternately contracting and relaxing different muscle groups. She should avoid becoming fatigued. Although travel in itself is not a cause of adverse outcomes such as miscarriage or preterm labor, certain precautions are recommended while traveling in a car. The woman should always use automobile restraints; a combination lap belt and shoulder harness is the most effective automobile restraint. Both shoulder and lap belts should be used. The lap belt should be worn low across the hip bones and as snug as is comfortable (Fig. 11-17). The shoulder belt should be worn above the pregnant uterus and below the neck to avoid chafing. The pregnant woman should sit upright. The headrest should be used to avoid a whiplash injury.

Maternal death as a result of injury is the most common cause of fetal death. The next most common cause is placental separation. This occurs because body contours change in reaction to the force of a collision. The uterus as a muscular organ can adapt its shape to that of the body, but the placenta lacks the resiliency to change. At the impact of collision, placental separation can occur.

Airline travel in large commercial jets usually poses little risk to the pregnant woman, but policies vary from airline to airline. The pregnant woman is advised to inquire about restrictions or recommendations from her carrier (Cunningham et al, 1997). Magnetometers (metal detectors) used at airport security checkpoints are not harmful to the fetus. The 8% humidity at which cabins are maintained in commercial airlines may result in some water loss; hydration (with water) should be maintained under these conditions. Sitting in the cramped seat of an airliner for prolonged periods may increase the risk of superficial and deep thrombophlebitis. A pregnant woman is encouraged to take a 15-minute walk around the aircraft during each hour of travel to minimize this risk (Patient Teaching box).

Medications. Although much has been learned in recent years about fetal drug toxicity, the possible teratogenicity of many drugs, both prescription and OTC, is still unknown. This is especially true for new medications and combinations of medications. Moreover, certain subclinical errors or deficiencies in intermediate metabolism in the fetus may cause an otherwise harmless drug to be converted into a hazardous one. The great-

Patient Teaching

SAFETY DURING PREGNANCY

Changes in the body due to pregnancy include relaxation of joints, alteration to center of gravity, faintness, and discomforts. Problems with coordination and balance are common. Therefore the woman should follow these guidelines:

- Use good body mechanics.
- Use safety features on tools/vehicles (safety seat belts, shoulder harnesses, headrests, goggles, helmets) as specified.
- Avoid activities requiring coordination, balance, and concentration.
- Take rest periods; reschedule daily activities to meet rest and relaxation needs.

Embryonic and fetal development is vulnerable to environmental teratogens. Many potentially dangerous chemicals are present in the home, yard, and workplace: cleaning agents, paints, sprays, herbicides, and pesticides. The soil and water supply may be unsafe. Therefore the woman should follow these guidelines:

- Read all labels for ingredients and proper use of product.
- Ensure adequate ventilation with clean air.
- Dispose of wastes appropriately.
- Wear gloves when handling chemicals.
- Change job assignments or workplace as necessary.
- Avoid high altitudes (not in pressurized aircraft), which could jeopardize oxygen intake.

est danger of drug-caused developmental defects in the fetus extends from the time of fertilization through the first trimester, a time when the woman may not realize she is pregnant. Self-treatment must be discouraged. The use of all drugs, including OTC medications and vitamins, should be limited and a careful record kept of all therapeutic agents used.

Immunization. Some concern has been raised over the safety of various immunization practices during pregnancy (Cunningham et al, 1997). Immunization with live or attenuated live viruses is contraindicated during pregnancy because of potential teratogenicity. Live virus vaccines include measles (rubeola and rubella), chickenpox, mumps, and the Sabin (oral) poliomyelitis vaccine. Vaccines with killed viruses that may be administered in pregnancy include tetanus, diphtheria, recombinant hepatitis B, rabies, and flu vaccines.

Alcohol, Cigarette Smoke, and Other Substances. A safe level of alcohol consumption during pregnancy has not yet been established. Although the consumption of occasional alcoholic beverages may not be harmful to the mother or her developing embryo or fetus, complete abstinence is strongly advised. Maternal alcoholism is associated with high rates of miscarriage and fetal alcohol syndrome; the risk for miscarriage is dose related (three or more drinks per day) in the first trimester. Growing evidence indicates that the pattern of drinking (i.e., frequency, timing, and duration), especially in the first trimester, is more predictive of fetal damage than the amount (Abel, 1996; Wagner et al, 1998). While nonpregnant women report more alcohol use than do those who are pregnant, the use of at least some alcohol among pregnant women is still too high. This finding underscores the need for more systematic public health efforts to educate women about the hazards of alcohol consumption in pregnancy (Ebrahim et al, 1998).

Cigarette smoking or continued exposure to second-hand smoke (even if the mother does not smoke) is associated with

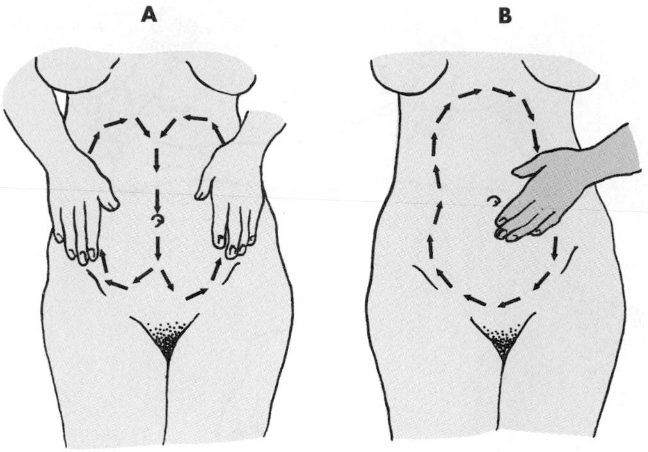

FIG. 11-18 • Patterns for effleurage, a light, rhythmic stroking useful for inducing relaxation. **A,** Self-effleurage. **B,** Effleurage by another.

fetal growth restriction (IUGR) and an increase in perinatal and infant morbidity and mortality. Smoking is associated with an increased frequency of preterm labor, PROM, abruptio placentae, placenta previa, and fetal death, possibly resulting from decreased placental perfusion.

All women who smoke should be strongly encouraged to quit or at least reduce the number of cigarettes they smoke. Pregnant women need to be told about the negative effects of even second-hand smoke on the fetus (American College of Obstetricians and Gynecologists, 1997). Efforts focused on preventing girls and women from beginning to smoke should be intensified (Johnson, 1998).

Most studies of human pregnancy have revealed no association between caffeine consumption and birth defects or low birth weight (LBW) (Cunningham et al, 1997). Because other effects are unknown, however, pregnant women are advised to limit their caffeine intake.

Any drug or environmental agent that enters the pregnant woman's bloodstream has the potential to cross the placenta and harm the fetus. Marijuana, heroin, and cocaine are common examples of such substances. Although substance abuse in pregnancy is a major public health concern, comprehensive care of drug-addicted women improves maternal and neonatal outcomes (Jansson et al, 1996).

Normal Discomforts. Women pregnant for the first time are confronted with symptoms that would be considered abnormal in the nonpregnant state. Much of prenatal care requested by such women is prompted by the need for explanations of the causes of the discomforts and for advice on ways to relieve the discomforts. The discomforts are fairly specific to each trimester of pregnancy. Table 11-2 provides information about the physiology, prevention, and self-care of discomforts (e.g., effleurage [Fig. 11-18]) experienced during the three trimesters. Nurses can do much to allay a first-time mother's anxiety about such symptoms by telling her about them in advance, using terminology that the woman (or couple) can understand. Women who understand the physical discomforts of pregnancy are less apt to become overly anxious about their health. In addition, understanding the rationale for treatment promotes their participation in their care. Interventions should

TABLE 11-2

Discomforts Related to Pregnancy

First Trimester		
Discomfort	**Physiology**	**Education for Self-Care**
Breast changes, new sensation; pain, tingling, tenderness	Hypertrophy of mammary glandular tissue and increased vascularization, pigmentation, and size and prominence of nipples and areolae caused by hormonal stimulation	Wear supportive maternity bras with pads to absorb discharge, may be worn at night; wash with warm water and keep dry; breast tenderness may interfere with sexual expression/foreplay but is temporary
Urgency and frequency of urination	Vascular engorgement and altered bladder function caused by hormones; bladder capacity reduced by enlarging uterus and fetal presenting part	Empty bladder regularly; perform Kegel exercises; limit fluid intake before bedtime; wear perineal pad; report pain or burning sensation to primary health care provider
Languor and malaise; fatigue (early pregnancy, most commonly)	Unexplained; may be caused by increasing levels of estrogen, progesterone, and hCG or by elevated BBT; psychologic response to pregnancy and its required physical/psychologic adaptations	Rest as needed; eat well-balanced diet to prevent anemia
Nausea and vomiting, morning sickness—occurs in 50%-75% of pregnant women; starts between first and second missed periods and lasts until about fourth missed period; may occur any time during day; fathers also may have symptoms	Cause unknown; may result from hormonal changes, possibly hCG; may be partly emotional, reflecting pride in, ambivalence about, or rejection of pregnant state	Avoid empty or overloaded stomach; maintain good posture—give stomach ample room; stop smoking; eat dry carbohydrate on awakening; remain in bed until feeling subsides, or alternate dry carbohydrate 1 hour with fluids such as hot herbal decaffeinated tea, milk, or clear coffee the next hour until feeling subsides; eat five to six small meals per day; avoid fried, odorous, spicy, greasy, or gas-forming foods; consult primary health care provider if intractable vomiting occurs
Ptyalism (excessive salivation) may occur starting 2 to 3 weeks after first missed period	Possibly caused by elevated estrogen levels; may be related to reluctance to swallow because of nausea	Use astringent mouth wash, chew gum, eat hard candy as comfort measures
Gingivitis and epulis (hyperemia, hypertrophy, bleeding, tenderness); condition will disappear spontaneously 1 to 2 months after birth	Increased vascularity and proliferation of connective tissue from estrogen stimulation	Eat well-balanced diet, with adequate protein and fresh fruits and vegetables; brush teeth gently and observe good dental hygiene; avoid infection; see dentist
Nasal stuffiness; epistaxis (nosebleed)	Hyperemia of mucous membranes related to high estrogen levels	Use humidifier; avoid trauma; normal saline nose drops or spray may be used
Leukorrhea: often noted throughout pregnancy	Hormonally stimulated cervix becomes hypertrophic and hyperactive, producing abundant amount of mucus	Not preventable; do not douche; wear perineal pads; perform hygienic practices such as wiping front to back; report to primary health care provider if accompanied by pruritus, foul odor, or change in character or color
Psychosocial dynamics, mood swings, mixed feelings	Hormonal and metabolic adaptations; feelings about female role, sexuality, timing of pregnancy, and resultant changes in life and lifestyle	Participate in pregnancy support group; communicate concerns to partner, family, and others; request referral for supportive services if needed (financial assistance)

Continued

TABLE 11-2
Discomforts Related to Pregnancy—cont'd

Discomfort	Physiology	Education for Self-Care
Second Trimester		
Pigmentation deepens, acne, oily skin	Melanocyte-stimulating hormone (from anterior pituitary)	Not preventable; usually resolves during puerperium
Spider nevi (angiomas) appear over neck, thorax, face, and arms during second or third trimester	Focal networks of dilated arterioles (end-arteries) from increased concentration of estrogens	Not preventable; they fade slowly during late puerperium; rarely disappear completely
Palmar erythema occurs in 50% of pregnant women; may accompany spider nevi	Diffuse reddish mottling over palms and suffused skin over thenar eminencies and fingertips; may be caused by genetic predisposition or hyperestrogenism	Not preventable; condition will fade within 1 week after giving birth
Pruritus (noninflammatory)	Unknown cause; various types as follows: nonpapular; closely aggregated pruritic papules	Keep fingernails short and clean; contact primary health care provider for diagnosis of cause
	Increased excretory function of skin and stretching of skin possible factors	Not preventable; symptomatic; Keri baths; mild sedation
		Distraction; tepid baths with sodium bicarbonate or oatmeal added to water; lotions and oils; change of soaps or reduction in use of soap; loose clothing
Palpitations	Unknown; should not be accompanied by persistent cardiac irregularity	Not preventable; contact primary health care provider if accompanied by symptoms of cardiac decompensation
Supine hypotension (vena cava syndrome) and bradycardia	Induced by pressure of gravid uterus on ascending vena cava when woman is supine; reduces uteroplacental and renal perfusion	Side-lying position or semisitting posture, with knees slightly flexed (see supine hypotension, p. 193)
Faintness and, rarely, syncope (orthostatic hypotension) may persist throughout pregnancy	Vasomotor lability or postural hypotension from hormones; in late pregnancy may be caused by venous stasis in lower extremities	Moderate exercise, deep breathing, vigorous leg movement; avoid sudden changes in position* and warm crowded areas; move slowly and deliberately; keep environment cool; avoid hypoglycemia by eating 5 to 6 small meals per day; wear elastic hose; sit as necessary; if symptoms are serious, contact primary health care provider
Food cravings	Cause unknown; craving determined by culture or geographic area	Not preventable; satisfy craving unless it interferes with well-balanced diet; report unusual cravings to primary health care provider
Heartburn (pyrosis or acid indigestion): burning sensation, occasionally with burping and regurgitation of a little sour-tasting fluid	Progesterone slows gastrointestinal (GI) tract motility and digestion, reverses peristalsis, relaxes cardiac sphincter, and delays emptying time of stomach; stomach displaced upward and compressed by enlarging uterus	Limit or avoid gas-producing or fatty foods and large meals; maintain good posture; sip milk for temporary relief; hot herbal tea; primary health care provider may prescribe antacid between meals; contact primary health care provider for persistent symptoms
Constipation	GI tract motility slowed because of progesterone, resulting in increased resorption of water and drying of stool; intestines compressed by enlarging uterus; predisposition to constipation because of oral iron supplementation	Drink six glasses of water per day; include roughage in diet; moderate exercise; maintain regular schedule for bowel movements; use relaxation techniques and deep breathing; do not take stool softener, laxatives, mineral oil, other drugs, or enemas without first consulting primary health care provider

*Caution woman to rise slowly and sit on edge of bed or to assume hands-and-knee posture before rising, and to get up slowly after sitting or squatting.

TABLE 11-2
Discomforts Related to Pregnancy—cont'd

Second Trimester—cont'd		
Discomfort	**Physiology**	**Education for Self-Care**
Flatulence with bloating and belching	Reduced GI motility because of hormones, allowing time for bacterial action that produces gas; swallowing air	Chew foods slowly and thoroughly; avoid gas-producing foods, fatty foods, large meals; exercise, maintain regular bowel habits
Varicose veins (varicosities): may be associated with aching legs and tenderness; may be present in legs and vulva; hemorrhoids are varicosities in perianal area	Hereditary predisposition; relaxation of smooth muscle walls of veins because of hormones causing tortuous dilated veins in legs and pelvic vasocongestion; condition aggravated by enlarging uterus, gravity, and bearing down for bowel movements; thrombi from leg varices rare but may be produced by hemorrhoids	Avoid obesity, lengthy standing or sitting, constrictive clothing, and constipation and bearing down with bowel movements; moderate exercises; rest with legs and hips elevated (see Fig. 11-15); wear support stockings; thrombosed hemorrhoid may be evacuated; relieve swelling and pain with warm sitz baths, local application of astringent compresses
Leukorrhea: often noted throughout pregnancy	Hormonally stimulated cervix becomes hypertrophic and hyperactive, producing abundant amount of mucus	Not preventable; do not douche; maintain good hygiene; wear perineal pads; report to primary health care provider if accompanied by pruritus, foul odor, or change in character or color
Headaches (through week 26)	Emotional tension (more common than vascular migraine headache); eye strain (refractory errors); vascular engorgement and congestion of sinuses resulting from hormone stimulation	Conscious relaxation; contact primary health care provider for constant "splitting" headache, to assess for PIH
Carpal tunnel syndrome (involves thumb, second, and third fingers, lateral side of little finger)	Compression of median nerve resulting from changes in surrounding tissues; pain, numbness, tingling, burning; loss of skilled movements (typing); dropping of objects	Not preventable; elevate affected arms; splinting of affected hand may help; regressive after pregnancy; surgery is curative
Periodic numbness, tingling of fingers (acrodysesthesia) occurs in 5% of pregnant women	Brachial plexus traction syndrome resulting from drooping of shoulders during pregnancy (occurs especially at night and early morning)	Maintain good posture; wear supportive maternity bra; condition will disappear if lifting and carrying baby does not aggravate it
Round ligament pain (tenderness)	Stretching of ligament caused by enlarging uterus	Not preventable; rest, maintain good body mechanics to avoid overstretching ligament; relieve cramping by squatting or bringing knees to chest, sometimes heat helps
Joint pain, backache, and pelvic pressure; hypermobility of joints	Relaxation of symphyseal and sacroiliac joints because of hormones, resulting in unstable pelvis; exaggerated lumbar and cervicothoracic curves caused by change in center of gravity resulting from enlarging abdomen	Maintain good posture and body mechanics; avoid fatigue; wear low-heeled shoes; abdominal supports may be useful; conscious relaxation; sleep on firm mattress; apply local heat or ice; get back rubs; do pelvic rock exercise; rest; condition will disappear 6 to 8 weeks after birth

Continued

TABLE 11-2
Discomforts Related to Pregnancy—cont'd

Third Trimester		
Discomfort	**Physiology**	**Education for Self-Care**
Shortness of breath and dyspnea occur in 60% of pregnant women	Expansion of diaphragm limited by enlarging uterus; diaphragm is elevated about 4 cm; some relief after lightening	Good posture; sleep with extra pillows; avoid overloading stomach; stop smoking; contact health care provider if symptoms worsen to rule out anemia, emphysema, and asthma
Insomnia (later weeks of pregnancy)	Fetal movements, muscle cramping, urinary frequency, shortness of breath, or other discomforts	Reassurance; conscious relaxation; back massage or effleurage (Fig. 11-18); support of body parts with pillows; warm milk or warm shower before retiring
Psychosocial responses: mood swings, mixed feelings, increased anxiety	Hormonal and metabolic adaptations; feelings about impending labor, birth, and parenthood	Reassurance and support from significant other and nurse; improved communication with partner, family, and others
Gingivitis and epulis (hyperemia, hypertrophy, bleeding, tenderness): condition will disappear spontaneously 1 to 2 months after birth	Increased vascularity and proliferation of connective tissue from estrogen stimulation	Well-balanced diet with adequate protein and fresh fruits and vegetables; gentle brushing and good dental hygiene; avoid infection; see dentist for teeth cleaning
Urinary frequency and urgency return	Vascular engorgement and altered bladder function caused by hormones; bladder capacity reduced by enlarging uterus and fetal presenting part	Empty bladder regularly, Kegel exercises; limit fluid intake before bedtime; reassurance; wear perineal pad; contact health care provider for pain or burning sensation
Perineal discomfort and pressure	Pressure from enlarging uterus, especially when standing or walking; multifetal gestation	Rest, conscious relaxation, and good posture; contact health care provider for assessment and treatment if pain is present
Braxton Hicks contractions	Intensification of uterine contractions in preparation for work of labor	Reassurance; rest; change of position; practice breathing techniques when contractions are bothersome; effleurage
Leg cramps (gastrocnemius spasm), especially when reclining	Compression of nerves supplying lower extremities because of enlarging uterus; reduced level of diffusible serum calcium or elevation of serum phosphorus; aggravating factors: fatigue, poor peripheral circulation, pointing toes when stretching legs or when walking, drinking more than 1 L (1 qt) of milk per day	Check for Homans' sign; if negative, use massage and heat over affected muscle; dorsiflex foot until spasm relaxes (Fig. 11-17); stand on cold surface; oral supplementation with calcium carbonate or calcium lactate tablets; aluminum hydroxide gel, 30 ml, with each meal removes phosphorus by absorbing it
Ankle edema (nonpitting) to lower extremities	Edema aggravated by prolonged standing, sitting, poor posture, lack of exercise, constrictive clothing (e.g., garters), or by hot weather	Ample fluid intake for natural diuretic effect; put on support stockings before arising; rest periodically with legs and hips elevated (see Fig. 11-15), exercise moderately; contact health care provider if generalized edema develops; *diuretics are contraindicated*

be individualized with attention given to the woman's lifestyle and culture (Davis, 1996).

Recognizing Potential Complications. One of the most important responsibilities of people involved in the care of the pregnant woman is to alert her to signs and symptoms that indicate a potential complication of pregnancy. The woman needs to know how and to whom such warning signs should be reported (see Box 11-4). It is difficult to remember specifics when stressed by a disturbing symptom. Therefore the woman and her family will be reassured if they receive a printed form listing the signs and symptoms that warrant an investigation and the phone numbers to call with questions or in an emergency.

The nurse needs to answer questions honestly when they arise during pregnancy. Pregnant women often have difficulty

Home Care

HOW TO RECOGNIZE PRETERM LABOR

Because the onset of preterm labor is subtle and often hard to recognize, it is important to know how to feel your abdomen for uterine contractions. You can feel for contractions in the following way. While lying down, place your fingertips on the top of your uterus. A contraction is the periodic tightening or hardening of your uterus. If your uterus is contracting, you will actually feel your abdomen get tight or hard and then feel it relax or soften when the contraction is over.

If you think you are having any of the other signs and symptoms of preterm labor, empty your bladder, drink three to four glasses of water for hydration, lie down tilted toward your side, and place a pillow at your back for support.

Check for contractions for 1 hour. To tell how often contractions are occurring, check the minutes that elapse from the beginning of one contraction to the beginning of the next.

It is *not normal* to have frequent uterine contractions (every 10 minutes or more often for 1 hour).

Contractions of labor are regular, frequent, and hard. They also may be felt as a tightening of the abdomen or a backache. This type of contraction causes the cervix to efface and dilate.

Call your doctor, nurse-midwife, clinic, or labor and birth unit, or go to the hospital if any of the following signs occur:

- You have uterine contractions every 10 minutes or more often for 1 hour or
- You have any of the other signs and symptoms for 1 hour or
- You have any bloody spotting or leaking of fluid from your vagina

It is often difficult to identify preterm labor. Accurate diagnosis requires assessment by the health care provider, usually in the hospital or clinic.

Post these instructions where they can be seen by everyone in the family.

deciding when to report signs and symptoms. The mother is encouraged to refer to the printed list of potential complications and to listen to her body (see Box 11-4). If she senses that something is wrong, she should call her care provider immediately.

Recognizing Preterm Labor. Teaching each expectant mother to recognize preterm labor is necessary. Preterm labor is that which occurs after the twentieth week but before the thirty-seventh week of pregnancy. It is a condition in which uterine contractions cause the cervix to open earlier than normal, and it can result in preterm birth. Although certain factors, such as multifetal pregnancy, may increase a woman's chances of going into preterm labor, the specific cause (or causes) is usually not known. It may be possible to prevent a preterm birth by knowing the warning signs and symptoms of preterm labor and by seeking care early if warning signs and symptoms should occur. Warning signs and symptoms of preterm labor are given in the Home Care box. Fig. 11-19 shows where in the body the signs and symptoms of preterm labor may be located.

Sexual Counseling. The sexual counseling of expectant couples includes countering misinformation, providing reassurance of normality, and suggesting alternative behaviors. The uniqueness of each couple is considered within a biopsychosocial framework (Guidelines box).

Many women merely need permission to be sexually active during pregnancy. Many other women, however, need information about the physiologic changes that occur during pregnancy and to have dispelled the myths associated with sex during

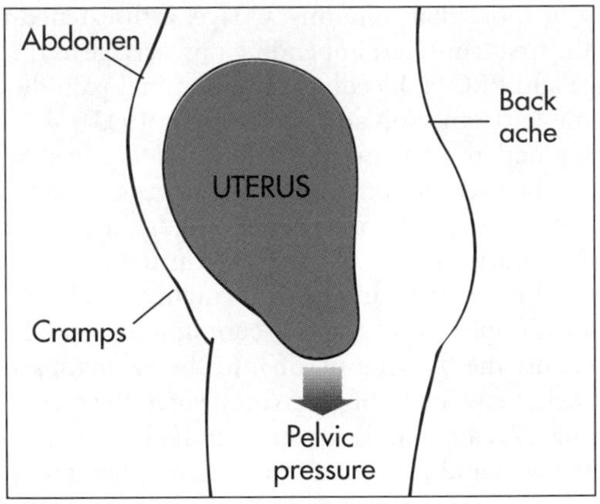

FIG. 11-19 • Symptoms of preterm labor.

Guidelines

SEXUALITY IN PREGNANCY

- Be aware that maternal physiologic changes, such as breast enlargement, nausea, fatigue, abdominal changes, perineal enlargement, leukorrhea, pelvic vasocongestion, and orgasmic responses, may affect sexuality and sexual expression.
- Discuss responses to pregnancy with your partner.
- Keep in mind that cultural prescriptions (dos) and proscriptions (don'ts) may affect your responses.
- Although your libido may be depressed during the first trimester, it often increases during the second and third trimesters.
- Discuss and explore with your partner:
  - Alternative behaviors (e.g., mutual masturbation, foot massage, cuddling)
  - Alternative positions (e.g., female superior, sidelying) for sexual intercourse
- Intercourse is safe as long as it is not uncomfortable. There is no correlation between intercourse and miscarriage, but observe the following precautions:
  - Abstain from intercourse if you experience uterine cramping or vaginal bleeding; report event to your caregiver as soon as possible.
  - Abstain from intercourse (or any activity that results in orgasm) if you have a history of cervical incompetence, until the problem is corrected.
- Continue to use "safer sex" behaviors. Women at risk for acquiring or conveying STIs are encouraged to use condoms during sexual intercourse throughout pregnancy.

pregnancy. Such tasks are within the purview of the maternity nurse and should be an integral component of the health care provided (Alteneder and Hartzell, 1997).

Some couples need to be referred for sex therapy or family therapy. Couples whose long-standing sexual dysfunction is intensified by pregnancy are good candidates for sex therapy. When a sexual problem is a symptom of a more serious relationship problem, the couple would benefit from family therapy.

Suggesting Alternative Behaviors. To date, research has not demonstrated that coitus and orgasm are contraindicated at any time during pregnancy for the obstetrically and medically healthy woman (Cunningham et al, 1997). Conditions that warrant precaution against coitus and orgasm include a history of more than one miscarriage; a threatened miscarriage in the first trimester; impending miscarriage in the second trimester; and PROM, bleeding, or abdominal pain during the third trimester (Rynerson and Lowdermilk, 1993).

Solitary and mutual masturbation and oral-genital intercourse may be used by couples as alternatives to penile-vaginal intercourse. Partners who enjoy cunnilingus (i.e., oral stimulation of the clitoris or vagina) may feel "turned off" by the normal increase in amount and odor of vaginal discharge during pregnancy. Couples who practice cunnilingus should be cautioned against the blowing of air into the vagina, particularly during the last few weeks of pregnancy, when the cervix may be slightly open. An air embolism can occur if air is forced between the uterine wall and fetal membranes and enters the maternal vascular system through the placenta.

It is often helpful to show the woman or couple illustrations of the possible variations of coital position (Fig. 11-20). The female-superior, side-by-side, rear-entry, and facing each other positions are alternatives to the traditional male-superior position. The woman astride (superior position) allows her to control the angle and depth of penile penetration and also protect her breasts and abdomen. The side-by-side position is preferred, especially during the third trimester, because it requires less energy and places less pressure on the pregnant abdomen.

Multiparous women sometimes experience significant breast tenderness in the first trimester. A coital position that avoids direct pressure on the woman's breasts, and decreased breast fondling during love play, can be recommended to such couples. The woman should also be reassured that this condition is normal and temporary.

Some women complain of lower abdominal cramping and backache after orgasm during the first and third trimesters. A back rub can often relieve some of the discomfort and provide a pleasant experience. A tonic uterine contraction, often lasting up to a minute, replaces the rhythmic contractions of orgasm during the third trimester. Changes in FHR without fetal distress have also been reported.

The objective of "safer sex" is to provide prophylaxis against the acquisition and transmission of STIs (e.g., HSV, HPV, and HIV). Because these diseases may be transmitted to the woman and her fetus, the use of condoms is recommended throughout pregnancy if the woman is at risk for an STI.

Psychosocial Support. Esteem, affection, trust, concern, consideration of cultural and religious responses, and listening are all components of the emotional support given to the pregnant woman and her family. The woman's satisfaction with her relationships and support, her feeling of competence, and her sense of being in control are important issues to be addressed in the third trimester. A discussion of fetal responses to stimuli (e.g., sound, light, maternal posture, and tension) as well as patterns of sleeping and waking can be helpful. Also discussed are emotional tensions that can arise in relation to the childbirth experience, such as those stemming from fear of pain, loss of control, and possible birth of the infant before reaching the hospital. Parents have anxieties about the responsibilities and tasks of parenthood, and concerns about the safety of the mother and unborn child; about siblings and their acceptance of the new baby; about social and economic responsibilities; and concerns arising from conflicts in cultural, religious, or personal value systems. Thorough assessment is

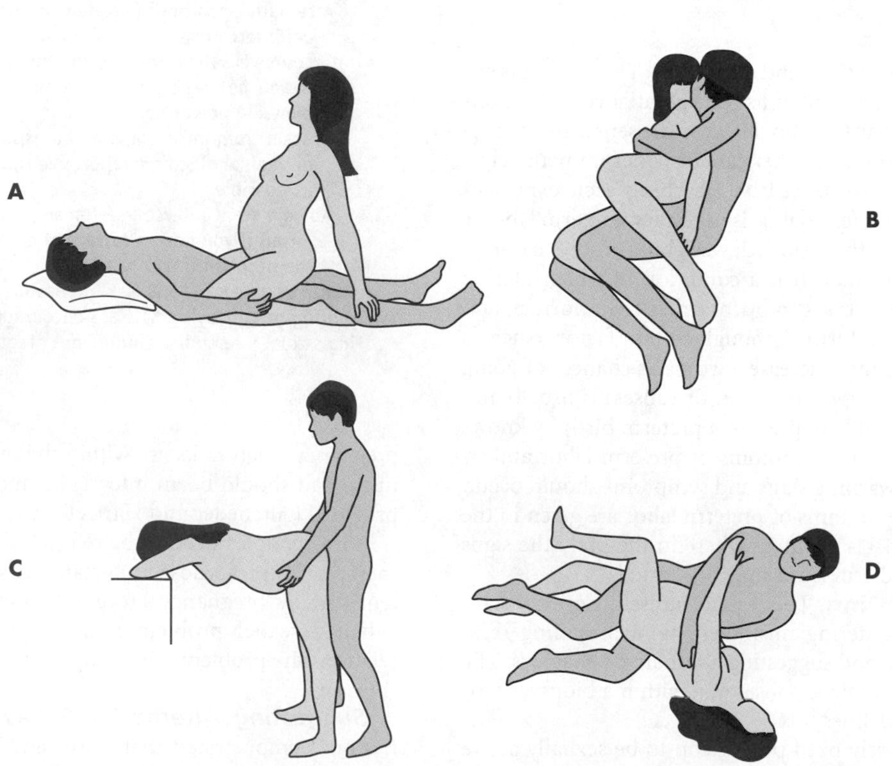

FIG. 11-20 • Positions for sexual intercourse during pregnancy. **A,** Female superior. **B,** Side by side. **C,** Rear entry. **D,** Facing each other.

promoted by guidelines that identify expected behavior and appropriate nursing interventions for each stage of psychosocial development in pregnancy (Malnory, 1996).

The father's or partner's commitment to the pregnancy, the couple's relationship, and their concerns about sexuality and sexual expression can emerge as issues for many expectant parents. Validation, feedback, and social comparison characterize the support given.

Providing the mother- and father-to-be with opportunities to discuss their concerns, simply listening, and validating the normality of their responses will all meet their needs to some degree. Nurses must also recognize that men feel more vulnerable during their partner's pregnancy. Female partners may also have these feelings. Anticipatory guidance and health promotion strategies can help partners cope with their concerns. Nursing intervention may help them to deal with such concerns either directly through counseling or indirectly through the education of the mothers. Health care providers can stimulate and encourage open dialogue between the couple.

➤ Evaluation

Evaluation of the effectiveness of care of the woman during pregnancy is based on the previously stated outcomes. More effort is needed in evaluating outcomes of nursing care during the prenatal period. A formal systematic follow-up on quality of care is not common but needs to be developed and incorporated in all settings (Nursing Care Plan).

Variations in Prenatal Care

The course of prenatal care described thus far may seem to suggest that the experiences of childbearing women are similar and that nursing interventions are uniform across all populations. Although typical patterns of response to pregnancy are easily recognized, and many aspects of prenatal care indeed are consistent, pregnant women enter the health care system with individual concerns and needs. The nurse's ability to assess unique needs and to tailor interventions to the individual are hallmarks of expertise in providing care. Variations that influence prenatal care include culture, age, and number of fetuses.

Cultural Influences. Prenatal care as North Americans know it is a phenomenon of Western medicine. In the Western biomedical model of care, women are encouraged to seek prenatal care as early as possible in their pregnancy by visiting a physician, nurse-midwife, office, or clinic. Such visits are usually routine and, as already mentioned, follow a systematic sequence, with the initial visit followed by monthly, then semimonthly, then weekly visits. Monitoring weight and blood pressure; testing blood and urine; teaching specific information about diet, rest, and activity; and preparing for childbirth are common components of prenatal care. This model is not only unfamiliar but may seem strange to many groups. Models for providing prenatal care for women in other parts of the world, however, are being explored (Al-Qutob, Mawajdeh, and Bin-Raad, 1996).

Many cultural variations in prenatal care exist. Even if the prenatal care described is familiar to a woman, some practices may conflict with the beliefs and practices of the subculture groups to which she belongs. Because of these and other factors (e.g., lack of money, lack of transportation, and poor communication on the part of health care providers), women from many such groups do not participate in the prenatal care system. The nurse may misinterpret their behavior as uncaring, lazy, or ignorant.

For many women, concern for modesty is a deterrent for seeking prenatal care. Some women consider exposing body parts, especially to a man, a major violation of their modesty. For many women, invasive procedures such as vaginal examination may be so threatening that they cannot be discussed even with their own husbands. Thus many women prefer a female over a male health care provider. Most women value and appreciate efforts to maintain their modesty.

Family Focus

COUPLE RELATIONSHIP AND SEXUALITY

Pregnancy is a time when the couple relationship can be strengthened or stressed. In addition to the physical changes during pregnancy, the pregnant woman and her partner face significant emotional, social, and cognitive changes. Expectant fathers/male partners often experience weight gain and nausea. They may be concerned about finances, their role as fathers, sexuality, and the child's effect on the couple's relationship. Fathers/partners often worry about their role during childbirth classes and during labor and birth, as well as about the safety of their partner and baby during the birth. Female partners may have the same concerns.

Sexual expression during pregnancy is highly individual. The sexual relationshp is affected by physical, emotional, and interactional factors, including myths about sex during pregnancy, sexual dysfunction problems, and physical changes in the woman.

Myths about body functions and fantasies about the influence of the fetus as a third party in lovemaking are commonly expressed. Anomalies, mental retardation, and other injuries to the mother and fetus may be attributed to sexual relations during pregnancy. Some couples fear that the woman's genitalia will be drastically changed by the birth process. Couples may not express their concerns to the health professional because of embarrassment or not wanting to appear foolish.

Discomfort during sexual activity may be caused by pressure on the woman's abdomen and deep penetration or thrusting. Postcoital cramping and backache during the first trimester have been reported.

As pregnancy progresses, changes in body shape, body image, and levels of discomfort influence both partners' desire for sexual expression. During the first trimester the woman's sexual desire may decrease, especially if she experiences breast tenderness, nausea, fatigue, and sleepiness. As she progresses into the second trimester, her combined sense of well-being and increased pelvic congestion may profoundly increase her desire for sexual release. In the third trimester, somatic complaints and physical bulkiness may increase her physical discomfort and decrease her interest in sex.

Partners need to feel free to discuss their sexual responses during pregnancy. Sensitivity to each other and a willingness to share concerns can strengthen their sexual relationship. Partners who do not understand the seemingly rapid physiologic and emotional changes of pregnancy can become confused by the other's behavior. By talking to each other about the changes they are experiencing, couples are able to define problems and offer the needed support. Nurses can facilitate communication between partners by talking to pregnant couples about possible changes in feelings and behaviors a couple may experience as pregnancy progresses.

Adapted from: Rynerson B, Lowdermilk D: Sexual intimacy in pregnancy. In Knuppel R, Drukker J: *High risk pregnancy: a team approach,* ed 2, Philadelphia, 1993, WB Saunders.

Nursing Care Plan: EDUCATING THE PREGNANT WOMAN ABOUT DISCOMFORTS OF PREGNANCY AND WARNING SIGNS

FIRST TRIMESTER
NURSING DIAGNOSIS Knowledge deficit related to schedule of prenatal visits throughout pregnancy as evidenced by patient questions and concerns

EXPECTED OUTCOME Patient will verbalize correct appointment schedule for the duration of the pregnancy.

Nursing Interventions/*Rationales*

Provide information regarding schedule of visits, tests, and other assessments and interventions that will be provided throughout the pregnancy *to empower patient to function in collaboration with the caregiver.*

NURSING DIAGNOSIS Altered nutrition: less than body requirements, related to nausea and vomiting as evidenced by patient report and weight loss

EXPECTED OUTCOME Patient will gain 1 kg to 2.5 kg during the first trimester.

Nursing Interventions/*Rationales*

Verify prepregnant weight *to plan a diet according to individual patient's nutritional needs.*
Obtain diet history *to identify current meal patterns and foods that may be implicated in nausea.*
Advise patient to consume small frequent meals and avoid having empty stomach *to avoid further nausea episodes.*
Suggest that patient eat a simple carbohydrate such as dry crackers before arising in the morning *to avoid empty stomach and decrease incidence of nausea and vomiting.*
Advise patient to call health care provider if vomiting is persistent and severe *to identify possible incidence of hyperemesis gravidarum.*

NURSING DIAGNOSIS Fatigue related to hormonal changes in the first trimester as evidenced by patient complaints

EXPECTED OUTCOME Patient will report a decreased number of episodes of fatigue.

Nursing Interventions/*Rationales*

Rest as needed *to avoid increasing feeling of fatigue.*
Eat a well-balanced diet *to meet increased metabolic demands and avoid anemia.*
Discuss the use of support systems to help with household responsibilities *to decrease workload at home and decrease fatigue.*

SECOND TRIMESTER
NURSING DIAGNOSIS Constipation related to progesterone influence on GI tract as evidenced by patient report of altered patterns of elimination

EXPECTED OUTCOME Patient will report a return to normal bowel elimination pattern following implementation of interventions.

Nursing Interventions/*Rationales*

Provide information to patient regarding pregnancy-related causes: progesterone slowing gastrointestinal motility, growing uterus compressing intestines, and influence of iron supplementation *to provide basic information for self-care during pregnancy.*
Assist patient to plan a diet that will promote regular bowel movements, such as increasing amount of oral fluid intake to at least six glasses of water a day, increasing the amount of fiber in daily diet, and to maintain moderate exercise *to promote self-care.*
Reinforce for patient that she should not take any laxatives, stool softeners, or enemas without first consulting the health care provider *to prevent any injuries to patient or fetus.*

NURSING DIAGNOSIS Knowledge deficit related to first pregnancy as evidenced by patient questions regarding possible complications of second and third trimesters

EXPECTED OUTCOME Patient will correctly list signs of potential complications that can occur during the second and third trimesters.

Nursing Interventions/*Rationales*

Provide information concerning the potential complications or warning signs that can occur during the second and third trimesters, including possible causes of signs and the importance of calling the health care provider immediately *to ensure identification and treatment of problems in a timely manner.*
Provide a written list of complications *to have a reference list for emergencies.*

In many cultural groups a physician is deemed appropriate only in times of illness, and because pregnancy is considered a normal process and the woman is in a state of health, the services of a physician are considered inappropriate. Even if there develops what Western medicine considers to be problems with the pregnancy, they may not be perceived as problems by members of other cultural groups.

Although many cultures consider pregnancy as a normal state, women of all cultures are expected to perform certain practices to ensure a good outcome. These cultural prescrip-

Critical Thinking

CULTURE AND CHILDBIRTH BELIEFS AND PRACTICES

Select an immigrant or other minority group and identify childbirth-related beliefs and practices that are unique to that group. Outline ways a childbirth education program might be modified to provide essential information while incorporating cultural patterns.

tions tell women what to do, while cultural proscriptions establish taboos. The purposes of these practices are to prevent maternal illness caused by a pregnancy-induced imbalanced state, and to protect the vulnerable fetus. Prescriptions and proscriptions regulate the woman's emotional response, clothing, physical activity and rest, sexual activity, and dietary practices. Exploration of the woman's beliefs, perceptions of the meaning of childbearing, and health care practices may help health care providers foster her self-actualization, promote attainment of the maternal role, and positively influence her relationship with her spouse (Callister, 1995).

To provide culturally sensitive care, the nurse must be knowledgeable about practices and customs, although it is not possible to know all there is to know about every culture and subculture, or the many lifestyles that exist. When exploring cultural beliefs and practices related to childbearing, the nurse can support and nurture those beliefs that promote physical or emotional adaptation. However, if potentially harmful beliefs or activities are identified, the nurse should carefully provide education and propose modifications.

Emotional Response. Virtually all cultures emphasize the importance of maintaining a socially harmonious and agreeable environment for the pregnant woman. An absence of stress is important in ensuring a successful outcome for mother and baby. Harmony with other people must be fostered, and visits from extended family members may be required to demonstrate pleasant and noncontroversial relationships. If discord exists in a relationship, it is usually dealt with in culturally prescribed ways.

Besides proscriptions regarding food, other proscriptions involve imitative magic. For example, some Mexicans believe pregnant women should not be allowed to witness an eclipse of the moon because it may cause a cleft palate in the infant. They also believe that exposure to an earthquake may precipitate preterm birth, miscarriage, or a breech presentation. In some cultures, a pregnant woman must not ridicule someone with an affliction for fear her child might be born with the same handicap. A mother should not hate a person lest her child resemble that person, and dental work should not be done during pregnancy because it may cause a baby to have a "harelip." A folk belief widely held in many cultures is that the pregnant woman should refrain from raising her arms above her head and from tying knots to prevent the umbilical cord from wrapping around the baby's neck or knotting. Other cultures believe that placing a knife under the bed of a laboring woman will "cut" her pain.

Clothing. Although most cultural groups do not prescribe specific clothing for pregnancy, modesty is an expectation for many. Some Mexican women of the Southwest wear a cord beneath the breast and knotted over the umbilicus. This cord, called a muneco, is thought to prevent morning sickness and ensure a safe birth. Amulets, medals, and beads also may be worn to ward off evil spirits (Spector, 1996).

Physical Activity and Rest. Norms that regulate physical activity of mothers during pregnancy vary tremendously. Many groups, including Native Americans and some Asian groups, encourage women to be active, to walk, and to engage in normal although not strenuous activities to ensure that the baby is healthy and not too large. Other groups, such as Filipinos, believe that any activity is dangerous, and others willingly take over the work of the pregnant woman. Some Filipinos believe that this inactivity protects the mother and child. The mother is encouraged simply to produce the succeeding generation. If health care providers do not know of this belief, they could misinterpret this behavior as laziness or noncompliance with the desired prenatal health care regimen. It is important for the nurse to find out the way each pregnant woman views activity and rest.

Sexual Activity. In most cultures, sexual activity is not prohibited until the end of pregnancy. Many Mexican-Americans view sexual activity as necessary to keep the birth canal lubricated. On the other hand, some Vietnamese may have definite proscriptions about sexual intercourse, requiring abstinence throughout the pregnancy because it is thought that sexual intercourse may harm the mother and the fetus.

Diet. Nutritional information given by Western health care providers may be a source of conflict for many cultural groups, but such a conflict commonly is not known by health care providers unless they understand the dietary beliefs and practices of the particular people for whom they are caring. Muslims, for example, must eat meat slaughtered in accordance with Muslim law. If this is not possible, they will accept kosher or vegetarian foods. Many cultures permit pregnant women to eat only warm foods.

Age.

The age of the childbearing couple may have a significant influence on their physical and psychosocial adaptation to pregnancy. Normal developmental processes that occur in both very young and older mothers are interrupted by pregnancy and require a different type of adaptation to pregnancy than that of the woman of typical childbearing age. Although the individuality of each pregnant woman is recognized, special needs of expectant mothers aged 15 years or younger or those aged 35 years or older are summarized here.

Adolescent Mothers. About 1 million adolescent females in the United States, or 4 out of every 10 girls, become pregnant each year (Alan Guttmacher Institute, 1998). Most of the pregnancies are unintended, and nearly 40% end in abortion. Nevertheless, adolescents are responsible for almost 500,000 births in the United States annually (Ventura, Curtin, and Mathews, 1998). Hispanic adolescents currently have the highest birth rate, although the rate for African-American adolescents also is high. Of girls who become pregnant, 1 in 6 will have a repeat pregnancy within 1 year (Cockey, 1997). Most of these young women are unmarried, and many are not ready for the emotional, psychosocial, and financial responsibilities of parenthood.

Despite these alarming statistics, and the fact that the United States has the highest adolescent birth rate in the industrialized world, the birth rate for adolescents has steadily declined since 1991 (Ventura et al, 1998). Concentrated national efforts have spawned a host of adolescent pregnancy prevention programs that have had varying degrees of success. Characteristics of programs that make a difference are those that have sustained commitment to adolescents over a long period, involve the parents and other adults in the community, promote abstinence and personal responsibility, and assist adolescents to develop a clear strategy for reaching future goals such as a college education or a career (Cockey, 1997).

When adolescents do become pregnant and decide to give birth, they are much less likely than older women to receive adequate prenatal care, with many receiving no care at all (Ventura, Curtin, and Mathews, 1998). These young women also are more likely to smoke and less likely to gain adequate weight during pregnancy. As a result of these and other factors, babies born to adolescents are at greatly increased risk of LBW, of serious and long-term disability, and of dying during the first year of life.

Delayed entry into prenatal care may be the result of late recognition of pregnancy, denial of pregnancy, or confusion about the services that are available. Such a delay in care may leave an inadequate time before birth to attend to correctable problems. The very young pregnant adolescent is at higher risk for each of the confounding variables associated with poor pregnancy outcomes (e.g., socioeconomic factors) and for those conditions associated with a first pregnancy regardless of age (e.g., pregnancy-induced hypertension [PIH]). However, when prenatal care is initiated early and consistently, and confounding variables are controlled, very young pregnant adolescents are at no greater risk (nor are their infants) for an adverse outcome than older pregnant women. Thus the role of the nurse in reducing the risks and consequences of adolescent pregnancy is twofold: first, to encourage early and continued prenatal care; and second to refer the adolescent, if necessary, for appropriate social support services, which can help reverse the effects of a negative socioeconomic environment (Fig. 11-21, Nursing Care Plan).

Older Mothers. Two groups have emerged in the population of women having a child late in their childbearing years. One group consists of women who have many children or who have an additional child during the menopausal period. The other group consists of relative newcomers to maternity care. These are women who have deliberately delayed childbearing until their late 30s or early 40s.

Multiparous Women. Multiparous women may have never used contraceptives because of personal choice or because of a lack of knowledge concerning contraceptives. They also may be women who have used contraceptives successfully during the childbearing years but, as menopause approaches, cease menstruating regularly, stop using contraception, and subsequently become pregnant. The older multiparous woman may feel that pregnancy separates her from her peer group and that her age is a hindrance to close associations with young mothers. Other parents welcome the unexpected infant as evidence of continuing maternal and paternal roles.

Nulliparous Women. The number of first-time pregnancies in women between ages 35 and 40 years has increased significantly over the last 10 years. It is common now to see women in their late 30s or even in their early 40s pregnant for the first time. Reasons for delaying pregnancy include advanced education, career priorities, better contraceptive measures, and infertility.

These women choose parenthood over a childfree lifestyle. They often are successfully established in a career and a lifestyle with a partner that includes time for self-attention, the establishment of a home with accumulated possessions, and freedom to travel. Questioned as to why they chose pregnancy later in life, many reply "Because time is running out."

The dilemma of choice includes recognition that being a parent will have both positive and negative consequences. Couples need to discuss the consequences of childbearing and childrearing before committing themselves to this lifelong venture. Partners in this group seem to share the preparation for parenthood, the planning for a family-centered birth, and the desire to be loving and competent parents. However, the reality of child care may prove difficult for such parents.

As with mothers of all ages, the mother over 35 who is accustomed to the stimulation of and contact with other adults may find isolation with her infant difficult to accept. Anger and resentment toward the father (or infant) can result, even with anticipatory guidance for these aspects of parenting.

First-time mothers older than 35 years select the "right time" for pregnancy; this time is influenced by their awareness of the increasing possibility of infertility or of genetic defects in the infant of older women. Such women seek information about pregnancy from books and friends. They actively try to prevent fetal disorders and are careful in searching for the best possible maternity care. They identify sources of stress in their lives. They have concerns about having enough energy and stamina to meet the demands of parenting and their new roles and relationships.

If they become pregnant after treatment for infertility, they may suddenly have negative or ambivalent feelings about the pregnancy. They may experience a multifetal pregnancy that may create emotional and physical problems. Adjusting to parenting two or more infants requires adaptability and additional resources.

During pregnancy, parents explore the possibilities and responsibilities of changing identities and new roles. They must prepare a safe and nurturing environment during pregnancy and after birth. They must integrate the child into an established family system and negotiate new roles (e.g., parent roles, sibling roles, and grandparent roles) for family members.

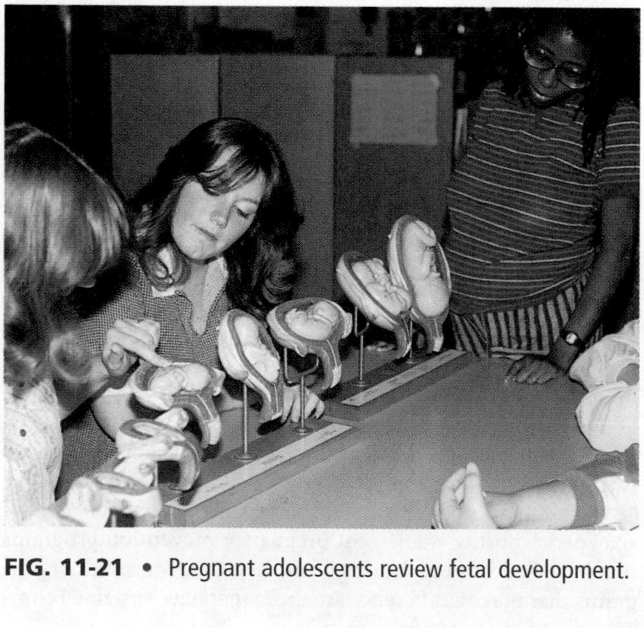

FIG. 11-21 • Pregnant adolescents review fetal development.

Adverse perinatal outcomes are more common in older primiparas than in younger women, even when they receive good prenatal care. Dollberg et al (1996) reported that women 35 years of age and older are more likely than younger primiparas to have LBW infants, premature birth, IUGR, and abruptio placentae. The incidence of malpresentation also is more common in older primiparas, and they are more likely to have a cesarean birth. In uncomplicated pregnancies, older mothers have significantly less fear of helplessness and loss of control in labor than younger women (Stark, 1997). Age and education are thought to balance the concerns of the older mothers related to age.

Multifetal Pregnancy. A multifetal pregnancy, or pregnancy with more than one fetus, places the mother and fetuses at risk. The maternal blood volume is increased, resulting in an increased strain on the maternal cardiovascular system. Anemia often develops because of a greater demand for iron by the fetuses. Marked uterine distention and increased pressure on the adjacent viscera and pelvic vasculature and diastasis of the two rectus abdominis muscles may occur (see Fig. 10-11). Placenta previa develops more commonly in multifetal pregnancies because of the large size or placement of the placentas (Cunningham et al, 1997). Premature separation of the placenta may occur before the second and any subsequent fetuses are born.

Twin pregnancies often end in prematurity. Spontaneous rupture of membranes before term is common. Congenital malformations are twice as common in monozygotic twins as in singletons. No increase is seen in the incidence of congenital anomalies in dizygotic twins. Two-vessel cords (i.e., cords with a single umbilical artery) occur more often in twins than in singletons; this abnormality is most common in monozygotic twins. The most serious problem for the fetus is the local shunting of blood between placentas (twin-to-twin transfusion); this causes the recipient twin to be larger and the donor twin to be

Nursing Care Plan — THE PREGNANT ADOLESCENT

NURSING DIAGNOSIS Altered nutrition: less than body requirements related to intake insufficient to meet metabolic needs of fetus and adolescent patient

EXPECTED OUTCOME Patient will gain weight as prescribed by age, take prenatal vitamins/iron as prescribed, and maintain normal hematocrit and hemoglobin.

Nursing Interventions/*Rationales*

Assess current diet history/intake *to determine prescriptions for additions or changes in present dietary pattern.*

Compare prepregnancy weight with current weight *to determine if pattern is consistent with appropriate fetal growth and development.*

Provide information concerning food prescriptions for appropriate weight gain, considering preferences for "fast food" and peer influences *to correct any misconceptions and increase chances for compliance with diet.*

Include patient's immediate family or support system during instruction *to ensure that person preparing family meals receives information.*

NURSING DIAGNOSIS Risk for injury, maternal or fetal, related to inadequate prenatal care and screening

EXPECTED OUTCOME Patient will experience uncomplicated pregnancy and deliver a healthy fetus at term.

Nursing Interventions/*Rationales*

Provide information, using therapeutic communication and confidentiality *to establish relationship and build trust.*

Discuss importance of ongoing prenatal and possible risks to adolescent patient and fetus *to reinforce that ongoing assessment is crucial to health and well-being of patient and fetus, even if patient feels well. The adolescent patient is more at risk for certain complications that may be avoided or managed early if prenatal visits are maintained.*

Discuss risks of alcohol, tobacco, and recreational drug use during pregnancy *to minimize risks to patient and fetus, since adolescent patient has a higher abuse rate than the rest of the pregnant population.*

Assess for evidence of sexually transmitted infection and provide information regarding safer sexual practice *to minimize risk to patient and fetus, since adolescent is more at risk for STIs.*

Screen for PIH on an ongoing basis *to minimize risk, since adolescent population is more at risk for PIH.*

NURSING DIAGNOSIS Social isolation related to body image changes of pregnant adolescent as evidenced by patient statements and concerns

EXPECTED OUTCOME Patient will identify support systems and report decreased feelings of social isolation.

Nursing Interventions/*Rationales*

Establish a therapeutic relationship *to listen objectively and establish trust.*

Discuss with patient changes in relationships that have occurred as a result of the pregnancy *to determine extent of isolation from family, peers, and father of the baby.*

Provide referrals and resources appropriate for developmental stage of patient *to give information for patient support.*

Provide information regarding parenting classes, breastfeeding classes, and childbirth preparation, classes *to give further information and group support, which lessens social isolation.*

small, pallid, dehydrated, malnourished, and hypovolemic. However, the larger twin may develop congenital heart failure during the first 24 hours after birth.

The clinical diagnosis of multifetal pregnancy is accurate in about 90% of cases. The likelihood of a multifetal pregnancy is increased if any one or a combination of the following factors is noted during a careful assessment:

- History of dizygotic twins in the female lineage
- Use of fertility drugs
- More rapid uterine growth for the number of weeks of gestation
- Hydramnios
- The palpation of more than the expected number of small or large parts
- Asynchronous fetal heartbeats or more than one fetal electrocardiographic tracing
- Ultrasonographic evidence of more than one fetus

The diagnosis of multifetal pregnancy can come as a shock to many expectant parents, and they may need additional support and education to help them cope with the changes they face. The mother will need nutrition counseling so that she gains more weight than that needed for a singleton birth. She should also be informed that maternal adaptations will probably be more uncomfortable, and about the possibility of a preterm birth.

If the presence of more than three fetuses is diagnosed, the parents may receive counseling regarding selective reduction of the fetuses to reduce the incidence of premature birth and improve the opportunities for the remaining fetuses to grow to term gestation (Berkowitz, 1998). This situation poses an ethical dilemma for many couples, especially those who have worked hard to overcome problems with infertility and those who harbor strong values regarding the right to life. The nurse able to engage the couple in discussion to identify what resources could help the couple (e.g., a minister, priest, rabbi, or mental health counselor) can make the process of making a decision somewhat less traumatic.

Prenatal care given to women with multifetal pregnancies includes changes in the pattern of care and modifications in other aspects such as the amount of weight gained and the nutritional intake observed. The prenatal visits of these mothers are scheduled at least every 2 weeks in the second trimester and weekly thereafter. No specific recommendation for weight gain for women with multifetal pregnancies has been made. In twin gestations, reported gains of 20 kg have been associated with positive outcomes. Iron and vitamin supplements are desirable.

The considerable uterine distention involved can cause the backache commonly experienced by pregnant women to be even worse. Elastic stockings or maternity tights may be worn to control leg varicosities. If there are risk factors for preterm birth (e.g., premature dilation of the cervix), abstinence from orgasm and nipple stimulation during the last trimester is recommended to help prevent preterm labor. Frequent ultrasound examinations and heart rate monitoring will occur. Some practitioners recommend bed rest beginning at 20 weeks to prevent preterm labor in women carrying multiple fetuses. Other practitioners question the value of prolonged bed rest. If bed rest is recommended, the mother needs to assume the lateral position to promote increased placental perfusion. If birth is delayed until after the thirty-sixth week, the risk of morbidity and mortality decreases for the neonates.

Multiple newborns will likely place a strain on finances, space, workload, and the mother's and family's coping abilities. Lifestyle changes may be necessary. Parents will need assistance in making realistic plans for the care of the babies, for example, whether to breastfeed and whether to raise them as "alike" or as separate individuals. Parents should be referred to national organizations such as Parents of Twins, Mothers of Multiples, and the La Leche League for further support.

Prebirth Education

The goal of childbirth education is to assist individuals and their family members to make informed decisions about pregnancy and birth. To accomplish this goal, the woman and her family need knowledge about the components of a healthy pregnancy, the process of labor and birth, and coping strategies to deal with the challenges of parenthood. Education should begin before pregnancy and continue through the postpartum period.

Some of the decisions the childbearing family must consider are the decision to have a baby, followed by choices of a care provider and type of care, the place for birth, and the type of infant feeding and care. If a woman has had a previous cesarean birth, she may consider having a vaginal birth. This section discusses these choices and the nurse's role in educating childbearing families to make informed decisions about them.

Previous pregnancy and childbirth experiences are important elements that influence current learning needs. The patient's (and support person's) age, cultural background, personal philosophy in regard to childbirth, socioeconomic status, spiritual beliefs, and learning styles all need to be assessed to develop the best plan to help the woman meet her needs.

Most childbirth education classes are attended by the pregnant woman and her partner, although a friend, teenage daughter, or parent may be the designated support person. Classes may also be held for grandparents and siblings to prepare them for their attendance at birth and/or the arrival of the baby (see Fig. 11-3). Siblings often see a film about birth and learn ways they can help welcome the baby. They also learn to cope with changes that include a reduction in parental time and attention. Grandparents learn about current child care practices and how to help their adult children adapt to parenting in a supportive way.

Childbirth Education Programs. Expectant parents and their families have different interests and information needs as the pregnancy progresses.

Early pregnancy ("early bird") classes provide fundamental information. Classes are developed around the following areas:

Family Focus

CHILDBIRTH EDUCATION CLASSES

A typical preparation-for-parenthood program recognizes that expectant parents and their families have different interests and information needs as the pregnancy progresses. Consequently, the program is designed to meet the informational needs of parents at the three major stages of pregnancy and after birth: first-trimester classes, second-trimester classes, third-trimester classes, lactation classes, and postpartum ("fourth-trimester") classes.

(1) early fetal development, (2) physiologic and emotional changes of pregnancy, (3) human sexuality, and (4) the nutritional needs of the mother and fetus. Environmental and workplace hazards may be addressed. Exercises, nutrition, warning signs, drugs, and self-medication are topics of interest and concern.

Midpregnancy classes emphasize the woman's participation in self-care. Classes provide information on preparation for breastfeeding and formula feeding, infant care, basic hygiene, common complaints and simple safe remedies, infant health, parenting, and updating and refining the birth plans.

Late pregnancy classes emphasize labor and birth. Different methods of coping with labor and birth have been developed and are often the basis for various prenatal classes. These include Lamaze, Bradley, and Dick-Read. A hospital tour is usually included.

Throughout the series of classes there is discussion of support systems that people can use during pregnancy and after birth. Such support systems help parents function independently and effectively. During all the classes the open expression of feelings and concerns about any aspect of pregnancy, birth, and parenting is welcomed.

Many fathers elect to participate actively during labor and the birth of their child. As noted earlier, however, some men, through personal or cultural conception of the father role, neither want nor intend to participate. It is important that the partners agree on each other's roles.

Recent Trends in Childbirth Education. A variety of approaches to childbirth education have evolved as childbirth educators attempt to meet learning needs. In addition to classes designed specifically for pregnant adolescents, their partners, and/or parents, classes exist for other groups with special learning needs. These include classes for first-time mothers over 35, single women, adoptive parents, and parents of twins. Refresher classes for parents with children not only review coping techniques for labor and birth but also help couples prepare for sibling reactions and adjustments to a new baby. Cesarean birth classes are offered for couples who have this kind of birth scheduled because of breech position or other risk factors. Other classes focus on vaginal birth after cesarean (VBAC), since many women successfully give birth vaginally after previous cesarean birth.

Strategies for Childbirth Education. Because of the multicultural composition of the population in North America, there is great diversity in attitudes, expectations, and behaviors judged appropriate during pregnancy and early parenthood. No one approach can meet all needs. For example, classes for new immigrants are particularly effective when taught in a native language (e.g., Spanish, Tagalog, and Cantonese). For classes to be meaningful, parent educators must understand the value systems in other cultures and their influence on issues such as nutrition, exercise, valuing of early prenatal care, maternal weight gain, and infant feeding practices. Parent educators must establish rapport, be understood, and build on cultural practices, reinforcing the positive and promoting change only if a practice, such as pica, is directly harmful. See Chapter 16 for more information on childbirth preparation classes.

Options for Care Providers. Often the first decision the woman makes is who will be her primary health care provider for the pregnancy and birth. This decision is doubly important because it usually affects where the birth will take place. The nurse can provide information about the different types of health care providers and what kind of care to expect from each type. Physicians (i.e., obstetricians and family practice physicians) attend about 93% of births in the United States and Canada (Ventura et al, 1998). They see low risk and high risk patients. Care often includes pharmacologic and medical management of problems as well as use of technologic procedures. Family practice physicians may need backup by obstetricians if a specialist is needed for a problem (e.g., a cesarean birth). Most physicians manage births in a hospital setting.

Nurse-midwives are registered nurses with advanced training in care of obstetric patients. They provide care for about 6% of the births in the United States and Canada (Ventura et al, 1998). Nurse-midwives may practice with physicians or independently and with an arrangement for physician backup. They usually see low risk obstetric patients. Care is often noninterventionist, and the woman and her family are encouraged to be active participants in the care. Nurse-midwives must refer patients to physicians for complications. Most births are managed in hospital settings or alternative birth centers; a few may be managed in a home setting.

Independent midwives, who also may be called lay midwives, are nonprofessional caregivers. Their training varies greatly, from formal training to self-teaching. They manage about 1% of births in the United States and Canada (Ventura et al, 1998). Patients who develop problems need to be seen by a physician. A majority (i.e., 61%) of births are managed in the home setting.

A doula is professionally trained to provide labor support, including physical, emotional, and informational support to women and their partners during labor and birth. The doula does not become involved with clinical tasks (Doulas of North America, 1999a, 1999b, 1999c). A doula typically meets with the mother and her partner before labor. Working collaboratively with other health care providers and the woman's supportive individuals, the doula focuses efforts on assisting the woman to achieve her goals. Box 11-6 provides questions to ask when interviewing a prospective doula. Box 11-7 includes organizations that offer information or referral services.

Birth Setting Choices. With careful thought, family-centered maternity care can be implemented in any setting. The three primary options for birth settings today are the hospital, birth center, and home. Women consider several factors in choosing a setting for childbirth, including the preference of their health care provider, characteristics of the birthing unit, and preference of their third-party payer. Approximately 99% of all births in the United States take place in a hospital setting (Ventura et al, 1998). However, the types of labor and birth services vary greatly, from the traditional labor and delivery rooms with separate postpartum and newborn units, to in-hospital birthing centers where all or almost all care takes place in a single unit.

Labor, Delivery, Recovery, Postpartum (Birthing) Rooms. Labor, delivery, and recovery (LDR) and labor, delivery, recovery, and postpartum (LDRP) rooms offer families a comfortable, private space for childbirth (Fig. 11-22). Women are admitted to LDR units, labor and give birth, and spend the first 1 to 2 hours postpartum there for immediate recovery and to have time with their families to bond with their newborns. After this period of recovery, the mothers and newborns are

Box 11-6

Questions to Ask When Choosing a Doula

To discover the specific training, experience, and services offered by anyone who provides labor support, potential patients, nursing supervisors, physicians, midwives, and others should ask the following questions of that person:

- What training have you had?
- Tell me about your experience with birth, personally and as a doula.
- What is your philosophy about childbirth and supporting women and their partners through labor?
- May we meet to discuss our birth plans and the role you will play in supporting me through childbirth?
- May we call you with questions or concerns before and after the birth?
- When do you try to join women in labor? Do you come to our home or meet us at the hospital?
- Do you meet with us after the birth to review the labor and answer questions?
- Do you work with one or more backup doulas for times when you are not available? May we meet them?
- What is your fee?

From Simkin P, Way K: *DONA position paper: The doula's contributions to modern maternity care,* Seattle, WA, 1998, Doulas of North America.

Box 11-7

Organizations that Offer Information or Referral Services for Doulas

DOULAS OF NORTH AMERICA (DONA)
1100 23rd Ave. East
Seattle, WA 98112
206-324-5440

ASSOCIATION OF LABOR ASSISTANTS AND CHILDBIRTH EDUCATORS (ALACE)
P.O. Box 382724
Cambridge, MA 02238
617-441-2500

INTERNATIONAL CHILDBIRTH EDUCATION ASSOCIATION (ICEA)
P.O. Box 20048
Minneapolis, MN 55420
800-624-4934

LAMAZE INTERNATIONAL
1200 19th St. NW, Suite 300
Washington, DC 20036
202-857-1100

transferred to a postpartum unit and nursery or mother-baby unit for the duration of their stay. In LDRP units, total care is provided from admission for labor through postpartum discharge in the same room and usually by the same nursing staff. The units are furnished in a homelike atmosphere.

Birth Centers. Free-standing birth centers are usually built in locations separate from the hospital but may be located nearby in case transfer of the woman or newborn is needed. These birth centers are intended to offer families a safe and cost-effective alternative to hospital or home birth. The centers are usually staffed by nurse-midwives or physicians who also have privileges at the local hospital. Only women at low risk for complications are included for care (Alden and Harris, 1995). Attendance at childbirth and parenting classes is required of all patients. The family is admitted to the birth center for labor and birth and will remain there until discharge, which often takes place within 6 hours of the birth.

Birth centers typically have homelike accommodations, including a double bed for the couple and a crib for the newborn (Fig. 11-23, *A*). Emergency equipment and drugs are stored discreetly within cupboards, out of view but easily accessible. Private bathroom facilities are incorporated into each birth unit. There may be an early labor lounge or a living room and small kitchen (Fig. 11-23, *B*). Services provided by the free-standing birth centers include those necessary for safe management during the childbearing cycle. Patients must understand that some situations require transfer to a hospital, and they must agree to abide by those guidelines. Expectant families develop birth plans, that is, the practices and procedures they would like to either include or exclude from their childbirth experience.

Birth centers may have resources for parents such as a lending library that includes books and videotapes; reference files on related topics; recycled maternity clothes, and baby clothes, and equipment; and supplies and reference materials for childbirth educators. The centers may also have referral files for community resources that offer services relating to childbirth and early parenting, including support groups (e.g., for single parents, for postbirth support, and for parents of twins), genetic counseling, women's issues, and consumer action. Fees vary with the services provided but typically are less than or equal to those charged by local hospitals. Some base fees on the ability of the family to pay (i.e., a reduced-fee sliding scale). Several third-party payers, as well as Medicaid and the Civilian Health and Medical Programs of the Uniformed Forces (CHAMPUS), recognize and reimburse these centers.

Home Birth. Home birth has always been popular in certain countries, such as Sweden and The Netherlands. In developing countries, hospitals or adequate lying-in facilities often are unavailable to most pregnant women, and home birth is a necessity. In North America, home births account for less than 1% of births (Ventura et al, 1998).

National groups supporting home birth are the Home Oriented Maternity Experience (HOME) and the National Association of Parents for Safe Alternatives in Childbirth (NAPSAC). These groups work to foster more humane childbearing practices at all levels, integrating the alternatives for childbirth to meet the needs of the total population. Medically directed home birth services with skilled nurse-midwives and medical backup have excellent outcome statistics.

With a home birth the family is in control of the experience, and the birth may be more physiologically natural in familiar surroundings. The mother may be more relaxed than she would be in the hospital environment. The family can assist in and be a part of the birth, and the mother-father/partner-infant (and sibling-infant) contact is immediate and sustained. Serious infection may be less likely (assuming strict aseptic principles are followed) since it is usual for people to be relatively immune to the bacteria in their own home.

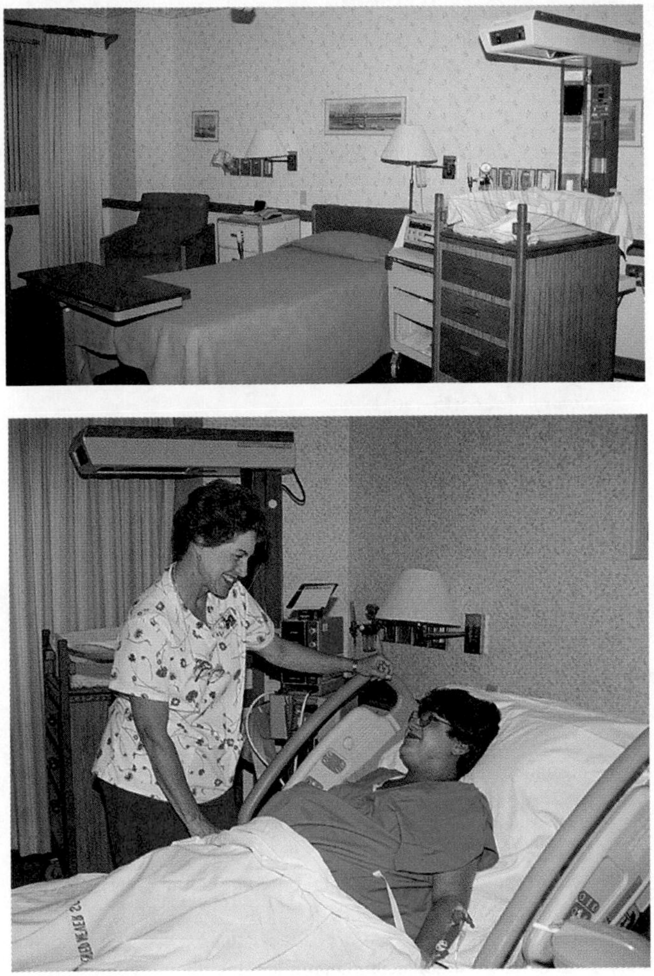

FIG. 11-22 • **A,** LDR unit. **B,** LDRP unit. (A, courtesy Marjorie Pyle, RNC, Lifecircle, Costa Mesa, CA.)

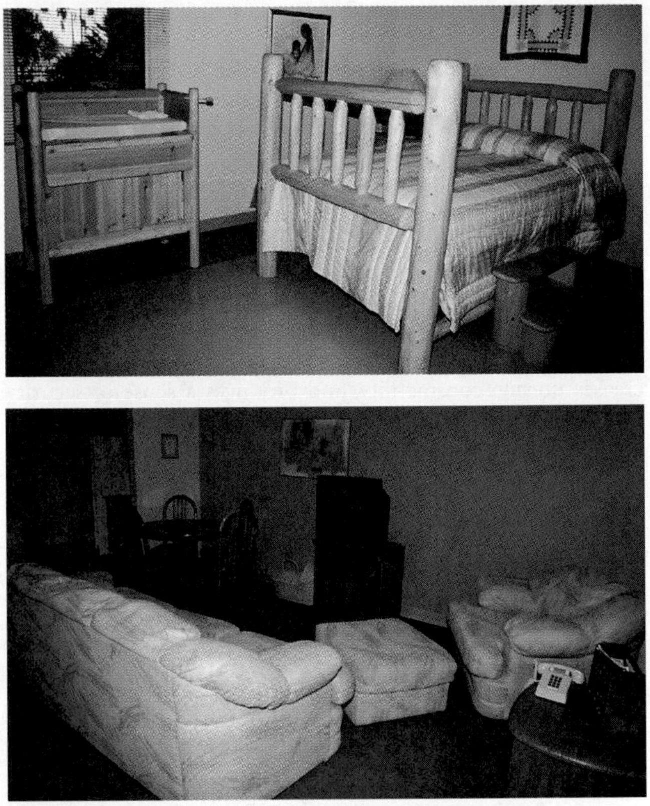

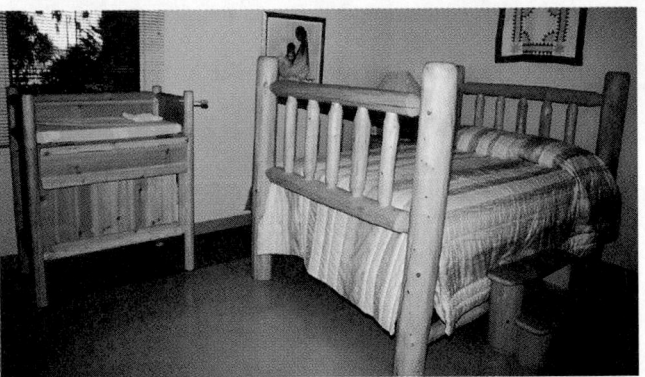

FIG. 11-23 • Birth center. **A,** Note double bed and crib. **B,** Lounge and kitchen. (Courtesy Michael S. Clement, MD, Mesa, AZ.)

Critical Thinking

HOME BIRTH

Millie, G1 P0, is interested in having a home birth. What assessments are necessary to identify whether it is feasible and safe for Millie to have a home birth? What supports are necessary for a home birth? Who in the area in which you live would attend a home birth? How would you identify providers who are willing to attend a home birth? In your setting, is home birth feasible and safe? By what criteria did you make that judgment?

Some disadvantages to a home birth need to be considered. Although some physicians and nurses support home births that use good medical and emergency backup systems, many regard this practice as exposing the mother and the fetus to unnecessary danger. Thus home births are not widely accepted by the medical community in the United States. This makes it difficult for a family to find a qualified health care provider willing to give prenatal care and to attend the birth. Backup emergency care by a physician in a hospital may be difficult to arrange in advance. If an emergency birth is necessary, no effective way exists to do this rapidly in the home setting.

Factors Increasing the Safety of Birth at Home. Most health care providers agree that if home birth is the woman's choice, certain criteria must be met for a safe home birth experience. The woman must be comfortable with her decision to have her baby at home. She should be in good health; home birth is not indicated for women with a high risk pregnancy. A drive to the hospital should take no more than 10 to 15 minutes. The woman should be attended by a well-trained physician or midwife with adequate medical supplies and resuscitation equipment, including oxygen.

Pain Management. Fear of pain is a key issue for pregnant women and the reason many give for attending childbirth education classes. Pain management strategies are an essential component of childbirth education. Couples need information about the advantages and disadvantages of pain medication and about other techniques for coping with labor. An emphasis on nonpharmacologic pain management strategies helps couples manage the labor and birth with dignity and increased comfort. Most instructors teach a flexible approach, which helps couples learn and master many techniques that can be used during labor. Couples are taught techniques such as massage, pressure on the palms or soles of the feet, hot compresses to the perineum, perineal massage, applications of heat or cold, breathing patterns, and focusing of attention on visual or other stimuli as ways to increase coping and decrease the distress from labor pain.

Other valuable tools are vocalization or "sounding" to relieve tension during pregnancy and labor; subdued lighting; warm water for showers or bathing during labor; and aromatherapy. Some hospitals have Jacuzzi bathtubs for use during labor (see Fig. 16-4). Childbearing couples are taught to recognize labor's start and to practice coping skills such as relaxation, slow breathing, and other nonpharmacologic strategies (see Chapter 16).

Relaxation counters the effects of sympathetic nervous system arousal. It produces a balance between the sympathetic and parasympathetic systems, slows heart and breathing rates, increases uterine contractility, and produces a sense of security and tranquility. To be effective, varied relaxation techniques must be incorporated into every class session. Paced breathing, biofeedback, therapeutic touch, acupressure, imagery and visualization, and music are relaxation techniques that can be used (see Chapter 16).

Key Points

- The prenatal period is a preparatory one, both physically and psychologically.
- Psychosocial aspects of care may affect pregnancy, childbirth, and the adjustment of the new family.
- The pregnant woman's readiness to learn is at a high level, making this an excellent time to help her expand her self-care skills.
- Maternal physical and familial adaptations to pregnancy generate needs that the nurse can anticipate and meet.
- Even with a normal pregnancy the nurse must remain alert to hazards such as supine hypotension, warning signs and symptoms, and signs of family maladaptations.
- Each pregnant woman needs to know how to recognize and report preterm labor.
- Parent-child, sibling-child, and grandparent-child relationships are affected by pregnancy.
- Cultural prescriptions and proscriptions influence responses to pregnancy and to the health care delivery system.
- Childbirth education is a process designed to help parents make the transition from the role of expectant parents to the role and responsibilities of parents of a new baby.
- *Healthy People 2010* provides goals for maternal and infant health.

References

Abel E: *Fetal alcohol syndrome,* Boca Raton, 1996, CRC Press.

Alan Guttmacher Institute: *Teen sex and pregnancy.* Retrieved 3/15/99 from www.agiusa.org/pubs/fb_teen_sex.html, 1998.

Alden K, Harris B: Choices in childbearing. In Fogel C, Woods N, editors: *Women's health care,* Thousand Oaks, CA, 1995, Sage.

Al-Qutob R, Mawajdeh S, Bin-Raad F: The assessment of reproductive health services: a conceptual framework for prenatal care, *Health Care Women Int* 17:423-434, 1996.

Alteneder R, Hartzell D: Addressing couples' sexuality concerns during the childbearing period: use of the PLISSIT model, *J Obstet Gynecol Neonatal Nurs* 26:651-658, 1997.

American College of Obstetricians and Gynecologists: *Smoking and women's health (ACOG Tech Bull No. 240),* Washington, DC, 1997, ACOG.

Beischer N, MacKay E, Colditz P: *Obstetrics and the newborn,* ed 3, Philadelphia, 1997, WB Saunders.

Bergsjo P, Villar J: Scientific basis for the content of routine antenatal care, *Acta Obstet Gynecol Scand* 76:15-25, 1997.

Berkowitz R: Ethical issues involving multifetal pregnancies, *Mt Sinai J Med* 65:15-190, 1998.

Callister L: Cultural meanings of childbirth, *J Obstet Gynecol Neonatal Nurs* 24:327-331, 1995.

Campbell-Brown M, Hytten F: Nutrition. In Chamberlain G, Broughton-Pipkin F, editors: *Clinical physiology in obstetrics,* Oxford, 1998, Blackwell Science.

Chestnut M: *High risk perinatal home care manual,* Philadelphia, 1998, JB Lippincott.

Cockey C: Preventing teen pregnancy, *AWHONN Lifelines* 1(3):32-40, 1997.

Crowley P: *Interventions to prevent, or improve outcome from, delivery at or beyond term.* Cochrane Library (Oxford) 3, CD-ROM, 1998.

Cunningham F et al: *Williams obstetrics,* ed 20, Stamford, CT, 1997, Appleton & Lange.

Davis D: The discomforts of pregnancy, *J Obstet Gynecol Neonatal Nurs* 25(1):73-81, 1996.

Dollberg S et al: Adverse perinatal outcome in the older primipara, *J Perinatol* 16(2 Pt 1):93-97, 1996.

Doulas of North America: *Do I need a doula?* (On-line). Available URL: www.dona.com.faq.html, 1999a.

Doulas of North America: *Doulas of North America position paper: the doula's contribution to modern maternity care* (On-line). Available URL: www.cona.com/positionpapers.html, 1999b.

Doulas of North America: *Mission statement* (On-line). Available URL: www.dona.com/mission.html, 1999c.

Ebrahim SH et al: Alcohol consumption by pregnant women in the United States during 1988-1995, *Obstet Gynecol* 92: 187-192, 1998.

Gilbert E, Harmon J: *Manual of high risk pregnancy and delivery,* ed 2, St Louis, 1998, Mosby.

Helewa M et al: Report of the Canadian Hypertension Society Consensus Conference: definitions, evaluation and classification of hypertensive disorders in pregnancy, *Can Med Assoc J* 157:715-725, 1997.

Jackson S, Soper D: Sexually transmitted diseases in pregnancy, *Obstet Gynecol Clin North Am* 24:631-644, 1997.

Jansson L et al: Pregnancy and addiction. A comprehensive care model, *J Subst Abuse Treat* 13:321-329, 1996.

Johnson C: Reducing smoking among women, *AWHONN Lifelines* 2(5):16, 1998.

Lawrence R: *Breastfeeding: a guide for the medical profession,* ed 5, St Louis, 1999, Mosby.

Lederman R: *Psychosocial adaptation in pregnancy,* ed 2, New York, 1996, Springer.

Malnory M: Developmental care of the pregnant couple, *J Obstet Gynecol Neonatal Nurs* 25:17-23, 1996.

May K: A typology of detachment and involvement styles adopted during pregnancy by first-time expectant fathers, *West J Nurs Res* 2(2):444-461, 1980.

May K: Three phases of father involvement in pregnancy, *Nurs Res* 31:337-342, 1982.

McFarlane J et al: Safety behaviors of abused women after an intervention during pregnancy, *J Obstet Gynecol Neonatal Nurs* 27:64-69, 1998.

Mercer R: *Becoming a mother,* New York, 1995, Springer.

Mvula M, Miller J: A comparative evaluation of collaborative prenatal care, *Obstet Gynecol* 91:169-173, 1998.

Neilson J: *Routine ultrasound in early pregnancy,* Cochrane Library (Oxford) 3, CD-ROM, 1998.

Oakley D et al: Comparison of outcomes of maternity care by obstetricians and certified nurse midwives, *Obstet Gynecol* 88:823-829, 1996.

Polivka B, Nickel J, Wilkins J: Urinary tract infection during pregnancy, *J Obstet Gynecol Neonatal Nurs* 26:405-413, 1997.

Rubin R: Maternal tasks in pregnancy, *Matern Child Nurs J* 4:143-153, 1975.

Rubin R: *Maternity identity and the maternal experience,* New York, 1984, Springer.

Rynerson B, Lowdermilk D: Sexual intimacy in pregnancy. In Knuppel R, Drukker J: *High risk pregnancy: a team approach,* ed 2, Philadelphia, 1993, WB Saunders.

Sampselle C et al: Effect of pelvic muscle exercise on transient incontinence during pregnancy and after birth, *Obstet Gynecol* 91:406-412, 1998.

Seidel H et al: *Mosby's guide to physical examination,* ed 4, St Louis, 1999, Mosby.

Simon N, Heaps K, Chodroff C: Improving the processes of care and outcomes in obstetrics/gynecology, *Joint Commission Journal on Quality Improvement* 23:485-497, 1997.

Skinner J et al: Transitions in infant feeding during the first year of life, *J Am Coll Nutr* 16:209-215, 1997.

Spector R: *Cultural diversity in health and illness,* ed 4, Stamford, CT, 1996, Appleton & Lange.

Stark M: Psychosocial adjustment during pregnancy: the experience of mature gravidas, *J Obstet Gynecol Neonatal Nurs* 26:206-211, 1997.

Ventura S, Curtin S, Mathews T: Teenage births in the United States: national and state trends, 1990-1996, *Nat Vital Stat Rep* 47(12):1-17, 1998.

Ventura S et al: Advance report of final natality statistics, 1996, *Monthly Vital Stat Rep* 46(11 suppl):1-99, 1998.

Wagner C et al: The impact of prenatal drug exposure on the neonate, *Obstet Gynecol Clin North Am* 25:169-194, 1998.

CHAPTER 12
Maternal and Fetal Nutrition

http://www.harcourthealth.com/MERLIN/Wong/maternal/

Learning Objectives

On completion of this chapter the reader will be able to:

- Explain recommended maternal weight gain during pregnancy.
- Compare the recommended level of intake of energy sources, protein, and key vitamins and minerals during pregnancy and lactation.
- Give examples of the food sources that provide the nutrients required for optimal maternal nutrition during pregnancy and lactation.
- Examine the role of nutrition supplements during pregnancy.
- List five nutritional risk factors during pregnancy.
- Compare the dietary needs of adolescent and mature pregnant women.
- Give examples of cultural food patterns and possible dietary problems for two ethnic groups or for two alternative eating patterns.

Nutrition is one of the many factors that influence the outcome of pregnancy (Fig. 12-1). However, maternal nutritional status is an especially significant factor, both because it is potentially alterable and because good nutrition before and during pregnancy is an important preventive measure for a variety of problems. These problems include birth of low-birth-weight and preterm infants. It is essential that the importance of good nutrition be emphasized to all women of childbearing potential. Nutrition assessment, intervention, and evaluation must be an integral part of the nursing care provided all pregnant women.

NUTRIENT NEEDS BEFORE CONCEPTION

A healthful diet before conception is the best way to ensure that adequate nutrients are available for the developing fetus. Folic acid (folate) intake is of particular concern before conception and during early gestation, because neural tube defects (i.e., failure in closure of the neural tube) are more common in infants of women with poor folic acid intake. It is estimated that the incidence of neural tube defects could be halved if all women had an adequate folic acid intake during this period (Butterworth and Bendich, 1996). All women capable of becoming pregnant are advised to consume 400 μg of folic acid daily in fortified foods (e.g., ready-to-eat cereals and enriched grain products) or supplements in addition to a diet rich in folic acid–containing foods such as green leafy vegetables, whole grains, and meats.

Both maternal and fetal risks in pregnancy are increased when the mother is significantly underweight or overweight when pregnancy begins. Ideally all women would achieve their desirable body weights before conception.

NUTRIENT NEEDS DURING PREGNANCY

Nutrient needs are determined, at least in part, by the stage of gestation in that the amount of fetal growth varies during the different stages of pregnancy. During the first trimester, when the embryo/fetus is very small, the synthesis of fetal tissues places relatively few demands on maternal nutrition. Therefore the first trimester needs are only slightly increased over those before pregnancy. In contrast, the last trimester is a period of noticeable fetal growth when most of the deposition of fetal stores of energy sources and minerals occurs. Basal metabolic rates (BMRs), when expressed as kilocalories (kcal) per minute, are approximately 20% higher in pregnant women than in nonpregnant women. This increase includes the energy cost for tissue synthesis.

Dietary Reference Intakes (DRIs) are a new approach that the Food and Nutrition Board of the National Academy of

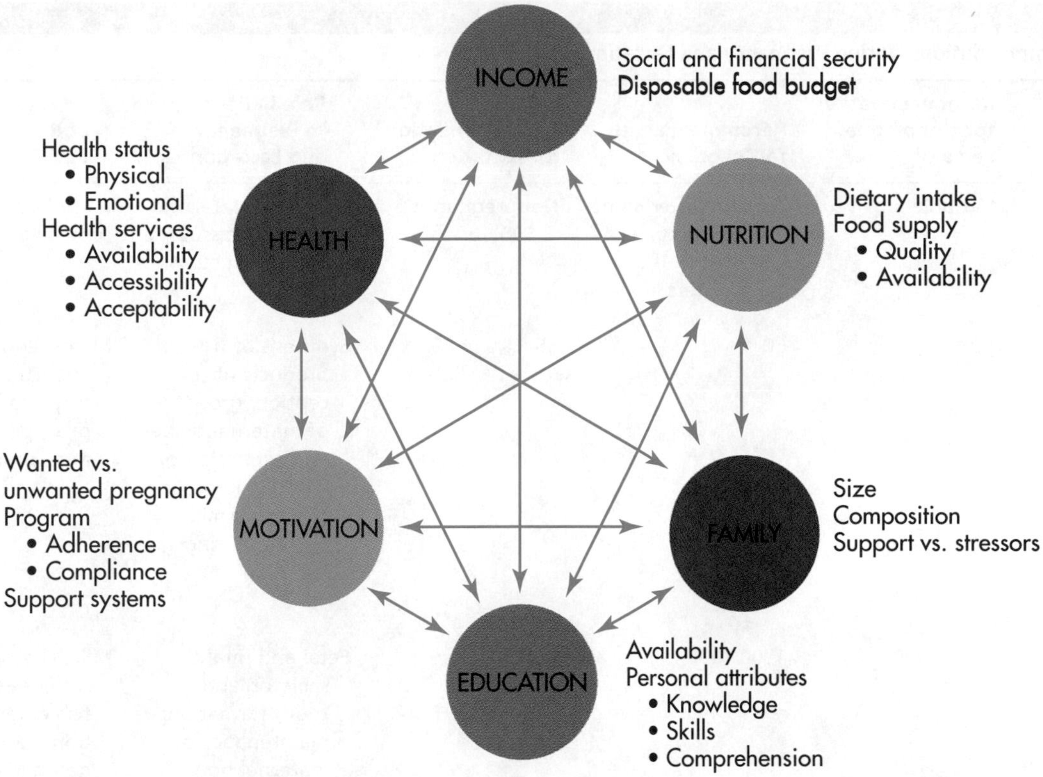

FIG. 12-1 • Web of influences that can affect outcome of pregnancy. (From Wardlaw G, Insel P: *Perspectives in nutrition,* St Louis, 1993, Mosby.)

Sciences has adopted to provide nutritional recommendations for the people of the United States. Health Canada is also involved in this effort (Yates, Schlicker, and Suitor, 1998). The DRIs consist of Recommended Dietary Allowances (RDAs) and Adequate Intakes (AIs), as well as guidelines for avoiding excessive nutrient intakes. RDAs are recommendations for daily nutritional intakes that meet the needs of almost all of the healthy members of the population. AIs are similar to the RDAs except that they are used when there are not enough data available to be certain that they meet the needs of the healthy population. The RDAs and the AIs include a wide variety of nutrients and food components, and are divided into age, sex, and life-stage categories (e.g., infancy, pregnancy, and lactation). They can be used as goals in planning the diets of individuals (Table 12-1).

Energy Needs

Energy (kilocalories or kcal) needs are met by carbohydrate, fat, and protein in the diet. No specific recommendations exist for the amount of carbohydrate and fat in the diet of the pregnant woman. However, intake of these nutrients should be adequate to support the recommended weight gain. Although protein can be used to supply energy, its primary role is to provide amino acids for the synthesis of new tissues (see the discussion on protein later in this chapter). The RDA during the second and third trimesters of pregnancy is 300 kcal greater than prepregnancy needs; very underweight or active women may require more than 300 additional kcal to sustain the desired rate of weight gain.

Weight Gain. The optimal weight gain during pregnancy is not known precisely. It is known, however, that the amount of weight gained by the mother during pregnancy has an important bearing on the course and outcome of pregnancy. Adequate weight gain reduces the risk of delivering a small-for-gestational age (SGA) or preterm infant.

The desirable weight gain during pregnancy varies among individual women. Maternal and fetal risks in pregnancy are increased when the mother is either significantly underweight or overweight before pregnancy, and when weight gain during pregnancy is either too low or too high. Women with inadequate weight gain have an increased risk of delivering an infant with intrauterine growth restriction (IUGR). Greater-than-expected weight gain during pregnancy may occur for many reasons, including multiple gestation, edema, pregnancy-induced hypertension (PIH), and overeating. When obesity is present (either preexisting or developed during pregnancy) there is an increased likelihood of macrosomia and fetopelvic disproportion, operative birth, birth trauma, and infant mortality. Obese women are more likely to have hypertension and di-

Critical Thinking

NUTRITION AND THE OVERWEIGHT PREGNANT WOMAN

Perform a nutrition assessment of a pregnant woman who appears to be overweight for her height. Calculate her prepregnancy BMI. With the woman, plan a diet that meets the minimum daily requirements and allows for growth of the pregnancy. Include consideration of personal preferences and cultural factors in your plan. With the woman, identify barriers to implementing the plan.

TABLE 12-1
Nutritional Recommendations During Pregnancy and Lactation

Nutrient (Unit)	Recommendation for Nonpregnant Female*	Recommendation for Pregnancy*	Recommendation for Lactation*	Role in Relation to Pregnancy and Lactation	Food Food Sources
Energy (kcal)	Variable	First trimester, same as nonpregnant; second and third trimesters, nonpregnant + 300	Nonpregnant + 500	Growth of fetal and maternal tissues; milk production	Carbohydrate, fat, protein
Protein (g)	50	60	65	Synthesis of the products of conception; growth of maternal tissue and expansion of blood volume; secretion of milk protein during lactation	Meats, eggs, cheese, yogurt, legumes (dry beans and peas, peanuts), nuts, grains
MINERALS					
Calcium (mg)	1300/1000	1300/1000	1300/1000	Fetal and infant skeleton and tooth formation; maintenance of maternal bone and tooth mineralization	Milk, cheese, yogurt, sardines or other fish eaten with bones left in, deep green leafy vegetables except spinach or Swiss chard, tofu, baked beans
Phosphorus (mg)	1250/700	1250/700	1250/700	Fetal and infant skeleton and tooth formation	Milk, cheese, yogurt, meats, whole grains, nuts, legumes
Iron (mg)	15	30	15	Maternal hemoglobin formation, fetal liver iron storage	Liver, meats, whole or enriched breads and cereals, deep green leafy vegetables, legumes, dried fruits
Zinc (mg)	12	15	19	Component of numerous enzyme systems; possibly important in preventing congenital malformations	Liver, shellfish, meats, whole grains, milk
Iodine (μg)	150	175	200	Increased maternal metabolic rate	Iodized salt, seafood, milk and milk products, commercial yeast breads, rolls, donuts
Magnesium (mg)	360/320	400/360	360/320	Involved in energy and protein metabolism, tissue growth, muscle action	Nuts, legumes, cocoa, meats, whole grains

Recommendations are the new Dietary Reference Intakes (RDA or AI, see text) where available (Food and Nutrition Board, National Academy of Sciences, Institute of Medicine: *Recommended levels for individual intake, B vitamins, and choline,* Washington, DC, 1998, National Academy Press; Standing Committee on the Scientific Evaluation of Dietary Reference Intakes, Food and Nutrition Board, Institute of Medicine: *Dietary reference intakes: Calcium, phosphorus, magnesium, vitamin D, and fluoride,* Washington, DC, 1997, National Academy Press.) Where DRI are not yet available, the values are taken from Food and Nutrition Board, 1989.
RBC, Red blood cells.
*When two values appear, separated by a diagonal slash, the first is for females <19 years and the second is for those 19 to 50 years old.

TABLE 12-1
Nutritional Recommendations During Pregnancy and Lactation—cont'd

Nutrient (Unit)	Recommendation for Nonpregnant Female*	Recommendation for Pregnancy*	Recommendation for Lactation*	Role in Relation to Pregnancy and Lactation	Food Food Sources
FAT-SOLUBLE VITAMINS					
A (RE)	800	800	1300	Essential for cell development, tooth bud formation, bone growth	Deep green leafy vegetables, dark yellow vegetables and fruits, chili peppers, liver, fortified margarine and butter
D (μg)	5	5	5	Involved in absorption of calcium and phosphorus, improves mineralization	Fortified milk and margarine, egg yolk, butter, liver, seafood
E (mg)	8	10	12	Antioxidant (protects cell membranes from damage), especially important for preventing breakdown of RBCs	Vegetable oils, green leafy vegetables, whole grains, liver, nuts and seeds, cheese, fish
WATER-SOLUBLE VITAMINS					
C (mg)	60	70	95	Tissue formation and integrity, formation of connective tissue, enhancement of iron absorption	Citrus fruits, strawberries, melons, broccoli, tomatoes, peppers, raw deep green leafy vegetables
Folic acid (μg)	400	600	500	Prevention of neural tube defects, support increased maternal RBC formation	Fortified ready-to-eat cereals and other grains, green leafy vegetables, oranges, broccoli, asparagus, artichokes, liver
Thiamine (mg)	1.0/1.1	1.4	1.5	Involved in energy metabolism	Pork, beef, liver, whole or enriched grains, legumes
Riboflavin (mg)	1.0/1.1	1.4	1.6	Involved in energy and protein metabolism	Meat, liver, deep green vegetables, whole grains
Niacin (mg)	14	18	17	Involved in energy metabolism	Meat, fish, poultry, liver, whole or enriched grains, peanuts
Pyridoxine (B_6) (mg)	1.2/1.3	1.9	2.0	Involved in protein metabolism	Meat, liver, deep green vegetables, whole grains
B_{12} (μg)	2.4	2.6	2.8	Production of nucleic acids and proteins, especially important in formation of RBC and neural functioning	Milk and milk products, egg, meat, liver, fortified soy milk

abetes, and their risk of giving birth to a child with a major congenital defect is double that of normal-weight women (Prentice and Goldberg, 1996). The cost of pregnancy in an obese woman has been estimated to be triple that of a normal-weight woman (Prentice and Goldberg, 1996).

The primary factor to consider in making a weight gain recommendation is the appropriateness of the prepregnancy weight for the woman's height. A commonly used method of evaluating the appropriateness of weight for height is the body mass index (BMI), which is calculated by the following formula:

$$\text{BMI} = \text{weight}/\text{height}^2$$

where the weight is in kilograms and height is in meters. Thus for a woman who weighed 51 kg before pregnancy and is 1.57 m tall:

$$\text{BMI} = 51/(1.57)^2, \text{ or } 20.7$$

BMI can be classified into the following categories: less than 19.8, underweight or low; 19.8 to 26.0, normal; 26.0 to 29.0, overweight or high; and greater than 29.0, obese.

For women with single fetuses, current recommendations are that women with a normal BMI should gain 11.5 to 16 kg during pregnancy, underweight women should gain 12.5 to 18 kg, overweight women should gain 7 to 11.5 kg, and obese women should gain at least 7 kg. Adolescents are encouraged to strive for weight gains at the upper end of the recommended range for their BMI because it appears that the fetus and the still-growing mother compete for nutrients. The risk of mechanical complications at birth is reduced if the weight gain of short adult women (i.e., less than 157 cm) is near the lower end of their recommended range. In twin gestations, gains of approximately 16 to 20 kg appear to be associated with the best outcomes (Ellings, Newman, and Bower, 1998).

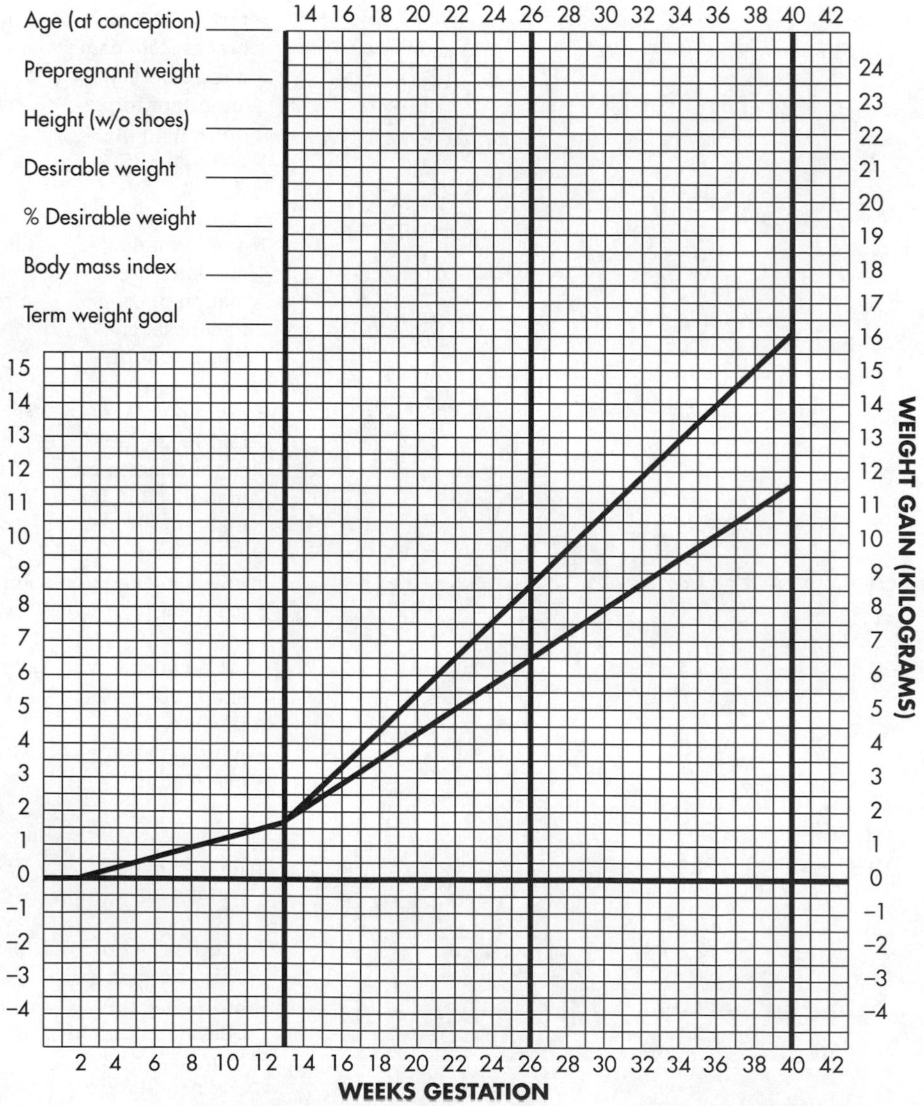

FIG. 12-2 • Prenatal weight gain chart for plotting weight gain of normal weight women. NOTE: Young adolescents, African-American women, and smokers should aim for the upper end of the recommended range; short women (<157 cm) should strive for gains at the lower end of the range.

Pattern of Weight Gain. Weight gain should take place throughout pregnancy. The risk of delivering an SGA infant is greater when the weight gain early in pregnancy has been poor. The likelihood of preterm birth is greater when the gains during the last half of pregnancy have been inadequate. These risks exist even when the total gain for the pregnancy is in the recommended range.

The optimal rate of weight gain depends on the stage of pregnancy. During the first and second trimesters, growth takes place primarily in maternal tissue; during the third trimester, growth occurs primarily in fetal tissues. During the first trimester there is an average total weight gain of only 1 to 2.5 kg. Thereafter the recommended weight gain increases to approximately 0.4 kg per week for a woman of normal weight (Fig. 12-2). The recommended weekly weight gain for overweight women during the second and third trimesters is 0.3 kg, and for underweight women it is 0.5 kg. The recommended caloric intake corresponds to this pattern of gain. For the first trimester there is no increment; during the second and third trimesters an additional 300 kcal/day over the prepregnant intake is recommended. The amount of food providing 300 kcal is not great. It can be provided by one additional serving from each of the following groups: milk, yogurt, or cheese (all skim milk products); fruits; vegetables; and bread, cereal, rice, or pasta.

The reasons for an inadequate weight gain (less than 1 kg per month for normal-weight women or less than 0.5 kg per month for obese women during the last two trimesters) or excessive weight gain (more than 3 kg per month) should be thoroughly evaluated. Possible reasons for deviations from the expected rate of weight gain include measurement or recording errors, differences in weight of clothing, time of day, and accumulation of fluids, as well as inadequate or excessive dietary intake. An exceptionally high gain is likely to be caused by an accumulation of fluids, and a gain of more than 3 kg in a month, especially after the twentieth week of gestation, often heralds the development of PIH.

Hazards of Restricting Adequate Weight Gain. An obsession with thinness and dieting permeates the North American culture. Slender, figure-conscious women may find it difficult to make the transition from guarding against weight gain before pregnancy to valuing weight gain during pregnancy. In counseling these women, the nurse can emphasize the positive effects of good nutrition, as well as the adverse effects of maternal malnutrition (as manifested by poor weight gain) on infant growth and development. This counseling includes information on the components of weight gain during pregnancy (Fig. 12-3) and the amount of this weight that will be lost at birth. Early in a woman's pregnancy, explaining ways to lose weight in the postpartum period helps relieve her concerns. Because lactation can help to reduce maternal energy stores gradually, this provides an opportunity to promote breastfeeding.

Pregnancy is not a time to diet. Even overweight or obese pregnant women need to gain at least enough weight to equal the weight of the products of conception (i.e., fetus, placenta, and amniotic fluid). If they limit their caloric intake to prevent weight gain, they may also excessively limit their intake of important nutrients. Moreover, dietary restriction results in catabolism of fat stores, which in turn augments the production of ketones. The long-term effects of mild ketonemia during pregnancy are not known, but ketonuria has been found to correlate with the occurrence of preterm labor. It should be stressed to obese women, and to all pregnant women, that the quality of the weight gain is important, with emphasis on the consumption of nutrient-dense foods and the avoidance of empty-calorie foods.

Weight gain is important, but pregnancy is not an excuse for uncontrolled dietary indulgence. Excessive weight gained during pregnancy may be difficult to lose after pregnancy, thus con-

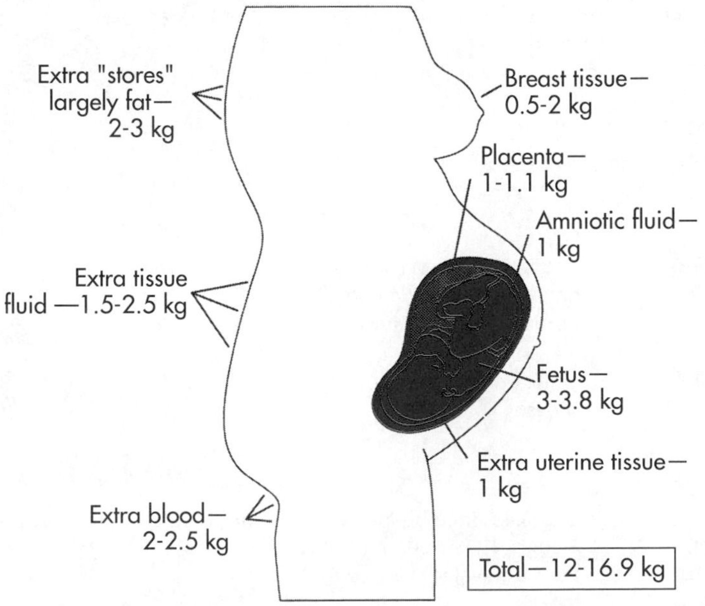

FIG. 12-3 • Components of maternal weight gain at 40 weeks of gestation. (Modified from Worthington-Roberts B, Williams S: *Nutrition in pregnancy and lactation,* ed 6, Dubuque, IA, 1997, Brown and Benchmark.)

tributing to chronic overweight or obesity, an etiologic factor in a host of chronic diseases including hypertension, diabetes mellitus, and arteriosclerotic heart disease. The woman who gains 18 kg or more during pregnancy is especially at risk.

Protein

Protein, with its essential constituent, nitrogen, is the nutritional element basic to growth. Adequate protein is essential to meet increasing demands in pregnancy. These demands arise from the rapid growth of the fetus; the enlargement of the uterus and its supporting structures, mammary glands, and placenta; an increase in maternal circulating blood volume and subsequent demand for increased amounts of plasma protein to maintain colloidal osmotic pressure; and the formation of amniotic fluid.

Milk, meat, eggs, and cheese are complete protein foods with a high biologic value. Legumes (dried beans and peas), whole grains, and nuts are also valuable sources of protein. In addition, these protein-rich foods are a source of other nutrients such as calcium, iron, and B vitamins; plant sources of protein often provide needed dietary fiber. The recommended daily food plan (Table 12-2) is a guide to the amounts of these foods that will supply the quantities of protein needed. The recommendations provide for only a modest increase in protein intake over the prepregnant levels in adult women. Protein intake in many people in the United States is relatively high, so many women may not need to increase their protein intake at all during pregnancy. Three servings of milk, yogurt, or cheese (four for adolescents) and 5 to 6 ounces (140 to 168 g) (two servings) of meat, poultry, or fish supply the recommended protein for the pregnant woman. Additional protein is provided by vegetables and breads, cereals, rice, and pasta. Pregnant adolescents, women from impoverished backgrounds, and women adhering to unusual diets such as a macrobiotic (highly restricted vegetarian) diet, are those most likely to have inadequate protein in-

TABLE 12-2
Daily Food Guide for Pregnancy and Lactation

		Suggested Number of Servings		
Food Group	**Serving Size**	**Nonpregnant, Nonlactating Woman**	**Pregnant Woman**	**Lactating Woman**
GRAIN PRODUCTS				
Include whole-grain and enriched breads, cereals, pasta, and rice.	1 slice bread; ½ bun, bagel, or English muffin; 1 oz ready-to-eat cereal; ½ c cooked grains	6-11	6-11	6-11
VEGETABLES				
Eat dark green leafy and deep yellow often. Eat dried beans and peas often; count ½ c cooked dried beans or peas as a serving of vegetables or 1 oz from meat group.	1 c raw leafy greens; ½ c of others	3-5	3-5	3-5
FRUITS				
Include citrus fruits, strawberries, or melons frequently.	1 medium apple, orange, banana, peach, etc; ½ c small or diced fruit; ¾ c juice	2-4	2-4	2-4
MILK AND MILK PRODUCTS	1 c milk or yogurt; 1½ oz cheese	2-3	3 or more	4 or more
MEAT, POULTRY, FISH, DRY BEANS, NUTS, AND EGGS				
Eat peanut butter or nuts rarely to avoid excessive fat intake. Limit egg intake to reduce cholesterol intake; trim fat from meat, and remove skin from poultry.	½ c cooked dried beans, 1 egg, or 1½ T peanut butter is equivalent to 1 oz of meat	Up to 6 oz total	Up to 6 oz total	Up to 6 oz total

c, Cup; *T*, tablespoon.

take. The use of high-protein supplements is not recommended, because these have been associated with an increased incidence of preterm births.

Fluids

Essential during the exchange of nutrients and waste products across cell membranes, water is the main substance of cells, blood, lymph, amniotic fluid, and other vital body fluids. It also aids in maintaining body temperature. A good fluid intake promotes good bowel function, which is sometimes a problem during pregnancy. Dehydration may increase the risk of cramping/contractions and preterm labor. The recommended daily intake is about 6 to 8 glasses (1500 to 2000 ml) of fluid. Water, milk, and juices are good fluid sources.

Women who consume more than 300 mg of caffeine daily (equivalent to about 500 to 750 ml of coffee) are at increased risk of miscarriage and of delivering infants with IUGR. Caffeine's ill effects have been supposed to result from vasoconstriction of the blood vessels supplying the uterus or interference with cell division in the developing fetus (Hinds et al, 1996). As a consequence, caffeine-containing products such as caffeinated coffee, tea, soft drinks, and cocoa beverages should be avoided or consumed only in limited quantities.

Aspartame (e.g., Nutrasweet and Equal) and acesulfame K (e.g., Sweet One), artificial sweeteners commonly used in low or no-calorie beverages, have not been found to have adverse effects on the normal mother or fetus; but aspartame use should be avoided by pregnant women who are homozygous for phenylketonuria (PKU).

Minerals and Vitamins

In general, the nutrient needs of pregnant women, except perhaps the need for iron, can be met through dietary sources. Counseling about the need for a varied diet rich in vitamins and minerals should be a part of every pregnant woman's early prenatal care and should be reinforced throughout pregnancy. However, supplements of certain nutrients (listed in the following discussion) are recommended whenever the woman's diet is very poor or whenever significant nutritional risk factors are present. Nutritional risk factors in pregnancy are listed in Box 12-1.

Box 12-1

Indicators of Nutritional Risk in Pregnancy

- Adolescence
- Frequent pregnancies: 3 within 2 years
- Poor fetal outcome in a previous pregnancy
- Poverty
- Poor diet habits with resistance to change
- Use of tobacco, alcohol, or drugs
- Weight at conception under or over normal weight
- Problems with weight gain
  - Any weight loss
  - Weight gain of less than 1 kg/mo after the first trimester
  - Weight gain of more than 1 kg/wk after the first trimester
- Multifetal pregnancy
- Low hemoglobin and/or hematocrit values

Iron. Iron is needed both to allow for transfer of adequate iron to the fetus and to permit expansion of the maternal RBC mass. Beginning in the latter part of the first trimester the blood volume of the mother increases steadily, peaking at about 1500 ml more than in the nonpregnant state. In twin gestations, the increase is at least 500 ml greater than in pregnancies with single fetuses. Plasma volume increases more than RBC mass. The relative excess of plasma causes a modest decrease in the hemoglobin concentration and hematocrit, known as physiologic anemia of pregnancy. This is a normal adaptation during pregnancy.

However, poor iron intake and absorption, which can result in iron deficiency anemia, is relatively common among women in the childbearing years. It affects nearly one fifth of the pregnant women in industrialized countries. The maternal mortality rate is increased among anemic women, who are poorly prepared to tolerate hemorrhage at the time of birth. In addition, anemic women may have a greater likelihood of cardiac failure during labor, postpartum infections, and poor wound healing. The fetus is also affected by maternal anemia. The risk of preterm birth is greater in anemic women, and fetal iron stores may also be reduced by maternal anemia (Allen, 2000). Anemia is more common among adolescents and African-American women than among adult Caucasian women.

Evidence supports the recommendation that all pregnant women receive a daily supplement of ferrous iron (Allen, 2000). (Iron supplements may be poorly tolerated during the nausea that is prevalent in the first trimester.) If iron deficiency anemia (as manifested by low levels of hematocrit or hemoglobin and serum ferritin) is present, higher dosages are required. Certain foods taken with an iron supplement can promote or inhibit absorption of iron. Even when a woman is taking an iron supplement, she should include good food sources of iron in her daily diet (see Table 12-1).

Calcium. There is no increase in the DRI of calcium during pregnancy and lactation, in comparison to the recommendation for the nonpregnant woman (see Table 12-1). The DRI (1000 mg daily for women 19 and older and 1300 mg for those younger than 19) appears to provide sufficient calcium for fetal bone and tooth development to proceed while maintaining maternal bone mass.

Milk and yogurt are especially rich sources of calcium, providing approximately 300 mg per cup (240 ml). Nevertheless, many women do not consume these foods or do not consume adequate amounts to provide the recommended intakes of calcium. One problem that can interfere with milk consumption is lactose intolerance; the inability to digest milk sugar (lactose) is caused by the absence of the lactase enzyme in the small intestine. Lactose intolerance is relatively common in adults, particularly African-Americans, Asians, Native Americans, and Eskimos. Milk consumption may cause abdominal cramping, bloating, and diarrhea in such people. Yogurt, sweet acidophilus milk, buttermilk, cheese, chocolate milk, and cocoa may be tolerated even when fresh fluid milk is not. Commercial products that contain the lactase enzyme (e.g., Lactaid) are available in pharmacies and many supermarkets. The lactase in these products hydrolyzes, or digests, the lactose in milk, making it possible for lactose-intolerant people to drink milk.

In some cultures, adults rarely drink milk. For example, Puerto Ricans and other Hispanic people may use milk only as an additive in coffee. Pregnant women from these cultures may need to consume nondairy sources of calcium. Vegetarian diets may also be deficient in calcium (Box 12-2). If calcium intake appears low, and the woman does not change her dietary habits despite counseling, a daily supplement containing 600 mg of elemental calcium may be needed. Calcium supplements may also be recommended when a pregnant woman experiences leg cramps caused by an imbalance in the calcium/phosphorus ratio.

Sodium. During pregnancy the need for sodium increases slightly, primarily because the body water is expanding (e.g., the expanding blood volume). Sodium is essential for maintaining body water balance. Grain, milk, and meat products, which are good sources of other nutrients needed during pregnancy, are significant sources of sodium.

In the past, dietary sodium was routinely restricted in an effort to control the peripheral edema that commonly occurs during pregnancy. However, it is now recognized that moderate peripheral edema is normal in pregnancy, occurring as a response to the fluid-retaining effects of elevated levels of estrogen. An excessive emphasis on sodium restriction may make it difficult for pregnant women to achieve an adequate diet. In addition, restriction of sodium intake may stress the adrenal glands and the kidney as they attempt to retain adequate sodium. In general, sodium restriction is necessary only if the woman has a medical condition such as renal or liver failure or hypertension.

Box 12-2

Calcium Sources for Women Who Do Not Drink Milk

Each of the following provides approximately the same amount of calcium as 1 cup of milk:

FISH
3 oz can of sardines
4$^1/_2$ oz can of salmon (if bones are eaten)

BEANS AND LEGUMES
3 cups of cooked dried beans
2$^1/_2$ cups of refried beans
2 cups of baked beans with molasses
1 cup of tofu (calcium is added in processing)

GREENS
1 cup of collards
1$^1/_2$ cups of kale or turnip greens

BAKED PRODUCTS
3 pieces of cornbread
3 English muffins
4 slices of French toast
2 (7 inch diameter) waffles

FRUITS
11 dried figs
1$^1/_8$ cups of orange juice with calcium added

SAUCES
3 oz of pesto sauce
5 oz of cheese sauce

Excessive intake of sodium is discouraged during pregnancy just as it is in nonpregnant women, because it may contribute to abnormal fluid retention and edema. Table salt (sodium chloride) is the richest source of sodium. Most canned foods contain added salt unless the label specifically states otherwise. Large amounts of sodium are also found in many processed foods, including meats (e.g., smoked or cured meats, cold cuts, and corned beef), baked goods, mixes for casseroles or grain products, soups, and condiments. Products low in nutritive value and excessively high in sodium include pretzels, potato and other chips, pickles, catsup, prepared mustard, steak and Worcestershire sauces, some soft drinks, and bouillon. A moderate sodium intake can usually be achieved by salting food lightly in cooking, adding no additional salt at the table, and by avoiding low-nutrient, high-sodium foods.

Zinc. Zinc is a constituent of numerous enzymes involved in major metabolic pathways. Zinc deficiency is associated with malformations of the central nervous system in infants. When large amounts of iron and folic acid are consumed, the absorption of zinc is inhibited and serum zinc levels are reduced as a result. Because iron and folic acid supplements are commonly prescribed during pregnancy, pregnant women should be encouraged to consume good sources of zinc daily (see Table 12-1). Women with anemia who receive high-dose iron supplements also need supplements of zinc (King, 2000).

Fluoride. The effect of prenatal fluoride supplementation on tooth development in the infant is not fully known. However, it appears that prenatal fluoride supplementation has little effect on the incidence and prevalence of tooth decay (Leverett et al, 1997). No increase in fluoride intake over the nonpregnant DRI is currently recommended during pregnancy (Standing Committee, 1997).

Fat-Soluble Vitamins. Fat-soluble vitamins (i.e., vitamins A, D, E, and K) are stored in the body tissues. With chronic overdoses, these vitamins can reach toxic levels. Because of the high potential for toxicity, pregnant women are advised to take fat-soluble vitamin supplements only as prescribed. Vitamins A and D deserve special mention.

Adequate intake of vitamin A is needed so that sufficient amounts can be stored in the fetus. However, dietary sources can readily supply sufficient amounts. Congenital malformations have occurred in infants of mothers who took excessive amounts of vitamin A during pregnancy, and thus supplements are not recommended for pregnant women. Vitamin A analogs such as isotretinoin (Accutane), which are prescribed for the treatment of cystic acne, are a special concern. Isotretinoin use during early pregnancy has been associated with an increased incidence of heart malformations, facial abnormalities, cleft palate, hydrocephalus, and deafness and blindness in the infant as well as an increased risk of miscarriage. Topical agents such as tretinoin (Retin-A) do not appear to enter the circulation in any substantial amounts, but their safety in pregnancy has not been confirmed.

Vitamin D plays an important role in absorption and metabolism of calcium. The main food sources of this vitamin are enriched or fortified foods such as milk and ready-to-eat cereals. Vitamin D is also produced in the skin by the action of ultraviolet light (in sunlight). Severe deficiency may cause neonatal hypocalcemia and tetany, as well as hypoplasia of the tooth enamel. Women with lactose intolerance and those who do not include milk in their diet for any reason are at risk for vitamin

D deficiency. Other risk factors are dark skin; habitual use of clothing that covers most of the skin; and living in northern latitudes where sunlight exposure is limited, especially during the winter.

Water-Soluble Vitamins. Body stores of water-soluble vitamins are much smaller than those of fat-soluble vitamins; the water-soluble vitamins, in contrast to fat-soluble vitamins, are readily excreted in the urine. Therefore good sources of water-soluble vitamins must be consumed frequently, and toxicity with overdose is less likely than with fat-soluble vitamins.

Because of the increase in RBC production during pregnancy, as well as the nutritional requirements of the rapidly growing cells in the fetus and placenta, pregnant women should consume about 50% more folic acid than nonpregnant women, or about 600 μg daily. This increased need for folic acid continues during lactation (Bailey and Gregory, 1999). In the United States, all enriched grain products (this includes most white breads, flour, and pasta) must contain folic acid at a level of 1.4 mg per kg of flour. This level of fortification supplies approximately 0.1 mg folic acid daily in the average American diet (USDHHS, FDA, 1996). All women of childbearing potential need careful counseling about including good sources of folic acid in their diet (Tinkle and Sterling, 1997).

Pyridoxine, or vitamin B_6, is involved in protein metabolism. Although levels of a pyridoxine-containing enzyme have been reported to be low in women with PIH, there is no evidence that supplementation prevents or corrects the condition. No supplement is recommended routinely, but women with poor diets and those at nutritional risk (see Box 12-1) may need a supplement. Supplementation is related to a lowered incidence of dental decay in pregnant women (Mahomed and Gulmezoglu, 2000).

Vitamin C, or ascorbic acid, plays an important role in tissue formation and enhances the absorption of iron. The vitamin C needs of most women are readily met by a diet that includes at least five servings per day of fruits and vegetables (Levine et al, 1999) (see Table 12-1), but women who smoke need more. For women at nutritional risk, a supplement is recommended. However, if the mother takes excessive doses of this vitamin during pregnancy, a vitamin C deficiency may develop in the infant after birth.

Nutrient Supplements. Food can and should be the normal vehicle to meet the additional needs imposed by pregnancy (excepting iron, for which a supplemental dose is recommended). However, some women chronically consume diets that are deficient in necessary nutrients and, for whatever reason, may be unable to change this intake. For these women a supplement should be considered. It is important that the pregnant woman understand that the use of a vitamin/mineral supplement does not lessen the need to consume a nutritious, well-balanced diet.

Other Nutritional Issues During Pregnancy

Pica and Food Cravings. Pica is the practice of consuming nonfood substances (e.g., clay, dirt, and laundry starch) or excessive amounts of foodstuffs low in nutritional value (e.g., cornstarch, ice, baking powder, and baking soda). Pica is often influenced by the woman's cultural background. In the United States it appears to be most common among African-American women, women from rural areas, and women with a family history of pica. Regular and heavy consumption of low-nutrient products may cause more nutritious foods to be displaced from the diet, and the items consumed may interfere with the absorption of nutrients, especially minerals. Women with pica have lower hemoglobin levels than those without pica (Rainville, 1998). The possibility of pica must be considered when pregnant women are found to be anemic, and the nurse should provide counseling about the health risks associated with pica. The existence of pica, as well as details of the type and amounts of products ingested, is likely to be discovered only by the sensitive interviewer who has developed a relationship of trust with the woman. It has been proposed that pica and food cravings (e.g., the urge to consume ice cream, pickles, or pizza) during pregnancy are caused by an innate drive to consume nutrients missing from the diet. However, research has not supported this hypothesis.

Adolescent Pregnancy. Many adolescent females have diets that fall below the recommended intakes of key nutrients, including energy, calcium, and iron. Sargent et al (1994) found 37% of African-American teens and 42% of Caucasian adolescents to be underweight when classified according to their BMI.

Pregnant adolescents and their infants are at increased risk of complications during pregnancy and parturition. Growth of the pelvis is delayed in comparison to growth in stature, and this helps to explain why cephalopelvic disproportion and other mechanical problems associated with labor are common among young adolescents. Competition between the growing adolescent and the fetus for nutrients may also contribute to some of the poor outcomes apparent in teen pregnancies. Pregnant adolescents are encouraged to choose a weight gain goal at the upper end of the range for their BMI.

NUTRIENT NEEDS DURING LACTATION

Nutritional needs during lactation are similar in many ways to those during pregnancy (see Table 12-1). Needs for energy (calories), protein, calcium, iodine, zinc, the B vitamins (i.e., thiamine, riboflavin, niacin, pyridoxine, and vitamin B_{12}), and vitamin C remain elevated over nonpregnant needs. The recommendations for some of these (e.g., vitamin C, zinc, and protein) is slightly to moderately higher than during pregnancy. This allowance covers the amount of the nutrients released in the milk, as well as the needs of the mother for tissue maintenance. In the case of iron and folic acid, the recommendation during lactation is lower than during pregnancy. Both of these nutrients are essential for RBC formation, and thus for maintaining the increase in the blood volume that occurs during pregnancy. With the decrease in maternal blood volume to nonpregnant levels after birth, maternal iron and folic acid needs also fall. Many lactating women experience a delay in the return of menses, and this also conserves blood cells and reduces iron and folic acid needs. It is especially important that the calcium intake be adequate; if it is not and the women does not respond to diet counseling, a supplement of 600 mg of calcium per day may be needed.

The recommended energy intake is an increase of 500 kcal more than the woman's nonpregnant intake. Lactating women should consume at least 1800 kcal/day; it is difficult to obtain adequate nutrients for maintenance of lactation at levels below that. Because of deposition of energy stores, the woman who has gained the optimal amount of weight during pregnancy is heavier after birth than at the beginning of pregnancy. As a result of the caloric demands of lactation, however, the lactating mother usually experiences a gradual but steady weight loss. Most women experience a rapid loss of several pounds during the first month postpartum whether or not they breastfeed. After the first month the average loss during lactation is 0.5 to 1.0 kg a month, and a woman who is overweight may be able to lose up to 2 kg without decreasing her milk supply.

Fluid intake must be adequate to maintain milk production, but the mother's level of thirst is the best guide to the right amount. There is no need to consume fluids in excess of the amount needed to satisfy thirst.

Care Management

During pregnancy, nutrition plays a key role in achieving an optimum outcome for the mother and her unborn baby. Motivation to learn about nutrition is usually higher during pregnancy as parents strive to "do what's right for the baby." Optimum nutrition cannot eliminate all problems that may arise in pregnancy, but it does establish a good foundation for supporting the needs of the mother and her unborn baby.

➤ Assessment

Assessment is based on a diet history (a description of the woman's usual food and beverage intake and factors affecting her nutritional status, such as medications being taken and adequacy of income to allow her to purchase the necessary foods) obtained from an interview and review of the woman's health records, physical examination, and laboratory results. Ideally a nutritional assessment is performed before conception so that any recommended changes in diet, lifestyle, and weight can be undertaken before the woman becomes pregnant.

Diet History

Obstetric and Gynecologic Impact on Nutrition. Nutritional reserves may be depleted in the multiparous woman or one who has had frequent pregnancies (especially 3 pregnancies within 2 years). A history of preterm birth or the birth of an LBW or SGA infant may indicate inadequate dietary intake. PIH may also be a factor in poor maternal nutrition. Birth of a large-for-gestational age (LGA) infant may indicate maternal diabetes mellitus. Previous contraceptive methods also may affect reproductive health. Increased menstrual blood loss often occurs during the first 3 to 6 months after placement of an intrauterine contraceptive device. Consequently the user may have low iron stores or even iron deficiency anemia. Oral contraceptive agents, on the other hand, are associated with decreased menstrual losses and increased iron stores; however, oral contraceptives may interfere with folic acid metabolism.

Medical History. Chronic maternal illnesses such as diabetes mellitus, renal disease, liver disease, cystic fibrosis or other malabsorptive disorders, seizure disorders and the use of anticonvulsant agents, hypertension, and PKU may affect nutritional status and dietary needs. In women with illnesses that have resulted in nutritional deficits or that require dietary treatment (e.g., diabetes mellitus and PKU), it is extremely important for nutritional care to be started and for the condition to be optimally controlled before conception. A registered dietitian can provide in-depth counseling for the woman who requires a therapeutic diet during pregnancy and lactation.

Usual Maternal Diet. The woman's usual food and beverage intake, adequacy of income and other resources to meet her nutritional needs, any dietary modifications, food allergies and intolerances, and all medications and nutrition supplements being taken, as well as pica and cultural dietary requirements, should be ascertained. In addition, the presence and severity of nutrition-related discomforts of pregnancy, such as morning sickness, constipation, and pyrosis (heartburn), should be determined. The nurse should be alert to any evidence of eating disorders such as anorexia nervosa, bulimia, or frequent and rigorous dieting before or during pregnancy.

The impact of food allergies and intolerances on nutritional status ranges from very important to almost nil. Lactose intolerance is of special concern in pregnant and lactating women because no other food group equals milk and milk products in terms of calcium content. If a woman suffers from lactose intolerance, the interviewer should explore her intake of other calcium sources (see Box 12-2).

The assessment must include an evaluation of the woman's financial status and her knowledge of sound dietary practices. The quality of the diet increases with increasing socioeconomic status and educational level. Poor women may not have access to adequate refrigeration and cooking facilities and may find it difficult to obtain adequate nutritious food.

Box 12-3 provides a simple tool for obtaining diet history information. When potential problems are identified, they should be followed up with a careful interview.

Physical Examination. Anthropometric (body) measurements provide both short- and long-term information on a woman's nutritional status and are thus essential to the assessment. At a minimum, the woman's height and weight must be determined at the time of her first prenatal visit and her weight should be measured at each subsequent visit (see earlier discussion of BMI).

A careful physical examination can reveal objective signs of malnutrition (Table 12-3). It is important to note, however, that some of these signs are nonspecific and that the physiologic changes of pregnancy may complicate the interpretation of physical findings. For example, lower extremity edema often occurs in calorie and protein deficiency, but it may also be a normal finding in the third trimester of pregnancy. Interpretation of physical findings is made easier by a thorough health history and by laboratory testing, if indicated.

Laboratory Testing. The only nutrition-related laboratory testing needed by most pregnant women is a hematocrit or hemoglobin measurement to screen for the presence of anemia. Because of the physiologic anemia of pregnancy, the reference values for hemoglobin and hematocrit must be adjusted during pregnancy. The lower limit of the normal range for hemoglobin during pregnancy is 11 g/dl in the first and third trimesters and 10.5 g/dl in the second trimester (compared with 12 g/dl in the nonpregnant state). The lower limit of the normal range for hematocrit is 33% during the first and third trimesters and 32% in the second trimester (compared with 36% in the nonpregnant state). Cutoff values for anemia are higher in women who smoke or who live at high altitudes, because the decreased oxygen-carrying capacity of their RBCs causes them to produce more RBCs than other women.

A woman's history or physical findings may indicate the need for additional testing, such as a complete blood cell count with a differential to identify megaloblastic or macrocytic ane-

Box 12-3

Food Intake Questionnaire

Which of the following did you eat or drink yesterday? If the way you ate yesterday wasn't the way you usually eat, choose a recent day that was typical for you.

FOOD OR DRINK	NUMBER OF SERVINGS	FOOD OR DRINK	NUMBER OF SERVINGS
Beer, wine, other alcoholic drinks		Orange or grapefruit juice	
Tea		Fruit juice other than orange or grapefruit	
Coffee		Soft drinks	
Fruit drink		Milk	
Water		Cereal with milk	
Cheese		Yogurt	
Macaroni and cheese		Pizza	
Other foods with cheese (such as lasagna, enchiladas, cheeseburgers)		Melon (such as watermelon, cantaloupe, honeydew)	
Orange or grapefruit		Berries (kind ________________)	
Bananas		Apples	
Peaches or apricots		Other fruit	
Green salad		Broccoli	
Spinach or greens		Green beans	
Green peas		Potatoes (other than fried)	
Sweet potatoes		Corn	
Carrots		Other vegetables	
Meat		Chicken or turkey	
Fish		Egg	
Peanut butter		Nuts	
Dried beans or peas		Hot dog	
Bacon or sausage		Cold cuts	
Bread		Roll	
Rice		Cereal	
Spaghetti or other pasta		Noodles	
Tortillas		Chips	
French fries		Cake	
Cookie		Donut or pastry	
Pie			

Are you often bothered by any of the following? (Circle all that apply)
Nausea Vomiting Heartburn Constipation
Are you on a special diet? No ________ Yes ________ If yes, what kind?
Do you try to limit the amount or kind of food you eat to control your weight? No ________ Yes ________
Do you avoid any foods for health or religious reasons? No ________ Yes ________ If yes, what foods?
Do you take any prescribed drugs or medications? No ________ Yes ________
If yes, what are they?
Do you take any over-the-counter medications (such as aspirin, cold medicines, Tylenol)?
No ________ Yes ________ If yes, what are they?
Do you ever have trouble affording the food you need? No ________ Yes ________
Do you have any help getting the food you need? No ________ Yes ________ (Circle all that apply)
Food stamps WIC School lunch or breakfast
Food from a food pantry, soup kitchen, or food bank

mia and measurement of levels of specific vitamins or minerals believed to be lacking in the diet.

The assessment gives a basis for making appropriate nursing diagnoses.

➤ Nursing Diagnoses

- Nutrition, altered: less than body requirements related to:
  —Inadequate information about nutritional needs and weight gain during pregnancy
  —Misperceptions regarding normal body changes during pregnancy and inappropriate fear of becoming fat
  —Inadequate income or skills in meal planning and preparation
- Nutrition, altered: more than body requirements related to:
  —Excessive intake of energy (calories) or decrease in activity during pregnancy
  —Use of unnecessary dietary supplements
- Constipation related to:
  —Decrease in GI motility because of elevated progesterone levels
  —Compression of intestines by the enlarging uterus
  —Oral iron supplementation

TABLE 12-3
Physical Assessment of Nutritional Status

Signs of Good Nutrition	Signs of Poor Nutrition
GENERAL APPEARANCE	
Alert, responsive, energetic, good endurance	Listless, apathetic, cachectic, easily fatigued, looks tired
MUSCLES	
Well developed, firm, good tone, some fat under skin	Flaccid, poor tone, undeveloped, tender, "wasted" appearance
NERVOUS CONTROL	
Good attention span, not irritable or restless, normal reflexes, psychologic stability	Inattentive, irritable, confused, burning and tingling of hands and feet, loss of position and vibratory sense, weakness and tenderness of muscles, decrease or loss of ankle and knee reflexes
GASTROINTESTINAL FUNCTION	
Good appetite and digestion, normal regular elimination, no palpable organs or masses	Anorexia, indigestion, constipation or diarrhea, liver or spleen enlargement
CARDIOVASCULAR FUNCTION	
Normal heart rate and rhythm, no murmurs, normal blood pressure for age	Rapid heart rate, enlarged heart, abnormal rhythm, elevated blood pressure
HAIR	
Shiny, lustrous, firm, not easily plucked, healthy scalp	Stringy, dull, brittle, dry, thin and sparse, depigmented, can be easily plucked
SKIN (GENERAL)	
Smooth, slightly moist, good color	Rough, dry, scaly, pale, pigmented, irritated, easily bruised, petechiae
FACE AND NECK	
Skin color uniform, smooth, pink, healthy appearance; no enlargement of thyroid gland; lips not chapped or swollen	Scaly, swollen, skin dark over cheeks and under eyes, lumpiness or flakiness of skin around nose and mouth; thyroid enlarged; lips swollen, angular lesions or fissures at corners of mouth
ORAL CAVITY	
Reddish pink mucous membranes and gums; no swelling or bleeding of gums; tongue healthy pink or deep reddish in appearance, not swollen or smooth, surface papillae present; teeth bright and clean, no cavities, no pain, no discoloration	Gums spongy, bleed easily, inflamed or receding; tongue swollen, scarlet and raw, magenta color, beefy, hyperemic and hypertrophic papillae, atrophic papillae; teeth with unfilled caries, absent teeth, worn surfaces, mottled
EYES	
Bright, clear, shiny, no sores at corners of eyelids, membranes moist and healthy pink color, no prominent blood vessels or mound of tissue (Bitot's spots) on sclera, no fatigue circles beneath	Eye membranes pale, redness of membrane, dryness, signs of infection, Bitot's spots, redness and fissuring of eyelid corners, dryness of eye membrane, dull appearance of cornea, soft cornea, blue sclerae
EXTREMITIES	
No tenderness, weakness, or swelling; nails firm and pink	Edema, tender calves, tingling, weakness; nails spoon-shaped, brittle
SKELETON	
No malformations	Bowlegs, knock-knees, chest deformity at diaphragm, beaded ribs, prominent scapulas

➤ Expected Outcomes

An individualized plan of care based on the nursing diagnoses should be developed in collaboration with the woman. For many women with uncomplicated pregnancies, the nurse can serve as the primary source of nutrition education during pregnancy. The registered dietitian, who has specialized training in diet evaluation and planning, nutritional needs during illness, and ethnic and cultural food patterns, as well as translating nutrient needs into food patterns, often serves as a consultant. Pregnant women with serious nutritional problems, those with intervening illnesses such as diabetes (either preexisting or gestational), and any others requiring in-depth dietary counseling should be referred to the dietitian. The nurse, dietitian, physician, and nurse-midwife collaborate in helping the woman achieve nutrition-related expected outcomes. Some common nutrition-related outcomes are that the woman will take the following actions:

- Achieve an appropriate weight gain during pregnancy. An appropriate goal for weight gain takes into account such factors as prepregnancy weight, whether she is overweight/obese or underweight, and whether the pregnancy is single or multifetal.
- Consume adequate nutrients from the diet and supplements to meet estimated needs.
- Cope successfully with nutrition-related discomforts associated with pregnancy, such as pyrosis (heartburn), morning sickness, and constipation.

➤ Plan of Care and Implementation

Nutritional care and teaching generally involves the following: (1) acquainting the woman with nutritional needs during pregnancy and, if necessary, the characteristics of an adequate diet; (2) helping her individualize her diet so that she achieves an adequate intake while satisfying her personal, cultural, financial, and health needs; (3) acquainting her with strategies for coping with the nutrition-related discomforts of pregnancy; (4) helping the woman use nutrition supplements appropriately; and (5) consulting with and making referrals to other professionals or services as indicated. Two programs that provide nutrition services are the food stamp program and the Special Supplemental Program for Women, Infants, and Children (WIC). These programs provide vouchers for selected foods to pregnant and lactating women, as well as infants and children at nutritional risk. WIC foods include items such as eggs, cheese, milk, juice, and fortified cereals—foods chosen because they provide iron, protein, vitamin C, and other vitamins.

Adequate Dietary Intake. Diet teaching can take place in a one-on-one interview or in a group setting. In either case it should emphasize the importance of choosing a varied diet composed of readily available foods, rather than specialized diet supplements. Good nutrition practices and avoidance of poor practices (e.g., smoking and alcohol or drug use) are essential content for prenatal classes designed for women in early pregnancy.

The food guide pyramid (Fig. 12-4) can be used as a guide to daily food choices during pregnancy and lactation, just as it is during other stages of the life cycle. The importance of consuming adequate amounts from the milk, yogurt, and cheese group needs to be emphasized, especially for adolescents and women under age 25, who are still actively adding calcium to their skeletons. Adolescents need at least 1 L of milk or the equivalent daily.

Pregnancy. The pregnant woman must understand what adequate weight gain during pregnancy means; must recognize the reasons for its importance; and must be able to evaluate her own gain in terms of the desirable pattern. Many women, particularly those who have worked hard to control their weight

Critical Thinking

NUTRITION EDUCATION IN THE PRENATAL CLINIC

Visit a prenatal clinic. Identify sources of nutrition education that are evident in the waiting room. Does the clinic employ a nutritionist/dietitian? Who provides nutrition counseling in the clinic? Are print materials available in multiple languages? Are translators available? Are there sources of free materials on nutrition that could be placed in the clinic? Identify strengths and weaknesses of nutrition education in that setting. Develop a feasible plan for improving nutrition education in the clinic.

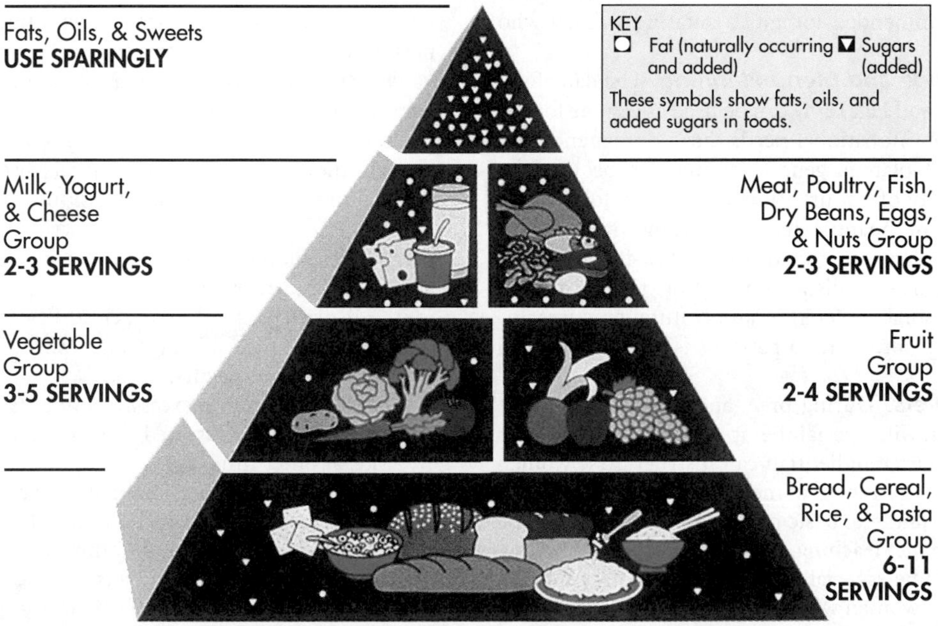

FIG. 12-4 • Food Guide Pyramid: A guide to daily food choices. (Courtesy Department of Agriculture, Washington, DC.)

before pregnancy, may find it difficult to understand why the weight gain goal is so high when a newborn infant is so small. The nurse can explain that maternal weight gain consists of increments in the weight of many tissues, not just the growing fetus.

On the other hand dietary overindulgence, which may result in excessive fat stores that persist after giving birth, should be discouraged. Nevertheless, it is best not to focus unduly on weight gain; this can result in feelings of stress and guilt in the woman who does not follow the preferred pattern of gain.

Postpartum. The need for a varied diet with portions of food from all food groups continues throughout lactation. As mentioned previously, the lactating woman should be advised to consume at least 1800 kcal daily, and she should receive counseling if her diet appears to be inadequate in any nutrients. Special attention should be given to her zinc, vitamin B_6, and folic acid intake because the recommendations for these remain higher than for nonpregnant women (see Table 12-1). Sufficient calcium is needed to allow for both milk formation and for maintenance of maternal bone mass. It may be difficult for lactating women to consume enough of these nutrients without careful diet planning.

The woman who does not breastfeed loses weight gradually if she consumes a balanced diet that provides slightly less than her daily energy expenditure. Lactating and nonlactating women should know that fat is the most concentrated source of calories in the diet (9 kcal/g vs. 4 kcal/g in carbohydrates and proteins), and fat calories are more efficiently converted into fat stores than are calories from carbohydrate or protein. Therefore the first step in weight reduction (or controlling excessive weight gain) is to evaluate sources of fat in the diet and to explore with the patient ways of reducing them. Even foods such as vegetables that are naturally low in fat can become high in fat when fried or sautéed, served with excessive amounts of salad dressing, consumed with high-fat dips or sauces, or seasoned with butter or bacon drippings. A reasonable weight loss goal for nonlactating women is 0.5 to 1 kg/week; a loss of 1 kg/month is recommended for most lactating women who need to lose weight.

Daily Food Guide and Menu Planning. The daily food plan (see Table 12-2 and Fig. 12-4) can be used as a guide for educating women about nutritional needs during pregnancy and lactation. This food plan is general enough to be used by women from a variety of cultures, including those following a vegetarian diet. One of the more helpful teaching strategies is to assist the patient to plan daily menus that follow the food plan and are affordable, have realistic preparation times, and are compatible with personal preferences and cultural practices. Information regarding cultural food patterns is provided later in this chapter.

Therapeutic Diets. During pregnancy and lactation, the food plan for women with special therapeutic diets may need to be modified. The registered dietitian can instruct these women about their diets and assist them in meal planning. However, the nurse should understand the basic principles of the diet and be able to reinforce the diet teaching.

The nurse should be especially aware of the dietary modifications necessary for women with diabetes mellitus (either gestational or preexisting) because this disease is relatively common and because fetal deformity and death occur more often in pregnancies complicated by hyperglycemia or hypoglycemia. Every effort should be made to maintain blood glucose levels in the normal range throughout pregnancy. The food plan of the woman with diabetes usually includes four to six meals and snacks daily, with the daily carbohydrate intake distributed fairly evenly among those meals and snacks. The complex carbohydrates (i.e., fibers and starches) should be well represented in the diet of the woman with diabetes. To maintain strict control of blood glucose, the pregnant woman with diabetes usually must monitor her own blood glucose daily. Urine glucose and ketone measurements are not sensitive enough to detect hyperglycemia accurately and provide no information about hypoglycemia. The nurse must teach the woman how to monitor her own blood glucose unless she was been doing so prior to becoming pregnant.

Iron Supplementation. As mentioned earlier, the nutritional supplement most commonly needed during pregnancy is iron. However, a variety of dietary factors can affect the completeness of absorption of an iron supplement. The following points should be addressed in patient education:

- Bran, milk, egg yolks, coffee, tea, or oxalate-containing vegetables such as spinach and Swiss chard will inhibit iron absorption if consumed at the same time as iron.
- Iron absorption is promoted by a diet rich in vitamin C (e.g., citrus fruits or melons) or "heme iron" found in red meats, fish, and poultry.
- Iron supplements are best absorbed on an empty stomach; thus they can be taken between meals with beverages other than milk, tea, or coffee.
- Some women have gastrointestinal discomfort when they take the supplement on an empty stomach; therefore a good time for them to take the supplement is just before bedtime.
- Constipation is common with iron supplementation.
- Iron supplements should be kept away from any children in the household because their ingestion could result in acute iron poisoning and even death.

Coping with Nutrition-Related Discomforts of Pregnancy. The most common nutrition-related discomforts of pregnancy are nausea and vomiting (or "morning sickness"), constipation, and pyrosis.

Nausea and Vomiting. Nausea and vomiting are most common during the first trimester. Usually, nausea and vomiting cause only mild to moderate problems nutritionally, although they may cause substantial discomfort. Antiemetic medications, vitamin B_6, and P6 acupressure may be effective in reducing the severity of nausea (Jewell and Young, 2000). The pregnant woman may find the following suggestions helpful in alleviating the problems:

- Eat dry, starchy foods such as dry toast, Melba toast, or crackers on awakening in the morning and at other times when nausea occurs.
- Avoid consuming excessive amounts of fluids early in the day or when nauseated (but compensate by drinking fluids at other times).
- Eat small amounts frequently (every 2 to 3 hours) and avoid large meals, which distend the stomach.
- Avoid skipping meals and thus becoming extremely hungry, which may worsen nausea. Have a snack such as cereal with milk, a small sandwich, or yogurt before bedtime.
- Avoid sudden movements. Arise from bed slowly.
- Decrease intake of fried and other fatty foods. Starches (e.g., pastas, rice, and breads) and low-fat protein foods

(e.g., skinless broiled or baked poultry, cooked dry beans or peas, lean meats, broiled or canned fish) are good choices.

- Some women find that tart foods or drinks (e.g., lemonade) or salty foods (e.g., potato chips) are tolerated during periods of nausea.
- Fresh air may help relieve nausea. Keep the environment well ventilated (e.g., open a window), go for a walk outside, or decrease cooking odors by using an exhaust fan.
- During periods of nausea, eat foods served at cool temperatures and foods that give off little aroma.
- Avoid brushing teeth immediately after eating.

Hyperemesis gravidarum (i.e., severe and persistent vomiting causing weight loss, dehydration, and electrolyte abnormalities) occurs in up to 1% of pregnant women. There is some evidence that ginger root may be effective in reducing nausea (Jewell and Young, 2000). Intravenous fluid and electrolyte replacement is usually necessary for women who lose 5% of their body weight. Often this is followed by improved tolerance of oral intake; therapy then consists of frequently consuming small amounts of low-fat foods. Enteral tube feeding using small-bore nasogastric tubes has been successful for some women. Because pulmonary aspiration of the feeding is a potential complication if vomiting occurs, antiemetic medications are sometimes used in conjunction with tube feedings. Tube feedings may be used to supplement oral intake, with the volume of the tube feeding gradually being decreased as oral intake improves. In some instances, total parenteral nutrition (balanced intravenous feedings of amino acids, carbohydrate, lipid, vitamins, and minerals) is used to nourish women with hyperemesis gravidarum when their nutritional status is severely impaired.

Constipation. Improved bowel function generally results from increasing the intake of fiber (e.g., wheat bran and whole-wheat products, popcorn, and raw or lightly steamed vegetables) in the diet because fiber helps to retain water within the stool, creating a bulky stool that stimulates intestinal peristalsis. The recommendation for adults for fiber is 25 g to 30 g per day. An adequate fluid intake (at least 50 ml/kg/day) helps to hydrate the fiber and increase the bulk of the stool. Making a habit of regular exercise that uses large muscle groups (e.g., walking, swimming, and cycling) also helps to stimulate bowel motility.

Pyrosis. Pyrosis, or heartburn, is usually caused by reflux of gastric contents into the esophagus. This condition can be minimized by eating small, frequent meals rather than two or three larger meals daily. Because fluids increase the distention of the stomach, they should not be consumed with foods. The woman needs to be sure to drink adequate amounts between meals. Avoiding spicy foods may help alleviate the problem. Lying down immediately after eating and wearing clothing that is tight across the abdomen can contribute to the problem of reflux.

Cultural Influences. Consideration of a woman's cultural food preferences enhances communication and provides a greater opportunity for following the agreed-upon pattern of intake. Women in most cultures are encouraged to eat a diet typical for them. The nurse needs to be aware of what constitutes a typical diet for each cultural or ethnic group. However, several variations may occur within one cultural group. Thus a careful exploration of individual preferences is needed. Although ethnic and cultural food beliefs may seem, at first glance, to conflict with the dietary instruction provided by physicians, nurses, and dietitians, it is often possible for the empathic health care provider to identify cultural beliefs that are congruent with the modern understanding of pregnancy and fetal development. Many cultural food practices have some merit or the culture would not have survived. Food cravings during pregnancy are considered normal by many cultures, but the kinds of cravings often are culturally specific. In most cultures women crave acceptable foods, such as chicken, fish, and greens among African-Americans. Cultural influences on food intake usually lessen if the woman and her family become more integrated into the dominant culture. Nutrition beliefs and the practices of selected cultural groups are summarized in Table 12-4.

Vegetarian Diets. Vegetarian diets represent another cultural effect on nutritional status. Foods basic to almost all vegetarian diets are vegetables, fruits, legumes, nuts, seeds, and grains. However, there are many variations in vegetarian diets. Semivegetarians, who are not truly vegetarians, include fish, poultry, eggs, and dairy products in their diets but do not eat beef or pork. Such a diet can be completely adequate for pregnant women. Besides plant products, lactoovovegetarians also eat dairy products and eggs. Iron and zinc intake may not be adequate in these women, but such diets can be otherwise nutritionally sound. Strict vegetarians, or vegans, consume only plant products. Because vitamin B_{12} is found only in foods of animal origin, this diet is therefore deficient in vitamin B_{12}. As a result, strict vegetarians should take a supplement or consume vitamin B_{12} fortified foods (e.g., soy milk) regularly. Vitamin B_{12} deficiency can result in megaloblastic anemia, glossitis, and neurologic deficits in the mothers. Infants born to affected mothers are likely to have megaloblastic anemia and exhibit neurodevelopmental delays. Iron, calcium, zinc, and vitamin B_6 intake may also be low in women on this diet, and some strict vegetarians have excessively low caloric intakes. The protein intake should be assessed especially carefully because plant proteins tend to be incomplete in that they lack one or more amino acids required for growth and the maintenance of body tissues. The daily consumption of a variety of different plant proteins (e.g., grains, dried beans and peas, nuts, and seeds) helps to provide all the essential amino acids.

➤ Evaluation

In evaluating the adequacy of nutritional intake during pregnancy, the patient's weight gain can be compared with standardized grids showing optimal patterns (see Fig. 12-2). It is helpful to remember that these grids are based on mean data and do not always account for factors such as ethnic or racial variations. To evaluate the adequacy of the woman's diet, it can be compared with the plan in Table 12-2. Again, it is essential that individual factors affecting nutritional needs and dietary intake be considered.

Physical examination and laboratory testing can be used to confirm that nutritional status is adequate (see the section on assessment). For example, a hematocrit greater than 35% and a hemoglobin concentration greater than 11.5 g/dl are indicators that iron intake is adequate to prevent anemia. When weight gain is inadequate or when nutritional deficits appear, the nurse must reassess the woman and her understanding of her nutritional needs, reinforce teaching as needed, and continue to reevaluate regularly (Nursing Care Plan).

TABLE 12-4

Characteristic Food Patterns of Selected Cultures

Milk Group	Protein Group	Fruits and Vegetables	Breads and Cereals	Possible Dietary Problems
NATIVE AMERICAN (MANY TRIBAL VARIATIONS; MANY "AMERICANIZED")				
Fresh milk Evaporated milk for cooking Ice cream Cream pie	Pork, beef, lamb, rabbit Fowl, fish, eggs Legumes Sunflower seeds Nuts: walnuts, acorn, pine, peanut butter Game meat	Green peas, beans Beets, turnips Leafy green and other vegetables Grapes, bananas, peaches, other fresh fruits Roots	Refined bread Whole wheat Cornmeal Rice Dry cereals "Fry" bread Tortillas	Obesity, diabetes, alcoholism, nutritional deficiencies expressed in dental problems and iron deficiency anemia Inadequate amounts of all nutrients Excessive use of sugar
MIDDLE EASTERN* (ARMENIAN, GREEK, SYRIAN, TURKISH)				
Yogurt Little butter	Lamb Nuts Dried peas, beans, lentils Sesame seeds	Peppers, tomatoes, cabbage, grape leaves, cucumbers, squash Dried apricots, raisins, dates	Cracked wheat and dark bread	Fry many meats and vegetables Lack of fresh fruits Insufficient foods from milk group High consumption of sweetenings, lamb fat, and olive oil
AFRICAN-AMERICAN				
Milk† Ice cream Cheese: longhorn, American	Pork: all cuts, plus organs, chitterlings Beef, lamb Chicken, giblets Eggs Nuts Legumes Fish, game	Leafy vegetables Green and yellow vegetables Potato: white, sweet Stewed fruit Bananas and other fresh fruit	Cornmeal and hominy grits Rice Biscuits, pancakes, white breads Puddings: bread, rice	Extensive use of frying, smothering in gravy, or simmering Fats: salt pork, bacon drippings, lard, and gravies High consumption of sweets Insufficient citrus Vegetables often boiled for long periods with pork fat and much salt Limited amounts from milk group†
CHINESE (CANTONESE MOST PREVALENT)				
Milk: water buffalo	Pork sausage‡ Eggs and pigeon eggs Fish Lamb, beef, goat Fowl: chicken, duck Nuts Legumes Soybean curd (tofu)	Many vegetables Radish leaves Bean, bamboo sprouts	Rice/rice flour products Cereals, noodles Wheat, corn, millet seed	Tendency of some immigrants to use large amounts of grease in cooking Limited use of milk and milk products Often low in protein, calories, or both Soy sauce (high sodium)
FILIPINO (SPANISH-CHINESE INFLUENCE)				
Flavored milk Milk in coffee Cheese: gouda, cheddar	Pork, beef, goat, rabbit Chicken Fish Eggs, nuts, legumes	Many vegetables and fruits	Rice, cooked cereals Noodles: rice, wheat	Limited use of milk and milk products Tendency to prewash rice Tendency to have only small portions of protein foods
ITALIAN				
Cheese Some ice cream	Meat Eggs Dried beans	Leafy vegetables Potatoes Eggplant, tomatoes, peppers Fruits	Pasta White breads, some whole wheat Farina Cereals	Prefer expensive imported cheeses; reluctant to substitute less expensive domestic varieties Tendency to overcook vegetables Limited use of whole grains

MSG, Monosodium L-glutamate.

*Religious holidays may involve fasting, which is believed to increase the likelihood of preterm labor. Fasting requirement may be waived during pregnancy.

†Lactose intolerance relatively common in adults.

‡Lower in fat content than Western sausage.

TABLE 12-4
Characteristic Food Patterns of Selected Cultures—cont'd

Milk Group	Protein Group	Fruits and Vegetables	Breads and Cereals	Possible Dietary Problems
ITALIAN—cont'd				
				High consumption of sweets Extensive use of olive oil Insufficient servings from milk group
JAPANESE (ISEI, MORE JAPANESE INFLUENCE; NISEI, MORE WESTERNIZED)				
Increasing amounts being used by younger generations	Pork, beef, chicken Fish Eggs Legumes: soys, red, lima beans Tofu Nuts	Many vegetables and fruits Seaweed	Rice, rice cakes Wheat noodles Refined bread, noodles	Excessive sodium: pickles, salty crisp seaweed, MSG, and soy sauce Insufficient servings from milk group May use prewashed rice
HISPANIC, MEXICAN-AMERICAN				
Milk Cheese Flan, ice cream	Beef, pork, lamb, chicken, tripe, hot sausage, beef intestines Fish Eggs Nuts Dry beans: pinto, chickpeas (often eaten more than once daily)	Spinach, wild greens, tomatoes, chilies, corn, cactus leaves, cabbage, avocado, potatoes Pumpkin, zapote, peaches, guava, papaya, citrus	Rice, cornmeal Sweet bread, pastries Tortilla: corn, flour Vermicelli (fideo)	Limited meats primarily due to cost Limited use of milk and milk products Large amounts of lard Abundant use of sugar Tendency to boil vegetables for long periods
PUERTO RICAN				
Limited use of milk products Coffee with milk (café con leche)	Pork Poultry Eggs (Fridays) Dried codfish Beans *(habichuelas)*	Avocado, okra Eggplant Sweet yams Starchy vegetables and fruits *(viandas)*	Rice Cornmeal	Small amounts of pork and poultry Extensive use of fat, lard, salt pork, and olive oil Lack of milk products
SCANDINAVIAN (DANISH, FINNISH, NORWEGIAN, SWEDISH)				
Cream Butter Cheeses	Wild game Reindeer Fish (fresh or dried) Eggs	Berries Dried fruit Vegetables: cole slaw, roots	Whole wheat, rye, barley, sweets (cookies and sweet breads)	Insufficient fresh fruits and vegetables High consumption of sweets, pickled or salted meats, and fish
SOUTHEAST ASIAN (VIETNAMESE, CAMBODIAN)				
Generally not taken Coffee with condensed cow's milk Plain yogurt Ice cream (rare) Soybean milk	Fish (daily): fresh, dried, salted Poultry/eggs: duck, chicken Pork Beef (seldom) Dry beans Tofu	Seasonal variety: fresh or preserved Green, leafy vegetables Yams Corn	Rice: grains, flour, noodles French bread "Cellophane" (bean starch) noodles	Fresh milk products generally not consumed Poultry/eggs may be limited Meat considered "unclean" is avoided Preference for a diet high in salt and pepper, as well as rice and pork High intake of MSG and soy sauce
JEWISH: ORTHODOX*				
Milk† Cheese†	Meat (bloodless; Kosher prepared): beef, lamb, goat, deer, poultry (all types), no pork Fish with fins and scales only No crustaceans	Wide variety	Wide variety	High intake of sodium in meat products

Nursing Care Plan NUTRITION DURING PREGNANCY

NURSING DIAGNOSIS Knowledge deficit related to nutritional requirements during pregnancy

EXPECTED OUTCOME The patient will delineate nutritional requirements and exhibit evidence of incorporating requirements into diet.

Nursing Interventions/*Rationales*

Review basic nutritional requirements for a healthy diet using recommended dietary guidelines and the food guide pyramid *to provide knowledge baseline for discussion.*

Discuss increased nutrient needs (calories, protein, minerals, vitamins) that occur as a result of being pregnant *to increase knowledge needed for altered dietary requirements.*

Discuss the relationship between weight gain and fetal growth *to reinforce interdependence of fetus and mother.*

Calculate the appropriate total weight gain range during pregnancy using the woman's body mass index as a guide and discuss recommended rates of weight gain during the various trimesters of pregnancy *to provide concrete measures of dietary success.*

Review food preferences, cultural eating patterns or beliefs, and prepregnancy eating patterns *to enhance integration of new dietary needs.*

Discuss how to fit nutritional needs into usual dietary patterns and how to alter any identified nutritional deficits or excesses *to increase chances of success with dietary alterations.*

Discuss food aversions or cravings that may occur during pregnancy and strategies to deal with these if they are detrimental to fetus (e.g., pica) *to ensure well-being of fetus.*

Have woman keep a food diary delineating eating habits, dietary alterations, aversions, and cravings *to track eating habits and potential problem areas.*

NURSING DIAGNOSIS Altered nutrition: more than body requirements related to excessive intake and/or inadequate activity levels

EXPECTED OUTCOME The patient's weekly weight gain will be reduced to the appropriate rate using her body mass index (BMI) and recommended weight gain ranges as guidelines.

Nursing Interventions/*Rationales*

Review recent diet history (including food cravings) using a food diary, 24-hour recall, or food frequency approach *to ascertain food accesses contributing to excess weight gain.*

Review normal activity and exercise routines *to determine level of energy expenditure;* discuss eating patterns and reasons that lead to increased food intake (e.g., cultural beliefs or myths, increased stress, boredom) *to identify habits that contribute to excess weight gain.*

Review optimal weight gain guidelines and their rationale *to ensure that woman is knowledgeable about healthful weight gain rates.*

Set target weight gains for the remaining weeks of the pregnancy *to establish set goals.*

Discuss with the woman what changes can be made in diet, activity, and lifestyle *to enhance chances of meeting weight gain goals and dietary needs.* Weight reduction diets should be avoided, since they may deprive the mother and fetus of needed nutrients and lead to ketonemia.

NURSING DIAGNOSIS Altered nutrition: less than body requirements related to inadequate intake of needed nutrients

EXPECTED OUTCOME The patient's weekly weight gain will be increased to the appropriate rate using her BMI and recommended weight gain ranges as guidelines.

Nursing Interventions/*Rationales*

Review recent diet history (including food aversions) using a food diary, 24-hour recall, or food frequency approach *to ascertain dietary inadequacies contributing to lack of sufficient weight gain.*

Review normal activity and exercise routines *to determine level of energy expenditure;* discuss eating patterns and reasons that lead to decreased food intake (e.g., morning sickness, pica, fear of becoming fat, stress, boredom) *to identify habits that contribute to inadequate weight gain.*

Review optimal weight gain guidelines and their rationale *to ensure that woman is knowledgeable about healthful weight gain rates.*

Set target weight gains for the remaining weeks of the pregnancy *to establish set goals.*

Review increased nutrient needs (calories, protein, minerals, vitamins) that occur as a result of being pregnant *to ensure woman is knowledgeable about altered dietary requirements.*

Review relationship between weight gain and fetal growth *to reinforce that adequate weight gain is needed to promote fetal well-being.*

Discuss with woman what changes can be made in diet, activity, and lifestyle *to enhance chances of meeting set weight gain goals and nutrient needs of mother and fetus.*

If woman has fear of being fat, if symptoms of an eating disorder are evident, or if problems in adjusting to a changing body image surface, refer woman to the appropriate mental health professional for evaluation, since intensive treatment and follow-up may be required *to ensure fetal health.*

Key Points

- A woman's nutritional status before, during, and after pregnancy contributes significantly to her and her infant's well-being.
- Many physiologic changes occurring during pregnancy influence the need for nutrients and the efficiency with which the body uses them.
- Both the total maternal weight gain and the pattern of weight gain are important determinants of the outcome of pregnancy.
- The recommended weight gain during pregnancy is determined by the appropriateness of the mother's prepregnancy weight for height (BMI).
- Nutritional risk factors include adolescent pregnancy, abuse of nicotine, alcohol or drugs, bizarre or faddish food habits, a low weight for height, and frequent pregnancies.
- Iron supplementation is routinely recommended during pregnancy. Other supplements may be warranted when nutritional risk factors are present.
- The nurse and the woman are influenced by cultural and personal values and beliefs during nutrition counseling.
- Pregnancy complications that may be nutrition-related include anemia, PIH, preterm birth, gestational diabetes, and IUGR.
- Dietary adaptation can be an effective intervention for some of the common discomforts of pregnancy, including nausea and vomiting, constipation, and heartburn.

References

Allen L: Anemia and iron deficiency: effects on pregnancy outcome, *Am J Clin Nutr* 71(5 Suppl):1280S-1284S, 2000.

Bailey L, Gregory J: Folate metabolism and requirements, *J Nutr* 129(4):779-782, 1999.

Butterworth C, Bendich A: Folic acid and the prevention of birth defects, *Annu Rev Nutr* 16:73-97, 1996.

Ellings J, Newman R, Bower N: Prenatal care and multiple pregnancy, *J Obstet Gynecol Neonatal Nurs* 27:457-465, 1998.

Hinds T et al: The effect of caffeine on pregnancy outcome variables, *Nutr Rev* 54(7):203-207, 1996.

Jewell D, Young G: Interventions for nausea and vomiting in early pregnancy, *Cochrane Database Syst Rev* (2):CD000145, 2000.

King J: Determinants of maternal zinc status during pregnancy, *Am J Clin Nutr* 71(5 Suppl):1334S-1343S, 2000.

Leverett D et al: Randomized clinical trial of the effect of prenatal fluoride supplements in preventing dental caries, *Caries Res* 31: 174-179, 1997.

Levine M et al: Criteria and recommendations for vitamin C intake, *JAMA* 281(15):1415-1423, 1999.

Mahomed K, Gulmezoglu A: Pyridoxine (vitamin B_6) supplementation in pregnancy, *Cochrane Database Syst Rev* (2):CD000179, 2000.

Prentice A, Goldberg G: Maternal obesity increases congenital malformations, *Nutr Rev* 54(5):146-150, 1996.

Rainville A: Pica practices of pregnant women are associated with lower maternal hemoglobin level at delivery, *J Am Diet Assoc* 98:293-296, 1998.

Sargent R et al: Black and white adolescent females' prepregnancy nutrition status. *Adolescence* 29 (116):845-858, 1994.

Standing Committee on the Scientific Evaluation of Dietary Reference Intakes, Food and Nutrition Board, Institute of Medicine: *Dietary Reference Intakes: calcium, phosphorus, magnesium, vitamin D, and fluoride,* Washington, DC, 1997, National Academy Press.

Tinkle M, Sterling B: Neural tube defects: a primary prevention role for nurses, *J Obstet Gynecol Neonatal Nurs* 26:503-512, 1997.

U.S. Department of Health and Human Services, Food and Drug Administration: Food standards: amendment of the standards of identity for enriched grain products to require addition of folic acid, *Federal Register* 61:87-91, 1996.

Yates A, Schlicker S, Suitor C: Dietary Reference Intakes: the new basis for recommendations for calcium and related nutrients, B vitamins, and choline, *J Am Diet Assoc* 98(6):699-706, 1998.

CHAPTER 13

Pregnancy at Risk: Preexisting Conditions

http://www.harcourthealth.com/MERLIN/Wong/maternal/

Learning Objectives

On completion of this chapter the reader will be able to:

- Differentiate the types of diabetes mellitus and their respective risk factors in pregnancy.
- Compare insulin requirements during pregnancy, postpartum, and lactation.
- Discuss care management for the pregnant woman with pregestational or gestational diabetes.
- Explain the effects of thyroid disorders on pregnancy.
- Differentiate the management of various cardiovascular disorders in pregnant women.
- Discuss the different types of anemia and their effects during pregnancy.
- Explain the care of pregnant women with pulmonary disorders.
- Describe the effect of gastrointestinal disorders on pregnancy.
- Review the effects of neurologic disorders on pregnancy.
- Describe the care of women whose pregnancies are complicated by autoimmune disorders.
- Explain the effects on and the management of pregnant women with human immunodeficiency virus (HIV).
- Discuss the care of pregnant women who use, abuse, or are dependent on alcohol or illicit or prescription drugs.

For most women, pregnancy represents a normal part of life. This chapter, however, will discuss the care of women for whom pregnancy represents a significant risk because it is superimposed on a chronic illness. With well-motivated patients who actively participate in the treatment plan, and with careful management from a multidisciplinary health care team, positive pregnancy outcomes are often possible today.

Providing safe and effective care for women experiencing high risk pregnancy and their fetuses is a challenge. While unique maternal and fetal needs prompted by these conditions exist, these women also experience many of the same pregnancy-related feelings, needs, and concerns as their "normal" counterparts. The primary objective of nursing care must be to guide and support the woman and her family in achieving optimal outcome for both the pregnant woman and the fetus.

This chapter focuses on metabolic disorders including diabetes mellitus and thyroid disorders; cardiovascular disorders; selected disorders of the respiratory, gastrointestinal, integumentary, and central nervous systems; and autoimmune disorders. Substance abuse and HIV are also discussed.

METABOLIC DISORDERS

Diabetes Mellitus

The perinatal mortality rate for well-managed diabetic pregnancies, excluding major congenital malformations, is about the same as for any other pregnancy (Landon, 1996b). The key to optimal pregnancy outcome is strict maternal glucose control before conception, as well as throughout the pregnancy. Consequently, much emphasis is placed on preconception counseling for women with diabetes.

Pregnancy complicated by diabetes is still considered high risk. It is most successfully managed with a multidisciplinary approach involving the obstetrician, internist or diabetologist, neonatologist, nurse, nutritionist, and social worker. Favorable outcome of pregnancy complicated by diabetes requires commitment and active participation by the woman and her family. The woman must comply with a schedule of frequent prenatal visits, strict adherence to the dietary regimen, regular self-monitoring of blood glucose level, frequent laboratory evaluation, intensive fetal surveillance, and possible hospitalization.

Care of the pregnant woman who has diabetes requires that the nurse fully understand the normal physiologic responses to pregnancy as well as the altered metabolism of diabetes. Furthermore, the nurse must understand the relationship between pregnancy and diabetes, including psychosocial implications, to assess the woman accurately, to plan for her care, and to intervene appropriately.

Pathogenesis. Diabetes mellitus is a group of metabolic diseases characterized by hyperglycemia resulting from defects in insulin secretion, insulin action, or both (Expert Committee on the Diagnosis and Classification of Diabetes Mellitus, 1997). Insulin, produced by beta cells in the islets of Langerhans in the pancreas, regulates blood glucose levels by enabling glucose to enter adipose and muscle cells where it is used for energy. Insulin also stimulates protein synthesis and storage of free fatty acids. When insulin is insufficient or ineffective in promoting glucose uptake by the muscle and adipose cells, glucose accumulates in the bloodstream and hyperglycemia results. Hyperglycemia causes hyperosmolarity of the blood, which attracts intracellular fluid into the vascular system, resulting in cellular dehydration and expanded blood volume. Consequently the kidneys function to excrete large volumes of urine (polyuria) in an attempt to regulate excess vascular volume and to excrete the unusable glucose (glycosuria). Polyuria and cellular dehydration cause excessive thirst (polydipsia).

The body compensates for its inability to convert carbohydrate (glucose) into energy by burning proteins (muscle) and fats. The end products of this metabolism are ketones and fatty acids, which in excess quantity produce ketoacidosis and acetonuria. Weight loss occurs because of the breakdown of fat and muscle tissue. This tissue breakdown causes a state of starvation that compels the individual to eat an excessive amount of food (polyphagia).

Over time, diabetes causes significant changes in both the microvascular and macrovascular circulations. These structural changes affect a variety of organ systems, primarily the heart, eyes, kidneys, and nerves. Complications resulting from diabetes include premature atherosclerosis, retinopathy, nephropathy, and neuropathy.

Diabetes may be caused by either impaired insulin secretion, when beta cells of the pancreas are destroyed by an autoimmune process; or by inadequate insulin action in target tissues at one or more points along the metabolic pathway. Both of these conditions are commonly present in the same person, and it is unclear which abnormality, if either, is the primary cause of the disease (Expert Committee on the Diagnosis and Classification of Diabetes Mellitus, 1997).

Classification. The classification and diagnosis of diabetes have been revised by an international Expert Committee working under the sponsorship of the American Diabetes Association (ADA) (1997). The revised classification system includes four groups: type 1 diabetes, type 2 diabetes, other specific types (e.g., diabetes caused by infection or drug-induced diabetes), and gestational diabetes mellitus.

Type 1 diabetes includes those cases that are primarily due to pancreatic islet beta cell destruction and that are prone to ketoacidosis. People with type 1 diabetes usually have an absolute insulin deficiency. Type 1 diabetes includes cases currently thought to be caused by an autoimmune process, as well as those for which the cause is unknown (Expert Committee on the Diagnosis and Classification of Diabetes Mellitus, 1997).

Type 2 diabetes is the most prevalent form of the disease and includes individuals who have insulin resistance and usually relative (rather than absolute) insulin deficiency. Specific etiologies for type 2 diabetes are unknown at this time. Type 2 diabetes often goes undiagnosed for years because hyperglycemia develops gradually and often is not severe enough for the person to recognize the classic signs of polyuria, polydipsia, and polyphagia. Many people who develop type 2 diabetes are obese or have an increased amount of body fat distributed primarily in the abdominal area. Other risk factors include aging, a sedentary lifestyle, hypertension, and prior gestational diabetes. Type 2 diabetes often has a strong genetic predisposition (Expert Committee on the Diagnosis and Classification of Diabetes Mellitus, 1997).

Pregestational diabetes is a label sometimes given to type 1 or type 2 diabetes that existed before pregnancy.

Gestational diabetes mellitus (GDM) is any degree of glucose intolerance with its onset or first recognition during pregnancy. This definition is appropriate whether or not insulin is used for treatment or whether the diabetes persists after pregnancy. It does not exclude the possibility that the glucose intolerance preceded the pregnancy. Women experiencing gestational diabetes should be reclassified 6 weeks or more after the pregnancy ends (Expert Committee on the Diagnosis and Classification of Diabetes Mellitus, 1997).

Metabolic Changes Associated with Pregnancy. Normal pregnancy is characterized by complex alterations in maternal glucose metabolism, insulin production, and metabolic homeostasis. During normal pregnancy, adjustments in maternal metabolism allow for adequate nutrition for both the mother and the developing fetus. Glucose, the primary fuel used by the fetus, is transported across the placenta through the process of carrier-mediated facilitated diffusion. This means that the glucose levels in the fetus are directly proportional to maternal levels. Although glucose crosses the placenta, insulin does not. By the tenth week of gestation the embryo or fetus secretes its own insulin at levels adequate to use the glucose obtained from the mother. Thus as maternal glucose levels rise, fetal glucose levels are increased, resulting in increased fetal insulin secretion.

During the first trimester of pregnancy, the pregnant woman's metabolic status is significantly influenced by the rising levels of estrogen and progesterone. These hormones stimulate the beta cells in the pancreas to increase insulin production, which promotes increased peripheral utilization of glucose and decreased blood glucose with fasting levels being reduced by approximately 10% (see Fig. 13-1, *A*). There is a concomitant increase in tissue glycogen stores and a decrease in hepatic glucose production, which further encourage lower fasting glucose levels. As a result of these normal metabolic changes of pregnancy, women with insulin-dependent diabetes are prone to hypoglycemia (low blood glucose) during the first trimester.

During the second and third trimesters, pregnancy exerts a "diabetogenic" effect on the maternal metabolic status. Because of the major hormonal changes, there is decreased tolerance to glucose, increased insulin resistance, decreased hepatic glycogen stores, and increased hepatic production of glucose. Rising levels of human placental lactogen (hPL), estrogen, progesterone, prolactin, cortisol, and insulinase increase insulin resistance through their actions as insulin antagonists. Insulin resistance is a glucose-sparing mechanism that ensures an abundant supply of glucose for the fetus. Maternal insulin requirements may double or quadruple by the end of pregnancy, usually leveling off or declining slightly after 36 weeks (Fig. 13-1, *B* and *C*).

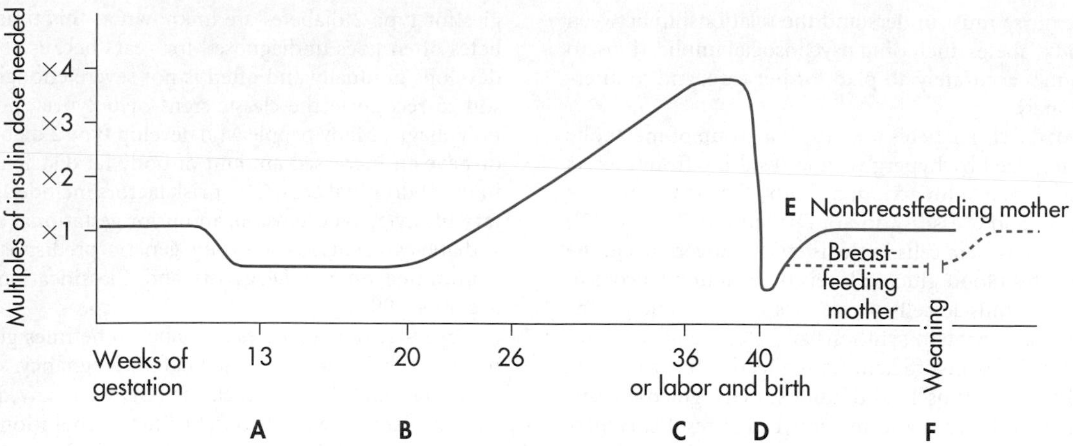

FIG. 13-1 • Changing insulin needs during pregnancy. **A,** First trimester: insulin need is reduced because of increased insulin production by the pancreas and increased peripheral sensitivity to insulin; nausea, vomiting, and decreased food intake by mother as well as glucose transfer to embryo/fetus contribute to hypoglycemia. **B,** Second trimester: insulin need increases as placental hormones, cortisol, and insulinase act as insulin antagonists, decreasing insulin's effectiveness. **C,** Third trimester: insulin need may double or even quadruple, but it usually levels off after 36 weeks. **D,** Day of delivery: maternal insulin requirements drop drastically to approach prepregnancy levels. **E,** Breastfeeding mother maintains lower insulin requirements, as much as 25% less than prepregnancy; insulin need of nonbreastfeeding mother returns to prepregnancy levels in 7 to 10 days. **F,** At weaning of breastfeeding infant, mother's insulin need returns to prepregnancy levels.

At birth, expulsion of the placenta prompts an abrupt drop in levels of circulating placental hormones, cortisol, and insulinase (Fig. 13-1, *D*). Maternal tissues quickly regain their prepregnancy sensitivity to insulin. For the nonbreastfeeding mother, prepregnancy insulin-carbohydrate balance usually returns in about 7 to 10 days (Fig. 13-1, *E*). Lactation uses maternal glucose; thus the breastfeeding mother's insulin requirements remain low for up to 6 to 9 months (Fig. 13-1, *E*). On completion of weaning, the mother's prepregnancy insulin requirement is reestablished (Fig. 13-1, *F*).

Pregestational Diabetes Mellitus. Women who have pregestational diabetes may have either type 1 or type 2 diabetes. These may or may not be complicated by vascular disease, retinopathy, nephropathy, or other diabetic sequelae. Almost all women with pregestational diabetes are insulin-dependent during pregnancy.

The diabetogenic state of pregnancy imposed on the compromised metabolic system of the woman with pregestational diabetes has significant implications. The normal hormonal adaptations of pregnancy affect glycemic control, and pregnancy may accelerate the progress of vascular complications.

During the first trimester, when maternal blood glucose levels are normally reduced and insulin response to glucose is enhanced, glycemic control is improved. Insulin dosage for the patient whose diabetes is well under control may need to be reduced to avoid hypoglycemia. There is an increased incidence of hypoglycemic episodes in women with type 1 diabetes during early pregnancy. Nausea, vomiting, and cravings typical of early pregnancy result in dietary fluctuations, which influence maternal glucose levels and necessitate reduction in insulin dosage.

Because insulin requirements steadily increase after the first trimester, insulin dosage must be adjusted accordingly to prevent episodes of hyperglycemia. Insulin resistance begins as early as 14 to 16 weeks and continues to rise until it stabilizes during the last few weeks of pregnancy.

In the past it was believed that pregnancy worsened microvascular complications. In fact, women who had diabetes and had vascular disease such as retinopathy or nephropathy were often encouraged to avoid or terminate pregnancy. With current management practices, however, women with vasculopathy other than coronary artery disease can achieve good pregnancy outcomes (Moore, 1999; Reece and Homko, 1994).

Diabetic neuropathy has more impact on perinatal outcome than any other vascular complication. Increased risks of preeclampsia, preterm labor, intrauterine growth restriction (IUGR), fetal distress, stillbirth, and neonatal death are associated with this condition (Moore, 1999).

Although neuropathic complications are common in type 1 and type 2 diabetes, little information exists about the effect of pregnancy on diabetic neuropathy. An autonomic neuropathy such as gastroparesis (e.g., anorexia, vomiting of undigested food, belching, early satiety, and weight loss) may affect diabetic control because of its effects on intake and absorption of adequate nutrition (Reece and Homko, 1993).

Preconception Counseling. Preconception counseling is recommended for all women of reproductive age with diabetes and is associated with improved pregnancy outcome (Landon, 1996b; Moore, 1999). Under ideal circumstances, the pregestational diabetic woman is counseled before conception to plan the optimal time for pregnancy, establish glycemic control before conception, and diagnose any vascular complications of diabetes. However, it is estimated that fewer than 20% of women with diabetes in the United States participate in preconception counseling (Landon, 1996b).

The woman's partner should be included in the counseling to assess the couple's level of understanding related to the effects of pregnancy on the diabetic condition and of the potential complications of pregnancy as a result of diabetes. The couple should also be informed of the anticipated alterations in management of diabetes during pregnancy and the need for a multidisciplinary team approach to health care. Financial implications of diabetic pregnancy and other demands related to frequent maternal and fetal surveillance should be discussed. Contraception is another important aspect of preconception counseling to assist the couple in planning for pregnancy.

Some types of oral hypoglycemic agents (e.g., sulfonylureas such as tolbutamide) may have teratogenic effects on the fetus and should be discontinued in the preconceptional period in women with type 2 diabetes (Hagay and Reece, 1999). These women are started on insulin before pregnancy when the pregnancy is planned, or as soon as the pregnancy is diagnosed when it is unplanned.

Maternal Risks and Complications. Although maternal morbidity and mortality rates have improved significantly, the pregnant woman with diabetes remains at risk for the development of complications. The best predictor of pregnancy outcome for the patient with diabetes and her neonate is the degree of maternal glycemic control during pregnancy.

Poor glycemic control around the time of conception and in the early weeks of pregnancy is associated with an increased incidence of spontaneous abortion in women who have diabetes. Those women with good glycemic control before conception and in the first trimester appear to be no more likely to have a miscarriage than women without diabetes (Moore, 1999).

Poor glycemic control later in pregnancy, particularly in women without vascular disease, increases the rate of fetal macrosomia, or excessive growth. Macrosomia occurs in 20% to 25% of diabetic pregnancies. These large infants tend to have a disproportionate increase in shoulder and trunk size; consequently, the risk of shoulder dystocia is greater in these babies than in other macrosomic infants. Thus women with diabetes face an increased likelihood of cesarean birth (because of failure to progress or descent) or of operative delivery (e.g., using episiotomy, forceps, or vacuum extraction) (Landon, 1996b; Moore, 1999).

Pregnancy-induced hypertension (PIH), or preeclampsia, occurs more often during diabetic pregnancy. The highest incidence occurs in women with preexisting vascular changes related to diabetes (Cunningham et al, 1997).

Hydramnios (polyhydramnios), or amniotic fluid in excess of 2000 ml, occurs about 10 times more often in diabetic pregnancies than in nondiabetic pregnancies. Overdistention of the uterus caused by hydramnios increases the risk of premature rupture of the membranes (PROM), preterm labor, and postpartum hemorrhage.

Infections are more common and more serious in pregnant women with diabetes. Disorders of carbohydrate metabolism alter the body's normal resistance to infection. The inflammatory response, leukocyte function, and vaginal pH are all affected. Vaginal infections, particularly monilial vaginitis, are more common. Urinary tract infections (UTIs) also are more prevalent. Infection is serious because it causes increased insulin resistance and may result in ketoacidosis. Postpartum infection is more common among women who are insulin-dependent.

Ketoacidosis occurs most often during the second and third trimesters when the "diabetogenic" effect of pregnancy is the greatest. When the maternal metabolism is stressed by illness or infection, the diabetic woman is at increased risk for diabetic ketoacidosis (DKA). The use of betasympathomimetic medications such as terbutaline (Brethine) may also contribute to the risk for hyperglycemia and subsequent DKA (Hagay and Reece, 1999). DKA may also occur because of the woman's failure to take insulin appropriately. The onset of previously undiagnosed diabetes during pregnancy is another cause of DKA. DKA may occur with blood glucose levels barely exceeding 200 mg/dl, compared with 300 to 350 mg/dl in the nonpregnant state. In response to stress factors such as infection or illness, hyperglycemia occurs as a result of increased hepatic glucose production and decreased peripheral glucose utilization. Stress hormones, which act to impair insulin action and further contribute to insulin deficiency, are released. Fatty acids are mobilized from fat stores into the circulation; as they are oxidized, ketone bodies are released into the peripheral circulation. The woman's buffering system is unable to compensate, and metabolic acidosis develops. The excessive blood glucose and ketone bodies result in osmotic diuresis with subsequent loss of fluid and electrolytes, volume depletion, and cellular dehydration. Prompt treatment of DKA is necessary to avoid maternal coma or death. Ketoacidosis occurring at any time during pregnancy can lead to intrauterine fetal death and is a cause of preterm labor. The perinatal mortality rate is about 20% with maternal ketoacidosis (Cunningham et al, 1997).

The risk of hypoglycemia is also increased. Early in pregnancy, when hepatic production of glucose is diminished and peripheral utilization of glucose is enhanced, hypoglycemia occurs frequently, often during sleep. Later in pregnancy, hypoglycemia may also result as insulin doses are adjusted to maintain normoglycemia. Women with a prepregnancy history of severe hypoglycemia are at increased risk for severe hypoglycemia during gestation. Mild to moderate hypoglycemic episodes do not appear to have significant deleterious effects on fetal well-being. The long-term fetal effects of severe maternal hypoglycemia are as yet uncertain (Hagay and Reece, 1999).

Fetal and Neonatal Risks and Complications. From the moment of conception, the infant of a mother with diabetes faces an increased risk of complications that may occur during the antenatal, intrapartal, or neonatal periods. These complications may be mild and transient, but are often life-threatening and may result in the infant's death. Infant morbidity and mortality associated with diabetic pregnancy are significantly reduced with strict control of maternal glucose levels before and during pregnancy.

Despite the improvements in care of pregnant women with diabetes, sudden and unexplained stillbirth is still a major concern. Typically this is observed in pregnancies after 36 weeks in women with vascular disease or poor glycemic control. It may also be associated with DKA, preeclampsia, hydramnios, or macrosomia. Although the exact cause of stillbirth is unknown, it may be related to chronic intrauterine hypoxia.

The most important cause of perinatal deaths in diabetic pregnancy is congenital anomalies. The incidence of congenital anomalies in infants born to women with diabetes is 6% to 10%, a twofold to fourfold increase over that of the general population. Up to 40% of all perinatal deaths among infants of women with diabetes are caused by congenital malformations

(Hagay and Reece, 1999). The incidence of congenital malformations is related to the severity and duration of the diabetes. In addition to hyperglycemia, hyperketonemia and hypoglycemia may play a role in the development of congenital anomalies (Landon, 1996b). Cardiac defects are the most common anomalies seen, followed by central nervous system and skeletal defects (Hagay and Reece, 1999).

Macrosomia is often defined as a weight of 4000 to 4500 g or greater. Macrosomia may also be defined as large-for-gestational age (LGA), that is, the infant weight is greater than the 90th percentile (Landon, 1996b). The fetal pancreas begins to secrete insulin at 10 to 14 weeks' gestation. The fetus responds to maternal hyperglycemia by secreting large amounts of insulin (hyperinsulinism). Insulin acts as a growth hormone, causing the fetus to produce excess stores of glycogen, protein, and adipose tissue, leading to increased fetal size. During birth, the macrosomic infant may incur fractured clavicle, liver or spleen laceration, brachial plexus injury, facial palsy, phrenic nerve injury, or subdural hemorrhage (Hagay and Reece, 1999; Moore, 1999) (see Chapter 27).

IUGR is often seen in infants of diabetic women with vascular disease. It is related to compromised uteroplacental circulation and may be worsened in the presence of ketoacidosis and preeclampsia. The amount of oxygen available to the fetus is decreased as a result of maternal vascular changes (Bernstein and Gabbe, 1996).

These infants are at increased risk for respiratory distress syndrome (RDS). Hyperglycemia and hyperinsulinemia may be instrumental in delaying pulmonary maturation in the fetus (Hagay and Reece, 1999).

For infants of a diabetic pregnancy, the transition to extrauterine life is often beset with metabolic abnormalities. Within the first 30 to 60 minutes after birth, neonatal hypoglycemia often occurs. This is caused by the effects of fetal hyperinsulinism and the rapid utilization of glucose after birth. The incidence of neonatal hypoglycemia is related to the mother's glycemic control during pregnancy and to her glucose levels during labor and birth. Hypocalcemia, hypomagnesemia, hyperbilirubinemia, and polycythemia also occur more often in infants of mothers with diabetes, which places these neonates at increased risk (Landon, 1996b).

Care Management

➤ Assessment

Interview. When a pregnant woman with diabetes initiates prenatal care, a thorough evaluation of her health status is completed. In addition to routine prenatal assessment, a detailed history regarding the onset and course of the diabetes and the degree of glycemic control before pregnancy is obtained. Effective management of diabetic pregnancy depends on the woman's adherence to a plan of care. For the woman to care for her diabetes on a daily basis, she must have an adequate understanding of her disease and the prescribed regimen. Thus with the initial prenatal visit, the woman's knowledge regarding diabetes and pregnancy, potential maternal and fetal complications, and the plan of care are assessed. With subsequent visits, follow-up assessments are completed. Data from these assessments are used to identify the woman's specific learning needs. The support person's knowledge of diabetes is also assessed, and teaching needs are identified.

The woman's emotional status is assessed to determine how she is coping with pregnancy superimposed on preexisting diabetes. Although normal pregnancy typically evokes some degree of stress and anxiety, pregnancy designated as "high risk" serves to compound anxiety and stress levels. Fear of maternal and fetal complications is a major concern. Strict adherence to the plan of care may necessitate alterations in patterns of daily living and be an additional source of stress.

The woman's support system is assessed to identify those people significant to her and their roles in her life. It is important to assess the reactions of family members or significant others to the pregnancy, to the strict management plan, and to their involvement in the treatment regimen. Any areas of emotional stress are identified because such stress can precipitate complications.

Physical Examination. At the initial visit, a thorough physical examination is performed to assess the woman's current health status. In addition to the routine prenatal examination, specific efforts are made to assess the effects of diabetes. A baseline electrocardiogram may be done to assess cardiovascular status. Evaluation for retinopathy is done, with follow-up as needed by an ophthalmologist each trimester and more often if retinopathy is diagnosed. Blood pressure is monitored carefully throughout pregnancy because of the increased risk for preeclampsia. The woman's weight gain is also monitored at each visit. Fundal height is measured, noting any abnormal increase in size for dates, which may indicate hydramnios or fetal macrosomia. Leopold's maneuvers may be performed to check for fetal size and possible hydramnios.

Laboratory Tests. Routine prenatal laboratory examinations are performed. In addition, baseline renal function may be assessed with a 24-hour urine collection for total protein excretion and creatinine clearance. Urinalysis and culture are performed on the initial prenatal visit and throughout the pregnancy to assess for the presence of urinary tract infection, which is common in diabetic pregnancy. At each visit, urine is also tested for the presence of glucose and ketones. Because of the risk of coexisting thyroid disease, thyroid function tests may also be performed (see later discussion of thyroid disorders).

For the woman with pregestational type 1 or type 2 diabetes, laboratory tests may be done to assess past glycemic control. At the initial prenatal visit, the glycosylated hemoglobin A_{1c} level may be measured. With prolonged hyperglycemia, some of the hemoglobin remains saturated with glucose for the life of the red cell. Therefore a test for glycosylated hemoglobin provides a measurement of glycemic control over time, indicating the level of glycemic control over the previous 4 to 6 weeks. Regular measurements of glycosylated hemoglobin provide data for altering the treatment plan and lead to improvement of glycemic control. Values for the measurement of hemoglobin A_{1c}, the most commonly used index of glycosylated hemoglobin, are as follows (Pagana and Pagana, 1997):

Adult/elderly	4% to 8%
Good diabetic control	7%
Fair diabetic control	10%
Poor diabetic control	13% to 20%

Fasting blood glucose and/or random (1 to 2 hours after eating) glucose levels may be assessed during antepartum visits (Fig. 13-2). Blood glucose self-monitoring records may also be reviewed.

➤ Nursing Diagnoses

Nursing diagnoses for the woman with pregestational diabetes include the following:

- Knowledge deficit related to:
  —Diabetic pregnancy, management, and potential effects on pregnant woman and fetus
  —Insulin administration and its effects
  —Hypoglycemia and hyperglycemia
  —Diabetic diet
- Anxiety, fear, dysfunctional grieving, powerlessness, body-image disturbance, situational low self-esteem, spiritual distress, altered role performance, altered family processes related to:
  —Stigma of being labeled "diabetic"
  —Effects of diabetes and its potential sequelae on the pregnant woman and the fetus
- Risk for injury to fetus related to:
  —Uteroplacental insufficiency
  —Birth trauma
- Risk for injury to mother related to:
  —Improper insulin administration
  —Hypoglycemia and hyperglycemia
  —Cesarean or operative vaginal birth
  —Postpartum infection

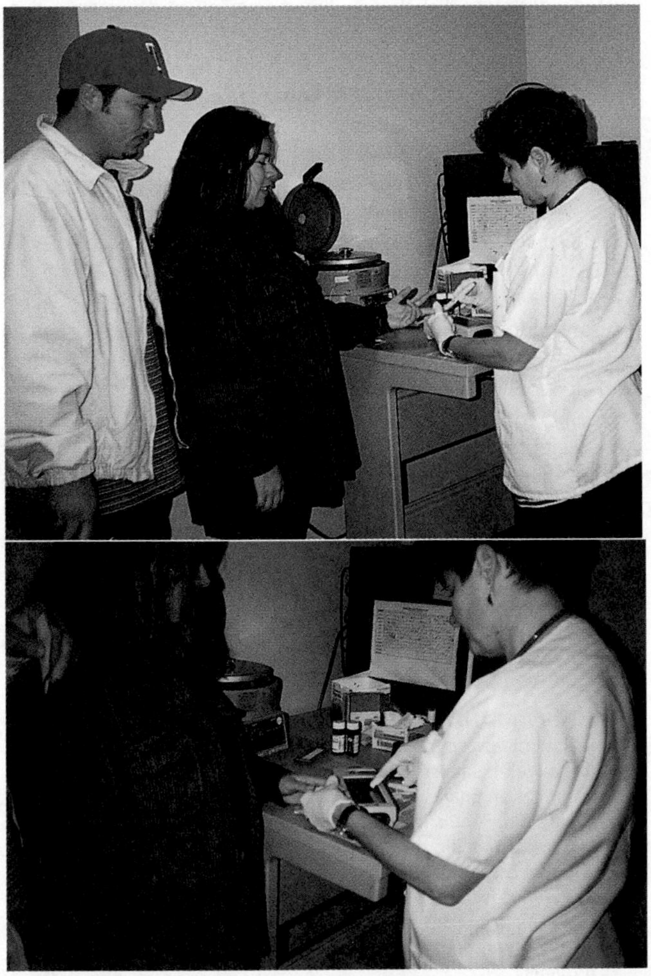

FIG. 13-2 • **A,** Clinic nurse collects blood to determine glucose level. **B,** Nurse interprets glucose value displayed by monitor. (Courtesy Dee Lowdermilk, UNC Ambulatory Care Clinics, Chapel Hill, NC.)

➤ Expected Outcomes

Expected outcomes of care for the pregnant woman with pregestational diabetes include that she will do the following:

- Demonstrate or verbalize understanding of diabetic pregnancy, the plan of care, and the importance of glycemic control.
- Achieve and maintain glycemic control.
- Demonstrate effective coping.
- Give birth to a healthy infant at term.

➤ Plan of Care and Implementation

Antepartum. Because of her high risk status, the woman with diabetes is monitored much more frequently and thoroughly than other pregnant women. During the first and second trimesters of pregnancy her routine prenatal care visits will be scheduled every 1 to 2 weeks; in the last trimester she will probably be seen one or two times each week. In the past, routine hospitalization was common for management of the diabetes, such as insulin dose changes. With the availability of better home glucose monitoring, and the growing reluctance of third-party payers to reimburse for hospitalization, pregnant women with diabetes are now generally managed as outpatients. Some patient and family education and maternal and fetal assessment may be done in the home, depending on the woman's insurance coverage and care provider preference.

Achieving and maintaining euglycemia, with blood glucose levels in the range of 65 to 130 mg/dl (Table 13-1), is the primary goal of medical therapy for the pregnant woman with diabetes. Euglycemia is achieved through a combination of diet, insulin, exercise, and blood glucose determinations. Providing the woman with the knowledge, skill, and motivation she needs to achieve and maintain excellent blood glucose control is the primary nursing goal.

Achieving euglycemia requires commitment of the woman and her family to make the necessary lifestyle changes, which can sometimes seem overwhelming. Maintaining tight blood glucose control necessitates that the woman follow a consistent daily schedule. She must go to bed and get up, eat, exercise, and take insulin at the same time every day. Blood glucose measurements are done frequently to determine how well the major components of therapy (i.e., diet, insulin, and exercise) are working together to control blood glucose levels.

TABLE 13-1
Target Blood Glucose Levels During Pregnancy

Time of Day	Target Glucose Level (mg/dl)
Premeal	>65 but <95
Postmeal (1 hour)	<130
Postmeal (2 hours)	<120
During hours of sleep	No less than 70

Source: Moore T: Diabetes in pregnancy. In Creasy R, Resnik R, editors: *Maternal-fetal medicine,* ed 4, Philadelphia, 1994, WB Saunders.

The woman should wear an identification bracelet at all times and carry insulin, syringes, and "glucose boosters" with her whenever she is away from home. She should be given written instructions for reporting the development of problems such as nausea, vomiting, and infections; and directions for reaching her health care provider by phone at night and on weekends and holidays (Guidelines box).

Because the diabetic woman is at risk for infections, eye problems, and neurologic changes, foot care and general skin care are important. A daily bath that includes good perineal care and foot care is important. Lotions, creams, or oils can be applied to dry skin. Tight clothing should be avoided. Shoes or slippers should be worn at all times, should fit properly, and are best worn with socks or stockings. Feet should be inspected regularly; toenails should be cut straight across; and professional help should be sought for any foot problems. Extremes of temperature should be avoided.

Diet. The woman with pregestational diabetes has usually had nutritional counseling regarding the management of diabetes. Because pregnancy precipitates special nutritional concerns and needs, the woman must be educated to incorporate these changes into dietary planning. Nutritional counseling is usually provided by a registered dietitian.

Dietary management during diabetic pregnancy must be based on blood (not urine) glucose levels. The diet is individualized to allow for increased fetal and metabolic requirements, with consideration of such factors as prepregnancy weight and dietary habits, overall health, ethnic background, lifestyle, stage of pregnancy, knowledge of nutrition, and insulin therapy. The dietary goal is to provide weight gain consistent with a normal pregnancy, to prevent ketoacidosis, and to minimize widely fluctuating blood glucose levels.

Energy needs are usually calculated on the basis of 30 to 35 calories per kilogram of ideal body weight, with the average diet including 2200 calories (first trimester) to 2500 calories (second and third trimesters). Total calories may be distributed among three meals and one evening snack, or more commonly, three meals and at least two snacks. Meals should be eaten on time and never skipped. Snacks must be carefully planned in accordance with insulin therapy to avoid fluctuations in blood glucose levels. A large bedtime snack of at least 25 g of carbohydrate with some protein is recommended to help prevent hypoglycemia and starvation ketosis during the night.

The ratio of carbohydrates, protein, and fat is important to meet the metabolic needs of the woman and the fetus. Approximately 50% to 60% of the total calories should be carbohydrates, with a minimum of 250 g per day. Simple carbohydrates are limited; complex carbohydrates that are high in fiber content are recommended because the starch and protein in these foods help regulate the blood glucose level by more sustained glucose release. Protein intake should constitute 12% to 20% of the total kilocalories; 20% to 30% of the daily caloric intake should come from fat, with no more than 10% from saturated fats (Home Care box). Weight gain for most women should be about 12 kg (22 to 30 lb) during the pregnancy (Gilbert and Harmon, 1998).

Exercise. Although exercise enhances the utilization of glucose and decreases insulin need in nonpregnant women with diabetes, there are limited data regarding exercise in the woman with pregestational diabetes. Any prescription of exercise during pregnancy for a woman with diabetes should be done by the primary health care provider and should be monitored closely to prevent complications. For those women with vasculopathy, only mild exercise is recommended because exercise causes a redistribution of blood flow, which increases the potential for ischemic injury to already compromised organs and the placenta. Also, women with vasculopathy typically depend completely on exogenous insulin and are at greater risk for wide fluctuations in blood glucose levels and ketoacidosis, which can be made worse by exercise.

Careful instructions for exercise are given. The exercise need not be vigorous to be beneficial: 15 to 30 minutes of walking four to six times a week is satisfactory for most pregnant women. Other exercises that may be recommended include non–weight-bearing activities such as arm ergometry or use of a recumbent bicycle. The best time for exercise is after meals when the blood sugar is rising. To monitor the effect of insulin on blood glucose levels, the woman can measure blood glucose before, during, and after exercise.

Guidelines

TREATMENT FOR HYPOGLYCEMIA

- **Be familiar with signs and symptoms of hypoglycemia (nervousness, headache, shaking, irritability, personality change, hunger, blurred vision, sweaty skin, tingling of mouth or extremities).**
- **Check blood glucose level immediately when hypoglycemic symptoms occur.**
- **If blood glucose is <60 mg/dl, immediately eat or drink something that contains 10 to 15 g of simple carbohydrate. Examples:**
  - **½ cup (4 oz) unsweetened fruit juice**
  - **½ cup (4 oz) regular (not diet) soda**
  - **5 to 6 Life Savers candies**
  - **1 tablespoon honey or corn (Karo) syrup**
  - **1 cup (8 oz) milk**
  - **2 to 3 glucose tablets**
- **Rest for 15 minutes, then recheck blood glucose.**
- **If glucose level is still <60 mg/dl, eat or drink another serving of one of the "glucose boosters" listed above.**
- **Wait 15 minutes, then recheck blood glucose. If it is still <60 mg/dl, notify health care provider immediately.**

Source: American Diabetes Association: *Medical management of pregnancy complicated by diabetes,* ed 2, Alexandria, VA, 1995, The Association; Becton Dickinson & Co: *Controlling low blood sugar reactions,* Franklin Lakes, NJ, 1997, Becton Dickinson.

Home Care

DIETARY MANAGEMENT OF DIABETIC PREGNANCY

- **Follow the prescribed diet plan.**
- **Eat a well-balanced diet, including daily food requirements for a normal pregnancy.**
- **Divide daily food intake among three meals and two to four snacks, depending on individual needs.**
- **Eat a substantial bedtime snack to prevent a severe drop in blood glucose level during the night.**
- **Limit the intake of fats if weight gain occurs too rapidly.**
- **Take daily vitamins and iron as prescribed by the health care provider.**
- **Avoid foods high in refined sugar.**
- **Eat consistently each day; never skip meals or snacks.**
- **Reduce the intake of saturated fat and cholesterol.**
- **Eat foods high in dietary fiber.**
- **Avoid alcohol and caffeine.**

Insulin Therapy. Adequate insulin is the primary factor in the maintenance of normoglycemia during pregnancy, thus ensuring proper glucose metabolism of the mother and fetus. Insulin requirements during pregnancy change dramatically as the pregnancy progresses, necessitating frequent adjustments in insulin dosage. In the first trimester, there is little or no change in prepregnancy insulin requirements; however, insulin dosage may need to be decreased because of hypoglycemia. During the second and third trimester, because of insulin resistance, the dosage must be increased to maintain target glucose levels.

For the woman with type 1 pregestational diabetes who has typically been accustomed to one injection per day of intermediate-acting insulin, multiple daily injections of mixed insulin are a new experience. The woman with type 2 diabetes previously treated with oral hypoglycemics is faced with the task of learning to self-administer injections of insulin. The nurse is instrumental in education and support with regard to insulin administration and the adjustment of insulin dosage to maintain normoglycemia (Patient Teaching box).

Patient Teaching

ADMINISTRATION OF INSULIN

Procedure for Mixing NPH (Intermediate-Acting) and Regular (Short-Acting) Insulin

- Wash hands thoroughly and gather supplies. Be sure the insulin syringe corresponds to the concentration of insulin you are using.
- Check insulin bottle to be certain it is the appropriate type and check the expiration date.
- Gently rotate (do not shake) the insulin vial to mix the insulin.
- Wipe off rubber stopper of each vial with alcohol.
- Draw into syringe the amount of air equal to total dose.
- Inject air equal to NPH (intermediate-acting) dose into NPH vial. Remove syringe from vial.
- Inject air equal to regular insulin dose into regular insulin vial.
- Invert regular insulin bottle and withdraw regular insulin dose.
- Without adding more air to NPH vial, carefully withdraw NPH dose.

Procedure for Self-Injection of Insulin

- Select proper injection site (remember to rotate sites).
- Injection site should be clean. Use of alcohol is not necessary. If alcohol is used, let it dry before injecting.
- Pinch the skin up to form a subcutaneous pocket and, holding the syringe like a pencil, puncture the skin at a 45- to 90-degree angle. If there is a great deal of fatty tissue at the site, spread the skin taut and inject the syringe at a 90-degree angle.
- Slowly inject the insulin.
- As you withdraw the needle, cover the injection site with sterile gauze and apply gentle pressure to prevent bleeding.
- Record insulin dosage and time of injection.

Many types of insulin are available today. Beef and pork insulin have largely been replaced by biosynthetic human insulin preparations (e.g., Humulin or Novolin), which are less likely to cause antibody formation. Patients with new onset of diabetes are almost always started on this type of insulin. Lispro (Humalog), a new rapid-acting insulin, is available. It has a faster onset and shorter duration of action than regular insulin. Because it is injected immediately before mealtime, there is less hypoglycemia following meals and fewer hypoglycemic episodes in some patients. Because its effects last 5 hours, most patients require a longer-acting insulin along with Lispro to maintain optimal glucose levels (Moore, 1999) (Table 13-2). Lispro can be used safely in pregnancy, but unlike other insulins, it is available only with a prescription.

Most women with insulin-dependent diabetes are managed with two or three injections per day. Usually, two-thirds of the daily insulin dose, with longer-acting (NPH) and short-acting (regular or Lispro) insulin combined in a 2:1 ratio, is given before breakfast. The remaining one third, again a combination of longer- and short-acting insulin, is sometimes administered in the evening before dinner. To reduce the risk of hypoglycemia during the night, separate injections may be administered, with short-acting insulin given before dinner, followed by longer-acting insulin at bedtime. An alternative insulin regime that works well for some women is to administer short-acting insulin before each meal and longer-acting insulin at bedtime (Hagay and Reece, 1999).

Although subcutaneous insulin injections are most common, continuous insulin infusion systems may be used during pregnancy. The insulin pump is designed to mimic more closely the function of the pancreas in secreting insulin (Fig. 13-3). This portable, battery-powered device infuses regular insulin at

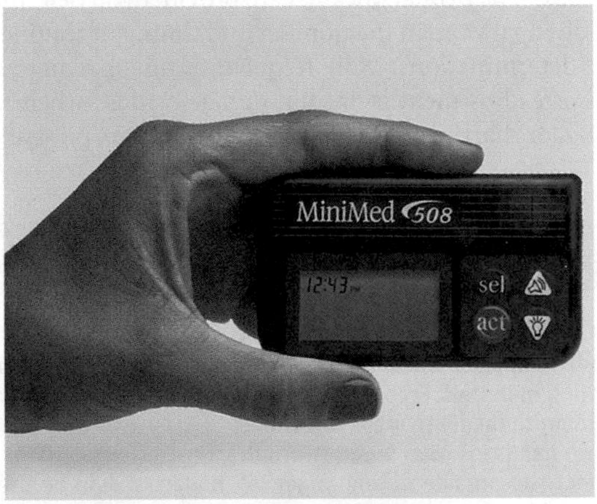

FIG. 13-3 • Insulin pump shows basal rate for pregnant women with diabetes. (Courtesy MiniMed, Inc., Sylmar, CA.)

TABLE 13-2

Insulin Administration During Pregnancy: Expected Time of Action

Type of Insulin	Onset	Peak	Duration
Lispro (rapid acting)	Within 15 min	30-90 min	3 hr
Regular (rapid acting)	30 min-1 hr	2-4 hr	5-8 hr
Intermediate acting	2-4 hr	5-10 hr	12-24 hr
Long acting	3-4 hr	14-24 hr	24-36 hr

a set basal rate and has the capacity to deliver up to four different basal rates in 24 hours. The pump also delivers bolus doses of insulin before meals to control postmeal blood glucose levels. The infusion tubing from the insulin pump can be left in place for several weeks without local complications. Although the insulin pump is convenient and generally provides good glycemic control, complications such as DKA, infection, or hypoglycemic coma can still develop. Use of the insulin pump requires a knowledgeable, motivated patient; skilled health care providers; and 24-hour availability of emergency assistance (Hagay and Reece, 1999; Moore, 1999).

Monitoring Blood Glucose Levels. Blood glucose testing at home with a glucose reflectance meter is the commonly accepted method for monitoring blood glucose levels. It is the most accurate method of documenting the degree of glycemic control in an out-of-hospital setting, and it enables the woman to adjust her insulin dosage on a 24-hour basis (Home Care box). Most insurance companies cover the cost of a meter and necessary supplies.

Meters that incorporate memory to store a large number of readings are available; however, the woman is encouraged to keep written records of glucose levels. She should bring her written records, her meter containing stored test results, or both with her to each appointment. It is important that the monitoring equipment be checked for accuracy at intervals by comparing the woman's results on her machine with the results of a laboratory test done at the same time on a capillary whole blood sample.

Blood glucose levels are routinely measured at various times throughout the day such as before breakfast, lunch, and dinner; 2 hours after meals; at bedtime; and in the middle of the night. Hyperglycemia will most likely be identified in the 2-hour postprandial values because blood glucose levels peak about 2 hours after a meal. The primary health care provider will determine for each individual woman the number and timing of routine blood glucose determinations. More frequent testing is required when there is a readjustment in insulin dosage or diet; when nausea, vomiting, or diarrhea occur; or when infection is present.

Home Care

TESTING BLOOD GLUCOSE LEVEL

- Gather supplies, check expiration date, and read instructions on testing materials. Prepare glucose reflectance meter for use according to manufacturer's directions.
- Wash hands in warm water (warmth increases circulation).
- Select site on side of any finger (all fingers should be used in rotation).
- Pierce site with lancet (may use automatic, spring-loaded, puncturing device). Cleaning the site with alcohol is not necessary.
- Drop hand down to side; with other hand gently squeeze finger from hand to fingertip.
- Allow blood to drop onto testing strip. Be sure to cover entire reagent area.
- Determine blood glucose value using the glucose reflectance meter, following manufacturer's instructions.
- Record results.
- Repeat daily as instructed by health care provider and as needed for signs of hypoglycemia or hyperglycemia.

Source: American Diabetes Association: *Medical management of pregnancy complicated by diabetes,* ed 2, Alexandria, VA, 1995, The Association.

Target levels of blood glucose during pregnancy are lower than nonpregnant values. Acceptable fasting levels are generally between 65 and 95 mg/dl, and 2-hour postprandial levels should be less than 120 mg/dl (Moore, 1999). The woman should be told to immediately report episodes of hypoglycemia (less than 60 mg/dl) and hyperglycemia (greater than 200 mg/dl) to her health care provider so that adjustments in diet or insulin therapy can be made.

Pregnant women with diabetes are much more likely to develop hypoglycemia than hyperglycemia, because the goal of therapy is to maintain the blood glucose in a narrow, low-normal range of 65 to 130 mg/dl. Most episodes of mild or moderate hypoglycemia can be treated with oral intake of 10 to 15 g of simple carbohydrates (see Guidelines box on p. 248). If severe hypoglycemia occurs in which the woman experiences a decrease in or loss of consciousness or an inability to swallow, she will require a parenteral injection of glucagon or intravenous (IV) glucose (Becton Dickinson & Co., 1997). Because hypoglycemia can develop rapidly, and because impaired judgment can be associated with even moderate episodes, it is vital that family members, friends, and work colleagues be able to quickly recognize signs and symptoms and initiate proper treatment if necessary.

Hyperglycemia is less likely to occur, but can rapidly progress to diabetic ketoacidosis. Women and family members should be alert for signs and symptoms of hyperglycemia, especially when infections or other illnesses occur (Home Care box).

Urine Testing. Urine testing for ketones continues to have a place in diabetic management, because it may provide vital information for the pregnant woman, such as the onset of DKA. Urine is tested daily with the first morning urine. Testing may also be done if a meal is missed or delayed, when illness occurs, or when blood glucose is greater than 200 mg/dl.

Spilling a trace or small amount of ketones requires no treatment. However, if ketones appear repeatedly at the same time each day, some adjustment in diet may be needed. If testing shows a large amount of ketones, the health care provider should be contacted immediately (ADA, 1995).

Complications Requiring Hospitalization. Occasionally hospitalization may be required to regulate insulin dosage

Home Care

WHAT TO DO WHEN ILLNESS OCCURS:

- Be sure to take insulin even though appetite and food intake may be less than normal (insulin needs are increased with illness or infection).
- Call the health care provider and relay the following information:
  - Symptoms of illness (e.g., nausea, vomiting, diarrhea)
  - Fever
  - Most recent blood glucose level
  - Urine ketones
  - Time and amount of last insulin dose
- Increase oral intake of fluids to prevent dehydration.
- Rest as much as possible.
- If unable to reach health care provider and blood glucose exceeds 200 mg/dL with urine ketones present, seek emergency treatment at the nearest health care facility. Do not attempt to self-treat for this.

and stabilize glucose levels. Hospitalization offers a controlled situation to initiate and regulate insulin therapy while providing opportunity for intensive education in self-administration of insulin and regulation of blood glucose. Infection, which can lead to hyperglycemia and diabetic ketoacidosis, is an indication for hospitalization, regardless of gestational age. Hospitalization during the third trimester for closer maternal and fetal observation may be indicated for women with vasculopathy because of the increased risk for renal impairment, hypertensive disorders, and fetal compromise (ADA, 1994).

Fetal Surveillance. Diagnostic techniques for fetal surveillance are often performed during a pregnancy complicated by diabetes to assess fetal growth and well-being. The goals of fetal surveillance are to detect fetal compromise as early as possible and to prevent intrauterine fetal death or unnecessary preterm birth. The majority of fetal surveillance measures are concentrated in the third trimester, when the risk of fetal death is greatest.

Early in pregnancy, the estimated date of birth (EDB) is determined. A baseline ultrasound is used during the first trimester to assess gestational age. Follow-up ultrasound examinations are usually performed during the pregnancy (as often as every 4 to 6 weeks) to monitor fetal growth, estimate fetal weight, and detect hydramnios, macrosomia, and congenital anomalies.

Because diabetic pregnancies are at greater risk for neural tube defects (e.g., spina bifida, anencephaly, and microcephaly), measurement of maternal serum alpha-fetoprotein is performed between 16 and 18 weeks of gestation. This is often done in conjunction with a detailed ultrasound study to examine the fetus for neural tube defects.

Fetal echocardiography may be performed between 18 and 22 weeks of gestation to detect cardiac anomalies. Some practitioners repeat this fetal surveillance test at 34 weeks. Doppler studies of the umbilical artery may be performed to detect placental compromise in women with vascular disease.

Maternal evaluation of fetal movements (kick counts) is used primarily as a screening technique in fetal surveillance. Nonstress tests (NSTs) to evaluate fetal well-being may be used weekly or more often, typically beginning around 28 to 32 weeks of gestation (see Chapter 8). After 32 weeks, testing may be done twice weekly. For the woman with vascular disease, testing may begin earlier and continue more frequently. In the presence of a nonreactive NST, a contraction stress test or fetal biophysical profile may be used to evaluate fetal well-being (Hagay and Reece, 1999; Landon, 1996b; Moore, 1999).

Determination of Birth Date and Mode of Delivery. Today the majority of diabetic pregnancies are allowed to progress to term (38 to 40 weeks), as long as good metabolic control is maintained and all parameters of antepartum fetal surveillance remain within normal limits. Reasons to proceed with delivery before term include poor metabolic control, worsening hypertensive disorders, fetal macrosomia, or fetal growth restriction (Hagay and Reece, 1999; Moore, 1999).

Many practitioners plan for elective labor induction between 38 and 40 weeks provided maternal glucose levels are well-controlled. To confirm fetal lung maturity before birth, an amniocentesis may be performed in pregnancies of less than 39 weeks. For the pregnancy complicated by diabetes, fetal lung maturation is better predicted by the amniotic fluid phosphatidylglycerol (PG) than by the lecithin/sphingomyelin (L/S) ratio. If the fetal lungs are still immature, birth should be postponed as long as the results of fetal assessment remain reassuring. Amniocentesis may be repeated to monitor lung maturity. Birth despite poor fetal lung maturity may be essential when testing suggests fetal compromise or if preeclampsia, rapidly worsening retinopathy, or renal failure develops (Landon, 1996b).

The mode of birth for women with pregestational diabetes is controversial. The rate of cesarean births for these women is high, around 45%. Cesarean birth is often performed when antepartum testing suggests fetal distress, an estimated fetal weight greater than 4000 g, or when an induction of labor is desired and the cervix fails to respond to prostaglandin ripening (Hagay and Reece, 1999; Landon, 1996b; Moore, 1999).

Intrapartum. During the intrapartum period the woman with pregestational diabetes must be monitored closely to prevent complications related to dehydration, hypoglycemia, and hyperglycemia. Most women use large amounts of energy (calories) to accomplish the work and manage the stress of labor and birth; however, this calorie expenditure varies with the individual. Blood glucose levels and hydration must be carefully controlled during labor. An intravenous (IV) line is inserted for infusion of a maintenance fluid such as lactated Ringer's solution or 5% dextrose/lactated Ringer's (D5LR) solution. Insulin may be administered by continuous infusion or by intermittent subcutaneous injection.

Determinations of blood glucose are made every hour, and fluids and insulin are adjusted to maintain blood glucose levels between 60 and 100 mg/dl. It is essential that these target glucose levels be maintained because hyperglycemia during labor can precipitate metabolic problems in the neonate, particularly hypoglycemia. Maternal hyperglycemia during labor can also lead to perinatal asphyxia and fetal/neonatal death.

During labor, continuous fetal heart monitoring is necessary. The mother should assume an upright or side-lying position during bed rest in labor to prevent supine hypotension because of a large fetus or polyhydramnios. Labor is allowed to progress, provided normal rates of cervical dilation, fetal descent, and fetal well-being are maintained. Failure to progress may indicate a macrosomic infant and cephalopelvic disproportion (CPD), which necessitates cesarean birth. The woman is observed and treated during labor for diabetic complications such as hyperglycemia, ketosis, ketoacidosis, and glycosuria. A pediatrician may be present at the birth to initiate assessment and neonatal care.

If a cesarean is the planned mode of birth, it should be scheduled in the early morning to facilitate glycemic control. The morning dose of insulin is withheld and the woman is allowed nothing by mouth. Epidural anesthesia is recommended because hypoglycemia can be detected earlier if the woman is awake. After surgery, glucose levels are closely monitored, at least every 2 hours, and an IV solution containing 5% dextrose is infused (Landon and Gabbe, 1995).

Postpartum. In the immediate postpartum period, insulin requirements decrease substantially because the major source of insulin resistance, the placenta, has been removed. Women with type 1 diabetes may require only one-half the prenatal insulin dose on the first postpartum day, provided that they are eating a full diet. It takes several days after delivery to reestablish carbohydrate homeostasis (see Fig. 13-1, *D* and *E*). Blood glucose levels are monitored in the postpartum period, and insulin dosage is adjusted accordingly. Usually insulin is not given until the blood glucose level is greater than 200 mg/dl (Hagay and Reece, 1999). The woman who is insulin-dependent must realize the importance of eating on time even if the baby needs feeding or other pressing demands exist. Women with type 2 diabetes often require no insulin in the postpartum period and are able to maintain normoglycemia through diet alone or with oral hypoglycemics.

Possible postpartum complications include preeclampsia-eclampsia, hemorrhage, and infection. Hemorrhage is a possibility if the mother's uterus was overdistended (e.g., by hydramnios or macrosomic fetus), or overstimulated (e.g., by oxytocin induction). Postpartum infections such as endometritis are more likely to occur in a postpartum woman with diabetes.

Mothers are encouraged to breastfeed. In addition to the advantages of maternal satisfaction and pleasure, breastfeeding has an antidiabetogenic effect. Insulin requirements may be half of prepregnancy levels because of the carbohydrate used in human milk production. Because glucose levels are lower, breastfeeding women are at increased risk for hypoglycemia, especially in the early postpartum period and after breastfeeding sessions (Hagay and Reece, 1999; Moore, 1999). Breastfeeding mothers with diabetes may be at increased risk for mastitis and yeast infections of the breast. Insulin dosage, which is decreased during lactation, must be recalculated at the time of weaning (Landon, 1996b) (see Fig. 13-1, *F*).

The diabetic mother may experience early breastfeeding difficulties. Poor metabolic control may delay lactogenesis and contribute to decreased milk production (Moore, 1999). Initial contact and opportunity to breastfeed the infant may be delayed if the infant is placed in a neonatal intensive care unit (NICU) or special care nursery for observation during the first few hours after birth. Support and assistance from nursing staff and lactation specialists can facilitate the mother's early experience with breastfeeding and encourage her to continue.

Recent evidence suggests that infants who are exclusively breastfed are less likely to develop diabetes, and that exposure to cow's milk products before 8 days of age is an important risk factor for the disease (Moore, 1999).

The new mother needs information about family planning and contraception. While family planning is important for all women, it is essential for the woman with diabetes to safeguard her own health and to promote optimal outcomes in any future pregnancies. The woman and her partner should be informed that the risks associated with pregnancy increase with the duration and severity of the diabetic condition, and that pregnancy may contribute to vascular changes associated with diabetes.

The risks and benefits of contraceptive methods should be discussed with the mother and her partner before discharge from the hospital. The barrier method is the preferred method of contraception for the woman who is insulin-dependent. Barrier methods such as the diaphragm or condom and spermicide pose the least risk. However, a problem with these methods is the inconsistency of use, which often leads to unplanned pregnancy (Landon, 1996b).

Use of oral contraceptives by diabetic women is controversial because of the risk of thromboembolic and vascular complications and the effect on carbohydrate metabolism. In women without vascular disease or other risk factors, low-dose oral contraceptives may be prescribed. Close monitoring of blood pressure and glucose levels is necessary to detect complications (Kjos, 1996; Landon and Gabbe, 1995).

Intrauterine contraceptive devices increase the risk of infection, especially during the first 4 months after insertion. However, they may be used for women who are older or who have hypertension or other vascular disease. Such individuals should be parous, in a monogamous relationship, at low risk for sexually transmitted infection, and have no history of pelvic infection. These women must be able to recognize the signs of pelvic infection and STIs and notify their health care provider promptly if they occur (Kjos, 1996).

There is no contraindication to use of the Norplant system in diabetic women without cardiovascular complications (Jovanovic-Peterson, 1993).

Sterilization should be discussed with the woman who has completed her family or who has significant vasculopathy (ADA, 1994).

➤ Evaluation

Evaluation of the care of the pregnant woman with pregestational diabetes is based on the previously stated expected outcomes, which are closely associated with the degree of maternal metabolic control during pregnancy (Nursing Care Plan).

Gestational Diabetes Mellitus

Gestational diabetes mellitus (GDM) complicates approximately 4% of all pregnancies in the United States and accounts for 90% of all cases of diabetic pregnancy. Prevalence varies by race and ethnicity. GDM occurs more commonly among Hispanic, Native American, Asian, and African-American populations than in Caucasians (Expert Committee on the Diagnosis and Classification of Diabetes Mellitus, 1997). Persons with GDM are at significant risk of developing glucose intolerance later in life; about 50% will be diagnosed as diabetic within 22 to 28 years. Classic risk factors include maternal age greater than 30 years; obesity; family history of type 2 diabetes; and an obstetric history of an infant weighing more than 4000 g, hydramnios, unexplained stillbirth, miscarriage, or an infant with congenital anomalies. Women at high risk for GDM are often screened at their initial prenatal visit and then rescreened later in pregnancy if the initial screen is negative.

The diagnosis of gestational diabetes is usually made during the second half of pregnancy. As fetal nutrient demands rise during the late second and third trimester, maternal nutrient ingestion induces greater and more sustained levels of blood glucose. At the same time, maternal insulin resistance is also increasing as a result of the insulin antagonistic effects of the placental hormones, cortisol, and insulinase. Consequently, maternal insulin demands rise as much as threefold. The majority of pregnant women are capable of increasing insulin production to compensate for the insulin resistance and to maintain normoglycemia. When the pancreas is unable to produce sufficient insulin or the insulin is not used effectively, gestational diabetes can result.

Maternal and Fetal Risks. Women with GDM have twice the risk of developing hypertensive disorders compared with normal pregnant women (Metzger and Coustan, 1998). They also have increased risk for fetal macrosomia, which can lead to increased rates of perineal lacerations, episiotomy, and cesarean birth (Jones and Stone, 1998). Infants born to women with GDM are at risk for macrosomia with associated shoulder dystocia and birth trauma. GDM also places the neonate at in-

Nursing Care Plan PREGNANCY COMPLICATED BY INSULIN-DEPENDENT DIABETES

NURSING DIAGNOSIS Knowledge deficit related to lack of recall of information as evidenced by patient questions and concerns

EXPECTED OUTCOME Patient will be able to verbalize important information regarding diabetes, its management, and potential effects on the pregnant woman and fetus.

Nursing Interventions/*Rationales*

Assess patient's current knowledge base regarding disease process, management, effects on pregnancy and fetus, and potential complications *to provide database for further teaching.*

Review the pathophysiology of diabetes, effects on pregnancy and fetus, and potential complications *to promote patient recall of information and compliance with treatment plan.*

Review procedure for insulin administration, demonstrate procedure for blood glucose monitoring and insulin measurement and administration, and obtain return demonstration *to establish patient comfort and competence with procedures.*

Discuss diet and exercise as prescribed by the diabetologist *to promote self-care.*

Review signs and symptoms of complications of hypoglycemia and hyperglycemia and appropriate interventions *to promote prompt recognition of complications and self-care.*

Provide contact numbers for health care team for prompt interventions and answers to questions on an ongoing basis *to promote patient comfort.*

NURSING DIAGNOSIS Risk for fetal injury related to elevated maternal glucose levels

EXPECTED OUTCOME Fetus will remain free of injury and be delivered at term in a healthy state.

Nursing Interventions/*Rationales*

Assess patient's current diabetic control *to identify risk for fetal mortality and congenital anomalies.*

Monitor fundal height during each prenatal visit *to identify appropriate fetal growth.*

Monitor for signs and symptoms of pregnancy-induced hypertension *to identify early manifestations because diabetic pregnant women are more at risk.*

Assess fetal movement and heart rate during each prenatal visit and perform weekly nonstress tests during the last 4 weeks of pregnancy *to assess for fetal well-being.*

Review procedure for blood glucose testing and insulin administration *to promote self-care.*

NURSING DIAGNOSIS Anxiety related to threat to maternal and fetal well-being as evidenced by patient verbal expressions of concern

EXPECTED OUTCOME Patient will identify sources of anxiety and report feeling less anxious.

Nursing Interventions/*Rationales*

Through therapeutic communication, promote an open relationship with patient *to promote patient trust.*

Listen to patient's feelings and concerns *to assess for any misconception or misinformation that may be contributing to anxiety.*

Review potential dangers by providing factual information *to correct any misconception or misinformation.*

Encourage patient to share concerns with her health care team *to promote patient and team collaboration in her care.*

Help woman identify and use appropriate coping strategies and support systems *to reduce fear/anxiety.*

Explore use of desensitization strategies such as progressive muscle relaxation, visual imagery, or thought stopping *to reduce fear-related emotions and related physical symptoms.*

creased risk for hypoglycemia, hypocalcemia, hyperbilirubinemia, thrombocytopenia, polycythemia, and respiratory distress syndrome (Jones and Stone, 1998; Metzger and Coustan, 1998).

The overall incidence of congenital anomalies among infants of women with gestational diabetes approaches that of the general population because gestational diabetes usually develops after the twentieth week of pregnancy—after the critical period of organogenesis (first trimester) has passed.

Screening for Gestational Diabetes Mellitus. Earlier recommendations from the ADA were that all pregnant women should be screened for the development of GDM. However the Expert Committee on the Diagnosis and Classification of Diabetes Mellitus stated in its 1997 report that it is neither cost-effective nor necessary to screen certain women who are at low risk for GDM. This low risk group includes normal-weight women younger than 25 years of age who have no family history of diabetes and who are not of an ethnic or racial group known to have a high prevalence of the disease. The American College of Obstetricians and Gynecologists (ACOG) (1994) stated that selective screening may be appropriate in some low risk settings (e.g., teen clinics), but that universal screening might be more appropriate for high risk populations. ACOG also states that women in certain groups with a high prevalence of GDM may be considered to have an abnormal screen and proceed directly to diagnostic testing.

The screening test used most often in North America (Glucola screening) consists of a 50 g oral glucose load, followed 1 hour later by a plasma glucose determination. Screening should be performed at 24 to 28 weeks of gestation. It is not necessary that the woman be fasting. A glucose value of 140 mg/dl is considered a positive screen and should be followed by a 3-hour oral glucose tolerance test (OGTT). The

3-hour OGTT is administered after an overnight fast and at least 3 days of unrestricted diet (at least 150 g carbohydrate) and physical activity. The woman is instructed to avoid caffeine because it tends to increase glucose levels, and to abstain from smoking for 12 hours before and during the test. A fasting blood glucose level is drawn before giving a 100 g glucose load. Blood glucose levels are then drawn 1, 2, and 3 hours later. The woman is diagnosed with gestational diabetes if two or more values are met or exceeded (Fig. 13-4).

Controversy exists over the management of women with only one abnormal OGTT value. Many experts believe that these women are at increased risk for fetal macrosomia. Some experts immediately diagnose and treat these women as if they had gestational diabetes. Other authorities prefer to retest them 1 month later with another 3-hour OGTT. Often women with one abnormal OGTT value will be placed on a modified diabetic diet that contains no concentrated sweets (e.g., candy, cookies, cake, pie, and sugar-sweetened drinks) for the remainder of the pregnancy.

Nursing diagnoses are similar to those identified for women with pregestational diabetes.

Expected outcomes of care for the woman with GDM are basically the same as for women with pregestational diabetes except that the time frame for planning may be shortened with GDM because the diagnosis is usually made later in pregnancy.

Interventions

Antepartum. When the diagnosis of gestational diabetes is made, treatment begins immediately, allowing little or no time for the woman and her family to adjust to the diagnosis before they are expected to participate in the treatment plan. This is in contrast to the woman with pregestational diabetes who may have had years to learn about the disease and adapt to dietary modifications, self-monitoring of glucose, and insulin administration. With each step of the treatment plan, the nurse and other health care providers should educate the woman and her family, providing detailed and comprehensive explanations to ensure understanding, participation, and adherence to the necessary interventions. Potential complications should be discussed, and the need for maintenance of normoglycemia throughout the remainder of the pregnancy is reinforced. It may be reassuring for the woman and her family to know that gestational diabetes typically disappears when the pregnancy is over.

As with pregestational diabetes, the aim of therapy in women with GDM is meticulous blood glucose control. Fasting blood glucose levels should be less than 105 mg/dl, and 2-hour postprandial blood levels should be less than 120 mg/dl (Hagay and Reece, 1999; Landon, 1996b).

Diet. Dietary modification is the mainstay of treatment for GDM. The woman with GDM is placed on a standard diabetic diet immediately upon diagnosis. The usual prescription is for 30 to 35 kcal/kg of present pregnancy weight, which translates into 2000 to 2500 calories per day for most women. Some authorities recommend fewer calories for overweight or morbidly obese women, believing that such a diet will cause less hyperglycemia and reduce the need for insulin (Landon, 1996b; Metzger and Coustan, 1998). Dietary counseling by a nutritionist is recommended. Most women with GDM do not require hospitalization for dietary instruction and management.

Exercise. Exercise in women with GDM appears to be safe. It helps lower blood glucose levels and may be instrumental in eliminating the need for insulin. Women with GDM who already have an active lifestyle should be encouraged to continue an exercise program. Brisk walking, use of a recumbent bicycle, and swimming are often recommended; exercises that use the upper body are ideal for most women because they are not associated with increased uterine contractions. Sedentary women may also be encouraged to increase their physical activity. They may be advised to begin by exercising three or four times a week for 15 to 39 minutes, gradually increasing intensity and duration (Jones and Stone, 1998). Of course, any exercise program should always be initiated or continued with the knowledge and consent of the primary health care provider.

Monitoring Blood Glucose Levels. Blood glucose monitoring is necessary to determine if euglycemia can be maintained by diet and exercise. Fasting and postprandial glucose levels

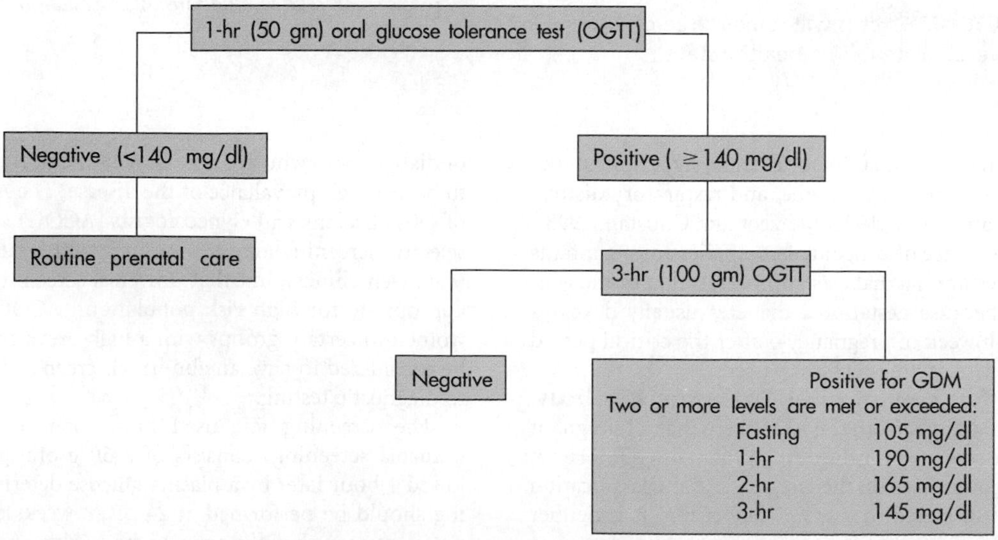

FIG. 13-4 • Screening and diagnosis for gestational diabetes. (From American Diabetes Association: Position statement: gestational diabetes mellitus, *Diabetes Care* 20 [suppl 1]:S44, 1997.)

should be monitored at least weekly (ACOG, 1994). Some women with GDM are provided with reflectance meters and encouraged to perform frequent self-monitoring at home, or monitoring may be done only at the clinic or office visit.

Insulin Therapy. Many women with GDM will require insulin during the pregnancy to maintain adequate blood glucose levels, despite compliance with the prescribed diet. This occurs because as pregnancy progresses, placental hormones increase blood glucose levels and cause insulin to work less effectively. Depending on the diet prescribed and the blood glucose thresholds used by the practitioner, as many as half of all women with GDM may require insulin at some point during pregnancy (Landon, 1996b). The nurse should never assume that increased blood glucose levels in the woman with GDM have been caused by dietary indiscretion alone; a thorough history must be taken to determine the cause.

ACOG (1994) recommends that women who repetitively exceed the glucose thresholds of 105 mg/dl fasting and 120 mg/dl 2 hours postprandial be started on insulin therapy. In practice, however, lower or higher thresholds for initiating insulin may be used (Landon, 1996b).

Fetal Surveillance. There is no standard recommendation for fetal surveillance in pregnancies complicated by GDM. Women whose blood glucose levels are well controlled by diet are a low risk for fetal death. Usually these women progress to term and spontaneous labor without intervention. Once the woman reaches 40 weeks gestation, fetal surveillance once or twice weekly is usually instituted (ACOG, 1994; Landon, 1996b; Metzger and Coustan, 1998).

Women with GDM whose blood glucose levels are not well controlled or who require insulin therapy, have hypertension, or have a history of previous stillbirth generally receive more intensive fetal biophysical monitoring. Nonstress tests and biophysical profiles are often performed weekly, beginning from 32 to 36 weeks of gestation (ACOG, 1994; Landon, 1996b; Metzger and Coustan, 1998).

Intrapartum. During the intrapartum period, blood glucose levels are monitored at least every 2 hours to maintain levels at 100 mg/dl or less. Glucose levels within this range will decrease the severity of neonatal hypoglycemia. IV fluids containing glucose are not given as a bolus to the woman who has gestational diabetes, although they may be necessary as maintenance fluids. Routine uterine activity and fetal heart rate assessments are done. Although gestational diabetes is not an indication for cesarean birth, it may be necessary in the presence of problems such as preeclampsia or macrosomia.

Postpartum. Most women with GDM return to normal glucose levels after childbirth (Metzger and Coustan, 1998). However, GDM is likely to recur in future pregnancies. Assessment for carbohydrate intolerance can be initiated 6 to 12 weeks postpartum or after breastfeeding has stopped and should be repeated at regular intervals throughout the woman's life (Metzger and Coustan, 1998). Obesity is a major risk factor for the later development of diabetes. Thus women with a history of GDM, particularly those who are overweight, should be encouraged to make lifestyle changes that include weight loss and exercise to reduce this risk (Hagay and Reece, 1999; Metzger and Coustan, 1998). Because offspring of women with GDM are at risk to develop obesity and diabetes in childhood or adolescence (Metzger and Coustan, 1998), regular health care for these children is essential.

Thyroid Disorders

Hyperthyroidism. Hyperthyroidism affects approximately 2 of every 1000 pregnancies (Landon, 1996b; Seely and Burrow, 1999). In 90% to 95% of pregnant women, it is caused by Graves disease. Other rare but possible causes include toxic nodular goiter and thyroiditis (Inzucchi and Burrow, 1999; Seely and Burrow, 1999). Clinical manifestations of hyperthyroidism are associated with an increased basal metabolism rate and increased sympathetic nervous system activity. Typical symptoms include fatigue, heat intolerance, warm skin, diaphoresis, emotional lability, tremulousness, and a wide pulse pressure. Many of these symptoms also occur with pregnancy, so the disorder can be difficult to diagnose. Signs that may help differentiate hyperthyroidism from normal pregnancy include unplanned weight loss, onycholysis (loose nails), and a pulse rate greater than 100 beats per minute that does not decrease with the Valsalva maneuver (Diehl, 1998; Seely and Burrow, 1999). Laboratory findings include elevated free thyroxine (T_4) level and a suppressed serum thyroid-stimulating hormone (TSH) level (Diehl, 1998; Seely and Burrow, 1999). Mild hyperthyroidism is not thought to impair fertility, although it is rare to find severe disease in early pregnancy. Hyperthyroidism should be treated during pregnancy; untreated or inadequately treated women give birth to infants with low birth weight and more minor fetal anomalies. Women with hyperthyroidism are also at increased risk to develop severe preeclampsia (Diehl, 1998: Seely and Burrow, 1999). Hyperemesis gravidarum is often associated with elevated thyroid hormone levels (Landon, 1996b; Seely and Burrow, 1999).

The primary treatment of hyperthyroidism during pregnancy is drug therapy; the medication of choice is propylthiouracil (PTU). The usual starting dosage is 100 to 150 mg every 8 hours. Patients generally show clinical improvement within 2 weeks of beginning therapy, but the medication requires 6 to 8 weeks to reach full effectiveness. During therapy the woman's free T_4 levels are measured monthly and the results used to taper the drug to the smallest effective dosage to prevent unnecessary fetal hypothyroidism (Diehl, 1998; Seely and Burrow, 1999). PTU is well tolerated by patients. Rare side effects include pruritus, skin rash, a metallic taste, nausea, bronchospasm, oral ulcerations, hepatitis, and a lupus-like syndrome (Seely and Burrow, 1999). The most severe side effect is agranulocytosis, which is more common in women over 40 years of age and in those taking high doses of PTU (Seely and Burrow, 1999). Symptoms of agranulocytosis are fever and sore throat, which should be reported immediately to the health care provider; at the same time, the woman should stop taking the PTU. Leukopenia of a transient and benign nature may occur as a result of PTU therapy. PTU readily crosses the placenta and may induce fetal hypothyroidism and goiter, although these complications rarely occur (Landon, 1996b; Seely and Burrow, 1999).

Beta-adrenergic blockers such as propranolol may be used in severe hyperthyroidism. Long-term use is not recommended because of the potential for IUGR and altered response to anoxic stress, postnatal bradycardia, and hypoglycemia (Seely and Burrow, 1999).

Radioactive iodine must not be used in diagnosis or treatment of hyperthyroidism because it may compromise the fetal thyroid. If a mother taking hyperthyroid medication chooses to breastfeed, she needs to be aware that physiologically significant doses of the drug are passed to the infant through the breast milk. The infant's thyroid status should be monitored periodically so hypothyroidism can be prevented (Cunningham et al, 1997; Seely and Burrow, 1999).

In severe cases, surgical treatment of hyperthyroidism (subtotal thyroidectomy) may be performed during the second or third trimester. Because of the increased risk of miscarriage and preterm labor associated with major surgery, this treatment is usually reserved for women with severe disease, those for whom drug therapy proves toxic, and those who are unable to adhere to the prescribed medical regimen. Postoperative hypothyroidism is common, occurring in at least 20% of women with hyperthyroidism.

A serious but uncommon complication of undiagnosed or partially treated hyperthyroidism is thyroid storm, which may occur in response to stresses such as infection, birth, or surgery. A woman experiencing this emergent condition may have fever, restlessness, tachycardia, vomiting, hypotension, or stupor. Prompt treatment is essential; IV fluids and oxygen are administered along with high doses of PTU. Potassium iodide, antipyretics, dexamethasone, and beta-adrenergic blockers may also be given; sedation may be necessary for extreme restlessness (Inzucchi and Burrow, 1999; Landon, 1996b).

Hypothyroidism. Hypothyroidism during pregnancy is rare because women with this condition are often infertile. Hypothyroidism is usually the result of Hashimoto's disease, thyroid gland ablation by radiation, previous surgery, or antithyroid medications. Reduced thyroid function because of hypothalamic or pituitary failure is rare, with only a few reported cases. Iodine deficiency in the United States is also rare (Diehl, 1998; Landon, 1996b).

Characteristic symptoms of hypothyroidism include fatigue, weight gain, cold intolerance, constipation, cool dry skin, coarsened hair, and muscle weakness. Laboratory findings during pregnancy include low or low-normal T_3 and T_4 levels and elevated levels of TSH (Diehl, 1998; Inzucchi and Burrow, 1999).

Pregnant women with untreated hypothyroidism are at risk for preeclampsia, placental abruption, and stillbirth. Infants born to mothers with hypothyroidism may be of low birth weight, but for the most part are healthy, without evidence of thyroid dysfunction (Diehl, 1998; Inzucchi and Burrow, 1999). Thyroid hormone supplements are used to treat hypothyroidism. Levothyroxine (e.g., L-thyroxine [Synthroid]) is most often prescribed during pregnancy. The usual beginning dose is 0.10 to 0.15 mg per day, in a single daily dose.

NURSE ALERT • Pregnant women should be told to take L-thyroxine 2 hours before or after iron tablets, because ferrous sulfate lowers the effectiveness of the medication (Diehl, 1998).

As pregnancy progresses, the woman usually requires increased amounts of L-thyroxine. The aim of drug therapy is to maintain the women's TSH level within the normal range for pregnant women. Dosage adjustments are made as necessary by measuring TSH levels periodically. Each dosage change should be followed 4 to 6 weeks later by determining the TSH level.

The fetus is dependent on maternal thyroid hormones until 12 weeks of gestation, when fetal production begins. Thus maternal hypothyroidism does not cause fetal hypothyroidism. However, maternal treatment of hypothyroidism may result in increased fetal levels of thyroid hormones. Careful monitoring of the neonate's thyroid status is important to detect any abnormalities.

Maternal Phenylketonuria

Phenylketonuria (PKU), a recognized cause of mental retardation, is an inborn error of metabolism caused by an autosomal recessive trait that creates a deficiency in the enzyme phenylalanine hydrolase. Absence of this enzyme impairs the body's ability to metabolize the amino acid phenylalanine, found in all protein foods. Consequently, there is toxic accumulation of phenylalanine in the blood, which interferes with brain development and function. PKU affects 1 in every 10,000 live births in the United States.

All newborns are tested for this disorder soon after birth; prompt diagnosis and therapy with a phenylalanine-restricted diet significantly decreases the incidence of mental retardation. Dietary therapy for PKU is recommended to continue throughout life (Acosta, 1995).

The key to prevention of fetal anomalies caused by PKU is the identification of women in their reproductive years who have the disorder. Screening programs during the school years and in the premarital period may help identify those individuals with PKU so that dietary therapy can be instituted before conception occurs. Screening for undiagnosed maternal PKU at the first prenatal visit may be warranted, especially in individuals with a family history of the disorder, with low intelligence of uncertain etiology, or who have given birth to microcephalic infants.

Infants diagnosed with PKU can be safely breastfed if the amount of breast milk ingested is monitored so that phenylalanine levels do not get too high. Mothers who choose to breastfeed must supplement the infant's diet with a special milk preparation that contains little or no phenylalanine (Kirby, 1999).

CARDIOVASCULAR DISORDERS

During a normal pregnancy the maternal cardiovascular system undergoes many changes that put a physiologic strain on the heart. The major cardiovascular changes that occur during a normal pregnancy and that affect the patient with cardiac disease are increased intravascular volume, decreased systemic vascular resistance, cardiac output changes occurring during labor and birth, and the intravascular volume changes that occur just after childbirth. The strain is present during pregnancy and continues for a few weeks after birth. The normal heart can compensate for the increased workload, and pregnancy, labor, and birth are generally well tolerated; but the diseased heart is challenged hemodynamically.

If the cardiovascular changes are not well tolerated, cardiac failure can develop during pregnancy, labor, or the postpartum period. In addition, if myocardial disease develops, if valvular disease exists, or a congenital heart defect is present, cardiac decompensation (i.e., inability of the heart to maintain a sufficient cardiac output) may occur.

About 1% of pregnancies are complicated by heart disease (Cunningham et al, 1997). Heart disease is the leading cause of nonobstetric maternal mortality and ranks fourth overall as a cause of maternal death. A maternal mortality rate of up to 50%

is anticipated in women with persistent cardiac decompensation. Box 13-1 lists maternal cardiac disease risk groups.

The degree of disability experienced by the woman with cardiac disease is often more important in the treatment and prognosis of cardiac disease complicating pregnancy than is the diagnosis of cardiac disease. The New York Heart Association's (NYHA, 1964) functional classification of organic heart disease, a widely accepted standard, is as follows:

Class I—Symptomatic at normal levels of activity
Class II—Symptomatic with increased activity
Class III—Symptomatic with ordinary activity
Class IV—Symptomatic at rest

No classification of heart disease can be considered rigid or absolute, but the NYHA classification offers a basic practical guide for treatment, assuming that frequent prenatal visits, good patient cooperation, and appropriate obstetric care occur. Medical therapy is conducted by a team approach that includes the cardiologist, obstetrical physician, and nurses. The functional classification may change over the course of the pregnancy because of the hemodynamic changes that occur in the cardiovascular system. There is a 30% to 50% increase in cardiac output compared to nonpregnancy resting values, with the majority of the increase in the first trimester and the peak in 20 to 24 weeks of gestation (Cunningham et al, 1997). The functional classification of the disease is determined at 3 months and again at 7 or 8 months of gestation.

There are contraindications to pregnancy in women with heart disease (Box 13-2). The incidence of miscarriage is increased, and preterm labor and birth is more prevalent in the pregnant woman with cardiac problems. In addition, IUGR is common, probably because of low oxygen pressure (Po_2) in the mother. The incidence (4% to 16%) of congenital heart lesions is increased in children of mother with congenital heart disease; thus preconception counseling is important (Mendelson, 1997).

A diagnosis of cardiac disease depends on the history, physical examination, x-ray findings, and if indicated, ultrasonogram results. The differential diagnosis of heart disease also involves ruling out respiratory problems and other potential causes of chest pain.

Maternal mortality of more than 50% during pregnancy has been associated with pulmonary hypertension; it is vital that the woman with cardiac disease be assessed and the diagnosis established as soon as possible (Mendelson, 1997).

Box 13-1

Maternal Cardiac Disease Risk Groups

GROUP I (MORTALITY 1%)
Corrected tetralogy of Fallot
Pulmonic/tricuspid disease
Mitral stenosis (classes I, II)
Patent ductus
Ventricular septal defect
Atrial septal defect
Porcine valve

GROUP II (MORTALITY 5%-15%)
Mitral stenosis with atrial fibrillation
Artificial heart valves
Mitral stenosis (classes III, IV)
Uncorrected tetralogy
Aortic coarctation (uncomplicated)
Aortic stenosis

GROUP III (MORTALITY 25%-50%)
Aortic coarctation (complicated)
Myocardial infarction
Marfan's syndrome
True cardiomyopathy
Pulmonary hypertension

From Gilbert E, Harmon J: *Manual of high risk pregnancy and delivery,* ed 2, St Louis, 1998, Mosby.

Peripartum Cardiomyopathy

The classical definition of peripartum cardiomyopathy is "congestive heart failure with cardiomyopathy found in the last month of pregnancy or in the first 5 months postpartum" (Landon, 1996a). The etiology of the disease in unknown; theories suggest genetic predisposition, autoimmunity, and viral infections.

Peripartum cardiomyopathy is more common in African-Americans, multiparous women age 30 and older, in twin pregnancies, and in women with preeclampsia (Mendelson and Lang, 1995). Maternal mortality has been estimated in the range of 25% to 50%, whereas infant mortality is approximately 10% (Jackson and Clark, 1993). Clinical findings are those of congestive heart failure (left ventricular failure). Symptoms include breathlessness, tachydysrhythmias, and edema, with radiologic findings of cardiomegaly. The prognosis is good if cardiomegaly does not persist after 6 months postpartum. Women whose hearts remain enlarged after 6 months postpartum will have peripartum cardiomyopathy in future pregnancies (Jackson and Clark, 1993). Sterilization should be considered because the mortality rate approaches 100%. Oral contraceptives are contraindicated because of the risk of thromboembolism.

Medical management of cardiomyopathy during pregnancy includes diuretics, potassium, anticoagulants, and digitalis. Bed rest is generally recommended, but its benefit is unclear (Jackson and Clark, 1993; Landon, 1996a).

Rheumatic Heart Disease

Rheumatic fever usually develops suddenly, often several symptom-free weeks after an inadequately treated group A beta-hemolytic streptococcal throat infection. Episodes of rheumatic fever create an autoimmune reaction in the heart tissue that leads to permanent damage of heart valves (usually the

Box 13-2

Contraindications to Pregnancy in a Woman with Heart Disease

Pulmonary hypertension
Shunt lesions associated with Eisenmenger's syndrome
Complex cyanotic congenital heart disease
Aortic coarctation complicated by aortic dissection
Poor ventricular function
Marfan's syndrome with marked aortic dilation

Adapted from Mendelson M: Congenital cardiac disease and pregnancy, *Clin Perinatol* 24(2):467-482, 1997.

mitral valve) and the chorda tendineae cordis. This damage is referred to as rheumatic heart disease (RHD). RHD may be evident during acute rheumatic fever or discovered years later. Recurrences of rheumatic fever are common; each has the potential to increase the severity of heart damage. If a woman has had rheumatic fever in the past, it can recur during pregnancy. The American Heart Association recommends lifelong prophylaxis with penicillin G benzathine, even during pregnancy. For those with penicillin allergies, erythromycin is an acceptable alternative during pregnancy. Heart murmurs, resulting from stenosis, valvular insufficiency, or thickening of the walls of the heart, characterize RHD. Abnormal pulse rate and rhythm, as well as congestive heart failure, are common.

Mitral Valve Stenosis

Mitral valve stenosis (narrowing of the opening of the mitral valve caused by stiffening of valve leaflets, thereby obstructing blood flow from the atrium to the ventricles) is associated with 90% of RHD seen in pregnancy (McAnulty, Metcalfe, and Ueland, 1995). Even though a history of rheumatic fever may be absent, it remains the most likely cause of mitral stenosis. As the mitral valve narrows, dyspnea worsens, occurring first on exertion and eventually at rest. A tight stenosis, plus the increase in blood volume and cardiac output of normal pregnancy, may cause ventricular failure and pulmonary edema; hemoptysis may occur.

The pregnant woman with mitral stenosis should be monitored clinically for symptoms and by echocardiograms to monitor the atrial and ventricular size as well as heart valve function. Prophylaxis for intrapartum endocarditis and pulmonary infections is provided (Box 13-3).

Mitral Valve Prolapse

Mitral valve prolapse (MVP) is a common, usually benign, condition occurring in nearly 10% of women of reproductive age (Cunningham et al, 1997). The mitral valve leaflets prolapse into the left atrium during ventricular systole, allowing some backflow of blood. Midsystolic click and late systolic murmur are hallmarks of this syndrome. Most cases are asymptomatic. A few women have atypical chest pain (i.e., sharp and located in the left side of the chest) that occurs at rest, is unrelated to exercise, and does not respond to nitrates. They may have anxiety, palpitations, dyspnea on exertion, and syncope. They are usually treated with beta blockers such as propranolol (Inderal).

Critical Thinking

THE WOMAN WITH DYSPNEA

You are assigned to admit a woman who is 26-weeks pregnant and is experiencing increasing dyspnea. She has a history of rheumatic fever as a child.

What would be your assessment questions? What physical assessments would you make? What lab values would you examine?

What is the likely origin of her respiratory distress? What is the usual antibiotic regimen for someone with her history? Patients in respiratory distress are often anxious. List interventions to reduce her anxiety. Identify home care concerns as you prepare to discharge your patient.

Pregnancy and its associated hemodynamic changes may change or alleviate the murmur and click of MVP, as well as its symptoms. As with RHD, antibiotic prophylaxis is given before invasive procedures for at-risk patients and for complicated vaginal deliveries in patients with MVP.

Infective Endocarditis

Infective endocarditis, or inflammation of the innermost lining (endocardium) of the heart caused by invasion of microorganism, is an uncommon disorder during pregnancy (Mendelson and Lang, 1995). It may be seen in women taking street drugs intravenously. Bacterial endocarditis, leading to incompetence of heart valves and thus congestive heart failure and cerebral emboli, can result in death. Treatment is the same as for the nonpregnant woman, that is, antibiotics (see Box 13-3).

Eisenmenger's Syndrome

Eisenmenger's syndrome is a "right-to-left or bi-directional shunting at either the atrial or ventricular level, combined with elevated pulmonary vascular resistance" (Landon, 1996a). The syndrome is associated with high mortality (12% to 70% in mothers and 50% in fetuses), and thus pregnancy is contraindicated. Contraception is essential and tubal ligation should be considered; oral contraceptives and intrauterine devices carry considerable risk (Mendelson and Lang, 1995). If pregnancy occurs, termination may be recommended if the woman has significant pulmonary hypertension (Landon, 1996a).

During pregnancy, physical activity should be limited and the supine position avoided; prophylactic anticoagulation is considered (Mendelson and Lang, 1995). During labor and birth, Swan-Ganz monitoring is essential. Central hypovolemia is avoided. If epidural analgesia is used, serial determinations of arterial oxygen concentrations should be done.

Box 13-3

Prophylaxis for Bacterial Endocarditis

DURING PREGNANCY FOR MINOR PROCEDURES

Low Risk Patients

Amoxicillin 3 g PO 1 hr before procedure; 1.5 g PO 6 hr after procedure

High Risk Patients

Vancomycin 1 g IV (over 1 hr) plus gentamicin 1.5 mg/kg (up to 80 mg) IM or IV 1 hr before procedure; repeat dose 8 hr after procedure

DURING LABOR AND BIRTH

Ampicillin 2 g IM or IV plus gentamicin 1.5 mg/kg (up to 80 mg) IM or IV during active labor and repeated 8 hr later and postpartum

Penicillin-Allergic Patients

Vancomycin 1 g IV may be substituted for the ampicillin

From Jackson G, Clark S: Cardiac and pulmonary disorders and pregnancy. In Moore T et al, editors: *Gynecology and obstetrics: a longitudinal approach,* New York, 1993, Churchill Livingstone; Landon M: Cardiac and pulmonary disease. In Gabbe S, Niebyl J, Simpson J, editors: *Obstetrics: normal and problem pregnancies,* ed 3, New York, 1996, Churchill Livingstone.

Care Management

Nursing care of the woman with a cardiovascular disorder combines routine peripartum care with care specific for the cardiac diagnosis. Cardiac conditions vary in their impact on pregnancy because of acuteness or chronicity.

The presence of cardiac disease makes the decision to become pregnant more difficult. Planned pregnancy requires that the woman understand the peripartum risks. If the pregnancy is unplanned, the nurse needs to explore the woman's desire to continue the pregnancy. The nurse should review with the woman options for pregnancy termination if her cardiac status is tenuous and abortion is an acceptable alternative.

➤ Assessment

The pregnant woman with cardiac disease requires detailed assessment throughout the peripartum period to determine the potential for optimal maternal health and a viable fetus. If she chooses to continue the pregnancy, the high risk pregnant woman's condition may be assessed as often as weekly.

The nurse elicits information from the woman regarding her personal medical history and that of her family; special notation is made of diseases of cardiovascular significance. The nurse assesses for factors that would increase stress on the heart (e.g., anemia, infection, and edema) and for how the woman is adapting to the physiologic changes of pregnancy.

In the assessment, special attention is given to the review of the cardiovascular and pulmonary systems. The nurse should determine whether the patient has experienced chest pain at rest or on exertion; edema of the face, hands, or feet; hypertension; heart murmurs; palpitations; paroxysmal nocturnal dyspnea; diaphoresis; and pallor or syncope. Pulmonary symptoms such as cough, hemoptysis, shortness of breath, and orthopnea also can be signs of cardiac disease. Table 13-3 lists the normal and abnormal cardiovascular signs and symptoms during pregnancy.

The nurse documents all medications taken by the woman—including over-the-counter medications such as supplemental iron—and is alert to their potential side effects and interactions. The woman is also assessed for undue emotional stress that might further compromise cardiac status. Examples of emotional stress are depression, anxiety or fear of morbidity or mortality for herself and the fetus, financial concerns related to extended hospitalization, anger because of impaired social interaction, and feelings of inadequacy regarding her inability to meet family and household demands.

The woman's cultural background may affect the amount of support that she is able to receive from significant others. Family size (i.e., number of children and extended family members in the home), and role expectations within the family, may be dictated by cultural norms. For the woman with cardiac impairment, family expectations may be a cause of major stress if she is unable to bear the expected number of children or if it is unacceptable to receive help with domestic chores.

Physical Examination. Routine assessments continue during the prenatal period, including monitoring the amount and pattern of edema, vital signs, discomforts of pregnancy, and amount and pattern of weight gain. The woman is observed for signs of cardiac decompensation (e.g., progressive generalized edema, crackles at the base of the lungs, or pulse irregularity) (Box 13-4). Medical intervention must be instituted immediately to maintain optimal cardiac status. Dyspnea, palpitations, syncope, and edema commonly occur in pregnant women and can mask the symptoms of a developing or worsening cardiovascular disorder. A woman's sudden inability to perform activities she previously was comfortable doing may indicate cardiovascular decompensation.

Laboratory and Diagnostic Tests. Routine urinalysis and blood work (i.e., complete blood count and blood chemistry) are done during the initial visit. A baseline electrocardio-

TABLE 13-3

Cardiovascular Signs and Symptoms During Pregnancy

Normal	Abnormal
SIGNS	
Neck vein pulsation	Neck vein distention
Diffuse/displaced apical pulse	Cardiomegaly; heave
Split S_1, accentuated S_2	Loud P_2; wide split of S_2
Third heart sound	Summation gallop
Systolic murmur (1-2/6)	Loud systolic murmur (4-6/6)
Venous hum	Diastolic murmur
Sinus dysrhythmia	Sustained dysrhythmia
Peripheral edema	Clubbing/cyanosis
SYMPTOMS	
Fatigue	Symptoms at rest
Chest pain	Exertional chest pain
Dyspnea	Exertional, severe dyspnea
Orthopnea	Orthopnea (progressive)
Hyperpnea	Paroxysmal nocturnal dyspnea
Palpitations	Tachycardia (>120 beats/min); dysrhythmia
Syncope (vasovagal)	Exertional syncope

Adapted from Mendelson M: Congenital cardiac disease and pregnancy, *Clin Perinatol* 24(2):467-482, 1997.

Box 13-4

Signs of Potential Complications

CARDIAC DECOMPENSATION

Pregnant Woman: Subjective Symptoms

- Increasing fatigue or difficulty breathing, or both, with her usual activities
- Feeling of smothering
- Frequent cough
- Palpitations; feeling that her heart is racing
- Swelling of face, feet, legs, fingers (e.g., rings do not fit anymore)

Nurse: Objective Signs

- Irregular weak, rapid pulse (≥100 beats/min)
- Progressive, generalized edema
- Crackles at base of lungs after two inspirations and exhalations
- Orthopnea: increasing dyspnea
- Rapid respirations (≥25 breaths/min)
- Moist, frequent cough
- Increasing fatigue
- Cyanosis of lips and nail beds

gram is done at the beginning of the pregnancy. Echocardiograms and pulse oximetry studies may be performed as indicated. Chest films may be necessary during late pregnancy. In addition, fetal ultrasound, fetal movement studies, or fetal nonstress tests may be used to determine fetal well-being.

➤ Nursing Diagnoses

The following examples are some nursing diagnoses that may be formulated. As always, individualizing diagnoses is vital.

- Fear related to:
  —Increased peripartum risk
- Knowledge deficit related to:
  —Cardiac condition
  —Pregnancy and how it affects cardiac condition
  —Requirements to alter self-care activities
- Risk for self-care deficit (bathing, grooming, and dressing) related to:
  —Fatigue or activity intolerance
  —Need for bed rest
- Impaired home maintenance management related to:
  —Mother's confinement to bed and/or limited activity level

➤ Expected Outcomes

The mother with cardiovascular problems faces curtailment of her activities. These restrictions can have physical and emotional implications. The community health nurse, social worker, and physical or occupational therapist are some of the resource people whose services may need to be incorporated into the plan of care. Appropriate expected outcomes might include the following:

The pregnant woman (and family, if appropriate) will:

- Verbalize understanding of the disorder, management, and probable outcome.
- Describe her role in management, including when and how to take medication, adjust diet, and prepare for and participate in treatment.
- Cope with emotional reactions to pregnancy and an infant at risk.
- Adapt to the physiologic stressors of pregnancy, labor and birth.
- Carry her fetus to viability or to term.

➤ Plan of Care and Implementation

Therapy for the pregnant woman with heart disease is focused on minimizing stress on the heart. This stress is greatest between 28 and 32 weeks as the hemodynamic changes reach their maximum. The workload of the cardiovascular system is reduced by appropriate treatment of any coexisting emotional stress, hypertension, anemia, hyperthyroidism, or obesity.

Signs and symptoms of cardiac decompensation are reviewed with the pregnant woman and her family. The woman with class I or II heart disease requires 8 to 10 hours of sleep every day and should take 30-minute naps after meals. Her activities are restricted, with housework, shopping, and exercise limited to the amount recommended for the functional classification of her heart disease.

The woman with class II cardiac disease should avoid heavy exertion and should stop any activity that causes even minor signs and symptoms of cardiac decompensation. She should be admitted to the hospital near term (or earlier if signs of cardiac overload or dysrhythmia develop) for evaluation and treatment.

Bed rest for much of the day is necessary for pregnant women with class III cardiac disease. About 30% of these women experience cardiac decompensation during pregnancy. These women may require hospitalization for the remainder of the pregnancy.

Because decompensation occurs even at rest in persons with class IV cardiac disease, a major initial effort must be made to improve the cardiac status of the pregnant woman in this category who chooses to continue her pregnancy (Patient Teaching box).

Infections are treated promptly. Women who have valvular disorders should receive prophylactic antibiotics against bacterial endocarditis during gestation (see Box 13-3).

Nutrition counseling is necessary, and optimally takes place with the woman's family present. The woman needs a diet that is well-balanced, high in iron and protein, and adequate in calories to gain weight. Iron supplements tend to cause constipation; the pregnant woman should increase her intake of fluids and fiber. A stool softener may be prescribed. It is important that the pregnant woman with cardiac disease avoid straining during defecation, thus causing the Valsalva maneuver (forced expiration against a closed airway, which when released causes blood to rush to the heart and overload the cardiac system) (Patient Teaching box). Sodium intake may be restricted; careful monitoring for hyponatremia is necessary. The sodium ion, with its ability to attract and hold fluid, affects the quality and amount of the circulating volume. Potassium intake is monitored with heart and other muscular weakness and dysfunction.

Patient Teaching

THE PREGNANT WOMAN AT RISK FOR CARDIAC DECOMPENSATION

- **Assess lifestyle patterns, emotional status, and environment of woman.**
- **Arrange for consultations as needed (i.e., dietitian, home care, child care, social work).**
- **Determine woman's and her family's understanding of her heart disease and how the disease affects her pregnancy.**
- **Determine stressors in the woman's life. Assist woman in identifying effective coping strategies.**
- **Instruct woman to report signs of cardiac decompensation or congestive heart failure: generalized edema, distention of neck veins, dyspnea, pulmonary crackles, cough, palpitations, weight gain of 4.4 kg in 1 day.**
- **Instruct woman to be watchful for signs of thromboembolism, such as redness, tenderness, pain or swelling of the legs. Instruct woman to seek medical help immediately if such symptoms occur.**
- **Instruct woman to avoid constipation and thus straining with bowel movements (Valsalva maneuver) by taking in adequate fluids and fiber. A stool softener may be ordered.**
- **Explore with woman ways to obtain the needed rest throughout the day. Depending on the level of her cardiac disease, she may need to sleep 10 hours per night and rest 30 minutes after meals (class I or II) or rest for most of the day (class III or IV).**
- **Help woman make use of community resources, including support groups, as indicated.**
- **Emphasize the importance of keeping her prenatal visits.**

From Gilbert E, Harmon J: *Manual of high risk pregnancy and delivery,* ed 2, St Louis, 1998, Mosby; Grohar J: Nursing protocols for antepartum home care, *J Obstet Gynecol Neonatal Nurs* 23(8):687-694, 1994; Health Care Resources: *Handbook of high risk perinatal home care,* St Louis, 1997, Mosby.

Cardiac medications are prescribed as needed for the pregnant woman, with attention given to fetal well-being. The hemodynamic changes that occur during pregnancy, such as increased plasma volume and increased renal clearance of drugs, can alter the amount of medication needed to establish and maintain a therapeutic drug level (Jackson and Clark, 1993). The woman's size and ethnic background must also be taken into consideration. For example, women of short stature and those of Asian descent require less medication for the desired physiologic response. Therefore the nurse must monitor the pregnant woman for adverse side effects as well as for the blood level of the medication.

If anticoagulant therapy is required during pregnancy, heparin should be used because this large-molecule drug does not cross the placenta (James et al, 1994). The nurse should closely monitor the woman's blood work, including clotting factors. The woman may need to learn to self-administer heparin. She also requires specific nutritional teaching to avoid foods high in vitamin K (e.g., raw dark green and leafy vegetables), which counteract the effects of the heparin. In addition, she will require a substitute source of folic acid in her diet.

Tests for fetal maturity and well-being and placental sufficiency may be necessary. Other therapy is directly related to the functional classification of heart disease. The nurse may need to reinforce the need for close medical supervision. Information about management of labor and birth and the postpartum period allows the woman time to plan for necessary extra care.

LEGAL TIP • Cardiac and Metabolic Emergencies The management of emergencies such as maternal cardiopulmonary distress or arrest or maternal metabolic crisis should be documented in policies, procedures, and protocols. Any independent nursing actions appropriate to the emergency should be clearly identified.

Intrapartum. For all pregnant women, the intrapartum period evokes the most apprehension in patients and caregivers. The woman with impaired cardiac function has additional reasons to be anxious because labor and giving birth place an additional burden on her already compromised cardiovascular system. The woman with class III or class IV cardiac disease will likely be hospitalized before the onset of labor.

If there are no obstetric problems, vaginal birth is recommended for the woman with cardiac disease. This is accomplished with the woman in a side-lying or upright position; if she is placed in the supine position, a pad is positioned under the hip to minimize the danger of supine hypotension. Epidural or pudendal block anesthesia is used. An episiotomy and the use of outlet forceps shortens the second stage of labor and decreases the work of the heart.

During labor, assessments for cardiac decompensation should be made. This includes taking vital signs at least every 10 to 30 minutes or according to institutional protocol or physician order. The color and temperature of the skin are noted. The woman is carefully watched for signs of emotional stress.

NURSE ALERT • The physician is alerted if the pulse is 100 beats per minute or greater or if the respirations are 25 breaths per minute or greater. Respiratory status is checked frequently for developing dyspnea, coughing, or crackles at the base of the lungs. Pale, cool, clammy skin may indicate cardiac shock.

Arterial blood gases (ABGs) may be needed to assess for adequate oxygenation. A Swan-Ganz catheter may be inserted to monitor hemodynamic status during labor and birth. ECG monitoring and continuous monitoring of blood pressure should be instituted. If evidence of cardiac decompensation appears, the physician may order deslanoside (Cedilanid-D) for rapid digitalization, furosemide (Lasix) for rapid diuresis, and oxygen by intermittent positive pressure to decrease the development of pulmonary edema.

Beta-adrenergic agents (e.g., ritodrine and terbutaline) should not be used for tocolysis. These agents are associated with myocardial ischemia. A synthetic oxytocin (Syntocinon) can be used for induction of labor. This drug does not appear to cause significant coronary artery constriction in the dosage prescribed for labor induction or control of postpartum uterine atony. Cervical ripening agents containing prostaglandins are not contraindicated, but reports of use in pregnant women with cardiac disease are not available.

Anxiety is decreased or alleviated through maintaining a calm atmosphere and by keeping the woman and her family informed. Discomfort is relieved with medication and supportive care. Epidural anesthesia is controversial in Eisenmenger's syndrome and pulmonary hypertension because it causes a decrease in cardiac output; it is avoided in idiopathic hypertrophic subaortic stenosis (IHSS) because it causes severe bradycardia (Thornhill and Camann, 1994).

Penicillin prophylaxis may be ordered for nonallergic pregnant women with class II or higher cardiac disease to protect against bacterial endocarditis in labor and during early puerperium. Ergot products should not be used because they tend to increase blood pressure. Dilute IV oxytocin immediately after birth may be employed to prevent hemorrhage.

Cesarean birth is not routinely recommended for women who have cardiovascular disease; there are risks of dramatic fluid shifts, hemodynamic changes that are sustained, and increased blood loss. There is increased mortality in women with Eisenmenger's syndrome who have cesarean birth (Mendelson, 1997). In class IV disease, maternal mortality approaches 50%; perinatal mortality is even higher.

Postpartum. Monitoring for cardiac decompensation in the postpartum period is essential. The first 24 to 48 hours postpartum are the most hemodynamically difficult for the woman. Cardiac output increases rapidly as extravascular fluid is remobilized into the vascular compartment. At the moment of birth, intraabdominal pressure is reduced drastically; pressure on veins is removed, the splanchnic vessels engorge, and blood flow to the heart is increased. When blood flow increases to the heart, a reflex bradycardia may result in response to the increased blood flow.

Special attention is given to the woman at risk for cardiac decompensation. The increased intravascular fluid can cause fluid volume excess in these women. Some physicians favor the application of an abdominal binder or alternating tourniquets on the extremities to minimize the effects of this rapid change in intraabdominal pressure. Hemorrhage and/or infection may worsen the cardiac condition. Monitoring for cardiac decompensation continues through the first weeks after birth because of hormonal shifts that affect hemodynamics. These shifts have been known to occur as late as the sixth postpartum week.

Care in the postpartum period is tailored to the woman's functional capacity. The woman is positioned with the head of the bed elevated and she is encouraged to lie on her side. Bed rest may be ordered, with or without bathroom privileges. She may need help to meet her grooming and hygiene needs. Progressive ambulation may be permitted as tolerated. Before and after walking the nurse assesses the woman's affect; pulse rate; breath sounds; coughing; edema; and skin color, temperature, and dryness.

The woman may direct a designated family member in the care of the infant. Breastfeeding is not contraindicated, but not all women with heart disease will be able to nurse their infants (Lawrence, 1999). The woman who chooses to breastfeed will need the support of her family and the nursing staff to be successful. To conserve the woman's energy, the infant may need to be brought to the mother and taken from her after the feeding.

If the woman is unable to breastfeed, and her energies do not allow her to bottle feed the infant, the baby can be brought after feeding to the mother. The infant should be held at the mother's eye level and near her lips and brought to her fingers so she can establish an emotional bond with her baby with a low expenditure of energy.

Preparation for discharge is carefully planned with the woman and family. Provision of help for the woman in the home by relatives, friends, and others must be addressed. The family is referred to community resources (e.g., homemaking services) as appropriate. Rest and sleep periods, activity, and diet must be planned. The couple may need information about reestablishing sexual relations and contraception or sterilization. Potential hazards of a subsequent pregnancy need to be examined by the woman and her partner. If sterilization is selected as a method

Nursing Care Plan — THE PREGNANT WOMAN WITH HEART DISEASE

NURSING DIAGNOSIS Activity intolerance related to effects of pregnancy on the patient with rheumatic heart disease with mitral valve stenosis

EXPECTED OUTCOME Woman will verbalize a plan to change lifestyle throughout pregnancy in order to avoid risk of cardiac decompensation.

Nursing Interventions/*Rationales*

Assist patient to identify factors that decrease activity tolerance and explore extent of limitations *to establish a baseline for evaluation.*

Help woman to develop an individualized program of activity and rest, taking into account the living and working environment as well as support of family and friends *to maintain sufficient cardiac output.*

Teach woman to monitor physiologic response to activity, (i.e., pulse rate, respiratory rate) and reduce activity that causes fatigue and/or pain *to maintain sufficient cardiac output and prevent potential injury to fetus.*

Enlist family and friends to assist woman in pacing activities and to provide support in performing role functions and self-care activities that are too strenuous *to increase chances of compliance with activity restrictions.*

Suggest that woman maintain an activity log that records activities, time, duration, intensity, and physiologic response *to evaluate effectiveness of and adherence to activity program.*

Discuss various quiet diversional activities which could be done by the woman *to decrease the potential for boredom during rest periods.*

NURSING DIAGNOSIS Therapeutic regimen: individual, risk for ineffective management related to woman's first pregnancy and perceived sense of wellness

EXPECTED OUTCOME Woman will participate in an effective therapeutic regimen for pregnancy complicated by heart disease.

Nursing Interventions/*Rationales*

Identify factors, such as insufficient knowledge about the effect of cardiac disease on pregnancy which could inhibit the woman from participating in a therapeutic regime *to promote early interventions, such as teaching about the importance of rest.*

Teach woman and family about factors, such as lack of rest or not taking prescribed medications which could adversely affect the pregnancy *to provide information and promote empowerment over the situation.*

Encourage expression of feelings about the disease and its potential effect on the pregnancy *to promote a sense of trust.*

Identify resources in the community *to provide a shared sense of common experiences.*

Encourage woman to verbalize her plan for carrying out the regime of care *to evaluate the effects of teaching.*

NURSING DIAGNOSIS Decreased cardiac output related to increased circulatory volume secondary to pregnancy and cardiac disease

EXPECTED OUTCOME The woman will exhibit signs of adequate cardiac output (i.e., normal pulse and blood pressure, normal heart and breath sounds, normal skin color, tone, and turgor, normal capillary refill, normal urine output, and no evidence of edema).

Nursing Interventions/*Rationales*

Reinforce the importance of activity/rest cycles *to prevent cardiac complications.*

Plan with woman a frequent visit schedule to caregiver *to provide adequate surveillance of high risk pregnancy.*

Teach woman to lie in lateral position *to increase uteroplacental blood flow* and to elevate legs while sitting *to promote venous return.*

Monitor intake and output and check for edema *to assess for renal complications or venous return problems.*

Monitor FHR and fetal activity, perform NST as indicated *to assess fetal status and detect uteroplacental insufficiency.*

of contraception, the risks of surgery, especially for the woman with class III or IV heart disease, need to be explained. Oral contraceptives are often contraindicated because of the risk of thromboembolism. Both the woman and her partner need to be involved in the decision-making process.

➤ Evaluation

The nurse knows that care was effective if expected outcomes of care have been met (Nursing Care Plan).

CARDIOPULMONARY RESUSCITATION OF THE PREGNANT WOMAN

Trauma, pulmonary embolism, anesthesia complications, drug overdose, hypovolemia, or septic shock may result in cardiopulmonary arrest. Preexisting disorders, such as heart or pulmonary disease, hypertension, or autoimmune collagen vascular disease, increase this risk (Luppi, 1999). Some modifications of the procedure for cardiopulmonary resuscitation (CPR) (Emergency box) and the Heimlich maneuver are needed during pregnancy (Fig. 13-5).

Various protocols exist for CPR during pregnancy. The most widely used guide is the American Heart Association's (AHA) advanced cardiac life support (ACLS) protocol (AHA, 1992). This protocol recommends 5 to 10 minutes of standard CPR with the uterus displaced laterally, fluid volume restoration, and defibrillation if indicated. If these measures are not successful within 15 minutes of the arrest, open chest heart massage is recommended if the fetus is viable. If there is still no change in maternal status after 15 minutes of open chest cardiac massage, or if there is fetal distress, immediate cesarean birth is recom-

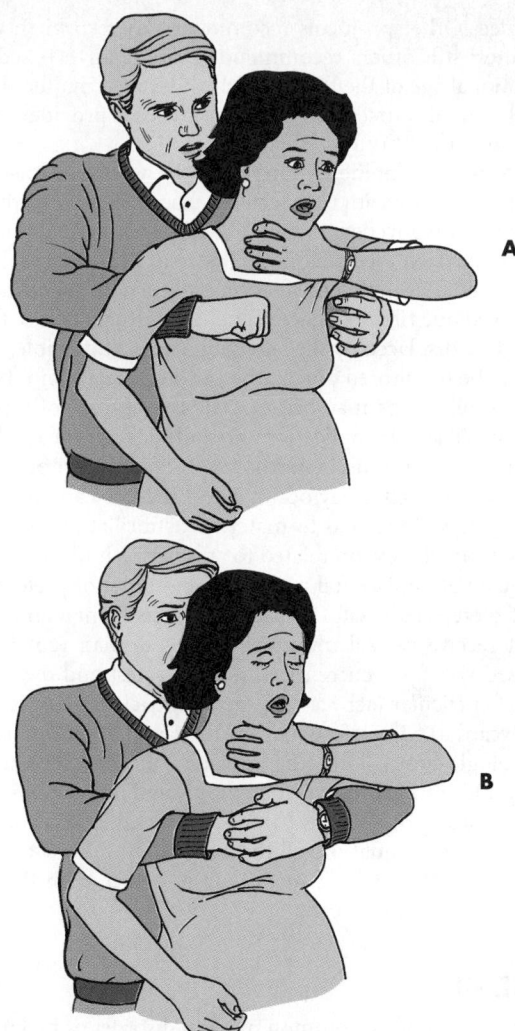

FIG. 13-5 • Clearing airway obstruction in a woman in the late stages of pregnancy. **A,** Standing behind the victim, place your arms under the woman's armpits and across the chest. Place thumb side of your clenched fist against the middle of the sternum; place other hand over fist. **B,** Perform backward chest thrusts until the foreign body is expelled or woman loses consciousness. If woman becomes unconscious because of foreign body airway obstruction, place her on her back (be sure the uterus is displaced laterally, e.g., a rolled blanket under her right hip), and kneel close to the victim's side. Open the mouth with the tongue-jaw lift, perform finger sweep, and attempt rescue breathing. If unable to ventilate, position hands as for chest compression. Deliver five chest thrusts firmly to remove the obstruction. Repeat the above sequence of Heimlich maneuver, finger sweep, and attempt to ventilate. Continue the above sequence until the pregnant woman's airway is clear of obstruction or help arrives to relieve you (Chandra N, Hazenski M, editors: *American Heart Association textbook of basic life support for health care providers,* Dallas, 1994, AHA). If woman is unconscious, give chest compressions as for woman without a pulse. (Data from American Heart Association: *Basic life support, heart saver guide,* Dallas, 1993, AHA.)

Emergency

CARDIOPULMONARY RESUSCITATION FOR THE PREGNANT WOMAN

CPR

Determine unresponsiveness.
Activate emergency medical system.
Position woman on a flat firm surface with the uterus displaced laterally with a wedge (e.g., a rolled towel placed under her right hip) or manually.

Airway

Open airway with head tilt-chin lift maneuver.

Breathing

Determine breathlessness (look, listen, feel).
If the woman is not breathing, give two slow breaths.

Circulation

Determine pulselessness by feeling carotid pulse.
If there is no pulse, begin chest compressions at a rate of 80 to 100/minutes.
After four cycles of fifteen compressions and two breaths, check her pulse. If pulse is not present, then continue CPR.

Heimlich Manuever (Fig. 13-5)

If the pregnant woman is unable to speak or cough, then perform chest thrusts. Stand behind the woman and place your arms under her armpits to encircle her chest. Press backwards with quick thrusts until the foreign body is expelled.

Data from American Heart Association: *Basic life support, heart saver guide,* Dallas, 1993, AHA.

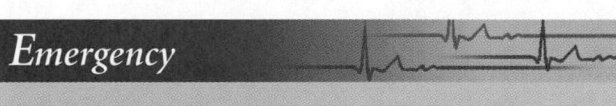

mended. Other protocols recommend cesarean birth within 5 minutes; still others recommend cesarean birth based on the gestational age of the fetus (Luppi, 1999). No matter what protocol is used, nurses and other health care providers must be prepared if CPR is to be successful.

To prevent supine hypotension, the woman is placed on a flat, firm surface with the uterus displaced laterally (either manually or with a wedge or rolled towel under her right hip) (Association of Women's Health, Obstetric, and Neonatal Nurses, 1998; Bajo, 1997). If defibrillation is needed, the paddles need to be placed one rib interspace higher than usual because the heart is slightly displaced by the enlarged uterus. If possible, the fetus should be monitored during the cardiac arrest (Bajo, 1997).

Complications may be associated with CPR of a pregnant woman. These complications include laceration of the liver, rupture of the uterus, hemothorax, and hemoperitoneum. Fetal complications also may occur. These include cardiac dysrhythmia or asystole related to maternal defibrillation and medications, CNS depression related to antidysrhythmic drugs and inadequate uteroplacental perfusion, and onset of preterm labor.

If there is successful resuscitation, the woman and her fetus must receive careful monitoring. The woman remains at increased risk for recurrent pulmonary arrest and dysrhythmias (e.g., ventricular tachycardia, supraventricular tachycardia, and bradycardia). Therefore her cardiovascular, pulmonary, and neurologic status should be assessed continuously. Uterine activity and resting tone must be monitored. Fetal status and gestational age should be determined and used in decision making regarding continuation of the pregnancy or the timing and route of birth. All assessment data influence both the medical and nursing plans of care.

ANEMIA

Anemia is the most common medical disorder of pregnancy, affecting at least 20% of pregnant women. Women with anemia have a higher incidence of puerperal complications such as infection than do pregnant women with normal hematologic values.

Anemia results in reduction of the oxygen-carrying capacity of the blood, and the heart tries to compensate by increasing the cardiac output. This effort increases the workload of the heart and stresses ventricular function. Therefore anemia that occurs with any other complication (e.g., preeclampsia) may result in congestive heart failure.

An indirect index of the oxygen-carrying capacity is the packed red blood cell volume (or hematocrit level). The normal hematocrit range in nonpregnant women is 38% to 45%. Normal values for pregnant women with adequate iron stores may be as low as 34%. This has been explained by hydremia (dilution of blood), also called the physiologic anemia of pregnancy.

At or near sea level, the pregnant woman in the first trimester is anemic when her hemoglobin level is less than 10 g/dl or the hematocrit is less than 33%. At high altitudes, much higher values indicate anemia; for example, at 1500 m (5000 ft) above sea level, a hemoglobin level less than 14 g/dl indicates anemia (Pagana and Pagana, 1997).

When a woman has anemia during pregnancy, the loss of blood at birth, even if minimal, is not well tolerated. She is at an increased risk for requiring blood transfusions. About 90% of cases of anemia in pregnancy are of the iron deficiency type. The remaining 10% embrace a considerable variety of acquired and hereditary anemias, including folic acid deficiency, sickle cell anemia, and thalassemia.

Nursing care of the pregnant woman with anemia requires that the nurse be able to distinguish between the normal physiologic anemia of pregnancy and the disease states. During prenatal visits the nurse should take a diet history and provide dietary teaching as appropriate. Pregnancy may cause increased fatigue, stress, and financial difficulties for a woman with anemia as she copes with her activities of daily living. The nurse should assess the pregnant woman's needs and provide her with appropriate resources or referral.

Iron Deficiency Anemia

Pathologic anemia of pregnancy is mainly the result of iron deficiency (James et al, 1994). Without iron therapy even pregnant women who enjoy excellent nutrition conclude pregnancy with an iron deficit. Iron for the fetus comes from the maternal serum (Duffy, 1995). Diet alone cannot replace gestational iron losses. Inadequate nutrition without therapy will certainly mean iron deficiency anemia during late pregnancy and the puerperium.

Successful iron therapy during pregnancy can be carried out in most cases with oral iron supplements (e.g., ferrous sulfate, 30 to 60 mg per day). It is important to teach the pregnant woman the significance of iron therapy (see Table 12-1). In addition, the woman should be instructed in dietary ways to decrease the gastrointestinal side effects of iron therapy. Some pregnant women cannot tolerate the prescribed oral iron because of nausea and vomiting. In such cases the woman should receive parenteral iron such as an iron-dextran complex (Imferon) (Duffy, 1995).

Folic Acid Deficiency Anemia

Folic acid deficiency during conception and early pregnancy increases the incidence of neural tube defects, cleft lip, and cleft palate (Letsky, 1995). It is common in multiple gestations. During pregnancy the recommended daily intake is 400 μg per day of folic acid, although women who have a deficiency may need 1 mg or more per day.

Poor diet, cooking with large volumes of water, or home canning of food (especially vegetables) may lead to folate deficiency. Malabsorption may play a part in the development of anemia caused by a lack of folic acid.

Since 1998, the U.S. Food and Drug Administration has required the addition of folic acid to cereals, pasta, breads, and other food that are labeled "enriched." However, the amount added is small and most pregnant women will need a supplement.

Sickle Cell Hemoglobinopathy

Sickle cell hemoglobinopathy is a disease caused by the presence of abnormal hemoglobin in the blood. Sickle cell trait (SA hemoglobin pattern), sickling of the red blood cells but with a normal red blood cell life span, usually causes only mild clinical symptoms. Sickle cell anemia (sickle cell disease) is a recessive, hereditary, familial hemolytic anemia that affects those of African-American or Mediterranean ancestry. These individu-

Critical Thinking

FOODS ENRICHED WITH FOLIC ACID

For foods to be labeled "enriched," they must include folic acid. Examine at least five items in a grocery store that are labeled enriched. How much folic acid does a single serving of each contain? Can a pregnant woman obtain the recommended amount of folic acid through eating these items? Plan a menu that includes foods high in folic acid.

als usually have abnormal hemoglobin types (SS or SC). People with sickle cell anemia have recurrent attacks (crises) of fever and pain in the abdomen or extremities beginning in childhood. These attacks are attributed to vascular occlusion (from abnormal cells), tissue hypoxia, edema, and red blood cell destruction. Crises are associated with normochromic anemia, jaundice, reticulocytosis, positive sickle cell test, and the demonstration of abnormal hemoglobin (usually SS or SC).

Almost 10% of African-Americans in North America have the sickle cell trait, but fewer than 1% have sickle cell anemia. The anemia often is complicated by iron and folic acid deficiency.

Nurses working in women's health clinics should encourage patients with sickle cell trait to undergo genetic counseling before pregnancy because pregnancy usually results in a worsening of most aspects of the disease (Scott et al, 1999). The anemia that occurs in normal pregnancies may aggravate sickle cell anemia and bring on more crises. Fetal loss is high because of impaired oxygen supply, sickling, and infarcts in the placental circulation (James et al, 1994). Pregnant women with sickle cell anemia are prone to pyelonephritis, leg ulcers, bone abnormalities, strokes, cardiopathy, congestive heart failure, and preeclampsia. UTIs and hematuria are common. An aplastic crisis may follow serious infection. Medical therapy may include prophylactic transfusions in the mother to decrease the sickle cells and to increase the hemoglobin (Duffy, 1995). Cesarean birth is warranted only for obstetric indications. Oral contraceptives are contraindicated.

Thalassemia

Thalassemia (Mediterranean or Cooley anemia) is a relatively common anemia in which an insufficient amount of globin is produced to fill the red blood cells (RBCs). The condition eventually manifests itself in severe bone deformities caused by massive marrow tissue expansion. For the infant with severe thalassemia, death from cardiac failure is common (Letsky, 1995). Thalassemia is a hereditary disorder that involves the abnormal synthesis of the alpha or beta chains of hemoglobin. β-thalassemia is the more common variety in the United States and often is diagnosed in individuals of Italian, Greek, southern Chinese, Mediterranean, North African, African-American, Middle Eastern, southern Asian, or Indo-Pakistani descent. The unbalanced synthesis of hemoglobin leads to premature RBC death, resulting in severe anemia. Thalassemia major is the homozygous form of the disorder; thalassemia minor is the heterozygous form. Couples with the thalassemia trait should seek genetic counseling.

Thalassemia major complicates pregnancy. Preeclampsia is more common in women with thalassemia major. Thalassemia major may be associated with LBW infants and increased fetal death. Placental weight often is increased, perhaps secondary to maternal anemia. The incidence of fetal distress from hypoxia is greater than in women without thalassemia major.

Pregnant women are managed similarly to those who have sickle cell disease. Folic acid should be given to avoid folate deficiency. The anemia will not respond to iron therapy; iron in any form is contraindicated. Prolonged parenteral iron can lead to harmful, excessive iron storage. Regular transfusion may be necessary.

Splenectomy may be necessary if enlargement and pain occur. Women with thalassemia major may die of chronic infection or progressive hepatic or cardiac failure—the result of excessive iron deposition—because much of the hemoglobin that is present is precipitated in the form of hard crystals.

Persons with thalassemia minor have a mild persistent anemia, but the RBC level may be normal or even elevated. However, no systemic problems are caused by the anemia. Thalassemia minor must be distinguished from iron deficiency anemia.

Pregnancy neither worsens thalassemia minor nor is compromised by the disease. As with thalassemia major, thalassemia minor will not respond to iron therapy and iron in any form is contraindicated. Persons with thalassemia minor should have a normal life span despite a moderately reduced hemoglobin level.

PULMONARY DISORDERS

As pregnancy advances and the uterus impinges on the thoracic cavity, any pregnant woman may have increased respiratory difficulty. This difficulty will be compounded by pulmonary disease.

A pregnant woman with a pulmonary disorder requires assessment, planning, and interventions specific to the disease process, in addition to the routine peripartum care. The nurse also must be alert to pulmonary complications precipitated by the pregnancy.

Asthma

Bronchial asthma is an acute respiratory illness caused by allergens, by marked change in ambient temperature, or by emotional tension. In many cases the actual cause may be unknown. A family history of allergy is common in people with asthma. In response to stimuli, there is widespread but reversible narrowing of the hyperreactive airways, making it difficult to breathe. The clinical manifestations are expiratory wheezing, productive cough, thick sputum, and/or dyspnea.

From 1% to 4% of pregnant women have asthma (Mabie, 1996). The effect of pregnancy on asthma is unpredictable; some improve, some stay the same, and some worsen. Physiologic alterations induced by pregnancy do not make the pregnant women more prone to asthmatic attacks; however, some adverse events are associated with asthma.

Therapy for bronchial asthma has three objectives: (1) relief of the acute attack, (2) prevention or limitation of later attacks, and (3) adequate maternal and fetal oxygenation. In all people with asthma, known allergens should be eliminated and a comfortable home temperature maintained.

TABLE 13-4
Medications Used in Pregnancy in Patients with Asthma

Stage/Condition of Pregnancy	Preferred Medication	Medication(s) to Avoid (Rationale)
Labor	Continue asthma medications	
Induction	Oxytocin	Prostaglandins (may cause bronchoconstriction or bronchospasm)
Pain relief	Fentanyl Epidural anesthesia	Morphine and Demerol (release histamine)
Preterm labor	Magnesium sulfate, nifedipine, β-agonist	β-Agonist if patient is already taking one for her asthma (may cause respiratory distress) NSAIDs (may exacerbate asthma)
Postpartum hemorrhage	Oxytocin	Methylergonovine and 15-methyl prostaglandin F_2-alpha (may worsen asthma)

NSAIDs, Nonsteroidal antiinflammatory drugs.
Data from Mabie W: Asthma in pregnancy, *Clin Obstet Gynecol* 39(1):56-69, 1996.

Respiratory infections should be treated and mist or steam inhalation employed to aid expectoration of mucus. Bronchial asthma therapy is initiated. Acute episodes may require albuterol, steroids, aminophylline, oxygen, β-adrenergic agents, and correction of fluid-electrolyte imbalance.

Asthma attacks can occur in labor; thus medications for asthma are continued in labor and postpartum. Some medications are to be avoided in pregnancy because they may precipitate or exacerbate an asthma attack (Table 13-4).

Cystic Fibrosis

Cystic fibrosis is a common autosomal-recessive genetic disorder in which the exocrine glands produce excessive viscous secretions, causing problems with both respiratory and digestive functions. An increase in pulmonary capillary permeability, decrease of lung volume, and shunting result in arterial hypoxemia. Respiratory failure and early death (in the early 20s) may occur.

In women with good nutrition, mild obstructive lung disease, and good chest x-rays, pregnancy is tolerated well (Hilman, Aitken, and Constantinescu, 1996). In those with severe disease, the pregnancy is often complicated by chronic hypoxia and frequent pulmonary infections. Women with cystic fibrosis show a decrease in their residual lung volume during pregnancy, as do normal pregnant women, and are unable to maintain vital capacity. Presumably, the pulmonary vasculature cannot accommodate the increased cardiac output of pregnancy. The results are decreased oxygen to the myocardium, decreased cardiac output, and increased hypoxia. A pregnant woman with less than 50% of expected vital capacity usually has a difficult pregnancy. Increased maternal and perinatal mortality is related to severe pulmonary infection.

Weight and symptoms of malabsorption should be monitored at each prenatal visit, and pancreatic enzymes adjusted as necessary. Oral supplements, including nasogastric feedings, may be necessary to maintain nutritional status (Hilman, Aitken, and Constantinescu, 1996).

During labor, monitoring for fluid and electrolyte balance is required. The amount of sodium lost through sweat can be significant, and hypovolemia can occur. Conversely, if the woman has any degree of cor pulmonale, fluid overload is a concern. Oxygen is given freely during labor, and monitoring by pulse oximetry is recommended (Hilman, Aitken, and Constantinescu, 1996). Epidural or local anesthesia is the preferred analgesic for birth.

Breastfeeding appears to be safe as long as the sodium content of the mother's milk is not abnormal (Lawrence, 1999). Pumping and discarding the milk is done until the sodium content has been determined.

GASTROINTESTINAL DISORDERS

Compromise of gastrointestinal function during pregnancy is a concern. Obvious physiologic alterations, such as the greatly enlarged uterus, and less apparent changes, such as hormonal differences and hypochlorhydria (deficiency of hydrochloric acid in the stomach's gastric juice), require understanding for proper diagnosis and treatment. Gallbladder disease and inflammatory bowel disease are two gastrointestinal disorders that may occur during pregnancy.

Cholelithiasis and Cholecystitis

Women are twice as likely to have cholelithiasis (presence of gallstones in the gallbladder) than are men (Baker, 1995), and pregnancy seems to make the woman more vulnerable to gallstone formation. Decreased muscle tone allows gallbladder distention, thickening of the bile, and prolongs emptying time. Increased progesterone levels result in a slight hypercholesterolemia. Nutritional counseling is important (Home Care box).

Cholecystitis (inflammation of the gallbladder) is also more common during pregnancy, probably because pressure of the enlarged uterus interferes with the normal circulation and drainage of the gallbladder. Acute cholecystitis occurs in about 1 in 4000 pregnancies, most often in older women who have been pregnant several times and who have a history of previous attacks (Depp, 1996).

Women with acute cholecystitis usually present with colicky abdominal pain, nausea, and vomiting. Fever and an increased

Home Care

NUTRITIONAL COUNSELING FOR THE PREGNANT WOMAN WITH CHOLECYSTITIS OR CHOLELITHIASIS

- Assess your diet for foods that cause discomfort and flatulence and omit foods that trigger episodes.
- Reduce dietary fat intake to 40 to 50 g per day.
- Limit protein to 10% to 12% of total calories.
- Choose foods so that most of the calories come from carbohydrates.
- Prepare food without adding fats or oils as much as possible.
- Avoid fried foods.

leukocyte count may also be present. Ultrasound is often used to detect the presence of stones or dilation of the common bile duct (Depp, 1996).

Meperidine (Demerol) or atropine alleviates ductal spasm and pain. Morphine stimulates the sphincter of Oddi and thus should be avoided. Generally, gallbladder surgery should be postponed until the puerperium.

INTEGUMENTARY DISORDERS

The skin surface may exhibit many physiologic and pathologic conditions during pregnancy. Dermatologic disorders induced by pregnancy include melasma (chloasma), herpes gestationis, noninflammatory pruritus of pregnancy, vascular "spiders," palmar erythema, and pregnancy granuloma (including epulides). Skin problems generally aggravated by pregnancy are acne vulgaris (acne) (in the first trimester), erythema multiforme, herpetiform dermatitis (fever blisters and genital herpes), granuloma inguinale (Donovan bodies), condylomata acuminata (genital warts), neurofibromatosis (von Recklinghausen's disease), and pemphigus. Dermatologic disorders usually improved by pregnancy include acne vulgaris (in the third trimester), seborrheic dermatitis (dandruff), and psoriasis. An unpredictable course during pregnancy may be expected in atopic dermatitis, lupus erythematosus, and herpes simplex.

NURSE ALERT • Isotretinoin (Accutane), commonly prescribed for acne, is contraindicated in pregnancy because of its high teratogenicity. Fetuses exposed to this medication are at increased risk for craniofacial, cardiac, and CNS anomalies.

Explanation, reassurance, and common sense measures should suffice for normal skin changes. Disease processes during and soon after pregnancy may be extremely difficult to diagnose and treat.

NEUROLOGIC DISORDERS

The pregnant woman with a neurologic disorder needs to deal with the potential teratogenic effects of prescribed medications, changes of mobility during pregnancy, and impaired ability to care for the baby. The nurse should be aware of all drugs the pregnant woman is taking and the associated potential for producing congenital anomalies. As the pregnancy progresses, the woman's center of gravity shifts and causes balance and gait changes. The woman should be advised of these expected changes and safety measures suggested as appropriate. Family and community resources should be assessed to provide child care for the neurologically impaired woman.

Epilepsy

Epilepsy is a disorder of the brain causing recurrent seizures and is the most common neurologic disorder accompanying pregnancy (Cartlidge, 1995). Epilepsy may result from developmental abnormalities or injury, or have no identified cause. Convulsive seizures may be more frequent or severe during complications of pregnancy such as edema, alkalosis, fluid-electrolyte imbalance, cerebral hypoxia, hypoglycemia, and hypocalcemia.

The effects of pregnancy on epilepsy are unpredictable. Up to 80% of women have no change in seizure activity during pregnancy, whereas 20% have an increase and up to 25% have a decrease in seizures (Gilmore, Pennell, and Stern, 1998).

The differential diagnosis between epilepsy and eclampsia may pose a problem. Epilepsy and eclampsia can coexist; however, a history of seizures and a normal plasma uric acid level, as well as the absence of hypertension, generalized edema, or proteinuria, point to epilepsy. Electroencephalography rarely is diagnostic.

During pregnancy, risk of vaginal bleeding is doubled, and there is a threefold risk of abruptio placentae. Abnormal presentations are more common in labor and delivery, as well as the increased possibility that the fetus will experience seizures in utero (Mishell and Brenner, 1994).

Metabolic changes in pregnancy usually alter pharmacokinetics. In addition, nausea and vomiting may interfere with ingestion and absorption of medication.

Failure to take medications is a common factor leading to worsening of seizure activity during pregnancy. This is largely due to the message that drugs are harmful to the fetus (Gilmore, Pennell, and Stern, 1998). Teratogenicity of antiepileptic drugs (AED) has been described thoroughly but the risks to the infant have been exaggerated. Congenital anomalies associated with AED include cleft lip or palate, congenital heart disease, urogenital defects, and neural tube defects (Gilmore, Pennell, and Stern, 1998).

Antiepileptic drugs should be monotherapeutic and used in the smallest therapeutic dose with the fewest side effects. Daily folic acid supplement is needed because of the depletion that occurs when taking anticonvulsants (Cartlidge, 1995).

Multiple Sclerosis

Multiple sclerosis (MS), a patchy demyelinization of the spinal cord and CNS, may be a viral disorder. Women are affected twice as often as men, with the most common onset occurring between the ages of 20 and 40 (Cartlidge, 1995). Infertility, miscarriage, stillbirth, and fetal anomalies do not appear to be increased in women with MS; however, most women with MS choose not to become pregnant (James et al, 1994).

MS may occasionally complicate pregnancy, but exacerbations and remissions are unrelated to the pregnant state. Steroids are commonly used to treat acute exacerbations. Nursing care of the pregnant woman with MS is similar to the care of the normal pregnant woman. Women with MS occasionally may have an almost painless labor, although the character of uterine contractions is unaffected by the disease.

Bell's Palsy

An association between Bell's palsy (idiopathic facial paralysis) and pregnancy was first cited by Bell in 1830. The incidence of Bell's palsy in pregnancy is about 57 per 100,000. The incidence usually peaks during the third trimester and the puerperium (Cartlidge, 1995). Blinking is impaired; eye pain is often the presenting symptom. A causative relationship does not seem to exist between the appearance of Bell's palsy and any complications of pregnancy.

No effects of maternal Bell's palsy have been observed in infants. Maternal outcome is generally good unless there is a complete block in nerve conduction. Steroids sometimes are prescribed for the condition, but they do not hasten recovery. In most affected women, 90% or more of facial function can be expected to return (Cunningham et al, 1997). Supportive care includes prevention of injury to the exposed cornea, facial muscle massage, careful chewing and manual removal of food from inside the affected cheek, and reassurance that return of total neurologic function is likely.

AUTOIMMUNE DISORDERS

Autoimmune disorders comprise a large group of diseases that disrupt the function of the immune system of the body. In these types of disorders, the body develops antibodies that attack its normally present antigens, causing tissue damage. Women in their reproductive years have a predilection for autoimmune disorders; therefore associations with pregnancy are not uncommon. Pregnancy may affect the disease process. Some disorders adversely affect the course of pregnancy or are detrimental to the fetus. Autoimmune disorders include rheumatoid arthritis (RA), systemic lupus erythematosus, and myasthenia gravis.

Systemic Lupus Erythematosus

One of the most common serious disorders in women of childbearing age, systemic lupus erythematosus (SLE), is a chronic multisystem inflammatory disease characterized by autoimmune antibody production that affects skin, joints, kidneys, lungs, CNS, liver, and other body organs (James et al, 1994). More than 250,000 people are known to have SLE, with an estimated 50,000 new cases per year. The exact cause is unknown, but viral infection and hormonal and genetic factors may be related.

Early symptoms such as fatigue, fever, skin rashes, weight loss, and arthralgias may be overlooked. Pericarditis is often the presenting symptom. Eventually all organs become involved. The condition is characterized by a series of exacerbations and remissions.

If the diagnosis has been established and the woman desires a child, she is advised to wait until she has been in remission for at least 6 months before attempting to get pregnant (Gilbert and Harmon, 1998). An exacerbation of SLE during pregnancy or postpartum occurs in 15% to 60% of women (James et al, 1994).

SLE during pregnancy is associated with increased rates of preterm deliveries, IUGR, stillbirth, and perinatal mortality (Cunningham et al, 1997). Complications such as preeclampsia and HELLP syndrome are common.

Medical therapy is kept to a minimum in women who are in remission or who have a mild form of SLE. Antiinflammatory medications such as prednisone and aspirin may be used. Immunosuppressive medications are not recommended during pregnancy but may be used in some situations. Nursing care focuses on early recognition of signs of SLE exacerbation and pregnancy complications, education and support of the woman and her family, and assessment of fetal well-being.

Women with SLE should limit their number of pregnancies because of increased adverse perinatal outcomes as well as the guarded maternal prognosis (Cunningham et al, 1997). Family planning is important; oral contraceptives are used with caution because vascular disease commonly accompanies SLE; tubal ligation may be the optimum means of managing fertility. Progestin implants have no known effects on flare-ups of lupus; intrauterine devices are prescribed cautiously (Cunningham et al, 1997).

Myasthenia Gravis

Myasthenia gravis, an autoimmune motor (muscle) end-plate disorder that involves acetylcholine use, affects the motor function at the myoneural junction. Muscle weakness results, particularly in the eyes, face, tongue, neck, limbs, and respiratory muscles. Myasthenia gravis occurs at the rate of 1 in 10,000 and twice as often in women as in men (Cunningham et al, 1997).

Pregnancy may complicate the disorder, although some women experience remission during gestation. Preterm births may be as high as 60% to 66% (Branch, 1993). If preterm labor occurs magnesium sulfate, which interferes with neuromuscular transmission, is absolutely contraindicated (Gilbert and Harmon, 1998).

Symptoms include easy fatigability, intermittent double vision (diplopia), upper eyelid drooping, and difficulty speaking, swallowing, and clearing secretions (James et al, 1994). In more serious cases, upper arm weakness and breathing difficulty are seen.

Women with myasthenia gravis usually tolerate labor well because of preexisting muscle relaxation. During the second stage, some women are unable to push effectively and may need a forceps or vacuum-assisted delivery. They may undergo myasthenic crisis during labor. Women with myasthenia gravis are extremely sensitive to narcotics and must be monitored closely if they are used for pain relief in labor. Epidural analgesia provides excellent analgesia and decreases the need for parenteral narcotics (Samuels, 1996). After birth, women must be carefully supervised because relapses often occur during the puerperium.

HUMAN IMMUNODEFICIENCY VIRUS AND ACQUIRED IMMUNODEFICIENCY SYNDROME

Infection with the human immunodeficiency virus (HIV) and the resultant acquired immunodeficiency syndrome (AIDS) are increasingly occurring in women. Although HIV and AIDS have been traditionally associated with homosexual populations, women are now the fastest-growing population of individuals with HIV infection and AIDS (Wortley and Fleming, 1997). Women are more likely to have acquired the infection through IV drug use or sexual contact with a high risk man. Women of color are disproportionately affected; about 75% of HIV-infected women are African-American or Hispanic. In the United States, AIDS is found 13 times more often in African-

American women than in Caucasian women; the occurrence rate in Hispanic women is 6 times greater than in Caucasian women (Duff, 1996; Flagler, Hughes, and Kovalesky, 1997). This section addresses management of the pregnant woman who is HIV positive or who has developed full-blown AIDS. See Chapter 6 for more information about the diagnosis and management of nonpregnant women with HIV and Chapter 28 for a discussion of HIV/AIDS in infants.

Preconception Counseling

Pregnancy is not encouraged in HIV-positive women; preconception counseling is recommended. Exposure to the virus has a significant impact on the pregnancy, neonatal feeding method, and neonatal health status. HIV-positive women should be counseled extensively about the risk of perinatal transmission and possible obstetric complications. Pregnancy itself does not appear to significantly accelerate the progression of HIV infection (Duff, 1996). HIV-positive women should be encouraged to seek prenatal care immediately if they suspect pregnancy in order to maximize chances for a positive outcome.

Incidence

In the general obstetric population in the United States, about 1 in 1000 women are HIV positive. In some inner-city populations, however, 1% to 1.5% of all pregnant women are infected with the virus (Duff, 1996).

Pregnancy Risks

Perinatal Transmission. About 90% of all pediatric AIDS cases are due to transmission of the virus from mother to child during the perinatal period. Exposure may occur to the fetus through the maternal circulation as early as the first trimester of pregnancy; to the infant during labor and birth by inoculation or ingestion of maternal blood and other infected fluids; or to the infant through breast milk. The frequency of perinatal transmission has been reported from a low of 5% to 10% to a high of 50% to 60%. Most researchers report transmission rates of 20% to 30% (Duff, 1996; Lamphear, 1994). Factors that increase the likelihood of perinatal viral transmission are listed in Box 13-5.

Treatment of HIV-infected women with the antiviral drug zidovudine (AZT) during pregnancy and intrapartum, and treatment of their infants for the first 6 weeks of life with zidovudine, decreases the rate of viral transmission from 25.5% to 8.3% (Connor et al, 1994). All women should be given the option of having a scheduled cesarean birth at 38 weeks to decrease the risk of transmission of HIV to their infant (American College of Obstetricians and Gynecologists, 1999).

Obstetric Complications. It is difficult to determine obstetric risk in persons with HIV infection because so many confounding variables are often present. Many HIV-positive women also suffer from drug and alcohol addiction, poor nutrition, limited access to prenatal care, and/or concurrent STIs. HIV-positive women are probably at risk for preterm labor and birth, PROM, IUGR, perinatal mortality, and postpartum endometritis (Duff, 1996).

Care Management

HIV counseling and testing should be offered to all women at their initial entry into prenatal care (Centers for Disease Control and Prevention, 1998). Most states in the United States have enacted legislation to ensure this is offered. If only those presumed to be at high risk are screened, about half of all HIV-positive women will not be detected (Duff, 1996). Identification of HIV-positive pregnant women is especially important because antepartum and intrapartum antiviral drug therapy has been shown to greatly decrease the risk of viral transmission to the fetus.

HIV-infected women should also be tested for other STIs such as gonorrhea; syphilis; chlamydial infection; hepatitis B, C, and D; and herpes. Cytomegalovirus (CMV) and toxoplasmosis antibody testing should be done because both infections can cause significant maternal and fetal complications and can be successfully treated with antimicrobial agents. Any history of vaccination and immune status should be documented, and chickenpox (varicella) and rubella titers should be determined. A tuberculin skin test should be performed; a positive test necessitates a chest x-ray film to identify active pulmonary disease. Also, a Papanicolaou (Pap) smear should be done (Duff, 1996).

All HIV-infected women should be treated with zidovudine during pregnancy regardless of the CD_4 counts (Boyer et al, 1994; Centers for Disease Control and Prevention, 1998). The major side effect of this drug is bone marrow suppression; periodic hematocrit, white blood cell (WBC) count, and platelet count assessments should be performed (Duff, 1996). Women

Box 13-5

Factors that Increase the Risk of Perinatal HIV Transmission

- Previous history of a child with HIV infection
- AIDS
- Preterm birth
- Decreased maternal CD_4 count
- Firstborn twin
- Chorioamnionitis
- Intrapartum blood exposure
- Failure to treat mother and fetus with zidovudine during the perinatal period

From Duff P: Maternal perinatal infection. In Gabbe S, Niebyl J, Simpson J, editors: *Obstetrics and problem pregnancies,* ed 3, New York, 1996, Churchill Livingstone.

Critical Thinking

THE PREGNANT WOMAN WHO IS HIV POSITIVE

Betsy is being seen in the prenatal clinic. She is HIV positive and has a past history of IV cocaine and heroin use. She has been drug free for the last 18 months. She tells you she is taking "some AIDS drug" during pregnancy but does not seem to know much about it. Which drug has Betsy most likely been taking and why? Will the therapy be continued during the intrapartum and postpartum periods? Will the infant receive any therapy? Describe the precautions you would take to protect yourself as you provide care for Betsy. What risk factors for acquiring HIV infection are present in Betsy's background? What information would you include in counseling her in terms of her lifestyle and future planning?

with CD_4 counts <200 cells/mm^3 should receive prophylactic treatment for *Pneumocystis carinii* pneumonia with daily trimethoprim-sulfamethoxazole (Duff, 1996). Any other opportunistic infections should be treated with medications specific for the infection; often dosages must be higher for women with HIV infection or AIDS.

Women who are HIV positive should also be vaccinated against hepatitis B, pneumococcal infection, hemophilus B influenza, and viral influenza. To support any pregnant woman's immune system, appropriate counseling is provided about optimal nutrition, sleep, rest, exercise, and stress reduction. The HIV-infected woman needs a greater amount of nutritional support and counseling about diet choices, food preparation, and food handling. Weight gain or maintenance in pregnancy is a challenge with the HIV-infected patient. The infected patient is counseled regarding "safer sex" techniques. Use of condoms and a spermicide is encouraged to minimize further exposure to HIV if her partner is the source. Orogenital sex is discouraged.

The woman is referred for drug rehabilitation as necessary to discontinue substance abuse. Abuse of alcohol, methamphetamines (e.g., "speed," "ice"), marijuana, cocaine, nitrites (e.g., "poppers," "snappers"), or other drugs compromises the body's immune system and increases the risks of AIDS and associated conditions. It also interferes with many medical and alternative therapies for AIDS. In addition, alcohol and other drugs affect the judgment of abusers, who may be more likely to engage in high risk activities that increase their exposure to HIV.

IV zidovudine is administered to the HIV-positive woman during the intrapartum period. A loading dose is initiated on her admission in labor, followed by a continuous maintenance dose throughout labor (Duff, 1996).

Every effort should be made during the birthing process to decrease the neonate's exposure to infected maternal blood and secretions. If feasible, the membranes should be left intact until the birth. Women who give birth within 4 hours after membrane rupture are less likely to transmit the virus to their neonates than are women who experience a longer interval between rupture and birth (Gilbert and Harmon, 1998). Fetal scalp electrode and scalp pH sampling should be avoided because these procedures may result in inoculation of the virus into the fetus. The use of forceps and vacuum extractor should also be avoided when possible. Episiotomy does not seem to greatly influence the infection rate (Gilbert and Harmon, 1998).

Immediately after birth, infants should be wiped free of all body fluids and then bathed as soon as they are in stable condition. All staff working with the mother or infant must adhere strictly to infection control techniques and observe Standard Precautions for blood and body fluid (Craven, Steger, and Jarek, 1994; Duff, 1996).

The postpartum period for the woman infected with HIV may be notable for infection, hemorrhage, or both. Women without symptoms may have an unremarkable postpartum course; on the other hand, immunosuppressed women with symptoms may be at increased risk for postpartum UTIs, vaginitis, postpartum endometritis, and poor wound healing. HIV-related thrombocytopenias may also increase the risk of hemorrhage (Mandelbrot et al, 1994).

The cleansed neonate can be with the mother after birth, but breastfeeding is discouraged because of the risk of transmission through breast milk. After discharge, the woman and her infant are referred to physicians who are experienced in the treatment of AIDS and associated conditions.

SUBSTANCE ABUSE

Substance abuse refers to the continued use of substances despite related problems in physical, social, or interpersonal areas. Any use of alcohol or illicit drugs during pregnancy is considered abuse (American Psychiatric Association, 1994). The damaging effects of alcohol and illicit drugs on pregnant women and their unborn babies are well documented (National Women's Health Resource Center, 1998). Alcohol and other drugs easily pass from a mother to her baby through the placenta. Smoking during pregnancy has serious health risks, including bleeding complications, miscarriage, stillbirth, prematurity, low birth weight, and sudden infant death syndrome (National Women's Health Resource Center, 1998). Congenital anomalies have occurred in infants of mothers who have taken drugs (Stuart and Laraia, 1998). The safest pregnancy is one in which the mother is drug- and alcohol-free.

Barriers to Treatment

Pregnant women who abuse substances commonly have little understanding of the ways in which these substances affect them, their pregnancies, and their babies. They often delay seeking prenatal care until labor begins. Stigma, shame, and guilt lead to a high denial of drinking or drug problems both by the woman herself and by family members and friends, who conceal the abuse from outsiders to protect the abuser (Finkelstein, 1994).

Legal Considerations

Because of the risks to the unborn children, pregnant women who abuse substances may face criminal charges under expanded interpretations of child abuse and drug-trafficking statutes. Some states are prosecuting pregnant women on charges of child abuse because they became pregnant while addicted to drugs. Some policymakers have proposed that pregnant women who abuse substances should be jailed, placed under house arrest, or committed to psychiatric hospitals for the remainder of their pregnancies (Stuart and Laraia, 1998).

LEGAL TIP • Drug Testing During Pregnancy There is no state requirement for a health care provider to test either the mother or the newborn for the presence of drugs. It is most important that nurses be aware of laws regarding prenatal drug use in the states in which they practice. In some states, a woman with a positive urine drug screen who is pregnant or who has just given birth must be referred to child protective services. If the mother is not in a drug treatment program or is judged unable to provide newborn care, her infant may be placed in foster care.

Care Management

Care of the pregnant substance abuser presents a tremendous nursing challenge. Many substance abusers are deeply depressed, sometimes because of previous life experiences. Often, substance abuse has provided a way for the woman to relieve psychologic distress and blunt the feelings of loneliness and emptiness that are part of depression. Sometimes, substance abusers have grown up in an environment where such behavior was considered normal; consequently, they may have had little opportunity to learn sober living skills. Inadequate role models, particularly coupled with continued substance abuse, greatly impact on a woman's ability to parent. She may require much assistance to care for, nurture, and form a warm, close intimate relationship with her child. The neonatal effects of maternal substance abuse are discussed in Chapter 28. The care needed by each woman varies according to her particular circumstances and the substance(s) abused. However, the nursing process is similar for all.

The care of the substance-dependent pregnant woman is based on historical data, symptoms, physical findings, and laboratory results. Screening questions for alcohol and drug abuse should be included in the overall assessment of the first prenatal visit of all women. Because women often deny or greatly underreport usage when asked directly about drug or alcohol consumption, it is crucial that the nurse display a non-judgmental and matter-of-fact attitude while taking the history in order to gain the woman's trust and elicit a reasonable accurate estimate (Cefalo and Moos, 1995). Information about drug use should be obtained by first asking about the woman's intake of OTC and prescribed medications. Next, her usage of "legal" drugs such as caffeine, nicotine, and alcohol should be ascertained. Finally, the woman should be questioned about her use of illicit drugs, such as cocaine, heroin, and marijuana. The approximate frequency and amount should be documented for each drug used.

Screening questionnaires generally ask about consequences of heavy drinking, alcohol intake, or both. The Michigan Alcoholism Screening Test (MAST) and the CAGE test are two well-known screens that are used. The T-ACE (Hankin and Sokol, 1995) (Box 13-6) and the TWEAK (Russell, 1994) (Box 13-7) have been developed to screen specifically for alcohol use during pregnancy. Urine screening is unreliable because alcohol is undetectable within a few hours following ingestion (Redding and Selleck, 1993). Abnormal liver function studies can provide diagnostic data about the physical effects of alcohol abuse.

Urine toxicology testing is often performed to screen for illicit drug use. Drugs may be found in urine days to weeks after ingestion, depending on how quickly they are metabolized and excreted from the body. Meconium (from the neonate) and hair can also be analyzed to determine past drug use over a longer period of time (Gilbert and Harmon, 1998).

In addition to screening for alcohol and drug abuse, the nurse should also screen for physical and sexual abuse and history of psychiatric illness, because these are risk factors in women who abuse substances.

Planning the care for a pregnant woman who is a substance abuser must take into consideration the woman's lifestyle and habits. While the ideal long-term outcome is total abstinence, it is not likely that the woman will either desire or be able to stop alcohol and drug use suddenly. Indeed, it may be harmful to the fetus for her to do so. A realistic goal may be to decrease substance use, and short-term outcomes will be necessary.

An interdisciplinary model is essential when planning the care for women who abuse substances. Major issues that must be addressed in treatment for women that generally are not part of treatment for men are low self-esteem, stigmatization, high probability of sexual abuse and physical abuse, lack of social support, need for social services and child care, need for women's health services, and need for support and education in the mothering role (Kearney, 1997). Pregnancy presents a window of opportunity for motivating women to stop their abuse of substances (Selleck and Redding, 1998).

Intervention with the pregnant substance abuser begins with education about specific effects on pregnancy, the fetus, and the newborn for each drug used. Consequences of perinatal drug use should be clearly communicated and abstinence recommended as the safest course of action. Women are often more receptive to making lifestyle changes during pregnancy than at any other time in their lives. The casual, experimental, or recreational drug user is often able to achieve and maintain sobriety when she receives education, support, and continued monitoring throughout pregnancy. Periodic screening during pregnancy of women who have admitted to drug use may help them to continue abstinence (Gilbert and Harmon, 1998).

Box 13-6

T-ACE Test

- How many drinks can you hold before getting sleepy or passing out? (TOLERANCE)
- Have people ANNOYED you by criticizing your drinking?
- Have you ever felt you ought to CUT DOWN on your drinking?
- Have you ever had a drink first thing in the morning to steady your nerves or get rid of a hangover? (EYE-OPENER)

Scoring: Two points are given for the TOLERANCE question for the ability to hold at least a six pack of beer or a bottle of wine. A "yes" answer to any of the other questions receives one point. An overall score of ≥2 indicates a high probability that the woman is a risk drinker.

From Hankin J, Sokol R: Identification and care of problems associated with alcohol ingestion in pregnancy, *Semin Perinatol* 19(4):286, 1995.

Box 13-7

TWEAK Test

- How many drinks can you hold before getting sleepy or passing out? (TOLERANCE)
- Have close friends or relatives WORRIED or complained about your drinking during the past year?
- Do you sometimes take a drink in the morning when you first get up? (EYE-OPENER)
- Has a friend or family member ever told you about things you said or did while you were drinking that you could not remember? (AMNESIA)
- Do you sometimes feel the need to KUT/CUT down on your drinking?

Scoring: Two points are given for the TOLERANCE question for the ability to hold more than five drinks. A "yes" answer to the WORRY question receives two points. A "yes" answer to any of the other questions receives one point. An overall score of ≥2 indicates the woman is likely to be a risk drinker.

From Russell M: New assessment tools for risk drinking during pregnancy: T-ACE, TWEAK, and others, *Alcohol Health Res World* 18(1):55, 1994.

Treatment for substance abuse will be individualized for each woman depending on the type of drug used and the frequency and amount of use. Detoxification, short-term inpatient or outpatient treatment, long-term residential treatment, aftercare services, and self-help support groups are all possible options. Women for Sobriety may be a more helpful organization for women than Alcoholics Anonymous or Narcotics Anonymous, which are based on the 12-step program. The emphasis on powerlessness over addiction and avoidance of codependency found in 12-step program may disempower and isolate women, particularly women of color (Saulnier, 1996).

In general, long-term treatment of any sort is becoming increasingly more difficulty to obtain, particularly for women who lack insurance coverage. Although some programs allow a woman to keep her child with her at the treatment facility, there are far too few available to meet the demand (Gilbert and Harmon, 1998).

Alcohol withdrawal treatment consists of the administration of benzodiazepines, an improvement in the woman's nutritional intake (by adding folic acid and other vitamins), and psychotherapy. Detoxification with disulfiram (Antabuse) is not used in pregnant women because of its teratogenic effects (Lewis and Woods, 1994).

Methadone treatment for pregnant women dependent on heroin or other narcotics is controversial. If women withdraw from heroin during pregnancy, blood flow to the placenta is impaired. The substitution of methadone for the heroin not only promotes withdrawal from heroin but also does not cause impaired blood flow to the placenta. Methadone, however, can cause detrimental fetal effects, and withdrawal from it after birth can be worse for the newborn than heroin withdrawal (Gilbert and Harmon, 1998; Glantz and Woods, 1993; Stuart and Laraia, 1998).

While cocaine is powerfully psychologically addictive, use of the drug does not result in physical dependence. Therefore women who abuse cocaine can stop its use abruptly without developing symptoms of withdrawal. Most cocaine abusers will need a great deal of assistance, such as an alcohol and drug treatment program, individual or group counseling, and participation in self-help support groups, in order to successfully accomplish this major lifestyle change.

Because of the lifestyle often associated with drug use, substance-abusing women are at risk for STIs including HIV. Laboratory assessments will likely include screening for STIs such as gonorrhea and chlamydial infection and antibody determinations for hepatitis B and HIV. A chest x-ray film may be taken to assess for pulmonary problems such as hilar lymphadenopathy, pulmonary edema, bacterial pneumonia, and foreign-body emboli. A skin test to screen for tuberculosis may also be ordered.

Initial and serial ultrasound studies are usually performed to determine gestational age because the woman may have had amenorrhea as a result of her drug use or may not know when her last menstrual period occurred. Because of concerns about stillbirth, an increased frequency of the birth of small-for-gestational-age (SGA) infant, and the potential for hypoxia, some experts recommend that nonstress testing be done in women who are known substance abusers (Glantz and Woods, 1993).

While substance abusers may be difficult to care for at any time, they are often particularly challenging during the intrapartum and postpartum periods because of manipulative and demanding behavior. Typically, these women display poor control over their behavior and a low threshold for pain. Increased dependency needs and poor parenting skills may also be apparent.

Nurses must understand that substance abuse is an illness and that these women deserve to be treated with patience, kindness, consistency, and firmness when necessary (Box 13-8). Even women who are actively abusing drugs will experience pain during labor and after giving birth. Withholding analgesia and/or anesthesia in an attempt to "punish" them for prenatal substance abuse is not helpful and should be avoided. It is helpful to develop a standardized plan of care so that patients have limited opportunities to play staff members against each other. Mother-infant attachment should be promoted by identifying the woman's strengths and by reinforcing positive maternal feelings and behaviors. Staffing should be sufficient to ensure strict surveillance of visitors and prevent unsupervised drug use.

Advice regarding breastfeeding must be individualized. Although all abuse substances appear in breast milk, some in greater amounts than others (Brody, Larner, and Minneman, 1998), breastfeeding is definitely contraindicated in women who continue to use amphetamines, alcohol, cocaine, heroin, or marijuana. The baby's nutrition and safety needs are of primary importance in this consideration. For some women, a desire to breastfeed may provide strong motivation to achieve and maintain sobriety.

Before a known substance abuser is discharged with her baby, the home situation must be assessed to determine that the environment is safe and that someone will be available to meet the infant's needs if the mother proves unable to do so. Usually the hospital's social services department will be involved in interviewing the mother before discharge to ensure that the infant's needs will be met. Sometimes family members or friends will be asked to become actively involved with the mother before discharge to ensure that the infant's needs will be met. A home care or public health nurse may be asked to make home visits to assess the mother's ability to care for the baby and provide guidance and support. If serious questions about the infant's well-being exist, the case will probably be referred to the state's child protective services agency for further action.

Box 13-8

Dealing with Pregnant Substance Abusers

- Realize that the decision to become and remain sober can *only* be made by the substance abuser.
- Understand that nurses do not have the power to cure anyone. We are only cheerleaders and supporters!
- Educate yourself about the effects of drug use in general and its effect on pregnancy and the newborn specifically.
- Treat substance abusers with the same respect and consideration you show other people.
- Become familiar with your local treatment centers. Learn which of them will accept pregnant women. Keep an up-to-date list of groups meeting in your community.
- Remember that there are no "hopeless cases." It is *never* too late to quit!
- Practice patience and persistence. It may take months or years to see the effects of your work.

Key Points

- Poor maternal glycemic control before conception and in the first trimester of pregnancy may be responsible for fetal congenital malformations and for maternal complications such as miscarriage, infection, pregnancy-induced hypertension, and dystocia (difficult labor) caused by macrosomia.
- Maternal insulin requirements increase as the pregnancy progresses and may quadruple by term as a result of insulin resistance created by placental hormones, insulinase, and cortisol.
- Careful monitoring of blood glucose levels, insulin administration when necessary, and dietary counseling are used to create a normal intrauterine environment for fetal growth and development in the pregnancy complicated by diabetes mellitus.
- Thyroid dysfunction during pregnancy requires close monitoring of thyroid hormone levels to regulate therapy and prevent fetal insult.
- High levels of phenylalanine in the maternal bloodstream cross the placenta and are teratogenic to the fetus. Damage can be prevented or minimized by dietary restriction of phenylalanine.
- The stress of the normal maternal adaptations to pregnancy on a heart whose functions are already taxed may cause cardiac decompensation.
- In the case of a cardiac arrest in a pregnant woman, the standard advanced cardiac life support (ACLS) guidelines should be implemented without modification.
- Anemia, the most common medical disorder of pregnancy, affects at least 20% of pregnant women.
- Women in their reproductive years show a predilection for autoimmune disorders (e.g., systemic lupus erythematosus and myasthenia gravis); therefore they may occur during pregnancy.
- Perinatal administration of zidovudine (AZT) is recommended to decrease transmission of the HIV virus from mother to fetus.
- Support from a variety of sources—including family and friends, health care providers, and the recovery community—is needed to help perinatal substance abusers achieve and maintain sobriety.

References

Acosta P: Nutrition support of maternal phenylketonuria, *Semin Perinat* 19(3):182-190, 1995.

American College of Obstetricians and Gynecologists: *Diabetes and pregnancy (ACOG Tech Bull No. 200)*, 1, Washington, DC, 1994, ACOG.

American College of Obstetricians and Gynecologists: ACOG recommends scheduled C-sections for HIV+ women, *ACOG News Release*, July 31, 1999.

American Diabetes Association: *Medical management of insulin-dependent (type 1) diabetes*, ed 2, Alexandria, VA, 1994, The Association.

American Diabetes Association: *Medical management of pregnancy complicated by diabetes*, ed 2, Alexandria, VA, 1995, The Association.

American Diabetes Association: Position statement: gestational diabetes mellitus, *Diabetes Care* 20 (suppl 1):S44, 1997.

American Heart Association Subcommittee on Emergency Cardiac Care: Standards and guidelines for cardiopulmonary resuscitation and emergency cardiac care, *JAMA* 268:2172, 2249, 1992.

American Psychiatric Association: *Diagnostic and statistical manual of mental disorders*, ed 4, Washington, DC, 1994, American Psychiatric Association Press.

Association of Women's Health, Obstetric, and Neonatal Nurses: *Standards and guidelines for professional nursing practice in the care of women and newborns*, ed 5, Washington, DC, 1998, The Association.

Bajo T: Cardiopulmonary resuscitation of the pregnant patient. In Foley M, Strong T, editors: *Obstetric intensive care*, Philadelphia, 1997, WB Saunders.

Baker A: Liver and bilary tract disease. In Barron W, Lindheimer M, editors: *Medical disorders during pregnancy*, St Louis, 1995, Mosby.

Becton Dickinson & Co.: *Controlling low blood sugar reactions*, Franklin Lakes, NJ, 1997, Becton Dickinson & Co.

Bernstein I, Gabbe S: Intrauterine growth restriction. In Gabbe S, Niebyl J, Simpson J, editors: *Obstetrics: normal and problem pregnancies*, ed 3, New York, 1996, Churchill Livingstone.

Boyer P et al: Factors predictive of maternal-fetal transmission of HIV-1: preliminary analysis of zidovudine given during pregnancy and/or delivery, *JAMA* 271(24):1925-1930, 1994.

Branch D: Autoimmune diseases in pregnancy. In Moore T et al, editors: *Gynecology and obstetrics: a longitudinal approach*, New York, 1993, Churchill Livingstone.

Brody T, Larner J, Minneman K: *Human pharmacology: molecular to clinical*, ed 3, St Louis, 1998, Mosby.

Cartlidge N: Neurologic disorders. In Barron W, Lindheimer M, editors: *Medical disorders during pregnancy*, St Louis, 1995, Mosby.

Cefalo R, Moos M: *Preconceptional health care, a practical guide*, ed 2, St Louis, 1995, Mosby.

Centers for Disease Control and Prevention: 1998 guidelines for treatment of sexually transmitted diseases, *MMWR* 47(RR-1):1, 1998.

Connor E et al: Reduction of maternal-infant transmission of human immunodeficiency virus type 1 with zidovudine treatment, *N Engl J Med* 331(18):1173-1180, 1994.

Craven D, Steger K, Jarek C: Human immunodeficiency virus infection in pregnancy: epidemiology and prevention of vertical transmission, *Infect Control Hosp Epidemiol* 15(1):36-47, 1994.

Cunningham F et al: *Williams obstetrics*, ed 20, Stamford, CT, 1997, Appleton & Lange.

Depp R: Cesarean delivery. In Gabbe S, Niebyl J, Simpson J, editors: *Obstetrics: normal and problem pregnancies*, ed 3, New York, 1996, Churchill Livingstone.

Diehl K: Thyroid dysfunction in pregnancy, *J Perinat Neonatal Nurs* 11(4):1-12, 1998.

Duff P: Maternal and perinatal infection. In Gabbe S, Niebyl J, Simpson J, editors: *Obstetrics: normal and problem pregnancies*, ed 3, New York, 1996, Churchill Livingstone.

Duffy T: Hematologic aspects of pregnancy. In Burrow G, Ferris T, editors: *Medical complications during pregnancy*, Philadelphia, 1995, WB Saunders.

Expert Committee on the Diagnosis and Classification of Diabetes Mellitus: Report of the Expert Committee, *Diabetes Care* 20(7):1183-1187, 1997.

Finkelstein N: Treatment issues for alcohol- and drug-dependent pregnant and parenting women, *Health Soc Work* 19(1):7-15, 1994.

Flagler S, Hughes T, Kovalesky A: Toward an understanding of addiction, *J Obstet Gynecol Neonatal Nurs* 26(4):441-448, 1997.

Gilbert E, Harmon J: *Manual of high risk pregnancy and delivery,* ed 2, St Louis, 1998, Mosby.

Gilmore J, Pennell P, Stern B: Medication use during pregnancy for neurologic conditions, *Neurol Clin North Am* 16:189-206, 1998.

Glantz C, Woods J: Cocaine, heroin, and phencyclidine: obstetric perspectives, *Clin Obstet Gynecol* 36(2):279, 1993.

Hagay A, Reece E: Diabetes mellitus in pregnancy. In Reece E, Hobbins J, editors: *Medicine of the fetus and mother,* ed 2, Philadelphia, 1999, Lippincott-Raven.

Hankin J, Sokol R: Identification and care of problems associated with alcohol ingestion in pregnancy, *Semin Perinatol* 19(4):286, 1995.

Hilman B, Aitken M, Constantinescu M: Pregnancy in patients with cystic fibrosis, *Clin Obstet Gynecol* 39:70-86, 1996.

Inzucchi S, Burrow G: Endocrine disorders in pregnancy. In Reece E, Hobbins J, editors: *Medicine of the fetus and mother,* ed 2, Philadelphia, 1999, Lippincott-Raven.

Jackson G, Clark S: Cardiac and pulmonary disorders and pregnancy. In Moore T et al, editors: *Gynecology and obstetrics: a longitudinal approach,* New York, 1993, Churchill Livingstone.

James D et al, editors: *High risk pregnancy: management options,* Philadelphia, 1994, WB Saunders.

Jones M, Stone L: Management of the woman with gestational diabetes mellitus, *J Perinat Neonatal Nurs* 11(4):13-24, 1998.

Jovanovic-Peterson L, editor: *Medical management of pregnancy complicated by diabetes,* Alexandria, VA, 1993, American Diabetes Association.

Kearney M: Drug treatment for women: traditional modes and new directions, *J Obstet Gynecol Neonatal Nurs* 26(4):459-468, 1997.

Kirby R: Maternal phenylketonuria: a new cause for concern, *J Obstet Gynecol Neonatal Nurs* 28(3):227-234, 1999.

Kjos S: Contraception in the diabetic woman, *Obstet Gynecol Clin North Am* 23(1):243-258, 1996.

Lamphear B: Trends and patterns in the transmisison of bloodborne pathogens to health care providers, *Epidemiol Rev* 16(2):437, 1994.

Landon M: Cardiac and pulmonary disease. In Gabbe S, Niebyl J, Simpson J, editors: *Obstetrics: normal and problem pregnancies,* ed 3, New York, 1996a, Churchill Livingstone.

Landon M: Diabetes mellitus and other endocrine disorders. In Gabbe S, Niebyl J, Simpson J, editors: *Obstetrics: normal and problem pregnancies,* ed 3, New York, 1996b, Churchill Livingstone.

Landon M, Gabbe S: Diabetes mellitus. In Barron W, Lindheimer M, editors: *Medical disorders during pregnancy,* ed 2, St Louis, 1995, Mosby.

Lawrence R: *Breastfeeding: a guide for the medical profession,* ed 5, St Louis, 1999, Mosby.

Letsky E: Hematologic disorders. In Barron W, Lindheimer M, editors: *Medical disorders during pregnancy,* ed 2, St Louis, 1995, Mosby.

Lewis D, Woods S: Fetal alcohol syndrome, *Am Fam Physician* 50(5):1025-1032, 1035-1036, 1994.

Luppi C: Cardiopulmonary resuscitation in pregnancy, *AWHONN's Lifelines* 3(3):41-45, 1999.

Mabie W: Asthma in pregnancy, *Clin Obstet Gynecol* 39(1):56-69, 1996.

Mandelbrot L et al: Thrombocytopenia in pregnant women infected with human immunodeficiency virus: maternal and neonatal outcome, *Am J Obstet Gynecol* 171(1):252-257, 1994.

McAnulty J, Metcalfe J, Ueland K: Cardiovascular disease. In Burrow G, Ferris T, editors: *Medical complications during pregnancy,* Philadelphia, 1995, WB Saunders.

Mendelson M: Congenital cardiac disease and pregnancy, *Clin Perinatal* 24(2):467-482, 1997.

Mendelson M, Lang R: Pregnancy and heart disease. In Barron W, Lindheimer M, editors: *Medical disorders during pregnancy,* St Louis, 1995, Mosby.

Metzger B, Coustan D: Summary and recommendations of the fourth international workshop-conference on gestational diabetes mellitus, *Diabetes* 21(suppl 2):B161-B167, 1998.

Mishell D, Brenner P, editors: *Management of common problems in obstetrics and gynecology,* ed 3, Boston, 1994, Blackwell Scientific Publications.

Moore T: Diabetes in pregnancy. In Creasy R, Resnik R, editors: *Maternal-fetal medicine,* ed 4, Philadelphia, 1999, WB Saunders.

National Women's Health Resource Center: Anxiety disorders and women's health, *Natl Womens Health Rep* 29(5):1-6, 1998.

New York Heart Association (NYHA): *Diseases of the heart and blood vessels: nomenclature and criteria for diagnosis,* ed 6, Boston, 1964, Little, Brown.

Pagana K, Pagana T: *Mosby's diagnostic and laboratory test reference,* ed 3, St Louis, 1997, Mosby.

Redding B, Selleck C: Perinatal substance abuse: assessment and management of the pregnant woman and her children, *Nurs Pract Forum* 4(4):216-223, 1993.

Reece E, Homko C: Assessment and management of pregnancies complicated by pregestational and gestational diabetes mellitus, *J Assoc Acad Minority Phys* 5(3):87-97, 1994.

Reece E, Homko C: Diabetes-related complications of pregnancy, *J Nat Med Assoc* 85(7):537, 1993.

Russell M: New assessment tools for risk drinking during pregnancy: T-ACE, TWEAK, and others, *Alcohol Health Res World* 18(1):55, 1994.

Samuels P: Collagen vascular diseases. In Gabbe S, Niebyl J, Simpson J, editors: *Obstetrics: normal and problem pregnancies,* ed 3, New York, 1996, Churchill Livingstone.

Saulnier C: Images of the twelve-step model and sex and love addiction in an alcohol intervention group for black women, *J Drug Issues* 26:95-123, 1996.

Scott J et al: *Danforth's obstetrics and gynecology,* ed 8, Philadelphia, 1999, Lippincott-Raven.

Seely L, Burrow G: Thyroid disease and pregnancy. In Creasy R, Resnik R, editors: *Maternal-fetal medicine,* ed 2, Philadelphia, 1999, WB Saunders.

Selleck C, Redding B: Knowledge and attitudes of registered nurses toward perinatal substance abuse, *J Obstet Gynecol Neonatal Nurs* 27(1):70-77, 1998.

Stuart G, Laraia M: *Stuart and Sundeen's principles and practice of psychiatric nursing,* ed 6, St Louis, 1998, Mosby.

Thornhill M, Camann W: Cardiovascular disease. In Chestnut D, editor: *Obstetric anesthesia: principles and practice,* St Louis, 1994, Mosby.

Wortley P, Fleming P: AIDS in women in the United States: recent trends, *JAMA* 278(11):911-916, 1997.

CHAPTER 14

Pregnancy at Risk: Gestational Conditions

http://www.harcourthealth.com/MERLIN/Wong/maternal/

Learning Objectives

On completion of this chapter the reader will be able to:

- Describe the pathophysiology of preeclampsia and eclampsia.
- Differentiate the management of the woman with mild preeclampsia and the woman with severe preeclampsia.
- Describe HELLP syndrome, including appropriate nursing actions.
- Explain the effects of hyperemesis gravidarum on maternal and fetal well-being.
- Compare and contrast placenta previa and abruptio placentae in relation to signs and symptoms, complications, and management.
- Discuss the diagnosis and management of disseminated intravascular coagulation (DIC).
- Explain the basic principles of care for a pregnant woman undergoing abdominal surgery.
- Discuss implications of trauma on mother and fetus during pregnancy.
- Identify priorities in assessment and stabilization measures for the pregnant trauma victim.
- Differentiate signs and symptoms; effects on pregnancy, fetus, and newborn; and management during pregnancy of common STIs.
- Describe signs, symptoms, and management of pregnant women with TORCH infections.
- Explain the basic principles of care for a pregnant woman having abdominal surgery.

Providing safe and effective care for the high risk patient requires a joint effort from all members of the health care team, with each member contributing unique skills and talents to provide optimum outcomes for mother and infant. This chapter discusses a wide range of disorders that did not exist before pregnancy, all of which have at least one thing in common: their occurrence in pregnancy puts the woman and fetus at risk. Hypertension in pregnancy, hyperemesis gravidarum, hemorrhagic complications of early and late pregnancy, surgery during pregnancy, trauma, and sexually transmitted infections (STIs) are discussed.

HYPERTENSION IN PREGNANCY

Significance and Incidence

Hypertension is the most common medical complication of pregnancy, with an incidence ranging from 1% to 5% (Ventura et al, 1999). A significant contributor to maternal and perinatal morbidity and mortality, preeclampsia complicates approximately 5% to 8% of all pregnancies not terminating in first-trimester miscarriage (American College of Obstetricians and Gynecologists, 1996; Sibai et al, 1997). In women with a history of chronic hypertension or renal disease predating pregnancy, the occurrence of preeclampsia is 25% (Jones and Hayslett, 1996). The prevalence rate for pregnancy-associated hypertension has risen among all age, racial, and ethnic groups since the early 1990s (Ventura et al, 1999).

Morbidity and Mortality

In the United States, when maternal deaths related to ruptured ectopic pregnancy are excluded, preeclampsia ranks second only to embolic events as a cause of maternal mortality. Preeclampsia/eclampsia predisposes the woman to potentially lethal complications such as eclampsia, abruptio placentae, disseminated intravascular coagulation (DIC), cerebral hemorrhage, hepatic failure, adult respiratory distress syndrome (ARDS), and acute renal failure (American College of Obstetricians and Gynecologists, 1996; Cunningham et al, 1997; Roberts, 1999).

Preeclampsia occurs primarily after the second trimester of pregnancy and contributes to intrauterine fetal death and perinatal mortality. Causes of perinatal death related to preeclampsia are placental insufficiency and abruptio placentae, which lead to intrauterine death, preterm birth, and low birth weight (Roberts, 1999).

Eclampsia (characterized by seizures) from profound cerebral effects of preeclampsia is the major maternal hazard. As a rule, maternal and perinatal morbidity and mortality are highest when eclampsia is seen early in gestation (before 28 weeks), maternal age is greater than 25 years, the woman is a multigravida, and chronic hypertension or renal disease is present. The fetus of the eclamptic woman is at increased risk from abruptio placentae, preterm birth, IUGR and acute hypoxia (Gilbert and Harmon, 1998).

Classification

The hypertensive disorders of pregnancy refer to a variety of conditions in which maternal blood pressure is elevated with a corresponding risk to maternal and fetal well-being. The two classification systems most commonly used in the United States today are based on reports from the American College of Obstetricians and Gynecologists (ACOG) (1996) and the Working Group on High Blood Pressure in Pregnancy (1990). These classification systems are summarized in Table 14-1.

TABLE 14-1
Classification of Hypertensive States of Pregnancy

Type	Description
GESTATIONAL HYPERTENSIVE DISORDERS: PREGNANCY-INDUCED HYPERTENSION (PIH)	
Transient hypertension	Development of mild hypertension during pregnancy in previously normotensive patient without proteinuria or pathologic edema
Gestational proteinuria	Development of proteinuria after 20 weeks of gestation in previously nonproteinuric patient without hypertension
Preeclampsia	Development of hypertension and proteinuria in previously normotensive patient after 20 weeks of gestation or in early postpartum period; in presence of trophoblastic disease it can develop before 20 weeks of gestation
Eclampsia	Development of convulsions or coma in preeclamptic patient
CHRONIC HYPERTENSIVE DISORDERS	
Chronic hypertension	Hypertension or proteinuria in pregnant patient with chronic hypertension
Superimposed preeclampsia/eclampsia	Development of preeclampsia or eclampsia in patient with chronic hypertension

From Gilbert E, Harmon J: *Manual of high risk pregnancy and delivery,* ed 2, St Louis, 1998, Mosby.

Clinically, there are two basic types of hypertension during pregnancy—chronic hypertension and pregnancy-induced hypertension (PIH)—with the distinction based on the onset of hypertension in relation to pregnancy. Chronic hypertension is hypertension that predates the pregnancy or hypertension continuing beyond 42 days postpartum (ACOG, 1996). PIH is the onset of hypertension, generally after the twentieth week of pregnancy, appearing as a marker of a pregnancy-specific vasospastic condition (ACOG, 1996; Roberts, 1999). Chronic hypertension and PIH may occur independently or simultaneously. PIH is further classified according to the maternal organ systems affected.

Preeclampsia. Preeclampsia is a pregnancy-specific condition in which hypertension develops after 20 weeks of gestation in a previously normotensive woman. It is a multisystem, vasospastic disease process characterized by hypertension and proteinuria. Preeclampsia is usually categorized as mild or severe in terms of management (Table 14-2).

An elevated blood pressure is often the first sign of preeclampsia. Hypertension is defined as a blood pressure equal to or exceeding 140/90 mm Hg. The Committee on Terminology of the American College of Obstetricians and Gynecologists has also defined hypertension as a mean arterial pressure (MAP) of 105 mm Hg or more.

Elevations over prepregnancy values are no longer considered diagnostic for hypertension. The blood pressure elevation must be present on at least two occasions 4 to 6 hours apart (Fairlie and Sibai, 1999). Techniques of measurement must be standardized (see Box 11-3).

Proteinuria is defined as a concentration of 0.1 g/L (1+ to 2+ on dipstick measurement) or more in at least two random urine specimens collected at least 6 hours apart. In a 24-hour specimen, proteinuria is defined as a concentration of 0.3 g/L per 24 hours.

Pathologic edema is clinically evident, generalized accumulation of fluid in the face, hands, or abdomen that is not responsive to 12 hours of bed rest. It may also be manifested as a rapid weight gain of more than 2 kg in 1 week. The presence of edema is no longer considered necessary for the diagnosis of preeclampsia (Sibai and Rodriguez, 1999).

Severe Preeclampsia. Severe preeclampsia is the presence of any one of the following in the woman diagnosed with preeclampsia: (1) systolic blood pressure of at least 160 mm Hg or a diastolic blood pressure of at least 110 mm Hg; (2) proteinuria of greater than 5 g protein excreted in a 24-hour specimen, or greater than 3+ to 4+ on dipstick measurement; (3) oliguria, less than 400 to 500 ml of urine output over 24 hours; (4) cerebral or visual disturbances, such as altered level of consciousness, headache, scotomata, or blurred vision; (5) hepatic involvement; (6) thrombocytopenia with a platelet count less than 150,000/mm^3; (7) pulmonary or cardiac involvement; (8) development of the HELLP syndrome; or (9) certain cases of severe fetal growth restriction (ACOG, 1996; Roberts, 1999, Sibai, 1996b; Working Group on High Blood Pressure in Pregnancy, 1990).

Eclampsia. Eclampsia is the onset of seizure activity or coma in the woman diagnosed with PIH, with no history of

TABLE 14-2
Differentiation Between Mild and Severe Preeclampsia

	Mild Preeclampsia	Severe Preeclampsia
MATERNAL EFFECTS		
Blood pressure	BP reading of 140/90 mm Hg × 2, 4-6 hr apart	Rise to ≥160/110 mm Hg on two separate occasions 4-6 hr apart with pregnant woman on bed rest
Mean arterial pressure (MAP)	>105 mm Hg	>105 mm Hg
Weight gain	Weight gain of more than 0.5 kg/wk during the second and third trimesters or sudden weight gain of 2 kg/wk at any time	Same as mild preeclampsia
Proteinuria Qualitative dipstick Quantitative 24 hr analysis	Proteinuria of 0.3 g/L in a 24 hr specimen or >0.1 g/L in a random daytime specimen on two or more occasions 6 hr apart (because protein loss is variable); with dipstick, values varying from 2+ to 3+	Proteinuria of >5 g/L in 24 hr or >4+ protein on dipstick
Edema	Dependent edema, some puffiness of eyes, face, fingers; pulmonary edema absent	Generalized edema, noticeable puffiness: eyes, face, fingers; pulmonary edema possibly present
Reflexes	May be normal	Hyperreflexia ≥3+, possible ankle clonus
Urine output	Output matching intake, ≥30 ml/hr or <650 ml/24 hr	<20 ml/hr or <400 ml to 500 ml/24 hr
Headache	Absent/transient	Severe
Visual problems	Absent	Blurred, photophobia, blind spots on funduscopy
Irritability/changes in affect	Transient	Severe
Epigastric pain	Absent	Present
Serum creatinine	Normal	Elevated
Thrombocytopenia	Absent	Present
AST elevation	Normal or minimal	Marked
FETAL EFFECTS		
Placental perfusion	Reduced	Decreased perfusion expressing as IUGR in fetus, FHR: late decelerations
Premature placental aging	Not apparent	At birth placenta appearing smaller than normal for duration of pregnancy, premature aging apparent with numerous areas of broken syncytia, ischemic necroses (white infarcts) numerous, intervillous fibrin deposition (red infarcts)

AST, Aspartate aminotransferase; *FHR,* fetal heart rate, *IUGR,* intrauterine growth restriction.

neurologic pathology (ACOG, 1996). A seizure can be the initial sign for a pregnancy complicated by PIH.

HELLP Syndrome. HELLP syndrome is a laboratory diagnosis for a variant of severe preeclampsia characterized by hemolysis (H), elevated liver enzymes (EL), and low platelets (LP) (Stone, 1998).

Chronic Hypertension. Chronic hypertension is defined as hypertension present before the pregnancy or diagnosed before the twentieth week of gestation. Hypertension that persists longer than 6 weeks postpartum is also classified as chronic hypertension. There is no widely accepted definition of mild hypertension. Severe hypertension is usually defined as a diastolic blood pressure of 110 mm Hg or higher (Sibai, 1996a). Preconception counseling is recommended about the increased risk of superimposed preeclampsia and lifestyle adjustments that may be necessary for women with chronic hypertension.

Chronic Hypertension with Superimposed Preeclampsia. Women with chronic hypertension may develop preeclampsia or eclampsia. Superimposed preeclampsia is defined as an increase in blood pressure (i.e., 30 mm Hg systolic or 15 mm diastolic >105 mm Hg MAP) along with proteinuria or generalized edema in women with chronic hypertension (Sibai, 1996b).

Transient Hypertension. Transient hypertension is the development of hypertension during pregnancy or during the first 24 hours postpartum without other signs of preeclampsia or preexisting hypertension. Blood pressure must return to normal levels by the tenth postpartum day (Sibai, 1996b). The presence of transient hypertension may be predictive of the eventual development of essential hypertension.

Etiology

Preeclampsia is a condition unique to human pregnancy; signs and symptoms develop only during pregnancy and disappear quickly after birth of the fetus and placenta. The cause is unknown. No one patient profile identifies the woman who will have preeclampsia. High risk factors associated with developing the disease are listed in Box 14-1.

Current theories regarding the etiology of PIH include increased vasocontrictor tone (Gilstrip and Gant, 1990), abnormal prostaglandin action (Friedman, 1988), endothelial cell activation (Dekker and Sibai, 1998; Friedman et al, 1995) and immunologic factors (Dekker and Sibai, 1998) (Fig. 14-1). Genetic predisposition may be another factor.

Box 14-1

Risk Factors Associated with the Development of Pregnancy-Induced Hypertension

- Chronic renal disease
- Chronic hypertension
- Family history of PIH
- Twin gestation
- Primigravidity
- Maternal age <19 years; >40 years
- Diabetes
- Rh incompatibility
- Obesity

Data from American College of Obstetricians and Gynecologists: *Hypertension in pregnancy* (*ACOG Tech Bull* 219), Washington, DC, 1996, ACOG; Caritis S et al: Predictors of preeclampsia in women at high risk, *Am J Obstet Gynecol* 179(4):946-951, 1998; Gilbert E, Harmon J: *Manual of high risk pregnancy and delivery,* ed 2, St Louis, 1998, Mosby; and Sibai B et al: Risk factors associated with preeclampsia in healthy nulliparous women, *Am J Obstet Gynecol* 177(5):1003-1010, 1997.

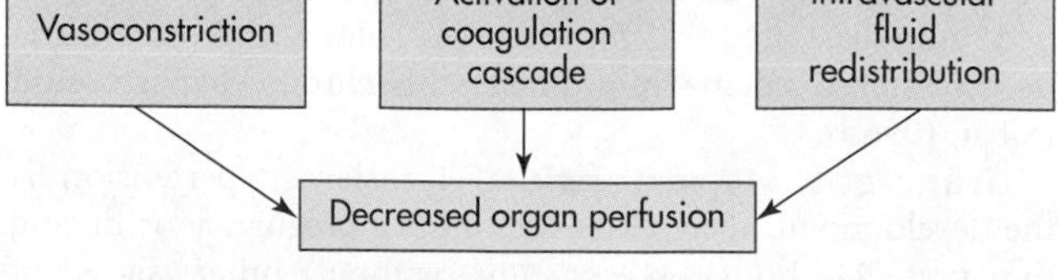

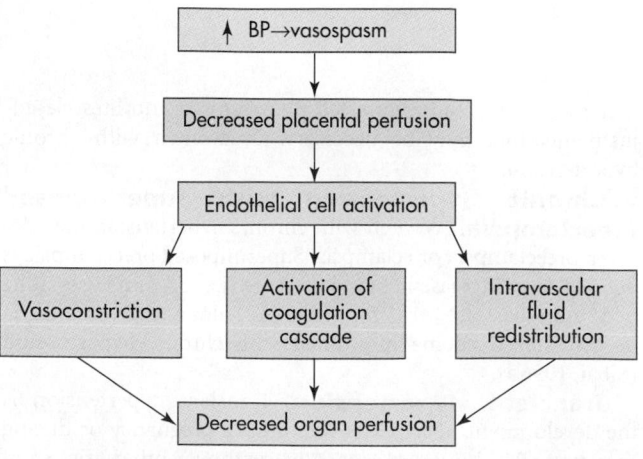

FIG. 14-1 • Etiology of PIH.

Pathophysiology

Preeclampsia progresses along a continuum from mild disease to severe preeclampsia, HELLP syndrome, or eclampsia. The pathophysiology of preeclampsia reflects alterations in the normal adaptations of pregnancy. Normal physiologic adaptations to pregnancy include increased blood plasma volume, vasodilation, decreased systemic vascular resistance, elevated cardiac output, and decreased colloid osmotic pressure.

Pathologic changes in the endothelial cells of the glomeruli are uniquely characteristic of preeclampsia, particularly in nulliparous women. The main pathogenic factor is not an increase in blood pressure but poor perfusion as a result of vasospasm. Arteriolar vasospasm diminishes the diameter of blood vessels, which impedes blood flow to all organs and raises blood pressure (Working Group on High Blood Pressure in Pregnancy, 1990). Function in organs such as the placenta, kidneys, liver, and brain is depressed by as much as 40% to 60%. The pathophysiologic sequelae are shown in Fig. 14-2.

HELLP Syndrome

HELLP syndrome appears only in 2% to 12% of severely preeclamptic women, or about 1 in 1000 pregnancies (Stone, 1998). Although the exact mechanism is unknown, HELLP syndrome is thought to occur secondary to changes occurring with preeclampsia (see Fig. 14-2). Arterial vasospasm, endothelial damage, and platelet aggregation with resultant tissue hypoxia are the underlying mechanisms for the pathophysiology of HELLP syndrome (Poole, 1993, 1997). A circulating immunologic component may be the underlying cause. Maternal mortality rates have been reported as high as 24%. Perinatal mortality rates range from 79 to 367 per 1000 live births (Portis et al, 1997).

Most commonly, HELLP syndrome is seen in older, Caucasian, multiparous women. About 90% of women report a history of malaise for several days. Many women (65%) experience epigastric or right upper quadrant abdominal pain (possibly related to hepatic ischemia), and approximately half develop nausea and vomiting. It is extremely important to understand that many women with HELLP syndrome may not have signs and symptoms of severe preeclampsia; many are normotensive and have no proteinuria. As a result, women with HELLP syndrome are often misdiagnosed with a variety of other medical or surgical disorders (Sibai, 1996b).

Critical Thinking

THE ADOLESCENT WITH PREECLAMPSIA

Marilyn, a 15-year-old, G1 P0, high school sophomore, is seen in the clinic for her routine prenatal visit at 30-weeks gestation. On examination, you note that she has gained 7 pounds since her last clinic visit 2 weeks ago, her blood pressure is 148/92, and on a urine dipstick she has 1+ proteinuria.

- **What is the likely diagnosis for Marilyn? What other signs and symptoms of this condition might you find? Develop a nursing care plan for Marilyn. What teaching about diet, rest, signs and symptoms to observe, and fetal assessment should be included in the plan?**

HELLP syndrome is a laboratory, not a clinical diagnosis. To be diagnosed as having HELLP syndrome, the woman's platelet count must be less than 100,000/mm³, her liver enzyme levels (aspartate aminotransferase [AST] and alanine aminotransferase [ALT]) must be elevated, and there must be some evidence of intravascular hemolysis (e.g., burr cells on peripheral smear or elevated bilirubin level) (Stone, 1998). A unique form of coagulopathy (not DIC) occurs with HELLP syndrome. The platelet count is low, but coagulation factor assays, prothrombin time (PT), partial thromboplastin time (PTT), and bleeding time remain normal (Stone, 1998).

Recognition of the clinical and laboratory findings associated with HELLP syndrome is important if early, aggressive therapy is to be initiated to prevent maternal and neonatal mortality. Complications reported with HELLP syndrome include renal failure, pulmonary edema, ruptured liver hematoma, DIC, and abruptio placentae (Sibai, 1996b).

Care Management

➤ Assessment

Hypertensive disorders of pregnancy can occur without warning or with the gradual development of symptoms. A key goal is early identification of pregnant women at risk for the development of preeclampsia (see Box 14-1). Therefore each woman is assessed for etiologic factors during the first prenatal visit. During each subsequent visit the woman is assessed for signs and symptoms that suggest the onset or presence of preeclampsia.

Interview. The nurse reviews the woman's admission form and prenatal record. When the nurse and pregnant woman are comfortable, the nurse begins with the interview to clarify, expand, or complete the form. Medical history is reviewed, especially the presence of diabetes mellitus, renal disease, and hypertension. Family history is explored for occurrence of preeclamptic or hypertensive conditions, diabetes mellitus, and other chronic conditions. The social and experi-

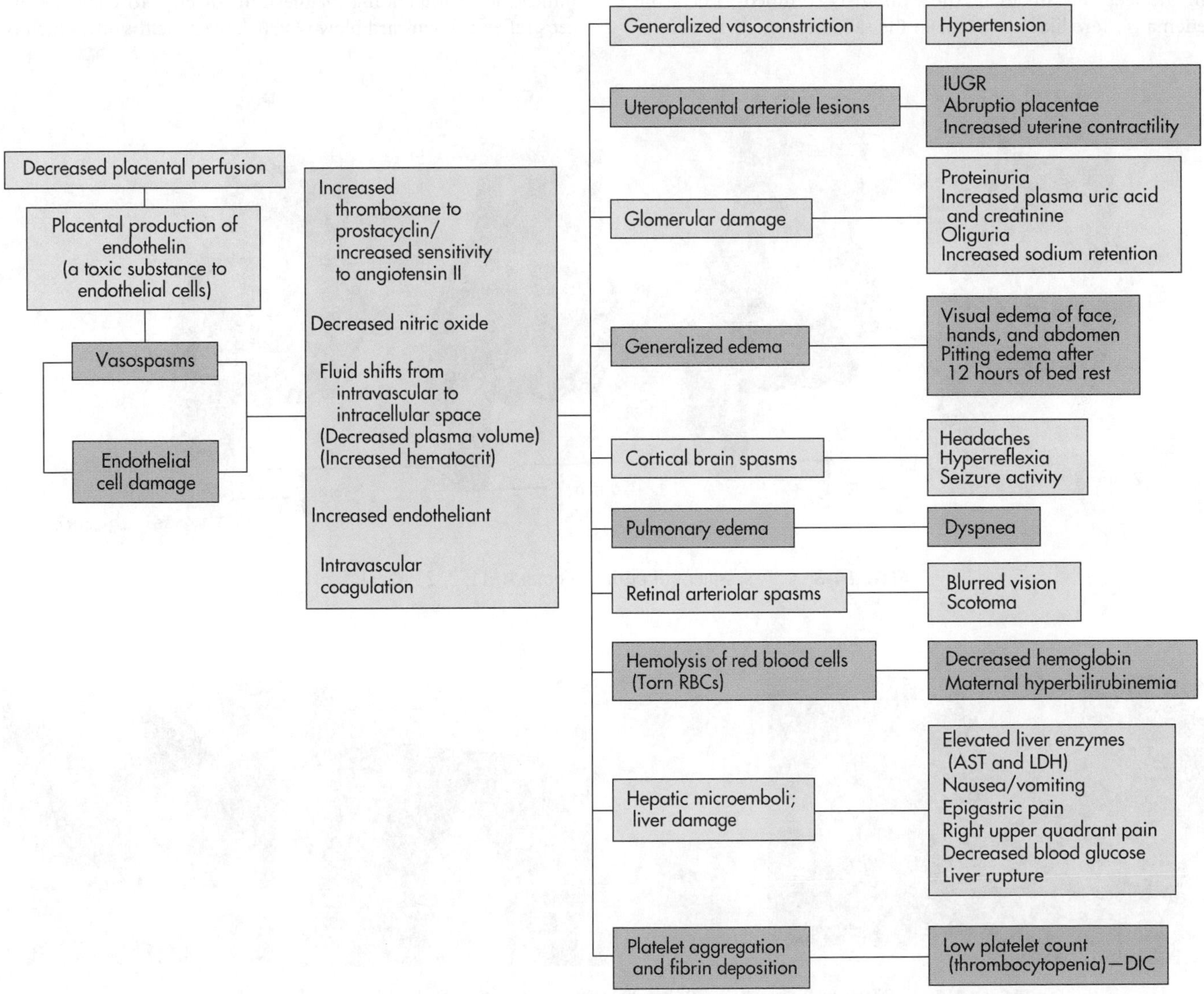

FIG. 14-2 • Pathophysiology of PIH. (Modified from Gilbert E, Harmon J: *Manual of high risk pregnancy and delivery,* ed 2, St Louis, 1998, Mosby.)

ential history provides information about the woman's marital status, nutritional status, cultural beliefs, activity level, and health habits such as smoking, drug use, and alcohol consumption.

A review of systems adds to the database for detecting blood pressure changes from baseline, abnormal weight gain and pattern of weight gain, increased signs of edema, and presence of proteinuria. It is also important to note whether the woman is having unusual, frequent, or severe headaches; visual disturbances; or epigastric pain.

Physical Examination. Accurate and consistent blood pressure assessment is important for establishing a baseline and monitoring subtle changes throughout pregnancy. Observation of edema in addition to hypertension warrants additional investigation. Edema is assessed for distribution, degree, and pitting. If periorbital or facial edema is not obvious, the pregnant woman is asked if it was present when she awoke. Edema may be described as dependent or pitting.

Dependent edema is edema of the lower or most dependent parts of the body, where hydrostatic pressure is greatest. If a pregnant woman is ambulatory, this edema may first be evident in the feet and ankles. If the woman is confined to bed, the edema is more likely to occur in the sacral region.

Pitting edema is edema that leaves a small depression or pit after finger pressure is applied to the swollen area. The pit, caused by movement of fluid away from the point of pressure to adjacent tissues, normally disappears within 30 seconds. Although the amount of edema is difficult to quantitate, the method shown in Fig. 14-3 may be used to record relative degrees of edema formation.

Symptoms reflecting CNS and visual system involvement usually accompany facial edema. Although it is not a routine assessment during the prenatal period, evaluation of the fundus of the eye yields valuable data. An initial baseline finding of normal eyegrounds assists in differentiating a preexisting from a new disease process. The woman may report no other symptoms such as epigastric pain or oliguria. Respirations are assessed for crackles, which may indicate pulmonary edema.

Deep tendon reflexes (DTRs) are evaluated if preeclampsia is suspected. The biceps and patellar reflexes and ankle clonus are assessed and the findings recorded (Fig. 14-4, Table 14-3). The evaluation of DTRs is especially important if the woman is being treated with magnesium sulfate; absence of DTRs is an early indication of impending magnesium toxicity. To elicit the biceps reflex a downward blow is struck over the thumb, which is

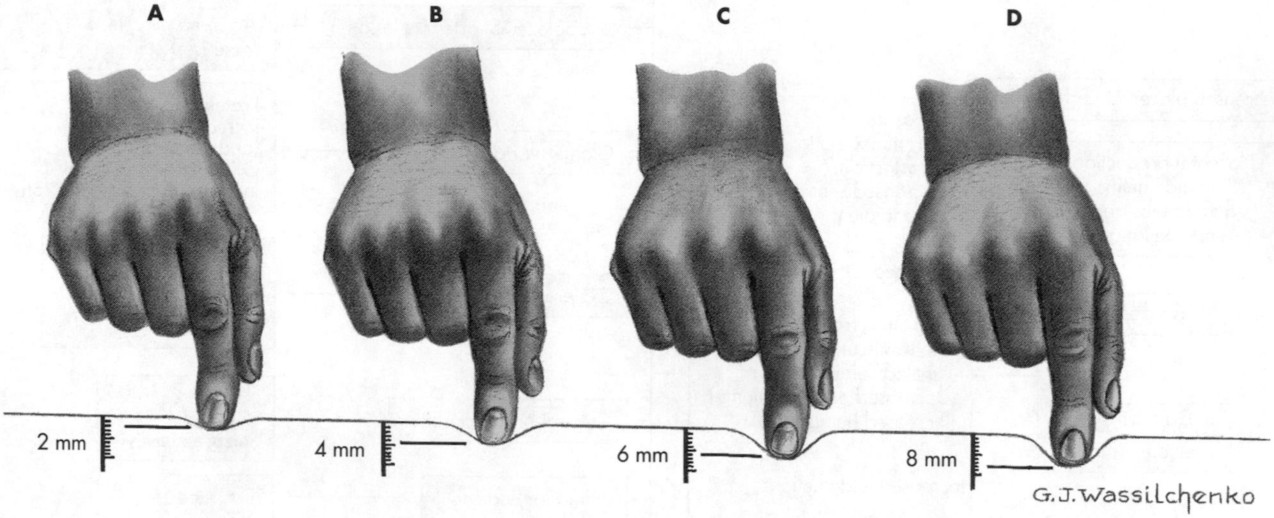

FIG. 14-3 • Assessment of pitting edema. **A,** 11; **B,** 21; **C,** 31; **D,** 41.

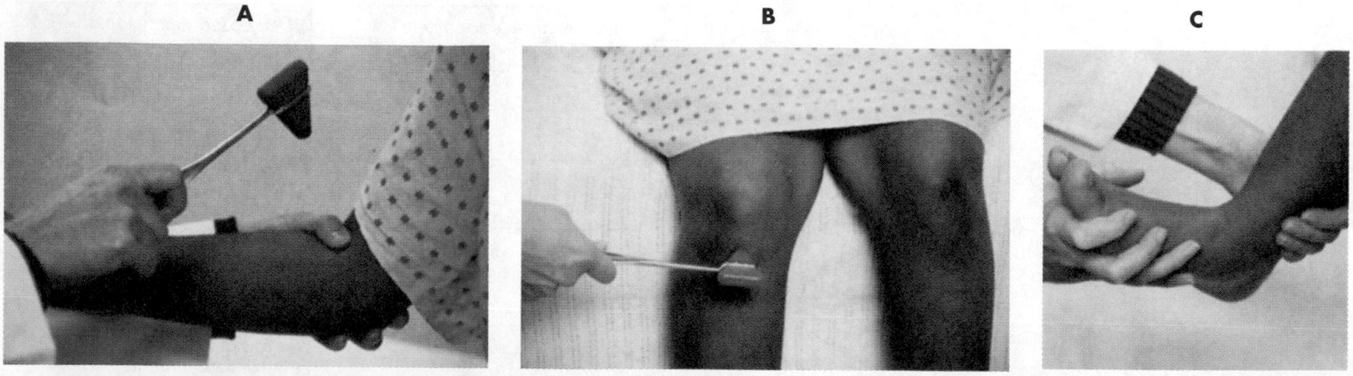

FIG. 14-4 • DTRs. **A,** Biceps reflex. **B,** Patellar reflex with woman's legs hanging freely over end of examining table. **C,** Test for ankle clonus. (From Seidel H et al: *Mosby's guide to physical examination,* ed 4, St Louis, 1999, Mosby.)

situated over the biceps tendon. Normal response is flexion of the arm at the elbow, described as a 2+ response (see Fig. 14-4, *A*, and Table 14-3). The patellar reflex is elicited with the woman's legs hanging freely over the end of the examining table, or with the woman lying on her side with the knee slightly flexed. A blow with a percussion hammer is dealt directly to the patellar tendon, inferior to the patella. Normal response is the extension or kicking out of the leg, which is recorded as 2+ (see Fig. 14-4, *B*, and Table 14-3). To assess for hyperactive reflexes (clonus) at the ankle joint, the examiner supports the leg with the knee flexed. With one hand, the examiner sharply dorsiflexes the foot, maintains the position for a moment, and then releases the foot (see Fig. 14-4, *C*). Normal (negative clonus) response is elicited when no rhythmic oscillations (jerks) are felt while the foot is held in dorsiflexion. When the foot is released, no oscillations are seen as the foot drops to the plantar-flexed position. Abnormal (positive clonus) response is recognized by rhythmic oscillations of one or more beats felt when the foot is in dorsiflexion and seen as the foot drops to the plantar-flexed position.

An important assessment is determination of fetal status. Uteroplacental perfusion is decreased in women with preeclampsia, placing the fetus in jeopardy. Biophysical or biochemical monitoring, such as nonstress testing, contraction stress testing, biophysical profile, and serial ultrasonography, is used to assess fetal status. The fetal heart rate (FHR) is assessed for baseline rate and the presence of variability and accelerations, which indicate an intact oxygenated fetal CNS. Abnormal baseline rate, decreased or absent variability, and late or variable decelerations are indications of fetal intolerance to the intrauterine environment.

Doppler flow velocimetry studies are used for evaluating maternal and fetal well-being (see Chapter 17). Uteroplacental perfusion is assessed by measuring the velocity of blood flow through the uterine artery, umbilical arteries, or both. A systolic/diastolic ratio greater than 3 after 26 weeks is considered abnormal, and ratios of 3.8 have been associated with preeclampsia and IUGR (Farmakides et al, 1994).

During the physical examination, the pregnant woman is examined for signs of deterioration of mild preeclampsia to severe preeclampsia or eclampsia. Signs of worsening liver involvement, renal failure, worsening hypertension, cerebral involvement, and developing coagulopathies must be assessed and documented. Respirations are assessed for crackles or diminished breath sounds, which may indicate pulmonary edema. (For warning signs of preeclampsia and the differentiation of mild from severe preeclampsia, see Table 14-2.) Noninvasive assessment parameters include level of consciousness, blood pressure, hemoglobin oxygen saturation (pulse oximetry), electrocardiographic findings, and urine output. Invasive hemodynamic monitoring may be indicated in selected patients. Eclampsia usually is preceded by various premonitory symptoms and signs, including headache, severe epigastric pain, hyperreflexia, and hemoconcentration. However, convulsions can appear suddenly and without warning in a seemingly stable woman with only minimum blood pressure elevations (Sibai, 1996b).

The convulsions that occur in eclampsia are frightening to observe. Increased hypertension and tonic contractions of all body muscles (arms flexed, hands clenched, and legs inverted) precede the tonic-clonic convulsions (Fig. 14-5). During this stage, muscles alternately relax and contract. Respirations are halted and then begin again with long, deep, stertorous inhalation. Hypotension follows, and coma ensues. Nystagmus and muscular twitching persist for a time. Disorientation and amnesia cloud the immediate recovery. Oliguria and anuria are notable. Seizures may recur within minutes of the first convulsion, or the woman may never have another. During the convulsions the mother and fetus are not receiving oxygen, so eclamptic seizures produce a marked metabolic insult to both mother and fetus.

Laboratory Tests. The nurse assists in obtaining a number of blood and urine specimens to aid in the diagnosis of preeclampsia, HELLP syndrome, or chronic hypertension. Baseline laboratory test information is useful in the early diagnosis of preeclampsia and for comparison with results obtained to evaluate progression and severity of disease. An initial blood specimen is obtained for the following tests to assess the disease process and its effect on renal and hepatic functioning:

- Complete blood cell count including a platelet count
- Clotting studies (including bleeding time, prothrombin time, partial thromboplastin time, and fibrinogen)
- Liver enzymes (lactic dehydrogenase [LDH], AST, ALT)
- Chemistry panel (BUN, creatinine, glucose, uric acid)
- Type and screen, possible crossmatch

TABLE 14-3
Assessing Deep Tendon Reflexes

Degree	Grading
Brisk with sustained clonus	5+
Hyperactive response (brisk with transient clonus)	4+
More than normal (brisk)	3+
Normal, active	2+
Low response (sluggish or dull)	1+
No response	0

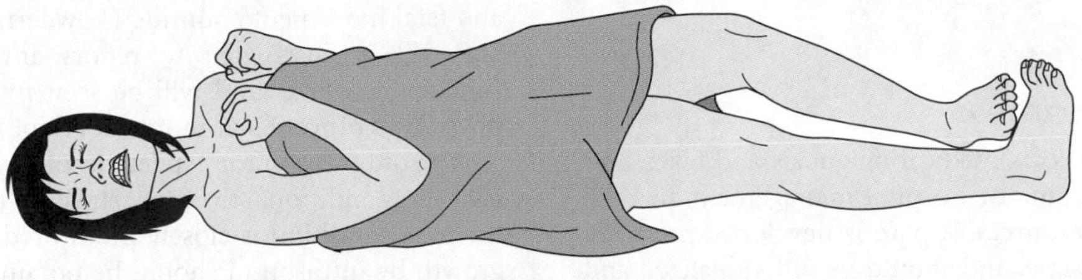

FIG. 14-5 • Eclampsia (convulsion or seizure).

The hematocrit, hemoglobin, and platelet levels are monitored closely for changes indicating a worsening of patient status. Because hepatic involvement is a possible complication, serum glucose levels are monitored if liver function tests indicate elevated liver enzymes. Once the platelet count drops below 100,000/mm³, coagulation profiles are needed to identify developing DIC.

Proteinuria is determined from dipstick testing of a clean-catch or catheterized urine specimen. A reading of 2+ on two or more occasions, at least 6 hours apart, should be followed by a 24-hour urine collection (Gilbert and Harmon, 1998). A 24-hour collection for protein and creatinine clearance is more reflective of true renal status. Proteinuria usually is a late sign in the course of preeclampsia. Protein readings are designated as follows:

0	Negative
Trace	Trace
+1	30 mg/dl (equivalent to 0.3 g/L)
+2	100 mg/dl
+3	300 mg/dl
+4	>1000 mg (1 g)/dl

Urine output is assessed for volume of at least 30 ml/hour or 120 ml in 4 hours.

Renal laboratory assessments include monitoring trends in serum creatinine and BUN levels. As renal function becomes compromised, renal excretion of creatinine and other waste products, including magnesium sulfate, decreases. As renal excretion decreases, serum levels for creatinine, BUN, uric acid, and magnesium rise.

➤ Nursing Diagnoses

Nursing diagnoses for the woman with hypertensive disorders in pregnancy include the following:

- Anxiety related to:
  —Preeclampsia and its effect on woman and infant
- Ineffective individual/family coping related to:
  —The woman's restricted activity and concern over a complicated pregnancy
  —The woman's inability to work outside the home
  —The transfer of the woman to a tertiary center for more intensive management
- Powerlessness related to:
  —Inability to prevent or control condition and outcomes
- Altered tissue/organ perfusion, decreased, related to:
  —Hypertension
  —Cyclic vasospasms
  —Cerebral edema
  —Hemorrhage
- Risk for injury to fetus related to:
  —Uteroplacental insufficiency
  —Preterm birth
  —Abruptio placentae

➤ Expected Outcomes

The planning of care follows medical diagnosis and takes into account the choice of home or hospital management and the woman's and family's resources. A plan is developed mutually with the woman, if possible, and should be individualized and related specifically to the needs of the patient and her family. Expected outcomes for care of patients with hypertensive disorders of pregnancy include that the woman will do the following:

- Recognize and immediately report abnormal signs and symptoms to prevent worsening of her condition.
- Adhere to the medical regimen to minimize risk to herself and her fetus.
- Identify and use available support systems.
- Verbalize her fears and concerns to cope with the condition and situation.
- With her fetus, will not suffer adverse sequelae from preeclampsia or its management.
- Develop no signs of eclampsia and its complications.
- Give birth to a healthy infant.

➤ Plan of Care and Implementation

Preeclampsia. Nursing actions are derived from medical management, health care provider directives, and nursing diagnoses. The most effective therapy is prevention. Early prenatal care, identification of at-risk women during pregnancy, and recognition and reporting of physical warning signs are essential components for optimizing maternal and perinatal outcomes. The nurse's skills in assessing the woman for factors and symptoms of preeclampsia and educating her about reporting symptoms cannot be overestimated.

The goals of therapy are to ensure maternal safety and to deliver a healthy newborn, as close to term as possible. At or near term, the woman with preeclampsia will most likely have an induction of labor, preceded if necessary by cervical ripening. When preeclampsia is diagnosed in a woman who is at less than 37 weeks of gestation, however, immediate delivery may not be in the best interest of the infant. In that instance, a thorough evaluation of the condition of both the mother and fetus will be done in the hospital, in a high risk clinic, or in a physician's office.

Emotional and psychologic support is essential to help the woman and her family cope. Their perceptions of the disease process, the reasons for it, and the care received will affect their compliance with and participation in treatment. The family will need to use coping mechanisms and support systems to help them through this crisis. A plan of care specifically designed for the woman with preeclampsia is superimposed on the nursing care all women need during labor and the birth process.

Mild Preeclampsia and Home Care. If the woman has mild preeclampsia (i.e., if blood pressure is stable, urine protein is less than 500 mg in a 24-hour collection, and no subjective complaints), she may be managed expectantly, usually at home. The maternal-fetal condition should be assessed two or three times per week. Many agencies are able to provide this assessment in the home. If the woman does not have insurance coverage, and home nursing is not possible, the woman may be asked to perform self-assessment daily, including weight, urine dipstick, protein determinations, blood pressure measurement, and fetal movement counting (Lowdermilk and Grohar, 1999). She will be instructed to report any subjective symptoms (Home Care box) and will be seen in the high risk clinic or physician's office if symptoms develop.

The only reason for expectant management of preeclampsia is to allow additional time for fetal growth and maturation; thus the fetal condition is closely monitored. An evaluation of fetal growth by ultrasound should be obtained every 3 weeks. Fetal movements are counted daily. Other fetal assessment tests include a nonstress test once or twice a week, and a biophysical profile as needed. Fetal jeopardy as evidenced by inappropriate growth or abnormal testing necessitates immediate delivery (Sibai, 1996b).

Activity Restriction. Bed rest in the lateral recumbent position is a traditional therapy for preeclampsia, and may improve uteroplacental blood flow during pregnancy. However, recommending bed rest for all high risk pregnant women is becoming more controversial. Maloni (1994) documented adverse physiologic outcomes related to complete bed rest, including cardiovascular deconditioning; diuresis with accompanying fluid, electrolyte, and weight loss; muscle atrophy; and psychologic stress. These changes begin on the first day of bed rest and continue for the duration of therapy. Sibai (1996b) recommends rest at home, rather than strict bed rest, and allows women hospitalized with mild preeclampsia to be out of bed.

Bed rest has been shown to be beneficial in decreasing blood pressure and promoting diuresis. Women with mild preeclampsia feel reasonably well; thus boredom from the restriction is common. Diversionary activities, visits from friends, telephone conversations, and creation of a comfortable and convenient environment are ways to cope with the boredom (Home Care box). Gentle exercise (e.g., range of motion, stretching, Kegel exercises, and pelvic tilts) is important in maintaining muscle tone, blood flow, regularity of bowel function, and a sense of well-being (Grohar, 1994; Maloni, 1998).

Relaxation techniques can help to reduce stress associated with the high risk condition and prepare the woman for labor and the birth.

Diet. Diet and fluid recommendations are much the same as for healthy pregnant women. Diets high in protein and low in salt have been suggested to prevent preeclampsia; however, the efficacy of this has not been proven. Sibai (1996a) recommends a regular diet with no salt restriction. Because pregnant women with hypertension have a lower plasma volume than do normotensive women, sodium restriction is not necessary. Women need salt for maintenance of blood volume and placental perfusion. The exception may be the woman with chronic hypertension that was successfully controlled with a low-salt diet before the pregnancy. Adequate fluid intake helps to maintain optimum fluid volume and aids in renal perfusion and filtration. The nurse uses assessment data regarding the woman's diet to counsel her in areas of deficiency, if needed (Guidelines box).

Successful home care requires that the woman be well educated about preeclampsia and motivated to follow the plan of care; she must be reliable about keeping appointments. The effects of illness, language, age, culture, beliefs, and support systems must be considered. Support systems must be mobilized and involved (Nursing Care Plan).

Severe Preeclampsia/HELLP Syndrome. If the woman's condition worsens, or if she already has severe preeclampsia or HELLP syndrome and is critically ill, she should receive appropriate management (usually in a tertiary care center) ranging from immediate birth to conservative management of the pregnancy (Leicht and Harvey, 1999). Recognition of the clinical and laboratory findings of severe preeclampsia or HELLP syndrome is important if early, aggressive therapy is to be initiated to prevent maternal and perinatal mortality. An unfavorable (i.e., uneffaced and undilated) cervix resulting from gestational age and the aggressive nature of this disorder supports cesarean birth. Prolonged induction of labor could increase maternal morbidity.

Antepartum care focuses on stabilization and preparation for birth. The woman may be admitted to an antepartum or a labor and birth unit, depending on the hospital. If the woman's

Home Care

ASSESSING AND REPORTING CLINICAL SIGNS OF PREECLAMPSIA

- Report immediately any increase in your blood pressure, protein in urine, weight gain greater than 1 pound/week, or edema.
- Take your blood pressure on the same arm in a sitting position each time for consistent and accurate readings. Support arm on a table in a horizontal position at heart level.
- Use the same scale, wearing the same clothes, at the same time each day, after voiding, before breakfast, for reliable daily weights.
- Dipstick your clean-catch urine sample for assessing proteinuria; report frequency or burning on urination.
- Report to your health care provider if proteinuria is +2 or more or if you have a decrease in urine output.
- Daily assess your baby's activity. Decreased activity (three or fewer movements per hour) may indicate fetal stress.
- It is important to keep your scheduled prenatal appointments so any changes in your or the baby's condition can be detected immediately.
- Keep a daily log/diary of your assessments for your home health care nurse, or bring it with you to your next prenatal visit.

Home Care

COPING WITH BED REST

- In bed, lie on your side (may alternate sides for comfort). This allows more blood to get to your uterus (womb) and baby.
- Increase your fluid intake to 8 glasses/day, and add roughage (e.g., bran, fruits, leafy vegetables) to your diet to decrease constipation.
- Include diversional activities such as puzzles, reading, and crafts to reduce boredom.
- Do gentle exercises such as circling your hands and feet or gently tensing and relaxing arm and leg muscles. This improves muscle tone, circulation, and sense of well-being.
- Encourage family participation in your care.
- Have significant others assist you with care of the house, children, etc.
- Use relaxation to help you cope with stress. Relax your body one muscle at a time or imagine some pleasant scene, word, or image. Soothing music can also help you to relax.

Guidelines

NUTRITION

- Eat a nutritious, balanced diet (e.g., 60 to 70 g protein, 1200 mg calcium, adequate zinc, magnesium, vitamins). Collaborate with registered dietitian for diet best suited for individual woman.
- There is no sodium restriction; however, avoid salty foods (e.g., canned foods, sodas, pretzels, potato chips, pickles, sauerkraut).
- Eat foods with roughage (e.g., whole grains, raw fruits, and vegetables).
- Drink 8 to 10 glasses of water per day.
- Avoid alcohol.

condition is severe, she may be placed in an intensive care unit for hemodynamic monitoring. Maternal and fetal surveillance, patient education regarding the disease process, and supportive measures directed toward the woman and her family are initiated. Assessments include review of the cardiovascular, pulmonary, renal, hematologic, and central nervous systems. Fetal assessments for well-being (e.g., NST, BPP, and Doppler velocimetry) are important because of the potential for hypoxia related to uteroplacental insufficiency. Baseline laboratory assessments include metabolic studies for liver enzyme (i.e., AST, ALT, and LDH) determination, CBC with platelets, coagulation profile to assess for DIC, and electrolyte studies to establish renal functioning.

Weight is measured on admission and every day thereafter. An indwelling urinary catheter facilitates monitoring of renal function and effectiveness of therapy. If appropriate, vaginal examination may be done to check for cervical changes. Abdominal palpation establishes uterine tonicity and fetal size, activity, and position. Electronic monitoring to determine fetal status is initiated at least once a day. The nurse's skill in implementing the techniques described here can be reassuring to the woman and her family. The woman's room must be close to staff and to emergency drugs, supplies, and equipment. Noise and external stimuli must be minimized. Seizure precautions are taken (Box 14-2).

Bed rest is commonly ordered. The nurse's ingenuity may be called on to help the woman cope physically and psychologically with the side effects of immobility and an environment limited in stimuli and support. Thromboembolic events, a risk factor during normal pregnancy, pose an even greater risk with preeclampsia (Nursing Care Plan).

Intrapartum nursing care of the woman with severe preeclampsia or the HELLP syndrome involves continuous maternal and fetal assessments as labor progresses. The assessment for and prevention of tissue hypoxia and hemorrhage, both of which can lead to permanent compromise of vital organs, continue throughout the intrapartum and postpartum periods (Leicht and Harvey, 1999).

Nursing Care Plan — THE WOMAN WITH PREECLAMPSIA

NURSING DIAGNOSIS **Risk for injury related to signs of preeclampsia**

EXPECTED OUTCOME Patient will demonstrate ability to assess self and fetus for signs of worsening preeclampsia; no adverse sequelae will occur as result of preeclamptic condition.

Nursing Interventions/*Rationales*

Review warning signs/symptoms of preeclampsia *to ensure adequate knowledge base exists for decision making.*

Assess home environment, including woman's ability to assume self-care responsibilities, support systems, language, age, culture, beliefs, and effects of illness, *to determine if home care is viable option.*

Teach woman how to do a self-assessment for clinical signs of preeclampsia (take and record blood pressure, measure urine protein, maintain daily weight log, assess edema formation, assess fetal activity) *to provide immediate evidence of a worsening condition.*

Teach woman to report any increases in blood pressure, +2 proteinuria, weight gain greater than 454 mg (1 lb) per week, presence of edema, and decreased fetal activity to her health care provider immediately *to prevent worsening of preeclamptic condition.*

Teach woman about use of bed rest, relaxation, and diet as palliative treatment options *to decrease blood pressure and promote diuresis.*

NURSING DIAGNOSIS **Fear/anxiety related to preeclampsia and its effect on the fetus**

EXPECTED OUTCOME Patient's feelings and symptoms of fear/anxiety will decrease/ease.

Nursing Interventions/*Rationales*

Provide a calm, soothing atmosphere and teach family to provide emotional support *to facilitate coping.*

Encourage verbalization of fears *to decrease intensity of emotional response.*

Involve woman and family in the management of her preeclamptic condition *to promote a greater sense of control.*

Help woman identify and use appropriate coping strategies and support systems *to reduce fear/anxiety.*

Explore use of desensitization strategies such as progressive muscle relaxation, visual imagery, or thought stopping *to reduce fear-related emotions and related physical symptoms.*

NURSING DIAGNOSIS **Diversional activity deficit related to imposed bed rest**

EXPECTED OUTCOME Patient will verbalize diminished feelings of boredom.

Nursing Interventions/*Rationales*

Assist woman to explore creatively personally meaningful activities that can be pursued from the bed *to ensure activities that have meaning, purpose, and value to the individual.*

Maintain emphasis on personal choices of woman *to promote control and minimize imposition of routines by others.*

Evaluate what support and system resources are available in the environment *to assist in providing diversional activities.*

Explore ways for woman to remain an active participant in home management and decision making *to promote control.*

Engage support of family and friends in carrying out chosen activities and making necessary environmental alterations *to ensure success.*

Teach woman about stress management and relaxation techniques *to help manage tension of confinement.*

Magnesium Sulfate. One of the important goals of care for the woman with severe preeclampsia or HELLP syndrome is preventing or controlling convulsions. Magnesium sulfate ($MgSO_4$) is the drug of choice in the prevention and treatment of convulsions caused by preeclampsia or eclampsia (American College of Obstetricians and Gynecologists, 1996). Benefits of $MgSO_4$ therapy include an increase in uterine blood flow to protect the fetus and an increase in prostacyclins to prevent uterine vasoconstriction (Gilbert and Harmon, 1998).

$MgSO_4$ is administered as a secondary infusion (i.e., "piggyback") to the main IV line by volumetric infusion pump. An initial loading dose of 4 to 6 g per protocol or physician's order is infused over 15 to 30 minutes. This dose is followed by a maintenance dose of $MgSO_4$ that is diluted in an IV solution per physician's order (e.g., 40 g $MgSO_4$ in 1000 ml lactated Ringer's solution) and administered by infusion pump at 1 to 3 g per hour (Gilbert and Harmon, 1998; Mandeville and Troiano, 1999). This dose should maintain a therapeutic serum magnesium level of 4 to 8 mg/dl. Serum magnesium levels are obtained after the patient has received magnesium sulfate for 4 to 6 hours. The infusion rate is adjusted to maintain the therapeutic level (Sisson and Sauer, 1996) (Box 14-3).

After the loading dose, there may be a transient lowering of the arterial blood pressure secondary to relaxation of smooth muscle.

NURSE ALERT • The woman's blood pressure, pulse, and respiratory status should be monitored closely while the loading dose is being administered by IV; and every 15 to 30 minutes at other times, depending on the stability of the woman's condition. Administration of magnesium sulfate is continued for at least the first 12 to 24 hours postpartum to prevent seizures.

Box 14-2

Hospital Precautionary Measures

- Environment
  - Quiet
  - Nonstimulating
  - Lighting subdued
- Seizure precautions
  - Padded side rails
  - Suction equipment tested and ready to use
  - Oxygen administration equipment tested and ready to use
- Call button within easy reach
- Emergency medication tray immediately accessible
  - Hydralazine and magnesium sulfate in or adjacent to woman's room
  - Calcium gluconate immediately available in a well-labeled syringe
- Emergency birth pack accessible

Box 14-3

Protocol for Care of Patient with Preeclampsia Receiving Magnesium Sulfate

MAGNESIUM SULFATE ADMINISTRATION

Patient and Family Teaching

Explain technique, rationale, and reactions to expect
- Route and rate
- Purpose of "piggyback"

Reasons for use
- Tailor information to patient's readiness to learn
- Explain that it is to prevent disease progression
- Explain that it is to prevent seizures

Reactions to expect from medication
- Initially patient will feel flushed, hot, sedated, especially during the bolus
- Sedation will continue

Monitoring to anticipate
- Maternal: blood pressure, pulse, DTRs, level of consciousness, urine output (indwelling catheter likely), presence of headache, visual disturbances, epigastric pain
- Fetal: FHR and activity

Administration
- Verify physician order
- Position woman in side-lying position
- Prepare solution and administer with an infusion control device (pump)
- Piggyback a solution of 40 g magnesium sulfate in 1000 ml of lactated Ringer's solution with an infusion control device at the ordered rates: loading dose—initial bolus of 4-6 g over 15 to 30 min; maintenance dose—1-3 g/hr

Maternal and Fetal Assessments
- Monitor blood pressure, pulse, respiratory rate, FHR, and contractions every 15-30 min, depending on patient condition
- Monitor intake and output, proteinuria, DTRs, presence of headache, visual disturbances, and epigastric pain at least hourly
- Restrict hourly fluid intake to a total of 100 to 125 ml/hr; urinary output should be at least 30 ml/hr

Reportable Conditions
- Blood pressure: systolic 160 mm Hg, diastolic 110 mm Hg, or both
- Respiratory rate: $\leq$12 breaths/min
- Urinary output <30 ml/hr
- Presence of headache, visual disturbances, or epigastric pain
- Increasing severity or loss of DTRs, increasing edema, proteinuria
- Any abnormal laboratory values (magnesium levels, platelet count, creatinine clearance, levels of uric acid, AST, ALT, prothrombin time, partial thromboplastin time, fibrinogen, fibrin split products)
- Any other significant change in maternal or fetal status

Emergency Measures
- Keep emergency drug tray at bedside with calcium gluconate and intubation equipment
- Keep side rails up
- Keep lights dimmed and maintain a quiet environment

Documentation
- All of the above

Intramuscular (IM) $MgSO_4$ is used rarely because the absorption rate cannot be controlled, the injections are painful, and tissue necrosis can occur. The IM route may be used with some women who are being transported to a tertiary care center. The IM dose is 4 to 5 g given in each buttock, or a total of 10 g (1% procaine may be ordered added to the solution to reduce injection pain) and can be repeated at 4-hour intervals. Z-track technique should be used for the deep IM injection, followed by gentle massage at the site.

$MgSO_4$ interferes with the release of acetylcholine at the synapses, decreasing neuromuscular irritability, depressing cardiac conduction, and decreasing CNS irritability. Because magnesium circulates free and unbound to protein and is excreted in the urine, accurate recordings of maternal urine output must be obtained.

Diuresis within 24 to 48 hours is an excellent prognostic sign. It is considered evidence that perfusion of the kidney has improved as a result of relaxation of arteriolar spasm. With improved perfusion, fluid moves from interstitial spaces to the intravascular bed and edema is reduced. Diuresis results in weight loss. While diuresis generally indicates improvement, diuresis in the presence of worsening clinical status may indicate impending renal failure. As renal function declines and serum creatinine levels rise, renal filtration is compromised. The woman can excrete large volumes of urine (e.g., >200 ml/hr) but will not excrete magnesium sulfate.

Because $MgSO_4$ is a CNS depressant, the nurse assesses for signs and symptoms of magnesium toxicity (see Box 14-3). Serum magnesium levels are obtained on the basis of the woman's response and if any signs of toxicity are present. Early symptoms of toxicity include nausea, a feeling of warmth, flushing, muscle weakness, decreased reflexes, and slurred speech.

NURSE ALERT • Loss of patellar reflexes, respiratory depression, oliguria, and cardiac arrest are signs of magnesium toxicity. Actions are needed to prevent respiratory or cardiac arrest. If magnesium toxicity is suspected, the infusion should be discontinued immediately. Calcium gluconate, the antidote for magnesium sulfate, may also be ordered (10 ml of a 10% solution, or 1 gm) and given by slow IV push (usually by the physician) over at least 3 minutes (Sibai, 1996b) to avoid undesirable reactions such as dysrhythmias, bradycardia, and ventricular fibrillation.

Because magnesium sulfate is also a tocolytic agent, its use may increase the duration of labor.

NURSE ALERT • The labor of a woman with preeclampsia receiving magnesium sulfate may need augmentation with oxytocin. The amount of oxytocin needed to stimulate labor may be more than that needed for a woman who is not on magnesium sulfate.

$MgSO_4$ does not seem to affect FHR variability in a healthy term fetus, and rarely is toxic in the healthy term newborn whose weight is within normal range for gestational age. Neonatal serum magnesium levels approximate those of the mother, and toxic levels can cause depressed respirations and hyporeflexia. The neonate with hypermagnesemia can be treated with calcium and exchange transfusion with citrated blood or may require assisted mechanical ventilation until serum levels normalize.

If eclampsia develops after the initiation of magnesium sulfate therapy, the treatment of choice is to administer an additional 2 g of magnesium sulfate IV push over 3 to 5 minutes (Leicht and Harvey, 1999) (Emergency box). Occasionally it is necessary to repeat the dose because the woman experiences

Emergency

MAGNESIUM SULFATE TOXICITY

Signs/Symptoms

Respirations <12/min
Hyporeflexia, absence of reflexes
Urine output <30 ml/hr
Toxic serum levels >9.6 mg/dl
Signs of fetal stress (e.g., fetal tachycardia or bradycardia)
Significant drop in maternal pulse or blood pressure

Interventions

Discontinue $MgSO_4$ immediately, and change to maintenance solution.
Call for assistance and notify health care provider for immediate care.
Administer calcium gluconate as ordered (e.g., 1 g for IV injection given over 3 minutes).
Monitor return of DTRs, respiratory rate and quality, pulse rate and quality, and urine output.
Monitor $MgSO_4$ level as indicated by patient response.

Emergency

ECLAMPSIA

Tonic-Clonic Convulsion Signs

Stage of invasion: 2 to 3 seconds; eyes fixed; twitching of facial muscles.
Stage of contraction: 15 to 20 seconds; eyes protrude and are bloodshot; all body muscles in tonic contraction.
Stage of convulsion: muscles relax and contract alternately (clonic). Respirations are halted and then begin again with long, deep, stertorous inhalation. Coma may ensue.

Interventions

Keep airway patent; turn head to one side; place pillow under one shoulder or back, if possible.
Call for assistance.
Protect with side rails up and padded.
Observe and record convulsion activity.

After Convulsion/Seizure

Observe for postconvulsion coma and incontinence.
Use suction as needed.
Administer oxygen via face mask at 10 L/min.
Start IV fluids and monitor for potential fluid overload.
Give $MgSO_4$ or anticonvulsant drug as ordered.
Insert indwelling catheter.
Monitor blood pressure.
Monitor fetal and uterine status.
Expedite laboratory work as ordered to monitor kidney function, liver function, coagulation system, and drug levels.
Provide hygiene and a quiet environment.
Support and keep woman and family informed.
Be prepared for birth when woman is stable.

additional seizures. Rarely, the woman will continue to experience seizures despite adequate blood magnesium levels. In that case, 250 mg of amobarbital sodium may be administered by slow IV push over 3 to 5 minutes (Sibai, 1996b). Diazepam is sometimes used to treat eclamptic seizures. However, this medication can cause phlebitis and venous thrombosis. If administered too rapidly, it can lead to apnea or cardiac arrest (Sibai, 1996b).

Both amobarbital sodium and diazepam have fetal and neonatal effects. FHR loses variability, a reflection of fetal oxygenation. High levels of these medications in the newborn depress sucking ability, cause hypotonia, and may result in temperature instability. The newborn's respiratory rate may be decreased. Careful surveillance of both maternal and fetal or neonatal status is warranted.

Control of Blood Pressure. For the severely hypertensive woman with preeclampsia, antihypertensive medications are usually ordered to lower the diastolic blood pressure. Initiation of antihypertensive therapy reduces maternal morbidity and mortality associated with left ventricular failure and cerebral hemorrhage. Because a degree of maternal hypertension is necessary to maintain uteroplacental perfusion, antihypertensive therapy must not decrease the arterial pressure too much or too rapidly. The target range for the diastolic pressure is 90 to 100 mm Hg (Leicht and Harvey, 1999).

Intravenous hydralazine remains the antihypertensive agent of choice for the treatment of hypertension in severe preeclampsia. Intravenous labetalol hydrochloride and oral methyldopa and nifedipine are also used (Cunningham et al, 1997; Sibai, 1996b; Sisson and Sauer, 1996). The choice of agent depends on patient response and physician preference.

Eclampsia

Immediate Care. The immediate care during a convulsion is to ensure a patent airway (see Emergency box on p. 286). When convulsions occur, the woman is turned to her side to prevent aspiration of vomitus and supine hypotension syndrome. After the convulsion ceases, food and fluid are suctioned from the glottis or trachea, and oxygen is given by face mask. $MgSO_4$ or another anticonvulsant is given for recurrent convulsions as ordered (Sibai, 1996b). If an IV infusion is not in place, one is begun with a large-bore needle. Time, duration, and a description of the convulsions is recorded, and any urinary or fecal incontinence is noted. The fetus is monitored for adverse effects. Transient bradycardia and decreased fetal heart rate variability are common.

Aspiration is a leading cause of maternal morbidity and mortality following an eclamptic seizure. After initial stabilization and airway management, the nurse should anticipate orders for a chest x-ray film and possibly arterial blood gases to determine whether aspiration occurred.

A rapid assessment of uterine activity, cervical status, and fetal status is performed after a convulsion. During the convulsion, membranes may rupture and the cervix may dilate because the uterus becomes hypercontractile and hypertonic; birth may be imminent. If not, once the woman's seizure activity and blood pressure are controlled, a decision should be made regarding whether birth should take place. The more serious the condition of the woman, the greater is the need to proceed to the birth, which is the definitive cure for the disease. The route of birth—induction of labor vs. cesarean birth—depends on the maternal and fetal condition. If fetal lungs are not mature, and the birth can be delayed for 48 hours, steroids such as betamethasone may be given.

The woman may have been incontinent of urine and stool or the membranes may have ruptured during the convulsion; she will need assistance with hygiene and a change of gown. Oral care with a soft toothbrush may be of comfort.

Immediately following a seizure, the woman may be very confused and can be combative, necessitating the temporary use of restraints. It may take several hours for the woman to regain her usual level of mental functioning. The health care provider explains procedures briefly and quietly. The woman is never left alone. The family is kept informed of management, the rationale for treatment, and the woman's progress.

Determination of central venous pressure (CVP) or pulmonary artery wedge pressure (PAWP) (Swan-Ganz catheter) may be required for accurate fluid monitoring in the presence of pulmonary edema or acute renal failure (ACOG, 1996). No oral intake is permitted if the woman is convulsing or has symptoms of severe preeclampsia. An indwelling catheter is required for accurate hourly measurement of urine output. For correction of hypovolemia, crystalloids (e.g., 0.9% saline or lactated Ringer's solution) are infused IV at a rate that maintains a urine output of at least 30 ml/hour. Maternal response to therapy is recorded.

Medications (e.g., $MgSO_4$ and antihypertensive agents) are given as directed. The woman's response is monitored and recorded, and all drugs, doses, and times are recorded. Laboratory tests are ordered to assess for HELLP syndrome and to have blood typed and crossmatched for administration of packed red blood cells as needed. Blood is kept available for emergency transfusion; abruptio placentae, with accompanying hemorrhage and shock, often occurs in women with eclampsia. Other tests include determination of electrolytes; liver function battery; and complete hemogram and clotting profile, including platelet count and fibrin split product levels (to assess for DIC).

Postpartum Nursing Care. After birth the symptoms of preeclampsia or eclampsia resolve quickly, usually within 48 hours; however, symptoms have been reported up to several weeks postpartum (Atterbury et al, 1998). The hematopoietic and hepatic complications of HELLP syndrome may persist longer. These patients often show an abrupt decrease in platelet count with a concomitant increase in LDH and AST levels after a trend toward normalization of values has begun. Generally, the laboratory abnormalities seen with HELLP syndrome resolve in 72 to 96 hours.

The nursing care of the woman with hypertensive disease differs in a number of respects from that required in a normal postpartum period. These variations in the nursing process are described in the following paragraphs.

Careful assessment of the woman with a hypertensive disorder continues throughout the postpartum period. Blood pressure is measured at least every 4 hours for 48 hours, or more often as the woman's condition warrants. Even if no convulsions occurred before the birth, they may occur within this period. $MgSO_4$ infusion may be continued up to 48 hours after the birth. The same assessments continue until the drug is discontinued.

NURSE ALERT • The woman is at risk for a boggy uterus and a large lochia flow as a result of $MgSO_4$ therapy. Uterine tone and lochial flow must be monitored closely.

The preeclamptic woman is hemoconcentrated and unable to tolerate excessive postpartum blood loss. Oxytocin or prostaglandin products are used to control bleeding. Ergot products (e.g., Ergotrate and Methergine) are contraindicated because they can increase blood pressure. The woman is asked to report symptoms such as headaches and blurred vision. The nurse assesses affect, level of consciousness, blood pressure, pulse, and respiratory status before an analgesic is given for headache. $MgSO_4$ potentiates the action of narcotics, CNS depressants, and calcium channel blockers; these medications need to be administered with caution. The woman may need to continue antihypertensive medication if her diastolic blood pressure exceeds 100 mm Hg at discharge.

The woman's and family's responses to labor, the birth, and the newborn are monitored. Interactions and involvement in the care of the newborn are encouraged as much as the woman and her family desire. In addition, the woman and her family need opportunities to discuss their emotional response to complications. The nurse also provides information concerning the prognosis. Preeclampsia and eclampsia do not necessarily recur in subsequent pregnancies (recurrence rate is approximately 30%), but careful prenatal care is essential.

If the outcome for the mother or baby is unfavorable, the family is assisted in coping with loss and grief.

Prevention. There have been numerous clinical trials describing various methods to prevent preeclampsia. The etiology continues to be unknown. Interventions used in the clinical trials include the use of low-dose aspirin, calcium, magnesium, zinc, and fish oil dietary supplementation. None of these interventions has proved beneficial. Nurses should be aware of what strategies are being studied and use the most reliable evidence about the results to counsel pregnant women about interventions that are likely to be beneficial. One resource is the Cochrane Pregnancy and Childbirth Database (Enkin et al, 1995).

➤ Evaluation

Evaluation of the effectiveness of care of the woman with preeclampsia is based on the expected outcomes.

HYPEREMESIS GRAVIDARUM

Nausea and vomiting complicates approximately 70% of all pregnancies, and is usually confined to the first trimester (Cruikshank et al, 1996). Although these manifestations are distressing, they are typically benign, with no significant alterations or risks to the mother or fetus.

When vomiting during pregnancy becomes excessive (i.e., enough to cause weight loss of at least 5% of prepregnancy weight) and is accompanied by dehydration, electrolyte imbalance, ketosis, and acetonuria, the disorder is termed hyperemesis gravidarum. The estimated incidence varies from 0.5 to 10 per 1000 births (Snell et al, 1998). Hyperemesis gravidarum usually begins during the first 10 weeks of pregnancy. Women with hyperemesis tend to be younger than 20 years of age, obese, and nonsmokers. They are also more likely to have multifetal or molar pregnancies (Riely, 1999).

Etiology

The etiology of hyperemesis gravidarum remains obscure. Several theories have been proposed as to the cause, although none of them adequately explains the disorder. Hyperemesis gravidarum may be related to high levels of estrogen or human chorionic gonadotropin and may be associated with transient hyperthyroidism during pregnancy. It may be accompanied by liver dysfunction manifested by elevated transaminase and abnormal bilirubin level and prothrombin time. Other possible causes include vitamin B deficiencies and increased sensitivity to circulating sex steroid hormones (Hill and Fleming, 1999; Riely, 1999; Snell et al, 1998).

Psychologic factors may also play a part in the development of hyperemesis gravidarum, at least in some women. Ambivalence toward the pregnancy, and difficult relationships with mothers or partners have been identified as causative factors. High stress levels are probably also associated with this condition (Hill and Fleming, 1999; Snell et al, 1998). Conflicting feelings regarding prospective motherhood, body changes, and lifestyle alterations—all normal reactions to pregnancy—may contribute to episodes of vomiting, particularly if these feelings are excessive or unresolved.

Clinical Manifestations

The woman with hyperemesis usually has significant weight loss and dehydration. She may have a decreased blood pressure, increased pulse rate, and poor skin turgor (Snell et al, 1998). She is almost always unable to keep down even clear liquids taken by mouth. Laboratory tests may reveal electrolyte imbalances.

Collaborative Care

Whenever a pregnant woman has a complaint of nausea and vomiting, the first priority is a thorough assessment to determine the severity of the problem. In most cases, the woman should be told to come immediately to the health care provider's office or to the emergency department, because the severity of illness is often difficult to determine by phone. Assessments should be made of the frequency, severity, and duration of episodes of nausea and vomiting. Other symptoms such as diarrhea, indigestion, and abdominal pain or distention are also identified. Pharmacologic and nonpharmacologic treatments should be recorded.

The woman's weight and vital signs are measured and a complete physical examination is performed, with attention to signs of fluid and electrolyte imbalance and nutritional status. The most important initial laboratory test to be obtained is a dipstick determination of ketonuria. Other laboratory tests that may be ordered include a urinalysis, CBC, electrolytes, liver enzymes, and bilirubin levels. These tests help rule out the presence of underlying diseases such a pyelonephritis, pancreatitis, cholecystitis, and hepatitis (Cruikshank et al, 1996). Because of the recognized association between hyperemesis gravidarum and hyperthyroidism, thyroid function may also be assessed.

Psychosocial assessment includes asking the woman about anxiety, fears, and concerns related to her own health and the effects on pregnancy outcome. Family members should be assessed both for anxiety and in regard to their role in providing support for the woman.

Initial Care. Initially the woman who is unable to keep down clear liquids by mouth will require IV therapy for correction of fluid and electrolyte imbalances. She should receive nothing by mouth until dehydration has been resolved and for at least 48 hours after vomiting has stopped (Cruikshank et al,

1996). In the past, women requiring IV therapy were admitted to the hospital. Today, they often are successfully managed at home. Antiemetic medications may be used if nausea and vomiting are uncontrolled; commonly used medications include pyridoxine, droperidol, diphenhydramine, and metoclopramide. Corticosteroids have also been used successfully to treat refractory hyperemesis gravidarum. Some women also benefit from psychotherapy or stress reduction techniques (Hill and Fleming, 1999; Snell et al, 1998). When the vomiting stops, feedings are started in small amounts at short intervals, and the diet is advanced slowly as tolerated. During therapy, the nurse observes the woman for signs of complications such as metabolic acidosis, jaundice, or hemorrhage, and alerts the physician should any of these occur.

In severe cases of hyperemesis gravidarum, enteral nutrition through a feeding tube or parenteral nutrition may be necessary to correct maternal nutritional deprivation. Total parenteral nutrition has also been used successfully (Hill and Fleming, 1999; Snell et al, 1998).

Accurate intake and output, including the amount of emesis, is an important aspect of nursing care. Oral hygiene while the woman is on NPO status and after episodes of vomiting helps allay associated discomforts. Assistance with positioning and providing a quiet, restful environment that is free from odors may increase the woman's comfort. When the woman begins responding to therapy, limited amounts of oral fluids and bland foods such as crackers and toast are begun. The diet is progressed slowly as tolerated by the woman until she is able to consume a nutritionally sound diet. Promoting adequate rest is important for the woman with hyperemesis; the nurse can assist in coordinating treatment measures and periods of visitation to provide opportunity for rest periods (Nursing Care Plan).

Nursing Care Plan — THE WOMAN WITH HYPEREMESIS GRAVIDARUM

NURSING DIAGNOSIS Altered nutrition: less than body requirements, related to nausea and persistent vomiting as evidenced by weight decrease as compared with prepregnant weight

EXPECTED OUTCOME Patient will exhibit no further weight losses and weight will stabilize. Patient will tolerate regular diet with adequate nutrients for pregnancy with no further nausea and vomiting.

Nursing Interventions/*Rationales*

Ascertain patient's prepregnant weight and monitor patient's current weight and intake and output *to provide a database for care planning.*

Resume oral diet as tolerated and prescribed by caregiver *to provide oral nutrition at optimum time.*

Provide small, frequent bland meals as patient tolerates *to assess patient's response to limited oral intake.*

Administer antiemetic medications as prescribed *to decrease or eliminate episodes of vomiting.*

Provide a quiet, restful environment *to decrease associated discomforts.*

Teach patient the importance of a low-fat, high-protein diet with fluids between meals *to provide optimum nutrition for fetal growth and keep nausea to a minimum.*

Refer to dietitian to develop optimum diet plan that is individualized to patient's current preferences, culture, and lifestyle *to encourage ongoing compliance.*

Discuss with patient the importance of contacting health care provider if intractable nausea and vomiting recur *to provide prompt treatment and avoid complications.*

NURSING DIAGNOSIS Fluid volume deficit related to excessive vomiting as evidenced by fluid and electrolyte imbalance

EXPECTED OUTCOME Patient's fluid and electrolyte balance will be restored.

Nursing Interventions/*Rationales*

Assess and document skin turgor, condition of mucous membranes, vital signs, and urine specific gravity *to provide database for planning care.*

Obtain daily weight *to provide ongoing evaluation of care.*

Monitor laboratory values and report deviations from normal *to prevent complications.*

Maintain accurate intake and output record *to assess for evidence of fluid deficit.*

Initiate and maintain IV therapy carefully *to maintain fluid balance.*

Administer antiemetics as prescribed *to inhibit nausea and vomiting.*

Begin oral fluids slowly and carefully *to slowly increase tolerance and restore fluid balance.*

NURSING DIAGNOSIS Anxiety related to effects of hyperemesis on fetal well-being as evidenced by patient statements of concern

EXPECTED OUTCOME Patient will exhibit decreased incidence of anxiety.

Nursing Interventions/*Rationales*

Use therapeutic communication to listen to patient concerns *to maintain a relationship and feeling of trust.*

Provide information regarding any potential risks to the fetus *to alleviate anxiety.*

Assist patient to identify personal strengths and previous coping mechanisms *to reinforce to patient those strengths and coping mechanisms that may be of assistance during this illness.*

Help patient identify sources of support and mobilize support person or group of her choice *to provide support as needed.*

Refer to social services as needed *to ensure ongoing evaluation and assistance.*

Home Care. Most women are able to take nourishment by mouth after several days of hospital or home care. Education at this time is important to prevent rapid recurrence of nausea and vomiting. Women should be encouraged to eat small, frequent meals consisting of low-fat, high-protein foods; to avoid greasy and highly seasoned foods; and to increase dietary intake of potassium and magnesium. Herbal teas such as chamomile and raspberry leaf may decrease nausea. Taking fluids between meals rather than with them sometimes helps decrease nausea. Many pregnant women find exposure to cooking odors nauseating; having other family members cook may decrease nausea. The woman is counseled to contact her health care provider immediately if the nausea and vomiting recurs, especially if accompanied by abdominal pain, dehydration, or weight loss greater than 2.3 kg in 1 week (Lowdermilk and Grohar, 1999).

A few women will continue to experience intractable nausea and vomiting throughout pregnancy. Rarely it may be necessary to maintain a woman on enteral, parenteral, or total parenteral nutrition in order to provide adequate nutrition for the mother and fetus. Many home health agencies are able to provide these services, and arrangements for service may be made depending on the woman's insurance coverage.

Regardless of the site of care, the woman needs calm, compassionate, and sympathetic care. Irritability, tearfulness, and mood changes are often consistent with this disorder. Fetal well-being is a primary concern of the woman. The family members should be included in the plan of care whenever possible. Their participation may help alleviate some of the emotional stress associated with this disorder. Psychologic counseling may be needed, as well as referral to a social worker. Usually hyperemesis gravidarum responds to therapy, and the prognosis is good.

HEMORRHAGIC DISORDERS

Bleeding in pregnancy may jeopardize maternal and fetal well-being. Maternal blood loss decreases oxygen-carrying capacity and predisposes the woman to increased risk for hypovolemia, anemia, infection, preterm labor, and preterm birth; and adversely affects oxygen delivery to the fetus. Fetal risks from maternal hemorrhage include blood loss or anemia, hypoxemia, hypoxia, anoxia, and preterm birth.

Hemorrhagic disorders in pregnancy are medical emergencies. It is estimated that 1 in 5 pregnancies is complicated by bleeding; the incidence and type of bleeding vary by trimester (Thorp, 1993). In the first trimester, most bleeding is a result of miscarriage and ectopic pregnancy. Approximately 50% of bleeding in the third trimester is caused by placenta previa and abruptio placentae (Cunningham et al, 1997). Antepartal hemorrhage is a leading cause of maternal death, with ectopic pregnancy rupture and abruptio placentae being responsible for

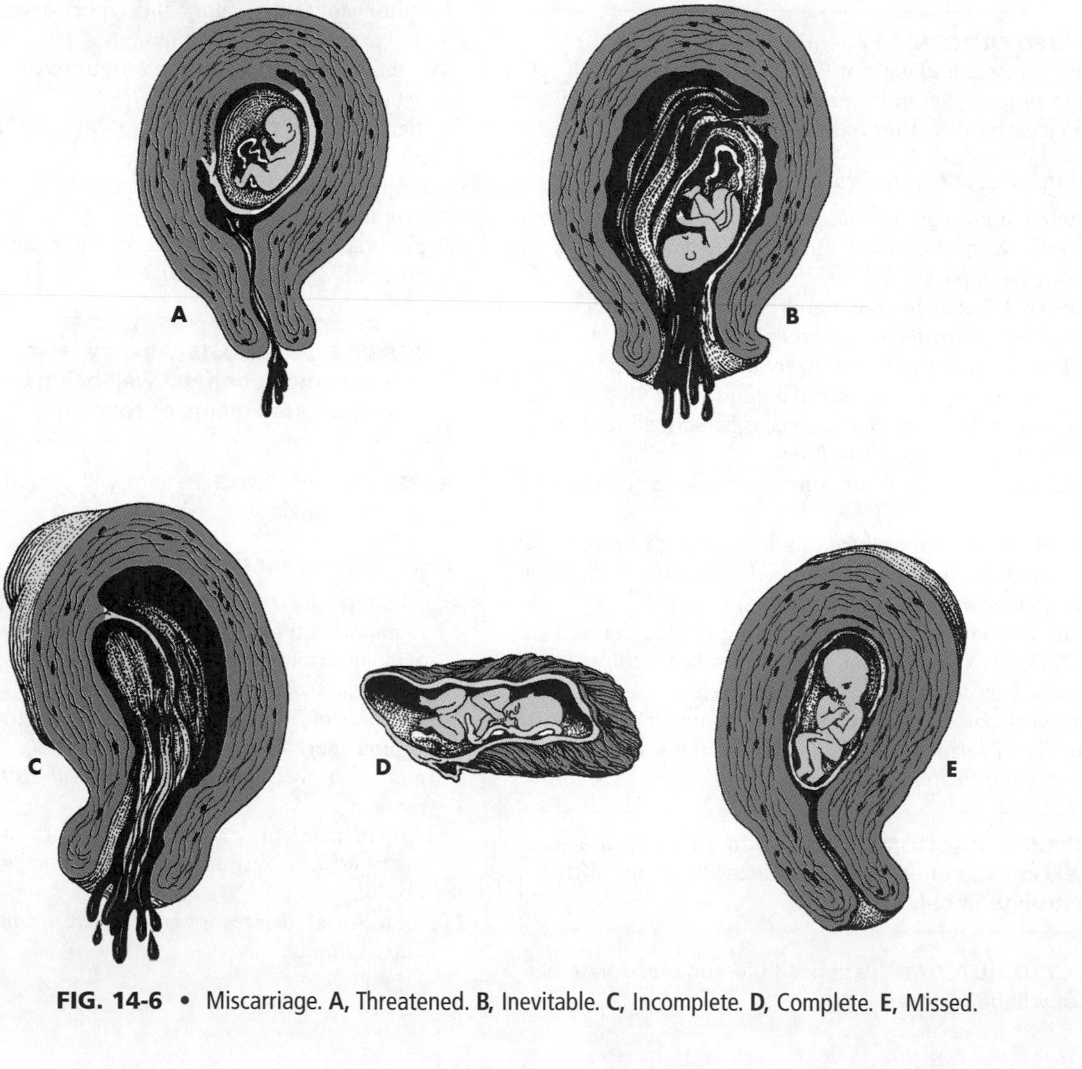

FIG. 14-6 • Miscarriage. **A,** Threatened. **B,** Inevitable. **C,** Incomplete. **D,** Complete. **E,** Missed.

most maternal deaths (Koonin et al, 1997). Blood loss can occur rapidly during pregnancy. With approximately 650 ml/minute (15% of maternal cardiac output) of blood flow to the uterine vasculature and placenta, disruption of vascular integrity has the potential for maternal exsanguination within 8 to 10 minutes (Knuppel and Hatangadi, 1995). Prompt, expert teamwork on the part of the health care providers is essential to save the lives of the mother and infant.

Early Pregnancy Bleeding

Bleeding during early pregnancy is alarming to the woman and of concern to health care providers. The common bleeding disorders of early pregnancy include miscarriage, premature dilation of the cervix, ectopic pregnancy, and hydatidiform mole (molar pregnancy).

Miscarriage. A pregnancy that ends before 20 weeks of gestation is defined as a miscarriage or spontaneous abortion. This 20-week marker is considered to be the point of viability, when a fetus may survive in an extrauterine environment. A fetal weight less than 500 g may also be used to define a miscarriage (Cunningham et al, 1997).

A miscarriage results from natural causes. Miscarriage is suggested as a more appropriate term to use with patients because abortion may be an insensitive term to use with families who are grieving a pregnancy loss (Freda, 1999). The term miscarriage is used throughout this discussion. The term abortion is used when discussing therapeutic or elective induced abortion (see Chapter 7).

Incidence and Etiology. Approximately 10% to 15% of all clinically recognized pregnancies end in miscarriage (Simpson, 1996). An early miscarriage is one that occurs before 12 weeks of gestation.

At least 50% of all clinically recognized pregnancy losses result from chromosomal abnormalities (Simpson, 1996). More than 90% of miscarriages occur early, before 8 weeks of gestation (Simpson, 1996). The causes of early abortion may include endocrine imbalance (as in women with luteal phase defects or who have insulin-dependent diabetes mellitus with high blood-glucose levels in the first trimester), immunologic factors (e.g., antiphospholipid antibodies), infections (e.g., bacteriuria and *Chlamydia trachomatis*), systemic disorders (e.g., systemic lupus erythematosus), and genetic factors (ACOG, 1995; Gilbert and Harmon, 1998).

A late miscarriage is one that occurs between 12 and 20 weeks of gestation. It usually results from maternal causes such as advancing maternal age and parity, chronic infections, premature dilation of the cervix and other anomalies of the reproductive tract, chronic debilitating diseases, inadequate nutrition, and recreational drug use (Cunningham et al, 1997). Little can be done to avoid genetic causes of pregnancy loss, but correction of maternal disorders, immunization against infectious diseases, adequate early prenatal care, and treatment of pregnancy complications can do much to prevent miscarriage.

Types. The types of miscarriage include threatened, inevitable, incomplete, complete, and missed (Fig. 14-6). All but the threatened miscarriage can lead to infection.

Clinical Manifestations. Signs and symptoms of miscarriage depend on the duration of the pregnancy. The presence of uterine bleeding, uterine contractions, or uterine pain is an ominous sign in early pregnancy that must be considered a threatened miscarriage until proven otherwise.

If miscarriage occurs before the sixth week of pregnancy, the woman may report a heavy menstrual flow. Miscarriage that occurs between the sixth and twelfth weeks of pregnancy causes moderate discomfort and blood loss. After the twelfth week, miscarriage is typified by more severe pain—similar to that of labor—because the fetus must be expelled. Diagnosis of the type of miscarriage is based on the signs and symptoms present (Table 14-4; see Fig. 14-6).

Symptoms of a threatened miscarriage (see Fig. 14-6, *A*) include spotting of blood and a closed cervical os. Mild uterine cramping may be present.

Inevitable (see Fig. 14-6, *B*) and incomplete (see Fig. 14-6, *C*) miscarriages involve a moderate to heavy amount of bleeding with an open cervical os. Tissue may be present with the bleeding. Mild to severe uterine cramping may be present. An inevitable miscarriage is often accompanied by rupture of membranes (ROM) and cervical dilation; passage of the products of conception will occur. An incomplete miscarriage involves the expulsion of the fetus with retention of the placenta (Cunningham et al, 1997).

TABLE 14-4
Types of Miscarriage and Usual Management

Type of Miscarriage	Management
Threatened	Bed rest, sedation, and avoidance of stress and orgasm are recommended. Further treatment depends on woman's response to treatment.
Inevitable and incomplete	Prompt termination of pregnancy is accomplished, usually by dilation and curettage (D&C).
Complete	No further intervention may be needed if uterine contractions are adequate to prevent hemorrhage and if there is no infection.
Missed	If spontaneous evacuation of uterus does not occur within 1 month, pregnancy is terminated by method appropriate to duration of pregnancy. Blood clotting factors are monitored until uterus is empty. DIC and incoagulability of blood with uncontrolled hemorrhage may develop in cases of fetal death after the twelfth week if products of conception are retained for longer than 5 weeks.
Septic	Immediate termination of pregnancy by method appropriate to duration of pregnancy. Cervical culture and sensitivity (C&S) studies are done, and broad-spectrum antibiotic therapy (e.g., ampicillin) is started. Treatment for septic shock is initiated if necessary.

In a complete miscarriage (see Fig. 14-6, *D*), all the fetal tissue is passed, the cervix is closed, and there may be slight bleeding. Mild uterine cramping may be present.

The term missed abortion (see Fig. 14-6, *E*) refers to a pregnancy in which the fetus has died but miscarriage does not occur. It may be diagnosed by ultrasonic examination after the uterus stops increasing in size or even decreases in size. There may be no bleeding or cramping, and the cervical os remains closed. If the products of conception are retained after a missed abortion, they may calcify, forming a uterine lithopedion or "womb stone" (see Fig. 14-6, *E*).

Recurrent early (habitual) miscarriage is the loss of three or more previable pregnancies.

Miscarriage can become septic, although this is not a common occurrence. Symptoms include fever and abdominal tenderness. Vaginal bleeding, which may be slight to heavy, is usually malodorous.

Care Management

➤ Assessment

A thorough assessment should be performed on the prenatal patient with vaginal bleeding in early pregnancy (Box 14-4). The data to be collected include pain, bleeding, and last menstrual period (LMP) to determine the approximate length of gestation. The initial database includes vital signs (a temperature higher than 38° C may indicate infection), previous pregnancies, previous pregnancy losses, type and location of pain, quantity and nature of bleeding, allergies, and emotional status.

Box 14-4

Assessment of Bleeding in Pregnancy

INITIAL DATABASE
Chief complaint
Vital signs
Gravidity, parity
LMP/Estimated date of birth (EDB)
Pregnancy history (previous and current)
Allergies
Nausea and vomiting
Pain (onset, quality, precipitating event)
Bleeding or coagulation problems
Level of consciousness
Emotional status

EARLY PREGNANCY
Confirmation of pregnancy
Bleeding (bright or dark, intermittent or continuous)
Pain (type, intensity, persistence)
Vaginal discharge

LATE PREGNANCY
EDB
Bleeding (quantity, associated pain)
Vaginal discharge
Amniotic membrane status
Uterine activity
Abdominal pain
Fetal status/viability

It is not uncommon for the woman and her family to be anxious and fearful regarding what may happen to her and to her pregnancy.

Various laboratory findings are characteristic of miscarriage. Evaluation of the placental hormone human chorionic gonadotropin (hCG) is used in the diagnosis of pregnancy and pregnancy loss. The β-subunit of hCG can be detected in maternal plasma and urine 8 to 9 days after ovulation if the woman is pregnant. In early pregnancy, the concentration of β-hCG should double every 1.4 to 2.0 days until about 60 or 70 days of gestation (Cunningham et al, 1997). Before 8 weeks of gestation, if miscarriage is suspected, two serum quantitative β-hCG levels are drawn 48 hours apart. If a normal pregnancy is present, the β-hCG level doubles within that time. Ultrasonography can then be used to determine the presence of a viable gestational sac. With considerable or persistent blood loss, anemia is likely (hemoglobin level less than 10.5 g/dl). If infection is present, the white blood cell count is greater than 12,000/mm^3. Sedimentation rate is not helpful for differential diagnostic purposes because an increased sedimentation rate occurs with pregnancy, anemia, or infection.

➤ Nursing Diagnoses

The following nursing diagnoses are appropriate for the woman experiencing a miscarriage:

- Anxiety/fear related to:
  —Unknown outcome and unfamiliarity with medical procedures
- Fluid volume deficit related to:
  —Excessive bleeding secondary to miscarriage
- Anticipatory grieving related to:
  —Unexpected pregnancy outcome
- Situational low self-esteem related to:
  —Inability to successfully carry a pregnancy to term gestation

➤ Expected Outcomes

Mutually determined expected outcomes for the woman experiencing miscarriage include that the woman will do the following:

- Discuss the impact of the loss on her and her family.
- Identify and use available support systems.
- Develop no signs and symptoms of complications (e.g., hemorrhage or infection).
- Verbalize relief from pain.

➤ Plan of Care and Implementation

Immediate nursing care focuses on physiologic stabilization. Typical orders to be followed would be initiation of an intravenous line, request for blood testing of hemoglobin and hematocrit, blood type and Rh, and indirect Coombs screen. An ultrasound is performed for diagnostic confirmation.

Medical Management. Medical management of miscarriage (see Table 14-4) depends on the classification and on signs and symptoms. Traditionally, threatened miscarriages have been managed with bed rest and supportive care. Follow-up treatment depends on whether the threatened miscarriage progresses to actual miscarriage, or symptoms subside and the pregnancy remains intact. Dilation and curettage (D&C) is a surgical procedure in which the cervix is dilated and a curette is inserted to scrape the uterine walls and remove uterine contents. A D&C is commonly used to treat inevitable and incomplete miscarriages. The nurse reinforces explanations, answers any questions or concerns, and prepares the woman for surgery.

Dilation and evacuation, performed after 16 weeks of gestation, consists of wide cervical dilation followed by instrumental removal of the uterine contents.

Before either surgical procedure is performed, a full history should be obtained, and general and pelvic examinations should be performed. General preoperative and postoperative care is appropriate for the woman requiring surgical intervention. Analgesia and anesthesia appropriate to the procedure are used.

For late incomplete or inevitable miscarriages (16 to 20 weeks) and missed abortions, prostaglandins may be administered into the amniotic sac or by vaginal suppository to augment or induce labor and cause the products of conception to be expelled. IV oxytocin may also be used.

Nursing care is similar to care for any woman whose labor is being induced (see Chapter 19). Special care may be needed for management of side effects of prostaglandin such as nausea and vomiting and diarrhea.

After evacuation of the uterus, 10 to 20 U of oxytocin in 1000 ml of fluids may be given to prevent hemorrhage. For excessive bleeding, ergot products (e.g., ergonovine) or a prostaglandin derivative (e.g., carboprost tromethamine) may be given to contract the uterus. Three or four doses of ergonovine (e.g., 0.2 mg orally or IM every 4 hours) may be given if the woman is normotensive. A 25-mg dose of carboprost may be given IM every 15 to 90 minutes for as many as eight doses (Cunningham et al, 1997). Antibiotics are given as necessary. Analgesics, such as antiprostaglandin agents, may decrease discomfort from cramping. Transfusion may be required for shock or anemia. If the woman is Rh negative and has not developed isoimmunization, she is given an intramuscular injection of Rh_o(D) immune globulin within 72 hours of the miscarriage.

Psychosocial aspects of care focus on what the pregnancy loss means to the woman and her family. How real the pregnancy and her baby are to the woman is thought to determine the intensity of grief response (Hutti, dePacheco, and Smith, 1998). Explanations of expected procedures, possible complications, and future implications for childbearing are provided.

As with other fetal or neonatal loss, the woman should be offered the option of seeing the products of conception. She may also want to know what the hospital does with the products of conception or whether she needs to make a decision about final disposition of fetal remains.

Home Care. The woman will be discharged home postoperatively after a D&C when vital signs are stable, vaginal bleeding remains minimal, and she is alert after anesthesia. Discharge teaching emphasizes the need for rest. If significant blood loss occurred, iron supplementation may be ordered. Teaching includes information about normal physical findings, such as cramping and type and amount of bleeding, resumption of sexual activity, and family planning. Follow-up care should assess the woman's physical and emotional recovery. Referrals to local support groups or counseling are provided as necessary (Patient Teaching box).

➤ Evaluation

Evaluation is based on the predetermined patient-centered outcomes.

Recurrent Premature Dilation of Cervix (Incompetent Cervix). Passive and painless dilation of the cervical os without labor or contractions of the uterus (incompetent cervix) may occur in the second trimester or early in the third trimester of pregnancy; miscarriage or preterm birth may result. This assumes an "all or nothing" role for the cervix; it is either "competent" or "incompetent." Current researchers contend that cervical competence is variable and exists as a continuum that is determined in part by cervical length. Other related causative factors include composition of the cervical tissue and the individual circumstances associated with the pregnancy in terms of maternal stress and lifestyle. Iams (1996) refers to this condition as abnormal or reduced cervical competence, whereas Freda (1999) prefers the term premature dilation of the cervix.

Etiology. Etiologic factors include a history of cervical lacerations during childbirth, excessive cervical dilation for curettage or biopsy, or ingestion of diethylstilbestrol (DES) by the woman's mother while pregnant with the woman. Other causes are a congenitally short cervix, and cervical or uterine anomalies. Reduced cervical competence is a clinical diagnosis based on history. Short labors and recurring loss of the pregnancy at progressively earlier gestational ages are characteristics of reduced cervical competence. Ultrasound is used for diagnosis; a short cervix (i.e., less than 20 mm in length) is indicative of reduced cervical competence. Often, but not always, the short cervix is accompanied by cervical funneling or effacement of the internal cervical os (Iams, 1996).

Collaborative Care. The nurse assesses the woman's feelings about her pregnancy and her understanding of reduced cervical competence. It is important to evaluate the woman's support systems. Because the diagnosis of reduced cervical competence is usually not made until the woman has lost one or two pregnancies, she may feel guilty or to blame for this impending loss. It is therefore important to assess for previous reactions to stress and for appropriateness of coping responses. The woman needs the support of her health care providers as well as that of her family.

Medical Management. Conservative management consists of bed rest, hydration, and tocolysis (inhibition of uterine con-

Patient Teaching

DISCHARGE TEACHING FOR WOMAN AFTER MISCARRIAGE

- Maintain appropriate perineal care; shower only for 2 weeks
- To reduce risk of infection, introduce nothing into the vagina until bleeding has stopped
- Notify physician of elevated temperature or foul-smelling vaginal discharge
- Eat foods high in iron and protein for RBC replacement and to promote tissue repair
- Notify physician if fatigue persists beyond 2 weeks
- Make appropriate referrals to community resources
- Provide supportive counseling, discuss importance of grieving the loss before becoming pregnant again
- Pregnancy should be postponed for at least 2 months to allow her body to recover

From Gilbert E, Harmon J: *Manual of high risk pregnancy and delivery,* ed 2, St Louis, 1998, Mosby.

tractions). A cervical cerclage may be performed. During pregnancy a McDonald cerclage, a band of homologous fascia, or nonabsorbable ribbon (Mersilene) may be placed around the cervix beneath the mucosa to constrict the internal os of the cervix (Fig. 14-7).

Prophylactic cerclage is placed at 10 to 14 weeks of gestation, after which the woman is told to refrain from intercourse, prolonged (i.e., more than 90 minutes) standing, and heavy lifting. She is followed during the course of her pregnancy with ultrasound scans to assess for cervical shortening and funneling.

The cerclage is electively removed (usually an office or a clinic procedure) when the woman reaches 37 weeks of gestation, or it may be left in place and a cesarean birth performed. Approximately 80% to 90% of pregnancies treated with cerclage result in live, viable births (Iams, 1996). If removed, the cerclage must be repeated with each successive pregnancy. Cerclage is rarely performed after 26 weeks of gestation (Iams, 1996).

A second method involves placement of a pursestring ligature to maintain a closed cervix. This procedure, the Shirodkar, allows for the suture to remain in place permanently for the woman that anticipates future pregnancies. Births are accomplished by cesarean.

Nursing Management. If a cervical cerclage is performed, the nurse monitors the woman postoperatively for contractions, ROM, and signs of infection. Discharge teaching focuses on continued monitoring of these aspects at home. Home uterine monitoring may be indicated with follow-up from a home health agency.

Antepartal Home Care. The woman must understand the importance of activity restriction at home and the need for close observation and supervision. Instruction includes the rationale for bed rest or activity restriction, and warning signs of preterm labor (Lowdermilk and Grohar, 1999).

Tocolytics may be given to prevent uterine contractions and further dilation of the cervix. The woman must be instructed on the importance of taking oral tocolytic medication as prescribed, on the expected response, and about possible side effects. If home monitoring is implemented, she is taught how to apply a uterine contraction monitor and transmit the monitor tracing by telephone to the monitoring center. Nurses at the monitoring center assess the tracing for contractions, answer questions, provide emotional support and education, and report information to the woman's physician or midwife. The woman should know the signs that warrant immediate transfer to the hospital, including strong contractions less than 5 minutes apart, rupture of membranes, severe perineal pressure, and an urge to push (Health Care Resources, 1997). If management is unsuccessful and the fetus is born before viability, appropriate grief support should be provided. If the birth is premature, appropriate anticipatory guidance and support are necessary.

Ectopic Pregnancy

Incidence and Etiology. An ectopic pregnancy is one in which the fertilized ovum is implanted outside the uterine cavity (Fig. 14-8). It accounts for 2% of all pregnancies in the United States (Flystra, 1998).

About 95% of ectopic pregnancies occur in the uterine (fallopian) tube, with most located on the ampullar or largest portion of the tube. Other sites include the ovary (1%), abdominal cavity (3% to 4%), and cervix (1%).

Ectopic pregnancy is responsible for 10% of all maternal mortality; it is the leading pregnancy-related cause of first trimester maternal mortality (Powell and Spellman, 1996; Simpson, 1996). Moreover, ectopic pregnancy is a leading cause of infertility. Only about 60% of women who have been treated for ectopic pregnancy are able to conceive afterward, and ap-

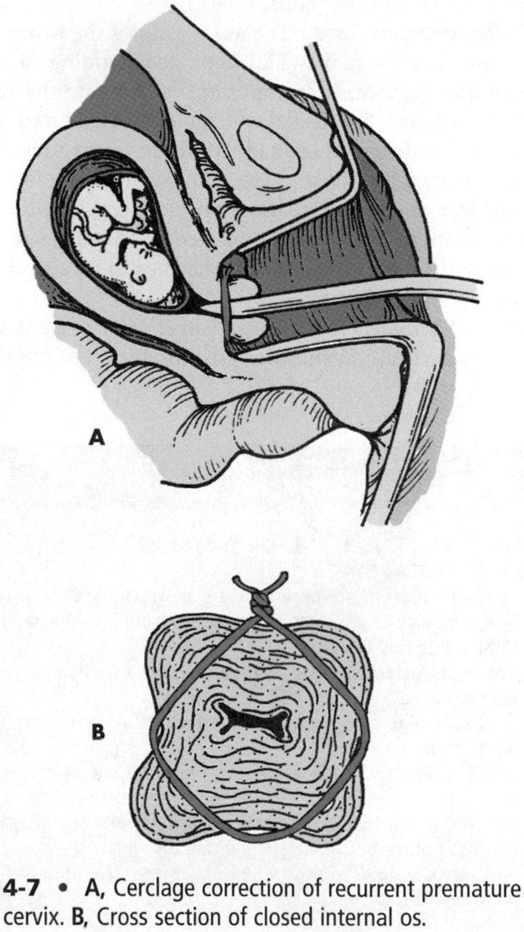

FIG. 14-7 • A, Cerclage correction of recurrent premature dilation of cervix. B, Cross section of closed internal os.

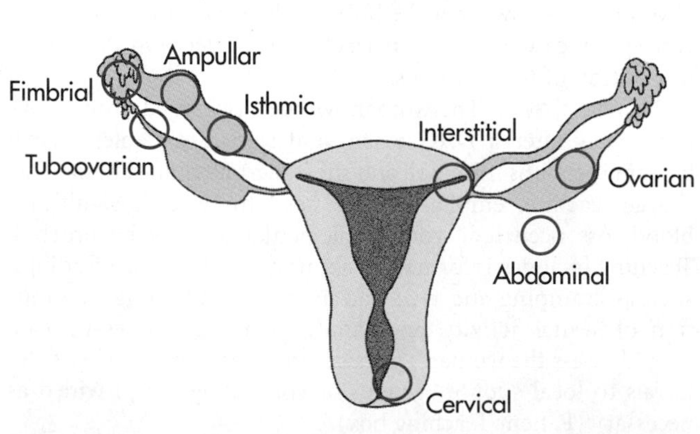

FIG. 14-8 • Sites of implantation of ectopic pregnancies. Order of frequency of occurrence is ampullar, isthmic, interstitial, fimbrial, tuboovarian ligament, ovarian, abdominal cavity, and cervical (external os).

proximately 40% of those pregnancies are ectopic (Powell and Spellman, 1996).

The incidence of ectopic pregnancy is rising due to improved diagnostic techniques and an increased incidence of STIs, better treatment of pelvic inflammatory disease (which formerly would have caused sterility), increased numbers of tubal sterilizations, and surgical reversal of tubal sterilizations (Simpson, 1996).

Ectopic pregnancy is classified according to the site of implantation (e.g., tubal or ovarian). The uterus is the only organ capable of containing and sustaining a term pregnancy. However, 5% to 25% of abdominal pregnancies, with birth by laparotomy, may result in a living infant (Fig. 14-9). The risk of deformity in these infants is as high as 40% (Gilbert and Harmon, 1998).

Clinical Manifestations. A missed menstrual period, adnexal fullness, and tenderness may suggest an unruptured tubal pregnancy. The tenderness can progress from a dull pain to a colicky pain when the tube stretches. Pain may be unilateral, bilateral, or diffuse over the abdomen. Abnormal vaginal bleeding occurs in 50% to 80% of women. If an ectopic pregnancy ruptures, pain increases. This pain may be generalized, unilateral, or acute deep lower quadrant pain caused by blood irritating the peritoneum. Referred shoulder pain can occur from diaphragmatic irritation caused by blood in the peritoneal cavity. The woman may exhibit signs of shock related to the amount of bleeding in the abdominal cavity and not necessarily related to obvious vaginal bleeding. An ecchymotic blueness around the umbilicus (Cullen's sign), indicating hematoperitoneum, may develop in a undiagnosed, ruptured intraabdominal ectopic pregnancy.

Diagnosis. The differential diagnosis of ectopic pregnancy involves consideration of numerous disorders that share many signs and symptoms. Miscarriage, ruptured corpus luteum cyst, appendicitis, salpingitis, ovarian cysts, torsion of the ovary, and urinary tract infection must be considered (Table 14-5). Diagnostic evaluation for ectopic pregnancy includes laboratory testing and vaginal sonography.

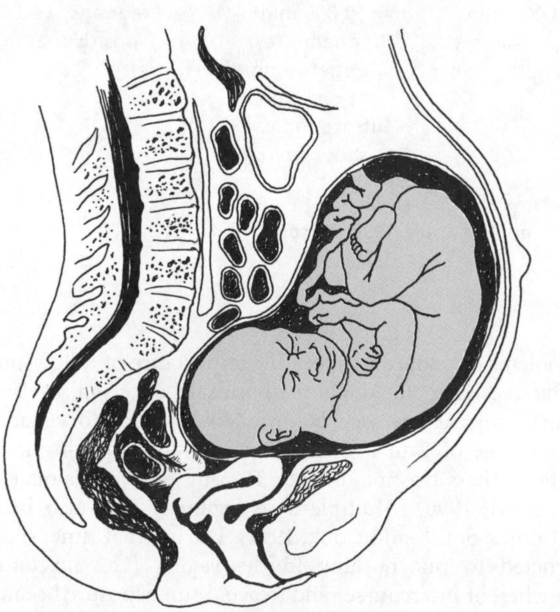

FIG. 14-9 • Ectopic pregnancy, abdominal.

Most ectopic pregnancies occur in the uterine tube; in the past, these were usually diagnosed at the time of rupture, when the major management problem was hemorrhage. Often laparotomy, followed by removal of the entire uterine tube, was the treatment necessary to control bleeding and save the woman's life.

Removal of the ectopic pregnancy by salpingostomy is possible before rupture. Residual tissue is dissolved with a dose of methotrexate postoperatively. Methotrexate is a folic acid analog that destroys the rapidly dividing cells (DeLoia, Stewart-Akers, and Creinin, 1998). It may also be used in a single-dose intramuscular injection to treat unruptured pregnancies (Lipscomb et al, 1998). It has been shown to produce results similar to those of surgical therapy in terms of high success rate, low complication rate, and good reproductive potential (Simpson, 1996).

Advanced ectopic abdominal pregnancy requires laparotomy as soon as the woman has been stabilized for surgery. If the placenta of a second- or third-trimester abdominal pregnancy is attached to a vital organ, such as the liver, separation and removal are usually not attempted because of risk of hemorrhage. The cord is cut flush with the placenta and the abdomen is closed, leaving the placenta in place. Degeneration and absorption of the placenta usually occur without complication, although infection and intestinal obstruction may occur. Methotrexate may be given to dissolve the residual tissue (Cunningham et al, 1997).

Collaborative Care. The key to early detection of ectopic pregnancy is having a high index of suspicion for this condition. Any woman with complaints of abdominal pain, vaginal spotting or bleeding, and a positive pregnancy test should undergo screening for ectopic pregnancy. Laboratory screening includes determination of serum progesterone and β-hCG levels. If either of these values is lower than would be expected for a normal pregnancy, the woman is asked to return within 48 hours for serial measurements. At this time, the woman will also undergo transvaginal ultrasound to confirm intrauterine or tubal pregnancy (Powell and Spellman, 1996).

The woman is also assessed for the presence of active bleeding, which is associated with tubal rupture. If internal bleeding is present, assessment may reveal vertigo, shoulder pain, hypotension, and tachycardia. A vaginal examination should be performed only once, and then with great caution. Approximately half of women with tubal pregnancies have a palpable mass on examination. It is possible to rupture the mass during a bimanual examination, so gentleness is critical (Simpson, 1996).

Hospital Care. Once an ectopic pregnancy is suspected, the physician is notified of assessment findings. Vital signs (i.e., pulse, respirations, and blood pressure) are assessed every 15 minutes or as needed based on severity of the bleeding and the woman's condition. Laboratory tests include determination of blood type and Rh factor, CBC, and serum quantitative β-hCG values. Ultrasonography is used to confirm an extrauterine pregnancy. General preoperative and postoperative care is appropriate for the woman requiring surgical intervention for an ectopic pregnancy. Blood replacement may be necessary. The nurse verifies the woman's Rh and antibody status and administers $Rh_o(D)$ immune globulin if appropriate. The woman

TABLE 14-5
Differential Diagnosis of Ectopic Pregnancy

	Ectopic Pregnancy	Appendicitis	Salpingitis	Ruptured Ovarian Cyst	Miscarriage
Pain	Unilateral cramps and tenderness before rupture May be colicky after rupture Sudden sharp abdominal pelvic pain Abdominal tenderness	Epigastric, periumbilical, then right lower quadrant pain, tenderness localizing at McBurney's point, rebound tenderness	Usually in both lower quadrants with or without rebound Mild to severe pelvic pressure	Unilateral, becoming general with progressive bleeding, dull cramping	Mild uterine cramps to severe uterine pain
Nausea and vomiting	Occasionally before, frequently after rupture	Usual, precedes shift of pain to right lower quadrant	Infrequent	Rare	Almost never
Menstruation	Some aberration, missed period, spotting	Unrelated to menses	Hypermenorrhea, metrorrhagia, or both	Period delayed, then bleeding, often with pain	Amenorrhea, then spotting, then brisk bleeding
Temperature, pulse, and blood pressure	37.2°-37.8° C, pulse variable, normal before and rapid after rupture, ↓BP after rupture	37.2°-37.8° C, pulse rapid	37.2°-40° C: pulse elevated in proportion to fever	Not over 37.2° C, pulse normal unless blood loss marked, then rapid	To 37.2° C Signs of shock related to obvious bleeding
Pelvic examination	Unilateral tenderness, especially on movement of cervix, crepitant mass on one side or in cul-de-sac; dark red or brown vaginal discharge	No masses, rectal tenderness high on right side No vaginal discharge	Bilateral tenderness on movement of cervix Purulent discharge	Tenderness over affected ovary, no masses	Cervix open or closed, uterus slightly enlarged, irregularly softened, tender with infection, vaginal bleeding
Laboratory findings	White blood cell count (WBC) to 15,000/mm³ Pregnancy test positive Ultrasound to rule out pregnancy after 6 weeks	WBC 10,000-18,000/mm³ (rarely normal) Pregnancy test negative	WBC 15,000-30,000/mm³ Pregnancy test negative	WBC normal to 10,000/mm³ Pregnancy test negative unless also pregnant Ultrasound will show ovarian cyst	WBC normal Pregnancy test positive

Modified from Gilbert E, Harmon J: *Manual of high risk pregnancy and delivery,* ed 2, St Louis, 1998, Mosby.

should be encouraged to verbalize her feelings related to the loss. Referral to community resources may be appropriate.

Home Care. Hemodynamically stable women with ectopic pregnancies are eligible for methotrexate therapy if the mass is unruptured and measures less than 4 cm in diameter by ultrasound (Simpson, 1996). Methotrexate therapy avoids surgery and is a safe, effective, and cost-effective way of managing many cases of tubal pregnancy. Management is almost always accomplished on an outpatient basis.

The woman is informed how the medication works, what adverse effects are possible, who to call if she has concerns or if problems develop, and about the importance of follow-up care. After receiving the single methotrexate injection, the woman must return at least weekly for follow-up laboratory studies for an average of 2 to 8 weeks. A repeat dose may be necessary if hCG titers do not drop to 15% by day 7 (Maiolatesi and Petticord, 1996). Multiple-dose regimens may also be given (Minnick-Smith and Cook, 1997). During that time, she is instructed to put nothing in the vagina (i.e., no tampons, douches, or intercourse) and to avoid sun exposure because the drug will make her more photosensitive (Powell and Spellman, 1996).

NURSE ALERT • The woman on methotrexate therapy who drinks alcohol and takes vitamins continuing folic acid (e.g., prenatal vitamins) increases her risk of experiencing side effects of the drug or of exacerbating the ectopic rupture.

Future fertility should be discussed. Any woman who has been diagnosed with an ectopic pregnancy should be told to contact her health care provider as soon as she suspects that she might be pregnant because of the increased risk for recurrent ectopic pregnancy. These women may need referral to grief or infertility support groups. In addition to the loss of the current pregnancy, they are faced with the possibility of future pregnancy losses and infertility.

Hydatidiform Mole. Hydatidiform mole (molar pregnancy) is a gestational trophoblastic disease. There are two distinct types: complete (or classic) mole; and partial mole.

Incidence and Etiology. Hydatidiform mole occurs in 1 in 1200 pregnancies in the United States, but a higher incidence has been reported in Asian countries (Berman, DiSaia, and Brewster, 1999). The etiology is unknown, although there may be an ovular defect or nutritional deficiency. Women at higher risk for hydatidiform mole are those who have undergone ovulation stimulation with clomiphene (Clomid) and those who are in their early teens or over age 40. The risk of developing a second mole is 1% to 2%.

Types. The complete mole results from fertilization of an egg whose nucleus has been lost or inactivated. The mole resembles a bunch of white grapes (Fig. 14-10). The hydropic (fluid-filled) vesicles grow rapidly, causing the uterus to be larger than expected for the duration of the pregnancy. Usually the complete mole contains no fetus, placenta, amniotic membranes, or fluid. Maternal blood has no placenta to receive it; therefore hemorrhage into the uterine cavity and vaginal bleeding occur. In about 20% of complete moles, progression toward choriocarcinoma occurs.

A partial mole occurs as a result of two sperm fertilizing an apparently normal ovum. Partial moles often have embryonic or fetal parts and an amniotic sac. Congenital anomalies are usually present. The potential for malignant transformation is about 2% to 4% (Copeland and Landon, 1996).

Clinical Manifestations. In the early stages the clinical manifestations of a complete hydatidiform mole cannot be distinguished from normal pregnancy. Later, vaginal bleeding occurs in almost 95% of patients. The vaginal discharge may be dark brown (resembling prune juice) or bright red, and either scant or profuse. It may continue for only a few days or intermittently for weeks. In early pregnancy, in about half of affected women, the uterus is significantly larger than expected from menstrual dates.

Anemia from blood loss, excessive nausea and vomiting (hyperemesis gravidarum), and abdominal cramps caused by uterine distention are relatively common findings. Preeclampsia occurs in about 15% of cases (usually between 9 and 12 weeks of gestation), but any symptoms of pregnancy-induced hypertension before 24 weeks of gestation may suggest hydatidiform mole. Hyperthyroidism and pulmonary embolization of trophoblastic elements occur less commonly but are serious complications of hydatidiform mole. Partial mole causes few of these symptoms and may be mistaken for an incomplete miscarriage or missed abortion.

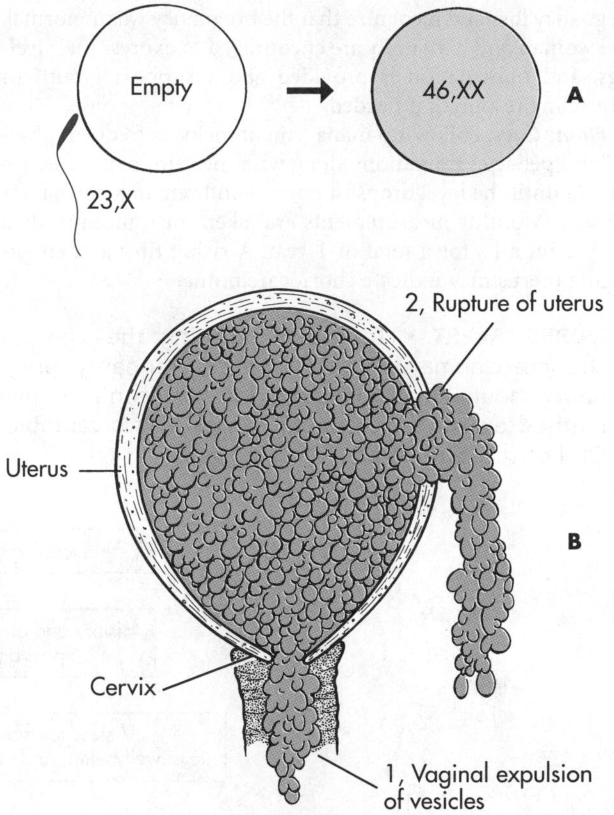

FIG. 14-10 • **A,** Chromosomal origin of complete mole. Single sperm (in color) fertilizes an "empty" ovum. Reduplication of sperm's 23,X set gives completely homozygous diploid 46,XX. Similar process follows fertilization of empty ovum by two sperm with two independently drawn sets of 23,X or 23,Y; both karyotypes of 46,XX and 46,YY can therefore result. **B,** Uterine rupture with hydatidiform mole. 1, Evacuation of mole through cervix. 2, Rupture of uterus and spillage of mole into peritoneal cavity (rare).

Collaborative Care. Nursing assessments during prenatal visits should include observation for signs of molar pregnancy during the first 24 weeks. If hydatidiform mole is suspected, ultrasonography and serial β-hCG immunoassays will be used to confirm the diagnosis. The sonographic pattern of a molar pregnancy is characterized by a diffuse snowstorm appearance. The hCG titer remains high or rises above the normal peak after the time it normally drops (i.e., 70 to 100 days) (Cunningham et al, 1997).

Medical-Surgical Management. Although most moles pass spontaneously, suction curettage offers a safe, rapid, and effective method of evacuation of hydatidiform mole if necessary (Gilbert and Harmon, 1998). Induction of labor with oxytocic agents or prostaglandins is not recommended because of the increased risk of embolization of trophoblastic tissue (Copeland and Landon, 1996). Administration of $Rh_o(D)$ immune globulin to women who are Rh negative is needed to prevent isoimmunization.

Nursing Care. The nurse provides the woman and her family with information about the disease process, the necessity for a long course of follow-up, and the possible consequences of the disease. The nurse helps the woman understand and cope with pregnancy loss and recognize that the pregnancy was abnormal. The woman and her family are encouraged to express their feelings, and information is provided about support groups or counseling resources if needed.

Home Care. Follow-up management includes frequent physical and pelvic examinations along with measurement of serum β-hCG until the level drops to normal and remains normal for 3 weeks. Monthly measurements are taken for 6 months, then every 2 months for a total of 1 year. A rising titer and an enlarging uterus may indicate choriocarcinoma.

NURSE ALERT • To avoid confusing the signs of choriocarcinoma with the signs of pregnancy, pregnancy should be avoided for 1 year. Any contraceptive method except the intrauterine device is acceptable. Oral contraceptives are highly effective.

Late Pregnancy Bleeding

Late pregnancy bleeding disorders include placenta previa, premature separation of placenta (abruptio placentae), and variations in the insertion of the cord and the placenta. Expedient assessment for and diagnosis of the cause of bleeding are essential to reduce maternal and perinatal morbidity and mortality (Fig. 14-11).

Placenta Previa. In placenta previa, the placenta is implanted in the lower uterine segment near or over the internal cervical os. The degree to which the internal cervical os is covered by the placenta has traditionally been used to classify three types of placenta previa (Fig. 14-12). Placenta previa often is described as complete, total, or central if the internal os is entirely covered by the placenta when the cervix is fully dilated. Partial placenta previa implies incomplete coverage of the internal os. Marginal placenta previa indicates that only an edge of the pla-

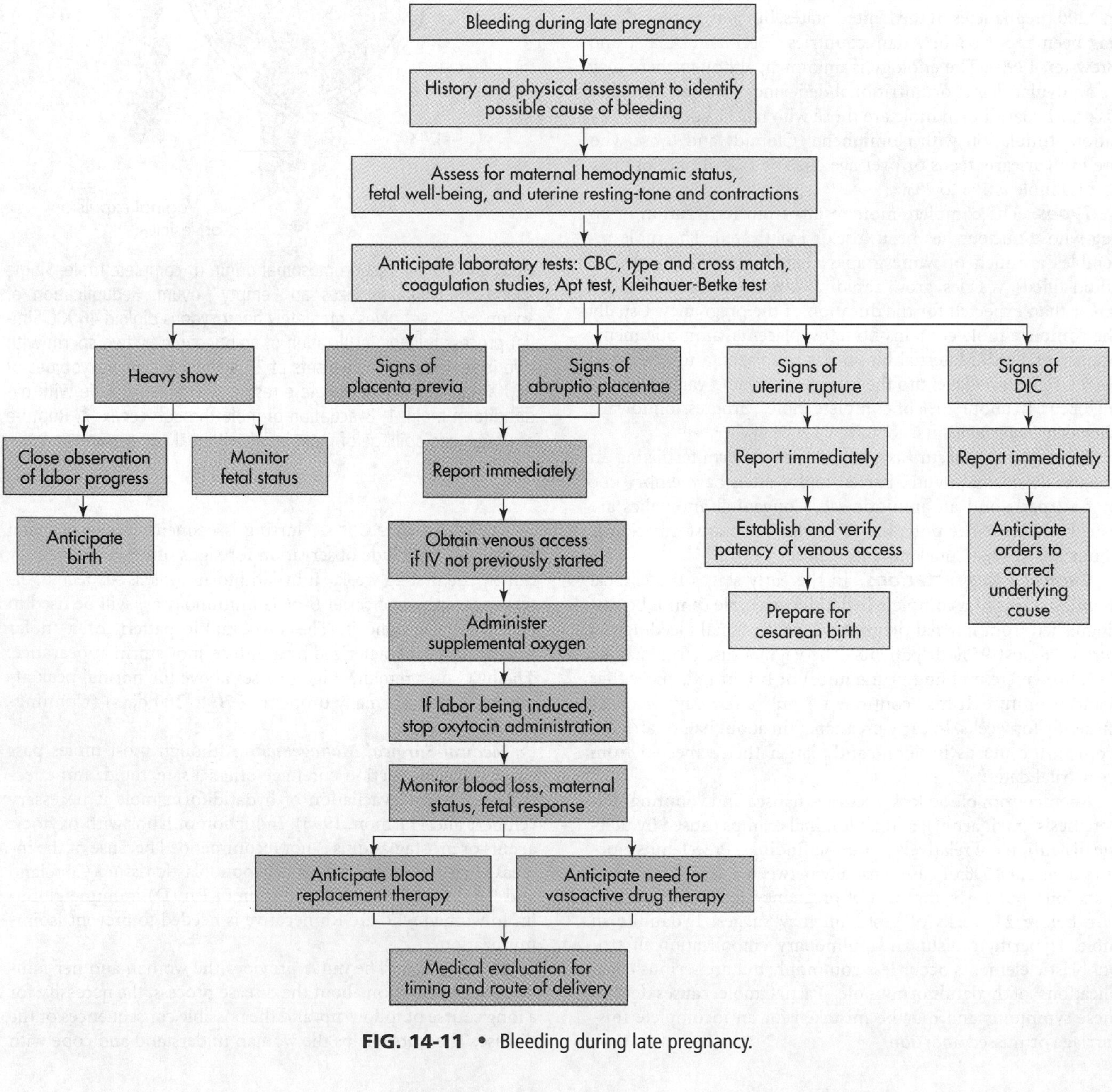

FIG. 14-11 • Bleeding during late pregnancy.

centa extends to the internal os, but may extend onto the os during dilation of the cervix during labor. The term low-lying placenta is used when the placenta is implanted in the lower uterine segment but does not reach the os.

Incidence and Etiology. The incidence of placenta previa is approximately 0.5% of births (Clark, 1999). The most important risk factors are previous placenta previa, previous cesarean birth, and induced abortion, possibly related to endometrial scarring (Ananth, Smulian, and Vintzileos, 1997). The risk also increases with multiple gestation (because of the larger placental area), closely spaced pregnancies, maternal age over 35 years, African or Asian ethnicity, smoking, and cocaine use (Clark, 1999).

Clinical Manifestations. About 70% of women with placenta previa have painless uterine bleeding; 20% have vaginal bleeding associated with uterine activity. Previa should be suspected whenever vaginal bleeding occurs after 24 weeks of gestation. This bleeding is associated with the stretching and thinning of the lower uterine segment that occurs during the third trimester. Placental attachment is gradually disrupted and bleeding occurs when the uterus is not able to contract adequately and stop blood flow from open vessels (Benedetti, 1996). The initial bleeding is usually a small amount and stops as clots form; however, it can recur at any time (Table 14-6). It is bright red in color.

Vital signs may be normal even with heavy blood loss, because a pregnant woman can lose up to 40% of blood volume without showing signs of shock. Clinical presentation and decreasing urinary output may be better indicators of acute blood loss than vital signs alone. The fetal heart rate is reassuring unless there is a major detachment of the placenta (Gilbert and Harmon, 1998).

Abdominal examination usually reveals a soft, relaxed, nontender uterus with normal tone. If the fetus is lying longitudinally, the fundal height is usually greater than expected for gestational age because the low placenta hinders descent of the presenting fetal part. Leopold's maneuvers may reveal a fetus in an oblique or breech position or lying transverse because of the abnormal site of placental implantation.

Diagnosis and Medical Management. The standard for the diagnosis of placenta previa is a transabdominal ultrasound examination. It is accurate 93% to 97% of the time. Transvaginal ultrasound examination may also be used in these situations. If ultrasound scanning reveals a normally implanted placenta, a speculum examination is performed to rule out local causes of bleeding (e.g., cervicitis, polyps, or carcinoma of the cervix). If expectant management is to be implemented, a vaginal speculum examination is postponed until fetal viability is reached (preferably after 34 weeks of gestation). If a pelvic examination is needed before that time, anticipate the possibility that an immediate cesarean birth may be required. The woman is taken to a delivery or operating room set up for cesarean birth because profound hemorrhage can occur during the examination. This type of vaginal examination, known as the double-setup procedure, is not often performed.

Management of placenta previa depends on the gestational age of the fetus and the amount of bleeding present. It includes expectant management and cesarean birth. Expectant management (observation and bed rest) usually is implemented when the fetus is not mature. Women may be placed in the hospital on complete bed rest or managed at home. If a woman is bleeding, she is usually placed in the labor and birth unit, where she and the fetus can be closely monitored.

Blood loss may not cease with the infant's birth. The large vascular channels in the lower uterine segment may continue to bleed because of the diminished muscle content of the lower uterine segment. The natural mechanism to control bleeding—the interlacing muscle bundles contracting around open vessels (the "living ligature" characteristic of the upper part of the uterus)—is absent in the lower part of the uterus. Therefore

Critical Thinking

PLACENTA PREVIA

Marta is a 26-year-old woman who is G6, P4 A1 at 26-weeks gestation seen in the emergency room with bright red vaginal bleeding.

- **What are the possible diagnoses for Marta? What physical assessment, laboratory tests, and diagnostic procedures would you anticipate that would be done to make a diagnosis? Under what circumstances could Marta be transferred to the antepartum unit or be discharged home?**

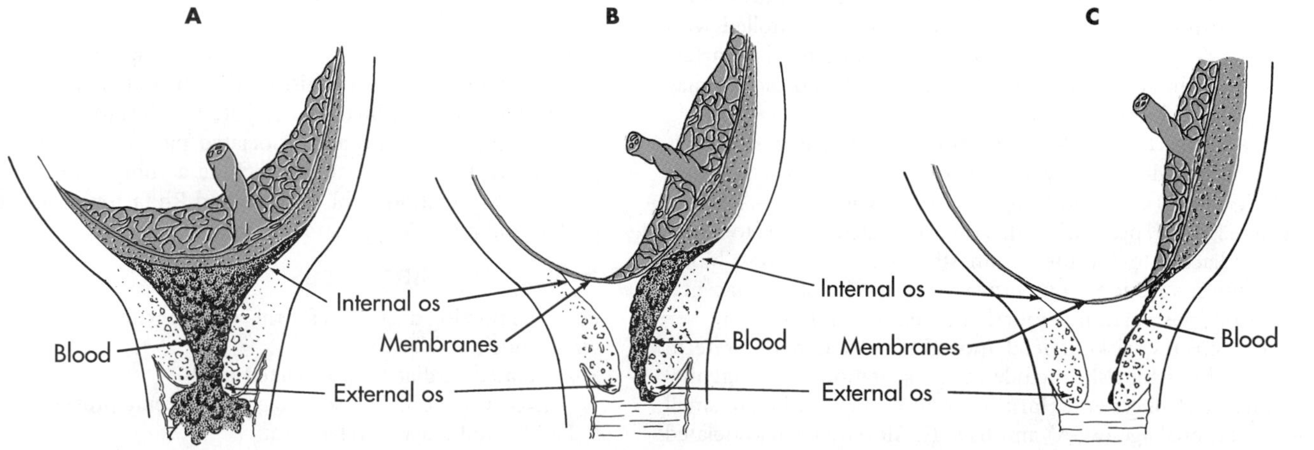

FIG. 14-12 • Types of placentae previa after onset of labor. **A,** Complete or total. **B,** Incomplete or partial. **C,** Marginal or low lying.

TABLE 14-6
Summary of Findings: Abruptio Placentae and Placenta Previa

	Abruptio Placentae			
	Grade 1 Mild Separation (10% to 20%)	Grade 2 Moderate Separation (20% to 50%)	Grade 3 Severe Separation (>50%)	Placenta Previa
Bleeding, external, vaginal	Minimal	Absent or moderate	Absent or moderate	Minimal to severe and life-threatening
Total amount of blood loss	<500 ml	1000-1500 ml	>1500 ml	Varies
Color of blood	Dark red	Dark red	Dark red	Bright red
Shock	Rare; none	Mild shock	Common, often sudden, profound	Uncommon
Coagulopathy	Rare, none	Occasional DIC	Frequent DIC	None
Uterine tonicity	Normal	Increased, may be localized to one region or diffuse over uterus, uterus fails to relax between contractions	Tetanic, persistent uterine contraction, boardlike uterus	Normal
Tenderness (pain)	Usually absent	Present	Agonizing, unremitting uterine pain	Absent
Ultrasonographic findings				
Location of placenta	Normal, upper uterine segment	Normal, upper uterine segment	Normal, upper uterine segment	Abnormal, lower uterine segment
Station of presenting part	Variable to engaged	Variable to engaged	Variable to engaged	High, not engaged
Fetal position	Usual distribution*	Usual distribution*	Usual distribution*	Commonly transverse, breech, or oblique
Pregnancy-induced or chronic hypertension	Usual distribution*	Commonly present	Commonly present	Usual distribution*
Fetal effects	Normal fetal heart rate pattern	Nonreassuring fetal heart rate pattern	Nonreassuring fetal heart rate pattern, death can occur	Normal fetal heart rate pattern

**Usual distribution* refers to the usual variations of incidence seen when there is no concurrent problem.

postpartum hemorrhage may occur even if the fundus is contracted firmly. If uterine bleeding cannot be controlled with oxytocic drugs, ligation of the hypogastric (internal iliac) arteries or even hysterectomy may be necessary. Hypovolemia may be treated with transfusion.

Maternal and Fetal Outcomes. Maternal morbidity is about 5% and mortality less than 1% with placenta previa (Clark, 1999). Complications associated with placenta previa include PROM, preterm birth, surgery-related trauma to structures adjacent to the uterus, anesthesia complications, blood transfusion reactions, overinfusion of fluids, other placental problems, postpartum hemorrhage, anemia, and infection.

The greatest risk of fetal mortality is caused by preterm birth. Other fetal risks include malpresentation and congenital anomalies (Gilbert and Harmon, 1998). Infants who are small for gestational age (SGA) and have IUGR have been associated with placenta previa; this association may be related to poor placental exchange or hypovolemia secondary to maternal blood loss and maternal anemia (Clark, 1999).

Care Management

➤ Assessment

A woman with third trimester vaginal bleeding requires immediate evaluation. Necessary history data include gravidity, parity, estimated date of birth, general status, bleeding (i.e., quantity, precipitating event, and associated pain), vital signs, and fetal status. Laboratory studies include a complete blood cell count, determination of blood type and Rh factor, coagulation profile, and possible type and crossmatch.

➤ Nursing Diagnoses

Potential nursing diagnoses for the woman with a placenta previa include the following:

- Decreased cardiac output related to:
  —Excessive blood loss secondary to placenta previa
- Fluid volume deficit related to:
  —Excessive blood loss secondary to placenta previa
- Altered peripheral tissue perfusion related to:
  —Hypovolemia and shunting of blood to central circulation

- Anxiety/fear related to:
  —Maternal condition and pregnancy outcome
- Anticipatory grieving related to:
  —Actual/perceived threat to self, pregnancy, or infant

➤ Expected Outcomes

Expected outcomes for the woman experiencing placenta previa may include the following. The woman will:

- Verbalize understanding of her condition and its management.
- Identify and use available support systems.
- Demonstrate compliance with prescribed activity limitations.
- Develop no complications related to bleeding.
- Give birth to a healthy term infant.

➤ Plan of Care and Implementation

Hospital Care

Active Management. Once placenta previa has been diagnosed, a management plan is developed based on gestational age, amount of bleeding, and fetal condition. If the woman is at term, and in labor or bleeding persistently, immediate delivery by cesarean is almost always indicated. In women with partial or marginal previas who have minimal bleeding, vaginal birth may be attempted. Vaginal birth may also be indicated for previable gestations or births involving intrauterine fetal demise (Benedetti, 1996).

Emotional support for the woman and her family is extremely important. The actively bleeding woman is concerned not only for her own well-being but also for the well-being of her fetus. All procedures should be explained, and a support person should be present. If the woman and her support person or family desire pastoral support, the nurse can notify the hospital chaplain service or provide information about other supportive resources.

Expectant Management. If the woman is less than 36 weeks gestation, is not in labor, and the bleeding is mild or has stopped, expectant management (i.e., rest and close observation) is generally the treatment of choice to give the fetus time to mature in utero. The woman may remain in the hospital on bed rest with bathroom privileges and perhaps limited activity (e.g., rides in a wheelchair). Bleeding is assessed by checking the amount of bleeding on perineal pads, bed pads, and linens. Weighing pads, although not often used, is one way to more accurately assess blood loss; one g is equal to 1 ml of blood.

No vaginal or rectal examinations are performed, and the woman is placed on pelvic rest (nothing in the vagina). Ultrasound examinations are done every 2 or 3 weeks. Fetal surveillance may include the use of a nonstress test (NST) or biophysical profile (BPP) once or twice a week.

The woman with placenta previa should always be considered a potential emergency because massive blood loss with resulting hypovolemic shock can occur quickly if bleeding resumes. Placenta previa in a preterm gestation may be an indication for admission to a tertiary perinatal center because many community hospitals are not equipped to perform emergency cesarean births 24 hours per day, 7 days per week.

If the fetus is at 36 weeks of gestation or more, if the bleeding continues, or if labor begins, birth will usually be by cesarean, preferably after fetal lung maturity is determined (L/S ratio of 2:1 or positive phosphatidylglycerol); but an emergency cesarean birth may be necessary at any time.

Home Care. Criteria for home care management vary among primary perinatal providers and home care agencies and are usually determined on a case-by-case basis. To be considered for home care referral, the woman must be in stable condition with no evidence of active bleeding and must have resources to be able to return to the hospital immediately if active bleeding resumes (Lowdermilk and Grohar, 1999). She must have close supervision by family or friends in the home. She should be taught how to assess fetal and uterine activity and bleeding; and told to avoid intercourse, douching, and enemas. She should limit her activities according to the advice of her physician; and be advised to keep all appointments for fetal testing, laboratory assessments, and prenatal care. Visits by a perinatal home care nurse may be arranged (Lowdermilk and Grohar, 1999).

➤ Evaluation

The expected outcomes of care are used to evaluate the care for the woman with placenta previa (see Nursing Care Plan).

Premature Separation of Placenta. Premature separation of the placenta, or abruptio placentae, is the detachment of part or all of the placenta from its implantation site (Fig. 14-13). Separation occurs in the area of the decidua basalis after 20 weeks of pregnancy and before birth of the baby.

Incidence and Etiology. Premature separation of the placenta is a serious event and accounts for significant maternal and fetal morbidity and mortality. One percent of all pregnancies are complicated by abruptio placentae; of these pregnancies, approximately 10% are severe enough to threaten fetal viability (Hunter and Weiner, 1996). Premature separation of the placenta accounts for about 15% of all perinatal deaths. Approximately one third of infants born to women with premature separation of the placenta die. More than 50% of these deaths are the result of preterm birth; many others are the result of intrauterine hypoxia.

Maternal hypertension is the most consistently identified risk factor for abruption (Benedetti, 1996). Cocaine is also a risk factor, likely in part because cocaine use is associated with the development of hypertension (Abu-Heija, al-Chalabi, and el-Iloubani, 1998). Blunt external abdominal trauma, most often the result of motor vehicle accidents or maternal battering, is an increasingly significant cause of placental abruption (Benedetti, 1996). Maternal smoking and poor nutrition may be associated with an increased risk (Kramer et al, 1997). There is a significant (i.e., 5% to 17%) recurrence risk for placental abruption. A woman who has had two previous premature separations has a recurrence risk of 25% in the next pregnancy (Benedetti, 1996).

Classification Systems. The most common classification of placental abruption is according to type and severity. This classification system is summarized in Table 14-6 (Clark, 1999; Hunter and Weiner, 1996).

Clinical Manifestations. The separation may be partial or complete, or only the margin of the placenta may be involved. Bleeding from the placental site may dissect (separate) the membranes from the decidua basalis and flow out through the vagina; it may remain concealed (retroplacental hemorrhage); or it may do both (see Fig. 14-13). Clinical symptoms vary with the degree of separation (see Table 14-6).

Nursing Care Plan — PLACENTA PREVIA

NURSING DIAGNOSIS **Decreased cardiac output related to bleeding secondary to placenta previa**

EXPECTED OUTCOME Patient will exhibit signs of increased blood volume and restoration of cardiac output (i.e., normal pulse and blood pressure; normal heart and breath sounds; normal skin color, tone, and turgor; normal capillary refill).

Nursing Interventions/*Rationales*

Palpate uterus for tenderness and tone; assess bleeding rate, amount, color, degree of bleeding, CBC values, and coagulation profile *to determine severity of situation.* Do not perform vaginal examination *because it may stimulate further bleeding.*

Establish baseline data for cardiac output (i.e., vital signs; heart and breath sounds; skin color, tone, turgor; capillary refill; level of consciousness; urinary output; pulse oximetry) *to use as basis for evaluating effectiveness of treatment.*

Initiate intravenous therapy or blood transfusions and medications per physician order *to restore blood volume and prevent organ compromise to mother and fetus.*

Place woman on bed rest *to decrease oxygen demands.*

Monitor vital signs, intake and output, hemodynamic status, and laboratory values *to evaluate treatment response.*

Provide emotional support to woman and her family (e.g., explain procedures and their rationale; explain what is happening and what to expect; keep support person present) *to allay fears and provide the family with some sense of control.*

After stabilization, teach woman home management, including bed rest, watching for spotting/bleeding, close follow-up with her health care provider, and preparation for immediate return to hospital if needed *to prevent or stem further complications.*

NURSING DIAGNOSIS **Risk for injury to the fetus related to decreased uterine/placental perfusion secondary to bleeding**

EXPECTED OUTCOME Patient will exhibit ongoing signs of fetal well-being (i.e., adequate fetal movement, normal fetal heart rate, reactive NST, normal biophysical profile [BPP]).

Nursing Interventions/*Rationales*

Monitor fetus daily for signs of tachycardia, decreased movement, loss of reactivity on NST *to identify and treat changes in fetal status early.*

Obtain BPP per physician order *to assess for signs of chronic asphyxia.*

Maintain maternal side-lying position *to prevent compression of aorta and vena cava.*

NURSING DIAGNOSIS **Risk for infection related to anemia and bleeding secondary to placenta previa**

EXPECTED OUTCOME Patient will show no signs of intrauterine infection.

Nursing Interventions/*Rationales*

Monitor vital signs for elevated temperature, pulse, and blood pressure; monitor laboratory results for elevated white blood cell count, differential shift; check for uterine tenderness and malodorous vaginal discharge *to detect early signs of infection resulting from exposure of placental tissue.*

Provide/teach perineal hygiene *to decrease the risk of ascending infection.*

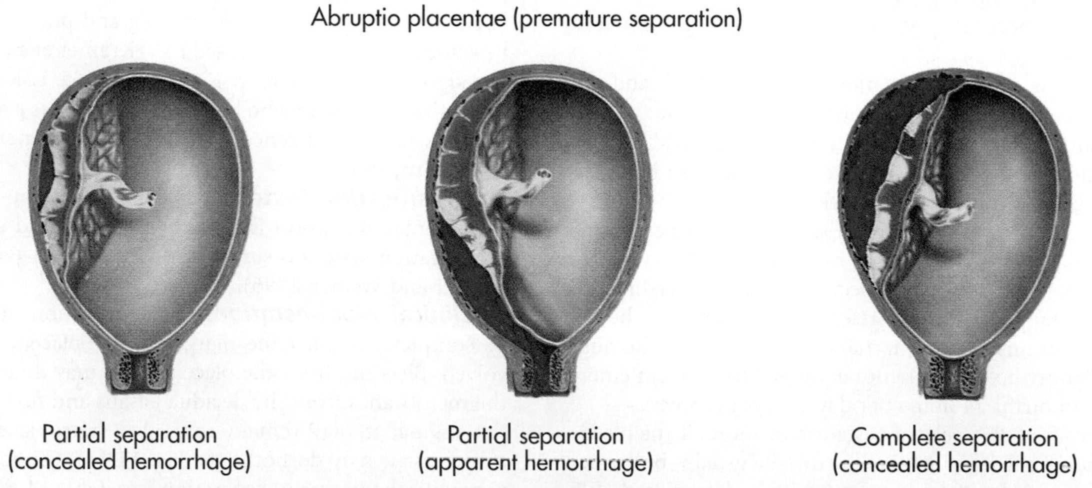

FIG. 14-13 • Abruptio placentae. Premature separation of normally implanted placenta.

Typically, vaginal bleeding, abdominal pain, and uterine tenderness and contractions are seen with abruptio placentae. Although abdominal pain and uterine tenderness are characteristic of abruption, either finding may be absent in the presence of a silent abruption (Konje and Walley, 1995). Bleeding may result in maternal hypovolemia (i.e., shock, oliguria, and anuria) and coagulopathy. Mild to severe uterine hypertonicity is present. Pain is mild to severe and localized over one region of the uterus or diffuse over the uterus with a boardlike abdomen.

Extensive myometrial bleeding damages the uterine muscle. If blood accumulates between the separated placenta and the uterine wall, it may produce a Couvelaire uterus. The uterus appears purplish and copper colored, it is ecchymotic, and contractility is lost. Shock may occur and is out of proportion to blood loss. The Apt test (for blood in amniotic fluid) is positive, hemoglobin and hematocrit levels drop, and coagulation factor levels drop. Clotting defects (DIC) develop in 10% to 30% of women, most within 8 hours of hospital admission. Renal failure and pituitary necrosis (Sheehan syndrome) may result from ischemia.

Maternal, Fetal, and Neonatal Outcomes. Maternal mortality rate approaches 1% in abruptio placentae; this condition remains a leading cause of maternal death. The mother's prognosis depends on the extent of placental detachment, overall blood loss, degree of DIC, and time between placental detachment and birth. Women who are Rh negative may become sensitized if the fetal Rh blood type is positive.

Perinatal mortality ranges from 15% to 30%; mortality occurs from fetal hypoxia, preterm birth, and SGA status. Risks of neurologic deficits are increased (Cunningham et al, 1997).

Collaborative Care. Abruptio placentae should be strongly suspected in the woman who has a sudden onset of intense (and usually localized) uterine pain, with or without vaginal bleeding. Initial assessment is much the same as for placenta previa. Physical examination usually reveals abdominal pain, uterine tenderness, and contractions. Approximately 60% of live fetuses exhibit nonreassuring signs on the electronic fetal heart monitor, such as loss of variability and late decelerations; uterine hyperstimulation and increased resting tone may also be noted on the monitor tracing (Benedetti, 1996). Many women have coagulopathy.

Nursing diagnoses and expected outcomes are similar to those described for placenta previa.

Hospital Care. Treatment depends on severity of blood loss and fetal maturity and status. If the abruption is mild, expectant management is implemented if the fetus is less than 36 weeks gestation and not in distress. The woman is hospitalized and closely observed for signs of bleeding and labor. The fetal status is monitored with intermittent FHR monitoring and NST or BPP until fetal maturity is achieved or until the woman's condition deteriorates and immediate birth is indicated. Use of corticosteroids to accelerate fetal lung maturity is appropriately included in the plan of care for the woman managed expectantly (ACOG, 1994; Hunter and Weiner, 1996). Women who are Rh negative may be given Rh_o(D) immune globulin if fetal-to-maternal hemorrhage occurs and the fetal blood is Rh positive.

If the mother is hemodynamically stable, a vaginal birth may be attempted if the fetus is alive and in no acute distress or if the fetus is dead. In the presence of fetal compromise, severe hemorrhage, coagulopathy, poor labor progress, or increasing uterine resting tone, a cesarean birth is performed. Maternal vital signs are monitored frequently to observe for signs of declining hemodynamic status. Continuous electronic fetal monitoring is mandatory. Fluid replacement must be aggressive in the presence of hemorrhage. Whole blood and Ringer's lactate are infused in quantities necessary to maintain a urine output of 30 to 60 ml/hour and a hematocrit of approximately 30%. An indwelling Foley catheter is inserted for continuous assessment of urine output. Fresh frozen plasma or cryoprecipitate may be given to maintain the fibrinogen level at a minimum of 100 to 150 mg/dl.

Emotional support for the woman and her family is extremely important. If actively bleeding, the woman is concerned not only for her own well-being but also for the well-being of her fetus. All procedures should be explained, and a support person should be present.

Home Care. Women with abruptio placentae are usually not managed out of the hospital because the placenta can separate at any time and immediate intervention or birth may be necessary.

Cord Insertion and Placental Variations. Velamentous insertion of the cord (vasa previa) is a rare placental anomaly associated with placenta previa and multiple gestation. The cord vessels begin to branch at the membranes and then course onto the placenta (Fig. 14-14, *A*). ROM or traction on the cord may tear one or more of the fetal vessels. As a result, the fetus may rapidly bleed to death. Battledore (marginal) insertion of the cord (Fig. 14-14, *B*) increases the risk of fetal hemorrhage, especially after marginal separation of the placenta.

Rarely, the placenta may be divided into two or more separate lobes, resulting in succenturiate placenta (Fig. 14-14, *C*). Each lobe has a distinct circulation: the vessels collect at the periphery, and the main trunks eventually unite to form the vessels of the cord. Blood vessels joining the lobes may be supported only by the fetal membranes and are therefore in danger of tearing during labor, birth, or expulsion of the placenta. During expulsion of the placenta, one or more of the separate lobes may remain attached to the decidua basalis, preventing uterine contraction and increasing the risk of postpartum hemorrhage.

Clotting Disorders in Pregnancy

Normal Clotting. Normally a delicate balance (homeostasis) is maintained between two opposing systems, the hemostatic system and the fibrinolytic system. The hemostatic system is involved in the life-saving process by stopping the flow of blood from injured vessels, in part through the formation of insoluble fibrin that acts as a hemostatic platelet plug. The coagulation process involves an interaction of the coagulation factors in which each factor sequentially activates the factor next in line in the so-called "cascade effect" sequence. The fibrinolytic system is the process by which the fibrin is split into fibrin degradation products and circulation is restored.

Clotting Problems. A history of abnormal bleeding, inheritance of unusual bleeding tendencies, or a report of significant aberrations of laboratory findings indicate a bleeding or clotting problem. For the pregnant woman, bleeding disorders are usually suspected if the woman has pregnancy-induced hypertension, HELLP syndrome, retained dead fetus syndrome, amniotic fluid embolism, sepsis, or hemorrhage. Determination of hemostasis is made by testing the usual mechanisms for the control of bleeding, the function of platelets, and the necessary clotting factors.

Disseminated Intravascular Coagulation. DIC is a pathologic form of clotting that is diffuse and consumes large amounts of clotting factors, causing widespread external and/or internal bleeding. DIC is an overactivation of the clotting cascade and the fibrinolytic system resulting in depletion of

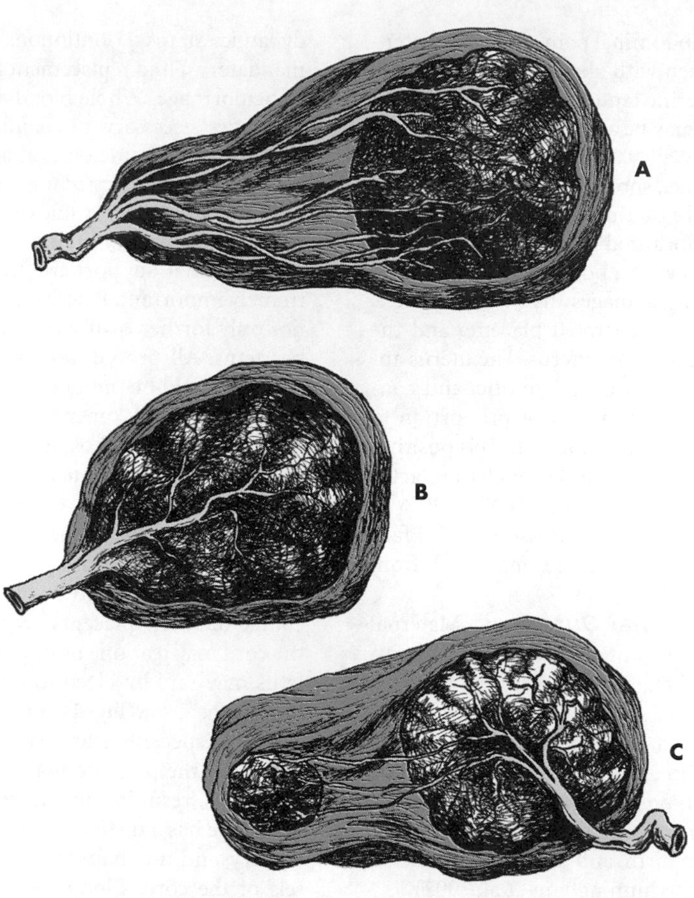

FIG. 14-14 • Cord insertion and placental variations. **A,** Velamentous insertion of cord. **B,** Battledore placenta. **C,** Succenturiate placenta.

platelets and clotting factors. This results in the formation of multiple fibrin clots throughout the body's vasculature, even in the microcirculation. Blood cells are destroyed as they pass through these fibrin-choked vessels. Thus DIC results in a clinical picture of hemorrhage, anemia, and ischemia.

DIC is always a secondary diagnosis. In the obstetric population, DIC is most often triggered by the release of large amounts of tissue thromboplastin; this occurs in abruptio placentae, retained dead fetus, and amniotic fluid embolus. Severe preeclampsia, HELLP syndrome, and gram-negative sepsis are examples of conditions that can trigger DIC because of widespread damage to vascular integrity.

Medical Management. The diagnosis of DIC is based on clinical findings and laboratory markers. Physical examination reveals unusual bleeding. Spontaneous bleeding from the woman's gums or nose may be noted. Petechiae may appear around the blood pressure cuff placed on her arm. Excessive bleeding may occur from the site of a slight trauma (e.g., venipuncture sites, IM or subcutaneous injection sites, or injury from insertion of urinary catheter). Maternal symptoms may include tachycardia and diaphoresis.

Laboratory tests reveal decreased platelets, fibrinogen, proaccelerin, antihemophilic factor, and prothrombin (the factors consumed during coagulation). Other factors should be normal. Fibrinolysis is first increased but is later severely depressed. Degradation of fibrin leads to the accumulation of fibrin-split products in the blood. Fibrin-split products have anticoagulant properties and thus prolong the PT. Bleeding time is normal; coagulation time shows no clot; clot retraction time shows no clot; and PTT is increased. DIC must be distinguished from other clotting disorders before therapy is initiated.

The primary management of DIC involves correction of the underlying cause, which may be removal of the dead fetus, treatment of existing infection or preeclampsia or eclampsia, or removal of a placental abruption. Concomitantly, treatment is directed toward support of maternal physiologic functioning and replacing essential factors faster than the body can consume them. Intravenous fluids are given to replace volume lost through severe bleeding. Packed red blood cells are administered to maintain enough circulating red blood cells to ensure tissue oxygenation. Fresh frozen plasma or cryoprecipitate is given to replace fibrinogen and coagulation factors. Platelets may also be administered.

Nursing Care Management. The nurse caring for the woman at risk for DIC must be aware of risk factors. Careful and thorough assessment is required, with particular attention to the signs of bleeding (e.g., petechiae, oozing from injection sites, and hematuria). Because renal failure is one consequence of DIC, urinary output is carefully monitored using an indwelling Foley catheter. Urine output must be maintained at more than 30 ml/hour. Vital signs are assessed frequently.

Supportive measures include keeping the pregnant woman's right hip elevated to maximize blood flow to the uterus. Oxygen may be administered through a tight-fitting rebreathing mask at 8 to 10 L/minute or per hospital protocol or physician order.

Blood and blood products must be administered safely. Fetal assessments are done to monitor fetal well-being.

The educational and emotional needs of the woman and her family must be recognized and supported. They need information about her condition and explanations of unfamiliar equipment and procedures and will most likely be very anxious about the health of the mother and baby.

von Willebrand Disease. von Willebrand disease, a type of hemophilia, is probably the most common of all hereditary bleeding disorders (Cunningham et al, 1997). It results from a factor VIII deficiency and platelet dysfunction. It is transmitted as an incomplete autosomal dominant trait to both sexes. Although von Willebrand disease is rare, it is one of the most common congenital clotting defects in American women of childbearing age. Symptoms include a familial bleeding tendency, previous bleeding episodes, prolonged bleeding time (the most important test), factor VIII deficiency (mild to moderate), and bleeding from mucous membranes. Factor VIII increases during pregnancy, and this increase may be sufficient to offset danger from hemorrhage during childbirth. von Willebrand disease is variable in its clinical course, severity, and laboratory values, so it is possible for this condition to go undetected throughout pregnancy until bleeding problems develop after birth. If the woman is known to have von Willebrand disease before labor, factor VIII levels should be monitored and cryoprecipitate given as needed to maintain activity at 40% of normal near term gestation (Benedetti, 1996).

INFECTIONS IN PREGNANCY

Sexually transmitted infections are responsible for significant morbidity and mortality in pregnancy. Some consequences of maternal infection, such as infertility and sterility, last a lifetime.

Psychosocial sequelae may include altered interpersonal relationships and lowered self-esteem. Congenitally acquired infection may affect the length and quality of a child's life.

Chapter 6 discusses the diagnosis and management of STIs. Chapter 28 discusses neonatal effects and management. This discussion focuses only on the effects of several common STIs on pregnancy and the fetus. Effects on the pregnancy and the fetus vary according to whether or not the infection has been treated at the time of labor and birth.

Factors that influence the development and management of STIs during pregnancy include previous history of STI or PID, number of current sexual partners, frequency of intercourse, and anticipated sexual activity during pregnancy. Lifestyle choices also may affect STIs in the perinatal period. Women who use intravenous drugs or who have partners that use intravenous drugs are at risk. Other lifestyle factors that increase susceptibility to STIs (through suppressive effects on the immune system) include smoking, alcohol use, inadequate or poor nutrition, and high levels of fatigue or personal stress.

Physical examination and laboratory studies to determine the presence of STIs in the pregnant woman are the same as those done in nonpregnant women (see Chapter 6).

Sexually Transmitted Infections

Treatment of specific STIs may be different for the pregnant woman and may even be different at different stages of pregnancy. Table 14-7 describes the maternal, fetal, and neonatal effects and treatment during pregnancy of common STIs (i.e., chlamydial infections, gonorrhea, syphilis, HIV, human papilloma virus, vaginal candidiasis, trichomonas vaginalis, and Group B streptococci). Varicella may also place a woman at risk during the childbearing cycle and is included in Table 14-7.

Infected women need instruction on how to take prescribed medications, information on whether their partner(s) also need to be evaluated and treated, and a review of preventive measures to avoid reinfection.

> *Critical Thinking*
>
> **SEXUALLY TRANSMITTED INFECTION IN PREGNANCY**
>
> **Veronica, a G2 P1 elementary school teacher, is admitted with diagnoses of vaginal bleeding and preterm labor at 28 weeks. Vaginal speculum examination reveals bleeding from the cervical os and a thick, mucopurulent discharge. Laboratory tests show the presence of *Chlamydia trachomatis,* and intravenous antibiotics are begun. The woman is told of the findings and is upset and angry to learn that she has an STI. She is also very worried about her baby.**
>
> - **What further assessment data do you need to develop a plan of care? What are some of the effects the situation may have on the patient's relationship with her partner? Examine your personal reactions in light of the information about the presence of an STI. How might these feelings affect your plan of care? Veronica expresses concern about how she will discuss the presence of an STI with her partner. Role play a situation in which you must tell a partner this information.**

TORCH Infections

*T*oxoplasmosis, *o*ther infections (e.g., hepatitis), *r*ubella virus, *c*ytomegalovirus, and *h*erpes simplex viruses, known collectively as TORCH infections, are a group of organisms capable of crossing the placenta and adversely affecting the development of the fetus. Generally, all TORCH infections produce influenza-like symptoms in the mother, but fetal and neonatal effects are more serious. TORCH infections and their maternal and fetal effects are presented in Table 14-8.

Infection Control

Infection control measures are essential to protect care providers and to prevent nosocomial infection of patients, regardless of the infectious agent. A consideration in the prevention of occupational disease transmission is that of cross-contamination. Health care providers may develop a false sense of security about the protection that gloves provide. For example, little is gained if gloves are worn to assess a newborn and those same gloved hands are used to answer the telephone, turn on a light, or document findings on the infant's chart. Cross-contamination of surfaces is common. Proper cleaning of contaminated surfaces is essential. The following guidelines are recommended: (1) cleanse washable surfaces with a solution of sodium hypochlorite and water (1 cup of household bleach to 9 cups of water) or a commercial disinfectant product; (2) remove all blood or other fluids before disinfection to avoid neutralizing the bleach solution. If a large spill has occurred, pour disinfectant over the spillage before removal, then disinfect as described.

TABLE 14-7

Maternal, Fetal, Neonatal Effects and Treatment of Common STIs

Infection	Maternal Effects	Fetal and/or Neonatal Effects	Management
Chlamydia trachomatis (bacteria)	Asymptomatic; may cause salpingitis, ectopic pregnancy, PID, infertility and sterility, postpartum endometritis	Preterm birth, low birth weight; stillbirth, neonatal death; conjunctivitis, pneumonia	Single dose of azithromycin or 7 days of doxycycline; amoxycillin or erythromycin may also be used. Use erythromycin in pregnancy. Test all sexual partners.
Gonorrhea (diplococci)	May cause PID and lead to ectopic pregnancy and sterility, PROM, and chorionitis. If untreated, may have postpartum gonoccal endometritis, acute salpingitis, dermatitis, and arthritis	Preterm birth, ophthalmia neonatorum and pneumonia	Spread by direct contact with lesions and indirectly by transfer by fomites. Treated with a single dose of ceftriaxone, cefixime, ciprofloxacin, or ofloxacin.
Syphilis (spirochete)	Primary: chancre Secondary: maculopopular rash on palms and soles, lymphadenopathy, fever, headache, malaise Tertiary: neurologic/cardiovascula musculoskeletal, or multiorgan system complications	Late miscarriage and stillbirth; congenital syphilis	Acquired through sexual contact. Parenteral penicillin is preferred for treatment of all stages of syphilis.
Human immunodeficiency virus/ Acquired immunodeficiency syndrome (virus)	Fatigue, anorexia, weight loss, chronic diarrhea, and fever Virus present in breast milk Postpartum: increased risk for URIs, vaginitis, postpartum endometritis, and poor wound healing	Maternal-fetal transmission of virus	Transmitted through contact with body fluids. Pregnancy is not recommended; preconception counseling is advised. Primary drug for treatment is zidovudine (AZT). Elective cesearean birth reduces rate of vertical transmission. Breastfeeding contraindicated.
Human papillomavirus (genital warts) (virus)	Proliferation and increased friability of lesions	Neonatal respiratory or laryngeal papillomatosis	Sexually transmitted. Recommend removal of large, outward-growing lesions; carbon dioxide laser treatments have been used.
Vaginal candidiasis (yeast)	Pain, itching, vaginal discharge; increased rate of infection during pregnancy May be present on nipples of breastfeeding mother	Oral candidiasis in newborns	Spread by direct contact. Mother treated with clotrimazole, miconazole, butoconazole, or terconazole. Newborn treated with oral nystatin.
Trichomonas vaginalis (protozoa)		Fever and irritability	Metronidazole should be administered to pregnant women only in the second and third trimesters.
Group B streptococci (diplococci)	Miscarriage, stillbirth, preterm birth, fever, septicemia, and puerperal infection	Sepsis and meningitis, blindness, deafness, mental retardation, learning disabilities, death	Normal flora; vertical transmission to newborn during passage through birth canal. Treated with penicillin, ampicillin, cephalothin, or erythromycin. Intrapartum treatment of women who are GBS carriers reduces the incidence of neonatal infection.
Varicella (virus)	Severe disseminated, epidemic type of varicella can be fatal to mother	Miscarriage; severe disseminated, epidemic type of varicella can be fatal to fetus. If maternal varicella occurs in the first trimester, fetus may develop rubella syndrome; chorioretinitis, hydrocephalus	Newborn may receive prophylactic treatment. Transmitted by direct contact. Give VZIG to exposed pregnant women. Treat severe infections with IV acyclovir or vidarabine.

TABLE 14-8
Maternal Infections: TORCH

Infection	Maternal Effects	Fetal Effects	Prevention, Identification, and Management
TOXOPLASMOSIS (PROTOZOA)	Acute infection similar to influenza, lymphadenopathy Woman immune after first episode (except in immunocompromised patients)	With maternal acute infection, parasitemia Less likely to occur with maternal chronic infection Miscarriage likely with acute infection early in pregnancy	Associated with eating raw or undercooked meat or with poor handwashing after handling infected cat litter. Use good handwashing technique. Avoid eating raw meat and exposure to litter used by infected cats; if cats in house, have toxoplasma titer checked. If titer is rising during early pregnancy, abortion may be considered an option. Treated with a combination of pyrimethamine and sulfadiazine.
OTHER			
Hepatitis A (infectious hepatitis) (virus)	Miscarriage, cause of liver failure during pregnancy Fever, malaise, nausea, and abdominal discomfort	Exposure during first trimester, fetal anomalies, fetal or neonatal hepatitis, preterm birth, intrauterine fetal death	Usually spread by droplet or hand contact especially by culinary workers; gamma globulin can be given as prophylaxis for hepatitis A.
Hepatitis B (serum hepatitis) (virus)	Symptoms variable—fever, rash, arthralgia, depressed appetite, dyspepsia, abdominal pain, generalized aching, malaise, weakness, jaundice, tender and enlarged liver	Infection occurs during birth Maternal vaccination during pregnancy should present no risk for fetus	Generally passed by contaminated needles, syringes, or blood transfusions; also can be transmitted orally or by coitus (but incubation period is longer); hepatitis B immune globulin can be given prophylactically after exposure. All pregnant women should be screened for HbsAg. Hepatitis B vaccine recommended for populations at risk (women from Asia, Pacific Islands, Indochina, Haiti, South Africa; Eskimos; health care providers, IV drug users, those sexually active with multiple partners or single partner with multiple risks).
Rubella (3-day or German measles) (virus)	Rash, fever, mild symptoms; suboccipital lymph nodes may be swollen; some photophobia Occasionally arthritis or encephalitis Miscarriage	Incidence of congenital anomalies—first month 50%, second month 25%, third month 10%, fourth month 4% Exposure during first 2 months—malformations of heart, eyes, ears, or brain, abnormal dermatoglyphics Exposure after fourth month—systemic infection, hepatosplenomegaly, IUGR, rash	Transmitted by droplets (sneezing). Vaccination of pregnant women contraindicated; pregnancy should be prevented for 3 months after vaccination; pregnant women nonreactive to hemagglutinin-inhibition antigen can be safely vaccinated after birth.
Cytomegalovirus (CMV) (a herpes virus)	May be asymptomatic or have mononucleosis-like syndrome, may have cervical discharge. No immunity develops	Fetal death or severe, generalized disease—hemolytic anemia and jaundice, hydrocephaly or microcephaly, pneumonitis, hepatosplenomegaly, deafness	Respiratory transmission; virus also in semen, cervical and vaginal secretions, breast milk, urine, feces, and banked blood.

Continued

TABLE 14-8
Maternal Infections: TORCH—cont'd

Infection	Maternal Effects	Fetal Effects	Prevention, Identification, and Management
Cytomegalovirus (CMV) (a herpes virus)—*cont'd*			Virus may be reactivated and cause disease in utero or during birth in subsequent pregnancies; fetal infection may occur during passage through infected birth canal. Treated by symptom management.
Herpes genitalis (herpes simplex virus, type 2 [HSV-2])	Primary blisters, rash, fever, malaise, nausea, headache; pregnancy risks include miscarriage, preterm labor, stillbirth	Transplacental infection is rare; congenital effects include skin lesions and scarring, IUGR, mental retardation, microcephaly	Risk of transmission is greatest during vaginal birth if woman has active lesions. Acyclovir not recommended in pregnancy; treat symptomatically. Thorough handwashing; wear gloves.

SURGERY DURING PREGNANCY

The incidence of surgery requiring anesthesia during pregnancy ranges from 0.2% to 2.2%, affecting an estimated 50,000 women each year. The need for immediate abdominal surgery occurs as often among pregnant women as among nonpregnant women of comparable age. However, diagnosis is more difficult in the pregnant woman. An enlarged uterus and displaced internal organs may make abdominal palpation more difficult, may alter the position of an affected organ, and/or may change the usual signs associated with a particular disorder. Reluctance to use conventional x-rays for diagnosis, coupled with a reluctance to operate during pregnancy, can delay diagnosis and increase morbidity for both the mother and the fetus (Sivanesaratnam, 2000). Common conditions necessitating abdominal surgery during pregnancy are appendicitis, intestinal obstruction, and gynecologic problems.

Appendicitis

Appendicitis is the most common acute surgical condition seen in pregnancy, occurring approximately once in 2000 pregnancies. Appendicitis occurs in approximately the same frequency during each trimester of pregnancy and in the postpartum period (Depp, 1996). The diagnosis is often delayed because the usual signs and symptoms mimic some normal changes of pregnancy such as nausea and vomiting and increased WBC count. As pregnancy progresses, the appendix is pushed upward and to the right from its usual anatomic location (see Fig. 13-6). Because of these changes, appendiceal rupture and peritonitis occur two to three times more often in pregnant women than in nonpregnant women.

The woman with appendicitis most commonly presents with abdominal pain, nausea and vomiting, and loss of appetite. Temperature may be normal or mildly increased (to 38.3° C). Because of the physiologic increase in WBCs that occurs in pregnancy, significant increases associated with appendicitis must be documented either by rising levels on serial samples or by an increasing left shift.

The diagnosis of appendicitis requires a high level of suspicion because the typical signs and symptoms are similar to those found in many other conditions, including pyelonephritis, round ligament pain, placental abruption, torsion of an ovarian cyst, cholecystitis, and preterm labor (Depp, 1996).

Appendectomy before rupture usually does not require either antibiotic or tocolytic therapy. If surgery is delayed until after rupture, multiple antibiotics are ordered. Rupture is likely to result in preterm labor and necessitate the use of tocolytic agents.

Intestinal Obstruction

The second most common nonobstetric abdominal emergency in pregnancy is intestinal obstruction. Any woman with a laparotomy scar is more likely to have an intestinal obstruction (adynamic ileus) during gestation. Adhesions as a result of previous surgery or pelvic inflammatory disease, an enlarging uterus, and displacement of the intestines are etiologic factors.

Constipation; persistent cramplike, abdominal pain; vomiting; auscultatory rushes within the abdomen; and "laddering" of the intestinal shadows on x-ray films aid in the diagnosis of intestinal obstruction. Immediate surgical intervention is required for release of the obstruction. Pregnancy is rarely affected by the surgery, assuming the absence of complications such as peritonitis.

Gynecologic Problems

Pregnancy predisposes a woman to ovarian problems, especially during the first trimester. Ovarian cysts and twisting of ovarian cysts or adnexal tissues may occur. Other problems include retained or enlarged cystic corpus luteum of pregnancy, and bacterial invasion of reproductive or other intraperitoneal organs.

Laparotomy or laparoscopy may be required to discriminate between ovarian problems and early ectopic pregnancy, appendicitis, or an infectious process.

Care Management

Initial assessment of the pregnant woman requiring surgery focuses on her presenting signs and symptoms. A thorough history and a physical examination are performed. Laboratory

Box 14-5

Discharge Teaching for Home Care

- Care of incision site
- Diet and elimination related to gastrointestinal function
- Signs and symptoms of developing complications: wound infection, thrombophlebitis, pneumonia
- Equipment needed and technique for assessing temperature
- Recommended schedule for resumption of activities of daily living
- Treatments and medications ordered
- List of resource persons and their telephone numbers
- Schedule of follow-up visits
- If birth has not occurred:
  Assessment of fetal activity (kick counts)
  Signs of preterm labor

testing includes, at a minimum, a complete blood count with differential and a urinalysis. Fetal heart rate and activity and uterine activity should be monitored; constant vigilance is maintained for symptoms of impending obstetric complications. The extent of preoperative assessment is determined by the immediacy of surgical intervention and the specific condition that requires surgery.

Hospital Care. The woman and her family are concerned about fetal well-being; their greatest fear related to surgery is the fear of losing the baby. An important part of preoperative nursing care is encouraging the woman to express her fears, concerns, and questions.

Preoperative care for a pregnant woman differs from that of a nonpregnant woman in one significant aspect: the presence of at least one other person—the fetus. Continuous FHR and uterine contraction monitoring should be performed if the fetus is considered viable. Food and fluids by mouth are restricted before a scheduled procedure or surgery; if the woman experiences a prolonged NPO status, IV fluids with dextrose should be given. Because of the danger of vomiting and aspirating, special precautions are taken before anesthesia is administered (e.g., administering an antacid). General preoperative and postoperative observations and ongoing care are the same as for any surgery.

Intraoperatively, perinatal nurses may collaborate with the surgical staff to provide for the special needs of pregnant women undergoing surgery. The woman should be positioned on the operating table with a lateral tilt to avoid maternal compression of the vena cava. Continuous fetal and uterine monitoring during the procedure is recommended since the risk of preterm labor is great. Monitoring can be accomplished using sterile Aquasonic gel and a sterile sleeve for the transducer. Uterine contractions may be palpated manually (Kendrick, 1994).

In the immediate recovery period, general observations and care pertinent to postoperative recovery are initiated. Frequent assessments are carried out for several hours after surgery. Whether the woman is cared for in the surgical postanesthesia recovery area or in labor and delivery, continuous fetal and uterine monitoring will likely be initiated or resumed because of the increased risk of preterm labor. Tocolysis may be necessary if preterm labor occurs.

Home Care. Plans for the woman's return home and for convalescent care should be completed as early as possible before discharge. The woman and other support persons need to be taught necessary skills and procedures, such as care of the incision and/or dressing changes. Provision should be made for supervised practice before discharge. Box 14-5 lists information that should be included in discharge teaching for the postoperative patient. The woman may also need referrals to various community agencies for evaluation of the home situation, child care, home health care, and financial or other assistance.

TRAUMA DURING PREGNANCY

Trauma is a common complication during pregnancy because the majority of pregnant women in the United States continue activities as usual. Thus pregnant women are at the same risk as others for vehicular crashes, falls, industrial mishaps, violence, and other injuries in the home and community. Treatment of pregnant trauma victims is complicated because doctors and nurses who have expertise in the care of trauma victims rarely have similar expertise in the care of pregnant women (Colburn, 1999).

Significance

Approximately 7% of pregnancies are complicated by physical trauma. As pregnancy progresses, the risk of trauma seems to increase because more cases of trauma are reported in the third trimester than earlier in gestation.

Acts of violence are increasing in record numbers throughout the United States. Violence is now viewed as a major public health problem (Saunders, 2000). About 17% (or 1 in 6) adult pregnant women are physically or sexually abused during pregnancy. Abuse that is already occurring often escalates during pregnancy (Greenberg et al, 1997).

The majority of maternal injuries are a result of motor vehicle crashes, followed by falls and direct assaults to the abdomen (Coleman, Trianfo, and Rund, 1997). Statistics show that trauma is the leading nonobstetric cause of maternal death (Depp, 1996). Maternal death caused by trauma is usually the result of head injury or hemorrhagic shock (Lavery and Staten-McCormick, 1995).

Trauma increases the incidence of miscarriage, preterm labor, abruptio placentae, and stillbirth (Greenberg et al, 1997). The effect of trauma on pregnancy is influenced by the length of gestation, type and severity of the trauma, and degree of disruption of uterine and fetal physiologic features. Fetal death as a result of trauma is more common than the occurrence of both maternal and fetal death. Careful evaluation of mother and fetus after all types of trauma is imperative.

Etiology

Motor vehicle accidents and battering most often result in blunt abdominal trauma. Maternal and fetal morbidity and mortality associated with motor vehicle accidents are directly correlated with whether the mother remains inside the vehicle or is ejected. Maternal death is usually the result of a head injury or exsanguination from a major vessel rupture. Maternal death usually results in fetal death. The most common fetal injury in severe trauma is skull fracture with subsequent intracranial hemorrhage (Pearlman and Tintinalli, 1991). Serious retroperitoneal hemorrhage after lower abdominal and pelvic trauma is reported more often during pregnancy. Serious maternal abdominal injuries are usually the result of splenic rupture or liver and renal injury.

When maternal survival of trauma occurs, fetal death is usually the result of abruptio placentae (Corsi et al, 1999; Rogers et al, 1999). It is imperative that all pregnant victims be carefully evaluated for signs and symptoms of abruptio placentae after even minor blunt abdominal trauma. Signs and symptoms of abruptio placentae include uterine tenderness or pain, uterine irritability, uterine contractions, vaginal bleeding, leaking of amniotic fluid, and a change in fetal heart rate characteristics. A second-generation fetal monitor with auto-correlation for continuous electronic fetal monitoring (EFM) may show early signs of abruptio placentae, including characteristics such as a change in the baseline rate, a loss of accelerations, or the presence of late decelerations.

Pelvic fracture may result from severe injury, and the usual two-point displacement of pelvic bones may produce bladder trauma or retroperitoneal bleeding. One point of displacement is commonly at the symphysis pubis and the second point is posterior because of the structure of the pelvis. Careful evaluation for clinical signs of internal hemorrhage is indicated.

Uterine rupture as a result of trauma is rare, occurring in only 0.6% of all reported cases of trauma during pregnancy. Uterine rupture depends on numerous factors, including gestational age; the intensity of the impact; and the presence of a predisposing factor such as a distended uterus caused by polyhydramnios or multiple gestation, or the presence of a uterine scar from previous uterine surgery. When uterine rupture occurs, the force responsible is usually a direct, high-energy blow. Fetal death is common with traumatic uterine rupture. However, maternal death occurs less than 10% of the time, and when it occurs it is usually the result of massive injuries sustained from an impact severe enough to rupture the uterus.

Care Management

Immediate priorities for stabilization of the pregnant woman after trauma should be identical to those of the nonpregnant trauma patient. Priorities of care for the pregnant woman after trauma must be to resuscitate the woman and stabilize her condition FIRST and then consider fetal needs. The perinatal nurse is often called on to function collaboratively with emergency department or trauma unit staff members in providing care for the pregnant trauma victim.

In cases of minor trauma, the woman is evaluated for vaginal bleeding, uterine irritability, abdominal tenderness, abdominal pain or cramps, and evidence of hypovolemia. A change in, or absence of, FHR or fetal activity; leakage of amniotic fluid; and presence of fetal cells in the maternal circulation are also included in the assessment.

In cases of major trauma, the systematic evaluation begins with a primary survey and the initial "ABCs" of resuscitation: establishment and maintenance of *a*irway, ensure adequate *b*reathing, and maintenance of an adequate *c*irculatory volume.

After immediate resuscitation and successful stabilization measures, a more detailed secondary survey of the mother and fetus should be accomplished. A complete physical assessment including all body systems is performed. The evaluation and care is usually performed by two teams of care providers, with the first team focusing on the mother and the second team focusing on the fetus and any pregnancy-related problems.

Findings from the injury must not be confused with the normal physiologic changes during pregnancy. The usual signs of organ rupture (e.g., guarding, rebound tenderness, and rigidity) may only be responses to stretching of the abdominal wall. An examination of the woman in a supine position results in hypotension and a systolic value as low as 80 mm Hg; changing her to a lateral position or simply moving the fetus raises the systolic value to more than 100 mm Hg. A silent abdomen, a sign of bowel trauma, may be a normal finding because of the decreased motility that occurs during pregnancy. A nasogastric tube is inserted, if indicated, because delayed emptying time of the stomach during pregnancy poses a threat of vomiting and possible aspiration if the woman has eaten within the last several hours. Fluid and electrolyte replacement is instituted and monitored. Oxygen needs are met.

During pregnancy the woman can sustain a significant blood loss (approximately a 30% reduction of circulating blood volume) without the usual signs and symptoms of hypovolemia. Pelvic blood vessels (e.g., the retroperitoneal and parametrial arteries) enlarge greatly during pregnancy; thus they are more easily damaged and ruptured. The large uterus can compartmentalize and hide a hemorrhage originating in the liver and spleen. A rapid pulse may reflect only the usual increase of 10 to 15 beats/min, or it may be a sign of hypovolemia.

Penetrating abdominal wounds, internal hemorrhage, and ruptured uterus are all indications for immediate surgical intervention. Wounds high in the abdomen are more likely to penetrate a vital structure because organs such as the bowel, liver, and spleen have been displaced upward by the enlarging uterus.

In addition to assisting with stabilization of the woman, the nurse provides emotional support for the injured woman and her family. If the trauma is the result of a motor vehicle accident, other family members may also have been critically injured or killed. The nurse collaborates with other staff to make sure that questions are answered and consistent information given. Grief support may be necessary.

Discharge Planning. The woman may be discharged home after several hours of evaluation following minor trauma. Her vital signs should be stable, with no evidence of bleeding at the time of discharge. The fetal tracing should be reassuring before monitoring is discontinued and the woman discharged. Education for the woman and her family is very important. She should be instructed to contact her health care provider immediately if changes in fetal movement or signs and symptoms indicative of preterm labor, of premature rupture of membranes, or of placental abruption develop. If the trauma occurred as a result of a motor vehicle accident, the importance of wearing a seat belt should be reinforced and she should be given directions for using it correctly during pregnancy (i.e., position the lap belt over hips and thighs rather than across the abdomen; see Fig. 11-17). If the trauma occurred as a result of domestic violence, the woman may need information about the abuse cycle; referral to a crisis center, law enforcement agency, or counseling center; and help in forming a safety plan (Greenberg et al, 1997; Huzel and Remsburg-Bell, 1996).

Key Points

- Hypertensive disorders during pregnancy are a leading cause of maternal and perinatal morbidity and mortality worldwide.
- The cause of preeclampsia is unknown, and there are no known reliable tests for predicting women at risk for developing preeclampsia/eclampsia.

- Preeclampsia/eclampsia is a multisystem disease, and the pathologic changes are present long before clinical manifestations, such as hypertension, are evident.
- Once preeclampsia becomes clinically evident, therapeutic interventions are palliative (e.g., bed rest and diet) and may slow the progression of the disease, allowing the pregnancy to continue, but the underlying pathology continues.
- The HELLP syndrome, which usually becomes apparent during the third trimester, is considered life-threatening.
- Magnesium sulfate, the anticonvulsant of choice for preventing eclampsia, requires careful monitoring of reflexes, respirations, and renal function; its antidote, calcium gluconate, should be at the bedside.
- Intent of emergency interventions for eclampsia is to prevent self-injury, ensure adequate oxygenation, reduce aspiration risk, and establish control with magnesium sulfate.
- Blood loss during pregnancy should always be regarded as a warning sign until ruled out by the woman's health care provider.
- Ectopic pregnancy is a significant cause of maternal morbidity and mortality even in developed countries.
- Abruptio placentae and placenta previa are differentiated by type of bleeding, uterine tonicity, and presence or absence of pain.
- Clotting disorders are associated with many obstetric complications.
- The physiologic adaptations of pregnancy mask warning signs and changes in vital signs during early shock states.
- The potential hazards of therapeutic interventions may further compromise the woman experiencing hemorrhagic disorders.
- Pregnancy confers no immunity against infection, and both mother and fetus must be considered when the pregnant woman contracts an infection.
- HIV is transmitted through blood, semen, and perinatal events.
- *Chlamydia trachomatis* is the most common sexually transmitted bacterial pathogen in the United States and is responsible for substantial morbidity, personal suffering, and a heavy economic burden.
- STIs often occur in groups; what appear to be resistant infections actually may be multiple infections or reinfections.
- Abuse of alcohol and drugs compromises the body's immune system and increases the risk for AIDS and associated conditions.
- Because medical history and examination cannot reliably identify all persons with HIV or other bloodborne pathogens, blood and body fluid precautions should be used consistently for everyone.
- STIs and genital and perigenital infections are biologic events, for which all individuals have a right to expect objective, compassionate, and effective health care.
- Preoperative care for a pregnant woman differs from that for a nonpregnant woman in one significant aspect: the presence of at least one other person—the fetus.
- Minor trauma is associated with major complications for the pregnancy, including abruptio placentae, fetomaternal hemorrhage, preterm labor and birth, and fetal death.

References

Abu-Heija A, al-Chalabi H, el-Iloubani N: Abruptio placentae: risk factors and perinatal outcome, *J Obstet Gynaecol Res* 24(2):141-144, 1998.

American College of Obstetricians and Gynecologists: *Antenatal corticosteroid therapy for fetal maturation (ACOG Tech Bull No. 147),* Washington, DC, 1994, ACOG.

American College of Obstetricians and Gynecologists: *Early pregnancy loss (ACOG Tech Bull No. 212),* Washington, DC, 1995, ACOG.

American College of Obstetricians and Gynecologists: *Hypertension in pregnancy (ACOG Tech Bull No. 219),* Washington, DC, 1996, ACOG.

Ananth C, Smulian J, Vintzileos A: The association of placenta previa with history of cesarean delivery and abortion: a meta-analysis, *Am J Obstet Gynecol* 177(5):1071-1078, 1997.

Atterbury J et al: Clinical presentation of women readmitted with postpartum severe preeclampsia or eclampsia, *J Obstet Gynecol Neonatal Nurs* 27(2):134-141, 1998.

Benedetti T: Obstetric hemorrhage. In Gabbe S, Niebyl J, Simpson J, editors: *Obstetrics: normal and problem pregnancies,* ed 3, New York, 1996, Churchill Livingstone.

Berman M, DiSaia P, Brewster W: Pelvic malignancy, gestational trophoblastic neoplasm, and nonpelvic malignancies. In Creasy R, Resnik R, editors: *Maternal-fetal medicine,* ed 4, Philadelphia, 1999, WB Saunders.

Clark S: Placenta previa and abruptio placenta. In Creasy R, Resnik R, editors: *Maternal-fetal medicine,* ed 4, Philadelphia, 1999, WB Saunders.

Colburn V: Trauma in pregnancy, *J Perinat Neonatal Nurs* 13(3):21-32, 1999.

Coleman M, Trianfo V, Rund D: Nonobstetric emergencies in pregnancy: trauma and surgical conditions, *Am J Obstet Gynecol* 177(3):497-502, 1997.

Copeland L, Landon M: Malignant diseases and pregnancy. In Gabbe S, Niebyl J, Simpson J, editors: *Obstetrics: normal and problem pregnancies,* ed 3, New York, 1996, Churchill Livingstone.

Corsi P et al: Trauma in pregnant women: analysis of maternal and fetal mortality, *Injury* 30(4):239-243, 1999.

Cruikshank D et al: Maternal physiology in pregnancy. In Gabbe S, Niebyl J, Simpson J, editors: *Obstetrics: normal and problem pregnancies,* ed 3, New York, 1996, Churchill Livingstone.

Cunningham F et al: *Williams obstetrics,* ed 20, Stamford, CT, 1997, Appleton & Lange.

Dekker G, Sibai B: Etiology and pathogenesis of preeclampsia: current concepts, *Am J Obstet Gynecol* 179(5):1359-1375, 1998.

DeLoia J, Stewart-Akers A, Creinin M: Effects of methotrexate on trophoblast proliferation and local immune responses, *Hum Reprod* 13(4):1063-1069, 1998.

Depp R: Cesarean delivery. In Gabbe S, Niebyl J, Simpson J, editors: *Obstetrics: normal and problem pregnancies,* ed 3, New York, 1996, Churchill Livingstone.

Enkin M et al: Effective care in pregnancy and childbirth: a synopsis, *Birth* 22(2):101-110, 1995.

Fairlie F, Sibai B: Hypertensive diseases in pregnancy. In Reece E et al, editors: *Medicine of the fetus and mother,* ed 2, Philadelphia, 1999, JB Lippincott.

Farmakides G et al: Doppler velocimetry. Where does it belong in evaluation of fetal status? *Clin Perinatol* 21(4):849-861, 1994.

Flystra D: Tubal pregnancy: a review of current diagnosis and treatment, *Obstet Gynecol Surv* 53(5):320-328, 1998.

Freda M: The power of words, *MCN Am J Matern Child Nurs* 24(2):63, 1999.

Friedman S: Preeclampsia: a review of the role of prostaglandins, *Obstet Gynecol* 71(1):122-137, 1988.

Friedman S et al: Biochemical corroboration of endothelial involvement in severe preeclampsia, *Am J Obstet Gynecol* 172:202-203, 1995.

Gilbert E, Harmon J: *Manual of high risk pregnancy and delivery,* ed 2, St Louis, 1998, Mosby.

Gilstrip L, Gant N: Pathophysiology of preeclampsia, *Semin Perinatol* 14(2):147-151, 1990.

Greenberg E et al: Vaginal bleeding and abuse: assessing pregnant women in the emergency department, *MCN Am J Matern Child Nurs* 22(4):182-186, 1997.

Grohar J: Nursing protocols for antepartum homecare, *J Obstet Gynecol Neonatal Nurs* 23(8):687-694, 1994.

Health Care Resources: *Handbook of high-risk prenatal home care,* St Louis, 1997, Mosby.

Hill W, Fleming A: Gastrointestinal diseases complicating pregnancy. In Reece E, Hobbins J, editors: *Medicine of the fetus and mother,* ed 2, Philadelphia, 1999, Lippincott-Raven.

Hunter S, Weiner C: Obstetric hemorrhage. In Repke J, editor: *Intrapartum obstetrics,* New York, 1996, Churchill Livingstone.

Hutti M, dePacheco M, Smith M: A study of miscarriage: development and validation of the Perinatal Grief Intensity Scale, *J Obstet Gynecol Neonatal Nurs* 27(5):547-555, 1998.

Huzel P, Remsburg-Bell E: Fetal complications related to minor maternal trauma, *J Obstet Gynecol Neonatal Nurs* 25(2):121-124, 1996.

Iams J: Preterm birth. In Gabbe S, Niebyl J, Simpson J, editors: *Obstetrics: normal and problem pregnancies,* ed 3, New York, 1996, Churchill Livingstone.

Jones D, Hayslett J: Outcome of pregnancy in women with moderate or severe renal insufficiency, *N Engl J Med* 335:226-232, 1996.

Kendrick J: Fetal and uterine response during maternal surgery, *MCN Am J Matern Child Nurs* 19(3):165-170, 1994.

Konje J, Walley R: Bleeding in late pregnancy. In James D et al, editors: *High risk pregnancy: management options,* Philadelphia, 1995, Saunders.

Knuppel R, Hatangadi S: Acute hypotension related to hemorrhage in the obstetric patient, *Obstet Gynecol Clin North Am* 22(1):111-129, 1995.

Koonin L et al: Pregnancy-related mortality surveillance—United States 1987-1990, *MMWR* 46(4):17-36, 1997.

Kramer M et al: Etiologic determinants of abruptio placentae, *Obstet Gynecol* 89(2):221-226, 1997.

Lavery J, Staten-McCormick M: Management of moderate to severe trauma in pregnancy, *Obstet Gynecol Clin North Am* 22(1):69-90, 1995.

Leicht T, Harvey C: Hypertensive disorders in pregnancy. In Mandeville L, Troiano N, editors: *AWHONN's high risk and critical care intrapartum nursing,* ed 2, Philadelphia, 1999, JB Lippincott.

Lipscomb G et al: Analysis of three hundred fifteen ectopic pregnancies treated with single-dose methotrexate, *Am J Obstet Gynecol* 178(6):1354-1358, 1998.

Lowdermilk D, Grohar J: *High risk antepartal home care,* White Plains, NY, 1999, March of Dimes.

Maiolatesi C, Petticord K: Methotrexate for nonsurgical treatment of ectopic pregnancy: nursing implications, *J Obstet Gynecol Neonatal Nurs* 25(2):205-208, 1996.

Maloni J: Home care of the high risk pregnant woman requiring bed rest, *J Obstet Gynecol Neonatal Nurs* 23:696-704, 1994.

Maloni J: *Antepartum bed rest: case studies, research and nursing care,* Washington, DC, 1998, AWHONN.

Mandeville L, Troiano N, editors: *AWHONN's high risk and critical care intrapartum nursing,* ed 2, Philadelphia, 1999, JB Lippincott.

Minnick-Smith K, Cook F: Current treatment options for ectopic pregnancy, *MCN Am J Matern Child Nurs* 22(10):21-25, 1997.

Pearlman M, Tintinalli J: Evaluation and treatment of the gravida and fetus following trauma during pregnancy, *Obstet Gynecol North Am* 18:371-381, 1991.

Poole J: HELLP syndrome and coagulopathies of pregnancy, *Crit Care Nurs Clin North Am* 5:457-487, 1993.

Poole J: Aggressive management of HELLP syndrome and preeclampsia, *AACN Clin Issues* 8(4):646-648, 1997.

Portis R et al: HELLP syndrome (hemolysis, elevated liver enzymes, and low platelets) pathophysiology and anesthetic considerations, *AANA J* 65(1):37-47, 1997.

Powell W, Spellman J: Medical management of the patient with an ectopic pregnancy, *J Perinat Neonatal Nurs* 9(4):31-43, 1996.

Riely C: Liver diseases in pregnancy. In Reece E, Hobbins J, editors: *Medicine of the fetus and mother,* ed 2, Philadelphia, 1999, Lippincott-Raven.

Roberts J: Pregnancy-related hypertension. In Creasy R, Resnik R, editors: *Maternal-fetal medicine,* ed 4, Philadelphia, 1999, WB Saunders.

Rogers F et al: A multi-institutional study of factors associated with fetal death in injured pregnant patients, *Arch Surg* 134(11):1274-1277, 1999.

Saunders E: Screening for domestic violence during pregnancy, *Int J Trauma Nurs* 6(2):44-47, 2000.

Sibai B: Drug therapy: treatment of hypertension in pregnant women, *N Engl J Med* 335(4):257-265, 1996a.

Sibai B: Hypertension in pregnancy. In Gabbe S, Niebyl J, Simpson J, editors: *Obstetrics: normal and problem pregnancies,* ed 3, New York, 1996b, Churchill Livingstone.

Sibai B et al: Risk factors associated with preeclampsia in healthy nulliparous women, *Am J Obstet Gynecol* 177(5):1003-1010, 1997.

Sibai B, Rodriguez J: Preeclampsia: diagnosis and management. In Reece E et al, editors: *Medicine of the fetus and mother,* Philadelphia, 1999, JB Lippincott.

Simpson J: Fetal wastage. In Gabbe S, Niebyl J, Simpson J, editors: *Obstetrics: normal and problem pregnancies,* ed 3, New York, 1996, Churchill Livingstone.

Sisson M, Sauer P: Pharmacologic therapy for pregnancy-induced hypertension, *J Perinatal Neonatal Nurs* 9(4):1-12, 1996.

Sivanesaratnam V: The acute abdomen and the obstetrician, *Baillieres Best Pract Res Clin Obstet Gynaecol* 14(1):89-102, 2000.

Snell L et al: Metabolic crisis: hyperemesis gravidarum, *J Perinat Neonatal Nurs* 12(2):26-37, 1998.

Stone J: HELLP syndrome: hemolysis, elevated liver enzymes, and low platelets, *JAMA* 280(6):559-562, 1998.

Thorp J: Third-trimester bleeding. In Moore T et al, editors: *Gynecology and obstetrics: a longitudinal approach,* New York, 1993, Churchill Livingstone.

Ventura S et al: Births: final data for 1997, *Natl Vital Stat Rep* 47(18):1-6, 1999.

Working Group on High Blood Pressure in Pregnancy: National high blood pressure education program working group report on high blood pressure in pregnancy, *Am J Obstet Gynecol* 163(5 pt 1):1689-1712, 1990.

CHAPTER 15

Labor and Birth Processes

http://www.harcourthealth.com/MERLIN/Wong/maternal/

Learning Objectives

On completion of this chapter the reader will be able to:

- Explain the five factors that affect the labor process.
- Describe the anatomic structure of the bony pelvis.
- Recognize the normal measurements of the diameters of the pelvic inlet, cavity, and outlet.
- Review the anatomy and measurements of the fetal skull.
- Explain the significance of molding of the fetal head during labor.
- Describe the cardinal movements of the mechanism of labor.
- Assess the maternal anatomic and physiologic adaptations to labor.
- Describe fetal adaptations to labor.

This chapter discusses the factors affecting labor, the process of labor, the normal progression of events, and the adaptations made by the woman and the fetus.

FACTORS AFFECTING LABOR

At least five factors affect the process of labor and birth. These are easily remembered as the five Ps: passenger (fetus and placenta), passageway (birth canal), powers (contractions), position of the mother, and psychologic response. The first four factors are presented here as the basis for understanding the physiologic process of labor. The fifth factor is discussed in Chapter 18.

Passenger

The movement of the passenger, or fetus, through the birth canal is a result of several interacting factors: size of the fetal head, fetal presentation, lie, attitude, and fetal position.

Because the placenta must also pass through the birth canal, it can be considered a passenger along with the fetus. However, the placenta rarely impedes the process of labor in normal vaginal birth.

Size of Fetal Head. The fetal head, because of its size and relative rigidity, has a major effect on the birth process. The fetal skull is composed of two parietal bones, two temporal bones, the frontal bone, and the occipital bone (Fig. 15-1, *A*).

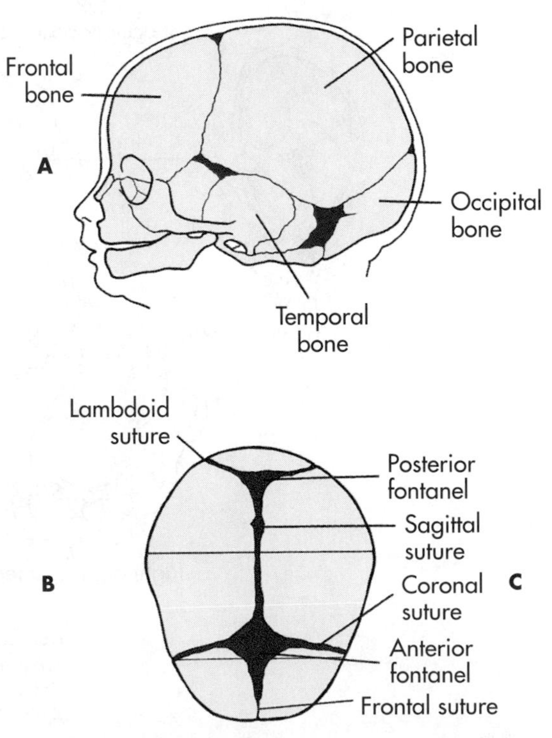

FIG. 15-1 • Fetal head at term. **A,** Bones. **B, C,** Sutures and fontanels.

These bones are united by membranous sutures: the sagittal, lambdoidal, coronal, and frontal (Fig. 15-1, *B*). Membrane-covered spaces called fontanels are located where the sutures intersect. After the rupture of amniotic membranes during labor, fetal presentation, position, and attitude may be assessed by palpating fontanels and sutures during vaginal examination.

The two most important fontanels are the anterior and posterior ones. The larger of these, the anterior fontanel, is diamond-shaped, about 2 cm by 3 cm in size, and lies at the junction of the sagittal, coronal, and frontal sutures. It closes by 18 months after birth. The posterior fontanel is triangular in shape, is about a 1 cm by 2 cm in size, and lies at the junction of the sutures of the two parietal bones and the occipital bone. It closes 6 to 8 weeks after birth.

Sutures and fontanels make the skull flexible to accommodate the infant brain, which continues to grow for some time after birth. Because the bones are not firmly united, however, slight overlapping of the bones, or molding of the shape of the head, occurs during labor. This capacity of the bones to slide over one another also permits adaptation to the various diameters of the maternal pelvis. Molding can be extensive, but with most newborns the head assumes its normal shape within 3 days of birth.

Although the size of the fetal shoulders may affect passage, their position can be altered relatively easily during labor so one shoulder occupies a lower level than the other. This creates a shoulder diameter that is smaller than that of the skull, facilitating passage through the birth canal. The circumference of the fetal hips is usually small enough not to create problems.

Fetal Presentation. Presentation refers to the part of the fetus that enters the pelvic inlet first and leads through the birth canal during labor at term. The three main presentations are cephalic (head first), occurring in 96% of births (Fig. 15-2); breech (buttocks first) occurring in 3% of births (Fig. 15-3, *A, B, C*); and shoulder, seen in 1% of births (Fig. 15-3, *D*). Presenting part refers to that part of the fetal body first felt by the examining finger during a vaginal examination. In a cephalic presentation, the presenting part is usually the occiput; in a breech presentation, it is the sacrum; in the shoulder presentation, it is the scapula of the shoulder. When the pre-

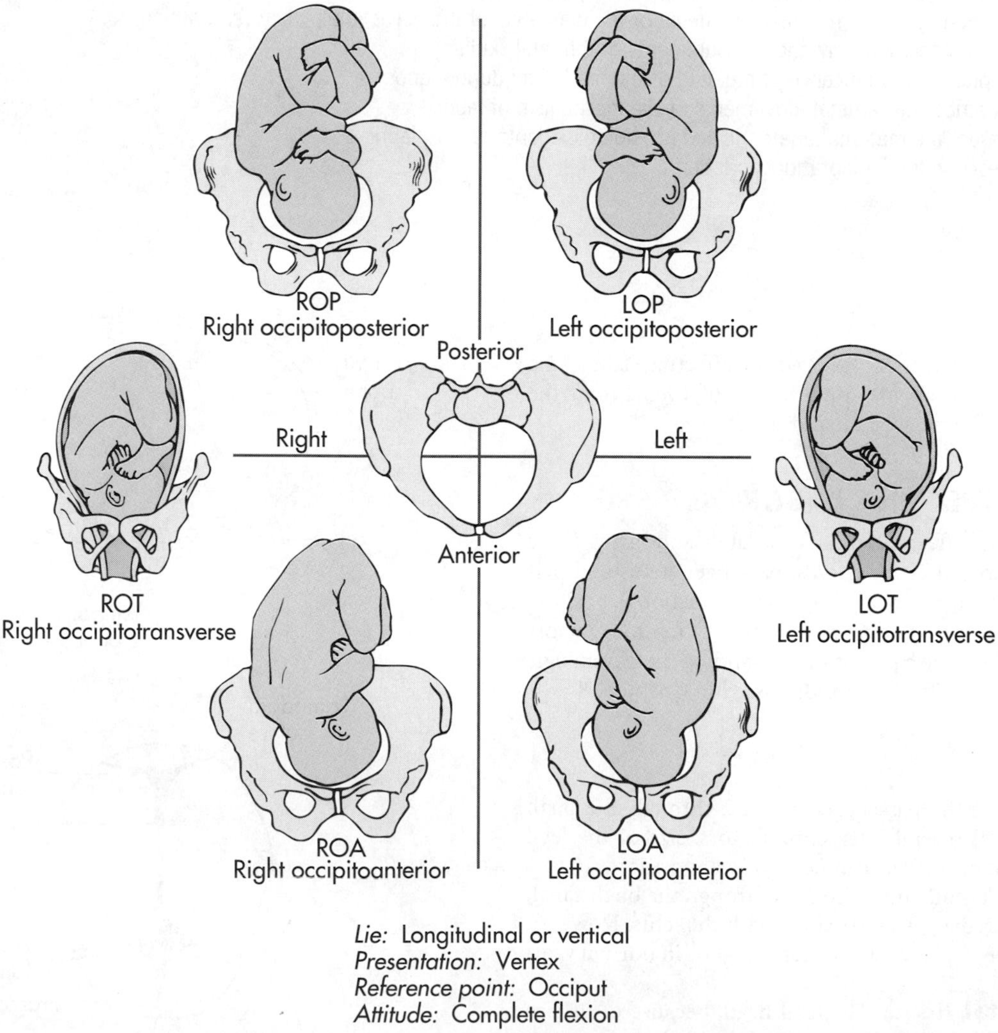

FIG. 15-2 • Examples of fetal vertex (occiput) presentations in relation to front, back, or side of maternal pelvis.

senting part is the occiput, the presentation is noted as vertex (Fig. 15-2). Factors that determine the presenting part include fetal lie, fetal attitude, and extension or flexion of the fetus's head.

Fetal Lie. Lie is the relationship of the long axis (spine) of the fetus to the long axis (spine) of the mother. There are two primary lies: longitudinal, or vertical, in which the long axis of the fetus is parallel with the long axis of the mother (see Figs. 15-2 and 15-3 *A, B, C*); and transverse, horizontal, or oblique, in which the long axis of the fetus is at a right angle to the long axis of the mother (see Fig. 15-3, *D*). Longitudinal lies are either cephalic or breech presentations, depending on the fetal structure that first enters the mother's pelvis. Vaginal birth cannot occur when the fetus stays in a transverse lie.

Fetal Attitude. Attitude is the relationship of the fetal body parts to each other. The fetus assumes a characteristic posture (attitude) in utero partly because of the mode of fetal growth and partly because of the way the fetus conforms to the shape of the uterine cavity. Normally, the back of the fetus is rounded so that the chin is flexed on the chest, the thighs are flexed on the abdomen, and the legs are flexed at the knees. The arms are crossed over the thorax, and the umbilical cord lies between the arms and the legs. This attitude is called general flexion (see Fig. 15-2).

Fetal Head Flexion. The biparietal diameter is the largest transverse diameter and measures about 9.25 cm at term (Fig. 15-4, *B*). In a well-flexed cephalic presentation, the biparietal diameter is the widest part of the head entering the pelvic inlet. There are several anteroposterior diameters, but the smallest and most important one is the suboccipitobregmatic diameter, which is about 9.5 cm at term. When the head is in complete flexion, this diameter allows the fetal head to pass through the true pelvis easily (Fig. 15-4, *A;* Fig. 15-5, *A*).When the head is more extended, the anteroposterior diameter widens and the head may not be able to enter the true pelvis (Fig. 15-5, *B, C*).

Fetal Position. The presentation or presenting part indicates that portion of the fetus that overlies the pelvic inlet. Position is the relationship of the presenting part (i.e., occiput, sacrum, mentum [chin], or sinciput [deflexed vertex]) to the four quadrants of the mother's pelvis (see Fig. 15-2). Position is

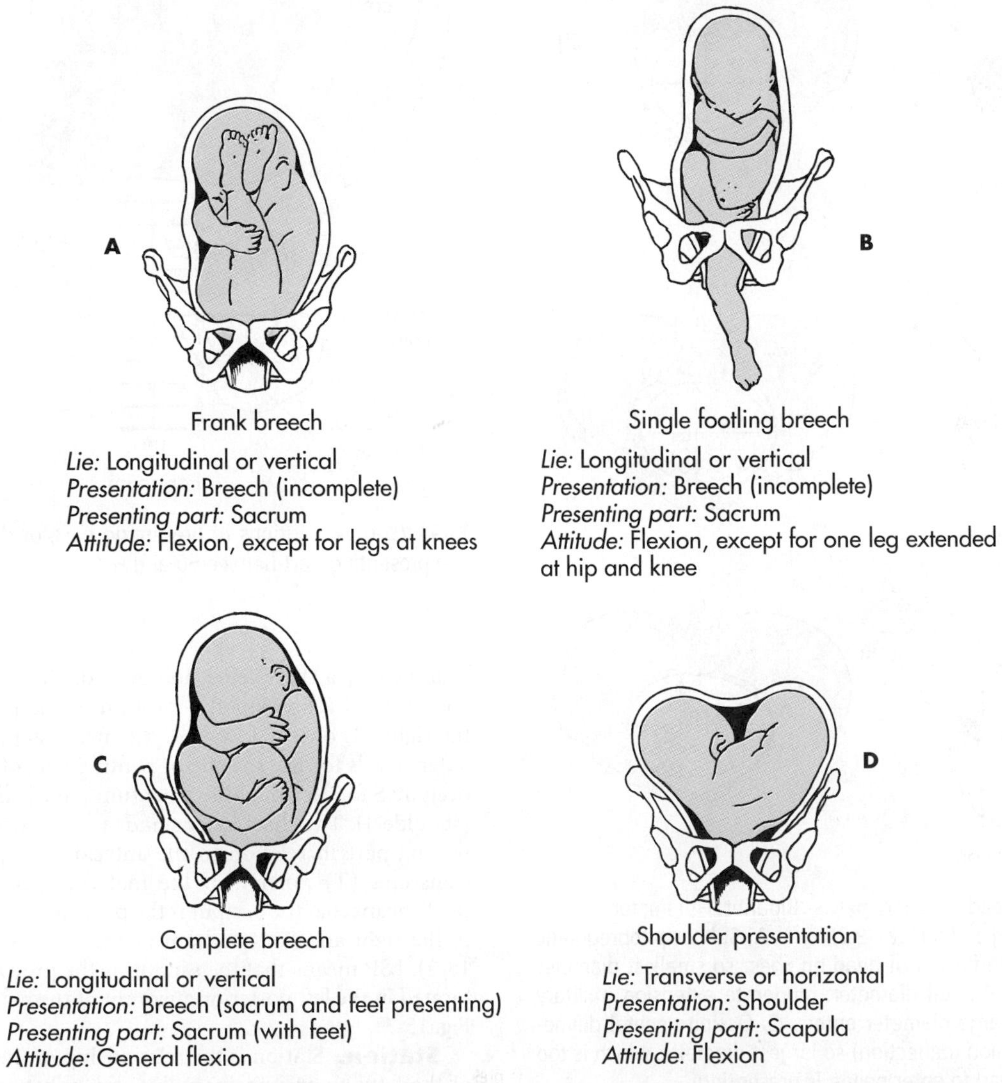
A
Frank breech
Lie: Longitudinal or vertical
Presentation: Breech (incomplete)
Presenting part: Sacrum
Attitude: Flexion, except for legs at knees
B
Single footling breech
Lie: Longitudinal or vertical
Presentation: Breech (incomplete)
Presenting part: Sacrum
Attitude: Flexion, except for one leg extended at hip and knee
C
Complete breech
Lie: Longitudinal or vertical
Presentation: Breech (sacrum and feet presenting)
Presenting part: Sacrum (with feet)
Attitude: General flexion
D
Shoulder presentation
Lie: Transverse or horizontal
Presentation: Shoulder
Presenting part: Scapula
Attitude: Flexion

FIG. 15-3 • Fetal presentations. **A, B, C,** Breech (sacral) presentation. **D,** Shoulder presentation.

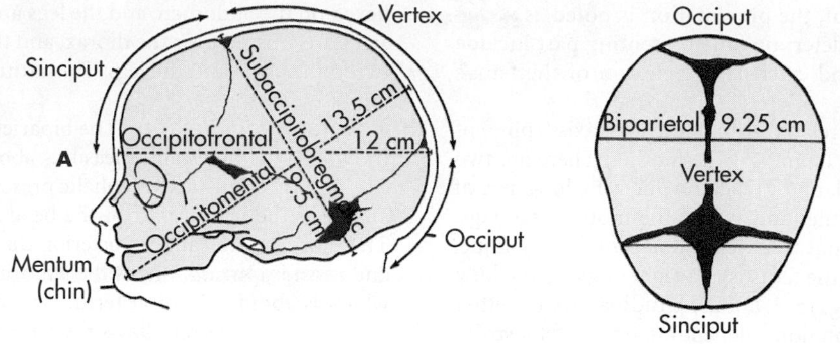

FIG. 15-4 • Diameters of the fetal head at term. **A,** Cephalic presentations: occiput, vertex, and sinciput; and cephalic diameters: suboccipitobregmatic, occipitofrontal, and occipitomental. **B,** Biparietal diameter.

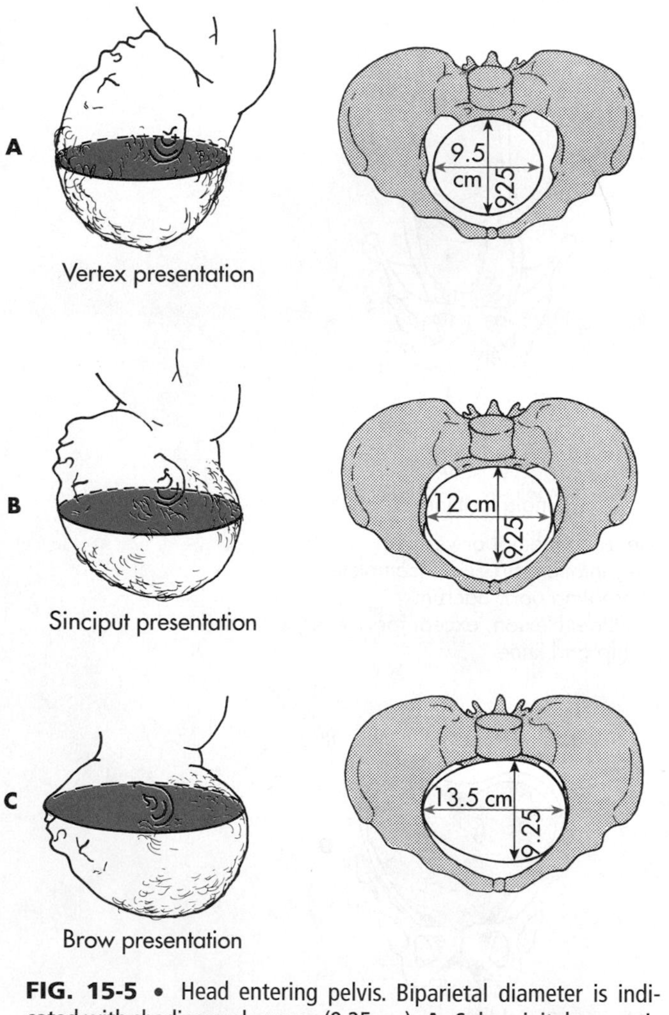

FIG. 15-5 • Head entering pelvis. Biparietal diameter is indicated with shading and arrows (9.25 cm). **A,** Suboccipitobregmatic diameter: complete flexion of head on chest so smallest diameter enters. **B,** Occipitofrontal diameter: moderate extension (military attitude) so that large diameter enters. **C,** Occipitomental diameter: marked extension (deflection) so largest diameter, which is too large to permit head to enter pelvis, is presenting.

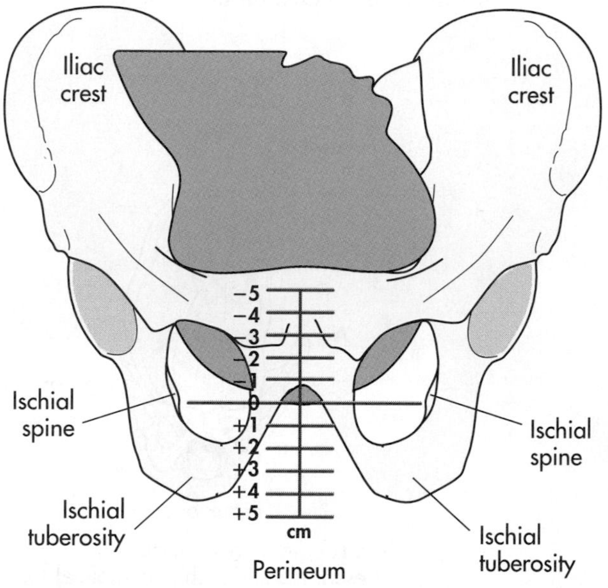

FIG. 15-6 • Stations of presenting part, or degree of descent. The presenting part between 0 and +1.

indicated by a three-letter abbreviation. The first letter of the abbreviation represents the location of the presenting part in the right (R) or left (L) side of the maternal pelvis. The middle letter stands for the specific presenting part of the fetus (O for occiput, S for sacrum, M for mentum [chin], and Sc for scapula [shoulder]). The third letter stands for the location of the presenting part in relation to the anterior (A), posterior (P), or transverse (T) portion of the maternal pelvis. For example, ROA means that the occiput is the presenting part and is located in the right anterior quadrant of the maternal pelvis (see Fig. 15-2). LSP means that the sacrum is the presenting part and is located in the left posterior quadrant of the maternal pelvis (see Fig. 15-3).

Station. Station is the relationship of the presenting part of the fetus to an imaginary line drawn between the maternal

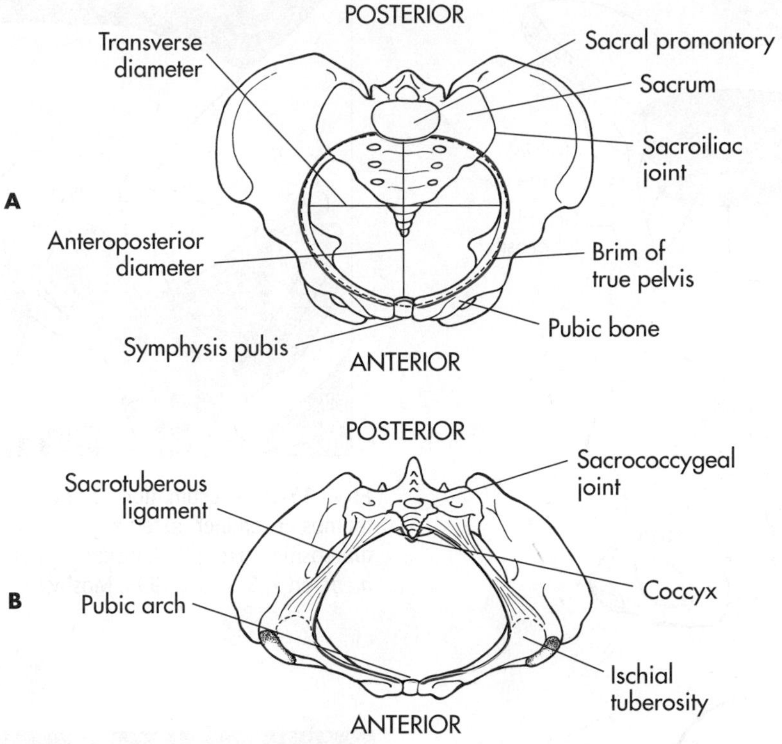

FIG. 15-7 • Female pelvis. **A,** Pelvic brim from above. **B,** Pelvic outlet from below.

ischial spines; it is a measure of the degree of descent of the presenting part of the fetus through the birth canal. Station is expressed in centimeters above or below the spines. For example, when the presenting part is 1 cm above the spines, it is noted as being minus 1 (-1) (Fig. 15-6). At the level of the spines, the station is referred to as zero (0). When the presenting part is 1 cm below the spines, the station is said to be plus 1 (+1). Birth is imminent when the presenting part is at +4 to +5 cm. The station of the presenting part should be assessed when labor begins so that the rate of descent of the fetus during labor can be determined accurately.

Engagement is the term used to indicate that the largest transverse diameter of the presenting part (usually the biparietal diameter) has passed through the maternal pelvic brim or inlet into the true pelvis; this usually corresponds to station. Engagement often occurs in the weeks just before labor begins in primigravidas and may occur before or during labor in multigravidas. Engagement can be determined by abdominal or vaginal examination.

Passageway

The passageway, or birth canal, is composed of the mother's rigid bony pelvis and the soft tissues of the cervix, pelvic floor, vagina, and introitus (the external opening to the vagina). Although the soft tissues (particularly the muscular layers of the pelvic floor) contribute to vaginal birth of the fetus, the maternal pelvis plays a far greater role in the labor process. The fetus must successfully accommodate itself to this relatively rigid passageway. Therefore the size and shape of the pelvis must be determined before childbirth begins.

Bony Pelvis. The anatomy of the bony pelvis is described in Chapter 5. The following discussion focuses on the importance of pelvic configurations as they relate to the labor process. (It may be helpful to refer to Figs. 5-5 and 5-6.)

The bony pelvis is formed by the fusion of the ilium, ischium, pubis, and sacrum bones. The bony pelvis is separated by the brim, or inlet, into two parts: the false pelvis and the true pelvis. The false pelvis is that part above the brim and plays no part in childbearing. The true pelvis is divided into three planes: the inlet or brim, the midpelvis or cavity, and the outlet.

The pelvic inlet, the upper border of the true pelvis, is formed anteriorly by the upper margins of the pubic bone; laterally by the iliopectineal lines along the innominate bones; and posteriorly by the anterior, upper margin of the sacrum and the sacral promontory.

The pelvic cavity, or midpelvis, is a curved passage with a short anterior wall and a much longer concave posterior wall. It is bounded by the posterior aspect of the symphysis pubis, the ischium, a portion of the ilium, the sacrum, and the coccyx.

The pelvic outlet is the lower border of the true pelvis. Viewed from below, it is ovoid and somewhat diamond-shaped. It is bounded by the pubic arch anteriorly, the ischial tuberosities laterally, and the tip of the coccyx posteriorly (Fig. 15-7, *B*). In the latter part of pregnancy the coccyx is movable (unless it has been broken in a fall during skiing or skating, for example, and has fused to the sacrum during healing).

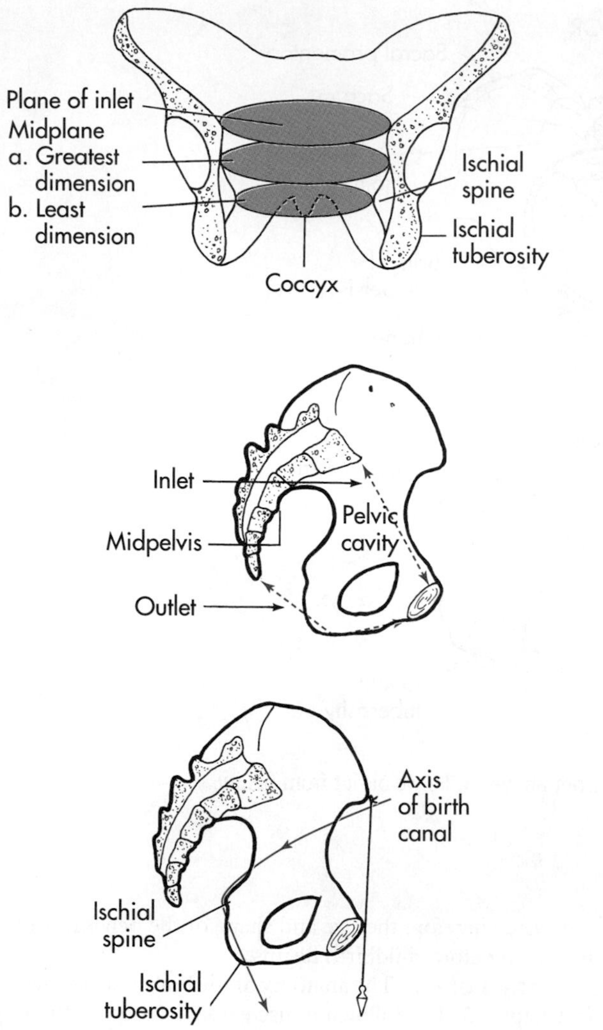

FIG. 15-8 • Pelvic cavity. **A,** Inlet and midplane. Outlet not shown. **B,** Cavity of true pelvis. **C,** Note curve of sacrum and axis of birth canal.

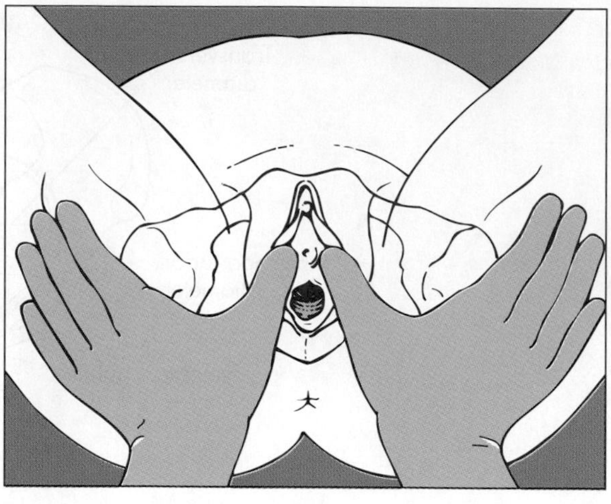

FIG. 15-9 • Estimation of angle of subpubic arch. Using both thumbs, examiner externally traces descending rami down to tuberosities. (From Barkauskas V et al: *Health and physical assessment,* ed 2, St Louis, 1998, Mosby.)

Critical Thinking

OBSTETRIC MEASUREMENTS

Examine three prenatal records for evidence of obstetric measurements. What measurements were done? By what method were the measurements assessed? Compare the findings with stated norms. Are the measurements adequate? Is a vaginal birth expected for these women? What patient teaching is necessary based on these findings?

The pelvic canal varies in size and shape at various levels. The diameters at the plane of the pelvic inlet, midpelvis, and outlet, plus the axis of the birth canal (Fig. 15-8) determine whether vaginal birth is possible and the manner by which the fetus may pass down the birth canal.

The subpubic angle, which indicates the type of pubic arch, together with the length of the pubic rami and the intertuberous diameter, is of great importance. Because the fetus must first pass beneath the pubic arch, a narrow subpubic angle is less favorable than a rounded, wide arch. Measurement of the subpubic arch is shown in Fig. 15-9. A summary of obstetric measurements is given in Table 15-1.

The four basic types of pelvis are gynecoid, android, anthropoid, and platypelloid. The gynecoid (classic female type) pelvis is the most common, with major gynecoid pelvic features present in 50% of all women. Anthropoid (resembling the pelvis of anthropoid apes) and android (resembling the male pelvis) features are less common, and platypelloid (the flat pelvis) pelvic features are the least common. Mixed types of pelves are more common than pure types (Cunningham et al, 1997). Examples of pelvic variations and their effects on mode of birth are given in Table 15-2.

Assessment of the bony pelvis can be performed during the first prenatal evaluation and need not be repeated if the pelvis is of adequate size and suitable shape. In the third trimester of pregnancy, the examination of the bony pelvis may be more thorough and the results more accurate because there is relaxation of the pelvic joints and ligaments due to hormonal influences. Widening of the joint of the symphysis pubis and the resulting instability may cause pain in any or all of the pelvic joints.

Because the examiner does not have direct access to the bony structures and because the bones are covered with varying amounts of soft tissue, estimates of size and shape are approximate. Precise bony pelvis measurements can be determined by using computed tomography, ultrasound, or x-ray films. X-ray examination is rarely done during pregnancy because the x-rays may damage the developing fetus.

Soft Tissues. The soft tissues of the passageway include the distensible lower uterine segment, cervix, pelvic floor muscles, vagina, and introitus (external opening to the vagina). Before labor begins, the uterus is composed of the uterine body (corpus) and cervix (neck). After labor has begun, uterine con-

TABLE 15-1
Obstetric Measurements

Plane	Diameter	Measurements
Inlet (superior strait)		
Conjugates		
Diagonal	12.5-13 cm	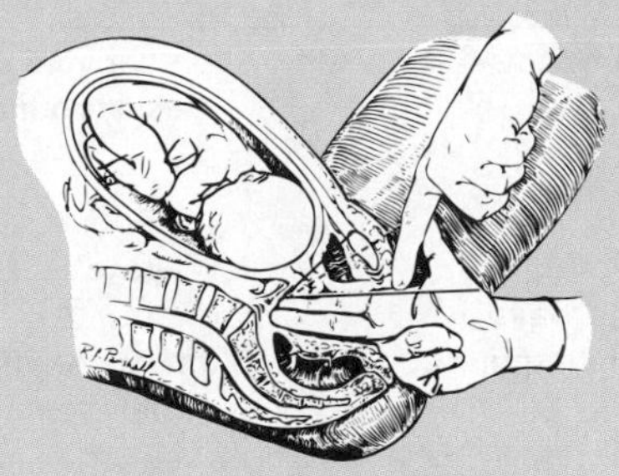
Obstetric: measurement that determines whether presenting part can engage or enter superior strait	1.5-2 cm less than diagonal (radiographic)	
True (vera) (anteroposterior)	≥11 cm (12.5) (radiographic)	Length of diagonal conjugate (solid colored line), obstetric conjugate (broken colored line), and true conjugate (black line)*
		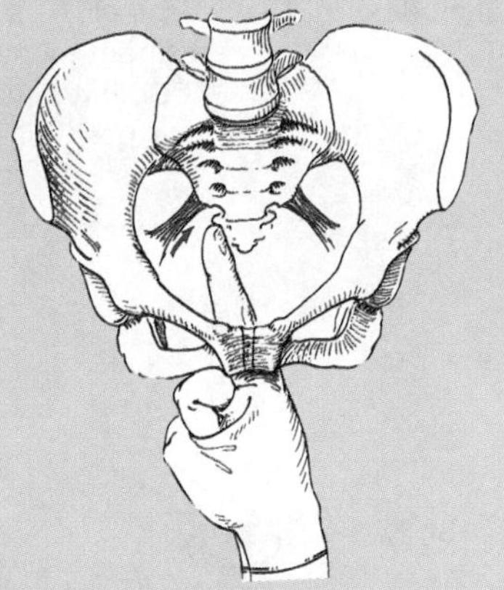
Midplane Transverse diameter (interspinous diameter) The midplane of the pelvis normally is its largest plane and the one of greatest diameter.	10.5 cm	Measurement of interspinous diameter*
		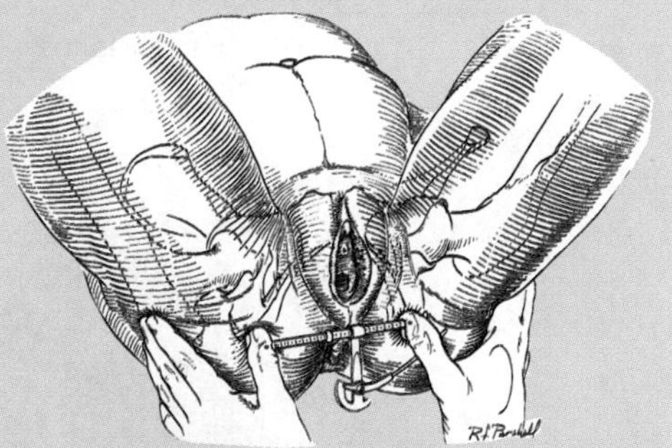
Outlet Transverse diameter (intertuberous diameter) (biischial) The outlet presents the smallest plane of the pelvic canal.	≥8 cm	Use of Thom's pelvimeter to measure intertuberous diameter*

*From Seidel H, et al: *Mosby's guide to physical examination,* ed 3, St Louis, 1995, Mosby.

tractions cause the uterine body to have a thick and muscular upper segment and a thin-walled, passive, muscular lower segment. A physiologic retraction ring separates the two segments (Fig. 15-10). The lower uterine segment gradually distends to accommodate the intrauterine contents as the wall of the upper segment thickens and its accommodating capacity is reduced. Contractions of the uterine body thus exert downward pressure on the fetus, pushing it against the cervix.

The cervix effaces (thins) and dilates (opens) sufficiently to allow descent of the first fetal portion into the vagina. As the fetus descends, the cervix is actually drawn upward and over this first portion.

TABLE 15-2
Comparison of Pelvic Types

	Gynecoid (50% of Women)	Android (23% of Women)	Anthropoid (24% of Women)	Platypelloid (3% of Women)
Brim	Slightly ovoid or transversely rounded Round	Heart shaped, angulated Heart	Oval, wider anteroposteriorly Oval	Flattened anteroposteriorly, wide transversely Flat
Depth	Moderate	Deep	Deep	Shallow
Side walls	Straight	Convergent	Straight	Straight
Ischial spines	Blunt, somewhat widely separated	Prominent, narrow interspinous diameter	Prominent, often with narrow interspinous diameter	Blunted, widely separated
Sacrum	Deep, curved	Slightly curved, terminal portion often beaked	Slightly curved	Slightly curved
Subpubic arch	Wide	Narrow	Narrow	Wide
Usual mode of birth	Vaginal Spontaneous Occipitoanterior position	Cesarean Vaginal Difficult with forceps	Forceps/spontaneous Occipitoposterior or occipitoanterior position	Vaginal Spontaneous

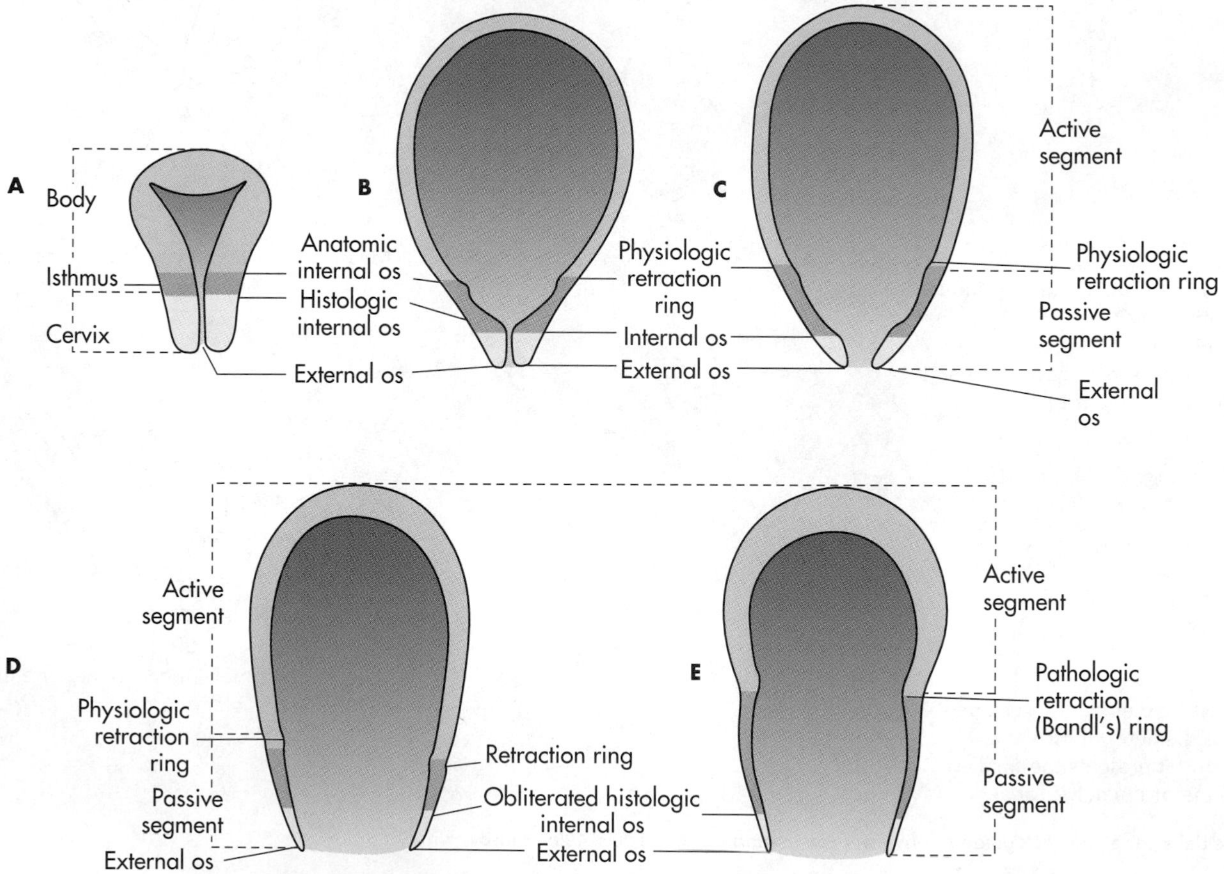

FIG. 15-10 • Progressive development of segments and rings of uterus at term. Note differences in **A,** nonpregnant uterus; **B,** uterus at term; **C,** uterus in normal labor in early first stage; and **D,** in second stage. Passive segment is derived from lower uterine segment (isthmus) and cervix, and physiologic retraction ring is derived from anatomic internal os. **E,** Uterus in abnormal labor in second-stage dystocia. Pathologic retraction (Bandl's) ring that forms under abnormal conditions develops from physiologic ring. (Modified from Willson J, Carrington E: *Obstetrics and gynecology,* ed 9, St Louis, 1991, Mosby.)

The pelvic floor is a muscular layer that separates the pelvic cavity above from the perineal space below. This structure helps the fetus rotate anteriorly as it passes through the birth canal. As noted earlier, the soft tissues of the vagina develop throughout pregnancy until at term the vagina can dilate to accommodate the fetus and permit passage of the fetus to the external world.

Powers

Involuntary and voluntary contractions combine to expel the fetus and the placenta from the uterus. Involuntary uterine contractions, called primary powers, signal the beginning of labor. Once the cervix has dilated, voluntary bearing-down efforts by the woman, called secondary powers, augment the force of the involuntary contractions.

Primary Powers. The involuntary contractions originate at certain pacemaker points in the thickened muscle layers of the upper uterine segment. From the pacemaker points, contractions move downward over the uterus in waves, separated by short rest periods.

The primary powers are responsible for the effacement and dilation of the cervix and descent of the fetus. Effacement of the cervix means the shortening and thinning of the cervix during the first stage of labor. The cervix, normally 2 to 3 cm in length and about 1 cm thick, is obliterated or "taken up" by a shortening of the uterine muscle bundles during the thinning of the lower uterine segment that occurs in advancing labor. Only a thin edge of the cervix can be palpated when effacement is complete. Effacement generally occurs in first-time pregnancy at term before more than slight dilation occurs. In subsequent pregnancies, effacement and dilation of the cervix tend to progress together. Degree of effacement is expressed in percentages from 0 to 100 (e.g., a cervix is 50% effaced) (Fig. 15-11 *A, B, C*).

Dilation of the cervix is the enlargement or widening of the cervical opening and the cervical canal that occurs once labor has begun. The diameter of the cervix increases from less than 1 cm to full dilation (approximately 10 cm) to allow birth of a term fetus. When the cervix is fully dilated (and completely retracted), it can no longer be palpated (Fig. 15-11, *D*). Full cervical dilation marks the end of the first stage of labor.

Dilation of the cervix occurs by the drawing upward of the musculofibrous components of the cervix as a result of strong uterine contractions. Pressure exerted by the amniotic fluid

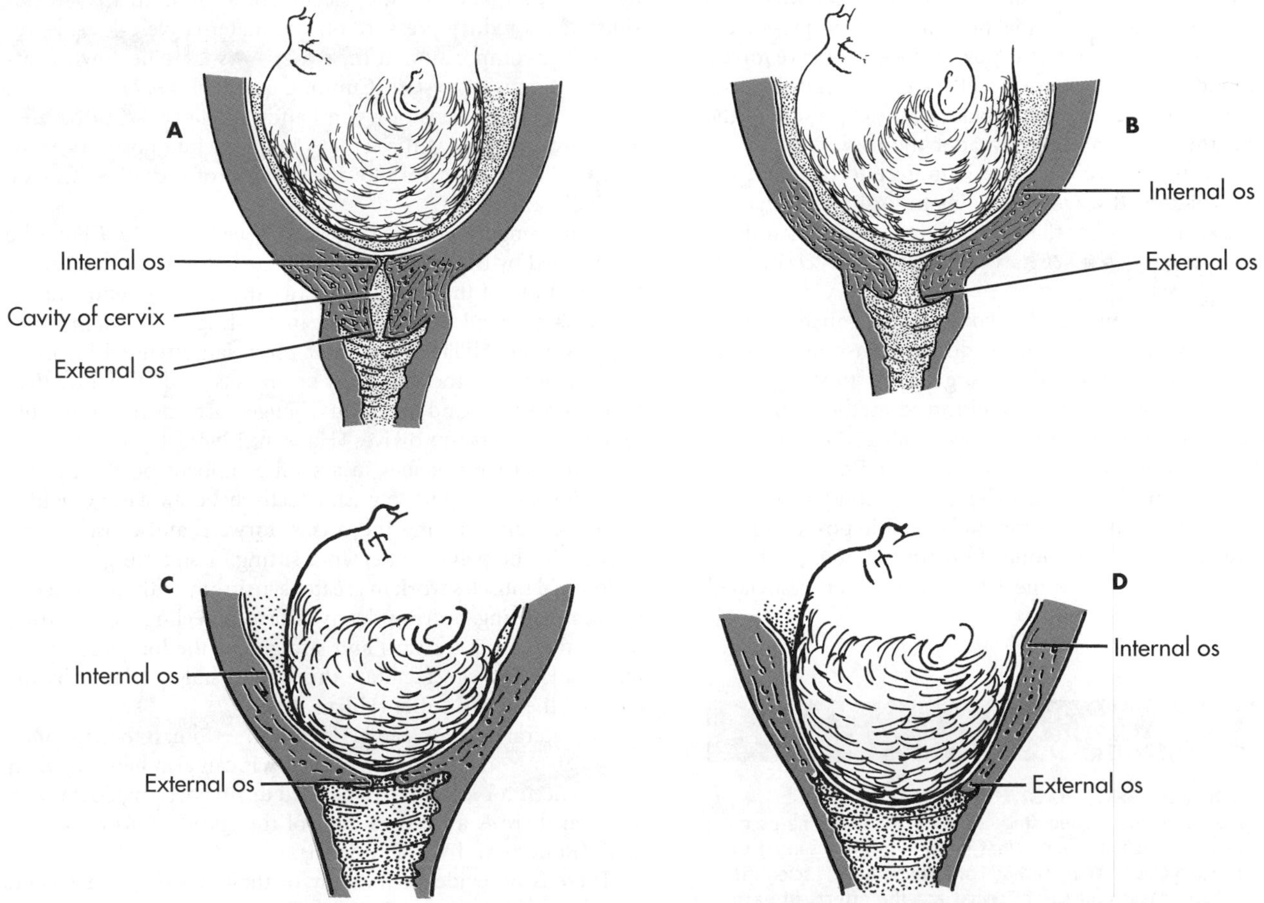

FIG. 15-11 • Cervical effacement and dilation. Note how cervix is drawn up around presenting part (internal os). Membranes are intact, and head is not well applied to cervix. **A,** Before labor. **B,** Early effacement. **C,** Complete effacement (100%). Head is well applied to cervix. **D,** Complete dilation (10 cm). There is some overlapping of cranial bones and membranes are intact.

while the membranes are intact, and the force applied by the presenting part also promote cervical dilation. Scarring of the cervix as a result of prior infection or surgery may slow cervical dilation.

In the first and second stages of labor, increased intrauterine pressure caused by contractions exerts pressure on the descending fetus and the cervix. When the presenting part of the fetus reaches the perineal floor, mechanical stretching of the cervix occurs. Stretch receptors in the posterior vagina cause release of exogenous oxytocin that triggers the maternal urge to bear down, or the Ferguson reflex.

Uterine contractions are involuntary and usually independent from external forces. For example, laboring women who are paraplegic have normal uterine contractions (Cunningham et al, 1997). Uterine contractions may decrease temporarily in frequency and intensity when narcotic analgesic medication or epidural analgesia is given early in labor (Alexander et al, 1998). There is continuing investigation of the relationship between prolonged labor and epidural analgesia (Thompson et al, 1998).

Secondary Powers. As soon as the presenting part reaches the pelvic floor the contractions change in character and become expulsive. The woman experiences an involuntary urge to push. She uses secondary powers (bearing-down efforts) to aid in expulsion of the fetus as she contracts her diaphragm and abdominal muscles and pushes. These bearing down efforts result in increased intraabdominal pressure that compresses the uterus on all sides and adds to the power of the expulsive forces.

The secondary powers have no effect on cervical dilation, but they are of considerable importance in the expulsion of the infant from the uterus and vagina after the cervix is fully dilated. Pushing in the second stage is more effective, and the woman is less fatigued when she begins to push only after she has the urge to do so rather than beginning to push when she is fully dilated but does not yet have the urge to do so (Roberts and Woolley, 1996).

The way a woman pushes in second stage is much debated. Spontaneous bearing-down efforts, directed pushing, Valsalva (closed glottis and prolonged bearing down) pushing, open glottis pushing, "mini" pushing, and forced methods of pushing have been investigated (Mayberry et al, 2000; Paine and Tinker, 1992; Thomson, 1995; Woolley and Roberts, 1995). While no significant differences in length of second-stage labor have been found among these methods, fetal hypoxia and acidosis are associated with prolonged breath holding and forceful pushing efforts, and perineal tears have been associated with directed pushing. Continued study is needed to determine the effectiveness and safety of various pushing techniques in relation to maternal and fetal outcomes (Peterson and Besuner, 1997).

Critical Thinking

EDUCATION FOR SECOND STAGE LABOR

Prepare a class on the second stage of labor for first-time pregnant women and their partners. What information is essential to include in such a class? What methods of pushing have a scientific base for effectiveness and safety? What are the effects of each type of pushing on the mother and the fetus? What types of pushing have you observed in the clinical setting? What types of coaching by nurses did you observe? To what extent do the nurses encourage pushing techniques that are scientifically sound?

Position of the Woman in Labor

Maternal position affects the woman's anatomic and physiologic adaptations to labor. Frequent changes in position relieve fatigue, increase comfort, and improve circulation. A woman in labor should be encouraged to find the positions that are most comfortable to her (Fig. 15-12, *A*).

An upright position (e.g., walking, sitting, kneeling, or squatting) offers a number of advantages. Gravity can promote the descent of the fetus. Uterine contractions are generally stronger and more efficient in effacing and dilating the cervix, resulting in shorter labor (Shermer and Raines, 1997).

An upright position is also beneficial to the mother's cardiac output, which normally increases during labor as uterine contractions return blood to the vascular bed. Increased cardiac output improves blood flow to the uteroplacental unit and the maternal kidneys. Cardiac output is compromised if the descending aorta and ascending vena cava are compressed during labor. Compression of these major vessels may result in supine hypotension that decreases placental perfusion. An upright position helps reduce pressure on the maternal vessels and prevents their compression. If the woman wishes to lie down, a lateral position is suggested (Cunningham et al, 1997).

The "all-fours" position (on hands and knees) may be used to relieve backache if the fetus is in an occipitoposterior position, and may assist in anterior rotation of the fetus (Coates, 1999; Simkin, 1995).

Positioning for second-stage labor (see Fig. 15-12, *B*) may be determined by the woman's preference, but it is constrained by the condition of the woman or fetus, the environment, and the health care provider's confidence in assisting in a birth in a specific position (Hillan, 1999). For physician-attended births in the United States, the lithotomy position is predominant. Alternative positions and position changes are more commonly practiced by nurse-midwives (Hanson, 1998).

A woman who pushes in a semirecumbent position needs adequate body support to push effectively because her weight is on her sacrum, moving the coccyx forward and causing a reduction in the pelvic outlet. In a sitting or squatting position, abdominal muscles work in greater synchrony with uterine contractions during bearing-down efforts. Kneeling or squatting moves the uterus forward and straightens the long axis of the birth canal and can facilitate the second stage of labor by increasing the pelvic outlet (Hillan, 1999).

The lateral position can be used by the woman to help rotate a fetus that is in a posterior position. It can also be used when there is need for less force to be used during bearing down such as when there is a need to control the speed of a precipitous birth (Roberts and Woolley, 1996).

There is no evidence that any of these positions for second stage-labor increase the need for operative techniques (e.g., forceps- or vacuum-assisted birth, cesarean birth, and episiotomy) or cause perineal trauma. There is also no evidence that use of any of these positions adversely affects the newborn (Biancuzzo, 1993; Golay, Vedam, and Sorger, 1993; Mayberry et al, 1999).

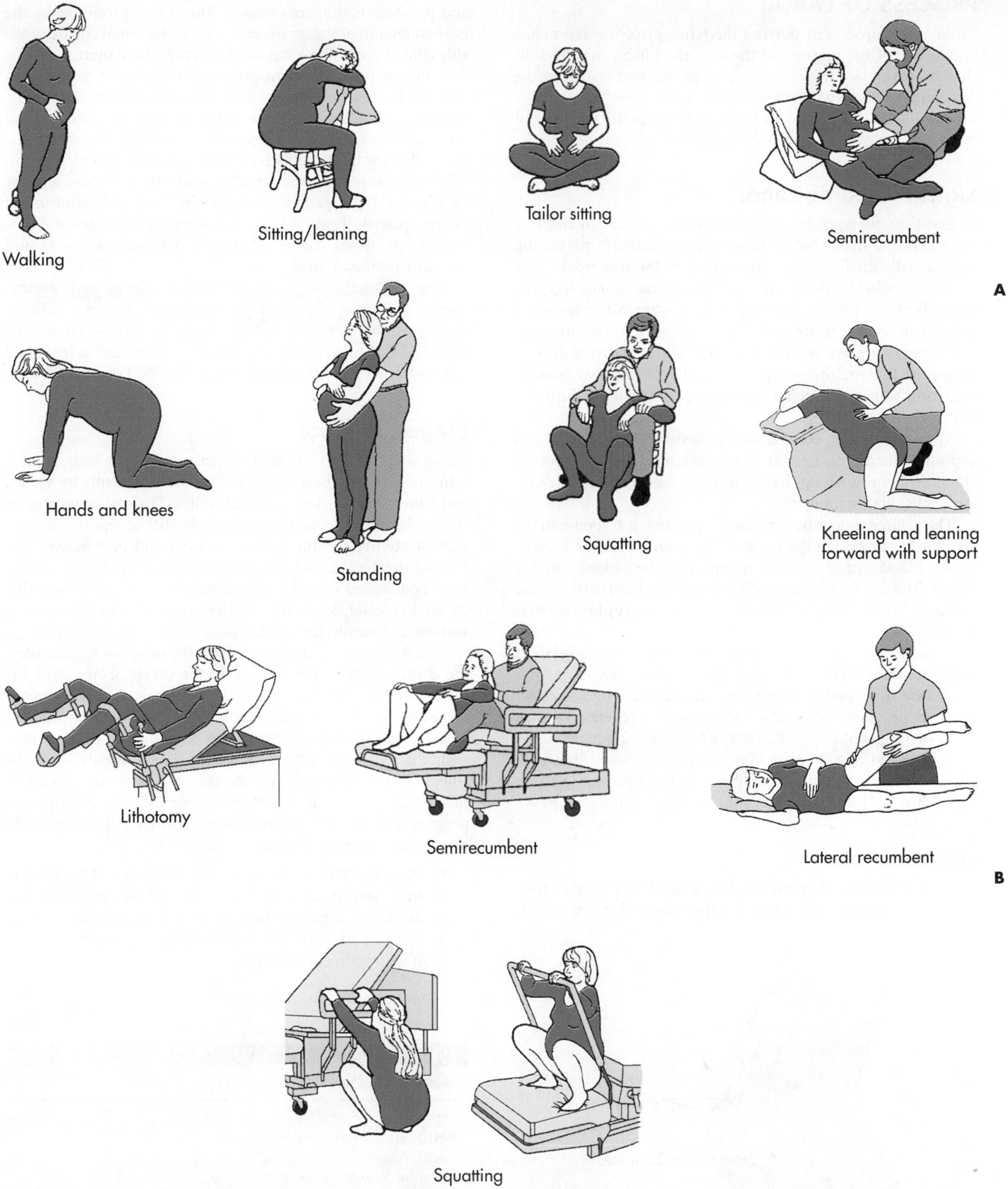

FIG. 15-12 • Positions for labor and birth. **A,** Positions for labor. **B,** Positions for birth.

PROCESS OF LABOR

Labor is the process of moving the fetus, placenta, and membranes out of the uterus and through the birth canal. Various changes take place in the woman's reproductive system in the days and weeks before labor begins. Labor itself can be discussed in terms of the mechanisms involved in the process and the stages the woman moves through.

Signs Preceding Labor

In first-time pregnancies, the uterus sinks downward and forward about 2 weeks before term, when the fetus's presenting part (usually the fetal head) descends into the true pelvis. This settling is called lightening or "dropping" and usually happens gradually (Fig. 15-13). After lightening, women feel less congested and breathe more easily. However, there is usually more bladder pressure as a result of this shift, and a return of urinary frequency. In a multiparous pregnancy, lightening may not take place until after uterine contractions are established and true labor is in progress.

The woman may complain of persistent low backache and sacroiliac distress as a result of relaxation of the pelvic joints. She may identify strong, frequent, but irregular uterine (Braxton Hicks) contractions.

The vaginal mucus becomes more profuse in response to the extreme congestion of the vaginal mucous membranes. Brownish or blood-tinged cervical mucus may be passed (bloody show). The cervix becomes soft (ripens) and partially effaced and may begin to dilate. The membranes may rupture spontaneously.

Other phenomena are common in the days preceding labor: a weight loss of 0.5 to 1.5 kg, caused by water loss resulting from electrolyte shifts that in turn are produced by changes in estrogen and progesterone levels; and a surge of energy. Women speak of a burst of energy that they often use to clean the house and put everything in order. Less commonly, some women experience diarrhea, nausea, vomiting, and indigestion (Varney, 1997). Box 15-1 lists signs that may precede labor.

Onset of Labor

The onset of true labor cannot be ascribed to a single cause. Many factors, including changes in the maternal uterus, cervix, and pituitary gland, are involved. Hormones produced by the normal fetal hypothalamus, pituitary, and adrenal cortex probably contribute to the onset of labor. Progressive uterine distention, increasing intrauterine pressure, and aging of the placenta seem to be associated with increasing myometrial irritability. This is a result of increased concentrations of estrogen and prostaglandins, as well as decreasing progesterone levels. The mutually coordinated effects of these factors are strong, regular, rhythmic uterine contractions. Normally, the outcome of these factors working together is birth of the fetus and expulsion of the placenta; however, it is still not completely understood how certain alterations trigger others and how proper checks and balances are maintained.

Fetal fibronectin is a protein found in plasma and cervicovaginal secretions of pregnant women before the onset of labor. Assessment of the presence of fetal fibronectin is used to predict the likelihood of preterm labor in women who are at increased risk for this complication (Coleman et al, 1998; Lukes et al, 1997).

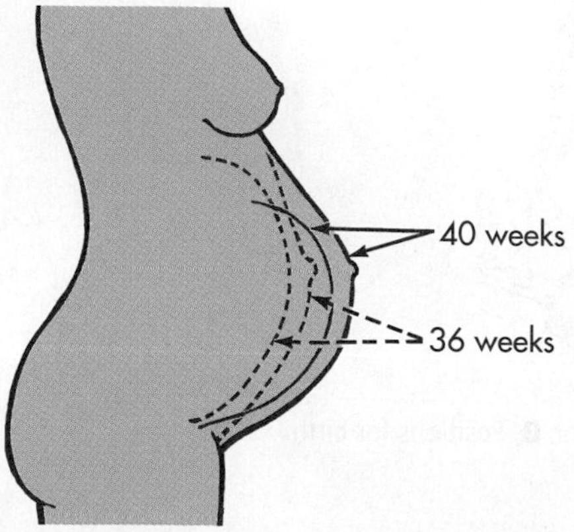

FIG. 15-13 • Lightening.

Stages of Labor

Labor is considered "normal" when the woman is at or near term, no complications exist, a single fetus presents by vertex, and labor is completed within 24 hours. The course of normal labor, which is remarkably constant, consists of regular progression of uterine contractions, effacement and progressive dilation of the cervix, and progress in descent of the presenting part. Four stages of labor are recognized. These stages are discussed in greater detail, along with nursing care for the laboring woman and family, in Chapter 18.

The first stage of labor lasts from the onset of regular uterine contractions to full dilation of the cervix. Commonly the onset of labor is difficult to establish; the woman may be admitted to the birthing unit in active labor and the beginning of labor may be only an estimate. The first stage is much longer than the second and third combined. Great variability is the rule, however, depending on the factors discussed earlier. Full dilation may occur in less than 1 hour in some multiparous pregnancies. In first-time pregnancy, complete dilation of the cervix can take up to 20 hours.

NURSE ALERT • There are no absolute values for the normal length of the first stage of labor (American College of Obstetricians and Gynecologists, 1995). Variations may reflect differences in patient population or in clinical practice.

Box 15-1

Signs Preceding Labor

- Lightening
- Return of urinary frequency
- Backache
- Stronger Braxton Hicks contractions
- Weight loss of 0.5 kg to 1.5 kg
- Surge of energy
- Increased vaginal discharge; bloody show
- Cervical ripening
- Rupture of membranes

The first stage of labor is divided into three phases: a latent phase, an active phase, and a transition phase. During the latent phase there is more progress in effacement of the cervix and little increase in descent. During the active phase and the transition phase, there is more rapid dilation of the cervix and increased rate of descent of the presenting part.

The second stage of labor lasts from full dilation of the cervix to birth of the fetus. The second stage takes an average of 20 minutes for a multiparous woman and 50 minutes for a nulliparous woman. Labor of up to 2 hours is considered within the normal range for the second stage, but there can be significant variations. For example, a woman who has received epidural analgesia may take up to 3 hours (Johnson and Rosenfeld, 1995). As long as there is progress and the fetal status is reassuring, the length of the second stage is usually not related to adverse perinatal outcomes (American College of Obstetricians and Gynecologists, 1995).

The third stage of labor lasts from the birth of the fetus until the placenta is expelled. The placenta normally separates with the third or fourth strong uterine contraction after the infant has been born. After it has separated, the placenta can be delivered with the next uterine contraction. The duration of the third stage may be as short as 3 to 5 minutes, although up to 1 hour is considered within normal limits (Bennett and Brown, 1993). The risk of hemorrhage increases as the length of the third stage increases (Cunningham et al, 1997).

The fourth stage of labor arbitrarily lasts about 2 hours after delivery of the placenta. It is the period of immediate recovery when homeostasis is reestablished. It serves as an important period of observation for complications such as abnormal bleeding (see Chapter 23).

Mechanism of Labor

The female pelvis has varied contours and diameters at different levels, and the presenting part of the passenger is large in proportion to the passageway. For vaginal birth to occur, the fetus must adapt to the birth canal during descent. Turns and other adjustments necessary in the human birth process are termed the mechanism of labor (Fig. 15-14). The seven cardinal move-

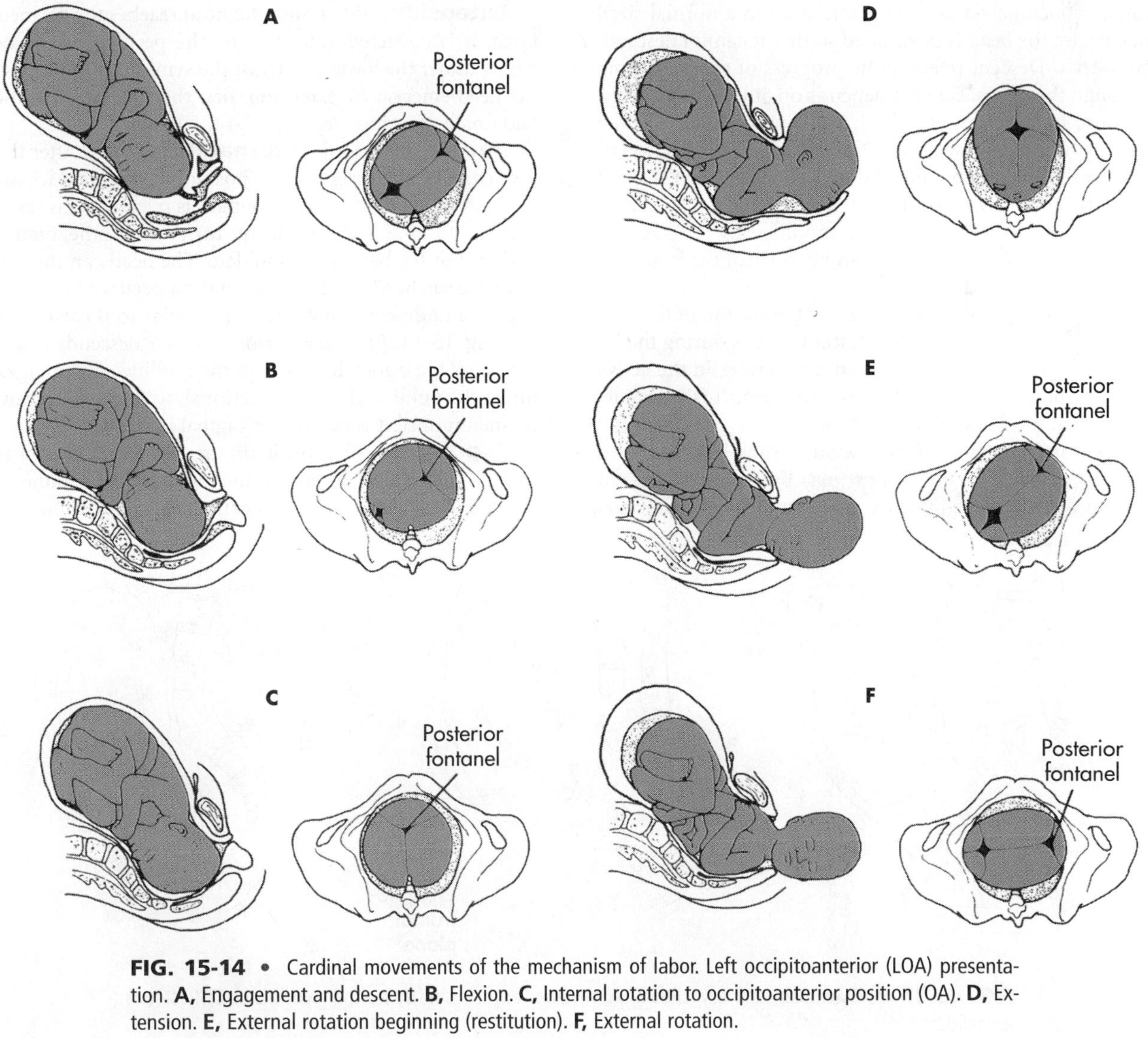

FIG. 15-14 • Cardinal movements of the mechanism of labor. Left occipitoanterior (LOA) presentation. **A,** Engagement and descent. **B,** Flexion. **C,** Internal rotation to occipitoanterior position (OA). **D,** Extension. **E,** External rotation beginning (restitution). **F,** External rotation.

ments of the mechanism of labor that occur in a vertex presentation are engagement, descent, flexion, internal rotation, extension, external rotation (restitution), and finally birth by expulsion. Although these phases are discussed separately, a combination of movements occurs simultaneously. For example, engagement involves both descent and flexion.

Engagement. When the biparietal diameter of the head passes the pelvic inlet, the head is said to be engaged in the pelvic inlet (see Fig. 15-14, *A*). In most nulliparous pregnancies this occurs before the onset of active labor because the firmer abdominal muscles direct the presenting part into the pelvis. However, Diegmann, Chez, and Danclair (1995) found almost 70% of study participants who were nulliparas in early labor had unengaged fetal heads. In multiparous pregnancies, in which the abdominal musculature is more relaxed, the head often remains freely movable above the pelvic brim until labor is established.

Asynclitism. The head usually engages in the pelvis in a synclitic position, one that is parallel to the anterior-posterior plane of the pelvis. Often asynclitism occurs (i.e., the head is deflected anteriorly or posteriorly in the pelvis); this can facilitate descent because the head is being positioned to accommodate to the pelvic cavity (Fig. 15-15). However, extreme asynclitism can cause cephalopelvic disproportion, even in a normal sized pelvis, because the head is positioned so that it cannot descend.

Descent. Descent refers to the progress of the presenting part through the pelvis. Descent depends on at least four forces: (1) pressure by the amniotic fluid; (2) direct pressure by the contracting fundus on the fetus; (3) force of the contraction of the maternal diaphragm and abdominal muscles in second stage labor; and (4) extension and straightening of the fetal body. The effects of these forces are modified by the size and shape of the maternal pelvic planes and the size of the fetal head and its capacity to mold.

The degree of descent is measured by the station of the presenting part (see Fig. 15-9). Little descent occurs during the latent phase of first stage labor. Descent accelerates in the active phase when the cervix has dilated to 5 to 7 cm. It is especially apparent when membranes have ruptured.

In first-time pregnancy, this descent is slow but steady; in subsequent pregnancies, the descent may be rapid. Progress in the descent of the presenting part is determined by abdominal palpation (Leopold's maneuvers) and vaginal examination until the presenting part can be seen at the introitus.

Flexion. As soon as the descending head meets resistance from the cervix, pelvic wall, or pelvic floor, it normally flexes so that the chin is brought into closer contact with the fetal chest (see Fig. 15-14, *B*). Flexion permits the smaller suboccipitobregmatic diameter (9.5 cm) rather than the larger diameters to present to the outlet.

Internal Rotation. The maternal pelvic inlet is widest in the transverse diameter. Therefore the fetal head passes the inlet into the true pelvis in the occipitotransverse position. The outlet is widest in the anteroposterior diameter, however. To exit, the fetal head must rotate. Internal rotation begins at the level of the ischial spines but is not completed until the presenting part reaches the lower pelvis. As the occiput rotates anteriorly, the face rotates posteriorly. With each contraction the fetal head is guided by the bony pelvis and the muscles of the pelvic floor. Eventually the occiput is in the midline beneath the pubic arch. The head is almost always rotated by the time it reaches the pelvic floor (see Fig. 15-14, *C*). Both the levator ani muscles and the bony pelvis are important for achieving anterior rotation. Previous childbirth injury or regional anesthesia compromises the function of the levator sling.

Extension. When the fetal head reaches the perineum for birth, it is deflected anteriorly by the perineum. The occiput passes under the lower border of the symphysis pubis first, then the head emerges by extension: first the occiput, then the face, and finally the chin (see Fig. 15-14, *D*).

Restitution and External Rotation. After the head is born, it rotates briefly to the position it occupied when it was engaged in the inlet. This movement is referred to as restitution (see Fig. 15-14, *E*). The 45-degree turn realigns the infant's head with her or his back and shoulders. The head can then be seen to rotate further. This external rotation occurs as the shoulders engage and descend in maneuvers similar to those of the head (see Fig. 15-14, *F*). The anterior shoulder descends first. When it reaches the outlet, it rotates to the midline and emerges from under the pubic arch. The posterior shoulder is guided over the perineum until it is free of the vaginal introitus.

Expulsion. After birth of the shoulders, the head and shoulders are lifted up toward the mother's pubic bone and the trunk of the baby is born by flexing it laterally in the direction

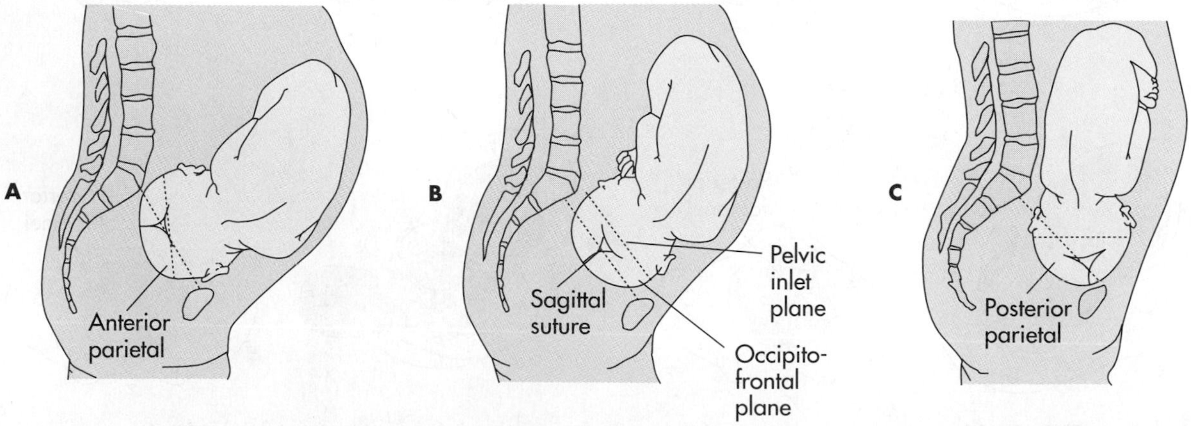

FIG. 15-15 • Synclitism and asynclitism. **A,** Anterior asynclitism. **B,** Normal synclitism. **C,** Posterior asynclitism.

of the symphysis pubis. When the baby has completely emerged, birth is complete and the second stage of labor ends.

PHYSIOLOGIC ADAPTATION TO LABOR

In addition to the maternal and fetal anatomic adaptations that occur during birth, physiologic adaptations must also occur. Accurate assessment of the mother and fetus requires knowledge of expected adaptations.

Fetal Adaptation

Several important physiologic adaptations occur in the fetus. These changes occur in fetal heart rate, fetal circulation, respiratory movements, and other behaviors.

Fetal Heart Rate. Fetal heart rate (FHR) monitoring provides reliable and predictive information about the condition of the fetus related to oxygenation. Stresses to the uteroplacental unit result in characteristic FHR patterns. It is important that the nurse have a basic understanding of the factors involved in fetal oxygenation and of fetal responses that reflect adequate fetal oxygenation (see Chapter 17 for further discussion).

The average FHR at term is 140 beats per minute. The normal range is 110 to 160 beats/min. The rate decreases progressively as the maturing fetus reaches term. Temporary accelerations and slight early decelerations of the FHR can be expected in response to spontaneous fetal movement, vaginal examination, fundal pressure, uterine contractions, abdominal palpation, and fetal head compression.

Fetal Circulation. Fetal circulation can be affected by many factors, including maternal position, uterine contractions, blood pressure, and umbilical cord blood flow. Uterine contractions during labor tend to decrease circulation through the spiral arterioles and subsequent perfusion through the intervillous space. Most healthy fetuses are well able to compensate for this stress and to their exposure to increased pressure while moving passively through the birth canal during labor. Umbilical cord blood flow is usually undisturbed by uterine contractions or fetal position (Lowe and Reiss, 1996).

Fetal Respiration. Certain changes stimulate chemoreceptors in the aorta and carotid bodies to prepare the fetus for initiating respirations immediately after birth (Lowe and Reiss, 1996). These changes include the following:

- Fetal lung fluid is cleared from the air passages during labor and vaginal birth.
- Fetal oxygen pressure (Po_2) falls.
- Arterial carbon dioxide pressure (Pco_2) rises.
- Arterial pH falls.
- Bicarbonate level falls.
- Fetal respiratory movements decrease during labor.

Maternal Adaptation

Changes occur as the woman progresses through the stages of labor. Various body systems adapt to the process of labor, exhibiting both objective and subjective symptoms.

Cardiovascular Changes. Changes in the woman's cardiovascular system occur during labor. During each contraction, 400 ml of blood is emptied from the uterus into the maternal vascular system. This increases cardiac output by about 10% to 15% in the first stage and by about 30% to 50% in the second stage. Heart rate increases slightly.

Changes in the woman's blood pressure also occur. Blood flow, reduced in the uterine artery by contractions, is redirected to peripheral vessels. Peripheral resistance increases and blood pressure rises (Chamberlain and Pipkin, 1998). During first stage labor, uterine contractions cause systolic readings to rise by about 10 mm Hg. Therefore assessing blood pressure between contractions provides more accurate readings (Varney, 1997). During second stage, contractions may cause systolic pressures to increase by 30 mm Hg and diastolic readings to increase by 25 mm Hg, with both systolic and diastolic pressures remaining somewhat elevated even between contractions. Therefore the woman already at risk for hypertension is at increased risk for complications such as cerebral hemorrhage.

Supine hypotension occurs when the ascending vena cava and descending aorta are compressed. The laboring woman is at greater risk for supine hypotension if the uterus is particularly large because of multifetal pregnancy, hydramnios, obesity, or if the woman is dehydrated or hypovolemic. In addition, anxiety and pain, as well as some medications, can cause hypotension.

The woman should be discouraged from using the Valsalva maneuver (holding one's breath and tightening abdominal muscles) during the second stage. The Valsalva maneuver increases intrathoracic pressure, reduces venous return, and increases venous pressure. The cardiac output and blood pressure increase, and the pulse rate slows temporarily. During the Valsalva maneuver, fetal hypoxia may occur. The process is reversed when the woman takes a breath.

The white blood cell (WBC) count can increase to 25,000/mm^3, although the average increase is to between 14,000 and 16,000/mm^3 (Cunningham et al, 1997). The mechanism leading to this increase in WBCs is unknown; it may be secondary to physical or emotional stress or to tissue trauma. Labor is strenuous and physical exercise alone can increase WBC count.

Some peripheral vascular changes occur, perhaps in response to cervical dilation or to compression of maternal vessels by the fetus passing through the birth canal. Flushed cheeks, hot or cold feet, and eversion of hemorrhoids may result (Box 15-2).

Respiratory Changes. Respiratory system adaptations also are seen. Increased physical activity with greater oxygen

Box 15-2

Maternal Physiologic Changes During Labor

- Cardiac output increases 10% to 15% in first stage, 30% to 50% in second stage.
- Heart rate increases slightly in first and second stage.
- Systolic blood pressure increases during uterine contractions in first stage; systolic and diastolic pressures increase during uterine contractions in second stage.
- White blood cell count increases.
- Respiratory rate increases.
- Temperature may be slightly elevated.
- Proteinuria of +1 may occur.
- Gastric motility and absorption of solid food is decreased; nausea, vomiting may occur in transition to second stage labor.
- Blood glucose level decreases.

consumption is reflected by an increase in the respiratory rate. Hyperventilation may cause respiratory alkalosis (an increase in pH), hypoxia, and hypocapnia (decrease in carbon dioxide). In the unmedicated woman in the second stage, oxygen consumption almost doubles. Anxiety also increases oxygen consumption.

Renal Changes. Several renal system changes occur. In the second trimester, the urinary bladder becomes an abdominal organ. When filling, it is palpable above the symphysis pubis. During labor, spontaneous voiding may be difficult for various reasons: tissue edema caused by pressure from the presenting part, discomfort, analgesia, and embarrassment. Proteinuria of +1 is a normal finding; it can occur in response to breakdown of muscle tissue from the physical work of labor.

Integumentary Changes. The integumentary system changes are evident, especially in the great distensibility (stretching) in the area of the vaginal introitus. The degree of distensibility varies with the individual. Despite this ability to stretch, even in the absence of episiotomy or lacerations, minute tears in the skin around the vaginal introitus do occur.

Musculoskeletal Changes. The musculoskeletal system is stressed during labor. Diaphoresis, fatigue, proteinuria (of +1), and possibly an increased temperature accompany the marked increase in muscle activity. Backache and joint aches (unrelated to fetal position) occur as a result of increased joint laxity at term. The labor process itself and pointing of her toes by the woman can cause leg cramps.

Neurologic Changes. The neurologic system reflects the stress and discomfort of labor. Sensorial changes occur as the woman moves through the phases of the first stage of labor and as she moves from one stage to the next. Initially she may be euphoric. Euphoria gives way to increased seriousness; then to amnesia between contractions during second stage; and, finally, to elation or fatigue after giving birth. Endogenous endorphins (morphine-like chemicals produced naturally by the body) raise the pain threshold and produce sedation. In addition, physiologic anesthesia of perineal tissues, caused by pressure of the presenting part, decreases perception of pain.

Gastrointestinal Changes. Labor affects the woman's gastrointestinal system. Dry lips and mouth may result from mouth breathing, dehydration, and emotional response to labor. During labor, gastrointestinal motility and absorption of solid foods are decreased, and stomach emptying time is slowed. Nausea, and the vomiting of undigested food eaten after onset of labor, are common. Nausea and belching also occur as a reflex response to full cervical dilation. The mother may state that diarrhea accompanied the onset of labor, or the nurse may palpate the presence of hard or impacted stool in the rectum.

Endocrine Changes. The endocrine system is active during labor. The onset of labor may be triggered by decreasing levels of progesterone and increasing levels of estrogen, prostaglandins, and oxytocin. Metabolism increases, and blood glucose levels may decrease with the work of labor.

Key Points

- Labor and birth are affected by the 5 Ps: passenger, passageway, powers, position of the mother, and psychologic responses.
- Because of its size and relative rigidity, the fetal head has a major effect on the birth process.
- Diameters at the plane of the pelvic inlet, midpelvis, and outlet, plus the axis of the birth canal, determine whether vaginal birth is possible and the manner by which the fetus may pass down the birth canal.
- Involuntary uterine contractions act to expel the fetus and placenta during first stage of labor; these are augmented by voluntary bearing-down efforts during second stage.
- First stage of labor is from the onset of regular contractions to when the cervix is fully dilated. Second stage of labor lasts from full dilation to birth of the infant. Third stage of labor lasts from the infant's birth to the expulsion of the placenta. The fourth stage is the first 2 hours after birth.
- The cardinal movements of the mechanism of labor are engagement, descent, flexion, internal rotation, extension, restitution and external rotation, and expulsion of the infant.
- Although the events precipitating the onset of labor are unknown, many factors, including changes in the maternal uterus, cervix, and pituitary gland, are thought to be involved.
- A healthy fetus with an adequate uterofetoplacental circulation will be able to compensate for the stress of uterine contractions.

References

Alexander J et al: The course of labor with and without epidural analgesia, *Am J Obstet Gynecol* 17(3):516-520, 1998.

American College of Obstetricians and Gynecologists: *Dystocia, and the augmentation of labor (ACOG Tech Bull No. 218),* Washington, DC, 1995, ACOG.

Bennett V, Brown L: *Myles textbook for midwives,* ed 12, Edinburgh, 1993, Churchill Livingstone.

Biancuzzo M: Six myths of maternal posture during labor, *MCN Am J Matern Child Nurs* 18(5):264-269, 1993.

Chamberlain G, Pipkin F: *Clinical physiology in obstetrics,* ed 3, Oxford, 1998, Blackwell Scientific.

Coates T: Malpositions of the occiput and malpresentations. In Bennett V, Brown L: *Myles textbook for midwives,* New York, 1999, Churchill Livingstone.

Coleman M et al: Fetal fibronectin detection in preterm labor: evaluation of a prototype bedside dipstick technique and cervical assessment, *Am J Obstet Gynecol* 179(6):1553-1558, 1998.

Cunningham F et al: *Williams obstetrics,* ed 20, Stamford, CT, 1997, Appleton & Lange.

Diegmann E, Chez R, Danclair W: Stations in early labor in nulliparous women at term, *J Nurse Midwifery* 40(4):382-385, 1995.

Golay J, Vedam S, Sorger L: The squatting position for the second stage of labor: effects on labor and on maternal and fetal well-being, *Birth* 20(2):73-78, 1993.

Hanson L: Second-stage pushing in nurse-midwifery practices. Part 2. Factors affecting use, *J Nurse Midwifery* 43(4):326-330, 1998.

Hillan E: Physiology and management of the second stage of labour. In Bennett V, Brown L: *Myles textbook for midwives,* New York, 1999, Churchill Livingstone.

Johnson S, Rosenfeld J: The effect of epidural anesthesia on the length of labor, *J Fam Pract* 40(4):244-247, 1995.

Lowe N, Reiss R: Parturition and fetal adaptation, *J Obstet Gynecol Neonatal Nurs* 25(1):339-349, 1996.

Lukes A et al: Predictors of positivity for fetal fibronectin in patients with symptoms of preterm labor, *Am J Obstet Gynecol* 176(3):639-641, 1997.

Mayberry L et al: Managing second-stage labor: exploring the variables during the second stage. *AWHONN Lifelines* 3(6):28-34, 1999/2000.

Paine L, Tinker D: The effect of maternal bearing-down efforts on the actual umbilical cord pH and length of second stage labor, *J Nurse Midwifery* 37(1):61-63, 1992.

Peterson L, Besuner P: Pushing techniques during labor: issues and controversies, *J Obstet Gynecol Neonatal Nurs* 26(6):719-726, 1997.

Roberts J, Woolley D: A second look at the second stage of labor, *J Obstet Gynecol Neonatal Nurs* 25(5):415-423, 1996.

Shermer R, Raines D: Positioning during the second stage of labor: moving back to basics, *J Obstet Gynecol Neonatal Nurs* 26(6):727-734, 1997.

Simkin P: Reducing pain and enhancing progress in labor: a guide to nonpharmacologic methods for maternity caregivers, *Birth* 22(3):161-171, 1995.

Thompson T et al: Does epidural analgesia cause dystocia? *J Clin Anesth* 10(1):58-65, 1998.

Thomson A: Maternal behaviors during spontaneous and directed pushing in the second stage of labour, *J Adv Nurs* 22(6):1027-1034, 1995.

Varney H: *Varney's midwifery,* ed 3, Sudbury, MA, 1997, Jones & Bartlett.

Woolley D, Roberts J: Second stage pushing: a comparison of Valsalva-style with "mini" pushing, *J Perinatal Educ* 4(4):37-43, 1995.

CHAPTER

16 Management of Discomfort

http://www.harcourthealth.com/MERLIN/Wong/maternal/

Learning Objectives

On completion of this chapter the reader will be able to:

- Compare various childbirth preparation methods.
- Describe breathing and relaxation techniques used for each stage of labor.
- Identify nonpharmacologic strategies to enhance relaxation and decrease discomfort during labor.
- Discuss types of analgesia and anesthesia used during labor.
- Compare pharmacologic methods of relief of discomfort in different stages of labor and for different methods of birth.
- Describe nursing responsibilities appropriate for a woman receiving analgesia and anesthesia during labor.

Pregnant women commonly worry about the pain they will experience during labor and birth and how they will react to and deal with that pain. A variety of childbirth preparation methods can assist the woman or couple cope with the discomfort of labor. The interventions selected depend on the situation and the preference of both the woman and her health care provider. The discomforts experienced during labor are discussed in this chapter, as are nonpharmacologic and pharmacologic interventions to relieve the discomforts possible during the different stages of labor. This information provides the basis for understanding the nurse's role in management of maternal discomfort during labor.

DISCOMFORT DURING LABOR AND BIRTH

Neurologic Origins

The discomfort experienced during labor has two origins (Lowe, 1996). During the first stage of labor, uterine contractions cause cervical dilation and effacement, and uterine ischemia (decreased blood flow and therefore local oxygen deficit) results from contraction of the arteries supplying the myometrium. Pain impulses during the first stage of labor are transmitted through the T11 and T12 spinal nerve segment and accessory lower thoracic and upper lumbar sympathetic nerves. These nerves originate in the uterine body and cervix.

The discomfort from cervical changes and uterine ischemia is visceral pain. It is located over the lower portion of the abdomen and radiates to the lumbar area of the back and down the thighs. Usually the woman experiences discomfort only during contractions and is free of pain between contractions.

During the second stage of labor, the stage of expulsion of the baby, the woman experiences perineal or somatic pain. Perineal discomfort results from stretching of perineal tissues to allow passage of the fetus and from traction on the peritoneum and uterocervical supports during contractions. Discomfort also can be produced by expulsive forces or by pressure exerted by the presenting part on the bladder, bowel, or other sensitive pelvic structures. Pain impulses during the second stage of labor are carried from perineal tissues via the S1 to S4 spinal nerve segments and the parasympathetic system.

Pain experienced during the third stage of labor and the so-called afterpains are uterine, similar to that experienced early in the first stage of labor. Areas of discomfort during labor are illustrated in Fig. 16-1.

Pain may be local, with cramping and a tearing or bursting sensation because of distention and laceration of the cervix, vagina, or perineal tissues. This discomfort is commonly perceived as an intense burning sensation as the tissue stretches. Pain also may be referred (i.e., referred pain), in which the discomfort is felt in the back, flanks, or thighs.

Factors Influencing Pain Response

A woman's pain during childbirth is unique to each woman and is influenced by a variety of factors. These factors include culture, anxiety and fear, previous birth experience, childbirth preparation, and support.

Culture. As nurses care for women and families from a variety of cultural backgrounds, they must have knowledge and understanding of how culture mediates pain (Lee and Essoka, 1998; Weber, 1996). An understanding of the beliefs, values, and practices of various cultures helps the nurse provide appropriate culturally sensitive care (Cultural Considerations box).

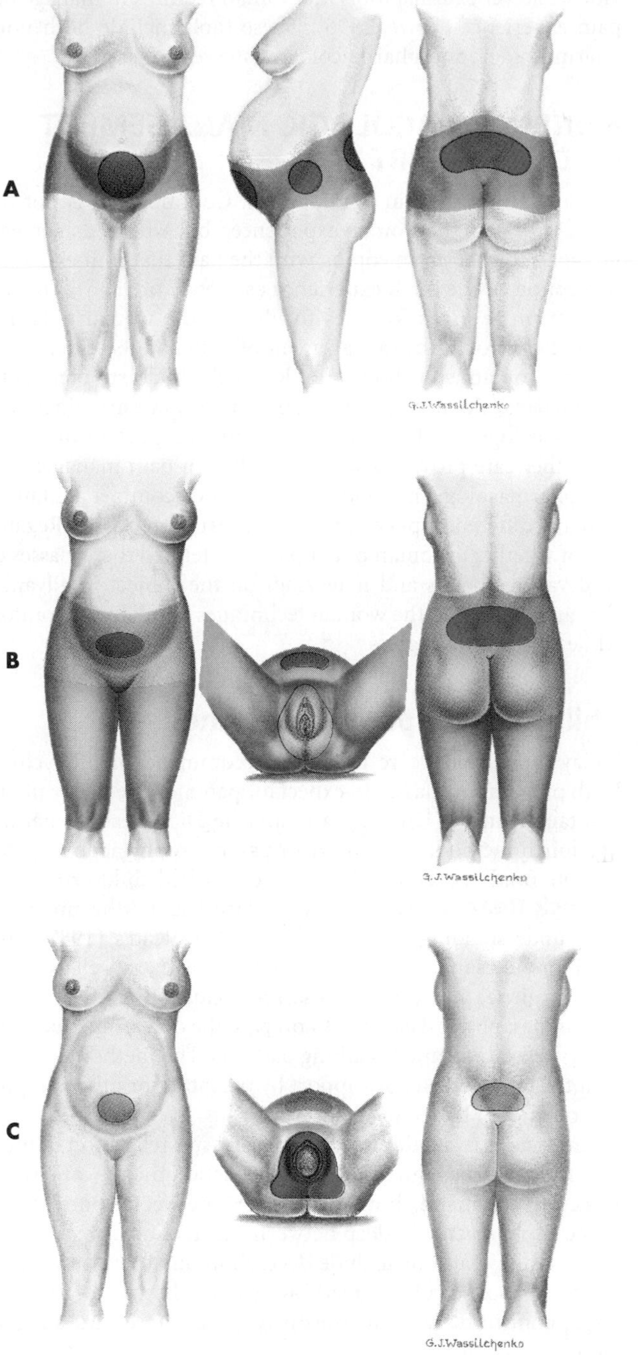

FIG. 16-1 • Discomfort during labor. **A,** Distribution of labor pain during first stage. **B,** Distribution of labor pain during later phase of first stage and early phase of second stage. **C,** Distribution of labor pain during later phase of second stage and actual birth. (*Gray shading* indicates areas of mild discomfort; *light colored shading* indicates areas of moderate discomfort; *dark colored areas* indicate intense discomfort.)

Anxiety and Fear. Anxiety and fear are commonly associated with increased pain during labor. Mild anxiety is considered normal for a woman during labor and birth. However, excessive anxiety and fear cause more catecholamine secretion, which increases the stimuli to the brain from the pelvis because

Cultural Considerations

SOME CULTURAL BELIEFS ABOUT PAIN

The following are only examples of how women of different cultural backgrounds may react to pain. Because they are generalizations, the nurse must assess each woman experiencing pain related to childbirth.

Chinese women may not exhibit reactions to pain, although it is acceptable to exhibit pain during childbirth. They consider it impolite to accept something when it is first offered; therefore pain interventions may need to be offered more than once. Acupuncture may be used for pain relief.

Arab or Middle Eastern women may be vocal in response to labor pain. They may prefer medication for pain relief.

Japanese women may be stoic in response to labor pain, but they may request medication when pain becomes severe.

Southeast Asian women may endure severe pain before requesting relief.

Hispanic women may be stoic until late in labor, when they may become vocal and request pain relief.

Native American women may use medications or remedies made from indigenous plants. They are often stoic in response to labor pain.

African-American women may express pain openly. Use of medication for pain relief varies.

Critical Thinking

CULTURE AND PAIN

Talk to a woman from a culture different from your own who has experienced childbirth. Ask her to describe her reactions to pain, how she sought relief of pain, the atmosphere of the childbirth setting, and the attitudes of the health care providers. How did her culture influence her response to labor and the associated pain? What expressions of pain are "acceptable" in her culture? What is the role of support persons in the labor process?

of decreased blood flow and increased muscle tension; this in turn magnifies pain (Lowe, 1996). Thus as fear and anxiety heighten, muscle tension increases, the effectiveness of the uterine contractions decreases, the experience of discomfort increases, and a cycle of increased fear and anxiety begins.

Previous Experience. For women who have had a difficult and painful previous birth experience, anxiety and fear from this past experience may lead to increased pain. Conversely, a woman who experienced a labor and birth where pain coping skills were successful may have increased anxiety because those previous coping skills no longer work due to a more difficult labor and birth.

Women with a history of substance abuse experience as much pain during labor as other women. Although it is usually unnecessary to withhold pain medications, close monitoring for complications associated with each substance is part of the nursing assessment.

Pain is a personal response in each individual. As pain is experienced, people develop various coping mechanisms to deal with it. Emotional tension from anxiety and fear may increase pain and perception of pain during labor (see the discussion of the Dick-Read method later in this chapter). Pain, or the possi-

Critical Thinking

PAIN MANAGEMENT

You are assigned to a woman in active labor who has a history of substance abuse. She is thrashing about in her bed and is requesting something for "this terrible pain." Examine the assumptions you may have about how women who abuse substances exhibit reactions to pain. Examine assumptions that both you and the patient may have about pain relief. Analyze arguments for and against use of narcotics for control of discomfort in someone who is or has been addicted to narcotics. Formulate a plan of care for pain relief in this situation, and justify your choice of interventions.

bility of pain, can induce fear in which anxiety borders on panic. Fatigue and sleep deprivation magnify pain. Parity may affect perception of labor pain because primiparous women have longer labors and thus greater fatigue, causing a vicious circle of increased pain and a more likely use of pharmacologic support.

Childbirth Preparation. Even pain stimuli that are particularly intense can, at times, be ignored. This is because certain nerve cell groupings within the spinal cord, brainstem, and cerebral cortex have the ability to modulate the pain impulse through a blocking mechanism. The gate-control theory helps explain the way hypnosis and the pain relief techniques taught in childbirth preparation classes work to relieve the pain of labor. According to this theory, pain sensations travel along sensory nerve pathways to the brain, but only a limited number of sensations, or messages, can travel through these nerve pathways at one time. By using distraction techniques such as massage or stroking, music, and imagery, the capacity of nerve pathways to transmit pain is reduced or completely blocked. These distractions are thought to work by closing down a hypothetic gate in the spinal cord, thus preventing pain signals from reaching the brain. Perception of pain stimuli is thereby diminished.

In addition, when the woman in labor engages in neuromuscular and motor activity, activity within the spinal cord itself further modifies the transmission of pain. Cognitive work involving concentration on breathing and relaxation requires selective and directed cortical activity that activates and closes the gating mechanism as well. The gate-control theory therefore underscores the need for a supportive birth setting that allows the laboring woman to relax and use various higher mental activities.

Comfort. While the predominant medical approach to labor is that it is painful and the pain must be removed, an alternative view is that labor is a natural process and women can experience comfort and transcend the discomfort or pain (Schuiling and Sampselle, 1999). Having needs and desires met engenders a feeling of comfort. Comfort may be viewed as strengthening; this represents a paradigm shift in the interpretation of pain in labor (Schuiling and Sampselle, 1999). The most helpful interventions in enhancing comfort are a caring nursing approach and a supportive presence (Collins et al, 1994).

Support. The pain occurring during childbirth and the management of this pain belongs to the woman experiencing the pain; the nurse must engage in a cooperative effort to provide whatever external tools the woman requires to manage her pain experience (Lowe, 1996). These tools include both nonpharmacologic and pharmacologic interventions.

NONPHARMACOLOGIC MANAGEMENT OF DISCOMFORT

The alleviation of pain is important. Commonly it is not the amount of pain the woman experiences, but whether she meets her goals for herself in coping with the pain that influences her perception of the birth experience as "good" or "bad." The observant nurse looks for cues to identify the woman's desired level of control in the management of pain and its relief.

The woman who chooses to deal with childbirth pain using nonpharmacologic or a combination of nonpharmacologic and pharmacologic methods needs care and support from nurses and other care providers who are skilled in pain management. Nonpharmacologic methods for relief of discomfort are taught in many different types of prenatal preparation classes. Regardless of whether a woman or couple has attended these classes or read various books and magazines on the subject in advance, the nurse can teach the woman techniques to relieve discomfort while labor is in progress.

Childbirth Preparation Methods

Today most health care providers recommend or offer childbirth preparation classes to expectant parents. The major methods taught in the United States are the Dick-Read or natural childbirth method; the Lamaze or psychoprophylactic method; and the Bradley method, or husband-coached childbirth.

Dick-Read Method. To replace fear of the unknown with understanding and confidence, Dick-Read's (1987) program provides information on labor and birth, as well as nutrition, hygiene, and exercise. Classes include practice in three techniques: physical exercise to prepare the body for labor; conscious relaxation; and breathing patterns. The method has been adapted to include labor support by the father or other support person chosen by the mother.

Conscious relaxation involves progressive relaxation of muscle groups in the entire body. With practice, many women can relax on command, both during and between contractions. Some woman actually sleep between contractions.

Breathing patterns include deep abdominal respirations for most of labor; shallow breathing toward the end of the first stage; and, until recently, breath-holding for second stage of labor.

Teachers of the Dick-Read method contend that the weight of the abdominal musculature of the contracting uterus increases pain. The woman is taught to force her abdominal muscles to rise as the uterus rises forward during a contraction, thus lifting the abdominal muscles off the contracting uterus.

Lamaze Method. The Lamaze (psychoprophylaxis) method grew out of Pavlov's work on classical conditioning. According to Lamaze, pain is a conditioned response. Therefore, women can also be conditioned not to experience pain in labor. The Lamaze method does this by conditioning women to respond to mock uterine contractions with controlled muscular relaxation and breathing patterns instead of crying out and losing control (Lamaze, 1972). Coping strategies also include concentrating on a focal point, such as a favorite picture or pattern,

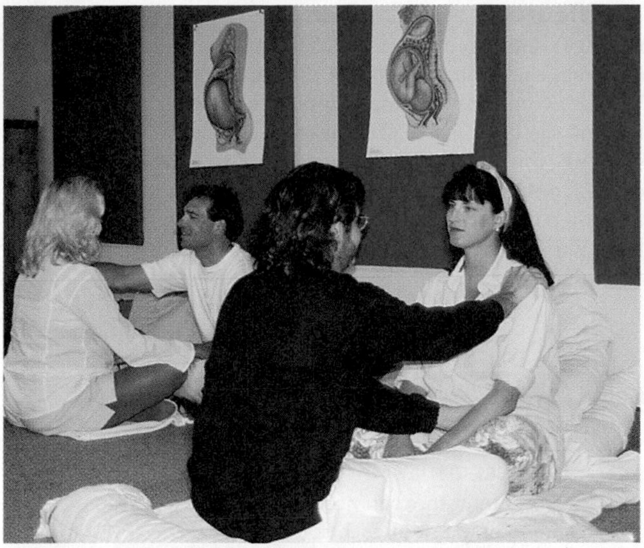

FIG. 16-2 • Expectant parents learning relaxation techniques. (Courtesy Marjorie Pyle, RNC, Lifecircle, Costa Mesa, CA.)

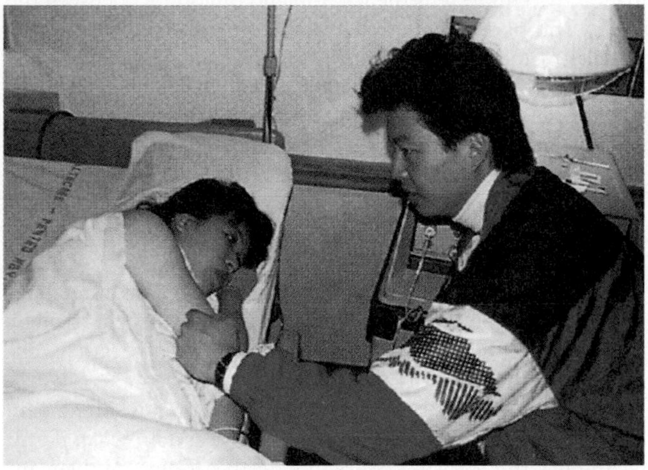

FIG. 16-3 • Laboring woman using focusing and breathing techniques during contraction with coaching from her partner. (Courtesy Marjorie Pyle, RNC, Lifecircle, Costa Mesa, CA.)

to keep nerve pathways occupied so they cannot respond to painful stimuli.

The woman is taught to relax uninvolved muscle groups while she contracts a specific muscle group (Fig. 16-2). She applies this in labor by relaxing uninvolved muscles while her uterus contracts. The perception of maintaining control is closely associated with satisfaction with the birth experience.

Lamaze teachers believe that chest breathing lifts the diaphragm off the contracting uterus, thus giving it more room to expand. Chest-breathing patterns vary according to the intensity of the contractions and the progress of labor. Teachers also seek to eliminate fear by increasing the woman's understanding of her body functions and the neurophysiology of pain. Support in labor is provided by the father or other support person or by a specially trained labor attendant called a monitrice.

Bradley Method. The Bradley method, also called husband-coached childbirth, was devised based on observations of animal behavior during birth. It emphasizes working in harmony with the body, using breath control and abdominal breathing, and promoting general body relaxation (Bradley, 1981).

The husband or partner takes an active role in assisting the woman to relax and use correct breathing techniques. This method also stresses environmental factors such as darkness, solitude, and quiet to make childbirth a more natural experience.

Comparison of Childbirth Methods. Most proponents of prepared childbirth agree that the major causes of pain in labor are fear and tension. All childbirth methods attempt to reduce these two factors and eliminate pain by increasing the woman's knowledge of the labor and birth process, enhancing her self-confidence and sense of control, preparing a support person, and training the woman in physical conditioning and relaxation breathing.

There are a few fine differences in approach. For example, in the Bradley method, women are discouraged from using medication and encouraged to focus inwardly and to take direction from their own body. In the Lamaze method, external focusing and distraction are stressed. In reality, few instructors adhere strictly to one particular method but instead incorporate a variety of strategies aimed at increasing the woman's ability to cope with labor and minimize her need for medication.

Relaxing and Breathing Techniques

Focusing and Feedback Relaxation. Some women bring a favorite object such as a photograph to the labor room; then focus their attention on this object during contractions. Others choose to fix their attention on some object in the labor room. In either event, as the contraction begins, they focus on the object to reduce their perception of pain.

With imagery, the nurse encourages the woman to focus on a pleasant scene, a place where she feels relaxed, or an activity she enjoys. She can imagine a walk through a restful garden; or breathing in light, energy, and healing color and breathing out worries and tension (Hoffart and Pross-Keene, 1998). These techniques, coupled with feedback relaxation, help the woman work with her contractions rather than against them. The support person monitors this process, telling the woman when to begin the breathing techniques (Fig. 16-3).

In a common feedback mechanism, the woman and her coach say the word "relax" at the onset of each contraction and throughout it as needed. The nurse can assist the woman by providing a quiet environment and offering cues as needed.

Music. Music can also enhance relaxation during labor. Women should be encouraged to bring their musical preferences and tape or compact disc players to the hospital or birthing center. Use of a headset or earphones may increase the effectiveness of the music because other sounds will be shut out. Ocean waves, Baroque, and New Age music assist in relaxation (Wiand, 1997).

Breathing Techniques. Different approaches to childbirth preparation use varying breathing techniques to help the woman maintain control through contractions. In the first stage of labor, such breathing techniques can promote relaxation of abdominal muscles and thereby increase the size of the abdominal cavity. This lessens the friction and discomfort between the uterus and abdominal wall during contractions. Because the muscles of the genital area also become more relaxed, they do not interfere with descent. In the second stage, breathing is used to increase abdominal pressure and thereby assist in expelling the fetus. It also is used to relax the pudendal muscles to prevent precipitate expulsion of the fetal head.

For those couples who have prepared for labor by practicing such relaxing and breathing techniques, occasional reminders may be all that is necessary to help them along. For those who have had no preparation, instruction in simple breathing and relaxation can be given early in labor and often is surprisingly successful. Motivation is high, and readiness to learn is enhanced by the reality of labor.

There are various breathing techniques for controlling pain during contractions. The nurse needs to ascertain what, if any, techniques the laboring couple knows before giving them instruction. Simple patterns are more easily learned. Paced breathing is the technique most associated with prepared childbirth. The Lamaze method uses a slow-paced, modified, and patterned breathing technique with the understanding that each labor is different and that couples need to adapt breathing techniques to their individual birth experience.

All patterns begin with the routine cleansing breath and end with a deep breath exhaled to "blow the contraction away." In general, slow abdominal breathing, approximately half the woman's normal breathing rate, is initiated when the woman can no longer walk or talk through contractions (Box 16-1). As contractions increase in frequency and intensity, the woman may need to change to chest breathing, which is more shallow and approximately twice her normal rate of breathing.

The most difficult time to maintain control during contractions comes when the cervix dilates to 8 to 10 cm. This period is also called the transition period. Even for the woman who has prepared for labor, concentration on breathing techniques is difficult to maintain. The type of technique used at this stage may be the 4:1 pattern: breath, breath, breath, breath, blow (as though blowing out a candle). This ratio may be increased to 6:1 or 8:1. However, an undesirable side effect of this type of breathing may be hyperventilation. The woman and her support person must be aware of and watch for symptoms of the resultant respiratory alkalosis: lightheadedness, dizziness, tingling of fingers, or circumoral numbness. Such alkalosis may be eliminated by having the woman breathe into a paper bag held tightly around the mouth and nose. This enables her to rebreathe carbon dioxide and replace the bicarbonate ion. She can also breathe into her cupped hands if no bag is available.

As the fetal head reaches the pelvic floor, the woman may experience the urge to push and may automatically begin to exert downward pressure by contracting her abdominal muscles. Nurses guide couples in the application of breathing and relaxation methods during labor, adapting methods to their particular needs, and using pushing techniques for birth that avoid a Valsalva response. Such techniques often involve moaning or other noise as women push without holding their breath.

The woman can control the urge to push by taking panting breaths or by slowly exhaling through pursed lips. This is good practice for the type of breathing to be used as the fetal head is slowly born.

Effleurage and Counterpressure. Effleurage (light massage) and counterpressure are two methods that have brought relief to many women during the first stage of labor. The gate-control theory may supply the reason for the effectiveness of these measures. Effleurage (see Fig. 11-18) is a light stroking, usually of the abdomen, in rhythm with breathing during contractions. It is used to distract the woman from contraction pain. Often the presence of monitor belts makes it difficult to perform effleurage on the abdomen; thus a thigh or the chest may be used.

Box 16-1

Breathing Techniques

CLEANSING BREATH

Relaxed breath in through nose and out mouth. Used at the beginning and end of each contraction.

SLOW-PACED BREATHING (APPROXIMATELY 6 TO 8 BREATHS PER MINUTE)

Not less than half normal breathing rate (no. breaths/min divided by 2)

In-2-3-4/Out-2-3-4/In-2-3-4/Out-2-3-4 . . .

MODIFIED-PACED BREATHING (APPROXIMATELY 32 TO 40 BREATHS PER MINUTE)

Not more than twice normal breathing rate (no. breaths/min times 2)

In-Out/In-Out/In-Out/In-Out . . .

For more flexibility and variety, the woman may combine the slow and modified breathing by using the slow breathing for beginnings and ends of contractions and modified breathing for more intense peaks. This technique conserves energy and lessens fatigue.

PATTERNED-PACED BREATHING (SAME RATE AS MODIFIED)

Enhances concentration

a. 3:1 Patterned breathing
   In-Out/In-Out/In-Out/In-Blow
   (repeat through contraction)
b. 4:1 Patterned breathing
   In-Out/In-Out/In-Out/In-Out/In-Blow
   (repeat through contraction)
   You may do any pattern desired, although ratios of 5:1 or higher tend to be very tiring. Some people like to do patterned breathing to a tune ("Yankee Doodle," "Old McDonald"), to a repeated phrase ("I think I can, I think I can"), or in a pyramid pattern such as 1:1, 2:1, 3:1, 4:1, 5:1—5:1, 4:1, 3:1, 2:1, 1:1.
c. *Coach call:* May be used when the woman needs more distraction and concentration (e.g., during transition). The woman's coach signals the breathing ratio with his or her fingers or by verbal cues, changing the ratio after each "IN-BLOW."
   Example:
   In-Out/In-Out/In-Blow
   In-Out/In-Out/In-Out/In-Out/In-Blow
   In-Out/In-Blow

From Shapiro H, et al: *The Lamaze ready reference guide for labor and birth*, ed 2, Washington, DC, 1997, Chapter ASPO/Lamaze.

Counterpressure is steady pressure in the sacral area with the fist or heel of the hand, which may help the woman cope with the sensations of internal pressure and pain in the lower back.

Water Therapy. Although not universally accepted or implemented, bathing, showering, or jet hydrotherapy (whirlpool baths) using warm water are other nonpharmacologic measures that can be used to promote comfort and relaxation during labor (Fig. 16-4). Many new birthing units have baths with air jets. With or without air jets, however, the buoyancy of warm water provides support for tense muscles.

Water therapy has several immediate benefits. The relief from discomfort and general body relaxation reduce the woman's anxiety, which in turn decreases adrenalin production. This triggers an increase in the levels of oxytocin (to stimulate labor) and endorphins (to reduce pain perception). In addition, the bubbles and gentle lapping of the water stimulate the nipples, which increases oxytocin production; this has not been observed to cause hyperstimulation. The cervix has often been observed to dilate 2 to 3 cm in 30 minutes of whirlpool therapy. In addition, it promotes diuresis and a decrease in blood pressure (Simkin, 1995). Whirlpool baths during labor have also been found to have positive effects on analgesia requirements, instrumentation rates, condition of the perineum, and personal satisfaction with labor (Rush et al, 1996).

If the woman is experiencing "back labor" secondary to an occiput posterior or transverse position, she is encouraged to assume the hands-and-knees or the side-lying position in the tub. Because this position decreases pain and increases relaxation and the production of oxytocin, the fetus can rotate spontaneously to the occiput anterior position.

In some settings, jet hydrotherapy may need to be approved by the woman's primary health care provider. The woman's vital signs must be within normal limits and she should be in the active phase of the first stage of labor. If she is in the latent phase, her contractions may slow down. Fetal well-being must also be documented.

Fetal heart rate (FHR) monitoring is done by Doppler device, fetoscope, or wireless external monitor device (see Fig. 16-4, *C*). Placement of internal electrodes is contraindicated for jet hydrotherapy. The woman's membranes may be intact or ruptured. If ruptured, the fluid must be clear or only lightly stained with meconium.

There is no limit to the time women can stay in the bath, and often women are encouraged to stay in it as long as desired. However, most women use jet hydrotherapy for 30 to 60 minutes (Schorn, McAllister, and Blanco, 1993).

During the bath, if the woman's temperature and the FHR increase, the water is cooled down or she is asked to step out of the bath to cool down. The bath water is kept between 36.7° C and 37.8° C (Simkin, 1995). The mother's temperature may remain slightly elevated for a short time after the bath. Fluids and ice chips and a cool face cloth are offered during the bath.

The tub must be kept meticulously clean. Cleansing solutions used vary with institutions; however, household bleach (e.g., Clorox) is commonly used.

Transcutaneous Electrical Nerve Stimulation. Transcutaneous electrical nerve stimulation (TENS) involves placing two pairs of electrodes on either side of the woman's thoracic and sacral spine (Fig. 16-5). These electrodes provide continuous mild electrical current from a battery-operated device. During a contraction, the woman increases the stimulation

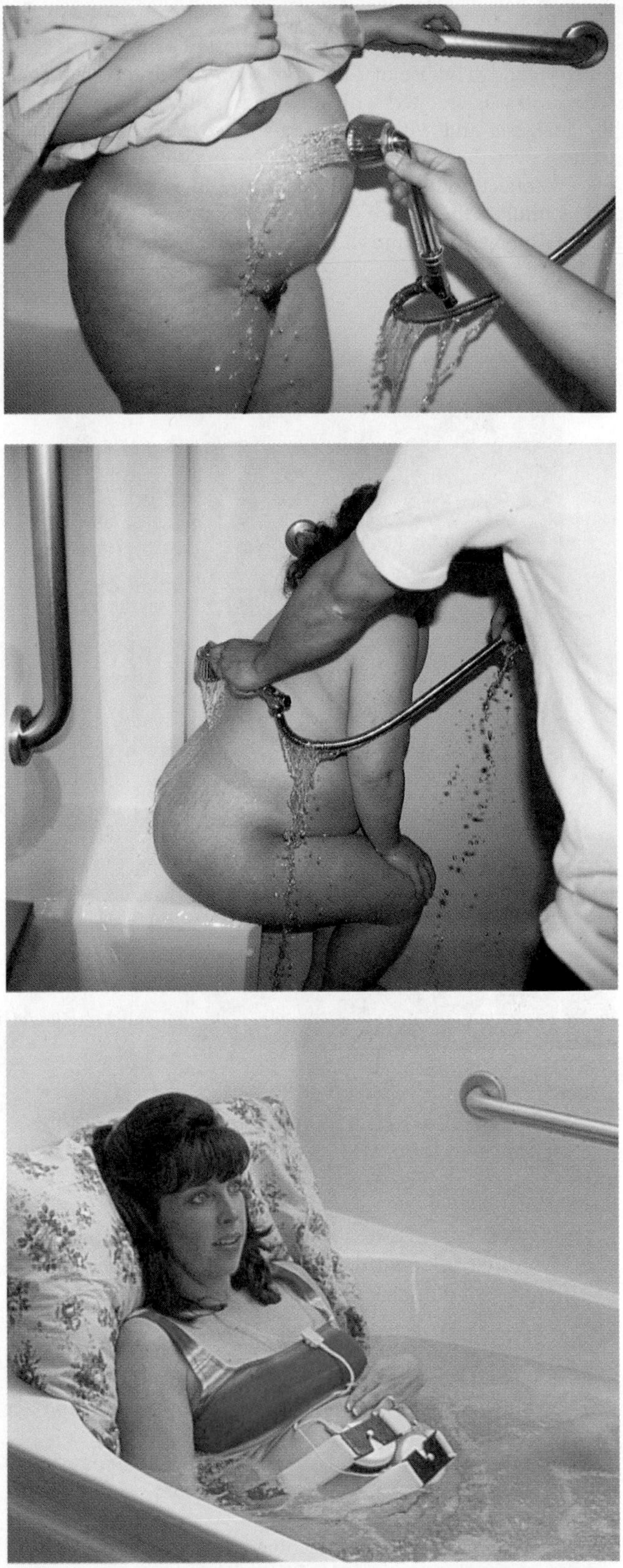

A

B

C

FIG. 16-4 • Water therapy during labor. **A,** Use of shower during labor. **B,** Woman experiencing back labor relaxes as husband sprays warm water on her back. **C,** Woman relaxing in Jacuzzi. (A, B, Courtesy Marjorie Pyle, RNC, Lifecircle, Costa Mesa, CA; C, courtesy Spacelabs Medical, Redmond, WA.)

by turning control knobs on the device. Women describe the resulting sensation as a tingling or buzzing and pain relief as good or very good. The use of TENS poses no risk to the mother or fetus, and it is credited with reducing or eliminating the need for analgesia and with increasing the woman's perception of control over the experience. It may be effective because of the placebo effect; that is, confidence in the effectiveness of TENS may stimulate the release of endogenous opiates (enkephalins) in the woman's body and thus alleviate the discomfort (Scott et al, 1999).

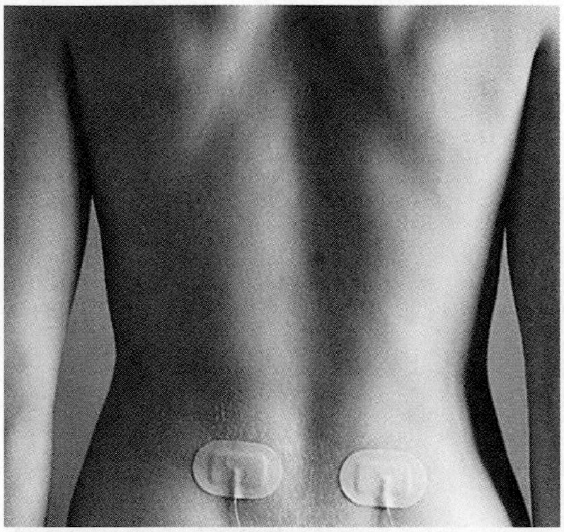

FIG. 16-5 • Placement of TENS electrodes on back for relief of labor pain.

The nurse assists the mother in using TENS by explaining the device and its use, by carefully placing and securing the electrodes, and by closely evaluating its effectiveness (Nursing Care Plan).

Other Nonpharmacologic Methods

There are various other nonpharmacologic methods for control of the discomfort of labor (Box 16-2). Many of these are taught in childbirth preparation classes. Most need practice for best results, although the nurse may use some of them successfully without the woman having prior knowledge.

Acupressure. Acupressure techniques can be used in pregnancy, labor, and postpartum to relieve pain and other discomforts. Pressure, heat, or cold is applied to acupuncture points called *tsubos.* These points have an increased density of neuroreceptors and increased electrical conductivity. Acupressure is best applied over the skin without using lubricants. Pressure is usually applied with the pads of the thumbs and fingers (Fig. 16-6). Synchronized breathing by the caregiver and the woman is suggested for greater effectiveness. Acupressure points include shoulders, low back, hips, ankles, nails on the small toes, soles of the foot, and sacral points.

Application of Heat and Cold. Warmed blankets, warm compresses, a warm bath or shower, or use of a moist heating pad can reduce pain during labor. Heat acts to relieve muscle ischemia and increase blood flow to the area of discomfort. Heat application is effective for back pain caused by a posterior presentation or general backache from fatigue (Simkin, 1995).

Cold application such as cool cloths or ice packs may be effective in increasing comfort when the woman feels warm, and

Nursing Care Plan — NONPHARMACOLOGIC MANAGEMENT OF DISCOMFORT

NURSING DIAGNOSIS Pain related to physiologic response to labor

EXPECTED OUTCOME Woman will express decrease in intensity of discomfort and experience satisfaction with her labor and pain performance.

Nursing Interventions/*Rationales*

Assess whether woman and significant other have attended childbirth classes, her knowledge of labor process, and her current level of anxiety *to plan supportive strategies.*

Encourage support person to remain with woman in labor *to provide support and increase probability of response to comfort measures.*

Teach or review nonpharmacologic techniques available to decrease anxiety and pain during labor (e.g., focusing and feedback, breathing techniques, effleurage, and sacral pressure) *to enhance chances of success in using techniques.*

Explore other techniques that the woman or significant other may have learned in childbirth classes (e.g., hypnosis, yoga, acupressure, biofeedback, therapeutic touch, aromatherapy, imaging, vocalizations) *to provide largest repertoire of coping strategies.*

Explore use of jet hydrotherapy if ordered by physician and if woman meets use criteria (i.e., vital signs within normal limits [WNL], cervix 4 to 5 cm dilated, active phase of first stage labor) *to aid relaxation and stimulate production of natural oxytocin.*

Explore use of transcutaneous nerve stimulation per physician order *to provide an increased perception of control over pain and an increase in release of endogenous opiates.*

Assist woman to change positions and to use pillows *to reduce stiffness, aid circulation, and promote comfort.*

Assess bladder for distention and encourage voiding often *to avoid bladder distention and subsequent discomfort.*

Encourage rest between contractions *to minimize fatigue.*

Keep woman and significant other informed about progress *to allay anxiety.*

Guide couple through the labor stages and phases, helping them use and modify comfort techniques that are appropriate to each phase *to ensure greatest effectiveness of techniques employed.*

may also be applied to areas of pain. Cooling relieves pain by lowering the muscle temperature and relieving muscle spasms (Simkin, 1995).

Heat and cold may be used alternately for a greater effect. Neither heat nor cold should be applied over ischemic or anesthetized areas because tissues can be damaged.

Therapeutic Touch. Therapeutic touch uses the concept of energy fields within the body called *prana.* Prana are thought to be deficient in some people who are in pain. Therapeutic touch uses the laying on of hands by a specially trained person to redirect energy fields associated with pain (Mackey, 1995). Little is known about the use or effectiveness of therapeutic touch for relieving labor pain.

Hypnosis. Hypnosis, while not commonly used for pain management in the United States, is associated with shorter labors and less analgesia (Jenkins and Pritchard, 1993). Hypnosis techniques used for labor and birth place an emphasis on relaxation. The woman may be given direct suggestions about pain relief or indirect suggestions that she is experiencing diminished sensations. The woman receives posthypnotic suggestions, such as "you will be able to push the baby out easily," to increase her confidence.

Biofeedback. Biofeedback is another relaxation technique that can be used for labor. Biofeedback is based on the theory that if a person can recognize physical signals, certain internal physiologic events can be changed (i.e., whatever signs the woman has that are associated with her pain). A woman must be educated to become aware of her body and its responses and how to relax for biofeedback to be effective (Alexander and Steeful, 1995). Informal biofeedback helps couples develop awareness of their bodies and learn strategies to change their responses to stress. If the woman responds to pain during a contraction with tightening muscles, frowning, moaning, and breath holding, her partner uses verbal and touch feedback to help her relax (Alexander and Steeful, 1995). Formal biofeedback, which uses machines to detect skin temperature, blood flow, or muscle tension, can also prepare women to intensify their relaxation response.

Aromatherapy. Aromatherapy uses oils distilled from plants, flowers, herbs, and trees to promote health and well-being and to treat illnesses. The use of herbal teas and vapors is reported to have good effects in pregnancy and labor for some women (Burns and Blamey, 1994). Lavender, clary sage, and bergamot promote relaxation and can be used by adding a few drops to a warm bath, to warm water used for soaking compresses that can be applied to the body, to an aromatherapy lamp to vaporize a room, or to oil for a back massage (Tiran, 1996).

NURSE ALERT • Caution: Never apply the oils used for aromatherapy full-strength directly to the skin.

Box 16-2

Nonpharmacologic Strategies to Encourage Relaxation and Relieve Pain

CUTANEOUS STIMULATION STRATEGIES
- Counterpressure
- Effleurage (light massage)
- Therapeutic touch
- Walking
- Rocking
- Changing positions
- Application of heat or cold
- TENS
- Acupressure
- Showers, baths

SENSORY STIMULATION STRATEGIES
- Aromatherapy
- Breathing techniques
- Music
- Imagery
- Use of focal points

COGNITIVE STRATEGIES
- Childbirth education
- Hypnosis

PHARMACOLOGIC MANAGEMENT OF DISCOMFORT

Sedatives

Sedatives such as barbiturates relieve anxiety and induce sleep only in prodromal or early latent labor and in the absence of pain. If the woman is experiencing pain, sedatives given without an analgesic may increase apprehension and cause the mother to become hyperactive and disoriented. Undesirable side effects include respiratory and vasomotor depression of both the mother and newborn. Because of these disadvantages, barbiturates are seldom used (Scott et al, 1999).

Analgesia and Anesthesia

Nursing management of obstetric analgesia and anesthesia combines the nurse's expertise in maternity care with a knowledge and understanding of anatomy and physiology and of medications and their desired and undesired side effects and methods of administration.

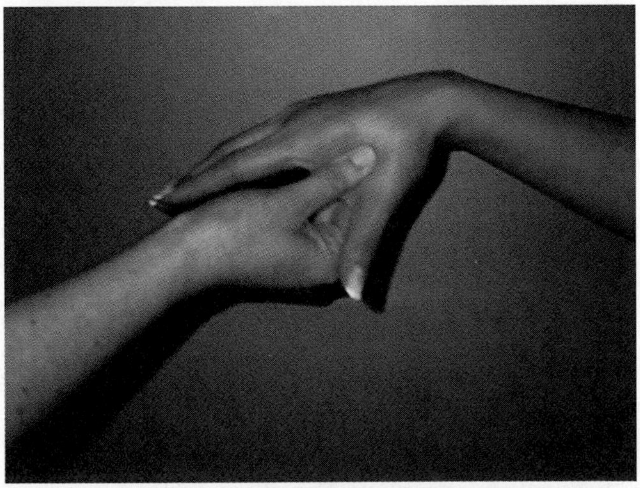

FIG. 16-6 • Ho-Ku acupressure point (back of hand where thumb and index finger come together) used to enhance uterine contractions without increasing pain. (From Dickason E, Silverman B, Kaplan J: *Maternal-infant nursing care,* ed 3, St Louis, 1998, Mosby.)

Box 16-3

Pharmacologic Control of Discomfort by Stage of Labor and Method of Birth

FIRST STAGE
- Systemic analgesia
  - Narcotic analgesic compounds
  - Mixed narcotic agonist-antagonist compounds, analgesic potentiators
- Nerve block analgesia/anesthesia
- Lumbar epidural analgesia

SECOND STAGE
- Nerve block analgesia/anesthesia
  - Local infiltration anesthesia
  - Pudendal block
  - Subarachnoid (spinal) anesthesia
  - Epidural block
  - Epidural and spinal narcotics
- Inhalation analgesia/anesthesia
  - Nitrous oxide-oxygen
  - General anesthesia

VAGINAL BIRTH
- Local infiltration
- Pudendal block
- Lumbar epidural block
  - Analgesia
  - Anesthesia
- Subarachnoid block
  - Analgesia
  - Anesthesia

CESAREAN BIRTH
- Subarachnoid block
  - Spinal block
  - Saddle block (low spinal)
- Lumbar epidural block
  - Anesthesia
- Inhalation
  - General anesthesia

Anesthesia encompasses analgesia, amnesia, relaxation, and reflex activity. Anesthesia abolishes pain perception by interrupting the nerve impulses going to the brain. The loss of sensation may be partial or complete, sometimes with the loss of consciousness.

The term analgesia is best reserved to describe the alleviation of the sensation of pain or the raising of the threshold for pain perception but without loss of consciousness.

The type of analgesic or anesthetic chosen is determined in part by the stage of labor and by the method of birth (Box 16-3).

Systemic Analgesia. Systemic analgesia remains the major method of analgesia for the woman in labor when personnel trained in regional analgesia are not available (Scott et al, 1999). Systemic analgesics cross the blood-brain barrier to provide central analgesic effects. They also cross the placental barrier. Effects on the fetus depend on the maternal dosage, the pharmacokinetics of the specific medication, and the route and timing of administration. Intravenous (IV) administration is often preferred over intramuscular (IM) administration because the onset of the medication's effect is faster and more reliable. Classes of analgesic medications used to relieve the pain of childbirth include narcotics, narcotic agonist-antagonist compounds, and tranquilizers such as analgesic-potentiating medications (ataractics).

Narcotic Analgesic Compounds. Narcotic analgesics such as meperidine (Demerol) and fentanyl (Sublimaze) are especially effective for the relief of severe, persistent, or recurrent pain. They have no amnesic effect (Box 16-4).

Meperidine is the most commonly used narcotic for women in labor (Scott et al, 1999). It overcomes inhibitory factors in labor and may even relax the cervix. After IV injection, onset is rapid (30 seconds), maximum effect is reached in 5 to 10 minutes, and effects last about 3 hours. Peak effect after IM injection of meperidine is reached in 40 to 50 minutes. Ideally, birth should occur less than 1 or more than 4 hours after IM injection to minimize neonatal depression. Because tachycardia is a possible side effect, meperidine is used cautiously in women with cardiac disease.

Fentanyl is a potent, short-acting narcotic analgesic (Box 16-5). Onset of the drug effect after IV injection occurs within 2 minutes and lasts about 30 to 60 minutes. Onset of the drug effect occurs in 7 to 15 minutes after IM injection, reaches its peak effect in 20 to 30 minutes, and lasts for 1 to 2 hours. Additive CNS and respiratory depression occurs if fentanyl is given with alcohol, antihistamines, antidepressants, or other sedative/hypnotics.

Mixed Narcotic Agonist-Antagonist Compounds. An *agonist* is an agent that activates something; an *antagonist* is an agent that prevents something from happening. Mixed narcotic agonist-antagonist compounds such as butorphanol (Stadol) and nalbuphine (Nubain), in the doses used during labor, provide analgesia without causing respiratory depression in the mother or the neonate (see Box 16-4). Both IM and IV routes are used for administration. Butorphanol or nalbuphine may be given during the first stage of labor.

Analgesic-Potentiators (Ataractics). Phenothiazines, so-called tranquilizers, have the property of augmenting most of the desirable but few of the undesirable effects of analgesics or general anesthetics. These ataractics do not relieve pain but decrease anxiety and apprehension, as well as potentiate narcotic effects. This potentiation effect causes the two drugs to work together more effectively, so that the narcotic dose can be reduced. Analgesic potentiators include compounds such as promethazine (Phenergan), propiomazine (Largon), hydroxyzine (Vistaril), and promazine (Sparine).

In addition to potentiating the effects of the analgesic, the ataractic (tranquilizer) also acts as an antinauseant and antiemetic. The combination of agents can be administered safely until the end of the first stage of labor. Since hydroxyzine is given only by IM injection, the onset of effect is slower and less predictable. Fetal or neonatal problems rarely develop when mothers are given the recommended doses.

Narcotic Antagonists. Narcotics such as meperidine and fentanyl can cause excessive CNS depression in the mother or newborn. Narcotic antagonists such as naloxone (Narcan) or naltrexone (Trexan) can promptly reverse the narcotic effects (Box 16-6).

A narcotic antagonist is especially valuable if labor is more rapid than expected and birth is anticipated when the narcotic is at its peak effect. The antagonist may be given through the woman's IV line or it can be administered IM. Narcotic antagonists can counteract maternal and neonatal narcotic effects. Therefore, the mother must be told that with the administration of an antagonist the pain will return.

Box 16-4

Medication Guide: Opioid Analgesics for Labor

MEDICATION	Meperidine (Demerol)	Butorphanol tartrate (Stadol)	Nalbuphine (Nubain)
ACTION	Opioid agonist analgesic; decreases pain impulse transmission via opioid receptors	Mixed agonist-antagonist analgesic; mechanism of action not determined	Mixed agonist-antagonist analgesic
INDICATION	Labor pain; postoperative pain after cesarean birth	Labor pain	Labor pain; postoperative pain after cesarean birth
DOSAGE AND ROUTE	25 mg IV; 50 mg IM May repeat in 2-3 hr; use of adjunctive medications such as promethazine may potentiate the narcotic effects and decrease nausea and vomiting	1-2 mg IV/IM May repeat in 3-4 hr	10 mg IV; 10-20 mg IM q3-6 hr
ADVERSE EFFECTS	Nausea and vomiting, sedation, drowsiness, tachycardia, hypotension, dry mouth, pruritis, respiratory depression (woman and newborn), decreased FHR variability, decreased uterine activity	See meperidine; may cause transient sinusoidal-like FHR rhythm	See meperidine
NURSING CONSIDERATIONS	Assess FHR and uterine activity; observe for respiratory depression; if birth occurs within 4 hr of dose, observe newborn for respiratory depression; naloxone available as antidote; side rails up	See meperidine; may precipitate withdrawal in opiate-dependent women	See butorphanol

NURSE ALERT • Narcotic antagonists must be administered cautiously to a substance-dependent woman because they may precipitate withdrawal symptoms (Box 16-7).

A narcotic antagonist can be given to the newborn to treat neonatal narcosis, which is a state of CNS depression in the newborn caused by a narcotic. Affected infants may exhibit respiratory depression, hypotonia, lethargy, and a delay in temperature regulation. Alterations in neurologic and behavioral responses may be evident for 72 hours after birth. Meperidine may be present in the neonate's urine for up to 3 weeks. Some depression of attention and social responsiveness can be evident for up to 6 weeks after birth.

In addition, the antagonist also counters the effect of stress-induced levels of endorphins. It is thought that endorphins increase during pregnancy and birth in humans and may increase the ability of women in labor to tolerate acute pain.

Nerve Block Analgesia and Anesthesia. A variety of compounds are used in obstetrics to produce regional analgesia (some pain relief and motor block) and anesthesia (pain relief and motor block). Most of these drugs are related chemically to cocaine and end with the suffix -caine. This helps identify a local anesthetic.

The principal pharmacologic effect of local anesthetics is the temporary interruption of the conduction of nerve impulses, notably pain. Examples of common agents given in 0.25% to 1% solutions are lidocaine (Xylocaine), bupivacaine (Marcaine), chloroprocaine (Nesacaine), tetracaine (Pontocaine), and mepivacaine (Carbocaine).

Rarely, people are sensitive (allergic) to one or more local anesthetics. Such a reaction may include respiratory depression, hypotension, and other serious adverse effects. Atropine, antihistamines, oxygen, and supportive measures should reverse these effects. Sensitivity may be identified by using minute amounts of the medication to test for an allergic reaction.

Box 16-5

Medication Guide: Fentanyl (Sublimaze) and Sufentanil (Sufenta)

ACTION	Opioid analgesics, rapid action with short duration (1-2 hr)
INDICATION	For epidural or intrathecal analgesia, usually in combination with a local anesthetic
DOSAGE AND ROUTE	Fentanyl—IM 50 to 100 μg; IV 25 to 50 μg Epidural—fentanyl, 1 to 2 μg with 0.125% bupivacaine at rate of 8 to 10 ml/hr; sufentanil, 1 μg with 0.125% bupivacaine at rate of 10 ml/hr
ADVERSE EFFECTS	Dizziness, drowsiness, allergic reactions, rash, respiratory depression
NURSING CONSIDERATIONS	Assess for respiratory depression; naloxone should be available as antidote

Local Infiltration Anesthesia. Local infiltration anesthesia of perineal tissues is commonly used when an episiotomy is

Box 16-6

Medication Guide: Naloxone (Narcan) and Naltrexone (Trexan)

ACTION	Opioid antagonists
INDICATION	Naloxone—reverses opioid-induced respiratory depression in woman or newborn; naltrexone—counteracts effects of epidural or intrathecal morphine; both may be used to reverse pruritis from epidural opioids
DOSAGE AND ROUTE	Naloxone—adult, 0.4 to 2 mg IV/IM/SC, repeat in 2 to 3 min up to 2 times if needed; newborn, 0.1 mg/kg IV (umbilical vein or endotracheal); repeat q2-3 min up to 3 times if needed, may also be given IM or SC Naltrexone—adult, 3 to 6 mg PO one dose
ADVERSE EFFECTS	Maternal hypotension, tachycardia, nausea and vomiting
NURSING CONSIDERATIONS	Woman should delay breastfeeding until medication is out of system; do not give if woman is using drugs of abuse—may cause abrupt withdrawal; if given to woman for reversal of respiratory depression due to opioid analgesic, pain will return

Box 16-7

Signs of Potential Complications

MATERNAL NARCOTIC WITHDRAWAL

Nausea, vomiting
Headache
Irritability
Fatigue
Perspiration, chills
Tremors, weakness, restlessness
Anxiety, apprehension, jittery feeling
Convulsions (seizures)

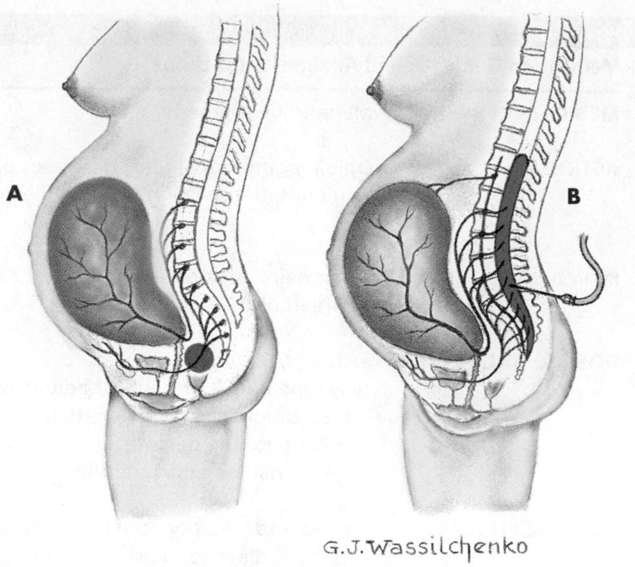

FIG. 16-7 • Pain pathways and sites of pharmacologic nerve blocks. **A,** Pudendal block; suitable during second and third stages of labor and for repair of episiotomy. **B,** Epidural block; suitable during all stages of labor and for repair of episiotomy.

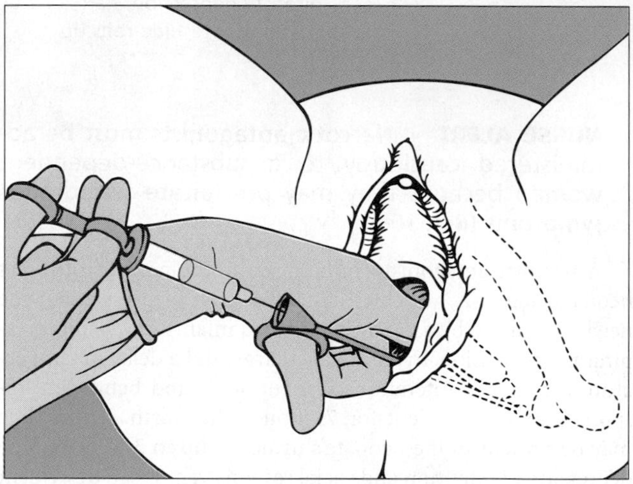

FIG. 16-8 • Pudendal block. Use of needle guide ("Iowa trumpet") and Luer-Lok syringe to inject medication.

to be done and when time or the fetal head position does not permit a pudendal block to be administered (Scott et al, 1999). Rapid anesthesia is produced by injecting 1% lidocaine or 2% chloroprocaine into the skin and then subcutaneously into the region to be anesthetized. Epinephrine often is added to the solution to intensify the anesthesia in a limited region and to prevent excessive bleeding and systemic effects by constricting local blood vessels (Clark, Queener, and Karb, 1993). Repeated injection will prolong the anesthesia as long as needed.

Pudendal Block. Pudendal block is useful for the second stage of labor, for episiotomy, and for birth. Although it does not relieve pain from uterine contractions, it does relieve pain in the lower vagina, vulva, and perineum (Fig. 16-7, *A*).

The pudendal nerve traverses the sacrosciatic notch just medial to the tip of the ischial spine on each side. Injection of an anesthetic solution at or near these points anesthetizes the pudendal nerves peripherally (Fig. 16-8). The transvaginal approach is generally used because it is less painful for the woman, has a higher success rate, and tends to cause fewer fetal complications (Chestnut, 1994). Pudendal block does not change maternal hemodynamic or respiratory functions, vital signs, or FHR. However, the bearing-down reflex is lessened or lost completely.

If all branches of the pudendal nerve are anesthetized, analgesia is sufficient for a spontaneous vaginal birth or for outlet (low) forceps-assisted birth. A pudendal block does not provide analgesia for uterine exploration or manual removal of the placenta (Scott et al, 1999).

Spinal Anesthesia. In spinal block, local anesthetic is injected through the third, fourth, or fifth lumbar interspace into the subarachnoid space (Fig. 16-9), where the medication mixes

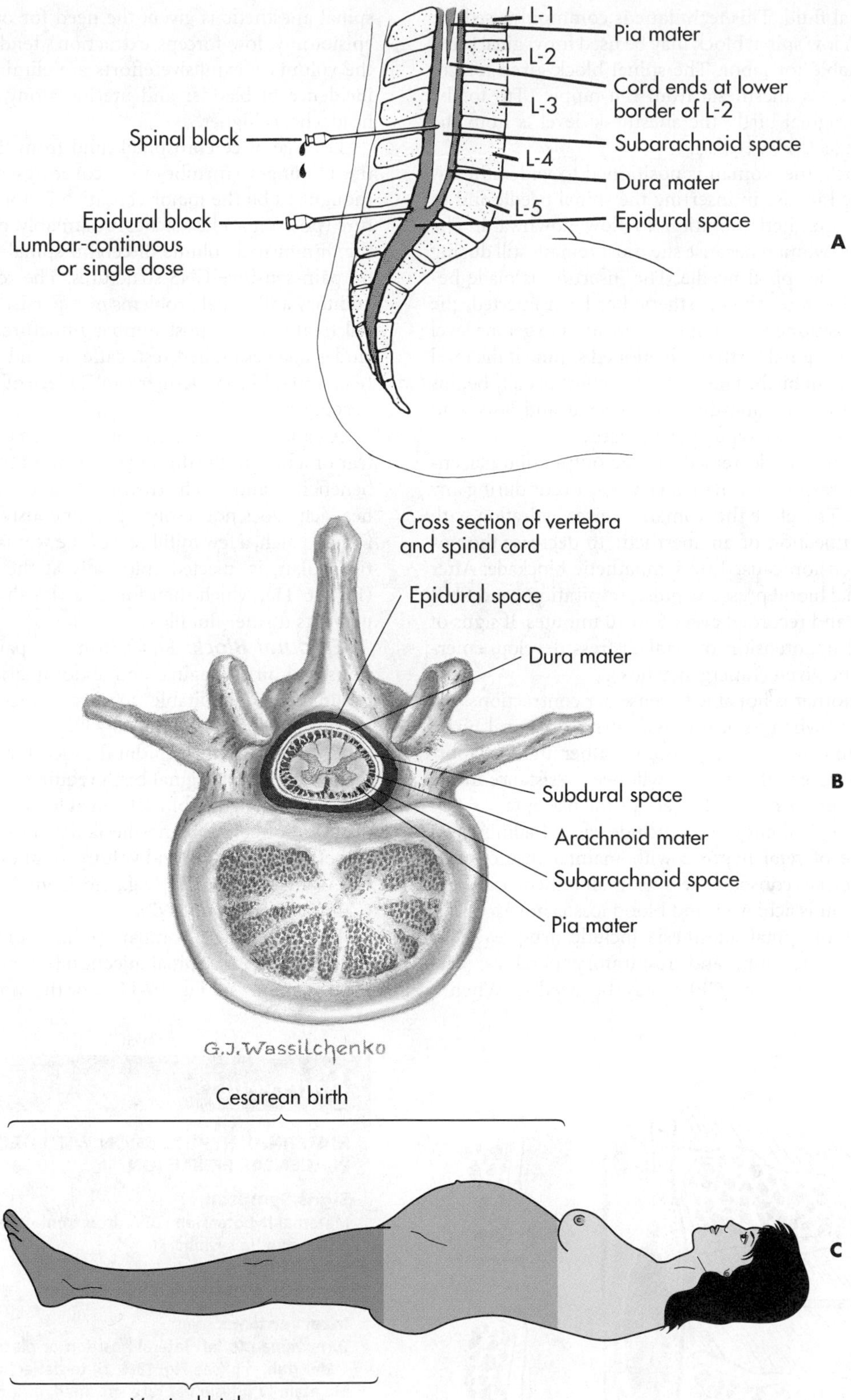

FIG. 16-9 • **A,** Membranes and spaces of spinal cord and levels of sacral, lumbar, and thoracic nerves. **B,** Cross section of vertebra and spinal cord. **C,** Levels of anesthesia necessary for cesarean and vaginal births.

with cerebrospinal fluid. This technique is commonly used for cesarean births. A low spinal block may be used for vaginal birth but it is not suitable for labor. The spinal block given for cesarean birth provides anesthesia from the nipple (T6) to the feet. If used for vaginal birth, the anesthesia level is from the hips (T10) to the feet (Fig. 16-10).

For spinal block, the woman is positioned to widen the intervertebral space for ease in inserting the spinal needle and to allow the heavy anesthetic solution to flow downward. The nurse supports the woman because she must remain still during the placement of the spinal needle. The insertion is made between contractions. After the anesthetic has been injected, the woman may be positioned in an upright position to get the level of anesthesia for a vaginal birth or positioned supine if the level desired is for cesarean birth. The anesthetic effect usually begins 1 to 2 minutes after the anesthetic is injected and lasts 1 to 3 hours, depending on the type of agent used.

Marked hypotension, decreased cardiac output and placental perfusion, and respiratory inadequacy may occur during any spinal anesthesia. Therefore the woman receives hydration with IV fluids before injection of an anesthetic to decrease the potential for hypotension caused by sympathetic blockade. After injection, maternal blood pressure, pulse, respirations, and FHR must be checked and recorded every 5 to 10 minutes. If signs of serious maternal hypotension or fetal distress develop, emergency care must be given (Emergency box).

Because the mother is not able to sense her contractions, she must be instructed when to bear down during a vaginal birth. If the birth occurs in a delivery room (rather than a labor-delivery-recovery room) the mother will need assistance in the transfer to a recovery bed after delivery of the placenta.

Advantages of spinal anesthesia include ease of administration and absence of fetal hypoxia with maintenance of normotension. Maternal consciousness is maintained, excellent muscular relaxation is achieved, and blood loss is not excessive.

Disadvantages of spinal anesthesia include drug reactions (e.g., allergy), hypotension, and respiratory paralysis; cardiopulmonary resuscitation (CPR) may be needed. When a spinal anesthetic is given, the need for operative delivery (i.e., episiotomy, low forceps extraction) tends to increase because the voluntary expulsive efforts are eliminated. After birth, the incidence of bladder and uterine atony, as well as postspinal headache, is higher.

Leakage of cerebrospinal fluid from the site of puncture of the meninges (membranous coverings of the spinal cord) is thought to be the major causative factor in postlumbar puncture (postspinal) headache. Presumably, postural changes cause the diminished volume of cerebrospinal fluid to exert traction on pain-sensitive CNS structures. The resulting headache and auditory and visual problems may persist for days or weeks. Initial treatment for post-lumbar puncture headache usually includes analgesics, bed rest, caffeine, and increased fluid intake (e.g., 150 ml/hr IV) (American College of Obstetricians and Gynecologists, 1996).

An autologous epidural blood patch (i.e., a patch repairing a tear or a hole in the dura mater around the spinal cord) is often beneficial, and such treatment may be considered if the headache does not resolve spontaneously (Scott et al, 1999). To form a patch, a few milliliters of the woman's blood without anticoagulant is injected epidurally at the site of the spinal tap (Fig. 16-11), which then forms a clot that covers the hole and prevents further fluid loss.

Epidural Block. Relief from the pain of uterine contractions and birth (vaginal and abdominal) can be accomplished by injecting a suitable local anesthetic into the epidural (peridural) space (see Fig. 16-11).

Complete lumbar epidural block for relieving the discomfort of labor and vaginal birth requires a block from T10 to S5. For cesarean birth, a block from at least T8 to S1 is essential. The diffusion of epidural anesthesia depends on the location of the catheter tip, the dose and volume of anesthetic agent used, and the woman's position (e.g., horizontal or head-up position) (Cunningham et al, 1997).

For induction of lumbar epidural anesthesia, the woman is positioned as for a spinal injection (i.e., sitting) or in a modified Sims position (see Fig. 16-11). For the modified lateral Sims po-

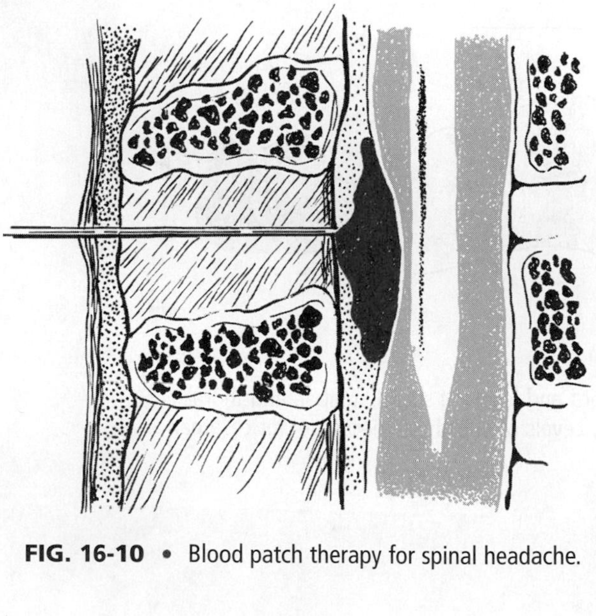

FIG. 16-10 • Blood patch therapy for spinal headache.

Emergency

MATERNAL HYPOTENSION WITH DECREASED PLACENTAL PERFUSION

Signs/Symptoms

- Maternal hypotension (20% drop from preblock level or less than 100 mm Hg systolic)
- Fetal bradycardia
- Decreased beat-to-beat FHR variability

Interventions

- Turn woman to left lateral position or place pillow or wedge under right hip (see Fig. 18-4, *D*) to deflect uterus.
- Maintain IV infusion at rate specified, or increase prn per hospital protocol.
- Administer oxygen by face mask at 10-12 L/min or per protocol.
- Elevate the woman's legs.
- Notify the physician/midwife/anesthesiologist/nurse anesthetist.
- Administer IV vasopressor (e.g., ephedrine) per protocol.
- Remain with woman; continue to monitor maternal blood pressure and FHR every 5 minutes until her condition is stable or per primary health care provider's order.

sition, the woman is placed on her side with her shoulders parallel, legs slightly flexed, and back arched.

After the epidural has been placed, the woman is preferably positioned on her side so that the uterus does not compress the ascending vena cava and descending aorta, which can impair venous return and decrease placental perfusion. Oxygen should be available to treat hypotension should it occur despite maintenance of hydration with IV fluid and displacement of the uterus to the side. Ephedrine (a vasopressor used to increase maternal blood pressure) and increased IV fluid infusion may be needed (see Emergency box). The FHR and progress in labor must be monitored carefully because the woman in labor may not be aware of changes in strength of uterine contractions or of descent of the presenting part.

A single injection or continuous infusion (via pump) through an indwelling plastic catheter results in excellent epidural analgesia-anesthesia. The advantages of an epidural are numerous: the mother experiences excellent pain relief and remains alert and cooperative, good relaxation is achieved, airway reflexes remain intact, only partial motor paralysis develops, gastric emptying is not delayed, and blood loss is not excessive. Fetal distress is rare but may occur with rapid absorption or marked maternal hypotension. The dose, volume, and type of anesthetic can be modified to allow the mother to push, to produce perineal anesthesia, and to permit use of forceps or even cesarean birth if required (Cunningham et al, 1997).

The disadvantages of an epidural block for the woman include the need for an IV line, occasional dizziness, weakness of the legs, difficulty emptying the bladder, and shivering (Buggy and Bardiner, 1995; Youngstrom, Baker, and Miller, 1996). Because a considerable amount of the drug must be used, adverse reactions or rapid absorption of the anesthetic agent may result in maternal hypotension, convulsions, or paresthesia. The length of labor and the incidence of operative delivery (e.g., episiotomy, use of forceps) may be increased if the woman cannot bear down effectively (Alexander et al, 1998; Howell, 1998). Occasionally, accidental high-spinal anesthesia (and later, postspinal headache) may follow inadvertent perforation of the dural membrane during administration of lumbar epidural anesthesia.

For some women the anesthetic selected is not effective, and a second form of anesthesia is required to establish effective pain relief. For women who progress rapidly in labor, pain relief may not be obtained before birth occurs (Nursing Care Plan).

Epidural and Intrathecal Narcotics. There is a high concentration of narcotic receptors along the pain pathway in the spinal cord, in the brainstem, and in the thalamus. Because these receptors are highly sensitive to narcotics, a small quantity of narcotic produces marked analgesia that lasts for several hours. Medication is injected through a catheter placed in the epidural or subarachnoid space, which reaches these narcotic receptors, and pain transmission is blocked without compromising motor ability. This so-called "walking epidural" restores

A
B
C

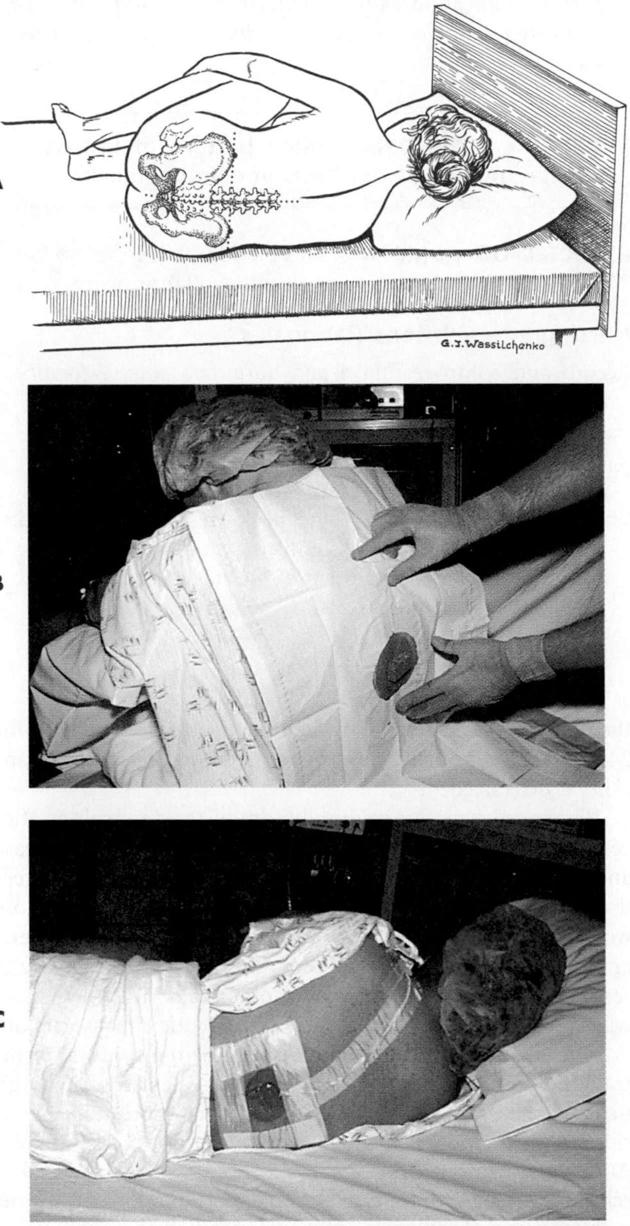

FIG. 16-11 • Position for spinal and epidural blocks. **A,** Lateral position. **B,** Upright position. **C,** Catheter is taped to woman's back with port segment located near her shoulder. (B and C, Courtesy Michael S. Clement, MD, Mesa, AZ.)

Community Focus

EPIDURAL VS. NON-EPIDURAL ANALGESIA FOR PAIN RELIEF IN LABOR

Epidural analgesia provides effective pain relief in labor, but has a number of possible adverse effects. For example, the first and second stages of labor are longer with epidural analgesia; the incidence of fetal malposition is increased; and the use of oxytocin and of instrumental vaginal deliveries is increased. Women must be provided information so that they can give informed consent for the use of labor epidurals. In addition, childbirth education and labor support are important to provide means for women to cope with the pain of contractions. Nurses can promote community efforts to provide a homelike environment conducive to a comfortable and safe childbirth experience.

Data from Howell C: Epidural versus no-epidural analgesia for pain relief in labour (Cochrane Review), *The Cochrane Library,* Issue 3, 2000. Oxford: Update Software.

Nursing Care Plan — LUMBAR EPIDURAL BLOCK DURING LABOR

NURSING DIAGNOSIS Coping, risk for ineffective individual, related to new experience with labor and epidural block

EXPECTED OUTCOME Woman will perform activities to maintain control over the situation.

Nursing Interventions/*Rationales*

Assess woman's understanding of the benefits and risks of epidural block procedure *to provide baseline for providing information.*

Encourage woman to express feelings *to provide clarification and verify any needs.*

Reinforce use of positive coping mechanisms *to assist in increasing control over the situation and promote self-esteem.*

Encourage participation of significant other during administration of epidural block and throughout the rest of the labor process *to assist in optimum use of coping mechanisms.*

NURSING DIAGNOSIS Risk for maternal/fetal injury related to maternal hypotension secondary to epidural block

EXPECTED OUTCOME No fetal or maternal injury will occur as the result of maternal hypotension for the duration of labor.

Nursing Interventions/*Rationales*

Assess fetal heart rate and maternal vital signs prior to initiation of block *to establish baseline data.*

Administer intravenous bolus solution as per physician's orders *to increase circulating blood volume and cardiac output.*

Place the woman in the lateral position *to avoid supine hypotensive syndrome and maintain placental perfusion.*

Monitor fetal heart rate and maternal vital signs *to provide indication of any deviations from the baseline and promote early intervention.*

If hypotension occurs, elevate the woman's legs, increase rate of IV solution as per protocol, administer oxygen by mask at 10 to 12 L per minute, notify the primary care provider, anesthesiologist, or nurse anesthetist, and administer vasopressor medication as per physician orders *to quickly increase maternal blood pressure and maintain placental perfusion.*

NURSING DIAGNOSIS Altered pattern of urinary elimination related to effects of epidural block

EXPECTED OUTCOME Woman's bladder will show no evidence of distention throughout the labor process.

Nursing Interventions/*Rationales*

Record and compare intake and output *to observe for decreased output as a result of decreased sensation.*

Palpate the bladder anterior to the symphysis pubis frequently *to assess if the bladder is distended as a result of increased fluid intake and decreased sensation.*

Encourage frequent voiding and perform catheterization if unable to empty bladder completely *to avoid interference with labor process and descent of presenting part as well as potential bladder trauma.*

the woman's confidence in her ability to master labor no longer dominated by pain (Youngstrom, Baker, and Miller, 1996).

The use of epidural or intrathecal narcotics during labor has several advantages. These narcotics do not cause maternal hypotension or affect vital signs. The woman feels contractions but not pain. Her ability to bear down during the second stage of labor is preserved because the pushing reflex is not lost and motor power remains intact.

Fentanyl, sufentanil, or preservative-free morphine may be used. Fentanyl and sufentanil produce short-acting analgesia (i.e., 1.5 to 3.5 hours), and morphine may provide pain relief for 4 to 7 hours. Morphine may be combined with fentanyl or sufentanil. The short-acting narcotics are often used with multiparous women, and the morphine may be used with nulliparous women or women with a history of long labors (Manning, 1996). For most women, intrathecal narcotics do not provide adequate analgesia for second-stage labor pain, episiotomy, or birth (Cunningham et al, 1997).

A more common indication for the administration of epidural or intrathecal narcotics is for relief of postoperative pain. For example, women who give birth by cesarean receive fentanyl or morphine through the catheter. The catheter may then be removed, and the women are usually free of pain for 24 hours. Occasionally the catheter is left in place in case another dose is needed.

Women who receive epidurally administered morphine after cesarean birth are up soon after surgery with surprising ease and are able to care for their babies. Early ambulation and freedom from pain also facilitate bladder emptying. To those women who have had a previous cesarean birth and experienced the usual postoperative pain, the effects of this approach seem miraculous. However, the mother may not understand why she may experience pain after the narcotic effect wears off.

Side effects of narcotics administered by the epidural or intrathecal route include nausea, vomiting, pruritus (itching), urinary retention, and delayed respiratory depression. These side effects are more common when morphine is administered. Antiemetics, antipruritics, and narcotic antagonists are used to relieve these symptoms. For example, naloxone or naltrexone, nalbuphine hydrochloride (Nubain), promethazine, or metoclopramide (Reglan) may be administered. Hospital protocols should provide specific instructions for treatment of these side effects. Use of epidural narcotics is not without risks. Respiratory depression is a serious concern; for this reason, the woman's respiratory rate should be assessed and documented every hour for 24 hours or per hospital protocol. Naloxone hydrochloride should be readily available for use if the respiratory rate falls below 10 breaths per minute or if the oxygen saturation rate drops below 89%. Administration of oxygen by face mask may also be initiated, and the anesthesiologist/anesthetist should be notified.

Drug Effects on Neonate. Debate persists concerning the effects of epidural anesthesia on the neonate's neurobehavioral responses. Findings from studies that examine associations between neurobehavioral outcome and epidural anesthesia are far from consistent. For example, studies comparing the neonatal neurobehavioral scores for infants born to mothers who did and mothers who did not receive epidural analgesia have shown either little or no difference in the scores (Hamza, 1994; Scherer and Holzgreve, 1995) or have shown that infants of mothers who received epidural anesthesia did not score as well on neurobehavioral tests (Sepkoski et al, 1992).

Paracervical (Uterosacral) Block. Paracervical block can be used to relieve pain from the lower uterine segment and cervix to the upper third of the vagina. It is rarely used for labor because of the potential fetal complications related to rapid absorption of the drug. Paracervical block may be used for anesthesia during abortion or other gynecologic procedures.

General Anesthesia. General anesthesia is rarely used for uncomplicated vaginal birth and is infrequently used for cesarean birth. It may be necessary if there is a contraindication to nerve block analgesia or anesthesia or if fetal indications necessitate a rapid birth (vaginal or cesarean).

If general anesthesia is being considered, the nurse gives the woman nothing by mouth and sees that an IV infusion is established. If time allows, the nurse premedicates the woman with a nonparticulate oral antacid such as sodium citrate (30 ml) to neutralize the acidic contents of the stomach. If there is sufficient time, some nurse anesthetists/anesthesiologists and physicians also order the administration of a histamine blocker such as cimetidine to decrease production of gastric acid and metoclopramide to increase gastric emptying (Scott et al, 1999). Before the anesthesia is given, a wedge should be placed under the woman's right hip to displace the uterus to the left. Uterine displacement prevents aortocaval compression, which interferes with placental perfusion. Sometimes the nurse is asked to assist with applying cricoid pressure before intubation (Fig. 16-12).

Priorities for recovery room care are to maintain an open airway, maintain cardiopulmonary functions, and prevent postpartum hemorrhage. Routine postpartum care is organized to facilitate parent-infant attachment as soon as possible and to answer the mother's questions. When appropriate, the nurse assesses the mother's readiness to see the baby, as well as her response to the anesthesia and to the event that necessitated general anesthesia (e.g., cesarean birth when vaginal birth was anticipated).

Inhalation Analgesia and Anesthesia. Nitrous oxide is the only inhalation agent used for obstetrics in the United States. It is rarely used for labor in the United States, but may be used for this purpose in other countries.

Nitrous oxide is commonly used for cesarean births when inhalation anesthesia is needed. It is usually combined with oxygen in a 50:50 mixture. Thiopental, a short-acting barbiturate, combined with succinylcholine, a muscle relaxant, is given intravenously before tracheal intubation.

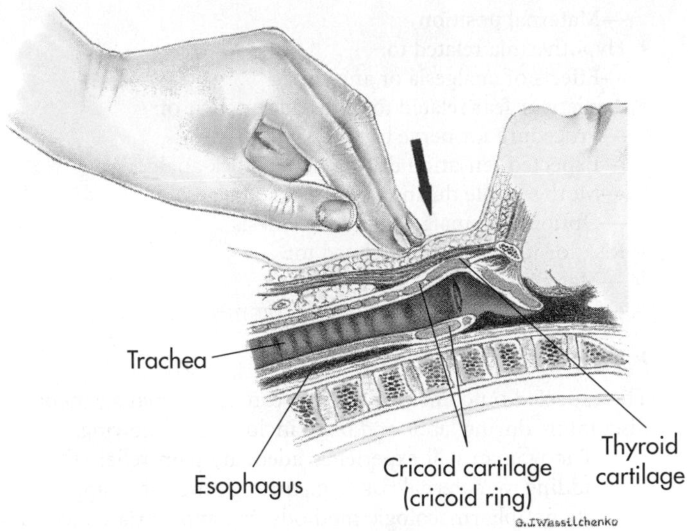

FIG. 16-12 • Technique of applying pressure on cricoid cartilage to occlude esophagus to prevent pulmonary aspiration of gastric contents during induction of general anesthesia.

Other inhalation agents include halothane, enflurane or isoflurane, and methoxyflurane. These agents relax the uterus quickly and facilitate intrauterine manipulation, version, and extraction. However, these agents cross the placenta readily and can produce narcosis in the fetus. They are rarely used today in the United States.

Care Management

➤ Assessment

The assessment of the woman, her fetus, and her labor is a joint effort of the nurse and the primary health care providers, who consult with the woman regarding their findings and recommendations. The needs of each woman are different, and many factors must be considered before deciding whether nonpharmacologic, a combination of nonpharmacologic and pharmacologic, or pharmacologic methods of pain management are used. A self-assessment tool, such as an analog scale, allows the woman to indicate on a line how severe she perceives her pain experience to be. Self-assessment is recommended to ensure that pain management is based on the subjective nature of the woman's pain rather than just on the nurse's judgment.

The woman is asked whether she attended childbirth preparation classes, and the extent of her preparation and preferences for management of discomfort are noted. Her knowledge of the options for management of discomfort is assessed. Information on the woman's perception of discomfort and about her expressed need for medication are added to the database. If verbal and physical signs indicate the existence of substance abuse, the nurse should ask the woman to identify the type of drug used, the last time the drug was taken, and the method of administration.

➤ Nursing Diagnoses

The following nursing diagnoses are relevant in the management of discomfort during labor and birth:

- Risk for altered tissue perfusion related to:
  —Effects of analgesia or anesthesia

—Maternal position
- Hypothermia related to:
  —Effects of analgesia or anesthesia
- Anxiety or fear related to knowledge deficit of:
  —Procedure for nerve block analgesia
  —Expected sensation during nerve block analgesia
  —Mother's role during nerve block analgesia
  —Options for analgesia and anesthesia
- Risk for injury to fetus related to:
  —Maternal hypotension
  —Maternal position (aortocaval compression)

➤ Expected Outcomes

The expected outcomes for nursing care in the management of discomfort during labor and birth include the following:

- The woman will experience adequate pain relief without adding to maternal risk (e.g., through the use of appropriate nonpharmacologic methods and appropriate medication, including the appropriate dose, timing, and route of administration).
- The fetus will maintain well-being, and the neonate will adjust to extrauterine life.
- The family/significant others will verbalize understanding of their needs in relation to the use of nonpharmacologic methods, analgesia, or anesthesia.

➤ Plan of Care and Implementation

A plan of care is developed for each woman and should address her particular clinical and nursing problems. The nurse collaborates with the primary health care provider and laboring woman to select those aspects of care relevant to the woman and her family.

Nonpharmacologic Interventions. The nurse supports and assists the woman as she uses nonpharmacologic interventions for pain relief and relaxation. Verbal and nonverbal acceptance of her behavior is given as necessary by the nurse, and reinforced by discussion and reassurance after birth when possible. Explanations about fetal response to maternal discomfort, the effects of maternal fatigue, and the medication itself are supportive measures. The woman may also be experiencing anxiety and stress related to the anticipated or actual pain. Stress can cause increased maternal catecholamine production. Raised levels of catecholamines have been linked to dysfunctional labor and fetal and neonatal distress and illness. Nurses must be able to implement strategies aimed at reducing this stress.

Informed Consent. The primary health care provider and anesthesia care provider are responsible for informing women of the alternative methods of pharmacologic pain relief available in the hospital setting. A description of the various anesthetic techniques and what they entail is essential to informed consent, even if the woman has received information about analgesia and anesthesia earlier in her pregnancy. This interview should take place just before or early in labor so the woman has time to consider alternatives. Nurses play a part in the informed consent process by clarifying and describing procedures and by acting as a patient's advocate and asking the primary health care provider for further explanations. The procedure and its advantages and disadvantages must be thoroughly explained.

LEGAL TIP • Informed Consent for Anesthesia

The woman receives (in an understandable manner):

- Explanation of the alternative methods of analgesia and anesthesia available
- Description of anesthetic and procedure for administration
- Description of the benefits, discomfort, risks, and consequences of the selected anesthetic for the mother and the fetus
- Explanation of how complications can be treated
- Information that the anesthetic is not always effective
- Indication that the woman may withdraw consent at any time
- Opportunity to have any questions answered
- Opportunity to explain in her own words components of the consent

The consent form will be:

- Written in the woman's primary language
- Have the woman's signature
- Have the date of consent
- Carry the signature of anesthesia caregiver certifying that the woman has received and appears to understand the explanation

Timing of Administration. It is often the nurse who notifies the primary health care provider that the woman is in need of pharmacologic measures to relieve her discomfort. Therefore the primary health care provider often writes orders for the administration of pain medication as needed based on the nurse's clinical judgment. (See Box 16-1 for the pharmacologic measures used to manage the discomfort of labor, summarized by the stage of labor and method of birth.)

Preparation for Procedures. The nurse reviews the methods of pain relief available to the woman (or validates her choices) and clarifies information for the mother as necessary. The procedure and what will be asked of the woman (e.g., to maintain flexed position during insertion of epidural needle) must be explained. The woman can also benefit from knowing the way that the medication is to be given, the degree of discomfort to expect from administration of the medication, the sensations she can expect, the time required for administration, and the interval before medication takes effect. The nurse explains the need for emptying the bladder before analgesic or anesthetic is given, and explains the reason for keeping the bladder empty. When an indwelling epidural catheter is to be threaded, the woman should be told that she may experience a momentary twinge down her leg, hip, or back and that this feeling is not a sign of injury.

A long needle is used for pudendal blocks (see Fig. 16-8). The sight of this needle may be frightening, and the woman can be reassured that only the tip of the needle will be inserted.

Administration of Medication. Accurate monitoring of the progress of labor forms the basis for the nurse's judgment that a woman needs pharmacologic control of discomfort. Knowledge of the medications used during childbirth is essential. The most effective route of administration is selected for each woman; then the medication is prepared and administered correctly.

Signs of Potential Problems. Any medication can cause an allergic reaction that may be minor or as severe as anaphylaxis. Minor reactions can consist of a rash, rhinitis, fever, asthma, or pruritus. Management of the less acute allergic response is not an emergency. As part of the assessment for such allergic reactions, the nurse should monitor the woman's vital signs, respiratory status, cardiovascular status, platelet count, and white blood cell count. The woman is observed for side effects of medications, especially drowsiness.

Severe allergic reactions may occur suddenly and lead to shock. The most dramatic form of anaphylaxis is sudden severe bronchospasm, vasospasm, severe hypotension, and death. Signs of anaphylaxis are largely caused by contraction of smooth muscles and may begin with irritability, extreme weakness, nausea, and vomiting. This may then lead to dyspnea, cyanosis, convulsions, and cardiac arrest. The acute allergic reaction—anaphylaxis—must be diagnosed and treated immediately. Treatment usually consists of 1:1000 epinephrine injected subcutaneously or intramuscularly, followed by parenteral administration of antihistamines. Supportive care is given to alleviate symptoms; the type of care is determined by the rapidly assessed cardiovascular and respiratory response of the woman to primary interventions; CPR may be necessary. The nurse must also be alert to fetal well-being: any FHR decelerations should be noted and reported to the primary health care provider.

Intravenous Route. The preferred route of administration of medications such as meperidine or fentanyl is through IV tubing, administered into the port nearest the woman while the infusion of IV solution is stopped. The medication is given slowly in small doses at the beginning of a contraction and over three to five consecutive contractions. Because uterine blood vessels are constricted during contractions, the medication stays within the maternal vascular system for several seconds before the uterine blood vessels reopen. The IV infusion is then restarted slowly to prevent a bolus of medication from forming. Using this method of injection, the amount of medication crossing the placenta to the fetus is minimized. With decreased placental transfer, the mother's degree of pain relief is maximized. The IV route has the following advantages:

- Onset of pain relief is more predictable.
- Pain relief is obtained with small doses of the drug.
- Duration of effect is more predictable.

Intramuscular Route. IM injections of analgesics, although still used, are not the preferred route of administration for the woman in labor. Identified disadvantages of the IM route include the following:

- Onset of pain relief is delayed.
- Higher doses of medication are required.
- Medication is released at an unpredictable rate from the muscle tissue and is available for transfer across the placenta to the fetus.

IM injections are given in the upper portion of the arm (deltoid site) if regional anesthesia is planned later in labor. This is the preferred site because the autonomic blockage from the regional (e.g., epidural) anesthesia causes blood flow to the gluteal region to be increased and accelerates absorption of the drug. The maternal plasma level of the drug necessary to bring pain relief usually is reached 45 minutes after IM injection, followed by a decline in plasma levels. The maternal drug levels (after IM injections) are unequal because of uneven distribution (maternal uptake) and metabolism. The advantage of using the IM route is quick administration.

Nerve Blocks. An IV line is established before induction of nerve blocks such as epidural, spinal, and general anesthesia. Anesthesia protocols usually include the administration of a bolus of IV fluid before epidural and spinal anesthesia for blood volume expansion to prevent maternal hypotension.

Lactated Ringer's or Plasma-Lyte A and normal saline solutions are the preferred infusion solutions. Infusion solutions without dextrose are preferred, especially when the solution must be infused rapidly (e.g., to treat severe dehydration or to maintain blood pressure) because solutions containing dextrose rapidly raise maternal blood glucose levels. The fetus responds to high blood glucose levels by increasing insulin production; fetal or neonatal hypoglycemia may result. In addition, dextrose changes osmotic pressure so that fluid is excreted from the kidneys more rapidly.

The woman needs assistance in assuming and maintaining the correct position for epidural and spinal anesthesia (see Fig. 16-12).

Safety and General Care. After administration of a nerve block, the woman is protected from injury by raising the side rails and, when the nurse is not in attendance, by placing a call bell within easy reach. Oxygen and suction should be readily available at the bedside. The nurse must make sure that there is no prolonged pressure on an anesthetized part (e.g., no lying on one side with weight on one leg; no tight bedclothes on feet). If stirrups are used for birth, the nurse should pad them, adjust both stirrups at the same level and angle, place both of the woman's legs into them while avoiding putting pressure to the popliteal angle, and apply restraints without restricting circulation.

The nurse monitors and records the woman's response to nonpharmacologic pain relief methods and to medication. This includes the level of pain relief, the level of apprehension, the return of sensations and perception of pain, and allergic or untoward reactions (e.g., hypotension, respiratory depression, and hypothermia). The nurse continues to monitor maternal vital signs, blood pressure, strength and frequency of uterine contractions, changes in the cervix and station of the presenting part, presence of the bearing-down reflex, bladder filling, and state of hydration. Determining the fetal response after the administration of analgesia or anesthesia is vital. The woman is asked if she (or the family) has any questions. The nurse assesses the woman's and her family's understanding of the need to ensure her safety (e.g., keeping side rails up, and calling for assistance as needed).

The time that elapses between the administration of a narcotic and the baby's birth is noted. Medication given to the newborn to reverse narcotic effects is recorded. Postpartum, the woman who has had spinal, epidural, or general anesthesia is assessed for return of sensory and motor sensation in addition to the usual postpartum assessments.

➤ Evaluation

Evaluation of the effectiveness of care of the woman needing management of discomfort during labor and birth is based on the previously stated outcomes.

Key Points

- The expected outcome of preparation for childbirth and parenting is "education for choice."
- Nonpharmacologic pain and stress-management strategies are valuable for managing labor discomfort alone or in combination with pharmacologic methods.
- The type of analgesic or anesthetic to be used is determined in part by the stage of labor and the method of birth.
- Narcotic effects can be potentiated with ataractics.
- Naloxone and naltrexone are narcotic antagonists that can reverse narcotic effects, especially respiratory depression.
- Pharmacologic control of discomfort during labor requires collaboration among the health care providers and the woman in labor.
- The nurse must understand medications, their expected effects, their potential side effects, and their methods of administration.
- An IV line and maternal hydration are essential during regional nerve blocks.
- Maternal analgesia or anesthesia potentially affects neonatal neurobehavioral response.
- The use of narcotic agonist-antagonist compounds in women with preexisting narcotic dependency may cause symptoms of narcotic withdrawal.
- General anesthesia is rarely used for vaginal birth but may be used for cesarean birth or whenever rapid anesthesia is needed in an emergency childbirth situation.

References

Alexander J et al: The course of labor with and without epidural analgesia, *Am J Obstet Gynecol* 178(3):516-520, 1998.

Alexander C, Steeful L: Biofeedback: listen to the body, *RN* 58(8):51-52, 1995.

American College of Obstetricians and Gynecologists: *Obstetric analgesia and anesthesia (ACOG Tech Bull No. 225)*, Washington, DC, 1996, ACOG.

Bradley R: *Husband-coached childbirth*, ed 3, New York, 1981, Harper & Collins.

Buggy D, Bardiner J: The space blanket and shivering during extradural anesthesia in labour, *Acta Anaesthesia Scand* 39(4): 551-553, 1995.

Burns E, Blamey C: Complementary medicine: using aromatherapy in childbirth, *Nurs Times* 90(9):54-60, 1994.

Chestnut D: Alternative regional anesthetic techniques: paracervical block, lumbar sympathetic block, pudendal block and perineal infiltration. In Chestnut D, editor: *Obstetrics anesthesia: principles and practices*, St Louis, 1994, Mosby.

Clark J, Queener S, Karb V: *Pharmacological basis of nursing practice*, ed 4, St Louis, 1993, Mosby.

Collins B et al: Descriptions of comfort by substance-using and nonusing postpartum women, *J Obstet Gynecol Neonatal Nurs* 23:293-300, 1994.

Cunningham F et al: *Williams obstetrics*, ed 20, Norwalk, CT, 1997, Appleton & Lange.

Dick-Read G: *Childbirth without fear*, ed 5, New York, 1987, Harper & Collins.

Hamza J: Effect of epidural anesthesia on the fetus and the neonate, *Cahiers d Anesthesiologie* 42(2):265-273, 1994.

Hoffart M, Pross-Keene E: The benefits of visualization, *Am J Nurs* 98(12):44-47, 1998.

Howell C: Epidural vs. nonepidural analgesia in labour, *The Cochrane Library* (3):110, Oxford CD-ROM, 1998.

Jenkins M, Pritchard M: Hypnosis: practical applications and theoretical considerations, *Br J Obstet Gynecol* 100(3):221-226, 1993.

Lamaze F: *Painless childbirth*, New York, 1972, Pocket Books.

Lee M, Essoka G: Continuing education. Patient's perception of pain: comparison between Korean-American and Euro-American obstetric patients, *J Cultural Diversity* 5(1):29-40, 1998.

Lowe N: The pain and discomfort of labor and birth, *J Obstet Gynecol Neonatal Nurs* 25(1):82-92, 1996.

Mackey R: Discovering the healing power of therapeutic touch, *Am J Nurs* 95(4):26-32, 1995.

Manning J: Intrathecal narcotics: new approach for labor anesthesia, *J Obstet Gynecol Neonatal Nurs* 25(3):221-224, 1996.

Rush J et al: The effects of whirlpool baths in labor: a randomized, controlled trial, *Birth* 23(3):136-143, 1996.

Scherer R, Holzgreve W: Influence of epidural analgesia on fetal and neonatal well-being, *Eur J Obstet Gynecol Reprod Biol* 59(suppl):S17-S29, 1995.

Schorn M, McAllister J, Blanco J: Water immersion and the effect on labor, *J Nurse Midwifery* 38:336-342, 1993.

Schuiling K, Sampselle C: Comfort in labor and midwifery art, *Image* 31(1):77-81, 1999.

Scott J et al: *Danforth's obstetrics and gynecology*, ed 8, Philadelphia, 1999, JB Lippincott.

Sepkoski C et al: The effects of maternal epidural anesthesia on neonatal behavior during the first month, *Dev Med Child Neurol* 34:1072-1080, 1992.

Simkin P: Reducing pain and enhancing progress in labor: a guide to nonpharmacologic methods of maternity caregivers, *Birth* 22(3):161-191, 1995.

Tiran D: Aromatherapy therapy in midwifery: benefits and risks, *Complementary Therapies in Nursing and Midwifery* 2(4):88-92, 1996.

Weber S: Cultural aspects of pain in childbearing women, *J Obstet Gynecol Neonatal Nurs* 25(1):67-72, 1996.

Wiand N: Relaxation levels achieved by Lamaze-trained pregnant women listening to music and ocean sound tapes, *J Perinatal Educ* 6(4):1-8, 1997.

Youngstrom P, Baker SW, Miller JL: Epidurals redefined in analgesia and anesthesia: a distinction with a difference, *J Obstet Gynecol Neonatal Nurs* 25(4):350-354, 1996.

CHAPTER 17

Fetal Assessment

http://www.harcourthealth.com/MERLIN/Wong/maternal/

Learning Objectives

On completion of this chapter the reader will be able to:

- Explain the baseline fetal heart rate (FHR) and evaluate periodic changes.
- Identify typical signs of nonreassuring FHR patterns.
- Describe preventive measures that can be used to maintain FHR patterns within normal limits.
- Compare nursing interventions used for managing specific FHR patterns, including tachycardia and bradycardia, increased and decreased variability, and late and variable decelerations.
- Compare FHR monitoring done by intermittent auscultation and external and internal electronic methods.

Electronic fetal monitoring (EFM) was first introduced in the 1970s. Since then considerable expertise has been gained in the assessment of fetal hemodynamic and oxygen status. Evaluation of the fetal heart rate (FHR) remains complex, however, because of the number of factors that must be considered and the variations in the "normal" fetal response to labor. Ways of describing FHR patterns have been based on terminology coined by equipment manufacturers, researchers, and authors and have varied by region, institution, and health care provider.

The lack of agreement on definitions and interpretations of FHR patterns has limited the study of efficacy and validity of EFM. In 1995 a research-planning workshop was held to develop research guidelines for EFM interpretation. A proposed nomenclature system for EFM interpretation with standardized definitions for fetal heart rate monitoring was published (National Institute of Child Health and Human Development Research Planning Workshop, 1997). These definitions are being tested for reliability and accuracy and will be refined based on results of the tests.

Even though testing of the definitions has not yet been completed, some effect on clinical practice is likely. Thus, this chapter includes the new definitions and a discussion of the current systems of interpretation of EFM. Practitioners who use the new terminology need to communicate with other health care providers so that a common nomenclature is ensured in any one setting. Those who wish to use established terminology should continue to use guidelines developed by the Association of Women's Health, Obstetric, and Neonatal Nurses (AWHONN, 1993b) and the American College of Obstetricians and Gynecologists (ACOG, 1995) All perinatal health care providers must keep abreast of new developments in EFM technology and knowledge to ensure the best possible outcomes for mothers and newborns.

BASIS FOR MONITORING

Fetal Response

Because labor is a period of physiologic stress for the fetus, frequent monitoring of fetal health is part of the nursing care during labor. The fetal oxygen supply must be maintained during labor to prevent fetal compromise and promote newborn health after birth. The fetal oxygen supply can decrease in a number of ways, including the following:

- Reduction of blood flow through the maternal vessels as a result of maternal hypertension (chronic hypertension or pregnancy-induced hypertension), hypotension (caused by supine maternal position, hemorrhage, or related to epidural analgesia or anesthesia), or hypovolemia (caused by hemorrhage)
- Reduction of the oxygen content of the maternal blood as a result of hemorrhage or severe anemia
- Alterations in fetal circulation, occurring with compression of the umbilical cord (transient during uterine contractions or prolonged as a result of cord prolapse), placental separation or complete abruption, or head compression (head compression causes increased intracranial pressure and vagal nerve stimulation with a decrease in the FHR)
- Reduction in blood flow to the intervillous space in the placenta secondary to uterine hypertonus (generally caused by excessive exogenous oxytocin), or secondary to deterioration of the placental vasculature from maternal disorders such as hypertension or diabetes mellitus

Fetal well-being during labor can be measured by the response of the FHR to uterine contractions. In general, reassuring FHR patterns are characterized by the following:

- A baseline FHR in the normal range of 110 and 160 beats/min with no periodic changes and a moderate baseline variability
- Accelerations of FHR with fetal movement

A normal uterine activity pattern in labor is characterized by contractions occurring every 2 to 5 minutes and lasting less than 90 seconds. Such contractions are moderate to strong in intensity, as assessed by palpation, or the intensity is less than 100 mm Hg, as measured by an intrauterine pressure catheter (IUPC); 30 seconds or more should elapse between the end of one contraction and the beginning of the next contraction. Between contractions, uterine relaxation should be detected by palpation or by an average intrauterine pressure of 15 mm Hg or less.

Fetal Compromise

The goals of intrapartum FHR monitoring are to identify and differentiate the reassuring patterns from the nonreassuring patterns, which can be indicative of fetal compromise.

Nonreassuring FHR patterns are those associated with fetal hypoxemia, which is a deficiency of oxygen in the arterial blood. If uncorrected, hypoxemia can deteriorate to severe fetal hypoxia, which is an inadequate supply of oxygen at the cellular level. Nonreassuring FHR patterns include the following:

- Progressive increase or decrease in baseline rate
- Tachycardia of 160 beats per minute or above
- Progressive decrease in baseline variability
- Severe variable decelerations (FHR less than 60 beats per minute lasting longer than 30 to 60 seconds, with rising baseline, decreasing variability, or slow return to baseline)
- Late decelerations of any magnitude, especially those that are repetitive and uncorrectable, with decreasing variability or a rising baseline FHR
- Absence of FHR variability
- Prolonged deceleration (greater than 60 to 90 seconds)
- Severe bradycardia (less than 70 beats per minute

MONITORING TECHNIQUES

Intermittent Auscultation

Intermittent auscultation of the fetal heart can be performed with a Leff scope, a DeLee-Hillis fetoscope, or an ultrasound device. If a Leff scope is used, the domed side should be opened to the connective tubing to the earpieces. The domed side is then applied to the maternal abdomen. The fetoscope is applied over the listener's head because bone conduction amplifies the fetal heart sounds for counting. The ultrasound device transmits ultrahigh frequency sound waves reflecting movement of the fetal heart and converts these sounds into an electronic signal that can be counted (Fig. 17-1).

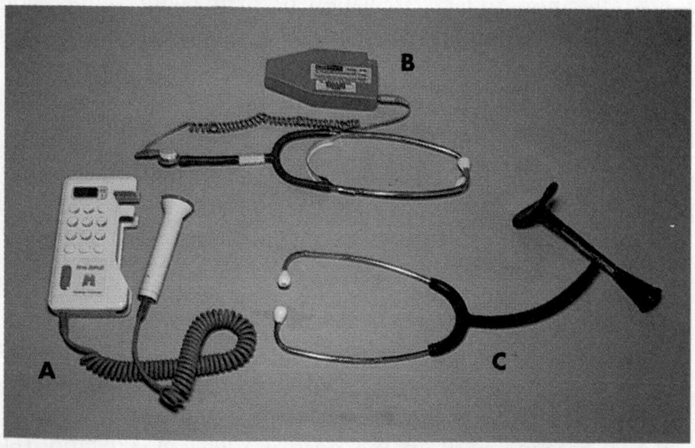

FIG. 17-1 • **A,** Ultrasound fetoscope. **B,** Ultrasound stethoscope. **C,** DeLee-Hillis fetoscope. (Courtesy Michael S. Clement, MD, Mesa, AZ.)

The procedure for performing auscultation is as follows:

1. Perform Leopold's maneuvers by palpating the maternal abdomen to identify fetal presentation and position.
2. Place the listening device over the area of maximum intensity and clarity of the fetal heart sounds to obtain the clearest and loudest sound, which is easiest to count.
3. Palpate the abdomen for the absence of uterine activity to be able to count the FHR between contractions.
4. Count the maternal radial pulse while listening to the FHR to differentiate it from the fetal rate.
5. Count the FHR for 30 to 60 seconds between contractions to identify the baseline rate. This rate can only be assessed in the absence of uterine activity.
6. Auscultate the FHR during a contraction and for 30 seconds after the end of the contraction to identify any increases or decreases in FHR in response to the contraction.

The method and frequency of fetal surveillance during labor will vary depending on maternal-fetal risk factors and on the preference of the personnel in a facility. The standard practice for auscultating the FHR, in the absence of risk factors, is described in Box 17-1.

NURSE ALERT • When the FHR is auscultated and documented, it is inappropriate to use the descriptive terms associated with electronic fetal monitoring because most of the terms are visual descriptions of the patterns produced on the monitor tracing. However, terms that are numerically defined, such as bradycardia and tachycardia, can be used.

Debate continues over the ideal method of fetal assessment during labor. Multiple research studies indicate that similar outcomes are associated with both intermittent auscultation of the FHR at the frequencies just given and electronic fetal heart

Box 17-1

Standard Practice of Fetal Heart Rate (FHR) Auscultation

FIRST STAGE
Latent phase every 60 minutes
Active phase every 30 minutes

SECOND STAGE
Every 15 minutes

When risk factors are present during labor, the FHR is auscultated as follows:

FIRST STAGE
Latent phase every 30 minutes
Active phase every 15 minutes

SECOND STAGE
Every 5 minutes

monitoring (American College of Obstetricians and Gynecologists, 1995; Thacker, Stoup, and Peterson, 1998). The advantages of intermittent auscultation are that it is a high-touch, low-technology method of assessing fetal status during labor and that it places fewer restrictions on maternal activity. Because childbirth is a natural process, most women and fetuses do well with minimal intervention and periodic assessment. In spite of that fact, almost 85% of women in labor in the United States are monitored electronically (Haggerty, 1999).

Every effort should be made to use the method of fetal assessment the woman desires when possible. However, auscultation of the FHR according to the frequency guidelines just given may be difficult in today's busy labor and birth units. When used as the primary method of fetal assessment, auscultation requires a one-to-one nurse-to-patient staffing ratio. If acuity and census change so that auscultation standards are no longer met, the nurse must notify the physician or nurse-midwife that continuous EFM will be used until staffing can be arranged to meet the standards.

The woman can become anxious if the examiner cannot readily count the FHR. It often takes time for the inexperienced listener to locate the heartbeat and find the area of maximum intensity. To allay the mother's concerns, she can be told that the nurse is "finding the spot where the sounds are loudest." The examiner can reassure the mother by offering her an opportunity to listen, too. If the examiner cannot locate the fetal heartbeat, assistance should be requested. In some cases ultrasound can be used to help locate the fetal heartbeat. Seeing the FHR on the ultrasound screen will be reassuring to the mother if there was initial difficulty in locating the best area for auscultation.

When using palpation to assess uterine activity, the examiner should keep his or her hand placed over the fundus before, during, and after contractions. Contraction intensity is usually described as mild, moderate, or strong. Contraction duration is measured in seconds, from beginning to end of the contraction. Frequency of contractions is measured in minutes, from the beginning of one contraction to the beginning of the next contraction. The examiner also evaluates the uterine resting tone or relaxation between contractions. Resting tone between contractions is usually described as soft or relaxed.

Accurate and complete documentation of fetal status and uterine activity is especially important when using intermittent auscultation because there is no paper tracing to record these assessments, as occurs continuously with electronic monitoring. Labor flow records or computer charting systems that prompt notations of all assessments are useful for comprehensive documentation.

Electronic Fetal Monitoring (EFM)

There are two modes of electronic fetal monitoring. The external mode involves the use of external transducers placed on the maternal abdomen to assess FHR and uterine activity. The internal mode involves the use of a spiral electrode applied to the fetal presenting part to assess the fetal electrocardiogram (ECG) and an IUPC to assess uterine activity and pressure. The differences between the external and internal modes of EFM are summarized in Table 17-1.

External Monitoring. Separate transducers are used to monitor the FHR and uterine contractions (Fig. 17-2). The ultrasound transducer works by reflecting high-frequency sound waves from a moving interface, in this case the fetal heart and valves. Therefore short-term variability and beat-to-beat changes in the FHR cannot be assessed accurately by this method. It is also difficult to reproduce a continuous and precise record of the FHR by this method because of artifacts introduced by fetal and maternal movement. The FHR is printed on specially formatted monitor paper. The standard paper speed is 3 cm/min. Once the area of maximum intensity of FHR has been located, conduction gel is applied to the surface of the ultrasound transducer and the transducer is positioned over this area.

TABLE 17-1
External and Internal Modes of Monitoring

External Mode	Internal Mode
FHR	
Ultrasound transducer: High-frequency sound waves reflect mechanical action of the fetal heart. Used during the antepartum and intrapartum period. Noninvasive. Does not require rupture of membranes or cervical dilation.	*Spiral electrode:* This electrode converts the fetal ECG as obtained from the presenting part to the FHR via a cardiotrachometer. This method can be used only when membranes are ruptured and the cervix is sufficiently dilated during the intrapartum period. Electrode penetrates into fetal presenting part by 1.5 mm and must be attached securely to ensure a good signal.
UTERINE ACTIVITY	
Tocotransducer: This instrument monitors frequency and duration of contractions by means of pressure-sensing device applied to the maternal abdomen. Used during both the antepartum and intrapartum periods.	*Intrauterine pressure catheter (IUPC):* This instrument monitors the frequency, duration, and intensity of contractions. There are two types of IUPCs: a fluid-filled system and a solid catheter. Both measure intrauterine pressure at the catheter tip and convert the pressure into millimeters of mercury on the uterine activity panel of the strip chart. Both can be used only when membranes are ruptured and the cervix is sufficiently dilated during the intrapartum period.

A

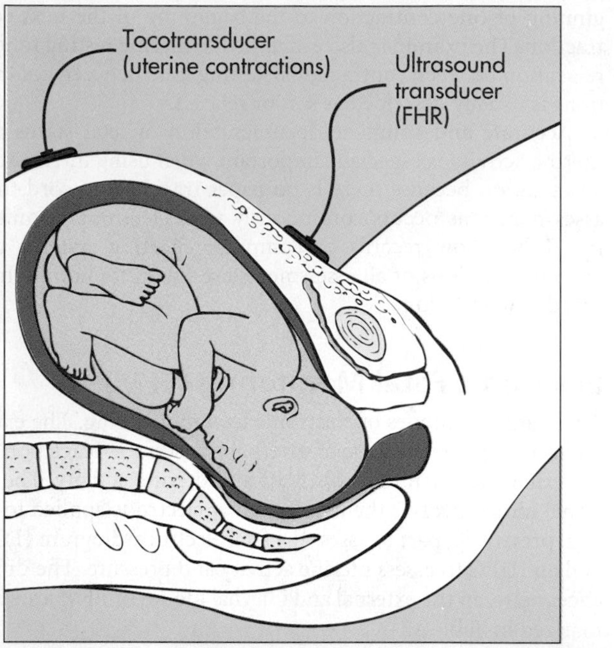

B

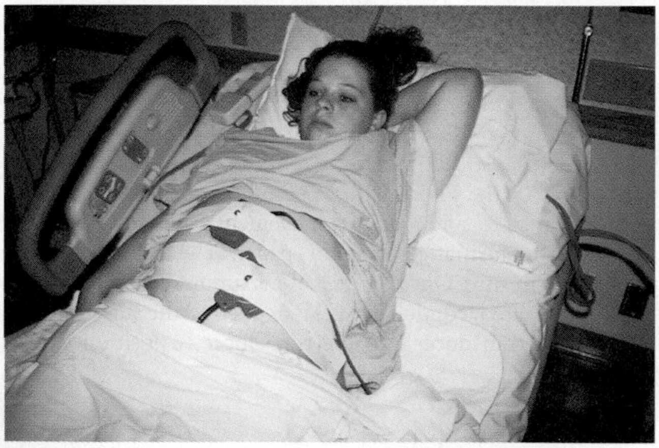

FIG. 17-2 • A, External noninvasive fetal monitoring using tocotransducer and ultrasound transducer. B, Ultrasound transducer is placed below umbilicus, over the area where fetal heart is heard best, and tocotransducer is placed on uterine fundus. (Courtesy Marjorie Pyle, RNC, Lifecircle, Costa Mesa, CA.)

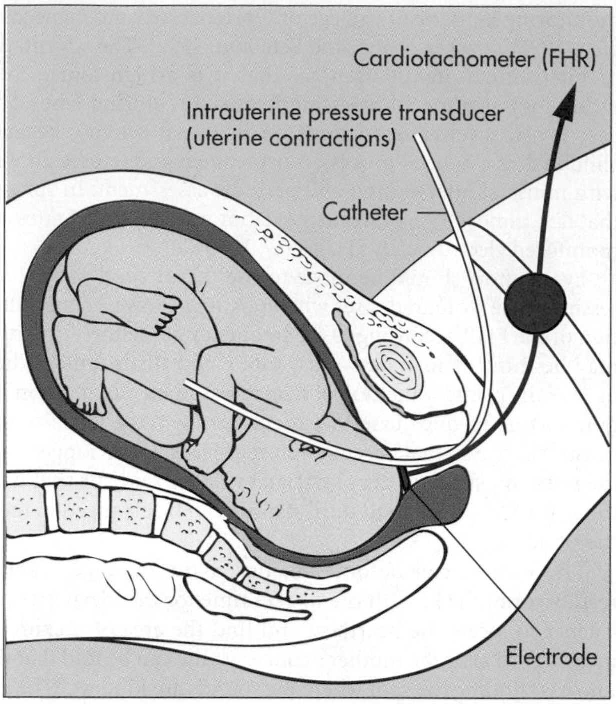

FIG. 17-3 • Diagrammatic representation of internal invasive fetal monitoring with intrauterine pressure catheter and spiral electrode in place (membranes ruptured and cervix dilated).

Critical Thinking

EXTERNAL FETAL MONITORING IN LABOR: PATIENT EDUCATION

You are assigned to a woman who is in the first stage of labor. She wonders why the fetal heart rate (FHR) is sometimes not being recorded on the monitor paper. She asks if there is "something wrong with the baby" when the FHR is not recording continuously. Based on your knowledge of how the external monitor works, how would you explain the lack of continuous tracing of the FHR? What actions can you take to improve the tracing? What type of documentation is appropriate about this tracing?

The tocotransducer (tocodynamometer) measures uterine activity transabdominally. The device is placed over the fundus above the umbilicus. Uterine contractions or fetal movements depress a pressure-sensitive surface on the side next to the abdomen. The tocotransducer can measure and record the frequency, regularity, and approximate duration of uterine contractions; but not their intensity. This method is especially valuable for measuring uterine activity during the first stage of labor in women with intact membranes and for antepartum testing. Because the tocotransducer of most electronic fetal monitors is designed for assessing uterine activity in the term pregnancy, it may not be sensitive enough to detect preterm uterine activity (Afriat, 1996). When monitoring the woman experiencing preterm labor, it is important to remember that the fundus may be located below the level of the umbilicus. The nurse also may need to rely on the woman to indicate when uterine activity is occurring, and may need to use palpation as an additional way of assessing contraction frequency.

The equipment is easily applied by the nurse, but it must be repositioned as the woman or fetus changes position (see Fig. 17-2, *B*). The woman is asked to assume a semisitting or lateral position. The equipment is removed periodically to wash the applicator sites and to give back rubs. This type of monitoring confines the woman to bed. Portable telemetry monitors allow observation of the FHR and uterine contraction patterns by means of centrally located electronic display stations. These portable units permit the woman to walk around during electronic monitoring.

Internal Monitoring. The technique of continuous internal monitoring provides an accurate appraisal of fetal well-being during labor (Fig. 17-3). For this type of monitoring, the membranes must be ruptured, the cervix sufficiently dilated,

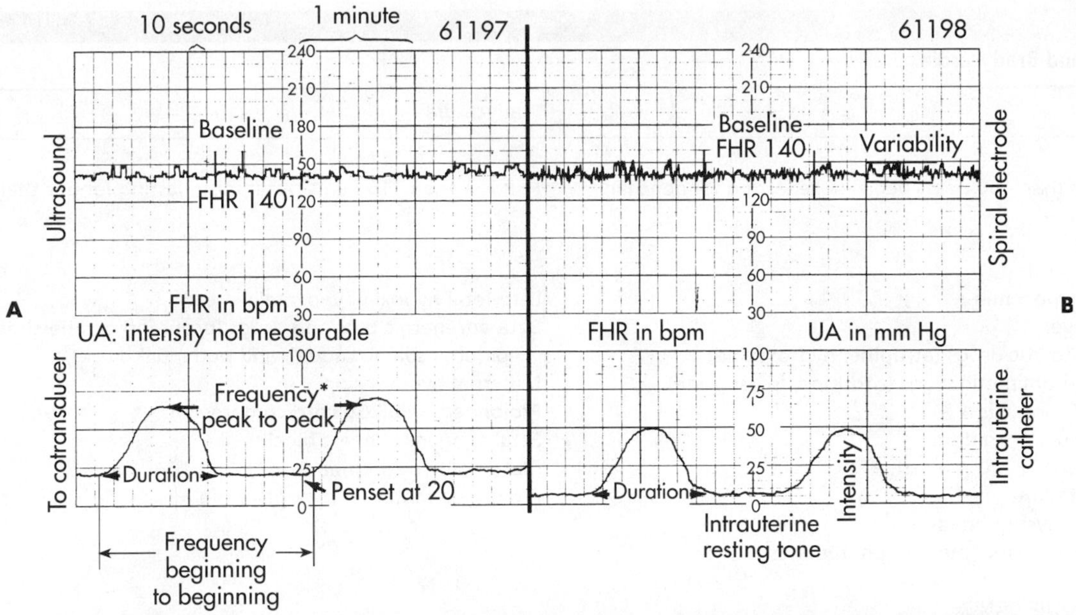

FIG. 17-4 • Display of FHR and uterine activity on monitor paper. **A,** External mode with ultrasound and tocotransducer as signal source. **B,** Internal mode with spiral electrode and intrauterine catheter as signal source. Frequency of contractions is measured from the beginning of one contraction to the beginning of the next. Peak-to-peak measurement is sometimes used when electronic uterine activity monitoring is done. (From Tucker S: *Pocket guide to fetal monitoring and assessment,* ed 4, St Louis, 2000, Mosby.)

and the presenting part low enough to allow placement of the electrode. A small spiral electrode attached to the presenting part shows a continuous FHR on the fetal monitor strip.

Internal monitoring of the FHR may be implemented without internal monitoring of uterine activity. To monitor uterine activity, a solid or fluid-filled IUPC is introduced into the uterine cavity. A solid catheter has a pressure-sensitive tip that measures changes in intrauterine pressure. A catheter filled with sterile water can also be used. As the catheter is compressed during a contraction, pressure is placed on the strain gauge or pressure transducer; this pressure is then converted into a pressure reading in millimeters of mercury. The average pressure range during a contraction is 50 to 85 mm Hg. The IUPC can measure the frequency, duration, and intensity of uterine contractions. The way in which the FHR and uterine activity are displayed on the monitor paper differs for the two modes of electronic monitoring (Fig. 17-4). Note that each small square represents 10 seconds; each larger box of six squares equals 1 minute (when paper is moving through the monitor at 3 cm/min).

FETAL HEART RATE PATTERNS

Baseline Fetal Heart Rate

The intrinsic rhythmicity of the fetal heart and the fetal autonomic nervous system control the FHR. An increase in sympathetic response results in acceleration of the FHR. An augmentation in parasympathetic response produces a slowing of the FHR. Usually, a balanced increase of sympathetic and parasympathetic response occurs during contractions, with no observable change in the FHR.

Baseline fetal heart rate is the average rate during a 10-minute segment that excludes periodic or episodic changes, periods of marked variability, and segments of the baseline that differ by more than 25 beats per minute (National Institute, 1997). The normal range at term is 110 to 160 beats per minute.

Tachycardia is a baseline FHR above 160 beats per minute. It can be considered an early sign of fetal hypoxia and can result from maternal or fetal infection, such as prolonged rupture of membranes with amnionitis; from maternal hyperthyroidism or fetal anemia; or in response to drugs such as atropine, hydroxyzine (Vistaril), terbutaline, or street drugs such as cocaine or methamphetamines.

Bradycardia is a baseline FHR below 110 beats per minute. (Bradycardia should be distinguished from prolonged deceleration patterns, which are periodic changes that are described later in this chapter.) Bradycardia can be considered a later sign of fetal hypoxia and is known to occur before fetal death. It can result from placental transfer of drugs such as anesthetics, prolonged compression of the umbilical cord, maternal hypothermia, and maternal hypotension. Maternal supine hypotensive syndrome, caused by uterine pressure (i.e., the weight of the gravid uterus) on the vena cava, decreases blood flow return to the maternal heart, which then reduces maternal cardiac output and blood pressure. These responses in the mother result in a decrease in the FHR and bradycardia. Table 17-2 contrasts tachycardia with bradycardia.

Variability of the FHR can be described as irregular fluctuations in the baseline FHR of 2 cycles per minute or greater (National Institute, 1997). Variability has been described as short-term (beat to beat) or long-term (rhythmic waves or cycles from baseline). The current definition for research does not distin-

TABLE 17-2
Tachycardia and Bradycardia

Tachycardia	Bradycardia
DEFINITION	
FHR greater than 160 beats per minute lasting longer than 10 min	FHR less than 110 beats per minute lasting longer than 10 min
CAUSE	
Early fetal hypoxemia Maternal fever Parasympatholytic drugs (atropine, hydroxyzine) Beta-sympathomimetic drugs (ritodrine, isoxsuprine) Intraamniotic infection Maternal hyperthyroidism Fetal anemia Fetal heart failure Fetal cardiac dysrhythmias Street drugs (cocaine, methamphetamines)	Late fetal hypoxia/hypoxemia Beta-adrenergic blocking drugs (propranolol; anesthetics for epidural, spinal, caudal, and pudendal blocks) Maternal hypotension Prolonged umbilical cord compression Fetal congenital heart block Maternal hypothermia Prolonged maternal hypoglycemia
CLINICAL SIGNIFICANCE	
Persistent tachycardia in absence of periodic changes does not appear serious in terms of neonatal outcome (especially true if tachycardia is associated with maternal fever); tachycardia is a nonreassurring sign when associated with late decelerations, severe variable decelerations, or absence of variability.	Bradycardia with moderate variability and absence of periodic changes is not a sign of fetal compromise if FHR remains greater than 80 beats per minute; bradycardia caused by hypoxia is a nonreassuring sign when associated with loss of variability and late decelerations.
NURSING INTERVENTION	
Dependent on cause; reduce maternal fever with antipyretics as ordered and cooling measures; oxygen at 8 to 10 L/min per face mask may be of some value; carry out health care provider's orders based on alleviating cause.	Dependent on cause; intervention not warranted in fetus with heart block diagnosed by ECG; oxygen at 8 to 10 L/min per face mask may be of some value; carry out health care provider's orders based on alleviating cause. Scalp stimulation may be performed to determine whether the fetus has the ability to compensate physiologically for stress (FHR will accelerate).

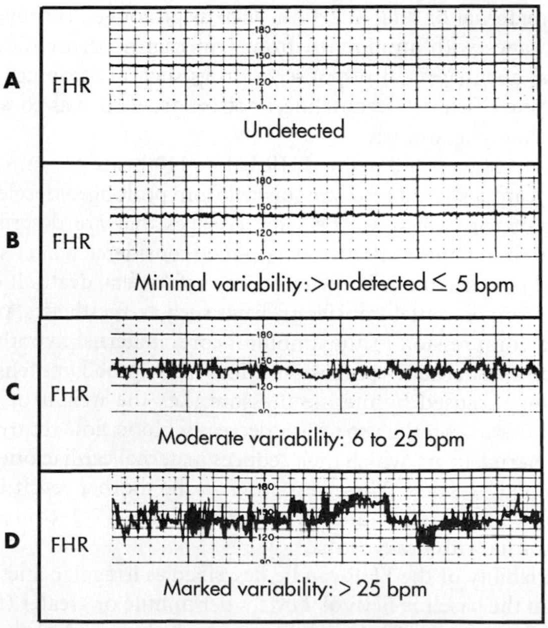

FIG. 17-5 • FHR variability. **A,** Undetected. **B,** Minimal. **C,** Moderate. **D,** Marked. (Modified from Tucker S: *Pocket guide to fetal monitoring and assessment,* ed 4, St Louis, 2000, Mosby.)

guish between short-term and long-term variability because in actual practice they are viewed together (National Institute, 1997). This definition does identify four ranges of variability as seen in Fig. 17-5. These are based on visualization of the amplitude in the peak-to-trough segment in beats per minute and include the following:

Absent or undetected variability
Minimal variability (greater than undetected but not more than 5 beats per minute)
Moderate variability (6 to 25 beats per minute)
Marked variability (greater than 25 beats per minute)

In clinical practice, short-term and long-term variability continue to be used to describe the FHR.

A sinusoidal pattern (i.e., a regular, smooth, wavelike pattern) is not included in the current research definition of FHR variability.

Absence of or undetected variability is considered nonreassuring. Decreased variability can result from fetal hypoxemia and acidosis, as well as from certain drugs that depress the central nervous system, including analgesics, narcotics (meperidine [Demerol]), barbiturates (secobarbital [Seconal] and pentobarbital [Nembutal]), tranquilizers (diazepam [Valium]), ataractics (promethazine [Phenergan]), and general anesthetics. In addition, a temporary decrease in variability can occur when the fetus is in a sleep state. These sleep states do not usually last

TABLE 17-3
Increased and Decreased Variability

Increased Variability	Decreased Variability
CAUSE	
Early mild hypoxemia Fetal stimulation by the following: Uterine palpation Uterine contractions Fetal activity Maternal activity Street drugs (e.g., cocaine and methamphetamines)	Hypoxia/acidosis CNS depressants Analgesics/narcotics Meperidine (Demerol) Alphaprodine (Nisentil) Morphine Pentazocine (Talwin) Barbiturates Secobarbital (Seconal) Pentobarbital (Nembutal) Amobarbital (Amytal) Tranquilizers Diazepam (Valium) Ataractics Promethazine (Phenergan) Propiomazine (Largon) Hydroxyzine (Vistaril) Promazine (Sparine) Parasympatholytics Atropine General anesthetics Prematurity—less than 24 wk Fetal sleep cycles Congenital abnormalities Fetal cardiac dysrhythmias
CLINICAL SIGNIFICANCE	
Significance of marked variability not known; increased variability from a previous average variability is earliest FHR sign of mild hypoxemia	Benign when associated with periodic fetal sleep states, which last 20 to 30 min; if caused by drugs, variability usually increases as drugs are excreted. Decreased variability considered nonreassuring if caused by hypoxia/asphyxia: occurring with late decelerations, decreased variability is associated with fetal acidosis and low Apgar scores
NURSING INTERVENTION	
Observe FHR tracing carefully for any nonreassuring patterns, including decreasing variability and late decelerations; if using external mode of monitoring, consider using internal mode (spiral electrode) for a more accurate tracing	Dependent on cause; intervention not warranted if associated with fetal sleep states or temporarily associated with CNS depressants; consider performing external stimulation of scalp stimulation during a vaginal examination to elicit an acceleration of FHR or return to average variability; consider application of internal mode (spiral electrode); assist health care provider with fetal blood sampling for pH if ordered; prepare for birth if so indicated by the primary health care provider

longer than 30 minutes. Table 17-3 contrasts key differences between increased and decreased variability.

Periodic and Episodic Changes in Fetal Heart Rate

Changes from baseline patterns in FHR are categorized as periodic or episodic. Periodic changes are those that occur with uterine contractions. Episodic (nonperiodic) changes are those that are not associated with uterine contractions. These patterns include accelerations and decelerations (National Institute, 1997).

Accelerations. Acceleration of the FHR is defined as a visually apparent abrupt increase in FHR above the baseline rate. The increase is 15 beats per minute or greater and lasts 15 seconds or more, with the return to baseline less than 2 minutes from the beginning of the acceleration. In preterm gestations, the definition of an acceleration is a peak of 10 beats per minute or more above baseline for at least 10 seconds. Acceleration of the FHR for more than 10 minutes is considered a baseline change.

Accelerations can be periodic or episodic. Accelerations that are periodic are caused by dominance of the sympathetic nervous response and are usually encountered with breech presentations (Fig. 17-6, *A*). Pressure of the contraction applied to the fetal buttocks results in accelerations, whereas pressure applied to the head results in decelerations. Accelerations may occur, however, during the second stage of labor in cephalic presentations.

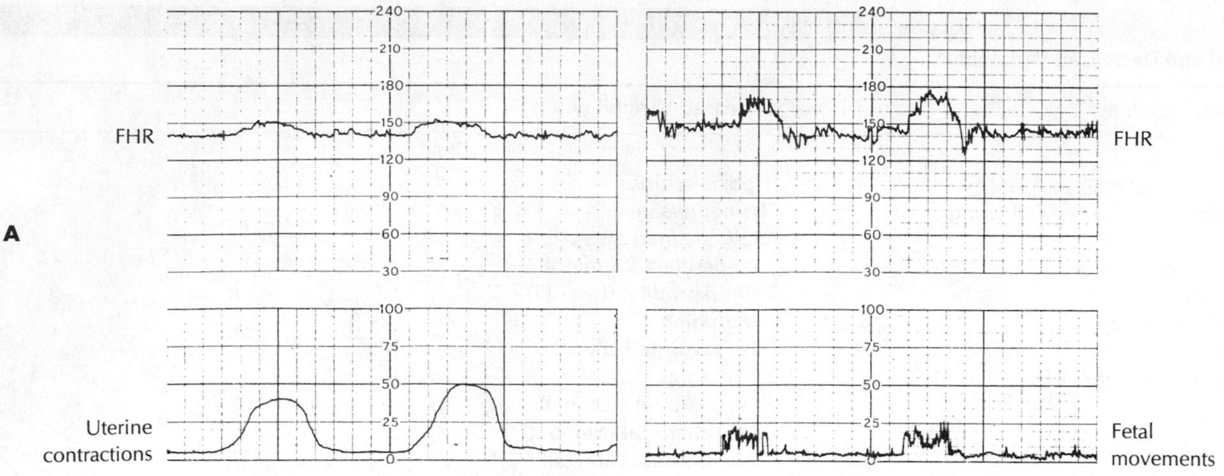

FIG. 17-6 • A, Acceleration of FHR with uterine contractions. **B,** Acceleration of FHR with fetal movement. (From Tucker S: *Pocket guide to fetal monitoring and assessment,* ed 4, St Louis, 2000, Mosby.)

Accelerations (Fig. 17-6, *B*) of the FHR that are episodic occur during fetal movement; these are indications of fetal well-being.

Decelerations. A deceleration (caused by dominance of parasympathetic response) may be benign or nonreassuring. The three types of decelerations that are encountered during labor are early, late, and variable. FHR decelerations are described by their relation to the onset and end of a contraction and by their shape.

Early deceleration of the FHR is a visually apparent gradual decrease in and return to baseline FHR in response to compression of the fetal head. It is a normal and usually benign finding (Fig. 17-7, *A*) (National Institute, 1997). This deceleration is characterized by a uniform shape and an early onset corresponding to the rise in intraamniotic pressure as the uterus contracts. When present, it usually occurs during the first stage of labor when the cervix is dilated 4 to 7 cm. Early decelerations sometimes are seen during the second stage when the woman is pushing. They may also occur in response to fetal head compression during uterine contractions, during vaginal examinations, as a result of fundal pressure, and during placement of the internal mode for fetal monitoring.

Because early decelerations are considered to be benign, interventions are not necessary. The value of identifying early decelerations is so that they can be distinguished from late or variable decelerations, which can be nonreassuring and for which interventions are appropriate. The different characteristics of acceleration of the FHR and early decelerations are contrasted in Table 17-4.

Uteroplacental insufficiency causes late deceleration. Late deceleration of the FHR is a visually apparent gradual decrease in and return to baseline FHR associated with uterine contractions (National Institute, 1997). The deceleration begins after the contraction has started, and the lowest point of the deceleration occurs after the peak of the contraction. Usually the deceleration does not return to baseline until after the contraction is over (see Fig. 17-7, *B*).

Persistent and repetitive late decelerations usually indicate the presence of fetal hypoxemia stemming from insufficient placental perfusion. They can be associated with fetal hypoxemia progressing to hypoxia and acidemia progressing to acidosis. They should be considered an ominous sign when they are uncorrectable, especially if they are associated with decreased variability and tachycardia. Late decelerations caused by maternal supine hypotensive syndrome are usually correctable when the woman turns on her side to displace the weight of the gravid uterus off the vena cava. Such lateral positioning allows better return of maternal blood flow to the heart, which in turn increases cardiac output and blood pressure.

Late decelerations caused by uteroplacental insufficiency can result from uterine hyperstimulation with oxytocin, pregnancy-induced hypertension, post date or postterm pregnancy, amnionitis, small-for-gestational-age (SGA) fetus, maternal diabetes, placenta previa, abruptio placentae, conduction anesthetics (producing maternal hypotension), maternal cardiac disease, and maternal anemia.

Variable deceleration is defined as a visual abrupt decrease in FHR below baseline. The decrease is usually more than 15 beats per minute, lasts at least 15 seconds, and usually returns to baseline in less than 2 minutes from the time of onset (National Institute, 1997). Variable decelerations occur any time during the uterine contracting phase and are caused by compression of the umbilical cord (see Table 17-5).

The pattern of variable deceleration patterns differs from that of early and late decelerations, which closely approximates the shape of the corresponding uterine contraction. Instead, variable decelerations often have a U or V shape, characterized by a rapid descent to and ascent from the nadir (or depth) of the deceleration (see Fig. 17-7, *C*). Some variable decelerations are preceded and followed by brief accelerations of the FHR; this "shouldering" is an appropriate compensatory response to compression of the umbilical cord.

Variable decelerations may be related to partial, brief compression of the cord. If encountered in the first stage of labor, they usually can be resolved by changing the mother's position, such as from one side to the other. Oxygen administration by face mask to the mother is sometimes helpful. Variable decelerations encountered during the second stage of labor are a result of umbilical cord compression during fetal descent. If repetitive variable decelerations occur during the second stage, it is important to discourage the woman from pushing with every contraction, so that the fetus has time to recover. Variable decelera-

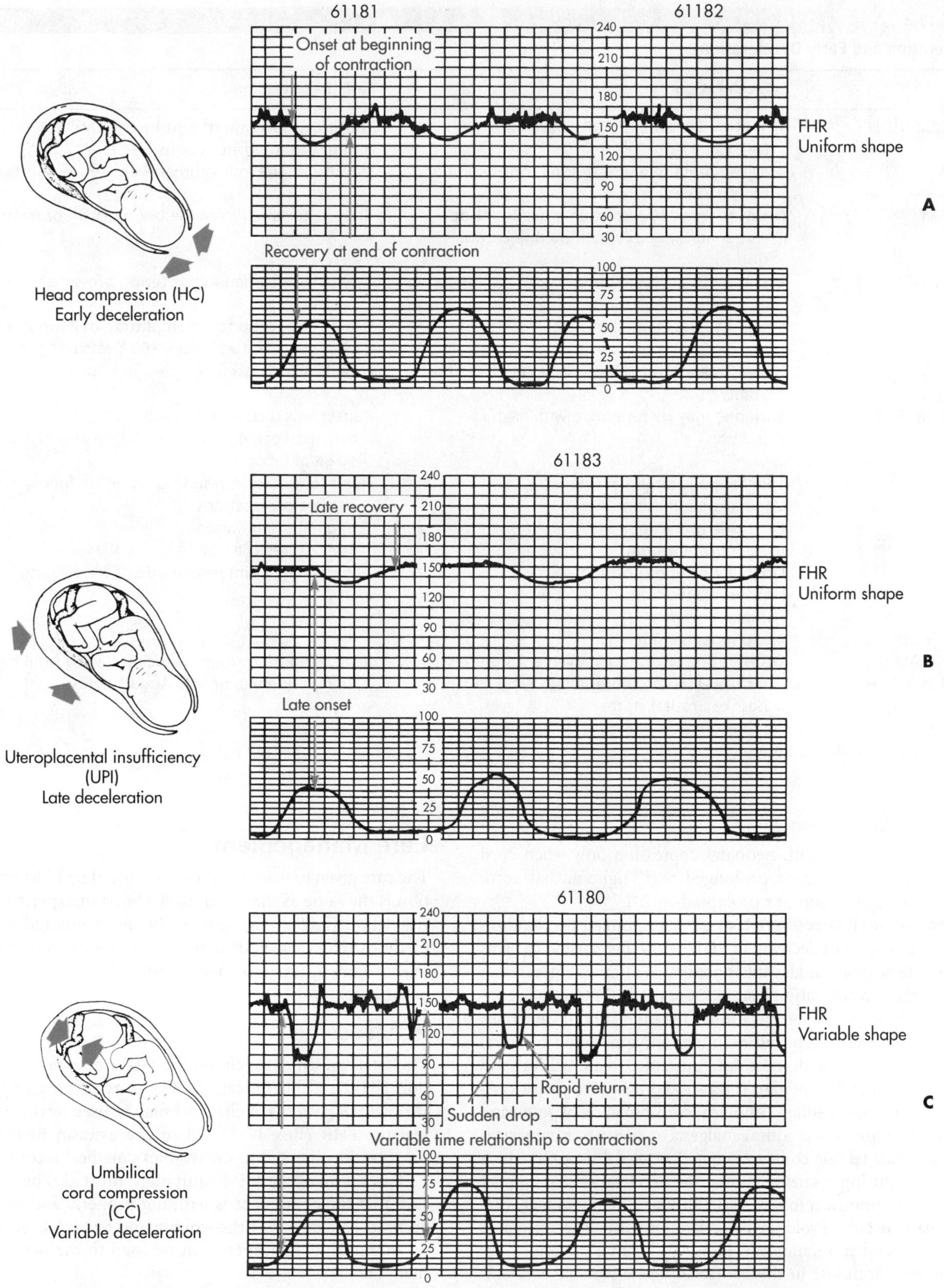

FIG. 17-7 • **A,** Early decelerations caused by head compression. **B,** Late decelerations caused by uteroplacental insufficiency. **C,** Variable decelerations caused by cord compression. (From Tucker S: *Pocket guide to fetal monitoring and assessment,* ed 4, St Louis, 2000, Mosby.)

TABLE 17-4
Acceleration and Early Deceleration

	Acceleration	Early Deceleration
DESCRIPTION	Transitory increase of FHR above baseline (see Fig. 17-6)	Transitory decrease of FHR below baseline concurrent with uterine contractions (see Fig. 17-7, *A*)
SHAPE	May resemble shape of uterine contraction or be spikelike	Uniform shape; mirror image of uterine contraction
ONSET	Onset to peak 30 sec; often precedes or occurs simultaneously with uterine contraction	Early in contraction phase before peak of contraction
RECOVERY	Less than 2 min from onset	By end of contraction as uterine pressure returns to its resting tone
AMPLITUDE	Usually 15 beats per minute above baseline	Usually proportional to amplitude of contraction; rarely decelerates below 100 beats per minute
BASELINE	Usually associated with average baseline variability	Usually associated with average baseline variability
OCCURRENCE	Variable; may be repetitive with each contraction	Repetitious (occurs with each contraction); usually occurs between 4 and 7 cm dilation and in second stage of labor
CAUSE	Spontaneous fetal movement Vaginal examination Electrode application Breech presentation Occiput posterior position Uterine contractions Fundal pressure Abdominal palpation	Head compression resulting from the following: Uterine contractions Vaginal examination Fundal pressure Placement of internal mode of monitoring
CLINICAL SIGNIFICANCE	Acceleration with fetal movement signifies fetal well-being representing fetal alertness or arousal states	Reassuring pattern not associated with fetal hypoxemia, acidemia, or low Apgar scores
NURSING INTERVENTION	None required	None required

tions are associated with neonatal depression only when cord compression is severe or prolonged (e.g., tight nuchal cord, short cord, knot in cord, or prolapsed cord).

Prolonged Decelerations. A prolonged deceleration is a visually apparent decrease in FHR below the baseline 15 beats per minute or more and lasting more than 2 minutes but less than 10 minutes. A deceleration lasting more than 10 minutes is considered a baseline change (National Institute, 1997). Generally, the benign causes are pelvic examination, application of spiral electrode, rapid fetal descent, and sustained maternal Valsalva maneuver. Other, less benign causes are progressive severe variable decelerations; sudden umbilical cord prolapse; hypotension produced by spinal or epidural analgesia or anesthesia; paracervical anesthesia; tetanic contraction; and maternal hypoxia, which may occur during a seizure. When the deceleration lasts longer than 1 to 2 minutes, a loss of variability with rebound tachycardia usually occurs. Prolonged decelerations usually are isolated events that end spontaneously. However, when a prolonged deceleration is seen late in the course of severe variable decelerations or during a prolonged series of late decelerations, the prolonged deceleration may occur just before fetal death.

NURSE ALERT • Nurses should notify the physician or nurse-midwife immediately and initiate appropriate treatment when they see a prolonged deceleration.

Care Management

The care given to women being monitored by EFM or auscultation is the same as that given to the woman experiencing a low risk labor. Care of the woman being monitored by internal methods may vary. FHR pattern recognition and intervention may require a nurse to have additional education and clinical experience.

➤ Assessment

The fetal assessment includes the fetal presentation, fetal position, FHR, and identification of both reassuring and nonreassuring FHR patterns. A checklist may be used by the nurse to assess the FHR (Box 17-2). All of the assessment information must be documented in the woman's medical record.

Evaluation of the EFM equipment must also be done to ensure that the equipment is working properly and to enable an accurate assessment of the woman and fetus. A checklist for fetal monitoring equipment can be used to evaluate the equipment (Box 17-3).

➤ Nursing Diagnoses

Nursing diagnoses for the woman who is being monitored electronically for fetal status are based on assessment findings. Possible diagnoses include the following:

- Decreased maternal cardiac output related to:
  —Supine hypotension secondary to maternal position

Box 17-2

Fetal Heart Rate Assessment Checklist

Client's name ____________________

Date/time ____________________

1. What is the baseline fetal heart rate (FHR)?

____ Beats per minute

Check one of the following as observed on the monitor strip:

____ Average baseline FHR (110 to 160 beats per minute)

____ Tachycardia (>160 beats per minute)

____ Bradycardia (<100 beats per minute)

2. What is the baseline variability?

____ Moderate variability (6 to 25 beats per minute)

____ Minimal variability (>5 beats per minute)

____ Absence of variability

____ Marked variability (>25 beats per minute)

3. Are there any periodic or episodic changes in FHR?

____ Accelerations with fetal movement

____ Repetitive accelerations with each contraction

____ Early decelerations (head compression)

____ Late decelerations (uteroplacental insufficiency)

____ Variable decelerations (cord compression)

____ Mild

____ Moderate

____ Severe

____ Prolonged deceleration

4. What does the uterine activity panel show?

____ Frequency (peak to peak or beginning to beginning)

____ Duration (beginning to end)

____ Intensity (in mm Hg only with intrauterine catheter)

____ Resting time at least 30 seconds

____ Resting tone (<15 mm Hg pressure)

COMMENTS ____________________

____

PANEL NUMBER ____________________

WHAT CAN BE OR SHOULD HAVE BEEN DONE

____

____

Modified from Tucker S: *Pocket guide to fetal monitoring and assessment,* ed 4, St Louis, 2000, Mosby.

Box 17-3

Checklist for Fetal Monitoring Equipment

PREPARATION OF MONITOR

1. Is the paper inserted correctly?
2. Are transducer cables plugged into the appropriate outlet of the monitor?

ULTRASOUND TRANSDUCER

1. Has ultrasound transmission gel been applied to the transducer?
2. Was the FHR tested and noted on the monitor paper?
3. Does a signal light flash or an audible beep occur with each heartbeat?
4. Is the belt secure and snug but comfortable for the laboring woman?

TOCOTRANSDUCER

1. Is the tocotransducer firmly positioned at the site of the least maternal tissue?
2. Has it been applied without gel or paste?
3. Was the pen-set knob adjusted between the 10 and 20 mm Hg marks and noted on the monitor paper?
4. Was this setting done between contractions?
5. Is the belt secure and snug but comfortable for the laboring woman?

SPIRAL ELECTRODE

1. Are the wires attached firmly to the leg plate?
2. Is the spiral electrode attached to the presenting part of the fetus?
3. Is the inner surface of the leg plate covered with electrode gel, if necessary?
4. Is the leg plate properly secured to the woman's thigh?

INTERNAL CATHETER/STRAIN GAUGE

1. Is the length line on the catheter visible at the introitus?
2. Is it noted on the monitor paper that a calibration was done?
3. Was the uterine activity tested?

Modified from Tucker S: *Pocket guide to fetal monitoring and assessment,* ed 4, St Louis, Mosby.

- Impaired fetal gas exchange related to:
  —Umbilical cord compression
  —Placental insufficiency
- Risk for fetal injury related to:
  —Unrecognized hypoxemia and hypoxia or anoxia
  —Infection secondary to internal monitoring or blood sampling
- Pain related to:
  —Use of belts to position transducers
  —Maternal position
  —Application of internal electrode or the obtaining of blood sample

➤ Expected Outcomes

The woman's and family's concerns and questions are considered in planning. Expected outcomes are set for the pregnant woman and family and the fetus and include the following:

- The pregnant woman and family will verbalize their understanding of the need for monitoring.
- The pregnant woman and family will recognize and avoid situations that compromise maternal and fetal circulation.
- The fetus will not suffer any hypoxemic, hypoxic, or anoxic episodes.
- Should fetal compromise occur, it will be identified promptly and appropriate nursing interventions such as intrauterine resuscitation will be initiated and the physician or nurse-midwife notified.

➤ Plan of Care and Implementation

It is the responsibility of the nurse providing care to the woman in labor to assess FHR patterns, perform independent nursing interventions, document observations and actions according to the established standard of care, and report nonreassuring patterns to the physician or certified nurse-midwife. Box 17-4 has a sample protocol for FHR monitoring.

Box 17-5 lists summary guidelines for the care of the woman being monitored electronically for fetal status during labor. (See also the Nursing Care Plan on p. 362.)

Box 17-4

Protocol for Fetal Heart Rate Monitoring

PATIENT/FAMILY TEACHING

Explain purpose of monitoring
Explain procedure
Provide rationale for maternal position other than supine

CARE

Assist woman to a comfortable position other than supine
Change maternal position at least every 2 hours
Change placement of external monitor belts every 2 hours when possible
Provide perineal care as needed when internal monitoring is implemented

MATERNAL/FETAL ASSESSMENTS

Obtain a 20-minute strip of EFM for all patients admitted to labor unit

Low Risk Patient

Auscultate or assess tracing every 30 minutes in active phase of first stage of labor
Auscultate or assess tracing every 15 minutes in second stage.

High Risk Patient

Auscultate or assess tracing every 15 minutes in active phase and every 5 minutes in second stage

Auscultation—All Patients

Count baseline FHR in between contractions
Assess FHR during the contraction and for at least 30 seconds after the contraction
Note increases or decreases of FHR
Assess FHR before ambulation
Interpret FHR data, nursing interventions, and patient responses
Notify primary health care provider

EFM—All Patients

Assess and interpret baseline FHR, variability of FHR (long term for external monitoring; long and short term for internal monitoring), and presence or absence of decelerations and accelerations

Assessments for All Patients

Assess uterine activity for frequency and duration, the intensity of contractions, and uterine resting tone
Assess FHR immediately after rupture of membranes, vaginal examinations, and any invasive procedure

REPORTABLE CONDITIONS

Presence of nonreassurring patterns
Worsening of any pattern
Presence of any fetal dysrhythmias
Difficulty in obtaining adequate FHR tracing or inadequate audible FHR

EMERGENCY MEASURES

Implement the following measures immediately in the event of the nonreassuring patterns:
- Reposition patient in lateral position to increase uteroplacental perfusion or relieve cord compression
- Administer oxygen at 8 to 10 L/min or per hospital protocol via face mask
- Discontinue oxytocin if infusing
- Correct maternal hypovolemia by increasing IV rate per protocol or as ordered
- Assess for bleeding or other cause of pattern change, such as maternal hypotension
- Notify primary health care provider
- Anticipate emergency preparation for surgical intervention if nonreassuring pattern continues despite interventions

DOCUMENTATION

Patient Record—Auscultation

FHR baseline, rate and rhythm, increases or decreases

Patient Record—EFM

Method of monitoring, change in method, and adjustments to equipment
FHR range, variability, presence of decelerations or accelerations
Uterine activity as determined by palpation or by external or internal monitoring
Interpretation of FHR data, nursing interventions, and patient responses
Notification of primary health care provider

Monitor Strip

Patient identification data
Assessments, procedures, and interventions (medications, etc.)
Notification of primary health care provider
Significant occurrences (sterile vaginal examination, rupture of membranes, etc.)
Adjustments of the monitor equipment

It is important to remember that although the use of EFM can be reassuring to many parents, it can be a source of anxiety to some. Therefore the nurse must be particularly sensitive to and respond appropriately to the emotional, information, and comfort needs of the woman in labor and those of her family (Fig. 17-8).

Electronic Fetal Monitoring Pattern Recognition. Nurses must evaluate many factors to determine whether an FHR pattern is reassuring or nonreassuring. A complete description of FHR tracings includes both qualitative and quantitative descriptions of baseline rate and variability, presence of accelerations, periodic or episodic decelerations, and changes in the FHR pattern over time (National Institute, 1997). Nurses evaluate these factors based on other obstetric complications, progress in labor, and analgesia or anesthesia. They must also consider the estimated time interval until birth. Interventions are therefore based on clinical judgment of a complex, integrated process.

NURSE ALERT • Fetal Monitoring Standards
Nurses who care for women during childbirth are legally responsible for correctly interpreting FHR

Box 17-5

Care of the Woman Using Electronic Fetal Monitoring

The following guidelines relate to patient teaching and the functioning of the monitor:

Explain that fetal status can be continuously assessed by EFM, even during contractions.

Explain that the lower tracing on the monitor strip paper shows uterine activity; the upper tracing shows the FHR.

Reassure woman and partner that prepared childbirth techniques can be implemented without difficulty.

Explain that, during external monitoring, effleurage can be performed on sides of abdomen or upper portion of thighs.

Explain that breathing patterns based on the time and intensity of contractions can be enhanced by the observation of uterine activity on the monitor strip paper, which shows the onset of contractions.

Note peak of contraction; knowing that contraction will not get stronger and is half over usually is helpful.

Note diminishing intensity.

Coordinate with appropriate breathing and relaxation techniques.

Reassure woman and partner that the use of internal monitoring does not restrict movement, although she is confined to bed.*

Explain that use of external monitoring usually requires the womans cooperation during positioning and movement.

Reassure woman and partner that use of monitoring does not imply fetal jeopardy.

Reassure her that the equipment is removed periodically to permit the applicator sites to be washed and other care to be given.

EXTERNAL MONITORING

Ultrasound Transducer

Function

Monitors FHR with high-frequency sound waves.

Nursing Care

Tap transducer before use to ensure sound transmission.

Apply ultrasound transmission gel to transducer, clean abdomen and transducer, and reapply gel q2hr and prn.

Massage reddened skin areas gently and reposition belt or adhesive device q2hr and prn.

Auscultate FHR with stethoscope or fetoscope if in doubt as to validity of tracing.

Position and reposition transducer prn to ensure receipt of clear, interpretable FHR data.

Tocotransducer

Function

Monitors uterine activity via a pressure-sensing device placed on the maternal abdomen.

Nursing Care

Position and reposition q2hr and prn on the fundus, where there is the least maternal tissue.

Keep abdominal strap snug but comfortable for the laboring woman.

Adjust pen-set between contractions to print between 10 and 20 mm Hg on the monitor strip paper.

Palpate fundus every 30 to 60 minutes to assess strength of contraction; only frequency and duration of contractions can be assessed with tocotransducer.

Do not determine woman's need for analgesia based on uterine activity displayed on monitor strip.

Gently massage reddened areas under transducer and belt qhr and prn.

INTERNAL MONITORING

Spiral Electrode

Obtains fetal ECG from presenting part and converts it into FHR.

Nursing Care

Ensure that wires are appropriately attached to leg plate.

Reapply electrode paste to leg plate if needed.

Observe FHR tracing on monitor strip for variability.

Turn electrode counterclockwise to remove; never pull straight cut from presenting part.

Administer perineal care after the woman voids during labor and prn.

Intrauterine Catheter

Function

Catheter (solid or fluid filled) that monitors intraamniotic pressure internally.

Nursing Care

Flush open system catheter with sterile water before insertion and prn.

Ensure that the length line on catheter is visible at introitus.

For closed system catheters, set baseline rate between uterine contractions when uterus is relaxed.

For open system catheters, turn stopcock off to woman, then with pressure valve of strain gauge released, flush strain gauge, remove syringe, and set stylus to 0 line of chart paper; test further according to manufacturer's instructions q3-4 hr and prn.

Check proper functioning by tapping catheter, asking woman to cough, or applying fundal pressure; observe appropriate inflection on strip chart.

Keep catheter taped to woman's leg to prevent dislodgment.

Modified from Tucker S, et al: *Patient care standards,* ed 7, St Louis, 2000, Mosby.

*Portable telemetry monitors allow the FHR and uterine contraction patterns to be observed on centrally located electronic display stations. These portable units permit ambulation during electronic monitoring.

patterns, initiating appropriate nursing interventions based on those patterns, and documenting the outcome of those interventions. Perinatal nurses are responsible for timely notification of the physician or nurse-midwife of nonreassuring FHR patterns. Perinatal nurses are also responsible for initiating the institutional chain of command should differences in opinion arise among health care providers concerning the interpretation of the FHR pattern and the intervention required.

Nursing Management of Nonreassuring Patterns. *Intrauterine resuscitation* is sometimes used to refer to those interventions initiated when a nonreassuring FHR pattern is noted. These interventions are directed primarily toward improving uterine and intervillous space blood flow and secondarily toward increasing maternal oxygenation and cardiac output (Fanaroff and Martin, 1997). These preventive interventions are described in the following sections: avoiding the supine position and encouraging maternal position changes; encouraging spontaneous short bursts of pushing in response to involuntary bearing-down urges; and encouraging pushing with the mouth and glottis open with vocalizing.

Previously it was thought that the left lateral maternal position preferentially promoted maternal cardiac output, thereby enhancing blood flow to the fetus. It is now known that either right or left lateral maternal position effectively enhances uteroplacental blood flow. The key issue is to avoid positioning the laboring woman on her back to reduce the risk of supine hypotension leading to decreased fetal perfusion.

Compression of the umbilical cord vessels results in variable decelerations. Amnioinfusion is an intervention that can help to relieve pressure on the nonprolapsed umbilical cord. If maternal hypotension is caused by acute hemorrhage (hypovolemia), the rapid infusion of blood volume expanders may be ordered.

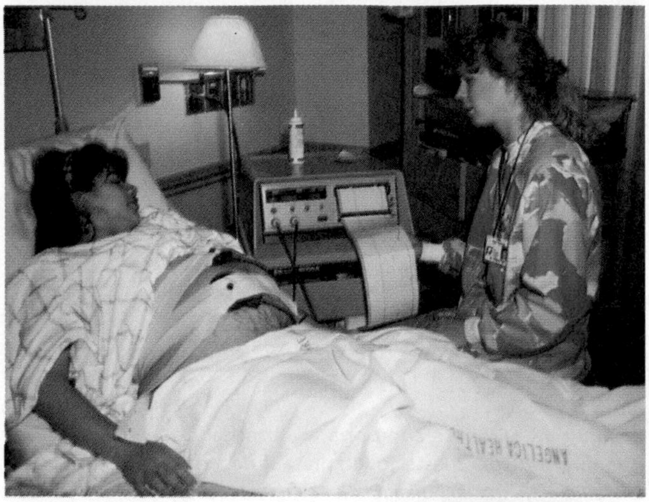

FIG. 17-8 • Nurse explains EFM as ultrasound transducer monitors the FHR. (Courtesy Marjorie Pyle, RNC, Lifecircle, Costa Mesa, CA.)

Critical Thinking

INTERPRETING FETAL HEART RATE (FHR) AND VARIABILITY

Review three sample or actual fetal monitor strips. Determine the baseline rate and variability of the FHR, periodic changes, if any, and the contraction interval, duration, intensity, as well as the resting tone. Discuss your findings in clinical conference. Describe appropriate nursing actions for the following periodic changes: accelerations, early decelerations, late decelerations, and variable decelerations.

Nursing Care Plan THE WOMAN BEING MONITORED ELECTRONICALLY DURING LABOR

NURSING DIAGNOSIS Maternal anxiety related to lack of knowledge about use of electronic monitor

EXPECTED OUTCOME The patient will exhibit increased understanding about fetal monitoring and signs of reduced anxiety (i.e., absence of physical indicators, absence of perceived threat, and absence of feelings of dread).

Nursing Interventions/*Rationales*

Explain and demonstrate to woman and labor support partner how the electronic monitor (internal or external) works in assessing FHR and in detecting and assessing quality of uterine contractions *to remove fear of unknown and ensure that woman can move with the monitor.*

When making adjustment to the monitor, explain to the couple what is being done and why *to increase understanding and allay anxiety.*

Explain that although a side-lying position or Fowler's position provides for optimum monitoring, position changes decrease discomfort; therefore encourage frequent changes in position (other than supine) and explain any monitoring adjustments that are being made as a result *to reduce discomfort and allay anxiety.*

NURSING DIAGNOSIS Risk for fetal injury related to inaccurate placement of transducers/electrodes, misinterpretation of results, or failure to use other assessment techniques to monitor fetal well-being

EXPECTED OUTCOME Fetal well-being is adequately assessed, and any fetal compromise is identified immediately.

Nursing Interventions/*Rationales*

Carefully follow guidelines and checklist for application and initiation of monitoring *to ensure proper placement of monitoring devices and production of accurate output from monitoring device.*

Check placement throughout monitoring process *to ensure that devices remain correctly placed.*

Regularly assess and record results of EFM (FHR and variability, decelerations, accelerations, uterine activity, contractions, uterine resting tone) *to provide consistent and timely evaluation of fetal well-being and progress of labor.*

Auscultate FHR and palpate contractions on a regular basis *to provide a cross-check on the EFM output and ensure fetal well-being.*

TABLE 17-5
Late Deceleration Vs. Variable Deceleration

	Late Deceleration	Variable Deceleration
DESCRIPTION	Transitory gradual decrease in FHR below baseline rate in contracting phase (see Fig. 17-7, *B*)	Abrupt decrease in FHR that is variable in duration, intensity, and timing related to onset of contractions (Fig. 17-7, *C*)
SHAPE	Uniform; mirror images of uterine contraction; may be deep or shallow	Variable; characterized by sudden drop in FHR in V, U, or W shape
ONSET	Late in contraction phase; after peak of contraction; nadir of deceleration occurs after peak of contraction	Onset of deceleration to the beginning of nadir <30 sec; decrease in FHR baseline is ≥15 beats per minute, lasting ≥15 sec; variable times in contracting phase; often preceded by transitory acceleration
RECOVERY	Well after end of contraction	Return to baseline is rapid and less than 2 min from onset, sometimes with transitory acceleration or acceleration immediately preceding and following deceleration (shouldering or "overshoot"); slow return to baseline with severe variable decelerations
DECELERATION	Usually proportional to amplitude of contraction; rarely decelerates below 100 beats per minute	*Mild:* decelerates to any level, less than 30 sec with abrupt return to baseline *Moderate:* decelerates no lower than 80 beats per minute, any duration with abrupt return to baseline *Severe:* decelerates below 60 beats per minute for longer than 60 sec, with slow return to baseline
BASELINE	Often associated with loss of variability and increasing baseline rate	Mild variables usually associated with average baseline variability; moderate and severe variables often associated with decreasing variability and increasing baseline rate
OCCURRENCE	Occurs with each contraction; may be observed at any time during labor	Variable; commonly observed late in labor with fetal descent and pushing
CAUSE	Uteroplacental insufficiency caused by the following: Uterine hyperactivity or hypertonicity Maternal supine hypotension Epidural or spinal anesthesia Placenta previa Abruptio placentae Hypertensive disorders Postmaturity Intrauterine growth restriction Diabetes mellitus Intraamniotic infection	Umbilical cord compression caused by the following: Maternal position with cord between fetus and maternal pelvis Cord around fetal neck, arm, leg, or other body part Short cord Knot in cord Prolapsed cord
CLINICAL SIGNIFICANCE	Nonreassuring worrisome pattern associated with fetal hypoxemia, acidemia, and low Apgar scores; considered ominous if persistent and uncorrected, especially when associated with fetal tachycardia and loss of variability	Variable decelerations occur in about 50% of all labors and usually are transient, correctable, and not associated with low Apgar scores; mild variable decelerations are reassuring; decelerations progressing from moderate to severe are associated with fetal acidemia, hypoxemia, and low Apgar scores; severe variable decelerations with average baseline variability just before birth are usually well tolerated
NURSING INTERVENTION	Change maternal position (lateral) Correct maternal hypotension by elevating legs Increase rate of maintenance IV; administer vasopressors Discontinue oxytocin if infusing Administer oxygen at 8 to 10 L/min with tight face mask Fetal scalp or acoustic stimulation Assist with birth (cesarean or vaginal assisted) if pattern cannot be corrected	Change maternal position (side to side); if decelerations are severe, proceed with following measures: Discontinue oxytocin if infusing Administer oxygen at 8 to 10 L/min with tight face mask Assist with vaginal or speculum examination If cord is prolapsed, examiner will elevate fetal presenting part with cord between gloved fingers until cesarean birth is accomplished Assist with amnioinfusion if ordered Assist with birth (vaginal assisted or cesarean) if pattern cannot be corrected

Until the infusion is established, the nurse can elevate the woman's legs. Blood pooled in the legs, especially with sympathetic blockade (e.g., epidural anesthesia), will then drain quickly into the central venous circulation and augment the effective intravascular volume (Fanaroff and Martin, 1997).

Oxytocin should always be infused as a piggyback connection near the indwelling needle (AWHONN, 1993a). If FHR patterns change for any reason, oxytocin stimulation of uterine muscle activity must be discontinued. This is accomplished by turning off the IV line from the piggyback (containing oxytocin) and opening the primary infusion line.

Some interventions are specific to the FHR pattern. (For nursing interventions appropriate for the management of tachycardia and bradycardia, see Table 17-2; for those appropriate for the management of increased or decreased variability, see Table 17-3.) No specific nursing interventions are required for the management of FHR acceleration or early deceleration (see Table 17-4); however, late and some types of variable FHR decelerations require aggressive intervention (Table 17-5). The physician or nurse-midwife decides whether medical intervention should be instituted, what intervention is indicated, or whether immediate vaginal or cesarean birth should be performed.

Other Methods of Assessment and Intervention

Assessment Techniques. Other methods of assessment are designed to be used in conjunction with EFM in an effort to identify and intervene on behalf of the fetus that is hypoxemic or acidotic. These methods include fetal blood sampling, FHR response to stimulation, and pulse oximetry monitoring of fetal oxygen saturation. Umbilical cord acid-base determination is an assessment technique that is a useful adjunct to the Apgar score in assessing the immediate condition of the newborn.

Fetal Scalp Blood Sampling. Sampling of the fetal scalp blood was designed to assess the fetal pH, Po_2, and Pco_2. The procedure is performed by obtaining a sample of fetal scalp blood through the dilated cervix after the membranes have ruptured. The scalp is swabbed with a disinfecting solution before making the puncture, and the sample is then collected. However, the blood gas values vary so rapidly with transient circulatory changes that fetal blood sampling is seldom performed. When used, it is usually in tertiary centers with the capability for repetitive sampling and rapid report of results. The circulatory changes that cause the variability and thus undermine the utility of this procedure are maternal acidosis or alkalosis, caput succedaneum, stage of labor, and timing of scalp sampling in relation to uterine contractions.

Fetal Heart Rate Response to Stimulation. Stimulation of the fetus, to elicit an acceleration of the FHR of 15 beats per minute for at least 15 seconds, is sometimes used as an alternative to fetal blood sampling (Tucker, 2000). The two methods of fetal stimulation currently in practice are scalp stimulation (using digital pressure during a vaginal examination) and vibroacoustic stimulation (using an artificial larynx or fetal acoustic stimulation device over the fetal head for 1 to 2 seconds). An FHR acceleration usually indicates fetal well-being. If the fetus does not have an acceleration, it does not necessarily indicate fetal compromise; however, further evaluation of fetal well-being is needed.

Fetal Pulse Oximetry. Continuous monitoring of fetal oxygen saturation by pulse oximetry is a method of fetal assessment currently in the clinical investigation stage (Luttkus and Dudenhausen, 1998). Fetal pulse oximetry works in a way similar to pulse oximetry used in children and adults. During a vaginal examination in a laboring woman with ruptured membranes, with the fetal head at a −2 station, a sensor is inserted next to the fetal cheek or temple area to assess oxygen saturation. The sensor is then connected to a monitor and the data displayed on the uterine activity panel of the fetal monitoring tracing. The normal range of oxygen saturation in the adult is 95% to 100%. The normal range for the healthy fetus is 30% to 70% (Lien and Garite, 1997), with the cutoff value for the critical threshold of $FSao_2$ (fetal oxygen saturation) at 30% (Carbonne et al, 1997).

The value of pulse oximetry is that in the event of nonreassuring FHR patterns, it could support the decision of whether labor should continue or intervention performed with an expeditious assisted vaginal or cesarean birth of the fetus. Multicenter randomized clinical trial testing in the United States and Europe is currently under way.

Umbilical Cord Acid-Base Determination. In assessing the immediate condition of the newborn after birth, a sample of cord blood is a useful adjunct to the Apgar score. The procedure is generally done by withdrawing blood from the umbilical artery and having the blood tested for pH, Pco_2, and Po_2. Metabolic acidosis can cause a low Apgar score.

Other Interventions. In addition to the emergency measures for nonreassuring FHR patterns, amnioinfusion and tocolysis may prevent fetal compromise.

Amnioinfusion. Amnioinfusion is a procedure used during labor to either supplement inadequate amounts of amniotic fluid or dilute meconium-stained amniotic fluid with saline or lactated Ringer's solution (Schmidt, 1997). The procedure to supplement amniotic fluid is indicated for patients with oligohydramnios (secondary to uteroplacental insufficiency, premature rupture of membranes, or postmaturity) who are at risk for variable decelerations because of umbilical cord compression.

Oligohydramnios is an abnormally small amount of amniotic fluid or the absence of amniotic fluid. Without the buffer of amniotic fluid, the umbilical cord can easily become compressed during contractions or fetal movement, diminishing the flow of blood between the fetus and placenta as evidenced by variable decelerations. Amnioinfusion replaces the "cushion" for the cord and relieves both the frequency and intensity of variable decelerations.

Amnioinfusion is also indicated in the presence of moderate to thick meconium to dilute and flush out the meconium with the intent of avoiding meconium aspiration syndrome in the neonate (Strong, 1995).

Risks associated with amnioinfusion are overdistention of the uterine cavity and increased muscle tone. Techniques of amnioinfusion treatment vary, but usually fluid is administered through an IUPC. The woman's membranes must be ruptured for the IUPC placement. The fluid is administered by attaching plastic (intravenous) tubing to a liter of normal saline or lactated Ringer's solution through a port in the IUPC. Double-lumen IUPCs are best because the intrauterine pressure can be monitored without stopping the procedure. The fluid is usually warmed with a blood warmer before administration, especially for the preterm or small-for-gestational-age fetus (American College of Obstetricians and Gynecologists, 1995).

Intensity and frequency of uterine contractions should be continually assessed during the procedure. The recorded uterine resting tone during amnioinfusion will appear higher than normal because of resistance to outflow and turbulence at the end of the catheter. The true resting tone can be checked by discontinuing the amnioinfusion (Afriat, 1996; Tucker, 2000).

Tocolytic Therapy. Tocolysis can be achieved through the administration of medications that inhibit uterine contractions. This therapy can be used as an adjunct to other interventions in the management of fetal compromise when the fetus is exhibiting nonreassuring patterns associated with increased uterine activity. Tocolysis improves blood flow through the placenta by inhibiting uterine contractions (Brown, 1998). Tocolysis may be considered by the primary health care provider and implemented when other interventions to reduce uterine activity, such as maternal position change and discontinuance of an oxytocin infusion, have no effect on diminishing the uterine contractions. A tocolytic medication such as magnesium sulfate or terbutaline can be administered intravenously to decrease uterine activity. If the FHR pattern improves, the woman may be allowed to continue labor; if there is no improvement, immediate surgical delivery may be needed.

Patient and Family Teaching. The nurse's role includes partnering with the woman to achieve a high-quality birthing experience. In addition to teaching and supporting the woman and her family in understanding of the laboring and birth process, breathing techniques, use of equipment, and pain management techniques, two factors can have an effect on fetal status: pushing and positioning. The nurse should provide information and support to the woman in regard to these two factors.

Discouraging the Valsalva Maneuver. The Valsalva maneuver can be described as the process of making a forceful bearing down attempt while holding one's breath with a closed glottis and tightening the abdominal muscles. This process stimulates the parasympathetic division of the autonomic nervous system producing a vagal response and results in the decrease of the maternal heart rate and blood pressure. Prolonged pushing in this manner can decrease placental blood flow, alter maternal and fetal oxygenation, decrease fetal pH and PO_2, increase fetal PCO_2, and increase the likelihood of fetal hypoxemia as reflected in FHR pattern changes.

Maternal Positioning. The nurse should solicit the woman's cooperation in avoiding the supine position. The woman should be encouraged to maintain a side-lying position or semi-Fowler's position with a lateral tilt to the uterus.

Documentation. Documentation is initiated and updated according to institutional protocol as monitoring progresses. In some institutions, observations noted and interventions implemented are recorded on the monitor strip to provide a comprehensive document that chronicles the course of labor and the care rendered. In other institutions, this documentation is confined to the labor flow record or computer chart. Advocates of documenting on both the medical record and the EFM strip cite as advantages of this approach the ease of writing directly on the strip while at the bedside and improved accuracy in documenting the critical events that occur and the interventions implemented. Others believe that charting on the EFM strip constitutes duplicate documentation of the same information noted in the medical record and thus is unnecessary additional paperwork for the nurse. Many of the aspects of care and events that can be documented on the monitor strip are listed in Box 17-6.

➤ Evaluation

Evaluation is a continuous process. The nurse can assume that care was effective when the outcomes for care have been achieved (see Nursing Care Plan on p. 362).

Box 17-6

Documentation: Monitor Strip

OBSERVATIONS
- Maternal vital signs
- Maternal position/repositioning
- Vaginal examinations and findings
- Medications (such as oxytocin); anesthesia/analgesia
- Voidings; emesis
- Pushing/bearing down
- Fetal movement
- Baseline FHR or periodic changes

ADJUSTMENTS
- Relocation of transducers
- Flushing or adjustment of catheter
- Replacement of electrode
- Replacement of catheter
- Time lapsed while changing monitor strip paper
- Reason for interruption/removal

INTERVENTIONS
- Position change
- Parenteral fluids
- Discontinuance of oxytocin
- Oxygen administration
- Amnioinfusion
- Fetal scalp stimulation
- Primary health care provider notification and response

Key Points

- Fetal well-being during labor is measured by the response of the FHR to uterine contractions.
- FHR characteristics include the baseline FHR and periodic changes in FHR.
- Monitoring of fetal well-being includes FHR assessment and watching for the presence of meconium-stained fluid.
- It is the responsibility of the nurse to assess FHR patterns, perform independent nursing interventions, and report nonreassuring patterns to the physician or nurse-midwife.
- The emotional, informational, and comfort needs of the woman and her family must be addressed when the mother and her fetus are being monitored.

References

Afriat C: Intrapartum fetal monitoring. In Simpson K, Creehan P, editors: *AWHONN's perinatal nursing,* Philadelphia, 1996, JB Lippincott.

American College of Obstetricians and Gynecologists: *Fetal heart rate patterns: monitoring, interpretation, and management (ACOG Tech Bull No. 207),* Washington, DC, 1995, ACOG.

Association of Women's Health, Obstetric, and Neonatal Nurses: *Cervical ripening and induction and augmentation of labor* (Practice Resource), Washington, DC, 1993a, AWHONN.

Association of Women's Health, Obstetric, and Neonatal Nurses: *Didactic content and clinical skills verification for professional nurse providers of basic, high risk, and critical-care intrapartum nursing,* Washington, DC, 1993b, AWHONN.

Brown C: Intrapartal tocolysis: an option for acute intrapartal fetal crisis, *J Obstet Gynecol Neonatal Nurs* 27(3):257-261, 1998.

Carbonne B et al: Multicenter study on the clinical value of fetal pulse oximetry: II. Compared predictive values of pulse oximetry and fetal blood analysis, *Am J Obstet Gynecol* 177: 593-598, 1997.

Fanaroff A, Martin R: *Neonatal-perinatal medicine: diseases of the fetus and infant,* ed 6, St Louis, 1997, Mosby.

Haggerty L: Continuous electronic fetal monitoring: contradictions between practice and research, *J Obstet Gynecol Neonatal Nurs* 28(4):409-416, 1999.

Lien J, Garite T: A better way of assessing fetal oxygenation? *Contemp Ob Gyn* 4:53-58, 62-65, 1997.

Luttkus A, Dudenhausen J: Fetal pulse oximetry, *Obstet Gynecol* 10(6):481-486, 1998.

National Institute of Child Health and Human Development Research Planning Workshop: Electronic fetal heart rate monitoring: research guidelines for interpretation, *Am J Obstet Gynecol* 177(6):1385-1390, 1997.

Schmidt J: Fluid check: making the case for intrapartum amnioinfusion, *AWHONN Lifelines* 1(5):46-51, 1997.

Strong T: Amnioinfusion, *J Reprod Med* 49(2):108-114, 1995.

Thacker S, Stroup D, Peterson H: Intrapartum electronic fetal monitoring data for clinical decisions, *Clinical Obstet Gynecol* 41(2):362-368, 1998.

Tucker S: *Pocket guide to fetal monitoring and assessment,* ed 4, St Louis, 2000, Mosby.

CHAPTER

18

Nursing Care During Labor and Birth

http://www.harcourthealth.com/MERLIN/Wong/maternal/

Learning Objectives

On completion of this chapter the reader will be able to:

- Review the factors included in the initial assessment of the woman in labor.
- Describe the ongoing assessment of maternal progress during the first, second, and third stages of labor.
- State the physical and psychosocial findings indicative of maternal progress during labor.
- Discuss fetal assessment during labor.
- Identify signs of developing complications during labor.
- Examine the influence of cultural and religious beliefs and practices on the process of labor and birth.
- Discuss the importance of support (family, doula) in labor.
- Describe the role and responsibilities of the nurse in an emergency childbirth situation.
- Identify the impact of perineal trauma on the woman.
- Discuss the nurse's role in reducing the incidence of routine episiotomy.

For most women, labor begins with the first uterine contraction, continues with hours of hard work during cervical dilation and birth, and ends as the woman and her family begin the attachment process with the infant. Nursing care focuses on supporting the woman and her family throughout the labor process with the goal of ensuring the best possible outcome for all involved.

FIRST STAGE OF LABOR

Care Management

The first stage of labor begins with the onset of regular uterine contractions and ends with complete effacement and full cervical dilation. Care begins when the woman reports one or more of the following:

- Onset of progressive, regular uterine contractions that increase in frequency, strength, and duration
- Blood-tinged vaginal discharge (bloody or pink show) indicating that the mucus plug has passed
- Fluid discharge from the vagina (spontaneous rupture of membranes)

The first stage of labor consists of three phases: the latent phase (up to 3 cm of dilation), the active phase (4 to 7 cm of dilation), and the transition phase (8 to 10 cm of dilation). Most nulliparous women seek admission to the hospital in the latent phase because they have not experienced labor before and are unsure of the "right" time to come in. Multiparous women usually do not come to the hospital until they are in the active phase. Even though no two labors are identical, women who have given birth before appear less anxious about the process, unless their previous experience has been negative.

Involving the woman as a partner in formulating the plan of care helps preserve the woman's sense of control, furthers participation in her own childbirth experience, and enhances her self-esteem and level of satisfaction (Proctor, 1998).

➤ Assessment

Assessment begins at the first contact with the woman, whether by telephone or in person. Many women call the hospital or birthing center to receive validation that it is all right for them to come in for evaluation or admission. The manner in which the nurse communicates with the woman during this initial contact can set the tone for a positive birth experience. A caring attitude encourages the patient to verbalize her questions and concerns. If possible, the nurse should have the woman's prenatal record in hand when speaking to her or admitting her for evaluation of labor. Copies of records are usually filed on the perinatal unit sometime during the third trimester.

Certain factors are assessed initially to determine if the woman is in true labor and should come to the hospital or be admitted (Varney, 1997) (Patient Teaching box). When a woman calls and there is a question about whether she is in labor (or in labor advanced enough to be admitted), the nurse should suggest that she call either her physician or certified nurse-midwife, or come to the hospital. This call may occur when the woman is in false labor or early in the latent phase of the first stage of labor. She may feel discouraged upon learning that the contractions that feel so strong and regular are not true contractions because they are not causing cervical dilation, or that they are still not strong or frequent enough for admission.

If the woman lives near the hospital, she may be asked to stay home or return home to allow labor to progress (i.e., until the contractions are more frequent and intense). The ideal setting for low risk women in early labor is the familiar environment of the home. The nurse can use a telephone interview (Box 18-1) to assess the woman's status, to give instructions regarding the optimum timing for admission, and to reinforce teaching of the signs that require immediate notification of the physician or nurse-midwife. Measures the woman and her significant others can use to enhance the progress of labor, reduce anxiety, and maintain comfort should be described.

A warm shower can be relaxing for the woman in early labor. Soothing back, foot, and hand massages, or a warm drink of preferred liquids such as tea or milk can help the woman to rest and even to sleep, especially if false or early labor is occurring at night. Diversional activities such as walking, reading, watching television, doing needlework, or talking with friends can reduce the perception of early discomfort, help the time pass, and reduce anxiety (Varney, 1997).

The woman who lives at a considerable distance from the hospital may be admitted in early labor. The same measures used by the woman at home should be offered to the hospitalized woman in early labor.

Patient Teaching

HOW TO DISTINGUISH TRUE LABOR FROM FALSE LABOR

True Labor

Contractions
- Occur regularly, becoming stronger, lasting longer, and occurring closer together.
- Become more intense with walking.
- Usually felt in lower back, radiating to lower portion of abdomen.
- Continue despite use of comfort measures.

Cervix (by vaginal examination)
- Shows progressive change (softening, effacement, and dilation signaled by the appearance of bloody show).
- Moves to an increasingly anterior position.

Fetus
- Presenting part usually becomes engaged in the pelvis. This results in increased ease of breathing; at the same time, the presenting part presses downward and compresses the bladder, resulting in urinary frequency.

False Labor

Contractions
- Occur irregularly or become regular only temporarily.
- Often stop with walking or position change.
- Can be felt in the back or abdomen above the navel.
- Often can be stopped through the use of comfort measures.

Cervix (by vaginal examination)
- May be soft but there is no significant change in effacement or dilation or evidence of bloody show.
- Is often in a posterior position.

Fetus
- Presenting part is usually not engaged in the pelvis.

Critical Thinking

TELEPHONE ADVICE FOR EARLY LABOR

A nulliparous woman calls the birthing center and anxiously tells the nurse, "I am in labor. My husband is going to bring me in right now to be admitted." Role play the approach the nurse should take in responding to this woman's report.

Box 18-1

Telephone Interview with Woman in Latent Phase of Labor

The perinatal nurse performs the following steps of the nursing process:

ASSESSMENT
- Gathers data regarding the woman's status, including signs and symptoms indicative of true or false labor.
- Discusses instructions given by the woman's primary health care provider regarding when to come for admission.

PLANNING AND IMPLEMENTATION
- Decides whether the woman will come for labor assessment and admission or be encouraged to stay at home until contractions increase in duration, frequency, and intensity.
- Assures the woman that she is welcome to call the perinatal unit at any time to discuss her labor status.
- Answers questions the woman and her family may have regarding labor or provides instruction as needed (e.g., which entrance of the hospital to enter).
- Suggests a variety of positions she can assume to maximally enhance uteroplacental and renal blood flow (e.g., side-lying position) and enhance the progress of labor (e.g., upright positions and ambulation).
- Suggests diversional activities, such as walking, reading, watching, television, talking to friends.
- Suggests measures to maintain comfort, such as a warm shower, back or foot massage.
- Discusses the oral intake of foods and fluids appropriate for early labor (light foods or fluids or clear liquids depending on the preference of her primary health care provider).
- Instructs the woman to come in immediately if membranes rupture, bleeding occurs, or fetal movements change.

EVALUATION
- Evaluates whether instructions and information have been understood by the woman by asking her to verbalize her understanding.

Admission to Labor Unit. When the woman arrives at the perinatal unit, assessment is the top priority (Fig. 18-1). The nurse first performs a screening assessment, using the techniques of interview and physical assessment, and reviews laboratory findings to determine the health status of the woman and her fetus and the progress of her labor. The physician or nurse-midwife is notified, and if the woman is admitted, a detailed systems assessment is done.

Admission Data. Admission forms such as the one in Fig. 18-2 can provide guidelines for the acquisition of important assessment information when a woman in labor is being evaluated or admitted. Additional sources of data include the following: (1) prenatal record, (2) initial interview, (3) physical examination to determine baseline physiologic parameters, (4) laboratory results, (5) expressed psychosocial and cultural factors, and (6) clinical evaluation of labor status.

Prenatal Data. The nurse should review the prenatal record to identify the woman's individual needs and risks. Incomplete information regarding the woman's prenatal health status could adversely affect the quality and safety of the care provided to her and her fetus/newborn during labor and birth and in the postpartum period.

If the woman has not had any prenatal care, certain baseline information must be obtained. If the woman is experiencing discomfort, the nurse asks questions between contractions when the woman can concentrate more fully on her responses.

It is important to know the woman's age so that the plan of care can be tailored to the needs of her age group. For example, a 14-year-old and a 40-year-old have different but specific needs, and their ages place them at risk for different problems. Height and weight relationships are important to identify the potential risk for cephalopelvic disproportion; a weight gain greater than that recommended may increase this risk. Other factors to consider are general health, any current medical conditions or allergies she may have, her respiratory status, and surgical procedures she has undergone.

Her past and present obstetric and pregnancy history are carefully noted. These include gravidity and parity and problems such as history of vaginal bleeding, pregnancy-induced hypertension (PIH), anemia, gestational diabetes, infections (e.g., bacterial or sexually transmitted), and immunodeficiencies.

If this is not the woman's first labor and birth experience, it is important to note the characteristics of her previous experiences. This information includes the duration of previous labors, the type of anesthesia used, the kind of birth (e.g., spontaneous vaginal, forceps- or vacuum-assisted, or cesarean birth), and condition of the baby.

It is important to confirm that the expected date of birth (EDB) is as accurate as possible. Other data in the prenatal record include patterns of maternal weight gain; physiologic measurements such as maternal vital signs (e.g., blood pressure, temperature, pulse, and respiration), fundal height, and baseline fetal heart rate (FHR); and laboratory test results. These tests include the woman's blood type and Rh factor, a complete or partial blood cell count (CBC or hemoglobin and hematocrit), the 50 g blood glucose test, determination of the rubella titer, serologic findings (Venereal Disease Research Laboratories [VDRL] or rapid plasma reagin [RPR]) for syphilis, surface antigen (HBsAG) for hepatitis B, culture for group B streptococci, and urinalysis. Additional tests may include tuberculosis screen with purified protein derivative (PPD), screening for human immunodeficiency virus (HIV), and screening for the sickle cell trait or other genetic disorders (e.g., maternal serum alpha-fetoprotein).

Questioning about physical abuse and substance abuse should form an integral part of the initial and ongoing assessment.

Interview. The woman's primary complaint or reason for coming to the hospital is determined in the interview. Her primary complaint may be that her bag of waters (BOW, or amniotic membranes) ruptured, with or without contractions. The woman may have come in for an obstetric check, which is a period of observation reserved for women who are unsure about the onset of labor. This allows time on the unit for diagnosis of labor without official admission, and minimizes or avoids cost to the patient when used by the hospital and approved by the woman's health insurance plan.

Even the experienced mother may have difficulty determining the onset of labor. The woman is asked to recall the events of the previous days and to describe the following:

- Time of onset of regular contractions
- Frequency and duration of uterine contractions
- Location and character of discomfort from the contractions (e.g., back pain or suprapubic discomfort)

Community Focus

ETHICAL ISSUES IN PERINATAL CARE IN COMMUNITY SETTINGS

Ethical issues for perinatal nurses are complex; both a mother and fetus are involved. There are at least six areas where ethical conflict may occur: "conflict between the mother and fetus, informed consent, confidentiality, cultural conflicts, conflicts associated with managed care, and conflicts in childbirth education." To resolve ethical issues, the principles of autonomy, beneficence, and justice are used. Perinatal nurses must become informed about ethical principles; they must be willing to advocate for their patients in all settings. Continued dialogue among nurses and other health care providers, attorneys, ethicists, and lay people must take place. There are no easy answers to complex ethical questions.

Data from Moore M: Ethical issues for nurses providing perinatal care in community settings, *J Perinat Neonat Nurs* 14(2):25-35, 2000.

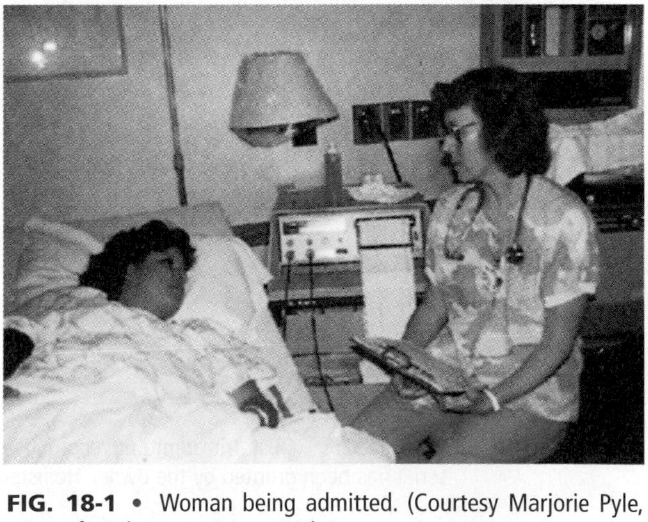

FIG. 18-1 • Woman being admitted. (Courtesy Marjorie Pyle, RNC, Lifecircle, Costa Mesa, CA.)

Obstetric Admitting Record Page 1 of 2

Basic Admission Data Date ___ / ___ / ___ Time ________
☐ Ambulatory ☐ Direct admit ☐ Stretcher
☐ Wheelchair ☐ Transfer from ________

G	T	Pt	A	L	LMP	EDD	Age
					/ /	/ /	
						EDD By fetal assessment / /	

Race/Ethnicity ________
Occupation ________ Education ________
Marital status S M Sep D W Religion ________

MD/CNM Tel no	Support person/Relationship Tel no

Reasons for Admission
☐ **Onset of labor**
☐ Induction of labor
☐ Spontaneous abortion
☐ Cesarean section
☐ Primary ☐ Repeat
(reason for primary ________)
☐ VBAC
☐ Tubal ligation
☐ Vaginal bleeding
☐ PROM
☐ Preterm labor
Detail reasons for admission ________

Observation evaluation
☐ Fetal status
☐ Ultrasound
☐ Amniocentesis
☐ NST
☐ CST
☐ Medical complications ________
☐ Obstetric complications ________

Patient Triage Data
Contractions ☐ **None** ☐ Palpation ☐ Tocotransducer
Frequency ________ Duration ________ Intensity ________
Began on ___ / ___ / ___ Time ________
Membranes ☐ **Intact** ☐ Bulging
☐ Ruptured (Date ___ / ___ / ___ Time ________)
Fluid ☐ Clear ☐ Bloody ☐ Foul smelling
☐ Meconium stained ☐ No foul odor
Vaginal bleeding ☐ **None** ☐ Normal show
☐ Bleeding (describe ________)

Cervical Exam
Station ________ Effacement ________ Dilatation ________ cms
Presentation
☐ Vertex ☐ Transverse lie
☐ Face/Brow ☐ Compound
☐ Breech (type ________) ☐ Unknown
Medication allergy/Sensitivity ☐ **None**
☐ Identify ________
Other allergy/Sensitivity ☐ **None**
☐ Identify ________

Patient Care Data

Personal Effects	Disposition		
Item	With patient	With support person	Other (describe)

Illness (≤ 14 days prior to admission) ☐ **None**
☐ Type/Treatment ________
Recent Exposure to Communicable Disease ☐ **None**
☐ Type/Date ________ ___ / ___ / ___
Last Oral Intake
Fluids ___ / ___ / ___ Time ________
Solids ___ / ___ / ___ Time ________
Medications ☐ **None**

Type/Dose	Last taken	With patient No	With patient Yes	Disposition
________	________	☐	☐	________

Alcohol/Drug use ☐ No ☐ Yes
Substances Amt/Day Last used
________ ________ ___ / ___ / ___ Time ________
________ ________ ___ / ___ / ___ Time ________

Plans for Birth and Hospital Stay
Support person present in L&D ☐ No ☐ Yes ________
Other family members in L&D ☐ No ☐ Yes ________
Anesthesia ☐ **None**
☐ Local ☐ Epidural ☐ Spinal ☐ General
Delivery site
☐ DR ☐ Birthing room ☐ LDR ☐ LDRP ☐ OR
Personal requests ________
Adoption ☐ No
☐ Yes Contact with infant ☐ No ☐ Yes
Adoption contact ________
Feeding preference ☐ Breast ☐ Bottle
Room preference ☐ Private ☐ Semi-Private
☐ Rooming-In
☐ Tubal ligation Authorization signed ☐ Yes ☐ No
☐ Circumcision Authorization signed ☐ Yes ☐ No

Psychosocial Data
Communication Deficit ☐ **None**
☐ Identify ________
Other children ☐ No ☐ Yes Age/Sex ________
________, ________, ________, ________

Partner involved ☐ Yes ☐ No

Admitting signature ________ Time ________

FIG. 18-2 • Obstetric admitting record. (Permission to use and/or reproduce this copyrighted material has been granted by the owner, Hollister, Inc., Libertyville, IL.)

Obstetric Admitting Record **Page 2 of 2**

Psychosocial Data (Cont'd.)

Basic needs met	Yes	No	If no, explain
Housing	☐	☐	
Clothing	☐	☐	
Food	☐	☐	
Transportation	☐	☐	

Free from apparent physical/emotional abuse ☐Yes ☐No
If no, explain____

Life Stress	No	Yes	If no, explain
Living	☐	☐	
Working	☐	☐	
Serious illness	☐	☐	

Self Care Needs ☐None ☐Needs help with____

Emotional status ☐Happy ☐Ambivalent
☐Anxious ☐Depressed ☐Angry

Discharge Planning Data

Discharge planning initiated ☐**Yes** ☐No
Discharge needs identified____

Social service referral ☐No ☐Yes __/__/__
Planned length of stay____days

Significant Prenatal Data

Prenatal Records Available on Admission
☐**Yes** ☐No
Source of prenatal data____
First prenatal visit__/__/__
Attended prenatal classes ☐**Yes** ☐No
Infant care provider:____

Lab Findings
☐**None**
Blood type & Rh____
Rubella titer____
Serology____
HbSAg____

Fetal Assessment Tests
☐**None**

Date	Test	Result
/		
/		
/		
/		

Maternal Problems Identified ☐**None**

	Active	Resolved
1.____	☐	☐
2.____	☐	☐
3.____	☐	☐

Fetal Problems Identified ☐**None**

	Active	Resolved
1.____	☐	☐
2.____	☐	☐
3.____	☐	☐

Physical Assessment

Detail all abnormal findings

Height	Wt pregrav/grav		
Temp	Pulse	Resp	BP

System	Normal	Abnormal
HEENT	☐	☐
Neurologic	☐	☐
Skin	☐	☐
Breasts	☐	☐
Extremities	☐	☐
Cardiovascular	☐	☐
Respiratory	☐	☐
Abdomen	☐	☐
Gastrointestinal	☐	☐
Urinary	☐	☐
Genitalia	☐	☐

Specimens obtained (check all that apply)

Urine test	Time	Results	Blood test	Time	Results
☐Urinalysis			☐Hgb		
☐C + S			☐Hct		
☐Glucose			☐VDRL/RPR		
☐Albumin			☐Type/Screen		
☐Ketones			☐		
☐pH			☐		
☐Blood			☐		

Fetal Evaluation Data

Fundal height____cms FHR____
Estimated fetal weight____
☐Fetoscope
☐Doppler
☐Fetal monitor
☐Other
Weeks gestation (est)
By dates____wks
By ultrasound____wks
Date__/__/__
Multiple gestation ☐**No** ☐Yes

Infant	Presentation	Position
1.		
2.		
3.		

Initial Problems Identified ☐**None**
1.____
2.____
3.____

Physician/CNM____
Notified by____
Date__/__/__Time____

____
Admitting signature

____
Examiner signature
Date__/__/__Time____

FIG. 18-2, cont'd • For legend see opposite page.

- Persistence of contractions despite changes in maternal position and activity (e.g., walking or lying down)
- Presence and character of vaginal discharge or show
- Status of amniotic membranes, such as gush or seepage of fluid (rupture of membranes, ROM). If there is a discharge that may be amniotic fluid, she is asked the date and time the fluid was first noted and the fluid's characteristics (e.g., amount, color, or unusual odor). In many instances a sterile speculum examination and a nitrazine (pH) or fern test can confirm that the membranes are ruptured (Box 18-2).

These descriptions help the nurse assess the degree of progress by determining the character of the contractions and the nature of the vaginal discharge. Bloody show is distinguished from bleeding in that it is pink in color and feels sticky because of its mucoid nature. It is scant to begin with and increases with effacement and dilation of the cervix. A woman may report a scant brownish discharge that may be attributed to cervical trauma as a result of vaginal examination or coitus within the last 48 hours.

In case general anesthesia is required in an emergency, it is important to assess the woman's respiratory status. The nurse determines this by asking the woman if she has a "cold" or related symptoms, "stuffy nose," sore throat, or cough. The status of allergies is rechecked, including allergies to medications routinely used in obstetrics such as meperidine (Demerol) or lidocaine (Xylocaine). Some allergic responses cause swelling of mucous membranes of the respiratory system, which could interfere with breathing and the administration of inhalation anesthetics.

Because vomiting and subsequent aspiration into the respiratory tract can complicate an otherwise normal labor, the nurse records the type and time of the woman's last solid food and liquid intake.

Any information not found in the prenatal record is obtained during the admission assessment. Pertinent data include the birth plan (Box 18-3), the choice of infant feeding method, anesthesia desired (if any), and the name of the pediatrician.

The nurse uses the birth plan information to plan individualized care for the woman's labor. The nurse prepares the

Box 18-2

Procedure: Tests for Rupture of Membranes

NITRAZINE TEST FOR pH

Explain procedure to woman/couple

Procedure

Wash hands

Use **nitrazine test** paper, a dye-impregnated test paper for determining pH. (Differentiates amniotic fluid, which is slightly alkaline, from urine and purulent material [pus], which are acidic)

Wearing a sterile glove lubricated with water, place a piece of test paper at the cervical os

OR

Use a sterile, cotton-tipped applicator to dip deep into vagina to pick up fluid; touch applicator to test paper. (Procedure may be done during speculum examination)

Read results:

Membranes probably intact: identifies vaginal and most body fluids that are acidic:

Yellow	pH 5.0
Olive-yellow	pH 5.5
Olive-green	pH 6.0

Membranes probably ruptured: identifies amniotic fluid that is alkaline:

Blue-green	pH 6.5
Blue-gray	pH 7.0
Deep blue	pH 7.5

Realize that false test results are possible because of presence of bloody show, insufficient amniotic fluid, or semen

Remove gloves and wash hands

Document Results

Positive or negative

TEST FOR FERNING OR FERN PATTERN

Explain procedure to woman/couple

Wash hands, apply sterile gloves, obtain specimen of fluid (usually during sterile speculum examination)

Spread a drop of fluid from vagina on a clean glass slide with a sterile, cotton-tipped applicator

Allow fluid to dry

Examine slide under microscope: observe for appearance of ferning (a frondlike crystalline pattern) (Do not confuse with cervical mucus test, when high levels of estrogen are responsible for causing the ferning.)

Observe for absence of ferning. (Alerts staff to possibility that amount of specimen was inadequate or that specimen was urine, vaginal discharge, or blood.)

Remove gloves and wash hands

Document Results

Positive or negative

Box 18-3

The Birth Plan

The birth plan should include the woman's/couple's preferences related to the following:

- Presence of birth companions such as the partner, older children, parents, friends, a doula, and the role each will play
- Presence of other persons such as students, male attendants, interpreters
- Clothing to be worn
- Environmental modifications such as lighting, music, privacy, focal point, items from home such as pillows
- Labor activities such as preferred positions for labor and for birth, ambulation, birth balls, showers and whirlpool baths, oral food and fluid intake
- Repertoire of comfort and relaxation measures
- Labor and birth medical interventions such as pharmacologic pain relief measures, intravenous therapy, electronic monitoring, induction or augmentation measures, episiotomy
- Care and handling of the newborn immediately after birth such as cutting of the cord, eye care, breastfeeding
- Cultural and religious requirements related to the care of the mother, newborn, and placenta.

The childbirth.org website (http://www.childbirth.org) provides couples with a interactive birth plan along with examples of birth plans.

woman for the possibility that changes may be needed in her plan as labor progresses, and assures her that information will be provided so that she can make informed decisions.

The nurse should discuss with the woman and her family their plans for preserving childbirth memories using photography and videotaping (Cesario, 1998). Health care agencies and insurance companies have voiced concerns that this type of recording of childbirth events could be used in court should the couple sue the health care agency or health care providers. The nurse can promote the appropriate use of cameras during the birth. Protection of privacy and safety are major concerns. Policies should be formulated to address issues such as the use of flash photography in the presence of combustible gases and where the person who is recording the birth can stand (Cesario, 1998). The fact that the birth was recorded should be entered in the patient's record.

Psychosocial Factors. The woman's general appearance and behavior (and that of her partner) provide valuable clues to the type of supportive care she will need. However, the nurse should keep in mind that general appearance and behavior may vary depending on the stage and phase of labor.

Women with a History of Sexual Abuse. Memories of sexual abuse can be triggered during labor by intrusive procedures such as vaginal examination; loss of control; being confined to bed and "restrained" by monitors, intravenous (IV) lines, and epidurals; being watched by students; and experiencing intense sensations in the uterus and genital area, especially at the time when the woman must push the baby out. Women who are survivors of abuse may fight the labor process by reacting in panic or anger toward care providers, may take control of every one and everything related to their childbirth, may surrender by being submissive and dependent, or may retreat by mentally dissociating themselves from the sensations of labor and birth (Rhodes and Hutchinson, 1994).

The nurse can help these women to associate the sensations they are experiencing with the process of childbirth and not their past abuse. The woman's sense of control should be maintained by explaining all procedures and why they are needed, validating her needs and paying close attention to her requests, proceeding at the woman's pace by waiting for her permission to touch her, accepting her reactions to labor, and protecting her privacy by limiting the exposure of her body and the number of persons involved in her care. It is recommended that all laboring women be cared for in this manner, because it is not unusual for a woman to choose not to reveal a history of sexual abuse (Heritage, 1998; Waymire, 1997).

Stress in Labor. Usually women in labor have a variety of concerns that they will voice if asked but rarely volunteer. To correct misinformation, it is important for the nurse to ask the woman what she expects or to suggest that the woman ask her primary health care provider about an issue. The following are common concerns that women in labor have: Will my baby be all right? Will I be able to stand labor? Will my labor be long? How will I act? Will I need medication? Will it work for me? Will my partner/someone be there to support me? Do I have to have an IV?

The nurse's responsibility to the woman in labor in relation to these concerns is to answer her questions or find out the answers, to provide support for her and her support persons and family, to take care of her in partnership with those persons the woman wants as her support team, and to serve as their advocate. The nurse communicates to the woman that she is not expected to act in any particular way and that the process will end in the birth of her baby, which is the only expectation she should have. Nursing support should reflect respect for and acceptance of a woman's individuality and behaviors. Nurses are perceived as supportive when they explain things in detail using positive terms and provide accurate information and specific directions. Women feel empowered when they are given information they can understand and that reflects support of their efforts. This feeling of empowerment contributes to a positive perception of the birth experience.

The father, coach, or significant other also experiences stress during labor. The nurse can assist and support these individuals by identifying their needs and expectations and by helping make sure these are met. The nurse can ascertain what role the support person intends to fulfill and whether he or she is prepared for that role by making observations and asking herself such questions as: Has the couple attended childbirth classes? What role does this person expect to play? Is he or she nervous, anxious, aggressive, or hostile? Does he or she look hungry, tired, worried, or confused? Does he or she watch television, sleep, or stay out of the room instead of paying attention to the woman? Does he or she touch the woman? What is the character of the touch? The nurse should be sensitive to needs of support persons and provide teaching and support as appropriate. Often the support this person is able to give the laboring woman is in direct proportion to the support he or she receives from nurses and other health care providers (Nichols, 1993).

Cultural Factors. It is important to note the woman's ethnic or cultural and religious background to anticipate nursing interventions that may need to be added or eliminated to individualize the plan of care (Fig. 18-3). The woman should be encouraged to request specific caregiving behaviors and practices that are important to her. If a special request contradicts usual practices in that setting, the woman or nurse can ask her primary health care provider to write an order to accommodate the special request. For example, in many cultures it is unacceptable to have a male caregiver examine a pregnant woman. In some cultures it is traditional to take the placenta home; in others the woman is given only certain nourishments during labor (Cultural Considerations box). Cultural beliefs and values can influence a woman's reliance on her primary health care provider during labor, as well as her desire to participate in making decisions about the care she receives (Callister, Vehvilainen-Julkunen, and Lauri, 1996).

When assessing a woman's cultural and religious preferences, Callister (1995) suggests that the nurse ask questions regarding the following:

- The value and meaning placed on the childbirth experience
- The view of childbirth as a wellness or illness experience, and as a private or social event
- Practices regarding diet, medications, activity, and emotional and physical support
- Appropriate maternal and paternal behaviors
- Birth companions—who they should be and what they should do
- Views regarding the newborn and newborn care immediately after birth

Within cultures, women may learn the "right" way to behave in labor and to react to the pain experienced in that way. These behaviors can range from total silence to moaning or screaming,

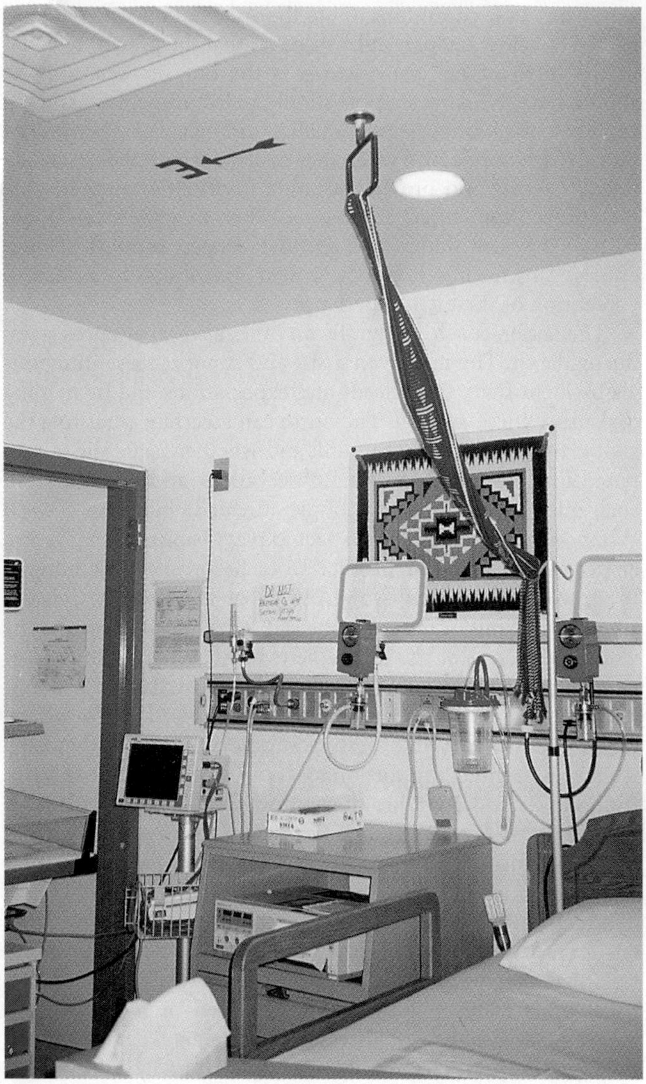

FIG. 18-3 • Birthing room specific to a Native American population. Note the arrow pointing east, the rug on the wall, and the cord hanging from the ceiling. (Chinle Comprehensive Health Care Center, Chinle, AZ; photo courtesy Patricia Hess, San Francisco, CA.)

but they are not in and of themselves a reflection of the degree of pain. A woman who moans with contractions may not be in as much physical pain as a woman who is silent but winces during contractions (Table 18-1). Some women feel it is shameful to scream or cry out in pain if a man is present (D'Avanzo, 1992). If the woman's support person is her mother, she may perceive the need to "behave" more strongly than if her support person is the father of the baby. She will perceive herself as failing or succeeding on the basis of her ability to adhere to these "standards" of behavior. Conversely, a woman's behavior in response to pain may influence the support received from significant others. In some cultures women who lose control and cry out in pain may be scolded, whereas in other cultures support persons will become more helpful (Choudhry, 1997; Weber, 1996).

The Non–English-Speaking Woman in Labor. A woman's level of anxiety in labor rises when she does not understand what is happening to her or what is being said (McKay and Smith, 1993). Some misunderstanding may occur with English-speaking women and cause some stress; but the effect of misunderstanding on non–English-speaking women is much more dramatic. These women often feel a complete loss of control over their situation if there is no health care provider present who speaks their language. They can panic and withdraw or become physically abusive when someone tries to do something they perceive might harm them or their babies. Sometimes a support person is able to serve as a translator. However, this must be done with caution because the translator may not be able to convey exactly what the nurse or others are saying or what the woman is saying, and this may raise the woman's stress level even more.

Ideally, a bilingual nurse will care for the woman. Alternatively, an employee or volunteer translator may be contacted for assistance. If no one in the hospital is able to translate, a translation service can be called so that a translation can take place over the telephone. For some women, a female translator may be more acceptable. If no translator is available, the labor and birth staff can prepare a set of cards with graphic depictions that illustrate common situations. These cards then can be used to communicate with non–English-speaking women. Even when the nurse has limited ability to communicate orally with the woman, in most instances the nurse's efforts to communicate are meaningful and appreciated by the woman.

Physical Examination. The initial physical examination includes a general systems assessment; performance of Leopold's maneuvers to determine fetal presentation, position, and point of maximum intensity (PMI) for auscultating the FHR; assessment of fetal status; assessment of uterine contractions; and vaginal examination to assess cervical effacement and dilation, fetal descent, and amniotic membranes and fluid. The most vital aspect of assessment is that of fetal status. Expected maternal progress and minimum assessment guidelines during the first stage of labor are presented in Tables 18-2 and 18-3. Standard Precautions should be used for all assessment and care measures (Box 18-4).

Cultural Considerations

BIRTH PRACTICES IN DIFFERENT CULTURES

South Korea
Stoic response to labor pain; fathers usually not present.

Japan
Natural childbirth methods practiced; may labor silently; may eat during labor; father may be present.

China
Stoic response to pain; fathers usually not present; side-lying position preferred for labor and birth, because this position is thought to reduce infant trauma.

India
Natural childbirth methods preferred; father is usually not present; female relatives usually present.

Iran
Father not present, prefers female support and female caregivers.

Mexico
May be stoic about discomfort until second stage, then may request pain relief; fathers and female relatives may be present.

Laos
May use squatting position for birth; fathers may or may not be present; prefer female attendants.

Modified from Geissler E: *Pocket guide to cultural assessment,* St Louis, 1999, Mosby.

TABLE 18-1

Sociocultural Basis of Pain Experience

Woman in Labor	Nurse
PERCEPTION OF MEANING	
Origin: Cultural concept of and personal experience with pain; for example: Pain in childbirth is inevitable, something to be endured. Pain in childbirth can be avoided completely. Pain in childbirth is punishment for sin. Pain in childbirth can be controlled.	Origin: Cultural concept of and personal experience with pain; in addition, nurse becomes accustomed to working with certain "expected" pain trajectories. For example, in obstetrics, pain is expected to increase as labor progresses, be intermittent, and have an end point; relief can be derived from medications once labor is well established and fetus or newborn can cope with amount and elimination of medications; relief can also come from woman's knowledge, attitude, and support from family or friends.
COPING MECHANISMS	
Woman may exhibit the following behaviors: Be traditionally vocal or nonvocal; crying out or groaning, or both, may be part of her ritual response to pain. Use counterstimulation to minimize pain (e.g., rubbing, applying heat, or applying counterpressure). Use relaxation, distraction, or autosuggestion as pain-countering techniques. Resist any use of "needles" as modes of administering pain relief agents.	Nurse may respond by Using self effectively (e.g., using tone of voice, closeness in space, and touch as media for conveying message of interest and caring). Using avoidance, belittling, or other distracting actions as protective device for self. Using pharmacologic resources at hand judiciously. Using comfort measures. Assuming accountability for control and management of pain.
EXPECTATIONS OF OTHERS	
Nurse may be seen as someone who will accept woman's statement of pain and act as her advocate. Medical personnel may be expected to relieve woman of all pain sensations. Nurse may be expected to be interested, gentle, kind, and accepting of behavior exhibited.	Only certain verbal or nonverbal responses to pain may be accepted as appropriate responses. Couple that is prepared for childbirth may be expected to refuse medication and to wish to "do everything on their own." Woman's definition of pain may not be accepted; that is, woman may wish to experience and participate in controlling pain or may not be able to accept any pain as reasonable.

TABLE 18-2

Expected Maternal Progress in First Stage of Labor

	Phases Marked by Cervical Dilation*		
Criterion	**0-3 cm (Latent)**	**4-7 cm (Active)**	**8-10 cm (Transition)**
Duration†	About 6-8 hr	About 3-6 hr	About 20-40 min
Contractions			
Strength	Mild to moderate	Moderate to strong	Strong to very strong
Rhythm	Irregular	More regular	Regular
Frequency	5-30 min apart	3-5 min apart	2-3 min apart
Duration	30-45 sec	40-70 sec	45-90 sec
Descent			
Station of presenting part	Nulliparous: 0 Multiparous: 0 to −2 cm	Varies: +1 to +2 cm Varies: +1 to +2 cm	Varies: +2 to +3 cm Varies: +2 to +3 cm
Show			
Color	Brownish discharge, mucus plug, or pale pink mucus	Pink to bloody mucus	Bloody mucus
Amount	Scant	Scant to moderate	Copious
Behavior and appearance‡	Excited; thoughts center on self, labor, and baby; may be talkative or silent, calm or tense; some apprehension; pain controlled fairly well; alert, follows directions readily; open to instructions	Becomes more serious, doubtful of control of pain, more apprehensive; desires companionship and encouragement; attention more inner directed; fatigue evidenced; malar (cheeks) flush; has some difficulty following directions	Pain described as severe; backache common; frustration, fear of loss of control, and irritability surface; vague in communications; writhing with contractions; nausea and vomiting, especially if hyperventilator; hyperesthesia; circumoral pallor, perspiration of forehead and upper lips; shaking tremor of thighs; feeling of need to defecate, pressure on anus

*In the nullipara, effacement is often complete before dilation begins; in the multipara, it occurs simultaneously with dilation. Average total duration: nullipara, 10 to 16 hr; multipara, 6 to 10 hr.

†Duration of each phase is influenced by such factors as parity, maternal position, and level of activity. For example, the labor of a nullipara tends to last longer, on average, than the labor of a multipara. Women who ambulate and assume upright positions or change positions frequently during labor tend to experience a shorter first stage.

‡Women who have epidural analgesia for pain relief may not demonstrate these behaviors.

TABLE 18-3

Minimum Assessment of the Low Risk Woman During the First Stage of Labor*

Variables	Cervical Dilation 0-3 cm (Latent)	4-7 cm (Active)	8-10 cm (Transition)
Blood pressure, pulse, respiration	q 30-60 min	q 30 min	q 15-30 min
Temperature†	q 4 hrs	q 4 hrs	q 4 hrs
Uterine activity	q 30-60 min	q 15-30 min	q 10-15 min
FHR	q 30-60 min	q 15-30 min	q 15-30 min
Vaginal show	q 30-60 min	q 30 min	q 15 min
Behavior, appearance, energy level	q 30 min	q 15 min	q 5 min

Vaginal examination‡ as necessary to identify progress of labor:

- To confirm change when symptoms indicate (e.g., increase in strength, duration, or frequency of contractions; increase in amount of bloody show; ROM; or woman feels pressure on her rectum)
- To determine whether dilation and descent are sufficient for administration of analgesic or anesthetic
- To reassess progress if labor takes longer than expected
- To determine station of presenting part

*Frequency of assessment is determined by the risk status of the maternal-fetal unit. More frequent assessment is required in high-risk situations. Frequency of assessment and method of documentation are also determined by agency policy, which is usually based on the recommended standards of medical and nursing organizations.
†If membranes have ruptured, check temperature every 2 hours; assess orally or tympanically between contractions.
‡In presence of vaginal bleeding, physician performs vaginal examination, usually under double setup, or ultrasonography.

Box 18-4

Standard Precautions During Childbirth

Birth is a time when nurses and other health care providers are exposed to a great deal of maternal and newborn blood and body fluids. Observation of Standard Precautions is necessary to prevent the transmission of infection. Perinatal infections most often are transmitted through contact with body fluids. The Standard Precautions applicable to childbirth include the following:

- Wash hands before and after putting on gloves and performing procedures.
- Wear gloves (clean or sterile, as appropriate) when performing procedures that require contact with the woman's genitalia and body fluids, including bloody show (e.g., during vaginal examination, amniotomy, hygienic care of the perineum, insertion of an internal scalp electrode and intrauterine pressure monitor, and catheterization).
- Wear cap, a mask that has a shield or protective eyewear, shoe covers, and cover gown during the birth. Gowns worn by the primary health care provider who is attending the birth should have a waterproof front and sleeves and should be sterile.
- Drape the woman with sterile towels and sheets as appropriate. Explain to the woman what can and cannot be touched.
- Help the woman's partner put on appropriate coverings for the birth, such as cap, mask, gown, and shoe covers. Show the partner where to stand and what can and cannot be touched.
- Wear gloves and gown when handling the newborn immediately after birth.
- Use an appropriate method to suction the newborn's airway, such as a bulb syringe, mechanical wall suction, or De Lee oral suction device that prevents the newborn's mucus from getting into the user's airway.

General Systems Assessment. A brief systems assessment is performed. This includes assessment of the heart, lungs, and skin; an examination to determine the presence and extent of edema of the legs, face, hands, or sacrum; and testing of deep tendon reflexes and clonus.

Vital signs (i.e., TPR and blood pressure) are assessed on admission, and initial values are used for comparison with subsequent values. If blood pressure is elevated, it should be reassessed 30 minutes later, between contractions, using a correct-size blood pressure cuff to obtain a reading after the woman has relaxed. To prevent supine hypotension and fetal distress, the woman should be encouraged to lie on her side and not supine (Fig. 18-4). Her temperature is monitored so that signs of infection or fluid deficit (e.g., dehydration associated with inadequate intake of fluids) can be identified. The woman's intake and output should be measured at least every 8 hours. Urinary protein and ketone levels should be determined using a dipstick each time the woman voids.

Leopold's Maneuvers (Abdominal Palpation). Leopold's maneuvers are performed with the woman briefly lying on her back (Box 18-5, Fig. 18-5). These maneuvers help identify the following: (1) number of fetuses; (2) the presenting part, fetal lie, and fetal attitude; (3) the degree of the presenting part's descent into the pelvis; and (4) the expected location of the PMI of the FHR on the woman's abdomen.

Assessment of FHR and Pattern. It is important for the nurse to understand the relationship between the location of the PMI of the FHR and fetal presentation, lie, and position. A high risk for childbirth complications may be revealed by variations in these findings. The PMI of the FHR is the location on the maternal abdomen where the FHR is heard the loudest. It is usually directly over the fetal back. The PMI is also an aid in determining the fetal presentation and position (Fig. 18-6). In a vertex presentation, the FHR is heard below the mother's umbilicus in either the right or the left lower quadrant of the abdomen. In a breech presentation, the FHR is heard above the

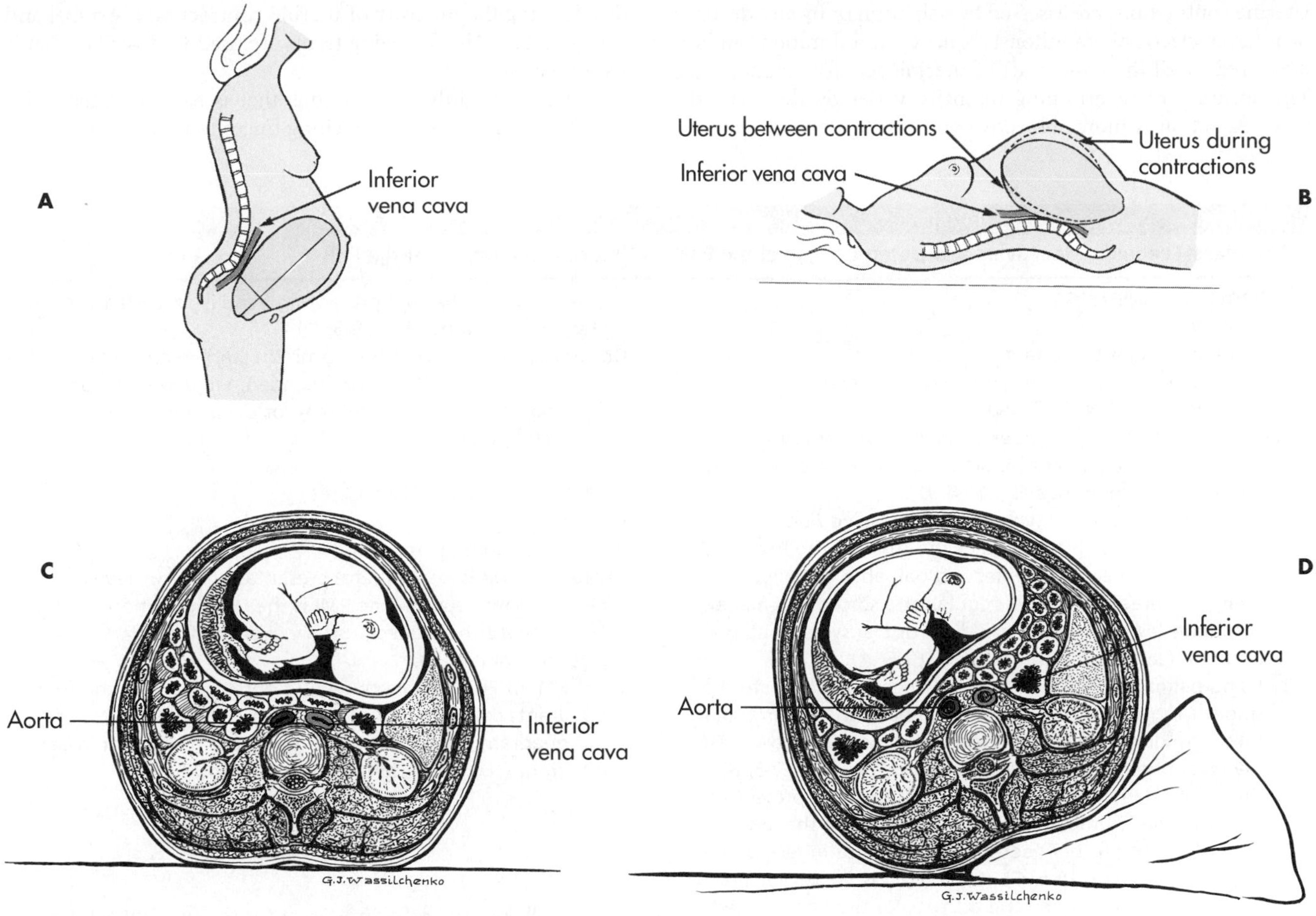

FIG. 18-4 • Supine hypotension. Note relationship of gravid uterus to ascending vena cava in standing posture (**A**) and in supine posture (**B**). **C,** Compression of aorta and inferior vena cava with woman in supine position. **D,** Relieved by use of a wedge pillow placed under woman's right side.

mother's umbilicus (Fig. 18-6, *A;* Fig. 18-7, *C*). As the fetus descends and rotates internally, the FHR is heard lower and closer to the midline of the maternal abdomen. The PMI of the fetus in the right occipitoanterior (ROA) position moves to the midline just over the symphysis pubis (Fig. 18-7, *A* and *B*). Just before birth the fetal position is occipitoanterior (OA) and the fetal back is directly above the symphysis pubis. Diagrams of the PMI for different presentations and positions are presented in Fig. 18-6. The assessment recommended for determining fetal status in the low risk woman during the second and third stages of labor is summarized in Table 18-4. The FHR must also be assessed (1) immediately after ROM because this is the most common time for the umbilical cord to prolapse; (2) after any change in the contraction pattern or maternal status; and (3) before and after medicating the woman or performing a procedure.

Assessment of Uterine Contractions. A general characteristic of effective labor is regular uterine activity; however, uterine activity is not directly related to labor progress. Uterine contractions are the primary powers that act involuntarily to expel the fetus and placenta from the uterus. Several methods are used to evaluate uterine contractions. These include the woman's subjective description, palpation and timing of the contraction by a health care provider, and electronic monitoring.

Each contraction exhibits a wavelike pattern. It begins with a slow increment (the "building up" of a contraction from its onset); gradually reaches an acme (the peak, with intrauterine pressure 50 to 75 mm Hg); and then diminishes rapidly (decrement, the "letting down" of the contraction). An interval of rest follows (intrauterine pressure is 5 to 15 mm Hg) that ends when the next contraction begins. The outward appearance of the woman's abdomen during and between contractions and the pattern of a typical uterine contraction are shown in Fig. 18-8.

The following characteristics are used to describe a uterine contraction:

- **Frequency**—How often uterine contractions occur; the time that elapses from the beginning of one contraction to the beginning of the next, or from the peak of one contraction to the peak of the next (if using electronic monitoring)
- **Intensity**—The strength of a contraction at its peak
- **Duration**—The time that elapses between the onset and the end of a contraction
- **Resting tone**—The tension in the uterine muscle between contractions

Uterine contractions are assessed by palpation or by an external or internal electronic monitor. Frequency and duration can be measured by all three methods of uterine activity monitoring. The accuracy of determining intensity varies by the method used. Palpation is more subjective and is a less precise way of determining the intensity of uterine contractions (Arrabal and Naegy, 1996). The following terms are used to describe what is felt on palpation:

- **Mild**—Slightly tense fundus that is easy to indent with fingertips (feels like touching finger to tip of nose)

Box 18-5

Procedure: Leopold's Maneuvers and Determination of the Points of Maximum Intensity of the FHR

LEOPOLD'S MANEUVERS

Wash hands.

Ask woman to empty bladder.

Position woman supine with one pillow under her head and with her knees slightly flexed.

Place small rolled towels under woman's right or left hip to displace uterus off major blood vessels (prevents supine hypotensive syndrome; see Fig. 18-4, *D*).

If right-handed, stand on woman's right, facing her:

1. Identify fetal part that occupies the fundus. The head feels round, firm, freely moveable, and palpable by ballottement; the breech feels less regular and softer. This maneuver identifies fetal lie (longitudinal or transverse) and presentation (cephalic or breech) (Fig. 18-5, *A*).
2. Using palmar surface of one hand, locate and palpate the smooth convex contour of the fetal back and the irregularities that identify the small parts (feet, hands, elbows). This maneuver helps identify fetal presentation (Fig. 18-5, *B*).
3. With right hand, determine which fetal part is presenting over the inlet to the true pelvis. Gently grasp the lower pole of the uterus between the thumb and fingers, pressing in slightly (Fig. 18-5, *C*). If the head is presenting and not engaged, determine the attitude of the head (flexed or extended).
4. Turn to face the woman's feet. Using both hands, outline the fetal head (Fig. 18-5, *D*) with the palmar surface of the fingertips. When the presenting part has descended deeply, only a small portion of it may be outlined. Palpation of the cephalic prominence helps identify the attitude of the head. If the cephalic prominence is bound on the same side as the small parts, this means that the head must be flexed and the vertex is presenting (Fig. 18-5, *D*). If the cephalic prominence is on the same side as the back, this indicates that the presenting head is extended and the face is presenting (Fig. 18-5, *D*).

Document fetal presentation, position, and lie and whether presenting part is flexed or extended, engaged, or free floating. Use hospital's protocol for documentation (e.g., "Vtx, LOA, floating").

DETERMINATION OF PMI OF FHR

Wash hands.

Perform Leopold's maneuvers.

Auscultate FHR based on fetal presentation identified with Leopold's maneuvers. The PMI is the location where the FHR is heard the loudest, usually over the fetal back (see Figs. 18-6 and 18-7).

Chart PMI of FHR using a two-line figure to indicate the four quadrants of the maternal abdomen, as follows: right upper quadrant (RUQ), left upper quadrant (LUQ), left lower quadrant (LLQ), and right lower quadrant (RLQ):

RUQ	LUQ
RLQ	LLQ

The umbilicus is the reference point for the quadrants (point where the lines cross). The PMI for the fetus in vertex presentation, in general flexion with the back on the mother's right side, commonly is found in the mother's right lower quadrant and is recorded with an "X" or with the FHR, as follows:

X	

or

140	

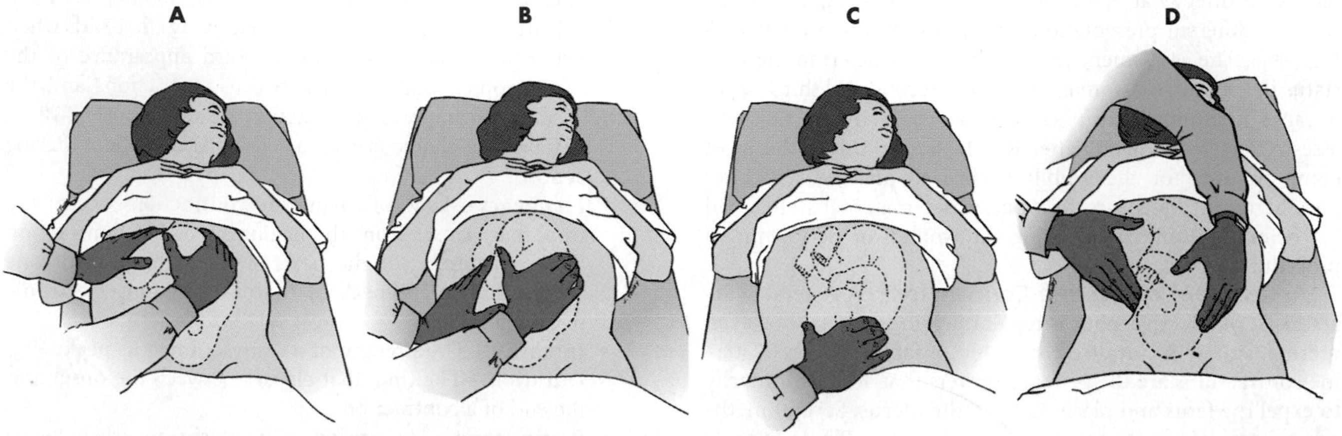

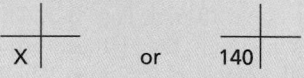

FIG. 18-5 • Leopold's maneuvers.

- **Moderate**—Firm fundus that is difficult to indent with fingertips (feels like touching finger to chin)
- **Strong**—Rigid, boardlike fundus that is almost impossible to indent with fingertips (feels like touching finger to forehead)

Women in labor tend to describe the pain of contractions in terms of their sensations in the lower abdomen or in the back, which may be unrelated to the firmness of the uterine fundus. Thus their assessment of the strength of their contractions can be less valid than that of an experienced health care provider, although the amount of discomfort reported is valid.

External electronic monitoring provides information about the relative strength of the uterine contractions. Internal electronic monitoring using an intrauterine pressure catheter is the most reliable way of assessing the intensity of uterine contractions.

On admission, a 20- to 30-minute baseline monitoring of uterine contractions and the FHR usually is done (Scott et al, 1999). (For the findings expected as labor progresses, see Tables 18-2, 18-3, and 18-4.)

The nurse's responsibility in monitoring uterine contractions is to ascertain whether they are powerful and frequent enough to accomplish the work of expelling the fetus and the placenta.

NURSE ALERT • If the characteristics of contractions are found to be abnormal, either exceeding or falling below what is considered acceptable in terms of the standard characteristics, the nurse should report this to the primary health care provider.

Vaginal Examination. The vaginal examination reveals whether the woman is in true labor, and enables the examiner to determine whether the membranes have ruptured (Fig. 18-9). Because this examination is often stressful and uncomfortable for the woman, it should be performed only when indicated by the status of the woman and her fetus. For example, a vaginal examination should be performed on admission, when significant change has occurred in uterine activity, on maternal perception of perineal pressure or the urge to bear down, when membranes rupture, or when variable decelerations of the FHR are noted. A full explanation of the examination and support of the woman are important factors in reducing the stress and discomfort associated with the examination.

Cervical Effacement, Dilation, and Fetal Descent. Uterine activity must be considered in the context of its effect on cervical effacement and dilation and on the degree of descent of the presenting part. The effect on the fetus must also be considered. Progress of labor can be effectively verified by the use

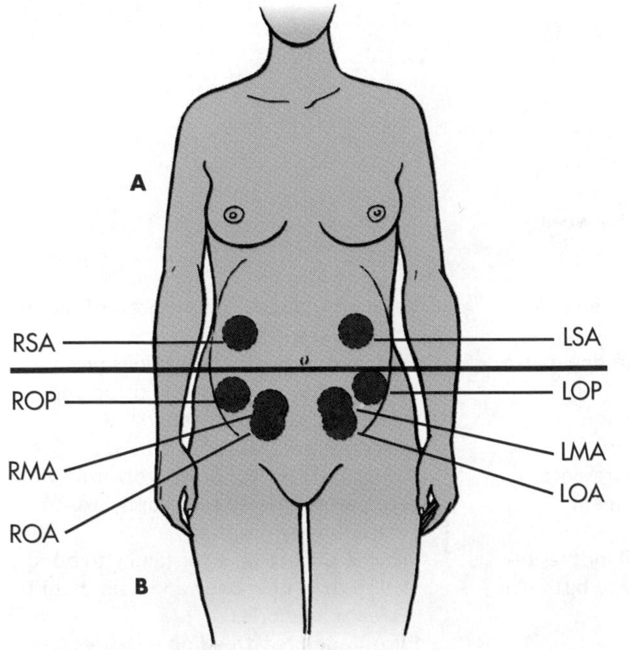

FIG. 18-6 • Areas of maximum intensity of FHR for differing positions: *RSA,* right sacrum anterior; *ROP,* right occipitoposterior; *RMA,* right mentum anterior; *ROA,* right occipitoanterior; *LSA,* left sacrum anterior; *LOP,* left occipitoposterior; *LMA,* left mentum anterior; and *LOA,* left occipitoanterior. **A,** Presentation is *breech* if FHR is heard *above* umbilicus. **B,** Presentation is *vertex* if FHR is heard *below* umbilicus.

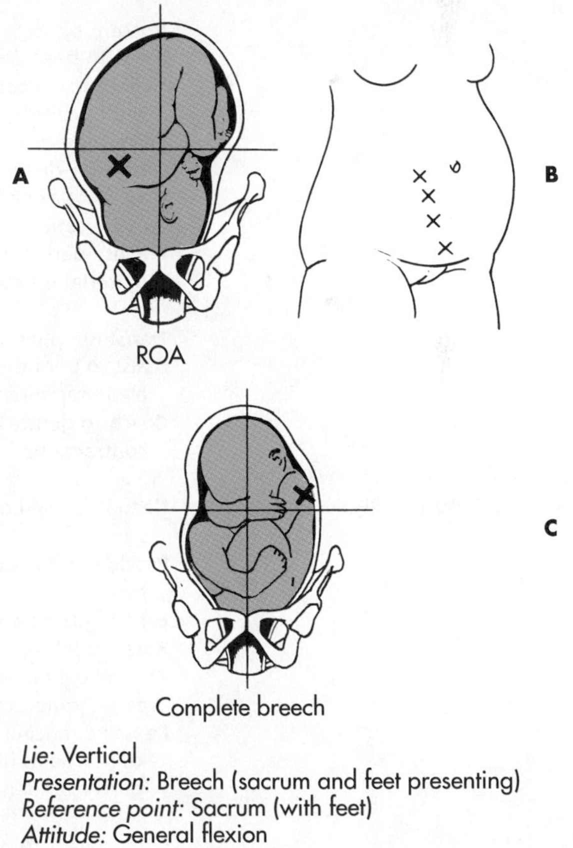

FIG. 18-7 • Location of the FHR. **A,** With fetus in ROA position. **B,** Changes in location of PMI of FHR as fetus undergoes internal rotation from ROA to OA for birth. **C,** With fetus in left sacrum posterior position. (A and C, courtesy Ross Laboratories, Columbus, OH.)

TABLE 18-4

Low Risk Woman in Second and Third Stages of Labor

Care Management	Second Stage of Labor	Third Stage of Labor
I. ASSESSMENT MEASURES*	**FREQUENCY**	**FREQUENCY**
• Blood pressure, pulse, respirations	Every 5-30 min	Every 15 min
• Uterine activity	Assess every contraction	Assess for placental separation
• Bearing-down effort	Assess each effort	
• Fetal heart rate (FHR)	Every 5-15 min	Perform Apgar at 1 and 5 min
• Vaginal show	Every 15 min	Assess bleeding until placental expulsion
• Signs of fetal descent: urge to bear down, perineal bulging, crowning	Every 10-15 min	
• Behavior, appearance, mood, energy level of woman; condition of partner	Every 10-15 min	Assess response to completion of childbirth process, reaction to newborn
II. PHYSICAL CARE MEASURES†	**Latent phase:** Assist to rest in position of comfort Encourage relaxation to conserve energy Promote urge to push; if delayed: ambulation, shower, pelvic rock, position changes **Descent phase:** Assist to bear down effectively Help to use recommended positions that facilitate descent Encourage correct breathing during bearing-down efforts Help to relax between contractions Provide comfort measures as needed Cleanse perineum immediately if fecal material is expelled **Transition phase:** Assist to pant during contraction to avoid rapid birth of head Coach to gently bear down between contractions	Assist to bear down to facilitate delivery of separated placenta Administer oxytocic as ordered Provide pain relief as needed Provide hygiene and comfort measures as needed
III. EMOTIONAL SUPPORT	Keep informed of progress of fetal descent Provide feedback for bearing-down efforts Explain purpose if medications given Role model comfort measures Provide continuous nursing presence Create a quiet, calm environment Reassure, encourage, praise Take charge as needed, until mother regains confidence in ability to birth her baby Offer mirror to watch birth	Keep informed about progress of placental separation Explain purpose if medications given Describe status of perineal tissue and inform if repair is needed Introduce parents to their baby Assess and care for newborn within view of parents; delay eye prophylaxis to facilitate eye contact Provide private time for family to bond with their new baby and help them to create memories Encourage breastfeeding if desired

*Frequency of assessment is determined by the risk status of the maternal-fetal unit. More frequent assessment is required in high risk situations. Frequency of assessment and method of documentation are also determined by agency policy, which is usually based on the recommended care standards of medical and nursing organizations.

†Physical care measures are performed by the nurse working together with the woman's partner and significant others.

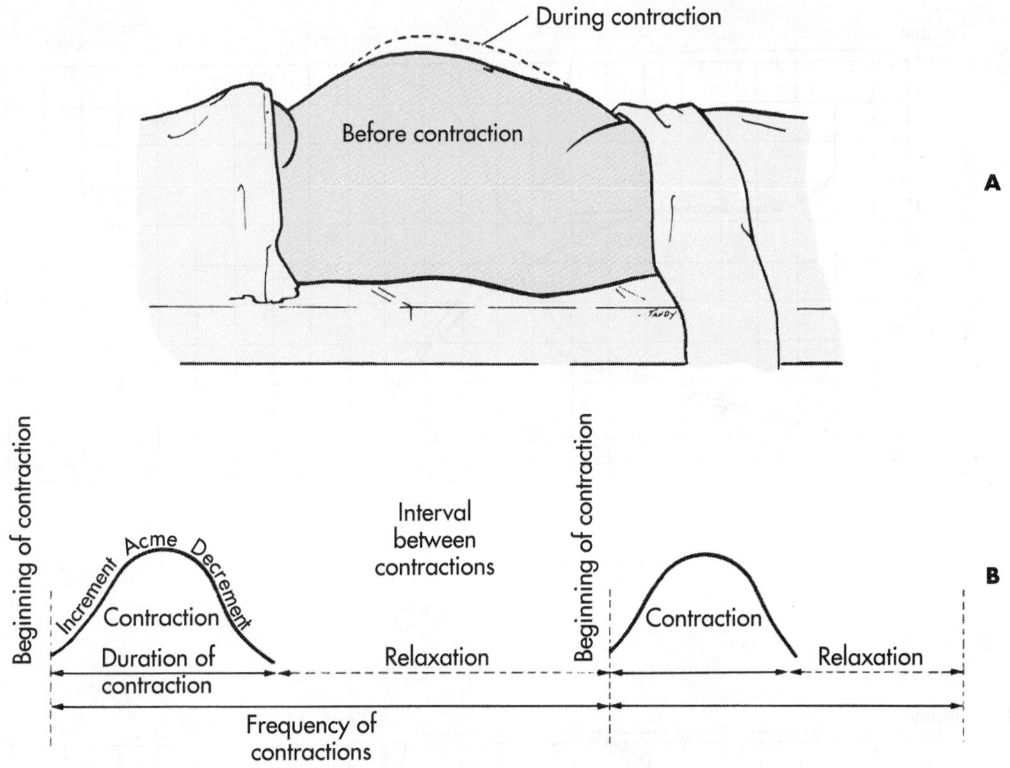

FIG. 18-8 • Assessment of uterine contractions. **A,** Abdominal contour before and during uterine contractions. **B,** Wavelike pattern of contractile activity.

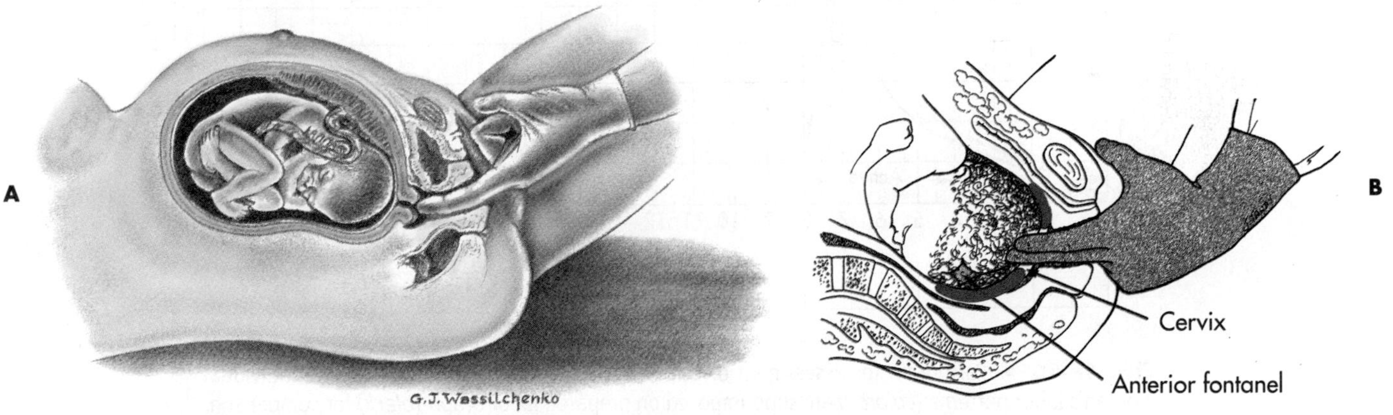

FIG. 18-9 • Vaginal examination. **A,** Undilated, uneffaced cervix; membranes intact. **B,** Palpation of sagittal suture line. Cervix effaced and partially dilated.

of graphic charts (partograms) on which cervical dilation and station (descent) are plotted. This type of graphic charting assists an early identification of deviations from expected labor patterns. Fig. 18-10 provides an example of one type of partogram; however, hospitals and birthing centers may develop their own graphs for recording assessments. Such graphs may include data not only on dilation and descent but also on maternal vital signs, FHR, and uterine activity. (See also Chapter 11.)

LEGAL TIP • Regardless of which charting format is used, complete documentation must include assessment findings, action(s) taken based on analysis of the findings, and response to the action(s) taken.

It is important for the nurse to recognize that active labor can actually last longer than the expected labor patterns. This finding should not be a cause for concern unless the maternal-fetal unit exhibits signs of distress.

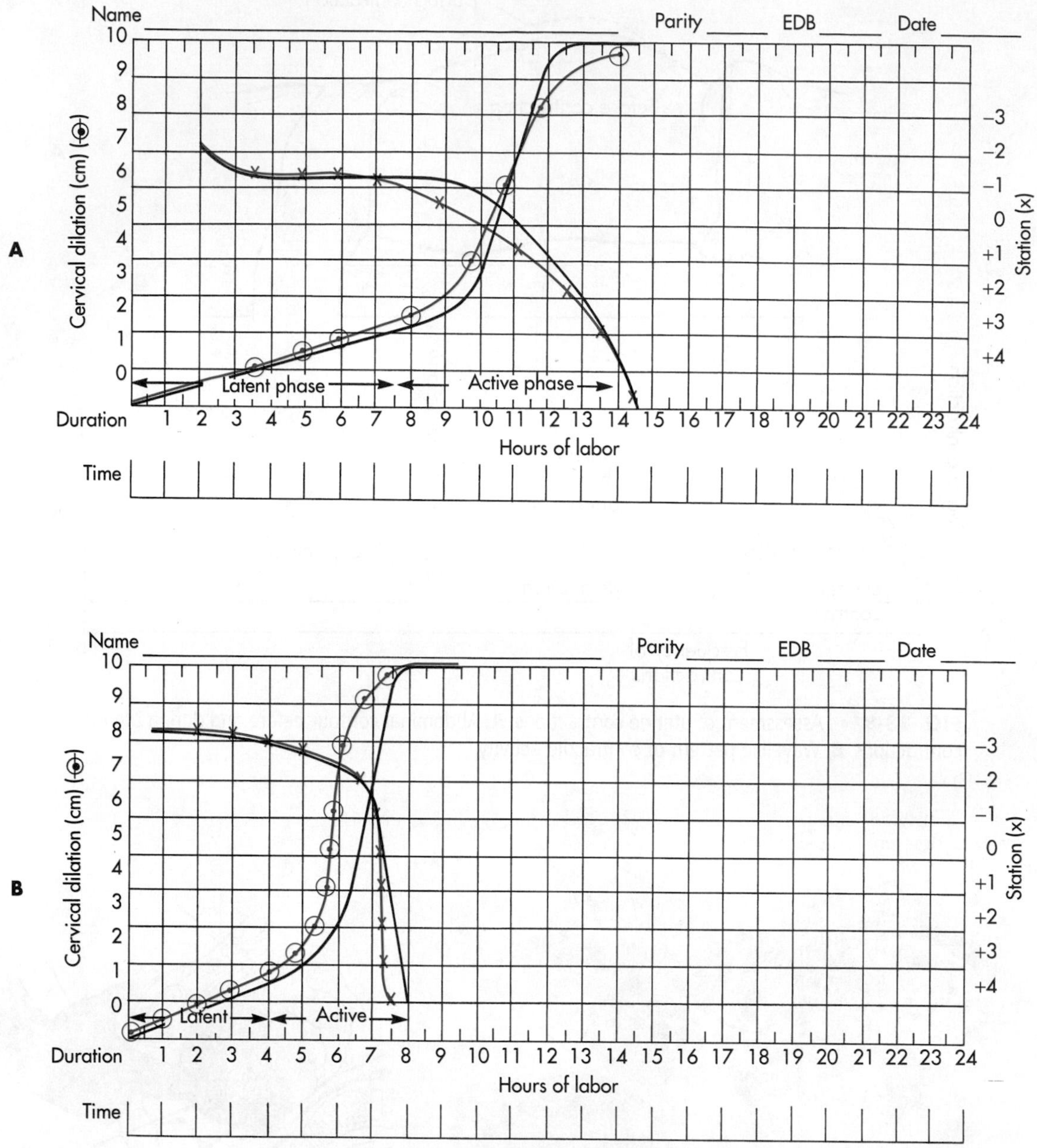

FIG. 18-10 • Partogram for assessment of patterns of cervical dilation and descent. Individual woman's labor patterns *(colored)* are superimposed on prepared labor graph *(black)* for comparison. **A,** Nulliparous labor. **B,** Multiparous labor. The rate of cervical dilation is indicated by the symbol "O." A line drawn through the symbols depicts the slope of the curve. Station is indicated with an "X." A line drawn through the Xs reveals the pattern of descent.

Laboratory and Diagnostic Tests

Analysis of Urine Specimen. A clean-catch urine specimen may be obtained to gather data about the pregnant woman's health. It is a convenient and simple procedure that can provide information about her hydration status (e.g., by specific gravity, color, and amount), nutritional status (e.g., ketones), infection (e.g., the presence of leukocytes), or the status of possible complications such as pregnancy-induced hypertension (PIH, shown by finding protein in the urine). The results can be obtained quickly and help the nurse determine appropriate interventions to implement.

Blood Tests. Blood tests performed vary with hospital protocol and the woman's health status. An example of minimum assessment is a hematocrit determination, in which the specimen is centrifuged on the perinatal unit. Blood can be obtained by a finger stick or from the hub of a catheter used to start an IV line. More comprehensive assessments such as white blood cell count, red blood cell count, hemoglobin level, hematocrit,

TABLE 18-5
Assessment of Amniotic Fluid

Characteristic of Fluid	Normal Finding	Deviation from Normal Finding	Cause of Deviation from Normal
Color	Pale, straw colored; may contain white flecks of vernix caseosa	Greenish brown color	Hypoxic episode in fetus; meconium in fluid May be normal finding in breech presentation
		Yellow-stained fluid	Fetal hypoxia ≥36 hrs before ROM; fetal hemolytic disease; intrauterine infection
		Port wine–colored	Bleeding associated with abruptio placentae
Viscosity and odor	Watery; no strong odor	Thick, cloudy, foul-smelling	Intrauterine infection Large amount of meconium can make fluid thick
Amount	500 to 1200 ml	≥200 ml	Hydramnios; associated with congenital anomalies of the fetus when fetus cannot drink fluid
		≤500 ml	Oligohydramnios; associated with incomplete or absent kidney; obstruction of urethra; infant cannot secrete or excrete urine

and platelet values are included in a complete blood cell count (CBC). A CBC may be ordered for women with a history of infection, anemia, PIH, or other disorders.

If the woman's blood type has not been verified, blood is drawn to determine the type and Rh factor. If blood typing has already been done, the primary health care provider may choose not to repeat the test. If obvious signs of immunocompromise or substance abuse are present, other diagnostic blood tests may be ordered.

Assessment of Amniotic Membranes and Fluid. Labor is initiated at term by spontaneous rupture of membranes (SROM, SRM) in approximately 25% of pregnant women. A lag period, rarely exceeding 24 hours, may precede the onset of labor. Membranes (the bag of waters) can also rupture spontaneously at any time during labor.

NURSE ALERT • The umbilical cord may prolapse when the membranes rupture. It is the nurse's responsibility to monitor the FHR for several minutes immediately after ROM, to ascertain fetal well-being, and then to document the findings.

Artificial rupture of membranes (AROM, ARM) or amniotomy may be done to augment or induce labor or to facilitate placement of internal monitors when fetal status indicates the need for some form of direct assessment method (e.g., attachment of a cardiotachometer to the presenting part and insertion of an intrauterine pressure catheter). (For the tests used to assess ROM, see Box 18-2.) Assessment of amniotic fluid characteristics is described in Table 18-5.

Infection. When membranes rupture, microorganisms from the vagina can ascend into the amniotic sac, causing chorioamnionitis and placentitis to develop. For this reason, maternal temperature and vaginal discharge are assessed frequently (every 1 to 2 hours) so that an infection developing after ROM can be identified early. Even when membranes are intact, however, microorganisms may ascend and cause premature ROM. There is controversy regarding whether prophylactic antibiotic therapy can protect against infection (i.e., chorioamnionitis) that involves both the maternal and fetal sides of the membrane.

The nurse's responsibility is to report findings promptly to the physician or nurse-midwife and to document findings in the labor record and on the monitor strip (if that is agency policy). If abnormal findings are obtained, continuous electronic monitoring is usually used for the duration of labor. The presence of meconium-stained amniotic fluid alerts the nurse to the necessity of observing fetal status more closely. After birth the newborn may be at high risk for alteration in respiratory status if meconium is aspirated into the lungs with the first breath.

Assessment findings serve as a baseline for evaluating the woman's progress during labor. Although some problems of labor are anticipated, others may appear unexpectedly during the clinical course of labor (Box 18-6).

Box 18-6
Signs of Potential Complications

LABOR
- Intrauterine pressure of more than 75 mm Hg (determined by intrauterine pressure catheter monitoring) or resting tone of more than 15 mm Hg
- Contractions consistently lasting 90 seconds or more
- Contractions consistently occurring 2 minutes or less apart
- Fetal bradycardia, tachycardia, or persistently decreased variability
- Irregular FHR; suspected fetal dysrhythmias
- Appearance of meconium-stained or bloody fluid from the vagina
- Arrest in progress of cervical dilation or effacement, descent of the fetus, or both
- Maternal temperature of 38° C or more
- Foul-smelling vaginal discharge
- Persistent bright or dark-red vaginal bleeding

➤ Nursing Diagnoses

Nursing diagnoses appropriate for the woman in first stage labor include the following:

- Anxiety related to:
  - —Negative experience with previous childbirth
  - —Cultural differences
- Altered urinary elimination related to:
  - —Reduced intake of oral fluids
  - —Diminished sensation of bladder fullness associated with epidural anesthesia/analgesia
- Impaired fetal gas exchange related to:
  - —Maternal hypotension
  - —Compression of umbilical cord
- Situational low self-esteem (maternal) related to:
  - —Inability to meet self-expectations
  - —Loss of control during labor

Nursing diagnoses that represent potential areas for concern during the second stage of labor include the following:

- Risk for injury to mother and fetus related to:
  - —Persistent use of Valsalva maneuver
- Situational low self-esteem related to:
  - —Knowledge deficit of normal, beneficial effects of vocalization during bearing-down efforts
  - —Inability to carry out plan for birth without medication
- Ineffective individual coping related to:
  - —Coaching that contradicts woman's physiologic urge to push
- Anxiety related to:
  - —Inability to control defecation with bearing-down efforts
  - —Knowledge deficit regarding inexperience with perineal sensations associated with the urge to bear down

Examples of nursing diagnoses relevant to the third stage of labor include the following:

- Risk for fluid volume deficit related to:
  - —Blood loss occurring following placental separation and expulsion
  - —Inadequate contraction of the uterus
- Anxiety related to:
  - —Lack of knowledge regarding birth of the placenta
  - —Occurrence of perineal trauma and the need for repair
- Fatigue related to:
  - —Energy expenditure associated with childbirth and the bearing-down efforts of the second stage

➤ Expected Outcomes

The nurse and woman set and prioritize expected outcomes that focus on the woman/couple. Expected outcomes for the woman in labor are that the woman will accomplish the following:

- Continue normal progression of labor while the FHR remains within normal range and without signs of distress
- Maintain adequate hydration status through oral and/or intravenous intake
- Actively participate in the labor process
- Verbalize discomfort and indicate the need for measures that help reduce discomfort and promote relaxation
- Accept comfort and support measures from significant others and health care providers as needed
- Sustain no injury to herself or the fetus during labor
- Expel the placenta with maternal blood loss of less than 500 ml or less than 1% of body weight
- Initiate, along with the partner and family, the processes of bonding and attachment with the newborn
- Express satisfaction with her performance during labor

➤ Plan of Care and Implementation

Standards of Care. Standards of care guide the nurse in preparing for and implementing procedures with the expectant mother. Protocols for care based on standards include the following:

- Check the primary health care provider's orders
- Assess the orders for appropriateness and correctness (e.g., the analgesic to be administered to relieve discomfort)
- Check labels on IV solutions, medications, and other materials used for nursing care
- Check the expiration date on any packs of supplies used for procedures
- Ensure that information on the woman's identification band is correct. Also check that the identification band is accurate (e.g., if she has allergies, ensure that the band is of the appropriate color)
- Employ an empathic approach when giving care:
  - —When explaining procedures, use words the woman can understand
  - —Respect the woman's individual needs and behaviors
  - —Establish rapport with the woman and her support person(s)/family
  - —Be kind, caring, and competent when performing necessary procedures
  - —Be aware that pain and discomfort are as the woman describes them
  - —Repeat instructions as necessary and ensure that the woman understands them
  - —Carry out appropriate comfort measures such as mouth care and back care, and ensure that the support person is coping
  - —Recognize that a woman's current childbirth experience and the actions of nurses and other health care providers can have a positive or negative effect on the woman's future childbirth experiences
- Use Standard Precautions, including precautions for invasive procedures as needed
- Document care according to hospital guidelines and communicate information to the primary health care provider when indicated

Physical Nursing Care During Labor. Physical nursing care of the woman in labor is an essential component of her care. The current emphasis on evidence-based practice has led to the following labeling of care measures used during labor and birth:

- Demonstrably beneficial (useful) or likely to be beneficial ■■
- A trade-off between beneficial and having a potentially adverse effect or of unknown effectiveness with insufficient evidence to support use
- Unlikely to be beneficial or likely to be harmful or ineffective

Managing care using this approach will enhance the safety, effectiveness, and acceptability of the physical care measures chosen to support the woman during labor and birth (Enkin et al, 1995; Technical Working Group of the World Health Organization, 1997). The various physical needs, the requisite nursing actions, and the rationale for care are presented in Table 18-6 and the Nursing Care Plan (see also Table 18-4).

General Hygiene. Women in labor should be offered the use of showers or Jacuzzis, if they are available, to enhance the feeling of well-being and to minimize the discomfort of contractions. Women should also be encouraged to wash their

TABLE 18-6
Woman's Responses and Support Person's Actions During First Stage of Labor

Woman's Responses	Nurse/Support Persons's Actions*
DILATION OF CERVIX 0-3 cm (LATENT) (contractions 10-30 sec long, 5-30 min apart, mild to moderate)	

Mood: alert, happy, excited, mild anxiety
Settles into labor room; selects focal point
Rests or sleeps, if possible
Uses breathing techniques
Uses effleurage, focusing, and relaxation techniques
	Provides encouragement, feedback for relaxation, companionship
	Assists to cope with contractions
	  Encourages use of focusing techniques
	  Helps to concentrate on breathing techniques
	Uses comfort measures
	  Assists woman into comfortable position
	  Informs woman of progress; explains procedures and routines
	  Gives praise
	  Offer fluids, ice chips as ordered

DILATION OF CERVIX 4-7 cm (ACTIVE) (contractions 30-45 sec long, 3-5 min apart, moderate to strong)	

Mood: seriously labor oriented, concentration and energy needed for contractions, alert, more demanding
Continues relaxation, focusing techniques
Uses breathing techniques
	Acts as buffer; limits assessment techniques to between contractions
	Assists with contractions
	  Encourages woman as needed to help her maintain breathing techniques
	Uses comfort measures
	  Assists with frequent position changes, emphasizing side-lying and upright positions
	  Encourages voluntary relaxation of muscles of back, buttocks, thighs, and perineum; effleurage
	  Applies counterpressure to sacrococcygeal area
	  Encourages and praises
	  Keeps woman aware of progress
	  Offers analgesics as ordered
	  Checks bladder; encourages her to void
	  Gives oral care; offers fluids, ice chips as ordered

DILATION OF CERVIX 8-10 cm (TRANSITION) (contractions 45-90 sec long, 2-3 min apart, strong)	

Mood: irritable, intense concentration, symptoms of transition (e.g., nausea, vomiting)
Continues relaxation, needs greater concentration to do this
Uses breathing techniques
Uses 4:1 breathing pattern if using psychoprophylactic techniques
Uses panting to overcome response to urge to push
	Stays with woman; provides constant support
	Assists with contractions
	  Reminds, reassures, and encourages woman to reestablish breathing pattern and concentration as needed
	  Alerts woman to begin breathing pattern before contraction becomes too intense if she is sedated or drowsy
	  Prompts panting respirations if woman begins to push prematurely
	Uses comfort measures
	  Accepts woman's inability to comply with instructions
	  Accepts irritable response to helping, such as counterpressure
	  Supports woman who has nausea and vomiting; gives oral care as needed; gives reassurance regarding signs of end of first stage
	Uses relaxation techniques (effleurage and voluntary relaxation)
	Keeps woman aware of progress

*Provided by nurses and support persons in collaboration with the nurse.

hands after voiding and to perform self-hygiene measures. Linen should be changed if it becomes wet or stained with blood, and linen savers (Chux) should be used and changed as needed.

Oral Intake. Traditionally the laboring woman has been offered only clear liquids or ice chips, or given nothing by mouth during the active phase of labor. This is to minimize the risk of anesthesia complications and their sequelae should general anesthesia be required in an emergency. These sequelae include aspiration of gastric contents and resultant compromise in oxygen perfusion, which may endanger the lives of the mother and fetus. This practice is being challenged today because regional anesthesia is used more often than general anesthesia, even for emergency cesarean births. Women are awake during regional anesthesia and are able to participate in their own care and protect their airway. Withholding of food and drink from women in labor has been identified as a form of care unlikely to be beneficial (Enkin et al, 1995).

Nursing Care Plan LABOR AND BIRTH

NURSING DIAGNOSIS Anxiety related to labor and the birthing process

EXPECTED OUTCOME Woman exhibits decreased signs of anxiety.

Nursing Interventions/*Rationales*

Orient woman and significant others to labor and birth unit and explain admission protocol *to allay initial feelings of anxiety.*

Assess woman's knowledge, experience, and expectations of labor; note any signs or expressions of anxiety, nervousness, or fear *to establish a baseline for intervention.*

Discuss the expected progression of labor and describe what to expect during the process *to allay anxiety associated with the unknown.*

Actively involve woman in care decisions during labor, interpret sights and sounds of environment (monitor sights and sounds, unit activities), and share information on progression of labor (vital signs, FHR, dilation, effacement) *to increase her sense of control and allay fears.*

NURSING DIAGNOSIS Pain related to increasing frequency and intensity of contractions

EXPECTED OUTCOME Woman exhibits signs of ability to cope with discomfort.

Nursing Interventions/*Rationales*

Assess woman's level of pain and strategies that she has used to cope with pain *to establish a baseline for intervention.*

Encourage significant other to remain as support person during labor process *to assist with support and comfort measures, because measures are often more effective when delivered by a familiar person.*

Instruct woman and support person in use of specific techniques such as conscious relaxation, focused breathing, effleurage, massage, and application of sacral pressure *to increase relaxation, decrease intensity of contractions, and promote use of controlled thought and direction of energy.*

Provide comfort measures such as frequent mouth care to prevent dry mouth, application of damp cloth to forehead, and changing of damp gown or bed covers *to relieve discomfort associated with diaphoresis; positioning to reduce stiffness.*

Encourage conscious relaxation between contractions *to prevent fatigue, which contributes to increased pain perceptions.*

Explain what analgesics and anesthesia are available for use during labor and birth *to provide knowledge to help woman make decisions about pain control.*

NURSING DIAGNOSIS Risk for altered pattern of urinary elimination related to sensory impairment secondary to labor

EXPECTED OUTCOME Bladder does not show signs of distention.

Nursing Interventions/*Rationales*

Palpate the bladder superior to the symphysis on a frequent basis *to prevent distention that occurs from increased fluid intake and inability to feel urge to void.*

Encourage frequent voiding (at least every 2 hours) and catheterize if necessary *to avoid bladder distention because it impedes progress of fetus down birth canal and may result in trauma to the bladder.*

Assist to bathroom or commode to void if appropriate and provide privacy *to facilitate bladder emptying with an upright position (natural) and relaxation.*

NURSING DIAGNOSIS Risk for ineffective individual coping related to birthing process

EXPECTED OUTCOME Woman actively participates in the birth process with no evidence of injury to her or her fetus.

Nursing Interventions/*Rationales*

Constantly monitor events of second-stage labor and birth, including physiologic responses of woman and fetus, emotional responses of woman and partner, *to ensure maternal, partner, and fetal well-being.*

Provide ongoing feedback to woman and partner *to allay anxiety and enhance participation.*

Continue to provide comfort measures such as positioning; mouth care; clean, dry bedding; cool cloth on forehead; and minimizing distractions *to decrease discomfort and aid in focus on the birth process.*

Encourage woman to experiment with various positions *to assist downward movement of fetus.*

Ensure that woman takes deep cleansing breaths before and after each contraction *to enhance gas exchange and oxygen transport to the fetus.*

Encourage woman to push spontaneously when urge to bear down is perceived during a contraction *to aid descent and rotation of fetus.*

Encourage woman to exhale, taking only short breath holds while bearing down *to avoid holding breath and triggering a Valsalva maneuver and increasing intrathoracic and cardiovascular pressure and decreasing perfusion of placental oxygen, placing the fetus at risk.*

Nursing Care Plan LABOR AND BIRTH—cont'd

Have woman take deep breaths and relax between contractions *to reduce fatigue and increase effectiveness of pushing efforts.*
Have mother pant as fetal head crowns *to control birth of head.*
Explain to woman and labor partner what is expected in the third stage of labor *to enlist cooperation.*
Have woman maintain her position *to facilitate delivery of the placenta.*
Ask mother if she wishes to dispose of the placenta in any specific manner *to comply with certain cultural customs.*

NURSING DIAGNOSIS Fatigue related to energy expenditure required during labor and birth

EXPECTED OUTCOME Mother's energy levels are restored.

Nursing Interventions/*Rationales*

Educate mother and partner about need for rest and help them plan strategies (e.g., restricting visitors, increasing role of support systems performing functions associated with daily routines) that allow specific times for rest and sleep *to ensure that woman can restore depleted energy levels in preparation for caring for a new infant.*
Monitor woman's fatigue level and the amount of rest received *to ensure restoration of energy.*

NURSING DIAGNOSIS Risk for fluid volume deficit related to decreased fluid intake and blood loss during the birth

EXPECTED OUTCOME Fluid balance is maintained, and there are no signs of dehydration.

Nursing Interventions/*Rationales*

Monitor fluid loss (i.e., blood, urine, perspiration) and vital signs; inspect skin turgor and mucous membranes for dryness *to evaluate hydration status.*
Administer oral/parenteral fluid per physician/nurse-midwife orders *to maintain hydration.*
Monitor the fundus for firmness after placental separation *to ensure adequate contraction and prevent further blood loss.*
Administer medications per physician/nurse-midwife orders *to aid contractions of the uterus.*

Critical Thinking

IMPLEMENTING EVIDENCE-BASED APPROACHES TO CHILDBIRTH

You are the nurse manager of a labor and birth unit of a hospital. After attending a national nursing education meeting regarding evidence-based approaches to enhance the progress of childbirth, you determine that these measures should be implemented on your unit. Acting as an advocate for your patients and a catalyst for change on your unit, outline the approach you would use to convince the nursing and medical staff to include these approaches when managing the care of laboring women.

Offering oral fluids is demonstrably useful and should be encouraged.

Although gastric emptying is slowed as a result of labor, stress, and the use of narcotics or sedatives, fasting does not cause gastric contents to be eliminated and may even cause them to be more acidic. In addition, fasting is identified by many laboring women as a stressor with which they must cope and a source of frustration during labor related to a loss of control with regard to meeting their own nourishment needs (Fowles, 1998).

Adequate intake of fluids and calories is required to meet the energy demands and fluid losses associated with childbirth. The progress of labor slows and ketosis develops if these demands are not met and fat is metabolized. This is most likely to occur in women who begin to labor early in the morning after a night without caloric intake. When women are permitted to consume fluids and food freely, they typically regulate their own oral intake, eating light foods (e.g., eggs, yogurt, ice cream, dry toast and jelly, or fruit) and drinking fluids during early labor, then tapering off to an intake of clear fluid and sips of water or ice chips as labor intensifies and the second stage approaches. Common practice is to allow clear liquids (e.g., water, tea, apple juice, clear sodas, gelatin, and broth) during early labor, tapering off to ice chips and sips of water as labor progresses and becomes more active. Food and fluid consumed orally during labor can meet a laboring woman's hydration and energy demands more effectively and safely than fluid administered intravenously.

Intravenous Intake. Fluids are administered intravenously to the laboring woman to maintain hydration, especially when a labor is long and the woman is unable to ingest a sufficient amount of fluid orally or if she is receiving epidural or intrathecal analgesia. However, routine use of intravenous fluids during labor is a form of care that is unlikely to be beneficial and may be harmful (Enkin et al, 1995; Technical Working Group of the World Health Organization, 1997). In most cases, an electrolyte solution without glucose is adequate and does not introduce excess glucose into the bloodstream. The latter is important because an excessive maternal glucose level results in fetal hyperglycemia and fetal hyperinsulinism. After birth, the neonate's high level of insulin will then deplete his or her glucose stores and hypoglycemia will result. If maternal ketosis occurs, the primary health care provider may order an IV solution containing a small amount of dextrose to provide the glucose needed to assist in fatty acid metabolism.

NURSE ALERT • Nurses should carefully monitor the intake and output of laboring women receiving IV fluids because they also face an increased danger of hypervolemia as a result of the fluid retention that occurs during pregnancy.

Voiding. Voiding every 2 hours should be encouraged by the nurse, especially if the bladder is distended. A distended bladder may impede descent of the presenting part, inhibit uterine contractions, and lead to decreased bladder tone or atony after birth. Women who receive epidural analgesia or anesthesia are especially at risk for retention of urine, and the need to void should be assessed more frequently in them.

The woman should be assisted to the bathroom to void unless the primary health care provider has ordered bed rest; the woman is receiving epidural analgesia or anesthesia; or, in the nurse's judgment, ambulation would compromise the status of the laboring woman or her fetus. If external monitoring is being used and the cords will reach, monitoring can continue while the woman uses the bathroom; otherwise, the cords are unplugged from the monitor while the woman is in the bathroom and monitoring is interrupted for that time.

Catheterization. If the woman is unable to void and her bladder is obviously distended, she may need to be catheterized. Most hospitals have protocols that rely on the nurse's judgment concerning the need for catheterization. During the catheterization, if there appears to be an obstacle that prevents advancement of the catheter, this is most likely the presenting part. If the catheter cannot be advanced, the nurse should stop the procedure and notify the primary health care provider of the difficulty.

Bowel Elimination. Most women do not have bowel movements during labor because of decreased intestinal motility. Stool that has formed in the large intestine often is moved downward toward the anorectal area by the pressure exerted by the fetal presenting part as it descends. This stool is often expelled during second-stage pushing and birth. However, the passage of stool with bearing-down efforts increases the risk of infection and may embarrass the woman, thereby reducing the effectiveness of these efforts. To prevent these problems, the nurse should immediately cleanse the perineal area to remove any stool, while at the same time reassuring the woman that the passage of stool at this time is a normal and expected event, because the same muscles used to expel the baby also expel stool. Routine use of an enema to empty the rectum is considered to be harmful or ineffective and should be eliminated (Enkin et al, 1995; Technical Working Group of the World Health Organization, 1997).

When the presenting part is deep in the pelvis, even in the absence of stool in the anorectal area, the woman may feel rectal pressure and think she needs to defecate. When the woman expresses the need to defecate, the nurse should perform a vaginal examination to assess cervical dilation and station. When a multiparous woman experiences the urge to defecate, this often means that birth will follow quickly.

Ambulation and Positioning. Freedom of maternal movement and choice of position through labor are forms of care likely to be beneficial for the laboring woman and should be encouraged (Enkin et al, 1995; Technical Working Group of the World Health Organization, 1997).

The potential advantages of ambulation include enhanced uterine activity, distraction from the discomfort of labor, enhanced maternal control, and an opportunity for close interaction with the woman's partner and care provider as they help her to walk. Ambulation is associated with a reduced rate of operative delivery (i.e., cesarean birth, use of forceps, and vacuum extraction) and less frequent use of narcotic analgesia (Albers et al, 1997). Walking, sitting, or standing during early labor is more comfortable than lying down and facilitates the progress of labor (Melzack, Belanger, and Lacroix, 1991). Ambulation is encouraged if membranes are intact, if the fetal presenting part is engaged after rupture of membranes, and if the woman has not received medication for pain (Fig. 18-11).

When the woman lies in bed she will usually change her position spontaneously as labor progresses (Albers et al, 1997). If she does not change position every 30 to 60 minutes, she should be assisted to do so. The side-lying (lateral) position promotes optimal uteroplacental and renal blood flow and increases oxygen saturation (Fig. 18-12, *B*). If the woman wants to lie supine, the nurse may place a pillow under one hip as a wedge to prevent the uterus from compressing the aorta and vena cava. Sitting is not contraindicated unless it adversely affects fetal status, which can be determined by checking the fetal heart rate. If the fetus is in the occiput posterior position, it may be helpful to encourage the woman to squat during contractions since this position increases pelvic diameter, allowing the head to rotate to a more anterior position (Fig. 18-12, *A*). A hands-and-knees position during contractions is also recommended to facilitate the rotation of the fetal occiput from a posterior to an anterior position as gravity pulls the fetal back forward (Fig. 18-13, *B*). Fetal presentation and the mechanisms of labor may be helped or hindered by maternal posture (Carbonne et al, 1996; Simkin, 1995). A variety of positions recommended for the laboring woman are described in Box 18-7.

A birth ball (gymnastic ball, also used in physical therapy) can be used to support a woman's body as she assumes a variety of labor and birth positions (McCartney, 1998) (Fig. 18-14). The woman can sit on the ball while leaning over the bed, or she can lean over the ball to support her upper body and reduce stress on her arms and hands when she assumes a hands-and-knees position. The birth ball can encourage pelvic mobility and pelvic and perineal relaxation when the woman sits on the firm yet pliable ball and rocks in rhythmic movements. Warm compresses applied to the perineum can maximize this relax-

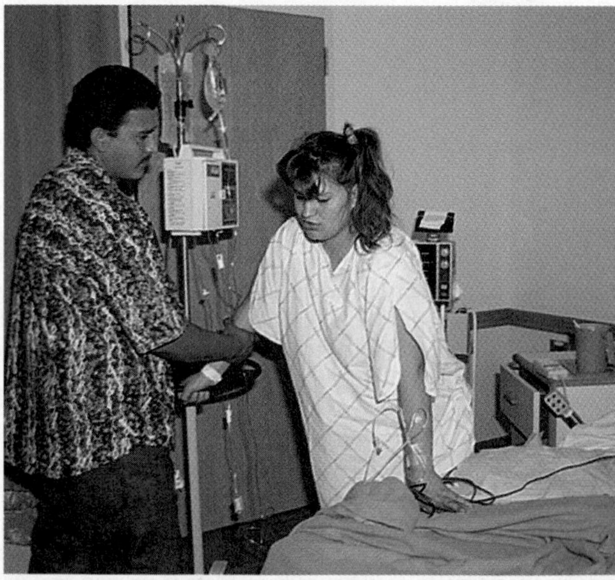

FIG. 18-11 • Woman preparing to walk with partner. (Courtesy Marjorie Pyle, RNC, Lifecircle, Costa Mesa, CA.)

ation effect. The birth ball should be large enough so that when the woman sits, her knees are bent at a 90-degree angle and her feet are flat on the floor and approximately 2 feet apart (Perez, 1998).

Support Measures. Effective physical and emotional support provided to women during labor can result in shorter labors, reduced rates of complications and surgical or obstetric interventions (e.g., cesarean births, labor augmentations and inductions, episiotomies, and forceps-assisted births), and enhanced self-esteem and satisfaction (Gagnon and Waghorn, 1999; Kennell et al, 1991).

Labor rooms should be airy, clean, and homelike. To enhance relaxation, bright overhead lights should be turned off when not needed. The temperature is controlled to ensure the laboring woman's comfort. The room should be large enough to accommodate a comfortable chair for the woman's partner, the monitoring equipment, and hospital personnel. Couples may be encouraged to bring extra pillows to make the hospital surroundings more homelike and to facilitate position changes.

The nurse can alleviate a woman's anxiety by explaining unfamiliar terms, providing information and explanations without her having to ask, and preparing her for sensations she will experience and procedures that will follow. By encouraging the woman or couple to ask questions and by providing honest, understandable answers, the nurse can play a significant role in helping the woman achieve a satisfying birth experience (Proctor, 1998; Tomlinson and Bryan, 1996).

Supportive nursing care for a woman in labor includes (1) helping the woman to maintain control and participate to the extent she wishes in the birth of her infant; (2) meeting the woman's expected outcomes for her labor; (3)

A

B

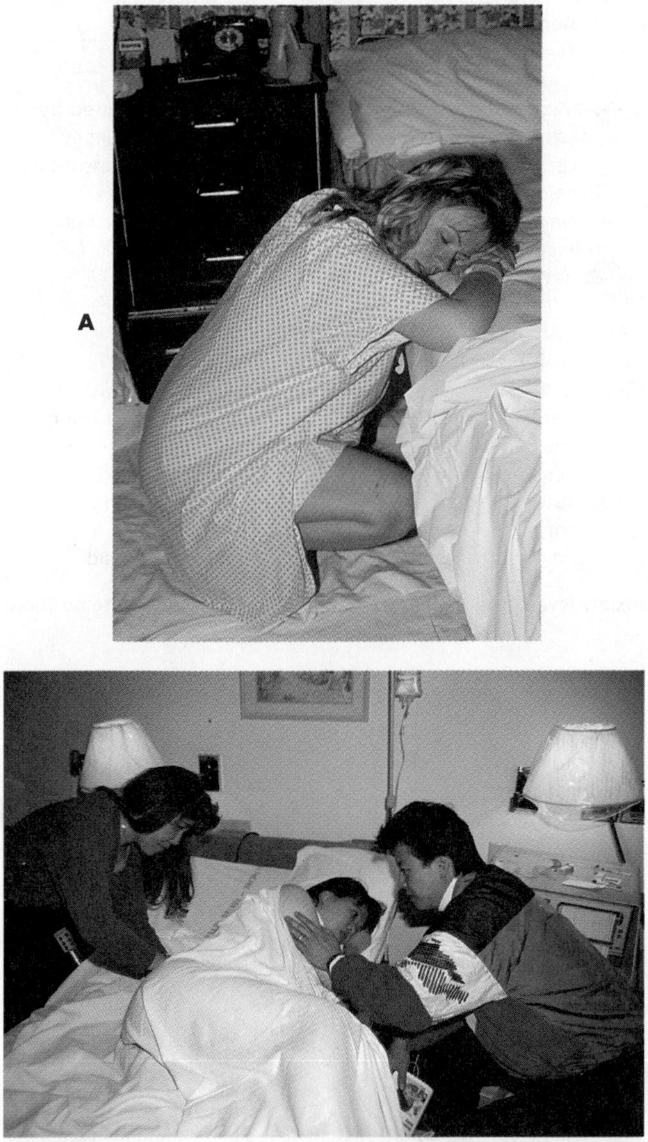

FIG. 18-12 • Maternal positions for labor. **A,** Squatting. **B,** Lateral position. Support person is applying sacral pressure while partner provides encouragement. (Courtesy Marjorie Pyle, RNC, Lifecircle, Costa Mesa, CA.)

A

B

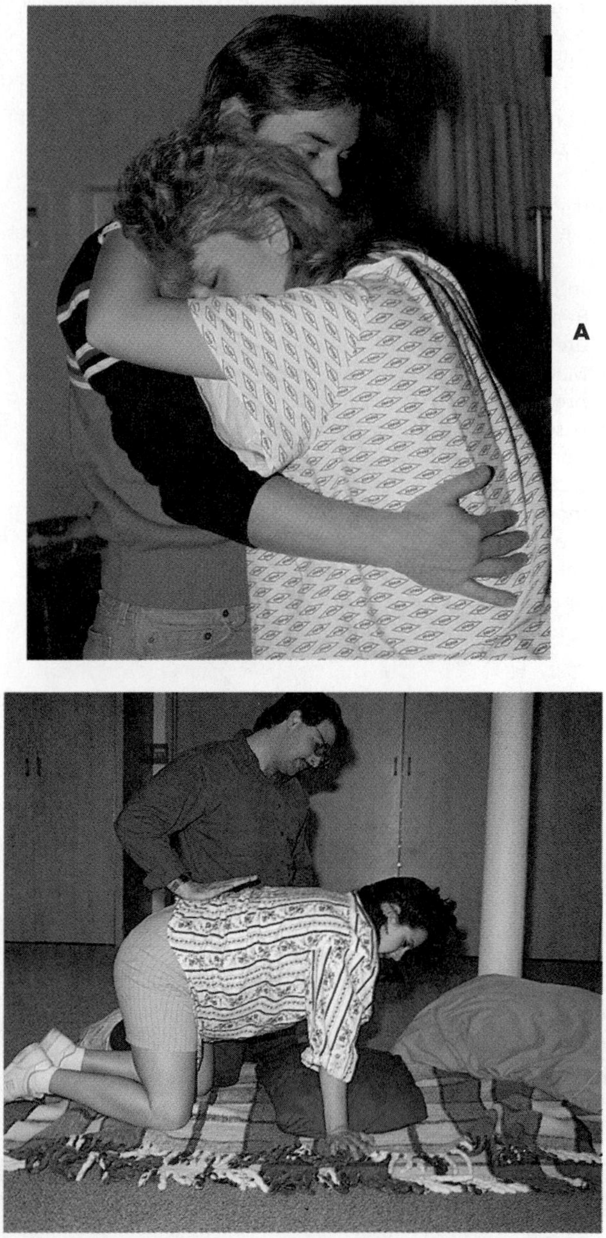

FIG. 18-13 • **A,** Woman standing and leaning forward with support. **B,** Woman in hands-and-knees position. (Courtesy Marjorie Pyle, RNC, Lifecircle, Costa Mesa, CA.)

acting as the woman's advocate, supporting her decisions and respecting her choices as appropriate and relating her wishes as needed to other health care providers; (4) helping the woman conserve her energy; (5) helping control the woman's discomfort; (6) acknowledging and providing positive reinforcement for the woman's efforts, as well as those of her partner, during labor; and (7) protecting the woman's privacy and modesty.

Couples who have attended childbirth education programs that teach the psychoprophylactic approach will know something about the labor process, coaching techniques, and comfort measures (Fig. 18-15). Even when expectant parents have

Box 18-7

Some Maternal Positions* During Labor and Birth

SEMIRECUMBENT POSITION

With woman sitting with her upper body elevated to at least a 30° angle, place wedge or small pillow under hip to prevent vena caval compression and reduce likelihood of supine hypotension (see Fig. 18-4, *B*)

- The greater the angle of elevation, the more gravity or pressure is exerted that promotes fetal descent, the progress of contractions, and the widening of pelvic dimensions.
- Convenient for rendering care measures and for external fetal monitoring.

LATERAL POSITION (SEE FIG. 18-12, *B*)

Have woman alternate between left and right side-lying position, and provide abdominal and back support as needed for comfort.

- Removes pressure from the vena cava and back; enhances uteroplacental perfusion and relieves backache.
- Makes it easier to perform back massage or counterpressure.
- Associated with less frequent, but more intense, contractions.
- Obtaining good external fetal monitor tracings may be more difficult.
- May be used as a birthing position.
- Takes pressure off perineum.

UPRIGHT POSITION

The gravity effect enhances the contraction cycle and fetal descent: the weight of the fetus places increasing pressure on the cervix; the cervix is pulled upward, facilitating effacement and dilation; impulses from the cervix to the pituitary gland increase, causing more oxytocin to be secreted; and contractions are intensified, thereby applying more forceful downward pressure on the fetus, but they are less painful.

- Fetus is aligned with pelvis, and pelvic diameters are widened slightly.
- Effective upright positions include the following:
  —Ambulation (see Fig. 18-11).
  —Standing and leaning forward with support provided by coach, end of bed, back of chair, or birth ball; relieves backache and facilitates application of counterpressure or back massage (see Fig. 18-13, *A*).
  —Sitting up in bed, chair, birthing chair, on toilet or bedside commode
  —Squatting (see Fig. 18-12, *A*).

HANDS-AND-KNEES POSITION—IDEAL POSITION FOR POSTERIOR POSITIONS OF THE PRESENTING PART (SEE FIG. 18-13, *B*).

Assume an "all fours" position in bed or on a covered floor; allows for pelvic rocking.

- Relieves backache characteristic of "back labor."
- Facilitates internal rotation of the fetus by increasing mobility of the coccyx, increasing the pelvic diameters, and using gravity to turn the fetal back and rotate the head.

*Assess the effect of each position on the laboring woman's comfort and anxiety level, progress of labor, and FHR pattern. Alternate positions every 30 to 60 minutes.

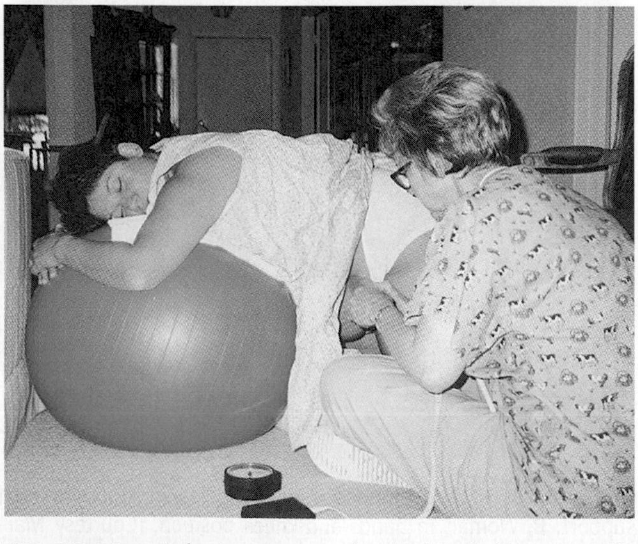

FIG. 18-14 • Laboring woman using birth ball. (Courtesy Polly Perez, Cutting Edge Press, Johnson, VT.)

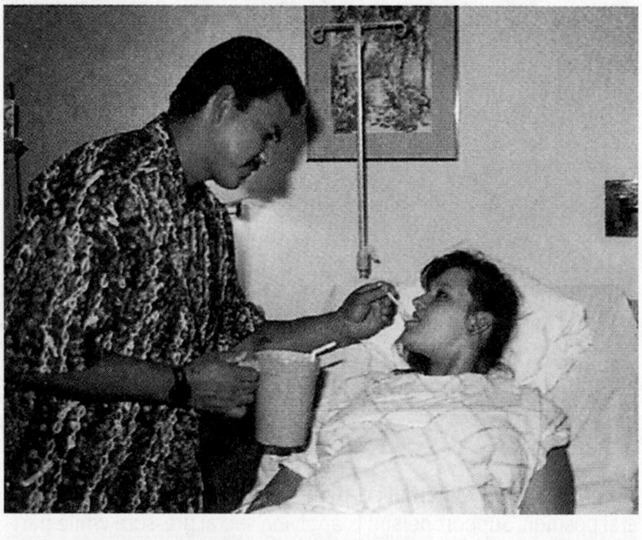

FIG. 18-15 • Partner providing comfort measures. (Courtesy Marjorie Pyle, RNC, Lifecircle, Costa Mesa, CA.)

not attended childbirth education classes, the nurse can teach them various techniques during the early phase of labor. In this case the nurse may provide more of the coaching and supportive care. Breathing and relaxation techniques and comfort measures as described in Chapter 16 can be implemented.

Many women become more sensitive to touch (hyperesthesia) as labor progresses; this is a typical response during transition (see Table 18-2). They may tell their coach to leave them alone or not to touch them. The partner who is unprepared for this normal response may feel rejected and may react by withdrawing active support. The nurse can reassure them that this response is a positive indication that the first stage is ending and the second stage is approaching.

Emergency Interventions. Emergency conditions that require immediate nursing intervention can arise with startling speed. Interventions for nonreassuring FHR, inadequate

Emergency

INTERVENTIONS FOR EMERGENCIES

Signs	Interventions*
Nonreassurring FHR Pattern • Fetal bradycardia (FHR <110 beats/min for >10 min)† • Fetal tachycardia (FHR >160 beats/min for >10 min in term pregnancy)§ • Irregular FHR, abnormal sinus rhythm shown by internal monitor • Persistent decrease in baseline FHR variability without any identified cause • Late, severe variable, and prolonged deceleration patterns • Absence of FHR	Notify primary health care provider‡ Change woman to side-lying position Discontinue oxytocin (Pitocin) infusion, if being infused Increase IV fluid rate, if fluid being infused per protocol order Administer oxygen at 8 to 10 L/min by tight face mask Check maternal temperature for elevation Start an IV line if one is not in place Administer amnioinfusion if ordered Stimulate fetal scalp or use acoustic stimulation
Inadequate Uterine Relaxation • Intrauterine pressure >75 mm Hg (shown by intrauterine pressure catheter monitoring) • Contractions consistently lasting >90 sec • Contraction interval <2 min	Notify primary health care provider‡ Discontinue oxytocin infusion, if being infused Change woman to side-lying position Increase IV fluid rate, if fluid is being infused Administer oxygen at 8 to 10 L/min by tight face mask Start an IV line if one is not in place Palpate and evaluate contractions Give tocolytics (terbutaline), as ordered
Vaginal Bleeding • Vaginal bleeding (bright red, dark red, or in amount in excess of that expected during normal cervical dilation) • Continuous vaginal bleeding with FHR changes • Pain; may or may not be present	Notify primary health care provider‡ Anticipate emergency (stat) cesarean birth *Do NOT perform a vaginal examination*
Infection • Foul-smelling amniotic fluid • Maternal temperature >38° C in presence of adequate hydration (straw-colored urine) • Fetal tachycardia >160 beats/min for >10 min	Notify primary health care provider‡ Institute cooling measures for laboring woman Start an IV line if one is not in place Assist with or perform collection of catheterized urine specimen and amniotic fluid sample and send to the laboratory for urinalysis and cultures
Prolapse of Cord • Fetal bradycardia with variable deceleration during uterine contraction • Woman reports feeling the cord after membranes rupture • Cord lies alongside or below the presenting part of the fetus; can be seen or felt in or protruding from the vagina • Major predisposing factors: —Rupture of membranes with a gush —Loose fit of presenting part in lower uterine segment —Presenting part not yet engaged	Call for assistance Have someone notify the primary health care provider immediately Glove the examining hand quickly and insert two fingers into the vagina to the cervix; with one finger on either side of the cord or both fingers to one side, exert upward pressure against the presenting part to relieve compression of the cord Place a rolled towel under the woman's hip Place woman in extreme Trendelenburg or modified Sims position or knee-chest position Wrap the cord loosely in a sterile towel saturated with warm sterile normal saline if the cord is protruding from the vagina Administer oxygen at 8 to 10 L/min by face mask until birth is accomplished Start IV fluids or increase existing drip rate Continue to monitor FHR by internal fetal scalp electrode, if possible Do not attempt to replace cord into cervix Prepare for immediate birth (vaginal or cesarean)

*Because emergency situations are often frightening events, it is important for the nurse to explain to the woman and her support person what is happening and how it is being managed.
†Practice is to intervene within 2 to 30 min of FHR <110 beats/min.
‡In most emergency situations, nurses take immediate action, following a protocol and standards of nursing practice. Another person can notify the primary health care provider, or this can be done by the nurse as soon as possible.
§Nonreassuring sign when associated with late decelerations or absence of variability, especially of >180 beats/min.

uterine relaxation, vaginal bleeding, infection, and prolapse of the cord are listed in the Emergency box.

Preparation for Giving Birth. The first stage of labor ends with complete dilation of the cervix. The nurse begins to prepare for birth when a multiparous woman is 6 to 8 cm dilated because progression through the last few centimeters of dilation can occur rapidly. Factors that influence the process are fetal position and size of the baby in relation to the size of previous babies.

Birth Setting. To prepare for birth in any setting, the birth table or case cart is usually set up during the transition phase of nulliparous women and during the active phase for multiparous women. (See Fig. 18-20 for an instrument table setup.) A radiant warmer for the newborn is turned on when crowning begins to occur in the nulliparous woman and when the multiparous woman is 8 to 9 cm dilated. If a traditional delivery room is used, a multiparous woman is usually transferred near the end of the first stage of labor. Transfer of the nulliparous woman takes place when the presenting part begins to distend the perineum between contractions during the second stage of labor (Fig. 18-16, *A*). Transfer to the delivery room is unnecessary in labor-delivery rooms (LDRs), labor-delivery-recovery-postpartum (LDRP) rooms, and birth centers.

Women in labor may use a whirlpool bath or Jacuzzi for the relaxing effects. Most authorities recommend that birth occur out of the water even though newborns do not begin to breathe until removed from the water. If birth occurs while in the water, the newborn should be removed immediately (Odent, 1997) (Fig. 18-17).

A

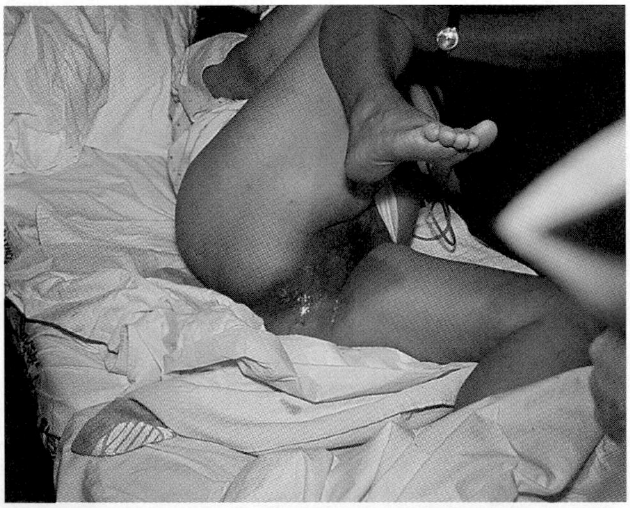

B

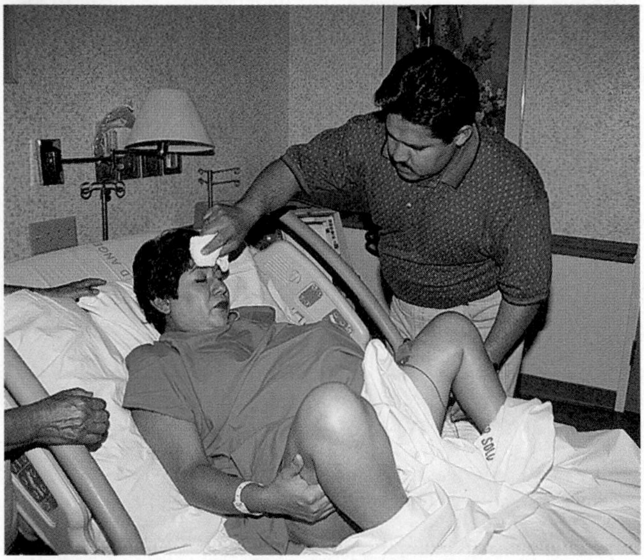

FIG. 18-16 • **A,** Pushing, side-lying position, perineal bulging. **B,** Pushing, semi-sitting. Partner wiping woman's face with cool cloth between contractions. (A, Courtesy Michael S. Clement, MD, Mesa, AZ; B, courtesy Marjorie Pyle, RNC, Lifecircle, Costa Mesa, CA.)

SECOND STAGE OF LABOR

The second stage of labor is the stage in which the infant is born. This stage begins with full cervical dilation (10 cm) and complete effacement (100%) and ends with the baby's birth. The force exerted by uterine contractions, gravity, and maternal bearing-down efforts facilitates achievement of the expected outcome of a spontaneous, uncomplicated, vaginal birth.

The second stage comprises three phases: latent, descent, and transition. These phases are characterized by maternal verbal and nonverbal behaviors, uterine activity, the urge to bear down, and fetal descent. The latent phase is a period of rest and relative calm. The woman is quiet and often relaxes with her eyes closed between contractions. The urge to bear down is not well established and is experienced primarily during the acme of a contraction. The descent phase is characterized by strong urges to bear down as the Ferguson reflex is activated by pressure of the presenting part on the stretch receptors of the pelvic floor. This stimulation causes the release of oxytocin from the posterior pituitary gland, which stimulates stronger, expulsive uterine contractions. The woman becomes more focused on bearing-down efforts, which become rhythmic. She changes positions frequently to find a more comfortable pushing position. The woman frequently announces the onset of contractions and becomes more vocal as she bears down. In the transition

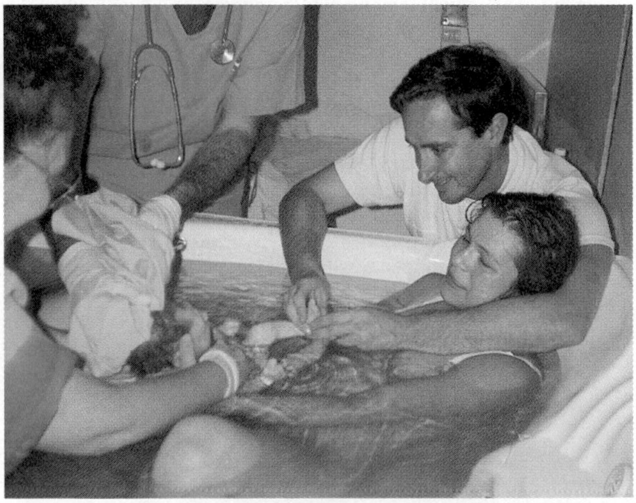

FIG. 18-17 • Waterbirth. (Courtesy Global Maternal/Child Health Association, Inc., Wilsonville, OR.)

phase the presenting part is on the perineum, and bearing-down efforts are most effective for promoting birth. The woman may be more verbal about pain, may scream or swear, and may act out of control. The nurse encourages the woman to "listen" to her body as she progresses through the phases of the second stage of labor. When a woman listens to her body to tell her when to bear down, her efforts become more effective.

If a woman is confined to bed in a recumbent position, the rhythmic urge to bear down is suppressed, since gravity is not being used to press the presenting part against the pelvic floor. Being moved to another room and placed on a delivery table in the lithotomy position, as has been the custom in North America for the past 30 years, also has an inhibiting effect on the urge to bear down. In most non-Western societies, labor and birth occur in the same room and women use various positions for labor, such as kneeling, sitting, standing, or squatting.

The only certain objective sign that the second stage of labor has begun is the inability to feel the cervix during vaginal examination, indicating that the cervix is fully dilated and effaced. Other signs that suggest the onset of the second stage include the following:

- Sudden appearance of perspiration on upper lip
- An episode of vomiting
- Increased bloody show
- Shaking of extremities
- Increased restlessness; verbalization that "I can't go on"
- Involuntary bearing-down efforts

These signs commonly appear at the time the cervix reaches full dilation (Scott et al, 1999). However, women with an epidural block may not exhibit such signs. Other indicators for each phase of the second stage are given in Tables 18-7 and 18-8.

Women can begin to experience an irresistible urge to bear down before full dilation. This is often related to the station of the presenting part below the level of the ischial spines of the maternal pelvis. Some health care providers believe that pushing the presenting part against a partially dilated cervix will result in cervical edema and damage. Research is needed to determine the consequences of pushing against a partially dilated cervix.

Assessment is continuous during the second stage of labor. Hospital protocol determines the specific type and timing of assessments as well as the way in which findings are documented. Signs and symptoms of impending birth (see Table 18-8) may appear unexpectedly, requiring immediate action by the nurse (Box 18-8).

Duration of Second Stage

The duration of the second stage is influenced by several factors such as the effectiveness of the primary and secondary powers

TABLE 18-7

Expected Maternal Progress in Second Stage of Labor

Criterion	Latent Phase (Average Duration, 10-30 min)	Descent Phase (Average Duration Varies)*	Transition Phase (Average Duration 5-15 min)
Contractions Magnitude (intensity)	Period of physiologic lull for all criteria; period of peace and rest	Significant increase	Overwhelmingly strong Expulsive
Frequency		2-2.5 min	1-2 min
Duration		90 sec	90 sec
Descent, station	0 to +2	Increases and Ferguson reflex† activated, +2 to +4	Rapid, +4 to birth Fetal head visible in introitus
Show: color and amount		Significant increase in dark red bloody show	Bloody show accompanies birth of head
Spontaneous bearing-down efforts	Slight to absent, except during acme of strongest contractions	Increased urge to bear down	Greatly increased
Vocalization	Quiet; concern over progress	Grunting sounds or expiratory vocalization; announces contractions	Grunting sounds and expiratory vocalizations continue; may scream or swear
Maternal behavior	Experiences sense of relief that transition to second stage is finished Feels fatigued and sleepy Feels a sense of accomplishment and optimism, because the "worst is over" Feels in control	Senses increased urge to push Alters respiratory pattern: has short 4 to 5 sec breath holds with regular breaths in between, 5 to 7 times per contraction Makes grunting sounds or expiratory vocalizations Frequent repositioning	Describes extreme pain Expresses feelings of powerlessness Shows decreased ability to listen or concentrate on anything but giving birth Describes *ring of fire* (burning sensation of acute pain as vagina stretches and fetal head crowns) Often shows excitement immediately after birth of head

From Anderhold K, Roberts J: Phases of second stage labor: four descriptive case studies, *J Nurse Midwifery* 36(5):267-275, 1991; Mahan C, McKay S: Are we overmanaging second stage labor? *Contemp OB/GYN* 24:37-63, 1984.

*Duration of descent phase can vary depending on maternal parity, effectiveness of bearing-down effort, and presence of spinal anesthesia or epidural analgesia.

†Pressure of presenting part on stretch receptors of pelvic floor stimulates release of oxytocin from posterior pituitary, resulting in more intense uterine contractions.

TABLE 18-8
Woman's Responses and Support Person's Action During Second Stage of Labor

Woman's Responses	Nurse/Support Person's Actions*
LATENT PHASE	
Experiences a short period of peace and rest	Encourages woman to "listen" to her body Continues support measures Suggests an upright position to encourage progression of descent if descent phase does not begin after 20 min
DESCENT PHASE	
Senses increased urgency to bear down as Ferguson reflex is activated Notes increase in intensity of uterine contractions—alters respiratory pattern: short 4- to 5-sec breath holds, 5 to 7 times per contraction Makes grunting sounds or expiratory vocalizations	Encourages respiratory pattern of short breath holds Stresses normality and benefits of grunting sounds and expiratory vocalizations Encourages bearing-down efforts with urge to push Encourages/suggests maternal movement and position changes (upright, if descent is not occurring) Encourages woman to "listen" to her body regarding movement and position change if descent is occurring Discourages long breath holds If birth is to occur in a delivery room, transfers woman to delivery room early to avoid rushing or, if permitted, offers her option of walking to delivery room Places woman in lateral recumbent position to slow descent if descent is too fast
TRANSITIONAL PHASE	
Behaves in manner similar to behavior during transition in first stage (8-10 cm) Experiences a sense of severe pain and powerlessness Shows decreased ability to listen Concentrates on birth of baby until head is born Experiences contractions as overwhelming in intensity Reports feeling ring of fire as head crowns Maintains respiratory pattern of three to five 7-sec breath holds per contraction, followed by forced expiration Eases head out with short expirations Responds with excitement and relief after head is born	Encourages slow, gentle pushing Explains that "blowing-away the contraction" facilitates a slower birth of the head Provides mirror to help woman see or touch the emerging fetal head (best to extend over two to three contractions) to help her understand the perinatal sensations Coaches woman to relax mouth, throat, and neck to promote relaxation of pelvic floor Applies warm compress to perineum to promote relaxation

*Provided by nurses and support persons in collaboration with the nurse.

of labor; the type and amount of analgesia or anesthesia used; the physical and emotional condition, position, activity level, and parity of the laboring woman; and the nature and source of support the woman receives. For many multiparous women, birth occurs within minutes of complete dilation, perhaps only one push later. Nulliparous women usually push for 1 to 2 hours before giving birth. If the woman has been given epidural anesthesia, pushing can last more than 2 hours.

Epidural analgesia blocks or reduces the urge to bear down and limits the woman's ability to attain an upright position to push. By adjusting dosages to the lowest effective level, allowing the epidural to wear off, or using mixtures containing a narcotic and a local anesthetic, the woman is able to more fully perceive the urge to bear down, to move more freely, and to attain an upright position. This enhances the ability to bear down effectively and achieve an uncomplicated vaginal birth (Shermer and Raines, 1997).

Commonly, a second stage of more than 2 hours in a first pregnancy and 1½ hours in subsequent pregnancies is considered prolonged in women without regional analgesia and is reported to the physician or nurse-midwife. However, the American College of Obstetricians and Gynecologists (ACOG, 1994) supports efforts to place less emphasis on a defined time limit. Using assessment tools such as the FHR and pattern, the descent of the presenting part, the quality of the uterine contractions, and status of the woman, a fetus who is not tolerating labor can be identified and premature intervention with episiotomies, forceps- and vacuum-assisted birth can be avoided.

If the status of the maternal-fetal unit is reassuring and progress is continuing, interventions to end the second stage of labor are unwarranted. The duration of active pushing is more relevant to the newborn's condition at birth than the duration of the second stage of labor itself (d'Entremont, 1996; Peterson and Besuner, 1997; Roberts and Woolley, 1996).

The nurse continues to monitor the FHR and the events of the second stage and provide comfort measures for the mother such as positioning; providing mouth care; maintaining clean, dry bedding; and removing extraneous noise, conversation, or other distractions (e.g., laughing and talking by attending personnel in or outside the labor area). The woman is encouraged

Box 18-8

Guidelines for Assistance at the Emergency Birth of a Fetus in the Vertex Presentation

1. The woman usually assumes the position most comfortable for her. A lateral position is often recommended.
2. Reassure the woman that birth is usually uncomplicated and easy in these situations. Use eye-to-eye contact and a calm, relaxed manner. If there is someone else available, such as the partner, that person could help support the woman in the position, assist with coaching, and compliment her on her efforts.
3. Wash your hands and put on gloves, if available.
4. Place under woman's buttocks whatever clean material is available.
5. Avoid touching the vaginal area to decrease the possibility of infection.
6. As the head begins to crown, you should do the following:
   a. Tear the amniotic membrane if it is still intact.
   b. Instruct the woman to pant or pant-blow, thus minimizing the urge to push.
   c. Place the flat side of your hand on the exposed fetal head and apply *gentle* pressure toward the vagina to prevent the head from "popping out." The mother may participate by placing her hand under yours on the emerging head. Note: Rapid delivery of the fetal head must be prevented because a rapid change of pressure within the molded fetal skull follows, which may result in dural or subdural tears and may cause vaginal or perineal lacerations.
7. After the birth of the head, check for the umbilical cord. If the cord is around the baby's neck, try to slip it over the baby's head or pull it *gently* to get some slack so that you can slip it over the shoulders.
8. Support the fetal head as restitution (external rotation) occurs. After restitution, with one hand on each side of the baby's head, exert *gentle* pressure downward so that the anterior shoulder emerges under the symphysis pubis and acts as a fulcrum; then, as *gentle* pressure is exerted in the opposite direction, the posterior shoulder, which has passed over the sacrum and coccyx, emerges.
9. Be alert! Hold the baby securely because the rest of the body may emerge quickly. The baby will be slippery!
10. Cradle the baby's head and back in one hand and the buttocks in the other. Keep the head down to drain away the mucus. Use a bulb syringe, if one is available, to remove mucus from the baby's mouth.
11. Dry the baby quickly to prevent rapid heat loss. Keep the baby at the same level as the mother's uterus until the end of the cord stops pulsating. Note: It is important to keep the baby at the same level as the mother's uterus to prevent the baby's blood from flowing to or from the placenta and the resultant hypovolemia or hypervolemia. Also, do not "milk" the cord.
12. Place the baby on the mother's abdomen, cover the baby (remember to keep the head warm, too) with the mother's clothing, and have her cuddle the baby. Compliment her (them) on a job well done, and on the baby, if appropriate.
13. *Wait* for the placenta to separate; *do not* tug on the cord. Note: Injudicious traction may tear the cord, separate the placenta, or invert the uterus. Signs of placental separation include a slight gush of dark blood from the introitus, lengthening of the cord, and change in the uterine contour from a discoid to globular shape.
14. Instruct the mother to push to deliver the separated placenta. Gently ease out the placental membranes using an up-and-down motion until the membranes are removed. If birth occurs outside a hospital setting, to minimize complications, do not cut the cord without proper clamps and a sterile cutting tool. Inspect the placenta for intactness. Place the baby on the placenta and wrap the two together for additional warmth.
15. Check the firmness of the uterus. Gently massage the fundus and demonstrate to the mother how she can massage her own fundus properly.
16. If supplies are available, clean the mother's perineal area and apply a peripad.
17. In addition to gentle massage of the fundus, the following measures can be taken to prevent or minimize hemorrhage:
   a. Put the baby to the mother's breast as soon as possible. Sucking or nuzzling and licking the nipple stimulates the release of oxytocin from the posterior pituitary. Note: If the baby does not or cannot nurse, manually stimulate the mother's nipples.
   b. Do not allow the mother's bladder to become distended. Assess the bladder for fullness and encourage her to void if fullness is found.
   c. Expel any clots from the mother's uterus.
18. Comfort or reassure the mother and her family or friends. Keep the mother and the baby warm. Give her fluids if available and tolerated.
19. If this is a multifetal birth, identify the infants in order of birth (using letters *A, B,* etc.).
20. Make notations regarding the following aspects of the birth:
   a. Fetal presentation and position
   b. Presence of cord around neck (nuchal cord) or other parts and number of times cord encircled part
   c. Color, character, and amount of amniotic fluid, if rupture of membranes occurs immediately before birth
   d. Time of birth
   e. Estimated time of determination of Apgar score (e.g., 1 and 5 minutes after birth), resuscitation efforts implemented, and ultimate condition of baby
   f. Sex of baby
   g. Time of placental expulsion, as well as the appearance and completeness of the placenta
   h. Maternal condition: affect, amount of bleeding, and status of uterine tonicity
   i. Any unusual occurrences during the birth (e.g., maternal or paternal response, verbalizations, or gestures in response to birth of baby)

to indicate other support measures she would like (see Table 18-6 and Nursing Care Plan on pp. 386-387).

Maternal Position

There is no single position for childbirth. Labor is a dynamic, interactive process involving the woman's uterus, pelvis, and voluntary muscles. In addition, angles between the baby and the woman's pelvis constantly change as the fetus turns and flexes down the birth canal. The woman may want to assume various positions for childbirth, and she should be encouraged and assisted in attaining and maintaining her positions of choice. Hanson (1998a) found that sitting and side lying are the two most common positions assumed by women for their bearing-down efforts and birth.

Birth attendants play a major role in influencing a woman's choice of position for birth, with midwives tending to advocate the nonlithotomy positions for the second stage of labor (Hanson, 1998b). Upright positions facilitate birth in the following ways:

- Straighten the longitudinal axis of the birth canal
- Use gravity to direct the fetal head toward the pelvic inlet, thereby facilitating descent
- Enlarge pelvic dimensions and restrict the encroachment of the sacrum and coccyx into the pelvic inlet
- Increase uteroplacental circulation, resulting in more intense, efficient uterine contractions
- Enhance the woman's ability to bear down effectively, thereby minimizing maternal exhaustion (Shermer and Raines, 1997)

Squatting is highly effective in facilitating the descent and birth of the fetus (Roberts and Woolley, 1996). Women should assume a modified, supported squat until the fetal head is engaged, at which time a deep squat can be used. A firm surface is required, and the woman will need side support. A birth ball can help a woman maintain the squatting position. In a birthing bed a squat bar is available for the woman to use to support herself.

When a woman uses the standing position for bearing down, her weight is borne on both femoral heads, allowing the pressure in the acetabulum to increase the transverse diameter of the pelvic outlet by up to 1 cm. This can be helpful if descent of the head is delayed because the occiput has not rotated from the lateral (transverse diameter of pelvis) to the anterior position (Biancuzzo, 1993). Birthing chairs/stools or rocking chairs may be used to provide women with a good physiologic position to enhance bearing-down efforts during childbirth. The upright position allows the mother to see the birth as it occurs and to maintain eye contact with the attendant. Most birthing chairs are designed so that if an emergency occurs, the chair can be adjusted to the horizontal or Trendelenburg position.

Oversized beanbag chairs and large floor pillows may be used for both labor and birth. They can mold around and support the mother in whatever position she selects.

Women may want to sit on the toilet to push because they are concerned about stool incontinence during this stage. They must be closely monitored and removed from the toilet before birth is imminent.

Because sitting on chairs, stools, toilets, or commodes can increase perineal edema and blood loss, it is important to assist the woman to change her position every 10 to 15 minutes (Shermer and Raines, 1997).

Side-lying is an effective position for the second stage, with the upper part of the woman's leg held by the nurse or coach or placed on a pillow (see Fig. 18-16, *A*). Some women prefer a semisitting position. To maintain good uteroplacental circulation and to enhance the woman's bearing-down efforts in this position, the woman's back and shoulders should be elevated to at least a 30-degree angle and a wedge should be placed under one hip (see Fig. 18-16, *B*)

The hands-and-knees position is an effective position for birth because it enhances placental perfusion, helps rotate a fetus from a posterior to an anterior position, and may facilitate the birth of the shoulders, especially if the fetus is large. Perineal trauma may also be reduced.

The nurse should frequently assess the effect of maternal positions on fetal status. If the woman is reluctant or afraid to try different positions, the nurse can actively encourage and assist the woman to do so. Information regarding the variety of effective childbirth positions should be an essential component of prepared childbirth classes.

The birthing bed is commonly used today and can be set for different positions according to the woman's needs (Figs. 18-18 and 18-19). The woman can squat, kneel, sit, recline, or lie on her side, choosing the position most comfortable for her without having to climb into bed for the birth. At the same time, there is excellent exposure for examination, electrode placement, and birth. Squat bars, over-the-bed tables, birth balls, and pillows can be used for support. The bed can be positioned for the administration of anesthesia and can be used to transport the woman to the operating room if a cesarean birth is necessary.

Bearing-Down Efforts. As the fetal head reaches the pelvic floor, most women experience the urge to bear down. Reflexively the woman will begin to exert downward pressure by contracting her abdominal muscles while relaxing her pelvic floor. This bearing down is an involuntary response to the

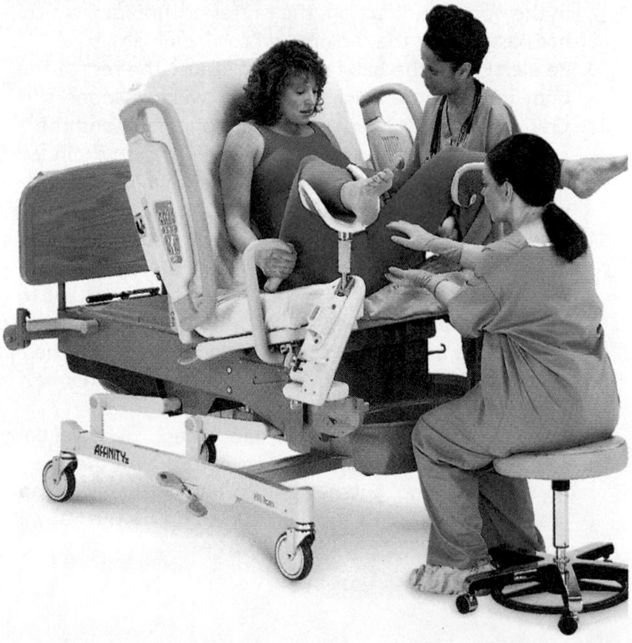

FIG. 18-18 • Birth bed. (Courtesy Hill-Rom, Batesville, IN.)

Ferguson reflex, which is activated by the pressure of the presenting part on stretch receptors of the pelvic musculature.

A strong expiratory grunt (vocalization) often accompanies pushing when the woman exhales as she pushes. This natural vocalization by women during open-glottis bearing-down efforts is likely to be discouraged by nurses in part to "conserve the woman's energy" but also as a result of concern that it will seem to other nurses and patients that the woman has lost control or the nurse has lost control of her patient (Peterson and Besuner, 1997).

When coaching women to push, the nurse should encourage them to push as they feel like pushing (i.e., instinctive, spontaneous pushing) rather than to give a prolonged push on command (Thomson, 1993), and encourage them to vocalize. The nurse monitors the woman's breathing so that the woman does not hold her breath for more than 5 to 7 seconds at a time (Hodnett, 1996; Roberts and Woolley, 1996). Bearing down while exhaling (open-glottis pushing) and taking breaths between bearing-down efforts help maintain adequate oxygen levels for the mother and fetus. Women who use spontaneous pushing are less likely to have second- or third-degree perineal lacerations or episiotomies (Sampselle and Hines, 1999).

Prolonged breath-holding, or sustained, directed bearing down (still a common practice) may trigger the Valsalva maneuver. This maneuver occurs when the woman closes the glottis (closed-glottis pushing), thereby increasing intrathoracic and cardiovascular pressure. This approach to bearing down is harmful or ineffective and should be discouraged (Enkin et al, 1995; Technical Working Group of the World Health Organization, 1997).

Women who receive epidural analgesia during labor often experience difficulty pushing because of a decreased bearing down reflex (Mayberry et al, 1999/2000). Delayed pushing, that is, waiting for fetal descent prior to initiating directed pushing, results in shorter periods of pushing, less fatigue, fewer variable heart rate decelerations, and similar Apgar scores as compared to women who are directed to begin pushing when dilation is complete (reported in Mayberry et al, 1999/2000).

A woman may reach the second stage of labor and then experience a lack of readiness to complete the process and give birth to her child. McKay and Barrows (1991) identified several factors that may inhibit the woman's voluntary bearing-down efforts. These factors include the following:

- Doubts about her readiness to be a mother
- Reluctance to care for another baby
- Desire to wait for support person or physician or midwife to arrive
- Fear or anxiety regarding the unfamiliar or painful sensations of the second stage of labor and pushing
- Embarrassment regarding behaviors during pushing, including sounds made and passage of stool
- Giving up and not wanting to proceed any further toward vaginal birth
- Fear that the baby will be in danger once it emerges from the protective intrauterine environment

By recognizing that a woman may experience a need to hold back the birth of her baby, the nurse can address the woman's concerns and effectively coach her through this stage of labor.

To ensure slow birth of the fetal head, the nurse should encourage the woman to control the urge to bear down by coaching her to take panting breaths or to exhale slowly through pursed lips as the baby's head crowns. At this point, the woman needs simple, clear directions from one person.

Amnesia between contractions is often pronounced in the second stage, and the woman may have to be roused to cooperate in the bearing-down process. Parents who have attended childbirth education classes may have devised a set of verbal cues for the laboring woman to follow. It is helpful to have these cues printed on a card that can be attached to the head of the bed so that the nurse can better substitute as coach if the partner has to leave.

Fetal Heart Rate and Pattern. As noted previously, the FHR must be checked. If the rate begins to slow or if there is a loss of variability, prompt treatment must be initiated. The woman can be turned on her side to reduce the pressure of the uterus against the ascending vena cava and descending aorta,

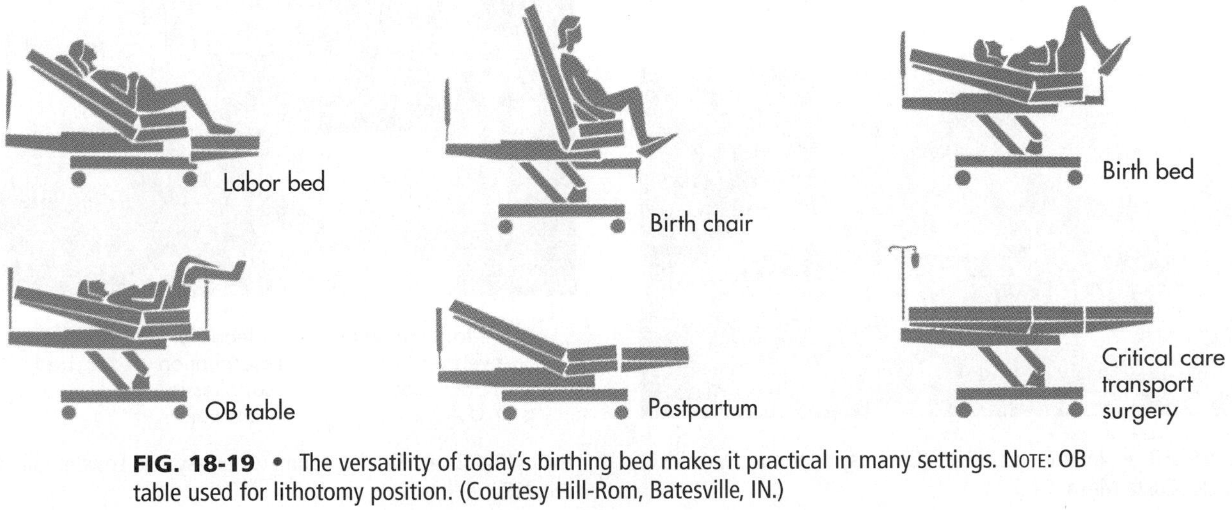

FIG. 18-19 • The versatility of today's birthing bed makes it practical in many settings. NOTE: OB table used for lithotomy position. (Courtesy Hill-Rom, Batesville, IN.)

and oxygen can be administered by mask at 8 to 10 L/min. This is often all that is required to restore the normal rate. If the FHR does not return to a normal rate immediately, the physician or nurse-midwife should be notified quickly because medical intervention may be indicated to hasten birth.

LEGAL TIP • Documentation Documentation of all observations (e.g., maternal vital signs, FHR and pattern, progress of labor) and nursing interventions, including patient response, should be done concurrently with care. The course of labor and maternal-fetal response may change without warning. It is important that all documentation be accurate, complete, and timely, and according to agency policy.

Supplies, Instruments, and Equipment. To prepare for birth in any setting, the birthing table or case cart is usually set up during the transition phase for nulliparous women and during the active phase for multiparous women.

The birthing table is prepared, and instruments are arranged on the instrument table (Fig. 18-20). Standard procedures are followed for gloving, identifying and opening sterile packages, adding sterile supplies to the instrument table, and unwrapping and handing sterile instruments to the physician or nurse-midwife. The crib and equipment are readied for the support and stabilization of the infant. A radiant warmer for the newborn is turned on when crowning begins to occur in the nulliparous woman and when the multiparous woman is 8 to 9 cm dilated.

The items used for birth may vary among different facilities; therefore each facility's procedure manual should be consulted to determine the protocols specific to that facility.

The nurse estimates the time until the birth will occur and notifies the physician or nurse-midwife if he or she is not in the room. Even the most experienced nurse can miscalculate the time left before birth occurs; thus, every nurse who attends a woman in labor must be prepared to assist with an emergency birth if the physician or nurse-midwife is not present (see Box 18-8).

Birth in a Delivery Room or Birthing Room

The woman will need assistance if she must move from the labor bed to the delivery table (Fig. 18-21). The woman can help if this is done between contractions, but because of her awkwardness, she cannot be rushed. In a birthing room, no such transfer is necessary (Fig. 18-22).

The various positions assumed for birth in a delivery room are the Sims position (in which the attendant will need to support the upper part of the woman's leg), the dorsal position, and the lithotomy position.

The lithotomy position has been the position most commonly used for birth in Western cultures, although this practice is changing slowly. The lithotomy position makes it more convenient for the physician or nurse-midwife to deal with any complications that arise. To place the woman in this position, her buttocks are brought to the edge of the table and her legs are placed in stirrups. Care must be taken to pad the stirrups, to raise and place both legs simultaneously, and to adjust the

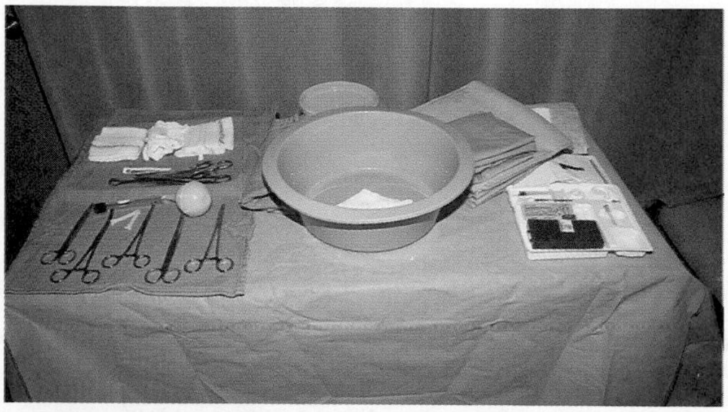

FIG. 18-20 • Instrument table. (Courtesy Marjorie Pyle, RNC, Lifecircle, Costa Mesa, CA.)

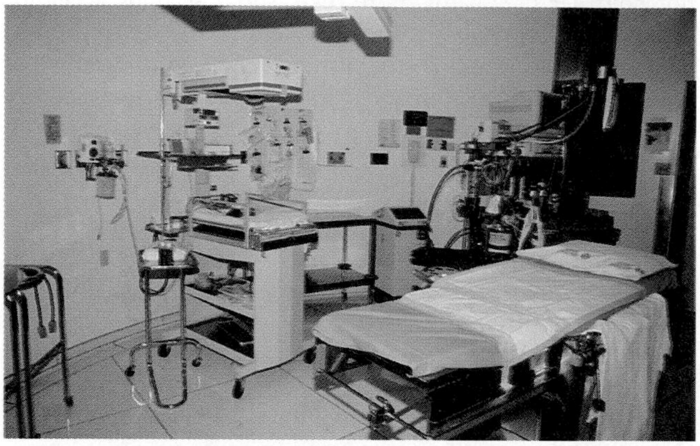

FIG. 18-21 • Delivery room. (Courtesy Michael S. Clement, MD, Mesa, AZ.)

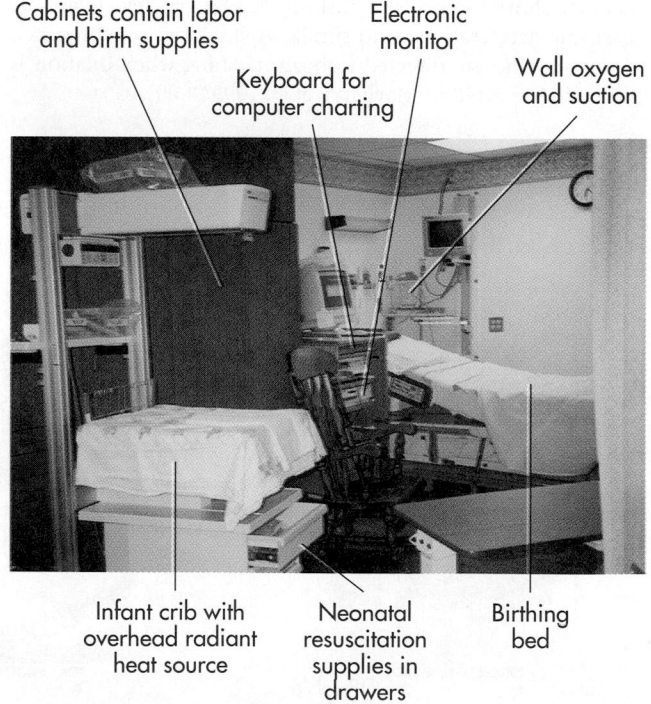

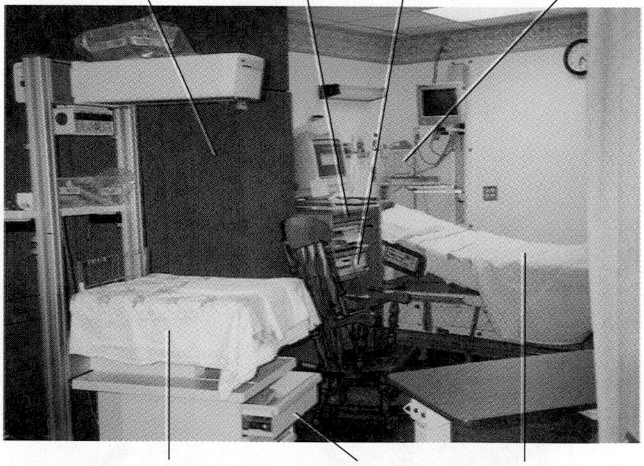

FIG. 18-22 • Birthing room. (Courtesy Dee Lowdermilk, Chapel Hill, NC.)

shanks of the stirrups so that the calves of the legs are supported. There should be no pressure on the popliteal space. If the stirrups are not the same height, ligaments in the woman's back can be strained as she bears down, leading to considerable discomfort in the postpartum period. The lower portion of the table may be dropped down and rolled back under the table.

It should be noted that the routine use of a supine or lithotomy position for labor and birth has been identified as a clearly harmful or ineffective practice and should be discouraged (Enkin et al, 1995; Technical Working Group of the World Health Organization, 1997).

Birth in an LDR or LDRP Room

The maternal position for birth varies from a lithotomy position with the woman's legs in stirrups; to one in which her feet rest on footrests while she holds onto a squat bar; to a side-lying position with the woman's upper leg supported by the coach, nurse, or squat bar. The foot of the bed can be removed so that the physician or nurse-midwife attending the birth can gain better perineal access for performing an episiotomy, delivering a large baby, or getting access to the emerging head to facilitate suctioning. Otherwise the foot of the bed is left in place and lowered slightly to form a ledge that allows access for birth and that also serves as a place to lay the newborn.

Once the woman is positioned for birth, the vulva and perineum are cleansed. Hospital protocols and preferences of the physician or nurse-midwife for cleansing may vary and can involve washing the area thoroughly with warm soapy water or a soapy povidone-iodine (Betadine) solution and then rinsing the area. Next the area may be sprayed with a disinfectant to prevent bacterial growth.

The circulating nurse (usually the same nurse as the labor nurse) continues to coach and encourage the woman. The nurse auscultates the FHR or checks the electronic monitor tracing every 5 to 15 minutes, depending on whether the woman is at low or high risk for problems or per protocol. She keeps the physician or nurse-midwife informed of the rate and pattern of the FHR (Tucker, 2000). The equipment for measuring blood pressure should be readied for instant use should signs of shock develop. Blood pressure readings taken while the woman pushes will be distorted (increased) by the increase in thoracic and abdominal pressures. A reading is obtained after birth before the woman is transferred to the recovery room. An oxytocic medication such as Pitocin may be prepared so that it is ready to administer after expulsion of the placenta. Standard Precautions should always be followed while care is administered during the process of labor and birth (see Box 18-4).

The physician or nurse-midwife puts on a cap, a mask that has a shield or protective eyewear, and shoe covers. Hands are then scrubbed and a sterile gown (with waterproof front and sleeves) and gloves are put on. Nurses attending the birth may also need to wear caps, protective eyewear, masks, gowns, and gloves. The woman may then be draped with sterile sheets and towels. The partner can help the woman remember not to touch the sterile drapes.

Nursing contact with the parents is maintained by touching, verbal comforting, explaining the reasons for care, and sharing the parents' joy at the birth of their child.

Mechanism of Birth: Vertex Presentation

The three phases of spontaneous birth of a fetus in a vertex presentation are (1) birth of the head, (2) birth of the shoulders, and (3) birth of the body and extremities (see Chapter 15).

With voluntary pushing, the head can be seen at the introitus (Fig. 18-23). Crowning occurs when the widest part of the head (the biparietal diameter) distends the vulva just before birth.

Prevention of Meconium Aspiration. If meconium has been present in the amniotic fluid during labor, a DeLee suction apparatus is placed on the sterile field and preparations are made for wall suction. Fluids are withdrawn from the infant's mouth and nose before the first breath is taken to prevent meconium aspiration. The primary health care provider should refrain from using the DeLee device with oral suction to withdraw fluid from the infant unless the suction device is designed to keep mucus from entering the user's airway.

The time of birth is the precise time when the entire body is out of the mother. This time must be noted on the record.

If the condition of the newborn is not compromised, it may be placed on the mother's abdomen immediately after birth and covered with a warm, dry blanket. The cord may be clamped at this time, and the physician or nurse-midwife may ask if the

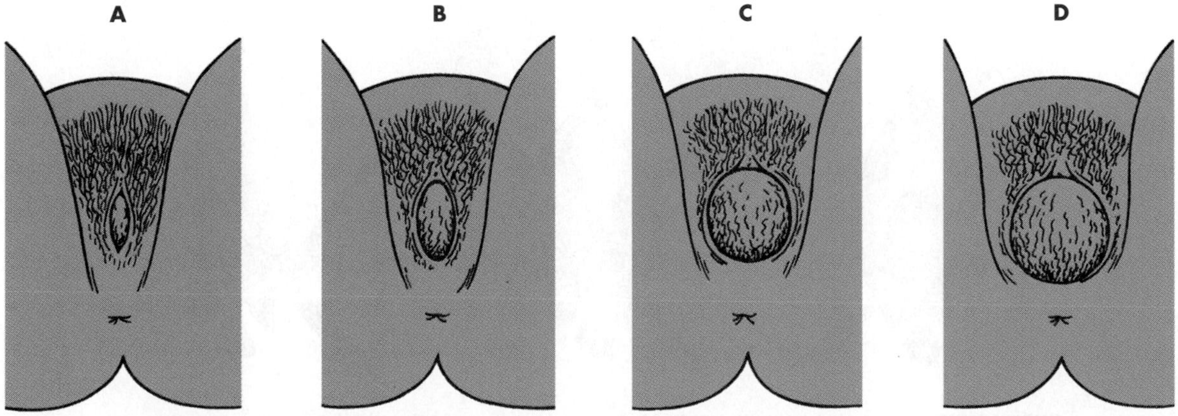

FIG. 18-23 • Beginning birth with vertex presenting. **A,** Anteroposterior slit. **B,** Oval opening. **C,** Circular shape, **D,** Crowning.

woman's partner would like to cut the cord. If so, the partner is given a sterile pair of scissors and instructed to cut the cord 1 inch (2.5 cm) above the clamp.

Use of Fundal Pressure. Fundal pressure is the application of gentle, steady pressure against the fundus of the uterus to facilitate vaginal birth. Historically it has been used when the administration of analgesia and anesthesia decreased the woman's ability to push during the birth, in cases of shoulder dystocia, and when second-stage fetal bradycardia or other nonreassuring FHR pattern was present. Use of fundal pressure by the nurse is not advised because there is no standard technique available for this maneuver and no current legal, professional, or regulatory standards for its use exist. In cases of shoulder dystocia, the all-fours position (the Gaskin maneuver) (Bruner et al, 1998), suprapubic pressure, and maternal position changes are among the recommended interventions (Cosner, 1996; Piper and McDonald, 1994).

Immediate Assessment and Care of the Newborn

Care given immediately after the birth focuses on assessing and stabilizing the newborn. The nurse's primary responsibility at this time is the infant, because the physician or nurse-midwife is involved with the expulsion of the placenta and care of the mother. The nurse must watch the infant for signs of distress and initiate appropriate interventions should these appear.

A brief assessment of the infant can be performed while the mother is holding him or her. This includes checking the infant's airway and Apgar score. Maintaining a patent airway, supporting respiratory effort, and preventing cold stress by drying and covering the newborn with a warm blanket or placing him or her under a radiant warmer are the major priorities for the newborn's immediate care. Further examination, identification procedures, and care can be postponed until later in the third stage of labor or early in the fourth stage.

Perineal Trauma Related to Childbirth

Lacerations. Most acute injuries and lacerations of the perineum, vagina, uterus, and their support tissues occur during childbirth. Some injuries to the supporting tissues, whether they were acute or nonacute and whether they were repaired or not, may lead to gynecologic problems later in life (e.g., pelvic relaxation, uterine prolapse, cystocele, and rectocele). Immediate repair promotes healing, limits residual damage, and decreases the possibility of infection.

The tendency to sustain lacerations varies with each woman; that is, the soft tissue in some women may be less distensible. Heredity may be a factor in this. For example, the tissue of light-skinned women, especially those with reddish hair, is not as readily distensible as that of darker-skinned women, and healing may be less efficient.

Perineal Lacerations. Perineal lacerations usually occur when the fetal head is being born. The extent of the laceration is defined in terms of its depth:

First degree—Laceration extends through the skin and structures superficial to muscles

Second degree—Laceration extends through muscles of perineal body

Third degree—Laceration continues through anal sphincter muscle

Fourth degree—Laceration also involves the anterior rectal wall

Perineal injury is often accompanied by small lacerations on the medial surfaces of the labia minora below the pubic rami and to the sides of the urethra and clitoris. Lacerations in this very vascular area often result in profuse bleeding; such lacerations must be repaired with absorbable suture (Fig. 18-24).

Special attention must be paid to third- and fourth-degree lacerations so that the woman retains fecal continence. Measures are taken to promote soft stools for a few days to increase the woman's comfort and to foster healing. Antimicrobial therapy may be used in some cases.

Vaginal and Urethral Lacerations. Vaginal lacerations often occur in conjunction with perineal lacerations. Vaginal lacerations tend to extend up the lateral walls (sulci) and, if deep enough, involve the levator ani. Additional injury may occur high in the vaginal vault near the level of the ischial spines. Vaginal vault lacerations may be circular and may result from forceps rotation, especially in the presence of cephalopelvic disproportion, rapid fetal descent, or precipitous birth. Lacerations can also occur around the urethra (periurethral) and in the area of the clitoris.

Cervical Injuries. Cervical injuries occur when the cervix retracts over the advancing fetal head. These cervical lacerations occur at the lateral angles of the external os; most are shallow, and bleeding is minimal. Larger lacerations may extend

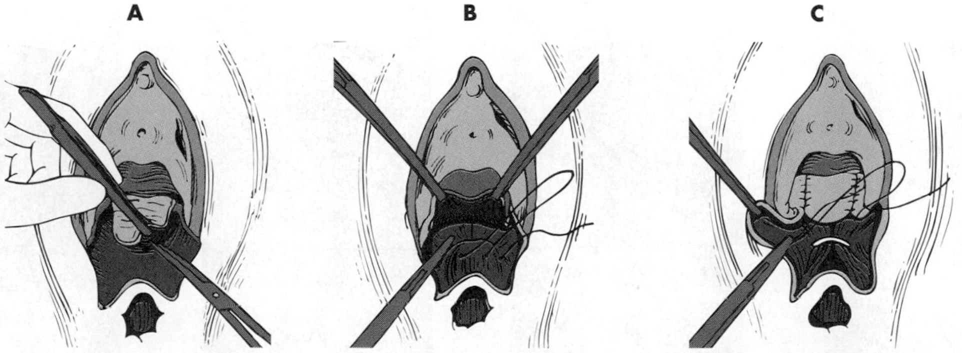

FIG. 18-24 • Perineal lacerations. **A,** Bilateral sulcus tears, periurethral tear, and separation of anal sphincter. **B,** Exposure and approximation of levator ani structures. **C,** Approximation of torn bulbocavernous muscle.

to the vaginal vault or beyond the vault into the lower uterine segment; serious bleeding may occur. Extensive lacerations may follow hasty attempts to enlarge the cervical opening artificially or to deliver the fetus before full cervical dilation is achieved. Injuries to the cervix can have adverse effects on future pregnancies and childbirths.

Episiotomy. An episiotomy is an incision made in the perineum to enlarge the vaginal outlet. It is performed more commonly in the United States and Canada than in Europe. Because the side-lying position causes less tension on the perineum, making it possible for a gradual stretching of the perineum, with this position there are fewer indications for the use of episiotomies. There is clear evidence that routine or liberal performance of an episiotomy for birth is a form of care that is likely to be harmful or ineffective (Enkin et al, 1995). Currently, the practice in many settings is to manually support the perineum during birth and allow the perineum to tear rather than perform an episiotomy. Tears are often smaller than an episiotomy, are repaired easily, and heal quickly. The rate of episiotomies is lower when nurse-midwives rather than obstetricians attend births.

Alternative measures for perineal management, such as warm compresses, manual support, and massage, have been shown to reduce, to varying degrees, the incidence of episiotomies, but further research is recommended (Albers et al, 1996; Lydon-Rochelle, Albers, and Teaf, 1995; Renfrew et al, 1998).

The type of episiotomy is designated by the site and direction of the incision (Fig. 18-25). Midline (median) episiotomy is most commonly used in the United States. It is effective, easily repaired, and generally the least painful. However, it can extend through the rectal sphincter (third-degree laceration/extension) or even into the anal canal (fourth-degree laceration/extension). Sphincter tone is usually restored following primary healing and a good repair.

Mediolateral episiotomy is used in operative births when the need for posterior extension is likely. Although a fourth-degree laceration may be prevented, a third-degree laceration may occur. Also, the blood loss is greater and the repair more difficult and painful than with midline episiotomies.

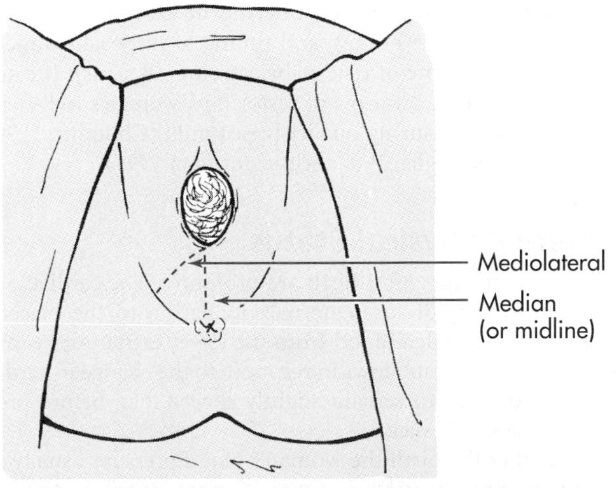

FIG. 18-25 • Types of episiotomies.

Emergency Childbirth

Even under the best of circumstances there probably will come a time when the perinatal nurse will be required to assist with the birth of an infant without medical assistance. Since it is neither possible nor desirable to prevent an impending birth, the perinatal nurse must be able to function independently and be skilled in the safe birth of a vertex fetus (see Box 18-8).

A lateral Sims posture may be the position of choice for birth when (1) the birth is progressing rapidly and there is insufficient time for slow distention of the perineum; (2) the fetal head seems too large to pass through the introitus without laceration, and episiotomy is not possible; or (3) the apparent size of the fetus is consistent with possible shoulder dystocia. In the lateral Sims position, less stress is placed on the perineum and better visualization of the perineum is possible as the upper leg is supported by the woman's partner or the nurse (see Fig. 18-16, *A*). In the event of shoulder dystocia, lateral Sims position increases the space needed for birth.

THIRD STAGE OF LABOR

The third stage of labor lasts from the birth of the baby until the delivery of the placenta. The goal in the management of the third stage of labor is the prompt separation and expulsion of the placenta, achieved in the easiest, safest manner.

The placenta is attached to the decidual layer of the basal plate's thin endometrium by numerous, randomized, fibrous anchor villi—much like a postage stamp is attached to a sheet of postage stamps. After the birth of the fetus, strong uterine contractions occur that cause the placental site to shrink markedly. This causes the anchor villi to break and the placenta to separate from its attachments. Normally the first few strong contractions 5 to 7 minutes after the baby's birth cause the placenta to be sheared from the basal plate. A placenta cannot detach itself from a flaccid (relaxed) uterus because the placental site is not reduced in size.

Placental separation is indicated by the following signs (Fig. 18-26):

- A firmly contracting fundus
- A change in the uterus from a discoid to a globular ovoid shape as the placenta moves into the lower uterine segment
- A sudden gush of dark blood from the introitus
- Apparent lengthening of the umbilical cord as the placenta draws closer to the introitus
- The finding of vaginal fullness (the placenta) on vaginal or rectal examination, or of fetal membranes at the introitus

Whether the placenta first appears by its shiny fetal surface (Schultze mechanism) or turns to show its dark roughened maternal surface (Duncan mechanism) is of no clinical importance. After the placenta and the amniotic membranes emerge, the physician or nurse-midwife examines them for intactness to ensure that no portion remains in the uterine cavity (i.e., no fragments of the placenta or membranes are retained) (Fig. 18-27).

Some women and their families may have culturally based beliefs regarding the care of the placenta and the manner of its disposal after birth, viewing the care and disposal of the placenta as a way of protecting the newborn from bad luck and illness. Requests by the woman to take the placenta home and dis-

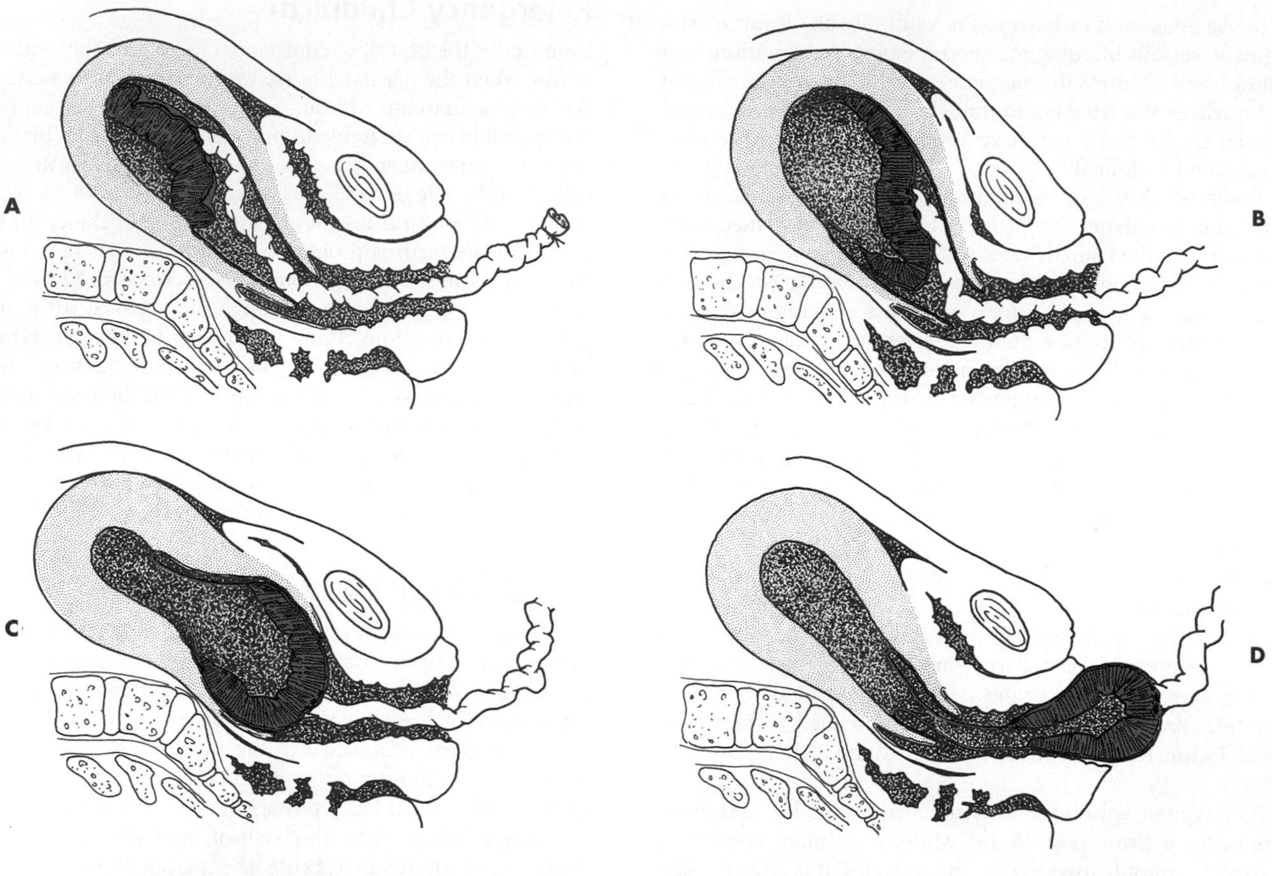

FIG. 18-26 • Third stage of labor. **A,** Placenta begins the separation process in central portion with retroplacental bleeding. Uterus changes from discoid to globular shape. **B,** Placenta completes separation and enters lower uterine segment. Uterus is globular in shape. **C,** Placenta enters vagina, cord is seen to lengthen, and there may be increased bleeding. **D,** Expulsion (birth) of placenta and completion of third stage.

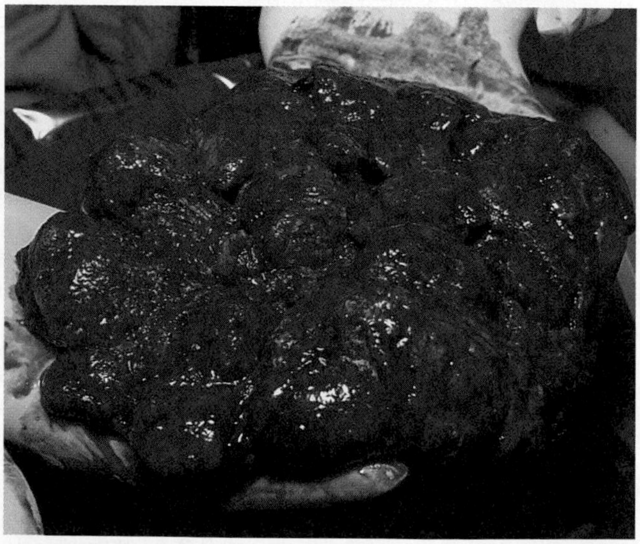

FIG. 18-27 • Examination of the placenta. (Courtesy Michael S. Clement, MD, Mesa, AZ.)

pose of it according to her customs may be at odds with health care agency policies, especially those related to infection control and the disposal of biologic wastes. Many cultures follow specific rules regarding the disposal of the placenta in terms of method (e.g., burning, drying, burying, or eating); site for disposal (in or near the home); and timing of disposal (immediately after birth, time of day, or by astrological signs). If eaten, the placenta can be a means of restoring a woman's well-being after birth or of ensuring quality breast milk (Choudhry, 1997; Howard and Berbiglia, 1997; Schneiderman, 1998).

Maternal Physical Status

Physiologic changes after birth are profound. The cardiac output increases rapidly as maternal circulation to the placenta ceases and the pooled blood from the lower extremities is mobilized. The pulse rate slows in response to the change in cardiac output and tends to remain slightly slower than before pregnancy for about 1 week.

Soon after the birth the woman's blood pressure usually returns to prepregnancy levels. Several factors contribute to an elevated blood pressure at this time: the excitement of the second stage, certain medications, and the time of day (blood pressure is highest during the late afternoon). Analgesics and anesthetics may also cause hypotension to develop in the hour after birth.

The major risk for women during the third stage of labor is postpartum hemorrhage. While the physician or nurse-midwife completes the delivery of the placenta, the nurse observes the mother for signs of excessive blood loss, including alteration in vital signs, pallor, lightheadedness, restlessness, decreased urinary output, and alteration in level of consciousness and orientation.

Because of the rapid cardiovascular changes taking place (e.g., the increased intracranial pressure during pushing and the rapid increase in cardiac output), the risk of rupture of a preexisting cerebral aneurysm and the risk of formation of pulmonary emboli are greater than usual during this period. Another dangerous, unpredictable problem is amniotic fluid embolism (see Chapter 19).

Women with a history of cardiac disorders are at increased risk for cardiac decompensation and pulmonary edema as a result of circulatory changes associated with the birth of the fetus and expulsion of the placenta.

To assist in the birth of the placenta, the woman is instructed to push when signs of separation have occurred. If possible, the placenta should be expelled by maternal effort during a uterine contraction. Alternate compression and elevation of the fundus, plus minimum, controlled traction on the umbilical cord, may be used to facilitate delivery of the placenta and amniotic membranes. Oxytocics may be administered after the placenta is removed because they stimulate the uterus to contract, thereby helping to prevent hemorrhage.

When the third stage is complete, and any lacerations are repaired or an episiotomy is sutured, the vulvar area is gently cleansed with warm, sterile water or normal saline solution and a sterile perineal pad is applied to the perineum. The birthing table or bed is repositioned and the woman's legs are lowered simultaneously if she gave birth in the lithotomy position. Drapes are removed and dry linen is placed under the woman's buttocks; she is provided with a clean gown and a warmed blanket. She is assisted into her bed if she is to be transferred from the birthing area to the recovery area. The side rails are raised during transfer. She may be given the baby to hold during the transfer, or the father or partner may carry the baby or transport it in a crib, either to the recovery area or to the nursery. Maternal and neonatal assessments for the fourth stage of labor are instituted. Box 18-9 summarizes normal vaginal childbirth.

Supportive Care During Labor and Birth

Doulas. A doula is a specially trained, experienced female labor attendant who provides a continuous, one-on-one, caring presence through the labor and birth of the woman she is attending. The doula also supports the woman's partner, who often feels unqualified to be the sole labor support. Doulas facilitate communication between the laboring woman and her partner, as well as between the couple and the health care team (Perez and Herrick, 1998; Simkin and Way, 1998). Continuous care provided by doulas reduces the cesarean birth rate; duration of labor; use of oxytocin, analgesics, and forceps; and requests for epidural anesthesia (Klaus, Kennell, and Klaus, 1993).

Support of the Father or Coach. Partners are encouraged to be present at the birth of their infants if this is in keeping with their cultural and personal expectations and beliefs. In this way, the psychologic closeness of the family unit is maintained and the partner can continue the supportive care given during labor. During the second stage the woman needs continuous support and coaching (Table 18-9). Because the coaching process can be physically and emotionally tiring for support persons, the nurse offers nourishment and fluids, and encourages them to take short breaks. If birth occurs in an LDR or LDRP room, the partner may be allowed to wear street clothes or be required to wear a clean scrub outfit, cap, and mask (for the birth). The support person who attends the birth in a delivery room is instructed to put on a cover gown or scrub clothes, mask, hat, and shoe covers as required. The nurse also specifies support measures that can be used for the laboring woman, and points out areas of the room in which the partner can move freely.

Although a woman or a man other than the father may be the woman's partner during labor, in North America the father of the baby is most often the support during labor. He often is able to provide the comfort measures and touch that the laboring woman needs. When the woman becomes focused on her pain, sometimes the partner can persuade her to try nonpharmacologic variations of comfort measures. In addition, he usually is able to interpret the woman's needs and desires to staff members.

Throughout the last 20 years, childbirth preparation education has been widely available. The father's ideal role was thought to be that of labor coach, and he was expected to actively help the woman cope with labor. However, this expectation may be unrealistic, because some men have concerns about their labor-coaching abilities. A father may actively assist the woman during and after contractions; act as a companion and give emotional and moral support; or watch the woman labor and give birth, and sleep, watch television, or leave the room for long periods of time. The degree of mutuality (i.e., level of interdependency and sharing) and understanding (i.e., the ability to know each other's needs) in a couple's relationship will determine which role the father adopts. Since a father or partner can participate in labor and birth in different ways, nurses need to encourage him to adopt the role most comfortable for him and for the woman, rather than an artificial role.

The feelings of a first-time father change as labor progresses. Often calm at the onset of labor, feelings of fear and helplessness begin to dominate as labor becomes more active and the father realizes that labor is more work than he anticipated. The first-time father may feel excluded as birth preparations begin during the transition phase. Once the second stage begins and birth nears, the father's focus changes from the woman to the baby who is about to be born (Chandler and Field, 1997).

The father will be exposed to many sights and smells that he may never before have experienced. It is important to tell him what to expect, and to make him feel comfortable about leaving the room to gather his composure should something occur that surprises him. Before he leaves the room, provision should be made for someone else to support the woman during his absence. Staff members should tell the father that his presence is helpful and encourage him to be involved in the care of the woman to the extent that he is comfortable.

Participation in the birth is ego building. The father can be of assistance; his presence is important. Support of the father/partner reflects the nurse's orientation and commitment

Box 18-9

Normal Vaginal Childbirth

FIRST STAGE

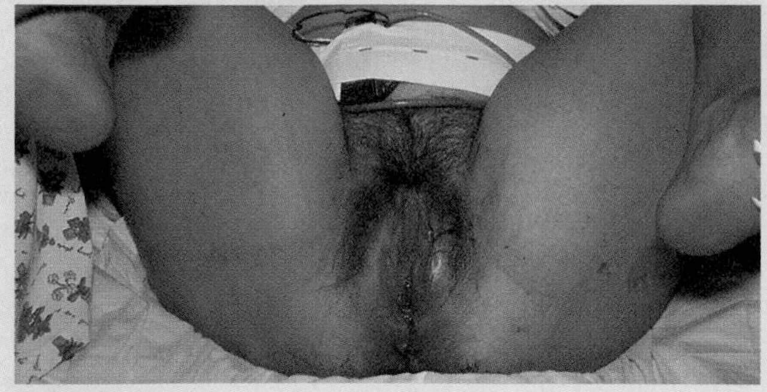

Anteroposterior slit. Vertex visible during contraction.

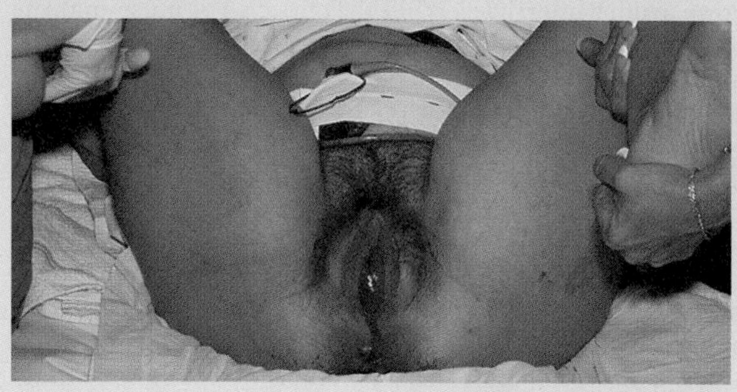

Oval opening. Vertex presenting. NOTE: Nurse *(on left)* is wearing gloves but support person *(on right)* is not.

SECOND STAGE

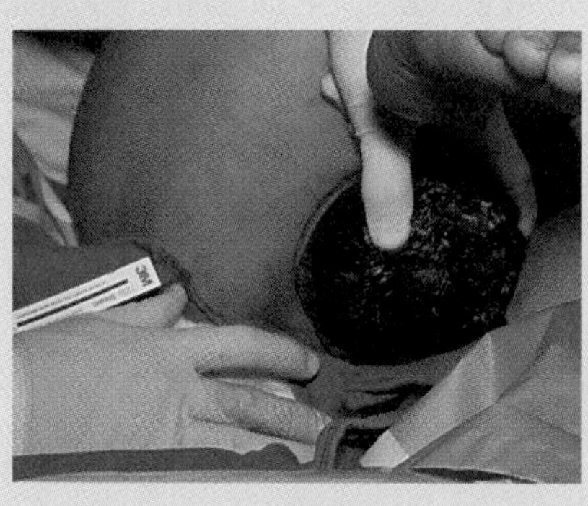

Crowning.

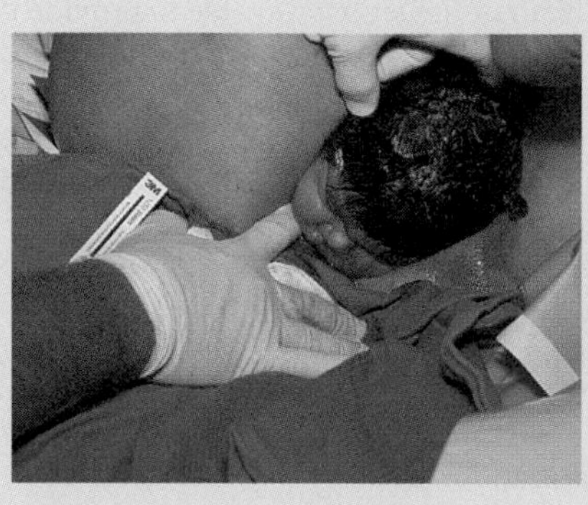

Nurse-midwife using Ritgen maneuver as head is born by extension.

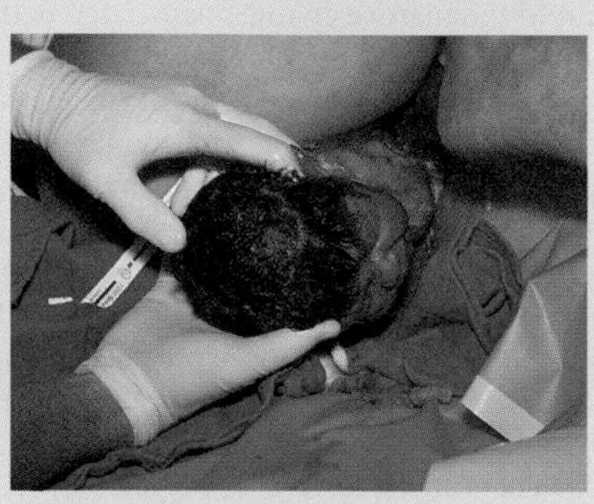

After nurse-midwife checks for nuchal cord, she supports head during external rotation and restitution.

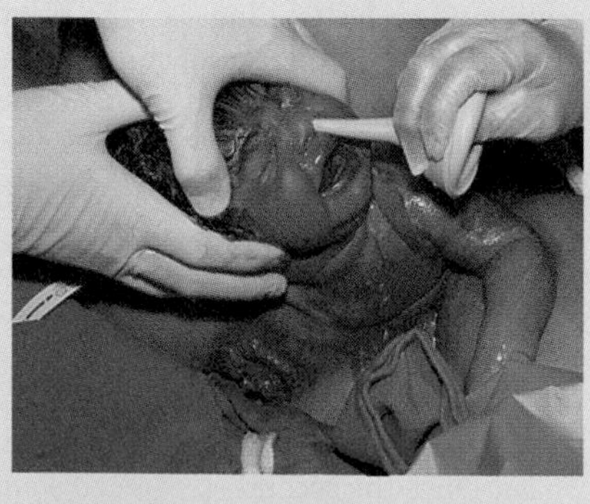

Use of bulb syringe to suction mucus.

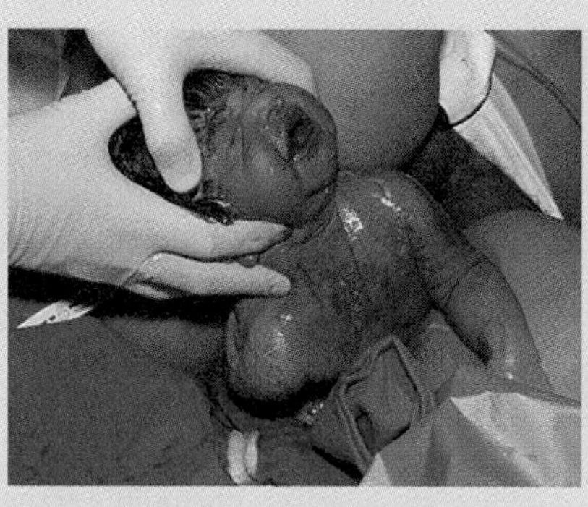

Birth of posterior shoulder.

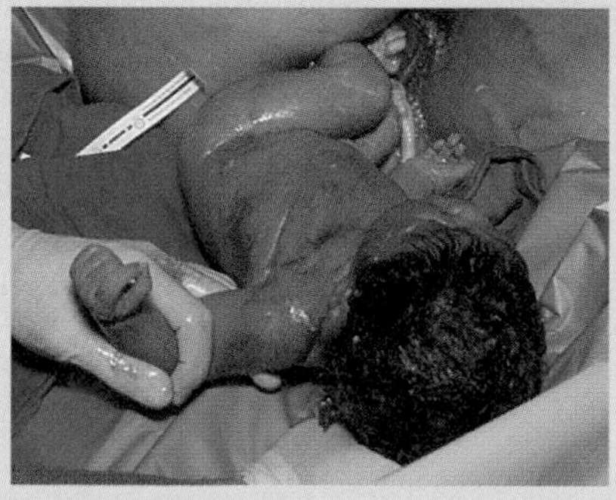

Birth of newborn by slow expulsion.

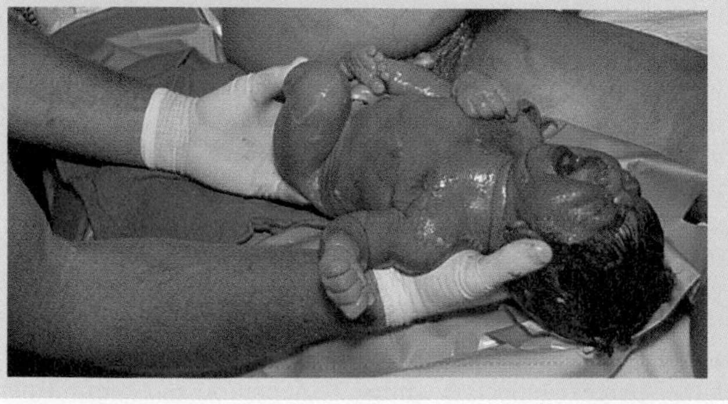

Second stage complete. Note that newborn is not completely pink yet.

Courtesy Michael S. Clement, MD, Mesa, AZ.

Box 18-9
Normal Vaginal Childbirth—cont'd

THIRD STAGE

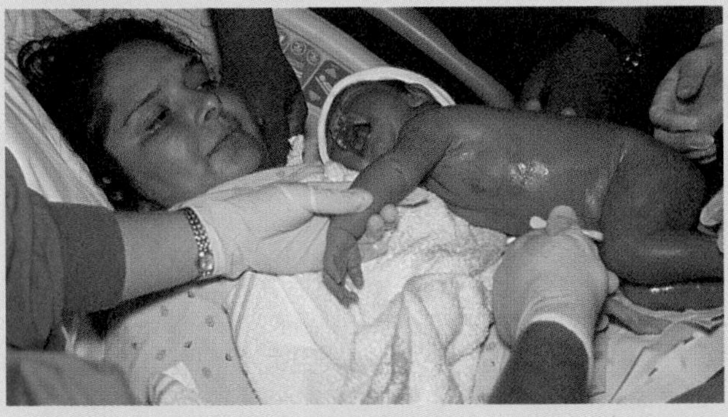

Newborn placed on mother's abdomen while cord is clamped and cut.

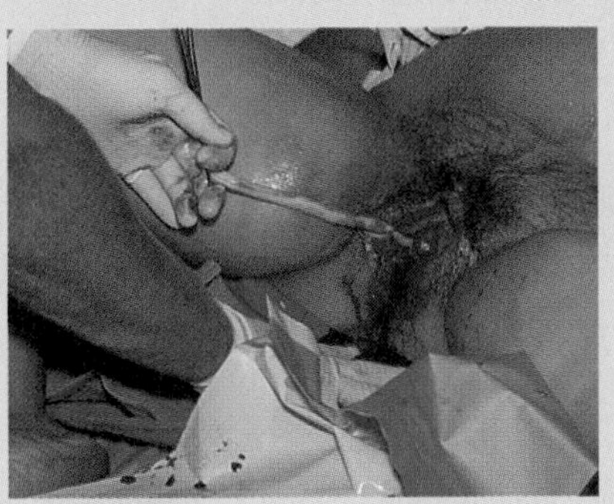

Note increased bleeding as placenta separates.

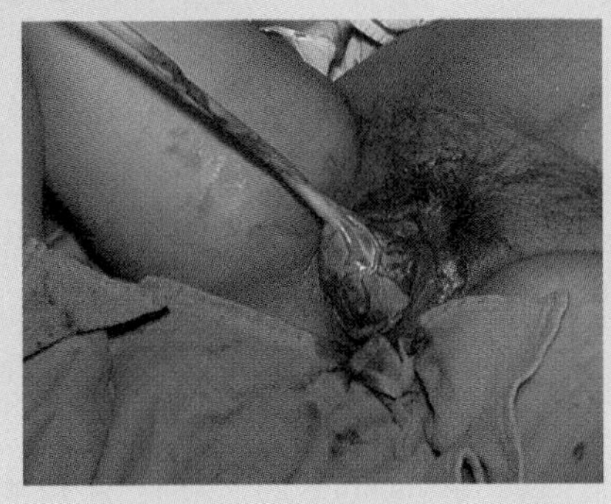

Expulsion of placenta

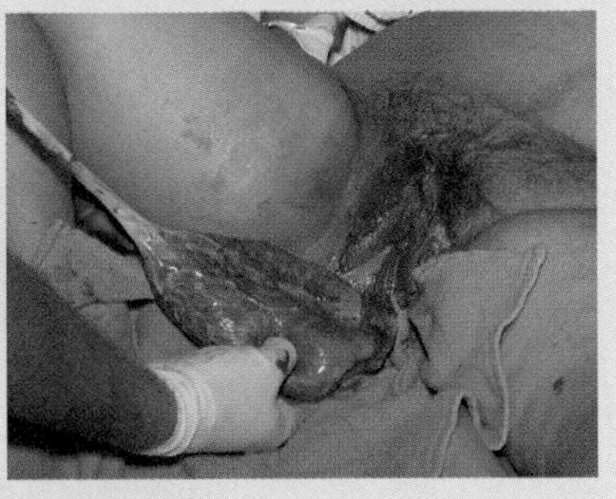

Expulsion is complete, marking the end of the third stage.

THE NEWBORN

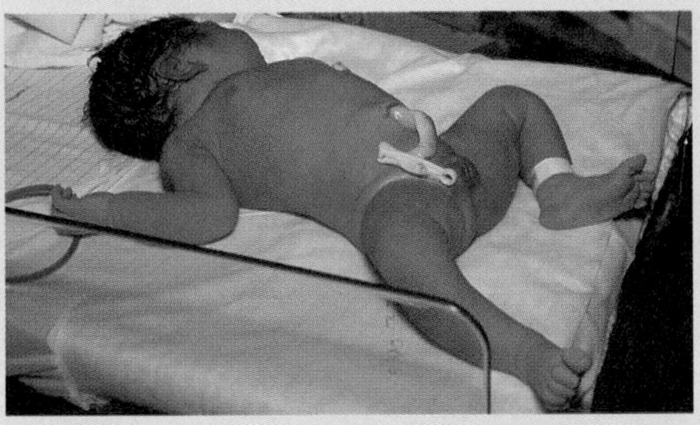

Newborn awaiting assessment. Note that color is almost completely pink.

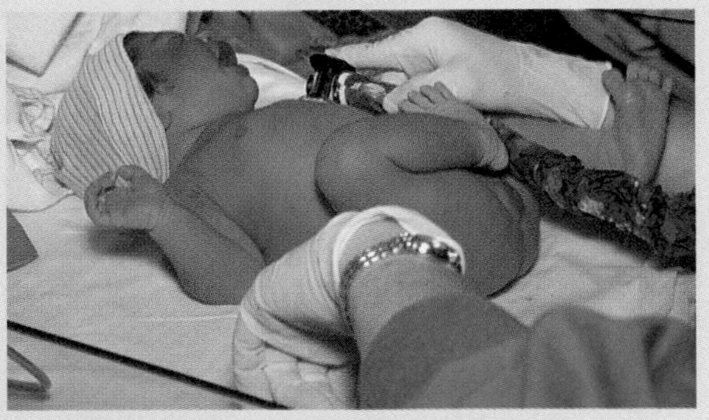

Newborn assessment under radiant warmer.

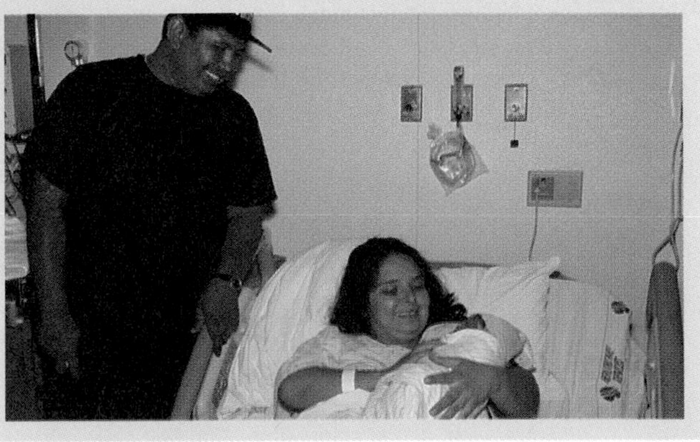

Parents admiring their newborn.

TABLE 18-9
Physical Nursing Care During Labor

Need	Nursing Actions	Rationale
GENERAL HYGIENE		
Showers/bed baths, Jacuzzi bath	Assess for progress in labor	Determines appropriateness of the activity
	Supervise showers closely if woman is in true labor	Prevents injury from fall; labor may be accelerated
	Suggest allowing warm water to flow over back	Aids relaxation; increases comfort
Perineum	Cleanse frequently, especially after rupture of membranes and when show increases	Enhances comfort and reduces risk of infection
Oral hygiene	Offer toothbrush or mouthwash or wash the teeth with ice-cold, wet washcloth as needed	Refreshes mouth; improves morale; helps counteract dry, thirsty feeling
Hair	Brush, braid per woman's wishes	Improves morale; increases comfort
Handwashing	Offer washcloths before and after voiding and as needed	Maintains cleanliness; improves morale and comfort
Face	Offer cool washcloth	Improves morale; provides relief from diaphoresis
Gowns/linens	Change prn; fluff pillows	Improves morale and comfort
NUTRIENT AND FLUID INTAKE		
Oral	Offer fluids and solid foods, following orders of primary health care provider and desires of laboring woman	Provides hydration and calories; enhances positive emotional experience and maternal control
IV	Establish and maintain IV as ordered	Maintains hydration; provides venous access for medications
ELIMINATION		
Voiding	Encourage voiding at least every 2 hours	A full bladder may impede descent of presenting part; overdistention may cause bladder atony and injury, as well as postpartum voiding difficulty
Ambulatory woman	Allow ambulation to bathroom according to orders of primary health care provider, if:	
	The presenting part is engaged	Reinforces normal process of urination
	The membranes are not ruptured	Precautionary measure to protect against prolapse of umbilical cord
	The woman is not medicated	Precautionary measure to protect against injury
Woman on bed rest	Offer bedpan	Prevents complications of bladder distention and ambulation
	Allow tap water to run; pour warm water over the vulva; give positive-suggestion	Encourages voiding
	Provide privacy	Shows respect for woman
	Put up side rails on bed	Prevents injury from fall
	Place call bell within reach	
	Offer washcloth for hands	Maintains cleanliness and comfort
	Wash vulvar area	Maintains standard of care
Catheterization	Catheterize according to orders of primary health care provider or hospital protocol if measures to facilitate voiding are ineffective	Prevents complications of bladder distention
	Insert catheter between contractions	Minimizes discomfort
	Avoid force if obstacle to insertion is noted	"Obstacle" may be caused by compression on urethra by presenting part
Bowel elimination—sensation of rectal pressure	Help the woman ambulate to bathroom or offer bedpan, after careful assessment	Prevents misinterpretation of rectal pressure from the presenting part as the need to defecate
	Perform vaginal examination	Determine degree of descent of presenting part
	Cleanse perineum immediately after passage of stool	Reduces risk of infection and sense of embarrassment

Box 18-10

Guidelines for Supporting the Father

- Orient to the labor room and the unit; explain location of the cafeteria, toilet, waiting room, and nursery; visiting hours; names and functions of personnel present.
- Inform him of sights and smells he can expect to encounter; encourage him to leave the room if necessary.
- Respect his or the couple's decision about the degree of his involvement. Offer them freedom to make decisions.
- Tell him when his presence has been helpful and continue to reinforce this throughout labor.
- Offer to teach him comfort measures.
- Inform him frequently of the progress of the labor and the woman's needs. Keep him informed about procedures to be performed.
- Prepare him for changes in the woman's behavior and physical appearance.
- Remind him to eat; offer him snacks and fluids if possible.
- Relieve him of the job of support person as necessary. Offer him blankets if he is to sleep in a chair by the bedside.
- Acknowledge the stress experienced by each partner during labor and birth and identify normal responses.
- Attempt to modify or eliminate unsettling stimuli, such as extra noise and extra light.

to each person, the family, and the community. Ways in which the nurse can support the father/partner are detailed in Box 18-10. A significantly lower percentage of women suffer postpartum emotional upsets when their partners receive support and assistance from parent education classes, physicians, midwives, and nurses throughout the childbearing cycle.

Culture and Father Participation. The choice of birth companion is influenced by the woman's cultural and religious background and by trends occurring within the society in which she lives. In Western societies, the father is viewed as the ideal birth companion (Chalmers and Meyer, 1994), whereas in other cultures a female companion is preferred (see Cultural Considerations, p. 374; and Chapter 2).

Support of the Grandparents. When grandparents act as labor coaches, it is important to support them and treat them with respect. They may have ways to deal with pain based on their experience. They should be encouraged to help as long as their actions do not compromise the status of the mother or the fetus. One example of an acceptable practice would be giving the woman herbal tea during labor. The nurse acts as a role model for parents by acknowledging the value of the grandparent's contributions to parental support, and by recognizing the difficulty parents have in witnessing their child's discomfort or crisis, regardless of the age of that child. If they have never witnessed a birth, the nurse may need to provide explanations about what is happening. Nursing actions that provide support for the grandparents can have a therapeutic effect on all members of the family.

Siblings During Labor. The preparation of siblings for acceptance of the new child helps promote attachment. The age and developmental level of children influence their responses; therefore preparation to be present during labor is adjusted to meet each child's needs. The child younger than 2 years of age shows little interest in pregnancy and labor; for the older child, the preparation may reduce fears and misconceptions. Most parents have a feel for their children's maturational level and ability to cope. Preparation can include a description of anticipated sights, smells, and sounds; a birth demonstration; a tour of the birthing unit; and an opportunity to be around a real newborn (Jonquil, 1993). Children must learn that their mother will be working hard during labor and birth and that she will not be able to talk to them during contractions, and that she may groan and pant at times. They can be told that labor is uncomfortable, but that their mother's body is made for the job. Storybooks about the birth process can be read to or by younger children to prepare them for the event. Films for preparing older preschool and school-age children to participate in the birth experience are available. Most facilities require that a specific person be designated to watch over the children who are participating in their mother's childbirth experience.

Interactions with the Newborn

Most parents enjoy being able to handle, hold, explore, and examine the baby immediately after birth. Both parents can assist with the thorough drying of the infant. The infant may be wrapped in a receiving blanket and placed on the woman's abdomen. If skin-to-skin contact is desired, the unwrapped infant may be placed on the woman's abdomen and then covered with a warm blanket.

Holding the newborn next to her skin helps the mother maintain the baby's body heat and provides skin-to-skin contact; care must be taken to keep the head warm as well. Stockinette caps are sometimes used to cover the newborn's head. It is the nurse's responsibility to make sure the infant stays warm and is in no danger of slipping from the parent's grasp.

Many women wish to begin breastfeeding their newborns at this time to take advantage of the infant's alert state (first period of reactivity) and to stimulate the production of oxytocin, which promotes contraction of the uterus. Others prefer to wait until the newborn, parents, and older siblings are together in the recovery area. In some cultures, breastfeeding is not considered acceptable until the milk comes in.

The woman usually feels some discomfort while the physician or nurse-midwife carries out the postbirth vaginal examination. The nurse can assist the woman to use breathing and relaxation techniques or use distraction to assist her in dealing with the discomfort. During this time the nurse can assess the newborn's physical condition; the baby can be weighed and measured, given eye prophylaxis and a vitamin K injection, given an identification bracelet, wrapped in warm blankets, and then given to the partner or back to the mother to hold when she is ready.

Parent-Newborn Relationships

The woman's reaction to the sight of her newborn may range from excited outbursts of laughing, talking, and even crying to apparent apathy. A polite smile and nod may be her only acknowledgment of the comments of nurses and the physician or nurse-midwife. Occasionally the reaction is one of anger or indifference; the woman turns away from the baby, concentrates on her own pain, and may make hostile comments. These varied reactions can arise from pleasure, exhaustion, or deep disappointment. When evaluating parent-newborn interactions after birth, the nurse should also consider the cultural characteristics of the woman and her family and the expected behaviors of that culture. In some cultures, the birth of a male child is preferred and women may grieve when a female child is born (Choudhry, 1997).

Whatever the reaction and its cause may be, the woman needs continuing acceptance and support from all staff. Notation regarding the parents' reaction to the newborn can be made in the recovery record. Nurses can assess this reaction by asking themselves questions such as: How do the parents look? What do they say? What do they do? Further assessment of the parent-newborn relationship can be conducted as care is given during the period of recovery. This is especially important if warning signs (e.g., passive or hostile reactions to newborn, disappointment with sex or appearance of newborn, absence of eye contact, or limited interaction of parents with each other) were noted immediately after birth. The nurse may find it helpful to discuss any warning signs that may have been noted with the woman's physician or nurse-midwife.

Siblings, who may have appeared only remotely interested in the final phases of the second stage, tend to experience renewed interest and excitement when the newborn appears. They can then be encouraged to hold the baby (Fig. 18-28).

Parents usually respond to praise of their newborn. Many need to be reassured that the dusky appearance of the baby's extremities immediately after birth is normal until circulation is well established. If appropriate, the nurse should explain the reason for the molding of the newborn's head. Information about hospital routine can be communicated. It is important, however, for nurses to recognize that the cultural background of the parents may influence expectations regarding care and handling of their newborn immediately after birth. For example, some traditional Southeast Asians believe that the head should not be touched because it is the most sacred part of a person's body. They also believe that praise of the baby is dangerous because jealous spirits may cause the baby harm or take it away (D'Avanzo, 1992). Hospital staff members, by their interest and concern, can provide an environment for making this time a satisfying experience for parents, family, and significant others.

➤ Evaluation

Evaluation is an ongoing process and is based on expected outcomes of care (see the Nursing Care Plan on pp. 386-387).

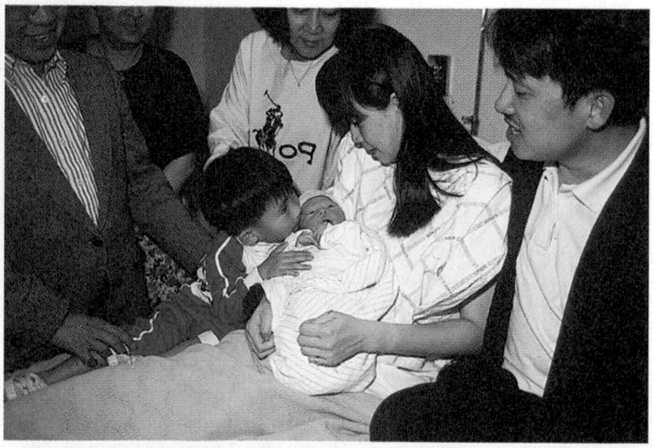

FIG. 18-28 • Big brother becomes acquainted with new baby sister. (Courtesy Marjorie Pyle, RNC, Lifecircle, Costa Mesa, CA.)

Key Points

- The onset of labor may be difficult to determine for both nulliparous and multiparous women.
- The familiar environment of her home is most often the ideal place for a woman during the latent phase of the first stage of labor.
- The nurse assumes much of the responsibility for assessing the progress of labor and for keeping the physician or nurse-midwife informed about progress in labor and deviations from expected findings.
- The fetal heart rate and pattern reveal the fetal response to the stress of the labor process.
- Meconium-staining of amniotic fluid is not always indicative of fetal distress associated with hypoxia.
- The woman's level of anxiety may rise when she does not understand what is being said to her about her labor because of the medical terminology used or because of a language barrier.
- Coaching, emotional support, and comfort measures assist the woman to use her energy constructively in relaxing and working with the contractions.
- Doulas provide a continuous supportive presence during labor that can have a positive effect on the process of childbirth and its outcome.
- The nurse who is aware of sociocultural aspects of helping and coping acts as an advocate or protective agent for the woman or couple during labor.
- Objective signs indicate that the placenta has separated and is ready to be expelled; excessive traction (pulling) on the umbilical cord, before the placenta has separated, can result in maternal injury.
- Siblings present for labor and birth need preparation and support for the event.
- Most parents/families enjoy being able to handle, hold, explore, and examine the baby immediately after birth.
- Nurses should observe progress in the development of parent-child relationships and be alert for warning signs that may appear during the immediate postpartum period.
- Following an emergency childbirth out of the hospital, the neonate sucking on the mother's nipple can stimulate the release of natural oxytocin from the maternal posterior pituitary gland; oxytocin stimulates the uterus to contract, thereby preventing postpartum hemorrhage.

References

Albers L et al: Factors related to perineal trauma in childbirth, *J Nurse Midwifery* 41(4):269-276, 1996.

Albers L et al: The relationship of ambulation in labor to operative delivery, *J Nurse Midwifery* 42(1):4-8, 1997.

American College of Obstetricians and Gynecologists: *Operative vaginal delivery (ACOG Tech Bull No. 196)*, Washington, DC, 1994, ACOG.

Arrabal P, Naegy D: Is manual palpation of uterine contractions accurate? *Am J Obstet Gynecol* 114(1 pt 1):217-219, 1996.

Biancuzzo M: Six myths of maternal posture during labor, *MCN Am J Matern Child Nurs* 18(5):264-269, 1993.

Bruner J et al: All-fours maneuver for reducing shoulder dystocia during labor, *J Reprod Med* 43(5):439-443, 1998.

Callister L: Cultural meanings of childbirth, *J Obstet Gynecol Neonatal Nurs* 24(4):327-331, 1995.

Callister L, Vehvilainen-Julkunen K, Lauri S: Cultural perceptions of childbirth, *J Holistic Nurs* 14(1):66-78, 1996.

Carbonne B et al: Maternal position during labor: effects on fetal oxygen saturation measured by pulse oximetry, *Obstet Gynecol* 88(5):797-800, 1996.

Cesario S: Should cameras be allowed in the delivery room? *MCN Am J Matern Child Nurs* 23(2):87-91, 1998.

Chalmers B, Meyer D: Companionship in the perinatal period: a cross-cultural survey of women's experiences, *J Nurse Midwifery* 39(4):265-272, 1994.

Chandler S, Field P: Becoming a father—first-time fathers' experience of labor and delivery, *J Nurse Midwifery* 42(1):17-24, 1997.

Choudhry U: Traditional practices of women from India: pregnancy, childbirth, and newborn care, *J Obstet Gynecol Neonatal Nurs* 26(5):533-539, 1997.

Cosner K: Use of fundal pressure during second-stage labor: a pilot study, *J Nurse Midwifery* 41(4):334-337, 1996.

D'Avanzo C: Bridging the cultural gap with Southeast Asians, *MCN Am J Matern Child Nurs* 17(4):204-208, 1992.

d' Entremont M: Directed pushing in the second stage of labour, *Modern Midwife* 6(6):12-16, 1996.

Enkin M et al: Effective care in pregnancy and childbirth: a synopsis, *Birth* 22(2):101-110, 1995.

Fowles E: Labor concerns of women 2 months after delivery, *Birth* 25(4):235-240, 1998.

Gagnon A, Waghorn K: One-to-one nurse labor support of nulliparous women stimulated with oxytocin, *J Obstet Gynecol Neonatal Nurs* 28 (4):371-376, 1999.

Hanson L: Second stage positioning in nurse midwifery practices. Part 1: Position use and preferences, *J Nurse Midwifery* 43(5):320-324, 1998a.

Hanson L: Second stage positioning in nurse midwifery practices. Part 2: Factors affecting use, *J Nurse Midwifery* 43(5):326-330, 1998b.

Heritage C: Working with childhood sexual abuse survivors during pregnancy, labor, and birth, *J Obstet Gynecol Neonatal Nurs* 27(6):671-677, 1998.

Hodnett E: Nursing support of the laboring woman, *J Obstet Gynecol Neonatal Nurs* 25(3):257-264, 1996.

Howard J, Berbiglia V: Caring for childbearing Korean women, *J Obstet Gynecol Neonatal Nurs* 26(6):665-671, 1997.

Jonquil S: Preparing siblings, *Midwifery Today Childbirth Education* 28(Winter):34-35, 1993.

Kennell J et al: Continuous emotional support during labor in a US hospital: a randomized controlled trial, *JAMA* 265(17):2197-2201, 1991.

Klaus M, Kennell J, Klaus P: *Mothering the mother,* Redwood City, CA, 1993, Addison-Wesley.

Lydon-Rochelle M, Albers L, Teaf D: Perineal outcomes and nurse-midwifery management, *J Nurse Midwifery* 40(1): 13-18, 1995.

Mayberry L et al: Managing second stage labor, *AWHONN Lifelines* 3(6):28-34, 1999/2000.

McCartney P: The birth ball—are you using it in your practice setting? *MCN Am J Matern Child Nurs* 23(4):218, 1998.

McKay S, Barrows T: Holding back: maternal readiness to give birth, *MCN Am J Matern Child Nurs* 16(5):250-254, 1991.

McKay S, Smith S: "What are they talking about? Is something wrong?" Information sharing during the second stage of labor, *Birth* 20(3):142-147, 1993.

Melzack R, Belanger E, Lacroix R: Labor pain: effects of maternal position on front and back pain, *J Pain Symptom Manage* 6(8):476-480, 1991.

Nichols M: Paternal perspectives of the childbirth experience, *Matern Child Nurs* J 21(3):99-108, 1993.

Odent M: Can water immersion stop labor? *J Nurse Midwifery* 42(5):414-416, 1997.

Perez P: *Using the Gymnastik Ball in pregnancy, labor, birth and postpartum,* Katy, TX, 1998, Cutting Edge Press.

Perez P, Herrick L: Doulas: exploring their roles with parents, hospitals, and nurses, *AWHONN Lifelines* 2(2):54-55, 1998.

Peterson L, Besuner P: Pushing techniques during labor: issues and controversies, *J Obstet Gynecol Neonatal Nurs* 26(6): 719-726, 1997.

Piper D, McDonald P: Management of anticipated and actual shoulder dystocia, *J Nurse Midwifery* 39(2 suppl):91S-105S, 1994.

Proctor S: What determines quality in maternity care? Comparing the perceptions of childbearing women and midwives, *Birth* 25(2):85-93, 1998.

Renfrew M et al: Practices that minimize trauma to the genital tract in childbirth: a systematic review of the literature, *Birth* 25(3):143-160, 1998.

Rhodes N, Hutchinson S: Labor experiences of childhood sexual abuse survivors, *Birth* 21(4):213-220, 1994.

Roberts J, Woolley D: A second look at the second stage of labor, *J Obstet Gynecol Neonatal Nurs* 25(5):415-423, 1996.

Sampselle C, Hines S: Research exchange. Spontaneous pushing during birth: relationship to perineal outcomes, *J Nurse Midwifery* 44(1):36-39, 1999.

Schneiderman J: Rituals of placenta disposal, *MCN Am J Matern Child Nurs* 23(3):142-143, 1998.

Scott J et al: *Danforth's obstetrics and gynecology,* ed 8, Philadelphia, 1999, Lippincott/Williams & Wilkins.

Shermer R, Raines D: Positioning during the second stage of labor: moving back to basics, *J Obstet Gynecol Neonatal Nurs* 26(6):727-734, 1997.

Simkin P: Reducing pain and enhancing progress in labor: a guide to nonpharmacologic methods for maternity caregivers *Birth* 22(3):161-171, 1995.

Simkin P, Way K: *Doulas of North American position paper: the doula's contribution to modern maternity care,* Seattle, 1998, DONA.

Technical Working Group, World Health Organization: Care in normal birth: a practical guide, *Birth* 24(2):121-123, 1997.

Thomson A: Pushing techniques in the second stage of labor, *J Adv Nurs* 18(2):171-177, 1993.

Tomlinson P, Bryan A: Family centered intrapartum care: revisiting an old concept, *J Obstet Gynecol Neonatal Nurs* 25(4):331-337, 1996.

Tucker S: *Pocket guide to fetal monitoring,* ed 4, St Louis, 2000, Mosby.

Varney H: *Varney's midwifery,* ed 3, Sudberry, MA, 1997, Jones & Bartlett.

Waymire V: A triggering time: childbirth may recall sexual abuse memories, *AWHONN Lifelines* 1(2):47-50, 1997.

Weber S: Cultural aspects of pain in childbearing women, *J Obstet Gynecol Neonatal Nurs* 25(1):67-72, 1996.

CHAPTER 19

Labor and Birth at Risk

http://www.harcourthealth.com/MERLIN/Wong/maternal/

Learning Objectives

On completion of this chapter the reader will be able to:

- Differentiate between preterm birth and low birth weight.
- Identify risk factors for preterm birth.
- Discuss current interventions to prevent preterm birth.
- Discuss the use of tocolytics and antenatal glucocorticoids in preterm birth.
- Describe deleterious effects of bed rest on pregnant women.
- Define preterm premature rupture of membranes.
- Describe nursing management of a trial of labor, induction and augmentation of labor, forceps- and vacuum-assisted birth, cesarean birth, and vaginal birth after a cesarean birth.
- Discuss the criteria for evaluating the nursing care of women experiencing labor and birth complications.
- Discuss the care of a woman experiencing postterm pregnancy.
- Discuss obstetric emergencies and their appropriate management.

When complications arise during labor and birth, perinatal morbidity and mortality increase. Some complications are anticipated, especially if the mother is identified as high risk during the antepartum period; others are unexpected or unforeseen. The woman, her family, and the obstetric team can feel devastated when things go wrong. Nurses must recognize these feelings if they are to provide effective support. It is crucial for nurses to understand the normal birth process to prevent and detect deviations from normal labor and birth and to implement nursing measures when complications arise. Optimum care of the laboring woman, the fetus, and the family experiencing complications is possible only when the nurse and other members of the obstetric team use their knowledge and skills in a concerted effort to provide care. This chapter focuses on labor and birth problems related to preterm labor and birth, dystocia, and postdate (i.e., postterm) pregnancy and obstetric emergencies.

PRETERM LABOR AND BIRTH

Preterm birth is any birth that occurs before the completion of 37 weeks of pregnancy. Preterm labor is defined as cervical changes and uterine contractions occurring between 20 weeks and 37 weeks of pregnancy (American College of Obstetricians and Gynecologists and American Academy of Pediatrics [ACOG/AAP], 1997). Preterm labor and birth are the most serious complications of pregnancy because they lead to about 75% of the perinatal mortality today (March of Dimes, 1997). Preterm labor and birth also affect infant mortality rates and are second only to congenital anomalies as leading causes of infant mortality in the United States (March of Dimes, 1997). Despite the fact that infant mortality rates in the United States have dropped precipitously since 1950 (e.g., 29.2% in 1950 vs. 7.1% in 1997), preterm birth rates have continued to rise. In 1996, the preterm birth rate in the United States was 11%, having steadily risen over a 15-year period from 7.5% in 1982 (March of Dimes, 1997).

Preterm Birth Vs. Low Birth Weight

Although they have distinctly different meanings, the terms "preterm birth" and "low birth weight" are often used interchangeably. Preterm birth describes length of gestation (i.e., $<$37 weeks), whereas low birth weight describes only weight at the time of birth (i.e., $\leq$2500 g). Low birth weight is far easier to measure than preterm birth, and thus in many settings and publications, low birth weight has been used as a substitute term for preterm birth. Preterm birth, however, is a more dangerous health condition for an infant because length of time in the uterus correlates with immaturity of body systems. Low-birth-weight babies can be, but are not necessarily, preterm; low birth weight can be caused by conditions other than preterm labor, such as intrauterine growth restriction (IUGR), a condition of fetal growth not necessarily related with initiation of labor; and pregnancy induced hypertension (PIH).

The incidence of preterm birth in the United States varies considerably according to race; the 1996 rate for African-

Americans (18.1%) was almost double the rate for Caucasians (9.6%) (March of Dimes, 1997). Anecdotal evidence suggests that sociodemographics may play a part in this difference.

Predicting Preterm Labor and Birth. The known risk factors for preterm birth were compiled by the Institute of Medicine (1985) and are shown in Box 19-1. Using these risk factors, researchers have tried to determine which women might go into labor prematurely. Risk assessment schema were developed and risk scoring systems were used (Collaborative Group on Preterm Birth Prevention, 1993). None of these risk scoring systems have resulted in lowering the preterm birth rate in the United States, however, because at least 50% of all women who ultimately give birth prematurely have no identifiable risk factors (U.S. Public Health Service, 1989).

Box 19-1

Risk Factors for Preterm Labor and Birth

DEMOGRAPHIC RISKS
- African-American race (doubles the risk)
- Below 17 or above 34 years
- Low socioeconomic status
- Unmarried
- Low level of education

MEDICAL RISKS PREDATING THIS PREGNANCY
- History of previous preterm birth (triples the risk)
- Multiple abortions (miscarriage or elective)
- Uterine anomalies
- Low prepregnancy weight for height
- Parity (0 or >4)
- Diabetes
- Hypertension

MEDICAL RISKS IN CURRENT PREGNANCY
- Multiple gestation
- Infection (e.g., bacterial vaginosis)
- Incompetent cervix
- Short interpregnancy interval
- Urinary tract infection
- Bleeding in first trimester
- Placenta previa or abruptio placentae
- Anemia
- Fetal anomalies
- Premature rupture of membranes (PROM)

BEHAVIORAL AND ENVIRONMENTAL RISKS
- Diethylstilbestrol (DES) exposure
- Smoking
- Poor nutrition
- Alcohol or other substance use, especially cocaine
- Late or no prenatal care

OTHER RISKS
- Stress
- Uterine irritability
- Long working hours
- Inability to rest

Data from Institute of Medicine. *Preventing low birthweight,* Washington, DC, 1985, National Academy Press.

Biochemical Markers. The two most common biochemical markers used in an effort to predict who might experience preterm labor are fetal fibronectin and salivary estriol.

Fetal fibronectins are glycoproteins found in plasma and produced during fetal life. They appear in the cervical canal early in pregnancy and then again in late pregnancy. Their appearance between 24 and 34 weeks of gestation predicts labor (Lockwood et al, 1991). The negative predictive value of fetal fibronectin is high (up to 95%); the positive predictive value is lower (25% to 40%) (Moore, 1999). This means that it may be possible to predict who will *not* go into preterm labor, but not who will. The test is done during a vaginal examination. The cost of the test ($180 to $215) limits the usefulness of this marker for the general public.

Salivary estriol is a form of estrogen produced by the fetus that is present in plasma at 9 weeks of gestation. Levels of salivary estriol have been shown to increase before preterm birth. Specimens of salivary estriol are collected by the woman in the home, at a cost of about $90 per test, with the testing done every 2 weeks for about 10 weeks for a total of about $450 per woman. This marker also has a high negative predictive value (98%) and a lower positive predictive value (7% to 25%) (Moore, 1999).

Endocervical Length. Some studies have suggested that a shortened cervix precedes preterm labor and can be determined by ultrasound measurement (Crane et al, 1997). A cervical length of less than 30 mm in a singleton pregnancy can predict some instances of preterm labor.

Causes of Preterm Labor and Birth. The cause of preterm labor is unknown and is assumed to be multifactorial (Goldenberg and Rouse, 1998) (Box 19-2). Infection is thought to be a major etiologic factor in some preterm labors. When cervical, bacterial, or urinary tract infections are present, the risk of preterm birth is increased (Box 19-3). Thus early continuous and comprehensive prenatal care, which can detect and treat infection, is essential in dealing with this aspect of preterm birth prevention.

Not all preterm births can or even should be prevented. About 25% of all preterm births are iatrogenic; that is, babies are intentionally delivered prematurely because of pregnancy complications that put the life or health of the fetus or the mother in danger, not because of preterm labor. Another 25% of all preterm births are preceded by spontaneous rupture of membranes followed by labor. These births are not known to be preventable. About 50% of preterm births, therefore, are possibly amenable to prevention efforts and are considered idiopathic preterm births (Goldenberg and Rouse, 1998).

Sociodemographic factors such as poverty, low educational level, lack of social support, smoking, little or no prenatal care, domestic violence, and stress are thought to contribute to the 50% of the preterm births that may be preventable.

Care Management

➤ Assessment

Because all pregnant women must be considered at risk for preterm labor (as they are for any other pregnancy complication), nursing assessment begins at the time of entry to prenatal care. Since the onset of preterm labor is often insidious and can be easily mistaken for normal discomforts of pregnancy, it is essential that nurses teach pregnant women how to detect the early symptoms of preterm labor (Box 19-4) (Freston et al, 1997).

Pregnant women need to be taught what to do if symptoms of preterm labor occur. Some women wait hours or days before contacting a health care provider after preterm labor symptoms have begun (Freston et al, 1997). Waiting too long to see a health care provider could result in inevitable preterm birth without the benefit of the administration of antenatal glucocorticoids (i.e., medication given to accelerate fetal lung maturity). In this event, the infant is born at higher risk for respiratory distress syndrome and intraventricular hemorrhage.

Patient education regarding any symptoms of contractions or cramping between 20 and 36 weeks of gestation should be directed toward telling the woman that these symptoms are not normal discomforts of pregnancy, and that contractions or cramping which do not go away should prompt the woman to contact her primary health care provider (Freda and Patterson, 1995). Since no one can distinguish between Braxton Hicks contractions and the contractions of early preterm labor, nurses should eliminate the term "Braxton Hicks contractions" from their teaching about pregnancy expectations.

Women who have risk factors for preterm birth are often offered special care with more frequent visits. Telephone support to at-risk women by nurses resulted in a 26% decrease in low-birth-weight births and a 27% decrease in preterm births in African-American women (Moore et al, 1998).

Box 19-2
Multifactorial Etiology of Preterm Labor and Birth

MATERNAL BEHAVIORS
Smoking
Substance use (alcohol or illegal drugs)
Poor nutrition
Work/fatigue
Short interpregnancy interval
Sexual activity

MATERNAL CHARACTERISTICS
Young or old age
Previous preterm birth
Short stature
Short cervix
Uterine anomalies
DES exposure
Incompetent cervix
Low prepregnancy weight
African-American
Unmarried
Low socioeconomic status
Victim of domestic violence

OTHER FACTORS
Inadequate support systems
Stress
Uterine irritability
Multiple gestation
Late or no prenatal care
Preterm premature rupture of membranes (PPROM)
Anemia
Infection
Catecholamine release
Decreased progesterone production
Decidual cell disruption
Prostaglandin synthesis
Cytokine release

➤ Nursing Diagnoses

Nursing diagnoses relevant for women at risk for preterm birth include the following:

- Knowledge deficit related to:
  —Recognition of preterm labor symptoms
- Risk for maternal or fetal injury related to:
  —Preterm labor and birth
- Impaired mobility related to:
  —Prescribed bed rest
- Anticipatory grieving related to:
  —Preterm labor and birth

➤ Expected Outcomes

Expected outcomes include that the woman will do the following:

- Learn the symptoms of preterm labor and be able to assess herself and her need for intervention
- Follow teaching suggestions and call her provider if symptoms occur
- Not experience preterm symptoms, or if she does, take appropriate action
- Maintain her pregnancy for at least 37 completed weeks
- Give birth to a healthy, full-term infant

➤ Plan of Care and Implementation

Prevention

The most important nursing intervention aimed at preventing preterm birth is the education of pregnant women about the early symptoms of preterm labor, so that if symptoms occur the woman can be referred promptly to her provider of care for more intensive care. (See Box 19-4 for the symptoms of preterm labor and what the woman should do if the symptoms appear.) All pregnant women should be taught this information and told to act on it if they are between 20 and 37 weeks of pregnancy (Fig. 19-1).

Box 19-3
Infections and Risk of Preterm Labor

Bacterial vaginosis	40% increased risk
Syphilis and gonorrhea	50% increased risk
Asymptomatic bacteriuria	50% increased risk

Source Fiscella K: Racial disparity in preterm births: the role of urogenital infections, *Public Health Rep* 111:104-113, 1996; Hillier S, et al: Association between bacterial vaginosis and preterm delivery of a low birthweight infant, *N Engl J Med* 333:1732-1742, 1995.

Box 19-4
Symptoms of Preterm Labor (Occurring Between 20 and 37 Weeks of Pregnancy)

Pelvic pressure (feels like the baby is pushing down)
Low, dull backache
Menstrual-like cramps
Change or increase in vaginal discharge
Uterine contractions (hardness) occurring every 10 minutes or more often, with or without pain
Intestinal cramping, with or without diarrhea

Early Recognition and Diagnosis. Early recognition of preterm labor is essential to implement interventions such as tocolytic therapy and administration of antenatal glucocorticoids. According to the ACOG/AAP Guidelines for Perinatal Care (1997), the diagnostic criteria for preterm labor are:

- 20 to 36 weeks gestation; and
- Documented uterine contractions; and either
- Documented cervical change with cervical effacement of 80%; or cervical dilation of greater than 1 cm

Therefore the pregnant woman at 30 weeks gestation with an irritable uterus but no documented cervical change is not in preterm labor. Misdiagnosis of preterm labor can lead to inappropriate use of pharmacologic agents that can be dangerous to the health of the woman and fetus.

Lifestyle Modifications. Nurses caring for women who exhibit symptoms of preterm labor should question the women about whether they have symptoms when they are engaged in any of the following activities:

- Sexual activity
- Riding long distances in automobiles, trains, or buses
- Carrying heavy loads such as laundry, groceries, or a small child
- Standing more than 50% of the time
- Heavy housework
- Climbing stairs
- Hard physical work
- Being unable to stop and rest when tired

If symptoms occur when the woman is engaged in any of these activities, the woman should consider what she was doing when the symptoms began, and then consider stopping those activities until 37 weeks of pregnancy, when preterm birth is no longer a risk. Counseling about lifestyle modifications should be individualized; only women who have symptoms of preterm labor when they are engaged in certain activities need to alter their lifestyles. There are no specific rules for which activities are safe for pregnant women and which are not. Each pregnant woman must understand which lifestyle factors might be contributing to her symptoms and be taught to modify only those factors.

Bed Rest. Bed rest is a commonly used intervention for the prevention of preterm labor. There is no evidence in the literature to support the efficacy of this intervention, however. Maloni and others (1993) have shown that there are deleterious effects of bed rest on women: after 3 days there is decreased muscle tone, weight loss, calcium loss, and glucose intolerance. Weeks of bed rest lead to bone demineralization, constipation, fatigue, isolation, anxiety, and depression.

Home Care. Despite the fact that bed rest has not been shown to reduce preterm birth, it is still commonly prescribed, and women who are at high risk for preterm birth are told that it would be best if they were at home on bed rest for weeks or months. The home care of the woman at risk for preterm birth is a challenge for the nurse. The scope of care given to women in their homes ranges from occasional visits to monitor the maternal and fetal condition to daily telephone consultation and reading of uterine monitoring strips. Families may need help in learning how to organize time and space or to restructure family routines so that the pregnant woman can remain a part of family activity while still maintaining bed rest (Fig. 19-2; Home Care and Family Focus boxes).

Home Uterine Activity Monitoring. Home care companies provide uterine monitoring services for women diagnosed with preterm labor, and nurses are usually an integral part of the systems developed by companies to educate the patients they serve. However, from the body of research over the past 15 years, researchers have concluded that home uterine activity monitoring does not prevent preterm birth, and its prohibitive cost makes it an unacceptable intervention in the larger scheme of prenatal care (Dyson et al, 1998).

Some research suggests that it is the nursing care offered by the home care nurse that helps women the most (Iams, Johnson, and O'Shaughnessy, 1988; Moore et al, 1998).

Suppression of Uterine Activity

Tocolytics. Should preterm labor occur, women are usually admitted to the hospital for assessment; fetal monitoring; cervical/vaginal cultures; and assessment of cervical status, amniotic fluid leakage, and maternal temperature (an early sign of

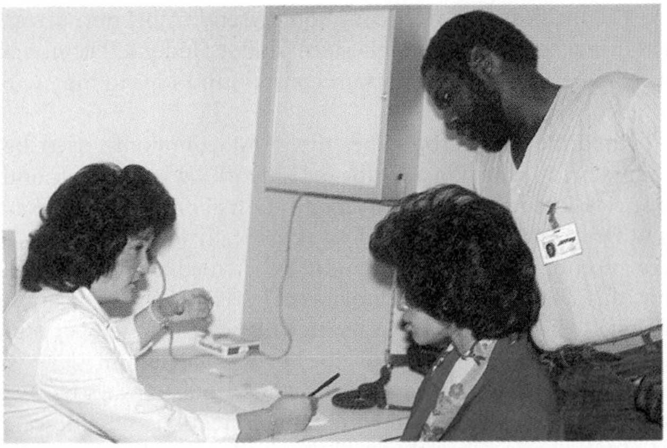

FIG. 19-1 • Nurse teaching woman signs and symptoms of preterm labor. (Courtesy Marjorie Pyle, RNC, Lifecircle, Costa Mesa, CA.)

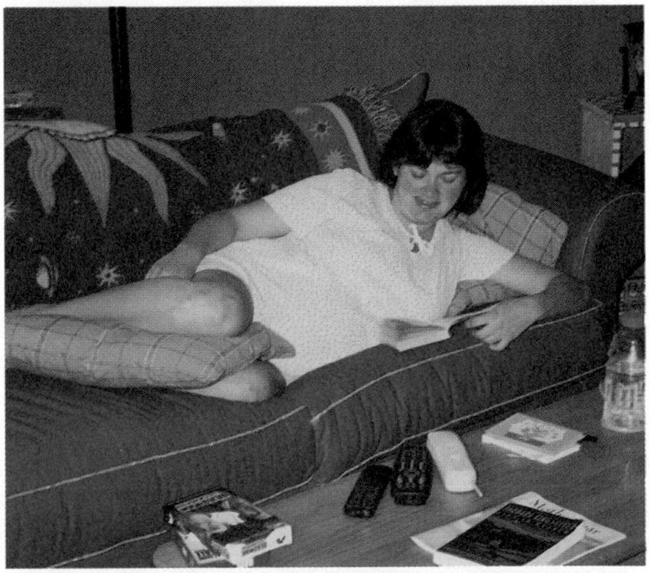

FIG. 19-2 • Woman at home on restricted activity for preterm labor prevention. Note how she has arranged her daytime resting area so that needed items are close at hand. (Courtesy Amy Turner, Cary, NC.)

Home Care

SUGGESTED ACTIVITIES FOR WOMEN ON BED REST

- **Set a routine for daily activities (e.g., getting dressed, moving from the bedroom to a "day bed rest place," [see Fig. 19-2] having social time, eating meals, self-monitoring fetal and uterine activity)**
- **Do passive exercises as allowed**
- **Review childbirth education information or have a childbirth class at home, if this can be arranged**
- **Plan menus and make up grocery shopping lists**
- **Shop by phone**
- **Read books about high risk pregnancy or other topics**
- **Keep a journal of the pregnancy**
- **Keep a calendar of your progress**
- **Reorganize files, recipes, household budget**
- **Update address book**
- **Do mending, sewing**
- **Listen to audiotapes, watch videos or TV**
- **Do crossword puzzles, jigsaw puzzles, etc.**
- **Do craft projects; make something for the baby**
- **Put pictures in photo albums**
- **Call a friend, family member, or support person each day or use e-mail**
- **Treat yourself to a facial, manicure, neck massage, or other special treat when you need a life.**

From Gilbert E, Harmon J: *Manual of high risk pregnancy and delivery,* ed 2, St Louis, 1998, Mosby; Isennock P: *Bed rest before baby: what's a mother to do?* Perry Hall, MD, 1992, Mustard Seed Publications; and Maloni J: *Antepartum bedrest: case studies, research, & nursing care,* Washington, DC, 1998, AWHONN.

Family Focus

ACTIVITIES FOR CHILDREN OF WOMEN ON BED REST

- **Schedule brief play periods throughout the day**
- **Keep a few favorite toys in a box or basket close to the bed or couch**
- **Read to the child(ren)**
- **Put puzzles together**
- **Watch videos, play video games (remote control for TV is ideal)**
- **Play cards or board games**
- **Color in coloring books**
- **Cut out pictures from magazines and paste on cardboard**
- **Play bed basketball with a soft (sponge) ball or rolled up sock and a trash can or empty laundry basket**

Adapted from Isennock P: *Bed rest before baby: what's a mother to do?* Perry Hall, MD, 1992, Mustard Seed Publications; Bolane J, Furlong J: *Coping with bedrest in pregnancy,* Waco, TX, 1994, Childbirth Graphcis.

chorioamnionitis). The initiation of tocolytic therapy might be considered at this time. Tocolytic therapy, the administration of pharmaceutical agents that suppress uterine activity, has been studied since the late 1970s (Viamantes, 1996). At first it was thought that tocolytic therapy could prolong a threatened pregnancy indefinitely; research has demonstrated that a gain of 24 hours to several days is the best outcome that can be expected (Goldenberg and Rouse, 1998). It is now thought that the best reason to use tocolytics is that they afford the opportunity to begin administering antenatal glucocorticoids to accelerate fetal lung maturity and reduce the severity of sequelae in infants born preterm (Goldenberg and Rouse, 1998).

Box 19-5
Contraindications to Tocolysis

MATERNAL

Severe PIH or eclampsia
Active vaginal bleeding
Intrauterine infection
Cardiac disease
Medical or obstetric condition that contraindicates continuation of pregnancy

FETAL

Estimated gestational age over 37 weeks
Dilation over 4 cm
Estimated birth weight greater than 2500 g
Fetal demise
Lethal fetal anomaly
Chorioamnionitis
Acute fetal distress
Chronic IUGR

Box 19-6
Nursing Care for Woman Receiving Tocolytic Therapy

Position woman on side for better placental perfusion
Explain the purpose, side effects, and contraindications of the drug
Assess blood pressure, pulse, and respirations regularly, according to institution's policies (in many institutions q15 min)
Notify provider if maternal pulse exceeds 120
Assess for signs of pulmonary edema (chest pain, shortness of breath, crackles, rhonchi)
Assess urinary output q1 hr; monitor for ketonuria
Limit fluid intake to 2500 to 3000 ml/day
Monitor electrolytes, blood glucose levels
Provide psychosocial support and opportunities for woman to express anxiety

The medications most commonly used for this purpose are ritodrine, terbutaline, magnesium sulfate, indomethacin, and nifedipine. There are important contraindications to the use of all tocolytics (Box 19-5).

Ritodrine and terbutaline, the most commonly used betamimetic medications for tocolysis, work by relaxing smooth muscles. Ritodrine is the only medication approved by the Food and Drug Administration (FDA) specifically for the purpose of cessation of uterine contractions. Other medications are used for this purpose on an "unlabeled" basis (i.e., medications known to be effective for a specific purpose though not specifically developed and tested for this purpose). Betamimetics have many maternal and fetal side effects and must always be used with extreme caution and careful, conscientious nursing care. Medication administration and nursing care is aimed at maintaining a therapeutic level of medication and avoiding the most serious side effects while maintaining optimal health of the fetus (Box 19-6, Table 19-1).

TABLE 19-1
Medication Guide: Tocolytic Therapy for Preterm Labor

Medication	Action	Indication	Dosage and Route	Adverse Reactions	Nursing Considerations
Ritodrine (Yutopar)	β-Adrenergic receptor stimulant; relaxes smooth muscles, inhibiting uterine activity and causing bronchodilation	Stop preterm labor	0.1 mg/min (IV); increase by 0.05 mg q10 min until contractions stop; maximum dose: 0.35 mg/min; PO dose: 5-10 mg q4 hr	Tachycardia, dysrhythmias, tremors, headache, nausea and vomiting, hyperglycemia, hypokalemia, fetal tachycardia, hypoxia	Close supervision necessary See Box 19-6. Women should be screened with ECG before therapy begins Start PO dose 30 min before IV dose is discontinued
Terbutaline (Brethine)	See ritodrine	Stop preterm labor May also be used to reduce hypertonic contractions	0.25 mg SC q30 min for 2 hr; maximum dose: 0.5 mg q4-6 hr; PO dose: 2.5-5 mg q4-6 hr	Tachycardia, flushing, palpitations, tremors, headache, nausea and vomiting, hypokalemia, ketonuria, altered glucose metabolism, fetal tachycardia	Close supervision necessary See Box 19-6 Caution: not FDA approved for use in preterm labor (unlabeled use) Subcutaneous pump may be used for continuous SC therapy
Magnesium sulfate	CNS depressant relaxes smooth muscles; competes with calcium entry into muscles and decreases intensity	Stop preterm labor	Initially 4-6 g IV over 20 min; then 1-3 g/hr until contractions stop	Hot flushes, sweating, nausea and vomiting, drowsiness, ↓ respirations, ↓ DTRs, ↓ urine output, ↓ BP	Assess for side effects; monitor magnesium levels; assess BP, respirations, urine output, DTRs; monitor FHR and uterine activity; antidote is calcium gluconate
Nifedipine (Procardia, Adalat)	Calcium channel blocker, relaxes smooth muscles	Stop preterm labor	Initially 10 mg (sublingual), then 10-20 mg q6 hr PO	Dizziness, headache, nervousness, nausea, palpitations, peripheral edema, hypotension	Do not use with magnesium sulfate; assess BP, pulse before giving; assess for signs of PTL Caution: not FDA approved for PTL (unlabeled use)
Indomethacin	Prostaglandin inhibition, relaxes smooth muscles	Stop preterm labor	100 mg (rectally), then 25-50 mg q4-6 hr (PO) up to 48 hr	Nausea and vomiting; dyspepsia, dizziness; fetal: premature closure of ductus arteriosus, oligohydramios	Uncommon use Do not use for woman with any bleeding potential; fetal assessment includes serial ultrasound to determine amniotic fluid levels and any change in ductus arteriosus; may cause hyperbilirubinemia in neonate Caution: not FDA approved for PTL (unlabeled use)

BP, Blood pressure; *DTRs,* deep tendon reflexes; *ECG,* electrocardiogram; *FHR,* fetal heart rate; *PTL,* preterm labor; *SC,* subcutaneous.

NURSE ALERT • Caution must be used when administering intravenous fluids to women in preterm labor because this practice can increase the risk for tocolytic-induced pulmonary edema. It is recommended that the total oral and intravenous fluid intake in 24 hours be restricted to 2400 to 3000 ml. Strict intake and output measurement, daily weight determination, and assessment of pulmonary function should be instituted (ACOG, 1995c; Freda and DeVore, 1996; Hill, 1995).

Magnesium sulfate is the most commonly used tocolytic agent, although its exact mechanism of action on uterine muscle is unclear. It has been used for decades for seizure control in women with preeclampsia, and began to be used for tocolysis in the 1970s (Iams, 1996). Indomethacin, a nonsteroidal antiinflammatory drug (NSAID), has been shown in some trials to cause a cessation of uterine contractions (Besinger et al, 1991). Nifedipine, a calcium channel blocker, is another tocolytic agent that can suppress contractions (Read and Wellby, 1986). It works by inhibiting calcium from entering smooth muscle cells, thus reducing uterine contractions. (For information on administration and nursing care of women receiving these medications, see Box 19-6 and Table 19-1.)

Promotion of Fetal Lung Maturity

Antenatal Glucocorticoids. Antenatal glucocorticoids given as intramuscular injections to the mother accelerate fetal lung maturity. This class of medications also seems to decrease rates of intraventricular hemorrhage in preterm infants (Goldenberg and Rouse, 1998). All women between 24 and 34 weeks of gestation should be given antenatal glucocorticoids when preterm birth is threatened, unless there is a medical indication for immediate delivery such as cord prolapse, chorioamnionitis, or abruptio placentae (National Institutes of Health, 1995). The regimen for administration of antenatal glucocorticoids is given in Box 19-7.

Management of Inevitable Preterm Birth. Labor that has progressed to a cervical dilation of 4 cm is likely to lead to inevitable preterm birth. Preterm births that occur in tertiary care centers lead to better neonatal and maternal outcomes. Women considered at risk for inevitable preterm birth, therefore, should be transferred quickly to such a facility to ensure the best possible outcome. The first dose of antenatal glucocorticoids should be given before transfer because these medications require 24 hours to take effect.

Maternal transport, while helping to ensure a better health outcome for the mother and the baby, may have its complications. Women may be transported to tertiary centers far from home, making visits by the family difficult and increasing the anxiety levels of the woman and her family.

Box 19-7

Medication Guide: Antenatal Glucocorticoid Therapy with Betamethasone, Dexamethasone

ACTION

Stimulates fetal lung maturation by promoting release of enzymes that induce production and/or release of lung surfactant. NOTE: The FDA has not approved these medications for this use (i.e., this is an unlabeled use for obstetrics).

INDICATION

To prevent or reduce the severity of respiratory distress syndrome in preterm infants between 24 and 34 weeks of gestation

DOSAGE AND ROUTE

Betamethasone: 12 mg IM × 2 doses 12 hr apart
Dexamethasone: 6 mg IM × 2 doses 12 hr apart
May be repeated in 7 days if birth has not occurred.

ADVERSE REACTIONS

Possible maternal infection, pulmonary edema (if given with β-adrenergic medications), may worsen maternal condition (diabetes, hypertension)

NURSING CONSIDERATIONS

Give deep IM in gluteal muscle. Teach signs of pulmonary edema. Assess blood glucose levels and lung sounds. Do not give if woman has infection. Use in women with PPROM not universally recommended.

Critical Thinking

PRETERM LABOR

You are assigned to a woman who is experiencing preterm labor at 28 weeks' gestation. She has a 2-year-old-son at home. This is the woman's third admission for preterm labor during this pregnancy. What impact might her history have on the nursing care she receives this time? Discuss the pros and cons of home management vs. hospital management for the prevention of preterm birth for this woman. Develop a teaching plan to reduce the frustration and boredom that the woman will experience if she is restricted to bed rest for the next several weeks. What resources are available to assist with care of her 2-year-old-son?

Family Focus

IMPACT OF PRETERM BIRTH

Parental concern for the well-being of the infant is apparent during labor. Parents need to be aware of the interest and support of staff members. However, false assurance of fetal health must be avoided. For some parents the reality of the situation is not appreciated until they see their daughter or son in the intensive care unit. For those who experience fetal or neonatal death, the loss intensifies once the stress of labor and childbirth is over.

During the postpartum period, physical care of the mother is similar to that required after any vaginal birth. However, the family will be very anxious concerning the health and prognosis of the infant. Care of the preterm infant involves not only medical and nursing personnel but also participation of the parents. The nurse must be aware of the impact that a preterm birth may have on family dynamics. Parents must accept that the infant has special needs, and they must learn to meet these needs before discharge so that they have more realistic expectations when they are at home*.

*Weingarten C et al: Married mothers' perceptions of their premature or term infants and the quality of their relationships with their husbands, *J Obstet Gynecol Neonatal Nurs* 19(1):64-73, 1990.

➤ Evaluation

Evaluation of the nursing care provided a woman at risk for preterm labor is based on the expected outcomes of care (see Nursing Care Plan).

PRETERM PREMATURE RUPTURE OF MEMBRANES

Premature rupture of membranes (PROM) is the rupture of the amniotic sac and leakage of amniotic fluid beginning at least 1 hour before the onset of labor at any gestational age. Preterm premature rupture of membranes (PPROM) (i.e., membranes rupture before 37 weeks of gestation) occurs in up to 25% of all cases of preterm labor. Infection often precedes PPROM, but the etiology of PPROM remains unknown. PPROM is diagnosed after the woman complains of either a sudden gush of fluid from the vagina, or a slow leak of fluid from the vagina.

Infection is the serious side effect of PPROM that makes it a major complication of pregnancy. Chorioamnionitis is an intraamniotic infection of the chorion and amnion that is potentially life-threatening for the fetus and the woman. Most cases of intrauterine infection respond well to antibiotics, yet sepsis can occur and can lead to maternal death. Fetal complications from chorioamnionitis include congenital pneumonia, sepsis, and meningitis (Mercer et al, 1997). Even in the absence of infection, PPROM can precipitate cord prolapse, a potentially life-threatening complication for the fetus.

Care Management: Home Vs. Hospital

Whenever PPROM is suspected, strict sterile technique should be used in any vaginal examination to avoid introduction of infection.

Women with PPROM should be taught how to count fetal movements daily because a slowing of fetal movement has been shown to be a precursor to severe fetal compromise. Several methods are commonly used to count fetal movements; one method is described in the Guidelines box.

Expectant management continues as long as there are no signs of infection or fetal distress. This care includes all the assessments previously described, as well as other tests of fetal well-being, such as biophysical profile, especially measurement of amniotic fluid index.

Guidelines

INSTRUCTIONS FOR SELF-CARE: COUNTING FETAL MOVEMENTS (KICK COUNTS)

Choose a time of day when you can sit or lie quietly.

Choices for counting strategies:

- **Starting at 9 AM, count the baby's movements until you have counted 10. If you have not counted 10 movements in 12 hours, notify your primary health care provider immediately.**
- **Count 4 movements, three times a day after meals. Most people count 4 movements in 1 hour. If you don't, then count for 1 more hour. If at the end of 2 hours you still haven't felt 4 movements, call your primary health care provider immediately.**

Dystocia

Dystocia is defined as long, difficult, or abnormal labor; it is caused by various conditions associated with the five factors affecting labor. It is estimated that dystocia occurs in approximately 8% to 11% of women during the first stage of labor when the fetus is in a vertex presentation. Second stage dystocia is equally as common (Wiznitzer, 1995). Dystocia can be caused by any of the following:

- Dysfunctional labor, resulting in ineffective uterine contractions or maternal bearing-down efforts (the powers). It is the most common cause of dystocia (Cunningham et al, 1997).
- Alterations in the pelvic structure (the passage)
- Fetal causes, including abnormal presentation or position, anomalies, excessive size, and number of fetuses (the passenger)
- Maternal position during labor and birth
- Psychologic responses of the mother to labor related to past experiences, preparation, culture and heritage, and support system

These five factors are interdependent. In assessing the woman for an abnormal labor pattern, the nurse must consider the way in which these factors interact and influence labor progress. Dystocia is suspected when there is an alteration in the characteristics of uterine contractions, a lack of progress in the rate of cervical dilation, or a lack of progress in fetal descent and expulsion.

Dysfunctional Labor. Dysfunctional labor is described as abnormal uterine contractions that prevent the normal progress of cervical dilation, effacement (primary powers), or descent (secondary powers). Dysfunction of uterine contractions can be further described as being hypertonic or hypotonic.

Several factors seem to increase a woman's risk for uterine dystocia, including:

- Body build (e.g., 30 pounds or more overweight, short stature)
- Uterine abnormalities (e.g., congenital malformations, over-distention as with multiple gestation or hydramnios)
- Malpresentations and positions of the fetus
- Cephalopelvic disproportion
- Overstimulation with oxytocin
- Maternal fatigue, dehydration and electrolyte imbalance, and fear
- Inappropriate timing of analgesic or anesthetic administration

Hypertonic Uterine Dysfunction. The woman experiencing hypertonic uterine dysfunction, or primary dysfunctional labor, is often an anxious first-time mother who is having painful and frequent contractions that are ineffective in causing cervical dilation or effacement to progress. These contractions usually occur in the latent stage (cervical dilation of <4 cm) and usually are uncoordinated (Fig. 19-3). The force of the contraction may be in the midsection of the uterus rather than in the fundus, and the uterus is therefore unable to apply downward pressure to push the presenting part against the cervix. The uterus may not relax completely between contractions.

Women experiencing hypertonic uterine dysfunction may be exhausted and express concern about loss of control because of the intense pain they are experiencing and the lack of progress. Therapeutic rest, which is achieved with a warm

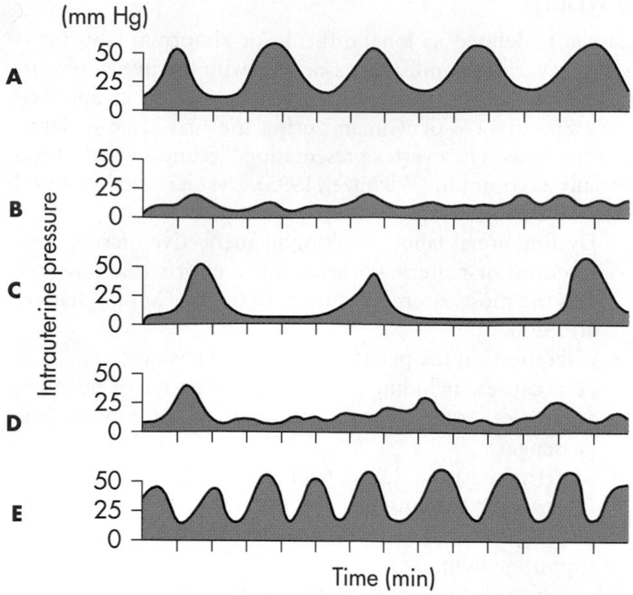

FIG. 19-3 • Uterine contractility patterns in labor. **A,** Typical normal labor. **B,** Subnormal intensity, with frequency greater than needed for optimum performance. **C,** Normal contractions but too infrequent for efficient labor. **D,** Incoordinate activity. **E,** Hypercontractility.

bath or shower and the administration of analgesics such as morphine, meperidine, or Nubain to inhibit uterine contractions, reduce pain and encourage sleep, is usually prescribed for the management of hypertonic uterine dysfunction. After a 4- to 6-hour rest, these women are likely to awaken in active labor with a normal uterine contraction pattern (Gilbert and Harmon, 1998).

Hypotonic Uterine Dysfunction. The second and more common type of uterine dysfunction is hypotonic uterine dysfunction, or secondary uterine inertia. The woman, who may be either in her first or a subsequent pregnancy, initially makes normal progress into the active stage of labor; then the contractions become weak and inefficient or stop altogether (see Fig. 19-3, *B*). The uterus is easily indented, even at the peak of contractions. Intrauterine pressure during the contraction (usually <25 mm Hg) is insufficient for progress of cervical effacement and dilation (Gilbert and Harmon, 1998). Cephalopelvic disproportion and malpositions are common causes of this type of uterine dysfunction.

A woman experiencing hypotonic uterine dysfunction may become exhausted and be at increased risk for infection. Management usually consists of performing an ultrasound or x-ray examination to rule out cephalopelvic disproportion and assessing the fetal heart rate pattern, characteristics of amniotic fluid if membranes are ruptured, and maternal well-being. If findings are normal, then measures such as ambulation, hydrotherapy, enema, stripping or rupture of membranes, nipple stimulation, and oxytocin infusion, can be used to augment labor (Varney, 1997).

Secondary Powers. Secondary powers, or bearing-down efforts, are compromised when large amounts of analgesic are given. Anesthesia may also block the bearing-down reflex and, as a result, alter the effectiveness of voluntary efforts. Exhaustion from lack of sleep or a long labor and fatigue from inadequate hydration and food intake affect the woman's voluntary efforts. Maternal position can work against the forces of gravity and decrease the strength and efficiency of the contraction (Nursing Care Plan). Table 19-2 summarizes dysfunctional labor.

Alterations in Pelvic Structure

Pelvic Dystocia. Pelvic dystocia can occur whenever there are contractures of the pelvic diameters that reduce the capacity of the bony pelvis, including the inlet, midpelvis, outlet, or any combination of these planes.

Disproportion of the pelvis is the least common cause of dystocia (Cunningham et al, 1997). Pelvic contractures may be caused by congenital abnormalities, maternal malnutrition, neoplasms, or lower spinal disorders. An immature pelvic size predisposes some adolescent mothers to pelvic dystocia. Pelvic deformities may also be the result of automobile or other accidents.

An inlet contracture occurs in 1% to 2% of term births and is diagnosed when the diagonal conjugate is less than 11.5 cm. The incidence of face and shoulder presentation is increased. Because these presentations prevent engagement and fetal descent, the risk of prolapse of the umbilical cord is increased. Inlet contracture is associated with maternal rickets and a flat pelvis. Weak uterine contractions may be noted during the first stage of labor in affected women.

Midplane contracture, the most common cause of pelvic dystocia, is diagnosed when the sum of the interischial spinous and posterior sagittal diameters of the midpelvis is 13.5 cm or less. Fetal descent is arrested (transverse arrest of the fetal head) because the head cannot rotate internally. These infants are usually born by cesarean, but vacuum extraction has been used safely when the cervix is fully dilated. Midforceps-assisted birth usually is not done because of the increased perinatal morbidity associated with this intervention.

Outlet contracture exists when the interischial diameter is 8 cm or less. It rarely occurs in the absence of midplane contracture. Women with outlet contracture have a long, narrow pubic arch and an android pelvis, and this causes fetal descent to be arrested. Maternal complications include extensive perineal lacerations during vaginal birth because the fetal head is pushed posteriorly.

Soft-Tissue Dystocia. Soft-tissue dystocia results from obstruction of the birth passage by an anatomic abnormality other than that involving the bony pelvis. The obstruction may result from placenta previa (i.e., low-lying placenta) that partially or completely obstructs the internal os of the cervix. Other causes such as leiomyomas (uterine fibroids) in the lower uterine segment, ovarian tumors, and a full bladder or rectum, may prevent the fetus from entering the pelvis. Occasionally, cervical edema occurs during labor when the cervix is caught between the presenting part and the symphysis pubis or when the woman begins bearing-down efforts prematurely, inhibiting complete dilation.

Bandl's ring, a pathologic retraction ring, is associated with prolonged rupture of membranes and protracted labor (Cunningham et al, 1997).

Fetal Causes. Dystocia of fetal origin may be caused by anomalies, excessive fetal size and malpresentation, malposition, or multifetal pregnancy. Complications associated with dystocia of fetal origin include neonatal asphyxia, fetal injuries

Nursing Care Plan DYSFUNCTIONAL LABOR: SECONDARY INERTIA

NURSING DIAGNOSIS Risk for injury to mother and/or fetus related to oxytocin stimulation secondary to dysfunctional labor

EXPECTED OUTCOME Maternal-fetal well-being is maintained; labor progresses and birth occurs.

Nursing Interventions/*Rationales*

Explain oxytocin protocol to woman and her labor partner *to allay apprehensions and enhance participation.*

Encourage woman to void before beginning protocol *to prevent discomfort and remove a barrier to labor progress.*

Apply the electronic fetal monitor per hospital protocol and obtain a 15- to 20-minute baseline strip *to ensure adequate assessment of FHR and contractions.*

Position woman in a side-lying position and administer the oxytocin per physician order using an IV infusion pump *to stimulate uterine activity and provide adequate control of the flow rate.*

Regulate the oxytocin per protocol and advancing the dose in increments of 1 to 2 mU/min every 15 to 60 minutes *to allow adequate evaluation of the woman's response to stimulation and to prevent hyperstimulation and fetal hypoxia.*

Maintain oxytocin dose and rate when contractions occur every 2 to 3 minutes with a duration of 40 to 90 seconds and intrauterine pressures of 40 to 90 mm Hg *to produce effective uterine stimulation without risk of hyperstimulation.*

If infusion rate is advanced to 20 mU/min without achieving the desired contractility pattern, notify physician *to avoid hyperstimulation and water intoxication.*

Monitor maternal vital signs every 30 to 60 minutes *to assess for oxytocin-induced hypertension.*

Monitor contractility pattern and FHR pattern every 15 minutes *to assess uterine activity for possible hypertonicity or ineffective uterine response to oxytocin and to detect evidence of fetal distress.*

Monitor intake, output, and specific gravity (limit intake to 1000 ml/8 hr; output should be at least 120 ml/4 hr) *to assess for urinary retention and prevent water intoxication.*

Monitor cervical dilation, effacement, and station *to assess progress of labor.*

If hypertonicity or signs of fetal distress are detected, discontinue oxytocin immediately *to arrest the progress of hypertonicity;* turn woman on her side *to increase placental blood flow;* increase primary IV rate to 200 ml/hr (unless signs of water toxicity are present); administer oxygen per face mask *to enhance placental perfusion,* notify physician; and continuously monitor maternal vital signs and FHR *to provide ongoing assessment of maternal/fetal status.*

NURSING DIAGNOSIS Pain related to increasing frequency, regularity, intensity, and prolonged peak of contractions

EXPECTED OUTCOME The woman exhibits signs of decreased discomfort.

Nursing Interventions/*Rationales*

Prepare woman and labor partner for the change in the nature of the contractions once the oxytocin drip is initiated *to prepare them and allow for more effective coping.*

Remind woman and labor partner that analgesics are available for use during labor *to provide knowledge to help them make decisions about pain control.*

Review the use of specific techniques such as conscious relaxation, focused breathing, effleurage, massage, and application of sacral pressure *to increase relaxation, decrease intensity of pain of contractions, and promote use of controlled thought and direction of energy.*

Provide comfort measures such as frequent mouth care *to prevent dry mouth,* application of damp cloth to forehead and changing of damp gown or bed covers *to relieve discomfort of diaphoresis,* and positioning *to reduce stiffness.*

Encourage conscious relaxation between contractions *to prevent fatigue, which contributes to increased pain perceptions.*

NURSING DIAGNOSIS Anxiety/ineffective coping related to prolonged labor, increased pain, and fatigue

EXPECTED OUTCOME Woman's anxiety is reduced; woman actively participates in the labor process.

Nursing Interventions/*Rationales*

Provide ongoing feedback to woman and partner *to allay anxiety and enhance participation.*

Present care options when possible *to increase feelings of control.*

Continue to provide comfort measures *to maintain a posture of support and caring and to aid woman in focusing on the labor process.*

Encourage woman and partner to continue to use those mechanisms that promote effective labor (e.g., breathing, positioning) *to keep woman and partner actively involved in process.*

NURSING DIAGNOSIS Risk for maternal/fetal infection related to prolonged rupture of membranes or possible invasive procedures (e.g., use of fetal scalp electrodes, use of forceps, episiotomy, cesarean birth)

EXPECTED OUTCOME There is no evidence of infection.

Nursing Interventions/*Rationales*

Monitor temperature *to assess for elevation as early indicator of infection*

Monitor FHR/variability *to assess for rates greater than 160 beats/min and minimal variability that is indicative of maternal fever and infection.*

Continued

Nursing Care Plan DYSFUNCTIONAL LABOR: SECONDARY INERTIA—cont'd

Monitor intake and output for dehydration *to assess for signs of infection that closely resemble those of dehydration, and differentiation is needed.*

Maintain Standard Precautions and use scrupulous handwashing techniques when providing care *to prevent spread of infection.*

Use strict aseptic technique when performing invasive procedures such as urinary catheterization, insertion of intravenous lines, or application of scalp electrodes *to reduce risk of nosocomial infection.*

Monitor IV sites, electrode sites, and incision sites for signs such as pain, redness, edema, heat, and drainage *to assess for infection.*

Monitor urine for color, concentration, odor, clouding, casts, and sediment *to assess for a urinary tract infection.*

When membranes rupture, assess fluid for color, amount, and odor, and for the presence of meconium stain *to assess for alterations that may be indicative of intrauterine infection.*

After membrane rupture, keep vaginal examinations to a minimum and use sterile gloves *to decrease risk of uterine infection.*

Assist woman to maintain good personal hygiene habits (e.g., wiping perineal region from front to back, keeping area dry *to reduce introduction of bacteria.*

Monitor laboratory values (e.g., white blood cell count, culture) *to assess for indicators of infection.*

TABLE 19-2
Dysfunctional Labor: Primary and Secondary Powers

Hypertonic Uterine Dysfunction	Hypotonic Uterine Dysfunction	Inadequate Voluntary Expulsive Forces
DESCRIPTION		
Usually occurs before 4 cm dilation; cause unknown, may be related to fear and tension (primary powers)	Cause may be contracture and fetal malposition, overdistention of uterus (e.g., twins), or unknown (primary powers)	Involves abdominal and levator animuscles Occurs in second stage of labor; cause may be related to conduction anesthetic, heavy analgesic, exhaustion
CHANGE IN PATTERN OF PROGRESS		
Pain out of proportion to intensity of contraction Pain out of proportion to effectiveness of contraction in effacing and dilating the cervix Contractions increase in frequency Contractions uncoordinated Uterus is contracted between contractions, cannot be indented	Contractions decrease in frequency and intensity Uterus easily indentable even at peak of contraction Uterus relaxed between contractions (normal)	No voluntary urge to push or bear down or inadequate/ineffective pushing
POTENTIAL MATERNAL EFFECTS		
Loss of control related to intensity of pain and lack of progress Exhaustion	Infection Exhaustion Psychologic trauma	Spontaneous vaginal birth prevented
POTENTIAL FETAL EFFECTS		
Fetal asphyxia with meconium aspiration	Fetal infection Fetal and neonatal death	Fetal asphyxia
CARE MANAGEMENT		
Initiate therapeutic rest measures • Administer analgesic (e.g., morphine, nubain, meperidine) if membranes not ruptured or cephalopelvic disproportion not present • Relieve pain to permit mother to rest • Assist with measures to enhance rest and relaxation (e.g., hydrotherapy)	Rule out cephalopelvic disproportion Stimulate labor with oxytocin (augmentation) Perform amniotomy Assist with measures to enhance the progress of labor (e.g., position changes, ambulation, hydrotherapy)	Coach mother in bearing down with contractions; assist with relaxation between contractions Position mother in favorable position for pushing Reduce epidural infusion rate Apply low forceps or vacuum if assistance is needed Schedule cesarean birth only if nonreassuring fetal status occurs

or fractures, and maternal vaginal lacerations. Although spontaneous vaginal birth is possible in these instances, a low-forceps or vacuum-assisted or cesarean birth often is necessary.

Anomalies. Gross ascites, large tumors, and open neural tube defects such as myelomeningocele and hydrocephalus are fetal anomalies that can cause dystocia. The anomalies affect the relationship of the fetal anatomy to the maternal pelvic capacity, with the result that the fetus is unable to descend through the birth canal.

Cephalopelvic Disproportion. Cephalopelvic disproportion (CPD), also called fetopelvic disproportion (FPD), is related to excessive fetal size (i.e., 4000 g or more). It occurred at the rate of 23 per 1000 live births in 1996 (Ventura et al, 1998).

When CPD is present, the fetus cannot fit through the maternal pelvis to be born vaginally. Excessive fetal size, or macrosomia, is associated with maternal diabetes mellitus, obesity, multiparity, or the large size of one or both parents. If the maternal pelvis is too small, abnormally shaped, or deformed, CPD may be of maternal origin. In this case, the fetus may be of average size or even smaller.

Malposition. The most common fetal malposition is persistent occipitoposterior position (i.e., right occipitoposterior [ROP] or left occipitoposterior [LOP]) (see Fig. 15-2), occurring in about 25% of all labors. Labor, especially the second stage, is prolonged; the woman typically complains of severe back pain from the pressure of the fetal head pressing against her sacrum. Box 19-8 contains suggested measures to relieve back pain and facilitate rotation of the fetal occiput to an anterior position, which will facilitate birth (Gilbert and Harmon, 1998).

Malpresentation. Breech presentation is the most common form of malpresentation and occurs in 3% to 4% of all births and in up to 25% of all preterm births. There are four main types of breech presentation: frank breech (thighs flexed, knees extended); complete breech (thighs and knees flexed); and two types of incomplete breech, one in which the knee extends below the buttocks and the other in which the foot extends below the buttocks (Fig. 19-4). Breech presentations are associated with multifetal gestation, preterm birth, fetal and maternal anomalies, hydramnios, and oligohydramnios. Diagnosis is made by abdominal palpation and vaginal examination and usually is confirmed by ultrasound scan (Laros, Flanagan, and Kilpatrick, 1995; Ventura et al, 1998).

During labor, fetal descent may be slow because the breech is not as good a dilating wedge as the fetal head; but the labor itself usually is not prolonged. There is risk of prolapse of the cord if the membranes rupture in early labor. The presence of meconium in amniotic fluid is not necessarily a sign of fetal distress because it results from pressure on the fetal abdominal

Box 19-8

Back Labor—Occiput Posterior Position

MEASURES TO RELIEVE BACK PAIN AND FACILITATE ROTATION OF FETAL HEAD

Measures to Reduce Back Pain During a Contraction

- *Counterpressure:* apply fist or heel of hand to sacral area
- *Heat or cold applications:* apply to sacral area
- *Double hip squeeze:*
  Woman assumes a position with hip joints flexed such as knee-chest
  Partner, nurse, or doula places hands over gluteal muscles and presses with palms of hands up and inward toward the center of the pelvis
- *Knee press:*
  Woman assumes a sitting position with knees a few inches apart and feet flat on the floor or on a stool
  Partner, nurse, or doula cups a knee in each hand with heels of hands on top of tibia then presses the knees straight back toward the woman's hips while leaning forward toward the woman

Measures to Facilitate the Rotation of the Fetal Head (May Also Relieve Back Pain)

- *Lateral abdominal stroking:* stroke the abdomen in direction that the fetal head should rotate
- *Hands-and-knees position* (all-fours): can also be accomplished by kneeling while leaning forward over a birth ball, padded chair seat, bed, or over-the-bed table
- *Squatting*
- *Pelvic rocking*
- *Stair climbing*
- *Lateral position:* lie on side toward which the fetus should turn
- *Lunges:* widens pelvis on side toward which woman lunges
  Woman stands, facing forward, next to/alongside a chair so that she can lunge toward the side the fetal back is on or in the direction of the fetal occiput
  Places foot on seat of chair with toes pointed toward the back of the chair then lunges
  Alternative position for lunge: kneeling

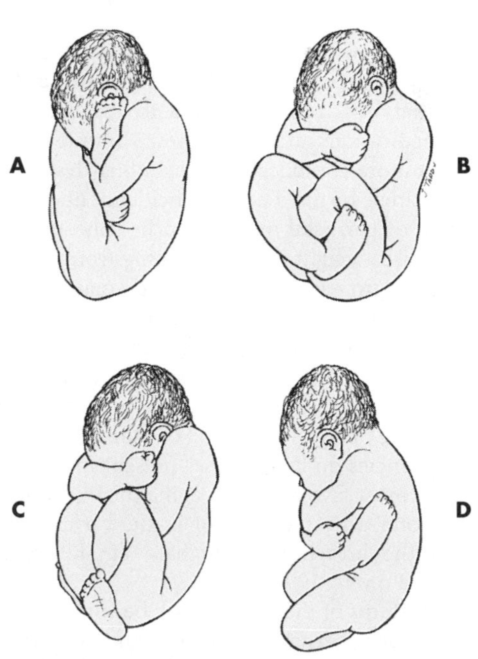

FIG. 19-4 • Types of breech presentation. **A,** Frank breech: thighs are flexed on hips; knees are extended. **B,** Complete breech: thighs and knees are flexed. **C,** Incomplete breech: foot extends below the buttocks. **D,** Incomplete breech: knee extends below the buttocks.

wall as it traverses the birth canal. Assessment of FHR and pattern should be used to determine if the passage of meconium is an expected finding associated with breech presentation or is a nonreassuring sign associated with fetal hypoxia. The fetal heart tones of infants in a breech position are best heard at or above the umbilicus.

Vaginal birth is accomplished by mechanisms of labor that manipulate the buttocks and lower extremities as they emerge from the birth canal (Varney, 1997). Piper forceps sometimes are used to deliver the head (see Fig. 19-8). External cephalic version (ECV) may be tried to turn the fetus to a vertex presentation. Cesarean birth may be necessary (Laros, Flanagan, and Kilpatrick, 1995).

Although opinions vary, a cesarean birth is commonly performed when the fetus is estimated to be larger than 3800 g or smaller than 1500 g, if this is a first pregnancy, if labor is ineffective, or if complications occur (Scott, 1999). Although cesarean birth reduces the risks to the fetus, the maternal risks are increased. ECV also poses risks and is not always successful. Women whose breech presentation occurs late in pregnancy need to be informed about the options for birth, including the risks associated with each option.

Face and brow presentations are uncommon and are associated with fetal anomalies, pelvic contractures, and CPD. Vaginal birth is possible if the fetus flexes to a vertex presentation, although forceps often are used. Cesarean birth is indicated if the presentation persists, if there is fetal distress, or if labor stops progressing.

Cesarean birth is usually necessary for a fetus in a shoulder presentation (i.e., the fetus is in a transverse lie), although external cephalic version may be attempted after 38 weeks' gestation (Cunningham et al, 1997; Varney, 1997).

Multifetal Pregnancy. Multifetal pregnancy is the gestation of twins, triplets, quadruplets, or more infants.

Since 1980, the twin birth rate has increased by 37%, and the higher order multiple rate has quadrupled (Ventura et al, 1998). It is likely that this trend is related to the use of fertility-enhancing medications and procedures. Multiple births are associated with more complications, including dysfunctional labor, than are single births. The high incidence of complications and high risk of perinatal mortality primarily stems from the birth of low-birth-weight infants resulting from preterm birth and intrauterine growth restriction. Fetuses may experience distress and asphyxia during birth as a result of cord prolapse and the onset of placental separation with the birth of the first fetus.

In addition, fetal complications such as congenital anomalies and abnormal presentations can lead to dystocia and an increased incidence of cesarean birth. For example, in only half of all twin pregnancies do both fetuses present in the vertex presentation, the most favorable for vaginal birth; in one third of pregnancies, one twin may present in the vertex presentation and one in the breech (Cunningham et al, 1997; Ellings, Newman, and Bowers, 1998).

The health status of the mother may be compromised by an increased risk for hypertension, anemia, and hemorrhage associated with uterine atony; abruptio placentae; and multiple or adherent placentas. Early detection and care of the maternal/fetal/newborn complications associated with multiple births are essential to achieve a positive outcome for mothers and babies. Maternal positioning and active support are used to enhance labor progress and placental perfusion. Teamwork and planning are essential in the management of childbirth in multiple pregnancies.

Position of the Woman. The functional relationships between the uterine contractions, the fetus, and the mother's pelvis are altered by the maternal position. In addition, the position can provide either a mechanical advantage or disadvantage to the mechanisms of labor by altering the effects of gravity and the body part relationships important to the progress of labor. For example, the hands-and-knees position facilitates rotation from a posterior occiput position more effectively than does the lateral position. Sitting and squatting facilitate fetal descent during pushing and shorten the second stage of labor (Biancuzzo, 1993). Discouraging maternal movement or restricting labor to the recumbent or lithotomy position may compromise labor. The incidence of dystocia in women confined to these positions is increased, resulting in increased need for augmentation of labor, the use of forceps, and vacuum-assisted or cesarean birth.

Psychologic Responses. Hormones released in response to stress can cause dystocia. Sources of stress vary for each woman, but pain and the absence of a support person are two recognized factors. Confinement to bed and restriction of maternal movement can be a source of psychologic stress that compounds the physiologic stress caused by immobility in the unmedicated, laboring woman. When anxiety is excessive, it can inhibit normal cervical dilation and result in prolonged labor and increased pain perception. Anxiety also causes increased levels of stress-related hormones (e.g., β-endorphin, adrenocorticotropic hormone, cortisol, and epinephrine). These hormones act on the smooth muscles of the uterus; increased levels can cause dystocia by reducing uterine contractility (Biancuzzo, 1993).

Abnormal Labor Patterns. In 1996, prolonged labor patterns occurred at the rate of 8.9 per 1000 live births, with the incidence slightly higher among women 40 to 49 years of age (Ventura et al, 1998).

Six abnormal labor patterns have been identified and classified by Friedman (1989) according to the nature of cervical dilation and fetal descent. The labor patterns seen in normal and abnormal labor are described in Table 19-3.

These patterns may result from a variety of causes that include ineffective uterine contractions, pelvic contractures, CPD, abnormal fetal presentation or position, early use of analgesics, conduction anesthesia, and anxiety and stress. Progress in either the first or second stage of labor can be protracted (prolonged) or arrested (stopped).

Health care providers must be careful when diagnosing a labor pattern as prolonged and when intervening based on this diagnosis. Criteria defining the differences between false, latent, and active labor should be established. Using hospital or unit admission areas to evaluate a woman's labor status is helpful in preventing the premature implementation of labor interventions such as induction of epidural analgesia.

Maternal morbidity and mortality may occur as a result of uterine rupture, infection, serious dehydration, and postpartum hemorrhage. A long, difficult labor also can have an adverse psychologic effect on the mother, father, and family.

Precipitous Labor. Precipitous labor is defined as labor that lasts less than 3 hours from the onset of contractions to the time of birth. Precipitous labor may result from hypertonic uterine contractions that are tetanic in intensity. Maternal and

TABLE 19-3
Labor Patterns in Normal and Abnormal Labor

NORMAL LABOR
1. Dilation: continues
   a. Latent phase: <4 cm and low slope
   b. Active phase: >5 cm or high slope
   c. Deceleration phase: ≥9 cm
2. Descent: active at ≥9 cm dilation

ABNORMAL LABOR

Pattern	Nulliparas	Multiparas
Prolonged latent phase	>20 hr	>14 hr
Protracted active phase dilation	<1.2 cm/hr	<1.5 cm/hr
Secondary arrest: no change	≥2 hr	≥2 hr
Protracted descent	<1 cm/hr	<2 cm/hr
Arrest of descent	≥1 hr	≥½ hr
Failure of descent	No change during deceleration phase and second stage	
Precipitous labor	>5 cm/hr	10 cm/hr

fetal complications can occur as a result. Maternal complications include uterine rupture, lacerations of the birth canal, amniotic fluid embolism, and postpartum hemorrhage. Fetal complications include hypoxia caused by decreased periods of uterine relaxation between contractions, and intracranial hemorrhage related to rapid birth (Cunningham et al, 1997).

Care Management

➤ Assessment

Risk assessment is a continuous process in the laboring woman. Review of the findings obtained during the initial interview conducted at the woman's admission to the labor unit, and ongoing observations of her psychologic response to labor may reveal factors that can be a source of dysfunctional labor. These factors may include anxiety or fear, a complication of pregnancy, or previous labor complications. The initial physical assessment and ongoing assessments provide information about maternal well-being; status of labor in terms of the characteristics of uterine contractions and progress of cervical effacement and dilation; fetal well-being in terms of FHR and pattern, presentation, station, and position; and status of the amniotic membranes.

Ultrasound scanning can identify potential dysfunctional labor problems related to the fetus or maternal pelvis. All of these assessments contribute to accurate identification of potential and actual nursing diagnoses related to dystocia and maternal-fetal compromise.

➤ Nursing Diagnoses

Potential or actual nursing diagnoses that might be identified for women experiencing dystocia include the following:

- Risk for maternal injury related to:
  —Interventions implemented for dystocia
- Powerlessness related to:
  —Loss of control
- Risk for infection related to:
  —Rupture of membranes
  —Operative procedures
- Sensory/perceptual alterations related to:
  —Numerous interventions for dystocia
- Ineffective individual coping related to:
  —Exhaustion
  —Lack of support system

➤ Expected Outcomes

Expected outcomes for the woman who is experiencing dystocia include the following. The woman will:

- Understand the causes and treatment of dysfunctional labor
- Use positive patterns of coping to maintain a positive self-concept
- Express relief of pain
- Experience labor and birth with minimal or no complications such as infection, injury, or hemorrhage
- Give birth to a healthy infant who has not experienced fetal distress

➤ Plan of Care and Implementation

Nurses assume many caregiving roles when labor is complicated. They also work collaboratively with other health care providers in providing care. Interventions that the nurse may be implement or assist with include external cephalic version, trial of labor, induction or augmentation with oxytocin, amniotomy, and operative procedures. The nursing role is identified with each of the procedures described.

LEGAL TIP • Standard of Care-Labor and Birth at Risk

- Document all assessments, interventions, and patient responses on patient record and monitor strips according to unit protocols, procedures, and policies and professional standards.
- Assess whether the woman (and family, if appropriate) is fully informed about procedures for which she is consenting.
- Maintain safety in administering medications and treatments correctly.
- Have verbal orders signed as soon as possible.
- Provide care at the acceptable standard (e.g., according to hospital protocols or professional standards).
- If short staffing occurs in the unit, and the nurse is assigned additional patients, the nurse should document that rejecting the additional assignment would have placed these patients in danger as a result of abandonment.
- Maternal and fetal monitoring continues until birth according to policies, procedures, and protocols of the birthing facility, even when a decision for cesarean birth is made.

Version. Version is the turning of the fetus artificially from one presentation to another. Version may be done externally or internally.

External Cephalic Version. External cephalic version (ECV) is used to attempt to turn the fetus from a breech or shoulder presentation to a vertex presentation for birth. It may be attempted in a labor and birth setting after 37 weeks of gestation. Before it is attempted, ultrasound scanning is done to determine the fetal position; locate the umbilical cord; rule out placenta previa; and assess the amount of amniotic fluid, the fetal age, and the presence of any anomalies. A nonstress test is performed to confirm fetal well-being, or the FHR is monitored for a time (usually 10 to 20 minutes). Informed consent is obtained. Contraindications to ECV include uterine anomalies, previous cesarean birth, CPD, placenta previa, multifetal gestation, and oligohydramnios (Cunningham et al, 1997; Laros, Flanagan, and Kilpatrick, 1995).

ECV is accomplished by gentle, constant pressure on the abdomen (Fig. 19-5). A tocolytic agent such as magnesium sulfate or terbutaline often is given to relax the uterus and to facilitate the maneuver. Ultrasound scanning is done to identify potential problems such as cord entanglement and placental separation (Cunningham et al, 1997; Laros, Flanagan, and Kilpatrick, 1995).

During an attempted ECV, the nurse continuously monitors the FHR, especially for bradycardia; checks maternal vital signs; and assesses the woman's level of comfort because the procedure may cause discomfort. After the procedure is completed, the nurse continues to monitor maternal vital signs, uterine activity, and FHR; and assesses for vaginal bleeding until the woman's condition is stable. Women who are Rh negative should receive Rh immune globulin because the manipulation

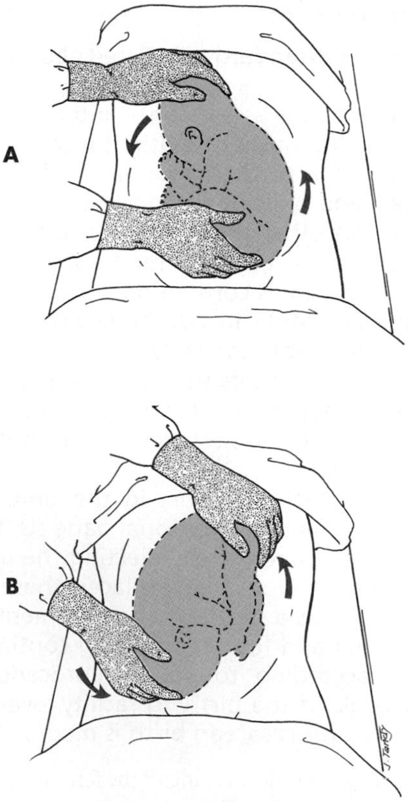

FIG. 19-5 • External version of fetus from breech to vertex presentation. This must be achieved without force. **A,** Breech is pushed up out of pelvic inlet while head is pulled toward inlet. **B,** Head is pushed toward inlet while breech is pulled upward.

can cause fetomaternal bleeding (Cunningham et al, 1997; Laros, Flanagan, and Kilpatrick, 1995).

Internal Version. With internal version, the fetus is turned by the physician, who inserts a hand into the uterus and changes the presentation to cephalic (head) or podalic (foot). Internal version may be used in multifetal pregnancies to deliver the second fetus. The safety of this procedure has not been documented; maternal and fetal injury is possible. Cesarean birth is the usual method for managing malpresentation in multifetal pregnancies. The nurse's role is to monitor the status of the fetus and to provide support to the woman.

Trial of Labor. A trial of labor (TOL) is the observance of a woman and her fetus for a reasonable period (e.g., 4 to 6 hours) of spontaneous active labor to assess the safety of vaginal birth for the mother and infant. TOL may be initiated if the mother's pelvis is of questionable size or shape, if she wishes to have a vaginal birth after a previous cesarean birth, or if the fetus is in an abnormal presentation. Fetal sonography or maternal pelvimetry (or both) may be done before a TOL to rule out CPD. The cervix must be soft and dilatable. During TOL, the woman is evaluated for the occurrence of active labor, including adequate contractions, engagement and descent of the presenting part, and effacement and dilation of the cervix.

Induction of Labor. Induction of labor is the chemical or mechanical initiation of uterine contractions before their spontaneous onset for the purpose of bringing about the birth. Induction may be indicated for a variety of medical and obstetric reasons. These include pregnancy-induced hypertension, diabetes mellitus and other maternal medical problems, postdate gestation, suspected fetal jeopardy (e.g., intrauterine growth restriction), logistic factors such as history of previous rapid birth or distance of the woman's home from the hospital, and fetal death. Under such conditions the risk to the mother or fetus is less than the risk of continuing the pregnancy (Mathews, 1998).

Both chemical and mechanical methods are used to induce labor. Intravenous oxytocin and amniotomy are the most common methods used in the United States. Less commonly used methods include nipple stimulation (manual or with a breast pump), the ingestion of castor oil or herbal preparations, a soapsuds enema, stripping of membranes, and acupuncture (Summers, 1997). Prostaglandins are also used for inducing labor.

Success rates for induction of labor are higher when the cervix is favorable, or inducible. A rating system such as the Bishop score (Table 19-4) can be used to evaluate inducibility. For example, a score of 9 or more on this 13-point scale indi-

TABLE 19-4
Bishop Score

	Score			
	0	1	2	3
Dilation (cm)	0	1-2	3-4	5-6
Effacement (%)	0-30	40-50	60-70	80
Station (cm)	−3	−2	−1	−1
Cervical consistency	Firm	Medium	Soft	
Cervix position	Posterior	Midline	Anterior	

cates that the cervix is soft, anterior, 50% or more effaced, and dilated 2 cm or more; and that the presenting part is engaged. Induction of labor is likely to be more successful if the score is 5 or more for nulliparas and 9 or more for multiparas (Gilbert and Harmon, 1998).

Cervical Ripening Methods

Chemical Agents. A prostaglandin gel has been approved by the FDA since 1993 as a cervical ripening agent (ACOG, 1995b). Various prostaglandins (hormones) have also been applied to the cervix before induction to "ripen" (soften and thin) the cervix (Box 19-9 and Box 19-10). This treatment usually results in a higher success rate for the induction of labor, the need for lower dosages of oxytocin during the induction, and shorter induction times. In some cases, women will go into labor after the application of prostaglandin, thereby eliminating the need to administer oxytocin to induce labor. Oxytocin induction usually is not started until 6 to 12 hours later to avoid hyperstimulation (ACOG, 1995b).

Mechanical Methods. Hygroscopic dilators (substances that absorb fluid from surrounding tissues and enlarge) also can be used for cervical ripening. Laminaria tents (natural cervical dilators made from seaweed) and synthetic dilators are inserted into the cervix. As they absorb fluid, they expand and cause cervical dilation. These dilators are left in place for 6 to 12 hours before being removed to assess cervical dilation. Fresh dilators are inserted if further cervical dilation is necessary. Synthetic dilators swell faster than natural dilators and become larger with less discomfort (ACOG, 1995b; Simpson and Poole, 1998; Summers, 1997).

Amniotomy. Amniotomy (i.e., artificial rupture of membranes [AROM]) can be used to induce labor when the condition of the cervix is favorable (ripe) or to augment labor if progress begins to slow. Labor usually begins within 12 hours of the rupture; however, if amniotomy does not stimulate labor, the resulting prolonged rupture may lead to infection. Once an amniotomy is performed, the woman is committed to giving birth. For this reason, amniotomy often is used in combination with oxytocin induction. Before the procedure, the woman should be told what to expect; she should also be assured that the actual rupture of membranes is painless for her and the fetus, though she may experience some discomfort when the Amnihook or other sharp instrument is inserted through the vagina and cervix (Box 19-11).

The presenting part of the fetus should be engaged and well applied to the cervix to reduce the risk of cord prolapse (ACOG, 1995b; Summers, 1997). The membranes are ruptured with an Amnihook or other sharp instrument and the amniotic fluid is allowed to drain slowly. The color, odor, and consistency of the

Box 19-9

Medication Guide: Cervical Ripening Using Prostaglandin E_2 (PGE_2): Dinoprostone (Cervidil Insert; Prepidil Gel)

ACTION

PGE_2 ripens the cervix, making it softer and causing it to begin to dilate and efface; stimulates uterine contractions.

INDICATIONS

PGE_2 is used for preinduction cervical ripening (ripen cervix before oxytocin induction of labor when the Bishop score is 4 or less), and to induce labor or abortion (abortifacient agent)

DOSAGE

Place Cervidil insert (10 mg dinoprostone gradually released over 12 hours) intravaginally into the posterior fornix. Insert Prepidil gel (2.5-ml syringe containing 0.5 mg of dinoprostone) into cervical canal just below internal cervical os. Repeat gel insertion in 6 hours as needed to a maximum of 1.5 mg in a 24-hour period. Continue treatment until maximum dosage is administered or until an effective contraction pattern is established (3 or more uterine contractions in 10 minutes), cervix ripens (Bishop score of 8 or greater), or significant adverse reactions occur.

ADVERSE REACTIONS

Potential adverse reactions include headache, nausea and vomiting, diarrhea, fever, hypotension, tachysystole (12 or more uterine contractions in 20 minutes without alteration of FHR pattern), hyperstimulation of the uterus (tachysystole with nonreassuring FHR patterns), or fetal passage of meconium.

NURSING CONSIDERATIONS

- Explain procedure to woman and her family. Ensure that an informed consent has been obtained as per agency policy.
- Assess maternal-fetal unit, before each insertion and during treatment following agency protocol for frequency. Assess maternal vital signs and health status, FHR pattern, and status of pregnancy, including indications for cervical ripening or induction of labor, signs of labor or impending labor, and the Bishop score. Recognize that a nonreassuring FHR pattern; maternal fever, infection, vaginal bleeding, or hypersensitivity; and regular, progressive uterine contractions contraindicate the use of dinoprostone.
- Use caution if the woman has a history of asthma; glaucoma; or renal, hepatic, or cardiovascular disorders.
- Bring gel to room temperature before administration. Do not force warming process by using a warm water bath or other source of external heat (e.g., microwave).
- Assist woman to maintain a supine position with lateral tilt or a side-lying position for 30 to 60 minutes after insertion of gel or for 2 hours after placement of insert.
- Prepare to swab vagina to remove remaining gel using a saline-soaked gauze wrapped around fingers or pull string to remove insert and to administer terbutaline 0.25 mg subcutaneously or intravenously if significant adverse reactions occur.
- Initiate oxytocin for induction of labor within 6 to 12 hours after last instillation of gel or within 30 minutes after removal of the insert.
- Follow agency protocol for induction if ripening has occurred and labor has not begun.
- Document all assessment findings and administration procedures.

Dinoprostone is the only FDA-approved medication for cervical ripening or labor induction.

Box 19-10

Medication Guide: Cervical Ripening Using Prostaglandin E_1 (PGE_1): Misoprostol (Cytotec)

ACTION

PGE_1 ripens the cervix, making it softer and causing it to begin to dilate and efface; stimulates uterine contractions.

INDICATIONS

PGE_1 is used for preinduction cervical ripening (ripen cervix before oxytocin induction of labor when the Bishop score is 4 or less) and to induce labor or abortion (abortifacient agent).

DOSAGE

Insert 25 to 50 μg (¼ to ½ of a 100-μg tablet) intravaginally into the posterior fornix using the tips of index and middle fingers without the use of a lubricant. Repeat every 3 to 6 hours as needed to a maximum of 300 to 400 μg in a 24-hour period or until an effective contraction pattern is established (3 or more uterine contractions in 10 minutes), cervix ripens (Bishop score of 8 or greater), or significant adverse reactions occur.

ADVERSE REACTIONS

Higher dosages are more likely to result in adverse reactions such as nausea and vomiting, diarrhea, fever, tachysystole (12 or more uterine contractions in 20 minutes without alteration of FHR pattern), hyperstimulation of the uterus (tachysystole with nonreassuring FHR patterns), or fetal passage of meconium.

NURSING CONSIDERATIONS

- Explain procedure to woman and her family. Ensure that an informed consent has been obtained as per agency policy.
- Assess maternal-fetal unit, before each insertion and during treatment following agency protocol for frequency. Assess maternal vital signs and health status, FHR pattern, and status of pregnancy, including indications for cervical ripening or induction of labor, signs of labor or impending labor, and the Bishop score. Recognize that a nonreassuring FHR pattern; maternal fever, infection, vaginal bleeding, or hypersensitivity; and regular, progressive uterine contractions contraindicate the use of misoprostol.
- Use caution if the woman has a history of asthma, glaucoma, or renal, hepatic, or cardiovascular disorders.
- Assist woman to maintain a supine position with lateral tilt or a side-lying position for 30 to 40 minutes after insertion.
- Prepare to swab vagina to remove unabsorbed medication using a saline soaked gauze wrapped around fingers and to administer terbutaline 0.25 mg subcutaneously or intravenously if significant adverse reactions occur.
- Initiate oxytocin for induction of labor no sooner than 4 hours after last dose of misoprostol was administered, following agency protocol, if ripening has occurred and labor has not begun.
- Document all assessment findings and administration procedures.

Misoprostol (Cytotec) has not yet been approved by the FDA for cervical ripening or labor induction.

Box 19-11

Procedure: Assisting with Amniotomy

PROCEDURE

Explain to the woman what will be done.

Assess FHR before procedure begins to obtain a baseline reading.

Place several underpads under the woman's buttocks to absorb the fluid.

Position the woman on a padded bed pan, fracture pan, or rolled up towel to elevate her hips.

Assist the health care provider who is performing the procedure by providing sterile gloves and lubricant for the vaginal examination.

Unwrap sterile package containing Amnihook or Allis clamp and pass instrument to the primary health care provider, who inserts it alongside the fingers and then hooks and tears the membranes.

Reassess the FHR.

Assess the color, consistency, and odor of the fluid.

Assess the woman's temperature every 2 hours or per protocol.

Evaluate the woman for signs and symptoms of infection.

DOCUMENTATION

Record the following:

Time of rupture

Color, odor, and consistency of the fluid

FHR before and after the procedure

Maternal status (how well procedure was tolerated)

fluid is assessed (i.e., for the presence or absence of meconium or blood). The time of rupture is recorded.

NURSE ALERT • The FHR is assessed before and immediately after the amniotomy to detect any changes (e.g., decelerations) that may indicate cord compression or prolapse.

The woman's temperature should be checked at least every 2 hours to rule out possible infection. If her temperature is 38° C or greater, the physician or nurse-midwife is notified. The nurse assesses for other signs and symptoms of infection such as maternal chills, fetal tachycardia, uterine tenderness on palpation, and foul-smelling vaginal drainage (Simpson and Poole, 1998). Comfort measures such as frequently changing the woman's underpads and perineal cleansing are implemented.

Oxytocin. Oxytocin is a hormone normally produced by the posterior pituitary gland; it stimulates uterine contractions. It may be used either to induce labor or to augment a labor that is progressing slowly because of inadequate uterine contractions.

The indications for oxytocin induction of labor may include but are not limited to the following:
- Suspected fetal jeopardy (e.g., intrauterine growth restriction)
- Inadequate uterine contractions; dystocia
- Premature rupture of membranes
- Postterm pregnancy
- Maternal medical problems (e.g., woman with severe Rh isoimmunization, diabetes, renal disease, or chronic pulmonary disease)
- Pregnancy-induced hypertension
- Fetal demise (death)
- Multiparous women with a history of precipitous labor who live far from the hospital

The management of stimulation of labor is the same regardless of indication. Because of the potential dangers associated with the injection of oxytocin in the prenatal and intranatal periods, the FDA has issued restrictions on its use.

Contraindications to oxytocic stimulation of labor include but are not limited to the following:
- CPD, prolapsed cord, transverse lie
- Nonreassurring FHR
- Placenta previa or vasa previa
- Prior classic uterine incision or uterine surgery
- Active genital herpes infection
- Invasive cancer of the cervix

Certain maternal and fetal conditions, although not contraindications to the use of oxytocin to stimulate labor, do require special caution during its administration. These conditions include the following:
- Multifetal presentation
- Breech presentation
- Presenting part above the pelvic inlet
- Abnormal FHR pattern not requiring emergency birth
- Polyhydramnios
- Grand multiparity
- Maternal cardiac disease; hypertension

Oxytocin use can present hazards to the mother and the fetus. These hazards are primarily dose related, with most problems caused by high doses that are given rapidly. Maternal hazards include water intoxication and tumultuous labor with tetanic contractions, which may cause premature separation of the placenta, rupture of the uterus, lacerations of the cervix, or postbirth hemorrhage. These complications can lead to infection, disseminated intravascular coagulation, or amniotic fluid embolism. Women may become anxious or fearful if the induction is not successful because they may then have concerns about the method of birth.

Uterine hyperstimulation reduces the blood flow through the placenta and results in FHR decelerations (e.g., bradycardia, diminished variability, late decelerations), fetal asphyxia, and neonatal hypoxia. If the estimated date of birth is inaccurate, physical injury, neonatal hyperbilirubinemia, and prematurity are other hazards.

Initiation of induction or augmentation of labor with oxytocin is the responsibility of the physician or nurse-midwife, although the medication often is administered by a nurse through a secondary IV line according to agency protocol and professional standards (Fig. 19-6; Box 19-12).

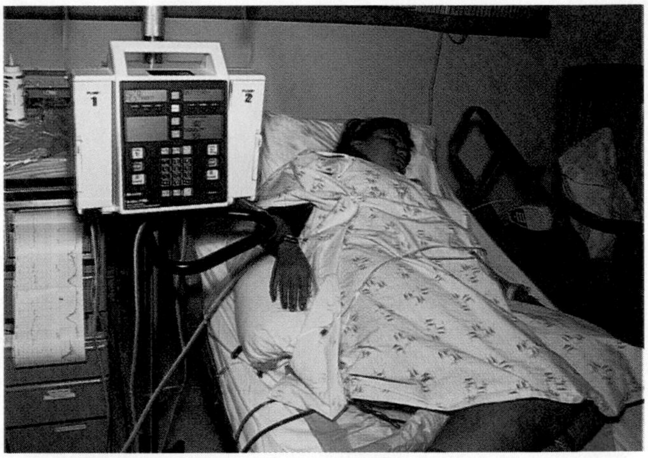

FIG. 19-6 • Woman in side-lying position receiving oxytocin. (Courtesy Michael S. Clement, MD, Mesa, AZ.)

Nursing Considerations. A written protocol for the preparation and administration of oxytocin should be established by the obstetric department (physicians and nurses) in each institution. Procedures that are recommended for a woman who is eligible for induction of labor are discussed in Boxes 19-12 and 19-13. Policies, protocols, and procedures of individual institutions will also dictate set-up and administration, the frequency of administration, and documentation.

NURSE ALERT • Oxytocin is discontinued immediately and the primary health care provider notified if uterine hyperstimulation or a nonreassuring FHR pattern occurs.

Other nursing interventions, such as administering oxygen by face mask, positioning the woman on her side, and infusing more intravenous fluids, are implemented immediately (Emergency box). Based on the status of the maternal-fetal unit, the physician or nurse-midwife may restart the infusion once the FHR and uterine activity return to acceptable levels (ACOG, 1995b).

Augmentation of labor refers to the stimulation of uterine contractions after labor has started spontaneously but progress is unsatisfactory. Common augmentation methods include oxytocin infusion, amniotomy, and nipple stimulation. Augmentation is usually implemented for the management of hypotonic uterine dysfunction resulting in a slowing of labor (protracted active phase). Noninvasive methods such as emptying the bladder, ambulation and position changes, relaxation measures, nourishment and hydration, and hydrotherapy should be attempted before invasive interventions are initiated. The procedures and nursing assessments are similar to those used for oxytocin induction of labor.

Some physicians advocate active management of labor: that is, the augmentation of labor to establish efficient labor with aggressive use of oxytocin (e.g., a starting dose of 6 mU/min with increases of 6 mU/min every 15 minutes to a maximum dose of 40 mU/min) to shorten labor. Active management of labor continues to be under study in the United States to determine effectiveness and impact on perinatal morbidity and mortality.

Forceps-Assisted Birth. A forceps-assisted birth is one in which an instrument with two curved blades is used to assist

Box 19-12

Protocol: Induction of Labor with Oxytocin

PATIENT/FAMILY TEACHING

Explain technique, rationale, and reactions to expect:

- Route and rate for administration of medication
- What "piggyback" is for
- Reasons for use:
  Induce labor, improve labor
- Reactions to expect concerning the nature of contractions: the intensity of contraction increases more rapidly, holds the peak longer, and ends more quickly; contractions will come regularly and more often
- Monitoring to anticipate:
  Maternal: blood pressure, pulse, uterine contractions, uterine tone
  Fetal: heart rate, activity
- Success to expect: a favorable outcome will depend on inducibility of the cervix (Bishop score of 9 for nulliparas and 5 for multiparas)
- Keep woman and support person informed of progress

ADMINISTRATION

Position woman in side-lying or upright position

Assess status of maternal fetal unit

Prepare solutions and administer with pump delivery system according to prescribed orders:

- Infusion pump and solution are set up (e.g., 10 U/1000 ml isotonic electrolyte solution)
- Piggyback solution is connected to IV line at proximal port (port nearest point of venous insertion)
- Solution with oxytocin is flagged with a medication label
- Begin induction at 0.5 to 2 mU/min
- Increase dose 1 to 2 mU/min at intervals of 15 to 60 minutes until either a dose of up to 20-40 mU/min or 300 Montevideo units (MVUs) is reached (see Box 19-13)

MAINTAIN DOSE IF:

- Intensity of contractions results in intrauterine pressures of 40 to 90 mm Hg (shown by internal monitor)
- Duration of contractions is 40 to 90 seconds
- Frequency of contractions is 2- to 3-minute intervals
- Cervical dilation of 1 cm/hr in the active phase

MATERNAL/FETAL ASSESSMENTS

- Monitor blood pressure, pulse, and respirations every 30 to 60 minutes and with every increment in dose
- Monitor contraction pattern and uterine resting tone every 15 minutes and with every increment in dose
- Assess intake and output; limit IV intake to 1000 ml/8 hr; output should be 120 ml or more every 4 hours
- Perform vaginal examination as indicated
- Monitor for nausea, vomiting, headache, hypotension
- Assess fetal status using electronic fetal monitoring; evaluate tracing every 15 minutes and with every increment in dose
- Observe emotional responses of woman and her partner

REPORTABLE CONDITIONS

- Uterine hyperstimulation
- Nonreassuring FHR pattern
- Suspected uterine rupture
- Inadequate uterine response at 20 mU/min

EMERGENCY MEASURES

Discontinue use of oxytocin per hospital protocol:

- Turn woman on her side
- Increase primary IV rate up to 200 ml/hr; unless patient has water intoxication, in which case, the rate is decreased to one that keeps the vein open
- Give woman oxygen by face mask at 8 to 10 L/min or per protocol or physician's order

DOCUMENTATION

- Medications: kind, amount, time of beginning, increasing dose, maintaining dose, and discontinuing medication in patient record and on monitor strip
- Reactions of mother and fetus
- Pattern of labor
- Progress of labor
- FHR
- Maternal vital signs
- Nursing interventions and woman's response
- Notification of primary health care provider

From American College of Obstetricians and Gynecologists (ACOG): Induction of labor, *(Tech Bull No. 217),* 1995, Washington, DC, ACOG; Pozaic S: Induction and augmentation of labor. In Mandeville L, Troiano N, editors: *High-risk and critical care intrapartum nursing,* ed 2, Philadelphia, 1999, Lippincott; Simpson K, Poole J: *Cervical ripening and induction and augmentation of labor,* Washington, DC, 1998, AWHONN; Summers L: Methods of cervical ripening and labor induction, *J Nurse Midwifery* 42(2):71-85, 1997.

Box 19-13

Calculation of Montevideo Units

Montevideo units (MVUs) can be used to describe uterine intensity when an intrauterine pressure gauge is being used. To calculate MVUs, the baseline uterine pressure (resting tone) is first subtracted from the peak contraction pressure for each contraction recorded on a 10-minute monitor tracing. These adjusted pressures are then added, and the sum is the number of Montevideo units (average, 180 to 240 MVUs).

For example, if the resting tone is 5 mm Hg and 3 contractions occur in 10 minutes with peaks of 80, 85, and 90 mm Hg, the resulting numbers are 80 − 5 + 85 − 5 + 90 − 5, which total 240 MVUs.

in the birth of the fetal head. The cephalic-like curve of the forceps commonly used is similar to the shape of the fetal head, with a pelvic curve to the blades conforming to the curve of the pelvic axis. The blades are joined by a pin, screw, or groove arrangement. These locks prevent the forceps from compressing the fetal skull. Maternal indications for forceps-assisted birth include the need to shorten the second stage in dystocia (difficult labor), to compensate for the woman's deficient expulsive efforts (e.g., if she is tired or has been given spinal or epidural anesthesia), or to reverse a dangerous condition (e.g., cardiac decompensation).

Fetal indications include the birth of a fetus in distress, certain abnormal presentations, arrest of rotation, as well as to deliver an aftercoming head in a breech presentation.

Emergency

UTERINE HYPERSTIMULATION WITH OXYTOCIN

Signs

Uterine contractions lasting more than 90 seconds and occurring more frequently than every 2 minutes
Uterine resting tone greater than 20 mm Hg
Nonreassuring FHR:
- Abnormal baseline ($<$110 or $>$160 beats/min)
- Absent variability
- Repeated late decelerations or prolonged decelerations

Interventions

Maintain woman in side-lying position
Turn off oxytocin infusion; keep maintenance IV line open; increase rate
Start administering oxygen by face mask, per protocol or physician's order
Notify primary health care provider
Prepare to administer terbutaline (Brethine) 0.25 mg subcutaneously if ordered to decrease uterine activity
Continue monitoring FHR and uterine activity
Document responses to actions

Certain conditions are required for a forceps-assisted birth to be successful. The woman's cervix must be fully dilated to avoid lacerations and hemorrhage. The bladder should be empty. The presenting part must be engaged, and a vertex presentation is desired. Membranes must be ruptured so that the position of the fetal head can be determined and the forceps can firmly grasp the head during birth. CPD should not be present.

The different definitions of forceps applications (ACOG, 1994a) include the following:

Outlet forceps—Appropriate when fetal scalp is visible on the perineum without manually separating the labia: used to shorten the second stage of labor (Fig. 19-7)

Low forceps—Application of forceps to a fetal head that is at least at a +2 cm station

Midforceps—Application of forceps to the fetal head that is engaged (no higher than station 0) but above the +2 cm station

There are no circumstances in which forceps should be applied to an unengaged presenting part.

Nursing Considerations. The nurse obtains the type of forceps requested by the physician (Fig. 19-8). The nurse may explain to the mother that the forceps blades fit like two tablespoons around an egg, with the blades coming over the baby's ears.

NURSE ALERT • Because compression of the cord between the fetal head and the forceps would cause a drop in FHR, the FHR is checked, reported, and recorded before and after forceps are applied.

If a drop in FHR occurs, the physician would remove and reapply the forceps. Ordinarily traction is applied during contractions.

After birth, the mother is assessed for vaginal and cervical lacerations (e.g., bleeding that occurs even with a contracted uterus) and urine retention, which may result from bladder injuries. The infant should be assessed for bruising or abrasions at the site of the blade applications, facial palsy resulting from pressure of the blades on the facial nerve (cranial VII), and subdural hematoma. Newborn and postpartum caregivers should be told that the birth was forceps-assisted.

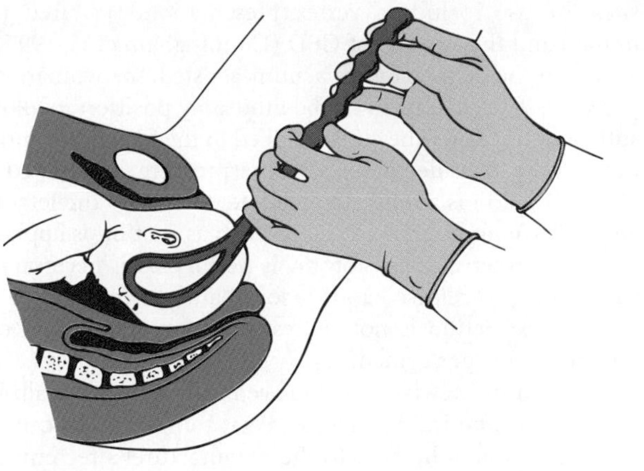

FIG. 19-7 • Outlet forceps-assisted extraction of the head.

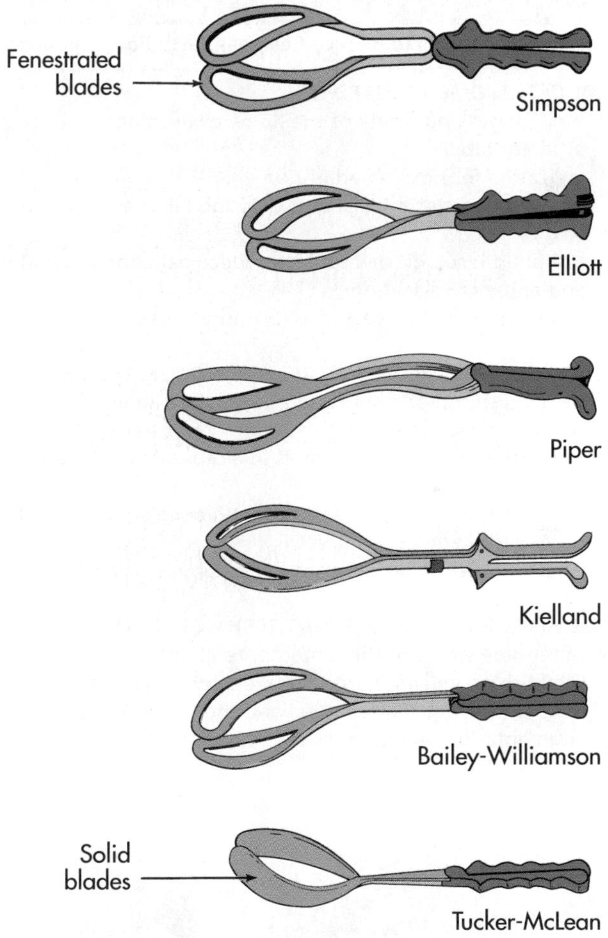

FIG. 19-8 • Types of forceps. Piper forceps are used to assist delivery of the head in a breech birth.

Vacuum-Assisted Birth. Vacuum-assisted birth, or vacuum extraction, is a birth method involving the attachment of a vacuum cup to the fetal head using negative pressure. Indications for use are similar to those for outlet forceps. Prerequisites for use include a vertex presentation, ruptured membranes, and the absence of CPD (Cunningham et al, 1997).

When the birth is to be vacuum-assisted, the woman is prepared for a vaginal birth in the lithotomy position to allow for sufficient traction. The cup is applied to the fetal head, and a caput develops inside the cup as the pressure is initiated (Fig. 19-9). Traction is applied to facilitate descent of the fetal head, and the woman is encouraged to push as suction is applied. As the head crowns, an episiotomy is performed if necessary. The vacuum cup is released and removed after birth of the head. If vacuum extraction is not successful, a forceps-assisted or cesarean birth is performed.

Risks to the newborn include cephalhematoma, scalp lacerations, and subdural hematoma. Fetal complications can be reduced by strict adherence to the manufacturer's recommendations for method of application, degree of suction, and duration of application. Maternal complications are uncommon but can include perineal, vaginal, and cervical lacerations.

Nursing Considerations. The nurse's role for the woman who has a vacuum-assisted birth is one of support person and educator. The nurse can prepare the woman for birth and encourage her to remain active in the birth process by pushing during contractions. The FHR should be assessed frequently during the procedure. After birth, the newborn should be observed for signs of infection at the application site and for cerebral irritation (e.g., poor sucking or listlessness). The newborn may be at risk for cephalhematoma and neonatal jaundice as bruising resolves, as well as for infection at the application site. The parents may need to be reassured that the caput succedaneum will begin to disappear in a few hours. Neonatal caregivers should be alerted that the birth was by vacuum extraction.

Box 19-14

Selected Measures to Reduce Cesarean Birth Rate and Increase Rate of VBACs

EDUCATE WOMEN REGARDING

- Advantages and safety of the home environment for early or latent labor
- Indicators for hospital admission
- Management techniques to use during labor to enhance progress
- Nonpharmacologic measures to reduce pain and discomfort and enhance relaxation
- Safety and effectiveness of TOLs and VBACs

ESTABLISH ADMISSION CRITERIA FOR WOMEN IN LABOR

- Distinguish clinical manifestations for false labor, latent/early labor, and active labor
- Conduct admission assessments in a separate admissions area
- Send women in false or early/latent labor home or keep them in the admissions area
- Admit women in active labor to the labor and birth unit

USE APPROPRIATE ASSESSMENT TECHNIQUES TO

- Determine status of the maternal-fetal unit
- Establish an individualized rationale for initiating labor interventions such as epidural anesthesia, induction/augmentation, amniotomy, cesarean birth

INITIATE A DOULA PROGRAM THAT PROVIDES ONE-TO-ONE SUPPORT FOR WOMEN IN LABOR

DEVELOP A PHILOSOPHY OF LABOR MANAGEMENT THAT

- Schedules admission during active labor
- Avoids automatic interventions such as routine induction for spontaneous rupture of membranes at term or postterm pregnancy and cesarean birth for breech presentation, twin gestation, genital herpes, or failure to progress
- Relies on assessment findings reflective of the status of the maternal-fetal unit rather than strict adherence to set ranges for the duration of the stages and phases of labor
- Employs intermittent rather than continuous electronic fetal monitoring of low risk pregnant women
- Focuses on measures that are known to enhance the progress of labor such as upright positions, frequent position changes, ambulation, oral nutrition and hydration, relaxation techniques, hydrotherapy
- Emphasizes nonpharmacologic measures to relieve pain
- Uses nonpharmacologic measures in a manner that reduces their labor-inhibiting effects
- Establishes criteria for elective cesarean birth and TOL
- Encourages women who have had a previous cesarean birth to participate in TOL to attempt a vaginal birth

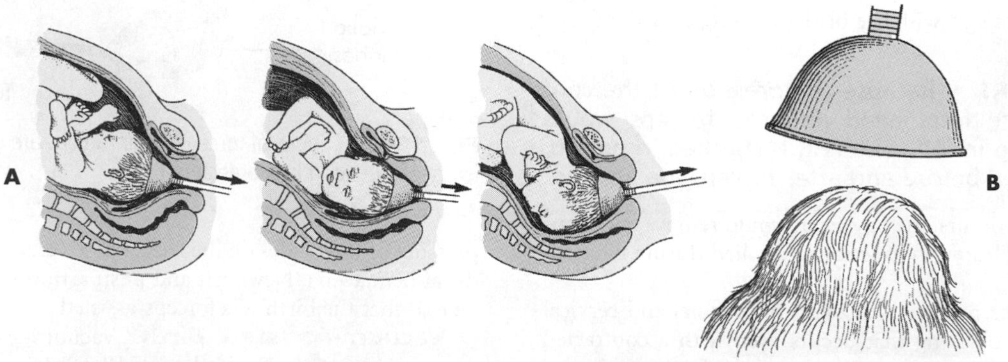

FIG. 19-9 • Use of vacuum extraction to rotate fetal head and assist with descent. **A,** Arrow indicates direction of traction on the vacuum cup. **B,** Caput succedaneum formed by the vacuum cup.

Cesarean Birth. Cesarean birth is the birth of a fetus through a transabdominal incision of the uterus. Whether a cesarean birth is planned (scheduled) or unplanned (emergency), the loss of the experience of giving birth to an infant in the traditional manner may have a negative effect on a woman's self-concept. An effort is made to maintain the focus on the birth of a child rather than on the operative procedure.

The purpose of cesarean birth is to preserve the life or health of the mother and her fetus; it may be the best choice when there is evidence of maternal or fetal complications. Since the advent of modern surgical methods and care, and the use of antibiotics, maternal and fetal morbidity and mortality have decreased. In addition, incisions are made into the lower uterine segment rather than into the muscular body of the uterus and thus promote more effective healing. However, despite these advances, cesarean birth still poses threats to the health of both mother and infant.

The incidence of cesarean births increased from less than 5% in 1965 to more than 20% in 1997 (Guyer et al, 1998). Factors cited in this increase include use of electronic fetal monitoring and epidural anesthesia; an increase in the number of first-time pregnancies, as well as pregnancies at an older age; and the high incidence of repeat cesarean births. Women 35 years of age and older have a total cesarean birth rate of 30%, or almost twice the rate for teenage women (15.7%) (Curtin and Kozak, 1998). A slight decline in the rate since 1990 may be attributed, in part, to more attempts at vaginal birth in mothers who have previously given birth by cesarean.

Women who have private insurance, are of a higher socioeconomic status, or who deliver in a private hospital are more likely to experience cesarean birth than are women who are poor, have no insurance, are receiving public assistance (e.g., Medicaid), or who give birth in public hospitals (DiMatteo et al, 1996; Porreco and Thorp, 1996; Scott, 1999).

Approaches for the management of labor and birth to reduce the rate of cesarean births while increasing the rate of vaginal births after cesarean (VBAC) are presented in Box 19-14.

The type of nursing care may also influence the rate of cesarean births. Radin, Harmon, and Hanson (1993) found that cesarean rates were lower for women whose nurses provided supportive care during labor. A labor management approach that uses one-to-one support and emphasizes ambulation, maternal position changes, relaxation measures, oral fluids and nutrition, hydrotherapy and nonpharmacologic pain relief, facilitates the progress of labor and reduces the incidence of dystocia (Albers, Lydon-Rochelle, and Krulewitch, 1995; Porreco and Thorp, 1996).

Indications. There are few absolute indications for a cesarean birth. Today most are performed primarily for the benefit of the fetus. The most common indications for cesarean birth are related to labor and birth complications. The complications most closely associated with cesarean births include fetal distress, CPD, malpresentations such as breech and shoulder, placental abnormalities (previa, abruptio), umbilical cord prolapse, dysfunctional labor pattern, and multiple gestation. Medical risk factors most closely associated with cesarean birth include hypertensive disorders, active genital herpes, and diabetes (Porreco and Thorpe, 1996; Ventura et al, 1998).

Forced Cesarean Birth. A woman's refusal to undergo cesarean birth for fetal reasons is often described as a maternal-fetal conflict. Health care providers are ethically obliged to protect the well-being of both the mother and the fetus; a decision for one affects the other. If a woman refuses a cesarean birth that is recommended because of fetal jeopardy, health care providers need to make every effort to find out why she is refusing and provide information that may persuade her to change her mind. If the woman continues to refuse surgery, the health care providers must decide if it is ethical to get a court order for the surgery; however, every effort should be made to avoid this legal step.

Surgical Techniques. The two main types of cesarean operation are the classic and the lower segment cesarean incisions. Classic cesarean birth is rarely performed today, although it may be used when rapid birth is necessary and in some cases of shoulder presentation and placenta previa. The incision is made vertically into the upper body of the uterus (Fig. 19-10, *A*). Because the procedure is associated with a higher incidence of blood loss, infection, and uterine rupture in subsequent pregnancies than is lower-segment cesarean birth, vaginal birth after a classic cesarean is contraindicated.

Lower-segment cesarean birth can be achieved through a vertical or transverse incision into the uterus (Fig. 19-10, *B* and *C*). The transverse incision is more popular, however, because it is easier to perform, is associated with less blood loss and fewer postoperative infections, and is less likely to rupture in subsequent pregnancies (Cunningham et al, 1997; Scott, 1999).

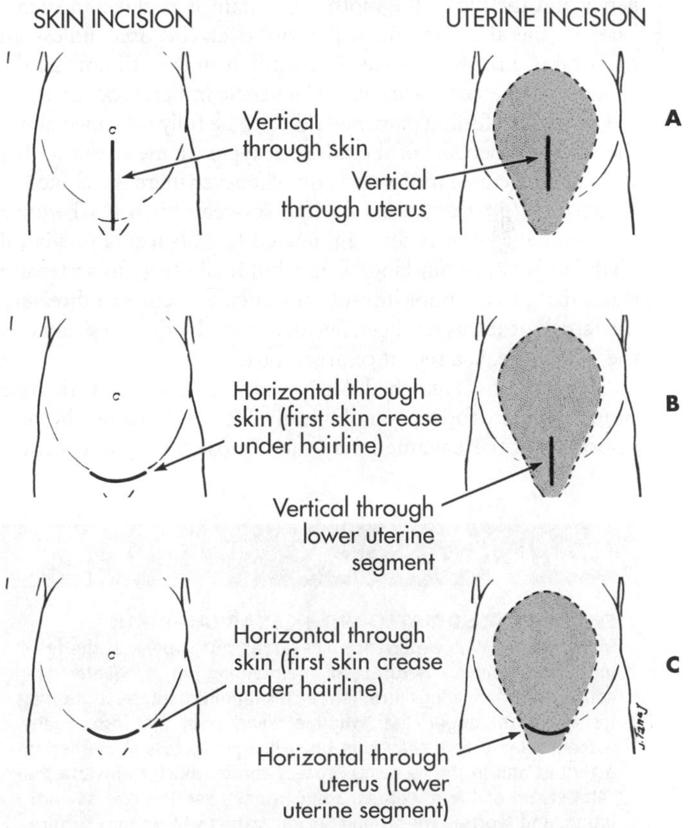

FIG. 19-10 • Cesarean birth: skin and uterine incisions. **A,** Classic: vertical incisions of skin and uterus. **B,** Low cervical: horizontal incision of skin; vertical incision of uterus. **C,** Low cervical: horizontal incisions of skin and uterus.

Complications and Risks. Cesarean births are not without complications for both the mother and fetus. Maternal complications occur in 25% to 50% of cesarean births; these include aspiration, pulmonary embolism, wound infection, wound dehiscence, thrombophlebitis, hemorrhage, urinary tract infection, injuries to bladder or bowel, and complications related to anesthesia. There also is a risk that the fetus will be born prematurely if gestational age is not accurately determined; fetal injuries can occur during the surgery (Scott, 1999). Besides these risks, the woman is at economic risk because the cost of a cesarean birth is higher than that of a vaginal birth, and a longer recovery period may require additional expenditures.

Women who experience cesarean birth may feel frustration (at losing control), disappointment, anger, and loss of self-esteem. Often the ability to interact with their newborn after birth is delayed; they are less likely to breastfeed. They often are less satisfied with their childbirth experience and report more fatigue and poor physical functioning during the first few weeks after discharge. Parents should be given opportunities to discuss the experience to try to understand and resolve concerns after the birth.

Anesthesia. Spinal, epidural, and general anesthetics are used for cesarean births. Epidural blocks are popular because women want to be awake for and aware of the birth experience. However, the choice of anesthetic depends on several factors. The mother's medical history or present condition, such as a spinal injury or hemorrhage, may rule out the use of regional anesthesia. Time is another factor, especially if there is an emergency and the life of the mother or infant is at stake. In such a case a general anesthetic will most likely be used unless an epidural is already in place. The woman may not know all the options or may have fears about "a needle in her back" or of being awake and feeling pain. She needs to be fully informed about the risks and benefits of the different types of anesthesia so that she can participate in the decision whenever there is a choice.

Scheduled Cesarean Birth. Cesarean birth is scheduled or planned if labor is contraindicated (e.g., placenta previa), if birth is necessary but labor is not inducible (e.g., hypertensive states that cause a poor intrauterine environment that threatens the fetus), or if this has been decided upon by the physician and the woman (e.g., a repeat cesarean birth).

Women who are scheduled to have a cesarean birth have time to prepare for it psychologically. However, the psychologic responses of these women may vary. Those having a repeat cesarean birth may have disturbing memories of the conditions preceding the initial surgical birth and of their experiences in the postoperative recovery period. They may be concerned about the added burden of caring for an infant and perhaps other children while recovering from a surgical operation. Others may feel glad to have been relieved of the uncertainty about the date and time of birth and to be free from the pain of labor.

Unplanned Cesarean Birth. The psychosocial outcomes of unplanned or emergency cesarean birth are usually more pronounced and negative in nature when compared with the outcomes associated with a scheduled or planned cesarean birth (DiMatteo et al, 1996). Women and their families experience abrupt changes in their expectations for birth, postbirth care, and the care of the new baby at home. This may be an extremely traumatic experience for all.

The woman usually approaches the procedure tired and discouraged after an ineffective and difficult labor. Fear predominates as she worries about her own safety and well-being and that of her fetus. She may be dehydrated, with low glycogen reserves. Because preoperative procedures must be done quickly and competently, the time available for explanation of the procedures and operation is often short. Because maternal and family anxiety levels are high at this time, much of what is said may be forgotten or misunderstood. The woman may experience feelings of anger or guilt in the postpartum period. Fatigue is often noticeable in these women, and they need much supportive care.

After surgery, therefore, time must be spent reviewing the events preceding the operation and the operation itself to ensure that the woman understands what has happened and that gaps in her recollections are filled. This approach will help create more realistic memories of the childbirth experience, thereby having a more positive influence on future pregnancies and labors (Ryding, Wijma, and Wijma, 1998).

Prenatal Preparation. Concerned professional and lay groups in the community have established councils for cesarean birth to meet the needs of these women and their families. Such groups advocate that a discussion of cesarean birth be included in all parenthood preparation classes. No woman can be guaranteed a vaginal birth, even if she is in good health and there is no indication of danger to the fetus before the onset of labor. For this reason, every woman needs to be aware of and prepared for this eventuality.

Childbirth educators stress the importance of emphasizing the similarities and differences between a cesarean and vaginal

Family Focus

FEELINGS ASSOCIATED WITH CESAREAN BIRTH

Many women who experience a cesarean birth speak of the feelings that interfere with their maintaining an adequate self-concept. These feelings include fear, disappointment, frustration at losing control, anger (the "why me" syndrome), and loss of self-esteem related to a change in body image. Success in mothering activities and in the recovery process can do much to restore the self-esteem of these women. Some women see the scar as mutilating, and worries concerning sexual attractiveness may surface. Some men are fearful of resuming intercourse because of the fear of hurting their mates. Parents will wonder if a cesarean birth was absolutely necessary. Such feelings may surface even years later. Parents should be provided opportunities to discuss the experience to try to understand and resolve concerns.

Critical Thinking

UNPLANNED CESAREAN BIRTH

You are preparing a woman and her partner for an unplanned cesarean birth because of nonreassuring fetal status. Examine the possible reactions of the woman and her partner to this situation. How would these reactions affect the effectiveness of nursing care? How would your preparation in this situation differ from preparing a woman for a planned cesarean? Explain the differences in postpartum needs between the woman who has had a planned cesarean and the woman who has experienced an unplanned one. Develop a teaching plan for the woman and her partner for her care after discharge. What supports in the community might be available to the family?

birth. In support of the philosophy of family-centered birth, many hospitals have policies that permit fathers and other partners to share in these births as they do in vaginal ones. Women who have undergone cesarean birth agree that the continued presence and support of their partners helped them respond positively to the entire experience.

Preoperative Care. Family-centered care is the goal for the woman who is to undergo cesarean birth and for her family. The preparation of the woman for cesarean birth is the same as that done for other elective or emergency surgery. The primary health care provider discusses with the woman and her family the need for the cesarean birth and the prognosis for mother and infant. The anesthesiologist assesses the woman's cardiopulmonary system and describes the options for anesthesia. Informed consent is obtained for the procedure.

Maternal vital signs and blood pressure and FHR continue to be assessed per hospital routine until the operation begins. Physical preoperative preparation usually includes inserting a retention catheter to keep the bladder empty, and administering prescribed preoperative medications. An abdominal-mons shave or a clipping of pubic hair may be performed. An antacid is administered orally to neutralize gastric secretions in case of aspiration. Intravenous fluids are started to maintain hydration and to provide an open line for the administration of blood or medications if needed. Blood and urine samples are collected and sent to the laboratory for analysis. Laboratory tests, which are usually ordered to establish baseline data, include a complete blood cell count and chemistry, blood typing and crossmatching, and urinalysis.

Removal of dentures, nail polish, and jewelry may be optional, depending on hospital policies. If the woman wears glasses and is going to be awake, the nurse should make sure her glasses accompany her to the operating room so she can see her infant. If the woman wears contact lenses, the nurse can find out whether they can be worn for the birth.

During preoperative preparation the support person is encouraged to remain with the woman as much as possible to provide continuing emotional support (if this is culturally acceptable to the woman and support person). The nurse provides essential information about the preoperative procedures during this time. Although the nursing actions may be carried out quickly if a cesarean birth is unplanned, verbal communication, particularly explanations, is important. Silence can be frightening to the woman and her support person. The nurse's use of touch can communicate feelings of care and concern for the woman. The nurse can assess the woman's and her partner's perceptions about cesarean birth.

If there is time before the birth, the nurse can teach the woman about postoperative expectations and about pain relief, turning, coughing, and deep breathing measures.

Intraoperative Care. Cesarean births occur in operating rooms in the surgical suite or in the labor and birth unit. Once the woman has been taken to the operating room, her care becomes the responsibility of the obstetric team, surgeon, anesthesiologist, pediatrician, and surgical nursing staff (Fig. 19-11). If possible, the partner, who is gowned appropriately, accompanies the mother to the surgical unit and remains close to her so that continued support and comfort can be provided.

The nurse who is circulating may assist with positioning the woman on the birth (surgical) table. It is important to position her so that the uterus is displaced laterally to prevent compressing the inferior vena cava, which causes decreased placental perfusion. This is usually accomplished by placing a wedge under the hip. A Foley catheter is inserted into the bladder at this time if one is not already in place.

If the partner either is not allowed or chooses not to be present, the nurse can stay in communication with him or her and

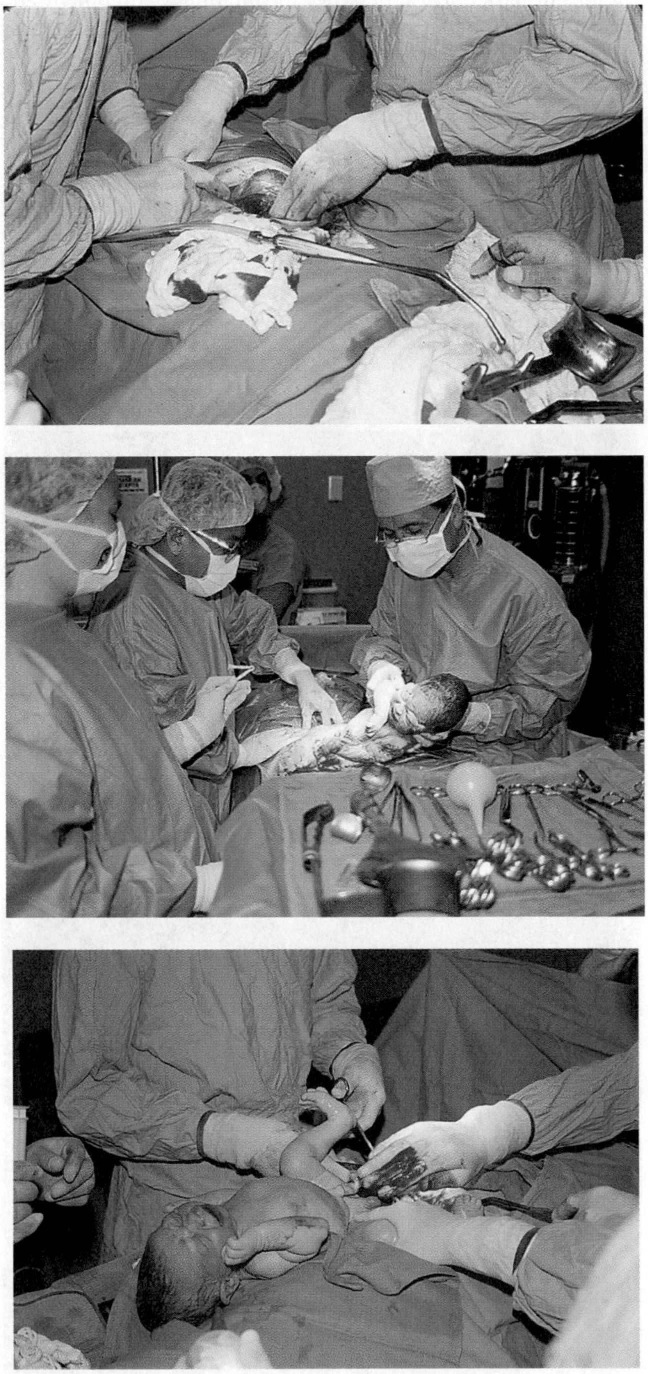

A

B

C

FIG. 19-11 • Cesarean birth. **A,** "Bikini" incision has been made, the muscle layer is separated, the abdomen entered, the uterus has been exposed and incised; suctioning of amniotic fluid continues as head is brought up through the incision. Note small amount of bleeding. **B,** The neonate's birth through the uterine incision is nearly complete. **C,** A quick assessment is performed; note extreme molding of head resulting from cephalopelvic disproportion. (Courtesy Marjorie Pyle, RNC, Lifecircle, Costa Mesa, CA.)

give progress reports whenever possible. If the mother is awake during the birth, the nurse can tell her what is happening and provide support. The mother may be anxious about the sensations she is experiencing, such as the coldness of solutions used to prepare the abdomen, and pressure or pulling during the actual birth of the infant. She also may be apprehensive because of the bright lights or the presence of unfamiliar equipment and masked and gowned personnel in the room. Explanations by the nurse can help to decrease the woman's anxiety.

Care of the infant usually is delegated to a pediatrician or a nurse team skilled in neonatal resuscitation, because these infants are considered to be at risk until there is evidence of physiologic stability after the birth.

A crib with resuscitation equipment is readied before surgery. Those responsible for care are expert not only in resuscitative techniques but also in their ability to detect normal and abnormal infant responses. After birth, if the infant's condition permits, the baby can be given to the woman's partner to hold. If the mother is awake, she can see and touch the baby (Fig. 19-12). The infant whose condition is compromised is transported after initial stabilization to the nursery for observation and the implementation of appropriate interventions. In some institutions the partner may accompany the infant; if not, personnel keep the family informed of the infant's progress, and parent-infant contacts are initiated as soon as possible.

If the family cannot accompany the woman during surgery, the family is directed to the surgical or obstetric waiting room. The physician then reports on the condition of the mother and child to family members after the birth is completed. Family members may accompany the infant as he or she is transferred to the nursery, giving them an opportunity to see and admire the new baby.

Immediate Postoperative Care. Once surgery is completed, the mother is transferred to a recovery room or back to her labor room. Women who have experienced a cesarean birth have both postoperative and postpartum needs that must be addressed. They are surgical patients as well as new mothers (Eakes and Brown, 1998). Nursing assessments in this immediate postbirth period include degree of recovery from the effects of anesthesia, postoperative and postbirth status, and degree of pain. A patent airway is maintained, and the woman is positioned to prevent possible aspiration. Vital signs are taken every 15 minutes for 1 to 2 hours, or until stable. The condition of the incisional dressing, the fundus, and the amount of lochia are assessed, as well as intravenous intake and urine output through the Foley catheter. The woman is helped to turn and do deep breathing and leg exercises. Medications to relieve pain may be administered.

If the baby is present, the mother and her partner are given some time alone with him or her to facilitate bonding and attachment. Breastfeeding can be initiated if the mother feels like trying. The woman usually is transferred to the postpartum unit after 1 to 2 hours, or once her condition is stable and the effects of anesthesia have worn off (i.e., she is alert, oriented, and able to feel and move extremities) (see Table 19-5).

Postpartum Care. The attitude of the nurse and other health team members can influence the woman's perception of herself after a cesarean birth. The caregivers should stress that the woman is a new mother first and a surgical patient second. This attitude helps the woman perceive herself as having the same problems and needs as other new mothers while at the same time requiring supportive postoperative care.

The woman's physiologic concerns for the first few days may be dominated by pain at the incision site and pain resulting from intestinal gas, and hence the need for pain relief. If epidural anesthesia was used for the surgery, epidural narcotics can be given in the recovery period to provide pain relief for approximately 24 hours. Otherwise, pain medications usually are given every 3 to 4 hours, or patient-controlled analgesia may be ordered instead. Other comfort measures such as position changes, splinting the incision with pillows, and relaxation techniques may be implemented. Women are often the best judges of what their bodies need and can tolerate, including the postoperative ingestion of foods and fluids. If desired by the woman, early introduction of solid food is safe. Women who eat early have been found to require less analgesia, and gastrointestinal problems do not occur (Burrows et al, 1995). Ambulation and rocking in a rocking chair may relieve gas pains, and avoiding consumption of gas-forming foods and carbonated

A

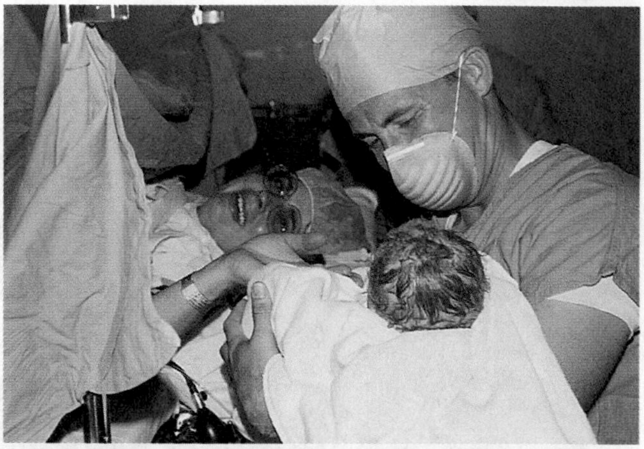

B

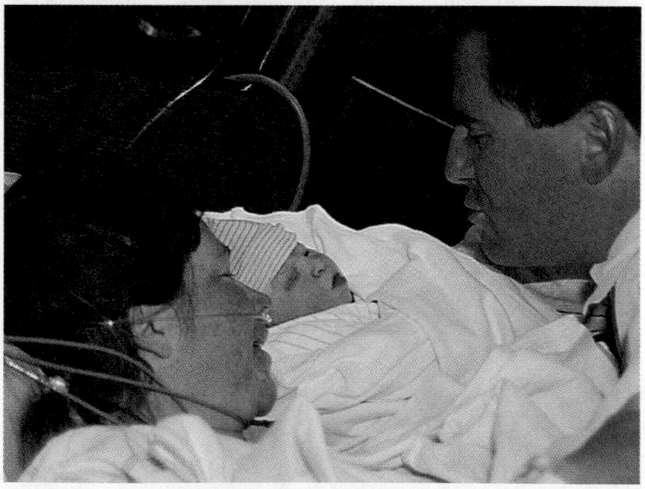

FIG. 19-12 • **A,** Parents and their newborn. The physician manually removes the placenta, suctions the remaining amniotic fluid and blood from the uterine cavity, and closes the uterine incision, peritoneum, muscle layer, fatty tissue, and finally the skin, while the new family shares some private time. **B,** Parents become better acquainted with their newborn while mother rests after surgery. (Courtesy Marjorie Pyle, RNC, Lifecircle, Costa Mesa, CA.)

Patient Teaching

POSTPARTUM PAIN RELIEF AFTER CESAREAN BIRTH

Incisional

Splint incision with a pillow when moving or coughing.
Use relaxation techniques such as music, breathing, and dim lights.
Apply a heating pad to the abdomen.

Gas

Walk as often as you can.
Do not eat or drink gas-forming foods, carbonated beverages, or whole milk.
Do not use straws for drinking fluids.
Take antiflatulence medication if prescribed.
Lie on your left side to expel gas.
Rock in a rocking chair.

Home Care

SIGNS OF POSTOPERATIVE COMPLICATIONS AFTER DISCHARGE

Report the following signs to your health care provider:
- Temperature exceeding 38° C
- Painful urination
- Lochia heavier than a normal period
- Wound separation
- Redness or oozing at the incision site
- Severe abdominal pain

beverages may help minimize them (Thomas et al, 1990) (Patient Teaching box).

Other physiologic concerns of women after a cesarean birth may include fatigue, activity intolerance, and incisional problems (Miovech et al, 1994). Nurses need to manage care to ensure adequate rest and pain relief.

Daily care includes perineal care, breast care, and routine hygienic care, including showering after the dressing has been removed (if showering is acceptable according to the woman's cultural prescriptions). The nurse assesses the woman's vital signs, incision, fundus, and lochia according to hospital policies, procedures, or protocols. Breath sounds, bowel sounds, circulatory status of lower extremities, and urinary and bowel elimination also are assessed. It is also important to note maternal affect.

During the postpartum period the nurse can provide care that meets the psychologic and teaching needs of mothers who have had cesarean births. The nurse can explain postpartum procedures to help the woman participate in her recovery from surgery. The nurse can help the woman plan care and visits from family and friends that allow for adequate rest periods. Information and assistance with infant care can facilitate adjustment to the mothering role. The woman should be encouraged to breastfeed her baby by receiving individualized assistance to comfortably hold and position the baby at her breast. The partner can be included in infant teaching sessions and in explanations about the woman's recovery. The couple should be encouraged to express their feelings about the birth experience. Some parents are angry, frustrated, or disappointed that a vaginal birth was not possible. Some women express feelings of low self-esteem or negative self-image. Others express relief and gratitude that the baby is healthy and safely born. It may be helpful to have the nurse who was present during the birth visit and help fill in "gaps" about the experience. Other psychologic and lifestyle concerns that have been reported include depression, feeling limited in activities, and changes in family interactions (Miovech et al, 1994; Ryding, Wijma, and Wijma, 1998).

Discharge after cesarean birth is usually by the third postoperative day (Curtin and Kozak, 1998). This time is often determined by criteria established by the woman's insurance carrier or the federal government (e.g., diagnosis-related groups).

The Newborn's and Mother's Health Protection Act of 1996 provides for a length of stay of up to 96 hours for cesarean births. These criteria may not coincide with the woman's physical or psychosocial readiness for discharge. Some states have added home-care provisions for mothers who meet appropriate criteria for discharge and choose to leave sooner than the allowed length of stay. This policy recognizes that home care is less costly than hospital care and in most cases is more beneficial for recovery (Carpenter, 1998).

The nurse must provide discharge teaching to prepare women for self-care and newborn care in a limited time, while trying to ensure that the woman is comfortable and able to rest. The nurse needs to assess the woman's information needs and coordinate the health care team's efforts to meet them.

Discharge teaching and planning should include information about nutrition; measures to relieve pain and discomfort; exercise and specific activity restrictions; time management that includes periods of uninterrupted rest and sleep; hygiene, breast and incision care; timing for resumption of sexual activity and contraception; signs of complications (see the Patient Teaching box and the Home Care box); and infant care. The nurse assesses the woman's need for continued support or counseling to facilitate her emotional recovery from the birth. Referrals to support groups or to community agencies may be indicated to further promote the recovery process.

Vaginal Birth after Cesarean. Indications for primary cesarean birth such as dystocia, breech presentation, or fetal distress, often are nonrecurring. Therefore a woman who has had a cesarean birth may subsequently become pregnant and not have any contraindications to labor and vaginal birth in that pregnancy.

ACOG (1994b) recommends that a TOL and vaginal birth after cesarean (VBAC) be routinely attempted in women who have had one previous cesarean birth by low transverse incision. Vaginal birth is relatively safe, with only a 0.5% risk of uterine rupture through a lower uterine segment scar (Knuppel and Drukker, 1993). Labor and a vaginal birth are not recommended if there are contraindications such as a previous fundal classic cesarean scar or evidence of CPD.

According to Scott (1999), 60% to 88% of women can give birth vaginally after a TOL. Women are most often the primary decision makers with regard to choice of birth method. During the antepartal period, the woman should be given information about VBAC and encouraged to choose it as an alternative to a repeat cesarean, as long as no contraindications exist. VBAC support groups and prenatal classes can help prepare the woman psychologically for labor and vaginal birth.

This labor should occur in a hospital facility that has the equipment and personnel available to begin surgery within

TABLE 19-5
Care Path: Cesarean Birth without Complications: Expected Length of Stay—48 to 72 Hours

	Immediate Post-op Cesarean	By 4th Hour After Admission to PP Unit	5 to 24 Hours	25 to 48 Hours	By Discharge
ASSESSMENTS	Recovery room/ PACU admission assessment completed	PP admission assessment and care plan completed			
Vital Signs	q15min × 1 hr; q30min × 4 hr, WNL	q1hr × 3, WNL	q4-8hr, WNL	q8hr, WNL	q8hr, WNL
Postpartum Assessment	q15min × 1 hr, WNL	q1hr × 3, WNL	q8hr, WNL	q8-12hr, WNL	q8-12hr, WNL
Abdominal Incision	Dressing dry and intact	Dressing dry and intact	Dressing dry and intact	Dressing off or changed, incision intact	Incision intact; staples may be removed and steri-strips in place, incision WNL
Genitourinary	Retention catheter output >30 ml/hr	Retention catheter output <30 ml/hr	Retention catheter output >30 ml/hr	Catheter discontinued, output >100 ml/void or 240 ml/8 hr	Urine output >240 ml/8 hr
Gastrointestinal		Absent or hypoactive BS	Hypoactive to active BS	Active BS + flatus	Active BS + flatus; may or may not have BM
Musculoskeletal	Alert or easily aroused, can move legs	Alert and oriented, moving all extremities	Ambulating with help	Ambulating unassisted	Ambulating ad lib
Bonding	Evidence of parent-infant bonding; first breastfeeding if desired		Parent-infant bonding continues	Parent-infant bonding progressing	
Laboratory Tests			Intrapartal CBC results on chart/ computer; determine Rh status and need for anti-Rh globulin; check for rubella immunity	PP HCT WNL, all lab results on chart, give anti-Rh globulin if indicated	Give rubella vaccine if indicated
INTERVENTIONS					
IV	IV continues	IV continues	IV continues	IV may be discontinued	
Diet	NPO	Ice chips, sips of clear liquids	Clear liquids	Regular diet or as tolerated	Regular diet

ADLs, Activities of daily living; *BM,* bowel movement; *BS,* bowel sounds; *CBC,* complete blood count; *HCT,* hematocrit; *IV,* intravenous; *NPO,* nothing by mouth; *NSAIDs,* nonsteroid antiinflammatory drugs; *OOB,* out-of-bed; *PCA,* patient-controlled analgesia; *PNV,* prenatal vitamins; *PP,* postpartum; *TCDB,* turn, cough, deep breathe; *WNL,* within normal limits.

TABLE 19-5—cont'd

Care Path: Cesarean Birth without Complications: Expected Length of Stay—48 to 72 Hours

	Immediate Post-op Cesarean	By 4th Hour After Admission to PP Unit	5 to 24 Hours	25 to 48 Hours	By Discharge
Perineal Care		Peri-care by nurse	Peri-care with help	Self-pericare	
Activity	Bed rest	Bed rest	OOB × 3 with help, ADLs assisted, assisted to comfortable position to hold and feed baby	Holds baby comfortably, ambulates without assistance, ADLs unassisted	Activity ad lib
Pulmonary Care	Patent airway; O_2 discontinued	TCDB q2hr with splinting, incentive spirometry q1hr if ordered, lungs clear	TCDB q2hr while awake; lungs clear	TCDB as needed; lungs clear	
Medications	Oxytocin added to IV Pain control: analgesics, IV, or epidural narcotic	Oxytocin continued Pain control: analgesics—PCA, IM, PO, or epidural narcotic	Oxytocin may be discontinued Pain control: IM, PO, PCA narcotics or analgesics	Oxytocin discontinued Pain control: PO analgesics, NSAIDs; PCA discontinued; stool softener, PNV	Rx filled or given to take home
Teaching, Discharge Plan	Breastfeeding, positioning, leg exercises	Verbalize understanding/unit routines, how to achieve rest, TCDB, involution, pain control	*Self:* comfort measures and care; reinforce TCDB and positioning; introduce teaching videos, lactation promotion or suppression *Infant:* handwashing, infant safety, positioning for feeding and burping, if breastfeeding, then positioning baby, latching on, timing, removing from breast	*Self:* diet; activity/rest; bowel/bladder function *Infant:* bonding; parent concerns; feeding, infant bath, cord care; need for car seat; newborn characteristics; circumcision, if requested; answer questions	*Self:* home care, signs of complications (infections, bleeding), normal psychologic adjustments, normal ADLs; resumption of sexual activities; contraception; identification of support system at home; self-concept issues related to cesarean birth. Inform whom to call if problems; review need to keep follow-up appointment; provide information about community resources; provide copy of home care *Infant:* parents to demonstrate infant care; reinforce use of booklets for infant care, whom to call if problems; discuss immunization needs; review need to keep follow-up appointments

30 minutes from the time a decision is made for cesarean birth. Ideally, the woman is admitted to the labor and birth unit at the onset of spontaneous labor. In the latent phase of labor, the nurse encourages normal activities such as ambulation. In the active phase of labor, FHR and uterine activity usually are monitored electronically, and intravenous access such as a heparin lock may be established. Collaboration among the woman in labor, the nurse, and other health care providers often results in a successful VBAC.

There is no evidence that administering oxytocin to induce or augment labor or the use of epidural anesthesia is contraindicated, although some physicians may not elect to use these procedures (Cunningham et al, 1997).

Attention should be given to the woman's psychologic and physical needs during the TOL. Anxiety can inhibit the release of oxytocin, delaying labor progress and perhaps leading to a repeat cesarean birth. To alleviate anxiety, the nurse can encourage the woman to use breathing and relaxation techniques and to change position to promote labor progress. The woman's partner can be encouraged to provide comfort measures and emotional support (Fawcett, Tulman, and Spedden, 1994). If a trial of labor does not proceed to vaginal birth, the woman will need support and encouragement to express her feelings about having another cesarean birth.

➤ Evaluation

Evaluation of the effectiveness of nursing care for a woman experiencing dystocia is based on the expected outcomes.

POSTTERM PREGNANCY, LABOR, AND BIRTH

A postterm or postdate pregnancy is one that extends beyond the end of week 42 of gestation, or more than 294 days from the first day of the last menstrual period. The incidence of postdate pregnancy is estimated to be between 4% and 14% (Cunningham et al, 1997).

Clinical manifestations of postterm pregnancy include maternal weight loss, decreased uterine size, meconium in the amniotic fluid, and advanced bone maturation of the fetal skeleton with an exceptionally hard fetal skull (Gilbert and Harmon, 1998).

Maternal and Fetal Risks

Maternal risks are often related to the birth of an excessively large infant. The woman is at increased risk for dysfunctional labor; birth canal trauma, including lacerations and extension of episiotomy related to vaginal birth; postpartum hemorrhage; and infection. Interventions such as induction of labor with oxytocin, vacuum- or forceps-assisted birth, and cesarean birth are more likely to be necessary. The woman also may experience fatigue and psychological reactions such as depression, frustration, and feelings of inadequacy as she passes her estimated date of birth (Arulkumarian, 1997; Freeman and Lagrew, 1996; Gilbert and Harmon, 1998).

Fetal risks appear to be twofold. The first is the possibility of prolonged labor, shoulder dystocia, birth trauma, and asphyxia from macrosomia. The second risk is the compromising effects on the fetus of an "aging" placenta. Spellacy (1999) notes that placental function gradually decreases after 37 weeks of gestation. Amniotic fluid volume declines to approximately 800 ml by 40 weeks, and to about 400 ml by 42 weeks of gestation. The resulting oligohydramnios can lead to fetal hypoxia related to cord compression. If placental insufficiency is present, there is a high likelihood of fetal distress occurring during labor. Neonatal problems may include asphyxia, meconium aspiration syndrome, dysmaturity syndrome, hypoglycemia, polycythemia, and respiratory distress (Gilbert and Harmon, 1998).

Care Management

The management of postdate pregnancy is still controversial. The induction of labor at 41 to 42 weeks is suggested by some authorities as a means of reducing the rate of cesarean birth and stillbirth or neonatal death (Hannah et al, 1996). Others follow a more individualized approach, allowing the pregnancy to proceed to 43 weeks as long as assessment of fetal well-being using a combination of tests is performed and the results of the tests are normal.

LEGAL TIP • Informed Consent Regarding Care During Postterm Pregnancy The woman with a postterm pregnancy should be informed about the risks and benefits of both treatment and nontreatment. The standard of practice for postterm pregnancy is to begin antepartal surveillance (e.g., maternal assessments and tests of fetal well-being) by 14 days after the EDB, no matter how the date was derived. The woman and her primary health care provider should mutually agree on a plan of care (Wood, 1994).

Antepartum assessments for postterm pregnancy may include daily fetal movement counts, nonstress tests, amniotic fluid volume assessments, contraction stress tests, biophysical profiles, and Doppler flow measurement.

The amniotic fluid volume (AFV) should be greater than 8 with at least one pocket of amniotic fluid greater than 2 cm and amniotic fluid present throughout the uterine cavity (Gilbert and Harmon, 1998; Schmidt, 1999). The biophysical profile may be the best way of gauging fetal well-being because it combines nonstress testing with real-time ultrasound scanning to assess fetal movements, fetal breathing movements, and AFV. Determining the AFV is critical in women with a postterm pregnancy because decreased AFV has been associated with fetal stress.

Cervical checks usually are performed weekly after 40 weeks of gestation to assess whether the condition of the cervix is favorable for induction (>5 on the Bishop score for multiparas and >9 for nulliparas; see Table 19-4). Vaginal secretions may be assessed for the amount of fetal fibronectin; a low concentration may predict increased risk for prolonged pregnancy. Amniocentesis or amnioscopy may be performed to detect meconium in the amniotic fluid (Spellacy, 1999).

During the postdate period the woman is encouraged to assess fetal activity daily, assess for signs of labor, and keep appointments with her primary health care provider (Home Care box). The woman and her family should be encouraged to express their feelings about the prolonged pregnancy. Referral to a support group or other supportive resource may be needed.

If the woman's cervix is ripe, labor is usually induced with oxytocin. If her cervix is not ripe, fetal surveillance is continued and a cervical ripening agent (e.g., prostaglandin gel or insert) may be administered followed by oxytocin induction (Gilbert and Harmon, 1998).

The fetus of a woman with a postterm pregnancy should be monitored electronically for a more accurate assessment of the FHR pattern. If oligohydramnios is present, amnioinfusion may be implemented to restore amniotic fluid volume in order to maintain a cushioning of the cord. Inadequate fluid volume leads to compression of the cord, which results in fetal hypoxia reflected in variable or prolonged deceleration patterns and passage of meconium. Accurate assessment of the woman's labor pattern also is important because dysfunctional labor is common (Spellacy, 1999).

Emotional support is essential for the woman with a postterm pregnancy and her family. A vaginal birth is anticipated, but the couple should be prepared for a forceps- or vacuum-assisted birth or cesarean birth if complications arise.

Home Care

POSTTERM PREGNANCY

Perform daily fetal movement counts.
Assess for signs of labor.
Call your primary health care provider if your membranes rupture, or if you perceive a decrease in or no fetal movement
Keep appointments for fetal assessment tests or cervical checks.
Come to the hospital soon after labor begins.

OBSTETRIC EMERGENCIES

Shoulder Dystocia

Shoulder dystocia is a rare obstetric emergency that increases the risk for fetal/neonatal and maternal morbidity and mortality during the attempt to deliver the fetus vaginally. Shoulder dystocia is a condition in which the head is born but the anterior shoulder cannot pass under the pubic arch. Fetopelvic disproportion related to excessive fetal size or maternal pelvic abnormalities may be a cause of shoulder dystocia (Hall, 1997; Wiznitzer, 1995).

Care Management

Many maneuvers such as suprapubic pressure and maternal position changes have been suggested and tried to free the anterior shoulder, although no one particular maneuver has been found to be most effective (Naef and Morrison, 1994). Suprapubic pressure can be applied to the anterior shoulder using the Mazzanti or Rubin technique (Fig. 19-13) in an attempt to push the shoulder under the symphysis pubis (Naef and Morrison, 1994). Having the woman move to a hands-and-knees position or a squatting position has also been used to resolve cases of shoulder dystocia (Piper and McDonald, 1994).

In the McRoberts maneuver (Fig. 19-14), the woman's legs are flexed apart with her knees on her abdomen (Piper and

A

B

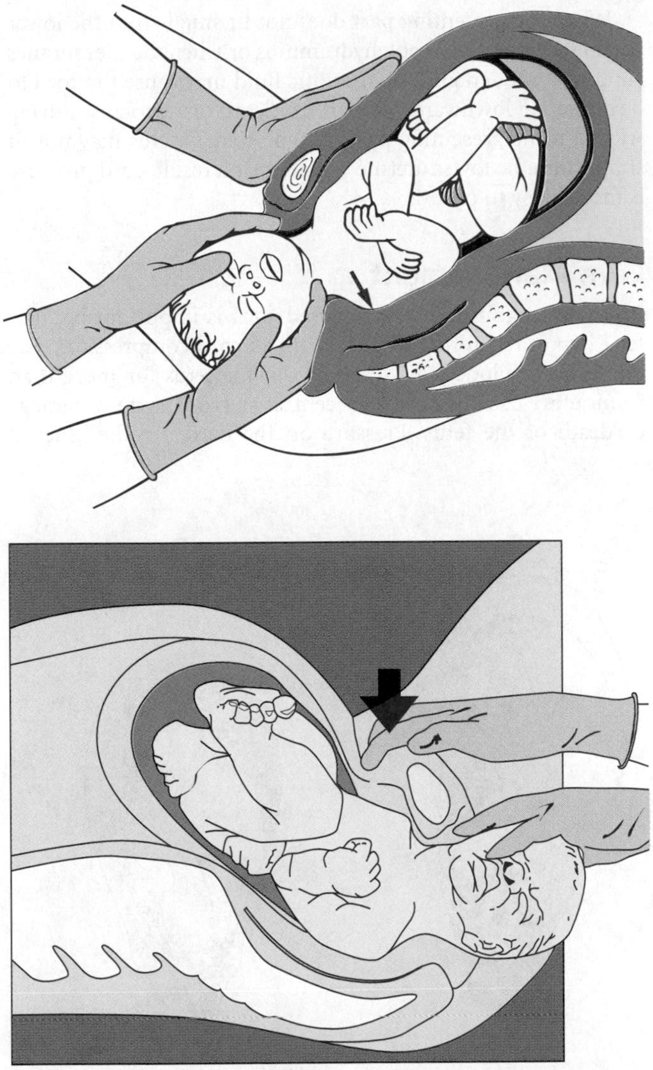

FIG. 19-13 • Application of suprapubic pressure. **A,** Mazzanti technique: pressure is applied directly posteriorly and laterally above the symphysis pubis. **B,** Rubin technique: pressure is applied obliquely posteriorly against the anterior shoulder.

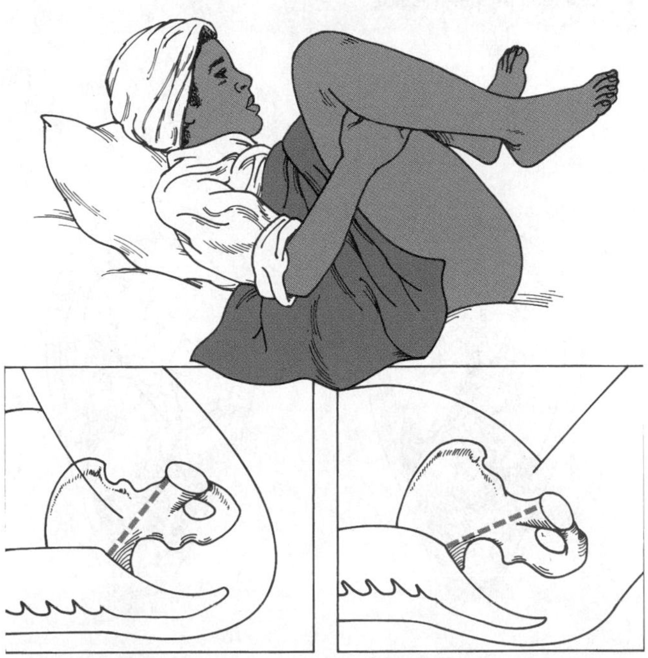

FIG. 19-14 • McRoberts maneuver. (Modified from Gabbe S, Niebyl J, Simpson J: *Obstetrics: normal and problem pregnancies,* ed 3, New York, 1996, Churchill Livingstone.)

McDonald, 1994). This maneuver causes the sacrum to straighten, and the symphysis pubis rotates toward the mother's head; the angle of pelvic inclination is decreased, freeing the shoulder. The Gaskin maneuver requires that the woman assume an all-fours position on her hands and knees (Bruner et al, 1998).

The nurse helps the woman assume the position(s) that may facilitate birth of the shoulders, and assists the primary health care provider with these maneuvers. The nurse also provides encouragement and support to reduce anxiety and fear.

Newborn assessment should include examination for fracture of the clavicle or humerus, as well as brachial plexus injuries and asphyxia (Hall, 1997). Maternal assessment should focus on early detection of hemorrhage.

Emergency

PROLAPSED CORD

Signs

- Fetal bradycardia with variable deceleration during uterine contraction.
- Woman reports feeling the cord after membranes rupture.
- Cord is seen or felt in or protruding from the vagina.

Interventions

- Call for assistance.
- Notify primary health care provider immediately.
- Glove the examining hand quickly and insert two fingers into the vagina to the cervix. With one finger on either side of the cord or both fingers to one side, exert upward pressure against the presenting part to relieve compression of the cord (Fig. 19-16, *A* and *B*). Place a rolled towel under the woman's right or left hip.
- Place woman into the extreme Trendelenburg or a modified Sims' position (Fig. 19-16, *C*), or a knee-chest position (Fig. 19-16, *D*).
- If cord is protruding from vagina, wrap loosely in a sterile towel saturated with warm sterile normal saline solution.
- Administer oxygen to the woman by mask at 8 to 10 L/min until birth is accomplished.
- Start IV fluids or increase existing drip rate.
- Continue to monitor FHR by internal fetal scalp electrode, if possible.
- Explain to woman and support person what is happening the way it is being managed.
- Prepare for immediate vaginal delivery if cervix is fully dilated or cesarean birth if it is not.

Prolapsed Umbilical Cord

Prolapse of the umbilical cord occurs when the cord lies below the presenting part of the fetus. Umbilical cord prolapse may be occult (hidden, not visible) at any time during labor whether or not membranes are ruptured (Fig. 19-15, *A* and *B*). It is most common to see frank (visible) prolapse directly after rupture of membranes, when gravity washes the cord in front of the presenting part (Fig. 19-15, *C* and *D*). Frank prolapse occurs in 1 out of 400 births. Contributing factors are a long cord (i.e., >100 cm), malpresentation (breech), transverse lie, or unengaged presenting part.

When the presenting part does not fit snugly into the lower uterine segment, as in polyhydramnios or when the membranes rupture, a sudden gush of amniotic fluid may cause the cord to be displaced downward. Similarly, the cord may prolapse during AROM if the presenting part is high. A small fetus may not fit snugly into the lower uterine segment; as a result, cord prolapse is more likely to occur.

Care Management

Prompt recognition of a prolapsed cord is important because fetal hypoxia resulting from prolonged cord compression (i.e., occlusion of blood flow to and from the fetus for more than 5 minutes) usually results in central nervous system damage or death of the fetus. Pressure on the cord may be relieved

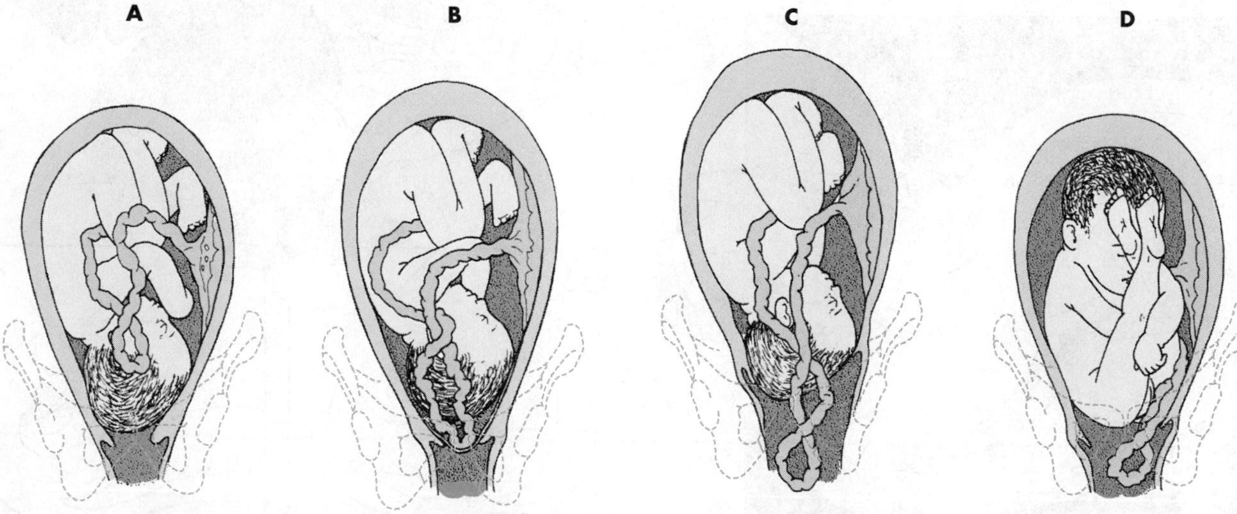

FIG. 19-15 • Prolapse of umbilical cord. Note pressure of presenting part on umbilical cord, which endangers fetal circulation. **A,** Occult (hidden) prolapse of cord. **B,** Complete prolapse of cord. Note membranes are intact. **C,** Cord presenting in front of fetal head may be seen in vagina. **D,** Frank breech presentation with prolapsed cord.

by the examiner putting a sterile gloved hand into the vagina and holding the presenting part off of the umbilical cord (Fig. 19-16, *A* and *B*). The woman is assisted into a position such as a modified Sims (Fig. 19-16, *C*), Trendelenburg, or knee-chest (Fig. 19-16, *D*), in which gravity keeps the presenting part off the cord. If the cervix is fully dilated, a forceps- or vacuum-assisted birth can be performed for the fetus in a cephalic presentation; otherwise a cesarean birth is likely to be performed. Nonreassuring fetal status, inadequate uterine relaxation, and bleeding can also occur as a result of a prolapsed umbilical cord. Indications for immediate interventions are presented in the Emergency box.

Rupture of the Uterus

Rupture of the uterus is a rare but very serious obstetric injury that occurs once in every 1500 to 2000 births. The most common causes of uterine rupture during pregnancy are separation of the scar of a previous classical cesarean birth, uterine trauma (e.g., accidents or surgery), and congenital uterine anomaly. During labor and birth, uterine rupture may be caused by intense spontaneous uterine contractions, labor stimulation (e.g., oxytocin), an overdistended uterus, (e.g., multifetal gestation), malpresentation, external or internal version, or a difficult forceps-assisted birth. It occurs more commonly in multigravidas than primigravidas.

A uterine rupture may be classified as complete or incomplete. A complete rupture extends through the entire uterine wall into the peritoneal cavity or broad ligament. An incomplete rupture extends into the peritoneum but not into the peritoneal cavity or broad ligament. Bleeding is usually internal. An incomplete rupture may also be a partial separation of an old cesarean scar and may go unnoticed unless the woman has a subsequent cesarean birth or other uterine surgery.

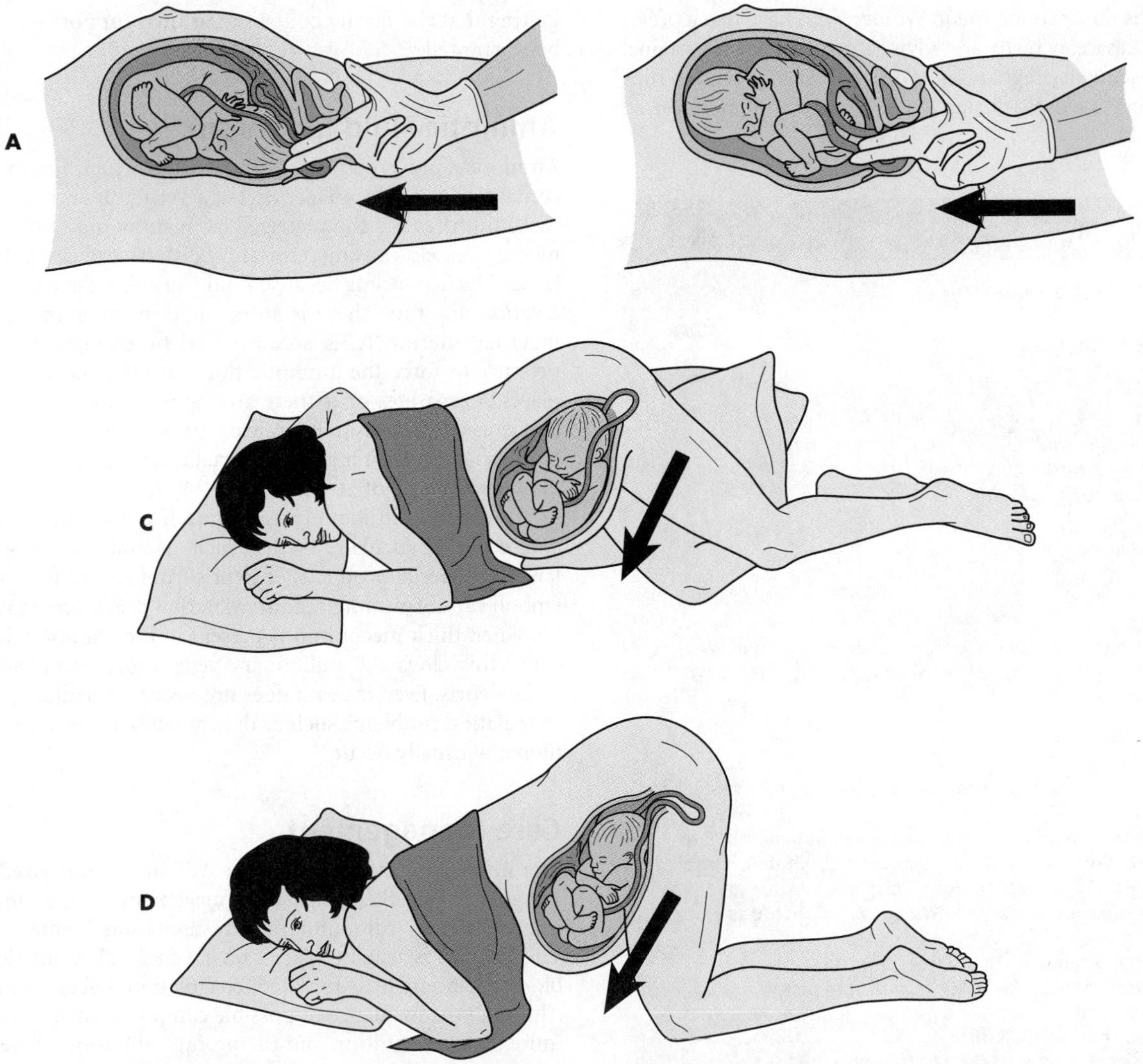

FIG. 19-16 • Arrows indicate direction of pressure against presenting part to relieve compression of prolapsed umbilical cord. Pressure exerted by examiner's fingers in **A,** vertex presentation, and **B,** breech presentation. **C,** Gravity relieves pressure when woman is in modified Sims' position with hips elevated as high as possible with pillows. **D,** Knee-chest position.

Signs and symptoms vary with the extent of the rupture and may be silent or dramatic. In an incomplete rupture, pain may not be present. The fetus may or may not have late decelerations, decreased variability, an increased or decreased heart rate, or other nonreassuring signs. The woman may experience vomiting, faintness, increased abdominal tenderness, hypotonic uterine contractions, and lack of progress. Eventually, bleeding and the effects of blood loss will be noted. Fetal heart tones may be lost. In a complete rupture, the woman may complain of a sudden, sharp abdominal pain and may state that "something gave way." If she is in labor, her contractions will cease and pain is relieved. She may exhibit signs of hypovolemic shock caused by hemorrhage (i.e., hypotension; tachypnea; pallor; and cool, clammy skin). If the placenta separates, the fetal heart rate will be absent. Fetal parts may be palpable through the abdomen. The nurse should suspect pulmonary embolism if the woman complains of chest pain (Varney, 1997).

Care Management

Prevention is the best treatment. Women who have had a previous classic cesarean birth are advised not to attempt vaginal birth in subsequent pregnancies. Women at risk for uterine rupture are assessed closely during labor. Women who are induced with oxytocin are monitored for signs of uterine hyperstimulation because this can precipitate uterine rupture. If hyperstimulation occurs, the oxytocin infusion is discontinued or decreased and a tocolytic medication may be given to decrease the intensity of uterine contractions. After giving birth, women are assessed for excessive bleeding, especially if the fundus is firm and there are signs of hemorrhagic shock.

If rupture occurs, medical management depends on the severity. A small rupture may be managed with a laparotomy and birth of the infant, repair of the laceration, and blood transfusions if needed. For a complete rupture, hysterectomy and blood replacement is the usual treatment.

The nurse's role may include starting intravenous fluids, transfusing blood products, and assisting with preparation for immediate surgery. Supporting the woman's family and providing information about the treatment is important during this emergency (Varney, 1997). The associated fetal mortality rates are high (i.e., >80%) and the maternal mortality rate may be as high as 50% to 75% (Cunningham et al, 1997). Providing information about spiritual support services or suggesting that the family contact their own support system may be warranted.

Emergency

AMNIOTIC FLUID EMBOLISM

Signs

Respiratory distress
- Restlessness
- Dyspnea
- Cyanosis
- Pulmonary edema
- Respiratory arrest

Circulatory collapse
- Hypotension
- Tachycardia
- Shock
- Cardiac arrest

Hemorrhage
- Coagulation failure: bleeding from incisions, venipuncture sites, trauma (lacerations); petechiae, ecchymoses, purpura
- Uterine atony

Interventions

Oxygenate
- Administer oxygen by face mask (8 to 10 L/min) or resuscitation bag delivering 100% oxygen
- Prepare for intubation and mechanical ventilation
- Initiate or assist with cardiopulmonary resuscitation; tilt pregnant woman 30 degrees to side to displace uterus

Maintain cardiac output and replace fluid losses
- Position woman on her side
- Administer IV fluids
- Administer blood: packed cells, fresh frozen plasma
- Insert indwelling catheter, and measure hourly urine output

Correct coagulation failure

Monitor fetal and maternal status

Prepare for emergency birth once woman's condition is stabilized

Provide emotional support to woman, her partner, and family

Amniotic Fluid Embolism

Amniotic fluid embolism (AFE) occurs when amniotic fluid containing particles of debris (e.g., vernix, hair, skin cells, or meconium) enters the maternal circulation and obstructs pulmonary vessels, causing respiratory distress and circulatory collapse. This can occur because fluid can enter the maternal circulation any time there is an opening in the amniotic sac or maternal uterine veins accompanied by enough intrauterine pressure to force the amniotic fluid into the veins (e.g., if the placenta separates or if there are rapid or strong contractions that cause the uterus to lacerate or rupture). AFE is estimated to be associated with a maternal mortality as high as 86% and a fetal mortality rate of 50% (Martin, 1996).

Amniotic fluid is more damaging if it contains meconium and other particulate matter such as mucus, fat globules, lanugo, bacterial products, or debris from a dead fetus because emboli can form more readily. Maternal death occurs most often when thick meconium is present in the amniotic fluid, because this clogs the pulmonary veins more completely than other debris. Even if death does not occur immediately, serious coagulation problems such as disseminated intravascular coagulopathy usually occur.

Care Management

The immediate interventions for AFE are summarized in the Emergency box. Such medical management must be instituted immediately. Cardiopulmonary resuscitation is often needed. The woman is usually placed on mechanical ventilation, and blood replacement is initiated; coagulation defects are treated. Although the incidence of possible complications is small, their immediate recognition and the prompt initiation of treatment is important.

The nurse's immediate responsibility is to assist with the resuscitation efforts. If the woman survives, she is usually moved to a critical care unit where hemodynamic monitoring, blood replacement, and coagulopathy treatment are implemented.

Support of the woman's partner and family is needed; they will be anxious and distressed. Brief explanations of what is happening are important during the emergency and can be reinforced after the immediate crisis is over. If the woman dies, emotional support and involvement of the perinatal loss support team or other resource for grief counseling is needed. Referral to grief and loss support groups would be appropriate.

Key Points

- Preterm labor is cervical change and uterine contractions occurring between 20 weeks and 37 weeks of pregnancy; preterm birth is any birth that occurs before the completion of 37 weeks of pregnancy.
- The incidence of preterm birth in the United States varies considerably by race.
- The cause of preterm labor is unknown, and is assumed to be multifactorial.
- Betamimetics are a class of medications that have many maternal and fetal side effects and must always be used with extreme caution.
- Bed rest, a commonly prescribed intervention for preterm labor, has many deleterious side effects and has never been shown to decrease preterm birth rates.
- Preterm birth that occurs in a tertiary care center leads to better neonatal and maternal outcomes.
- Vigilance for signs of infection is a major part of the care for women with PPROM.
- Dystocia results from differences in the normal relationships among any of the five factors affecting labor.
- Dysfunctional labor occurs as a result of hypertonic uterine dysfunction, hypotonic uterine dysfunction, or inadequate voluntary expulsive forces.
- The functional relationships between the uterine contractions, the fetus, and the mother's pelvis are altered by maternal positioning.
- Uterine contractility is increased by oxytocin and prostaglandin and is decreased by tocolytic agents.
- Cervical ripening using chemical or mechanical measures can increase the success of labor induction.
- Expectant parents benefit from learning about operative obstetrics (e.g., forceps-assisted or cesarean birth) during the prenatal period.
- The basic purpose of cesarean birth is to preserve the life or health of the mother and her fetus.
- Unless contraindicated, a vaginal birth is possible after a previous cesarean birth.
- Labor management that emphasizes one-to-one support of the laboring woman by another female (e.g., doula, nurse, or nurse-midwife) can reduce the rate of cesarean birth and increase the rate of VBACs.
- Postterm pregnancy poses a risk to both the mother and the fetus.
- Obstetric emergencies (e.g., shoulder dystocia, prolapsed cord, rupture of the uterus, and amniotic fluid embolism) occur rarely but require immediate intervention.

References

Albers L, Lydon-Rochelle M, Krulewitch C: Maternal age and labor complications in healthy primigravidas at term, *J Nurse Midwifery* 40(1):4-11, 1995.

American College of Obstetricians and Gynecologists (ACOG): *Operative vaginal delivery (Tech Bull No. 196),* Washington, DC, 1994a, ACOG.

American College of Obstetricians and Gynecologists (ACOG): *Committee opinion: vaginal delivery after a previous cesarean birth* (Committee on Obstetrics Practice 143), Washington, DC, 1994b, ACOG.

American College of Obstetricians and Gynecologists (ACOG): *Induction of labor (Tech Bull No. 217),* Washington, DC, 1995b, ACOG.

American College of Obstetricians and Gynecologists (ACOG): *Preterm labor (Tech Bull 206),* Washington, DC, 1995c, ACOG.

American College of Obstetricians and Gynecologists and American Academy of Pediatrics (ACOG/AAP): *Guidelines for perinatal care,* ed 4, Washington, DC, 1997, ACOG.

Arulkumarian S: Prolonged pregnancy. In James D et al, editors: *High risk pregnancy management options,* London, 1997, WB Saunders.

Besinger R et al: A randomized comparative trial of indomethacin and ritodrine for the long-term treatment of preterm labor, *Am J Obstet Gynecol* 164:981-986, 1991.

Biancuzzo M: Six myths of maternal posture during labor, *MCN Am J Matern Child Nurs* 18(5):264-269, 1993.

Bruner J et al: All-fours maneuver for reducing shoulder dystocia during labor, *J Reprod Med* 43(5):439-443, 1998.

Burrows W et al: Safety and efficacy of early postoperative solid food consumption after cesarean section, *J Reprod Med* 40(6):463-467, 1995.

Carpenter J: Shortening the short stay, *AWHONN Lifelines* 2(1):28-34, 1998.

Collaborative Group on Preterm Birth Prevention: Multicenter randomized controlled trial of a preterm birth prevention program, *Am J Obstet Gynecol* 169:352-366, 1993.

Crane J et al: Transvaginal ultrasound in the prediction of preterm delivery: singleton and twin gestations, *Obstet Gynecol* 90(3):357-363, 1997.

Cunningham F et al: *Williams obstetrics,* ed 20, Stamford, CT, 1997, Appleton & Lange.

Curtin S, Kozak L: Decline in U. S. cesarean delivery rate appears to stall, *Birth* 25(4):259-262, 1998.

DiMatteo M et al: Cesarean childbirth and psychosocial outcomes: a meta-analysis, *Health Psychol* 15(4):303-314, 1996.

Dyson D et al: Monitoring women at risk for preterm labor, *N Engl J Med* 338:15-19, 1998.

Eakes M, Brown H: Home alone-meeting the needs of mothers after cesarean birth, *AWHONN Lifelines* 2(1):36-40, 1998.

Ellings J, Newman R, Bowers N: Intrapartum care for women with multiple pregnancy, *J Obstet Gynecol Neonatal Nurs* 27(4):466-472, 1998.

Fawcett J, Tulman L, Spedden J: Responses to vaginal birth after cesarean section, *J Obstet Gynecol Neonatal Nurs* 23(3): 253-259, 1994.

Freda M, DeVore J: Should intravenous hydration be the first line of defense with threatened preterm labor? A critical review of the literature, *J Perinatol* 16(5):385-389, 1996.

Freda M, Patterson E: *Preterm birth: prevention and nursing management. Nursing module.* New York, 1995, March of Dimes.

Freeman R, Lagrew D: Post date pregnancy. In Gabbe S, Niebyl J, Simpson J, editors: *Obstetrics: normal and problem pregnancies,* ed 3, New York, 1996, Churchill Livingstone.

Freston M et al: Responses of pregnant women to potential preterm labor symptoms, *J Obstet Gynecol Neonatal Nurs* 26:35-41, 1997.

Friedman E: Normal and dysfunctional labor. In Cohen W et al, editors: *Management of labor,* ed 2, Rockville, MD, 1989, Aspen.

Gilbert E, Harmon J: *Manual of high risk pregnancy and delivery,* ed 2, St Louis, 1998, Mosby.

Goldenberg R, Rouse D: Prevention of premature birth, *N Engl J Med* 339:313-320, 1998.

Guyer B et al: Annual summary of vital statistics, 1997, *Pediatrics* 102(6):333-349, 1998.

Hall S: The nurse's role in the identification of risks and treatment of shoulder dystocia, *J Obstet Gynecol Neonatal Nurs* 26(1):25-32, 1997.

Hannah M et al: Postterm pregnancy: putting the merits of a policy of induction of labor into perspective, *Birth* 23(1): 13-19, 1996.

Hill W: Risks and complications of tocolysis, *Clin Obstet Gynecol* 38(4):725-745, 1995.

Iams J: Preterm birth. In Gabbe S, Niebyl J, Simpson J, editors: *Obstetrics: normal and problem pregnancies,* ed 3, New York, 1996, Churchill Livingstone.

Iams J, Johnson F, O'Shaughnessy R: A prospective randomized trial of home uterine monitoring in pregnancies at increased risk of preterm labor, *Am J Obstet Gynecol* 159:595-603, 1988.

Institute of Medicine: *Preventing low birthweight,* Washington, DC, 1985, National Academy Press.

Knuppel R, Drukker J: *High risk pregnancy: a team approach,* ed 2, Philadelphia, 1993, WB Saunders.

Laros R, Flanagan T, Kilpatrick J: Management of term breech presentation: a protocol of external cephalic version and selective trial of labor, *Am J Obstet Gynecol* 172(6):1916-1923, 1995.

Lockwood C et al: Fetal fibronectin in cervical and vaginal secretions as a predictor of preterm delivery, *N Engl J Med* 325:669-674, 1991.

Maloni J et al: Physical and psychosocial side effects of antepartum bed rest, *Nurs Res* 42(4):197-203, 1993.

March of Dimes: *Stat book,* White Plains, NY, 1997, March of Dimes Birth Defects Foundation.

Martin R: Amniotic fluid embolism, *Clin Obstet Gynecol* 39(1):101-106, 1996.

Mathews T: Trends in stimulation and induction of labor, 1989-1995, *Stat Bull* 78(4):20-26, 1998.

Mercer B et al: Antibiotic therapy for reduction of infant morbidity after preterm premature rupture of the membranes, *JAMA* 278(12):989-995, 1997.

Miovech S et al: Major concerns of women after cesarean delivery, *J Obstet Gynecol Neonatal Nurs* 23(1):53-59, 1994.

Moore M: Biochemical markers for preterm birth, *MCN Am J Matern Child Nurs* 24:66-74, 1999.

Moore M et al: A randomized trial of nurse intervention to reduce preterm and low birthweight births, *Obstet Gynecol* 91:656-661, 1998.

Naef R, Morrison J: Guidelines for the management of shoulder dystocia, *J Perinatol* 14(6):435-441, 1994.

National Institutes of Health Consensus Development Conference Group: Effect of corticosteroids for fetal maturation on perinatal outcomes, *Am J Obstet Gynecol* 173:246-252, 1995.

Piper D, McDonald P: Management of anticipated and actual shoulder dystocia: interpreting the literature, *J Nurse Midwifery* 39(suppl 2):91S-105S, 1994.

Porreco R, Thorp J: The cesarean birth epidemic: trends, causes, and solutions, *Am J Obstet Gynecol* 175(2):369-374, 1996.

Radin T, Harmon J, Hanson D: Nurses' care during labor: its effects on the cesarean birth rate of healthy nulliparous women, *Birth* 20(1):14-21, 1993.

Read M, Wellby D: The use of a calcium antagonist (nifedipine) to suppress preterm labor, *Br J Obstet Gynaecol* 93:933-937, 1986.

Ryding E, Wijma K, Wijma B: Experiences of emergency cesarean section: a phenomenological study of 53 women, *Birth* 25(4):246-251, 1998.

Schmidt J: Prolonged pregnancy. In Mandeville L, Troiano N, editors: *High risk and critical care intrapartum nursing,* ed 2, Philadelphia, 1999, Lippincott.

Scott J: Cesarean delivery. In Scott J et al, editors: *Danforth's obstetrics and gynecology,* ed 8, Philadelphia, 1999, Lippincott, Williams & Wilkins.

Simpson K, Poole J: *Cervical ripening and induction and augmentation of labor,* Washington, DC, 1998, AHWONN.

Spellacy W: Postdate pregnancy. In Scott J et al, editors: *Danforth's obstetrics and gynecology,* ed 8, Philadelphia, 1999, Lippincott, Williams & Wilkins.

Summers L: Methods of cervical ripening and labor induction, *J Nurse Midwifery* 42(2):71-85, 1997.

Thomas L et al: The effects of rocking, diet modifications, and antiflatulent medication of postcesarean section gas pain, *J Perinat Neonatal Nurs* 4(3):12-24, 1990.

U.S. Public Health Service: *Caring for our future: the content of prenatal care,* Washington, DC, 1989, USPHS.

Varney H: *Varney's textbook for midwives,* ed 3, Sudberry, MA, 1997, Jones & Bartlett.

Ventura J et al: Report of Final Natality Statistics, 1996, *Monthly Vital Statistics Report* 46(11 suppl):1-100, 1998.

Viamantes C: Pharmacologic intervention in the management of preterm labor: an update, *J Perinatal Neonatal Nurs* 9(4):13-30, 1996.

Wiznitzer A: Obstructed labor and shoulder dystocia, *Curr Opin Obstet Gynecol* 7(6):486-491, 1995.

Wood C: Postdate pregnancy update, *J Nurse Midwifery* 39(supp 2):110S-122S, 1994.

CHAPTER 20

Maternal Physiologic Changes

http://www.harcourthealth.com/MERLIN/Wong/maternal/

Learning Objectives

On completion of this chapter the reader will be able to:

- Describe the anatomic and physiologic changes that occur during the postpartum period.
- Identify characteristics of uterine involution and lochial flow and describe ways to measure them.
- List expected values for vital signs and blood pressure, deviations from normal findings, and probable causes of the deviations.

The postpartum period is the 6-week interval between the birth of the newborn and the return of the reproductive organs to their normal nonpregnant state. This period is sometimes referred to as the puerperium, or fourth trimester of pregnancy. The physiologic changes that occur during the reversal of the processes of pregnancy, though distinctive, are normal. To provide care during the recovery period that is beneficial to the mother, her infant, and her family, the nurse must synthesize knowledge of maternal anatomy and physiology of the recovery period, the newborn's physical and behavioral characteristics, infant care activities, and family response to the birth of the infant. This chapter focuses on anatomic and physiologic changes that occur in the mother during the postpartum period.

REPRODUCTIVE SYSTEM AND ASSOCIATED STRUCTURES

Uterus

Involution Process. The return of the uterus to a nonpregnant state following birth is known as involution. This process begins immediately after expulsion of the placenta by contraction of the uterine smooth muscle.

At the end of the third stage of labor the uterus is in the midline, approximately 2 cm below the level of the umbilicus, with the fundus resting on the sacral promontory. At this time, the uterus is approximately the size it was at 16 weeks of gestation (about the size of a grapefruit), and weighs approximately 1000 g.

Within 12 hours the fundus may be approximately 1 cm above the umbilicus (see Fig. 20-1). Involution progresses rapidly during the next few days. The fundus descends 1 to 2 cm every 24 hours. By the sixth postpartum day the fundus is normally located halfway between the umbilicus and the symphysis pubis. A week after birth the uterus once again lies in the true pelvis. The uterus should not be palpable abdominally after the ninth postpartum day.

The uterus, which at full term weighs approximately 11 times its prepregnancy weight, involutes to approximately 500 g by 1 week after birth and to 350 g by 2 weeks after birth. At 6 weeks it weighs 50 to 60 g (Fig. 20-1).

Increased estrogen and progesterone levels are responsible for stimulating the massive growth of the uterus during pregnancy. Prenatal uterine growth results from both hyperplasia, an increase in the number of muscle cells; and from hypertrophy, an enlargement of the existing cells. Postpartally, the decrease in these hormones causes autolysis, the self-destruction of excess hypertrophied tissue. The additional cells laid down during pregnancy remain and account for the slight increase in uterine size after each pregnancy.

Subinvolution is the failure of the uterus to return to a nonpregnant state. The most common causes of subinvolution are retained placental fragments and infection.

Contractions. Postpartum hemostasis is achieved primarily by compression of intramyometrial blood vessels as the uterine muscle contracts, rather than by platelet aggregation and clot formation. The hormone oxytocin, released from the pituitary gland, strengthens and coordinates these uterine contractions, which compress blood vessels and promote hemostasis. During the first 1 to 2 postpartum hours, uterine contractions may decrease in intensity and become uncoordinated. Because it is vital that the uterus remain firm and well contracted, exogenous oxytocin (Pitocin) is usually administered

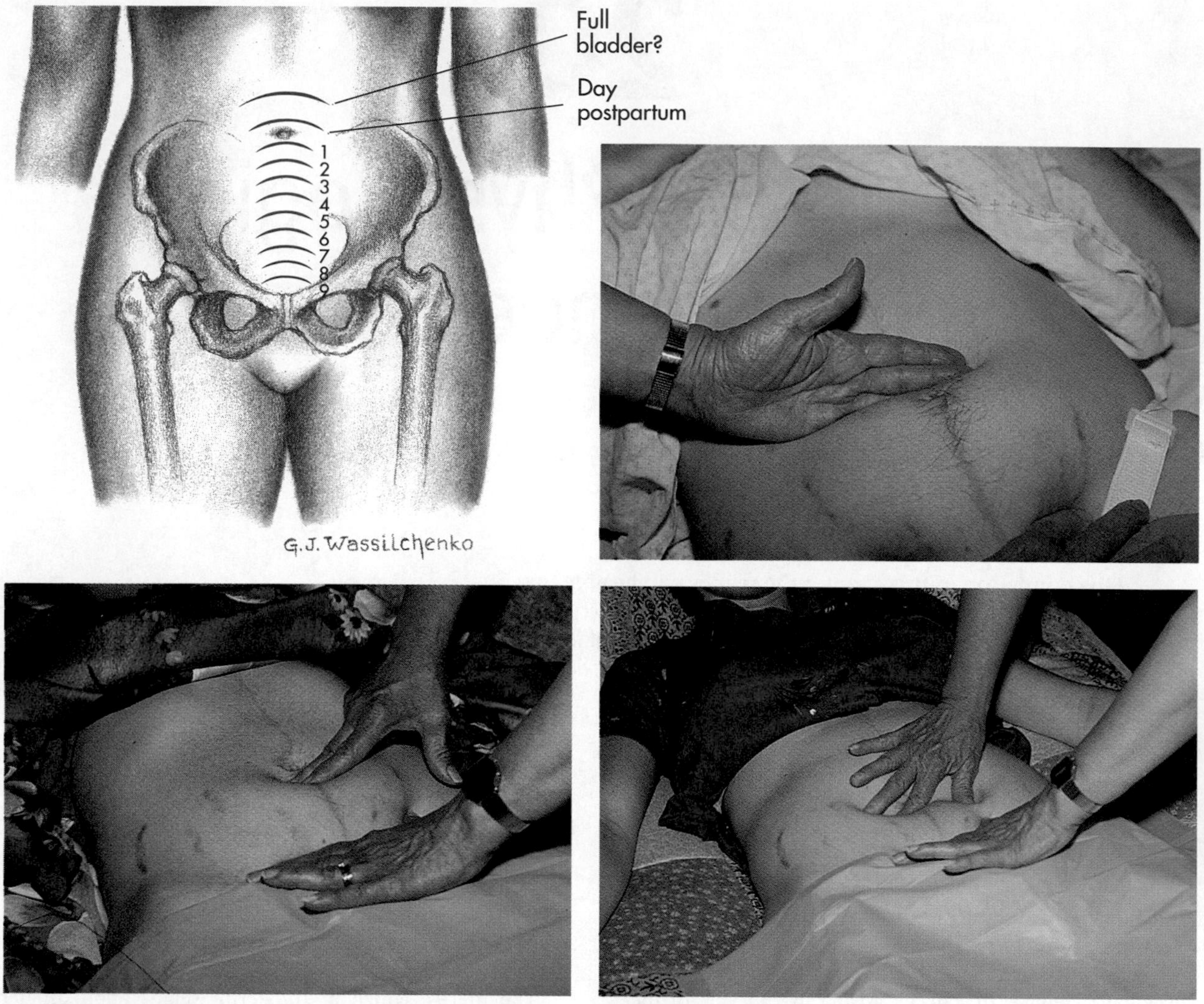

FIG. 20-1 • Assessment of involution of uterus after childbirth. **A,** Normal progress, days 1 through 9. **B,** Size and position of uterus 2 hours after childbirth. **C,** Two days after childbirth. **D,** Four days after childbirth. (B, C, and D courtesy Marjorie Pyle, RNC, Lifecircle, Costa Mesa, CA.)

intravenously or intramuscularly immediately after expulsion of the placenta. Mothers who plan to breastfeed may also be encouraged to put the baby to breast immediately after birth because suckling stimulates oxytocin release.

Afterpains. In first-time mothers, uterine tone is good, the fundus generally remains firm, and the mother does not perceive uterine cramping. Periodic relaxation and vigorous contractions are more common in subsequent pregnancies and may cause uncomfortable cramping called afterpains, which persist throughout the early puerperium. Afterpains are more noticeable after births in which the uterus was overdistended (e.g., large baby, multifetal gestation, or polyhydramnios). Breastfeeding and exogenous oxytocic medication usually intensify these afterpains because both stimulate uterine contractions.

Placental Site. Immediately after the placenta and membranes are expelled, vascular constriction and thromboses reduce the placental site to an irregular nodular and elevated area. Upward growth of the endometrium causes sloughing of necrotic tissue and prevents the scar formation that is characteristic of normal wound healing. This unique healing process enables the endometrium to resume its usual cycle of changes and to permit implantation and placentation in future pregnancies. Endometrial regeneration is completed by the end of the third postpartum week, except at the placental site. Regeneration at the placental site usually is not complete until 6 weeks after birth.

Lochia. Postbirth uterine discharge, commonly called lochia, initially is bright red and changes later to a pinkish red or reddish brown. It may contain small clots. For the first 2 hours after birth the amount of uterine discharge should be about that of a heavy menstrual period. After that time, the lochia flow should steadily decrease.

Lochia rubra consists mainly of blood and decidual and trophoblastic debris. The flow pales, becoming pink or brown (lochia serosa) after 3 to 4 days. Lochia serosa consists of old blood, serum, leukocytes, and tissue debris. About 10 days after childbirth the drainage becomes yellow to white (lochia alba).

Lochia alba consists of leukocytes, decidua, epithelial cells, mucus, serum, and bacteria. Lochia alba may continue for 2 to 6 weeks after the birth.

If the woman receives an oxytocic medication, the flow of lochia is usually scant until the effects of the medication wear off. The amount of lochia is usually less after cesarean births. Flow of lochia usually increases with ambulation and breastfeeding. Lochia tends to pool in the vagina when the woman is lying in bed; the woman then may experience a gush of blood when she stands. This gush should not be confused with hemorrhage.

Persistence of lochia rubra early in the postpartum period suggests continued bleeding as a result of retained fragments of the placenta or membranes. Recurrence of bleeding about 10 days after birth is from the healing placental site. However, any bleeding occurring 3 to 4 weeks after birth may be caused by infection or subinvolution. Continued flow of lochia serosa or lochia alba may indicate endometritis, particularly if fever, pain, or abdominal tenderness is associated with the discharge. Lochia should smell like normal menstrual flow; an offensive odor usually indicates infection.

Not all postpartal vaginal bleeding is lochia; vaginal bleeding after birth may be due to unrepaired vaginal or cervical lacerations. Table 20-1 distinguishes between lochial and nonlochial bleeding.

TABLE 20-1
Lochial and Nonlochial Bleeding

Lochial Bleeding	Nonlochial Bleeding
Lochia usually trickles from the vaginal opening. The steady flow is greater as the uterus contracts.	If the bloody discharge spurts from the vagina, there may be cervical or vaginal tears in addition to the normal lochia.
A gush of lochia may result as the uterus is massaged. If it is dark in color, it has been pooled in the relaxed vagina, and the amount soon lessens to a trickle of bright red lochia (in the early puerperium).	If the amount of bleeding continues to be excessive and bright red, a tear may be the source.

Cervix

The cervix is soft immediately after birth. By 18 hours postpartum it has shortened, become firm, and regained its form. The cervix up to the lower uterine segment remains edematous, thin, and fragile for several days after birth. The ectocervix (portion of the cervix that protrudes into the vagina) appears bruised and has some small lacerations—optimal conditions for the development of infection. The cervical os, which dilated to 10 cm during labor, closes gradually. Two fingers may still be introduced into the cervical os for the first 4 to 6 days postpartum; however, only the smallest curette can be introduced by the end of 2 weeks. The external cervical os never regains its prepregnant appearance; it is no longer shaped like a circle but appears as a jagged slit that is often described as a "fish mouth." Lactation delays the production of cervical and other estrogen-influenced mucus and mucosal characteristics.

Vagina and Perineum

Postpartum estrogen deprivation is responsible for the thinness of the vaginal mucosa and the absence of rugae. The greatly distended, smooth-walled vagina gradually returns to its prepregnancy size by 6 to 8 weeks after childbirth. Rugae reappear by about the fourth week, but they are never as prominent as they are in the nulliparous woman. Most rugae are permanently flattened. The mucosa remains atrophic in the lactating woman, at least until menstruation resumes. Thickening of the vaginal mucosa occurs with the return of ovarian function. Estrogen deficiency is also responsible for a decreased amount of vaginal lubrication. Localized dryness and coital discomfort (dyspareunia) may persist until ovarian function returns and menstruation resumes. The use of a water-soluble lubricant during sexual intercourse is usually recommended.

Initially the introitus is erythematous and edematous, especially in the area of the episiotomy or laceration repair. Later it is barely distinguishable from that of a nulliparous woman if lacerations and an episiotomy have been carefully repaired, hematomas are prevented or treated early, and the woman observes good hygiene during the first 2 weeks after birth.

Most episiotomies are visible only if the woman is lying on her side with her upper buttock raised or if she is placed in the lithotomy position. A good light source is essential for visualization of some episiotomies. Healing of an episiotomy is the same as any surgical incision. Signs of infection (i.e., pain, redness, warmth, swelling, or discharge) or loss of approximation (i.e., separation of the edges of the incision) may occur. Healing should occur within 2 to 3 weeks.

Hemorrhoids (anal varicosities) are commonly seen. Internal hemorrhoids may evert while the woman is pushing during birth. Women often experience associated symptoms such as itching, discomfort, and bright red bleeding upon defecation. Hemorrhoids usually decrease in size within 6 weeks of childbirth.

Pelvic Muscular Support. The supporting structure of the uterus and vagina may be injured during childbirth and may contribute to later gynecologic problems. Supportive tissues of the pelvic floor that are torn or stretched during childbirth may require up to 6 months to regain tone. Kegel exercises, which help to strengthen perineal muscles and encourage healing, are recommended after childbirth. Pelvic relaxation refers to the lengthening and weakening of the fascial supports of pelvic structures. These structures include the uterus, upper posterior vaginal wall, urethra, bladder, and rectum. Although relaxation can occur in any woman, it is commonly a direct but delayed complication of childbirth.

ENDOCRINE SYSTEM

Placental Hormones

Significant hormonal changes occur during the postpartal period. Expulsion of the placenta results in dramatic decreases of the hormones produced by that organ. Decreases in human chorionic somatomammotropin (hCS), estrogens, cortisol, and the placental enzyme insulinase reverse the diabetogenic effects of pregnancy, resulting in significantly lower blood sugar levels in the immediate puerperium. Mothers with type 1 diabetes will likely require much less insulin for several days after birth. Because these normal hormonal changes make the puerperium a transitional period for carbohydrate metabolism, it is more difficult to interpret glucose tolerance tests.

Estrogen and progesterone levels drop markedly after expulsion of the placenta, and reach their lowest levels 1 week postpartum. Decreased estrogen levels are associated with breast engorgement and with the diuresis of excess extracellular fluid accumulated during pregnancy. In nonlactating women, estrogen levels begin to rise by 2 weeks after birth and by postpartum day 17 are higher than in women who breastfeed (Bowes, 1996).

Pituitary Hormones and Ovarian Function

Lactating and nonlactating women differ considerably in the timing of their first ovulation and when menstruation resumes. The persistence of elevated serum prolactin levels in breastfeeding women appears to be responsible for suppressing ovulation. Because levels of follicle-stimulating hormone (FSH) have been shown to be identical in lactating and nonlactating women, it is thought that the ovulation is suppressed in lactating women because the ovary does not respond to FSH stimulation when increased prolactin levels are present (Bowes, 1996).

Prolactin levels in blood rise progressively throughout pregnancy. In women who breastfeed, prolactin levels remain elevated into the sixth week after birth (Rebar, 1999). Serum prolactin levels are influenced by the frequency of breastfeeding, the duration of each feeding, and the degree to which supplementary feedings are used. Individual differences in the strength of an infant's sucking stimulus probably also affect prolactin levels. In nonlactating women, prolactin levels decline after birth and reach the prepregnant range in 4 to 6 weeks (Rebar, 1999).

Ovulation occurs as early as 27 days after birth in nonlactating women, with a mean time of 70 to 75 days. About 70% of nonbreastfeeding women resume menstruating by 3 months after birth. In women who breastfeed, the mean length of time to initial ovulation is 17 weeks. In lactating women, both resumption of ovulation and return of menses are determined in large part by breastfeeding patterns (Resnik, 1999). Many women ovulate before their first postpartum menstrual period occurs; thus there is need to discuss contraceptive options early in the puerperium (Rebar, 1999).

The first menstrual flow after childbirth is usually heavier than normal. Within 3 or 4 cycles the amount of menstrual flow returns to the woman's prepregnancy volume.

ABDOMEN

When the woman stands up during the first days after birth, her abdomen protrudes and gives her a still-pregnant appearance. During the first 2 weeks after birth the abdominal wall is relaxed. It takes about 6 weeks for the abdominal wall to return almost to its nonpregnancy state. The skin regains most of its previous elasticity, but some striae may persist. The return of muscle tone depends on previous tone, proper exercise, and the amount of adipose tissue. Occasionally, with or without overdistention because of a large fetus or multiple fetuses, the abdominal wall muscles separate, a condition termed diastasis recti abdominis (see Fig. 10-11). Persistence of this defect may be disturbing to the woman, but surgical correction rarely is necessary. With time, the defect becomes less apparent.

URINARY SYSTEM

The hormonal changes of pregnancy (i.e., high steroid levels) contribute to an increase in renal function; diminishing steroid levels after childbirth may partly explain the reduced renal function that occurs during the puerperium. Kidney function returns to normal within 1 month after birth. From 2 to 8 weeks are required for the pregnancy-induced hypotonia and dilation of the ureters and renal pelves to return to the nonpregnant state (Resnik, 1999). In a small percentage of women, dilation of the urinary tract may persist for 3 months, increasing the chances of developing a urinary tract infection.

Urine Components

The renal glycosuria induced by pregnancy disappears, but lactosuria may occur in lactating women. The blood urea nitrogen increases during the puerperium as autolysis of the involuting uterus occurs. This breakdown of excess protein in the uterine muscle cells also results in a mild (+1) proteinuria for 1 to 2 days after childbirth in approximately 50% of women (Simpson and Creehan, 1996). Ketonuria may occur in women with an uncomplicated birth or after a prolonged labor with dehydration.

Postpartal Diuresis

Within 12 hours of birth, women begin to lose excess tissue fluid accumulated during pregnancy. Profuse diaphoresis often occurs, especially at night, for the first 2 or 3 days after childbirth. Postpartal diuresis, caused by decreased estrogen levels, removal of increased venous pressure in the lower extremities, and loss of the remaining pregnancy-induced increase in blood volume, also aids the body to rid itself of excess fluid. Fluid loss through perspiration and increased urinary output accounts for a weight loss of approximately 2.25 kg during the puerperium.

Urethra and Bladder

Birth-induced trauma, increased bladder capacity following childbirth, and the effects of conduction anesthesia combine to cause a decreased urge to void. In addition, pelvic soreness caused by the forces of labor, vaginal lacerations, or the episiotomy reduces or alters the voiding reflex. Decreased voiding combined with postpartal diuresis may result in bladder distention. Immediately after birth, excessive bleeding can occur if the bladder becomes distended because it pushes the uterus up and to the side and prevents the uterus from firmly contracting. Later in the puerperium, overdistention can make the bladder more susceptible to infection and impede the resumption of normal voiding (Resnik, 1999). With adequate emptying of the bladder, bladder tone is usually restored by 5 to 7 days after childbirth.

GASTROINTESTINAL SYSTEM

Appetite

The mother usually is hungry shortly after the birth and can tolerate a light diet. Most new mothers are very hungry after full recovery from analgesia, anesthesia, and fatigue. Requests for double portions of food and frequent snacks are not uncommon.

Bowel Evacuation

A spontaneous bowel evacuation may not occur for 2 to 3 days after childbirth. This delay can be explained by decreased muscle tone in the intestines during labor and the immediate puerperium, prelabor diarrhea, lack of food, or dehydration. The mother often anticipates discomfort during the bowel movement because of perineal tenderness as a result of episiotomy, lacerations, or hemorrhoids and resists the urge to defecate. Regular bowel habits should be reestablished when bowel tone returns.

Obstetric trauma (e.g., direct injury to the sphincter muscle or damage to the innervation of the pelvic floor) is perhaps the leading cause of anal incontinence in otherwise healthy women (Toglia, 1996). Women should be taught during pregnancy about episiotomy and its possible sequelae. Pelvic floor (Kegel) exercises should be encouraged.

BREASTS

Promptly after birth, there is a decrease in the concentrations of hormones that stimulated breast development during pregnancy (i.e., estrogen, progesterone, human chorionic gonadotropin, prolactin, cortisol, and insulin). The time it takes for these hormones to return to prepregnancy levels is determined in part by whether the mother breastfeeds her infant.

Breastfeeding Mothers

As lactation is established, a mass (lump) may be felt in the breast. Unlike the lumps associated with fibrocystic breast disease or cancer (which may be consistently palpated in the same location), a filled milk sac shifts position from day to day. Before lactation begins, the breasts feel soft and a yellowish fluid, colostrum, can be expressed from the nipples. After lactation begins, the breasts feel warm and firm. Tenderness may persist for about 48 hours after the start of lactation. Bluish-white milk with a skim-milk appearance (true milk) can be expressed from the nipples. The nipples are examined for erectility and signs of irritation such as cracks, blisters, or reddening.

Nonbreastfeeding Mothers

The breasts generally feel nodular in contrast to the granular feel of breasts in nonpregnant women. The nodularity is bilateral and diffuse. Prolactin levels drop rapidly. Colostrum is present for the first few days after childbirth. Palpation of the breast on the second or third day, as milk production begins, may reveal tissue tenderness in some women. On the third or fourth postpartum day, engorgement may occur. The breasts are distended (swollen), firm, tender, and warm to the touch (because of vasocongestion). Breast distention is caused primarily by the temporary congestion of veins and lymphatics rather than by an accumulation of milk. Milk is present but should not be expressed. Axillary breast tissue (the tail of Spence) and any accessory breast or nipple tissue along the milk line may be involved. Engorgement resolves spontaneously, and discomfort decreases usually within 24 to 36 hours. A breast binder or tight bra, ice packs, or mild analgesics may be used to relieve discomfort. Nipple stimulation is avoided. If suckling is never begun (or is discontinued), lactation ceases within a few days to a week.

CARDIOVASCULAR SYSTEM

Blood Volume

Changes in blood volume after birth depend on several factors such as blood loss during childbirth and the amount of extravascular water (physiologic edema) mobilized and excreted. Blood loss results in an immediate but limited decrease in total blood volume. Thereafter, most of the blood volume increase during pregnancy (1000 to 1500 ml) is eliminated within the first 2 weeks after birth, with return to nonpregnancy values by 6 months postpartum (Simpson and Creehan, 1996).

Pregnancy-induced hypervolemia (an increase in blood volume of at least 40% over prepregnancy values near term) allows most women to tolerate considerable blood loss during childbirth. Many women lose about 300 to 400 ml of blood during vaginal birth of a single fetus, and about twice this much during cesarean birth.

Readjustments in the maternal vasculature after childbirth are dramatic and rapid. The woman's response to blood loss during the early puerperium differs from that in a nonpregnant woman. Three postpartal physiologic changes protect the woman by increasing the blood volume: (1) elimination of uteroplacental circulation reduces the size of the maternal vascular bed by 10% to 15%; (2) loss of placental endocrine function removes the stimulus for vasodilation; and (3) mobilization of extravascular water stored during pregnancy occurs. Thus hypovolemic shock usually does not occur in women who experience a normal blood loss.

Cardiac Output

Pulse rate, stroke volume, and cardiac output increase throughout pregnancy. Immediately after the birth they remain elevated or rise even higher for 30 to 60 minutes as the blood that was shunted through the uteroplacental circuit suddenly returns to the maternal systemic venous circulation. Data regarding the exact time cardiac hemodynamic levels return to normal are not available, but cardiac output values remain elevated for at least 48 hours after birth, decrease rapidly in the first 2 weeks postpartum, and return to prepregnancy level by 24 weeks postpartum. Stroke vol-

> *Critical Thinking*
>
> **MATERNAL POSTPARTUM BLOOD LOSS**
>
> **Review the records of four women on the postpartum unit, two of whom had vaginal births and two who had cesarean births. Compare the estimated blood loss and hemoglobin and hematocrit values between women who gave birth vaginally and by cesarean and with stated postpartum norms. Examine the nurses' notes and the intake and output records; is there evidence of postpartum diaphoresis and diuresis? What conclusions can you draw based on your findings? What nursing interventions were required to establish normal urinary output?**

ume, cardiac output, end-diastolic volume, and systemic vascular resistance values have been shown to remain greatly elevated for as long as 12 weeks postpartum (Resnik, 1999).

Vital Signs

Few alterations in vital signs are seen under normal circumstances. There may be a small, transient rise in both systolic and diastolic blood pressure that lasts approximately 4 days after the birth (Table 20-2). Respiratory function returns to nonpregnant levels by 6 to 8 weeks after birth. After the uterus is emptied, the diaphragm descends, the normal cardiac axis is restored, and the point of maximal impulse (PMI) and the electrocardiogram (ECG) are normalized.

Blood Components

Hematocrit and Hemoglobin. During the first 72 hours after childbirth, there is a greater loss of plasma volume than in the number of blood cells. This results in a rise in hematocrit and hemoglobin levels by the seventh day after birth. There is no increased red blood cell (RBC) destruction during the puerperium, but any excess will disappear gradually in accordance with the life span of the RBC. The exact time at which RBC volume returns to prepregnancy values is not known, but it is within normal limits when measured 8 weeks after childbirth (Bowes, 1996).

White Blood Cell Count. Normal leukocytosis of pregnancy averages approximately 12,000/mm^3. During the first 10 to 12 days after childbirth, values between 20,000 and 25,000/mm^3 are common. Neutrophils are the most numerous white blood cells (WBCs). Leukocytosis coupled with the normal increase in erythrocyte sedimentation rate that occurs may obscure the diagnosis of acute infections at this time.

Coagulation Factors. Clotting factors and fibrinogen are normally increased during pregnancy and remain elevated in the immediate puerperium. When combined with vessel damage and immobility, this hypercoagulable state causes an increased risk of thromboembolism (blood clots), especially after a cesarean birth. Fibrinolytic activity also increases during the first few days after childbirth (Bowes, 1996). Factors I, II, VIII, IX, and X decrease within a few days to nonpregnant levels. Fibrin split products, probably released from the placental site, can also be found in maternal blood.

Varicosities

Varicosities (varices) of the legs and around the anus (hemorrhoids) are common during pregnancy. Varices, even the less common vulvar varices, regress (empty) rapidly immediately after childbirth. Surgical repair of varicosities is not considered during pregnancy. Total or nearly total regression of varicosities is expected after childbirth.

NEUROLOGIC SYSTEM

Neurologic changes during the puerperium are those that result from a reversal of maternal adaptations to pregnancy and those resulting from trauma during labor and childbirth.

Pregnancy-induced neurologic discomforts abate after birth. Elimination of physiologic edema through the diuresis that follows childbirth relieves carpal tunnel syndrome by easing compression of the median nerve. The periodic numbness and tingling of fingers that afflict 5% of pregnant women usually disappear after the birth unless lifting and carrying the baby aggravates the condition. Headache requires careful assessment. Postpartum headaches may be caused by various conditions, including pregnancy-induced hypertension (PIH), stress, and leakage of cerebrospinal fluid into the extradural space during placement of the needle for epidural or spinal anesthesia. Depending on the cause and effectiveness of the treatment, the duration of the headaches can vary from 1 to 3 days to several weeks.

MUSCULOSKELETAL SYSTEM

Adaptations of the mother's musculoskeletal system that occur during pregnancy are reversed in the puerperium. These adaptations include the relaxation and subsequent hypermobility of the joints and the change in the mother's center of gravity in response to the enlarging uterus. The joints are completely stabilized by 6 to 8 weeks after birth. However, although all other joints return to their normal prepregnancy state, those in the parous woman's feet do not. The new mother may notice a permanent increase in her shoe size.

INTEGUMENTARY SYSTEM

Chloasma of pregnancy usually disappears at the end of pregnancy. Hyperpigmentation of the areolae and linea nigra may not regress completely after childbirth. Some women will have permanent darker pigmentation of those areas. Striae gravidarum (stretch marks) on the breasts, abdomen, and thighs may fade but usually do not disappear.

Vascular abnormalities such as spider angiomas (nevi), palmar erythema, and epulis generally regress in response to the rapid decline in estrogens after the end of pregnancy. For some woman, spider nevi persist indefinitely.

The abundance of fine hair seen during pregnancy usually disappears after giving birth; however, any coarse or bristly hair that appears during pregnancy usually remains. Fingernails return to their prepregnancy consistency and strength.

Profuse diaphoresis that occurs in the immediate postpartum period is the most noticeable change in the integumentary system.

IMMUNE SYSTEM

No significant changes in the maternal immune system occur during the postpartum period. The mother's need for a rubella vaccination or for RhoGAM for prevention of Rh isoimmunization should be determined.

Critical Thinking

POSTPARTUM PHYSIOLOGIC CHANGES

Interview two women in their early postpartum recovery phase regarding normal physiologic changes experienced during that time. What knowledge deficits did you identify? Prepare simple educational materials describing postpartum physiologic changes that are designed for women with limited reading ability or for those who do not speak English.

TABLE 20-2
Vital Signs After Childbirth

Normal Findings	Deviations from Normal Findings and Probable Causes
TEMPERATURE	
During first 24 hours may rise to 38° C as a result of dehydrating effects of labor. After 24 hours the woman should be afebrile.	A diagnosis of puerperal sepsis is suggested if a rise in maternal temperature to 38° C is noted after the first 24 hours after childbirth and recurs or persists for 2 days. Other possibilities are mastitis, endometritis, urinary tract infections, and other systemic infections.
PULSE	
Pulse, along with stroke volume and cardiac output, remains elevated for the first hour or so after childbirth. It then begins to decrease. By 8 to 10 weeks after childbirth the pulse has returned to a nonpregnant rate.	A rapid pulse rate or one that is increasing may indicate hypovolemia as a result of hemorrhage.
RESPIRATIONS	
Respirations should decrease to within the woman's normal prebirth range by 6 to 8 weeks after birth.	Hypoventilation may follow an unusually high subarachnoid (spinal) block or epidural narcotic after a cesarean birth.
BLOOD PRESSURE	
Blood pressure is altered *slightly* if at all. Orthostatic hypotension, as indicated by feelings of faintness or dizziness immediately after standing up, can develop in the first 48 hours as a result of the splanchnic engorgement that may occur after birth.	A low or decreasing blood pressure may reflect hypovolemia secondary to hemorrhage. However, it is a late sign, and other symptoms of hemorrhage usually alert the staff. An increased reading may result from excessive use of vasopressor or oxytocic medications. Because pregnancy-induced hypertension (PIH) can persist into or occur first in the postpartum period, routine evaluation of blood pressure is needed. If a woman complains of headache, hypertension must be ruled out as a cause before analgesics are administered.

Key Points

- The uterus involutes rapidly after birth and returns to the true pelvis within 1 week.
- The rapid drop in estrogen and progesterone levels after expulsion of the placenta is responsible for triggering many of the anatomic and physiologic changes in the puerperium.
- Assessment of lochia and fundal height is essential to monitor the progress of normal involution and to identify potential problems.
- Few alterations in vital signs are seen after birth under normal circumstances.
- Activation of blood clotting factors, immobility, and sepsis predispose the woman to thromboembolism.
- Marked diuresis, decreased bladder sensitivity, and overdistention of the bladder can lead to problems with urinary elimination.
- Postpartum physiologic changes allow the woman to tolerate considerable blood loss at birth.

References

Bowes W: Postpartum care. In Gabbe S, Niebyl J, Simpson J, editors: *Obstetrics: normal and problem pregnancies,* ed 2, New York, 1996, Churchill Livingstone.

Rebar R: The breast and the physiology of lactation. In Creasy R, Resnik R, editors: *Maternal-fetal medicine,* ed 4, Philadelphia, 1999, WB Saunders.

Resnik R: The puerperium. In Creasy R, Resnik R, editors: *Maternal-fetal medicine,* ed 4, Philadelphia, 1999, WB Saunders.

Simpson K, Creehan P: *AWHONN's perinatal nursing,* Philadelphia, 1996, JB Lippincott.

Toglia M: Anal incontinence: an underrecognized, undertreated problem, *The Female Patient* 21(1):17-30, 1996.

CHAPTER 21

Nursing Care During the Fourth Trimester

http://www.harcourthealth.com/MERLIN/Wong/maternal/

Learning Objectives

On completion of this chapter the reader will be able to:

- Identify the priorities of maternal care given during the fourth stage of labor.
- Identify common selection criteria for safe early postpartum discharge.
- Summarize nursing interventions to prevent infection and excessive bleeding; to promote normal bladder and bowel patterns; and to care for the breasts of women who are breast- or bottle-feeding.
- Explain the influence of cultural expectations on postpartum adjustment.
- Discuss discharge teaching and postpartum care.

The goal of nursing care in the immediate postpartum period is to assist women and their partners during their initial transition to parenting. The approach to the care of women after birth has changed from one modeled on sick care to one that is wellness oriented. Consequently, in the United States most women remain hospitalized no more than 1 or 2 days after giving birth, and some for as few as 6 hours. Because there is so much important information to be shared with these women in a very short time, it is vital that their care be thoughtfully planned and provided. Care is focused on the woman's physiologic recovery, her psychologic well-being, and her ability to care for herself and her new baby, and it includes other family members.

FOURTH STAGE OF LABOR

The first 1 to 2 hours after birth, sometimes called the fourth stage of labor, is a crucial time for mother and newborn. Both are not only recovering from the physical process of birth but are also becoming acquainted with each other and additional family members. During this time, maternal organs undergo their initial readjustment to the nonpregnant state and the functions of body systems begin to stabilize. Meanwhile, the newborn continues the transition from intrauterine to extrauterine existence.

The fourth stage of labor is an excellent time to begin breastfeeding because the infant is in an alert state and ready to nurse. Breastfeeding at this time also aids in the contraction of the uterus and the prevention of maternal hemorrhage. In most centers the mother remains in the labor and birth area during this recovery time. In an institution where labor, delivery, and recovery (LDR) rooms are used, the woman stays in the same room where she gave birth. In traditional settings, women are taken from the delivery room to a separate recovery area for observation. Arrangements for care of the newborn vary during the fourth stage of labor. In many settings, the baby remains at the mother's bedside and the labor/birth nurse cares for both of them. In other institutions the baby is taken to the nursery for several hours of observation after an initial bonding period with the parents (Fig. 21-1).

Assessment

If the recovery nurse has not previously cared for the new mother, her assessment begins with an oral report from the nurse who attended the woman during labor and birth and a review of the prenatal, labor, and birth records. Of primary importance are conditions that could predispose the mother to hemorrhage, such as precipitous labor, large baby, grand multiparity (having given birth 7 or more times), or induced labor. For healthy women, hemorrhage is probably the most dangerous potential complication during the fourth stage of labor.

During the first hour in the recovery room, physical assessments of the mother are frequent. All factors except temperature are assessed every 15 minutes for 1 hour. Temperature is assessed at the beginning and end of the recovery period. After the fourth 15-minute assessment, if all parameters have stabilized within the normal range, the process is usually repeated once in the sec-

Box 21-1

Assessment During Fourth Stage of Labor

Before beginning the assessment, wash hands thoroughly, assemble necessary equipment, and explain the procedure to the patient.

BLOOD PRESSURE

Measure blood pressure per assessment schedule.

PULSE

Assess rate and regularity.

TEMPERATURE

Determine temperature.

FUNDUS

Put on clean examination gloves.
Position woman with knees flexed and head flat.
Just below umbilicus, cup hand and press firmly into abdomen. At the same time, stabilize the uterus at the symphysis with the opposite hand.
If fundus is firm (and bladder is empty), with uterus in midline, measure its position relative to woman's umbilicus. Lay fingers flat on abdomen under umbilicus; measure how many fingerbreadths (fb) or centimeters (cm) fit between umbilicus and top of fundus. If the fundus is above the umbilicus, this is recorded as plus fb or cm; if below, as minus fb or cm.
If fundus is not firm, massage it gently to contract and expel any clots before measuring distance from umbilicus.
Place hands appropriately; massage gently only until firm.
Expel clots while keeping hands placed as in Fig. 21-2. With upper hand, firmly apply pressure downward toward vagina; observe perineum for amount and size of expelled clots.

BLADDER

Assess distention by noting location and firmness of uterine fundus and by observing and palpating bladder. Distended bladder is seen as a suprapubic rounded bulge that is dull to percussion and fluctuates like a water-filled balloon. When the bladder is distended, the uterus is usually boggy in consistency, well above the umbilicus, and to the woman's right side.
Assist woman to void spontaneously. Measure amount of urine voided.
Catheterize as necessary.
Reassess after voiding or catheterization to make sure the bladder is not palpable and the fundus is firm and in the midline.

LOCHIA

Observe lochia on perineal pads and on linen under the mother's buttocks. Determine amount and color, note size and number of clots; note odor.
Observe perineum for source of bleeding (e.g., episiotomy, lacerations).

PERINEUM

Ask or assist woman to turn on her side and flex upper leg on hip.
Lift upper buttock.
Observe perineum in good lighting.
Assess episiotomy site or laceration repair for intactness, hematoma, edema, bruising, redness, and drainage.
Assess for presence of hemorrhoids.

ond hour. Box 21-1 and Fig. 21-2 describe the physical assessment of the mother during the fourth stage of labor. Fig. 21-3 demonstrates an easy-to-use flow sheet that combines the essential immediate postpartum and anesthesia recovery assessments.

During the fourth stage of labor, intense tremors that resemble shivering from a chill are commonly seen; they are not related to infection. Several theories have been offered to explain these tremors or shivering, such as their being the result of a sudden release of pressure on pelvic nerves after birth, a response to a fetus-to-mother transfusion that occurred during placental separation, a reaction to maternal adrenaline production during labor and birth, or a reaction to epidural anesthesia. Warm blankets and reassurance that the chills or tremors are common, self-limiting, and last only a short while are useful interventions.

The nutritional status of the woman is assessed. Restriction of food and fluid intake and the loss of fluids (e.g., blood, perspiration, or emesis) during labor cause many women to express a strong desire to eat or drink soon after birth. In the absence of complications, a woman who has given birth vaginally has recovered from the effects of the anesthetic and has stable vital signs, a firm uterus, and small to moderate lochial flow may have fluids and a regular diet as desired (American Academy of Pediatrics and American College of Obstetricians and Gynecologists, 1997).

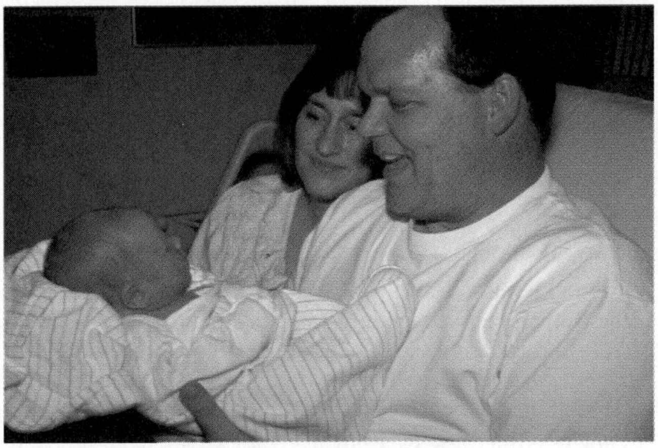

FIG. 21-1 • Mother and father get acquainted with their newborn. (Courtesy Michael S. Clement, MD, Mesa, AZ.)

Postanesthesia Recovery

The woman who has given birth by cesarean or who has received regional anesthesia for a vaginal birth requires special attention during the recovery period. Recovery from anesthesia requires that cardiopulmonary support and emergency supplies

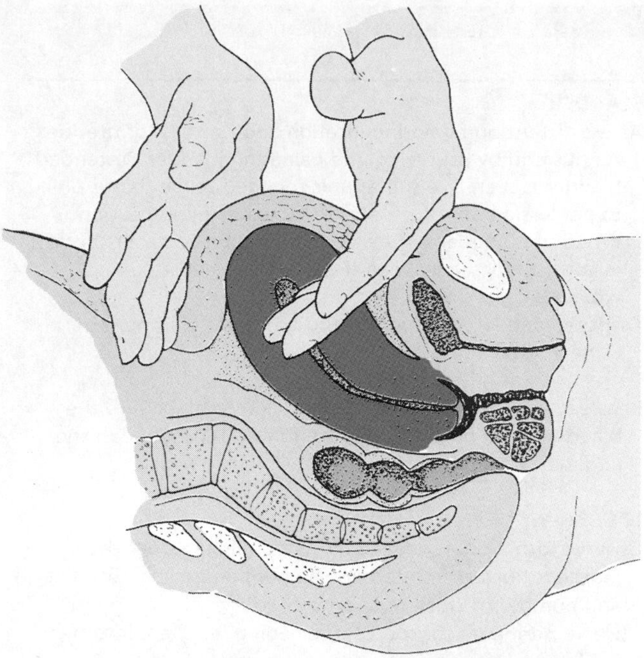

FIG. 21-2 • Palpating fundus of uterus during the fourth stage of labor. Note that upper hand is cupped over fundus; lower hand dips in above symphysis pubis and supports uterus while it is massaged gently.

(e.g., resuscitation bag and face mask) be available (Johnson & Johnson, 1996). A postanesthesia recovery (PAR) score is determined for each patient on arrival, and is updated as part of every 15-minute assessment. Components of the PAR score include activity, respirations, blood pressure, level of consciousness, and color.

NURSE ALERT • Regardless of her obstetric status, no woman should be discharged from the recovery area until she has completely recovered from the effects of anesthesia.

If the woman received general anesthesia, she should be awake and alert and oriented to time, place, and person. Her respiratory rate should be within normal limits, and her oxygen saturation levels at least 95%, as measured by a pulse oximeter. If the woman received epidural or spinal anesthesia, she should be able to raise her legs, extended at the knees, off the bed; or to flex her knees, place her feet flat on the bed, and raise her buttocks well off the bed. The numb or tingling, prickly sensation should be entirely gone from her legs. Often it takes 1½ to 2 hours for these anesthetic effects to disappear.

Transfer from the Recovery Area

After the initial recovery period of 1 to 2 hours has been completed, the woman may be transferred to a postpartum room in the same or another nursing unit. In facilities with labor, delivery, recovery, postpartum (LDRP) rooms, the nurse who provides care during the recovery period usually continues caring for the woman. Women who have received general or regional anesthesia must be cleared for transfer from the recovery area by a member of the anesthesia care team.

In preparing the transfer report the recovery nurse uses information from the records of admission, birth, and recovery. Information that must be communicated to the postpartum nurse includes identity of the health care provider; gravidity and parity; age; anesthetic used; any medications given; duration of labor and time of rupture of membranes; oxytocin induction or augmentation; type of birth and repair; blood type and Rh status; group B streptococcus (GBS) status; status of rubella immunity; syphilis and hepatitis serology test results; intravenous infusion of any fluids; physiologic status since birth; description of fundus, lochia, bladder, and perineum; sex and weight of infant; time of birth; pediatrician; chosen method of feeding; any abnormalities noted; and assessment of initial parent-infant interaction.

Most of this information is also documented for the nursing staff in the newborn nursery. In addition, specific information should be provided regarding the infant's Apgar scores, weight, voiding, stooling, and whether fed since birth. Nursing interventions that have been completed (e.g., eye prophylaxis and vitamin K injection) must also be recorded.

Women who give birth in birthing centers may go home within a few hours, after the woman's and infant's conditions are stable.

DISCHARGE—BEFORE 24 HOURS AND AFTER 48 HOURS

Early postpartum discharge, shortened hospital stays, and 1-day maternity stays are all terms for the decreasing length of hospital stays of mothers and their babies after a low risk birth. The trend of shortened hospital stays is based largely on efforts to reduce health care costs, coupled with consumer demands to have less medical intervention and more family-focused experiences (Ferguson and Englehard, 1997; Wilkerson, 1996).

Laws Relating to Discharge

Health care providers expressed concern with shortened stays since some medical problems do not show up in the first 24 hours after birth and because new mothers do not have sufficient time to learn how to care for their newborns and identify newborn health problems such as jaundice and dehydration related to breastfeeding difficulties (Havens and Hannan, 1996).

The concern for the potential increase in adverse maternal-infant outcomes from hospital early discharge practices led the American College of Obstetricians and Gynecologists, the American Academy of Pediatrics, and other professional health care organizations to promote the enactment of federal and state maternity length-of-stay bills to ensure adequate care for both the mother and the newborn. The passage of the Newborns' and Mothers' Health Protection Act of 1996 provided minimum federal standards for health plan coverage for mothers and their newborns (Ferguson and Engelhard, 1997). Under the Act, all health plans are required to allow the new mother and newborn to remain in the hospital for a minimum of 48 hours after a normal vaginal birth and for 96 hours after a cesarean birth unless the attending provider, in consultation with the mother, decides upon early discharge.

Procedure: ______
Diagnosis: ______
Physician: ______
Anesthesia: ______
Anesthetist: ______
Armbands: ______ mother ______ infant
Clothing: c̄ family c̄ patient

Maternity Recovery Room Record

Admission note:

Activity	
Able to move 4 extremities voluntarily or on command	2
Able to move 2 extremities voluntarily or on command	1
Able to move 0 extremities voluntarily or on command	0
Respiration	
Able to deep breathe and cough freely	2
Dyspnea or limited breathing	1
Apneic	0
Blood pressure	
BP ± mm Hg of preanesthetic level	2
BP ± 25-50 mm Hg of preanesthetic level	1
BP ± Greater than 50 mm Hg of preanesthetic level	0
Conscious level	
Fully aware	2
Arousable on calling	1
Not responding	0
Color	
Pink	2
Pale, dusky, blotchy, jaundiced, other	1
Cyanotic	0

Par score: ADM: DC: Homan's Sign Pos☐ Neg☐

								Bonding	Teaching
Activity								☐Appropriate	☐Fundal massage
Respiration								☐Inappropriate	☐TC & DB
Blood pressure								☐NA (explain)	☐Breastfeeding
Conscious level									☐Assistance on 1st ambulation
Color									
Total									☐

											Meds / IV / Rate	Time / Initial
Vital signs: Initial hour: q 15 min then Routine: q 4 other per protocol Tox: *q 1	Time											
	BP											
	Pulse											
	Resp / O_2Sat											
Fundus: FB-Fingerbreadth B-Boggy FM-Firm MD-Midline	Fundus											
Lochia: CL-Clots MOD-Moderate SM-Small LG-Large	Lochia											
Bladder: D-Distended F-Foley ND-Nondistended	Bladder											
Episiotomy/Incision: NL-Normal D-Dry ABNL-Abnormal I-Intact	Epis / Inc											
q 4°	Temp											
Clear CL, Wheezing W, Diminished D	Breath sounds											
q 1° / q 4°	DTR / Protein											
Admission intake Total												
Admission output Total											Intake total Shift 7A 3P 11P	Signature
Initials												
Discharge note											Output total Shift 7A 3P 11P	

Report called to:

Anesthesia D/C:
Epidural catheter: In Out NA

IV ____cc LTC @ D/C

*Toxemia (preeclampsia) LTC, left to count.

FIG. 21-3 • An example of a maternity recovery room record. (Courtesy The Regional Medical Center at Memphis [The Med], Memphis, TN.)

Criteria for Discharge

Early discharge and postpartum home care can be a safe and satisfying option for women and their families when it is comprehensive and based on individual needs (Wilkerson, 1996). Hospital stays need to be long enough to identify problems and to ensure that the woman is sufficiently recovered and prepared to care for herself and the baby at home.

It is essential that nurses consider the medical needs of the woman and her baby and provide care that is coordinated to meet those needs in order to provide timely physiologic interventions and treatment to prevent morbidity and hospital readmission. With predetermined criteria for identifying low risk in the mothers and newborns (Box 21-2), the length of hospitalization can be based on medical need for care in an acute care setting or in consideration of the ongoing care needed in the home environment (AAP/ACOG, 1997; Weekly and Neumann, 1997).

Care paths provide the nurse with an organized approach toward meeting essential maternal-newborn care and teaching goals within a limited time frame (Table 21-1). Care paths can be developed for vaginal or cesarean births. Other methods such as postpartum order sets and maternal-newborn teaching checklists (Fig. 21-4) can be used to accomplish patient care and educational outcomes.

Hospital-based maternity nurses continue to play invaluable roles as caregivers, teachers, and patient and family advocates in developing and implementing effective home care strategies. The nurse participates in the determination of whether the mother and newborn meet the criteria for early discharge.

LEGAL TIP • Early Discharge Whether or not the woman and her family have chosen early discharge, the nurse and the primary health care provider are held responsible if the woman is discharged before her condition has stabilized within normal limits. If complications occur, the medical and nursing staff could be sued for abandonment.

Care Management—Physical Needs

➤ Assessment

A complete physical assessment, including measurement of vital signs, is performed upon admission to the postpartum unit. If the woman's vital signs are within normal limits, they are usually assessed every 4 to 8 hours for the remainder of her hospitalization. Other components of the initial assessment include the mother's emotional status, energy level, degree of physical discomfort, hunger, and thirst. Intake and output assessments should always be included if an intravenous infusion or a urinary catheter is in place. If the woman gave birth by cesarean, her incisional dressing should also be assessed. To some degree, her knowledge level concerning self-care and infant care can also be determined at this time.

Ongoing Physical Assessment. The new mother should be evaluated thoroughly each shift throughout hospitalization. Physical assessments include evaluation of the breasts, uterine fundus, lochia, perineum, bladder and bowel function, vital signs, and legs. If a woman has an intravenous line in place, her fluid and hematologic status should be evaluated before it is

Box 21-2

Criteria for Early Discharge

MOTHER

- Uncomplicated pregnancy, labor, vaginal birth, and postpartum course
- No evidence of premature rupture of membranes
- Blood pressure, temperature stable and within normal limits
- Ambulating unassisted
- Voiding adequate amounts without difficulty
- Hemoglobin >10 g
- No significant vaginal bleeding; perineum intact or no more than second-degree episiotomy or laceration repair; uterus is firm
- Received instructions on postpartum self-care

INFANT

- Term infant (38 to 42 weeks) with weight appropriate for gestational age
- Normal findings on physical assessment
- Temperature respirations, and heart rate within normal limits and stable for the 12 hours preceding discharge
- At least two successful feedings completed (normal sucking and swallowing)
- Urination and stooling have occurred at least once
- No evidence of significant jaundice in the first 24 hours after the birth
- No excessive bleeding at the circumcision site for at least 2 hours
- Screening tests performed according to state regulations; tests to be repeated at follow-up visit if done before the infant is 24 hours old
- Initial hepatitis B vaccine given or scheduled for first follow-up visit
- Laboratory data reviewed: maternal syphilis and hepatitis B status; infant or cord blood type and Coombs test results if indicated

GENERAL

- No social, family, or environmental risk factors identified
- Family or support person available to assist mother and infant at home
- Follow-up scheduled within 1 week if discharged before 48 hours after the birth
- Documentation of skill of mother in feeding (breast or bottle), cord care, skin care, perineal care, infant safety (use of car seat, sleeping positions), and recognizing signs of illness and common infant problems

Source: American Academy of Pediatrics: Hospital stay for healthy term infants, *Pediatrics* 96(4):788-790, 1995; Weekly S, Neumann M: Speaking up for baby: the case for individualized neonatal discharge plans, *AWHONN Lifelines* 1(1):24-29, 1997.

Abbott Northwestern Hospital
A HealthSpan™ Organization
SELF/FAMILY LEARNING CHECKLIST

Patient Name, Social Security #, Date of Birth

I learn best by: ☐ *Group classes* ☐ *Individual instruction* ☐ *Video instruction* ☐ *Reading it myself*

Please indicate your desired learning needs by placing a check in one of the columns next to each topic.

KEY *1 = Most important to learn before I go home*
2 = I already know

(Please DATE when learning need is met.)

CARING FOR YOURSELF	1	2	DATE
Episiotomy and perineal care			
Vaginal discharge			
Hemorrhoids/Constipation			
Breast care			
Nutrition			
Activity			
Post partal exercises			
Return of menstruation			
Family planning			
Blood clots			
Post partum emotions			
Post partum warning signs			
Cesarean Birth			
Incisional care			
AFTER DISCHARGE			
When to call health care provider			
OTHER			
Working mothers			
Day care			
Sibling adjustment			
Single parent support			
Time out for parents			
Infant safety and security			
Infant As A Person Class			
New Parent Connection			

CARING FOR BABY	1	2	DATE
Diapering			
Baby bath, skin and cord care			
Circumcised/uncircumcised care			
Burping			
Bowel movements/wet diapers			
Sleeping habits			
Newborn behavior			
Jaundice			
Signs of illness			
Car seat safety			
General infant safety/poison control			
Signs/symptoms of dehydration			
Bulb syringe			
BREAST FEEDING			
Sore nipples			
Positioning			
Frequency of feedings			
Expressing/storing milk			
Engorgement			
Feeding water			
Nursing while working			
Weaning			
BOTTLE FEEDING			
Types of formula			
Preparing formula			
Frequency of feedings			

MEDICATIONS AT HOME

MEDICATIONS	STRENGTH	DOSAGE	FREQUENCY	PURPOSE/SPECIAL INSTRUCTIONS
			times per day	
			times per day	
			times per day	

RESOURCES
REFERRALS
☐ *Physician Discharge Instructions* ______
☐ *Home Care Agency* ______
☐ *Other Referrals* ______

VALUABLES: ☐ *Returned* ☐ *None* **MEDICATIONS:** ☐ *Returned* ☐ *None* ☐ *Room checked for belongings*

Patient verbalized understanding of discharge information received.

PATIENT OR SUPPORT PERSON ______ *NURSE'S SIGNATURE* ______ *DATE* ______

SELF/FAMILY LEARNING CHECKLIST

SELF/FAMILY LEARNING CHECKLIST

FIG. 21-4 • Self/family learning checklist. (Copyright Abbott Northwestern Hospital of Allina Health System, Minneapolis and St Paul, MN.)

TABLE 21-1

Care Path: 24-Hour Vaginal Birth without Complications

Date of Birth: ____________________

Hour of Birth: ____________________

The uncomplicated vaginal birth patient's admission/discharge is based on a 24-hour length of stay postbirth based on individual needs.

Time: ____________

	Recovery	**Adm. to PP Unit—8 Hour**	**9-16 Hours**	**17-24 Hours/Discharge**
Primary Physiologic Focus	Woman will have normal vital signs (VS) as documented on flowsheet	Woman will have normal VS and moderate lochia rubra	Woman will have normal VS and minimal lochia rubra	Woman will have normal VS and minimal lochia rubra
	NA MET Variance	**NA MET Variance**	**NA MET Variance**	**NA MET Variance**
	Vital signs every 15 min × 1 hour, then hourly Assess perineum/episiotomy Ice pack prn Assess lochia	Vital signs every 4 hours. Assess perineum/episiotomy Ice pack prn Assess lochia	Vital signs every shift. Assess perineum/episiotomy Ice pack prn Assess lochia	Vital signs every shift. Assess perineum/episiotomy Ice pack prn Assess lochia
	Recovery	**Adm. to PP Unit—8 Hours**	**9-16 Hours**	**17-24 Hours/Discharge**
IVs/Labwork/ Medications	Woman will have appropriate lab work done and medication given by time of transfer to mother/baby unit	Woman will begin to verbalize understanding of hepatitis status and medication requirements	Woman will have appropriate lab work done by 16 hours PP	Woman will have appropriate lab work done and appropriate meds initiated
	NA MET Variance	**NA MET Variance**	**NA MET Variance**	**NA MET Variance**
	CBC, if not done before birth Urine drug screen if ordered U/A—dipstick (Send to lab, if abnormal)	Review hepatitis B status Medication regimen initiated	CBC Review rubella status Review Hgb and Hct	Fe Tab Prenatal vitamin Rubella vaccine, if appropriate RhoGAM, if indicated Laxative
	Recovery	**Adm. to PP Unit—8 Hours**	**9-16 Hours**	**17-24 Hours/Discharge**
Nutrition/ Elimination	Parent will be up to bathroom before transfer	Woman will resume normal nutritional status and bladder function	Woman will resume normal nutritional status and bladder function	Woman will have normal bowel and bladder function
	NA MET Variance	**NA MET Variance**	**NA MET Variance**	**NA MET Variance**
	Assess bladder fullness Assist to bathroom Assess for tolerance of PO intake	Encourage ambulation Encourage PO fluids Assist to bathroom as needed Assess bladder function Encourage PO intake	Encourage ambulation Encourage PO fluids Assist to bathroom as needed Assess bladder function Encourage PO intake	Encourage ambulation Encourage PO fluids Assist to bathroom as needed. Laxative prn
	Recovery	**Adm. to PP Unit—8 Hours**	**9-16 Hours**	**17-24 Hours/Discharge**
Psychosocial	Woman/family will begin attachment behaviors with newborn	Woman/family will demonstrate appropriate attachment behaviors	Family will verbalize comfort with new infant	Family will verbalize comfort with new infant
	NA MET Variance	**NA MET Variance**	**NA MET Variance**	**NA MET Variance**
	Encourage mother/family members to hold and touch infant Provide skin-to-skin contact of mother/infant Provide mother the opportunity to breastfeed, if applicable	Offer flexible rooming-in with infant Allow for verbalization of woman's feelings Assess discharge needs and need for Social Service consult	Reinforce interventions	Reinforce interventions Completion of birth certificate Arrange for home visit

TABLE 21-1—cont'd
Care Path: 24-Hour Vaginal Birth without Complications

Date of Birth: ____________________
Hour of Birth: ____________________
The uncomplicated vaginal birth patient's admission/discharge is based on a 24-hour length of stay postbirth based on individual needs.
Time: ____________

	Recovery	Adm. to PP Unit—8 Hours	9-16 Hours	17-24 Hours/Discharge
Self-Care Activity	Woman will begin self-care activities as tolerated	Woman will be up to bathroom/shower with assistance	Woman will be up to bathroom/shower independently	Woman will be up to bathroom/shower independently
	NA MET Variance	**NA MET Variance**	**NA MET Variance**	**NA MET Variance**
	Instruct woman in pericare and pad changes	Reinforce proper pericare Instruct on use of sitz bath Encourage woman to shower	Reinforce proper pericare. Reinforce use of sitz bath	Reinforce proper pericare Reinforce use of sitz bath
	Recovery	**Adm. to PP Unit—8 Hours**	**9-16 Hours**	**17-24 Hours/Discharge**
Teaching/ Discharge Planning	Woman will begin to verbalize and/or demonstrate self-care and infant care activities	Woman will begin to verbalize and/or demonstrate infant and self-care activities	Woman/family will demonstrate appropriate infant care activities	Woman/family will demonstrate appropriate infant care activities
	NA MET Variance	**NA MET Variance**	**NA MET Variance**	**NA MET Variance**
	Date. Initials: Teaching to include: Breastfeeding latch-on and positioning, if applicable Appropriate handwashing techniques Cough and deep breathing exercises Instruct in pain relief techniques/medication	Teaching to include: Breastfeeding/formula initial feeding information Breast care Perineal care Proper nutrition Safety issues reviewed	Teaching to include: Attendance at mother/baby care class Breast care or formula information Newborn channel Lactation consult prn Appropriate handwashing techniques	Teaching to include: Reinforcement of teaching from mother/baby class Plans for self/infant follow-up. Review IHSP* Review Baby Net program Telephone number for follow-up questions Home-going meds and purposes
	1.	1.	1.	1.
	2.	2.	2.	2.
	3.	3.	3.	3.
	4.	4.	4.	4.

Variance Documentation: ____________________

*IHSP denotes a test done to determine whether follow-up is needed in the Infant Hearing Screening Program (IHSP).

removed. Signs of potential problems that may be identified during the assessment process are listed in Box 21-3.

Routine Laboratory Tests. Several laboratory tests may be performed in the immediate postpartum period. Hemoglobin and hematocrit values are often evaluated on the first postpartum day to assess blood loss during childbirth, especially after cesarean birth. In some hospitals a clean-catch or catheterized urine specimen may be obtained and sent for routine urinalysis or culture and sensitivity, especially if an indwelling urinary catheter was inserted during the intrapartum period. In addition, if the woman's rubella and Rh status are unknown, tests to determine her status and need for possible treatment should be performed at this time.

Although all women experience similar physiologic changes during the postpartum period, certain factors act to make each woman's experience unique. From a physiologic standpoint the length and difficulty of the labor, type of birth (i.e., vaginal or cesarean), presence of episiotomy or lacerations, parity, and whether the mother plans to breastfeed or bottle-feed are factors to be considered with each woman.

Box 21-3

Signs or Potential Complications

PHYSIOLOGIC PROBLEMS

Temperature
More than 38° C after the first 24 hr

Pulse
Tachycardia or marked bradycardia

Blood Pressure
Hypotension or hypertension

Energy Level
Lethargy, extreme fatigue

Uterus
Deviated from the midline, boggy consistency, remains above the umbilicus after 24 hr

Lochia
Heavy, foul odor, bright red bleeding that is not lochia

Perineum
Pronounced edema, not intact, signs of infection, marked discomfort

Legs
Homans sign positive; painful, reddened area; warmth on posterior aspect of calf

Breasts
Redness, heat, pain, cracked and fissured nipples, inverted nipples, palpable mass

Appetite
Lack of appetite

Elimination
Urine: inability to void, urgency, frequency, dysuria; bowel; constipation, diarrhea

Rest
Inability to rest or sleep

➤ Nursing Diagnoses

After analyzing the data obtained during the assessment process, the nurse establishes nursing diagnoses that will provide a guide for planning care. Examples of nursing diagnoses commonly established for the postpartum patient include the following:

- Risk for fluid volume deficit (hemorrhage) related to:
  —Uterine atony after childbirth
- Urinary retention or constipation related to:
  —Postchildbirth discomfort
  —Childbirth trauma to tissues
- Pain related to:
  —Uterine involution
  —Trauma to perineum
  —Episiotomy
  —Hemorrhoids
  —Engorged breasts
- Sleep pattern disturbance related to:
  —Discomforts of postpartum period
  —Long labor process
  —Infant care and hospital routine
- Ineffective breastfeeding related to:
  —Maternal discomfort
  —Infant positioning

➤ Expected Outcomes

The nursing plan of care includes both the postpartum woman and her infant, even if the nursery nurse retains primary responsibility for the infant. In many hospitals, couplet care (also called mother and baby care or single-room maternity care) is practiced. Nurses in these settings have been educated in both mother and infant care and function as primary nurses for both mother and infant, even if the infant is kept in the nursery. This approach is a variation of rooming-in, in which the mother and infant room together and mother and nurse share the care of the infant. The organization of the mother's care must take the newborn into consideration. The day actually revolves around the baby's feeding and care times.

Once the nursing diagnoses are formulated, the nurse plans with the woman what nursing measures are appropriate and which are to be given priority.

The nursing plan of care includes periodic assessments to detect deviations from normal physical changes, measures to relieve discomfort or pain, safety measures to prevent injury or infection, and teaching and counseling measures designed to promote the woman's feelings of competence in self-care and baby care. Family members are included in the teaching. The nurse evaluates continuously and is ready to change the plan if indicated. Almost all hospitals use standardized care plans as a base. The nurse's adaptation of the standardized plan to specific medical and nursing diagnoses results in individualized patient care.

Expected outcomes for the postpartum period are based on the nursing diagnoses identified for the individual patient. Examples of common expected outcomes for physiologic needs are that the woman will:

- Demonstrate normal involution and lochial characteristics
- Remain comfortable and injury free

- Demonstrate normal bladder and bowel patterns
- Demonstrate knowledge of breast care, whether breastfeeding or bottle-feeding
- Integrate the newborn into the family

➤ Plan of Care and Implementation

Nurses assume many roles while implementing the nursing plan of care. They provide direct physical care, teach mother and baby care, and provide anticipatory guidance and counseling. Perhaps most important of all, they nurture the woman by providing encouragement and support as the woman begins to assume the many tasks of motherhood. Nurses who take the time to "mother the mother" do much to increase feelings of self-confidence in new mothers.

The first step in providing individualized care is to confirm the woman's identity by checking her wristband. At the same time the infant's identification number is matched with the corresponding band on the mother's wrist, and, in some instances, the father's wrist. The nurse determines how the mother wishes to be addressed and then notes her preference in her record and in her nursing care plan.

The woman and her family are oriented to their surroundings. Familiarity with the unit, routines, resources, and personnel reduces one potential source of anxiety—the unknown. The mother is reassured through knowing whom and how she can call for assistance and what she can expect in the way of supplies and services. If the woman's usual daily routine before admission differs from the facility's routine, the nurse works with the woman to develop a mutually acceptable routine.

Infant abduction from hospitals in the United States has increased over the past few years. The mother should be taught to check the identity of any person who comes to remove the baby from her room. Hospital personnel usually wear picture identification badges. On some units, all staff members wear matching scrubs or special badges. Other units use closed circuit television, computer monitoring systems, or fingerprint identification pads. As a rule, the baby is never carried in a staff member's arms between the mother's room and the nursery but is always wheeled in a bassinet, which also contains baby care supplies. Patients and nurses must work together to ensure the safety of newborns in the hospital environment (Nursing Care Plan).

Nursing Care Plan THE WOMAN WHO HAS HAD A SPONTANEOUS VAGINAL BIRTH

NURSING DIAGNOSIS Risk for fluid volume deficit related to uterine atony

EXPECTED OUTCOME Woman's fundus will remain firm and lochia rubra moderate.

Nursing Interventions/*Rationales*

Review woman's history for risk factors, such as uterine overdistention, *to identify and assess women who may be more at risk for postpartum hemorrhage.*
Assess fundal character and location frequently as well as response to gentle massage *to promote contraction of the uterus.*
Express clots. Demonstrate to woman how to assess and massage her own fundus *to promote self-care.*
Evaluate bladder character and promote voiding if full *to avoid uterine relaxation and displacement of uterine fundus.*
Assess amount and color of lochia *to indicate amount of blood loss.*
Monitor vital signs *to determine extent of fluid loss.*
Administer medications to enhance uterine contractility as prescribed, such as Pitocin and Methergine, *to prevent hemorrhage.*
Initiate or increase IV therapy *to replace fluid loss..*

NURSING DIAGNOSIS Pain related to perineal trauma and hormonal influences as evidenced by patient report

EXPECTED OUTCOME Woman will report lessening of discomfort and identify methods effective in decreasing discomfort.

Nursing Interventions/*Rationales*

Assess character, location, and pain scale as reported by woman *to identify appropriate interventions.*
Inspect perineum for redness, edema, ecchymoses, discharge, and approximation (REEDA scale) *to identify any complications.*
Apply ice pack to perineum during the first 12 to 24 hours postbirth *to decrease edema and promote comfort by local anesthesia.*
Administer analgesics as prescribed *to decrease perception of painful impulses.*
Teach women to contract gluteal muscles when sitting *to avoid direct pressure on perineum.*

NURSING DIAGNOSIS Risk for altered urinary elimination related to perineal trauma and effects of anesthesia

EXPECTED OUTCOME Woman will void within 6 to 8 hours postbirth and empty bladder completely.

Nursing Intervention/*Rationales*

Assess position and character of uterine fundus and bladder *to ascertain if any further interventions are indicated because of displacement of the fundus or distention of the bladder.*
Measure intake and output *to assess any evidence of dehydration and subsequent decreased anticipated urine output.*
Encourage voiding by walking woman to bathroom, running water over perineum, running water in sink, providing privacy *to use a variety of interventions to encourage voiding.*
Encourage oral intake *to replace any fluids lost at delivery and prevent dehydration.*
Catheterize as necessary with indwelling or straight method *to ensure bladder emptying and allow for uterine involution.*

Prevention of Infection. One important means of preventing infection is maintenance of a clean environment. Bed linens should be changed as needed. Disposable pads and draw sheets may need to be changed frequently. By not walking about barefoot, women avoid contaminating the linens when they return to bed. A sitz bath or heat lamp used in common must be scrubbed after each woman's use. Personnel must be conscientious about their handwashing techniques to prevent cross infection. Standard Precautions must be practiced. Staff members with colds, coughs, or skin infections (e.g., a cold sore on the lips [herpes simplex virus type I]) must follow hospital protocol when in contact with postpartum patients. In many hospitals, staff with open herpetic lesions, strep throat, conjunctivitis, upper respiratory infections, or diarrhea are encouraged to avoid contact with mothers and infants by staying home until the condition is no longer contagious.

Proper care of the episiotomy site and any perineal lacerations prevents infection in the genitourinary area and aids the healing process. Educating the woman to wipe from front to back (urethra to anus) after voiding or defecating is a simple first step. In many hospitals a squeeze bo ttle filled with warm water or an antiseptic solution is used after each voiding to cleanse the perineal area (see Box 21-4). The woman should change her perineal pad from front to back each time she voids or defecates, and wash her hands thoroughly before and after doing so.

Prevention of Excessive Bleeding. The most common cause of excessive bleeding following birth is uterine atony, or failure of the uterine muscle to contract firmly. The two most important interventions for preventing excessive bleeding are maintaining good uterine tone and preventing bladder distention.

NURSE ALERT • If uterine atony occurs, the relaxed uterus distends with blood and clots, blood vessels in the placental site are not clamped off, and excessive bleeding results.

Excessive blood loss following childbirth may also be caused by vaginal or vulvar hematomas, unrepaired lacerations of the vagina or cervix, and retained placental fragments.

NURSE ALERT • A perineal pad saturated in 15 minutes or less, or pooling of blood under the buttocks, are indications of excessive blood loss, requiring immediate assessment, intervention, and notification of the physician or nurse-midwife.

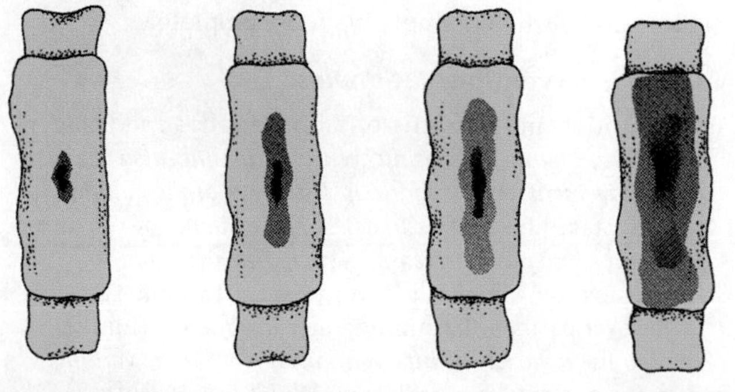

FIG. 21-5 • Blood loss after birth is assessed by the extent of perineal pad saturation as *(from left to right)* scant (<2.5 cm); light (<10 cm); moderate (>10 cm); or heavy (one pad saturated within 2 hours).

Accurate visual estimation of blood loss is an important nursing responsibility. Blood loss is usually described subjectively as scant, light, moderate, or heavy (profuse). Fig. 21-5 shows examples of perineal pad saturation corresponding to each of these descriptions.

It is difficult to judge the amount of lochial flow based only on observation of perineal pads. Postpartal blood loss may be estimated by observing the amount of staining on a perineal pad (see Fig. 21-5). More objective estimates of blood loss include weighing blood clots and item saturated with blood (1 ml equals 1 g); using devices that catch and measure blood flowing from the vagina; and establishing the milliliters it takes to saturate perineal pads being used (Johnson & Johnson, 1996; Luegenbiehl, 1997), however, these methods are not common in practice.

Any estimation of lochial flow is inaccurate and incomplete without consideration of the time factor. The woman who saturates a peripad in 1 hour or less is bleeding much more than the woman who saturates one peripad in 8 hours.

Luegenbiehl (1997) found that nurses in general tend to overestimate, rather than underestimate, blood loss. Different brands of peripads vary in their saturation volume and soaking appearance. For example, blood placed on some brands tends to soak down into the pad, whereas on other brands it tends to spread outward. Nurses should determine saturation volume and soaking appearance for the peripad brands used in their institution in order to improve accuracy of blood loss estimation.

Blood pressure is not a reliable indicator of impending shock from early hemorrhage. More sensitive means of identifying shock are provided by respirations, pulse, skin condition, urinary output, and level of consciousness. The frequent physical assessments performed during the fourth stage of labor are designed to provide prompt identification of excessive bleeding (Emergency box).

Maintenance of Uterine Tone. A major intervention to restore good tone is stimulation by gently massaging the uterine fundus until firm (see Fig. 21-2). Fundal massage may cause a temporary increase in the amount of vaginal bleeding seen as pooled blood leaves the uterus. Clots may also be expelled. The uterus may remain boggy even after massage and expulsion of clots.

Fundal massage can be a very uncomfortable procedure. Understanding the causes and dangers of uterine atony and the purpose of fundal massage can help the woman to be more cooperative. Teaching the patient to massage her own fundus enables her to maintain some control and decreases her anxiety.

Critical Thinking

ASSESSMENT OF BLEEDING POSTPARTUM

Two hours ago, Ms. Ratzinger gave birth to a baby who weighed 3450 g. Her pregnancy was complicated with polyhydramnios. During her assessment, you note that her peripad is saturated and there is blood pooled under her buttocks. How can you determine how much blood is present? What additional assessments should you make? What are likely causes of this amount of bleeding? Is there reason for concern? What interventions can you implement immediately? Who should you notify? What interventions can you expect the primary health care provider to order? What information should you record on her medical record?

Additional interventions likely to be used are administration of intravenous fluids and oxytocic medications (i.e., drugs that stimulate contraction of the uterine smooth muscle). (See Table 23-1 for information about common oxytocic medications.)

Prevention of Bladder Distention. A full bladder causes the uterus to be displaced above the umbilicus and well to one side of midline in the abdomen. It also prevents the uterus from contracting normally. Nursing interventions focus on helping the woman to empty her bladder spontaneously as soon as possible. The first priority is to assist the woman to the bathroom or onto a bedpan if she is unable to ambulate. Having the woman listen to running water, placing her hands in warm water, or pouring water from a squeeze bottle over her perineum may stimulate voiding. Other techniques include assisting the woman into the shower or sitz bath and encouraging her to void; and placing oil of peppermint in a bedpan under the woman (the vapors may relax the urinary meatus and trigger spontaneous voiding). Administering analgesics, if ordered, may be indicated because some women may fear voiding because of anticipated pain. If these measures are unsuccessful, a sterile catheter may be inserted to drain the urine.

Promotion of Comfort, Rest, Ambulation, and Exercise

Comfort. Most women experience some degree of discomfort during the postpartum period. Common causes of discomfort include afterbirth pains, episiotomy or perineal lacerations, hemorrhoids, and breast engorgement. The woman's description of the type and severity of her pain is the best guide in choosing an appropriate intervention. To confirm the location and extent of discomfort, the nurse inspects and palpates areas of pain as appropriate for redness, swelling, discharge, and heat; and observes for body tension, guarded movements, and facial tension. Blood pressure, pulse, and respirations may be elevated in response to acute pain. Diaphoresis may accompany severe pain. A lack of objective signs does not necessarily mean there is no pain, because there may also be a cultural component to the expression of pain. Nursing interventions are intended to eliminate the pain sensation entirely or reduce it to a tolerable level that allows the woman to care for herself and her baby. Nurses may use both nonpharmacologic and pharmacologic interventions to promote comfort. Pain relief is enhanced by using more than one method or route.

Nonpharmacologic Interventions. Afterbirth pains are menstrual-like cramps experienced by many women as the uterus contracts following childbirth. Warmth, distraction, imagery, therapeutic touch, relaxation, and interaction with the infant may decrease the discomfort associated with these uterine contractions.

Simple interventions that can decrease the discomfort associated with an episiotomy or perineal lacerations include encouraging the woman to lie on her side whenever possible and to use a pillow when sitting. Other interventions include application of an ice pack; topical application (if ordered); dry heat; cleansing with a squeeze bottle; and a cleansing shower, tub bath, or sitz bath (Fig. 21-6). Many of these interventions are also effective for hemorrhoids, especially ice packs, sitz baths, and topical applications (such as witch hazel pads). Box 21-4 gives more specific information about these interventions.

The discomfort associated with engorged breasts may be lessened by applying either ice, heat, or cabbage leaves to the breasts; and wearing a well-fitted support bra. Decisions about specific interventions for engorgement are based on whether the woman chooses breastfeeding or bottle-feeding (see Chapter 26).

Emergency

HYPOVOLEMIC SHOCK

Signs and Symptoms

Persistent significant bleeding—perineal pad soaked within 15 minutes; *may not be accompanied by a change in vital signs or maternal color or behavior.*
Woman states she feels weak, light-headed, "funny," "sick to my stomach," or "sees stars."
Woman begins to act anxious or exhibits air hunger.
Woman's skin turns ashen or grayish.
Skin feels cool and clammy.
Pulse rate increases.
Blood pressure declines.

Interventions

Notify primary health care provider.
If uterus is atonic, massage gently and expel clots to cause uterus to contract; compress uterus manually, as needed, using two hands. Add oxytocic agent to IV drip, as ordered.
Give oxygen by face mask or nasal prongs at 8 to 10 L/min.
Tilt the woman to her side or elevate the right hip; elevate her legs to at least a 30-degree angle.
Provide additional or maintain existing IV infusion of lactated Ringer's solution or normal saline solution to restore circulatory volume.
Administer blood or blood products, as ordered.
Monitor vital signs.
Insert an indwelling urinary catheter to monitor perfusion of kidneys.
Administer emergency drugs, as ordered.
Prepare for possible surgery or other emergency treatments or procedures.
Chart incident, medical and nursing interventions instituted, and results of treatments.

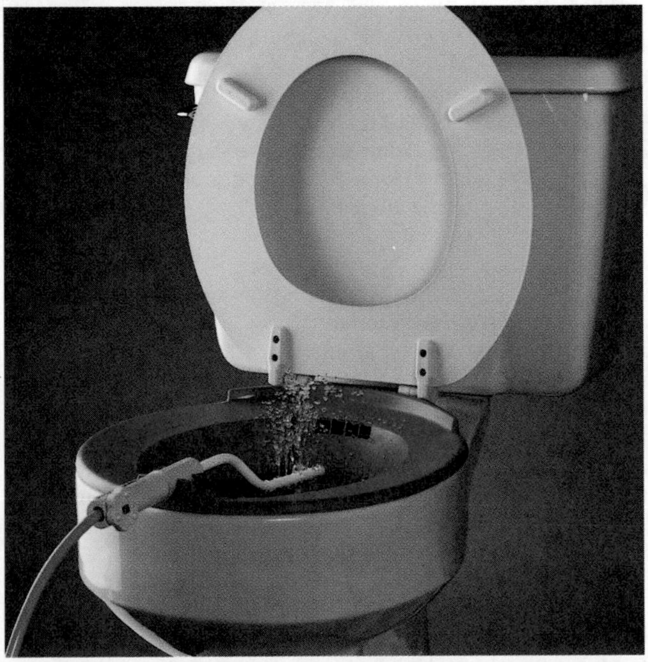

FIG. 21-6 • Hygienic sitz bath (Surgi-Gator) for perineal care. (Courtesy Andermac, Inc., Yuba City, CA.)

Box 21-4

Interventions for Episiotomy, Lacerations, and Hemorrhoids

Explain both procedure and rationale before implementation.

CLEANSING

Wash hands before and after cleansing perineum and changing pads.
Wash perineum with mild soap and warm water at least once daily.
Cleanse from symphysis pubis to anal area.
Apply peripad from front to back, protecting inner surface of pad from contamination.
Wrap soiled pad and place in covered waste container.
Change pad with each void or defecation or at least 4 times per day.
Assess amount and character of lochia with each pad change.

ICE PACK

Apply a covered ice pack to perineum from front to back

1. During first 2 hours to decrease edema formation and increase comfort
2. After the first 2 hours following the birth to provide anesthetic effect

SQUEEZE BOTTLE

Demonstrate for and assist woman; explain rationale.
Fill bottle with tap water warmed to approximately 38° C (comfortably warm on the wrist).
Instruct woman to position nozzle between her legs so that squirts of water reach perineum as she sits on toilet seat. Explain that it will take whole bottle of water to cleanse perineum.
Remind her to blot dry with toilet paper or clean wipes.
Remind her to avoid contamination from anal area.
Apply clean pad.

SITZ BATH

Built-in Type

Prepare bath by thoroughly scrubbing with cleaning agent and rinsing.
Pad with towel before filling.
Fill one-half to one-third full with water of correct temperature 38° to 40.6° C. Some women prefer cool sitz baths. Ice is added to water to lower the temperature to the level comfortable for the woman.
Encourage woman to use at least twice a day for 20 minutes.
Place call bell within easy reach.
Teach woman to enter bath by tightening gluteal muscles and keeping them tightened and then relaxing them after she is in the bath.
Place dry towels within reach.
Ensure privacy.
Check woman in 15 minutes; assess pulse as needed.

Disposable Type

Clamp tubing and fill bag with warm water.
Raise toilet seat, place bath in bowl with overflow opening directed toward back of toilet.
Place container above toilet bowl.
Attach tube into groove at front of bath.
Loosen tube clamp to regulate rate of flow: fill bath to about one-half full; continue as above for built-in sitz bath.

SURGI-GATOR

Assemble Surgi-Gator (Fig. 21-6).
Instruct woman regarding use and rationale.
Follow package directions.
Instruct woman to sit on toilet with legs apart and to put nozzle so tip is just past the perineum, adjusting placement as needed.
Remind her to return her applicator to her bedside stand.

DRY HEAT

Inspect lamp for defects.
Cover lamp with towels.
Position lamp 50 cm from perineum; use 3 times a day for 20-minute periods.
Teach regarding use of 40-W bulb at home.
Provide draping over woman.
If same lamp is being used by several women, clean it carefully between uses.

TOPICAL APPLICATIONS

Apply anesthetic cream or spray: use sparingly 3 to 4 times per day.
Offer witch hazel pads (Tucks) after voiding or defecating; woman pats perineum dry from front to back, then applies witch hazel pads.

Pharmacologic Interventions. Most health care providers routinely order a variety of analgesics to be administered as needed, including both narcotic and nonnarcotic (nonsteroidal antiinflammatory medications) choices, with their dosage and time frequency ranges. Topical applications of antiseptic or anesthetic ointments or sprays is a common pharmacologic intervention. Patient-controlled analgesia (PCA) pumps and continuous epidural analgesia infusions are technologies commonly used to provide pain relief after cesarean birth.

NURSE ALERT • The nurse should carefully monitor all women receiving opioids because respiratory depression and decreased intestinal motility are side effects.

Many women want to participate in decisions about analgesia. Severe pain, however, may interfere with active participation in choosing pain relief measures. If an analgesic is to be given, the nurse must make a clinical judgment of the type, dosage, and frequency from the medications ordered. The woman is informed of the prescribed analgesic and its common side effects; this teaching is documented.

Breastfeeding mothers often have concerns about the effects of an analgesic on the infant. Although nearly all drugs present in maternal circulation are also found in breast milk, many analgesics commonly used during the postpartum period are considered relatively safe for breastfeeding mothers. Often the timing of medications can be adjusted to minimize infant exposure. A mother may be given pain medication immediately after breastfeeding so that the interval between medication administration and the next nursing period is as long as possible. The decision to administer medications of any type to a breastfeeding mother must always be made by carefully weighing the woman's need against actual or potential risks to the infant.

If acceptable pain relief has not been obtained in 1 hour, and there has been no change in the initial assessment, the nurse may need to contact the primary care provider for additional pain relief orders or further directions. Unrelieved pain results in fatigue, anxiety, and a worsening perception of the pain. It might also indicate the presence of a previously unidentified or untreated problem.

Rest. The excitement and exhilaration experienced after the birth of the infant may make rest difficult. The new mother, who is often anxious about her ability to care for her infant or is uncomfortable, may also have difficulty sleeping. The demands of the infant, the hospital environment and routines, and the frequent presence of visitors contribute to alterations in her sleep pattern.

Fatigue. Fatigue is common in the postpartum period (Pugh et al, 1999) and involves both physiologic components associated with long labors, cesarean birth, anemia, and breastfeeding; and psychologic components related to depression and anxiety. Infant behavior can also be related to fatigue, particularly for mothers of more difficult infants.

Interventions must be planned to meet the woman's individual needs for sleep and rest. Backrubs, other comfort measures, and medication for sleep for the first few nights may be necessary. The side-lying position for breastfeeding minimizes fatigue in nursing mothers (Milligan, Flenniken and Pugh, 1996). Support and encouragement in mothering behaviors help reduce anxiety. Hospital and nursing routines may be adjusted to meet individual needs. In addition, the nurse can help the family limit visitors and provide a comfortable chair or bed for the partner.

Ambulation. Early ambulation is successful in reducing the incidence of thromboembolism and in promoting the woman's more rapid recovery of strength. Free movement is encouraged once anesthesia wears off unless an analgesic has been administered. After the initial recovery period is over, the mother is encouraged to ambulate frequently.

NURSE ALERT • Having a hospital staff or family member present the first time the woman gets out of bed after birth is wise because she may feel weak, dizzy, faint, or light-headed.

Critical Thinking

FATIGUE AND REST AFTER CHILDBIRTH

Mrs. Johnson gave birth to her third baby; she has two children at home ages 3 years and 18 months. Her husband travels frequently with his job. She is breastfeeding the baby without difficulty but is concerned about how she will care for all three of her children, stating "I remember how tired I was after my last baby." Develop a plan of care with Mrs. Johnson to promote adequate rest. What assessments would be relevant for identifying causes of fatigue? What community resources are available to her? What role does nutrition play in fatigue?

The rapid decrease in intraabdominal pressure after birth results in a dilation of blood vessels supplying the intestines (splanchnic engorgement) and causes blood to pool in the viscera. This condition contributes to the development of orthostatic hypotension when the woman who has recently given birth sits or stands up, first ambulates, or takes a warm shower or sitz bath. The nurse needs also to consider the baseline blood pressure, amount of blood loss, and type, amount, and timing of analgesic or anesthetic medications administered when assisting a woman to ambulate.

Prevention of clot formation is important. Women who must remain in bed after giving birth are at increased risk for the development of a thrombus. If a woman remains in bed longer than 8 hours (e.g., for postpartum $MgSO_4$ therapy for preeclampsia), exercise to promote circulation in the legs is indicated using the following routine:

- Alternate flexion and extension of feet
- Rotate ankle in circular motion
- Alternate flexion and extension of legs
- Press back of knee to bed surface; relax

If the woman is susceptible to thromboembolism, she is encouraged to walk about actively for true ambulation and is discouraged from sitting immobile in a chair. Women with varicosities are advised to wear support hose. If a thrombus is suspected, as evidenced by a positive Homans' sign (complaint of pain in calf muscles when the foot is dorsiflexed) or warmth, redness, or tenderness in the suspected leg, the primary health care provider should be notified immediately; meanwhile the woman should be confined to bed, with the affected limb elevated on pillows.

Exercise. Most women who have just given birth are extremely interested in regaining their nonpregnant figures. Postpartum exercise can begin soon after birth, although the woman should be encouraged to start with simple exercises and gradually progress to more strenuous ones. Fig. 21-7 illustrates a number of exercises appropriate for the new mother. Abdominal exercises are postponed until about 4 weeks after cesarean birth.

Kegel pelvic exercises to strengthen muscle tone are extremely important, particularly after vaginal birth. To perform them, the woman alternately contracts and relaxes the muscles around the vagina. Kegel exercises help women regain the muscle tone that is often lost as pelvic tissues are stretched and torn during pregnancy and birth. Women who maintain muscle strength may benefit years later by maintaining urinary continence.

It is essential that women learn to perform Kegel exercises correctly (see Patient Teaching box on p. 39). Approximately one fourth of all women who learn Kegel exercises do them incorrectly and may increase their risk of incontinence (Sampselle and Miller, 1996). This may occur when women inadvertently bear down on the pelvic floor muscles, thrusting the perineum outward. The woman's technique can be assessed during the pelvic examination at the 6-week check-up by inserting two fingers intravaginally and checking whether the pelvic floor muscles correctly contract and relax.

Promotion of Nutrition. During the hospital stay, most women display a good appetite and eat well; nutritious snacks are usually welcomed. Women may request that family members bring to the hospital favorite or culturally appropriate foods (Fig. 21-8). Cultural dietary preferences must be re-

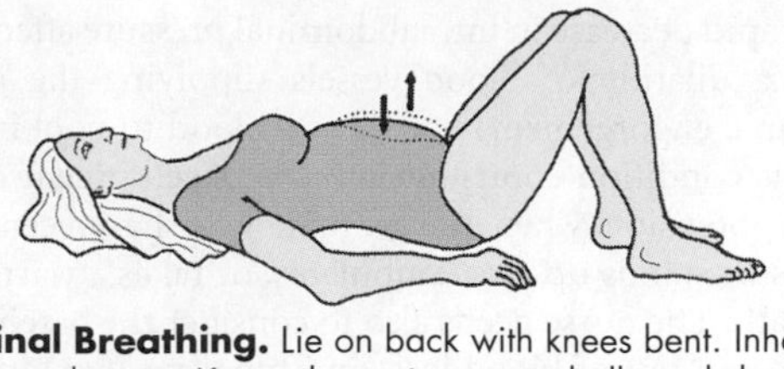

Abdominal Breathing. Lie on back with knees bent. Inhale deeply through nose. Keep ribs stationary and allow abdomen to expand upward. Exhale slowly but forcefully while contracting the abdominal muscles; hold for 3 to 5 seconds while exhaling. Relax.

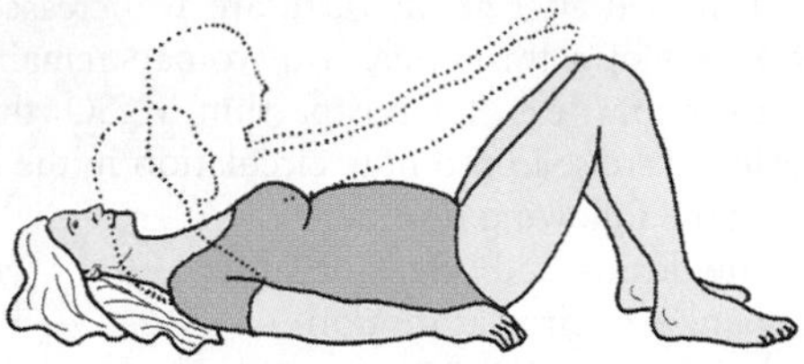

Reach for the Knees. Lie on back with knees bent. While inhaling, deeply lower chin onto chest. While exhaling, raise head and shoulders slowly and smoothly and reach for knees with arms outstretched. The body should only rise as far as the back will naturally bend while waist remains on floor or bed (about 6 to 8 inches). Slowly and smoothly lower head and shoulders back to starting position. Relax.

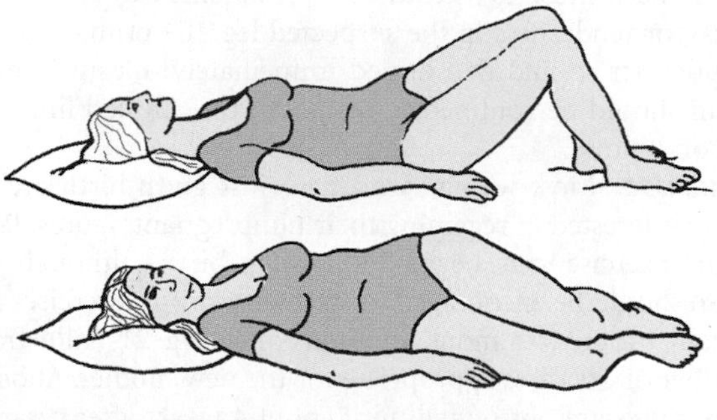

Double Knee Roll. Lie on back with knees bent. Keeping shoulders flat and feet stationary, slowly and smoothly roll knees over to the left to touch floor or bed. Maintaining a smooth motion, roll knees back over to the right until they touch floor or bed. Return to starting position and relax.

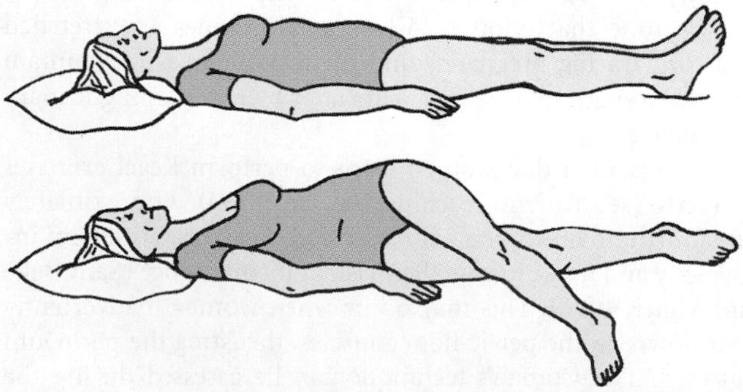

Leg Roll. Lie on back with legs straight. Keeping shoulders flat and legs straight, slowly and smoothly lift left leg and roll it over to touch the right side of floor or bed and return to starting position. Repeat, rolling right leg over to touch left side of floor or bed. Relax.

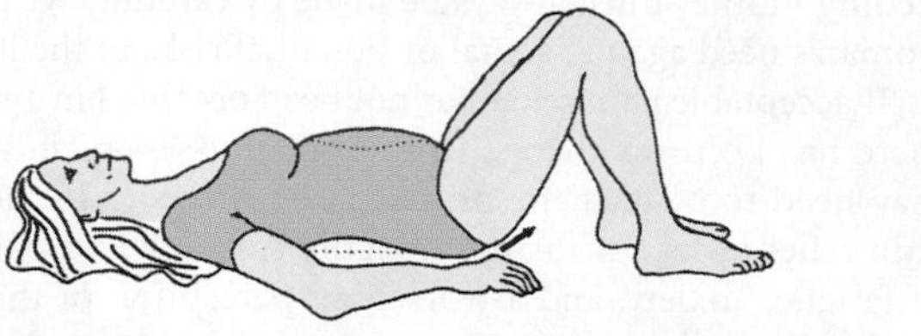

Combined Abdominal Breathing and Supine Pelvic Tilt (Pelvic Rock). Lie on back with knees bent. While inhaling deeply, roll pelvis back by flattening lower back on floor or bed. Exhale slowly but forcefully while contracting abdominal muscles and tightening buttocks. Hold for 3 to 5 seconds while exhaling. Relax.

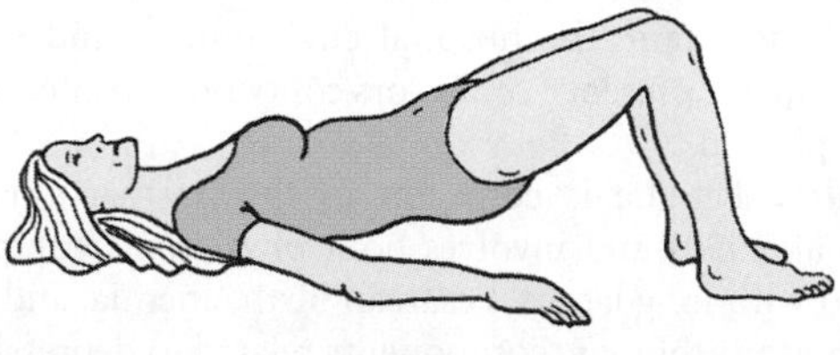

Buttocks Lift. Lie on back with arms at sides, knees bent, and feet flat. Slowly raise buttocks and arch back. Return slowly to starting position.

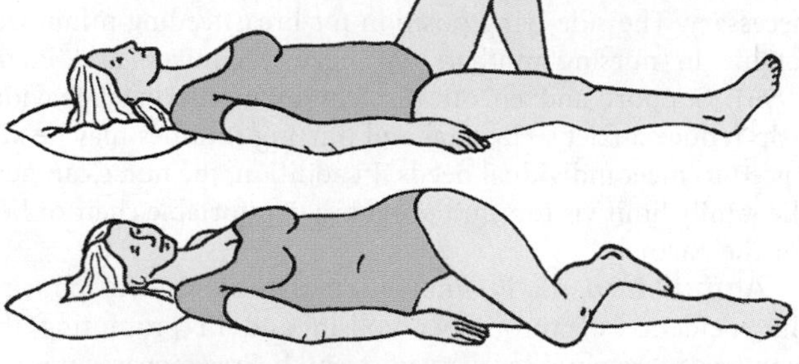

Single Knee Roll. Lie on back with right leg straight and left leg bent at the knee. Keeping shoulders flat, slowly and smoothly roll left knee over to the right to touch floor or bed and then back to starting position. Reverse position of legs. Roll right knee over to the left to touch floor or bed and return to starting position. Relax.

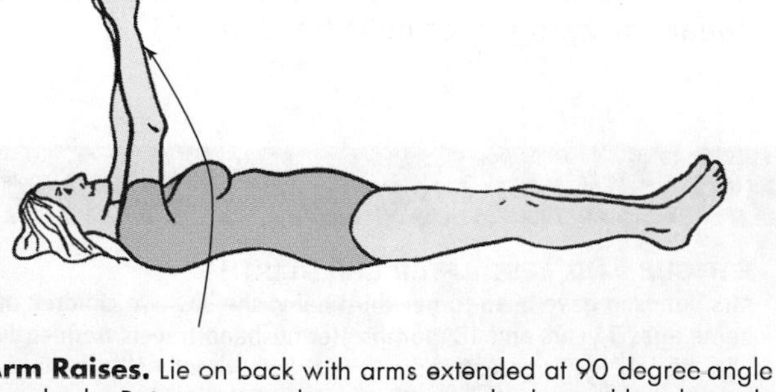

Arm Raises. Lie on back with arms extended at 90 degree angle from body. Raise arms so they are perpendicular and hands touch. Lower slowly.

FIG. 21-7 • Postpartum exercise should begin as soon as possible. The woman should start with simple exercises and gradually progress to more strenuous ones.

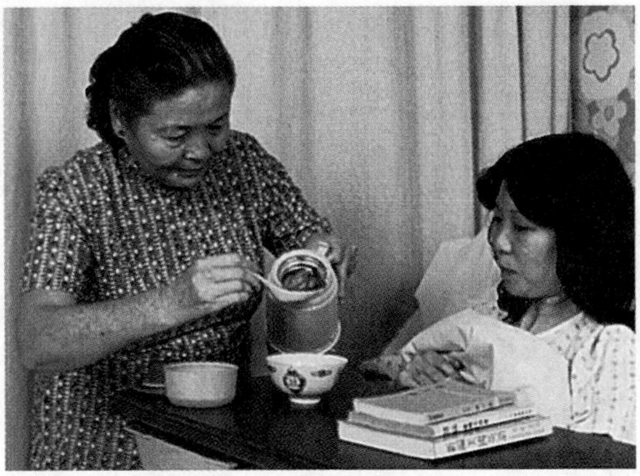

FIG. 21-8 • Special foods are considered essential for recovery in the Asian culture. (Courtesy Concept Media, Irvine, CA.)

spected. This interest in food presents an ideal opportunity for nutritional counseling on dietary needs after pregnancy, such as for breastfeeding, preventing constipation and anemia, promoting weight loss, and promoting healing and well-being (see Chapter 12). Prenatal vitamins and iron supplements are often continued until 6 weeks postpartum or until the ordered supply has been used.

Promotion of Normal Bladder and Bowel Patterns

Bladder Function. After giving birth the mother should void spontaneously within 6 to 8 hours. The first several voidings should be measured to document adequate emptying of the bladder. A volume of at least 150 ml is expected for each voiding. Some women experience difficulty in emptying the bladder, possibly a result of diminished bladder tone, edema from trauma, or fear of discomfort.

Bowel Function. Interventions to promote normal bowel elimination include educating the woman about measures to avoid constipation such as ensuring adequate roughage and fluid intake and promoting exercise. Alerting the woman to side effects of medications such as narcotic analgesics (e.g., decreased gastrointestinal tract motility) may encourage her to implement measures to reduce the risk of constipation. Stool softeners or laxatives may be necessary during the early postpartum period. With early discharge a new mother may be home before having a bowel movement. Some mothers experience gas pains. Ambulation or rocking in a rocking chair may stimulate passage of flatus and relief of discomfort.

Breastfeeding Promotion and Lactation Suppression

Breastfeeding Promotion. The first 2 hours after childbirth are an excellent time to encourage the mother to breastfeed. The infant is in an alert state and ready to breastfeed. Breastfeeding aids in the contraction of the uterus and prevention of maternal hemorrhage. This is an opportune time to instruct the mother in breastfeeding and to assess the physical appearance of the breasts. (See Chapter 26 for further information on assisting the breastfeeding woman.)

Lactation Suppression. Suppression of lactation is necessary when the woman has decided not to breastfeed or in the case of neonatal death. Wearing a well-fitted support bra or breast binder continuously for at least the first 72 hours after giving birth is important. Women should avoid breast stimulation, including running warm water over the breasts, newborn suckling, or pumping of the breasts. A few nonbreastfeeding mothers experience severe breast engorgement (swelling of breast tissue caused by increased blood and lymph supply to the breasts preceding lactation). If breast engorgement occurs, it can usually be managed satisfactorily with nonpharmacologic interventions.

Ice packs to the breasts are also helpful in decreasing the discomfort associated with engorgement. The woman should use a 15 minutes on, 45 minutes off, schedule (to prevent the rebound swelling that can occur if ice is used continuously), or she can place fresh cabbage leaves inside her bra. The leaves are replaced each time they wilt. Cabbage leaves have been used to treat swelling in other cultures for years (Roberts, 1995). The exact mechanism of action is not known, but it is thought that naturally occurring plant estrogens or salicylates may be responsible for the effects. A mild analgesic may also be necessary to help the mother through this uncomfortable time. Medications that were once prescribed for lactation suppression (e.g., estrogen, estrogen and testosterone, and bromocriptine) are no longer used.

Health Promotion of Future Pregnancies and Children

Rubella Vaccination. For women who have not had rubella (10% to 20% of all women) or women who are serologically not immune (titer of 1:8 or enzyme immunoassay [EIA] level <0.8), a subcutaneous injection of rubella vaccine is recommended in the immediate postpartum period to prevent the possibility of contracting rubella in future pregnancies. Seroconversion occurs in approximately 90% of women vaccinated after birth. The live attenuated rubella virus is not communicable in breast milk; therefore breastfeeding mothers can be vaccinated. However, because the virus is shed in urine and other body fluids, the vaccine should not be given if the mother or other household members are immunocompromised. Rubella vaccine is made from duck eggs, so women who have allergies to these eggs may develop a hypersensitivity reaction to the vaccine, for which they will need adrenaline. A transient arthralgia or rash is common in vaccinated women but is benign. Because the vaccine may be teratogenic, women must be informed about the vaccine.

LEGAL TIP • Rubella Vaccination Informed consent for rubella vaccination in the postpartum period includes information about possible side effects and the risk of teratogenic effects. Women must understand that they must practice contraception to avoid pregnancy for 2 to 3 months after being vaccinated.

Prevention of Rh Isoimmunization. Injection of Rh immune globulin (a solution of gamma globulin that contains Rh antibodies) within 72 hours after birth prevents sensitization in the Rh-negative woman who has had a fetomaternal transfusion of Rh-positive fetal red blood cells (RBCs) (Box 21-5). Rh immune globulin promotes lysis of fetal Rh-positive blood cells before the mother forms her own antibodies against them.

NURSE ALERT • After birth, Rh immune globulin is administered to all Rh-negative, antibody (Coombs)-negative women who give birth to Rh-positive infants.

Box 21-5

Medication Guide for Rh Immune Globulin, RhoGAM, Gamulin Rh, HypRho-D

ACTION

Suppression of immune response in nonsensitized women with Rh-negative blood who receive Rh-positive blood cells because of fetomaternal hemorrhage, transfusion, or accident

INDICATIONS

Suppress antibody formation in women with Rh-negative blood after birth, miscarriage/pregnancy termination, abdominal trauma, ectopic pregnancy, amniocentesis, version, or chorionic villi sampling

DOSAGE/ROUTE

Standard dose 1 vial (300 μg) IM in deltoid or gluteal muscle; microdose 1 vial (50 μg) IM in deltoid muscle

ADVERSE EFFECTS

Myalgia, lethargy, localized tenderness and stiffness at injection site, possible allergic response

NURSING CONSIDERATIONS

- Give standard dose to mother within 72 hours after birth if baby is Rh positive, at 28 weeks of gestation as prophylaxis, or after an incident or exposure risk that occurs after 28 weeks of gestation (e.g., amniocentesis, second trimester miscarriage or abortion, after version).
- Give microdose for first trimester miscarriage or abortion, ectopic pregnancy, chorionic villi sampling.
- Verify that the woman is Rh negative and has not been sensitized, that Coombs test is negative, and that baby is Rh positive. Provide explanation to the woman about procedure, including the purpose, possible side effects, and effect on future pregnancies. Have the woman sign a consent form if required by agency. Verify correct dosage and confirm lot number and woman's identity before giving injection (verify with another RN or other procedure per agency policy); document administration per agency policy.

The administration of 300 μg (1 vial) of Rh immune globulin is usually sufficient to prevent maternal sensitization. If a large fetomaternal transfusion is suspected, however, the dosage needed should be determined by performing a Kleihauer-Betke test, which detects the amount of fetal blood in the maternal circulation. If more than 15 ml of fetal blood is present in maternal circulation, the dosage of Rh immune globulin must be increased.

A 1:1000 dilution of Rh immune globulin is crossmatched to the mother's RBCs to ensure compatibility. Because Rh immune globulin is usually considered a blood product, precautions similar to those used for transfusing blood are necessary when it is given. The identification number on the patient's hospital wristband should correspond to the identification number found on the laboratory slip. The nurse must also check to see that the lot number of the laboratory slip corresponds to the lot number on the vial. Finally, the expiration date on the vial should be checked to ensure it is a usable product.

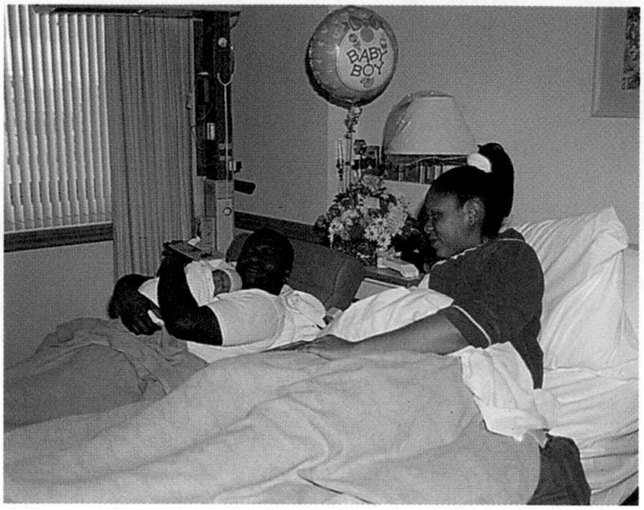

FIG. 21-9 • Bonding and attachment begun early after birth are fostered in the postpartum period. (Courtesy Marjorie Pyle, RNC, Lifecircle, Costa Mesa, CA.)

NURSE ALERT • Rh immune globulin is administered to the mother intramuscularly. It should never be given to an infant.

Rh immune globulin suppresses the immune response. Therefore the woman who receives both Rh immune globulin and rubella vaccine must be tested in 3 months to see if she has developed rubella immunity. If not, the woman will need another dose of rubella vaccine.

There is some disagreement about whether Rh immune globulin should be considered a blood product. Health care providers need to discuss the most current information about this issue with women whose religious beliefs conflict with having blood products administered to them.

➤ Evaluation

The nurse can be reasonably assured that care was effective when the expected outcomes of care for physical needs have been achieved.

Care Management—Psychosocial Needs

Meeting the psychosocial needs of new mothers involves assessing the parents' reactions to the birth experience, their feelings about themselves, and their interactions with the new baby (Fig. 21-9) and other family members. Specific interventions are then planned to increase the parents' knowledge and self-confidence as they assume the care and responsibility of the new baby and integrate a new member into their existing family structure in a way that meets their cultural expectations.

➤ Assessment

Impact of the Birth Experience. Many women indicate a need to examine the birth process itself and look at their own intrapartal behavior in retrospect. Their partners may express similar desires. If their birth experience was different from that included in their birth plan (e.g., induction, epidural anesthesia, or cesarean birth), both partners may need to mourn the loss of their expectations before they can adjust to the reality of their birth experience. Inviting them to review the events and describe how they feel helps the nurse assess how well they understand what happened and how well they have been able to put their childbirth experience into perspective.

Maternal Self-Image. An important assessment concerns the woman's self-concept, body image, and sexuality. How this new mother feels about herself and her body during the puerperium may affect her behavior and adaptation to parenting. The woman's self-concept and body image may also affect her sexuality.

Feelings related to sexual adjustment after childbirth are often a cause of concern for new parents. Women who have recently given birth may be reluctant to resume sexual intercourse for fear of pain, or they may worry that coitus could damage healing perineal tissue. Because many new parents are anxious for information but reluctant to bring up the subject, postpartum nurses should matter-of-factly include the topic of postpartum sexuality during their routine physical assessment. While examining the episiotomy site, for example, the nurse can say, "I know you're sore right now, but it probably won't be long until you (or you and your partner) are ready to make love again. Have you thought about what that might be like? Would you like to ask me questions?" This approach assures the woman and her partner that resuming sexual activity is a legitimate concern for new parents and indicates the nurse's willingness to answer questions and share information.

Adaptation to Parenthood/Parent-Infant Interactions. The psychosocial assessment also includes evaluating adaptation to parenthood, as evidenced by mother's and father's reactions to and interactions with the new baby. Clues indicating successful adaptation begin to appear early in the postbirth period as parents react positively to the newborn infant and continue the process of establishing a relationship with him or her.

Parents are adapting well to their new role when they exhibit a realistic perception and acceptance of their newborn's needs and his or her limited abilities, immature social responses, and helplessness. Examples of positive parent-infant interactions include taking pleasure in their infant and in the tasks done for and with him or her; understanding their infant's emotional states and providing comfort; and reading their infant's cues for new experiences and sensing his/her fatigue level.

Family Structure and Functioning. A woman's adjustment to her role as mother is affected greatly by her relationships with her partner, her mother and other relatives, and any other children. Nurses can help to ease the new mother's return home by identifying possible conflicts among family members and helping the woman plan strategies for dealing with these problems before discharge. Such a conflict could arise when couples have very different ideas about parenting. Dealing with the stresses of sibling rivalry and unsolicited grandparent advice can also affect the woman's transition to motherhood. Only by asking about other nuclear and extended family members can the nurse discover potential problems in such relationships and help to plan workable solutions for them.

Impact of Cultural Diversity. The final component of a complete psychosocial assessment is the woman's cultural beliefs and values. Much of a woman's behavior during the postpartum period is strongly influenced by her cultural background. Nurses are likely to come into contact with women from many different countries and cultures. All cultures have developed safe and satisfying methods of caring for new mothers and babies. Only by understanding and respecting the values and beliefs of each woman can the nurse design a plan of care to meet their individual needs.

Sometimes the psychosocial assessment indicates serious actual or potential problems that must be addressed. Box 21-6 lists several psychosocial needs that, at a minimum, warrant ongoing evaluation following hospital discharge. Patients exhibiting these needs should be referred to appropriate community resources for assessment and management.

Box 21-6
Signs of Potential Complications

PSYCHOSOCIAL NEEDS
Unable or unwilling to discuss labor and birth experience.
Refers to self as ugly and useless.
Excessively preoccupied with self (body image).
Markedly depressed.
Lacks a support system.
Partner and/or other family members react negatively to the baby.
Refuses to interact with or care for baby. For example, does not name baby, does not want to hold or feed baby, is upset by vomiting and wet or dirty diapers. (Cultural appropriateness of actions needs to be considered.)
Expresses disappointment over baby's sex.
Sees baby as messy or unattractive.
Baby reminds mother of family member or friend she doesn't like.

➤ Nursing Diagnoses

After analyzing the data obtained during the assessment process, the nurse establishes nursing diagnoses to provide a guide for planning care. Nursing diagnoses related to psychosocial issues that are often established for the postpartum patient include the following:

- Altered family processes related to:
  —Unexpected birth of twins
- Impaired verbal communication related to:
  —Patient's hearing impairment
  —Nurse's language not the same as patient's
- Altered parenting related to:
  —Long, difficult labor
  —Unmet expectations of labor and birth
- Anxiety related to:
  —Newness of parenting role, sibling rivalry, or response of grandparent
- Risk for situational low self-esteem related to:
  —Body image changes

➤ Expected Outcomes

Expected psychosocial outcomes during the postpartum period are based on the nursing diagnoses identified for the individual woman and her family. Examples of common expected outcomes include that the woman (family) will do the following:

- Identify measures that promote a healthy personal adjustment in the postpartum period.
- Maintain healthy family functioning based on cultural norms and personal expectations.

➤ Plan of Care and Implementation

The nurse functions in the roles of teacher, encourager, and supporter rather than doer while implementing the psychosocial plan of care for a postpartum woman. Implementation of the psychosocial care plan involves carrying out specific activities to achieve the expected outcome of care planned for each individual woman. Several topics that should be included in the psychosocial plan of care include promotion of parenting skills and family member adjustment to the newest member. These topics are discussed in Chapter 22.

Cultural issues must also be considered when planning care. There are many traditional health beliefs and practices among the different cultures within the American population. Traditional health practices that are used to maintain health or to avoid illnesses deal with the whole person (i.e., body, mind, and spirit) and tend to be culturally based.

Women from various cultures may view health as a balance between opposing forces (e.g., yin versus yang), being in harmony with nature, or just "feeling good." Traditional practices may include the observance of certain dietary restrictions, clothing, or taboos for balancing the body; participation in certain activities such as sports and art for maintaining mental health; and use of silence, prayer, or meditation for developing spiritually. Practices (e.g., using religious objects or eating garlic) are used to protect oneself from illness and may involve avoiding people who are believed to create hexes, spells, or who have an "evil eye." Restoration of health may involve a person taking folk medicines (e.g., herbs or animal substances) or using a traditional healer.

Childbirth occurs within this sociocultural context. Rest, seclusion, dietary restraints, and ceremonies honoring the mother are all common traditional practices that are followed for the promotion of the health and well-being of the mother and baby.

There are several common traditional health practices used and beliefs held by women and their families during the postpartum period. In Asia, for example, pregnancy is considered to be a hot (yang) condition, then childbirth results in a sudden loss of yang forces (Mattson, 1995). Therefore balance needs to be restored by increasing the return of yang forces present physically or symbolically in hot food, hot water, and warm air.

Another common belief is that the mother and baby remain in a weak and vulnerable state for a period of several weeks following birth. During this time the mother may remain in a passive role, take no baths or showers, and stay in bed to prevent cold air from entering her body.

Women who have immigrated to the United States or other Western nations without their extended families may not have much help at home, making it difficult for them to observe these activity restrictions. Box 21-7 lists some common cultural beliefs about the postpartum period and family planning.

It is important that nurses consider all cultural aspects when planning care and not use their own cultural beliefs as the framework for that care. Although the beliefs and behaviors of other cultures may seem different or strange, they should be encouraged as long as the mother wants to conform to them and she and the baby suffer no ill effects. The nurse needs to determine whether a woman is using any folk medicine during the postpartum period because active ingredients in folk medicine may have adverse physiologic effects on the woman when ingested with prescribed medicines. The nurse should not assume that a mother desires to use traditional health practices that represent a particular cultural group merely because she is a member of that culture. Many young women who are first-generation or second-generation Americans may follow their cultural traditions only when older family members are present, or not at all.

➤ Evaluation

The nurse can be reasonably assured that care was effective if expected outcomes of care for psychosocial needs have been met.

Discharge Teaching

Self-Care, Signs of Complications. Discharge planning begins at the time of admission to the unit and should be reflected in the plan of care developed for each individual woman. For example, a great deal of time during the hospital stay is usually spent in teaching about maternal and newborn

Box 21-7

Some Cultural Beliefs About the Postpartum Period and Family Planning

POSTPARTUM CARE

Chinese, Mexican, Korean, and Southeast Asian women may wish to eat only warm foods and drink hot drinks to replace blood loss and to restore the balance of hot and cold in their bodies. These women may also wish to stay warm and avoid bathing, exercises, and hair washing for 7 to 30 days after childbirth. Self-care may not be a priority; care by family members is preferred. The woman has respect for elders and authority. These woman may wear abdominal binders. They may prefer not to give their babies colostrum.

Haitian women may request to take the placenta home to bury or burn.

Muslim women follow strict religious laws on modesty and diet. A Muslim woman must keep her hair, body, arms to the wrist, and legs to the ankles covered at all times. She cannot be alone in the presence of a man other than her husband or a male relative. Observant Muslims will not eat pork or pork products and are obligated to eat meat slaughtered according to Islamic laws (halal meat). If halal meat is not available, kosher meat, seafood, or a vegetarian diet is usually accepted.

FAMILY PLANNING

Birth control is government mandated in mainland *China.* Most *Chinese women* will have an IUD inserted after the birth of their first child. Women do not want hormonal methods of contraception because they fear putting these medications in their bodies.

Saudi Arabian and Hispanic women will likely choose the rhythm method because most are Catholic.

(East) Indian men are encouraged to have voluntary sterilization by vasectomy.

Muslim couples may practice contraception by mutual consent as long as its use is not harmful to the woman. Acceptable contraceptive methods include foam and condoms, the diaphragm, and natural family planning.

Hmong women highly value and desire large families, which limits birth control practices.

care, because all women must be capable of providing basic care for themselves and their infants at the time of discharge. It is also crucial that every woman be taught to recognize the physical signs and symptoms that might indicate problems and how to obtain advice and assistance quickly if these signs appear. Before discharge, women need basic instruction regarding the resumption of sexual intercourse, prescribed medications, routine mother-baby checkups, and contraception.

Just before the time of discharge the nurse reviews the woman's chart to see that laboratory reports, medications, signatures, and other items are in order. Some hospitals have a checklist to use before the woman's discharge. The nurse verifies that medications, if ordered, have arrived on the unit; that any valuables kept secured during the woman's stay have been returned to her and that she has signed a receipt for them; and that the infant is ready to be discharged.

No medication that would make the mother sleepy should be administered if she is the one who will be holding the baby on the way out of the hospital. In most instances the woman is seated in a wheelchair and is given the baby to hold. Some families leave unescorted and ambulatory, depending on hospital protocol. The woman's possessions are gathered and taken out with her and her family. The woman's and the baby's identification bands are carefully checked. Babies must be secured in a car seat for the drive home.

Sexual Activity/Contraception. Many couples resume sexual activity before the traditional postpartum checkup 6 weeks after childbirth. Risk of hemorrhage and infection are minimal approximately 2 weeks postpartum. Couples may be anxious about the topic but uncomfortable and unwilling to bring it up. It is important that the nurse discuss the physical and psychologic effects that giving birth can have on sexual activity (Home Care box). Contraceptive options should also be discussed with women (and their partners if present) before discharge so that they can make informed decisions about fertility management before resuming sexual activity. Waiting to discuss contraception at the 6-week checkup may be too late. It is possible, particularly in women who bottle-feed, for ovulation to occur as soon as 1 month after birth. A woman who engages in unprotected sex risks becoming pregnant. Current contraceptive options are discussed in detail in Chapter 7. Women who are undecided about contraception at the time of discharge need information about using condoms with foam or creams until the first postpartum checkup.

Prescribed Medications. Women routinely continue to take their prenatal vitamins and iron during the postpartum period. It is especially important that women who are breastfeeding or who are discharged with a lower than normal hematocrit take these medications as prescribed. Women with extensive episiotomies or vaginal lacerations (third or fourth degree) are usually prescribed stool softeners to take at home. Pain relief medications (analgesics or nonsteroidal antiinflammatory medications) may be prescribed, especially for women who had cesarean birth. The nurse should make certain that the woman knows the route, dosage, frequency, and common side effects of all ordered medications.

Routine Mother and Baby Checkups. Women who have experienced uncomplicated vaginal births are still commonly scheduled for the traditional 6-week postpartum examination. Women who have had a cesarean birth are often seen in the physician's/nurse-midwife's office or clinic 2 weeks after hospital discharge. The date and time for the follow-up appointment should be included in the discharge instructions. If an appointment is not made before the woman leaves the hospital, she should be encouraged to call the physician's/nurse-midwife's office or clinic and schedule an appointment herself.

Parents who have not already done so need to make plans for newborn follow-up at the time of discharge. Most offices and clinics like to see newborns for an initial examination within the first week or by 2 weeks of age. If an appointment for a specific date and time was not made for the infant before leaving the hospital, the parents should be encouraged to call the office or clinic right away.

Dealing with Activities of Daily Life at Home. Even the small details of daily life may become stressful, given the demands of a newborn and the discomfort or fatigue associated with birth and a busy homecoming day, or both. The parents may wish to buy disposable diapers for the first hours at home even if they plan to use cloth diapers. During pregnancy, the woman is encouraged to freeze extra casseroles or leftovers to use for the first few meals at home; family, friends and neighbors can be encouraged to bring prepared food during this time.

Planning for discharge soon after an infant feeding ensures that the couple will have adequate time to get home and relatively settled before the next feeding. Offering a sample carton of premixed bottles for the formula-fed infant prevents need for rushed preparation of formula.

Dealing with Visitors. A newborn in the family or neighborhood draws visitors. The nurse can help the parents

Home Care

RESUMPTION OF SEXUAL INTERCOURSE

You can safely resume sexual intercourse by the second to fourth week after birth when bleeding has stopped and the episiotomy has healed. For the first 6 weeks to 6 months, the vagina does not lubricate well.

Your physiologic reactions to sexual stimulation for the first 3 months after birth will be slower and less intense. The strength of the orgasm is reduced.

A water-soluble gel, cocoa butter, or a contraceptive cream or jelly might be recommended for lubrication. If some vaginal tenderness is present, your partner can be instructed to insert one or more clean, lubricated fingers into the vagina and rotate them within the vagina to help relax it and to identify possible areas of discomfort. A position in which you have control of the depth of the insertion of the penis also is useful. The side-by-side or female-on-top position may be more comfortable.

The presence of the baby influences postbirth lovemaking. Parents hear every sound made by the baby; conversely you may be concerned that the baby hears every sound you make. In either case, any phase of the sexual response cycle may be interrupted by hearing the baby cry or move, leaving both of you frustrated and unsatisfied. In addition, the amount of psychologic energy expended by you in child care activities may lead to fatigue. Newborns require a great deal of attention and time.

Some women have reported feeling sexual stimulation and orgasms when breastfeeding their babies. Breastfeeding mothers often are interested in returning to sexual activity before non-breastfeeding mothers.

You should be instructed to correctly perform the Kegel exercises to strengthen your pubococcygeal muscle. This muscle is associated with bowel and bladder function and with vaginal feeling during intercourse.

explore ways in which they can assert their needs in such situations. When family or friends ask what they can do to help, the family can respond with "Please bring us a casserole or a meal" or "Could you please pick up some items at the grocery store?" The couple may want to work out a signal for alerting the partner that the new mother is becoming tired or uncomfortable and needs to have the partner invite the visitors into another part of the house. Some new mothers have found that if they remain in their robe and do not appear ready for company, visitors stay for a shorter time. A "Please Do Not Disturb" sign on the front door may be useful.

Follow-Up After Discharge

Home Visits. Home visits to new mothers and babies within a few days of discharge can help bridge the gap between hospital care and routine visits to health care providers. Nurses are able to assess the mother, infant, and home environment; answer questions and provide education; and make referrals to community resources if necessary. Home visits may also help reduce the need for more expensive health care, such as nonroutine health care visits and rehospitalization, and decrease stress in new families (Brown and Johnson, 1998). Immediate follow-up contact and home visits must be available 7 days a week.

A referral form containing information about both mother and baby should be completed at hospital discharge and sent immediately to the home care agency. Fig. 21-10 is an example of such a referral form.

The home visit is most commonly scheduled on the woman's second day home from the hospital, but it may be scheduled on any of the first 4 days at home, depending on the individual family's situation and needs. Additional visits are planned throughout the first week, as needed. The home visits may be extended beyond that time if the family's needs warrant it and if a home visit is the most appropriate option for carrying out the follow-up care required to meet the specific needs identified.

During the home visit the nurse conducts a systematic assessment of mother and newborn to determine physiologic adjustment, identify any existing complications, and answer any questions the mother/family has about herself or newborn care. Conducting the assessment in a separate room provides private time for the mother to ask questions on topics such as breast care, family planning, and constipation. The assessment focuses on the mother's emotional adjustment and her knowledge of self- and infant care.

During the newborn assessment, the nurse can demonstrate and explain normal newborn behavior and capabilities and encourage the mother/family to ask questions or express concerns they may have. The home care nurse must verify if the newborn screen for phenylketonuria and other inborn errors of metabolism has been drawn. If the baby was discharged from the hospital before 24 hours of age, the newborn screen will need to be done by the home care or clinic nurse.

Telephone Follow-Up. As part of the routine follow-up of a woman and her infant after discharge from the hospital, many providers are implementing one or more postpartum telephone follow-up calls to their patients for assessment, health teaching, identification of complications to effect timely intervention, and referrals. Telephone follow-up may be part of the services offered by the hospital, private physician or clinic, or a private agency; it may be either a separate service, or combined with other strategies for extending postpartum care. Telephonic nursing assessments are commonly used after a postpartum home care visit to reassess a woman's knowledge about the signs and symptoms of adequate hydration in breastfeeding or, after initiating home phototherapy, to assess the caregiver's knowledge regarding equipment complications.

The "warm line" represents another type of telephone link between the new family and concerned caregivers or experienced parent volunteers. A warm line is a helpline or consultation service, not a crisis intervention line. The warm line is appropriately used for dealing with less extreme concerns that may seem urgent at the time the call is placed but are not actual emergencies. Calls to warm lines commonly relate to infant feeding, prolonged crying, or sibling rivalry. Warm line services may extend beyond the fourth trimester. Families need to call when concerns arise, and be given phone numbers for ready access to answers to their questions.

Support Groups. A special group experience is sometimes sought by the woman adjusting to motherhood. On occasion, postpartum women who have met earlier in prenatal clinics or on the hospital unit may begin to associate for mutual support. Members of Lamaze classes who attend a postpartum reunion may decide to extend their relationship during the fourth trimester.

A postpartum support group enables mothers and fathers to share with and support each other as they adjust to parenting. Many new parents find it reassuring to discover that they are not alone in their feelings of confusion and uncertainty. An experienced parent can often impart concrete information that can be valuable to other members in a postpartum support group. Inexperienced parents may find themselves imitating the behavior of others in the group whom they perceive as particularly capable.

Referral to Community Resources. To develop an effective referral system, it is important that the nurse have an understanding of the needs of the woman and family and of the organization and community resources available for meeting those needs. Locating and compiling information about available community services contributes to the development of a referral system. It is important for the nurse to develop his or her own resource file of services that are commonly used by health care providers.

Community Focus

BREASTFEEDING SUPPORT

Women breastfeed longer if they have support in their breastfeeding efforts. Nurses and lactation consultants provide support during inpatient stays after childbirth. Women can find support in the community in various groups. Social support interventions that include peer support are successful in increasing the duration of exclusive breastfeeding and satisfaction with breastfeeding. Nurses in their discharge planning can refer breastfeeding mothers to community groups for support. Community and home health nurses can facilitate breastfeeding efforts through organizing or facilitating support groups. Mothers experienced in breastfeeding can facilitate these efforts.

Data from Vari P, Camburn J, Henly S: Professionally mediated peer support and early breastfeeding success, *J Perinat Educ* 9(1):22-30, 2000.

OB Homecare
Phone: 612-863-4478
Fax: 612-863-4568

POSTPARTUM HOME CARE REFERRAL

☐PHN Referral Made to ____________ County

Mother's Name: ____________________

Address/Phone where mother will be staying:

Address: ____________________

City: ____________________

Phone #:(_____)__________

☐ Address & Phone Verified

Language Spoken: ☐ English ☐ Other: __________

Understands English: ☐ Well ☐ Poor

☐ Mother Needs Interpreter ☐ Hearing Impaired

Who interpreted in hospital: ____________

Phone: (_____)__________

Mom's MD/Midwife: (Full Name) ____________

Phone #: (_____)__________

Next Appt: ____________

MOTHER:

Gravida _____ T___ P___ A___ L___

Marital Status: S M W D Sep

Normal Maternal Exam: ☐Yes ☐No (explain below)

☐ Vaginal Birth ☐ C/Birth

Epis/Incision: ____________

Meds: ____________

Allergies: ____________

☐ Needs Large BP Cuff

OTHER ISSUES:

Diabetic: ____________

Hgb pp, if abnormal: ____________

Psycho/Social Issues:

☐ Parent/Child Interaction ☐ Limited Support System
☐ Mental Health Status ☐ Drug Use/Dependency
☐ Previous Losses ☐ Hx of Domestic Violence
☐ Other: ____________

Husband/Significant Other: ____________

Baby's Name: ____________ ☐ M ☐ F

Delivery Date/Time: _________@_______

Mother's Discharge Date/Time: _________@_______

Baby's MD (Full Name): ____________

Phone #: (_____)__________

Next Appt: ____________

BABY:

Gestation: _______weeks ☐ Fetal Loss

Birth Weight: ________ Discharge wt: ________

Apgars: 1" _____ 5" _____

Feedings: ☐ Breast ☐ Bottle ☐ Both

Feeding Issues: ____________

Normal Infant Exam: ☐ Yes ☐ No (explain below)

Circumcised: ☐ Yes ☐ No

Additional Order:

☐ Home care to draw newborn screen
****Must send lab-slip home with family.**

ADDITIONAL COMMENTS or ABNORMAL FINDINGS FOR MOTHER OR BABY:

____
____
____
____
____
____
____

Mom aware of referral: ☐Yes ☐No **REFERRAL COMPLETED BY:** ____________

☐ Faxed to OB Homecare @-612-863-4568: ☐ Facesheet ☐ Referral
☐ Faxed to PHN __________ County: ☐ Facesheet ☐ Referral
Currently being seen by PHN: ☐ Yes ☐ No

FIG. 21-10 • Referral form. (Courtesy OB Homecare of Allina Hospitals and Clinics, Minneapolis, MN.)

The nurse can begin by gathering existing information from community resources such as the local health department, library, or church; local resource agencies such as Planned Parenthood, HAND, or La Leche League; and major service organizations such as March of Dimes, American Red Cross, and WIC Supplemental Nutrition Program. Also, national perinatal organizations such as Nursing Mothers Council; Depression After Delivery—National; Postpartum Support, International; Positive Parenting and Parenting Fitness; National Perinatal Association; and Child Welfare League of America can be helpful. These services can provide published resource guides and lists of community service agencies specific to the group or condition that they represent (Clemen-Stone, McGuire, and Eigsti, 1998; Perinatal Resources, 1997).

Key Points

- Postpartum care is modeled on the concept of health.
- Cultural beliefs and practices affect the patient's response to the puerperium.
- The nursing care plan includes assessments to detect deviations from normal, comfort measures to relieve discomfort or pain, and safety measures to prevent injury or infection.
- Teaching and counseling measures are designed to promote the woman's feelings of competence in self-care and baby care.
- Common nursing interventions in the postpartum period include evaluating and treating the boggy uterus and the full urinary bladder; providing for nonpharmacologic and pharmacologic relief of pain and discomfort associated with the episiotomy, lacerations, or breastfeeding; and instituting measures to promote or suppress lactation.
- Meeting the psychosocial needs of the new mother involves taking into consideration the composition and functioning of the entire family.
- Early postpartum discharge will continue to be the trend as a result of consumer demand, medical necessity, discharge criteria for low risk childbirth, and cost-containment measures.
- Early discharge classes, telephone follow-up, home visits, warm lines, and support groups are effective means of facilitating physiologic and psychologic adjustments in the postpartum period.

References

American Academy of Pediatrics and American College of Obstetricians and Gynecologists: *Guidelines for perinatal care,* ed 3, Elk Grove Village, IL, 1997, AAP.

Brown S, Johnson B: Enhancing early discharge with home follow-up: a pilot project, *J Obstet Gynecol Neonatal Nurse* 27(1):33-38, 1998.

Clemen-Stone S, McGuire S, Eigsti D: *Comprehensive community health nursing,* ed 5, St Louis, 1998, Mosby.

Ferguson S, Engelhard C: Short stay: the art of legislating quality and economy, *AWHONN Lifelines* 1(1):17-23, 1997.

Havens D, Hannan C: Legislation to mandate maternal and newborn length of stay, *J Pediatr Health Care* 10(3):141-144, 1996.

Johnson & Johnson: *Compendium of postpartum care,* Skillman, NJ, 1996, Johnson & Johnson Consumer Products, Inc.

Luegenbiehl D: Improving visual estimation of blood volume on peripads, *MCN Am J Matern Child Nurs* 22(6):294-298, 1997.

Mattson S: Culturally sensitive perinatal care for Southeast Asians, *J Obstet Gynecol Neonatal Nurs* 24(4):335-341, 1995.

Milligan R, Flenniken P, Pugh L: Positioning intervention to minimize fatigue in breastfeeding women, *Appl Nurs Res* 9(2):67-70, 1996.

Perinatal Resources: Publications and organizations: *J Perinatal Educ* 6(2):61-68, 1997.

Pugh L et al: Clinical approaches in the assessment of childbearing fatigue, *J Obstet Gynecol Neonatal Nurs* 28(1):74-80, 1999.

Roberts K: A comparison of chilled cabbage leaves and chilled gelpaks in reducing breast engorgement, *J Hum Lact* 11(1):17-20, 1995.

Sampselle C, Miller J: Pelvic muscle exercise: effective patient teaching, *The Female Patient* 21(5):29-36, 1996.

Weekly S, Neumann M: Speaking up for baby: the case for individualized neonatal discharge plans, *AWHONN Lifelines* 1(1):24-29, 1997.

Wilkerson N: Appraisal of early postpartum discharge programs, *J Perinatal Educ* 5(2):1-5, 1996.

CHAPTER

22

Transition to Parenthood

http://www.harcourthealth.com/MERLIN/Wong/maternal/

Learning Objectives

On completion of this chapter the reader will be able to:

- Discuss ways to facilitate parent-infant adjustment.
- Describe sensual responses that strengthen attachment.
- Identify infant behaviors that facilitate and that inhibit parental attachment.
- Differentiate the three periods in parental role change after childbirth.
- Identify behaviors of the three phases of maternal adjustment.
- Discuss paternal adjustment.
- Discuss the effects of the following on parental response: parental age (e.g., adolescence and over 35 years), social support, culture, socioeconomic conditions, personal aspirations, and sensory impairment.
- Describe sibling adjustment.
- Describe grandparent adaptation.

Becoming a parent creates a period of change and instability for men and women who decide to have children. This occurs whether parenthood is biologic or adoptive and whether the parents are married husband-wife couples, cohabiting couples, single mothers, single fathers, lesbian couples with one woman as biologic mother, or gay male couples who adopt a child. This period of developmental change is referred to as the transition to parenthood.

This chapter reviews the transition to parenthood, including the parenting process and the adjustment of parents, siblings, and grandparents.

PARENTING PROCESS

Biologic parenthood begins with the union of ovum and sperm. During the prenatal period the mother provides an environment in which the unborn child develops and grows. This close symbiotic union ends with birth. At this point, other people assume partial or complete involvement in the infant's care. The biologic or substitute woman or man parent then enters into a crucial relationship with the child that persists throughout the life of each. Parenthood can serve as a maturation factor for women and men regardless of whether it is biologically based. For children, parenthood is all-important; their continued existence depends on the quality of care they receive. Sank (1991) described parenting as a process of role attainment and role transition that begins during pregnancy. The transition ends when the parent develops a sense of comfort and confidence in performing the parental role.

Nurses can help inexperienced parents feel confident and competent in their new roles. They can provide opportunities for parents to practice child care tasks in the hospital, birth setting, or in the home, where assistance and feedback are available. Nurses can enhance parents' self-concept by helping them feel more comfortable and confident in their parenting skills.

Parental Attachment, Bonding, and Acquaintance

The process by which a parent comes to love and accept a child, and a child comes to love and accept a parent, is referred to as attachment. Using the terms attachment and bonding, Klaus et al (1972) proposed that the period shortly after birth is important to mother-to-infant attachment. They defined the phenomenon of bonding as a sensitive period in the first minutes and hours after birth, when mothers and fathers must have close contact with their infants for optimal later development (Klaus and Kennell, 1976). Klaus and Kennell (1982) later revised their theory of parent-infant bonding, modifying their claim of the critical nature of immediate contact with the infant after birth. They acknowledged the adaptability of human parents, stating it took longer than minutes or hours for parents to form an emotional relationship with their infants. The terms attachment and bonding continue to be used interchangeably.

Attachment is developed and maintained by proximity and interaction with the infant; through this the parent becomes acquainted with the infant, identifies the infant as an individual, and claims the infant as a member of the family. Attachment is facilitated by positive feedback (i.e., social, verbal, and nonverbal responses, whether real or perceived, that indicate acceptance of one partner by the other). Attachment occurs through a mutually satisfying experience. A mother commented on her son's grasp reflex, "I put my finger in his hand, and he grabbed right on. It is just a reflex, I know, but it felt good anyway" (Fig. 22-1).

The concept of attachment has been extended to include mutuality; that is, the infant's behaviors and characteristics call forth a corresponding set of maternal behaviors and characteristics. The infant displays signaling behaviors such as crying, smiling, and cooing that initiate the contact and bring the caregiver to the child. These behaviors are followed by executive behaviors such as rooting, grasping, and postural adjustments that maintain the contact. The caregiver is attracted to an alert, responsive, cuddly infant and repelled by an irritable, apparently disinterested infant. Attachment occurs more readily with the infant whose temperament, social capabilities, appearance, and sex fit the parent's expectations. If the child does not meet these expectations, resolution of the parent's disappointment can delay the attachment process.

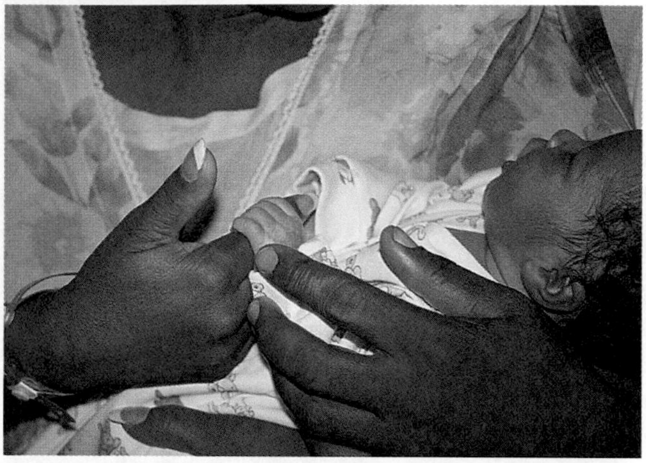

FIG. 22-1 • Hands. (Courtesy Marjorie Pyle, RNC, Lifecircle, Costa Mesa, CA.)

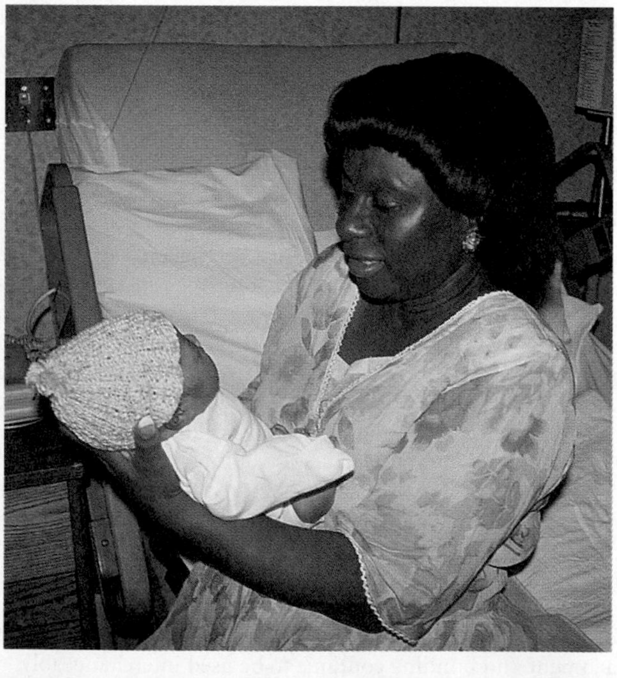

FIG. 22-2 • Mother and baby make eye contact in en face position. (Courtesy Marjorie Pyle, RNC, Lifecircle, Costa Mesa, CA.)

An important part of attachment is acquaintance (Klaus and Kennell, 1983). Parents use eye contact (Fig. 22-2), touching, talking, and exploring to become acquainted with their infant during the immediate postpartum period. Adoptive parents undergo the same process when they first meet their new child. During this period families engage in the claiming process, which is the identification of the new baby (Fig. 22-3). The child is first identified in terms of "likeness" to other family members, then in terms of "differences," and finally in terms of "uniqueness." The unique newcomer is thus incorporated into the family. Mother and father scrutinize their infant carefully and point out characteristics that the child shares with other family members and that are indicative of a relationship between them. The claiming process is revealed by maternal comments such as the following: "Russ held him close and said, 'He's the image of his father,' but I found one part like me—his toes are shaped like mine."

On the other hand, some mothers react negatively. They "claim" the infant in terms of the discomfort or pain the baby causes. The mother interprets the infant's normal responses as being negative toward her, and reacts to her child with dislike or indifference. She does not hold the child close or touch the child to be comforting; for example, "The nurse put the baby into Marie's arms. She promptly laid him across her knees and glanced up at the television. 'Stay still until I finish watching—you've been enough trouble already.'"

Nursing interventions related to the promotion of parent-infant attachment are numerous and varied (Table 22-1). They can enhance positive parent-infant contacts by heightening parental awareness of an infant's responses and ability to communicate. As the parent attempts to become competent and loving in that role, nurses can bolster the parent's self-confidence and ego. Nurses are in prime positions to identify actual and potential problems and collaborate with other health

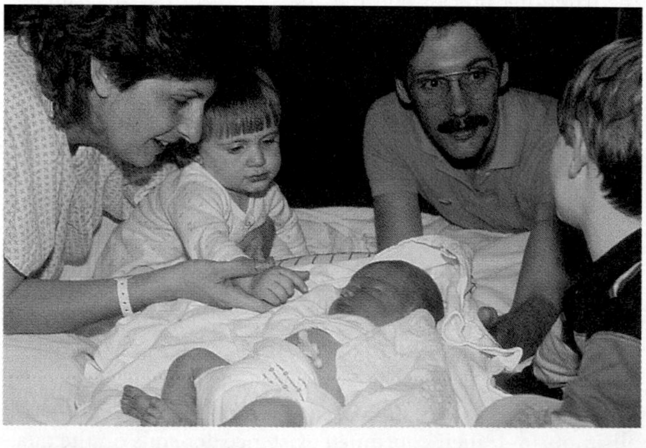

FIG. 22-3 • Family members examine the new baby. They discuss how she resembles them and other family members. (Courtesy Marjorie Pyle, RNC, Lifecircle, Costa Mesa, CA.

care professionals who will provide care for the parents after discharge. Nursing considerations for fostering maternal-infant bonding among special populations may vary (Cultural Considerations box).

Assessment of Attachment Behaviors. One of the most important areas of assessment is careful observation of those behaviors thought to indicate the formation of emotional bonds between the newborn and family, especially the mother. Unlike physical assessment of the neonate, which has concrete guidelines to follow, assessment of parent-infant attachment requires much more skill in terms of observation and interviewing. Rooming-in of mother and infant and liberal visiting privileges for father, siblings, and grandparents facilitate recognition of behaviors that demonstrate positive or negative attachment. An excellent opportunity exists during feeding. Guidelines for assessment of bonding behaviors are presented in the Patient Teaching box.

During pregnancy, and often even before conception occurs, parents develop an image of the "ideal" or "fantasy" infant. At birth the fantasy infant becomes the real infant. How closely the dream child resembles the real child influences the bonding process. Assessing such expectations during pregnancy and at the time of the infant's birth allows identification of discrepancies in the parents' view of the fantasy child versus the real child.

The labor process significantly affects the immediate attachment of mothers to their newborn infants. Factors such as a long labor, feeling tired or "drugged" after birth, and problems with breastfeeding can delay the development of initial positive feelings toward the newborn.

Parent-Infant Contact

Early Contact. Early close contact may facilitate the attachment process between parent and child. This does not mean that a delay will inhibit this process (humans are too resilient for that), but additional psychologic energy may be needed to achieve the same effect. To date, no scientific evidence has

TABLE 22-1
Examples of Parent-Infant Attachment Interventions

Intervention Label/Definition	Critical Activities	Supporting Activities
ATTACHMENT PROMOTION		
Facilitation of development of parent-infant relationship	Give parents opportunity to hold infant soon after birth Keep infant with parents after birth when possible	Provide rooming-in in hospital Provide pain relief for mother Provide opportunity for parents to see, hold, and examine newborn immediately after birth
ENVIRONMENTAL MANAGEMENT: ATTACHMENT PROCESS		
Manipulation of environment that facilitates development of parent-infant relationship	Allow for family visitation as desired Create environment that fosters privacy	Permit father/significant other to sleep in room with mother Provide rocking chair
FAMILY INTEGRITY PROMOTION: CHILDBEARING FAMILY		
Facilitation of growth of individuals or families who are adding infant to family	Convey accepting attitude (for nonthreatening environment for family to express feelings) Reinforce parenting behaviors	Offer to be listener for significant other Discuss sibling's reaction to newborn, as appropriate
LACTATION COUNSELING		
Use of interactive helping process to assist in maintenance of successful breastfeeding	Educate parents about infant feeding for informed decision making Give parents recommended education material, as needed	Provide information about advantages and disadvantages of breastfeeding Inform parents about appropriate classes or groups for breastfeeding
PARENT EDUCATION: CHILDBEARING FAMILY		
Preparation of individuals to perform their role as parents	Reinforce skills parent does well in caring for infant to promote confidence Assist parents in interpreting infant cues	Monitor learning needs of family Appraise parents' learning styles (how they learn best)
RISK IDENTIFICATION: CHILDBEARING FAMILY		
Identification of individuals or families who are likely to have difficulties in parenting and prioritization of strategies to prevent parenting problems	Review maternal history of chemical dependency, noting duration, type of drug(s), and time and strength of last dose before birth Monitor behaviors indicative of problem with attachment	Determine parents' feelings about unplanned pregnancy Determine economic, marital, and educational status of parents

Modified from McCloskey J, Bulechek G: *Nursing interventions classification*, ed 2, St Louis, 1996, Mosby.

Cultural Considerations

FOSTERING BONDING IN SPECIFIC POPULATIONS

Women in Economically Disadvantaged Situations

Low-income mothers may have to contend with stressors that distract them from developing a relationship with their babies. Inability to pay for infant supplies or child care, chaotic home situations, and worry over eligibility for social and health care services deplete these women's psychologic energy

Nurses need to conduct nonjudgmental, individual assessments of resources and social networks to avoid inaccurate and stereotypical assumptions. Nurses can help economically disadvantaged mothers access social services, such as the Women, Infants, and Children (WIC) program and Medicaid. For mothers whose home environments provide little or no support and multiple stressors, early discharge may not be optimal. Nurses can advocate for longer hospital stays for these mothers when the hospital environment is more conducive to bonding.

Economically disadvantaged mothers, especially adolescents, are not as likely to be aware of the benefits of bonding or to be knowledgeable of normal infant behaviors. These women may not be aware of maternity care options, such as rooming-in, or may be less assertive in asking for such options. The nurse needs to be a patient educator and advocate, explaining the choices and the potential benefits. The nurse should ensure a supportive, encouraging environment that will help mothers engage in positive interactions with their infants. By use of the Brazelton Neonatal Behavioral Assessment Scale, the nurse can capture the mother's attention with a mother-infant interactional experience and, at the same time, increase the mother's knowledge of infant behavior. Written material can be provided after the assessment to reinforce the behavioral concepts.

Examples, from sections of an individualized handout written as if from the baby, include "My strengths: great motor maturity—I stretch my arms way up over my head" and "How you can help: swaddle my arms so I can suck on my hands" (Tedder, 1991).

Women of Varying Ethnic and Cultural Groups

Childbearing practices and rituals of other cultures may not be congruent with standard practices associated with bonding in the Anglo-American culture. For example, Chinese families traditionally use extended family members to care for the newborn so that the mother can rest and recover, especially after a cesarean birth. Some Native American, Asian, and Hispanic women do not initiate breastfeeding until their breast milk comes in. Haitian families do not name their babies until after the confinement month. Amount of eye contact varies among cultures, too. Yup'ik Eskimo mothers almost always position their babies so that eye contact can be made.

Nurses should become knowledgeable of the childbearing beliefs and practices of diverse cultural and ethnic groups. Because individual cultural variations exist within groups, nurses need to clarify with the patient and family members or friends what cultural norms the client follows. Incorrect judgments may be made about mother-infant bonding if nurses do not practice culturally sensitive care.

Modified from Geissler E: *Pocket guide to cultural assessment,* St. Louis, 1994, Mosby; Symanski M: Maternal-infant bonding: practice issues for the 1990s, *J Nurse Midwifery 37*(2 Suppl):67S-73S, 1992; Tedder J: Using the Brazelton Neonatal Assessment Scale to facilitate the parent-infant relationship in a primary care setting, *Nurse Pract* 16(3):26-30, 35-36, 1991.

Patient Teaching

ASSESSING ATTACHMENT BEHAVIORS

When the infant is brought to the parents, do they reach out for the infant and call the infant by name? (Recognize that in some cultures, parents may not name the infant in the early newborn period.)

Do the parents speak about the infant in terms of identification—whom the infant looks like; what appears special about their infant over other infants?

When parents are holding the infant, what kind of body contact is there—do parents feel at ease in changing the infant's position; are fingertips or whole hands used; are there parts of the body they avoid touching or parts of the body they investigate and scrutinize?

When the infant is awake, what kinds of stimulation do the parents provide—do they talk to the infant, to each other, or to no one; how do they look at the infant—direct visual contact, avoidance of eye contact, or looking at other people or objects?

How comfortable do the parents appear in terms of caring for the infant? Do they express any concern regarding their ability or disgust for certain activities, such as changing diapers?

What type of affection do they demonstrate to the newborn, such as smiling, stroking, kissing, or rocking?

If the infant is fussy, what kinds of comforting techniques do the parents use, such as rocking, swaddling, talking, or stroking?

demonstrated that immediate contact after birth is essential for the human parent-child relationship.

Parents who desire but are unable to have early contact with their newborn can be reassured that such contact is not essential for optimal parent-infant interactions. Otherwise, adopted infants would not form the usual affectional ties with their parents. Nor does the mode of infant-mother contact after birth (i.e., skin-to-skin versus wrapped) appear to have any important effect. Nurses need to counsel parents that the emotional bond to the infant is not necessarily weaker because they missed early contact or because the contact was not skin-to-skin. Opportunities for parents to be with the infant in the intensive care nursery, to touch or hold the baby (if at all possible), and to receive reports of the infant's progress must be part of the nursing plan of care. Nurses need to stress that the parent-infant relationship is a process that occurs over time.

Extended Contact. The provision of rooming-in facilities for the mother and her baby is common in family-centered care. The infant is transferred to the area from the transitional nursery (if the facility uses one) after showing satisfactory extrauterine adjustment. The father is encouraged to participate in the care of the infant, and siblings and grandparents are also encouraged to visit and become acquainted with the infant. Whether the method of family-centered care is rooming-in or a family birth unit, mothers and their partners are considered equal and integral parts of the developing family. Partners are encouraged to take as active a role as they wish. Some hospitals arrange for the discharge of the mother and infant any time from 2 to 24 hours after the birth if the condition of the mother and that of the child warrant it. Follow-up care with nursing personnel from a home health care agency is usually part of this plan.

Extended contact with the infant should be available for all parents but especially for those at risk for parenting inadequacies, such as adolescents and low-income women. Any activity that optimizes family-centered care is worthy of serious consideration by postpartum nurses. Baby Friendly status for a hospital is one means to promote family-centered care.

The Baby Friendly Hospital Initiative, sponsored by the World Health Organization and UNICEF, was founded to encourage institutions to offer optimal levels of care for lactating mothers. When a hospital achieves *The Ten Steps to Successful Breastfeeding for Hospitals,* it is recognized as a Baby Friendly Hospital. The steps include the following: having a written breastfeeding policy, training staff, informing pregnant women about the benefits of breastfeeding, initiating breastfeeding within 1 hour of birth, helping mothers maintain lactation even when separated from their infants, giving newborns only breastmilk to drink, rooming-in 24 hours a day, breastfeeding on demand, avoiding pacifiers, and promoting the establishment of breastfeeding support groups and referring mothers to them. For further information contact Baby-Friendly USA at 8 Jan Sebastian Way, No. 13, Sandwich, MA 02563; by phone at (508) 888-8044; or by e-mail at hea@capecod.net.

Communication Between Parent and Infant

The parent-infant relationship is strengthened through the use of sensual responses and abilities by both partners in the interaction. The nurse should keep in mind that there may be cultural variations in these interactive behaviors.

Touch. Touch, or the tactile sense, is used extensively by parents and other caregivers as a means of becoming acquainted with the newborn. Many mothers reach out for their infants as soon as they are born and the cord is cut. They lift them to their breasts, enfold them in their arms, and cradle them. Once the infant is close to them, they begin the exploration process with their fingertips, one of the most touch-sensitive areas of the body. Within a short time the caregiver uses the palm to caress the baby's trunk, and eventually enfolds the infant. Gentle stroking motions are used to soothe and quiet the infant; patting or gently rubbing the infant's back is a comfort after feedings. Infants also pat the mother's breast as they nurse. Both seem to enjoy sharing each other's body warmth. There is a desire by parents to touch, pick up, and hold the infant (Fig. 22-4). They comment on the softness of the baby's skin and are aware of milia and rashes. As parents become increasingly sensitive to the infant's like or dislike of different types of touch, they draw closer to their baby.

Variations in touching behaviors have been noted in mothers from different cultural groups (Galanti, 1991; Inman, 1996; Jambunathan and Stewart, 1995; Jiménez, 1995). For example, minimal touching and cuddling is a traditional Southeast Asian practice thought to protect the infant from evil spirits. Because they hold different traditions and spiritual beliefs, women in India and Bali have practiced infant massage since ancient times.

Eye-to-Eye Contact. Interest in having eye contact with the baby has been demonstrated repeatedly by parents. Some mothers remark that once their babies have looked at them, they feel much closer to them. Parents spend much time getting their babies to open their eyes and look at them. In American culture, eye contact appears to cement the development of a trusting relationship, and is an important factor in human relationships at all ages. In other cultures, eye-to-eye contact may be perceived differently. For example, in Mexican culture, sustained direct eye contact is considered to be rude, immodest, and dangerous for some. This danger may arise from the *mal ojo* ("evil eye"), resulting from excessive admiration. Women and children are thought to be more susceptible to the mal ojo (Geissler, 1994).

As newborns become functionally able to sustain eye contact with their parents, time is spent in mutual gazing, often in the en face position. In this position, the parent's face and the infant's face are approximately 8 inches apart and on the same plane (Fig. 22-5). Nursing and medical practices need to be implemented that encourage this interaction. Immediately after birth, for example, the infant can be positioned on the mother's abdomen or breasts with the mother's and the infant's faces on the same plane so that they can easily make eye contact. Lights can be dimmed so that the infant's eyes will open. Instillation of prophylactic antibiotic ointment in the infant's eyes can be de-

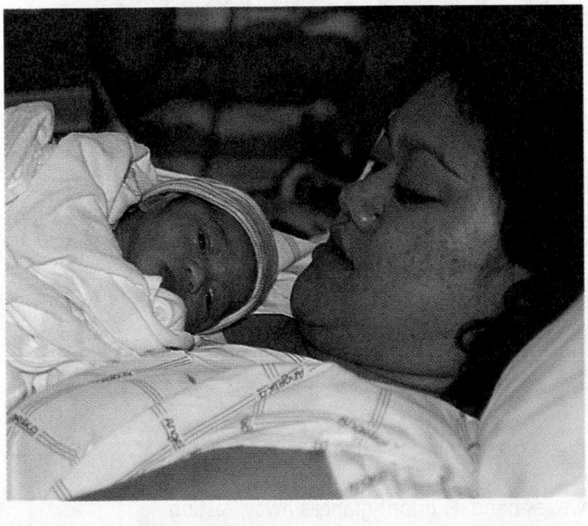

FIG. 22-4 • Mother interacts with newborn. (Courtesy Judy Bamber, San Jose, CA.)

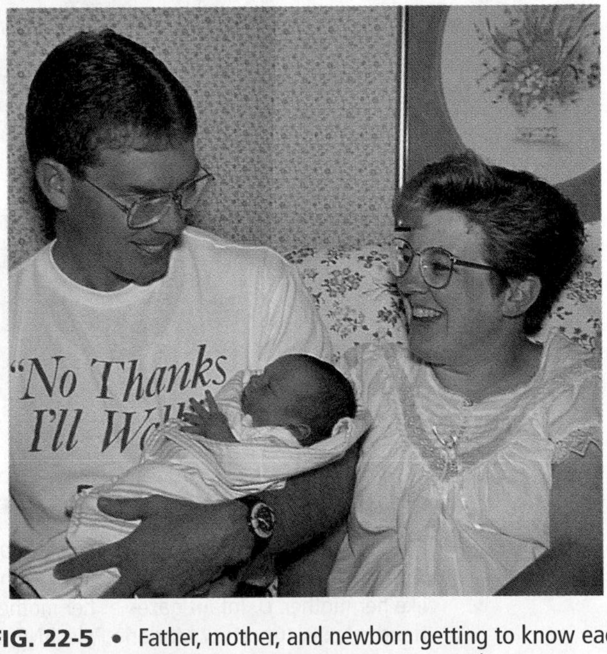

FIG. 22-5 • Father, mother, and newborn getting to know each other. (Courtesy Michael S. Clement, MD, Mesa, AZ.)

layed until the infant and parents have had some time together in the first hour after birth.

Voice. The shared response of parents and infants to each other's voices is also remarkable. Parents wait tensely for the first cry. Once that cry has reassured them of the baby's health, they begin comforting behaviors. As the parents talk in high-pitched voices, the infant is alerted and turns toward them.

The infant responds to higher-pitched voices, and can distinguish the mother's voice from others soon after birth. Infants use their cries to signal hunger, pain, boredom, and tiredness. With experience, parents learn to distinguish such cries.

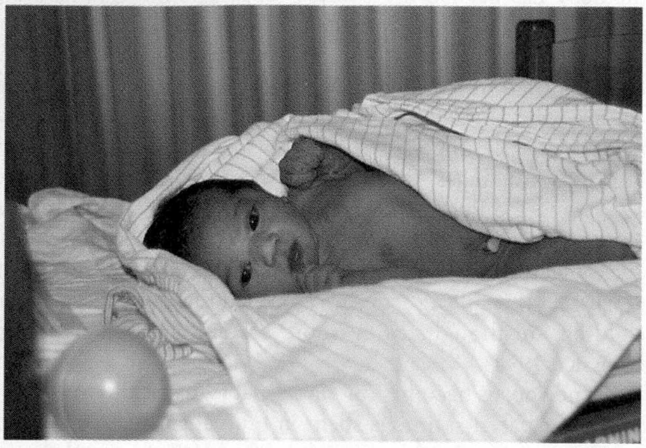

FIG. 22-6 • Infant in alert state. (Courtesy Marjorie Pyle, RNC, Lifecircle, Costa Mesa, CA.)

Odor. Another behavior shared by parents and infants is a response to each other's odor. Mothers comment on the smell of their babies when first born, and have noted that each infant has a unique odor. Infants learn rapidly to distinguish the odor of their mother's breast milk.

Entrainment. Newborns move in time with the structure of adult speech. They wave their arms, lift their heads, and kick their legs, seemingly "dancing in tune" to a parent's voice. Culturally determined rhythms of speech are ingrained in the infant long before spoken language is used to communicate. This shared rhythm also gives the parent positive feedback and establishes a positive setting for effective communication.

Biorhythmicity. The fetus is in tune with the mother's natural rhythms, such as heartbeats. After birth, a crying infant may be soothed by being held in a position where the mother's heartbeat can be heard or by hearing a recording of a heartbeat. One of the newborn's tasks is to establish a personal biorhythm. Parents can help in this process by giving consistent loving care and by using their infant's alert state to develop responsive behavior and thereby increase social interactions and opportunities for learning (Fig. 22-6). The more quickly parents become competent in child care activities, the more quickly their psychologic energy can be directed toward observing the communication cues the infant gives them.

Reciprocity and Synchrony. Reciprocity is a type of body movement or behavior that provides the observer with cues. The observer or receiver interprets those cues and responds to them. Reciprocity often takes several weeks to develop with a new baby. For example, when the newborn fusses and cries, the mother responds by picking up and cradling the

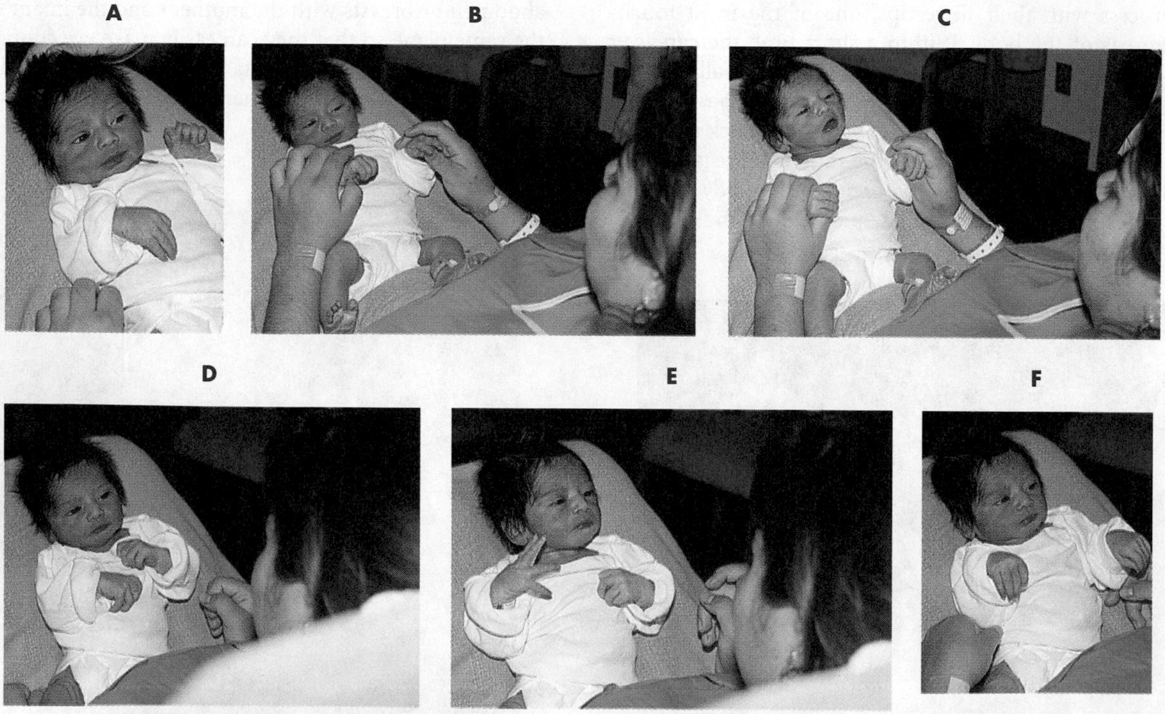

FIG. 22-7 • Holding newborn in en face position, mother works to alert her daughter, 6 hours old. **A,** Infant is quiet and alert. **B,** Mother begins talking to daughter. **C,** Infant responds, opens mouth like her mother. **D,** Infant gazes at her mother. **E,** Infant waves hand. **F,** Infant glances away, resting. Hand relaxes. (Courtesy Marjorie Pyle, RNC, Lifecircle, Costa Mesa, CA.)

infant; the baby becomes quiet and alert and establishes eye contact; the mother verbalizes, sings, and coos while the baby maintains eye contact. The baby then averts the eyes and yawns; the mother decreases her active response (Fig. 22-7). If the parent continues to stimulate the infant, the baby may become fussy.

Synchrony refers to the "fit" between the infant's cues and the parent's response. When parent and infant experience a synchronous interaction, it is mutually rewarding (Fig. 22-8). Parents need time to interpret the infant's cues correctly. For example, after a certain time the infant develops a specific cry in response to different situations such as boredom, loneliness, hunger, and discomfort. The parent may need assistance in deciphering these cries, along with trial and error interventions, before synchrony develops.

Parental Role After Childbirth

Adaptation involves a stabilizing of tasks, a coming to terms with commitments. Parents demonstrate growing competence in child care activities and are more attuned to their infant's behavior. Typically, the period from the decision to conceive through the first months of having a child is termed the transition to parenthood.

Transition to Parenthood. Historically, the transition to parenthood was viewed as a crisis. The current perspective is that parenthood is a developmental transition (Tomlinson, 1996) rather than a major life crisis for the majority of families. The transition to parenthood is described as a time of disorder and disequilibrium, as well as satisfaction, for mothers and their partners (Rogan et al, 1997; Sethi, 1995; Tomlinson, 1996). Usual methods of coping often seem ineffective. Some parents can be so distressed that they are unable to be supportive of each other. Since men typically identify their spouses as their primary or only source of support, the transition can be harder for the fathers, who feel deprived because the mothers, who are also experiencing stress, cannot provide their usual level of support. Strong emotions such as the helplessness, inadequacy, and anger that arise when dealing with a crying infant catch many parents unprepared. On the other hand, parenthood allows adults to develop and display a selfless, warm, and caring side of themselves that may not be expressed in other adult roles. To view the world through the eyes of a child and to be childlike (not childish) are two rich rewards of parenthood.

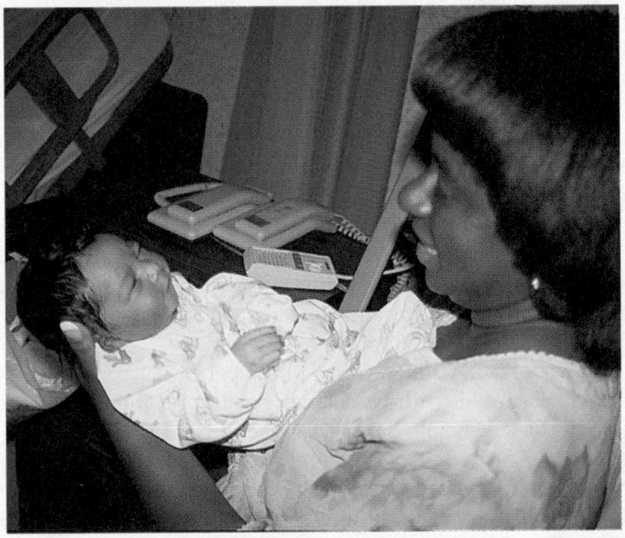

FIG. 22-8 • Sharing a smile: example of synchrony. (Courtesy Marjorie Pyle, RNC, Lifecircle, Costa Mesa, CA.)

For the majority of mothers and their partners, the transition to parenthood is viewed as an opportunity rather than a time of danger. Parents are stimulated to try new coping strategies as they work to master their new roles and reach new developmental levels. As they work through the transition, personal strength and resourcefulness are revealed (Rogan et al, 1997).

Parental Tasks and Responsibilities. Parents need to reconcile the actual child with the fantasy and dream child. This means coming to terms with the infant's physical appearance, sex, innate temperament, and physical status. If the real child differs greatly from the fantasy child, parents may delay acceptance of the child. In some instances, they may never accept the child.

Some parents are startled by the normal appearance of the neonate—the size, color, molding of the head, or bowed appearance of the legs. Many fathers have commented that they thought the odd shape of the infant's head (molding) meant the infant would be mentally retarded.

Many parents know the sex of the infant before birth because of ultrasound assessments; for those who do not have this information, disappointment over the sex of the infant can take time to resolve. The parents may provide adequate physical care but find it difficult to be sincerely involved with the infant until this internal conflict has been resolved. As one mother remarked, "I really wanted a boy. I know it is silly and irrational, but when they said, 'She's a lovely little girl,' I was so disappointed and angry—yes, angry—I could hardly look at her. Oh, I looked after her okay, her feedings and baths and things, but I couldn't feel excited. To tell the truth, I felt like a monster not liking my child. Then one day she was lying there and she turned her head and looked right at me. I felt a flooding of love for her come over me, and we looked at each other a long time. It's okay now. I wouldn't change her for all the boys in the world."

Parents need to become adept in the care of the infant, including caregiving activities, noting the communication cues given by the infant to indicate needs, and responding appropriately to the infant's needs. Self-esteem grows with competence. Breastfeeding makes mothers feel they are contributing in a unique way to the welfare of the infant. The infant's response to the parental care and attention may be interpreted by the parent as a comment on the quality of that care. Infant behaviors that are interpreted by parents as positive responses to their care include being consoled easily, enjoying being cuddled, and making eye contact. Spitting up frequently after feedings, crying, and being unpredictable may be perceived as negative responses to parental care. Continuation of these infant responses that are viewed as negative can result in alienation of parent and infant to the detriment of the infant.

Assistance, including advice by husbands, partners, wives, mothers, mothers-in-law, and professional workers, can either be seen as supportive or an indication of how inept these others judge the new parents to be. Criticism, real or imagined, of the new parents' ability to provide adequate physical care, nutrition, or social stimulation for the infant can prove devastating. By providing encouragement and praise for parenting efforts, nurses can bolster the new parents' confidence.

Parents must establish a place for the newborn within the family group. Whether the infant is the firstborn or the last born, all family members must adjust their roles to accommodate the newcomer. The firstborn child needs support to accept a rival for parental affections. An older child needs help dealing with losing a favored position in the family hierarchy. The parents are expected to negotiate these changes.

Maternal Adjustment. Three phases are evident as the mother adjusts to her parental role. These phases are characterized by dependent behavior, dependent-independent behavior, and interdependent behavior (Table 22-2).

Dependent Phase. During the first 24 to 48 hours after childbirth the mother's dependency needs predominate. To the extent that these needs are met by others, the mother is able to divert her psychologic energy to her infant rather than to focus it on herself. She needs "mothering" herself to "mother." Rubin (1961) aptly described these few days as the taking-in phase, a time when nurturing and protective care are required by the new mother. In Rubin's classic description, the taking-in phase lasted 2 to 3 days. Later studies found that women move more rapidly through the taking-in phase (Ament, 1990; Wrasper, 1996). Evans and colleagues (1998), in a study of women giving birth vaginally, found that both taking-in and taking-hold (see next section) were present on the evening of birth. There were small decreases in taking-in and small increases in taking-hold between the evening of birth and the first morning after.

TABLE 22-2
Phases of Maternal Postpartum Adjustment

Phase	Characteristics
Dependent: taking-in*	• First 24 hours (range of 1 to 2 days) • Focus: self and meeting of basic needs • Reliance on others to meet needs for comfort, rest, closeness, and nourishment • Excited and talkative • Desire to review birth experience
Dependent-independent: taking-hold*	• Starts second or third day; lasts 10 days to several weeks • Focus: care of baby and competent mothering • Desire to take charge • Still need for nurturing and acceptance by others • Eagerness to learn and practice—optimal period for teaching by nurses • Handling of physical discomforts and emotional changes • Possible experience with "blues"
Interdependent: letting go*	• Focus: forward movement of family as unit with interacting members • Reassertion of relationship with partner • Resumption of sexual intimacy • Resolution of individual roles

*From Rubin R: Basic maternal behavior, *Nurs Outlook 9*, 683-686, 1961.

This dependent phase is a time of great excitement during which parents need to verbalize their experience of pregnancy and birth. Focusing on, analyzing, and accepting these experiences helps the parents move on to the next phase. Some parents use staff members or other mothers as an audience, whereas others are more comfortable talking with family and friends about the pregnancy and birth experience.

Because anxiety and preoccupation with her new role often narrow a mother's perceptions, information may have to be repeated. The new mother may require reminders to rest or, conversely, to ambulate enough to promote recovery.

Physical discomfort can interfere with the mother's need for rest and relaxation. The selective use of comfort measures and medication depends on the nurse. Many women hesitate to ask for medication, believing that any pain they experience is normal and to be expected; breastfeeding mothers may fear the effects of medication on the infant.

Dependent-Independent Phase. If the mother has received adequate nurturing in the first few hours or days, by the second or third day, her desire for independent action reasserts itself. In the dependent-independent phase, the mother alternates between a need for extensive nurturing and acceptance by others and the desire to "take charge" once again. She responds enthusiastically to opportunities to learn and to practice baby care or, if she is an accomplished mother, to carry out or direct this care (Mercer and Ferketich, 1995). Rubin (1961) described this phase as the taking-hold phase, and noted that it lasts approximately 10 days. Evans and associates (1998) found that taking-hold behaviors began increasing between the evening of birth and the first morning despite high levels of sleep disturbance. Childbirth preparation classes, early contact with the newborn, rooming-in, and early discharge are some of the current obstetric practices that seem to enhance taking-hold behaviors (Martell, 1996; Wrasper, 1996).

Most mothers are discharged home during this dependent-independent phase. Once home, mothers must continue to cope with physical adaptations and psychologic adjustments.

Prenatally and postnatally, nurses can discuss common postpartal concerns that mothers experience. They can provide anticipatory guidance on coping strategies, such as resting when the infant sleeps or planning with an extended family member or friend to do the housework for the first week or two after the baby is born. Once a mother is home, periodic phone calls from a nurse who cared for her in the birth setting can provide the mother with an opportunity to vent her concerns and get support and advice from "her" nurse. First-time mothers inexperienced in child care, women whose careers had provided outside stimulation, women who lack friends or family members with whom to share delights and concerns, and adolescent mothers may need additional supportive counseling.

Postpartum Blues. The "pink" period surrounding the first day or two after birth, characterized by heightened joy and feelings of well-being, is often followed by a "blue" period. Approximately 75% to 80% of women experience the postpartum blues or "baby blues" (Albright, 1993; Wood et al, 1997) that occur in women of all ethnic and racial groups (Campbell, 1992). During the blues, women are emotionally labile, often crying easily and for no apparent reason. This lability seems to peak around the fifth day, subsiding by the tenth day. Other symptoms of postpartum blues include depression, a let-down feeling, restlessness, fatigue, insomnia, headache, anxiety, sadness, and anger. Biochemical, psychologic, social, and cultural factors have been explored as possible causes of the postpartum depressive state; however, the etiology remains unknown. Whatever the cause, the early postpartum period appears to be one of emotional and physical vulnerability for new mothers, who may be psychologically overwhelmed by the reality of parental responsibilities. The mother may feel deprived of the supportive care she received from family members and friends during pregnancy. Some mothers regret the loss of the mother-unborn child relationship and mourn its passing. Still others experience a let-down feeling when labor and birth are complete. Fatigue after childbirth is compounded by the around-the-clock demands of the new baby and can accentuate the feelings of depression. A lowered level of circulating glucocorticoids or a subclinical hypothyroidism may exist during the puerperium. Postpartum depressive symptoms can have a negative effect on maternal role attainment (Fowles, 1998). To help mothers cope with postpartum blues, nurses can suggest various strategies (Patient Teaching box).

"Am I Blue?" (Johnson & Johnson, 1996), a self-administered questionnaire, can help mothers to assess their level of "blues" and to decide when to seek advice from their nurse, nurse-midwife, or physician (Fig. 22-9). Home visits and telephone follow-up calls by the nurse are important to assess the mother's pattern of "blue" feelings and behavior over time.

Although the postpartum blues are usually mild and short lived, approximately 10% to 15% of women experience a more severe syndrome called postpartum depression (PPD) (Wood et al, 1997) (see Chapter 23). The symptoms can range from mild to severe, with women having "good days" and "bad days." All symptoms can be equally distressing and make the woman feel as if she is "going mad." PPD leaves the woman with feelings of failure, overwhelming guilt, loneliness, and low self-esteem. Nurses need to teach women how to differentiate symptoms of the "blues" and PPD, and should urge women to report depressive symptoms promptly if they occur.

Patient Teaching

COPING WITH POSTPARTUM BLUES

- Remember that the "blues" are normal.
- Get plenty of rest; nap when the baby does if possible. Go to bed early, and let friends know when to visit.
- Use relaxation techniques learned in childbirth classes (or ask the nurse to teach you and your partner some techniques).
- Do something for yourself. Take advantage of the time your partner or family members care for the baby—soak in the tub or go for a walk.
- Plan a day out of the house—go to the mall with the baby, being sure to take a stroller or carriage, or go out to eat with friends without the baby. Many communities have churches or other agencies that provide child care programs such as Mothers' Morning Out.
- Talk to your partner about the way you feel—for example, about feeling tied down, how the birth met your expectations, and things that will help you.
- If you are breastfeeding, give yourself and your baby time to learn.
- Seek out and use community resources such as La Leche League or community mental health centers. One nationally recognized resource is:
  Postpartum Support International
  927 North Kellogg Avenue
  Santa Barbara, CA 93111
  (805) 967-7636

Interdependent Phase. In this phase, interdependent behavior reasserts itself, and the mother and her family move forward as a unit with interacting members. The relationship of the partners, although altered by the introduction of a baby, resumes many of its former characteristics. A primary need is to establish a lifestyle that includes but in some respects also excludes the baby. The couple needs to share interests and activities that are adult in scope.

The couple may begin to engage in sexual intercourse during the second to fourth week after the baby is born. Some couples begin earlier, as soon as it can be accomplished without discomfort, depending on factors such as timing, amount of vaginal dryness, and breastfeeding status. Sexual intimacy enhances the adult aspect of the family, and the adult pair shares a closeness denied to other family members. Many new fathers speak of the alienation experienced when they observe the intimate mother-infant relationship, and some are frank in expressing feelings of jealousy toward the infant. The resumption of sexual intimacy seems to bring the parents' relationship back into focus.

The interdependent phase, termed the letting-go phase, is often stressful for the parental pair. Interests and needs often diverge during this time. Women and their partners must resolve the effects on their relationship of their individual roles related to child rearing, homemaking, and careers. Mothers (and partners) may take a more traditional role in an effort to adapt to parenthood; however, traditional women have reported more family disorganization months into parenthood (Tomlinson and Irwin, 1993). A special continuing effort has to be made to strengthen the adult-adult relationship as a basis for the family unit.

Little is known about postpartum maternal adjustment in the lesbian couple. Relationship satisfaction in first-time lesbian parent couples appears related to egalitarianism, commitment, sexual compatibility, and communication skills, as well as to the birth mother's decision for insemination by an anonymous sperm donor (Osterwell, 1991). Similar to heterosexual parent couples, most lesbian parent couples voice concern about less time and energy for their relationship after the arrival of the baby (Gartrell et al, 1996). Both partners consider themselves to be equal parents of the baby when they share actively in child rearing (Brewaeys et al, 1995).

Paternal Adjustment. Research on paternal adjustment to parenthood indicates that fathers go through predictable phases during their transition to parenthood (Henderson and Brouse, 1991). During this period, fathers experience intense emotions (Box 22-1). Many fathers acknowledge that their expectations were of limited value once they were immersed in the reality of parenthood. Feelings that often accompany this reality are sadness, ambivalence, jealousy, frustration at not being able to participate in breastfeeding, and an overwhelming desire to be more involved; most of these are different from the feelings mothers report. On the other hand, some fathers are pleasantly surprised at the ease and fun of parenting. In their transition to mastery, fathers take control and become more actively involved in the infant's life.

Am I Blue?

Many new mothers feel anxious, sad, or angry about the changes in their lives after the birth of their new baby. It is perfectly normal to feel this way, but sometimes the feelings grow so strong that they make life difficult. This quiz lists many feelings and experiences of "blue" or depressed mothers. Mark how strong each of these feelings or experiences is for you, compared with what is normal for you. For example: Do you feel no anger [0]; mild (very little) anger [1]; moderate (some) anger [2]; or severe (very strong) anger [3] compared with the way you usually feel? Add up your total score when you are finished, and discuss the results with your health care provider.

0 = Not there at all 1 = Mild 2 = Moderate 3 = Severe	0	1	2	3
Anger				
Anxiety attacks: periods of very strong fear, shortness of breath, rapid heartbeat				
Increased or decreased appetite and/or weight gain or loss that doesn't seem normal				
Strong feeling that you need to get away, need more time for your own interests				
Problems in a relationship with a family member, lover, close friend, etc.				
Crying spells				
Less interest in your personal appearance				
Less motivation—less energy or interest in accomplishing goals				
Depression				
Fatigue—feeling tired or exhausted				
Fear of harming yourself or your baby				
Loss of your sense of humor				
Nervousness, feeling tense or edgy				
Feelings of guilt				
Feelings of panic				
Feeling alone or lonely; without the support of others				
Feeling no love, or not enough love, for your baby				
Feeling forgetful, distracted, absent-minded—having trouble concentrating				
Frustration				
Hopelessness				
Insomnia				
Feeling irritable, bad-tempered				
Loss of sexual desire and/or pleasure in sex				
Loss of self-respect or confidence—feeling like you don't count or can't do anything right				
Feeling confused, uncertain				
Mood swings—your moods and emotions change all the time				
Obsessive thoughts—ideas or feelings you can't stop from repeating in your mind				
Odd or frightening thoughts—thoughts or images that scare you or that you can't control				
Thoughts of suicide, feeling like you want to die				
Feeling sad, unhappy				
				TOTAL

SCORE:

0 – 31 = MILD BLUES
This will probably pass, but pay attention to your feelings and needs.

32 – 64 = MODERATE BLUES
You may want to ask for help from a close friend or family member, or ask the advice of your health care provider.

65 – 98 = SEVERE BLUES
You could be depressed; see your health care provider for a check-up and advice as soon as possible.

If you are afraid you might harm yourself or your baby—ask a health care provider you trust for help— you don't have to be alone!

FIG. 22-9 • Am I Blue? (Courtesy Johnson & Johnson Consumer Products, Skillman, NJ.)

Box 22-1

Paternal Adjustment to Fatherhood

Fathers as well as mothers are affected emotionally by the birth of an infant. For example, *The News Tribune* of Tacoma reported that Vin Baker, a professional basketball player, is receiving counseling for depression. Baker said that he is "fighting a lot of depression now and coping with a lot of different things." He has been removed from the starting lineup, which has been difficult. He also cites that becoming a father was stressful. "I was sitting at home, I was in tears, I was crying all day."

Modified from the *Richmond Times-Tribune,* April 17, 2000, p. C9.

Community Focus

FATHERS' EXPERIENCE OF LABOR AND POSTPARTUM

In Western industrialized countries, the trend is for fathers to be present at childbirth. Fathers who attended childbirth classes, and who use avoidance when confronted with threat, experience childbirth as less fulfilling than fathers who cope similarly but do not attend classes. Fathers who reported childbirth as being fulfilling and a delight were less depressed at 6 weeks postpartum. Babies born by cesarean were described more negatively at 6 weeks postpartum when compared with babies born vaginally. More married fathers attended classes and were less depressed than unmarried fathers. Thus it appears that for some fathers, attending prenatal classes is beneficial; for others it may not be. In addition, fathers' experience of childbirth may influence later emotional well-being. Nurses involved in prenatal preparation of families for childbirth need to take into consideration various needs and wishes of individual members. Whereas education may be encouraged to reduce anxiety and fear related to the unknown, attending classes is not the best strategy for some men. For these men, childbirth preparation must be individualized based on expressed needs and wishes.

Data from Greenhalgh R, Slade P, Spiby H: Fathers' coping style, antenatal preparation, and experiences of labor and the postpartum, *Birth* 27(3):177-184, 2000.

First-time fathers perceive the first 4 to 10 weeks of parenthood in much the same way that mothers do, that is, as a period characterized by uncertainty, increased responsibility, disruption of sleep, and inability to control time needed to care for the infant and reestablish the marital dyad. Fathers express concern about decreased attention from their partners relative to their personal relationship, the mother's lack of recognition of the father's desire to participate in decision making for the infant, and limited time available to establish a relationship with their infants. These concerns can precipitate feelings of jealousy of the infant. Discussing their needs with the partner and becoming more involved with their infants and partner can help alleviate such feelings of jealousy.

Father-Infant Relationship. In American culture, neonates have a powerful impact on their fathers, who become intensely involved with their babies (Fig. 22-10). The term used for the father's absorption, preoccupation, and interest in the infant is engrossment. Characteristics of engrossment include some of the sensual responses relating to touch and eye-to-eye contact that have been discussed earlier; and also the father's keen awareness of features both unique and similar to himself that validate his claim to the infant. An outstanding response is one of strong attraction to the newborn. Fathers spend considerable time "communicating" with the infant and taking delight in the infant's response to them. A sense of increased self-esteem and a sense of being proud, bigger, more mature, and older are all experienced by fathers after seeing their baby for the first time.

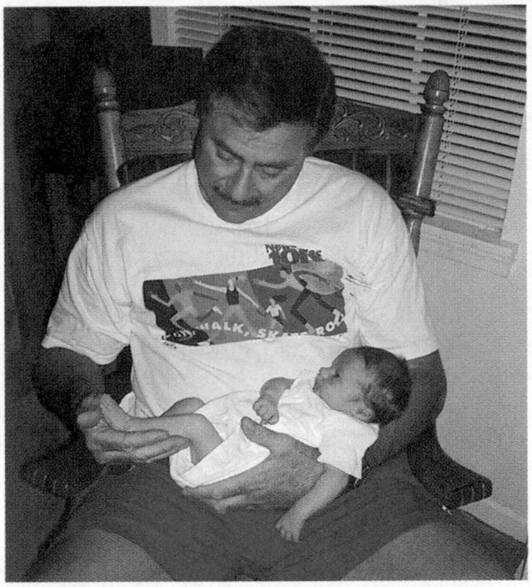

FIG. 22-10 • Engrossment. Father absorbed in looking at his newborn. (Courtesy Leslie Canerday, Phoenix, AZ.)

Fathers spend less time than mothers with infants, and fathers' interactions with their infants tend to be characterized by stimulating social play rather than caretaking. The subtle and more open differences in stimulation from two sources, mother and father, provide a wider social experience for the infant.

Impact of Fatherhood. For Caucasian, middle-class, American males, first-time fatherhood is seen as a maturing event during which increased responsibility is assumed. Fathers report taking their work more seriously while trying to balance work and family demands. These men experience an identity change, developing an image of themselves as fathers. Over time, they develop strong bonds with their infants and feel a sense of fulfillment and purpose in life.

Despite their active involvement in the perinatal period, fathers tend to gravitate toward a more traditional division of family responsibilities. One reason for this return to more traditional roles may be the new father's concerns about his ability to financially support his new family. As a first-time father explained: "[Child care] costs much more than I expected. The cost was amazing. I would have never guessed how much of a drain child care could put on our income" (Leventhal-Belfer, Cowan, and Cowan, 1992).

Fathers can benefit from nursing interventions during the postpartum period just as mothers can. Nurses can arrange to teach infant care when the father is present, and provide anticipatory guidance for fathers about the transition to parenthood. Separate prenatal and parenting classes and parenting support groups for fathers can provide them with an opportunity to discuss their concerns and have some of their needs met. Postpartum phone calls and home visits by the nurse should include time for assessment of the father's adjustment and needs.

Factors Influencing Parental Responses

The way parents respond to the birth of their child is influenced by various factors, including age, social networks, socioeconomic conditions, and personal aspirations of the future.

Age. Maternal age has a definite effect on the outcome of pregnancy. The mother, fetus, and newborn are at highest risk when the mother is an adolescent or is more than 35 years old.

The Adolescent Mother. Although it is biologically possible for the adolescent female to become a parent, her egocentricity and concrete thinking interfere with her ability to parent effectively. The very young adolescent mother is inexperienced and unprepared to recognize the early signs of illness, potential danger, or household hazards. She may inadvertently neglect her child. The higher mortality rates among the infants of adolescent mothers are attributed to the inexperience, lack of knowledge, and immaturity of the mothers, causing them to be unable to recognize a problem and obtain the necessary resources to rectify the situation. Nevertheless, in most instances, with adequate support and developmentally appropriate teaching, adolescents can learn effective parenting skills.

The transition to parenthood may be difficult for adolescent parents. Coping with the developmental tasks of parenthood is often complicated by the unmet developmental needs and tasks of adolescence. Some young parents may experience difficulty accepting a changing self-image and adjusting to new roles related to the responsibilities of infant care. Other adolescent parents, however, may have higher self-concepts than their non-parenting peers (Alpers, 1998).

As adolescent parents move through the transition to parenthood, they may feel different from their peers, excluded from fun activities, and prematurely forced to enter an adult social role. The conflict between their own desires and the infant's demands, in addition to the low tolerance for frustration that is typical of adolescence, further contribute to the normal psychosocial stress of childbirth. Lower maternal education is associated with less favorable maternal responses to distress and infant behavior (Diehl, 1997).

Maintaining a relationship with the baby's father is beneficial for the teen mother and her infant. A close and satisfying relationship is positively correlated with maternal-fetal and maternal-infant attachment (Bloom, 1998). The involvement of the baby's father is related to appropriate maternal behaviors and positive mother-infant relationship (Diehl, 1997).

> ## Critical Thinking
>
> **POSTPARTUM ADJUSTMENT FOR THE ADOLESCENT**
>
> **Carol is a 15-year-old first time mother of a 5-day old girl; she lives with her mother. The father of the baby, Robert, is 17 years old and attended childbirth classes with Carol. She is breastfeeding the baby, but told the nurse the baby sucks too slowly and takes too much time to eat. She also said she thinks the baby should know enough to sleep longer at night. Robert would like to feed the baby some cereal, since he heard that will make a baby sleep longer at night. What teaching does this couple need? How will you determine their knowledge deficits? Whose assistance can you solicit to assist this young couple? To whom can you refer them?**

Adolescent mothers provide warm and attentive physical care; however, they use less verbal interaction than do older parents, and adolescents tend to be less responsive and to interact less positively with their infants than do older mothers (Barratt and Roach, 1995; Thompson et al, 1995). Interventions emphasizing verbal and nonverbal communication skills between mother and infant are important. Such intervention strategies must be concrete and specific because of the cognitive level of adolescents. Although some observers suggest that some adolescents may use more aggressive behaviors, a higher incidence of child abuse has not been documented. In comparison with adult mothers, teenage mothers have a limited knowledge of child development. They tend to expect too much of their children too soon, and often characterize their infants as being fussy. This limited knowledge may cause teenagers to respond to their infants inappropriately.

The need for continued assessment of the new mother's parenting abilities during this postbirth period is essential. In addition, continued support should also be provided by involving the grandparents and other family members, as well as through home visits and group sessions for discussion of infant care and parenting problems. Outreach programs concerned with self-care, parent-child interactions, child injuries, and failure to thrive—in addition to programs that provide prompt and effective community intervention—prevent more serious problems from occurring. As the adolescent performs her mothering role within the framework of her family, she may need to address dependency versus independency issues. The adolescent's family members may also need help adapting to their new roles.

The Adolescent Father. The adolescent father and mother face immediate developmental crises, which include completing the developmental tasks of adolescence, making a transition to parenthood, and sometimes adapting to marriage. These transitions can be stressful. The nurse may initiate interaction with the adolescent father by asking him to be present when postpartum home visits are made, and to accompany the mother and the baby to well-baby checks at the clinic or pediatrician's office. With the adolescent mother's agreement, the nurse may contact the father directly. Adolescent fathers need support to discuss their emotional responses to the pregnancy. The father's feelings of guilt, powerlessness, or bravado should be recognized because of their negative consequences for both the parents and the child. Counseling of adolescent fathers needs to be reality oriented. Topics such as finances, child care, parenting skills, and the father's role in the birth experience need to be discussed. Teenage fathers also need to know about reproductive physiology and birth control options as well as safer sex practices.

The adolescent father may continue to be involved in an ongoing relationship with the young mother and his baby. In many instances he also plays an important role in the decisions about child care and raising the child. He may need help to develop realistic perceptions of his role as father to a child. He is encouraged to use coping mechanisms that are not detrimental to his own, his partner's, or his child's well-being. The nurse enlists support systems, parents, and professional agencies on his behalf.

Maternal Age Greater Than 35 Years. Older mothers have unique needs related to increased biologic risk. Higher rates of gestational diabetes, pregnancy-induced hypertension, gestational bleeding, abruptio placentae, and intrapartal fetal distress have been reported (Berkowitz et al, 1990; Fretts et al, 1995; Gilbert, Nesbitt and Danielson, 1999). Many of these mothers, because they are less physically resilient than younger women, may have a longer recovery period.

Adjustment of older mothers to changes involved in becoming a parent and seeing themselves as competent is aided by support from their partners. Support from other family members and friends is also important for positive self-evaluation of parenting, for a sense of well-being and satisfaction, and will help in dealing with stress.

Changes in the sexual aspect of a relationship can create a stressor for new midlife parents. Mothers report that finding time and energy for a romantic rendezvous is more difficult. They attribute much of this to the reality of caring for an infant, but the decreasing libido that normally accompanies getting older contributes.

Work/career issues are sources of conflict for older mothers (Reese and Harkless, 1996). Conflicts emerge over being disinterested in work, worrying about giving enough attention to work with the distractions of a new baby, and anticipating what it will be like to return to work. Child care is a major factor causing stress about work.

Another major issue for older mothers with careers is the perception of loss of control (Reese and Harkless, 1996). Mothers older than 35, when compared with younger mothers, are at a different stage in their careers, having attained high levels of education, career, and income. The loss of control experienced when going from the consistency of a work role to the inconsistency of the parent role comes as a surprise to many. Helping the older mother have realistic expectations of herself and of parenthood is essential.

New mothers who are also perimenopausal may find it hard to distinguish fatigue, loss of sleep, decreased libido, or other physiologic symptoms as the causes of the change in their sex lives. Although many women view menopause as a natural stage of life, for midlife mothers this cessation of menstruation coincides with the state of parenthood. The changes of midlife and menopause can add more emotional and physical stress to older mothers' lives because of the time- and energy-consuming aspects of raising a young child (Cain, 1994). Resources that older parents may find helpful are listed in Box 22-2.

Paternal Age Greater Than 35 Years. Looking back, older fathers described their experience of midlife parenting as wonderful but not without drawbacks. What they saw as positive aspects of parenthood in older years included increased love and commitment between the spouses, a reinforcement of why one married in the first place, a feeling of being complete, experiencing of "the child" in oneself again, more financial stability than in younger years, and more freedom to focus on parenting rather than on career. A common theme expressed was sharing: sharing joy, sharing in raising the child, sharing as a family. The main drawback of midlife parenting that these men reported was the change that it made in the relationships with their partners. They missed the deeper and more selfish couple relationship, and looked forward to the time when they could have that again (Cain, 1994).

Culture. Cultural beliefs and practices are important determinants of parenting behaviors. Culture defines what is socially acceptable in terms of eye contact, touch, and space (Lipson, Dibble, and Minarik, 1996). Culture influences the interactions with the baby as well as the parent's or family's caregiving style. For example, the provision for a period of rest and recuperation for the mother after birth is important in several cultures. Asian mothers must remain at home with the baby at least 30 days after birth, and are not supposed to engage in household chores, including care of the baby. Many times the grandmother takes over the baby's care immediately, even before discharge from the hospital (Geissler, 1994). Likewise, Jordanian mothers have a 40-day lying-in after birth, during which their mothers or sisters care for the baby (Geissler, 1994). Hispanics practice an intergenerational family ritual, *la cuarentena.* For 40 days after birth, the mother is expected to recuperate and get acquainted with her infant. Traditionally this involves many restrictions concerning food (e.g., spicy or cold foods, fish, pork, and citrus are avoided; tortillas and chicken soup are encouraged); exercise; and activities, including sexual intercourse. Abdominal binding is a traditional practice, and many women avoid tub bathing and washing their hair. Traditional Hispanic husbands do not expect to see their wives or infants until both have been cleaned and dressed after birth. La cuarentena incorporates individuals into the family, instills parental responsibility, and integrates the family during a critical life event (Geissler, 1994; Niska, Snyder, and Lia-Hoagberg, 1998).

Desire for and valuing of children is salient in all cultures. In Asian families, children are valued as a source of family strength and stability, are perceived as wealth, and are objects of parental love and affection. Infants almost always are given an affection-

Critical Thinking

POSTPARTUM ADJUSTMENT FOR THE OLDER MOTHER

Audrey is a 36-year-old attorney who has been practicing law for 7 years. She just gave birth to her first baby; she and her husband delayed parenting by choice until their careers were well established. She had an uneventful pregnancy, labor, and birth. During a telephone call 48 hours after discharge, when the nurse asks how things are going, Audrey bursts into tears and says, "I didn't expect it to be like this! Nothing is going right." What is likely to be the cause of Audrey's statement? What assessments should the nurse make? What resources are available for Audrey? Is a home visit necessary? Is a referral necessary? What patient teaching in the hospital could have been done to help Audrey deal with her feelings and the stress of being a new parent?

Box 22-2

Resources for Older Parents

FEMALE (Formerly Employed Mother at the Leading Edge)
P.O. Box 31
Elmhurst, IL 60126
(630) 941-3553

Mothers at Home
8310A Old Courthouse Road
Vienna, VA 22182
(703) 827-5903

National Council for Adoption
(202) 328-8072

ate "cradle" name that is used during the first years of life; for example, a Filipino girl might be called "Ling-Ling" and a boy "Bong-Bong." Refer to Table 2-2 for examples of some traditional cultural beliefs that may be important to parents from African-American, Asian, and Hispanic cultures.

Knowledge of cultural beliefs can help the nurse make more accurate assessments and diagnoses of observed parenting behaviors. For example, nurses may become concerned when they observe cultural practices that appear to reflect poor maternal-infant bonding. Algerian mothers may not unwrap and explore their infants as part of the acquaintance process because in Algeria, babies are wrapped tightly in swaddling clothes to protect them physically and psychologically (Geissler, 1994). The nurse may observe a Vietnamese woman who gives minimal care to her infant but refuses to cuddle or further interact with her baby. This apparent lack of interest in the newborn is this cultural group's attempt to ward off "evil spirits," and actually reflects an intense love and concern for the infant (Galanti, 1991). An Asian mother might be criticized for almost immediately relinquishing the care of the infant to the grandmother and not even attempting to hold her baby when it is brought to her room. However, in Asian extended families, members show their support for a new mother's rest and recuperation by assisting with the care of the baby. Contrary to the guidance given to mothers in the United States about "nipple confusion," a mix of breastfeeding and bottle-feeding is standard practice for Japanese mothers. This is out of concern for the mother's rest during the first 2 to 3 months and does not lead to any problems with lactation; breastfeeding is widespread and successful among Japanese women (Sharts-Hopko, 1995).

Socioeconomic Conditions. Socioeconomic conditions often determine access to available resources. Parents whose economic condition is made worse with the birth of each child and who are unable to use an effective method of fertility management may find childbirth complicated by concern for their own health and a sense of helplessness. Mothers who are single; separated or divorced from their husbands; or without a partner, family, and friends for whatever reason may view the birth of a child with dread. Serious financial problems may override any desire for mothering the infant.

Parental Sensory Impairment

In the early dialogue between the parent and child, all senses—sight, hearing, touch, taste, and smell—are used by each to initiate and sustain the attachment process. A parent who has an impairment of one of the senses needs to maximize use of the remaining senses.

Visually Impaired Parent. Although parents who are visually impaired need the presence and the support of another responsible person, they can become adept in many child care activities. A strength that visually impaired people have is a heightened sensitivity to other sensory outputs. A blind mother can tell when her infant is facing her because she can feel the baby's breath on her face.

One of the major difficulties that visually impaired parents experience is the skepticism, open or hidden, of health care professionals. Blind people sense a reluctance on the part of others to acknowledge that they have a right to be parents. All too often, nurses and doctors lack the experience to deal with the childbearing and child-rearing needs of visually impaired mothers, as well as mothers with other disabilities (such as the hearing impaired, physically impaired, and mentally challenged). The best approach by the nurse is to assess the mother's capabilities. From that basis, the nurse can make plans to assist the woman, often in much the same way as for a mother with sight. Visually impaired mothers have made suggestions for providing care for women such as themselves during childbearing (Box 22-3). This kind of approach by the nurse can help avoid a sense of increased vulnerability on the mother's part.

Eye-to-eye contact is considered important in American culture. With a parent who is visually impaired, this critical factor in the parent-child attachment process is obviously missing. However, the blind parent, who may never have experienced this method of strengthening relationships, does not miss it. The infant will need other sensory input from that parent. An infant looking into the eyes of a mother who is blind may not be aware that the eyes are unseeing. Other people in the newborn's environment can also participate in active eye-to-eye contact to supply this need. A problem may arise, however, if the visually impaired parent has an impassive facial expression. Her infant, making repeated unsuccessful attempts to engage in face play with the mother, will abandon the behavior with her and intensify it with the father or other people in the household. Nurses can provide anticipatory guidance regarding this situation and help the mother learn to nod and smile while talking and cooing to the infant.

Hearing-Impaired Parent. The parent who has a hearing impairment faces another set of problems, particularly if the deafness dates from birth or early childhood. The mother and her partner are likely to have established an independent household. A number of devices that transform sound into light flashes are now marketed and can be fitted into the infant's room to permit immediate detection of crying. Even if the parent is not speech trained, vocalizing can serve as both a stimulus and a response to the infant's early vocalizing. Deaf parents can provide additional vocal training by use of recordings and television, so that from birth the child is aware of the full range

Box 22-3

Nursing Approaches for Working with Visually Impaired Parents

1. Parents who are blind need verbal teaching by health care providers because printed maternity information is not accessible to blind people.
2. A visually impaired parent needs an orientation to the hospital room that allows the parent to move about the room independently. For example, "Go to the left of the bed and trail the wall until you feel the first door. That is the bathroom."
3. Parents who are blind need explanations of routines.
4. Parents who are blind need to feel devices (e.g., monitors, pelvic models) and to hear descriptions of the devices.
5. Visually impaired parents need a chance to ask questions.
6. Visually impaired parents need the opportunity to hold and touch the baby after birth.
7. Nurses need to demonstrate baby care by touch and to follow with, "Now let me see you do it."
8. Nurses need to give instructions such as, "I'm going to give you the baby. The head is to your left side."

of the human voice. Sign language is acquired readily by young children, and the first sign used is as varied as the first word.

Section 504 of the Rehabilitation Act of 1973 requires that hospitals and other institutions receiving funds from the U.S. Department of Health and Human Services use various communication techniques and resources with the deaf, including having staff members or certified interpreters who are proficient in sign language. For example, provision of written materials with demonstrations and having nurses stand where the parent can read their lips (if the parent practices lipreading) are two techniques that can be used. A creative approach is for the nursing unit to develop videotapes in which information on postpartum care, infant care, and parenting issues is signed by an interpreter and spoken by a nurse. A videotape in which a nurse signs while speaking would be ideal.

SIBLING ADAPTATION

Because the family is an interactive, open unit, the addition of a new family member affects everyone in the family. Siblings have to assume new positions within the family hierarchy. The older child's goal is to maintain the lead position. Parents are faced with the task of caring for a new child while not neglecting the others. Parents need to distribute their attention in an equitable manner.

Reactions of siblings may result from temporary separation from the mother, changes in the mother's or father's behavior, or the siblings' response to the infant's coming home (Bartlett and McGrath, 1999). Positive behavioral changes of siblings include interest in and concern for the baby and increased independence. Regression in toileting and sleep habits, aggression toward the baby, and increased seeking of attention and whining are examples of negative behaviors.

The parents' attitudes toward the arrival of the baby can set the stage for the other children's reactions (Fig. 22-11). Because the baby absorbs the time and attention of the important people in the other children's lives, jealousy is to be expected once the initial excitement of having a new baby in the home is over.

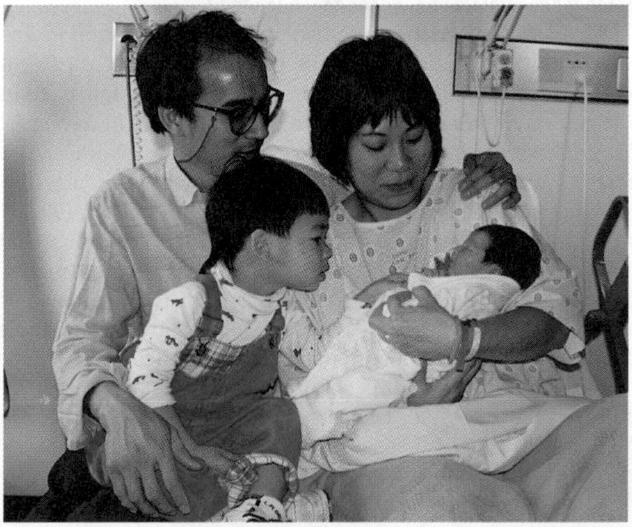

FIG. 22-11 • Parents introducing big brother to infant daughter. (Courtesy Kim Molloy, Knoxville, IA.)

Parents, especially mothers, spend much time and energy promoting sibling acceptance of a new baby. Participating in sibling preparation classes makes a difference in the ability of mothers to cope with sibling behavior. Older children are actively involved in preparing for the infant, and this involvement intensifies after the birth of the child. Parents have to manage their feelings of guilt that the older children are being deprived of parental time and attention. Parents have to monitor the behavior of older children toward the more vulnerable infant and divert aggressive behavior. Strategies that parents have used to facilitate acceptance of a new baby by siblings are presented in the Family Focus box.

Siblings demonstrate acquaintance behaviors with the newborn. The acquaintance process depends on the information given to the child before the baby is born and on the child's cognitive development level. The initial behaviors of siblings with the newborn include looking at the infant and touching the head (Fig. 22-12). The initial adjustment of older children to a newborn takes time, and children should be allowed to interact at their own pace rather than be forced to do so. To expect a young child to accept and love a rival for the parents' affection assumes an unrealistic level of maturity. Sibling love grows as does other love, that is, by being with another person and sharing experiences (Fig. 22-13). The relationship that develops between siblings has been conceptualized as sibling attachment. This bond between siblings involves a secure base in which one child provides support for the other, is missed when absent, and is looked to for comfort and security.

Family Focus

STRATEGIES FOR FACILITATING SIBLING ACCEPTANCE OF A NEW BABY

1. Take your firstborn child on a tour of your hospital room and point out similarities to his or her birth. This is like the room I was in with you, and the baby is in the same kind of bassinet that you were in.
2. Have a small gift from the baby to give to your older child each day.
3. Give the older child a T-shirt that says, "I'm a big brother" (or "sister").
4. Arrange for your children to be in the first group (grandparents, sister) to see the newborn. Let them hold the baby in the hospital. One mother and father arranged for their firstborn son to be present at the births of his three brothers and to be the first one to hold them.
5. Plan time for both children. "When I get home, I'll arrange my day so that I can have the baby's care done in the morning while Sam (first child) is at school. Maybe the baby will sleep part of the afternoon and I can spend some time with Sam."
6. Fathers can spend time with the older sibling while mothers are taking care of the baby and vice versa. Siblings like to have time and attention from both parents.
7. Give preschool and early school-age siblings a newborn doll as "their baby" to care for. Give sibling a photograph of the new baby to take to school to show off "his" or "her" baby. Older siblings may enjoy the responsibility of helping care for the newborn, such as learning how to give the baby a bottle or change a diaper. One mother let her preschooler help burp the new baby by patting on the baby's back. She figured her son could pat the baby fairly firmly without harming him and at the same time get out some pent-up aggressive feelings.

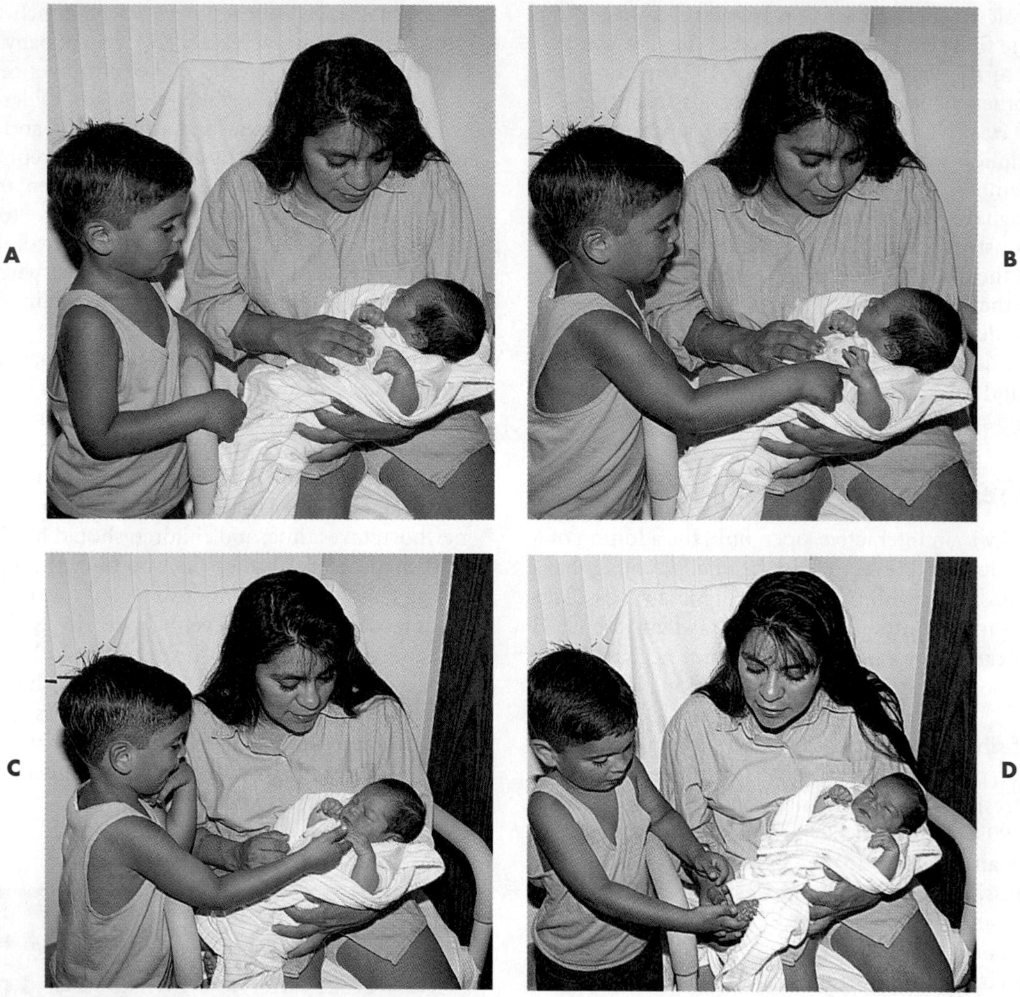

FIG. 22-12 • First meeting. **A,** Boy with mother during first meeting with new sibling. **B,** First tentative touch. **C,** Testing with fingertip. **D,** Relationship more secure: it is now okay to hold with whole hand. (Courtesy Marjorie Pyle, RNC, Lifecircle, Costa Mesa, CA.)

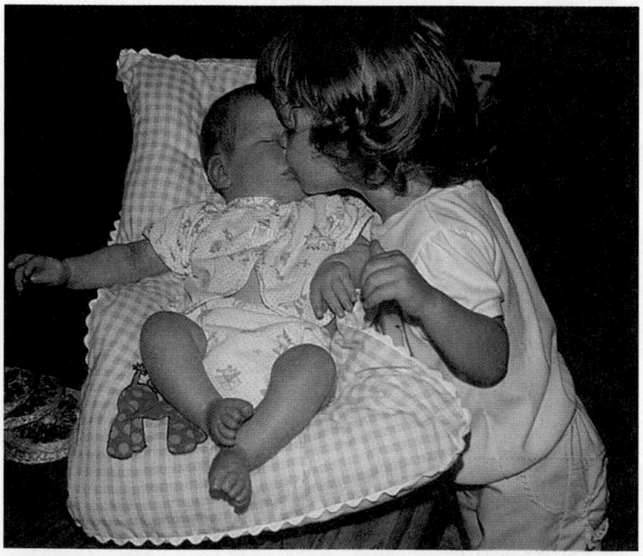

FIG. 22-13 • Sister kisses her new brother. Family contacts are important for newborn and siblings. (Courtesy Marjorie Pyle, RNC, Lifecircle, Costa Mesa, CA.)

GRANDPARENT ADAPTATION

Grandparents experience a transition to grandparenthood. Intergenerational relationships shift and grandparents must deal with changes in practices and attitudes toward childbirth, child rearing, and men's and women's roles at home and in the workplace. The degree to which grandparents understand and accept current practices can influence how supportive they are perceived to be by their adult children (Hansen and Jacob, 1992).

At the same time that they are adjusting to grandparenthood, the majority of grandparents are experiencing normative middle- and old-age life transition issues such as retirement and a move to smaller housing, and need support from their adult children. Some may feel regret about their limited involvement because of poor health or geographic distance. Maternal grandmothers, more so than the other three grandparents, may have high expectations of themselves that cause them to be very self-critical (Hansen and Jacob, 1992).

The extent of involvement of grandparents in the care of the newborn depends on many factors, for example, the willingness of the grandparents to become involved, the proximity of the grandparents, and ethnic and cultural expectations of the grandparent's role. If the new parents live in the United States,

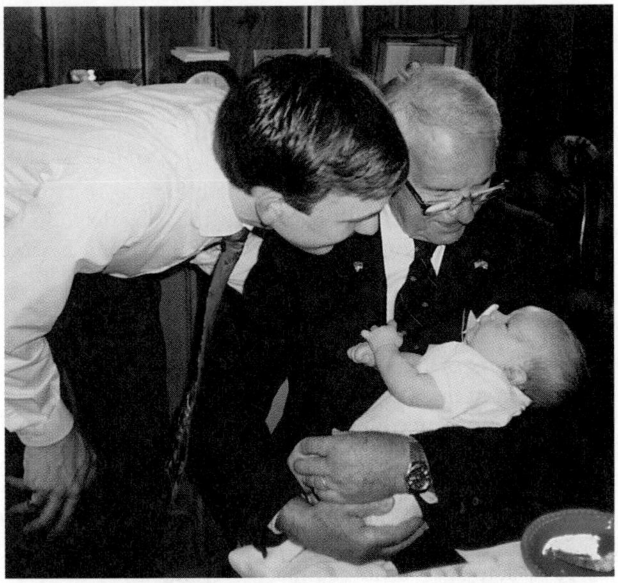

FIG. 22-14 • Father, grandfather, and new grandson get acquainted. (Courtesy Eric Schult.)

Asian grandparents typically are asked to come to the United States to care for the baby and the mother after birth and to care for the children once the parents return to work. In the United States, paternal grandparents, in contrast to those in other cultures, often consider themselves secondary to the maternal grandparents; less seems expected of them, and they are initially less involved. Nevertheless, these grandparents are eager to help and express great pleasure in their son's fatherhood and his involvement with the baby (Fig. 22-14).

For first-time parents, pregnancy and parenthood can reawaken old issues related to dependence versus independence. Couples often do not plan on their parents' help immediately after the baby arrives. They want time "to be a family," inferring a couple-baby unit, not the intergenerational family network. Contrary to their expectations, however, new parents do call on their parents for help. The majority of maternal grandmothers are present soon after the birth, being called in on short notice by the parents after several nights with a crying baby.

A simple technique to help people span the generation gap is through a printed "letter to new parents" (written from the grandparents' perspective), which can be included in prenatal kits distributed in childbirth preparation classes and made available to all family members on the postpartum unit. Grandparents' classes can be used to bridge the generation gap and to help the grandparents understand their adult children's parenting concepts. The classes include information on up-to-date childbearing practices; family-centered care; infant care, feeding, and safety (car seats); and exploration of roles that grandparents play in the family unit.

CARE MANAGEMENT: PRACTICAL SUGGESTIONS FOR THE FIRST WEEKS AT HOME

Numerous changes occur during the first weeks of parenthood. Care management should be directed toward helping parents cope with infant care, role changes, altered lifestyle, and change in family structure resulting from the addition of a new baby. Parents may have inadequate or incorrect understanding of what to expect in the early postpartum weeks. Developing skill and confidence in caring for an infant can be especially anxiety provoking.

Nurses, especially those making postpartum visits to parents' homes, are in a prime position to help new families. The nurse's role becomes primarily one of teacher-supporter, focusing on enabling new parents to become capable of self-care and infant care and of meeting the needs of the family unit.

➤ Assessment

Assessment should include a psychosocial assessment focusing on parent-infant attachment, adjustment to the parental role, sibling adjustment, social support, and education needs, as well as mother's and baby's physical adaptation. Early home visits are an excellent opportunity for the nurse to assess beginnings of successful or harmful parenting behaviors and to provide positive reinforcement for loving and nurturing behaviors with the infant. Parents who interact in inappropriate or abusive ways with their infants should be followed more closely, and an appropriate mental health practitioner or professional social worker should be notified (Johnson & Johnson, 1996).

➤ Nursing Diagnoses

Nursing diagnoses pertinent to transition to parenthood include:

- Family coping: potential for growth related to:
  - —Positive attitude and realistic expectations for newborn and adapting to parenthood
  - —Nurturing behaviors with newborn
  - —Verbalizing positive factors in lifestyle change
- Risk for altered parenting related to:
  - —Lack of knowledge in infant care
  - —Feelings of incompetence and/or lack of confidence
  - —Unrealistic expectations of newborn/infant
  - —Fatigue from interrupted sleep
- Parental role conflict related to:
  - —Role transition and role attainment
  - —Unwanted pregnancy
  - —Lack of resources to support parenting (e.g, no paid leave)
- Risk for altered parent-infant attachment related to:
  - —Difficult labor and birth
  - —Postpartum complications
  - —Neonatal complications/anomalies

➤ Expected Outcomes

A plan of care is formulated in collaboration with the family, incorporating their priorities and preferences, to meet their specific needs. Expected outcomes for effective transition to parenthood include that the parents will:

- Demonstrate behaviors that reflect appreciation of sensory and behavioral capacities of the infant.
- Verbalize increasing confidence and competence in feeding, diapering, dressing, and sensory stimulation of the infant.
- Identify deviations from normal in the infant that should be brought to the immediate attention of the primary health care provider.
- Relate effectively to the newborn's siblings and grandparents.

➤ Plan of Care and Implementation

Instructions for the First Days at Home. Parents, especially first-time parents, must be helped to anticipate what the transition from hospital to home will be like. Anticipatory guidance can help prevent a shock of reality that might negate the parents' joy or cause them undue stress. Even the simplest strategies can provide enormous support. Written information reinforcing education topics is helpful to provide to parents, as is a list of available community resources, both local and national (Box 22-4). Classes in the prenatal period or during the postpartum stay are helpful. Instructions for the first days at home should minimally include activities of daily living, dealing with visitors, and activity and rest.

Infant Care. Providing practical suggestions for infant care can help parents adjust to parenthood. Mothers and fathers want to feel capable and confident in the physical care of their 'infant. The nurse should assess each parent's need for instruction on care such as bathing, clothing, and safety.

Anticipatory Guidance Regarding the Newborn. Anticipatory guidance helps prepare new parents for what to expect as their newborn grows and develops. Parents with realistic expectations of infant needs and behavior are better prepared to adjust to the demands of a new baby and to parenthood itself.

New parents can be overwhelmed by a large volume of information and become anxious. Anticipatory guidance needs to include the following: newborn sleep-wake cycles, interpretation of crying and quieting techniques, infant developmental milestones, sensory enrichment/infant stimulation, recognizing signs of illness, and well-baby follow-up and immunizations.

Development of Day-Night Routines. Nurses can help prepare new parents for the fact that most newborns cannot tell the difference between night and day and must learn the rhythm of day-night routines. Nurses should provide basic suggestions for settling a newborn and for helping him or her develop a predictable routine. Examples of such suggestions include:

- In the late afternoon, bring the baby out to the center of family activity. Keep the baby there for the rest of the evening. If the baby falls asleep, let the baby do so in the infant seat or in someone's arms. Save the crib or bassinet for nighttime sleep.
- Give the baby a bath right before bedtime. This soothes the baby and helps him or her expend energy.
- Feed the baby for the last evening time around 11 PM and put him or her to bed in the crib or bassinet.
- For nighttime feedings and diaper changes, keep a small night-light on to avoid turning on bright lights. Talk in soft whispers (if at all) and handle the baby gently and only as absolutely necessary to feed and diaper. Nighttime feedings should be all business and no play! Babies usually go back to sleep if the room is quiet and dark.

A predictable, stable routine gradually develops for most babies; however, there will be some babies who never develop one. New parents will find it easier if they are willing to be flexible and to give up some control during those early weeks.

Interpretation of Crying and Quieting Techniques. Crying is an infant's first social communication. Some babies cry more than others, but all babies cry. They cry to communicate that they are hungry, uncomfortable, wet, ill, or bored, and sometimes for no apparent reason at all. The longer parents are around their infants, the easier it becomes to interpret what a cry means. Many infants have a fussy period during the day, often in the late afternoon or early evening when everyone is naturally tired. Environmental tension adds to the length and in-

Box 22-4

Resources for New Parents

The Fatherhood Project at the Families and Work Institute
330 Seventh Avenue
New York, NY 10001
(212) 465-2044

The Institute for Responsible Fatherhood and Family Revitalization
1146 19th Street NW
Suite 800
Washington, DC 20036
(800) 7-FATHER or (800) 732-8437

At-Home Dad (newsletter for fathers who stay at home)
61 Brightwood Avenue
North Andover, MA 01845-1702
E-mail: athomedad@aol.com

Postpartum Support International
927 North Kellogg Avenue
Santa Barbara, CA 93111
(805) 967-7636

La Leche League International
1400 North Meacham Road
Schaumburg, IL 60173
(847) 519-7730
(Local La Leche League groups are usually listed in city and town phone books)

Motherhood Maternity Health and Fitness Program
SBI Corporation
1106 Stratford Drive
Carlisle, PA 17013
(717) 258-4641

Single Parent Resource Center
141 West 28th Street
Suite 302
New York, NY 10001
(212) 947-0221

Pink Inc.! Publishing
P.O. Box 866
Atlantic Beach, FL 32233-0866
(904) 731-7120

tensity of crying spells. Babies also have periods of vigorous crying when no comforting can help. These periods of crying may last for long stretches until the infants seem to cry themselves to sleep. Possibly the infants are trying to discharge enough energy so that they can settle themselves down. The nurse needs to reinforce for new parents that time and infant maturation will take care of these types of cries.

Crying because of colic is a common concern of new parents. Babies with colic cry inconsolably for several hours, pull their legs up to their stomach, and pass large amounts of gas. No one really knows what colic is or why babies get it. Parents can be encouraged to contact their nurse practitioner or pediatrician if they are concerned that their baby has colic.

Certain types of sensory stimulation can calm and quiet infants and help them get to sleep. Important characteristics of this sensory stimulation—whether tactile, vestibular, auditory, or visual—appear to be that the stimulation is mild, slow, rhythmic, and consistently and regularly presented. Tactile stimulation can include warmth, patting, back rubbing, and covering the skin with textured cloth. Swaddling to keep arms and legs close to the body (as in utero) provides widespread and constant tactile stimulation and a sense of security. Vestibular stimulation is especially effective and can be accomplished by mild rhythmic movement such as rocking or holding the infant upright, as on the parent's shoulder.

The nurse can teach parents a number of strategies that help quiet a fussy baby, prevent crying, and induce quiet attention or sleep (Boxes 22-5 and 22-6).

Developmental Milestones. Knowledge of infant growth and development helps parents have realistic expectations of what an infant can do. When parents understand and appreciate the limitations and developing abilities of their infant, adjustment to parenthood can go more smoothly. Emphasizing the individuality of the infant enhances the capacity of the family to offer their infant an optimally nurturing environment (Brazelton, 1995).

Brazelton (1995) suggests the concept of "touch-points" for intervention: that is, points at which a change in the system (i.e., baby, parent, and family) is brought about by the baby's spurts in development (e.g., cognitive, motor, or emotional). Immediately before each spurt in development, there is a predictable short period of disorganization in the baby. Parents are likely to feel disorganized and stressed as well. Because these periods of disorganization are predictable, nurses can offer parents anticipatory guidance to help them understand what happens with infant development and to prepare them for the subsequent spurts in development.

Box 22-5

How to Swaddle an Infant

1. Fold down the top corner of the blanket. Position the infant on the blanket with the infant's neck near the fold.
2. Bring the blanket around the infant's right side and across the infant, tucking the corner under the left side.
3. Bring the bottom of the blanket up to the infant's chest.
4. Bring the remaining corner of the blanket across the infant, tucking the corner under the infant's right side. The infant should be wrapped securely but not tightly; some room should be left for the infant to move.

Box 22-6

Infant Quieting Techniques

- Many newborns feel insecure in the center of a large crib. They prefer a small, warm, soft space that reminds them of intrauterine life. Try a smaller bed, such as a bassinet, portable crib, buggy, or cradle, or use a rolled-up blanket to turn a corner of the big crib into a smaller place.
- Carry your baby in a frontpack or backpack.
- Swaddle your newborn snugly in a receiving blanket. Swaddling keeps your newborn's arms and legs close to his or her body, similar to the intrauterine position. It makes the newborn feel more secure.
- Prewarm the crib sheets with a hot water bottle or heating pad that you remove before putting your baby to bed. Some babies startle when placed on a cold sheet.
- Some newborns need extra sucking to soothe themselves to sleep. Breastfeeding mothers may prefer to let their infant suckle at the breast as a soothing technique. Other mothers choose to use a pacifier. Stroke the pacifier against the roof of the baby's mouth to encourage him or her to suck it during the first 2 weeks. Around 3 months of age, infants become able to consistently find and suck their thumbs as a way of self-consoling.
- A rhythmic, monotonous noise simulating the intrauterine sounds of your heartbeat and blood flow may help your infant settle down. Some parents have found that putting the baby in a portable crib beside the dishwasher or washing machine helps settle a fussy baby.
- Movement often helps quiet a baby. Take your baby for a ride in the car, or take your baby for an outing in a stroller or carriage. Rock your baby in a rocking chair or cradle.
- Place your baby on his or her stomach across your lap; pat and rub his or her back while gently bouncing your legs or swaying them from left to right.
- Babies enjoy close skin-to-skin contact. A combination of this and warm water often helps soothe a fussy baby. Fill your tube with warm water. Get in and let the baby lie on your chest so that the baby is immersed in the water up to his or her neck. Cuddle the baby close.
- Let your baby see your face. Talk to your baby in a soothing voice.
- Your baby may simply be bored. Bring him or her into the room where you and the rest of the family are. Change your baby's position; many babies like to be upright, such as being held up on your shoulder.

Two touchpoints occur during the early postpartum-newborn period: one soon after birth and another at 2 to 3 weeks (Brazelton, 1995). In the hospital or at a home visit during the first week, the nurse can use Brazelton's Neonatal Behavioral Assessment Scale (Brazelton and Nugent, 1996) to demonstrate to parents their baby's amazing repertoire of abilities. In this way, parents begin to appreciate their baby's individuality and become more sensitive to their baby's behavioral cues. At 2 to 3 weeks, the home care nurse or pediatric office nurse should assess for the regular end-of-the-day fussy period that most infants have between 3 and 12 weeks of age. Helpful topics to include in the anticipatory guidance are the normalcy and positive value of the fussy period, how to settle a fussy baby, and ways to help a baby develop a predictable schedule.

Infant Stimulation. Interacting with their parents is an important way in which infants learn about themselves and their environment. Home health nurses are in a prime position to evaluate the home environment and to make suggestions to parents for promotion of their baby's physical, cognitive, and emotional development. Box 22-7 and Table 36-1 presents suggestions for visual, auditory, tactile, and kinetic stimulation.

Another method of sensory enrichment that parents can learn to use is infant massage. This type of nurturing touch can help create a loving bond between the infant and parent and has been shown to contribute to the physical and emotional well-being of both the massage giver and receiver (Schneider, 1996, 1997). Infant massage is a gentle, warm communication done *with* the infant, not *to* the infant. The focus is on reciprocal interaction between infant and parent; the parent talks to the infant, asks permission to start the massage, questions the infant, and facilitates dialogue.

One of the most important benefits of infant massage (Box 22-8) for the parents is the improved ability to read their infant's cues (Schneider, 1997). Positive cues include eye contact, smiling, looking at the parent's face, babbling or cooing, and smooth movements of arms and legs. Negative cues from the infant include pulling away, frowning, grimacing, turning the head away, arching the back, crying, squirming, and flailing

Box 22-7
Teaching Your Newborn

- Newborns learn things every day. You can teach your newborn by playing with him or her and giving your newborn toys that help him or her to learn.
- Talk to your baby a lot. Tell your baby what is going on in the room ("Listen to the dog barking."). Label objects that you see or use ("Here's the washcloth.") and describe things you are doing ("Let's put the shirt over Kerry's head!").
- Look at your baby's face and make eye contact. Play face-making games: smile, stick out your tongue, open your eyes wide. As your baby gets older, he or she will try to imitate these facial expressions.
- Babies like music and rhythmic movement. Rock or swing your baby as you sing to him or her in a gentle voice.
- Acknowledge your baby's attempts to "answer" your talking and singing. He or she will respond to you by looking in your direction, making eye contact, moving his or her arms and legs, and/or making sounds.
- Babies like bright colors and vivid contrasts. Show your baby pictures and objects that are black and white, bright primary colors (red, blue, yellow), and/or large patterns. Keep colorful mobiles and toys where your baby can see them.
- Babies like to be held upright. Holding your newborn on your shoulder lets your baby look around his or her world and provides vestibular stimulation. Let your baby lift his or her head for a few seconds. Keep your hand ready to support your baby's head.

Box 22-8
Benefits of Infant Massage

IN THE PSYCHOSOCIAL DOMAIN

Benefits to the Infant of Receiving Massage
- Promotes bonding and attachment
- Promotes body/mind/spirit connection
- Increases self-esteem
- Increases sense of love, acceptance, respect, and trust
- Enhances communication

Benefits to the Parent of Giving Massage
- Improves ability to read infant cues
- Improves synchrony between caregiver and infant
- Promotes bonding
- Increases confidence in parenting
- Increases communication—verbal and nonverbal
- Improves relaxation
- Provides time to share and quality time
- Promotes parenting skills

IN THE PHYSIOLOGICAL/PHYSICAL GROWTH DOMAIN

Benefits to the Infant of Receiving Massage
- Improves relaxation and release of accumulated stress
- Stimulates circulation
- Strengthens digestive, circulatory, and gastrointestinal systems, which can lead to weight gain
- Reduces discomfort from teething, congestion, gas, colic, and emotional stress
- Improves muscle tone/coordination
- Increases elimination, circulation, and respiration
- Improves sleep patterns
- Increases hormonal function

Benefits to the Parent of Giving Massage
- Improves sense of well-being
- Reduces blood pressure
- Reduces stress
- Improves overall health

From Schneider E: Touch communication: the power of infant massage, *Massage Magazine* 68:40, 1997.

the arms and legs. Increased ability to read their infant's cues can increase parental confidence and self-esteem, thereby assisting adaptation to parenthood.

Recognizing Signs of Illness. As well as explaining the need for well-baby follow-up visits, the nurse should discuss with parents the signs of illness in newborns. Parents should be advised to call their nurse-practitioner or pediatrician immediately if they notice such signs, and to ask about over-the-counter medications, such as Tylenol for infants, to keep at home (Nursing Care Plan).

➤ Evaluation

Evaluation is based on the expected outcomes of care. The plan is revised as needed based on the evaluation findings.

Nursing Care Plan HOME CARE FOLLOW-UP: TRANSITION TO PARENTHOOD

NURSING DIAGNOSIS Risk for infant care deficit related to lack of experience/lack of support

EXPECTED OUTCOME Infant care routines are adequate, and infant appears healthy.

Nursing Interventions/*Rationales*

Observe infant care routines (bathing, diapering, feeding, play) *to evaluate parental ease with care and adequacy of techniques.*

Observe infant appearance (height-weight ratio, head circumference, fontanels, skin tone and turgor); assess infant's vital signs, overall tone, reflexes, and age-appropriate developmental skills *to evaluate for signs indicative of inadequate care.*

Explore available support systems for infant care *to determine adequacy of existing system.*

Provide ongoing follow-up as needed *to ensure amelioration of identified potential and actual care deficits.*

NURSING DIAGNOSIS Sleep pattern disturbance related to infant demands and environmental interruptions

EXPECTED OUTCOME Woman sleeps for uninterrupted periods and feels rested on waking.

Nursing Interventions/*Rationales*

Discuss woman's routine and specify things that interfere with sleep *to determine scope of problem and direct interventions.*

Explore ways woman and significant others can make environment more conducive to sleep (i.e., privacy, darkness, quiet, back rubs, soothing music, warm milk); teach use of guided imagery and relaxation techniques *to promote optimal conditions for sleep.*

Eliminate things or routines (i.e., caffeine, foods that induce heartburn, strenuous mental/physical activity) *to avoid interference with sleep.*

Advise family to limit visitors and activities *to avoid further taxation and fatigue.*

NURSING DIAGNOSIS Risk for impaired home maintenance management related to addition of new family member/inadequate resources/inadequate support systems

EXPECTED OUTCOME Home exhibits signs of safe and functional environment.

Nursing Interventions/*Rationales*

Observe the home environment (i.e., available living space and sleeping arrangements; adequacy of facilities for food preparation and storage, hygiene and toileting; overall state of repair; cleanliness; presence of safety hazards) *to determine adequacy and effective use of resources.*

Observe arrangements for the newborn, such as sleeping space, care equipment and supplies (bathing, changing, feeding, transportation) *to determine adequacy of resources.*

Explore who is responsible for cooking, cleaning, child care, and newborn care and determine whether the mother seems adequately rested *to determine adequacy of support systems.*

Identify and arrange referrals to needed social agencies (i.e., Aid to Families with Dependent Children [AFDC], Women, Infants, and Children [WIC] program, food pantries) *to ameliorate resource deficits (finances, supplies, equipment).*

NURSING DIAGNOSIS Risk for altered family processes related to inclusion of new family member

EXPECTED OUTCOME Infant is successfully assimilated into family structure.

Nursing Interventions/*Rationales*

Observe family interaction with the newborn and note degree of bonding, evidence of sibling rivalry, and involvement in newborn care *to evaluate acceptance of newest family member.*

Clarify identified misinformation and misperceptions *to promote clear communication.*

Support family efforts as they move toward adjusting and incorporating the new member *to reinforce new functions and roles.*

If needed, make referrals to appropriate social services or community agencies *to ensure ongoing support and care.*

Key Points

- The birth of a child necessitates changes in the existing interactional structure of a family.
- Attachment is the process by which the parent and infant come to love and accept each other.
- Attachment is strengthened through the use of sensual responses or interactions by both partners in the parent-infant interaction.
- In adjusting to the parental role, the mother moves from a dependent state (taking in) to an interdependent state (letting go).
- Mothers may exhibit signs of postpartum blues (baby blues) or postpartum depression (PPD).
- Fathers experience emotions and adjustments during the transition to parenthood that are similar to, and also distinctly different from, those of mothers.
- Modulation of rhythm, modification of behavioral repertoires, and mutual responsivity facilitate infant-parent adjustment.
- Many factors (e.g., age, culture, socioeconomic level, and expectations of what the child will be like) influence adaptation to parenthood.
- Parents face a number of tasks related to sibling adjustment that require creative parental interventions.
- Grandparents can have a positive influence on the postpartum family.

References

Albright A: Postpartum depression: an overview, *J Counseling Development* 71: 316, 1993.

Alpers R: The changing self-concept of pregnant and parenting teens, *J Prof Nurs* 14(2):111-118, 1998.

Ament L: Maternal tasks of the puerperium re-identified, *J Obstet Gynecol Neonatal Nurs* 19(4):330-335, 1990.

Barratt M, Roach M: Early interactive processes: parenting by adolescent and adult single mothers, *Infant Behavior and Development* 18:97-109, 1995.

Bartlett L, McGrath J: Children's responses to the birth of a sibling: interventions to assist the family in transition, *Mother Baby J* 4(4):19-25, 1999.

Berkowitz G et al: Delayed childbearing and the outcome of pregnancy, *N Engl J Med* 322:659-664, 1990.

Bloom K: Perceived relationship with the father of the baby and maternal attachment in adolescents, *J Obstet Gynecol Neonatal Nurs* 27(4):420-430, 1998.

Brazelton T: Working with families: opportunities for early intervention, *Pediatr Clin North Am* 42(1):1, 1995.

Brazelton T, Nugent J: *Neonatal behavioural assessment scale,* ed 3, London, 1996, MacKeith.

Brewaeys A et al: Lesbian mothers who conceived after donor insemination: a follow-up study, *Hum Reprod* 10(10): 2731-2735, 1995.

Cain M: *First time mothers, last chance babies: parenting at 35+,* Far Hills, NJ, 1994, New Horizon Press.

Campbell J: Maternity blues: a model for biological research. In Hamilton J, Harberger P, editors: *Postpartum psychiatric illness: a picture puzzle,* Philadelphia, 1992, University of Pennsylvania Press.

Diehl K: Adolescent mothers: what produces positive mother-infant interaction? *MCN Am J Matern Child Nurs* 22:89-95, 1997.

Evans M et al: Postpartum sleep in the hospital: relationship to taking-in and taking-hold, *Clin Nurs Res* 7(4):379-389, 1998.

Fowles E: The relationship between maternal role attainment and postpartum depression, *Health Care Women Int* 19(1): 83-94, 1998.

Fretts R et al: Increased maternal age and the risk of fetal death, *N Engl J Med* 333:953-957, 1995.

Galanti G: *Caring for patients from different cultures,* Philadelphia, 1991,University of Pennsylvania Press.

Gartrell N et al: The National Lesbian Family Study: interview with prospective mothers, *Am J Orthopsychiatry* 66(2): 272-281, 1996.

Geissler E: *Pocket guide to cultural assessment,* St Louis, 1994, Mosby.

Gerson E: *Infant behavior in the first year of life,* New York, 1993, Raven Press.

Gilbert W, Nesbitt T, Danielsen B: Childbearing beyond age 40: pregnancy outcome in 24,032 cases, *Obstet Gynecol* 93:9-14, 1999.

Hansen L, Jacob E: Intergenerational support during the transition to parenthood: issues for new parents and grandparents, *Families in Society: J Contemporary Human Services* 73(8):471-479, 1992.

Henderson A, Brouse A: The experiences of new fathers during the first three weeks of life, *J Adv Nurs* 16(3):293-298, 1991.

Inman M: The power of touch: infant massage therapy, *Childbirth Instructor Magazine* 4th quarter, 1996.

Jambunathan J, Stewart S: Hmong women in Wisconsin: what are their concerns in pregnancy and childbirth? *Birth* 22(4):204-210, 1995.

Jiménez S: The Hispanic culture, folklore, and perinatal health, *J Perinat Educ* 4(1):9, 1995.

Johnson & Johnson: *Compendium of postpartum care,* Skillman, NJ, 1996, Johnson & Johnson Consumer Products.

Klaus M et al: Maternal attachment: importance of first postpartum days, *N Engl J Med* 286:460-463, 1972.

Klaus M, Kennell J: *Bonding: the beginnings of parent-infant attachment,* St Louis, 1983, Mosby.

Klaus M, Kennell J: *Maternal-infant bonding,* St Louis, 1976, Mosby.

Klaus M, Kennell J: *Parent-infant bonding,* ed 2, St Louis, 1982, Mosby.

Leventhal-Belfer L, Cowan P, Cowan C: Satisfaction with child care arrangements: effects on adaptation to parenthood, *Am J Orthopsychiatry* 62(2):165-177, 1992.

Lipson J, Dibble S, Minarik P: *Culture and nursing care: a pocket guide,* San Francisco, 1996, UCSF Nursing Press.

Martell L: Is Rubin's "taking-in" and "taking-hold" a useful paradigm? *Health Care Women Int* 17(1):1-13, 1996.

Mercer R, Ferketich S: Experienced and inexperienced mothers maternal competence during infancy, *Res Nurs Health* 18: 333-343, 1995.

Niska K, Snyder M, Lia-Hoagberg B: Family ritual facilitates adaptation to parenthood, *Public Health Nurs* 15(5):329-337, 1998.

Osterwell D: *Correlates of relationship satisfaction in lesbian couples who are parenting their first child together.* Doctoral dissertation, Berkeley, 1991, California School of Professional Psychology.

Reese S, Harkless G: Divergent themes in maternal experience in women older than 35 years of age, *Appl Nurs Res* 9(3): 148-153, 1996.

Rogan F et al: 'Becoming a mother'—Developing a new theory of early motherhood, *J Adv Nurs* 25:877-885, 1997.

Rubin R: Basic maternal behavior, *Nurs Outlook* 9:683-686, 1961.

Sank J: *Factors in the prenatal period that affect parental role attainment during the postpartum period in Black American mothers and fathers.* Doctoral dissertation, 1991, University of Texas at Austin.

Schneider E: The power of touch: massage for infants, *Infants and Young Children* 8(3):40-55, 1996.

Schneider E: Touch communication: the power of infant massage, *Massage Magazine* 68:40, 1997.

Sethi S: The dialectic in becoming a mother: experiencing a postpartum phenomenon, *Scandinavian J Caring Sciences* 9(4):235-244, 1995.

Sharts-Hopko N: Birth in the Japanese context, *J Obstet Gynecol Neonatal Nurs* 24(14):343-351, 1995.

Thompson P et al: Adolescent parenting: outcomes and maternal perceptions, *J Obstet Gynecol Neonatal Nurs* 24:713-718, 1995.

Tomlinson P: Marital relationship change in the transition to parenthood: a reexamination as interpreted through transition theory, *J Fam Nurs* 2(3):286-305, 1996.

Tomlinson P, Irwin B: Qualitative study of women's reports of family adaptation pattern four years following transition to parenthood, *Issues Ment Health Nurs* 14:119-139, 1993.

Wood A et al: The downward spiral of postpartum depression: *MCN Am J Matern Child Nurs* 22:308-316, 1997.

Wrasper C: Discharge timing and Rubin's concept of puerperal change, *J Perinat Educ* 5(2):13-23, 1996.

CHAPTER

23 Postpartum Complications

http://www.harcourthealth.com/MERLIN/Wong/maternal/

Learning Objectives

On completion of this chapter the reader will be able to:

- Identify causes, signs and symptoms, possible complications, and medical and nursing management of postpartum hemorrhage.
- Differentiate among the causes of postpartum hemorrhage.
- Describe thromboembolic disorders including incidence, etiology, signs and symptoms, and management.
- Summarize the role of the nurse in assessing potential problems and managing care of women with postpartum complications in the home setting.
- Discuss emotional complications of pregnancy, including management of mood disorders.
- Differentiate among postpartum emotional complications including incidence, risk factors, signs and symptoms, and management.
- Describe emotional, behavioral, cognitive, and physical responses commonly experienced during the grieving process associated with perinatal loss.
- Identify specific nursing interventions to meet the special needs of parents and their families related to perinatal loss and grief.
- Differentiate among helpful and unhelpful responses in caring for parents experiencing loss and grief.

Providing safe and effective care of the woman and family experiencing postpartum physical and psychologic complications, sequelae of childbirth trauma, or grief related to perinatal loss requires a joint effort from all members of the health care team. This chapter focuses on the postpartum complications of hemorrhage and infection, sequelae of childbirth trauma, psychologic complications, and loss and grief.

POSTPARTUM HEMORRHAGE

Postpartum hemorrhage (PPH), traditionally defined as the loss of 500 ml or more of blood after vaginal birth and 1000 ml or more after cesarean birth, is a leading cause of maternal morbidity and mortality in the United States today. Postpartum hemorrhage may be classified as early, within the first 24 hours after birth, or late, more than 24 hours after birth but less than 6 weeks postpartum (American College of Obstetricians and Gynecologists [ACOG], 1998). Shortened hospital stays increase the potential for acute episodes of PPH to occur outside the traditional hospital or birth center setting.

Etiology and Risk Factors

The most common cause of PPH is uterine atony, which complicates approximately 1 in 20 births (Gonik, 1999). Other causes include retained placenta, placenta accreta, cervical or vaginal lacerations, uterine rupture or inversion, lower genital tract lacerations and hematomas, infection and coagulopathies (ACOG, 1998; Varner, 1998). Late postpartum hemorrhage most commonly is the result of subinvolution of the placenta site, retained placental tissue, or endometritis (ACOG, 1998).

Excessive bleeding can be considered with reference to the stages of labor. From birth of the fetus until separation of the placenta, the character and quantity of blood passed may suggest excessive bleeding. For example, dark blood is probably of venous origin, perhaps from varices or superficial lacerations of the birth canal. Bright blood is arterial and may indicate deep lacerations of the cervix. Spurts of blood with clots may indicate partial placental separation. Failure of blood to clot or remain clotted indicates coagulopathy.

Excessive bleeding may occur during the period between the separation of the placenta and its expulsion or removal. Commonly such bleeding is the result of incomplete placental separation, undue manipulation of the fundus, or excessive traction on the cord. After the placenta has been expelled, persistent or excessive blood loss most commonly is a result of atony of the uterus (i.e., failure to contract well or maintain contraction) or prolapse of the uterus into the pelvis.

Uterine Atony. Uterine atony is marked hypotonia of the uterus. Normally, placental separation and expulsion are facilitated by contraction of the uterus; this also prevents hemorrhage from the placental site. If the uterus is flaccid after detachment of all or part of the placenta, brisk venous bleeding occurs and normal coagulation of the open vasculature is impaired and continues until the uterine muscle is contracted.

Uterine atony is the leading cause of PPH accounting for more than 90% of all cases of PPH (Norris, 1997). It is associated with high parity, hydramnios, a macrosomic fetus, and multifetal gestation. In such conditions the uterus is overstretched and contracts poorly after birth. Other causes of atony include traumatic birth, use of halogenated anesthesia or magnesium sulfate, rapid or prolonged labor, chorioamnionitis, and use of oxytocin for labor induction or augmentation (ACOG, 1998; Varner, 1998).

Lacerations of the Genital Tract. Lacerations of the cervix, vagina, and perineum are also causes of postpartum hemorrhage. Hemorrhage related to lacerations should be suspected if bleeding continues despite a firm, contracted uterine fundus. This bleeding can be a slow trickle, an oozing, or frank hemorrhage.

Factors that influence the causes and incidence of obstetric lacerations of the lower genital tract include operative birth, precipitous birth, congenital abnormalities of the maternal soft parts, and contracted pelvis. Size, abnormal presentation, and position of the fetus; relative size of the presenting part and the birth canal; prior scarring from infection, injury, or surgery; and vulvar, perineal, and vaginal varicosities can also cause lacerations.

Extreme vascularity in the labia and periclitoral areas often results in profuse bleeding if laceration occurs. Hematomas may also be present.

Lacerations of the perineum are the most common of all injuries in the lower portion of the genital tract. These are classified as first, second, third, and fourth degree (see Chapter 18).

Pelvic hematomas (i.e., a collection of blood in the connective tissue) may be vulvar, vaginal, or retroperitoneal in origin. Vulvar hematomas are the most common. Pain is the most common symptom, and most vulvar hematomas are visible. Vaginal hematomas occur more commonly in association with a forceps-assisted birth, an episiotomy, or primigravidity (Ridgeway, 1995). Retroperitoneal hematomas are the least common but are life threatening. They are caused by laceration of one of the vessels attached to the hypogastric artery, usually associated with rupture of a cesarean scar during labor (Benedetti, 1996).

Cervical lacerations usually occur at the lateral angles of the external os. Most are shallow, and bleeding is minimal. More extensive lacerations may extend into the vaginal vault or into the lower uterine segment.

Retained Placenta

Nonadherent Retained Placenta. Retained placenta may result from partial separation of a normal placenta, entrapment of the partially or completely separated placenta by an hourglass constriction ring of the uterus, mismanagement of the third stage of labor, or abnormal adherence of the entire placenta or a portion of the placenta to the uterine wall. Placental retention because of poor separation is common in very preterm births (i.e., 20 to 24 weeks of gestation).

Management of nonadherent retained placenta is by manual separation and removal by the primary care provider. Supplementary anesthesia is usually not needed for women who have had regional anesthesia for birth. For other women, administration of light nitrous oxide and oxygen inhalation anesthesia or IV thiopental facilitates intrauterine exploration and placental separation. After this removal, the woman is at continued risk for PPH or for infection.

Adherent Retained Placenta. Abnormal adherence of the placenta occurs for unknown reasons, but it is thought to result from zygote implantation in an area of defective endometrium so that there is no zone of separation between the placenta and the decidua. Attempts to remove the placenta in the usual manner are unsuccessful, and laceration or perforation of the uterine wall may result, putting the woman at great risk for severe PPH and infection (Cunningham et al, 1997).

Inversion of the Uterus. Inversion (turning inside out) of the uterus after birth is a potentially life-threatening complication. The incidence of uterine inversion is approximately 1 in 2000 to 2500 births (ACOG, 1998), and may recur with a subsequent birth.

Uterine inversion may be partial or complete. Complete inversion of the uterus is obvious; a large, red, rounded mass (perhaps with the placenta attached) protrudes 20 to 30 cm outside the introitus. Incomplete inversion cannot be seen but must be felt; a smooth mass will be palpated through the dilated cervix.

Contributing factors to uterine inversion include fundal implantation of the placenta, vigorous fundal pressure, excessive traction applied to the cord, uterine atony, leiomyomas, and abnormally adherent placental tissue (Bowes, 1999; Cunningham et al, 1997). Uterine inversion occurs most often in multiparous women and with placenta accreta or increta. Although proper management of the third stage of labor prevents the majority of uterine inversions, some are unavoidable.

The primary presenting signs of uterine inversion are hemorrhage, shock, and pain. Hemorrhage is the primary presenting sign in up to 94% of women with uterine inversion, with blood loss estimated to range from 800 to 1800 ml. Up to 40% of these women may also be in shock (Wendel and Cox, 1995).

Prevention—always the easiest, cheapest, and most effective therapy—is especially appropriate for uterine inversion. The umbilical cord should not be pulled on unless the placenta has definitely separated.

Subinvolution of the Uterus. Late postpartum bleeding may occur as a result of subinvolution of the uterus. Subinvolution is defined as the delayed return of the enlarged uterus to normal size and function. Recognized causes of subinvolution include retained placental fragments and pelvic infection.

Signs and symptoms include prolonged lochial discharge, irregular or excessive bleeding, and sometimes hemorrhage. A pelvic examination usually reveals a uterus that is larger than normal and one that may be boggy.

Care Management

➤ Assessment

The nurse must be alert to the symptoms of hemorrhage and hypovolemic shock and be prepared to act quickly to minimize blood loss (Box 23-1). The woman's history should be reviewed

Box 23-1

Noninvasive Assessments of Cardiac Output in Postpartum Patients Who Are Bleeding

Palpation of pulses (rate, quality, equality)
- Arterial
- Blood pressure

Auscultation
- Heart sounds/murmurs
- Breath sounds

Inspection
- Skin color, temperature, turgor
- Level of consciousness
- Capillary refill
- Urinary output
- Neck veins
- Pulse oximetry
- Mucous membranes

Presence or absence of anxiety, apprehension, restlessness, disorientation

for factors that predispose the woman to postpartum hemorrhage. The fundus is assessed to determine whether it is firmly contracted at or near the level of the umbilicus. Bleeding should be assessed for color and amount. The perineum is inspected for signs of lacerations or hematomas to determine the possible source of bleeding.

Vital signs may not be reliable indicators of shock immediately postpartum because of physiologic adaptations of this period. However, frequent vital sign measurements in the first 2 hours after birth may identify trends that are related to blood loss (e.g., tachycardia, tachypnea, and falling blood pressure).

Assessment for bladder distention is important because a distended bladder can displace the uterus and prevent uterine contraction. The skin is assessed for warmth and dryness; nail beds are checked for color and promptness of capillary refill. Laboratory studies include evaluation of hemoglobin and hematocrit levels.

Late PPH may develop within 24 hours of birth or later in the postpartum period. The woman may be at home when the symptoms occur. Discharge teaching should emphasize the signs of normal involution, as well as potential complications.

➤ Nursing Diagnoses

Nursing diagnoses for women experiencing PPH include the following:
- Fluid volume deficit (immediate) related to:
  —Excessive blood loss secondary to uterine atony, lacerations, or uterine inversion
- Risk for injury (maternal) related to:
  —Attempted manual removal of retained placenta
  —Administration of blood products
  —Operative procedures
- Altered parenting related to:
  —Separation from infant secondary to treatment regimen
- Altered peripheral tissue perfusion related to:
  —Excessive blood loss and shunting of blood to central circulation

➤ Expected Outcomes

Expected outcomes for the woman experiencing postpartum hemorrhage may include the following. The woman will:
- Identify and use available support systems
- Maintain normal vital signs and laboratory values
- Not experience complications related to excessive bleeding
- Verbalize understanding of the condition, its management, and discharge instructions

➤ Plan of Care and Implementation

Medical Management. Early recognition and diagnosis of postpartum hemorrhage is critical to care management. The first step is to evaluate the contractility of the uterus. If the uterus is hypotonic, management is directed toward increasing contractility and minimizing blood loss.

Hypotonic Uterus. The initial management of excessive postpartum bleeding is firm massage of the uterine fundus, expression of any clots in the uterus, eliminating bladder distention, and continuous intravenous (IV) infusion of 10 to 40 units of oxytocin in 1000 ml Ringer's lactate or normal saline solution. If the uterus fails to respond to oxytocin, a dose of 0.2 mg ergonovine (Ergotrate) or methylergonovine (Methergine) may be given intramuscularly (IM) to produce sustained uterine contractions. If these first-line drugs are not effective, a derivative of prostaglandin F_{2a} (carboprost tromethamine) 0.25 mg is given intramuscularly. It can also be given intramyometrially at cesarean birth or intraabdominally after vaginal birth. Most hemorrhage can be controlled after one or two injections of 0.25 mg intramuscularly (ACOG, 1998). See Table 23-1 for a comparison of medications used to manage PPH. In addition to the medications used to contract the uterus, rapid administration of crystalloid solutions and or blood will be needed to restore the intravascular volume.

NURSE ALERT • Use of ergonovine or methylergonovine is contraindicated in the presence of hypertension or cardiovascular disease. Prostaglandin F_{2a} should be used cautiously in women with cardiovascular disease or asthma (Bowes, 1999).

If bleeding persists, bimanual compression may be considered by the obstetrician or nurse-midwife. This procedure involves inserting a fist into the vagina and pressing the knuckles against the anterior side of the uterus while placing the other hand on the abdomen and massaging the posterior uterus. If the uterus still does not become firm, manual exploration of the uterine cavity for retained placental fragments is implemented. If the preceding procedures are ineffective, surgical management may be the only alternative. Surgical management options include vessel ligation (i.e. uteroovarian, uterine, and hypogastric), angiographic embolization, and hysterectomy (ACOG, 1998).

Bleeding with a Contracted Uterus. If the uterus is firmly contracted and bleeding continues, the source of bleeding still needs to be identified and treated. Assessment may include visual or manual inspection of the perineum, vagina, cervix, or rectum; and laboratory studies (e.g., hemoglobin, hematocrit, coagulation studies, and platelet count) (ACOG, 1998). Treatment depends on the source of the bleeding. Lacerations are usually sutured. Hematomas may be managed with observation, application of cold therapy, or ligation of the bleeding vessel. Fluids and or blood replacement may be needed (Akins, 1994; Druelinger, 1994; Roberts, 1995).

TABLE 23-1
Medications Used to Manage Postpartum Hemorrhage

	Oxytocin (Pitocin)	Methylergonovine (Methergine)	Prostaglandin $F_{2\alpha}$ (Prostin/15M; Hemabate)
ACTION	Contraction of uterus; decreases bleeding	Contraction of uterus	Contraction of uterus
SIDE EFFECT	Infrequent; water intoxication; nausea and vomiting	Hypertension, nausea, vomiting, headache	Headache, nausea, vomiting, fever
CONTRAINDICATIONS	None for PPH	Hypertension, cardiac disease	Asthma, hypersensitivity
DOSAGE; ROUTE	10-40 U/L diluted in lactated Ringer's solution or normal saline at 125-200 mU/min IV or 10-20 U IM	0.2 mg IM q2-4 hr up to 5 doses; 0.2 mg IV only for emergency	0.25 mg IM or intramyometrially q15-90 min up to 8 doses
NURSING CONSIDERATIONS	Continue to monitor vaginal bleeding and uterine tone	Check blood pressure before giving and do not give if >140/90; continue monitoring vaginal bleeding and uterine tone	Continue to monitor vaginal bleeding and uterine tone

Uterine Inversion. Uterine inversion is an emergency situation requiring immediate recognition, replacement of the uterus within the pelvic cavity, and correction of associated clinical conditions. Medical management involves treating shock, repositioning the uterus, giving oxytocic medications after the uterus is positioned, and initiating broad-spectrum antibiotic therapy. A nasogastric tube may be inserted to minimize the risk of paralytic ileus.

Subinvolution. Treatment of subinvolution depends on the cause. Ergonovine 0.2 mg every 4 hours for 2 or 3 days and antibiotic therapy are the most common medications used (Cunningham et al, 1997). Dilation and curettage (D&C) may be needed to remove retained placental fragments or to débride the placental site.

Herbal Remedies. Herbal remedies to control PPH have been used with some success in some settings. Some herbs have homeostatic actions, while others work as oxytocic agents to contract the uterus (Akins, 1994; Weed, 1986). Box 23-2 lists herbs that have been used and their actions. However, published evidence of the safety and efficacy of herbal therapy is lacking.

Box 23-2
Herbal Remedies for Postpartum Hemorrhage

HERBS	ACTION
Witch hazel	Homeostatic
Lady's mantle	Homeostatic
Blue cohosh	Oxytocic
Cotton root bark	Oxytocic
Motherwort	Promotes uterine contraction; vasoconstrictive
Shepherd's purse	Promotes uterine contraction
Alfalfa leaf	Increases availability of vitamin K; increases hemoglobin
Nettle	Increases availability of vitamin K; increases hemoglobin
Red raspberry leaves	Homeostatic, promotes uterine contraction

Source Schirmer G: *Herbal medicine,* Bedford TX, 1998, MED2000; Weed S: *Wise woman herbal for the childbearing year,* Woodstock, NY, 1986, Ash Tree Publishing Co.

Nursing Interventions. Immediate nursing care of the woman with PPH includes assessment of vital signs and uterine consistency and administration of oxytocin or other drugs to stimulate uterine contraction according to standing orders or protocols. The primary health care provider, if not present, is notified.

The woman and her family will be anxious about her condition. The nurse can intervene by calmly providing explanations about interventions being performed and the need to act quickly.

After the bleeding has been controlled, the care of the woman with lacerations of the perineum is similar to that for women with episiotomies (i.e., analgesia as needed for pain and hot or cold applications as necessary). The need for increased roughage in the diet and increased intake of fluids is emphasized. Stool softeners may be used to assist the woman in reestablishing bowel habits without straining and putting stress on the suture lines.

NURSE ALERT • To avoid injury to the suture line, a woman with third- or fourth-degree lacerations is not given rectal suppositories or enemas.

The care of the woman who has experienced an inversion of the uterus focuses on immediate stabilization of hemodynamic status. This requires close observation of her response to treatment to prevent shock or fluid overload. If the uterus has been repositioned manually, care must be taken after the birth to avoid aggressive fundal massage.

Discharge instructions for the woman who has had PPH are similar to those for any postpartum woman. In addition, she should be told that she will probably feel fatigue or even exhaustion, and will need to limit her physical activities to conserve her strength. She may need instructions in increasing her dietary iron and protein intake and iron supplementation to rebuild lost red cell volume. She may need assistance with infant care and household activities until she has regained strength. Some women have problems with delayed or insufficient lactation and also postpartum depression. Referrals for home care follow-up or to community resources may be needed (Nursing Care Plan).

➤ Evaluation

The nurse can be reasonably assured that care was effective to the extent that the expected outcomes have been achieved.

Hemorrhagic (Hypovolemic) Shock

Hemorrhage may result in hemorrhagic (hypovolemic) shock. Shock is an emergency situation in which the perfusion of body organs may become severely compromised; death may occur. Physiologic compensatory mechanisms are activated in response to hemorrhage. The adrenal glands release catecholamines, causing arterioles and venules in the skin, lungs, gastrointestinal tract, liver, and kidneys to constrict. The available blood flow is diverted to the brain and heart and away from other organs, including the uterus. If shock is prolonged, the continued reduction in cellular oxygenation results in an accumulation of lactic acid and acidosis (from anaerobic glucose metabolism). Acidosis (lowered serum pH) causes arteriolar vasodilation; venule vasoconstriction persists. A circular pattern is established; that is, decreased perfusion, increased tissue anoxia and acidosis, edema formation, and pooling of blood further decrease the perfusion; cellular death occurs. The Emergency box presents the assessments and interventions for hemorrhagic shock.

Nursing Care Plan — POSTPARTUM HEMORRHAGE

NURSING DIAGNOSIS Fluid volume deficit related to postpartum hemorrhage

EXPECTED OUTCOME Patient will demonstrate fluid balance as evidenced by stable vital signs, prompt capillary refill time, and balanced intake and output.

Nursing Interventions/*Rationales*

Monitor vital signs, oxygen saturation, urine specific gravity, and capillary refill *to provide baseline data.*

Measure and record amount and type of bleeding by weighing and counting saturated pads. If woman is at home, teach her to count pads and save any clots or tissue. If woman is admitted to hospital, save any clots and tissue for further examination *to estimate type and amount of blood loss for fluid replacement.*

Provide quiet environment *to promote rest and decrease metabolic demands.*

Give explanation of all procedures *to reduce anxiety.*

Begin IV access with 18-gauge or larger needle for infusion of isotonic solution as ordered *to provide fluid or blood replacement.*

Administer medications as ordered, such as oxytocin, methergine, or prostin *to increase contractility of the uterus.*

Insert indwelling urinary catheter *to provide most accurate assessment of renal function and hypovolemia.*

Prepare for surgical intervention as needed *to stop the source of bleeding.*

NURSING DIAGNOSIS Tissue perfusion, altered, related to hypovolemia

EXPECTED OUTCOME Woman will have stable vital signs, oxygen saturation, arterial blood gases, and adequate hematocrit and hemoglobin.

Nursing Interventions/*Rationales*

Monitor vital signs, oxygen saturation, arterial blood gases, and hematocrit and hemoglobin *to assess for hypovolemic shock and decreased tissue perfusion.*

Assess for any changes in level of consciousness *to assess for evidence of hypoxia.*

Assess capillary refill, mucous membranes, skin temperature *to note indicators of vasoconstriction.*

Give supplementary oxygen as ordered *to provide additional oxygenation to tissues.*

Suction as needed, insert oral airway, *to maintain clear, open airway for oxygenation.*

Monitor arterial blood gases *to provide information about acidosis or hypoxia.*

Administer sodium bicarbonate if ordered *to reverse metabolic acidosis.*

NURSING DIAGNOSIS Anxiety related to sudden change in health status

EXPECTED OUTCOME Woman will verbalize the anxious feelings are diminished.

Nursing Interventions/*Rationales*

Using therapeutic communication, evaluate woman's understanding of events *to provide clarification of any misconceptions.*

Provide calm, competent attitude and environment *to aid in decreasing anxiety.*

Explain all procedures *to decrease anxiety about the unknown.*

Allow woman to verbalize feelings *to permit clarification of information and promote trust.*

Continue to assess vital signs or other clinical indicators of hypovolemic shock *to evaluate if psychologic response of anxiety intensifies physiologic indicators.*

Medical Management. Vigorous treatment is necessary to prevent adverse sequelae. Medical management of hypovolemic shock involves restoring circulating blood volume and eliminating the cause of the hemorrhage (e.g., lacerations, uterine atony, or inversion). To restore circulating blood volume, a rapid IV infusion of crystalloid solution is given at a rate of 3 ml infused for every 1 ml of estimated blood loss. Packed RBCs are usually infused if the woman is still actively bleeding and no improvement in her condition is noted after the initial crystalloid infusion. Infusion of fresh frozen plasma may be needed if clotting factors and platelet counts are below normal values (Cunningham et al, 1997).

Nursing Interventions. Hemorrhagic shock often occurs rapidly, but the classic signs of shock may not appear until the postpartum woman has lost 30% to 40% of blood volume. The nurse continues to reassess the woman's condition and mobilizes appropriate resources.

Most interventions are instituted to improve or monitor tissue perfusion. The nurse continues to monitor the woman's pulse and blood pressure. If invasive hemodynamic monitoring is ordered, the nurse may assist with placement of a central venous pressure (CVP) or pulmonary artery (Swan-Ganz) catheter and monitor CVP, pulmonary artery pressure, or pulmonary artery wedge pressure as ordered.

Additional assessments to be made include evaluation of skin temperature, color, and turgor, as well as assessment of the woman's mucous membranes. Breath sounds should be auscultated before fluid volume replacement, if possible, to provide a baseline for future assessment. Inspection for oozing at the sites of incisions or injections, and assessment of the presence of petechiae or ecchymosis in areas not associated with surgery or trauma, are critical in the evaluation for disseminated intravascular coagulopathy.

Oxygen is administered, preferably by a nonrebreathing face mask, at 10 to 12 L/min to maintain oxygen saturation. Oxygen saturation should be monitored with a pulse oximeter, although measurements may not always be accurate in a patient with hypovolemia or decreased perfusion. Level of consciousness is assessed frequently and provides additional indications of blood volume and oxygen saturation. In early stages of decreased blood flow, the woman may report "seeing stars" or feeling dizzy or nauseated. She may become restless and orthopneic. As cerebral hypoxia increases, she may become confused and react slowly to stimuli or not at all. Some women complain of headaches. An improved sensorium is an indicator of improved perfusion.

Continuous electrocardiographic monitoring may be indicated for the woman who is hypotensive or tachycardic, who continues to bleed profusely, or who is in shock. A Foley catheter with a urometer is inserted to allow hourly assessment of urine output. The most objective and least invasive assessment of adequate organ perfusion and oxygenation is a urine output of at least 30 ml/hr. Blood may need to be drawn and sent to the laboratory for studies that include hemoglobin and hematocrit level, platelet count, and coagulation profile.

Fluid or Blood Replacement Therapy. Critical to successful management of the woman experiencing a hemorrhagic complication is establishment of venous access, preferably with a large-bore IV catheter. The establishment of two IV lines facilitates fluid resuscitation. Vigorous fluid resuscitation includes the administration of crystalloids (lactated Ringer's, normal saline solution), colloids (albumin), blood, and blood components. Fluid resuscitation must be carefully monitored because fluid overload can occur. Intravascular fluid overload occurs most often with colloid therapy.

Transfusion reactions may follow administration of blood or blood components including cryoprecipitates. Even in an emergency, each unit should be checked per hospital protocol. Complications include hemolytic reactions, febrile reactions, allergic reactions, circulatory overloading, and air embolism.

LEGAL TIP • Standard of Care for Bleeding Emergencies The standard of care for obstetric emergency situations such as postpartum hemorrhage or hypovolemic shock is that provision should be made for the nurse to implement independent nursing actions. Policies, procedures, standing orders or protocols, and clinical guidelines should be established by each health care facility in which births occur and should be agreed upon by health care providers involved in the care of obstetric patients.

Emergency

HEMORRHAGIC SHOCK

Assessments	Characteristics
Respirations	Rapid and shallow
Pulse	Rapid, weak, irregular
Blood pressure	Decreasing (late sign)
Skin	Cool, pale, clammy
Urinary output	Decreasing
Level of consciousness	Lethargy → coma
Mental status	Anxiety → coma
Central venous pressure	Decreased

Intervention

- Summon assistance and equipment
- Start IV infusion per standing orders
- Ensure patent airway; administer oxygen
- Continue to monitor status

Coagulopathies

When bleeding is continuous and there is no identifiable source, a coagulopathy may be the cause. The woman's coagulation status needs to be assessed quickly and continuously. The nurse may draw and send blood to the laboratory for studies. Abnormal results depend on the cause and may include increased prothrombin time, increased partial thromboplastin

Critical Thinking

PROTOCOLS FOR EMERGENCY SITUATIONS

Review protocols in a labor and birth unit for care of obstetric patients during emergency situations such as PPH or pulmonary embolism. Interview nurses for their role during these emergencies. Evaluate whether the protocols allow the nurses to function as needed in the emergency. Suggest changes in the protocols based on your interview.

time, decreased platelets, decreased fibrinogen level, increased fibrin degradation products, and prolonged bleeding time. Causes of coagulopathies may be pregnancy complications such as idiopathic thrombocytopenic purpura or von Willebrand's disease.

Disseminated Intravascular Coagulation. Disseminated intravascular coagulation (DIC) is a pathologic form of clotting that is diffuse and consumes large amounts of clotting factors, including platelets, fibrinogen, prothrombin, and factors V and VII. Widespread external bleeding, internal bleeding, or both can result. DIC also causes vascular occlusion of small vessels resulting from small clots forming in the microcirculation. In the obstetric population, DIC may occur as a result of abruptio placentae, amniotic fluid embolism, dead fetus syndrome (i.e., fetus dies but is retained in utero for at least 6 weeks), severe preeclampsia, septicemia, cardiopulmonary arrest, and hemorrhage.

Primary medical management in all cases of DIC involves correction of the underlying cause (e.g., removal of the dead fetus, treatment of existing infection or of preeclampsia or eclampsia, or removal of a placental abruption). Volume replacement, blood component therapy, optimization of oxygenation and perfusion status, and continued reassessment of laboratory parameters are the usual forms of treatment. Plasma levels usually return to normal within 24 hours after birth. Platelet counts usually return to normal within 7 days (Kilpatrick and Laros, 1999).

Nursing interventions include assessment for signs of bleeding and for signs of complications from the administration of blood and blood products. Because renal failure is one consequence of DIC, urinary output is monitored, usually by insertion of an indwelling urinary catheter. Urinary output must be maintained at more than 30 ml/hr.

The woman and her family will be anxious or concerned about her condition and prognosis. The nurse offers explanations about care and provides emotional support to the woman and her family through this critical time.

THROMBOEMBOLIC DISEASE

A thrombosis is the formation of a blood clot or clots inside a blood vessel and is caused by inflammation (thrombophlebitis) or partial obstruction of the vessel. Three thromboembolic conditions are of concern in the postpartum period:

- Superficial venous thrombosis—Involvement of the superficial saphenous venous system
- Deep venous thrombosis—Involvement varies but can extend from the foot to the iliofemoral region
- Pulmonary embolism—Complication of deep venous thrombosis occurring when part of a blood clot dislodges and is carried to the pulmonary artery where it occludes the vessel and obstructs blood flow to the lungs

Incidence and Etiology

The incidence of thromboembolic disease in the postpartum period varies from about 1 in 1000 to 1 in 2000 women (Cunningham et al, 1997). The incidence has declined in the last 20 years because early ambulation after childbirth has become the standard practice. The major causes of thromboembolic disease are venous stasis and hypercoagulation, both of which are present in pregnancy and continue into the postpartum period. Other risk factors include cesarean birth, history of venous thrombosis or varicosities, obesity, maternal age over 35, multiparity, and smoking (Falter, 1997).

Clinical Manifestations

Superficial venous thrombosis is the most common form of postpartum thrombophlebitis. It is characterized by pain and tenderness in the lower extremity. Physical examination may reveal warmth; redness; and an enlarged, hardened vein over the site of the thrombosis. Deep vein thrombosis is more common in pregnancy and is characterized by unilateral leg pain, calf tenderness, and swelling (Fig. 23-1). Physical examination may reveal redness and warmth, but women may also have a large clot with few symptoms (Mishell et al, 1997). A positive Homans sign may be present, but further evaluation is needed because the calf pain may be attributed to other causes such as a strained muscle resulting from the birthing position. Pulmonary embolism is characterized by dyspnea and tachypnea.

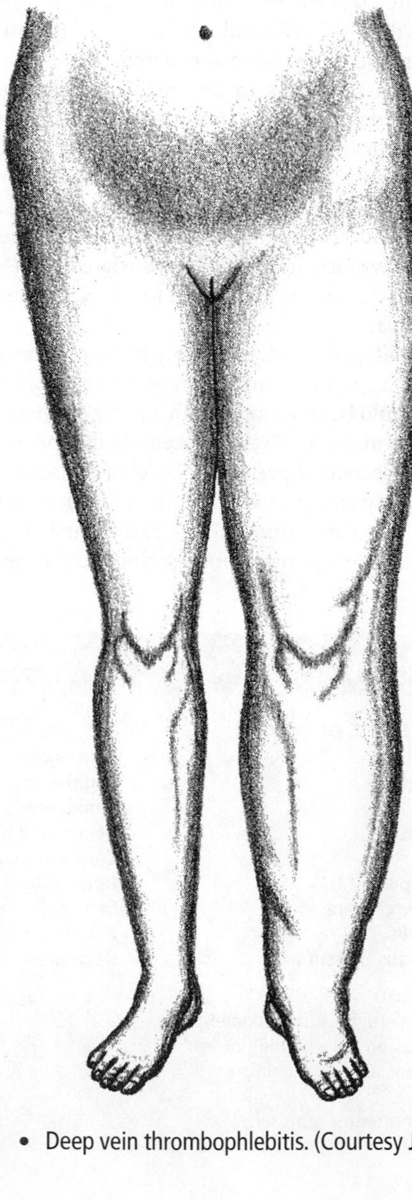

FIG. 23-1 • Deep vein thrombophlebitis. (Courtesy Julie L. Perry.)

Other signs and symptoms commonly seen include apprehension, cough, tachycardia, hemoptysis, elevated temperature, and pleuritic chest pain (Laros, 1999).

Venography is the most accurate method for diagnosing deep venous thrombosis; however, it is an invasive procedure that exposes the woman and fetus to ionizing radiation and is associated with serious complications. Noninvasive diagnostic methods such as real time and color Doppler ultrasound are more commonly used (Cunningham et al, 1997). With pulmonary embolism, murmurs may be heard on cardiac auscultation. Electrocardiograms are usually normal. Arterial Po_2 may be lower than normal. A ventilation/perfusion scan, Doppler ultrasound, and pulmonary arteriogram may be used for diagnosis (Laros, 1999).

Medical Management

Superficial venous thrombosis is treated with analgesia (nonsteroidal antiinflammatory agents), rest with elevation of the affected leg, and elastic stockings (Falter, 1997). Local application of heat may also be used. Deep venous thrombosis is usually treated with anticoagulant therapy (usually continuous intravenous heparin for 5 to 7 days), bed rest with the affected leg elevated, and analgesia. After the symptoms have decreased, the woman may be fitted with elastic stockings to use when she is allowed to ambulate. Oral anticoagulant therapy (warfarin) is started and will be continued for about 3 months. For pulmonary embolism, continuous intravenous heparin therapy is used until symptoms have resolved. Intermittent subcutaneous heparin or oral anticoagulant therapy is usually continued for 6 months.

Nursing Interventions

In the hospital, nursing care of the woman with a thrombosis consists of assessments: inspection and palpation of the affected area; palpation of peripheral pulses; checking Homans sign; measurement and comparison of leg circumferences; inspection for signs of bleeding; monitoring for signs of pulmonary embolism including chest pain, coughing, dyspnea, and tachypnea; and checking respiratory status for presence of crackles. Laboratory reports are monitored for prothrombin or partial thromboplastin times. The woman and her family are assessed for their level of understanding about the diagnosis and their ability to cope during the unexpected extended period of recovery.

Interventions include explanations and education about the diagnosis and the treatment. The woman will need assistance with personal care as long as she is on bed rest; the family should be encouraged to participate in the care if they wish. While the woman is on bed rest, she should be encouraged to change positions frequently, but not to place the knees in a sharply flexed position that could cause pooling of blood in the lower extremities. She should also be cautioned not to rub the affected areas because this action could cause the clot to dislodge. Once the woman is allowed to ambulate, she is taught how to prevent venous congestion by putting on the elastic stockings before getting out of bed.

Heparin and warfarin are administered as ordered; the physician is notified if clotting times are outside the therapeutic level. If the woman is breastfeeding, she is assured that neither heparin nor warfarin is excreted in significant amounts in breastmilk. If the infant has been discharged, the family is encouraged to bring the infant for feedings as permitted by hospital policy; the mother can also express milk to be sent home.

Pain can be managed with a variety of measures. Position changes, elevating the leg, and application of moist warm heat may decrease discomfort. Administration of analgesics and antiinflammatory medications may be needed.

NURSE ALERT • Medications containing aspirin are not given to women on anticoagulant therapy because aspirin inhibits synthesis of clotting factors and can lead to prolonged clotting time and increased risk of bleeding.

The woman is usually discharged home on oral anticoagulants and will need an explanation of the treatment schedule and possible side effects. If subcutaneous injections are to be given, the woman and family are taught how to administer the medication and about site rotation. The woman and her family should also be given information about safe care practices to prevent bleeding and injury while she is on anticoagulant therapy, such as using a soft toothbrush and using an electric razor. She will also need information about the need for follow-up with her health care provider to monitor clotting times and to make sure the correct dose of anticoagulant therapy is maintained. The woman should also use a reliable form of contraception if taking warfarin because this medication is considered teratogenic (Toglia and Nolan, 1997).

POSTPARTUM INFECTIONS

Postpartum infection (i.e., puerperal sepsis or childbed fever) is any clinical infection of the genital canal that occurs within 28 days after miscarriage, induced abortion, or childbirth. The first symptom of postpartum infection is usually a fever of 38° C or more on 2 successive days of the first 10 postpartum days (not counting the first 24 hours after birth). Puerperal infection is one of the major causes of morbidity and mortality throughout the world; however, it occurs in only 6% of births in the United States (3% after vaginal births; 5 to 10 time higher after cesarean births)(Gibbs and Sweet, 1999). Common postpartum infections include endometritis, wound infections, mastitis, urinary tract infections, and respiratory tract infections.

The most common infecting organisms are the numerous streptococcal and anaerobic organisms. *Staphylococcus aureus*, gonococci, coliform bacteria, and clostridia are less common but serious pathogenic organisms that also cause postpartum infection. Postpartum infections are more common in women who have concurrent medical or immunosuppressive conditions or who had a cesarean or other operative delivery. Intrapartal factors such as prolonged rupture of membranes, prolonged labor, and internal maternal or fetal monitoring also increase the risk of infection (Varner, 1998). Factors that predispose the woman to postpartum infection are listed in Box 23-3.

Endometritis

Endometritis (infection of the lining of the uterus) is the most common postpartum infection. It usually begins as a localized infection at the placental site, but can spread to the entire en-

Box 23-3
Predisposing Factors for Postpartum Infection

PRECONCEPTION OR ANTEPARTAL FACTORS
History of previous venous thrombosis, urinary tract infection, mastitis, pneumonia
Diabetes mellitus
Alcoholism
Drug abuse
Immunosuppression
Anemia
Malnutrition

INTRAPARTAL FACTORS
Cesarean birth
Prolonged rupture of membranes
Chorioamnionitis
Prolonged labor
Bladder catheterization
Internal fetal/uterine pressure monitoring
Multiple vaginal examinations after rupture of membranes
Epidural anesthesia
Retained placental fragments
Postpartum hemorrhage
Episiotomy or lacerations
Hematomas

dometrium. Incidence is higher after cesarean birth. Signs of endometritis include fever (usually greater than 38° C); increased pulse; chills; anorexia; nausea; fatigue and lethargy; pelvic pain; uterine tenderness; and foul-smelling, profuse lochia (Calhoun and Brost, 1995). Leukocytosis and a markedly increased red blood cell sedimentation rate are typical laboratory findings of postpartum infections. Anemia may also be present. Blood cultures or intracervical or intrauterine bacterial cultures (aerobic and anaerobic) should reveal the offending pathogens within 36 to 48 hours.

Wound Infections

Wound infections are also common postpartum infections but often develop after the woman is at home. Sites of infection include the cesarean incision and the episiotomy or repaired laceration site. Predisposing factors are similar to those for endometritis (see Box 23-3). Signs of wound infection include erythema, edema, warmth, tenderness, seropurulent drainage, and wound separation. Fever and pain may also be present.

Urinary Tract Infections

Urinary tract infections (UTIs) occur in 2% to 4% of postpartum women. Risk factors include urinary catheterization, frequent pelvic examinations, epidural anesthesia, genital tract injury, history of UTI, and cesarean birth. Signs and symptoms include dysuria, frequency and urgency, low grade fever, urinary retention, hematuria, and pyuria. Costovertebral angle (CVA) tenderness or flank pain may indicate upper UTI. Urinalysis results may reveal *Escherichia coli,* although other gram-negative aerobic bacilli may also cause UTIs.

Critical Thinking

POSTPARTUM INFECTION
What is the rate of postpartum infection in your facility? Interview the infection control nurse for possible sources of postpartum infections and suggestions for control of such infections. Examine discharge teaching instructions for evidence of topics related to postpartum infection. Identify resources for patient education on postpartum infection.

Mastitis

Mastitis, or breast infection, affects about 1% of women soon after childbirth, most of whom are first-time mothers who are breastfeeding. Mastitis almost always is unilateral and develops well after the flow of milk has been established. The infecting organism generally is the hemolytic *Staphylococcus aureus.* An infected nipple fissure usually is the initial lesion, followed by ductal system involvement. Inflammatory edema and engorgement of the breast soon obstruct the flow of milk in a lobe; regional, then generalized, mastitis follows. If treatment is not prompt, mastitis may progress to a breast abscess. Symptoms rarely appear before the end of the first postpartum week and are more common in the second to fourth weeks. Chills, fever, malaise, and local breast tenderness are noted first. Pain, swelling, redness, and axillary adenopathy may also occur. Antibiotics are prescribed. Lactation is maintained (if desired) by emptying the breasts every 2 to 4 hours by manual expression or a breast pump.

Care Management

Prenatal and intrapartal factors that predispose a woman to postpartum infection are listed in Box 23-3. Signs and symptoms associated with postpartum infection were discussed with each infection. Laboratory tests usually performed include a complete blood count, venous blood cultures, and uterine tissue cultures.

➤ Nursing Diagnoses

Nursing diagnoses for women experiencing postpartum infection include the following:

- Knowledge deficit related to:
  —Etiology, management, course of infection
  —Transmission and prevention of infection
- Impaired tissue integrity related to:
  —Effects of infection process
- Pain related to:
  —Mastitis
  —Puerperal infection
  —Urinary tract infection
- Altered family processes related to:
  —Unexpected complication to expected postpartum recovery
  —Possible separation from newborn
  —Interruption in process of realigning relationships after the addition of the new family member
- Risk for altered parenting related to:
  —Fear of spread of infection to newborn

The most effective and cheapest treatment of postpartum infection is prevention. Preventive measures include good prenatal nutrition to control anemia and intrapartal hemorrhage. Good maternal perineal hygiene is emphasized. Strict adherence by all health care personnel to aseptic techniques during childbirth and the postpartum period is very important.

Management of endometritis consists of intravenous broad-spectrum antibiotic therapy (i.e., cephalosporins, penicillins, or clindamycin and gentamicin) and supportive care, including hydration, rest, and pain relief. Antibiotic therapy is usually discontinued 24 hours after the woman is asymptomatic (Gibbs and Sweet, 1999). Assessments of lochia, vital signs, and changes in the woman's condition continue during treatment. Comfort measures depend on the symptoms and may include cool compresses, warm blankets, perineal care, and sitz baths. Teaching should include side effects of therapy, prevention of spread of infection, signs and symptoms of worsening condition, and adherence to the treatment plan and the need for follow-up care. Women may need to be encouraged or assisted to maintain mother-infant interactions and breastfeeding (if allowed during treatment).

Postpartum women are usually discharged to home by 48 hours after birth. This is often before signs of infection are evident. Nurses in birth centers and hospital settings need to be able to identify women at risk for postpartum infection and to provide anticipatory teaching and counseling before discharge. After discharge, telephone follow-up, hot lines, support groups, lactation counselors, home visits by nurses, and teaching materials (e.g., videos and written materials) are all interventions that can be implemented to decrease the risk of postpartum infections. Home care nurses need to be able to recognize signs and symptoms of postpartum infection so that the woman can be instructed to contact her primary health care provider. These nurses must also be able to provide the appropriate nursing care for women who need follow-up home care.

Treatment of wound infections may combine antibiotic therapy with wound débridement. Wounds may be opened and drained. Nursing care includes frequent wound and vital sign assessments and wound care. Comfort measures include sitz baths, warm compresses, and perineal care. Teaching includes good hygiene techniques, including good handwashing techniques, self-care measures, and which signs of worsening conditions to report to the primary health care provider. The woman is usually discharged to home for self-care or home nursing care after treatment is initiated in the inpatient setting.

Medical management for UTIs consists of antibiotic therapy, analgesia, and hydration. Postpartum women are usually treated on an outpatient basis; therefore, teaching should include instructions on how to monitor temperature, bladder function, and appearance of urine. The woman should also be taught about signs of potential complications and the importance of taking all antibiotics as prescribed. Other suggestions for prevention of UTIs include proper perineal care, wiping from front to back after urinating or having a bowel movement, and increasing fluid intake.

Because mastitis rarely occurs before the postpartum woman is discharged, teaching should include warning signs of mastitis and counseling about prevention of cracked nipples. Management includes intensive antibiotic therapy (e.g., cephalosporins and vancomycin, which are particularly useful in staphylococcal infections), support of breasts, local heat or cold, adequate hydration, and analgesics.

Almost all instances of acute mastitis can be avoided by using proper breastfeeding technique to prevent cracked nipples. Missed feedings, waiting too long between feedings, and abrupt weaning may lead to clogged nipples and mastitis. Cleanliness practiced by all who have contact with the newborn and new mother also reduces the incidence of mastitis.

SEQUELAE OF CHILDBIRTH TRAUMA

Women are at risk for problems related to the reproductive system from the age of menarche through menopause and the older years. These problems, which include structural disorders of the uterus and vagina related to pelvic relaxation and urinary incontinence, are often the delayed but direct result of childbearing.

With fetopelvic disproportion, prolonged labor, or a precipitous birth, structures of the vesical and vaginal walls are stretched and may be injured. The bladder neck and urethra may be compressed between the presenting part and the pubic bones, or forced downward ahead of the presenting part. Since soft tissue damage usually occurs behind an intact vaginal epithelium, there is nothing visible to repair. However, defects may also occur in women who have never been pregnant.

Structural disorders can have far-reaching effects for the woman and her family. Beyond the obvious physiologic alterations, the woman also experiences threats to her self-concept and her ability to cope. A woman's concept of herself as a sexual being can be affected by the condition and its treatments. A woman's family is also challenged in the way it responds to her diagnosis.

Uterine Displacement and Prolapse

Normally the round ligaments hold the uterus in anteversion, and the uterosacral ligaments pull the cervix backward and upward. Uterine displacement is a variation of this normal placement. The most common type of displacement is posterior displacement, or retroversion, in which the uterus is tilted posteriorly and the cervix rotates anteriorly. Other variations include retroflexion and anteflexion (Fig. 23-2).

By 2 months postpartum, the ligaments should return to normal length; but in about one third of women, the uterus remains retroverted. This condition is rarely symptomatic, but conception may be difficult because the cervix points toward the anterior vaginal wall and away from the posterior fornix, where seminal fluid pools after coitus. If symptoms occur, they may include pelvic and low back pain, exaggeration of premenstrual tension, and dyspareunia.

Uterine prolapse is a more serious type of displacement. Degrees of prolapse can vary from mild to complete. In complete prolapse, the cervix and body of the uterus protrude through the vagina and the vagina is inverted (Fig. 23-3).

Uterine displacement and prolapse can be caused by congenital or acquired weakness of the pelvic support structures (often referred to as pelvic relaxation). Although extensive damage may be noted and repaired shortly after birth, symptoms related to pelvic relaxation most often appear during the perimenopausal period, when the effects of ovarian hormones on pelvic tissues are lost and atrophic changes begin. Pelvic

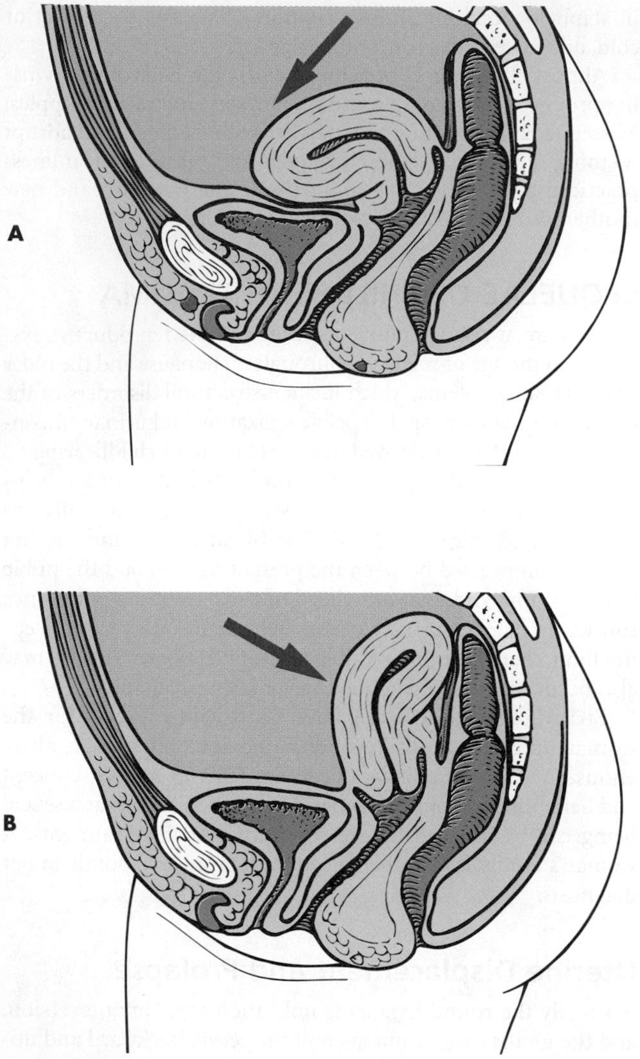

FIG. 23-2 • Types of uterine displacement. **A**, Anterior displacement. **B**, Retroversion (backward displacement of uterus).

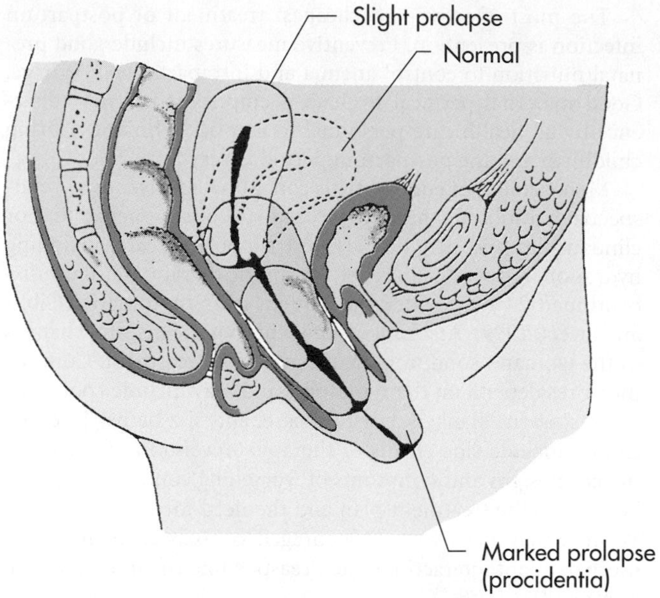

FIG. 23-3 • Prolapse of uterus

trauma, stress and strain, and the aging process are contributing causes. Other causes of pelvic relaxation include reproductive surgery and pelvic radiation.

Clinical Manifestations. Generally, symptoms of pelvic relaxation relate to the structure involved: urethra, bladder, uterus, vagina, cul-de-sac, or rectum. The most common complaints are pulling and dragging sensations, pressure, protrusions, fatigue, and low backache. Symptoms may be worse after prolonged standing or deep penile penetration during intercourse. Stress urinary incontinence may be present.

Cystocele and Rectocele

Cystocele and rectocele often occur with uterine prolapse (although they can occur independently), causing the uterus to sag even further backward and downward into the vagina. Cystocele (Fig. 23-4, *A*) is the protrusion of the bladder downward into the vagina that develops when supporting structures in the vesicovaginal septum are injured. Anterior wall relaxation develops gradually over time as a result of congenital defects of supports, childbearing, obesity, or advanced age. When the woman stands, the weakened anterior vaginal wall cannot support the weight of the urine in the bladder; the vesicovaginal septum is forced downward, the bladder is stretched, and its capacity is increased. With time the cystocele enlarges until it protrudes into the vagina. Complete emptying of the bladder is difficult because the cystocele sags below the bladder neck. Rectocele is the herniation of the anterior rectal wall through the relaxed or ruptured vaginal fascia and rectovaginal septum; it appears as a large bulge that may be seen through the relaxed introitus (Fig. 23-4, *B*).

Clinical Manifestations. Cystoceles and rectoceles often are asymptomatic. If symptoms of cystocele are present, they may include complaints of a bearing-down sensation or that "something is in my vagina." Other symptoms include urinary frequency, retention, incontinence, and possible recurrent cystitis and urinary tract infections. On pelvic examination there is a bulging of the anterior wall of the vagina when the woman is asked to bear down. Unless the bladder neck and urethra are damaged, urinary continence is unaffected. Women with large cystoceles complain of having to push upward on the sagging anterior vaginal wall to be able to void.

Rectoceles may be small and produce few symptoms, but some are so large that they protrude outside of the vagina when the woman stands. Symptoms are absent when the woman is lying down. A rectocele causes a disturbance in bowel function, a sensation of bearing down, or a sensation that the pelvic organs are falling out. With a very large rectocele it may be difficult to have a bowel movement. Each time the woman strains during bowel evacuation, the feces are forced against the thinned rectovaginal wall, stretching it even more. Some women facilitate evacuation by applying digital pressure vaginally to hold up the rectal pouch.

Urinary Incontinence

About 20% of women between ages 25 and 64 years have urinary incontinence (UI) (uncontrollable leakage of urine). Although nulliparous women can have UI, the incidence is higher in women who have given birth and also increases with parity (Sampselle et al, 1997). Conditions that disturb urinary control include stress urinary incontinence, which is due to sudden increases in intraabdominal pressure such as those caused by sneezing or coughing; urge incontinence, caused by disorders of the bladder and urethra such as urethritis and urethral stricture, trigonitis, and cystitis; neuropathies such as multiple sclerosis, diabetic neuritis, and pathologic conditions of the spinal cord; and congenital and acquired urinary tract abnormalities.

Stress urinary incontinence may follow injury to bladder neck structures. A sphincter mechanism at the bladder neck compresses the upper urethra, pulls it upward behind the symphysis, and forms an acute angle at the junction of the posterior urethral wall and the base of the bladder (Fig. 23-5). To empty the bladder, the sphincter complex relaxes and the trigone contracts to open the internal urethral orifice and pull the contracting bladder wall upward, forcing urine out. The angle between the urethra and the base of the bladder is lost or increased if the supporting pubococcygeus muscle is injured; this change, coupled with a urethrocele, causes incontinence. Urine spurts out when the woman is asked to bear down or cough while she is in the lithotomy position.

Genital Fistulas

A fistula is an abnormal communication between one hollow viscus and another, or from one hollow viscus to the outside. Genital fistulas may occur between the bladder and the genital tract (e.g., vesicovaginal); between the urethra and the vagina (urethrovaginal); and between the rectum or sigmoid colon and the vagina (rectovaginal) (Fig. 23-6). Fistulas may be a result of a congenital anomaly, gynecologic surgery, obstetric trauma, cancer, radiation therapy, gynecologic trauma, or infection.

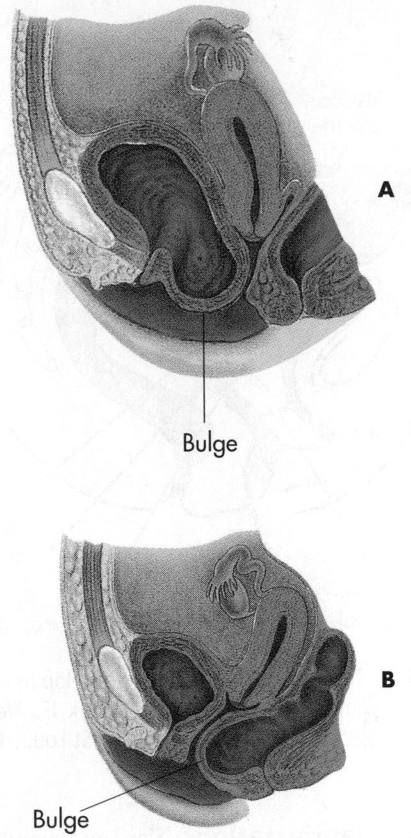

FIG. 23-4 • Side views of **A**, cystocele and **B**, rectocele. (From Seidel H et al: *Mosby's guide to physical examination,* ed 4, St Louis, 1999, Mosby.)

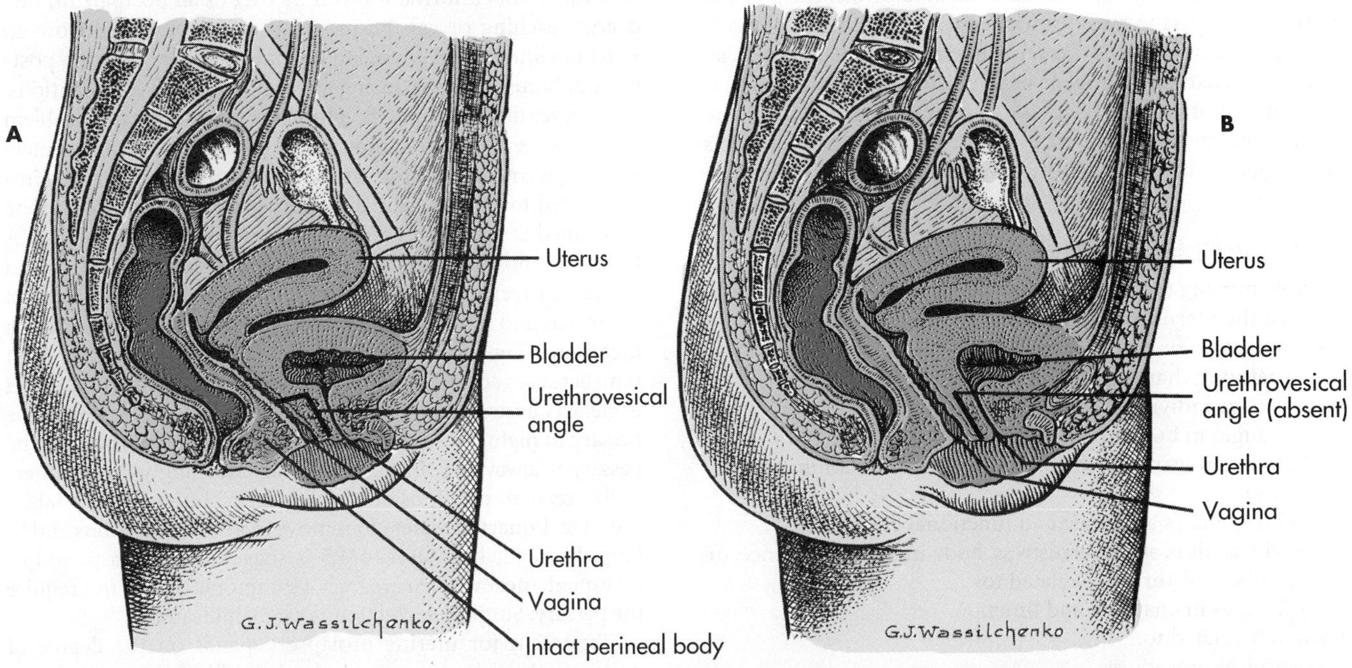

FIG. 23-5 • Urethrovesical angle. **A,** Normal angle. **B,** Widening (absence) of angle.

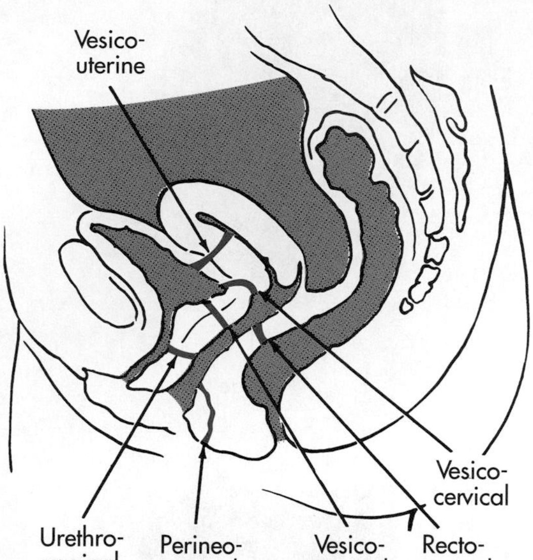

FIG. 23-6 • Types of fistulas that may develop in vagina, uterus, and rectum. (From Phipps WJ, Sands JK, Marek JF: *Medical-surgical nursing: concepts and clinical practice*, ed 6, St Louis, 1999, Mosby.)

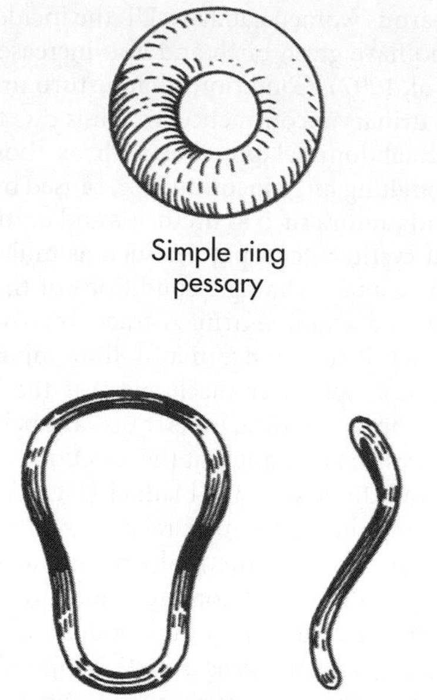

FIG. 23-7 • Examples of pessaries (simple ring and Smith-Hodge).

Clinical Manifestations. Signs and symptoms of vaginal fistulas depend on the site but may include the presence of urine, flatus, or feces in the vagina; odors of urine or feces in the vagina; and irritation of vaginal tissues.

Care Management

➤ Assessment

Assessment for problems related to structural disorders of the uterus and vagina focuses primarily on the genitourinary tract, the reproductive organs, bowel elimination, and psychosocial and sexual factors. A complete health history, physical examination, and laboratory tests are done to support the appropriate medical diagnosis. The nurse needs to assess the woman's knowledge of the disorder, its management, and the possible prognosis.

➤ Nursing Diagnoses

Possible nursing diagnoses for the patient with a structural disorder of the uterus or vagina include the following:

- Constipation or diarrhea related to:
  —Anatomic changes
- Ineffective individual coping related to:
  —Changes in body image
- Altered family processes or interpersonal relationships related to:
  —The woman's anatomic and functional changes
- Social isolation, spiritual distress, body image disturbance, or self-esteem disturbance related to:
  —Changes in anatomy and function
- Anxiety related to:
  —Surgical procedure
  —Prognosis

➤ Plan of Care and Implementation

The health care team works together to treat the disorders related to alterations in pelvic support and to assist the woman in management of her symptoms. In general, nurses working with these women can provide information and self-care education to prevent problems before they occur; to manage or reduce symptoms and to promote comfort and hygiene if symptoms are already present; and to recognize when further intervention is needed. This information can be part of all postpartum discharge teaching or can be provided at postpartum follow-up visits in clinics or in physician or midwife offices, during postpartum home visits, or during gynecologic health examinations.

Interventions for specific problems depend on the problem and the severity of the symptoms. If discomfort related to uterine displacement is a problem, several interventions can be implemented to treat uterine displacement. Kegel exercises can be performed several times a day to increase muscular strength. A knee-chest position performed for a few minutes several times a day can correct a mildly retroverted uterus. A pessary to support the uterus and hold it in the correct position may be inserted in the vagina (Fig. 23-7). Usually a pessary is used only for a short time because it can lead to pressure necrosis and vaginitis. Good hygiene is important; some women can be taught to remove the pessary at night, cleanse it, and replace it in the morning. If the pessary is always left in place, regular douching with commercially prepared solutions or weak vinegar solutions (e.g., 1 tablespoon to 1 quart of water) to remove increased secretions and to keep the vaginal pH at 4 to 4.5 is suggested. After a period of treatment, most women are free of symptoms and do not require the pessary. Surgical correction is rarely indicated.

Treatment for uterine prolapse depends on the degree of prolapse. Pessaries may be useful in mild prolapse. Estrogen therapy also may be used in the older woman to improve tissue tone. If these conservative treatments do not correct the problem, or there is a significant degree of prolapse, abdominal or vaginal hysterectomy is usually recommended.

Treatment for a cystocele includes use of a vaginal pessary or surgical repair. Pessaries may not be effective. Anterior repair (colporrhaphy) is the usual surgical procedure, and is usually done for large symptomatic cystoceles. This involves a surgical shortening of pelvic muscles to provide better support for the bladder. An anterior repair is often combined with a vaginal hysterectomy.

Small rectoceles may not need treatment. The woman with mild symptoms may get relief from a high-fiber diet and adequate fluid intake, stool softeners, or mild laxatives. Vaginal pessaries usually are not effective. Large rectoceles that are causing significant symptoms are usually repaired surgically. A posterior repair (colporrhaphy) is the usual procedure. This surgery is performed vaginally and involves shortening the pelvic muscles to provide better support for the rectum. Anterior and posterior repairs may be performed at the same time and with vaginal hysterectomy.

Mild to moderate urinary incontinence can be significantly decreased or relieved in many women by bladder training and pelvic muscle (Kegel) exercises (Czarapata and McKillips, 1997; Sampselle et al, 1997). Other management strategies include insertion of a bladder neck support prosthesis, estrogen therapy, and surgery (Mishell et al, 1997).

Nursing care of the woman with pelvic relaxation problems or a fistula requires great sensitivity because the woman's reactions are often intense. She may become withdrawn or, conversely, hostile because of embarrassment about odors and soiling of her clothing that are beyond her control. The nurse should be tactful in suggesting hygienic practices that reduce odor. Commercial deodorizing douches are available, or noncommercial solutions such as diluted chlorine (e.g., 1 teaspoon of chlorine household bleach to 1 quart of water) may be used. The chlorine solution is also useful for external perineal irrigation. Sitz baths and thorough washing of the genitalia with unscented, mild soap and warm water also help. Sparse dusting with deodorizing powders can be useful. If a rectovaginal fistula is present, enemas given before leaving the house may provide temporary relief from oozing of fecal material until corrective surgery is performed. Irritated skin and tissues may benefit from use of a heat lamp or application of vitamins A and D ointment. Hygienic care is time consuming and may need to be repeated frequently throughout the day; protective pads or pants may need to be worn. All of these activities can be demoralizing to the woman and frustrating to her and her family.

Many of the nurse's efforts with these problems are directed toward participating in a team effort to prepare the woman for surgery. Preoperative teaching involves the primary nurse, operating room nurse, surgeon, and anesthesiologist. The nurse in the health promotion setting is usually most aware of the woman's living circumstances, physical limitations, and social problems and therefore may be best suited to coordinate continuity of care after discharge.

POSTPARTUM PSYCHOLOGIC COMPLICATIONS

Mental health disorders in the postpartum period have implications for the mother, the newborn, and the entire family. Such conditions can interfere with attachment to the newborn and family integration, and some may threaten the safety and well-being of the mother, newborn, and other children.

In the Diagnostic and Statistical Manual of Mental Disorders (American Psychiatric Association [APA], 1994), postpartum psychologic disorders are categorized (from less severe to most severe, respectively) as postpartum blues (discussed in Chapter 22), postpartum depression without psychotic features, and postpartum depression with psychotic features (postpartum psychosis).

Postpartum Depression without Psychotic Features

Postpartum depression (PPD) is an intense and pervasive sadness with severe and labile mood swings and is more serious and persistent than postpartum blues. Intense fears, anger, anxiety, and despondency that persist past the baby's first few weeks are not a normal part of postpartum blues. Occurring in approximately 10% to 15% of new mothers, these symptoms rarely disappear without outside help.

The symptoms of postpartum major depression do not differ from symptoms of nonpostpartum mood disorders except that the mother's ruminations of guilt and inadequacy feed her worries about being an incompetent and inadequate parent. In PPD, there may be odd food cravings (often, sweet desserts) and binges with abnormal appetite and weight gain. New mothers report an increased yearning for sleep; sleeping heavily, but awakening instantly with any infant noise; and an inability to go back to sleep after infant feedings.

A distinguishing feature of PPD is irritability. These episodes of irritability may flare up with little provocation, and they may sometimes escalate to violent outbursts or dissolve into uncontrollable sobbing. Many of these outbursts are directed against significant others ("He never helps me") or the baby ("She cries all the time and I feel like hitting her"). Women with postpartum major depressive episodes often have severe anxiety, panic attacks, and spontaneous crying long after the usual duration of baby blues.

Many women feel especially guilty about having depressive feelings at a time when they believe they should be happy. They may be reluctant to discuss their symptoms or their negative feelings toward the infant. A prominent feature of PPD is rejection of the infant, often caused by abnormal jealousy. The mother may be obsessed by the notion that the baby may take her place in her partner's affections. Attitudes toward the infant may include disinterest, annoyance with care demands, and blaming because of her lack of maternal feeling. When observed, she may appear awkward in her responses to the baby. Obsessive thoughts about harming the infant are very frightening to her. Often she does not share these thoughts because of embarrassment, but when she does, other family members become very frightened.

Medical Management. The natural course is one of gradual improvement over the 6 months after birth. Support treatment alone is not efficacious for major postpartum depression. Pharmacologic intervention is needed in most instances. Treatment options include antidepressants, anxiolytic agents, and electroconvulsive therapy. Psychotherapy focuses on her fears and concerns regarding her new responsibilities and roles, as well as monitoring for suicidal or homicidal thoughts. For some women, hospitalization is necessary.

Postpartum Depression with Psychotic Features

Postpartum psychosis is a syndrome most often characterized by depression (as described previously), delusions, and thoughts by the mother of harming either the infant or herself (Kaplan and Sadock, 1998).

A postpartum mood disorder with psychotic features occurs in 1 to 2 per 1000 births (Kaplan and Sadock, 1998). Once a woman has had one postpartum episode with psychotic features, there is a 35% to 60% likelihood of recurrence with each subsequent birth (APA, 1994).

Symptoms often begin within days after the birth (although the mean time to onset is 2 to 3 weeks) and almost always within 8 weeks of birth (Kaplan and Sadock, 1998). Characteristically, the woman begins to complain of fatigue, insomnia, and restlessness, and may have episodes of tearfulness and emotional lability. Complaints regarding the inability to move, stand, or work are also common. Later, suspiciousness, confusion, incoherence, irrational statements, and obsessive concerns about the baby's health and welfare may be present (Kaplan and Sadock, 1998). Delusions may be present in 50% of all women and hallucinations in about 25%. Auditory hallucinations that command the mother to kill the infant can also occur in severe cases. When delusions are present, they are often related to the infant. The mother may think the infant is possessed by the devil, has special powers, or is destined for a terrible fate (APA, 1994). Grossly disorganized behavior may be manifested as a disinterest in the infant or an inability to provide care. Some will insist that something is wrong with the baby, or accuse nurses or family of hurting or poisoning their child. Nurses are advised to be alert for mothers who are agitated, overactive, confused, complaining, or suspicious.

Medical Management. A favorable outcome is associated with a good premorbid adjustment (before the onset of the disorder) and a supportive family network (Kaplan and Sadock, 1998). The course of the syndrome is similar to that seen in patients with mood disorders. Because mood disorders are usually episodic, women may experience another episode of symptoms within a year or two of the birth. Postpartum psychosis is a psychiatric emergency. Antidepressants and lithium are the treatments of choice. If the mother is breastfeeding, some sources say no pharmacologic agents should be prescribed (Kaplan and Sadock, 1998), but other sources advise caution while prescribing some agents (Schatzberg and Nemeroff, 1998). The mother will probably need psychiatric hospitalization. It is usually advantageous for the mother to have contact with her baby if she

Box 23-4

Suggested Questions to Elicit Responses from the Postpartum Depression Checklist

LACK OF CONCENTRATION
Are you experiencing difficulty concentrating?
Does your mind seem to be filled with cobwebs?
Does it seem at times like fogginess sets in?

LOSS OF INTERESTS
Do you feel your life is empty of your previous interests and goals?
Have you lost interest in your hobbies that used to bring you pleasure and enjoyment?

LONELINESS
Are you experiencing feelings of loneliness?
Do you feel as though no one really understands what you are experiencing?
Do you feel uncomfortable around other people?
Have you been isolating yourself from other people?

INSECURITY
Have you been feeling insecure, fragile, or vulnerable?
Does the responsibility of motherhood seem overwhelming?

OBSESSIVE THINKING
Is your mind constantly filled with obsessive thinking, such as "What's wrong with me?" "Am I going crazy?" "Why can't I enjoy being with my baby?"
When trying to fall asleep at night, is your mind still racing with repetitive thoughts?

LACK OF POSITIVE EMOTIONS
Are you experiencing feelings of emptiness?
Do you feel like a robot just going through the motions?
When caring for your infant/child, do you feel any joy or love?

LOSS OF SELF
Do you feel as though you are not the same person you used to be?
Are you afraid that your life will never be normal again?

ANXIETY ATTACKS
Are you experiencing uncontrollable anxiety attacks?
Are you experiencing periods of palpitations, chest pains, sweating, or tingling hands?
When going through an anxiety attack, do you feel as though you're losing your mind?

LOSS OF CONTROL
Do you feel you are in control of your emotions and thoughts?
Are you experiencing loss of control in any aspects of your life?

GUILT
Are you feeling guilty because you are not giving your infant/child the love and attention he or she needs?
Are you experiencing guilt over thoughts of harming your infant/child?
Do you feel you are a good mother?

CONTEMPLATING DEATH
Have you ever experienced thoughts of harming yourself?
Have you been feeling so low that the thought of leaving this world is appealing to you?

Source: Beck C: Screening methods for postpartum depression, *J Obstet Gynecol Neonatal Nurs* 24(4):308-312, 1995.

so desires, but visits must be closely supervised. Psychotherapy is indicated after the period of acute psychosis is past.

Even though the prevalence of PPD is fairly well established, few women are referred to a mental health care provider. Those identified are often treated inappropriately with benzodiazepines or subtherapeutic doses of antidepressants.

➤ Assessment

In order to recognize symptoms of PPD as early as possible, the nurse should be an active listener and demonstrate a caring attitude. Nurses cannot depend on women to volunteer unsolicited information about their depression or to ask for help. The nurse should observe for signs of depression and ask appropriate questions to determine moods, appetite, sleep, energy and fatigue levels, and ability to concentrate. If the nurse assesses that the new mother is depressed, she or he must ask if the mother has thought about hurting herself or the baby.

Nurses can use screening tools such as the Postpartum Depression Checklist (Beck, 1995, 1998) (Box 23-4) and the Edinburgh Postnatal Depression Scale (Cox, Holden and Savogsky, 1989) in assessing whether the depressive symptoms have progressed from postpartum blues to PPD. If the initial screening indicates that the woman may be depressed, a formal screening is helpful in determining the urgency of the referral and the type of provider. It is also important to assess the woman's family; they may be able to offer valuable information as well as have a need to express how they have been affected by the woman's emotional disorder.

➤ Nursing Diagnoses

Possible nursing diagnoses for the woman experiencing postpartum depression include the following:

- Risk for injury to newborn related to:
  —Mother's depression (inattention to infant's needs for hygiene, nutrition, safety) and psychotropic medications via breast milk
- Ineffective family coping related to:
  —Increased care needs of mother and infant
- Risk for altered parenting related to:
  —Inability of depressed mother to attach to infant
- Anxiety in mother related to:
  —Postpartum hormonal fluctuation
- Risk for violence toward self (mother) or children related to:
  —Postpartum depression

On the Postpartum Unit. The postpartum nurse must observe the new mother carefully for any signs of tearfulness, and conduct further assessments as necessary. PPD must be discussed by nurses to prepare new parents for potential problems in the postpartum period. The family must be able to recognize the symptoms and know where to go for help. Written materials that explain what the woman can do to prevent depression are useful. Nurses can also educate women about normal newborn/infant growth and development and help the women develop realistic expectations about infant behavioral cues (Wood et al, 1997).

Mothers are often discharged before the blues or PPD occurs. If the postpartum nurse is concerned about the mother, a mental health consult should be requested before the mother leaves the hospital. Routine instructions regarding PPD should be given to whoever comes to take the patient home; for example, "If you notice that your wife (or daughter) is upset or crying a lot, please call the postpartum care provider immediately—don't wait for the routine postpartum appointment."

In the Home and Community. Postpartum home visits can reduce the incidence of or complications from depression; however, home visits are not always feasible. Supervision of the mother with emotional complications may become a prime concern. Because depression can greatly interfere with her mothering functions, family and friends may need to participate in the infant's care. This supervision can be planned by the collaborative efforts of the nurse and family members.

Even if the woman is severely depressed, hospitalization can be avoided if adequate resources can be mobilized to ensure safety for both mother and infant. The nurse in home care will need to make frequent phone calls or home visits to do assessment and counseling. Community resources that may be helpful are temporary child care or foster care, homemaker service, meals on wheels, parenting guidance centers, mother's-day-out programs, and telephone support groups.

Women with moderate to severe cases of PPD should be referred to a mental health therapist, such as an advanced practice psychiatric nurse, for evaluation and therapy. Inpatient psychiatric hospitalization may be necessary. This decision is made when the safety needs of the mother or child are threatened.

PPD is usually treated with antidepressant medications. The woman taking mood stabilizers (Box 23-5) must be taught about the many side effects, and especially, for those on lithium, the need to have serum lithium levels drawn every 6 months. Women with severe psychiatric syndromes will probably require antipsychotic medications (Box 23-6).

Patient education is important for those taking antipsychotic medications; most of these medications can cause seda-

Box 23-5

Mood Stabilizers

Carbamazepine (Tegretol)
Clonazepam (Klonopin)
Divalproex (Depakote)
Lithium carbonate (Eskalith)

Box 23-6

Commonly Used Antipsychotic Medications

PHENOTHIAZINES
Chlorpromazine (Thorazine)
Fluphenazine (Prolixin)
Perphenazine (Trilafon)
Thioridazine (Mellaril)
Trifluoperazine (Stelazine)

OTHER
Clozapine (Clozaril)
Haloperidol (Haldol)
Loxapine (Loxitane)
Olanzapine (Zyprexa)
Pimozide (Orap)
Quetiapine (Seroquel)
Risperidone (Risperdal)
Thiothixene (Navane)

tion and orthostatic hypotension—both of which could interfere with the mother being able to safely care for her baby. The medications can also cause parasympathetic nervous system (PNS) effects such as constipation, dry mouth, blurred vision, tachycardia, urinary retention, weight gain, and agranulocytosis. CNS effects may include akathisia, dystonias, Parkinsonism-like symptoms, tardive dyskinesia (irreversible), and neuroleptic malignant syndrome (potentially fatal).

When breastfeeding women have emotional complications and need psychotropic medications, referral to a psychiatrist who specializes in postpartum disorders is preferred. Depressed women who are not breastfeeding will need supervision to take antidepressants as ordered. Because they do not exert any effect before about 2 weeks and usually do not reach full effect before 4 to 6 weeks, many women discontinue taking the medication on their own (Nursing Care Plan).

LOSS AND GRIEF

Situational life crises can be superimposed on the experiences of childbearing. These may include infertility, premature labor/premature birth, a cesarean birth, any perception of loss of control during the birthing experience, birth of a boy when the parents wanted a girl, the birth of a handicapped child, a maternal death, and/or fetal or neonatal death. All of these situations have a common denominator—they are losses of what was hoped for, dreamed about, and/or planned.

From the perspective of health care providers, these crises vary in degree. However, from the perspective of the parents, the perceived loss may be the most terrible thing that has ever happened to them. At the birth they are mourning instead of celebrating life.

The statistics on perinatal loss and death of an infant are grim. Each year, approximately 5 of every 1000 births end in stillbirth or fetal death. Newborn death accounts for almost 27,000 deaths per year in the United States (Guyer et al, 1998); 18,000 infants die in the early postpartum period from prematurity, birth defects, and other acute illnesses (Guyer et al, 1998). Thus parents can experience grief before or during the childbearing experience. In addition, 7 to 8 women per 100,000 die in the United States of childbirth related causes.

The focus of this section is to prepare the beginning nurse to provide sensitive, supportive, and therapeutic interventions to parents and families experiencing perinatal loss in a variety of settings.

Critical Thinking

COMMUNITY RESOURCES FOR LOSS AND GRIEF

Investigate what resources and support groups exist in your community to assist parents who have experienced a maternal death, birth of a "less-than-perfect" child, a cesarean birth, the death of a baby through miscarriage, stillbirth, or newborn death. Are sources available? Are there enough of these sources to assist parents? How difficult was it for you to identify these sources? What could you do to make sources more known to bereaved parents and families?

Nursing Care Plan POSTPARTUM DEPRESSION

NURSING DIAGNOSIS Risk for injury to the newborn and patient related to patient's emotional state as evidenced by maternal behaviors and increased score on a postpartum depression scale

EXPECTED OUTCOME The patient and newborn will remain free of injury.

Nursing Interventions/*Rationales*

Assess the postpartum patient for risk factors for depression; use assessment scale to determine which patient may be most at risk *to identify patients needing prompt interventions.*

Maintain frequent contact with patient by telephone calls and home visits *to determine if further interventions are necessary because most patients are discharged early from the inpatient setting.*

Assess patient for any suicidal thoughts or plans *to provide for safety of patient and neonate.*

Refer mild cases of depression to support groups *to provide group interaction with women having similar problems.*

Refer moderate to severe cases of depression to mental health therapist *to provide for individualized psychiatric care.*

Refer breastfeeding mother to lactation consultant *to provide information regarding effects of antidepressant and antipsychotic medications.*

NURSING DIAGNOSIS Ineffective family coping, disabling, related to postpartum maternal depression as evidenced by family members' denial of patient's illness

EXPECTED OUTCOME Family will identify positive coping mechanisms and initiate a plan to cope with the patient's depression.

Nursing Interventions/*Rationales*

Provide opportunity for family and significant others to verbalize feelings and concerns *to establish a trusting relationship.*

Give information to the family regarding postpartum depression *to clarify any misconceptions or misinformation.*

Assist family to identify positive coping mechanism that have been effective during past crises *to promote active participation in care.*

Assist family to identify community sources of support *to provide additional resources as needed.*

Refer family to mental health counselor as needed *to provide further expertise from a mental health professional.*

Conceptual Model of Parental Grief. Miles (1984) and Miles and Demi (1986, 1997) proposed a conceptual model of parental grief, based on the work of Lindemann (1944), Parkes (1972), Parkes and Weiss (1983), and Worden (1991). The model proposes that the grief responses of a parent are closely linked to that parent's self-image as a mother or father. Parental grief responses occur in three overlapping phases of grief—acute distress, intense grief, and reorganization.

Acute Distress. The loss of a pregnancy, or the death of an infant, is an acute and distressing experience for mothers and fathers who planned for and expected a normal healthy infant as the outcome. The loss encompasses a loss of their identity as a mother or father and the loss of their many dreams related to parenthood. The immediate reaction to news of a perinatal loss or infant death is a period of acute distress. Parents generally are in a state of shock and numbness. They may feel a sense of unreality and confusion, as though they were in a bad dream or in a fog or trancelike state. Disbelief and denial can occur. Parents also feel very sad and depressed; intense outbursts of emotion and crying are common. However, lack of affect, euphoria, and calmness may occur and may reflect numbness, denial, or a personal way of coping with stress.

It is during this time of acute distress that parents face the first task of grief: accepting the reality of the loss. The pregnancy has ended or the baby has died and their lives have changed. While parents are often required to make many decisions, such as naming the infant or making funeral arrangements, normal functioning is impeded and decisions are difficult to make. Grandparents, friends, clergy, or other relatives may be available to help the couple cope. However, it is important that the mother and father ultimately make the decisions that are right for them.

Intense Grief. The phase of intense grief encompasses many difficult emotions, including loneliness, emptiness, and yearning; guilt, anger, and fear; disorganization and depression; and physical symptoms. Being able to adjust to the environment after the loss means learning how to accommodate the changes that the loss has brought. Deciding what to do about the nursery and baby clothes, how to handle comments of co-workers when returning to work, and how to cope with insensitive family members and friends are among the problems bereaved parents face during this phase of grief.

Parents often experience feelings of loneliness, emptiness, and yearning. The mother may report that her arms ache to hold or nurse her baby, and that she wakes to the sound of a baby crying. When her milk comes in, it is particularly poignant when there is no baby to take to breast. Some parents cope with these feelings by avoiding memories and by not talking about the baby, whereas others want to reminisce and discuss their loss over and over.

During this phase of intense grief, guilt may emerge from the deep feelings of helplessness in not somehow preventing the pregnancy loss or the death of the infant. With many perinatal losses, there is no clear cause of the event, leaving the woman to speculate about what she might have done or not done to cause the loss. Guilt may be intense if the mother thinks she is being punished for some unrelated event such as having had a prior induced abortion.

Other common responses during this phase are anger, resentment, bitterness, and irritability. Anger may be focused on the health care team who failed to save the pregnancy or infant, toward a God who allowed the loss to occur; or toward family, friends, or peers when they do not provide the support the bereaved parents need and want.

Deep sadness and depression occur when the parent is faced with the full awareness of the reality of the loss. This may occur several months after the perinatal loss and can continue for some time. Sadness and depression may be accompanied by disorganization and problems with cognitive processing; parents may have difficulty getting things done, be unable to concentrate, be restless, have confused thought processes, have difficulty solving problems, and make poor decisions.

Physical symptoms of grief include fatigue, headaches, dizziness, and backaches. Developing health problems such as colds or hypertension is not uncommon. It may be difficult to sleep; the appetite may be depressed or voracious. Lack of sleep and inadequate nutrition and fluids can complicate other grief responses.

Reorganization. From the time of the pregnancy loss or infant death, parents attempt to understand "why?" This leads to a long and intense search for meaning. At first the "why" is focused on the cause of death. Parents next focus on "why me, why mine?" These questions lead some parents into an existential search about the meaning of life and death. This search continues into the phase of reorganization and may lead to profound changes in the parents' view of the fragility of life.

Time helps to slowly ease the painful feelings of grief. Over time, the pain becomes less frequent. Reorganization occurs when the parent is better able to function at home and work, experiences a return of self-esteem and confidence, can cope with new challenges, and has placed the loss in perspective. Reorganization begins to peak sometime after the first year as parents begin to achieve the task of moving on with their lies. Enjoying the simple pleasures of life without feeling guilty, nurturing self and others, developing new interests, and reestablishing relationships are all signs of moving on. For some women and families, another pregnancy and the birth of a subsequent child is an important step to be able to move on with their lives. Parents will never forget the baby who died, and they are not the same persons as before the loss. The term "bittersweet grief," coined by Kowalski (1984), refers to the grief response that occurs with reminders of the loss. This typically happens on birthdays, death days, and anniversaries; at school events; during changes in the seasons; and during the time of the year when the loss occurred. Grief feelings also can be triggered after a subsequent live birth.

Anticipatory Grief. Some parents experience anticipatory grief; that is, they have knowledge of an impending loss, such as when a baby is admitted to a neonatal intensive care unit (NICU) with problems or when a diagnosis of an anacephalic fetus is made by ultrasound examination. The fetus is still alive, but the prognosis is poor. Being able to anticipate the loss gives families an opportunity to plan, feel more in control of their situation, and be able to say good-bye in a special way. However, some individuals or family members may distance or detach themselves from the experience or the baby as a way of protecting themselves or avoiding the pain of loss and grief.

Care Management

Nursing care of mothers and fathers experiencing a perinatal loss begins the first time they are faced with the potential loss of their pregnancy or death of their infant. Supportive interventions are important both at the time of the loss and after the parents have returned home.

Families that experience loss may have many and varied feelings and responses. Some people view an early pregnancy as the union of cells; others have visions of a baby; and still others are wrapped up in the thrill of being pregnant.

➤ Assessment

Assessment of family members' perceptions of the loss and their perceptions of the events surrounding the loss is crucial before intervention. This assessment is as important for families experiencing a miscarriage or ectopic pregnancy as it is for those experiencing stillbirth or neonatal loss.

Support during a perinatal loss is important to most couples. However, it is important to assess the amount and type of support from others that a couple wants. Some prefer to handle the tragedy alone for awhile; others want assistance in calling other family members, friends, and clergy to be with them and to help them with decisions.

➤ Nursing Diagnoses

Examples of nursing diagnoses for a couple experiencing perinatal grief include the following:

- Altered family processes related to:
  - —Maternal depression leading to changes in role function
  - —Inadequate communication of feelings between the grieving mother and father
  - —Lack of attention and support to siblings
- Fatigue and sleep pattern disturbance related to:
  - —Inability to fall asleep because of grief
  - —Waking in the night and thinking about the loss
- Self-esteem disturbance related to:
  - —Prolonged feelings of poor self-worth because of the loss
  - —Feeling unworthy of having a child
- Spiritual distress related to:
  - —Anger with God
  - —Confusion about why prayers were not answered
- Altered thought processes related to:
  - —Difficulty making decisions
  - —Inability to get organized
  - —Poor work performance
  - —Confused thinking

➤ Expected Outcomes

Expected outcomes are set and prioritized in patient-centered terms according to the mutual goals chosen by the patient and the nurse. Expected outcomes may include that the woman/famly will do the following:

- Actualize the loss
- Share experiences and verbalize feelings of grief
- Understand the normal grief responses they may experience at the time of and following the loss
- Identify family and community resources for support

➤ Plan of Care and Implementation

Interventions and support for parents from the nursing and medical staff following a perinatal loss or infant death are extremely important in their healing. While parents often cannot recall details of their experiences at the time of death, they may recall vividly a minor event that was perceived as particularly painful or particularly helpful. The interventions provided below are general ideas about what may be helpful to parents. However, care must be individualized to each parent and family.

Communicating and Caring Techniques. Mothers, fathers, and extended families look to the medical and nursing staff for support and understanding during the time of loss. Therapeutic communication and counseling techniques help the mother, father, and other family members express their feelings and emotions, understand their responses to the loss, and make decisions.

The nurse should listen patiently while people tell their story of loss and grief. Asking questions that help people talk about their grief and the experiences surrounding the loss may be needed. However, grief responses in the initial days of crisis make it difficult for individuals to concentrate on what is being asked, to think about what the question means, and to respond to the question. The use of silence often gives the bereaved person the opportunity to collect thoughts and to respond to questions. The nurse should resist the temptation to give advice or to use clichés in offering support (Box 23-7).

Nurses need to become comfortable with their own feelings of grief and loss to effectively support and care for the bereaved. It is appropriate to express feelings with the bereaved families and to share the moment with them.

Worden (1991) identified several counseling techniques the nurse might use in helping the family share and express their grief. These include the following:

Actualize the Loss. Ask the bereaved questions that help them to express the experience of the loss. Use the name of their baby, and view the body of the baby before speaking with family members.

Help the survivor identify and express feelings. Expressed grief can be overwhelming to health care professionals. Feelings of anger, guilt, and sadness are paramount in the early days and months following a loss. When the bereaved express feelings of anger, it can be helpful to identify the feeling by simply saying, "You sound angry," or "You look angry. Where is this anger

Box 23-7

What to Say and What Not to Say to Bereaved Parents

WHAT TO SAY

"I'm sad for you."
"How are you doing with all of this?"
"This must be hard for you."
"What can I do for you?"
"I'm sorry."
"I'm here, and I want to listen."

WHAT NOT TO SAY

"God had a purpose for her."
"Be thankful you have another child."
"The living must go on."
"I know how you feel."
"It's God's will."
"You have to keep on going for her sake."
"You're young, you can have others."
"We'll see you back here next year, and you'll be happier."
"Now you have an angel in heaven."
"This happened for the best."
"Better for this to happen now, before you knew the baby."
"There was something wrong with the baby anyway."

Used with permission of Bereavement Services. Copyright Lutheran Hospital—La Crosse, Inc., a Gundersen Lutheran Affiliate, La Crosse, WI.

coming from?" Being willing to sit down and talk about their anger can help the survivors to move past the anger and identify feelings of powerlessness and helplessness in not being able to control many aspects of the situation.

The bereaved have many questions about their loss. "What did I do?" "What caused this to happen?" "Do you think I should have, could have done . . . ?" Part of the grief process is for the bereaved to figure out what happened, what their role was in the loss. The nurse needs to recognize that the answers to these questions must come from the bereaved. It is part of their healing. When a bereaved mother asks, "Do you think that I shouldn't have painted the baby's room? Did that cause my baby to die?" An appropriate response might be, "I understand you need to find an answer for why your baby died. What are some of the other things you've been thinking about?"

Being with someone who is terribly sad, crying, or sobbing can be extremely difficult. The initial impulse is to touch them and/or hand them a tissue. While this action may seem supportive, it may stop or stifle the expression of emotion. The bereaved will indicate when they are ready for a tissue by beginning to wipe their eyes or nose, raising their head, and looking around or reaching for a tissue.

Careful assessment before using touch as a therapeutic technique is important. If touch is used inappropriately, the bereaved will stiffen, pull away, look at where they were touched, or stop expressing their feelings and emotions.

Provide Time to Grieve. Families become unaware of time frames when they first learn of and come to grips with their loss. They do not care about the change of shifts or the needs that the hospital system might have in "moving things along." When families are pushed or rushed into making decisions, they may make a decision based on the needs of the health care system, not their own. Nurses must be sensitive to the need that families might have to spend time with their baby. Providing time to see and hold their baby in private, making arrangements for their baby to be returned to them for further viewing, and delaying the processing of consent forms for autopsy or removal from the hospital are ways to give the family the opportunity to say good-bye.

Interpret Normal Feelings. Many parents have feelings of losing control when they express the normal feelings and emotions of grief. They may feel like they are "going crazy" because of thoughts that plague them about the baby. It is essential for the nurse to reassure and educate bereaved parents about the grief process, including the physical, social, and emotional responses of individuals and families.

After discharge, providing information/education on the grief process can be done by making follow-up phone calls to bereaved families; offering them the opportunity to talk with other bereaved parents in one-on-one support over the phone; referring them to a mutual, self-help perinatal bereavement support group; or providing a list of publications or websites intended for helping parents who have experienced a perinatal loss. As with any referral, the nurse should read the materials or check out the websites first (Box 23-8).

Allow for Individual Differences. Grief is very personal and private. How people respond to loss and grief depends on such things as age, gender, culture, religion, and socioeconomic

Box 23-8

Web Resources for When a Baby Dies

AAPC
American Association of Pastoral Counselors
http://www.aapc.org

GROWTH HOUSE, INC.
Page to grief related to pregnancy, including miscarriage, stillbirth, termination of pregnancy, and neonatal death
http://www.growthhouse.org

GRIEFNET
A collection of resources of value to those who are experiencing loss and grief
http://www.griefnet.org

HAND
Houston's Aid in Neonatal Death: Supporting grieving parents in the greater Houston area with the rest of the world via the Internet
http://www.hern.org/~hand

HANNAH'S PRAYER
Christian support for fertility challenges
http://www.hannah.org

HYGEIA™
An on-line journal for pregnancy and neonatal loss: Dr. Michael Berman
http://www.connix.com/~hygeia/

MISCARRIAGE SUPPORT AND INFORMATION RESOURCES
Comprehensive resource list
http://www.pinelandpress.com/support/miscarriage.html

OBGYN.net
List of resources for loss and bereavement
http://www.obgyn.net/woman/loss/loss.htm

PEN-PARENTS, INC.
An international nonprofit support network for bereaved parents
http://www.penparents.org

A PLACE TO REMEMBER
Uplifting resources for those who have been touched by a crisis in pregnancy or the birth of a baby
http://www.aplacetoremember.com

SHARE
Pregnancy and Infant Loss Support, Inc.
http://www.nationalshareoffice.com

SIDS NETWORK
Sudden infant death syndrome (SIDS) information website
http://www.sids-network.org

THE COMPASSIONATE FRIENDS
A self-help organization for bereaved parents and siblings
http://www.compassionatefriends.org

status; how others around them respond to their loss; and how they coped with prior losses. Within a family, many different types of responses may occur. Typically, men want to protect their partner from further pain, and parents/grandparents want to protect their children from more hurt. The underlying feelings of powerlessness and helplessness can be hidden behind expressions of anger, resistance to ideas, overcontrol of situations, or blame. These feelings can leave the partner or grandparent feeling isolated and alone, when in fact it is the care and concern for their loved one(s) that perpetuates the expression of the feelings. The nurse can respond to these underlying feelings by recognizing what a difficult time this is for the mother, father, parent, grandparents, and/or child. He or she can acknowledge how hard it must be for them to feel so responsible about making sure everything and everyone is taken care of. The nurse can ask them about their own hopes, dreams, and subsequent feelings of loss. These communication techniques can help the nurse move the resistive person to a position of support where the person's needs can also be met.

Families need to be given the opportunity to change their minds, to express their needs to each other, and to make decisions based on their needs as individuals and as family members.

Cultural and Spiritual Needs of Parents. Many of the responses to perinatal loss described in this section are based on Euro-American views of perinatal grief and loss. Although there may be no particular differences in individual, intrapersonal experiences of grief based on culture, ethnicity, or religions, there are many differences in mourning rituals, traditions, and behavioral expressions of grief (Cowles, 1996). Thus, the practices suggested earlier may not be appropriate for parents from other cultural, ethnic, and religious groups, and the nurse must consider the potential unique responses and needs of parents from different groups (Hebert, 1998). This involves understanding the cultural orientation and beliefs of the individual parent, the partner, the extended family, and the larger community to which they belong.

Cultural and religious differences can affect the way parents respond to a perinatal loss. This includes their way of communicating with health care professionals, as well as their emotional and behavioral responses and family interaction patterns. With perinatal loss, culture and religious beliefs can affect issues such as seeing the infant, naming the infant, taking pictures, allowing autopsies, and baptism or other rituals performed at death.

Physical Comfort. Coping with loss and grief after childbirth can be an overwhelming experience for the woman and her family. Often these families request that the mother be moved off the maternity unit or be discharged to home; the thought of being on the same unit with healthy mothers and babies is more than they can cope with. Other mothers, however, may want to remain on the maternity unit, where the staff nurses are better prepared to meet their physical and emotional needs. It should be the mother's choice as to where she wants to spend her postpartum stay.

The physical needs of a bereaved mother are the same as those of any mother who has given birth, but with an unhappy twist: the milk may come in, but there is no baby to nurse; the afterpains remind the mother of her emptiness; and gas pains feel like there is still a baby moving inside her. Many struggle with the frustration of having to go through all the pain of childbearing, only to return home with empty arms.

Options for Parents. It is sometimes difficult for the nurse to offer the bereaved information about their rights regarding options without making them feel guilty if they do not choose to exercise that right. Communicating with parents that options are their right, not their obligation, is vitally important.

Seeing and Holding. One of the first options to be discussed is whether the family wants to see their baby or, in the case of miscarriage or ectopic pregnancy, the products of conception. A statement such as "Some parents have found it helpful to see their baby" (or "the products of conception") gives the parents permission to do what might seem odd or distasteful. Responses can vary greatly between someone who experiences a miscarriage or ectopic pregnancy and someone who has experienced stillbirth or newborn death, as well as between family members.

Parents appreciate explanations as to how their baby looks (e.g., red, peeling skin like a bad sunburn, dark discoloration similar to bruises, molding of the head that makes the head look soft and swollen, or any defects). This helps them know what to expect. The nurse should make the baby look as normal as possible. Actions such as bathing the baby, applying lotion to the baby's skin, combing the hair, placing identification bands on the arm and leg, dressing the baby in a diaper and special outfit, sprinkling powder in the baby's blanket, and wrapping the baby in a pretty blanket convey to the parents that their baby is cared for as carefully as any baby in the nursery.

Caring for a baby who has died can be a difficult task for the nurse. It can be even more difficult if the fetus has been dead for several days or weeks in utero. In some cases decapitation or dismemberment may have occurred. If the baby has been in the morgue, the baby can be placed underneath a warmer for 20 to 30 minutes and wrapped in a warm blanket before being brought to the parents. Cold cream rubbed over stiffened joints can help in repositioning the baby.

When bringing the baby to the parents, it is important to hold the baby close, touch a hand or cheek, use the baby's name, and talk with the parents about the special features of their child to convey that it is all right for them to do likewise. If a baby has a congenital anomaly, the nurse can have a perfect hand or foot showing.

Parents need to be offered time alone with their baby. They need to know when the nurse will return and how to call should they require anything. It is difficult to predict how much time parents will need to spend with their baby. These moments are the only ones they will have with this child. Some parents need only a few minutes; others need hours. With the current practice of short-stay postpartum care, the nurse may need to advocate for patients who have experienced a loss to give them the time they need to grieve.

Bathing and Dressing. When possible, families should be given the opportunity to bathe, dress, and/or anoint their baby. This can be a very symbolic ritual for many families. The skin of some babies is fragile and may crack or ooze when touched. Parents can still apply lotion with cotton balls, sprinkle powder, tie ribbons, fasten the diaper, and place amulets, medallions, rosaries, or special toys or mementos in their baby's hands or alongside their baby. They may want to do other parenting functions, such as combing hair, wrapping the baby in a blanket, placing the baby in a bassinet, or carrying their baby to the nursery. They may have special clothes for the baby at home, or they may want to purchase a special outfit for the baby.

Privacy. If at all possible, the mother should be admitted to a private room. Marking the door to the room with a special card that denotes to hospital staff that this family has experienced a loss can be helpful (Fig. 23-8).

Visitation with Other Family Members or Friends. Families need to be offered the opportunity to have their children, grandparents, extended family members, and friends visit with them during hospitalization, as well as to see and hold their baby. This affords others the opportunity to become acquainted with the baby, to understand the parents' loss, to offer their support, and to say good-bye. This experience also helps parents explain to their surviving children who their brother or sister was and what death means; it offers the children answers to their questions in a concrete manner and helps them in expressing their grief.

Religious Rituals/Funeral Arrangements. Support from the clergy is an option that should be offered to all parents. Parents may wish to have their own pastor, priest, rabbi, or spiritual leader contacted; they may wish to see the hospital's chaplain; or they may choose neither option. A member of the clergy may offer the parents the opportunity for baptism, when appropriate (Box 23-9). Parents should be given information about the choices for the final disposition of their baby, regardless of gestational age. In the instance of a baby under 20 weeks of gestation, many hospitals offer to make the final disposition arrangements. Babies under 20 weeks of gestation are considered to be products of conception. Embryos, fallopian tubes removed in an ectopic pregnancy, tissue from a pregnancy obtained during a D&C, and fetuses under 20 weeks of gestation are all considered tissue. Should parents want to know what arrangements the hospital makes for their babies, the nurse should answer the parents' questions as honestly as possible. In most states if a baby is over 20 weeks and 1 day of gestation or is born alive, it is the parents' responsibility to make the final arrangements for their baby.

LEGAL TIP • Live Birth In all states there are laws that govern what constitutes a live birth. In most states a "live birth" is considered to be any product of conception expelled from a woman that shows any signs of life. Signs of life are considered to be any muscle irritability, respiratory effort, or heart rate regardless of gestational age. Nurses should be knowledgeable about their state laws regarding what constitutes a live birth and what forms need to be completed and filed in the case of fetal death, stillbirth, or newborn death.

Special Memories. Parents need tangible mementos of their baby. A lock of hair may be an important keepsake. Parents need to be asked first, for permission, before a lock of hair is cut. Hair can be removed from the nape of the baby's neck, where it is not noticeable. Parents may also bring in a baby book that had already been purchased. In addition, special memory books, cards, and information on grief and mourning are available through national perinatal bereavement organizations for purchase by parents or hospitals/clinics (Fig. 23-9).

Box 23-9

Infant Baptism

In an emergency, baptism may be performed by anyone by pouring water over the forehead (or products of conception) and saying "I baptize you in the name of the Father and of the Son and of the Holy Spirit." The person performing the baptism needs only to have the intention of baptizing and does not necessarily have to believe in infant baptism for the baptism to be valid. If the infant has no signs of life, the person performing the baptism can add "If you are alive, I baptize you . . ."

In the Greek Orthodox tradition, baptism is only for the living; thus a miscarried or stillborn infant would not be baptized. If the infant is born alive and in serious danger of death, the infant can be lifted up while saying "The servant of God is baptized in the name of the Father and the Son and Holy Spirit."*

*From: Harakas S (RHarakas@aol.com): *E-mail to M. Miles* (mmiles@email.unc.edu), May 17, 1999.

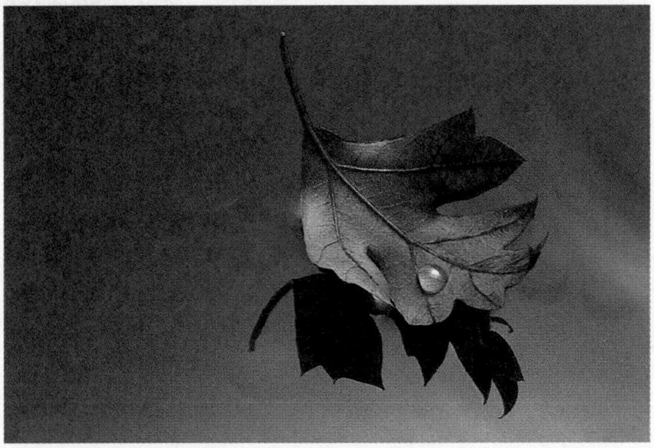

FIG. 23-8 • Door card for room of mother who has experienced perinatal loss. (Used with permission of Bereavement Services. Copyright Lutheran Hospital—La Crosse, Inc., a Gundersen Lutheran Affiliate, La Crosse, WI.)

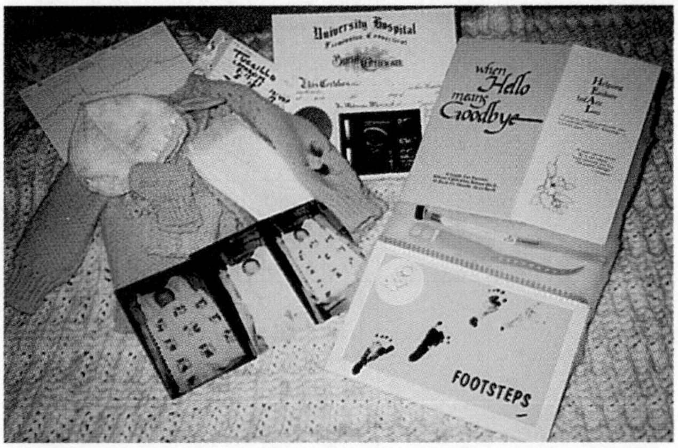

FIG. 23-9 • A memory kit assembled at the University of Connecticut Health Center, Farmington, CT. It includes pictures of the infant, clothing, death certificate, footprints, ID bands, fetal monitor printout, and ultrasound picture. (From Dickason E, Silverman B, Kaplan J: *Maternal-infant nursing care,* ed 3, St Louis, 1998, Mosby.)

SAMPLE

RTS Bereavement Services

CHECKLIST FOR ASSISTING PARENT(S) EXPERIENCING STILLBIRTH OR NEWBORN DEATH

Mother's discharge date: ______	Age ____ Gr ___ Para ___ L.C. ___ Due date ____
Mother's name: ______	Previous loss: ______
Address: ______	Date/Time delivered: ______
Phone number: ( ) ______	Date/Time death: ______
Father's name: ______	Baby's name: ______ Sex: ____
Address: ______	Children's name(s): ______ Age: ____
Phone number: ( ) ______	______ Age: ____
Optimal call time:	______ Age: ____
RTS Counselor: ______	Support people
Unit: ______ Ext ____	Attending MD &/or Pediatrician ______
Regular OB MD/Midwife: ______	Notify Peds Nurse Practitioner ______
Religion: ______	

Date	Time		Comments	Initials
		Notify/Assign RTS counselor ☐ Yes ☐ No		
		Pastoral Care notified ☐ Yes ☐ No		
		Funeral Home notified: ☐ Yes ☐ No Family Burial: ☐ Yes ☐ No		
		Saw baby when born and/or after delivery: ☐ Mother ☐ Father		
		Touched and/or held baby: ☐ Mother ☐ Father ☐ Siblings ☐ Grandparents ☐ Friends		
		Offered private time with their baby: ☐ Yes ☐ No		
		Baptism offered: (use seashell as vessel, give to parents) ☐ Yes ☐ No		
		Remembrance of Blessing offered: ☐ Yes ☐ No (can offer for any perinatal loss) ☐ Given to parents		
		Given option to transfer off Maternity Unit: ☐ Yes ☐ No		
		Patient's room flagged with door card ☐ Yes ☐ No		
		Autopsy: ☐ Yes ☐ No Genetic studies: ☐ Yes ☐ No Genetic Associate notified: ☐ Yes ☐ No		
		Regular Physician/Midwife notified of death: ☐ Yes ☐ No Memo sent to Physician/Midwife: ☐ Yes ☐ No		
		Section of Fetal monitor strip: ☐ Given to parents ☐ On file		
		ID Bands/Crib cards/Tape measure: ☐ Given to parents ☐ On file		
		Footprints/Handprints/Weight/Length recorded on "In Memory Of" sheet: ☐ Given to parents ☐ On file		
		Lock of hair offered: (ask permission) ☐ Yes ☐ No ☐ Given to parents ☐ On file		
		Mementos (clothing, hat , blanket, pacifier, crib cards, basin, baby ring, bear, thermometer, silk flower) ☐ Given to parents ☐ On file		
		Complimentary birth keepsake ☐ Given to parents ☐ On file		
		RTS Photos taken: (clothed, unclothed, w. props, family photo) 1) Polaroid - 3 or more ☐ Given to parents ☐ On file 2) 35 mm (6-12 pictures) ☐ Given to parents ☐ On file 3) Medical photos: ☐ Yes ☐ No		

FIG. 23-11 • Checklist for assisting parents experiencing stillbirth or newborn death. (Used with permission of Bereavement Services. Copyright Lutheran Hospital—La Crosse, Inc., a Gundersen Lutheran Affiliate, La Crosse, WI.)

Date	Time		Comments	Initials
		Informed about postponing funeral until mother is able to attend: ☐ Yes ☐ No		
		Services/Funeral arrangements, options discussed: ☐ Self-transport ☐ Gravesite service ☐ Visitation ☐ Hospital chapel ☐ Cremation ☐ Funeral home ☐ Burial at foot or head of relative's grave ☐ Specific area for babies in cemetery ☐ Plan own service		
		Funeral arrangements made by: ☐ Mother ☐ Father Discussed: ☐ Seeing baby at funeral home ☐ Taking pictures there ☐ Providing outfit/toy for baby ☐ Dressing baby at funeral home		
		Grief information packet given to: ☐ Mother ☐ Father		
		Discussed grief process/incongruent grief with: ☐ Mother ☐ Father		
		Discussed grief conference: ☐ Yes ☐ No		
		RTS Parents Support Group brochure given to: ☐ Mother ☐ Father		
		RTS business card given to: ☐ Mother ☐ Father		
		Pregnancy & Infant Loss Card sent to RTS secretary: ☐ Yes ☐ No		
		Follow-up calls: 1 week: . . . . 3 weeks: . . . . Due date: . . . . 6-10 months: . . . . Anniversary date:		
		Grief conference planned with parents: Date ________ Time ________ Place ________ Letter of confirmation sent: ☐ Yes ☐ No		
		Parent Support Group, first meeting attended: Date: ________ Follow-up meetings attended: Dates ________		
		Would like another parent to call: ☐ Yes ☐ No ☐ Ask later Parent contact: ________		

Forms Needed: Report of fetal death (Photocopy and save for mother.)
Autopsy if ordered
Record of death
Genetics protocol (folder) if ordered
Notice of removal of a human corpse from an institution
Final disposition form
If funeral home involved - Final disposition will be completed by them.
Original certificate of death (for NB death only)

Note: Family Burial - Check with your funeral home.

** You may wish to list your hospital and state forms that are necessary, as required by your state laws and your institution.

FIG. 23-11, cont'd • For legend see p. 520.

The nurse provides information about the baby's weight, length, and head circumference to the family. Footprints and handprints are taken and placed with the other information on a special card or memory/baby book. Sometimes it is difficult to obtain good handprints or footprints. Using alcohol or acetone on the palms or soles first can help the ink adhere to make the prints clearer, especially for small babies.

Any article that comes in contact or is used in caring for the baby should be saved, placed in a sealable bag, and given to the parents. Articles should not be washed or cleaned beforehand, since the parents may want to be able to keep the smell of their baby. Some examples of articles that can be given to parents are the tape measure used to measure the baby, lotions, combs, clothing, hats, blankets, pacifier, crib cards, and identification bands. Identification bands should be placed on the baby before they are given to the parents. These bands help the parents to remember the size of the baby and enable them to touch something their baby touched.

Pictures. Pictures are the most important memento a parent can have. Photographs should be taken whenever there is an identifiable baby. It does not matter how tiny the baby is, what the baby looks like, or how long the baby has been deceased.

Pictures can be taken with an instant print camera, as well as with a 35-mm camera. Every effort should be made to make the baby appear special. Pictures should include close-ups of the baby's face, hands, and/or feet. The baby should be clothed or wrapped in a blanket with a hat or gown in some of the pictures and unclothed in other pictures. If there are any congenital anomalies, close-ups of the anomalies should also be taken. Flowers, blocks, stuffed animals, or toys can also be placed in the background to make the picture more special, like a portrait. The parents or siblings may also want to have their picture taken holding the baby. Keeping a camera nearby and taking pictures when parents are spending special time with their baby can provide wonderful memories for later on (Fig. 23-10).

Documentation. Many hospitals have a checklist that is used in providing care, mobilizing members of the multidisciplinary health care team, communicating options the family has chosen, and keeping track of all the details in meeting the needs of bereaved parents (Fig. 23-11). The checklists may or may not be a permanent part of the chart. Documentation in the nursing notes includes primary concerns, grief responses, health teaching, health care advice, and referrals of the mother or any other family members.

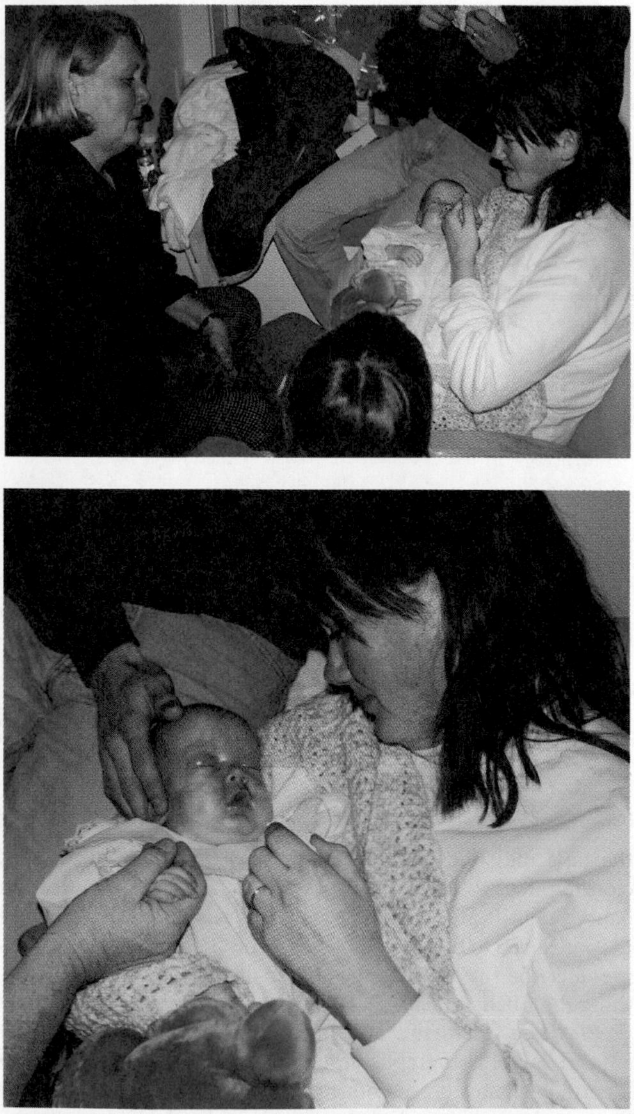

FIG. 23-10 • Laura's family members say a special good-bye. (Courtesy Amy and Ken Turner, Cary, NC.)

Follow-up After Discharge. Follow-up phone calls after a loss occurs are important. The grief of the mother and her family does not end with discharge but really begins once they return home, attend the funeral, and start to live their life without the baby. The calls are made to let the parents know they are still thought of and cared about. The calls are made at predictably difficult times, such as the first week at home; 1 month to 6 weeks later (parents should be invited to attend a support group at this time); 4 to 6 months after the loss; on the due date (for families who experienced a miscarriage, ectopic pregnancy, or death of a premature baby); and/or on the anniversary of the death. The calls are an opportunity for parents to ask questions, share their feelings, seek advice, and receive information to help them in processing their grief.

A grief conference is an opportunity for families to sit down with their health care providers and receive information about the baby's autopsy report or genetic studies, or just to ask questions they have had since their baby's death. Parents appreciate the opportunity to review the events of hospitalization, to go over the baby's and/or mother's chart with their primary health care provider, and to talk with those who cared for them during hospitalization. The grief conference gives health care professionals the opportunity to assess how the family is coping with their loss and to provide additional information/education on grief.

MATERNAL DEATH

It is rare for a woman to die in childbirth; the incidence of maternal deaths is between 7 and 8 per 100,000 (Centers for Disease Control and Prevention, 1998). The father and extended family, who are faced with not only mourning the death of a wife and mother but also the death of the baby, have a particularly difficult time. On the other hand, the father may be faced with parenting a baby without a surviving mother. Death of a mother disrupts the family structure and leaves the father with the care of a baby at a time when he is greatly distressed. Thus the father and extended family, especially other children and grandparents, need supportive grief counseling at the time of death and following discharge to be able to heal after such a devastating loss.

The nursing care of families at this time is similar to that already described. Options need to be offered, memories made, and mementos obtained and held for the family until they are ready for them. These families are at risk for developing complicated bereavement and altered parenting of the surviving baby and other children in the family. Referral to social services to help the family mobilize support systems, as well as for counseling, can help to combat potential problems before they develop and can be beneficial not only at the time of the loss but also in the future.

The emotional toll that a maternal death can take on the nursing and medical staff must also be addressed. Guilt, anger, fear, sadness, and depression are all common responses to a maternal death. The staff may want to review the situation surrounding the events, the medical record, and their responses in the forum of a mortality/morbidity review and a critical incident debriefing to help in coping with the feelings and emotions that result from a maternal death. Attending memorial or funeral services may benefit staff and family.

Critical Thinking

REDUCING MATERNAL MORTALITY AND COMPLICATIONS

One of the *Healthy People 2010* objectives is to reduce the maternal mortality rate to no more than 3.3 per 100,000 live births. What is the maternal mortality rate in your community? What efforts are being made in your community to reduce the maternal mortality rate? If possible, attend a morbidity/mortality review where a maternal death is discussed. Discuss in your clinical group the potential impact of current health care reform initiatives in achieving the *Healthy People 2010* goal.

➤ Evaluation

Evaluation is based on the expected outcomes of care. The plan is revised as needed based on evaluation findings.

Key Points

- Postpartum hemorrhage is the most common and most serious type of excessive obstetric blood loss.
- Hemorrhagic (hypovolemic) shock is an emergency situation in which the perfusion of body organs may become severely compromised and death may ensue.
- The potential hazards of therapeutic interventions may further compromise the woman with hemorrhagic disorders.
- Postpartum infection is the major cause of maternal morbidity and mortality throughout the world.
- Postpartum urinary tract infections are common because of trauma experienced during labor.
- Breast infection affects about 1% of women soon after childbirth.
- Structural disorders of the uterus and vagina related to pelvic relaxation are often the delayed but direct result of childbearing.
- An understanding of grief responses and the bereavement process is fundamental in the implementation of the nursing process.
- Therapeutic communication and counseling techniques can help families in identifying their feelings and in feeling comfortable in expressing their grief.
- Follow-up after discharge is an essential component in providing care to families who have experienced a loss.
- Nurses need to be aware of their own feelings of grief and loss to provide a nonjudgmental environment of care and support for bereaved families.

References

Akins S: Postpartum hemorrhage: a 90s approach to an age-old problem, *J Nurse Midwifery* 39(2suppl):123S-134S, 1994.

American College of Obstetricians and Gynecologists (ACOG): *Postpartum hemorrhage (ACOG Ed Bull No. 243),* Washington, DC, 1998, ACOG.

American Psychiatric Association (APA): *Diagnostic and statistical manual of mental disorders,* ed 4, Washington, DC, 1994, American Psychiatric Association Press.

Beck C: A checklist to identify women at risk for developing postpartum depression, *J Obstet Gynecol Neonatal Nurs* 27:39-46, 1998.

Beck C: Screening methods for postpartum depression, *J Obstet Gynecol Neonatal Nurs* 24(4):308-312, 1995.

Benedetti T: Obstetric hemorrhage. In Gabbe S, Niebyl J, Simpson J, editors: *Obstetrics: normal and problem pregnancies,* ed 3, New York, 1996, Churchill Livingstone.

Bowes W: Clinical aspects of normal and abnormal labor. In Creasy R, Resnick R, editors: *Maternal-fetal medicine,* ed 4, Philadelphia, 1999, WB Saunders.

Calhoun B, Brost B: Emergency management of sudden puerperal fever, *Obstet Gynecol Clin North Am* 22(2):357-367, 1995.

Centers for Disease Control and Prevention: Maternal mortality—United States, 1982-1996, *MMWR* 47(34):705-707, 1998.

Cowles K: Cultural perspectives of grief: an expanded concept analysis, *J Adv Nurs* 23:287-294, 1996.

Cox J, Holden J, Sagovsky R: Edinburgh Postnatal Depression Scale, *Br J Psychiatry* 150:782-786, 1989.

Cunningham F et al: *Williams obstetrics,* ed 20, Stamford, CT, 1997, Appleton & Lange.

Czarapata B, McKillips K: Silent suffering: helping women find the path to continence, *AWHONN Lifelines* 1(2):28-34, 1997.

Druelinger L: Postpartum emergencies, *Emerg Med Clin North Am* 12(1):219-237, 1994.

Falter H: Deep vein thrombosis in pregnancy and the puerperium: a comprehensive review, *J Vasc Nurs* 15(2):58-62, 1997.

Gibbs R, Sweet R: Maternal and fetal infectious disorders. In Creasy R, Resnick R, editors: *Maternal-fetal medicine,* ed 4, Philadelphia, 1999, WB Saunders.

Gonik B: Intensive care monitoring of the critically ill pregnant patient. In Creasy R, Resnick R, editors: *Maternal-fetal medicine,* ed 4, Philadelphia, 1999, WB Saunders.

Guyer B et al: Annual summary of vital statistics—1997, *Pediatrics* 102(6):1333-1347, 1998.

Hebert M: Perinatal bereavement in its cultural context, *Death Studies* 22:61-78, 1998.

Kaplan H, Sadock B: *Synopsis of psychiatry,* ed 8, Baltimore, 1998, Williams & Wilkins.

Kilpatrick S, Laros R: Maternal hematologic disorders. In Creasy R, Resnick R, editors: *Maternal-fetal medicine,* ed 4, Philadelphia, 1999, WB Saunders.

Kowalski K: *Perinatal death: an ethnomethodological study of factors influencing perinatal bereavement,* Unpublished doctoral dissertation, Denver, 1984, University of Colorado.

Laros R: Thromboembolic disease. In Creasy R, Resnick R, editors: *Maternal-fetal medicine,* ed 4, Philadelphia, 1999, WB Saunders.

Lindemann E: Symptomatology and management of acute grief, *Am J Psychiatry* 101:141-148, 1944.

Miles M: Helping adults mourn the death of a child. In Wass H, Corr C, editors: *Children and death,* Washington, DC, 1984, Hemisphere Publishing.

Miles M, Demi A: Guilt in bereaved parents. In Rando T, editor: *Parental loss of a child: clinical and research considerations,* Champaign, IL, 1986, Research Press.

Miles M, Demi A: Historical and contemporary theories of grief. In Corless I, Germino B, Pittman-Lindemann M, editors: *Dying, death and bereavement,* Boston, MA, 1997, Jones & Bartlett.

Mishell D et al: *Comprehensive gynecology,* ed 3, St Louis, 1997, Mosby.

Norris T: Management of postpartum hemorrhage, *Am Fam Physician* 55(2):635-640, 1997.

Parkes C: *Bereavement: studies of grief in adult life,* New York, 1972, International Universities Press.

Parkes C, Weiss R: *Recovery from bereavement,* New York, 1983, Basic Books.

Ridgeway L: Puerperal emergency: vaginal and vulvar hematomas, *Obstet Gynecol Clin North Am* 22(2):275-282, 1995.

Roberts W: Emergent obstetric management of postpartum hemorrhage, *Obstet Gynecol Clin North Am* 22(2):283-302, 1995.

Sampselle C et al: Continence for women: evidence-based practice, *J Obstet Gynecol Neonatal Nurs* 26(4):375-385, 1997.

Schatzberg A, Nemeroff C: *The American Psychiatric Press textbook of psychopharmacology,* ed 2, Washington, DC, 1998, American Psychiatric Press.

Toglia M, Nolan T: Venous thromboembolism during pregnancy: a review of diagnosis and management, *Obstet Gynecol Survey* 52(1):60-72, 1997.

Varner M: Medical conditions of the puerperium, *Clin Perinatol* 25(2):403-416, 1998.

Weed S: *Wise woman herbal for the childbearing year,* Woodstock, NY, 1986, Ash Tree Publishing Co.

Wendel P, Cox S: Emergent obstetric management of uterine inversion, *Obstet Gynecol Clin North Am* 22(2):261-274, 1995.

Wood A et al: The downward spiral of postpartum depression, *MCN Am J Matern Child Nurs* 22:308-316, 1997.

Worden W: *Grief counseling and grief therapy: a handbook for the mental health practitioner,* New York, 1991, Springer.

CHAPTER

24 Physiologic Adaptations of the Newborn

http://www.harcourthealth.com/MERLIN/Wong/maternal/

Learning Objectives

On completion of this chapter the reader will be able to:

- Describe the changes in the biologic system of the neonate during the transition to extrauterine life.
- Describe the sequence to follow in assessment of the newborn.
- Recognize deviations from normal physiologic findings during examination of the newborn.
- Compare and contrast the four types of heat loss in a neonate and describe how to prevent heat loss.
- Describe the behavioral adaptations of the newborn, including periods of reactivity and sleep-wake states.
- Describe the sensory and perceptual functioning of the neonate.

The neonatal period includes the time from birth through the twenty-eighth day of life. By term gestation, the fetus' various anatomic and physiologic systems have reached a level of development and functioning that permits a separate existence from the mother. At birth the newborn infant manifests behavioral competencies and a readiness for social interaction. These adaptations set the stage for future growth and development.

TRANSITION TO EXTRAUTERINE LIFE

Infants undergo phases of instability during the first 6 to 8 hours after birth. These phases collectively are termed the transition period between intrauterine and extrauterine existence. The first phase of the transition period lasts up to 30 minutes after birth and is called the first period of reactivity. The newborn's heart rate increases rapidly to 160 to 180 beats/min but gradually falls by 30 minutes to a baseline rate between 100 to 120 beats/min. Respirations are irregular, with a rate between 60 and 80 breaths/min. Crackles may be present on auscultation; audible grunting, nasal flaring, and retractions of the chest may also be noted. Brief periods of apnea may occur; the body temperature may decrease. The infant is alert and may have spontaneous startles, tremors, crying, and movement of the head from side to side. Bowel sounds become audible and meconium may be passed.

After the first period of reactivity, the newborn either sleeps or has a marked decrease in motor activity. This period of unresponsiveness, often accompanied by sleep, lasts from 60 to 100 minutes and is followed by a second period of reactivity.

The second period of reactivity occurs roughly between 4 and 8 hours after birth and lasts from 10 minutes to several hours. Periods of tachycardia and tachypnea occur, associated with increased muscle tone, skin color, and mucus production. Meconium is commonly passed at this time. All newborns experience this transition, regardless of gestational age or type of birth.

Physiologic Adjustments

Respiratory System. With the cutting of the umbilical cord, the infant must undergo rapid and complex changes. The most critical and immediate adjustment a newborn must make at birth is the establishment of respirations. During normal vaginal birth some lung fluid is squeezed or drained from the newborn's trachea and lungs. With the first breath of air, the newborn begins a sequence of cardiopulmonary changes.

Initial breathing is probably the result of a reflex triggered by pressure changes, chilling, noise, light, and other sensations related to the birth process. In addition, the chemoreceptors in the aorta and carotid bodies initiate neurologic reflexes when arterial oxygen pressure (Po_2) falls, arterial carbon dioxide pressure (Pco_2) rises, and arterial pH falls. In most cases an exaggerated respiratory reaction follows within 1 minute of birth, and the infant takes the first gasping breath and cries.

After respirations are established, respirations are shallow and irregular, ranging from 30 to 60 breaths per minute, with short periods of apnea (less than 15 seconds). These short periods of apnea occur most often during the active (rapid eye movement [REM]) sleep cycle and decrease in frequency and duration with age. Apneic periods over 15 seconds in duration should be evaluated.

Signs of Respiratory Distress. Most term infants breathe spontaneously and continue to have normal respirations (Fig. 24-1, *A*). Signs of respiratory distress may include nasal flaring, retractions (i.e., indrawing of tissue between the ribs, below the rib cage, or above the sternum and clavicles), or grunting with respirations. Any increased use of intercostal muscles may be a sign of distress. Seesaw respirations (Fig. 24-1, *B*) instead of normal abdominal respirations are not normal and should be reported. A respiratory rate less than 30 or greater than 60 breaths/min with the infant at rest needs to be reported to the physician. The respiratory rate can be negatively influenced (slowed or depressed) by analgesics or anesthetics administered to the mother during birth. Apneic episodes can be related to rapid warming or cooling of the infant; tachypnea may result from aspiration or a diaphragmatic hernia.

Maintaining Adequate Oxygen Supply. During the first hour of life the pulmonary lymphatics continue to remove large amounts of fluid. Removal of fluid is also a result of the pressure gradient from alveoli to interstitial tissue to blood capillary. Reduced vascular resistance accommodates this flow of lung fluid. Retention of fluid interferes with the infant's ability to maintain adequate oxygenation.

The chest circumference is approximately 30 to 33 cm at birth. Auscultation of the chest of a newborn infant reveals loud, clear breath sounds that seem very near because little chest tissue intervenes. The ribs of the infant articulate with the spine at a horizontal rather than a downward slope; consequently the rib cage cannot expand with inspiration as readily as an adult's. Neonatal respiratory function is largely a matter of diaphragmatic contraction. The newborn infant's chest and abdomen rise simultaneously with inspiration.

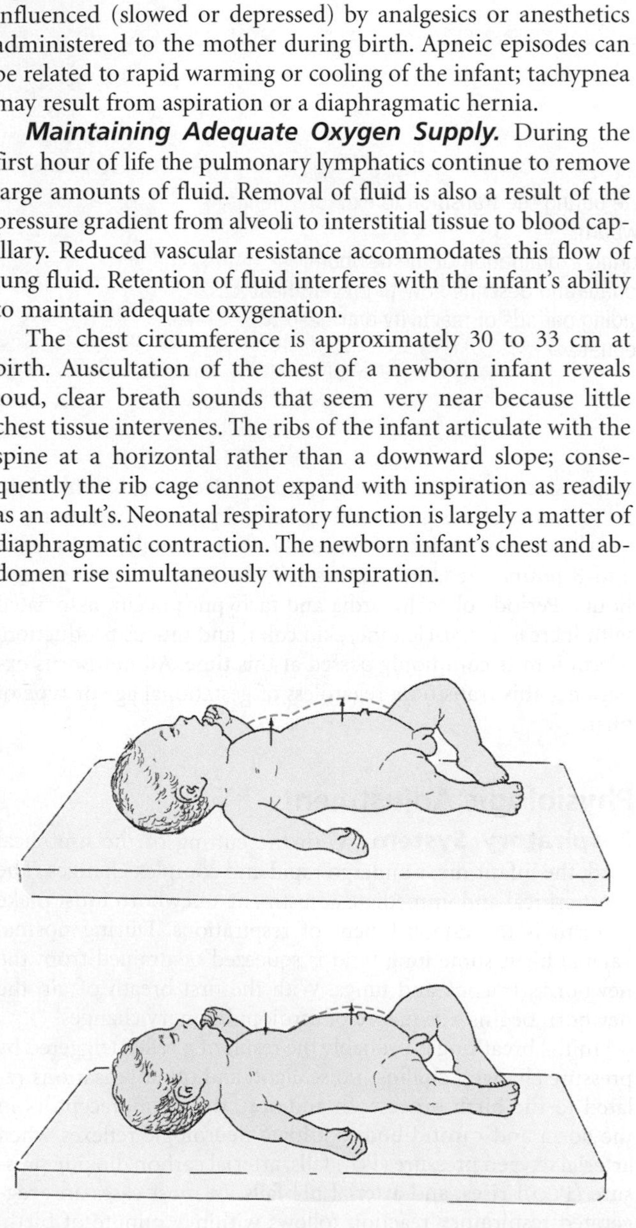

FIG. 24-1 • Comparison of normal and seesaw respirations. **A,** Normal respiration. Chest and abdomen rise with inspiration. **B,** Seesaw respiration. Chest wall retracts and abdomen rises with inspiration. (Courtesy Mead Johnson & Co, Evansville, IN.)

The alveoli of the infant's lungs are lined with surfactant. Lung expansion augments surfactant secretion. Surfactant lowers surface tension, thereby requiring less pressure to keep the alveolus open, and maintains alveolar stability by changing surface tension as the size of the alveolus changes.

Cardiovascular System. The cardiovascular system changes markedly after birth. The infant's first breath inflates the lungs and reduces pulmonary vascular resistance to pulmonary blood flow. The pulmonary artery pressure drops. This sequence is the major mechanism by which pressure in the right atrium declines. The increased pulmonary blood flow returned to the left side of the heart increases the pressure in the left atrium. This change in pressures causes a functional closure of the foramen ovale. During the first few days of life, crying may reverse the flow through the foramen ovale temporarily and lead to mild cyanosis.

In utero, fetal PO_2 is 27 mm Hg. After birth, when the PO_2 level in the arterial blood approximates 50 mm Hg, the ductus arteriosus constricts. Later, the ductus arteriosus occludes and becomes a ligament. With the clamping and severing of the cord, the umbilical arteries, umbilical vein, and ductus venosus close immediately and are converted into ligaments. The hypogastric arteries also occlude and become ligaments.

Heart Rate and Sounds. The heart rate averages 140 beats/min at birth, with variations noted during sleeping and waking states. Shortly after the first cry the infant's heart rate may be as high as 175 to 180 beats/min. The range of the heart rate in the full-term infant is 80 to 100 beats/min during sleep and 120 to 160 beats/min while awake. It is not unusual to find a heart rate of 180 beats/min when the infant cries. A heart rate that is either high (>160 beats/min) or low (<120 beats/min) should be reevaluated within an hour or when the activity of the infant changes.

The apical impulse (point of maximal impulse [PMI]) in the newborn is at the fourth intercostal space and to the left of the midclavicular line. The PMI is often visible.

Apical pulse rates should be obtained on all infants. Auscultation should be for a full minute, preferably when the infant is asleep. Sinus dysrhythmia (irregular heart rate) may be considered a physiologic phenomenon in infancy and an indication of good heart function.

Heart sounds during the neonatal period are of higher pitch, shorter duration, and greater intensity than during adult life. The first sound is typically louder and duller than the second sound, which is sharp. Most heart murmurs heard during the neonatal period have no pathologic significance, and more than half of the murmurs disappear by 6 months.

Blood Pressure. The newborn infant's average systolic blood pressure (BP) is 60 to 80 mm Hg, and the average diastolic pressure is 40 to 50 mm Hg. The blood pressure varies from day to day during the first month of life. A drop in systolic blood pressure (about 15 mm Hg) in the first hour of life is common. Crying and movement usually cause increases in the systolic blood pressure. The measurement of BP is best accomplished with a Doppler device and while the infant is at rest. The correct size cuff must be used for accurate measurement of an infant's BP. Unless there is a specific indication, blood pressure is not usually measured in the newborn.

Blood Volume. Blood volume in the newborn is about 80 to 85 ml/kg of body weight. Immediately after birth the total blood volume averages 300 ml, but this volume can increase by as much as 100 ml, depending on the length of time the infant is attached to the placenta (Wong, 1999). The infant born prematurely has a relatively greater blood volume than the term newborn. This occurs because the preterm infant has a proportionately greater plasma volume, not a greater red blood cell (RBC) mass.

Early or late clamping of the cord changes circulatory dynamics of the newborn. Late clamping expands the blood volume from the so-called placental transfusion. This, in turn, causes an increase in heart size, higher systolic blood pressure, and increased respiratory rate.

Hematopoietic System. The hematopoietic system of the newborn exhibits certain variations from that of the adult. Levels of RBCs and leukocytes differ, but platelets levels are relatively the same.

Red Blood Cells and Hemoglobin. At birth the average levels of RBCs and hemoglobin are higher than those in the adult. Cord blood of the term newborn may have a hemoglobin concentration from 14 to 24 g/dl (mean 17 g/dl). The hematocrit ranges from 44% to 64% (mean 55%). The RBC count is correspondingly elevated, ranging from 4.8 to 7.1/ mm^3. These values fall and reach the average levels of 11 to 17 g/dl and 4.2 to 5.2/ mm^3, respectively, by the end of the first month. The blood values may be affected by delayed clamping of the cord, which results in a rise in hemoglobin, RBCs, and hematocrit. The source of the sample is a significant factor because capillary blood will yield higher values than venous blood. The time after birth when the blood sample is obtained is also significant; the slight rise in RBCs after birth is followed by a substantial drop. At birth the infant's blood contains about 80% fetal hemoglobin, but because of the shorter life span of the cells containing fetal hemoglobin, the percentage falls to 55% by 5 weeks and to 5% by 20 weeks. Iron stores generally are sufficient to sustain normal RBC production for 5 months in the term infant; thus mild, brief anemia is not serious.

Leukocytes. Leukocytosis, with the white blood cell (WBC) count of approximately 18,000 per mm^3 (range 9,000 to 30,000 per mm^3), is normal at birth. The number of WBCs increases to 23,000 to 24,000/mm^3 during the first day after birth. The initial high WBC count of the newborn decreases rapidly, and a resting level of 11,500/mm^3 is normally maintained during the neonatal period. Serious infection is not well tolerated by the newborn, and marked increase in the WBC count is unlikely, even in critical sepsis (infection). In most instances, sepsis is accompanied by a decline in WBCs, particularly in neutrophils. The activity of the bone marrow is accurately reflected by the number of circulating cells, both erythrocytes and leukocytes.

Platelets. Platelet count ranges between 200,000 and 300,000/mm^3 and is essentially the same in newborns as in adults. The level of factors II, VII, IX, and X, found in the liver, is decreased during the first few days of life because the newborn cannot synthesize vitamin K. However, bleeding tendencies in the newborn are rare, and unless the vitamin K deficiency is great, clotting is sufficient to prevent hemorrhage.

Blood Groups. The infant's blood group is genetically determined and established early in fetal life. However, during the neonatal period there is a gradual increase in the strength of the agglutinogens present in the RBC membrane. Cord blood samples may be used to identify the infant's blood type and Rh status.

Thermogenic System. Next to establishing respirations, heat regulation is most critical to the newborn's survival. Thermoregulation is the maintenance of balance between heat loss and heat production. Newborns attempt to stabilize their internal body temperatures within a narrow range. Hypothermia from excessive heat loss is a common and dangerous problem in neonates. The newborn's ability to produce heat (thermogenesis) often approaches that of the adult; however, the tendency toward rapid heat loss in a cold environment is increased in the newborn and poses a hazard.

Thermogenesis. The shivering mechanism of heat production is rarely operable in the newborn. Nonshivering thermogenesis is accomplished primarily by brown fat, which is unique to the newborn; and secondarily by increased metabolic activity in the brain, heart, and liver. Brown fat is located in superficial deposits in the interscapular region and axillae, as well as in deep deposits at the thoracic inlet, along the vertebral column, and around the kidneys. Brown fat has a richer vascular and nerve supply than ordinary fat. Heat produced by intense lipid metabolic activity in brown fat can warm the neonate by increasing heat production as much as 100%. Reserves of brown fat, usually present for several weeks after birth, are rapidly depleted with cold stress. The less mature the infant, the less reserve of this essential fat is available at birth.

Heat Loss. Heat loss in the newborn occurs by four modes:

1. *Convection* is the flow of heat from the body surface to cooler ambient air. Because of heat loss by convection, the ambient temperature in the nursery is kept at 24° C and newborns are wrapped to protect them from the cold.
2. *Radiation* is the loss of heat from the body surface to a cooler solid surface not in direct contact but in relative proximity. To prevent this type of loss, cribs and examining tables are placed away from outside windows.
3. *Evaporation* is the loss of heat that occurs when a liquid is converted to a vapor. In the newborn, heat loss by evaporation occurs as a result of vaporization of moisture from the skin. The process is invisible and is known as insensible water loss. This heat loss is intensified by failure to dry the newborn directly after birth or by drying the infant too slowly after a bath.
4. *Conduction* is the loss of heat from the body surface to cooler surfaces in direct contact. When admitted to the nursery, the newborn is placed in a warmed crib to minimize heat loss.

Loss of heat must be controlled to protect the infant. Control of such modes of heat loss is the basis of caregiving policies and techniques.

Temperature Regulation. Anatomic and physiologic differences among the newborn, child, and adult are notable. The newborn's thermal insulation is less than that of an adult; the blood vessels are closer to the surface of the skin. Newborns have larger body surface to body weight (mass) ratios than children and adults. The flexed position of the newborn helps guard against heat loss because it diminishes the amount of body surface exposed to the environment. Infants can also reduce the loss of internal heat through the body surface by constricting peripheral blood vessels.

Cold stress imposes metabolic and physiologic problems on all infants, regardless of gestational age and condition. The respiratory rate increases in response to the increased need for oxygen. In the cold-stressed infant, oxygen consumption and energy are diverted from maintaining normal brain cell and cardiac function and growth to thermogenesis for survival. If the infant cannot maintain an adequate oxygen tension, vasoconstriction follows and jeopardizes pulmonary perfusion. As a consequence, the partial pressure of arterial oxygen (PaO_2) is decreased, and the blood pH drops. These changes aggravate existing respiratory distress syndrome (RDS). Moreover, decreased pulmonary perfusion and oxygen tension may maintain or reopen the right-to-left shunt across the patent ductus arteriosus.

The basal metabolic rate increases with cold stress (Fig. 24-2). If cold stress is protracted, anaerobic glycolysis occurs, resulting in increased production of acids. Metabolic acidosis develops, and if a defect in respiratory function is present, respiratory acidosis also develops. Excessive fatty acids displace the bilirubin from the albumin-binding sites. The resulting increased level of circulating unbound bilirubin heightens the risk of kernicterus even at serum bilirubin levels of 10 mg/dl or less.

Hyperthermia develops more rapidly in the newborn than in the adult because of decreased ability to increase evaporative skin water losses. Although newborn infants have 6 times as many sweat glands per unit area as adults, these glands do not function sufficiently to allow the infant to sweat. Serious overheating of the newborn can cause cerebral damage from dehydration or heat stroke and death.

Renal System. At term the kidneys occupy a large portion of the posterior abdominal wall. The bladder lies close to the anterior abdominal wall and is an abdominal as well as a pelvic organ. In the newborn almost all palpable masses in the abdomen are renal in origin.

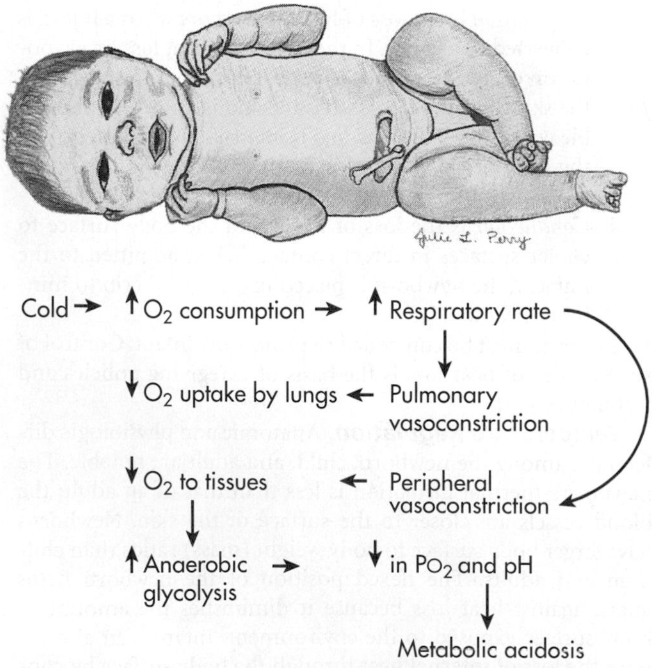

FIG. 24-2 • Effects of cold stress. When an infant is stressed by cold, oxygen consumption increases and pulmonary and peripheral vasoconstriction occur, thereby decreasing oxygen uptake by the lungs and oxygen to the tissues; anaerobic glycolysis increases; and there is a decrease in PO_2 and pH, leading to metabolic acidosis.

A small quantity (approximately 40 ml) of urine is usually present at birth in the bladder of a full-term infant. The frequency of voiding varies from 2 to 6 times during the first and second days of life and from 5 to 25 times during the subsequent 24 hours. About 6 to 10 voidings per day of pale straw-colored urine are indicative of adequate fluid intake. Generally, term infants void 15 to 60 ml of urine per kilogram per day (Fanaroff and Martin, 1997).

Full-term infants have limited capacity to concentrate urine; therefore the specific gravity ranges from 1.001 to 1.020 (Pagana and Pagana, 2000). The ability to concentrate urine fully is attained by about 3 months of age. After the first voiding the infant's urine may appear cloudy (because of mucus content) and have a much higher specific gravity. This decreases as fluid intake increases. Normal urine during early infancy is usually straw-colored and almost odorless. Sometimes pink-tinged uric crystal stains appear on the diaper; these stains are normal.

Loss of fluid through urine, feces, lungs, increased metabolic rate, and limited fluid intake results in a 5% to 10% loss of the birth weight. This usually occurs over the first 3 to 5 days of life. If the mother is breastfeeding and her milk supply has not come in yet (which occurs by the third or fourth day after birth), the neonate is protected from dehydration by its increased extracellular fluid volume. The neonate should regain the birth weight within 10 days.

Because renal thresholds are low in the infant, bicarbonate concentration and buffering capacity are decreased. This may lead to acidosis and electrolyte imbalance.

Fluid and Electrolyte Balance. About 40% of the body weight of the newborn is extracellular fluid. Each day the newborn takes in and excretes roughly 600 to 700 ml of water, which is 20% of the total body fluid or 50% of the extracellular fluid. The glomerular filtration rate (GFR) of a newborn is about 30% to 50% that of the adult. This results in a decreased ability to remove nitrogenous and other waste products from the blood. However, the newborn's ingested protein is almost totally metabolized for growth.

Sodium reabsorption is decreased as a result of a lowered sodium, potassium-activated adenosine triphosphate (ATPase) activity. The decreased ability to excrete excessive sodium results in hypotonic urine compared with plasma. There is a higher concentration of sodium, phosphates, chloride, and organic acids and a lower concentration of bicarbonate ions. The infant has a higher renal threshold for glucose.

Gastrointestinal System. The full-term newborn is capable of swallowing, digesting, metabolizing, absorbing proteins and simple carbohydrates, and emulsifying fats. With the exception of pancreatic amylase the characteristic enzymes and digestive juices are present even in low-birth-weight neonates.

In the adequately hydrated infant, the mucous membrane of the mouth is moist and pink; the hard and soft palates are intact. Drooling of mucus is common in the first few hours after birth. Small whitish areas (Epstein's pearls) may be found on the gum margins and at the juncture of the hard and soft palate. The cheeks are full because of well-developed sucking pads. These, like the labial tubercles (sucking calluses) on the upper lip, disappear around the age of 12 months, when the sucking period is over.

Even though in utero sucking motions have been recorded by ultrasound, these motions are not coordinated in any infant who is less than 1500 g at birth or born before 32 weeks of gestation. Sucking behavior is influenced by neuromuscular maturity, maternal medications received during labor and birth, and the type of initial feeding.

A special mechanism present in healthy term newborns coordinates the breathing, sucking, and swallowing reflexes necessary for oral feeding. Sucking in the newborn takes place in small bursts of three or four sucks at a time. The infant is unable to move food from the lips to the pharynx; therefore placing the nipple (breast or bottle) well inside the baby's mouth is necessary. Peristaltic activity in the esophagus is uncoordinated in the first few days of life. It quickly becomes a coordinated pattern in normal infants and they swallow easily.

Teeth begin developing in utero with enamel formation continuing until about 10 years of age. Tooth development is influenced by neonatal or infant illnesses, medications, and illnesses of or medications taken by the mother during pregnancy. The fluoride level in the water supply also influences tooth development. Occasionally an infant may be born with one or more teeth. Native American infants are commonly born with teeth.

Bacteria are not present in the infant's gastrointestinal tract at birth. Soon after birth, oral and anal orifices permit entrance of bacteria and air. Generally the highest bacterial concentration is found in the lower portion of the intestine, particularly in the large intestine. Normal colonic bacteria are established within the first week after birth, and normal intestinal flora help synthesize vitamin K, folate, and biotin. Bowel sounds can usually be heard shortly after birth.

Stomach capacity varies from 30 to 90 ml, depending on the size of the infant. Emptying time for the stomach is highly variable. Several factors, such as time and volume of feedings or type and temperature of food, may affect the emptying time. The cardiac sphincter and nervous control of the stomach are immature, so some regurgitation may occur. Regurgitation during the first day or two of life can be decreased by avoiding overfeeding, by burping the infant, and by positioning the infant with the head slightly elevated.

Digestion. The infant's ability to digest carbohydrates, fats, and proteins is regulated by the presence of certain enzymes. Most of these are functional at birth. One exception is amylase, produced by the salivary glands after about 3 months and by the pancreas at about 6 months of age. This enzyme is necessary to convert starch into maltose. The other exception is lipase, also secreted by the pancreas; it is necessary for the digestion of fat. Thus the normal newborn is capable of digesting simple carbohydrates and proteins, but has a limited ability to digest fats.

Further digestion and absorption of nutrients occurs in the small intestine in the presence of pancreatic secretions, secretions from the liver through the common bile duct, and secretions from the duodenal portion of the small intestine.

Stools. At birth the lower intestine is filled with meconium. Meconium is formed during fetal life from the amniotic fluid and its constituents, intestinal secretions (including bilirubin), and cells (shed from the mucosa). Meconium is greenish black and viscous and contains occult blood. The first meconium passed is usually sterile, but within hours all meconium passed contains bacteria. The majority of normal term infants pass meconium within 12 hours of life and almost all do so by 24 hours. The number of stools passed varies during the first week, being most numerous between the third and sixth days. Newborns fed early pass stools sooner. Progressive changes in the stooling pattern indicate a properly functioning gastrointestinal tract (Box 24-1).

Hepatic System. The liver and gallbladder are formed by the fourth week of gestation. In the newborn the liver can be palpated about 1 cm below the right costal margin because it is enlarged and occupies about 40% of the abdominal cavity. The infant's liver plays an important role in iron storage, carbohydrate metabolism, conjugation of bilirubin, and coagulation.

Iron Storage. The fetal liver (which serves as the site for production of hemoglobin after birth) begins storing iron in utero. The infant's iron store is proportional to total body hemoglobin content and length of gestation. At birth the term neonate has iron store sufficient to last 4 to 6 months; the preterm infant's iron stores will be depleted sooner.

Carbohydrate Metabolism. At birth the newborn is cut off from its maternal glucose supply and as a result experiences an initial decrease in serum glucose levels. The newborn's increased energy needs, decreased hepatic release of glucose from glycogen stores, increased RBC volume, and increased brain size may initially contribute to the rapid depletion of stored glycogen within the first 24 hours after birth. In most healthy term newborns, blood glucose levels stabilize at 50 to 60 mg/dl during the first several hours after birth; by the third day of life, the blood glucose levels should be approximately 60 to 70 mg/dl. The initiation of feedings assists in the stabilization of the newborn's blood glucose levels.

Conjugation of Bilirubin. Bilirubin is a yellow pigment derived from the hemoglobin released with the breakdown of RBCs and the myoglobin in muscle cells. The hemoglobin is phagocytized by the reticuloendothelial cells, converted to bilirubin, and released in an unconjugated form. Unconjugated (indirect bilirubin) is relatively insoluble and almost entirely bound to circulating albumin, a plasma protein. The unbound bilirubin can leave the vascular system and permeate other ex-

Box 24-1

Change in Stooling Patterns of Newborns

MECONIUM

Infant's first stool; composed of amniotic fluid and its constituents, intestinal secretions, shed mucosal cells, and possibly blood (ingested maternal blood or minor bleeding of alimentary tract vessels).

Passage of meconium should occur within the first 24 to 48 hours, although it may be delayed up to 7 days in very low-birth-weight infants.

TRANSITIONAL STOOLS

Usually appear by third day after initiation of feeding; greenish brown to yellowish brown, thin, and less sticky than meconium; may contain some milk curds.

MILK STOOL

Usually appears by fourth day.

In *breastfed infants,* stools are yellow to golden, are pasty in consistency, and have an odor similar to that of sour milk.

In *formula-fed infants* stools are pale yellow to light brown, are firmer in consistency, and have a more offensive odor.

travascular tissues (e.g., skin, sclera, and oral mucous membranes). The resulting yellow coloring is termed jaundice.

In the liver the unbound bilirubin is conjugated with glucuronide in the presence of the enzyme glucuronyl transferase. The conjugated form of bilirubin (direct bilirubin) is soluble and is excreted from liver cells as a constituent of bile. Along with other components of bile, direct bilirubin is excreted into the biliary tract system that carries the bile into the duodenum. Bilirubin is converted to urobilinogen and stercobilinogen within the duodenum through the action of the bacterial flora. Urobilinogen is excreted in urine and feces; stercobilinogen is excreted in the feces (Fig. 24-3). The total serum bilirubin level is the sum of the levels of both conjugated and unconjugated bilirubin.

Adequate serum albumin–binding sites are available unless the infant experiences asphyxia neonatorum (respiratory failure in the newborn), cold stress, or hypoglycemia. A mother's prebirth ingestion of medications such as sulfa drugs and aspirin can reduce the amount of serum albumin–binding sites in the newborn. Although the neonate has the functional capacity to convert bilirubin, physiologic hyperbilirubinemia commonly occurs in infants.

Physiologic Jaundice. Physiologic jaundice or neonatal hyperbilirubinemia occurs in 50% of full-term and 80% of preterm newborns. The incidence and severity of physiologic jaundice is increased in Asian, Native American, and Eskimo infants (Merenstein and Gardner, 1998). Although neonatal jaundice is considered benign, bilirubin may accumulate to hazardous levels and lead to a pathologic condition. Neonatal jaundice occurs because the newborn has a higher rate of bilirubin production and the reabsorption of bilirubin from the neonatal small intestine is considerable (Guyton and Hall, 1995).

Physiologic jaundice fulfills the following specific criteria (Korones, 1995):

- The infant is otherwise well.
- In term infants, jaundice first appears after 24 hours and disappears by the end of the seventh day.
- In preterm infants, jaundice is first evident after 48 hours and disappears by the ninth or tenth day.
- The serum concentration of unconjugated bilirubin usually does not exceed 12 mg/dl in term infants and 15 mg/dl in preterm infants.
- Hyperbilirubinemia is almost exclusively of the unconjugated variety, and conjugated (direct) bilirubin does not exceed 1 to 1.5 mg/dl.
- Daily increments of bilirubin concentration should not surpass 5 mg/dl. Bilirubin levels in excess of 12 mg/dl may indicate either an exaggeration of the physiologic handicap or the presence of disease.

NURSE ALERT • At any serum bilirubin level, the appearance of jaundice during the first day of life or persistence beyond the ages previously delineated usually indicates a pathologic process.

Jaundice is generally first noticed in the head, especially the sclera and mucous membranes, and then progresses gradually to the thorax, abdomen, and extremities.

Feeding practices may influence the appearance and degree of physiologic jaundice. Early feeding (within the first hour) tends to keep the serum bilirubin level low by stimulating intestinal activity (the gastrocolic reflex) and the passage of meconium.

Cold stress of the newborn may result in acidosis and raise the level of free fatty acids. In the presence of acidosis, albumin binding of bilirubin is weakened and bilirubin is freed.

Kernicterus, the most serious complication of neonatal hyperbilirubinemia, is caused by the precipitation of bilirubin in neuronal cells, resulting in their destruction. Cerebral palsy, epilepsy, and mental retardation may occur if the infant survives kernicterus.

Jaundice Associated with Breastfeeding. Breastfeeding-associated jaundice (early-onset jaundice) is associated with the breastfeeding pattern and occurs 2 to 4 days after birth. Breast milk jaundice (late-onset jaundice) is a progressive indirect hyperbilirubinemia beyond the first week of life. (See Chapter 26 for a discussion of these conditions.)

Coagulation. Coagulation factors, which are synthesized in the liver, are activated by vitamin K. The lack of intestinal bacteria needed to synthesize vitamin K results in transient blood coagulation deficiency between the second and fifth days of life. An injection of vitamin K on the day of birth helps prevent clotting problems.

Immune System. The cells that provide the infant with immunity are developed early in fetal life; however, they are not activated for several months. For the first 3 months of life, the infant is protected by passive immunity received from the mother. Natural barriers such as the acidity of the stomach and the production of pepsin and trypsin, which maintain sterility of the small intestine, are not fully developed until 3 to 4 weeks

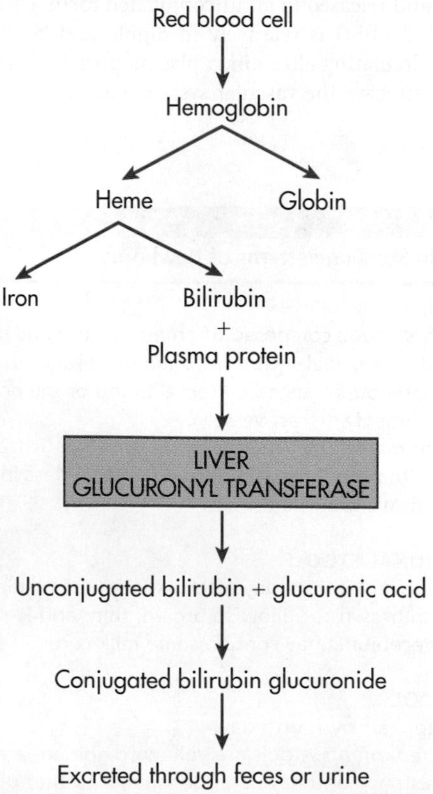

FIG. 24-3 • Formation and excretion of bilirubin. (From Wong D: *Whaley & Wong's nursing care of infants and children,* ed 6, St Louis, 1999, Mosby.)

of age (Guyton and Hall, 1995). The membrane-protective IgA is missing from the respiratory and urinary tracts and, unless the newborn is breastfed, is also absent from the gastrointestinal tract. The infant begins to synthesize IgG, and levels reach about 40% of adult levels by 1 year of age (Guyton and Hall, 1995). Significant amounts of IgM are produced at birth, and adult levels are reached by 9 months of age. The production of IgA, IgD, and IgE is much more gradual, and maximum levels are not attained until early childhood. The infant who is breastfed receives passive immunity through the colostrum and breast milk.

Integumentary System. All skin structures are present at birth. The epidermis and dermis are bound loosely and are very thin. Vernix caseosa (a cheeselike whitish substance) is fused with the epidermis and serves as a protective covering. The infant's skin is very sensitive and can be easily damaged. The term infant has an erythematous (red) skin for a few hours after birth, after which it fades to its normal color. The skin often appears blotchy or mottled, especially over the extremities. The hands and feet appear slightly cyanotic (acrocyanosis); this is caused by vasomotor instability, capillary stasis, and a high hemoglobin level. Acrocyanosis is normal and appears intermittently over the first 7 to 10 days, especially with exposure to cold.

The healthy term infant is plump. Subcutaneous fat accumulated during the last trimester acts as insulation. The newborn's skin may be slightly tight, suggesting fluid retention. Fine lanugo hair may be noted over the face, shoulders, and back. Actual edema of the face and ecchymosis (bruising) may be noted as a result of face presentation or forceps-assisted birth.

Creases can be found on the palms of the hands. The simian line, a single palmar crease, is often found in Asian infants or in infants with Down syndrome. The soles of the feet should be inspected for the number of creases. Premature newborns have few if any creases. Increasing numbers of creases correlate with a greater maturity rating.

Caput Succedaneum. Caput succedaneum is a generalized, easily identifiable edematous area of the scalp, most commonly found on the occiput (Fig. 24-4, *A*). The sustained pressure of the presenting vertex against the cervix results in compression of local vessels, thereby slowing venous return. The slower venous return causes an increase in tissue fluids within the skin of the scalp, and an edematous swelling develops. This boggy edematous swelling, present at birth, extends across the suture lines of the skull and disappears spontaneously within 3 to 4 days. Infants who are born with the assistance of vacuum extraction usually have a caput in the area where the cup was applied.

Cephalhematoma. Cephalhematoma is a collection of blood between a skull bone and its periosteum. Therefore a cephalhematoma does not cross a cranial suture line (Fig. 24-4, *B*). Often caput succedaneum and cephalhematoma occur simultaneously.

Bleeding may occur with spontaneous birth from pressure against the maternal bony pelvis. Low forceps birth and difficult forceps rotation and extraction may also cause bleeding. This soft, fluctuating, irreducible fullness does not pulsate or bulge when the infant cries. It appears several hours or the day after birth and may not become apparent until a caput succedaneum is absorbed. A cephalhematoma is usually largest on the second or third day, by which time the bleeding stops. The fullness of a cephalhematoma spontaneously resolves in 3 to 6 weeks. It is not aspirated because infection may develop if the skin is punctured. As the hematoma resolves, hemolysis of RBCs occurs and jaundice may result. Hyperbilirubinemia (jaundice) may occur after the newborn is home.

Desquamation. Desquamation (peeling) of the skin of the term infant does not occur until a few days after birth. Its presence at birth is an indication of postmaturity.

Sweat and Oil Glands. Sweat glands are present at birth but do not respond to increases in ambient or body temperature. Some fetal sebaceous (oil) gland hyperplasia and secretion of sebum results from the hormonal influences of pregnancy. Vernix caseosa is a product of the sebaceous glands. Removal of the vernix is followed by desquamation of the epidermis in most infants. Distended, small, white sebaceous glands, noticeable on the newborn face, are known as milia.

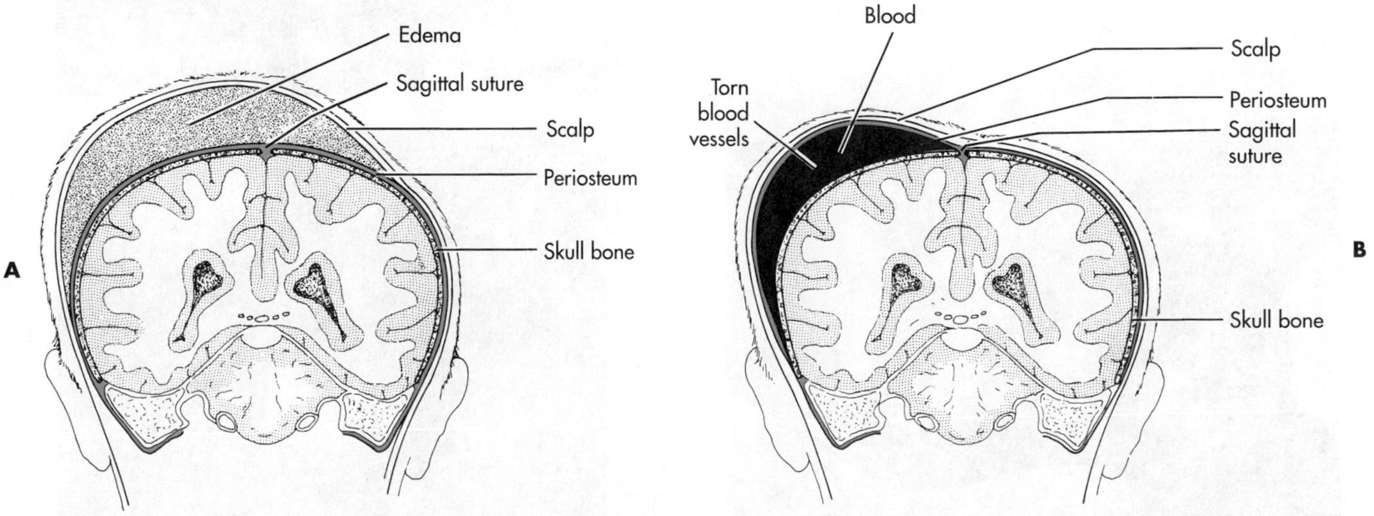

FIG. 24-4 • Differences between caput succedaneum and cephalhematoma. **A,** Caput succedaneum. Edema of scalp is noted at birth and crosses suture lines. **B,** Cephalhematoma. Bleeding between periosteum and skull bone appears within first 2 days and does not cross suture lines.

Mongolian Spots. Mongolian spots, bluish-black areas of pigmentation, may appear over any part of the exterior surface of the body, including the extremities. They are more commonly noted on the back and buttocks (Fig. 24-5). These pigmented areas are most frequently noted in babies whose ethnic origins are in the Mediterranean area, Latin America, Asia, or Africa. They are more common in dark-skinned individuals, regardless of race. They fade gradually over months or years.

Nevi. Known as "stork bites," telangiectatic nevi are pink and easily blanched (Fig. 24-6, *A*). They appear on the upper eyelids, nose, upper lip, lower occiput bone, and nape of the neck. They have no clinical significance and fade between the first and second year of life.

The strawberry mark, or nevus vasculosus, is a common type of capillary hemangioma. It consists of dilated, newly formed capillaries occupying the entire dermal and subdermal layers with associated connective tissue hypertrophy. The typical lesion is a raised, sharply demarcated, bright or dark red, rough-surfaced swelling that resembles a strawberry. Lesions are usually single but may be multiple, with 75% occurring on the head. These lesions can remain until the child is of school age or sometimes even longer.

A port-wine stain, or nevus flammeus, is usually observed at birth and is composed of a plexus of newly formed capillaries in the papillary layer of the corium. It is red to purple; varies in size, shape, and location; and is not elevated. True port-wine stains do not blanch on pressure or disappear. They are most commonly found on the face.

Erythema Toxicum. Erythema toxicum, a transient rash, is also called erythema neonatorum, "newborn rash" or "flea bite" dermatitis. It is found in term neonates during the first 3 weeks of age. It has lesions in different stages: erythematous macules, papules, and small vesicles (Fig. 24-6, *B*). The lesions may appear suddenly anywhere on the body. The rash is thought to be an inflammatory response. Eosinophils, which help decrease inflammation, are found in the vesicles. Although the appearance is alarming, the rash has no clinical significance and requires no treatment.

Reproductive System

Female. At birth the ovaries contain thousands of primitive germ cells. These represent the full complement of potential ova; no oogonia form after birth in term infants. The ovarian cortex, which is made up primarily of primordial follicles, occupies a larger portion of the ovary in the female newborn than in the adult. From birth to sexual maturity, the number of ova decreases by approximately 90%.

An increase in estrogen during pregnancy, followed by a drop after birth, results in a mucoid vaginal discharge and even some slight bloody spotting (pseudomenstruation). External genitals (i.e., labia majora and minora) are usually edematous, with increased pigmentation. In term neonates, the labia majora and minora cover the vestibule (Fig. 24-7, *A*). In preterm infants the clitoris is prominent and the labia majora are small and widely separated. Vaginal or hymenal tags are common findings and have no clinical significance. Vernix caseosa may be present between the labia.

If the female was born in the breech position, the labia may be edematous and bruised. The edema and bruising resolve in a few days; no treatment is necessary.

Male. The testes descend into the scrotum by birth in 90% of newborn boys. Although this percentage drops with premature birth, by 1 year of age the incidence of undescended testes in all males is less than 1%.

A tight prepuce (foreskin) is common in newborns. The urethral opening may be completely covered by the prepuce, which may not be retractable for 3 to 4 years. Smegma, a white cheesy

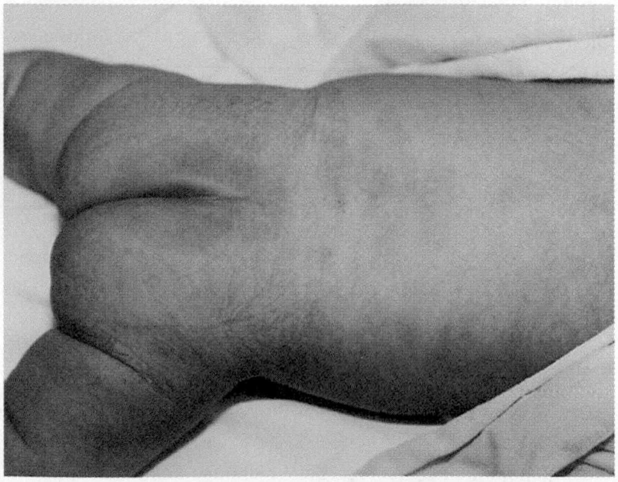

FIG. 24-5 • Mongolian spot.

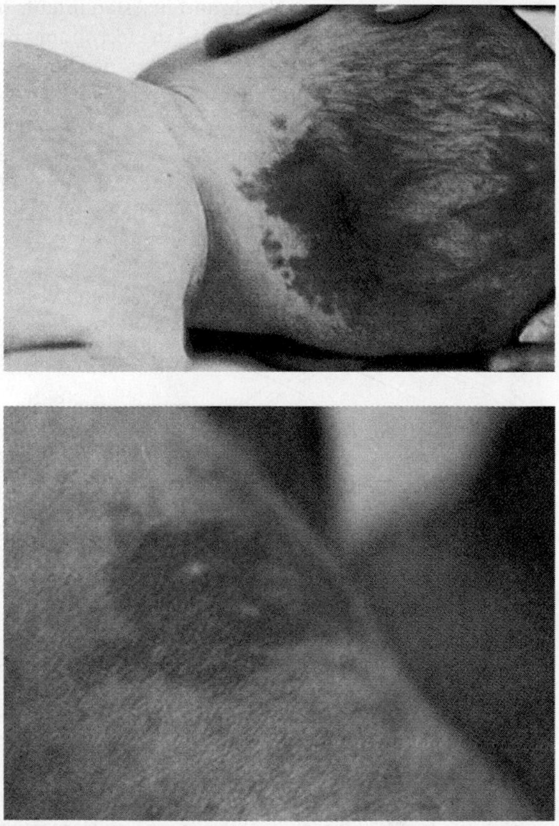

A

B

FIG. 24-6 • **A,** Telangiectatic nevus (stork bite). **B,** Erythema toxicum. (Courtesy Mead Johnson & Co., Evansville, IN.)

substance, is commonly found under the foreskin. Small, white, firm cysts called epithelial pearls may be seen at the tip of the prepuce. In the preterm male of less than 28 weeks' gestation, the testes remain within the abdominal cavity and the scrotum appears high and close to the body. By 28 to 36 weeks' gestation, the testes can be palpated in the inguinal canal and a few rugae appear on the scrotum. At 36 to 40 weeks' gestation, the testes are palpable in the upper scrotum and rugae appear on the anterior portion. After 40 weeks the testes can be palpated in the scrotum and rugae cover the scrotal sac. The postterm neonate has deep rugae and a pendulous scrotum. The scrotum is usually more deeply pigmented than the rest of the skin (see Fig. 24-7, *B*) and is especially apparent in darker-skinned infants. This pigmentation is a response to maternal estrogen. Hydroceles, caused by an accumulation of fluid around the testes, may be found. They can be transilluminated with a light and usually decrease in size without treatment.

If the male infant is born in a breech presentation, the scrotum is edematous and may be bruised. The swelling and discoloration subside within a few days.

Swelling of Breast Tissue. Swelling of the breast tissue in term infants of both sexes is caused by the hyperestrogenism of pregnancy. In a few infants a thin discharge (witch's milk) can be seen. This finding has no clinical significance, requires no treatment, and subsides within a few days as the maternal hormones are eliminated from the infant's body.

The nipples should be symmetric on the chest. Breast tissue and areola size increase with gestation. The areola appears slightly elevated at 34 weeks' gestation. By 36 weeks a breast bud of 1 to 2 mm is palpable and increases to 12 mm by 42 weeks.

Skeletal System. The infant's skeletal system undergoes rapid development during the first year of life. At birth, more cartilage is present than ossified bone. Because of cephalocaudal (head-to-rump) development, the newborn looks somewhat out of proportion.

The head at term is one fourth of the total body length. The arms are slightly longer than the legs. In the newborn the legs are one third of the total body length but only 15% of the total body weight. As growth proceeds, the midpoint in head-to-toe measurements gradually descends from the level of the umbilicus at birth to the level of the symphysis pubis at maturity.

The face appears small in relation to the skull. The skull appears large and heavy. Cranial size and shape can be distorted by molding (the shaping of the fetal head by overlapping of the cranial bones to facilitate movement through the birth canal during labor) (Fig. 24-8).

A

B

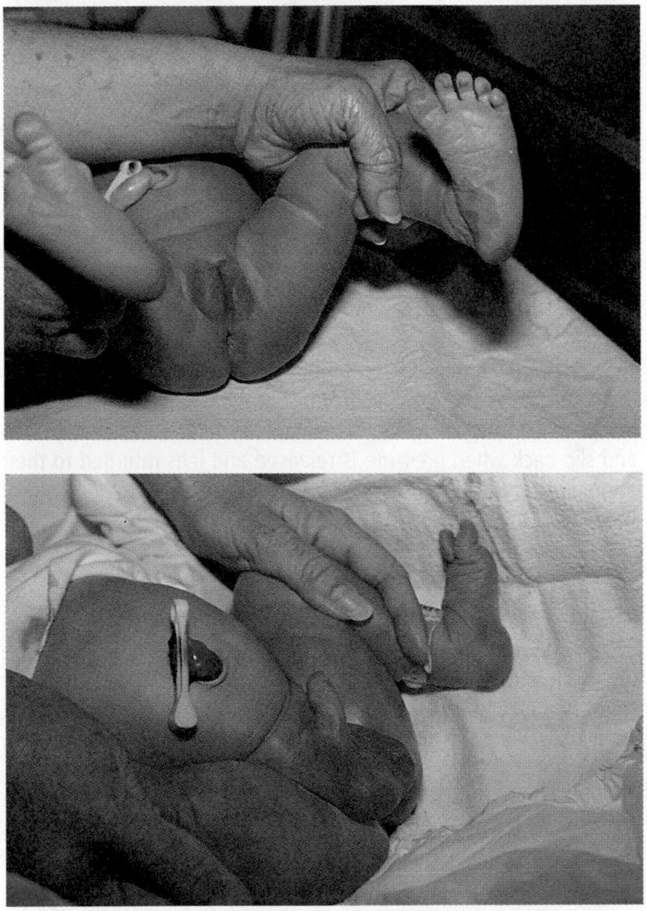

FIG. 24-7 • External genitalia. **A,** Genitalia in female term infant. **B,** Genitalia in male infant (uncircumcised penis). Rugae cover scrotum, indicating term gestation. Cord has been swabbed with ethylene blue to prevent infection. (Courtesy Marjorie Pyle, RNC, Lifecircle, Costa Mesa, CA.)

A

B

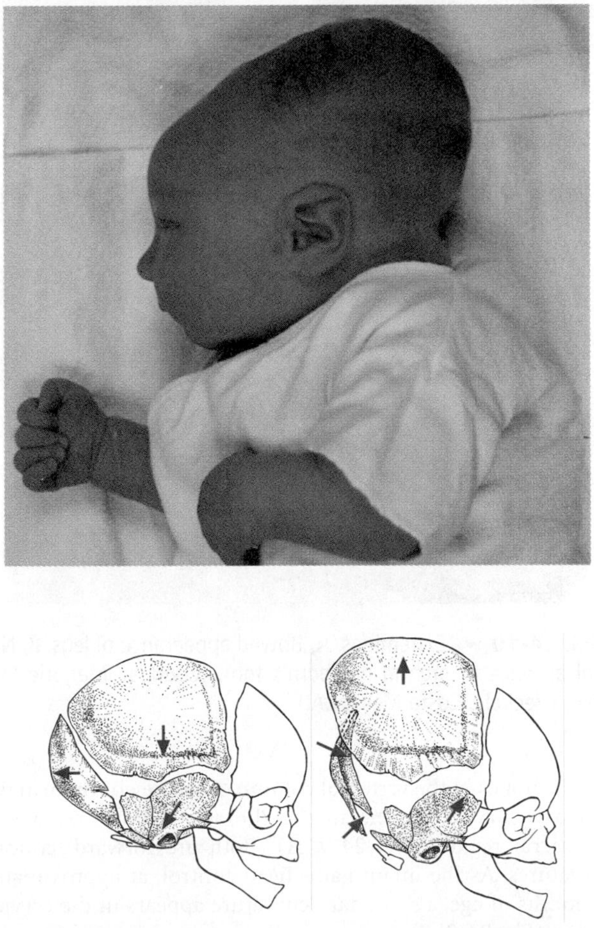

FIG. 24-8 • Molding. **A,** Significant molding after vaginal birth. **B,** Schematic of bones of skull when molding is present. (A, courtesy Kim Molloy, Knoxville, IA.)

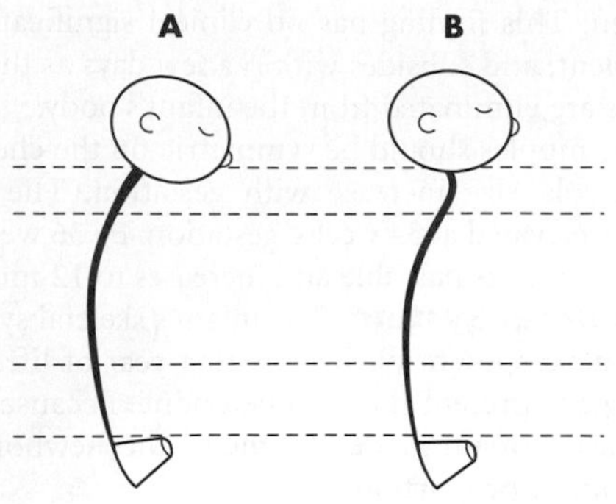

FIG. 24-9 • Development of spinal curvatures. **A,** Newborn infant. **B,** Cervical secondary curvature. (From Wong D: *Whaley & Wong's nursing care of infants and children,* ed 5, St Louis, 1995, Mosby.)

A

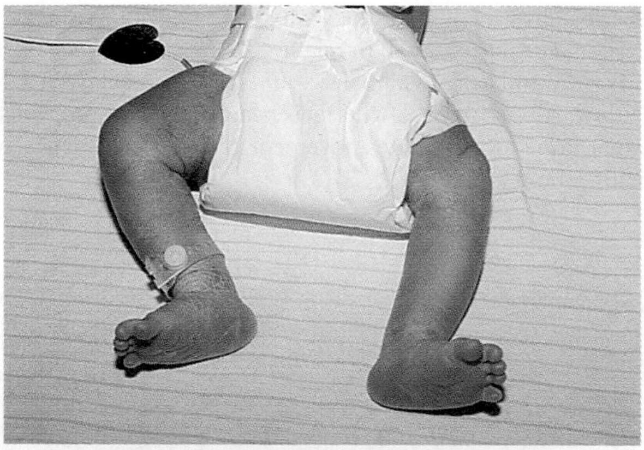

B

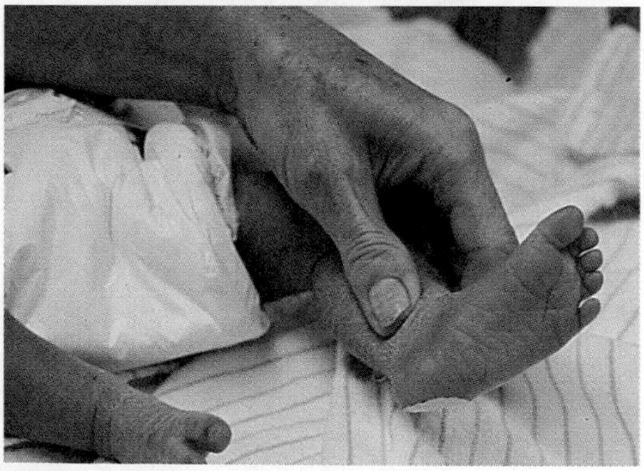

FIG. 24-10 • Extremities. **A,** Bowed appearance of legs. **B,** Normal absence of arch in newborn's foot. (Courtesy Marjorie Pyle, RNC, Lifecircle, Costa Mesa, CA.)

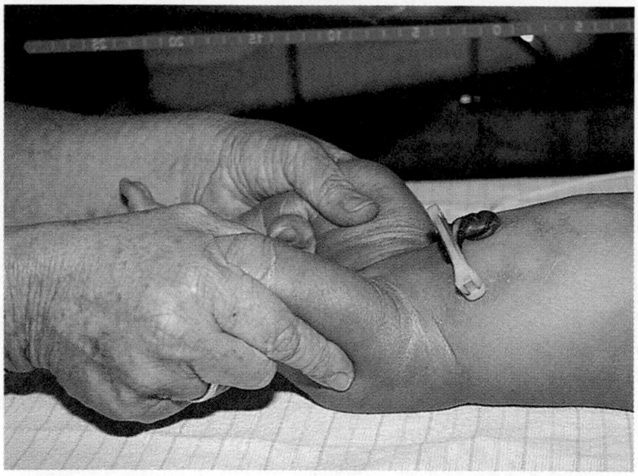

A

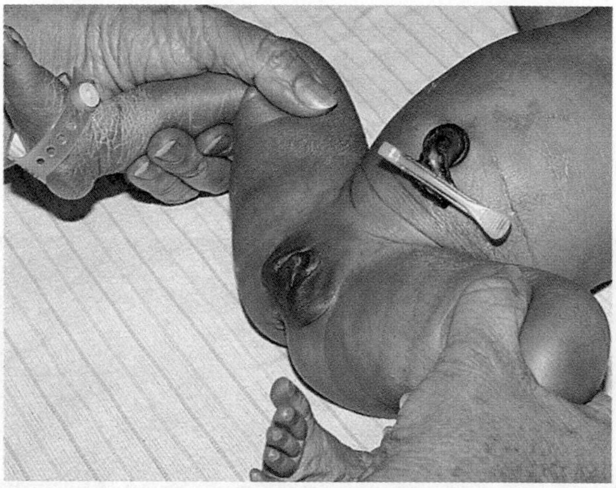

B

FIG. 24-11 • Method of assessing for hip dysplasia or dislocation using Ortolani's maneuver. **A,** Examiner's index fingers are placed over greater trochanter and thumbs over inner thigh opposite lesser trochanter. **B,** Gentle pressure is exerted to further flex thigh on hip, and thighs are rotated outward. If hip dysplasia is present, head of femur can be felt to slip forward in acetabulum and slip back when pressure is released and legs returned to their original position. A click is sometimes heard (Ortolani's sign). (Courtesy Marjorie Pyle, RNC, Lifecircle, Costa Mesa, CA.)

The bones in the vertebral column of the newborn form two primary curvatures, one in the thoracic region and one in the sacral region (Fig. 24-9, *A*). Both are forward, concave curvatures. As the infant gains head control, at approximately 3 months of age, a secondary curvature appears in the cervical region (Fig. 24-9, *B*).

In some newborn infants, there is a significant separation of the knees when the ankles are held together, resulting in an appearance of bowlegs (Fig. 24-10, *A*). At birth, there is no apparent arch to the foot. The extremities should be symmetric and of equal length. Skin folds should be equal and symmetric. The hips should be checked for dysplasia using Ortolani's maneuver (Fig. 24-11). Fingers and toes should be equal in number and have nails. Extra digits (polydactyly) are sometimes found on the hands and feet. Fingers or toes may be fused (syndactyly). Creases can be found on the palms of the hands and cover the soles of the term newborn's feet. If the infant's presentation was breech, the knees may remain extended and the infant will maintain the in utero position for several weeks.

The newborn's spine appears straight and can be flexed easily. The vertebrae should appear straight and flat. The base of the spine should be free from a dimple. If a dimple is noted, further inspection is required to determine whether a sinus is present. A pilonidal dimple, especially with a sinus along with a nevus pilosis (hairy nevus), may be associated with spina bifida.

Critical Thinking

EXPLAINING THE TRANSITION TO EXTRAUTERINE LIFE

Prepare parent education materials that explain the transition to extrauterine life. What information is essential for parents to understand? Who is your audience? Prepare materials for parents who are non–English speaking and for those who have limited education. How will your approach differ for parents of different ethnic or cultural groups?

Neuromuscular System. The neuromuscular system is almost completely developed at birth. The term newborn is a vital, responsive, and reactive being with a remarkable capacity for social interaction and self-organization (Fanaroff and Martin, 1997).

Growth of the brain after birth follows a predictable pattern of rapid growth during infancy and early childhood; growth becomes more gradual during the remainder of the first decade and minimal during adolescence. The cerebellum ends its growth spurt, which began at about 30 gestational weeks, by the end of the first year. This may be the reason the brain is vulnerable to nutritional deficiencies and trauma in early infancy.

The brain requires glucose as a source of energy, and a relatively large supply of oxygen for adequate metabolism. Such requirements signal a need for careful assessment of the infant's respiratory status. The necessity for glucose requires attentiveness to those neonates who may have hypoglycemic episodes.

Spontaneous motor activity may be seen as transient tremors of the mouth and chin, especially during crying episodes; and of the extremities, notably the arms and hands. Transient tremors are normal and can be observed in nearly every newborn. These tremors should not be present when the infant is quiet and should not persist beyond 1 month of age. Persistent tremors or tremors involving the entire body may indicate pathologic conditions. Marked tonicity, clonicity, and twitching of facial muscles are signs of convulsions. Normal tremors, tremors of hypoglycemia, and central nervous system (CNS) disorders need to be differentiated so corrective care can be instituted as necessary.

Neuromuscular control in the newborn, although very limited, can be noted. If newborns are placed face down on a firm surface, they will turn their heads to the side to maintain an airway. They attempt to hold their heads in line with their bodies if they are raised by their arms. Various reflexes serve to promote safety and adequate food intake.

Newborn Reflexes. The newborn infant has many primitive reflexes. The times at which these reflexes appear and disappear reflect the maturity and intactness of the developing nervous system. The most common reflexes found in the normal newborn are described in Table 24-1.

PHYSICAL ASSESSMENT

The assessment of the newborn should progress systematically from head to toe, with evaluation and assessment of each system (e.g., respiratory and cardiovascular). The findings provide a database for implementing the nursing process with newborns, and for providing anticipatory guidance for the parents. An immediate assessment of the newborn is carried out in the room where the birth occurred. The Apgar score (see Chapter 25), determined at 1 and 5 minutes, provides information that must be considered in the context of data from the total assessment.

A complete physical examination should be done within 24 hours after birth, after the newborn's temperature stabilizes or under a radiant warmer. The area used for examination should be well-lighted, warm, and free from drafts. The infant is undressed as needed and placed on a firm, warmed, flat surface. The physical assessment should begin with a review of the maternal history and prenatal and intrapartal records. This provides a background for the recognition of any potential problems. This assessment also includes general appearance, behavior, vital signs measurements, and maternal-infant interactions. Descriptions of any variations from normal, and all abnormal findings are included (Table 24-2). After birth, ongoing assessments of the newborn are made and an evaluation is performed before discharge.

General Appearance

The neonate's maturity level can be gauged by assessment of general appearance. Features to assess in the general survey include posture, head size, lanugo, vernix caseosa, breast tissue, sole creases, cry, and state of alertness. The normal resting position of the neonate is one of general flexion. The umbilicus is the center of the newborn's body and the abdomen is prominent.

Vital Signs

The temperature, heart rate, and respiratory rate are always obtained. BP may not be routinely assessed unless cardiac problems are possible. An irregular, very slow, or very fast heart rate may indicate a need for BP measurement.

The axillary temperature is a safe, accurate substitute for the rectal temperature. Electronic thermometers have expedited this task and provide a reading within 1 minute. Standard mercury thermometers should be held in place for at least 3 minutes. Taking an infant's temperature may cause the infant to cry and struggle against the placement of the thermometer in the axilla. Tympanic thermometers may be used after the newborn's ear canals are free of vernix. Before taking the temperature the examiner may determine the apical heart rate and respiratory rate while the infant is quiet and at rest. The normal axillary temperature averages 37° C with a range from 36.5° to 37.2° C.

The respiratory rate varies with the state of alertness after birth. Respirations are abdominal in nature and can be counted by observing or by lightly feeling the rise and fall of the abdomen. Neonatal respirations are shallow and irregular. It is important to count the respirations for a full minute to obtain an accurate count because of normal short periods of apnea. The examiner should also observe for symmetry of chest movement. The average respiratory rate is 40 breaths/min but will vary between 30 and 60 breaths/min or may be higher than 60 breaths/min if the newborn is very active or crying (see Table 24-2).

Apical pulse rates should be obtained on all infants. Auscultation should be for a full minute, preferably when the infant is asleep. The infant may need to be held and comforted during assessment. Heart rate may range from 100 to 180 beats/min

Text continued on p. 551

TABLE 24-1
Assessment of Newborn's Reflexes

Reflex	Eliciting the Reflex	Characteristic Response	Comments
Sucking and rooting	Touch infant's lip, cheek, or corner of mouth with nipple	Infant turns head toward stimulus, opens mouth, takes hold, and sucks	Response is difficult if not impossible to elicit after infant has been fed; if response weak or absent, consider prematurity or neurologic defect Parental guidance: Avoid trying to turn head toward breast or nipple, allow infant to root; response disappears after 3 to 4* mo but may persist up to 1 yr
Swallowing	Feed infant, swallowing usually follows sucking and obtaining fluids	Swallowing is usually coordinated with sucking and usually occurs without gagging, coughing, or vomiting	If response is weak or absent, this may indicate prematurity or neurologic defect Sucking and swallowing are often uncoordinated in preterm infant
Grasp			
Palmar Plantar	Place finger in palm of hand Place finger at base of toes	Infant's fingers curl around examiner's fingers, toes curl downward	Palmar response lessens by 3 to 4 mo, parents enjoy this contact with infant; plantar response lessens by 8 mo
Extrusion	Touch or depress tip of tongue	Newborn forces tongue outward	Response disappears about fourth month of life
Glabellar (Myerson's)	Tap over forehead, bridge of nose, or maxilla of newborn whose eyes are open	Newborn blinks for first four or five taps	Continued blinking with repeated taps is consistent with extrapyramidal disorder
Tonic neck or "fencing"	With infant falling asleep or sleeping, turn head quickly to one side	With infant facing left side, arm and leg on that side extend; opposite arm and leg flex (turn head to right, and extremities assume opposite postures)	Responses in leg are more consistent Complete response disappears by 3 to 4 mo, incomplete response may be seen until third or fourth year After 6 wk, persistent response is sign of possible cerebral palsy

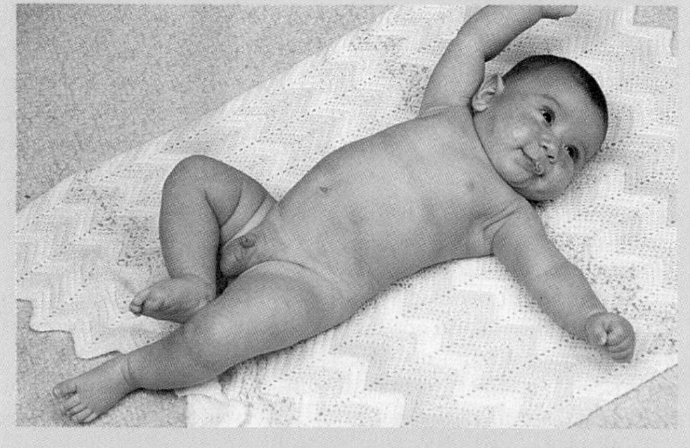

Classic pose in spontaneous tonic neck reflex. (Courtesy Marjorie Pyle, RNC, Lifecircle, Costa Mesa, CA.)

*All durations for persistence of reflexes are based on time elapsed after 40 weeks of gestation, that is, if newborn was born at 36 weeks of gestation, add 1 month to all time limits given.

TABLE 24-1—cont'd
Assessment of Newborn's Reflexes

Reflex	Eliciting the Reflex	Characteristic Response	Comments
Moro's	Hold infant in semisitting position, allow head and trunk to fall backward to an angle of at least 30 degrees Place infant on flat surface, strike surface to startle infant	Symmetric abduction and extension of arms are seen; fingers fan out and form a C with thumb and forefinger; slight tremor may be noted; arms are adducted in embracing motion and return to relaxed flexion and movement Legs may follow similar pattern of response Preterm infant does not complete "embrace"; instead, arms fall backward because of weakness	Response is present at birth; complete response may be seen until 8 wk; body jerk only is seen between 8 and 18 wk; response is absent by 6 mo if neurologic maturation is not delayed; response may be incomplete if infant is deeply asleep; give parental guidance about normal response Asymmetric response may connote injury to brachial plexus, clavicle, or humerus Persistent response after 6 mo indicates possible brain damage

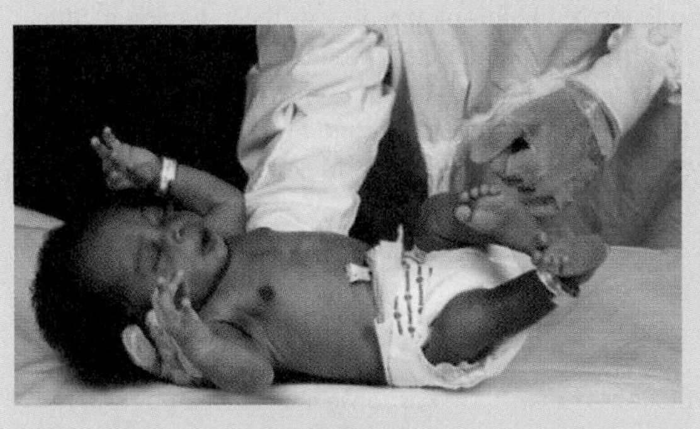

A, Moro's reflex.

Reflex	Eliciting the Reflex	Characteristic Response	Comments
Stepping or "walking"	Hold infant vertically, allowing one foot to touch table surface	Infant will simulate walking, alternating flexion and extension of feet; term infants walk on soles of their feet, and preterm infants walk on their toes	Response is normally present for 3 to 4 wk

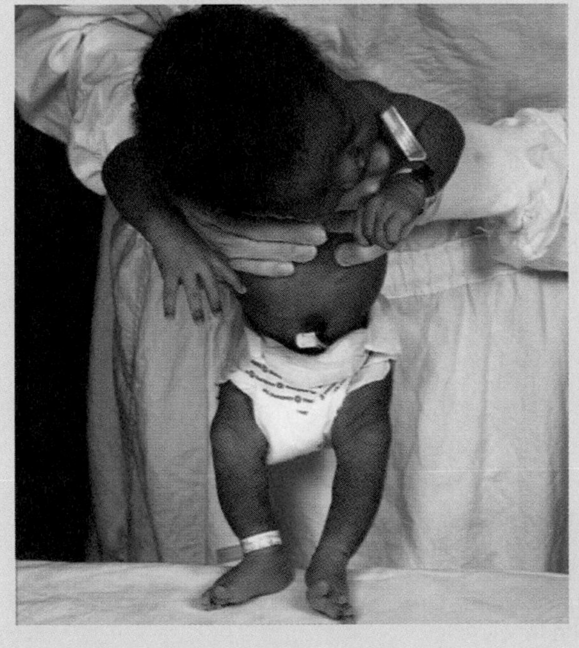

B, Stepping reflex. (From Dickason E, Silverman B, and Kaplan J: *Maternal-infant nursing care,* ed 3, St Louis, 1998, Mosby.)

Continued

TABLE 24-1—cont'd

Assessment of Newborn's Reflexes

Reflex	Eliciting the Reflex	Characteristic Response	Comments
Crawling	Place newborn on abdomen	Newborn makes crawling movements with arms and legs	Response should disappear about 6 wk of age
Deep tendon	Use finger instead of percussion hammer to elicit patellar, or knee jerk, reflex; newborn must be relaxed	Reflex jerk is present; even with newborn relaxed, nonselective overall reaction may occur	
Crossed extension	Infant should be supine; extend one leg, press knee downward, stimulate bottom of foot; observe opposite leg	Opposite leg flexes, adductus, and then extends	

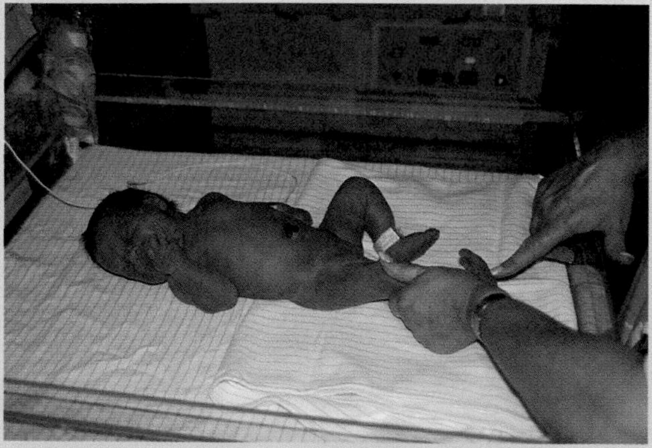

Crossed extension reflex. With the infant in supine position, examiner extends one leg of the infant and presses the knee down. Stimulation of sole of foot of fixated limb should cause free leg to flex, adduct, and extend as if attempting to push away stimulating agent. This reflex should be present during newborn period. (Courtesy Marjorie Pyle, RNC, Lifecircle, Costa Mesa, CA.)

Startle	Perform sharp hand clap; best elicited if newborn is 24 to 36 hr old or older	Arms abduct with flexion of elbows, hands stay clenched	Response should disappear by 4 mo of age Response is elicited more readily in preterm newborn (inform parents of this characteristic)
Babinski's sign (plantar)	On sole of foot, beginning at heel, stroke upward along lateral aspect of sole, then move finger across ball of foot	All toes hyperextend, with dorsiflexion of big toe—recorded as a positive sign	Absence requires neurologic evaluation, should disappear after 1 yr of age Response depends on general muscle tone and maturity and condition of infant

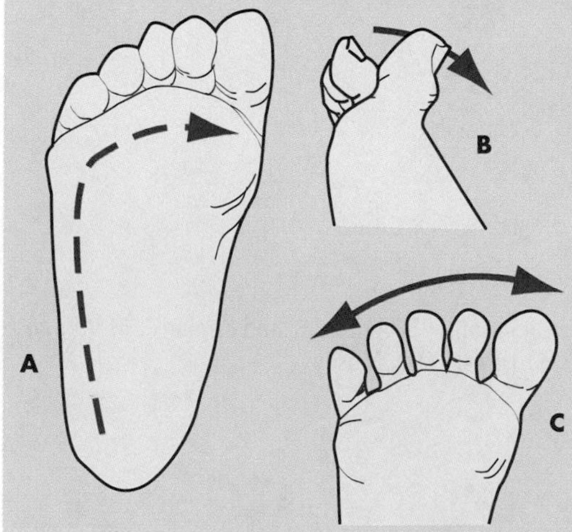

Babinski's reflex. **A,** Direction of stroke. **B,** Dorsiflexion of big toe. **C,** Fanning of toes. (From Wong D: *Whaley & Wong's nursing care of infants and children,* ed 6, St Louis, 1999, Mosby.)

Pull-to-sit (traction)	Pull infant up by wrists from supine position with head in midline	Head will lag until infant is in upright position, then head will be held in same plane with chest and shoulder momentarily before falling forward; infant will attempt to right head	Response disappears by fourth week

TABLE 24-1—cont'd

Assessment of Newborn's Reflexes

Reflex	Eliciting the Reflex	Characteristic Response	Comments
Trunk incurvation (Galant)	Place infant prone on flat surface, run finger down back about 4 to 5 cm lateral to spine, first on one side and then down other	Trunk is flexed and pelvis is swung toward stimulated side	Absence suggests general depression of nervous system

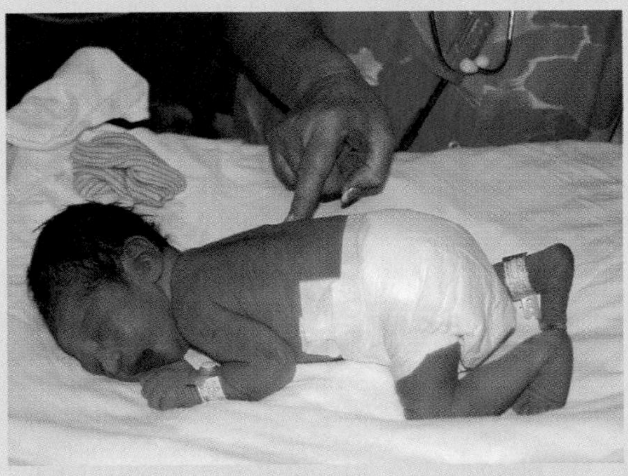

Trunk incurvation reflex. In prone position, infant responds to linear skin stimulus (blunt end of pin or finger) along paravertebral area by flexing the trunk and swinging the pelvis toward stimulus. With transverse lesions of cord, no response below the level of the lesion is present. Response may vary but should be obtainable in all infants, including preterm ones. If not seen in the first few days, it is usually apparent by 5 to 6 days. (Courtesy Marjorie Pyle, RNC, Lifecircle, Costa Mesa, CA.)

Reflex	Eliciting the Reflex	Characteristic Response	Comments
Magnet	Place infant in supine position, partially flex both lower extremities and apply pressure to soles of feet	Both lower limbs should extend against examiner's pressure	Absence suggests damage to spinal cord or malformation Reflex may be weak or exaggerated after breech birth.

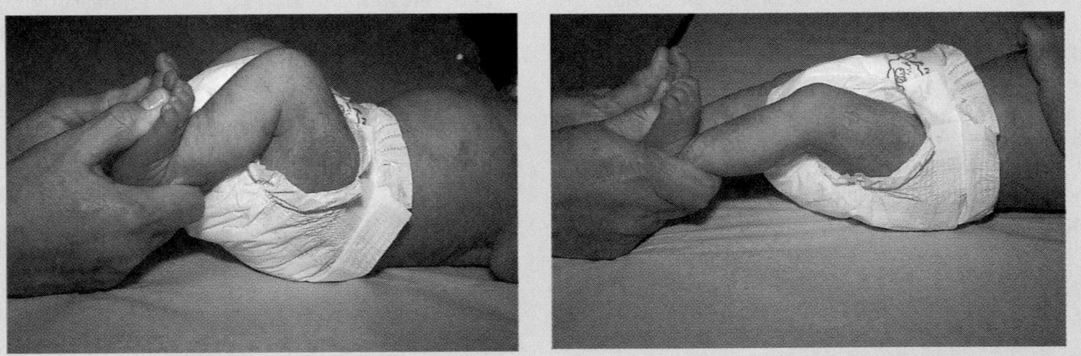

Magnet reflex. With child in supine position and lower limbs semiflexed, light pressure is applied with fingers to both feet. Normally, while the examiner's fingers maintain contact with the soles of the feet, the lower limbs extend. Weak reflex may be seen after breech presentation *without* extended legs or may indicate sciatic nerve stretch syndrome. Breech presentation *with* extended legs may evoke exaggerated response. (Courtesy Michael S. Clement, MD, Mesa, AZ.)

Reflex	Eliciting the Reflex	Characteristic Response	Comments
Additional newborn responses Yawn, stretch, burp, hiccup, sneeze	These are spontaneous behaviors	May be slightly depressed temporarily because of maternal analgesia or anesthesia, fetal hypoxia, or infection	Parental guidance: Most of these behaviors are pleasurable to parents Parents need to be assured that behaviors are normal Sneeze is usually response to lint, etc., in nose and not an indicator of a cold No treatment is needed for hiccups; sucking may help

TABLE 24-2
Physical Assessment of Newborn

Area Assessed and Appraisal Procedure	Normal Findings: Average Findings	Normal Findings: Normal Variations	Deviations From Normal Range: Possible Problems (Etiology)
POSTURE			
Inspect newborn before disturbing for assessment Refer to maternal chart for fetal presentation, position, and type of birth (vaginal, surgical), since newborn readily assumes prenatal position	Vertex: arms, legs in moderate flexion; fists clenched Resistance to having extremities extended for examination or measurement, crying possible when attempted Cessation of crying when allowed to resume curled-up fetal position Normal spontaneous movement bilaterally asynchronous (legs moving in bicycle fashion) but equal extension in all extremities	Frank breech: legs straighter and stiff, newborn assuming intrauterine position in repose for a few days Prenatal pressure on limb or shoulder possibly causing temporary facial asymmetry or resistance to extension of extremities	Hypotonia, relaxed posture while awake (prematurity or hypoxia in utero, maternal medications) Hypertonia (drug dependence, central nervous system [CNS] disorder) Opisthotonos (CNS disturbance) Limitation of motion in any of extremities (see Skeletal System, p. 533)
VITAL SIGNS			
Check heart rate and pulses: Thorax (chest) Inspection Palpation Auscultation Apex: mitral valve Second interspace, left of sternum: pulmonic valve Second interspace, right of sternum: aortic valve Junction of xiphoid process and sternum: tricuspid valve	Visible pulsations in left midclavicular line, fifth intercostal space Apical pulse, fourth intercostal space 120-160 beats/min Quality: *first sound* (closure of mitral and tricuspid valves) and *second sound* (closure of aortic and pulmonic valves) sharp and clear	100 beats/min (sleeping) to 160 beats/min (crying); possibly irregular for brief periods, especially after crying Murmurs, especially over base or at left sternal border in interspace 3 or 4 (foramen ovale anatomically closing at about 1 yr)	Tachycardia: persistent, ≥160 beats/min (respiratory distress syndrome [RDS]) Bradycardia: persistent, ≤120 beats/min (congenital heart block) Murmurs (possibly functional) Arrhythmias: irregular rate Sounds Distant (pneumomediastinum) Poor quality Extra Heart on right side of chest (dextrocardia, often accompanied by reversal of intestines)
For femoral pulse palpation, place fingers along inguinal ligament about midway between symphysis pubis and iliac crest; feel bilaterally simultaneously	Femoral pulses equal and strong		Weak or absent femoral pulses (hip dysplasia, coarctation of aorta, thrombophlebitis)
Obtain temperature: Axillary: method of choice until 6 yr of age Electronic thermistor probe (avoid taping over bony area)	Axillary: 37° C Temperature stabilized by 8-10 hr of age Undeveloped shivering mechanism	36.5°-37.2° C Heat loss: 200 kcal/kg/min from evaporation, conduction, convection, radiation	Subnormal (prematurity, infection, low environmental temperature, inadequate clothing, dehydration) Increased (infection, high environmental temperature, excessive clothing, proximity to heating unit or in direct sunshine, drug addiction, diarrhea and dehydration)

TABLE 24-2—cont'd
Physical Assessment of Newborn

Area Assessed and Appraisal Procedure	Normal Findings: Average Findings	Normal Findings: Normal Variations	Deviations From Normal Range: Possible Problems (Etiology)
VITAL SIGNS—cont'd Obtain temperature—cont'd			Temperature not stabilized by 10 hr after birth (if mother received magnesium sulfate, newborn less able to conserve heat by vasoconstriction; maternal analgesics possibly reducing thermal stability in newborn)
Check respiratory rate and effort: Observe respirations when infant is at rest Count respirations for full minute Check apnea monitor Listen for sounds audible without stethoscope Observe respiratory effort	40/min Tendency to be shallow and irregular in rate, rhythm, and depth when infant is awake No sounds audible on inspiration and expiration Breath sounds: bronchial; loud, clear, near	30-60/min Possibly appearing to be Cheyne-Stokes with short periods of apnea and no evidence of respiratory distress First period (reactivity): 50-60/min Second period: 50-70/min Stabilization (1-2 days): 30-40/min	Apneic episodes: >15 sec (preterm infant: "periodic breathing," rapid warming or cooling of infant) Bradypnea: <25/min (maternal narcosis from analgesics or anesthetics, birth trauma) Tachypnea: >60/min (RDS, aspiration syndrome, diaphragmatic hernia) Sounds Crackles, rhonchi, wheezes (fluid in lungs) Expiratory grunt (narrowing of bronchi) Distress evidenced by nasal flaring, retractions, chin tug, labored breathing (RDS, fluid in lungs)
Obtain blood pressure (BP) (usually assessed only if a problem is suspected) Check electronic monitor BP cuff: BP cuff width affects readings, use cuff 2.5 cm wide and palpate radial pulse	78/42 (approximately) At birth Systolic: 60-80 mm Hg Diastolic: 40-50 mm Hg At 10 days Systolic: 95-100 mm Hg Diastolic: slight increase	Variation with change in activity level: awake, crying, sleeping	Difference between upper and lower extremity pressures (coarctation of aorta) Hypotension (sepsis, hypovolemia) Hypertension (coarctation of aorta)
WEIGHT* Put protective liner cloth or paper in place and adjust scale to 0 (see Fig. 24-12) Weigh at same time each day Protect newborn from heat loss	Female 3400 g Male 3500 g Regaining of birth weight within first 2 weeks	2500-4000 g Acceptable weight loss: 10% or less Second baby weighing more than first	Weight ≤2500 g (prematurity, small for gestational age, rubella syndrome) Weight ≥4000 g (large for gestational age, maternal diabetes, heredity—normal for these parents) Weight loss over 10% (dehydration)

*NOTE: Weight, length, and head circumference should all be close to the same percentile for any child.

Continued

TABLE 24-2—cont'd

Physical Assessment of Newborn

Area Assessed and Appraisal Procedure	Normal Findings: Average Findings	Normal Findings: Normal Variations	Deviations From Normal Range: Possible Problems (Etiology)
LENGTH			
Measure length from top of head to heel, measuring is difficult in term infant because of presence of molding, incomplete extension of knees (see Fig. 24-13, *D*)	50 cm	45-55 cm	<45 cm or >55 cm (chromosomal aberration, heredity—normal for these parents)
HEAD CIRCUMFERENCE			
Measure head at greatest diameter: occipitofrontal circumference (see Fig. 26-13, *A*) May need to remeasure on second or third day after resolution of molding and caput succedaneum	33-35 cm Circumference of head and chest approximately the same for first 1 or 2 days after birth	32-36.8 cm	Small head ≤32 cm: microcephaly (rubella, toxoplasmosis, cytomegalic inclusion disease) Hydrocephaly: sutures widely separated, circumference ≥4 cm more than chest circumference (maldevelopment, infection) Increased intracranial pressure (hemorrhage, space-occupying lesion)
CHEST CIRCUMFERENCE			
Measure at nipple line (see Fig. 24-13, *B*)	2-3 cm less than head circumference, averages 30-33 cm		≤30 cm (prematurity)
ABDOMINAL CIRCUMFERENCE			
Measure below umbilicus (see Fig. 26-13, *C*) (not usually measured unless specific indication)	Abdomen enlargement after feeding because of lax abdominal muscles Same size as chest		Enlarging abdomen between feedings (abdominal mass or blockage in intestinal tract)
SKIN			
Check color: Inspect and palpate Inspect naked newborn in well-lighted, warm area without drafts; natural daylight best Inspect newborn when quiet and when active	Generally pink Varying with ethnic origin, skin pigmentation beginning to deepen right after birth in basal layer of epidermis Acrocyanosis, especially if chilled	Mottling Harlequin sign Plethora Telangiectases ("stork bites" or capillary hemangiomas) Erythema toxicum/neonatorum ("newborn rash") Milia	Dark red (prematurity, polycythemia) Gray (hypotension, poor perfusion) Pallor (cardiovascular problem, CNS damage, blood dyscrasia, blood loss, twin-to-twin transfusion, nosocomial infection) Cyanosis (hypothermia, infection, hypoglycemia, cardiopulmonary diseases, cardiac, neurologic, or respiratory malformations)
		Petechiae over presenting part	Petechiae over any other area (clotting factor deficiency, infection)
		Ecchymoses from forceps in vertex births or over buttocks, genitalia, and legs in breech births	Ecchymoses in any other area (hemorrhagic disease, traumatic birth)

TABLE 24-2—cont'd
Physical Assessment of Newborn

Area Assessed and Appraisal Procedure	Normal Findings: Average Findings	Normal Findings: Normal Variations	Deviations From Normal Range: Possible Problems (Etiology)
SKIN—cont'd			
Check for jaundice	None at birth	Physiologic jaundice in 50% of term infants after first 24 hr	Jaundice within first 24 hr (Rh isoimmunization)
Check birthmarks:			
Inspect and palpate for location, size, distribution, characteristics, color	Transient hyperpigmentation Areolae Genitals Linea nigra	Mongolian spotting Infants of African-American, Asian, and Native American origin: 70% Infants of Caucasian origin: 9%	Hemangiomas Nevus flammeus: port-wine stain Nevus vasculosus: strawberry mark Cavernous hemangiomas
Check condition:			
Inspect and palpate for intactness, smoothness, texture, edema	No skin edema Opacity: few large blood vessels visible indistinctly over abdomen	Slightly thick; superficial cracking, peeling, especially of hands, feet No visible blood vessels, a few large vessels clearly visible over abdomen Some fingernail scratches	Edema on hands, feet; pitting over tibia (over hydration) Texture thin, smooth, or of medium thickness; rash or superficial peeling visible (prematurity, postmaturity) Numerous vessels very visible over abdomen (prematurity) Texture thick, parchmentlike; cracking, peeling (postmaturity) Skin tags, webbing Papules, pustules, vesicles, ulcers, maceration (impetigo, candidiasis, herpes, diaper rash)
Assess hydration and consistency			
Weigh infant routinely Inspect and palpate Gently pinch skin between thumb and forefinger over abdomen and inner thigh to check for turgor Check subcutaneous fat deposits (adipose pads) over cheeks, buttocks	Dehydration: loss of weight best indicator After pinch released, skin returns to original state immediately	Normal weight loss after birth: up to 10% of birth weight Possibly puffy Variation in amount of subcutaneous fat	Loose, wrinkled skin (prematurity, postmaturity, dehydration: fold of skin persisting after release of pinch) Tense, tight, shiny skin (edema, extreme cold, shock, infection) Lack of subcutaneous fat, prominence of clavicle or ribs (prematurity, malnutrition)
Check voiding	Voiding within 24 hours of birth Voiding six to ten times per day		
Check vernix caseosa:			
Observe amount		Variation in amount; usually more found in creases, folds	Absent or minimal (postmaturity) Excessive (prematurity)
Observe its color and odor before bath or wiping	Whitish, cheesy, odorless		Yellow color (possible fetal anoxia more than 36 hr before birth, Rh or ABO incompatibility)

Continued

TABLE 24-2—cont'd
Physical Assessment of Newborn

Area Assessed and Appraisal Procedure	Normal Findings: Average Findings	Normal Findings: Normal Variations	Deviations From Normal Range: Possible Problems (Etiology)
SKIN—cont'd			
Check vernix caseosa—cont'd			Green color (possible in utero release of meconium or presence of bilirubin) Odor (possible intrauterine infection)
Assess lanugo: Inspect for this fine, downy hair, its amount and distribution	Over shoulders, pinnas of ears, forehead	Variation in amount	Absent (postmaturity) Excessive (prematurity, especially if lanugo abundant, long and thick over back)
HEAD			
Palpate skin	(See Skin)	Caput succedaneum, possibly showing some ecchymosis	Cephalhematoma
Inspect shape, size	Making up one fourth of body length Molding (see Fig. 24-8)	Slight asymmetry from intrauterine position Lack of molding (prematurity, breech presentation, cesarean birth)	Molding Severe molding (birth trauma) Indentation (fracture from trauma)
Palpate, inspect, measure fontanels	Anterior fontanel 5-cm diamond, increasing as molding resolves Posterior fontanel triangle, smaller than anterior	Variation in fontanel size with degree of molding Difficulty in feeling fontanels possible because of molding	Fontanels Full, bulbing (tumor, hemorrhage, infection) Large, flat, soft (malnutrition, hydrocephaly, retarded bone age, hypothyroidism) Depressed (dehydration)
Palpate sutures	Palpable and unjoined sutures	Possible overlap of sutures with molding	Sutures Widely spaced (hydrocephaly) Premature closure
Inspect pattern, distribution, amount of hair; feel texture	Silky, single strands lying flat; growth pattern toward face and neck	Variation in amount	Fine, wooly (prematurity) Unusual swirls, patterns, or hairline; or coarse, brittle (endocrine or genetic disorders)
EYES			
Check placement on face	Eyes and space between eyes each one third the distance from outer-to-outer canthus (Fig. 24-14)	Epicanthal folds: normal racial characteristic	Epicanthal folds when present with other signs (chromosomal disorders such as Down, cri-du-chat syndromes)
Check for symmetry in size, shape	Symmetric in size, shape		
Check eyelids for size, movements, blink	Blink reflex	Edema if silver nitrate instilled; also may occur if erythromycin or tetracycline instilled	
Assess for discharge	None No tears	Some discharge if silver nitrate used Occasional presence of some tears	Discharge: purulent (infection)
Evaluate eyeballs for presence, size, shape	Both present and of equal size, both round, firm	Subconjunctival hemorrhage	Agenesis or absence of one or both eyeballs

TABLE 24-2—cont'd
Physical Assessment of Newborn

Area Assessed and Appraisal Procedure	Normal Findings: Average Findings	Normal Findings: Normal Variations	Deviations From Normal Range: Possible Problems (Etiology)
EYES—cont'd			Small eyeball size (rubella syndrome) Lens opacity or absence of red reflex (congenital cataracts, possibly from rubella) Lesions: coloboma, absence of part of iris (congenital) Pink color of iris (albinism) Jaundiced sclera (hyperbilirubinemia)
Check pupils	Present, equal in size, reactive to light		Pupils: unequal, constricted, dilated, fixed (intracranial pressure, medications, tumors)
Evaluate eyeball movement	Random, jerky, uneven, focus possible briefly, following to midline	Transient strabismus or nystamus until third or fourth month	Persistent strabismus Doll's eyes (increased intrancranial pressure) Sunset (increased intracranial pressure)
Assess eyebrows: amount of hair, pattern	Distinct (not connected in midline)		Connection in midline (Cornelia de Lange syndrome)
NOSE			
Observe shape, placement, patency, configuration of bridge of nose	Midline Apparent lack of bridge, flat, broad Some mucus but no drainage Preferential nose breather Sneezing to clear nose	Slight deformity from passage through birth canal	Copious drainage, with or without regular periods of cyanosis at rest and return of pink color with crying (choanal atresia, congenital syphilis) Malformed (congenital syphilis, chromosomal disorder) Flaring of nares (respiratory distress)
EARS			
Observe size, placement on head, amount of cartilage, open auditory canal	Correct placement line drawn through inner and outer canthi of eyes reaching to top notch of ears (at junction with scalp) (Fig. 24-15) Well-formed, firm cartilage	Size: small, large, floppy Darwin's tubercle (nodule on posterior helix)	Agenesis Lack of cartilage (prematurity) Low placement (chromosomal disorder, mental retardation, kidney disorder) Preauricular tags Size: possibly overly prominent or protruding ears
Assess hearing	Responds to voice and other sounds	State (e.g., alert, asleep) influencing response	Deaf: no response to sound
FACIES			
Observe overall appearance of face	"Normal" appearance, well-placed, proportionate, symmetric features	Positional deformities	Infant appearance "odd" or "funny" Usually accompanied by other features such as low-set ears, other structural disorders (hereditary, chromosomal aberration)

Continued

TABLE 24-2—cont'd
Physical Assessment of Newborn

Area Assessed and Appraisal Procedure	Normal Findings: Average Findings	Normal Findings: Normal Variations	Deviations From Normal Range: Possible Problems (Etiology)
MOUTH			
Inspect and palpate Check placement on face Assess lips for color, configuration, movement	Symmetry of lip movement	Transient circumoral cyanosis	Gross anomalies in placement, size, shape (cleft lip and/or palate, gums) Cyanosis, circumoral pallor (respiratory distress, hypothermia) Asymmetry in movement of lips (seventh cranial nerve paralysis)
Check gums	Pink gums	Inclusion cysts (Epstein's pearls—Bohn's nodules, whitish, hard nodules on gums or roof of mouth)	Teeth: predeciduous or deciduous (hereditary)
Assess tongue for attachment, mobility, movement, size	Tongue not protruding, freely movable, symmetric in shape, movement	Short frenulum	Macroglossia (prematurity, chromosomal disorder)
Evaluate cheeks	Sucking pads inside cheeks		Thrush: white plaques on cheeks or tongue that bleed if touched *(Candida albicans)*
Assess palate (soft, hard): Arch Uvula	Soft and hard palates intact Uvula in midline	Anatomic groove in palate to accommodate nipple, disappearance by 3 to 4 yr of age Epstein's pearls	Cleft hard or soft palate
Assess chin	Distinct chin		Micrognathia (Pierre Robin or other syndrome)
Evaluate saliva for amount, character	Mouth moist		Excessive saliva (esophageal atresia, tracheoesophageal fistula)
Check reflexes: Rooting Sucking Extrusion	Reflexes present	Reflex response dependent on state of wakefulness and hunger	Absent (prematurity)
NECK			
Inspect and palpate length	Short, thick, surrounded by skin folds; no webbing		Webbing (Turner's syndrome)
Check sternocleidomastoid muscles, movement and position of head	Head held in midline (sternocleidomastoid muscles equal), no masses Freedom of movement from side to side and flexion and extension, no movement of chin past shoulder	Transient positional deformity apparent when newborn is at rest: passive movement of head possible	Restricted movement, holding of head at angle (torticollis [wryneck], opisthotonos) Absence of head control (prematurity, Down syndrome)
Assess trachea for position and thyroid gland	Thyroid not palpable		Masses (enlarged thyroid) Distended veins (cardiopulmonary disorder) Skin tags
CHEST			
Inspect and palpate Shape	Almost circular, barrel shaped	Tip of sternum possibly prominent	Bulging of chest, unequal movement (pneumothorax, pneumomediastinum) Malformation (funnel chest—pectus excavatum)

TABLE 24-2—cont'd
Physical Assessment of Newborn

Area Assessed and Appraisal Procedure	Normal Findings: Average Findings	Normal Findings: Normal Variations	Deviations From Normal Range: Possible Problems (Etiology)
CHEST—cont'd			
Check respiratory movements	Symmetric chest movements, chest and abdominal movements synchronized during respirations	Occasional retractions, especially when crying	Retractions with or without respiratory distress (prematurity, RDS)
Evaluate clavicles	Clavicles intact		Fracture of clavicle (trauma); crepitus
Assess ribs	Rib cage symmetrical, intact; moves with respirations		Poor development of rib cage and musculature (prematurity)
Assess nipples for size, placement, number	Nipples prominent, well formed; symmetrically placed		Nipples Supernumerary, along nipple line Malpositioned or widely spaced
Check breast tissue	Breast nodule: approximately 6 mm in term infant	Breast nodule: 3-10 mm Secretion of witch's milk	Lack of breast tissue (prematurity)
Auscultate: Heart sounds and rate and breath sounds (see Vital Signs)			Sounds: bowel sounds (see Abdomen)
ABDOMEN			
Inspect, palpate, and smell umbilical cord	Two arteries, one vein Whitish gray Definite demarcation between cord and skin, no intestinal structures within cord Dry around base, drying Odorless Cord clamp in place for 24 hr		One artery (renal anomalies) Meconium stained (intrauterine distress) Bleeding or oozing around cord (hemorrhagic disease) Redness or drainage around cord (infection, possible persistence of urachus)
		Reducible umbilical herniation	Hernia: herniation of abdominal contents into area of cord (e.g., omphalocele); defect covered with thin, friable membrane, possibly extensive
Inspect size of abdomen and palpate contour (see Fig. 24-13, *C*)	Rounded, prominent, dome shaped because abdominal musculature not fully developed Liver possibly palpable 1-2 cm below right costal margin No other masses palpable No distention	Some diatasis of abdominal musculature	Gastroschisis: fissure of abdominal cavity Distention at birth (ruptured viscus, genitourinary masses or malformations: hydronephrosis, teratomas, abdominal tumors) Mild (overfeeding, high gastrointestinal tract obstruction) Marked (lower gastrointestinal tract obstruction, imperforate anus) Intermittent or transient (overfeeding) Partial intestinal obstruction (stenosis of bowel)

Continued

TABLE 24-2—cont'd
Physical Assessment of Newborn

Area Assessed and Appraisal Procedure	Normal Findings: Average Findings	Normal Findings: Normal Variations	Deviations From Normal Range: Possible Problems (Etiology)
ABDOMEN—cont'd			Visible peristalsis (obstruction) Malrotation of bowel or adhesions Sepsis (infection)
Auscultate bowel sounds and note number, amount, and character of stools; note behavior (e.g., crying fussiness) before or during elimination	Sounds present within 1-2 hr after birth Meconium stool passing within 24-48 hr after birth		Scaphoid, with bowel sounds in chest and respiratory distress (diaphragmatic hernia)
Assess color		Linea nigra possibly apparent and caused by hormone influence during pregnancy	
Check movement with respiration	Respirations primarily diaphragmatic, abdominal and chest movement synchronous		Decreased abdominal breathing (intrathoracic disease, diaphragmatic hernia) "Seesaw" (respiratory distress)
GENITALIA			
Female (see Fig. 24-7, *A*)			
Inspect and palpate			
General appearance	Female genitals	Increased pigmentation caused by pregnancy hormones	Ambiguous genitals—enlarged clitoris with urinary meatus on tip, fused labia (chromosomal disorder, maternal drug ingestion)
Clitoris	Usually edematous		
Labia majora	Usually edematous, covering labia minora in term newborns	Edema and ecchymosis after breech birth	
Labia minora	Possible protrusion over labia majora	Blood-tinged discharge from pseudomenstruation caused by pregnancy hormones	Stenosed meatus Labia majora widely separated and labia minora prominent (prematurity)
Discharge	Smegma	Some vernix caseosa between labia possible	
Vagina	Open orifice Mucoid discharge Hymenal/vaginal tag		Absence of vaginal orifice or imperforate hymen Fecal discharge (fistula)
Urinary meatus	Beneath clitoris, difficult to see	Rust-stained urine (uric acid crystals)*	
Male (see Fig. 24-7, *B*)			
Inspect and palpate			
General appearance	Male genitals		
Penis		Increased size and pigmentation caused by pregnancy hormones	Ambiguous genitals
Urinary meatus appears as slit	Meatus at tip of penis		Urinary meatus not on tip of glans penis (hypospadias, epispadias) Round meatal opening
Prepuce (foreskin)	Prepuce covering glans penis and not retractable	Prepuce removed if circumcised Wide variation in size of genitals	

*To determine whether rust color is caused by uric acid or blood, wash urine under running warm tap water; uric acid washes out, blood does not.

TABLE 24-2—cont'd
Physical Assessment of Newborn

Area Assessed and Appraisal Procedure	Normal Findings: Average Findings	Normal Findings: Normal Variations	Deviations From Normal Range: Possible Problems (Etiology)
GENITALIA—cont'd			
Male—cont'd			
Scrotum Rugae (wrinkles)	Large, edematous, pendulous in term infant; covered with rugae	Scrotal edema and ecchymosis if breech birth Hydrocele, small, noncommunicating	Scrotum smooth and testes undescended (prematurity, cryptorchidism) Hydrocele Inguinal hernia
Testes	Palpable on each side	Bulge palpable in inguinal canal	Undescended (prematurity)
Check urination	Voiding within 24 hr, stream adequate, amount adequate	Rust-stained urine (uric acid crystals)*	
Check reflexes:			
Erection	Erection possibly occurring spontaneously and when genitals touched		
Cremasteric	Testes retracted, especially when newborn is chilled		
EXTREMITIES			
Make a general check: Inspect and palpate Degree of flexion Range of motion Symmetry of motion Muscle tone	Assuming of position maintained in utero Attitude of general flexion Full range of motion, spontaneous movements	Transient (positional) deformities	Limited motion (malformations) Poor muscle tone (prematurity, maternal medications, CNS anomalies) Positive scarf sign
Check arms and hands: Inspect and palpate Color Intactness Appropriate placement	Longer than legs in newborn period Contours and movements symmetric	Slight tremors sometimes apparent Some acrocyanosis, especially when chilled	Asymmetry of movement (fracture/crepitus, brachial nerve trauma, malformations) Asymmetry of contour (malformations, fracture) Amelia or phocomelia (teratogens) Palmar creases Simian line with short, incurved little fingers (Down syndrome)
Check number of fingers	Five on each hand Fist often clenched with thumb under fingers		Webbing of fingers: syndactyly Absence or excess of fingers Strong, rigid flexion; persistent fists; positioning of fists in front of mouth constantly (CNS disorder) Yellowed nail beds (meconium staining)
Palpate humerus	Intact		Fractured humerus
Evaluate joints Shoulder Elbow Wrist Fingers	Full range of motion, symmetric contour		Increased tonicity, clonicity, prolonged tremors (CNS disorder)
Check reflex: grasp			

Continued

TABLE 24-2—cont'd
Physical Assessment of Newborn

Area Assessed and Appraisal Procedure	Normal Findings: Average Findings	Normal Findings: Normal Variations	Deviations From Normal Range: Possible Problems (Etiology)
EXTREMITIES—cont'd			
Check legs and feet:			
Inspect and palpate Color Intactness Length in relation to arms and body and to each other	Appearance of bowing because lateral muscles more developed than medial muscles	Feet appearing to turn in but can be easily rotated externally, positional defects tending to correct while infant is crying Acrocyanosis	Amelia, phocomelia (chromosomal defect, teratogenic effect) Temperature of one leg differing from that of the other (circulatory deficiency, CNS disorder)
Number of toes	Five on each foot		Webbing, syndactyly (chromosomal defect) Absence or excess of digits (chromosomal defect, familial trait)
Femur	Intact femur		Femoral fracture (difficult breech birth)
Head of femur as legs are flexed and abducted, placement in acetabulum (see Fig. 24-11)	No click heard, femoral head not overriding acetabulum		Congenital hip dysplasia/dislocation
Major gluteal folds	Major gluteal folds even		
Soles of feet	Soles well lined (or wrinkled) over two thirds of foot in term infants Planter fat pad giving flat-footed effect		Soles of feet Few lines (prematurity) Covered with lines (postmaturity) Congenital clubfoot
Evaluate joints Hip Knee Ankle Toes	Full range of motion, symmetric contour		Hypermobility of joints (Down syndrome)
Check reflexes			Asymmetric movement (trauma, CNS disorder)
BACK			
Assess anatomy:			
Inspect and palpate Spine Shoulders Scapulae Iliac crests	Spine straight and easily flexed Infant able to raise and support head momentarily when prone	Temporary minor positional deformities, correction with passive manipulation	Limitation of movement (fusion or deformity of vertebra)
Base of spine—pilonidal area	Shoulders, scapulae, and iliac crests lining up in same plane		Spina bifida cystica (meningocele, myelomeningocele) Pigmented nevus with tuft of hair, location anywhere along the spine, often associated with spina bifida occulta
Check reflexes (spinal related) Test trunk incurvation reflex	Trunk flexed and pelvis swings to stimulated side	May not be apparent in first few days but is usually present in 5-6 days	If transverse lesion is present, no response below lesion; absence of response: nervous system abnormality or general depression
Test magnet reflex	Lower limbs extend as pressure applied to feet with legs in semiflexed position	Weak or exaggerated response with breech presentation	Absence: suggestive of spinal cord damage or malformation

TABLE 24-2—cont'd
Physical Assessment of Newborn

Area Assessed and Appraisal Procedure	Normal Findings: Average Findings	Normal Findings: Normal Variations	Deviations From Normal Range: Possible Problems (Etiology)
ANUS			
Inspect and palpate Placement Number Patency Test for sphincter response (active "wink" reflex) Observe for following: Abdominal distention Passage of meconium Fecal drainage from surrounding orifices	One anus with good sphincter tone Passage of meconium within 24 hr after birth Good "wink" reflex of anal sphincter	Passage of meconium within 48 hr of birth	Low obstruction: and membrane High obstruction: anal or rectal atresia Drainage of fecal material from vagina in female or urinary meatus in male (rectal fistula)
STOOLS			
Observe frequency, color, consistency	Meconium followed by transitional and soft yellow stools		No stool (obstruction) Frequent watery stools (infection, phototherapy)

Text continued from p. 535.
shortly after birth and, when the infant's condition has stabilized, from 120 to 140 beats/min.

If blood pressure is measured, a Doppler (electronic) monitor facilitates this procedure. Neonatal BP usually is highest immediately after birth and falls to a minimum by 3 hours after birth. It then begins to rise steadily and reaches a plateau between 4 and 6 days after birth. This measurement is usually equal to that of the immediate postbirth BP. The BP varies with the neonate's activity.

BP may be measured in both the arms and the legs to detect any discrepancy between the two sides or between the upper and lower body. A discrepancy of 10 mm Hg or more between the arms and legs may signal a cardiac defect such as coarctation of the aorta.

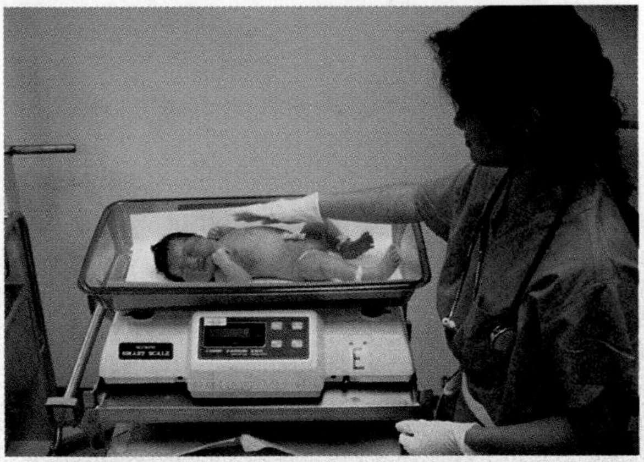

FIG. 24-12 • Weighing the infant. Note that a hand is held over infant as a safety measure. The scale is covered to protect against cross infection. (Courtesy Kim Molloy, Knoxville, IA.)

Baseline Measurements of Physical Growth

Baseline measurements are taken and recorded to help assess the progress and determine the growth patterns of the neonate. These may be recorded on growth charts. The following measurements are made when the neonate is assessed.

Weight. The newborn is usually weighed shortly after birth. This may be done in the labor and birthing area or on admission to the nursery. Care must be taken to ensure the scales are balanced. The totally unclothed neonate is placed in the center of the scale, which is usually covered with a disposable pad or diaper to prevent heat loss via conduction and cross infection. The nurse should place one hand over (but not touching) the neonate to prevent the infant from falling off the scales (Fig. 24-12). It is common to weigh the infant at the same time every day during the hospital stay. Birth weight of a term infant typically ranges from 2500 to 4000 g.

Circumferences and Length. The head is measured at the widest part, which is the occipitofrontal diameter (Fig. 24-13, *A*). The tape measure is placed around the head just above the infant's eyebrows. The term neonate's head circumference ranges from 32 to 36.8 cm.

The chest circumference usually measures about 2 cm less than head circumference. The chest may be the same size as the head but should not exceed it. The tape is placed around the infant's chest at the nipple line (Fig. 24-13, *B*).

Abdominal circumference is measured by placing the tape around the abdomen just above the umbilicus (Fig. 24-13, *C*). Measurements vary with the size of the infant. The abdomen should be cylindrical in shape and protrude slightly. Abdominal measurements are not always taken but should be measured when there is suspicion of abdominal distention.

The length may be difficult to obtain because of the flexed posture of the newborn (Fig. 24-13, *D*). The examiner places the

A

B

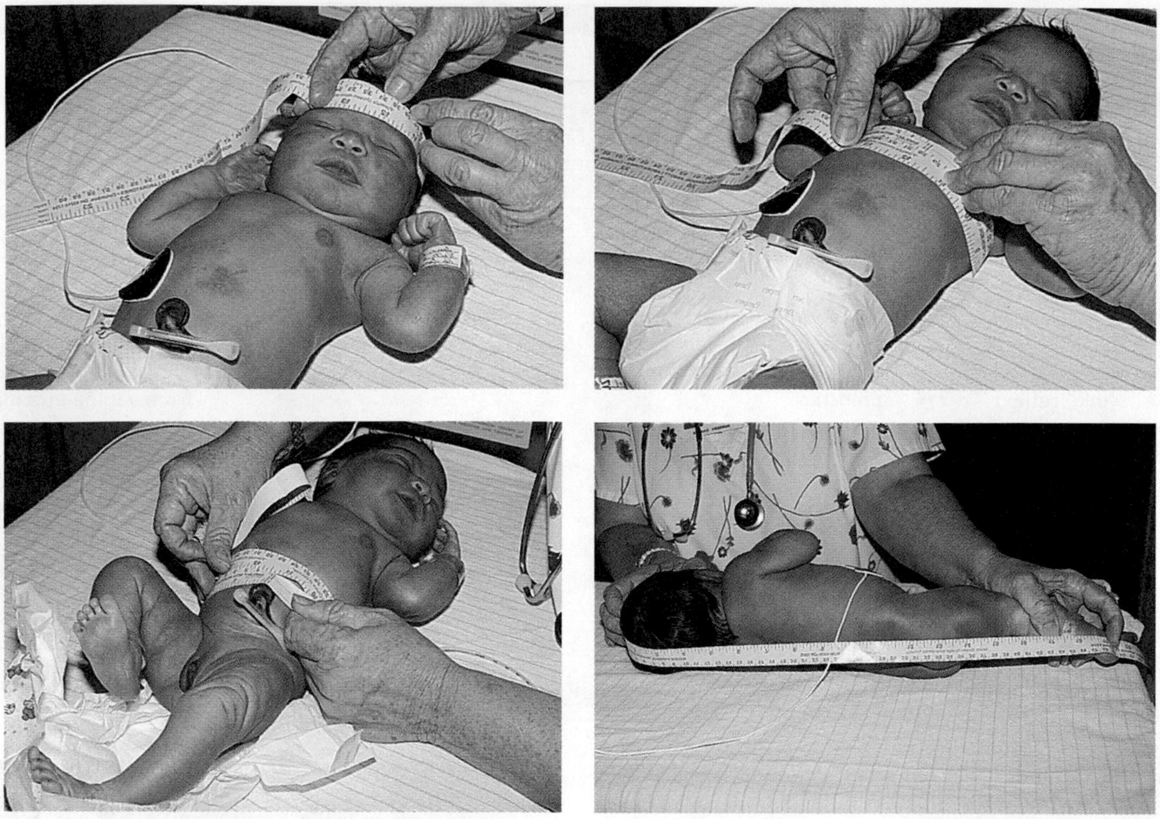

C

D

FIG. 24-13 • Measurements. **A,** Circumference of head. **B,** Circumference of chest. **C,** Abdominal circumference. **D,** Length, crown to rump. To determine total length, include length of legs. If measurements are taken before the infant's initial bath, the nurse must wear gloves. (Courtesy Marjorie Pyle, RNC, Lifecircle, Costa Mesa, CA.)

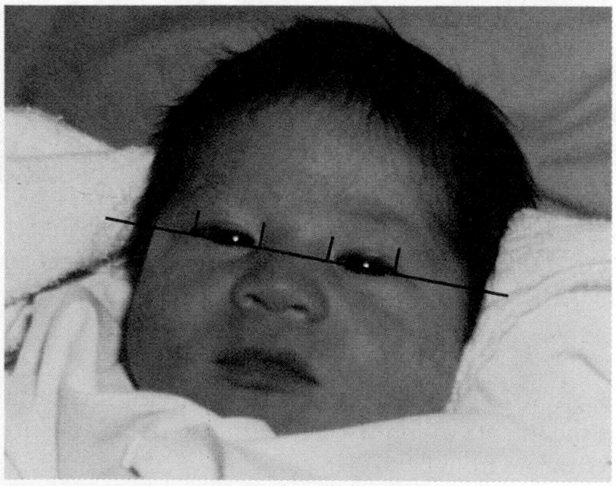

FIG. 24-14 • Eyes. In pseudostrabismus, inner epicanthal folds cause the eyes to appear misaligned; however, corneal light reflexes are perfectly symmetric. Eyes are symmetric in size and shape and are well placed.

newborn on a flat surface and extends the leg until the knee is flat against the surface. Placing the head against a perpendicular surface and extending the leg may assist with this measurement. In the term neonate, head-to-heel length ranges from 45 to 55 cm.

Neurologic Assessment

The physical assessment includes a neurologic assessment of the newborn's reflexes (see Table 24-1). This provides useful information about the infant's nervous system and state of neurologic maturation. Many reflex behaviors (e.g., sucking and rooting) are important for survival. Other reflexes such as gagging, coughing, and sneezing, act as safety mechanisms. The assessment needs to be carried out as early as possible because abnormal signs present in the early neonatal period may disappear. They may reappear months or years later as abnormal functions.

BEHAVIORAL CHARACTERISTICS

The healthy infant must accomplish behavioral and biologic tasks to develop normally. Behavioral characteristics form the basis of the social capabilities of the infant. Normal newborns differ in their activity levels, feeding and sleeping patterns, and responsiveness. Parents' reactions to their newborns are often determined by these differences. Showing parents the unique characteristics of their infant assists parents to develop a more positive perception of the infant with increased interaction between infant and parent (Nursing Care Plan).

Behavioral responses, as well as physical characteristics, change during the period of transition. The Brazelton Neonatal Behavioral Assessment Scale (BNBAS) can be used to systemat-

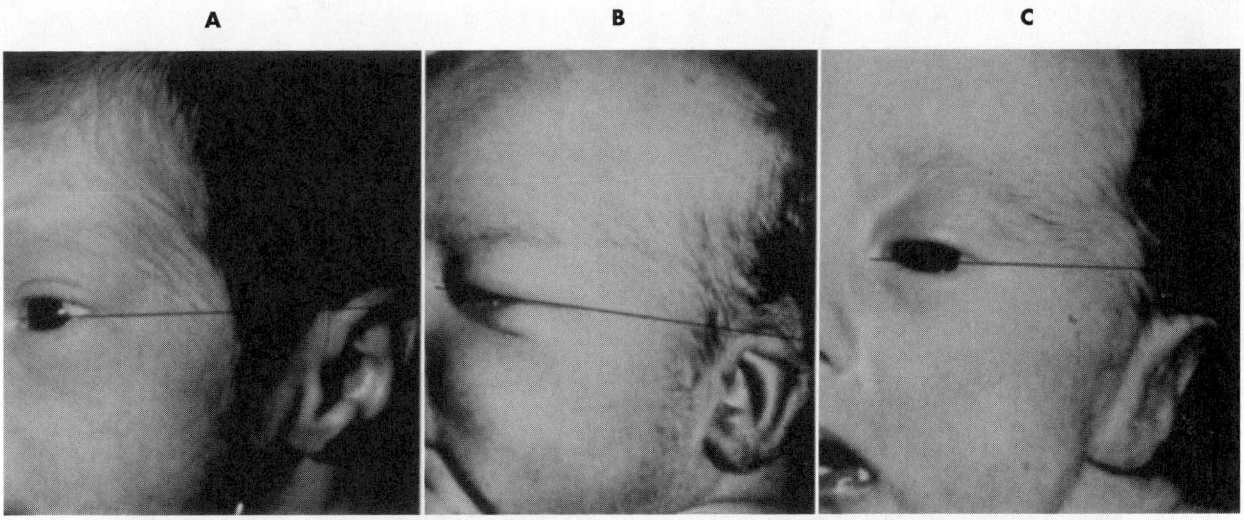

FIG. 24-15 • Placement of ear on head in relation to line drawn from inner to outer canthus of eye. **A,** Normal position. **B,** Abnormally angled ear. **C,** True low-set ear. (Courtesy Mead Johnson & Co., Evansville, IN.)

Nursing Care Plan IMMEDIATE CARE OF THE NEWBORN

NURSING DIAGNOSIS Risk for injury related to birth trauma as evidenced by caput succadaneum or cephalhematoma

EXPECTED OUTCOME Neonate will be free of injury as a result of the birth process.

Nursing Interventions/*Rationales*

Assess neonate thoroughly for any evidence of birth trauma *to provide ongoing identification of potential complications.*

Evaluate neonate often for evidence of jaundice *to promote early interventions.*

Monitor bilirubin levels, if ordered by physician, *to detect rising levels as a result of cephalhematoma.*

Keep neonate clean, dry, and wrapped securely in blanket *to promote comfort and security.*

Provide explanations to parents that any scalp trauma or hematoma will subside without treatment *to alleviate anxiety.*

Give information to parents regarding potential jaundice *to increase awareness upon discharge of neonate.*

Encourage parents to report any evidence or increase of jaundice to health care provider *to provide early intervention if necessary.*

NURSING DIAGNOSIS Knowledge deficit related to caput succadaneum or cephalhematoma as evidenced by parent's statements

EXPECTED OUTCOME Parents will verbalize correct information regarding neonate's condition at time of discharge.

Nursing Interventions/*Rationales*

Provide information to parents regarding alterations in appearance of head and scalp *to alleviate anxiety.*

Instruct parents to observe for evidence of jaundice or increase in jaundice *to provide early interventions if necessary.*

Teach parents to report any evidence of infant pain or discomfort to care provider *to give information that may require further assessment.*

Encourage expression of feelings of parents *to provide clarification and correct any misconceptions regarding severity of these benign newborn deviations.*

Provide parents with contact number for health care provider *to ensure that parents have opportunity to have questions answered and concerns addressed.*

ically assess the infant's behavior (Brazelton and Nugent, 1996). The BNBAS is an interactive examination that assesses the infant's response to 28 areas organized according to the clusters in Box 24-2. It is generally used as a research or diagnostic tool and requires special training.

In addition to their use as initial and ongoing tools to assess neurologic and behavioral responses, the scales can be used to assess initial parent-infant relationships and as a guide for parents to help them focus on their infant's individuality and to develop a deeper attachment to their child. See Chapter 22 for further discussion of attachment.

Sleep-Wake States

Variations in the state of consciousness of infants are called sleep-wake states (Brazelton and Nugent, 1996). The six states

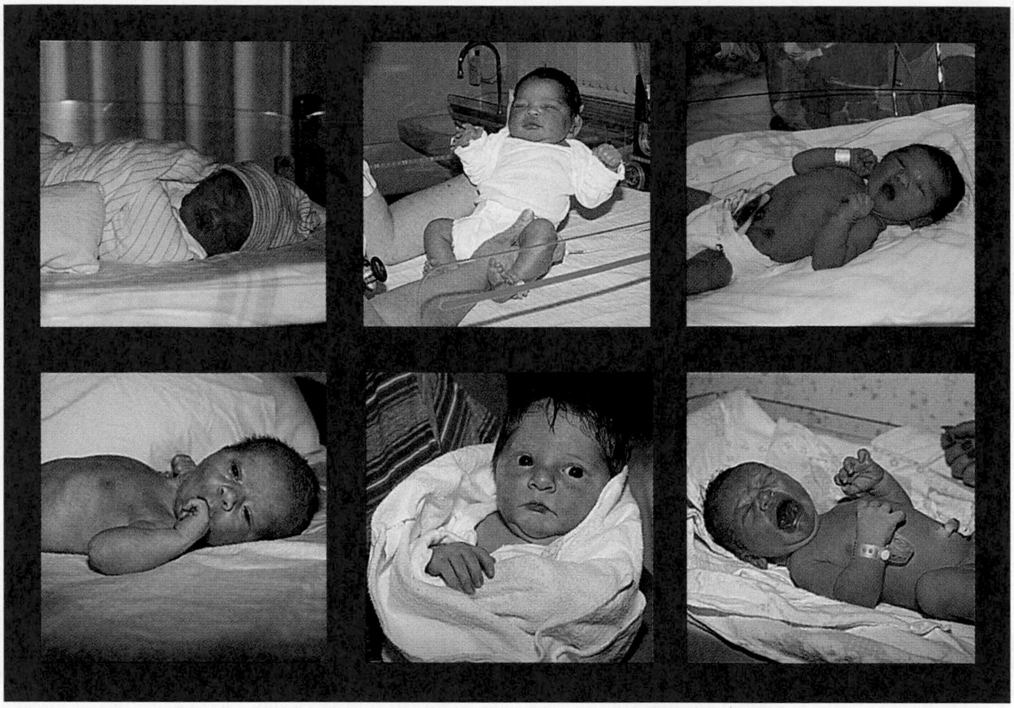

FIG. 24-16 • Newborn sleep-wake states. States of consciousness: **A,** deep sleep; **B,** light sleep; **C,** drowsy; **D,** quiet alert; **E,** active alert; **F,** crying. (Courtesy Marjorie Pyle, RNC, Lifecircle, Costa Mesa, CA.)

Box 24-2

Clusters of Neonatal Behaviors in BNBAS

Habituation—Ability to respond to and then inhibit responding to discrete stimulus (e.g., light, rattle, bell, pinprick) while asleep
Orientation—Quality of alert states and ability to attend to visual and auditory stimuli while alert
Motor performance—Quality of movement and tone
Range of state—Measure of general arousal level or arousability of infant
Regulation of state—How infant responds when aroused
Autonomic stability—Signs of stress (e.g., tremors, startles, skin color) related to homeostatic (self-regulator) adjustment of the nervous system
Reflexes—Assessment of several neonatal reflexes

form a continuum from deep sleep to extreme irritability (Fig. 24-16). There are two sleep states (i.e., deep sleep and light sleep) and four wake states (i.e., drowsy, quiet alert, active alert, and crying). Each state has specific characteristics and state-related behaviors. The optimum state of arousal is the quiet alert state. During this state infants smile, vocalize, move in synchrony with speech, watch their parents' faces, and respond to people talking to them. The infant's reaction to internal and external stimuli and ability to control their responses while in these sleep-wake states reflect the ability to organize behavior.

Infants use purposeful behavior to maintain the optimum arousal state as follows: (1) actively withdrawing by increasing physical distance; (2) rejecting by pushing away with hands and feet; (3) decreasing sensitivity by falling asleep or breaking eye contact by turning head; or (4) using signaling behaviors, such as fussing and crying. These behaviors permit infants to quiet themselves and reinstate readiness to interact.

Critical Thinking

PLANNING ACTIVITIES THAT PROMOTE ATTACHMENT

Based on your knowledge of the physiologic adaptations and behavioral characteristics of newborn infants, plan activities that promote parent-infant attachment in a parent at risk for altered parenting. Risk for altered parenting could include such factors as adolescence, substance abuse, or postpartum depression.

The first 6 weeks of life involve a steady decrease in the proportion of active REM sleep to total sleep. A steady increase in the proportion of quiet sleep to total sleep also occurs. Periods of wakefulness increase. For the first few weeks the wakeful periods seem dictated by hunger, but soon a need for socializing appears as well. The newborn sleeps approximately 17 hours a day, with periods of wakefulness gradually increasing. By the fourth week of life, some infants stay awake from one feeding to the next.

Other Factors Influencing Behavior of Newborns

Gestational Age. The gestational age of the infant and level of CNS maturity affect the observed behavior. In an infant with an immature CNS, the entire body responds to a pinprick of the foot; the mature infant withdraws only the foot. CNS immaturity is reflected in reflex development and sleep-wake cycles. Preterm infants have brief periods of alertness but have difficulty maintaining this state. Premature or sick infants show fatigue or stress sooner than full-term healthy infants do.

Time. The time elapsed since labor and birth affects the behavior of infants as they attempt to become organized initially. Time elapsed since the previous feeding and time of day may also influence infants' responses.

Stimuli. Environmental events and stimuli affect the behavioral responses of infants. The newborn responds to animate and inanimate stimuli. Nurses in intensive care nurseries observe that infants respond to loud noises, bright lights, monitor alarms, and tension in the unit. If a mother is tense and has a rapid heart rate while feeding her infant, the infant will have an increase in heart rate that is similar to the mother's.

Medication. Controversy surrounds the effects on infant behavior of maternal medication (e.g., analgesia, and anesthesia) during labor. Some researchers note that infants of mothers given medications may continue to demonstrate poor state organization after the fifth day; medication effects have been noted as long as 30 days after birth. Other researchers maintain that the effect can be beneficial or nonexistent.

Sensory Behaviors

From birth, infants possess sensory capabilities that indicate a state of readiness for social interaction. Infants effectively use behavioral responses in establishing their first dialogues. These responses, coupled with the newborn's "baby appearance" (e.g., facial proportions of forehead and eyes larger than the lower part of the face) and their small size and helplessness, rouse feelings of wanting to hold, protect, and interact with them.

Vision. At birth the eye is structurally incomplete and the muscles are immature. The pupils react to light, the blink reflex is easily stimulated, and the corneal reflex is activated by light touch. The clearest visual distance is 17 to 20 cm, which is about the distance the infant's face is from the mother's face as she breastfeeds or cuddles. Infants are sensitive to light; they will frown if a bright light is flashed in their eyes, and will turn toward a soft, red light. If the room is darkened, they will open their eyes wide and look about. By 2 months of age, they can detect color; but at 5 days of age and younger seem more attracted by black-and-white patterns (Kenner, Lott, and Flandermeyer, 1997).

Response to movement is noticeable. If a bright light is shown to newborns (even at 15 minutes of age), they will follow it visually; some will even turn their heads to do so. Because human eyes are bright, shiny objects, newborns will track their parents' eyes. Parents often comment on how exciting this behavior is. The development of eye-to-eye contact is very important for parent-infant attachment. Children of blind parents, and parents who have blind children, must circumvent this obstacle for the formation of a relationship.

Visual acuity is surprising; even at 2 weeks of age, infants can distinguish patterns with stripes 3 mm apart. By 6 months their vision is as acute as that of an adult. They prefer to look at patterns rather than plain surfaces, even if the latter are brightly colored. They prefer more complex patterns to simple ones. They prefer novelty (changes in pattern) by 2 months of age. The infant of a few weeks of age is therefore capable of responding actively to an enriched environment.

Hearing. As soon as the amniotic fluid drains from the ears, the infant's hearing is similar to that of an adult. Loud sounds of about 90 decibels cause the infant to react with a startle reflex. The newborn responds to low frequency sounds such as a heartbeat or lullaby by decreasing motor activity or stopping crying. High-frequency sound elicits an alerting response.

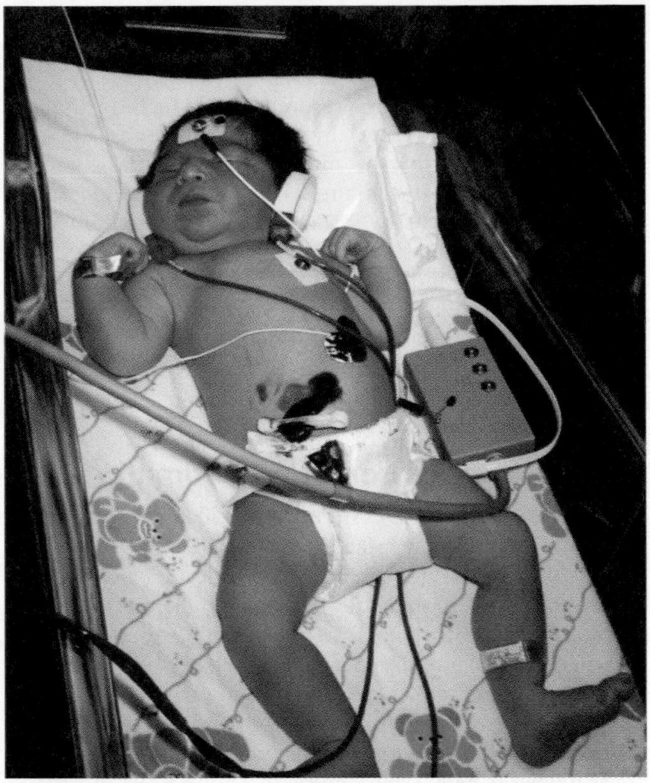

FIG. 24-17 • Hearing screening in the newborn nursery. (Courtesy Dee Lowdermilk, Chapel Hill, NC.)

The infant responds readily to the mother's voice. Studies indicate a selective listening to maternal voice sounds and rhythms during intrauterine life that prepares newborns for recognition and interaction with their primary caregivers—their mothers. Newborns are accustomed to hearing the regular rhythm of the mother's heartbeat. As a result, they respond by relaxing and ceasing to fuss and cry if a regular heartbeat simulator is placed in their cribs.

Hearing loss is a common major abnormality at birth; approximately 1 to 3 in 1000 normal term infants have bilateral hearing loss (American Academy of Pediatrics [AAP], 1999). To identify affected infants, the hearing of all infants is screened in the newborn nursery (Fig. 24-17).

Smell. Newborns react to strong odors such as alcohol or vinegar by turning their heads away. Breastfed infants are able to smell breast milk and can differentiate their mother from other lactating women by the smell (Lawrence, 1999).

Taste. The newborn can distinguish between tastes, and various types of solutions elicit differing facial expressions. A tasteless solution produces no response; a sweet solution elicits eager sucking. A sour solution causes puckering of the lips, and a bitter liquid produces a grimace. Newborns prefer glucose water to plain water (Lawrence, 1999).

Young infants are particularly oriented toward the use of their mouths, both for meeting their nutritional needs for rapid growth and for releasing tension through sucking. The early development of circumoral sensation, muscle activity, and taste would seem to be preparation for survival in the extrauterine environment.

Touch. The newborn is responsive to touch on all parts of the body. The face (especially the mouth), hands, and soles of the feet seem to be the most sensitive. Reflexes can be elicited by stroking the infant. The newborn's responses to touch suggest this sensory system is well prepared to receive and process tactile messages. Touch and motion are essential to normal growth and development. However, each infant is unique, and variations can be seen in newborns' responses to touch. Birth trauma or stress and depressant drugs taken by the mother decrease the infant's sensitivity to touch or painful stimuli.

Response to Environmental Stimuli

Temperament. Classic studies have identified individual variations in the primary reaction pattern of newborns and described them as temperament. Their style of behavioral response to stimuli is guided by the temperament affecting the newborn's sensory threshold, ability to habituate, and response to maternal behaviors. The newborn possesses individual characteristics that affect selective responses to various stimuli present in the internal and external environments.

The three major patterns of behavioral style or temperament are as follows (Chess, 1969; Chess and Thomas, 1977):

1. The *easy child,* who demonstrates regularity in bodily functions, readily adapts to change, has a predominantly positive mood and moderate sensory threshold, and approaches new situations or objects with a moderate response
2. The *slow-to-warm-up child,* who has a low activity level, withdraws on first exposure to new stimuli, is slow to adapt and low in intensity of response, and is somewhat negative in mood
3. The *difficult child,* who is irregular in bodily functions, intense in reactions, generally negative in mood, and resistant to change or new stimuli and often cries loudly for long periods

Habituation. Habituation is a protective mechanism that allows the infant to become accustomed to environmental stimuli. Habituation is a psychologic and physiologic phenomenon in which the response to a constant or repetitive stimulus is decreased. In the term newborn, this can be demonstrated in several ways. Shining a bright light into a newborn's eyes will cause a startle or squinting the first two or three times. The third or fourth flash will elicit a diminished response, and by the fifth or sixth flash, the infant ceases to respond (Brazelton and Nugent, 1996). The same response pattern holds true for the sounds of a rattle or for a pinprick to the heel.

The ability to habituate allows the newborn to select stimuli that promote continued learning about the social world, thus avoiding overload. The intrauterine environment seems to have programmed the newborn to be especially responsive to human voices, soft lights, soft sounds, and sweet tastes.

The newborn quickly learns the sounds in a newborn nursery and the home and is able to sleep in their midst. The selective responses of the newborn indicate cerebral organization capable of memory and making choices. The ability to habituate depends on the state of consciousness, hunger, fatigue, and temperament. These factors also affect consolability, cuddliness, irritability, and crying.

Consolability. Barr (1990) described variations in the ability of newborns to console themselves or to be consoled. In the crying state, most newborns initiate one of several ways to reduce their distress. Hand-to-mouth movements are common, with or without sucking, as well as alerting to voices, noises, or visual stimuli.

Cuddliness. Cuddliness is especially important to parents because they often gauge their ability to care for the child by the child's responses to their actions. The degree to which newborns mold into the contours of the person holding them varies. Barr (1990) tested the effect of body contact and vestibular stimulation in both soothing babies and creating alertness. The vestibular stimulation of being picked up and moved had the greater effect.

Irritability. Some newborns cry longer and harder than others. For some the sensory threshold seems low. They are readily upset by unusual noises, hunger, wetness, or new experiences, and thus respond intensely. Others with a high sensory threshold require a great deal more stimulation and variation to reach the active, alert state.

Crying. Crying in an infant may signal hunger, pain, desire for attention, or fussiness. Some mothers state that they learn to distinguish among the cries. The duration of crying is also highly variable in each infant; newborns may cry for as little as 5 minutes or as much as 2 hours or more per day. The amount of crying peaks in the second month and then decreases. There is a diurnal rhythm of crying, with more crying occurring in the evening hours. Crying does not seem to differ with different caretakers.

Key Points

- By term the infant's various anatomic and physiologic systems have reached a level of development and functioning that permits a physical existence apart from the mother.
- The term infant has sensory capabilities that indicate a state of readiness for social interaction.
- At any serum bilirubin level the appearance of jaundice during the first day of life or persistence of jaundice beyond 7 to 8 days may indicate a pathologic process.
- Loss of heat in a newborn, even a healthy newborn, may result in acidosis and raise the level of free fatty acids, leading to cold stress.
- Assessment of the newborn requires data from the prenatal, intrapartal, and postpartal periods.
- The newborn assessment should proceed systematically so that each system is thoroughly evaluated.
- Many reflex behaviors are important for the newborn's survival.
- Individual personalities and behavioral characteristics of infants play a major role in the ultimate relationship between infants and their parents.
- Each newborn has a predisposed capacity to handle the multitude of stimuli in the external world.

References

American Academy of Pediatrics (AAP) Task Force on Newborn and Infant Hearing: Newborn and infant hearing loss: detection and intervention, *Pediatrics* 103(2):527-530, 1999.

Barr R: The normal crying curve: What do we really know? *Dev Med Child Neurol* 32:356-362, 1990.

Brazelton T, Nugent J: *Neonatal behavioural assessment scale,* ed 3, London, 1996, MacKeith.

Chess S: Individuality and baby care, *Dev Med Neurol* 11: 749-754, 1969.

Chess S, Thomas A: Temperament and the parent-child interaction, *Pediatr Ann* 6(9):574-582, 1977.

Fanaroff A, Martin R: *Neonatal-perinatal medicine diseases of the fetus and infant,* ed 6, St Louis, 1997, Mosby.

Guyton A, Hall J: *Textbook of medical physiology,* ed 9, Philadelphia, 1995, WB Saunders.

Kenner C, Lott J, Flandermeyer A: *Comprehensive neonatal nursing,* ed 2, Philadelphia, 1997, WB Saunders.

Korones S: *High-risk newborn infants: the basis for intensive care,* ed 5, St Louis, 1995, Mosby.

Lawrence R: *Breastfeeding: a guide for the medical profession,* ed 5, St Louis, 1999, Mosby.

Merenstein G, Gardner S: *Handbook of neonatal intensive care,* ed 4, St Louis, 1998, Mosby.

Pagana K, Pagana T: *Mosby's diagnostic and laboratory test reference,* ed 5, St Louis, 2000, Mosby.

Wong D: *Whaley & Wong's nursing care of infants and children,* ed 6, St Louis, 1999, Mosby.

CHAPTER 25

Nursing Care of the Newborn

http://www.harcourthealth.com/MERLIN/Wong/maternal/

Learning Objectives

On completion of this chapter the reader will be able to:

- Identify the purpose and components of the Apgar score.
- Compare and contrast the characteristics of preterm, term, postterm, and postmature neonates.
- Estimate the gestational age of newborns.
- Explain what is meant by a safe environment.
- Discuss phototherapy and the guidelines for teaching parents about this treatment.
- Explain purposes and methods of circumcision, the postoperative care of the circumcised infant, and parent teaching information regarding circumcision.
- Review procedures for a heel stick, collecting urine specimens, assisting with venipuncture, and restraining the newborn.
- Evaluate pain in the newborn based on physiologic changes and behavioral observations.
- Review anticipatory guidance nurses provide parents before discharge.

Although most infants make the necessary biopsychosocial adjustment to extrauterine existence without undue difficulty, their well-being depends on the care they receive from others. This chapter describes the assessment and care of the infant from immediately after birth until discharge. A discussion of pain in the neonate and its management is included.

BIRTH THROUGH THE FIRST 2 HOURS

Care Management

Care begins immediately after the birth and focuses on assessing and stabilizing the condition of the newborn. The nurse has primary responsibility for the infant during this period, because the physician or midwife is involved with delivery of the placenta and care of the mother. The nurse must be alert for any signs of distress and initiate appropriate interventions.

Initial Assessment and Apgar Scoring. The first assessment of the newborn is done immediately after birth by using the Apgar score (Table 25-1) and a brief physical examination (Box 25-1). A gestational age assessment is done within 2 hours of birth (Fig. 25-1). A more comprehensive physical examination may be completed within 24 hours of birth (see Table 24-2).

Apgar Score. The Apgar score permits a rapid assessment of the need for resuscitation based on five signs that indicate the physiologic state of the newborn: (1) heart rate based on auscultation with a stethoscope; (2) respiratory rate based on observed movement of the chest wall; (3) muscle tone based on degree of flexion and movement of the extremities; (4) reflex irritability based on response to gentle slaps on the soles of the feet; and (5) color described as pallid, cyanotic, or pink (see Table 25-1). Evaluations are made at 1 and 5 minutes after birth and can be done by the nurse or birth attendant. Scores of 0 to 3 indicate severe distress, scores of 4 to 6 indicate moderate difficulty, and scores of 7 to 10 indicate that the infant should not have difficulty adjusting to extrauterine life. Apgar scores do not predict future neurologic outcome, but the 5-minute score does correlate with the degree of risk for neonatal morbidity and mortality.

Initial Physical Assessment. The initial physical assessment includes a brief review of systems (see Box 25-1).

a. **External**—Notes skin color, staining, peeling, or wasting (dysmaturity); notes length of nails and development of creases on soles of feet; checks for presence of breast tissue; assesses nasal patency by closing one nostril at a time while observing respirations and color; notes meconium staining of cord, skin, fingernails, or amniotic fluid (staining may indicate fetal hypoxia; offensive odor may indicate intrauterine infection)

TABLE 25-1
Apgar Score

	Score		
Sign	**0**	**1**	**2**
Heart rate	Absent	Slow (<100)	Over 100
Respiratory rate	Absent	Slow, weak cry	Good cry
Muscle tone	Flaccid	Some flexion of extremities	Well flexed
Reflex irritability	No response	Grimace	Cry
Color	Blue, pale	Body pink, extremities blue	Completely pink

Box 25-1
Initial Physical Assessment by Body System

CNS [ ] moves extremities, muscle tone good
[ ] symmetric features, movement
[ ] suck, rooting, Moro response, grasp reflexes good
[ ] anterior fontanel soft and flat
CV [ ] heart auscultation, strong and regular
[ ] no murmurs heard
[ ] pulses strong/equal bilaterally
RESP [ ] lungs auscultated, clear bilaterally
[ ] respiratory rate <60 breaths/min
[ ] chest expansion symmetric
[ ] no upper airway congestion
GU [ ] male: urethral opening at tip of penis; testes descended bilaterally
female: vaginal opening apparent
GI [ ] abdomen soft, no distention
[ ] cord attached and clamped
[ ] anus appears patent
ENT [ ] eyes clear
[ ] palates intact
[ ] nares patent
SKIN Color [ ] pink [ ] acrocyanotic
[ ] no lesions or abrasions
[ ] no peeling
[ ] birthmarks ______________
[ ] caput/molding
[ ] vacuum "cap"
[ ] forceps marks
[ ] other
Comments: ______________

Community Focus

SIGNIFICANCE OF THE APGAR SCORE

The Apgar score was developed to provide a systematic method of assessing an infant's condition at birth. Researchers have tried to correlate Apgar scores with various outcomes such as development, intelligence, and neurologic development. In some instances, researchers have attempted to attribute causality to the Apgar score; that is, to suggest that the low Apgar score caused or predicted later problems. This is an inappropriate use of the Apgar score. Instead the score should be used to ensure that infants are systematically observed at birth to ascertain the need for immediate care. Either a physician or a nurse may assign the score; however, to avoid the real or perceived appearance of bias, the person assisting with the birth should not assign the score. Lack of consistency in the assigned scores limits studies of the Apgar's long-term predictive value. Prospective parents and the public need education on the significance of the Apgar as well as its limits. Since infants rarely receive the maximum score of 10, parents need to know that scores of 7 to 10 are within normal limits. Attorneys involved in litigation related to injury of an infant at birth or negative outcomes, either short term or long term, also need education about the Apgar, its significance and limits. This useful tool needs to be used appropriately; health care providers, parents, and the public may need education to ensure appropriate use of the score.

Data from Montgomery K: Apgar scores: examining the long-term significance, *J Perinat Educ* 9(3):5-9, 2000.

b. **Chest**—Palpates for PMI and auscultates for rate and quality of heart tones and murmurs; notes character of respirations and presence of crackles; notes equality of breath sounds on each side of chest by holding stethoscope in each axilla
c. **Abdomen**—Verifies presence of a rounded abdomen and absence of anomalies; notes number of vessels in cord
d. **Neurologic**—Checks muscle tone and reflex reaction and assesses Moro reflex; palpates anterior fontanel for fullness or bulge; notes by palpation the presence and size of the fontanels and sutures
e. **Other observations**—Notes gross structural malformations obvious at birth

The nurse responsible for the care of the newborn immediately after birth verifies that respirations have been established, dries the infant, assesses temperature, and places identical identification bracelets on the infant and the mother. In some settings, the father or partner also wears an identification bracelet. The infant may be wrapped in a warm blanket and placed in the arms of the mother, given to the partner to hold, or kept undressed under a radiant warmer. In some settings, immediately after birth the infant is placed on the mother's abdomen to allow skin-to-skin contact. This contributes to maintenance of the infant's optimum temperature and parental bonding. The infant may be admitted to a nursery or remain with the parents throughout the hospital stay.

The initial examination of the newborn can occur while the nurse is drying and wrapping the infant, or observations can be made while the infant is lying on the mother's abdomen or in

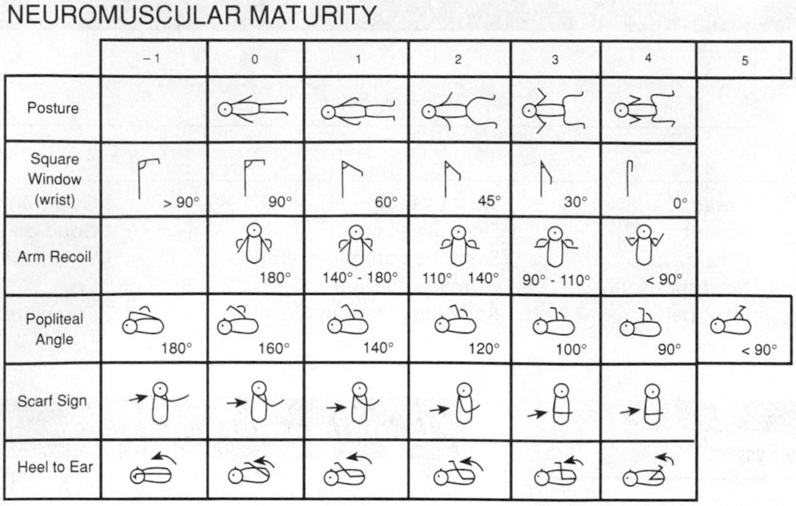
NEUROMUSCULAR MATURITY
-1
0
1
2
3
4
5
Posture
Square Window (wrist)
> 90°
90°
60°
45°
30°
0°
Arm Recoil
180°
140° - 180°
110° 140°
90° - 110°
< 90°
Popliteal Angle
180°
160°
140°
120°
100°
90°
< 90°
Scarf Sign
Heel to Ear

A PHYSICAL MATURITY

Skin	sticky friable transparent	gelatinous red, translucent	smooth pink, visible veins	superficial peeling or rash, few veins	cracking pale areas rare veins	parchment deep cracking no vessels	leathery cracked wrinkled
Lanugo	none	sparse	abundant	thinning	bald areas	mostly bald	
Plantar Surface	heel-toe 40-50 mm: -1 <40 mm: -2	>50 mm no crease	faint red marks	anterior transverse crease only	creases ant. 2/3	creases over entire sole	
Breast	imperceptible	barely perceptible	flat areola no bud	stippled areola 1-2 mm bud	raised areola 3-4 mm bud	full areola 5-10 mm bud	
Eye/Ear	lids fused loosely: -1 tightly: -2	lids open pinna flat stays folded	sl. curved pinna; soft; slow recoil	well-curved pinna; soft but ready recoil	formed & firm instant recoil	thick cartilage ear stiff	
Genitals (male)	scrotum flat, smooth	scrotum empty faint rugae	testes in upper canal rare rugae	testes descending few rugae	testes down good rugae	testes pendulous deep rugae	
Genitals (female)	clitoris prominent labia flat	prominent clitoris small labia minora	prominent clitoris enlarging minora	majora & minora equally prominent	majora large minora small	majora cover clitoris & minora	

MATURITY RATING

score	weeks
-10	20
-5	22
0	24
5	26
10	28
15	30
20	32
25	34
30	36
35	38
40	40
45	42
50	44

FIG. 25-1 • Estimation of gestational age. **A,** New Ballard Scale for newborn maturity rating. Expanded scale includes extremely premature infants and has been refined to improve accuracy in more mature infants. (From Ballard J et al: New Ballard Score, expanded to include extremely premature infants, *J Pediatr* 119(3):417, 1991.)

her arms immediately after birth. Efforts should be directed to minimizing interference in the initial parent-infant acquaintance process. If the infant is breathing easily, has good color, and is normal in appearance, then further examination can be delayed until after the parents have had an opportunity to interact with the infant. Routine procedures and the admission process can be carried out in the mother's room or in a separate nursery. Box 25-2 shows an example of newborn routine orders.

➤ Nursing Diagnoses

Nursing diagnoses are established after analysis of the findings of the physical assessment. Nursing diagnoses for the newborn include the following:

- Ineffective airway clearance related to:
  —Airway obstruction with mucus
- Impaired gas exchange related to:
  —Hypothermia
- Ineffective thermoregulation related to:
  —Heat loss to the environment
- Risk for infection related to:
  —Umbilical cord stump
  —Fetal scalp electrode sites

➤ Expected Outcomes

Expected outcomes can apply both to the infant and the parents. Expected outcomes for the newborn during the immediate recovery period include that the infant will achieve the following:

- Maintain effective breathing patterns
- Maintain effective thermoregulation

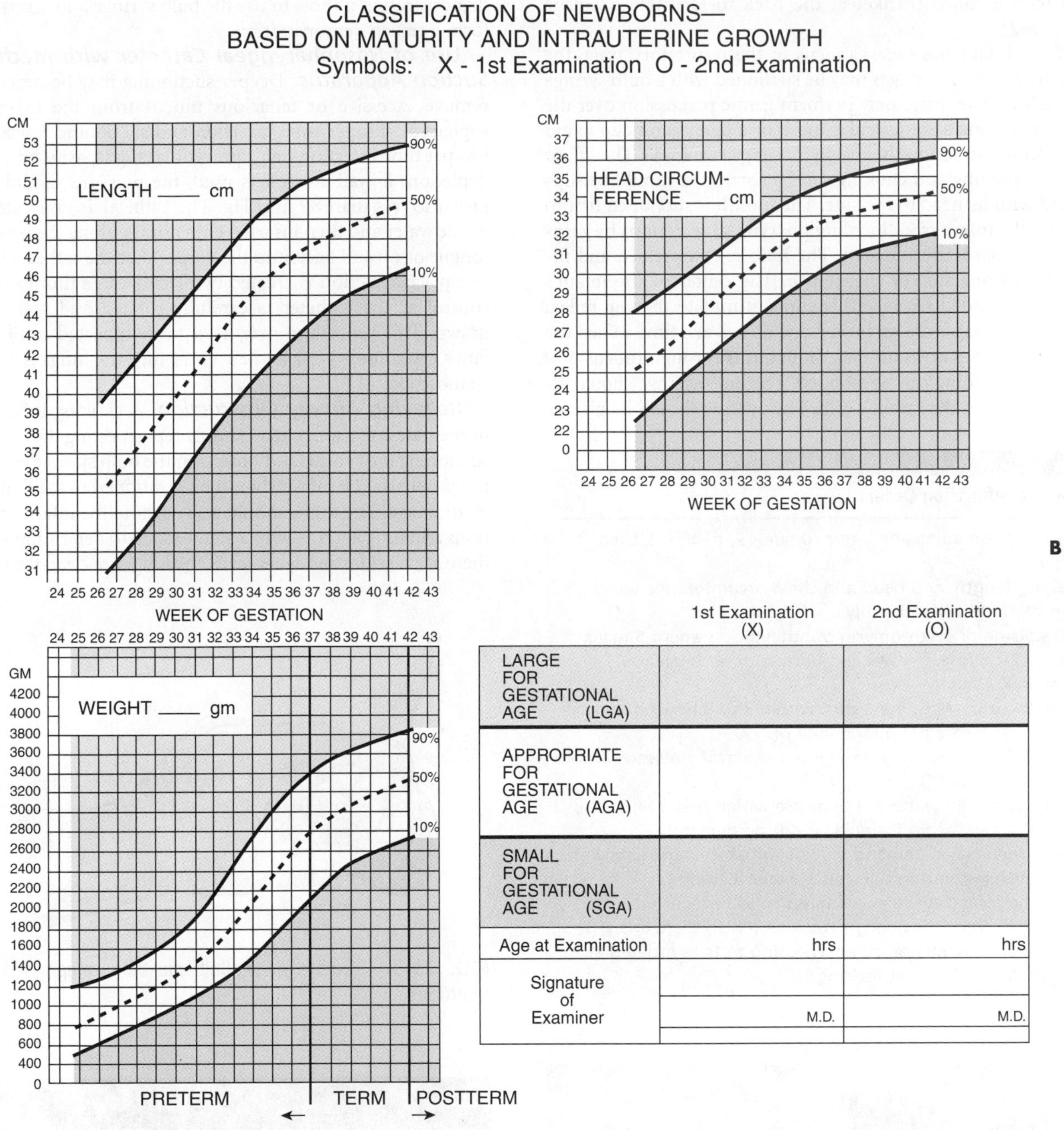

FIG. 25-1, cont'd • B, Newborn classification based on maturity and intrauterine growth. Modified from Lubchenco L, Hansman C, Boyd E: Intrauterine growth in length and head circumference as estimated from live births at gestational ages from 26 to 42 weeks, *J Pediatr* 37(3):403, 1996; and Battaglia F, Lubchenko L: A practical classification of newborn infants by weight and gestational age, *J Pediatr* 71(2):159, 1967.)

- Remain free from infection
- Receive necessary nutrition for growth

Expected outcomes for the parents include that they will do the following:

- Attain knowledge, skill, and confidence relevant to infant care activities
- State understanding of biologic and behavioral characteristics of the newborn
- Begin to integrate the infant into the family

➤ Plan of Care and Implementation

Changes can occur rapidly in newborns immediately after birth. Assessment must be followed quickly by implementation of appropriate care.

Stabilization and Resuscitation. Generally, the normal term infant born vaginally has little difficulty clearing the air passages. Most secretions are moved by gravity and brought by the cough reflex to the oropharynx to be drained or swallowed. The infant is maintained in a side-lying position with a rolled blanket at the back to facilitate drainage (Fig. 25-2).

If the infant has excess mucus in the respiratory tract, the mouth and nasal passages may be suctioned with a bulb syringe (Fig. 25-3). The nurse may perform gentle percussion over the chest wall using a soft circular mask or a percussion cup to aid in loosening secretions before suctioning (Fig. 25-4). The infant who is coughing and choking on the secretions should be supported with its head to the side. The mouth is suctioned first to prevent the infant from inhaling pharyngeal secretions by gasping as the nares are touched. The bulb is compressed and inserted into one side of the mouth. The center of the infant's mouth is avoided because this could stimulate the gag reflex. The nasal passages are suctioned one nostril at a time. When the infant's cry does not sound as though it is through mucus or a bubble, suctioning can be stopped. The bulb syringe should always be kept in the infant's crib. The parents should be given a demonstration of how to use the bulb syringe and asked to perform a return demonstration.

Use of Nasopharyngeal Catheter with Mechanical Suction Apparatus. Deeper suctioning may be necessary to remove excessive or tenacious mucus from the infant's nasopharynx. Proper tube insertion and suctioning 5 seconds or less per tube insertion helps prevent laryngospasms and oxygen depletion. If wall suction is used, the pressure should be adjusted to less than 80 mm Hg. The catheter is lubricated with sterile water and then inserted either orally along the base of the tongue or up and back into the nares. After the catheter is properly placed, suction is created by placing one's thumb over the control as the catheter is carefully rotated and gently withdrawn. This procedure may need to be repeated until the infant's cry sounds clear and air entry into the lungs is heard by stethoscope.

Relieving Airway Obstruction. A choking infant needs immediate attention. Often, simply repositioning the infant and suctioning the mouth and nose with the bulb syringe eliminates the problem. The infant should be positioned to facilitate gravity drainage. The nurse should also listen to the infant's respirations and lung sounds with a stethoscope to determine whether there are crackles and wheezes. If the lungs are clear, the bulb sy-

Box 25-2

Routine Admission Orders

- Vital signs on admission and q30min × 2, q1hr × 2, then q8hr
- Weight, length, and head and chest circumference on admission; then weigh daily
- Tetracycline or erythromycin ophthalmic ointment 5 mg/g 1- to 2-cm line in lower conjunctiva of each eye (ou)
- Vitamin K 1 mg IM
- Hematocrit by warm heel stick within 3 to 8 hours of age; call health care provider if <44 or >72
- Dextrostix prn; notify health care provider if <40 mg/dl; offer early D_5W PO
- Feedings: sterile water × 1 by nurse within first 4 hr of life; if tolerated, begin formula q3-4hr on demand
- (Breastfeeding on demand may be initiated immediately after birth without initial sterile water feeding.)
- Rooming-in as desired and infant's condition permits
- Newborn screen for phenylketonuria (PKU), thyroxine (T_4) and galactosemia or other screening tests as ordered at least 24 hr after first feeding

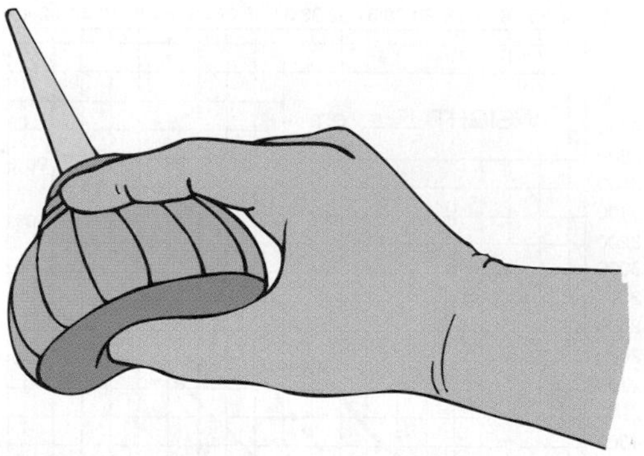

FIG. 25-3 • Bulb syringe. Bulb must be compressed before insertion.

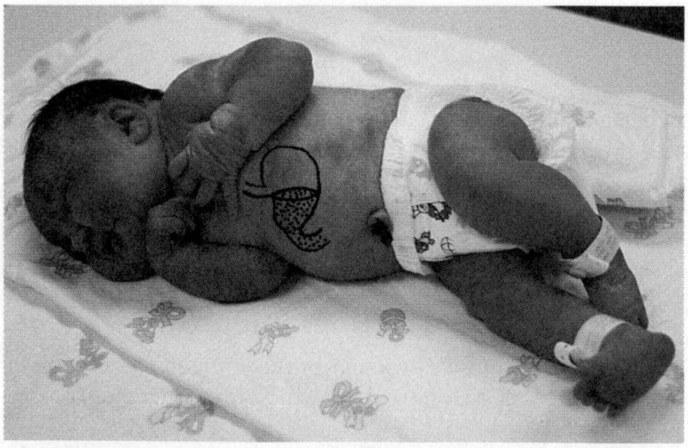

FIG. 25-2 • Side-lying position. Infant is turned to right side and supported in this position to facilitate drainage from mouth and to promote emptying of stomach contents into the small intestine. (From Wong D: *Whaley & Wong's nursing care of infants and children,* ed 6, St Louis, 1999, Mosby.)

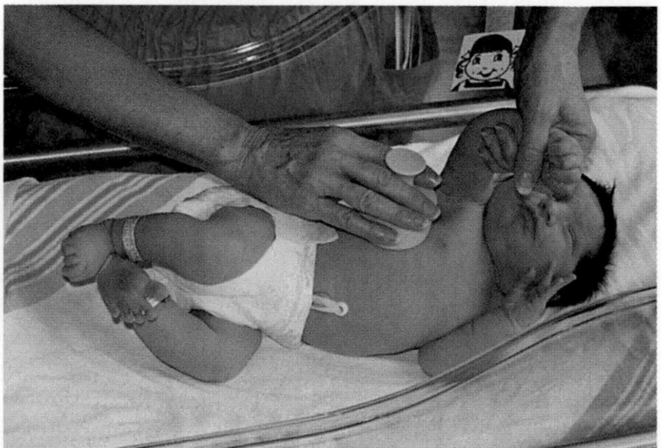

FIG. 25-4 • Chest percussion. Nurse performs gentle percussion over the chest wall using a percussion cup to aid in loosening secretions before suctioning.

ringe is used to clear the mouth and nose. If the bulb syringe does not provide relief, mechanical suction can be used.

If these measures do not relieve the obstruction, the nurse gives the infant back blows and chest thrusts (Fig. 25-5). All personnel working with infants must have current infant CPR certification. Many institutions offer infant CPR courses to new parents before discharge. Because cardiac and respiratory arrest can occur in infants, careful monitoring is necessary so that rapid treatment can be initiated.

Maintaining an Adequate Oxygen Supply. Four conditions are essential for maintaining an adequate oxygen supply:

- A clear airway
- Respiratory efforts
- A functioning cardiopulmonary system
- Heat support (exposure to cold stress increases oxygen needs)

Signs of potential complications related to abnormal newborn breathing are shown in Box 25-3.

Maintenance of Body Temperature. Effective neonatal care includes maintenance of an optimal thermal environment. Cold stress increases the need for oxygen and can upset the acid-base balance. The infant may react by increasing the respiratory rate and may become cyanotic. Ways to stabilize the newborn's body temperature include placing the infant directly on the mother's abdomen and covering with a warm

Box 25-3

Abnormal Newborn Breathing

- Bradypnea: respirations (≤25/min)
- Tachypnea: respirations (≥60/min)
- Abnormal breath sounds: crackles, rhonchi, wheezes, expiratory grunt
- Respiratory distress: nasal flaring, retractions, chin tug, labored breathing

Emergency

RELIEVING AIRWAY OBSTRUCTION

Back blow and chest thrusts are used to clear an airway obstructed by a foreign body.

Back Blows (Fig. 25-5, *A*)

Position the infant prone over forearm with the head down and the infant's jaw firmly supported.

Rest the supporting arm on the thigh.

Deliver four back blows forcefully between the infant's shoulder blades with the heel of the free hand.

Turn Infant

Place the free hand on the infant's back to sandwich the baby between both hands; one hand supports the neck, jaw, and chest while the other supports the back.

Turn the infant over and place the head lower than the chest, supporting the head and neck.

Alternative position: Place the infant face down on your lap with the head lower than the trunk; firmly support the head. Apply back blows and then turn the infant as a unit.

Chest Thrusts (Fig. 25-5, *B*)

Provide four downward chest thrusts on the lower third of the sternum.

Remove foreign body, if it is visible.

Open Airway

Open airway with the head tilt-chin lift maneuver and attempt to ventilate.

Repeat the sequence of back blows, turning, and chest thrusts.

Continue these emergency procedures until signs of recovery occur:

Palpable peripheral pulses return.

The pupils become normal in size and are responsive to light.

Mottling and cyanosis disappear.

Record the time and duration of the procedure and the effects of this intervention.

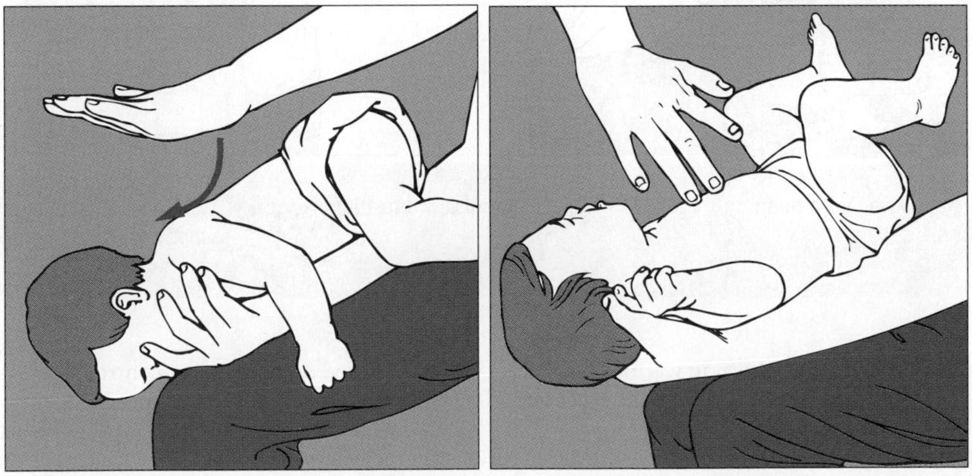

FIG. 25-5 • Back blows and chest thrust in infant to clear airway obstruction. **A,** Back blow. **B,** Chest thrust.

Emergency

CARDIOPULMONARY RESUSCITATION

Wash hands before and after touching infant and equipment. Wear gloves, if possible.

Assess Responsiveness

Observe color; tap or gently shake shoulders.
Yell for help; if alone, perform CPR for 1 min before calling for help again.

Position Infant

Turn the infant onto back, supporting the head and neck.
Place the infant on firm, flat surface.

Airway

Open the airway with the head tilt-chin lift method (Fig. 1).
Place one hand on the infant's forehead and tilt the head back.
Place the fingers of other hand under the bone of the lower jaw at the chin.

Breathing

Assess for evidence of breathing:
- Observe for chest movement.
- Listen for exhaled air.
- Feel for exhaled air flow.

To breathe for infant:
- Take a breath.
- Place mouth over the infant's nose and mouth to create a seal.

NOTE: When available, a mask with a one-way valve should be used.
Give two slow breaths (1 to 1.5 sec/breath), pausing to inhale between breaths.
NOTE: Gently puff the volume of air in your cheeks into infant. Do not force air.
The infant's chest should rise slightly with each puff; keep fingers on the chest wall to sense air entry.

Circulation

Assess circulation:
- Check pulse of the brachial artery (Fig. 2) while maintaining the head tilt.
- If the pulse is present, initiate rescue breathing. Continue doing once every 3 sec or 20 times/min until spontaneous breathing resumes.
- If the pulse is absent, initiate chest compressions and coordinate them with breathing.

Chest compression. There are two systems of chest compression. Nurses should know both methods.
Maintain the head tilt and:
1. Place thumbs side-by-side in the middle third of the sternum with fingers around the chest and supporting the back (Fig. 3).
   —Compress the sternum 1.25 to 2 cm. OR
2. Place index finger of hand just under an imaginary line drawn between the nipples. Place the middle and ring fingers on the sternum adjacent to the index finger.
   —Using the middle and ring fingers, compress the sternum approximately 1.25 to 2.5 cm.

Avoid compressing the xiphoid process.
Release the pressure without moving the thumbs/fingers from the chest.
Repeat at least 100 times/min, doing five compressions in 3 sec or less.
Perform 10 cycles of five compressions and one ventilation.
After the cycles, check the brachial artery to determine whether there is a pulse.
Discontinue compressions when the infant's spontaneous heart rate reaches or exceeds 80 beats/min.
Record the time and duration of the procedures and the effects of intervention.

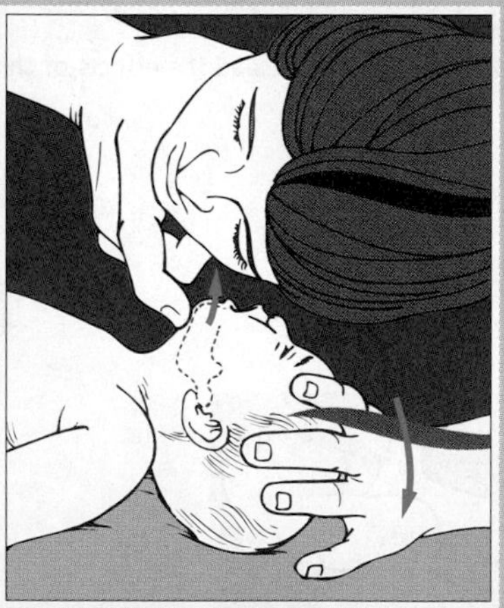

FIG. 1 • Opening airway with head tilt-chin lift method.

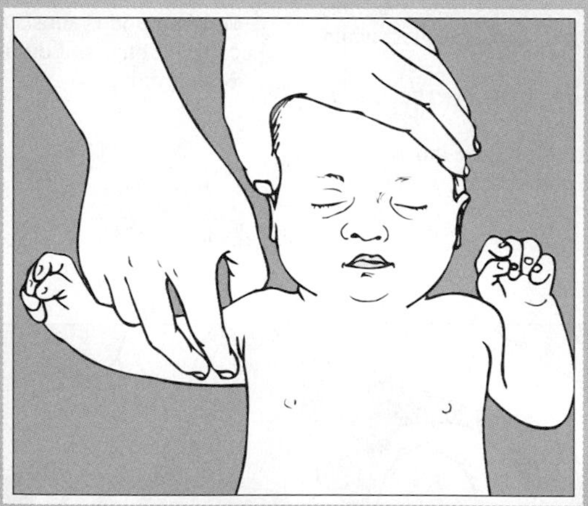

FIG. 2 • Checking pulse of brachial artery.

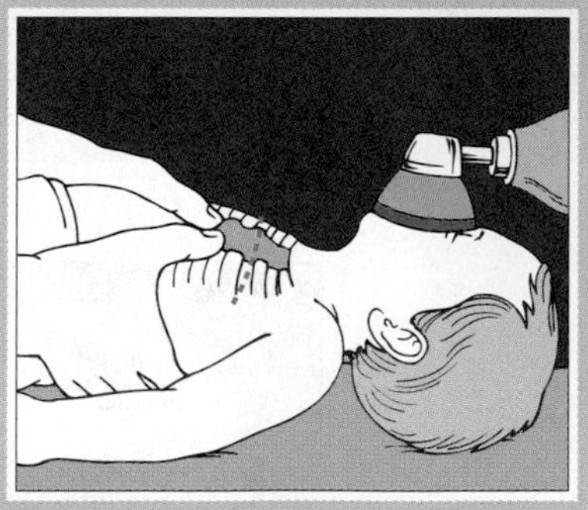

FIG. 3 • Side-by-side thumb placement for chest compressions in newborn.

blanket; drying and wrapping the newborn in warmed blankets immediately after birth; keeping the head well covered; and keeping the ambient temperature at 24° C.

If the infant does not remain with the mother during the first 1 to 2 hours after birth, the nurse places the thoroughly dried, unclothed baby under a radiant heat panel or warmer until the body temperature stabilizes. The infant's skin temperature is used as the point of control when using a warmer with a servocontrolled mechanism. The control panel usually is maintained between 36° and 37° C. This setting should maintain the healthy term infant's skin temperature around 36.5° C. A thermistor probe (automatic sensor) is taped to the right upper quadrant of the abdomen immediately below the right costal margin (never over a bone). This will ensure detection of

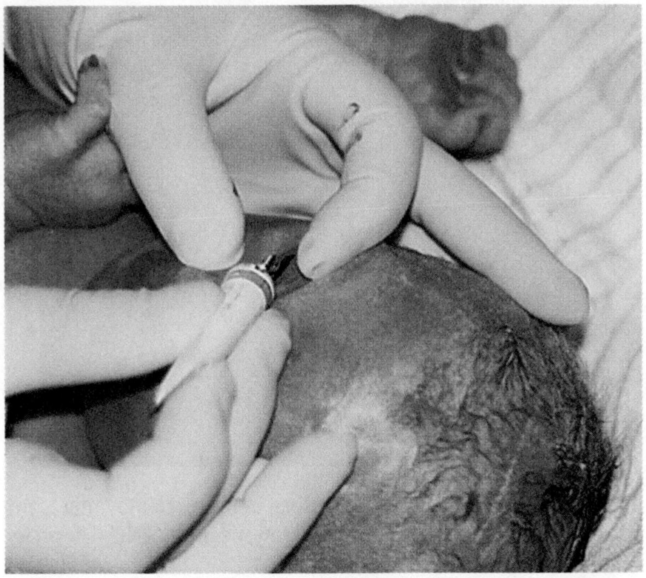

FIG. 25-6 • Instillation of medication into eye of newborn. Thumb and forefinger are used to open the eye; medication is placed in the lower conjunctiva from the inner to the outer canthus. (Courtesy Marjorie Pyle, RNC, Lifecircle, Costa Mesa, CA.)

Box 25-4

Medication Guide: Eye Prophylaxis With Erythromycin Ophthalmic Ointment 0.5% and Tetracycline Ophthalmic Ointment 1%

ACTION

These antibiotic ointments are both bacteriostatic and bactericidal. They provide prophylaxis against *Neisseria gonorrhoeae* and *Chlamydia trachomatis.*

INDICATION

These medications are for the prevention of ophthalmia neonatorum in newborns of mothers who are infected with gonorrhea; and conjunctivitis in newborns of mothers infected with chlamydia.

Neonatal Dosage

Apply a 1- to 2-cm ribbon of ointment to the lower conjunctival sac of each eye; may also be used in drop form.

ADVERSE REACTIONS

May cause chemical conjunctivitis that lasts 24 to 48 hours; vision may be blurred temporarily.

Nursing Considerations

Administer within 1 to 2 hours of birth. Wear gloves. Cleanse eyes if necessary before administration. Open eyes by putting a thumb and finger at the corner of each lid and gently pressing on the periorbital ridges. Squeeze the tube and spread the ointment from the inner canthus of the eye to the outer canthus. Do not touch the tube to the eye. After 1 minute, excess ointment may be wiped off. Observe eyes for irritation. Explain treatment to parents.

Eye prophylaxis for ophthalmia neonatorum is required by law in all states of the United States.

minor temperature changes resulting from peripheral vasoconstriction, vasodilation, or increased metabolism long before a change in core body temperature develops. The other end of the probe cord is attached to the control panel. The sensor needs to be checked periodically to make sure that it is securely attached to the infant's skin. The axillary temperature of the newborn is checked every hour until the newborn's temperature stabilizes. By the twelfth hour, the newborn's temperature should stabilize within the normal range.

During all procedures, heat loss must be avoided or minimized for the newborn; examinations and activities are performed with the newborn under a heat panel. The initial bath is postponed until the newborn's skin temperature reaches 36.5° C (Penny-MacGillivray, 1996).

Even a normal term infant in good health can become hypothermic. Birth in a car on the way to the hospital, a cold birthing room, or inadequate drying and wrapping immediately after birth may cause the infant's temperature to fall below normal range (hypothermia). Warming the hypothermic baby is accomplished with care. Rapid warming may cause apneic spells and acidosis in an infant. The warming process is therefore monitored to progress slowly over a period of 2 to 4 hours.

Immediate Interventions. It is the nurse's responsibility to perform certain interventions immediately after birth to provide for the safety of the newborn.

Eye Prophylaxis. The instillation of a prophylactic agent in the eyes of all neonates (Fig. 25-6) is mandatory in the United States as a precaution against ophthalmia neonatorum, which is an inflammation of the eyes from gonorrheal or chlamydial infection contracted by the newborn during passage through the mother's birth canal. In some Canadian institutions the parents may sign a form refusing eye prophylaxis. In the United States, if the family objects to this treatment, the primary care provider may ask that the parents sign an informed refusal form, and their refusal will be noted in the neonate's record. The agent used for prophylaxis varies according to hospital protocols, but usual agents include forms of erythromycin and tetracycline. Canadian hospitals have not recommended the use of silver nitrate since 1986. Its use in the United States is minimal because silver nitrate does not protect against chlamydial infection and can cause chemical conjunctivitis. In some institutions instillation of eye prophylaxis is delayed until an hour or so after birth so that eye contact and parent-infant attachment and bonding are facilitated. The Centers for Disease Control and Prevention specify that a delay of up to 2 hours is safe (Box 25-4).

Vitamin K Prophylaxis. Administering vitamin K intramuscularly is routine in the newborn period. A single injection of 0.5 to 1 mg of vitamin K is given soon after birth to prevent hemorrhagic disorders. Vitamin K is produced in the gastrointestinal tract by bacteria starting soon after microorganisms are introduced. By day 8, normal newborns are able to produce their own vitamin K (Box 25-5).

Umbilical Cord Care. The care of the umbilical cord is the same as that for any surgical wound (Krebs, 1998). The goal of care is prevention and early detection of hemorrhage or infection. The umbilical cord stump is an excellent medium for bacterial growth and can easily become infected.

Box 25-5

Medication Guide: Vitamin K: Phytonadione (AquaMEPHYTON, Konakion)

ACTION

This intervention provides vitamin K because the newborn does not have the intestinal flora to produce this vitamin in the first week after birth. It also promotes formation of clotting factors (II, VII, IX, and X) in the liver.

INDICATION

Vitamin K is used for prevention and treatment of hemorrhagic disease in the newborn.

NEONATAL DOSAGE

Administer a 0.5- to 1-mg (0.25- to 0.5-ml) dose intramuscularly within 2 hours of birth; may be repeated if newborn shows bleeding tendencies.

ADVERSE REACTIONS

Edema, erythema, and pain at injection size may occur rarely; hemolysis, jaundice, and hyperbilirubinemia have been reported, particularly in preterm infants.

NURSING CONSIDERATIONS

Wear gloves. Administer in the middle third of the vastus lateralis muscle using a 25-gauge, 5/8-inch needle. Inject into skin that has been cleaned, or allow alcohol to dry on puncture site for 1 minute to remove organisms and prevent infection. Stabilize leg firmly and grasp muscle between the thumb and fingers. Insert the needle at a 90-degree angle; aspirate and inject medication slowly if there is no blood return. After removing needle, massage the site with a dry gauze square to increase absorption. Observe for signs of bleeding from the site.

NURSE ALERT • If bleeding from the blood vessels of the cord is noted, the nurse checks the clamp (or tie) and applies a second clamp next to the first one. If bleeding is not stopped immediately, the nurse calls for assistance.

Hospital protocol directs the time and technique for routine cord care. The stump and base of the cord should be assessed for edema, redness, and purulent drainage with each diaper change. The nurse cleanses the cord and skin area around the base of the cord with the prescribed preparation (e.g., erythromycin solution, triple-blue dye, or alcohol). The cord clamp is removed after 24 hours when the cord is dry (Fig. 25-7).

Promote Parent-Infant Bonding. Today's childbirth practices strive to promote the family as the focus of care. Parents generally desire to share in the birth process and to have early contact with their infants. Early contact between mother and newborn can be important in developing future relationships. It also has a positive effect on the duration of breastfeeding. There are physiologic benefits of early mother-infant contact. Oxytocin and prolactin levels rise in the mother while sucking reflexes are activated in the infant. The process of developing active immunity begins as the infant ingests flora from the mother's skin.

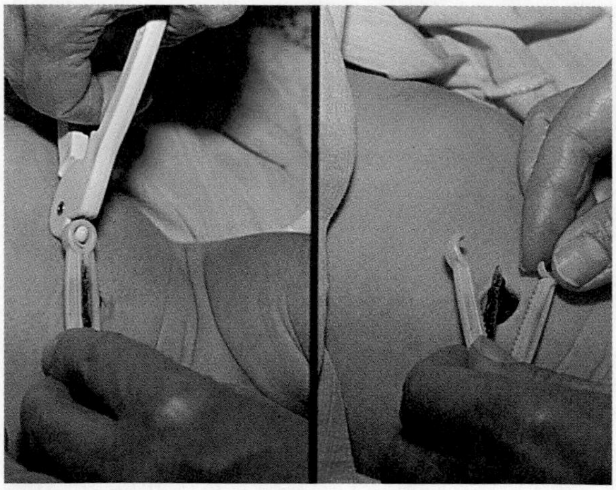

FIG. 25-7 • Using special scissors, remove clamp after cord dries (about 24 hours). (Courtesy Marjorie Pyle, RNC, Lifecircle, Costa Mesa, CA.)

➤ Evaluation

Evaluation of the effectiveness of care of the newborn is based on the previously stated outcomes.

FROM 2 HOURS AFTER BIRTH UNTIL DISCHARGE

Care Management

The infant's admission to the nursery may be delayed or it may never actually occur. Depending upon the routine of the hospital, the infant often remains in the labor area and is transferred to the nursery/postpartum unit with the mother. Many hospitals have adopted variations of single-room maternity care (SRMC). One nurse provides care for both the mother and the newborn. SRMC allows the infant to remain with the parents after the birth. Many of the procedures, such as assessment of weight and measurement, instillation of eye medications, intramuscular administration of vitamin K, and physical assessment, may be carried out in the labor and birth unit. Nurses who work in an SRMC unit; labor, delivery, recovery room (LDR); or labor, delivery, recovery, postpartum room (LDRP) need to be educated in intrapartal, neonatal, and postpartum nursing care and be competent in providing it. If the infant is transferred to the nursery, the infant's identification is verified by the nurse receiving the infant, who places the baby in a warm environment and begins the admission process.

Regardless of the physical organization for care, many hospitals have a small holding nursery, which is available for procedures or on request by the mother who wishes her infant to be placed there. This arrangement promotes parent-infant bonding while still allowing the new parents some time to be alone.

➤ Assessment

Assessment of Gestational Age. The assessment of physical and neurologic findings to determine gestational age should optimally be done between 2 and 12 hours after birth. If the tests are done earlier, while the infant is recovering from the stress of birth, muscle movements may reflect fatigue; for example, the arm recoil is slower. After 48 hours, there are some significant changes. The plantar creases on the soles of the feet appear to be more numerous and visible as the skin loses fluid and dries.

Assessment of gestational age is important because perinatal morbidity and mortality are related to gestational age and birth weight. The simplified *Assessment of Gestational Age* (Ballard, Novak, and Driver, 1979) is commonly used to assess gestational age of infants between 35 and 42 weeks. It assesses six external physical and six neuromuscular signs. Each sign has a number score, and the cumulative score correlates with a maturity rating of 26 to 42 weeks. The score is accurate to plus or minus 2 weeks and is accurate for infants of all races.

The *New Ballard Scale,* a revision of the original scale, can be used with newborns as young as 20 weeks of gestation. The tool has the same physical and neuromuscular sections but includes −1 to −2 scores that reflect signs of extremely premature infants, such as fused eyelids; imperceptible breast tissue; sticky, friable, transparent skin; no lanugo; and square window (flexion of wrist) angle greater than 90 degrees (see Fig. 25-1, *A*). The scale overestimates gestational age by 2 to 4 days in infants younger than 37 weeks of gestation, especially at gestational ages of 32 to 37 weeks (Ballard et al, 1991).

Classification of Newborns by Gestational Age and Birth Weight. There is a normal range of birth weights for each gestational week (see Fig. 25-1, *B*), but the birth weights of preterm, term, postdate, or postmature newborns may also be outside these normal ranges. Birth weights are classified in the following ways:

- **Large-for-gestational-age (LGA)**—Weight is above the 90th percentile (or two or more standard deviations above the norm) at any week
- **Appropriate-for-gestational-age (AGA)**—Weight falls between the 10th and the 90th percentile for the infant's age
- **Small-for-gestational-age (SGA)**—Weight is below the 10th percentile (or two or more standard deviations below the norm) at any week
- **Low birth weight (LBW)**—Weight of 2500 g or less at birth. These newborns have had either less than the expected rate of intrauterine growth or a shortened gestation period. Preterm birth and LBW commonly occur together (e.g., less than 32 weeks of gestation and birth weight of less than 2500 g).
- **Very low birth weight (VLBW)**—Weight of 1500 g or less at birth
- **Intrauterine growth restriction (IUGR)**—Term applied to the fetus whose rate of growth does not meet expected norms

Newborns are classified according to their gestational ages in the following ways:

- **Preterm or premature**—Born before completion of 37 weeks of gestation, regardless of birth weight
- **Term**—Born between the beginning of week 38 and the end of week 42 of gestation
- **Postterm (postdate)**—Born after completion of week 42 of gestation
- **Postmature**—Born after completion of week 42 of gestation and showing the effects of progressive placental insufficiency

Maternal Effects on Gestational Age Assessment. Some maternal conditions can affect the results of the gestational assessment. For example, any infant who has experienced oxygen deprivation during labor will have poor muscle tone. Infants in respiratory distress tend to be flaccid and assume a "frog-leg" posture. Even though an infant may appear large, such as the infant of a diabetic mother, it may respond in the same way as a premature infant. The infant of a mother who has been on magnesium sulfate will tend to be somewhat lethargic.

ASSESSMENT OF COMMON PROBLEMS IN THE NEWBORN

Physical Examination

A complete physical examination is done within 24 hours, after the infant's temperature has stabilized. See Chapter 24 for a detailed description of this examination.

Physical Injuries

Birth trauma includes any physical injury sustained by a newborn during labor and birth. Many injuries are minor and readily resolve in the neonatal period without treatment. Other types of trauma require some form of intervention. A few are serious enough to be fatal. Several factors predispose an infant to birth trauma (Fanaroff and Martin, 1997). Maternal factors include uterine dysfunction that leads to prolonged or precipitous labor, preterm or postterm labor, and cephalopelvic disproportion. Injury may result from dystocia caused by fetal macrosomia, multifetal gestation, abnormal or difficult presentation, and congenital anomalies. Intrapartum events that can result in scalp injury include the use of intrapartum monitoring of the fetal heart rate and fetal scalp sampling. Obstetric birth techniques can also cause injury. These include forceps birth, vacuum extraction, external version and extraction, and cesarean birth.

Soft-Tissue Injuries. Caput succedaneum and cephalhematoma are described in Chapter 24 (see Fig. 24-4).

Subconjunctival and retinal hemorrhages result from rupture of capillaries caused by increased pressure during birth. The hemorrhages clear within 5 days after birth and usually present no further problems. Parents need explanation and reassurance that these injuries are harmless.

Erythema, ecchymoses, petechiae, abrasions, lacerations, or edema of buttocks and extremities may be present. Localized discoloration may appear over presenting parts and may result from application of forceps or the vacuum extractor. Ecchymoses and edema may appear anywhere on the body. Petechiae, or pinpoint hemorrhagic areas, acquired during birth may extend over the upper trunk and face. These lesions are benign if they disappear within 2 or 3 days of birth and no new lesions appear. Ecchymoses and petechiae may be signs of a more serious disorder, such as thrombocytopenic purpura. To differentiate hemorrhagic areas from skin rashes and discolorations, try to blanch the skin with two fingers. Petechiae and ecchymoses do not blanch because extravasated blood remains within the tissues, whereas skin rashes and discolorations do blanch.

Trauma secondary to dystocia occurs to the presenting fetal part. Forceps injury and bruising from the vacuum cup occur at the site of application of the instruments. In a forceps injury there is commonly a linear mark across both sides of the face that is in the shape of the blades of the forceps. The affected areas are kept clean to minimize risk of infection. With the increased use of the vacuum extractor and use of padded forceps blades, the incidence of these lesions may be significantly reduced (Fanaroff and Martin, 1997).

Accidental lacerations may be inflicted with a scalpel during cesarean birth. These cuts may occur on any part of the body but are most often found on the scalp, buttocks, and thighs. Usually they are superficial and only need to be kept clean. Butterfly adhesive strips will hold together the edges of more serious lacerations. Rarely are sutures needed.

Skeletal Injuries. Fracture of the clavicle, or collarbone, is the most common fracture during birth; the break usually occurs in the middle third of the bone. It is often associated with difficult vertex or breech birth of infants of greater than average size. Limitation of the motion of the arm, crepitus of the bone, and an absent Moro's reflex on the affected side are diagnostic findings. Except for the use of gentle rather than rigorous handling of the infant, there is no accepted treatment for a fractured clavicle. The infant may be positioned in bed with the fractured side up. The figure-eight bandage, which is appropriate for the older child with a fractured clavicle, is not used for the newborn. The prognosis is good.

Fracture of the humerus and femur may occur during a difficult birth, but such fractures in newborns generally heal rapidly. Immobilization is accomplished with slings, splints, swaddling, and other devices.

The infant's immature, flexible skull can withstand a great deal of molding before fracture results. Unless a blood vessel is involved, linear fractures heal without special treatment. These fractures account for 70% of all fractures in this age group. Depressed skull fractures may occur without laceration of either the skin or the dural membrane (Fig. 25-8). These fractures may occur during difficult births from pressure of the head on the bony pelvis or from injudicious application of forceps. Spontaneous or nonsurgical elevation of the indentation using a hand breast pump or vacuum extractor has been reported (Fanaroff and Martin, 1997).

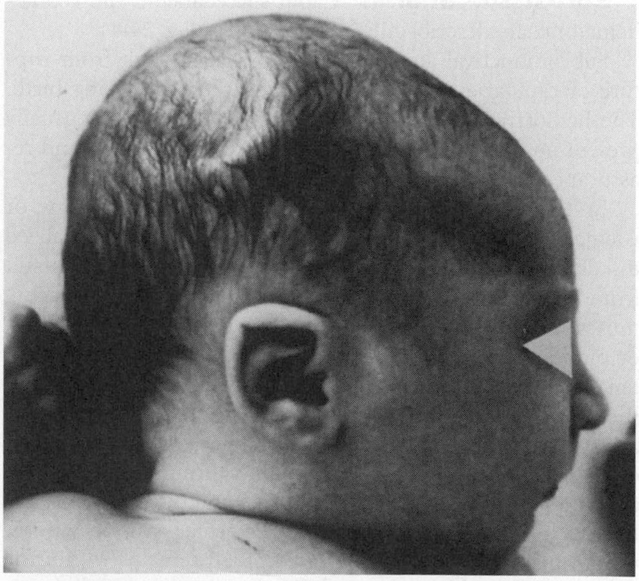

FIG. 25-8 • Depressed skull fracture in a full-term male after rapid (1-hour) labor. The infant was delivered by occiput-anterior presentation after rotation from occiput-posterior position. (From Fanaroff A, Martin R: *Neonatal-perinatal medicine: diseases of the fetus and infant,* ed 6, St Louis, 1997, Mosby.)

Congenital dislocation of the hip, or congenital hip dysplasia, is often a hereditary disorder and occurs more commonly in girls because of the structure of the female pelvis. In this condition, the acetabulum is abnormally shallow; this allows the head of the femur to become dislocated upward and backward so that it lies on the dorsal aspect of the ilium. The pressure of the displaced femoral head may then form a false acetabulum on the ilium. A stretched joint capsule results, and ossification of the femoral head is delayed.

Reduced movement, splinting of the affected hip, limited abduction, and asymmetry of the hip may be noted before dislocation occurs. After dislocation, all of these signs are present, together with external rotation and shortening of the leg. A clicking sound may be heard on gentle forced abduction of the leg (Ortolani's sign; see Fig. 24-11), and a bulge of the femoral head is felt or seen.

Treatment involves pressing the femoral head into the acetabulum to form an adequate socket before ossification is complete. Thick diapers may be applied to abduct and externally rotate the leg and flex the hip; the anterior flaps of the diapers are pinned under the posterior flaps. Alternatively, a Frejka pillow may be applied over a diaper and plastic pants. A Pavlik harness is also used commonly in treatment of congenital hip dislocation (Fig. 54-14). Later a spica cast may be applied to maintain abduction, extension, and internal rotation, usually with the infant in a "frog-leg" position.

Parents need support in handling an infant with skeletal injuries because they are often fearful of hurting their newborn. Parents are encouraged to practice handling, changing, and feeding the injured newborn under the guidance of the nursing staff. This increases the parents' knowledge and confidence, in addition to facilitating attachment. A plan for follow-up therapy is developed with the parents so that the times and arrangements for therapy are convenient for them.

Physiologic Problems

Physiologic Jaundice. Approximately 50% to 80% of all full-term newborns are visibly jaundiced (yellowish) during the first 3 days of life. Serum bilirubin levels less than 5 mg/dl usually are not reflected in visible skin jaundice. Physiologic jaundice is characterized by a progressive increase in serum levels of unconjugated bilirubin from 2 mg/dl in cord blood to a mean peak of 6 mg/dl by 72 hours of age, followed by a decline to 5 mg/dl by day 5, and not exceeding 12 mg/dl. These serum values are considered to be the normal physiologic limits for the healthy term newborn who has not been exposed to perinatal complications such as hypoxia. No bilirubin toxicity develops under these conditions. For the normal term newborn, a serum bilirubin level of 12 to 15 mg/dl is usually the cut-off point for the use of phototherapy, and 20 mg/dl is the cut-off point for exchange transfusion.

Every newborn is assessed for jaundice. The blanch test helps differentiate cutaneous jaundice from skin color. To do the test, pressure is applied with a finger over a bony area (e.g., nose, forehead, and sternum) for several seconds to empty all the capillaries in that spot. If jaundice is present, the blanched area will look yellow before the capillaries refill. The conjunctiva and buccal mucosa are also assessed, especially in darker-skinned infants. It is better to assess for jaundice in natural light because artificial lighting and the reflection from nursery walls can distort the actual skin color.

Jaundice is noticeable first in the head and then progresses gradually toward the abdomen and extremities because of the newborn infant's circulatory pattern (i.e., cephalocaudal developmental progression).

Hypoglycemia. Hypoglycemia during the early newborn period of a term infant is defined as a blood glucose concentration of less than 35 mg/dl or a plasma concentration of less than 40 mg/dl. It occurs because the newborn abruptly loses its glucose supply when the cord is cut. Because hypoglycemia may be asymptomatic, a blood glucose test is often done soon after birth and repeated at 4 hours of age. More frequent testing is required if the newborn is in an at-risk group (i.e., LGA, SGA, or LBW) or has been exposed to stressors such as cold, perinatal asphyxia, or tocolysis to inhibit preterm labor.

Signs of hypoglycemia include jitteriness; irregular respiratory effort; cyanosis; apnea; weak, high-pitched cry; feeding difficulty; lethargy; twitching; eye rolling; and seizures. The signs may be transient but recurrent.

Hypoglycemia in the low risk term infant is usually eliminated by feeding the infant. Occasionally the intravenous administration of glucose is required.

Hypocalcemia. Hypocalcemia (blood calcium levels less than 7 mg/dl) may occur in newborns of diabetic mothers, in those who experienced perinatal asphyxia or trauma, and in LBW and preterm infants. Early-onset hypocalcemia occurs within the first 72 hours after birth. Signs of hypocalcemia include jitteriness, edema, apnea, intermittent cyanosis, and abdominal distention.

In most instances, early-onset hypocalcemia is self-limiting and resolves within 1 to 3 days. Treatment includes early feeding and, occasionally, administration of calcium supplements.

Jitteriness is a symptom of both hypoglycemia and hypocalcemia. Therefore, hypocalcemia must be considered if therapy for hypoglycemia is ineffective. In many newborns, jitteriness remains despite therapy and cannot be explained by either hypoglycemia or hypocalcemia (Fanaroff and Martin, 1997).

LABORATORY AND DIAGNOSTIC TESTS

Blood glucose levels are measured and urinalysis is performed commonly in newborns. Other tests may be performed as needed, including measurement of bilirubin levels, newborn screening tests (e.g., phenylketonuria [PKU], thyroid [T_4], and galactosemia), hematocrits, and drug tests. Box 25-6 lists standard laboratory values in a term newborn.

Some states require newborns to be tested for up to nine disorders. Information about which tests are required in a state can be obtained from state health departments. About 30 states require testing for sickle cell anemia, and some states now require testing for cystic fibrosis (March of Dimes, 1994) and HIV (Frank, Esch, and Margeson, 1998). Some of the major disorders for which infants are screened are described in Table 25-2.

Collection of Specimens

Ongoing evaluation of a newborn often requires obtaining blood by heel stick or venipuncture or the collection of a urine specimens.

Heel Stick. Most blood specimens are drawn by laboratory technicians. However, nurses may be required to perform heel sticks to obtain blood for glucose monitoring and to measure hematocrit levels. The same technique is needed to complete the PKU form or to test for galactosemia and hypothyroidism or other inborn errors of metabolism (see Table 25-2).

It may be helpful to warm the heel before the sample is taken; application of heat for 5 to 10 minutes helps dilate the blood vessels in the area. A cloth soaked with warm water and wrapped loosely around the foot provides effective warming (Fig. 25-9, *A*). Disposable heel warmers are available from a variety of companies; they should be used with care to prevent burns. Nurses should wear gloves when collecting any specimen. The nurse cleanses the area with alcohol, restrains the infant's foot with a free hand, and then punctures the site. A spring-loaded automatic puncture device causes less pain and requires fewer punctures than a manual lance blade.

The most serious complication of infant heel stick is necrotizing osteochondritis from lancet penetration of the bone (Meehan, 1998). To prevent this, the penetration should be made at the outer aspect of the heel and should be no deeper than 2.4 mm (Wong, 1999). To identify the appropriate puncture site, the nurse should draw an imaginary line running from between the fourth and fifth toes and parallel to the lateral aspect of the foot to the heel where the stick should be made; a second line can also be drawn from the great toe to the medial aspect of the heel (Fig. 25-9, *B*). Repeated trauma to the walking surface of the heel can cause fibrosis and scarring that may lead to problems with walking later in life.

After the specimen has been collected, pressure is applied with a dry gauze square. No further alcohol should be applied because this will cause the site to continue to bleed. The site is then covered with an adhesive bandage. The nurse ensures proper disposal of equipment used, reviews the laboratory slip for correct identification, and checks the specimen for adequate labeling and routing.

A heel stick is traumatic for the infant and causes pain. After several heel sticks, infants have been observed to withdraw their feet when they are touched. To reassure the infant and to promote feelings of safety, the neonate should be cuddled and comforted when the procedure is complete.

Venipuncture. Venous blood samples can be drawn from the antecubital, saphenous, superficial wrist, and, rarely, scalp veins. If an intravenous (IV) site is used to obtain a blood spec-

Box 25-6
Standard Laboratory Values in a Term Newborn

Hemoglobin	14-24 g/dl
Hematocrit	44%-64%
Glucose	40-60 mg/dl
Bilirubin, direct	0-1 mg/dl
Blood gases	
Arterial	pH 7.32-7.49
	Pco_2 26-41 mm Hg
	Po_2 60-70 mm Hg
Venous	pH 7.31-7.41
	Pco_2 40-50 mm Hg
	Po_2 40-50 mm Hg

TABLE 25-2
Newborn Screening Summary

Disorder/Evidence	Symptoms	Screening Incidence	Treatment
PKU (classic) Elevated phenylalanine	Severe mental retardation, eczema, seizures, behavior disorders, decreased pigmentation, distinctive "mousey" odor	1:10,000 to 1:15,000 More common in Caucasians	Lifelong dietary management with low-phenylalanine diet; possible tyrosine supplementation
Congenital hypothyroidism (primary) Low T_4, elevated TSH	Mental and motor retardation, short stature, coarse, dry skin and hair, hoarse cry, constipation	Overall 1:4000 with ethnic variation 1:12,000 African-American 1:1000 Native American	Maintain-l-thyroxine levels in upper half of normal range; periodic bone age to monitor growth
Galactosemia (transferase deficiency) Elevated galactose; low or absent fluorescence	Neonatal death from severe dehydration, sepsis, or liver pathology; mental retardation, jaundice, blindness, cataracts	1:10,000 to 1:90,000	Eliminate galactose and lactose from the diet; soy formulas in infancy; lactose-free solid foods
Maple syrup urine disease (MSUD) Elevated leucine	Acidosis; hypertonicity and seizures, vomiting, drowsiness, apnea, coma; infant death or severe mental retardation and neurologic impairment; behavioral disorders	1:90,000 to 1:200,000	Diet low in leucine, isoleucine, and valine; thiamine supplement if responsive
Homocystinuria Elevated methionine	Mental retardation, seizures, behavioral disorders, early-onset thromboses, dislocated lenses, tall lanky body habitus	1:200,000	Methionine-restricted diet; cystine supplement; vitamin B_6 supplement if responsive
Congenital adrenal hyperplasia (CAH) Elevated 17-hydroxyprogesterone; abnormal electrolytes	Hyponatremia, hypokalemia, hypoglycemia, dehydration, and early death; ambiguous genitalia in females; progressive virilization in both sexes	1:15,000 to 1:3000 Native Eskimos	Replace corticosteroids; plastic surgery to correct ambiguous genitalia
Biotinidase deficiency Deficient or absent activity of biotinidase on colorimetric assay	Mental retardation, seizures, ataxia, skin rash, hearing loss, alopecia, optic nerve atrophy, coma, and death	1:60,000 to 1:100,000	10 mg biotin daily

Data from Wright L, Brown A, and Davidson-Mundt A: Newborn screening: the miracle and the challenge, *J Pediatr Nurs* 7(1):26-42, 1992.

A

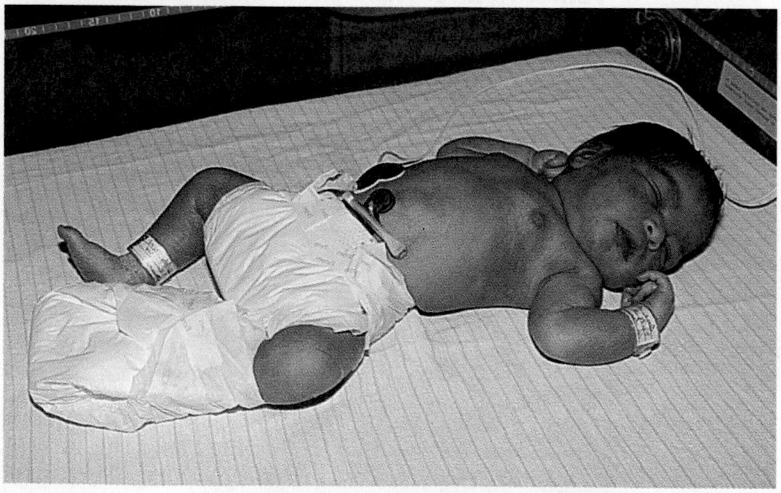

B

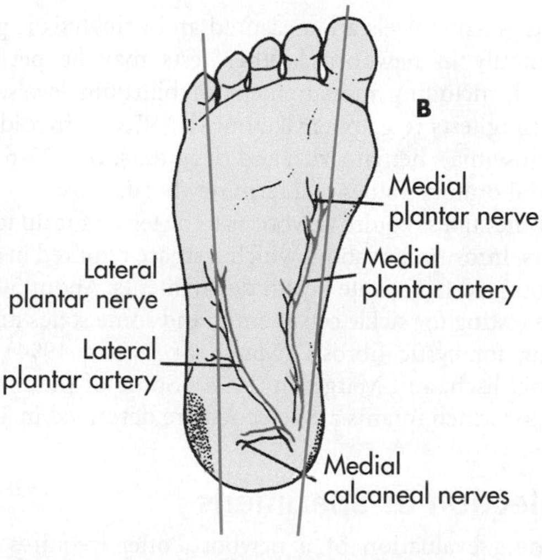

FIG. 25-9 • Heel stick. **A,** Newborn with foot wrapped for warmth to increase blood flow to extremity before heel stick. **B,** Heel stick sites (shaded areas) on infant's foot for obtaining samples of capillary blood. (A, Courtesy Marjorie Pyle, RNC, Lifecircle, Costa Mesa, CA.)

imen, it is important to consider the type of infusion fluid; contamination of the blood with the fluid can alter results.

When venipuncture is required, positioning of the needle is extremely important. Although regular venipuncture needles may be used, some individuals prefer butterfly needles. It is necessary to be very patient during the procedure because the blood return from small veins is slow, and consequently the small needle must remain in place longer. The mummy restraint commonly is used to help secure the infant (see Fig. 45-8).

If venipuncture or arterial puncture is being performed for blood gas studies, crying, fear, and agitation will affect the values. Therefore every effort must be made to keep the infant quiet during the procedure. For blood gas studies the blood sample tubes are packed in ice (to reduce blood cell metabolism) and are taken immediately to the laboratory for analysis.

Pressure must be maintained over an arterial or femoral puncture with a dry gauze square for at least 3 to 5 minutes to prevent bleeding from the site. The nurse should observe the infant frequently for evidence of bleeding or hematoma at the puncture site for at least an hour after any venipuncture. The infant's tolerance of the procedure should be noted and recorded. The infant should be cuddled and comforted (e.g., rocked, given a pacifier) when the procedure is completed.

Obtaining a Urine Specimen. Examination of urine is a valuable laboratory tool for infant assessment; the way in which the specimen is collected may influence the results. The urine sample should be fresh and examined within 1 hour of collection.

A variety of urine collection bags are available, including the Hollister U-Bag (Fig. 25-10). These are clear plastic, single-use bags with adhesive material around the opening at the point of attachment.

To prepare the infant, the nurse removes the diaper and places the infant in a supine position. The genitalia, perineum, and surrounding skin are washed and thoroughly dried because the adhesive of the bag will not stick to moist, powdered, or oily skin surfaces. The protective paper is removed to expose the adhesive (Fig. 25-10, *A*). In female infants, the perineum is stretched to flatten skin folds, then the adhesive area is pressed firmly to the skin all around the urinary meatus and vagina. (NOTE: Start with the narrow portion of the butterfly-shaped adhesive patch.) The nurse must be sure to start at the bridge of skin separating the rectum from the vagina and work upward (Fig. 25-10, *B*). In male infants the penis and scrotum are tucked through the opening of the collector before the nurse removes the protective paper from the adhesive; then the protective paper is removed, and the flaps pressed firmly to the perineum, making sure the entire adhesive coating is firmly attached to skin and the edges of the opening do not pucker (Fig. 25-10, *C*). This helps ensure a leak-proof seal and decreases the chance of contamination from stool. Cutting a slit in the diaper and pulling the bag through the slit may also help prevent leaking.

The diaper is carefully replaced and the bag is checked frequently. When a sufficient amount of urine (this amount varies according to the test done) has been obtained, the bag is removed. The infant's skin is observed for signs of irritation while the bag is in place. The specimen can be aspirated with a syringe or drained directly from the bag. For draining, the bag is held in one hand and tilted to keep urine away from the tab. The tab is then removed and the urine is drained into a clean receptacle (Fig. 25-10, *D*).

Collection of a 24-hour specimen can be a challenge; the infant may need to be restrained. The 24-hour urine bag is applied in the manner just described, and the urine is drained into a receptacle. The collection tube can be shortened or capped (Fig. 25-10, *E*). The infant's skin is watched closely for signs of irritation and for lack of a proper seal.

For some types of urine testing, urine can be aspirated directly from the diaper by means of a syringe without a needle. If the diaper has absorbent gelling material that traps urine, a small gauze pad or cotton balls are placed inside the diaper and the urine is aspirated from them (Wong, 1999).

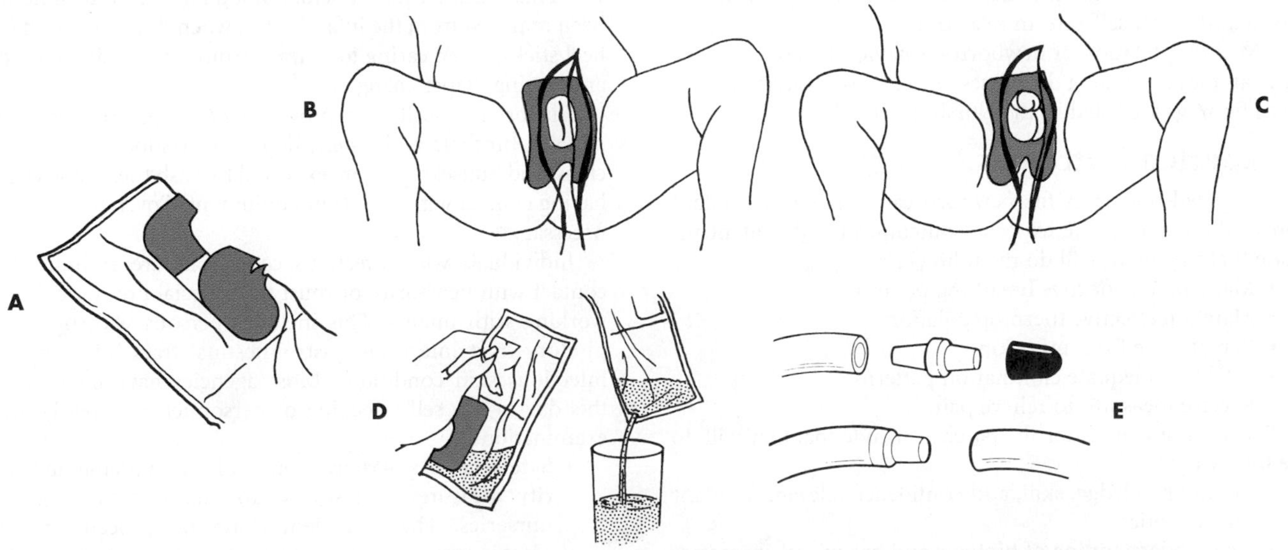

FIG. 25-10 • Collection of urine specimen. **A,** Protective paper is removed from the adhesive surface. **B,** Applied to females. **C,** Applied to males. **D,** Cut to drain urine. **E,** Collection tube. (Permission to use and/or reproduce this copyrighted material has been granted by the owner, Hollister, Inc., Libertyville, IL.)

Restraining the Infant. The infant may need to be restrained to (1) protect the infant from injury; (2) facilitate examinations; and (3) limit discomfort during tests, procedures, and specimen collections. The following special considerations must be kept in mind when restraining an infant:

- Apply restraints and check them to make sure they are not irritating the skin or impairing circulation.
- Maintain proper body alignment.
- Apply restraints without using knots or pins if possible. If knots are used, make the kind that can be released quickly. Use pins with care so that there is no danger of their puncturing or pressing against the infant's skin.
- Check the infant hourly or more often if indicated.

The mummy restraint may be used during examinations, treatments, or specimen collections that involve the head and neck (see Fig. 45-8).

Although the blanket support is not a true restraint, it controls the infant's position and movement. The blanket may be rolled or folded and placed at the infant's sides.

Restraint without Appliance. The infant may be restrained with the nurse's own hands and body. Fig. 45-13 illustrates restraint of the infant in position for lumbar puncture.

➤ Nursing Diagnoses

Possible nursing diagnoses for the newborn include the following:

- Ineffective breathing pattern related to:
  —Obstructed airway
- Impaired gas exchange related to:
  —Hypothermia (cold stress)
- Risk for ineffective thermoregulation related to:
  —Heat loss to environment
- Pain related to:
  —Circumcision
  —Heel sticks, venipuncture
  —Possible nursing diagnoses for the parent(s) are as follows:
- Family coping, potential for growth related to:
  —Knowledge of newborn's social capabilities
  —Knowledge of newborn's dependency needs
  —Knowledge of biologic characteristics of the newborn
- Situational low self-esteem related to:
  —Misinterpretation of newborn's behavioral cues

Examples of nursing diagnoses derived from specific assessment findings are listed in the Nursing Care Plan.

➤ Expected Outcomes

The expected outcomes for newborn care relate to the infant and to the parents. The expected outcomes for the infant include that the infant will do the following:

- Maintain an effective breathing pattern
- Maintain effective thermoregulation
- Remain free from infection
- Establish adequate elimination patterns
- Receive measures to relieve pain

Expected outcomes for the parents include that they will do the following:

- Attain knowledge, skill, and confidence relevant to infant care activities
- State understanding of biologic and behavioral characteristics of the newborn
- Have opportunities to intensify their relationship with the newborn
- Begin to integrate the infant into the family

➤ Plan of Care and Implementation

In the inpatient setting, priorities of care must be established and a systematic teaching plan for infant care devised. One way to achieve this is to use critical path case management. A care path may be developed that covers the changes expected in the infant during the first several days of life. Table 25-3 is an example of a care path for neonatal adaptation to extrauterine life. When variations from the care path occur, further assessment and intervention may be necessary.

Protective Environment. The provision of a protective environment is basic to the care of the newborn. The construction, maintenance, and operation of nurseries in accredited hospitals is monitored by national professional organizations, such as the American Academy of Pediatrics, and local or state governing bodies. In addition, hospital personnel develop their own policies and procedures for protecting the newborns under their care. Prescribed standards cover areas such as the following:

- **Environmental factors**—Provision of adequate lighting, elimination of potential fire hazards, safety of electric appliances, adequate ventilation, and controlled temperature (i.e., warm and free of drafts) and humidity (i.e., lower than 50%)
- **Measures to control infection**—Adequate floor space to permit positioning bassinets at least 60 cm apart, handwashing facilities, and areas for cleaning and storing equipment and supplies

Only those personnel directly involved in the care of mothers and infants are allowed in this area, thereby reducing the opportunities for the introduction of pathogenic organisms.

NURSE ALERT • Personnel are instructed to use good handwashing techniques. The most important single measure in the prevention of neonatal infection is hand washing between handling different infants.

Health care workers must wear gloves during the following: when handling the infant before blood and amniotic fluid have been removed from the infant's skin; when drawing blood (e.g., heel stick); when caring for a fresh wound (e.g., circumcision); and during diaper changes.

Visitors and health care providers such as nurses, physicians, parents, brothers and sisters, department supervisors, electricians, and housekeepers are expected to wash their hands before having contact with infants or equipment. Cover gowns are not necessary.

Individuals with infectious conditions are excluded from contact with newborns, or must take special precautions when working with infants. This includes persons with upper respiratory tract infections, gastrointestinal tract infections, and infectious skin conditions. Most agencies have now coupled this day-to-day self-screening of personnel with yearly health examinations.

- **Safety factors**—Many agencies have implemented security measures in response to infant abductions from nurseries. These incidents have been occurring with greater frequency. Examples of measures taken include placing matching identification bracelets on infants and their parents; and footprinting or taking identification pictures after birth, before the infant leaves the mother's side.

Nursing Care Plan THE NORMAL NEWBORN

NURSING DIAGNOSIS Risk for ineffective airway clearance related to excess mucus production/improper positioning

EXPECTED OUTCOME Neonate's airway remains patent; breath sounds are clear and no respiratory distress is evident.

Nursing Interventions/*Rationales*

Suction mouth and nasopharynx with bulb syringe as needed; clean nares of crusted secretions *to clear airway and prevent aspiration and airway obstruction.*

Position neonate on right side after feeding *to prevent aspiration* and on back or side when sleeping *to prevent suffocation.*

Teach parents that gagging, coughing, and sneezing are normal neonatal responses *that assist the neonate in clearing airways.*

Teach parents how to hold, suction, feed, and position the neonate with return demonstration *to ensure parental skill at airway clearance and maintenance.*

NURSING DIAGNOSIS Risk for altered body temperature related to larger body surface in relationship to mass

EXPECTED OUTCOME Neonate temperature remains in range of 36.5° C to 37.2° C.

Nursing Interventions/*Rationales*

Maintain neutral thermal environment *to identify any changes in neonate's temperature that may be related to other causes.*

Monitor neonate's temperature often *to identify any changes promptly and ensure early interventions.*

Bathe neonate efficiently when temperature is stable, using warm water, drying carefully, and avoiding exposing neonate to drafts *to avoid losses from evaporation and convection.*

Report any alterations in temperature findings promptly *to assess and treat for possible infection.*

NURSING DIAGNOSIS Risk for infection related to immature immunologic defenses/environmental exposure

EXPECTED OUTCOME The neonate will be free from signs of infection.

Nursing Interventions/*Rationales*

Review maternal record for evidence of any risk factors *to ascertain whether the neonate may be predisposed to infection.*

Monitor vital signs *to identify early possible evidence of infection, especially temperature instability.*

Have all care providers, including parents, practice good handwashing techniques before handling newborn *to prevent spread of infection.*

Monitor and instruct parents to monitor visitors and personnel for evidence of infection and limit contact as needed *to prevent spread of infection.*

Keep genital area clean and dry using proper cleansing techniques *to prevent skin irritation, cross-contamination, and infection.*

Keep umbilical stump clean and dry and keep exposed to air *to allow to dry and minimize chance of infection.*

If circumcised, keep site clean and dressed with prescribed ointment and diaper applied loosely *to prevent trauma and infection and to promote healing.*

Teach parents to keep neonate away from crowds and environmental irritants *to reduce potential sources of infection.*

NURSING DIAGNOSIS Risk for injury related to sole dependence on caregiver

EXPECTED OUTCOME Neonate remains free of injury.

Nursing Interventions/*Rationales*

Monitor environment for hazards such as sharp objects, long fingernails of caretaker and neonate, and jewelry of caretaker that may be sharp *to prevent injury.*

Handle neonate gently and support head, transport only in crib, ensure use of car seat by parents, teach parents never to place neonate on high surface unsupervised, and to supervise pet and sibling interactions *to prevent injury.*

Assess neonate often for any evidence of jaundice *to identify rising bilirubin levels, treat promptly, and prevent kernicterus.*

NURSING DIAGNOSIS Coping, family; potential for growth related to anticipatory guidance regarding responses to neonate's crying

EXPECTED OUTCOME Parents will verbalize understanding of methods of coping with neonate's crying and describe increased success in interpreting neonate's cries.

Nursing Interventions/*Rationales*

Alert parents to crying as neonate's form of communication and that cries can be differentiated to indicate hunger, wetness, pain, and loneliness *to provide reassurance that crying is not indicative of neonate's rejection of parents and that parents will learn to interpret different cries.*

Differentiate self-consoling behaviors from fussing/crying *to give parents concrete examples of interventions.*

Discuss methods of consoling a neonate such as changing diapers; showing parent's face to neonate; talking softly to neonate; swaddling; rocking; using a pacifier, feeding, or burping; or going for a car ride *to provide anticipatory guidance.*

TABLE 25-3
Care Path: Neonatal Adaptation to Extrauterine Life

	Day 1	Day 2	Day 3	Day 4	Day 7	Day 14
WEIGHT		Loss of 5%-10% of birth weight	Gain of 150-300 g per day			Birth weight regained
TEMPERATURE	Stabilized at 37° C					
FEEDINGS						
Volume						
Formula	15-60 ml	60-90 ml	60-90 ml	60-90 ml	60-90 ml	60-90 ml
Breast		Softening of at least one breast at each feeding				
Frequency						
Formula	6-10 times/24 hr		6-10 times/24 hr		6-10 times/24 hr	
Breast	8-12 times/24 hr		8-12 times/24 hr		8-12 times/24 hr	
VOIDING	At least 1 time in first 24 hr	2-6 times/24 hr	6-10 times/24 hr			6-10 times/24 hr
STOOLS		Meconium; at least 1 time in first 48 hr	Transitional stool: 1-5/day	Yellow stool: 1-5/day		Yellow stool: 1-2/day
SLEEP	16-20 hr/24 hr					16-20 hr/24 hr
UMBILICAL CORD	Moist; clamped	Dry; clamp removed				Cord off
CIRCUMCISION	Red; sore	Yellow exudate covers glans	Healing	Healing		Healed
COLOR	Pink; acrocyanotic	Pink; slight jaundice	Peak of jaundice		Pink	
BILIRUBIN LEVEL	0-6 mg/dl	≤8 mg/dl	≤12 mg/dl		≤2 mg/dl	
LABORATORY TESTS	Glucose when required; HCT	PKU, T_4 galactose				Repeat PKU, if needed
MEDICATIONS	Eye prophylaxis and vitamin K within 2 hr of birth; HBV within 12 hr of birth					

HBV, Hepatitis B vaccine; *HCT,* hematocrit, *PKU,* phenylketonuria.

Personnel wear picture identification badges or other badges that identify them as newborn personnel. Mother-baby units may have infant tracking systems that will set off an alarm if a baby is left alone or with unauthorized personnel. Mothers are instructed to be certain they know the identity of anyone who cares for the infant and never to release the infant to anyone who is not wearing appropriate identification.

SUPPORTING PARENTS IN THE CARE OF THEIR INFANT

The sensitivity of the caregiver to the social responses of the infant is basic to the development of a mutually satisfying parent-child relationship (Leitch, 1999). Sensitivity increases over time as parents become more aware of their infant's social capabilities (Cultural Considerations box).

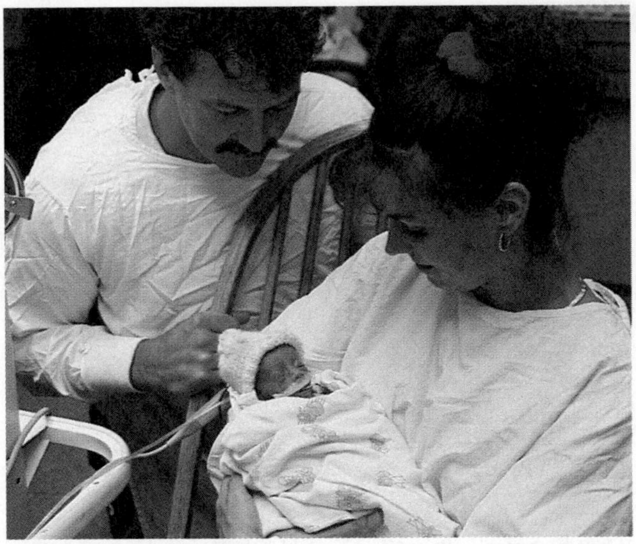

FIG. 25-11 • Mother-father-baby interaction. (From Wong D: *Whaley & Wong's nursing care of infants and children,* ed 6, St Louis, 1999, Mosby.)

Cultural Considerations

CULTURAL BELIEFS AND PRACTICES

Nurses working with childbearing families from other cultures and ethnic groups must be aware of cultural beliefs and practices that are important to individual families. People with a strong sense of heritage may hold on to traditional health beliefs long after adopting other American lifestyle practices. These health beliefs may involve practices regarding the newborn. For example, some Asians, Hispanics, eastern Europeans, and Native Americans delay breastfeeding because they believe that colostrum is "bad." Some Hispanics and African-Americans place a belly band over the infant's navel. The birth of a male child is generally preferred by Asians and Indians, and some Asians and Haitians delay naming their infant.

Source Geissler, E: *Pocket guide to cultural assessment,* St Louis, 1994, Mosby.

Social Interactions

The activities of daily care during the neonatal period present the best times for infant and family interactions. While caring for their baby, the mother and father can talk to the infant, play baby games, caress and cuddle the child, and perhaps use infant massage. In Fig. 25-11, a mother, father, and infant are shown engaging in arousal, imitation of facial expression, and smiling. Too much stimulation should be avoided after feeding and before a sleep period. Older children's contact with a newborn needs to be supervised in terms of strength of hugs, the exploring of eyes and nose, and attempts to feed the baby. Parents often keep baby books that record their infant's progress.

Infant Feeding

The infant may be put to breast shortly after birth, or at least within 4 hours of birth. If the infant is to be bottle-fed, a nurse may offer a few sips of sterile water to be certain that the infant's sucking and swallowing reflexes are intact and that there are no anomalies such as a tracheoesophageal fistula. Most infants are on demand feeding schedules and are allowed to feed when they awaken. Ordinarily mothers are encouraged to feed their infants every 3 to 4 hours during the day and only when the infant awakens during the night in the first few days after birth. Breastfed babies nurse more often than bottle-fed babies because breast milk is digested faster than formulas made from cow's milk and the stomach empties sooner as a result. Water supplements are usually not recommended. For a thorough discussion of infant feeding, see Chapter 26.

Family Focus

FAMILY RELATIONSHIPS AND SOCIAL SUPPORT

The family's ethnic and cultural background is important in determining the health status, genetic or familial risk factors present, and social support available to the woman throughout pregnancy and in the postpartum period. Family relationships, including husband-wife roles, vary among individuals and groups. The husband may be the decision-maker, and his consent may be necessary before the woman agrees to prenatal treatment. Female rather than male family members may be involved in the pregnancy and birth. Mothers and mothers-in-law may be present and supportive during pregnancy, birth, and the early postnatal period to provide advice and care. In such instances, they need to be included in teaching sessions. Community and church support may be available. Assessment of family and community resources is an essential component of care.

THERAPEUTIC AND SURGICAL PROCEDURES

Intramuscular Injection

As discussed previously, it is routine to administer a single dose of 0.5 to 1 mg of vitamin K intramuscularly (see Box 25-5).

Hepatitis B (Hep B) vaccination is recommended for all infants. Infants at highest risk of contracting hepatitis B are those born to women who come from Asia, Africa, South America, the South Pacific, and southern and eastern Europe. If the infant is born to an infected mother or to a mother who is a chronic carrier, hepatitis vaccine and hepatitis B immune globulin (HBIG) should be given within 12 hours of birth (Boxes 25-7 and 25-8). The hepatitis vaccine is given in one site and the HBIG in another. For infants born to healthy women, the first dose of the vaccine may be given at birth or at 1 or 2 months of age. Parental consent should be obtained before administering these medications.

In most cases a 25-gauge, ⅝-inch needle should be used for the vitamin K and hepatitis vaccine injections. A 22-gauge needle may be necessary if thicker medications such as some penicillins are to be given.

Selection of the site for injection is important. Injections must be given in muscles large enough to accommodate the medication, and major nerves and blood vessels must be avoided. The muscles of newborns may not tolerate more than 0.5 ml per IM injection. The injection site for newborns is the vastus lateralis (Fig. 25-12). The dorsogluteal muscle is very small, poorly developed, and dangerously close to the sciatic nerve, which occupies a larger proportion of space in infants

Box 25-7

Medication Guide: Hepatitis B Vaccine (Recombivax HB, Engerix-B)

Hepatitis B vaccine (HBV) induces protective anti–hepatitis B antibodies in 95% to 99% of healthy infants who receive the recommended three doses. The duration of protection of the vaccine is unknown.

INDICATION
HBV is for immunization against infection caused by all known subtypes of hepatitis B virus.

NEONATAL DOSAGE
The usual dosage is Recombivax HB 5 μg/0.5 ml or Engerix-B 10 μg/0.5 ml at 0, 1, and 6 months. An alternate dosing schedule is 0, 1, 2, and 12 months and is usually for newborns whose mothers were HBsAg positive.

ADVERSE REACTIONS
Common adverse reactions are rash, fever, erythema, swelling, and pain at injection site.

NURSING CONSIDERATIONS
Parental consent must be obtained before administration. Wear gloves. Administer in the middle third of the vastus lateralis muscle using a 25-gauge, ⅝-inch needle. Inject into skin that has been cleaned, or allow alcohol to dry on puncture site for 1 minute to remove organisms and prevent infection. Stabilize leg firmly and grasp muscle between the thumb and fingers. Insert the needle at a 90-degree angle; aspirate and inject medication slowly if there is no blood return. After removing needle, massage the site with a dry gauze square to increase absorption. If the infant was born to HBsAg-positive mother, hepatitis B immune globulin (HBIG) should be given within 12 hours of birth in addition to the HB vaccine. Separate sites must be used.

Box 25-8

Medication Guide: Hepatitis B Immune Globulin (HBIG)

ACTION
HBIG provides a high titer of antibody to hepatitis B surface antigen (HBsAg).

INDICATION
The HBIG vaccine provides prophylaxis against infection in infants born of HBsAg-positive mothers.

NEONATAL DOSAGE
Administer one 0.5 ml dose intramuscularly within 12 hours of birth.

ADVERSE REACTIONS
Hypersensitivity may occur.

NURSING CONSIDERATIONS
Must be given within 12 hours of birth. Wear gloves. Administer in the middle third of the vastus lateralis muscle using a 25-gauge, ⅝-inch needle. Inject into skin that has been cleaned, or allow alcohol to dry on puncture site for 1 minute to remove organisms and prevent infection. Stabilize leg firmly and grasp muscle between the thumb and fingers. Insert the needle at a 90-degree angle; aspirate and inject medication slowly if there is no blood return. After removing needle, massage the site with a dry gauze square to increase absorption. May be given at same time as hepatitis B vaccine, but at a different site.

than in older children. Therefore it is not recommended as an injection site until the child has been walking for at least 1 year.

Newborn infants offer little, if any, resistance to injections. Although they squirm and may be difficult to hold in position if they are awake, they can usually be restrained without the need for assistance from a second person if the nurse is experienced.

The neonate's leg should be stabilized. Gloves are worn for the injection. The nurse cleanses the injection site with alcohol and then pinches up the infant's muscle with the thumb and forefinger. The needle is inserted into the vastus lateralis at a 90-degree angle. The muscle is released and the plunger of the syringe is gently withdrawn. If no blood is aspirated, the medication is injected. If blood is aspirated, the needle is withdrawn and the injection is given in another site. The needle is withdrawn quickly and the site massaged with a gauze square to hasten absorption unless contraindicated. It is not uncommon for blood to ooze from the injection site, but it is not necessary to cover the site with an adhesive bandage. Pressure should be applied until oozing stops.

The nurse should always remember to comfort the infant after an injection and to properly discard equipment. It is important to record medication, date and time, amount, route, and site of injection.

Therapy for Hyperbilirubinemia

The best therapy for hyperbilirubinemia is prevention. Because bilirubin is excreted in meconium, prevention can be facilitated by early feeding, which stimulates passage of meconium. However, despite early passage of meconium, the term infant may have trouble conjugating the increased amount of bilirubin derived from disintegrating fetal red blood cells. As a result, the serum levels of unconjugated bilirubin may rise beyond normal limits, causing hyperbilirubinemia (see Chapter 24). The goal of treatment of hyperbilirubinemia is to help reduce the newborn's serum levels of unconjugated bilirubin. There are two principal ways of doing this: phototherapy and exchange blood transfusion. Exchange transfusion is used to treat those infants whose raised levels of bilirubin cannot be controlled by phototherapy.

Phototherapy. During phototherapy the infant is placed, unclothed, approximately 45 to 50 cm under a bank of lights. The distance may vary based on unit protocol and type of light used. The infant is turned every 2 hours to expose all body surfaces to the light. This is done for several hours or days until the infant's serum bilirubin level decreases to within acceptable range. The decision to discontinue therapy is based on a definite downward trend in the bilirubin values. After therapy has been terminated, the infant may have a rebound of bilirubin level, which is usually harmless.

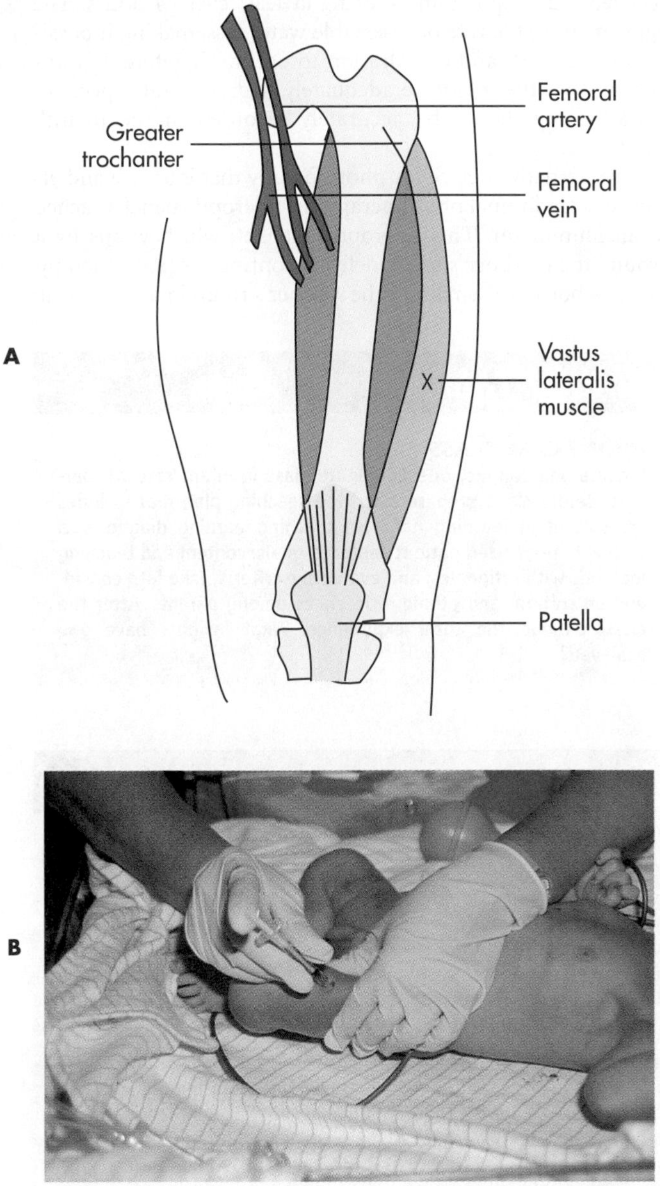

FIG. 25-12 • Intramuscular injection. **A,** Acceptable intramuscular injection site (*X*) for newborn infant. **B,** Infant's leg stabilized for intramuscular injection. Nurse is wearing gloves to give injection. (B, Courtesy Marjorie Pyle, RNC, Lifecircle, Costa Mesa, CA.)

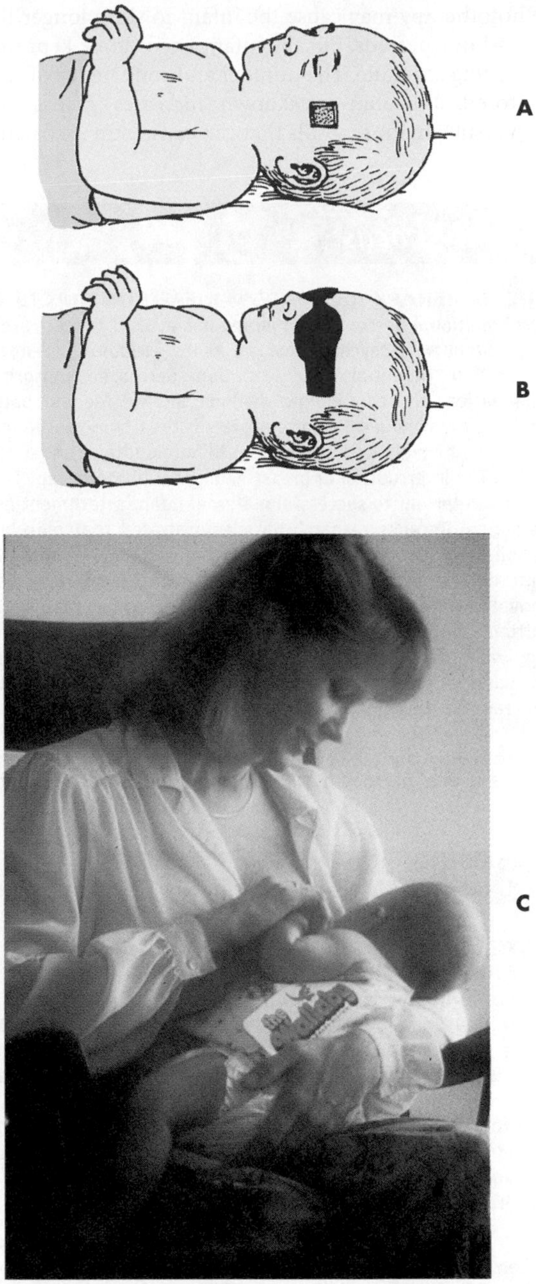

FIG. 25-13 • Eye patches for newborns receiving phototherapy. **A,** Small Velcro patch stuck to both sides of head. **B,** Eye cover sticks to Velcro patch, which reduces movement of eye cover and facilitates removal for feedings. **C,** A mother can breastfeed her baby without interrupting phototherapy. (C, Courtesy Respironics, Inc., Pittsburgh, PA.)

Several precautions must be taken while the infant is undergoing phototherapy. The lamp energy output should be monitored routinely during treatment with a photometer (Fanaroff and Martin, 1997). The infant's eyes must be protected by an opaque mask to prevent overexposure to the light; the eye shield should cover the eyes completely but not occlude the nares. Before the mask is applied, the infant's eyes should be closed gently to prevent excoriation of the corneas. The mask should be removed during infant feedings so that the eyes can be checked and the parents can have visual contact with the infant (Fig. 25-13, *A* and *B*).

Often a "string bikini" made from a disposable face mask is used instead of a diaper. This allows optimal skin exposure, yet provides sufficient protection to the genitals and bedding. Before its application, the metal strip must be removed from the mask to prevent burning the infant. Lotions and ointments should not be used because they absorb heat and can cause burns.

Phototherapy may cause the infant to sleep longer than the usual 4-hour periods, but the infant needs to be kept on a regular feeding schedule. The number and consistency of stools are monitored. Bilirubin breakdown increases gastric motility, which results in loose stools that can cause skin excoriation and breakdown; the infant's buttocks must be cleaned after each stool to help maintain skin integrity.

During phototherapy, the infant's temperature may become elevated; this requires monitoring at least every 4 hours. The lights increase the rate of insensible water loss, making it possible for fluid loss and dehydration to occur. Therefore it is important that the infant be adequately hydrated. All aspects of phototherapy should be accurately recorded in the infant's chart.

An alternative device for phototherapy that is as safe and effective as traditional phototherapy is a fiberoptic panel attached to an illuminator. This fiberoptic blanket, which wraps light around the newborn's torso, delivers continuous phototherapy. The newborn can remain in the mother's room in an open crib

Family Focus

PHOTOTHERAPY AND PARENT-INFANT INTERACTION

The traditional use of phototherapy has evoked concerns regarding a number of psychobehavioral issues, including parent-infant separation, potential social isolation, decreased sensorineural stimulation, altered biologic rhythms, altered feeding patterns, and activity changes. Parental anxiety is greatly increased, particularly at the sight of the newborn blindfolded and under special lights. The interruption of breastfeeding for phototherapy is a potential deterrent to successful maternal-infant attachment and interaction. Because research has demonstrated that bilirubin catabolism occurs primarily within the first few hours of the initiation of phototherapy, there is increased support for the removal of the infant from treatment for feeding and holding. Intermittent phototherapy may be just as effective as continuous therapy when used correctly. The benefits of stopping phototherapy for parental feeding and holding outweigh concerns related to the clearance of bilirubin.

Data from Blackburn S, Loper D: *Maternal, fetal, and neonatal physiology: a clinical perspective,* Philadelphia, 1992, WB Saunders.

Critical Thinking

INFANT CARE CLASS

Prepare and conduct one 20-minute class in infant care for parents. Before class, prepare a written teaching plan that includes assessment of learning needs; a teaching-learning diagnosis; a plan with prioritized patient-centered goals; content and teaching methods with rationales; and evaluative criteria. Take into consideration cultural and ethnic differences among parents. After the class, critique the total experience. What insights have you achieved?

Guidelines

HYPERBILIRUBINEMIA

Definitions

Hyperbilirubinemia—Higher levels of bilirubin than normal
Bilirubin—End product of RBCs when they mature and break down
RBCs—Red blood cells
Jaundice—Yellow skin, sclerae, and mucous membranes caused by circulating bilirubin
Phototherapy—The use of fluorescent light to break down the bilirubin in the skin into substances that can be excreted in the feces (stool) and urine
Bililites—Fluorescent lights used for phototherapy

How Jaundice Happens

When RBCs break down, they release bilirubin, which then circulates in the blood. The bilirubin combines with another substance in the liver. This combined substance moves through the blood to the kidneys and the intestines, where it is eliminated in the urine and the stool. The bilirubin gives the yellow color to urine and the brown color to the stool.

Before birth, babies have more RBCs in each ounce of blood than adults have. The RBCs of the unborn infant also have a shorter life span (70 to 90 days) than RBCs formed after birth (120 days). When the RBCs of a fetus break down, the bilirubin produced by this is carried by the fetus's blood, through the placenta and to the mother's liver to be excreted.

After birth, the infant's liver must get rid of the bilirubin. Even though a baby's liver functions well, it may not be able to get rid of all the bilirubin produced by breakdown of RBCs. Bilirubin then seeps out of the blood and into the tissues, coloring them yellow (jaundice). The blood level of bilirubin rises quickly up to the fifth day and then it declines; the jaundice usually clears up by the end of the first week.

The Danger of Excess Bilirubin

Some newborns seem to have extra bilirubin to excrete. High levels of bilirubin may cause damage to the brain. According to the American Academy of Pediatrics guidelines (1994), phototherapy is considered in a healthy term infant who is 1 to 2 days old if the total bilirubin level is 12 mg/dl or more; it is instituted if the bilirubin level is 15 mg/dl or more. The infant is placed under phototherapy lights or on a bili blanket. This helps the infant eliminate the extra bilirubin and prevents damage to the brain.

Caring for the Infant

The newborn is placed in an incubator under phototherapy lights so that it can be kept warm and the nurse can observe it.
The infant wears an eye mask to keep the light out of the eyes.
The infant is undressed so that as much light as possible can reach the skin. The newborn may wear a "string bikini" made out of a paper face mask as a diaper.
The infant's temperature is taken often so that any changes in temperature can be noted and the infant is not allowed to become too hot or too cold.
The infant may be given extra water to drink or extra breastfeedings because infants have watery, green stools resulting from excretion of the extra bilirubin, and this can lead to dehydration.
The newborn is taken out from under the lights for feedings and cuddling unless a bili blanket is being used. There is no need to remove the bili blanket for feeding.
Blood is taken from the heel to check the amount of bilirubin still in the newborn's blood, and the nurse updates the parents about the results.

After the Newborn Goes Home

The parents should be encouraged to ask any questions that they might have. The nurse gives them a telephone number to call at any hour with their questions. If therapy is continued at home, referral is made to home care.

or in her arms during treatment; follow unit protocol for the use of eye patches (Fig. 25-13, *C*). The blanket may also be used for home phototherapy.

Parent Education. Serum levels of bilirubin in the newborn continue to rise until the fifth day of life. Many parents leave the hospital within 24 hours, and some as early as 6 hours after birth. Therefore parents must be able to assess the newborn's degree of jaundice. They should have written instructions for assessing the infant's condition, and the name of a contact person to whom they should report their findings. Some hospitals have a nurse make a home visit to evaluate the infant's condition. If it proves necessary to measure bilirubin levels after discharge from the hospital, the home care nurse may draw the blood for the specimen, or the parents may take the baby to a laboratory (Guidelines box).

Circumcision

Circumcision of male infants is commonly performed in the United States. The American Academy of Pediatrics (AAP) Task Force on Circumcision (1999) noted that, although there is scientific evidence of potential medical benefits of circumcision, the data are not sufficient to recommend routine circumcision. The Task Force further recommended that if circumcision is performed, analgesia should be used.

Circumcision is a matter of personal parental choice. Parents usually decide to have their newborn circumcised for one or more of the following factors: hygiene, religious conviction, tradition, culture, or social norms. Regardless of the reason for the decision, parents should be given unbiased information and the opportunity to discuss the benefits and risks (Van Ryzin, 2000).

Expectant parents need to begin learning about circumcision during the prenatal period, but circumcision often is not discussed with the parents before labor. In many instances, it is only when the mother is being admitted to the hospital or birth unit that she is first confronted with the decision regarding circumcision. Because the stress of the intrapartal period makes this a difficult time for parental decision making, this is not an ideal time to broach the topic of circumcision and expect a well-thought-out decision.

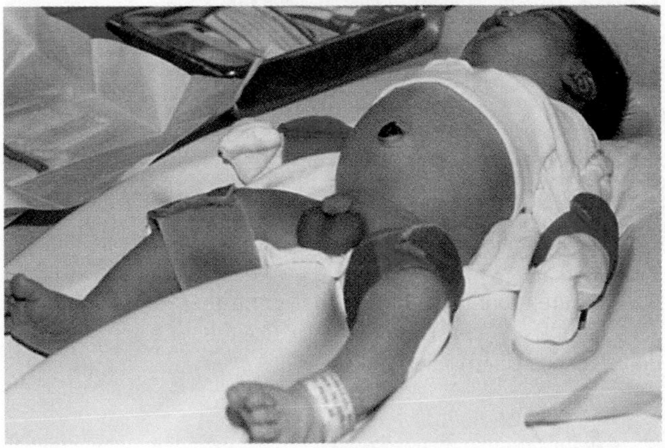

FIG. 25-14 • "Circ board" restrains infant during circumcision. (Courtesy Marjorie Pyle, RNC, Lifecircle, Costa Mesa, CA.)

Procedure. Circumcision involves removing the prepuce (foreskin) of the glans. The procedure is not usually done immediately after birth because of the danger of cold stress, but it is performed in the hospital before the infant's discharge. The circumcision of a Jewish male is performed on the eighth day after birth and is done at home in a ceremony called a bris, unless the infant is unwell. This is logical from a physiologic standpoint because clotting factors drop somewhat immediately after birth and do not return to prebirth levels until the end of the first week.

Feedings are usually withheld up to 4 hours before the circumcision to prevent vomiting and aspiration. To prepare the infant for the circumcision, he is positioned on a plastic restraint form (Fig. 25-14) and his penis is cleansed with soap and water or other prep solution such as povidone-iodine. The infant is draped to provide warmth and a sterile field, and the sterile equipment is readied for use.

Although some circumcision procedures require no special equipment or appliances (Fig. 25-15), numerous instruments have been designed for this purpose. Use of the Yellen or Mogen clamps (Fig. 25-16) may make this an almost bloodless operation. The procedure itself takes only a few minutes to perform. After it is completed, a small petrolatum gauze dressing or a generous amount of petrolatum or A & D ointment may be applied to the penis for the first day to prevent the diaper from adhering the site. A PlastiBell may also be used for the circumcision. The advantages to its use are that it applies constant direct pressure to prevent hemorrhage during the procedure and afterwards protects against infection, keeps the site from sticking to the diaper, and prevents pain with urination. When using the bell for circumcision, it is first fitted over the glans; the suture is tied around the rim of the bell; and excess prepuce is cut away. The plastic rim remains in place for about a week; it falls off af-

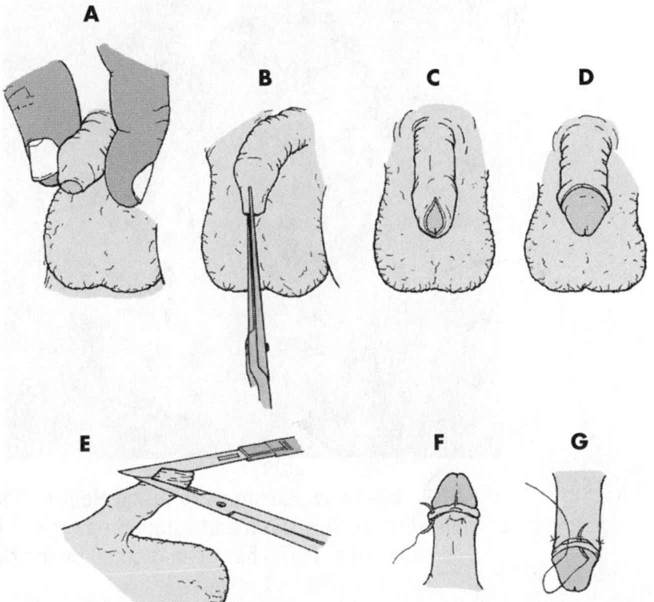

FIG. 25-15 • Technique of circumcision. **A** to **D**, Prepuce is stripped and slit to facilitate its retraction behind glans penis. **E**, Prepuce is now clamped and excessive prepuce cut off. **F** and **G**, A very small needle with plain 2-0 or 3-0 catgut is used for suture material; some physicians prefer silk.

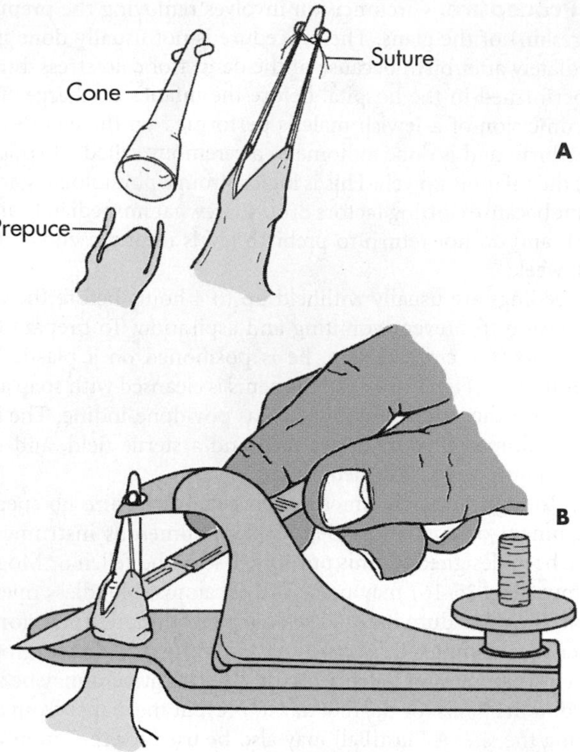

FIG. 25-16 • Circumcision with Yellen clamp. **A,** Prepuce drawn over cone. **B,** Yellen clamp is applied, hemostasis occur, then prepuce (over cone) is cut away.

Patient Teaching

CIRCUMCISION

- Wash hands before touching the newly circumcised penis

Check for Bleeding

- Check circumcision for bleeding every hour for the first 12 hours after the procedure
- If bleeding occurs, apply gentle pressure with a folded sterile gauze square. If bleeding does not stop with pressure, notify primary health care provider

Observe for Urination

- Check to see that the infant urinates after being circumcised
- Infant should have a wet diaper 6 to 10 times per 24 hours

Keep Area Clean

- Change diaper and inspect circumcision at least every 4 hours
- Wash penis gently with warm water to remove urine and feces. Apply petrolatum to the glans with each diaper change (omit petrolatum if Plastibell was used)
- Use soap only after circumcision is healed
- Fanfold diaper to prevent pressure on the circumcised area

Check for Infection

- Glans penis is dark red after circumcision, then becomes covered with yellow exudate in 24 hours. This is normal and will persist for 2 to 3 days. Do not attempt to remove it
- Redness, swelling, or discharge indicate infection. Notify primary health care provider if you think the circumcision area is infected

Provide Comfort

- Circumcision is painful. Handle the area gently
- Provide extra holding, feeding, and opportunities for nonnutritive sucking for a day or two

A

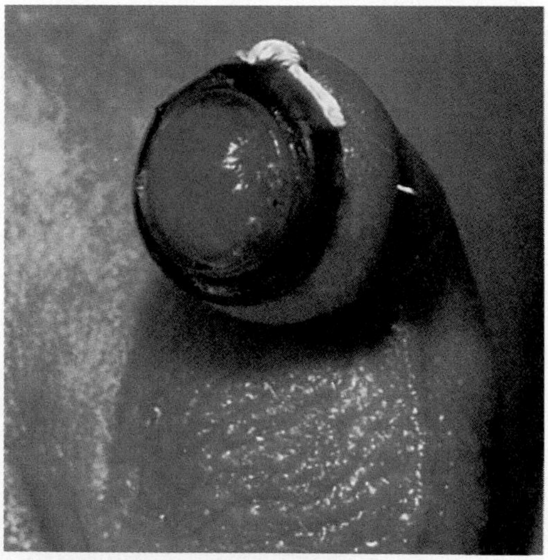

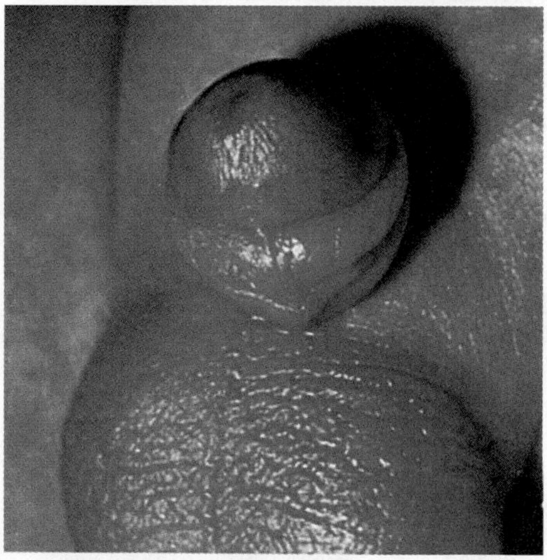

B

FIG. 25-17 • Circumcision using Hollister PlastiBell. **A,** Suture around rim of PlastiBell controls bleeding. **B,** Plastic rim and suture drop off in 7 to 10 days. (Permission to use and/or reproduce this copyrighted material has been granted by the owner, Hollister, Inc., Libertyville, IL.)

ter healing has taken place (Fig. 25-17). Petrolatum is not needed when the bell is used.

Discomfort. Circumcision is painful; the pain is manifested by both physiologic and behavioral changes in the infant (see discussion that follows). Three types of anesthesia/analgesia are used in newborns who undergo circumcisions. These include (from most effective to less effective) ring block, dorsal penile nerve block (DPNB), and topical anesthetic (Williamson, 1997).

A ring block is the injection of buffered lidocaine administered subcutaneously on each side of the penile shaft. A DPNB includes subcutaneous injections of buffered lidocaine at the 2 o'clock and 10 o'clock positions at the base of the penis. The circumcision should not be done for at least 5 minutes after these injections.

A topical cream containing prilocaine-lidocaine such as EMLA (eutectic mixture of local anesthetics) can be applied to the base of the penis at least 1 hour before the circumcision. The area where the prepuce attaches to the glans is well coated with the cream and then covered with a transparent occlusive dressing or finger cot. After the procedure, the cream is removed. Blanching or redness of the skin may occur.

Oral acetaminophen and comfort measures such as having the infant suck on a pacifier and talking to the infant in a soothing voice have not proved to be effective in pain reduction (Williamson, 1997); however, pacifiers dipped in a concentrated glucose solution have been used during the procedure with varying levels of effectiveness.

After the circumcision, the infant is comforted until he is quieted. If the parents were not present during the procedure, the infant is returned to them. The infant may be fussy for several hours and may refuse a feeding.

Care of the Newly Circumcised Infant. The nurse checks the infant hourly for the next 12 hours to make sure that no bleeding is occurring and that voiding is normal. If bleeding is noted from the circumcision, the nurse applies gentle pressure to the site of bleeding with a folded sterile gauze pad, or sprinkles powdered gel foam on it. If bleeding is not easily controlled, a blood vessel may need to be ligated. In this event, one nurse notifies the physician and prepares the necessary equipment (i.e., circumcision tray and suture materials) while another nurse maintains intermittent pressure until the physician arrives. If the parents take the baby home before the end of the 12-hour observation period, they must be taught the proper home care (Patient Teaching box). Before the infant is discharged, the nurse checks to see that the parents have the physician's telephone number.

Nursing actions are planned and implemented to prevent infection. Prepackaged wipes for cleaning the diaper area should not be used because they contain alcohol, which delays healing and causes discomfort. Instead, the nurse washes the penis gently with water to remove urine and feces and, if necessary, applies fresh petrolatum around the glans after each diaper change. The glans penis, normally dark red during healing, becomes covered with a yellow exudate in 24 hours. This is part of normal healing, not an infective process; no attempt should be made to remove the exudate, which persists for 2 to 3 days. Parents should be taught to fan-fold the diaper so that it does not press on the circumcised area. They should be encouraged to change the diaper at least every 4 hours to prevent it from sticking to the penis.

PAIN IN NEONATES

Pain has physiologic and psychologic components. The psychologic component of pain, and the diffuse total body response to pain exhibited by the neonate, led many health care providers to believe that infants, especially preterm infants, do not experience pain (Franck and Gregory, 1993). However, the central nervous system is well-developed as early as 24 weeks' gestation. The peripheral and spinal structures that transmit pain information are present and functional between the first and second trimester. The pituitary-adrenal axis is also well developed at this time, and a fight-or-flight reaction is observed in response to the catecholamines released in response to stress (Franck, 1998).

The physiologic response to pain in the neonate can be life-threatening. Pain response can decrease tidal volume, increase demands on the cardiovascular system and increase metabolism and neuroendocrine imbalance. The hormonal-metabolic response to pain in a term infant has a greater magnitude and shorter duration than in adults. The newborn's sympathetic response to pain is less mature and thus less predictable than an adult's (Franck and Gregory, 1993).

Assessment

Pain can be assessed in behavioral, physiologic/autonomic, and metabolic categories (Franck and Gregory, 1993).

Behavioral Responses. The most common behavioral sign of pain is a vocalization or cry. The pain cry is distinctive: high-pitched and shrill. A cry face is characteristic for an infant experiencing pain. Other facial features exhibited during a pain stimulus include eye squeeze, brow contraction, deepened nasolabial furrows, taut and quivering tongue, and open mouth. The infant will flex and adduct the upper body and lower limbs in an attempt to withdraw from the painful stimulus (Anand, Gruneau, and Oberlander, 1997; Hadjistavropoulos et al, 1997). The preterm infant has a lower threshold for initiation of this flex response. An infant who receives a muscle-paralyzing agent such as vecuronium will be unable to mount a behavioral or visible pain response.

Physiologic/Autonomic Responses. Significant changes in heart rate, blood pressure (increased or decreased), intracranial pressure, vagal tone, respiratory rate, and oxygen saturation occur during noxious stimulation (Franck and Gregory, 1993; Lynam, 1995).

Metabolic Responses. Infants release epinephrine, norepinephrine, glucagon, corticosterone, cortisol, 11-deoxycorticosterone, lactate, pyruvate, and glucose in response to pain (Franck and Gregory, 1993; Lynam, 1995).

Several pain assessment tools have been developed for the assessment of pain in the neonate. One pain assessment tool used by nurses in the NICU is the CRIES (Table 25-4). This tool was developed for use by nurses who work with preterm and full-term infants. CRIES is an acronym for the physiologic and behavioral indicators of pain used in the tool. The indicators include crying, requiring increased oxygen, increased vital signs, expression, and sleeplessness. Each indicator is scored from 0 to 2. The total possible pain score, which represents the worst pain, is 10. A pain score greater than 4 should be considered significant. This tool can be used on infants between the ages of 32 weeks of gestation and 20 weeks postterm (Bildner and Krechel, 1996; Krechel and Bildner, 1995).

Management of Neonatal Pain

The goals of management of neonatal pain are to (1) minimize intensity, duration, and physiologic cost of the pain, and (2) maximize the neonate's ability to cope and recover from the pain (Franck and Gregory, 1993). Nonpharmacologic and pharmacologic strategies are used.

Nonpharmacologic Management. Containment, also known as swaddling, is effective in reducing excessive, im-

TABLE 25-4
CRIES Neonatal Postoperative Pain Scale

	0	1	2
Crying	No	High pitched	Inconsolable
Requires O_2 for sat >95%	No	<30%	>30%
Increased vital signs	Heart rate and blood pressure equal or less than preoperative state	Heart rate and blood pressure <20% of preoperative state	Heart rate and blood pressure >20% of preoperative state
Expression	None	Grimace	Grimace/grunt
Sleepless	No	Wakes at frequent intervals	Constantly awake

CODING TIPS FOR USING CRIES

Crying	The characteristic cry of pain is *high pitched* If no cry or cry that is not high pitched, score 0 If cry high pitched but infant is easily consoled, score 1 If cry is high pitched and infant is inconsolable, score 2
Requires O_2 for sat >95%	Look for *changes* in oxygenation. Infants experiencing pain manifest decreases in oxygenation as measured by tCO_2 or oxygen saturation. (Consider other causes of changes in oxygenation, such as atelectasis, pneumonothorax, oversedation) If no oxygen is required, score 0 If <30% O_2 is required, score 1 If >30% O_2 is required, score 2
Increased vital signs	NOTE: Measure blood pressure last because this may wake child, causing difficulty with other assessments. Use baseline preoperative parameters from a nonstressed period Multiply baseline HR × 0.2, then add this to baseline HR to determine the HR that is 20% over baseline. Do likewise for BP. Use mean BP If HR and BP are both unchanged or less than baseline, score 0 If HR or BP is increased but increase is <20% of baseline, score 1 If either one is increased >20% over baseline, score 2
Expression	The facial expression most often associated with pain is a grimace This may be characterized by brow lowering, eyes squeezed shut, deepening of the nasolabial furrow, open lips and mouth If no grimace is present, score 0 If grimace alone is present, score 1 If grimace and noncry vocalization grunt is present, score 2
Sleepless	This is scored based on the infant's state during the hour preceding this recorded score If the child has been continuously asleep, score 0 If he/she has awakened at frequent intervals; score 1 If he/she has been awake constantly, score 2

BP, Blood pressure; *HR,* heart rate.
Neonatal pain assessment tool developed at the University of Missouri-Columbia.
From Krechel S, Bildner J: CRIES: a new neonatal postoperative pain measurement score: initial testing of validity and reliability, *Pediatr Anaesth* 5:53-61, 1995.

mature motor responses. This may provide comfort through other senses such as thermal, tactile, and proprioceptive senses (Franck and Gregory, 1993; Lynam, 1995). Nonnutritive sucking (NNS) is the most common comfort measure used. However, the effectiveness of NNS on the pain response is limited and confined to the pain caused by certain procedures (Lynam, 1995; Mohan et al, 1998). Distraction with visual, oral, auditory, or tactile stimulation may be helpful in term or older infants (Franck and Gregory, 1993).

Pharmacologic Management. Pharmacologic agents are routinely used for adults during painful procedures. These same agents are now being routinely used for neonates to alleviate pain with procedures. Local anesthesia has become routine during certain invasive procedures such as chest tube insertion and may be used for circumcision. Topical anesthesia has been used for circumcision, lumbar puncture, venipuncture, and heel sticks (Franck, 1998; Mohan et al, 1998). Opioids have been used as preprocedural analgesia. If the infant is not ventilated, the use of opioids is of concern because of the potential for these agents to cause respiratory depression (Franck, 1998; Franck and Gregory, 1993).

DISCHARGE PLANNING AND TEACHING

Infant care activities can cause much anxiety for the new parent (see Nursing Care Plan). Support from nursing staff members can be an important factor in determining whether new mothers seek and accept help in the future. Whether this is the woman's or couple's first baby, or an adolescent whose mother will be the primary caregiver, or whether they attended parenthood preparation classes, parents appreciate anticipatory guidance in the care of their infant. The nurse should not try to cover all the content at one time because the parents can be overwhelmed by too much information and become anxious. However, because of the early discharge of new mothers that is currently common practice, it may be a problem for the nurse to teach all the content that is necessary. As a result, many institutions have developed home visitation programs that take the necessary teaching to the new parents, although the hospital nurse still provides most of the essential information for newborn care.

To set priorities for teaching, the nurse follows parental cues. Knowledge deficits should be identified before beginning to teach. Normal growth and development and the changing needs of the infant (e.g., for stimulation, exercise, and social contacts) as well as the topics that follow should be included during discharge planning with parents.

Temperature

The following topics should be reviewed:

- The causes of elevation in body temperature (e.g., overwrapping, cold stress with resultant vasoconstriction, or minimum response to infection) and the body's response to extremes in environmental temperature
- Signs to be reported, such as high or low temperatures with accompanying fussiness, stuffy nose, lethargy, irritability, poor feeding, and crying
- Ways to promote normal body temperature, such as giving a tepid tub bath, dressing the infant appropriately for the air temperature, and protecting the infant from long exposure to sunlight
- Use of warm wraps or extra blankets in cold weather
- Technique for taking the baby's axillary temperature

Respirations

Review the following points:

- Normal variations in the rate and rhythm
- Reflexes such as sneezing to clear the air passage
- Need to protect the infant from the following:
  —People with upper respiratory tract infections
  —Pollution from a smoke-filled environment (second-hand smoke)
  —Suffocation from loose bedding, water beds, and bean bag chairs; drowning (in bath water); entrapment under excessive bedding; anything tied around the infant's neck; poorly constructed playpens, bassinets, or cribs
- Sleep position—on side or back when put to sleep
- Aspiration pneumonia: a commonly aspirated substance is baby powder, which usually is a mixture of talc (hydrous magnesium silicate) and other silicates. Parents are advised that, if they prefer to use a powder, a corn starch preparation can be substituted. Whenever a powder is used, it should be placed in the caregiver's hand and then applied to the skin, never sprinkled directly onto the skin.
- Symptoms of the common cold: nasal congestion, coughing, sneezing, difficulty in swallowing or breathing, low-grade fever. Advise the parents on measures to help the infant, for example:
  —Feeding smaller amounts more often to prevent overtiring the infant
  —Holding the baby in an upright position to feed
  —For sleeping, raising the infant's head and chest by raising the mattress 30 degrees (do not use pillow)
  —Avoiding drafts; not overdressing the baby
  —Using only medications prescribed by a physician
  —Covering the upper lip with a light film of petrolatum to minimize excoriation from nasal secretions

> ### *Critical Thinking*
>
> **SIDS AND INFANT SLEEP POSITION**
>
> **Prepare a display on SIDS and infant sleep position for a well-baby clinic. Identify the age, education, and ethnicity of patients who come to the clinic. Outline content that is important to include. Describe how you would adapt the display based on the demographics of the patients who come to the clinic.**

Feeding Schedules

Feeding practices and schedules for newborns are discussed in Chapter 26.

Elimination

A review includes the following reminders:

- Changes to be expected in the color of the stool (i.e., meconium to transitional to soft yellow/golden yellow) and the number of bowel evacuations, plus the odor of stools for breastfed or bottle-fed infants (see Chapter 26)
- Color of normal urine and number of voidings (6 to 10) to expect each day

Positioning and Holding

Positioning the infant on the right side after feeding promotes gastric emptying into the small intestine (see Fig. 25-2). Placing the infant in the crib in a side-lying position also promotes drainage of mucus from the mouth and applies no pressure to the cord or the sensitive circumcised penis. The American Academy of Pediatrics advises against placing the infant in the prone position during the first few months of life; the supine position is recommended (AAP, 1996). The prone position has been associated with an increased incidence of sudden infant death syndrome (SIDS). Parents can be referred to "Back to Sleep," P.O. Box 29111, Washington, DC 20040; 1-800-505-CRIB for further information about infant position for sleep.

Anatomically the infant's shape—a barrel chest and flat, curveless spine—makes it easy for the child to roll and startle. The placement of a folded or rolled blanket against the infant's spine will prevent rolling to the supine position and promote a feeling of security. Care must be taken to prevent the infant from rolling off flat, unguarded surfaces. When an infant is on such a surface, the parent or nurse who must turn away from the infant even for a moment should always keep one hand placed securely on the infant. The infant is always held securely with its head supported because newborns are unable to maintain an erect head posture for more than a few moments. Fig. 25-18 illustrates various positions for holding an infant with adequate support.

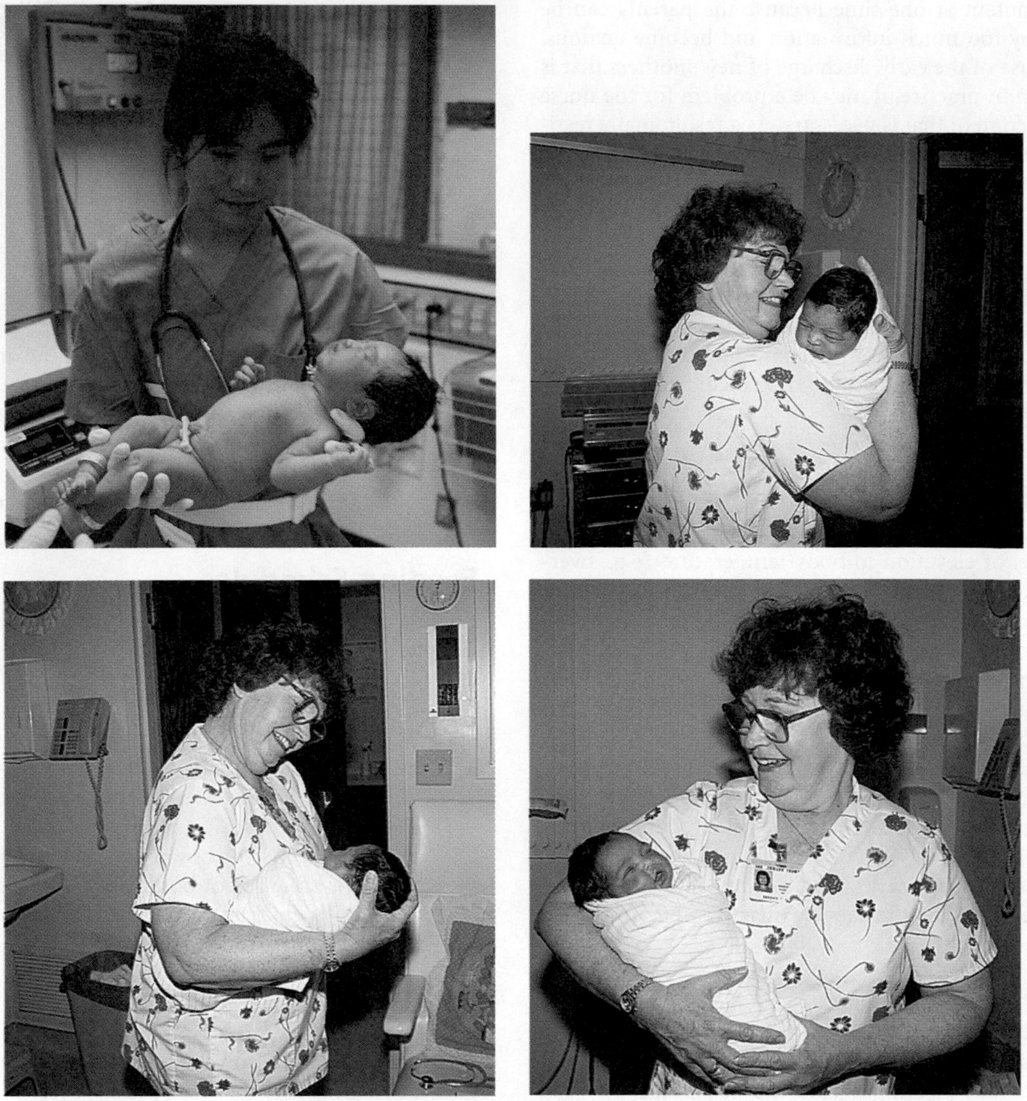

A B C D

FIG. 25-18 • Holding baby securely with support for head. **A,** Holding infant while moving infant from one place to another. Baby is undressed to show posture. **B,** Holding baby upright in "burping" position. **C,** "Football" hold. **D,** Cradling hold. (A, courtesy Kim Molloy, Knoxville, IA; B, C, and D, courtesy Marjorie Pyle, RNC, Lifecircle, Costa Mesa, CA.)

Rashes

Diaper Rash. The warm, moist atmosphere in the diaper area provides an optimal environment for candidal growth; dermatitis appears in the perianal area, inguinal folds, and lower abdomen. The affected area is intensely erythematous with a sharply demarcated, scalloped edge, often with numerous satellite lesions that extend beyond the larger lesion. The usual source of infection is through the gastrointestinal tract when organisms are swallowed from the birth canal during delivery. It may also appear 2 to 3 days after an oral infection.

Therapy consists of applications of an anticandidal ointment, such as nystatin or clotrimazole, with each diaper change. Sometimes the infant also is given an oral antifungal preparation to eliminate any gastrointestinal source of infection.

Washing and drying the wet and soiled area and changing the diaper immediately after voiding or stooling will prevent and help treat diaper rash. Parents can be taught that placing the infant in a warm room with the buttocks exposed to air or even filtered sunlight can help dry up diaper rash. Warmth can also be achieved with a 25-watt bulb placed 45 cm from the affected area for brief periods (i.e., 15 minutes) several times a day. Disposable diapers and plastic pants should be avoided until healing occurs.

Other Rashes. A rash on the face may result from the infant's scratching (excoriation) or from rubbing the face against the sheets, particularly if regurgitated stomach contents are not washed off promptly. Newborn rash, erythema toxicum, is a common finding (see Chapter 24).

Clothing

Parents commonly ask how warmly they should dress their infant. A simple rule of thumb is to dress the child as they dress themselves, adding or subtracting clothes and wraps for the child as necessary. A shirt or diaper may be sufficient clothing for the young infant. A cap or bonnet is needed to protect the scalp and minimize heat loss if the weather is cool, or to protect against sunburn and shade the eyes if it is sunny and hot. Wrapping the infant snugly in a blanket maintains body temperature and promotes a feeling of security. Overdressing in warm temperatures can cause discomfort, as can underdressing in cold weather.

Safety: Use of Car Seat

Infants should travel only in federally approved, rear-facing safety seats secured in the rear seat (Fig. 25-19). The safest area of the car is the back seat. A car seat that faces the rear gives the best protection for the disproportionately weak neck and heavy head of an infant. In this position, the force of a frontal crash is spread over the head, neck, and back; the back of the car seat supports the spine.

NURSE ALERT • Infants should use a rear-facing car seat from birth to 20 pounds and to 1 year of age.

The car seat is secured using the vehicle seat belt; the infant is secured using the harness system in the car seat. If the infant must ride in the front seat, the air bag must be turned off to prevent injury from the air bag.

NURSE ALERT • In cars equipped with air bags, rear-facing infant seats must not be placed in the front seat. Serious injury can occur if the air bag inflates because these types of infant seats fit closer to the dashboard (Fig. 25-19).*

Infants less than 37 weeks of gestation should be observed in a car seat for a period of time before discharge. The infant is monitored for apnea, bradycardia, and a decrease in SaO_2. It may be necessary to place blanket rolls on either side of the infant for support of the head and trunk. To prevent slumping, the back-to-crotch strap distance should be 14 cm. If necessary, a rolled blanket can be placed between the infant and the crotch strap.

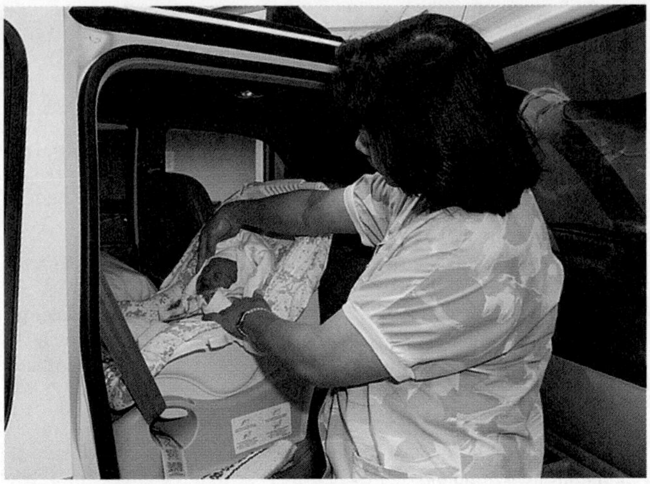

FIG. 25-19 • Rear-facing infant seat in rear seat of car. Infant is placed in seat when going home from the hospital. (Courtesy Marjorie Pyle, RNC, Lifecircle, Costa Mesa, CA.)

Nonnutritive Sucking

Sucking is the infant's chief pleasure. However, sucking needs may not be satisfied by breastfeeding or bottle-feeding alone. In fact sucking is such a strong need that infants who are deprived of sucking, such as those with a cleft lips, will suck on their tongues. Some newborns are born with sucking pads on their fingers that developed during in utero sucking. Several benefits of nonnutritive sucking have been demonstrated, such as an increased weight gain in premature infants and decreased crying.

Problems arise when parents are concerned about the sucking of fingers, thumb, or pacifier and try to restrain this natural tendency. Before giving advice, nurses should investigate the parents' feelings and base the guidance they give on the information solicited. For example, some parents may see no problem with the use of a finger but may find the use of a pacifier objectionable. In general, there is no need to restrain either practice, unless thumb sucking persists past 4 years of age or past the time when the permanent teeth erupt. Parents are advised to consult with their pediatrician and pediatric nurse practitioner about this topic.

To decrease an infant's dependence on nonnutritive sucking, the feeding time can be prolonged. One way of doing this is to use a bottle with a small-holed, firm nipple because this necessitates stronger sucking and slows the feeding. A parent's excessive use of the pacifier to calm the child should also be explored, however. It is not unusual for parents to place a pacifier in their infant's mouth as soon as it begins to cry, thus only reinforcing a pattern of distress-relief.

If parents choose to let their child use a pacifier, they need to be aware of certain safety considerations before purchasing one. A homemade or poorly designed pacifier can be dangerous because the entire object may be aspirated, if it is small, or a portion may become lodged in the pharynx. Improvised pacifiers, such as those commonly made in hospitals from a padded nipple, also pose dangers because the nipple may separate from the plastic collar and be aspirated. Safe pacifiers are made of one piece that includes a shield or flange large enough to prevent entry into the mouth and a handle that can be grasped (see Fig. 36-12).

Sponge Bathing, Cord Care, and Skin Care

Bathing serves a number of purposes. It provides opportunities for (1) completely cleansing the infant, (2) observing the infant's condition, (3) promoting comfort, and (4) parent-child-family socializing.

An important consideration in skin cleansing is a preservation of the skin's acid mantle, which is formed from the uppermost horny layer of the epidermis, sweat, superficial fat, metabolic products, and external substances such as amniotic fluid and microorganisms. At birth, the skin has a pH of 6.4. Within 4 days, the pH of the newborn's skin surface falls to within the bacteriostatic range ($pH < 5$) (Krebs, 1998). Consequently, only plain, warm water should be used for the bath during that 4-day period. Alkaline soaps (such as Ivory) and oils, powder, and lotions should not be used during this time because they al-

*Air bag safety sheets are available from the American Academy of Pediatrics, 141 Northwest Point Blvd., Elk Grove Village, IL 60007; phone 1-800-433-9016; fax 847-228-1281; or access the website at www.aap.org.

Home Care

SPONGE BATHING

Fit Baths into the Family Schedule

Give a bath at any time convenient to you, but not immediately after a feeding period because the increased handling may cause regurgitation.

Prevent Heat Loss

The temperature of the room should be 24° C, and the bathing area should be free of drafts.

Control heat loss during the bath to conserve the infant's energy. Bathing the infant quickly, exposing only a portion of the body at a time, and thorough drying are all important parts of the bathing technique.

Gather Supplies and Clothing Before Starting

Clothing suitable for wearing indoors: diaper, shirt; stretch suit or nightgown optional

Unscented, mild soap

Pins, if needed for diaper, keep them closed and placed well out of baby's reach

Cotton balls

Towels for drying infant and a clean washcloth

Receiving blanket

Tub for water, or use a sink

Bathe the Baby

Bring infant to bathing area when all supplies are ready.

Never leave the infant alone on bath table or in bath water, not even for a second! If you have to leave, take the infant with you or put back into crib.

Test temperature of the water. It should feel pleasantly warm to the inner wrist 36.6° to 37.2° C.

Do not hold infant under running water—water temperature may change, and infant may be scalded or chilled rapidly.

Wash infant's head before unwrapping and undressing the body to prevent heat loss.

Cleanse the eyes from the inner canthus outward, using separate parts of a clean washcloth for each eye. For the first 2 to 3 days there may be a discharge resulting from the reaction of the conjunctiva to the ointment (erythromycin) used as a prophylactic measure against infection. Any discharge should be considered abnormal and reported to the health care provider.

Wash the scalp with water and mild soap; rinse well and dry thoroughly (Fig. 25-20). Scalp desquamation, called *cradle cap,* often can be prevented by removing any scales with a fine-toothed comb or brush after washing. If condition persists, the health care provider may prescribe an ointment to massage into the scalp.

Creases under the chin and arms and in the groin may need daily cleansing. The crease under the chin may be exposed by elevating the infant's shoulders 5 cm and letting the head drop back.

Cleanse ears and nose with twists of moistened cotton or a corner of the washcloth. Do not use cotton-tipped swabs because they may cause injury.

Undress baby and wash body and arms and legs. Pat dry gently. Baby may be tub bathed after the cord drops off and umbilicus and circumcised penis are completely healed.

Prevent Skin Trauma

The fragile skin can be injured by too vigorous cleansing.

If stool or other debris has dried and caked on the skin, soak the area to remove it. Do not attempt to rub it off, because abrasion may result. Gentleness, patting dry rather than rubbing, and use of a mild soap without perfumes or coloring are recommended. Chemicals in the coloring and perfume can cause rashes on sensitive skin.

Care of the Cord

Use a cotton swab. Dip swab in solution the health care provider has ordered and cleanse around base of the cord where it joins the skin. Notify the health care provider of any odor, discharge, or skin inflammation around the cord. The clamp is removed when the cord is dry (approximately 24 hours). The diaper should not cover the cord because a wet or soiled diaper will slow or prevent drying of the cord and foster infection. When the cord drops off after a week to 10 days, small drops of blood may be seen when the baby cries. This will heal by itself. It is not dangerous.

Care of Hands and Feet

Wash and dry between the fingers and toes.

Do not cut fingernails and toenails immediately after birth. The nails have to grow out far enough from the skin so that the skin is not cut by mistake. If the baby scratches himself or herself, apply loosely fitted mitts over each of the baby's hands. Do so as a last resort, however, because it interferes with the baby's ability for self-consolation sucking on thumb or finger. When the nails have grown, the fingernails and toenails can be cut more easily with manicure scissors (preferably scissors with rounded tips) when the infant is asleep. Nails should be kept short.

Cleanse Genitals

Cleanse the genitals of infants daily and after voiding or defecating. For girls, the genitals may be cleansed by separating the labia and gently washing from the pubic area to the anus. For uncircumcised boys, gently pull back (retract) the foreskin. Stop when resistance is felt. Wash and rinse the tip (glans) with soap and warm water and replace the foreskin. The foreskin must be returned to its original position to prevent constriction and swelling. In most newborns the inner layer of the foreskin adheres to the glans and the foreskin cannot be retracted. By the age of 3 years in 90% of boys, the foreskin can be retracted easily without causing pain or trauma. For others, the foreskin is not retractable until adolescence. As soon as the foreskin is partly retractable and the child is old enough, he can be taught self-care. Once healed, the circumcised penis does not require any special care other than cleansing with diaper changes.

ter the acid mantle, thus providing a medium for bacterial growth. Although the sponging technique is generally used, bathing the newborn by immersion has been found to allow less heat loss and provoke less crying; this is not advised, however, until the umbilical cord falls off.

Until the initial bath is completed, personnel must wear gloves to handle the newborn.

The umbilical cord begins to dry, shrivel, and blacken by the second or third day of life. The umbilicus should be inspected often for signs of infection (e.g., foul odor, redness, and purulent discharge), granuloma (i.e., small, red, raw-appearing polyp where the umbilical cord separates), bleeding, and discharge. The cord clamp is removed when the cord is dry, in about 24 hours (see Fig. 25-8). The cord normally falls off in 10 to 14 days after birth.

In the hospital the umbilicus is usually cleansed with alcohol or other designated solution with each assessment and with diaper changes if the cord is moist.

The Home Care box contains information regarding sponge bathing, skin care, cord care, cutting nails, and dressing the infant.

Home Care

NEWBORN HOME CARE FOLLOWING EARLY DISCHARGE

Wet diapers: 6 to 10 per day
Breastfeeding: Successful latch-on and feeding every 1½ to 3 hr daily
Formula feeding: Successfully, voiding as noted above, taking 3 to 4 oz every 3 to 4 hr daily
Circumcision: Wash with warm water only; yellow exudate forming, nonbleeding, Plastibell intact 48 hr
Stools: At least one every 48 hr (bottle-feeding) or two to three per day (breastfeeding)
Color: Pink to ruddy when crying; pink centrally when at rest or asleep
Activity: Has four or five wakeful periods per day and alerts to environmental sounds and voices
Jaundice: Physiologic jaundice (not appearing in first 24 hr), feeding, voiding, and stooling as noted above or practitioner notification for suspicion of pathologic jaundice (appears within 24 hr of birth, ABO/Rh problem suspected); decreased activity; poor feeding; dark orange skin color persisting beyond fifth day in light-skinned newborn
Cord: Kept above diaper line; nonodorous; drying
Vital signs: Heart rate 120 to 140 beats/min at rest; respiratory rate 30 to 55 at rest without evidence of sternal retractions, grunting, or nasal flaring; temperature 36.5° to 37.2° C axillary
Position of sleep: Back

From Wong D: *Whaley & Wong's nursing care of infants and children,* ed 6, St Louis, 1999, Mosby.
*Any deviation from the above and/or suspicion of poor newborn adaptation should be reported to the practitioner at once.

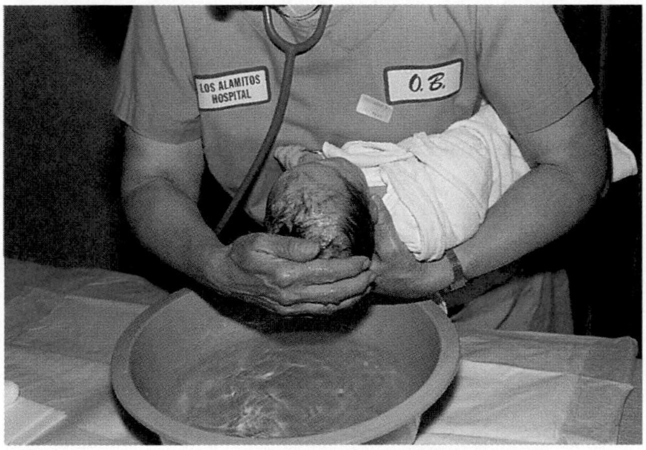

FIG. 25-20 • Wash hair with baby wrapped to prevent heat loss from wet scalp. (Courtesy Marjorie Pyle, RNC, Lifecircle, Costa Mesa, CA.)

Infant Follow-Up Care

With shorter hospital stays, the focus and site of infant care is changing. Home care may be provided either by a nurse as part of the follow-up of patients, or through a visiting nurse or community health nurse referral service. For infants discharged early, newborn home care is essential (Home Care box) (see also Chapter 3).

Parents should plan for their infant's health follow-up care at the following ages: 2 to 4 weeks of age; then every 2 months until 6 to 7 months of age; then every 3 months until 18 months; at 2 years; at 3 years; at preschool; and every 2 years thereafter.

Immunizations

The schedule for immunizations should be reviewed with the parents. HBV (hepatitis B vaccine) is currently administered to newborns before hospital discharge with parental permission. See Chapter 36 for a complete discussion of infant immunizations.

➤ Evaluation

The nurse can be reasonably assured that care was effective to the extent that the expected outcomes for care have been achieved.

Key Points

- Assessment of the newborn requires data from the prenatal, intrapartal, and postnatal periods.
- Knowledge of biologic and behavioral characteristics is essential for guiding assessment and interpreting data.
- Providing a protective environment is a key responsibility of the nurse, and includes such measures as careful identification procedures, support of physiologic functions, measures to prevent infection, and restraining techniques.
- Maintenance of adequate ventilation includes ensuring an adequate airway and body temperature within the normal range.
- Parent education is a major responsibility of the nurse and includes involvement of parents in all phases of the nursing process.
- The newborn has social as well as physical needs.
- Circumcision is an elective surgical procedure.
- Pain in neonates must be assessed and managed.
- Whether or not this is the couple's first baby, parents appreciate anticipatory guidance in the care of their child.

References

American Academy of Pediatrics (AAP) Task Force on Circumcision: Circumcision policy statement, *Pediatrics* 103(3): 686-693, 1999.

American Academy of Pediatrics (AAP): Task force on infant positioning: positioning and sudden infant death syndrome (SIDS) update, *Pediatrics* 98(6):1216-1218, 1996.

Anand K, Gruneau R, Oberlander T: Developmental character and long-term consequences of pain in infants and children, *Child and Adolescent Psychiatric Clinics of North America* 6(4):703-724, 1997.

Ballard J, Novak K, Driver M: A simplified score for assessment of fetal maturity of newly born infants, *J Pediatr* 95(5 Pt. 1):769-774, 1979.

Ballard J et al: New Ballard score, expanded to include extremely premature infants, *J Pediatr* 119(3):417-423, 1991.

Bildner J, Krechel S: Increasing staff nurse awareness of postoperative pain management in the NICU, *Neonatal Netw* 15: 11-16, 1996.

Fanaroff A, Martin R: *Neonatal-perinatal medicine: diseases of the fetus and infant,* ed 6, St Louis, 1997, Mosby.

Franck L: Identification, management, and prevention of pain in the neonate. In Kenner C, Lott J, Flandermeyer A, editors: *Comprehensive neonatal nursing: a physiologic perspective,* ed 2, Philadelphia, 1998, WB Saunders.

Franck L, Gregory G: Clinical evaluation and treatment of infant pain in the neonatal intensive care unit. In Schechter M, Berde C, Yaster M, editors: *Pain in infants, children and adolescents,* Baltimore, 1993, Williams & Wilkins.

Frank S, Esch J, Margeson N: Mandatory HIV testing of newborns: the impact on women, *Am J Nurs* 98(10):49-51, 1998.

Hadjistavropoulos H et al: Judging pain in infants: behavioural, contextual, and developmental determinants, *Pain* 7(3): 319-324, 1997.

Krebs T: Cord care: is it necessary? *Mother Baby J* 3(2):5-12, 18-20, 1998.

Krechel S, Bildner J: CRIES: a new neonatal postoperative pain measurement score: initial testing of validity and reliability, *Pediatr Anesth* 5:53-61, 1995.

Leitch D: Mother-infant interaction: achieving synchrony, *Nurs Res* 48(1):55-58, 1999.

Lynam L: Research utilization: nonpharmacological management of pain in neonates, *Neonatal Netw* 14(5):59-62, 1995.

March of Dimes: *Public health information sheet: newborn screening tests,* White Plains, NY, 1994, March of Dimes.

Meehan R: Heelsticks in neonates for capillary blood sampling, *Neonatal Netw* 17(1):17-24, 1998.

Mohan C et al: Comparison of analgesics in ameliorating the pain of circumcision, *J Perinat* 18(1):13-14, 1998.

Penny-MacGillivray T: A newborn's first bath: when? *J Obstet Gynecol Neonat Nurs* 25(6):481-487, 1996.

Van Ryzin L: The circumcision debate, *Am J Nurs* 100(7): 24A-24B, 2000.

Williamson M: Circumcision anesthesia: a study of nursing implications for dorsal penile nerve block, *Pediatr Nurs* 23: 59-63, 1997.

Wong D: *Whaley & Wong's nursing care of infants and children,* ed 6, St Louis, 1999, Mosby.

CHAPTER 26

Newborn Nutrition and Feeding

http://www.harcourthealth.com/MERLIN/Wong/maternal/

Learning Objectives

On completion of this chapter the reader will be able to:

- Describe current recommendations for feeding infants.
- Discuss benefits of breastfeeding for infants, mothers, families, and society.
- Describe nutritional needs of infants.
- List newborn feeding readiness cues.
- Describe the anatomy and physiology of breastfeeding.
- Identify nursing interventions to facilitate and promote successful breastfeeding.
- List signs of adequate intake in the breastfed infant.
- Identify common problems associated with breastfeeding and nursing interventions to help resolve them.
- Discuss patient teaching for the family using formula-feeding.

Good nutrition in infancy fosters optimal growth and development. Infant feeding is more than the provision of nutrition; it represents an opportunity for social and psychologic interactions between parent and infant. It can also establish a basis for lasting development of good eating habits. The health supervision of infants requires knowledge of their nutritional needs. This chapter focuses on meeting nutritional needs for normal growth and development from birth to 6 months of age, with emphasis on the neonatal period when feeding practices and patterns are being established. Both breastfeeding and formula-feeding are addressed.

RECOMMENDED INFANT NUTRITION

The American Academy of Pediatrics (AAP) recommends that infants be breastfed exclusively for the first 6 months of life, and that breastfeeding continue for at least 12 months (AAP, 1997). If infants are weaned before 12 months, they should receive iron-fortified infant formula. *Healthy People 2010* goals include that 75% of women will breastfeed at birth, 50% will breastfeed for 6 months, and 25% of women will continue to breastfeed to 1 year of age (Department of Health and Human Services, 2000). Currently in the United States, approximately 60% of infants are breastfed at birth but fewer than 25% are still breastfeeding at 6 months of age.

Benefits of Breastfeeding

Human milk is designed specifically for human infants and is nutritionally superior to any alternative. Breast milk is considered a living tissue because it contains almost as many live cells as does blood. It is bacteriologically safe and is always fresh. The nutrients in breast milk are more easily absorbed than those in formula.

Benefits of breastfeeding for the infant include the following:

- Breast milk enhances maturation of the GI tract and contains immune factors that contribute to a lower incidence of diarrheal illness, necrotizing enterocolitis, Crohn's disease, and celiac disease (Barnard, 1997; Lopez-Alarcon, Villalpando, and Fajardo, 1997; Scariati, Grummer-Strawn, and Fein, 1997).
- Breastfed infants receive specific antibodies and cell-mediated immunologic factors that help protect against otitis media, respiratory illnesses such as respiratory syncytial virus and pneumonia, urinary tract infections, bacteremia, and bacterial meningitis (Cushing et al, 1998; Lopez-Alarcon, Villalpando, and Fajardo, 1997).
- There is a lower incidence of allergies among breastfed infants from families at high risk. Allergic manifestations occur at a greater rate and are more severe in formula-fed infants (Halken and Host, 1996).
- Breastfed infants are less likely to die from SIDS (Ford et al, 1993).

- Breast milk may have a protective effect against childhood lymphoma and insulin-dependent diabetes (Davis, 1998; Gerstein, 1994).
- Breast milk may enhance cognitive development (Horwood and Fergusson, 1998).

Maternal benefits include the following:

- Women who have breastfed have a decreased risk of ovarian, uterine, and breast cancer (Enger et al, 1998; Rosenblatt and Thomas, 1995).
- Breastfeeding promotes uterine involution and is associated with a decreased risk of postpartum hemorrhage (Lawrence, 1999).
- Mothers who are breastfeeding tend to return to their prepregnancy weight more quickly (Dewey, Heinig, and Nommsen, 1993).
- Breastfeeding may provide some protection against the development of osteoporosis (Eisman, 1998).
- Breastfeeding provides a unique bonding experience and increases maternal role attainment (Lawrence, 1999).

Benefits to families and society include the following:

- Breastfeeding is convenient; there are no bottles or other equipment to purchase, clean, or dispose of.
- Breastfed babies are portable; when traveling, there are fewer supplies to take along.
- Breastfeeding saves money. The cost of formula far exceeds the cost of extra food for the lactating mother. Breastfeeding families who are eligible for WIC represent a cost savings to the government. Because breastfed babies have a lower incidence of illness and infection, health care costs are lower for families and federal, state, and local governments. Less time is lost from work because parents do not have to stay home with sick infants, which is a benefit to employers (Riordan, 1997).

Choosing an Infant Feeding Method

Women who elect to breastfeed usually do so because they are aware of the benefits to the infant. Many seek the unique bonding experience between mother and infant that is characteristic of breastfeeding. The support of her partner and family is a major factor in a mother's decision to breastfeed and in her ability to do so successfully. Prenatal preparation ideally includes the father of the baby, providing information about the benefits of breastfeeding and how he can participate in infant care and nurturing (Bar-Yam and Darby, 1997).

Prenatal breastfeeding classes are an excellent vehicle to relay important information to expectant parents. Each encounter with an expectant mother is an opportunity to dispel myths, clarify misinformation, and address personal concerns. Connecting expectant mothers with women who are breastfeeding or who have successfully breastfed and are from similar backgrounds may be helpful. Peer counseling programs, such as those instituted by WIC programs, are beneficial, particularly in low socioeconomic groups where bottle-feeding is common (Arlotti et al, 1998). To provide effective support for the mother, health care professionals must be knowledgeable about the benefits of breastfeeding, the basic process of breastfeeding, breastfeeding management, and interventions for common problems (Box 26-1).

Cultural Influences on Infant Feeding. Cultural beliefs and practices are significant influences on infant feeding methods. As many as 50 of 120 cultures studied typically do not give colostrum to newborns and only begin breastfeeding after the milk has "come in" (Morse, Jehle, and Gamble, 1990). Some Filipinos, Mexican-Americans, Vietnamese, Hmong, Koreans, and Nigerians are among these groups. When breastfeeding is delayed until the milk is in, babies are given prelacteal food. In India, infants may be fed liquids such as honey, tea, water, or sugar water before the initiation of breastfeeding (Choudhry, 1997). Other cultures begin breastfeeding immediately and offer the breast each time the infant cries. Cultural attitudes regarding modesty and breastfeeding are important considerations.

Nutrient Needs

Energy. Infants require adequate caloric intake to provide energy for growth, digestion, physical activity, and maintenance of organ metabolic function. For the first 3 months, the infant needs 110 kcal/kg/day. From 3 months to 6 months, the requirement is 100 kcal/kg/day. This decreases slightly to 95 kcal/kg/day from 6 to 9 months, and increases to 100 kcal/kg/day from 9 months to 1 year (AAP, 1998).

Human milk provides approximately 67 kcal/100 ml or 20 kcal/oz; the greatest amount of energy is provided by the fat content of breast milk. Infant formulas are made to simulate the caloric content of human milk; standard formulas contain 20 kcal/oz.

Carbohydrate. Because newborns have only small hepatic glycogen stores, carbohydrates should provide at least 40% to 45% of the total calories in the diet. Moreover, newborns may have limited ability for gluconeogenesis (formation of glucose from amino acids and other substrates) and ketogenesis (formation of ketone bodies from fat), which are mechanisms that provide alternative energy sources.

As the primary carbohydrate in human milk, lactose is the most abundant carbohydrate in the diet of infants up to 6 months of age. Lactose provides calories in an easily available

Box 26-1

Guidelines for Breastfeeding Support

- During pregnancy a breast assessment is performed that includes a breastfeeding history, a breast examination, and a medication use history
- A prenatal plan of care is developed to prepare the woman for lactation
- Immediately after birth, the newborn is kept with the mother when possible so that breastfeeding can be initiated when the newborn is most receptive
- After birth:
  - —Assistance with latch-on and positioning are given as needed
  - —Encouragement of frequent feedings is reinforced
  - —Discharge instructions for knowing criteria for successful breastfeeding are given
  - —Information about community resources for breastfeeding is given
- Especially for premature and low-birth-weight infants, breastfeeding is encouraged

Adapted from AWHONN: *Standards and guidelines for professional nursing practice in the care of women and newborns,* ed 5, Washington, DC, 1998, The Association.

form; its slow breakdown and absorption probably also increase calcium absorption. Corn syrup solids or glucose polymers are added to infant formulas to supplement the lactose in the cow's milk and provide sufficient carbohydrates.

Fat. For infants to acquire adequate calories from the limited amount of human milk or formula they are able to consume, at least 15% of the calories provided must come from fat (triglycerides). The fat must be easily digestible. Fat in human milk is easier to digest and absorb than that in cow's milk because of the arrangement of the fatty acids on the glycerol molecule and because of the presence of the enzyme lipase.

Cow's milk is used in most infant formulas, but the milk fat is removed and replaced by another fat source, such as corn oil, that can be digested and absorbed by the infant. If whole milk or evaporated milk without added carbohydrate is fed to infants, the resulting fecal loss of fat (and therefore loss of energy) may be excessive because the milk moves through the infant's intestines too quickly for adequate absorption to take place. This can lead to poor weight gain.

In addition to its energy contributions, fat also furnishes essential fatty acids (EFAs) which are required for growth and tissue maintenance. EFAs are components of cell membranes and precursors of some hormones. Inadequate intake of EFAs results in eczema and growth failure. The lack of EFAs in skim and low-fat milk is another reason infants should not be fed these products.

Protein. The protein requirement per unit of body weight is greater in the newborn than at any other time of life. The RDA for protein during the first 6 months is 2.2 g/kg.

The protein content of human milk, which is lower than that of unmodified cow's milk, is ideal for the newborn. Human milk contains far more lactalbumin in relation to casein than does cow's milk, and lactalbumin is more easily digested than casein. In addition, the amino acid composition of human milk is suited to the newborn's metabolic capabilities. For example, phenylalanine and methionine levels are low, and cystine and taurine levels are high. The protein in some commercial formulas is modified to increase the amount of lactalbumin (or whey protein) and to decrease the relative proportion of casein to more closely approximate human milk.

Fluids. The fluid requirement for normal infants is about 80 to 100 ml of water per kilogram of body weight per 24 hours (Behrman, Kliegman, and Arvin, 1996). In general, neither breastfed nor formula-fed infants need to be fed water, not even those living in very hot climates. Breast milk contains 87% water, which easily meets fluid requirements. Feeding water to infants may only decrease caloric consumption at a time when infants are growing rapidly.

Infants have room for little fluctuation in fluid balance and should be monitored closely for fluid intake and water loss. Infants lose water through excretion of urine and through insensible losses such as respiration. Under normal circumstances, infants are born with some fluid reserve, and some of the weight loss during the first few days is related to loss of this fluid.

Vitamins. Human milk contains all the vitamins required for infant nutrition, with individual variations based on maternal diet and genetic differences. Vitamins are added to cow's milk formulas to approximate the levels in breast milk. While cow's milk contains adequate amounts of vitamin A and vitamin B complex, vitamin C (ascorbic acid) and vitamin E must be added.

Vitamin D is also added to commercial infant formulas. While human milk may be somewhat deficient in vitamin D, supplementation may not be necessary provided that the infant is exposed to sunlight for 30 minutes per week wearing only a diaper, or for 2 hours per week fully clothed but without a hat. To prevent rickets, supplementation may be recommended for preterm infants and for dark-skinned infants with limited exposure to the sun, as well as for infants whose mothers eat vegetarian diets that exclude meat, fish, and dairy products.

Vitamin K, required for blood coagulation, is produced by intestinal bacteria. However, the gut is sterile at birth, and a few days are needed for intestinal flora to become established and produce vitamin K. To prevent hemorrhagic problems in the newborn, an injection of vitamin K is routinely given at birth.

Minerals. The mineral content of commercial infant formula is designed to reflect that of breast milk. Unmodified cow's milk is much higher in mineral content than human milk, which makes it unsuitable for infants in the first year of life. Minerals are typically highest in human milk during the first few days after birth and decrease slightly throughout lactation.

The ratio of calcium to phosphorus in human milk is 2:1, a proportion optimal for bone mineralization. Although cow's milk is high in calcium, the calcium-to-phosphorus ratio is low, resulting in decreased absorption. Consequently, young infants fed unmodified cow's milk are at risk for hypocalcemia, tetany, and seizures. The calcium-to-phosphorus ratio in commercial infant formulas is between that of human and cow's milk.

Milk of all types is low in iron; however, iron from human milk is better absorbed than that from cow's milk, iron-fortified formula, or infant cereals. Breastfed infants benefit from the high lactose and vitamin C levels in human milk, which facilitate iron absorption. The infant who is totally breastfed normally maintains adequate hemoglobin levels for the first 6 months of life. After that time, iron-fortified cereals and other iron-rich foods are added to the diet. Infants weaned from the breast before 6 months of age and all formula-fed infants should receive an iron-fortified commercial infant formula until 12 months of age.

The fluoride levels in human milk and in commercial formulas are low. This mineral, which is important in the prevention of dental caries, may cause spotting of the permanent teeth (fluorosis) in excess amounts. It is recommended that a fluoride supplement be given only to those infants not receiving fluoridated water after 6 months of age (American Academy of Pediatrics, 1997).

OVERVIEW OF LACTATION

Milk Production

Each female breast is composed of 15 to 20 segments (lobes) embedded in fat and connective tissue and well-supplied with blood vessels, lymphatic tissue, and nerves (Fig. 26-1). Within each lobe are alveoli (the milk-producing cells) surrounded by myoepithelial cells, which contract to send the milk forward into the ductules. Each ductule enlarges into lactiferous ducts and the sinuses, where milk collects just behind the nipple. Each nipple has 15 to 20 pores through which milk is transferred to the suckling infant.

Although nearly every woman can lactate, some mothers have insufficient glandular development to exclusively breastfeed their infants. Typically these women experienced few breast

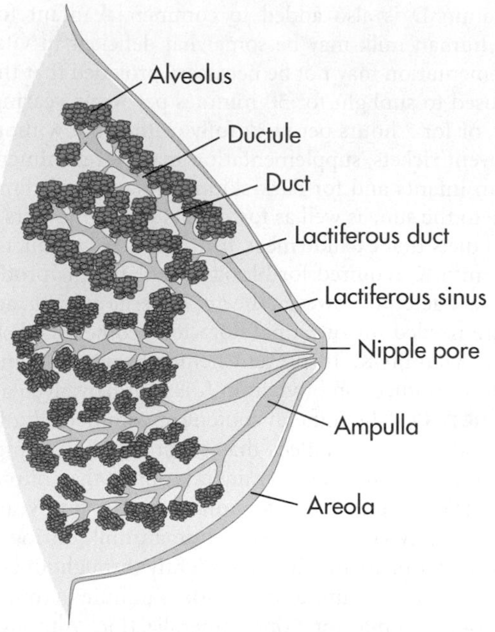

FIG. 26-1 • Detailed structural features of human mammary gland.

changes during either puberty or early pregnancy. In some cases, women may still be able to breastfeed and offer supplemental nutrition to support optimal infant growth. There are devices available to allow mothers to offer supplements while the baby is at the breast (Fig. 26-2).

After the mother gives birth, there is a precipitous fall in her estrogen and progesterone levels, which triggers release of prolactin from the anterior pituitary. During pregnancy, prolactin prepares the breasts to secrete milk and, during lactation, to synthesize and secrete milk. Prolactin levels are highest during the first 10 days after birth; they gradually decline over time, but remain above baseline levels for the duration of lactation. Prolactin is produced in response to infant suckling and emptying of the breasts (lactating breasts are never completely empty; milk is constantly being produced by the alveoli as the infant feeds) (Fig. 26-3, *A*). Milk production is a supply-meets-demand system; that is, as milk is removed from the breast, more is produced. Incomplete emptying of the breasts with feedings can lead to a decrease in milk production.

Oxytocin is the other hormone essential to lactation. As the nipple is stimulated by the suckling infant, the posterior pituitary is prompted by the hypothalamus to produce oxytocin. This hormone is responsible for the milk ejection reflex (MER), or let-down reflex (Fig. 26-3, *B*). The myoepithelial cells surrounding the alveoli respond to oxytocin by contracting and sending the milk forward through the ducts to the nipple. Many "let-downs" can occur with each feeding session. The milk ejection reflex can be triggered by thoughts, sights, sounds, or odors that the mother associates with her baby (or other babies), such as hearing the baby cry. Many women report a tingling "pins and needles" sensation in the breasts as let-down occurs, although some mothers can detect milk ejection only by observing the sucking and swallowing of the infant. Let-down may also occur during sexual activity, since oxytocin is released during orgasm.

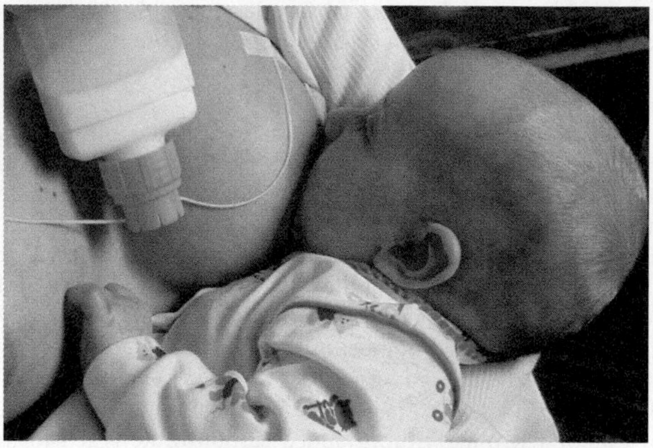

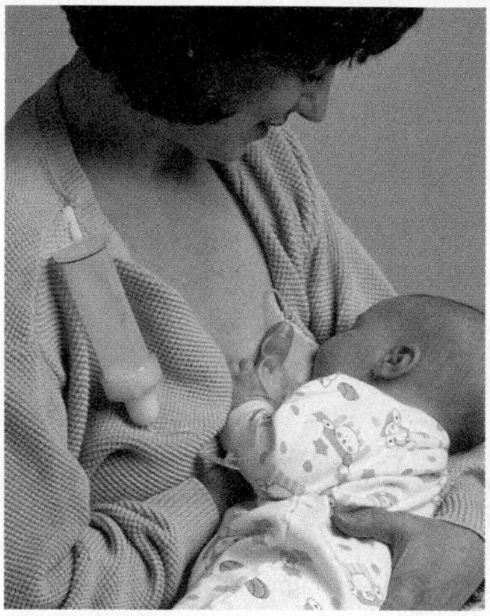

FIG. 26-2 • Supplemental nursing system. (Courtesy Medela, Inc., McHenry, IL.)

Oxytocin is the same hormone that stimulates uterine contractions during labor. Oxytocin contracts the mother's uterus after birth to control postpartum bleeding and to promote uterine involution. Thus mothers who breastfeed are at decreased risk for postpartum hemorrhage. These uterine contractions that occur with breastfeeding can be painful during and after the feeding, particularly in multiparas, for 3 to 5 days after giving birth.

Prolactin and oxytocin have been referred to as the "mothering hormones" since they are known to affect the postpartum woman's emotions as well as her physical state. Many women report feeling thirsty or very relaxed during breastfeeding, probably as a result of these hormones.

The nipple erection reflex is an integral part of lactation. When the infant cries, suckles, or rubs against the breast, the nipple becomes erect. This assists in the propulsion of milk through the lactiferous sinuses to the nipple pores. Nipple sizes, shapes, and their ability to become erect vary with individuals. Some women have flat or inverted nipples that do not become erect with stimulation; however, they are usually able to learn to breastfeed successfully. It is important that these infants are not offered bottles or pacifiers until breastfeeding is well established.

A

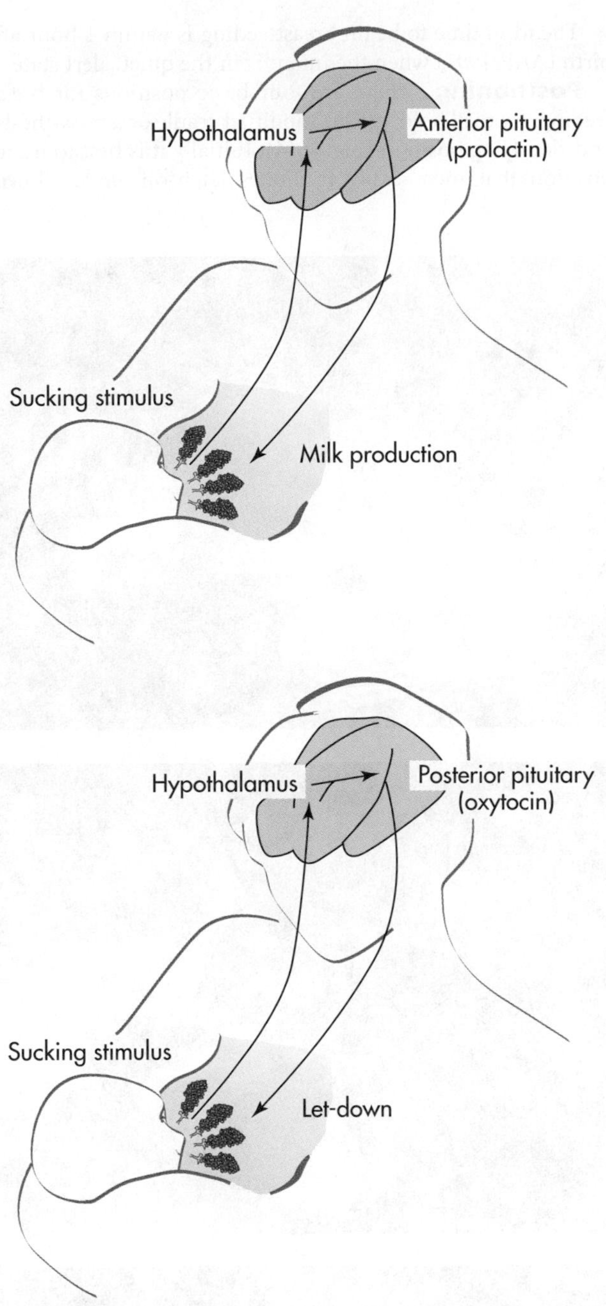

B

FIG. 26-3 • Maternal breastfeeding reflexes. **A,** Milk production. **B,** Let-down.

Uniqueness of Human Milk

Human milk is a highly complex species-specific fluid uniquely designed to meet the needs of the human infant. It is specific to the needs of each newborn; for example, the milk of the mothers of preterm infants differs in composition from that of mothers who give birth at term.

Human milk contains antibodies that provide some protection against a broad spectrum of bacterial, viral, and protozoan infections. Secretory IgA is the major antibody in human milk.

Human milk composition and volumes vary according to the stage of lactation. In lactogenesis stage I, beginning in pregnancy, the breasts are preparing for milk production. Colostrum, a clear, yellowish fluid, is present in the breasts at this time. Colostrum is more concentrated than mature milk and is extremely rich in immunoglobulins. It has higher concentrations of protein and minerals, but less fat than mature milk. The high protein level of colostrum facilitates binding of bilirubin, and the laxative action of colostrum promotes early passage of meconium. Colostrum gradually changes to mature milk; this is referred to as "the milk coming in" or lactogenesis stage II. By the third to fifth day after birth, most women have experienced this onset of copious milk secretion. Breast milk continues to change in composition for approximately 10 days, when the mature milk is established in stage III of lactogenesis (Lawrence, 1999).

Composition of mature milk changes during each feeding. As the infant nurses, the fat content of breast milk increases. Initially there is a release of bluish white foremilk that is part skim milk (about 60% of the volume), and part whole milk (about 35% of the volume). It provides primarily lactose, protein, and water-soluble vitamins. The hindmilk, or cream (about 5%), is usually let down 10 to 20 minutes into the feeding, although it may occur sooner. It contains the denser calories from fat necessary for optimal growth and contentment between feedings. Because of this changing composition of human milk during each feeding, it is important to breastfeed the infant long enough to supply a balanced feeding. Milk production gradually increases, so that by the time her infant is 2 weeks old, the mother produces 720 to 900 ml of milk every 24 hours. Babies experience fairly predictable growth spurts (i.e., at about 10 days, 3 weeks, 6 weeks, 3 months, and 4 to 6 months), when more frequent feedings stimulate increased milk production. These more frequent feedings usually last 24 to 48 hours, and then the infants resume their usual feeding pattern.

Care Management: The Breastfeeding Mother and Infant

➤ Assessment

Infant. Before the initiation of breastfeeding, the nurse needs to consider several factors to effectively assist the breastfeeding infant. Maturity level, experience during labor and birth, any birth trauma or maternal risk factors, congenital defects or physical instability, and state of alertness all affect the readiness and ability of the infant to breastfeed.

During feeding, the infant is assessed by direct observation for latch-on, position and alignment, and sucking and swallowing. After the feeding, the infant is observed for behavior such as contentment or sleepiness. Elimination patterns are noted: within 24 hours after birth, at least 1 wet diaper and 1 stool; by day 3, 3 or 4 wet diapers and 1 or 2 stools that are beginning to change from meconium to yellowish; after day 4 (and mother's milk has "come in"), 6 to 8 wet diapers and at least 3 stools per 24 hours (AAP, 1998). Other factors to assess include the presence of jaundice, weight loss $<10\%$, and a regain of birth weight by 10 to 14 days of age.

Mother. Before breastfeeding is begun, the nurse should carefully assess the mother's knowledge of breastfeeding and her physical and psychologic readiness to breastfeed. Factors to include are her previous experience with breastfeeding, knowledge about breastfeeding, cultural factors, physical features of the breasts or nipples or other physical limitations, psychologic readiness (time since birth, mood and energy level), and support of the father of the baby or other family members.

During the time in the hospital, the nurse can help the mother view each breastfeeding session as a "feeding lesson" or "practice session" that will foster maternal confidence and a satisfying breastfeeding experience for mother and infant. Assessment includes condition of nipples, transition to mature milk, breasts feeling lighter or softer after feeding, mother feeling relaxed or sleepy after feeding, uterine cramping and/or increased lochia flow during and after a feeding, and mother's appearance of comfort with breastfeeding techniques.

➤ Nursing Diagnoses

Nursing diagnoses for the breastfeeding woman include the following:

- Effective breastfeeding related to:
  —Mother's knowledge of breastfeeding techniques
  —Mother's appropriate response to infant's feeding readiness cues
  —Mother's ability to facilitate efficient breastfeeding
- Risk for ineffective breastfeeding pattern related to:
  —Insufficient knowledge regarding newborn's reflexes and breastfeeding techniques
  —Lack of support by father of baby, family, friends
  —Lack of maternal self-confidence; presence of anxiety, fear of failure
  —Poor infant sucking reflex
  —Difficulty waking sleepy baby
- Risk for altered nutrition: less than body requirements related to:
  —Increased caloric and nutrient needs for breastfeeding (mother)
  —Incorrect latch-on and inability to transfer milk (infant)
- Risk for fluid volume deficit related to:
  —Ineffective sucking (infant)

➤ Expected Outcomes

The expected outcomes include that the infant will do the following:

- Latch on and feed effectively at least eight times per day
- Gain weight appropriately
- Remain well-hydrated (have 6 to 8 wet diapers and at least 3 bowel movements every 24 hours after day 4)
- Sleep or seem contented between feedings

Examples of expected outcomes for the mother include that she will do the following:

- Verbalize/demonstrate understanding of breastfeeding techniques, including positioning and latch-on, signs of adequate feeding, and self-care
- Report no nipple discomfort with breastfeeding
- Express satisfaction with the breastfeeding experience
- Consume a nutritionally balanced diet with appropriate caloric and fluid intake to support breastfeeding

➤ Plan of Care and Implementation

In the early days after birth, interventions focus on helping the mother and the newborn initiate breastfeeding and achieve some degree of success/satisfaction before discharge from the hospital. Interventions to promote breastfeeding progress from basics such as latch-on and positioning to signs of adequate feeding and self-care measures such as prevention of engorgement.

The ideal time to begin breastfeeding is within 1 hour after birth (AAP, 1997) when the infant is in the quiet, alert state.

Positioning. There are four basic positions for breastfeeding: football hold, cradle, modified cradle or across-the-lap, and side-lying position (Fig. 26-4). Initially it is best to use the position that most easily facilitates latch-on while allowing

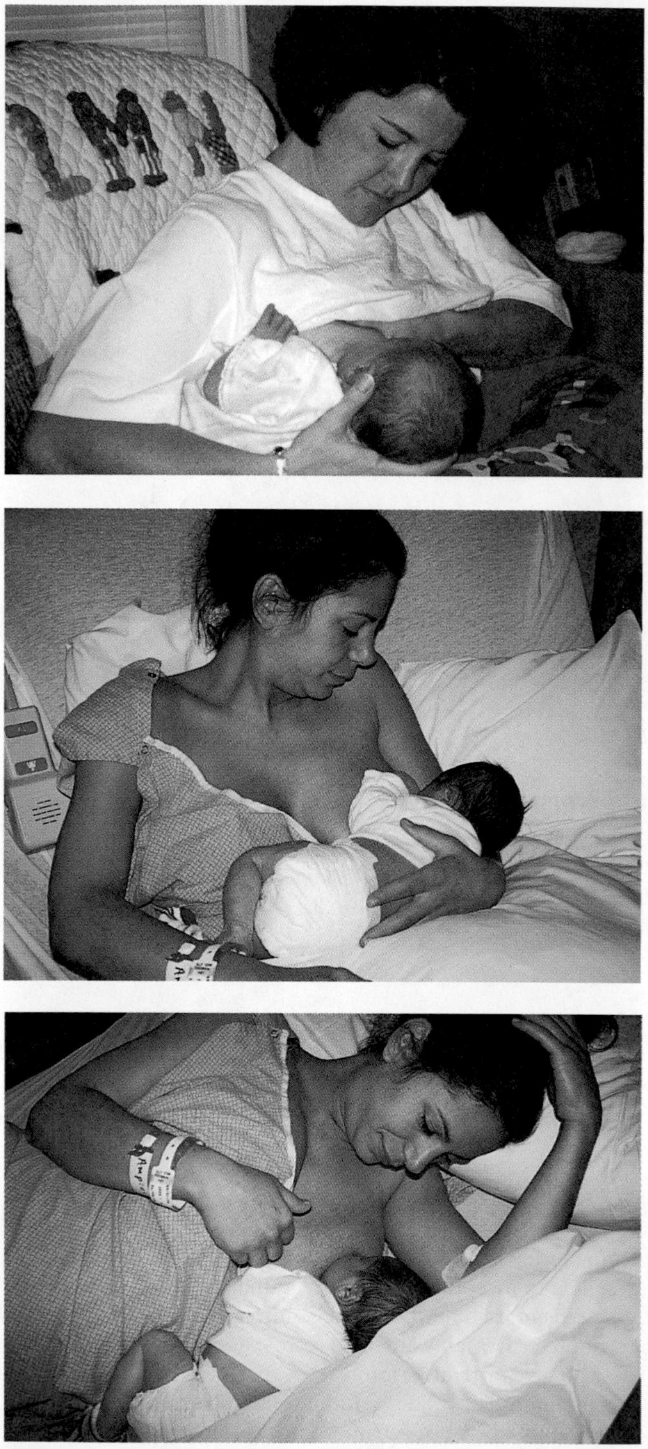

A

B

C

FIG. 26-4 • Breastfeeding positions. **A,** Football hold. **B,** Cradling. **C,** Lying down. (B and C, courtesy Marjorie Pyle, RNC, Lifecircle, Costa Mesa, CA.)

maximum comfort for the mother. The football hold is usually preferred by mothers who gave birth by cesarean. The modified cradle or across-the-lap hold also works well for early feedings. The side-lying position allows the mother to rest while breastfeeding and is often preferred by women experiencing perineal pain and swelling. Cradling is the most common breastfeeding position for infants who have learned to latch on easily and feed effectively. Before discharge from the hospital, the mother should be assisted to try all of the positions so that she will feel confident in her ability to vary positions at home.

Whichever position is used, the mother should be comfortable, with pillows used as needed to provide support for her back and arms. The infant is placed at the level of the breast, supported by pillows or folded blankets; turned completely on his or her side; and facing the mother so that the infant is "belly to belly" with the arms "hugging" the breast. The baby's mouth is directly in front of the nipple. It is important that the mother support the baby's neck and shoulders with her hand and not push on the occiput. The baby's body is held in correct alignment (i.e., ears, shoulders, and hips are in a straight line) during latch-on and feeding (Fig. 26-5).

Latch-On. In preparation for latch-on, it may be helpful for the mother to manually express a few drops of colostrum or milk and spread it over the nipple. This lubricates the nipple and may entice the baby to open the mouth as the milk is tasted.

To facilitate latch-on, the mother supports her breast in one hand with the thumb on top and the fingers underneath at the back edge of the areola. The breast is compressed slightly so that an adequate amount of breast tissue is taken into the mouth with latch-on (Weissinger, 1998). Most mothers need to support the breast during feeding for at least the first few weeks until the baby can stay latched on easily.

The mother lightly touches the baby's lower lip with her nipple, stimulating the mouth to open. When the mouth is open wide and the tongue is down, the mother quickly pulls the baby onto the nipple. She brings the baby to the breast, not the breast

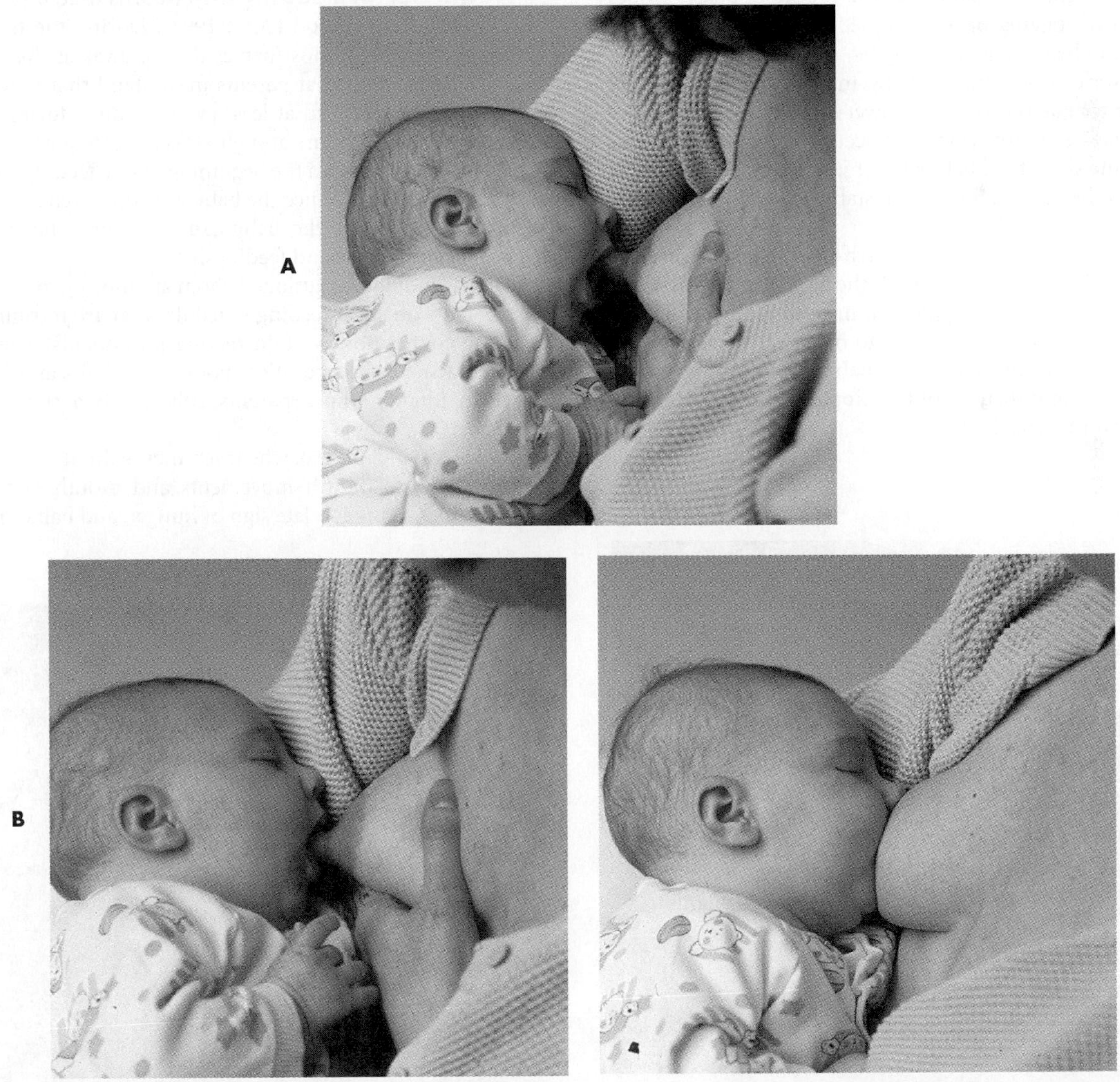

FIG. 26-5 • Latching on. **A,** Tickle baby's lip with your nipple until he or she opens wide. **B,** Once baby's mouth is opened wide, quickly pull baby onto breast. **C,** Baby should have as much areola (dark area around nipple) in his or her mouth as possible, not just the nipple. (Courtesy Medela, Inc., McHenry, IL.)

to the baby. If the breast is pushed into the baby's mouth, the baby often closes the mouth too soon and does not latch on correctly.

The amount of the areola in the baby's mouth with correct latch-on depends on the size of the baby's mouth and the size of the areola and nipple. In general, the baby's mouth should cover the nipple and an areolar radius of approximately 2 to 3 cm all around the nipple.

When the baby is latched on correctly, the nose, cheeks, and chin should all be touching the breast (Fig. 26-6). The mother should not pull the nipple out of the mouth when trying to create a breathing space for the baby's nose. Depressing the breast tissue around the baby's nose is not necessary. If the mother is worried about the baby's breathing, she can raise the baby's hips slightly to change the angle of the baby's head at the breast. If the baby cannot breathe, reflexes will prompt the baby to move the head and pull back to breathe.

Sucking creates a vacuum in the intraoral cavity as the breast is compressed between the tongue and the palate. If the mother experiences pinching or pain after the first few sucks, or does not feel a firm tugging on the nipple, the latch-on and positioning should be evaluated.

If each suck is painful, the baby may be having difficulty keeping the tongue out over the lower gum ridge. Clicking or smacking may be audible when this occurs. The nurse can place a finger on the side of the baby's lower jaw, pulling down gently but firmly as the baby sucks, to help stabilize the jaw so that the tongue stays in place.

Any time the signs of adequate latch-on and sucking are not present, the baby should be taken off the breast and latch-on attempted again. To prevent nipple trauma as the baby is taken off the breast, the mother is instructed to break the suction by inserting her finger in the side of the baby's mouth between the gums and keeping it there until the nipple is completely out of the baby's mouth (Fig. 26-7).

When the baby is latched on correctly and is sucking appropriately, (1) the mother reports a firm tug on her nipple, but no pinching or pain, (2) the baby sucks with cheeks rounded, not dimpled, (3) the baby's jaw glides smoothly with sucking, and (4) swallowing is audible.

Milk Ejection or Let-Down. As the baby begins sucking on the nipple, the let-down, or milk ejection reflex is stimulated. The hormone oxytocin causes milk to be sent forward from the milk ducts to the nipple. The following signs indicate that let-down has occurred:

- The mother may feel a tingling sensation in the nipples, although many women do not feel their milk let down.
- The baby's suck changes from quick, shallow sucks to a slower, more drawing, sucking pattern.
- Swallowing is heard as the baby sucks.
- The mother feels relaxed, even sleepy, during feedings.
- The mother experiences uterine cramping and increased lochia flow during or after the feeding.
- The opposite breast may leak.

Frequency of Feedings. Newborns need 8 to 12 feedings in a 24 hour period (AAP, 1997). During the first 24 to 48 hours after birth, most babies do not awaken this often to feed. It is important that parents understand that they should awaken the baby to feed at least every 3 hours during the day and at least every 4 hours at night. (Feeding frequency is determined by counting from the beginning of one feeding to the beginning of the next.) Once the baby is feeding well and gaining weight appropriately, the baby can determine the timing of feedings through demand feedings.

Parents should be cautioned about attempting to place newborn infants on strict feeding schedules that are recommended by some contemporary child-rearing proponents. There have been incidences of dehydration, poor weight gain, and failure to thrive in infants whose parents adhered to a strict feeding schedule.

Babies should be fed whenever they exhibit feeding cues such as hand-to-mouth movements and mouth and tongue movements. Crying is a late sign of hunger, and babies may be-

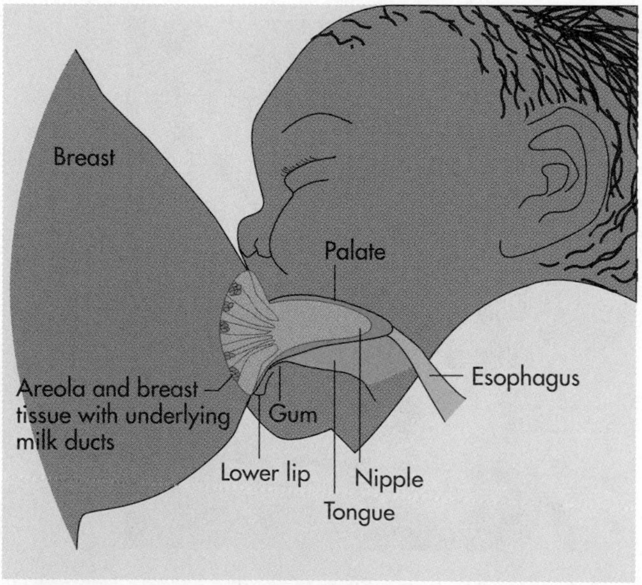

FIG. 26-6 • Correct attachment (latch on) of infant at breast.

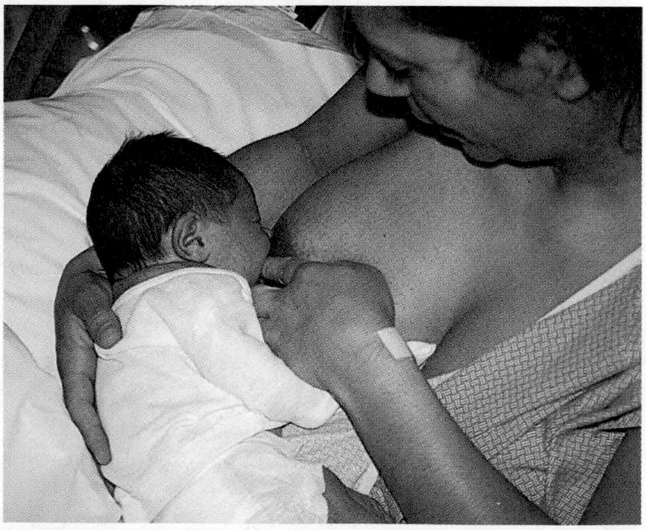

FIG. 26-7 • Removing infant from the breast. (Courtesy Marjorie Pyle, RNC, Lifecircle, Costa Mesa, CA.)

come frantic when they have to wait too long to feed. Some infants will shut down or go into a deep sleep when their needs are not met. Keeping the baby close is the best way to observe and respond to infant feeding cues.

Duration of Feedings. The duration of breastfeeding sessions is highly variable, since the timing of milk transfer differs for each mother-baby pair. While some infants may complete a feeding in 5 or 10 minutes, others may require 45 minutes or longer. The average time for feeding is 30 minutes, or approximately 15 minutes per breast. Instructing mothers to feed for a set number of minutes in inappropriate. It is better to teach mothers how to determine when a baby has finished a feeding: the baby's suck/swallow pattern has slowed, the breast is softened, and the baby appears content and may fall asleep or release the nipple.

If a baby seems to be feeding effectively, and is having adequate urine output but not gaining weight well, the mother may be switching to the second breast too soon. The high lactose content in foremilk may cause the baby to have explosive stools, gas pains, and inconsolable crying. Keeping the baby on the first breast until it is soft ensures that the baby receives the more calorie-dense, high-fat hindmilk, which usually results in increased weight gain.

Supplements, Bottles, and Pacifiers. The American Academy of Pediatrics (1997) recommends that, unless a medical indication exists, no supplements be given to breastfeeding infants. Supplements and pacifiers, if used at all, should be used only when breastfeeding is well established.

Situations related to the infant that may necessitate supplemental feedings include low birth weight, hypoglycemia, dehydration, or inborn errors of metabolism. Mothers may be unable to feed because of severe illness, or they may be taking medications incompatible with breastfeeding.

Offering a bottle after breastfeeding "just to make sure the baby is getting enough" is normally unnecessary and should be avoided. This can contribute to nipple confusion (i.e., difficulty knowing how to latch on to the breast) and to low milk supply because the baby becomes overly full and does not breastfeed often enough. Supplementation interferes with the supply-meets-demand cycle of milk production. The parents may interpret the baby's willingness to take a bottle to mean that the mother's milk supply is inadequate. They need to know that a baby will automatically suck from a bottle as the nipple triggers the suck/swallow reflex.

Babies can become confused going from breast to bottle or bottle to breast. Breastfeeding and bottle-feeding require different skills. The way babies use their tongues, cheeks, and lips, as well as the swallowing patterns, are very different. While some babies can transition easily between breast and bottle, some experience considerable difficulty. It is impossible to predict which babies will adapt well and which ones will not. Therefore, it is best to avoid bottles until breastfeeding is well established, usually after 3 to 4 weeks. If supplementation is needed, there are mechanisms such as supplemental nursing systems that allow the infant to breastfeed while being supplemented (see Fig. 26-3). Although some parents combine breastfeeding and bottle-feeding, many babies never take a bottle and go directly from the breast to a cup as they grow.

Pacifiers are not recommended until breastfeeding is well established. Their use has been associated with early termination of breastfeeding (Aarts et al, 1999; Howard et al, 1999). Newborns need to learn the association between sucking and satiation. Although some infants have nonnutritive sucking needs between feedings, it is best to wait to introduce a pacifier until the infant is proficient at breastfeeding.

Special Considerations

Sleepy Baby. During the first few days of life, some babies need to be awakened for feedings. If the infant is awakened from a sound sleep, attempts at feeding are more likely to be unsuccessful. Unwrapping the baby, changing the diaper, sitting the baby upright, talking to the baby with variable pitch, gently massaging the baby's chest or back, and stroking the palms or soles may bring the baby to an alert state.

Fussy Baby. Babies sometimes awaken from sleep crying frantically. Although they may be hungry, they cannot focus on feeding until they are calmed. Calming techniques include swaddling the baby, holding the baby close, talking soothingly, and allowing the baby to suck on a clean finger.

Some infants cry as soon as they are positioned for feeding. This may be due to a bruised head or previously undetected fractured clavicle. Changing the feeding position may solve the problem.

If an infant required extensive suctioning at birth, there may be an aversion to oral stimulation and the baby may scream and stiffen if anything approaches the mouth. Parents may need to spend time holding and cuddling the baby before attempting to breastfeed.

Fussiness may be related to gastrointestinal distress (i.e., cramping and gas pains). This may occur in response to an occasional feeding of infant formula or it may be related to something the mother has ingested. Although most mothers can consume their normal diet without affecting the baby, foods such as cabbage, broccoli, or onions may aggravate some babies. Others may react to cow's milk products ingested by the mother. There are no standard foods that all mothers should avoid when breastfeeding; each mother/baby couple responds individually. If gas is a problem, giving the baby liquid simethicone drops before a feeding may be helpful.

Persistent crying or refusing to breastfeed can indicate illness and the health care provider should be notified. Ear infections, sore throat, or oral thrush may cause the infant to be fussy and not breastfeed well.

Slow Weight Gain. Commonly newborns lose 8% to 10% of their birth weight during the first 3 to 5 days after birth as they eliminate amniotic fluid and meconium. Thereafter, they should begin to gain weight at the rate of 110 to 200 g per week or 20 to 28 g per day. The infant who continues to lose weight after 5 days, who does not regain birth weight by 2 weeks, or whose weight is below the 10th percentile by 1 month should be evaluated and closely monitored by a health care provider.

Most often, slow weight gain is related to inadequate breastfeeding. Feedings may be short or infrequent, or the infant may be latching on incorrectly or sucking ineffectively or inefficiently. Other causes are illness; infection; malabsorption; or circumstances that increase the baby's energy needs, such as congenital heart disease, cystic fibrosis, or being small-for-gestational-age.

Maternal factors may contribute to slow weight gain. There may be inadequate emptying of the breasts, pain with feeding, or inappropriate timing of feedings. Inadequate glandular breast tissue or previous breast surgery may affect milk supply. Severe intrapartum or postpartum hemorrhage, illness, or medications may decrease milk supply. Stress and fatigue may also negatively affect milk production.

Usually the solution to slow weight gain is to improve the feeding technique. Positioning and latch-on are evaluated and adjustments made. It may help to add a feeding or two in a 24-hour period. Massaging alternate breasts during feedings may help increase the amount of milk going to the infant. With this technique, the mother massages her breast from the chest wall to the nipple whenever the baby has sucking pauses. Some think this technique may also increase the fat content of the milk, which aids in weight gain.

When babies are calorie-deprived and need supplementation, the extra breast milk or formula can be given with a spoon or cup, a nursing supplementer, or a bottle. If there are latch-on problems, it is best to avoid bottles. In most cases, supplementation is needed only for a short time until the baby gains weight and is feeding adequately.

Jaundice. Jaundice (hyperbilirubinemia) in the newborn is discussed in detail in Chapter 24. Physiologic jaundice usually occurs after 24 hours of age and peaks by the third day. This is referred to as early-onset jaundice, which in the breastfed infant may be associated with insufficient feeding and infrequent stooling. Colostrum has a natural laxative effect and promotes early passage of meconium. Bilirubin is excreted from the body primarily (98%) through the intestines. Infrequent stooling allows bilirubin in the stool to be reabsorbed into the infant's system, thus promoting hyperbilirubinemia. Infants who receive water or glucose water supplements are more likely to have hyperbilirubinemia, since only 2% of bilirubin is excreted through the kidneys. Decreased caloric intake (less milk) is associated with decreased stooling and increased jaundice.

To prevent early-onset breastfeeding jaundice, babies should be breastfed early and often during the first several days of life. More frequent feedings are associated with lower bilirubin levels.

If the infant's intake of milk needs to be increased, a supplemental feeding device may be used to deliver additional breast milk or formula while the infant is nursing. Hyperbilirubinemia may reach levels that require treatment with phototherapy administered with a light or a blanket (see Chapter 25).

Late-onset jaundice affects few breastfed infants; it develops in the second week of life, peaking at about 10 days of age. These infants are typically thriving, gaining weight, and stooling normally, and all pathologic causes of jaundice have been ruled out. It was once postulated that an enzyme in the milk of some mothers caused the bilirubin level to increase. It now appears that a factor in human milk increases the intestinal absorption of bilirubin. In most cases no intervention is necessary, although some experts recommend temporary interruption of breastfeeding for 12 to 24 hours to allow bilirubin levels to decrease. During this time, the mother pumps her breasts and the baby is offered alternative nutrition, usually formula (Lawrence, 1999).

Preterm Infants. Human milk is the ideal food for preterm infants, with benefits that are unique and in addition to those received by term, healthy infants. Breast milk enhances retinal maturation in preterm infants and improves neurologic outcome. There is also greater physiologic stability with breastfeeding as compared to bottle-feeding (Brown et al, 1996; Meier and Brown, 1996).

Mothers of preterm infants should begin pumping their breasts as soon as possible after birth with a hospital-grade electric pump. To establish an optimal milk supply, the mother should use a dual collection kit and pump 8 to 10 times daily for 10 to 15 minutes and/or until the milk flow has ceased for a few minutes (Meier, 1997). These women are taught proper handling and storage of breast milk to minimize bacterial contamination and growth.

Breastfeeding Twins. Caring for twins takes some planning, but breastfeeding means that feedings are always ready instantly; no one has to wash bottles and fix formula; and, for some mothers, both babies can be fed at once. The mother with twins will need extra nourishment (200 to 500 kcal/day for each baby).

Each baby feeds from one breast per feeding, usually for about 20 to 30 minutes. Some mothers assign each baby a breast; others switch babies from one breast to the other, either on a schedule or randomly. The mother may find it easiest to use a modified demand feeding schedule; that is, feeding the first baby who wakes up and then waking the second baby for feeding.

During the early weeks, parents may find it helpful to keep a record of feeding times and which breast was used first by which baby. If one twin nurses more vigorously than the other, that baby should be alternated between breasts to equalize breast stimulation.

If the mother wants to feed the babies simultaneously, she may wish to experiment with positions. For example, one baby can be held in the football hold and the other in the cradle hold, or the babies can each be held in a cradling position. Each baby can be supported on firm pillows while in the football hold. At first, some mothers using this position (Fig. 26-8) may require assistance to get the babies off the breasts.

Expressing and Storing Breast Milk. There are situations when expression of breast milk (Fig. 26-9) is necessary or desirable, such as when engorgement occurs, the mother and baby are separated (e.g., preterm or sick infant is in neonatal intensive care), the mother is employed outside the home and wants to maintain her milk supply, the nipples are severely sore or cracked, or the mother leaves the infant with a caregiver and will not be present for feeding.

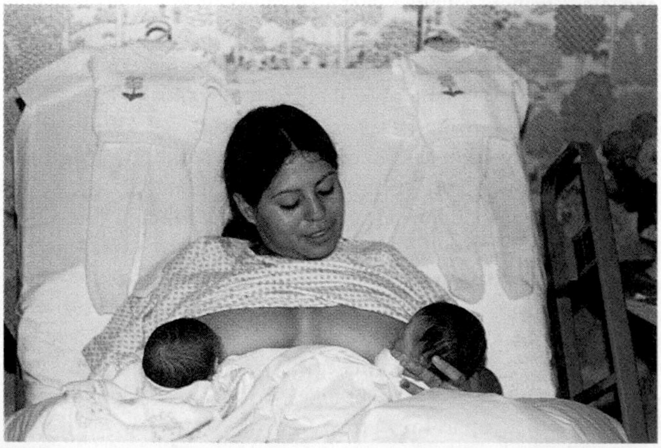

FIG. 26-8 • Breastfeeding twins. (Courtesy Marjorie Pyle, RNC, Lifecircle, Costa Mesa, CA.)

Because pumping and hand expression are rarely as effective as a baby in removing milk from the breast, the milk supply should never be judged based on the volume expressed.

Hand Expression. To manually express milk, after thoroughly washing her hands, the mother places one hand on her breast at the edge of the areola. With her thumb above and fingers below, she presses in toward her chest wall and gently compresses the breast while rolling her thumb and fingers forward. These motions are repeated rhythmically until the milk begins to flow. While the milk is flowing easily, the mother maintains a steady, light pressure. The thumb and fingers should not pinch the breast or slip down to the nipple. The hand should be rotated to reach all sections of each breast. After expressing milk from the second breast, she should return to the first breast and then repeat until all readily available milk is expressed.

Pumping. There are numerous ways to approach pumping. Some women pump when they first wake up in the morning or when the baby has fed but did not completely empty the breast. Others prefer to pump just before going to sleep. Some pump one breast while the baby is feeding from the other. Double pumping (pumping both breasts at the same time) saves time (Fig. 26-10).

The amount of milk obtained when pumping depends on the type of pump being used, the time of day, how long it has been since the baby breastfed, the mother's milk supply, how practiced she is at pumping, and her comfort level (pumping is uncomfortable for some women). Breast milk may vary in color and consistency, depending on the time of day, the age of the baby, and foods the mother has eaten (e.g., the milk may appear green after the mother eats spinach).

Types of Pumps. There are many types of breast pumps (see Fig. 26-10). Some are more effective than others, and they vary in price. Manual pumps are the least expensive and may be the most appropriate where portability and quietness of operation are critical, or when a mother is pumping only for an occasional bottle (see Fig. 26-10, *B*).

Full-service electric pumps, or hospital-grade pumps, are similar to the sucking action and pressure of the breastfeeding infant. These are expensive and therefore are usually rented. When breastfeeding is delayed after birth (e.g., the infant is preterm or ill), or when mother and baby are separated for lengthy periods, these pumps are most appropriate (Fig. 28-10, *A*). Electric, self-cycling double pumps are efficient and easy to use. Some of these pumps come with carry bags containing coolers to store pumped milk (see Fig. 26-9).

Smaller battery-operated or electric pumps are also available. Some have automatic suck/release cycling and others require use of a finger to regulate strength and speed of suction. These are typically used when pumping is done occasionally, but some models are satisfactory for working mothers or others who pump on a regular basis.

Storage of Breast Milk. Breast milk can be stored safely in any clean glass or plastic container. Disposable bottle liners are easy and inexpensive to use when storing milk. When using bottle liners, double bagging is recommended to protect the milk most effectively.

Breast milk can be refrigerated safely for 48 hours after it is expressed. If it is not used within that time, it can be frozen (at 0° C) for up to 6 months; it should be kept in the middle or toward the back of the freezer to avoid variations in temperature. Milk can be stored for 1 year in a freezer at −20° C. When storing breast milk, the container should be dated and the oldest milk used first.

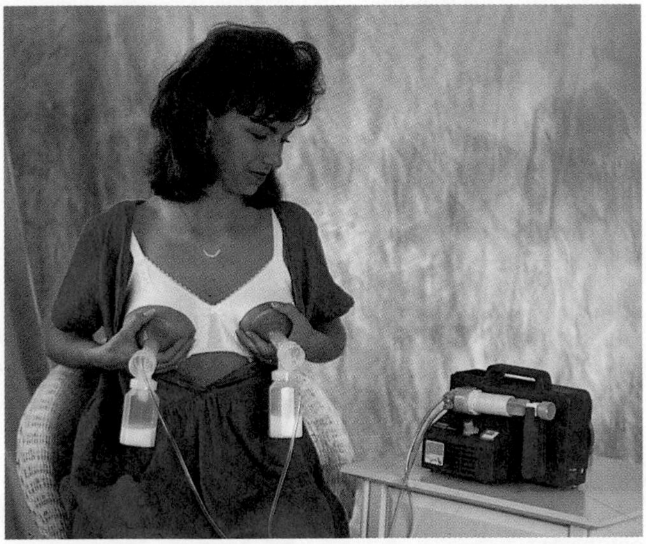

FIG. 26-9 • Bilateral breast pumping. (Courtesy Medela, Inc., Mchenry, IL.)

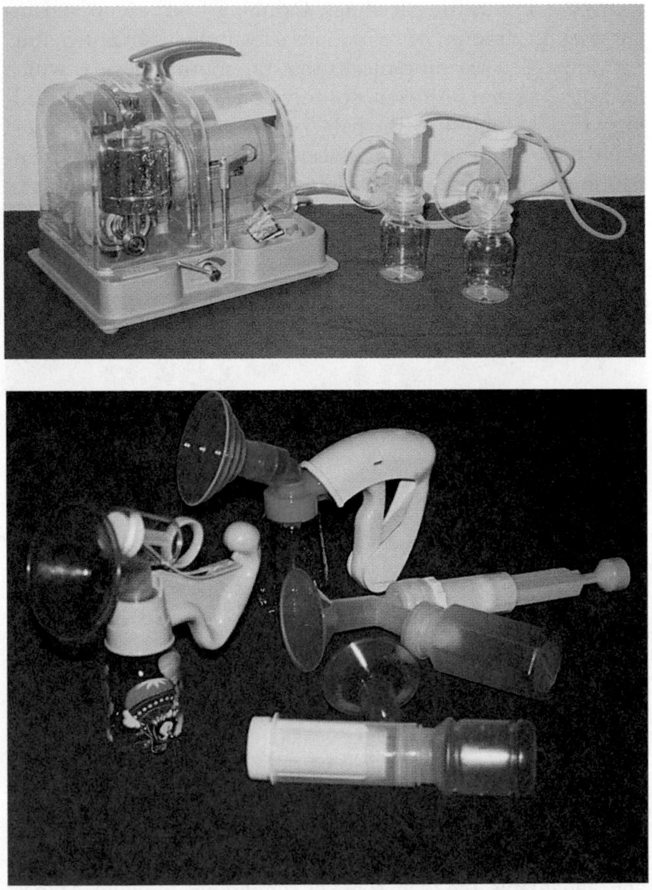

A

B

FIG. 26-10 • **A,** Hospital-grade electric breast pump. **B,** Manual breast pumps. (B, courtesy Marjorie Pyle, RNC, Lifecircle, Costa Mesa, CA.)

Frozen milk is thawed by placing the container in warm water or in the refrigerator. It cannot be refrozen, and should be used within 24 hours. After thawing, the container should be shaken gently to mix the layers that have separated.

NURSE ALERT • Frozen milk is never thawed or heated in a microwave oven. Microwaving does not heat evenly and can cause encapsulated boiling bubbles to form in the center of the liquid. This may not be detected when checking drops of milk for temperature. Babies have sustained severe burns to the mouth, throat, and upper GI tract as a result of microwaved milk (Lawrence, 1999).

Being Away From the Baby. Many women successfully combine breastfeeding with employment, attending school, or other commitments. If feedings are missed, the milk supply may be affected. Some women's bodies adjust the milk supply to the times she is with the baby for feedings. Other mothers must pump while away or their supply diminishes rapidly. Businesses are increasingly making available rooms where mothers can nurse their infants or use breast pumps (Fig. 26-11).

Weaning. Typically, weaning is initiated at a time chosen by the mother or the infant. Weaning can be accomplished with little effort and no discomfort when it is done gradually. Abrupt weaning is likely to be distressing for both mother and baby, as well as physically uncomfortable for the mother.

Infant-led weaning means that the baby moves at his or her own pace in omitting feedings. Drinking from a cup and increasing the amount of solid foods substitute for breastfeeding.

Mother-led weaning means that the mother decides which feedings to drop. This is most easily done by omitting the feeding of least interest to the baby or the one the infant is most likely to sleep through. It can also be the feeding most convenient for the mother to omit. After a week or more, another feeding is dropped, and so on, until the infant is weaned from the breast. Allowing time for the milk supply to adjust before omitting another feeding prevents discomfort for the mother as her supply gradually decreases.

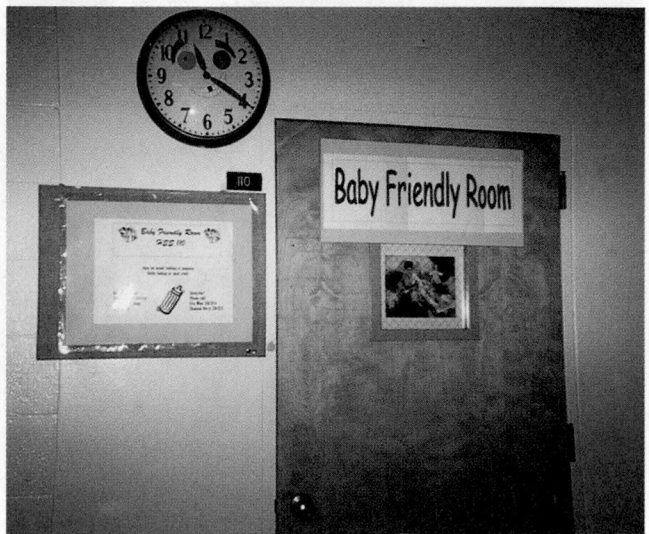

FIG. 26-11 • Room on a university campus dedicated to parents and infants. The room contains comfortable furniture, a breast pump, a refrigerator, a baby changing table, and a television and VCR for instructional purposes. The room is available to students, faculty, and staff. (Courtesy Shannon Perry, San Jose, CA.)

Infants can be weaned directly from the breast to a cup. Bottles are usually offered to infants less than 6 months of age. If the infant is weaned before 1 year of age, formula should be offered instead of cow's milk.

If abrupt weaning is necessary, breast engorgement often occurs. The mother is instructed to take mild analgesics, wear a supportive bra, apply ice packs or cabbage leaves to the breasts, and pump if needed to increase comfort. The pump should not be used to empty the breasts, since they should remain full enough to promote a decrease in milk production.

Milk Banking. For those infants who cannot be breastfed but who also cannot survive except on human milk, banked donor milk is critically important. Because of the antiinfective and growth-promoting properties of human milk—as well as its superior nutrition—donor milk is used in many neonatal intensive care units for preterm or sick infants when the mother's own milk is not available. Donor milk is also used therapeutically for medical purposes, such as in transplant recipients who are immunocompromised.

The Human Milk Banking Association of North America (HMBANA) has established guidelines for the operation of donor human milk banks (Arnold and Tully, 1996). Donor milk banks collect, screen, process, and distribute milk donated by breastfeeding mothers who are feeding their own infants and pumping a few extra ounces each day for the milk bank. All donors are screened both by interview and serologically for communicable diseases. Donor milk is stored frozen until it is heat processed to kill potential pathogens, then it is refrozen for storage until it is dispensed for use. The heat processing adds a level of protection for the recipient that is not possible with any other donor tissue or organ. Milk is dispensed only by prescription. There is a per-ounce fee charged by the bank for processing, but the HMBANA guidelines prohibit payment to donors.

Care of the Mother

Diet. The composition of human milk varies slightly among women, regardless of their diets. The mother's milk automatically contains everything the baby needs, except in rare cases of maternal nutrient deficiencies. For most women, only 200 to 500 extra calories per day need to be added to the diet to provide adequate nutrients for the infant while also protecting the mother's body stores.

There are no specific foods or drinks that all breastfeeding mothers must either consume or avoid. Lactating mothers should ideally consume a balanced diet of nutrient-dense foods. Adequate amounts of calcium, minerals, and fat-soluble vitamins are important.

If the breastfeeding mother is drinking enough fluids to quench her thirst, she is likely drinking enough to support lactation. Typically, women find that they are drinking as much as 2 to 3 quarts of fluid each day, with the choice of fluid depending on the mother's preference. Because of her increased need for fluids, the breastfeeding mother may wish to keep a drink within reach during breastfeeding. An indicator of adequate fluid intake is the color of the mother's urine. If she is drinking enough fluids, her urine should be clear to light yellow throughout the day.

Weight Loss. Because it takes energy to produce milk, many mothers experience a gradual weight loss while breastfeeding as fat stores deposited during pregnancy are used. For the mother who is overweight, this fact can present an added incentive for breastfeeding. However, the mother who wants to diet while lactating should avoid losing large amounts of weight quickly because fat-soluble environmental contaminants to which she has been exposed are stored in her body's fat reserves and these may be released into her milk. In addition, some mothers find that their milk supply decreases when caloric intake is severely restricted. Most mothers find that they can lose about 1 kg per week without affecting their milk supply.

Exercise. There is no reason for a breastfeeding woman to restrict her physical activity. Women continue activities such as hiking, jogging, swimming, and aerobics with no detrimental effect on milk supply or composition. Women often find they are more comfortable if they engage in exercise soon after breastfeeding when their breasts are as empty as possible. Wearing a well-designed, supportive bra may also be helpful.

Rest. It is important for the breastfeeding mother to rest as much as possible, especially in the first 1 or 2 weeks after birth. Fatigue, stress, and worry can interfere with milk production and let-down. The nurse can encourage the mother to sleep when the baby sleeps. Breastfeeding in a side-lying position promotes rest for the mother. Assistance with household chores and caring for other children can be done by the father, grandparents or other relatives, and friends.

Breast Care. The breastfeeding mother's normal bathing routine is all that is required to keep her breasts clean. Soap can have a drying effect on nipples, so she should be instructed to avoid washing the nipples with soap. The small amount of soap that runs down her breasts while washing her face and neck or shampooing her hair is of no concern.

Breast creams should not be used routinely because they may block the natural oil secreted by the Montgomery glands on the areola. Some breast creams contain alcohol, which may dry the nipples. Vitamin E oil or cream is not recommended for use on nipples because it is a fat-soluble vitamin and a breastfeeding infant might consume enough vitamin E from the nipple to reach toxic levels. In addition, some people are allergic to vitamin E oil.

Modified lanolin with reduced allergens can be used safely on dry or sore nipples. Lanolin is beneficial in moist wound healing of sore nipples (Brent et al, 1998; Huml, 1995). Because lanolin is made from sheep's wool, the nurse should ask the mother if she is allergic to wool before applying the ointment. Lanolin is not recommended if it is suspected that nipple soreness may be due to a monilial infection. Antifungal creams are used to treat yeast infections on nipples.

The mother with flat or inverted nipples will likely benefit from wearing breast shells in her bra. These hard plastic devices exert mild pressure around the base of the nipple to encourage nipple eversion. They are also useful for sore nipples to keep the mother's bra or clothing from touching the nipples (Fig. 26-12).

If a mother needs breast support, she will be uncomfortable unless she wears a bra, because the ligament that supports the breast (Cooper's ligament) will otherwise stretch and be painful. If she is comfortable without a bra, there is no reason for her to wear one. If a woman prefers to wear a bra, it should fit well, offer nonbinding support, and feel comfortable. Underwire bras or improperly fitting bras may contribute to clogged milk ducts. Mothers should be encouraged to breastfeed at least once daily without a bra on so that all milk ducts can empty well.

Leakage of milk between feedings is a problem for some women. Using breast pads (washable or disposable) inside a bra and wearing layered or printed tops can help camouflage the leakage. Plastic-lined pads are not recommended because they trap moisture and may lead to sore nipples. To stop leakage, the mother can be alert to any sensation, such as tingling, that her milk is letting down. If this happens, she can usually stop the let-down by pressing straight back on her nipples. In public the mother can fold her arms across her chest to apply pressure unobtrusively.

Breast Self-Examination. Although only 1% to 2% of cases of breast cancer is diagnosed during pregnancy or lactation, the breastfeeding woman should perform breast self-examination (BSE) (see Chapter 5). The woman who is not menstruating should choose a convenient date on which to do her BSE every month. She needs to become familiar with the normal nodularity of her lactating breasts so that she can detect anything unusual on examination. Nodules that match in location in both breasts are almost always breast tissue. Nodules that increase and decrease in size are probably milk glands or ducts. Because lactating breasts are very dense, mammography is of limited diagnostic value. Should a suspicious nodule be discovered, a biopsy can usually be done without interrupting breastfeeding.

Effect of Menstruation. The return of menstrual periods varies among lactating women. The majority will resume menstruation by 6 months postpartum. Menstruation has no effect on breastfeeding. There are no hormonal effects on the infant, although some babies may seem fussy for the first day. The quality of milk is not affected (Lawrence, 1999).

Sexual Sensations. Some women experience rhythmic uterine contractions during breastfeeding. Such sensations are not unusual because uterine contractions and milk ejection are both triggered by oxytocin; but they may be disturbing to some mothers who perceive them to be similar to orgasm.

Breastfeeding and Contraception. Although breastfeeding confers a period of infertility, it is not considered an effective method of contraception. Breastfeeding delays the return of ovulation and menstruation; however, ovulation may occur before the first menstrual period after birth. Thus the breastfeeding woman who is relying on the lactational amenorrhea (LAM) method of birth control needs to be knowledgeable about ways to determine when ovulation occurs (i.e., basal body temperature, presence of cervical mucus, and cervical position). Hormonal contraceptives, including pills, injectables, and im-

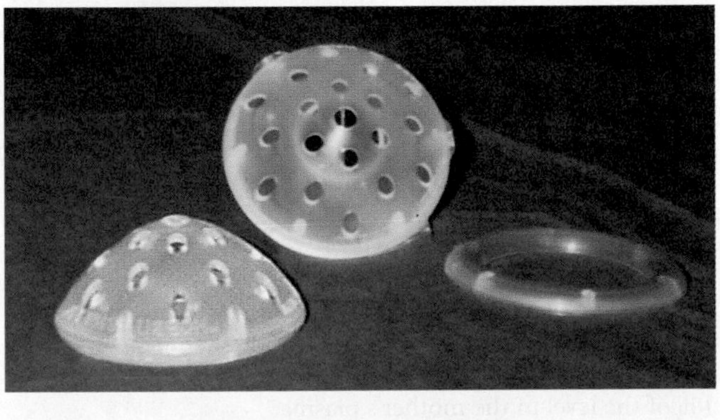

FIG. 26-12 • Breast shells.

plants, may cause a decrease in the milk supply and are best avoided during the first 6 weeks postpartum. Oral contraceptives containing estrogen are not recommended for breastfeeding mothers. Progestin-only birth control pills are less likely to interfere with the milk supply. Some mothers find that the progestin-only injection (Depo-Provera) or the implantable Norplant interferes with milk production, although others notice no alteration in the milk supply. Nonhormonal contraceptive methods (e.g. foam, condoms, nonhormonal intrauterine device [IUD], natural family planning, or sterilization) are less likely to have a detrimental effect on breastfeeding (Kelsey, 1996).

Breastfeeding During Pregnancy. It is possible for a breastfeeding woman to conceive and continue breastfeeding throughout the subsequent pregnancy if there are no medical contraindications (e.g., risk of preterm labor). When the second baby is born, colostrum is produced. The practice of breastfeeding a newborn and an older child is called tandem nursing. The nurse should remind the mother to always feed the newborn first to ensure that the newborn is receiving adequate nutrition. The supply-meets-demand principle works just as with breastfeeding multiple babies.

Diabetic Mother. The diabetic mother is encouraged to breastfeed. In addition to benefits for the infant and maternal satisfaction, breastfeeding has an antidiabetogenic effect. Blood glucose levels and insulin requirements are lower because of the carbohydrate used in milk production. During lactation, the diabetic woman may be able to eat more food and still take less insulin. However, insulin dosage must be adjusted as the baby is weaned. Some diabetic women are at increased risk for sore nipples caused by monilial infections and may have an increased risk for mastitis (Lawrence, 1999).

Drugs and Breastfeeding. Although there is much concern about the compatibility of drugs and breastfeeding, there are in fact few drugs that are contraindicated during lactation (Appendix A). Considerations in evaluating the safety of a specific medication during breastfeeding include the pharmacokinetics of the drug in the maternal system, as well as the absorption, metabolism, distribution, storage, and excretion in the infant. The gestational and chronological age of the infant, body weight, and breastfeeding pattern are also considered (Lawrence, 1997). Most medications do not cause problems for the infant, but breastfeeding mothers should be cautioned about taking any but essential ones. In certain instances (e.g., radioactive diagnostic agents) the mother is instructed to pump her breasts and discard the pumped milk until the drug has cleared her body.

Smoking may impair milk production; it also exposes the infant to the risks of secondhand smoke. Mothers who continue to smoke tobacco when lactating should be advised not to smoke within 2 hours before breastfeeding and to never smoke in the same room with the infant (Lawrence, 1997). If a mother chooses to consume alcohol, she should be advised to minimize its effects by having only one drink and consuming it immediately after a feeding. Alcoholic beverages may impair the milk ejection reflex. The mother who is pumping for a preterm or sick infant should avoid alcohol until her baby is healthy.

Coffee intake may lead to a reduced iron concentration in milk, and consequently contibute to the development of anemia in the infant. The caffeine concentration in milk is only about 1% of the level in the mother's plasma.

The infant's immature renal system limits the ability to excrete the caffeine; caffeine accumulates in the infant's system and can cause irritability and poor sleeping patterns. Some infants are sensitive to even small amounts of caffeine; mothers of such infants should limit caffeine intake. Caffeine is found in coffee, tea, chocolate, and many soft drinks (Lawrence, 1999).

Herbs and herbal teas are becoming more widely used during lactation. Although some are considered safe, others contain pharmacologically active compounds that may have detrimental effects. A thorough history should include the composition of any herbal remedies. Each remedy should then be evaluated for its compatibility with breastfeeding. A regional poison control center may provide information on the active properties of herbs (Lawrence, 1997).

Environmental Contaminants. Except under unusual circumstances, breastfeeding is not contraindicated because of exposure to environmental contaminants such as DDT (an insecticide) and tetrachloroethylene (used in dry cleaning) (Lawrence, 1997).

Special Considerations. The breastfeeding mother may experience some common problems. In the majority of cases, these complications are preventable if the mother receives appropriate education about breastfeeding. Early recognition and resolution of these problems is important to prevent interruption of breastfeeding and to promote the mother's comfort and sense of well-being. Emotional support provided by the nurse or lactation consultant is essential to help allay the mother's frustration and anxiety and to prevent early cessation of breastfeeding.

Engorgement. Engorgement is a common response of the breasts to the sudden change in hormones and the presence of increased volume of milk. It usually occurs on the third to fifth day postpartum when the "milk comes in" and lasts about 24 hours. Blood supply to the breasts increases and causes swelling of tissues surrounding the milk ducts. The duct may be pinched shut, so that the milk does not flow. The breasts are firm, tender, swollen, hot, and may appear shiny and red. The tenderness and swelling extends into the axilla. The areolae are firm and the nipples may flatten making it difficult for the baby to latch on. Because back pressure on full milk glands inhibits milk production, if milk is not removed from the breasts, the milk supply may diminish.

When engorgement occurs, the nurse should assure the mother that this is a temporary condition usually resolved within 24 hours. The mother is instructed to feed every 2 hours, softening at least one breast, and pumping the other breast to soften. Pumping during engorgement will not cause a problematic increase in milk supply.

Because of the swelling of breast tissue surrounding the milk glands' ducts, ice packs are recommended in a 15 to 20 minutes on, 45 minutes off rotation between feedings. The ice packs should cover both breasts. Large bags of frozen peas or corn make easy packs and can be refrozen between uses.

Raw cabbage leaves placed over the breasts in between feedings may help reduce the swelling (Roberts, 1995). The mother washes the cabbage leaves and places them in her freezer until they are cold, then places them over her breasts. The leaves are replaced when they begin to wilt. Although the exact mechanism of action of cabbage leaves in treatment of engorgement is not understood, it is thought that continuous application might decrease milk supply. Raw cabbage leaves are often very effective for formula-feeding mothers who want their milk to "dry up."

Antiinflammatory medications such as ibuprofen may help reduce pain and swelling associated with engorgement. Mothers often have an elevated temperature and experience achiness in their breasts; ibuprofen can help remedy this.

Because heat increases blood flow, application of heat to an already congested breast is usually counterproductive. Occasionally, however, standing in a warm shower will start the milk leaking or the mother may be able to manually express enough milk to soften the areola enough for the baby to be able to latch on and feed.

Sore Nipples. Mild nipple discomfort at the beginning of feedings or mild nipple tenderness during the first few days of breastfeeding is common. Severe soreness and abraded, cracked, or bleeding nipples are not normal and most often result from poor positioning, incorrect latch-on, improper suck, or a monilial infection. Many women expect breastfeeding to be painful based on stories they have heard from family and friends, however, breastfeeding is not supposed to be painful. Limiting the time at the breast will not prevent sore nipples; the key to preventing sore nipples is correct breastfeeding technique.

For the first few days after birth, the mother may experience some tenderness with the infant's initial sucks. This should quickly dissipate as the milk begins to flow and acts as a lubricant. To make the initial sucks less painful, the mother can express a few drops of milk to moisten the nipple and areola before latch-on. The mother should ensure that the baby is well-supported, is in straight body alignment, and has no pressure on the back of her or his head. The baby's nose, cheeks, and chin should be touching the breast, and the mother should be supporting the breast with her hand during the early feedings. The nurse helps to reposition as necessary to try to resolve the nipple discomfort.

If the mother reports a pinching sensation of the nipple as the baby sucks, it may be helpful to gently pull down on the side of the baby's jaw while he or she is sucking to increase the amount of breast tissue in the baby's mouth. If the nipple pain continues, the mother needs to remove the baby from the breast, breaking suction with her finger in the baby's mouth. She then attempts latch-on again, making sure the baby's mouth is open wide before the baby is pulled quickly to the breast (see Fig. 26-5).

The infant's suck can be assessed by the nurse or lactation consultant by inserting a clean gloved finger in the baby's mouth and stimulating the baby to suck. If the baby is not extruding his tongue over the lower gum, and the mother reports pain or pinching with sucking, the baby may have a short frenulum (commonly referred to as being "tongue-tied"). Sometimes this is corrected surgically to free the tongue for less painful, more effective breastfeeding.

The treatment for sore nipples is first to correct the cause. Once the problem is identified and corrected, sore nipples should heal within a few days, even though the baby continues to breastfeed regularly.

When sore nipples occur, it is more comfortable to start the feeding on the least sore nipple. Applying ice to the nipple for 2 to 3 minutes provides a numbing effect that increases comfort with latch-on. After feeding, the nipples are wiped with water to remove the baby's saliva. A few drops of milk can be expressed, rubbed into the sore area, and allowed to air dry. It is usually soothing to apply a cooled, steeped caffeinated tea bag to sore nipples (tannic acid may help promote healing). The tea bag is "dabbed" on the nipples, and should not be left in place for longer than 1 to 2 minutes. Warm water compresses may also be comforting (Lavergne, 1997).

If nipples are extremely sore or damaged and the mother cannot tolerate breastfeeding, she may be advised to use an electric breast pump for 24 to 48 hours to allow the nipples to begin healing before resuming breastfeeding. It is important that the mother use a pump that will effectively empty the breasts.

Sore nipples should be open to air as much as possible. Breast shells worn inside the bra allow for air to circulate while keeping clothing off sore nipples.

Flexible nipple shields have been marketed as a treatment for sore nipples; however, they do not protect the nipples and can actually chafe the nipple as the infant sucks. There is also danger of the baby not receiving adequate milk flow through the shield because it is difficult for most infants to get far enough back on the breast to adequately compress the lactiferous sinuses and get the milk to flow. There are special situations in which nipple shields are useful; however, they should be used only by trained lactation consultants who closely monitor the infant's intake of milk and growth.

Monilial Infections. Sore nipples that occur after the newborn period are often due to a monilial (yeast) infection. The mother usually reports severe nipple pain and tenderness, burning or stinging, and may have sharp, shooting, burning pains in the breasts during and after feedings. The nipples appear somewhat pink and shiny or may be scaly or flaky; there may be a visible rash, small blisters, or thrush. Most often, the pain is out of proportion to the appearance of the nipple. Yeast infections of the nipples and breast can be excruciatingly painful and can lead to early cessation of breastfeeding if not recognized and treated promptly.

Babies may or may not exhibit symptoms of monilial infection. Oral thrush and a red, raised diaper rash are common indications of a yeast infection. An affected infant is often very fussy and gassy. When feeding, the baby is likely to pull off the breast soon after starting to feed, crying with apparent pain. The infant may be biting or gumming at the breast.

The most common predisposing factors for yeast infections of the breast include previous antibiotic use, vaginal yeast infections, and nipple damage.

Mothers and babies must be treated simultaneously, even if the infant has no visible signs of infection. Treatment for mother is typically an antifungal cream applied to the nipples after feedings. Most pediatricians prescribe an oral antifungal medication, such as Nystatin, for infants. Treatment should

Critical Thinking

SORE NIPPLES IN BREASTFEEDING MOTHER

Role play how you could determine whether a mother's telephone call for help with sore nipples requires teaching about positioning and correct latch-on or if she might have a monilial infection on her nipples. What specific questions would you ask? To whom might you refer her?

continue for at least 7 days after symptoms begin to improve. Careful handwashing is essential to prevent the spread of yeast.

Plugged Milk Ducts. A milk duct may become plugged or clogged, causing an area of the breast to become swollen and tender. This area typically does not empty or soften with feeding or pumping. There may also be a small white pearl on the tip of the nipple; this is the curd of milk blocking the flow. The mother is afebrile and has no generalized symptoms.

Plugged ducts are most often the result of inadequate emptying of the breast. This may be due to clothing that is too tight, a poorly fitting or underwire bra, or always using the same position for feeding. Application of warm compresses to the affected area and to the nipple before feeding helps promote emptying of the breast and release of the plug. (A disposable diaper filled with warm water makes an easy compress.)

Frequent feeding is recommended, with the baby beginning the feeding on the affected side to foster more complete emptying. The mother is advised to massage the affected area while the baby nurses or while she is pumping. Varying feeding positions and feeding without wearing a bra may be useful in resolving a plugged duct.

If the mother develops fever or flu-like symptoms, she may have developed mastitis and should notify her health care provider. Plugged milk ducts do not necessarily cause mastitis, but milk stasis may increase susceptibility to breast infection.

Mastitis. A breast infection or mastitis is characterized by the sudden onset of flu-like symptoms, including fever, chills, body aches, and headache. (Flu-like symptoms in a breastfeeding mother should be considered indicative of mastitis, until proven otherwise.) There is localized breast pain and tenderness and a hot, reddened area on the breast, often resembling the shape of a pie wedge. Mastitis most commonly occurs in the upper outer quadrant of the breast; it may affect one or both breasts.

There are certain factors that may predispose a woman to mastitis. Inadequate emptying of the breasts is common, related to engorgement, plugged ducts, a sudden decrease in the number of feedings, abrupt weaning, or wearing underwire bras. Sore, cracked nipples may lead to mastitis by providing a portal of entry for causative organism (*Staphylococcus, Streptococcus,* and *E. coli* are most common). Stress and fatigue, ill family members, breast trauma, and poor maternal nutrition are also predisposing factors for mastitis (Fetherston, 1998).

Breastfeeding mothers should be taught the signs of mastitis before they are discharged from the hospital, and they need to know to call the health care provider promptly if the symptoms occur. Treatment includes antibiotics such as cephalexin or dicloxacillin, and analgesics/antipyretic medications such as ibuprofen. Rest is extremely important; the mother is advised to sleep whenever the baby sleeps. The mother should feed the baby or pump frequently, striving to adequately empty the affected side. Warm compresses to the breast before feeding or pumping may be useful. Adequate fluid intake and a balanced diet are important for the mother with mastitis.

Complications of mastitis include breast abscess, chronic mastitis, or fungal infections of the breast. Most complications can be prevented by early recognition and treatment.

Hepatitis C. The infection rate of infants born to mothers with hepatitis C is 4% in both bottle-fed and breastfed infants. Therefore, there is no increased risk of transmission with breastfeeding (ACOG, 1999).

Role of the Nurse in Promoting Successful Lactation

Nurses play a major role in breastfeeding education and support for new parents. Nurses often work with lactation consultants in hospitals, physicians' offices, or community settings. Although the vast majority are registered nurses, lactation consultants come from a variety of educational backgrounds such as nutrition, physical and occupational therapy, home economics, psychology, social work, education, or the basic sciences. Lactation consultants have had specialized postbaccalaureate education, training, and clinical experience working with breastfeeding mothers, and have passed a certifying examination that requires meeting defined academic and clinical experience criteria.

Nurses in prenatal settings can educate the mother and her partner about the advantages of breastfeeding and explore reasons why they may prefer bottle-feeding. They can provide expectant parents with current reading materials and information about prenatal classes. At each encounter, the nurse can answer questions and provide additional information as needed.

Assessment of the mother's breasts and nipples during pregnancy is important. Flat or inverted nipples are identified. The mother may be offered breast shells (see Fig. 26-12) to wear during the last trimester of pregnancy to encourage eversion of the nipples, although antepartal use may be ineffective. These breast shells can also be worn postpartum between feedings.

The nurse should determine if the woman has had any breast surgery. Breast reduction or augmentation may interfere with the ability to produce milk and transfer it successfully to the baby.

There is no special nipple preparation necessary during pregnancy. Efforts to "toughen" the nipples by pulling on them or rubbing them with a rough towel are to be avoided. Such stimulation can cause release of oxytocin and result in preterm labor; or damage the outer layer of protective skin cells, which may increase the risk of sore nipples.

In the immediate postpartum period, the nurse is instrumental in helping the mother initiate breastfeeding as soon as possible after birth. Encouraging parents to keep the baby in the mother's room (rooming in) allows the opportunity for the mother to learn to recognize feeding cues and to feed the baby when these cues are present. The nurse provides help with positioning and latch-on until the mother can accomplish this independently. Explanations are given early regarding frequency and duration of feedings, how to wake a sleepy baby, and how to determine if the baby is getting enough milk. Information about the transition to mature milk (milk coming in) and how to prevent or deal with engorgement is needed. The mother is informed about the prevention and treatment of sore nipples and about signs of mastitis (including the importance of contacting the primary health care provider if these occur).

Parents often expect that because breastfeeding is "natural" that it will come naturally for both mother and baby. This misconception needs to be clarified early so that parents may view breastfeeding as a learning process and not have unrealistic expectations. All health care providers who are knowledgeable about breastfeeding can offer needed support and encouragement to parents, helping to instill a sense of confidence.

Follow-Up After Hospital Discharge. Problems with sore nipples, engorgement, and jaundice are likely to occur after discharge. Thus it is the role of the hospital nurse to educate and prepare the mother for problems she may encounter once she is home. It is critical that the mother be given a list of resources for help with breastfeeding concerns, and that she realizes when to call for assistance. Community resources for breastfeeding mothers include lactation consultants in hospitals, physicians' offices, or in private practice; nurses in pediatric or obstetric offices; support groups such as La Leche League; and peer counseling programs (such as those offered through WIC).

Telephone follow-up by hospital or office nurses within the first day or two after discharge can provide a means to identify any problems and offer needed advice and support. The AAP recommends that infants discharged before 48 hours of age be seen by a health care provider within 48 hours and have an office visit within 7 days after discharge. In some settings and circumstances, home care follow-up is available for mothers after hospital discharge.

➤ Evaluation

Evaluation is based on the expected outcomes, and the plan of care is revised as needed based on the evaluation (Nursing Care Plan).

FORMULA-FEEDING

Reasons for Formula-Feeding

The decision to feed a baby infant formula may be the result of the mother's or partner's personal preference, the influence of other significant family members, or simply a lack of familiarity with breastfeeding. Occasionally there is no other option: the mother may have extensive breast scarring or may have had a bilateral mastectomy; the mother may be taking medications that preclude breastfeeding; or the baby may be adopted. Some mothers are able to induce lactation for an adopted baby. Rarely, an infant may have galactosemia and must be fed a lactose-free formula.

Infant formula may be used to supplement breastfeeding if the mother's milk supply is inadequate. It may also be fed to the baby if the mother will be away and wishes to leave a bottle of formula instead of expressed breast milk.

Formula-feeding is also recommended for mothers who are infected with the human immunodeficiency virus (HIV).

Parent Education

Inexperienced mothers and fathers who are formula-feeding their infants usually need teaching, counseling, and support. They may need assistance with the feeding process and with any problems they may experience. Some parents who are formula-feeding express concern that the baby will suffer as a result of their decision. Emphasis on the beneficial use of feeding times for close contact and socializing with the infant can help relieve some of this concern.

Readiness for Feeding. The first feeding of formula is ideally given after the initial transition to extrauterine life is made. Feeding readiness cues include such things as stability of vital signs, presence of bowel sounds, an active sucking reflex, and those cues described earlier for breastfed babies. Before the first formula feeding, some institutions have a policy of offering sips of water to the newborn to assess patency of the GI tract and absence of tracheoesophageal fistula. If the infant sucks and swallows the water without difficulty, formula is then offered.

Feeding Patterns. Typically a newborn at first will drink 10 to 15 ml of formula at a feeding. Intake gradually increases during the first week of life. Most babies are drinking 90 to 150 ml at a feeding by the end of the second week, or sooner. Generally a baby who weighs less than 4.5 kg takes in about 840 ml of formula every 24 hours after the newborn period. A baby who weighs more than 4.5 kg ingests about 960 ml in 24 hours.

The newborn infant should be fed at least every 3 to 4 hours, even if that requires waking the baby for the feedings. The infant showing an adequate weight gain can be allowed to sleep at night and fed only on awakening. Most newborns need 6 to 8 feedings in 24 hours, and the number of feedings decreases as

Nursing Care Plan — THE NEWBORN WITH INSUFFICIENT INTAKE OF NUTRIENTS

NURSING DIAGNOSIS **Ineffective breastfeeding related to knowledge deficit of mother as evidenced by ongoing incorrect latch-on technique**

EXPECTED OUTCOME Patient will express increased satisfaction with breastfeeding, and neonate will exhibit satisfaction of hunger and sucking needs.

Nursing Interventions/*Rationales*

Assess patient's knowledge and motivation for breastfeeding *to acknowledge patient's desire for effective outcome and provide starting point for teaching.*

Observe a breastfeeding session *to provide database for positive reinforcement and problem identification.*

Describe and demonstrate ways to stimulate the sucking reflex, various positions for breastfeeding, and the use of pillows during a session *to promote patient and neonatal comfort and effective latch-on.*

Monitor neonatal position of mouth on areola and position of head and body *to give positive reinforcement for correct latch-on position or to correct poor latch-on position.*

Teach patient ways to stimulate neonate to maintain an awake state by diapering, unwrapping, massaging, or burping *to complete a breastfeeding thoroughly and satisfactorily.*

Give patient information regarding lactation diet, expression of milk by hand or pump, and storage of expressed breast milk *to provide basic information.*

Make sure patient has written information on all aspects of breastfeeding *to reinforce verbal instructions and demonstrations.*

Refer to support group and lactation consultant if needed *to provide further information and group support.*

the infant matures. Usually by 3 to 4 weeks after birth a fairly predictable feeding pattern has developed. Scheduling feedings arbitrarily at predetermined intervals may not meet a baby's needs, but initiating feedings at convenient times often moves the baby's feedings to times that work for the family.

Mothers will usually notice an increase in the infant's appetite at the ages of 7 to 10 days, 3 weeks, 6 weeks, 3 months, and 6 months. These appetite spurts correspond to growth spurts. The amount of formula per feeding should be increased by about 30 ml at these times to meet the baby's needs.

Feeding Techniques. Parents who choose formula-feeding often need education regarding feeding techniques. Formula can be fed at room temperature or warmed. Formula should never be heated in a microwave oven. Microwaving does not heat evenly and can cause encapsulated boiling bubbles to form in the center of the liquid. This may not be detected when checking drops of milk for temperature. Babies have sustained severe burns to the mouth, throat, and upper GI tract as a result of microwaved milk (Lawrence, 1999). If it is warmed, the formula's temperature should be tested before it is given to the baby.

During feedings parents should be encouraged to sit comfortably, holding the infant closely in a semi-upright position. Feedings provide an opportunity to bond with the baby through touching, talking, singing, or reading to the infant. Parents should consider feedings as a time of peaceful relaxation with their baby (Figs. 26-13 and 26-14).

A bottle should never be propped with a pillow or other inanimate object and left with the infant. This practice may result in choking, and it deprives the infant of important interaction during feeding. Moreover, propping the bottle has been implicated in causing nursing bottle caries, or decay of the first teeth resulting from continuous bathing of the teeth with carbohydrate-containing fluid as the infant sporadically sucks the nipple.

The bottle should be held so that fluid fills the nipple and none of the air in the bottle is allowed to enter the nipple (Fig. 26-14). After the newborn period the infant who falls asleep, turns aside the head, or ceases to suck usually is signaling that enough formula has been taken. Parents should be taught to look for these cues and avoid overfeeding, which could contribute to obesity.

Most infants swallow air when fed from a bottle and should be given a chance to burp several times during a feeding (Fig. 26-15).

Bottles and Nipples. There are various brands and styles of bottles and nipples available to parents. Most babies will feed well with any bottle and nipple. It is important that the bottles and nipples be washed in warm, soapy water using a bottle and nipple brush to facilitate thorough cleansing. Careful rinsing is necessary. Boiling of bottles and nipples is not needed unless there is some question about the safety of the water supply.

Infant Formulas

Commercial Formulas. Because human milk is species-specific to meet the needs of the human infant, it is used as the standard for all infant formulas. Commercial infant formulas are designed to resemble human milk as closely as possible, although none has ever duplicated it.

Infants who are not breastfed should be given commercial formulas. If this is too expensive, the family would likely be eligible for services through the WIC program, which provides iron-fortified infant formula. Cow's milk is the basis for most infant formulas, although soy-based and other specialized formulas are available for the infant who cannot tolerate cow's milk.

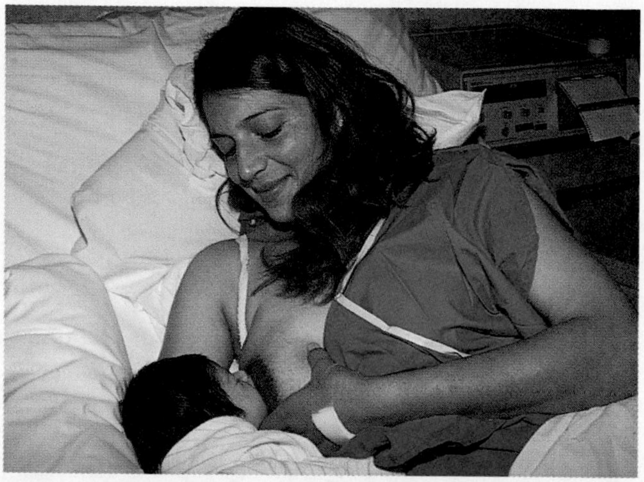

FIG. 26-13 • Mother and infant enjoying breastfeeding. (Courtesy Marjorie Pyle, RNC, Lifecircle, Costa Mesa, CA.)

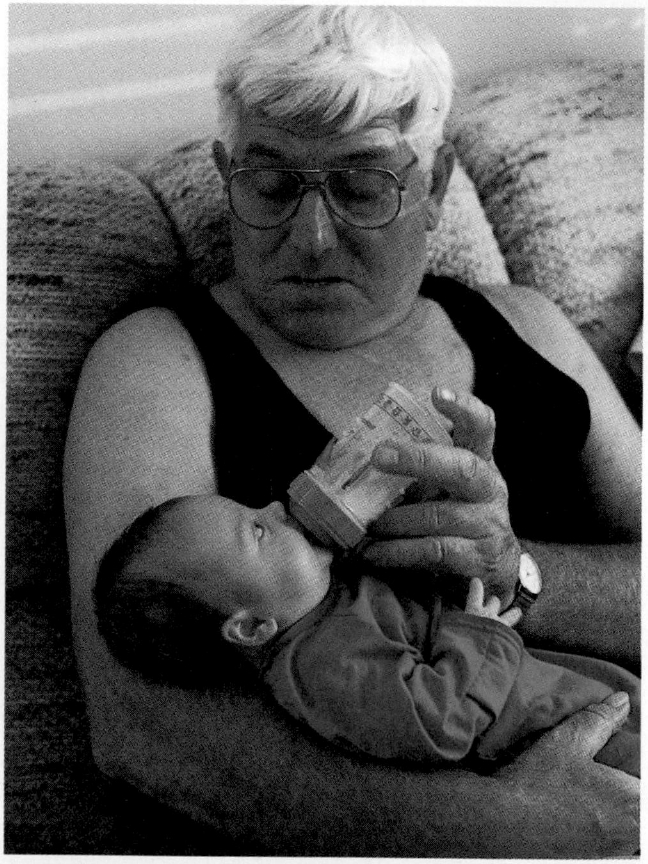

FIG. 26-14 • Grandfather feeding infant granddaughter. Note angle of bottle, which ensures milk covers nipple area. (Courtesy Kim Molloy, Knoxville, IA.)

Commercial formulas are available in three forms: powder, concentrate, and ready-to-feed. All are equivalent in nutritional content, but they vary considerably in price. Powdered formulas are least expensive and are convenient because they are lightweight and require no refrigeration before mixing with water. Concentrated liquid formula is more expensive than powder. It is diluted with water and can be stored in the refrigerator for 24 hours after opening. Ready-to-feed formula is most expensive but easiest to use. The desired amount is poured into the bottle. The opened can is safely refrigerated for 24 hours. This type of formula can also be purchased in individual disposable bottles for the most convenient feeding.

Special Formulas. Some infants have an allergic reaction to cow's milk formula. They may experience diarrhea, rash, colic, vomiting, and in extreme cases, fail to thrive. Some of these infants may be able to tolerate a soy milk formula; however, some are allergic to soy protein. If hypersensitivity to cow's milk protein is suspected, a hydrolyzed casein formula may be effective. However, these special formulas are very expensive. Some women may be able to begin breastfeeding or, in life-threatening cases, obtain human milk through a milk bank, at least temporarily.

Formula Preparation. The commercial infant formula must include label directions for preparation and use of the formula with pictures and symbols for the benefit of individuals who cannot read. Some manufacturers are translating the directions into languages such as Spanish, French, Vietnamese, Chinese, and Arabic to prevent misunderstanding and errors in formula preparation. It is important to impress on families that the proportions must not be altered—that is, neither diluted to extend the amount of formula nor concentrated to provide more calories.

Although manufacturers of commercial formulas include directions for preparing their products, the nurse should review formula preparation with the mother. It is especially important that formula be mixed properly. The newborn's kidneys are immature; giving the infant overly concentrated formula may provide protein and minerals in amounts that exceed the kidneys' excretory ability. In contrast, if the formula is diluted too much (sometimes done to save money), the infant does not consume sufficient calories and does not grow well.

Sterilization of formula rarely is recommended when families have access to a safe public water supply. Instead, formula is prepared with attention to cleanliness. When water from a private well is used, parents should be advised to contact the health department to have a chemical and bacteriologic analysis of the water done before using the water in formula preparation. The presence of nitrates, excess fluoride, or bacteria may be harmful to the infant.

Critical Thinking

BOTTLE-FEEDING MOTHER—SLOW WEIGHT GAIN

A mother brings her baby in for a 1-month well-baby examination. She mentions to you that her mother-in-law told her the baby looks "skinny," so she has been putting less water in the formula to increase the caloric intake of each feeding. Identify assessment data that must be collected to deal with this situation. Develop a plan of care for an infant whose weight gain is (1) within normal limits or (2) less than recommended.

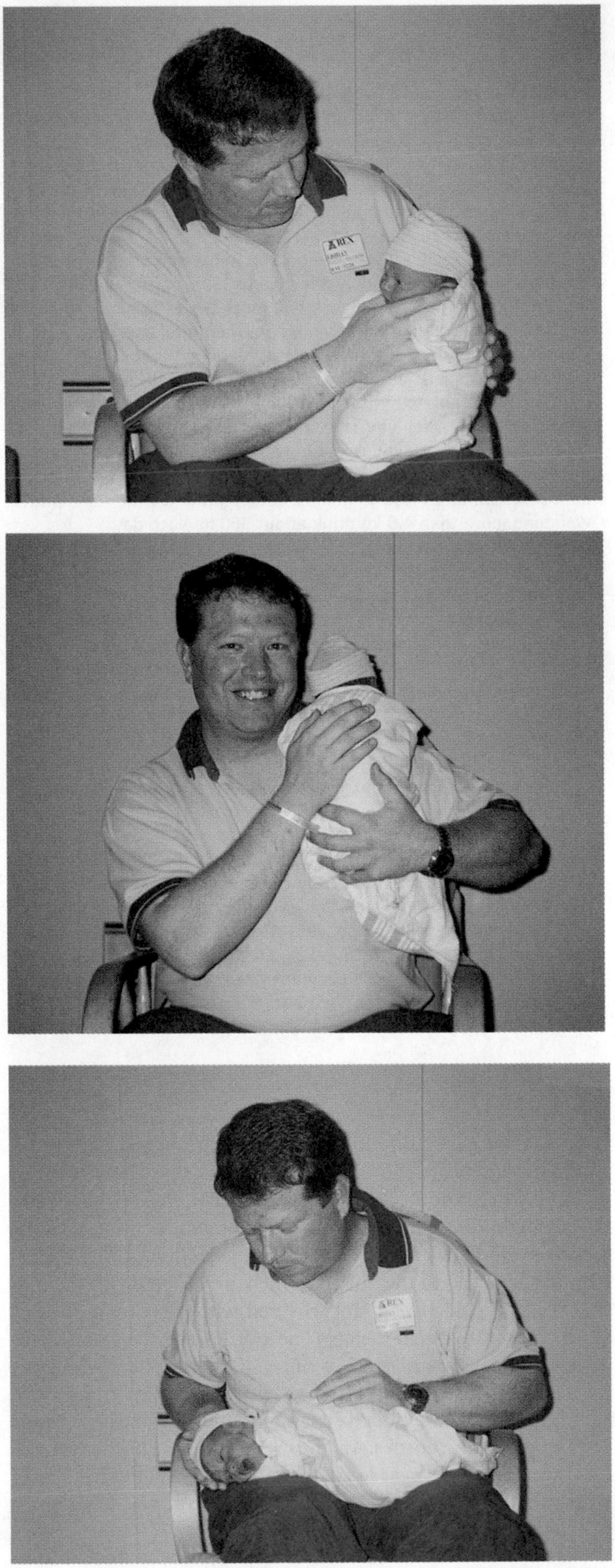

A

B

C

FIG. 26-15 • Positions for burping an infant. **A,** Sitting. **B,** On the shoulder. **C,** Across the lap.

Home Care

FORMULA PREPARATION AND FEEDING

Your newborn baby will be hungry about every 2½ to 3 hours, but sometimes may go 3 to 4 hours between feedings. The newborn should not go longer than 4 hours between feedings until a weight gain pattern is established—usually in about 2 weeks. Your baby needs to be awake before being fed. If your baby is sleepy, massage the baby's back and chest and talk to him or her.

Your baby's feedings will change a lot in the first week after birth. The first day, most babies only drink 7.5 to 15 ml of formula at a feeding. By the time they are a week old, most babies drink 30 to 60 ml at a feeding and then gradually increase their intake as they grow. If you do not use all of the formula at a feeding, throw away what is left because it spoils once it has mixed with the baby's saliva.

You may want to write down how many milliliters your baby drinks each day. When you take the baby in for a checkup, the physician or nurse will ask you about how much formula the baby drinks. By 1 week of age, most babies who weigh 3 to 4.5 kg are drinking about 840 ml in 24 hours. Smaller babies drink a little less. Babies weighing more than 4.5 kg drink about 960 ml each day.

To feed your baby, place the nipple in the baby's mouth on the tongue. It should touch the roof of the mouth to stimulate the baby's sucking reflex. Hold the bottle like a pencil. Keep the bottle tipped so that the nipple stays filled with milk and the baby does not suck in air.

Hold your baby close for feedings. This should be a pleasant time for social interaction and cuddling. Some newborns take longer to feed than others: be patient. It may be necessary to keep the baby awake and encourage continued sucking. Moving the nipple gently in the baby's mouth may stimulate more sucking.

Some newborns swallow air when sucking. Give your baby a chance to burp several times during early feedings. As your baby gets older and you get more experienced you will know when to stop for burping.

If your baby fusses or cries between feedings, check the diaper to see if he or she needs to be changed and see if the baby needs to be picked up and cuddled. If the baby continues to cry and acts hungry, then he or she needs to be fed. Babies do not get hungry on a schedule.

Place your baby on the right side after feedings so that air bubbles can come up easily. A rolled-up receiving blanket or small towel against the baby's back will keep him or her in the side-lying position. Some babies sleep better on their backs. To decrease the risk of SIDS, however, it is important not to put your baby to sleep stomach down.

The stools (bowel movements) of a formula-fed newborn are yellow and soft but formed. The baby will probably have a stool during or after each feeding in the first 2 weeks, but this will then gradually decrease to 1 or 2 stools each day.

Safety Tips

- Babies should be held and never left alone while feeding. Do not prop the bottle: the baby could inhale formula or choke on any that was spit up.
- Know how to use the bulb syringe in case your baby should choke.
- Drinking bottles of formula or juice while falling asleep can cause tooth decay (nursing bottle caries) in young children.

Formula Preparation

- Wash your hands and clean the bottle, nipple, and can opener carefully before preparing formula.
- If new nipples seem too hard, they can be softened by boiling them in water for 5 minutes before use.
- Read the label on the container of formula and mix it exactly according to the directions.
- Use tap water to mix concentrated or powdered formula unless directed otherwise by your baby's physician or nurse.
- Test the size of the nipple hole by holding a prepared bottle upside down. The formula should drip from the nipple. If it runs in a stream, the hole is too big and should not be used. If it has to be shaken for the formula to come out, the hole is too small. You can either buy a new nipple or enlarge the hole by boiling the nipple for 5 minutes with a sewing needle inserted in the hole.
- If a nipple collapses when your baby sucks, loosen the nipple ring a little to let in air.
- Opened cans of ready-to-feed or concentrated formula should be covered and refrigerated. Any unused portions must be discarded after 48 hours.
- Unopened bottles or cans of formula can be stored at room temperature.
- If the formula is refrigerated, warm it by placing the bottle in a pan of hot water. Never use a microwave to warm any food to be given to a baby. Test the temperature of the formula by letting a few drops fall on the inside of your wrist. If the formula feels comfortably warm to you, it is the correct temperature.

If the sanitary conditions in the home appear unsafe, it would be better to recommend the use of ready-to-feed formula or to teach the mother to sterilize the formula. The two traditional methods for sterilization are terminal heating and the aseptic method. In the terminal heating method, the prepared formula is placed in the bottles, which are topped with the nipples placed upside down and covered with the caps, and then sealed loosely with the rings. The bottles are then boiled together in a water bath for 25 minutes. In the aseptic method, the bottles, rings, caps, nipples, and any other necessary equipment, such as a funnel, are boiled separately, after which the formula is poured into the bottles. Any formula left in the bottle after the feeding should be discarded because the baby's saliva has mixed with it. (Instructions for formula preparation and feeding are provided in the Home Care box.)

Vitamin and Mineral Supplementation. Commercial iron-fortified formula contains all the nutrients needed by the infant for the first 6 months of life. After 6 months the only mineral supplementation required is 0.25 mg of fluoride per day if the local water supply is not fluoridated (AAP, 1997).

Weaning. The bottle-fed baby will gradually learn to use a cup, and the parents will find that they are preparing fewer bottles. Commonly the feeding before bedtime is the last one to remain. Babies have a strong need to suck, and the baby who has had the bottle taken away too early or abruptly will compensate with nonnutritive sucking on his or her fingers, thumb, a pacifier, or even his or her own tongue. Weaning from a bottle should therefore be done gradually because the baby has learned to rely on the comfort that sucking provides.

Key Points

- Human milk is species-specific and is the recommended form of nutrition for infant. It provides immunologic protection against many infections and diseases.
- Breast milk changes in composition with each stage of lactation, during each feeding, and as the infant grows.

- During the prenatal period, parents should be informed of the benefits of breastfeeding for infants, mothers, families, and society.
- Infants should be breastfed as soon as possible after birth and at least 8 to 12 times per day thereafter.
- There are objective, measurable indicators that the infant is breastfeeding effectively.
- Breast milk production is based on a supply-meets-demand principle; the more the infant nurses, the greater the milk supply.
- Commercial infant formulas provide satisfactory nutrition for most infants.
- All infants should be held for feedings.
- Parents should be instructed about the types of commercial infant formulas, proper preparation for feeding, and correct feeding technique.
- Unmodified cow's milk is not appropriate for feeding the infant during the first year of life.

References

Aarts C et al: Breastfeeding patterns in relation to thumb sucking and pacifier use, *Pediatrics* 104(4):E50, 1999.

American Academy of Pediatrics (AAP): *Pediatric nutrition handbook,* ed 4, Elk Grove Village, IL, 1998, American Academy of Pediatrics.

American Academy of Pediatrics Work Group on Breastfeeding: Breastfeeding and the use of human milk, *Pediatrics* 100(6):1035-1039, 1997.

American College of Obstetricians and Gynecologists (ACOG): *ACOG recommends scheduled C-sections for HIV+ women* [Press release, 1999, July 31]. Available online at: http://www.acog.com/from-home/publications/press-releases/nr7 31-99-2.htm.

Arlotti J et al: Breastfeeding among low-income women with and without peer support, *J Community Health Nurs* 15(3):163-178, 1998.

Arnold L, Tully M: *Guidelines for the establishment and operation of a donor human milk bank,* ed 6, West Hartford, CT, 1996, Human Milk Banking Association of North America.

Barnard J: Gastrointestinal disorders due to cow's milk consumption, *Pediatr Ann* 26(4):244-250, 1997.

Bar-Yam N, Darby L: Fathers and breastfeeding: a review of the literature, *J Hum Lact* 13(1):45-50, 1997.

Behrman R, Kliegman R, Arvin A, editors: *Nelson's textbook of pediatrics,* ed 15, Philadelphia, 1996, WB Saunders.

Brent N et al: Sore nipples in breastfeeding women: a clinical trial of wound dressings vs. conventional care, *Arch Pediatr Adolesc Med* 152(11):1077-1082, 1998.

Brown L et al: Use of human milk for low-birth-weight infants, *Online J Know Synth Nurs* 3(27):1-9, 1996.

Choudhry U: Traditional practices of women from India: pregnancy, childbirth, and newborn care, *J Obstet Gynecol Neonatal Nurs* 26(5):533-539, 1997.

Cushing A et al: Breastfeeding reduces risk of respiratory illness in infants, *Am J Epidemiol* 147(9):863-870, 1998.

Davis M: Review of the evidence for an association between infant feeding and childhood cancer, *Int J Cancer* (Suppl)11: 29-33, 1998.

Department of Health and Human Services: *Healthy People 2010,* conference edition, vol 2, Objectives for improving health, Washington, DC, 2000, Author. Available online at: http://www.health.gov/healthypeople/document/default.htm.

Dewey K, Heinig M, Nommsen L: Maternal weight-loss patterns during prolonged lactation, *Am J Clin Nutr* 58:162-166, 1993.

Eisman J: Relevance of pregnancy and lactation to osteoporosis, *Clin Perinatol* 25(2):303-326, 1998.

Enger S et al: Breastfeeding experience and breast cancer risk among postmenopausal women, *Cancer Epidemiol Biomarkers Prev* 7(5):365-369, 1998.

Fetherston C: Risk factors for lactational mastitis, *J Hum Lact* 14(2):101-109, 1998.

Ford R et al: Breastfeeding and the risk of sudden infant death syndrome, *Int J Epidemiol* 22(5):885-890, 1993.

Gerstein H: Cow's milk exposure and type I diabetes mellitus, *Diabetes Care* 17:13-19, 1994.

Halken S, Host A: Prevention of allergic disease: exposure to food allergens and dietetic intervention, *Pediatr Allergy Immunol* 7(9 suppl):102-107, 1996.

Horwood L, Fergusson D: Breastfeeding and later cognitive and academic outcomes, *Pediatrics* 101(1):E9, 1998.

Howard C et al: The effects of early pacifier use on breastfeeding duration, *Pediatrics* 103(3):E33, 1999.

Huml S: Cracked nipples in the breastfeeding mother, *Adv Nurs Pract:* 1, April 1995.

Kelsey J: Hormonal contraception and lactation, *J Hum Lact* 12(4):315-318, 1996.

Lavergne N: Does application of tea bags to sore nipples while breastfeeding provide effective relief? *J Obstet Gynecol Neonatal Nurs* 26(1):53-58, 1997.

Lawrence R: A review of the medical benefits and contraindications to breastfeeding in the United States, *Maternal and child health technical information bulletin,* Arlington, VA, 1997, National Center for Education in Maternal and Child Health.

Lawrence R: *Breastfeeding: A guide for the medical profession,* ed 5, St Louis, 1999, Mosby.

Lopez-Alarcon M, Villalpando S, Fajardo A: Breastfeeding lowers the frequency and duration of acute respiratory infections and diarrhea in infants under six months of age, *J Nutr* 127(3):436-443, 1997.

Meier P: *Professional guide to breastfeeding premature infants,* Columbus, OH, 1997, Ross Products Division, Abbott Laboratories.

Meier P, Brown L: State of the science: breastfeeding for mothers and low-birth-weight infants, *Nurs Clin North Am* 31(2):351-365, 1996.

Morse J, Jehle C, Gamble D: Initiating breastfeeding: a world survey of the timing of postpartum breastfeeding, *Int J Nurs Stud* 27(3):303-313, 1990.

Riordan J: The cost of not breastfeeding: a commentary, *J Hum Lact* 13(2):93-97, 1997.

Roberts K: A comparison of chilled cabbage leaves and chilled gel-paks in reducing breast engorgement, *J Hum Lact* 11(1):17-20, 1995.

Rosenblatt K, Thomas D: Prolonged lactation and endometrial cancer. WHO collaborative study of neoplasia and steroid contraceptives, *Int J Epidemiol* 24:499-503, 1995.

Scariati P, Grummer-Strawn L, Fein S: A longitudinal analysis of infant morbidity and the extent of breastfeeding in the United States, *Pediatrics* 99(6):E5, 1997.

Weissinger D: A breastfeeding teaching tool using a sandwich analogy for latch-on, *J Hum Lact* 14(1):51-56, 1998.

CHAPTER 27

Infants with Gestational Age–Related Problems

http://www.harcourthealth.com/MERLIN/Wong/maternal/

Learning Objectives

On completion of this chapter the reader will be able to:

- Compare and contrast the characteristics of preterm, term, postterm, and postmature neonates.
- Discuss respiratory distress syndrome and the approach to treatment.
- Compare methods of oxygen therapy.
- Describe nursing interventions for nutritional care of the preterm infant.
- Discuss the pathophysiology of retinopathy of prematurity and bronchopulmonary dysplasia, and identify risk factors that predispose preterm infants to these problems.
- List the signs and symptoms of perinatal asphyxia.
- Describe meconium aspiration syndrome.
- Describe assessment of infants for birth trauma and for sequelae of a diabetic pregnancy.
- Plan developmentally appropriate care.
- Examine the needs of parents of high risk infants.
- Evaluate a neonatal transport plan.

Modern technology and expert nursing care have made important contributions to improving the health and overall survival of high risk infants. However, infants who are born considerably before term and survive are particularly susceptible to the development of sequelae related to their preterm birth. These conditions include necrotizing enterocolitis, bronchopulmonary dysplasia, intraventricular and periventricular hemorrhage, and retinopathy of prematurity. The focus of this chapter is on care of the preterm infant, but care of other high risk infants with gestational age-related problems is also discussed. Care of infants of mothers with diabetes is included because these infants experience many of the same problems.

High risk infants are most often classified according to birth weight, gestational age, and predominant pathophysiologic problems (Box 27-1). Intrauterine growth rates are not the same for all infants, and other factors (e.g., heredity, placental insufficiency, and maternal disease) influence intrauterine growth and birth weight. The classification system in the box encompasses birth weight and gestational age.

PRETERM INFANTS

Preterm infants, those born before 37 weeks of gestation, are at risk because their organ systems are immature and they lack adequate reserves of bodily nutrients. Preterm birth is responsible for almost two thirds of infant deaths. The cause of preterm birth is largely unknown; however, the incidence of preterm birth is highest among low socioeconomic groups. This is likely a result of the lack of comprehensive prenatal health care. Other factors found to be associated with preterm birth include preeclampsia, maternal infection, multifetal pregnancy, incompetent cervix, and placental accidents.

The potential problems and care needs of the preterm infant weighing 2000 g differ from those of the term, postterm, or postmature infant of equal weight. The presence of physiologic disorders and anomalies affects the infant's response to treatment. In general, the closer infants are to term, the easier their adjustment to the external environment.

There are varying opinions about the practical and ethical dimensions of resuscitation of extremely-low-birth-weight infants (those infants whose birth weight is 1000 g or less). Ethical issues associated with resuscitation of these infants include whether to resuscitate, who should make that decision, whether the cost of resuscitation is justified, and if the bene-

Box 27-1

Classification of High Risk Infants

CLASSIFICATION ACCORDING TO SIZE

Low-birth-weight (LBW) infant—An infant whose birth weight is less than 2500 g regardless of gestational age

Very-very-low-birth-weight (VVLBW) or extremely-low-birth-weight (ELBW) infant—An infant whose birth weight is less than 1000 g

Very-low-birth-weight (VLBW) infant—An infant whose birth weight is less than 1500 g

Moderately-low-birth-weight (MLBW)—An infant whose birth weight is 1501 to 2500 g

Appropriate-for-gestational-age (AGA) infant—An infant whose weight falls between the 10th and 90th percentiles on intrauterine growth curves

Small-for-date (SFD) or small-for-gestational-age (SGA) infant—An infant whose rate of intrauterine growth was slowed and whose birth weight falls below the 10th percentile on intrauterine growth curves

Intrauterine growth restriction (IUGR)—Found in infants whose intrauterine growth is restricted (sometimes used as a more descriptive term for the SGA infant)

Large-for-gestational-age (LGA) infant—An infant whose birth weight is above the 90th percentile on intrauterine growth charts

CLASSIFICATION ACCORDING TO GESTATIONAL AGE

Premature (preterm) infant—An infant born before completion of 37 weeks of gestation, regardless of birth weight

Full term infant—An infant born between the beginning of 38 weeks and the completion of 42 weeks of gestation, regardless of birth weight

Postmature (postterm) infant—An infant born after 42 weeks of gestational age, regardless of birth weight

fits of technology outweigh the burdens in relation to quality of life.

Care Management

➤ Assessment

For the high risk infant, an accurate assessment of gestational age (see Chapter 25) is critical in helping the nurse identify the potential problems the newborn is likely to experience. The response of the preterm or postterm infant to extrauterine life is different from that of the term infant. By understanding the physiologic basis of these differences, the nurse can assess these infants, determine the response of the preterm or postterm infant, and discern which of the potential problems are most likely to occur.

Respiratory Function. Pink color, adequate tissue perfusion, and respiratory patterns are quickly established in nonstressed newborns, and they are soon vigorous and show appropriate muscle tone. However, infants with a potential for respiratory depression at birth because of asphyxia, prematurity, or congenital malformations may exhibit cyanosis, decreased tissue perfusion, retractions, nasal flaring, or a combination of these problems.

The preterm infant is likely to have difficulty making the pulmonary transition from intrauterine to extrauterine life. Numerous problems may affect the respiratory systems of preterm infants and may include the following:

- Decreased number of functional alveoli
- Deficient surfactant levels
- Smaller lumen in the respiratory system
- Greater collapsibility or obstruction of respiratory passages
- Insufficient calcification of the bony thorax
- Weak or absent gag reflex
- Immature and friable capillaries in the lungs
- Greater distance between functional alveoli and capillary bed

In combination, these deficits severely hinder the infant's respiratory efforts and can produce respiratory distress or apnea. Early signs of respiratory distress include flaring of the nares and an expiratory grunt. Depending on the cause, retractions may begin as subcostal, suprasternal, or clavicular retractions. If the infant shows increasing respiratory effort (e.g., seesaw breathing patterns, retraction, flaring of the nares, expiratory grunts, and apneic spells) this indicates deepening distress. A compromised infant's color progresses from pink to circumoral cyanosis and then to generalized cyanosis. Acrocyanosis deepens. (Acrocyanosis is a normal finding in the neonate, but central cyanosis indicates the existence of an underlying problem.)

Periodic breathing is a respiratory pattern commonly seen in premature infants. Such infants exhibit 5- to 10-second respiratory pauses followed by 10 to 15 seconds of compensatory rapid respirations. Such periodic breathing should not be confused with apnea, which is a 15- to 20-second cessation of respirations. The nurse needs to be prepared to provide oxygen and ventilation as necessary (Cloherty and Stark, 1997).

Cardiovascular Function. Evaluation of heart rate and rhythm, skin color, blood pressure, perfusion, pulses, oxygen saturation, and acid-base status provides information on the cardiovascular status. The nurse must be prepared to intervene if symptoms of hypovolemia or shock (or both) are found. These symptoms include hypotension, slow capillary refill (>3 seconds), and continued respiratory distress despite the provision of oxygen and ventilation.

An accurate and timely blood pressure reading can assist in making an early diagnosis of cardiorespiratory disease and in monitoring the effects of fluid therapy. Blood pressure readings can be obtained by the Doppler method or by an electronic monitor.

Maintaining Body Temperature. Preterm infants are susceptible to temperature instability as a result of numerous factors. Preterm infants are at high risk for heat loss because of the large surface area in relation to body weight. Other factors that place preterm infants at risk for temperature instability include the following:

- Minimal insulating subcutaneous fat
- Limited stores of brown fat (an internal source for the generation of heat present in normal term infants)
- Decreased or absent reflex control of skin capillaries (shiver response)
- Inadequate muscle mass activity (therefore the preterm infant is unable to produce its own heat)
- Poor muscle tone, resulting in more body surface area being exposed to the cooling effects of the environment

- Friable (easily damaged) capillaries
- An immature temperature regulation center in the brain

The goal of thermoregulation is a neutral thermal environment (NTE), which is the environmental temperature at which oxygen consumption is minimal but adequate to maintain the body temperature (Cloherty and Stark, 1997). With knowledge of the four mechanisms of heat transfer (i.e., convection, conduction, radiation, and evaporation), the nurse can create an environment for the preterm infant that prevents temperature instability (see Chapter 24). The infant is kept in a radiant warmer or incubator with control settings at a temperature to maintain the NTE. Since overheating produces an increase in oxygen and calorie consumption, the infant is also jeopardized if he or she becomes hyperthermic.

Central Nervous System Function. The preterm infant's central nervous system (CNS) is susceptible to injury as a result of the following problems:

- Birth trauma with damage to immature structures
- Bleeding from fragile capillaries
- Impaired coagulation process, including prolonged prothrombin time
- Recurrent anoxic episodes
- Predisposition to hypoglycemia

The developing nervous system has the ability to reorganize neural connection after injury, therefore some injuries that would be permanent in adults are not so in infants. Certain neurologic signs appear to be predictive of later abnormal neurologic abnormalities. These signs include hypotonia, a decreased level of activity, weak cry for more than 24 hours, and inability to coordinate suck and swallow (Fanaroff and Martin, 1997). Ongoing assessment and documentation of these neurologic signs is needed for the purposes of discharge teaching and making follow-up recommendations, as well as for their predictive value.

Maintaining Adequate Nutrition. The goal of neonatal nutrition is to promote normal growth and development (Cloherty and Stark, 1997). However, the maintenance of adequate nutrition in the preterm infant is complicated by problems with intake and metabolism. The preterm infant has the following disadvantages with regard to intake: weak or absent suck, swallow, and gag reflexes; a small stomach capacity; and weak abdominal muscles. The preterm infant's metabolic functions are compromised by a limited store of nutrients, a decreased ability to digest proteins and absorb nutrients, and immature enzyme systems.

The nurse must continuously assess the infant's ability to take in and digest nutrients. Some preterm infants require gavage or intravenous (IV) feedings instead of oral feedings.

Maintaining Renal Function. The preterm infant's immature renal system is unable to (1) adequately excrete metabolites and drugs; (2) concentrate urine; or (3) maintain acid-base, fluid, or electrolyte balances (Cloherty and Stark, 1997). Therefore intake and output, as well as specific gravity, must be assessed. Laboratory tests must be done to assess acid-base and electrolyte balances. Medication levels are also monitored in preterm infants because certain medications can overwhelm the immature system's ability to excrete them.

Maintaining Hematologic Status. The preterm infant is predisposed to hematologic problems due to the following conditions:

- Increased capillary friability
- Increased tendency to bleed (prolonged prothrombin time and partial thromboplastin time)
- Slowed production of red blood cells resulting from rapid decrease in erythropoiesis after birth
- Loss of blood due to frequent blood sampling for laboratory tests
- Decreased red blood cell survival related to relatively larger size of the red blood cell and its increased permeability to sodium and potassium

The nurse assesses such infants for any evidence of bleeding from puncture sites and the gastrointestinal (GI) tract. Infants are also examined for signs of anemia (e.g., decreased hemoglobin and hematocrit levels, pale skin, increased apnea, lethargy, tachycardia, and poor weight gain) (Fanaroff and Martin, 1997).

Resisting Infection. Preterm infants are at increased risk for infection because they have a shortage of stored maternal immunoglobulins, an impaired ability to make antibodies, and a compromised integumentary system (i.e., thin skin and fragile capillaries). Preterm infants exhibit various nonspecific signs and symptoms of infection (Box 27-2). Early identification and treatment of sepsis is essential.

Protection from Infection. Protection from infection is an integral part of all newborn care, but preterm and sick infants are particularly susceptible to infectious organisms. As with all aspects of care, strict handwashing is the single most important measure to prevent nosocomial infections. Personnel with known infectious disorders are barred from the unit until they are no longer infectious. Standard Precautions are instituted in all nursery areas as a method of infection control to protect the infants and staff.

Skin Care. The skin of preterm infants is characteristically immature relative to that of full-term infants. Because of its increased sensitivity and fragility, the use of alkaline-based soap that might destroy the "acid mantle" of the skin is avoided. The increased permeability of the skin facilitates absorption of ingredients. All skin products (e.g., alcohol or povidone-iodine)

Box 27-2

Signs and Symptoms of Infection

Temperature instability
- Hypothermia
- Hyperthermia

CNS changes
- Lethargy
- Irritability

Changes in color
- Cyanosis, pallor
- Jaundice

Cardiovascular instability
- Poor perfusion
- Hypotension
- Bradycardia/tachycardia

Respiratory distress
- Tachypnea
- Apnea
- Retractions, nasal flaring, grunting

Gastrointestinal problems
- Feeding intolerance
- Vomiting
- Diarrhea
- Glucose instability

Metabolic acidosis

are used with caution, and the skin is rinsed with water afterward because these substances may cause severe irritation and chemical burns in LBW infants. Adhesives used after heel sticks or to secure monitoring equipment or intravenous infusions may excoriate the skin or adhere to the skin surface so firmly that the skin can be separated from understructures and pulled away with the tape. The use of skin barriers protects healthy skin and helps excoriated skin heal. Solvents used to remove tape are avoided because they tend to dry and burn the delicate skin.

Growth and Development Potential

Although it is impossible to predict with complete accuracy the growth and development potential of each preterm newborn, some findings support an anticipated favorable outcome in the absence of ongoing medical sequelae that can affect growth, such as bronchopulmonary dysplasia, necrotizing enterocolitis, and CNS problems. The lower the birth weight, the greater the likelihood of negative sequelae. The growth and development milestones (e.g., motor milestones, vocalization, and growth) are corrected for gestational age until the child is approximately 2½ years of age.

The age of a preterm newborn is corrected by adding the gestational age and the postnatal age. For example, an infant born at 32 weeks of gestation 4 weeks ago would now be considered 36 weeks of age. The infant's corrected age 6 months after the birth date is then 4 months, and the infant's responses are accordingly evaluated against the norm expected for a 4-month-old infant.

There are certain measurable factors that predict normal growth and development. The preterm infant experiences catch-up body growth during the first 2 to 3 years of life, with maximum growth occurring between 36 and 40 weeks of postconceptional age (Fanaroff and Martin, 1997). The head is the first to experience catch-up growth, followed by a gain in weight and height (Cloherty and Stark, 1997). At the infant's discharge from the hospital, which usually occurs between 37 and 40 weeks of postconceptional age, the infant should exhibit the following characteristics:

- An ability to raise the head when prone and hold the head parallel with the body when tested for head lag response
- An ability to cry with vigor when hungry
- An appropriate amount and pattern of weight gain according to a growth grid
- Neurologic responses appropriate for corrected age

At 39 to 40 weeks of postconceptual age the infant should be able to focus on the examiner's or parent's face and to follow with his or her eyes.

Parental Adaptation to Preterm Infant

Parents who experience the preterm birth of their infant have a different experience from parents giving birth to a full-term infant (Shields-Poe and Pinelli, 1997). Because of this difference, parental attachment and adaptation to the parental role may differ as well.

Parental Tasks. Parents must accomplish a number of psychologic tasks before effective relationships and parenting patterns can evolve. These tasks include the following:

- Experiencing anticipatory grief over the potential loss of an infant. The parent grieves in preparation for the infant's possible death, although the parent clings to the hope that the child will survive. This begins during labor and lasts until the infant dies or shows evidence of surviving.
- Acceptance by the mother of her failure to give birth to a healthy, full-term infant. Grief and depression typify this phase, which persists until the infant is out of danger and is expected to survive.
- Resuming the process of relating to the infant. As the baby's condition begins to improve and the baby gains weight, feeds by nipple, and is weaned from the incubator, the parent can begin the process of developing an attachment to the infant that was interrupted by the infant's critical condition at birth.
- Learning how this baby differs in special needs and growth patterns, caregiving needs, and growth and development expectations.
- Adjusting the home environment to the needs of the new infant. Visitors may be limited to reduce the risk of exposure to pathogens; the environmental temperature may be altered to optimize conditions for the infant. Grandparents and siblings also react to the birth of the preterm infant. Parents must deal with the grief of grandparents and the bewilderment and anger of the infant's siblings at the apparent disproportionate amount of parental time spent on the newborn.

Parental Responses. Parents progress through stages as they interact with their infants, from maintaining an en face position and stroking and touching their infant (Fig. 27-1) to assuming some child care activities such as feeding, bathing, and diapering the infant.

Parenting Disorders. The incidence of physical and emotional abuse is greater in infants who, because of preterm birth or illness, are separated from their parents for a time after birth (Fanaroff and Martin, 1997). Physical abuse includes varying degrees of poor nutrition, poor hygiene, and battering. Emotional abuse ranges from subtle disinterest to outright dislike of the child.

Factors surrounding the birth may predispose parents to subconsciously or overtly reject the child. These factors might include parental pain and anxiety, a heavy financial burden because of the cost of the infant's care, unresolved anticipatory grief, threat to self-esteem, or the fact that the infant was the product of an unwanted pregnancy. The goal of health professionals is early identification of abuse and neglect so that further problems can be prevented and, in turn, the incidence of such abuse can be reduced.

➤ Nursing Diagnoses

Potential nursing diagnoses for high risk infants and their parents include the following:

- Impaired gas exchange related to:
  —Decreased number of functional alveoli
  —Deficiency of surfactant
- Ineffective breathing pattern related to:
  —Inadequate chest expansion secondary to infant's position
- Ineffective thermoregulation related to:
  —Immature thermoregulation center
- Risk for infection related to:
  —Invasive procedures
  —Decreased immune response
- Parental anxiety related to:
  —Lack of knowledge regarding infant's condition
  —Lack of knowledge regarding infant's cues

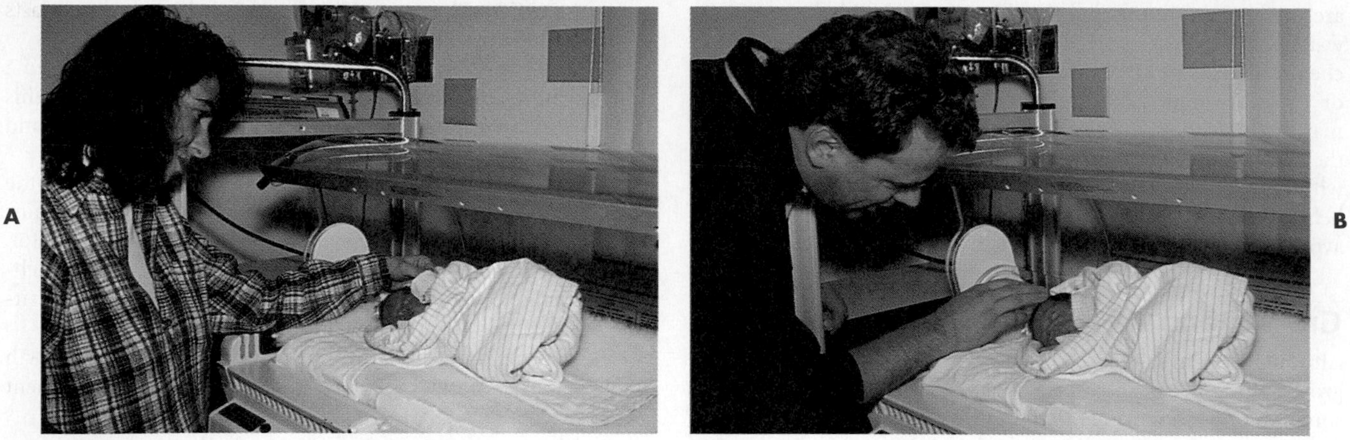

FIG. 27-1 • A, Mother interacts with her premature infant by touch. B, Father interacts with his baby by stroking and touching baby with fingertips. (Courtesy Michael S. Clement, MD, Mesa, AZ.)

➤ Expected Outcomes

The nursing plan of care for the preterm infant is dictated by the physiologic needs of the infant's immature systems, and often involves emergency treatments and procedures. Nursing care is a critical element in the infant's chances for survival. In addition to meeting the infant's physical needs, nursing care is planned in conjunction with parents to promote parent-infant attachment and interaction. Expected outcomes are presented in patient-centered terms and include that the infant will do the following:

- Maintain physiologic functioning
- Maintain adequate nutrition
- Experience no or minimal hematologic problems
- Remain free of infection
- Become attached to parents

Expected outcomes for the parents include that they will do the following:

- Perceive the child as potentially normal (if this is medically substantiated)
- Provide care comfortably
- Experience pride and satisfaction in the care of the infant
- Organize their time and energies to meet the love, attention, and care needs of the other members of the family as well as their own needs.

➤ Plan of Care and Implementation

The best environment for fetal growth and development is in the uterus of a healthy, well-nourished woman. The goal of care for the preterm infant is to provide an extrauterine environment that approximates a healthy intrauterine environment in order to promote normal growth and development. Medical and nursing personnel and respiratory therapists work as a team to provide the intensive care needed.

The admission of a preterm newborn to the intensive care nursery is usually an emergency situation. Resuscitation is started in the birthing unit, and warmth and oxygen is provided during transport to the nursery. A rapid initial assessment is done to determine the infant's need for lifesaving treatment.

The nurse uses many technologic support systems to monitor body responses and maintain body functions in the infant. Technical skill needs to be combined with a gentle touch and concern about the traumatic effects of harsh lighting and the volume of machinery noise. The neonatal intensive care unit (NICU) environment may be a major contributing factor to learning and behavioral problems in preterm infants (Blackburn, 1998).

Physical Care. The preterm infant's environmental support typically consists of the following equipment and procedures:

- Incubator or overhead heat panel to control body temperature (NTE)
- Oxygen administration, depending on infant's cardiopulmonary and circulatory status
- Electronic monitors as needed for observation of respiratory and cardiac functions
- Assistive devices for positioning the infant in neutral flexion
- Clustering of care and minimization of stimulation

Various metabolic support measures that may be instituted consist of the following:

- Parenteral fluids to support nutrition and maintain normal arterial blood gas (ABG) levels and acid-base balance
- IV access to facilitate antibiotic therapy if sepsis is a concern
- Blood work to monitor ABG levels, pH, blood glucose level, electrolytes, and the status of blood cultures

Maintaining Body Temperature. The high risk infant is susceptible to heat loss and its complications (see Fig. 24-2). In addition, LBW infants may be unable to increase their metabolic rate because of impaired gas exchange, caloric intake restrictions, or poor thermoregulation. Transepidermal water loss is greater because of skin immaturity in very premature infants (i.e., those at less than 28 weeks of gestation) and can contribute to temperature instability.

High risk infants are cared for in the thermoneutral environment created by use of an external heat source. A probe applied to the infant is attached to an external heat source supplied by a radiant warmer or a servocontrolled incubator. Maintaining an infant's body temperature between 36.5° and 37.2° C decreases oxygen consumption (Blake and Murray, 1998).

Warming the Hypothermic Infant. Rapid changes in body temperature may cause apnea and acidosis in the neonate.

A B

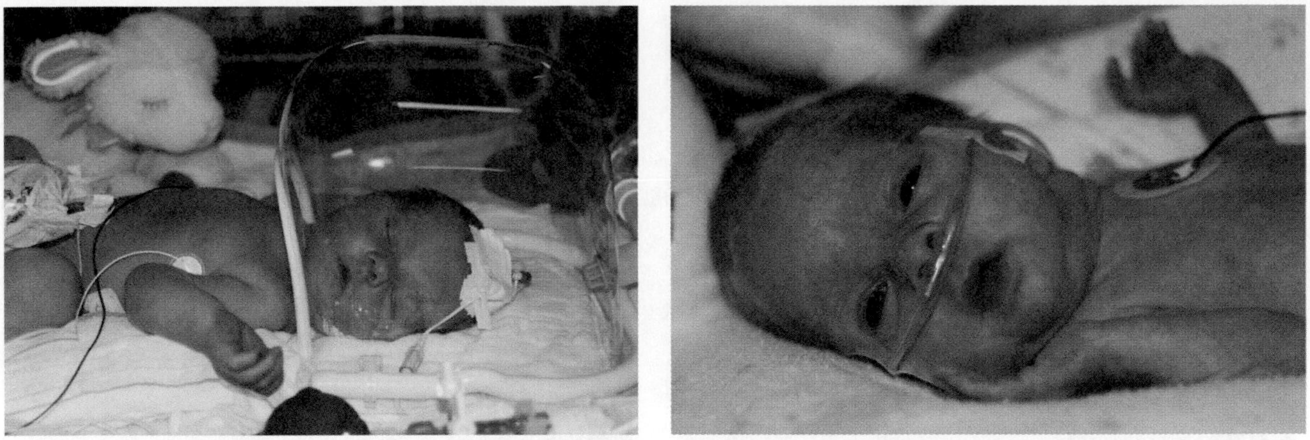

FIG. 27-2 • **A,** Infant under hood. **B,** Infant with nasal cannula. (Courtesy Victoria Langer, RNC, MSN, NNP: from Dickason E, Silverman B, Kaplan J: *Maternal-infant nursing care,* ed 3, St Louis, 1998, Mosby.)

Therefore the warming of a hypothermic infant should occur over a 2- to 4-hour period. To accomplish this, the infant is placed either under a radiant warmer or in an incubator with a servocontrol mechanism. To ensure an optimal response during warming, the servocontrol thermostat should be increased incrementally by 0.3° C more than each skin temperature measured. When the skin temperature reaches at least 36.5° C, the servocontrol thermostat is then reset to maintain a thermoneutral environment.

Weaning the Infant from the Incubator. To wean the infant from the incubator, the incubator heat is decreased slowly over at least several hours. Infants weighing more than 1500 g who show stable self-regulation of their temperatures are candidates for weaning. The nurse carries out the following measures to wean the infant from the incubator:

- Dresses the infant in a diaper, shirt, and double-thickness cap
- Lowers the incubator temperature by no more than 0.5° C per each 2-hour period
- Records the temperature of both the infant and incubator
- Assesses the infant's responses to the changes every 15 minutes until four stable readings are obtained
- Monitors the infant's temperature and other vital signs

This procedure is repeated until the incubator temperature is the same as the room temperature and the infant's skin temperature consistently remains above 36.5° C (Meier, 1994). The infant is placed in an open bassinet when the axillary temperature is stable, after which it is reassessed in conjunction with the delivery of routine care. If necessary, the infant may be returned to the incubator and weaning repeated once the infant is able to regulate its temperature.

Oxygen Therapy. Clinical criteria indicating the need for oxygen administration include increased respiratory effort, respiratory distress with apnea, tachycardia, bradycardia, and central cyanosis with or without hypotonia. The need for supplemental oxygen should be substantiated by biochemical data (i.e., arterial oxygen pressure [$Pa{O_2}$] of less than 60 mm Hg or an oxygen saturation of less than 92%). High risk infants often require saturations of more than 95% to maintain respiratory stability because their hemoglobin levels are commonly low. As the $Pa{O_2}$ falls, less oxygen is released from the hemoglobin, which increases the risk for cellular hypoxia (Hagedorn, Gardner, and Abman, 1998).

Oxygen administered to an infant is warmed and humidified to prevent cold stress and drying of the respiratory mucosa. During the administration of oxygen the concentration, volume, temperature, and humidity of the gas are carefully controlled. Delivery of oxygen for more than a few minutes requires the use of special equipment (i.e., hood, nasal cannula, positive-pressure mask, or endotracheal tube) because the concentration of free-flow oxygen cannot be monitored accurately (Hagedorn, Gardner, and Abman, 1998). The indiscriminant use of oxygen may be hazardous. Possible complications of oxygen therapy include retinopathy of prematurity and bronchopulmonary dysplasia.

Infants who need oxygen should have their respiratory status assessed accurately every 1 to 2 hours; this includes a continuous pulse oximetry reading and at least one ABG measurement (Hagedorn, Gardner, and Abman, 1998). The interventions implemented range from hood oxygen administration to ventilator therapy. They are determined on the basis of the findings yielded by the clinical assessment, including telemetry (pulse oximetry or $tcP{O_2}$ monitoring) and laboratory tests (Hagedorn, Gardner, and Abman, 1998).

Hood Therapy. Oxygen in a specified concentration can be administered by hood to infants who do not require mechanical pressure support. The hood is a clear plastic cover that is sized to fit over the head and neck of the infant (Fig. 27-2, *A*). The oxygen level is checked every 1 to 2 hours and the concentration adjusted in response to the infant's condition.

Nasal Cannula. Low-flow amounts of oxygen can be administered by nasal cannula (Fig. 27-2, *B*). Nasal cannula are used for older infants who are recuperating but still require supplemental oxygen; they are the preferred method for home oxygen administration (Hagedorn, Gardner, and Abman, 1998). The infant receives an adequate, continuous flow of oxygen while allowing optimal vision, positioning, and parental holding. Infants can also breastfeed while receiving oxygen by this method. The nasal prongs must be inspected often to ensure that they are not partially obstructed by milk or secretions.

Continuous Positive Airway Pressure Therapy. Infants who are unable to maintain an adequate $Pa{O_2}$ despite the

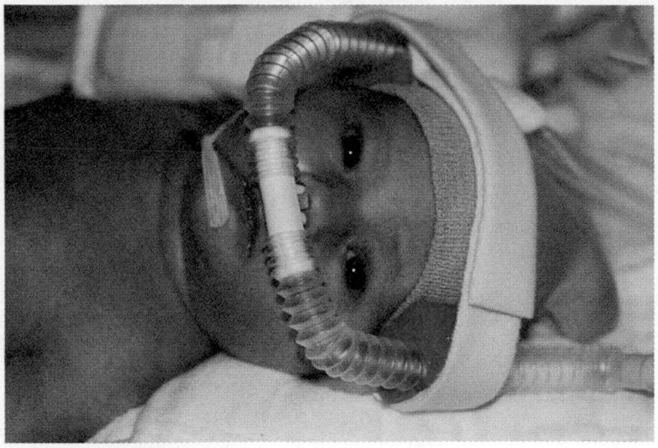

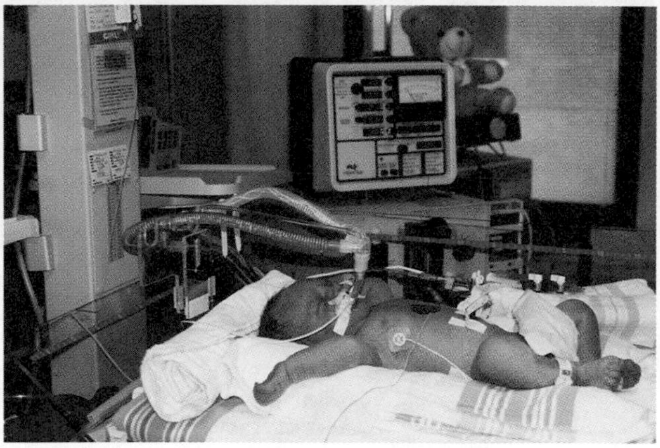

FIG. 27-3 • **A,** Infant receiving ventilatory assistance with continuous positive airway pressure (CPAP). **B,** Infant intubated and on ventilator. (Courtesy Victoria Langer, RNC, MSN, NNP: from Dickason E, Silverman B, Kaplan J: *Maternal-infant nursing care,* ed 3, St Louis, 1998, Mosby.)

administration of oxygen by hood or nasal cannula may require the delivery of oxygen using continuous positive airway pressure (CPAP). CPAP infuses oxygen or air under a preset pressure (Fig. 27-3, *A*) by means of nasal prongs, a face mask, or an endotracheal tube. An orogastric tube should be used for decompression of the stomach during use of nasal prongs (Hagedorn, Gardner, and Abman, 1998). CPAP increases the functional residual capacity; improves the diffusion time of pulmonary gases, including oxygen; and can decrease pulmonary shunting. If implemented early enough, CPAP may preclude the need for mechanical ventilation. CPAP can cause vascular shunting in the pulmonary beds, which can lead to persistent pulmonary hypertension and severe respiratory distress.

Mechanical Ventilation. Mechanical ventilation must be implemented if other methods of therapy cannot correct abnormalities in oxygenation. Its use is indicated whenever blood gas values reveal the existence of severe hypoxemia or severe hypercapnia (Fig. 27-3, *B*). The condition of the infant experiencing apnea with bradycardia, ineffective respiratory effort, shock, asphyxia, infection, meconium aspiration syndrome, respiratory distress syndrome, or congenital defects that affect ventilation may also deteriorate and require intubation to reverse the process. Dexamethasone may be administered to prevent chronic lung disease (Garland et al, 1999).

Ventilator settings are determined by the infant's particular needs. The ventilator is set to provide a predetermined amount of oxygen to the infant during spontaneous respirations and also to provide mechanical ventilation in the absence of spontaneous respirations. See Box 27-3 for an explanation of ventilator terminology.

Surfactant Administration. Surfactant can be administered as an adjunct to oxygen and ventilation therapy. Before 34 weeks of gestation, most infants do not produce enough surfactant to survive extrauterine life (American Academy of Pediatrics, 1999; Hagedorn, Gardner, and Abman, 1998). As a result, lung compliance is decreased, and not enough gas exchange occurs as the lungs become atelectatic and require greater pressures to expand. By administering artificial surfactant, respiratory compliance is improved until the infant can generate enough surfactant on his or her own. Exogenous surfactant is manufactured from human or bovine amniotic fluid and is given in several doses through an endotracheal tube (Hagedorn, Gardner, and Abman, 1998). The infant must be monitored for the occurrence of potential side effects such as patent ductus arteriosus and pulmonary hemorrhage. Use of this medication has been associated with a significantly reduced length of time on ventilators and oxygen therapy, and an increased survival rate in premature infants (Box 27-4).

Extracorporeal Membrane Oxygenation Therapy (ECMO). Infants with severe pulmonary dysfunction who are at more than 34 weeks of gestation may be candidates for extracorporeal membrane oxygenation therapy. ECMO uses cardiopulmonary bypass to oxygenate the infant's blood outside the body through a membrane oxygenator. The membrane oxygenator serves as an artificial lung while the infant's lungs heal. Because of the massive systemic anticoagulation therapy required in the pump tubing, and the increased risk for hemorrhage, the criteria for the use of ECMO is very strict (Donovan, Schwartz, and Moles, 1998). The risk for intraventricular hemorrhages in premature infants is particularly high, and for this reason ECMO therapy cannot be used in them.

High-Frequency Ventilation. Other modes of ventilator therapy include high-frequency oscillator ventilation, jet ventilation, flow interruption ventilation, and liquid ventilation (Cools and Offringa, 1999; Donovan, Schwartz, and Moles, 1998; Plavka et al, 1999). These methods of high-frequency ventilation work by providing smaller volumes of oxygen at a significantly more rapid rate (more than 300 breaths/min) than traditional mechanical ventilators do. As a result, the intrathoracic pressure and the risk of barotrauma is decreased. In liquid ventilation, the surface tension is reduced while oxygenation is improved through the recreation of a fetal lung environment. Instead of air pressure, an experimental oxygenated lipid solution is pumped continuously through the lungs.

Weaning from Respiratory Assistance. The infant is ready to be weaned from respiratory assistance when the ABG and oxygen saturation levels are maintained within normal limits. A spontaneous, adequate respiratory effort must be present, and the infant must show improved muscle tone during increased activity. Weaning is done in a stepwise and gradual manner. This may consist of the infant being extubated, placed on continuous positive airway pressure, and then

Box 27-3

Definitions of Ventilator Terminology

Peak inspiratory pressure (PIP)	The peak level of pressure on inspiration. High pressures may cause overdistention, which can cause complications such as a pneumothorax.
Positive end-expiratory pressure (PEEP)	Creates mechanical continuous positive airway pressure (CPAP). The therapeutic range is 3 to 8 cm H_2O (Wong, 1999).
Rate	The frequency with which the ventilator delivers the specified volume of gases (oxygen and air) to the infant. This provides the minimal number of breaths per minute needed for adequate oxygenation.
Inspiration/expiration ratio (I:E)	The amount of time during each breath spent on inspiration versus expiration.
Mean airway pressure (MAP)	The amount of pressure exerted on the airway throughout the respiratory cycle. The average pressure is constant on high-frequency ventilators but varies during inspiratory and expiratory cycles on the conventional mode of ventilation.

From Hagedorn M, Gardner S, Abman S: Respiratory distress. In Merenstein G, Gardner S, editors: *Handbook of neonatal intensive care,* ed 3, St Louis, 1993, Mosby; and Wong D: *Whaley & Wong's nursing care of infants and children,* ed 6, St Louis, 1999, Mosby.

Box 27-4

Medication Guide: Surfactant Replacement: Bovine Lung Extract: Beractant (Survanta) Artificial Surfactant: Colfosceril (Exosurf)

ACTION

These medications provide exogenous surfactant to correct deficiency in lung immaturity.

INDICATIONS

Surfactants are used in the prevention and treatment of respiratory distress syndrome in premature infants.

- For *prevention,* drug is administered within 15 minutes of birth to infants with clinical manifestations of surfactant deficiency or with a birth weight less than 1250 g.
- For *treatment,* drug is administered to infants with confirmed diagnosis of respiratory distress syndrome, preferably within 8 hours of birth.

DOSAGE

Dosage depends on drug used. Administer via endotracheal tube.

ADVERSE REACTIONS

Adverse reactions include respiratory distress immediately after administration and bradycardia and oxygen desaturation.

NURSING CONSIDERATIONS

Observe infant's condition for changes. Diuresis may occur with improvement. Ventilator settings may need changing as the infant's ability to oxygenate increases.

weaned to oxygen by means of a hood or nasal cannula. Throughout the weaning process the infant's oxygen levels are monitored by pulse oximetry, $tcPo_2$ monitoring, and blood gas levels.

Some infants are not able to be weaned from all oxygen support by the time of discharge from the hospital and may require home oxygen therapy for several months. Bronchopulmonary dysplasia, a patent ductus arteriosus, or CNS damage may underlie intolerance of weaning (Hagedorn, Gardner, and Abman, 1998).

The parents need to be given consistent information and be reassured about the infant's respiratory progress. Decisions regarding the nature of continued interventions should be included in a multidisciplinary plan of care, and the therapy should be frequently explained to the family.

Nutritional Care. High risk infants may be too ill or weak to breastfeed or bottle-feed because of respiratory distress or sepsis (Townsend, Johnson, and Hay, 1998). Early enteral feeding of the asphyxiated neonate with a low Apgar score is also avoided to prevent bowel necrosis. In such cases, nutrition is provided parenterally. Infants who require parenteral nutrition may have one or more of the following problems (Townsend, Johnson, and Hay, 1998):

- Lack of a coordinated suck-and-swallow reflex
- Inability to suck because of a congenital anomaly
- Respiratory distress requiring aggressive ventilator support
- Asphyxiation with a potential for necrotizing enterocolitis

Type of Nourishment. The types of formulas used, the mode and volume of feeding, and the feeding schedule of the infant are based on the findings yielded by assessment of the following variables:

- Weight of the infant
- Pattern of weight gain or loss (infants weighing less than 1500 g require more energy for growth and thermoregulation)
- Presence or absence of suck and swallow reflexes
- Behavioral readiness to take oral feedings
- Physical condition, including presence or absence of bowel sounds, abdominal distention, or bloody stools, as well as presence and degree of respiratory distress or apneic episodes
- Residual from previous feeding, if being gavage fed
- Malformations (especially GI defects)
- Renal function, including urinary output and laboratory values (e.g., nitrogen balance, electrolyte balance, and glucose level)

Weight and Fluid Loss or Gain. The caloric, nutrient, and fluid requirements of high risk infants are greater than those of the normal term newborn. Premature or dysmature (malnourished) newborns often have limited stores of nutrients and fluids. Symptomatic or asymptomatic hypoglycemia, electrolyte imbalances, or other metabolic disturbances can develop in an infant whose nutritional intake is poor. Hypoglycemia may cause serious damage to carbohydrate-dependent brain cells.

The infant's weight is measured and recorded daily and the rate of weight loss or gain is calculated. Further depletion of weight and metabolic stores can occur as a result of one or a combination of the following factors:

- Birth asphyxia
- Increased respirations or respiratory effort
- Patent ductus arteriosus
- Hypothermic environment
- Insensible fluid loss caused by evaporation (with radiant heat or phototherapy)
- Vomiting, diarrhea, and dysfunctional absorption from the GI tract
- Growth demands (a preterm infant's growth is at least two times faster than a term infant's growth rate after birth)
- Inability of the renal system to concentrate urine and maintain an adequate rate of urea excretion

The high risk newborn is predisposed to have weight and fluid losses because of the greater amount of fluid needed to meet demands of the increased cellular metabolic processes (resulting from stress, repair, or growth). Even with the early institution of fluid and nutrition intake, the premature infant's weight and fluid losses seem exaggerated. Inadequate fluid intake, resulting from either delayed administration or insufficient volume, can cause further weight and fluid losses in the premature infant.

Insensible water loss (IWL) is an evaporative loss that occurs largely through the skin. Approximately 30% of this IWL comes from the respiratory tract. During the first week of extrauterine life, the premature infant can lose up to 15% of his or her birth weight. After the initial week, weight loss or gain during each 24-hour period should not exceed 2% of the previous day's weight. (The way to calculate a weight loss or gain is detailed in Box 27-5.) Weight loss may be caused by increased stooling or voiding, increased evaporative losses, inadequate volume or incorrect fluid administration, and problems with malabsorption. Weight gain may be due to overfeeding or fluid retention.

Elimination Patterns. Frequency of urination, as well as the amount, color, pH, and specific gravity of the urine is assessed. The assessment of bowel movements includes frequency of stooling and character of the stool, as well as whether there is constipation, diarrhea, or loss of fats (steatorrhea). Infants with unexplained abdominal distention are assessed carefully to rule out the presence of hypomotility or obstructions of the GI tract.

Box 27-5

Calculation of a Weight Loss or Gain

EXAMPLE 1

Day 4 1,750 g
Day 5 1,730 g
20 g loss

$$\frac{20}{1,750} = \frac{X\%}{100\%}$$

$$1,750X = 2,000$$

$$1,750\overline{)2,000.0} \quad 1.1$$

X = 1.1% weight loss

EXAMPLE 2

Day 4 1,750 g
Day 5 1,790 g
40 g gain

$$\frac{40}{1,750} = \frac{X\%}{100\%}$$

$$1,750X = 4,000$$

$$1,750\overline{)4,000.00} \quad 2.3$$

X = 2.3% weight gain

Oral Feeding. Nourishment by the oral route is preferred for the infant who has adequate strength and GI function. The best milk for an infant is that of its mother. Breast milk may be fed by breast or bottle. Formula may be fed by bottle or a supplementer.

Many high risk infants cannot suck well enough to breastfeed or bottle-feed until they have recovered from their initial illness or matured physically; infants may be put to breast for practice feeds as soon as medically stable. Mothers of high risk infants are encouraged to continue pumping breast milk. Because of the significant breastfeeding attrition rates among these mothers, they need support and frequent encouragement to continue pumping while their infant is not yet able to nurse.

Gavage Feeding. Gavage feeding is a method of providing breast milk or formula through a nasogastric or orogastric tube (Fig. 27-4). Gavage feeding can be done either with a tube inserted at each feeding or continuously through an indwelling catheter. Infants who cannot tolerate large-bolus feedings (e.g., those on ventilators for more than a week) are given continuous feedings. Breast milk or formula can be supplied intermittently using a syringe with gravity-controlled flow, or can be given continuously using an infusion pump. The type of fluid instilled is recorded with every syringe change. The volume of the continuous feedings is recorded hourly, and the residual gastric aspirate is measured every 4 hours. Residuals of less than a quarter of a feeding can be refed to the infant to prevent the loss of gastric electrolytes. Feeding is stopped if the residual is greater than a quarter of the feeding, and is not resumed until the infant can be assessed for a possible feeding intolerance (Townsend, Johnson, and Hay, 1998).

The orogastric route of gavage feedings is preferred because most infants are preferential nose breathers. However, some infants do not tolerate oral tube placement. The procedure for inserting a gavage feeding tube is described in Box 27-6.

To begin the feeding, the nurse connects the barrel of a syringe to the gavage tube. While crimping the feeding tube, the nurse pours the specified amount of breast milk or formula into the syringe. The crimp in the tube is then released and the feeding allowed to flow by gravity at a rate that approximates that of an oral feeding (about 1 ml/min). The infant can be held or swaddled to help the infant associate the feeding with positive interactions.

Once the prescribed volume has been delivered, the tube is crimped or pinched and the syringe removed. The gavage tube is capped (or the nurse continues to pinch it) while removing it in one steady motion. Capping or pinching the tube prevents breast milk or formula from leaking from the tube and being aspirated during removal of the tube.

After the feeding, the infant is positioned to prevent aspiration. The documentation of the procedure includes the size of the feeding tube, the amount and quality of the residual from the previous feeding, the type and quantity of fluid instilled, and the infant's response to the procedure.

Gastrostomy Feeding. Gastrostomy feeding involves the surgical placement of a tube through the skin of the abdomen into the stomach. The tube is then taped in an upright position to prevent trauma to the incision site. After the site heals, small bolus feedings are initiated per physician's orders. Feedings by gravity are done slowly over 20 to 30 minutes. Special care must be taken to prevent rapid bolusing of the fluid because this may lead to abdominal distention, GI reflux into the esophagus, or respiratory compromise. Meticulous skin care at the tube insertion site is necessary to prevent skin breakdown or infection. Intake and output are monitored scrupulously because these infants are prone to diarrhea until regular feedings are established.

Parenteral Fluids. Feeding supplemental parenteral fluids is indicated for infants who are unable to obtain sufficient fluids or calories by enteral feedings. Some of these infants are dependent on total parenteral nutrition (TPN) for extensive periods.

The physician orders TPN per hospital protocol. The orders must specify the electrolytes and nutrients desired, as well as the volume and rate of infusion. The amounts of calories, protein, and fat are determined on the basis of the individual infant's energy needs (Lefrak and Dowling, 1998).

Nursing interventions include securing and protecting the insertion site, observing principles of asepsis and neonatal skin care, inspecting the infusion site for signs of infiltration and repositioning the infant often to maintain body alignment and protect the site. Parents need information about TPN and the equipment used.

Advancing Infant Feedings. Feedings are advanced from passive (parenteral and gavage) to active (nipple and breastfeeding) as assessment data and the infant's ability to tol-

Box 27-6

Procedure: Inserting a Gavage Feeding Tube

1. Measure the length of the gavage tube from the tip of the nose to the lobe of the ear to the midpoint between the xiphoid process and the umbilicus (Fig. 27-4, *A*). Mark the tube with a piece of tape.
2. Lubricate the tip of the tube with sterile water and insert gently through the nose or mouth (Fig. 27-4, *B*) until the predetermined mark is reached. Placement of the tube in the trachea will cause the infant to gag, cough, or become cyanotic.
3. Check correct placement of the tube by:
   a. Pulling back on the plunger to aspirate stomach contents. Lack of fluid is not necessarily evidence of improper placement. Aspiration of respiratory secretions may be mistaken for stomach contents; however, the pH of the stomach contents is much lower (more acidic) than the pH of respiratory secretions.
   b. Injecting a small amount of air (1 to 3 ml) into the tube while listening for gurgling by using a stethoscope placed over the stomach. Ensure that the tube is inserted to the mark; it is possible to hear air entering the stomach even if the tube is positioned above the gastroesophageal (cardiac) sphincter.
4. Tape the tube in place and also tape it to the cheek to prevent accidental dislodgement and incorrect positioning (Fig. 27-4, *C*)
   a. Assess the infant's skin integrity before taping the tube.
   b. Edematous or very premature infants should have a pectin barrier placed under the tape to prevent abrasions.*
5. Tube placement must be assessed before each feeding.

*Lund C, Durand D: Skin and skin care. In Merenstein G, Gardner S, editors: *Handbook of neonatal intensive care,* ed 4, St Louis, 1998, Mosby.

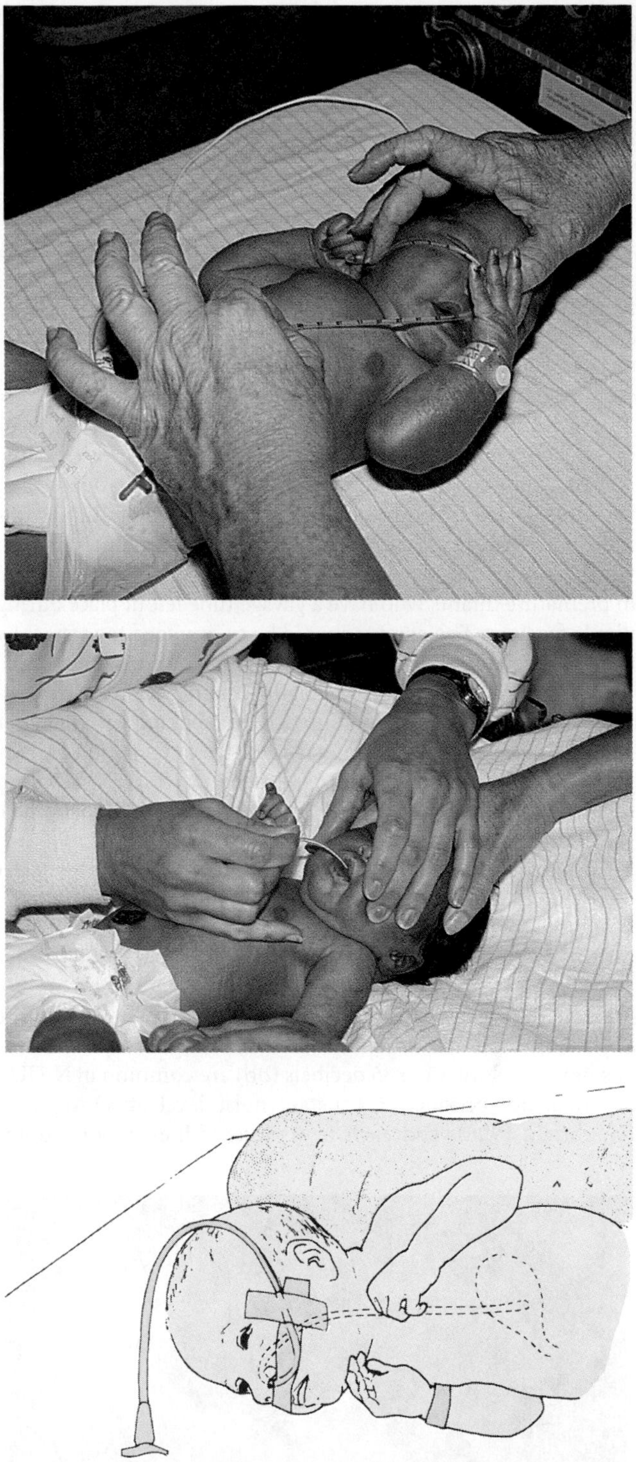

FIG. 27-4 • Gavage feeding. **A,** Measurement of gavage feeding tube from tip of nose to earlobe and to midpoint between end of xiphoid process and umbilicus. Tape may be used to mark correct length on tube. **B,** Insertion of gavage tube using orogastric route. **C,** Indwelling gavage tube, nasogastric route. After feeding by orogastric or nasogastric tube, infant is propped on right side for 1 hour to facilitate emptying of stomach into small intestine. Note rolled towel for support. (A and B, courtesy Marjorie Pyle, RNC, Lifecircle, Costa Mesa, CA.)

erate feedings warrant it. The infant's sucking patterns can also be used to determine readiness to nipple feed.

The infant receiving nutrition parenterally is gradually weaned off this type of nutrition. The nourishment given by gavage feedings is increased while the parenteral fluids are decreased. Feedings are advanced slowly and cautiously; if feedings are advanced too rapidly, vomiting, diarrhea, abdominal distention, and apneic episodes may result.

A commercial human milk fortifier can be added to the gavaged breast milk, or the number of calories per 30 ml of commercial formula can be increased if the infant needs additional calories. Calories in breast milk can be lost if the cream separates and adheres to the tubing during continuous infusion. Microbore tubing decreases the risk of this happening.

The infant receiving gavage feedings progresses to bottle-feeding or breast milk feedings. Gavage feedings are decreased as the infant's ability to suckle breast milk or formula improves. Often the infant is fed by both nipple and gavage feeding during this transition; this ensures intake of the prescribed volumes of both fluid and nutrients. An increased respiratory effort is a problem in premature infants who have a gavage tube left in place during nipple feedings. The parents should be encouraged to interact by talking and making eye contact with the infant during feedings.

Nonnutritive Sucking. For the infant who requires gavage or parenteral feedings, nonnutritive sucking on a pacifier during the gavage procedure may improve oxygenation and facilitate earlier transition to nipple feeding (Fig. 27-5). Such nonnutritive sucking may lead to decreased energy expenditure with less restlessness.

Mothers of premature infants should be encouraged to let their infant start sucking at the breast during kangaroo care; some infant's suck and swallow reflexes may be coordinated as early as 32 weeks of gestation.

Environmental Concerns. Infants in NICUs are exposed to high levels of auditory input from the various machine alarms, and this can have adverse effects (Fig. 27-6). Continuous noise levels of 45 to 85 decibels (db) are common in NICUs. An incubator produces a constant noise level of 60 to 80 db (Haubrich, 1998), and each new piece of life-support equipment used adds another 20 db to the background noise. The infant's hearing may be damaged if it is exposed to a constant decibel level of 90 db or frequent decibel swings higher than 110 db.

The infant's vision may be altered by respiratory equipment or a phototherapy mask, making it difficult for the infant to interact with caregivers and family members. The infant may be unable to establish diurnal and nocturnal rhythms because of the continuous exposure to overhead lighting. In addition, sedation or pain medications affect the way in which the infant perceives the environment.

Effects of environmental hazards can be potentiated by some drugs used for infant therapy. Diuretics (especially furosemide [Lasix]), antibiotics (gentamicin), and antimalarial agents can potentiate noise-induced hearing loss (Haubrich, 1998). Routine hearing screening should be performed on all infants before discharge (see Fig. 24-17).

Nurses can modify the environment to provide a developmentally supportive milieu. In that way, the infant's neurobehavioral and physiologic needs can be better met, the infant's developing organization can be supported, and growth and development fostered (Blackburn, 1998).

Developmental Care. The goal of developmental care is to support each infant's efforts to become as well-organized, competent, and stable as possible. Developmental care includes all care procedures and the physical and social aspects of care in the NICU (Als, 1998). The caregiver uses the infant's own behavior and physiologic functioning as the basis for planning care and providing interventions. Through caregiver observation, the infant's strengths, thresholds for disorganization, and areas in which the infant is vulnerable can be identified (Als, 1998). The family is included in developmental care as the primary coregulators (Als, 1998; Heermann and Wilson, 2000). Working together, the family and other caregivers provide opportunities to enhance the strengths of the family and the infant and to reduce the stress that is associated with the birth and care of high risk infants.

Lowering light and noise levels by instituting "quiet hours" during each 8-hour shift and positioning are just two of the ways in which nurses can support infants in their development (Gray et al, 1998). Sleep interruptions are minimized and positioning and bundling the infant help promote self-regulation and prevent disorganization (Petryshen et al, 1997).

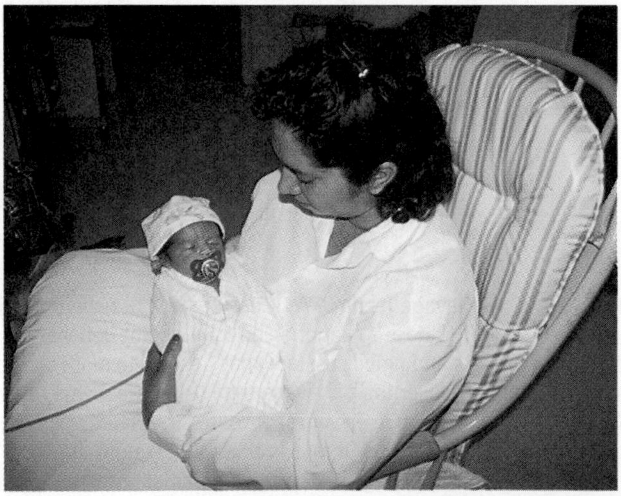

FIG. 27-5 • Nonnutritive sucking by infant. (Courtesy Marjorie Pyle, RNC, Lifecircle, Costa Mesa, CA.)

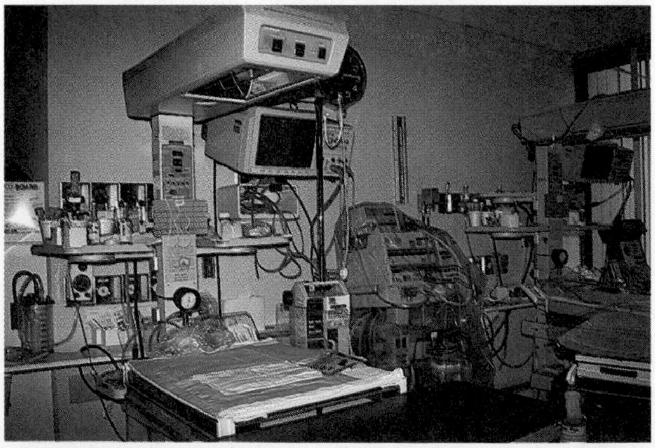

FIG. 27-6 • Significant environmental stimulation. Note bed, wall oxygen attachments, monitor, ventilator, incubator, and pumps, all of which have alarm systems. (Courtesy Marjorie Pyle, RNC, Lifecircle, Costa Mesa, CA.)

Positioning. The motor development of preterm infants permits less flexion than their full-term counterparts. Caregivers can provide a variety of positions for infants; side-lying and prone are preferred to supine. Body containment with use of blanket rolls, swaddling, holding the infant's arms in a crossed position, and secure holding provide boundaries and promote self-regulation during feeding, procedures, and other stressful interventions (Gardner and Lubchenco, 1998). The prone position encourages flexion of the extremities; a sling or hiproll assists in maintenance of flexion. Use of a sheepskin prevents abrasion of the knees (Gardner and Lubchenco, 1998). Holding the limbs close to the body when the infant is moved decreases stimulation that produces jerky, uncoordinated movements (Wong, 1999). Proper body alignment is necessary to prevent developmental problems that may affect the ability to walk as the child matures.

Reducing Inappropriate Stimuli. Staff can reduce unnecessary noise by the following: closing doors or portholes on incubators quietly, placing gently on top of incubators only those objects necessary, keeping radios at low volume, speaking quietly, and handling equipment noiselessly. Earmuffs may also reduce auditory input (Wong, 1999).

Nursing care affects sleep-wake behaviors in preterm infants (Brandon, Holditch-Davis, and Beylea, 1999). Infants can be protected from light by dimming the lights during the night, placing a blanket over the incubator (Fig. 27-7), or by covering the infant's eyes with a mask. Sleep-wake cycles can be induced with such measures. Infants need periods when they are completely undisturbed (Wong, 1999).

Infant Communication. Infants communicate their needs and ability to tolerate sensory stimulation through physiologic responses. The nurses and parents of high risk infants must therefore be alert to such cues. Although full-term infants may thrive on stimulation, this same stimulation in high risk infants can instead provoke physical symptoms of stress and anxiety (Blackburn, 1998; Gardner and Lubchenco, 1998).

Problems with noxious stimuli and barriers to normal contact may cause anxiety and tension. Clues to overstimulation include averting the gaze, hiccupping, gagging, or regurgitating food. Term infants exhibit a startle reflex, and premature infants move all of their limbs in an uncoordinated fashion in response to noxious stimuli. An irregular respiratory rate or an increased heart rate may develop in severely distressed infants, and they may then be unable to regain a calm state.

A relaxed infant state is indicated by stabilization of vital signs, closed eyes, and a relaxed posture. Nonintubated infants may make soothing verbal sounds when they are relaxed. Infants requiring artificial ventilation cannot cry audibly and often show their distress through posturing; they then relax once their needs are met. As high risk infants heal and mature, they increasingly respond to stimuli in a self-regulated manner rather than with a dissociated response. Infants who do not show increased self-regulation should be evaluated for a neurologic problem.

Infant Stimulation. A neonatal individualized development care and assessment program (NIDCAP) routinely integrates aspects of neurodevelopmental theory with caregivers' observations, environmental interventions, and parental support (Gardner and Lubchenco, 1998). Routine reassessment is built into the program's design. Developmental stimuli may consist of such simple measures as placing a waterbed on top of the infant's mattress, or kangaroo (skin-to-skin) holding. The simplest calming technique is to contain the infant's extremities close to the body using both hands. The care of the infant is organized to allow extended periods of undisturbed rest and sleep. Pain medications or sedatives should be administered consistently per the unit's protocol.

Infants acquire a sense of trust as they learn the feel, sound, and smell of their parents (Gardner and Lubchenco, 1998). High risk infants must also learn to trust their caregivers to obtain comfort. However, caregivers in the nursery may inflict pain as part of the care they must give. For this reason, it is important for both the parents and the caregivers to employ comforting interventions such as removing painful stimuli, stopping hunger, and changing wet or soiled clothing to foster trust.

When the infant is ready for stimulation, the nurse has many options. All infants can tolerate being held, even if only for short periods. Additional ways for the nurse or parents to stimulate infants include cuddling, rocking, singing, and talking to the infant (Fig. 27-8). These activities are beneficial, increase weight gain, and decrease time to discharge (Standley, 1998).

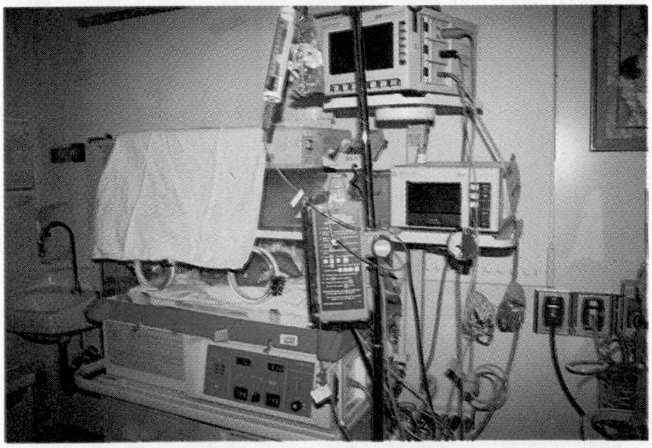

FIG. 27-7 • Infant in double-walled incubator with a blanket for a light shield. (Courtesy Marjorie Pyle, RNC, Lifecircle, Costa Mesa, CA.)

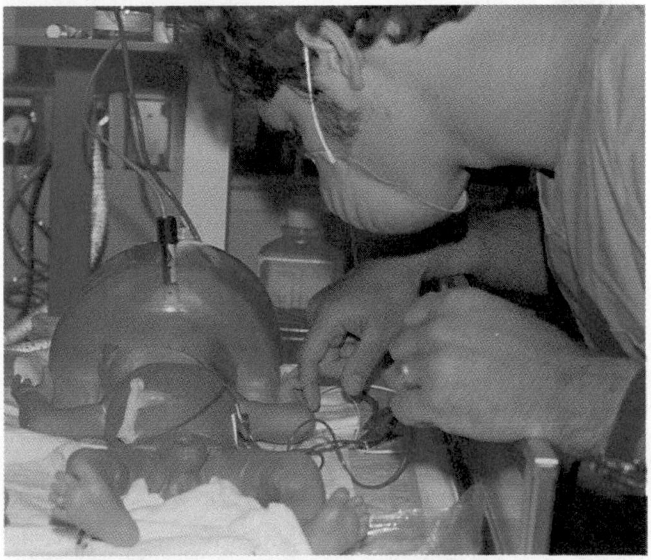

FIG. 27-8 • A father caresses his tiny preterm infant in the NICU. (Courtesy Marjorie Pyle, RNC, Lifecircle, Costa Mesa, CA.)

Stroking the infant's skin during medical therapy can provide tactile stimulation. The caregiver responds to the infant's cues by offering reassurance, providing for nonnutritive sucking, stroking the infant's back, and talking to the infant.

Mobiles and decals that can be changed frequently may also be placed within the infant's visual range to stimulate the infant visually. Wind-up musical toys provide rhythmic distractions as long as they are not too loud. If the infant is receiving phototherapy, the protective eye patches are removed periodically (e.g., during feeding) so that the infant can see the caregiver's face for short, comforting sessions.

Kangaroo Care. Kangaroo care (skin-to-skin holding) helps infants to directly interact with their parents (Gale and VandenBerg, 1998). In this technique the infant, dressed only in a diaper, is placed directly on the parent's bare chest and then covered with the parent's clothing or a warmed blanket (Fig. 27-9). In this way, the parent's body temperature also functions as an external heat source that enhances the infant's temperature regulation. Even ventilator-dependent infants weighing under 1 kg have been found to benefit from this measure, although they usually tolerate it for 30 minutes or less at a time (Neu, 1999).

Preterm infants experiencing kangaroo care recover rapidly from birth-related fatigue (Ludington-Hoe et al, 1999). Infants and parents who participate in kangaroo care have been observed to have dramatically better outcomes. The mothers report increased breast milk output and fewer feelings of helplessness related to their experiences in the NICU. The infants have been found to maintain their temperatures and oxygenation levels better and to experience fewer episodes of crying, apnea, and periodic respirations (Neu, Browne, and Vojir, 2000). They have also been observed to be alert and quiet longer and to have slightly higher heart rates. Kangaroo care also meets developmental needs by fostering neurobehavioral development.

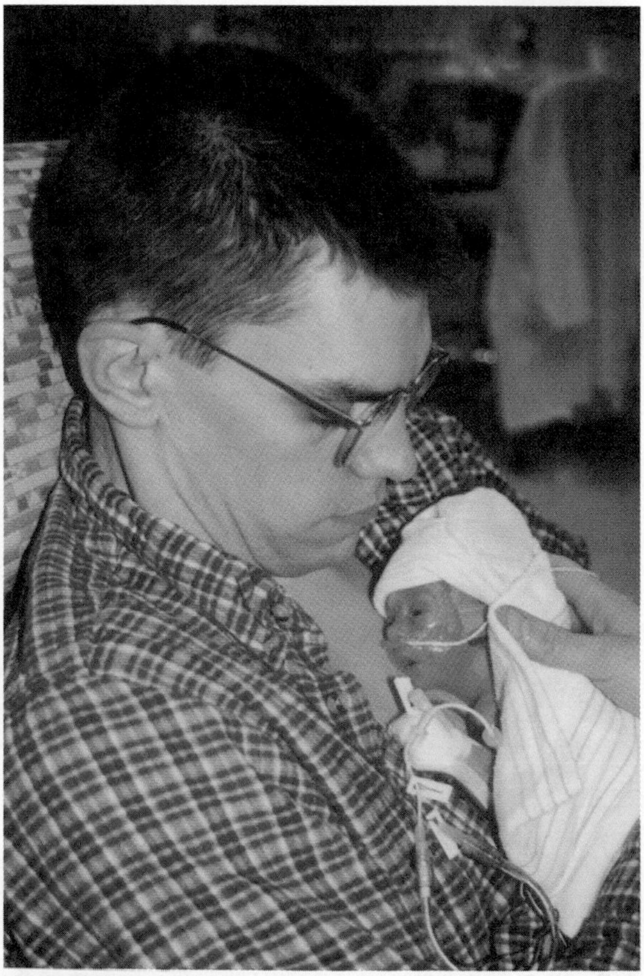

FIG. 27-9 • Father providing kangaroo care. (Courtesy Judy Meyr, St. Louis, MO.)

Parental Support. The nurse as support person and teacher shapes the environment and makes caregiving more responsive to the needs of parents and infant. Nurses are instrumental in helping parents learn who their infant is and to recognize behavioral cues in his or her development (VandenBerg, 1999).

If a high risk birth is anticipated, the family can be given a tour of the NICU or shown a video to prepare them for the sights and activities of the unit. After the birth, the parents can be given a booklet, be shown a video, or have someone describe what they will see when they go to the unit to see their infant. As soon as possible, the parents should see and touch their infant so that they can begin to acknowledge the reality of the birth and the infant's true appearance and condition. They will need encouragement to begin to accomplish the psychologic tasks imposed by the preterm birth. A nurse and/or physician should be present during the parent's first visit to see the infant for the following reasons:

- To help them "see" the infant rather than focus on equipment. The significance and function of the apparatus that surrounds the infant should be explained.
- To explain the characteristics normal for an infant of their baby's gestational age. In this way, parents do not compare their infant with a full-term healthy baby.
- To encourage the parent to express feelings about the pregnancy, labor, and birth and the experience of having a preterm infant.
- To assess the parent's perceptions of the infant and determine the appropriate time for them to become actively involved in care.

Community Focus

NUTRITION GUIDANCE FOR FAMILIES OF LOW-BIRTH-WEIGHT INFANTS

Low-birth-weight infants are often discharged from the hospital when they weigh approximately 2200 g. Many of these infants are small-for-gestational-age, and continued attention to their nutrition is important. In a study, monthly telephone-based nutrition guidance and support was successful in reducing stress of mothers and assisting to normalize growth of the infants. To achieve this catch-up growth, the daily intake of the infants was above the Recommended Daily Allowance (RDA) for age during the first few months of life. Community and home health nurse nurses must be cognizant of the importance of nutrition in this vulnerable population. Providing consistent information and support to assist mothers to ensure that their infants maintain an intake exceeding the RDA will decrease problems of inadequate growth and development experienced by low-birth-weight infants.

Data from Kennedy T, Oakland M, Shaw R: A nutrition intervention with families of low-birth-weight infants, *Nutr Clin Pract* 15(1):30-35, 2000.

As soon after the birth as possible, the parents are given the opportunity to meet the infant in the en face position, to touch the infant, and to see his or her favorable characteristics. The mother is encouraged to visit the nursery as desired and help with the infant's care. When the family cannot be present physically, staff members devise appropriate methods to keep the family in frequent touch with the newborn, such as daily phone calls, notes written as if from the infant, or photographs of the baby.

Some hospitals have support groups for parents of infants in intensive care nurseries. These groups encourage parents experiencing anxiety and grief to share their feelings. A parent with NICU experience often makes contact with a new member and provides additional support. These parents provide support for the new NICU parent through hospital visits, phone contact, and home visits.

Some high risk infants can be discharged earlier than expected (Gamblian, Hess, and Kenner, 1998). Criteria for early discharge require the infant to be stable physiologically, be receiving adequate nutrition, and have a stable body temperature. The parents or other caregivers must exhibit physical, emotional, and educational readiness to assume care of the infant. Ideally, the home environment is adequate for meeting the needs of the infant. The parents need to show that they know the way to take the infant's temperature, signs and symptoms to report, and that they understand the dietary needs of the infant.

Parent Education

Cardiopulmonary Resuscitation. Sudden infant death syndrome (SIDS) is more likely to develop in preterm infants than in term infants; infants discharged from an NICU are about twice as likely to die unexpectedly during the first year of life as infants in the general population. Instruction in cardiopulmonary resuscitation (CPR) is essential for parents of all infants but especially for parents of infants at risk for life-threatening events. Risk factors include prematurity, apnea and/or bradycardia spells, and the tendency to choke. Before taking the infant home, parents must be able to administer CPR. All parents should be encouraged to obtain instruction in CPR at their local Red Cross or other community agency.

➤ Evaluation

The nurse uses the previously stated outcomes of care to evaluate the effectiveness of the physical and psychosocial aspects of care (Nursing Care Plan).

Critical Thinking

PRETERM INFANT

A multiparous woman has a preterm infant who was born at 28 weeks of gestation and was transported to a special care nursery. The woman does not live in the city where the tertiary center is located, and she is to be discharged tomorrow. It is anticipated that the infant will require a stay in the NICU for at least 8 more weeks and will likely require oxygen therapy at home after discharge. What information should the transport team provide the parents? What kinds of assistance will this mother need now and after the infant goes home? Identify resources in the community that may have services she can use.

Complications Associated with Prematurity

Respiratory Distress Syndrome. Respiratory distress syndrome (RDS) is a lung disorder usually affecting premature infants. The incidence of RDS in infants weighing less than 1500 g is 56% (Hack et al, 1995). Maternal and fetal conditions associated with a decreased incidence and severity of RDS include female infant; African-American race; maternal steroid (betamethasone) therapy; and stressors such as maternal pregnancy-induced hypertension, maternal drug abuse, chronic retroplacental abruption, prolonged rupture of membranes, and IUGR (Hagedorn, Gardner, and Abman, 1998). The incidence and severity of RDS increase with a decrease in gestational age. Perinatal asphyxia, hypovolemia, male infant, Caucasian race, maternal diabetes, second-born twin, familial predisposition, maternal hypotension, cesarean birth without labor, hydrops fetalis, and third-trimester bleeding are all factors that place an infant at increased risk for RDS (Hagedorn, Gardner, and Abman, 1998).

RDS is caused by a lack of pulmonary surfactant, which leads to progressive atelectasis, loss of functional residual capacity, and ventilation-perfusion imbalance with an uneven distribution of ventilation. Surfactant deficiency may be caused by insufficient surfactant production, abnormal composition and function, disruption of surfactant production, or a combination of these factors. The sequence of events that occurs is further compromised by weak respiratory muscles and an overly compliant chest wall, which is common to premature infants. Lung capacity is compromised by the presence of proteinaceous material and epithelial debris in the airways. The resulting decreased oxygenation, cyanosis, and metabolic or respiratory acidosis can increase pulmonary vascular resistance (PVR). This increased PVR can lead to right-to-left shunting and a reopening of the ductus arteriosus and foramen ovale (Merenstein and Gardner, 1998).

Clinical symptoms of RDS include tachypnea; grunting; nasal flaring; intercostal, supraclavicular, or subcostal retractions; hypercapnia; respiratory or mixed acidosis; hypotension; and shock. These respiratory symptoms usually present immediately after birth or within 6 hours of birth. Physical examination reveals crackles, poor air exchange, pallor, use of accessory muscles (retractions), and occasionally apnea. Radiographic findings include uniform reticulogranular appearance and air bronchograms (Fanaroff and Martin, 1997). The infant's clinical course is variable. There is usually an increased oxygen requirement and increased respiratory effort as atelectasis, loss of functional residual capacity, and ventilation-perfusion imbalance worsen.

Severe respiratory distress syndrome is often associated with a shocklike state, as manifested by diminished cardiac inflow and low arterial blood pressure. The ELBW or VLBW infant, as a result of extreme pulmonary immaturity, decreased glycogen stores, and lack of accessory muscles, may have severe RDS at birth.

RDS is a self-limiting disease with respiratory symptoms abating after 72 hours. The disappearance of respiratory symptoms coincides with the production of surfactant in type 2 cells of the alveoli.

The treatment for RDS is supportive. Adequate ventilation and oxygenation must be established and maintained in an attempt to prevent ventilation-perfusion mismatch and atelectasis. Exogenous surfactant, which alters the typical course of RDS, may be administered at or shortly after birth. Positive-pressure ventilation, CPAP, and oxygen therapy may be needed

Nursing Care Plan THE HIGH RISK PREMATURE NEWBORN

NURSING DIAGNOSIS Ineffective breathing pattern related to pulmonary and neuromuscular immaturity, decreased energy, fatigue

EXPECTED OUTCOME Infant exhibits adequate oxygenation (i.e., ABGs and acid-base balance within normal limits [WNL], oxygen saturations 92% or greater, respiratory rate and pattern WNL, breath sounds clear, absence of grunting, nasal flaring, minimal retractions, skin color WNL).

Nursing Interventions/*Rationales*

Position neonate prone or supine, avoiding neck hyperextension *to promote optimum air exchange.* Use a side-lying position after feeding or in cases of excessive mucus production *to avoid aspiration.* Avoid Trendelenburg position *because it can cause increased intracranial pressure and reduce lung capacity.*

Suction nasopharynx, trachea, and endotracheal tube as indicated *to remove mucus.* Avoid oversuctioning *because it can cause bronchospasm, bradycardia, hypoxia, and predispose neonate to intraventricular hemorrhage.*

Administer percussion, vibration, and postural drainage as prescribed *to facilitate drainage of secretions.*

Administer oxygen and monitor neonatal response *to maintain oxygen saturation.*

Maintain a neutral thermal environment *to conserve oxygen use.*

Monitor arterial blood gases, acid-base balance, oxygen saturation, respiratory rate and pattern, breath sounds, and airway patency; observe for grunting, nasal flaring, retractions, and cyanosis *to detect signs of respiratory distress.*

NURSING DIAGNOSIS Ineffective thermoregulation related to immature temperature regulation and minimal subcutaneous fat stores

EXPECTED OUTCOME Infant exhibits maintenance of stable body temperature within normal range for postconceptional age (36.5° to 37.2° C).

Nursing Interventions/*Rationales*

Place neonate in a prewarmed radiant warmer *to maintain stable temperature.*

Place temperature probe on neonatal abdomen *to control heat levels in radiant warmer.*

Take axillary temperature periodically *to monitor temperature and cross-check functioning of warmer unit.*

Avoid infant exposure to cool air and drafts, cold scales, cold stethoscopes, cold examination tables, and prolonged bathing *that predispose the infant to heat loss.*

Monitor probe often *because detachment can cause overheating or warmer-induced hyperthermia.*

Transfer infant to a servocontrolled open warmer bed or incubator *when temperature has stabilized.*

NURSING DIAGNOSIS Risk for infection related to immature immune system

EXPECTED OUTCOME Infant exhibits no evidence of nosocomial infection.

Nursing Interventions/*Rationales*

Institute scrupulous handwashing techniques before and after handling neonate; ensure all supplies and/or equipment are clean before use; and ensure strict aseptic technique with invasive procedures *to minimize exposure to infective organisms.*

Prevent contact with persons who have communicable infections; and instruct parents in infection control procedures *to minimize infection risk.*

Administer prescribed antibiotics *to provide coverage for infection during sepsis workup.*

Continuously monitor vital signs for stability *because instability, hypothermia, or prolonged temperature elevations serve as indicators of infection.*

NURSING DIAGNOSIS Risk for altered nutrition, less than body requirements related to inability to ingest nutrients secondary to immaturity

EXPECTED OUTCOMES Infant receives adequate amount of nutrients with sufficient caloric intake to maintain positive nitrogen balance; demonstrates steady weight gain.

Nursing Interventions/*Rationales*

Administer parenteral fluid/total parenteral nutrition (TPN) as prescribed *to provide adequate nutrition and fluid intake.*

Monitor for signs of intolerance to TPN, *which can interfere with effective replenishment of nutrients.*

Periodically assess readiness to orally feed (i.e., strong suck, swallow, and gag reflexes) *to provide appropriate transition from TPN to oral feeding as soon as neonate is ready.*

Advance volume and concentration of formula when orally feeding per unit protocol *to avoid overfeeding and feeding intolerance.*

If mother desires to breastfeed when neonate is stable, demonstrate how to express milk *to establish and maintain lactation until infant can breastfeed.*

NURSING DIAGNOSIS Risk for fluid volume deficit/excess related to immature physiology

EXPECTED OUTCOME Infant exhibits evidence of fluid homeostasis.

Nursing Interventions/*Rationales*

Administer parenteral fluids as prescribed and regulate carefully *to maintain fluid balance.* Avoid hypertonic fluids

Nursing Care Plan THE HIGH RISK PREMATURE NEWBORN—cont'd

such as undiluted medications and concentrated glucose *becaue they can cause excess solute load on immature kidneys.*

Implement strategies (e.g., use of plastic covers and increase of ambient humidity) *that minimize insensible water loss.*

Monitor hydration status (i.e., skin turgor, blood pressure, edema, weight, mucous membranes, fontanels, urine specific gravity, and electrolytes) and intake and output *to evaluate for evidence of dehydration or overhydration.*

NURSING DIAGNOSIS Risk for impaired skin integrity related to immature skin structure, immobility, or invasive procedures

EXPECTED OUTCOME Infant's skin remains intact with no evidence of irritation or injury.

Nursing Interventions/*Rationales*

Cleanse skin as needed with plain warm water and apply moisturizing agents to skin *to prevent dryness and reduce friction across skin surface.*

When performing procedures: minimize use of tape and apply a skin barrier between tape and skin; use transparent elastic film for securing central and peripheral lines; use limb electrodes for monitoring or attach with hydrogel and rotate electrodes often; remove adhesives with soap and water rather than alcohol or acetone-based adhesive removers *to minimize skin damage.*

Monitor use of thermal devices such as warmers or heating pads carefully *to prevent burns.*

Monitor skin closely for evidence of redness, rash, irritation, bruising, breakdown, ischemia, and infiltration *to detect and treat potential complications early.*

NURSING DIAGNOSIS Risk for injury related to increased intracranial pressure and intraventricular hemorrhage secondary to immature central nervous system

EXPECTED OUTCOME Infant will exhibit normal intracranial pressure (ICP) with no evidence of intraventricular hemorrhage.

Nursing Interventions/*Rationales*

Institute minimum stimulation protocol (i.e., minimal handling, clustering care techniques, avoidance of sudden head movements to one side, undisturbed sleep periods, light variations to simulate day and night, limiting personnel and equipment noise in environment) *to decrease stress responses, which can increase ICP.*

Institute ordered pharmacologic and nonpharmacologic pain control methods *to manage pain and reduce physical stress.*

Avoid hypertonic solutions and medications *because they increase cerebral blood flow.*

Elevate head of bed 15 to 20 degrees *to decrease ICP.*

Monitor vital signs *for evidence of ICP.*

Recognize signs of overstimulation (i.e., flaccidity, yawning, irritability, crying, staring, and active averting) *so stimulation can be stopped to allow rest.*

NURSING DIAGNOSIS Altered parenting related to separation and interruption of parent/infant attachment secondary to premature birth

EXPECTED OUTCOMES Parents establish contact with neonate; demonstrate competent parenting skills and willingness to care for neonate.

Nursing Interventions/*Rationales*

Before parents' first visit to the NICU, prepare them by explaining what the neonate will look like, what the equipment will look like, and its function *to diminish fear and decrease sense of shock.*

Keep parents informed about infant's condition (e.g., improvements and setbacks) and important aspects of infant's care; encourage and answer parental questions; actively listen to parent concerns *to establish trust, open communication, and caring atmosphere to aid in coping.*

Encourage parents to visit the NICU often; to name infant; to touch, hold, or caress infant as physical condition permits; to be actively involved in infant's care; to bring personal items (e.g., clothing, stuffed animals, or pictures of family) *to allow formation of emotional bond.*

Reinforce parent involvement and praise care endeavors *to increase self-confidence in their contribution.*

Encourage parents to bring other siblings to visit; explain to siblings what they are seeing; encourage siblings to draw pictures or write letters for infant and place in or near infant's crib *to promote family involvement, help ease sibling fears, and let them contribute to infant's care.*

Refer parents to social services as needed *to ensure comprehensive care.*

during the respiratory illness. Prevention of complications associated with mechanical ventilation is critical. These complications include pulmonary interstitial emphysema (PIE), pneumothorax, pneumomediastinum, and pneumopericardium.

Acid-base balance is evaluated by monitoring ABG values (Table 27-1). Frequent blood sampling requires arterial access either by umbilical artery catheterization (UAC) or by a peripheral arterial line. Pulse oximetry and transcutaneous carbon dioxide and oxygen monitors document trends in ventilation and oxygenation. Capillary blood gas values may be used to evaluate pH and P_{CO_2} in infants whose condition is more stable (Cloherty and Stark, 1997).

The maintenance of an NTE continues to be of critical importance in infants with RDS; infants with hypoxemia are unable to increase their metabolic rate when cold stressed (Fanaroff and Martin, 1997).

TABLE 27-1
Normal Arterial Blood Gas Values for Neonates

Value	Range
pH	7.33-7.42
Arterial oxygen pressure (Pao_2)	50-80 mm Hg
Carbon dioxide pressure ($Paco_2$)	38-48 mm Hg
Bicarbonate (HCO_3)	20-24 mEq/L
Oxygen saturation	>90%

From Dickason E, Silverman B, and Kaplan J: *Maternal-infant nursing care,* ed 3, St Louis, 1998, Mosby.

The clinical and radiographic presentation of neonatal pneumonia may be similar to that of RDS. Fluid in the minor tissue may also be noted in infants with neonatal pneumonia. Therefore sepsis evaluation, including blood culture, complete blood count (CBC) with differential, and occasionally a lumbar puncture, is done in infants with RDS to rule out neonatal pneumonia. Broad-spectrum antibiotics are begun while the results of cultures are awaited (Cloherty and Stark, 1997).

Fluid and nutrition must be maintained for the infant critically ill with RDS. Parenteral nutrition can provide protein and fats to promote a positive nitrogen balance. Daily monitoring of electrolytes, urine output, specific gravity, and weight assists in the evaluation of hydration status (Cloherty and Stark, 1997; Fanaroff and Martin, 1997).

The need for frequent blood sampling may make blood transfusions necessary. A venous hematocrit of more than 40% is usually needed by the critically ill infant to maintain adequate oxygen-carrying capacity (Fanaroff and Martin, 1997).

NURSE ALERT • Directed-donor blood is often requested. Directed-donor blood is usually obtained from a family member or close friend of the family who has the same blood type as the infant or a compatible type. It may be necessary to notify the infant's family of the potential need for blood transfusion on admission to allow for the processing of directed-donor blood.

Reassuring the family that stringent testing of all blood products is done may alleviate some of their anxiety about blood-borne pathogens. Because some religions prohibit the use of blood transfusions, it is critical to obtain a complete history from the family, including their religious preference. Alternative strategies for maintaining the hematocrit may be needed in these instances.

Complications Associated with Oxygen Therapy

Retinopathy of Prematurity. Retinopathy of prematurity (ROP) is a complex, multicausal disorder that affects the developing retinal vessels of premature infants. The normal retinal vessels begin to form in utero at approximately 16 weeks' gestation in response to an unknown stimulus. The retinal vessels continue to develop until they reach maturity at approximately 42 to 43 weeks after conception. Once the retina is completely vascularized, the retinal vessels are not susceptible to ROP. The mechanism of injury in ROP is unclear. Oxygen tensions that are too high for the level of retinal maturity initially result in vasoconstriction. After oxygen therapy is discontinued, neovascularization occurs in the retina and vitreous, with capillary hemorrhages, fibrotic resolution, and possible retinal detachment. Scar tissue formation and consequent visual impairment may be mild or severe. The entire disease process in severe cases may take as long as 5 months to evolve. Examination by an ophthalmologist before discharge and a schedule for repeat examinations thereafter are recommended for the parents' guidance.

The key to management of ROP is prevention and early detection of premature birth. Circumferential cryopexy, laser photocoagulation, vitamin E therapy, and decreasing the intensity of ambient light are used in the treatment of ROP with varying results (Fanaroff and Martin, 1997).

Bronchopulmonary Dysplasia. Bronchopulmonary dysplasia (BPD) is a chronic pulmonary iatrogenic condition caused by barotrauma from pressure ventilation and oxygen toxicity (Hagedorn, Gardner, and Abman, 1998). The etiology of BPD is multifactorial and includes pulmonary immaturity, surfactant deficiency, lung injury and stretch, barotrauma, inflammation caused by oxygen exposure, fluid overexposure, ligation of a patent ductus arteriosus, and genetic predisposition (Hagedorn, Gardner, and Abman, 1998). The incidence of BPD in infants weighing less than 1500 g who require mechanical ventilation for RDS ranges from 5% to 38% (Fanaroff and Martin, 1997).

Clinical symptoms of BPD include tachypnea, retractions, nasal flaring, increased work of breathing, exercise intolerance (to handling and feeding), and tachycardia (Hagedorn, Gardner, and Abman, 1998). Auscultation of lung fields in affected infants reveals crackles, decreased air movement, and occasionally expiratory wheezing.

Treatment for BPD includes oxygen therapy, nutrition, fluid restriction, and medications (e.g., diuretics, corticosteroids, and bronchodilators). The key to the management of BPD is prevention by reducing the incidence of prematurity and RDS and by using surfactant and other less toxic therapies.

The prognosis for infants with BPD depends on the degree of pulmonary dysfunction. Most deaths occur within the first year of life as a result of cardiorespiratory failure, sepsis, or respiratory infection; in some infants the deaths are sudden and unexplained (Bancalari, 1997).

Patent Ductus Arteriosus. The ductus arteriosus is a muscular contractile structure in the fetus connecting the left pulmonary artery and the dorsal aorta. The ductus constricts after birth as oxygenation, the levels of circulating prostaglandins, and the muscle mass increase. Other factors that promote ductal closure include catecholamines, low pH, bradykinin, and acetylcholine (Zahka and Patel, 1997). When the fetal ductus arteriosus fails to close after birth, patent ductus arteriosus (PDA) occurs. The incidence of PDA in premature infants weighing less than 1500 g is 30% (Fanaroff and Martin, 1997).

The clinical presentation in an infant with a PDA includes systolic murmur, active precordium, bounding peripheral pulses, tachycardia, tachypnea, crackles, and hepatomegaly. The systolic murmur is heard best at the second or third intercostal space at the upper left sternal border. An active precordium is caused by an increased left ventricular stroke volume. A widened pulse pressure may result in an increase in peripheral pulses (Daberkow-Carson and Washington, 1998; Zahka and Patel, 1997).

Radiographic studies of infants with PDA typically show cardiac enlargement and pulmonary edema. ABG findings reveal hypercarbia and metabolic acidosis. Echocardiography can demonstrate a PDA and can quantitate the amount of blood shunting across the PDA (Daberkow-Carson and Washington, 1998).

The PDA can be managed medically or surgically. Medical management consists of ventilatory support, fluid restriction, and the administration of diuretics and indomethacin. Indomethacin is a prostaglandin synthetase inhibitor that blocks the effect of the arachidonic acid products on the ductus and causes the PDA to constrict (Daberkow-Carson and Washington, 1998). Ventilatory support is adjusted based on ABG levels. Fluid restriction is implemented to decrease cardiovascular volume overload in association with the diuretic therapy. Surgical ligation is done when PDA is clinically significant and medical management has failed (Daberkow-Carson and Washington, 1998).

Nursing care of the infant with PDA focuses on supportive care. The infant needs an NTE, adequate oxygenation, meticulous fluid balance, and parental support.

Periventricular-Intraventricular Hemorrhage. Periventricular-intraventricular hemorrhage (PV-IVH) is one of the most common types of brain injury that occurs in neonates and is among the most severe in both short-term and long-term outcomes. The true incidence of PV-IVH is unknown, but the general estimate is 20% to 30% in infants less than 32 weeks of gestation or under 1500 g; approximately 50% of infants who die in the first few days of life experience hemorrhage (Moe and Paige, 1998). Use of prenatal corticosteroids can reduce the incidence to about 25% (Reed and Blumer, 1997).

The pathogenesis of PV-IVH includes intravascular factors (e.g., fluctuating or increasing cerebral blood flow, increases in cerebral venous pressures, and coagulopathy), vascular factors, extravascular factors, and nursery care. PV-IVH events typically occur within the first week of life. PV-IVH is classified according to severity, which determines long-term neurodevelopmental outcomes.

Nursing care focuses on recognition of factors that increase the risk of PV-IVH, interventions to decrease the risk of bleeding, and supportive care to infants who have bleeding episodes. The infant is positioned with the head in midline and the head of the bed elevated slightly to prevent or minimize fluctuations in intracranial blood pressure. NTE is maintained, as well as oxygenation. Rapid infusions of fluids should be avoided. Blood pressure is monitored closely for fluctuations. The infant is monitored for signs of pneumothorax because it often precedes PV-IVH.

Necrotizing Enterocolitis. Necrotizing enterocolitis (NEC) is an acute inflammatory disease of the gastrointestinal mucosa, commonly complicated by perforation. This often fatal disease occurs in about 2% to 5% of newborns in NICUs. Although the cause of NEC is unknown, the following factors contribute to its development: asphyxia, RDS, umbilical artery catheter, exchange transfusion, early enteral feedings, PDA, congenital heart disease, polycythemia, anemia, shock, and gastrointestinal infection. Breastfeeding seems to lower the incidence of NEC, as does nonnutritive sucking during gavage feedings (Pickler and Terrell, 1994).

Reversal of perinatal asphyxia within 30 minutes may prevent GI tract insult and thus prevent the pathophysiologic events that trigger NEC. After 30 minutes, the distribution of cardiac output tends to be directed more toward the heart and brain and away from the abdominal organs. Therefore prompt birth of the intrauterine-asphyxiated fetus or ventilation of the asphyxiated newborn may be beneficial to the GI tract as well as to other organs.

The onset of NEC in the full-term infant usually occurs between 4 and 10 days after birth. In the preterm infant the onset may be delayed for up to 30 days. Signs of developing NEC are nonspecific, which is characteristic of many neonatal disease processes. Some generalized signs include decreased activity, hypotonia, pallor, recurrent apnea and bradycardia, decreased oxygen saturation, respiratory distress, metabolic acidosis, oliguria, hypotension, decreased perfusion, temperature instability, and cyanosis. GI symptoms include abdominal distention, increasing or bile-stained residual gastric aspirates, vomiting (bile or blood), grossly bloody stools, abdominal tenderness, and erythema of the abdominal wall (Holland, Price, and Bensard, 1998).

Diagnosis of NEC is confirmed by radiographic examination that reveals bowel loop distention, pneumatosis intestinalis, pneumoperitoneum, portal air, or a combination of these findings. The abnormal radiographic findings are caused by the bacterial colonization of the GI tract associated with NEC, resulting in an ileus. Pneumatosis intestinalis, pneumoperitoneum, and portal air are caused by gas produced by the bacteria that invade the wall of the intestines and escape into the peritoneum and portal system when perforation occurs. Laboratory evaluation includes a complete blood cell count with differential, coagulation studies, ABG analysis, serum electrolyte levels, and blood culture. The white blood cell (WBC) count may be either increased or decreased. The platelet count and coagulation studies may be abnormal, with thrombocytopenia and disseminated intravascular coagulation (DIC). Electrolyte levels may be abnormal, with leaking capillary beds and fluid shifts with the infection.

Treatment of infants with NEC is supportive. Oral or tube feedings are discontinued to rest the GI tract. An orogastric tube is placed and attached to low suction to provide gastric decompression. Parenteral therapy (often by TPN) is begun. NEC is an infectious disease; control of infection is imperative, with an emphasis on careful handwashing before and after infant contact. Antibiotic therapy may be instituted, and surgical resection is performed if perforation or clinical deterioration occurs. Therapy may be prolonged and recovery may be delayed by adhesions, complications of bowel resection, short gut syndrome (especially if the ileocecal valve is removed), and intolerance of oral feedings.

POSTMATURE INFANTS

Postterm infants are those whose gestation is prolonged beyond 42 weeks, regardless of birth weight; the infant is called postmature. These infants may be large-for-gestational-age (LGA) or small-for-gestational-age (SGA), but most often their weight is appropriate-for-gestational-age (AGA). It is important to determine whether the pregnancy is actually prolonged and also whether there is any evidence of fetal jeopardy as a result. The cause of prolonged pregnancy is unknown. Postmaturity can be associated with placental insufficiency, resulting in a newborn who has a wasted appearance (dysmature) at birth due to loss of subcutaneous fat and muscle mass. There may be meconium staining of the fingernails, the hair and nails may be long, and vernix may be absent. The skin may peel off. Not all postmature infants show signs of dysmaturity; some continue to grow in utero and are large at birth.

Perinatal mortality is significantly higher in the postmature fetus and neonate. During labor and birth, increased oxygen demands of the postmature fetus may not be met. Insufficient gas exchange in the postmature placenta increases the likelihood of intrauterine hypoxia, which may result in the passage of meconium in utero, thereby increasing the risk for meconium aspiration syndrome. Of all the deaths of postmature newborns, one half occur during labor and birth, about one third occur before the onset of labor, and one sixth occur in the newborn period.

Meconium Aspiration Syndrome

Meconium staining of the amniotic fluid can be indicative of nonreassuring fetal status, especially in a vertex presentation. It appears in from 8% to 20% of all births. Many infants with meconium staining exhibit no signs of depression at birth; however, the presence of meconium in the amniotic fluid necessitates careful supervision of labor and close monitoring of fetal well-being. The presence of a team skilled in neonatal resuscitation is required at the birth of any infant with meconium-stained amniotic fluid. The mouth and nares of the infant should be suctioned on the perineum before the infant's first breath.

If meconium is not removed from the airway at birth, it can migrate down to the terminal airways, causing mechanical obstruction leading to meconium aspiration syndrome (MAS). The fetus may have aspirated meconium in utero; this can cause a chemical pneumonitis. These infants may develop pulmonary hypertension of the newborn (PPHN), further complicating their management.

Persistent Pulmonary Hypertension of the Newborn

PPHN is a term applied to the combined findings of pulmonary hypertension, right-to-left shunting, and a structurally normal heart. PPHN may present either as a single entity or as the main component of MAS, congenital diaphragmatic hernia, RDS, hyperviscosity syndrome, or neonatal pneumonia or sepsis. PPHN is also called persistent fetal circulation (PFC) because the syndrome includes reversion to fetal pathways for blood flow.

A brief review of fetal blood flow can help in the visualization of the problems with PPHN (see Fig. 8-11). In utero, oxygen-rich blood leaves the placenta via the umbilical vein, goes through the ductus venosus, and enters the inferior vena cava. From here, it empties into the right atrium and is mostly shunted across the foramen ovale to the left atrium, effectively bypassing the lungs. This blood enters the left ventricle, leaves through the aorta, and preferentially perfuses the carotid and coronary arteries. Thus the heart and brain receive the most oxygenated blood. Blood drains from the brain into the superior vena cava, reenters the right atrium, proceeds to the right ventricle, and exits through the main pulmonary artery. The lungs are a high-pressure circuit, needing only enough perfusion for growth and nutrition. The ductus arteriosus (connecting the main pulmonary artery and the aorta) is the path of least resistance for the blood leaving the right side of the fetal heart, shunting most of the cardiac output away from the lungs and toward the systemic system. This right-to-left shunting is the key to fetal circulation.

After birth, both the foramen ovale and the ductus arteriosus close in response to various biochemical processes, pressure changes within the heart, and dilation of the pulmonary vessels. This dilation allows virtually all of the cardiac output to enter the lungs, become oxygenated, and provide oxygen-rich blood to the tissues for normal metabolism. Any process that interferes with this transition from fetal to neonatal circulation may precipitate PPHN. PPHN characteristically proceeds into a downward spiral of exacerbating hypoxia and pulmonary vasoconstriction. Prompt recognition and aggressive intervention are required to reverse this process.

The infant with PPHN is typically born at term or postterm and presents with tachycardia and cyanosis. Management depends on the underlying etiology of the persistent pulmonary hypertension. The use of extracorporeal membrane oxygenation (ECMO) has improved the chances of survival of these infants.

Another mode of treatment for PPHN and other respiratory disorders of the newborn is high-frequency ventilation, a group of assisted-ventilation methods that deliver small volumes of gas at high frequencies and limit the development of high airway pressure, thus reducing barotrauma (Fanaroff and Martin, 1997).

OTHER PROBLEMS RELATED TO GESTATION

Small-for-Gestational-Age and Intrauterine Growth Restriction

Infants who are small-for-gestational-age (i.e., weight is below the 10th percentile expected at term) or infants who have IUGR (i.e., rate of growth does not meet expected growth pattern) are considered high risk, with the perimortality rate 5 to 20 times greater than that for the normal term infant (Kliegman, 1997).

Various conditions can affect and impede growth in the developing fetus. Conditions occurring in the first trimester that affect all aspects of fetal growth (e.g., infections, teratogens, and chromosomal abnormalities), or extrinsic conditions early in pregnancy result in symmetric IUGR (i.e., head circumference, length, and weight are all less than 10%). Conditions causing symmetric growth retardation result in a short, SGA infant, usually with a smaller head circumference and reduced brain capacity. Growth restriction in later stages of pregnancy, as a result of maternal or placental factors, results in asymmetric growth restriction (with respect to gestational age, weight will be less than the tenth percentile whereas length and head circumference will be greater than the tenth percentile). Infants with asymmetric IUGR have the potential for normal growth and development. Abnormal fetal size may indicate an adaptive response, with diminished fetal weight-sparing brain growth (Fanaroff and Martin, 1997).

Care of the SGA infant is based on the clinical problems present and is the same given to preterm infants with the same problems. Gas exchange is supported by maintaining a clear airway and preventing cold stress. Hypoglycemia is treated with oral feedings (e.g., breast, formula, or dextrose solution) per hospital protocol. Parenteral infusions may be necessary. An external heat source (radiant warmer or incubator) is used until the infant's temperature is stabilized. Nursing support of parents is similar to that given to parents of preterm infants.

Common problems that affect small-for-gestational-age IUGR infants are perinatal asphyxia, meconium aspiration (discussed previously), hypoglycemia, and heat loss.

Perinatal Asphyxia. Commonly, IUGR infants have been exposed to chronic hypoxia for varying periods before labor and birth. Labor is a stressor to the normal fetus; it is an even greater stressor for the growth-restricted fetus. The chronically hypoxic infant is severely compromised by even a normal labor and has difficulty compensating after birth. The alert, wide-eyed appearance of the newborn is attributed to prolonged fetal hypoxia. Appropriate management and resuscitation are essential for the depressed infant.

The birth of SGA babies with perinatal asphyxia may be associated with a maternal history of heavy cigarette smoking; preeclampsia; low socioeconomic status; multifetal gestation; gestational infections such as rubella, cytomegalovirus, and toxoplasmosis; advanced diabetes mellitus; and cardiac problems. Sequelae to perinatal asphyxia include MAS and hypoglycemia.

Hypoglycemia. All stressed infants are at risk for the development of hypoglycemia. Stress may include perinatal asphyxia and IUGR. The definition of hypoglycemia differs for the term and the preterm infant. Hypoglycemia occurring within the first 3 days of life is defined as a blood glucose level of less than 40 mg/dl in the term infant or less than 25 mg/dl in the preterm infant. Symptoms of hypoglycemia include poor feeding, hypothermia, and diaphoresis. CNS symptoms can include tremors and jitteriness, weak cry, lethargy, floppy posture, seizures, or coma. Diagnosis is confirmed by laboratory blood glucose determinations or with reagent strips such as Chemstrip-BG or Dextrostix (McGowan, Hagedorn, and Hay, 1998).

Heat Loss. For numerous reasons, SGA infants are particularly susceptible to temperature instability, and close attention must be paid to them to maintain thermoneutrality. These reasons include the fact that they have less muscle mass, less brown fat, less heat-preserving subcutaneous fat, and little ability to control skin capillaries. Nursing considerations focus on maintenance of thermoneutrality to promote recovery from perinatal asphyxia because cold stress jeopardizes such recovery (Blake and Murray, 1998).

Large-for-Gestational-Age

The large-for-gestational-age, or oversized, infant traditionally has been one who weighs 4000 g or more at birth. An infant is considered LGA despite gestation when the weight is above the 90th percentile on growth charts or two standard deviations above the mean weight for gestational age. Certain fetal disorders can also result in LGA infants. These include transposition of the great vessels and Beckwith-Wiedemann syndrome.

Maternal pelvic diameters have not kept pace with the better maternal health and nutrition that results in larger babies; thus fetopelvic disproportion often occurs, particularly in obese women, women who gain 16 kg or more during gestation, and women with undiagnosed and/or uncontrolled diabetes, who are prone to have large babies. Birth trauma, especially associated with breech or shoulder presentation, is a serious hazard for the oversized neonate. Asphyxia, CNS injury, or both may occur.

All pregnancies of longer than 42 weeks' gestation must be carefully evaluated. All large fetuses are monitored during a trial of labor, and preparation is made for a cesarean birth if nonreassuring fetal status or poor progress of labor occurs. LGA newborns may be preterm, term, or postdate; they may be infants of diabetic (or prediabetic) mothers; or they may be postmature. Each of these problems carries special concerns. Regardless of coexisting potential problems, the oversized infant is at risk by virtue of size alone.

The nurse assesses the LGA infant for gestational age, hypoglycemia, and trauma resulting from vaginal or cesarean birth. The blood glucose levels of LGA infants are monitored, and hypoglycemia is corrected. Any specific birth injuries are identified and treated appropriately.

Infants of Diabetic Mothers

All infants born to mothers with diabetes are at some risk for complications. The degree of risk is affected by the severity and duration of maternal disease. Problems seen in IDMs include congenital anomalies, macrosomia, birth trauma and perinatal asphyxia, RDS, hypoglycemia, hypocalcemia and hypomagnesemia, cardiomyopathy, hyperbilirubinemia, and polycythemia. Because some of these problems are also seen in infants with gestational age–related problems, discussion of infants of mothers with diabetes is included here.

Pathophysiology. The mechanisms responsible for the problems seen in IDMs are not fully understood. Congenital anomalies are believed to be caused by fluctuations in blood glucose levels and episodes of ketoacidosis in early pregnancy. Later in pregnancy, when the mother's pancreas cannot release sufficient insulin to meet increased demands, maternal hyperglycemia results. The high levels of glucose cross the placenta and stimulate the fetal pancreas to release insulin. The combination of the increased supply of maternal glucose and other nutrients, the inability of maternal insulin to cross the placenta, and increased fetal insulin results in excessive fetal growth called macrosomia (see the discussion that follows).

Hyperinsulinemia accounts for many of the problems the fetus or infant develops. In addition to fluctuating glucose levels, maternal vascular involvement or superimposed maternal infection adversely affect the fetus. Normally, maternal blood has a more alkaline pH than does carbon dioxide–rich fetal blood. This phenomenon encourages the exchange of oxygen and carbon dioxide across the placental membrane. When the maternal blood is more acidotic than the fetal blood, such as during ketoacidosis, little carbon dioxide or oxygen exchange occurs at the level of the placenta. The mortality for the unborn baby resulting from an episode of maternal ketoacidosis may be as high as 50% or more (Fanaroff and Martin, 1997).

There are indications that some neonatal conditions (e.g., macrosomia, hypoglycemia, polyhydramnios, preterm birth, and perhaps fetal lung immaturity) may be eliminated, or the incidence decreased, by maintaining control over maternal glucose levels within narrow limits (Reece et al, 1998). Good control is defined as the maintenance of maternal blood glucose levels between 100 and 120 mg/dl.

Congenital Anomalies. Congenital anomalies occur in about 7% to 10% of IDMs. Their incidence is two to four times that for infants born to mothers without diabetes (Tyrala, 1996). The incidence is greatest among SGA newborns. IUGR leading to SGA infants is seen in IDMs with severe vascular disease. The most commonly occurring anomalies involve the cardiac, musculoskeletal, and central nervous systems. In most defects associated with diabetic pregnancies, the structural abnormality occurs before the eighth week after conception. This reinforces the importance of control of blood glucose both before conception and in the early stages of pregnancy.

The incidence of congenital heart lesions in these infants is five times higher than that in the general population. Coarctation of the aorta, transposition of the great vessels, and atrial or ventricular septal defects are the most common lesions encountered in the IDM. Maternal diabetic control is correlated with the incidence of lesions; that is, the better the control, the fewer the lesions.

CNS anomalies include anencephaly, encephalocele, meningomyelocele, and hydrocephalus. The musculoskeletal system may be affected by caudal regression syndrome (i.e., sacral agenesis, with weakness or deformities of the lower extremities, malformation and fixation of the hip joints, and shortening or deformity of the femurs). Hypertrichosis on the pinnae (excessive hair growth on the external ear) has been added to the list of characteristic clinical features (Fanaroff and Martin, 1997). Other defects noted in this population include gastrointestinal atresia and urinary tract malformations.

Macrosomia. Despite improvements in the control of maternal blood sugar levels, the incidence of macrosomia in the insulin-dependent diabetic is higher than in infants born of mothers who are not diabetic. At birth the typical LGA infant has a round, cherubic ("tomato" or cushingoid) face, chubby body, and a plethoric or flushed complexion (Fig. 27-10). The infant has enlarged internal organs (i.e., hepatosplenomegaly, splanchnomegaly, and cardiomegaly) and increased body fat, especially around the shoulders. The placenta and umbilical cord are larger than average. The brain is the only organ that is not enlarged. IDMs may be LGA but physiologically immature.

The macrosomic infant is at risk for hypoglycemia, hypocalcemia, hyperviscosity, and hyperbilirubinemia. The excessive shoulder size in these infants often leads to dystocia, particularly because the head may be smaller in proportion to the shoulders than in a nonmacrosomic infant. Macrosomic infants, who may be born vaginally or by cesarean birth after a trial of labor, may incur birth trauma.

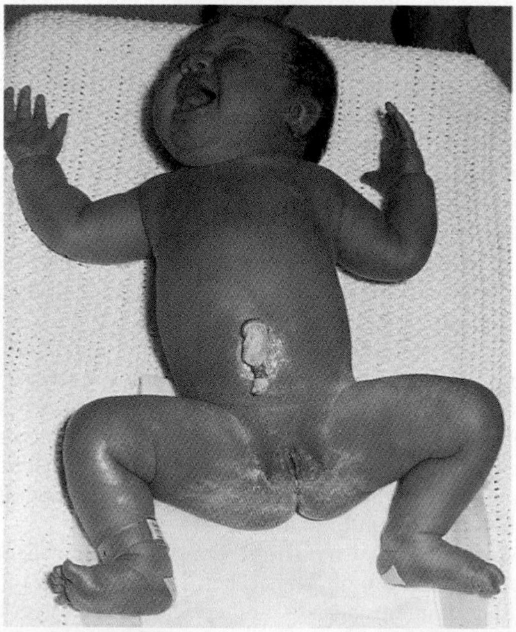

FIG. 27-10 • Macrosomia. (From O'Doherty N: *Neonatology: micro atlas of the newborn,* Nutley, NJ, 1986, Hoffmann-La Roche.)

Birth Trauma and Perinatal Asphyxia. Birth injury (resulting from macrosomia or method of birth) and perinatal asphyxia occur in 20% of IGDMs and 35% of IDMs. Examples of birth trauma include cephalhematoma; paralysis of the facial nerve (seventh cranial nerve) (see Fig. 28-4); fracture of the clavicle or humerus; brachial plexus paralysis, usually Duchenne-Erb (right upper arm) palsy (see Figs. 28-5 and 28-6); and phrenic nerve paralysis, invariably associated with diaphragmatic paralysis.

Respiratory Distress Syndrome. IDMs or IGDMs are 4 to 6 times more likely than normal infants to develop RDS. With improved maternal glucose control, this risk has been substantially reduced. In the fetus exposed to high levels of maternal glucose, synthesis of surfactant may be delayed because of the high fetal serum level of insulin (Tyrala, 1996). Fetal lung maturity, as evidenced by a lecithin/sphingomyelin (L/S) ratio of 2:1, is not reassuring if the mother has diabetes mellitus or gestation-induced diabetes mellitus. For the infants of such mothers, an L/S ratio of 3:1 or more or the presence of phosphatidylglycerol in the amniotic fluid is more indicative of adequate lung maturity.

Hypoglycemia. Hypoglycemia affects many IDMs. After constant exposure to high circulating levels of glucose, hyperplasia of the fetal pancreas occurs, resulting in hyperinsulinemia. Disruption of the fetal glucose supply occurs with the clamping of the umbilical cord, and the neonate's blood glucose level falls rapidly in the presence of fetal hyperinsulinism. Hypoglycemia is most common in the macrosomic or preterm infant, but blood glucose levels should be monitored in all infants of known or suspected diabetic mothers.

Asymptomatic or symptomatic hypoglycemia most commonly presents within the first 1 to 3 hours after birth. Signs of hypoglycemia include jitteriness, apnea, tachypnea, and cyanosis. Significant hypoglycemia may result in seizures. Hypoglycemia is worsened by the presence of hypothermia or respiratory distress.

Hypocalcemia and Hypomagnesemia. Hypocalcemia occurs in as many as 50% of IDMs. A number of these cases are related to hypoxia or prematurity; however the overall incidence of hypocalcemia is higher than in nondiabetic pregnancies (Tyrala, 1996). Hypomagnesemia is believed to develop because of maternal renal losses that occur in diabetes. Hypocalcemia is associated with preterm birth, birth trauma, and perinatal asphyxia. Signs of hypocalcemia, a prevalent finding in IDMs and IGDMs, are similar to those of hypoglycemia, but they occur between 24 and 36 hours of age. Hypocalcemia must be considered if therapy for hypoglycemia is ineffective.

Cardiomyopathy. All IDMs need careful observation for cardiomyopathy because an increased heart size is often found among these infants. Two types of cardiomyopathy can occur. Clinicians must be alert to identify correctly the type of lesion so that appropriate therapy is instituted. Both types of lesions are associated with respiratory symptoms and congestive heart failure.

Hypertrophic cardiomyopathy (HCM) is characterized by a hypercontractile and thickened myocardium. The ventricular walls are thickened, as is the septum, which in severe cases results in outflow tract obstructions. The mitral valve is poorly functioning. In nonhypertrophic cardiomyopathy (non-HCM) the myocardium is poorly contractile and overstretched. The ventricles are increased in size, and there is no outflow obstruction. Most infants are asymptomatic, but severe outflow obstruction may cause left ventricular heart failure. HCM may be treated with a beta-adrenergic blocker (such as propranolol to decrease contractility and heart rate). A cardiotonic agent is used to treat non-HCM (such as digoxin to increase contractility and decrease heart rate). The abnormality usually resolves in 3 to 12 months (Fanaroff and Martin, 1997).

Hyperbilirubinemia and Polycythemia. IDMs are at increased risk of developing hyperbilirubinemia. Many IDMs are also polycythemic. Polycythemia increases blood viscosity, thereby impairing circulation. In addition, this increased number of RBCs to be hemolyzed increases the potential bilirubin load that the neonate must clear. The excessive RBCs are produced in extramedullary foci (liver and spleen) in addition to the usual sites in bone marrow. Therefore both liver function and bilirubin clearance may be adversely affected. Bruising associated with birth of a macrosomic infant will contribute further to high bilirubin levels.

Nursing Care. Ideally, planning for the IDM begins during the antenatal period. Pediatric staff members are present at the birth. Implementation of care depends on the neonate's particular problems. If the maternal blood glucose level was well controlled throughout the pregnancy, the infant may require only monitoring. Because euglycemia is not always possible, the nurse must promptly recognize and treat any consequences of maternal diabetes that arise (Nursing Care Plan).

Nursing Care Plan — THE INFANT OF MOTHER WITH GESTATIONAL DIABETES

NURSING DIAGNOSIS Risk for injury related to hypoglycemia, hypocalcemia, polycythemia, or hyperbilirubinemia secondary to maternal gestational diabetes

EXPECTED OUTCOME Infant will exhibit blood glucose, serum calcium, hematocrit, and serum bilirubin levels that are within normal limits.

Nursing Interventions/*Rationales*

Monitor blood glucose levels (less than 40 mg/dl indicative of hypoglycemia); serum calcium levels (less than 7 mg/dl indicative of hypocalcemia); and serum bilirubin levels (over 15 mg/dl indicative of hyperbilirubinemia) *to assess and detect early onset to prevent complications.*

Observe for signs of hypoglycemia (e.g., jitteriness, twitching, lethargy, apathy, convulsions, cyanosis, sweating, eye rolling, and refusal to eat); hypocalcemia (e.g., jitters, apnea, high-pitched cry, and abdominal distention); polycythemia (e.g., plethora); and hyperbilirubinemia (e.g., jaundice) *to assess and detect signs of onset to prevent complications.*

Institute early feeding of infant or glucose supplements as prescribed *to prevent or treat early hypoglycemia;* increased milk feedings/calcium supplements per physician order *to prevent or treat early hypocalcemia;* early and frequent feedings *to reduce hematocrit and enhance excretion of bilirubin in stool;* or phototherapy for bilirubin over 12 to 15 mg/dl.

Reduce adverse environmental factors (e.g., stimuli such as jarring or shaking, cold stress, and respiratory distress), *which can predispose infant to hypoglycemia or precipitate a seizure.*

NURSING DIAGNOSIS Risk for impaired gas exchange related to lung immaturity or cardiomyopathy secondary to maternal gestational diabetes

EXPECTED OUTCOME Infant will exhibit signs of adequate oxygen supply (i.e., respiratory rate, rhythm, and amplitude and blood gas levels within normal limits).

Nursing Interventions/*Rationales*

Monitor infant vital signs, blood gas levels per order, and patency of airway *to evaluate pulmonary and circulatory status.*

Avoid activities that may lower body temperature and lead to cold stress, *which can induce respiratory distress.*

Suction as needed *to keep airway patent and prevent aspiration.*

Position infant on side *to facilitate mucus drainage.*

Have resuscitation equipment and oxygen available *for quick treatment of respiratory distress.*

NURSING DIAGNOSIS Risk for ineffective thermoregulation related to physiologic immaturity; risk for infection related to immature immunologic defenses/environmental exposure

See the Nursing Plan of Care for the normal newborn in Chapter 25.

NURSING DIAGNOSIS Anxiety (risk for powerlessness, situational low self-esteem, ineffective coping) related to neonate's condition, management, and prognosis

EXPECTED OUTCOME Parents demonstrate understanding of prognosis and therapy for infant.

Nursing Interventions/*Rationales*

Explain potential effects of maternal diabetic condition on newborn *to relieve fear of unknown and support ability to cope.*

Encourage open communication (e.g., inform parents of ongoing condition, procedures, and treatment; answer questions; correct misperceptions; actively listen to parental concerns) *to provide support and help provide sense of control.*

Encourage parents to interact with infant and to become involved in care routines *to foster emotional connection.*

DISCHARGE PLANNING

Discharge planning for the high risk newborn begins at the time of admission. Throughout the infant's hospitalization, the discharge planning coordinator gathers information from all of the health care team members. This information is used to determine the infant's and family's readiness for discharge.

As home care needs of the infant's parents are assessed, steps are taken to eliminate any knowledge deficits. Discharge teaching for the high risk newborn is extensive, requires time, and cannot be adequately accomplished on the day of discharge. Information is provided about infant care, especially as it pertains to the particular infant's home needs (e.g., the administration of oxygen or gastrostomy feedings). Parent education includes having them give return demonstrations of their infant care skills to show whether they are becoming increasingly independent in the provision of this care. Parents should also obtain an age-appropriate car seat before the discharge of their infant.

Successful discharge of high risk infants to their homes or community hospital requires a multidisciplinary approach. Medical, nursing, and social services are crucial to the smooth transition of these infants and their families to the community and home. If the infant is transported back to the community hospital that referred either the mother before birth or the infant after birth, interfacility communication is essential to continuity of care.

Discharge to home for high risk infants does not mean they can be treated like normal newborns. Follow-up by a pediatrician or nurse practitioner familiar with the complications common to the high risk newborn is essential. Further follow-up of specific complications by qualified specialists and referral to high risk centers for developmental interventions can help ensure the best outcome possible for these fragile infants.

Referrals for appropriate resources also need to be made. Infants with developmental disabilities, or those infants who may be at risk for further problems (premature infants), are referred to appropriate community programs. Social service involvement is especially important for young or psychosocially high risk parents (e.g., substance abusers or those with a mental illness).

TRANSPORT TO A REGIONAL CENTER

If a hospital is not equipped to care for a high risk mother and fetus or a high risk infant, transfer to a specialized perinatal or regional tertiary care center is arranged. Maternal transport ideally occurs with fetus in utero because this has two distinct advantages: (1) neonatal morbidity and mortality decrease, and (2) the mother and infant are not separated at birth.

For a variety of reasons, it is not always possible to transport the mother before the birth. Therefore, physicians and nurses in all facilities must have the skills and equipment necessary for making an accurate diagnosis and implementing emergency interventions to stabilize the infant's condition until transport can occur (Pettett, Sewell, and Merenstein, 1998). The goal of these interventions is to maintain the infant's condition within the normal physiologic range. Specific attention is given to vital signs, oxygen and ventilation, thermoregulation, acid-base balance, fluid and electrolyte levels, glucose level, and developmental interventions.

Arrangements for transport to an intensive care facility are made as soon as the high risk infant is identified. Each hospital that delivers infants should be able to provide for appropriate neonatal stabilization and arrange for transport to a tertiary care facility. The infant must be kept warm and adequately oxygenated (including intubation if indicated); have vital signs and oxygen saturation monitored; and, when indicated, receive an intravenous infusion. The infant is transported in a specially designed incubator unit containing a complete life-support system and other emergency equipment that can be carried by ambulance, van, or helicopter.

The transport team may consist of physicians, nurse-practitioners, nurses, and respiratory therapists. Commonly a nurse trained in neonatal intensive care and a respiratory therapist constitute the team. The team must have experience in resuscitation, stabilizations, and provision of critical care during the transport. Teams provide information for the parents about the tertiary center (Box 27-7).

The birth of any high risk infant can cause profound parental stress. Parents can grieve the loss of the ideal infant. They are fearful of the possible eventual outcomes for the infant. They must also deal with the technologic world surrounding their infant; amid all the equipment, it is sometimes difficult for them to perceive the infant and respond to its needs. Parents of high risk infants who have been transported to regional centers therefore need special support.

Box 27-7

Information for Parents About the Tertiary Center

- Exact location of the unit—address, map
- Visiting hours and hospital rules
- Telephone numbers
- Names of individual likely to be involved with the baby's care
- Information of the special care unit—what it is, what it does
- Location of parking facilities, nearby lodging, and rules regarding young children (siblings)
- Any particular rules or regulations regarding the special care unit

From Pettett G, Sewell S, and Merenstein G: Regionalization and transport in perinatal care. In Merenstein G, Gardner S, editors: *Handbook of neonatal intensive care,* ed 4, St Louis, 1998, Mosby.

Critical Thinking

NEONATAL TRANSPORT

During a scheduled clinical experience in the NICU or a special care nursery, observe a transport team leaving to pick up an infant from a referring hospital or bringing in an infant to the special care nursery. Who are the transport team members? What equipment are they using? How was the referral made? What communication links are there between the special care nursery and the community hospitals in the surrounding area? How are parents kept informed of the condition of the infant?

TRANSPORT FROM A REGIONAL CENTER

Infants may need to be transferred back to the referring facility. Often premature infants who require thermoregulation and gavage feedings can be cared for in community hospitals

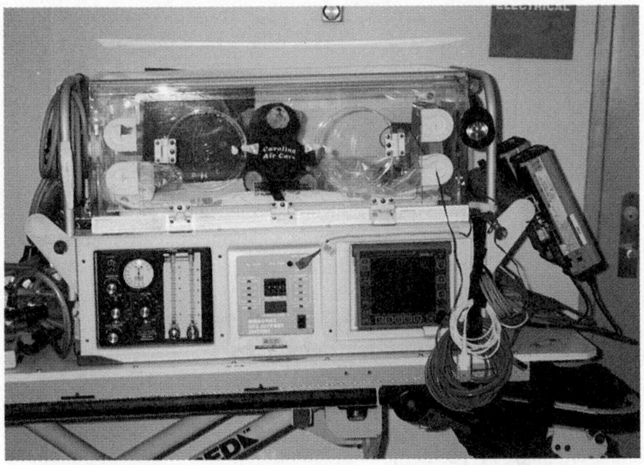

FIG. 27-11 • Total life support system for transport of high risk newborns. (Courtesy UNC Hospitals, Carolina Air Care, Chapel Hill, NC.)

closer to the parents' home. This allows parents to visit their infant more easily and to work with their personal health care provider on the long-range expected outcomes for the infant. Specialized incubators make these trips possible (Fig. 27-11). However, parents may express mixed feelings about such return transports and may be reluctant to adapt to a different facility and group of caregivers. To minimize some of these concerns, it is important to give the parents very clear information about return transports during the initial discharge planning.

Although at the time of discharge parents may not recognize the need for information on the various resources available to help them in the care of their infant, they can be given such lists of agencies and telephone numbers for later use. Providing them with a patient-specific directory covering special programs, social support, community, and funding resources can help them make the transition to the home care of their infants. As the nurse continually reinforces the idea that the infant will go home, this prompts the parents to plan for the days ahead and therefore be ready to take their infant home when the time comes.

Key Points

- Preterm infants are at risk for problems related to the immaturity of their organ systems.
- Respiratory distress syndrome, retinopathy of prematurity, and bronchopulmonary dysplasia are associated with prematurity.
- High risk infants must be observed for respiratory distress and other early signs of physiologic disorders.
- Metabolic abnormalities of diabetes mellitus in pregnancy adversely affect embryonic and fetal development.
- The adaptation of parents to preterm or high risk infants differs from that of parents to normal full-term infants.
- Parents need special instruction (e.g., CPR, oxygen therapy, suctioning, developmental care) before they take a high risk infant home.
- All infants born to mothers with diabetes are at risk for complications.
- SGA infants are considered to be at risk because of fetal growth restriction.
- Nonreassuring fetal status among postmature infants is related to the progressive placental insufficiency that can occur in a postterm pregnancy.
- Specially trained nurses may transport high risk infants to and from special care units.

References

Als H: Developmental care in the newborn intensive care unit, *Curr Opin Pediatr* 10(2):138-142, 1998.

American Academy of Pediatrics Committee on Fetus and Newborn: Surfactant replacement therapy for respiratory distress syndrome, *Pediatrics* 103(3):684-685, 1999.

Bancalari E: The respiratory system: neonatal chronic lung disease. In Fanaroff A, Martin R, editors: *Neonatal-perinatal medicine: diseases of the fetus and infant,* St Louis, 1997, Mosby.

Blackburn S: Environmental impact of the NICU on developmental outcomes, *J Pediatr Nurs* 13(5):279-289, 1998.

Blake W, Murray J: Heat balance. In Merenstein G, Gardner S, editors: *Handbook of neonatal intensive care,* ed 4, St Louis, 1998, Mosby.

Brandon D, Holditch-Davis D, Beylea M: Nursing care and the development of sleeping and waking behaviors in preterm infants, *Res Nurs Health* 22(3):217-229, 1999.

Cloherty J, Stark A: *Manual of neonatal care,* ed 4, Boston, 1997, Little, Brown.

Cools F, Offringa M: Meta-analysis of elective high frequency ventilation in preterm infants with respiratory distress syndrome, *Arch Dis Chld Fetal Neonatal Ed* 80(1):F15-20, 1999.

Daberkow-Carson E, Washington R: Cardiovascular diseases and surgical interventions. In Merenstein G, Gardner S, editors: *Handbook of neonatal intensive care,* ed 4, St Louis, 1998, Mosby.

Donovan E, Schwartz J, Moles L: New technologies applied to the management of respiratory dysfunction. In Kenner C, Lott J, Flandermeyer A, editors: *Comprehensive neonatal nursing: a physiologic perspective,* ed 2, Philadelphia, 1998, WB Saunders.

Fanaroff A, Martin R: *Neonatal-perinatal medicine: diseases of the fetus and infant,* ed 6, St Louis, 1997, Mosby.

Gale G, VandenBerg K: Kangaroo care, *Neonatal Netw* 17(5): 69-71, 1998.

Gamblian V, Hess D, Kenner C: Early discharge from the NICU, *J Pediatr Nurs* 13(5):296-301, 1998.

Gardner S, Lubchenco L: The neonate and the environment: impact on development. In Merenstein G, Gardner S, editors: *Handbook of neonatal intensive care,* ed 4, St Louis, 1998, Mosby.

Garland J et al: A three-day course of dexamethasone therapy to prevent chronic lung disease in ventilated neonates: a randomized trial, *Pediatrics* 104(1 pt 1):91-99, 1999.

Gray K et al: Developmentally supportive care in a neonatal intensive care unit: a research utilization project, *Neonatal Netw* 17(2):33-38, 1998.

Hack M et al: Very-low-birth-weight outcomes of the National Institute of Child Health and Human Development Neonatal Network, November 1989 to October 1990, *Am J Obstet Gynecol* 172(2 pt 1):457-464, 1995.

Hagedorn M, Gardner S, Abman S: Respiratory diseases. In Merenstein G, Gardner S, editors: *Handbook of neonatal intensive care,* ed 4, St Louis, 1998, Mosby.

Haubrich K: Assessment and management of auditory dysfunction. In Kenner C, Lott J, Flandermyer A, editors: *Comprehensive neonatal nursing: a physiologic perspective,* ed 2, Philadelphia, 1998, WB Saunders.

Heermann J, Wilson M: Nurses' experiences working with families in an NICU during implementation of family-focused developmental care, *Neonatal Netw* 19(4):23-29, 2000.

Holland R, Price F, Bensard D: Neonatal surgery. In Merenstein G, Gardner S, editors: *Handbook of neonatal intensive care,* ed 4, St Louis, 1998, Mosby.

Kliegman R: Intrauterine growth retardation. In Fanaroff A, Martin R, editors: *Neonatal-perinatal medicine: diseases of the fetus and infant,* St Louis, 1997, Mosby.

Lefrak L, Dowling D: Nutrition: Physiologic basis of metabolism and management of enteral and parental nutrition. In Kenner C, Lott J, Flandermeyer A, editors: *Comprehensive neonatal nursing: a physiologic perspective,* ed 2, Philadelphia, 1998, WB Saunders.

Ludington-Hoe S et al: Birth-related fatigue in 34-36 week preterm neonates: rapid recovery with very early kangaroo (skin-to-skin) care, *J Obstet Gynecol Neonatal Nurs* 28(1):94-103, 1999.

McGowan J, Hagedorn M, Hay W: Glucose homeostasis. In Merenstein G, Gardner S, editors: *Handbook of neonatal intensive care,* ed 4, St Louis, 1998, Mosby.

Meier P: Transition of the preterm infant to an open crib: process of the project group, *J Obstet Gynecol Neonatal Nurs* 23(4):321-326, 1994.

Merenstein G, Gardner S, editors: *Handbook of neonatal intensive care,* ed 4, St Louis, 1998, Mosby.

Moe P, Paige P: Neurologic disorders. In Merenstein G, Gardner S, editors: *Handbook of neonatal intensive care,* ed 4, St Louis, 1998, Mosby.

Neu M: Parents' perception of skin-to-skin care with their preterm infants requiring assisted ventilation, *J Obstet Gynecol Neonatal Nurs* 28(2):157-164, 1999.

Neu M, Browne J, Vojir C: The impact of two transfer techniques used during skin-to-skin care on the physiologic and behavioral responses of preterm infants, *Nurs Res* 49(4):215-223, 2000.

Petryshen P et al: Comparing nursing costs for preterm infants receiving conventional vs. developmental care, *Nurs Econ* 15(3):138-145,150, 1997.

Pettett G, Sewell S, Merenstein G: Regionalization and transport in perinatal care. In Merenstein G, Gardner S, editors: *Handbook of neonatal intensive care,* ed 4, St Louis, 1998, Mosby.

Pickler R, Terrell B: Nonnutritive sucking and necrotizing enterocolitis, *Neonatal Netw* 13(8):15-18, 1994.

Plavka R et al: A prospective randomized comparison of conventional mechanical ventilation and very early high frequency oscillatory ventilation in extremely premature newborns with respiratory distress syndrome, *Intensive Care Med* 25(1):68-75, 1999.

Reece E et al: Pregnancy outcomes among women with and without diabetic microvascular disease (White's classes B to FR) versus nondiabetic controls, *Am J Perinatol* 15(9):549-555, 1998.

Reed M, Blumer J: Pharmacologic treatment of the fetus. In Fanaroff A, Martin R, editors: *Neonatal-perinatal medicine: diseases of the fetus and infant,* St Louis, 1997, Mosby.

Shields-Poe D, Pinelli J: Variables associated with parental stress in neonatal intensive care units, *Neonatal Netw* 16(1):29-37, 1997.

Standley J: The effect of music and multimodal stimulation on responses of premature infants in neonatal intensive care, *Pediatr Nurs* 24(6):532-538, 1998.

Townsend S, Johnson C, and Hay W: Enteral nutrition. In Merenstein G, Gardner S, editors: *Handbook of neonatal intensive care,* ed 4, St Louis, 1998, Mosby.

Tyrala E: The infant of the diabetic mother, *Obstet Gynecol Clin North Am* 23(1):221-240, 1996.

VandenBerg K: What to tell parents about the developmental needs of their baby at discharge, *Neonatal Netw* 18(1):57-59, 1999.

Wong D: *Whaley & Wong's nursing care of infants and children,* ed 6, St Louis, 1999, Mosby.

Zahka K, Patel C: The cardiovascular system: congenital defects. In Fanaroff A, Martin R, editors: *Neonatal-perinatal medicine: diseases of the fetus and infant,* St Louis, 1997, Mosby.

CHAPTER

28

The Newborn at Risk: Acquired and Congenital Problems

http://www.harcourthealth.com/MERLIN/Wong/maternal/

Learning Objectives

On completion of this chapter the reader will be able to:

- Summarize assessment and care of the newborn with soft tissue, skeletal, and nervous system injuries due to birth trauma.
- Describe the assessment of a newborn for infection.
- Assess the effects of maternal use of alcohol, heroin, methadone, marijuana, cocaine, and smoking tobacco on the fetus and newborn.
- Describe the assessment of a newborn experiencing drug withdrawal.
- Describe assessment, prevention, and management of hyperbilirubinemia.
- Compare Rh and ABO incompatibility.
- Review prenatal diagnosis of neonatal disorders.
- Describe preoperative and postoperative nursing care of the newborn.
- Describe each congenital disorder presented in this chapter and identify the priority of nursing care for each.

A challenge for the nurse is the birth of an infant at risk because of conditions or circumstances that are superimposed on the normal course of events associated with birth and the adjustment to extrauterine existence. The infant may be considered high risk because of birth trauma, maternal substance abuse, infection, or congenital anomalies. Birth trauma includes physical injuries sustained by a neonate during labor and birth. Congenital anomalies include such conditions as esophageal atresia, anencephaly, omphalocele, and heart defects.

At times, the nurse is able to anticipate problems, such as when a woman is admitted in premature labor or a congenital anomaly is diagnosed by ultrasound before birth. At other times, birth of a high risk infant is unanticipated. In either case, the personnel and equipment necessary for immediate care of the infant must be available.

BIRTH TRAUMA

Birth trauma (injury) is physical injury sustained by a neonate during labor and birth. It remains an important source of neonatal morbidity.

In theory, most birth injuries may be avoidable, especially if careful assessment of risk factors and appropriate planning of birth occur. The use of ultrasonography allows antepartum diagnosis of macrosomia, hydrocephalus, and unusual presentations. Elective cesarean birth can be chosen for some pregnancies to prevent significant birth injury (Merenstein and Gardner, 1998). A small percentage of significant birth injuries are unavoidable despite skilled and competent obstetric care, such as in especially difficult or prolonged labor or when the infant is in an abnormal presentation (Fanaroff and Martin, 1997). Some injuries cannot be anticipated until the specific circumstances are encountered during childbirth. Emergency cesarean birth may provide a last-minute salvage, but in these circumstances the injury may be truly unavoidable. The same injury might be caused in several ways; for example, a cephalhematoma could result from an obstetric technique such as forceps birth or vacuum extraction or from pressure of the fetal skull against the maternal pelvis.

Many injuries are minor and resolve readily in the neonatal period without treatment. Other traumas require some degree of intervention. A few are serious enough to be fatal. The nurse's contributions to the welfare of the newborn begin with early observation and accurate recording. The prompt reporting of signs that indicate deviations from normal permits early initiation of appropriate therapy. Table 28-1 provides an overview of neurologic birth injuries and the sites in which they occur.

Care Management

The Apgar score may alert the caregiver to birth injuries and help in identifying infants in need of immediate resuscitation. Flaccid muscle tone, regardless of cause, increases the risk of joint dislocations and separation during the birth process. Flaccid tone in extremities may be traced to nerve plexus injuries or long-bone fractures. A weak or hoarse cry is characteristic of laryngeal nerve palsy as a result of excessive traction on the neck during birth. Pronounced bruising of the skin may preclude accurate assessment for color.

TABLE 28-1
Types of Birth Injuries

Site of Injury	Type of Injury
Scalp	Caput succedaneum Subgaleal hemorrhage Cephalhematoma
Skull	Linear fracture Depressed fracture Occipital osteodiastasis
Intracranial	Epidural hematoma Subdural hematoma (laceration of falx, tentorium, or superficial veins) Subarachoid hemorrhage Cerebral contusion Cerebellar contusion Intracerebellar hematoma
Spinal cord (cervical)	Vertebral artery injury Intraspinal hemorrhage Spinal cord transection or injury
Plexus	Erb's palsy Klumpke's paralysis Total (mixed) brachial plexus injury Horner syndrome Diaphragmatic paralysis Lumbosacral plexus injury
Cranial and peripheral nerve	Radial nerve palsy Medial nerve palsy Sciatic nerve palsy Laryngeal nerve palsy Diaphragmatic paralysis Facial nerve palsy

From Moe P, Paige L: Neurologic disorders. In Merenstein G, Gardner S, editors: *Handbook of neonatal intensive care,* ed 4, St Louis, 1998, Mosby.

A complete physical assessment of the newborn is performed soon after birth. Because evidence of birth injury may not be apparent at the initial examination, assessment continues during each contact with the neonate.

Meeting the unique needs of the birth-injured newborn requires constant vigilance. Nursing actions are selected in terms of the particular disorder and the individual needs of the infant and family.

Soft Tissue Injuries. Caput succedaneum is a localized edematous swelling of the scalp that is not confined within the suture lines of the skull. The swelling persists for a few days after birth and then disappears without treatment. It is most often seen after vertex vaginal births and has no pathologic significance (see Fig. 24-4, *A*).

Cephalhematoma is a collection of blood from ruptured blood vessels between the periosteum and the surface of the skull. Because blood collects beneath the periosteum, it does not cross the cranial suture lines (see Fig. 24-4, *B*). The swelling may appear unilaterally or bilaterally, usually is minimal or absent at birth, increases over the first 3 days of life, and disappears gradually in 2 to 3 weeks. Occasionally, hyperbilirubinemia may result from breakdown of the accumulated blood.

Subconjunctival (scleral) and retinal hemorrhages result from rupture of capillaries caused by increased intracranial pressure (ICP) during birth. They clear up within 5 days after birth and usually present no problems. However, parents need reassurance about their presence.

Erythema, ecchymoses, petechiae, abrasions, lacerations, and edema of buttocks and extremities may be present. Localized discoloration may appear over presenting or dependent parts. Ecchymoses and edema may appear anywhere on the body and on the presenting body part from the application of forceps. They also may result from manipulation of the infant's body during birth.

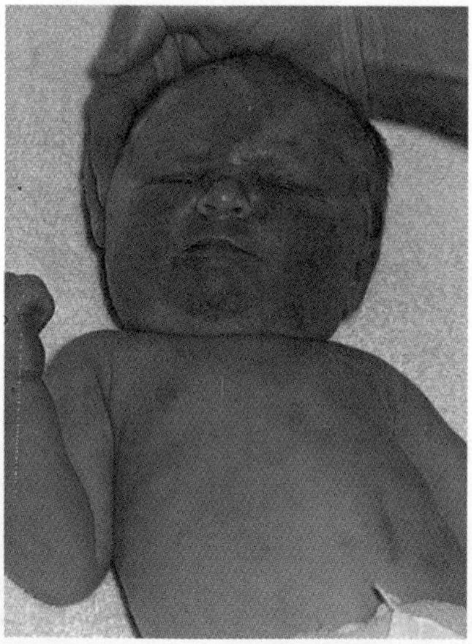

FIG. 28-1 • Marked bruising on the entire face of an infant born vaginally after face presentation. Less severe ecchymoses were present on the extremities. Phototherapy was required for treatment of jaundice resulting from the breakdown of accumulated blood. (From O'Doherty N: *Neonatology: micro atlas of the newborn,* Nutley, NJ, 1986, Hoffmann-La Roche.)

Bruises over the face may be the result of face presentation (Fig. 28-1). In a breech presentation, bruising and swelling may be seen over the buttocks or genitalia (Fig. 28-2). The skin over the entire head may be ecchymotic and covered with petechiae caused by a tight nuchal cord. Petechiae, or pinpoint hemorrhagic areas, acquired during birth may extend over the upper portion of the trunk and face. These lesions are benign if they disappear within 2 days of birth and no new lesions appear. Ecchymoses and petechiae may be signs of a more serious disorder, such as thrombocytopenia. If the hemorrhagic areas do not disappear spontaneously in 2 days, the physician is notified. To differentiate hemorrhagic areas from skin rashes and discolorations such as Mongolian spots, the nurse blanches the skin with two fingers. Because extravasated blood remains within the tissues, petechiae and ecchymoses do not blanch.

Forceps injury occurs at the site of application of the instrument. Forceps injury typically has a linear configuration across both sides of the face, outlining the placement of the forceps. The affected areas are kept clean to minimize the risk of secondary infection. These injuries usually resolve spontaneously within several days with no specific therapy. The increased use of padded forceps blades and vacuum-assisted birth may reduce the incidence of these lesions (Fanaroff and Martin, 1997).

Accidental lacerations may be inflicted with a scalpel during cesarean birth or with scissors during an episiotomy. These cuts may occur on any part of the body but most often are found on the scalp, buttocks, and thighs. Usually they are superficial, needing only to be kept clean. Butterfly adhesive strips will hold the edges of more serious lacerations together. Rarely, sutures are needed.

Skeletal Injuries. The newborn's immature, flexible skull can withstand a great degree of deformation (molding) before fracture results. Considerable force is required to fracture the newborn's skull. Two types of skull fractures typically are identified in the newborn: linear fractures and depressed fractures. The location of the fracture and involvement of underlying structures determine its significance.

If an artery lying in a groove on the undersurface of the skull is torn as a result of the fracture, increased ICP will follow. Unless a blood vessel is involved, linear fractures (which account for 70% of all fractures for this age group) heal without special treatment. The soft skull may become indented without laceration of either the skin or the dural membrane. These depressed fractures, or "ping-pong ball" indentations, may occur during difficult births from pressure of the head on the bony pelvis (see Fig. 25-9). They also can occur as a result of injudicious application of forceps.

The clavicle is the bone most often fractured during birth. Generally the break is in the middle third of the bone (Fig. 28-3). Dystocia, particularly shoulder impaction, may be the predisposing problem. Limitation of motion of the arm, crepitus over the bone, and the absence of the Moro reflex on the affected side are diagnostic. Except for use of gentle rather than vigorous handling, no accepted treatment for fractured clavicle exists, and the prognosis is good. The figure-eight bandage appropriate for the older child should not be used for the newborn.

The humerus and femur are other bones that may be fractured during a difficult birth. Fractures in newborns generally heal rapidly. Immobilization is accomplished with slings, splints, swaddling, and other devices.

The parents need support in handling these infants because they often are fearful of hurting them. Parents are encouraged to practice handling, changing, and feeding the affected neonate under the guidance of nursery personnel. This increases their confidence and knowledge and facilitates attachment. A plan for follow-up therapy is developed with the parents so that the times and arrangements for therapy are acceptable to them.

Peripheral Nervous System Injuries. Erb-Duchenne paralysis (brachial paralysis of the upper portion of the arm) is the most common type of paralysis associated with a difficult birth, occurring at rates of 0.5 to 1.9 per 1000 live births (Moe and Paige, 1998) (Fig. 28-4). Injury to the upper plexus results from stretching or pulling the head away from the

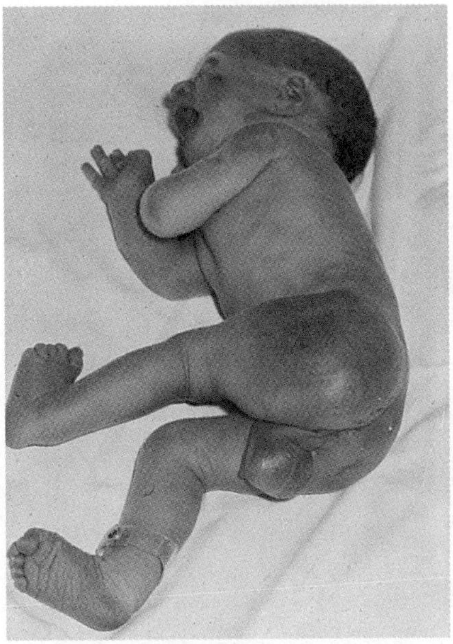

FIG. 28-2 • Swelling of genitalia and bruising of the buttocks after a breech delivery. (From O'Doherty N: *Neonatology: micro atlas of the newborn,* Nutley, NJ, 1986, Hoffmann-La Roche.)

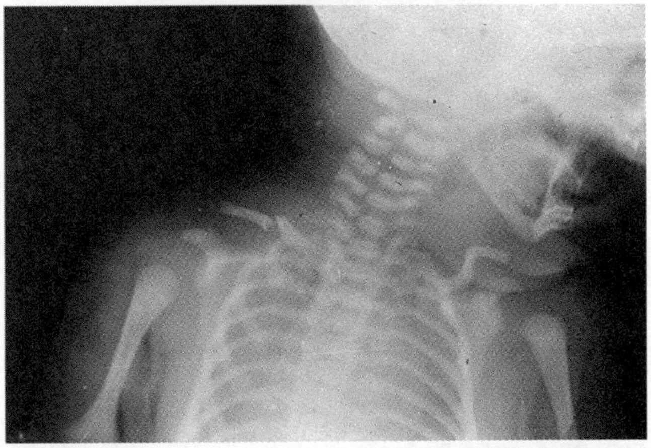

FIG. 28-3 • Fractured clavicle after shoulder dystocia. (From O'Doherty N: *Neonatology: micro atlas of the newborn,* Nutley, NJ, 1986, Hoffmann-La Roche.)

shoulder during a difficult birth. Typical symptoms are a flaccid arm with the elbow extended and the hand rotated inward, absence of the Moro reflex on the affected side, sensory loss over the lateral aspect of the arm, and an intact grasp reflex.

Treatment is by intermittent immobilization, proper positioning, and range of motion (ROM) exercises. Gentle manipulation and ROM exercises are delayed until about the tenth day to prevent additional injury to the brachial plexus.

Immobilization may be accomplished with a brace or splint or by pinning the infant's sleeve to the mattress. The infant should be positioned for 2 or 3 hours at a time as follows (Fig. 28-5):

- Abduct the arm 90 degrees
- Externally rotate the shoulder
- Flex the elbow 90 degrees
- Supinate the wrist with the palm directed slightly toward the face

Damage to the lower plexus (Klumpke's paralysis) is less common. With lower arm paralysis the wrist and hand are flaccid, the grasp reflex is absent, deep tendon reflexes are present, and dependent edema and cyanosis may be apparent (in the affected hand). Treatment consists of placing the hand in a neutral position, padding the fist, and gently exercising the wrist and fingers.

Parents are taught to position and immobilize the arm or wrist (or both). They can gently massage and manipulate the muscles to prevent contractures while the arm is healing. If edema or hemorrhage is responsible for the paralysis, the prognosis is good and recovery may be expected in a few weeks. If laceration of the nerves has occurred and healing does not result in return of function within a few months (i.e., 3 to 6 months or 2 years at the most), surgery may be indicated; however, little or no function will return. Full recovery is expected in 88% to 92% of infants (Moe and Paige, 1998).

Facial palsy or paralysis (Fig. 28-6) generally is caused by pressure on the facial nerve during birth. The face on the affected side is flattened and unresponsive to the grimace that accompanies crying or stimulation; the eye remains open and the forehead will not wrinkle. Often the condition is transitory, resolving within hours or days of birth. Permanent paralysis is rare.

Treatment involves assistance with feeding, prevention of damage to the cornea of the open eye, and supportive care of

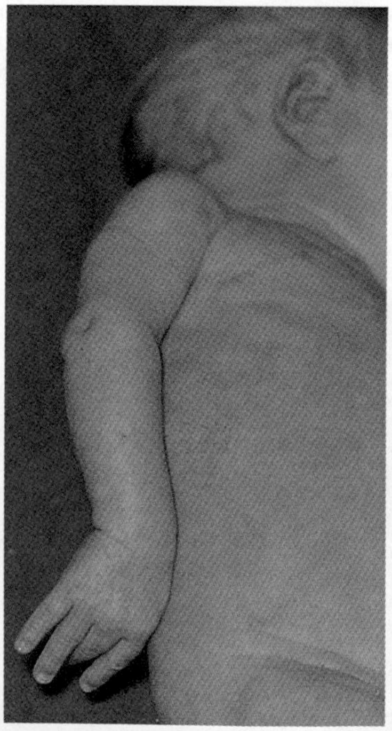

FIG. 28-4 • Erb-Duchenne paralysis in newborn infant. Moro's reflex was absent in right upper extremity. Recovery was complete. (From O'Doherty N: *Neonatology: micro atlas of the newborn,* Nutley, NJ, 1986, Hoffmann-La Roche.)

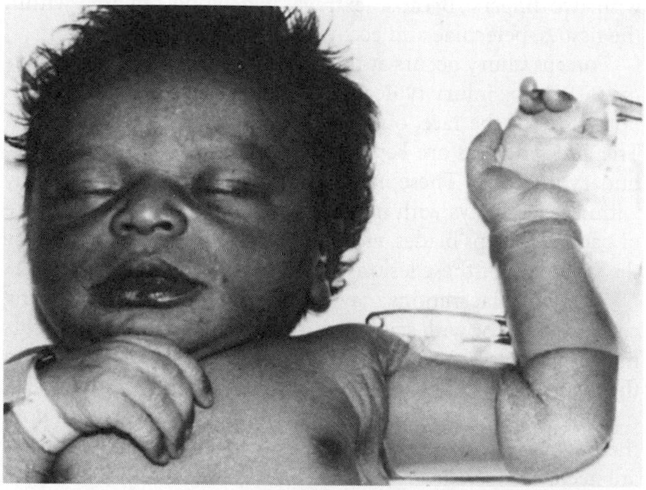

FIG. 28-5 • Recommended corrective positioning for treatment of Erb-Duchenne paralysis. Note abduction and external rotation at shoulder, flexion at elbow, supination of forearm, and slight dorsiflexion at wrist. (From Behrmann R: *Neonatology: diseases of the fetus and infant,* St Louis, 1973, Mosby.)

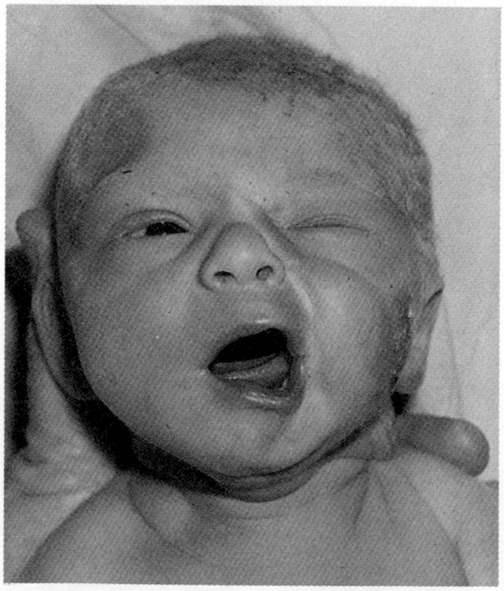

FIG. 28-6 • Facial paralysis 15 minutes after forceps birth. Absence of movement on affected side is especially noticeable when infant cries. (From O'Doherty N: Neonatology: *Micro atlas of the newborn,* Nutley, NJ, 1986, Hoffmann-La Roche.)

the parents. Usually the infant's face appears distorted, especially when crying. Feeding may be prolonged, with the milk flowing out the newborn's mouth around the nipple on the affected side. The mother needs understanding and sympathetic encouragement while learning how to feed and care for the infant, as well as how to hold and cuddle the baby.

Phrenic nerve injury almost always occurs as a component of brachial plexus injury rather than as an isolated problem. Injury to the phrenic nerve results in diaphragmatic paralysis. Cyanosis and irregular thoracic respirations, with no abdominal movement on inspiration, are characteristic of paralysis of the diaphragm. Babies with diaphragmatic paralysis usually require mechanical ventilatory support, at least for the first few days after birth. Other treatments include diaphragmatic pacing or surgical correction.

Central Nervous System Injuries. All types of intracranial hemorrhage (ICH) occur in newborns. ICH as a result of birth trauma is more likely to occur in the full-term, large infant. The frequency and degree of severity of ICH are different in the newborn than in older children or adults. In the newborn, more than one type of hemorrhage can and does commonly occur (Fanaroff and Martin, 1997; Wong, 1999).

Subdural hemorrhages (hematomas), or life-threatening collections of blood in the subdural space, most often are produced by the stretching and tearing of the large veins in the tentorium of the cerebellum, the dural membrane that separates the cerebrum from the cerebellum. When this type of bleeding occurs, the typical history includes a nulliparous mother, with the total labor and birth occurring in less than 2 or 3 hours; a difficult birth involving high or midforceps application; or a large-for-gestational-age infant. Subdural hematoma occurs infrequently today because of improvements in obstetric care. However, it is especially serious because of its inaccessibility to aspiration by subdural tap (Fanaroff and Martin, 1995; Wong, 1999).

Subarachnoid hemorrhage, the most common type of ICH, occurs in term infants as a result of trauma and in preterm infants as a result of hypoxia. Small hemorrhages are the most common. Bleeding is of venous origin, and underlying contusion also may occur (Wong, 1999).

The clinical presentation of hemorrhage in the full-term infant can vary considerably. In many infants, signs are absent, and hemorrhaging is diagnosed only because of abnormal findings on lumbar puncture, for example, RBCs in the cerebrospinal fluid (CSF). The initial clinical manifestations of neonatal subarachnoid hemorrhage may be the early onset of alternating depression and irritability, with refractory seizures (Fanaroff and Martin, 1997). Occasionally the infant appears normal initially and then has seizures on the second or third day of life, followed by no apparent sequelae.

In general, nursing care of an infant with ICH is supportive and includes monitoring of ventilatory and intravenous therapy, observation and management of seizures, and prevention of increased ICP. Minimal handling to promote rest and reduce stress should guide nursing care (Wong, 1999).

Spinal cord injuries almost always result from breech births, especially difficult ones in which version and extraction are used. This type of injury is rarely seen today because cesarean birth is often used for breech presentation (Fanaroff and Martin, 1997).

Critical Thinking

COMPARING NORMAL AND HIGH RISK NEONATES

After you have spent an observation day in either a nursery for term newborns or a maternal-newborn unit and are familiar with basic newborn behaviors and care, observe infants in an intermediate care nursery. Compare the different feeding methods in the two units. Discuss with a nurse the various feeding policies and the unit's plan to implement full breastfeedings or bottle-feedings for several infants. Assess an infant requiring oxygen support during a nipple feeding. Why would a premature infant require oxygen support during nipple feedings but not during gavage feedings?

NEONATAL INFECTIONS

Sepsis

Sepsis (presence of microorganisms or their toxins in the blood or other tissues) continues to be one of the most significant causes of neonatal morbidity and mortality. The newborn infant is susceptible to infection. Maternal immunoglobulin M (IgM) does not cross the placenta. Immunoglobulin A (IgA) and IgM require time to reach optimum levels after birth. Phagocytosis is less efficient. Serum complement levels are inadequate; serum complement (C1 through C6) is involved in immunologic reactions, some of which kill or lyse bacteria and enhance phagocytosis. Dysmaturity seen with IUGR and preterm and postdate birth further compromises the neonate's immune system.

Table 28-2 outlines risk factors for neonatal sepsis. Special precautions for preventing infection, as well as prompt recognition when it occurs, are necessary for optimum newborn care.

TABLE 28-2
Risk Factors for Neonatal Sepsis

Source	Risk Factors
Maternal	Low socioeconomic status
	Poor prenatal care
	Poor nutrition
	Substance abuse
Intrapartum	Premature rupture of fetal membranes
	Maternal fever
	Chorioamnionitis
	Prolonged labor
	Premature labor
	Maternal urinary tract infection
Neonatal	Twin gestation
	Male
	Birth asphyxia
	Meconium aspiration
	Congenital anomalies of skin or mucous membranes
	Galactosemia
	Absence of spleen
	Low birth weight or prematurity
	Malnourishment
	Prolonged hospitalization

Adapted from Askin D: Bacterial and fungal sepsis in the neonate. *J Obstet Gynecol Neonatal Nurs* 24(7):635-643, 1995.

Neonatal infections may be acquired in utero, during birth, during resuscitation, and nosocomially (Fanaroff and Martin, 1997).

Neonatal bacterial infection is classified into two patterns according to the time of presentation. Early-onset or congenital sepsis usually manifests within 24 hours of birth, progresses more rapidly than later-onset infection, and carries a mortality rate of 10% to 25% (Klein and Marcy, 1995). Early-onset infection is usually caused by microorganisms from the normal flora of the maternal vaginal tract, including group B streptococci, *Haemophilus influenzae, Listeria monocytogenes, Escherichia coli,* and *Streptococcus pneumoniae* (Merenstein, Adams, and Weisman, 1998). It is associated with a history of obstetric complications such as preterm labor, premature rupture of membranes, maternal fever during labor, and chorioamnionitis (Klein and Marcy, 1995).

Acquired infection is most commonly seen after 2 weeks of age and is slower in progression. Bacteria responsible for late-onset sepsis are varied, may be acquired from the birth canal or from the external environment, and include *Staphylococcus aureus, Staphylococcus epidermidis, Pseudomonas organisms,* and group B streptococci.

Viral infections may cause miscarriage, stillbirth, intrauterine infection, congenital malformations, and acute disease. These pathogens also may cause chronic infection, with subtle manifestations that may be recognized only after a prolonged period. It is important to recognize the manifestations of infections in the neonatal period to be able to treat the acute infection, to prevent nosocomial infections in other infants, and to anticipate effects on the infant's subsequent growth and development.

Fungal infections are of greatest concern in the immunocompromised or premature infant. Occasionally, fungal infections such as thrush are found in otherwise healthy term infants.

Septicemia refers to a generalized infection in the bloodstream. Pneumonia, the most common form of neonatal infection, is one of the leading causes of perinatal death (Fanaroff and Martin, 1997). Bacterial meningitis affects 1 in 2500 liveborn infants. Gastroenteritis is sporadic, depending on epidemic outbreaks. Local infections such as conjunctivitis and omphalitis occur commonly, but incidence rates are unavailable. Infection continues to be a significant factor in fetal and neonatal morbidity and mortality.

Care Management

➤ Assessment

The prenatal record is reviewed for risk factors associated with infection and the signs and symptoms suggestive of infection. Maternal vaginal or perineal infection may be transmitted directly to the infant during passage through the birth canal. Psychosocial history and history of sexually transmitted infections (STIs) may indicate possible human immunodeficiency virus (HIV), hepatitis B virus (HBV), or cytomegalovirus (CMV) infection.

Perinatal events also are reviewed. Premature rupture of membranes (PROM) may be caused by maternal or intrauterine infection. Ascending infection may occur after prolonged PROM, prolonged labor, or intrauterine fetal monitoring. A maternal history of fever during labor or the presence of foul-smelling amniotic fluid may also indicate the presence of infection. Antibiotic therapy initiated during labor should be noted. Resuscitation that requires intubation and deep suctioning may result in infection. The neonate's gestational age, maturity, birth weight, and sex all affect the incidence of infection. Sepsis occurs about twice as often and results in a higher mortality in male than in female infants. The neonate is assessed for respiratory distress, skin abscesses, rashes, and other indications of infection.

During the postnatal period the time of onset of suspicious signs is noted. Onset within the first 48 hours of life is more often associated with prenatal or perinatal predisposing factors. Onset after 2 or 3 days more often reflects disease acquired at or subsequent to birth (Fanaroff and Martin, 1997).

The earliest clinical signs of neonatal sepsis are characterized by a lack of specificity. The nonspecific signs include lethargy, poor feeding, poor weight gain, and irritability. The nurse or parent may simply note that the infant is just not doing as well as before. Differential diagnosis may be difficult because signs of sepsis are similar to signs of noninfectious neonatal problems such as anemia and hypoglycemia. Additional clinical and laboratory information and appropriate cultures supplement the findings described. Table 28-3 outlines signs of sepsis.

Laboratory studies are important. Specimens for cultures include blood, CSF, stool, and urine. Direct (conjugated) bilirubin levels may be increased, especially if the infecting microorganism is gram-negative. Complete blood cell count with differential is performed to determine the presence of anemia or increased or decreased WBC count (the latter is an ominous sign). C-reactive protein may or may not be elevated (Table 28-4).

TABLE 28-3
Signs of Sepsis*

System	Signs
Respiratory	Apnea, bradycardia Tachypnea Grunting, nasal flaring Retractions Decreased oxygen saturation Acidosis
Cardiovascular	Decreased cardiac output Tachycardia Hypotension Decreased perfusion
Central nervous	Temperature instability Lethargy Hypotonia Irritability, seizures
Gastrointestinal	Feeding intolerance Abdominal distention Vomiting, diarrhea
Integumentary	Jaundice Pallor Petechiae

Adapted from Askin D: Bacterial and fungal sepsis in the neonate. *J Obstet Gynecol Neonatal Nurs* 24(7):635-643, 1995.
*Laboratory findings include neutropenia, increased bands, hypoglycemia or hyperglycemia, metabolic acidosis, and thrombocytopenia.

Vigilant assessment continues during and after treatment. The newborn continues to be assessed for sequelae to septicemia, which include meningitis, DIC, and septic shock.

Septic shock results from the toxins released into the bloodstream. The most common sign is a drop in blood pressure, a vital sign often overlooked in the care of the neonate. Other signs are rapid, irregular respirations and pulse (similar to septicemia in general).

➤ Nursing Diagnoses

Any number of nursing diagnoses are possible, depending on the infant's gestational age and birth weight, the organ systems involved, and the nature of the infection. Examples of nursing diagnoses related to neonatal infections include the following:

Newborn

- Infection related to:
  - —Maternal vaginal (or other) infection
  - —Resuscitation or ventilation therapy
  - —Indwelling umbilical catheters, TPN, parenteral fluids
  - —Intrauterine electronic fetal monitoring
  - —Dysmaturity, IUGR, gestational age
- Ineffective thermoregulation related to:
  - —Infection
- Impaired tissue integrity related to:
  - —Use of multiple supportive measures (e.g., biometric monitoring, TPN, inhalation therapy)
- Pain related to:
  - —Multiple supportive measures

Parents and family

- Anxiety, fear, or anticipatory grieving related to:
  - —Uncertainty about infant's prognosis
  - —Poor prognosis
- Risk for altered parent-infant attachment related to:
  - —Separation of parent and newborn
  - —Feelings of inadequacy in caring for infant
- Powerlessness or spiritual distress related to:
  - —Perinatal events or newborn's condition

➤ Expected Outcomes

Planning begins with the development of standards for preventive measures in nurseries, and protocols for the diagnosis and treatment of infections. Individual assessment findings are used to plan care for each infant. Parents and family are encouraged to participate in planning. Expected outcomes include the following:

- The newborn will remain free of sepsis
- The newborn's early signs of sepsis will be recognized, and appropriate therapy will be instituted
- If therapy is necessary, the newborn will suffer no harmful sequelae
- Parents will begin bonding and attachment to newborn
- Parents will maintain self-esteem

➤ Plan of Care and Implementation

Preventive Measures. Virtually all controlled clinical trials have demonstrated that effective handwashing is responsible for the prevention of nosocomial infection in nursery units

TABLE 28-4
Suspected Neonatal Sepsis

ASSESSMENTS	**1.** Potential maternal risk factors and unstable vital signs, especially temperature instability **2.** Sepsis screen in first hour (CBC with differential, platelets, and CRP level) if there are significant maternal risk factors (prolonged rupture of membranes, maternal temperature) or if infant demonstrates physiologic signs of sepsis
TREATMENT	**1.** Start IV administration of antibiotics by peripheral IV **2.** Provide other treatments as needed for additional physiologic problems (ventilator for respiratory distress, incubator for temperature instability)
POSSIBLE CONSULTATIONS	**1.** Neonatologists and advanced practice nurses for care of unstable infants **2.** Medical specialists for care of infants with additional problems (congenital deformities) **3.** Lactation consultant, interpreter, social worker, and chaplain as needed or requested
ADDITIONAL ASSESSMENTS	**1.** Weight and measurements **2.** Blood culture, chest x-ray study, urinalysis, and lumbar puncture, if infant is symptomatic or CRP level is positive **3.** Repeat determination of CRP level in the morning for 2 days. If negative and infant not symptomatic, stop antibiotic treatment **4.** Continuous cardiac and saturation monitor assessment if infant's condition is unstable
DIRECT INFANT CARE	**1.** Vital signs every 1 to 2 hours for the first 4 hours, then every 4 hours **2.** Advance oral feedings as tolerated (infant NPO only if condition is physiologically unstable) **3.** Bath and cord care done per unit protocols
TEACHING AND DISCHARGE PLANNING	**1.** Initiate on admission. Provide parents with written and oral information on suspected sepsis **2.** Reinforce information and determine parents' understanding of information before discharge. Include information on well-baby care and community follow-up with the family's primary health care provider

From Lucile Salter Packard Children's Hospital at Stanford, CA.

(Fanaroff and Martin, 1997). Nursing is directly or indirectly responsible for minimizing or eliminating environmental sources of infectious agents in the nursery. Measures to be taken include Standard Precautions, careful and thorough cleaning, frequent replacement of used equipment (e.g., changing intravenous tubing per hospital protocol, and cleaning resuscitation and ventilation equipment), and disposal of excrement and linens in an appropriate manner. Overcrowding must be avoided in nurseries.

Antibiotic is instilled into newborns' eyes 1 to 2 hours after birth to prevent infection. The skin, its secretions, and normal flora are natural defenses that protect against invading pathogens. Warm water may be used to remove blood and meconium from the neonate's face, head, and body. A mild nonmedicated soap (in single-use container or in a small bar reserved for a single newborn) can be used with careful water rinsing. The vernix caseosa is left in place. No single method of cord care has been shown to prevent colonization and subsequent disease. Alcohol, triple dye, or an antimicrobial agent are typically used. Cords cleaned with sterile water or those left to dry naturally separate more quickly than those cleaned with alcohol, and resulted in no increase in number of infections (Dores et al, 1998; Medves and O'Brien, 1997). Nurses must follow agency protocols for cord care; they can recommend revision of protocols based on research.

Curative Measures. Breastfeeding or feeding the newborn breast milk from the mother is encouraged. Protective mechanisms exist in breast milk. Colostrum contains IgA, which offers protection against infection in the gastrointestinal tract. Human milk contains iron-binding protein that exerts a bacteriostatic effect on *E. coli.* Human milk also contains macrophages and lymphocytes. The vulnerability of infants to common mucosal pathogens such as respiratory syncytial virus (RSV) may be reduced by passive transfer of maternal immunity in the colostrum and breast milk.

Administering medications, taking precautions when performing treatments, and following isolation procedures are also interventions to be considered when a newborn has an infection.

Monitoring the intravenous infusion rate and administering antibiotics are nursing responsibilities. It is important to administer the prescribed dose of antibiotic within 1 hour after it is prepared to avoid loss of drug stability. If the intravenous fluid the infant is receiving contains electrolytes, vitamins, or other medications, the nurse should check with the hospital pharmacy before adding antibiotics. The antibiotic (or other medication) may be deactivated or may form a precipitate when combined with other substances. In that case a piggyback solution of the prescribed fluid is attached with a three-way stopcock at the infusion site.

Care must be taken in suctioning secretions from any newborn's oropharynx or trachea. These secretions may be infected.

Isolation procedures are implemented as indicated according to hospital policy. Isolation protocols are changing rapidly, and the nurse is urged to participate in continuing education and in-service programs to remain up to date.

Rehabilitative Measures. Rehabilitative measures vary with the individual needs of the neonate. Some neonates need to be weaned from ventilatory support systems. Those who suffer sequelae such as mental retardation and epilepsy require a knowledgeable family and supportive community resources. Some children will require corrective care for problems with dentition, vision, and hearing.

➤ Evaluation

The nurse can be reasonably assured that care was effective if the outcomes for care are achieved.

TORCH Infections

The occurrence of certain maternal infections during early pregnancy is known to be associated with various congenital malformations and disorders. The most common and best understood infections are represented by the acronym TORCH, for toxoplasmosis, other (gonorrhea, syphilis, varicella, HBV, and HIV), rubella, cytomegalovirus, and herpes simplex virus (HSV) (Box 28-1). HSV may result in a severe, often fatal systemic illness in neonates. Survivors of herpetic infection may have residual neurologic defects and chorioretinitis. The other congenital infections also may result in encephalopathy with various anomalies, including microcephaly, chorioretinitis, intracranial calcifications, microphthalmus, and cataracts. To a certain extent the varied clinical manifestations of these infections overlap, but a specific diagnosis can be made by the clustering of clinical findings, as well as specific antibody studies (Fanaroff and Martin, 1997).

Toxoplasmosis. Toxoplasmosis is a multisystem disease caused by the protozoan *Toxoplasma gondii.* Cats who hunt infected birds and mice harbor the parasite and excrete the infective oocysts in their feces. Human infection follows hand-to-mouth contact, such as after disposal of cat litter or after handling or ingesting raw meat from cattle or sheep that grazed in contaminated fields. About 30% of women who contract toxoplasmosis during gestation transmit the disease to their offspring (Lynfield and Guerina, 1997). Fetal infection occurs in 0.07% to 0.11% of all pregnancies (Beazley and Egerman, 1998; Boyer, 1996). The diagnosis of toxoplasmosis in the neonate is supported by elevated levels of cord blood serum IgM.

More than 70% of affected infants are free of symptoms. The clinical features of toxoplasmosis resemble cytomegalic inclusion disease (CMID) in the infant. Both diseases are responsible for serious perinatal mortality and morbidity: 10% to 15% die, 85% have severe psychomotor problems or mental retardation by age 2 to 4 years, and 50% have visual problems by age 1 year.

Severe toxoplasmosis is associated with preterm birth, growth restriction, microcephaly or hydrocephaly, microphthalmus, chorioretinitis, CNS calcification, thrombocytopenia, jaundice, and fever. Petechiae or a maculopapular rash may also be evident. Some clinical manifestations do not develop until later in life. The affected infant may be treated with

Box 28-1

TORCH Infections Affecting Newborns

T	Toxoplasmosis
O	Other: gonorrhea, syphilis, varicella, hepatitis B virus (HBV), human immunodeficiency virus (HIV)
R	Rubella
C	Cytomegalovirus (CMV) infections or cytomegalic inclusion disease (CMID)
H	Herpes simplex virus (HSV) infection

pyrimethamine, as well as oral sulfadiazine, but folic acid supplement will be required to prevent anemia.

Gonorrhea. The incidence of gonococcal infection in pregnant women ranges from 2.5% to 7.3% (Fanaroff and Martin, 1997). With this high incidence, it is not surprising that neonatal infection with *Neisseria gonorrhoeae* often occurs. After rupture of membranes, ascending infection can result in orogastric contamination of the fetus. The organism also may invade mucosal surfaces such as the conjunctiva (ophthalmia neonatorum), rectal mucosa, and pharynx. Contamination may occur as the infant passes through the birth canal, or it may occur postnatally from an infected adult. Neonatal gonococcal arthritis, septicemia, meningitis, vaginitis, and scalp abscesses can also develop.

Eye prophylaxis (e.g., with 0.5% erythromycin ointment) is administered at or shortly after birth to prevent ophthalmia neonatorum. The infant with a mild infection often recovers completely with appropriate treatment (e.g., neonatal ceftriaxone). Occasionally, infants die of overwhelming infection in the early neonatal period.

Syphilis. Congenital and neonatal syphilis have reemerged in recent years as significant health problems. It is estimated that for every 100 women diagnosed with primary or secondary disease, 2 to 5 infants will contract congenital syphilis. If syphilis during pregnancy is untreated, 40% to 50% of neonates born to these women will have symptomatic congenital syphilis. Treatment failure can occur, particularly when treatment is given in the third trimester; therefore infants born to women treated after 20 weeks' gestation should be investigated for congenital syphilis.

Fetal infestation with the spirochete *Treponema pallidum* is blocked by Langhans' layer in the chorion until this layer begins to atrophy between 16 and 18 weeks' gestation. If spirochetemia is untreated, it will result in fetal death by midtrimester miscarriage or stillbirth (in 1 in 4 cases). All neonates in whom the infection occurs before 7 months' gestation are affected. Only 60% are affected if the infection occurs late in pregnancy. If maternal infection is treated adequately before the eighteenth week, neonates seldom demonstrate signs of the disease. Although treatment after the eighteenth week may cure fetal spirochetemia, pathologic changes may not be prevented completely.

Because the fetus becomes infected after the period of organogenesis (first trimester), maldevelopment of organs does not result. Congenital syphilis may stimulate preterm labor, but no evidence indicates that it causes IUGR. Stigmas of congenital syphilis may include inflammatory and destructive changes in the placenta; in organs such as the liver, spleen, kidneys, and adrenal glands; and in bone covering and marrow. Disorders of the CNS, teeth, and cornea may not become evident until several months after birth.

The most severely affected infants may be hydropic (edematous) and anemic, with enlarged liver and spleen. Hepatosplenomegaly probably results from extramedullary hematopoietic activity stimulated by the severe anemia. In some infants, signs of congenital syphilis do not appear until late in the neonatal period. In these newborns, early signs such as poor feeding, slight hyperthermia, and snuffles may be nonspecific. Snuffles refers to the copious, clear, serosanguineous mucus discharge from the obstructed nose. A mucopurulent discharge indicates secondary infection, usually by streptococci or staphylococci.

By the end of the first week of life, a copper-colored maculopapular dermal rash appears in untreated newborns. The rash is characteristically first noticeable on the palms of the hands, soles of the feet, the diaper area, and around the mouth and anus. The maculopapular lesions may become vesicular and confluent and extend over the trunk and extremities. Condylomata (i.e., elevated, wartlike lesions) may be seen around the anus. Rough, cracked, mucocutaneous lesions of the lips heal to form circumoral radiating scars known as rhagades.

If the mother was adequately treated before giving birth, and serologic testing of the infant does not show syphilis, generally the infant is not treated with antibiotics. The infant is checked for antibody titer (received from the mother via the placenta) every 2 weeks for 3 months, at which time the test result should be negative. Some physicians recommend antibiotic therapy for asymptomatic or inconclusive cases.

Penicillin is the usual treatment (Hollier and Cox, 1998). Erythromycin is the substitute antibiotic of choice for infants sensitive to penicillin.

NURSE ALERT • The infant with syphilis is contagious until treated. Care providers should use Standard Precautions (contact isolation) in caring for the infant until the infant has been on antibiotics for at least 24 hours.

In general, treatment of syphilis is more effective if it is begun early rather than later in the course of the disease. However, a recurrence rate of 5% can be expected. Even adequate treatment of congenital syphilis after birth does not always prevent late complication (e.g., 5 to 15 years after initial infection). Potential complications include neurosyphilis, deafness, Hutchinson's teeth (notched incisors), saber shins, joint involvement, saddle nose (depressed bridge), gummas (soft, gummy tumors) over the skin and other organs, and interstitial keratitis (inflammation of the cornea).

Varicella Zoster. The varicella zoster virus responsible for chickenpox and shingles is a member of the herpes family. About 90% of women in their childbearing years are immune; therefore the risk of infection in pregnancy is low, 0.7 to 3 per 1000 births (Birthhistle and Carrington, 1998; Chapman, 1998).

Varicella transmission to the fetus may occur across the placenta when the disease is contracted in the first half of pregnancy, but this is relatively infrequent. When transmission to the fetus does occur in the early part of pregnancy, the effects on the fetus include limb atrophy, neurologic abnormalities, eye abnormalities, and IUGR.

When maternal infection occurs in the last 3 weeks of pregnancy, 25% of infants born to these mothers will develop clinical varicella (Nathwani et al, 1998). The severity of the infant's illness increases greatly if maternal infection occurred within 5 days before or 2 days after birth. The mortality in severe illness is 30% (Chapman, 1998).

Infants born to mothers who develop chickenpox between 5 days before birth and 48 hours after birth should be given VZIG at birth because of the risk of severe disease. Acyclovir can be used to treat infants with generalized involvement and pneumonia (Chapman, 1998; Nathwani et al, 1998).

Term infants exposed to chickenpox after birth will have either a mild infection or no infection if they are born to immune mothers. Those born to nonimmune mothers may develop chickenpox, but the course is not usually severe. Experts are divided as to whether this group of infants should receive VZIG. Infants less than 28 weeks of age are at risk regardless of their mother's status and probably benefit from VZIG if exposed to chickenpox.

Hepatitis B Virus. Hepatitis B virus (HBV) infection during pregnancy is not associated with an increase in malformations, stillbirths, or IUGR; however, about a 32% increase in risk exists for preterm birth (Fanaroff and Martin, 1997). The transmission rate of HBV to the newborn is as high as 90% when the mother is seropositive for both hepatitis B surface antigen (HbsAg) and hepatitis B e antigen (HbeAg) (Duff, 1998). Transmission occurs transplacentally; serum to serum; and by contact with contaminated urine, feces, saliva, semen, or vaginal secretions during birth. Infants are most commonly infected during birth or in the first few days of life. The rate of transmission is highest when the mother contracts the virus immediately before birth. These mothers will be positive for HBsAg. Transmission may occur through breast milk, but antigens also develop in formula-fed infants at the same or higher rate. Diagnosis is made by viral culture of amniotic fluid as well as the presence of HBsAg and IgM in the cord blood or baby's serum.

Neonatal and fetal effects are serious. Preterm birth exposes the neonate to the problems of prematurity. Infants may be symptom free at birth, or show evidence of acute hepatitis with changes in liver function. The mortality for full-blown hepatitis is 75%. Infants who become carriers are at high risk for chronic hepatitis, cirrhosis of the liver, or liver cancer even years later (Fanaroff and Martin, 1997).

Infants whose mothers have antibodies for HBsAg or who have developed hepatitis during pregnancy or the postpartum period should be treated with hepatitis B immunoglobulin (HBIG), 0.5 ml intramuscularly, as soon as possible after birth or within the first 12 hours of life. The vaccine should also be given concurrently, but at a different site (Fanaroff and Martin, 1997). The second dose of vaccine is given at 1 month and the third dose at 6 months. The vaccine should protect the child for up to 9 years. After the infant has been cleansed thoroughly and has received the vaccine, breastfeeding may be initiated. Vaccination for infants not exposed to HBV is recommended before discharge; breastfeeding for these infants may begin before the vaccine is given.

Human Immunodeficiency Virus and Acquired Immunodeficiency Syndrome. It is estimated that globally, more than 1 million children born to HIV-infected women will acquire the virus (Mofenson, 1997). Since 1994, when research demonstrated that prenatal treatment of HIV-positive women reduced the vertical transmission of HIV to the fetus, there has been a drop in the risk of transmission from 25% to 8%, an almost 70% decrease (Minkoff, 1998). The majority of cases of pediatric AIDS result from maternal-to-fetal transmission. Universal counseling and screening of pregnant women is recommended in the United States and Canada (American College of Obstetrics and Gynecologists [ACOG], 1997; Centers for Disease Control and Prevention [CDC], 1998).

Transmission of HIV from the mother to the infant may occur transplacentally at various gestational ages. Transmission close to or at the time of birth is thought to account for 50% to 80% of cases (Franck and Johnson, 1998; Mofenson, 1997; Scarlatti, 1996). Postnatal transmission through breastfeeding may also occur with an additional risk of 14% attributed to breast milk contact (Scarlatti, 1996).

Diagnosis of HIV infection in the neonate is complicated by the presence of maternal IgG antibodies, which cross the placenta after 32 weeks of gestation. The accuracy of all HIV tests varies according to the infant's age and is dependent on the viral load in the blood.

Typically the HIV-infected neonate is asymptomatic at birth. These infants tend to be of lower birth weight than those born to noninfected mothers. Some will have physical stigma from concurrent exposure to injectable drugs or other STIs. Early-onset HIV disease (i.e., virus detected within 48 hours of birth) is attributed to prenatal infection and occurs in 10% to 15% of infected infants (Franck and Johnson, 1998). These babies develop opportunistic infections (caused by an organism that does not usually cause illness) and rapid progression of immunodeficiency, which progresses to death in the first 1 to 2 years of life (Franck and Johnson, 1998).

The remainder of infants develop AIDS more slowly. Eighty to ninety percent of perinatally infected infants show signs by 1 year of life. Some children infected at birth show no signs of disease 8 to 10 years later (Scarlatti, 1996). The age of onset of symptoms predicts the length of survival.

The presenting signs and symptoms of HIV infection vary from severe immunodeficiency to nonspecific findings such as failure to thrive, parotitis, and recurrent or persistent upper respiratory infections. In the first year of life, lymphadenopathy and hepatosplenomegaly are common (Scarlatti, 1996). The infant may have fever, chronic diarrhea, chronic dermatitis, interstitial pneumonitis, persistent thrush, and AIDS-defining secondary infections. Common secondary infections include *Pneumocystis carinii* pneumonia, candidiasis, CMV infection, cryptosporidiosis, herpes simplex or herpes zoster, and disseminated varicella.

Care Management. Although it is rare for an infant to be born with symptoms of HIV infection, all infants born to seropositive mothers should be presumed to be HIV positive. Management begins by implementing Standard Precautions. Measures should also be undertaken to protect the infant from further exposure to maternal blood and body fluids. The infant's skin should be cleansed with soap and water and alcohol before invasive procedures such as vitamin K administration or heel punctures. Umbilical cord stumps are cleaned meticulously every day until healing is complete. Isolation is not required, and the infant can usually be cared for in the normal nursery. The use of gloves is not required for care activities such as dressing or feeding the infant.

Regimens for the prevention of HIV transmission include treatment of the neonate with zidovudine for 6 weeks following birth until the infant's HIV status is determined (CDC, 1998; Tuomala, 1997). If the infant is diagnosed with HIV infection, the family should be counseled about conventional and investigational treatment options.

Counseling regarding the care of the mothers themselves, the family's care of the infant, and future pregnancies challenges the caregiver. Some parents opt to place infected infants in foster homes despite the low risk for transmission among members of the same household. Social services are required in these cases. If the parent chooses to keep the infant, home health care may be arranged. For more information and updated information, parents are offered the following resource: the National AIDS hotline, 1-800-342-AIDS.

The family must be counseled about vaccinations. Children with symptomatic or asymptomatic HIV infection should receive all routine vaccines except oral poliovirus and varicella vaccines. The family should be advised that household contacts should not receive oral polio vaccine (OPV) because the virus can be transmitted to the immunocompromised child. Inactivated poliomyelitis vaccine (IPV) can be given (Franck and Johnson, 1998; Wong, 1999).

Rubella Infection. Since rubella vaccination was begun in 1969, cases of congenital rubella have been reduced dramatically; however, it is still seen occasionally in the newborn. Vaccination failures, lack of compliance, and the migration of nonimmunized persons result in periodic outbreaks of rubella, also known as German or 3-day measles.

The risk for congenital anomalies varies with the gestational age of the fetus at the time maternal infection occurs. Abnormalities are most severe if the mother contracts the virus during the first trimester.

More than two thirds of infected infants have no symptoms apparent at birth, but sequelae may develop years later. Hearing loss, the most common result, appears to be progressive after birth. Congenital rubella syndrome comprises cataracts or glaucoma, hearing loss, and cardiac defects (i.e., pulmonary artery stenosis, patent ductus arteriosus, or coarctation of the aorta) (Rosa, 1998). Multiple other abnormalities may also be present, including IUGR, microphthalmia, hypotonia, hepatosplenomegaly, thrombocytopenic purpura, dermatoglyphic abnormalities, bony radiolucencies, and brain wave abnormalities (Burchett, 1998). Severe infections may result in fetal death. Delayed effects of infection manifest as thyroid dysfunction, diabetes mellitus, growth hormone deficiency, myocarditis, glaucoma, microcephaly, and polycystic kidney disease (Fanaroff and Martin, 1997).

The rubella virus has been cultured in infants for up to 18 months after their birth. These infants are a serious source of infection to susceptible individuals, particularly women in the childbearing years. Extended pediatric isolation is mandatory until the noncontagious stage of rubella has been reached (i.e., the infant should be isolated until pharyngeal mucus and the urine are free of virus).

Cytomegalovirus Infection. CMV infection during pregnancy may result in miscarriage, stillbirth, or congenital or neonatal cytomegalic inclusion disease (CMID). It is the most common cause of congenital viral infections in humans, occurring in 1% of all newborns (Fanaroff and Martin, 1997). Most (90% to 95%) of the affected infants are asymptomatic at birth; however, hearing loss and learning disabilities have been reported in previously asymptomatic infants (Brown and Abernathy, 1998).

The neonate with classic, full-blown CMID displays IUGR and has microcephaly. The neonate also has a rash, jaundice, and hepatosplenomegaly (Fig. 28-7). Anemia, thrombocytopenia, and hyperbilirubinemia are to be expected. Intracranial, periventricular calcification often is noted on x-ray films. Inclusion bodies ("owl's eye" figures) in cells sedimented from freshly voided urine or in liver biopsy specimens are typical.

Elevated levels of cord blood IgM are suggestive of disease. The virus may be isolated from urine or saliva of the newborn. Differential diagnosis includes other causes of jaundice, syphilis (positive Venereal Disease Research Laboratories [VDRL] findings), toxoplasmosis (positive Sabin-Feldman dye test result), hemolytic disease of the newborn (positive Coombs test reaction), or coxsackievirus infection (positive culture).

Despite the extensive, endemic nature of the disease in women and men and its potential for havoc in perinatal life, only occasionally are critically affected newborns seen. Milder forms of the disease often result when the fetus is affected late in pregnancy. CMV can be transmitted through breast milk while the mother is experiencing acute CMV syndrome. CMV infections acquired after birth are often asymptomatic and have no sequelae. Exceptions to this occur in preterm infants, in whom postnatal acquisition of CMV can result in pneumonia, hepatitis, thrombocytopenia, and long-term neurologic sequelae.

Antenatally infected infants who are asymptomatic at birth are at risk for late sequelae. Hearing loss may not be apparent until after the first year of life. Chorioretinitis, microcephaly, mental retardation, and neuromuscular deficits may occur by 2 years of age. Some children are at risk for a defect in tooth enamel, resulting in severe caries.

Herpes Simplex Virus. HSV infections among newborns are being diagnosed more frequently. HSV infection is estimated to occur in as many as 1 in 2000 to 1 in 5000 births (Fanaroff and Martin, 1997).

The neonate may acquire the virus by any of four modes of transmission:

- Transplacental infection
- Ascending infection by way of the birth canal
- Direct contamination during passage through an infected birth canal
- Direct transmission from infected personnel or family (Riley, 1998)

Congenital infection is rare and is characterized by in utero destruction of normally formed organs. Affected infants are growth restricted. They have severe psychomotor restriction, with intracranial calcifications, microcephaly, hypertonicity, and seizures. They suffer eye involvement, including microphthalmus, cataracts, chorioretinitis, blindness, and retinal dysplasia. Some infants have patent ductus arteriosus, limb anomalies, and recurrent skin vesicles, with a short life expectancy.

Most infants are infected directly during passage through the birth canal. The risk of infection during vaginal birth in the presence of genital herpes has not been clearly delineated. It

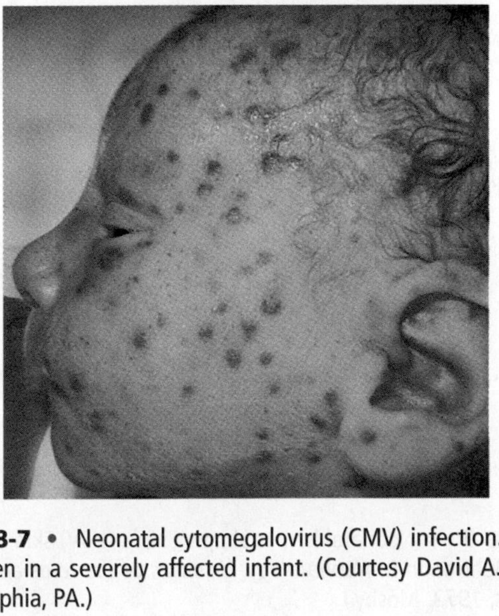

FIG. 28-7 • Neonatal cytomegalovirus (CMV) infection. Typical rash seen in a severely affected infant. (Courtesy David A. Clarke, Philadelphia, PA.)

may be as high as 40% to 60%, with active primary infection at term. Primary maternal infections after 32 weeks' gestation carry a higher risk for the fetus and newborn than do recurrent infections (Fanaroff and Martin, 1997). The transmission rate of chronic vaginal herpes from the pregnant woman to her newborn is low. Passive intrauterine immunity to herpes may be responsible.

Postnatal acquisition of the virus and spread within a nursery have been documented by DNA analysis. Both mother and father, as well as maternal breast lesions, have been implicated in neonatal infections. There also is concern regarding symptomatic and asymptomatic shedding among hospital personnel. Nursery personnel with cold sores should practice strict handwashing and wear a mask, but no evidence indicates they should be removed from the nursery unless they have a herpetic whitlow (primary HSV infection of the terminal segment of a finger) (Fanaroff and Martin, 1997).

Clinically, neonatal HSV infections are classified as disseminated infection, encephalitis, or localized infection of the skin, eye, or mouth. Disseminated infections may involve virtually every organ system, but those primarily involved are the liver, adrenal glands, and lungs. Affected infants exhibit initial symptoms usually in the first week of life but sometimes in the second week, with signs of bacterial sepsis or shock. Clinical manifestations include skin vesicles in about 50% of infants (Fig. 28-8). Death results from progression of CNS involvement, respiratory distress and pneumonitis, shock, DIC, and bleeding. Overall, the mortality without antiviral therapy is 57% (Riley, 1998).

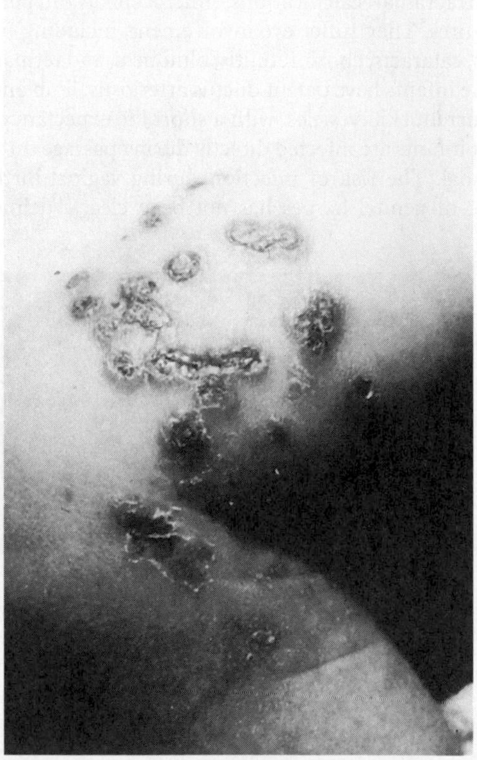

FIG. 28-8 • Neonatal herpes simplex virus (HSV) skin infection. (From Behrmann R: *Neonatology: diseases of the fetus and infant,* St Louis, 1973, Mosby.)

Care Management. Gloves should be worn when caregivers are in contact with these infants. The neonate's eyes, oral cavity, and skin are inspected carefully for the presence of any lesions (Fig. 28-9). Cultures are obtained from the mouth, eyes, and any lesions. Circumcision, if performed, is delayed until the infant is ready to be discharged. The infant may be discharged with the mother if the infant's cultures are negative for the virus. As long as no suspicious lesions are on the mother's breasts, breastfeeding is allowed. For the infant at risk, prophylactic topical eye ointment (vidarabine) is administered for 5 days to prevent keratoconjunctivitis. No current recommendations exist for prophylactic systemic therapy; each case should be considered individually. Blood, urine, and CSF specimens should be cultured when indicated clinically. If herpetic lesions first occur after 6 weeks of life, the risk of dissemination and severe illness is very low (Fanaroff and Martin, 1997).

Therapy includes general supportive measures, as well as treatment with vidarabine or acyclovir. Acyclovir is the most commonly used drug. It is considered safe because only viral replication is inhibited, although long-term sequelae are not yet known. Acyclovir is easier to administer; there is no difference between vidarabine and acyclovir for treatment of HSV (Jacobs, 1998). Continuing therapy may be required in recurrences. Ophthalmic ointment should be administered simultaneously (Fanaroff and Martin, 1997).

Bacterial Infections

Group B Streptococcus. The most common cause of neonatal sepsis and meningitis in the United States is the group B streptococcus (GBS) (Lieu et al, 1998).The incidence of early-onset GBS infection is 0.7 to 4 per 1000 live births (Adriaanse et al, 1996; Guerina, 1998). Early-onset GBS infection in the neonate occurs in the first 7 days of life but most commonly manifests in the first 24 hours following birth. Risk factors for the development of early-onset GBS include low birth weight, preterm birth, rupture of membranes of more than 18 hours, maternal fever, previous GBS infant, maternal GBS bacteriuria, and multiple gestation (Adriaanse et al, 1996; Guerina, 1998). Usually resulting from vertical transmission from the birth

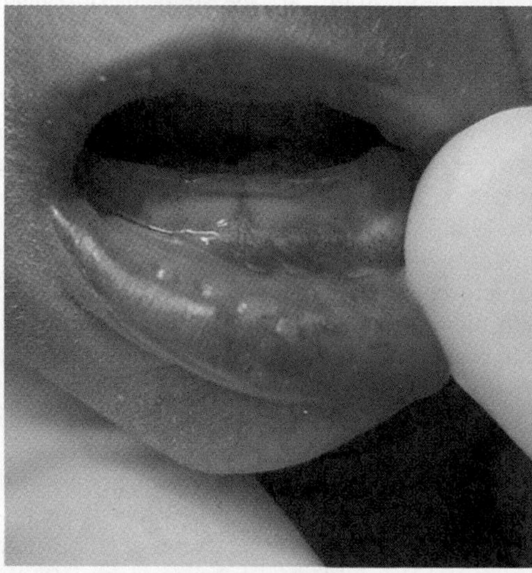

FIG. 28-9 • HSV oral lesions. (Courtesy David A. Clarke, Philadelphia, PA.)

canal, early-onset disease results in a respiratory illness that mimics the symptoms of severe respiratory distress. The infant may rapidly develop septic shock, which has a significant mortality rate. Prophylactic antibiotics given to mothers with risk factors during labor significantly reduces the incidence and severity of early-onset GBS infection in the newborn (CDC, 1996; Lieu et al, 1998).

Late-onset GBS infection presents between 1 week and 3 months of age with an average age of onset of 24 days. Eighty-five percent of infants with late-onset GBS have meningitis; this population has a mortality rate of 0% to 23%. Fifty percent of the survivors develop neurologic damage (Adriaanse et al, 1996).

Escherichia Coli. E. coli is the second most common cause of neonatal sepsis and meningitis in the United States (Guerina, 1998). *E. coli* is found in the gastrointestinal tract soon after birth and makes up the bulk of human fecal flora. In addition to meningitis, *E. coli* can also cause infections in other body systems, including the urinary tract. There is concern that increasing the use of ampicillin in labor as prophylaxis against GBS infection will result in more virulent *E. coli* infection due to ampicillin-resistant organisms (Joseph, Pyati, and Jacobs, 1998).

Tuberculosis. The incidence of tuberculosis (TB), which is caused by *Mycobacterium tuberculosis,* is increasing in Canada and the United States. Congenitally acquired TB, although rare, can cause otitis media, pneumonia, hepatosplenomegaly, enlarged lymph glands, or disseminated disease. After birth, exposed infants contract TB through droplets expelled by infected individuals, which results in pneumonia and necrosis of lung tissue. Untreated neonatal tuberculosis is almost always fatal.

Chlamydia Infection. *Chlamydia trachomatis* is an intracellular bacterium that causes neonatal conjunctivitis and pneumonia. The conjunctivitis (congestion and edema), with minimal discharge, develops 5 days to 2 weeks after birth. Inclusion conjunctivitis is usually self-limiting but if untreated, chronic follicular conjunctivitis, with conjunctival scarring and corneal microgranulations, has been reported (Schachter and Grossman, 1995).

The neonate is treated with oral erythromycin for 2 to 3 weeks. Silver nitrate is not effective against *C. trachomatis,* but erythromycin or tetracycline ointment may prevent ophthalmic infection (Fanaroff and Martin, 1997). Eye prophylaxis is not sufficient to prevent the development of chlamydial pneumonia; therefore infants at risk should also be treated with systemic antibiotics such as oral erythromycin syrup.

Fungal Infections

Candidiasis. Candida infections, formerly known as moniliasis, may occur in the newborn. *Candida albicans,* the organism usually responsible, may cause disease in any organ system. It is a yeastlike fungus (producing yeast cells and spores) that can be acquired from a maternal vaginal infection during birth; by person-to-person transmission; or from contaminated hands, bottles, nipples, or other articles. It usually is a benign disorder in the neonate, often confined to the oral and diaper regions (Wong, 1999).

Candidal diaper dermatitis appears on the perianal area, inguinal folds, and lower portion of the abdomen. The affected area is intensely erythematous, with a sharply demarcated, scalloped edge, often with numerous satellite lesions that extend beyond the larger lesion. The source of the infection is through the gastrointestinal tract. Treatment is with applications of an anticandidal ointment such as nystatin (Mycostatin) or miconazole 2% (Monistat) with each diaper change. The infant also may be given an oral antifungal preparation to eliminate any gastrointestinal source of infection (Wong, 1999).

Oral candidiasis (thrush, or mycotic stomatitis) is characterized by the appearance of white plaques on the oral mucosa, gums, and tongue. The white patches are easily differentiated from milk curds; the patches cannot be removed and tend to bleed when touched. In most cases the infant does not seem to be in discomfort from the infection. A few infants may have some difficulty swallowing.

Infants who are sick, debilitated, or receiving antibiotic therapy are more susceptible to thrush. Those with conditions such as cleft lip or palate, neoplasms, and hyperparathyroidism seem to be more vulnerable to mycotic infection.

Care Management. The objectives of management are to eradicate the causative organism, to control exposure to *C. albicans,* and to improve the infant's resistance. Interventions include maintenance of scrupulous cleanliness (by nursing personnel, parents, and others) to prevent reinfection. Good handwashing technique is always essential. Clean surfaces should be provided for neonates. Proper cleanliness of the equipment and environment is critical. If the infant is breastfeeding, the mother is also treated with topical nystatin.

Medications are administered as ordered. Nystatin is instilled into the newborn's mouth with a medicine dropper after the infant is given sterile water to wash out any residual milk. Nystatin may also be swabbed over mucosa, gums, or tongue. Less often, an aqueous solution of gentian violet (1% to 2%) is applied with a swab to oral mucosa, gums, and tongue. The nurse should guard against staining the skin, clothes, and equipment and should warn parents about the purple staining of the baby's mouth.

SUBSTANCE ABUSE

Certain maternal behaviors result in perinatal risk. Maternal habits hazardous to the fetus and neonate include drug addiction, smoking, and alcohol abuse. Occasional withdrawal reactions have been reported in neonates of mothers who use to excess such drugs as barbiturates, alcohol, or amphetamines. Serious reactions are seen in neonates whose mothers abuse psychoactive drugs or are treated with methadone. Almost 50% of pregnancies of women addicted to opioids result in LBW infants who are not necessarily preterm. Alcohol is a teratogen. Maternal ethanol abuse during gestation can lead to a readily identifiable fetal alcohol syndrome.

The adverse effects of exposure of the fetus to drugs are varied. They include transient behavioral changes such as fetal breathing movements; and irreversible effects such as fetal death, IUGR, structural malformations, and mental retardation. Critical determinants of the effect of the drug on the fetus include the specific drug, the dosage, the route of administration, the genotype of the mother or fetus, and the timing of the drug exposure. Fig. 28-10 shows critical periods in human embryogenesis and the teratogenic effects of drugs. Table 28-5 summarizes the effects of commonly abused substances on the fetus and neonate.

Alcohol

The incidence of fetal alcohol syndrome (FAS) in the United States is about 2 per 10,000 live births (Church and Abel, 1998).

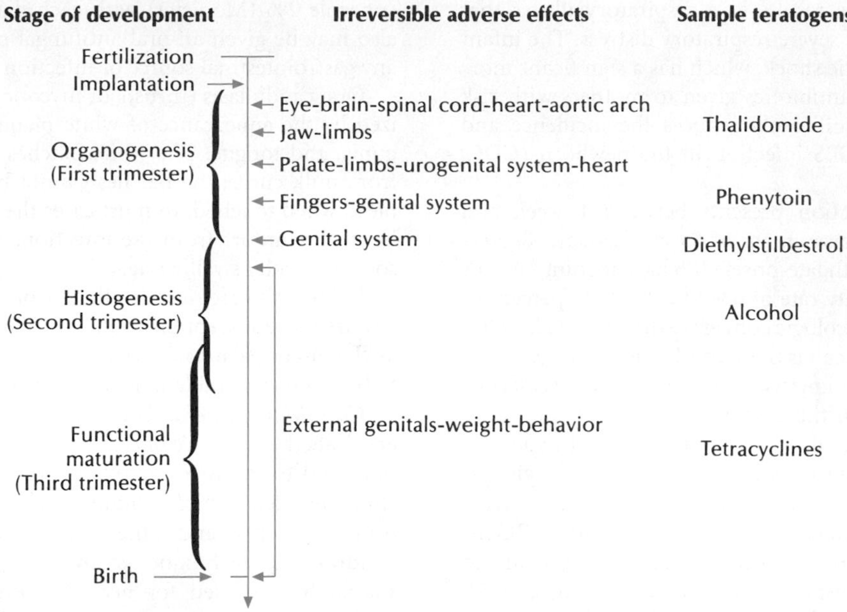

FIG. 28-10 • Critical periods in human embryogenesis. (From Fanaroff A, Martin R: *Neonatal-perinatal medicine: diseases of the fetus and infant,* ed 5, St Louis, 1995, Mosby.)

TABLE 28-5
Summary of Neonatal Effects of Commonly Abused Substances

Substance	Neonatal Effects
Alcohol	*Fetal alcohol syndrome* (FAS): craniofacial anomalies, including short eyelid opening, flat midface, flat upper lip groove, thin upper lip; microcephaly; hyperactivity; developmental delays; attention deficits *Fetal alcohol effects:* milder forms of FAS, cardiac anomalies, failure to thrive
Cocaine	Prematurity, small-for-gestational-age, microcephaly, poor feeding, irregular sleep patterns, diarrhea, visual attention problems, hyperactivity, difficult to console, hypersensitivity to noise and external stimuli, irritability, developmental delays, congenital anomalies such as prune belly syndrome (i.e., distended, flabby, wrinkled abdomen caused by lack of abdominal muscles)
Heroin	Low birth weight, small-for-gestational-age, neonatal abstinence syndrome (see Table 28-7)
Amphetamines	Small for gestational age, prematurity, poor weight gain, lethargy
Tobacco	Prematurity, low birth weight, increased risk for sudden infant death syndrome, increased risk for bronchitis, pneumonia, developmental delays
Marijuana	Possible neonatal tremors, possible low birth weight

According to Abel (1997), FAS is based on minimum criteria of signs in each of three categories: prenatal and postnatal growth restriction; CNS malfunctions, including mental retardation; and craniofacial features such as microcephaly, small eyes or short palpebral fissures, thin upper lip, flat midface, and an indistinct philtrum. Neurologic problems in FAS children include some degree of IQ deficit, attention deficit disorder, diminished fine motor skills, and poor speech (D'Apolito, 1998). Infants exposed prenatally to alcohol who are affected but do not meet the criteria for FAS may be said to have fetal alcohol effects (FAEs) (D'Apolito, 1998). These effects range from learning disabilities and behavioral problems to speech or language problems and hyperactivity. Often these problems are not detected until the child goes to school and learning problems become evident. FAEs can be seen with other disorders, such as fetal hydantoin syndrome; therefore a careful history is needed.

Predictable abnormal patterns of fetal and neonatal morphogenesis are attributed to severe, chronic alcoholism in women who continue to drink heavily during pregnancy. The pattern of growth deficiency begun in prenatal life persists after birth, especially in the linear growth rate, rate of weight gain, and growth of head circumference.

Ocular structural anomalies are common findings (Fig. 28-11). Limb anomalies and various cardiocirculatory anomalies, especially ventricular septal defects, pose problems for the child. Table 28-6 outlines physical findings in FAS. Mental retardation (e.g., IQ of 79 or below at 7 years of age), hyperactivity, and fine motor dysfunction (e.g., poor hand-to-mouth coordination, weak grasp) add to the handicapping problems that maternal alcoholism can impose. Genital abnormalities are seen in daughters of alcohol-addicted mothers. Two thirds of newborns with FAS are girls; the cause of this altered fetal sex ratio

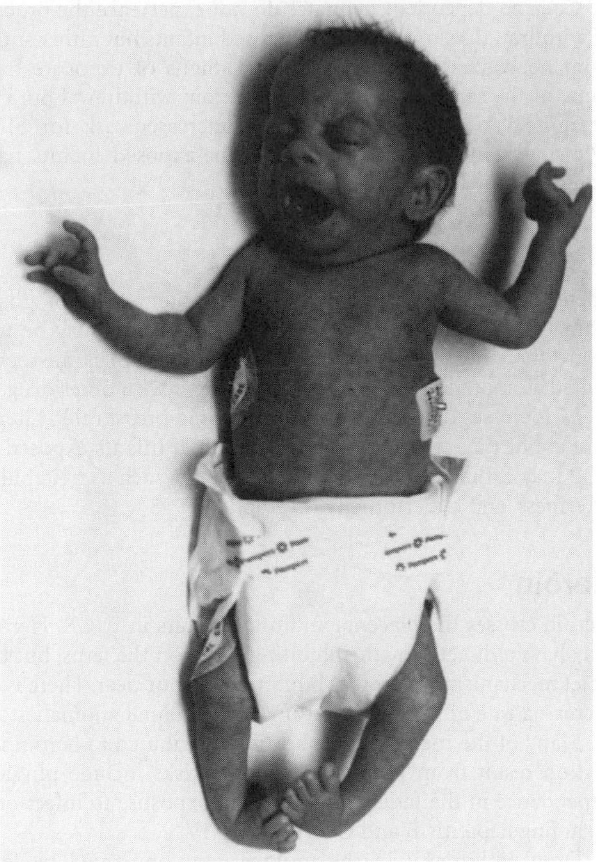

FIG. 28-11 • Infant with fetal alcohol syndrome. (From Wong D: *Whaley & Wong's nursing care of infants and children,* ed 6, St Louis, 1999, Mosby.)

is unknown. Severe and chronic alcoholism (ethanol toxicity), not maternal malnutrition, is responsible for the severity and consistency of postnatal performance problems (Fanaroff and Martin, 1997). High alcohol levels are lethal to the developing embryo. Lower levels cause brain and other malformations. Long-term prognosis is discouraging even in an optimum psychosocial environment, when one considers the combination of growth failure and mental retardation.

Alcohol effects depend not only on the amount of alcohol consumed but also on the interaction of quantity, frequency, type of alcohol, and other drug abuse. Other drugs, such as cigarettes, caffeine, and marijuana, may potentiate the fetal effects of alcohol consumption during gestation (Fanaroff and Martin, 1997).

The infant of a mother who abuses alcohol is faced with many clinical problems. Identification of the problems leads to the medical diagnosis of FAS. The infant may suffer respiratory distress related to preterm birth, neurologic damage, and a "floppy" epiglottis and small trachea. Tracheoepiglottal anomalies may cause cardiopulmonary arrest. Other disorders include recurrent otitis media and hearing loss. Craniofacial features may be important in diagnosing craniofacial and oral anomalies, dental development abnormalities, and long-term body growth patterns. Feeding difficulties are related to preterm birth, poor sucking ability, and possible cleft palate. The infant

TABLE 28-6
Features of Fetal Alcohol Syndrome

Affected Part	Characteristics
Eyes	Epicanthal folds, strabismus, ptosis, hypoplastic retinal vessels
Mouth	Poor suck, cleft lip, cleft palate, small teeth
Ears	Deafness
Skeleton	Radioulnar synostosis, fusion of cervical vertebrae, restricted bone growth
Heart	Atrial and ventricular septal defects, tetralogy of Fallot, patent ductus arteriosus
Kidney	Renal hypoplasia, hydronephrosis, urogenital sinus
Liver	Extrahepatic biliary atresia, hepatic fibrosis
Immune system	Increased infections: otitis media, upper respiratory infections, immune deficiencies
Tumors	Nonspecific neoplasms
Skin	Abnormal palmar creases, irregular hair, whorls

From Weiner L, Morse B: FAS: clinical perspectives and prevention. In Chasnoff I, editor: *Drugs, alcohol, pregnancy and parenting,* Boston, 1991, Kluwer.

Critical Thinking

DEVELOPMENT OF HIGH RISK INFANT

Describe the environment in which the infant is cared for. Include the incubator/bassinet as well as the nursery itself. Observe the way in which a high risk infant interacts with nursing staff and family members. Are the interactions the same with both? What time-out signals does the infant display when distressed? Discuss the implications of nursing care for the neonate and family on the basis of your findings.

may exhibit brain dysfunction, microcephaly, and grand mal seizures.

Long-term effects into childhood may include impaired visuomotor perception and performance, lowered IQ scores, and delayed receptive and expressive language, as well as reduced capacity to process and store factual data (Church and Abel, 1998). It is now recognized as one of the leading causes of mental retardation in the United States. Although the distinctive facial features of the infant tend to become less evident, the mental capacities never become normal.

Nursing care involves many of the same strategies used for the care of preterm infants. Special efforts are made to involve the parents in their child's care and to encourage opportunities for parent-child attachment.

Placing infants in a warm, caring environment with understanding caregivers who can deal with the infant's hyperirritability can lead to improved emotional development and social functioning (D'Apolito, 1998; Wagner et al, 1998). These caregivers provide extensive cuddling and human contact and can deal with the eating problems that typically lead to a diagnosis of failure to thrive. However, these infants may not go home to an optimal environment because many such families are dysfunctional.

Tobacco

Cigarette smoking in pregnancy is associated with birth weight deficits of up to 250 g for a full-term neonate (Fanaroff and Martin, 1997). Maternal cigarette smoking is implicated in 21% to 39% of LBW infants. Passive exposure to secondhand smoke by a pregnant woman may also result in the birth of an LBW infant.

The rate of miscarriage and preterm birth is increased in the smoking population (Lee, 1998). Nicotine and cotinine, the two pharmacologically active substances in tobacco, are found in higher concentrations in infants whose mothers smoke. These substances can be secreted in breast milk for up to 2 hours after the mother has smoked. Cigarette smoke contains more than 2000 compounds, including carbon monoxide, dioxin, cyanide, and cadmium. Deficits in growth, in intellectual and emotional development, poor auditory responsiveness, increased fine motor tremors, hypertonicity, and decreased verbal comprehension have been observed in infants exposed to smoke.

Pregnant women must be informed about the harmful effects of smoking on their unborn baby's health. These include IUGR, miscarriage, PROM, placenta previa, perinatal death, LBW, deficits in learning and behavior, and SIDS (Bennett, 1999; Lee, 1998). There is a positive association between maternal smoking and SIDS (Lee, 1998; Milerad et al, 1998). It is not clear whether this association reflects in utero exposure, passive exposure postnatally, or both. Mothers and all others should refrain from smoking near the infant.

Marijuana

Marijuana crosses the placenta. Its use during pregnancy may result in a shortened gestation and a higher incidence of IUGR (Wagner et al, 1998). Some investigators have found a higher incidence of meconium staining (Fanaroff and Martin, 1997). Some association has been reported between the use of marijuana and a decrease in infant birth weight and length and the occurrence of congenital anomalies; however, the findings have been inconsistent (Lee, 1998). Compounding the issue of the effects of marijuana, especially among adolescents, is multidrug use, which combines the harmful effects of marijuana, tobacco, alcohol, and cocaine. Long-term follow-up studies on exposed infants are needed.

Cocaine

Antenatal effects of maternal cocaine ingestion include infarctions to developing organs; these result in defects such as hydronephrosis, hypospadias, prune belly syndrome (distended flabby abdomen and renal anomalies), congenital heart disease, skull defects, ileal atresia, and limb reduction. Infants born to cocaine-abusing mothers show a high rate of meconium staining, perinatal morbidity, IUGR, preterm birth, small head circumference, and neurologic abnormalities (Bennett, 1999; Chiriboga et al, 1999). Cocaine crosses the placenta and is found in breast milk.

Cocaine-dependent neonates do not experience the process of withdrawal seen in narcotic-exposed infants but rather suffer from neurotoxic effects of the drug. Signs of exposure have some of the same characteristics as heroin withdrawal but can be quite varied. There may be an increased risk for SIDS (Plessinger and Woods, 1998). Cocaine-exposed infants have limited ability to habituate to stimuli.

Phencyclidine ("Angel Dust")

Phencyclidine (PCP) increases the risk of injury to the pregnant woman and therefore also to her fetus. The user may be unaware that she is ingesting PCP because it often is misrepresented as another drug of abuse or is mixed with other drugs.

PCP crosses the placenta and is found in breast milk. Literature about the effects on infants is limited. Infants exposed to PCP may exhibit abnormal motor behavior such as irritability, jitteriness, and hypertonicity (D'Apolito, 1998).

Heroin

Heroin crosses the placenta and often results in IUGR. Heroin may have a direct growth-inhibiting effect on the fetus, but the exact mechanisms of growth inhibition are not clear. There is an increased rate of stillbirths but not of congenital anomalies.

Many of the medical complications attributed to heroin ingestion result from prematurity. Other risks include physical dependence in the fetus and the risk of exposure to infections, including hepatitis B and C virus and HIV.

Drug withdrawal in the mother is accompanied by fetal withdrawal, which can lead to fetal death (Kaltenbach, Berghella, and Finnegan, 1998; Wagner et al, 1998). Maternal detoxification in the first trimester carries an increased risk of miscarriage. Detoxification is not recommended after the thirty-second week because of possible withdrawal-induced fetal distress (Kaltenbach, Berghella, and Finnegan, 1998).

Heroin withdrawal occurs in 50% to 80% of infants born to addicted mothers, usually within the first 24 to 72 hours of life (Wagner et al, 1998). The signs depend on the length of maternal addiction, the amount of drug taken, and the time of injection before birth. The infant whose mother is taking methadone may not demonstrate signs of withdrawal until a week or so after birth. The symptoms of infants whose mothers used heroin or methadone are similar. Initially the infant may be depressed. The withdrawal syndrome may manifest as a combination of any of the following signs. The infants may be jittery and hyperactive. Usually the infant's cry is shrill and persistent. The infant may yawn or sneeze frequently. The tendon reflexes are increased, but the Moro reflex is decreased. The neonate may exhibit poor feeding and sucking, tachypnea, vomiting, diarrhea, hypothermia or hyperthermia, and sweating. In addition, an abnormal sleep cycle, with absence of quiet sleep and disturbance of active sleep, has been described in these infants (Fanaroff and Martin, 1997). The risk of SIDS is 5 to 10 times higher for infants with significant withdrawal problems than for infants in the general population.

If withdrawal is not treated, vomiting, diarrhea, dehydration, apnea, and convulsions may develop. Death may follow. Therapy is individualized. Dehydration and electrolyte imbalance are prevented or treated. Usually the following drugs are ordered, singly or in combination: phenobarbital, paregoric (compound tincture of opium), or diazepam.

NURSE ALERT • The use of naloxone (Narcan) is contraindicated in infants born to narcotic addicts because it may cause severe signs of narcotic abstinence syndrome and seizures.

Methadone

Methadone, a synthetic opiate, has been the therapy of choice for heroin addiction since 1965. Methadone crosses the placenta. An increasing number of infants have been born to methadone-maintained mothers, who seem to have better prenatal care and a somewhat better lifestyle than those taking heroin (Fanaroff and Martin, 1997).

Some question exists concerning the benefits of methadone therapy during pregnancy because of its effect on the fetus. Methadone withdrawal resembles heroin withdrawal but tends to be more severe and prolonged. In addition, the incidence of seizures is higher. Seizures usually occur between days 7 and 10. These infants exhibit a disturbed sleep pattern similar to that seen in heroin withdrawal. They have a higher birth weight than those infants in heroin withdrawal, usually AGA. No increased incidence of congenital anomalies is seen.

Late-onset withdrawal occurs at age 2 to 4 weeks and may continue for weeks or months. A higher incidence of SIDS also has been reported in these infants (Wagner et al, 1998). This factor is important for perinatal nurses who coordinate follow-up care for the infant and education for the mother or other caregiver. Community health nurses must know about the potential for withdrawal symptoms to occur.

Therapy for methadone withdrawal is similar to that for heroin withdrawal. The few available follow-up studies of these infants reveal a high incidence of hyperactivity, learning and behavior disorders, and poor social adjustment (Fanaroff and Martin, 1997).

Miscellaneous Substances

Methamphetamines. The fetal and neonatal effects of maternal use of methamphetamines in pregnancy are not well known. The effects appear to be dose related. LBW, preterm birth, and perinatal mortality may be consequences of higher doses used throughout pregnancy. A higher incidence of cleft lip and palate and cardiac defects has been reported in infants exposed to amphetamines in utero (Plessinger, 1998). Following birth, infants may experience bradycardia or tachycardia that resolves as the drug is cleared from the infants' system. Lethargy may continue for several months, along with frequent infections and poor weight gain. Emotional disturbances and delays in gross and fine motor coordination may be seen during early childhood.

Phenobarbital. Phenobarbital crosses the placenta readily and is subsequently found in high levels in the fetal liver and brain. Because of its slow metabolic rate, withdrawal onset is generally 2 to 14 days after birth and duration is about 2 to 4 months. Irritability, crying, hiccups, and sleepiness mark the initial response. During the second stage the infant is extremely hungry, regurgitates and gags frequently, and demonstrates episodic irritability, sweating, and a disturbed sleep pattern.

Treatment consists of swaddling, frequent feedings, and protection from noxious external stimuli. If no improvement occurs, the neonate should be given phenobarbital and then slowly withdrawn from this drug after control of symptoms (Fanaroff and Martin, 1997).

Caffeine. Caffeine has not been implicated as a teratogen in humans. Fernandes and colleagues (1998) reported that caffeine consumption greater than 150 mg per day was associated with IUGR and LBW. Santos and co-workers (1998) reported no adverse effects in the fetus with consumption of less than 300 mg of caffeine a day.

Care Management

➤ Assessment

Assessment of the newborn requires a review of the mother's prenatal record. A medical and social history of drug abuse and detoxification is noted. The infant may have IUGR or be preterm with LBW.

The woman who is addicted to narcotics may have infections that compound the risk to the infant, including hepatitis; septicemia; and STIs, including AIDS (Wagner et al, 1998).

The nurse often is the first to observe the signs of drug dependence in the infant. The nurse's observations help the physician differentiate between drug dependence and other conditions, such as tracheoesophageal fistula, CNS disorder, sepsis, hypoglycemia, and electrolyte imbalance.

The infant is assessed by means of the guidelines discussed in Chapter 25. The infant's gestational age and maturity are noted. In utero exposure to some drugs results in observable malformations or dysmorphism (abnormality of shape). Neonatal behavior may arouse suspicion. Neonatal abstinence syndrome is the term given to the group of signs and symptoms associated with drug withdrawal in the neonate (Table 28-7). Fig. 28-12 provides an example of a scoring system for assessing withdrawal symptoms. Because many women are multidrug users, the newborn initially may exhibit a confusing complex of signs.

Urine or meconium screening may be used to identify substances abused by the mother. Although initially costly and of limited availability, tests of meconium collected on the first or

TABLE 28-7
Signs of Neonatal Abstinence Syndrome

System	Signs
Gastrointestinal	Poor feeding, vomiting, regurgitation, diarrhea, excessive sucking
Central nervous	Irritability, tremors, shrill cry, incessant crying, hyperactivity, little sleep, excoriations on knees and face, convulsions
Metabolic, vasomotor, respiratory	Nasal congestion, tachypnea, sweating, frequent yawning, increased respiratory rate >60/min, fever >37.2° C

NEONATAL ABSTINENCE SCORING SYSTEM

SYSTEM	SIGNS AND SYMPTOMS	SCORE	AM	PM	COMMENTS
CENTRAL NERVOUS SYSTEM DISTURBANCES	Excessive High Pitched (Or Other)Cry Continuous High Pitched (Or Other)Cry	2 3			Daily Weight:
	Sleeps <1 Hour After Feeding Sleeps <2 Hours After Feeding Sleeps <3 Hours After Feeding	3 2 1			
	Hyperactive Moro Reflex Markedly Hyperactive Moro Reflex	2 3			
	Mild Tremors Disturbed Moderate-Severe Tremors Disturbed	1 2			
	Mild Tremors Undisturbed Moderate-Severe Tremors Undisturbed	3 4			
	Increased Muscle Tone	2			
	Excoriation (Specific Area)	1			
	Myoclonic Jerks	3			
	Generalized Convulsions	5			
METABOLIC/VASOMOTOR/RESPIRATORY DISTURBANCES	Sweating	1			
	Fever <101° (99-100.8° F./37.2-38.2° C.) Fever >101° (38.4° C. and Higher)	1 2			
	Frequent Yawning (>3 or 4 Times/Interval)	1			
	Mottling	1			
	Nasal Stuffiness	1			
	Sneezing (>3 or 4 Times/Interval)	1			
	Nasal Flaring	2			
	Respiratory Rate >60/min Respiratory Rate >60/min with Retractions	1 2			
GASTROINTESTINAL DISTURBANCES	Excessive Sucking	1			
	Poor Feeding	2			
	Regurgitation Projectile Vomiting	2 3			
	Loose Stools Watery Stools	2 3			
	TOTAL SCORE				
	INITIALS OF SCORER				

FIG. 28-12 • Neonatal Abstinence Scoring (NAS) system, developed by L. Finnegan. (From Nelson N: *Current therapy in neonatal-perinatal medicine*, ed 2, St Louis, 1990, Mosby.)

second day of life have been shown to be both sensitive and reliable in detecting the metabolites of several street drugs, including cocaine (Buchi, 1998; Kwong and Shearer, 1998).

➤ Nursing Diagnoses

Nursing diagnoses, which depend on the assessment findings, are tailored to the individual needs of the neonate and the family. Following are examples of nursing diagnoses:

Neonate

- Risk for infection related to:
  —Maternal risk behaviors
  —PROM
- Altered growth and development related to:
  —Effects of maternal substance abuse
- Sleep pattern disturbance related to:
  —Drug withdrawal
- Disorganized infant behavior related to:
  —Effects of maternal substance abuse

Parents

- Altered parenting related to:
  —Continuation of substance abuse or detoxification program
  —Guilt about infant's condition
  —Inability to cope with care needs of a special infant
- Anxiety related to knowledge deficit regarding:
  —Care needs of an affected infant
- Violence: self-directed or directed toward infant related to:
  —Drug-dependent lifestyle

➤ Plan of Care and Implementation

Planning for care of the infant born to a substance-abusing mother presents a challenge to the health care team. Parents are included in the planning for the newborn's care and are also encouraged to plan for their own care. A multidisciplinary approach is needed that includes home health or community resource personnel (e.g., regulatory agencies such as child protective services).

Education and social support to prevent the abuse of drugs provide the ideal approach. However, given the scope of the drug abuse problem, total prevention is unrealistic.

Nursing care of the drug-dependent neonate involves supportive therapy for fluid and electrolyte balance, nutrition, infection control, and respiratory care. Swaddling, holding, reducing stimuli, and feeding as necessary may be helpful in easing withdrawal (Nursing Care Plan). Specific suggestions for providing care to infants experiencing withdrawal are listed in the Patient Teaching box.

Pharmacologic treatment is usually based on the severity of withdrawal symptoms, as determined by an assessment tool (see Fig. 28-12). When indicated, medications are given as ordered. Neonatal morphine solution or phenobarbital, and occasionally paregoric, may be given until symptoms are under control. Dosing may be determined according to the abstinence score (Schechner, 1998). The dose is reduced over approximately 2 weeks, at the end of which time treatment is discontinued.

Drug dependence in the neonate is physiologic, not psychologic. Thus a predisposition to dependence later in life is not believed to be a factor. However, the psychosocial environment in which the infant may be raised can create a tendency to addiction.

Patient Teaching

CARE OF THE INFANT EXPERIENCING WITHDRAWAL

- **Place the infant in a side-lying position with the spine and legs flexed.**
- **Position the infant's hands in midline with the arms at the side**
- **Carry the infant in a flexed position.**
- **When interacting with the infant, introduce one stimulus at a time when the infant is in a quiet, alert state. Watch for time-out or distress signals (e.g., gaze aversion, yawning, sneezing, hiccups, arching, mottled color).**
- **When the infant is distressed, swaddle in a flexed position and rock in a slow, rhythmic fashion.**
- **Put the infant in a sitting position with chin tucked down for feeding.**

The issue of breastfeeding in this population is difficult. Although breast milk remains the optimum source of nutrition for these infants, care must be taken to avoid exposing the infant to additional drugs through the breast milk. The American Academy of Pediatrics (1994) published a list of drugs of abuse contraindicated in breastfeeding (Table 28-8).

HEMOLYTIC DISORDERS

Hyperbilirubinemia

Hyperbilirubinemia is a condition in which the bilirubin level in the blood is increased. It is characterized by a yellow discoloration of the skin, mucous membranes, sclera, and various organs. This yellow discoloration is referred to as jaundice or icterus. Jaundice is caused primarily by the accumulation in the skin of unconjugated bilirubin, a breakdown product of hemoglobin forming after its release from hemolyzed RBCs. Physiologic jaundice, discussed in Chapter 24, is the most common variation in newborns and is usually benign. The challenge in the care of neonates with hyperbilirubinemia is to distinguish physiologic jaundice from a serious clinical pathologic condition.

Physiologic Jaundice. Physiologic jaundice occurs in about half of all healthy full-term newborns and typically arises more than 24 hours after birth. Physiologic jaundice is more common and typically more severe in preterm infants, in whom the serum bilirubin level typically reaches a mean peak of 10 to 12 mg/dl by the fifth day of life.

Pathologic Jaundice. Pathologic jaundice, or hyperbilirubinemia, is that level of serum bilirubin which, if left untreated, can result in kernicterus, or the deposition of bilirubin in the brain and in other body cells. Following are findings that support a diagnosis of pathologic jaundice and that, if encountered in an infant, warrant further investigation (Fanaroff and Martin, 1997):

- Serum bilirubin concentrations of greater than 4 mg/dl in cord blood
- Clinical jaundice evident within 24 hours of birth
- Total serum bilirubin levels increasing by more than 5 mg/dl in 24 hours or increasing at a rate of 0.5 mg/dl or greater over a 4- to 8-hour period
- A serum bilirubin level in a full-term newborn that exceeds 15 mg/dl at any time, or clinical jaundice lasting more than 10 days

Nursing Care Plan — THE INFANT UNDERGOING DRUG WITHDRAWAL

NURSING DIAGNOSIS Risk for injury related to hyperactivity, seizures secondary to passive narcotic addiction resulting from maternal substance abuse during pregnancy

EXPECTED OUTCOME Infant exhibits no signs of seizure activity.

Nursing Interventions/*Rationales*

Administer phenobarbital, diazepam per physician order *to decrease CNS irritability and control seizure activity.*

Decrease environmental stimuli *that may trigger irritability and hyperactive behaviors.*

Plan care activities carefully *to allow for minimum stimulation.*

Wrap infant snugly and hold infant tightly *to reduce self-stimulation behaviors and protect skin from abrasions.*

If infant is cocaine addicted, position to avoid eye contact, swaddle infant, use vertical rocking techniques, and use a pacifier *to counter poor organizational response to stimuli and depressed interactive behaviors.*

Monitor activity level, note the relationship between activity level and external stimulation, and stop external stimulation *if it causes activity increase.*

NURSING DIAGNOSIS Altered nutrition, less than body requirements related to CNS irritability, poor suck reflex, vomiting, and diarrhea

EXPECTED OUTCOME Infant exhibits ingestion and retention of adequate nutrients and appropriate weight gain.

Nursing Interventions/*Rationales*

Feed in frequent small amounts, elevate head during and after feeding, and burp well *to diminish vomiting and aspiration.*

Experiment with various nipples *to find one most effective in compensating for poor suck reflex.*

Monitor weight daily and maintain strict intake and output *to evaluate success of feeding.*

If intake is insufficient, feed by oral gavage per physician order *to ensure ingestion of needed nutrients.*

Have suction available as required *to reduce chances of aspiration.*

NURSING DIAGNOSIS Risk for fluid volume deficit related to diarrhea and vomiting

EXPECTED OUTCOME Infant exhibits evidence of fluid homeostatsis.

Nursing Interventions/*Rationales*

Administer oral and parenteral fluids per physician order and regulate *to maintain fluid balance.*

Monitor hydration status (i.e., skin turgor, weight, mucous membranes, fontanels, urine specific gravity, electrolytes) and intake and output *to evaluate for evidence of dehydration.*

NURSING DIAGNOSIS Ineffective maternal coping, anxiety, powerlessness, related to drug use, infant distress during withdrawal, and single-parent status

EXPECTED OUTCOMES Mother will accept newborn's condition and participate in care activities, showing evidence of maternal-infant bonding process.

Nursing Interventions/*Rationales*

Explain effects of maternal drug use on newborn and the withdrawal process *to provide understanding and reality concerning effects of drug use.*

Encourage open communication (e.g., inform mother of ongoing condition, procedures, and treatment; answer questions; correct misperceptions; actively listen to her concerns) *to provide a sense of respect, provide support, and encourage a sense of control.*

Encourage mother to interact with infant and to become involved in care routines *to foster emotional connection.*

Explain how to do care procedures, how to avoid excess stimulation, and how to hold and rock infant *to enhance mother's care abilities and her sense of confidence and control.*

If the mother is addicted to cocaine, explain infant's inability to interact, gaze aversion, arching back, and lack of response to cuddling *to enhance understanding of infant behaviors.*

Make appropriate referrals to social agencies for treatment of maternal drug addiction, infant development programs, and other needed support services *to ensure adequate resources for care of self and infant.*

- A serum bilirubin level in a preterm newborn that exceeds 10 mg/dl at any time
- Any case of visible jaundice that persists for more than 10 days of life in a full-term infant or 21 days in a preterm infant, unless the infant is receiving breast milk

There are many potential causes of pathologic hyperbilirubinemia in neonates (Box 28-2). The most common are hemolytic diseases of the newborn.

Hemolytic Disease of the Newborn. Hemolytic disease occurs when the blood groups of the mother and baby are different; the most common of these are Rh factor and ABO incompatibilities. Hemolytic disorders occur when maternal antibodies are present naturally or form in response to an antigen from the fetal blood crossing the placenta and entering the maternal circulation. The maternal antibodies of the IgG class cross the placenta, causing hemol-

TABLE 28-8

Drugs of Abuse Contraindicated During Breastfeeding*

Drug	Reported Effect or Reasons for Concern
Amphetamine†	Irritability, poor sleeping pattern
Cocaine	Cocaine intoxication
Heroin	Tremors, restlessness, vomiting, poor feeding
Marijuana	Only one report in literature; no effect mentioned; at risk for inhaling smoke
Nicotine (smoking)	Shock, vomiting, diarrhea, rapid heart rate, restlessness; decreased milk production
Phencyclidine	Potent hallucinogen

Modified from American Academy of Pediatrics: The transfer of drugs and other chemicals into human milk, *Pediatrics* 93(1):137-150, 1994; also in Lawrence R: *Breastfeeding: a guide for the medical profession,* ed 5, St Louis, 1999, Mosby.

*AAP Committee on Drugs strongly believes that breastfeeding mothers should not ingest any substances listed here. Not only are they hazardous to the nursing infant, but they are also detrimental to the physical and emotional health of the mother. This list is obviously not complete; no drug of abuse should be ingested by breastfeeding mothers even though adverse reports are not in the literature.

†Drug is concentrated in human milk.

ysis of the fetal RBCs, resulting in hyperbilirubinemia and jaundice.

Rh Incompatibility. Rh incompatibility, or isoimmunization, occurs when an Rh-negative mother has an Rh-positive fetus who inherits the dominant Rh-positive gene from the father. If the mother is Rh negative, and the father is Rh positive and homozygous for the Rh factor, all the offspring will be Rh positive. If the father is heterozygous for the factor, there is a 50% chance that each infant born of the union will be Rh positive and a 50% chance that each will be Rh negative. An Rh-negative fetus is in no danger because it has the same Rh factor as the mother. An Rh-negative fetus with an Rh-positive mother is also in no danger. Only the Rh-positive offspring of an Rh-negative mother is at risk. From 10% to 15% of all Caucasian couples and about 5% of African-American couples have Rh incompatibility. Incompatibility is rare in Asian couples. The incidence of Rh sensitization and resulting hemolytic disease of the newborn have decreased dramatically since the development of Rh_o(D) immune globulin in 1968. However, hemolytic disease of the fetus or newborn resulting from isoimmunization continues to be a significant problem in the United States.

The pathogenesis of Rh incompatibility is as follows: hematopoiesis in the fetus, or the formation of blood cells, begins as early as the eighth week of gestation; in up to 40% of pregnancies, these cells pass through the placenta into the maternal circulation. When the fetus is Rh positive and the mother Rh negative, the mother forms antibodies against the fetal blood cells: first IgM antibodies that are too large to pass through the placenta; and then IgG antibodies that can cross the placenta. The process of antibody formation is called maternal sensitization. Sensitization may occur during pregnancy, birth, abortion, or amniocentesis. Usually women become sensitized in their first pregnancy with an Rh-positive fetus but do not

Box 28-2

Potential Causes of Pathologic Hyperbilirubinemia in Neonates

MATERNAL FACTORS

Rh and ABO incompatibility
Maternal infections
Maternal diabetes
Oxytocin administration during labor
Maternal ingestion of sulfonamides, diazepam, or salicylates near time of birth

FETAL/NEWBORN FACTORS

Prematurity
Hepatic cell damage by infection or drugs
Neonatal hyperthyroidism
Polycythemia
Intestinal obstruction such as meconium ileus
Pyloric stenosis
Biliary atresia
Sequestered blood (e.g., from cephalhematomas, ecchymosis or hemangiomas)
Maternal blood swallowed by neonate

produce enough antibodies to cause lysis (destruction) of the fetal blood cells. In subsequent pregnancies, antibodies form in response to repeated contact with the antigen from the fetal blood, and lysis results.

Severe Rh incompatibility results in marked fetal hemolytic anemia because the fetal erythrocytes are destroyed by maternal Rh-positive antibodies. Although the placenta usually clears the bilirubin generated by the RBC breakdown, in extreme cases fetal bilirubin levels increase. This results in fetal jaundice, also known as icterus gravis.

The fetus compensates for the anemia by producing large numbers of immature erythrocytes to replace those hemolyzed, thus the name for this condition: erythroblastosis fetalis. In hydrops fetalis, the most severe form of this disease, the fetus has marked anemia, together with cardiac decompensation, cardiomegaly, and hepatosplenomegaly. Hypoxia results from the severe anemia. In addition, because of the decreased intravascular oncotic pressure involved, fluid leaks out of the intravascular space, resulting in generalized edema as well as effusions into the peritoneal (ascites), pericardial, and pleural (hydrothorax) spaces. The placenta is often edematous, which, along with the edematous fetus, can cause the uterus to rupture.

Intrauterine or early neonatal death may occur as a result of hydrops fetalis, although intrauterine exchange transfusions and early birth of the fetus may avert this. Intrauterine transfusion involves the infusion of Rh-negative, type O blood into the umbilical vein. Such transfusions are administered as needed until birth.

ABO Incompatibility. ABO incompatibility is more common than Rh incompatibility, but causes less severe problems in the affected infant. It occurs if the fetal blood type is A, B, or AB and the maternal type is O. It occurs rarely in infants with type B blood born to mothers with type A blood. The incompatibility arises because naturally occurring anti-A and anti-B antibodies are transferred across the placenta to the fetus. Unlike the situation that pertains to Rh incompatibility, first-born infants may be affected because mothers with type O blood already have anti-A and anti-B antibodies in their blood. Such a newborn may show a weakly positive result to a direct Coombs test. The cord bilirubin level usually is less than 4 mg/dl, and any resulting hyperbilirubinemia usually can be treated with phototherapy. Exchange transfusions are required only occasionally. Although ABO incompatibility is a common cause of hyperbilirubinemia, it rarely precipitates significant anemia resulting from the hemolysis of RBCs.

Kernicterus. The goal of the care given the infant with hyperbilirubinemia is the prevention of kernicterus. Kernicterus, or bilirubin encephalopathy, is caused by the deposition of bilirubin in the brain, especially within the basal ganglia, cerebellum, and hippocampus. This deposition can occur because unconjugated bilirubin is highly lipid soluble, making it capable of crossing the blood-brain barrier if it is not bound to protein. If the concentration of unconjugated bilirubin reaches toxic levels, it results in the yellowish staining of the brain tissue and the necrosis of neurons.

Kernicterus, which can develop in newborns who show no apparent signs of clinical jaundice, is generally considered to be directly related to the total serum bilirubin level, although these levels alone do not predict the risk of brain injury. In a full-term infant, a serum bilirubin level of 25 mg/dl is considered the upper limit beyond which the risk for kernicterus increases, although the condition may occur at much lower levels in premature infants or infants with other complications. In some high risk, low-birth-weight infants, a mean peak level of unconjugated bilirubin of even 10 to 12 mg/dl may be associated with the development of kernicterus (Fanaroff and Martin, 1997). Some of the perinatal events that increase the likelihood of kernicterus developing, even at these lower bilirubin levels, include hypoxia, asphyxia, acidosis, hypothermia, hypoglycemia, sepsis, treatment with certain medications, and hypoalbuminemia. These conditions either interfere with the conjugation of bilirubin or compete for albumin-binding sites. The resulting unconjugated bilirubin can then pass through the blood-brain barrier and enter the brain, resulting in kernicterus.

Kernicterus has been associated with acute and long-term symptoms of neurologic damage; it is never present at birth. The clinical manifestations typically appear between 2 and 6 days after birth and go through several phases as the disease progresses, generally beginning after the bilirubin level has peaked. About half of the affected infants survive, although they often suffer permanent neurologic sequelae such as choreoathetoid cerebral palsy or ataxia, sensorineural hearing loss, perceptual problems, mental retardation, or attention deficit disorder.

There have been recent reports of several cases of kernicterus in infants of mothers who were discharged early after birth. The follow-up of infants who are discharged early is therefore imperative (Home Care box).

Care Management

At the first prenatal visit of an Rh-negative woman with a fetus who may be Rh-positive, an indirect Coombs test should be done to determine whether she has antibodies to the Rh antigen. In this test the maternal blood serum is mixed with Rh-positive RBCs. If the Rh-positive RBCs agglutinate or clump, this indicates that maternal antibodies are present. The dilution of the specimen of blood at which clumping occurs determines the titer, or level, of maternal antibodies. This titer indicates the degree of maternal sensitization. A level of 1:8 rarely results in fetal jeopardy. If the titer reaches 1:16, amniocentesis is performed to determine delta optical density (delta OD) of amniotic fluid to estimate fetal hemolytic process. Rising bilirubin levels may indicate the need for an intrauterine transfusion.

The indirect Coombs test is repeated at 28 weeks. If the result remains negative, indicating that sensitization has not occurred, the woman is given an intramuscular injection of $Rh_o(D)$ immune globulin. If the test result is positive, showing that sensitization has occurred, the test is repeated at 4 to 6 week intervals to monitor the maternal antibody titer as just described.

At birth, the neonate's cord blood is sent to the laboratory to determine the infant's blood type and Rh status. A direct Coombs test is performed on this cord blood to determine whether there are maternal antibodies in the fetal blood. If antibodies are present, the titer, which indicates the degree of maternal sensitization, is measured. If the titer is 1:64, an exchange transfusion is indicated. In addition, the prevention of or prompt therapy for perinatal asphyxia, acidosis, cold stress, sepsis, and hypoglycemia will decrease the newborn's risk for severe hemolytic disease and his or her susceptibility to kernicterus. Early feeding is also initiated to stimulate the gastrocolic reflex and thus facilitate the removal of bilirubin through stooling.

If pathologic jaundice is present, the cause is determined and therapeutic management is begun. Phototherapy is used to reduce the serum bilirubin levels, particularly if the jaundice is physiologic rather than pathologic, if the jaundice occurs past the 24-hour period after birth, and if the bilirubin levels are generally less than 15 mg/dl. Phototherapy using bililights or a phototherapy blanket is carried out in the normal newborn nursery (see Chapter 25 and Fig. 25-16).

Exchange transfusions are needed less often today because of the decrease in the incidence of hemolytic disease in newborns resulting from isoimmunization. Other factors must always be considered as well, particularly the clinical condition of the infant, because it is a procedure with many potential complications and a mortality risk of about 0.5% (Frank, Cooper, and Merenstein, 1998).

Exchange transfusion is accomplished by alternately removing a small amount of the infant's blood and replacing it with an equal amount of donor blood. If the infant has Rh incompatibility, type O Rh-negative blood is used for transfusion, so the maternal antibodies still present in the infant do not hemolyze the transfused blood. Depending on the infant's size,

Home Care

MONITORING FOR JAUNDICE AFTER EARLY DISCHARGE

If the infant is discharged from the hospital before 48 hours of age, the parents should receive teaching regarding adequate hydration and assessment of the infant for the appearance of jaundice. Appropriate testing and follow-up of the infant should be available. A program of home phototherapy, where available, allows infants to receive treatment of uncomplicated hyperbilirubinemia following discharge from the hospital. For these infants, nurses provide monitoring of treatment and of serum bilirubin levels as outlined by hospital or agency policy.

Nursing Care Plan THE INFANT WITH HYPERBILIRUBINEMIA

NURSING DIAGNOSIS Risk for injury related to hemolytic disease and treatment effects

EXPECTED OUTCOME Bilirubin levels decrease with treatment, there is no evidence of harmful effects from phototherapy (i.e., no eye irritation, dehydration, temperature instability, or skin breakdown), and there are no complications from exchange transfusions.

Nursing Interventions/*Rationales*

Initiate early feedings *to enhance excretion of bilirubin in stools.*

Observe skin and mucous membranes for signs of jaundice, *indicative of rising bilirubin-levels;* monitor serum bilirubin levels *to determine rate of rise and treatment response.*

Note time of jaundice onset *to help distinguish physiologic from other causes of jaundice.*

Observe for signs of hypoxia, hypothermia, hypoglycemia, and metabolic acidosis, *which occur as a result of hyperbilirubinemia and increase the risk of brain damage.*

Initiate phototherapy per physician order *to decrease bilirubin levels.*

During phototherapy, shield infant's eyes *to prevent damage to corneas and retinas;* keep infant nude and change positions often *for maximum body surface exposure;* cleanse skin often *to prevent irritation;* maintain adequate fluid intake *to prevent dehydration;* monitor body temperature *to prevent hyperthermia.*

Before exchange transfusion, keep infant on nothing-by-mouth (NPO) status for 2 to 4 hours *to prevent aspiration;* check donor blood for compatibility *to prevent transfusion reaction;* have resuscitation equipment (i.e., oxygen, Ambu bag, endotracheal tube, and laryngoscope) at bedside *in preparation for emergency action.*

Assist physician with exchange transfusion procedure; track amounts of blood withdrawn and transfused *to maintain balanced blood volumes;* maintain body temperature *to avoid hypothermia and cold stress;* monitor vital signs and observe for rash, *which are indicators of transfusion reaction.*

After transfusion, continue to monitor vital signs *to discover transfusion reaction or other complications;* check umbilical cord to discuss bleeding or signs of infection.

NURSING DIAGNOSIS Risk for knowledge deficit related to administration of home phototherapy

EXPECTED OUTCOME Family demonstrates ability to provide home therapy.

Nursing Interventions/*Rationales*

Explore family's willingness to try home phototherapy *to evaluate feasibility of home therapy option.*

Explore family's understanding of jaundice and proposed therapy *to establish baseline for teaching.*

Teach family with demonstration–return demonstration, allowing for several practice sessions, and supplement with written materials with pictorial representations *to ensure safe and optimum results.*

Include the following in your instructions: placement of lamp or fiberoptic unit; proper eye care and patching; proper skin care; proper positioning under lamp; provision of increased fluid intake; monitoring of time under lamp; monitoring of vital signs, skin, eyes, feeding patterns, stooling and voiding patterns; observation *to prevent complications.*

Stress importance of obtaining the prescribed bilirubin tests on schedule *to track success of therapy.*

Give parents contact if they have any questions while carrying out therapy *to offer ongoing support and increase parent comfort.*

maturity, and condition, amounts of 5 to 20 ml of the infant's blood are removed at one time and replaced with donor blood. The total amount of blood exchanged approximates 170 ml/kg of body weight, or 75% to 85% of the infant's total blood volume. Preservatives in donor blood that lower the infant's serum calcium level may trigger symptoms of hypocalcemia, such as jitteriness, irritability, convulsions, tachycardia, and electrocardiogram changes. This may necessitate an infusion of calcium gluconate to correct the deficit (Nursing Care Plan).

CONGENITAL ANOMALIES

Congenital defects occur in 2% to 3% of all live births (Steele, 1997), but this number increases to about 6% by 5 years, when more anomalies are diagnosed. In addition, the incidence of congenital malformations in fetuses that are aborted is higher than that in infants who are born alive, thus also adding to the overall incidence. Major congenital defects are the leading cause of death in infants younger than 1 year of age in the United States and account for 20% of neonatal deaths. Although there has been a decrease in the incidences of other causes of neonatal mortality, the death rate associated with most congenital anomalies has essentially remained stable since 1932.

The most common major congenital anomalies that cause serious problems in the neonate are congenital heart disease, neural tube defects, cleft lip or palate, clubfoot, and congenital hip dysplasia. These are thought to result from the interaction of multiple genetic and environmental factors. Some of the most common malformations include lack of a helical fold of the pinna, complete or incomplete simian creases, and a capillary hemangioma other than on the face or posterior aspect of the neck.

Ways of preventing and detecting these anomalies are being improved continuously, as are techniques for the care of the fetus with certain anomalies. Promoting the availability of these services to populations at risk challenges community health care systems. An interdisciplinary team approach is vital for providing holistic care: the surgical treatment, rehabilitation, and education of the child, as well as psychosocial and financial assistance for the parents. Parental disappointment and disillusion add to the complexity of the nursing care needed for these infants.

Central Nervous System Anomalies

Most congenital anomalies of the CNS result from defects in the closure of the neural tube during fetal development. Although the cause of neural tube defects is unknown, they are thought to stem from the interaction of many genes that may be influenced by factors in the fetal environment. Environmental influences such as treatment with valproic acid (an anticonvulsant), methotrexate (a chemotherapeutic agent), and alcohol consumption have been implicated. Maternal folic acid deficit has a direct bearing on failure of the neural tube to close; therefore folic acid supplementation is recommended for women of childbearing age. Although a neural tube defect is usually an isolated defect, it can occur with some chromosomal abnormalities and syndromes and also with other defects such as cleft palate, ventricular septal defect, tracheoesophageal fistula, diaphragmatic hernia, imperforate anus, and renal anomalies. Some neural tube defects can be diagnosed prenatally by ultrasound studies and the finding of elevated levels of alphafetoprotein in the amniotic fluid and maternal serum.

Encephalocele and Anencephaly. Encephalocele and anencephaly are abnormalities resulting from failure of the anterior end of the neural tube to close. An encephalocele is a herniation of the brain and meninges through a skull defect. Treatment consists of surgical repair and shunting to relieve hydrocephalus, unless a major brain malformation is present. Some of these infants will have some degree of cognitive deficit. Anencephaly is the absence of both cerebral hemispheres and of the overlying skull. It is a condition that is incompatible with life; many of the infants are stillborn or die within a few days of birth. Comfort measures are provided until the infant eventually dies of respiratory failure.

Spina Bifida. Spina bifida, the most common defect of the CNS, results from failure of the neural tube to close at some point. There are two categories of spina bifida: spina bifida occulta and spina bifida cystica. Spina bifida occulta is a malformation in which the posterior portion of the laminas fails to close but the spinal cord or meninges do not herniate or protrude through the defect (Fig. 28-13, *B*). It is usually asymptomatic and may not be diagnosed unless there are associated problems. Spina bifida cystica includes meningocele and myelomeningocele. A meningocele is an external sac that contains meninges and CSF and that protrudes through a defect in the vertebral column. A myelomeningocele is similar, except that it also contains nerves; therefore the infant has motor and sensory deficits below the lesion. In the United States, myelomeningocele occurs in approximately 1 in 1000 live births (Ball and Bindler, 1999).

A myelomeningocele is visible at birth, most often in the lumbosacral area. It is usually covered with a very fragile, thin membrane (Fig. 28-13, *A*). The sac can tear easily, allowing CSF to leak out and providing an entry for infectious agents into the CNS. Myelomeningocele usually is associated with an Arnold-Chiari malformation, which results from the improper development and downward displacement of part of the brain into the cervical spinal canal. This in turn results in the development of hydrocephalus, which affects about 90% of children with myelomeningocele, although it may not be present at birth. The long-term prognosis in an affected infant can be determined to a large extent at birth, with the degree of neurologic dysfunction related to the level of the lesion, which determines the nerves involved. Many physicians recommend that treatment be instituted regardless of the level of the lesion unless there is a severe CNS anomaly, advanced hydrocephalus at birth, severe anoxic brain damage, active CNS infection, or a malformation or syndrome incompatible with long-term survival. Prenatal diagnosis makes possible a scheduled cesarean birth allowing for more careful delivery of the infant's back to try to prevent rupture of the meningeal sac.

A major preoperative nursing intervention for a neonate with a myelomeningocele is to protect the protruding sac from injury, rupture, and resultant risk of CNS infection. Such infants should be positioned in a side-lying or prone position to prevent pressure on the sac until surgical repair is done. If the infant is able to be held, the nurse or parent must be careful to

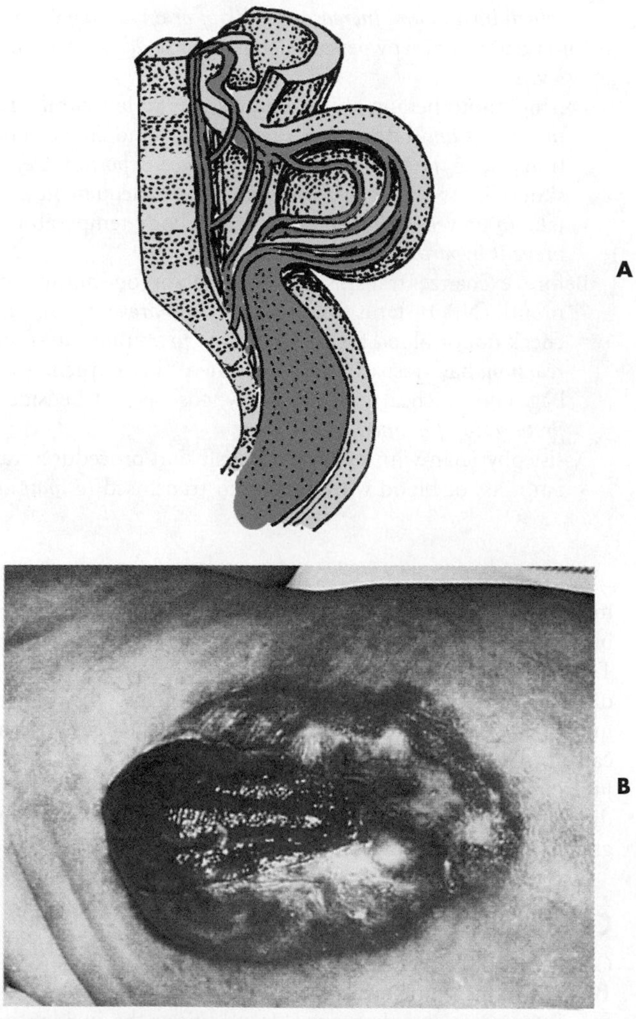

FIG. 28-13 • **A,** Myelomeningocele. Note absence of vertebral arches. **B,** Myelomeningocele (spina bifida). (From Zitelli B, Davis H: *Atlas of pediatric physical diagnosis,* ed 3, St Louis, 1997, Mosby.)

keep the defect from being injured. The sac should be covered with a sterile, moist, nonadherent dressing and be cared for using sterile technique. The skin around the defect must be cleansed and dried carefully to prevent breakdown, which would establish a portal of entry for infectious agents. Because a lack of normal innervation may prevent the bladder from emptying completely, the nurse should use Credé's method at regular intervals to express urine from the bladder.

A major nursing intervention is providing support and needed information to parents as they begin to learn to cope with an infant who has immediate needs for intensive care and who probably will have long-term needs as well. Surgical repair is often done in the neonatal period, preferably within the first 24 hours. Very early closure can prevent CNS infection and trauma to the exposed nerves. It can also prevent stretching of other nerve roots, which can occur as the sac continues to enlarge after birth. Surgical shunt procedures to prevent increasing hydrocephalus may be needed. Other problems, such as infection, are treated as they occur.

Hydrocephalus. Hydrocephalus is a condition in which the ventricles of the brain are enlarged as a result of an imbalance between the production and absorption of the CSF. Congenital hydrocephalus usually arises as a result of a malformation in the brain or an intrauterine infection. It occurs in approximately 3 to 4 per 1000 live births (Jackson and Harvey, 1996). About one third of all cases of congenital hydrocephalus result from stenosis of the aqueduct of Sylvius in the brain. Hydrocephalus often occurs in conjunction with a myelomeningocele, which blocks the flow of CSF.

An infant with congenital hydrocephalus initially has a bulging anterior fontanel and a head circumference that increases at an abnormal rate, resulting from the increase in CSF pressure (Fig. 28-14). Enlargement of the forehead with depressed eyes that are rotated downward, causing a "setting sun" sign, occurs as the condition worsens. If the surgical shunting of excess CSF from the brain is not done soon after birth, the resulting increasing ICP will lead to irreversible neurologic damage, as evidenced by palpably widening sutures and fontanels; lethargy; poor feeding; vomiting; irritability; opisthotonos; and a high-pitched, shrill cry.

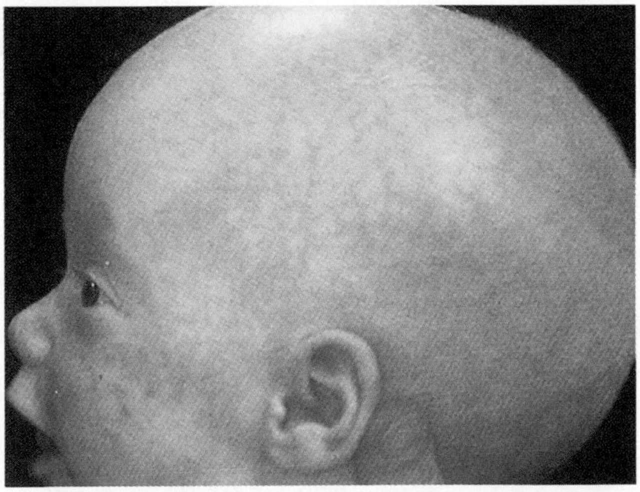

FIG. 28-14 • Infantile hydrocephalus. The characteristic appearance is an enlarged head, thinning of the scalp, distended scalp veins, and a full fontanel. (From Booth I, Wozniak E: *Pediatrics,* Baltimore, 1984, Williams & Wilkins.)

Nursing actions appropriate to the needs of a newborn with hydrocephalus include careful documentation of the ongoing observations. Measurement of the head circumference and other neurologic assessments are done frequently. If the infant's head is large, the placement of sheepskin or a flotation mattress under the infant and frequent position changes are necessary to prevent skin breakdown. Chapter 51 contains a more detailed description of the evaluation and management of the child with hydrocephalus.

Microcephaly. Microcephaly refers to a small brain in a generally normally formed head. It can be the result of an autosomal-recessive disorder; a chromosomal abnormality; exposure of the woman to x-rays; or rubella, cytomegalovirus, or other maternal infections. Microcephalic infants require supportive nursing care and medical observation to determine the extent of the psychomotor retardation that almost always accompanies this abnormality. There is no treatment. Parents need support to learn to care for a child with such cognitive impairment.

Cardiovascular System Anomalies

Congenital heart defects (CHDs) are anatomic abnormalities of the heart that are present at birth, although they may not be diagnosed immediately. Some type of pediatric cardiovascular problem is present in 10 of every 1000 live births (Daberkow-Carson and Washington, 1998). Ventricular septal defects, constituting more than 20% of all CHDs, are the most common type of acyanotic lesion. Tetralogy of Fallot, constituting 10% of all CHDs, is the most common type resulting in cyanosis. After prematurity, CHDs are the next major cause of death in the first year of life.

The etiology of CHDs is unknown in more than 90% of the cases. Maternal factors associated with a higher incidence of CHD include maternal rubella, alcoholism, diabetes, poor nutrition, or age over 40 years. The maternal ingestion of folic acid antagonists, anticonvulsants, progesterone, estrogen, lithium, or Coumadin, or the use of the acne medication Accutane (isotretinoin), are thought to be involved in the cause of heart defects, as is radiation exposure.

Genetic factors are implicated in the pathogenesis of CHD. As a general rule, these defects are thought to be multifactorial in origin, involving both genetic and environmental influences; however, a familial occurrence of virtually all forms of CHD has been noted.

Chromosomal abnormalities may also be associated with CHDs. For example, 45% of children with trisomy 21, or Down syndrome, have a cardiac defect. All children who have trisomy 18, the second most common chromosomal abnormality, have cardiac anomalies. See Chapter 48 for a discussion of classifications of CHDs.

Severe CHDs are often evident immediately after birth, especially those defects that cause cyanosis (e.g., transposition of the great vessels). Infants with these anomalies are transferred directly to special care nurseries or pediatric units.

If symptoms are present at birth, they may be obvious with the first cry, which may be weak and muffled or loud and breathless. Affected newborns may be cyanotic and unrelieved by oxygen treatment, with the cyanosis increasing whenever the child is in the supine position or cries. The bluish gray, dusky color of cyanotic infants may be mild, moderate, or severe. Other infants may be acyanotic and pale, with or without mottling upon exertion, such as crying, feeding, or stooling.

The affected newborn's activity level varies from restlessness to lethargy and possible unresponsiveness, except to pain. Persistent bradycardia (i.e., resting heart rate of less than 80 to 100 beats/min) or tachycardia (i.e., rate exceeding 160 to 180 beats/min) may be noted (Wong, 1999). The cardiac rhythm may be abnormal, and murmurs may be heard. Signs of congestive heart failure, diminished cardiac output, and decreased tissue perfusion may be evident.

Because the cardiac and respiratory systems function together, cardiac disease may be manifested by respiratory signs and symptoms. The respiratory rate should be determined when the newborn is in a resting state. Abnormal findings may include tachypnea, which is a rate of 60 breaths/min or more; retractions with nasal flaring; grunting occurring with or without exertion; and dyspnea, which may worsen when the infant is supine or exerting itself.

A major role of the nurse is to assess infants for abnormal findings, which, if observed, must be reported immediately. Newborns exhibiting these symptoms require prompt diagnosis and appropriate therapy in a neonatal or pediatric intensive care unit. Interventions planned if a nursing diagnosis of decreased cardiac output is made include: administering oxygen as ordered; administering cardiotonic and other medications, such as diuretics, that rid the body of accumulated fluid; decreasing the work load of the heart by maintaining a thermoneutral environment; feeding using the gavage method if necessary; and preventing crying, if this precipitates cyanosis. Various diagnostic tests such as echocardiography and cardiac catheterization are performed to obtain specific information about the defect and the need for surgical intervention.

Respiratory System Anomalies

Screening for congenital anomalies of the respiratory system is necessary even in infants who are apparently normal at birth. Respiratory distress at birth or shortly thereafter may be the result of lung immaturity or anomalous development. Congenital laryngeal web and bilateral choanal atresia are readily apparent at birth. Respiratory distress caused by diaphragmatic hernia and tracheoesophageal fistula may appear immediately or be delayed, depending on the severity of the defect.

Laryngeal Web and Choanal Atresia. A laryngeal web, which is uncommon, results from the incomplete separation of the two sides of the larynx and is most often between the vocal cords. Choanal atresia (Fig. 28-15) is the most common congenital anomaly of the nose; it is a bony or membranous septum located between the nose and the pharynx. Inability to pass a suction catheter through the nose into the pharynx usually leads to its detection. Nearly half of the infants with choanal atresia have other anomalies. Infants with either a laryngeal web or choanal atresia require emergency surgery.

Diaphragmatic Hernia. Diaphragmatic hernia results from a defect in the formation of the diaphragm, allowing the abdominal organs to be displaced into the thoracic cavity. It occurs in approximately 1 in 3000 to 4000 live births (Finer et al, 1998); however, if stillbirths resulting from this defect are included, the incidence increases to 1 in 2000. Herniation of the abdominal viscera into the thoracic cavity may cause severe respiratory distress and represent a neonatal emergency (Fig. 28-16). The defect and herniation may be minimal and easily repaired,

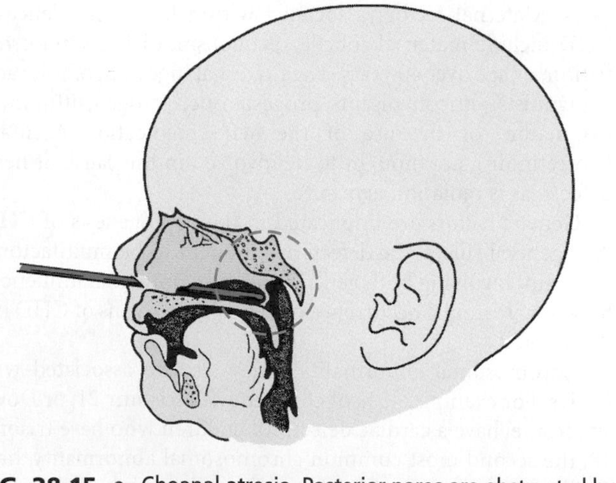

FIG. 28-15 • Choanal atresia. Posterior nares are obstructed by membrane or bone, either bilaterally or unilaterally. Infant becomes cyanotic at rest. With crying, newborn's color improves. Nasal discharge is present. Snorting respirations often are observed with increased respiratory effort. Newborn may be unable to breathe and eat at the same time. Diagnosis is made by noting inability to pass small feeding tube through one or both nares. (Used with permission of Ross Products Division, Abbott Laboratories, Inc., Columbus, OH 43216. From Clinical Education Aid No. 6, Copyright 1963, Ross Products Division, Abbott Laboratories, Inc.)

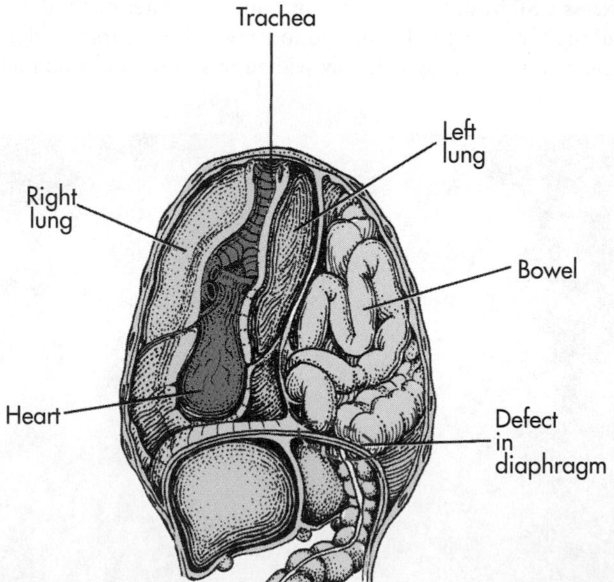

FIG. 28-16 • Diaphragmatic hernia. (Used with permission of Ross Products Division, Abbott Laboratories, Inc., Columbus, OH 43216. From Clinical Education Aid No. 6, Copyright 1963, Ross Products Division, Abbott Laboratories, Inc.)

or the defect may be so extensive that the viscera present in the thoracic cavity during embryonic life have prevented the normal development of pulmonary tissue. The defect is usually on the left because that is the side of the diaphragm that fuses last.

Most congenital diaphragmatic hernias are discovered prenatally on ultrasound studies; this may be repaired by fetal surgery in some research institutions. At birth, most affected infants have severe respiratory distress, and respiratory assessment reveals worsening distress as the bowel fills with air. Typically the breath sounds are diminished and bowel sounds are heard in the chest. Heart sounds may be heard on the right side of the chest because the heart has been displaced there by the abdominal contents. Physical examination reveals a flat or scaphoid abdomen and a prominent ipsilateral chest. Diagnosis can be made on the basis of the x-ray finding of loops of intestine in the thoracic cavity and the absence of intestine in the abdominal cavity.

Preoperative nursing interventions include participating in the stabilization of the infant's condition until surgical repair can be done. The infant should be positioned with the head and chest elevated and the affected side downward to allow the normal lung to expand. Gastric contents are aspirated and suction applied to decompress the GI tract and prevent further cardiothoracic compromise. Oxygen therapy, mechanical ventilation, and the correction of acidosis are necessary in infants with large defects. Extracorporeal membrane oxygenation (ECMO) may be used in infants with severe circulatory and respiratory complications.

The prognosis depends largely on the degree of pulmonary development and the success of diaphragmatic closure, but the prognosis in severe cases is poor. The overall survival rate for infants who are symptomatic within the first few hours of life is about 50%, although it has improved recently with the advent of ECMO.

Gastrointestinal System Anomalies

Anomalies in the gastrointestinal system can occur anywhere along the gastrointestinal tract, from the mouth to the anus. Some anomalies, such as cleft lip, omphalocele, and gastroschisis, are apparent at birth. Others, including cleft palate, esophageal atresia, pyloric stenosis, intestinal obstructions, and imperforate anus become apparent as the infant is further assessed or becomes symptomatic.

Cleft Lip and Palate. Cleft lip or palate is a commonly occurring congenital midline fissure, or opening, in the lip or palate resulting from failure of the primary palate to fuse (Fig. 28-17). One or both deformities may occur. Multiple genetic and, to a lesser extent, environmental factors (e.g., maternal infection, radiation exposure, alcohol ingestion, and treatment with medications such as corticosteroids, some tranquilizers, and anticonvulsants) appear to be involved in their development. Pathophysiology, evaluation, and treatment are addressed in Chapter 47.

Feeding is difficult because the cleft lip renders the newborn unable to maintain a seal around a nipple; the cleft palate renders the infant unable to form a vacuum to maintain suction when feeding. In addition, the inability to suck and swallow normally allows milk to pool in the nasopharynx, which increases the likelihood of aspiration. Furthermore, as the infant attempts to suck, milk often comes out through the cleft and out of the nares. Although the degree of difficulty depends on the size of the cleft, feeding problems are greater in infants with a cleft palate than in those with a cleft lip. Breastfeeding can be successful in some infants (Darzi, Chowdri, and Bhat, 1996). There are special nipples, bottles, and appliances available to aid in feeding (Fig. 28-17, *D*). In general, parents of infants with these defects need a great deal of education and support as they learn to feed their baby, to prevent what should be a normal part of infant care from becoming a very frustrating experience.

Parents of infants with a cleft lip or palate need much support, particularly in the case of a cleft lip because this is both a cosmetic and functional defect. Recognizing that this may interfere with normal parent-infant bonding in the neonatal period, the nurse must assess for this and intervene appropriately.

Esophageal Atresia and Tracheoesophageal Fistula. Esophageal atresia (EA) and tracheoesophageal fistula (TEF), the most life-threatening anomalies of the esophagus, often occur together, although they can also occur singly. EA is a congenital anomaly in which the esophagus ends in a blind pouch or narrows into a thin cord, thus failing to form a continuous passageway to the stomach (Fig. 28-18). TEF is an abnormal connection between the esophagus and trachea.

Hydramnios is a common finding in pregnancy, particularly if the fetus has an EA without TEF. Variations of the anomalies are possible, depending on the presence or absence of a TEF, the site of the fistula, and the location and degree of the esophageal obstruction.

Infants with the life-threatening anomaly EA with TEF show significant respiratory difficulty immediately after birth. EA with or without TEF results in excessive oral secretions, drooling, and feeding intolerance. When fed, the infant may swallow, but then cough and gag and return the fluid through the nose and mouth. Respiratory distress can result from aspiration or from the acute gastric distention produced by the TEF. Choking, coughing, and cyanosis occur after even a small amount of fluid is taken by mouth.

Nursing interventions are supportive until surgery is performed. Any infant with excessive oral secretions and respiratory distress should not be fed orally until further evaluation is carried out. The infant is placed in a semi-Fowler's position, which facilitates respiratory efforts and diminishes the reflux of

Family Focus

BREASTFEEDING THE INFANT WITH CLEFT LIP AND/OR CLEFT PALATE

Many health professionals assume that successful breastfeeding is impossible because of the cleft lip and/or cleft palate. On the contrary, breastfeeding is not only possible, it has several benefits, including the normal integration of the infant into the family, decreased problems with otitis media, and passive immunity to upper respiratory tract infections. In addition, breastfeeding enhances normal muscular movements of the mouth and face, and benefits normal speech development.*

If the mother intended to breastfeed before delivery, she is encouraged and helped to do so as soon as possible after birth. If available, the services of a lactation expert or of La Leche League International, Inc., should be used.

*Danner S: Breastfeeding the infant with a cleft palate, *NAACOG Clin Issues Perinat Womens Health Nurs* 3:634, 1992.

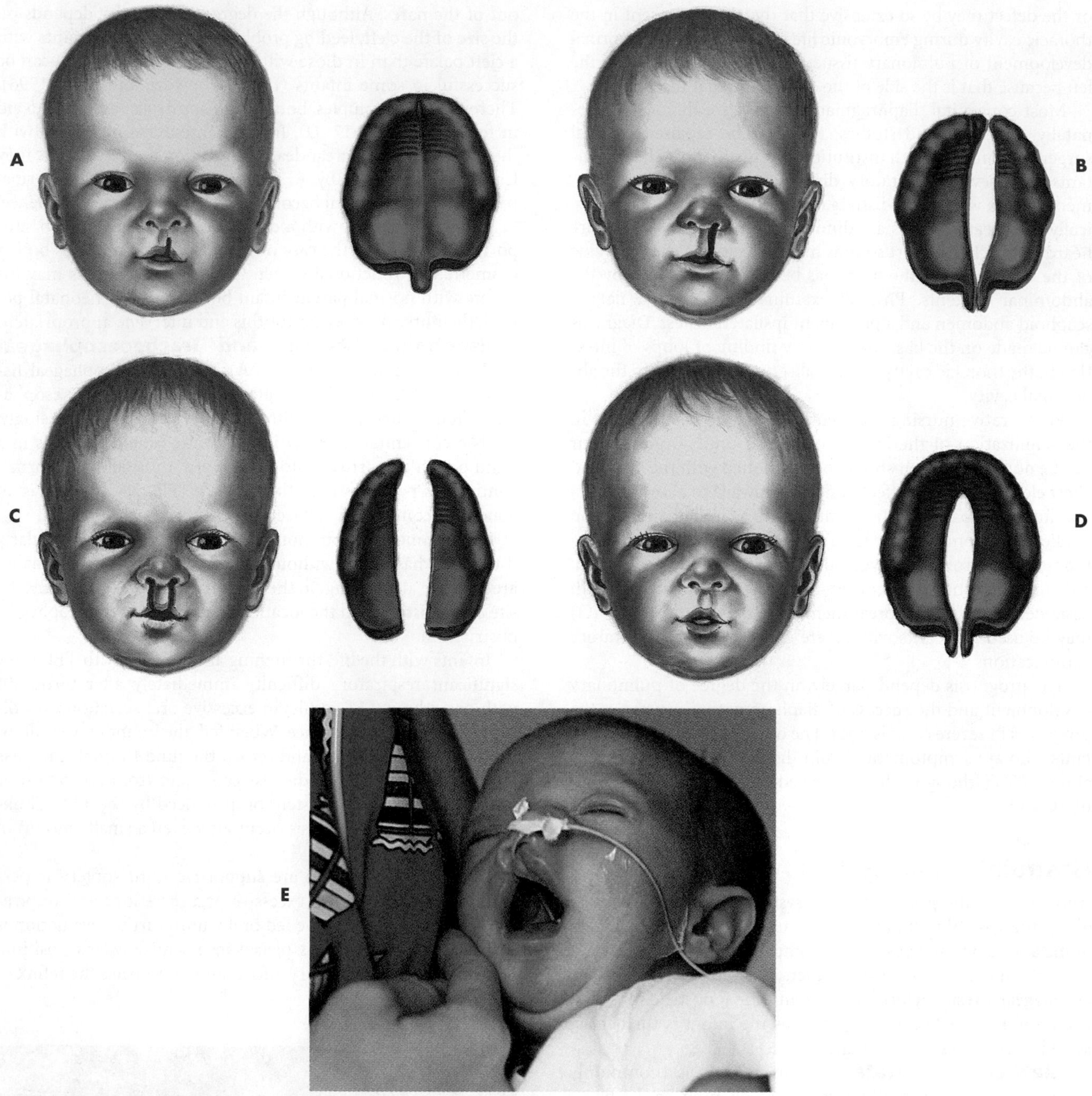

FIG. 28-17 • Variations in clefts of lip and palate at birth. **A,** Notch in vermilion border. **B,** Unilateral cleft lip and cleft palate. **C,** Bilateral cleft lip and cleft palate. **D,** Cleft palate. **E,** Infant with complete unilateral cleft lip. Note the feeding tube. (A-D, From Wong D: *Whaley & Wong's nursing care of infants and children,* ed 5, St Louis, 1995, Mosby; E, from Dickason E, Silverman B, Kaplan J: *Maternal-infant nursing care,* ed 3, St Louis, 1998, Mosby.)

gastric contents into the trachea. A double-lumen catheter is placed in the proximal esophageal pouch and attached to continuous suction to remove secretions and decrease the possibility of aspiration. Other supportive measures include maintaining fluid and electrolyte balance intravenously, and thermoregulation. Surgical correction, done in one stage if possible, consists of ligating the fistula and anastomosing the two segments of the esophagus. The chances for survival in those infants in a good-risk category exceed 95%. (See Chapter 47 for further discussion of surgical treatment and nursing care.)

Omphalocele and Gastroschisis. Omphalocele and gastroschisis are two of the more common congenital defects that occur in the abdominal wall. They are rare, however, with omphalocele occurring in approximately 1 in 5000 live births. The incidence of gastroschisis is 1 to 3 in 10,000 live births (Wong, 1999).

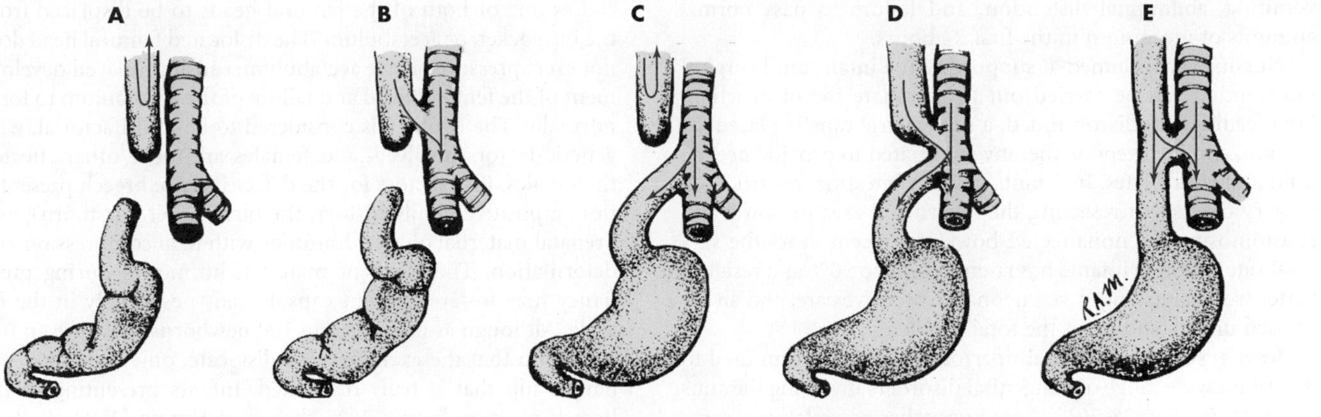

FIG. 28-18 • Congenital atresia of esophagus and tracheoesophageal fistula. A, Upper and lower segments of esophagus end in blind sac, occurring in 5% to 8% of such infants. **B,** Upper segment of esophagus ends in atresia and connects to trachea by fistulous tract, occurring rarely. **C,** Upper segment of esophagus ends in blind pouch; lower segment connects with trachea by small fistulous tract, occurring in 80% to 95% of such infants. **D,** Both segments of esophagus connect by fistulous tracts to trachea, occurring in less than 1% of such infants. Infant may aspirate with first feeding. **E,** Esophagus is continuous but connects by fistulous tact to trachea; known as *H-type.* (From Wong D: *Whaley & Wong's nursing care of infants and children,* ed 6, St Louis, 1999, Mosby.)

An omphalocele is a covered defect of the umbilical ring into which varying amounts of the abdominal organs may herniate (Fig. 28-19). Although it is covered with a peritoneal sac, the sac may rupture during or after birth. Many infants born with an omphalocele are premature, and more than half have other serious syndromes or anomalies involving the gastrointestinal, cardiac, genitourinary, musculoskeletal, and nervous systems.

Gastroschisis is the herniation of the bowel through a defect in the abdominal wall to the right of the umbilical cord. No membrane covers the contents, as occurs with an omphalocele. Unlike infants with omphalocele, these infants rarely have associated anomalies.

The preoperative nursing care is similar for infants with either defect. Exposure of the viscera causes problems with thermoregulation and fluid and electrolyte balance. Before closure is performed, the exposed viscera are covered with moistened saline gauze and plastic wrap. Antibiotics, fluid and electrolyte replacement, gastric decompression, and thermoregulation are needed for physiologic support. If complete closure is impossible because of the small size of the defect and the large amount of viscera to be replaced, a Silastic silo pouch (Dow Corning, Midland, MI) is created and sewn to the fascia of the abdominal defect. The defect is closed surgically after the reduction of contents is complete, which usually takes 7 to 10 days. Gastric decompression is necessary preoperatively to prevent aspiration pneumonia and to allow as much bowel as possible to be placed into the abdomen during surgery. Surgery is usually performed soon after birth. With surgical treatment, nutritional support, and medical management, the prognosis has improved for infants born with an abdominal wall defect. It is estimated that more than 80% of infants born with omphalocele survive, as do more than 90% of those born with gastroschisis (Wong, 1999).

Gastrointestinal Obstruction. Congenital intestinal obstruction can occur anywhere in the gastrointestinal tract and take one of the following forms: atresia, which is a complete obliteration of the passage; partial obstruction, in which the symptoms may vary in severity and sometimes not be detected in the neonatal period; or malrotation of the intestine, which leads to twisting of the intestine (volvulus) and obstruction. EA, discussed previously, is a type of gastrointestinal obstruction. Meconium ileus is an obstruction caused by impacted meconium and is the earliest symptom of cystic fibrosis, a life-threatening chronic illness. Infants with this type of obstruction should be tested for cystic fibrosis because 95% of infants with meconium ileus have cystic fibrosis.

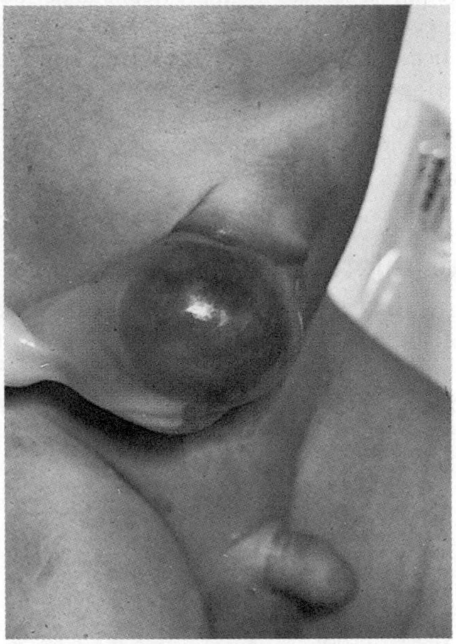

FIG. 28-19 • Omphalocele. (From O'Doherty N: *Neonatology: micro atlas of the newborn,* Nutley, NJ, 1986, Hoffmann-La Roche.)

In addition to hydramnios in the pregnant woman, the infant shows the following cardinal signs and symptoms: bilious vomiting, abdominal distention, and failure to pass normal amounts of meconium in the first 24 hours.

Nursing care is aimed at supporting the infant until surgical intervention can be carried out to eliminate the obstruction. Oral feedings are discontinued, a nasogastric tube is placed for suction, and intravenous therapy is initiated to provide needed fluid and electrolytes. In infants with an intestinal obstruction, surgery consists of resecting the obstructed area of bowel and anastomosing the nonaffected bowel. In recent years the survival rate for these infants has risen to 85% to 90% as a result of better treatments, improved neonatal intensive care, and an increased understanding of the total problem.

Imperforate Anus. Imperforate anus is a term used to describe a wide range of congenital disorders involving the anus and rectum (Fig. 28-20). These anomalies are relatively common, with an incidence of approximately 1 in 5000 live births (Holland, Price, and Bensard, 1998). Occurring more in male than in female infants, they result from the failure of anorectal development in weeks 7 and 8 of gestational life. Such infants have no anal opening, and commonly there is also a fistula from the rectum to the perineum or genitourinary system. The anomalies can be further classified according to the location of the defect into "high" or "low" types, which determine the treatments necessary as well as the prognosis. Infants with high anomalies require a colostomy in the neonatal period, with corrective surgery done in stages over time. Low anomalies may involve stenotic areas, or there may be a thin translucent membrane covering the anal opening. Treatment for such a membrane is excision followed by daily dilation, which parents are taught to do. See Chapter 47 for further discussion of surgical treatment.

Musculoskeletal System Anomalies

Developmental Dysplasia of the Hip. Developmental dysplasia of the hip (DDH) consists of disorders that result from the abnormal development of one or all of the components of the hip joint, resulting in instability of the hip. This causes one or both of the femoral heads to be displaced from the hip socket, or acetabulum. The dislocated femoral head does not exert pressure on the acetabulum, causing delayed development of the femoral head and failure of the acetabulum to form normally. The etiology is considered to be multifactorial, with genetic factors involved, and females are more often affected than males. Risk factors for the defect include breech presentation, a positive family history, the birth order (firstborn), and prenatal maternal oligohydramnios with fetal compression and deformation. The effect of maternal hormones during pregnancy may foster hip joint capsule laxity, especially in the female. Although as many as 1 in 100 newborns will have an unstable hip that the examiner can dislocate, only 1 in 1000 will have a hip that is truly dislocated. Infants presenting in the breech position have a 20% chance of having DDH (Ballock and Richards, 1997; Novacheck, 1996).

The examiner tests for an unstable or actually dislocated femoral head by abducting the hips and feeling for a click when the femoral head passes back into the acetabulum (see Fig. 24-11). Other diagnostic clues include an asymmetric number of skinfolds, one knee higher than the other when the hips and knees are flexed to 90 degrees, and limited hip abduction (Fig. 28-21).

Early detection, often by the nurse during a routine newborn assessment, allows for early treatment, which is more effective than later treatment and can prevent complications. Treatment involves the use of a Pavlik harness, a device that keeps the hips and knees flexed, the hips abducted, and the femoral head in the acetabulum (Fig. 28-22). Worn continuously for 3 to 6 months, it promotes the development of muscle and cartilage, resulting in a stable hip. Although the harness is effective up to 90% of the time, traction, casting, and even surgery may be necessary to stabilize the hip. See Chapter 54 for more detailed discussion of developmental dysplasia of the hip.

Clubfoot. Clubfoot is a congenital deformity in which portions of the foot and ankle are twisted out of normal position. There are varying degrees of severity and various combinations of abnormal positions. The most common, seen in

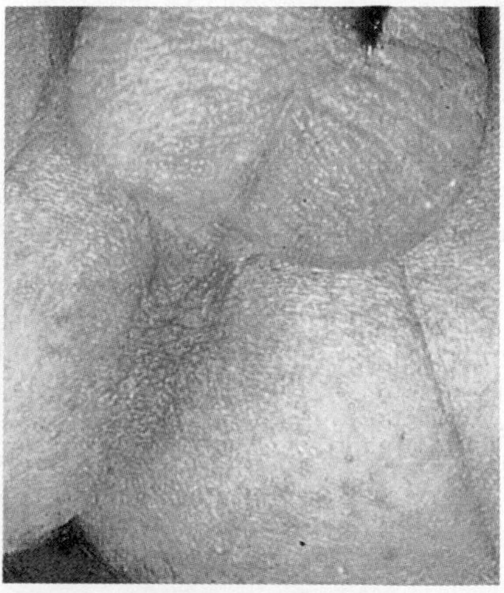

FIG. 28-20 • Imperforate anus. (From Chessell G et al: *Diagnostic picture tests in clinical medicine* (vol. 2), St Louis, 1984, Mosby.)

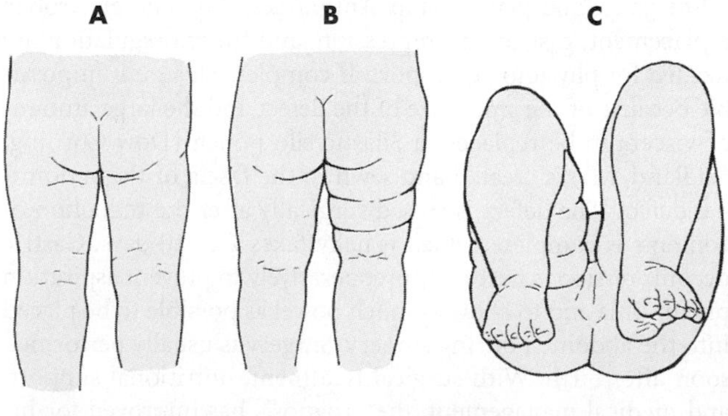

FIG. 28-21 • Congenital dysplasia of hip. **A,** Normal gluteal and popliteal skin creases. **B,** Abnormal skin creases and asymmetry of skinfolds. **C,** Apparent shortening of femur. Femoral head is displaced. (Used with permission of Ross Products Division, Abbott Laboratories, Inc., Columbus, OH 43216. From Clinical Education Aid No. 6, Copyright 1963, Ross Products Division, Abbott Laboratories, Inc.)

approximately 95% of infants with clubfoot, is talipes equinovarus. In this abnormality the foot points downward and inward, the ankle is inverted, and the Achilles tendon is shortened. Unless treated, further stiffening occurs, and bony changes result.

Clubfoot is one of the most common congenital anomalies, occurring in approximately 1 per 1000 live births, with 2 times more males than females affected (Grover, 1996). The condition is bilateral in approximately 50% of cases. The exact cause is unknown, but possibilities include a genetic predisposition, in utero compression, and abnormal embryonic development. Treatment begins soon after birth. This consists of manipulation and frequent serial casting, which is necessary because of the rapid growth of the infant. If this is ineffective, surgical correction is necessary.

Because these infants are often placed in a cast before they are discharged, the nurse must teach the parents the way to care for an infant in a cast, including protecting the cast and assessing the toes for neurovascular compromise. This is particularly important because growth could cause the child to outgrow the cast. See Chapter 54 for a discussion of the correction of this anomaly.

Polydactyly. Occasionally hands or feet are seen with extra digits. In some instances, polydactyly is hereditary. If there is little or no bone involvement, the extra digit is tied with silk suture soon after birth. The finger falls off within a few days, leaving a small scar. When there is bone involvement, surgical repair is indicated.

Genitourinary System Anomalies

Hypospadias and Epispadias. Hypospadias constitutes a range of penile anomalies associated with an abnormally located urinary meatus. The meatus can open below the glans penis or anywhere along the ventral surface of the penis, the scrotum, or the perineum. It is the most common anomaly of the penis, affecting approximately 1 in 250 male infants (Paulozzi, Erickson, and Jackson, 1997). It is classified according to the location of the meatus and the presence or absence of chordee, which is a ventral curvature of the penis.

Mild cases of hypospadias are often repaired for cosmetic reasons and involve a single surgical procedure. In more severe cases, several operations are required to reconstruct the urethral opening and correct the chordee, thereby straightening the penis. The goals are to improve the appearance of the genitalia and make it possible for the child to be able to urinate in a standing position and have a sexually adequate organ. These infants are not circumcised because the foreskin may be needed during surgical repair. Repair is done early, often during or soon after the first year of life.

Epispadias, a rare anomaly, results from failure of urethral canalization. About 55% of the affected infants are males who have a widened pubic symphysis and a broad spadelike penis with the urethra opened on its dorsal surface (Bellinger, 1997). In females there is a wide urethra and a bifid clitoris. Severity ranges from mild anomaly to a severe one that is associated with exstrophy of the bladder. Surgical correction is necessary, and affected male infants should not be circumcised.

Exstrophy of the Bladder. The most common bladder anomaly is exstrophy (Fig. 28-23), which often occurs in conjunction with epispadias. It is rare, occurring only in about 1 in 40,000 live births (Bellinger, 1997). It results from the abnormal development of the bladder, abdominal wall, and the symphysis pubis that causes the bladder, urethra, and ureteral orifices to all be exposed. The bladder is visible in the suprapubic area as a red mass with numerous folds, with urine draining from it onto the infant's skin.

Immediately after birth the exposed bladder is covered with a sterile, nonadherent dressing to protect it until closure can be performed. It is recommended that reconstructive surgery be started in the neonatal period, preferably with the bladder being closed during the first or second day of life.

Sexual Ambiguity. Sexual ambiguity in the newborn (Fig. 28-24) often is discovered by the nurse during a physical assessment. Erroneous or abnormal sexual differentiation may be a genetic aberration, such as congenital adrenal hypoplasia, which can be life-threatening because it involves deficiency of all adrenocortical hormones. Other possible causes of sexual ambiguity include chromosomal abnormalities, defective sex

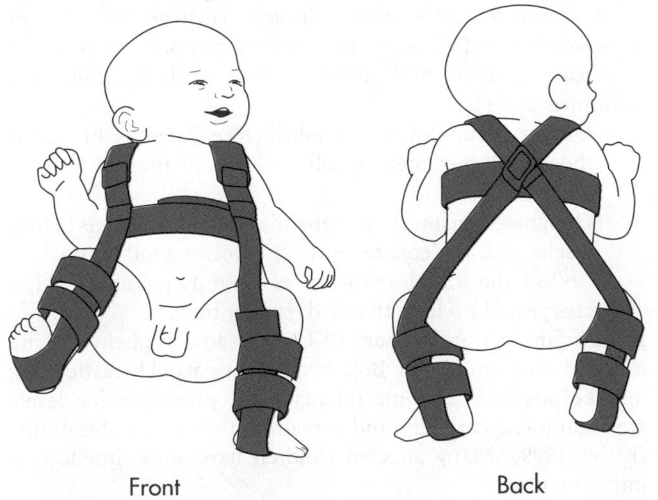

FIG. 28-22 • Treatment for congenital hip dislocation by application of the Pavlik harness. (From Ball J: *Mosby's pediatric patient teaching guides,* St Louis, 1998, Mosby.)

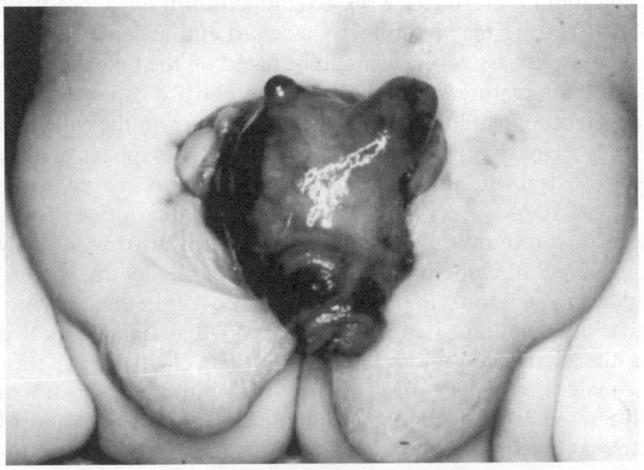

FIG. 28-23 • Exstrophy of bladder. (Courtesy Edward S. Tank, MD, Division of Urology, Oregon Health Sciences University, Portland, OR.)

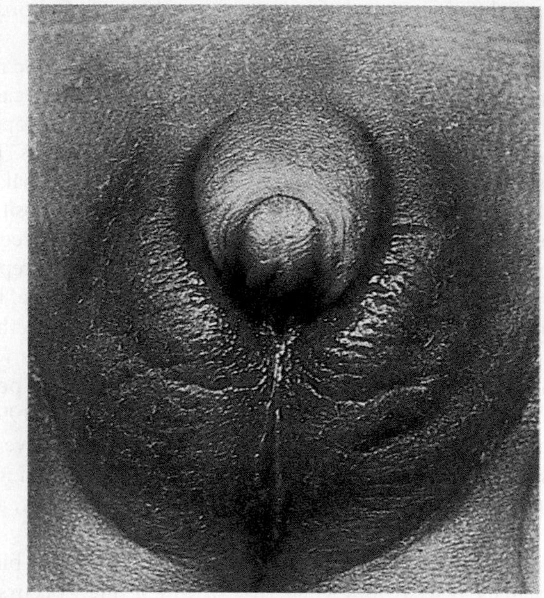

FIG. 28-24 • Ambiguous external genitalia (i.e., structure can be enlarged clitoral hood and clitoris or malformed penis). (Courtesy Edward S. Tank, MD, Division of Urology, Oregon Health Sciences University, Portland, OR.)

hormone synthesis in males, and the placental transfer of masculinizing agents to female fetuses. Gender assignment should be based on data gathered from the following sources: maternal and family history, including the ingestion of steroids during pregnancy and relatives with ambiguous genitalia or who died during the neonatal period; physical examination; chromosomal analysis (results are available in 2 to 3 days); endoscopy, ultrasonography, and radiographic contrast studies; biochemical tests, such as analysis of urinary steroid excretion, which helps detect several of the adrenal cortical syndromes; and, in some instances, laparotomy or gonad biopsy.

Therapeutic intervention, including any surgery, should be started as soon as possible. Any child born with ambiguous genitalia should not receive a sex assignment until the appropriate sex of rearing may be properly assessed and assigned. An appropriate sex assignment should be based on the following: potential for mature sexual function, potential fertility, and the long-term psychologic and intellectual impact on the child and family (Finegold, 1997). Parents need much support as they learn to deal with this very challenging situation.

Teratoma. A teratoma is an embryonal tumor that may be solid, cystic, or mixed. It is composed of at least two and usually three types of embryonal tissue: ectoderm, mesoderm, and endoderm. A teratoma in the newborn may occur in the skull, mediastinum, abdomen, or sacral area; more than half are located in the sacrococcygeal area. The treatment of choice for such neonates is complete surgical resection. Approximately 80% of all teratomas are benign, and no additional therapy is needed after complete resection done in the neonatal period. If the tumor is not surgically resected before the infant is 1 to 2 months old, the likelihood of the teratoma becoming malignant increases rapidly.

Care Management

Apgar scoring and a brief assessment are completed for all neonates after birth. Any deviations from normal are reported to the physician or nurse-midwife immediately. A thorough assessment of all body systems follows, with identification of both visible anomalies and those that might not be visible.

Some infants have multiple congenital anomalies. A recognized pattern of malformations is referred to as a syndrome. The most common is Down syndrome, with the diagnosis confirmed early in the neonatal period.

Genetic Diagnosis. Diagnostic procedures for the detection of genetic disorders are performed after birth at any time from the postnatal period through adulthood. There are many tests for various disorders; only the most commonly used ones are discussed here.

Biochemical Tests. The most widespread use of postnatal testing for genetic disease is the routine screening of newborns for inborn errors of metabolism such as phenylketonuria (PKU), galactosemia, and hypothyroidism; this is mandatory in most states in the United States. An inborn error of metabolism is the term applied to a large group of disorders caused by a metabolic defect that results from the absence of or change in a protein, usually an enzyme, and mediated by the action of a certain gene. These defects can involve any substrate produced from protein, carbohydrate, or fat metabolism. Inborn errors of metabolism are recessive disorders, and a person must receive a defective gene from each parent for them to occur. The parents usually are unaffected because their normal dominant gene directs the synthesis of sufficient protein to meet their metabolic needs under normal circumstances. With the advent of new biochemical techniques, it is now possible to detect the abnormal gene responsible for causing an increasing number of these disorders.

PKU results from a deficiency of the enzyme phenylalanine dehydrogenase. The test for PKU is not reliable until the newborn has ingested an ample amount of the amino acid phenylalanine, a constituent of both human and cow's milk. The nurse must document the initial ingestion of milk and perform the test at least 24 hours after that time. The current trend toward early infant discharge from the hospital has the potential to cause neonates with a disorder such as PKU not to be screened as often as in the past. In response to this, the American Academy of Pediatrics (1996) made the following recommendations:

- Obtain a subsequent sample before 2 weeks of age if the initial specimen is collected before the newborn is 24 hours old
- Designate a primary care provider for all newborns before discharge for adequate newborn screening follow-up
- Collect the initial specimen as close as possible to discharge and no later than 7 days after birth

If the infant is found to have PKU, a diet low in phenylalanine is begun soon after birth. Breastfeeding or partial breastfeeding may be possible for some infants if the phenylalanine levels are monitored carefully and remain within acceptable limits (Kirby, 1999). Many affected children have some intellectual impairment.

Galactosemia, caused by a deficiency of the enzyme galactose-1-phosphate uridyltransferase, results in the inability to convert galactose to glucose. Galactosemia can be detected by measuring the blood levels of galactose in the urine of newborns suspected of having the disease who have ingested formula containing galactose. Early symptoms are vomiting, weight loss, and CNS symptoms, including poor feeding, drowsiness, and seizures. If the disorder goes untreated, the galactose levels will continue to increase and the affected infant will show failure to thrive, mental retardation, cataracts, jaundice, hepatomegaly, and cirrhosis of the liver, with death possibly occurring in the first month of life. Therapy consists of eliminating galactose from the diet.

Congenital hypothyroidism results from a deficiency of thyroid hormones; it affects approximately 1 of every 3600 to 5000 newborns (American Academy of Pediatrics [AAP], 1996). All states in the United States routinely screen for hypothyroidism. This involves measuring thyroxine (T_4) in a drop of blood obtained from a heel stick at 2 to 5 days of age. At this time the normally expected increase in T_4 would be lacking in newborns with hypothyroidism. It is more often included as part of the newborn screen done in the first 24 to 48 hours or before discharge. Early screening may have false-positive results. Treatment is thyroid replacement.

Cytologic Studies. Abnormalities can occur in either the autosomes or the sex chromosomes. Chromosomal disorders often can be diagnosed on the basis of the clinical manifestations alone. However, an infant may have a clinical appearance that is only suggestive of a problem. Cytologic studies then need to be done to confirm or rule out a suspected diagnosis.

Disorders in the number or structure of chromosomes can be diagnosed by a karyotype (see Fig. 8-1, *B*), which is a photographic enlargement of the chromosomes arranged by their numbered pairs.

Dermatoglyphics. Dermatoglyphics is the study of the patterns formed by the ridges in the skin on the digits, palms, and soles. These patterns, formed early in development, are strongly correlated with the effects of chromosomes. Many disorders that affect multiple body systems also affect these dermal ridges. The addition or deletion of genetic material produces alterations in the loops, swirls, and arches of the finger and toe prints, in the palm lines, and in the flexion creases on the palms of the hands and soles of the feet. Characteristic dermatoglyphic patterns have been noted for almost all the chromosomal abnormalities, such as Down syndrome.

An infant with Down syndrome may have a single, palmar crease (Fig. 28-25, *B*); a single flexion crease of the fifth digit; and an open-field pattern on the ball of the foot (Subjansky and Matthews, 1998). The characteristic dermatoglyphic feature in a child with Turner syndrome is the large size of the dermal patterns on the fingers and toes. Certain fingerprint patterns may also be found in those people who have cardiac valvular problems later in life. Asymmetry of palmar ridges has been reported in congenital anomalies such as cleft lip and palate and congenital vertebral anomaly (Goldberg et al, 1997).

Nursing Care

Newborn. A collaborative health team approach that includes specialists (e.g., orthodontists, physical therapists, and geneticists) and community service representatives is needed in the care of infants with some disorders. Surgical intervention in the neonatal period may be necessary for the infant requiring either immediate correction or a palliative procedure to relieve the symptoms of the anomaly until definitive correction can be done. However, the complications induced by the stress of surgery may upset the delicate metabolic balance in a neonate already attempting to adapt to its extrauterine environment. This is compounded by the fact that there is only a limited amount of nutrient reserves normally present in the neonate, and these reserves are already being drawn on by the energy-expending processes involved in rapid growth. Any surgical procedures performed during this time of growth place additional demands on these reserves. There is also a higher morbidity and mortality in neonates than in older children or adults undergoing similar procedures. However, despite these problems unique to neonates, advances in surgical techniques, anesthesia, and the nursing care given in intensive care nurseries have together been responsible for lessening the risk of surgery in neonates.

The health care team must be highly skilled to meet the needs of these infants. These needs are similar to those of other

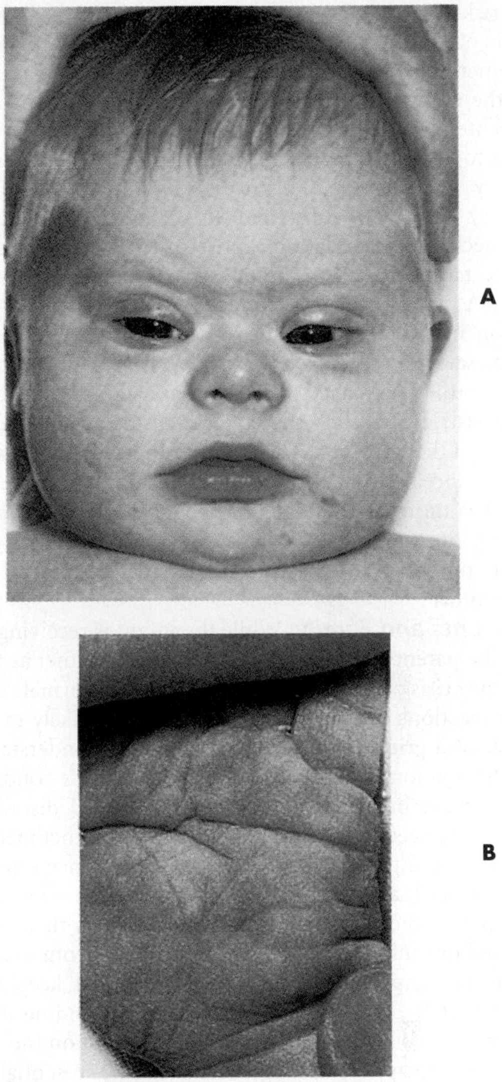

FIG. 28-25 • A, Clinical features of Down syndrome. **B,** Simian crease. (From Zitelli B, Davis H: *Atlas of pediatric physical diagnosis,* ed 3, St Louis, 1997, Mosby.)

high risk infants. In addition to stabilization of the infant's condition, other preoperative interventions, such as orogastric tube placement for abdominal decompression, pain management, and the maintenance of fluid and electrolyte balance, are implemented to manage specific problems.

Postoperatively, the infant is returned to the intensive care nursery, where close monitoring is maintained. The infant's respiratory efforts are supported; this often requires suctioning and mechanical ventilation. Constant surveillance is necessary to detect any respiratory complications resulting from the anesthesia. A pulse oximeter is attached to measure the oxygen saturation in hemoglobin, which closely correlates with arterial oxygen saturation. Oxygen is provided as needed. An indwelling gastric catheter attached to intermittent suction is placed to remove gastric secretions, thereby preventing aspiration and distention of the abdomen. The infant's fluid, electrolyte, and acid-base balances are monitored and adjusted as needed. Urinary output is monitored and should equal 1 to 2 ml/kg/hr. Other nursing interventions are focused on caring for the surgical site, maintaining thermoregulation, pain management, and promoting comfort.

Parents and Family. While the infant is receiving optimal care, the parents also have needs that must be met as they deal with the crisis of having an infant with an abnormal condition. Their reactions are carefully assessed and are likely to be those typical of a grief response. Facilitating their understanding of the information given them about their infant's condition is a vital nursing intervention. A newly diagnosed disorder often implies the need for the implementation of a therapeutic regimen. For example, the disorder may be an inborn error of metabolism, such as PKU, which requires consistent and rigid adherence to a diet. The family may need help with securing the required formula and in receiving counseling from a clinical dietitian. The importance of maintaining the diet, keeping an adequate supply of special preparations, and avoiding the use of unauthorized substitutions must be impressed on the family.

Referral to appropriate agencies is another essential component of the follow-up management, and the nurse should make the parents aware of all possible sources of aid, including pertinent literature, parent groups, and national organizations. Many organizations and foundations, such as the Cystic Fibrosis Foundation and the Muscular Dystrophy Association, provide services and equipment for affected children. There are also numerous parent groups the family can join. There they can share experiences and derive mutual support in coping with problems similar to those of other group members. Nurses must be familiar with the services available in their community that provide assistance and education to families with these special problems.

A major nursing function is providing emotional support to the family during all aspects of the care of the child born with a defect or disorder. The feelings stemming from the real or imagined threat posed by a congenital anomaly are as varied as the people being counseled. Responses may include apathy, denial, anger, hostility, fear, embarrassment, grief, and loss of self-esteem.

Parents benefit from seeing before-and-after pictures of other babies born with the same defect. Coupled with other verbal and nonverbal supportive care, this visual reassurance may be effective in allaying their concerns.

Critical Thinking

BIRTH OF A CHILD WITH A CONGENITAL ANOMALY

Emilie, an 18-year-old single mother, has just given birth to a son, John, who has a cleft lip and palate. You are bringing the baby to the mother for the first time. Identify your feelings about the infant and his physical defect. Anticipate how the mother is likely to react to this encounter. Rehearse how you will describe the infant to his mother. Describe the surgical treatment of the defects. Describe care necessary for John, including feeding and preoperative and postoperative care.

Families need much information, guidance, and support as they make decisions regarding the care of their infant. Once they have been given the facts and possible consequences and all the assistance they need in problem solving, the final decision regarding a course of action must be their own. It is then incumbent on health care providers to support the decision of the family.

Key Points

- The identification of maternal and fetal risk factors in the intrapartum period is vital for planning adequate care of high risk infants.
- A small percentage of significant birth injuries may occur despite skilled and competent obstetric care.
- Metabolic abnormalities of diabetes mellitus in pregnancy adversely affect embryonic and fetal development.
- Infection in the newborn may be acquired in utero, during birth, during resuscitation, and from within the nursery.
- The most common maternal infections during early pregnancy that are associated with various congenital malformations are represented by the acronym TORCH.
- HIV transmission from mother to infant occurs transplacentally at various gestational ages, perinatally by maternal blood and secretions, and by breast milk.
- Preterm infants are at risk for problems related to the immaturity of organ systems.
- Hyperbilirubinemia has a variety of etiologic factors, including maternal-fetal Rh and ABO incompatibility.
- The injection of $Rh_o(D)$ immune globulin in Rh-negative and Coombs test–negative women bestows passive immunity and also minimizes the possibility of isoimmunization.
- The nurse often first observes signs of newborn drug withdrawal and acquires information from the maternal history.
- Major congenital defects are now the leading cause of death in term neonates born to mothers who had good perinatal care.

- The curative and rehabilitative problems of a child with a congenital disorder are often complex, requiring a multidisciplinary approach to care.
- Parents need special instruction (e.g., CPR, oxygen therapy, or suctioning) before they take a high risk infant home.
- The supportive care given to the parent of infants with an abnormal condition must begin at birth or at the time of diagnosis and continue for years.

References

Abel E: *Fetal alcohol abuse syndrome revisited,* New York, 1997, Plenum Press.

Adriaanse A et al: Neonatal early onset group B streptococcal infection. A nine-year retrospective study in a tertiary care hospital, *J Perinat Med* 24(5):531-538, 1996.

American Academy of Pediatrics Committee on Drugs: The transfer of drugs and other chemicals into human milk, *Pediatrics* 93(1):137-150, 1994.

American Academy of Pediatrics Committee on Genetics: Newborn screening facts, *Pediatrics* 98:473-481, 1996.

American College of Obstetricians and Gynecologists: Human immunodeficiency virus infection in pregnancy, *Int J Gynecol Obstet* 57:73-80, 1997.

Ball J, Bindler R: *Pediatric nursing: caring for children,* ed 2, Stamford, CT, 1999, Appleton & Lange.

Ballock R, Richards B: Hip dysplasia: early diagnosis makes a difference, *Contemp Pediatr* 15:108-117, 1997.

Beazley D, Egerman R: Toxoplasmosis, *Semin Perinatol* 22(4):332-338, 1998.

Bellinger M: Urologic disorders. In Zitelli B, Davis H, editors: *Atlas of pediatric physical diagnosis,* ed 3, St Louis, 1997, Mosby.

Bennett A: Perinatal substance abuse and the drug-exposed neonate, *Adv Nurse Pract* 7(5):32-36, 1999.

Birthhistle K, Carrington D: Fetal varicella syndrome-a reappraisal of the literature, *J Infect* 36(S1):25-29, 1998.

Boyer K: Diagnosis and treatment of congenital toxoplasmosis, *Adv Pediatr Infect Dis* 11:449-457, 1996.

Brown H, Abernathy M: Cytomegalovirus infection, *Semin Perinatol* 22(4):260-266, 1998.

Buchi K: The drug exposed infant in the well baby nursery, *Clin Perinatol* 25(2):335-348, 1998.

Burchett S: Viral infections. In Cloherty J, Stark A, editors: *Manual of neonatal care,* ed 4, Boston, 1998, Little, Brown.

Centers for Disease Control and Prevention: Prevention of perinatal group B streptococcal disease: a public health perspective, *MMWR* 45(RR-7):1-24, 1996.

Centers for Disease Control and Prevention: *CDC working group on antiretroviral therapy and medical management of HIV-infected children: guidelines for the use of antiretroviral agents in pediatric HIV infection* (On-line), 1998, Available on-line at: www.cdc.gov/epo/mmwr/preview.

Chapman S: Varicella in pregnancy, *Semin Perinatol* 22(4): 339-346, 1998.

Chiriboga C et al: Dose-response of fetal cocaine exposure on newborn neurologic function, *Pediatrics* 103(6):79-85, 1999.

Church M, Abel E: Fetal alcohol syndrome: hearing, speech and vestibular disorders, *Obstet Gynecol Clin North Am* 25(1): 85-97, 1998.

Daberkow-Carson E, Washington R: Cardiovascular diseases and surgical interventions. In Merenstein G, Gardner S, editors: *Handbook of neonatal intensive care,* ed 4, St Louis, 1998, Mosby.

D'Apolito K: Substance abuse: infant and childhood outcomes, *J Pediatr Nurs* 13(5):307-316, 1998.

Darzi M, Chowdri N, Bhat A: Breastfeeding or spoon feeding after cleft lip repair: a prospective, randomized study, *Br J Plast Surg* 49:24-26, 1996.

Dores S et al: Alcohol versus natural drying for newborn cord care, *J Obstet Gynecol Neonatal Nurs* 27(6):621-627, 1998.

Duff P: Hepatitis in pregnancy, *Semin Perinatol* 22(4):277-283, 1998.

Fanaroff A, Martin R: *Neonatal-perinatal medicine: diseases of the fetus and infant,* ed 6, St Louis, 1997, Mosby.

Fernandes O et al: Moderate to heavy caffeine consumption during pregnancy and relationship to spontaneous abortion and abnormal fetal growth: a meta-analysis, *Reprod Toxicol* 12(4):435-444, 1998.

Finegold D: Endocriology. In Zitelli B, Davis H, editors: *Atlas of pediatric physical diagnosis,* ed 3, St Louis, 1997, Mosby.

Finer N et al: Congenital diaphragmatic hernia: developing a protocolized approach, *J Pediatr Surg* 33:31-37, 1998.

Franck L, Johnson L: Recognition and management of neonates at risk for perinatally acquired infection with human immunodeficiency virus, *Crit Care Nurse* 18(4):74-85, 1998.

Frank C, Cooper S, Merenstein G: Jaundice. In Merenstein G, Gardner S, editors: *Handbook of neonatal intensive care,* ed 4, St Louis, 1998, Mosby.

Goldberg C et al: Fluctuating asymmetry and vertebral malformation: a study of dermatolyphics in congenital spine deformities, *Spine* 22:775-779, 1997.

Grover G: Rotational problems of the lower extremity: in-toeing and out-toeing. In Berkowitz C, editor: *Pediatrics: a primary care approach,* Philadelphia, 1996, WB Saunders.

Guerina N: Bacterial and fungal infections. In Cloherty J, Stark A, editors: *Manual of neonatal care,* ed 4, Boston, 1998, Little, Brown.

Holland R, Price F, Bensard D: Neonatal surgery. In Merenstein G, Gardner S, editors: *Handbook of neonatal intensive care,* ed 4, St Louis, 1998, Mosby.

Hollier L, Cox S: Syphilis, *Semin Perinatol* 22(4):323-331, 1998.

Jackson P, Harvey J: Hydrocephalus. In Jackson P, Vessey J, editors: *Primary care of the child with a chronic condition,* ed 2, St Louis, 1996, Mosby.

Jacobs R: Neonatal herpes simplex virus infections, *Semin Perinatol* 22(1):64-71, 1998.

Joseph T, Pyati S, Jacobs N: Neonatal early-onset *Escherichia coli* disease, *Arch Pediatr Adolesc Med* 152(1):35-40, 1998.

Kaltenbach K, Berghella V, Finnegan L: Opioid dependence during pregnancy. Effects and management, *Obstet Gynecol Clin North Am* 25(1):139-151, 1998.

Kirby R: Maternal phenylketonuria: a new cause for concern, *J Obstet Gynecol Neonatal Nurs* 28(3):227-234, 1999.

Klein J, Marcy S: Bacterial sepsis and meningitis. In Remington S, Klein J, editors: *Infectious diseases of the fetus and newborn infant,* Philadelphia, 1995, WB Saunders.

Kwong T, Shearer D: Detection of drug use during pregnancy, *Obstet Gynecol Clin North Am* 25(1):43-64, 1998.

Lee M: Marihuana and tobacco use in pregnancy, *Obstet Gynecol Clin North Am* 25(1):65-83, 1998.

Lieu T et al: Neonatal group B streptococcal infection in a managed care population, *Obstet Gynecol* 92(1):21-27, 1998.

Lynfield R, Guerina N: Toxoplasmosis, *Pediatr Rev* 18(3):75-83, 1997.

Medves J, O'Brien B: Cleaning solutions and bacterial colonization in promoting healing and early separation of the umbilical cord in healthy newborns, *Can J Public Health* 88(6): 380-382, 1997.

Merenstein G, Adams K, Weisman L: Infection in the neonate. In Merenstein G, Gardner S, editors: *Handbook of neonatal intensive care,* ed 4, St Louis, 1998, Mosby.

Merenstein G, Gardner S, editors: *Handbook of neonatal intensive care,* ed 4, St Louis, 1998, Mosby.

Milerad J et al: Objective measurements of nicotine exposure in victims of sudden infant death syndrome and in other unexpected child deaths, *J Pediatr* 133(2):232-236, 1998.

Minkoff H: Human immunodeficiency virus infection in pregnancy, *Semin Perinatol* 22(4):293-308, 1998.

Moe P, Paige L: Neurologic disorders. In Merenstein G, Gardner S, editors: *Handbook of neonatal intensive care,* ed 4, St Louis, 1998, Mosby.

Mofenson L: Mother-child HIV-1 transmission: timing and determinants, *Obstet Gynecol Clin North Am* 24(4):759-784, 1997.

Nathwani D et al: Varicella infections in pregnancy and the newborn, *J Infect* 36(S1):59-71, 1998.

Novacheck T: Developmental dysplasia of the hip, *Pediatr Clin North Am* 43:829-848, 1996.

Paulozzi L, Erickson D, Jackson R: Hypospadias trends in two U. S. surveillance systems, *Pediatrics* 100:831-834, 1997.

Plessinger M: Prenatal exposure to amphetamines, *Obstet Gynecol Clin North Am* 25(1):119-138, 1998.

Plessinger M, Woods J: Cocaine in pregnancy, *Obstet Gynecol Clin North Am* 25(1):99-118, 1998.

Riley L: Herpes simplex virus, *Semin Perinatol* 22(4):284-292, 1998.

Rosa C: Rubella and rubeola, *Semin Perinatol* 22(4):318-322, 1998.

Santos I et al: Caffeine intake and low birth weight: a population-based case-control study, *Am J Epidemiol* 147(7):620-627, 1998.

Scarlatti G: Pediatric HIV infection, *Lancet* 348(9031):863-867, 1996.

Schachter J, Grossman M: Chlamydia. In Remington J, Klein J, editors: *Infectious diseases of the fetus and newborn,* Philadelphia, 1995, WB Saunders.

Schechner S: Drug abuse and withdrawal. In Cloherty J, Stark A, editors: *Manual of neonatal care,* ed 4, Boston, 1998, Little, Brown.

Steele M: Common chromosomal disorders. In Zitelli B, Davis H, editors: *Atlas of pediatric physical diagnosis,* ed 3, St Louis, 1997, Mosby.

Subjansky E, Matthews A: Genetic disorders, malformations, and inborn errors of metabolism. In Merenstein G, Gardner S, editors: *Handbook of neonatal intensive care,* ed 4, St Louis, 1998, Mosby.

Tuomala R: Prevention of transmission, *Obstet Gynecol Clin North Am* 24(4):785-795, 1997.

Wagner C et al: The impact of prenatal drug exposure on the neonate, *Obstet Gynecol Clin North Am* 25(1):169-194, 1998.

Wong D: *Whaley & Wong's nursing care of infants and children,* ed 6, St Louis, 1999, Mosby.

CHAPTER 29

Contemporary Pediatric Nursing

http://www.harcourthealth.com/MERLIN/Wong/maternal/

Learning Objectives

On completion of this chapter the reader will be able to:

- Define the terms mortality and morbidity.
- Identify two ways that knowledge of mortality and morbidity can improve child health.
- List three major causes of death during infancy, early childhood, later childhood, and adolescence.
- List two major causes of illness during childhood.
- Outline four events that were significant in the evolution of child health care in the United States.
- Describe five broad functions of the pediatric nurse in promoting the health of children.
- Define critical thinking.
- List the five steps of the nursing process.
- Define nursing diagnosis.
- Differentiate among three domains of nursing practice: dependent, independent, and interdependent.
- Differentiate standard care plan from individualized care plan.

HEALTH DURING CHILDHOOD

Health, as defined by the World Health Organization (WHO), is "a state of complete physical, mental, and social well-being and not merely the absence of disease." Despite this broad definition, health is traditionally assessed by observing mortality (death) and morbidity (illness) over time. Therefore the balance between physical, mental, and social well-being and the presence of disease becomes a prime indicator of health.

Information concerning mortality and morbidity is important to nurses. Such data yield significant information about (1) the causes of death and illness, (2) high risk age groups for certain disorders or hazards, (3) advances in treatment and prevention, and (4) specific areas of health counseling.

Healthy People 2000 and 2010

Although the health of people, including children, in the United States improved dramatically during the twentieth century, there remains cause for concern. There is a growing awareness that many of the serious domestic problems, such as acquired immunodeficiency syndrome (AIDS), drug abuse, violence, and unwanted pregnancies, have a direct effect on the health of the nation. The solutions to these problems do not lie in better or more innovative medical treatment, but in prevention.

In 1990, *Healthy People 2000* established three broad goals for public health in the 1990s: (1) increase the span of healthy life for Americans, (2) reduce health disparities among Americans, and (3) achieve access to preventive services for all Americans.

Healthy People 2000 included the following objectives pertaining to pediatrics: improving nutritional and infant health, reducing unintentional injuries, improving oral health, reducing and controlling human immunodeficiency virus (HIV) infection, preventing sexually transmitted infectons (STIs), increasing immunization against and preventing infectious diseases, and improving clinical preventive services by reducing barriers to health care.

Healthy People 2010 builds on the initiatives pursued in *Healthy People 2000. Healthy People 2010* is committed to the single focus of promoting health and preventing illness, disability and premature death (U.S. Department of Health and Human Services, 2000). Two overriding goals have been proposed for *Healthy People 2010:* (1) increase quality years of healthy life, and (2) eliminate health disparities. These two goals will be supported by four enabling goals concerned with promoting healthy behaviors, protecting health, ensuring access to quality health care, and strengthening community prevention. New focus areas have been added in response to changes in health care and public health during the last 10 years. These areas include impairment and disability, people with low income, race and ethnicity, chronic diseases, and public health infrastructure (Office of Disease Prevention and Health Promotion, 1997).

Mortality

Figures describing rates of occurrence for events such as death in children are often referred to as *vital statistics. Mortality statistics* describe the incidence or number of individuals who have died over a specific period. They are usually presented as rates per 100,000 because of their lower frequency of occurrence. Mortality rates are calculated from a sample of death certificates.

Beginning in 1989, several important changes have taken place in the reporting of health statistics. Figures for birth and death are based on the person's state of residence, not the state in which the event occurred. The tabulation of race for live births has changed from the race of the child to the race of the mother. As a result of these changes, figures for births and deaths, as well as infant mortality rates by race cannot be compared to statistics reported before these changes (Murphy, 2000).

NURSE ALERT • Because of the complexity of compiling such data, statistics may vary in different reports and should be interpreted cautiously. For example, figures may be *estimated* (from previously collected data), *provisional* (from temporary current data), or *final* (from complete provisional data). Final statistics are often published 2 or more years after data collection.

TABLE 29-1

Death Rates by Age and Sex: United States, 1998 (Rates Per 100,000 Population)

	All Races		
Age	**Both Sexes**	**Male**	**Female**
All ages*	864.7	876.4	853.5
Under 1 year†	751.3	818.2	681.3
1-4	34.6	37.6	31.4
5-9	17.7	20.0	15.3
10-14	22.1	26.9	17.2
15-19	70.6	98.7	40.8

From Murphy SL: Deaths: final data for 1998. *National Vital Statistics Reports* 48(11), 2000.
*Includes all age groups >19 years.
†Death rate for "Under 1 year" (based on population estimates) differ from infant mortality rates (based on live births).

TABLE 29-2

Death Rates for Children, Canada, 1995 (Rates per 100,000 Population)

	Rate	
Age (Years)	**Male**	**Female**
Under 1	672.5	552.5
1-4	29.5	24.7
5-9	17.7	14.0
10-14	21.6	18.8
15-19	80.3	33.1
20-24	104.8	32.5

Data from Statistics Canada, 1995.

Infant Mortality. The *infant mortality rate* is the number of deaths per 1000 live births during the first year of life. It may be further divided into *neonatal mortality* (<28 days of life) and *postneonatal mortality* (28 days to 11 months of life). In the United States there has been a dramatic decrease in infant mortality. At the beginning of the twentieth century, the rate was approximately 200 infant deaths per 1000 live births. Final data for 1998 indicate the rate was 7.2 deaths per 1000 live births, remaining unchanged from 1997 (Murphy, 2000). This decrease has resulted primarily from improvements in perinatal care, such as treatment of respiratory distress syndrome; and fewer deaths from sudden infant death syndrome (SIDS).

From a worldwide perspective, the United States lags behind other developed countries. Statistics for 1997 indicate that it ranked second-to-last among the 24 developed nations with the lowest infant death rates, far behind Sweden, which had the lowest rate. The United States lags behind its neighbor Canada, which ranked sixteenth. Although the reason is unknown, a major difference between the United States and the other 23 countries is that the latter all have a national health program.

TABLE 29-3

Mortality Rates for the 10 Leading Causes of Infant Death in 1998 (Rates per 100,000 Live Births)

Rank	Cause of Death (Based on Ninth Revision, International Classification of Diseases)	Percent	Rate
...	All races, all causes	100	719.8
1	Congenital anomalies	21.9	157.6
2	Disorders relating to short gestation and unspecified low birth weight	14.5	104.0
3	Sudden Infant Death Syndrome	9.9	71.6
4	Newborn affected by maternal complications of pregnancy	4.7	34.1
5	Respiratory distress syndrome	4.6	32.9
6	Newborn affected by complications of placenta, cord, and membranes	3.4	24.4
7	Infections specific to the perinatal period	2.9	20.7
8	Accidents and adverse effects	2.7	19.1
9	Intrauterine hypoxia and birth asphyxia	1.6	11.7
10	Pneumonia and influenza	1.6	11.2

Modified from Murphy SL: Deaths: final data for 1998. *National Vital Statistics Reports,* 48(11), 2000.

Birth weight is considered the major determinant of neonatal death in technologically developed countries and is closely related to gestational age (Ventura et al, 1998). The relationship between birth weight (and gestational age) and mortality shows that the lower the birth weight, the higher the mortality. The relatively high incidence of *low birth weight (LBW)* (i.e., <2500 g) in the United States is considered a key factor in its higher neonatal mortality rates when compared with other countries. Access to and use of high-quality prenatal care is the single most promising preventive strategy to decrease early delivery and infant mortality. Other factors that increase the risk of infant mortality include African-American race, male gender, short or long gestation, maternal age (younger or older), and lower level of maternal education (Murphy, 2000).

Although there has been a steady and significant decline in infant mortality, the number of deaths occurring in the first year of life is still proportionately high when compared with death rates at other ages (Table 29-1). This is also true of other countries, such as Canada (Table 29-2). In the United States and Canada the death rate for infants under 1 year of age is greater than the rate for individuals ages 1 through 54 years. It is not until age 55 and over that the death rate begins to exceed the rate for infants.

During the first half of the 1900s, neonatal mortality rates did not show the remarkable reduction observed in postneonatal infant mortality. In the early 1960s attention was focused on perinatal health care in an effort to decrease the number of neonatal deaths. As a result, neonatal mortality declined from 29 per 1000 live births in 1950 to 7.2 per 1000 live births in 1997 (Guyer et al, 1999). As Table 29-3 demonstrates, most of the 10 leading causes of death during infancy continue to occur during the perinatal period. The first four causes—congenital anomalies, disorders related to short gestation and unspecified low birth weight, sudden infant death syndrome, and maternal complications of pregnancy—accounted for almost half of all deaths of infants under 1 year of age in 1998 (Murphy, 2000).

Although a number of perinatal problems have benefited from improved treatment, congenital anomalies continue to be a leading cause of infant mortality. The incidences of most birth defects have remained substantially the same. Heart defects have been rising, but the increase is the result of improved methods of detection, not increased births of affected infants. Anencephaly and spina bifida are expected to decrease as much as 50% with the recommendation of folic acid supplementation for all women of childbearing age (see Spina Bifida [Myelomeningocele], Chapter 55). Most birth defects are associated significantly with LBW; therefore, prevention of congenital anomalies depends on reducing the number of LBW infants.

When infant death rates are categorized according to race, a disturbing difference is seen. The infant mortality for Caucasians is considerably lower than for all other races in the United States, with African-Americans having twice the rate for Caucasians. Although the infant mortality of both groups has declined, the gap has remained fairly constant. Unfortunately, data on minority groups are less readily available.

One encouraging note is that the gap in mortality rates between all non-Caucasian races has been narrowing. Since the Indian Health Service assumed responsibility for the health of Native Americans, infant mortality for Native Americans has declined. This improvement, however, is primarily the result of declines in neonatal mortality. The postneonatal death rate for Native Americans remains more than twice the rate for Caucasians (Mathews, Curtin, and MacDorman, 2000). This suggests that Native American infants leave the hospital healthy but go to environments that may decrease their chances of survival past the first year.

Childhood Mortality. For children older than 1 year of age, the death rate has always been less than that for infants. Children ages 5 to 14 years have the lowest rate of death (Table 29-4). However, a sharp rise occurs during later adolescence, primarily from injuries, homicide, and suicide. In 1998, these conditions were responsible for about 75% of deaths in

TABLE 29-4
Deaths and Death Rates for the Five Leading Causes of Childhood Death in Specific Age Groups in 1998*

Cause of Death and Age	1998 Rate†
TOTAL: 1-19 YEARS	
All causes	35.9
Accidents and adverse effects	15.3
Homicide and legal intervention	4.1
Malignant neoplasms	2.8
Suicide	2.7
Congenital anomalies	1.4
1-4 YEARS	
All causes	34.2
Accidents and adverse effects	12.4
Congenital anomalies	3.5
Homicide and legal intervention	2.4
Malignant neoplasms	2.3
Diseases of the heart	1.3
5-9 YEARS	
All causes	17.6
Accidents and adverse effects	7.5
Malignant neoplasms	2.4
Congenital anomalies	1.0
Homicide and legal intervention	0.8
Diseases of the heart	0.7
10-14 YEARS	
All causes	21.8
Accidents and adverse effects	8.5
Malignant neoplasms	2.8
Suicide	1.6
Homicide and legal intervention	1.4
Diseases of the heart	0.8
15-19 YEARS	
All causes	69.7
Accidents and adverse effects	32.4
Homicide and legal intervention	11.3
Suicide	8.7
Malignant neoplasms	3.6
Diseases of the heart	1.9

Modified from Guyer B et al: Annual summary of vital statistics—1998, *Pediatrics* 104(6):1243, 1999.
*Preliminary data.
†Rate per 100,000 population in specified group.

teenagers and young adults 15 to 19 years old. A general trend in racial differences that occurs in infant mortality is also apparent in childhood deaths for all ages and for both sexes. Caucasians have fewer deaths for all ages; for both Caucasians and African-Americans, male deaths outnumber female deaths (see Table 29-5).

After 1 year of age there is a dramatic change in the cause of death, with unintentional injuries being the leading cause from the youngest ages to the adolescent years. In addition, *violent deaths* have been steadily increasing among young people ages 10 through 25 years, especially African-Americans and males (Rachuba, Stanton, and Howard, 1995). Homicide is the second leading cause of death in the 15- to 19-year age group (see Table 29-4). Children 12 years of age and older tend to be killed by nonfamily members (acquaintances and gangs, typically of the same race) and most frequently by firearms.

Firearm homicide is the leading cause of death among African-American males ages 15 to 19 years. Suicide, a form of self-violence, is the third leading cause of death among teenagers and young adults 15 to 19 years old (see Table 29-4).

The causes of increased violence against children and self-inflicted violence are not fully understood. In young children the increase in homicide may represent more accurate identification of child abuse. In all cases the problem of child homicides is an extremely complex one, involving numerous social, economic, and other influences. Prevention lies in a better understanding of the social and psychologic factors that lead to the high rates of homicide and suicide. Nurses need to be aware of young people who are depressed, are repeatedly in trouble with the criminal justice system, or are associated with groups known to be violent. Prevention requires identification of these young people and therapeutic intervention by qualified professionals. Pediatric nurses can assess children and adolescents for indications that they are at risk for violence and educate all individuals about the importance of maintaining safe, nonviolent homes, schools, and communities.

The major declines in death rates during childhood have been in deaths caused by gastrointestinal diseases, infectious diseases, perinatal conditions, neoplasms, and injuries. The absence of infectious diseases as a leading cause of death is testimony to the role antibacterial agents and immunizations have played in the declining mortality rates. More effective treatment of severe infections has resulted in other disorders becoming more prominent in the list of leading killers. Most notable among these are the neoplasms, although fewer children die from cancer than ever before (see Leukemias, Chapter 49). Deaths caused by infectious diseases declined by 45% between 1995 and 1998; they now account for a small percentage of overall deaths. In 1987, a special cause of death category was created in the United States to classify deaths related to HIV in-

TABLE 29-5

Mortality from Leading Types of Unintentional Injuries, United States, 1996 (Rates per 100,000 Population in Each Age Group)

	Age (Years)			
Type of Accident	Under 1	1-4	5-14	15-24
MALES				
All causes	828.0	42.2	25.4	130.6
Unintentional injuries (all types)	23.2	16.2	11.1	55.2
Motor vehicle	5.7 (2)	5.7 (1)	6.0 (1)	40.7 (1)
Drowning	1.5 (5)	4.0 (2)	1.7 (2)	3.4 (2)
Fires and burns	1.8 (4)	3.0 (3)	0.8 (3)	—
Firearms	—	—	0.5 (4)	2.0 (4)
Ingestion of food/object	2.3 (3)	0.7 (4)	—	—
Falls	—	—	—	1.1 (5)
Mechanical suffocation	8.8 (1)	0.6 (5)	0.4 (5)	—
Poisoning	—	—	—	2.4 (3)
All other unintentional injuries	3.3	2.2	1.6	5.6
Accidents as a percent of all deaths	2.8%	38.4%	43.7%	42.3%
FEMALES				
All causes	680.0	34.3	17.8	46.2
Unintentional injuries (all types)	19.3	11.3	6.7	20.1
Motor vehicle	5.8 (2)	4.8 (1)	4.2 (1)	17.1 (1)
Drowning	1.5 (4)	2.0 (3)	0.6 (3)	0.5 (3)
Fires and burns	1.6 (3)	2.2 (2)	0.7 (2)	—
Firearms	—	—	0.1 (4)	0.2 (4)
Ingestion of food/object	1.5 (4)	0.5 (4)	—	—
Falls	—	—	—	0.2 (4)
Mechanical suffocation	6.3 (1)	0.4 (5)	0.1 (4)	—
Poisoning	—	—	—	0.6 (2)
All other unintentional injuries	2.6	1.4	0.9	1.6
Accidents as a percent of all deaths*	2.8%	32.9%	37.6%	43.5%

Modified from National Safety Council: *Injury Facts,* Itaska, IL, 1999, National Safety Council.
Data from National Center for Health Statistics.
*Indicates rank among the leading types of accidents.

fection. Since 1995, mortality related to HIV infection has decreased by 71%; HIV was no longer one of the 15 leading causes of death in 1998 (Guyer et al, 1999).

Injuries. Injuries, the leading cause of death in children over 1 year of age, are responsible for more deaths and disabilities in children than all causes of disease combined. As children grow older, the percentage of deaths from injuries increases (Table 29-5). Injuries have not shown the dramatic declines seen in other areas of childhood mortality, because an injury has traditionally been regarded as an unavoidable accident or a behavioral problem rather than a health problem. The term *accident* suggests a chaotic, random event that is "luck" or "chance"; the term *injury* is preferred because it connotes a sense of responsibility and control. In addition, injury control, including research, has not received high priority or sufficient financial support. Research on injuries has not been based on a theoretic framework, as has been done with diseases. There is a need to view injuries and their prevention in terms of *host* (the affected person), *environment* (the time and place), and *agent* (the object that is the direct cause).

The pattern of deaths caused by unintentional injuries (especially from motor vehicles, drowning, and burns) is remarkably consistent in most Western societies. However, the United States far exceeds other countries in the number of violent deaths. (For the leading causes of deaths from injuries for each age group according to sex, see Table 29-5.) Fortunately, prevention strategies such as use of car restraints, bicycle helmets, and smoke detectors have resulted in a significant decrease in fatalities for children. Currently, all states have enacted legislation requiring young children to be properly restrained in motor vehicles. Despite safety efforts, the overwhelming cause of death in children over 1 year of age is motor vehicle (MV)-related fatalities, including occupant, pedestrian, bicycle, and motorcycle deaths (Fig. 29-1). The majority of deaths from injuries occur in males. Even though the percentage of infants dying from MV injuries is small compared with the total number of deaths in that age group, children under 1 year of age still have a high death rate from MV occupant deaths, primarily from failure to be properly restrained.

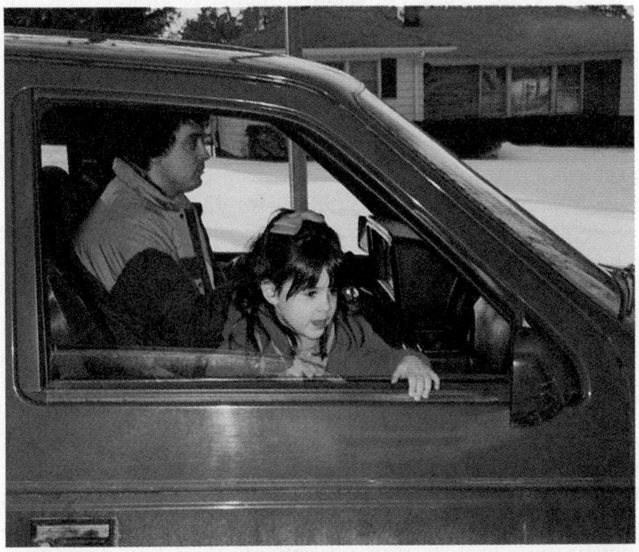

FIG. 29-1 • Motor vehicle injuries are the leading cause of death in children over 1 year of age. The majority of the fatalities involve occupants who are unrestrained.

When deaths from injuries are compared according to sex and age, the causes of death differ. The developmental stage of the child determines the type of injury that is most likely to occur at a specific age. For example, a child between the ages of 1 and 4 years is equally likely to die as an occupant or as a pedestrian in MV injuries. However, a child between the ages of 5 and 9 years is more likely to die from pedestrian crashes, and adolescents are more likely to die as an occupant in a crash. Children ages 5 to 14 are at greatest risk of bicycling fatalities. The majority of bicycling deaths are from head injuries. Helmets reduce the risk of head injury by 85%, but few children wear them (National Safety Council, 1999).

Drowning and burns are the second and third leading causes of death in boys ages 1 to 14, but the order is reversed in girls (Fig. 29-2). Drowning continues to be a significant cause of death in older teenagers. In addition, firearms are a major cause of death in males (Fig. 29-3). During infancy, mechanical suffocation often ranks as the leading cause of death, but is infrequent in older children (Fig. 29-4). More than half of all poisonings causing injury occur in children under 2 years of age (Fig. 29-5). By age 4 to 5 years, nonintentional poisonings are uncommon. Another increase occurs in the 15- to 24-year age group, where poisoning is the third leading cause of death in males and second in females. Poisoning in this age group is typically intentional and usually represents death from suicide (especially in females) or drug abuse.

Not all injuries are unintentional. Some may be intentional and represent abuse or suicide. An important nursing consideration when injuries do occur is to help determine if they were intentional.

Injury Prevention. Analyzing deaths from specific types of injuries by age and sex is useful in identifying high risk groups. When comparing deaths from injuries with other causes of childhood mortality, it is clear that preventing injuries offers the greatest promise for improving survival. Recent data indicate that advanced physical development poses additional risks for 5- to 8-year-olds. Nurses play a major role in providing anticipatory guidance to parents and older children regarding the hazards during each age period (Christoffel et al, 1996).

Injury prevention is discussed in each chapter on health promotion of the various age groups.

In theory, all injuries are preventable. A primary nursing responsibility is to anticipate and recognize when safety measures apply. The preventive aspects of child care are an ongoing part of health promotion throughout childhood. Anticipatory guidance regarding developmental expectations serves to alert parents to the types of injuries that are most likely to occur at any given age. Early in the parent-child relationship, parents need advice on how to provide a safe environment for their child. It cannot be assumed that parents of one or more children are familiar with all areas of child safety. The addition of a new infant may cause sibling rivalry, and the new child may be at risk from a jealous sibling. The American Academy of Pediatrics has developed an injury prevention program (*TIPP*) that provides useful information and anticipatory guidance on safety issues for parents and health care providers.* Another resource devel-

*For more information, contact the American Academy of Pediatrics, 141 Northwest Point Boulevard, Elk Grove Village, IL 60007; 1-888-227-1770; fax (847) 228-1281; website: www.aap.org.

A

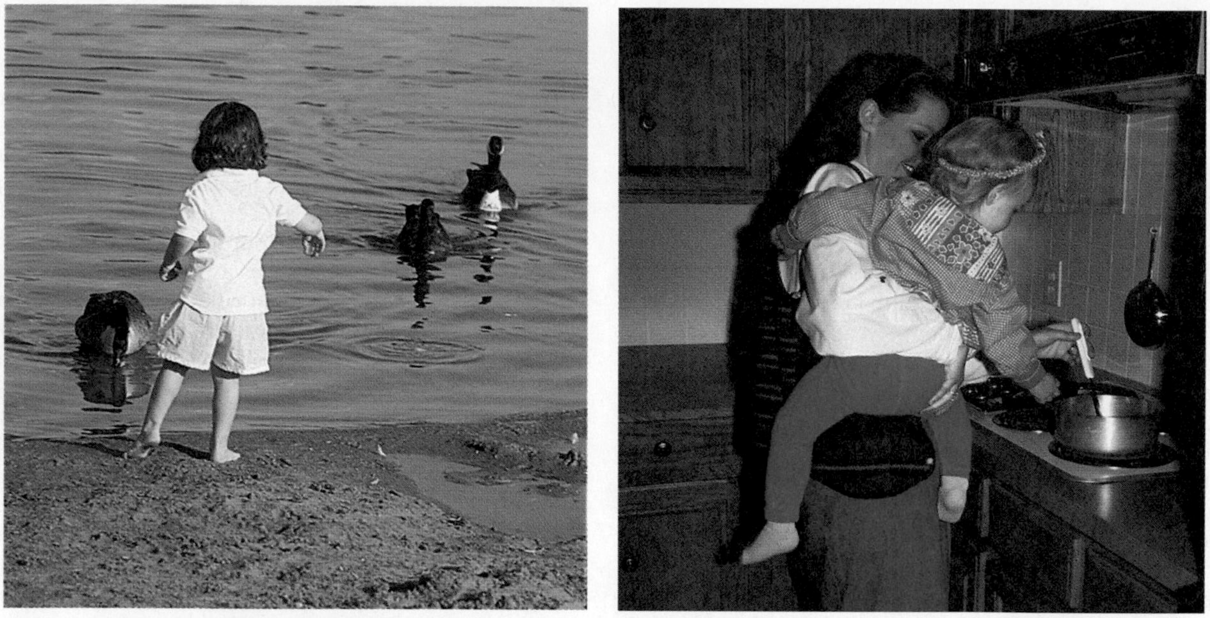

B

FIG. 29-2 • **A,** Drowning is the second leading cause of death from injury in boys and the third in girls ages 1 to 14 years. **B,** Burns are the second leading cause of death from injury in girls and the third in boys ages 1 to 14 years.

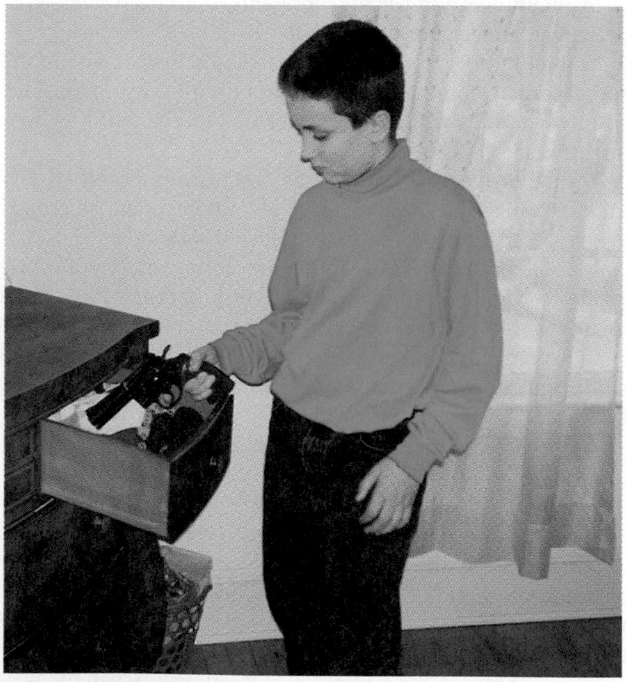

FIG. 29-3 • Improper use of firearms is the fourth leading cause of death from injury in boys and girls ages 5 to 24 years.

oped to decrease injuries is the Consumer Product Safety Commission (CPSC) of the United States Government. This agency provides a number of publications that recommend various areas of safety concerns for children.*

Morbidity

The prevalence of a specific illness in the population at a particular time is known as *morbidity statistics.* These are generally presented as rates per 1000 population because of their greater frequency of occurrence. Unlike mortality statistics, morbidity is very difficult to define and may denote acute illness, chronic disease, or disability. Common sources of data for morbidity statistics include reasons for visits to physicians, diagnoses for hospital admission, or household interviews. Unlike death rates, which are updated annually, morbidity statistics are revised less often and do not necessarily represent the general population.

The types of diseases that children contract during childhood vary according to age. For example, upper respiratory tract infections tend to decrease with age, and other disorders such as acne and headaches tend to increase with age. Children who have had a particular type of problem are more likely to have that problem again. Morbidity is not distributed randomly in children. Children from poor families tend to have more health problems. This finding suggests the need exists to heighten efforts to improve access to health care for low-income children.

Recent concern has focused on specific groups of children who have increased morbidity: homeless children, children living in poverty, children of LBW, children with chronic illnesses, foreign-born adopted children, and children in day care centers. A number of factors place these groups at risk for poor health. A major cause is limited access to health care, especially for the homeless, the poverty stricken, and children with chronic health problems. Other reasons include improved survival of children with chronic health problems, particularly infants of very LBW. Children living in or exposed to at-risk environments such as country of origin (for adopted children) and day care centers may be more likely to have a variety of medical conditions, especially infections (Lears, Guth, and Lewandowski, 1998; Loubiala et al, 1997).

---

*For more information, call 1-800-638-CPSC or 1-800-638-2272.

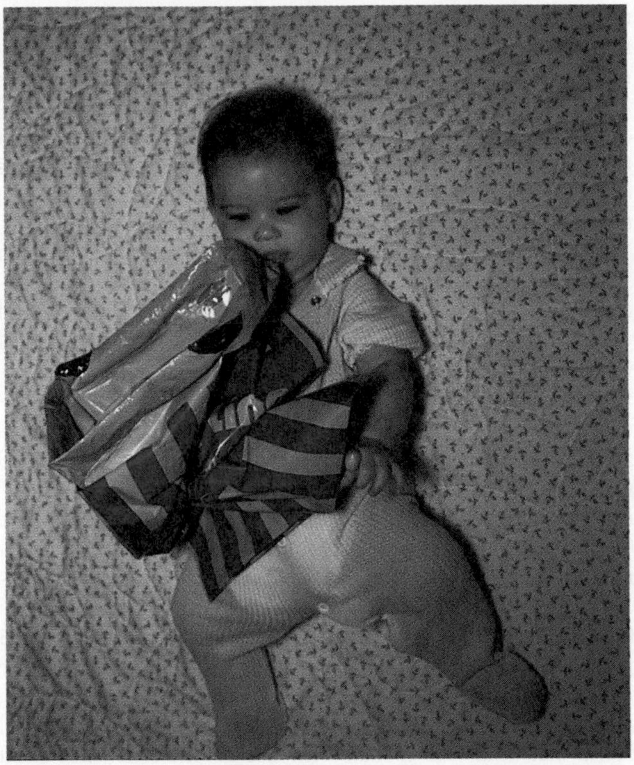

FIG. 29-4 • Aspiration/suffocation is often the leading cause of death from injury in infants.

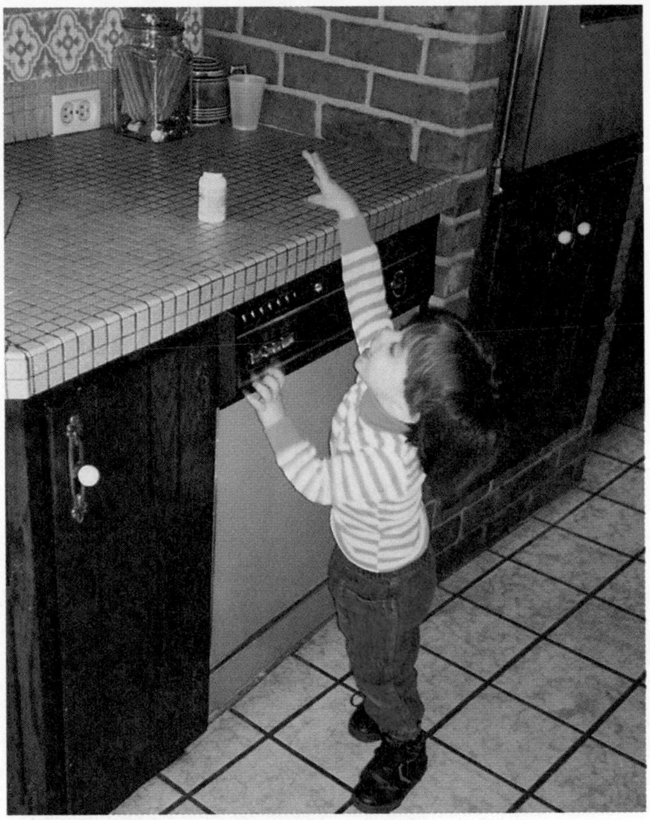

FIG. 29-5 • Poisoning causes a considerable number of injuries in children under 4 years of age, but it is the third leading cause of death from injury in males and second in females (usually from suicide) in young people ages 15 to 24 years.

Injuries are an additional factor influencing morbidity. Each year 40,000 to 50,000 children are injured permanently, and at least one million children seek medical care because of unintentional injuries (Mofenson and Greensher, 1997).

The most important aspect of morbidity is the degree of disability it produces. *Disability* can be measured in days absent from school or days confined to bed. On an average, children lose 5.3 days per year because of injury or illness. Approximately 6% of all children ages 0-17 have limitation in activities resulting from chronic conditions lasting at least 3 months (Guyer, Minkovitz, and Strobino, 2001). (The incidence of chronic conditions is discussed in Chapter 41).

For many children, childhood is a time of relative health; however, it is the rare child who never becomes ill. Education of parents regarding the usual types of childhood illnesses and recognition of symptoms requiring treatment is an important part of nursing care. Future progress in decreasing childhood morbidity and mortality rests more on parent education than on discoveries such as antibiotics. Nurses play a vital role in advancing child care through health promotion.

Evolution of Child Health Care in the United States

Children in colonial America were born into a world with many hazards to their health and survival. Epidemics were common. Physicians were few, and only a small number had any formal training. Midwives were untrained, basing their practice on past experiences. Books providing information on child care and feeding were scarce and, when available, were useful only to a minority of literate parents.

Medical care by physicians was limited to wealthy families who lived in or could travel to more developed cities. Children who lived on farms were mainly cared for by another family member or by a competent neighbor. Traveling medicine men, with their various forms of quackery, were common. Children who were bought as slaves or born to slaves had only as much care as their owner was able or willing to provide. Native American children were treated according to the tradition of each tribe, which was often a mixture of medicine, magic, and religion. With the colonization of America, Native Americans were exposed to many new, often fatal, diseases.

Statistics on childhood mortality during the colonial period are largely unavailable. Epidemic diseases included smallpox, measles, mumps, chickenpox, influenza, diphtheria, yellow fever, cholera, and whooping cough. However, the disease that surpassed all others as a cause of childhood death was dysentery. Sometimes entire families succumbed to this illness. Other diseases that were major contributors to childhood illness were the "slow epidemics" of tuberculosis, nutritional diseases, and injuries.

Although scientific knowledge was accumulating, especially from work done in Europe, there were no organized efforts in the United States to apply that knowledge to the care of the sick.

It was not until the Industrial Revolution was well under way in the nineteenth century that the consequences of childhood illness and injury and the effects of child labor, poverty, and neglect became more widely recognized. The end of the nineteenth century is often regarded as the dark ages of pediatrics, and the first half of the twentieth century as the dawn of improved health care for children.

The study of pediatrics began in the late 1800s under the influence of a Prussian-born physician, *Abraham Jacobi* (1830-1919), who is referred to as the *Father of Pediatrics.* At this time new advances in the scientific and clinical investigation of childhood diseases were made. One outstanding achievement was the establishment of "milk stations," where mothers could bring sick children for treatment and learn the importance of pure milk and its proper preparation.

The crusade for pure milk helped bring the dairy industry under legal control and led to the establishment of infant welfare stations. The remarkable decline in infant mortality since 1900 has been achieved through prevention and health-promoting measures such as improved sanitation and pasteurization of milk. Before these regulations existed, the unsanitary milk supply was a chief source of infantile diarrhea and bovine tuberculosis. Cows were often kept in filthy stables and fed garbage and distillery wastes. Milk from cows fed distillery wastes was reported to make infants "tipsy." Some of the cows were so diseased with tuberculosis that they had to be raised on cranes to be milked.

At the same time, increasing concern developed for the social welfare of children, especially those who were homeless or employed as factory laborers. The work of *Lillian Wald* (1867-1940) had far-reaching effects on child health and nursing. She founded the Henry Street Settlement in New York City, which eventually provided nursing service, social work, and an organized program of social, cultural, and educational activities. Wald is regarded as the *founder of public health* or *community nursing.* She was instrumental in establishing the role of the first full-time school nurse, *Lina Rogers.* Soon other nurses were employed to teach parents and children about the prevention or need for treatment of minor skin conditions, malnutrition, and other impairments or illnesses identified in the school. An outgrowth of nursing involvement in school health was the development of pediatric courses and specialized clinical experience in schools of nursing.

As more causes of disease were identified, there was an emphasis on isolation and asepsis. In the early 1900s children with contagious diseases were isolated from adult patients. Parents were prohibited from visiting because they might transmit disease to and from the home. Even toys and personal articles of clothing were kept from the child. It was not until the 1940s and the famous works of Spitz and Robertson on institutionalized children that the effects of isolation and maternal deprivation were recognized. This research brought forth a surge of interest in the psychologic health of children and resulted in changes for hospitalized children, such as rooming-in, sibling visitations, child life (play) programs, pre-hospitalization preparation, parent education, and hospital schooling.

Influenced by social reformers such as Lillian Wald, national leaders began to take action to improve children's living conditions. In 1909 President Theodore Roosevelt called the first *White House Conference on Children.* It focused on care of dependent children and attempted to address the deplorable working conditions of youngsters. As a result of this conference, the *U.S. Children's Bureau* was established in 1912. This marked the beginning of a period of studies of economic and social factors related to infant mortality, maternal deaths, and maternal and infant care in rural areas, all of which created the basis for stimulating better standards of care for mothers and children. This helped lead to the first Maternity and Infancy Act (Sheppard-Towner Act) in 1921, which provided grants to states to develop a division of maternal and child health as a unit of the health department.

With the passage of *Title V of the Social Security Act (SSA)* in 1935, a federal-state partnership was established under the administration of the Children's Bureau. Title V included federal grants-in-aid to states (matched by state funds) for three types of work: *maternal and child health (MCH), Crippled Children's Services (CCS),* and *child welfare services.* The first programs provided by Title V were prenatal, postnatal, and child health clinics, and training of personnel. The early emphasis of the CCS was on orthopedic care. With the recognition that a child's ability to function also could be limited by a chronic illness, state CCS programs became involved with children who had developmental, behavioral, and educational problems and, more recently, with home care of children with complex medical conditions. This broadened concept was officially reflected in the 1985 passage of legislation that changed the name of the CCS to the *Program for Children with Special Health Needs (CSHN).*

Numerous other federal programs have been developed. Some that have had a major impact on maternal and child health include the following:

Medicaid—In 1965 Medicaid was created under Title XIX of the Social Security Act to reduce financial barriers to health care for the poor. It is the largest maternal-child health program. A major project under Medicaid is the Child Health Assessment Program (CHAP), which provides services for a large number of pregnant women and children. Not all poor children are eligible for Medicaid; financial eligibility varies considerably from state to state.

Aid to Families with Dependent Children (AFDC)—AFDC was established by the Social Security Act of 1935 as a cash grant program to enable states to aid needy children without fathers.

MCH Services Block Grant—The MCH Services Block Grant provides health services to mothers and children, particularly those with low income or limited access to health services. Its primary purposes are to reduce infant mortality; reduce the incidence of preventable disease and handicapping conditions among children; and increase the availability of prenatal, delivery, and postpartum care to eligible mothers.

Alcohol, Drug Abuse, and Mental Health Block Grant—Established by the Omnibus Budget Reconciliation Act of 1981, this block grant provides funds to states for (1) projects to support prevention, treatment, and rehabilitation related to substance abuse and (2) grants to community mental health centers for the identification, assessment, and treatment of severely mentally disturbed children and adolescents.

Social Services Block Grant—Established under Title XX of the Social Security Act, this block grant provides states with funds for child day care, protective and emergency services, counseling, family planning, home-based services, information and referral, and adoption and foster care services.

Women, Infants, and Children (WIC)—In 1974 the WIC Special Supplemental Food Program was started. It provides nutritious food and nutrition education to low-income, pregnant, postpartum, and lactating women and to infants and children up to age 5 years. Other nutrition programs include Food Stamps; National School Lunch Program; School Breakfast Program; and Child Care Food Program, which provides financial assistance for nutritious meals to children in day care centers, family and group day care homes, and Head Start centers.

Education for All Handicapped Children Act (P.L. 94-142)—In 1975 P.L. 94-142 was passed to provide free appropriate public education to all handicapped children from ages 3 to 21 years and to provide for supportive services (e.g., speech and counseling) that ensure the benefit of special education.

Education of the Handicapped Act Amendments of 1986 (P.L. 99-457)—In 1986, P.L. 99-457 was passed to allow for the provision of federal funding to states to develop and implement a statewide, comprehensive, coordinated, and multidisciplinary program of early intervention services for handicapped infants and toddlers and their families.

Family and Medical Leave Act (FMLA)—Signed into law in 1993, FMLA allows eligible employees to take up to 12 weeks of unpaid leave from their jobs every year to care for newborn or newly adopted children; to care for children, parents, or spouses who have serious health conditions; or to recover from their own serious health conditions. After the leave, the law entitles employees to return to their previous jobs or to equivalent jobs with the same pay, benefits, and other conditions.

Despite the number of federal and state programs available to assist children and families, there remain serious barriers to health care in the United States, including (1) *financial barriers,* such as not having insurance, having insurance that does not cover certain services, or being unable to pay for services; (2) *system barriers,* such as having to travel great distances for health care, or state-to-state variations in Medicaid benefits; and (3) *knowledge barriers,* such as a lack of understanding of the need for prenatal or child health supervision or an unawareness of the services available. The current thrust in health care is to improve children's and families' access to health care.

One of the major changes in health care delivery has been the establishment of a *prospective payment system* based on *diagnosis-related groups (DRGs).* The DRG categories define *pretreatment (prospective) billing* for almost all United States hospitals reimbursed by Medicare. With hospitals now financially responsible when Medicare patients exceed the allotted admission stay, more patients are being discharged early. This has created an immense need for home care and other sources of community-based services. Because health care cost containment remains a national priority, some form of prospective payment will affect children and adults. Nurses need to be aware of the changing economics and be prepared to meet the challenges of managed care companies and health maintenance organizations (HMOs).*

*For information on managed care references and resources, access the website: www.nursingworld.org.

PEDIATRIC NURSING

Philosophy of Care

Nursing of infants and children is consistent with the *definition of nursing* as "the diagnosis and treatment of human responses to actual or potential health problems." This definition incorporates the four essential features of contemporary nursing practice:

1. Attention to the full range of human experiences and responses to health and illness without restriction to a problem-focused orientation
2. Integration of objective data with knowledge gained from an understanding of the patient's or group's subjective experience
3. Application of scientific knowledge to the processes of diagnosis and treatment
4. Provision of a caring relationship that facilitates health and healing (American Nurses Association, 1995)

Family-Centered Care. The philosophy of family-centered care recognizes the family as the constant in a child's life. Service systems and personnel must support, respect, encourage, and enhance the strength and competence of the family through an empowerment approach and effective giving of help (Dunst and Trivette, 1996). Families are supported in their natural caregiving and decision-making roles by building on their unique strengths as individuals and families. They are encouraged to develop their own means of self-care at home and in the community (Hockenberry-Eaton and Diamond, 1994). Patterns of living at home and in the community are promoted. The needs of all family members, not just the child's, are considered (Box 29-1). The philosophy acknowledges diversity among family structures and backgrounds; family goals, dreams, strategies, and actions; and family support, service, and information needs (Ahmann, 1994).*

Two basic concepts in family-centered care are enabling and empowerment. Professionals *enable* families by creating opportunities and means for all family members to display their present abilities and competencies and to acquire new ones that are necessary to meet the needs of the child and family. *Empowerment* describes the interaction of professionals with families in such a way that families maintain or acquire a sense of control over their lives and make positive changes that result from helping behaviors that foster their own strengths, abilities, and actions (Dunst and Trivette, 1996).

The *parent-professional partnership* is a powerful mechanism for enabling and empowering families. Parents serve as respected equals with professionals† and have the right to decide what is important for themselves and their family. The professional's role is to support and strengthen the family's ability

*Resources on family-centered care are available from the Institute for Family-Centered Care, 7900 Wisconsin Avenue, Suite 405, Bethesda, MD 20814; (301) 652-0281, fax (301) 652-0186; website: www.familycenteredcare.org; and the Kennedy Krieger Institute, 707 N. Broadway, Baltimore, MD 21205; 1-888-554-2080; website: www.kennedykrieger.org.

For additional information, please view "Family-Centered Care" in ***Whaley and Wong's Pediatric Nursing Video Series,*** St Louis, 1996, Mosby; 1-800-426-4545; website: www.mosby.com.

†For information about parent-professional partnerships, a free pamphlet *Equals in This Partnership* is available from The National Center for Infants, Toddlers and Families, 734 15th Street NW, Suite 1000, Washington, DC 20005-1013; phone (202) 638-1144; website: www.zerotothree.org.

Box 29-1

The Key Elements of Family-Centered Care

Incorporating into policy and practice the recognition that the ***family is the constant*** in a child's life whereas the service systems and the support personnel within those systems fluctuate

Facilitating ***family/professional collaboration*** at all levels of hospital, home, and community care:
Care of an individual child
Program development, implementation, and evaluation
Policy formation

Exchanging complete and unbiased information between family members and professionals in a supportive manner at all times

Incorporating into policy and practice the recognition and ***honoring of cultural diversity,*** strengths, and individuality within and across all families, including ***ethnic, racial, spiritual, social, economic, educational,*** and ***geographic diversity***

Recognizing and respecting ***different methods of coping*** and implementing comprehensive policies and programs that provide ***developmental, educational, emotional, environmental,*** and ***financial support*** to meet the diverse needs of families

Encouraging and facilitating ***family-to-family support*** and networking

Ensuring that ***home, hospital,*** and ***community service*** and ***support systems*** for children needing specialized health and developmental care and their families are ***flexible, accessible,*** and ***comprehensive*** in responding to diverse family-identified needs

Appreciating families as families and children as children, recognizing that they possess a wide range of strengths, concerns, emotions, and aspirations beyond their need for specialized health and developmental services and support

From Shelton TL, Stepanek JS: *Family-centered care for children needing specialized health and developmental services,* Bethesda, MD, 1994, Association for the Care of Children's Health.

to nurture and promote its members' development in a way that is both enabling and empowering. Professionals must also work together as a team to benefit children and their families (Patterson, 1996).

Partnerships imply the belief that partners are capable individuals who become more capable by sharing knowledge, skills, and resources in a manner that benefits all participants. Collaboration is viewed as a continuum. Families have the option of being anywhere along that continuum, depending on their strengths and needs and the professionals who are involved. The nurse can help every family, including those with a previous history of serious personal and/or family problems, to identify its strengths, build on them, and assume a comfortable level of participation. Although caring for the family is strongly emphasized throughout the text, it is highlighted in features such as Cultural Awareness, Family Focus, and Family Home Care boxes.

Atraumatic Care. Although tremendous advances have been made in pediatric care, many changes that have cured illness and prolonged life are traumatic, painful, upsetting, and frightening. Unfortunately, minimizing the trauma of medical interventions has not kept pace with the technologic advances. With knowledge of the stressors imposed on ill children and their families, and armed with interventions that are safe and effective in eliminating or reducing these stressors, health professionals must direct their efforts to providing atraumatic care.

Atraumatic care is the provision of therapeutic care in settings, by personnel, and through the use of interventions that eliminate or minimize the psychologic and physical distress experienced by children and their families in the health care system. *Therapeutic care* encompasses the prevention, diagnosis, treatment, or palliation of chronic or acute conditions. *Setting* refers to whatever place that care is given (e.g., the home, the hospital, or any other health cares setting). *Personnel* include anyone directly involved in providing therapeutic care. *Interventions* range from psychologic approaches, such as preparing children for procedures, to physical interventions, such as providing space for a parent to room-in with a child. *Psychologic distress* may include anxiety, fear, anger, disappointment, sadness, shame, and guilt. *Physical distress* may range from sleeplessness and immobilization to the experience of disturbing sensory stimuli such as pain, temperature extremes, loud noises, bright lights, or darkness. Atraumatic care is concerned with the who, what, when, where, why, and how of any procedure performed on a child for the purpose of preventing or minimizing psychologic and physical stress (Wong, 1989).

The overriding goal in providing atraumatic care is *first, do no harm.* Three principles provide the framework for achieving this goal: (1) prevent or minimize the child's separation from the family; (2) promote a sense of control; and (3) prevent or minimize bodily injury and pain. Examples of providing atraumatic care include fostering the parent-child relationship during hospitalization, preparing the child before any unfamiliar treatment or procedure, controlling pain, allowing the child privacy, providing play activities for expression of fear and aggression, providing choices to children, and respecting cultural differences.

Throughout the text the concept of atraumatic care is an integral part of all discussions of nursing care. Selected examples are highlighted in Atraumatic Care boxes. Many other boxes and tables focusing on culture, family teaching, research, and critical thinking incorporate aspects of providing care as atraumatically as possible. Chapter 44, Reaction to Illness and Hospitalization, is organized according to the principles of providing atraumatic care.

Case Management. Case management has a rich history of coordinating care to control costs (Kersbergen, 1996). The movement to case management began in adult care but was quickly adapted to pediatric care. Benefits to case management, such as improved patient/family satisfaction, decreased fragmentation of care, and the ability to describe and measure outcomes for a homogeneous group of patients, became apparent.

Case managers have responsibility and accountability for a particular group of patients and use a system of paths or timelines derived from standards of care to plan care (Kaufman and Blanchon, 1996).

These timelines have a variety of names: critical paths, guidelines for care, case management plans, Caremaps,* coordi-

*Caremap is a registered trademark of the Center for Case Management, Inc., South Natick, MA 01760; phone (508) 651-2600.

nated care plans, or other titles that are agreed on within a specific agency. Regardless of the name given to the timeline, these are multidisciplinary plans that include all the components of care for an episode or multiple episodes of illness, as well as the outcomes that are expected as a result of delivering that care. They can be confined to inpatient care or can include the entire continuum of care, including home care (see also Chapter 43). Care paths are the tools of case management. Many nursing skills that are not acknowledged are made visible by the numerous responsibilities outlined by the care path (MacPhee and Hoffenberg, 1996).

Concurrent with the movement to provide care in a systematic manner are efforts by professional and government organizations to develop *clinical practice guidelines* for the care of an illness, disease, or related problems. Although timelines for care are usually developed within an institution and reflect local practice patterns, clinical guidelines are developed on a national level and reflect the research that has been conducted relative to a specific disease or illness. A federal agency that has developed clinical guidelines is the Agency for Health Care Research and Quality (AHRQ).*

As the movement for providing care based on guidelines continues, institutions are challenged to incorporate clinical guidelines into the timelines for care that are developed locally. The result of this effort has been professionally developed clinical guidelines that can be integrated into practice at the local level.

It is expected that future payment for health care will be tied to clinical guidelines. This effort will provide encouragement for care to be provided in the most cost-effective manner while ensuring care that is based on guidelines that reflect state-of-the-art care rather than traditional practice.

Role of the Pediatric Nurse

Therapeutic Relationship. The establishment of a therapeutic relationship is the essential foundation for providing quality nursing care. Pediatric nurses need to be meaningfully related to children and their families and yet separate enough to distinguish their own feelings and needs. In a *therapeutic relationship,* caring, well-defined boundaries separate the nurse from the child and family. These boundaries are positive and professional and promote the family's control over the child's health care (McKlindon and Barnsteiner, 1999; Rushton, McEnhill, and Armstrong, 1996). Both the nurse and the family are empowered, and open communication is maintained. In a *nontherapeutic relationship* these boundaries are blurred, and many of the nurse's actions may serve personal needs (e.g., a need to feel wanted and involved) rather than the family's needs.

Although relevant in all settings, a family-centered approach to nursing practice is most obvious in the home care arena. However, it is in the home care setting that nurses face the greatest challenge in determining the boundary between a collaborative relationship with the family and becoming part of the family system. Several factors challenge the maintenance of such clear boundaries: the informal home environment, the casual social conversations that occur with family members throughout the day, the participation by family members in care of the child, and the attempt by some families to reduce the stress of having a stranger in the home by incorporating the nurse as a member of the family.

Exploring whether relationships with patients are therapeutic or nontherapeutic can help nurses identify problem areas early in their interactions with children and families. Although questions for exploring types of involvement can be labeled negative or positive, no one action makes a relationship therapeutic or nontherapeutic. For example, nurses may spend additional time with the family but still recognize their own needs and maintain professional separateness. An important clue to nontherapeutic relationships is the staff's concerns about their peer's actions with the family.*

Family Advocacy/Caring. Although nurses are responsible to themselves, the profession, and the institution of employment, their primary responsibility is to the consumer of nursing services, the child, and the family. The nurse must work with members of the family, identify their goals and needs, and plan interventions that best meet the defined problems. As an advocate, the nurse assists children and their families in making informed choices and acting in the child's best interest. Advocacy involves ensuring that families are aware of all available health services, are informed adequately of treatments and procedures, are involved in the child's care, and are encouraged to change or support existing health care practices. The United Nations Declaration of the Rights of the Child (Box 29-2) provides guidelines for nursing practice to ensure that every child receives optimum care. The nurse uses this knowledge to adapt care for the child's optimum physical and emotional well-being.

As nurses care for children and families, they must demonstrate *caring* by expressing compassion and empathy for others. Aspects of caring embody the concept of atraumatic care and the development of a therapeutic relationship with patients. Parents perceive caring as a sign of quality nursing care, which is often focused on the nontechnical needs of the child and family. Parents describe "personable" care as actions by the nurse, including acknowledging the parents' presence, listening, mak-

*To order guidelines, contact AHRQ Publications Clearinghouse, P.O. Box 8547, Silver Spring, MD 20907; 1-800-358-9295; website: www.guideline.gov.

*For information on one hospital's guidelines for establishing therapeutic relationships between nurses and children and families, contact Jane H. Barnsteiner, PhD, RN, FAAN, Director of Nursing Practice and Research, Children's Hospital of Philadelphia, 34th and Civic Center Blvd., Philadelphia, PA 19104-4399; (215) 590-3147; e-mail barnsteiner@email.chop.edu.

Box 29-2

United Nations' Declaration of the Rights of the Child

All children need:
- To be free from discrimination
- To develop physically and mentally in freedom and dignity
- To have a name and nationality
- To have adequate nutrition, housing, recreation, and medical services
- To receive special treatment if handicapped
- To receive love, understanding, and material security
- To receive an education and develop his or her abilities
- To be the first to receive protection in disaster
- To be protected from neglect, cruelty, and exploitation
- To be brought up in a spirit of friendship among people

ing the parent feel comfortable in the hospital environment, involving the parent and child in the nursing care, showing interest and concern for their welfare, showing affection and sensitivity to the parent and child, communicating with them, and individualizing the nursing care. Parents perceive "personable" nursing care as being integral to establishing a positive relationship.

The nurse is aware of the needs of children and works with all caregivers to ensure that these fundamental requirements are met. This often necessitates that the nurse expand the boundaries of practice to less traditional settings. The nurse may be involved in education, political/legislative change, rehabilitation, screening, administration, and even engineering and architecture. Regardless of how removed from direct patient care individual nurses become, they continue to foster health care practices that promote the well-being of children by incorporating knowledge of child growth and development into particular roles of practice. For example, as an educator the nurse has the primary responsibility of helping others learn about and care for children. The nurse's audience may be other nurses, parents, schoolteachers, other members of the health team, or the general public.

Disease Prevention/Health Promotion. The trends toward health care have been prevention of illness and maintenance of health, rather than treatment of disease or disability. Nursing has kept pace with this change, especially in the area of child care. In 1965 specialized *pediatric nurse practitioner (PNP)* programs began to be developed, and have led to several specialized ambulatory or primary care roles for nurses. The thrust of these programs has been to educate nurses beyond the basic preparational stage in areas of child health maintenance so that all children can receive high-quality care. The practitioner programs have expanded to prepare specialized PNPs such as oncology pediatric nurse practitioners. Although the curriculum varies, the course content generally includes history-taking, physical diagnosis, growth and development, health education, pharmacology, counseling, common childhood problems, and planning care for individuals and groups. These programs are now part of graduate nursing education.

The *clinical nurse specialist (CNS)* role has been developed in an attempt to provide expert nursing care. In addition, the CNS serves as a role model for the staff's clinical practice, as a researcher to validate nursing observations and interventions, as a change agent within the health care system, and as a consultant/teacher to the health care team. The clinical specialist is competent in providing nursing care during all stages of illness or wellness, and functions in any of the settings where patients may be found (e.g., the hospital, home, community, clinic, or long-term facility). The CNS role has developed within each of the traditional specialty areas and includes subspecialties such as cardiovascular, oncologic, and neurologic pediatric CNS. The educational preparation includes a graduate degree in nursing. Several graduate programs now combine the PNP and CNS roles, an issue that continues to receive much attention (Page and Mackowiak, 1997). Although the title for the merged roles varies, these nurses are commonly called *advanced nurse practitioners (ANPs)*. Advanced practice nurses staff and manage health care clinics (Segal-Isaacson, 1996).

Every nurse involved with child care must practice preventive health care. Regardless of the identified problem, the role of the nurse is to plan care that fosters every aspect of growth and development. In a thorough assessment process, problems related to nutrition, immunizations, safety, dental care, development, socialization, discipline, or schooling often become obvious. Once the problem is identified, the nurse acts to intervene directly or to refer the family to other health persons or agencies.

The best approach to prevention is education and anticipatory guidance. The chapters on health promotion that follow include sections on anticipatory guidance. An appreciation of the hazards or conflicts of each developmental period enables the nurse to guide parents regarding childrearing practices aimed at preventing potential problems. One of the most significant examples is safety. Because each age group is at risk for special types of injuries, preventive teaching can help prevent most injuries and significantly lower permanent disability and mortality from injuries in children.

Prevention also involves less obvious aspects of child care. Besides preventing physical disease or injury, the nurse's role is also to promote mental health. For example, it is not sufficient to administer immunizations without regard for the psychologic trauma associated with the procedure. Optimum health involves the practice of good medicine with a humane approach to health care; the nurse is often the one professional capable of ensuring "humanity."

Health Teaching. Health teaching is inseparable from family advocacy and illness prevention. Health teaching may be a direct goal of the nurse, such as during parenting classes; or may be indirect, such as helping parents and children understand a diagnosis or medical treatment, encouraging children to ask questions about their bodies, referring families to health-related professional or lay groups, supplying patients with appropriate literature, and providing anticipatory guidance.

Health teaching is often one area in which nurses need preparation and practice with competent role models, because it involves transmitting information at the child's and family's level of understanding and desire for information. As an effective educator, the nurse focuses on giving appropriate health teaching with generous feedback and evaluation to promote learning.

Support/Counseling. Attention to emotional needs requires support and sometimes counseling. The role of child advocate or health teacher is supportive by the very nature of the individualized approach. Support can be offered in the following ways: listening, touching, and physical presence. Touching and physical presence are most helpful with children because they facilitate nonverbal communication.

Counseling involves a mutual exchange of ideas and opinions that provides the basis for mutual problem solving. It involves support, teaching, techniques to foster expression of feelings or thoughts, and approaches to help the family cope with stress. Optimally, counseling not only helps to resolve a crisis or problem but also enables the family to attain a higher level of functioning, greater self-esteem, and closer relationships. Although counseling is often the role of nurses in more specialized areas, counseling techniques are discussed in various sections of this text to help students and nurses cope with immediate crises and refer families for additional professional assistance.

Restorative Role. The most basic of all nursing roles is the restoration of health through caregiving activities. Nurses are intimately involved with meeting the physical and emotional needs of children, including feeding, bathing, toileting, dressing, security, and socialization. Although they are responsible for instituting physicians' orders, they are also held singularly accountable for their own actions and judgments regardless of written orders.

A significant aspect of restoration of health is continual assessment and evaluation of physical status. In the chapters that follow, the concentrated focus on physical assessment, pathophysiology, and scientific rationale for therapy assist the nurse in decision making regarding health status. The nurse must be aware of normal findings in order to identify and document deviations. In addition, the pediatric nurse never loses sight of the child's individual emotional and developmental needs, which can significantly influence the course of the disease process.

Coordination/Collaboration. The nurse, as a member of the health team, collaborates and coordinates nursing services with the activities of other professionals. Working in isolation does not serve the child's best interest. The concept of "holistic care" can only be realized through a unified interdisciplinary approach. Being aware of individual contributions and limitations to the child's care, the nurse must collaborate with other specialists to provide high-quality health services. Failure to recognize limitations can be nontherapeutic and perhaps destructive. For example, the nurse who feels competent in counseling but who is really inadequate in this area may not only prevent the child from dealing with a crisis but may also impede future success with a qualified professional.

Even nurses who practice in isolated geographic areas, widely separated from other health professionals, cannot be considered independent. Every nurse works interdependently with the child and family, collaborating on needs and interventions so that the final care plan is one that truly meets the child's needs. Unfortunately, this aspect of collaboration and coordination is often lacking in health care planning. Numerous disciplines often work together to formulate a comprehensive approach without consulting patients regarding their ideas or preferences. The nurse is in a vital position to include consumers in their care, either directly or indirectly, by communicating their thoughts to the health team.

Ethical Decision Making. Ethical dilemmas arise when competing moral considerations underlie various alternatives. Parents, nurses, physicians, and other health care team members may reach different but morally defensible decisions by assigning different weights to the competing moral values. These competing moral values may include *autonomy,* the patient's right to be self-governing; *nonmaleficence,* the obligation to minimize or prevent harm; *beneficence,* the obligation to promote the patient's well-being; and *justice,* the concept of fairness (Cornelison, 1998; Salvatore and Baxter, 1998). Nurses must determine the most beneficial or least harmful action within the framework of societal mores, professional practice standards, the law, institutional rules, religious traditions, the family's value system, and the nurse's personal values.

When ethical conflicts occur, nurses may experience conflicting loyalties to their profession, colleagues, patients and families, institutions, and society. The nurse's role in ethical decision making can be ambiguous; a nurse may be obliged to carry out procedures that are based on physician orders or hospital policy but inconsistent with the patient's best interest. At times, members of the health care team do not seek the nurse's input or involvement, leaving the nurse with incomplete information about the clinical situation or without a voice in decision making.

The role of nurses as members of the health care team justifies their participation in collaborative ethical decision making. Nurses routinely use a systematic problem-solving method known as the *nursing process* to resolve clinical problems. Each decision requires the nurse to collect pertinent physiologic and psychosocial data, assess relevant values held by the patient and family, and incorporate those data into a plan of care. Each of these activities is a crucial component of ethical decision making.

Furthermore, because nurses spend the most time directly caring for the child, they are in a unique position to provide insight about the patient's condition and response to therapy. In addition, they assist families in dealing with their grief and stress and often interpret information regarding the child's condition, prognosis, and treatment options to help families make informed decisions. Because of their relationship to families, nurses are able to represent the child's and parents' values, beliefs, and preferences, thus serving as an important liaison for communication between the family and other health team members.

The nurse also uses the professional code of ethics for guidance and as a means for professional self-regulation. The Code for Nurses by the American Nurses Association focuses on the nurse's accountability and responsibility to the patient and emphasizes the nursing role as an independent, professional one that upholds its own legal liability (Box 29-3).

Box 29-3

Code of Nurses

1. The nurse provides services with respect for human dignity and the uniqueness of the patient unrestricted by considerations of social or economic status, personal attributes, or the nature of health problems.
2. The nurse safeguards the patient's right to privacy by judiciously protecting information of a confidential nature.
3. The nurse acts to safeguard the patient and the public when health care and safety are affected by the incompetent, unethical, or illegal practice of any person.
4. The nurse assumes responsibility and accountability for individual nursing judgments and actions.
5. The nurse maintains competence in nursing.
6. The nurse exercises informal judgment and uses individual competence and qualifications as criteria in seeking consultation, accepting responsibilities, and delegating nursing activities to others.
7. The nurse participates in activities that contribute to the ongoing development of the profession's body of knowledge.
8. The nurse participates in the profession's efforts to implement and improve standards of nursing.
9. The nurse participates in the profession's efforts to establish and maintain conditions of employment conducive to high quality nursing care.
10. The nurse participates in the profession's effort to protect the public from misinformation and misrepresentation and to maintain the integrity of nursing.
11. The nurse collaborates with members of the health professions and other citizens in promoting community and national efforts to meet the health needs of the public.

American Nurses Association, 1997. Reproduced with permission of the American Nurses Association.

Nurses must prepare themselves systematically for collaborative ethical decision making. This can be accomplished through formal coursework, continuing education, contemporary literature, and working to establish an environment conductive to ethical discourse. Nurses must be knowledgeable about mechanisms for dispute resolution, case review by ethics committees, procedural safeguards, state statutes, and case law.

Nurses often face ethical issues regarding patient care, such as the use of lifesaving measures for very-low-birth-weight newborns or the terminally ill child's right to refuse treatment. They may struggle with questions regarding truthfulness, balancing their rights and responsibilities in caring for children with AIDS, whistle-blowing, or resource allocation.

Research. Practicing nurses should contribute to research because they are the individuals observing human responses to health and illness. Unfortunately, few nurses systematically record or analyze such observations. For example, pediatric nurses devise innovative methods to encourage children to comply with treatments. If these interventions are clinically evaluated and shared with other nurses in research publications, nursing practice can be based primarily on science, not tradition or trial and error.

The current emphasis on measurable outcomes to determine the efficacy of interventions (often in relation to the cost) demands that nurses know whether clinical interventions result in positive outcomes for their patients. This demand has influenced the current trend toward *evidence-based practice.* Evidence-based practice implies questioning why something is effective and if there is a better approach. The concept of evidence-based practice also involves analyzing and translating published clinical research into the everyday practice of nursing. When nurses base their clinical practice on science and research, and document their clinical outcomes, they will be able to validate their contributions to health, wellness, and cure not only to their patients, third-party payers, and institutions, but also to the nursing profession (Freda, 1998). Evaluation is essential to the nursing process, and research is one of the best ways to accomplish this.

Health Care Planning. In recent years the nurse's role has expanded beyond the nucleus of the family to include the community (Kerfoot, 1996). Traditionally nurses have been involved in public health care, either on a continuous or an episodic basis. Rarely, however, have nurses been involved in health care planning, especially on a political or legislative level.

In the future, nurses must incorporate a political component into their professional identity and attempt to influence the decision-making body of government (Brown, 1996).*

As the largest health care profession, nursing needs to have a voice, especially as family/consumer advocate. This suggests a knowledge and awareness of community needs, interest in government formulation of bills, support of politicians to ensure passage (or rejection) of significant legislation, and active involvement in groups dedicated to the welfare of children (e.g., professional nursing societies, parent-teacher organizations, parent support groups, religious organizations, and voluntary organizations).

*The following are sources of information on government issues: White House Comment Line, (202) 456-1119 (9 AM-5 PM EST); White House fax (202) 456-2461; White House e-mail: president@whitehouse.gov.

Health care planning involves not only providing new services but also promoting the highest quality of existing ones. Nursing needs to ensure the excellence of its own profession through each individual member, who practices according to the Code of Nurses and standards of practice. A standard of practice is the level of performance that is expected of a professional. Pediatric nurses are obligated to follow the Standards of Maternal-Child Health Nursing (Box 29-4) and specific standards for their specialty, such as pediatric oncology nursing or school nursing.* They should also be involved in making certain their colleagues implement the standards through education, role modeling, and supervision.

Throughout the following chapters, the highest standards of nursing practice are continually reflected in the emphasis on thorough assessment, focus on scientific rationale as the basis for care, summary of nursing care goals and responsibilities, and comprehensive discussion of growth and development. Family-centered principles are continually evident in the consideration of dynamics affecting the child, parents, siblings, and

*Available from the Association of Pediatric Oncology Nurses, 4700 W. Lake Avenue, Glenview, IL 60025-1485; (847) 375-4700; fax (847) 375-4777; website: www.apon.org; and the National Association of School Nurses, Lamplighter Lane, P.O. Box 1300, Scarborough, ME 04074-1300; (207) 883-2117; website: www.nasn.org.

Box 29-4

American Nurses Association Standards of Maternal and Child Health Nursing Practice

Standard I: The nurse helps children and parents attain and maintain optimum health.

Standard II: The nurse assists families to achieve and maintain a balance between the personal growth needs of individual family members and optimum family functioning.

Standard III: The nurse intervenes with vulnerable patients and families at risk to prevent potential developmental and health problems.

Standard IV: The nurse promotes an environment free of hazards to reproduction, growth and development, wellness and recovery from illness.

Standard V: The nurse detects changes in health status and deviations from optimum development.

Standard VI: The nurse carries out appropriate interventions and treatment to facilitate survival and recovery from illness.

Standard VII: The nurse assists patients and families to understand and cope with developmental and traumatic situations during illness, childbearing, childrearing, and childhood.

Standard VIII: The nurse actively pursues strategies to enhance access to and utilization of adequate health care services.

Standard IX: The nurse improves maternal and child health nursing practice through evaluation of practice, education, and research.

From American Nurses Association: *Standards of maternal and child health nursing practice,* Washington, DC, 1983, The Association. (As of this writing, unrevised and out of print.)

extended members. The nurse is viewed as a vital component of the health care delivery system.

Future Trends

The present shift in focus from treatment of disease to promotion of health will expand nurses' roles in ambulatory care, with prevention and health teaching receiving a major emphasis. As prospective payment becomes more obvious in pediatric care, the need for home care and community health services will require nurses to be more independent and highly skilled beyond the traditional care settings. Both of these trends are illustrated throughout the following chapters, with increased emphasis on prevention through anticipatory guidance, child health and family assessment, and discharge planning and care in the home and community. As changing social policy shapes the expanding health care arena, the focus of nursing care is no longer what we *do for* families, but rather what we *do in partnership with* them (Plotnick and Presler, 1996). Therefore the philosophy of family-centered care is no longer an option, but a mandate.

Technologic advances related to patient care, as well as the demand for computer knowledge in the work setting, are inevitable future trends. As more positions are created in the health care system that do not require a nursing background (e.g., "patient care educator" and unlicensed assistive personnel), nurses will be required to continually update their knowledge and demonstrate their unique contribution. *Unlicensed assistive personnel (UAP)* "are individuals who are trained to function in an assistive role to the registered professional nurse in the provision of [student] care activities as delegated by and under the supervision of the registered professional nurse" (American Nurses Association, 1994).

NURSE ALERT • When the registered nurse (RN) determines that someone who is not licensed to practice nursing can safely provide a selected nursing activity or task for a patient, and delegates that activity to the individual, the RN remains responsible and legally accountable for the care provided.

Changing demographics will also impact pediatric nursing. Although the actual number of children under age 18 years will increase from 64.3 million in 1990 to an estimated 78 million in 2020, their relative importance in terms of proportion of the total population will decrease from 26% to 24%. In other words, the adult population is growing faster than the pediatric population. Accompanying this trend is a decrease in younger children and an increase in older children, as well as a decrease in the Caucasian population with an increase in minority groups. For example, Caucasian births are expected to decline, African-American births are projected to rise, and the largest increases will occur in Hispanic and Asian births. Such changes will impact the delivery of health care, with problems of adolescents and minority groups taking on more significance. As the elderly make up a larger percentage of the population, health care dollars will be split between the youngest and oldest groups, with shrinking resources having to meet the needs of both. Nurses will need to keep abreast of developments in adolescent medicine and continually adapt their care to the cultural milieu in which they practice. An ever-present challenge will be cost containment without sacrificing quality care.

Key Points

- *Healthy People 2010* broadened the health care objectives achieved in the 1990s and focuses on prevention as the method of achieving its goals.
- Although the infant mortality rate in the United States is at an all-time low, the United States lags significantly behind most other major industrialized countries such as Canada.
- Low birth weight, which is closely related to early gestational age, is considered the leading cause of neonatal death in the United States.
- Injuries are the leading cause of death in children over age 1 year, with the majority being motor vehicle injuries.
- Childhood morbidity encompasses acute illness, chronic disease, and disability.
- Eighty percent of childhood illness is attributable to infections, with respiratory tract infections occurring two to three times as often as all other illnesses combined.
- The "new morbidity" refers to behavioral, social, and educational problems that can significantly alter a child's health.
- Developmental stage and environment are important factors in the prevalence of injuries at a given age and help to direct preventive measures.
- During the first half of the 1980s public health initiatives such as environmental strategies to control infection and the development of antibiotics were the major advances leading to decreased childhood deaths.
- During the latter half of the 1990s the advancement and application of medical knowledge and technology, specifically in the care of high risk and low-birth-weight newborns, lowered the number of deaths in children, especially the neonatal mortality rate.
- The work of Lillian Wald, a social reformer, has had far-reaching effects on child health and nursing. She started visiting nurse services in New York City and was instrumental in establishing the role of the first full-time school nurse.
- The philosophy of family-centered care recognizes the family as the constant in a child's life, and that service systems and personnel must support, respect, encourage, and enhance the strength and competence of the family.
- Atraumatic care is the provision of therapeutic care in settings, by personnel, and through the use of interventions that eliminate or minimize the psychologic and physical distress experienced by children and their families in the health care system.
- Managed care is a health care delivery system that attempts to balance cost and quality through a network of health care providers and predetermined prospective payment for services.
- The pediatric nurse's roles include a therapeutic relationship, family advocacy, disease prevention/health promotion, health teaching, support-counseling, coordination/collaboration, ethical decision making, research, and health care planning.

- With the shift in focus from treatment of disease to promotion of health, nurses' roles have expanded in ambulatory care and community, with emphasis on prevention and health teaching.
- Changing demographics will result in greater significance of adolescents' and minority groups' problems and decreasing resources for health care.
- Critical thinking is purposeful, goal-directed thinking based on rational and deliberate thought.
- The process of nursing children and families includes accurate and complete assessment, analysis of assessment data to arrive at a nursing diagnosis, planning of care, implementation of the plan, and evaluation of interventions.

References

Ahmann E: Family-centered care; the time has come, *Pediatr Nurs* 20(1):52-53, 1994.

American Nurses Association: *Nursing's social policy statement,* Washington, DC, 1995, American Nurses Publishing.

American Nurses Association: *Registered professional nurses and unlicensed assistive personnel,* Washington, DC, 1994, American Nurses Publishing.

Brown SG: Incorporating political socialization theory into baccalaureate nursing education, *Nurs Outlook* 44(3):120-123, 1996.

Christoffel K et al: Psychosocial factors in childhood pedestrian injury: a matched case-control study, *Pediatrics* 97(1):33-42, 1996.

Cornelison AH: A profile of ethical principles, *J Pediatr Nurs* 13(6):383-386, 1998.

Dunst CJ, Trivette C: Empowerment, effective help-giving practices and family centered care, *Pediatr Nurs* 22(4):334-337, 1996.

Freda MC: Toward evidence-based practice, *MCN* 23:177, 1998.

Guyer B et al: Annual summary of vital statistics—1998, *Pediatrics* 104(6):1229-1245, 1999.

Guyer B, Minkovitz CS, Strobino D: Morbidity and mortality among the young. In Hoekelman A: *Primary pediatric care,* ed 4, St Louis, 2001, Mosby.

Hockenberry-Eaton M, Diamond J: Family centered care for children with chronic illnesses, *J Pediatr Health Care* 8: 196-197, 1994.

Kaufman J, Blanchon D: Managed care for children with special needs: a care coordination model, *J Care Manage* 2(2):46-59, 1996.

Kersbergen AL: Case management: a rich history of coordinating care to control costs, *Nurs Outlook* 44(4):169-172, 1996.

Kerfoot K: The new nursing leader for the new world order of health care, *Pediatr Nurs* 22(4):349-350, 1996.

Lears MK, Guth KJ, Lewandowski L: International adoption: a printer for pediatric nurses, *Pediatr Nurs* 24:578-586, 1998.

Loubiala PJ et al: Day-care centers and diarrhea: a public health perspective, *J Pediatr* 131:476-479, 1997.

MacPhee M, Hoffenberg E: Nursing case management for children with failure to thrive, *J Pediatr Health Care* 10(2):63-73, 1996.

Mathews TS, Curtin SC, MacDorman MF: Infant mortality statistics from the 1998 period linked birth/infant death data set, *Natl Vital Stat Rep* 48(12):1-25, 2000.

McKlindon D, Barnsteiner JH: Therapeutic relationships. Evolution of the Children's Hospital of Philadelphia model, *MCN Am J Matern Child Nurs* 24(5):237-243, 1999.

Mofenson HC, Greensher J: Injury prevention. In Hoekelman RA: *Primary pediatric care,* ed 3, St Louis, 1997, Mosby.

Murphy SL: Deaths: final data for 1998, *Natl Vital Stat Rep* 48(11):1-105, 2000.

National Safety Council: *Injury facts,* Itaska, IL, 1999, National Safety Council.

Office of Disease Prevention and Health Promotion: *Developing objectives for* Healthy People 2010, Washington, DC, September 1997, U.S. Department of Health and Human Services.

Page ME, Mackowiak L: The clinical nurse specialist and nurse practitioner: complementary roles, *J Soc Pediatr Nurs* 2(4): 188-190, 1997.

Patterson E: Nursing children with disabilities: a conceptual framework for organizing services, *Aust J Adv Nurs* 13(3): 32-39, 1996.

Plotnick J, Presler B: Rugged individualism and compassion: the foundation of public policy, *MCN* 21(1):20-33, 1996.

Rachuba L, Stanton B, Howard D: Violent crime in the United States, *Arch Pediatr Adolesc Med* 149(9):953-960, 1995.

Rushton CH, McEnhill M, Armstrong L: Establishing therapeutic boundaries as patient advocates, *Pediatr Nurs* 22(3): 185-189, 1996.

Salvatore T, Baxter T: *Administrative ethics: a guide for home care providers,* Springfield, PA, 1998, HCMA Ltd.

Segal-Isaacson AE: Negotiating the reimbursement morass, *Adv Pract Nurs Sourcebook* 1:4-6, 1996.

U.S. Department of Health and Human Services: *Healthy People 2010* (Conference Edition in Two Volumes). Washington, DC: January 2000, USDHHS.

Ventura SJ et al: Births and deaths: preliminary data for 1997, *National Vital Statistic Reports* 47(4), 1998.

Wong D: Principles of atraumatic care. In Feeg V, editor: *Pediatric nursing: forum on the future: looking toward the 21st century,* Pitman, NJ, 1989, Anthony J Jannetti.

CHAPTER

30 Community-Based Nursing Care of the Child and Family

http://www.harcourthealth.com/MERLIN/Wong/maternal/

Learning Objectives

On completion of this chapter the reader will be able to:

- Define community nursing.
- Identify a target population.
- Describe selected aspects of the epidemiologic process.
- Discuss the pediatric continuum of care.
- Explain the components of the community nursing process.

DEFINITION OF COMMUNITY

A *community* can be defined as a group of people living in a specific geographic area (Hitchcock, Schubert, and Thomas, 1999). A community is also a system that includes children and families, the physical environment, educational facilities, safety and transportation resources, political and governmental agencies, health and social services, communication resources, economic resources, and recreational facilities (Anderson and McFarlane, 1996). Community health initiatives are directed at either the general health of the community as a whole, or at specific populations within the community that have unique needs. *Populations* are defined as groups of people with common values such as religion, age, ethnicity, culture, or beliefs (see Chapter 31 for specific cultures). These common values often guide various behaviors of populations such as health promotion activities. *Target populations* are groups of people toward whom health care workers direct their activities to improve the health status of individuals in the group.

Community care encompasses an alliance of health care providers, advocates, government agencies, managed care organizations, businesses, and the children and families within a specific community. The mission of an alliance that provides community care is to collaboratively provide access to services that promote the child health initiatives of *Healthy People 2010** (Velsor-Friedrich, 2000). The alliance collaborates to identify, plan, implement, and evaluate the health system within a community. Community care is "without walls" in that the services of the health care system are often redesigned to meet the changing needs of the community. *Community nursing* empowers children and families to advocate effectively for the resources they need to maintain optimal health. Community nursing and community care are practiced in the following settings within the community: home health agencies, schools, doctors' offices, ambulatory health clinics, emergency rooms, triage call centers, insurance agencies, health departments, international relief agencies, health education agencies, juvenile detention facilities, camps, day care centers, foster care facilities, and rehabilitation agencies. The American Nurses Association has established nine standards for community health nursing related to the following categories: theory, data collection, diagnosis, planning, intervention, evaluation, quality assurance and professional development, interdisciplinary collaboration, and research. An understanding of the processes that guide nursing care in a community is essential for all nurses. These processes include the epidemiologic process, continuity of care, and the community nursing process.

*The *Healthy People 2010* website can be accessed at: www.health.gov/

EPIDEMIOLOGIC PROCESS

Epidemiology is the science of community health applied to the detection and identification of causes of morbidity and mortality. The epidemiologic process identifies the distribution and causes of disease, injury, or illness and determines the levels of prevention. *Healthy People 2010** is an example of a health promotion and disease prevention program that was developed using the epidemiologic process. (Lurie, 2000).

Measuring the Distribution of Disease, Injury, or Illness

Morbidity rates are used to measure illness and accidents; along with natality and mortality rates, they present an objective picture of the health status of a community. There are two types of rates: incidence and prevalence. *Incidence* measures the occurrence of new events in a population over a time. *Prevalence* measures existing events in a population over a time (Hitchcock, Schubert, and Thomas, 1999). For example, the incidence of type 1 diabetes in a particular community is estimated by counting the new cases of type 1 diabetes in a population and dividing that figure by the population at risk. The prevalence of type 1 diabetes is estimated by counting the existing cases of type 1 diabetes in a population and dividing that figure by the population at risk. Both incidence and prevalence are usually given as rates per 1000, 10,000, or 100,000 population, depending on their frequency.

Causative Agents

Causative agents are classified into the following three general categories (Lancaster and Lancaster, 1996):

1. **Environmental**—Includes agents such as pollution of air, water, or food; noise hazards; presence of toxic wastes; and exposure to toxic substances such as lead or carbon monoxide
2. **Behavioral**—Includes agents such as alcohol and drug abuse, violence, smoking, high risk lifestyles, stress, lack of exercise, crime, noncompliance with treatment regimens, and accidental injuries
3. **Biologic**—Includes genetic or familial predisposition to diseases such as asthma or diabetes; genetically inherited disorders such as hemophilia or Down syndrome; and exposure to infectious diseases such as human immunodeficiency virus, mumps, tuberculosis, or hepatitis

Levels of Prevention

Three levels of intervention are included in the epidemiologic process: primary, secondary, and tertiary. Community health programs are based on these three levels of prevention (Hitchcock, Schubert, and Thomas, 1999). *Primary prevention* interventions are interventions that protect children from disease or injury. Examples of these interventions include well-child care clinics, immunization programs, safety programs (e.g., bike helmets, car seats, seat belts, and childproof containers), nutrition programs, environmental efforts (e.g., recycling and clean air programs), sanitation measures (e.g., fluoridated water, garbage removal, and sewage treatment), and community parenting classes. *Secondary level interventions* are interventions that promote early detection and treatment of illness or efforts to prevent the spread of contagious diseases, progression of disease, or disability. Examples of secondary interventions include tuberculosis and lead screening programs; isolation or restricting of children from school when they have communicable diseases; early intervention developmental services (e.g., Head Start); and mental health counseling for stressful events such as separation, divorce, death, or community natural disasters (e.g., earthquakes, floods, and hurricanes). *Tertiary prevention* interventions optimize function for children with a disability or chronic disease. Tertiary interventions include rehabilitation and disease management programs for asthma, sickle cell disease, cancer, anorexia, and special education programs for children.

CONTINUUM OF CARE

Community health services are provided within a continuum of care system (Fig. 30-1). The continuum of care system has subsystems for each of the four dimensions of health status: wellness, acute illness, chronic illness, and end of life of a child (Leyden, 1996). Continuity of care provides anticipatory guidance for the dimensions of health in a comprehensive manner. The physical, mental, and social aspects of care are integrated services provided along a continuum based on the family's needs. The continuum of care approach empowers families to advocate for the optimal health of their children. The continuum begins with the healthy infant, child, or adolescent for whom a family-centered care approach is provided for health promotion activities (e.g., growth and development, immunizations, safety, or screening). All children and families may experience an acute illness or injury of an episodic nature and seek acute health care services. An altered state of wellness requires immediate case management by a primary care provider. Case management is similar to the nursing process but integrates the available community resources and health insurance benefits in a manner that promotes continuity of care in order to achieve optimal health status (Leyden, 1997).

In the event a child is diagnosed during the acute phase with a chronic illness, the approach to care is disease management. Disease management encompasses an aggressive continuity of care plan that depicts the life care needs that may occur as a result of the altered phases of health that may accompany a

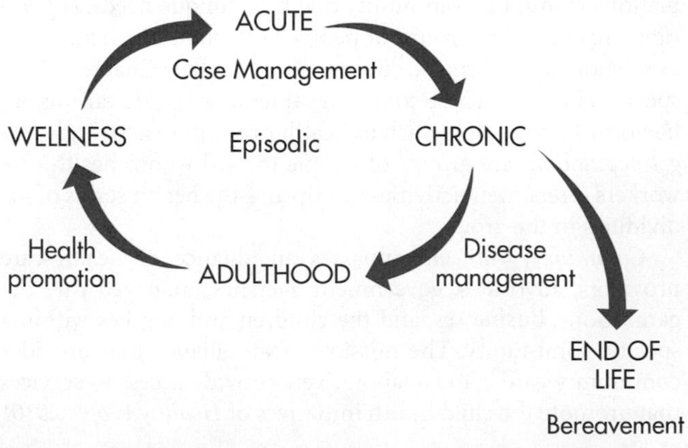

FIG. 30-1 • Pediatric continuum of care. (Christine Golazeski-Leyden. Copyright 1996. Used with permission.)

*The *Healthy People 2010* website can be accessed at: www.health.gov/

chronic illness. The altered phases of health include acute episodes requiring intensive services through home care, ambulatory care, or inpatient hospitalization; rehabilitation therapy for maximizing functional ability; wellness and maintenance care monitored by the primary care provider and school nurse; and end-of-life care for terminal disease progression at home or inpatient hospice. Disease management is provided by an interdisciplinary team (e.g., primary care provider, school nurse, insurance case manager, inpatient nurse, home care nurse, ambulatory care nurse, rehabilitation therapist, counselor or social worker, and pharmacist) that empowers the family to be the leader and outcome manager of the plan. The end-of-life care of the continuum may be expected or a result of sudden death. A family bereavement plan is initiated if possible before death. The end-of-life care plan addresses pain management, spirituality, cultural beliefs, level of participation at the time of death for dressing the child's body if desired, saying goodbye, funeral preparation, and bereavement counseling (see Chapter 41). Bereavement counseling is essential and continues throughout the life of the surviving family members.

COMMUNITY NURSING PROCESS

In community nursing the focus of the nursing process shifts from the individual child and family to the community or target population. The stages of the process are similar whether the patient is one child or a population of children; only the indicators of wellness and illness differ (Anderson and McFarlane, 1996). *Assessment* is focused on collecting subjective and objective information about the target population in order to diagnose problems based on community needs. *Planning* involves the description of community-centered goals and objectives. The nurse works with the community to *implement* a program that enables members to reach their goals and to *evaluate* whether the goals were met. Community nursing is collaborative; the nurse is one member of a community alliance that includes other health professionals, educators, politicians, religious leaders, members of public and voluntary organizations, and consumers (Bushy, 1997). The role of the nurse depends on the scope of the project, the target population, and the expertise of alliance members. For example, the school nurse may assume a leadership role in planning for the health needs of elementary school children and serve as a panel member on a citywide committee assessing environmental pollution.

Community Needs Assessment

The assessment phase of the community nursing process is called a *community needs assessment.* Assessment involves the collection of subjective and objective information about a community. *Subjective information* indicates what community members say are their most important needs, and can be determined in a number of ways. One way is to distribute questionnaires to a sample of the people living in the community. Another way is to interview community members directly, phoning or meeting with individuals who represent the group or who have a special role in the group. Community leaders are an example of people who have a special role.

Objective information is data that the nurse collects by direct observation. A windshield tour is one method of direct observation. The nurse drives through a neighborhood and takes notes about the environment, including the appearance of houses, the presence of sidewalks and gutters, or the number of public areas. Objective information about the health of the community can also be obtained from such sources as the Chamber of Commerce, the Census Bureau, libraries, state health departments, and the Internet sites of voluntary health organizations or government agencies. Information about service agencies can be found in resource directories. Resource directories include the local telephone book, community resource directories compiled by such organizations as the United Way, and population-specific books provided by public and voluntary agencies.

One way to organize an assessment is to use a guide that lists community systems that need to be examined. This process is similar to using a physical assessment guide to examine the different body systems in an individual patient. Anderson and McFarlane (1996) described eight community systems that the nurse needs to examine: health and social services, communication, recreation, physical environment, education, safety and transportation, politics and government, and economics. During the assessment the nurse studies how well each component in the community functions and interacts to meet the health needs of children, and whether any barriers disrupt the components and prevent access to care for children and their families.

Once the assessment is completed, the community nurse analyzes the information. The nurse evaluates the results of surveys and questionnaires; determines if the needs described by community members can be met by existing community agencies; and identifies individuals who may be at highest risk because of an environmental, behavioral, or biologic agent. The nurse determines the mortality and morbidity rates in the community and compares them to a standard. Comparisons can be made on the basis of time or place. In comparisons of time, the nurse contrasts mortality and morbidity rates in the current year with the rates during an earlier period of time. In comparisons of place, the nurse contrasts the rates in the community with a standard population to find out if the mortality and disease rates are higher in the target population. Standard rates may come from another community or from city, state, or national rates.

A *community health diagnosis* is the reflection of health status, risks, or needs as determined by a causative agent. The format of a community diagnosis is similar to that of an individual nursing diagnosis with a problem (need) and etiology related to that problem (causative agent). An example of a community nursing diagnosis is "Child abuse related to a violent environment."

Community Planning

The nurse collaborates with community members to develop a plan that addresses the needs and problems of the target population. To maximize the use of community resources, problems should first be prioritized on the basis of their severity, the felt needs of the community, and the ability of the community nurse to bring about change. Once the problems are prioritized, the nurse works with community members to develop at least one goal for each problem the members will address. *Goals* are outcomes that give direction to interventions and provide a measure of the change the interventions produced. Community interventions often take the form of *health programs* for improving the health status of the target population. Community health programs are based on the three levels of prevention: primary, secondary, and tertiary. For example, a goal for preventing bicycle injuries is, "Within 1 year all students in the first grade will wear bicycle helmets." The nurse and community members then plan a program that includes a health education program about bicycle safety for students and their parents (primary prevention) and a screening program to determine how many students need helmets (secondary prevention).

The planning group considers the resources that are already available in the community and the resources that will be needed for implementing a health program, including personnel, supplies and equipment, office space, phones, and computers. Decisions are made about the timeline of the program, the budget, and strategies that can be used to obtain funding. The nurse may also contact health professionals who have implemented successful programs in other communities; they can provide valuable time-saving tips and suggestions. Program descriptions are found through professional contacts and on-line resources and by reviewing the literature.

Community Implementation

During implementation the nurse and community members carry out the intervention. Whether the program is simple or complex, oversight is needed to ensure that everyone involved is communicating with each other, following the guidelines of the plan, keeping within the timeline, and documenting daily activities and expenses. This documentation will be invaluable during the evaluation phase of the process.

Community Evaluation

Evaluation identifies whether the goals and program objectives were met. There are various models of program evaluation. The structure, process, and outcome method is commonly used by health care organizations. Donabedian (1966) first described this approach, which is appropriate for community program evaluation in the twenty-first century.

1. *Structure:* Where and by whom is the care delivered in a program?
2. *Process:* Was the care delivered using the operational standards and within the financial guidelines of the program?
3. *Outcomes:* What was the impact to health status? Was there an improvement?

Structure focuses on the qualifications of personnel; the adequacy of buildings, offices, supplies, and equipment; and the characteristics of the target population. Process focuses on the interaction of patients and providers. Process indicators include the number of people who attended a health education program, the number of pamphlets distributed, and the efficiency of the program. Outcome focuses on whether program objectives and community goals were met. Program evaluation should be ongoing so that performance improvement initiatives are monitored and so that an improvement in the way health care is delivered will affect the health status of the target population.

Key Points

- Caring for children within a community requires a multi-disciplinary approach to care.
- The science of epidemiology provides evaluation for the factors associated with morbidity and mortality within a community.
- Causes associated with disease and illness within a community include environmental, behavioral, and biologic influences.
- Community health programs are based on three levels of intervention: primary, secondary, and tertiary intervention.
- Within a community, health care services are provided from a continuum of care, including wellness, acute illness, chronic illness, and end-of-life care.
- A community needs assessment involves collection of subjective and objective information about the community.
- A community health diagnosis is similar to a nursing diagnosis, identified by a problem with defined etiology related to the problem.
- Program planning and implementation in the community requires collaboration between the nurse and community members who are in positions to promote change.
- Evaluation of effective community programs includes consideration of the structure, process, and outcomes related to the program.

References

Anderson ET, McFarlane JM: *Community as partner: theory and practice in nursing,* Philadelphia, 1996, JB Lippincott.

Bushy, A: Empowering initiatives to improve a community health status, *J Nurs Care Qual* 11(4):32-42, 1997.

Donabedian A: Measuring the effectiveness of medical interventions: new expectations of health services research, *Health Serv Res* 25:697-708, 1966.

Hitchcock JE, Schubert PE, Thomas SA: *Community health nursing: caring in action,* New York, 1999, Delmar Publishers.

Lancaster J, Lancaster W: Economics of health care delivery. In Stanhope M, Lancaster J, editors: *Community health nursing,* ed 5, St Louis, 1996, Mosby.

Leyden CG: *Pediatric case management,* poster presented at Pediatric Nursing Conference, New Orleans, October 1996.

Leyden CG: Preventing insurance denials: disease management, *Pediatr Nurs* 23(5):516-517, 1997.

Lurie, N: *Healthy People 2010:* Setting the nation's public health agenda, *Academic Medicine* 75(1):12-13, 2000.

Velsor-Friedrich, B: *Healthy People 2000/2010:* Health appraisal of the nation and future objectives, *J Pediatr Nurs* 15(1): 47-48, 2000.

CHAPTER

31 Family Influences on Child Health Promotion

http://www.harcourthealth.com/MERLIN/Wong/maternal/

Learning Objectives

On completion of this chapter the reader will be able to:

- Discuss definitions of family.
- Describe three major family theories.
- Identify different family structures found in the United States.
- Discuss the effect of family size and configuration on personality development.
- Discuss the role transition experienced by new parents.
- Explain various parenting behaviors such as parenting styles, disciplinary patterns, and communication skills.
- Demonstrate an understanding of special parenting situations such as adoption, divorce, single-parenting, parenting in reconstituted families, and dual-earner families.

GENERAL CONCEPTS

Definition of Family

The term *family* has been defined in a number of ways and for a number of purposes according to the individual's own frame of reference, value judgment, or discipline. For example, biology describes the family as fulfilling the biologic function of perpetuation of the species. Psychology emphasizes the interpersonal aspects of the family and its responsibility for personality development. Economics views the family as a productive unit providing for material needs; and sociology depicts it as the social unit that reacts with the larger society. Others define family in relation to the persons who make up the family unit; the most common type of relationships are *consanguineous* (blood relationships), *affinal* (marital relationships), and *family of origin* (family unit a person is born into).

Traditionally, a family has been conceptualized as a group of individuals with the belief that both a mother and father are needed to rear a child. Nearly all societies grant a very high rank to the married status, but in today's society a broad definition of the family is needed, such as "a group of people, living together or in close contact, who take care of one another and provide guidance for their dependent members." Most important for any given patient, "family" is whatever the patient considers it to be (Patterson, 1995) (Critical Thinking box). These important people in the family's life may be related, unrelated, immediate family, or extended family members.

A great deal of emotion has been generated about some of the newer concepts of family, such as communal families, single-parent families, and homosexual families. To accommodate these and other varieties of family styles, the descriptive term *household* is being used more often. Whatever form the family takes, children need to feel that their family is acceptable and valuable (Visher and Visher, 1995).

Nursing of infants and children is intimately involved with care of the child *and* the family. Consequently, nurses must be aware of the functions of the family, various types of family structures, and theories that provide a foundation for understanding the changes within a family and for directing family-oriented interventions.

Family Nursing Interventions

In working with children, nurses must include family members in their plan of care. In essence, *the patient is the family.* To discover family dynamics and the unit's strengths and weaknesses, a thorough family assessment is needed (see Chapter 34). The interventions that nurses use with families depend on their theoretic model of the family. In family systems theory, for example, the focus is on the interactions of the members rather than on an individual member. In this case, using group dynamics to involve all members in the intervention process and being a skillful communicator are essential (Critical Thinking box). Systems theory also presents an excellent opportunity for anticipatory guidance. Because each member of the family reacts to every stress experienced by that system (e.g., the birth of a child), nurses can intervene to help the family prepare for and

Critical Thinking

FAMILY STRUCTURE

As the nurse, you are interviewing the mother of John, a school-age boy. The mother says their family consists of herself, her son, her lesbian partner, and two foster children. John's father lives in another state and has no contact with him. John has one grand-parent, who lives in another city in a nursing home. When planning care for John and his family, John's family should be considered to be which of the following?

First, Think About It . . .

- **Within what point of view are you thinking?**
- **What concepts or ideas are central to your thinking?**

1. **Nuclear family of mother, father, and son**
2. **Single-parent family of mother and son**
3. **Extended family of mother, father, grandparent, and son**
4. **Family members identified by the mother**

The best response is 4. The general point of view exists that the family defines its members. In this situation John's family consists of those people who live in his home at the present time. Traditionally, the idea is that family composition has referred to either nuclear or extended families. However, many alternative family structures such as John's occur. The nurse needs to recognize that not all families are traditional in their membership.

Critical Thinking

FAMILY THEORIES

As the school nurse, you are working with a family that consists of a mother, father, and their 10-year-old son and 16-year-old daughter. The daughter, Jenny, has stopped going to school this week. Although she has had many conflicts with her parents, her relationship with her father is strained. He recently took away her driving privileges because of curfew violations. Jenny says she is quitting school if she cannot drive. Which of the following three family theories would you apply when working with this family?

First, Think About It . . .

- **What concepts or ideas are central to your thinking?**
- **What conclusions are you coming to?**

1. **Developmental theory**
2. **Family stress theory**
3. **Family systems theory**

The best response is 3. In family systems theory the family is viewed as a system that continually interacts with its members. Family interactions, rather than individual members, are viewed as the source of the problems. The conclusion that developmental or family stress theory could be applied is not conceptually accurate, since the family is experiencing an interaction problem more than a developmental or stress-related problem.

cope with the change. Also, at each stress point there is an opportunity for change and learning because families are more open to interventions at this time (Brazelton, 1995).

In the family stress theory, crisis intervention strategies are employed, and the chief focus is on helping members cope with the challenging event. In the developmental theory, a primary nursing function is to provide anticipatory guidance that prepares members for transition to the next family stage.

Nurses use a variety of strategies when working with families (Box 31-1). It is important for nurses to be aware of their degree

Box 31-1
Family Nursing Interventions

Behavior modification
Contracting
Case management, including coordination and advocacy
Collaboration
Consultation
Counseling, including support, cognitive reappraisal (reframing), crisis intervention, and group work
Empowerment strategies
Environmental modification
Family advocacy
Lifestyle modification, including stress management
Networking, including use of self-help groups and social support
Referring
Role modeling
Role supplementation
Teaching strategies
Values clarification

From Friedman MM: *Family nursing: theory and practice,* ed 4, Norwalk, CT, 1999, Appleton & Lange.

of professional competence in using family nursing interventions. An important nursing role is to recognize situations where referral to more specialized services is required.

FAMILY ROLES, RELATIONSHIPS, AND STRENGTHS

Each individual has a position, or status, in the family structure, and plays culturally and socially defined roles in interactions within the family group. Each family has its own traditions and values, and sets its own standards for interaction within and outside the group. Each family determines the experiences its children should have, those experiences they are to be shielded from, and how each of these experiences meets the needs of family members. Where family ties are strong, social control is highly effective, and most members conform to their roles willingly and with commitment. Conflicts arise when people do not fulfill their roles in ways that meet other family members' expectations, either because they are unaware of the expectations or because they choose not to meet them.

Parental Roles

In all family groups the socially recognized status of father and mother exists with socially sanctioned roles that prescribe appropriate sexual behavior and childrearing responsibilities. The guides for behavior in these roles serve to control sexual conflict in society and provide for prolonged care of children. The degree to which parents are committed and the way they play their roles are influenced by their unique socialization experience.

Role definitions are changing as a result of the changing economy and the women's liberation movement. Women are achieving equality with men in education; more are entering the labor force; and the number of women who choose to have fewer children, or none at all, is increasing. During childhood, particularly in the upper and middle classes, the trend is toward deemphasizing the basic male-female characteristics of aggression, dependence, and achievement. As the role of the woman changes, there must necessarily be a change in the complementary role of the man. Fathers are taking a more active role in childrearing and household activities, particularly in middle-class families. Marital roles remain most segregated in the lower classes. Redefinition of sex roles in the American family is taking place, but a cultural lag of the persisting traditional role definitions creates conflicts in many of these families.

Role Learning

Roles are learned through the socialization process. During all stages of development children learn and practice, through interaction with others and in their play, a set of social roles and something of the characteristics of the roles of others. They behave in patterned and more or less predictable ways because they learn roles that define mutual expectations in typical and recurring social relationships. Although role definitions are changing, the basic determinants of parenting remain the same. These three determinants of parenting infants and young children are: (1) the parental personality and psychologic well-being, (2) contextual subsystems of support, and (3) child characteristics (Foss, 1996). These determinants have been consistent measurements in determining a person's success in fulfilling the parental role.

Role conceptions are transmitted by socializing agents (e.g., parents, peers, and authority figures) who use positive and negative sanctions to ensure conformity to their norms. Role behaviors positively reinforced by rewards such as love, affection, friendship, and honors are strengthened. Negative reinforcement takes the form of ridicule, withdrawal of love, expressions of disapproval, or banishment.

In some cultures the role behavior expected of children conflicts with desirable adult behavior. For example, in the United States, children are expected to be submissive in childhood but dominant as adults. This conflict of expectations is known as *role discontinuity.* Other cultures value the same behaviors, such as courage and aggression, both in children and in adults; this provides *role continuity.*

One responsibility of the family is to develop culturally appropriate role behavior in the children. At a very early age children learn to perform in expected ways consistent with their position in the family and culture. The observed behavior of each child is a single manifestation—a combination of social influences, as well as individual psychologic processes. In this way the uniting of the child's intrapersonal system (the self) with the interpersonal system (the family) is simultaneously understood as the conduct of the child.

Role structuring initially takes place within the family unit, where the children fulfill a set of roles and respond to the complementary roles of their parents and other family members. The roles of the children are shaped primarily by the parents, who apply direct or indirect pressures in an attempt to induce or force children into the desired patterns of behavior or direct their efforts toward modification of the role responses of the child on a mutually acceptable basis. Parents have their own techniques and will determine the course that the process of socialization is to follow (see Guidelines box on p. 698).

Children respond to life situations according to behaviors learned in reciprocal transactions. As they acquire important role-taking skills, their relationships with others change. For instance, when a teenager is also the mother but lives in a household where the grandmother is a co-resident, the adolescent mother may experience more support for the adolescent role than for the parenting role (Black and Nitz, 1996). Children become proficient at understanding others as they acquire the ability to discriminate their own perspectives from those of others. Children who get along well with others and attain status in the peer group have well-developed role-taking skills.

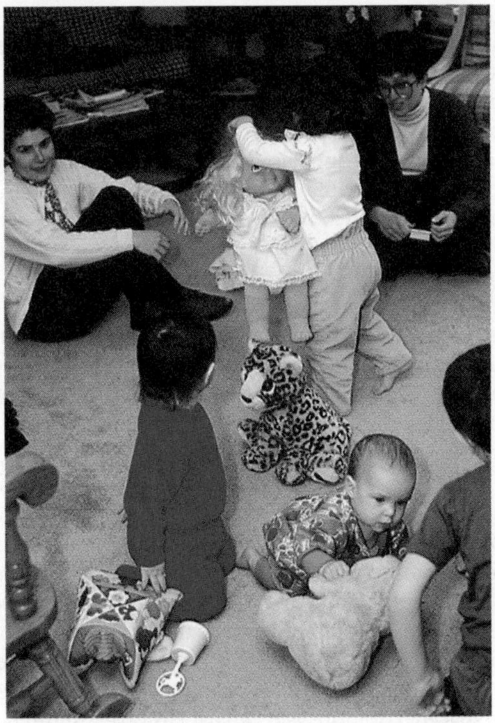

FIG. 31-1 • Innumerable relationships and activities are possible in a large family.

Family Size and Configuration. Parenting practices differ between small and large families. In small families more emphasis is placed on the individual development of the children. Parenting is intensive rather than extensive, and there is constant pressure to measure up to family expectations. Children's development and achievement are measured against that of other children in the neighborhood and social class. In small families there is more democratic participation by the children than in larger families. Adolescents in small families identify more strongly with their parents and rely more on their parents for advice. They have well-developed, autonomous inner controls as contrasted with adolescents from larger families, who rely more on adult authority.

Children in a large family are able to adjust to a variety of changes and crises. There is more emphasis on the group and less on the individual (Fig. 31-1). Cooperation is essential, often because of economic necessity. The large number of persons sharing a limited amount of space requires a greater degree of organization, administration, and authoritarian control. The control is wielded by a dominant family member—a parent or an older child. The number of children reduces the intimate, one-to-one contact between the parent and any individual child. Consequently, children turn to each other for what they cannot get from their parents. The reduced parent-child contact encourages individual children to adopt specialized roles in an attempt to gain recognition in the family.

Discipline is often administered by older siblings in large families. Siblings are usually better attuned to what constitutes misbehavior, and sibling disapproval or ostracism is often a more meaningful disciplinary measure than parental interventions. In situations such as the death or illness of a parent, an older sibling assumes responsibility for the family at considerable personal sacrifice. Large families seem to generate a sense of security in the children that is fostered by sibling support and cooperation. However, adolescents from a large family are more peer oriented than family oriented.

Spacing of Children and Ordinal Position. Age differences between siblings affect the childhood environment, but to a lesser extent than does the sex of the siblings. The arrival of a sibling has the greatest impact on the older child, and a 2- to 4-year difference in age appears to be most threatening to the older child. When the older child is very young, the self-image is too immature to be threatened. At an older age the child is better able to understand the situation and therefore is less likely to see the newcomer as a threat, although the child does feel the loss of the only-child status. Studies reveal that there is more affection and less rivalry or hostility when children are spaced 3 or more years apart. However, findings are not consistent (Newman, 1996).

In general, the narrower the spacing between siblings, the more the children influence one another, especially in emotional characteristics; the wider the spacing, the greater the influence of the parents.

For a number of years, sibling relationships were viewed from a Freudian perspective that emphasizes the concept of sibling rivalry; however, researchers in recent decades have viewed siblings through developmental or ecologic frameworks and have focused on interactions within family systems. Results of these broader perspectives reveal rich and varied sibling interaction.

Perhaps the sibling relationship's most unique feature is its duration. Likely the longest relationship one will share with another human being, the sibling relationship lasts through a lifetime, often 50 to 80 years, as compared with the child-parent relationship of approximately 30 to 50 years. Siblings spend long periods together and come to know each other—at their best and worst—extremely well.

It has been observed for some time that the birth position of children affects their personalities. Parents treat children differently, and sibling interactions are different depending on the children's position within the family. Also, power is unequally distributed among siblings. Older siblings attempt to dominate younger ones; therefore younger siblings develop interpersonal skills, the ability to negotiate, and an ability to accept unfavorable outcomes to a greater extent than older siblings. Later-born children are obliged to interact with other siblings from birth and seem to be more outgoing and make friends more easily than first-borns. However, children vary tremendously; these generalizations represent averages and do not apply in all situations. General characteristics of children in the various ordinal positions are presented in Box 31-2.

Sibling Functions. Siblings exert power, exchange services, and express feelings in reciprocal ways that are often not revealed explicitly in the presence of parents. They see themselves in their brother or sister, experience life vicariously through their sibling's behavior, and begin to expand on their own possibilities. Siblings can also be touchstones for what the other would not like to be, and they tend to use each other as yardsticks for comparison. They are sounding boards for one another; they offer a safe forum for experimenting with new behaviors and roles before using either with parents or nonfamily peers.

Brothers and sisters provide each other with tangible services (e.g., lending money, clothing, toys, sports equipment; or teaching a skill), help each other with childhood problems, provide support for each other in dealing with parents or others outside the family, and may provide introductions for each other to new friendship groups. Children learn to negotiate and bargain, and sometimes to manipulate. Many opportunities

Box 31-2

Influence of Ordinal Position on Children

FIRSTBORN CHILDREN

Are more achievement oriented
Are more dominant
Receive more physical punishment
Are allowed to show more aggression to siblings
Have stronger consciences, are more self-disciplined and inner directed
Are more socially anxious
Are prone to feelings of guilt
Identify more with parents than with peers
Are more conservative
Are subject to greater parental expectations
Begin to speak earlier in life
Demonstrate higher intellectual achievement
Plan better and experience fewer frustrations
Are likely to be most wanted

MIDDLE CHILDREN

Have more demands made on them for household help
Are praised less often
Receive less of the parents' time
Learn to compromise and be adaptable
Are less stimulated toward achievement
Are more difficult to characterize because of a variety of positions in the family

YOUNGEST CHILDREN

Are less dependent than firstborn children
Are less tense, more affectionate, and more good-natured
Tend to identify more with peer group than with parents
Are more flexible in their thinking
Are popular with classmates
Have fewer demands placed on them for household help

ONLY CHILDREN

Resemble firstborn children
Are more mature and cultivated
Experience greater parental pressure for mature behavior and achievement
Demonstrate superiority in language facility
Rarely develop into the stereotype of a spoiled, selfish child
Often enjoy a rich fantasy life as a result of isolation

Box 31-3
Characteristics of Twins

MONOZYGOTIC (MZ, IDENTICAL TWINS)	DIZYGOTIC (DZ, FRATERNAL TWINS)
Result of one fertilized ovum that became separated early in development	Result of fertilization of two ova
Alike physically and genetically	Differ physically and genetically
Same sex	May be like or opposite sex
Frequency:	Frequency:
Occurs uniformly in all populations	Varies among races (highest—African Americans, lowest—Asians, intermediate—Caucasians)
Unaffected by maternal age	More common with advancing maternal age (maximum at age 35-39, then decreases rapidly)
Tendency unaffected by heredity	Marked familial tendency Expressed only in the female Fathers appear to transmit disposition toward double ovulation to daughters
Similar behavior	Dissimilar behavior; more sibling rivalry

arise for conflict and conflict resolution. Siblings learn about sharing, competition, rivalry, and compromise. They can also protect one another from parental-executive abuse of power and can form a coalition to deal with the issues of authority, power, and emotional support. Negotiating with parents is stronger when siblings act together rather than singly.

Siblings interpret the outside world for each other and perform genuine educative functions for the parents. A related function is *pioneering,* wherein one sibling initiates a process, thereby giving permission to the others to follow accordingly. Patterns may include breaking explicit family rules, taking new developmental pathways (such as leaving the family), or adopting different moral/political codes and lifestyles.

Tattling can be an important lever in sibling interactions; on the other hand, there is often a conspiracy of silence among siblings that can leave the parents feeling isolated and excluded. A willingness to make and maintain each other's privacy often serves as a powerful bond of loyalty among the children. It is this loyalty that often distinguishes the relationship between siblings from that between friends.

More Active Sibling Relationships. Sibling relationships vary among cultures. Certain factors, however, may be giving the sibling relationship greater significance in North America than in the past. Shrinking family size, longer life spans, divorce and remarriage, geographic mobility, maternal employment and alternative sources of child care, competitive pressures, stress, and various forms of parental insufficiency may be propelling siblings into greater contact and emotional interdependence than ever before.

For example, siblings often join forces to confront the trauma of divorce. They often rely on each other for support when parents remarry. The large number of working mothers means that many young siblings today have large amounts of time when their relationship is not monitored by a personally committed adult. Often an older sibling is required to baby-sit, resulting in children spending more and more time together unsupervised. In a worried, mobile, small-family, high-stress, fast-paced, parent-absent society, children often turn to a brother or sister to meet their needs for contact, constancy, and permanency.

Multiple Births. A deviation in early development that occurs with variable frequency is multiple births. Twins are not uncommon in the population, but triplets are rare and quadruplets or quintuplets are extremely unusual. In any of these situations the offspring can be of the like or unlike gender (i.e., derived from a single ovum; from multiple ova; or a combination of the two, which can involve one or more cell divisions). The cause of twinning is unknown, but the increase in the number of larger multiples (e.g., quintuplets and sextuplets) during recent years has been associated with fertility-enhancing techniques (i.e., ovulation-inducing drugs and assisted reproductive techniques such as in vitro fertilization) (Ventura et al, 1997). Because women in their 30s are almost 2½ times as likely as women in their 20s to have higher-order plural births, the rise in the multiple-birth ratio has been associated with increased childbearing among older women as well as the expanded use of fertility drugs (Guyer et al, 1999).

Twins are of two distinct type: *identical,* or *monozygotic (MZ);* and *fraternal,* or *dizygotic* (*DZ*) (Box 31-3). In the United States the overall twinning rate is approximately 1 in 80 pregnancies; one third are MZ twins, and two thirds are DZ twins.

A special kind of sibling relationship is observed in twins, although getting along with each other and quarreling are not much different from those behaviors in any other two siblings, especially if they are different-sex fraternal twins. Twins generally tend to work out a relationship that is reasonably satisfactory to both and demonstrate early independence from parental attention. They develop a remarkable capacity for cooperative play and considerable loyalty and generosity toward each other. It is not uncommon for them to evolve a private language between themselves that may interfere with development of the family language.

In a twinship, one member of the pair, to a greater or lesser extent, is more dominant, outgoing, and assertive than the other, often to the consternation of their parents. However, the seemingly more passive twin is able to accomplish as much and get his or her way as often as the more assertive twin.

It has also been observed that there is a difference in behavior between identical and fraternal twins. Whereas there is near unison in the actions of identical twins (although they alternate in assuming the leadership), fraternal twins, even of the same sex, do not display this quality. Sibling rivalry can be quite pronounced in fraternal twins, especially in different-sex twins.

Identical twins also differ in their response to the tendency of some parents to treat twins exactly alike. The present philosophy is to determine the degree to which the children demonstrate an inclination toward togetherness. Some twins thrive best when they are constantly in each other's company; others prefer more individuality and separateness. The conservative approach is to allow the children to follow their natural inclinations. Early years of togetherness are often the basis of the twins' security; to separate them too early may produce unnecessary stresses. The tendency is to foster individual differences as they are evidenced in order to ease the process of separation when it becomes advisable.

Parental Adjustment. The entrance of any new member into a household creates a number of stresses, but with multiple births two or more new members must be incorporated into the family at the same time. The problems are obvious. Two infants must be provided with physical care, including twice the feeding, diapering, and all of the purchasing and preparation that accompany the care of an infant. Scheduling becomes crucial, and each advancement in development brings new problems and adjustments (e.g., space and sleeping arrangements, selecting a stroller and other equipment). Care must be observed in selecting toys. As play becomes a serious business, some toys that would be safe and appropriate for a single child become weapons when two infants share a playpen. It is a good idea to select different toys for the children as they grow older, and encourage sharing.

PARENTING

Motivation for Parenthood

A dominant characteristic in all societies is that adults are expected to become parents and to be gratified by the experience. Pressures of tradition, sentiment regarding the state of parenthood, and religious exhortations to fulfill divine commands of fertility profoundly influence decision making, because conformity to social-role expectations is a strong influence in family planning.

Factors that are likely to influence family size include social class, religion, race, financial stability, type of conjugal-role relationships, and the social-psychologic aspects of sexual relations. Of course, how effectively the couple practices contraception may determine whether the family size remains as planned. Also, in the case of divorce and remarriage, an individual may decide to have more children with the new spouse.

Preparation for Parenthood

The basic goals of parenting are to promote the physical survival and health of the children, to foster the skills and abilities necessary to be a self-sustaining adult, and to foster behavioral capabilities for maximizing cultural values and beliefs. However, new parents approach parenthood with meager experience and scant knowledge, although no other task can compare, in overall consequences, with that of rearing a human being. Parents learn by trial and error, committing the same mistakes that have been committed by countless other parents; but they somehow manage to accomplish the task, becoming more skilled with each additional child. Tradition, rather than rational planning, furnishes the chief norms for childrearing. Experience in having been nurtured as a child is an essential component of successful parenting.

Their own parents are probably the only persons who parents observe intimately in the parental role; this results in a *generational continuity*—parents rear their own children in much the same way as they themselves were reared. Other essential skills and knowledge parents need in order to feel more comfortable in the parenting role include a basic understanding of childhood growth and development, bathing, feeding, use of play, and interpersonal communication skills. All of this information is integrated throughout this text.

Transition to Parenthood

Although there is disagreement as to whether or not the birth of a couple's first child should be labeled a crisis, the early weeks of an infant's life call for a couple to make drastic adjustments. Although the parents have anticipated and perhaps prepared for the child's arrival, the birth means the sudden imposition of totally dependent care 24 hours a day for the new member of the family. It may very well be a crisis if the event is perceived as disturbing old habits and relationships and eliciting new responses. It requires role changes, destroys or significantly modifies former relationships, and means adjusting to new role realignments. Whereas previously the roles of a couple were husband and wife, they now become, in addition, father and mother. It is difficult to adjust to being parents, but it is a normal human experience and a tool for personal growth.

The advent of a new family member requires that the family cope with greater financial responsibilities, a possible loss of income, changes in sleeping habits, and less time for the husband and wife to spend with each other (especially if it is a firstborn) and/or with other children. If the events are perceived as aversive, it could well disrupt the couple's bond. Some investigators find that the birth of a first child results in a reduction of the couple's intimacy and affection, whereas others report that the adjustment to parenthood is only mildly stressful.

Other factors influencing the transition to the parental role include:

- Parents with previous experience, such as another child, appear to be more relaxed and have less conflict in disciplinary relationships, and they are more aware of normal growth and development expectations.
- The amount of stress experienced by one or both parents may interfere with their ability to exhibit patience and understanding or otherwise cope with their children's behavior.
- Special characteristics of the infant, such as being temperamentally difficult, can cause the parents to lose confidence and doubt their abilities. Also, an infant with special care needs, such as those associated with a disability, can be a significant source of added stress.
- Fathers who are highly involved with their child often feel more comfortable in the parenting role (Fig. 31-2).
- Marital relationships can have a negative effect on parental transition, because marital tension or strife can alter caregiving routines and interfere with enjoyment of the infant. Conversely, parents who support and encourage one another serve as a positive influence on establishing a satisfying parental role.

Support Systems. Successful adaptation to the stress of transition to parenthood involves at least two types of family resources (McCubbin and McCubbin, 1989). First are the *internal resources* of the family, such as adaptability and integration. Changing from an orderly, predictable life to a relatively disordered, unpredictable one is a universal adaptation that families must make. Rigid schedules are impossible to maintain, and former activities must be curtailed or abandoned. *Adaptation* is reflected in learning to be patient, becoming better organized,

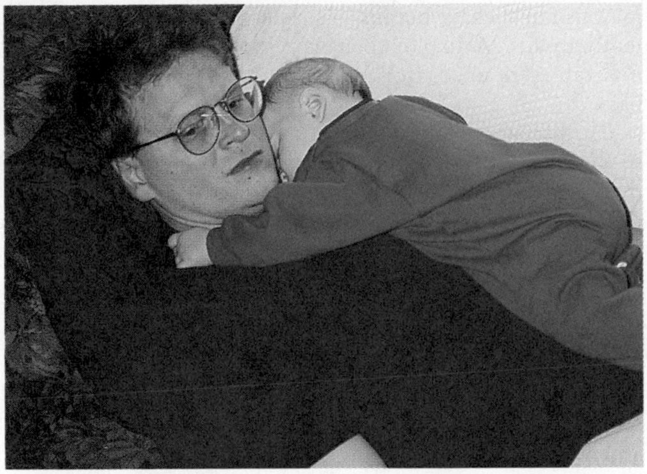

FIG. 31-2 • The role of the father is essential to a family's health and well-being.

and becoming more flexible. *Integration* involves an attempt of the couple to continue some activities they engaged in before they became parents. In this way couples are able to maintain a sense of continuity and appreciate the importance of the husband-wife relationship.

The second kind of resource for coping with stress is the use of *coping strategies* that strengthen the organization and functioning of the family. These include the use of community resources, the use of social support, and the adoption of a future orientation. Interpersonal supports that provide information, advice, and caretaking are derived from friends, relatives, and neighbors. Relationships with family, friends, and community are essential. Arranging for time away from the child or children is beneficial. Fathers can assume care of the family to allow the mother some time to herself at home or away from the home, even if just for an afternoon or evening. Adoption of a future orientation provides reassurance to parents that things will get better, that they will cope, and that it is realistic to plan for the time when they will be able to engage in self-fulfilling activities.

It is also reassuring to know that others experience ambivalent feelings toward parenthood and share the same difficulties and frustrations. Exchanging ideas and experiences with other parents provides an opportunity to voice concerns and to learn new ways of coping with the multiple problems of childrearing. Whether it is family, friends, or community resources, parents need persons to whom they can turn for advice, comfort, and assistance—persons with whom they can share the joys and difficulties of childrearing.

Parenting Behaviors

Parental Styles of Control. Although there are variations and degrees in parenting styles, they can generally be described as either authoritarian, permissive, or authoritative. *Authoritarian,* or *dictatorial* parents try to control their children's behavior and attitudes through unquestioned mandates. They establish rules and regulations or a standard of conduct that they expect to be followed rigidly and unquestioningly. They value and reward absolute obedience, mute acceptance of their word, and unfailing respect for the family's principles and beliefs. They forcefully punish any behavior that is contrary to parental standards. Parental authority is exercised with little explanation and little involvement of the child in decision making. The message is: "Do it because I say so."

Punishment need not be corporal but may be stern, such as withdrawal of love and approval. Careful training often results in rigidly conforming behavior in the children, who tend to be sensitive, shy, self-conscious, retiring, and submissive. They are more apt to be courteous, loyal, honest, and dependable—but docile. These behaviors are more typically observed when parental arbitrary power assertion is accompanied by close supervision and a reasonable level of affection. If not, arbitrary power assertion is more likely to be associated with both defiant and antisocial behavior.

Permissive, or *laissez faire* parents exert little or no control over their children's actions. These well-meaning parents sometimes confuse permissiveness with license. They avoid imposing their own standards of conduct and allow their children to regulate their own activity as much as possible. These parents consider themselves to be resources for the children, not role models. If rules do exist, the parents explain the underlying reason, encourage the children's opinions, and consult them in decision-making processes. They employ lax, inconsistent discipline, do not set sensible limits, and do not prevent the children from upsetting the home routine. The parents rarely punish the children, because most behavior is considered acceptable. Consequently, the children, in effect, control the parents. Children of permissive parents are often disobedient, disrespectful, irresponsible, aggressive, and generally defiant of authority.

Authoritative, or *democratic* parents combine some childrearing practices from both the foregoing extremes. They direct their children's behavior and attitudes by emphasizing the reason for rules and by negatively reinforcing deviations. They respect the individuality of each of their children, and allow them to voice their objections to family standards or regulations. Parental control is firm and consistent but tempered with encouragement, understanding, and security. Control is focused on the issue, not on withdrawal of love or the fear of punishment. These parents foster "inner-directedness," a conscience that regulates behavior based on feelings of guilt or shame for wrongdoing, not on fear of being caught or punished. Parents' realistic standards and reasonable expectations produce children with high self-esteem who are self-reliant, assertive, inquisitive, content, and highly interactive with other children.

The most successful type of childrearing seems to be the authoritative method. Parents do not set rigid, arbitrary limits but maintain firm control, particularly in areas of parent-child disagreement. Permissiveness is tempered with reasonable and consistent setting of limits. Parental power is shared, and both parents provide leadership but listen to what the children think.

Limit Setting and Discipline

In its broadest sense, *discipline* means to teach or it simply refers to a set of rules governing conduct. In a narrower sense, it refers to the actions taken to enforce the rules following noncompliance. *Limit setting* refers to establishing the rules or guidelines for behavior. Generally, the clearer the limits that are set and the more consistently they are enforced, the less need there is for disciplinary action. For example, it is often suggested that parents should set limits on the amount of time children spend watching television (Trost et al, 1996).

Therefore the initial goal for the family is for the nurse to help parents establish realistic and concrete "rules." Limit setting and discipline are positive, necessary components of childrearing and serve several useful functions as they help children:

- Test their limits of control
- Achieve in areas appropriate for mastery at their level
- Channel undesirable feelings into constructive activity
- Protect themselves from danger
- Learn socially acceptable behavior

Children want and need limits. Unrestricted freedom is a tremendous threat to their security and safety. Through testing the limits imposed on them, children learn the extent to which they can manipulate their environment, as well as gain reassurance from knowing that others will be there to protect them from potential harm.

Minimizing Misbehavior. The goals of or reasons for misbehavior may include attention, power, defiance, and a display of inadequacy (e.g., the child misses classes because of a fear that he or she is unable to do the work). Children may also misbehave because the rules are not clear or consistently applied. Acting out behavior, such as a temper tantrum, may represent uncontrolled frustration, anger, depression, or pain.

The best approach is to structure interactions with children so that unacceptable behavior is prevented or minimized. Although many parents devise strategies that are most effective for their child, general guidelines include those listed in the Home Care box.

Types of Discipline. To deal with misbehavior, parents need to implement appropriate disciplinary action. Numerous approaches are available, and some have definite advantages over others (Guidelines box).

Reasoning involves explaining why an act is wrong; it is usually appropriate for older children, especially when moral issues are involved. However, young children cannot be expected to "see the other side" because of their egocentrism. Children in the preoperative stage of cognitive development (i.e., toddlers and preschoolers) have a limited ability to distinguish between their point of view and those of others (Blum et al, 1995).

Sometimes children use the "reasoning" as a way of gaining attention: for example, they may misbehave in order for the parents to give them a lengthy explanation of the wrongdoing, because negative attention is better than none. When children use this technique, parents may have to end the explanation by stating, "This is the rule, and this is how I expect you to behave. I won't explain it any further."

Unfortunately, reasoning is often combined with *scolding*, which sometimes takes the form of shame or criticism. For example, the parent may state, "You are a bad boy for hitting your brother." Children take such remarks seriously and personally, believing that *they* are bad.

Home Care

MINIMIZING MISBEHAVIOR

Set realistic goals for acceptable behavior and expected achievements.

Structure opportunities for small successes to lessen feelings of inadequacy.

Praise children for desirable behavior with attention and verbal approval.

Structure the environment to prevent unnecessary difficulties (e.g., place fragile objects in inaccessible area).

Set clear and reasonable rules; expect the same behavior regardless of the circumstances, and if exceptions are made, clarify that the change is for one time only.

Teach desirable behavior through own example, such as using a quiet, calm voice rather than screaming.

Review expected behavior before special or unusual events, such as visiting a relative or having dinner in a restaurant.

Phrase requests for appropriate behavior positively, such as "Put the book down," rather than "Don't touch the book."

Call attention to unacceptable behavior as soon as it begins; use distraction to change the behavior or offer alternatives to annoying actions, such as a quiet toy for one that is excessively noisy.

Give advance notice or "friendly reminders," such as "When the TV program is over, it is time for dinner" or "I'll give you to the count of three and then we have to go."

Be attentive to situations that increase the likelihood of misbehaving, such as overexcitement or fatigue, or decreased personal tolerance to minor infractions.

Offer sympathetic explanations for not granting a request, such as "I am sorry I can't read you a story now, but I have to finish dinner. Then we can spend time together."

Keep any promises made to children.

Avoid outright conflicts; temper discussions with statements such as "Let's talk about it and see what we can decide together" or "I have to think about it first."

Provide children with opportunities for power and control.

Guidelines

IMPLEMENTING DISCIPLINE

Consistency. Implement disciplinary action exactly as agreed on and for each infraction.

Timing. Initiate discipline as soon as child misbehaves; if delays are necessary, such as to avoid embarrassment, verbally disapprove of the behavior and state that disciplinary action will be implemented.

Commitment. Follow through with the details of the discipline, such as timing of minutes; avoid distractions that may interfere with the plan, such as telephone calls.

Unity. Make certain that all caregivers agree on the plan and are familiar with the details to prevent confusion and alliances between child and one parent.

Flexibility. Choose disciplinary strategies that are appropriate to child's age, temperament, and the severity of the misbehavior.

Planning. Plan discipline strategies in advance and prepare child if feasible (e.g., explain use of time-out); for unexpected misbehavior, try to discipline when you are calm.

Behavior-orientation. Always disapprove of the behavior, not the child, with such statements as "That was a wrong thing to do. I am unhappy when I see behavior like that."

Privacy. Administer discipline in private, especially with older children, who may feel ashamed in front of others.

Termination. Once the discipline is administered, consider child as having a "clean slate" and avoid bringing up the incident or lecturing.

NURSE ALERT • When reprimanding children, focus only on the misbehavior, not on the child. Use of "I" messages rather than "you" messages expresses personal feelings without accusation or ridicule. For example, an "I" message attacks the behavior ("I am upset when Johnny is punched; I don't like to see him hurt"), not the child.*

Positive and negative reinforcement is the basis of *behavior modification* theory—behavior that is rewarded will be repeated; behavior that is not rewarded will be extinguished. Using *rewards* is a positive approach; by encouraging children to behave in specified ways, the tendency to misbehave is lessened. With young children, using paper stars is a very effective method. For older children the "token system" is appropriate, especially if a certain number yields a special reward, such as a trip to the movies or a new book. For a reward system to be effective, the expected behaviors must be explained to the child and the rewards must be reinforcing. A chart should be used to record the stars or tokens, and every earned reward should be promptly given. Verbal approval should always accompany material rewards.

Consistently *ignoring* behavior will eventually extinguish or minimize the act. Although this approach sounds very simple, it is often difficult to implement consistently. Parents often "give in" and resort to previous patterns of discipline. Consequently, the behavior is actually reinforced because the child learns that persistence gains parental approval.

For ignoring to be effective, health professionals must devote a fair amount of time toward (1) explaining the approach in detail, (2) recording behavior before the extinction process is instituted to see if a problem exists and to compare results after ignoring is begun, (3) making certain that the parent's attention is the reinforcer, and (4) warning parents of a phenomenon called "response burst," which refers to an *increase* in the child's behavior soon after the process is initiated because the child is testing the parents to see if they are serious about the plan.

The strategy of *consequences* involves allowing children to experience the results of their misbehavior and includes three types:

1. **Natural**—Those that occur without any intervention, such as being late and missing dinner
2. **Logical**—Those that are directly related to the rule, such as not being allowed to play with another toy until the used ones are put away
3. **Unrelated**—Those that are imposed deliberately, such as no playing until homework is completed or the use of time-out

Natural or logical consequences are preferred but are effective only when they are meaningful to children. For example, the natural consequence of living in a messy room may do little to encourage cleaning up, but allowing no friends over until the room is neat can be very motivating! Withdrawing privileges is often an unrelated consequence. After the child experiences the consequence, the parent should refrain from any comment, because the usual tendency is for the child to try to place blame for imposing the rule.

Time-out is actually a refinement of the common practice of "sending the child to his or her room" and is a type of unrelated consequence. It is also based on the premise of removing the reinforcer (i.e., the satisfaction or attention the child is receiving from the activity). When placed in an unstimulating and isolated place, children become bored and consequently agree to behave in order to reenter the family group (Fig. 31-3). Time-out avoids many of the problems of other disciplinary approaches, because no physical punishment is involved, no reasoning or scolding is given, and the parent is usually not present for all of the time-out, facilitating his or her ability to consistently apply the punishment. It also offers both the child and the parent a "cooling off" time. To be effective, time-out must be planned in advance (Home Care box).

Corporal, or *physical punishment* most often takes the form of spanking. Based on the principles of aversive therapy, inflicting pain through spanking causes a dramatic short-term decrease in the behavior. However, there are some serious flaws in this approach: (1) it teaches children that violence is acceptable; (2) many times the spanking is the result of parental rage and may physically harm the child; and (3) children become "accustomed" to spanking, requiring more severe corporal punishment each time (American Academy of Pediatrics, 1998).

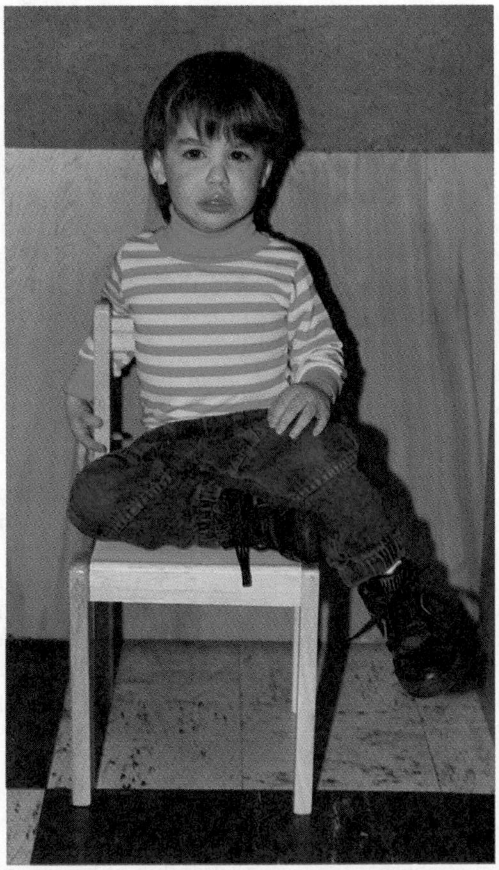

FIG. 31-3 • Time-out is an excellent disciplinary strategy for young children.

*For more information contact: Active Parenting Publishers, 810 Franklin Ct., Suite B, Marietta, GA 30067; phone 1-800-825-0060; or visit the website: www.active-parenting.com. For parents of adolescents, the pamphlet *Parents* can point out what to look for and where to seek help with emotional and behavior issues. It can be ordered from: Parents, P.O. Box 9538, Washington, DC 20016.

Home Care

USING TIME-OUT

- Select an area for time-out that is safe, convenient, and unstimulating, but where the child can be monitored, such as the bathroom, hallway, or laundry room; avoid frightening areas such as a cellar or a dark closet.
- Determine what behaviors warrant a time-out.
- Make sure children understand the "rules" and how they are expected to behave.
- Explain to children the process of time-out:
  - When they misbehave, they will be given one warning.
  - If they do not obey, they will be sent to the place designated for time-out.
  - They are to sit there for a specified period of time.
  - If they cry, refuse, or display any disruptive behavior, the time-out period will begin after they quiet down.
  - When they are quiet for the duration of the time, they can then leave the room.
- A rule for the length of time-out is *1 minute per year of age;* use a kitchen timer with an audible bell to record the time rather than a watch.
- Implement time-out in a public place by selecting a suitable area or explain to children that time-out will be spent immediately on returning home.

Spanking can result in severe physical injury. Nevertheless, corporal punishment is often exempted from the category of assault, even when it produces specific injuries, which may be treated as "accidental" or "incidental" to discipline.

Even when corporal punishment does not involve serious physical damage to children, the psychologic impact may be great (Bauman and Friedman, 1998; Smith and Brooks-Gunn, 1997). It can also interfere with effective parent-child interaction; children who receive corporal punishment are less likely to learn what they *should* do, because the focus is on what they *should not* do (American Academy of Pediatrics, 1998). In addition, when the parent is not around, the misbehavior is likely to occur, for children have not learned to behave well for their own sake. Parental use of corporal punishment may also interfere with the child's development of moral reasoning.

SPECIAL PARENTING SITUATIONS

Parenting is a demanding task under the most ideal circumstances, but when parents and children are faced with situations that deviate from what is considered to be the norm, the potential for family disruption is increased. Some of the issues that are encountered frequently are divorce, single parenthood, blended families, adoption, and dual-career families. The problems associated with children of alcoholic parents, parents with physical disabilities, homeless parents, or incarcerated parents are ones that are not addressed in the following discussions but may be topics that the reader may wish to investigate.

Parenting the Adopted Child

Adoption establishes the legal relationship of parent and child between persons who are not so related by birth, with the same rights and obligations that exist between children and their biological parents. In the past the biologic mother alone made the decision to relinquish the rights to her child. In recent years, however, the courts have acknowledged the legal rights of the biologic father regarding the decision. Concerned child advocates have questioned decisions that honor the father's rights when the decision may not be in the best interests of the child. As the rights of the child have become recognized, older children have successfully dissolved their legal bond with their biologic parents to pursue adoption by adults of their choice. Furthermore, there is a growing interest and demand within the gay and lesbian community to adopt. Agencies have developed few specific policies in this regard and face questions about the legal and social ramifications of adopting in a relationship not based on marriage, as well as possible consequences of not developing policies (Sullivan, 1995).

Unlike biologic parents who prepare for their child's birth with prenatal classes and the support of friends and relatives, adoptive parents have few sources of support and preparation for the new addition to their family. Nurses who offer services to adoptive parents can provide the information, support, and reassurance needed to reduce parental anxiety regarding the adoptive process, and make referrals to state parental support groups that provide guidance for adoptive parents. Such sources can be contacted through a state or county welfare office. Prospective parents seeking information on international adoptions can contact Families Adopting Children Everywhere, Inc. (FACE).*

Most problems faced by adoptive parents are no different from those encountered by natural parents. All parents want to be good parents, but this desire is often intensified in adoptive parents. Adoptive parents have been portrayed as being more apprehensive and insecure than biologic parents and in need of more assistance. However, adoptive parents may feel the need for less assistance than biologic parents. This feeling is probably due to the adoptive parents' completely voluntary decision to become parents, the relatively long time they have to prepare for parenting, and the maturity associated with adopting.

The sooner infants enter their adoptive home, the better for purposes of parent-infant attachment; the more caregivers the infant has before adoption, the more problems are likely to be encountered in attachment. The infant must break the bond with the previous caregiver and form a new bond with the adoptive parents. The difficulties in forming an attachment will depend on the amount of time the infant has spent with earlier caregivers, such as the birth mother, nurse, or adoption agency personnel.

Siblings, adopted or biologic, who are old enough to understand should be included in decisions regarding the commitment to adopt, with reassurance that they are not being replaced. Ways that the siblings can interact with the adopted child should be stressed (Fig. 31-4).

Issues of Origin. The task of telling children that they are adopted is a cause of deep concern and anxiety. There are no clear-cut guidelines for parents to follow in determining precisely when and at what age children are ready for the information, and parents are naturally reluctant to present the children with such unsettling news. However, it is an important aspect of

*P.O. Box 28058, Northwood Station, Baltimore, MD 21239; (410) 488-2656.

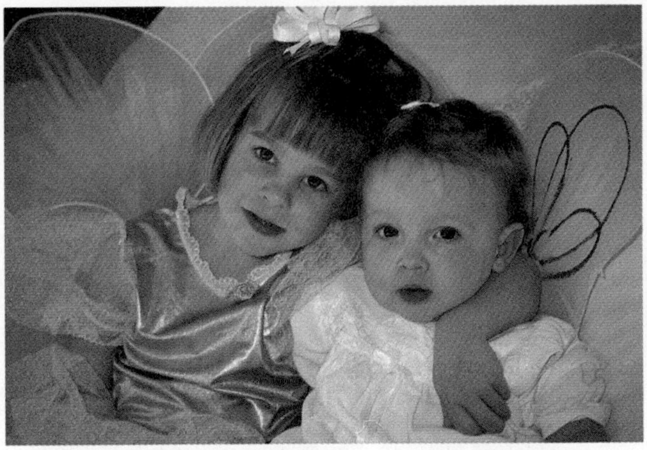

FIG. 31-4 • An older adopted sister lovingly embraces her adopted sister.

their parental responsibilities, and although they may be tempted to withhold the fact from the child, it is an essential component of the child's identity (Critical Thinking box).

The timing seems to arise naturally as parents become aware of the child's readiness. Most authorities believe that children should be informed at an age young enough so that as they grow older, they do not remember a time when they did not know that they were adopted. The time must be right for both the parents and the child and is highly individual; it may be when children ask where babies come from, at which time children can also be told the facts of their adoption. If they are told in such a way as to convey the idea that they were active participants in the selection process, they will be less apt to feel that they were abandoned victims in a helpless situation. For example, parents can tell children that their personal qualities drew the parents to them. It is wise for parents who have not previously discussed adoption to tell children that they are adopted before the children enter school to avoid third parties inadvertently telling the children before the parents have had the opportunity to do so. Complete honesty between parents and children usually strengthens the relationship.

Parents can anticipate some behavior changes following the disclosure—especially in children who are older. One study found that children who were adopted were two to five times more likely to be referred for psychologic treatment than nonadopted peers (Grotevant and McRoy, 1996). Children may use the fact of their adoption as a weapon to manipulate and threaten parents. There is the inevitable "My real mother would not treat me like this," or "You don't love me as much because I'm adopted." Statements such as these hurt parents and increase their feelings of insecurity, so that as parents they may become overpermissive. Adopted children need the same undemanding love, combined with firm discipline and limit setting, as any other child (Critical Thinking box).

Adolescence may be an especially trying time for parents of adopted children. The normal confrontations between adolescents and parents may assume more painful aspects in adoptive families. Adolescents may use their adoption as a tool in defying parental authority, or as a justification for aberrant behavior. As they attempt to master the task of identity formation, the feeling of abandonment by their biologic parents may come to awareness or may be intensified. Gender differences in reacting to adoption may surface. It has been shown that girls have more difficulty accepting their sexuality, because they may not be able to identify with a nonfertile female parent.

The children fantasize about their biologic parents, and may feel the need to discover their identify in order to define themselves and their own identity—one of the major tasks of adolescent development. It is important for adoptive parents to keep lines of communication open and to reassure the youngsters that they understand the feelings of needing to search for their identities. In some states birth certificates are made legally available to adopted children when they come of age. It is important for parents to be honest with questioning adolescents and to tell them of this possibility (the parents themselves are unable to obtain the birth certificate; it is the child's responsibility if he or she desires it).

Cross-Racial and International Adoption. Adoption of children of racial backgrounds different from that of the family is relatively commonplace. In addition to the problems faced by adopted children of any age, children of a cross-racial adoption must deal with their differentness. It is advised that parents who adopt such children do everything to preserve the adopted children's racial heritage.

Critical Thinking

PARENTING THE ADOPTED CHILD

Twelve-month-old Justin was adopted at birth. His parents tell you that they wonder when they should tell Justin that he is adopted. As the nurse, what nursing actions would you provide for Justin's parents?

First, Think About It . . .

- **What precise questions are you trying to answer?**
- **What would the consequences be if you put your thoughts into action?**

1. **Reassure them that because Justin was adopted at birth, they do not need to tell him he was adopted.**
2. **Give Justin's parents some books, pamphlets, and community resources on adoption so that they can decide on their own what to do.**
3. **Discuss the general understanding that they should tell Justin in a matter-of-fact manner at an early age so that he will always know he was adopted.**
4. **Recommend that they not tell Justin until he reaches early adolescence and can better understand this information.**

The best response is 3. Being adopted can be viewed by the adoptee as part of his unique heritage. Justin's parents chose to have him join the family as a welcomed member. Children join families in many ways, such as biologic heritage or blending of families. Sharing the story of adoption is an important parental responsibility and can be handled much like one shares birth experiences with a biologic child. Most authorities believe that children should be informed at a young enough age so that as they grow older, they do not remember a time when they did not know they were adopted. Waiting until adolescence is too late. Children have a more difficult adjustment if disclosure occurs when they are older. Giving Justin's parents resources about adoption is appropriate; however, because they have asked you, as the nurse, for guidance, a more direct approach is best.

NURSE ALERT • As a health care provider, it is important not to ask the wrong questions, such as "Is she yours, or is she adopted?" "What do you know about the 'real' mother?" "Are they really brother and sister?" or "How much did she cost?" (Hostetter and Johnson, 1996).

Although the children are full-fledged members of an adopting family and citizens of the adopted country, if they have a foreign appearance or other decided racial characteristics, problems may be encountered outside the family. Bigotry may appear among relatives and friends. Strangers may make thoughtless comments and talk about the children as though they were not members of the family. It is vital that the family make it clear to others that this is their child and a cherished member of the family.

In international adoptions* the medical information the parents receive may be either quite complete or very sketchy: weight, height, and head circumference are often the only objective information present in the child's medical record (Hostetter and Johnson, 1996). Many internationally adopted children were born prematurely, and common health problems such as infant diarrhea and malnutrition may delay growth and development. Some children may have serious or multiple health problems, and this can be very stressful for the parents.

Parenting and Divorce

Since the mid-1960s there has been a marked change in the stability of families; this is reflected in increased rates of divorce, single parenthood, and remarriage. In 1999 (June 1998 to June 1999) the divorce rate for the United States was 4.2 per 1000 total population (U.S. Department of Health and Human Services, 2000). The divorce rate has changed very little since 1987. In the previous decade the rate increased almost yearly, with a peak in 1979. Although almost half of all divorcing couples are childless, over 1 million children experience divorce each year, and most of the children are very young.

The process of divorce begins with a period of marital conflict of varying length and intensity, followed by a separation, the actual legal divorce, and the reestablishment of different living arrangements. Because a function of parenthood is to provide for the security and emotional welfare of children, disruption of the family structure often engenders strong feelings of guilt in the parents.

During a divorce, parents' coping abilities may be compromised. The parents may be much too preoccupied with their own feelings, needs, and life changes to be available and supportive to their children. Newly employed parents, usually mothers, are likely to leave children with new caregivers, in strange settings, or alone after school. The parent may also spend more time away from home, searching for or establishing new relationships. Sometimes, however, the adult feels frightened and alone and begins to depend on the child as a substitute for the absent parent. This dependence places an enormous burden on the child.

Common characteristics in the custodial household following separation and divorce include disorder, coercive types of control, inflammable tempers in both parents and children, reduced parental competence, a greater sense of parental helplessness, poorly enforced discipline, and diminished regularity in enforcing household routines. Noncustodial parents also are seldom prepared for the role of visitor, may assume the role of recreational and "fun" parent, and may not have a residence suitable for children's visits. They may be concerned about maintaining the arrangement over the years to follow.

Impact of Divorce on Children. The results of numerous studies show that divorce has a profound effect on children. Long-term studies indicate that many youngsters suffer from psychologic and social difficulties associated with continuing and/or new stresses in the postdivorce family. A main outcome is heightened anxiety about forming enduring relationships as young adults (Thompson, 1998). Even when a divorce is amiable and open, children may recall parental separation with the same emotions felt by victims of a natural disaster: loss, grief, and vulnerability to forces beyond their control.

The impact of divorce on children depends on a variety of factors, including the age and sex of the children, the outcome of the divorce, and the quality of the parent-child relationship and parental care during the years following the divorce. Family characteristics appear to be more crucial to children's well-being than specific child characteristics, such as age or sex. The most damaging factor is continuing conflict between the divorced parents (Thompson, 1998). High levels of ongoing family conflict are related to problems of social development, emotional stability, and cognitive skills for the child.

Complications sometimes associated with divorce include efforts on the part of one parent to subvert the child's loyalties to the other, abandonment to other caregivers, and adjustment to a stepparent. A major problem occurs when children become the middle person between the divorced parents. They become the message bearer between the parents, are often quizzed about the activities of the other parent, and have to listen to criticisms from one parent about the other. A nurse may be able to intercede by helping the child get out of the middle by stating "I messages" based on the formula of "I feel. . . ." This approach may empower the child to feel more in control. For example, the "I message" may be: "I feel uncomfortable when you ask me all those questions about Mom. I would like it if you would talk to her yourself" (Arbuthnot and Gordon, 1995).

Children may feel a sense of shame and embarrassment concerning the family situation. Feelings experienced by children of different ages are found in Box 31-4. Such feelings cause children to see themselves as different, inferior, or unworthy of love, especially if they feel any responsibility for the family dissolution. Although the social stigma attached to divorce no longer produces the emotions it did in the past, it may still exist in some areas and can reinforce children's negative self-image. The lasting effects of divorce depend on the children's and the parents' adjustment to the transition from an intact family to a single-parent family and, often, to a reconstituted family.

Although most studies have concentrated on the negative effects of divorce on youngsters, positive outcomes of divorce have been reported. A successful postdivorce family, either as a single-parent or as a reconstituted family, can improve the quality of life for adults and children. Living with conflict is resolved, and a better relationship with one or both parents may

*For more information contact the International Adoption Clinic, Fairview University Medical Center, P.O. Box 211, 420 Delaware St. SE, Minneapolis, MN 55455; 1-800-688-5252.

Box 31-4

Feelings and Behaviors of Children Related to Divorce

INFANCY
- Effects of reduced mothering or lack of mothering
- Increased irritability
- Disturbance in eating, sleeping, and elimination
- Interference with attachment process

EARLY PRESCHOOL CHILDREN (AGES 2-3 YEARS)
- Frightened and confused
- Blame themselves for the divorce
- Fear of abandonment
- Increased irritability, whining, tantrums
- Regressive behaviors (e.g., thumb sucking, loss of elimination control)
- Separation anxiety

LATER PRESCHOOL CHILDREN (AGES 3-5 YEARS)
- Fear of abandonment
- Blame themselves for the divorce; decreased self-esteem
- Bewilderment regarding all human relationships
- Become more aggressive in relationships with others (e.g., siblings, peers)
- Engage in fantasy to seek understanding of the divorce

EARLY SCHOOL-AGE CHILDREN (AGES 5-6 YEARS)
- Depression and immature behavior
- Loss of appetite and sleep disorders
- May be able to verbalize some feelings and understand some divorce-related changes
- Increased anxiety and aggression
- Feel abandoned by departing parent

MIDDLE SCHOOL-AGE CHILDREN (AGES 6-8 YEARS)
- Panic reactions
- Feelings of deprivation—loss of parent, attention, money, and secure future
- Profound sadness, depression, fear, and insecurity
- Feelings of abandonment and rejection
- Fear regarding the future
- Difficulty expressing anger at parents
- Intense desire for reconciliation of parents
- Impaired capacity to play and enjoy outside activities
- Decline in school performance
- Altered peer relationships—become bossy, irritable, demanding, and manipulative
- Frequent crying, loss of appetite, sleep disorders
- Disturbed routine, forgetfulness

LATER SCHOOL-AGE CHILDREN (AGES 9-12 YEARS)
- More realistic understanding of divorce
- Intense anger directed at one or both parents
- Divided loyalties
- Able to express feelings of anger
- Ashamed of parental behavior
- Feel the need for revenge; may wish to punish the parent they hold responsible
- Feel lonely, rejected, and abandoned
- Altered peer relationships
- Decline in school performance
- May develop somatic complaints
- May engage in aberrant behavior such as lying, stealing
- Temper tantrums
- Dictatorial attitude

ADOLESCENTS (AGES 12-18 YEARS)
- Able to disengage themselves from parental conflict
- Feel a profound sense of loss—of family, childhood
- Feelings of anxiety
- Worry about themselves, parents, siblings
- Express anger, sadness, shame, embarrassment
- May withdraw from family and friends
- Disturbed concept of sexuality
- May engage in acting-out behaviors

result. Children may also have less contact with a disturbed parent.

Age- and Sex-Related Responses to Divorce. Previously it was believed that divorce had a greater impact on younger children, but more recent observations indicate that divorce constitutes a major disruption for children in all age groups. The feelings and behaviors of children may differ according to age (see Box 31-4) and sex, but all suffer stresses second only to the stress produced by the death of a parent.

Although considerable research has looked at sex differences in children's adjustments to divorce, the findings are not conclusive. Some studies have indicated an unstable masculinity in boys, and precocious sexual activity and difficulty in establishing lasting relationships in girls (Thompson, 1998).

Telling the Children. Parents are understandably hesitant to tell children about their decision to divorce. A vast majority of parents neglect to discuss with their preschool children either the divorce or the inevitable changes it brings. Without preparation, even children who remain in the family home may be confused by the parental separation.

Most likely, the children are already experiencing vague, uneasy feelings that are more difficult to cope with than being told truthfully about the situation. If possible, the initial disclosure should include both parents and siblings, followed by later discussions with each child individually. Ample time should be set aside for the discussions, and they should take place during a period of calm, not after an argument. Parents who physically hold or touch their children provide them with a feeling of warmth that is reassuring. The discussions should include the reason for the divorce—while minimizing blame—and reassurance that the divorce is not the fault of the children. Children may feel guilty, as though they have somehow failed or are being punished for misbehavior. They wonder what role they played in the divorce or failure to keep the family together.

Parents need not fear crying in front of the children; it gives the children permission to cry also. Children need to ventilate their feelings. They normally feel anger and resentment and should be allowed to communicate these feelings without punishment. They also have feelings of terror and abandonment and long for consistency and order in their lives. They need to know where they will live, who will take care of them, if they will be with their siblings, and if there will be enough money to live on. The children may also fear that if the parents stopped loving each other, they could stop loving them as well. Their need for assurance of love is tremendous at this time.

Further issues a child may ponder include questions about what will happen on special days like birthdays and holidays, whether both parents will come to school events, and whether the child will still have the same friends (Arbuthnot and Gordon, 1995).

Custody and Parenting Partnerships. Traditionally, when parents separated, the mother was given custody of the children. Now both parents and the courts are seeking alternatives. The present belief is that neither fathers nor mothers should be awarded custody automatically. Rather, custody should be awarded to the parent who is best able to provide for the children's welfare. In certain situations children experience severe stress when living or spending time with a parent. In most divorce cases the mother still receives custody of the child with visitation agreements for the father. However, more courts are now awarding custody to fathers. Men usually make more money and can offer more material benefits than many women are able to provide. The incidence of delinquent support payments to custodial mothers is a matter of universal knowledge and concern.

Often overlooked are the changes that may occur in the children's relationships with other relatives, especially grandparents. Grandparents on the noncustodial side are often kept from their grandchildren; those on the custodial side may be overwhelmed by their adult child's return to the household with grandchildren.*

Two other, less common, custody arrangements are divided custody and joint custody. *Divided,* or *split custody* means that each parent is awarded custody of one or more of the children, thereby separating siblings. For example, sons might live with the father and daughters with the mother. Joint custody takes one of two forms. In *joint physical custody* the parents alternate the physical care and control of the children on a reasonably equitable basis while maintaining shared parenting responsibilities legally. This type of custody arrangement works well for families who live close to each other and whose occupations allow an active role in the care and rearing of the children. In *joint legal custody* the children reside with one parent but both parents are the children's legal guardians and both participate in childrearing.

Co-parenting offers substantial benefits for the family: children can be close to both parents, and life with each parent can be more normal as opposed to a disciplinarian mother and a recreational father. However, to be successful, the parents must place a high value on the commitment to provide as normal parenting as possible and be able to separate their marital conflicts from the parenting roles. No matter what type of custody arrangement is awarded, the primary consideration is the welfare of the children.

**Grandparents,* a newsletter for grandparents in divided families, is published by Scarsdale Family Counseling Service, 405 Harwood Building, Scarsdale, NY 10583; phone (914) 723-3281.

Single Parenting

Single-parent status is acquired by means of divorce, separation, or death, or through birth or adoption of a child by a single person. Although divorce rates have stabilized, the number of single-parent households continues to rise. Today, 1 child in 4 lives in a single-parent family, with the majority of single parents being women (Fuller, 1997). It is estimated that at least half of the children born during the 1990s will spend part of their time in a family headed by a divorced, separated, widowed, or never-married mother. Although some women are single parents by choice, most of these women never planned on being single parents, and many feel pressure to marry or remarry. In one study it was noted that when young African-American grandmothers serve as a parental replacement, their surrogate role supports early pregnancies and may contribute to repeated pregnancies (Camblin, Odulana, and White, 1996).

Managing shortages of money, time, and energy are major concerns of single parents. Studies repeatedly confirm the financial difficulties of single-parent families, particularly in the case of single mothers. In addition, these families are often forced by their financial status to live in communities where inadequate housing and personal safety are concerns. Moreover, single parents may feel guilty about the time spent away from their children. Divorced mothers from marriages where the father assumed the breadwinning role and the mother the household maintenance and parenting roles have been found to have the most difficulty in adjusting to becoming the breadwinner for the family (Youngblut et al, 2000). Many single parents have trouble arranging for adequate child care, and care for sick children is especially difficult to obtain.

Literature on the subject of single parents is diverse. Several authors (Elshtain, 1997; Mackey, 1997; Whitehead, 1997) suggest that such large-scale distribution of single parents is harmful to the society as a whole because the children are more likely to be poor and stay poor, commit crime, and be a source of discipline problems in public education. Zinsmeister (1997) thinks that because of the absence of the father in most single-parent homes the mother is overtaxed as both nurturer and disciplinarian, and that a lack of a male role model may lead to poor educational performance, truancy, criminal activity, and psychologic problems for these children. However, Skolnick and Rosencranz (1997) state that single-parent families have been unfairly stigmatized, that the harm caused by single or unwed mothers is exaggerated and unfair, and that single motherhood is a legitimate choice.

Fathers who have custody of their children have many of the same problems as divorced mothers. They feel overburdened by the responsibility, are depressed, and are concerned about their ability to cope with the emotional needs of the children, especially the needs of the girls. A lack of homemaking skills is characteristic of most fathers. They find it difficult at first to coordinate household tasks, school visits, and other activities associated with managing a household alone. Fathers often demand more assistance with household tasks and more independence from their children than custodial mothers do, and they are likely to make use of alternative caregiving and support systems.

Supports and resources for single-parent families include health care services that are open evenings and weekends; high-quality child care; respite child care to relieve parental exhaustion and burnout; and parent enhancement centers for advancing education and job skills, providing recreational activities, and offering parenting education. Groups for single-parent fathers and grandparents who are primary caregivers are also important. There is a need on the part of the parent for social contacts and a life separate from the children for the emotional growth of both parent and child. The single parent can find support and encouragement from Parents Without Partners, Inc.,* an organization designed to meet the needs of this increasingly important group.

Parenting in Reconstituted Families

In the United States, approximately 1 in 8 dependent children in homes where parents have divorced will experience yet another major change in their lives after divorce—a return to a nuclear family and the sudden acquisition of a stepparent when the custodial parent remarries (Dunn, 1995). The entry of a stepparent into a ready-made family requires adjustments for all of the family members. Some obstacles to the role adjustments and family problem solving include disruption of previous lifestyles and interaction patterns, complexity in the formation of new ones, and lack of social supports. Despite these problems, most children from divorced families want to live in a two-parent home.

Cooperative parenting relationships can allow more time for each set of parents to be alone to establish their own relationships with the children. Under ideal circumstances, power conflicts between the two households can be reduced, and tension and anxiety can be lessened for all family members. In addition, the children's self-esteem can be increased, and there is a greater likelihood of continued contact with grandparents. Flexibility, mutual support, and open communication are critical in successful relationships in stepfamilies and stepparenting situations.

Unfortunately, stepfamilies usually do not seek help to prevent problems from arising. Typically, information and counseling are sought only when problems have surfaced and can no longer be ignored. A preventive rather than remedial approach to stepfamilies and stepparenting is needed (Dunn, 1995) (Family Focus box).

Parenting in Dual-Earner Families

No change in family lifestyle has had more impact then the large numbers of women entering the workplace. As women moved away from the traditional homemaker pattern, the numbers of dual-earner families increased dramatically. This trend is unlikely to diminish. As a result, the family is subjected to considerable stress as members attempt to meet the challenge of the often competing demands of occupational needs and those regarded as necessary for a rich family life.

Role definitions are often altered to arrange an equitable division of time and labor, as well as to resolve conflicts between earlier and later norms, especially those related to the traditional norms of the culture. Overload is a common source of stress in a dual-earner family, and social activities are significantly curtailed. Time demands and scheduling are major problems, and when there are children, the demands can be even more intense; dual-earner couples may increase the strain on themselves to avoid creating stress for their children, although there is no evidence to indicate that the dual-earner lifestyle, as such, is stressful to children. However, the stress experienced by the parents may affect the children indirectly.

Working Mothers. Even though working mothers have become the norm in the United States, disapproving attitudes from some health care workers and some child care books, lack of a national policy on child care, and memories from their own childhood of being cared for by an at-home mother contribute to the torn and guilty feelings many working mothers experience.

Child care is critical to the working mother's well-being. The quality of child care is a persistent concern for all working parents. Determinants of child care quality are based on health and safety requirements, responsive and warm interaction between staff and children, developmentally appropriate activities and trained staff, limited group size, age-appropriate caregivers, child ratios, and adequate indoor and outdoor space (Scarr, 1998). In general, the quality of child care is affected by lower ratios, smaller group sizes, and better-qualified teachers.

Any research on the effects of day care must be examined carefully; the characteristics of the day care setting and the measures used for child outcomes, such as attachment, must be taken into consideration. Also, the economic background of the family interacts with the effects of the type of child care and its psychologic outcomes (Friedman et al, 1994).

Nurses play an important role in helping families to find suitable sources of child care and to prepare children for this experience. Although many types of families exist, it is more important to know and understand how a particular family functions (Acock and Demo, 1996).

Family Focus

BLENDED FAMILIES AND LIVING "IN STEP"

Let relationships develop slowly and naturally. Don't expect too much too soon, from the children, from your spouse, or from yourself.

Don't criticize or belittle lost (or new) parents, or try to erase or replace them. Stepparents are additional parents.

Expect confused feelings, anxieties, competition for attention, bids for loyalty. Decide on standards of discipline and behavior and stick to them.

Communicate. Don't pretend everything is fine if it isn't. Look at problems squarely and deal with them openly.

If you need help, admit it and get it. Read a book, get counseling, join a support group, call a family meeting.

From Stein B: Yours, mine, and ours: a look at stepfamilies, *Growing Parent* 12(9):1-5, 1984.

Key Points

- Because there is no agreement about the definition of family, a family is what a patient considers it to be.

*International Headquarters, 401 N. Michigan Ave., Chicago, IL 60611-4267; phone (312) 644-6610; or visit the website: www.parentswithoutpartners.org.

- Although the traditional family structure has been nuclear or extended, in recent years other forms, such as the single-parent family, have emerged.
- Family size and positioning within the family structure have a strong impact on a child's development.
- Interpersonal skills and a basic understanding of childhood growth and development are two essential areas of focus for parents.
- Parental control tends to be predominantly one of three types: authoritarian, permissive, or authoritative.
- Three areas of special concern to adoptive families include the initial attachment process, the task of telling the children they are adopted, and identity formation during adolescence.
- Marital factors within the home significantly influence a child's development. The impact of divorce on a child depends on the child's age and sex, and the quality of the parent-child relationship and parental care following the divorce.
- Single-parenting and stepparenting create adjustment difficulties and stress that is added to the already-demanding parental role. Significant numbers of children will live in a single-parent or reconstituted family at some point.

References

Acock A, Demo D: Family structure, family process, and adolescent well-being, *J Res Adolesc* 6(4):457-488, 1996.

American Academy of Pediatrics, Committee on Psychosocial Aspects of Child and Family Health: Guidance for effective discipline, *Pediatrics* 101(4):723-728, 1998.

Arbuthnot J, Gordon D: *Surviving divorce: a student's companion to children in the middle,* Athens, OH, 1995, Center for Divorce Education.

Bauman LJ, Friedman SB: Corporal punishment, *Pediatr Clin North Am* 45(2):403-415, 1998.

Black M, Nitz K: Grandmother co-residence, parenting and child development among low income, urban teen mothers, *J Adolesc Health* 18:218-226, 1996.

Blum NJ et al: Disciplining young children: the role of verbal instructions and reasoning, *Pediatrics* 96(2):336-341, 1995.

Brazelton TB: Working with families: opportunities for early intervention, *Pediatr Clin North Am* 42(1):1-10, 1995.

Camblin L, Odulana J, White P: Cultural roles and health status of contemporary African American young grandmothers, *J Multicult Nurs Health* 2(4):28-35, 1996.

Dunn J: Stepfamilies and children's adjustment, *Arch Dis Child* 73(6):487-489, 1995.

Elshtain JB: Single-parent families contribute to the breakdown of society. In Swisher KL, editor: *Single-parent families,* San Diego, CA, 1997, Greenhaven Press.

Foss G: A conceptual model for studying parenting behaviors in immigrant populations, *Adv Nurs Sci* 19(2):74-87, 1996.

Friedman SL et al: Effects of child care on psychological development: issues and future directions for research, *Pediatrics* 94(6, suppl 2):1069-1070, 1994.

Fuller L: Single-parent families: a unique challenge, *Nurse Pract* 22(11):116-120, 1997.

Grotevant H, McRoy R: Emotional disorders in adopted children and youth. In McManus M, editor: Adoption: a lifelong journey for children and families, *Focal Point* 10(1), 1996.

Guyer B et al: Annual summary statistics—1998, *Pediatrics* 104(8):1229-1245, 1999.

Hostetter M, Johnson D: Medical supervision of internationally adopted children, *Pediatr Basics* 77:10-17, 1996.

Mackey WC: Single-parent families contribute to violent crime. In Swisher KL, editor: *Single-parent families,* San Diego, CA, 1997, Greenhaven Press.

McCubbin M, McCubbin H: Theoretical orientation to family stress and coping. In Figley C, editor: *Treating families under stress,* New York, 1989, Brunner/Mazel.

Newman J: The more the merrier? Effects of family size and sibling spacing on sibling relationships, *Child Care Health Dev* 22(5):285-302, 1996.

Patterson J: Promoting resilience in families experiencing stress, *Pediatr Clin North Am* 42(1):47-63, 1995.

Scarr S: American child care today, *Am Psychol* 53(2);95-108, 1998.

Skolnick A, Rosencranz S: The harmful effects of single-parent families are exaggerated. In Swisher KL, editor: *Single-parent families,* San Diego, CA, 1997, Greenhaven Press.

Smith J, Brooks-Gunn J: Correlates and consequences of harsh discipline for young children, *Arch Pediatr Adolesc Med* 15(8):777-786, 1997.

Sullivan A: Policy issues in gay and lesbian adoption, *Adopt Foster* 19(4):21-25, 1995.

Thompson P: Adolescents from families of divorce: vulnerability to physiological and psychological disturbances, *J Psychosoc Nurs Ment Health Serv* 36(3):34-39, 1998.

Trost S et al: Gender differences in physical activity and determinants of physical activity in rural fifth grade children, *J Sch Health* 66(4):145-150, 1996.

U.S. Department of Health and Human Services: Births, marriages, divorces, and deaths: provisional data for June 1999, *Natl Vital Stat Rep* 48(8):1-2, 2000.

Ventura SJ et al: Advance report of final natality statistics, 1995, *Monthly Vital Statistics Report* 44(3, suppl), 1997.

Visher E, Visher J: Beyond the nuclear family: resources and implications for pediatricians, *Fam Focused Pediatr* 42(1):31-43, 1995.

Whitehead BD: Single-parent families are harmful. In Swisher KL, editor: *Single-parent families,* San Diego, CA, 1997, Greenhaven Press.

Youngblut, JM et al: Factors influencing single mothers' employment status, *Health Care for Women International* 21: 125-136, 2000.

Zinsmeister K: Divorce harms children. In Swisher KL, editor: *Single-parent families,* San Diego, CA, 1997, Greenhaven Press.

CHAPTER 32

Social, Cultural, and Religious Influences on Child Health Promotion

http://www.harcourthealth.com/MERLIN/Wong/maternal/

On completion of this chapter the reader will be able to:

- Define culture, culture shock, ethnicity, and race.
- Describe the subcultural influences on child development in the areas of socialization, education, and aspiration.
- Compare and contrast the advantages and disadvantages encountered in the educational system by children from lower- and middle-class backgrounds.
- Characterize family life in present-day America.
- Identify common diseases or disorders that affect certain ethnic or cultural groups.
- Identify areas of potential conflict of values and customs for a nurse interacting with a family from a different cultural/ethnic group.
- Describe three religious groups whose beliefs significantly affect their health practices.

CULTURE

The future of any society depends on its children. Therefore society must provide for their care, nurturance, and socialization. Culture plays a critical role in the socialization agenda of children through particular views of parenting and child development (Yoos et al, 1995). The customs and values of the culture help to organize a society's childrearing system and are transmitted from one generation to the next through the medium of the family.

Culture is the context of the child's experience of health and illness, wellness and sickness (Talabere, 1996). A holistic view of any child requires that nurses develop some understanding of the ways that culture contributes to the development of social and emotional relationships and influences childrearing practices and attitudes toward health.

Transcultural nursing knowledge has become imperative during the past decade because of the increased migration of people worldwide. Professional nurses are providing care to diverse populations from almost every point of the globe (Cooper, 1996). This orientation to transcultural nursing includes an awareness of the nurse's own frame of reference. With a conscious effort to recognize and appreciate the views and beliefs of health care recipients, nurses can provide culturally competent nursing care (Phillips and Lobar, 1995; Yoos et al, 1997).

Culture is a pattern of assumptions, beliefs, and practices that unconsciously frames or guides the outlook and decisions of a group of people. Culture differs from both race and ethnicity. *Race* is defined as a division of mankind possessing traits that are transmissible by descent and that are sufficient to characterize it as a distinct human type. One classification of race, based on skin color, is Caucasoid (white), Negroid (black), and Mongoloid (yellow). *Ethnicity* is the affiliation of a set of persons who share a unique cultural, social, and linguistic heritage. *Socialization* is the process by which children acquire the beliefs, values, and behaviors of a given society in order to function within the group.

Culture is a complex whole in which each part is interrelated (Spector, 2000). A culture is composed of individuals who share a set of values, beliefs, practices (e.g., language, dress, diet, and health care), social relationships, law, politics, economics, and norms of behavior that are learned, integrative, social, and satisfying (Habayeb, 1995). Culture is not a surface veneer that covers a basic outlook shared by all human beings; rather it is an ingrained orientation to life that serves as a frame of reference for individual perception and judgment. People from one culture differ from those in other cultures in the ways they think, solve problems, and perceive and structure the world. Culture is, essentially, the way of life of a group of people that incorporates experiences of the past, that influences thought and action in the present, and that transmits these traditions to future group members. Adaptation is necessary, however, for the culture to survive in an ever-changing world. Consciously and unconsciously, the members abandon, modify, or assume new patterns to meet the needs of the group.

The observable components of a culture, such as material objects (e.g., dress, art, utensils, and other artifacts) and actions, are sometimes termed the *material overt* or *manifest culture; nonmaterial covert culture* refers to those aspects that cannot be observed directly, such as the ideas, beliefs, customs, and feelings of the culture. Related to the large culture are many *subcultures,* each with an identity of its own. Children are socialized into a particular subculture rather than into the culture as a whole. Subcultural influences, such as ethnicity and social class, are discussed in more detail later in this chapter.

The culture in which children are reared determines the type of food they will eat, the language they will speak, the ideals of behavior they will follow, and the way they will conduct themselves in social roles (Yoos et al, 1995). To be acceptable members of the culture, children must learn how the culture expects them to behave toward others in the group. In turn, they learn how they can expect others to behave toward them.

Cultures and subcultures contribute to the uniqueness of child members in such a subtle way and at such an early age that children grow up to feel that their beliefs, attitudes, values, and practices are the "correct," and "normal" ones; those of other cultures may be viewed as "deviant" or "wrong." A set of values learned in childhood is apt to characterize children's attitudes and behavior for life, guiding their long-range strivings and monitoring their short-range, impulsive inclinations. Thus every ongoing society socializes each succeeding generation to its cultural heritage.

The manner and sequence of the growth and development phenomenon are universal and fundamental features of all children; however, the variations in behavioral responses that children display to similar events are believed to be determined by their culture. Inborn temperament and modes of behavior that prompt children to behave in their own preferred and highly individual manner may be in harmony or in conflict with the culture. Such forces as heredity and maturation impose limits on the influence that parents and other social groups may bring to bear.

Standards and norms vary from culture to culture and from location to location; a practice that is accepted in one area may meet with disapproval or create tension in another. The extent to which cultures tolerate divergence from the established norm varies among cultures and subcultural groups. Although conformity provides a degree of security, it is a decided deterrent to change.

Social Roles

Much of children's self-concept is derived from their ideas about their social roles. *Roles* are cultural creations; therefore the culture prescribes patterns of behavior for persons in a variety of social positions. All persons who hold similar social positions have an obligation to behave in a particular manner. A role prohibits some behaviors and allows others. Because it delineates and clarifies roles, the culture is a significant influence on the development of children's self-concept (i.e., attitudes and beliefs they have about themselves).

A social group consists of a system of roles carried out in both primary and secondary groups. A *primary group* is characterized by intimate, continued, face-to-face contact; mutual support of members; and the ability to order or constrain a considerable proportion of individual members' behavior. Two such groups are the family and the peer group, both of which exert a great deal of influence on the child.

Secondary groups are groups that have limited, intermittent contact and in which there is generally less concern for members' behavior. These groups offer little in terms of support or pressure toward conformity except in rigidly limited areas. Examples of secondary groups are professional associations and church organizations (also considered in relation to subgroups). The childrearing orientation in a secondary-group environment, such as an urban community, differs considerably from that of a primary-group community. An urban community is dynamic and rapidly changing; therefore many of the traditional behaviors and values do not meet its needs. Consequently, parents are often uncertain about what to teach their children. They may wish to rear their children with values consistent with their own, but the differences in experience between the generations are too great. As a result, they often grant their children autonomy in some areas of decision making early in the developmental process, and other secondary groups assume a greater influence. The children are exposed to an assortment of social groups with diverse sets of values and expectations. None of the groups is highly dominant in its influence; therefore the children are exposed to an eclectic set of values, some in agreement and some at conflict with the others. From there they must ultimately select those that they determine to be best for them and adopt them to form a consistent set of roles and behaviors to be incorporated into the self-concept.

Guilt and Shame Orientation. Conditioning children to feel either guilt or shame for misdeeds is a technique used by a culture to control social behavior—to internalize the norms and expectations of others. Some cultural groups value a well-developed conscience (superego) and condition their children to feel guilt following wrongdoing. Offenders get an uncomfortable physical feeling and want to purge themselves. Since guilt is based within the individual, successful conditioning produces self-regulated persons who punish themselves without their being caught in the act of wrongdoing.

In many cultural groups guilt is lacking and social controls are based on the use of shame. Offenders do not want anyone to see them when they have been found guilty of a wrongful deed. Sometimes children in these groups learn that anything is acceptable as long as one is not caught; the shame results when the forbidden act is found out by others.

Although both techniques are used by members of both primary- and secondary-group communities, shame is apt to be more successful in a primary-group community because most behaviors are quite public. In secondary-group communities it is less effective; persons are not as apt to be caught and, if caught, can withdraw and join a group that is unaware of the misdeed. Guilt probably has a greater influence on behavior in urban communities, although many authorities believe that the trend in urban North America is shifting away from a guilt orientation. Rapid changes in the North American culture leave parents unsure of their own values; therefore much of their function is abandoned to the school and peers. Peers are notorious for using shame as a disciplinary technique.

Subcultural Influences

Except in rare situations, children grow and develop in a blend of cultures and subcultures. In a large, complex society such as the United States, different groups have their own set of standards, values, and expectations within the collective ways of the large culture. Although many cultural differences are related to geographic boundaries, subcultures are not always restricted by location.

Children's membership in a cultural subgroup is, for the most part, involuntary; they are born into a family with a specific ethnic and/or racial heritage, socioeconomic level, and religious beliefs. Although in the complex North American society there are countless subcultures and considerable variation in the way of life, those subcultures that seem to exert the greatest influence on childrearing are ethnicity, social class, and occupational role. In addition, schools and peer-group subcultures are strong influences in the socialization of the child.

Ethnicity. *Ethnicity* is the classification of or affiliation with any of the basic groups or divisions of mankind or any heterogeneous population differentiated by customs, characteristics, language, or similar distinguishing factors. Ethnic differences extend to many areas and include such manifestations as family structure, language, food preferences, moral codes, and expression of emotion. Some standards of behavior result from the cultural heritage of the specific ethnic group. The term *ethnic* has aroused strong negative feelings and is often rejected by the general population (Spector, 2000).

To establish their place in the group, children learn how to adhere to a mode of behavior that is in accordance with standards distinctive to the group, and learn how they can expect others to behave toward them. They take their cues from observing and imitating those to whom they are exposed. For example, children of a racial minority form a perception of their role as a group member by observing the manner in which role models within the subgroup respond to treatment by people outside the subgroup. When they see group members display an attitude of inferiority, they assume this to be the appropriate behavior. These perceptions are then incorporated into their own self-concept.

In the United States the cross-cultural lines are becoming blurred as subcultures are assimilated and blended into the larger culture (Fig. 32-1). Although ethnic differences in childrearing are probably diminishing, they remain important. It is particularly difficult for persons to attempt to maintain an identity with a subculture while living and conforming to the requirements of the dominant culture. Universal customs and language used in commercial and educational systems are different from those of the minority culture. Often the values are in conflict. Consequently, children reared in this environment are confused about roles and values, and they usually adopt those of the more influential or higher status culture. Youth, in particular, are influenced by the locally dominant group.

Ethnocentrism is the emotional attitude that one's own ethnic group is superior to others; that one's values, beliefs, and perceptions are the correct ones; and that the group's ways of living and behaving are the best way (Rogers, 1995). *Ethnic stereotyping* or labeling stems from ethnocentric views of people. Ethnocentrism implies that all other groups are inferior and that their ways are not in the best interests of the group. It is a common attitude among a dominant ethnic group and strongly influences the ability of one person to evaluate the beliefs and behaviors of others objectively. This inherent viewpoint of individuals tends to bias their interpretation and understanding of the behavior of others. Sometimes nurses have a tendency to have ethnocentric attitudes when giving care to people from different cultures (Petersen, 1995). Ethnocentric differences are valid, and culturally competent nurses recognize and acknowledge these differences and work toward desirable outcomes for the family, the child, and the nurse (Phillips and Lobar, 1995).

Social Class/Occupation. Although there are exceptions, probably the greatest influence on childrearing practices and their consequences is the social class of the family into which a child is born. Differences in childrearing goals and practices, as well as in attitudes toward health, have been found to be greater between social classes than between races or ethnic groups. In North America, social class and socioeconomic level are essentially synonymous and are most easily determined by occupation; for example, the upper middle class consists primarily of professional and business people, almost all with a college education. The working class includes employees in manufacturing, trades, and service occupations (such as barbers or hairdressers) who have a high school education. In the lower class the breadwinners are typically unskilled laborers or unem-

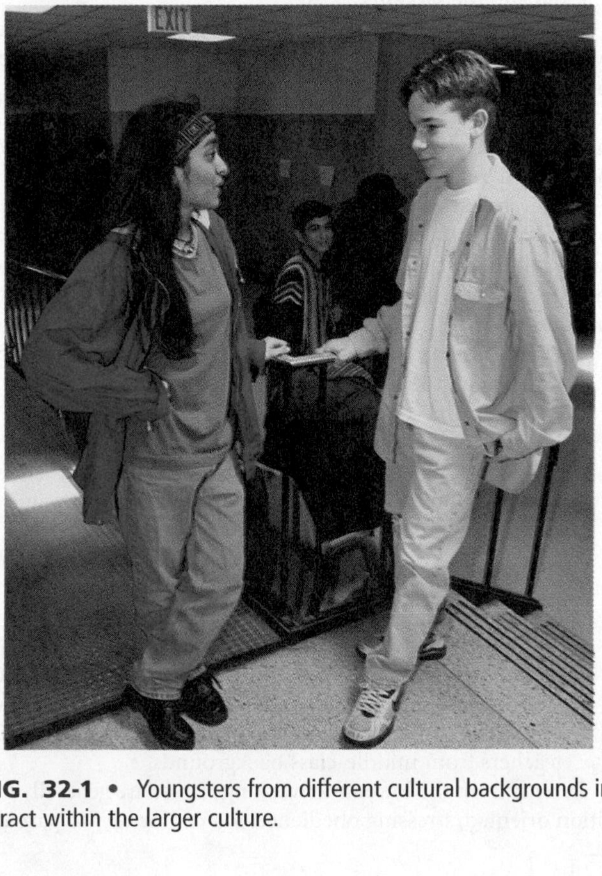

FIG. 32-1 • Youngsters from different cultural backgrounds interact within the larger culture.

ployed, and families may or may not be receiving public assistance. Since children are reared differently by parents who vary in respect to these factors, social class can be expected to produce substantial variation in their upbringing.

Middle and Upper Classes. Middle- and upper-class children live in an enriched environment that provides material comforts and broader opportunities. The parents are usually educated beyond high school and have occupations that require judgment, creativity, and resourcefulness. These attributes are fostered in their children. Other authority figures, such as teachers with whom the children are routinely in contact, are usually from a middle-class background and have activities and expectations for the children that are similar to those of the parents.

Most middle-class parents are future oriented, have higher educational and occupational aspirations for their children, and use long-range planning to meet these goals. Middle-class parents typically encourage their children to participate in activities that foster achievement (e.g., dancing lessons, athletics, and scouting) in the belief that this will make them well-rounded, self-directed adults.

In the area of discipline, middle-class parents are more apt to use manipulative techniques such as reasoning and drawing on the child's sense of guilt. They tend to scold and use isolation rather than physical punishment. There is more concern regarding the *intent* of the act rather than the *consequences* of the act.

It is believed that upper-class parents are more permissive and foster desirable behavior through positive reinforcement. However, much of the actual child care in upper-class families is delegated to surrogates, such as housekeepers, governesses, or private schools. The parent serves as an arbitrator between the children and the servants.

Lower and Working Classes. The uncertainty of their lives leads members of the lower classes to be present oriented; that is, to take advantage of gratification when possible. This orientation is distinctly different from that of most members of the middle class, who may be more willing to delay gratification to achieve a long-term goal.

Children in lower-class families encounter major educational disadvantages, reflected in the high incidence of academic failure and dropout rates. The major educational disadvantages many children from the lower social class encounter include:

- Parents are more likely to value the concrete and tangible rather than the abstract, and are therefore less inclined to encourage these qualities in their children.
- Parents are less likely to read to the child or encourage educational play because of their own educational level.
- No role models may be available to support the value of education.
- Inadequate funding and/or poor quality of education may exist in neighborhood schools.
- Poor health and inadequate nutrition of the children is common.
- Parents are more likely to have limited communication skills such as simple grammar; inability to express abstractions; and ethnic dialects, which hamper interactions with teachers from middle-class backgrounds.

Parents from the lower and working classes are generally tradition oriented, stressing obedience and conformity to parental values and external regulations. The most commonly used form of discipline for undesirable behavior is physical punishment. Parents are usually less interested in the direction of children's activities than with conduct; they are more concerned that children stay out of trouble.

Poverty. A subcultural influence closely related to, but different from, social class is the condition known as poverty. It is a relative concept and is usually associated with the general standards of a population. The term *poverty* implies both visible and invisible impoverishment. *Visible poverty* refers to lack of money or material resources, including insufficient clothing, poor sanitation, and deteriorating housing. *Invisible poverty* refers to social and cultural deprivation, such as limited employment opportunities, inferior educational opportunities, lack of or inferior medical services and health care facilities, and an absence of public services.

An *absolute standard* of poverty attempts to delimit some basic set of resources needed for adequate existence; a *relative standard* reflects the median standard of living in a society, and is the term used in referring to childhood poverty in the United States. That is, what appears to be deprivation in one area may be a standard or norm in another.

Despite the enormous wealth in the United States, there was no change in the poverty rate of children between 1985 and 1994. Presently, it is estimated that 1 in 5 children (21%) live in poverty (income of $16,655 or less for a family of 4 in 1998 [U.S. Census Bureau, 1999]). This rate is substantially higher than the rate in other industrialized countries. Although Caucasian children saw their poverty rate increase the most during the 1980s (1 in 7 are poor), minority children are more likely to be poor. Almost 50% of African-American children and more than one third of Hispanic children live in families with incomes below the poverty level (Annie E. Casey Foundation, 1999). Large numbers of Native American children also live in poverty, with unemployment rates on one reservation estimated at 80%. Some children on the reservation claim that their main source of food is the school-based free breakfast and lunch program (Rollins, 1993).

Many Americans picture the typical child who is poor as a city dweller with unemployed parents, usually living in a single-parent home. Although chronic poverty is more concentrated in central city areas, 60% of the nation's poor children live in the suburbs or rural areas of the country (Bennett et al, 1999). The chances of being poor increase substantially when children are born to parents who have not graduated from high school. The poverty rate for children living with parents who dropped out of high school was 57% in 1995, compared with 4% for children who had at least one parent with a college degree (Annie E. Casey Foundation, 1999).

Factors Related to Poverty. Throughout the United States there are groups of people, geographically segregated, who constitute what are known as "pockets of poverty." These are seen in the dense urban areas, such as the ghettos; and many rural areas, especially those that are geographically isolated from needed facilities and services. The nonurbanized regions identified as poverty areas in the United States are Appalachia, the deep South, the lower Southwest, and northern New England.

Certain ethnic or racial groups are overrepresented in the impoverished population. The most obvious of these are African-Americans, Latinos, Hispanics, and Native Americans.

Homelessness. One of the most pressing problems in the United States is the growing number of homeless families. *Homeless individuals* are those persons who lack resources and community ties necessary to provide for their own adequate shelter. In the past the homeless population traditionally included single adults, mostly men. Currently, the fastest growing segment of the homeless consists of families, most commonly single mothers with two or three children.

Homeless children have increased in numbers as poverty has become feminized, minorities have become poorer, and low-income housing has become less accessible. Estimates on the number of homeless children in the United States at any given time range from 68,000 to 100,000. The majority of homeless children are less than 5 years of age and are predominantly from minority groups.

Many families are becoming homeless because of physical and substance abuse. Other reasons include job layoffs, low income, parental mental illness, domestic conflict, disagreements with the landlord, poor living conditions, and unexpected family or economic crises. Many families move into homelessness gradually after family members and friends are no longer willing to provide housing.

Other groups of homeless children are "runaway" and "throwaway" adolescents. Many runaways are victims of physical and sexual abuse, and leave home because of long-term family or school problems. Poor parent-child relationships, extreme family conflict, feelings of alienation from parents, inconsistency in supervision, and unpredictability in discipline are other factors often cited.

Lack of a permanent dwelling deprives children of the most basic necessities for proper growth and development. Homelessness disrupts a child's friendships and schooling (Strehlow and Amos-Jones, 1999). Homeless children suffer from physical and mental disorders exceeding those found in poor children who have a permanent residence.

Migrant Families. One of the most disadvantaged population groups is migrant farmworkers and their children. Indications suggest that in the United States there are between 3 and 5 million migrant and seasonal workers and their dependents, whose average yearly income is well below the poverty level. In addition, most of these families have no health care insurance.

The low position of these families on the economic scale—and their rootless, mobile existence—subject them to inadequate sanitation, substandard housing, social isolation, and lack of educational and medical facilities (Sandhaus, 1998). This lifestyle is especially deleterious to the children. Schooling and health care are inadequate. Children are apt to live in a number of localities and attend a variety of schools in the course of a year, with no continuity in either education or health care. Because both parents work in the fields, children receive little adult supervision; therefore injury rates are high, and meals are erratic. Except where prohibited and enforced by law, children are even recruited to work in the fields along with the adults.

Some migrants have a home base to which they return at the end of growing season; others travel continuously, migrating north in summer and south in winter. With most there is little if any integration into the dominant culture; therefore migrant groups suffer social isolation. Groups who travel together, especially those with the same ethnic background, develop a cohesiveness and form their own set of values and customs. Sometimes a migrant family will leave the migration stream and become part of a permanent community. However, this involves adaptation to a new environment and lifestyle that can be stress provoking to these families.

Affluence. On the opposite end of the socioeconomic spectrum are the children of affluent members of society. Although they can live within the warmth of a positive family relationship, many of them appear to be just as deprived as poverty-stricken children. Wealth does not provide protection against many of life's problems and disappointments, especially in the area of parent-child relationships. Like their counterparts in the poverty groups, children of the affluent may suffer from discrimination, inadequate parenting, or unsatisfactory role models.

Children of the wealthy suffer most from lack of parental contact. There may be long separations from loving, caring parents because of social or business interests. Some have a cold, sometimes hostile parent, who is rarely available to them. Even their places of residence contribute to their isolation and loneliness. Paid parent surrogates, including servants, sports professionals (such as tennis or swimming instructors), and private school personnel, provide them with adult companionship and authority. During their early years, many wealthy children form stronger attachments to these people than to their parents. However, as these children grow older, they become aware of class distinctions. They realize that they must separate from these early relationships to form bonds with individuals in their class. Parents may begin involving the older adolescent in the family business and in adult social activities. But for many young people, a meaningful life with their family has come too late and they feel lonely, isolated, and unloved.

Many children from wealthy families, like those from poor families, seem to thrive and flourish, making positive contributions to their families and society. However, some grow up to display a lack of motivation or self-discipline, and boredom. They are suspicious of others, finding it difficult to believe they are liked for themselves and not for their money or position, and they do not trust others enough to enter into true friendships. Affluent children may also fail to acquire skills to handle responsibility and money.

Religion. Probably the most influential factor in shaping the culture of the United States is the Judeo-Christian faith. Many immigrants came to the United States for religious freedom, and established a religious and moral atmosphere that persists today. However, there are individual differences that are part of the general culture.

The religious orientation of the family dictates a code of morality, and influences the family's attitudes toward education, male and female role identity, and beliefs regarding their ultimate destiny (Fig. 32-2). It may also determine the school that the children attend, the companions with whom they associate, and often their mate selection. In a few instances, such as in the Mennonite and Amish communities, religion is the basis for a common way of life that determines where the children are reared and their lifestyle (see also Religious Beliefs, p. 721).

Schools. Next to the family, the schools exert the major force in providing continuity between generations by conveying a vast amount of culture from the older members to the young. In this way children are prepared to carry out the traditional so-

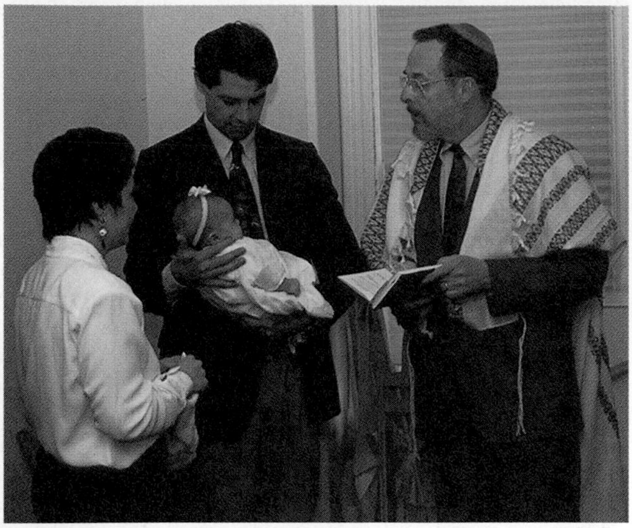

FIG. 32-2 • Soon after an infant is born, many families have special religious ceremonies.

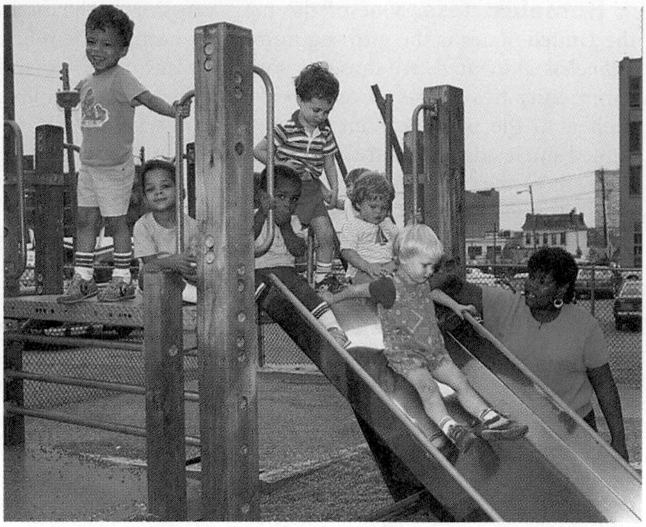

FIG. 32-3 • Children from a variety of cultural and ethnic backgrounds begin to socialize in the child care setting.

cial roles they are expected to assume as adults in society. School rules and regulations regarding attendance, authority relationships, and the system of sanctions and rewards based on achievement transmit to the child the behavioral expectations of the adult world of employment and relationships. School is often the only institution in which children systematically learn about the negative consequences of behaviors that deviate from social expectations. Teachers are expected to stimulate and guide the intellectual development of children, develop their sense of esthetics, and foster their capacity for creative problem solving. Through education, individuals in the lower classes are offered the opportunity for further education and the opportunity to move up in the social strata.

Traditionally, the socialization process of school has begun when the child enters kindergarten or first grade. Today, with more than 60% of mothers of preschool children working outside the home, this socialization process begins much earlier for a significant number of children in a variety of child care settings.

Peer Cultures. Peer groups also have an impact on the socialization of children (Fig. 32-3). Peer relationships become increasingly important and influential as children proceed through school. In school, children have what can be regarded as a culture of their own. This culture is also represented in a much purer form in the unsupervised play group than in the school, which is partly produced by adults.

Children are exposed to value systems such as those of the family, ethnic group, and social class. In peer-group interaction they are confronted with a variety of these sets of values. The values imposed by the peer group are especially compelling because children must accept and conform to them to be accepted as members of the group. When the peer values are not too different from those of family and teachers, the mild conflict created by these small differences serves to separate children from the adults in their lives and to strengthen the feeling of belonging to the peer group.

The kind of socialization provided by the peer group depends on the special subculture that develops from the background, interests, and capabilities of its members. Some groups support school achievement; others focus on athletic prowess; and still others are decidedly antithetical to educative goals. Scholastic achievement is strongly related to the value system of the peer groups. Many conflicts between teachers and students, and between parents and students, can be attributed to fear of rejection by peers. A conflict between what is expected from parents regarding academic achievement and what is expected from the peer culture is especially pronounced in high school.

Although it has neither the traditional authority of the parents nor the legal authority of the schools, the peer group manages to convey a substantial amount of information to its members, especially about taboo subjects such as sex and drugs. Through peer relationships, children learn ways to deal with dominance and hostility and to relate with persons in positions of leadership and authority. The peer subculture relieves boredom and provides recognition that individual members do not receive from teachers and other authority figures.

The peer-group culture has secrets, mores, and codes of ethics with which members promote feelings of group solidarity and detachment from adults. Traditions and folkways are transferred from "generation to generation" of schoolchildren, and have a great influence over the behavior of all group members. There are age-related games and other activities, and as children move from one level to the next, folkways of the younger group are discarded as those of the older group are adopted. For example, a school-age child rides a bicycle to school; the high school student prefers to drive a car. As they advance, children are forward oriented only—they look forward with anticipation but look backward with contempt.

Biculture. Some children are exposed to the values, role relationships, and lifestyles of two or more cultures. The virtual "straddling" of two cultures is referred to as *biculturation* and involves the ability to efficiently bridge the gap between an individual's culture of origin and the dominant culture (Rogers, 1995). This may occur because the child's parents are from two or more different cultures. In Hawaii, for example, it is common for children to be of four or more cultures. Other children straddle cultures as members of a minority culture within the dominant culture. This biculture is sometimes observed in the play group, but usually is not a significant factor until children enter school. Then they must unlearn some of the established practices of one culture in order to become socialized in the other, especially in role relationships. For example, children from Hispanic and Oriental cultures are taught to look away when scolded; in American schools the teacher expects direct eye contact: "Look at me when I speak to you." Children learn new roles and social behavior more rapidly than their adult counterparts.

The biculture is particularly marked in language differences. The bilingual child is said to be at a disadvantage in school situations of the dominant culture, in which there is controversy over bilingual education. Those supporting bilingual education adhere to the principle that children will understand more readily and perform more realistically (especially in testing situations) if learning is directed in their own language; others contend that children living in a dominant culture should adopt the ways of that culture, including language. There is less conflict for children when their language and culture are supported by the school, even if the dominant language is used.

The Child and Family in North America

America's orientation toward homogenization—"the great melting pot"—is changing. Increased awareness of the growing proportion of ethnic minorities that make up the United States population, coupled with a new positive value and emphasis being placed on ethnic diversity, has resulted in a renewed interest in cultural variation.

The frontier background of the North American culture has contributed to the overall orientation to life and childrearing. There has always been a basic optimistic view of the world, a belief that things can be better and that the children can and will be better off than the parents. This hopeful outlook and a general future orientation, together with the possibility of upward social mobility, have created a pervasive overall attitude of optimism. Increasing development of self-confidence and autonomy in children is fostered and encouraged. Children in North America are generally permitted a greater degree of freedom than in more tradition-oriented cultures, where individuals remain in one class for life.

Family life in North America is characterized by increasing geographic and economic mobility. There is less reliance on tradition, families are fragmented, and there is limited opportunity to transmit and acquire the traditional and accepted customs of a culture. Consequently, young adults rely to a greater extent on the professed experts, on their peers, and on the mass media for acquisition of acceptable patterns of behavior, including childrearing practices. Conflicting information can be a source of confusion and frustration as parents attempt to determine the comparatively stable, essential components of the culture and transmit these to their children.

Children in North America grow up with a number of different adults who all provide input as role models, teachers, and standards for behavior. Most children live in some form of nuclear family, located in sharply differentiated neighborhoods determined by income and ethnic status within a highly technical, largely urban society. Class differences in childrearing persist, but they are becoming less divergent as a result of the increased homogeneity of the culture.

Cultural Considerations

CLASSIFICATION OF MINORITY GROUPS

According to the 1990 U.S. Census Group Profiles, African-Americans are referred to as *blacks* and defined as "any persons whose lineage included ancestors who originated from any of the black racial groups of Africa." An *Asian* or *Pacific Islander* is any person with "origins in any of the original peoples of the Far East, Southeast Asia, the Indian subcontinent, or the Pacific Islands." Native Americans are referred to as *American Indians* and *Alaska Natives* and defined "as persons having origins in the original peoples of North America, and who maintain cultural identification through tribal affiliations or community recognition." *Hispanics* are defined as "persons of Mexican, Puerto Rican, Cuban, Central or South American, or other Spanish culture or origin, regardless of race." The term *Latino* is often used to describe individuals in this group (Council of Economic Advisers, 1998).

Minority-Group Membership. The United States has more racial, ethnic, and religious minority groups than any other country as a result of high immigration rates and high birth rates among these groups. Ethnic minority groups are becoming increasingly important because it is anticipated that these groups will produce children at a faster rate than will the majority Caucasian population. Consequently, the minority population is increasing while the majority Caucasian population is decreasing. The term cultural diversity refers to the differences that exist among these various groups of people (Habayeb, 1995; Talabere, 1996).

African-Americans are the largest minority group, followed closely by Hispanics. Currently, Hispanics are the fastest-growing minority in the United States and have many health care needs that are not being met (Warda, 2000). By the year 2010, Hispanics will surpass non-Hispanic African-Americans as the largest racial or ethnic group in the United States. In 2050, 22% of the American population is expected to be Hispanic (Council of Economic Advisers, 1998) (Cultural Considerations box).

NURSE ALERT • Because American cultures and subcultures can be so diverse, it is essential that nurses be aware of and knowledgeable about the predominant groups in their work community and apply this knowledge in their practice.

NURSE ALERT • Generalizations made about an ethnic group may not apply to certain subgroups and individuals.

When minority groups arrive in another country, a certain degree of cultural/ethnic blending occurs through the involuntary process of *acculturation;* this is gradual change produced in a culture by the influence of another culture, and that increases similarity between the cultures. However, these changes occur to various degrees in different families and groups. Many groups continue to identify with their traditional heritage while adapting to the ill-defined concept of the "American way." Acculturation may be referred to as *assimilation,* which is the process of developing a new cultural identity (Spector, 2000).

Studies in the past have indicated that early in life, children become aware of their racial or ethnic status and of the discriminatory attitudes of the majority culture toward their group. The direct effects of discrimination are anger and low self-esteem, which become manifest in a variety of behaviors. Inner conflicts and suppressed hostility that focus children's attention inward may be factors in the failure of many children to achieve in other areas.

Evidence indicates that changes in attitudes are slowly taking place in some groups and in some places. *Cultural pluralism* supports the rights of group differences and promotes a mutual respect for the existence of cultural differences (Culley, 1996; Rogers, 1995). With growing awareness, interest, and understanding by increasing numbers of the majority group (accompanied by the recent emergence of racial and ethnic pride), minority-group children are becoming more secure and confident in their racial or ethnic identities. Individuals vary in their reactions to membership in a minority group, and much of this variation can be attributed to familial factors. As with all children, the most important influences on development of a positive self-image are warm, understanding parents who take an active interest in fostering their children's growth. Parents who accept their children and react positively and constructively, rather than in a negative and self-defeating manner, help their children develop feelings of self-worth, self-esteem, and self-acceptance. The more adequate that children feel, the more positive will be their attitudes toward both majority and minority children, the greater will be their ability to withstand prejudice and intolerance, and the less will be their need for counter-aggressive behavior.

Critical Thinking

REDUCING CULTURAL SHOCK

A woman from the Middle East is visiting her child who is hospitalized for a serious illness. Her husband left for home a short time ago to wash and change clothes. She speaks little English. You need to obtain consent from her for an emergency procedure. She is hesitant and refuses to sign the consent form. What should you do?

First, Think About It . . .

- **Within what point of view are you thinking?**
- **If you accept your conclusions, what are the implications?**

1. **Document that the mother refuses to sign the consent form and inform the physician that the procedure cannot be done.**
2. **Realize that she may be hesitant to sign for consent without her husband present because her culture requires the man to make the decisions for the welfare of the family members.**
3. **Explain to her that you cannot help her child unless she signs for permission to do so.**
4. **Realize that she may not understand what you're saying and try to find an interpreter.**

The best response is 2. Typically, in the Arab culture the point of view exists that men make the decisions and wives are expected to support those decisions. Trying to find an interpreter or intimidating the mother to sign does not address the main issue of the Arab cultural tradition. The implications may be that in emergency cases treatment is often approved by the institution or state if a physician documents that treatment is necessary and that any delay in treatment may jeopardize the health of the child. In this situation, contacting the father first is appropriate.

Cultural Shock

The term *cultural shock* describes the "feelings of helplessness and discomfort and a state of disorientation experienced by an outsider attempting to comprehend or effectively adapt to a different cultural group because of differences in cultural practices, values, and beliefs" (Leininger, 1978). This state occurs with both patients and health care providers who move from one cultural setting to another. It can happen to persons who immigrate to a new country (such as Asian refugees), or to persons from a subcultural group who must adjust to the ways of an unfamiliar subgroup (such as children entering the school subculture or consumers who enter the hospital subculture). Cultural shock is characterized by the inability to respond to or function in a new or strange situation (Critical Thinking box.)

Numerous factors influence reactions to a new environment. Language barriers, including dialects and jargon specific to a subcultural group, inhibit effective communication. Habits and customs (such as different role behaviors or etiquette) and differences in attitudes and beliefs are puzzling to the stranger in the new environment. The outsider experiences an intense sense of isolation and feelings of loneliness and nonrelatedness.

Nurses are challenged to overcome cultural shock and develop the dynamics of *cultural sensitivity,* an awareness of cultural similarities and differences. In doing so, the nurse is helped to practice *culturally competent* care that goes beyond cultural sensitivity to implementation (Talabere, 1996). Becoming more culturally sensitive will enhance valuable knowledge of various cultural groups. Suggestions to gain cultural insights include (Boyer, 1996; Sekhon, 1996):

- Set a language goal.
- Use note cards when conversing, if necessary.
- Do not be afraid to mix a little English with your new language.
- Start by asking "yes" and "no" questions.
- Tour an ethnic grocery store.
- Have dinner at an ethnic restaurant.
- Attend cultural events and celebrations in your community.

CULTURAL/RELIGIOUS INFLUENCES ON HEALTH CARE

Susceptibility to Health Problems

Some groups of people are more susceptible than others to certain illnesses. An innate susceptibility is acquired through generations of evolutionary changes that take place within constrained or segregated populations. The proximity to disease, environmental factors, and the general physical status are significant factors associated with health problems.

Hereditary Factors. Historically, the increased health risks associated with ethnicity have been explained in terms of genetic differences or related factors such as socioeconomic status (Scribner, 1996). The genetic constitution of individuals as groups influences the degree to which they are susceptible to a specific disorder. It may be a result of an inherent lack of resistance to a disease organism (a trait that is an advantage in one environment but places the possessor at a disadvantage in another), or it may be a consequence of intermarriage within a relatively narrow range of geographic, ethnic, or religious restrictions.

A classic example of a geographic constraint is the common communicable disease rubeola (measles). The rubeola virus, or the populations that were continually exposed to it, became altered in such a way that the disease was considered to be a universal disease of childhood from which the majority of children suffered no ill effects. When other populations (e.g., the inhabitants of the Hawaiian Islands) were exposed to the virus by explorers and missionaries, they experienced a violent response that resulted in high mortality.

A number of conditions show ethnic or racial differences. For example, Tay-Sachs disease, characterized by early neurologic deterioration and mental retardation, affects primarily Ashkenazi Jewish families, particularly those of northeastern European origin, whereas Sephardic Jewish families appear to be no more at risk for the disease than are other populations. The incidence of cystic fibrosis is highest in Caucasians and almost nonexistent in Asians, and the rare affected African-Americans are usually in areas where there is apt to be mixed ancestry. A classic disorder of blacks, especially Africans, is sickle cell disease (see Chapter 49); however, the incidence of cardiovascular disease, pneumonia, and diabetes is also high among this population. Native Americans have particularly high rates of tuberculosis, diarrhea, alcoholism, and suicide. Racial and ethnic differences are further considered in relation to diseases and defects as they are discussed throughout the text.

Common food items and drugs may cause health problems in certain ethnic groups. For example, persons of Mediterranean, African, Near Eastern, and Asian origin often have glucose-6-phosphate dehydrogenase (G-6-PD) deficiency. They may develop acute hemolytic anemia after they ingest fava (horse or broad) beans or certain drugs such as aspirin preparations, sulfonamides, or primaquine. Other groups, especially southern Europeans, Jews, Arabs, African-Americans, Asians, and Native Americans, have a deficiency of lactase, the enzyme needed to metabolize lactose. Ingestion of lactose can cause abdominal distention, flatus, and diarrhea. Unknowing but well-meaning health workers may be responsible for these symptoms in their patients when they prescribe foods or food supplements containing lactose as nutrients.

Physical Characteristics. Among racial groups there are observable differences in physical appearance. The most obvious are skin and hair coloring and texture. Skin color is determined by the amount of melanin pigment present in the skin. Persons from countries located near the equator have darkly pigmented skin, which serves to protect the skin from the year-round exposure to the sun's rays; persons from the northern countries have very light skin, which provides for maximum exposure to the sun's rays (necessary for vitamin D metabolism) during the shorter daylight hours. There can be wide variations in skin color between these two extremes in terms of geographic origin or from intermixing of dark and light skin color. When dark pigmentation is present, the detection of skin color changes (e.g., vasomotor alterations, cyanosis, and jaundice) can be difficult; this requires modification of assessment techniques (see Table 35-8).

Variations in the newborn are often related to racial or ethnic origin. For example, newborn infants of Asian and African-American parents are smaller than infants of Caucasian parentage, and bluish pigmented areas (mongolian spots) on the sacral region are a common observation in Asian, African-American, Native American, and Hispanic infants.

Evaluation of stature and body build reveals some racial tendencies. Children from Asian countries are commonly smaller, falling below the 10th percentile on weight and height charts used for children in the United States. This difference in stature can lead to misinterpretation of health status and capabilities. A small child may appear very intelligent for body size but may be of average mental ability for age.

Socioeconomic Factors. The most overwhelming adverse influence on health is socioeconomic status. At any one time, a higher percentage of lower-class individuals are suffering from some health problem than are individuals in any other group. The sum of all aspects of their situation contributes to and compounds health problems; this includes crowded living conditions and poor sanitation, which facilitate transfer of disease (e.g., tuberculosis). There is a higher incidence of lead poisoning in children from families from the lower classes, where there is more ready access to lead in the environment, especially lead-based paint in old housing (Centers for Disease Control and Prevention, 1997).

In the lower classes children are less likely to be immunized against preventable diseases than are children in the upper and middle classes. Lack of funds or inaccessibility to health services inhibits treatment for any but severe illness or injury. Sometimes health care is inadequate because of ignorance. In some areas a disorder is so commonplace that it is looked on as unavoidable; it is not recognized as something that requires (or is amenable to) treatment. The parents may not have information regarding causes, treatment, outcome of the illness, or preventive measures. The nurse can use the limited opportunities when the family does come into contact with the health care system to inquire about immunization, screen for vision problems, provide nutritional information, and offer additional prevention and health promotion resources.

Poverty. A high correlation between poverty and the prevalence of illness has long been observed. Impoverished families suffer from poor nutrition; without medical insurance they have little if any preventive health care, inadequate health maintenance, and very limited access to medical treatment. One of the most significant health problems related to poverty is a high infant mortality rate (Annie E. Casey Foundation, 1999). Day-to-day needs of food, clothing, and lodging take precedence over health care as long as the ailing person feels able to perform activities of daily living.

Poor families are denied access to many health institutions for emergency or other hospital care. Often they must travel long distances to use service centers that are willing to assume their care. In an emergency they must find money for taxi fare, borrow an automobile, or seek other means of transportation. They must find care for dependents, such as other infants and small children, or have them accompany them when taking the ill child for care. Families tend to delay preventive care indefinitely unless health services are relatively accessible. They are more likely to consult folk practitioners or other persons within their community.

Poor nutrition accounts for many health problems in the lower classes. Lack of funds and knowledge results in a diet that may be seriously lacking in essential food substances, especially protein, vitamins, and iron. This inadequate diet often leads to nutritional deficiency disorders and growth retardation in children; in many, the total intake is insufficient to support normal growth. Unstructured eating patterns and irregularly scheduled mealtimes can also contribute to erratic food intake and a proportionately larger consumption of nonnourishing snacks, which can result in excessive weight gain.

Because of deficient preventive care, dental problems are more prevalent. Lack of standard immunizations, together with reduced resistance from poor nutrition, renders the exposed children in poor segments of the population vulnerable to communicable diseases. Poor sanitation and crowded living conditions also contribute to the higher incidence and perpetuation of illness. In general, poor people become ill more often and remain ill for longer periods than do persons in the general population.

Homelessness. Research indicates that families are the fastest-growing subgroup of the homeless population. Rural homeless families have been found to be similar to other homeless families in that the majority are headed by women. Unfortunately, rural families are less likely to escape from poverty (Wagner, Menke, and Ciccone, 1995).

Homeless children experience all of the health problems associated with poverty, as well as other types of disorders. Their families have fewer resources with which to control the environment or to promote rehabilitation and prevent disease. Preventive health care, especially immunization and dental care, is seriously lacking. Impaired vision is common among homeless children, perhaps reflecting missed opportunities for vision screening. Homeless children have been found to experience poorer health status and more emergency department visits than low-income, housed children (Weinreb et al, 1998).

Migrant Families. Migrants generally suffer more illness, both acute and chronic, than the general population. They are subject to unhealthy environments, poverty, and insufficient medical care; their health-seeking behavior, in general, is an illness- or injury-oriented recourse to medical care. Affected persons will postpone seeking care for themselves or their children until physical pain or suffering is almost unbearable. The health problems of migrant children appear to be dental caries, upper respiratory tract infections, tuberculosis, otitis media, scabies and lice, intestinal parasites, pesticide exposure, injuries, teenage pregnancy, and growth and development delay.

Tuberculosis rates among migrant families are high. A risk factor for the increased incidence of tuberculosis in children has been the migration of families from high risk prevalence areas of tuberculosis, such as Asia, Africa, and Latin America (Castiglia, 1997). Also, farmworkers are approximately six times more likely to develop the disease than the general population of employed adults. Drug-resistant tuberculosis is an important consideration among this population; it requires altered treatment regimens, and higher rates of resistance have been found in the ethnic and social groups constituting much of the migrant farm workforce (Advisory Council for the Elimination of Tuberculosis, 1992).

When medical care is provided to a migrant family, follow-up care is usually impossible because of their transient lifestyle. Compliance with medical therapies is primarily related to accessibility and availability; for example, medications provided by health workers are more likely to be taken than those that must be obtained at a pharmacy. In addition, medications are often discontinued following self-perceived recovery.

Customs and Folkways

Nurses must be aware of the need to consider cultural differences in patients when providing health care. An understanding of the various beliefs regarding the causation of illness and disease, as well as traditional health practices, is essential to successful intervention. The more nurses know about the values, beliefs, and customs of other ethnic groups, the better able they are to meet the needs of these families and to gain their cooperation and compliance.

Cultural Relativity. Although clinical characteristics of a disease or condition are essentially the same across cultures, how a child or family interprets or experiences it varies. Culture as an influence is one obvious explanation for variance. *Cultural relativity* is the concept that any behavior must be judged first in relation to the context of the culture in which it occurs. Nurses must first relate to the family's perceptions and interpretations of experiences from the family's background and cultural belief system before they can effectively intervene.

Some cultures, for example, may view a chronic illness or disability as affecting only particular aspects of a child's life, and the child as a whole is viewed as normal. In contrast, Chinese families often describe the illness as having global effects on many aspects of the child's present and future life (Martinson, Armstrong, and Qiao, 1997). These contrasting views may result in a difference in goals and expectations that parents have for their children.

In some cultures the child's gender may influence a family's perception of the implications of an illness or disability. For example, in the Arabic and Asian cultures the male child is held in higher esteem than the female child. This also holds true for some families of Jewish, Italian, Greek, and Indian origin. The male child may receive better health care and more food, because this is the child who will take care of his parents in their old age.

Defining disease or signs and symptoms of illness is also influenced by culture. Some cultures, for example, perceive diarrhea as a cleansing of the body that is essential for health maintenance and illness prevention and/or cure. Furthermore, signs or symptoms resulting from diarrhea and ensuring dehydration (e.g., malaise, fever, anorexia, and irritability) may be viewed as separate illness entities.

Nurses can often recognize a family's health-related cultural perceptions and interpretations through discussion and observation. Implications of these perceptions should be explored and considered when planning effective, culturally appropriate interventions.

Relationships with Health Care Providers. The manner of relating with health care providers differs considerably among cultural groups. One area of conflict to some nurses is the attitude toward time and waiting that is part of some cultures. For example, African-Americans are very flexible in their time orientation; an African-American family may be late for or miss appointments because other issues take precedence over the appointment, and they may not communicate this to the health agency. Hispanics, too, have a very relaxed view of time. Whereas the dominant culture in the United States says that "time flies," the Hispanic says, "time walks." The Japanese, on the other hand, consider time to be valuable and something to be used wisely. They tend to be punctual for medical appointments, and persistent in following prescribed regimens. A Vietnamese family will subordinate time to values considered to be more significant, such as propriety. They may be late for an appointment because of an overextended visit by a friend in their home. In general, Asian-Americans view the American focus on time as offensive. They spend hours getting to know people and view predetermined, abrupt endings as rude. Introductory small talk is considered good manners.

In many cultural groups the mother assumes the responsibility for health care; in others both parents are involved equally in relationships with health workers. A somewhat different approach is apparent in some of the Asian cultures. For example, the father in Vietnamese families, as unquestioned head of the family, is traditionally the family member who interacts with persons, including health care providers, outside the family unit (Fig. 32-4).

In the Hispanic family the father, as head of the house, makes decisions regarding illness and treatment of family members, but the grandmother in the extended family is consulted regarding child care. Usually the family confers with other members before reaching a decision regarding treatment or hospitalization of a child. The Arab family also relies on others to give advice and guidance in a time of crisis. A Japanese father may appear to be passive and uninvolved but actually is involved according to his own cultural standards.

NURSE ALERT • In working with families, it is essential for nurses to identify key members. Failure to include these significant individuals in teaching can seriously hinder adherence to the plan of care.

Nurses should make themselves aware of any specific attitudes regarding the manner of approach to a child in a given culture. Navajo Indians do not like a stranger near their infants. It is feared that the stranger may "witch" the child and cause him or her harm. On the other hand, if a stranger, particularly a woman, lavishes attention on a Latino infant but fails to touch the child, the child will develop symptoms of the "evil eye" (see p. 719). Vietnamese and Korean families may become upset if a newborn is admired at length for fear that evil spirits will overhear and desire the infant.

Some ethnic groups, such as the Amish, consider a child's admission to the hospital a family affair, with all members gathering to support and console the child and parents. In others, such as the Samoan culture, the family is willing to relinquish the care of the child to the hospital authority without interference. Their visits with the child are short, although intense; this behavior may be misinterpreted by the hospital staff as disinterest or abandonment.

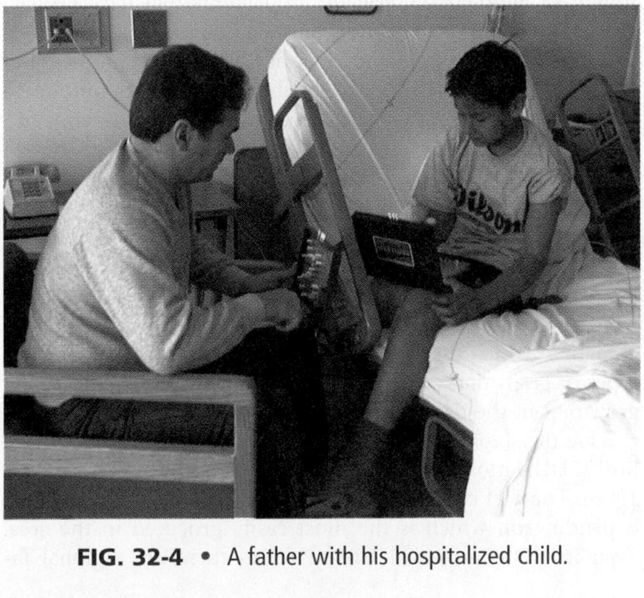

FIG. 32-4 • A father with his hospitalized child.

Nurses who are members of a majority culture may encounter tension and distrust in a child from a minority culture as a result of the child's learned perception or relationship with other persons in the majority group. Based on these perceptions, minority children often suspect that nurses may have hostile feelings toward them and fear ill treatment. When such children are hospitalized, this feeling compounds the feelings of loneliness, helplessness, and retribution that accompany fearful happenings and separation from families. The reverse situation may be encountered by a nurse from a minority culture attempting to meet the needs of a child who has been conditioned to view the nurse's cultural or ethnic group as inferior.

Communication. Communication may be a source of distress and misunderstanding between persons from different ethnic groups, especially if the languages are different. Also, prejudice has been found to be one of the biggest barriers to cross cultural communication (Taylor, 1998). Ideally, conversations with families who are unable to speak the dominant language are best conducted by a health care worker who speaks the language of the family. If this is not possible, it may be necessary to use an interpreter. However, use of an interpreter can be a source of misunderstanding if the interpreter is unfamiliar with medical terminology or if there are no corresponding words in the second language to express the ideas and concepts under discussion (see Communicating with Families through an Interpreter, Chapter 34).

Some persons with poor or limited language comprehension may simply smile and nod in agreement if they do not understand the questions or directives. It is vital that the family fully understand all implications of a child's care and management before they sign permits for special procedures or assume responsibility for the child's care. It is not uncommon for a Vietnamese or a Japanese family to indicate "yes" when in fact they mean "no" in order to avoid social disharmony. They tend to use indirectness rather than confrontation, and may become evasive when direct questioning makes them feel uncomfortable.

NURSE ALERT • Helpful Communication Tools

- Have a series of audio and audiovisual recordings in several languages designed to greet the family and familiarize them with the hospital.
- In the event that an interpreter is not available, develop a multilingual booklet containing commonly used phrases and illustrations of hospital routines.
- Have legal consent forms and explanations of common diagnostic tests available in several languages.
- Keep cards with common greetings, phrases, and names of body parts in the family's language with the patient's chart (e.g., *miseries* [pain] and *locked bowels* [constipation] in African-Americans; and *caida de la mollera* [fallen fontanel from dehydration], *susto* [fright], *dolor, duele,* or *lele* [pain], and *la diarrhea* [diarrhea] in Hispanics).

Nonverbal communication is a practiced art in many Native American tribes, and the members are highly sensitive to body language. They emphasize periods of silence to formulate thoughts in preparation for speech, and often remain silent after listening to statements by others in order to assimilate properly what has been said. Interruption, interjection, or haste to arrive at abrupt conclusions is perceived as immature behavior.

The level of comfort with body space or distance from others varies among cultures. Anglos are generally comfortable at an arm's length; Hispanics tend to get closer; and Asians prefer a greater distance.

Eye contact is viewed differently among cultures. Although Anglos are advised to look people straight in the eye, it is not uncommon for persons in some ethnic groups to avoid eye contact and become uncomfortable when conversing with health workers. A Vietnamese patient may not look directly into the nurse's eyes, as a sign of respect. Some Native Americans will make eye contact during the initial greeting, but continued, unwavering eye contact is considered insulting and disrespectful. Asians may consider eye contact a sign of hostility or impoliteness.

Gestures also may have different meanings. For example, some Asians consider finger or foot pointing disrespectful. Native Americans consider vigorous handshaking a sign of aggression, whereas to Anglos the gesture is a sign of good will.

Families may be reluctant to question or otherwise initiate contact with health professionals. In the Asian cultures, for example, it is considered a sign of disrespect to question those who are viewed as persons of authority. A Japanese family may wait silently rather than ask or question. They believe that the health professionals know best and will meet their needs without being asked. It is also important to avoid criticism. Criticism can cause Asians to "lose face," to feel ashamed, which is highly undesirable.

Language has been considered the biggest barrier to the use of health care services by many families, especially Southeast Asians (Mattson, 1995). Often families may have poor language comprehension, so it is necessary to speak slowly and carefully (not loudly) when conversing with them. Many persons are able to read and write English better than they can speak or understand it. Also, the dominant language usually takes over in anxiety-provoking situations, even in persons who are able to communicate satisfactorily under ordinary circumstances.

Terms of address and use of first and last names vary among cultures and can create confusion. For example, in Asian cultures the family name is given first in respect for the family and the given name follows. Therefore all siblings in a family have the same first name. Ethiopians have a very complex system whereby women retain their last names after marriage and the paternal grandfather's name becomes the child's last name.

The expression of emotion also varies ethnically. In some cultures (e.g., Hispanic or Jewish) emotions are expressed openly and members are accustomed to sharing their sorrows and joys with family and friends. Conversely, Nordic and Asian groups are more restrained.

Health care providers generally ask questions and use handouts, booklets, and—particularly with children—dolls and pictures as communication aids. This is uncommon in some cultures. For example, Native American healers ask few questions and do not use forms. In some cultures it is inappropriate or considered taboo to look at the inside of the body, even in pictures, or to use dolls or puppets (Malach and Segel, 1990). Nurses need to consider both verbal and nonverbal communication techniques to interact effectively with children from different cultures and their families (Guidelines box).

Guidelines

CULTURALLY SENSITIVE INTERACTIONS

Nonverbal Strategies

Invite family members to choose where they would like to sit or stand, allowing them to select a comfortable distance.
Observe interactions with others to determine which body gestures (e.g., shaking hands) are acceptable and appropriate. Ask when in doubt.
Avoid appearing rushed.
Be an active listener.
Observe for cues regarding appropriate eye contact.
Learn appropriate use of pauses or interruptions for different cultures.
Ask for clarification if nonverbal meaning is unclear.

Verbal Strategies

Learn proper terms of address.
Use a positive tone of voice to convey interest.
Speak slowly and carefully, not loudly, when families have poor language comprehension.
Encourage questions.
Learn basic words and sentences of family's language, if possible.
Avoid professional terms.
When asking questions, tell family why the questions are being asked, the way in which the information they provide will be used, and how it might benefit their child.
Repeat important information more than once.
Always give the reason or purpose for a treatment or prescription.
Use information written in family's language.
Offer the services written in family's language.
Offer the services of an interpreter when necessary (see Chapter 34).
Learn from families and representatives of their culture methods of communicating information without creating discomfort.
Address intergenerational needs (e.g., family's need to consult with others).
Be sincere, open, and honest and, when appropriate, share personal experiences, beliefs, and practices to establish rapport and trust.

Food Customs. Food customs and symbolism are an integral part of various cultural, ethnic, and religious groups. Although in a large country such as the United States most persons have adopted the eclectic food habits that have evolved over generations, many ethnic and geographic food traditions and preferences are retained. Special holidays, ceremonies, and life experiences such as births, birthdays, weddings, and death are often marked by special food items or feasts. In many cultures specific food practices are followed during pregnancy in the belief that certain foods damage the developing fetus.

The distinctive food customs of ethnic groups are a product of their native environment, often determined by availability. Fish is a staple food of persons living near the ocean, such as people from Japan, Polynesia, southern Europe, and Scandinavia. Fruit and vegetable preferences are directly related to the climate in which they grow naturally or can be cultivated. The types of grain that are ethnically associated are also those that grow best in the native lands. For example, wheat and basmati rice are the staple grains of South Asians, and roti (unleavened bread) is the most commonly eaten bread in the home (Sekhon, 1996). The diet of the Eskimo is predominantly fish and meat, depending on which is the most easily procured in the area. Even in the continental United States there are regional fa-

TABLE 32-1
Foods Common to Most Ethnic Food Patterns

Meat and Alternatives	Milk and Milk Products	Grain Products	Vegetables	Fruits	Others
Pork*	Milk	Rice	Carrots	Apples	Fruit juices
Beef	Ice cream	White bread	Cabbage	Bananas	
Chicken	Yogurt	Noodles, macaroni, spaghetti	Green beans	Oranges	
Eggs		Dry cereal	Greens (especially spinach)	Peaches	
Beans			Sweet potatoes or yams	Pears	
			Tomatoes		

From Endres JB, Rockwell RE: *Food, nutrition, and the young child,* St Louis, 1980, Mosby.
*May be restricted because of religious custom.

vorites, such as rice, hominy grits, and okra in the southern states. In some cultures food is highly spiced; in others, foods tend to be bland. Table 32-1 lists the food items common to most cultures and can be used to select foods that most children know and like.

There are a number of restrictions related to food items. Some have a physiologic origin, such as lack of dairy foods in the diets of some persons of African or Asian ancestry in whom a hereditary lactase deficiency prevents digestion of foods containing lactose. Others have religious restrictions, such as kosher foods and food preparation of the Orthodox Jewish faith and the vegetarian diet of Seventh-Day Adventists (see Vegetarian Diets, Chapter 47).

Children in a strange environment, such as the hospital, feel much more comfortable when they are served familiar foods (Fig. 32-5). Hospital food often tastes strange and bland. The family may be concerned that their child is not receiving foods appropriate to their culture and beliefs. Where possible, it is advisable to provide children's ethnic foods or allow families to bring favorite foods. Concern for differences in food habits and patterns projects an attitude of respect for the family's ethnic or religious heritage.

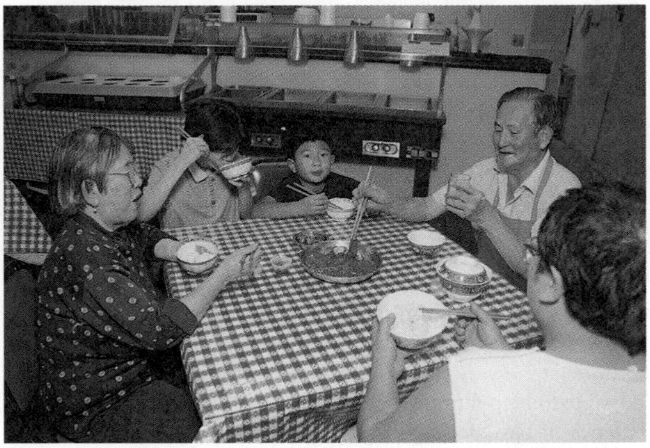

FIG. 32-5 • Food customs outside the home can differ significantly from traditional cultural practices.

Health Beliefs and Practices

Health Beliefs. Beliefs related to the causes of illness and the maintenance of health are an integral part of the cultural heritage of families. Often inseparable from religious beliefs, they influence the way that families cope with health problems and the way that they respond to health care providers. Predominant among most cultures are beliefs related to natural forces, supernatural forces, and imbalance between forces.

Natural Forces. The most common natural forces held responsible for ill health if the body is not adequately protected include cold air entering the body, impurities in the air, or other natural sources. For example, a Chinese mother may overdress her infant in an effort to keep cold wind from entering the child's body. The Chinese believe that cold weather, rain, and wind are responsible for "cold" conditions.

In the African-American culture, natural phenomena such as phases of the moon, seasons of the year, and planet positions are believed to affect the body and its processes. Therefore health maintenance is strongly associated with the ability to read "the signs." Most Native Americans consider health to be a state of harmony with nature and the universe.

Supernatural Forces. High on the list of causes of illness are forces beyond comprehension and logical explanation. Evil influences such as voodoo, witchcraft, or evil spirits are viewed in some cultures as causes of adverse health, especially those illnesses that cannot be explained by other means.

A health belief that is common among people from Latin American, Mediterranean, Near Eastern, some Asian, and some African societies is the concept of the "evil eye" (*mal ojo* is the Hispanic term). It is part of the concept of health as a state of balance; illness is a state of imbalance (see Imbalance of Forces). Strength and power are associated with the evil eye. Therefore, as long as an individual's strength and weakness remain in balance, he or she is unlikely to become a victim of the evil eye. Weaknesses are not necessarily physical. For example, an excess of some emotion (e.g., envy) can create a weakness. Infants and small children, because of immature development of their internal strength-weakness states, are especially vulnerable to the gaze of the evil eye. Consequently, the evil eye concept serves to rationalize an inexplicable onset of illness in children who display such symptoms as restlessness, crying, diarrhea, vomiting, and fever.

Although seldom expressed to health care providers, the belief that a witch can cast a spell over others at the request of someone who wishes them ill is found in Hispanic, African, and Australian aboriginal cultures. The victim is often tortured in effigy by pins driven into a doll at the location where the intended victim is to be hurt. "Voodoo deaths" have occurred from the victim's belief in the curse, and may result from dehydration as the victim gives up the will to live and refuses to drink.

Imbalance of Forces. The concept of balance or equilibrium is widespread throughout the world. One of the most common imbalances supported by the Hispanic, Filipino, Chinese, and Arab cultures is that which exists between "hot" and "cold." This belief is reputedly derived from the Hippocratic theory of humoral pathology, which states that illness is caused by an imbalance of the four humors: phlegm, blood, black bile, and yellow bile. Hot and cold describe certain properties and conditions completely unrelated to temperature. Diseases, areas of the body, foods, and illnesses are classified as either "hot" or "cold." In Chinese health belief the forces are termed *yin* (cold) and *yang* (hot). To maintain health, these hot and cold forces must be kept in balance.

Illness is treated by restoring normal balance through the application of appropriate "hot" or "cold" remedies. A "cold" condition such as a respiratory disease is believed to be caused by exposure to cold weather, rain, or cold wind entering the body; it is treated by administration of "hot" foods, herbs, or drugs. Menstruation is considered to be a "hot" condition; therefore, women are cautioned against ingesting "hot" foods, which might increase menstrual flow or produce cramping. Ingesting too much of either "hot" or "cold" foods can also be interpreted as a cause of illness.

Health care workers who are aware of this belief are better able to understand why some persons refuse to eat certain foods. It is possible to help families devise a diet that contains the necessary balance of basic food groups prescribed by the medical subculture while conforming to the beliefs of the ethnic subculture.

Health Practices. There are many similarities among cultures regarding prevention and treatment of illness. All cultures have some types of home remedies that they apply before seeking help from other persons. Within the ethnic community, folk healers who are endowed with the ability to "cure" maladies are sought for special situations and when home remedies are unsuccessful. There is the *curandero* (male) or *curandera* (female) of the Mexican-American community, whose healing powers are believed to be a gift from God. The Asian consults an herbalist, knowledgeable in medicines; and/or an ethnic practitioner practiced in Asian therapies, including *acupuncture* (insertion of needles), *acupressure* (application of pressure), and *moxibustion* (application of heat). Native Americans consult a variety of healers with specific skills and knowledge. Specialized medicine persons diagnose illness, provide nonsacred treatments (usually by way of massage and herbs), and care for souls. Other specialists perform services or affect cures through spiritual means. Native Hawaiians consult *kahunas* and practice *ho'oponopono* to heal family imbalance or disputes.

The folk healers are very powerful persons in their community. They "speak the language" of the family who seeks help, and often combine their rituals and potions with prayer and entreaties to God. They also are able to create an atmosphere conducive to successful management. Furthermore, they exhibit a sincere interest in the family and their problems.

Some folk remedies are compatible with the medical regimen and can be used to reinforce the treatment plan. For example, most of the foods contraindicated for persons with peptic ulcers are "hot" foods and would be avoided because of their belief systems. Also, aspirin (a "hot" medication) is an appropriate therapy for "cold" diseases such as the common cold and arthritis. It is not uncommon to discover that a folk prescription has a scientific basis. However, numerous health remedies or preventive practices have no scientific basis, such as the use of garlic or *asafetida* (a piece of rotten flesh that looks like a dried sponge), which is worn around the neck to prevent contagious diseases. Also, the wearing of copper or silver bracelets to protect the wearer as he or she grows has no scientific basis. Practices that do no harm should be respected.

Overcoming the effect of the evil eye usually requires specialized rituals conducted by the appropriate practitioner. For example, the Chicano curandera ascertains that the condition is truly the result of the evil eye by performing an assessment ritual and then, with a confirmed diagnosis, performs a curative ritual. Sometimes the faith in the folk practitioner results in a delay in obtaining needed medical treatment, although the practitioner will usually suggest medical care if his or her ministrations are unsuccessful.

Health practices of different cultures may also present problems in assessment and interpretation. For example, certain cultural practices or remedies can be misdiagnosed as evidence of "child abuse" by uninformed professionals (Box 32-1). It is important to explain why these and other familiar remedies may now be considered harmful. Families need to understand how such practices can place them in jeopardy with child protective

Box 32-1

Cultural Practices Possibly Considered Abusive by the Dominant Culture

Coining—A Vietnamese practice that may produce weltlike lesions on the child's back when a coin, held on edge, is repeatedly rubbed lengthwise on the oiled skin to rid the body of the disease.

Cupping—An Old World practice (also practiced by the Vietnamese) of placing a container (e.g., tumbler, bottle, jar) containing steam against the skin surface to "draw out the poison" or other evil element. When the heated air within the container cools, a vacuum is created that produces a bruiselike blemish on the skin directly beneath the mouth of the container.

Burning—A practice of some Southeast Asian groups whereby small areas of skin are burned to treat enuresis and temper tantrums.

Female genital mutilation (female circumcision)—Removal of or injury to any part of the female genital organ; practiced in Africa, the Middle East, Latin America, India, the Far East, North America, Australia, and Western Europe.*

Forced kneeling—A child discipline measure of some Caribbean groups where a child is forced to kneel for a long period of time.

Topical garlic application—A practice of Yemenite Jews in which crushed garlic cloves or garlic-petroleum jelly plaster is applied to the wrists to treat infectious disease; the practice can result in blisters or garlic burns.

Traditional remedies that contain lead—***Greta*** and ***azarcon*** (Mexico; used for digestive problems), ***paylooah*** (Southeast Asia; used for rash or fever), and ***suma*** (India; used as a cosmetic to improve eyesight).

*Wright J: Female genital mutilation: an overview, *J Adv Nurs* 24(2):251-259, 1996.

services and to explore alternative measures that are more acceptable to the dominant culture.

Cultural health remedies that are detrimental to health include eating clay, excessive amounts of salt, or compounds that contain lead or mercury. A careful history can reveal these remedies, but it may require the collaboration of a folk healer to convince a user to stop the practice.

Faith healing and religious rituals are closely allied with many folk-healing practices. Wearing of amulets, medals, and other religious relics believed by the culture to protect the individual and facilitate healing is a common practice. It is important for health workers to recognize the value of this practice and to keep the items where the family has placed them or nearby. It offers comfort and support and rarely impedes medical and nursing care. If an item must be removed during a procedure, it should be replaced, if possible, when the procedure is completed. The reason for its temporary removal is explained to the family, and they are reassured that their wishes will be respected (Family Focus box).

Nurses can be most effective by operating from a multicultural perspective. Adopting a multicultural perspective means using appropriate aspects of each health cultural orientation under consideration to develop culturally acceptable health care interventions.

NURSE ALERT • Avoid directly criticizing traditional health cultural beliefs and practices as wrong or harmful, or implying that biomedical measures are uniformly correct and effective and the only way to prevent illness or treat sickness. Such criticisms usually result in rejection of both biomedical health care practitioners and their health teaching. When folk practices do not interfere with the welfare of the patient, they need not be discouraged. Often a compromise can be reached that accomplishes the goal of the nurse while maintaining the dignity and self-esteem of the child and family.

Family Focus

ON CULTURAL AWARENESS

I am a pediatric emergency nurse with a high regard for cultural diversities and a respect for healing practices and beliefs. I even made a manual for my emergency department that contains some of the information needed to help us to understand and communicate with subcultures in the urban community that we serve. Although I learned a great deal putting this manual together, it doesn't come close to the lesson I learned with the following experience.

A 15-month-old Bosnian child in status epilepticus was carried in by her parents. They were very frightened and spoke very little English. I learned that the child had received a measles, mumps, and rubella (MMR) immunization the day before. As I proceeded to unwrap her from the blanket she was in, I quickly assessed the ABCs (airway, breathing, and circulation). I noticed that she was very warm (probably a febrile seizure) and that a rag soaked in alcohol was tied around each thigh. Focusing on her potential airway compromise and trying to calm the parents, I proceeded to put an oxygen mask on her, undress her for a full assessment, and remove the alcohol rags. I spoke to the parents all the while in a calm, soothing voice. Once an IV was established and I gave her Ativan, the seizures stopped. So did the communication between her parents and me. I noticed that they would no longer give me eye contact, and the mother would not even speak to me after the seizures stopped. It wasn't until I was returning to the department from admitting her that I realized why they might have stopped communicating with me . . . I had removed the rags! Had I only thought to ask their permission to remove the rags, things may have been different.

Laura L. Kuensting, MSN(R), RN
Cardinal Glennon Children's Hospital
St. Louis, Missouri

Religious Beliefs

Religious and spiritual dimensions of life are among the most important influences in many people's lives. The terms *religion* and *spirituality* are often used interchangeably; however, spirituality subsumes religion. Both religion and spirituality give meaning to life and provide a source of love and relatedness between individuals and their God (Lukoff, Lu, and Turner, 1995). Holistic nursing care is promoted through an integration of spiritual and psychosocial care. The care focuses on activities that support a person's system of beliefs and worship, such as prayer, reading religious materials, and assisting with religious rituals. Meeting the spiritual needs of the child and family can provide strength, whereas unmet spiritual needs can result in spiritual distress and debilitation (Fulton and Moore, 1995). In practice, application of the nursing process for spiritual care can provide for the spiritual well-being of the child and family.

Among many groups illness, injury, or death is believed to be sent by God as a punishment for sin. Some may believe that health workers will be unable to help a person whom God is punishing and may express a fatalistic attitude toward treatment, stating it is "the will of God." Others view it as a test of strength, like the testing of Job in the Bible, and strive to remain faithful and overcome the conflicts.

Religious affiliation has implications for many health-related functions and procedures. It is comforting for the family of an ill child to have this need recognized and respected. Nurses need to determine if there are any special considerations, including dietary restrictions, related to spiritual practices that are important to the family. Family members are asked whether they want a clergy member present and whether they prefer hospital staff to call or prefer to do this on their own.

It is also important to determine the wishes of the family regarding baptism, rites or practices related to death, and other religious rituals (e.g., circumcisions, communion, or use of amulets or icons). Religion, which offers families understanding and spiritual support, is a valuable asset to health care. Characteristics of selected religions with beliefs that affect health care are outlined in Table 32-2.

Importance of Culture and Religion to Nurses

A general agreement exists among nurses to raise the cultural competence of professional nursing practice (Lester, 1998). To begin to understand and to deal effectively with families in a multicultural community or in a unicultural community that is different from one's own, nurses must be aware of their own attitudes and values regarding a way of life, including health practices (Ahmann, 1994; Phillips and Lobar, 1995). Nurses, too, are products of their own cultural backgrounds. They also need to recognize that they are part of the "nursing culture." Nurses

Text continued on p. 727

TABLE 32-2
Religious Beliefs that Affect Nursing Care

Beliefs About Birth and Death	Beliefs About Diet and Food Practices	Beliefs Regarding Medical Care	Comments
BAPTIST (27 GROUPS)			
Birth: No infant baptism Believers are baptized by immersion as adults **Death:** Clergy seeks to minister by counsel and prayer with patient and family **Organ donation/ transplantation:** Both organ donation and transplantation are generally approved of when they do not seriously endanger donor and when they offer medical hope for recipient	Some groups discourage coffee, tea, and alcohol	May encounter some resistance to some therapies, such as abortion Some believe in predestination; may respond passively to care	Fundamentalist and conservative groups accept Bible as inspired word of God
BUDDHIST			
Birth: No infant baptism Infant presentation **Death:** Last rite chanting is often practiced at bedside soon after death; the deceased's family or Buddhist priest should be contacted **Organ donation/ transplantation:** Believe that organ donation is a matter of individual conscience	No requirements or restrictions Some sects are strictly vegetarian Discourage use of alcohol and drugs	Illness is believed to be a trial to aid development of soul; illness due to Karmic causes May be reluctant to have surgery or certain treatments on holy days Cleanliness is believed to be of great importance Family may request Buddhist priest for counseling	Optimistic outlook; teach ways to overcome fears, anxieties, apprehension
CHURCH OF CHRIST SCIENTIST (CHRISTIAN SCIENCE)			
Birth: No baptism **Death:** No last rites; autopsy is not permitted except in cases of sudden death; it is an individual's decision to choose burial or cremation **Organ donation/ transplantation:** Church takes no specific position on transplantation or donation as distinct from other medical or surgical procedures	No requirements or restrictions	Oppose human intervention with drugs or other therapies; however, accept legally required immunizations Many adhere to belief that disease is human mental concept that can be dispelled by spiritual truth to extent that they refuse all medical treatment	Many desire services of practitioner or reader; will sometimes refuse even emergency treatment until they have consulted a reader
CHURCH OF JESUS CHRIST OF LATTER DAY SAINTS (MORMON)			
Birth: No baptism at birth Infant is blessed by church official at first opportunity after birth (in church)	Prohibit tea, coffee, alcohol Some individuals avoid chocolate and other products that contain caffeine	Devout adherents believe in divine healing through anointment with oil and laying on of hands by	May request ***Sacrament*** on Sunday while in hospital

From Carpenito LJ: *Nursing diagnosis: application to clinical practice,* ed 4, Philadelphia, 1992, JB Lippincott; Conley L: Childbearing and childrearing practices in Mormonism, *Neonatal Network* 9(3):41-48, 1990; Kozier B, Erb G: *Fundamentals of nursing,* ed 5, Menlo Park, CA, 1995, Addison-Wesley; McQuay JE: Cross cultural customs and beliefs related to health crisis, death, and organ donation/transplantation, *Crit Care Nurs Clin North Am* 7(3):581-594, 1995; and Spector RE: *Cultural diversity in health and illness,* ed 5, Upper Saddle River, NJ, 2000, Prentice Hall Health.

TABLE 32-2—cont'd
Religious Beliefs that Affect Nursing Care

Beliefs About Birth and Death	Beliefs About Diet and Food Practices	Beliefs Regarding Medical Care	Comments
CHURCH OF JESUS CHRIST OF LATTER DAY SAINTS (MORMON)—cont'd			
Baptism by immersion at 8 years **Death:** Believe that it is proper to bury the dead in the ground, and cremation is discouraged **Organ donation/ transplantation:** Question of whether one should will his or her organs to be used as transplants is left to the individual	Encourage sparing use of meats Fasting for 24 hours on first Sunday of each month (from after evening meal Saturday until evening meal Sunday)	church officials (appointed church members) Medical therapy is not prohibited	Financial support for sick is available through well-funded welfare system Discourage cremation Discourage use of tobacco Married adults wear special undergarments
EPISCOPAL (ANGLICAN)			
Birth: Infant baptism is mandatory; urgent if poor prognosis **Death:** Last rites (Rite for Anointing of the Sick) are not mandatory for all members; when death is imminent, family and pastor are gathered, and it is usually highly desirable to have Litany at the Time of Death read **Organ donation/ transplantation:** No objections to organ donation/transplantation as long as moral integrity of donor is not violated	Abstain from meat on fast days May fast on Wednesday, Friday, during Lent, and before Christmas Some fast for 6 hours before receiving Holy Communion	Some believe in spiritual healing Rite for anointing of the sick is available but not mandatory	Religious icons are very important Communion four times yearly: Christmas, Easter, June 30, and August 15; may be mandatory for some
FRIENDS (QUAKERS)			
Birth: No baptism Infant's name is recorded in official book **Death:** Do not believe in life after this life; each individual has a divine nature **Organ donation/ transplantation:** No formal statement; both are permitted	No requirements or restrictions Most practice moderation Avoid alcohol and illicit drugs	No special rites or restrictions	Believe in plain speech and dress Pacifists
HINDU			
Birth: No ritual **Death:** Certain prescribed rites are followed after death; priest may tie thread around neck or wrist to signify blessing; family will wash the body; are particular about who touches their dead; bodies are to be cremated	Many dietary restrictions Beef and veal are not eaten Some are strict vegetarians	Illness or injury is believed to represent sins committed in previous life Accept most modern medical practices	Cremation is preferred

Continued

TABLE 32-2—cont'd
Religious Beliefs that Affect Nursing Care

Beliefs About Birth and Death	Beliefs About Diet and Food Practices	Beliefs Regarding Medical Care	Comments
HINDU—cont'd			
Organ donation/transplantation: No religious laws prohibiting donation; individual decision			
ISLAM (MUSLIM/MOSLEM)			
Birth: At birth, the first words said to the infant in his/her right ear are Allah-o-Akbar (Allah is great) and the remainder of the Call for Prayer is recited. An Aqeeqa (party) to celebrate the birth of the child is arranged by the parents. Circumcision of the male child is practiced. **Death:** In Islam, life is seen as a test in preparation for the everlasting life in the hereafter; therefore, according to Islam, death is simply a transition. Islam teaches that God has prescribed the time of death for everyone and only He knows when, where, or how a person is going to die. Islam encourages making the best use of all of God's gifts including the precious gift of life in this world. At the time of death, there are specific rituals (e.g., bathing, wrapping the body in cloth) that must be done. Before moving and handling the body, it is preferable to contact someone from the person's Mosque or the local Islamic Society to perform these rituals **Organ donation/transplantation:** Permitted; however, there are some stipulations depending on the type of transplant/donation and its effect on the donor and recipient. It is advisable to contact the individual's Mosque or the local Islamic Society for further consultation	Prohibit all pork products; fasting is practiced during the ninth month of the Islamic year (Ramadan)	Believers are encouraged in the Qu'ran to seek treatment. It is taught that only Allah cures; however, Muslims are taught not to refuse treatment in the belief that Allah will take care of them because he also chooses at times to work through the efforts of humans	Muslims do not use alcohol or mind-altering drugs

From Carpenito LJ: *Nursing diagnosis: application to clinical practice,* ed 4, Philadelphia, 1992, JB Lippincott; Conley L: Childbearing and childrearing practices in Mormonism, *Neonatal Network* 9(3):41-48, 1990; Kozier B, Erb G: *Fundamentals of nursing,* ed 5, Menlo Park, CA, 1995, Addison-Wesley; McQuay JE: Cross cultural customs and beliefs related to health crisis, death, and organ donation/transplantation, *Crit Care Nurs Clin North Am* 7(3):581-594, 1995; and Spector RE: *Cultural diversity in health and illness,* ed 5, Upper Saddle River, NJ, 2000, Prentice Hall Health.

TABLE 32-2—cont'd
Religious Beliefs that Affect Nursing Care

Beliefs About Birth and Death	Beliefs About Diet and Food Practices	Beliefs Regarding Medical Care	Comments
JEHOVAH'S WITNESS			
Birth: No baptism **Death:** No official last rites practiced when death occurs **Organ donation/ transplantation:** No definite statement related to this issue; do not encourage organ donation but believe it is a matter for individual conscience	Eat nothing to which blood has been added; can eat animal flesh that has been drained	Adherents are generally absolutely opposed to transfusions, including banking of own blood May be opposed to use of albumin, globulin, factor replacement (hemophilia), vaccines Not opposed to nonblood plasma expanders	Often possible to obtain a court order appointing a hospital official as temporary guardian to consent to a child's transfusion when parents refuse consent Autopsy is approved only as required by law No restrictions on giving blood sample
JUDAISM (ORTHODOX AND CONSERVATIVE)			
Birth: No baptism Ritual circumcision of male infants on eighth day; performed by Mohel (ritual circumciser familiar with Jewish law and aseptic technique) **Death:** According to tradition, during last moments of life, relatives and close friends remain with the deceased **Organ donation/ transplantation:** This is permitted and considered a Mitzuah (good deed)	Numerous dietary kosher laws exist Are allowed only meat from animals that are vegetable eaters and are ritually slaughtered; fish that have scales and fins Milk products served first can be followed by meat in a few minutes, but milk may not be consumed for several hours after eating meat Fasting for 24 hours is part of Yom Kippur observance Matzo replaces leavened bread during Passover week	May resist surgical procedures during Sabbath, which extends from sundown Friday until sundown Saturday Seriously ill and pregnant women are exempt from fasting Illness is grounds for violating dietary laws (e.g., patient with congestive heart failure does not have to use kosher meats, which are high in sodium)	Oppose all forms of mutilation, including autopsy; amputated limbs, organs, or surgically removed tissues should be made available to family for burial Donation or transplantation of organs requires rabbinical consent May oppose prolongation of life after irreversible brain damage
LUTHERAN			
Birth: Baptize infants shortly after birth **Death:** Last rites are optional **Organ donation/ transplantation:** Considered a matter of personal choice	No requirements or restrictions	Church or pastor may be notified of hospitalization Communion may be given before or after surgery or similar crisis	Accept scientific developments
METHODIST			
Birth: Infant baptism is practiced but is usually done within the community of the Church after counseling and guidance from clergy. However, in emergency situations, a request for baptism would not be seen as inappropriate **Death:** In the case of perinatal death, there are prayers within the United Methodist Book of worship that could be said by anyone. Prayer, scripture, and singing are often seen as appropriate and desirable	No requirements or restrictions	In the Methodist tradition, it is believed that every person has the right to death with dignity and has the right to be involved in all medical decisions. Refusal of aggressive treatment is seen as an appropriate option.	Some encourage donation of body or body parts to science

Continued

TABLE 32-2—cont'd

Religious Beliefs that Affect Nursing Care

Beliefs About Birth and Death	Beliefs About Diet and Food Practices	Beliefs Regarding Medical Care	Comments
METHODIST—cont'd			
Organ donation/ transplantation: This is supported and encouraged; It is considered a part of good stewardship			
NAZARENE			
Birth: Baptism optional **Death:** No last rites	No requirements or restrictions Alcohol is prohibited	Church official administers Communion and laying on of hands Adherents believe in divine healing but not exclusive of medical treatment	Cremation is permitted
PENTECOSTAL (ASSEMBLY OF GOD, FOUR-SQUARE)			
Birth: No baptism at birth Baptism by complete immersion after age of accountability **Death:** No official last rites practiced when death occurs **Organ donation/ transplantation:** No official position	Abstain from alcohol, eating blood, strangled animals, or anything to which blood has been added Some individuals may not consume pork	No restrictions regarding medical care Deliverance from sickness is provided for in atonement; may pray for divine intervention in health matters and seek God in prayer for themselves and others when ill	Some insist illness is divine punishment; most consider it an intrusion of Satan Practice glossolalia (speaking in tongues)
PRESBYTERIAN			
Birth: Infant baptism by sprinkling **Death:** Last rites are not a sacramental procedure; instead, they read scripture and pray **Organ donation/transplantation:** individual conscience and a person's right to make decisions regarding his or her own body	No requirements or restrictions	Communion is administered when appropriate and convenient Blood transfusion is accepted Believe science should be used for relief of suffering	Full forgiveness is granted for any illness connected with a sin
ROMAN CATHOLIC			
Birth: Infant baptism is mandatory; especially urgent if poor prognosis, when it may be performed by anyone **Death:** Rite for Anointing of the Sick is a sacrament for the living; if prognosis is poor while patient is alive, patient or his or her family may request it **Organ donation/ transplantation:** Transplantation of organs is viewed by Catholics as ethically and morally acceptable to Vatican; organ donation is viewed as an act of charity	Fasting (eating only one full meal and no eating between meals) and abstaining from meat are mandatory on Ash Wednesday and Good Friday; fasting is optional during Lent; no meat on Fridays during Lent as a general rule Children and most hospital patients are exempt from fasting Some older Catholics may adhere to rule of no meat on Friday	Encourage anointing of the sick Traditional church teaching does not approve of contraceptives or abortion	Family may request that major amputated limb be buried in consecrated ground Autopsy is acceptable Religious articles are important

From Carpenito LJ: *Nursing diagnosis: application to clinical practice,* ed 4, Philadelphia, 1992, JB Lippincott; Conley L: Childbearing and childrearing practices in Mormonism, *Neonatal Network* 9(3):41-48, 1990; Kozier B, Erb G: *Fundamentals of nursing,* ed 5, Menlo Park, CA, 1995, Addison-Wesley; McQuay JE: Cross cultural customs and beliefs related to health crisis, death, and organ donation/transplantation, *Crit Care Nurs Clin North Am* 7(3):581-594, 1995; and Spector RE: *Cultural diversity in health and illness,* ed 5, Upper Saddle River, NJ, 2000, Prentice Hall Health.

Box 32-2

Exploring Your Cultural Heritage

To provide culturally sensitive care to children and their families from cultures that are different from your own, you must first become aware of your own cultural values and beliefs and recognize how they influence your attitudes and behaviors. As you begin to understand the values that culture instills, you become better prepared to assess another culture objectively. The following questions have no right or wrong answers. They should help you clarify your attitudes and beliefs and how they influence your ability to work with people from diverse cultural backgrounds.

What ethnic group, socioeconomic class, religion, age-group, and community do you belong to?

- What about these groups do you find embarrassing or would like to change? Why?
- What socioculture factors in your background might be rejected by members of other cultures?
- What did your parents and significant others say about people who were different from your family?

What do you believe or value?

- How do you define health, disease, illness?
- Are you usually on time? Early? Late?
- How do you feel if others are late? Frustrated? Angry? Not respected?
- What are your views on childhood education?
- Are you comfortable with physical contact (touching, embracing)? How much and with whom?
- What are your religious views and biases? Do you adhere to religious rituals?
- What are your feelings on child-rearing practices (including nutrition, discipline, play, roles)?

What experiences have you had with people from ethnic groups, socioeconomic classes, religions, age-groups, or communities different from your own?

- What were those experiences like?
- How did you feel about them?

What personal qualities do you have that will help you establish interpersonal relationships with persons from other cultural groups?

What personal qualities may be detrimental?

Data from Randall-David E: *Strategies for working with culturally diverse communities and clients,* Washington, DC, 1989, Association for the Care of Children's Health; and Niederhauser V: Health care of immigrant children: incorporating culture into practice, *Pediatr Nurs* 15(6):569-574, 1989.

Text continued from p. 721

function within the framework of a professional culture with its own values and traditions and, as such, become socialized into their professional culture in their educational program and later in their work environments and professional associations.

Often nurses and other health care workers are not aware of their own cultural values and how those values influence their thoughts and actions. Those who are aware of their own culturally founded behavior are more sensitive to cultural behavior in others (Box 32-2). Recognizing that a behavior may be characteristic of a culture rather than an "abnormal" behavior places nurses at an advantage in their relationships with families. When nurses respect the cultural differences of a family, they are better able to determine whether the behavior is distinctive to the individual or a characteristic of the culture.

Critical Thinking

CULTURAL PRACTICES

Knowledge of cultural practices in a locality can be as important as knowledge of communicable diseases. What is true about this knowledge?

First, Think About It . . .

- **What is the purpose of your thinking?**
- **Within what point of view are you thinking?**

1. **It is not valuable unless the nurse uses it to assess contributing cultural factors that may aid or hinder the care of the child and family.**
2. **It is not helpful unless the nurse is part of the culture.**
3. **It is valuable only in making nurses aware of diversity in care.**
4. **It is learned only from reading about the traditional beliefs and practices of cultural groups.**

The best response is 1. Information about a culture serves no purpose and is not valuable unless you apply the knowledge to the situation. A nurse does not need to be a part of a culture to be aware of differences and to respect its practices. Although cultural knowledge may be helpful in awareness of diversities in practices and care, putting the knowledge to use is the challenge and the goal. Information about cultures is learned from a variety of methods such as observation, previous experience/interactions, television, journals, textbooks, and travel. Also, it is important to remember that the nurse interprets cultural knowledge from within the nurse's own point of view.

Cultural standards and values, the family structure and function, and past experiences with health care influence a family's feelings and attitudes toward health, their children, and health care delivery systems. It is often difficult for nurses to be nonjudgmental and objective in working with families whose behaviors and attitudes differ from or conflict with their own. Being aware of one's own feelings and attitudes and respecting those of the family are essential to a helping relationship and achievement of nursing goals. Relying on one's own values and experiences for guidance can result only in frustration and disappointment. It is one thing to know what is needed to deal with a health problem; it is often quite another to implement a fruitful course of action unless nurses work within the cultural and socioeconomic framework of the family (Critical Thinking box).

It is beneficial to adapt ethnic practices to the health needs of the family rather than attempt to change long-standing beliefs. To aid their efforts to understand and respect the cultural beliefs of families, nurses should have a readily available resource file containing pertinent information about the cultural and subcultural characteristics of the community in which they practice (e.g., traditional practices related to infant feeding and the time and manner of weaning and toilet training). Bridging cultural gaps in delivery of health care to children requires the establishment of a close relationship with families and other influential persons in the community (such as the local folk healer) and periodic assessment of one's own attitudes and behaviors—and those of other health workers—toward people of other racial or ethnic origins.

Some characteristics of selected cultures are outlined in Table 32-3. Tables 32-2 and 32-3 are presented as beginning frameworks for practicing transcultural nursing. Nurses must

Text continued on p. 734

TABLE 32-3
Cultural Characteristics Related to Health Care of Children and Families

Cultural Group	Health Beliefs	Health Practices
ASIANS		
Chinese	A healthy body is viewed as gift from parents and ancestors and must be cared for Health is one of the results of balance between the forces of ***yin*** (cold) and ***yang*** (hot)—energy forces that rule the world Illness caused by imbalance Believe blood is source of life and is not regenerated ***Chi*** is innate energy Lack of chi and blood results in deficiency that produces fatigue, poor constitution, and long illness	Goal of therapy is to restore balance of yin and yang Acupuncturist applies needles to appropriate meridians identified in terms of yin and yang Acupressure and ***tai chi*** replacing acupuncture in some areas ***Moxibustion*** is application of heat to skin over specific meridians Wide use of medicinal herbs procured and applied in prescribed ways Folk healers are herbalist, spiritual healer, temple healer, fortune healer Meals may or may not be planned to balance hot and cold Milk intolerance relatively common Use of condiments (e.g., monosodium glutamate and soy sauce) may create difficulty with some diet regimens (e.g., low-salt diets)
Japanese	Three major belief systems: ***Shinto*** religious influence Humans inherently good Evil caused by outside spirits Illness caused by contact with polluting agents (e.g., blood, corpses, skin diseases) Chinese and Korean influence Health achieved through harmony and balance between self and society Disease caused by disharmony with society and not caring for body Portuguese influence Uphold germ theory of disease	Believe evil removed by purification Energy restored by means of acupuncture, acupressure, massage, and moxibustion along affected meridians ***Kampō*** medicine—use of natural herbs Believe in removal of diseased parts Trend is to use both Western and Oriental healing methods Care for disabled viewed as family's responsibility Take pride in child's good health Seek preventive care, medical care for illness May avoid some food combinations (e.g., milk and cherries, watermelon and crab) and believe pickled plums to have special properties
Vietnamese	Good health considered to be balance between yin and yang Believe person's life has been predisposed toward certain phenomena by cosmic forces Health believed to be result of harmony with existing universal order; harmony attained by pleasing good spirits and avoiding evil ones Belief in ***am duc,*** the amount of good deeds accumulated by ancestors Many use rituals to prevent illness Practice some restrictions to prevent incurring wrath of evil spirits	Family uses all means possible before using outside agencies for health care Fortune-tellers determine event that caused disturbance May visit temple to procure divine instruction Use astrologer to calculate cyclic changes and forces Regard health as family responsibility; outside aid sought when resources run out Certain illnesses considered only temporary (such as pustules, open wounds) and ignored Seek generalist health healers May use special diets to prevent illness and promote health Lactose intolerance prevalent

From Anderson P, Fenichel D: *Serving culturally diverse families of infants and toddlers with disabilities,* Washington, DC, 1989, National Center for Clinical Infant Programs; Clark AL, editor: *Culture and childrearing,* Philadelphia, 1981, FA Davis; DeSantis L: Cultural factors affecting newborn and infant diarrhea, *J Pediatr Nurs* 3(6):391-398, 1988; Geissler EM: *Pocket guide to cultural assessment,* St Louis, 1994, Mosby; Giger J, Davidhizar R: *Transcultural nursing: assessment and intervention,* ed 2, St Louis, 1995, Mosby; Holland S, Sweeney E: *Vietnamese children and families: the impact of culture,* Washington, DC, 1985, Association for the Care of Children's Health; Hollingsworth AO, Brown LP, Brooten DA: The refugees and childbearing: what to expect, *RN* 43(11):45-48, 1980; Orgue MS, Bloch B, Monrroy LSA: *Ethnic nursing care,* St Louis, 1983, Mosby; Randall-David E: *Strategies for working with culturally diverse communities and clients,* Washington, DC, 1989, Association for the Care of Children's Health; and Sodetaini-Shibata AE: The Japanese American. In Clark AL, editor: *Culture and childrearing,* Philadelphia, 1981, FA Davis.

Family Relationships	Communication	Comments
Extended family pattern common Strong concept of loyalty of young to old Respect for elders taught at early age—acceptance without questioning or talking back Children's behavior a reflection on family Family and individual honor and "face" important Self-reliance and self-restraint highly valued; self-expression repressed Males valued more highly than females; women submissive to men in family	Open expression of emotions unacceptable Often smile when do not comprehend	Do not react well to painful diagnostic workup; are especially upset by drawing of blood Deep respect for their bodies and believe it best to die with bodies intact; therefore may refuse surgery Believe in reincarnation Older members fear hospitals; often believe hospital is a place to go to die Children sometimes breastfed for up to 4 or 5 years*
Close intergenerational relationships Family provides anchor Family tends to keep problems to self Value self-control and self-sufficiency Concept of ***haji*** (shame) imposes strong control; unacceptable behavior of children reflects on family Many adopt practices of contemporary middle class Concern for child's missing school may result in sending to school before fully recovered from illness	Issei—born in Japan; usually speak Japanese only Nisei, Sansei, and Yomsei have few language difficulties New immigrants able to read and write English better than able to speak or understand it Make significant use of nonverbal communication with subtle gestures and facial expression Tend to suppress emotions Will often wait silently	Generational categories: ***Issei***—1st generation to live in United States ***Nisei***—2nd generation ***Sansei***—3rd generation ***Yonsei***—4th generation Issei and Nisei are tolerant and permissive in childbearing until child is 5 or 6; then emphasis is on emotional reserve and control Cleanliness highly valued Time considered valuable and used widely Tendency to practice emotional control may make assessment of pain more difficult
Family is revered institution Multigenerational families Family is chief social network Children highly valued Individual needs and interests are subordinate to those of a family group Father is main decision maker Women taught submission to men Parents expect respect and obedience from children	Many immigrants are not proficient in speaking and understanding English May hesitate to ask questions Questioning authority is sign of disrespect; asking questions considered impolite Use indirectness rather than forthrightness in expressing disagreement May avoid eye contact with health professionals as a sign of respect	Consider status more important than money Children taught emotional control Time concept more relaxed—consider punctuality less significant than other values (e.g., propriety) Place high value on social harmony

*Most Asian cultures consider the child 1 year old at the time of birth. Traditional Chinese custom adds 1 year on January 1 regardless of the birthday: for example, a child born in December is 2 years old the next January.

Continued

TABLE 32-3—cont'd
Cultural Characteristics Related to Health Care of Children and Families

Cultural Group	Health Beliefs	Health Practices
ASIANS—cont'd		
Filipinos	Believe God's will and supernatural forces govern universe Illness, accidents, and other misfortunes are God's punishment for violations of His will Widely accept "hot" and "cold" balance and imbalance as cause of health and illness	Some use amulets as a shield from witchcraft or as good luck pieces Catholics substitute religious medals and other items
AFRICAN-AMERICANS	Illness classified as: Affected by forces of nature without adequate protection (e.g., cold air, pollution, food and water) Unnatural evil influences (e.g., witchcraft, voodoo, hoodoo, hex, fix, root work); symptoms often associated with eating Believe serious illness sent by God as punishment (e.g., parents punished by illness or death of child) Believe serious illness can be avoided May resist health care because illness is "the will of God"	Self-care and folk medicine very prevalent Folk therapies usually religious in origin Attempt home remedies first; poorer people do not seek help until illness serious Usually seek help from: "Old lady"—woman in community with a common knowledge of herbs; consulted regarding pediatric care Spiritualist—has received gift from God for healing incurable diseases or solving personal problems; strongly based in Christianity Priest (voodoo priest/priestess)—most powerful healer Root doctor meets need for herbs, oils, candles, and ointments Prayer is common means for prevention and treatment
HAITIANS*	Illnesses have a supernatural or natural origin Supernatural illnesses are caused by angry voodoo spirits, enemies, or the dead, especially deceased ancestors Natural illnesses are based on conceptions of natural causation: Irregularities of blood volume, flow, purity, viscosity, color, and/or temperature (hot/cold) Gas (***gaz***) Movement and consistency of mothers' milk "Hot/cold" imbalance in the body Bone displacement Movement of diseases Health is maintained by good dietary and hygienic habits	Health is a personal responsibility Foods have properties of "hot"/"cold" and "light"/"heavy" and must be in harmony with one's life-cycle and bodily states Natural illnesses are treated by home remedies first Supernatural illness treated by healers: voodoo priest (***houngan***) or priestess (***mambo***), midwife (***fam saj***), and herbalist or leaf doctor (***dokte fey***) Amulets and prayer used to protect against illness due to curses or willed by evil people
HISPANICS		
Mexicans (Latinos, Chicanos, Raza-Latinos)	Health beliefs have strong religious association Believe in body imbalance as a cause of illness, especially imbalance between ***caliente*** ("hot") and ***frio*** ("cold") or "wet" and "dry")	Seek help from ***curandero*** or ***curandera,*** especially in rural areas Curandero(a) receives his or her position by birth, apprenticeship, or a "calling" via dream or vision

From Anderson P, Fenichel D: *Serving culturally diverse families of infants and toddlers with disabilities,* Washington, DC, 1989, National Center for Clinical Infant Programs; Clark AL, editor: *Culture and childrearing,* Philadelphia, 1981, FA Davis; DeSantis L: Cultural factors affecting newborn and infant diarrhea, *J Pediatr Nurs* 3(6):391-398, 1988; Geissler EM: *Pocket guide to cultural assessment,* St Louis, 1994, Mosby; Giger J, Davidhizar R: *Transcultural nursing: assessment and intervention,* ed 2, St Louis, 1995, Mosby; Holland S, Sweeney E: *Vietnamese children and families: the impact of culture,* Washington, DC, 1985, Association for the Care of Children's Health; Hollingsworth AO, Brown LP, Brooten DA: The refugees and childbearing: what to expect, *RN* 43(11):45-48, 1980; Orgue MS, Bloch B, Monrroy LSA: *Ethnic nursing care,* St Louis, 1983, Mosby; Randall-David E: *Strategies for working with culturally diverse communities and clients,* Washington, DC, 1989, Association for the Care of Children's Health; and Sodetaini-Shibata AE: The Japanese American. In Clark AL, editor: *Culture and childrearing,* Philadelphia, 1981, FA Davis.
*This section was written by Lydia De Santis, PhD, RN.

Family Relationships	Communication	Comments
Family is highly valued, with strong family ties Multigenerational family structure common, often with collateral members as well Personal interests are subordinate to family interests and needs Members avoid any behavior that would bring shame on the family	Immigrants and older persons may not be able to speak or understand English	Tend to have a fatalistic outlook on life Believe time and providence will solve all
Strong kinship bonds in extended family; members come to aid of others in crisis Less likely to view illness as a burden Augmented families common (unrelated persons living in same household) Place strong emphasis on work and ambition Sex-role sharing among parents Elderly members respected	Alert to any evidence of discrimination Place importance on nonverbal behavior May use nonstandard English or "Black English" Use testing behaviors to assess personnel in health care situations before seeking active care Best to use simple, direct, but caring approach	High level of caution/distrust of majority group Social anxiety related to tradition of humiliation, oppression, and loss of dignity Will elect to retain dignity rather than seek care if values are compromised Strong sense of peoplehood High incidence of poverty Minister a strong influence in community Visits by family minister are sought, expected, and valued in helping to cope with illness and suffering
Maintenance of family reputation is paramount Lineal authority supreme; children in a subordinate position in family hierarchy Children valued for parental social security in old age and expected to contribute to family welfare at an early age Children viewed as gifts from God and treated with indulgence and affection	Recent immigrants and older persons may speak only Haitian creole May prefer family/friends to act as translators and confidants Often smile and nod in agreement when do not understand Quiet and gentle communication style and lack of assertiveness lead health care providers to falsely believe they comprehend health teaching and are compliant Will not ask questions if health care provider is busy or rushed	Will use biomedical and ethnomedical (folk) systems simultaneously Resistant to dietary and work restrictions Adherence to prescribed treatments directly related to perceived severity of illness
Traditionally men considered breadwinners and key decision makers in matters outside the home; women considered homemakers Males considered big and strong (***macho***)	May use nonstandard English Some bilingual; many speak only Spanish May have a strong preference for native language and revert to it in times of stress	High degree of modesty—often a deterrent to seeking medical care and open discussions of sex Youngsters often reluctant to take communal showers in schools

Continued

TABLE 32-3—cont'd
Cultural Characteristics Related to Health Care of Children and Families

Cultural Group	Health Beliefs	Health Practices
HISPANICS—cont'd		
Mexicans (Latinos, Chicanos, Raza-Latinos) —cont'd	Some maintain good health is a result of "good luck"—a reward for good behavior Illness prevented by performing properly, eating proper foods, and working proper amount of time; accomplished through prayer, wearing religious medals or amulets, and sleeping with relics at home Illness is a punishment from God for wrongdoing, forces of nature, and the supernatural	Treatments involve use of herbs, rituals, and religious artifacts Practice for severe illness—make promises, visit shrines, offer medals and candles, offer prayers Adhere to "hot" and "cold" food prescriptions and prohibitions for prevention and treatment of illness
Puerto Ricans	Subscribe to the "hot-cold" theory of causation of illness Believe some illness caused by evil spirits and forces	Infrequent use of health care systems Seek folk healers—use of herbs, rituals Consult spiritualist medium for mental disorders ***Santeria*** is system, and practitioners are called ***santeros*** Treatments classified as "hot" or "cold"
Cubans*	Prevention of good nutrition are related to good health	Diligent users of the medical model Eclectic health-seeking practices, including preventive measures and, in some instances, folk medicine of both religious and nonreligious origins; home remedies; in many instances seek assistance of santeros and spiritualists to complement medical treatment Nutrition is important; parents show overconcern with eating habits of their children and spend a considerable part of the budget on food; traditional Cuban diet is rich in meat and starch; consumption of fresh vegetables added in United States
NATIVE AMERICANS (numerous tribes)	Believe health is state of harmony with nature and universe Respect of bodies through proper management All disorders believed to have aspects of supernatural Violation of a restriction or prohibition thought to cause illness Fear of witchcraft May carry objects believed to guard against witchcraft Theology and medicine strongly interwoven	Medicine persons: Altruistic persons who must use powers in purely positive ways Persons capable of both good and evil—perform negative acts against enemies Diviner-diagnosticians—diagnose but do not have powers or skill to implement medical treatment Specialists—use herbs and curative but nonsacred medical procedures Medicine persons—use herbs and ritual Singers—cure by the power of their song obtained from supernatural beings; effect cures by laying on of hands

From Anderson P, Fenichel D: *Serving culturally diverse families of infants and toddlers with disabilities,* Washington, DC, 1989, National Center for Clinical Infant Programs; Clark AL, editor: *Culture and childrearing,* Philadelphia, 1981, FA Davis; DeSantis L: Cultural factors affecting newborn and infant diarrhea, *J Pediatr Nurs* 3(6):391-398, 1988; Geissler EM: *Pocket guide to cultural assessment,* St Louis, 1994, Mosby; Giger J, Davidhizar R: *Transcultural nursing: assessment and intervention,* ed 2, St Louis, 1995, Mosby; Holland S, Sweeney E: *Vietnamese children and families: the impact of culture,* Washington, DC, 1985, Association for the Care of Children's Health; Hollingsworth AO, Brown LP, Brooten DA: The refugees and childbearing: what to expect, *RN* 43(11):45-48, 1980; Orgue MS, Bloch B, Monrroy LSA: *Ethnic nursing care,* St Louis, 1983, Mosby; Randall-David E: *Strategies for working with culturally diverse communities and clients,* Washington, DC, 1989, Association for the Care of Children's Health; and Sodetaini-Shibata AE: The Japanese American. In Clark AL, editor: *Culture and childrearing,* Philadelphia, 1981, FA Davis.
*This section was written by Mercedes Sandaval, PhD.

Family Relationships	Communication	Comments
Strong kinship; extended families include ***compadres*** (godparents) established by ritual kinship Children valued highly and desired, taken everywhere with family Many homes contain shrines with statues and pictures of saints Elderly treated with respect	May shake hands or engage in introductory embrace Interpret prolonged eye contact as disrespectful	Relaxed concept of time—may be late for appointments More concerned with present than with future and therefore may focus on immediate solutions rather than long-term goals Magicoreligious practices common May view hospital as place to go to die
Family usually large and home centered—the core of existence Father has complete authority in family—family provider and decision maker Wife and children subordinate to father Children valued—seen as a gift from God Children taught to obey and respect parents; corporal punishment to ensure obedience	May use nonstandard English Spanish speaking or bilingual Strong sense of family privacy—may view questions regarding family as impudent	Relaxed sense of time Pay little attention to *exact* time of day Suspicious and fearful of hospitals
Strong family ties with mother and father kinships Children supported and assisted by parents long after becoming adults Elderly cared for at home	Most are bilingual (English/Spanish) except for segments of the senior population	In less than 30 years Cubans have been able to obtain a higher standard of living than other Hispanic groups in United States Have been able to retain many of their former social institutions (e.g., bilingual and private schools, clinics, social clubs, the family as an extended network of support) Many do not feel discriminated against or harbor feelings of inferiority with respect to Anglo-Americans or mainstream population
Extended family structure—usually includes relatives from both sides of family Elder members assume leadership roles	Most continue to speak their tribal language, as well as English Nonverbal communication	Time orientation—present Respect for age Going to hospital associated with illness or disease; therefore may not seek prenatal care, since pregnancy viewed as natural process Tend to take time to form an opinion of professionals Sexual matters not openly discussed with members of opposite sex

Text continued from p. 727

assess the cultural and religious practices of families to identify how these practices are similar to and different from those of their own cultural and religious backgrounds. Guidelines for assessing cultural and religious practices of families are described in Box 34-7.

NURSE ALERT • These generalizations are presented to help nurses learn the unique beliefs and practices of various groups and are not meant to be stereotypes of any group. It is critical to remember that no cultural group is homogeneous; every racial and ethnic group contains great diversity, and knowledge of a culture may not reflect an individual member's beliefs (Nance, 1995).

Key Points

- Culture is the sum total of mores, traditions, and beliefs about how people function; it encompasses other products of human works and thoughts specific to members of an intergenerational group, community, or population.
- Nurses have a responsibility to understand the influence of culture, race, and ethnicity on the development of social and emotional relationships, child-rearing practices, and attitudes toward health.
- A child's self-concept evolves from ideas about his or her social roles.
- Guilt and shame are two behaviors commonly conditioned in children to control social behavior.
- Important subcultural influences on children include ethnicity, social class, occupation, poverty, affluence, religion, schools, peers, and biculture.
- A trend that has significantly influenced the American family is increasing geographic and economic mobility.
- Membership in a minority group presents special challenges for children, although changes in societal attitudes are slowly taking place.
- A child's physical characteristics and susceptibility to health problems are strongly related to ethnic and cultural variations of hereditary and socioeconomic forces.
- Groups of children suffering from greater physical and mental health problems are those living in poverty, those who are homeless, and those who have migrant families.
- Because verbal and nonverbal communication is an important cultural consideration, nurses need to acknowledge and respect their patient's practices in order for productive interaction to occur.
- Cultural beliefs related to cause of illness and maintenance of health may focus on natural forces, supernatural forces, or imbalance of forces.
- In planning and implementing patient care, nurses need to strive to adapt ethnic practices to the family's health needs rather than attempt to change long-standing beliefs.
- No cultural group is homogeneous; every racial and ethnic group contains great diversity.

References

Advisory Council for the Elimination of Tuberculosis: Prevention and control of tuberculosis in migrant farm workers, *MMWR* 41(RR-10):1-15, 1992.

Ahmann E: "Chunky stew": appreciating cultural diversity while providing health care for children, *Pediatr Nurs* 20:320-324, 1994.

Annie E. Casey Foundation: *Kids count data book: state profiles of child well-being,* Washington, DC, 1999, Center for the Study of Social Policy.

Bennett NG et al: *Young children in poverty: a statistical update,* New York, 1999, National Center for Children in Poverty, Columbia University.

Boyer K: A little Spanish goes a long way, *Nurs Spectrum* 4:13, 1996.

Castiglia PT: Tuberculosis, a pediatric concern, *J Pediatr Health Care* 11(2):75-77, 1997.

Centers for Disease Control and Prevention: *Preventing lead poisoning in young children,* Atlanta, 1997, The Centers.

Cooper TP: Culturally appropriate care: optional or imperative, *Adv Pract Nurs Q* 2(2):1-6, 1996.

Council of Economic Advisers for the President's Initiative on Race: *Changing America: indicators of social and economic well-being by race and Hispanic origin,* Washington, DC, 1998, Executive Office of the President, Council of Economic Advisers.

Culley L: A critique of multiculturalism in health care: the challenge for nurse education, *J Adv Nurs* 23:564-570, 1996.

Fulton RA, Moore CM: Spiritual care of the school-age child with a chronic condition, *Pediatr Nurs* 10(4):224-231, 1995.

Habayeb GL: Cultural diversity: a nursing concept not yet reliably defined, *Nurs Outlook* 43(5):224-227, 1995.

Leininger M: *Transcultural nursing,* New York, 1978, John Wiley & Sons.

Lester L: Cultural competence: a nursing dialogue 2, *Am J Nurs* 98(9):36-43, 1998.

Lukoff D, Lu FG, Turner R: Cultural considerations in the assessment and treatment of religious and spiritual problems, *Psychiatr Clin North Am* 18(3):467-485, 1995.

Malach F, Segel N: Perspectives on health care delivery systems for American Indian families, *Child Health Care* 19(4): 219-228, 1990.

Martinson IM, Armstrong V, Qiao J: The experience of the family of children with chronic illness at home in China, *Pediatr Nurs* 23(4):371-375, 1997.

Mattson S: Culturally sensitive perinatal care for Southeast Asians, *JOGNN* 24(4):335-341, 1995.

Nance TA: Intercultural communications: finding common ground, *JOGNN* 24(3):249-255, 1995.

Petersen B: Surviving culture shock: lessons learned as a medical missionary in Jamaica, *J Emerg Nurs* 21(6):505-506, 1995.

Phillips S, Lobar S: Performing a culturally competent child health assessment, *Fla Nurse* 43(6);23, 1995.

Rogers G: Educating case managers for culturally competent practice, *J Case Manage* 4(2):60-65, 1995.

Rollins J: *Project Taking Charge field test site reports: August 1992-March 1993,* Manuscript submitted for publication, 1993.

Sandhaus S: Migrant health: a harvest of poverty, *Am J Nurs* 98(9):52-54, 1998.

Scribner R: Paradox as paradigm: the health outcomes of Mexican Americans, *Am J Public Health* 86(3):303-304, 1996.

Sekhon SK: Insights into South Asian culture: food and nutritional values, *Top Clin Nutr* 11(4):47-56, 1996.

Spector RE: *Cultural diversity in health and illness,* ed 5, Upper Saddle River, NJ, 2000, Prentice Hall Health.

Strehlow AJ, Amos-Jones T: The homeless as a vulnerable population, *Nurs Clin North Am* 34(2):261-274, 1999.

Talabere LR: Meeting the challenge of cultural care in nursing diversity, sensitivity, competence, and congruence, *J Cult Diversity* 3(2):53-61, 1996.

Taylor R: Check your cultural competence, *Nurs Manage* 29(8):30-32, 1998.

U.S. Census Bureau: *Preliminary estimate of poverty thresholds for 1998,* www.census.gov/hhes/poverty/threshld/98prelim.html, 1999.

Wagner J, Menke EM, Ciccone MA: What is known about the health of rural homeless families, *Public Health Nurs* 12(6): 400-408, 1995.

Warda MR: Mexican Americans' perceptions of culturally competent care, *West J Nurs Res* 22(2):203-224, 2000.

Weinreb L et al: Determinants of health and service use patterns in homeless and low-income housed children, *Pediatrics* 102(3):554-562, 1998.

Yoos HL et al: Child rearing beliefs in the African-American community: implications for culturally competent pediatric care, *J Pediatr Nurs* 10(6):343-353, 1995.

Yoos HL et al: An asthma management program for urban minority children, *J Pediatr Health Care* 11(2):66-74, 1997.

CHAPTER 33 Developmental Influences on Child Health Promotion

http://www.harcourthealth.com/MERLIN/Wong/maternal/

Learning Objectives

On completion of this chapter the reader will be able to:

- Describe major trends in growth and development.
- Explain the alterations in the major body systems that take place during the process of growth and development.
- Discuss the development and relationships of personality, cognitive, language, moral, spiritual, and self-concept development.
- Describe the role of play in the growth and development of children.
- Demonstrate an understanding of the roles of innate and environmental factors in the physical and emotional development of children.

GROWTH AND DEVELOPMENT

Foundations of Growth and Development

Growth and development is usually referred to as a unit; it expresses the sum of the numerous changes that take place during the lifetime of an individual. The entire course is a dynamic process that encompasses several interrelated dimensions:

Growth—An increase in number and size of cells as they divide and synthesize new proteins; results in increased size and weight of the whole or any of its parts

Development—A gradual change and expansion; advancement from lower to more advanced stages of complexity, the emerging and expanding of the individual's capacities through growth, maturation, and learning

Maturation—An increase in competence and adaptability; aging; usually used to describe a qualitative change; a change in the complexity of a structure that makes it possible for that structure to begin functioning; to function at a higher level

Differentiation—Processes by which early cells and structures are systematically modified and altered to achieve specific and characteristic physical and chemical properties; sometimes used to describe the trend of mass to specific; development from simple to more complex activities and functions

All of these processes are interrelated, simultaneous, and ongoing; none occurs apart from the others. The processes depend on a sequence of endocrine, genetic, constitutional, environmental, and nutritional influences (Seidel et al, 1999). The child's body becomes larger and more complex; the personality simultaneously expands in scope and complexity. Very simply, growth can be viewed as a *quantitative* change, and development as a *qualitative* change.*

Stages of Development. Most authorities in the field of child development conveniently categorize child growth and behavior into approximate age stages or in terms that describe the features of an age group. The age ranges of these stages are admittedly arbitrary and, because they do not take into account individual differences, cannot be applied to all children with any degree of precision. However, this categorization affords a convenient means to describe the characteristics associated with the majority of children at periods when distinctive developmental changes appear and specific developmental tasks must be accomplished. (A *developmental task* is a set of skills and competencies specific to each developmental stage that children must accomplish or master in order to deal effectively with their environment.) It is also significant for nurses to know that there are characteristic health problems specific to each major phase of development. The sequences of descriptive age periods and subperiods that are used here, and that are elaborated in subsequent chapters, are listed in Box 33-1.

*For additional information, please view "Growth and Development" in ***Whaley and Wong's Pediatric Nursing Video Series,*** St Louis, 1996, Mosby; 1-800-426-4545; website: www.mosby.com

Box 33-1

Developmental Age Periods

Prenatal period: Conception to birth

Germinal: Conception to approximately 2 weeks

Embryonic: 2 to 8 weeks

Fetal: 8 to 40 weeks (birth)

A rapid growth rate and total dependency make this one of the most crucial periods in the developmental process. The relationship between maternal health and certain manifestations in the newborn emphasizes the importance of adequate prenatal care to the health and well-being of the infant.

Infancy period: Birth to 12 months

Neonatal: Birth to 27 or 28 days

Infancy: 1 to approximately 12 months

The infancy period is one of rapid motor, cognitive, and social development. Through mutuality with the caregiver (parent), the infant establishes a basic trust in the world and the foundation for future interpersonal relationships. The critical first month of life, although part of the infancy period, is often differentiated from the remainder because of the major physical adjustments to extrauterine existence and the psychologic adjustment of the parent.

Early childhood: 1 to 6 years

Toddler: 1 to 3 years

Preschool: 3 to 6 years

This period, which extends from the time the children attain upright locomotion until they enter school, is characterized by intense activity and discovery. It is a time of marked physical and personality development. Motor development advances steadily. Children at this age acquire language and wider social relationships, learn role standards, gain self-control and mastery, develop increasing awareness of dependence and independence, and begin to develop a self-concept.

Middle childhood: 6 to 11 or 12 years

Frequently referred to as the "school age," this period of development is one in which the child is directed away from the family group and centered around the wider world of peer relationships. There is steady advancement in physical, mental, and social development, with emphasis on developing skill competencies. Social cooperation and early moral development take on more importance with relevance for later life stages. This is a critical period in the development of a self-concept.

Later childhood: 11 to 19 years

Prepubertal: 10 to 13 years

Adolescence: 13 to approximately 18 years

The tumultuous period of rapid maturation and change known as adolescence is considered to be a transitional period that begins at the onset of puberty and extends to the point of entry into the adult world—usually high school graduation. Biologic and personality maturation are accompanied by physical and emotional turmoil, and there is redefining of the self-concept. In the late adolescent period the young person begins to internalize all previously learned values and to focus on an individual, rather than a group, identity.

Beck C: Screening methods for postpartum depression, *J Obstet Gynecol Neonatal Nurs* 24(4):308-312, 1995.

Patterns of Growth and Development. There are definite and predictable patterns in growth and development that are continuous, orderly, and progressive. These patterns or trends are universal and basic to all human beings, but each human being accomplishes them in a manner and time unique to that individual.

Directional Trends. Growth and development proceed in regular, related directions or gradients and reflect the physical development and maturation of neuromuscular functions (Fig. 33-1). The first pattern is the *cephalocaudal,* or *head-to-tail,* direction. The head end of the organism develops first and is very large and complex, whereas the lower end is small and simple and takes shape at a later period. The physical evidence of this trend is most apparent during the period before birth, but it also applies to postnatal behavior development. Infants achieve structural control of the head before they have control of the trunk and extremities, hold their backs erect before they stand, use their eyes before their hands, and gain control of their hands before they have control of their feet.

Second, the *proximodistal,* or *near-to-far* trend applies to the midline-to-peripheral concept. A conspicuous illustration is the early embryonic development of limb buds, which is followed by rudimentary fingers and toes. In the infant, shoulder control precedes mastery of the hands, the whole hand is used as a unit before the fingers can be manipulated, and the central nervous system develops more rapidly than the peripheral nervous system.

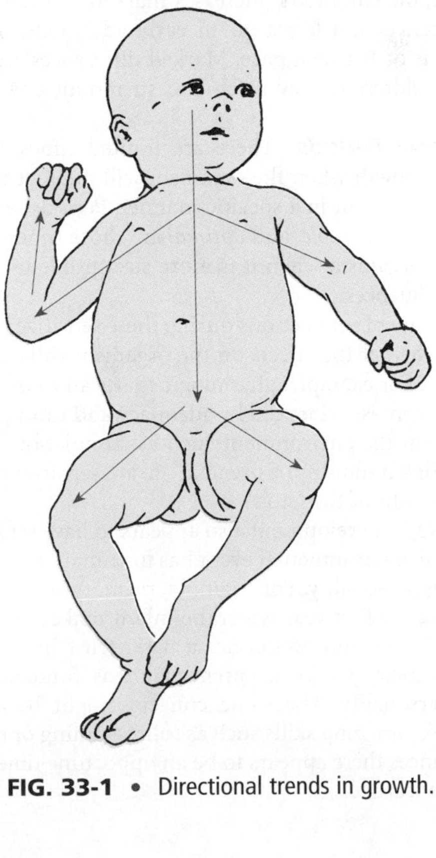

FIG. 33-1 • Directional trends in growth.

These trends or patterns are bilateral and appear symmetric—each side develops in the same direction and at the same rate as the other. For some of the neurologic functions, this symmetry is only external because of unilateral differentiation of function at an early stage of postnatal development. For example, by the age of approximately 5 years the child has demonstrated a decided preference for the use of one hand over the other, although previously either one had been used.

The third trend, differentiation, describes development from simple operations to more complex activities and functions. From very broad, global patterns of behavior, more specific, refined patterns emerge. All areas of development (i.e., physical, mental, social, and emotional) proceed in this direction. Through the process of development and differentiation, early embryonal cells with vague, undifferentiated functions progress to an immensely complex organism composed of highly specialized and diversified cells, tissues, and organs. Generalized development precedes specific or specialized development; gross, random muscle movements take place before fine muscle control.

Sequential Trends. In all dimensions of growth and development there is a definite, predictable sequence, with each child normally passing through every stage. Children crawl before they creep, creep before they stand, and stand before they walk. Later facets of the personality are built on the early foundation of trust. The child babbles, then forms words and, finally, sentences; writing emerges from scribbling.

Developmental Pace. Although there is a fixed, precise order to development, it does not progress at the same rate or pace. There are periods of accelerated growth and periods of decelerated growth in both total body growth and the growth of subsystems. The rapid growth before and after birth gradually levels off throughout early childhood. Growth is relatively slow during middle childhood, increases markedly at the beginning of adolescence, and levels off in early adulthood. Each child grows at his or her own pace. Marked differences are observed between children as they reach and surmount developmental milestones.

Sensitive Periods. There are limited times during the process of growth when the organism will interact with a particular environment in a specific manner. Periods termed *critical, sensitive, vulnerable,* and *optimal* are those times in the lifetime of an organism when it is more susceptible to positive or negative influences.

The quality of interactions during these sensitive periods determines whether the effects on the organism will be beneficial or harmful. For example, physiologic maturation of the central nervous system is influenced by adequacy and timing of contributions from the environment such as stimulation and nutrition. The first 3 months of prenatal life are sensitive periods for physical growth of the fetus.

Psychologic development also appears to have sensitive periods when an environmental event has maximal influence on the developing personality. For example, primary socialization occurs during the first year when the infant makes the initial social attachments and establishes a basic trust in the world. A warm relationship with a parent figure is fundamental to a healthy personality. The same concept might be applied to readiness for learning skills such as toilet training or reading. In these instances there appears to be an opportune time when the skill is best learned.

Individual Differences. Each child grows in his or her own unique and personal way. Great individual variation exists in the age at which developmental milestones are reached. The sequence is predictable; the exact timing is not. Rates of growth vary, and measurements are defined in terms of ranges to allow for individual differences. Some children are fast growers, others are moderate, and still others are slower to reach maturity. Periods of fast growth, such as the pubescent growth spurt, may begin earlier or later in some children. Children may grow quickly or slowly during the spurt, and may finish sooner or later than others. Gender is an influential factor because girls seem to be more advanced in physiologic growth at all ages.

Biologic Growth and Physical Development

As children grow, their external dimensions change. These changes are accompanied by corresponding alterations in structure and function of internal organs and tissues that reflect the gradual acquisition of physiologic competence. Each part has its own rate of growth, which may be directly related to alterations in the size of the child (e.g., the heart rate). Skeletal muscle growth approximates whole body growth; brain, lymphoid, adrenal, and reproductive tissues follow distinct and individual patterns. When there has been a secondary cause of growth deficiency, such as severe illness or acute malnutrition, recovery from the illness or the establishment of an adequate diet will produce a dramatic acceleration of the growth rate that usually continues until the child's individual growth pattern is resumed.

External Proportions. Variations in the growth rate of different tissues and organ systems produce significant changes in body proportions during childhood. The cephalocaudal trend of development is most evident in total body growth as indicated by these changes (Fig. 33-2). During fetal development the head is the fastest growing body part, and at 2 months of gestation the head constitutes 50% of total body length. During infancy growth of the trunk predominates; the legs are the most rapidly growing part during childhood; in adolescence the trunk once again elongates. In the newborn infant the lower limbs are one third the total body length but only 15% of the total body weight; in the adult the lower limbs constitute one half of the total body height and 30% or more of the total body weight. As growth proceeds, the midpoint in head-to-toe measurements gradually descends from a level even with the umbilicus at birth to the level of the symphysis pubis at maturity.

Biologic Determinants of Growth and Development. The most prominent feature of childhood and adolescence is physical growth. Throughout development various tissues in the body undergo changes in growth, composition, and structure. In some tissues the changes are continuous (e.g., bone growth and dentition); in others, significant alterations occur at specific stages (e.g., appearance of secondary sex characteristics). When these measurements are compared with standardized norms, a child's developmental progress can be determined with a high degree of confidence (Table 33-1).

Linear growth, or *height* occurs almost entirely as a result of skeletal growth and is considered a stable measurement of general growth. Growth in height is not uniform throughout life, and it ceases when maturation of the skeleton is complete. The maximum growth in length occurs before birth, but the newborn continues to grow at a rapid, though slower, rate.

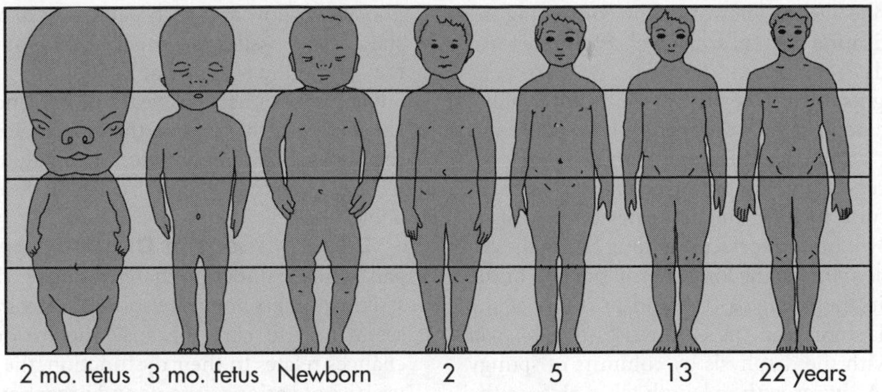

FIG. 33-2 • Changes in body proportions from before birth to adulthood. (From Crouch JE, McClintic JR: *Human anatomy and physiology,* ed 2, New York, 1976, Wiley & Sons.)

TABLE 33-1
General Trends in Height and Weight Gain During Childhood

Age Group	Weight*	Height*
Infants		
Birth-6 months	Weekly gain: 140-200 g (5-7 oz) Birth weight doubles by end of first 4-7 months	Monthly gain: 2.5 cm (1 inch)
6-12 months	Weight gain: 85-140 g (3-5 oz) Birth weight triples by end of first year	Monthly gain: 1.25 cm (½ inch) Birth length increases by approximately 50% by end of first year
Toddlers	Birth weight quadruples by age 2½ Yearly gain: 2-3 kg (4½-6½ lb)	Height at age 2 years is approximately 50% of eventual adult height Gain during second year: about 12 cm (4¾ inches) Gain during third year: about 6-8 cm (2⅜-3¼ inches)
Preschoolers	Yearly gain: 2-3 kg (4½-6½ lb)	Birth length doubles by age 4 years Yearly gain: 5-7.5 cm (2-3 inches)
School-age children	Yearly gain: 2-3 kg (4½-6½ lb)	Yearly gain after age 7: 5 cm (2 inches) Birth length triples by about age 13 years
Pubertal growth spurt		
Females—10-14 years	Weight gain: 7-25 kg (15-55 lb) Mean: 17.5 kg (38⅛ lb)	Height gain: 5-25 cm (2-10 inches); approximately 95% of mature height achieved by onset of menarche or skeletal age of 13 years Mean: 20.5 cm (8¼ inches)
Males—11-16 years	Weight gain: 7-30 kg (15-65 lb) Mean: 23.7 kg (52⅛ lb)	Height gain: 10-30 cm (4-12 inches); approximately 95% of mature height achieved by skeletal age of 15 years Mean: 27.5 cm (11 inches)

*Yearly height and weight gains for each age group represent averaged estimates from a variety of sources.

NURSE ALERT • **Double the child's height at the age of 2 years to estimate how tall he or she may be as an adult.**

At birth, *weight* is more variable than height and is, to a greater extent, a reflection of the intrauterine environment. The average newborn weighs from 3175 to 3400 g (7 to 7½ pounds). In general, the birth weight doubles by 4 to 7 months of age and triples by the end of the first year. By the end of the second year it usually quadruples. After this point the "normal" rate of weight gain, just as the growth in height, assumes a steady annual increase of approximately 2 to 2.75 kg (4⅖ to 6 pounds) per year until the adolescent growth spurt.

Both *bone age* determinants and state of *dentition* are used as indicators of development. Because both are discussed elsewhere, neither is elaborated here (see next section for bone age; see also Chapter 36 for dentition).

Skeletal Growth and Maturation. The most accurate measure of general development is *skeletal* or *bone age,* the radiologic determination of osseous maturation. Skeletal age appears to correlate more closely with other measures of physiologic maturity (e.g., onset of menarche) than with chronologic age or height. This "bone age" is determined by comparing the mineralization of ossification centers and advancing bony form to age-related standards.

Bone formation begins during the second month of fetal life when calcium salts are deposited in the intracellular substance (matrix) to form first calcified cartilage and then true bone. There are some differences in this bone formation. In small bones the bone continues to form in the center and cartilage continues to be laid down on the surfaces. In long bones the ossification begins in the *diaphysis* (the long central portion of the bone) and continues in the *epiphysis* (the end portions of the bone). Between the diaphysis and the epiphysis, an *epiphyseal cartilage plate* unites with the diaphysis by columns of spongy tissue, the *metaphysis.* Active growth in length takes place in the epiphyseal growth plate. Interference with this growth site by trauma or infection can result in deformity.

The first centers of ossification appear in the 2-month-old embryo, and at birth the number is approximately 400, or about half the number at maturity. New centers appear at regular intervals during the growth period and provide the basis for assessment of bone age. Postnatally the earliest centers to appear (at 5 to 6 months of age) are those of the capitate and hamate bones in the wrist. Therefore radiographs of the hand and wrist provide the most useful areas for screening to determine skeletal age, especially before age 6 years. These centers appear earlier in girls than in boys.

Nurses must understand that the growing bones of children possess many unique characteristics. Bone fractures occurring at the growth plate may be difficult to discover and may significantly affect subsequent growth and development (Urbanski and Hanlon, 1996).

Factors that may influence skeletal muscle injury rates and types in children and adolescents include (Kaczander, 1997):

- Less protective sports equipment for children
- Less emphasis on conditioning, especially flexibility
- In adolescents, fractures are more common than ligamentous ruptures because of the rapid growth rate of the physeal zone of hypertrophy (i.e., the segment of tubular bone that is concerned mainly with growth)

Neurologic Maturation. In contrast to other body tissues, which grow rapidly after birth, the nervous system grows proportionately more rapidly before birth. Two periods of rapid brain cell growth occur during fetal life: a dramatic increase in the number of neurons between 15 and 20 weeks of gestation, and another increase at 30 weeks, which extends to 1 year of age. The rapid growth of infancy continues during early childhood and then slows to a more gradual rate during later childhood and adolescence.

It is believed that no new nerve cells appear after the sixth month of fetal life. Postnatal growth consists of increasing the amount of cytoplasm around the nuclei of existing cells, increasing the number and intricacy of communications with other cells, and advancing their peripheral axons to keep pace with expanding body dimensions. This allows for increasingly complex movement and behavior. Neurophysiologic changes also provide the foundation for language, learning, and behavior development. Neurologic or electroencephalographic development is sometimes used as an indicator of maturational age in the early weeks of life.

Lymphoid Tissues. Lymphoid tissues contained in the lymph nodes, thymus, spleen, tonsils, adenoids, and blood lymphocytes follow a growth pattern unlike that of other body tissues. These tissues are small in relation to total body size, but they are well developed at birth. They increase rapidly to reach adult dimensions by 6 years of age and continue to grow. At about age 10 to 12 years they reach a maximum development that is approximately twice their adult size. This is followed by a rapid decline to stable adult dimensions by the end of adolescence.

Development of Organ Systems. All tissues and organ systems undergo changes during development. Some are striking; others are more subtle. Many have implications for assessment and care. Because the major importance of these changes relates to their dysfunction, the developmental characteristics of various systems and organs are discussed throughout the book as they relate to these areas. Physical characteristics and physiologic changes that vary with age are included in age group descriptions.

Physiologic Changes

Physiologic changes that take place in all organs and systems are discussed as they relate to dysfunction. Others such as pulse and respiratory rates and blood pressure are an integral part of physical assessment (see Chapter 35). In addition, there are changes in basic functions, including metabolism, temperature, and patterns of sleep and rest.

Metabolism. The rate of metabolism when the body is at rest (*basal metabolic rate,* or *BMR*) demonstrates a distinctive change throughout childhood. Highest in the newborn infant, the BMR closely relates to the proportion of surface area to body mass, which changes as the body increases in size. In both sexes the proportion decreases progressively to maturity. The BMR is slightly higher in boys at all ages and during pubescence further increases over that in girls.

The rate of metabolism determines the caloric requirements of the child. The basal energy requirement of infants is about 108 kcal/kg of body weight and decreases to 40 to 45 kcal/kg at maturity (Table 33-2). Water requirements remain at approximately 1.5 ml per calorie of energy expended throughout life. Children's energy needs vary considerably at different ages and with changing circumstances. The energy requirement to build tissue steadily decreases with age, following the general growth curve; however, energy needs vary with the individual child and may be considerably higher. For short periods (e.g., during strenuous exercise) and more prolonged periods (e.g., illness), the needs can be very high.

Temperature. Body temperature, reflecting metabolism, displays the same decrement from infancy to maturity (see the Appendix). Thermoregulation is one of the most important adaptation responses of the infant during the transition from intrauterine to extrauterine life. Following the unstable regulatory ability in the neonatal period, heat production steadily declines as the infant grows into childhood. Individual differences of 0.5° to 1° F are normal, and occasionally a child normally displays an unusually high or low temperature. Beginning at approximately 12 years of age, girls display a temperature that remains relatively stable, whereas the temperature in boys continues to fall for a few more years. Females maintain a temperature slightly above that of males throughout life.

Even with improved temperature regulation, infants and young children are highly susceptible to temperature fluctua-

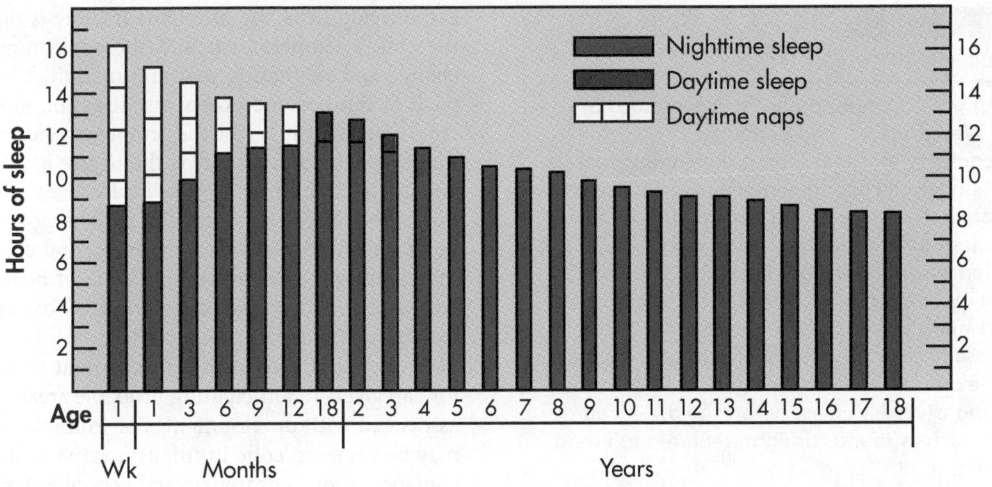

FIG. 33-3 • Changes in number of hours of sleep with increasing age. (Modified from Ferber R: *Solve your child's sleep problems,* New York, 1985, Simon & Schuster.)

tions. Body temperature responds to changes in environmental temperature and is increased with active exercise, crying, and emotional upset. Infections can cause a higher and more rapid temperature increase in infants and young children than in older children. In relation to body weight, an infant produces more heat per unit than children near maturity. Consequently, during active play or when heavily clothed, an infant or small child is likely to become overheated.

Sleep and Rest. Sleep, a protective function in all organisms, allows for repair and recovery of tissues following activity. As in most aspects of development, there is wide variation among individual children in the amount and distribution of sleep at various ages. As children mature, there is a change in the total time they spend in sleep and the amount of time they spend in deep sleep.

Newborn infants sleep much of the time that is not occupied with feeding and other aspects of their care. As infants grow older, the total time spent in sleep gradually decreases, they remain awake for longer periods, and they sleep longer at night. For example, the length of a sleep cycle increases from approximately 50 to 60 minutes in the newborn infant to approximately 90 minutes in adolescence (Anders, Sadeh, and Appareddy, 1995). During the latter part of the first year, most children sleep through the night and take one or two naps during the day. By the time they are 12 to 18 months old, most children have eliminated the second nap. After age 3 years the child has usually given up daytime naps, except in cultures in which an afternoon nap or siesta is customary. During ages 4 to 10 years, sleep time declines slightly and then increases somewhat during the pubertal growth spurt. The changes in length of sleep at different ages are shown in Fig. 33-3.

There is a change in the quality of sleep as children mature. The time spent in deep, restful sleep increases from 50% in infancy to 80% in the older child.

Temperament

Temperament is defined as "the manner of thinking, behaving, or reacting characteristic of an individual" (Chess and Thomas, 1985) and refers to the way in which a person deals with life. From the time of birth, children exhibit marked individual differences in the way that they respond to their environment and the way others, particularly the parents, respond to them and their needs. A genetic basis has been suggested for some differences in temperament. Nine characteristics of temperament have been identified through interviews with parents (Box 33-2). Temperament refers to behavioral tendencies, not to discrete behavioral acts. There are no implications of good or bad. Most children can be placed into one of three common

TABLE 33-2

Recommended Daily Requirements for Calories and Protein Through Adolescence*

Age (Years)	Energy Allowance (kcal/kg)	Protein (g)
INFANTS		
0-½	108	13
½-1	98	14
CHILDREN		
1-3	102	16
4-6	90	24
7-10	70	28
MALES		
11-14	55	45
15-18	45	49
FEMALES		
11-14	47	46
15-18	40	44

Data from Food and Nutrition Board: *Recommended daily allowances,* ed 10, Washington, DC, 1989, National Academy Press.
*See also Recommended Daily Allowances, p. 1236.

Box 33-2
Attributes of Temperament

Activity—level of physical motion during activity such as sleep, eating, play, dressing, and bathing
Rhythmicity—regularity in the timing of physiologic functions such as hunger, sleep, and elimination
Approach-withdrawal—nature of initial responses to a new stimulus such as people, situations, places, foods, toys, and procedures (***Approach*** responses are positive and are displayed by activity or expression; ***withdrawal*** responses are negative expressions or behaviors.)
Adaptability—ease or difficulty with which the child adapts or adjusts to new or altered situations
Threshold of responsiveness (sensory threshold)—amount of stimulation, such as sounds or light, required to evoke a response in the child
Intensity of reaction—energy level of the child's reactions, regardless of quality or direction
Mood—amount of pleasant, happy, friendly behavior compared with unpleasant, unhappy, crying, unfriendly behavior exhibited by the child in various situations
Distractibility—ease with which a child's attention or direction of behavior can be diverted by external stimuli
Attention span and persistence—length of time a child pursues a given activity ***(attention)*** and the continuation of an activity in spite of obstacles ***(persistence)***

categories based on their overall pattern of temperamental attributes:

The easy child. Easy-going children are even-tempered, are regular and predictable in their habits, and have a positive approach to new stimuli. They are open and adaptable to change and display a mild to moderately intense mood that is typically positive. Approximately 40% of children fall into this category.

The difficult child. Difficult children are highly active, irritable, and irregular in their habits. Negative withdrawal responses are typical, and they require a more structured environment. These children adapt slowly to new routines, people, or situations. Mood expressions are usually intense and primarily negative. They exhibit frequent periods of crying, and frustration often produces violent tantrums. This group makes up about 10% of children.

The slow-to-warm-up child. Slow-to-warm-up children typically react negatively and with mild intensity to new stimuli and, unless pressured, adapt slowly with repeated contact. They respond with only mild but passive resistance to novelty or changes in routine. They are quite inactive and moody, but show only moderate irregularity in functions. Fifteen percent of children demonstrate this temperament pattern.

Thirty-five percent of children either have some, but not all, of the characteristics of one of the categories or are inconsistent in their behavioral responses. Many normal children demonstrate this wide range of behavioral patterns.

Significance of Temperament. Observations indicate that children who display the difficult or slow-to-warm-up patterns of behavior are more vulnerable to the development of behavior problems in early and middle childhood. Any child can develop behavior problems if there is dissonance between the child's temperament and the environment. Demands for change and adaptation that are in conflict with the child's capacities can become excessively stressful. However, authorities emphasize that it is not the temperament patterns of children that place them at risk; it is the *degree of fit* between children and their environment, specifically their parents, that determines the degree of vulnerability. The potential for optimum development exists when environmental expectations and demands fit with the individual's style of behavior and the parents' ability to navigate this period (Gross and Conrad, 1995) (see Failure to Thrive, Chapter 36).

Early identification of temperament provides a useful tool for caregivers in anticipating probable areas of difficulty or risk associated with development. For example, "difficult" children may be prone to colic in infancy; active children require more vigilance to prevent injury; and school entry requires different approaches for children with different temperaments.

Research indicates that irritable and unadaptable infants can raise doubts in mothers about their competence (Beck, 1996). Studies on the relationship between temperament and the ability to perform a task successfully (mastery motivation) have found that infants with high mastery are more cooperative and less difficult (Morrow and Camp, 1996).

DEVELOPMENT OF PERSONALITY AND MENTAL FUNCTION

Personality and cognitive skills develop in much the same manner as biologic growth—new accomplishments build on previously mastered skills. Many aspects depend on physical growth and maturation. This is not a comprehensive account of the multiple facets of personality and behavior development. Many aspects are integrated with the child's emotional and social development in later discussion of various age groups. Table 33-3 summarizes some of the developmental theories.

Theoretic Foundations of Personality Development

Psychosexual Development (Freud). Freud considered the sexual instincts to be significant in the development of the personality. However, he used the term *psychosexual* to describe any *sensual pleasure.* During childhood certain regions of the body assume a prominent psychologic significance; this source of new pleasures and new conflicts gradually shifts from one part of the body to another at particular stages of development:

Oral stage (birth to 1 year)—During infancy the major source of pleasure seeking is centered on oral activities such as sucking, biting, chewing, and vocalizing. Children may prefer one of these over the others, and the preferred method of oral gratification can provide some indication of the personality they develop.

Anal stage (1 to 3 years)—Interest during the second year of life centers in the anal region as sphincter muscles develop and children are able to withhold or expel fecal material at will. At this stage the climate surrounding toilet training can have lasting effects on children's personalities.

Phallic stage (3 to 6 years)—During the phallic stage the genitals become an interesting and sensitive area of the body. Children recognize differences between the sexes

TABLE 33-3
Summary of Personality, Cognitive, and Moral Development Theories

Stage/Age	Psychosexual Stages (Freud)	Psychosocial Stages (Erikson)	Cognitive Stages (Piaget)	Moral Judgment Stages (Kohlberg)
I INFANCY Birth to 1 year	Oral-sensory	Trust vs. mistrust	Sensorimotor (birth to 2 years)	
II TODDLERHOOD 1-3 years	Anal-urethral	Autonomy vs. shame and doubt	Preoperational thought, preconceptual phase (transductive reasoning, e.g., specific to specific) (2-4 years)	Preconventional (premoral) level Punishment and obedience orientation
III EARLY CHILDHOOD 3-6 years	Phallic-locomotion	Initiative vs. guilt	Preoperational thought, intuitive phase (transductive reasoning) (4-7 years)	Preconventional (premoral) level Naive instrumental orientation
IV MIDDLE CHILDHOOD 6-12 years	Latency	Industry vs. inferiority	Concrete operations (inductive reasoning and beginning logic) (7-11 years)	Conventional level Good-boy, nice-girl orientation Law-and-order orientation
V ADOLESCENCE 12-18 years	Genitality	Identity and repudiation vs. identity confusion	Formal operations (deductive and abstract reasoning) (11-15 years)	Postconventional or principled level Social-contract orientation Universal ethical principle orientation (no longer included in revised theory)

and become curious about the dissimilarities. This is the period around which the controversial issues of the Oedipus and Electra complexes, penis envy, and castration anxiety are centered.

Latency period (6 to 12 years)—During the latency period children elaborate on previously acquired traits and skills. Physical and psychic energy are channeled into acquisition of knowledge and vigorous play.

Genital stage (age 12 and over)—The last significant stage begins at puberty with maturation of the reproductive system and production of sex hormones. The genital organs become the major source of sexual tensions and pleasures, but energies are also invested in forming friendships and preparation for marriage.

Psychosocial Development (Erikson). The most widely accepted theory of personality development is that advanced by Erikson (1963). Although built on Freudian theory, it is known as *psychosocial* development and emphasizes a healthy personality as opposed to a pathologic approach. Erikson also uses the biologic concepts of critical periods and epigenesis, describing key conflicts or core problems that the individual strives to master during critical periods in personality development. Successful completion or mastery of each of these core conflicts is built on the satisfactory completion or mastery of the previous core problem.

Each psychosocial stage has two components (i.e., the favorable and the unfavorable aspects of the core conflict), and progress to the next stage depends on resolution of this conflict. No core conflict is ever mastered completely but remains a recurrent problem throughout life. No life situation is ever secure. Each new situation presents the conflict in a new form. For example, when children who have satisfactorily achieved a sense of trust encounter a new experience (e.g., hospitalization), they must again develop a sense of trust in those responsible for their care in order to master the situation. Erikson's life span approach to personality development consists of eight stages; however, only the first five relating to childhood are included here:

Trust vs. mistrust (birth to 1 year)—The first and most important attribute to develop for a healthy personality is a basic trust. Establishment of basic trust dominates the first year of life and describes all the child's satisfying experiences at this age. Corresponding to Freud's oral stage, it is a time of "getting" and "taking in" through all the senses. It exists only in relation to something or someone; therefore consistent, loving care by a nurturing person is essential to development of trust. *Mistrust* develops when trust-promoting experiences are deficient or lacking or when basic needs are inconsistently or inadequately met. Although shreds of mistrust are sprinkled throughout the personality, from a basic trust in parents stems trust in the world, other people, and oneself. The result is *faith* and *optimism.*

Autonomy vs. shame and doubt (1 to 3 years)—Corresponding to Freud's anal stage, the problem of *autonomy* can be symbolized by the holding on and letting go of the sphincter muscles. The development of autonomy during the toddler period is centered around children's increasing ability to control their bodies, themselves, and their environment. They want to do things for themselves, using their newly acquired motor skills of walking, climbing, and manipulating and their mental powers of selection and decision making. Much of their learning is acquired through imitating the activities and behavior of others. Negative feelings of *doubt* and *shame* arise when children are made to feel small and self-conscious, when their choices are disastrous, when others shame them, or when they are forced to be dependent in areas in which they are capable of assuming control. The favorable outcomes are *self-control* and *willpower.*

Initiative vs. guilt (3 to 6 years)—The stage of *initiative* corresponds to Freud's phallic stage and is characterized by vigorous, intrusive behavior; enterprise; and a strong imagination. Children explore the physical world with all their senses and powers. They develop a conscience. No longer guided only by outsiders, there is an inner voice that warns and threatens. Children sometimes undertake goals or activities that are in conflict with those of parents or others, and being made to feel that their activities or imaginings are bad produces a sense of *guilt.* Children must learn to retain a sense of initiative without impinging on the rights and privileges of others. The lasting outcomes are *direction* and *purpose.*

Industry vs. inferiority (6 to 12 years)—The stage of industry is the latency period of Freud. Having achieved the more crucial stages in personality development, children are ready to be workers and producers. They want to engage in tasks and activities that they can carry through to completion; they need and want real achievement. Children learn to compete and cooperate with others, and they learn the rules. It is a decisive period in their social relationships with others. Feelings of *inadequacy* and *inferiority* may develop if too much is expected of them, or if they believe that they cannot measure up to the standards set for them by others. The ego quality developed from a sense of industry is *competence.*

Identity vs. role confusion (12 to 18 years)—Corresponding to Freud's genital period, the development of *identity* is characterized by rapid and marked physical changes. Previous trust in their bodies is shaken, and children become overly preoccupied with the way they appear in the eyes of others as compared with their own self-concept. Adolescents struggle to fit the roles they have played and those they hope to play with the current roles and fashions adopted by their peers, to integrate their concepts and values with those of society, and to come to a decision regarding an occupation. Inability to solve the core conflict results in *role confusion.* The outcome of successful mastery is *devotion* and *fidelity* to others and to values and ideologies.

Theoretic Foundations of Mental Development

Cognitive Development (Piaget). Cognitive development consists of age-related changes that occur in mental activities. The best-known theory regarding children's thinking, and a more comprehensive developmental theory than those already described, was developed by the Swiss psychologist Jean Piaget (1969). According to Piaget, intelligence enables individuals to make adaptations to the environment that increase the probability of survival, and through their behavior individuals establish and maintain equilibrium with the environment.

Piaget proposed three stages of reasoning: (1) intuitive, (2) concrete operational, and (3) formal operational. When they enter the stage of concrete logical thought at about age 7 years, children are able to make logical inferences, classify, and deal with quantitative relationships about concrete things. Not until adolescence are they able to reason abstractly with any degree of competence. Each stage is derived from and builds on the accomplishments of the previous stage in a continuous, orderly process. The course of intellectual development is both maturational and invariant and is divided into the following stages (ages are approximate):

Sensorimotor (birth to 2 years)—The sensorimotor stage of intellectual development consists of six substages (see pp. 832 and 882) that are governed by sensations in which simple learning takes place. Children progress from reflex activity through simple repetitive behaviors to imitative behavior. They develop a sense of "cause-and-effect" as they direct behavior toward objects. Problem solving is primarily trial and error. They display a high level of curiosity, experimentation, and enjoyment of novelty, and begin to develop a sense of self as they are able to differentiate themselves from their environment. They become aware that objects have *permanence*—that an object exists even though it is no longer visible. Toward the end of the sensorimotor period children begin to use language and representational thought.

Preoperational (2 to 7 years)—The predominant characteristic of the preoperational stage of intellectual development is *egocentrism,* which in this sense does not mean selfishness or self-centeredness, but the inability to put oneself in the place of another. Children interpret objects and events, not in terms of general properties, but in terms of their relationships or their use to them. They are unable to see things from any perspective other than their own; they cannot see another's point of view, nor can they see any reason to do so (see Cognitive Development [Piaget], Chapter 38).

Preoperational thinking is concrete and tangible. Children cannot reason beyond the observable, and they lack the ability to make deductions or generalizations. Thought is dominated by what they see, hear, or otherwise experience. However, they are increasingly able to use language and symbols to represent objects in their environment. Through imaginative play, questioning, and other interacting, they begin to elaborate concepts and to make simple associations between ideas. In the latter stage of the period their reasoning is intuitive (e.g., the stars have to go to bed just as they do) and they are only beginning to deal with problems of weight, length, size, and time. Reasoning is also transductive—because two events occur together, they cause each other, or knowledge of one characteristic is transferred to another (e.g., all women with big bellies have babies).

Concrete operations (7 to 11 years)—At this age thought becomes increasingly logical and coherent. Children are able to classify, sort, order, and otherwise organize facts about the world to use in problem solving. They develop a new concept of permanence—conservation (see Cognitive Development [Piaget], Chapter 39). That is, they realize that physical factors such as volume, weight, and number remain the same even though outward appearances are changed. They are able to deal with a number of different aspects of a situation simultaneously. They do not have the capacity to deal in abstraction; they solve problems in a concrete, systematic fashion based on what they can perceive. Reasoning is inductive. Through progressive changes in thought processes and relationships with others, thought becomes less self-centered. They can consider points of view other than their own. Thinking has become socialized.

Formal operations (11 to 15 years)—Formal operational thought is characterized by adaptability and flexibility. Adolescents can think in abstract terms, use abstract symbols, and draw logical conclusions from a set of observations. For example, they can solve the following question: If A is larger than B, and B is larger than C, which symbol is the largest? (The answer is A.) They can make hypotheses and test them; they can consider abstract, theoretic, and philosophic matters. Although they may confuse the ideal with the practical, most contradictions in the world can be dealt with and resolved.

Language Development. Children are born with the mechanism and capacity to develop speech and language skills. However, they will not speak spontaneously. The environment must provide a means for them to acquire these skills. Speech requires intact physiologic structure and function (including respiratory, auditory, and cerebral) plus intelligence, a need to communicate, and stimulation.

The rate of speech development varies from child to child and is directly related to neurologic competence and cognitive development. Gesture precedes speech, and in this way a small child communicates satisfactorily. As speech develops, gesture recedes but never disappears entirely. At all stages of language development, children's comprehension vocabulary (what they understand) is greater than their expressed vocabulary (what they can say), and this development reflects a continuing process of modification that involves both the acquisition of new words and the expanding and refining of word meanings previously learned. By the time they begin to walk, children are able to attach a name to objects and persons.

The first parts of speech used are nouns, sometimes verbs (e.g., "go"), and combination words (such as "bye-bye"). Responses are usually structurally incomplete during the toddler period, although the meaning is clear. Next they begin to use adjectives and adverbs to qualify nouns, followed by adverbs to qualify nouns and verbs. Later, pronouns and gender words are added (such as "he" and "she"). By the time children enter school, they are able to use simple, structurally complete sentences that average five to seven words.

Moral Development (Kohlberg). Children also acquire moral reasoning in a developmental sequence. Moral development, as described by Kohlberg (1968), is based on cognitive developmental theory and consists of the following three major levels, each of which has two stages:

Preconventional level—The preconventional level of moral development parallels the preoperational level of cognitive development and intuitive thought. Culturally oriented to the labels of good/bad and right/wrong, children integrate these in terms of the physical or pleasurable consequences of their actions. At first children determine the goodness or badness of an action in terms of its consequences. They avoid punishment and obey without question those who have the power to determine and enforce the rules and labels. They have no concept of the basic moral order that supports these consequences. Later children determine that the right behavior consists of that which satisfies their own needs (and sometimes the needs of others). Although elements of fairness, give and take, and equal sharing are evident, they are interpreted in a very practical, concrete manner without loyalty, gratitude, or justice.

Conventional level—At the conventional stage children are concerned with conformity and loyalty. They value the maintenance of family, group, or national expectations regardless of consequences. Behavior that meets with approval and pleases or helps others is considered to be good. One earns approval by being "nice." Obeying the rules, doing one's duty, showing respect for authority, and maintaining the social order is the correct behavior. This level is correlated with the stage of concrete operations in cognitive development.

Postconventional, autonomous, or principled level—At the postconventional level the individual has reached the cognitive stage of formal operations. Correct behavior tends to be defined in terms of general individual rights and standards that have been examined and agreed on by the entire society. Although procedural rules for reaching consensus become important with emphasis on the legal point of view, there is also emphasis on the possibility for changing law in terms of societal needs and rational considerations.

The most advanced level of moral development is one in which self-chosen ethical principles guide decisions of conscience. These are abstract and ethical but universal principles of justice and human rights with respect for the dignity of persons as individuals. It is believed that few persons reach this stage of moral reasoning.

Spiritual Development. Spiritual beliefs are closely related to the moral and ethical portion of the child's self-concept and, as such, must be considered as part of the child's basic needs assessment. Children need to have meaning, purpose, and hope in their lives. Also, the need for confession and forgiveness is present, even in very young children. Extending beyond religion (an organized set of beliefs and practices), spirituality affects the whole person: mind, body, and spirit (Clutter, 1991). Fowler (1974) has identified seven stages in the development of faith, four of which are closely associated with and parallel cognitive and psychosocial development in childhood:

Stage 0: Undifferentiated—This stage of development encompasses the period of infancy during which children have no concept of right or wrong, no beliefs, and no convictions to guide their behavior. However, the beginnings of a faith are established with the development of basic trust through their relationships with the primary caregiver.

Stage 1: Intuitive-projective—Toddlerhood is primarily a time of imitating the behavior of others. Children imitate the religious gestures and behaviors of others without comprehending any meaning or significance to the activities. During the preschool years children assimilate some of the values and beliefs of their parents. Parental attitudes toward moral codes and religious beliefs convey to children what they consider to be good and bad. Children still imitate behavior at this age and follow parental beliefs as part of their daily lives rather than through an understanding of their basic concepts.

Stage 2: Mythical-literal—Through the school-age years, spiritual development parallels cognitive development and is closely related to children's experiences and social interactions. Most children have a strong interest in religion during the school-age years. The existence of a deity is accepted, and petitions to an omnipotent being are important and expected to be answered; good behavior is rewarded, and bad behavior is punished. Their developing conscience bothers them when they disobey. They have a reverence for thoughts and matters and are able to articulate their faith. They may even question its validity.

Stage 3: Synthetic-convention—As children approach adolescence, however, they become increasingly aware of spiritual disappointments. They recognize that prayers are not always answered (at least on their own terms) and may begin to abandon or modify some religious practices. They begin to reason, to question some of the established parental religious standards, and to drop or modify some religious practices.

Stage 4: Individuating-reflexive—Adolescents become more skeptical and begin to compare the religious standards of their parents with those of others. They attempt to determine which to adopt and incorporate into their own set of values. They also begin to compare religious standards with the scientific viewpoint. It is a time of searching rather than reaching. Adolescents are uncertain about many religious ideas but will not achieve profound insights until late adolescence or early adulthood.

Development of Self-Concept

Self-concept is how an individual describes himself or herself (Willoughby, King, and Polatajko, 1996). The term *self-concept* includes all the notions, beliefs, and convictions that constitute an individual's relationships with others. It is not present at birth but develops gradually as a result of unique experiences within the self, with significant others, and with the realities of the world. However, an individual's self-concept may or may not reflect reality.

In infancy the self-concept is primarily an awareness of one's independent existence learned in part as a result of social contacts and experiences with others. The process becomes more active during toddlerhood as children explore the limits of their capacities and the nature of their impact on others. School-age children are more aware of differences among people, are more sensitive to social pressures, and become more preoccupied with issues of self-criticism and self-evaluation. During early adolescence children focus more on physical and emotional changes taking place and on peer acceptance. The self-concept is crystallized during later adolescence as young people organize their self-concept around a set of values, goals, and competencies acquired throughout childhood.

Body Image. A vital component of self-concept, *body image* refers to the subjective concepts and attitudes that individuals have toward their own bodies. It consists of the physiologic (the perception of one's physical characteristics), psychologic (values and attitudes toward the body, abilities, and ideals), and social nature of one's image of self (the self in relation to others). All three of the components interrelate with each other. Body image is a complex phenomenon that evolves and changes during the process of growth and development. Any actual or perceived deviation from the "norm" (no matter how this is interpreted) is cause for concern. The extent to which a characteristic, defect, or disease affects children's body image is influenced by the attitudes and behavior of those around them.

The significant others in their lives exert the most important and meaningful impact on children's body image. Labels that are attached to them (such as "skinny," "pretty," or "fat") or body parts (such as "ugly mole," "bug eyes," or "yucky skin") are incorporated into the body image. Because they lack the understanding of deviations from the physical standard or norm, children notice prominent differences in others and unwittingly make "rude" and often cruel remarks about such minor deviations as large or widely spaced front teeth, large or small eyes, moles, or extreme variations in height.

Infants receive input about their bodies through self-exploration and sensory stimulation from others. As they begin to manipulate their environment, they become aware of their bodies as separate from others. Toddlers learn to identify the various parts of their bodies and are able to use symbols to represent objects. Preschoolers become aware of the wholeness of their bodies and discover the genitals. Exploration of the genitals and the discovery of differences between the sexes become important. There is only a vague concept of internal organs and function (Stuart and Sundeen, 1998).

School-age children begin to learn about internal body structure and function and become aware of differences in body size and configuration. They are highly influenced by the cultural norms of society and current fads. Children whose bodies deviate from the norm are often criticized or ridiculed.

Adolescence is the age when children become most concerned about the physical self. The unfamiliar body changes and the new physical self must be integrated into the self-concept. Adolescents face conflicts over what they see and what they visualize as the ideal body structure. Body image formation during adolescence is a crucial element in the shaping of identity, the psychosocial crisis of adolescence.

The term *self-esteem* refers to a personal, subjective judgment of one's worthiness derived from and influenced by the social groups in the immediate environment and individuals' perceptions of how they are valued by others. Self-esteem changes with development. Highly egocentric toddlers are unaware of any difference between competence and social approval. On the other hand, preschool and early school-age children are increasingly aware of the discrepancy between their competencies and the abilities of more advanced children. Being accepted by adults and peers outside the family group becomes more important to them. Positive feedback enhances their self-esteem; they are vulnerable to feelings of worthlessness and are anxious about failure.

As children's competencies increase and they develop meaningful relationships, their self-esteem rises. This self-esteem is again at risk during early adolescence when they are defining an identity and sense of self in the context of their peer group. Unless children are continually made to feel incompetent and of little worth, any decrease in self-esteem during vulnerable times is only temporary. Children assess the following aspects of themselves in forming an overall evaluation of their self-esteem (Sieving and Zirbel-Donisch, 1990):

Competence—How adequate are my cognitive, physical, and social skills?

Sense of control—How well can I complete tasks needed to produce desired actions? Is someone or something specific vs. luck or chance responsible for my successes and failures?

Moral worth—How closely do my actions and behaviors meet moral standards that have been set?

Worthiness of love and acceptance—How worthy am I of love and acceptance from my parents, other significant adults, siblings, and peers?

Factors that influence the formation of a child's self-esteem include (1) the child's temperament and personality, (2) abilities and opportunities available to accomplish age-appropriate developmental tasks, (3) significant others, and (4) social roles assumed and the expectations of these roles (see also Psychosocial History, Chapter 34).

ROLE OF PLAY IN DEVELOPMENT

Through the universal medium of play children learn what no one can teach them. They learn about their world and how to deal with this environment of objects, time, space, structure, and people. They learn about themselves operating within that environment—what they can do, how to relate to things and situations, and how to adapt themselves to the demands society makes on them. Play is the *work* of the child. In play children continually practice the complicated, stressful processes of living, communicating, and achieving satisfactory relationships with other people.

Classification of Play

From a developmental point of view, patterns of children's play can be categorized according to content and social character. In both there is an additive effect; each builds on past accomplishments, and some element of each is maintained throughout life. At each stage in development the new predominates.

Content of Play

The content of play involves primarily the physical aspects of play, although social relationships cannot be ignored. The content of play follows the directional trend of the simple to the complex:

Social-affective play—Play begins with social-affective play, wherein infants take pleasure in relationships with people. As adults talk, touch, nuzzle, and in various ways elicit a response from an infant, the infant soon learns to provoke parental emotions and responses with such behaviors as smiling, cooing, or initiating games and activities. The type and intensity of the adult behavior with children varies among cultures.

Sense-pleasure play—Sense-pleasure play is a nonsocial stimulating experience that originates from without. Objects in the environment—light and color, tastes and odors, textures and consistencies—attract children's attention, stimulate their senses, and give pleasure. Pleasurable experiences are derived from handling raw materials (e.g., water, sand, and food), from body motion (e.g., swinging, bouncing, and rocking), and from other uses of senses and abilities (e.g., smelling and humming) (Fig. 33-4).

Skill play—Once infants have developed the ability to grasp and manipulate, they persistently demonstrate and exercise their newly acquired abilities through skill play, repeating an action over and over again. The element of sense-pleasure play is often evident in the practicing of a new ability; but all too often the determination to conquer the elusive skill produces pain and frustration (e.g., learning to ride a bicycle).

Unoccupied behavior—In unoccupied behavior children are not playful, but focus their attention momentarily on anything that strikes their interest. Children daydream, fiddle with clothes or other objects, or walk aimlessly. This role differs from that of onlookers, who actively observe the activity of others.

Dramatic, or pretend, play—One of the vital elements in children's process of identification is dramatic play, also known as symbolic or pretend play. It begins in late infancy (11 to 13 months) and is the predominant form of play in the preschool child. Once children begin to invest situations and people with meanings and to attribute affective significance to the world, they can pretend and fantasize almost anything. By acting out events of daily life, children learn and practice the roles and identities modeled by the members of their family and society. Children's toys, replicas of the tools of society, provide a

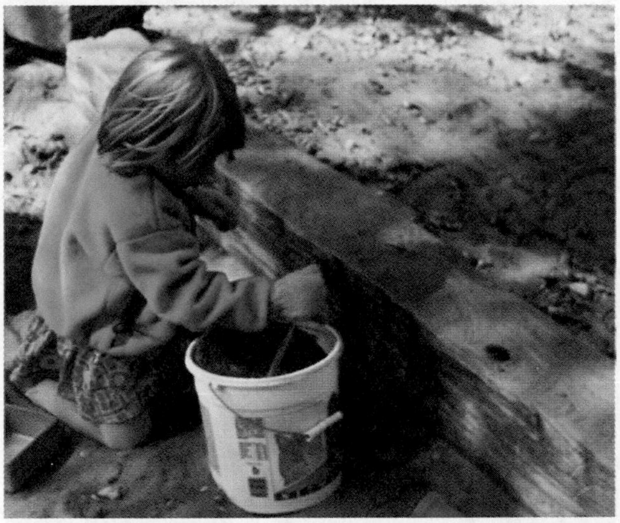

FIG. 33-4 • Children derive pleasure from handling raw materials.

medium for learning about adult roles and activities that may be puzzling and frustrating to them. Interacting with the world is one way children get to know it. The simple, imitative, dramatic play of the toddler, such as using the telephone, driving a car, or rocking a doll, evolves into more complex, sustained dramas of the preschooler, which extend beyond common domestic matters to the wider aspects of the world and the society, such as playing police officer, storekeeper, teacher, or nurse. Older children work out elaborate themes, act out stories, and compose plays (Fig. 33-5).

Games—Children in all cultures engage in games, alone and with others. Solitary activity involving games begins as very small children participate in repetitive activities and progress to more complicated games that challenge their independent skills, such as puzzle solving, solitaire, and computer or video games. Very young children participate in simple, *imitative games* such as pat-a-cake and peekaboo. Preschool children learn and enjoy *formal games* that begin with ritualistic, self-sustaining games such as ring-around-a-rosy and London Bridge. With the exception of some simple board games, preschool children do not engage in competitive games. Preschoolers hate to lose and will try to cheat, want to change rules, or demand exceptions and opportunities to change their moves. School-age children and adolescents enjoy *competitive games,* including cards, checkers, chess, and physically active games such as baseball.

Social Character of Play

The play interactions of infancy are between the child and an adult. Children continue to enjoy the company of an adult but are increasingly able to play alone. As age advances, interaction with age-mates increases in importance and becomes an essential part of the socialization process. Through interaction, highly egocentric infants, unable to tolerate delay or interference, ultimately acquire concern for others and the ability to delay or even reject their own gratification needs at the expense of another. A pair of toddlers engage in considerable combat because their personal needs cannot tolerate delay or compromise. By the time they reach age 5 or 6 years, children are able to arrive at a compromise or make use of arbitration, usually after they have attempted and failed to gain their own way. Through continued interaction with peers and the growth of conceptual abilities and social skills, children are able to increase participation with others in the following types of play:

Onlooker play—During onlooker play children watch what other children are doing but make no attempt to enter into the play activity. There is an active interest in observing the interaction of others but no movement toward participating. Watching an older sibling bounce a ball is a common example of the onlooker role.

Solitary play—During solitary play children play alone with toys different from those used by other children in the same area. They enjoy the presence of other children but make no effort to get close to or speak to them. Their interest is centered on their own activity, which they pursue with no reference to the activities of the others.

Parallel play—During parallel activities children play independently but among other children. They play with toys like those the children around them are using, but play as each child sees fit, neither influencing nor being influenced by the other children. Each plays beside, but not with, other children (Fig. 33-6). There is no group association. Parallel play is the characteristic play of toddlers, but it may also occur in other groups of any age. Individuals involved in a creative craft, with each person separately working on an individual project, are engaged in parallel play.

Associative play—In associative play children play together and are engaged in a similar or even identical activity, but there is no organization, division of labor, leadership assignment, or mutual goal. Children borrow and lend play materials, follow each other with wagons and tricycles, and sometimes attempt to control who may or may not play in the group. Each child acts ac-

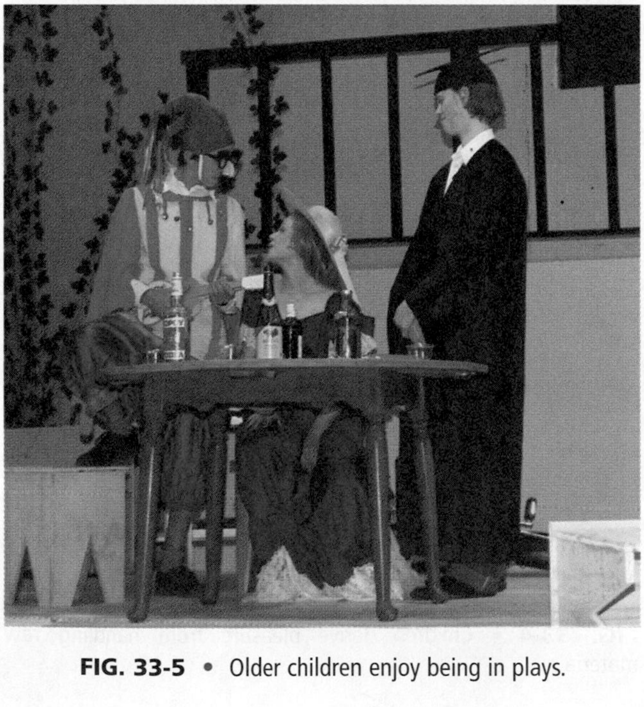

FIG. 33-5 • Older children enjoy being in plays.

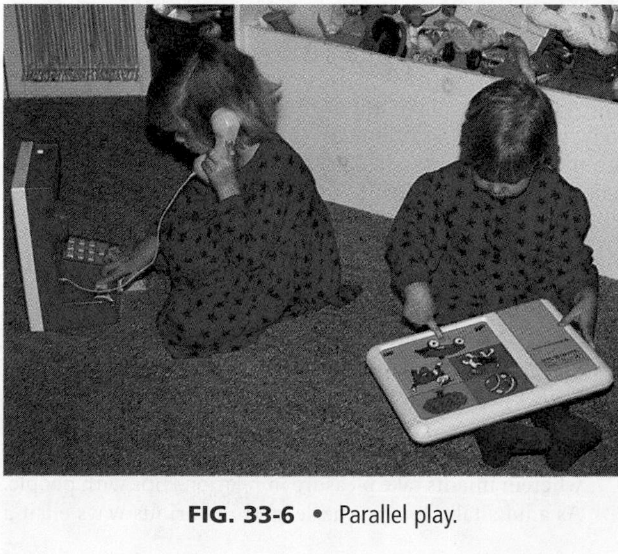

FIG. 33-6 • Parallel play.

cording to his or her own wishes; there is no group goal (Fig. 33-7). For example, two children play with dolls, borrowing articles of clothing from each other and engaging in similar conversation, but neither directs the other's actions or establishes rules regarding the limits of the play session. There is a great deal of behavioral contagion: when one child initiates an activity, the entire group follows the example.

Cooperative play—Cooperative play is organized, and children play in a group *with* other children (Fig. 33-8). They discuss and plan activities for the purposes of accomplishing an end—to make something, to attain a competitive goal, to dramatize situations of adult or group life, or to play formal games. The group is loosely formed, but there is a marked sense of belonging or not belonging. The goal and its attainment require organization of activities, division of labor, and playing roles. The leader-follower relationship is definitely established, and the activity is controlled by one or two members who assign roles and direct the activity of the others. The activity is organized to allow one child to supplement another's function in order to complete the goal.

Functions of Play

Sensorimotor Development. Sensorimotor activity is a major component of play at all ages and is the predominant form of play in infancy. Active play is essential for muscle development and serves a useful purpose as a release for surplus energy. Through sensorimotor play children explore the nature of the physical world. Infants gain impressions of themselves and their world through tactile, auditory, visual, and kinesthetic stimulation. Toddlers and preschoolers revel in body movement and exploration of things in space. With increasing maturity, sensorimotor play becomes more differentiated and involved. Whereas very young children run for the sheer joy of body movement, older children incorporate or modify the motions into increasingly complex and coordinated activities such as races, games, roller-skating, and bicycle riding.

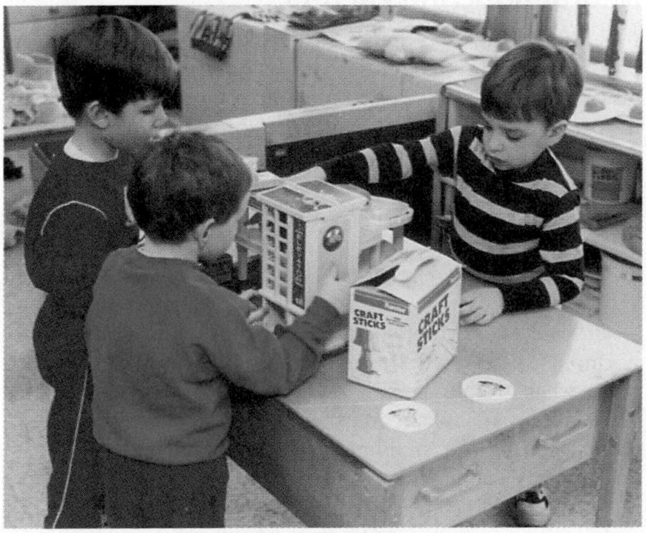

FIG. 33-7 • Associative play.

Intellectual Development. Through exploration and manipulation, children learn colors, shapes, sizes, textures, and the significance of objects. They learn the significance of numbers and how to use them; they learn to associate words with objects; and they develop an understanding of abstract concepts and spatial relationships, such as *up, down, under,* and *over.* Activities such as puzzles and games help them develop problem-solving skills. Books, stories, films, and collections expand knowledge and provide enjoyment as well. Play provides a means to practice and expand language skills. Through play children continually rehearse past experiences to assimilate them into new perceptions and relationships. Play helps children comprehend the world in which they live and distinguish between fantasy and reality.

The availability of play materials and the quality of parental involvement are two of the most important variables related to cognitive development during infancy and preschool (Chase, 1994).

NURSE ALERT • Toys need to have several levels of challenge to keep from becoming obsolete too quickly.

Socialization. From very early infancy children show interest and pleasure in the company of others. Their initial social contact is with the nurturing person, but through play with other children they learn to establish social relationships and to solve the problems associated with these relationships. They learn to give and take, which is more readily learned from critical peers than from the more tolerant adults. They learn the sex role that society expects them to fulfill, as well as approved patterns of behavior and conduct. Closely associated with socialization is development of moral values and ethics. Children learn right from wrong, the standards of the society, and to assume responsibility for their actions.

Creativity. In no other situation is there more opportunity to be creative than in play. Children can experiment and try

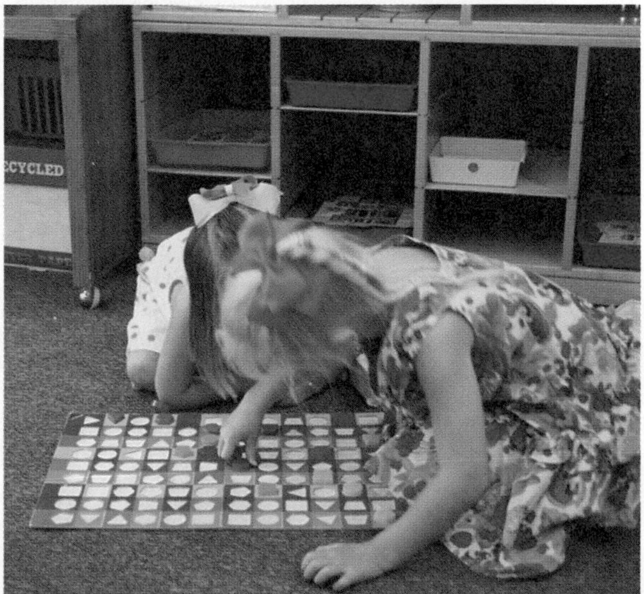

FIG. 33-8 • Cooperative play.

out their ideas in play through every medium at their disposal, including raw materials, fantasy, and exploration. Creativity is stifled by pressure toward conformity; therefore striving for peer approval may inhibit creative endeavors in the school-age or adolescent child. Creativity is primarily a product of solitary activity; yet creative thinking is often enhanced in group settings where listening to others' ideas stimulates further exploration of one's own ideas. Once children feel the satisfaction of creating something new and different, they transfer this creative interest to situations outside the world of play.

Self-Awareness. Beginning with active explorations of their bodies and awareness of themselves as separate from the mother, the process of self-identity is facilitated through play activities. Children learn who they are and their place in the world. They become increasingly able to regulate their own behavior, to learn what their abilities are, and to compare their abilities with those of others. Through play children are able to test their abilities, to assume and try out various roles, and to learn the effect their behavior has on others.

Therapeutic Value. Play is therapeutic at any age. It provides a means for release from the tension and stress encountered in the environment. In play children can express emotions and release unacceptable impulses in a socially acceptable fashion. Children are able to experiment and test fearful situations and can assume and vicariously master the roles and positions that they are unable to perform in the world of reality. Children reveal much about themselves in play. Through play children are able to communicate to the alert observer the needs, fears, and desires that they are unable to express with their limited language skills. Throughout their play children need the acceptance of adults and their presence to help them control aggression and to channel their destructive tendencies.

Moral Value. Although children learn at home and at school those behaviors considered right and wrong in the culture, the interaction with peers during play contributes significantly to their moral training. Nowhere is the enforcement of moral standards so rigid as in the play situation. If they are to be acceptable members of the group, children must adhere to the accepted codes of behavior of the culture (e.g., fairness, honesty, self-control, and consideration for others). Children soon learn that their peers are less tolerant of violations than are adults, and that to maintain a place in the play group they must conform to the standards of the group.

Toys

The types of toys chosen by and/or provided for children can facilitate their development in the areas just described. Toys that are small replicas of the culture and its tools help them assimilate their culture. Toys that require pushing, pulling, rolling, and manipulating teach them about physical properties of the items, and help to develop muscles and coordination. Rules and the basic elements of cooperation and organization are learned through board games.

Because they can be used in a variety of ways, raw materials with which children can exercise their own creativity and imaginations are sometimes superior to ready-made items. For example, building blocks can be used to construct a variety of things, to count, and to learn shapes and sizes.

Toy Safety. Selection of toys and play equipment is a joint effort between parents and children, but evaluation of their safety is the responsibility of the adult. Government agencies do not inspect and police all toys on the market. Therefore adults who purchase, supervise purchases, or allow children to use play equipment need to evaluate such equipment for its safety, including toys that are gifts or those that are purchased by the children themselves (Home Care box). They should also be alert to notices of toys determined to be defective and recalled by the manufacturers. Parents and health care workers can obtain information on a variety of recalled products and can report potentially dangerous toys and child products to the U.S. Consumer Product Safety Commission (CPSC)* or, in Canada, the Canadian Toy Testing Council.†

SELECTED FACTORS THAT INFLUENCE DEVELOPMENT

Heredity

Inherited characteristics have a profound influence on development. The sex of the child, determined at the time of conception, directs both the pattern of growth and the behavior of others toward the child. In all cultures, attitudes and expectations are different with respect to the sex of the child. Sex and other hereditary determinants strongly affect the end result of growth and the rate of progress toward it. There is a high correlation between parent and child with regard to traits such as height, weight, and rate of growth. Most physical characteristics, including shape and form of features, body build, and physical peculiarities, are inherited and can influence the way in which children grow and interact with their environment. Many dimensions of personality, such as temperament, activity level, responsiveness, and a tendency toward shyness, are believed to be inherited.

Differences in health and vigor of children may be attributed to hereditary traits. An inherited physical or mental disorder will alter or modify a child's physical and/or emotional growth and interactions. The extent to which disabling conditions interfere with the child's growth and well-being is considered in relation to numerous disabilities throughout the remainder of the text.

Neuroendocrine Factors

It has been suggested there may be a growth center in the hypothalamic region responsible for maintaining genetically determined growth patterns. Some functional relationship is believed to exist between the hypothalamus and the endocrine system that influences growth. There is also evidence, based on observations of denervated skeletal muscles, that the peripheral nervous system may influence growth, because muscles deprived of nerve supply degenerate. Many of these effects are not sufficiently explained by disuse or diminished blood supply.

Probably all hormones affect growth in some fashion. Three hormones (i.e., growth hormone, thyroid hormone, and androgens), when given to persons deficient in these hormones, stimulate protein anabolism and thereby produce retention of elements essential for building protoplasm and bony tissue. It

*CPSC hotline: 1-800-638-CPSC; website: www.cpsc.gov.

†22 Hamilton Ave North, Ottowa, Ontario, Canada K1Y 1V6; (613) 729-7101.

Home Care

TOY SAFETY*

Selection

Select toys that suit the skills, abilities, and interests of children.

Select toys that are safe for the specific child; look for a label that indicates the intended age-group. Toys that are safe for one age may not be safe for another.

For infants, toddlers, and all children who still mouth objects, avoid toys with small parts that may pose a fatal choking or aspiration hazard. Toys in this category are usually labeled, "Not recommended for children under 3 years."

For infants avoid toys with strings or cords that are 7 inches or longer because they may cause strangulation.

For all children under 8 years avoid electric toys with heating elements.

For children under 5 years avoid arrows or darts.

Check for safety labels such as "flame retardant" or "flame resistant."

Select toys durable enough to survive rough play; look for sturdy construction such as tightly secured eyes, nose, or any small parts.

Select toys light enough that they will not cause harm if one falls on a child.

Look for toys with smooth, rounded edges. Avoid toys with sharp edges that can cut or that have sharp points. Points on the inside of the toy can puncture if the toy is broken.

Avoid toys with any shooting or throwing objects that can injure eyes.

This includes toys with which other missiles such as sticks or pebbles might be used as substitutes for the intended projectiles.

Arrows and darts used by children should have blunt tips and be manufactured from resilient materials; make certain the tips are securely attached.

Make certain that materials in toys are nontoxic.

Avoid toys that make loud noises that might be damaging to a child's hearing.

Even some squeaking toys are too loud when held close to the ear.

If selecting caps for cap guns, look for the label required by federal law to be on boxes or packages of caps, which states: "Warning—Do not fire closer than 1 foot to the ear. Do not use indoors."

If selecting a toy gun, be certain that the barrel or the entire gun is brightly colored to avoid being mistaken for a real gun.

Check toy instructions for clarity. They should be clear to an adult and, when appropriate, to the child.

Supervision

Maintain a safe play environment.

Remove and discard plastic wrappings on toys immediately; they could suffocate a child.

Remove large toys, bumper pads, and boxes from playpens; an adventuresome child can use such items as a means of climbing or falling out.

Set "ground rules" for play.

Supervise young children closely during play.

Teach children how to use toys properly and safely.

Instruct older children to keep their toys away from younger brothers, sisters, and friends.

Keep children who are playing with riding toys away from stairs, hills, traffic, and swimming pools.

Establish and enforce rules regarding protective gear.

Insist that children wear helmets when using bicycles, skateboards, or in-line skates.

Insist that children wear gloves and wrist, elbow, and knee pads when using skateboards or in-line skates.

Instruct children on electrical safety.

Teach children the proper way to unplug an electric toy—pull on the plug, not the cord.

Teach children to beware of electrical appliances and even electrically operated playthings; often children are unfamiliar with the hazards of electricity in association with water.

Teach children the safe use of utensils that under certain circumstances can cause injury—scissors, knives, needles, heating elements, or loops, long string, or cord.

Maintenance

Inspect old and new toys regularly for breakage, loose parts, and other potential hazards.

Look for jagged or sharp edges or broken parts that might constitute a choking hazard.

Check moveable parts to make certain they are attached securely to the toys; sometimes pieces that are safe when attached to the toy become a danger when detached.

Examine all outdoor toys regularly for rust and weak or sharp parts that could become a danger to a child.

Check electrical cords and plugs for cracked or fraying parts.

Maintain toys in good repair, without signs of possible hazards such as sharp edges, splinters, weak seams, or rust.

Make repairs immediately, or discard out of reach of children.

Sand sharp wooden toys or splintered surfaces so they are smooth.

Use only paint labeled "nontoxic" to repaint toys, toy boxes, or children's furniture.

Storage

Provide a safe place for children to store toys.

Select a toy chest or toy box that is ventilated, is free of self-locking devices that could trap a child inside, and has a lid designed not to pinch a child's fingers or fall on a child's head.

To avoid entrapment and suffocation, containers other than toy chests used for storage purposes should be fitted with spring-loaded support devices if they have a hinged lid.

Teach children to store toys safely to prevent accidental injury from stepping, tripping, or falling on a toy.

Playthings meant for older children and adults should be safely stowed away on high shelves, in locked closets, or in other areas unavailable to younger children.

*Another helpful resource is *Toy safety: guidelines for parents,* from American Academy of Pediatrics, Division of Publications, 141 Northwest Point Blvd, Elk Grove Village, IL, 60007; (888) 227-1770; fax (847) 228-1281; website: www.aap.org.

appears that each of the hormones that has a significant influence on growth manifests its major effect at a different period of growth (see Chapter 52).

Nutrition

Nutrition is probably the single most important influence on growth. Dietary factors regulate growth at all stages of development, and their effects are exerted in numerous and complex ways. During the rapid prenatal growth period, poor nutrition may influence development from the time of implantation of the ovum until birth. During infancy and childhood the demand for calories is relatively great, as evidenced by the rapid increase in both height and weight. At this time protein and caloric requirements are higher than at almost any period of postnatal development. As the growth rate slows with its concomitant decrease in metabolism, there is a corresponding reduction in caloric and protein requirements (see Table 33-2).

Growth is uneven during the periods of childhood between infancy and adolescence when there are plateaus and small growth spurts. The child's appetite will fluctuate in response to these variations until the turbulent growth spurt of adolescence, when adequate nutrition is extremely important but may be subjected to numerous emotional influences. Adequate nutrition is closely related to good health throughout life, and an overall improvement in nourishment is evidenced by the gradual increase in size and early maturation of children in the last century.

Interpersonal Relationships

Relationships with significant others play a critical role in development, particularly in emotional, intellectual, and personality development. Not only do the quality and quantity of contacts with other persons exert an influence on the growing child, but also the widening range of contacts is essential to learning and the development of a healthy personality.

The nurturing person is unquestionably the single most influential person during early infancy. This person is the one who meets the infant's basic needs of food, warmth, comfort, and love. He or she provides stimulation for the child's senses, and facilitates his or her expanding capacities. Through this person the child learns to trust the world and to feel secure to venture in increasingly wider relationships.

It is generally the parents who are most influential in helping the child to assume sex-role identification. Parents define and reinforce acceptable sex-role behavior and provide sex-appropriate role models for the child. In the absence of a sex-role model in the family setting, the child may adopt some characteristics of the opposite-sex parent or sibling. Often the child identifies with a teacher or other significant person of the same sex.

Siblings are children's first peers, and the way in which they learn to relate to each other affects later interactions with peers outside the family group. The sphere of persons from whom children seek approval widens to include other members of their family, their peers, and, to a lesser extent, other authority figures (e.g., teachers). The increasing importance of the peer group in determining the behavior of school-age children and adolescents is well documented (Fig. 33-9).

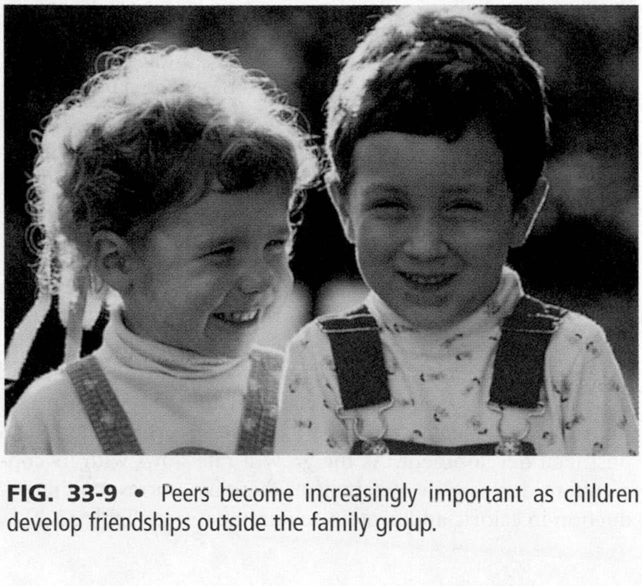

FIG. 33-9 • Peers become increasingly important as children develop friendships outside the family group.

When children fail to have quality interpersonal relationships with nurturing persons, they experience *emotional deprivation.* The most prominent feature of emotional deprivation, particularly during the first year, is developmental delays. Much of the information regarding the adverse effects of interpersonal influences on development has been acquired through retrospective studies of gross deprivation and trauma. The most notable instances involved homeless infants who were placed in institutions for care. Those infants who did not receive consistent mothers care failed to gain weight even with an adequate diet; they were pale, listless, and immobile, and were unresponsive to stimuli that usually elicit a response such as smiling or cooing in the normal infant. If emotional deprivation continues for a sufficient length of time, the child may not survive infancy.

Although the most remarkable examples of emotional deprivation were first recognized among infants in institutions, the term *masked deprivation* has been used to describe children reared in homes where there is a distorted parent-child relationship or otherwise disordered home environment. Infants do not thrive if the caregiving person is hostile, fearful of handling them, or indifferent to them and their needs. Such children exhibit poor growth even though they are apparently free of physical disease. Growth delays in these children are believed to be caused by a psychologically induced endocrine imbalance that interferes with growth. These same infants and children display "catch-up" growth in a changed environment (see Failure to Thrive, Chapter 36).

Socioeconomic Level

Evidence indicates that the socioeconomic level of a child's family has a significant impact on growth and development. At all ages children from upper- and middle-class families are taller than comparative children of families in the lower socioeconomic strata. The cause of these differences is less definite, although the poorer health and nutrition of lower socioeconomic levels are probably significant factors. Nutritious food sources (especially proteins) are scarce, and other factors (e.g., larger family size and irregularity in eating, sleeping, and exercise) may play a role.

Families from lower socioeconomic groups may lack the knowledge or resources needed to provide the safe, stimulating, and enriched environment that fosters optimum development for children. They may be unable to move from unsafe neighborhoods where drug traffic and drive-by shootings are the norm. The effects on the emotional development of children living under these conditions have been compared with those experienced by children living in war zones.

Disease

Altered growth and development is one of the clinical manifestations in a number of hereditary disorders. Growth impairment is particularly marked in skeletal disorders, such as the various forms of dwarfism and at least one of the chromosomal anomalies (i.e., Turner syndrome). Many of the disorders of metabolism (e.g., vitamin D-resistant rickets, the mucopolysaccharidoses, and the numerous endocrine disorders) interfere with the normal growth pattern. In other disorders the tendency for growth is toward the upper percentile of height (e.g., Klinefelter and Marfan syndromes).

Many chronic illnesses that are associated with varying degrees of growth failure are congenital cardiac anomalies and respiratory disorders such as cystic fibrosis. Any disorder characterized by the inability to digest and absorb body nutrients will have an adverse effect on growth and development.

Environmental Hazards

Hazards in the environment are a source of concern to health care providers and others interested in health and safety. Physical injuries are the most prevalent consequences of environmental dangers; these are discussed extensively throughout the text as they apply in relation to age, specific hazards, and selected physical disabilities.

Children are at a high risk for harm resulting from the chemical residues of modern life present in the environment. The hazards of these chemical residues relate to their potential carcinogenicity, enzymatic effects, and accumulation (Holland et al, 2000; Kaiser, 2000). The harmful agents most often associated with health risks are chemicals and radiation. Water, air, and food contamination from a variety of origins is well documented. Significant sources of exposure are substances in the immediate environment such as lead and asbestos; chemicals secreted in breast milk (especially prescribed drugs and nicotine); and contamination within well-insulated homes (especially from disinfectants or burning of substances that produce toxic fumes). Passive inhalation of tobacco smoke by infants and children is a hazard at all stages of development. The harmful effects of large doses of radiation are unquestioned, although the effects of low-dose or short-term radiation are debatable, as are the safe vs. harmful dosage levels.

Stress in Childhood

Although all children experience stress, some youngsters appear to be more vulnerable than others. Children's age, temperament, life situation, and state of health affect their vulnerability, reactions, and ability to handle stress. Also, the responses to a stressor can be behavioral, psychologic, or physiologic. It is impossible, unrealistic, and undesirable to protect children from stress; but providing them with interpersonal security helps them develop coping strategies for dealing with stress.

Parents and other caregivers can try to recognize signs of stress to help children deal with stresses before they become overwhelming. Signs of stress take many forms but are typically the same ones seen in children who are abused (see Chapter 37) or depressed (see Chapter 39). If a number of stresses are imposed on children at the same time, the children are more vulnerable. When a succession of stresses produces an excessive stress load, children may experience a serious change in health and/or behavior.

It is most important that parents and persons working with children understand the nature of childhood stress and the ways it can be recognized or anticipated. Caregivers must *listen* to children so they are aware of children's fears and concerns, and must let them know that they are important and that what they say matters. Physical contact is comforting and reassuring to children. Simply holding, touching, or hugging children is both relaxing and comforting and facilitates communication. Spending unhurried time with children; family outings and vacations; and exposing children to positive influences all help build children's strength and security. Supportive interpersonal relationships are essential to the psychologic well-being of children.

Coping. *Coping* refers to a special class of individual reactions to stressors: specifically, a reaction to a stressor that resolves, reduces, or replaces the affect state classified as stressful. *Coping strategies* are the specific ways in which children cope with stressors, as distinguished from *coping styles,* which are relatively unchanging personality characteristics or outcomes of coping (Boyd and Hunsberger, 1998; Ryan-Wenger, 1992). Research indicates that as children age they tend toward a more internal locus of control and use more vigilant modes of coping (LaMontagne et al, 1996). Children, like adults, respond to everyday stress by trying to change the circumstances or by trying to adjust to circumstances the way they are. Any strategy that provides relaxation is effective in reducing stress, and most children have their own natural methods such as withdrawal, physical activity, reading, listening to music, working on a project, or taking a nap. Some turn to parents to solve their problems, or they may develop socially unacceptable strategies, such as cheating, stealing, or lying.

Children can be taught stress-reduction techniques to use in coping. First, they must be helped to recognize signs of tension in themselves; they can then be taught any of a variety of appropriate strategies—special exercises, relaxation and breathing, mental imagery, and numerous other simple activities. Also, parents and other caregivers can anticipate possible stress-provoking events and prepare children for coping by role playing a scenario or by "talking it through" beforehand. Most of the stress-reducing strategies discussed in Chapter 44 in relation to managing pain are effective for any stress situation.

Probably the most useful tool that children can learn is how to solve problems. When children can view any new situation as a problem to be solved and an opportunity to learn, they are not vulnerable to the control of others. It provides them with a sense of mastery over their own lives and reinforces the fact that they have within themselves the ability and information to handle whatever comes their way. Problem-solving skill gives them the confidence to know where and how to seek help when they need it.

Influence of the Mass Media

Media can have an enormous influence on the developing child. There is no doubt that the media provide children with a means for extending their knowledge about the world in which they live, and have contributed to narrowing the differences between classes. However, there is growing concern regarding the enormous influence the media can have on the developing child, because today's children are just as captivated as they were decades ago (Rowitz, 1996). Linkages have been established between mass media use and risk-taking behaviors in adolescents (Strasburger and Donnerstein, 1999). The images of risky behavior presented by the media may serve to establish or reinforce teenagers' perceptions of their social environment. Also, media content may directly influence risk perception; media protagonists seldom suffer adverse consequences of their behaviors despite their grossly distorted experiences with violence, illness, or crime. Children may identify closely with people or characters portrayed in reading materials, movies, videos, and television programs and commercials.

Reading Materials. Books, newspapers, and magazines are the oldest forms of mass media. They contribute to children's competence in almost every direction and also provide enjoyment. Recognition of the impact that reading matter used in the schools has on the value system and socialization processes has prompted reevaluation of the content of textbooks in terms of the biased presentation of male and female role models, the sugar-coated view of life situations, and the biased history of minority groups.

Fairy tales, for generations the mainstay of young children's literature, for a time suffered condemnation as being sexist; overly violent in content; and riddled with unfavorable stereotypes, such as the wicked stepmother, dwarfs, and physical unattractiveness associated with evil. They are now believed to provide an excellent medium for explaining puzzling and important topics such as death, stepparents, and inner feelings and turmoils. Although they do not provide solutions, fairy tales confront children with emotional predicaments and offer suggestions for dealing with them.

Comic books and other pulp reading materials have been popular in every generation, usually at the expense of literature provided by schools, libraries, and parents. Many children have nothing else to read. The easy reading, quick action, and adventure in brief episodes seem to fulfill a need for children who are striving to understand both aggression in others and their own impulses. Reading ability, intelligence, and school adjustment apparently have no relationship to the number and type of comic books read. Most comic books appear to be relatively harmless to the majority of children and may be beneficial. Comic books seem to have only a minor influence on acquisition of beliefs, values, and behaviors. The popularity of this medium has prompted some educators to encourage translations of literature into comic book form to stimulate students' interest in the classics.

Movies. Movies that are closely bound to reality and often portray an assortment of socially approved behaviors perhaps make a contribution to children's value systems and do provide opportunities for desirable social learning. On the other hand children, especially adolescents, flock to the "macho" movies where heroes resort to violent resolution of problems, such as karate and wild automobile chases. The carryover of these influences into daily life and relationships may account in part for the increase in violent behavior of young persons. Also, research indicates that videos may desensitize the viewer to violence (Rowitz, 1996).

Another concern is the plethora of "slasher" and R-rated movies available to children and teenagers in theaters and through cable television and videocassettes. The content of movies has changed markedly during the past few years, with violence and mutilation being major themes. To children who are unable to distinguish between reality and fantasy, these films play on their deepest fears and result in bedtime fears, nightmares, and a fearful view of the world.

Young children can be frightened by some of the movies considered safe for family viewing. For example, *Bambi* can be frightening to young children, and the villainous witches in *Snow White* and the *Wizard of Oz* are terrifying figures. Also, certain classic Disney movies, such as *Snow White* and *Cinderella*, depict stepmothers as evil, destructive persons; such portrayals can have a deleterious effect on children-stepmother relationships or can be confusing to children who have developed a positive relationship with a stepmother.

Television. The medium with the most impact on children in North America today is television, which has become one of the most significant socializing agents in the lives of young children. The content of programs and commercials provides multiple sources for acquiring information, modeling behaviors, and observing value orientations. Besides producing a leveling effect on class differences in general information and vocabulary, TV exposes children to a wider variety of topics and events than they encounter in day-to-day life. Television always has time to talk to children and is a form of access to the adult world.

NURSE ALERT • It has been reported that the television is on for more than 6 hours per day in more than half of American homes, and that children watch an average of 21 to 28 hours of television per week (Clarke-Pearson, 1997; Vessey, Yim-Chiplis, and MacKenzie, 1998).

Controversy continues to be generated regarding the favorable vs. deleterious influence of television on child development and behavior. Derksen and Strasburger (1994) found that television has a powerful influence on the development of unhealthy behaviors and negative attitudes in children. Several factors encourage the learning or performing of television-influenced behaviors (Box 33-3).

Box 33-3

Factors that Encourage Learning or Performing Television-Influenced Behaviors

Age: Younger children focus on behaviors rather than on motives or consequences. They view alternatives in a concrete manner, and they are unable to differentiate between central and peripheral plot information. Small children remember various assorted items in the program; for example, they remember the act, not the motive or consequences.

Identification with characters or situations. Children will more often imitate behaviors of persons and situations similar to those in their own lives.

Reward and punishment syndrome. Children will imitate behaviors they see rewarded or *not* punished when it is expected. They are less likely to repeat an act they see punished; their attention is immediately attracted when they see an act committed that they know should be punished but is not.

Opportunity to reproduce behaviors. Children will imitate behaviors when given the right environment or when violence seems an accepted solution. When children see a situation on television, they will use this information when they encounter a similar situation that requires a solution.

Motivation to reproduce behaviors. Children will imitate behavior when given the appropriate incentives: expectation of reward or lack of punishment. Some children have self-control; others do not.

Most researchers have concluded that protracted television viewing can have detrimental effects on children. Increased verbal and physical aggressive behavior, reduced persistence at problem solving, greater sex-role stereotyping, and reduced creativity have been reported repeatedly.

The passive activity associated with television watching is often accompanied by eating—in many cases, high-caloric snacks. Furthermore, children may expend tremendous mental energy processing the audiovisual messages from television, which may be very exhausting and make them less likely to engage in physical activity later. Television viewing has a fairly profound effect of lowering the metabolic rate and may be a mechanism for the relationship between obesity and the amount of television viewing. Andersen and colleagues (1998) found that the incidence of body fat increased in direct proportion to the amount of hours of television watched by children in the United States; as the number of hours of television viewing increased, children were less likely to participate in vigorous physical activities.

Television programs and commercials, like movies, contain many implicit and explicit messages that promote alcohol consumption, smoking, violence, and promiscuous or unsafe sexual activity. An area of increasing concern is Music Television (MTV), especially when heavy metal rock groups, whose lyrics and videos sensationalize violent sex, suicide, and satanism, are featured. There is now clear evidence documenting a relationship between television viewing and the use of alcohol or tobacco, violence and aggressive behavior, the use of guns to commit violent acts, and early sexual activity (Strasburger and Donnerstein, 1999). Media advertisement has increasingly been scrutinized out of concern for its effects in encouraging young people to purchase and use alcohol and tobacco.

On the positive side, television has been shown to be a positive influence on children's abilities to deal with a variety of social issues such as divorce, the arrival of a new baby, discrimination, honesty, and helpfulness. Children who view educational programming (e.g., *Mister Rogers' Neighborhood* and *Sesame Street*) for a long period become more affectionate, considerate, cooperative, and helpful toward their playmates. The ways that minority and ethnic characters are portrayed on television can have an impact on the way the majority culture views minority persons and on the self-image of minority children.

Many parents are concerned about the effects of television viewing on their children, and most would like information regarding its use. Parents need to supervise the amount and type of TV programs their children watch, and to teach their children how to watch TV (Home Care box).

Computers/Internet. The use of computers in both the classroom and household has impacted childhood learning and development. Schools offer a variety of computer programs that enable children of all ages to broaden their world views. Computers offer the advantage of interactive learning and hand-eye coordination. Parents have a wide variety of computer software choices for learning and gaming.

Although computer technology has enhanced many forms of learning and recreation, there are potential dangers to children. The Internet and electronic mailing have made correspondence and information available to children from around the world in minutes. Some activities such as "cybersex" and "kiddie porn," as well as some "chat rooms," may expose children to individuals who may attempt to take advantage of the child's naiveté for illicit purposes. Government officials are working to curb illegal activities on the Internet that involve children, yet at the same time maintain freedom of speech. Filtered Internet service providers are available that may serve to protect children from objectionable sites.* Nurses must be involved in encouraging parents to be knowledgeable of their children's Internet activities while providing appropriate learning activities unique to computers. One helpful strategy is to locate the computer in a public area of the home such as the kitchen or family room, which enables parents to easily monitor its use.

**FamilyConnect, Inc.* provides a filtering system that prevents access to pornographic and illegal websites. For more information call (888) 400-0239; or visit the website at: www.familyconnect.com. An excellent book that explains the dangers of the Internet and strategies to protect children is *Wicked Wild Web* by J.R. Robison and C. Ophus (2000), Autumn Sky Publishing, P.O. Box 702252, Tulsa, OK 74170; (888) 400-0239 (then dial 0 for operator); website: www.wickedwildweb.com.

Home Care

TELEVISION VIEWING

Provide a positive role model by developing television substitutes such as reading, athletics, physical conditioning, and hobbies.
Construct a time chart of child's activities (homework, television viewing, scheduled outside activities, playing with a friend).
Discuss with child what you both believe to be a balanced set of activities.
At the beginning of each week, select appropriate programs for television schedules.
Allow child to select programs from this approved list.
Limit child's viewing to 2 hours or less per day.
Rule out television at specific times (e.g., before breakfast or on school nights).
Make a list of alternative activities (e.g., riding a bicycle, reading a book, or working on a hobby).
Require that child choose to do something from this list before watching television.
Watch programs with child.
- **Discuss program and commercial content with child:**
- **Distinguish between the real and the unreal.**
- **Correlate consequences with actions.**
- **Point out subtle messages.**
- **Explore alternatives to aggressive conflict resolution.**
- **Stress purpose of program (e.g., entertainment, education).**
- **Explain likes and dislikes.**

Turn the television off after the selected program is over.
Monitor cable and pay television selections; use a lockbox if necessary.
Limit use of television as a safe distraction to potentially stressful times (e.g., keeping the children occupied while the parent gets organized after a difficult day).

Key Points

- Growth describes a change in quantity and occurs when cells divide and synthesize new proteins.
- Maturation, a qualitative change, describes the aging process or an increase in competence and adaptability.
- Differentiation refers to a biologic description of the processes by which early cells and structures are modified and altered to achieve specific and characteristic physical and chemical properties.
- Development involves change from a lower to a more advanced stage of complexity.
- The five major developmental periods are prenatal, infancy, early childhood, middle childhood, and later childhood (pubescence and adolescence).
- Growth and development proceed in predictable patterns of direction, sequence, and pace.
- The directional trends in growth and development are cephalocaudal, proximodistal, and mass to specific.
- Physical development includes increase in height and weight and changes in body proportion, dentition, and some body tissues.
- The three broad classifications of child temperament are the easy child, the difficult child, and the slow-to-warm-up child.
- The developmental theories most widely used in explaining child growth and development are Freud's psychosexual stages, Erikson's stages of psychosocial development, Piaget's stages of cognitive development, and Kohlberg's stages of moral development.
- To develop a positive self-concept, children need recognition for their achievements and the approval of others.
- Through play, children learn about their world and how to relate to things, people, and situations.
- Play provides a means of development in the areas of sensorimotor and intellectual progress, socialization, creativity, self-awareness, and moral behavior; it serves as a means for release of tension and expression of emotions.
- Growth and development are affected by a variety of conditions and circumstances including heredity, physiologic function, gender, disease, physical environment, nutrition, and interpersonal relationships.
- Children's vulnerability and reactions to stress depend to a large extent on their age, coping behaviors, and support systems.
- The mass media can be influential in children's learning and behavior.

References

Anders TF, Sadeh A, Appareddy V: Normal sleep in neonates and children. In Ferber R, Kryger M, editors: *Principles and practice of sleep medicine in the child,* Philadelphia, 1995, WB Saunders.

Andersen RE et al: Relationship of physical activity and television watching with body weight and level of fatness among children, *JAMA* 279(12):938-943, 1998.

Beck CT: A meta-analysis of the relationship between postpartum depression and infant temperament, *Nurs Res* 45(4): 225-230, 1996.

Boyd JR, Hunsberger M: Chronically ill children coping with repeated hospitalizations: their perceptions and suggested interventions, *J Pediatr Nurs* 13(6):330-341, 1998.

Chase RA: Toys, play, and infant development, *J Perinat Educ* 3(2):7-19, 1994.

Chess S, Thomas A: Temperamental differences: a critical concept in child health care, *Pediatr Nurs* 11:167-171, 1985.

Clarke-Pearson KM: Children-media violence-solutions, *NC Med J* 58(4):265-268, 1997.

Clutter L: Fostering spiritual care for the child and family. In Smith DP et al, editors: *Comprehensive child and family nursing skills,* St Louis, 1991, Mosby.

Derksen DJ, Strasburger VC: Children and the influence of the media, *Prim Care* 21(4):747-759, 1994.

Erikson EH: *Childhood and society,* ed 2, New York, 1963, WW Norton.

Fowler JW: Toward a developmental perspective on faith, *Relig Educ* 69:207-219, 1974.

Gross D, Conrad B: Temperament in toddlerhood, *J Pediatr Nurs* 10(3):146-151, 1995.

Holland P et al: Life course accumulation of disadvantage: Childhood health and hazard exposure during adulthood, *Social Science and Medicine* 50:1285-1295, 2000.

Kaczander BI: Pediatric sports medicine: a unique perspective, *Pediatr Manage* 16(2):53-60, 1997.

Kaiser J: Hazards of particles, PCBs focus of Philadelphia meeting, *Science* 288:424-425, 2000.

Kohlberg L: Moral development. In Sills DL, editor: *International encyclopedia of the social sciences,* New York, 1968, Macmillan.

LaMontagne LL et al: Children's preoperative coping and its effects on postoperative anxiety and return to normal activity, *Nurs Res* 45(3):141-147, 1996.

Morrow JD, Camp BW: Mastery motivation and temperament of 7-month-old infants, *Pediatr Nurs* 22(3):211-217, 1996.

Piaget J: *The theory of stages in cognitive development,* New York, 1969, McGraw-Hill.

Rowitz M: Heavy metal: do videos and lyrics alter attitudes? *AAP News* 12(1):20-21, 1996.

Ryan-Wenger N: A taxonomy of children's coping strategies: a step toward theory development, *Am J Orthopsychiatry* 62(2):256-263, 1992.

Seidel HM et al: *Mosby's guide to physical examination,* ed 4, St Louis, 1999, Mosby.

Sieving R, Zirbel-Donisch S: Development and enhancement of self-esteem in children, *J Pediatr Health Care* 4(6):290-296, 1990.

Strasburger VC, Donnerstein E: Children, adolescents, and the media: issues and solution, *Pediatrics* 103(1):129-139, 1999.

Stuart GW, Sundeen SJ: *Principles and practice of psychiatric nursing,* ed 6, St Louis, 1998, Mosby.

Urbanski LF, Hanlon DP: Pediatric orthopedics, *Top Emerg Med* 18(2):73-90, 1996.

Vessey JA, Yim-Chiplis PK, MacKenzie NR: Effects of television viewing on children's development, *Pediatric Nurs* 23(5): 483-486, 1998.

Willoughby C, King G, Polatajko H: A therapist's guide to chil dren's self-esteem, *Am J Occup Ther* 50(2):124-132, 1996.

CHAPTER 34

Communication and Health Assessment of the Child and Family

http://www.harcourthealth.com/MERLIN/Wong/maternal/

Learning Objectives

On completion of this chapter the reader will be able to:

- Describe guidelines for communication and interviewing.
- Identify communication strategies for interviewing parents.
- Formulate guidelines for using an interpreter.
- Identify communication strategies for communicating with children of different age groups.
- Describe four communication techniques that are useful with children.
- State the components of a complete health history.
- Describe two strategies for structural and functional assessment of the family.
- List three areas that are evaluated as part of a nutritional assessment.

COMMUNICATION

Forms of communication may be verbal, nonverbal, or abstract. *Verbal communication* may involve language and its expression; vocalizations in the form of laughs, moans, or squalls; or the implications of what is not said in light of what has been said. *Nonverbal communication* is often called body language and includes gestures, movements, facial expressions, postures, and reactions. *Abstract communication* takes the form of play, artistic expression, symbols, photographs, and choice of clothing. Because it is possible to exert greater conscious control over verbal communication, it is a less reliable indicator of true feelings, especially with children.

Many factors influence the communication process. To be successful (i.e., gratifying), communication must be appropriate to the situation, properly timed, and clearly delivered. This implies that nurses understand and use the techniques of effective communication, including listening. Verbal and nonverbal messages must be congruent; that is, two or more messages sent via different levels must not be contradictory. The essential issue in communication is to keep lines open and to check perceptions often to assess the quality of understanding (Nance, 1995).

Verbal Communication—The Power of Words

Words shape reality, and thus hold tremendous power. A person can change another's perception of reality by the choice of words that are used. For example, if the diagnosis of cancer is always referred to as a tumor, cyst, malignancy, or carcinoma, patients may never really know that they have cancer. Consequently, they may assume less responsibility for their care than if they were aware of the seriousness of the condition. By learning to recognize how patients and health professionals use language to manipulate reality, one can also learn how to change perceptions and communicate more effectively.

Avoidance Language. The most common way that people try to alter reality is by avoiding words that truly describe it. For example, euphemisms such as "passed on" are used instead of "death." Avoidance language indicates that a person wants to hide something, particularly feelings. As a rule, accepting a person's use of euphemisms only serves to perpetuate the fears and never helps the person deal with them. In contrast, use of straightforward, precise, descriptive language lends perspective to the situation and allows the person to discuss the fears. Most often, imagined fears are much worse than reality.

Distancing Language. People may use impersonal words, such as "it" or "others," to shield themselves from the painful reality of a situation. For example, parents may state that they know *someone* with a child who is slow, when they may actually be talking about personal fears regarding *their* child. By realizing that the parents may need to talk about this difficult subject, the nurse can provide sensitive statements that ease them into discussing their situation.

One of the dangers in supporting distancing language is that the person may effectively deny that a problem exists. To return to the previous example, if the issue of retardation is never approached directly but is allowed to be "someone else's problem," the parents may not be able to make decisions for special schools or individualized training. Sometimes distancing is desirable because the topic may be too painful to discuss directly. The use of the third person technique may be therapeutic in allowing an individual the opportunity to indirectly approach a subject and receive feedback but still remain in control.

Nonverbal Communication—Paralanguage

In addition to the spoken word, messages are also relayed through nonverbal means, or *paralanguage*—the pitch, pause, intonation, rate, volume, and stress apparent in speech. Young children become very adept at understanding paralanguage; long before they know the meaning of words, they sense anxiety or fear by the rise in pitch or the accelerated rate of the parent's voice. By careful observation of the spoken word, nurses can better understand the meaning of another's verbal message and more accurately control their own paralanguage.

Because most people do not exert conscious control over their paralanguage, it is a valuable clue to feelings and concerns. For example, *pausing* may signify a need to formulate thoughts, recall information, or fabricate a story. Frequent pauses often make the speaker sound unsure. Long pauses may mean that the individual needs more information.

Rate is another characteristic that gives unspoken messages. Talking too fast usually makes the speaker sound glib and insensitive. Talking slowly with a firm tone and appropriate pauses conveys authority. Therefore, a person is much more likely to "hear" instructions if the latter approach is used. Children in particular respond attentively to a slow, even, steady voice.

Confirming and Disconfirming Behaviors. People respond to each other through *confirming behaviors,* such as nodding the head, using direct eye contact, repeating or requesting clarification, and making appropriate comments; or *disconfirming behaviors,* such as tapping fingers or a foot, turning away from the speaker, avoiding eye contact, and interrupting (Seidel et al, 1999). Because there is a reciprocal relationship between such behaviors, nurses need to use confirming behaviors to receive confirmation in return. This "mirroring" effect is particularly evident in children because of their sensitivity to nonverbal cues.

GUIDELINES FOR COMMUNICATION AND INTERVIEWING

The most widely used method of communicating with parents on a professional basis is the interview process. Unlike social conversation, interviewing is a specific form of goal-directed communication. As nurses converse with children and adults, they focus on the individuals to determine the kind of person they are, their usual mode of handling problems, whether help is needed, and the way in which they react to counseling. Developing interviewing skills requires time and practice, but some guiding principles can facilitate this process.

Establishing a Setting for Communication

Appropriate Introduction. Introduce yourself to, and ask the name of, each family member who is present. Address parents or other adults by their appropriate titles, such as "Mr." and "Mrs.," unless they specify a preferred name. Record the preferred name on the medical record. Using formal address or their preferred names, rather than using first names or "mom" or "dad," conveys respect and regard for the parents and other caregivers and the critical roles they play in the lives of their children.

At the beginning of the visit, include children in the interaction by asking them their name, age, and other information. Nurses often direct all questions to adults, even when children are old enough to speak for themselves. This serves to terminate one extremely valuable source of information: the patient. Nurses must make every effort to sense the world of the child and family as they sense it (Seidel et al, 1999). When the child is included, follow the general rules for communicating with children in the Guidelines box on p. 763.

Role Clarification and Explanation of the Interview. During the introduction it is also necessary to clarify the nurse's particular role in the health setting. For example, nurses performing interviews may be pediatric nurse practitioners, inpatient staff nurses, clinic nurses, office nurses, visiting nurses, or school nurses. A parent is much more likely to reveal personal information about the child and family if the relevance and the importance of the interview are stressed. If this is not done, parents may refuse to elaborate on certain areas because they feel it has no bearing on the "problem." In addition, because more than one member of the health team may take a history during the course of a hospital admission, it is important to clarify the reason for each interview (Seidel et al, 1999).

Another reason for role clarification is education of the health consumer. With expanded roles in nursing, it is not unusual for families to think that the examiner is a physician rather than a nurse. Role clarification is especially important because some parents may feel deceived if they later are made aware of the nurse's identity. The general consumer acceptance of pediatric nurse practitioners (PNPs) has been very favorable, so it is also important to acknowledge their expertise by emphasizing the PNP's role.

Preliminary Acquaintance. To make the family feel at ease and to develop rapport, begin the interview with some general conversation. The opening statements should be general but still informative. Comments such as "How have things been since your last visit?" "Tell me about Johnny," or (to the child) "What do you think is going to happen today?" allow the parent or child to express the main concern in a casual, relaxed atmosphere.

The preliminary acquaintance conversation also reveals how responsive the informant may be to questions. For example, using open-ended statements such as "Tell me about the baby" may lead the parent into a lengthy, detailed discussion. In this case, direct questions toward specific answers to avoid irrelevant remarks. At other times a parent may respond to open-ended questions with only minimal information, in which case continue to use open-ended questions rather than questions with "yes" or "no" answers.

Ensuring Privacy and Confidentiality. The place where the interview is conducted is almost as important as the interview itself. The physical environment should allow for as much privacy as possible, with distractions (e.g., interruptions, noise, or visible activity) kept to a minimum. At times it is necessary to turn off a television or radio. The environment should also have some play provision for young children to keep them occupied during the parent-nurse interview (Fig. 34-1). Parents who are constantly interrupted by their children are unable to concentrate fully and tend to give short, brief answers to terminate the interview as quickly as possible (Critical Thinking box).

Confidentiality is also an essential component of the initial phase of the interview. Since the interview is usually shared with other members of the health team or the teacher (as in the case of students), be sure to inform the family of the limits regarding confidentiality. If there is concern regarding confidentiality in a situation, such as talking to a parent suspected of child abuse or a teenager contemplating suicide, deal with this directly and inform the person that in such instances confidentiality cannot be ensured. However, the nurse judiciously protects information of a confidential nature (Sullivan, 1997).

Computer Privacy and Applications in Nursing

The use of computer technology to store and retrieve health information has become widespread. The privacy and security of this health information is a growing concern throughout the health care community. Any person accessing health information of a confidential nature is charged with managing safeguards of disclosures, since violations might incur civil damages.

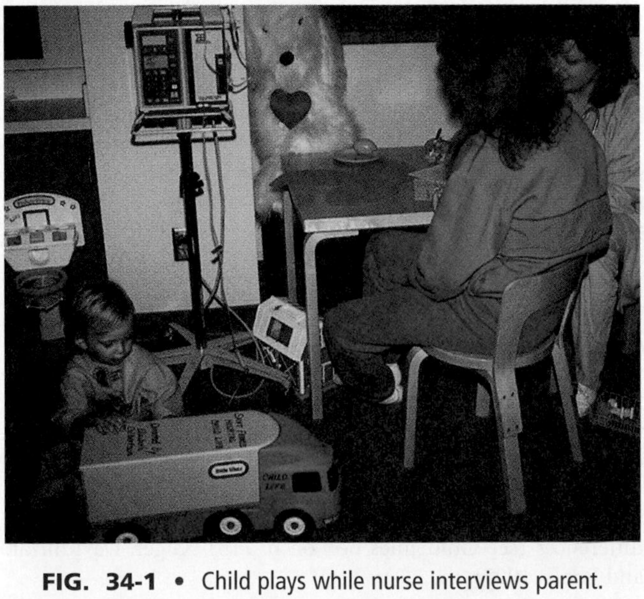

FIG. 34-1 • Child plays while nurse interviews parent.

In 1994 a committee of the Institute of Medicine recommended a national code of fair health information practices. The suggestion was made that health data organizations (HDOs) should establish data protection units to develop privacy policies and security practices for manual and automated data processing systems. Technologic safeguards and managerial procedures known as *computer security* can be applied to computer hardware to ensure that individual privacy is protected (Hoffman, 1995).

Computer and information applications in nursing *(nursing informatics)* are used by 75% of all nurses to record care, access information, and obtain library resources. Two important health care applications are record transmission, including facsimile (fax) and electronic mail (e-mail); and telemedicine. The telemedicine application is capable of two-way video conferencing, transmission of radiographs, and clinical consultation between remote sites and centralized resources. Nurses can use these computer applications to make unique interventions that contribute to the health care of families (Brennan, 1996).*

Telephone Triage and Counseling

Nurses are increasingly becoming responsible for assessment of children's symptoms and clinical judgment for further medical care (*triage*) via telephone report. Most often, health problems

*Resources include: Nicoll LH: *Nurses' guide to the Internet,* ed 2, Philadelphia, 1998, JB Lippincott; and the bimonthly publication, *Computers in Nursing* (to order, call 1-800-638-3030; fax (301) 714-2300; e-mail: lrorders@phl.lrpub.com; or visit the website at: www.lww.com.

Critical Thinking

THE INTERVIEW

During your interview with Ms. Gaines, 2½-year-old Jesse continually interrupts the conversation. Although Ms. Gaines has told her several times to be quiet, the interruptions continue. Frustrated, the mother states firmly, "If you don't be good, the nurse will give you a shot." Jesse begins to cry softly and hugs her mother's legs. What would be an appropriate response?

First, Think About It . . .

- **Within what point of view are you thinking?**
- **If you accept your conclusions, what are the implications?**

1. **State, "Ms. Gaines, don't threaten Jesse that way. Her behavior isn't bothering me."**
2. **Do nothing, because Jesse has become quiet.**
3. **State, "Jesse, nurses don't give needles because children are not being quiet. Here are paper and crayons to draw some pictures while your mom and I talk."**
4. **Hug Jesse and give her crayons and paper to draw.**

The best response is 3. The threat of injections or other painful or frightening procedures should never be used to gain a child's cooperation. You want to reassure Jesse about this but at the same time reinforce the need for her to be quiet. The point of view that providing play materials helps keep her occupied is developmentally sound.

Although the other responses may seem appropriate, they fail to remove the threat of a "shot" to Jesse and may bear negative implications for your future relationship. In particular, the first response can alienate your relationship with the parent. It also dismisses the issue that the interruptions do bother Ms. Gaines and most likely affect the quality of the interview.

are assessed and prioritized according to urgency, and treatment is judiciously provided via telephone services. Successful outcomes are based on the consistency and accuracy of the information provided, and parents are empowered to participate in their child's medical care. Telephone triage care management has increased access to quality health care services, and patient satisfaction has significantly improved. Unnecessary emergency department and clinic visits have decreased, saving medical costs and time (e.g., less work absence) for families in need of health care. The most common telephone triage call is for a fever (see Chapter 45). Approximately 37% of the triage calls related to fever require emergency care, and nearly 50% benefit from home management (Deadrick and Boggess, 1996).

NURSE ALERT • Legal issues can emerge from errors in telephone triage care management. Always advise that the child should be seen if there is any doubt as to the seriousness of the illness.

A well-designed telephone triage program is essential for safe, prompt, and consistent-quality health care. Telephone triage is more than "just a phone call," since a child's life is a high price to pay for poorly managed or incompetent telephone assessment skills. Typically, general guidelines for telephone triage include screening questions; determining when to immediately refer to Emergency Medicine Services (EMS) (dial 911); and determining when to refer to same-day appointments, appointments in 24 to 72 hours, appointments in 4 days or more, or home care (Gobis, 1997).

COMMUNICATING WITH FAMILIES

Communicating with Parents

Although the parent and child are separate and distinct individuals, relationships with the child are often mediated via the parent, particularly in the case of younger children. For the most part, information about the child is acquired by direct observation or is communicated to the nurse by the parents. Usually it can be assumed that because of the close contact with the child, the parent gives reliable information. Making an assessment of the child requires input from the child (both verbal and nonverbal), information from the parent, and the nurse's own observations of the child and interpretation of the relationship between the child and the parent. Counseling and guidance must be directed to the caregiver of infants and small children; when children are old enough to be active participants in their own health maintenance, the parent becomes a collaborator in health care.

Encouraging the Parent to Talk. Interviewing parents not only offers the opportunity to determine the health and developmental status of the child, but also offers information about factors that influence the child's life. Whatever the parent sees as a problem should also be a concern of the nurse. These problems are not always easy to identify. Nurses need to be alert for clues and signals by which a parent communicates worries and anxieties. Careful phrasing with broad, open-ended questions such as "What is Jimmy eating now?" provides more information than several single-answer questions such as "Is Jimmy eating what the rest of the family eats?"

Sometimes the parent will take the lead without prompting. At other times it may be necessary to direct another question on the basis of an observation, such as "Connie seems unhappy today" or "How do you feel when David cries?" If the parent appears to be tired or distraught, consider asking, "What do you do to relax?" or "What help do you have with the children?" A comment such as "You handle the baby very well. What kinds of experience have you had with babies?" to new parents who appear comfortable with their first child gives positive reinforcement and provides an opening for any questions they might have regarding the care of the infant. Often all that is required to keep parents talking is a nod or saying "yes" or "uh-huh."

When attempting to elicit feelings and uncover covert problem areas, avoid closed-ended questions that begin with "Does. . . . ," "Did . . . ," or "Is . . . ," which usually require only a single response. In addition, asking questions such as "Does your son have any problems at school?" subtly implies a lack of parental skills and evokes defensiveness. Instead, say, "What . . . ," "How . . . ," "Tell me about . . ." and encourage elaboration with "You were saying . . . ," "You say that . . . ," or reflecting back a key word. Open-ended questions are nonthreatening and encourage description.

Directing the Focus. The ability to direct the focus of the interview while allowing for maximum freedom of expression is one of the most difficult goals in effective communication. One approach is the use of open-ended or broad questions, followed by guiding statements. For example, if the parent proceeds to list the other children by name, say, "Tell me their ages, too." If the parent continues to describe each child in depth, something that is not the purpose of the interview, redirect the focus by stating, "Let's talk about the other children later. You were beginning to tell me about Paul's activities at school." This approach conveys interest in the other children but focuses the assessment on the patient.

In the event that the parent has suggested that a problem exists with one of the other children, reintroduce this subject at the end of the interview to assess the need for further family follow-up. Saying to the parent, "Before, you were mentioning that your older son is having trouble in school. Tell me what you see as the problem," reintroduces this subject but only in terms of the possible problem.

Listening and Cultural Awareness. Listening is the most important component of effective communication. When listening is truly aimed at understanding the patient, it is an active process that requires concentration and attention to all aspects of the conversation—verbal, nonverbal, and abstract. Major blocks to listening are environmental distraction and premature judgment.

The attitudes and feelings of the nurse are easily injected into an interview. Often nurses' perceptions of a parent's behavior are influenced by their own perceptions, prejudices, and assumptions, which may include racial, religious, and cultural stereotypes. What may be interpreted as passive hostility or disinterest in a parent may be shyness or an expression of anxiety. For example, in Western cultures eye contact and directness are signs of paying attention. However, in many non-Western cultures, including that of Native Americans, directness, such as looking someone in the eye, is considered rude. Children are taught to avert their gaze and to look down when being addressed by an adult, especially one with authority (Seidel et al, 1999). Therefore judgments about "listening," as well as verbal interactions, need to be made with an appreciation of cultural differences (see Guidelines box on p. 718) (Giger, Davidhizar, and Poole, 1997).

Although it is necessary to make some preliminary judgments, listen with as much objectivity as possible by clarifying meanings and by attempting to see the situation from the parent's point of view. Effective interviewers use conscious control over their reactions, responses, and the techniques they use.

Minimum verbal activity with active listening facilitates parent involvement. It is tempting to spend time explaining, describing, and interpreting health information when the opportunity presents itself. However, it is possible to provide effective health education by timing the information properly and presenting only as much as is necessary at the moment.

Careful listening facilitates the use of clues, verbal leads, or signals from the interviewee to move the interview along. Frequent references to an area of concern, repetition of certain key words, and/or a special emphasis on something or someone serve as cues to the interviewer for the direction of inquiry. Concerns and anxieties are usually mentioned in a casual, offhand manner. Even though they are casual, they are important and deserve careful scrutiny to identify problem areas. For example, a parent who is concerned about a child's habit of bedwetting may casually mention that the child's bed was "wet this morning."

Because the interview is almost always triangular—between the nurse, parent, and child—the parent may wish to convey information in such a way as to prevent the child from hearing it. This requires active listening on the part of the nurse to hear the unspoken message. The following example illustrates this point:

> During a routine health visit, the nurse performed a complete history and physical examination on a 4-year-old girl. The child was accompanied by her mother, who appeared to be a reliable, well-informed, and talkative informant. During the child's birth history, the mother gave all the information asked. However, during the family history, the mother stated to the nurse, "I had a hysterectomy 6 years ago." Because the nurse gave no indication of acknowledging the significance of this statement, the mother repeated it, only this time she stressed the "6 years." The nurse, who had not been listening as attentively as she should have, realized that the mother was telling her something very important. The mother raised her eyebrows and gently shook her head "no," warning the nurse not to explore this area too openly. The nurse correctly read the cues and stated, "Let's return to your health history later."
>
> At the completion of the physical examination, the nurse took the child to the health center's playroom and took the opportunity to investigate this contradictory information of a "4-year-old child born to a woman with a hysterectomy 6 years ago." The mother revealed that the child was adopted. The mother was greatly concerned about the fact that the child was unaware of this and requested the nurse's advice.
>
> Fortunately, the nurse had "listened" carefully enough to realize the significance of this woman's concern and allowed her the opportunity to discuss it in private.

Listening is also helpful in assessing reliability. For example, the answers elicited at the beginning of the interview may differ from those at the end, when the parent feels more confident in revealing problems. It is important to identify any discrepancies and reintroduce those topics for further investigation.

Using Silence. Silence as a response is often one of the most difficult interviewing techniques to learn. It requires a sense of confidence and comfort on the part of the interviewer to allow the interviewee space in which to think without interruptions. Silence permits the interviewee to sort out thoughts and feelings and to search for responses to questions. It also allows for sharing of feelings in which two or more people absorb the emotion to its depth.

Sometimes it is necessary to break the silence and reopen communication. Do this in a way that encourages the person to continue talking about what is considered important. Breaking a silence by introducing a new topic or by prolonged talking essentially terminates the interviewee's opportunity to use the silence. Suggestions for breaking the silence include statements such as "Is there anything else you wish to say?" "I see you find it difficult to continue; how may I help?" or "I don't know what this silence means. Perhaps there is something you would like to put into words but find difficult to say."

Being Empathic. *Empathy* is the capacity to understand what another person is experiencing from within that person's frame of reference; it is often described as the ability to put oneself in another's shoes. The essence of empathic interaction is accurately understanding another's feelings (Price and Archbold, 1997; White, 1997; Wright and Leahey, 1999). Empathy differs from *sympathy,* which is having feelings or emotions in common with another person, rather than understanding those feelings. Sympathy is not therapeutic in the helping relationship, because it leads to feeling emotionally overinvolved, and potentially leads to professional burnout.

Of the different types of support, such as empathy, encouragement, or reassurance, empathy is the most beneficial but least used form (Wissow, Roter, and Wilson, 1994). Some individuals are naturally empathic; however, empathy can be learned by attending to the verbal and nonverbal language of the interviewee. *Neurolinguistic programming (NLP)* is concerned with the manner of accessing and understanding information and is an excellent method of increasing empathic communication. Although people may use all of the following sensory modalities to communicate, usually one modality predominates: visual, auditory, or kinesthetic. The specific sensory mode is identified by observing the type of verbs, adjectives, and adverbs the person uses and then using this mode in responding to the individual. For example, if a person using the visual mode states, "I can't see why you have to perform these procedures on my child," a response using the same mode is, "What do you *see* as the reason for them?"

Defining the Problem. To arrive at a solution to a problem, the nurse and the parent must agree that a problem exists. Sometimes the parent may believe that there is a problem that the nurse is unable to see. For example, a mother was overly concerned about every small sniffle, sneeze, or cough in her infant, who had been carefully examined and found to be healthy with no evidence of a respiratory problem. On careful questioning, the nurse discovered that a previous child had died of pneumonia in infancy. Consequently, the nurse was better able to understand the mother's concern and could help the mother deal with her special anxieties about her infant; the nurse could also teach her how to recognize any need for concern.

Occasionally the nurse identifies a problem that the parent denies exists. In this case, pursue the situation and either find a way to deal with it or enlist the aid of other health team members. For example, the parents of a child with Down syndrome may refuse to believe that their child is different from any other child of the same age. They may say, "He is just a little slow," or "All the child needs to do is to try harder." A child with an obvious behavior problem may be described by the parents as "stubborn." Such statements may be clues that the parents have not progressed past the stage of denial in adjusting to the condition.

Solving the Problem. Once the problem is identified and agreed on by the parent and the nurse, they can begin to arrive at a solution. A parent who is included in the problem-solving process is more apt to follow through with a course of action. Such questions as "What have you tried so far?" or "What have you thought about doing?" provide leads for exploration and give the parents the feeling that their ideas and solutions are worthwhile. These can be followed by "What prevents you from trying that?" "That sounds like a good plan," and "You seem to be stumped. Have you considered trying this?" Such approaches encourage active participation and reinforce rather than belittle parents' efforts to solve their problems.

Sometimes the parents arrive at a solution that the nurse does not consider the best alternative. If it can be ascertained that it will do no harm and if the parents are convinced of its merits, it is usually best to allow them to continue with the plan. A course of action is more likely to be carried out when parents can reach their own conclusions. However, when parental decisions may be hazardous, nurses are obligated to discuss the risks with the family and try to reach a more beneficial solution. Whenever possible, decisions should be theirs, with the nurse serving as a facilitator in problem solving.

Providing Anticipatory Guidance. The ideal way to handle a situation is to deal with it before it becomes a problem. The best preventive measure is anticipatory guidance. Traditionally, anticipatory guidance has focused on providing families with information on normal growth and development, as well as nurturing childrearing practices. For example, one of the most significant areas in pediatrics is injury prevention. Beginning prenatally, parents need specific instructions on home safety. Because of the child's maturing developmental skills, home safety changes must be implemented early to minimize risks to the child.

Many normal developmental changes can disturb unprepared parents, such as a toddler's diminished appetite, negativism, altered sleeping patterns, and anxiety toward strangers. Such topics are discussed in the chapters on health promotion to provide the nurse with knowledge to counsel parents.

However, anticipatory guidance should extend beyond giving information and empower families to use the information as a means of building competence in their parenting abilities. Often parents need early guidance with their children, and anticipatory guidance builds confidence in their parenting skills. To achieve this level of anticipatory guidance, do the following (Desselle and Pearlmutter, 1997):

- Base interventions on needs identified by the family, not by the professional.
- View the family as competent or as having the ability to be competent.
- Provide opportunities for the family to achieve competence.

Avoiding Blocks to Communication. Some blocks to communication can adversely affect the quality of the helping relationship. Many of these blocks are initiated by the interviewer, such as giving unrestricted advice or forming prejudged conclusions. Another type of block occurs primarily with the interviewees and deals with information overload. When individuals are presented with too much information, or information that is overwhelming, they will often demonstrate signals of increasing anxiety or decreasing attention. Such signals should alert the interviewer to give less information or to clarify what has been said. Some of the more common blocks to communication, including signs of information overload, are listed in Box 34-1.

Communication blocks can be corrected by careful analysis of the interview process. One of the best methods for improving interviewing skills is audiotape and/or videotape feedback. With supervision and guidance, the interviewer can recognize the blocks and consciously avoid them.

Communicating with Families Through an Interpreter. Sometimes communication is impossible because two people speak different languages. In this case it is necessary to obtain information through a third party, the interpreter. When an interpreter is used, the same guidelines for interviewing are used. Specific guidelines for using an adult interpreter are presented in the Guidelines box.

Communicating with families through an interpreter requires sensitivity to cultural, legal, and ethical considerations. For example, in some cultures using a child as an interpreter is considered an insult to an adult, because children are expected to show respect by not questioning their elders. In some cultures, class differences between the interpreter and the family may cause the family to feel intimidated and less inclined to offer information. Therefore choose the translator carefully, and provide time for the interpreter and family to establish rapport.

Issues of legal and ethical concerns may also arise. For example, in obtaining informed consent through an interpreter, it is important that the family be fully informed of all aspects of the particular procedure that they are consenting to. Issues of confidentiality may arise when family members related to another patient are asked to interpret for the family, thus revealing sensitive information that may be shared with other families on the unit.

When no one else is available to translate, children within the family are often asked to assume this role. In this situation it is important to stress *literal* translation of parent responses.

Box 34-1

Blocks to Communication

Socializing
Giving unrestricted and sometimes unasked for advice
Offering premature or inappropriate reassurance
Giving overready encouragement
Defending a situation or opinion
Using stereotyped comments or clichés
Limiting expression of emotion by asking directed, closed-ended questions
Interrupting and finishing the person's sentence
Talking more than the interviewee
Forming prejudged conclusions
Deliberately changing the focus

SIGNS OF INFORMATION OVERLOAD

Long periods of silence
Wide eyes and fixed facial expression
Constant fidgeting or attempting to move away
Nervous habits (e.g, tapping, playing with hair)
Sudden disruptions (e.g., asking to go to the bathroom)
Looking around
Yawning, eyes drooping
Frequently looking at a watch or clock
Attempting to change topic of discussion

To maximize correct translations, it may be necessary to interrupt the parent and ask the child to translate every few sentences. When using children as interpreters, ask questions directed at specific answers and assess the interpreted translation in terms of nonverbal expressions of communication.*

NURSE ALERT • When using translated materials, such as a health history form, be sure the informant is literate in the foreign language.

Communicating with Children

Although the greatest amount of verbal communication may usually be carried out with the parent, do not exclude the child during the interview. Pay attention to infants and younger children through play or by occasionally directing questions or remarks to them. Include older children as active participants.

In communication with children of all ages, the nonverbal components of the communication process convey the most significant messages. It is difficult to disguise feelings, attitudes, and anxiety in relating to children. They are very alert to surroundings and attach meaning to every gesture and move that is made; this is particularly true of very young children.

Active attempts to make friends with children before they have had an opportunity to evaluate an unfamiliar person tend to increase their anxiety. It is helpful to talk to the child and parent but continue to go about activities that do not involve the child directly, thus allowing the child to observe from a safe position. If the child has a special toy or doll, "talk" to the doll first. Ask simple questions such as "Does your teddy bear have a special name?" to ease the child into conversation. Other guidelines for communicating with children are presented in the Guidelines box. Specific guidelines for preparing children for procedures, a common nursing function, are discussed in Chapter 45.

Communication Related to Development of Thought Processes. The normal development of language and thought offers a frame of reference in knowing how to communicate with children. Thought processes progress from sensorimotor to perceptual to concrete and finally to abstract, formal operations. The early social communicative development of children has been divided into three stages: (1) *perlocutionary stage*—unintentional communication behavior; (2) *illocutionary stage*—true intent in communication efforts; and (3) *locutionary stage*—intentional communication behaviors and use of symbols (Hoge and Parette, 1995). An understanding

*Interpreting services are also available through American Telephone and Telegraph (AT&T) by calling 1-800-628-8486 or 1-800-752-6096.

Guidelines

USING AN INTERPRETER

Explain to interpreter the reason for the interview and the type of questions that will be asked.

Clarify whether a detailed or brief answer is required and whether the translated response can be general or literal.

Introduce interpreter to family and allow some time before the actual interview so that they can become acquainted.

Communicate directly with family members when asking questions to reinforce interest in them and to observe nonverbal expressions, but do not ignore interpreter.

Pose questions to elicit only one answer at a time, such as "Do you have pain?" rather than "Do you have any pain, tiredness, or loss of appetite?"

Refrain from interrupting family member and interpreter while they are conversing.

Avoid commenting to interpreter about family members, since they may understand some English.

Be aware that some medical words, such as "allergy," may have no similar word in another language; avoid medical jargon whenever possible.

Respect cultural differences; it is often best to pose questions about sex, marriage, or pregnancy indirectly—ask about "child's father" rather than "mother's husband."

Allow time following the interview for interpreter to share something that he or she felt could not be said earlier; ask about interpreter's impression of nonverbal clues to communication and family members' reliability or ease in revealing information.

Arrange for family to speak with same interpreter on subsequent visits whenever possible.

Guidelines

COMMUNICATING WITH CHILDREN

Allow children time to feel comfortable.

Avoid sudden or rapid advances, broad smiles, extended eye contact, or other gestures that may be seen as threatening.

Talk to the parent if child is initially shy.

Communicate through transition objects such as dolls, puppets, stuffed animals before questioning a young child directly.

Give older children the opportunity to talk without the parents present.

Assume a position that is at eye level with child (Fig. 34-2).

Speak in a quiet, unhurried, and confident voice.

Speak clearly, be specific, use simple words, and short sentences.

State directions and suggestions *positively.*

Offer a choice only when one exists.

Be honest with children.

Allow them to express their concerns and fears.

Use a variety of communication techniques.

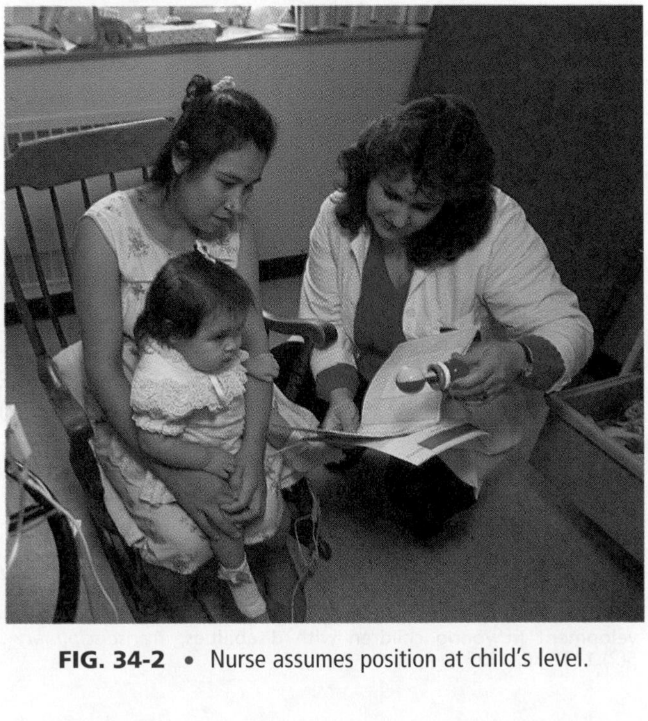

FIG. 34-2 • Nurse assumes position at child's level.

of the typical characteristics of these stages provides the nurse with a framework to facilitate social communication (Box 34-2).

Infancy. Because they are unable to use words, infants primarily use and understand nonverbal communication. Infants communicate their needs and feelings through nonverbal behaviors and vocalizations that can be interpreted by someone who is around them for a sufficient amount of time. Infants smile and coo when content and cry when distressed. Crying is provoked by unpleasant stimuli from inside or outside, such as hunger, pain, body restraint, or loneliness. Adults interpret this to mean that an infant needs something, and consequently try to alleviate the discomfort and reduce tension. Crying (or the desire to cry) persists as a part of everyone's communication repertoire.

Infants respond to adults' nonverbal behaviors. They become quiet when they are cuddled, patted, or receive other forms of gentle, physical contact. They derive comfort from the sound of a voice, even though they do not understand the words that are spoken. Until infants reach the age at which they experience stranger anxiety, they readily respond to any firm, gentle handling and quiet, calm speech. Loud, harsh sounds and sudden movements are frightening.

Older infants' attentions are centered on themselves and their parents; therefore any stranger is a potential threat until proved otherwise. Holding out the hands and asking the child to "come" is seldom successful, especially if the infant is with the parent. If infants must be handled, simply pick them up firmly without gestures. Observe the position in which the parent holds the infant. Most infants have learned to prefer a particular position and manner of handling. In general, infants are more at ease upright than horizontal. Also, hold infants so that they can see their parents. Until they have developed the understanding that an object (in this case the parent) removed from sight can still be present, they have no way of knowing that the object is still there.

Early Childhood. Children under 5 years of age are egocentric. They see things only in relation to themselves and from their point of view. Therefore focus communication on them. Tell them what they can do or how they will feel. Experiences of others are of no interest to them. It is futile to use another child's experience as an attempt to gain the cooperation of very small children. Allow them to touch and examine articles that will come in contact with them. A stethoscope bell will feel cold; palpating a neck might tickle. Although they have not yet acquired sufficient language skills to express their feelings and wants, toddlers are able to communicate effectively with their hands to transmit ideas without words. They push an unwanted object away, pull another person to show them something, point, and cover the mouth that is saying something they do not wish to hear.

Everything is direct and concrete to small children. They are unable to work with abstractions and interpret words literally. Analogies escape them because they are unable to separate fact from fantasy. For example, they attach literal meaning to such common phrases as "two-faced," "sticky fingers," or "coughing your head off." Children who are told they will get "a little stick in the arm" may not be able to envision an injection (Fig. 34-3). Therefore avoid using a phrase that might be misinterpreted by a small child (see Box 45-1).

Use language that is consistent with the child's developmental level. For example, in talking with a toddler, use simple, *short* sentences; repeat words that are *familiar* to the child; and limit descriptions to *concrete* explanations. Be certain that nonverbal messages are consistent with words and actions. For example, do not smile while doing something painful; children may think you enjoy hurting them.

Young children assign human attributes to inanimate objects. Consequently, they fear that objects may jump, bite, cut, or pinch all by themselves. Children do not know that these devices are unable to perform without human direction. To minimize their fears, keep unfamiliar equipment out of view until it is needed.

School-Age Years. Younger school-age children rely less on what they see and more on what they know when faced with new problems. They want explanations and reasons for every-

Box 34-2

Stages of Communicative Development in Young Children

PERLOCUTIONARY STAGE (0 TO 8-9 MONTHS)
Characteristics
Child is reflexive to stimuli
Increasing purpose in action

EMERGING ILLOCUTIONARY STAGE (8-9 TO 12-15 MONTHS)
Characteristics
Communicates intentionally with signals and gestures

CONVENTIONAL ILLOCUTIONARY/EMERGING LOCUTIONARY STAGE (12-15 TO 18-24 MONTHS)
Characteristics
Communicates intentionally with gestures, vocalizations, and verbalizations

Modifed from Hoge DR, Parette HP: Facilitating communicative development in young children with disabilities, *Transdisciplinary J* 5(2):113-130, 1995.

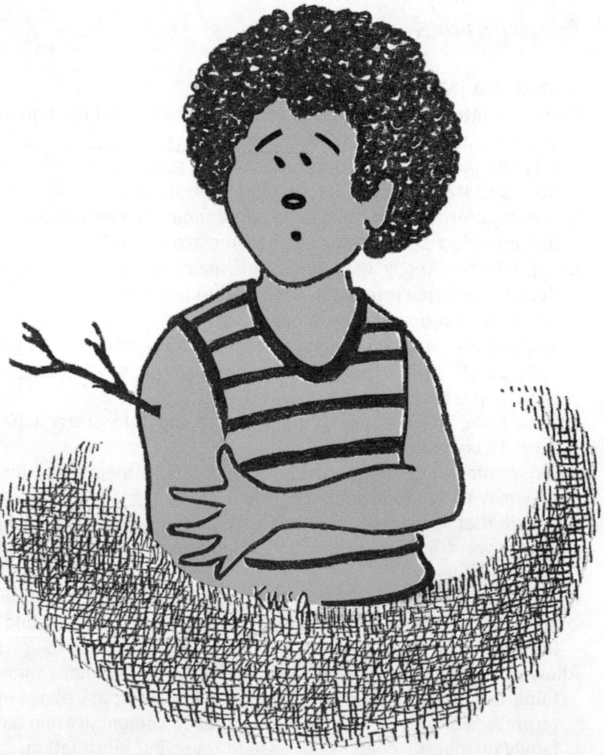

FIG. 34-3 • A young child may take the expression "a little stick in the arm" literally.

thing, but require no verification beyond that. They are interested in the functional aspect of all procedures, objects, and activities. They want to know why an object exists, why it is used, how it works, and the intent and purpose of its user. They need to know what is going to take place and why it is being done to *them* specifically. For example, to explain a procedure such as taking a blood pressure, show the child how squeezing the bulb pushes air into the cuff and makes the "silver" in the tube go up. Let the child operate the bulb. An explanation for the reason might be as simple as "I want to see how far the silver goes up when the cuff squeezes your arm." Consequently, the child becomes an enthusiastic participant.

School-age children have a heightened concern about body integrity. Because of the special importance and value they place on their body, they are overly sensitive to anything that constitutes a threat or suggestion of injury to it. This concern extends to their possessions also, so that they may appear to overreact to loss or threatened loss of treasured objects. Helping children to voice their concerns enables the nurse to provide reassurance and to implement activities that reduce their anxiety. For example, if a shy child dislikes being the center of attention, ignore that particular child by talking and relating to other children in the family or group. When children feel more comfortable, they will usually interject personal ideas, feelings, and interpretations of events.

Older children have an adequate and satisfactory use of language. They still require relatively simple explanations, but their ability to think correctly can facilitate communication and explanation. Commonly, they have sufficient experience with health and health workers to understand what is transpiring and generally what is expected of them.

Adolescence. As children move into adolescence, they fluctuate between child and adult thinking and behavior. They are riding a current that is moving them rapidly toward a maturity that may be beyond their coping ability. Therefore, when tensions rise, they may seek the security of the more familiar and comfortable expectations of childhood. Anticipating these shifts in identity allows the nurse to adjust the course of interaction to meet the needs of the moment. No single approach can be relied on consistently, and encountering cooperation, hostility, anger, bravado, and a variety of other behaviors and attitudes can be expected. It is as much a mistake to regard the adolescent as an adult with an adult's wisdom and control as it is to assume that the teenager has the concerns and expectations of a child.

Often adolescents are more willing to discuss their concerns with an adult outside the family, and they commonly welcome the opportunity to interact with a nurse. They are accepting of anyone who displays a genuine interest in them. However, adolescents are quick to reject persons who attempt to impose their values on them, whose interest is feigned, or who appear to have little respect for who they are and what they think or say.

As with all children, adolescents need to express their feelings. Generally, they talk quite freely when given an opportunity. However, what adolescents say cannot always be taken at face value. When emotional factors are involved, the feelings that are interjected into words are as significant as the words that are used. To give support, be attentive, try not to interrupt, and avoid comments or expressions that convey disapproval or surprise. Avoid prying and asking embarrassing questions, and resist any impulse to give advice. Often adolescents reveal their feelings or ask a question about a source of concern when they are involved in routine matters such as a physical assessment.

Teenagers characteristically have a language and culture all their own that further sets them apart. To avoid misinterpretation, clarify terms often. Occasionally adolescents refuse to answer or answer only in monosyllables. Usually this happens when they are opposed to the contact or do not yet feel safe enough to reveal themselves. In this instance confine discussions to irrelevant topics to reduce the element of threat until such time as they feel more secure. Be alert for signals indicating that they are ready to talk. The major sources of concern for adolescents are attitudes and feelings toward sex, substance abuse, relationships with parents, peer-group acceptance, and developing a sense of identity.

Interviewing the adolescent presents some special situations. The first may be whether to talk with the adolescent alone, with the adolescent and parents together, or with each person individually. Of course such questions don't arise if the adolescent is alone, except whether to suggest to the teenager that the parents may be interviewed at another time. If the parents and teenager are together, talking with the adolescent first has the advantage of immediately identifying with the young person, thus fostering the interpersonal relationship. However, talking with the parents initially may provide insight into the family relationship. In either case, give both parties an opportunity to be included in the interview. If time constraints are important, such as during history taking, clarify these at the onset to avoid appearing to "take sides" by talking more with one person than with the other.

Confidentiality is of great importance when interviewing adolescents. Explain to parents and teenagers the limits of confidentiality, specifically that young persons' disclosures will not be shared unless they indicate a need for intervention, as in the case of suicidal behavior.

Another dilemma in interviewing adolescents is that two views of a problem commonly exist—the teenager's and the parents'. Clarification of the problem is a major task. However, providing both parties with an opportunity to discuss their perceptions in an open and unbiased atmosphere can, by itself, be therapeutic. Demonstrating positive communication skills can help families communicate more effectively (Guidelines box).

Guidelines

COMMUNICATING WITH ADOLESCENTS

Build a Foundation

- Spend time together
- Encourage expression of ideas and feelings
- Respect their views
- Tolerate differences
- Praise good points
- Respect their privacy
- Set a good example

Communicate Effectively

- Give undivided attention
- Listen, listen, listen
- Be courteous, calm, and open-minded
- Try not to overreact. If you do, take a break
- Avoid judging or criticizing
- Avoid the "third degree" of continuous questioning
- Choose important issues when taking a stand
- After taking a stand:
  - Think through all options
  - Make expectations clear

Box 34-3

Creative Communication Techniques with Children

VERBAL TECHNIQUES

"I" Messages

Relate a feeling about a behavior in terms of "I."
Describe effect behavior had on the person.
Avoid use of "you."
"You" messages are judgmental and provoke defensiveness.
Example: "You" message—"You are being very uncooperative about doing your treatments."
Example: "I" message—"I am concerned about how the treatments are going because I want to see you get better."

Third-Person Technique

Involves expressing a feeling in terms of a third person ("he," "she," "they").
Is less threatening than directly asking children how they feel because it gives them an opportunity to agree or disagree without being defensive.
Example: "Sometimes when a person is sick a lot, he feels angry and sad because he cannot do what others can." Either wait silently for a response or encourage a reply with a statement such as "Did you ever feel that way?"
Approach allows children three choices: (1) to agree and, hopefully, express how they feel; (2) to disagree; or (3) to remain silent, in which case they probably have such feelings but are unable to express them at this time.

Facilitative Responding

Involves careful listening and reflecting back to patients the feelings and content of their statements.
Responses are empathic and nonjudgmental, and legitimize the person's feelings.
Formula for facilitative responses: "You feel __________ because __________."
Example: If child states, "I hate coming to the hospital and getting needles," a facilitative response is, "You feel unhappy because of all the things that are done to you."

Storytelling

Uses the language of children to probe into areas of their thinking while bypassing conscious inhibitions or fears.
Simplest technique is asking children to relate a story about an event, such as "being in the hospital."
Other approaches:
Show children a picture of a particular event, such as a child in a hospital with other people in the room, and ask them to describe the scene.
Cut out comic strips, remove words, and have child add statements for scenes.

Mutual Storytelling

Reveals child's thinking and attempts to change child's perceptions or fears by retelling a somewhat different story (more therapeutic approach than storytelling).
Begins by asking child to tell a story about something, followed by another story told by the nurse that is similar to child's tale but with differences that help child in problem areas.
Example: Child's story is about going to the hospital and never seeing his or her parents again. Nurse's story is also about a child (using different names but similar circumstances) in a hospital whose parents visit everyday, but in the evening after work until the child is better and goes home with them.

Bibliotherapy

Uses books in a therapeutic and supportive process.
Provides children with an opportunity to explore an event that is similar to their own but sufficiently different to allow them to distance themselves from it and remain in control.
General guidelines for using bibliotherapy are:
Assess child's emotional and cognitive development in terms of readiness to understand the book's message.
Be familiar with the book's content (intended message or purpose) and the age for which it is written.
Read the book to the child if child is unable to read.
Explore the meaning of the book with the child by having child:
Retell the story
Read a special section with the nurse or parent
Draw a picture related to the story and discuss the drawing
Talk about the characters
Summarize the moral or meaning of the story

Dreams

Often reveal unconscious and repressed thoughts and feelings
Ask child to talk about a dream or nightmare.
Explore with child what meaning dream could have.

"What If" Questions

Encourage child to explore potential situations and to consider different problem-solving options.
Example: "What if you got sick and had to go the hospital?" Children's responses reveal what they know already and what they are curious about, provide opportunity for helping children learn coping skills, especially in potentially dangerous situations.

Three Wishes

Involves asking, "If you could have any three things in the world, what would they be?"
If child answers. "That all my wishes come true," ask child for specific wishes.

Rating Game

Uses some type of rating scale (numbers, sad to happy faces) to rate an event or feeling.
Example: Instead of asking youngsters how they feel, ask how their day has been "on a scale of 1 to 10, with 10 being the best."

Word Association Game

Involves stating key words and asking children to say the first word they think of when they hear the word.
Start with neutral words and then introduce more anxiety producing words, such as "illness," "needles," "hospitals," and "operation."
Select key words that relate to some event in child's life that is relevant.

Box 34-3
Creative Communication Techniques with Children—cont'd

Sentence Completion

Involves presenting a partial statement and having child complete it. Some sample statements are:
- The thing I like best (least) about school is ________.
- The best (worst) age to be is ________.
- The most (least) fun thing I ever did was ________.
- The thing I like most (least) about my parents is ________.
- The one thing I would change about my family is ________.
- If I could be anything I wanted, I would be ________.
- The thing I like most (least) about myself is ________.

Pros and Cons

Involves selecting a topic, such as "being in the hospital," and having child list "five good things and five bad things" about it.

Is an exceptionally valuable technique when applied to relationships, such as things family members like and dislike about each other.

NONVERBAL TECHNIQUES

Writing

Is an alternative communication approach for older children and adults.

Specific suggestions include:
- Keep a journal or diary.
- Write down feelings or thoughts that are difficult to express.
- Write "letters" that are never mailed (a variation is making up a "pen pal" to write to).
- Keep an account of child's progress from both a physical and an emotional viewpoint.

Drawing

Is one of the most valuable forms of communication—both nonverbal (from looking at the drawing) and verbal (from child's story of the picture).

Children's drawings tell a great deal about them because they are projections of their inner selves.

Spontaneous drawing involves giving child a variety of art supplies and providing the opportunity to draw.

Directed drawing involves a more specific direction, such as "draw a person" or the "three themes" approach (state three things about child and ask child to choose one and draw a picture).

Guidelines for Evaluating Drawings

Use spontaneous drawings and evaluate more than one drawing whenever possible.

Interpret drawings in light of other available information about child and family.

Interpret drawings as a whole rather than on specific details of the drawing.

Consider individual elements of the drawing that may be significant:
- ***Sex of figure drawn first***—Usually relates to child's perception of own sex role.
- ***Size of individual figures***—Expresses importance, power, or authority.
- ***Order in which figures are drawn***—Expresses priority in terms of importance.
- ***Child's position in relation to other family members***—Expresses feelings of status or alliance.
- ***Exclusion of a member***—May denote feeling of not belonging or desire to eliminate.
- ***Accentuated parts***—Usually express concern for not belonging or desire to eliminate.
- ***Absence of or rudimentary arms and hands***—Suggest timidity, passivity, or intellectual immaturity; tiny, unstable feet may be an expression of insecurity, and hidden hands may mean guilt feelings.
- ***Placement of drawing on the page and type of stroke***—Free use of paper and firm, continuous strokes express security, whereas drawings restricted to a small area and lightly drawn in broken or wavering lines may be a sign of insecurity.
- ***Erasures, shading, or cross-hatching***—Expresses ambivalence, concern, or anxiety with a particular area.

Magic

Uses simple magic tricks to help establish rapport with child, encourage compliance with health interventions, and provide effective distraction during painful procedures.

Although "magician" talks, no verbal response from child is required.

Play

Is universal language and "work" of children.

Tells a great deal about children because they project their inner selves through the activity.

Spontaneous play involves giving child a variety of play materials and providing the opportunity to play.

Directed play involves a more specific direction, such as providing medical equipment or a dollhouse for focused reasons, such as exploring child's fear of injections or exploring family relationships.

Communication Techniques

In addition to such conventional interviewing methods as reflection and open-ended questions, a number of techniques encourage family members to express their thoughts and feelings in a less directive and confrontational manner. Several approaches are projective—they present nonspecific material that enables individuals to externalize or project inner aspects of themselves to others.

A variety of verbal techniques can be used to encourage communication. Some of these techniques can be used to pose questions or explore concerns in a less threatening manner. Others can be presented as "word games," which are often well received by children. For many children and adults, however, talking about feelings is difficult and verbal communication may be more stressful than supportive. In such instances several nonverbal techniques can be used to encourage communication.

Both verbal and nonverbal techniques are described in Box 34-3. Because of the importance of play in communicating with children, play is discussed more extensively later in this chapter. Any of the verbal or nonverbal techniques can give rise to strong feelings that surface unexpectedly. Be prepared to handle them or to recognize when issues go beyond your ability to deal with them. At that point, consider an appropriate referral.

Play. Play is a universal language of children. It is one of the most important forms of communication and can be an effective technique in relating to them. Clues about physical, intellectual, and social developmental progress can often be gleaned from the form and complexity of a child's play behaviors. Play requires a minimum of equipment or none at all. Therapeutic play is often used to reduce the trauma of illness and hospitalization (see Chapter 44) and to prepare children for therapeutic procedures (see Chapter 45).

Because their ability to perceive precedes their ability to transmit, small infants respond to activities that register on their senses. Patting, stroking, and other skin play convey messages. Repetitive actions, such as stretching infants' arms out to the side while they are lying on their back and then folding them across the chest or raising and revolving the legs in a bicycling motion, will elicit pleasurable sounds. Colorful items to catch the eye; or interesting sounds, such as a ticking clock, chimes, bells, or singing, can be used to attract children's attention.

Older infants respond to simple games. The old game of peekaboo is an excellent means of initiating communication with infants while maintaining a "safe," nonthreatening distance. After this intermittent eye-to-eye contact, the nurse is no longer viewed as a stranger but as someone who is a friend. This can be followed by touch games. Clapping an infant's hands together for pat-a-cake or wiggling the toes for "this little piggy" delights an infant or small child. Much of the nursing assessment can be carried out with the use of games and simple play equipment while the infant remains in the safety of the parent's arms or lap. Talking to a foot or other part of the child's body is an effective tactic.

The nurse can capitalize on the natural curiosity of small children by playing games such as "Which hand do you take?" and "Guess what I have in my hand," or by manipulating items such as a flashlight or stethoscope. Finger games are very useful. More elaborate materials, such as puppets and replicas of familiar or unfamiliar items, serve as excellent means of communicating with small children. The variety and extent are limited only by the nurse's imagination.

Through play, children reveal their perceptions of interpersonal relationships with their family, friends, or hospital personnel. Children may also reveal the wide scope of knowledge they have acquired from listening to others around them. For example, through needle play, children may disclose how carefully they have watched each procedure by precisely duplicating the technical skills. They may also reveal how well they remember those who performed procedures. One child who painstakingly reenacted every detail of a tedious medical procedure also played the role of the physician who had repeatedly shouted at her to be still for the long ordeal. Her anger at him was most evident during the play session and revealed the cause for her abrupt withdrawal and passive hostility toward the medical and nursing staff following the test.

Play sessions serve not only as assessment tools for determining children's awareness and perceptions of their illness, but also as methods of intervention and evaluation. In the previous example, when the child revealed anger toward the physician, the nurse acted the part of the patient but this time did not accept the physician's harsh commands to stay still. Instead, the nurse said to the physician all the things the child had wished she could say.

Subsequent play sessions can also be used to evaluate the child's progress. A change in the type of drawing or the theme of the play may indicate progression toward or away from the ability to deal with anxiety.

HISTORY TAKING

Performing a Health History

The format used for history taking may be (1) *direct*—the nurse asks for information via direct interview with the informant; or (2) *indirect*—the informant supplies the information by completing some type of questionnaire. The direct method is superior to either the indirect approach or a combination of approaches. However, in view of time constraints, the direct approach is not always practical. If the direct approach cannot be used, review parents' written responses and question them regarding any unusual answers. The categories listed in Box 34-4 encompass children's current and past health status and information about their psychosocial environment.

Identifying Information. Much of the identifying information may already be available from other recorded sources. However, if the parent and youngster seem anxious, use this opportunity to ask about such information to help them feel more comfortable.

Informant. One of the important elements of information is identifying the informant, the person(s) who furnished the information. Record (1) who the persons is (e.g., child, parent, or other); (2) an impression of this person's reliability and willingness to communicate; and (3) any special circumstances, such as the use of an interpreter or conflicting answers by more than one person.

Chief Complaint. The chief complaint is the specific reason for the child's visit to the clinic, office, or hospital. It may be viewed as the theme with the present illness as the description of the problem. The chief complaint is elicited by asking open-ended neutral questions such as "What seems to be the matter?" "How may I help you?" or "Why did you come here today?" Avoid labeling-type questions such as "How are you sick?" or "What is the problem?" since it is possible that the reason for the visit is not an illness or problem.

Occasionally it is difficult to isolate one symptom or problem as the chief complaint because the parent may identify many. In this situation be as specific as possible when asking questions. For example, asking informants to state which one problem or symptom prompted them to seek help now may help them focus on the most immediate concern.

Present Illness. The history of the present illness* is a narrative of the chief complaint from its earliest onset through its progression to the present. Its four major components are (1) the details of *onset,* (2) a complete *interval* history, (3) the *present* status, and (4) the reason for seeking help *now.* The focus of the present illness is on all factors relevant to the main problem, even if they have disappeared or changed during the onset, interval, and present.

*The term *illness* is used in its broadest sense to denote any problem of a physical, emotional, or psychosocial nature. It is actually a history of the chief complaint.

Box 34-4

Outline of a Pediatric Health History

IDENTIFYING INFORMATION

1. Name
2. Address
3. Telephone
4. Birthdate and place
5. Race/ethnic group
6. Sex
7. Religion
8. Date of interview
9. Informant

CHIEF COMPLAINT (CC)

To establish the major *specific* reason for the child's and parents' seeking professional health attention

PRESENT ILLNESS (PI)

To obtain *all* details related to the chief complaint.

PAST HISTORY (PH)

To elicit a profile of the child's previous illnesses, injuries, or operations

1. Birth history (pregnancy, labor, and delivery, perinatal history)
2. Previous illnesses, injuries, or operations
3. Allergies
4. Current medications
5. Immunizations
6. Growth and development
7. Habits

REVIEW OF SYSTEMS (ROS)

To elicit information concerning any potential health problem

1. General
2. Integument
3. Head
4. Eyes
5. Ears
6. Nose
7. Mouth
8. Throat
9. Neck
10. Chest
11. Respiratory
12. Cardiovascular
13. Gastrointestinal
14. Genitourinary
15. Gynecologic
16. Musculoskeletal
17. Neurologic
18. Endocrine

FAMILY MEDICAL HISTORY

To identify the presence of genetic traits or diseases that have familial tendencies and to assess exposure to a communicable disease in a family member and family habits that may affect the child's health, such as smoking and other chemical use.

PSYCHOSOCIAL HISTORY

To elicit information about the child's self-concept.

SEXUAL HISTORY

To elicit information concerning the child's sexual concerns and/or activities and any pertinent data regarding adults' sexual activity that influence the child

FAMILY HISTORY

To develop an understanding of the child as an individual and as a member of a family and a community

1. Family composition
2. Home and community environment
3. Occupation and education of family members
4. Cultural and religious traditions
5. Family function and relationships

NUTRITIONAL ASSESSMENT

To elicit information on the adequacy of the child's nutritional intake and need

1. Dietary intake
2. Clinical examination

Analyzing a Symptom. Because pain is often the most characteristic symptom denoting the onset of a physical problem, it is used as an example for analysis of a symptom. Assessment includes (1) type, (2) location, (3) severity, (4) duration, and (5) influencing factors (Guidelines box; see also Pain Assessment, Chapter 44).

Past History. The past history contains information relating to all previous aspects of the child's health status and concentrates on several areas that are ordinarily deleted in the history of an adult, such as birth history, detailed feeding history, immunizations, and growth and development. Since a great deal of information is included in this section, use a combination of open-ended and fact-finding questions. For example, begin interviewing for each section with an open-ended statement such as "Tell me about your child's birth" in order to provide the informants with the opportunity to relate what they think is most important. Ask fact-finding questions related to specific details whenever necessary to focus the interview on certain topics.

Birth History. The birth history includes all data concerning (1) the mother's health during pregnancy, (2) the labor and delivery, and (3) the infant's condition immediately after birth. Since prenatal influences have significant effects on a child's physical and emotional development, a thorough investigation of the birth history is essential. Because parents may question what relevance pregnancy and birth have on the child's present condition, particularly if the child is past infancy, explain why such questions are included. An appropriate statement may be, "I will be asking you some questions about your pregnancy and . . . (refer to child by name) birth. Your answers will give me a more complete picture of his (or her) overall health."

Because emotional factors also affect the outcome of pregnancy and the subsequent parent-child relationship, investigate (1) concurrent crises during pregnancy and (2) prenatal attitudes toward the fetus. It is best to approach the topic of parental acceptance of pregnancy through indirect questioning. Asking parents if the pregnancy was planned is a leading statement because they may respond affirmatively for fear of criticism if the pregnancy was unexpected. Rather, encourage parents to disclose their true reactions by referring to specific facts relating to the pregnancy, such as the spacing between offspring, an extended or short interval between marriage and conception, or the concurrent experience of pregnancy and adolescence. The parent can choose to explore such statements

Guidelines

ANALYZING THE SYMPTOM: PAIN

Type. Be as specific as possible. With young children, asking the parents how they know the child is in pain may help describe its type, location, and severity. For example, a parent may state, "My child must have a severe earache because she pulls at her ears, rolls her head on the floor, and screams. Nothing seems to help." Help older children describe the "hurt" by asking them if it is sharp, throbbing, dull, or stabbing. Record whatever words they use in quotes.

Location. Be specific. "Stomach pains" is too general a description. Children can better localize the pain if they are asked to "point with one finger to where it hurts" or to "point to where Mommy or Daddy would put a Band-Aid." Determine if the pain radiates by asking. "Does the pain stay there or move? Show me with your finger where the pain goes."

Severity. Severity is best determined by finding out how it affects the child's usual behavior. Pain that prevents a child from playing, interacting with others, sleeping, and eating is most often severe. Assess pain intensity using a rating scale, such as numeric scale or faces scale (see Table 44-2).

Duration. Include the duration, onset, and frequency. Describe this in terms of activity and behavior, such as "pain lasted all night, because child refused to sleep and cried intermittently."

Influencing factor. Include anything that causes a change in the type, location, severity, or duration of the pain: (1) precipitating events (those that cause or increase the pain), (2) relieving events (those that lessen the pain, such as medications), (3) temporal events (times when the pain is relieved or increased), (4) positional events (standing, sitting, lying down), and (5) associated events (meals, stress, coughing).

with further explanations or, for the moment, may not be able to reveal such feelings. If the parent remains silent, refocus on this topic later in the interview.

Dietary History. Because parental concerns are common and nursing interventions are important in ensuring optimum nutrition, the dietary history is discussed in detail at the end of this chapter under Nutritional Assessment.

Previous Illnesses, Injuries, and Operations. When inquiring about past illnesses, begin with a general statement such as "What other illnesses has your child had?" Since parents are most likely to recall serious health problems, ask specifically about colds; earaches; and childhood diseases such as measles, rubella (German measles), chickenpox, mumps, pertussis (whooping cough), diphtheria, tuberculosis, scarlet fever, strep throat, tonsillitis, and allergic manifestations.

In addition to illnesses, ask about injuries that required medical intervention, operations, and any other reason for hospitalization, including the dates of each incident. It is important to focus on injuries such as accidental falls, poisonings, chokings, or burns, since this may be a potential area for parental guidance.

Allergies. Ask about commonly known allergic disorders such as hay fever and asthma, as well as unusual reactions to drugs, food, or latex products, or other contact agents such as poisonous plants, animals, household products, or fabrics. If asked appropriate questions, most people can give reliable information about drug reactions. Documentation of a drug allergy must include the information found in the Guidelines box (Cantrill and Cottrell, 1997).

Guidelines

TAKING AN ALLERGY HISTORY

Has your child ever taken any drugs or tablets that have disagreed or caused an allergy? If yes, can you remember the name(s) of these drugs?
Can you describe the reaction?
Was the drug by mouth (as a tablet or medicine), or was it an injection?
How soon after starting the drug did the reaction happen?
How long ago did this happen?
Did anyone tell you it was an *allergic* reaction, or did you decide for yourself?
Has your child ever taken this drug, or a similar one, again? If yes, did your child experience the same problems?
Have you told the doctors or nurses about your child's reaction or allergy?

Modified from Cantrill JA, Cottrell WN: Accuracy of drug allergy documentation, *Am J Health Syst Pharm* 54:1627-1629, 1997.

NURSE ALERT • Information about allergic reactions to drugs or other products is essential. Failure to document a serious reaction places the child at risk if the agent is given.

Current Medications. Inquire about current drug regimens, including vitamins, antipyretics (especially aspirin), antibiotics, antihistamines, decongestants, or antitussives. List all medications, including name, dose, schedule, duration, and reason for administration. Often parents are unaware of the actual name of the drug. Whenever possible, ask parents to bring the containers with them to the next visit, or ask them for the name of the pharmacy and call for a list of all the child's recent prescription medications. However, this list will not include over-the-counter medications. Since parents may give their child medications not prescribed by the physician, a careful assessment must include all drugs or alternative medicines (Hocking and deMello, 1997).

Immunizations. A record of all immunizations is essential. Since many parents are unaware of the exact name and date of each immunization, the most reliable source of information is a hospital, clinic, or private practitioner's record. All immunizations and "boosters" are listed, stating (1) the name of the specific disease, (2) the number of injections, (3) the dosage (sometimes lesser amounts are given if a reaction is anticipated), (4) the ages when administered, and (5) the occurrence of any reaction following the immunization.

NURSE ALERT • Inquire about previous administration of any horse or other foreign serum, recent administration of gamma globulin or blood transfusion, and anaphylactic reactions to neomycin or chicken eggs.

Growth and Development. The most important previous growth patterns to record are (1) approximate weight at 6 months, 1 year, 2 years, and 5 years of age; (2) approximate length at ages 1 and 4 years; and (3) dentition, including age of onset, number of teeth, and symptoms during teething. Developmental milestones include (1) age of holding up head steadily; (2) age of sitting alone without support; (3) age of walking without assistance; (4) age of saying first words with meaning; (5) present grade in school; (6) scholastic grades; and (7) interaction with other children, peers, and adults.

Use specific and detailed questions when inquiring about each developmental milestone. For example "sitting up" can mean many different activities, such as sitting propped up, sitting in someone's lap, sitting with support, sitting up alone but in a hyperflexed position for assisted balance, or sitting up unsupported with the back slightly rounded. A clue to misunderstanding of the requested activity may be an unusually early age of achievement (see Developmental Assessment, Chapter 35).

Habits. Habits are an important area to explore (Box 34-5). Parents often express concerns during this part of the history. Encourage their input by saying, "Please tell me any concerns you have about your child's habits, activities, or development." Investigate further any concerns that are expressed.

One of the most common concerns relates to sleep. Many children develop a normal sleep pattern, and all that is required during the assessment is a general overview of nighttime sleep and nap schedules. However, a number of children also develop sleep problems (see Sleep Problems, Chapters 36 and 38). When sleep problems occur, a more detailed sleep history is required in order to guide appropriate interventions.*

Habits related to use of chemicals apply primarily to older children and adolescents. If a youngster admits to smoking, drinking, or drug use, ask about the quantity and frequency. Questions such as "Have you ever had a drinking or drug problem?" or "When was the last time you had a drink or took drugs?" may yield more reliable data than questions such as "How much do you drink?" or "How often do you drink or take drugs?" Clarify that "drinking" includes all types of alcohol, such as beer and wine. When quantities such as a "glass" of wine or a "can" of beer are given, ask about the size of the container.

If older children deny use of chemical substances, inquire about past experimentation. Asking, "You mean you never tried to smoke or drink?" implies that the nurse expects some such activity, and the youngster may be more inclined to answer truthfully. Be aware of the confidential nature of such questioning, the adverse effect that the parents' presence may have on the adolescent's willingness to answer, and that self-report may not be an accurate account of chemical abuse.

Review of Systems. The review of systems is a specific review of each body system, similar to the order of the physical examination (Box 34-6). Often the history of the present illness provides a complete review of the system involved in the chief complaint. Since asking questions about other body systems may appear unrelated and irrelevant to the parents or child, precede the questioning with an explanation of why the data are needed (similar to the explanation concerning the relevance of the birth history) and reassure the parents that the child's main problem has not been forgotten.

Begin the review of a specific system with a broad statement such as "How has your child's general health been?" or "Has your child had any problems with his eyes?" If the parent states that there have been past problems with some bodily function, pursue this with an encouraging statement such as "Tell me more about that." If the parent denies any problems, query for specific symptoms (e.g., "No headaches, bumping into objects, or squinting?"). If the parent reconfirms the absence of such symptoms, record positive statements in the history, such as "Mother denies headaches, bumping into objects, or squinting." In this way, anyone who reviews the health history is aware of exactly what symptoms were investigated.

*A sleep history and a sleep chart for the family to record the child's daily sleep and wake activities is available in Wong DL, Hess CS: ***Wong and Whaley's clinical manual of pediatric nursing,*** ed 5, St Louis, 2000, Mosby.

Box 34-5

Habits to Explore During the Health Interview

- Behavior patterns such as nail biting, thumb sucking, pica (habitual ingestion of nonfood substances), rituals ("security" blanket or toy), and unusual movements (head banging, rocking, overt masturbation, and walking on toes)
- Activities of daily living, such as hour of sleep and arising, duration of nighttime sleep and naps, type and duration of exercise, regularity of stools and urination, age of toilet training, and occurrences of daytime or nighttime bed-wetting
- Unusual disposition, as well as response to frustration
- Use or abuse of alcohol, drugs, coffee, or tobacco

Family Medical History. The family medical history is used primarily for the purpose of discovering the potential existence of hereditary or familial diseases in the parent and child. In general, it is confined to first-degree relatives (i.e., parents, siblings, grandparents, and immediate aunts and uncles). Information for each family member includes age, marital status, state of health if living, cause of death if deceased, and any evidence of the following conditions: heart disease, hypertension, cancer, diabetes mellitus, tuberculosis, sickle cell disease, mental retardation, mental disorders such as depression or psychosis, emotional problems, syphilis, or rheumatic fever. Confirm the accuracy of the reported disorders by inquiring about the symptoms, course, treatment, and sequelae of each diagnosis.

Geographic Location. One of the important areas to explore when assessing the family health history is geographic location, including the birthplace and travel to different areas in or outside of the country, for identification of possible exposure to endemic diseases. Although the primary interest focuses on the child's temporary residence in various localities, also inquire about close family members' travel, especially during tours of military service or business trips. Children are especially susceptible to parasitic infestation in areas of poor sanitary conditions and to vector-borne diseases, such as those from mosquitoes or ticks in warm and humid or heavily wooded regions.

Psychosocial History. The traditional medical history includes a personal and social section that concentrates on children's personal status (e.g., school adjustment and any unusual habits) and the family and home environment. Since several personal aspects are covered under development and habits, and the social aspects are discussed in detail under Family Assessment, only those issues related to children's ability to cope and their general view of themselves in terms of self-concept are presented here (see Development of Self-Concept, Chapter 33).

Through observation, obtain a general idea of how children handle themselves in terms of confidence in dealing with others, ability to answer questions, and coping with new situations. Observe the parent-child relationship for the types of messages sent to children about their coping skills and self-worth. Do the parents treat the child with respect, focusing on strengths; or is

Box 34-6

Guidelines for Review of Systems

General—Overall state of health, fatigue, recent and/or unexplained weight gain or loss (period of time for either), contributing factors (change of diet, illness, altered appetite), exercise tolerance, fevers (time of day), chills, night sweats (unrelated to climatic conditions), frequent infections, general ability to carry out activities of daily living

Integument—Pruritus, pigment or other color changes, acne, eruptions, rashes (location), tendency for bruising, petechiae, excessive dryness, general texture, disorders or deformities of nails, hair growth or loss, hair color change (for adolescent, use of hair dyes or other potentially toxic substances, such as hair straighteners)

Head—Headaches, dizziness, injury (specific details)

Eyes—Visual problems (ask about behaviors indicative of blurred vision, such as bumping into objects, clumsiness, sitting very close to television, holding a book close to face, writing with head near desk, squinting, rubbing the eyes, bending head in an awkward position), cross-eye (strabismus), eye infections, edema of lids, excessive tearing, use of glasses or contact lenses, date of last optic examination

Nose—Nosebleeds (epistaxis), constant or frequent runny or stuffy nose, nasal obstruction (difficulty in breathing), alteration or loss of sense of smell

Ears—Earaches, discharge, evidence of hearing loss (ask about behaviors, such as need to repeat requests, loud speech, inattentive behavior), results of any previous auditory testing

Mouth—Mouth breathing, gum bleeding, toothaches, toothbrushing, use of fluoride, difficulty with teething (symptoms), last visit to dentist (especially if temporary dentition is complete), response to dentist

Throat—Sore throats, difficulty in swallowing, choking (especially when chewing food—may be from poor chewing habits), hoarseness, or other voice irregularities

Neck—Pain, limitation of movement, stiffness, difficulty in holding head straight (torticollis), thyroid enlargement, enlarged nodes or other masses

Chest—Breast enlargement, discharge, masses, enlarged axillary nodes (for adolescent female, ask about breast self-examination)

Respiratory—Chronic cough, frequent colds (number per year), wheezing, shortness of breath at rest or on exertion, difficulty in breathing, sputum production, infections (pneumonia, tuberculosis), date of last chest x-ray examination, and skin reaction from tuberculin testing

Cardiovascular—Cyanosis or fatigue on exertion, history of heart murmur or rheumatic fever, anemia, date of last blood count, blood type, recent transfusion

Gastrointestinal (much of this in regard to appetite, food tolerance, and elimination habits has been asked elsewhere)—Nausea, vomiting (not associated with eating, may be indicative of brain tumor or increased intracranial pressure), jaundice or yellowing skin or sclera, belching, flatulence, recent change in bowel habits (blood in stools, change of color, diarrhea, or constipation)

Genitourinary—Pain on urination, frequency, hesitancy, urgency, hematuria, nocturia, polyuria, unpleasant odor to urine, force of stream, discharge, change in size of scrotum, date of last urinalysis (for adolescent, sexually transmitted disease, type of treatment; for male adolescent, ask about testicular self-examination)

Gynecologic—Menarche, date of last menstrual period, regularity or problems with menstruation, vaginal discharge, pruritus, date and result of last Pap smear (include obstetric history as discussed under birth history when applicable); if sexually active, type of contraception, sexually transmitted disease and type of treatment

Musculoskeletal—Weakness, clumsiness, lack of coordination, unusual movements, back or joint stiffness, muscle pains or cramps, abnormal gait, deformity, fractures, serious sprains, activity level

Neurologic—Seizures, tremors, dizziness, loss of memory, general affect, fears, nightmares, speech problems, any unusual habits

Endocrine—Intolerance to weather changes, excessive thirst and/or urination, excessive sweating, salty taste to skin, signs of early puberty

the interaction one of constant reprimands, with emphasis on weaknesses and faults? Do the parents help the child learn new coping strategies or support the ones the child uses?

Messages about body image are also conveyed through the parent-child interaction. Do the parents label the child and body parts, such as "bad boy," "skinny legs," or "ugly scar"? Do the parents handle the child gently, using soothing touch to calm an anxious child, or do they treat the child roughly, using slaps or restraint to force compliance? If the child touches certain parts of the body, such as the genitals, do the parents make comments that suggest a negative connotation?

With older children many of the communication strategies discussed earlier in the chapter are useful in eliciting more definitive information about their coping and self-concept. Children can write down five things they like and dislike about themselves. Sentence completion statements such as "The thing I like best (or worst) about myself is ____________," "If I could change one thing about myself, it would be ____________," or "When I am scared, I ____________," can be used.

Sexual History. The sexual history is an essential component of adolescents' health assessment. The history uncovers areas of concern related to sexual activity, alerts the nurse to circumstances that may indicate screening for sexually transmitted diseases or testing for pregnancy, and provides information related to the need for sexual counseling, such as safe sex practices (Wright, 1997).

One approach toward initiating a conversation about sexual concerns is to begin with a history of peer interactions. Open-ended statements such as "Tell me about your social life," or "Who are your closest friends?" generally lead into a discussion of dating and sexual issues. To probe further, include questions about the adolescent's attitudes on such topics as sex education, "going steady," "living together," and premarital sex. Phrase questions to reflect concern rather than judgment or criticism of sexual practices.

In any conversation regarding sexual history, be aware of the language that is used in either eliciting or conveying sexual information. For example, avoid asking if the adolescent is "sexually active," since this term is broadly defined. "Are you having sex with anyone?" is probably the most direct and best understood question. Since homosexual experimentation may occur, refer to all sexual contacts in nongender terms, such as "anyone" or "partners," rather than "girlfriends" or "boyfriends."

A detailed account of sexual partners is needed if the patient has a history of, displays any of the symptoms of, or asks for treatment of a sexually transmitted infection. A difficult but necessary part of the interview is to determine the sites of possible infection. Since sexual diseases can be contracted at any of the body orifices, inform the adolescent that a sexually transmitted disease can be acquired without visible signs of disease at nongenital sites.

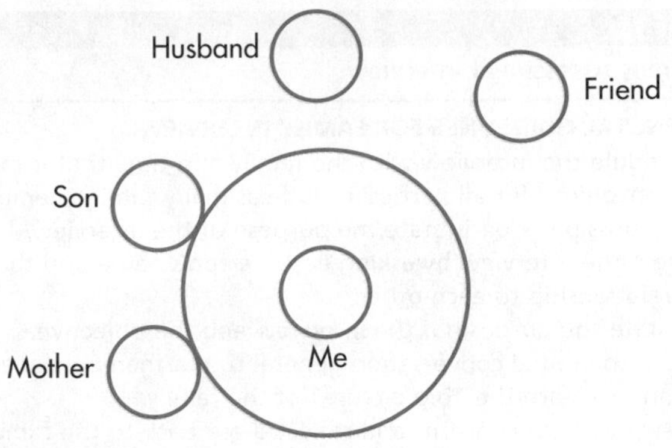

FIG. 34-4 • Sociogram of mother with strong, unresolved grief feelings regarding loss of child.

FAMILY ASSESSMENT

Assessment of the family, both its structure and function, is an important component of the history-taking process. Because the quality of the functional relationship between the child and family members is a major factor in emotional and physical health, family assessment is discussed separately and in greater detail apart from the more traditional health history.

Family assessment is the collection of data about the composition of the family and the relationships among its members. In its broadest sense, *family* refers to all those individuals who are considered by the family member to be significant to the nuclear unit, including relatives, friends, and other social groups such as the school and church. Although family assessment is not family therapy, it can and often is therapeutic. Involving family members in discussing family characteristics and activities often stimulates productive discussion and insight into family dynamics and relationships.

Because of the time involved in performing an in-depth family assessment as presented here, be selective in deciding when knowledge of family function may facilitate nursing care. During brief contacts with families, a full assessment is not appropriate, and screening with one or two questions from each category may reflect the health of the family system or the potential need for additional assessment.

Assessment of Family Structure

Family structure refers to the composition of the family—who lives in the home and those social, cultural, religious, and economic characteristics that influence the child's and family's overall psychobiologic health (Wright and Leahey, 1999) (see also Chapters 31 and 32). Since the information elicited in this part of the history is often the most personal and confidential, include it toward the end of the interview when rapport is well established.

The most common method of eliciting information on the family structure is to interview family members. The principal areas of concern (Box 34-7) are the following: (1) family composition, (2) home and community environment, (3) occupation and education of family members, and (4) cultural and religious traditions.

NURSE ALERT • **In assessing family composition, it is sometimes difficult to ascertain the status of the adult relationships. If the parent fails to mention the other parent, ask, "Where is the child's father (or mother)?" Avoid saying "husband" or "wife" because this assumes that only marital relationships exist.**

Several structural assessment tools can be used to collect and record data about the family composition and environment. Like the interview method, such tools also provide information about relationships, although several additional methods should be used to assess family function.

A *sociogram* is a drawing of circles that indicates the significant persons in an individual's life; its use is appropriate for adults and children as young as 5 years of age. The person is given blank paper and a pencil with the instructions: "Draw a circle to represent you. Around the circle draw circles to show the most significant persons in your life and label each. Draw the circles near to your circle to represent closeness. For example, the person who is most important is the circle closest to you." Family members can label the relationships as supportive with a plus sign or negative with a minus sign.

Not only is the sociogram a portrait of the person's significant relationships, it may also uncover unresolved relationships (Fig. 34-4). After completing the sociogram, encourage the family to explore their feelings further with questions such as:

- How would you change the circles to improve relationships?
- How do you think you could accomplish these changes?
- If one person in the circle were to change, what effect do you think that would have on others in the circle?

Assessment of Family Function

Family function is concerned with how the family behaves toward one another and with the quality of the relationships (see also Chapter 31). It is considered the most important component in determining "family health." Assessment of function requires more skill on the part of the interviewer than does assessment of structure and is best approached after structure is assessed. As in assessment of family structure, the more traditional method of eliciting information on family function is by interviewing family members. For principal areas of concern, see Box 34-7.

Box 34-7

Family Assessment Interview

GENERAL GUIDELINES FOR FAMILY INTERVIEW

Schedule the interview with the family at a time that is most convenient for all parties; include as many family members as possible; clearly state the purpose of the interview.
Begin the interview by asking each person's name and their relationship to each other.
Restate the purpose of the interview and the objective.
Keep the initial conversation general to put members at ease and to learn the "big picture" of the family.
Identify major concerns and reflect these back to the family to be certain that all parties perceive the same message.
Terminate the interview with a summary of what was discussed and a plan for additional sessions if needed.

STRUCTURAL ASSESSMENT AREAS

Family Composition

Immediate members of the household (names, ages, and relationships)
Significant extended family members
Previous marriages, separations, death of spouses, or divorces

Home and Community Environment

Type of dwelling/number of rooms/occupants
Sleeping arrangements
Number of floors, accessibility of stairs, elevators
Adequacy of utilities
Safety features (fire escape, smoke and carbon monoxide detectors, guardrails on windows, use of car restraint)
Environmental hazards (e.g., chipped paint, poor sanitation, pollution, heavy street traffic)
Availability and location of health facilities, schools, play areas
Relationship with neighbors
Recent crises or changes in home
Child's reaction/adjustment to recent stresses

Occupation and Education of Family Members

Types of employment
Work schedules
Work satisfaction
Exposure to environmental/industrial hazards
Sources of income and adequacy
Effect of illness on financial status
Highest degree or grade level attained

Cultural and Religious Traditions

Religious beliefs and practices
Cultural/ethnic beliefs and practices
Language spoken in home

Assessment Questions Include:

Does the family identify with a particular religious/ethnic group? Are both parents from that group?
How is religious/ethnic background part of family life?
What special religious/cultural traditions are practiced in the home (e.g., food choices and preparation)?
Where were family members born, and how long have they lived in this country?
What language does the family speak most frequently?
Do they speak/understand English?
What do they believe causes health or illness?
What religious/ethnic beliefs influence the family's perception of illness and its treatment?
What methods are used to prevent/treat illness?
How does the family know when a health problem needs medical attention?
Who is the person the family contacts when a member is ill?
Does the family rely on cultural/religious healers or remedies? If so, ask them to describe the type of healer or remedy.
Who does the family go to for support (clergy, medical healer, relatives)?
Does the family experience discrimination because of their race, beliefs, or practices? Ask them to describe.

FUNCTIONAL ASSESSMENT AREAS

Family Interactions and Roles

Interactions refer to ways family members relate to each other.
Chief concern is amount of intimacy and closeness among the members, especially spouses.
Roles refer to behaviors of people as they assume a different status or position.

Observations include:

Family members' responses to each other (cordial, hostile, cool, loving, patient, short-tempered)
Obvious roles of leadership vs submission
Support and attention shown to various members

Assessment Questions Include:

What activities do the family perform together?
Whom do family members talk to when something is bothering them?
What are members' household chores?
Who usually oversees what is happening with the children, such as at school or concerning their health?
How easy or difficult is it for the family to change or accept new responsibilities for household tasks?

Power, Decision Making, and Problem Solving

Power refers to individual member's control over others in family: manifested through family decision making and problem solving.
Chief concern is clarity of boundaries of power between parents and children.
One method of assessment involves offering a hypothetical conflict or problem, such as a child failing school, and asking family how they would handle this situation.

Assessment Questions Include:

Who usually makes the decisions in the family?
If one parent makes a decision, can the child appeal to the other parent to change it?
What input do children have in making decisions or discussing rules?
Who makes and enforces the rules?
What happens when a rule is broken?

Communication

Communication is concerned with clarity and directness of communication patterns.

Box 34-7

Family Assessment Interview—cont'd

Further assessment includes periodically asking family members if they understood what was just said and to repeat the message.

Observations Include:

Who speaks to whom
If one person speaks for another or interrupts
If members appear disinterested when certain individuals speak
If there is agreement between verbal and nonverbal messages

Assessment Questions Include:

How often do family members wait until others are through talking before "having their say?"
Do parents or older siblings tend to lecture and preach?
Do parents tend to talk "down" to the children?

Expression of Feelings and Individuality

Expressions are concerned with personal space and freedom to grow with limits and structure needed for guidance.
Observing patterns of communication offers clues to how freely feelings are expressed.

Assessment Questions Include:

Is it OK for family members to get angry or sad?
Who gets angry most of the time? What do they do?
If someone is upset, how do other family members try to comfort this person?
Who comforts specific family members?
When someone wants to do something, such as try out for a new sport or get a job, what is the family's response (offer assistance, discouragement, or no advice)?

Box 34-8

Family Apgar

DEFINITION	FUNCTIONS MEASURED BY THE FAMILY APGAR	RELEVANT OPEN-ENDED QUESTIONS
Adaptation is the use of intrafamilial and extrafamilial resources for problem solving when family equilibrium is stressed during a crisis.	How resources are shared, or the degree to which a member is satisfied with the assistance received when family resources are needed	How have family members aided each other in time of need? In what way have family members received help or assistance from friends and community agencies?
Partnership is the sharing of decision-making and nurturing responsibilities by family members.	How decisions are shared, or the member's satisfaction with mutuality in family communication and problem solving	How do family members communicate with each other about such matters as vacations, finances, medical care, large purchases, and personal problems?
Growth is the physical and emotional maturation and self-fulfillment that is achieved by family members through mutual support and guidance.	How nurturing is shared, or the member's satisfaction with the freedom available within the family to change roles and attain physical and emotional growth or maturation	How have family members changed during the past years? How has this change been accepted by family members? In what ways have family members aided each other in growing or developing independent lifestyles?
Affection is the caring or loving relationship that exists among family members.	How emotional experiences are shared, or the member's satisfaction with the intimacy and emotional interaction that exists in the family	How have family members reacted to your desire for change? How have members of your family responded to emotional expressions, such as affection, love, sorrow, or anger?
Resolve is the commitment to devote time to other members of the family for physical and emotional nurturing. It also usually involves a decision to share wealth and space.	How time (and space and money) is shared, or the member's satisfaction with the time commitment that has been made to the family by its members	How do members of your family share time, space, and money?

Modified from Smilkstein G: The Family Apgar: a proposal for a family function test and its use by physicians, *J Fam Pract* 6(6):1231-1239, 1978.

In addition to observing and interviewing the family to assess family function, several other methods are available and should be used as needed to obtain a comprehensive assessment. In the following section selected instruments are discussed that are reliable and valid, but that require little or no formal training and only minimal time to administer.

The *Family Apgar (FAPGAR)* is a brief screening questionnaire designed to reflect a family member's satisfaction with the functional state of the family (Smilkstein, Ashworth, and Montano, 1982) (see Appendix B). The acronym APGAR is for *A*daptation, *P*artnership, *G*rowth, *A*ffection, and *R*esolve (commitment). The acronym was chosen because it is familiar to health professionals, but it bears no relationship to the Apgar scoring system for newborns.

The questions in Box 34-8 can be used in the interview without the Apgar ratings to elicit similar types of information. It can be completed in about 5 minutes, can be used by families with traditional and alternative lifestyles and from different cultures, and is appropriate for children 10 years of age or older. Separate forms have been designed to assess relationships with friends and fellow workers, since these groups represent other significant sources of support.

The responses to the five questions are scored as follows: "Almost always"—2; "Some of the time"—1; and "Hardly ever"—0. Each score is totaled. Scores of 7 to 10 suggest a highly functional family; 4 to 6, a moderately dysfunctional family; and 0 to 3, a severely dysfunctional family. Also, a low score in any single item could signal family dysfunction. The family Apgar is not recommended for use with individuals from enmeshed (overly close) or "psychosomatic" families (Murphy et al, 1998). Persons with health problems, such as asthma, atopic dermatitis, or irritable bowel syndrome, may report falsely high scores (Smilkstein, 1993).

The *Feetham Family Functioning Survey* provides information about family members' *perception* of relationships that contribute to or are affected by family functioning* (Feetham, Perkins, and Carroll, 1992). Although recommended primarily as a research instrument, it can be used clinically without scoring the items to identify areas that may be of concern to the family. The survey consists of 25 ratings of family functioning (e.g., household tasks; child care; sexual and marital relationships; interaction with family, children, and friends; community involvement; and sources of emotional support) and two open-ended questions. Each of the questions on family functioning is rated on three 7-point scales of "How much is there now?" "How much should there be?" and "How important is this to me?" Discrepancy between the first two ratings, together with the rating of importance, contribute to an assessment of the members' perceptions of family functioning. The survey takes less than 10 minutes to complete and can be used with single-parent and two-parent families (Failla and Jones, 1991; Feetham, Perkins, and Carroll, 1992).

Undoubtedly the richest environment for observing a child's development and interactions with family members is the home. Two tools that can be used to assess the child's home environment are the *Home Observation for Management of the Environment (HOME)*† *Inventory* (Caldwell and Bradley, 1984) and the *Home Screening Questionnaire (HSQ)*‡ (Frankenburg and Coons, 1986). Both are divided into two age groups: birth to 3 years of age, and 3 to 6 years of age. HOME has an additional inventory for children ages 6 to 10 years. Forms are also available for children with moderate to severe disabilities in each of the three age groups for visual, auditory, orthopedic, and cognitive impairments. HOME assesses the quality and quantity of the social, emotional, and cognitive support that is available to children in their home environment, including low-income families and low-birth-weight children (Bradley et al, 1994).

Some of the HOME items require direct observation, whereas others necessitate questioning of the parents. Each item receives a "yes" or "no" response. The number of "yes" responses correlates with the amount of appropriate environmental stimulation. Any "no" responses indicate possible areas for intervention and counseling. Use of HOME requires about a 1-hour home visit with both the child and the major caregiver.

The HSQ was developed using HOME as a guide. The 0- to 3-year form consists of 30 items plus a checklist of toys available to the child in the home. The 3- to 6-year form has 34 items and a similar toy checklist. The questions are written at approximately a third- to sixth-grade reading level and, unlike the HOME, can be completed by the parents in any setting in about 15 to 20 minutes. Scoring directions are detailed in the manual and are based on credits for different answers. For each age group there is a minimum score for determining suspect or nonsuspect results.

NUTRITIONAL ASSESSMENT

Dietary Intake

Knowledge of child's dietary intake is a useful and practical component of a nutritional assessment. However, it is also one of the most difficult factors to assess. Individuals' recall of food consumption, especially amounts eaten, is often unreliable. In addition, people may be hesitant to reveal their eating patterns if they sense criticism from the nurse. People from different cultures may have difficulty adequately describing the types of food they eat. Despite these obstacles, a food intake record is essential. Several methods are available.

Regardless of the format used in recording food intake, every nutritional assessment should begin with a *dietary history.* The exact questions used to elicit a dietary history vary with the child's age. In general, the younger the child, the more specific and detailed the history should be. Box 34-9 provides a sample dietary history for children and includes additional questions regarding infant feeding.

The broad overview elicited from the dietary history can be helpful in evaluating food frequency records. It also is concerned with financial and cultural factors that influence food selection and preparation (Cultural Considerations box).

The most common and probably easiest method of assessing daily intake is the *24-hour recall.* The child or parent recalls every item eaten in the past 24 hours and the approximate amounts. The 24-hour recall is most beneficial when it represents a typical day's intake. Some of the difficulties with a daily recall are the family's inability to remember exactly what was eaten, and inaccurate estimation of portion size. To increase accuracy of reporting portion sizes, the use of food models and additional questioning are recommended. In general, this method is most useful in providing *qualitative* information about the child's diet.

To improve the reliability of the daily recall, the family can complete a *food diary* by recording every food and liquid con-

*The survey is available for a fee from Nursing Systems and Research, Children's National Medical Center, 111 Michigan Ave. NW, Washington, DC, 20010; phone (202) 939-4980.

†The forms and an administration manual are available for a fee from the Center for Research on Teaching and Learning, College of Education, University of Arkansas at Little Rock, 2801 S. University Ave., Little Rock, AK 72204; phone (501) 569-3422.

‡The forms and manual are available for a fee from Denver Developmental Materials, Inc., P.O. Box 371075, Denver, CO 80237-5075, phone (303) 355-4729 or 1-800-419-4729.

Box 34-9
Dietary History

What are the family's usual mealtimes?
Do family members eat together or at separate times?
Who does the family grocery shopping and meal preparation?
How much money is spent to buy food each week?
How are most foods prepared—baked, broiled, fried, other?
How often does the family or your child eat out?
- What kinds of restaurants do you go to?
- What kinds of food does your child typically eat at restaurants?

Does your child eat breakfast regularly?
Where does your child eat lunch?
What are your child's favorite foods, beverages, and snacks?
- What are the average amounts eaten per day?
- What foods are artificially sweetened?
- What are your child's snacking habits?
- When are sweet foods usually eaten?
- What are your child's toothbrushing habits?

What special cultural practices are followed? What ethnic foods are eaten?
What foods and beverages does your child dislike?
How would you describe your child's usual appetite (hearty eater, picky eater)?
What are your child's feeding habits (breast, bottle, cup, spoon, eats by self, needs assistance, any special devices)?
Does your child take vitamins or other supplements? Do they contain iron or fluoride?
Are there any known or suspected food allergies? Is your child on a special diet?
Has your child lost or gained weight recently?
Are there any feeding problems (excessive fussiness, spitting up, colic, difficulty sucking or swallowing)? Are there any dental problems or appliances, such as braces, that affect eating?
What types of exercise does your child do regularly?
Is there a family history of cancer, diabetes, heart disease, high blood pressure, or obesity?

ADDITIONAL QUESTIONS FOR INFANTS

What was the infant's birth weight? When did it double? Triple?
Was the infant premature?
Are you breast-feeding or have you breast-fed your infant? For how long?
If you use a formula, what is the brand?
- How long has the infant been taking it?
- How many ounces does the infant drink a day?

Are you giving the infant cow's milk (whole, low-fat, skimmed)?
- When did you start?
- How many ounces does the infant drink a day?

Do you give your infant extra fluids (water, juice)?
If the infant takes a bottle to bed at nap or nighttime, what is in the bottle?
At what age did you start cereal, vegetables, meat or other protein sources, fruit/juice, finger food, table food?
Do you make your own baby food or use commercial foods, such as infant cereal?
Does the infant take a vitamin/mineral supplement? If so, what type?
Has the infant shown an allergic reaction to any food(s)? If so, list the foods and describe the reaction.
Does the infant spit up frequently, have unusually loose stools, or have hard, dry stools? If so, how often?
How often do you feed your infant?
How would you describe your infant's appetite?

sumed for a certain number of days. A 3-day record consisting of 2 weekdays and 1 weekend day is representative for most people. Providing specific charts to record intake can improve compliance. The family should record items immediately after eating.

A *food frequency questionnaire* or *record* (Box 34-10) provides information about the number of times in a day, week, or month a child consumes items from the different food groups. In general, it provides a qualitative overview but has the advantage of avoiding recall based on a "typical" day. It can be especially useful when verifying a food history or diary.

Clinical Examination

A significant amount of information regarding nutritional deficiencies is elicited from a clinical examination, especially from assessing the skin, hair, teeth, gums, lips, tongue, and eyes. Hair, skin, and mouth are vulnerable because of the rapid turnover of epithelial and mucosal tissue. Table 34-1 summarizes clinical signs of possible nutritional deficiency or excess. Few are diagnostic for a specific nutrient, and if suspicious signs are found, they must be confirmed with dietary and biochemical data. Generally, the clinical examination does not reveal children *at risk* for a deficiency or excess.

Anthropometry, an essential parameter of nutritional status, is the measurement of height, weight, head circumference, proportions, skinfold thickness, and arm circumference in young children. Height and head circumference reflect past

Cultural Considerations

FOOD PRACTICES

Because cultural practices are very prevalent in food preparation, consider carefully the kinds of questions that are asked and the judgments made in regard to counseling. For example, some cultures, such as Hispanic, African-American, and Native American, include many vegetables, legumes, and starches in their diet that together provide sufficient essential amino acids, even though the actual amount of meat or dairy protein is low. (See Chapter 32 for cultural food practices.)

Box 34-10

Food Frequency Record*

Food Group	Number of Servings (day, week)	Serving Size (in cup, tablespoon, or ounce portions)	Food Group	Number of Servings (day, week)	Serving Size (in cup, tablespoon, or ounce portions)
BREADS/CEREALS/RICE/PASTA			**MILK/CHEESE/YOGURT**		
Bread, tortilla			Milk		
Cooked pasta, rice, hot cereal			Cheese		
Dry cereal (not presweetened)			Yogurt		
Crackers			Pudding		
Muffins			Ice cream		
Other			Other		
VEGETABLES			**OTHER PROTEIN FOODS**		
Yellow or orange			Meat		
Green/leafy			Fish		
Other			Poultry		
			Egg		
			Peanut butter		
			Soy legumes (dried beans, peas)		
			Nuts		
			Other		
FRUITS/JUICES			**FATS/OILS/SWEETS**		
Citrus (orange, grapefruit, strawberries, lemon, lime, tangerine)			Butter, oil, margarine, mayonnaise, salad dressing		
Noncitrus			Soda, punch		
Other			Cake/cookie, etc.		
			Candy		
			Presweetened cereal		

*For comparison of actual intake with recommended intake, see Food Guide Pyramid, Fig. 47-1.

nutrition, whereas weight, skinfold thickness, and arm circumference reflect present nutritional status, especially of protein and fat reserves. Skinfold thickness is a measurement of the body's fat content because approximately one half of the body's total fat stores are directly beneath the skin. The upper arm muscle circumference is correlated with measurements of total muscle mass. Since muscle serves as the body's major protein reserve, this measurement is considered an index of the body's protein stores. Ideally, growth measurements are recorded over time, and comparisons are made regarding the *velocity* of growth based on previous and present values. Techniques for anthropomorphic measurement are discussed in Chapter 35.

Numerous *biochemical tests* are available for assessing nutritional status; these include analysis of plasma, blood cells, and urine; or tissues from the liver, bone, hair, and fingernails. Many of these tests are complicated and are not performed routinely. Common laboratory procedures for nutritional status include measurement of hemoglobin, hematocrit, transferrin, albumin, creatinine, and nitrogen. Laboratory values for these tests and more specific nutrient measurements are given in Appendix I.

Evaluation of Nutritional Assessment

After collecting the data needed for a thorough nutritional assessment, evaluate the findings to plan appropriate counseling. From the data, assess if the child is (1) malnourished, (2) at risk for becoming malnourished, or (3) well nourished with adequate reserves.

Analyze the daily food diary for the variety and amounts of foods suggested in the Food Guide Pyramid (see Fig. 47-1). For example, If the list includes no vegetables, inquire about this rather than assuming that the child dislikes vegetables; it could be that none were served on that day. Also, evaluate the information in terms of the family's ethnic practices and financial resources. Encouraging increased protein intake with additional meat may be unfeasible for families on a limited budget or those with food practices that use meat sparingly, such as in Asian meal preparation.

Compare findings from clinical examination and anthropometry with the data obtained from the dietary intake. For example, signs of anemia and a dietary record of iron-poor foods suggest laboratory analysis of hemoglobin, hematocrit, and transferrin. Refer any suspicious findings for further evaluation.

TABLE 34-1
Clinical Assessment of Nutritional Status

Evidence of Adequate Nutrition	Evidence of Deficient or Excess Nutrition	Deficiency/Excess*
GENERAL GROWTH		
Within 5th and 95th percentiles for height, weight, and head circumference	Below 5th or above 95th percentiles for growth	Protein, calories, fats, and other essential nutrients, especially vitamin A, pyridoxine, niacin, calcium, iodine, manganese, zinc
Steady gain with expected growth spurts during infancy and adolescence	Absence of or delayed growth spurts; poor weight gain	
Sexual development appropriate for age	Delayed sexual development	Excess vitamin A, D
SKIN		
Smooth, slightly dry to touch	Hardening and scaling	Vitamin A
Elastic and firm	Seborrheic dermatitis	Excess niacin
Absence of lesions	Dry, rough, petechiae	Riboflavin
Color appropriate to genetic background	Delayed wound healing	Vitamin C
	Scaly dermatitis on exposed surfaces	Riboflavin, vitamin C, zinc
	Wrinkled, flabby	Niacin
	Crusted lesions around orifices, especially nares	Protein, calories, zinc
	Pruritus	Excess vitamin A, riboflavin, niacin
	Poor turgor	Water, sodium
	Edema	Protein, thiamine Excess sodium
	Yellow tinge (jaundice)	Vitamin B_{12} Excess vitamin A, niacin
	Depigmentation	Protein, calories
	Pallor (anemia)	Pyridoxine, folic acid, vitamins B_{12}, C, E (in premature infants), iron Excess vitamin C, zinc
	Paresthesia	Excess riboflavin
HAIR		
Lustrous, silky, strong, elastic	Stringy, friable, dull, dry, thin	Protein, calories
	Alopecia	Protein, calories, zinc
	Depigmentation	Protein, calories, copper
	Raised areas around hair follicles	Vitamin C
HEAD		
Even molding, occipital prominence, symmetric facial features	Softening of cranial bones, prominence of frontal bones, skull flat and depressed toward middle	Vitamin D
Fused sutures after 18 months	Delayed fusion of sutures	Vitamin D
	Hard tender lumps in occiput	Excess vitamin A
	Headache	Excess thiamine
NECK		
Thyroid not visible, palpable in midline	Thyroid enlarged; may be grossly visible	Iodine
EYES		
Clear, bright	Hardening and scaling of cornea and conjunctiva	Vitamin A
Good night vision	Night blindness	
Conjunctiva—Pink, glossy	Burning, itching, photophobia, cataracts, corneal vascularization	Riboflavin
EARS		
Tympanic membrane—Pliable	Calcified (hearing loss)	Excess vitamin D

*Nutrients listed are deficient unless specified as excess.

Continued

TABLE 34-1—cont'd
Clinical Assessment of Nutritional Status

Evidence of Adequate Nutrition	Evidence of Deficient or Excess Nutrition	Deficiency/Excess*
NOSE		
Smooth, intact nasal angle	Irritation and cracks at nasal angle	Riboflavin Excess vitamin A
MOUTH		
Lips—Smooth, moist, darker color than skin	Fissures and inflammation at corners	Riboflavin Excess vitamin A
Gums—Firm, coral pink color, stippled	Spongy, friable, swollen, bluish red or black color, bleed easily	Vitamin C
Mucous membranes—Bright pink, smooth, moist	Stomatitis	Niacin
Tongue—Rough texture, no lesions, taste sensation	Glossitis Diminished taste sensation	Niacin, riboflavin, folic acid Zinc
Teeth—Uniform white color, smooth, intact	Brown mottling, pits, fissures Defective enamel Caries	Excess fluoride Vitamins A, C, D, calcium, phosphorus Excess carbohydrates
CHEST		
In infants, shape is almost circular in children, lateral diameter increases in proportion to anteroposterior diameter	Depressed lower portion of rib cage Sharp protrusion of sternum	Vitamin D
Smooth costochrondral junctions	Enlarged costochondral junctions	Vitamins C, D
Breast development—Normal for age	Delayed development	See under General Growth; especially zinc
CARDIOVASCULAR SYSTEM		
Pulse and blood pressure (BP) within normal limits	Palpitations Rapid pulse Arrhythmias Increased BP Decreased BP	Thiamine Potassium Excess thiamine Magnesium, potassium Excess niacin, potassium Excess sodium Thiamine; excess niacin
ABDOMEN		
In young children, cylindric and prominent	Distended, flabby, poor musculature Prominent, large	Protein, calories Excess calories
Older children, flat	Potbelly, constipation	Vitamin D
Normal bowel habits	Diarrhea Constipation	Niacin Excess vitamin C Excess calcium, potassium
MUSCULOSKELETAL SYSTEM		
Muscles—Firm, well-developed, equal strength bilaterally	Flabby, weak, generalized wasting Weakness, pain, cramps Muscle twitching, tremors Muscular paralysis	Protein, calories Thiamine, sodium, chloride, potassium, phosphorus, magnesium Excess thiamine Magnesium Excess potassium
Spine—Cervical and lumbar curves (double S-curve)	Kyphosis, lordosis, scoliosis	Vitamin D
Extremeties—Symmetric; legs straight with minimum bowing	Bowing of extremities, knock-knees Epiphyseal enlargement Bleeding into joints and muscles, joint swelling, pain	Vitamin D, calcium, phosphorus Vitamin A, D Vitamin C
Joints—Flexible, full range of motion, no pain or stiffness	Thickening of cortex of long bones with pain and fragility, hard tender lumps in extremities Osteoporosis of long bones	Excess vitamin A Calcium; excess vitamin D

TABLE 34-1—cont'd
Clinical Assessment of Nutritional Status

Evidence of Adequate Nutrition	Evidence of Deficient or Excess Nutrition	Deficiency/Excess*
NEUROLOGIC SYSTEM		
Behavior—Alert, responsive, emotionally stable	Listless, irritable, lethargic, apathetic (sometimes apprehensive, anxious, drowsy, mentally slow, confused)	Thiamine, niacin, pyridoxine, vitamin C, potassium, magnesium, iron, protein, calories Excess vitamins A, D, thiamine, folic acid, calcium
Absence of tetany, convulsions	Masklike facial expression, blurred speech, involuntary laughing	Excess manganese
	Convulsions	Thiamine, pyridoxine, vitamin D, calcium, magnesium Excess phosphorus (in relation to calcium)
Intact peripheral nervous system	Peripheral nervous system toxicity (unsteady gait, numb feet and hands, fine motor clumsiness)	Excess pyridoxine
Intact reflexes	Diminished or absent tendon reflexes	Thiamine, vitamin E

*Nutrients listed are deficient unless specified as excess.

Key Points

- Communication, the most important skill nurses must possess in the care of children, has verbal, nonverbal, and abstract components.
- To effectively establish a setting for communication, nurses must make an appropriate introduction, clarify their role and the purpose of the interview, and ensure privacy and confidentiality.
- When communicating with parents, nurses need to encourage parental involvement, listen carefully, use silence, and be empathic.
- Communication with children must reflect their developmental stage.
- Verbal communication techniques that have proved to be effective include the third-person technique, facilitative responding, storytelling, bibliotherapy, the use of "what if" questions, and other word games.
- The objectives of performing a health history are to identify pertinent information, determine the chief complaint, analyze the present illness, secure the past history, review biologic systems, and record a family medical history and child psychosocial and sexual history.
- Family assessment is the collection of data about family composition and relationships among its members; it also focuses on home and community environment, occupation and education, and cultural and religious traditions.
- The family function interview examines interaction and roles, power, decision making, problem solving, communication, and expression of feelings and individuality.
- Nutritional assessment is performed by determination of dietary intake, clinical examination, and biochemical analysis.

References

Bradley RH et al: A reexamination of the association between HOME scores and income, *Nurs Res* 43(5):260-266, 1994.

Brennan PF: The future of clinical communication in an electronic environment, *Holistic Nurs Pract* 11(1):97-104, 1996.

Caldwell B, Bradley R: *Home observation for measurement of the environment,* rev ed, Little Rock, 1984, University of Arkansas.

Cantrill JA, Cottrell WN: Accuracy of drug allergy documentation, *Am J Health Syst Pharm* 54:1627-1629, 1997.

Deadrick D, Boggess P: *Pediatrics on telephone line.* Paper presented at the first Annual National Conference for Advanced Practice Nurses, Rutgers University, Nov 6-8, 1996.

Desselle DD, Pearlmutter L: Navigating two cultures: deaf children, self-esteem, and parents' communication patterns, *Soc Work Educ* 19(1):23-30, 1997.

Failla S, Jones LC: Families of children with developmental disabilities: an examination of family hardiness, *Res Nurs Health* 14:41-50, 1991.

Feetham S, Perkins M, Carroll R: Exploratory analysis: a technique for analysis of dyadic data in research of families. In Feetham S et al, editors: *The nursing of families: theory/research/education/practice,* Newbury Park, CA, 1992, Sage Publications.

Frankenburg W, Coons C: Home Screening Questionnaire: its validity in assessing home environment, *J Pediatr* 108(4):624-626, 1986.

Giger J, Davidhizar R, Poole VL: Health promotion among ethnic minorities: the importance of cultural phenomena, *Rehabil Nurs* 22(6):303-307, 1997.

Gobis LJ: Reducing the risks of phone triage, *RN* 60(4):61-63, 1997.

Hocking G, deMello WF: Taking a "drugs" history, *Anaesthesia* 52:904-905, 1997.

Hoffman LJ: Data security and privacy in health information systems, *Top Emerg Med* 17(4):24-26, 1995.

Hoge DR, Parette HP: Facilitating communicative development in young children with disabilities, *Transdisciplinary J* 5(2): 113-130, 1995.

Murphy JM et al: The family APGAR and psychosocial problems in children: a report from ASPN and PROS, *J Fam Pract* 46(1):54-63, 1998.

Nance TA: Intercultural communication: finding common ground, *JOGNN* 24(3):249-255, 1995.

Price V, Archbold J: What's it all about, empathy? *Nurs Educ Today* 17(2):106-110, 1997.

Seidel HM et al: *Mosby's guide to physical examination,* ed 4, St Louis, 1999, Mosby.

Smilkstein G: Family APGAR analyzed (letter), *Fam Med* 25(5): 293-294, 1993.

Smilkstein G, Ashworth C, Montano D: Validity and reliability of the family APGAR as a test of family function, *J Fam Pract* 15(2):303-311, 1982.

Sullivan GH: Protecting patient's privacy, *RN* 60(6):55-56, 58-59, 1997.

White SJ: Empathy: a literature review and concept analysis, *J Clin Nurs* 6(4):253-257, 1997.

Wissow LS, Roter DL, Wilson MEH: Pediatrician interview style and mother's disclosure of psychosocial issues, *Pediatrics* 93(2):289-295, 1994.

Wright K: Anticipatory guidance: developing a healthy sexuality, *Pediatr Ann* 26(2, suppl):S142-S144, 1997.

Wright LM, Leahey M: *Nurse and families: a guide to family assessment and intervention,* ed 3, Philadelphia, 1999, FA Davis.

CHAPTER 35

Physical and Developmental Assessment of the Child

http://www.harcourthealth.com/MERLIN/Wong/maternal/

Learning Objectives

On completion of this chapter the reader will be able to:

- Prepare a child for a physical examination based on his or her developmental needs.
- Perform a comprehensive physical examination in a sequence appropriate to the child's age.
- Recognize expected normal findings for children at various ages.
- Record the physical examination according to the head-to-toe format.
- Perform a developmental assessment using a standard screening test.

GENERAL APPROACH TOWARD EXAMINING THE CHILD

Sequence of the Examination

Ordinarily, the sequence for examining patients follows a head-to-toe direction. The main function of such a systematic approach is to provide a general guideline for assessment of each body area to minimize the chances of omitting segments of the examination. The standard recording of data also facilitates exchange of information among different professionals. The typical organization of a physical examination is indicated in the chapter outline. In examining children, this orderly sequence is often altered to accommodate the child's developmental needs, although the examination is recorded following the head-to-toe model.* Using developmental and chronologic age as the main criteria for assessing each body system accomplishes several goals:

- Minimizes stress and anxiety associated with assessment of various body parts
- Fosters a trusting nurse-child-parent relationship
- Allows for maximum preparation of the child
- Preserves the essential security of the parent-child relationship, especially with young children
- Maximizes the accuracy and reliability of assessment findings

Preparation of the Child

Although the physical examination consists of painless procedures, to a child the use of a tight arm cuff, probes in the ears and mouth, pressing on the abdomen, and listening to the chest with a cold piece of metal can be considerably stressful. Therefore the same considerations discussed in Chapter 45 for preparing children for procedures are followed here. In addition to that discussion, general guidelines related to the examining process are presented in Box 35-1. The physical examination should be as pleasant as possible, as well as educational. For example, the nurse can use a detailed drawing or anatomically correct doll to help preschoolers and older children learn about their bodies (Vessey, 1995). The paper-doll technique is a useful approach to teaching children about the part of the body that is being examined (Fig. 35-1). At the conclusion of the visit, the child can bring home the paper doll as a memento of the experience.

In most instances children cooperate best when their parents remain with them; however, there are occasions when older children, particularly adolescents, prefer to be examined alone, such as during the genital examination. Often the child being examined is also accompanied by a sibling, who may be disruptive because of boredom. A helpful tactic is to involve the sibling in the examination by allowing the child to hold the stethoscope or a tongue blade and praising the child for the "help" during the assessment.

Table 35-1 summarizes guidelines for positioning, preparing, and examining children at various ages. Because no child fits precisely into one age category, it may be necessary to vary the approach after a preliminary assessment of the child's develop-

*For additional information, please view "Pediatric Assessment" in ***Whaley and Wong's Pediatric Nursing Video Series,*** St Louis, 1996, Mosby; 1-800-426-4545; website: www.mosby.com.

Box 35-1

General Guidelines for Performing Pediatric Physical Examinations

Perform examination in appropriate, nonthreatening area.
- Have room well lighted and decorated with neutral colors.
- Have room temperature comfortably warm.
- Place all strange and potentially frightening equipment out of sight.
- Have some toys, dolls, stuffed animals, and games available for child.
- If possible, have rooms decorated and equipped for different-age children.
- Provide privacy, especially for school-age children and adolescents.

Provide time for play and becoming acquainted.

Observe behaviors that signal child's readiness to cooperate:
- Talking to the nurse
- Making eye contact
- Accepting the offered equipment
- Allowing physical touching
- Choosing to sit on examining table rather than parent's lap

If signs of readiness are not observed, use the following techniques:
- Talk to parent while essentially "ignoring" child; gradually focus on child or a favorite object, such as a doll.
- Make complimentary remarks about child, such as appearance, dress, or a favorite object.
- Tell a funny story or play a simple magic trick.
- Have a nonthreatening "friend" available, such as a hand puppet to "talk" to child for the nurse (see Fig. 35-22, *A*).

If child refuses to cooperate, use the following techniques:
- Assess reason for uncooperative behavior; consider that a child who is unduly afraid may have had a previous traumatic experience.
- Try to involve child and parent in process.
- Avoid prolonged explanations about examining procedure.
- Use a firm, direct approach regarding expected behavior.
- Perform examination as quickly as possible.
- Have attendant gently restrain child.
- Minimize any disruptions or stimulation.
  - Limit number of people in room.
  - Use isolated room.
  - Use quiet, calm, confident voice.

Begin examination in a nonthreatening manner for young children or children who are fearful:
- Use activities that can be presented as games, such as test for cranial nerves (see Table 35-11 or parts of developmental screening tests on p. 822).
- Use approaches such as Simon Says to encourage child to make a face, squeeze a hand, stand on one foot, and so on.
- Use paper-doll technique.
- Lay child supine on an examining table or floor that is covered with a large sheet of paper.
- Trace around child's body outline.
- Use body outline to demonstrate what will be examined, such as drawing a heart and listening with stethoscope before performing activity on child.

If several children in the family will be examined, begin with most cooperative child to provide modeling of desired behavior.

Involve child in examination process:
- Provide choices, such as sitting on table or in parent's lap.
- Allow child to handle or hold equipment.
- Encourage child to use equipment on a doll, family member, or examiner.
- Explain each step of the procedure in simple language.

Examine child in a comfortable and secure position:
- Sitting in parent's lap
- Sitting upright if in respiratory distress

Proceed to examine the body in an organized sequence (usually head to toe) with the following exceptions:
- Alter sequence to accommodate needs of different-age children (see Table 35-1).
- Examine painful areas last.
- In emergency situation, examine vital functions (airway, breathing, and circulation) and injured area first.

Reassure child throughout examination, especially about bodily concerns that arise during puberty.

Discuss findings with family at end of examination.

Praise child for cooperation during examination; give reward such as a small toy or sticker.

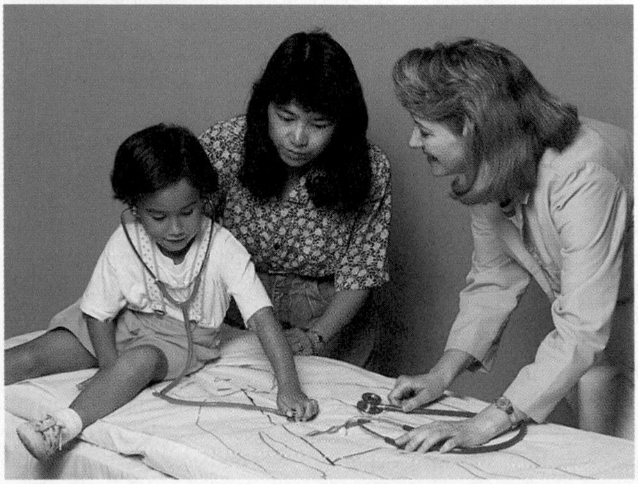

FIG. 35-1 • Using paper-doll technique to prepare child.

mental achievements and needs. Even when the best approach is used, many toddlers are uncooperative and unable to be consoled for much of the physical examination. However, some seem intrigued by the new surroundings and unusual equipment and respond more like preschoolers than toddlers. Likewise, some early preschoolers may require more of the "security measures" employed with younger children, such as continued parent-child contact, and less of the preparatory measures used with preschoolers, such as playing with the equipment before and during the actual examination (Fig. 35-2).

Although the variations in the general approaches are numerous, some of them are elaborated on here because they are more common. For example, the suggested sequence may change considerably when the child is in pain or when obvious physical defects are present. In either situation, examine the affected area last to minimize distress early in the examination and to focus on normal, healthy, or functioning body parts.

TABLE 35-1
Age-specific Approaches to Physical Examination During Childhood

Position	Sequence	Preparation
INFANT		
Before sits alone: supine or prone, preferably in parent's lap; before 4 to 6 months: can place on examining table After sits alone: use sitting in parent's lap whenever possible If on table, place with parent in full view	If quiet, auscultate heart, lungs, abdomen Record heart and respiratory rates Palpate and percuss same areas Proceed in usual head-to-toe direction Perform traumatic procedures last (eyes, ears, mouth [while crying]) Elicit reflexes as body part is examined Elicit Moro reflex last	Have child completely undressed if room temperature permits Leave diaper on male infant Gain cooperation with distraction, bright objects, rattles, talking Smile at infant; use soft, gentle voice Pacify with bottle of sugar water or feeding Enlist parent's aid for restraining to examine ears, mouth Avoid abrupt, jerky movements
TODDLER		
Sitting or standing on/by parent Prone or supine in parent's lap	Inspect body area through play: "count fingers," "tickle toes" Use minimal physical contact initially Introduce equipment slowly Auscultate, percuss, palpate whenever quiet Perform traumatic procedures last (same as for infant)	Have parent remove outer clothing Remove underwear as body part is examined Allow to inspect equipment; demonstrating use of equipment is usually ineffective If uncooperative, perform procedures quickly Use restraint when appropriate; request parent's assistance Talk about examination if cooperative; use short phrases Praise for cooperative behavior
PRESCHOOL CHILD		
Prefer standing or sitting Usually cooperative prone/supine Prefer parent's closeness	If cooperative, proceed in head-to-toe direction If uncooperative, proceed as with toddler	Request self-undressing Allow to wear underpants if shy Offer equipment for inspection; briefly demonstrate use Make up story about procedure: "I'm seeing how strong your muscles are" (blood pressure) Use paper-doll technique Give choices when possible Expect cooperation; use positive statements: "Open your mouth"
SCHOOL-AGE CHILD		
Prefer sitting Cooperative in most positions Younger child prefers parent's presence Older child may prefer privacy	Proceed in head-to-toe direction May examine genitalia last in older child Respect need for privacy	Request self-undressing Allow to wear underpants Give gown to wear Explain purpose of equipment and significance of procedure, such as otoscope to see eardrum, which is necessary for hearing Teach about body functioning and care
ADOLESCENT		
Same as for school-age child Offer option of parent's presence	Same as older school-age child	Allow to undress in private Give gown Expose only areas to be examined Respect need for privacy Explain findings during examination: "Your muscles are firm and strong" Matter-of-factly comment about sexual development: "Your breasts are developing as they should be" Emphasize normalcy of development Examine genitalia as any other body part; may leave to end

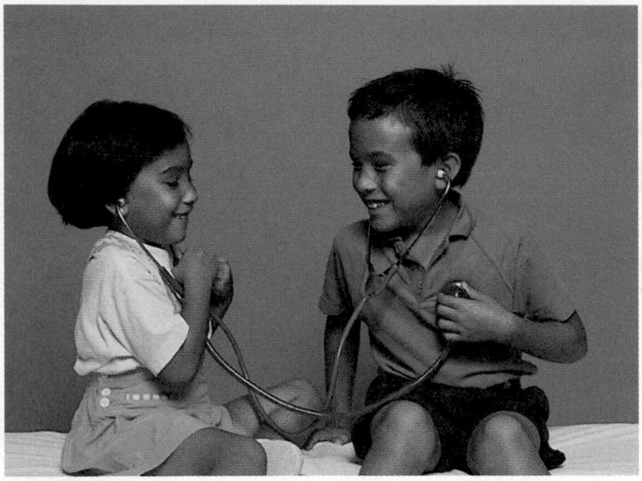

FIG. 35-2 • Preparing children for physical examination.

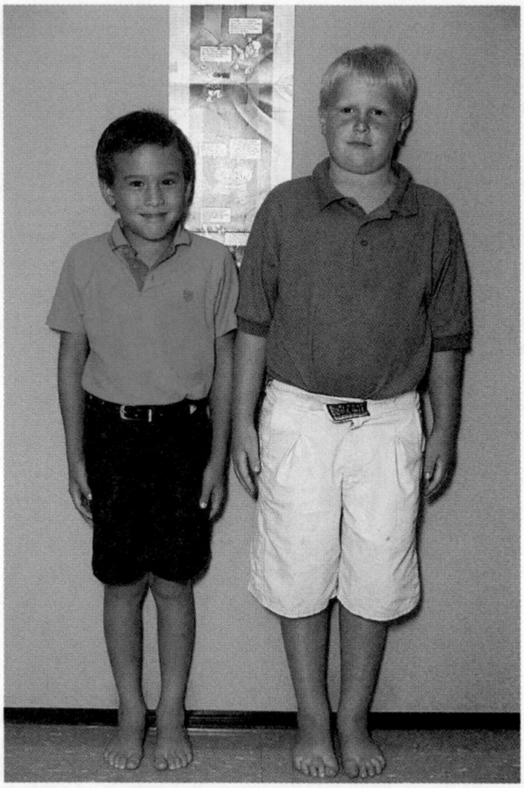

FIG. 35-3 • These children of identical age (8 years) are markedly different in size. The child on the left, of Asian descent, is at the 5th percentile for height and weight. The child on the right is above the 95th percentile for height and weight. However, both children demonstrate normal growth patterns.

Positioning may also be altered because of physical distress. For example, the child who is having difficulty breathing may not be able to lie down; therefore, perform as much of the physical examination as possible with the child in a sitting or slightly reclining position, or complete the examination at another time.

PHYSICAL EXAMINATION

Although the approach to and sequence of the physical examination differ according to the child's age, the following discussion outlines the traditional model for physical assessment. Although the focus includes all pediatric age groups, the reader is referred to Chapter 36 for a detailed discussion of a newborn assessment. Because the physical examination is a vital part of preventive pediatric care, a schedule for periodic health visits is given in Box 35-2.

Growth Measurements

Measurement of physical growth in children is a key element in evaluation of their health status. Physical growth parameters include weight, height (length), skinfold thickness, arm circumference, and head circumference. Values for these growth parameters are plotted on percentile charts, and the child's measurements in percentiles are compared with those of the general population (Fig. 35-3).

The most commonly used growth charts in the United States are from the *National Center for Health Statistics (NCHS)*. The growth charts have been revised to include the body mass index-for age (BMI-for-age) charts, 3rd and 97th smoothed percentiles for all charts, and the 85th percentile for the weight-for-stature and BMI-for-age charts (see Appendix E). The data was collected from five national surveys during 1963 to 1994. The revised charts have eliminated the disjunctions between the curves for infants and older children and have been extended for children and adolescents to age 20 years (Kuczmarski, 2000).

The weight-for-age percentile distributions are now continuous between the infant and the older child charts at 24 to 36 months. The length-for-age to stature-for-age, and the weight-for-length to weight-for-stature curves are parallel in the overlapping ages of 24 to 36 months. The revised weight-for-stature charts were developed to accommodate children 2 to 5 years of age. The weight-for-stature charts provide a smoother transition from the weight-for-length charts for preschool-aged children.

The most prominent change to the complement of growth charts for older children and adolescents is the addition of the BMI-for-age growth curves. The BMI-for-age charts were developed with national survey data (1963 to 1994) excluding data from the 1988 to 1994 NHANES III survey for children older than 6 years because an increase in body weight and BMI occurred between NHANES III and previous national surveys. Without this exclusion, the 85th and 95th percentile curves would have been higher, and fewer children and adolescents would have been classified at risk or overweight. Therefore, the BMI-for-age growth curves do not represent the current population of children over 6 years of age.

The sex-specific BMI-for-age charts for ages 2 to 20 years replace the 1977 NCHS weight-for-statures charts that were limited to prepubescent boys under 11.5 years of age and statures less than 145 cm, and to prepubescent girls under 19.0 years of age and statures less than 137 cm. BMI-for-age may be used to identify children and adolescents at the upper end of the distribution who are either overweight (i.e., ≥95th percentile) or at risk for overweight (i.e., ≥85th and <95th percentile). The formulas for determining BMI are available by accessing the website at: www.cdc.gov/nccdphp/dnpa/bmi/bmi-definition.htm.

Box 35-2

Child Preventive Care Time Line

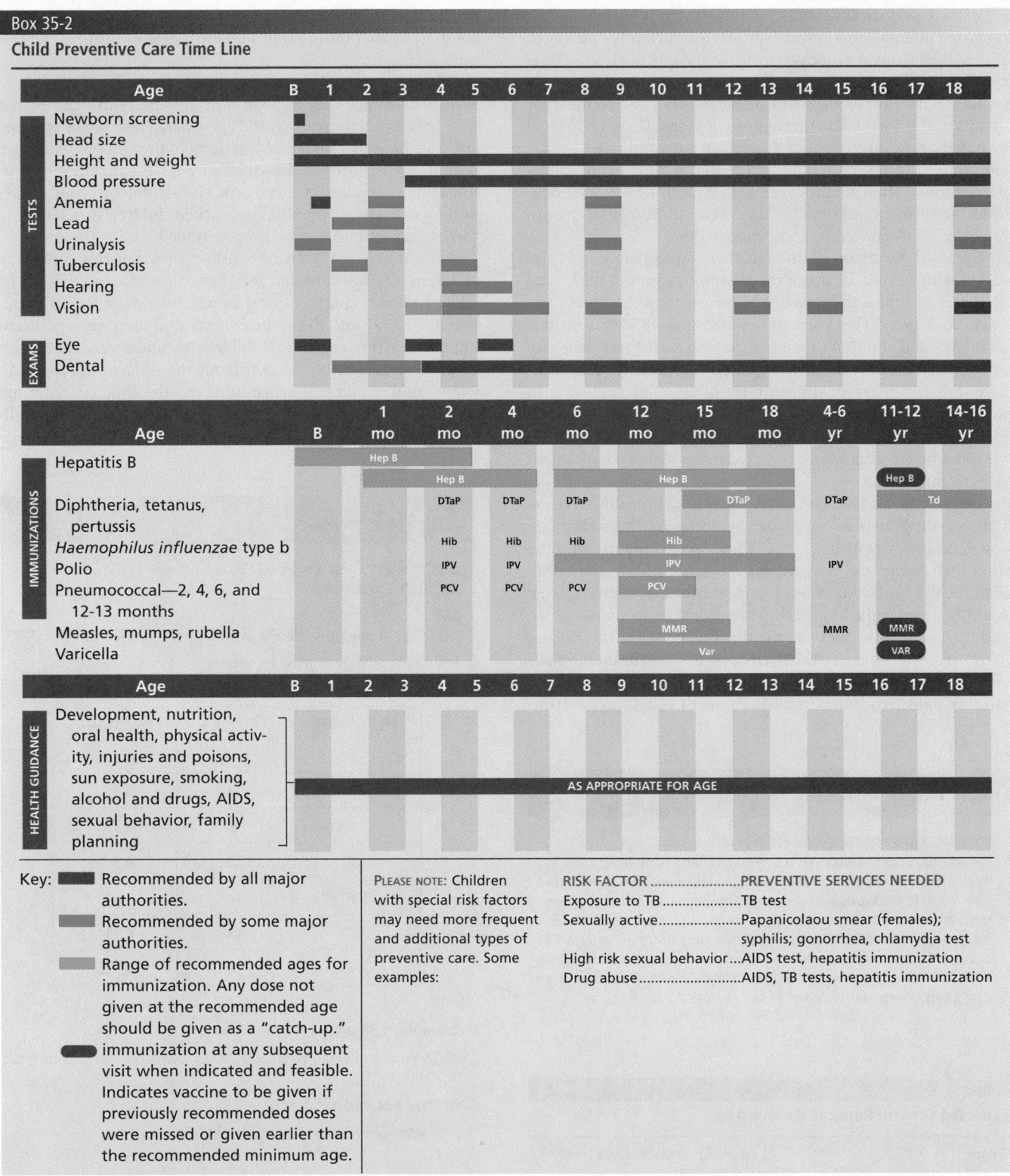

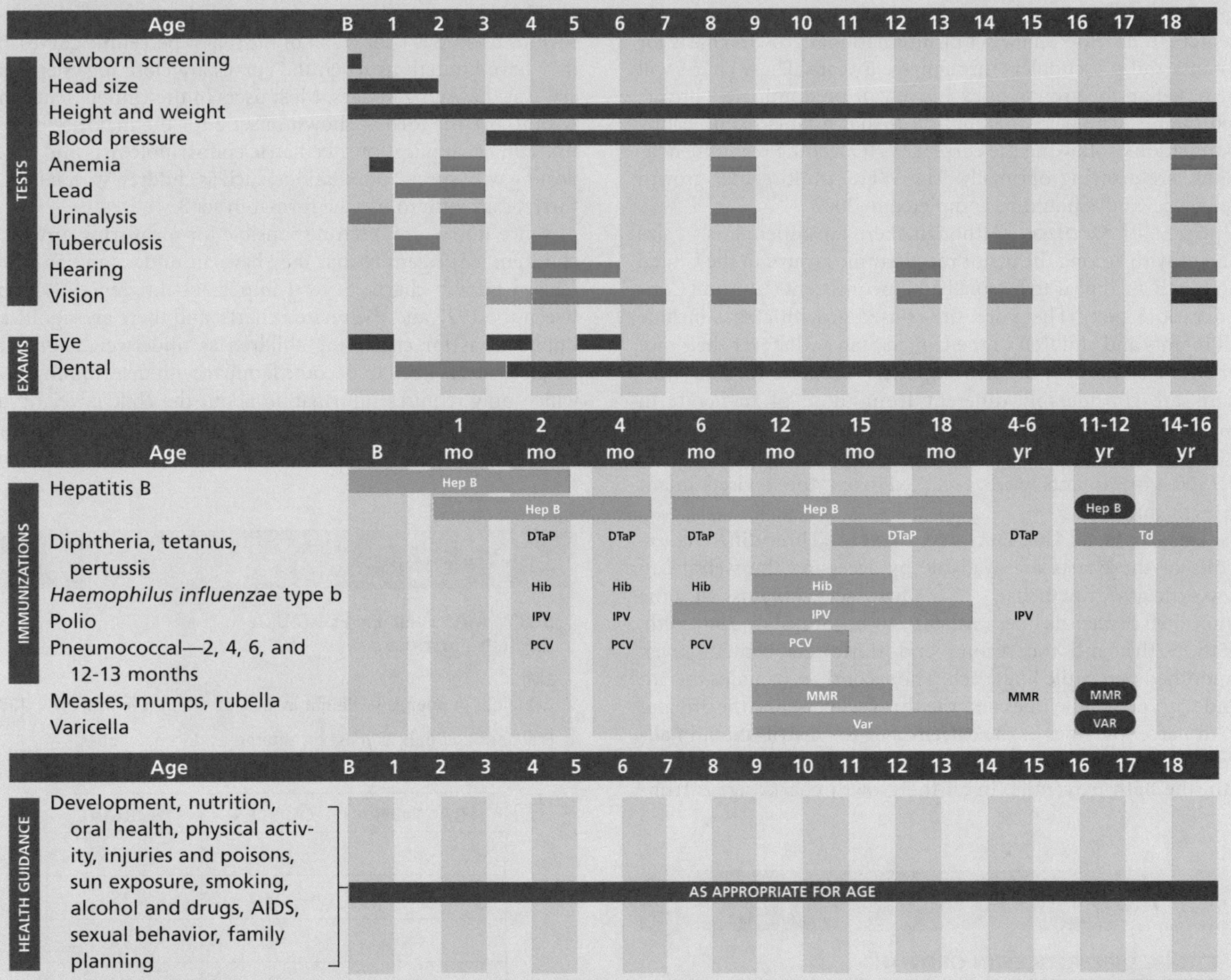

Key:
- (dark bar) Recommended by all major authorities.
- (medium bar) Recommended by some major authorities.
- (light bar) Range of recommended ages for immunization. Any dose not given at the recommended age should be given as a "catch-up."
- (rounded bar) immunization at any subsequent visit when indicated and feasible. Indicates vaccine to be given if previously recommended doses were missed or given earlier than the recommended minimum age.

PLEASE NOTE: Children with special risk factors may need more frequent and additional types of preventive care. Some examples:

RISK FACTOR	PREVENTIVE SERVICES NEEDED
Exposure to TB	TB test
Sexually active	Papanicolaou smear (females); syphilis; gonorrhea, chlamydia test
High risk sexual behavior	AIDS test, hepatitis immunization
Drug abuse	AIDS, TB tests, hepatitis immunization

Modified from *Child health guide: put prevention into practice,* U.S. Department of Health and Human Services, undated, pp. 20-21. Immunization schedule approved by the Advisory Committee on Immunization Practices, the American Academy of Pediatrics, and the American Academy of Family Physicians. Hepatitis A is recommended in selected areas. See also immunizations, Chapter 36.

Breast- and Formula-Fed Infants. The national survey data better represent the combined size and growth patterns of the general United States population (1971 to 1994). Over the past two decades in the United States, approximately one-half of all infants were reported to ever have been breastfed and approximately one-third were breastfed for 3 months or more. Therefore, compared with the 1977 NCHS growth charts, the nationally representative data on which the revised infant growth charts are based will better represent the combined growth patterns of breastfed and formula-fed infants in the United States.

With regard to differences in the growth of breast- or formula-fed infants, other research efforts are currently ongoing to address this issue. A Working Group of the World Health Organization (WHO) is collecting data at seven international study centers to develop a new set of international growth charts for infants and preschoolers through age 5 years. These charts will be based on the growth of exclusively or predominately breast-fed infants. The basic assumption is that infants from healthy populations, following the current WHO feeding recommendations, are growing optimally. The WHO multi-center growth reference study should be completed in 2002.

Special Groups. Although there are differences in size and growth among the major racial/ethnic groups in the United States, these appear to be small and inconsistent (Cultural Considerations box). Therefore, the revised growth charts include all infants and children in the United States whatever their race or ethnicity. Because the growth patterns of preterm, VLBW infants are considerably different from those of higher birth weight term infants, and because specialized growth charts exist to track the growth of VLBW infants, data for VLBW (i.e., <1500 gm) infants were excluded from the revised infant growth charts.

Versions of the Growth Charts. Three different versions of the charts are available by accessing the website at: www.cdc.gov/growthcharts. The first set contains all nine smoothed percentile lines (3rd, 5th, 10th, 25th, 50th, 75th, 90th, 95th, 97th), and the second and third sets contain seven smoothed percentile lines each. The second set contains the 5th and 95th percentile lines and the third set contains the 3rd and 97th percentile lines at the extremes of the distribution. In addition, the charts for weight-for-stature and BMI-for-age contain the 85th percentile. In all the growth charts, age is truncated to the preceding full month, for example, 1 month (1.0 to 1.9 mo), 11 months (11.0 to 11.9 mo), 23 months (23.0 to 23.9 mo), and so forth.

The three sets of charts are provided to meet the needs of various users. Set 1 shows all of the major percentile curves, but may have limitations when the curves are close together, especially at the youngest ages. Most users in the United States may wish to use the format shown in set 2 for the majority of routine clinical applications. Pediatric endocrinologists and others dealing with special populations, such as children with failure to thrive, may wish to use the format in set 3.

Since nurses are often responsible for measuring growth in children, it is essential that they have an understanding of the revised growth charts. Several important differences exist between the 1977 and the revised charts, and there are significant implications for classifying children as underweight or overweight. Nurses need to become familiar with determining BMI, which only requires information about the child's weight and height (Guidelines box). With the increasing number of children who are overweight in the United States, the BMI charts

Cultural Considerations

ETHNIC DIFFERENCES IN GROWTH

A potential concern with the U.S. growth charts is their accuracy in evaluating the growth of children from different ethnic and socioeconomic backgrounds. Research findings indicate that these growth charts can serve as a reference guide for all racial or ethnic groups if used from the perspective that different groups of children have varying normal distributions on the growth curves. The NCHS charts are accurate for African-American children because this group was included in the sample population.

TABLE 35-2

Expected Growth Rates at Various Ages

Age	Expected Growth Rate (cm/yr)
1 to 6 months	18-22
6 to 12 months	14-18
2nd year	11
3rd year	8
4th year	7
5th to 10th years	5-6

From *Human growth and growth disorders: an update,* South San Francisco, 1989, Genentech.

Guidelines

BODY MASS INDEX FORMULA
English Formula

BMI =
[Weight in pounds ÷ Height in inches ÷ Height in inches] × 703

Fractions and ounces must be entered as decimal values.

FRACTION	OUNCES	DECIMAL
1/8	2	0.125
1/4	4	0.25
3/8	6	0.375
1/2	8	0.5
5/8	10	0.625
3/4	12	0.75
7/8	14	0.875

Example: A 33-pound, 4-ounce child is 37⅝ inches tall.

33.25 pounds divided by 37.625 inches, divided by 37.625 inches × 703 = 16.5

Metric Formula

BMI = Weight in kilograms ÷ [Height in meters]^2

or

BMI =
[Weight in kilograms ÷ Height in cm ÷ Height in cm] × 10,000

Example: A 16.9 kg child is 105.2 cm tall.

16.9 divided by 105.2 cm divided by 105.2 cm × 10,000 = 15.3

Kuczmarski RJ et al: *CDC growth charts: United States. Advance data from vital and health statistics; no 314,* Hyattsville, MD: National Center for Health Statistics, June 8, 2000; may be accessed at: www.cdc.gov/nchs/about/major/nhanes/growthcharts/fullreport.htm

will increasingly become a critical component of children's physical assessment.

Children whose growth may be questionable include:

- Children whose height and weight percentiles are widely disparate (e.g., height in the 10th percentile and weight in the 90th percentile, especially with above-average skinfold thickness)
- Children who fail to show the expected growth rates in height and weight, especially during the rapid growth periods of infancy and adolescence (Table 35-2).
- Children who show a sudden increase, except during puberty, or a decrease in a previously steady growth pattern

Since growth is a continuous but uneven process, the most reliable evaluation lies in comparison of growth measurements over a prolonged time.

Length. The term *length* refers to measurements taken when children are supine (also referred to as *recumbent length*). Until children are 24 months old (36 months if the birth to 36-month chart is used), measure recumbent length. Because of the normally flexed position during infancy, fully extend the body by (1) holding the head in midline, (2) grasping the knees together gently, and (3) pushing down on the knees until the legs are fully extended and flat against the table. If using a measuring board, place the head firmly at the top of the board and the heels of the feet firmly against the footboard.

If such a measuring device is not available, measure length by placing the child on a paper-covered surface, marking the end points of the top of the head and the heels of the feet, and measuring between these two points (Fig. 35-4). For accurate measurement, hold the writing utensil at a right angle to the table when marking the cephalic point; position the feet with the toes pointing directly to the ceiling when marking the heel point. Regardless of the method used, have someone assist in holding the child's head in midline while you extend the legs and take the measurements.

Height. The term *height* (or *stature*) refers to the measurement taken when children are standing upright. Measure height by having the child, with shoes removed, stand as tall and straight as possible, with the head in midline and the line of vision parallel to the ceiling or floor. Be sure the child's back is to the wall or other vertical flat surface, with the heels, buttocks, and back of the shoulders touching the wall and the medial malleoli touching if possible (Fig. 35-5). Check for and correct bending of the knees, slumping of the shoulders, or raising of the heels of the feet.

For the most accurate measurement, use a wall-mounted unit (*stadiometer;* see Fig. 35-5). The moveable measuring rod of platform scales is accurate only if it maintains a parallel position to the floor and rests securely on the topmost part of the head. To improvise a flat surface for measuring length, attach a paper or metal tape or yardstick to the wall, position the child adjacent to the tape, and place a three-dimensional object, such as a thick book or box, on top of the head. Rest the side of the object firmly against the wall to form a right angle. Measure length or stature to the nearest 1 mm or ⅛ inch.

Weight. Weight is measured with an appropriately sized beam balance scale, which measures weights to the nearest 10 g or K ounce for infants and 100 g or ¼ pound for children. Before the child is weighed, the scale is balanced by setting it at

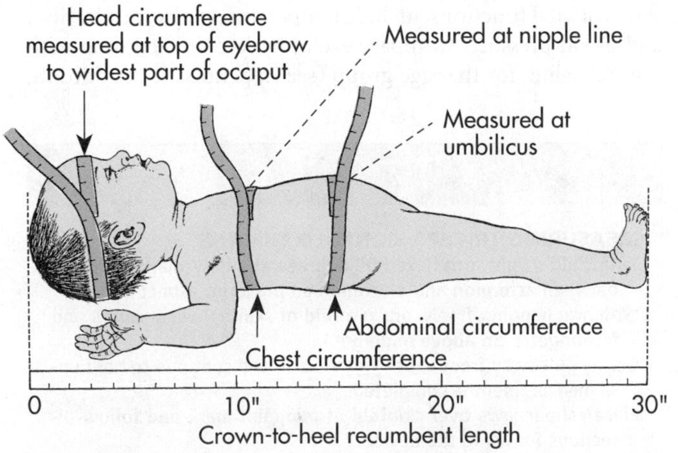

FIG. 35-4 • Measurement of head, chest, and abdominal circumference and crown-to-heel (recumbent) length.

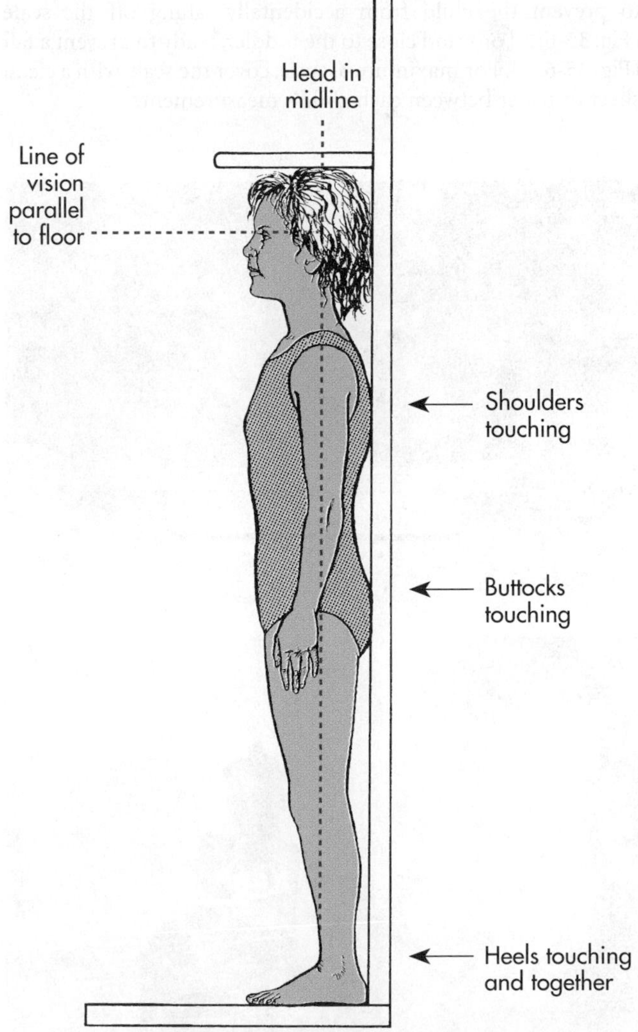

FIG. 35-5 • Measurement of height. (Redrawn from *Human growth and growth disorders: an update,* South San Francisco, 1989, Genentech.)

zero and noting if the balance registers exactly in the middle of the mark. If the end of the balance beam rises to the top or bottom of the mark, more or less weight, respectively, is added. Some scales are designed to allow for self-correction, but others need to be recalibrated by the manufacturer. Scales vary in their accuracy; infant scales tend to be more accurate than adult platform scales, and newer scales tend to be more accurate than older ones, especially at the upper levels of weight measurement. When precise measurements are needed, two nurses should take the weight independently, and if there is a discrepancy a third reading should be taken.

Take measurements in a comfortably warm room. When the birth to 36-month growth charts are used, children should be weighed nude. Older children are usually weighed while wearing their underpants or a light gown. However, always respect the privacy of all children. If the child must be weighed wearing some article of clothing, or some type of special device, such as a prosthesis or an armboard for an intravenous device, note this when recording the weight. Children who are measured for recumbent length are usually weighed on an infant platform scale and placed in a lying-down or sitting position. When weighing children, place your hand lightly above the body of the infant to prevent the child from accidentally falling off the scale (Fig. 35-6, *A*) or stand close to the toddler, ready to prevent a fall (Fig. 35-6, *B*). For maximum asepsis, cover the scale with a clean sheet of paper between each child's measurement.

A

B

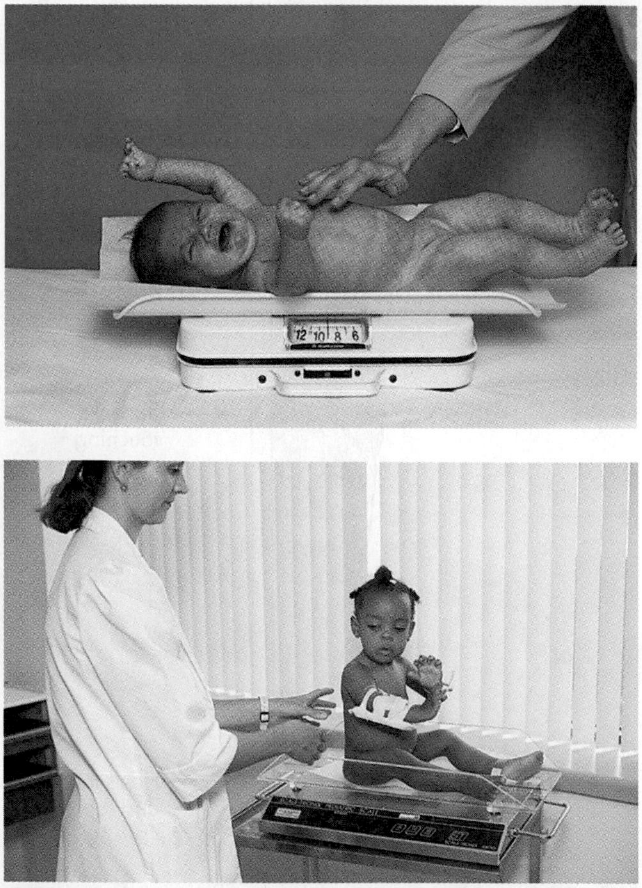

FIG. 35-6 • **A,** Infant on scale. **B,** Toddler on scale. Note position of nurse to prevent falls.

Skinfold Thickness and Arm Circumference. Measures of relative weight and stature cannot distinguish between adipose (fat) tissue and muscle. One convenient measure of body fat is *skinfold thickness.* Skinfold thickness is measured with special calipers, such as the Lange calipers. The most common sites for measuring skinfold thickness are the triceps (most practical for routine clinical use), subscapular, suprailiac, abdomen, and upper thigh. For greatest reliability the exact procedure for measurement must be followed and the average of at least two measurements of one site recorded (Guidelines box).

Arm circumference is an indirect measure of muscle mass. Measurement of arm circumference follows the same procedure for skinfold thickness, except the midpoint is measured with a paper or steel tape. Place the tape vertically along the posterior aspect of the upper arm to the acromial process and to the olecranon process; half the measured length is the midpoint. Percentiles for triceps skinfold and arm circumference in children are listed in Appendix E, and may be used as reference data. However, the percentiles are not standards or norms, because values between the 5th and 95th percentiles are not ranges of normal.

Head Circumference. Measure head circumference in children up to 36 months of age and in any child whose head size is questionable. Measure the head at its greatest circumference, usually slightly above the eyebrows and pinna of the ears and around the occipital prominence at the back of the skull (see Fig. 35-4). Since head shape can affect the location of the maximum circumference, more than one measurement at points above the eyebrows may need to be taken to obtain the most accurate measure. Use a paper or metal tape because a cloth tape can stretch and give a falsely small measurement. For greatest accuracy, use devices with tenths of a centimeter, because the percentile charts have only 0.5-cm increments.

Plot the head size on the appropriate growth chart under head circumference. Generally, head and chest circumferences are equal at about 1 to 2 years of age. During childhood, chest circumference exceeds head size by about 5 to 7 cm (2 to 3 inches). (For newborns, see Physical Assessment, Chapter 25.)

Physiologic Measurements

Physiologic measurements, key elements in evaluating physical status of vital functions, include temperature, pulse, respiration, and blood pressure. Compare each physiologic recording with normal values for that age group (see Appendix J). In addition,

Guidelines

MEASURING TRICEPS SKINFOLD THICKNESS

With child's right arm flexed 90 degrees at elbow, mark midpoint between acromion and olecranon on posterior aspect of arm.

With arm hanging freely, grasp a fold of skin between thumb and forefinger 1 cm above midpoint.

Gently pull away from underlying muscle and continue to hold until measurement is completed.

Place caliper jaws over skinfold at midpoint mark and follow directions for using the device.

Estimate reading to nearest 1 mm, 2 to 3 seconds after applying pressure.

Take measurements until duplicates agree within 1 mm.

compare the values taken on preceding health visits with present recordings. For example, a falsely elevated blood pressure reading may not indicate hypertension if previous recent readings have been within normal limits. The isolated recording may indicate some stressful event in the child's life.

As in most procedures carried out with children, older children and adolescents are treated much the same as are adults. However, special consideration must be given to preschool children (Atraumatic Care box).

For best results in taking vital signs of infants, count respirations first (before the infant is disturbed), take the pulse next, and measure temperature last. If vital signs cannot be taken without disturbing the child, record the child's behavior (e.g., crying) along with the measurement.

Atraumatic Care

REDUCING YOUNG CHILDREN'S FEARS

Young children, especially preschoolers, fear intrusive procedures because of their poorly defined body boundaries. Therefore avoid invasive procedures, such as measuring rectal temperature, whenever possible. Also, avoid using the word "take" when measuring vital signs, since young children interpret words literally and may think that their temperature or other function will be taken away. Instead, say, "I want to know how warm you are."

Temperature. Temperature can be measured at several sites in the body via the oral, rectal, axillary, skin, or tympanic membrane routes. Substitutes for the traditional mercury thermometer include the electronic thermometer, the tympanic membrane sensor (see Fig. 35-7), the liquid crystal contact thermometer, and the digital thermometer. These devices offer the advantages of measuring temperature rapidly and/or avoiding oral or rectal intrusion (Table 35-3). Although the accuracy of these instruments differs, accuracy is decreased to a greater extent if correct technique is not used, if the child is febrile, or if the child's age is not considered.

No universal agreement exists regarding the length of time mercury thermometers should be kept in place. Recommendations based on research are 7 minutes for an oral reading, 4 minutes for a rectal reading, and 5 minutes for an axillary reading. However, these times may vary widely within practice settings and may not represent clinically significant differences from temperature readings taken for shorter intervals.

Normal body temperature registers 37.0° C (98.6° F) via the oral route. Traditionally it has been assumed that rectal temperatures are 1° F higher and axillary temperatures are 1° F lower than oral temperatures. However, it has been demonstrated that this difference is considerably less (Pontious et al, 1994b). Because of these variations, chart the route along with the recorded temperature reading.

Whenever a child feels extra warm to the touch, measure the temperature, even if it was normal only a short time before.

A

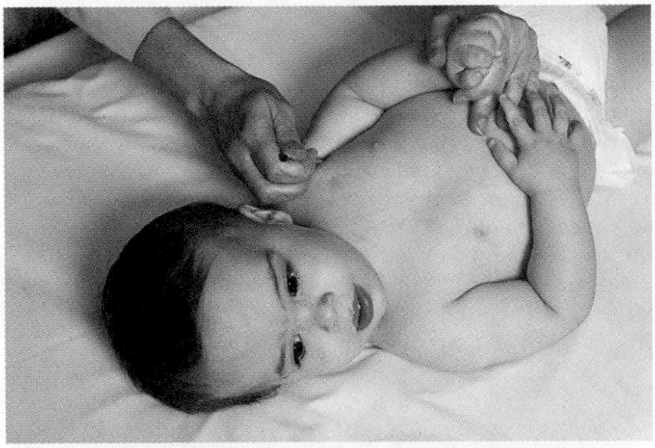

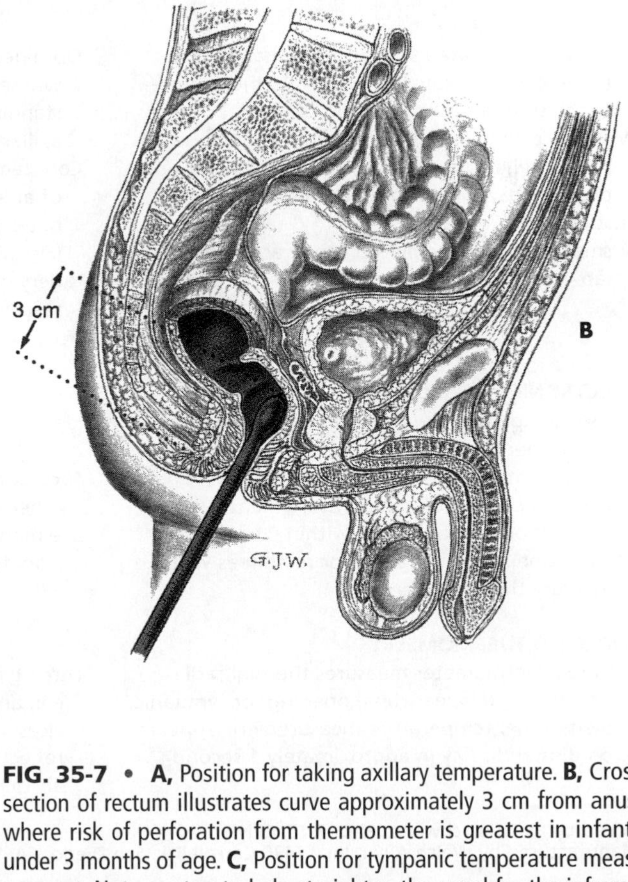

B

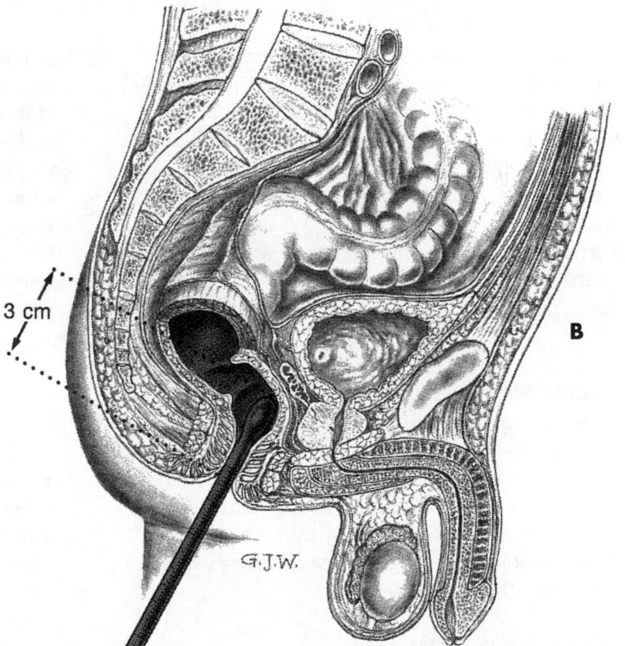

C

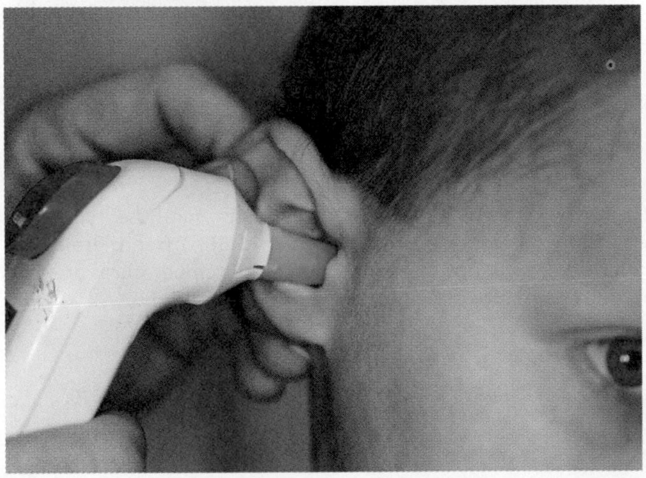

FIG. 35-7 • **A,** Position for taking axillary temperature. **B,** Cross section of rectum illustrates curve approximately 3 cm from anus, where risk of perforation from thermometer is greatest in infants under 3 months of age. **C,** Position for tympanic temperature measurement. Note ear tug to help straighten the canal for the infrared sensor to focus on the eardrum.

TABLE 35-3
Comparison of Body Temperature Techniques

Description/Procedure	Comments
MERCURY GLASS THERMOMETER	
Heat causes mercury to expand and rise in glass tube	Only difference in selection of mercury thermometers is that rectal type has more rounded tip as compared with oral type, which has more slender, elongated tip The appropriate length of time that mercury thermometer should remain in place for accurate measurement of temperature is controversial; a general rule is to leave thermometer in place approximately 3 minutes, or follow agency policy
Oral Temperature	
Place under tongue in right or left posterior sublingual pocket, not in front of tongue; have child keep mouth closed without biting on thermometer	Contrary to traditional belief, oral site indicates rapid changes in core body temperature better than rectal site, but accuracy may be an issue (Jensen et al, 1994) Several factors affect temperature of mouth, such as hot or cold beverages, smoking, open-mouth breathing, and ambient temperature (Hooker and Houston, 1996)
Axillary Temperature	
Place under arm with tip in center of axilla and kept close to skin, not clothing; hold child's arm firmly against side (Fig. 35-7, *A*)	Recommended for children who object strongly to rectal temperature but for whom an oral temperature is not feasible Has advantage of avoiding intrusive procedure and eliminating risk of rectal perforation and possible peritonitis May be affected by poor peripheral perfusion (lower value) or use of radiant warmers or brown fat in cold-stressed neonates (higher value) (Bliss-Holtz, 1995; Haddock, Merrow, and Swanson, 1996)
Rectal Temperature	
Place well-lubricated tip not more than 2.5 cm (1 inch) into rectum; securely hold thermometer close to anus May place child in side-lying, supine, or prone position (i.e., supine with knees flexed toward abdomen); cover penis because procedure often stimulates urination A small child may be placed prone across parent's lap	Obtained when no other route or device can be used (e.g., in children whose mental age or temperament prevents cooperation and understanding instructions, agitated children, and those who have had oral or axillary injuries or surgery) (Anagnostakis et al, 1993) Core temperature is not obtained unless thermometer is inserted to depth of at least 5 cm, which incurs risk of rectal perforation, especially in neonates younger than 3 months of age, since colon curves at depth of 3 cm (Fig. 35-7, *B*); also not recommended in anyone who has had rectal surgery or in children with diarrhea or those receiving chemotherapy that affects mucosa or causes neutropenia (Hockenberry-Eaton and Kline, 1997) Accuracy is affected by stool in rectum (higher value)
ELECTRONIC THERMOMETER	
Senses temperature with electronic component called thermistor mounted at tip of plastic and stainless steel probe, which is connected to electronic recorder; temperature measurement appears on digital display within 60 seconds Place probe in mouth, axilla, or rectum as with mercury thermometer	Ideally suited to pediatric use because plastic sheath is unbreakable and child's mouth can remain open when oral temperature is taken Accuracy for axillary temperature is supported by some research but not by other studies (Haddock, Merrow, and Swanson, 1996; Wilshaw et al, 1999) Use predictive mode for oral/rectal temperatures; use monitor mode for axillary temperatures unless axillary predictive mode available (SureTemp 678*)
INFRARED THERMOMETRY	
Infrared thermometer measures thermal radiation from axilla, ear canal opening, or tympanic membrane; temperature measurement appears on digital display in approximately 1 second	Three types of infrared thermometers are available for aural use: tympanic, ear, and arterial heat balance via the ear canal (AHBE); often these devices are referred to as tympanic thermometers; all temperatures are a reflection of arterial temperature (Pompei and Pompei, 1996; Wilshaw et al, 1999)

Revised by Patricia Schwartz, PhD, RNC, CPNP.
*Manufactured by Welch Allyn, Inc., 7420 Carroll Rd., San Diego, CA, 92121; phone 1-800-854-2904, (619) 621-6600; fax (619) 621-6610.

TABLE 35-3—cont'd
Comparison of Body Temperature Techniques

Description/Procedure	Comments
INFRARED THERMOMETRY—cont'd	
Tympanic Membrane Sensor	
Insert covered probe tip gently in ear canal pointing toward midpoint between opposite eyebrow and sideburns (Childs, Harrison, and Hodkinson, 1999) For most accurate results, straighten ear canal for sensor to measure heat from drum, not sides of canal (see Figs. 35-20 and 35-7, C); take three measurements; and record highest reading Most models use "offsets" or internal calculations that transform ear temperature into supposedly equivalent oral or rectal temperatures	Tympanic membrane is excellent site because both eardrum and hypothalamus (temperature-regulating center) are perfused by same circulation Warm, ambient temperature may increase aural temperature (Henker and Coyne, 1995) Although frequently used in pediatric settings, especially ambulatory clinics, debate continues on accuracy of tympanic thermometry in screening febrile child (Lanham et al, 1999; Modell et al, 1998; Prazer, 1998; Robinson et al, 1998) Because of difficulty with correct placement in young infants' ears, accuracy may be affected (Robinson et al, 1998; Houlder, 2000)
Ear Sensor (LighTouch LTX)*	
Measures infrared heat energy radiating from canal opening, scans canal for highest temperature reading, and then calculates arterial temperature (correlates highly with core or internal body temperature) Insert hemispherical probe in ear opening; ear tug is not necessary	Available in two sizes, smaller size of LighTouch Pedi-Q is for infants and toddlers (Wilshaw et al, 1999) Does not calculate offsets; therefore reading is only for arterial temperature (not equivalent to other sites)
Axillary Sensor (LighTouch LTN)*	
Measures infrared heat energy radiating from axilla Touch covered probe to axilla, depress and release button, remove and read	Can be used on wet skin; in incubators; or under radiant heaters, warming pads, or other heat sources
DIGITAL THERMOMETER	
Consists of probe that connects to microprocessor chip, which translates signals into degrees and sends temperature measurement to digital display Used like oral mercury thermometer	More accurate and easier to read but somewhat more expensive than mercury or plastic strip thermometer Often useful when single-patient use is needed (e.g., patients in isolation)
LIQUID CRYSTAL SKIN CONTACT THERMOMETER (CHEMICAL DOT THERMOMETER)	
Single-use disposable, flexible thermometer with specific chemical mixture in each circle that changes color to measure temperature increments of two tenths of a degree Two types: Used like mercury thermometer; kept in mouth (1 minute), axilla (3 minutes), or rectum (3 minutes); color change is read 10 to 15 seconds after removing thermometer Wearable, continuous-use thermometer, which is placed under axilla; may be read within 2 to 3 minutes after placement and continuously thereafter; remove and replace every 48 hours	May underestimate oral temperature and overestimate axillary temperature (Erickson, Meyer, and Woo, 1996) Found to be accurate and reliable for children with and without fever, especially for temperature less than 38°C (100.4°F) (Pontious et al, 1994a, 1994b; Payne et al, 1994) Easier to read than mercury or plastic strip thermometer Safer than glass thermometer Read thermometer away from heat source (e.g., radiant warmer) For older chemical dot thermometers, if unused thermometer changes color from storage in a warm area (greater than 35° C (95° F), place in freezer for 1 hour and then at room temperature for 24 hours before using (Py Ma H Corporation, 1994); newer types do not require special storage (Medical Indicators, Inc., 1999) Wearable, continuous-reading thermometer preferred by parents because it requires minimal disturbance to child (i.e., nurse can just lift child's arm to get a temperature reading (Rivera et al, 1997)
PLASTIC STRIP THERMOMETER (THERMOGRAPH)	
Changes color in response to sensed temperature changes Place strip on forehead until color change occurs; usually takes less than 15 seconds Some strips are used like oral mercury thermometer	Accuracy is variable; best used for screening (Shann and Mackenzie, 1996) Advantages for home and community use include simple instructions and minimal cost (Valadez, Elmore-Meegan, and Morley, 1995)

*Manufactured by Exergen Corporation, 51 Water St., Watertown, MA 02172, phone 1-800-422-3006, (617) 923-9900; fax (617) 923-9911; website: www.exergen.com.

Other signs of increased body temperature are flushed skin, increased respiratory and heart rates, malaise, and a "glassy look" to the eyes.

Pulse. A satisfactory pulse can be taken radially in children over 2 years of age. However, in infants and young children the apical impulse (heard through a stethoscope held to the chest at the apex of the heart) is more reliable (see Fig. 35-29 for location of pulses). Count the pulse for 1 full minute in infants and young children because of possible irregularities in rhythm. However, when frequent apical rates are needed, use shorter counting time (e.g., 15- or 30-second intervals). For greater accuracy, measure the apical rate while the child is asleep; record the child's behavior along with the rate. Pulses may be graded according to the criteria in Table 35-4. Compare radial and femoral pulses at least once during infancy to detect the presence of circulatory impairment, such as coarctation of the aorta. (See Appendix J for normal rates for pediatric age groups.)

TABLE 35-4
Grading of Pulses

Grade	Description
0	Not palpable
+1	Difficult to palpate, thready, weak, easily obliterated with pressure
+2	Difficult to palpate, may be obliterated with pressure
+3	Easy to palpate, not easily obliterated with pressure (normal)
+4	Strong, bounding, not obliterated with pressure

Respiration. Count the respiratory rate in the same manner as for the adult patient. In infants, however, observe abdominal movements because respirations are primarily diaphragmatic. Since the movements are irregular, count them for 1 full minute for accuracy (see Appendix J for normal respiratory rates in children).

Blood Pressure (BP). BP measurement by noninvasive methods is part of a routine vital sign determination. BP should be measured annually in children 3 years of age through adolescence; and in children with symptoms of hypertension, children in emergency departments and intensive care units, and high risk infants (National Institute of Health [NIH], 1996). Several authorities also recommend routine measurements in low risk neonates (Seidel, Rosenstein, and Pathak, 1997).

Measurement Devices. The most common method of measuring BP uses *auscultation* and either a *mercury-gravity* or an *aneroid sphygmomanometer.* Both types are reliable and accurate, but the mercury-gravity manometer does not require recalibration as does the aneroid type.

BP can also be measured using electronic devices that employ oscillometric or Doppler techniques. In *oscillometry,* pressure changes are transmitted through the arterial wall to the pressure cuff, and the oscillations are detected by a pressure-sensitive indicator. Oscillometers have digital read-outs for systolic, diastolic, and *mean arterial pressure (MAP),* and pulse. The MAP is not the same as the mean BP (i.e., the arithmetic average of systolic and diastolic pressures). Rather, it is a value somewhat lower than the arithmetic mean. BP readings that use oscillometry, such as DINAMAP, are generally higher and correlate better with direct radial artery values than measurements using auscultation (Amoore, 1998; Gillman and Cook, 1995; Ling et al, 1995; Wattigney et al, 1996) (see Table 35-5). Oscillometry also eliminates common problems found with the auscultation method, such as deflating the cuff too rapidly, not

TABLE 35-5
Normative Dinamap BP Values (Systolic/diastolic, mean arterial pressure in parentheses)

Age-Group	Mean	90th Percentile	95th Percentile
Newborn (1-3 days)	65/41 (50)	75/49 (59)	78/52 (62)
1 month to 2 years	95/58 (72)	106/68 (83)	110/71 (86)
2 to 5 years	101/57 (74)	112/66 (82)	115/68 (85)

From Park M, Menard S: Normative oscillometric blood pressure values in the first 5 years in an office setting, *Am J Dis Child* 143(7):860-864, 1989.

TABLE 35-6
Recommended Bladder Dimensions for Blood Pressure Cuffs

Arm Circumference at Midpoint (cm)	Cuff Name*	Bladder Width (cm)	Bladder Length (cm)
5-7.5	Newborn	3	5
7.5-13	Infant	5	8
13-20	Child	8	13
24-32	Adult	13	24
32-42	Wide adult	17	32
42-50	Thigh	20	42

From Frohlich ED et al: Recommendations for human blood pressure determination by sphygmomanometers: report of a special task force appointed by the Steering Committee, American Heart Association, *Circulation* 77:501A, 1988.
*Cuff name does not guarantee that cuff will be appropriate size for a child within that age range.

hearing the softest sounds, and rounding the numbers for the Korotkoff sounds.

Doppler ultrasound translates changes in ultrasound frequency caused by blood movement within the artery to audible sound by means of a transducer in the cuff. This technique is useful for systolic pressure measurement but is unreliable for diastolic pressure measurement. Oscillometric and Doppler instruments are very useful in measuring BP in infants and have largely replaced the flush method, which reflects only the mean BP; and the auscultatory method.

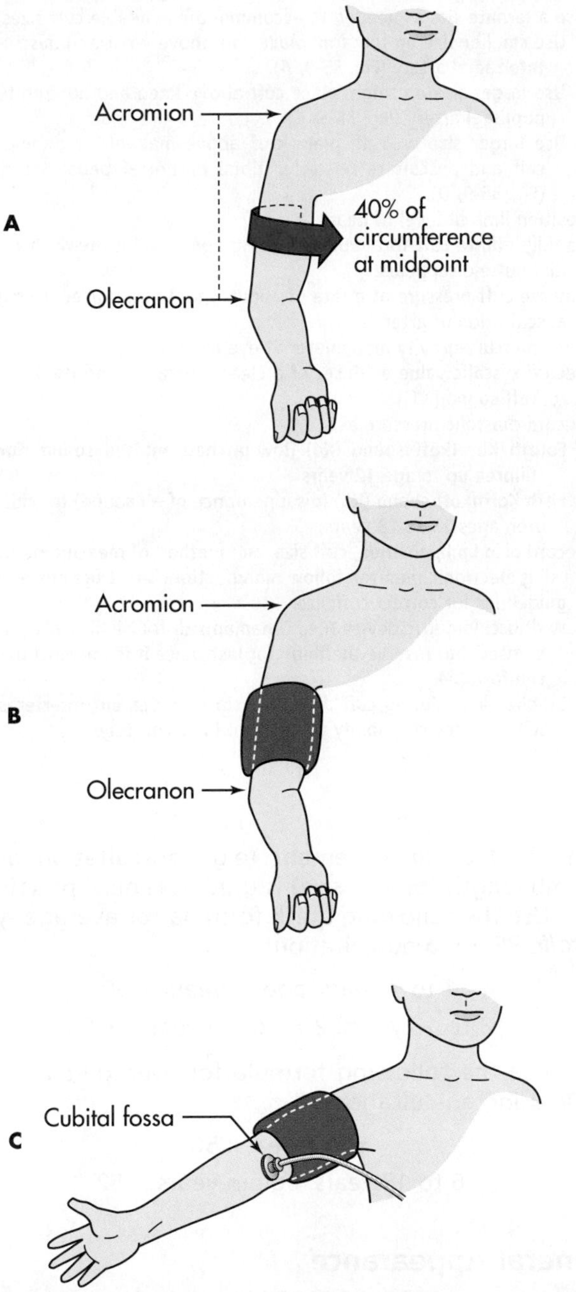

FIG. 35-8 • Determination of proper cuff size. **A,** The cuff bladder width should be approximately 40% of the circumference of the arm measured at a point midway between the olecranon and acromion. **B,** Cuff bladder length should cover 80% to 100% of the circumference of the arm. **C,** Blood pressure should be measured with cubital fossa at heart level. The arm should be supported. The stethoscope bell is placed over the brachial artery pulse, proximal and medial to the cubital fossa, and below the bottom edge of the cuff. (From NIH, National Heart, Lung, Blood Institute: NIH Pub No. 96-3790, Sept. 1996.)

Selection of Cuff. No matter what type of noninvasive technique is used, the most important factor in accurately measuring BP is the use of an appropriately sized cuff (cuff size refers only to the inner inflatable bladder, not the cloth covering). A technique to establish an appropriate cuff size is to choose a cuff having a bladder width that is approximately 40% of the arm circumference midway between the olecranon and the acromion. This will usually be a cuff bladder that covers 80% to 100% of the circumference of the arm (Fig. 35-8).

Using limb circumference for selecting cuff width more accurately reflects direct arterial BP than using limb length, because this method takes into account the variations in thickness of the arm and the amount of pressure required to compress the artery (Gillman and Cook, 1995). For measurement sites other than the upper arms, the limb circumference guidelines can be used, although the shape of the limb (i.e., conical shape of the thigh) may prevent appropriate placement of the cuff and may inaccurately reflect intraarterial BP (Table 35-6, Fig. 35-9).

Cuffs that are either too narrow or too wide affect the accuracy of BP measurements, although wide cuffs tend to affect BP readings less. If the cuff is too small, the reading on the device is falsely high. If the cuff is too large, the reading is falsely low.

NURSE ALERT • In choosing cuff sizes, use an appropriately sized cuff. When the correct size is not available, use an oversized cuff rather than an undersized one or use another site that more appropriately fits the cuff size. Do not choose a cuff based on the name of the cuff (e.g., an "infant" cuff may be too small for some infants).

When another site is used, BP measurements using noninvasive techniques may differ. Generally, systolic pressure in the lower extremities (i.e., thigh or calf) is greater than pressure in the upper extremities, and systolic BP in the calf is higher than that in the thigh. These differences, listed in Table 35-7, apply to oscillometric measurements taken on the right extremities with the child supine and with the cuff size based on the circumference method (Park, Lee, and Johnson, 1993).

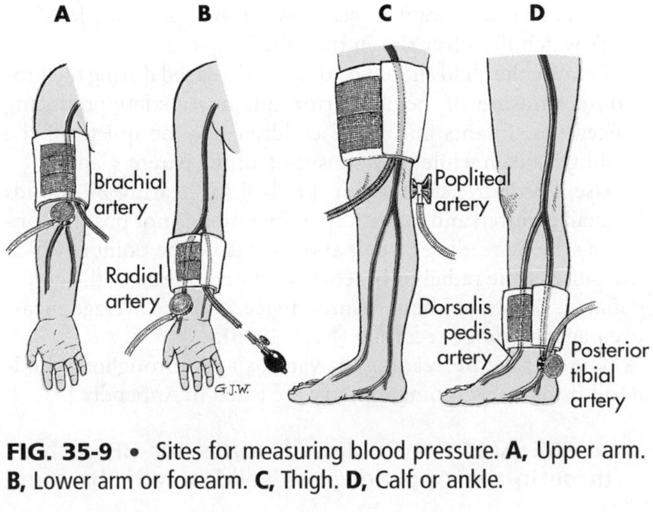

FIG. 35-9 • Sites for measuring blood pressure. **A,** Upper arm. **B,** Lower arm or forearm. **C,** Thigh. **D,** Calf or ankle.

TABLE 35-7
Differences in Oscillometric Systolic BP between Arm and Lower Extremity Sites in Normal Children

Age Group (Years)	Systolic BP × Mean + SD)	
	Arm-Thigh	Arm-Calf
4-8	−1.1 ± 6.8	−9.3 ± 7.4
9-16	−2.4 ± 7.7	−5.0 ± 26.9

From Park M, Lee D, Johnson GA: Oscillometric blood pressure in the arm, thigh, and calf in healthy children and those with aortic coarctation, *Pediatrics* 91(4):761-765, 1993.

NURSE ALERT • Compare blood pressure in the upper and lower extremities at least once to detect abnormalities such as coarctation of the aorta, in which the lower extremity pressure is less than the upper extremity pressure.

Measurement and Interpretation. Measuring and interpreting BP in infants and children requires additional attention to correct procedure because: (1) limb sizes vary and cuff selection must accommodate the circumference; (2) excessive pressure on the antecubital fossa affects the Korotkoff sounds; (3) children easily become anxious, which can elevate BP; and (4) BP values change with age and growth.

Age, height, weight, and body mass have been shown to be highly correlated with BP (NIH, 1996). Recent studies indicate that height is a more appropriate index of maturation than weight for use with normative BP data, and should be considered when evaluating BP in children. Tables are now available that indicate—when height is taken into account—that more short children (<10th percentile for age-sex-specific height) and fewer tall children (>90th percentile for age-sex-specific height) are likely to be classified as hypertensive. (See Appendix J for BP tables.)

Although the technique of BP measurement in children is generally the same as that used for adults (Guidelines box), some aspects of the procedure are especially important. Because children are easily upset by unfamiliar procedures, prepare them for BP measurement. For children of preschool age and above, explain each step of the procedure and tell them how the cuff will feel, such as a tight feeling or an arm hug. Use explanations such as "I want to see how strong your muscle is" or "Let's watch the silver rise in the tube."

Because the child should be quiet and relaxed during the procedure, measure BP before performing any anxiety-producing procedures. Infants and small children may be quieter if the reading is taken while they are sitting in the parent's lap.

Use a pediatric stethoscope and bell for hearing BP sounds in small children and infants. If auscultation is not possible, obtain a systolic reading by palpation; measure the point at which the pulse at the radial or brachial artery reappears as the cuff is deflated. BP should be measured twice, and the average measurement should be recorded (NIH, 1996).

The average BP readings at various ages throughout childhood using sphygmomanometry are listed in Appendix J.

NURSE ALERT • Published norms for BP, such as those in the Appendix, are valid only if the same method of measurement (e.g., auscultation and limb length for cuff size) is used in clinical practice.

Use the following quick formula for average *systolic BP* using auscultation:

1 to 7 years: age in years + 90

8 to 18 years: 2 × age in years) + 83

Use the following formula for average *diastolic BP* using auscultation:

1 to 5 years: 56

6 to 18 years: age in years + 52

Guidelines

MEASURING BLOOD PRESSURE

- Use an appropriately sized cuff.
- Use same position, preferably sitting, and right arm for brachial artery site (Figs. 35-8 and 35-9, *A*)
- Use alternate site as needed to accommodate available cuff sizes.
  - Use smaller size on forearm: place cuff above wrist and auscultate radial artery (Fig. 35-9, *B*).
  - Use larger size on thigh: place cuff above knee and auscultate popliteal artery (Fig. 35-9, *C*).
  - Use larger size on calf: place cuff above malleoli or at midcalf and auscultate posterior tibial or dorsal pedal artery (Fig. 35-9, *D*).
- Position limb at level of heart.
- Rapidly inflate cuff to about 20 mm Hg above point at which radial pulse disappears.
- Release cuff pressure at a rate of about 2 to 3 mm Hg/sec during auscultation of artery.
- Read mercury-gravity manometer at eye level.
- Record systolic value as onset of a clear tapping sound (first Korotkoff sound [K1]).
- Record diastolic pressure as:
  - Fourth Korotkoff sound (K4) (low-pitched, muffed sound) for children up to age 12 years
  - Fifth Korotkoff sound (K5) (disappearance of all sound) for children ages 13 to 18 years
- Record also limb, position, cuff size, and method of measurement.
- If using electronic monitor, follow manufacturer's instructions and guidelines for correct cuff size.
  - With oscillometric device (i.e., Dinamap), all four limb sites can be used, but reserve the thigh for last, since it is the most uncomfortable.
  - Stablize limb during cuff deflation, since movement interferes with the device's ability to measure BP accurately.

General Appearance

The general appearance of the child is a cumulative, subjective impression of the child's physical appearance, state of nutrition, behavior, personality, interactions with parents and nurse (also siblings if present), posture, development, and speech. Although general appearance is recorded at the beginning of the physical examination, it encompasses all of the observations of the child during the interview and physical assessment.

Note the *facies,* the facial expression and appearance of the child. For example, the facies may give clues to children who are in pain; have difficulty breathing; feel frightened, discontented, or happy; are mentally deficient; or are acutely ill.

Observe the *posture, position,* and types of *body movement.* The child with hearing or vision loss may characteristically tilt the head in an awkward position to hear or see better. The child in pain may favor a body part. The child with low self-esteem or a feeling of rejection may assume a slumped, careless, and apathetic pose or posture. Likewise, a child with confidence, a feeling of self-worth, and a sense of security usually demonstrates a tall, straight, well-balanced posture. While observing such "body language," do not interpret too freely but rather record objectively.

Note the child's *hygiene* in terms of cleanliness; unusual body odor; the condition of the hair, neck, nails, teeth, and feet; and the condition of the clothing. Such observations are excellent clues to possible instances of neglect, inadequate financial resources, housing difficulties (e.g., no running water), or lack of knowledge concerning children's needs.

General appearance includes an overall impression of the child's state of *nutrition.* This impression is more than a statement describing body weight or stature, such as "slender and tall." It is an estimation of the quality, as well as the quantity, of nutritional intake. For example, two children can be of the same height and weight, yet one can appear overweight because of flabby, loose skin, whereas the other child appears strong, robust, and well built because of firm, well-defined musculature. Likewise, a small, slender child may be well nourished with no signs of chronic undernutrition, such as bony prominences, a protuberant abdomen, flat buttocks, gaunt facies, and poor muscle tone with evidence of wasting.

Compare your impression of the nutritional state with the parents' history of feeding practices. Discrepancies between the two "impressions" may be a valuable area for nutritional counseling. For example, parents who believe that their child is too thin and eats too little, despite evidence of adequate growth and physical signs of proper nutrition, may find it helpful to keep a daily diary to calculate the child's cumulative food intake. Many parents are surprised at the quantity of food ingested, even though the amounts at each meal or snack are small.

Behavior includes the child's personality, level of activity, reaction to stress, requests, frustration, interactions with others (primarily the parent and nurse), degree of alertness, and response to stimuli. Some mental questions that serve as reminders for observing behavior include: What is the child's overall personality? Does the child have a long attention span or is he or she easily distracted? Can the child follow two or three commands in succession without the need for repetition? What is the youngster's response to delayed gratification or frustration? Is eye-to-eye contact used during conversation? What is the child's reaction to the nurse and family members? Is the child quick or slow to grasp explanations?

Development can be assessed by carefully observing the child, but verify your impressions with screening tests. Various tests for assessing development, speech, vision, and hearing are discussed later in this chapter and in Chapter 42.

Record an overall estimate of the child's speech development, motor skills, degree of coordination, and recent area of achievement under general appearance. For example, the following statement may apply to an 18-month-old child: "Motor development advanced for age; climbs, runs, jumps (most recent motor skill), manipulates small objects with ease; excellent coordination and balance; beginning to name many objects; uses two-word phrases; and enjoys talking to self and others."

Skin

Skin is assessed for color, texture, temperature, moisture, and turgor. Examination of the skin and its accessory organs primarily involves inspection and palpation. The normal *color* in light-skinned children varies from a milky white and rose color to a deeply hued pink color. Dark-skinned children, such as those of Native American, Hispanic, or African-American descent, have inherited various brown, red, yellow, olive green, and bluish tones in their skin. Oriental persons have skin that is normally of a yellow tone.

Several variations in skin color can occur, some of which warrant further investigation. These types of color changes and their appearance in children with light or dark skin are summarized in Table 35-8.

Normally the skin *texture* of young children is smooth, slightly dry, and not oily or clammy. Evaluate skin *temperature* by symmetrically feeling each part of the body and comparing upper areas with lower ones. Note any difference in temperature.

Determine *tissue turgor,* or the amount of elasticity in the skin, by grasping the skin on the abdomen between the thumb and index finger, pulling it taut, and quickly releasing it. Elastic tissue immediately assumes its normal position without residual marks or creases. In children with poor skin turgor the skin remains suspended or tented for a few seconds before slowly falling back on the abdomen. Skin turgor is one of the best estimates of adequate hydration and nutrition.

Accessory Structures. Inspection of the accessory structures of the skin may be performed while the skin is being examined or when the scalp and extremities are being assessed.

Inspect the *hair* for color, texture, quality, distribution, and elasticity. Children's scalp hair is usually lustrous, silky, strong, and elastic. Genetic factors affect the appearance of hair. For example, the hair of African-American children is usually curlier and coarser than that of Caucasian children. Hair that is stringy, dull, brittle, dry, friable, and depigmented may suggest poor nutrition. Record any bald or thinning spots. Loss of hair in infants may indicate lying in the same position, and may be a clue for counseling parents concerning the child's stimulation needs.

Inspect the hair and scalp for general cleanliness. Various ethnic groups condition their hair with oils or lubricants, which, if not thoroughly washed from the scalp, clog the sebaceous glands, causing scalp infections. Also examine the area for lesions; scaliness; evidence of infestation, such as lice or ticks; and signs of trauma, such as ecchymosis, masses, or scars.

In children who are approaching puberty, look for growth of secondary hair as a sign of normally progressing pubertal changes. Note precocious or delayed appearance of hair growth because, although not always suggestive of hormonal dysfunction, it may be of great concern to the early- or late-maturing adolescent.

Inspect the *nails* for color, shape, texture, and quality. Normally the nails are pink, convex, smooth, and hard but flexible (not brittle). The edges, which are usually white, should extend over the fingers. Dark-skinned individuals may have more deeply pigmented nail beds. Short, ragged nails are typical of habitual biting. Uncut, dirty nails are a sign of poor hygiene.

Each individual has a distinct set of handprints and footprints. The patterns, or *dermatoglyphics,* are unique to the individual and vary a great deal in detail and complexity. The palm normally shows three flexion creases (Fig. 35-10, *A*). In some

TABLE 35-8
Differences in Color Changes of Racial Groups

Description	Appearance in Light Skin	Appearance in Dark Skin
CYANOSIS		
Bluish tone through skin; reflects reduced (deoxygenated) hemoglobin	Bluish tinge, especially in palpebral conjunctiva (lower eyelid), nail beds, earlobes, lips, oral membranes, soles, and palms	Ashen gray lips and tongue
PALLOR		
Paleness may be a sign of anemia, chronic disease, edema, or shock	Loss of rosy glow in skin, especially face	Ashen gray appearance in black skin More yellowish brown color in brown skin
ERYTHEMA		
Redness may be result of increased blood flow from climatic conditions, local inflammation, infection, skin irritation, allergy, or other dermatoses or may be caused by increased numbers of red blood cells as a compensatory response to chronic hypoxia	Redness easily seen anywhere on body	Much more difficult to assess; rely on palpation for warmth or edema
ECCHYMOSIS		
Large, diffuse areas, usually black and blue, caused by hemorrhage of blood into skin; are typically result of injuries	Purplish to yellow-green areas; may be seen anywhere on skin	Very difficult to see unless in mouth or conjunctiva
PETECHIAE		
Same as ecchymosis except for size: small, distinct pinpoint hemorrhages 2 mm or less in size; can denote some type of blood disorder, such as leukemia	Purplish pinpoints most easily seen on buttocks, abdomen, and inner surfaces of the arms or legs	Usually invisible except in oral mucosa, conjunctiva of eyelids, and conjunctiva covering eyeball
JAUNDICE		
Yellow staining of the skin usually caused by bile pigments	Yellow staining seen in sclerae of eyes, skin, fingernails, soles, palms, and oral mucosa	Most reliably assessed in sclerae, hard palate, palms, and soles

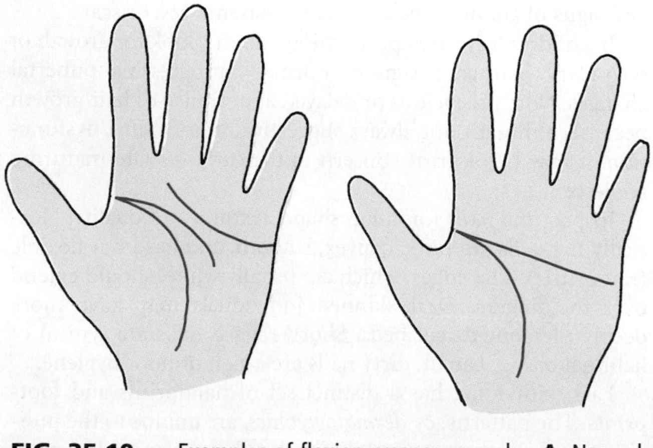

FIG. 35-10 • Examples of flexion creases on palm. **A,** Normal. **B,** Transpalmar crease.

situations, such as Down syndrome, the two distal horizontal creases are fused to form a single horizontal crease (the *single palmar crease,* or *transpalmar crease*) (Fig. 35-10, *B*). If grossly abnormal lines or folds are observed, sketch a picture to describe them and refer the finding to a specialist for further investigation.

Lymph Nodes

Lymph nodes are usually assessed when the part of the body in which they are located is examined. Although the body's lymphatic drainage system is extensive, the usual sites for palpating accessible lymph nodes are shown in Fig. 35-11.

Palpate nodes by using the distal portion of the fingers and gently but firmly pressing in a circular motion along the regions where nodes are normally present. During assessment of the nodes in the head and neck, tilt the child's head upward slightly but without tensing the sternocleidomastoid or trapezius muscles. This position facilitates palpation of the *submental, sub-*

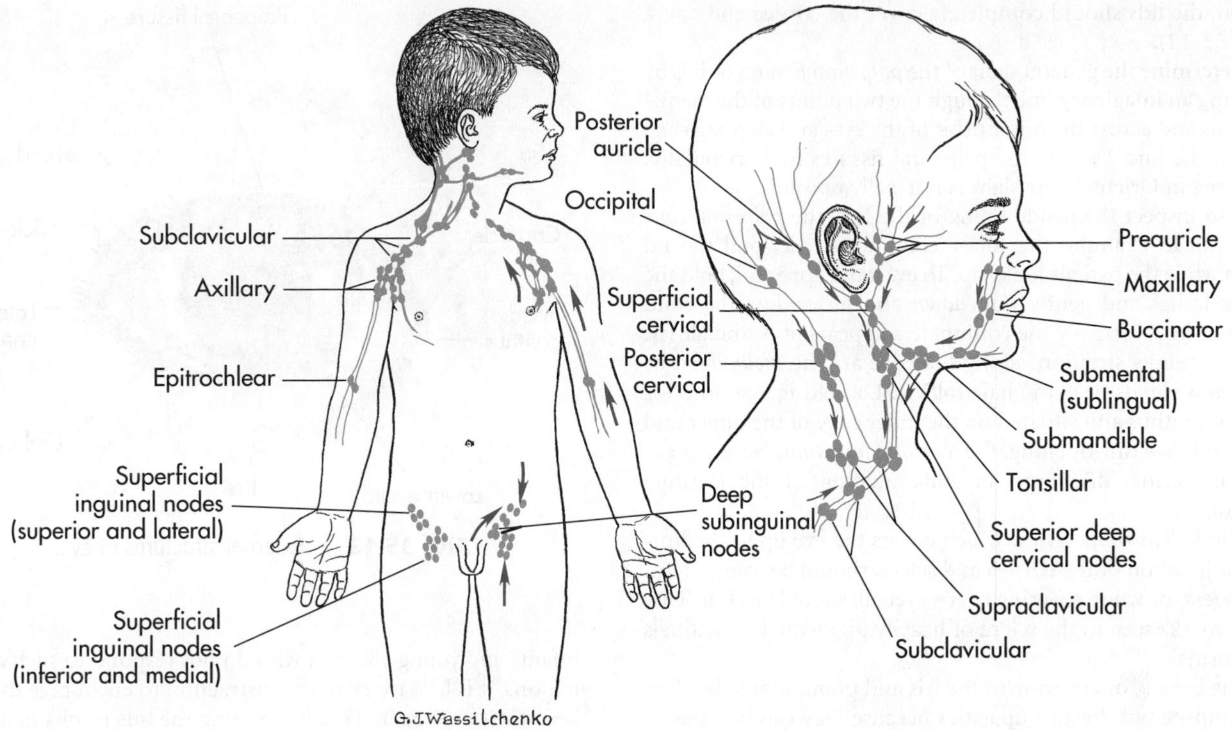

FIG. 35-11 • Location of superficial lymph nodes. Arrows indicate directional flow of lymph.

maxillary, tonsillar, and *cervical nodes.* Palpate the axillary nodes with the arms relaxed at the sides but slightly abducted. Assess the *inguinal nodes* with the child in the supine position. Note size, mobility, temperature, and tenderness, as well as reports by the parents regarding any visible change of enlarged nodes. In children small, nontender, moveable nodes are usually normal. Tender, enlarged, warm lymph nodes generally indicate infection or inflammation close to their location. Report such findings for further investigation.

Head and Neck

Observe the head for general *shape* and *symmetry.* A flattening of one part of the head, such as the occiput, may indicate that the child continually lies in this position. Marked asymmetry is usually abnormal and may indicate premature closure of the sutures (craniosynostosis).

Note *head control* in infants and *head posture* in older children. Most infants by 4 months of age should be able to hold their head erect and in midline when in a vertical position.

NURSE ALERT • Significant head lag after 6 months of age indicates cerebral injury and is referred for further evaluation.

Evaluate range of motion by asking the older child to look in each direction (i.e., to either side, up, and down); or by manually putting the younger child through each position. Limited range of motion may indicate *wryneck,* or *torticollis,* a result of injury to the sternocleidomastoid muscle in which the child holds the head to one side with the chin pointing toward the opposite side.

NURSE ALERT • Hyperextension of the head (opisthotonos) with pain on flexion is a serious indication of meningeal irritation and is referred for immediate medical evaluation.

Palpate the *skull* for patent sutures, fontanels, fractures, and swellings. Normally the posterior fontanel closes by the second month of life and the anterior fontanel fuses between 12 and 18 months of age. Early or late closure is noted, since either may be a sign of a pathologic condition. (For a more detailed discussion of the cranial bones, see Chapter 36.)

While examining the head, observe the *face* for symmetry, movement, and general appearance. Ask the child to "make a face" to assess symmetric movement and disclose any degree of paralysis. Note any unusual facial proportion such as an unusually high or low forehead; wide- or close-set eyes; or a small, receding chin.

In addition to assessment of the head and neck for movement, inspect the neck for size and palpate it for associated structures. The neck is normally short, with skinfolds between the head and shoulders during infancy; however, it lengthens during the next 3 to 4 years.

NURSE ALERT • If any masses are detected in the neck, report them for further investigation. Large masses can block the airway.

Eyes

Inspection of External Structures. Inspect the lids for proper placement on the eye. When the eye is open, the upper lid should fall near the upper iris. When the eyes are closed, the lids should completely cover the cornea and sclera (Fig. 35-12).

Determine the general slant of the *palpebral fissures* or lids by drawing an imaginary line through the two points of the medial canthus and across the outer orbit of the eyes and aligning each eye on the line. Usually the palpebral fissures lie horizontally; however, in Orientals the slant is normally upward.

Also inspect the inside lining of the lids, the *palpebral conjunctiva.* To examine the lower conjunctiva sac, pull the lid down while the patient looks up. To evert the upper lid, hold the upper lashes and gently pull *down* and *forward* as the child looks down. Normally the conjunctiva appears pink and glossy. Vertical yellow striations along the edge are the *meibomian* or *sebaceous glands* near the hair follicle. Located in the inner or medial canthus and situated on the inner edge of the upper and lower lids is a tiny opening, the *lacrimal punctum.* Note any excessive tearing, discharge, or inflammation of the lacrimal apparatus.

The *bulbar conjunctiva,* which covers the eye up to the limbus or junction of the cornea and sclera, should be transparent. The *sclera,* or white covering of the eyeball, should be clear. Tiny black marks seen in the sclera of heavily pigmented individuals are normal.

The *cornea,* or covering of the iris and pupil, should be clear and transparent. Record opacities because they can be signs of scarring or ulceration, which can interfere with vision. The best way to test for opacities is to illuminate the eyeball by shining a light at an angle (obliquely) toward the cornea.

Compare the *pupils* for size, shape, and movement. They should be round, clear, and equal. Test their *reaction to light* by quickly shining a source of light toward the eye and removing it. As the light approaches, the pupils should constrict; as the light fades, the pupils should dilate. Test the pupil response of *accommodation* by having the child look at a bright, shiny object at a distance and quickly moving the object toward the face. The pupils should constrict as the object is brought near the eye. Normal findings on examination of the pupils may be recorded as *PERRLA,* which means "*P*upils *E*qual, *R*ound, *R*eact to *L*ight and *A*ccommodation."

Inspect the *iris* and pupil for color, size, shape, and clarity. Permanent eye color is usually established by 6 to 12 months of age. As the iris and pupil are inspected, look for the *lens.* Normally the lens is not visible through the pupil.

Inspection of Internal Structures. The ophthalmoscope permits visualization of the interior of the eyeball with a system of lenses and a high-intensity light. The lenses permit clear visualization of eye structures at different distances from the nurse's eye and correct visual acuity differences in the examiner and child. Use of the ophthalmoscope requires practice to know which lens setting produces the clearest image.

The ophthalmic and otic head are usually interchangeable on one "body" or handle, which encloses the power source, either disposable or rechargeable batteries. The nurse should practice changing the heads, which snap on and are secured with a quarter turn; and replacing the batteries and lightbulbs. Nurses who are not directly involved in physical assessment are often responsible for ensuring that the equipment functions properly.

Preparing the Child. The nurse can prepare the child for the ophthalmoscopic examination by showing the child the instrument, demonstrating the light source and how it shines in the eye, and explaining the reason for darkening the room. For

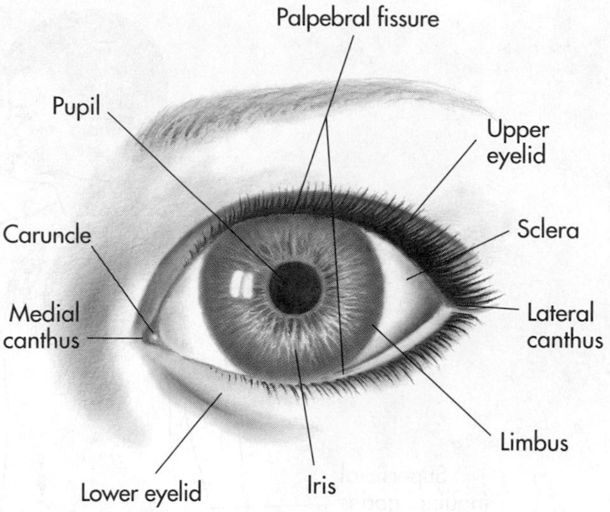

FIG. 35-12 • External structures of eye.

infants and young children who do not respond to such explanations, it is best to try to use distraction to encourage them to keep their eyes open. Forcibly parting the lids results in an uncooperative, watery-eyed child and a frustrated nurse. Usually, with some practice, the nurse can elicit a red reflex almost instantly while approaching the child and may also gain a momentary inspection of the blood vessels, macula, or optic disc.

Funduscopic Examination. Fig. 35-13 shows the structures of the back of the eyeball, or the *fundus.* The fundus is immediately apparent as the *red reflex.* The intensity of the color increases in darkly pigmented individuals.

NURSE ALERT • A brilliant, uniform red reflex is an important sign because it rules out many serious defects of the cornea, aqueous chamber, lens, and vitreous chamber. Any dark shadows or opacities are recorded because they indicate some abnormality in any of these structures.

As the ophthalmoscope is brought closer to the eye, the most conspicuous feature of the fundus is the optic disc, the area where the blood vessels and optic nerve fibers enter and exit from the eye. The color of the disc is creamy pink; it is lighter in color than the surrounding fundus; normally it is round or vertically oval.

After the optic disc is located, the area is inspected for *blood vessels.* The central retinal artery and vein appear in the depths of the disc and emanate outward with visible branching. The *veins* are darker in color and about one fourth larger in size than the *arteries.* Normally the branches of the arteries and veins cross each other.

Other structures that may be seen are the *macula,* the area of the fundus with the greatest concentration of visual receptors; and, in the center of the macula, a minute glistening spot of reflected light called the *fovea centralis;* this is the area of most perfect vision.

Vision Testing. Several tests are available for assessing vision. This discussion focuses on four areas: (1) ocular alignment, (2) visual acuity, (3) peripheral vision, and (4) color vision. Behavioral and physical signs that indicate visual impairment are discussed in Chapter 42.

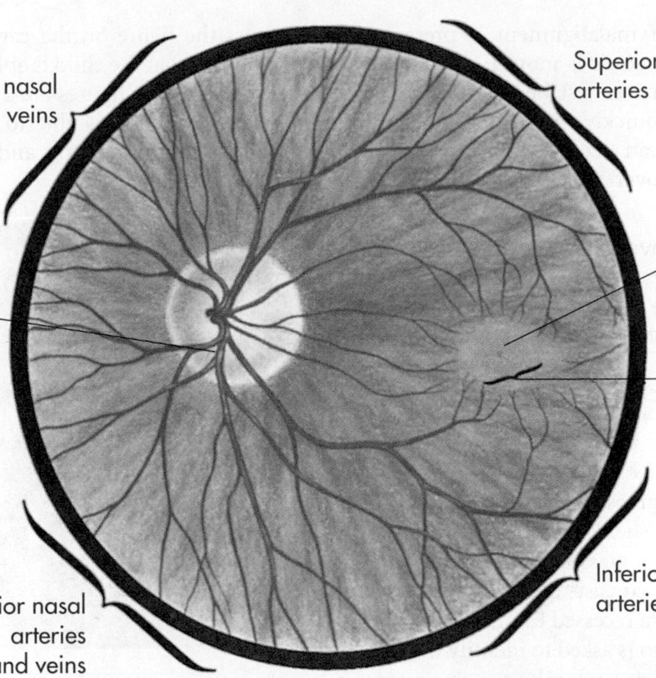

FIG. 35-13 • Structures of fundus. (From Seidel HM et al: *Mosby's guide to physical examination,* ed 4, St Louis, 1999, Mosby.)

Ocular Alignment. Normally, by the age of 3 to 4 months, children are able to fixate on one visual field with both eyes simultaneously (binocularity). One of the most important tests for binocularity is alignment of the eyes to detect nonbinocular vision, or *strabismus.* In strabismus, or cross-eye, one eye deviates from the point of fixation. If the malalignment is constant, the weak eye becomes "lazy," and the brain eventually suppresses the image produced by that eye. If strabismus is not detected and corrected by age 4 to 6 years, blindness from disuse, known as *amblyopia,* may result.

Tests commonly used to detect malalignment are the corneal light reflex and the cover tests. To perform the *corneal light reflex test,* or *Hirschberg test,* shine a flashlight or the light of the ophthalmoscope directly into the patient's eyes from a distance of about 40.5 cm (16 inches). If the eyes are *orthophoric,* or normal, the light falls symmetrically within each pupil (Fig. 35-14, *A*). If the light falls off center in one eye, the eyes are malaligned. *Epicanthal folds,* excess folds of skin that extend from the roof of the nose to the inner termination of the eyebrow and that partially or completely overlap the inner canthus of the eye, may give a false impression of malalignment (*pseudostrabismus*) (Fig. 35-14, *B*). Epicanthal folds are often found in Oriental children.

In the *cover test,* one eye is covered, and the movement of the *uncovered* eye is observed while the child looks at a near (33 cm, or 13 inches) or distant (6 m, or 20 feet) object. If the uncovered eye does not move, it is aligned. If the uncovered eye moves, a malalignment is present because when the stronger eye is temporarily covered, the misaligned eye attempts to fixate on the object.

In the *alternate cover test,* occlusion is shifted back and forth from one eye to the other, and movement of the eye that was *covered* is observed as soon as the occluder is removed while the child focuses on a point in front of him or her. If normal alignment is present, shifting the cover from one eye to the other will

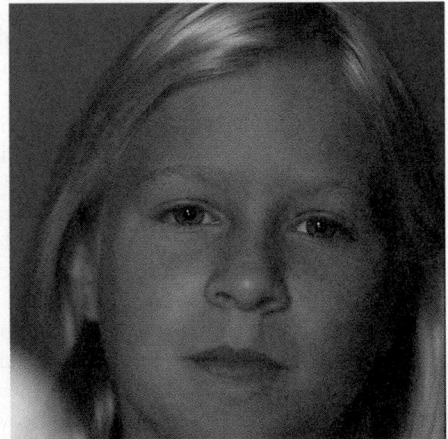

A

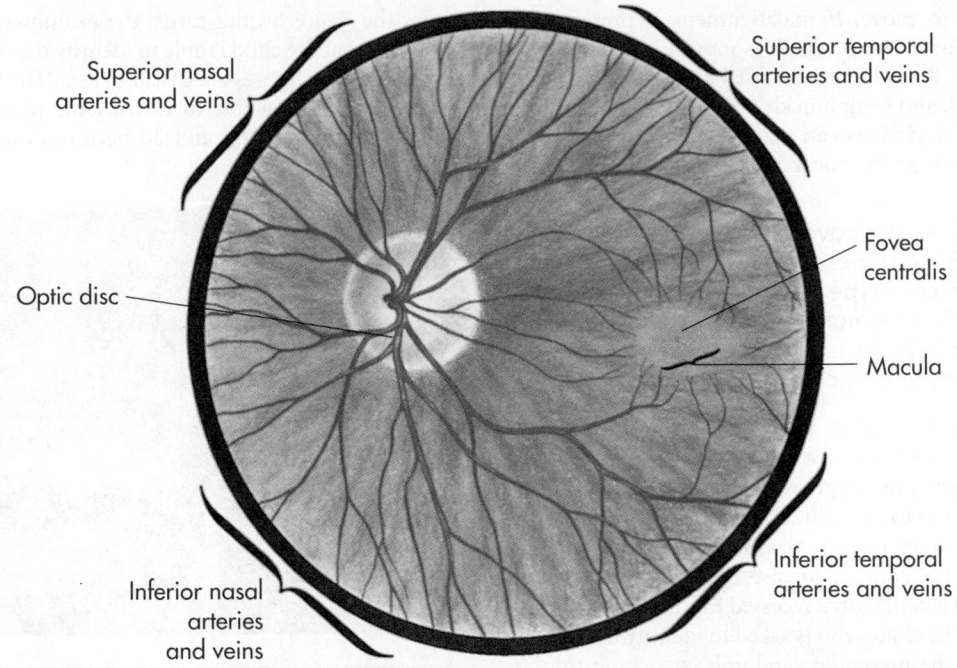

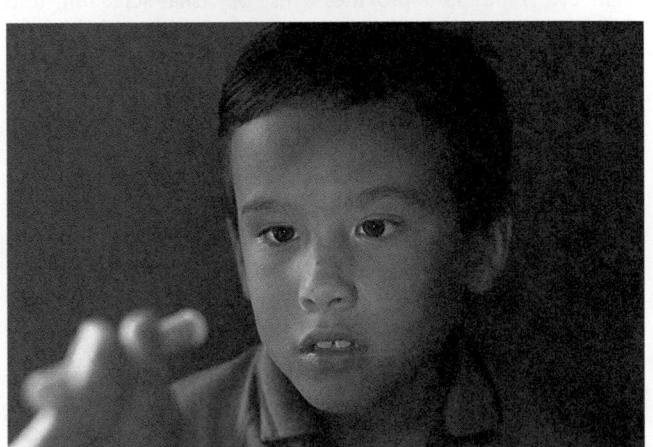

B

FIG. 35-14 • **A,** Corneal light reflex test demonstrating orthophoric eyes. **B,** Pseudostrabismus. Inner epicanthal folds cause eyes to appear malaligned; however, corneal light reflexes fall perfectly symmetrically.

not cause the eye to move. If malalignment is present, eye movement will occur when the cover is moved. This test takes more practice than the other cover test because the occluder must be moved back and forth quickly and accurately to see the eye move. Because deviations can occur at different ranges, it is important to perform the cover tests at both close and far distances.

NURSE ALERT • The cover test is usually easier to perform if the examiner uses his or her own hand rather than a card-type occluder (Fig. 35-15). Attractive occluders fashioned like an ice cream cone or happy-face lollipop cut from cardboard are also well received by young children.

In older children the *random-dot-E* **stereoscopic test** can be used to assess for stereoacuity (depth perception). This test is more likely to detect lesser degrees of eye muscle imbalance. The random-dot-E test cards are held 16 inches from the child's eyes. The child wears stereoscopic glasses while looking straight ahead at the cards. The card set consists of a blank card, a card with a raised E, and a card with a recessed E. The cards are held straight in front of the child, who is asked to identify the E card. The E card should be presented randomly, switching from a right, left, down, right, up, and left presentation of the letter. To pass the test, the child must identify the E correctly in 4 out of 6 attempts.

Visual Acuity Testing in Children Beyond Infancy. The most common test for measuring visual acuity is the *Snellen letter chart,* which consists of lines of letters of decreasing size (see Appendix D). The American Academy of Pediatrics (1996) now recommends that children, during testing, stand 10 feet from the chart with their heels at the 10-foot line. When screening for visual acuity in children, the child's right eye is tested first by covering the left. Children who wear glasses should be screened wearing the lenses. Tell the child to keep both eyes open during the examination. If the child fails the current line, move up the chart to the next larger line. Continue up the chart until a line is found that the child can pass. Then begin moving down the chart again until the child fails to read the line. To pass each line, the child must correctly identify 4 out of 6 symbols on the line. Repeat the procedure, covering the right eye. Table 35-9 provides a list of visual screening tests for children and guidelines for referral recommended by the American Academy of Pediatrics (1996).

For children unable to read letters and numbers, the *tumbling E* or *HOTV* is useful (Coats and Jenkins, 1997). The tumbling E test uses the capital letter E to point in four different directions. The child is then asked to point in the direction that the E is facing. The HOTV test consists of a wall chart composed of Hs, Os, Ts, and Vs. The child is given a board containing a large H, O, T, and V. The examiner points to a letter on the wall chart, and the child matches the correct letter on the board held in his or her hand. The tumbling E and HOTV are excellent tests for preschool-age children.

When a child is unable to perform the tumbling E or HOTV test, the LH symbol or Allen card test may be used. The Allen card test uses common figures to test the child's vision. It is important to assess whether the child is able to identify the pictures before actual vision testing. The examiner walks backward slowly, flipping through the cards and presenting different pictures to the child. The examiner continues to move backward as the child correctly calls out the figures. When the child begins to miss the figure on the cards, the examiner moves forward to confirm that the child is able to identify the figures at that point. All Allen card figures are 20/30 in size. The farthest distance at which the child is able to identify the pictures accurately becomes the numerator, and 30 becomes the denominator. For

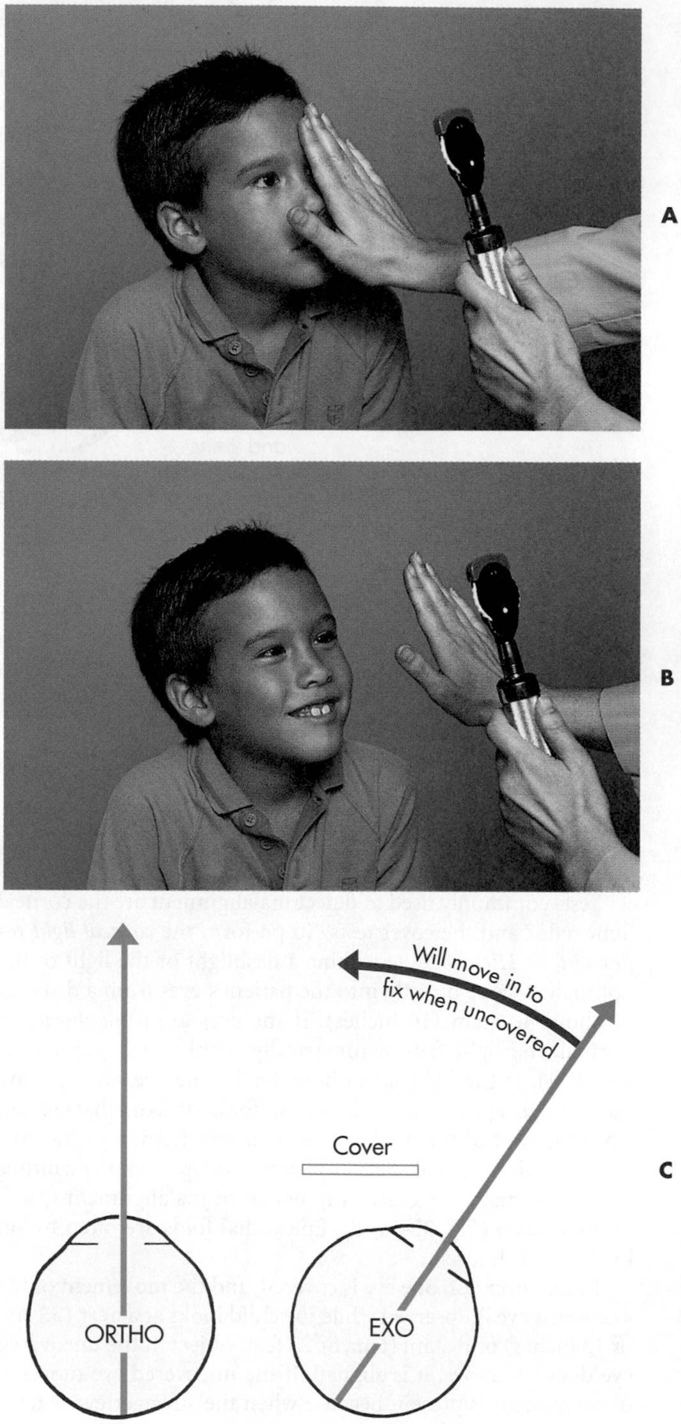

FIG. 35-15 • Cover/uncover test to detect amblyopia in patients with strabismus. **A,** Eye is occluded, child is fixating on light source. **B,** If eye does not move when uncovered, eyes are aligned. **C,** Exophoria. As eye is uncovered, it shifts to fixate on object. (C, from Prior JA, Silverstein JS, Stang JM: *Physical diagnosis: the history and examination of the patient,* ed 6, St Louis, 1981, Mosby.)

TABLE 35-9
Visual Screening Tests for Children

Test	Description	Comments*
TESTS FOR VISUAL ACUITY		
Snellen Letter†	Uses letters of English alphabet for testing	For most children above second grade who are familiar with reading the alphabet
Snellen Number†	Uses numbers for testing	For children who know their numbers
Snellen E (Tumbling E)†	Uses capital letter E pointing in four directions; children "read" chart by showing direction of E or using a large duplicate E to match E on chart	For illiterate or non–English-speaking people, preschoolers, and children in the first grade Preschoolers often have difficulty with direction despite adequate vision
Home Eye Test for Preschoolers‡	Uses large letter E for demonstration and E chart for testing at 10 feet	For use by parents for children ages 3 to 6 years
Blackbird Preschool Vision Screening System§	Uses a modified E to resemble a flying bird; children identify which way bird is flying Uses flash cards, storytelling, and disposable cardboard eyeglass occluders	Designed for children as young as 3 years
HOTV or Matching Symbol†	Uses the four letters H, O, T, and V on a chart for testing Child names letters on chart or matches them to a demonstration card	For children as young as 3 years Avoids problem with image reversal and eye-hand coordination that can occur with letter E
LH Symbol	Spiral-bound flash cards of house, apple, circle, and square in different sizes	
Denver Eye Screening Test (DEST)‖	Uses single cards for letter E, one for demonstration and one for testing Also uses **Allen cards** (pictures of a tree, birthday cake, horse and rider, telephone, car, house, and teddy bear) for testing	For children 2½ years and older May be reliably used with cooperative children beginning at age 24 months
TESTS FOR OCULAR ALIGNMENT		
Cover Test	As child looks at distant object, one eye is occluded to check for movement in uncovered eye; child is tested at 3 m or 10 feet	Can be performed on preschoolers without difficulty
Random-Dot-E Stereo Test	Uses stereoscopic glasses and E cards; child is tested at 40 cm	Used to assess for stereoacuity (depth perception)
REFERRAL CRITERIA¶		
Visual Acuity at 3-5 Years of Age	**Visual Aquity at 6 Years and Older**	**Ocular Alignment at Younger Than 3 Years**
<4 out of 6 correct at 20 feet; either eye tested at 10 feet monocularly (i.e., <10/20 or 20/40) *or* Two-line difference between eyes, even within pass range (i.e., 10/12.5 and 10/20 or 20/25 and 20/40)	<4 out of 6 correct at 15 feet with either eye tested at 10 feet monocularly (i.e., <10/15 or 20/30) *or* Two-line difference between eyes, even within pass range (i.e., 10/10 and 10/15 or 20/20 and 20/30)	Cover test: any movement Random-dot-E test: <4 out of 6 correct

*Ages for testing are based on published reports. Proper instruction of young children is essential for successful screening.
†Available from Good-Lite Co., 1540 Hannah Ave., Forest Park, IL 60130; phone (708) 366-3860.
‡Available from the National Society to Prevent Blindness, 500 E. Remington Rd., Schaumburg, IL 60173; phone 1-800-331-2020; website: www.prevent-blindness.org.
§Available from Blackbird Vision Screening System, P.O. Box 277424, Sacramento, CA 95827; phone 1-800-363-6884.
‖Available from Denver Developmental Materials, Inc., P.O. Box 6919, Denver, CO 80206-0919; phone (303) 355-4729; 1-800-419-4729.
¶From American Academy of Pediatrics: Eye examination and vision screening in infants, children, and young adults, *Pediatrics* 98(1):156, 1996.

example, if the child is able to identify the pictures accurately at 15 feet, the visual acuity is recorded as 15/30. This is equivalent to 20/40 or 10/20 visual acuity. The LH symbol test differs somewhat from the Allen card test because it is a spiral-bound set of flash cards. The flash cards contain large pictures of a house, apple, circle, and square. The LH symbol cards contains the symbol size and visual acuity value for a 10-foot testing distance. The visual acuity is determined by the smallest symbols that the child is able to identify at 10 feet.

The *Blackbird Preschool Vision Screening System* was developed by a nurse. The screening system uses a modified E that resembles a bird and a story about the Blackbird to help engage children's attention. Testing is done with flash cards or a wall-mounted chart, and the child is instructed to indicate the direction of the bird's flight. The Blackbird System also contains guidelines for vision screening of noncommunicative children, nonreaders, or non-English-speaking children to assist screeners with more difficult-to-test populations. The *Blackbird Storybook Home Eye Test* is designed for parents to prescreen young children at home.

Visual Acuity Testing in Infants and Difficult-to-Test Children. In newborns, vision is tested mainly by checking for *light perception* by shining a light into the eyes and noting responses such as pupillary constriction, blinking, following the light to midline, increased alertness, or refusal to open the eyes after exposure to the light. Although the simple maneuver of checking light perception and eliciting the pupillary light reflex indicates that the anterior half of the visual apparatus is intact, it does not confirm that the infant can see. In other words, this test does not assess whether the brain receives the visual message and interprets the signals.

Another test of visual acuity is the infant's ability to fix on and follow a target. Although any brightly colored or patterned object can be used, the human face is excellent. Hold the infant upright while moving your face slowly from side to side.

NURSE ALERT • If visual fixation and following are not present by 3 to 4 months of age, further ophthalmologic evaluation is needed.

Other signs that may indicate visual loss or other serious eye problems include fixed pupils, strabismus, constant nystagmus, the setting-sun sign, and slow lateral movements. Unfortunately, it is very difficult to test each eye separately; the presence of such signs in one eye could indicate unilateral blindness.

Special tests are available for testing infants and other difficult-to-test children to assess acuity and/or confirm blindness. For example, in *visually evoked potentials,* the eyes are stimulated with a bright light or pattern, and electrical activity to the visual cortex is recorded through scalp electrodes. Acuity is assessed by using progressively smaller patterns.

Peripheral Vision. In children who are old enough to cooperate, estimate *peripheral vision,* or the visual field of each eye, by having children fixate on a specific point directly in front of them while an object such as a finger or a pencil is moved from beyond the field of vision into the range of peripheral vision. Check each eye separately and for each quadrant of vision. As soon as children see the object, have them say "stop." At that point measure the angle from the anteroposterior axis of the eye (straight line of vision) to the peripheral axis (point at which the object is first seen). Normally children see about 50 degrees upward, 70 degrees downward, 60 degrees nasalward, and 90 degrees temporally. Limitations in peripheral vision may indicate blindness from damage to structures within the eye or damage to any of the visual pathways.

Color Vision. Another important test is for color vision. It is estimated that 8% to 10% of Caucasian males and less than half that percentage of African-American males inherit the X-linked disorder known as *color vision deficit* (or by the less acceptable term, *color blindness*). From 0.5% to 1% of Caucasian females are affected. Although the severity of impaired perception of color varies considerably, the two most common types are *protanomaly,* in which the child confuses gray with pink or pale blue with green; and *deuteranomaly,* in which the child confuses gray with pale purple or green. In most of these individuals the color vision deficit causes no major problems. However, some difficulties encountered by individuals with more severe deficits include the inability to distinguish amber or red traffic lights, failure to see a red brake light on a car, difficulty in distinguishing green traffic lights from certain types of incandescent street lamps, and a poor sense of color coordination of clothing. For school-age children the greatest difficulty lies in performance of academic skills that use color as a visual aid. Adolescents may be ineligible for certain vocational opportunities, such as electronics, photography, printing, interior decorating, pharmaceuticals, textiles, police work, and several types of military service.

The tests available for color vision include the *Ishihara test* and the *Hardy-Rand-Rittler (HRR) test.* Each consists of a series of cards (pseudoisochromatic) on which is printed a color field composed of spots of a certain "confusion" color. Against the field is a number or symbol similarly printed in dots but of a color likely to be confused with the field color by the person with a color vision deficit. As a result, the figure or letter is invisible to an affected individual but is clearly seen by a person with normal vision. By using the HRR test, which uses symbols rather than numbers, reliable testing can be done on young children (Birch and Platts, 1993). Nurses administering the test must be familiar with the testing materials and should be able to inform the parents of the disorder's effects on practical areas of living, its genetic transmission, and its irreversibility.

Ears

Inspection of External Structures. The entire external earlobe is called the *pinna,* or *auricle,* and is located on each side of the head. Measure the *height* alignment of the pinna by drawing an imaginary line from the outer orbit of the eye to the occiput, or most prominent protuberance of the skull. The top of the pinna should meet or cross this line. Low-set ears are commonly associated with renal anomalies or mental retardation. Measure the *angle* of the pinna by drawing a perpendicular line from the imaginary horizontal line and aligning the pinna next to this mark. Normally the pinna lies within a 10-degree angle of the vertical line (Fig. 35-16). If it falls outside this area, record the deviation and look for other anomalies.

Normally the pinna extends slightly outward from the skull. Except in newborn infants, ears that are flat against the head or protruding away from the scalp may indicate problems. Flattened ears in infants may suggest a frequent side-lying position and, just as with isolated areas of hair loss, may be a clue to investigating parents' understanding of the child's stimulation needs.

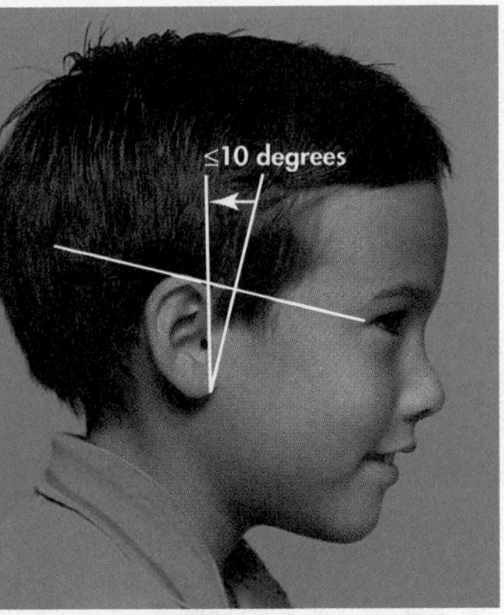

FIG. 35-16 • Ear alignment.

Atraumatic Care

REDUCING DISTRESS FROM OTOSCOPY IN YOUNG CHILDREN

Make examining the ear a game by explaining that you are looking for a "big elephant" in the ear. This kind of make-believe is an absorbing distraction and usually elicits cooperation. After the ear has been examined, clarify that "looking for elephants" was only pretend and thank the child for letting you look in his or her ear. You can also ask the child to put a finger on the opposite ear to keep the light from getting out, which is a great distraction technique.

Inspect the *skin* surface around the ear for small openings, extra tags of skin, or sinuses. If a sinus is found, note this because it may represent a fistula that drains into some area of the neck or ear. Cutaneous tags represent no pathologic process but may cause parents concern in terms of the child's appearance.

Also assess the ear for *hygiene.* An otoscope is not necessary for looking into the external canal to note the presence of *cerumen,* a waxy substance produced by the ceruminous glands in the outer portion of the canal. Cerumen is usually yellow-brown and soft. If an otoscope is used and any discharge is seen, its color and odor are noted. Prevent transmitting potentially infectious material to the other ear or to another child through handwashing and using disposable specula or sterilizing reusable specula between each examination.

Inspection of Internal Structures. The head of the otoscope permits visualization of the tympanic membrane by use of a bright light, a magnifying glass, and a speculum. Some otoscopes have an attachment for a pneumonic device to insert air into the canal to determine membrane compliance (movement). The speculum, which is inserted into the external canal, comes in a variety of sizes to accommodate different canal widths. The largest speculum that fits comfortably into the ear is used to achieve the greatest area of visualization. The lens, or magnifying glass, is moveable, allowing the examiner to insert an object, such as a curette, into the ear canal through the speculum while still viewing the structures through the lens.

Positioning the Child. Before beginning the otoscopic examination, position the child properly and restrain if necessary. Older children usually cooperate and do not need restraint. However, prepare them for the procedure by allowing them to play with the instrument, demonstrating how it works, and stressing the importance of remaining still. A helpful suggestion is to let them observe you examining the parent's ear. Restraint is needed for younger children because the ear examination upsets them (Atraumatic Care box).

As you insert the speculum into the meatus, move it around the outer rim to accustom the child to the feel of something entering the ear. If examining a painful ear, touch a nonpainful part of the affected ear, then examine the unaffected ear, and finally return to the painful ear. By this time the child is usually less fearful of anything causing discomfort to the ear and will cooperate more.

For their protection and safety, infants and toddlers must be restrained for the otoscopic examination. There are two general positions of restraint. In one the child is seated sideways in the parent's lap with one arm "hugging" the parent and the other arm at the side. The ear to be examined is toward the nurse. With one arm the parent holds the child's head firmly against his or her chest, and with the other arm "hugs" the child, thereby seeming the child's free arm. The ear is examined using the procedure for holding the otoscope described in the following paragraphs (Fig. 35-17, *A*).

The other position involves placing the child on the side, back, or abdomen with the arms at the side and the head turned so that the ear to be examined points toward the ceiling. Lean over the child using the upper part of the body to restrain the arm and upper trunk movements, and the examining hand to stabilize the head. This position is practical for young infants or for older children who need minimal restraining, but it may not be feasible for other children who protest vigorously. For safety, enlist the help of a parent or an assistant in immobilizing the head by firmly placing one hand above the ear and the other on the child's side, abdomen, or back (Fig. 35-17, *B*).

With cooperative children, examine the ear with the child in a side-lying, sitting, or standing position. One disadvantage to standing is that the child may "walk away" as the otoscope enters the canal. If the child is standing or sitting, tilt the head slightly toward the child's opposite shoulder to achieve a better view of the drum (Fig. 35-18).

With the thumb and forefinger of the free (usually nondominant) hand, grasp the auricle. For the two positions of restraint, hold the otoscope upside down at the junction of its head and handle with the thumb and index finger. Place the other fingers against the skull to allow the otoscope to move with the child in case of sudden movement. In examining a cooperative child, hold the handle with the otic head upright or upside down. Use the dominant hand to examine both ears; or reverse hands for each ear, whichever is more comfortable.

Before using the otoscope, visualize the external ear and the tympanic membrane as if superimposed on a clock (Fig. 35-19). The numbers become important geographic landmarks. Introduce the speculum into the meatus between the 3 and 9 o'clock positions in a downward and forward position. Because the canal is curved, the speculum does not permit a panoramic view of the tympanic membrane unless the canal is straightened. In infants the canal curves upward. Therefore, pull the

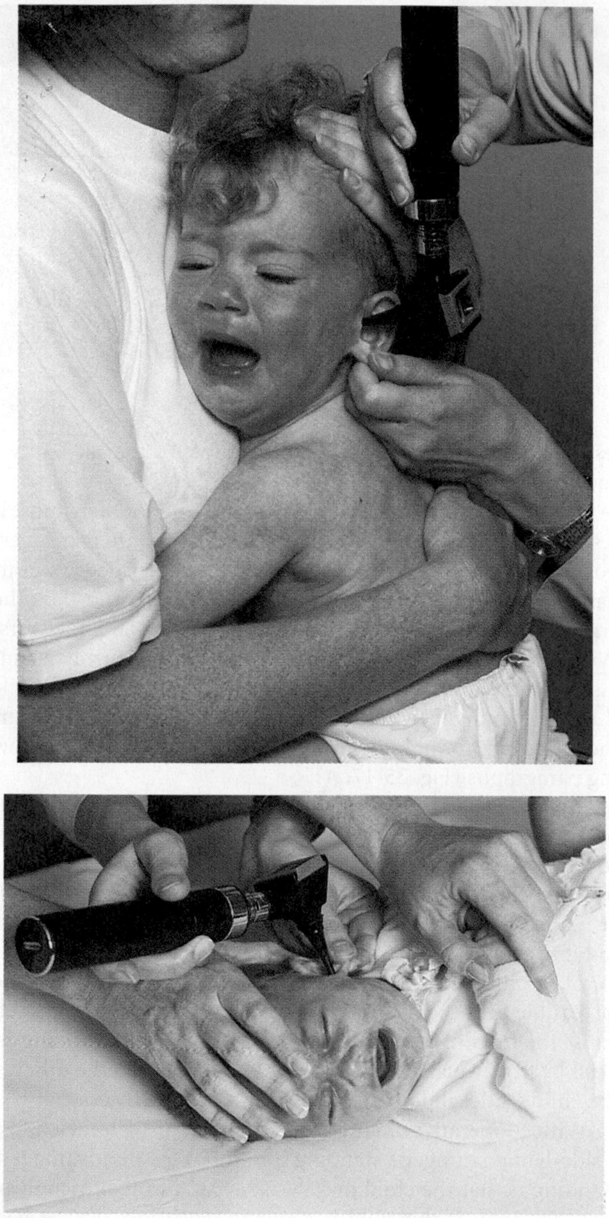

FIG. 35-17 • Position for restraining **A,** child, and **B,** infant during otoscopic examination.

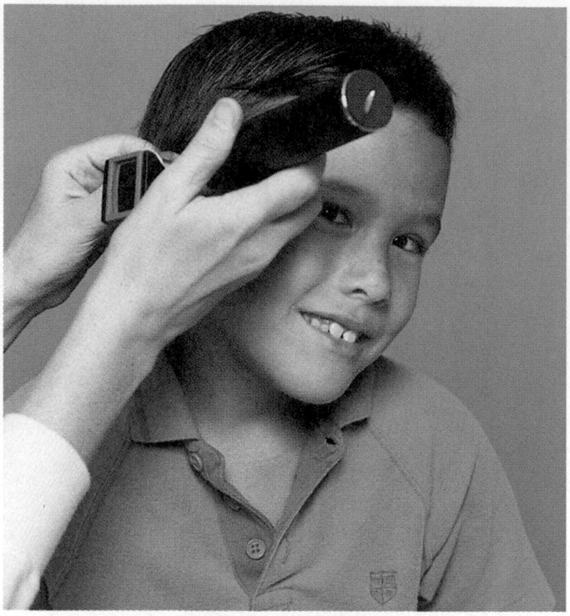

FIG. 35-18 • Positioning head by tilting it toward opposite shoulder for full view of tympanic membrane.

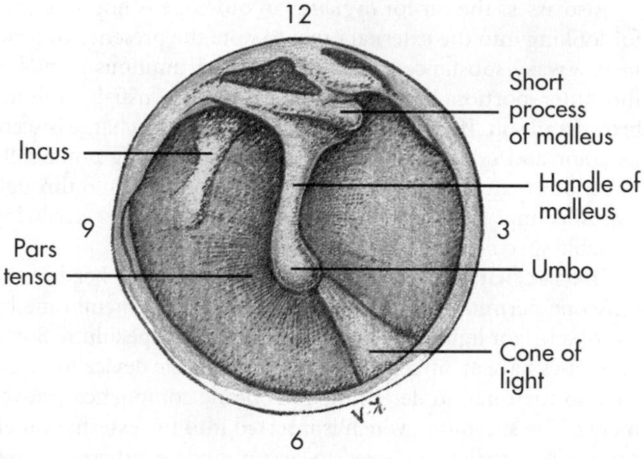

FIG. 35-19 • Landmarks of tympanic membrane with "clock" superimposed. (Modified from Potter PA, Perry AG: *Basic nursing: theory and practice,* ed 2, St Louis, 1991, Mosby.)

pinna down and back to the 6 to 9 o'clock range to straighten the canal (Fig. 35-20, *A*).

With older children, usually those over 3 years or age, the canal curves downward and forward. Therefore pull the pinna *up* and *back* toward a 10 o'clock position (Fig. 35-20, *B*). If there is difficulty in visualizing the membrane, try repositioning the head, introducing the speculum at a different angle, and pulling the pinna in a slightly different direction. Do not insert the speculum past the cartilaginous (outermost) portion of the canal, usually a distance of 0.60 to 1.25 cm (¼ to ½ inch) in older children. Insertion of the speculum into the posterior or bony portion of the canal causes pain.

In neonates and young infants, the walls of the canal are pliable and floppy because of the underdeveloped cartilaginous and bony structures. Therefore the very small 2-mm speculum usually needs to be inserted deeper into the canal than in older children. Great care must be exercised not to damage the walls or drum. For this reason, only an experienced examiner should insert an otoscope into the ears of very young infants.

Otoscopic Examination. As you introduce the speculum into the external canal, inspect the walls of the canal, the color of the tympanic membrane, the light reflex, and the usual landmarks of the bony prominences of the middle ear.

The *walls* of the external auditory canal are pink, although they are more pigmented in dark-skinned children. Minute hairs are evident in the outermost portion, where cerumen is produced. Note signs of irritation, foreign bodies, or infection.

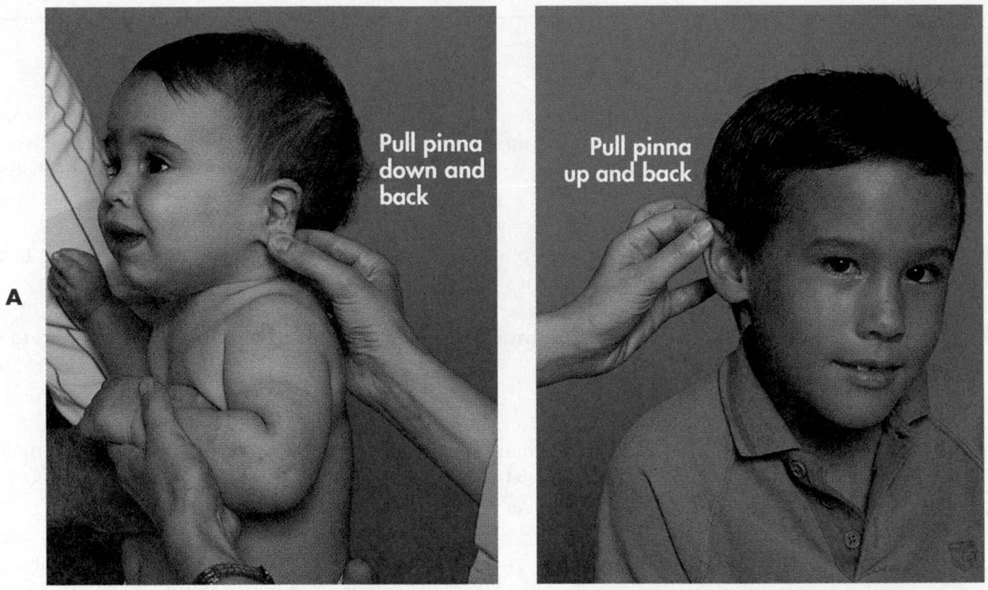

FIG. 35-20 • Positioning of eardrum **A,** in infant; and **B,** in child over 3 years of age.

Foreign bodies in the ear are not uncommon in children and range from erasers to beans. Symptoms may include pain, discharge, and affected hearing. Soft objects, such as paper or insects, can be removed with forceps. Small, hard objects, such as pebbles, can be removed with a suction tip, a hook, or irrigation. However, irrigation is contraindicated if the object is vegetative matter, such as beans or pasta, which might swell when in contact with fluid.

NURSE ALERT • If there is any doubt about the type of object in the ear, and the appropriate method to remove it, refer the child to the appropriate practitioner.

The *color* of the *tympanic membrane* is a translucent, light, pearly pink or gray. Note marked erythema (which may indicate suppurative otitis media); a dull, nontransparent grayish color (sometimes suggestive of serous otitis media), or ashen gray areas (signs of scarring from a previous perforation). A black area usually suggests a perforation of the membrane that has not healed.

The characteristic tenseness and slope of the tympanic membrane cause the light of the otoscope to reflect at about the 5 or 7 o'clock position. The *light reflex* is a fairly well-defined, cone-shaped reflection that normally points away from the face.

The *bony landmarks* of the drum are formed by the *umbo,* or tip of the malleus bone. It appears as a small, round, opaque, concave spot near the center of the drum. The *manubrium* (long process or handle) of the malleus appears to be a whitish line extending from the umbo upward to the margin of the membrane. At the upper end of the long process, near the 1 o'clock position (in the right ear), is a sharp, knoblike protuberance representing the *short process* of the malleus. Note the absence of the light reflex or the loss or abnormal prominence of any of these landmarks.

Auditory Testing. Several types of hearing tests are available (Table 35-10). Some of them, such as audiometric testing, involve specialized equipment that measures the degree of hearing loss. Others, such as tests for the startle reflex in neonates, are rough estimations of perception of sound. The nurse must operate under a high index of suspicion for those children who may have conditions associated with hearing loss and who may have developed behaviors that indicate auditory impairment. Types of hearing loss, causes, clinical manifestation, and appropriate treatment are discussed in Chapter 42.

Nose

Inspection of External Structures. The nose is located in the middle of the face just below the eyes and above the lips. Compare its placement and alignment by drawing an imaginary vertical line from the center point between the eyes down to the notch of the upper lip. The nose should lie exactly vertical to this line, with each side exactly symmetric. Note its location, any deviation to one side, and asymmetry in overall size and in diameter of the nares (nostrils). The *bridge* of the nose is sometimes flat in Asian and African-American children. Observe the *alae nasi* for any sign of flaring, which indicates respiratory difficulty. Always report any flaring of the alae nasi. Fig. 35-21 illustrates the usual landmarks used in describing the external structures of the nose.

Inspection of Internal Structures. Inspect the *anterior vestibule* of the nose by pushing the tip upward, tilting the head backward, and illuminating the cavity with a flashlight or otoscope without the attached ear speculum.

Note the *color* of the *mucosal lining,* which is normally redder than the oral membranes, as well as any swelling, discharge, dryness, or bleeding. There should be no discharge from the nose.

On looking deeper into the nose, inspect the *turbinates* or *concha,* plates of bone that jut into the nasal cavity and are enveloped by mucous membrane. The turbinates greatly increase the surface area of the nasal cavity as air is inhaled. The spaces or channels between the turbinates are called *meatus* and correspond to each of the three turbinates. Normally the front end of the inferior and middle turbinate and the middle meatus are seen. They should be the same color as the lining of the vestibule.

TABLE 35-10

Selected Hearing and Tympanic Membrane Compliance Tests*

Description	Comments
CLINICAL HEARING TESTS	
In newborns elicit the startle reflex and observe other neonatal responses to loud noises, such as facial grimaces, blinking, gross motor movement, quiet if crying or crying if quiet, opening the eyes, or ceasing sucking activity.	An objective sign of alerting to sound may be an increase in heart rate or respiratory rate. Absence of alerting behaviors suggests hearing loss. Eliciting the startle reflex is used only in infants from birth to 4 months.
During infancy note child's reaction to a noise. Stand approximately 18 inches away from infant, to the side, and out of child's peripheral field of vision. With the room silent and infant sitting in parent's lap, distracted by some object, make a voice sound such as "ps" or "phth" (high-pitched) or "oo" (low-pitched), ring a bell or a rattle, or rustle tissue paper.	Test is usually inadequate for children beyond infancy because of their tendency to ignore sounds or be distracted. Compare response of localizing sound to expected age response (see Biologic Development, Chapter 36).
TYMPANOMETRY	
Measures tympanic membrane compliance (or mobility) and estimates middle ear air pressure. A soft rubber cuff is pressed over the external canal to produce an airtight seal; an automatic reading of air pressure registers on the machine.	Detects middle ear disease and abnormalities but does not indicate the degree of hearing loss or the interpretation of sound. Difficult to perform in young children because of inability to maintain an adequate seal or excessive movement by the child.
CONDUCTION TESTS	
Rinne test. Stem of tuning fork is placed against the mastoid bone until the sound ceases to be audible. Tuning fork is then moved so that the prongs are held near, but not touching, the auditory meatus. Child should again hear the sound **(Rinne positive).** If sound is not again audible **(Rinne negative),** some abnormality is interfering with the conduction of air through the external and middle chambers.	Requires the cooperation and ability of the child to signal when the sound is no longer audible and when it is again heard. Not useful for most children before preschool age.
Weber test. Stem of tuning fork is held in the midline of the head. Child should hear the sound equally in both ears **(Weber positive).** With air conductive loss, child will hear the sound better in the affected ear **(Weber negative).**	Often not suitable for young children because of their difficulty in discriminating between "better, more, or less."
AUDIOMETRY	
Electrical audiometer measures the threshold of hearing for pure-tone frequencies and loudness. A sound is transmitted to the child's ear and reduced until child indicates that the sound is no longer heard; this procedure is repeated for several sounds covering the range found in conversation. In an air conduction audiogram the sounds are transmitted through earphones. In a bone conduction audiogram the sounds are passed through a plaque placed over the mastoid bone.	Provides valuable information regarding the severity of the hearing loss, the sound cycles involved, and the possible location of the defect. Requires specialized training of personnel, expensive equipment, and cooperation from the child in terms of confirming the perception of sound. For children ages 24 months to approximately 5 years, play audiometry can be used; it is based on behavior modification and involves reinforcement for correct response.
EVOKED OTOACOUSTIC EMISSIONS (EOAEs)	
Special OAE analyzer delivers a rapid series of clicks to the ear through a probe fitted with a tympanometry tip that is inserted closely in the external auditory canal. The presence of OAEs, defined as sound energy emitted by the cochlea that is believed to be generated by movement of the outer hairs of the organ of Corti, is usually associated with normal or near normal cochlear sensitivity; their absence indicates a hearing loss of at least 20-25 dB, provided there is no conductive dysfunction.†	Preferred method of screening neonates for sensorineural hearing loss (ototoxicity and noise-induced hearing loss). Requires specialized equipment. Minimal training is required. Infants must be in a quiet sleep for testing. Results do not indicate severity of cochlear damage; should be followed by BAER (see below).
BRAINSTEM-AUDITORY EVOKED RESPONSE (BAER)	
Through electrode wires attached to the infant's or child's scalp, electrical or brain wave potentials generated within the auditory system are transmitted to a computer for analysis. Following repetitive acoustic stimulation, the waveforms from a normal sleeping or quiet infant consist of several peaks and valleys that reflect activations of neural structures of the brain.	Requires expensive equipment and specialized training of personnel.

*Any child who is suspected of a hearing loss because of poor performance using screening tests is referred for special audiometric or BAER testing.
†Abdo MH, Feghali JG, Stapells DR: Transient evoked otoacoustic emissions: clinical applications and technical considerations, *Int J Pediatr Otorhinolaryngol* 25:61-71, 1993.

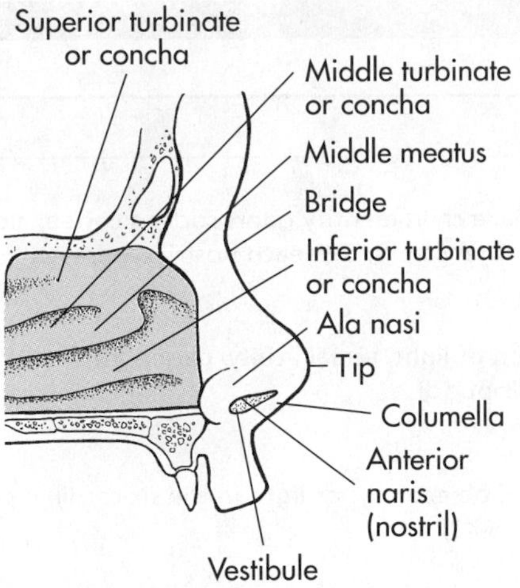

FIG. 35-21 • External landmarks and internal structures of nose.

Inspect the *septum,* which should divide the vestibules equally. Note any deviation, especially if it causes an occlusion of one side of the nose. A perforation may be evident within the septum. If this is suspected, shine the light of the otoscope into one naris and look for admittance of light through the perforation to the other nostril.

Since olfaction is an important function of the nose, testing for smell may be done at this point or as part of cranial nerve assessment (Table 35-11).

Mouth and Throat

With a cooperative child, almost the entire examination of the mouth and throat can be accomplished without the use of a tongue blade. Ask the child to open the mouth wide, to move the tongue in different directions for full visualization, and to say "ahh," which depresses the tongue for full view of the back of the mouth (tonsils, uvula, and oropharynx). For a closer look at the buccal mucosa, or lining of the cheeks, ask children to use their fingers to move the outer lip and cheek to one side (Atraumatic Care box).

Infants and toddlers, however, usually resist attempts to keep the mouth open. Because inspecting the mouth is an upsetting part of the examination, leave it for the end of the physical examination (along with examination of the ears) or do it during episodes of crying. However, the use of a tongue blade (preferably flavored) to depress the tongue is necessary. Place the tongue blade along the *side* of the tongue, not in the center back area where the gag reflex is elicited. Fig. 35-22, *B,* illustrates proper positioning of the child for the oral examination.

The major structure of the exterior of the mouth is the *lips.* The lips should be moist, soft, smooth, and pink, and colored a deeper hue than the surrounding skin. The lips should be symmetric when relaxed or tensed. Assess symmetry when the child talks or cries.

Inspection of Internal Structures. The major structures that are visible within the oral cavity and oropharynx are the mucosal lining of the lips and cheeks, gums or gingiva, teeth, tongue, palate, uvula, tonsils, and posterior oropharynx (Fig. 35-23). Inspect all areas lined with *mucous membranes* (i.e., inside the lips and cheeks, gingiva, underside of the tongue, palate, and back of the pharynx) for color, any areas of white patches of ulceration, bleeding, sensitivity, and moisture. The membranes should be bright pink, smooth, glistening, uniform, and moist.

Atraumatic Care

ENCOURAGING OPENING THE MOUTH FOR EXAMINATION

- Perform the examination in front of a mirror.
- Let child first examine someone else's mouth, such as the parent, the nurse, or a puppet (Fig. 35-22, *A*) and then examine child's mouth.
- Instruct child to tilt the head back slightly, breathe deeply through the mouth, and hold the breath; this action lowers the tongue to the floor of the mouth without the use of a tongue blade.
- Lightly brushing the palate with a cotton swab also may open the mouth for assessment.

Inspect the *teeth* for number in each dental arch, for hygiene, and for occlusion or bite (see also Teething, Chapter 36). Discoloration of tooth enamel with obvious plaque (whitish coating on the surface of the teeth) is a sign of poor dental hygiene and indicates a need for counseling. Brown spots in the crevices of the crown of the tooth or between the teeth may be caries (cavities). Chalky white to yellow or brown areas on the enamel may indicate fluorosis (excessive fluoride ingestion). Teeth that appear greenish black may be stained temporarily from ingestion of supplemental iron.

Examine the *gums (gingiva)* surrounding the teeth. The color is normally coral pink, and the surface texture is stippled, similar to the appearance of orange peel. In dark-skinned children, the gums are more deeply colored, and a brownish area is often observed along the gum line.

Inspect the *tongue* for the presence of papillae, small projections that contain several taste buds and give the tongue its characteristic rough appearance. Note the size and mobility of the tongue. Normally the tip of the tongue should extend to the lips or beyond.

The roof of the mouth consists of the *hard palate,* which is located near the front of the oral cavity; and the *soft palate,* which is located toward the back of the pharynx and has a small midline protrusion called the *uvula.* Carefully inspect the palates to be sure that they are intact. The arch of the palate should be dome shaped. A narrow, flat roof or a high, arched palate affects the placement of the tongue and can cause feeding and speech problems. Test movement of the uvula by eliciting a gag reflex. It should move upward to close off the nasopharynx from the oropharynx.

Examine the oropharynx and note the size and color of the *palatine tonsils.* They are normally the same color as the surrounding mucosa; glandular, rather than smooth in appearance; and barely visible over the edge of the palatoglossal arches. The size of the tonsils varies considerably during childhood. However, report any swelling, redness, or white areas on the tonsils.

Chest

Inspect the chest for size, shape, symmetry of movement, breast development, and the presence of the bony landmarks formed by the ribs and sternum. The *rib cage* consists of twelve ribs and the sternum, or breast bone, located in the midline of the trunk (Fig. 35-24). The *sternum* is composed of three main parts. The *manubrium,* the uppermost portion, can be felt at the base of the neck at the *suprasternal notch.* The largest segment of the ster-

TABLE 35-11
Assessment of Cranial Nerves

Description/Function	Tests
I—OLFACTORY NERVE	
Olfactory mucosa of nasal cavity Smell	With eyes closed, have child identify odors such as coffee, alcohol from a swab, or other smells; test each nostril separately
II—OPTIC NERVE	
Rods and cones of retina, optic nerve Vision	Check for perception of light, visual acuity, peripheral vision, color vision, and normal optic disc
III—OCULOMOTOR NERVE	
Extraocular muscles (EOM) of eye: Superior rectus (SR)—moves eyeball up and in Inferior rectus (IR)—moves eyeball down and in Medial rectus (MR)—moves eyeball nasally Inferior oblique (IO)—moves eyeball up and out	Have child follow an object (toy) or light in the six cardinal positions of gaze (see Fig. 35-43)
Pupil constriction and accommodation	Perform PERRLA
Eyelid closing	Check for proper placement of lid
IV—TROCHLEAR NERVE	
Superior oblique (SO) muscle—moves eye down and out	Have child look down and in (see Fig. 35-43)
V—TRIGEMINAL NERVE	
Muscles of mastication	Have child bite down hard and open jaw; test symmetry and strength
Sensory: face, scalp, nasal and buccal mucosa	With child's eyes closed, see if child can detect light touch in mandibular and maxillary regions Test corneal and blink reflex by touching cornea lightly (approach from side so that child does not blink before cornea is touched)
VI—ABDUCENS NERVE	
Lateral rectus (LR) muscle—moves eye temporally	Have child look toward temporal side (see Fig. 35-43)
VII—FACIAL NERVE	
Muscles for facial expression	Have child smile, make funny face, or show teeth to see symmetry of expression
Anterior two thirds of tongue (sensory)	Have child identify a sweet or salty solution; place each taste on anterior section and sides of protruding tongue; if child retracts tongue, solution will dissolve toward posterior part of tongue
VIII—AUDITORY, ACOUSTIC, OR VESTIBULOCOCHLEAR NERVE	
Internal ear Hearing/balance	Test hearing; note any loss of equilibrium or presence of vertigo
IX—GLOSSOPHARYNGEAL NERVE	
Pharynx, tongue	Stimulate posterior pharynx with a tongue blade; child should gag
Posterior one third of tongue (sensory)	Test sense of sour or bitter taste on posterior segment of tongue
X—VAGUS NERVE	
Muscles of larynx, pharynx, some organs of gastrointestinal system, sensory fibers of root of tongue, heart, lung, and some organs of gastrointestinal system	Note hoarseness of voice, gag reflex, and ability to swallow Check that uvula is midline; when stimulated with a tongue blade, should deviate upward and to stimulated side
XI—ACCESSORY NERVE	
Sternocleidomastoid and trapezius muscles of shoulder	Have child shrug shoulders while applying mild pressure; with examiner's hands placed on shoulders, have child turn head against opposing pressure on either side; note symmetry and strength
XII—HYPOGLOSSAL NERVE	
Muscles of tongue	Have child move tongue in all directions; have child protrude tongue as far as possible; note any midline deviation Test strength by placing tongue blade on one side of tongue and having child move it away

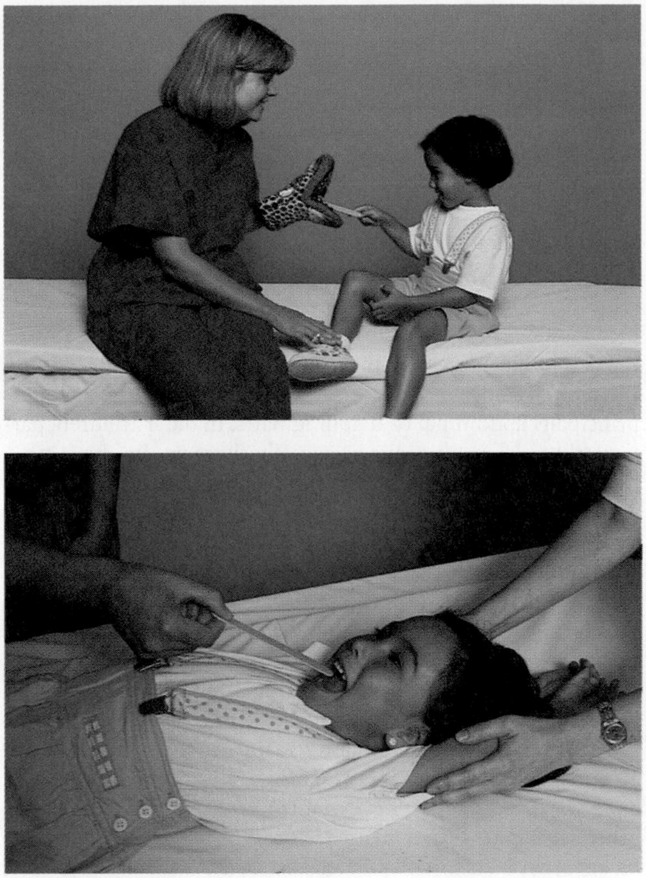

FIG. 35-22 • **A,** Encouraging child to cooperate. **B,** Positioning child for examination of mouth.

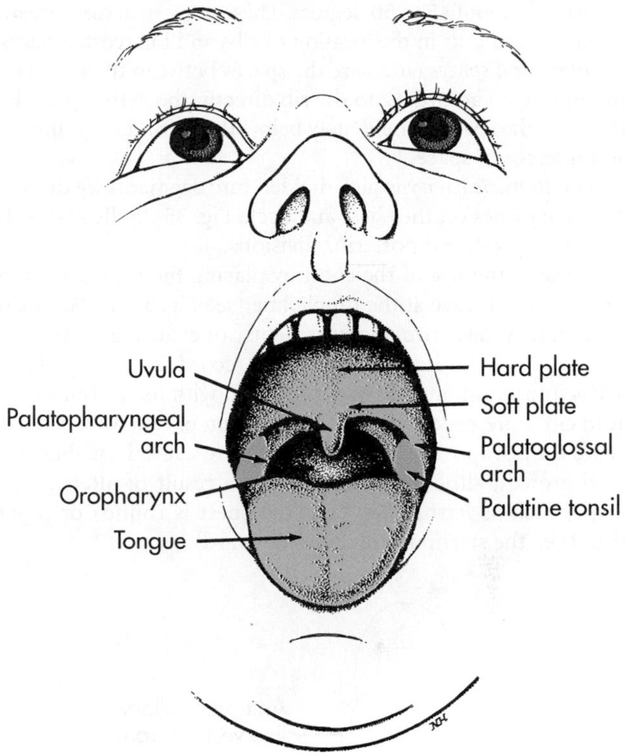

FIG. 35-23 • Interior structures of mouth.

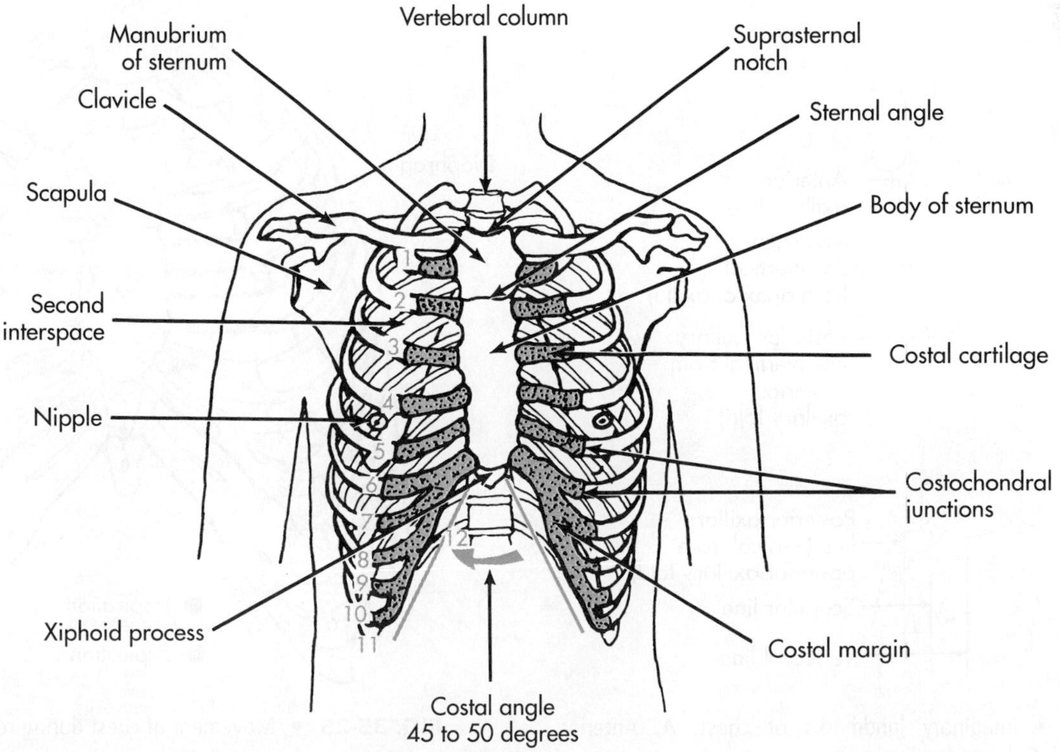

FIG. 35-24 • Rib cage.

num is the *body,* which forms the *sternal angle (angle of Louis)* as it articulates with the manubrium. At the end of the body is a small, moveable process called the *xiphoid.* The angle of the costal margin as it attaches to the sternum is called the *costal angle* and is normally about 45 to 50 degrees. These bony structures are important landmarks in the location of ribs and intercostal spaces.

Intercostal spaces (ICS) are the spaces between the ribs. They are numbered according to the rib directly above the space. For example, the space immediately below the second rib is the second intercostal space.

The *thoracic cavity* is also divided into segments by drawing imaginary lines on the chest and back. Fig. 35-25 illustrates the anterior, lateral, and posterior divisions.

Measure the *size* of the chest by placing the measuring tape around the rib cage at the nipple line (see Fig. 35-4). For greatest accuracy take two measurements, one during inspiration and the other during expiration, and record the average. Chest size is important, mainly in comparison with its relationship to head circumference, which is discussed on p. 790. Always report marked disproportions because most are caused by abnormal head growth, although some may be a result of altered chest shape, such as *barrel chest* (i.e., the chest is round) or *pigeon chest* (i.e., the sternum protrudes outward).

During infancy the *shape* of the chest is almost circular, with the anteroposterior (front-to-back) diameter equaling the transverse, or lateral (side-to-side), diameter. As the child grows, the chest normally increases in the transverse direction, causing the anteroposterior diameter to be less than the lateral diameter. Note the *angle* made by the lower costal margin and the sternum, and palpate the junction of the ribs with the costal cartilage (costochondral junction) and sternum, which should be fairly smooth.

Movement of the chest wall should be symmetric bilaterally and coordinated with breathing. During inspiration the chest rises and expands, the diaphragm descends, and the costal angle increases. During expiration the chest falls and decreases in size, the diaphragm rises, and the costal angle narrows (Fig. 35-26). In children under 6 or 7 years of age, respiratory movement is principally abdominal or diaphragmatic. In older children, particularly girls, respirations are chiefly thoracic. In either type, the chest and abdomen should rise and fall together. Always report any asymmetry of movement.

While inspecting the skin surface of the chest, observe the position of the *nipples,* as well as any evidence of *breast development.* Normally the nipples are located slightly lateral to the midclavicular line between the fourth and fifth ribs. Note symmetry of nipple placement and normal configuration of a darker pigmented areola surrounding a flat nipple in the prepubertal child.

Pubertal breast development usually begins in girls between 10 and 14 years of age (see Chapter 40). Record early (precocious) or delayed breast development, as well as evidence of any other secondary sexual characteristics. In males *breast enlargement (gynecomastia)* may be caused by hormonal or systemic disorders, but more commonly it is a result of adipose tissue from obesity or a transitory body change during early puberty. In either situation investigate the child's feelings regarding breast enlargement.

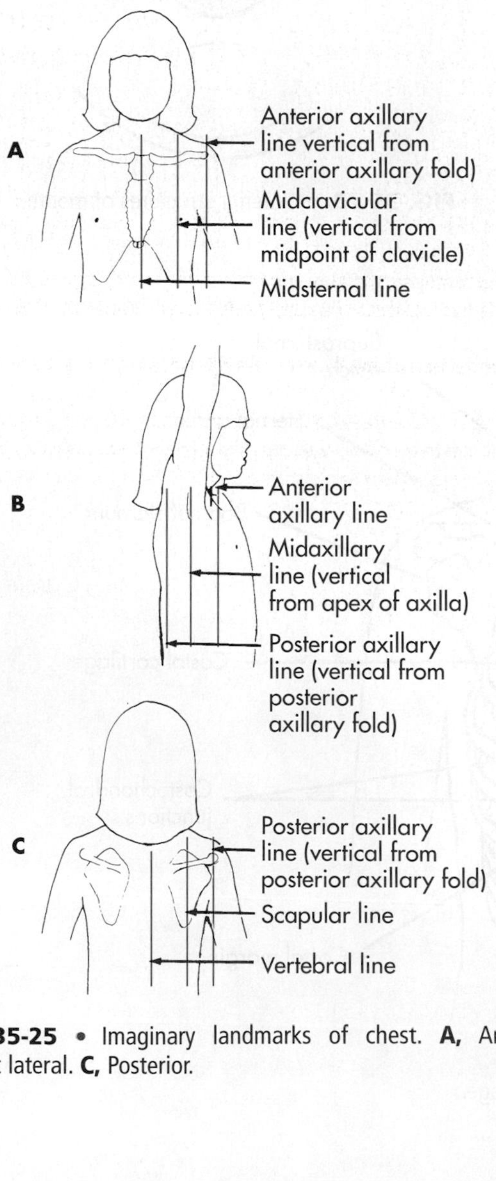

FIG. 35-25 • Imaginary landmarks of chest. **A,** Anterior. **B,** Right lateral. **C,** Posterior.

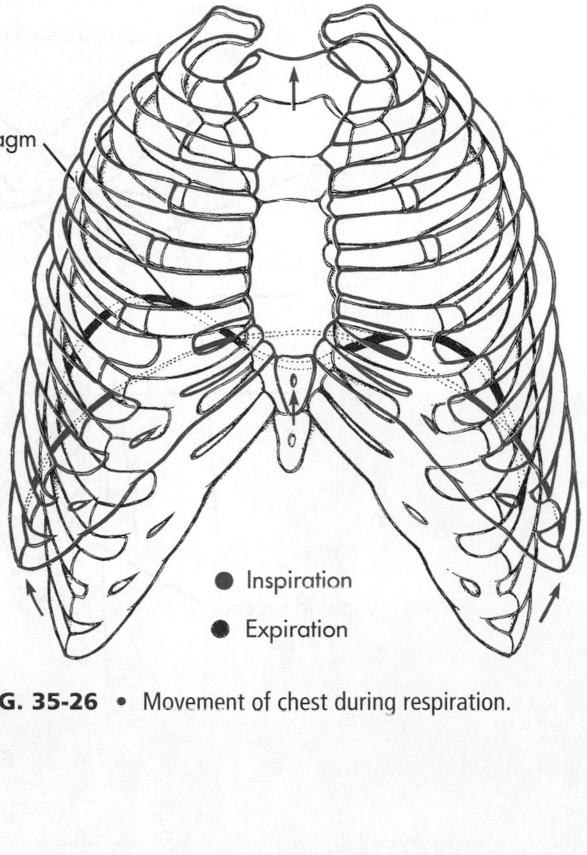

FIG. 35-26 • Movement of chest during respiration.

In adolescent females who have achieved sexual maturity, palpate the breasts for evidence of any masses or hard nodules. Use this opportunity to discuss the importance of routine self-breast examination. Emphasize that most palpable masses are benign to decrease any fear or concern that results when a mass is felt.

Lungs

The *lungs* are situated inside the thoracic cavity, with one lung on each side of the sternum. Each lung is divided into an *apex*, which is slightly pointed and rises above the first rib; a *base*, which is wide and concave and rides on the dome-shaped diaphragm; and a body, which is divided into lobes. The right lung has three lobes: the upper, middle, and lower. The left lung has only two lobes, the upper and lower, because of the space occupied by the heart (Fig. 35-27).

Inspection of the lungs primarily involves observation of respiratory movements, discussed previously. Evaluate respirations for rate (number per minute); rhythm (regular, irregular, or periodic); depth (deep or shallow); and quality (effortless, automatic, difficult, or labored). Note the character of breath sounds, such as noisy, grunting, snoring, or heavy.

Evaluate respiratory movements by placing each hand flat against the back or chest with the thumbs in midline along the lower costal margin of the lungs. The child should be sitting during this procedure and, if cooperative, should take several deep breaths. During respiration your hands will move with the chest wall. Assess the amount and speed of respiratory excursion and note any asymmetry of movement.

Experienced examiners may percuss the lungs. The anterior lung is percussed from apex to base, usually with the child in the supine or sitting position. Each side of the chest is percussed in sequence in order to compare the sounds. When the posterior lung is percussed, the procedure and sequence are the same, although the child should be sitting. Resonance is heard over all the lobes of the lungs that are not adjacent to other organs. Any deviation from the expected sound is recorded and reported.

Auscultation. Auscultation involves using the stethoscope to evaluate breath sounds (Guidelines box). Breath sounds are best heard if the child inspires deeply (Atraumatic Care box). In the lungs breath sounds are classified as vesicular, bronchovesicular, or bronchial (Box 35-3).

Guidelines

EFFECTIVE AUSCULTATION

Make sure child is relaxed and not crying, talking, or laughing. Record if child is crying.
Check that room is comfortable and quiet.
Warm stethoscope before placing it against skin.
Apply firm pressure on chestpiece but not enough to prevent vibrations and transmission of sound.
Avoid placing stethoscope over hair or clothing, moving it against skin, breathing on tubing, or sliding fingers over chestpiece, which may cause sounds that falsely resemble pathologic findings.
Use a symmetric and orderly approach to compare sounds.

Atraumatic Care

ENCOURAGING DEEP BREATHS

Ask child to "blow out" the light on an otoscope or pocket flashlight; discreetly turn off the light on the last try so that the child feels successful.
Place a cotton ball in child's palm; ask child to blow the ball into the air and have parent catch it.
Place a small tissue on the top of a pencil and ask child to blow the tissue off.
Have child blow a pinwheel, a party horn, or bubbles.

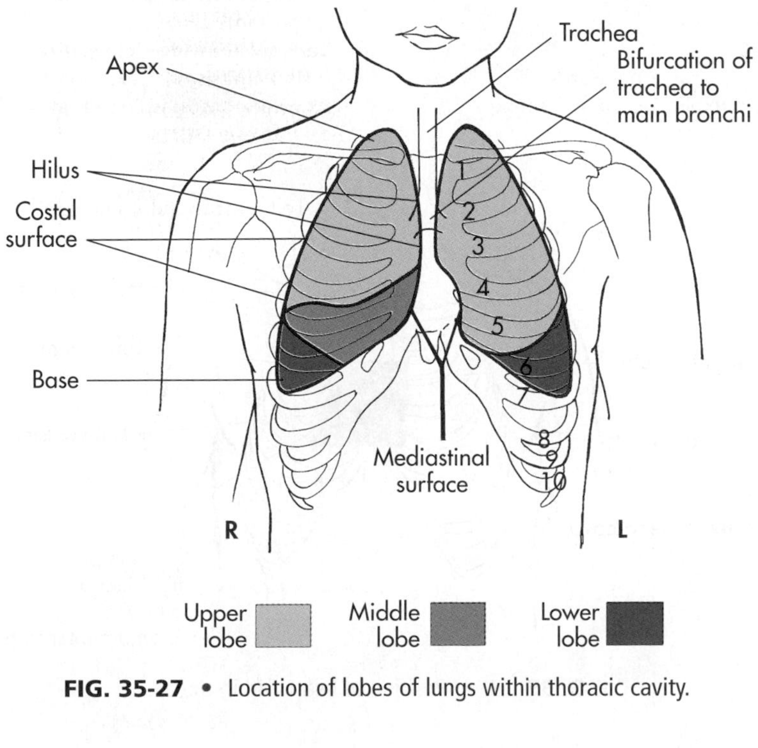

FIG. 35-27 • Location of lobes of lungs within thoracic cavity.

Absent or *diminished breath sounds* are always an abnormal finding and warrant investigation. Fluid, air, or solid masses in the pleural space all interfere with the conduction of breath sounds. Diminished breath sounds in certain segments of the lung can alert the nurse to pulmonary areas that may benefit from chest physiotherapy. Increased breath sounds following pulmonary therapy indicate improved passage of air through the respiratory tract. Terms used to describe various respiration patterns are found in Box 35-4.

Various pulmonary abnormalities produce *adventitious sounds* that are not normally heard over the chest. These sounds occur in addition to normal or abnormal breath sounds. They are classified into two main groups: *crackles,* which result from the passage of air through fluid or moisture; and *wheezes,* which are produced as air passes through narrowed passageways, regardless of the cause (e.g., exudate, inflammation, spasm, or tumor). Considerable practice with an experienced tutor is necessary to differentiate the various types of lung sounds. Often it is best to describe the type of sound heard in the lungs rather than trying to label it. Always report any abnormal sounds for further medical evaluation.

Box 35-3

Classification of Normal Breath Sounds

VESICULAR BREATH SOUNDS

Heard over entire surface of lungs, with exception of upper intrascapular area and area beneath manubrium.

Inspiration is louder, longer, and higher pitched than expiration.

Sound is soft, swishing noise.

BRONCHOVESICULAR BREATH SOUNDS

Heard over manubrium and in upper intrascapular regions where trachea and bronchial bifurcate.

Inspiration is louder and higher in pitch than in vesicular breathing.

BRONCHIAL BREATH SOUNDS

Heard only over trachea near suprasternal notch.

Inspiratory phase is short, and expiratory phase is long.

Heart

The heart is situated in the thoracic cavity between the lungs in the mediastinum and above the diaphragm (Fig. 35-28). About two thirds of the heart lies within the left side of the rib cage, with the other third on the right side as it crosses the sternum. The heart is positioned in the thorax like a trapezoid:

Vertically along the right sternal border (RSB) from the second to the fifth rib

Horizontally (long side) from the lower right sternum to the fifth rib at the left midclavicular line (LMCL)

Diagonally from the left sternal border (LSB) at the second rib to the LMCL at the fifth rib

Horizontally (short side) from the RSB and LSB or the second intercostal space (ICS)-base of the heart

Inspection is best done with the child sitting in a semi-Fowler's position. Look at the anterior chest wall from an angle, comparing both sides of the rib cage with each other; normally, they are symmetric. In children with thin chest walls, a pulsa-

Box 35-4

Various Patterns of Respiration

Tachypnea—Increased rate

Bradypnea—Decreased rate

Dyspnea—Distress during breathing

Apnea—Cessation of breathing

Hyperpnea—Increased depth

Hypoventilation—Decreased depth (shallow) and irregular rhythm

Hyperventilation—Increased rate and depth

Kussmaul breathing—Hyperventilation, grasping and labored respiration, usually seen in diabetic coma or other states of respiratory acidosis

Cheyne-Stokes respirations—Gradually increasing rate and depth with periods of apnea

Biot breathing—Periods of hyperpnea alternating with apnea (similar to Cheyne-Stokes except that depth remains constant)

Seesaw (paradoxic) respirations—Chest falls on inspiration and rises on expiration

Agonal—Last gasping breaths before death

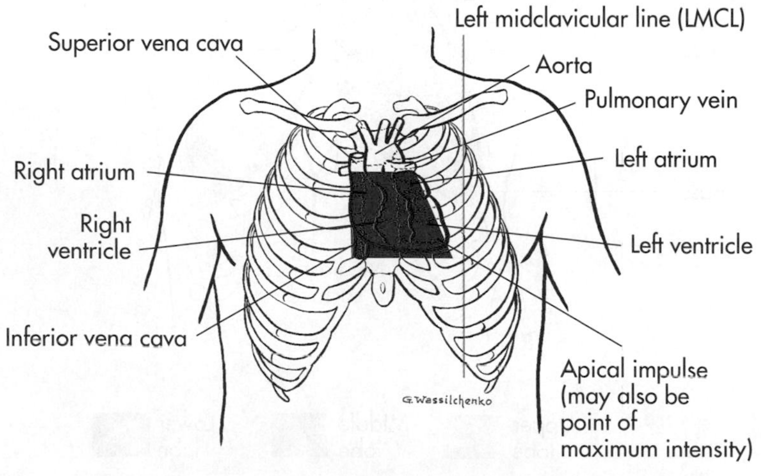

FIG. 35-28 • Position of heart within thorax.

tion may be visible. Because comprehensive evaluation of cardiac function is not limited to the heart, also consider other findings such as the presence of all pulses (especially the femoral pulses) (Fig. 35-29), distended neck veins, clubbing of the fingers, peripheral cyanosis, edema, blood pressure, and respiratory status.

Use palpation to determine the location of the *apical impulse (AI),* the most lateral cardiac impulse that may correspond to the apex. The AI is found:

- Just lateral to the left MCL and fourth ICS in children <7 years of age
- At the left MCL and fifth ICS in children >7 years of age

Although the AI gives a general idea of the size of the heart (with enlargement, the apex is lower and more lateral), its normal location is quite variable, making it a rather unreliable indicator of heart size.

The *point of maximum intensity (PMI),* as the name implies, is the area of most intense pulsation. Usually the PMI is located at the same site as the AI, but it can occur elsewhere. For this reason, the two terms should not be used synonymously.

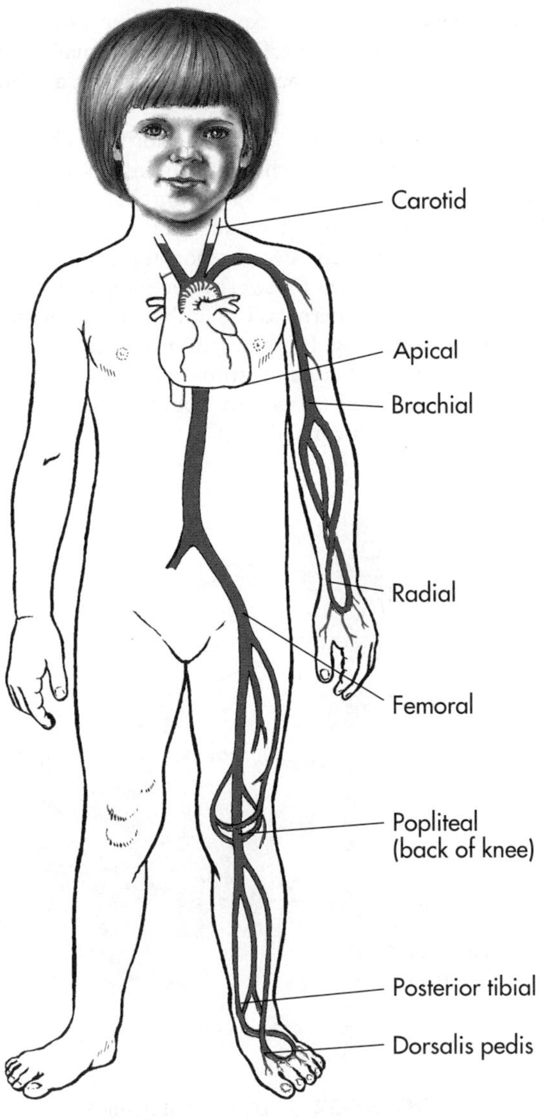

FIG. 35-29 • Location of pulses.

Assess *capillary refill time,* an important test for peripheral circulation. Press the skin lightly on a central site, such as the forehead; or a peripheral site, such as the top of the hand, to produce a slight blanching. The time it takes for the blanched area to return to its original color is the *capillary refill time.*

NURSE ALERT • Capillary refill should be brisk-in less than 2 seconds; prolonged refill may be associated with poor systemic perfusion, as well as a cool ambient temperature.

Auscultation

Origin of Heart Sounds. The heart sounds are produced by the opening and closing of the valves and the vibration of blood against the walls of the heart and vessels. Normally two sounds—S_1 and S_2—are heard, which correspond respectively to the familiar "lub dub" often used to describe the sounds. S_1 is caused by closure of the *tricuspid* and *mitral valves* (sometimes called the *atrioventricular valves*). S_2 is the result of closure of the *pulmonic* and *aortic valves* (sometimes called *semilunar valves*). Normally the split of the two sounds in S_2 is distinguishable and widens during inspiration. *Physiologic* splitting is a significant normal finding.

NURSE ALERT • "Fixed splitting," in which the split in S_2 does not change during inspiration, is an important diagnostic sign of atrial septal defect.

Two other heart sounds—S_3 and S_4—may be produced. S_3 is normally heard in some children; S_4 is rarely heard as a normal heart sound; usually it indicates the need for further cardiac evaluation.

Another important category of heart sounds is *murmurs,* sounds that are produced by vibrations within the heart chambers or in the major arteries from the back-and-forth flow of blood. The description and classification of murmurs are skills that require considerable practice and training. Consult with an experienced practitioner whenever a murmur is identified or suspected.

Differentiating Normal Heart Sounds. Fig. 35-30 illustrates the approximate anatomic position of the valves within

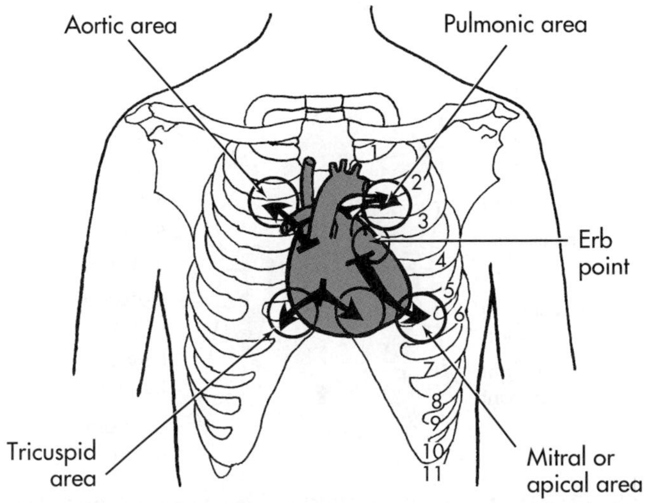

FIG. 35-30 • Direction of heart sounds for anatomic valve sites and areas *(circled)* for auscultation.

the heart chambers. Note that the anatomic location of valves does not correspond to the area where the sounds are heard best. The auscultatory sites are located in the direction of the blood flow through the valves.

Normally S_1 is louder at the apex of the heart in the mitral and tricuspid area, and S_2 is louder near the base of the heart in the pulmonic and aortic area. Listen to each sound by inching down the chest. The following areas should also be auscultated for sounds, such as murmurs, which may radiate to these sites: sternoclavicular area above the clavicles and manubrium, area along the sternal border, area along the left midaxillary line, and area below the scapulae.

Auscultate the heart with the child in at least two positions: sitting and reclining. If adventitious sounds are detected, further evaluate them with the child standing, sitting and leaning forward, and lying on the left side. For example, atrial sounds such as S_4 are heard best with the person in a recumbent position, and usually fade if the person sits or stands.

Evaluate heart sounds for (1) *quality* (should be clear and distinct, not muffled, diffuse, or distant); (2) *intensity,* especially in relation to the location or auscultatory site (should not be weak or pounding); (3) *rate* (should be the same as the radial pulse); and (4) *rhythm* (should be regular and even). A particular arrhythmia that occurs normally in many children is *sinus arrhythmia,* in which the heart rate increases with inspiration and decreases with expiration. Differentiate this rhythm from a truly abnormal arrhythmia by having children hold their breath. In sinus arrhythmia, cessation of breathing causes the heart rate to remain steady.

Abdomen

Examination of the abdomen involves inspection, followed by auscultation and then palpation. Perform palpation last because it may distort the normal abdominal sounds. Knowledge of the anatomic placement of the abdominal organs is essential to differentiate normal, expected findings from abnormal ones (Fig. 35-31).

For descriptive purposes the abdominal cavity is divided into four quadrants by drawing a vertical line midway from the sternum to the pubic symphysis and a horizontal line across the abdomen through the umbilicus. Each section is named as follows:

- Left upper quadrant (LUQ)
- Left lower quadrant (LLQ)
- Right upper quadrant (RUQ)
- Right lower quadrant (RLQ)

Inspection. Inspect the *contour* of the abdomen with the child erect and supine. Normally the abdomen of the infant and young child is quite cylindric and, in the erect position, fairly prominent because of the physiologic lordosis of the spine. In the supine position the abdomen appears flat. A midline protrusion from the xiphoid to the umbilicus or pubic symphysis is usually *diastasis recti,* or failure of the rectus abdominis muscles to join in utero. In a healthy child a midline protrusion is usually a variation of normal muscular development.

NURSE ALERT • A tense, boardlike abdomen is a serious sign of paralytic ileus and intestinal obstruction.

The *skin* covering the abdomen should be uniformly taut, without wrinkles or creases. Sometimes silvery, whitish striae ("stretch marks") are seen, especially if the skin has been stretched as in obesity. Superficial veins are usually visible in light-skinned, thin infants, but distended veins are an abnormal finding.

Observe *movement* of the abdomen. Normally chest and abdominal movements are synchronous. In infants and thin children *peristaltic waves* may be visible through the abdominal wall; they are best observed by standing at eye level to and across from the abdomen. Always report this finding.

Examine the *umbilicus* for size, hygiene, and evidence of any abnormalities, such as hernias. The umbilicus should be flat or only slightly protruding. If a herniation is present, palpate the sac for abdominal contents and estimate the approximate size of the opening. *Umbilical hernias* are common in infants, especially in African-American children.

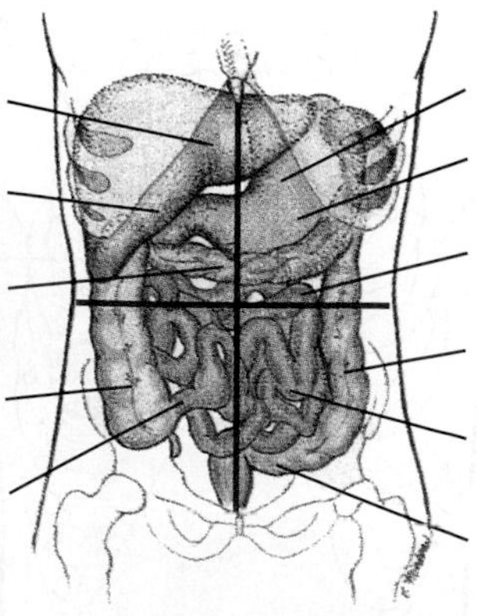

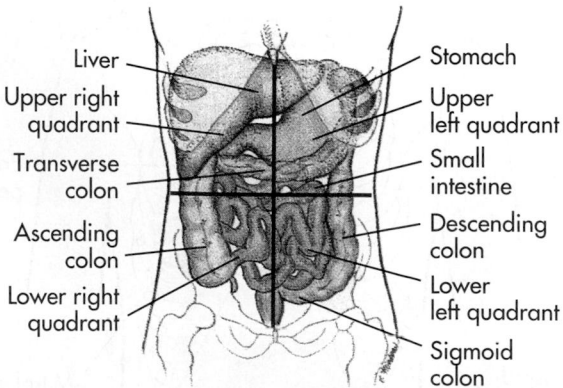

FIG. 35-31 • Location of structures in abdomen. Crossed lines divide cavity into quadrants. (From Potter PA, Perry AG: *Basic nursing: theory and practice,* ed 3, St Louis, 1995, Mosby.)

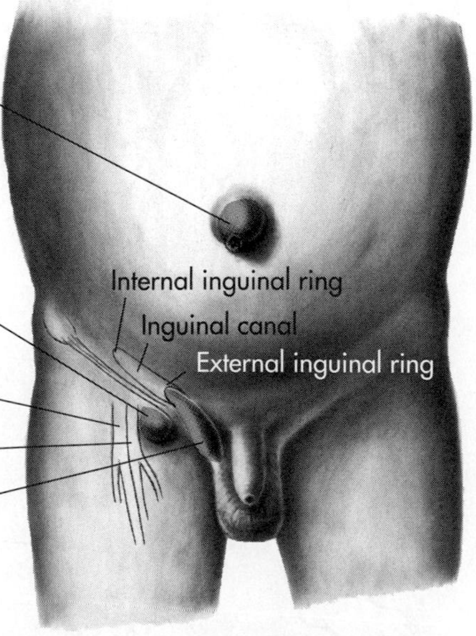

FIG. 35-32 • Location of hernias.

Hernias may exist elsewhere on the abdominal wall (Fig. 35-32). *An inguinal hernia* is a protrusion of peritoneum through the abdominal wall into the inguinal canal. It occurs mostly in males, is often bilateral, and may be visible as a mass in the scrotum. To locate a hernia, slide the little finger into the external inguinal ring at the base of the scrotum and ask the child to cough. If a hernia is present, it will hit the tip of the finger.

A *femoral hernia,* which occurs more commonly in girls, is felt or seen as a small mass on the anterior surface of the thigh just below the inguinal ligament in the femoral canal (a potential space medial to the femoral artery). Feel for a hernia by placing the index finger of your right hand on the child's right femoral pulse (left hand for left pulse) and the middle ring finger flat against the skin toward the midline. The ring finger lies over the femoral canal, where the herniation occurs. Palpation of hernias in the pelvic region is often part of the examination of genitalia.

Auscultation. The most important finding to listen for is *peristalsis,* or *bowel sounds,* which sound like short metallic clicks and gurgles. Their frequency per minute should be recorded (e.g., 5 sounds/min). Bowel sounds may be stimulated by stroking the abdominal surface with a fingernail. Report absence of bowel sounds or hyperperistalsis because either usually denotes an abdominal disorder.

Palpation. Two types of palpation are performed: superficial and deep. In superficial palpation, lightly place your hand against the skin and feel each quadrant, noting any areas of tenderness, muscle tone, and superficial lesions, such as cysts. Because *superficial palpation* is often perceived as tickling, several techniques can be used to minimize this sensation and provide relaxation (Atraumatic Care box). Admonishing the child to stop laughing only draws attention to the sensation and decreases cooperation.

Deep palpation is used for palpating organs and large blood vessels and for detecting masses and tenderness that were not discovered during superficial palpation. Palpation usually begins in the lower quadrants and proceeds upward to avoid missing the edge of an enlarged liver or spleen. Except for palpating the liver, successful identification of other organs, such as the spleen, kidney, and part of the colon, requires considerable practice with tutored supervision. Report any questionable mass.

The lower edge of the *liver* is sometimes felt in infants and young children as a superficial mass 1 to 2 cm ($\frac{4}{10}$ to $\frac{8}{10}$ inch) below the right costal margin (the distance is sometimes measured in fingerbreadths). Normally the liver descends during inspiration as the diaphragm moves downward. Do not mistake this downward displacement as a sign of liver enlargement.

NURSE ALERT • If the liver is palpable 3 cm below the right costal margin, or the spleen is palpable more than 2 cm below the left costal margin, these organs are enlarged, a finding that is always reported for further medical investigation.

Palpate the *femoral pulses* by placing the tips of two or three fingers (e.g., index, middle, and/or ring) along the inguinal ligament about midway between the iliac crest and pubic symphysis. Feel both pulses simultaneously to make certain that they are equal and strong (Fig. 35-33).

NURSE ALERT • Absence of femoral pulses is a significant sign of coarctation of the aorta and is referred for medical evaluation.

Atraumatic Care

PROMOTING RELAXATION DURING ABDOMINAL PALPATION

- Position child comfortably, such as in a semireclining position in the parent's lap, with knees flexed.
- Warm the hands before touching the skin.
- Use distraction, such as telling stories or talking to child.
- Teach child to use deep breathing and to concentrate on an object.
- Give infant a bottle or pacifier.
- Begin with light, superficial palpation and gradually progress to deeper palpation.
- Palpate any tender or painful areas last.
- Have child hold the parent's hand and squeeze it if palpation is uncomfortable.
- Use the nonpalpating hand to comfort child, such as placing the free hand on the child's shoulder while palpating the abdomen.
- To minimize sensation of tickling during palpation:
  - Have children "help" with palpation by placing their hand over the palpating hand.
  - Have them place their hand on the abdomen with the fingers spread wide apart, and palpate between their fingers.

Genitalia

Examination of genitalia conveniently follows assessment of the abdomen while the child is still supine. In adolescents inspection of the genitalia may be left to the end of the examination. The best approach is to examine the genitalia matter-of-factly, placing no more emphasis on this part of the assessment than on any other segment. It helps to relieve children's and parents' anxiety by telling them the results of the findings; for example, the nurse might say, "Everything looks fine here."

If it is necessary to ask questions, such as about discharge or difficulty in urinating, respect the child's privacy by covering the lower abdomen with the gown or underpants. To prevent embarrassing interruptions, keep the door or curtain closed and post a "do not disturb" sign. Have a drape ready to cover the genitalia if someone enters the room.

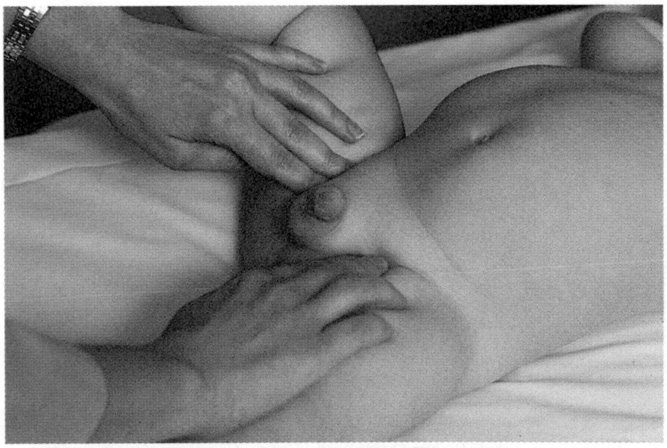

FIG. 35-33 • Palpating for femoral pulses.

In examining the genitalia, wear gloves whenever touching body surfaces. It might be helpful for the adolescent to know that wearing gloves also prevents skin-to-skin contact.

The genital examination is an excellent time for eliciting questions of concern about body functioning or sexual activity. Also use this opportunity to increase or reinforce the child's knowledge of reproductive anatomy by naming each body part and explaining its function. This part of the health assessment is an opportune time to teach testicular self-examination to boys.*

Male Genitalia. Note the external appearance of the glans and shaft of the penis, the prepuce, the urethral meatus, and the scrotum (Fig. 35-34). The *penis* is generally small in infants and young boys until puberty, when it begins to increase in both length and width. In an obese child the penis often looks abnormally small because of the folds of skin partially covering it at the base. Be familiar with normal pubertal growth of the external male genitalia in order to compare the findings with the expected sequence of maturation (see Chapter 40).

Examine the *glans* (head of the penis) and *shaft* (portion between the perineum and prepuce) for signs of swelling, skin lesions, inflammation, or other irregularities. Any of these signs may indicate underlying disorders, especially sexually transmitted diseases.

The *urethral meatus* is carefully inspected for location and evidence of discharge. Normally it is centered at the tip of the glans.

Hair distribution is also noted. Normally no pubic hair is present before puberty. Soft, downy hair at the base of the penis is an early sign of pubertal maturation. In older adolescents hair distribution is diamond-shaped from the umbilicus to the anus.

The location and size of the *scrotum* are noted. The scrota hang freely from the perineum behind the penis, and the left scrotum normally hangs lower than the right. In infants the scrota appear large in relation to the rest of the genitalia. The skin of the scrotum is loose and highly rugated (wrinkled). During early adolescence the skin normally becomes redder and coarser. In dark-skinned children the scrota are usually more deeply pigmented.

Palpation of the scrotum includes identification of the testes, epididymis, and, if present, inguinal hernias. The two *testes* are felt as small ovoid bodies about 1.5 to 2 cm (6/10 to 8/10 inch) long-one in each scrotal sac. They do not enlarge until puberty, when they approximately double in size.

When palpating for the presence of the testes, avoid stimulating the *cremasteric reflex,* which is stimulated by cold, touch, emotional excitement, or exercise. This reflex pulls the testes higher into the pelvic cavity. Several measures are useful in preventing the cremasteric reflex during palpation of the scrotum. First, warm the hands. Second, if the child is old enough, examine him in a tailor or "Indian" position, which stretches the muscle, preventing its contraction (Fig. 35-35, *A*). Third, block the normal pathway of ascent of the testes by placing the thumb and index finger over the upper part of the scrotal sac along the inguinal canal (Fig. 35-35, *B*). If there is any question concerning the existence of two testes, place the index and middle fingers in a scissors fashion to separate the right and left scrotum. If after using these techniques the testes have not been palpated, feel along the inguinal canal and perineum to locate masses that may be undescended testes. Although undescended testes may descend at any time during childhood and are checked at each visit, failure to palpate testes is reported.

Female Genitalia. The examination of female genitalia is limited to inspection and palpation of external structures. If a vaginal examination is required, an appropriate referral is made unless the nurse is qualified to perform the procedure. A convenient position for examination of the genitalia involves plac-

*For free information on testicular cancer, contact the Jason A. Struble Memorial Cancer Fund, Inc., 624 Kehrs Mill Rd., Ballwin, MO 63011.

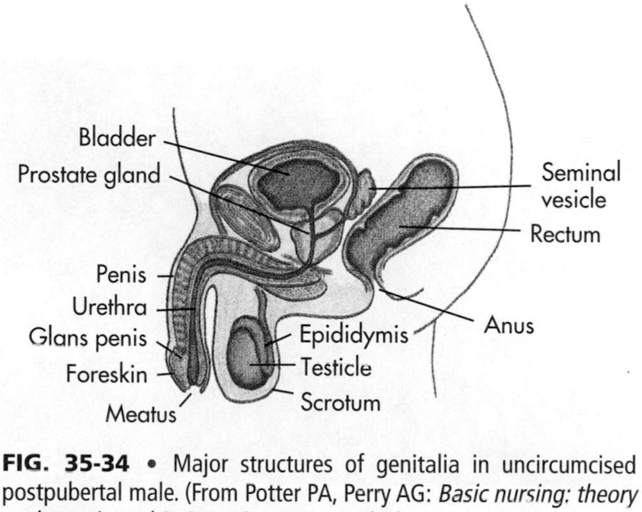

FIG. 35-34 • Major structures of genitalia in uncircumcised postpubertal male. (From Potter PA, Perry AG: *Basic nursing: theory and practice,* ed 3, St Louis, 1995, Mosby.)

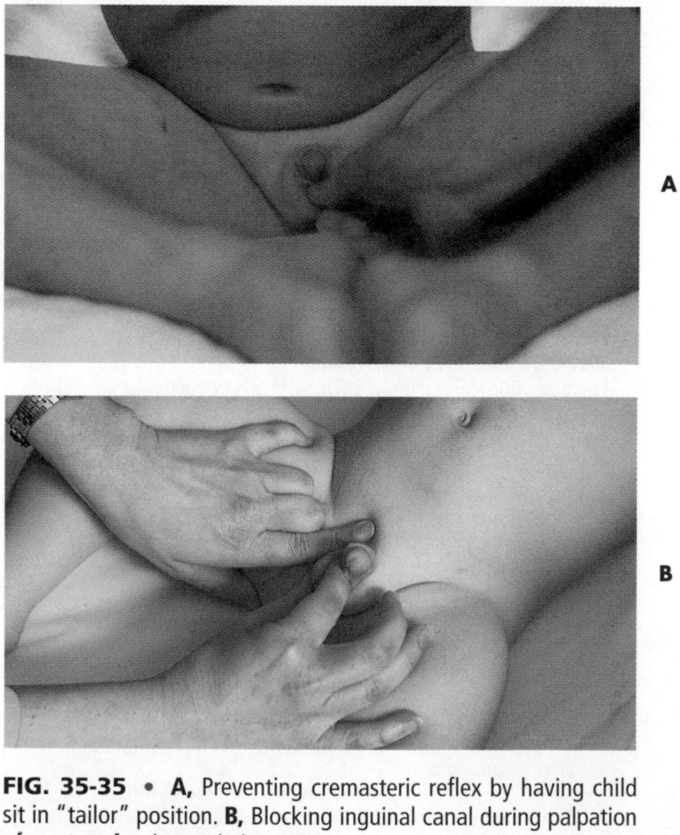

FIG. 35-35 • **A,** Preventing cremasteric reflex by having child sit in "tailor" position. **B,** Blocking inguinal canal during palpation of scrotum for descended testes.

ing the young child supine on the examining table or in a semireclining position on the parent's lap with the feet supported on your knees as you sit facing the child. Divert the child's attention from the examination by instructing her to try to keep the soles of her feet pressed against each other. Separate the labia majora with the thumb and index finger and retract outward to expose the labia minora, urethral meatus, and vaginal orifice.

Examine the female genitalia for size and location of the structures of the *vulva* or *pudendum* (Fig. 35-36). The mons pubis is a pad of adipose tissue over the symphysis pubis. At puberty the mons is covered with hair, which extends along the labia. The usual pattern of female *hair distribution* is an inverted triangle. The appearance of soft, downy hair along the labia majora is an early sign of sexual maturation.

Note the size and location of the *clitoris.* It is a small erectile organ located at the anterior end of the labia minora. It is covered by a small flap of skin, the *prepuce.*

The *labia majora* are two thick folds of skin running posteriorly from the mons to the posterior commissure of the vagina. Internal to the labia majora are two folds of skin called the *labia minora.* Although the labia minora are usually prominent in the newborn, they gradually atrophy, which makes them almost invisible until their enlargement during puberty.

The inner surface of the labia should be pink and moist. Note the size of the labia and any evidence of fusion, which may suggest male scrota. Normally no masses are palpable within the labia.

The *urethral meatus* is located posterior to the clitoris and is surrounded by Skene glands and ducts. Although not a prominent structure, the meatus appears as a small V-shaped slit. Note its location, especially if it opens from the clitoris or inside the vagina. Gently palpate the glands, which are common sites of cysts and sexually transmitted lesions.

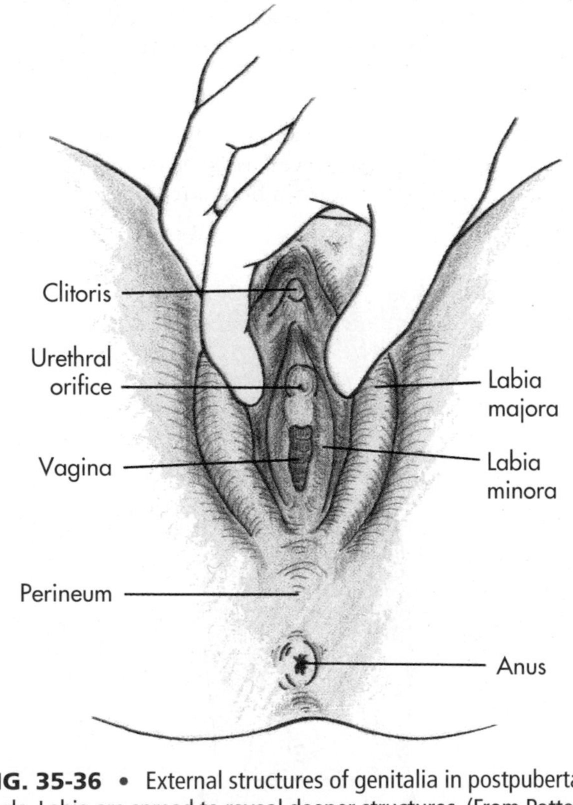

FIG. 35-36 • External structures of genitalia in postpubertal female. Labia are spread to reveal deeper structures. (From Potter PA, Perry AG: *Basic nursing: theory and practice,* ed 4, St Louis, 1999, Mosby.)

The *vaginal orifice* is located posterior to the urethral meatus. Its appearance varies depending on individual anatomy and sexual activity. Ordinarily, examination of the vagina is limited to inspection. In virgins a thin, crescent-shaped or circular membrane called the *hymen* may cover part of the vaginal opening. In some instances it completely occludes the orifice. After rupture, small, rounded pieces of tissue called *caruncles* remain. Although an imperforate hymen denotes lack of penile intercourse, a perforate one does not necessarily indicate sexual activity (see also Sexual Abuse, Chapter 38).

Surrounding the vaginal opening are *Bartholin glands,* which secrete a clear, mucoid fluid into the vagina for lubrication during intercourse. Palpate the glands for cysts. Also note the discharge from the vagina, which is usually clear or white.

NURSE ALERT • In females who have been circumcised, the genitalia will appear different. Do not show surprise or disgust, but note the appearance and discuss the procedure with the young woman.

Anus

Following examination of the genitalia, the anal area is easily examined, although the child should be placed on the abdomen. Note the general firmness of the *buttocks* and symmetry of the *gluteal folds.* Assess the tone of the anal sphincter by eliciting the *anal reflex.* Gently scratching the anal area results in an obvious quick contraction of the external anal sphincter.

Back and Extremities

Spine. The general *curvature* of the spine is noted. Normally the back of a newborn is rounded or C-shaped from the thoracic and pelvic curves. The development of the cervical and lumbar curves approximates development of various motor skills, such as cervical curvature with head control, and gives the older child the typical double S curve.

Marked curvatures in posture are abnormal (see Fig. 54-17). *Scoliosis,* lateral curvature of the spine, is an important childhood problem, especially in girls. Although scoliosis may be identified by observing and palpating the spine and noting a sideways displacement, more objective tests include:

- With the child standing erect, clothed only in underpants (and bra if older girl), observe from behind, noting asymmetry of the shoulders and hips.
- With the child bending forward so that the back is parallel to the floor, observe from the side, noting asymmetry or prominence of the rib cage.

A slight limp, a crooked hemline, or complaints of a sore back are other signs and symptoms of scoliosis.

Inspect the *back,* especially along the spine, for any tufts of hair, dimples, or discoloration. *Mobility* of the vertebral column is easily assessed in most children because of their propensity for constant motion during the examination. However, mobility can be tested by asking the child to sit up from a prone position or to do a modified sit-up exercise.

Movement of the cervical spine is an important diagnostic sign of neurologic problems, such as meningitis. Normally movement of the head in all directions is effortless.

NURSE ALERT • Hyperextension of the neck and spine, or opisthotonos, which is accompanied by pain when the head is flexed, is always referred for immediate medical evaluation.

Extremities. Inspect each extremity for symmetry of length and size; refer any deviation for orthopedic evaluation. Count the fingers and toes to be certain of the normal number. This is so often taken for granted that an extra digit (*polydactyly*) or fusion of digits (*syndactyly*) may go unnoticed.

Inspect the arms and legs for *temperature* and *color,* which should be equal in each extremity, although the feet may normally be colder than the hands.

Assess the *shape* of bones. Several variations of bone shape may be observed in children. Although many of them cause parents concern, most are benign and require no treatment. *Bowleg,* or *genu varum,* is lateral bowing of the tibia. It is clinically present when the child stands with the medial malleoli (rounded prominence on either side of the ankle) opposite each other and the space between the knees is greater than approximately 5 cm (2 inches) (Fig. 35-37). Toddlers are usually bowlegged after beginning to walk until all of their lower back and leg muscles are well developed. Unilateral or asymmetric bowlegs that are present beyond the age of 2 to 3 years, particularly in African-American children, may represent pathologic conditions requiring further investigation.

Knock-knee, or *genu valgum,* appears as the opposite of bowleg, in that the knees are close together but the feet are spread apart. It is determined clinically by using the same method as for genu varum but by measuring the distance between the malleoli, which normally should be less than 7.5 cm (3 inches) (Fig. 35-38). Knock-knee is normally present in children from about 2 to 7 years of age. Knock-knee that is excessive, asymmetric, accompanied by shortened stature, or evident in a child nearing puberty requires further evaluation.

Next inspect the *feet.* Infants' and toddlers' feet appear flat because the foot is normally wide and the arch is covered by a fat pad. Development of the arch occurs naturally from the action of walking. Normally, at birth the feet are held in a valgus (outward) or varus (inward) position. To determine whether a foot deformity at birth is a result of intrauterine position or development, scratch the outer, then inner, side of the sole. If the foot position is self-correctable, it will assume a right angle to the leg. As the child begins to walk, the feet turn outward less than 30 degrees and inward less than 10 degrees.

Toddlers have a "toddling" or broad-based gait, which facilitates walking by lowering the center of gravity. As the child reaches preschool age, the legs are brought closer together. By school age the walking posture is much more graceful and balanced.

The most common gait problem in young children is *pigeon toe,* or *toeing in,* which usually results from torsional deformities such as internal tibial torsion (abnormal rotation or bowing of the tibia). Tests for tibial torsion include measuring the thigh-foot angle, which requires considerable practice for accuracy.

Elicit the *plantar* or *grasp reflex* by exerting firm but gentle pressure with the tip of the thumb against the lateral sole of the foot from the heel upward to the little toe and then across to the big toe. The normal response in children who are walking is flexion of the toes. *Babinski sign,* dorsiflexion of the big toe and fanning of the other toes, is normal during infancy but abnormal after about 1 year of age or when locomotion begins (see p. 538).

Joints. Evaluate the joints for *range of motion.* Normally this requires no specific testing if the nurse has been observant of the child's movements during the examination. However, the hips should be routinely investigated in infants for congenital dislocation. Signs of congenital hip dislocation are shown in Fig. 28-21. Report any evidence of joint immobility or hyperflexibility.

Palpate the joints for *heat, tenderness,* and *swelling.* These signs, as well as redness over the joint, warrant further investigation.

Muscles. Note symmetry and quality of muscle development, tone, and strength. Observe *development* by looking at the shape and contour of the body in both a relaxed and a tensed

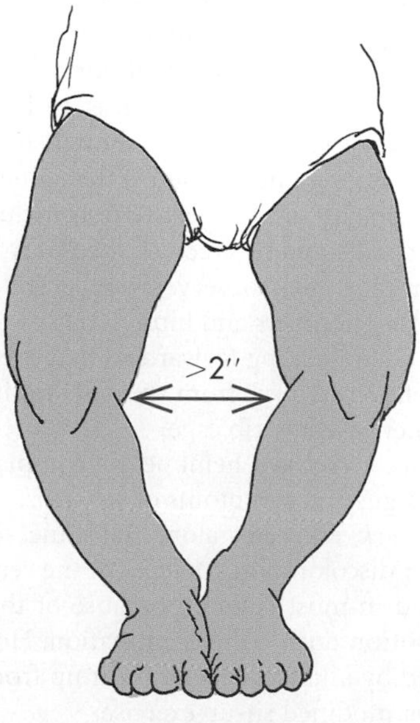

FIG. 35-37 • Bowleg.

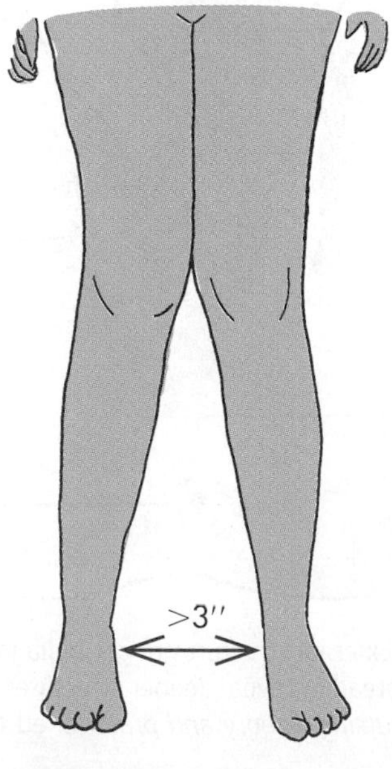

FIG. 35-38 • Knock-knee.

state. Estimate tone by grasping the muscle and feeling its firmness when it is relaxed and contracted. A common site for testing tone is the biceps muscle of the arm. Children are usually willing to "make a muscle" by clenching their fist.

Estimate *strength* by having the child use an extremity to push or pull against resistance, as in the following examples:

- **Arm strength**—Child holds the arms outstretched in front of the body and tries to raise the arms while downward pressure is applied
- **Hand strength**—Child shakes hands with nurse and squeezes one or two fingers of the nurse's hand
- **Leg strength**—Child sits on a table or chair with the legs dangling and tries to raise the legs while downward pressure is applied

Note symmetry of strength in the extremities, hands, and fingers, and report evidence of paresis or weakness.

Neurologic Assessment

The assessment of the nervous system is the broadest and most diverse part of the examining process, since every human function, both physical and emotional, is controlled by neurologic impulses. Much of the neurologic examination has already been discussed, such as assessment of behavior, sensory testing, and motor functioning. The following focuses on a general appraisal of cerebellar functioning, deep tendon reflexes, and the cranial nerves.

Cerebellar Functioning. The cerebellum controls balance and coordination. Much of the assessment of cerebellar functioning is included in observing the child's posture, body movements, gait, and development of fine and gross motor skills. Tests such as balancing on one foot and the heel-to-toe walk assess balance. Test *coordination* by asking the child to reach for a toy, button clothes, tie shoes, or draw a straight line on a piece of paper, provided that the child is old enough to do these activities. Coordination can also be tested by any sequence of rapid successive movements, such as quickly touching each finger with the thumb of the same hand.

Several tests for cerebellar function are described in Box 35-5 and can be performed as games. When the Romberg test is done, stay beside the child if there is a possibility that the child may fall. School-age children should be able to perform these tests, although, in the finger-to-nose test, preschoolers normally can only bring the finger within 5 to 7.5 cm (2 to 3 inches) of the nose. Difficulty in performing these exercises indicates poor sense of position (especially with the eyes closed) and incoordination (especially with the eyes opened).

Reflexes. Testing reflexes is an important part of the neurologic examination. Persistence of primitive reflexes (see Chapter 24), loss of reflexes, or hyperactivity of deep tendon reflexes is usually a result of a cerebral insult.

Elicit reflexes by using the rubber head of the reflex hammer, flat of the finger, or side of the hand. If the child is easily frightened by equipment, use your hand or finger. Although testing reflexes is a simple procedure to perform, the child may inhibit the reflex by unconsciously tensing the muscle. To avoid tensing, distract younger children with toys or talk to them. Older children can concentrate on the exercise of grasping their two hands in front of them and trying to pull them apart. This diverts their attention away from the testing and causes involuntary relaxation of the muscles.

Deep tendon reflexes are stretch reflexes of a muscle. The most common deep tendon reflex is the *knee jerk*, or *patellar reflex* (sometimes called the *quadriceps reflex*). The reflexes normally elicited are described in Figs. 35-39 to 35-42. Report any diminished or hyperreflexic response for further evaluation.

Box 35-5

Tests for Cerebellar Function

Finger-to-nose test—With child's arm extended, ask child to touch the nose with the index finger with eyes open and then closed.

Heel-to-shin test—While standing, have child run the heel of one foot down the shin or anterior aspect of the tibia of the other leg, both with eyes opened and then closed.

Romberg test—With eyes closed, have child stand with heels together; falling or leaning to one side is abnormal and is called ***Romberg sign.***

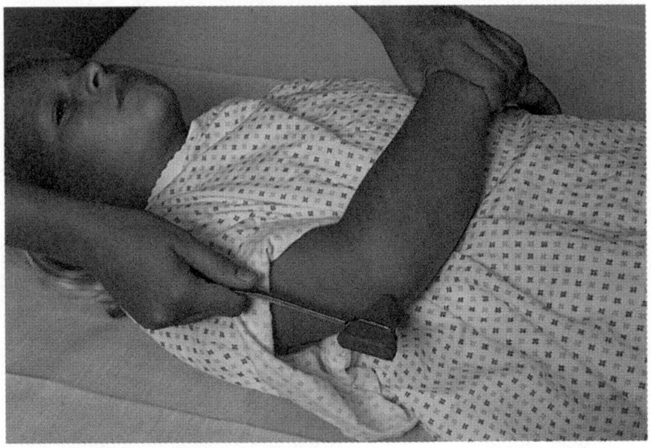

FIG. 35-39 • Testing for triceps reflex. Child is placed supine, with forearm resting over chest, and triceps tendon is struck. Alternate procedure: child's arm is abducted, with upper arm supported and forearm allowed to hang freely. Triceps tendon is struck. Normal response is partial extension of forearm.

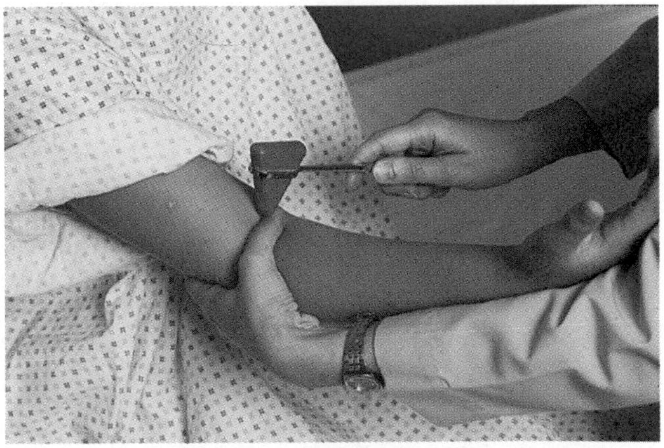

FIG. 35-40 • Testing for biceps reflex. Child's arm is held by placing partially flexed elbow in examiner's hand with thumb over antecubital space. Examiner's thumbnail is struck with hammer. Normal response is partial flexion of forearm.

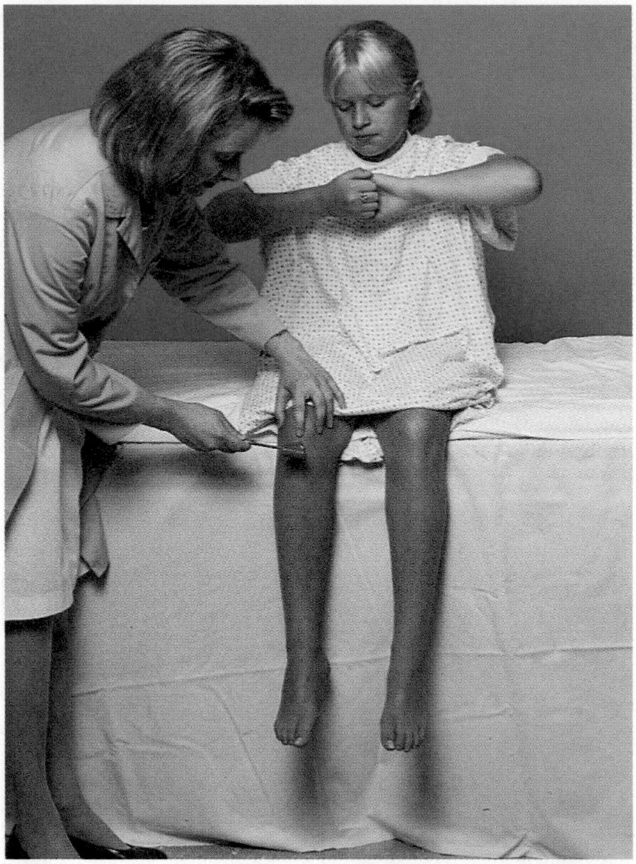

FIG. 35-41 • Testing for patellar, or knee jerk reflex using distraction. Child sits on edge of examining table (or on parent's lap) with lower legs flexed at knee and dangling freely. Patellar tendon is tapped just below kneecap. Normal response is partial extension of lower leg.

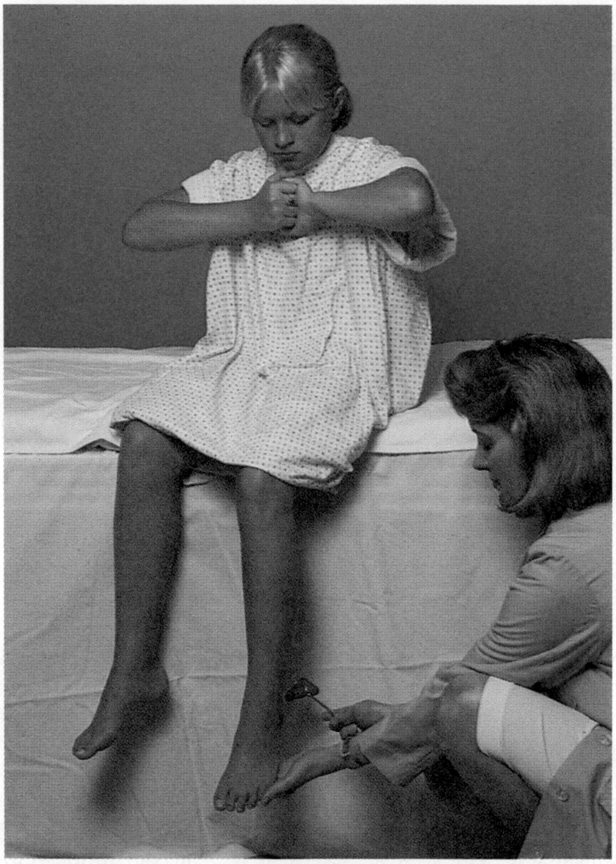

FIG. 35-42 • Testing for Achilles reflex. The child should be in the same position as for the knee jerk reflex. Foot is supported lightly in examiner's hand, and Achilles tendon is struck. Normal response is plantar flexion of foot (foot pointing downward).

Cranial Nerves. Assessment of the cranial nerves is an important area of neurologic assessment (Table 35-11). With young children, present the tests as games to encourage trust and security at the beginning of the examination. Or include the cranial nerve test when each "system" is examined, such as tongue movement and strength, gag reflex, swallowing, cardinal positions of gaze (Fig. 35-43), and position of the uvula during examination of the mouth.

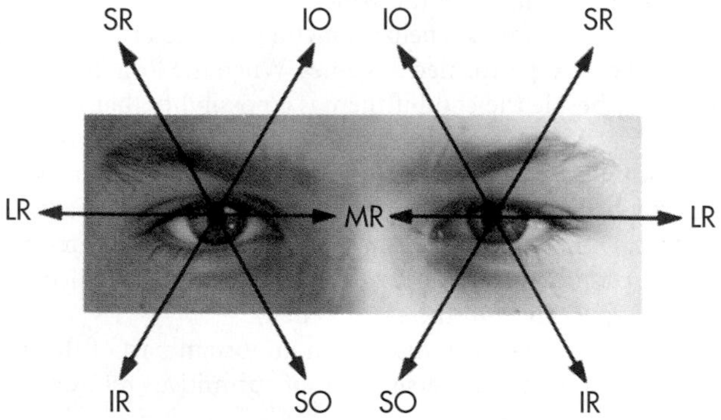

FIG. 35-43 • Testing cardinal position of gaze.

DEVELOPMENTAL ASSESSMENT

One of the most essential components of a complete health appraisal is assessment of developmental functioning. *Screening procedures* are designed to identify quickly and reliably those children whose developmental level is below normal for their age and who therefore require further investigation. They also provide a means of recording objective measurements of present developmental functioning for future reference. Since the passage of P.L. 99-457, the Education of the Handicapped Act Amendments of 1986, much greater emphasis is placed on developmental assessment of children with disabilities, and nurses can play a vital role in providing this service. All of the procedures discussed in this section can be administered in a variety of settings—home, school, day care center, hospital, practitioner's office, or clinic.

Denver II

The most widely used developmental screening tests for young children have been the series of tests developed by Dr. William Frankenburg and his colleagues in Denver, Colorado. The oldest and best known, the *Denver Developmental Screening Test*

(DDST) and its revision, the DDST-R, have been revised, restandardized, and renamed the *Denver II.* Before administering the Denver II, the examiner should be trained by, and receive a certificate from, a master instructor who has been trained by the Denver faculty.* The Denver II differs from the DDST in items, test form, interpretation, and referral (see Appendix D). The previous total of 105 items has been increased to 125, including an increase from 21 DDST to 39 Denver II language items. Previous items that were difficult to administer and/or interpret have been either modified or eliminated. Many items that were previously tested by parental report now require observation by the examiner.

Each item was evaluated to determine if significant differences exist on the basis of sex, ethnic group, maternal education, and place of residence. Items for which clinically significant differences exist were replaced or, if retained, are discussed in the Technical Manual. When evaluating children delayed on one of these items, the examiner can look up norms for the subpopulations to consider if the delay may be caused by sociocultural or environmental differences.

The items on the test form are arranged in the same format as the DDST-R The norms for the distribution bars were updated with the new standardization data but retain the 25th, 50th, 75th, and 90th percentile divisions. The test form contains a place to rate the child's behavioral characteristics (e.g., compliance, interest in surroundings, fearfulness, and attention span).

To determine relative areas of advancement and areas of delay, sufficient items should be administered to establish the basal and ceiling levels in each sector. By scoring appropriate items as "pass," "fail," "refusal," or "no opportunity," and relating such scores to the age of the child, each item can be interpreted as described in the accompanying box. To identify cautions, all items intersected by the age line are administered. To screen solely for developmental delays, only the items located totally to the left of the child's age line are administered. Criteria for referral are based on the availability of resources in the community (Box 35-6).

Research on the Denver II's validity and accuracy is in its beginning stages. One study found that most children with even subtle developmental problems were identified. However, almost half of the children without developmental problems received suspect scores, resulting in a high rate of overreferrals (Glascoe et al, 1992). To minimize overreferrals, a decision for referral depends not only on the results of the Denver II, but also on the practitioner's clinical judgment after considering the child's developmental history; general health status; social, cultural, and emotional environment; and the availability of local resources for diagnosis and treatment (Frankenburg, 1994a).

Although it is not the purpose of this discussion to detail the instruction manual, some points concerning preparation, administration, and interpretation of the Denver II are important to stress. Before beginning the screen, ask if the child was born prematurely and correctly calculate the adjusted age. Up to 24 months of age, allowances are made for infants born prematurely by subtracting the number of weeks of missed gestation from their present age and testing them at the adjusted age. For example, a 16-week-old infant who was born 4 weeks early is tested at a 12-week adjusted age level. Explain to the parents and child, if appropriate, that the screenings are not intelligence tests but a method of showing what the child can do at a particular age. Emphasize that the child is not expected to perform each item on the test.

Tell the parent before the screening begins that the results of the child's performance will be explained after all of the items have been concluded. It is the nurse's responsibility to properly inform parents of any testing or screening procedure before its administration so that they are fully aware of its purpose and intent.

Prepare toddlers and preschoolers for the procedure by presenting it as a game. The Denver I1 is an excellent way to begin a health appraisal because it is nonthreatening, requires no painful or unfamiliar procedures, and capitalizes on the child's natural activity of play. Because children are easily distracted, perform each item quickly and present only one toy from the kit at a time. After that toy's purpose is concluded, such as building a tower of blocks or identifying its color, replace the toy in the bag and take out another one. Other temporary factors that may interfere with the child's performance include fatigue, illness, fear, hospitalization, separation from the parent, or general unwillingness to perform the activities. In addition, undiagnosed mental retardation, hearing loss, vision loss, neurologic impairment, or a familial pattern of slow development greatly influences the child's performance.

Box 35-6

Denver II Scoring

INTERPRETATION OF DENVER II SCORES

Advanced—Passed an item completely to the *right* of the age line (passed by fewer than 25% of children at an age older than the child)

OK—Passed, failed, or refused an item intersected by the age line between the 25th and 75th percentiles

Caution—Failed or refused items intersected by the age line on or between the 75th and 90th percentiles

Delay—Failed an item completely to the *left* of the age line; refusals to the left of the age line may also be considered delays, since the reason for the refusal may be inability to perform the task

INTERPRETATION OF TEST

Normal—No delays and a maximum of one caution

Suspect—One or more delays and/or two or more cautions

Untestable—Refusals on one or more items completely to the left of the age line or on more than one item intersected by the age line in the 75th to 90th percentile.

RECOMMENDATIONS FOR REFERRAL FOR SUSPECT AND UNTESTABLE TESTS

Rescreen in 1 to 2 weeks to rule out temporary factors.

If rescreen is suspect or untestable, use clinical judgment based on the following: number of cautions and delays; which items are cautions and delays; rate of past development; clinical examination and history; availability of referral resources.

*Forms and complete instructions are available from Denver Developmental Materials, Inc., P.O. Box 6919, Denver, CO 80206-9019; phone (303) 355-4729 or 1-800-419-4729. The DDST and DDST-R are no longer available because they have been replaced by the Denver II.

Following completion of the Denver II, ask the parent if the child's performance was typical of behavior at other times. If the parent replies affirmatively and the child's cooperation was satisfactory, explain the results, emphasizing all successful items first, then those items failed but that the child was not expected to pass, and finally those items that were delays. If the parent replies that the child's performance was not typical of usual behavior, it is best to defer any scoring or discussion of results, especially if the refusals yield a suspect score. In this situation, reschedule testing for a time when the child is more likely to cooperate.

In explaining a normal score, focus on how well the child performed and reinforce the parents' efforts in satisfactorily stimulating their child. In addition to assessing the child's present developmental level, the Denver II can be used to guide parents toward those activities that are appropriate, although not necessarily expected, for the child's age. By testing for items to the right of the age line (ones the child is not expected to perform), children with advanced development, who may be gifted, can be identified.

In explaining delays, carefully note the parent's response, especially casual acceptance such as "He'll catch up" or questions such as "Does this mean my child is retarded?" Be aware of personal anxieties during these situations and refrain from giving reassurances such as "I'm sure he will do better next time." Rather, respond honestly to parents' questions, yet with appropriate flexibility and concern, stressing the need for further developmental testing.

Denver II Prescreening Developmental Questionnaire (PDQ-II)

The PDQ-II is a further revision of the PDQ and the R-PDQ. This version uses the norms (90th and 75th percentiles) from the DENVER II. The PDQ-II is a parent-answered prescreen consisting of 91 questions from the DENVER II, although only a subset of questions are asked for each age group. The form may be read to parents and caregivers who are less educated.

Four different forms are available and are selected based on age: orange (0 to 9 months), purple (9 to 24 months), cream (2 to 4 years), and white (4 to 6 years). The caregiver answers questions until (1) three "NOs" are circled (they do not have to be consecutive) or (2) all the questions on both sides of the form have been answered. Scoring is based on the number of delays or cautions (Box 35-6). Children who have no delays or cautions are considered to be developing normally. If a child has one delay or two cautions, the caregiver is provided with age-appropriate developmental activities to pursue with the child, and a rescreen with the PDQ-II is done 1 month later. If on rescreening the child has one or more delays, the DENVER II is administered as soon as possible. If a child has two or more delays or three or more cautions on the first screening with the PDQ-II, the DENVER II is administered as soon as possible (Bresnick, 2000).

Developmental Screening and Interpretation

Although screening tests are an effective method of applying the knowledge of children's expected rate of development to a large segment of the population, they are only as successful as the individual's expertise in administering them. Because many of the screening tests are devised to be used by paraprofessionals, there are inherent risks in screening if such individuals are not properly trained or supervised. For example, false-positive findings can label the child as developmentally delayed and cause problems that otherwise might not have existed. False-negative findings can prevent children with problems from receiving the help they need.

Nurses administering developmental screening or supervising paraprofessionals' testing need to assess the child's "whole picture" and not rely solely on any screening procedure. Development, like growth and health, is a dynamic process. Tests such as the Denver II should be used as part of *developmental surveillance,* a continuous comprehensive primary health care approach that includes the parents as partners with professionals (Frankenburg, 1994b). Evaluation of the child's total well-being is the result of evaluating data from a comprehensive health and family history, physical examination, and developmental screening.

Key Points

- The most common approach to examining children follows a head-to-toe sequence.
- Growth measurements during the physical examination focus on length, height, weight, skinfold thickness, and arm and head circumference. Assessment of growth is measured against standard growth charts to determine a child's status in comparison with other children of the same age.
- Measurements of temperature, pulse, respiration, and blood pressure constitute the physiologic approach to assessment.
- The general appearance of a child is a cumulative, subjective impression of physical appearance, state of nutrition, behavior, personality, interactions with parents and nurse, posture, development, and speech.
- Assessment of the skin, which primarily involves inspection and palpation, focuses on color, texture, temperature, moisture, and turgor. The nurse needs to be aware of both physiologic and ethnic factors that may affect these areas.
- In assessment of the lymph nodes, the nurse examines, by palpation, the part of the body in which the glands are located.
- The head is inspected for shape, symmetry, mobility, and head control.
- Examination of the eyes includes placement and alignment, inspection of external and internal structures, and vision testing.
- The ears are examined for placement and alignment, inspection of external and internal structures, and auditory testing.
- The lungs are examined by methods of inspection, palpation, percussion, and auscultation.
- Auscultation is the most important procedure for examining the heart.
- Abdominal assessment follows an orderly sequence of inspection, auscultation, and palpation, since palpation may distort normal abdominal sounds.
- Examination of the genitalia may provoke anxiety in the child, and the nurse must avoid any transference of anxiety.

- Neurologic assessment addresses behavior; motor, sensory, and cerebellar functioning; reflexes; and cranial nerves.
- The Denver II, a major revision and a restandardization of the DDST, differs from the DDST in items included in the test, the test form, and the interpretation of scoring.

References

American Academy of Pediatrics, Committee on Practice and Ambulatory Medicine, Section on Ophthalmology: Eye examination and vision screening in infants, children, and young adults (RE9625), *Pediatrics* 98(1):153-157, 1996.

Amoore JN: A comparative evaluation of the DINAMAP 8100 and DINAMAP Compact TS using a non-invasive blood pressure simulator, *Blood Press Monit* 3(5):309-314, 1998.

Anagnostakis D et al: Rectal-axillary temperature difference in febrile and afebrile infants and children, *Clin Pediatr* 32(5):268-272, 1993.

Birch J, Platts CE: Colour vision screening in children: an evaluation of three pseudoisochromatic tests, *Ophthalmic Physiol Opt* 13(4):344-349, 1993.

Bliss-Holtz J: Methods of newborn infant temperature monitoring: a research review, *Issues Compr Pediatr Nurs* 18(4): 287-298, 1995.

Bresnick B: *Personal communication,* February, 2000.

Childs C, Harrison R, Hodkinson C: Tympanic membrane temperature as a measure of core temperature, *Arch Dis Child* 80(3):262-266, 1999.

Coats DK, Jenkins RH: Vision assessment of the pediatric patient: refinements, *Am Acad Ophthalmol* 1(1):1-12, 1997.

Erickson RS, Meyer LT, Woo TM: Accuracy of chemical dot thermometers in critically ill adults and children, *Image J Nurs Sch* 28(1):23-28, 1996.

Frankenburg WK: Preventing developmental delays: is developmental screening sufficient? I. Developmental screening and the Denver II, *Pediatrics* 93(4):586-589, 1994a.

Frankenburg WK: Preventing developmental delays: is developmental screening sufficient? II. Partners in health care, *Pediatrics* 93(4):589-593, 1994b.

Gillman MW, Cook NR: Blood pressure measurement in childhood epidemiological studies, *Circulation* 92(4):1049-1057, 1995.

Glascoe FP et al: Accuracy of the Denver-II in developmental screening, *Pediatrics* 89:1221-1225, 1992.

Haddock B, Merrow DL, Swanson MS: The falling grace of axillary temperatures, *Pediatr Nurs* 22(2):121-125, 1996.

Henker R, Coyne C: Comparison of peripheral temperature measurements with core temperature, *AACN Clin Issues* 6(1):21-30, 1995.

Hockenberry-Eaton M, Kline NE: Nursing support of the child with cancer. In Pizzo, PA, Poplack DP, editors: *Principles and practices of pediatric oncology,* vol 3, Philadelphia, 1997, JB Lippincott.

Hooker EA, Houston H: Screening for fever in an adult emergency department: oral vs tympanic thermometry, *South Med J* 89(2):230-234, 1996.

Houlder LC: The accuracy and reliability of tympanic thermometry compared to rectal and axillary sites in young children, *Pediatr Nurs* 26(3):311-314, 2000.

Jensen BN et al: The superiority of rectal thermometry to oral thermometry with regard to accuracy, *J Adv Nurs* 20:660-665, 1994.

Kuczmarski RJ et al: CDC growth charts: United States. Advance data from vital and health statistics; no. 314, Hyattsville, MD: National Center for Health Statistics, June 8, 2000; may be accessed at: www.cdc.gov/nchs/about/major/nhanes/growthcharts/fullreport.htm

Lanham DM et al: Accuracy of tympanic temperature readings in children under 6 years of age, *Pediatr Nurs* 25(1):39-42, 1999.

Ling J et al: Clinical evaluation of the oscillometric blood pressure monitor in adults and children based on the 1992 AAMI SP-10 standards, *J Clin Monit* 11(2):123-130, 1995.

Medical Indicators, Inc: NexTemp™ single-use clinical thermometers: the quick, accurate, "no-hassle" way to take a temp, *NCF1,* Jan 1999.

Modell JG et al: Unreliability of the infrared tympanic thermometer in clinical practice: a comparative study with oral mercury and oral electronic thermometers, *South Med J* 191(7):649-654, 1998.

National Institutes of Health, National Heart, Lung, and Blood Institute: *Update on the Task Force Report (1987) on high blood pressure in children and adolescents: a working group report from the National High Blood Pressure Education Program,* NIH Pub. No. 96-3790, Sept 1996.

Park M, Lee D, Johnson CA: Oscillometric blood pressures in the arm, thigh and calf in healthy children and those with aortic coarctation, *Pediatrics* 92(4):761-765, 1993.

Payne D et al: Chemical and glass thermometers for axillary temperatures: how do they compare? *Arch Dis Child* 71(3): 259-260, 1994.

Pompei F, Pompei M: *Physicians reference handbook on temperature,* Watertown, MA, 1996, Exergen.

Pontious S et al: Accuracy and reliability of temperature measurement by instrument and site, *J Pediatr Nurs* 9(2):114-123, 1994a.

Pontious S et al: Accuracy and reliability of temperature measurement in the emergency department by instrument and site in children, *Pediatr Nurs* 20(1):58-63, 1994b.

Prazer GE: The aural infrared thermometer: a practitioner's perspective, *J Pediatr* 133:471-472, 1998.

Py Ma H Corporation: *Tempa Dot single use thermometer: technical information,* Flemington, NJ, 1994, The Corporation.

Rivera AY et al: Evaluation of a liquid crystal contact thermometer in children with fever, *J Invest Med* 45(1), 1997.

Robinson JL et al: Comparison of esophageal, rectal, axillary, bladder, tympanic, and pulmonary artery temperatures in children, *J Pediatr* 133:553-556, 1998.

Seidel HM, Rosenstein BJ, Pathak A: *Primary care of the newborn,* ed 2, St Louis, 1997, Mosby.

Shann F, Mackenzie A: Comparison of rectal, axillary and forehead temperatures, *Arch Pediatr Adolesc Med* 150:74-78, 1996.

Valadez JJ, Elmore-Meegan M, Morley D: Comparing liquid crystal thermometer readings and mercury thermometer readings of infants and children in a traditional African setting, *Trop Geogr Med* 47(3):130-133, 1995.

Vessey JA: Developmental approaches to examining young children, *Pediatr Nurs* 21(1):53-56, 1995.

Wattigney WA et al: Utility of an automatic instrument for blood pressure measurement in children: the Bogalusa Heart Study, *Am J Hypertens* 9(3):256-262, 1996.

Wilshaw R et al: A comparison of the use of tympanic, axillary, and rectal thermometers in infants, *J Pediatr Nurs* 14(2): 88-93, 1999.

CHAPTER
36 The Infant and Family

http://www.harcourthealth.com/MERLIN/Wong/maternal/

Learning Objectives

On completion of this chapter the reader will be able to:

- Identify the major biologic, psychosocial, cognitive, and social developments during the first year of life.
- Relate parent-child attachment, separation anxiety, and stranger fear to developmental achievements during infancy.
- Provide anticipatory guidance to parents regarding common parental concerns during infancy.
- Provide parents with feeding recommendations for infants.
- Outline immunization requirements during infancy.
- List general contraindications, precautions, and administration routes for immunizations.
- Provide anticipatory guidance to parents regarding injury prevention based on the infant's developmental achievements.
- List measures that can be used to alleviate colic.
- Plan nursing care that meets the physical and emotional needs of the nonorganic failure-to-thrive child and parent.
- Provide nursing care that meets the immediate and long-term needs of the family who lost a child from sudden infant death syndrome.
- Identify the stresses and needs of the family whose child is home monitored for apnea.
- Identify characteristics of children with autism.

PROMOTING OPTIMUM GROWTH AND DEVELOPMENT

Biologic Development

At no other time in life are physical changes and developmental achievements so dramatic as during infancy. All major body systems undergo progressive maturation, and there is concurrent development of skills that increasingly allows infants to respond to and cope with the environment. Acquisition of these fine and gross motor skills occurs in an orderly head-to-toe and center-to-periphery (cephalocaudal and proximodistal) sequence.

Proportional Changes. During the first year growth is very rapid, especially during the initial 6 months. Infants gain 150 to 210 g (5 to 7 ounces) weekly until approximately age 5 to 6 months, when the birth weight has at least doubled. An average weight for a 6-month-old child is 7.26 kg (16 pounds). Weight gain slows during the second 6 months. By 1 year of age the infant's birth weight has tripled, for an average weight of 9.75 kg (21.5 pounds). Infants who are breastfed beyond 4 to 6 months of age typically gain less weight than those who are bottle-fed (American Academy of Pediatrics, 1998b; Dewey et al, 1993). Because breastfed infants grow at a different rate than those who are bottle-fed, growth charts that reflect both patterns of infant weight gain are needed.

Height increases by 2.5 cm (1 inch) a month during the first 6 months and also slows during the second 6 months. Increases in length occur in sudden spurts, rather than in a slow, gradual pattern. Average height is 65 cm (25½ inches) at 6 months and 74 cm (29 inches) at 12 months. By 1 year the birth length has increased by almost 50%. This increase occurs mainly in the trunk, rather than in the legs, and contributes to the characteristic physique of the infant.*

Head growth is also rapid. During the first 6 months head circumference increases approximately 1.5 cm (6/10 inch) a month but decreases to only 0.5 cm (2/10 inch) monthly during the second 6 months. The average size is 43 cm (17 inches) at 6 months and 46 cm (18 inches) at 12 months. By 1 year, head size has increased by almost 33%. Closure of the cranial sutures occurs, with the posterior fontanel fusing by 6 to 8 weeks of age

*For additional information, please view "Growth and Development" in ***Whaley and Wong's Pediatric Nursing Video Series,*** St Louis, 1996, Mosby: 1-800-426-4545; access the website at: www.mosby.com.

and the anterior fontanel closing by 12 to 18 months of age (the average age being 14 months).

Expanding head size reflects the growth and differentiation of the *nervous system.* By the end of the first year the brain has increased in weight about 2½ times. Maturation of the brain is exhibited in the dramatic developmental achievements of infancy (see Table 36-2). Primitive reflexes are replaced by voluntary, purposeful movement, and new reflexes that influence motor development appear.

The *chest* assumes a more adult contour, with the lateral diameter becoming larger than the anteroposterior diameter. The chest circumference approximately equals the head circumference by the end of the first year. The heart grows less rapidly than does the rest of the body. Its weight is usually doubled by 1 year of age; in comparison, body weight triples during the same period. The size of the heart is still large in relation to the chest cavity; its width is approximately 55% of the chest width.

Maturation of Systems. Other organ systems also change and grow during infancy. The *respiratory* rate slows somewhat (see Appendix J) and is relatively stable. Respiratory movements continue to be abdominal. Several factors predispose the infant to more severe and acute respiratory problems. The close proximity of the trachea to the bronchi and its branching structures rapidly transmits infectious agents from one anatomic location to another. The short, straight eustachian tube closely communicates with the ear, allowing infection to ascend from the pharynx to the middle ear. In addition, the inability of the immune system to produce *immunoglobulin A (IgA)* in the mucosal lining provides less protection against infection in infancy than during later childhood.

The *heart rate* slows (see Appendix J), and the rhythm is often *sinus arrhythmia* (i.e., rate increases with inspiration and decreases with expiration). Blood pressure also changes during infancy (see Appendix J). Systolic pressure rises during the first 2 months as a result of the increasing ability of the left ventricle to pump blood into the systemic circulation. Diastolic pressure decreases during the first 3 months, then gradually rises to values close to those at birth. Fluctuations in blood pressure occur during varying states of activity and emotion.

Significant *hemopoietic changes* occur during the first year (see Appendix F). Fetal hemoglobin (HgbF) is present for the first 5 months, with adult hemoglobin steadily increasing through the first half of infancy. Fetal hemoglobin results in a shortened survival of red blood cells (RBCs) and thus a decreased number of RBCs. A common result at 2 to 3 months of age is *physiologic anemia.* High levels of HgbF are thought to depress the production of erythropoietin, a hormone released by the kidney that stimulates RBC production.

Maternal iron stores are present for the first 5 to 6 months and gradually diminish, which also accounts for lowered hemoglobin levels toward the end of the first 6 months. The occurrence of physiologic anemia is not affected by an adequate supply of iron. However, when erythropoiesis is stimulated, iron supplies are necessary for the formation of hemoglobin.

The *digestive processes* are immature at birth. Saliva is secreted in small amounts, but the majority of the digestive processes do not begin functioning until age 3 months, when drooling is common because of the poorly coordinated swallowing reflex. The enzyme *ptyalin* (also called *amylase*) is present in small amounts but usually has little effect on the foodstuffs because of the small amount of time the food stays in the mouth. Gastric digestion in the stomach consists primarily of the action of hydrochloric acid and rennin, an enzyme that acts specifically on the casein in milk to cause the formation of curds (i.e., coagulated semisolid particles of milk). The curds cause the milk to be retained in the stomach long enough for digestion to occur.

Digestion also takes place in the duodenum, where pancreatic enzymes and bile begin to break down protein and fat. Secretion of the pancreatic enzyme *amylase,* which is needed for digestion of complex carbohydrates, is deficient until about the fourth to sixth month of life. *Lipase* is also limited, and infants do not achieve adult levels of fat absorption until 4 to 5 months of age. *Trypsin* is secreted in sufficient quantities to catabolize protein into polypeptides and some amino acids.

The immaturity of the digestive processes is evident in the appearance of stools. During infancy, solid foods (e.g., peas, carrots, corn, and raisins) are passed incompletely broken down in the feces. An excess quantity of fiber easily disposes the child to loose, bulky stools.

During infancy the stomach enlarges to accommodate a greater volume of food. By the end of the first year the infant is able to tolerate three meals a day and an evening bottle and may have one or two bowel movements daily. With any type of gastric irritation, however, the infant is vulnerable to diarrhea, vomiting, and dehydration (see Chapter 47).

The *liver* is the most immature of all the gastrointestinal organs throughout infancy. The ability to conjugate bilirubin and secrete bile is achieved after the first couple of weeks of life. However, the capacities for gluconeogenesis, formation of plasma protein and ketones, storage of vitamins, and deaminization of amino acids remain relatively immature for the first year of life.

Maturation of the suckling, sucking, and swallowing reflexes and the eruption of teeth (see Teething, p. 845) parallel the changes in the gastrointestinal tract and prepare the infant for the introduction of solid foods.

The *immunologic system* undergoes numerous changes during the first year. The full-term newborn receives significant amounts of maternal IgG, which for approximately 3 months confers immunity against antigens to which the mother was exposed. During this time the infant begins to synthesize IgG; approximately 40% of adult levels are reached by 1 year of age. Significant amounts of IgM are produced at birth, and adult levels are reached by 9 months of age. The production of IgA, IgD, and IgE is much more gradual, and maximum levels are not attained until early childhood.

During infancy, *thermoregulation* becomes more efficient; the ability of the skin to contract and of muscles to shiver in response to cold increases. The peripheral capillaries respond to changes in ambient temperature to regulate heat loss. The capillaries constrict in response to cold, conserving core body temperature and decreasing potential evaporative heat loss from the skin surface. The capillaries dilate in response to heat, decreasing internal body temperature through evaporation, conduction, and convection. Shivering *(thermogenesis)* causes the muscles and muscle fibers to contract, generating metabolic heat that is distributed throughout the body. Increased adipose tissue during the first 6 months insulates the body against heat loss.

A shift in the *total body fluid* occurs. At birth 75% of the infant's body weight is water, and there is an excess of extracellular fluid (ECF). As the percentage of body water decreases, so does the amount of ECF—from 40% at term to 20% in adulthood. The high proportion of ECF, which is composed of blood plasma, interstitial fluid, and lymph, predisposes the infant to a more rapid loss of total body fluid and, consequently, dehydration.

The immaturity of the *renal structures* also predisposes the infant to dehydration. Complete maturity of the kidney occurs during the latter half of the second year, when the cuboidal epithelium of the glomeruli becomes flattened. Before this time the filtration capacity of the glomeruli is reduced. Urine is voided frequently and has a low specific gravity (i.e., 1.000 to 1.010).

Auditory acuity is at adult levels during infancy. Visual acuity begins to improve, and binocular fixation is established. *Binocularity,* or the fixation of two ocular images into one cerebral picture *(fusion),* begins to develop by 6 weeks of age and should be well established by age 4 months. *Depth perception (stereopsis)* begins to develop by age 7 to 9 months but may exist earlier as an innate safety mechanism against accidental falling.

Fine Motor Development. Fine motor behavior includes the use of the hands and fingers in the prehension (grasp) of an object. Grasping occurs during the first 2 to 3 months as a reflex and gradually becomes voluntary. At 1 month of age the hands are predominantly closed, and by 3 months they are mostly open. By this time infants demonstrate a desire to grasp an object, but they "grasp" it more with the eyes than with the hands. If a rattle is placed in the hand, the infant will actively hold onto it. By 4 months of age the infant regards both a small pellet and the hands and then looks from the object to the hands and back again. By 5 months the infant is able to voluntarily grasp an object.

Gradually the palmar grasp (using the whole hand) is replaced with a pincer grasp (using the thumb and index finger). By 8 to 9 months of age the infant uses a crude pincer grasp and by 11 months has progressed to a neat pincer grasp (Fig. 36-1).

By 6 months of age infants have increased manipulative skill: they hold their bottle, grasp their feet and pull them to their mouth, and feed themselves a cracker. By 7 months they transfer objects from one hand to the other, use one hand for grasping, and hold a cube in each hand simultaneously. They enjoy banging objects and will explore the moveable parts of a toy.

By 10 months of age the pincer grasp is sufficiently established to enable infants to pick up a raisin and other finger foods. They can deliberately let go of an object and will offer it

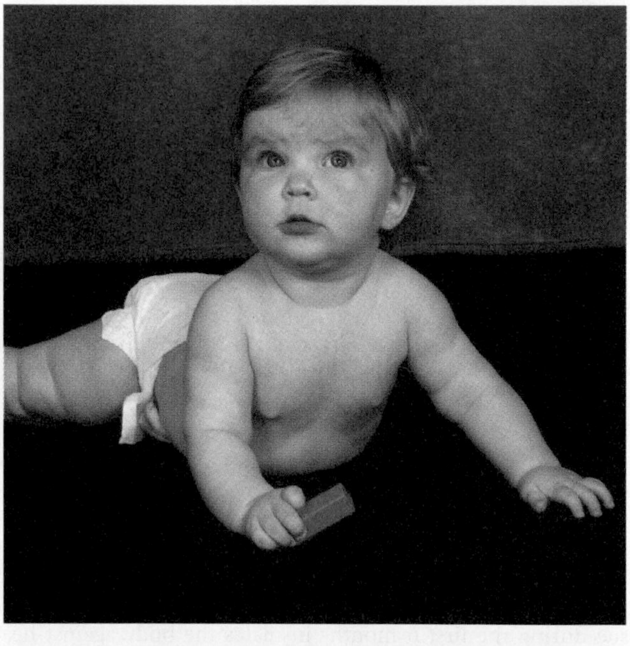

FIG. 36-1 • Crude pincer grasp at 8 to 10 months. (Photo by Paul Vincent Kuntz, Texas Children's Hospital.)

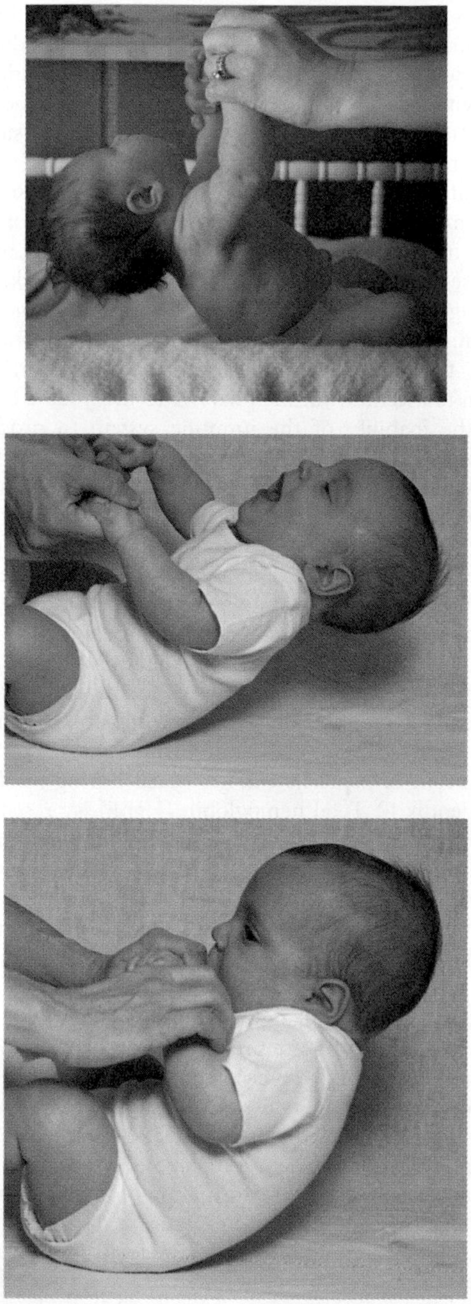

A

B

C

FIG. 36-2 • Head control while pulled to sitting position. **A,** Complete head lag at 1 month. **B,** Partial head lag at 2 months. **C,** Almost no head lag at 4 months.

to someone. By 11 months they put objects into a container and like to remove them. By age 1 year, infants try to build a tower of two blocks but fail.

Gross Motor Development

Head Control. The full-term newborn can momentarily hold the head in midline and parallel when the body is suspended ventrally and can lift and turn the head from side to side when prone. This is not the case when the infant is lying prone on a pillow or soft surface; infants do not have the head control to lift their head out of the depression of the object and therefore risk suffocation. Marked head lag is evident when the infant is pulled from a lying to a sitting position. By 3 months of age infants can hold their head well beyond the plane of the body. By 4 months of age infants can lift the head and front portion of the chest approximately 90 degrees above the table, bearing their weight on the forearms. Only slight head lag is evident when the infant is pulled from a lying to a sitting position, and by 4 to 6 months head control is well established (Figs. 36-2 and 36-3).

NURSE ALERT • Any child who displays head lag at 6 months of age should have a developmental/neurologic evaluation.

Rolling Over. Newborns may roll over accidentally because of their rounded back. The ability to willfully turn from the abdomen to the back occurs at 5 months, and the ability to turn from the back to the abdomen occurs at 6 months. Infants put to sleep on their sides may easily roll over to a prone (face-down) position, thus placing them at higher risk for SIDS (Willinger et al, 1998). It is therefore important to place infants in a supine position for sleep. While the infant is awake, a prone position is acceptable to enhance achievement of milestones such as head control, crawling, creeping, and turning over. It is noteworthy that the parachute reflex (Fig. 36-4), which elicits a protective response to falling, appears at 7 months.

A

B

C

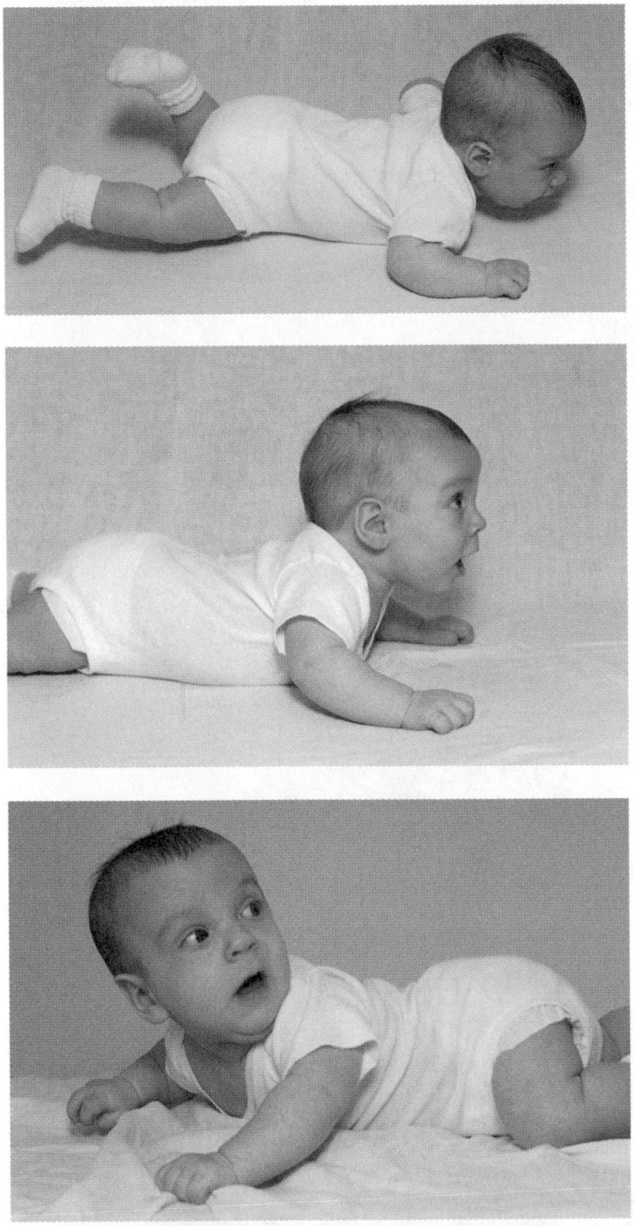

FIG. 36-3 • Head control while prone. **A,** Infant momentarily lifts head at 1 month. **B,** Infant lifts head and chest 90 degrees and bears weight on forearms at 4 months. **C,** Infant lifts head, chest, and upper abdomen and can bear weight on hands at 6 months. Note how this position facilitates turning from abdomen to back.

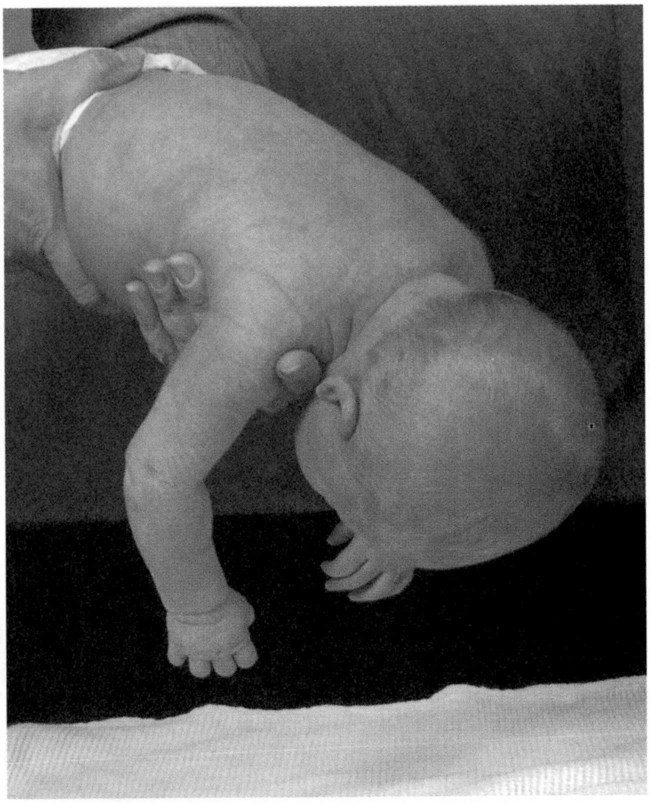

FIG. 36-4 • Parachute reflex. (Photo by Paul Vincent Kuntz, Texas Children's Hospital.)

Sitting. The ability to sit follows progressive head control and straightening of the back (Fig. 36-5). For the first 2 to 3 months the back is uniformly rounded. The convex cervical curve forms at approximately 3 to 4 months of age, when head control is established. The convex lumbar curve appears when the child begins to sit, at about age 4 months. As the spinal column straightens, the infant can be propped in a sitting position. By age 7 months infants can sit alone, leaning forward on their hands for support. By age 8 months they can sit well while unsupported and begin to explore their surroundings in this position rather than in a lying position. By 10 months they can maneuver from a prone to a sitting position.

Locomotion. Locomotion involves acquiring the ability to bear weight, propel forward on all four extremities, stand upright with support and, finally, walk alone (Fig. 36-6). Following a cephalocaudal pattern, infants 4 to 6 months old have increasing coordination in their arms. Initial locomotion results in infants propelling themselves backward by pushing with the

A B C D

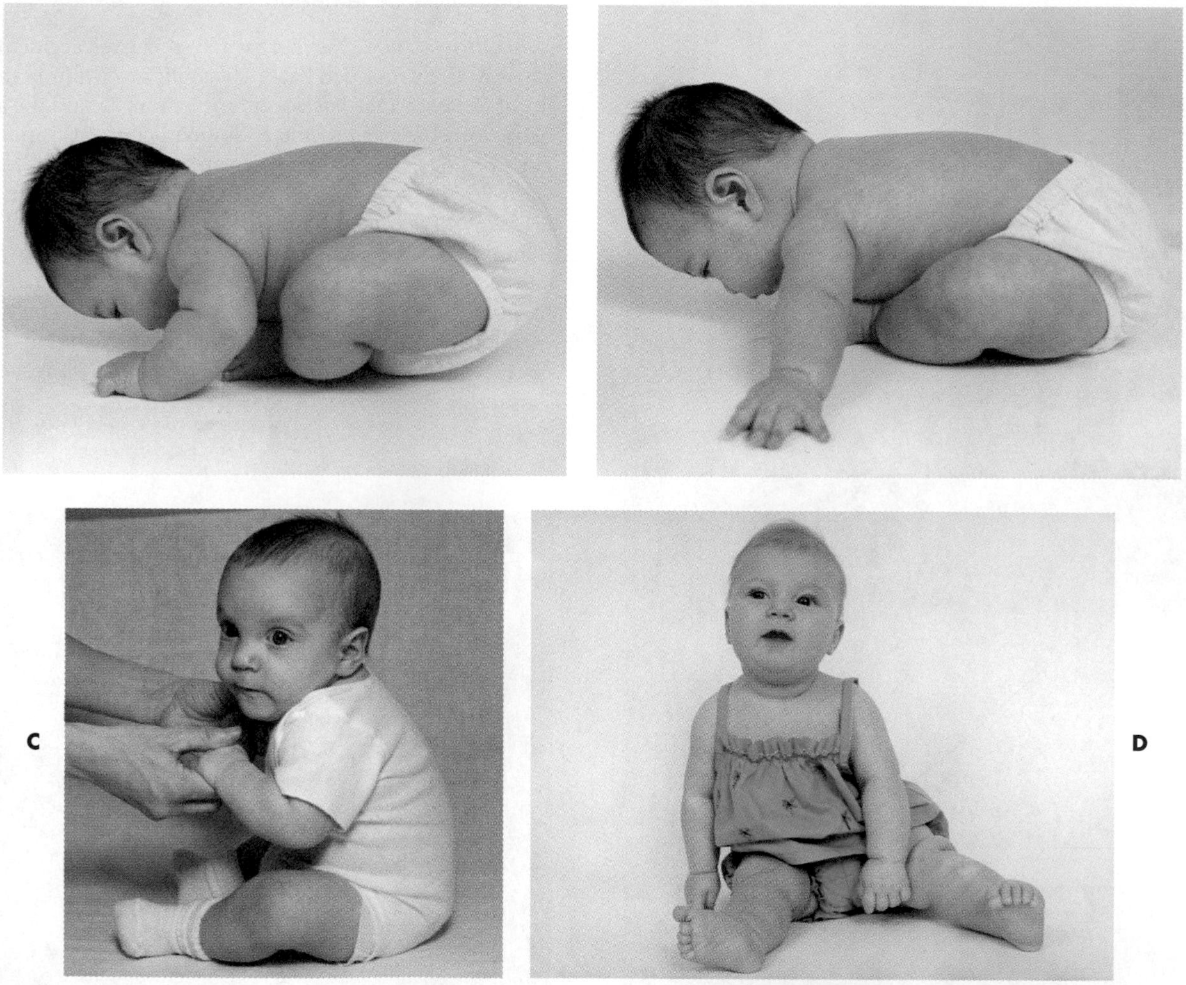

E

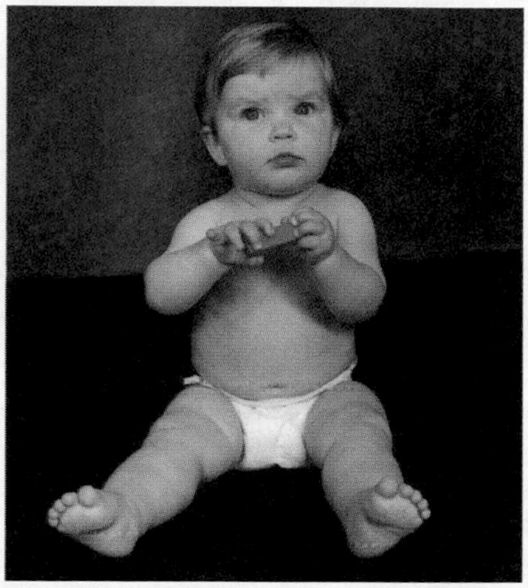

FIG. 36-5 • Development of sitting. **A,** Back is completely rounded, and infant has no ability to sit upright at 1 month. **B,** At 2 months, exhibits more control; back is still rounded, but infant can sit up momentarily with some head control. **C,** Back is rounded only in lumbar area, and infant is able to sit erect with good head control at 4 months. **D,** Infant can sit alone, leaning on hands for support, at 7 months. **E,** Infant sits without support at 8 months. Note the transferring of objects that occurs beginning at 7 months. (Photos by Paul Vincent Kuntz, Texas Children's Hospital.)

arms. By 6 to 7 months of age they are able to bear all their weight on their legs with assistance. *Crawling* (propelling forward with belly on floor) progresses to *creeping* (on hands and knees with belly off floor) by 9 months. At this time they stand while holding onto furniture and can pull themselves to the standing position, but they are unable to maneuver back down except by falling. By 11 months they walk while holding onto furniture or with both hands held, and by age 1 year they may be able to walk with one hand held. A number of infants attempt their first independent steps by their first birthday.

Psychosocial Development

Developing a Sense of Trust (Erikson). Erikson's phase I (birth to 1 year) is concerned with *acquiring a sense of trust* while *overcoming a sense of mistrust.* The trust that develops is a trust of self, of others, and of the world. Infants "trust" that their feeding, comfort, stimulation, and caring needs will be met. The crucial element for the achievement of this task is the quality of both the parent (caregiver)-child relationship and the care the infant receives. The provision of food, warmth, and shelter by itself is inadequate for the development of a strong

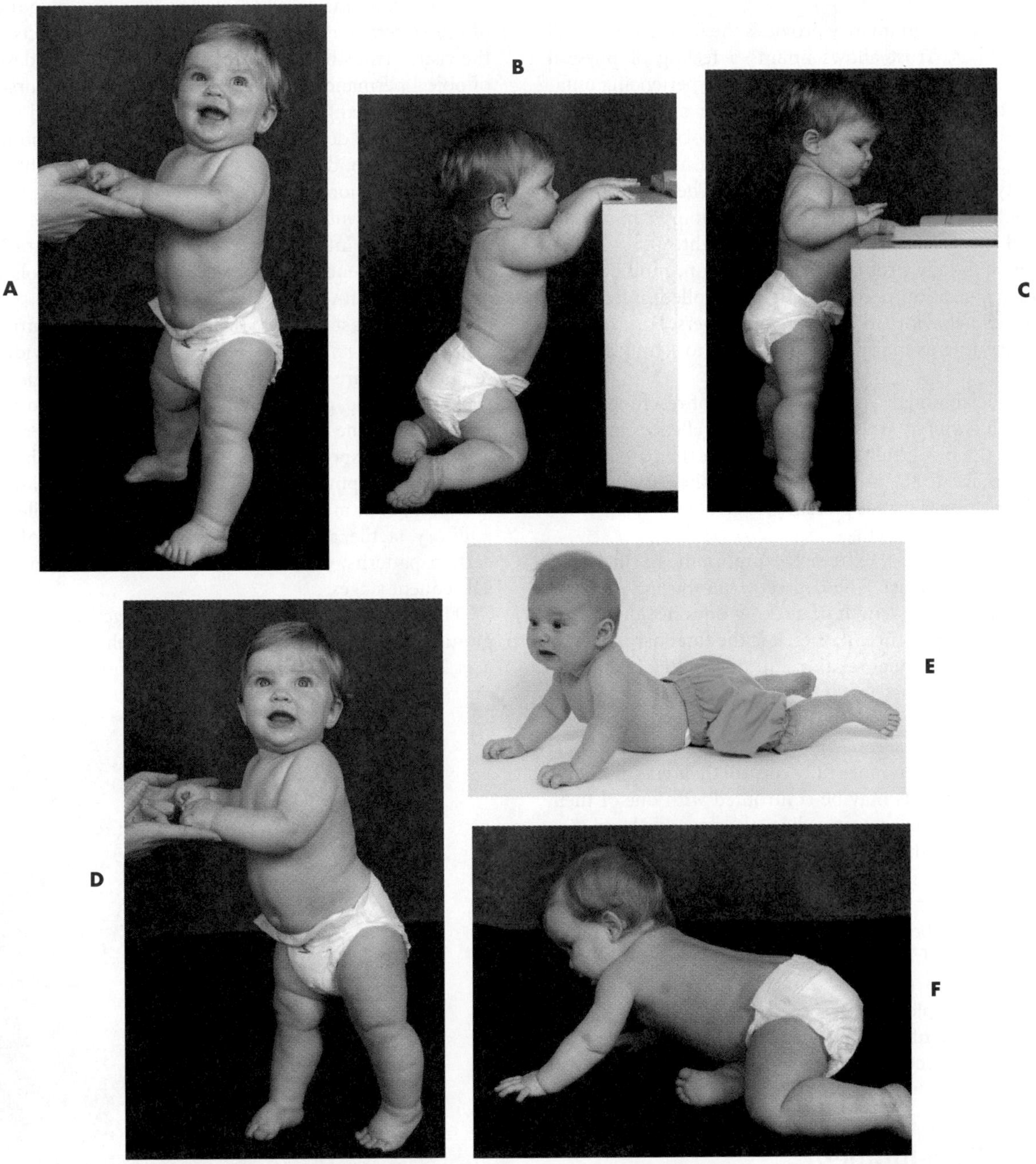

FIG. 36-6 • Development of locomotion. **A,** Infant bears full weight on feet by 7 months. **B,** Infant can maneuver from sitting to kneeling position. **C,** Infant can stand holding onto furniture at 9 months. **D,** While standing, infant takes deliberate step at 10 months. **E,** Infant crawls with abdomen on floor and pulls self forward, and then, **F,** creeps on hands and knees at 9 months. (Photos by Paul Vincent Kuntz, Texas Children's Hospital.)

sense of self. The infant and parent must jointly learn to satisfactorily meet their needs in order for mutual regulation of frustration to occur. When this synchrony fails to develop, mistrust is the eventual outcome.

Failure to learn "delayed gratification" leads to mistrust. Mistrust can result either from too much or too little frustration. If parents always meet their children's needs before the children signal their readiness, infants will never learn to test their ability to control the environment. If the delay is prolonged, infants experience constant frustration and eventually mistrust others in their efforts to satisfy them. Therefore consistency of care is essential.

The trust acquired in infancy provides the foundation for all succeeding phases. Trust allows infants a feeling of physical comfort and security, which assists them in experiencing unfamiliar, unknown situations with a minimum of fear. Erikson has divided the first year of life into two oral/social stages. During the first 3 to 4 months, food intake is the most important social activity in which the infant engages. The newborn can tolerate little frustration or delay of gratification. Primary *narcissism* (total concern for oneself) is at its height.

However, as bodily processes such as vision, motor movements, and vocalization become better controlled, infants use more advanced behaviors to interact with others. For example, rather than cry, infants may put their arms up to signify a desire to be held.

The next social modality involves a mode of reaching out to others through *grasping*. Grasping is initially reflexive, but even as a reflex it has a powerful social meaning for the parents. The reciprocal response to the infant's grasping is the parents' holding on and touching. There is pleasurable tactile stimulation for both the child and the parents.

Tactile stimulation is extremely important in the total process of acquiring trust. The degree of mothering skill, the quantity of food, or the length of sucking does not determine the quality of the experience. Rather, it is the total nature of the quality of the interpersonal relationship that influences the infant's formulation of trust.

During the second stage the more active and aggressive modality of *biting* occurs. Infants learn that they can hold onto what is their own and can more fully control their environment. During this stage infants may be confronted with one of their first conflicts. If they are breastfeeding, they quickly learn that biting causes the mother to become upset and withdraw the breast. Yet biting also brings internal relief from teething discomfort and a sense of power or control.

This conflict may be solved in a variety of ways. The mother may wean the infant from the breast and begin bottle-feeding, or the infant may learn to bite substitute "nipples," such as a pacifier, and retain pleasurable breastfeeding. The successful resolution of this conflict strengthens the mother-child relationship because it occurs at a time when infants are recognizing the mother as the most significant person in their life.

Cognitive Development

Sensorimotor Phase (Piaget). The theory most commonly used to explain *cognition,* or the ability to know, is that of Piaget. The period from birth to 24 months is termed the *sensorimotor phase* and is composed of six stages; however, because this discussion is concerned with ages birth to 12 months, only the first four stages are discussed. The last two stages occur during the toddler period of 12 to 24 months and are discussed in Chapter 37.

During the sensorimotor phase infants progress from reflex behaviors to simple repetitive acts to imitative activity. Three crucial events take place during this phase. The first event involves *separation,* in which infants learn to separate themselves from other objects in the environment. They realize that others besides themselves control the environment and that certain readjustments must take place for mutual satisfaction to occur. This coincides with Erikson's concept of the formation of trust.

The second major accomplishment is achieving the concept of *object permanence,* or the realization that objects that leave the visual field still exist. A typical example of the development of object permanence is when infants are able to pursue objects they observe being hidden under a pillow or behind a chair (Fig. 36-7). This skill develops at approximately 9 to 10 months of age, which corresponds to the time of increased locomotion skills.

The last major intellectual achievement of this period is the ability to use *symbols,* or *mental representation.* The use of symbols allows the infant to think of an object or situation without actually experiencing it. The recognition of symbols is the beginning of the understanding of time and space.

Piaget's first stage, from birth to 1 month, is identified by the infant's *use of reflexes.* At birth the infant's individuality and temperament are expressed through the physiologic reflexes of sucking, rooting, grasping, and crying. The repetitious nature of the reflexes is the beginning of associations between an act and a sequential response. When infants cry because they are hungry, a nipple is put in the mouth, and they suck, feel satisfaction, and sleep. They are assimilating this experience while perceiving auditory, tactile, and visual cues. This experience of perceiving certain patterns, or "ordering," provides a foundation for the subsequent stages.

The second stage, *primary circular reactions,* marks the beginning of the replacement of reflexive behavior with voluntary acts. During the period from 1 to 4 months, activities such as

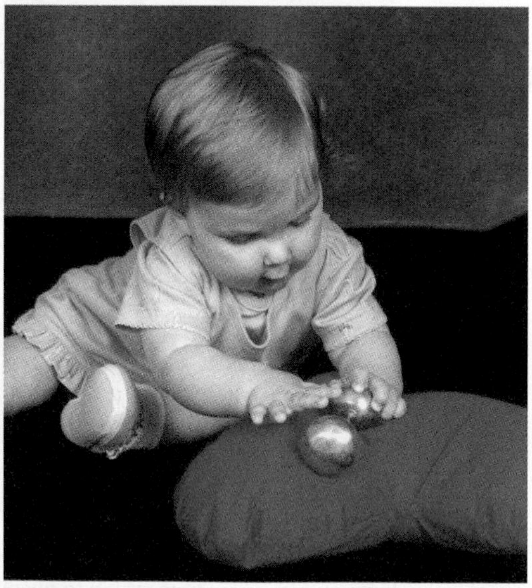

FIG. 36-7 • Nine-month-old infant actively searches for object hidden behind pillow. (Photo by Paul Vincent Kuntz, Texas Children's Hospital.)

sucking or grasping become deliberate acts that elicit certain responses. The beginning of accommodation is evident. Infants incorporate and adapt their reactions to the environment and recognize the stimulus that produced a response. Previously they would cry until the nipple was brought to the mouth. Now they associate the nipple with the sound of the parent's voice. They accommodate this new piece of information and adapt by ceasing to cry when they hear the voice—before receiving the nipple. What is taking place is a realization of causality and a recognition of an orderly sequence of events. The environment is taken in with all of the senses and with whatever motor ability is present.

The *secondary circular reactions* stage is a continuation of primary circular reactions and lasts until 8 months of age. In this stage the primary circular reactions are repeated and prolonged for the response that results. Grasping and holding now become shaking, banging, and pulling. Shaking is performed to hear a noise, not solely for the pleasure of shaking. The quality and quantity of an act become evident. More or less shaking produces different responses. Causality, time, deliberate intention, and separateness from the environment begin to develop.

Three new processes of human behavior occur. *Imitation* requires the differentiation of selected acts from several events. By the second half of the first year, infants can imitate sounds and simple gestures. *Play* becomes evident as they take pleasure in performing an act after they have mastered it. Many of the infant's waking hours are absorbed in sensorimotor play. *Affect* (the outward manifestation of emotion and feeling) is seen as infants begin to develop a sense of permanency. During the first 6 months infants believe that an object exists only for as long as they can visually perceive it. In other words, out of sight—out of mind. Affect to external objects is evident when the object continues to be present or remembered even though it is beyond the range of perception. Object permanence is a critical component of parent-child attachment and is seen in the development of stranger anxiety at 6 to 8 months of age (see p. 834).

During the fourth sensorimotor stage, *coordination of secondary schemas and their application to new situations,* infants use previous behavioral achievements primarily as the foundation for adding new intellectual skills to their expanding repertoire. This stage is largely transitional. Increasing motor skills allow for greater exploration of the environment. They begin to discover that hiding an object does not mean that it is gone but that removing an obstacle will reveal the object. This marks the beginning of intellectual reasoning. Furthermore, they can experience an event by observing it, and they begin to associate symbols with events (e.g., "bye-bye" with "Daddy goes to work"), but the classification is purely their own. In this stage they learn from the object itself; this is in contrast to the second stage, in which infants learn from the type of interaction between objects or individuals. Intentionality is further developed in that infants now actively attempt to remove a barrier to the desired (or undesired) action (see Fig. 36-7). If something is in their way, they attempt to climb over it or push it away. Previously an obstacle would cause them to give up any further attempt to achieve the desired goal.

Development of Body Image

The development of body image parallels sensorimotor development. Infants' kinesthetic and tactile experiences are the first perceptions of their body, and the mouth is the principal area of pleasurable sensations. Other parts of the body are primarily objects of pleasure—the hands and fingers to suck and the feet to play with. As physical needs are met, they feel comfort and satisfaction with their body. Messages conveyed by the caregivers reinforce these feelings. For example, when infants smile, they receive emotional satisfaction from others who smile back.

Achieving the concept of object permanence is basic to the development of self-image. By the end of the first year infants recognize that they are distinct from their parents. At the same time, there is increasing interest in their image, especially in the mirror (Fig. 36-8). As motor skills develop, they learn that parts of the body are useful; for example, the hands bring objects to the mouth, and the legs help them move to different locations. All of these achievements transmit messages to them about themselves. Therefore it is important to transmit positive messages to infants about their bodies.

Social Development

Infants' social development is initially influenced by their reflexive behavior, such as the grasp, and eventually depends primarily on the interaction between them and the principal caregivers. *Attachment* to the parent is increasingly evident during the second half of the first year. In addition, tremendous strides are made in communication and personal-social behavior. Whereas crying and reflexive behavior are methods to meet one's needs in the neonatal period, the social smile is an early step in social communication. This has a profound effect on family members and is a tremendous stimulus for evoking continued responses from others. By 4 months infants laugh aloud.

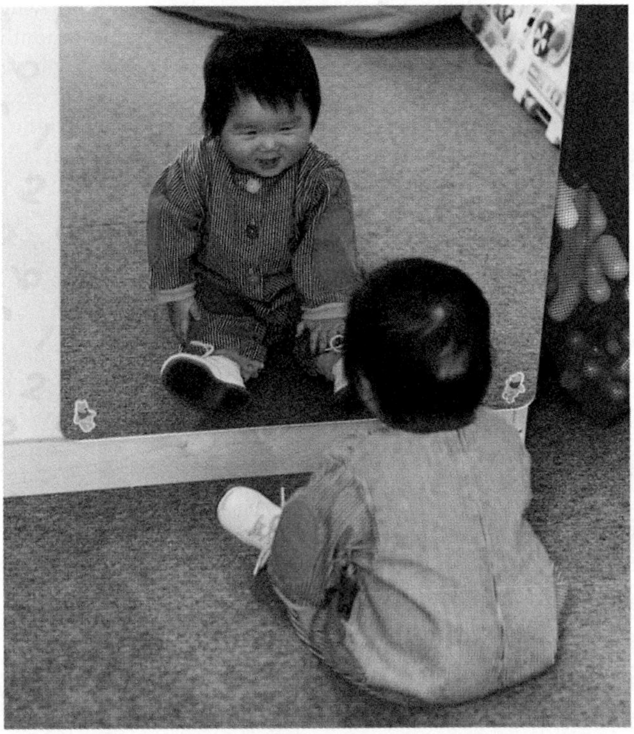

FIG. 36-8 • Nine-month-old infant enjoying own image in mirror.

Play is a major socializing agent and provides stimulation needed to learn from and interact with the environment. By age 6 months infants are very personable. They play games such as peekaboo when their head is hidden in a towel, they signal their desire to be picked up by extending their arms, and they show displeasure when a toy is removed or their face is washed.

Attachment. The importance of human physical contact to infants cannot be overemphasized. Parenting is not an instinctual ability but a learned, acquired process. The attachment of parent and child, which begins before birth and assumes even more importance at birth, continues during the first year. In the following discussion of attachment, the term mother is used in the broad context of the consistent caregiver with whom the child relates more than anyone else. However, in society's changing social climate and sex-role stereotypes, this person may very well be the father or a grandparent. Studies on father-child attachment demonstrate that stages similar to maternal attachment occur (Jones and Heermann, 1992).

Attachment progresses during infancy, with the child assuming an increasingly significant role. Two components of cognitive development are required for attachment: (1) the ability to discriminate the mother from other individuals; and (2) the achievement of object permanence. Both of these processes prepare the infant for an equally important aspect of attachment—separation from the parent. Separation-individuation should occur as a harmonious, parallel process with emotional attachment.

During the formation of attachment to the parent, the infant progresses through four distinct but overlapping stages. For the first few weeks infants respond indiscriminately to anyone. Beginning at approximately 8 to 12 weeks of age, they cry, smile, and vocalize more to the mother than to anyone else but continue to respond to others, whether familiar or not. At approximately 6 months of age, infants show a distinct preference for the mother. They follow her more, cry when she leaves, enjoy playing with her more, and feel most secure in her arms. About 1 month after showing attachment to the mother, many infants begin attaching to other members of the family, most often the father.

Infants acquire other developmental behaviors that influence the attachment process. These include: (1) differential crying, smiling, and vocalization (more to the mother than to anyone else); (2) visual-motor orientation (looking more at the mother, even if she is not close); (3) crying when the mother leaves the room; (4) approaching through locomotion (crawling, creeping, or walking); (5) clinging (especially in the presence of a stranger); and (6) exploring away from the mother while using her as a secure base. By 11 to 12 months they are able to anticipate her imminent departure by watching her behaviors, and they begin to protest before she leaves. At this point many parents learn to postpone alerting the child to their departure until just before leaving.

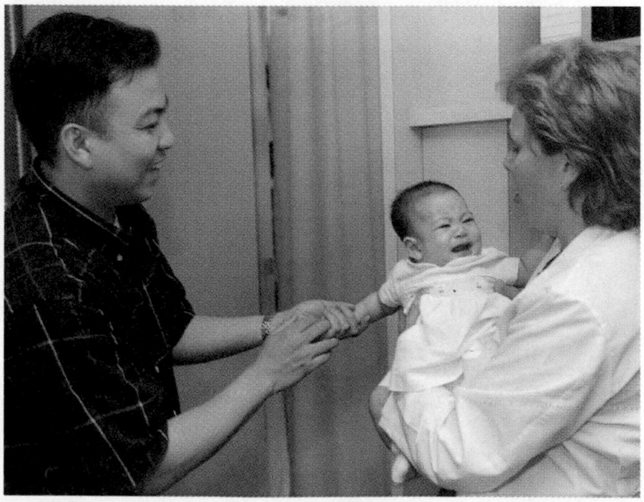

FIG. 36-9 • Behaviors related to fear of strangers include clinging to the parent and turning away from the stranger. (Photo by Paul Vincent Kuntz, Texas Children's Hospital.)

Stranger Fear. As infants demonstrate attachment to one person, they correspondingly exhibit less friendliness to others. Between ages 6 and 8 months, fear of strangers and stranger anxiety become prominent and are related to infants' ability to discriminate between familiar and nonfamiliar people. Behaviors such as clinging to the parent, crying, and turning away from the stranger are common (Fig. 36-9).

Language Development. The infant's first means of verbal communication is crying. Crying as a biologic sign conveys a message of urgency and signals displeasure, such as hunger. However, crying is also a social event that affects the development of the parent-infant relationship—either by its absence, which usually has a positive effect on parents, or its presence, which may involve a negative response or persuade parents to minister to the child's physical or emotional needs.

In the first few weeks of life, crying has a reflexive quality and is mostly related to physiologic needs. Infants cry for 1 to 1½ hours a day up to 3 weeks of age; then build up to 2 and even 4 hours by 6 weeks. Crying tends to decrease by 12 weeks of age. It is thought that the increase in crying for no apparent reason during the first few months may be related to the discharge of energy and the maturational changes in the central nervous system. During the end of the first year, infants cry for attention; from fear (especially stranger fear); and from frustration, usually in response to their developing but inadequate motor skills.

NURSE ALERT • Be alert to parents' reports about maternal postpartum depression and infant crying, because these concerns may indicate a stressed mother-infant relationship.

Vocalizations heard during crying eventually become syllables and words (e.g., the "mama" heard during vigorous crying). Infants vocalize as early as 5 to 6 weeks of age by making small throaty sounds. By 2 months they make single vowel sounds such as *ah, eh,* and *uh.* By 3 to 4 months the consonants *n, k, g, p,* and *b* are added, and the infants coo, gurgle, and laugh aloud. By 8 months they imitate sounds, add the consonants *t, d,* and *w,* and combine syllables (e.g., "dada"), but they do not ascribe meaning to the word until 10 to 11 months of age (Family Focus box). By 9 to 10 months they comprehend the meaning of

Family Focus

CHILD'S DEVELOPING LANGUAGE SKILLS

During the acquisition of new language skills the child temporarily may stop using other recently learned sounds or words. This is often distressing for parents, who have waited in anticipation for the words "dada" or "mama," because these sounds are commonly replaced by other vocalizations and may not be repeated for several weeks. Nurses can reassure parents that the child will again say these special words, and with increased meaning.

the word "no" and obey simple commands. By age 1 year they can say three to five words with meaning.

Play. Play during infancy represents the various social modalities observed during cognitive development. The activity of infants is primarily narcissistic and revolves around their own body. As discussed under Development of Body Image (p. 833), body parts are primarily objects of play and pleasure.

During the first year, play becomes more sophisticated and interdependent. From birth to 3 months, infants' responses to the environment are global and largely undifferentiated. Play is dependent; pleasure is demonstrated by a quieting attitude (1 month), a smile (2 months), or a squeal (3 months). From 3 to 6 months, infants show more discriminate interest in stimuli and begin to play alone with a rattle or a soft stuffed toy or with someone else. There is much more interaction during play. By 4 months of age they laugh aloud, show preference for certain toys, and become excited when food or a favorite object is brought to them. They recognize an image in a mirror, smile at it, and vocalize to it.

By 6 months to 1 year, play involves sensorimotor skills. Actual games such as peekaboo and pat-a-cake are played. Verbal repetition and imitation of simple gestures occurs in response to demonstration. Play is much more selective, not only in terms of specific toys, but also in terms of "playmates." Although play is solitary or one-sided, infants choose with whom they will interact. At 6 to 8 months they usually refuse to play with strangers. Parents are definite favorites, and infants know how to attract their attention. At 6 months they extend the arms to be picked up, at 7 months cough to make their presence known, at 10 months pull the parent's clothing, and at 12 months call them by name. This represents a tremendous advance from the newborn who signaled biologic needs by crying to express displeasure.

Stimulation is as important for psychosocial growth as food is for physical growth. Knowledge of developmental milestones allows nurses to guide parents regarding proper play for infants. It is not sufficient to place a mobile over a crib and toys in a playpen for a child's optimum social, emotional, and intellectual development. Play must provide interpersonal contact and recreational and educational stimulation. Infants need to be *played with,* not merely *allowed to play.* Although the type of play infants engage in is called *solitary,* this is a figurative, not literal, term to denote one-sided play. The types of toys given to the child are much less important than the quality of personal interaction that occurs.

Table 36-1 lists play activities appropriate for the developmental level of the infant in view of motor, language, and personal-social achievements. Although the activities are grouped according to the major mode of stimulation provided, there is overlap in many instances. In addition, play activities suggested for one age group may be appropriate for older infants but inappropriate for younger infants.

Temperament

The infant's temperament or behavioral style influences the type of interaction that occurs between the child and parents and other family members (see general discussion of temperament in Chapter 33). In assessing a child's temperament, it is the parents' perception of the child and the degree of fit between their expectations and the child's actual temperament that are important. The more dissonance or lack of harmony between the child's temperament and the parent's ability to accept and deal with the behavior, the more risk for subsequent parent-child conflicts.

The *Revised Infant Temperament Questionnaire (RITQ)* (Carey and McDevitt, 1978) can be used as a screening tool with parents. The questionnaire focuses on nine temperament variables, but the 95 questions relate specifically to activities such as sleep, feeding, play, diapering, and dressing. The scores from the RITQ help identify the child's temperamental style. Use of the RITQ is well accepted by parents and should be accompanied by an adequate explanation of the results. In discussing the results, it is best to avoid descriptors such as "difficult" by describing such infants in terms of characteristics such as "intense" or "less predictable." The Early Infancy Temperament Questionnaire (EITQ) is a 76-item parent questionnaire that was adapted from the RITQ to specifically evaluate temperament characteristics of infants 1 to 4 months old, whereas the RITQ is best suited for infants 4 months old and older (Medoff-Cooper, 1995; Medoff-Cooper, Carey, and McDevitt, 1993).

With knowledge of the infant's temperament, nurses are better able to (1) provide parents with background information that will help them see their child in a better perspective, (2) offer a more organized picture of their child's behavior and possibly reveal distortions in their perceptions of the behavior, and (3) guide parents regarding appropriate childrearing techniques.

Childrearing Practices Related to Temperament. Most parents realize that their infant is born with unique characteristics, and few parents of difficult infants need to be told of the challenge of caring for them. However, very few parents are aware of the significance of the temperamental characteristics and of constructive approaches to dealing with them. The following are examples of interventions that promote more positive parenting of infants with different temperament styles.*

"Difficult" children may respond better to scheduled feedings and structured caregiving routines than to demand feedings and frequent changes in daily routines. These children sleep less and may need more structured approaches to bedtime to prevent bedtime problems. "Highly distractible" children may require additional soothing measures such as swinging, rocking, or being carried in a pack that the parent wears across the chest or back. Children with "high activity" levels require vigilant watching, and parents need to take extra precautions in safeguarding the home. These children benefit from increased opportunities for gross motor activity to constructively channel their energy.

The child who is "slow to warm up" may demonstrate more stranger fear than other children and may require gradual and frequent preparation for new situations, such as substitute child care. Even the "easy child" can present problems in that the parents may need reminders to feed the child who sleeps for prolonged intervals and rarely cries. They may need to "retrain" the child because of the ease of developing habits such as keeping the child up late or sleeping with the youngster, which may later become troublesome.

Appropriate counseling based on awareness of the child's temperament can greatly enhance the quality of interaction be-

*A recommended resource for parents is *The Difficult Child* by S.K. Turecki and L. Tonner (1989, Bantam Books).

TABLE 36-1
Play During Infancy

Age (Months)	Visual Stimulation	Auditory Stimulation	Tactile Stimulation	Kinetic Stimulation
SUGGESTED ACTIVITIES				
Birth-1	Look at infant at close range Hang bright, shiny object within 20-25 cm (8-10 inches) of infant's face and in midline Hang mobiles with black-and-white designs	Talk to infant; sing in soft voice Play music box, tape, or CD Have ticking clock or metronome nearby	Hold, caress, cuddle Keep infant warm May like to be swaddled	Rock infant; place in cradle Use stroller for walks
2-3	Provide bright objects Make room bright with pictures or mirrors Take infant to various rooms while doing chores Place infant in infant seat for vertical view of environment	Talk to infant Include in family gatherings Expose to various environmental noises other than those of home Use rattles, wind chimes	Caress infant while bathing, at diaper change Comb hair with a soft brush Give massage	Use infant swing Take in car for rides Exercise body by moving extremities in swimming motion Use cradle gym
4-6	Place infant in front of unbreakable mirror Give brightly colored toys to hold (small enough to grasp)	Talk to infant; repeat sounds infant makes Laugh when infant laughs Call infant by name Crinkle different papers by infant's ear Place rattle or ball in hand	Give infant soft squeeze toys of various textures Allow to splash in bath Place nude on soft, furry rug and move extremities	Use swing or stroller Bounce infant in lap while holding in standing position Support infant in sitting position; let infant lean forward to balance self Place infant on floor to crawl, roll over, sit
6-9	Give infant large toys with bright colors, moveable parts, and noisemakers Place unbreakable mirror where infant can see self Play peekaboo, especially hiding face in a towel Make funny faces to encourage imitation Give ball of yarn or string to pull apart	Call infant by name Repeat simple words such as "dada," "mama," "bye-bye" Speak clearly Name parts of body, people, and foods Tell infant what you are doing Use "no" only when necessary Give simple commands Show how to clap hands, bang a drum	Let infant play with fabrics of various textures Have bowl with foods of different sizes and textures to feel Let infant "catch" running water Encourage "swimming" in large bathtub or shallow pool Give wad of sticky tape to manipulate	Hold upright to bear weight and bounce Pick up, say "up" Put down, say "down" Place toys out of reach; encourage infant to get them Play pat-a-cake
9-12	Show infant large pictures in books Take infant to places where there are animals, many people, different objects (shopping center) Play ball by rolling it to child, demonstrate "throwing" it back Demonstrate building a two-block tower	Read infant simple nursery rhymes Point to body parts and name each one Imitate sounds of animals	Give infant finger foods of different textures Let infant mess and squash food Let infant feel cold (ice cube) or warm objects, say what temperature each is Let infant feel a breeze (fan blowing)	Give large push-pull toys Place furniture in a circle to encourage cruising Turn in different positions
SUGGESTED TOYS				
Birth-6	Nursery mobiles Unbreakable mirrors See-through crib bumpers Contrasting colored sheets	Music boxes Musical mobiles Crib dangle bells Small-handled, clear rattle	Stuffed animals Soft clothes Soft or furry quilt Soft mobiles	Rocking crib/cradle Weighted or suction toy Infant swing

TABLE 36-1—cont'd
Play During Infancy

Age (Months)	Visual Stimulation	Auditory Stimulation	Tactile Stimulation	Kinetic Stimulation
SUGGESTED TOYS—cont'd				
6-12	Various colored blocks Nested boxes or cups Books with rhymes and bright pictures Strings of big beads Simple take-apart toys Large ball Cup and spoon Large puzzles Jack-in-the-box	Rattles of different sizes, shapes, tones, and bright colors Squeaky animals and dolls Light, rhythmic music	Soft, different-texture animals and dolls Sponge toys, floating toys Squeeze toys Teething toys Books with textures/objects, such as fur and zipper	Activity box for crib Push-pull toys Wind-up swing

tween parents and infant. Even just letting parents know that "difficult" traits are innate can relieve feelings of guilt and incompetence (Family Focus box).

Because of the complexity of the developmental process during the first 12 months, Table 36-2 is presented to help organize and clarify the data already discussed. Although all milestones are important, some represent essential integrative aspects of development that lay the foundation for achievement of more advanced skills. These essential milestones are designated by an asterisk in the table. The table represents the average monthly age at which various skills are attained. It must be remembered that although the sequence is the same, the rate will vary among children.

Coping with Concerns Related to Normal Growth and Development

Separation and Stranger Fear. A number of fears can appear during infancy. However, the fear that causes parents the most concern is fear related to strangers and separation. Although erroneously interpreted by some as a sign of undesirable, antisocial behavior, stranger fear and separation anxiety are important components of a strong, healthy, parent-child attachment. Nevertheless, this period can present difficulties for the parent and child. Parents may be more confined to the home because baby-sitters are violently protested by the infant. To accustom the infant to new people, parents are encouraged to have close friends or relatives visit often. This provides for other persons with whom the child is comfortable and who can give parents time for themselves.

Infants also need opportunities to safely experience strangers. Usually toward the end of the first year, infants begin to venture away from the parent and demonstrate curiosity about strangers. If allowed to explore at their own rate, many infants eventually "warm up." If parents hold the child away from their face, the infant can observe while maintaining close physical contact.

The best approach for the stranger (who may be the nurse) is to talk softly, meet the child at eye level (to appear smaller), maintain a safe distance from the infant, and avoid sudden, intrusive gestures, such as holding the arms out and smiling broadly.

Family Focus

DIFFICULT TEMPERAMENT AND PRETERM INFANTS

Parents typically rate preterm, low-birth-weight infants as being more difficult than full-term infant.* Parents are often concerned that the difficult temperament is permanent and results from the many negative and painful hospital experiences. The family can be reassured that although these infants may be difficult to parent for the first 6 months of corrected age (chronologic age minus amount of prematurity), over time the infants tend to become less difficult.† Most of the studies indicating that preterm infants are more difficult to console were performed before wide-scale implementation of individualized developmental care for such infants. Kangaroo care and assisting the infant in self-regulation behaviors may in fact change current thought. By enabling preterm infants to experience more positive caretaking and less stressful stimuli, such infants may be found in the future to be less temperamental.

Parents may find the following book helpful: *The Fussy Baby* by W. Sears (Franklin Park, IL, 1989, La Leche League International).

*Langkamp DL, Kim Y, Pascoe JM: Temperament of preterm infants at 4 months of age: maternal ratings and perceptions, *J Dev Behav Pediatr* 19(6):391-396, 1998.
†Medoff-Cooper B: Infant temperament: implications for parenting from birth through 1 year, *J Pediatr Nurs* 10(3):141-145, 1995.

Parents also may wonder whether they should encourage the child's clinging, dependent behavior, especially if there is pressure from others who view this as "spoiling" (see the following discussion). Parents need to be reassured that such behavior is healthy, desirable, and necessary for the child's optimum emotional development. If parents can reassure the infant of their presence, the infant will learn to realize that they are still there even if not physically present. Talking to infants when leaving the room, allowing them to hear one's voice on the telephone, and using transitional objects (e.g., a favorite blanket or toy) reassures them of the parent's continued presence.

Alternate Child Care Arrangements. For many parents, especially working mothers, the need for locating safe and competent child care facilities for the infant is an increasingly difficult problem—one that is compounded by the number of mothers working outside the home. Over the past 30 years there has been a marked shift in child care arrange-

Text continued on p. 842.

TABLE 36-2
Growth and Development During Infancy

Age (Months)	Physical	Gross Motor	Fine Motor
1	Weight gain of 150-210 g (5-7 ounces) weekly for first 6 months Height gain of 2.5 cm (1 inch) monthly for first 6 months Head circumference increases by 1.5 cm (½ inch) monthly for first 6 months Primitive reflexes present and strong Doll's eye reflexes and dance reflex fading Obligatory nose breathing (most infants)	Assumes flexed position with pelvis high but knees not under abdomen when prone (at birth, knees flexed under abdomen)* Can turn head from side to side when prone; lifts head momentarily from bed (see Fig. 36-3, *A*)* Has marked head lag, especially when pulled from lying to sitting position (see Fig. 36-2, *A*) Holds head momentarily parallel and in midline when suspended in prone position Assumes asymmetric tonic neck reflex position when supine When held in standing position, body is limp at knees and hips In sitting position, back is uniformly rounded, absence of head control	Hands predominantly closed Grasp reflex strong Hand clenches on contact with rattle
2	Posterior fontanel closed Crawling reflex disappears	Assumes less flexed position when prone—hips flat, legs extended, arms flexed, head to side* Less head lag when pulled to sitting position (see Fig. 36-2, *B*) Can maintain head in same plane as rest of body when held in ventral suspension When prone, can lift head almost 45 degrees off table When moved to sitting position, head is held up but bends forward (see Fig. 36-5, *B*) Assumes asymmetric tonic neck reflex position intermittently	Hands often open Grasp reflex fading
3	Primitive reflexes fading	Able to hold head more erect when sitting, but still bobs forward Has only slight head lag when pulled to sitting position Assumes symmetric body positioning Able to raise head and shoulders from prone position to a 45- to 90-degree angle from table; bears weight on forearms When held in standing position, able to bear slight fraction of weight on legs Regards own hand	Actively holds rattle but will not reach for it* Grasp reflex absent Hands kept loosely open Clutches own hand; pulls at blankets and clothes
4	Drooling begins Moro, tonic neck, and rooting reflexes have disappeared*	Has almost no head lag when pulled to sitting position (see Fig. 36-2, *C*)* Balances head well in sitting position (see Fig. 36-5, *C*)* Back less rounded, curved only in lumbar area	Inspects and plays with hands; pulls clothing or blanket over face in play* Tries to reach objects with hand but overshoots Grasps object with both hands

*Milestones that represent essential integrative aspects of development that lay the foundation for the achievement of more advanced skills.

Sensory	Vocalization	Socialization/Cognition
Able to fixate on moving object in range of 45 degrees when held at a distance of 20-25 cm (8-10 inches) Visual acuity approaches 20/100† Follows light to midline Quiets when hears a voice	Cries to express displeasure Makes small, throaty sounds Makes comfort sounds during feeding	Is in sensorimotor phase—stage I, use of reflexes (birth-1 month), and stage II, primary circular reactions (1-4 months) Watches parent's face intently as parent talks to infant
Binocular fixation and convergence to near objects beginning When supine, follows dangling toy from side to point beyond midline Visually searches to locate sounds Turns head to side when sound is made at level of ear	Vocalizes, distinct from crying* Crying becomes differentiated Coos Vocalizes to familiar voice	Demonstrates social smile in response to various stimuli*
Follows object to periphery (180 degrees)* Locates sound by turning head to side and looking in same direction* Begins to have ability to coordinate stimuli from various sense organs	Squeals aloud to show pleasure* Coos, babbles, chuckles Vocalizes when smiling "Talks" a great deal when spoken to Less crying during periods of wakefulness	Displays considerable interest in surroundings Ceases crying when parent enters room Can recognize familiar faces and objects, such as feeding bottle Shows awareness of strange situations
Able to accommodate to near objects Binocular vision fairly well established Can focus on a 1.25-cm (½-inch) block Beginning eye-hand coordination	Makes consonant sounds *n, k, g, p, b* Laughs aloud* Vocalization changes according to mood	Is in stage III, secondary circular reactions Demands attention by fussing; becomes bored if left alone Enjoys social interaction with people Anticipates feeding when sees bottle or mother if breastfeeding Shows excitement with whole body, squeals, breathes heavily

†Degree of visual acuity varies according to vision measurement procedure used.

Continued

TABLE 36-2—cont'd
Growth and Development During Infancy

Age (Months)	Physical	Gross Motor	Fine Motor
4—cont'd		Able to sit erect if propped up Able to raise head and chest off surface to angle of 90 degrees (see Fig. 36-3, *B*) Assumes predominant symmetric position Rolls from back to side*	Plays with rattle placed in hand, shakes it, but cannot pick it up if dropped Can carry objects to mouth
5	Beginning signs of tooth eruption Birth weight doubles	No head lag when pulled to sitting position When sitting, able to hold head erect and steady Able to sit for longer periods when back is well supported Back straight When prone, assumes symmetric positioning with arms extended Can turn over from abdomen to back* When supine, puts feet to mouth	Able to grasp objects voluntarily* Uses palmar grasp, bidextrous approach Plays with toes Takes objects directly to mouth Holds one cube while regarding a second one
6	Growth rate may begin to decline Weight gain of 90-150 g (3-5 ounces) weekly for next 6 months Height gain of 1.25 cm (½ inch) monthly for next 6 months Teething may begin with eruption of two lower central incisors* Chewing and biting occur*	When prone, can lift chest and upper abdomen off surface, bearing weight on hands (see Fig. 36-3, *C*) When about to be pulled to a sitting position, lifts head Sits in high chair with back straight Rolls from back to abdomen When held in standing position, bears almost all of weight Hand regard absent	Resecures a dropped object Drops one cube when another is given Grasps and manipulates small objects Holds bottle Grasps feet and pulls to mouth
7	Eruption of upper central incisors	When supine, spontaneously lifts head off surface Sits, leaning forward on hands (see Fig. 36-5, *D*)* When prone, bears weight on one hand Sits erect momentarily Bears full weight on feet (see Fig. 36-6, *A*) When held in standing position, bounces actively	Transfers objects from one hand to the other (see Fig. 36-5, *E*)* Has unidextrous approach and grasp Holds two cubes more than momentarily Bangs cube on table Rakes at a small object
8	Begins to show regular patterns in bladder and bowel elimination Parachute reflex appears (see Fig. 36-4)	Sits steadily unsupported (see Fig. 36-5, *E*)* Readily bears weight on legs when supported; may stand holding onto furniture Adjusts posture to reach an object	Has beginning pincer grasp using index, fourth, and fifth fingers against lower part of thumb Releases objects at will Rings bell purposely Retains two cubes while regarding third cube Secures an object by pulling on a string Reaches persistently for toys out of reach

*Milestones that represent essential integrative aspects of development that lay the foundation for the achievement of more advanced skills.

Sensory	Vocalization	Socialization/Cognition
		Shows interest in strange stimuli Begins to show memory
Visually pursues a dropped object Is able to sustain visual inspection of an object Can localize sounds made below ear	Squeals Makes cooing vowel sounds interspersed with consonant sounds (e.g., *ah-goo*)	Smiles at mirror image Pats bottle or breast with both hands More enthusiastically playful, but may have rapid mood swings Is able to discriminate strangers from family Vocalizes displeasure when object is taken away Discovers parts of body
Adjusts posture to see an object Prefers more complex visual stimuli Can localize sounds made above ear Will turn head to the side, then look up or down	Begins to imitate sounds* Babbling resembles one-syllable utterances—*ma, mu, da, di, hi** Vocalizes to toys, mirror image Takes pleasure in hearing own sounds (self-reinforcement)	Recognizes parents; begins to fear strangers Holds arms out to be picked up Has definite likes and dislikes Begins to imitate (cough, protrusion of tongue) Excites on hearing footsteps Laughs when head is hidden in a towel Briefly searches for a dropped object (object permanence beginning)* Frequent mood swings—from crying to laughing with little or no provocation
Can fixate on very small objects* Responds to own name Localizes sound by turning head in a curving arch Beginning awareness of depth and space Has taste preferences	Produces vowel sounds and chained syllables—*baba, dada, kaka** Vocalizes four distinct vowel sounds "Talks" when others are talking	Increasing fear of strangers; shows signs of fretfulness when parent disappears* Imitates simple acts and noises Tries to attract attention by coughing or snorting Plays peekaboo Demonstrates dislike of food by keeping lips closed Exhibits oral aggressiveness in biting and mouthing Demonstrates expectation in response to repetition of stimuli
	Makes consonant sounds *t, d,* and *w* Listens selectively to familiar words Utterances signal emphasis and emotion Combines syllables, such as *dada,* but does not ascribe meaning to them	Increasing anxiety over loss of parent, particularly mother, and fear of strangers Responds to word "no" Dislikes dressing, diaper change

Continued

TABLE 36-2—cont'd
Growth and Development During Infancy

Age (Months)	Physical	Gross Motor	Fine Motor
9	Eruption of upper lateral incisor may begin	Creeps on hands and knees Sits steadily on floor for prolonged time (10 minutes) Recovers balance when leans forward but cannot do so when leaning sideways Pulls self to standing position and stands holding onto furniture (see Fig. 36-6, *B* to *C*)*	Uses thumb and index fingers in crude pincer grasp (see Fig. 36-1)* Preference for use of dominant hand now evident Grasps third cube Compares two cubes by bringing them together
10	Labyrinth-righting reflex is strongest—when infant is in prone or supine position, is able to raise head	Can change from prone to sitting position Stands while holding onto furniture, sits by falling down Recovers balance easily while sitting While standing, lifts one foot to take a step (see Fig. 36-6, *D*)	Crude release of an object beginning Grasps bell by handle
11	Eruption of lower lateral incisor may begin	When sitting, pivots to reach toward back to pick up an object Cruises or walks holding onto furniture or with both hands held*	Explores objects more thoroughly (e.g., clapper inside bell) Has neat pincer grasp Drops object deliberately for it to be picked up Puts one object after another into a container (sequential play) Able to manipulate an object to remove it from tight-fitting enclosure
12	Birth weight tripled* Birth length increased by 50%* Head and chest circumference equal (head circumference 46 cm [18 inches]) Has total of six to eight deciduous teeth Anterior fontanel almost closed Landau reflex fading Babinski reflex disappears Lumbar curve develops; lordosis evident during walking	Walks with one hand held* Cruises well May attempt to stand alone momentarily; may attempt first step alone* Can sit down from standing position without help	Releases cube in cup Attempts to build two-block tower but fails Tries to insert a pellet into a narrow-necked bottle but fails Can turn pages in a book, many at a time

*Milestones that represent essential integrative aspects of development that lay the foundation for the achievement of more advanced skills.

Text continued from p. 837.

ments, with fewer children being cared for at home and more children being cared for in group centers or other settings.

The basic types of care are in-home care, either in the parents' or caregivers' home (family day care); and center-based care, usually in a day care center. *In-home care* may consist of a full-time baby-sitter who lives in the home, a full-time baby-sitter who comes to the home, cooperative arrangements such as exchange baby-sitting, and family day care. A licensed *family day care home* typically provides care and protection for up to five children for part of a day and does not include informal arrangements such as exchange baby-sitting or caregivers in the child's own home. The five children include the family day care provider's own children younger than 5 years of age living in the home. Unfortunately, many family day care homes operate

Sensory	Vocalization	Socialization/Cognition
Localizes sounds by turning head diagonally and directly toward sound Depth perception increasing	Responds to simple verbal commands Comprehends "no-no"	Parent (mother) is increasingly important for own sake Shows increasing interest in pleasing parent Begins to show fears of going to bed and being left alone Puts arms in front of face to avoid having it washed
	Says "dada," "mama" with meaning* Comprehends "bye-bye" May say one word (e.g., "hi," "bye," "no")	Inhibits behavior to verbal command of "no-no" or own name Imitates facial expressions; waves bye-bye Extends toy to another person but will not release it Develops object permanence* Repeats actions that attract attention and cause laughter Pulls clothes of another to attract attention Plays interactive game such as pat-a-cake Reacts to adult anger; cries when scolded Demonstrates independence in dressing, feeding, locomotive skills, and testing of parents Looks at and follows pictures in a book
	Imitates definite speech sounds	Experiences joy and satisfaction when a task is mastered Reacts to restrictions with frustration Rolls ball to another on request Anticipates body gestures when a familiar nursery rhyme or story is being told (e.g., holds toes and feet in response to "This little piggy went to market") Plays game up-down, "so big," or peekaboo Shakes head for "no"
Discriminates simple geometric forms (e.g., circle) Amblyopia may develop with lack of binocularity Can follow rapidly moving object Controls and adjusts response to sound; listens for sound to recur	Says three to five words besides "dada," "mama"* Comprehends meaning of several words (comprehension always precedes verbalization) Recognizes objects by name Imitates animal sounds Understands simple verbal commands (e.g., "Give it to me," "Show me your eyes")	Shows emotions such as jealousy, affection (may give hug or kiss on request), anger, fear Enjoys familiar surroundings and explores away from parent Is fearful in strange situation; clings to parent May develop habit of "security blanket" or favorite toy Has increasing determination to practice to locomotor skills Searches for an object even if it has not been hidden, but searches only where object was last seen*

without a license and may care for large numbers of infants without adequate staff and facilities.

Center-based care usually refers to a licensed day care facility that provides care for six or more children, for 6 or more hours in a day. *Work-based group care* is another option that is becoming increasingly popular as employers recognize the benefit of providing quality and convenient child care to their employees. *Sick-child care* may also be available for times when the youngster is ill. Such programs are often located in community hospitals or in work settings.

A major nursing responsibility is guiding parents in locating suitable facilities that have a well-qualified staff. State licensing agencies can help parents identify day care centers that accept children of specific age groups and that are convenient to home and work. Their records are available to the public and provide reports from the health, safety, and fire departments; periodic evaluations from the licensing agency; complaints filed against the center; and qualifications of the center's employees. State-licensed programs are supposed to abide by established standards, which represent the minimum requirements and safeguards; however, enforcement of the standards is sometimes inadequate. Early childhood programs may also belong to a voluntary accreditation system, the National Academy of Early Childhood Programs, which serves as a model for optimum care.* References from other parents are also helpful, provided that they have investigated the center carefully and have remained involved with the agency's activities.

The same attention should be applied to locating competent baby-sitters. References from other employers are essential, and there is no substitute for observing the interaction between the individual and the child. Although very young infants need little if any preparation for the introduction of a new caregiver, older infants may benefit from a gradual placement to reduce stranger anxiety. At all times the parent should have the right to visit the child, and regular conferences should be established to review the child's progress.

Limit Setting and Discipline. As infants' motor skills advance and mobility increases, parents are faced with the need to set safe limits to protect the child and establish a positive and supportive parent-child relationship (see Nurse's Role in Injury Prevention, p. 866). Although there are numerous disciplinary techniques, some are more appropriate for this age than others. An effective approach used in disciplining a child is the use of time-out. The basic principles are the same as those discussed in Chapter 31, except that the place for time-out needs to be commensurate with the child's abilities. For example, the playpen is better for most infants than a chair. Although parents may be concerned with instituting discipline during infancy, it is important to stress that the earlier effective disciplinary methods are employed, the easier it is to continue these approaches.

Parents must recognize the child's cognitive and behavioral limitations; adequate protection from hazards must be implemented because infants and toddlers do not understand a cause-effect relationship between dangerous objects and physical harm. Children will innately test limits and explore during the exploratory phase of growth; instead of discouraging exploration, safe alternatives should be provided, dangerous household items should be put away, and children should be given consistent discipline and nurturing.

Thumb-Sucking and Use of a Pacifier. Sucking is the infant's chief pleasure and may not be satisfied by breast- or bottle-feeding. It is such a strong need that infants who are deprived of sucking, such as those with a cleft lip repair, will suck on their tongue. Some newborns are born with sucking blisters on their hands from in utero sucking activity. The benefits of nonnutritive sucking, such as increased weight gain in preterm infants and decreased crying, have been documented (Pickler and Frankel, 1995).

Problems arise when parents are concerned about the sucking of the fingers, thumb, or pacifier and attempt to restrain this natural tendency. Before giving advice, nurses should investigate the parents' feelings and base guidance on this information (Critical Thinking box).

During infancy and early childhood there is no need to restrain nonnutritive sucking of the fingers. Malocclusion may occur if thumb-sucking persists past 4 years of age, or past 6 years as indicated by some authorities (Johns, Miller, and Hochstetler, 1998), or when the permanent teeth erupt. There is probably less dental displacement with the use of a pacifier than with the use of a hard, rigid finger. Pacifiers may be relinquished earlier than thumbs because they are less readily available.

There are studies linking the early introduction of a pacifier with early termination of breastfeeding and early weaning from the breast. Biancuzzo (1999) suggests that health care workers must maintain a commonsense approach to pacifier usage and breastfeeding. Parents should be informed of the relationship between pacifier use and early termination of breastfeeding so that an informed decision can be made. Furthermore, pacifier use should not replace actual feeding or suckling: prohibiting pacifier use will not ensure an increase in the length of breast-

Critical Thinking

THUMB-SUCKING

During a well-child visit you observe that Mrs. Lopez persistently takes the thumb out of her 10-month-old daughter, Maria's, mouth. You ask if she has concerns about the thumb-sucking. She replies, "Of course. Her teeth are coming in so nice and straight, and I don't want the thumb to make them crooked." What is an appropriate response?

First, Think About It . . .

- **What information are you using?**
- **How are you interpreting that information?**

1. **"Sucking on a thumb or pacifier is very common in young children, especially in infants. It satisfies their need to suck and helps them to comfort themselves. Sometimes, making an issue of the sucking can cause it to last longer."**
2. **"Thumb-sucking is perfectly normal, and children stop when they are ready. So don't worry about it."**
3. **"If thumb-sucking continues when most of her teeth are in, it will make them crooked. But we don't need to worry about it now."**
4. **"You are right to be concerned. Let her suck longer on the bottle to satisfy her sucking needs."**

The best response is 1. The response provides factual information in a nonjudgmental manner that invites further discussion. You may interpret options 2 and 3 as partly correct in regard to thumb-sucking, but they offer premature reassurance. Option 4 is incorrect, and at 10 months of age, infants should be relying less, not more, on bottle-feeding, which can lead to excessive intake of milk, juice, or other sweetened beverages in place of solid foods and to dental caries (see Weaning, p. 848, and Dental Health, p. 850).

*Information about the accreditation criteria and procedures of the National Academy of Early Childhood Programs is available from the National Association for the Education of Young Children, 1509 16th St. NW, Washington, DC 20036; 1-800-424-2460 or (202) 232-8777; fax (202) 328-1846; website: www.naeyc.org. These criteria are excellent guidelines for evaluating child care facilities. Other resources are *Child Care: What's Best for Your Family,* available from the American Academy of Pediatrics, 141 Northwest Point Blvd., Elk Grove Village, IL 60007; 1-800-433-9016 or (847) 228-5005; fax (847) 228-5097; website: www.aap.org; and *Parent's Guide to Day Care,* available from the National Association of Pediatric Nurse Associates and Practitioners (NAPNAP), 1101 Kings Highway North, Suite 206, Cherry Hill, NJ 08034-1912; (877) 662-7627 or (856) 667-1773; fax (856) 667-7187; website: www.napnap.org.

feeding, and there should be an emphasis on allowing the infant to control the pace, frequency, and termination of feeding rather than allowing the pacifier (or anything else) to become the focus of the interaction.

The use of a pacifier in infants has also been suggested as a causative factor in the increase in episodes of acute otitis media (Niemela, Uhari, and Mottonen, 1995); however, evidence is inconclusive. The effect of continual pacifier use on early speech and language development is unknown, but the pacifier may decrease the child's desire to imitate sounds and may affect intelligibility. Parents need to be alerted that continual dependency on a pacifier may influence social and speech development.

If the child uses a pacifier, safety considerations in purchasing one must be stressed. Parents should be cautioned against altering a pacifier, thus making it more dangerous (see Aspiration of Foreign Objects, p. 859). To decrease dependence on nonnutritive sucking in young infants, sucking pleasure can be increased by prolonging feeding time. A small-holed, firm nipple causes stronger sucking and slower feeding. Also, the parent's excessive use of the pacifier to calm the child should be explored. It is not unusual for parents to place a pacifier in the infant's mouth as soon as crying begins, thus reinforcing a pattern of distress-relief.

At the time of this writing, there is no evidence that pacifier use and nonnutritive sucking in preterm infants has any effect on the initiation and length of breastfeeding. Nonnutritive sucking should not be withheld from preterm infants, especially when performed in conjunction with the use of concentrated sucrose for pain management.

Thumb-sucking reaches its peak at age 18 to 20 months and is most prevalent when the child is hungry or tired. Persistent thumb-sucking in a listless, apathetic child always warrants investigation. It may be a sign of an emotional problem between parent and child; or of boredom, isolation, and lack of stimulation.

Teething. One of the more difficult periods in the infant's (and parents') life is the eruption of the deciduous (primary) teeth, often referred to as teething. The age of tooth eruption shows considerable variation among children, but the order of their appearance is fairly regular and predictable (Fig. 36-10). The first primary teeth to erupt are the lower central incisors, which appear at approximately 6 to 8 months of age. These are followed closely by the upper central incisors. A quick guide to assessment of deciduous teeth during the first 2 years is:

Age of the child in months − 6 = number of teeth
For example: 8 months of age − 6 = 2 teeth

Teething is a physiologic process; some discomfort is common as the crown of the tooth breaks through the periodontal membrane. Some children show minimum evidence of teething, such as drooling, increased finger sucking, or biting on hard objects. Others are very irritable, have difficulty sleeping, and refuse to eat. Generally, signs of illness such as fever, vomiting, or diarrhea are not symptoms of teething but of illness and may warrant further investigation. However, as many parents report, a low-grade temperature is common in the 4- to 19-day period before and on the day of tooth eruption.

Because teething pain is a result of inflammation, cold is soothing. Giving the child a frozen teething ring helps relieve the inflammation. Several nonprescription topical anesthetic ointments (e.g., Baby Ora-Jel) are available. The active ingredient in most of these is benzocaine. If such products are used, parents are advised to apply them correctly. In the event of persistent irritability that affects sleeping and feeding, systemic analgesics such as acetaminophen or ibuprofen can be given; however, parents should know that this is a temporary measure.

NURSE ALERT • Teething The use of teething powders or procedures, such as cutting the gums or rubbing them with aspirin, are discouraged because ingestion of the powder, infection or irritation of the tissue, or aspiration of the aspirin can occur. Hard candy may cause accidental choking or aspiration and should be avoided at this age.

Infant Shoes. Many parents are unaware of the type of shoes that are appropriate for the older infant and buy expensive infant shoes because of misleading advertising claims. Inflexible shoes that have hard soles can be detrimental. They can delay walking, aggravate intoeing or outtoeing, and impede the development of supportive foot muscles. Therefore, the counseling of parents regarding footwear should begin when infants are 6 months old—well before they are walking.

It is helpful to begin by explaining to parents that changes in the feet occur during infancy and early childhood as locomotion and weight bearing progress. At birth the feet are flat

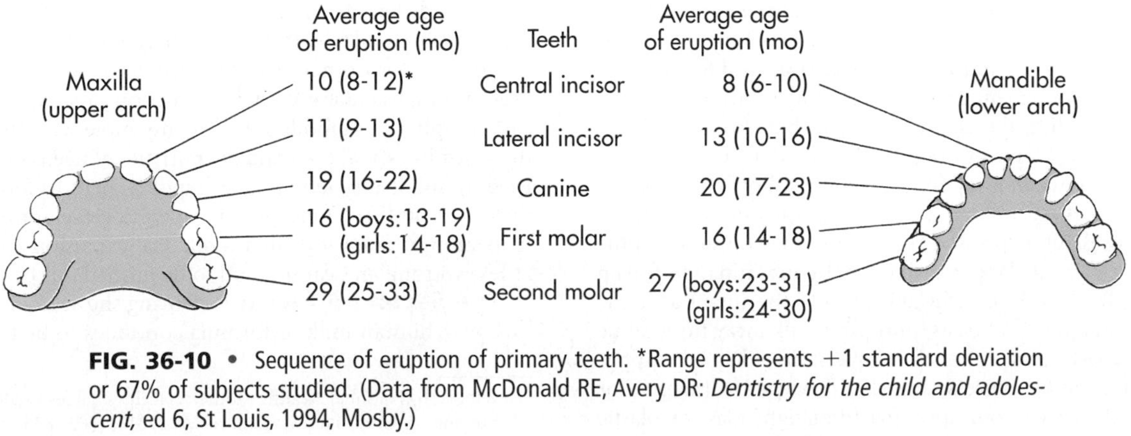

FIG. 36-10 • Sequence of eruption of primary teeth. *Range represents +1 standard deviation or 67% of subjects studied. (Data from McDonald RE, Avery DR: *Dentistry for the child and adolescent,* ed 6, St Louis, 1994, Mosby.)

because the arches are protected by fat pads on the soles of the feet. As the bones in the arches develop, the pads disappear and the feet begin to assume a mature shape. A normal arch is determined by proper alignment of all the bones and development of the surrounding musculature, not by the height of the arch.

When children begin walking, the main reason for shoes is protection. To provide *protection,* the shoe should retain its fit; be made of durable material with a smooth interior and few construction seams to irritate the skin; and be soft and flexible, especially in the toe area. A high-top shoe is not necessary for support but may be helpful in keeping the foot in the shoe.

A good shoe conforms to the anatomic shape of the foot, with a rounded toe and sufficient toe room. During weight bearing there should be at least the space of half the width of the thumbnail, or 1.25 cm (½ inch), between the end of the longest toe and the shoe. Roomy and square-toed socks allow for proper growth and alignment. Inexpensive but well-constructed sneakers or soft-leather moccasin-type shoes are suggested as adequate footgear for walking infants.

Even if the shoes are fitted properly, frequent changes are needed to accommodate the infant's rapidly growing feet. Shoe size changes at approximately 3-month intervals between 12 to 36 months; during this time the child's foot should be measured every 3 months. Curled toes when shoes are removed, and redness and irritation of the skin on the bottom of the toes, indicate the need for a larger shoe size.

PROMOTING OPTIMUM HEALTH DURING INFANCY

Nutrition

Ideally, discussion of optimum nutrition should begin prenatally with the decision to breast- or bottle-feed the infant. The choice for either is highly individual and is discussed in Chapter 11. This section is primarily concerned with infant nutrition during the next 12 months, when growth needs and developmental milestones ready the child for the introduction of solid foods.

The First 6 Months. Human milk is the most desirable complete diet for the infant during the first 6 months (American Academy of Pediatrics, 1998b). The normal infant receiving breast milk from a well-nourished mother needs no specific vitamin and mineral supplements, with the exception of iron by 4 to 6 months of age (when fetal iron stores are depleted). Iron supplementation is recommended at this time to offset the decrease in iron available in human milk and to enhance erythropoiesis. Daily supplements of vitamin D and vitamin B_{12} may be indicated if the mother's intake of these vitamins is inadequate.

Employed mothers can continue breastfeeding with guidance and encouragement. Mothers are encouraged to set realistic goals for employment and breastfeeding, with accurate information regarding the costs, risks, and benefits of available feeding options. Many mothers may find that a program of breast pumping when away from home and bottle-feeding the infant the expressed milk with or without formula supplementation is successful. Expressed breast milk may be stored in the refrigerator without danger of bacterial contamination for up to 8 days (Bocar, 1997). Although feeding the infant at home may occur on a demand basis, pumping milk away from home may be needed every 3 hours to maintain adequate supply. Breast milk may be expressed by hand or pump (manual or electric) and stored in an appropriate airtight glass or plastic container. Expressed breast milk may be frozen for up to 12 months, but care should be taken to prevent the typical freezer burn. Health care workers and new mothers may find the booklet *Working and Breastfeeding—Can You Do It? Yes, You Can!* by Johnson & Johnson helpful.*

In addition to efficient breast pumping, mothers also need child care by a trusted individual or agency and support and assistance from significant others. Like all breastfeeding mothers, these women must have proper nutrition and rest for adequate lactation. Maternal fatigue is considered the biggest threat to successful breastfeeding in employed mothers (Corbett-Dick and Bezek, 1997).

An acceptable alternative to breastfeeding is commercial iron-fortified formula. Like human milk, it supplies all of the nutrients needed by the infant for the first 6 months.

Unmodified whole cow's milk, low-fat cow's milk, skim milk, and imitation milks are not acceptable as a major source of nutrition for infants because of their altered ability to be digested, an increased risk of contamination, and a lack of components needed for appropriate growth. Whole milk can cause iron deficiency anemia in infants, possibly as a result of occult gastrointestinal blood loss. Pasteurized whole cow's milk is deficient in iron, zinc, and vitamin C and has a high renal solute load, which makes it undesirable for infants less than 12 months of age (American Academy of Pediatrics, 1998b).

NURSE ALERT • Whole milk should not be introduced to infants until after 1 year of age (American Academy of Pediatrics, 1998b).

The amount of formula per feeding and the number of feedings per day vary among infants. Infants on demand feeding usually determine their own feeding schedule, but some infants may need a more planned schedule based on average feeding patterns to ensure sufficient nutrients. In general, the number of feedings decreases from six at 1 month of age to four or five at 6 months. Regardless of the number of feedings, the total amount of formula ingested should not exceed 32 ounces (960 ml/day). Parents should be cautioned concerning the excessive use of juices and nonnutritive drinks such as fruit-flavored drinks or carbonated beverages (soda or pop) during this period. Many juices and nonnutritive drinks, although readily available to consumers, do not provide sufficient caloric intake for infants less than 12 months of age; such drinks may replace the nutrients in milk (formula) and lead to growth or health problems. Also, water supplementation is not recommended for healthy infants because it may lead to water intoxication (American Academy of Pediatrics, 1998b).

The addition of solid foods before 4 to 6 months of age is not recommended, although mothers may receive conflicting advice from other women (e.g., their mothers) who cared for children during the era of early introduction of solids. During the early months solid foods are not compatible with the ability of the gastrointestinal tract and the nutritional needs of the infant. Feeding solids to young infants exposes them to food antigens that may produce food-protein allergy. Developmentally, infants are not ready for solid food. The extrusion (protrusion) reflex is strong and causes food to be pushed out of the mouth.

The Second 6 Months. During the second half of the first year, human milk or formula continues to be the primary

*Developed by National Healthy Mothers, Healthy Babies Coalition, 121 W. Washington St., Suite 3400, Alexandria VA 22314; (703) 836-6110; website: www.hmhb.org.

source of nutrition. Fluoride supplementation should begin, depending on the infant's intake of fluoridated tap water (see Dental Health, p. 850). If breastfeeding is discontinued, a commercial iron-fortified formula should be substituted. Follow-up or transition formulas specially marketed for older infants offer no special advantages over other infant formulas (American Academy of Pediatrics, 1998b).

The major change in feeding habits is the addition of solid foods to the infant's diet. Physiologically and developmentally, the infant 4 to 6 months of age is in a transition period. By this time the gastrointestinal tract has matured sufficiently to handle more complex nutrients and is less sensitive to potentially allergenic foods. Tooth eruption is beginning and facilitates biting and chewing. The extrusion reflex has disappeared, and swallowing is more coordinated to allow the infant to accept solids easily. Head control is well developed, which permits infants to sit with support and purposely turn the head away to communicate disinterest in food. Voluntary grasping and improved eye-hand coordination gradually allow infants to pick up finger foods and feed themselves. Their increasing sense of independence is evident in their desire to hold the bottle and try to "help" during feeding.

Selection and Preparation of Solid Foods. The choice of solid foods to introduce first is variable but should meet the reasons for feeding solids, such as supplying nutrients not found in formula or breast milk. Iron-fortified infant cereal is generally introduced first because of its high iron content (i.e., 7 mg/3 tablespoons of prepared dry cereal). Commercially prepared ready-to-serve dry cereals for infants include rice, barley, oatmeal, and high-protein cereals; rice is usually suggested as an initial food because of its easy digestibility and low allergenic potential. Cereals such as cream of farina are not used because infant commercial cereals are a better source of iron.

Infant cereal (iron fortified) is mixed with formula until whole milk is given. If the infant is breastfed, the cereal is mixed with expressed breast milk or water. After 6 months of age, fruit juices can be mixed with the dry cereal; the vitamin C content of the juice enhances the absorption of iron in the cereal. Because of their benefit as a source of iron, infant cereals should be continued until the child is 18 months of age.

Fruit juice can be offered from a cup for its rich source of vitamin C and as a substitute for milk for one feeding a day. Large quantities of certain juices (e.g., apple, pear, prune, sweet cherry, peach, and grape) are avoided because they may cause abdominal pain, diarrhea, or bloating in some children. Some studies have shown that excessive fruit juice consumption (e.g., 12 or more oz/day) in young children increases the likelihood of short stature and childhood obesity (Dennison, Rockwell, and Baker, 1997) and nonorganic failure to thrive (Smith and Lifshitz, 1994); however, Skinner et al (1999) found no association between growth failure and the consumption of 12 ounces or more of 100% fruit juice in children 24 to 36 months of age. Because vitamin C is naturally destroyed by heat, juice is not warmed. Juice containers are always kept covered and refrigerated to prevent further vitamin loss.

NURSE ALERT • Offer fruit juice from a cup, rather than a bottle, to prevent the development of nursing caries (see Low-Cariogenic Diet, Chapter 37).

The addition of other foods is arbitrary. A common sequence is to introduce strained fruits followed by vegetables; and, finally, meats. If foods are introduced early, citrus fruits, meats, and eggs are delayed until after 6 months of age because of their potential to result in allergy. At 6 months, foods such as a cracker or zwieback can be offered as a type of finger and teething food. By 8 to 9 months, junior foods and nutritious finger foods such as a firmly cooked vegetable, raw pieces of fruit (except grapes), or cheese can be given. By 1 year, well-cooked table foods are served.

Commercially prepared baby foods are the most commonly used types of food served to infants in the United States. They are convenient and contain no added salt or sugar, but they are relatively expensive. An alternative is to prepare baby foods at home, which is a simple and inexpensive process. Fruits and vegetables can be steamed in a small amount of water and pureed in a blender or food processor. Many of them, such as ripe banana, can be mashed fine with a fork. Fruits such as apples or pears require little or no water in the cooking process. Vegetables such as carrots, potatoes, or string beans require additional water in the cooking and blending process.

Preferably, home-prepared infant foods should be fresh or frozen, because canned foods, other than those prepared for infants, may contain excessive sodium or sugar or be a source of lead from the container. If sweetening is needed, refined sugar can be used, but honey and corn syrup are avoided because of the risk of infant botulism. There is no evidence that the addition of salt to foods such as vegetables increases the infant's acceptance of the new food.

Low-calorie foods should be avoided in infants and toddlers unless a strict, medically prescribed diet is required. The infant's growth during this phase is crucial to future development, and curtailing dietary fat should be done with great caution. Many parents may be concerned that their child is getting too much dietary fat; in such cases the primary practitioner should be consulted before dietary substitutions are made. On the other hand, making an infant or toddler finish a bottle or "clean up the plate" may lead to unhealthy eating habits (see Obesity, Chapter, 40).

NURSE ALERT • Although microwaving of bottles and baby food is not recommended, it remains a common practice. Guidelines have been developed for microwave heating of refrigerated formula, and these should be given to the family (Home Care box).

Home Care

MICROWAVE HEATING OF REFRIGERATED INFANT FORMULA

Before heating:
- Heat only 4 ounces or more.
- Heat only *refrigerated* formula.
- Always *stand* the bottle up.
- Always leave the bottle top *uncovered* to allow heat to escape.

Heating instructions (full power):
- Heat 4-ounce bottles for no more than 30 seconds.
- Heat 8-ounce bottles for no more than 45 seconds.

Serving instructions:
- Always replace nipple assembly; *invert* 10 times (vigorous shaking is unnecessary).
- Formula should be cool to the touch; formula warm to the touch may be too hot to serve.

Always *test* formula; place several drops on your tongue or on the back of the hand (not the inside wrist).

Modified from Sigman-Grant M, Bush G, Anantheswaran R: Microwave heating of infant formula: a dilemma resolved, *Pediatrics* 90(3):414, 1992.

Introduction of Solid Foods. When the spoon is first introduced, infants often push it away and appear dissatisfied. Some patience and skill are required to overcome this initial response. A small-bowled, straight, long-handled spoon, similar to a demitasse spoon, allows a small portion of food to be placed toward the back of the tongue. Food that is placed on the front of the tongue and pushed out is simply scooped up and refed. As infants become accustomed to the spoon, they more eagerly accept the food and eventually will open the mouth in anticipation (or keep it closed in dislike). Because the first introduction of food is a new experience, spoon feeding should be attempted after ingestion of some breast milk or formula to associate this activity with a pleasurable and satisfying experience. Trying to introduce a food *after* the entire milk feeding is usually useless because the infant is satiated and has no inclination to try something new.

After several spoon feedings, food can be introduced at the beginning of a meal. It is best to introduce many foods during the first year, when the infant is more likely to eat them because of a hearty appetite resulting from a rapid growth rate. During the toddler years eating becomes less of an adventure, and strong food preferences become evident.

One food item is introduced at intervals of 4 to 7 days to allow for identification of food allergies. New foods are fed in small amounts, from 1 teaspoon to a few tablespoons. As the amount of solid food increases, the quantity of milk is decreased to less than 1 L daily to prevent overfeeding.

Because feeding is a learning process, as well as a means of nutrition, new foods are given alone to allow the child to learn new tastes and textures. Food should not be mixed in the bottle and fed through a nipple with a large hole: this deprives the child of the pleasure of learning new tastes and of developing a discriminating palate. It can also cause problems with poor chewing of food later in life because of lack of experience. Guidelines for the introduction of new foods are given in the Home Care box.

The infant's first, second, and often twentieth try at self-feeding or cup feeding is a sloppy experience. Finger foods such as soft fruits or vegetables are just as good playthings as food; they can be squeezed, smeared, squashed, and thoroughly painted on oneself, others, and the surrounding environment. However, all of this is part of learning, and mastery follows many accidents.

Home Care

INTRODUCING SOLID FOODS TO INFANTS

Introduce solids when infant is hungry.

Begin spoon-feeding by pushing food to back of tongue because of infant's natural tendency to thrust the tongue forward.

Use a small spoon with a straight handle; begin with 1 or 2 teaspoons of food; gradually increase to a couple of tablespoons per feeding.

Introduce one food at a time, usually at intervals of 4 to 7 days to allow for identification of food allergies.

As the amount of solid food increases, decrease the quantity of milk to prevent overfeeding.

Do not introduce foods by mixing them with formula in the bottle.

A recommended resource is *Starting solids: a guide for parents and child care providers,* available from the National Association of Pediatric Nurse Associates and Practitioners (NAPNAP), 1101 Kings Highway North, Suite 206, Cherry Hill, NJ 08034-1931.

If parents find this experience distressing, a few suggestions may prove helpful. The feeding area should have a floor that can be easily wiped and is relatively far from walls, upholstered furniture, or drapes. A handheld portable vacuum is helpful in cleaning up crumbs. Messes are confined to one area if the child is seated in a high chair rather than allowed to crawl or walk around while drinking or eating. Infants should be expected to get themselves covered with food; therefore a large bib (plastic can be wiped easily but needs to be removed after feeding) should be used, as well as washable clothes that are easily removed. In a carpeted eating area, a bedsheet or washable drop cloth can be spread under the high chair to save on cleanup time and avoid frustration; the infant can be expected to drop food at this stage. High chairs can be thoroughly cleaned in a shower. Outdoor dining provides an excellent opportunity for practicing with a cup, spoon, or fingers because accidents are simple to hose or sweep away. Children cannot be pressured into eating neatly or into developing table manners before manipulative skill is acquired.

Preventing Obesity. The selection of solid foods is also an important aspect of controlling obesity. Approximately 20% of commercial baby foods contain less than 50 kcal/100 g, whereas another 20% contain more than 100 kcal/100 g. Choosing low-calorie foods can significantly lower the daily caloric intake without actually decreasing the total quantity of food. The use of sweet foods is kept to a minimum by not adding sugar to the formula or cereal and avoiding finger foods such as cookies. Other foods rich in calories that should be restricted in serving size rather than eliminated include butter, cream, ice cream, pudding, and chocolate.

Parents are encouraged to interpret the infant's signals of discomfort and intervene in ways other than through feeding. Crying, fussiness, and sucking do not necessarily indicate hunger. Rocking, stroking, holding, and offering a toy or a pacifier may be more appropriate than automatically responding with food.

Weaning. Defined as the process of giving up one method of feeding for another, *weaning* usually refers to relinquishing the breast or bottle for a cup. In Western societies this is generally regarded as a major task for infants and is often seen as a potentially traumatic experience. It is psychologically significant because the infant is required to give up a major source of oral pleasure and gratification.

There is no one time for weaning that is best for every child, but generally most infants show signs of readiness during the second half of the first year. They have learned that good things come from a spoon. Their increasing desire for freedom of movement may lessen their desire to be held close for feedings. They are acquiring more control over their actions and can easily manipulate a cup to their lips (even if it is held upside down!). Imitation becomes a powerful motivator by age 8 or 9 months, and they enjoy using a cup or glass like others do.

Weaning should be gradual, replacing one bottle- or breast-feeding at a time. The nighttime feeding is usually the last feeding to be discontinued. It is advisable never to begin allowing a child to take a bottle of milk to bed—this is a major cause of nursing caries in deciduous teeth. If breastfeeding is terminated before 5 or 6 months of age, weaning should be to a bottle to provide for the infant's continued sucking needs. If discontinued later, weaning can be directly to a cup, especially by age

12 to 14 months. Any sweet liquid, such as fruit juice, should be given in a cup.

Sleep and Activity

Sleep patterns vary among infants, with active infants typically sleeping less than placid children. Generally, by 3 to 4 months of age most infants have developed a nocturnal pattern of sleep that lasts 9 to 11 hours. The total daily sleep is approximately 15 hours. The number of naps per day varies, but infants may take one or two naps by the end of the first year. Breastfed infants usually sleep for less prolonged periods, with more frequent waking, especially during the night, than do bottle-fed infants. Because of the trend toward breastfeeding, sleep norms such as those previously described, which were based primarily on bottle-fed infants, may not be relevant.

Most infants are naturally active and need no encouragement to be mobile. However, problems can arise when devices such as playpens, strollers, commercial swings, and walkers are used excessively. These items restrict movement and prevent infants from exploring and developing gross motor skills. Contrary to popular belief, walkers do not enhance coordination and are dangerous if tipped over or placed near stairs. The American Academy of Pediatrics (1995) recommend a ban on the sale of infant walkers because of the large number of injuries. Newer models of infant walkers have been designed to decrease infant injuries (see Falls, p. 864).

NURSE ALERT • Formal infant exercise programs do not provide any long-term benefit to normal infants, and the possibility for damage to the infant's skeletal system exists. For these reasons, such programs are not recommended (American Academy of Pediatrics, 1988).

Sleep Problems. Concerns regarding sleep are common during infancy. Sometimes these concerns are as basic as parents' questioning if the infant needs additional sleep. In this case it is best to investigate the reason for their concern, stressing the individual needs of each child. Infants who are active during wakeful periods and growing normally are sleeping a sufficient amount of time.

However, there are a number of more serious concerns that require intervention. The more common sleep disturbances are a learned pattern or developmental characteristic of some infants (Table 36-3). Although many families may report sleep problems typical of these patterns, interventions are offered only when the pattern is disruptive to the family (Cultural Considerations box).

When a sleeping problem is presented, a careful assessment is essential. Charting sleep habits both before and after interventions is also an important strategy.* Questions regarding the frequency and duration of waking, the usual bedtime routine, the number of nighttime feedings, the perceived problem (e.g., how much disruption the behavior generates), and the attempted interventions are important in planning effective approaches designed for the specific sleep problem. A common suggestion given for any type of sleep problem—"let the child cry until he or she falls asleep"—is very difficult to implement and is inappropriate for certain conditions. Once the parents relent and console the child, they have only reinforced the crying.

An equally effective and more atraumatic approach to night crying, known as *graduated extinction,* is to let the child cry for progressively longer times between brief parental interventions that consist only of reassurance—not rocking, holding, or using a bottle or pacifier. For example, the parents may check on the child every 5 minutes during the first night and progressively extend this interval by 5 minutes on successive nights (Ferber and Kryger, 1995).

Families who cannot tolerate unexpected crying spells while everyone else is asleep can try the two-step approach. Graduated extinction is used during naps and at bedtime until the parents retire. If the child cries during the night, the parents use comforting measures. However, once the child is partially trained, step 2 is initiated—the use of graduated extinction at all times.

The best way to prevent sleep problems is to encourage parents to establish bedtime rituals that do not foster problematic patterns. One of the most constructive is placing infants *awake* in their own crib. When infants are accustomed to falling asleep somewhere else, such as in their parent's arms, and then being transferred to their crib, they awaken in unfamiliar surroundings and are unable to fall asleep until the routine is repeated. Also, the bed should be used for sleeping only—not as a playpen. It is advisable not to hang playthings over or on the bed; in this way the child associates the bed with sleep, not with activity. Although the interventions described previously and in Table 36-3 are usually successful, it is much easier to prevent the

*A 2-week sleep record for families is available in Wong DL, Hess CS: ***Wong and Whaley's clinical manual of pediatric nursing,*** ed 5, St Louis, 2000, Mosby.

Cultural Considerations

THE FAMILY BED

Co-sleeping, or the "family bed," in which parents allow the children to sleep with them, is a relatively common and accepted practice, especially among African-American, Hispanic,* and Asian-American families, such as the Japanese. Other groups that are adopting co-sleeping include (1) single parents, whose need for company may encourage this practice; (2) working parents, who desire the closeness at night that was lost during the day; and (3) parents who have had an issue about sleep or separation in their own past.† Recent concerns about the association of sudden infant death syndrome (SIDS) and co-sleeping appear to be unfounded. There is no scientific evidence to support infant co-sleeping with the mother as a potential risk factor for SIDS or as a preventive measure against the occurrence of SIDS.‡ A recent study, however, has reported an increase in the number of infant deaths by suffocation associated with bed sharing and the use of adult beds, particularly in infants younger than 3 months old.§

*Schachter F et al: Cosleeping and sleep problems in Hispanic-American urban young children, *Pediatrics* 84(3):522-530, 1989.
†Brazelton T: Parent-infant cosleeping revisited, *The Brazelton Center Newsletter,* vol 2, Boston, 1990.
‡American Academy of Pediatrics, Task Force on Infant Positioning and SIDS: Does bed sharing affect the risk of SIDS? *Pediatrics* 109(2):272-273, 1997.
§Drago DA, Dannenberg AL: Infant mechanical suffocating deaths in the United States, 1980-1997, *Pediatrics* 103(5):e59, 1999.

TABLE 36-3
Selected Sleep Disturbances During Infancy and Early Childhood

Disorder/Description	Management
NIGHTTIME FEEDING*	
Child has a prolonged need for middle-of-night bottle-feeding or breastfeeding Child goes to sleep at breast or with a bottle Awakenings are frequent (may be hourly) Child returns to sleep after feeding; other comfort measures (e.g., rocking or holding) are usually ineffective	Increase daytime feeding intervals to 4 hours or more (may need to be done gradually) Offer last feeding as late as possible at night; may need to gradually reduce amount of formula or length of breastfeeding Offer no bottles in bed Put to bed *awake* When child is crying, check at progressively longer intervals each night; reassure child but do not hold, rock, take to parent's bed, or give bottle or pacifier
DEVELOPMENTAL NIGHT CRYING	
Child age 6-12 months with undisturbed nighttime sleep now awakes abruptly; may be accompanied by nightmares	Parents should be reassured that this phase is temporary Enter room immediately to check on child but keep reassurances *brief* Avoid feeding, rocking, taking to parent's bed, or any other routine that may initiate trained night crying
TRAINED NIGHT CRYING* (INAPPROPRIATE SLEEP ASSOCIATIONS)	
Child typically falls asleep in place other than own bed (e.g., rocking chair or parent's bed) and is taken to own bed while asleep; on awakening, cries until usual routine is instituted (e.g., rocking)	Put child in own bed when *awake* If possible, arrange sleeping area separate from other family members When child is crying, check at progressively longer intervals each night; reassure child but do not resume usual routine
REFUSAL TO GO TO SLEEP*	
Child resists bedtime and comes out of room repeatedly Nighttime sleep may be continuous, but frequent awakenings and refusal to return to sleep may occur and become a problem if parent allows child to deviate from usual sleep pattern	Evaluate if hour of sleep is too early (child may resist sleep if not tired) Parents should be assisted in establishing consistent before-bedtime routine and enforcing consistent limits regarding child's bedtime behavior If child persists in leaving bedroom, close door for progressively longer periods Use reward system with child to provide motivation
NIGHTTIME FEARS	
Child resists going to bed or wakes during the night because of fears Child seeks parent's physical presence and falls asleep easily with parent nearby, unless fear is overwhelming	Evaluate if hour of sleep is too early (child may fantasize when nothing to do but think in dark room) Calmly reassure the frightened child; keeping a night light on may be helpful Use reward system with child to provide motivation to deal with fears Avoid patterns that can lead to additional problems (e.g., sleeping with child or taking child to parent's room) If child's fear is overwhelming, consider desensitization (e.g., progressively spending longer periods of time alone; consult professional help for protracted fears) Distinguish between nightmares and sleep terrors (confused partial arousals)

Modified from Ferber R: Behavioral "insomnia" in the child, *Psychiatr Clin North Am* 10(4):641-653, 1987.
*Guidelines for parents in dealing with these sleep problems are in Wong DL, Hess CS: ***Wong and Whaley's clinical manual of pediatric nursing,*** ed 5, St Louis, 2000, Mosby.

problem with appropriate counseling during the early months of the infant's life.*

*An excellent resource for parents is *Solve Your Child's Sleep Problems* by Richard Ferber (1986, Simon & Shuster Trade; 1-800-223-2336; website: www.simonsays.com). Available in Spanish.

Dental Health

Good dental hygiene begins as soon as the primary teeth erupt. The teeth and gums are initially cleaned by wiping with a damp cloth; toothbrushing is too harsh for the tender gingiva. The caregiver can stabilize the infant by cradling the child with one arm and using the free hand to cleanse the teeth. Oral hygiene can be made pleasant by singing or talking to the infant. There are no clear guidelines regarding when toothbrushing should begin. It is generally recommended that a small, soft-bristled toothbrush be used as more teeth erupt and the infant adjusts to the routine of cleaning. Water is preferred to toothpaste, which the infant will swallow (and if the toothpaste is fluoridated, the infant will ingest excessive amounts of fluoride).

Fluoride, an essential mineral for building caries-resistant teeth, is needed beginning at 6 months of age if the infant does not receive water that has an adequate fluoride content. The American Academy of Pediatrics (1998b) and the American Academy of Pediatric Dentists no longer recommend fluoride supplementation from birth to 6 months. The fluoride dosage has been decreased from earlier recommendations because of an increased occurrence of dental fluorosis from excessive fluoride ingestion. The latest recommendation is to give children 6 months to 3 years of age 0.25 mg fluoride daily if water fluoride content is less than 0.3 ppm (parts per million) (American Academy of Pediatrics, 1998b).

Dietary considerations are also important because habits begun during infancy tend to continue into later years. Foods with concentrated sugar are used sparingly (if at all) in the infant's diet. The practice of coating pacifiers with honey or using commercially available hard-candy pacifiers is discouraged. Besides being cariogenic, honey also may cause infant botulism, and parts of the candy pacifier can be aspirated (see Aspiration of Foreign Objects, p. 859). Parents need to be counseled regarding the detrimental effects of frequent and prolonged bottle- or breastfeeding during sleep, when the sweet milk or other fluid, such as juice, bathes the teeth, producing *nursing caries.* (See also Chapter 37 for a more extensive discussion of dental care, including nursing caries.)

Immunizations

One of the most dramatic advances in pediatrics has been the decline of infectious diseases during the twentieth century because of the widespread use of immunization for preventable diseases. Although many of the immunizations can be given to individuals of any age, the recommended primary schedule begins during infancy and, with the exception of boosters, is completed during early childhood. Therefore the discussion of childhood immunizations for diphtheria, tetanus, pertussis (DTaP using acellular pertussis); polio; measles, mumps, rubella (MMR); *Haemophilus influenzae* type b (Hib); hepatitis B virus (HBV); pneumococcal; and chickenpox is included under health promotion during infancy. Selected vaccines generally reserved for children considered at high risk for the disease are discussed here and as appropriate throughout the text. (See also Communicable Diseases, Chapter 38, for a discussion of several of the diseases for which vaccines are available.)

Schedule for Immunizations. In the United States two organizations—the Advisory Committee on Immunization Practices (ACIP) of the Centers for Disease Control and Prevention (CDC), and the Committee on Infectious Diseases of the American Academy of Pediatrics (AAP)—govern the recommendations for immunization policies and procedures. In Canada, recommendations are from the National Advisory Committee on Immunization under the authority of the Minister of National Health and Welfare. The policies of each committee are *recommendations,* not rules, and they change as a result of advances in the field of immunology. Nurses need to keep informed of the latest advances and changes in policy.

In the United States the recommended age for beginning primary immunizations of infants is at birth (Table 36-4). Children born prematurely should receive the full dose of each vaccine at the appropriate chronologic age. Recommended schedules for children not immunized during infancy are included in Table 36-5. Table 36-6 describes immunization schedules for Canadian children.

Children who began primary immunization at the recommended age, but fail to receive all of the doses, do not need to begin the series again but instead receive only the missed doses. For situations in which there is doubt that the child will return for immunization according to the optimum schedule, any of the recommended vaccines can be administered simultaneously. Parenteral vaccines are given in separate syringes in different injection sites (American Academy of Pediatrics, 2000a).

Recommendations for Routine Immunizations

Hepatitis B Virus (HBV). HBV is an important pediatric disease because HBV infections that occur during childhood and adolescence can lead to fatal consequences from cirrhosis or liver cancer during adulthood. Up to 90% of infants infected perinatally and 25% to 50% of children infected before age 5 years become HBV carriers. In addition, the incidence of HBV infection increases rapidly during adolescence (American Academy of Pediatrics, 2000a). Both full-term and preterm infants born to mothers whose HBsAg status is positive or unknown should receive hepatitis B vaccine and hepatitis B immune globulin (HBIG) 0.5 ml within 12 hours of birth at two different injection sites. The American Academy of Pediatrics (2000a) also encourages immunization of all children by age 11 to 12 years.

The vaccine is given intramuscularly in the vastus lateralis in newborns or in the deltoid for older infants and children. Regardless of age, the dorsogluteal site is avoided because it has been associated with low antibody seroconversion rates, indicating a reduced immune response (Zuckerman, Cockcroft, and Zuckerman, 1992). No data exist regarding the seroconversion when the ventrogluteal site is used.

Hepatitis A Virus (HAV). HAV has recently been recognized as a significant child health problem, particularly in communities with unusually high infection rates. HAV is spread by the fecal-oral route and from person-to-person contact, mostly by ingestion of contaminated food or water, and only rarely by blood transfusion. The illness has an abrupt onset with fever, malaise, anorexia, nausea, abdominal discomfort, dark urine, and jaundice being the most common clinical signs of infection. In children under 6 years of age, who represent approximately one-third of all cases of HAV, the disease may be asymptomatic, and jaundice is rarely evident. Children living in communities with high infection rates should be immunized with either Havrix or Vaqta vaccine, given by the intramuscular route in the deltoid. These vaccines are recommended for children 2 years of age and older, in two doses administered at least 6 months apart (Prevention of hepatitis A, 1999). For further information, see footnote i in Table 36-4.

Diphtheria. Diphtheria vaccine is commonly administered: (1) in combination with tetanus and pertussis vaccines (DTaP) or DTaP and Hib vaccines for children younger than 7 years of age; (2) in combination with a conjugate *H. influenza* type B vaccine (see Table 36-4); (3) in a combined vaccine with tetanus (DT) for children younger than 7 years of age who have some contraindication to receiving pertussis vaccine; (4) in

TABLE 36-4

Recommended Childhood Immunization Schedule United States, January-December 2001[a]

Age ▶ / Vaccine ▼	Birth	1 mo	2 mo	4 mo	6 mo	12 mo	15 mo	18 mo	24 mo	4-6 yr	11-12 yr	14-16 yr
Hepatitis B[b]	Hep B											
			Hep B		Hep B						(Hep B[b])	
Diphtheria, Tetanus, Pertussis[c]			DTaP	DTaP	DTaP		DTaP[c]			DTaP	Td	
H. influenzae type b[d]			Hib	Hib	Hib	Hib						
Polio[e]			IPV	IPV	IPV[e]					IPV[e]		
Pneumococcal[f]			PCV	PCV	PCV	PCV						
Measles, Mumps, Rubella[g]						MMR				MMR[g]	(MMR[g])	
Varicella[h]						Var					(Var[h])	
Hepatitis A[i]									Hep A[i]-in selected areas			

Vaccines are listed under routinely recommended ages. [Bars] indicate range of recommended ages for immunization. Any dose not given at the recommended age should be given as a "catch-up" immunization at any subsequent visit when indicated and feasible. (Ovals) indicate vaccines to be given if previously recommended doses were missed or given earlier than the recommended minimum age.

From American Academy of Pediatrics, Committee on Infectious Diseases: Recommended childhood immunization schedule—United States, *Pediatrics* 107(1):202-203, 2001. Approved by the Advisory Committee on Immunization Practices (ACIP), the American Academy of Pediatrics (AAP), and the American Academy of Family Physicians (AAFP).

[a]This schedule indicates the recommended ages for routine administration of currently licensed childhood vaccines, as of 11/1/00, for children through 18 years of age. Additional vaccines may be licensed and recommended during the year. Licensed combination vaccines may be used whenever any components of the combination are indicated and its other components are not contraindicated. Providers should consult the manufacturer's package inserts for detailed recommendations.

[b]***Infants born to HBsAg-negative mothers*** should receive the 1st dose of hepatitis B (Hep B) vaccine by age 2 months. The 2nd dose should be at least one month after the 1st dose. The 3rd dose should be administered at least 4 months after the 1st dose and at least 2 months after the 2nd dose; but not before 6 months of age for infants.

Infants born to HBsAg-positive mothers should receive hepatitis B vaccine and 0.5 mL hepatitis B immune globulin (HBIG) within 12 hours of birth at separate sites. The 2nd dose is recommended at 1-2 months of age and the 3rd dose at 6 months of age.

Infants born to mothers whose HBsAg status is unknown should receive hepatitis B vaccine within 12 hours of birth. Maternal blood should be drawn at the time of delivery to determine the mother's HBsAg status; if the HBsAg test is positive, the infant should receive HBIG as soon as possible (no later than 1 week of age).

All children and adolescents who have not been immunized against hepatitis B should begin the series during any visit. Special efforts should be made to immunize children who were born in or whose parents were born in areas of the world with moderate or high endemicity of hepatitis B virus infection.

[c]The 4th dose of DTaP (diphtheria and tetanus toxoids and acellular pertussis vaccine) may be administered as early as 12 months of age, provided 6 months have elapsed since the 3rd dose and the child is unlikely to return at age 15-18 months. Td (tetanus and diphtheria toxoids) is recommended at 11-12 years of age if at least 5 years have elapsed since the last dose of DTP, DTaP or DT. Subsequent routine Td boosters are recommended every 10 years.

[d]Three *Haemophilus influenzae* type b (Hib) conjugate vaccines are licensed for infant use. If PRP-OMP (PedvaxHIB® or ComVax® [Merck]) is administered at 2 and 4 months of age, a dose at 6 months is not required. Because clinical studies in infants have demonstrated that using some combination products may induce a lower immune response to the Hib vaccine component, DTaP/Hib combination products should not be used for primary immunization in infants at 2, 4 or 6 months of age, unless FDA-approved for these ages.

[e]An all-IPV schedule is recommended for routine childhood polio vaccination in the United States. All children should receive four doses of IPV at 2 months, 4 months, 6-18 months, and 4-6 years of age. Oral polio vaccine (OPV) should be used only in selected circumstances. (See *MMWR* May 19, 2000/49[RR-5];1-22.)

[f]The heptavalent conjugate pneumococcal vaccine (PCV) is recommended for all children 2-23 months of age. It also is recommended for certain children 24-59 months of age. (See *MMWR* Oct. 6, 2000/49[RR-9]:1-35).

[g]The 2nd dose of measles, mumps, and rubella (MMR) vaccine is recommended routinely at 4-6 years of age but may be administered during any visit, provided at least 4 weeks have elapsed since receipt of the 1st dose and that both doses are administered beginning at or after 12 months of age. Those who have not previously received the second dose should complete the schedule by the 11-12 year old visit.

[h]Varicella (Var) vaccine is recommended at any visit on or after the first birthday for susceptible children, i.e., those who lack a reliable history of chickenpox (as judged by a health care provider) and who have not been immunized. Susceptible persons 13 years of age or older should receive 2 doses, given at least 4 weeks apart.

[i]Hepatitis A (Hep A) is recommended in selected states and/or regions, and for certain high risk groups; consult your local public health authority. (See *MMWR* Oct. 1, 1999/48[RR-12]; 1-37.)

For additional information about the vaccines listed above, please visit the National Immunization Program Home Page at www.cdc.gov/nip or call the National Immunization Hotline at 800-232-2522 (English) or 800-232-0233 (Spanish).

From AAP News, Jan 2001.

TABLE 36-5

Recommended Immunization Schedules for Children Not Immunized in the First Year of Life*

Recommended Time/Age	Immunization(s)†,‡	Comments
YOUNGER THAN 7 YEARS		
First visit	DTaP, Hib, HBV, MMR, PCV7§	If indicated, tuberculin testing may be done at same visit. If child is 5 years of age or older, Hib is not indicated in most circumstances.
Interval after first visit		
1 month (4 weeks)	DTaP, IPV, HBV, Var‖	The second dose of IPV may be given if accelerated poliomyelitis immunization is necessary, such as for travelers to areas where polio is endemic.
2 months	DTaP, Hib, IPV	Second dose of Hib is indicated only if first dose was received when younger than 15 months.
≥8 months	DTaP, HBV, IPV	IPV and HBV are not given if third doses were given earlier.
Age 4-6 years (at or before school entry)	DTaP, IPV, MMR¶	DTaP is not necessary if fourth dose was given after fourth birthday; IPV is not necessary if third dose was given after fourth birthday.
7-12 YEARS		
First visit	HBV, MMR¶, Td, IPV	
Interval after first visit	HBV, MMR, Var,‖ Td, IPV	IPV also may be given 1 month after first visit if accelerated poliomyelitis immunization is necessary.
2 months (8 weeks)		
8-14 months	HBV,** Td, IPV	IPV is not given if third dose was given earlier.
Age 11-12 years	See Table 36-4	

From American Academy of Pediatrics, Committee on Infectious Diseases, Pickering L, editor: *2000 Red Book: report of the Committee on Infectious Diseases,* ed 25, Elk Grove Village, IL 2000, The Academy.
*Table is not completely consistent with all package inserts. For products used, also consult manufacturer's package insert for instructions on storage, handling, dosage, and administration. Biologics prepared by different manufacturers may vary, and package inserts of the same manufacturer may change. Therefore the physician should be aware of the contents of the current package insert.
†If all needed vaccines cannot be administered simultaneously, priority should be given to protecting the child against those diseases that pose the greatest immediate risk. In the United States, these diseases for children younger than 2 years usually are measles and *H. influenzae* type b infection; for children older than 7 years, they are measles, mumps, and rubella. Before 13 years of age, immunity against hepatitis B and varicella should be ensured.
‡DTaP, HBV, Hib, MMR, and Var can be given simultaneously at separate sites if failure of the patient to return for future immunizations is a concern.
§PCV7 (Prevnar) is administered 6-8 weeks apart as follows: at 7-11 months 2 doses with booster, 12-15 months, and 12-23 months. Immunization with PCV7 and 23PS is recommended for children 24-59 months who are at ***high risk*** of invasive pneumococcal infection (see p. 855).
‖Varicella vaccine can be administered to susceptible children any time after 12 months of age. Unvaccinated children who lack a reliable history of chickenpox should be vaccinated before their thirteenth birthday.
¶Minimal interval between doses of MMR is 1 month (4 weeks).
**HBV may be given earlier in a 0-, 2-, and 4-month schedule.
HBV, Hepatitis B virus vaccine; *Var,* varicella vaccine; *DTaP,* diphtheria and tetanus toxoids and acellular pertussis vaccine; *Hib, Haemophilus influenzae* type b conjugate; *IPV,* inactivated poliovirus; *MMR,* live measles, mumps, and rubella; *Td,* adult tetanus toxoid (full dose) and diphtheria toxoid (reduced dose for children ≥7 years and adults); *PCV7,* pneumococcal vaccine for children <5 years.

smaller doses (15% to 20% of that in DTaP or DT) with tetanus vaccine (Td) for use in children age 7 years and older; or (5) as a single antigen when combined antigen preparations are not indicated. Although the diphtheria vaccine does not produce absolute immunity, protective antitoxin persists for 10 years or more when given according to the recommended schedule, and boosters are given every 10 years for life.

Tetanus. Three forms of tetanus vaccine are available: tetanus toxoid, tetanus immune globulin (TIG) (human), and tetanus antitoxin (usually horse serum). Tetanus toxoid is used for routine primary immunization, usually in one of the combinations listed for diphtheria, and provides protective antitoxin levels for 10 years or more.

For wound management, passive immunity is available with TIG. In persons with a history of two previous doses of tetanus toxoid, a booster dose of the toxoid can be given. Separate syringes and different sites are used when tetanus toxoid and TIG are given concurrently. Table 36-7 presents a summary of the recommended procedure for tetanus prophylaxis in wound management.

Pertussis. Pertussis vaccine is recommended for all children 6 weeks through 6 years of age (up to the seventh birthday) who have no neurologic contraindications to its use. It is not given to children 7 years or older because the risk of side effects from the vaccine increases as the incidence, severity, and fatality of the disease decrease.

Currently, two forms of pertussis vaccine are available in the United States. The *whole-cell pertussis vaccine* is prepared from inactivated cells of *Bordetella pertussis* and contains multiple antigens. In contrast, the *acellular* pertussis vaccine contains one or more immunogens derived from the *B. pertussis* organism. The highly purified acellular vaccine is associated with fewer local and systemic reactions than those occurring with the whole-cell vaccine in children of similar age. The acellular pertussis vaccine is recommended by the American Academy of Pediatrics (2000a, b) for the first three immunizations and is usually given

TABLE 36-6
Routine Immunization for Infants and Children—Provincial and Territorial Schedules, Canada

Province or Territory	DTaP (Months)	Polio-IPV (Months)	Hib (Months)	Td/Td-IPV (Years)	Hepatitis B (3 doses)	MMR (First Dose) (Months)	MMR/MR (Second (Dose)
Alberta	2, 4, 6, 18 (and 4-6 years)	2, 4, 6, 18 (and 4-6 years)	2, 4, 6, 18	Td, 14-16	Grade 5	12	MMR, 4-6 years
British Columbia	2, 4, 6, 18 (and 4-6 years)[a]	2, 4, 6, 18 (and 4-6 years)[a]	2, 4, 6, 18	Td, 14-16	Grade 6	12	MMR, 18 months
Manitoba	2, 4, 6, 18 (and 4-6 years)	2, 4, 6, 18 (and 4-6 years)	2, 4, 6, 18	Td, 14-16	Not planned	12	MMR, 5 years
Newfoundland	2, 4, 6, 18 (and 4-6 years)	2, 4, 6, 18 (and 4-6 years)	2, 4, 6, 18	Td-IPV, 14-16	Grade 4	12	MMR, 18 months
New Brunswick	2, 4, 6, 18 (and 4-6 years)[b]	2, 4, 6, 18 (and 4-6 years)[c]	2, 4, 6, 18	Td-IPV, 14-16[c]	Infants 0, 2, 12 months or grade 4[d]	12	MMR, 18 months
Northwest Territories	2, 4, 6, 18 (and 4-6 years)[e]	2, 4, 6, 18 (and 4-6 years)[e]	2, 4, 6, 18	Td-IPV, 14-16[f]	Infants 0, 1, 6 months or grade 4[g]	12	MMR, 18 months
Nova Scotia	2, 4, 6, 18 (and 4-6 years)	2, 4, 6, 18 (and 4-6 years)	2, 4, 6, 18	Td-IPV, 14-16	Grade 4	12	MMR, 4-6 years
Ontario	2, 4, 6, 18 (and 4-6 years)[h]	2, 4, 6, 18 (and 4-6 years)[h]	2, 4, 6, 18	Td-IPV, 14-16[i]	Grade 7	12	MMR, 4-6 years
Prince Edward Island	2, 4, 6, 18 (and 4-6 years)	2, 4, 6, 18 (and 4-6 years)	2, 4, 6, 18	Td-IPV, 14-16	Infants 2, 4, 15 months, or grade 3[j]	12	MMR, 18 months[k]
Quebec	2, 4, 6, 18 (and 4-6 years)	2, 4, 6, 18 (and 4-6 years)[l]	2, 4, 6, 18	Td-IPV, 14-16[l]	Grade 4	12	MMR, 18 months
Saskatchewan	2, 4, 6, 18 (and 4-6 years)[m]	2, 4, 6, 18 (and 4-6 years)[m]	2, 4, 6, 18	Td, 14-16[n]	Grade 6	12	MR, 18 months
Yukon Territory	2, 4, 6, 18 (and 4-6 years)	2, 4, 6, 18 (and 4-6 years)	2, 4, 6, 18	Td-IPV, 14-16	Grade 4	12	MMR, 18 months

From Health Canada: *Paediatr Child Health,* vol 3, supp B, March/April 1998; website: http://www.hc-sc.gc.ca/main/lcdc/web/publicat/paediatr/vol3supb/pche_j.html#tab6.

[a]In British Columbia a fifth dose of diphtheria, tetanus, and acellular pertussis (DTaP) and inactivated polio vaccine (IPV) at 4 to 6 years is not necessary if the fourth dose was given after the fourth birthday.
[b]In New Brunswick whole-cell pertussis vaccine was used through 1997.
[c]In New Brunswick polio vaccine at 14 to 16 years is not required if the child has completed the primary series and received 1 or more doses of oral polio vaccine (OPV) in the past.
[d]In New Brunswick hepatitis B vaccination is currently given to children in grade 4 who have not been vaccinated in infancy.
[e]In Northwest Territories a fifth dose of DTaP and IPV at 4 to 6 years is not necessary if the fourth dose was given after the fourth birthday.
[f]In Northwest Territories polio vaccine at 14 to 16 years is not required if the child has completed the primary series and received 1 or more doses of OPV in the past.
[g]In Northwest Territories hepatitis b vaccination is currently given to children in grade 4 who have not been vaccinated in infancy.
[h]In Ontario a fifth dose of DTaP and IPV at 4 to 6 years is not necessary if the fourth dose was given after the fourth birthday.
[i]In Ontario polio vaccine at 14 to 16 years is not required if the child has completed the primary series and received 1 or more doses of OPV in the past (OPV was used routinely from January 1990 through March 1993).
[j]In Prince Edward Island hepatitis B vaccination is currently given to children in grade 3 who have not been vaccinated in infancy.
[k]In Prince Edward Island a second measles, mumps, and rubella (MMR) vaccine dose is currently given to children 4 to 6 years of age who would not have received their second dose at 18 months.
[l]In Quebec polio vaccine doses at 4 to 6 years and at 14 to 16 years are omitted if OPV was used for earlier doses.
[m]In Saskatchewan a fifth dose of DTaP and a fifth dose of IPV at 4 to 6 years are not necessary if the fourth dose was given after the fourth birthday.
[n]In Saskatchewan polio vaccine at 14 to 16 years is given only if 1 dose of OPV was not received in the past.
Hib, Haemophilus influenzae b vaccine; *MR,* measles and rubella vaccine; *Td,* tetanus diphtheria toxoid adult-type.

TABLE 36-7
Guide to Tetanus Prophylaxis in Routine Wound Management, 1997

History of Adsorbed Tetanus Toxoid (Doses)	Clean, Minor Wounds		All Other Wounds*	
	Td†	TIG	Td†	TIG
Unknown or <three	Yes	No	Yes	Yes
≥Three‡	No§	No	No‖	No

Data from American Academy of Pediatrics, Committee on Infectious Diseases, Pickering L, editor: *2000 Red Book: report of the Committee on Infectious Diseases,* ed 25, Elk Grove Village, IL, 2000, The Academy.
*Such as, but not limited to, wounds contaminated with dirt, feces, soil, and saliva; puncture wounds; avulsions; and wounds resulting from missiles, crushing, burns, and frostbite.
†For children <7 years old: DTaP (DT, if pertussis vaccine is contraindicated) is preferred to tetanus toxoid alone. For persons ≥7 years of age, Td is preferred to tetanus toxoid alone.
‡If only three doses of *fluid* toxoid have been received, then a fourth dose of toxoid, preferably an adsorbed toxoid, should be given.
§Yes, if >10 years since last dose.
‖Yes, if >5 year since last dose. (More frequent boosters are not needed and can accentuate side effects.)

at 2, 4, and 6 months of age with diphtheria and tetanus (DTaP). Four forms of acellular pertussis vaccine are currently licensed for use in infants: Acel-Imune, Tripedia, Certiva, and Infanrix (diphtheria, tetanus toxoid, and acellular pertussis conjugate).

Polio. In July 1999 the ACIP recommended an all-IPV schedule for routine childhood polio vaccination. Since January 2000, all children should receive four doses of IPV (i.e., at 2 months, 4 months, 6 to 18 months, and 4 to 6 years of age) (Advisory Committee on Immunization Practices, 1999; American Academy of Pediatrics, 1999a).

The change from the exclusive use of OPV to the exclusive use of IPV is related to the rare occurrence of *vaccine-associated polio paralysis (VAPP)* from OPV. The exclusive use of IPV eliminates the risk of VAPP but is associated with an increased number of injections and increased cost.

Measles. The measles (rubeola) vaccine is given at 12 to 15 months of age. During the course of measles outbreaks, the vaccine can be given any time after 6 months of age, followed by a second inoculation after age 12 months.

Because of continued outbreaks of measles among unvaccinated preschool-age children and among vaccinated school-age children and college students, a second measles immunization is recommended at 4 to 6 years of age (at school entry) or revaccination by 11 to 12 years of age if only the measles vaccine has been administered (American Academy of Pediatrics, 1998a). Revaccination should include all individuals born after 1956 who have not received two doses of measles vaccine after 12 months of age. Individuals born before this date are thought to be immune from exposure to natural measles virus.

Mumps. Mumps virus vaccine is recommended for children at 12 to 15 months of age and is typically given in combination with measles and rubella. It should not be administered to infants younger than 12 months because persisting maternal antibodies can interfere with the immune response.

Because of recent outbreaks of the disease, especially in children 10 to 19 years of age, mumps immunization is recommended for all individuals born after 1957 who may be susceptible to mumps (i.e., those who have no history of having had the disease or vaccine and when there is no laboratory evidence of immunity).

Rubella. Rubella is a relatively mild infection in children, but in a pregnant woman the actual infection presents serious risks to the developing fetus. Therefore the aim of rubella immunization is actually to protect the unborn child rather than the recipient of the immunization.

Rubella immunization is recommended for all children at 12 to 15 months of age, and is administered in a combined form with measles and mumps vaccine. Increased emphasis should also be placed on vaccinating all unimmunized prepubertal children and susceptible adolescents and adult women in the childbearing age group.

Because the live attenuated virus may cross the placenta and theoretically may present a risk to the developing fetus, rubella vaccine is not given to any pregnant woman. Although this is standard practice, current evidence from women who received the vaccine while pregnant and delivered unaffected offspring indicates that the risk to the fetus is negligible. In addition, there is no reported danger of administering rubella vaccine to a child if the mother is pregnant.

Pneumococcal. Pneumococcal infections are the most common invasive bacterial infections in children in the United States. The incidence of invasive pneumococcal infections peaks in young children, reaching rates of 228 in 100,000 in children 6 to 12 months of age (Overturf, 2000). Children at *highest risk* include those with congenital or acquired asplenia or splenic dysfunction, human immunodeficiency virus, congenital immune deficiency, chronic cardiac or pulmonary disease, cerebrospinal fluid leaks, chronic renal insufficiency, diseases associated with immunosuppressive therapy, and diabetes mellitus. Children at moderate risk include all children 23 to 45 months of age, children 36 to 59 months attending out-of-home care, and children 36 to 59 months old who are of Native American or African-American descent (Overturf, 2000).

Heptavalent pneumococcal conjugate vaccine (PCV) is recommended for universal use in children 23 months and younger. The vaccine can be given concurrently with other childhood vaccines at 2, 4, 6, and 12 to 15 months of age. Children at *highest risk* for invasive pneumococcal infection should receive both PCV and 23PS vaccines.

Safety and efficacy of PCV and 23PS in children 24 months or older at *moderate or lower risk* of invasive pneumococcal infection remains under investigation. Current FDA indications are for administration of PCV only to children younger than 24 months. However, all children 24 to 59 months old, whether or not they are a low or moderate risk, may benefit from the administration of pneumococcal immunizations. Therefore, a single dose of PCV or 23PS vaccine may be given to children 24 months or older. The 23PS is an acceptable alternative to PCV, although an enhanced immune response and probable reduction of nasopharyngeal carriage favor the use of PCV.

Haemophilus Influenzae Type B (Hib). Hib conjugate vaccines provide protection against a number of serious infections caused by Hib, especially bacterial meningitis, epiglottitis, bacterial pneumonia, septic arthritis, and sepsis (Hib is not associated with the viruses that cause influenza, or "flu"). Several Hib vaccines are available; some are combination vaccines, such as *Comvax* (Hib and HBV). These conjugate vaccines connect Hib to a nontoxic form of another organism, such as meningococcal protein or diphtheria protein. There is *no* antibody response to these nontoxic proteins, but they significantly improve the antibody response to Hib, especially in infants. The use of combination vaccines provides equivalent immunogenicity and decreases the number of injections an infant receives; however, it is important that they be given to the appropriate-age child.

When possible, the Hib conjugate vaccine used at the first vaccination should be used for all subsequent vaccinations in the primary series. All Hib vaccines are administered by intramuscular injection using a separate syringe and at a separate site from any concurrent vaccinations.

Varicella. Administration of the cell-free live-attenuated varicella vaccine (*Varivax*) is recommended for healthy children 12 to 18 months of age. A single dose of 0.5 ml should be given by subcutaneous injection. From the age of 19 months to the thirteenth birthday, a single dose of varicella vaccine may be given at any time to children who may be susceptible, either by lack of proof of varicella vaccination or a reliable history of varicella infection (American Academy of Pediatrics, 2000a). The vaccine should be kept frozen in the lyophilized form (stable particles that readily go into solution) and used within 30 minutes of being reconstituted to ensure viral potency (American Academy of Pediatrics, 2000a).

Varicella vaccine may be administered simultaneously with MMR. However, separate syringes and injection sites should be used. If they are not administered simultaneously, the interval between administration of varicella vaccine and MMR should be at least 1 month. Varicella vaccine may also be given simultaneously with DTaP, IPV, HBV, and/or Hib (American Academy of Pediatrics, 2000a, b).

Recommendations for Selected Immunizations. Several additional vaccines are recommended for children at high risk for particular diseases. Most of these children have chronic disorders or impaired immune systems that make them more susceptible to certain infections than the general population. Selected immunizations are presented in Table 36-8. Others, such as the rabies vaccine, are discussed elsewhere in this text.

Reactions. Vaccines used for routine immunizations are among the safest and most reliable drugs available. However, minor side effects do occur following many of the immunizations and, rarely, a serious reaction may result from the vaccine.

With inactivated antigens, such as DTaP, side effects are most likely to occur within a few hours or days of administration and are usually limited to local tenderness, erythema, and swelling at the injection site; low-grade fever; and behavioral changes (e.g., drowsiness. fretfulness, eating less, and prolonged or unusual cry). Local reactions tend to be less severe when the del-

TABLE 36-8
Recommendations for Selected Nonmandated Vaccines

Description	Administration/Precautions
INFLUENZA VIRUS VACCINE (SEVERAL TRADE NAMES)	
Afford protection against strains of influenza. Recommended for children 6 months of age and older with chronic disorders of cardiovascular or pulmonary systems, including asthma, whose severity warranted regular medical care or hospitalization during preceding year. Other eligible children include those with diabetes mellitus, renal dysfunction, anemia, immunosuppression, human immunodeficiency virus (HIV) infection, or those receiving long-term aspirin therapy (because of risk of developing Reye syndrome after influenza infection).	Administered in fall, preferably November; repeated yearly Intramuscular injection; 2 doses of split vaccine at least 4 weeks apart for children 12 years of age or younger; 1 dose of split or whole vaccine for children older than 12 years of age Contraindicated in persons with anaphylactic hypersensitivity to eggs May be given simultaneously with other childhood immunizations but at separate site
MENINGOCOCCAL POLYSACCHARIDE VACCINE (MENOMUNE)	
Affords protection against *Neisseria meningitidis:* sero-groups A, C, Y, and W-135. Recommended for children 2 years of age and older with terminal complement deficiencies and anatomic or functional asplenia.	Subcutaneous injection Duration of protection unknown Safety during pregnancy not established
LYME DISEASE VACCINE (LYMErix)	
Affords protection against infection with the spirochete *Borrelia burgdorferi,* which causes Lyme disease (LD). Recommended for individuals 15 to 70 years of age who are at high risk for LD from significant exposure to tick habitats in endemic areas (northeast and north-central United States) and for those who have been infected with LD.	Intramuscular injection in deltoid muscle Administered on 0-, 1-, and 12-month schedule. Doses 2 and 3 should be given several weeks before *B. burgdorferi* season, which usually begins in April.

toid rather than the vastus lateralis site is used, and when a needle of sufficient length to deposit the vaccine in the muscle is used (Atraumatic Care box). Rarely, more severe reactions may occur, especially with pertussis (see Table 36-9). Reactions to DTaP tend to be more severe if they occurred with a previous immunization.

Hib vaccine is one of the safest vaccines available but may be associated with low-grade fever and mild local reactions at the site of injection, which resolve rapidly. Fever (i.e., temperature more than 38.5° C [101.3° F]) may rarely occur.

Unlike the inactivated antigens, live attenuated virus vaccines such as MMR and OPV multiply for days or weeks, and unfavorable reactions and "vaccine-associated" disorders can occur for 30 to 60 days. These reactions are usually mild, although reactions to rubella tend to be more troublesome in older children and adults.

Contraindications/Precautions. Nurses need to be aware of the reasons for withholding immunizations—both for the child's safety in terms of avoiding reactions and for the child's maximum benefit from receiving the vaccine. Unfounded fears and lack of knowledge regarding contraindications can needlessly prevent a child from having protection from life-threatening diseases. For the contraindications to the usual childhood vaccines, see Table 36-9.

Administration. The principal precautions in administering immunizations include proper storage of the vaccine to protect its potency and institution of recommended procedures for injection. The nurse must be familiar with the manufacturer's directions for storage and reconstitution of the vaccine. For example, if the vaccine is to be refrigerated, it should be stored on a center shelf and not in the door, where frequent temperature increases from opening the refrigerator can alter the vaccine's potency. For protection against light, the vial can be wrapped in aluminum foil. Periodic checks are established to ensure that no vaccine is used after its expiration date.

The DTaP vaccines contain the adjuvant alum to retain the antigen at the injection site and prolong the stimulatory effect. Because subcutaneous or intracutaneous injection of the adjuvant can cause local irritation, inflammation, or abscess formation, attention to excellent intramuscular injection technique must be used (Atraumatic Care box).

The total series requires several injections, and every attempt is made to rotate the sites and administer the injections as painlessly as possible (see discussion on intramuscular injections in Chapter 45). When two or more injections are given at separate sites, the order of injections is arbitrary. Some practitioners suggest injecting the less painful one first. Some believe this is DTaP, whereas others suggest the MMR or Hib vaccine. Still others advocate injecting at two sites simultaneously (which requires two operators).

A recent study found that children between the ages of 4 and 6 years rated sequential injections for immunizations vs. simultaneous injections as being equally successful (Horn and McCarthy, 1999). Parents in the study preferred simultaneous immunization injections.

Because allergic reactions can occur after injection of vaccines, appropriate precautions are taken (see Anaphylaxis, Chapter 48).

Another important nursing responsibility is accurate documentation. Each child should have an immunization record for parents to keep, especially for families who move often. A survey of the accuracy of parental recall of children's immunizations found that parents underestimated the number of polio, DTaP, and MMR vaccines. The accuracy rate was not related to ethnic background, education level, or insurance coverage. Although immunization rates have increased significantly, health professionals should use every opportunity to encourage complete immunization of all children.

The following information is documented on the medical record: day, month, and year of administration; manufacturer and lot number of vaccine; and the name, address, and title of the person administering the vaccine. Additional data to record are the site and route of administration and evidence that the parent or legal guardian gave informed consent before the immunization was administered. Any adverse reactions after the administration of any vaccine are reported to the Vaccine Adverse Event Reporting System (VAERS).*

An additional source of information that must be given to parents before the administration is the *vaccine information statement (VIS)* for the particular vaccine being administered. VISs are designed to provide updated information regarding the risks and benefits of each vaccine to the adult vaccinee or parents/legal guardians of children being vaccinated. Questions regarding the information in the VIS should be answered by the practitioner. VISs are available from state or local health departments or the following websites: Immunization Coalition—www.immunize.org/vis/; or Centers for Disease Control and Prevention—www.cdc·gov/nip/publications/vis/.

*For information call 1-800-822-7967; or access the website at: www.fda.gov/cber/vaers/vaers.htm.

Atraumatic Care

IMMUNIZATIONS

To minimize local reactions from vaccines:

- Select a needle of adequate length (1 inch [2.5 cm] in infants) to deposit the antigen deep in the muscle mass.
- Inject into the vastus lateralis or ventrogluteal muscle; the deltoid may be used in children 18 months of age or older or in infants receiving HBV vaccine.
- Use an air bubble to clear the needle after injecting the vaccine (theoretically beneficial but unproved).

To minimize pain:

- Apply the topical anesthetic EMLA to the injection site and cover with an occlusive dressing for 2½ hours.
- Apply a vapocoolant spray (i.e., ethyl chloride or FluoriMethane) directly to the skin or to a cotton ball, which is placed on the skin for 15 seconds immediately before the injection.*
- In preschool children use distraction, such as telling the child to "take a deep breath and blow and blow and blow until I tell you to stop."

Note: Changing the needle on the syringe after drawing up the vaccine and before injecting it has not been shown to decrease local reactions. In children 4 to 6 years of age, the administration of sequential injections or simultaneous injections of vaccines did not alter their perceptions of distress, but parents preferred the simultaneous method.†

*Reis EC, Holubkov R: Vapocoolant spray is equally effective as EMLA cream in reducing immunization pain in school-aged children, *Pediatrics* 100(6):1025, 1997.

†Horn MI, McCarthy AM: Children's responses to sequential versus simultaneous immunization injections, *J Pediatr Health Care* 13(1): 18-23, 1999.

TABLE 36-9
Contraindications and Precautions to Vaccinations[a]

True Contraindications and Precautions	Not Contraindications (Vaccines May Be Administered)
GENERAL FOR ALL VACCINES (DTaP, IPV, MMR, HiB, HEPATITIS B, VAR)	
Contraindications	**Not Contraindications**
Anaphylactic reaction to a vaccine contraindicates further doses of that vaccine	Mild to moderate local reaction (soreness, redness, swelling) following a dose of an injectable antigen
Anaphylactic reaction to a vaccine constituent contraindicates the use of vaccines containing that substance	Mild acute illness with or without low-grade fever
Moderate or severe illnesses with or without a fever	Current antimicrobial therapy
	Convalescent phase of illnesses
	Prematurity (same dosage and indications as for normal, full-term infants)
	Recent exposure to an infectious disease
	History of penicillin or other nonspecific allergies or family history of such allergies
DIPHTHERIA, TETANUS, PERTUSSIS OR ACELLULAR PERTUSSIS (DTaP)	
Contraindications	**Not Contraindications**
Encephalopathy within 7 days of administration of previous dose of DTaP	Temperature of <40.5° C (105° F) following a previous dose of DTaP
	Family history of seizures[b]
Precautions[b]	Family history of sudden infant death syndrome
Fever of ≥40.5° C (105° F) within 48 hours after vaccination with a prior dose of DTaP	Family history of an adverse event following DTaP administration
Collapse or shocklike state (hypotonic-hyporesponsive episode) within 48 hours of receiving a prior dose of DTaP	
Seizures within 3 days of receiving a prior dose of DTaP[c]	
Persistent, inconsolable crying lasting ≥3 hours within 48 hours of receiving a prior dose of DTaP	
ORAL POLIO (OPV)[d]	
Contraindications	**Not Contraindications**
Infection with HIV or a household contact with HIV	Breastfeeding
Known altered immunodeficiency (hematologic and solid tumors; congenital immunodeficiency; and long-term immunosuppressive therapy)	Current antimicrobial therapy
Immunodeficient household contact	Diarrhea
Precaution[b]	
Pregnancy	
INACTIVATED POLIO (IPV)	
Contraindication	
Anaphylactic reaction to neomycin or streptomycin	
Precaution[b]	
Pregnancy	

Modified from American Academy of Pediatrics, Committee on Infectious Diseases, Pickering L, editor: *2000 Red Book: report of the Committee on Infectious Diseases,* ed 25, Elk Grove Village, IL, 2000, The Academy.

[a]This information is based on the recommendations of the Advisory Committee on Immunization Practices (ACIP) and those of the Committee on Infectious Diseases (*Red Book* Committee) of the American Academy of Pediatrics (AAP). Sometimes these recommendations vary from those contained in the manufacturer's package inserts. For more detailed information, providers should consult the published recommendations of the ACIP, AAP, and the manufacturer's package inserts.

[b]The events or conditions listed as precautions although not contraindications, should be carefully reviewed. The benefits and risks of administering a specific vaccine to an individual under the circumstances should be considered. If the risks are believed to outweigh the benefits, the vaccination should be withheld; if the benefits are believed to outweigh the risks (e.g., during an outbreak or foreign travel), the vaccination should be administered. Whether and when to administer DTaP to children with proven or suspected underlying neurologic disorders should be decided on an individual basis. It is prudent on theoretic grounds to avoid vaccinating pregnant women.

[c]Acetaminophen given before administering DTaP and thereafter every 4 hours for 24 hours should be considered for children with a personal or family history of convulsions in siblings or parents.

[d]No data exist to substantiate the theoretic risk of a suboptimal immune response from the administration of OPV and MMR within 30 days of each other.

TABLE 36-9—cont'd
Contraindications and Precautions to Vaccinations[a]

True Contraindications and Precautions	Not Contraindications (Vaccines May Be Administered)
MEASLES, MUMPS, RUBELLA (MMR)[e]	
Contraindications Pregnancy Known altered immunodeficiency (hematologic and solid tumors, congenital immunodeficiency, and long-term immunosuppressive therapy)	**Not Contraindications**[e] Tuberculosis or positive PPD skin test Simultaneous TB skin testing[e] Breastfeeding Pregnancy of mother of recipient Immunodeficient family member or household contact Infection with HIV Nonanaphylactic reactions to eggs or neomycin
Precautions[b] Recent immune globulin administration Immune globulin products and MMR should not be given simultaneously; if unavoidable, give at different sites and revaccinate or test for seroconversion in 3 months; if IG is given first, MMR should not be given for at least 3-6 months, depending on dose; if MMR is given first, IG should not be given for 2 weeks Thrombocytopenia/thrombocytopenia purpura	
HAEMOPHILUS INFLUENZAE TYPE b (Hib)	
Contraindication Nonidentified	**Not a Contraindication** History of Hib disease
HEPATITIS B VIRUS (HBV)	
Contraindication Anaphylactic reaction to common baker's yeast	**Not a Contraindication** Pregnancy
VARICELLA (VAR)	
Contraindications Immunocompromised individuals (e.g., HIV, acute lymphocytic leukemia) Pregnancy Children receiving corticosteroids	**Not a Contraindication** Breastfeeding

Modified from American Academy of Pediatrics, Committee on Infectious Diseases, Pickering L, editor: *2000 Red Book: report of the Committee on Infectious Diseases,* ed 25, Elk Grove Village, IL, 2000, The Academy.
[b]The events or conditions listed as precautions although not contraindications, should be carefully reviewed. The benefits and risks of administering a specific vaccine to an individual under the circumstances should be considered. If the risks are believed to outweigh the benefits, the vaccination should be withheld; if the benefits are believed to outweigh the risks (e.g., during an outbreak or foreign travel), the vaccination should be administered. Whether and when to administer DTaP to children with proven or suspected underlying neurologic disorders should be decided on an individual basis. It is prudent on theoretic grounds to avoid vaccinating pregnant women.
[e]Measles vaccination may temporarily suppress tuberculin reactivity. If testing cannot be done the day of MMR vaccination, the test should be postponed for 4 to 6 weeks.

In response to the concerns of manufacturers, practitioners, and parents of children with serious vaccine-associated injuries, the *National Childhood Vaccine Injury Act (NCVIA)* of 1986 and the *Vaccine Compensation Amendments* of 1987 were passed. These laws are designed to provide fair compensation for children who are inadvertently injured and provide greater protection from liability for vaccine manufacturers and providers.

Injury Prevention

Injuries are a major cause of death during infancy, especially for children 6 to 12 months old. Constant vigilance, awareness, and supervision are essential as the child gains increased locomotor and manipulative skills that are coupled with an insatiable curiosity about the environment. Table 36-10 lists the major developmental achievements of each period during infancy and the appropriate injury prevention plan.

Aspiration of Foreign Objects. Asphyxiation by foreign material in the respiratory tract, combined with mechanical suffocation, is the leading cause of fatal injury in children younger than 1 year of age. The size, shape, and consistency of foods or objects are important determinants of fatal obstruction. For example, small spheric or cylindric and pliable objects (less than 3.2 cm, or 1¼ inches) are more likely to completely obstruct the airway. Unfortunately, common household items can be deadly to infants.

As soon as infants have the ability to find their mouth, they are vulnerable to aspiration of small objects, such as those left within reach or removeable parts of objects that may on initial inspection appear safe. All toys must be carefully inspected for potential danger. Rattles, for example, have small beads in them to produce noise. A broken or cracked rattle can be dangerous because the beads can easily be aspirated while the infant has the toy in the mouth. Stuffed animals are another potentially dangerous toy if any of the parts, such as the eyes or nose, are

TABLE 36-10
Injury Prevention During Infancy

AGE: BIRTH-4 MONTHS

Major Developmental Accomplishments

Involuntary reflexes, such as the crawling reflex, may propel infant forward or backward, and the startle reflex may cause the body to jerk
May roll over
Increasing eye-hand coordination with voluntary grasp reflex

Injury Prevention

Aspiration
Not as great a danger to this age group, but should begin practicing safeguarding early (see under Age: 4-7 Months)
Never shake baby powder directly on infant; place powder in hand and then on infant's skin; store container closed and out of infant's reach
Hold infant for feeding; do not prop bottle
Know emergency procedures for choking*
Use pacifier with one-piece construction and loop handle

Suffocation/drowning
Keep all plastic bags stored out of infant's reach; discard large plastic garment bags after tying in a knot
Do not cover mattress with plastic
Use firm mattress and loose blankets; no pillows
Make sure crib design follows federal regulations and mattress fits snugly—crib slats $<2\frac{3}{8}$ inches (6 cm) apart
Position crib away from other furniture and away from radiators
Do not tie pacifier on a string around infant's neck
Remove bibs at bedtime
Never leave infant alone in bath
Do not leave infant younger than 12 months alone on adult or youth mattress or "beanbag" type pillows

Falls
Always raise crib rails
Never leave infant on a raised, unguarded surface
When in doubt as to where to place child, use floor
Restrain child in infant seat and never leave child unattended while the seat is resting on a raised surface
Avoid using a high chair until child can sit well with support

Poisoning
Not as great a danger to this age group, but should begin practicing safeguards early (see under Age: 4-7 Months)

Burns
Install smoke detectors in home
Use caution when warming formula in microwave oven; always check temperature of liquid before feeding
Check bathwater
Do not pour hot liquids when infant is close by; such as sitting on lap
Beware of cigarette ashes that may fall on infant
Do not leave infant in sun for more than a few minutes; keep exposed areas covered
Wash flame-retardant clothes according to label directions
Use cool-mist vaporizers
Do not leave child in parked car
Check surface heat of car restraint before placing child in seat

Motor vehicles
Transport infant in federally approved, rear-facing car seat,* preferably in back seat
Do not place infant on seat (of car) or in lap
Do not place child in a carriage or stroller behind a parked car
Do not place infant or child in front passenger seat with an air bag

Bodily damage
Avoid sharp, jagged objects
Keep diaper pins closed and away from infant

AGE: 4-7 MONTHS

Major Developmental Accomplishments

Rolls over
Sits momentarily
Grasps and manipulates small objects
Resecures a dropped object
Has well-developed eye-hand coordination
Can focus on and locate very small objects
Mouthing is very prominent
Can push on hands and knees
Crawls backward

Injury Prevention

Aspiration
Keep buttons, beads, syringe caps, and other small objects out of infant's reach
Keep floor free of any small objects
Do not feed infant hard candy, nuts, food with pits or seeds, or whole or circular pieces of hot dog
Exercise caution when giving teething biscuits, because large chunks may be broken off and aspirated

Suffocation
Keep all latex balloons out of reach
Remove all crib toys that are strung across crib or playpen when child begins to push up on hands or knees or is 5 months old

Falls
Restrain in a high chair
Keep crib rails raised to full height

*Community and home care instructions for care of the choking infant and for use of child safety seats are available in Wong DL, Hess CS: ***Wong and Whaley's clinical manual of pediatric nursing***, ed 5, St Louis, 2000, Mosby.

TABLE 36-10—cont'd
Injury Prevention During Infancy

AGE: 4-7 MONTHS—cont'd

Injury Prevention—cont'd

Aspiration—cont'd
Do not feed infant while child is lying down
Inspect toys for removeable parts
Keep baby powder, if used, out of reach

Burns
Keep faucets out of reach
Place hot objects (cigarettes, candles, incense) on high surface
Limit exposure to sun; apply sunscreen

Motor vehicles
See under Age: Birth-4 Months

Poisoning
Avoid storing large quantities of cleaning fluid, paints, pesticides, and other toxic substances
Discard used containers of poisonous substances
Do not store toxic substances in food containers
Make sure that paint for furniture or toys does not contain lead
Place toxic substances on a high shelf or in locked cabinet
Hang plants or place on high surface rather than on floor
Discard used button-sized batteries; store new batteries in safe area
Know telephone number of local poison control center (usually listed in front of telephone directory)

Bodily damage
Give toys that are smooth and rounded, preferably made of wood or plastic
Avoid long, pointed objects as toys
Avoid toys that are excessively loud
Keep sharp objects out of infant's reach

AGE: 8-12 MONTHS

Major Developmental Accomplishments

Crawls/creeps
Stands, holding onto furniture
Stands alone
Cruises around furniture
Walks
Climbs
Pulls on objects
Throws objects
Is able to pick up small objects; has pincer grasp
Explores by putting objects in mouth
Dislikes being restrained
Explores away from parent
Increasing understanding of simple commands and phrases

Injury Prevention

Aspiration
Keep lint and small objects off floor, furniture, and out of reach of children
Take care in feeding solid table food to ensure that very small pieces are given
Do not use beanbag toys or allow child to play with dried beans
See also under Age: 4-7 Months

Suffocation/drowning
Keep doors of ovens, dishwashers, refrigerators, coolers, and front-loading clothes washers and dryers closed at all times
If storing an unused appliance, such as a refrigerator, remove the door
Supervise contact with inflated balloons; immediately discard popped balloons, and keep uninflated balloons out of reach
Fence swimming pools
Always supervise when near any source of water, such as cleaning buckets, drainage areas, toilets
Keep bathroom door closed
Eliminate unnecessary pools of water
Keep one hand on child at all times when in tub

Falls
Fence stairways at top and bottom if child has access to either end†
Dress infant in safe shoes and clothing (soles that do not "catch" on floor, tied shoelaces, pant legs that do not touch floor)
Avoid walkers, especially near stairs
Ensure that furniture is sturdy enough for child to pull self to standing position and cruise

Poisoning
Administer medications as a drug, not as a candy
Do not administer medications unless so prescribed by a practitioner
Replace medications and poisons immediately after use; replace caps properly if a child-protector cap is used
Have syrup of ipecac in home; use only if advised

Burns
Place guards in front of or around any heating appliance, fireplace, or furnace
Keep electrical wires hidden or out of reach
Place plastic guards over electrical outlets; place furniture in front of outlets
Keep hanging tablecloths out of reach (child may pull down hot liquids or heavy or sharp objects)

†Information on many items such as cribs or walkers available from U.S. Consumer Product Safety Commission, 1-800-638-CPSC; website: www.cpsc.gov/.

removeable buttons or plastic pieces. An active infant can grab a low-hanging mobile and quickly chew off a small piece. As soon as the infant crawls or plays on the floor, the floor must be kept free of any small articles that can be picked up and swallowed, such as coins.

When infant *clothes* are purchased, the type of closure is important. A front button can easily be pulled off and swallowed. Safety pins for diapers are kept closed and away from the dressing table. Even though a young infant may not search for them, practicing this good habit from the beginning prevents future injuries.

Food items are the second most common cause of aspiration, and the most common offenders are hot dogs, candy, nuts, and grapes. When new foods are given to the child, nuts, hard candies, marshmallows, large amounts of peanut butter, or fruits with pits or seeds are avoided. When traveling (especially in airplanes) or entertaining, snack foods such as peanuts and popcorn are kept away from young children. If given to young children, hot dogs must be cut into small, irregular pieces rather than served whole or sliced into sections, because their size (diameter), round shape, and consistency allow for complete occlusion of the airway. Perhaps the most dangerous foods are dried beans, which, if aspirated, enlarge when they come in contact with the wet mucosa and block the airway.

Pacifiers can also be dangerous because the entire object may be aspirated if it is small, or the nipple and shield may become detached from the handle and become lodged in the pharynx. Improvised pacifiers, such as those made in hospitals from a padded nipple, also present dangers. The nipple may separate from the plastic collar and be aspirated. In addition, parents may continue to offer this pacifier to the infant at home. To eliminate the hazards of improvised pacifiers, hospitals should use only safe, commercial types. Pacifiers should not be altered from their original shape to encourage or discourage usage. Candy pacifiers pose dangers because the candy portion can dislodge from the circular base and be aspirated. To be safe, pacifiers should have the following (Nowak, 1993) (Fig. 36-11):

- Sturdy, one-piece construction with material that is nontoxic, flexible, and firm but not brittle
- An easily grasped handle
- A mouthguard that cannot be separated from the nipple, that has two ventilating holes, and that is too large to be aspirated
- No detachable ribbon or string
- A label warning against tying the pacifier around the infant's neck

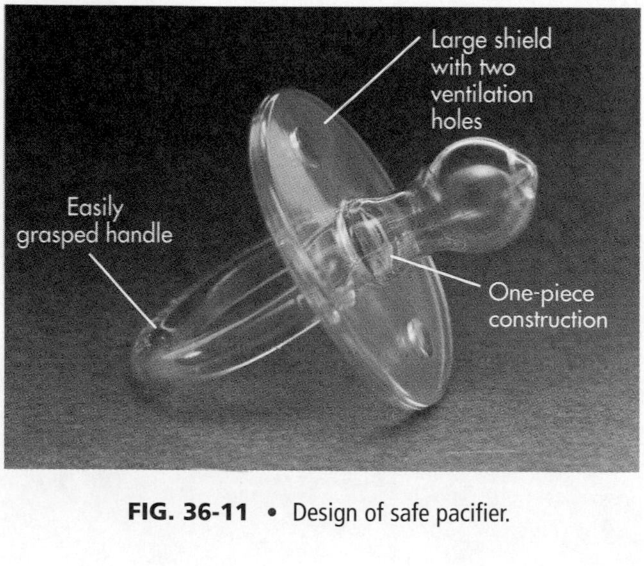

FIG. 36-11 • Design of safe pacifier.

Using a syringe to accurately measure and dispense oral liquid medications to young children has become common practice. However, the *syringe cap* is a potential aspiration hazard. As a precaution, keep parts of medication devices out of the reach of children and be certain the cap is removed before dispensing medication.

Another hazardous substance if aspirated is *baby powder*, which is usually a mixture of talc (hydrous magnesium silicate) and other silicates. Although the use of talc has been discouraged, it is a common baby care product that can cause severe and often fatal aspiration pneumonia. One of the factors involved in talc aspiration is the similar appearance of baby powder containers and nursing bottles. Talc containers often become favorite playthings and are placed in the mouth. Improperly using powder by sprinkling it directly on the skin creates a cloud of talc dust that is easily inhaled. Parents are advised of the danger of baby powder and are discouraged from using it. If they prefer to use a powder, a cornstarch preparation can be substituted (see Diaper Dermatitis, Chapter 53). Whenever a powder is used, it should be placed in the hand and then applied to the skin, never shaken directly from the container onto the skin. The container is kept closed and immediately stored in a safe place, especially away from curious toddlers, who often imitate caregiving activities and may accidentally shake it on the infant.

Suffocation. Mechanical suffocation includes suffocation by covering of the airway (i.e., mouth and nose); by pressure on the throat and chest; and by exclusion of air, such as by refrigerator entrapment. Nonfood items cause the majority of deaths in young children. *Latex balloons,* whether partially inflated, uninflated, or popped, are a leading cause of pediatric choking deaths from children's products (Holida, 1993). They should be kept away from infants and young children. Even the practice of inflating latex gloves to amuse children in health care settings may pose a danger, especially if the child is latex sensitive.

NURSE ALERT • Encourage adults to:
- Blow up balloons for children
- Supervise children's balloon play
- Pick up and dispose of broken balloon pieces
- Warn older children of dangers of chewing or sucking on balloons
- Substitute Mylar or paper balloons for latex balloons

In addition, the accessibility of the plastic linings of diapers used on the infant and/or on dolls is especially dangerous to young children.

The *bed* or *crib* poses a number of hazards. An infant who is placed in a bed under tucked-in blankets and sheets can be caught under them and unable to wriggle free. Baby pillows filled with plastic foam beads that make them resemble small beanbags are dangerous; very young infants are suffocated when the pillow contours to the face and blocks the airway. There are potential dangers when adults sleep with a small infant because of the possibility of rolling over and smothering the child. The incidence of infant suffocation by a bed sharing adult increased between 1980 and 1997 (Drago and Dannenberg, 1999). The most common causes of infant suffocation were wedging between a bed or mattress and a wall; and oronasal obstruction by a plastic bag.

Infant strangulation may occur if the infant's head becomes caught between the crib slats and mattress or other objects close to the crib. Suffocation deaths are not confined to cribs; ill-fitting mattresses in adult or youth beds, bunk beds, and waterbeds have also been reported. According to U.S. federal regulation, the distance between crib slats should not be more than 2⅜ inches (approximately 6 cm), roughly the width of three adult fingers. Mattresses and bumper pads should fit snugly against the slats. A general rule is that the mattress is too small if two adult fingers can be placed between the mattress and crib or bed side. A temporary solution is to place large, rolled towels in the space to create a snug fit.

Corner post extensions on cribs are another source of strangulation. Children have died when their clothing caught on raised corner posts as they climbed out of the crib. Voluntary manufacturing standards state that corner post extensions not exceed 1⁄16 inch; however, the safety of any extension is questionable. Decorative extensions need to be removed from cribs. Ideally, information regarding correct crib design should be given prenatally, before parents have purchased or borrowed a crib.*

Mesh-sided playpens and cribs can result in death if the sides are left in the lowered position. Infants have suffocated when they fell off the edge of the mattress and the head or chest was compressed between the floorboard and mesh side. Parents should be advised of this danger and encouraged to always keep the sides locked securely in the up position whenever the child is in the playpen or crib.

The crib should be positioned away from large furniture, because children who crawl out of the crib may become caught between the two objects. Cribs should also be located away from windows, where drape or blind cords can become wrapped around the infant's neck.

Another cause of suffocation is *plastic bags.* Large plastic bags used over garments are very lightweight and can easily and quickly be wrapped around the head of an active infant or pressed against the face. For this reason, pillows and mattresses should not be covered with plastic. Older infants may play with a plastic bag and accidentally pull it over their heads. Because plastic is nonporous, suffocation occurs in a matter of minutes.

Cords (e.g., drapery or window blinds) located near the infant are a potential cause of strangulation. Bibs are removed at bedtime, and objects such as pacifiers are never hung on a string around the infant's neck. This is a common practice in some cultures that can be remedied by tying a *short* string to a pacifier and clipping the string to the child's shirt.

Toys that have strings attached (e.g., a telephone) or toys that are tied to cribs or playpens can be hazards because the string can become wrapped around the child's neck or the child can become entrapped in the toy. As a precaution, all cords should be less than 30 cm (12 inches) long. Crib toys should be hung high enough that the infant cannot become entangled in them and should no longer be used once the child is able to reach them.

If applied too loosely or left unfastened, restraining straps can be a hazard. For example, a child may slide off a high chair beneath the tray and become strangled on the loose strap. All straps should be fastened securely.

Motor Vehicle Injuries. Automobile injuries are the leading cause of accidental death in children older than 1 year of age. However, a significant number of infants are injured or die from improper restraint within the vehicle, most often from riding on the lap of another occupant. Recent reports indicate that child restraint use decreases with increasing age of children and increasing number of occupants. Lack of proper child restraint continues to be a major factor in fatal accidents involving children (Murphy, 1999). All infants must be secured in a U.S. federally approved restraint rather than held or placed on the seat of the car. There is no safe alternative.

Infant restraints are designed either as an infant-only model (Fig. 36-12) or as a convertible infant-toddler model. Either restraint is a semireclined seat that faces the rear of the car. A rear-facing car seat provides the best protection for the disproportionately heavy head and weak neck of a young child. This position minimizes the stress on the neck by spreading the force of a frontal crash over the entire back, neck, and head; the spine is supported by the back of the car seat. If the seat were faced forward, the head would whip forward because of the force of the crash, creating enormous stress on the neck.

NURSE ALERT • Infants should use rear-facing car seats from birth to 20 pounds and as close to 1 year of age as possible.

The restraint is anchored to the vehicle with the vehicle's seat belt, and the restraint has a harness system for securing the infant. Some harness systems require a clip to keep the shoulder straps correctly positioned. Although many infant restraints can be recliners, they are used in the car only in the position specified by the manufacturer.

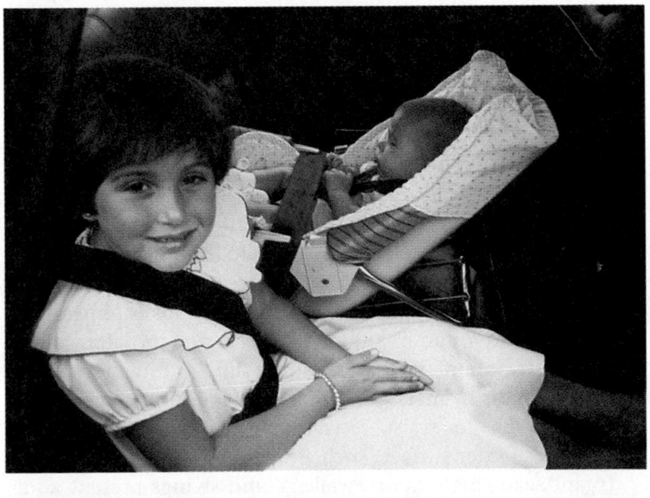

FIG. 36-12 • Federally approved infant car restraint. Note placement in middle of back seat and use of car lap/shoulder belt for older child.

*The booklet *It Hurts When They Cry* gives basic information on hazards, safety features, and proper use of nursery furniture and equipment. It is available at no charge from the U.S. Consumer Product Safety Commission, Publication Requests, Washington, DC 20207; 1-800-638-2772; website: www.cpsc.gov. Additional free information is available from the Danny Foundation, 3158 Danville Blvd., P.O. Box 680, Alamo, CA 94507; 1-800-83-DANNY; website: www.dannyfoundation.org.

Severe injuries and deaths in children have occurred from air bags deploying on impact in the front passenger seat. The back seat is the safest area of the car. If the back seat is not an option, an infant restraint may be positioned in the front seat provided that the seat belt can be locked into position and there is no passenger-side air bag. If there is a passenger-side air bag, and the child has special health care needs or constant observation is recommended by the practitioner and no other adult is available to ride in the back seat with the child, an on/off switch may be installed to prevent the air bag from deploying and injuring the child riding in the front seat. Another condition that may arise is the use of vehicles without a back seat; in such cases it is best that the front passenger seat be placed as far back as possible and appropriate child safety restraint employed.

NURSE ALERT • Rear-facing infant safety seats must not be placed in the front seats of cars equipped with an air bag on the passenger side. If an infant safety seat is placed in the passenger seat with an air bag, the child could be seriously injured if the air bag is released, because rear-facing infant seats extend closer to the dashboard.

For restraints to be effective, they must be used properly. Dressing the infant in an outfit with sleeves and legs allows the harness to hold the child securely in the seat without rubbing against the skin. A small blanket or towel rolled tightly can be placed on either side of the head to minimize movement. Padding between the infant's legs and crotch is added to prevent slouching and keep the infant's hips against the back of the seat. Thick, soft padding is not placed under the infant or behind the back because the padding will compress during the impact, leaving the harness straps loose. (For further discussion of restraints, see Chapter 37.)

Falls. Falls are most common after 4 months of age when the infant has learned to roll over, but they can occur at any age. The best advice is to never place a child of any age unattended on a raised surface that has no type of guardrails. When in doubt, the safest place is the floor. Even though young infants cannot climb over a partially raised crib rail, it is best to form a habit of raising the rail all the way, because someday that infant will be able to climb out. Crib sides should have a latching device that cannot be easily released. The welds attaching the crib corner locks to the corner posts should not be cracked or broken. If the welds are damaged, the bedspring could fall to the floor. Ideally, cribs should be placed on carpeted, not hard, floors.

Another danger area for falling is the *changing table,* which is usually high and narrow. Although these tables have a restraining belt, children are never left unattended, even when restrained. The best way to avoid needing to leave is to arrange the area with all necessary articles within easy reach so that the child is always in full sight of the caregiver. It takes only a fraction of a second for an infant to fall off. During the latter half of the first year, infants usually resist dressing and diapering and may be difficult to manage. If there is danger that the child is strong enough to resist restraining, the infant should be changed on a safer surface, such as a clean floor.

Infant seats, high chairs, walkers, and swings present additional opportunities for falls. If the *infant seat* is placed on a table, the child should never be left unrestrained or unattended. The same rule is essential for other baby equipment, particularly when the child has learned to crawl and to stand up. *High chairs* are designed for older infants who can sit well and who are tall enough to have the tray at the level of their chest or abdomen. Small infants can slip through a high chair if a protective harness is not used. *Infant walkers* are responsible for a number of different types of injuries that occur because the walker tipped over or fell down stairs. Parents need to be warned of these dangers and encouraged to keep a constant vigil on their child's activities. The use of older-model walkers should be discouraged. The American Academy of Pediatrics (1995) does not recommend the use of walkers. In response to the large number of accidents and deaths associated with infant walkers, several manufacturers made modifications on these products to prevent falls down stairs. The new models should have a label or sign indicating "meets new safety standard." Infant walkers may still pose a risk for climbing up to reach dangerous objects and should be carefully supervised. One alternative is to use a stationary play station with a seat similar to a walker. There is no evidence that using infant walkers helps infants walk sooner.

Once infants are mobile, they should not be allowed to crawl unsupervised on any raised surface, near stairs, or near any water reservoir. Gates should be used at the *bottom* and *top of stairs,* because both present dangers to the crawling and climbing infant. However, certain types of gates can present hazards. Freestanding enclosures constructed of crisscrossed wood slats that expand and contract can trap the head or neck when children attempt to climb over them. If these types of gates are used, they must be securely fastened to prevent mobility of the slats.

As children begin to pull themselves to a standing position, *heavy objects,* such as unsturdy furniture or any freestanding item (e.g., wrought iron fish tank stands or televisions), can be extremely dangerous if pulled down on top of the child. To prevent such injury, televisions should be placed on lower furniture and as far back as possible, and angle braces or anchors can secure furniture to walls.

Even when the environment is made safe, infants may sometimes literally trip over their own feet from *clothing.* Slippery socks; hard, slick soles on shoes or rubber soles that can catch, especially on a carpet; and long pants or pajama bottoms can easily upset a child's balance. Such dangers need to be pointed out to parents, especially when infants are taking their first steps.

Poisoning. Poisoning is one of the major causes of death in children younger than 5 years of age. The highest incidence occurs in the 2-year-old group, with the second highest incidence occurring in 1-year-old children. Infants who do not crawl are relatively free from danger of poisonous agents by virtue of immobility. However, once locomotion begins, danger from poisoning is present almost everywhere. There are more than 500 toxic substances in the average home, and approximately one third of all poisonings occur in the kitchen.

The major reason for ingestion of poisons is *improper storage.* To protect the infant, toxic agents should not be placed on a low shelf, low table, or on the floor. Drugs that are kept in a purse pose additional dangers; if the handbag is given to infants to play with, they may open it and ingest the drug. Another unrecognized hazard occurs during diaper changes, when infants are near many toxic substances such as ointments, creams, oils, and talc. Parents may even hand infants a potentially poisonous object to quiet them. Such dangers need to be stressed to parents, and toys need to be kept at diapering areas to minimize risks.

Plants are another source of poisoning for infants. Plants are commonly placed on the floor, and the leaves or flowers are attractive and easy to pull off. More than 700 species of plants are known to have caused illness or death.

Another danger is ingestion of the *button-sized batteries* used in devices such as hearing aids, calculators, watches, and cameras. Because they are bright and shiny, they are attractive to children. However, they can cause severe morbidity, even death, if lodged in the esophagus. The strong alkali in a battery can leak and cause a severe caustic burn. As a precaution, small batteries must be safely stored and discarded where young children cannot easily retrieve them.

Not all poisonings result from ingestion—*inhalation* is another possible route, such as inhaling chlorine vapors from household cleaning or pool supplies. Passive cocaine toxicity has occurred in young children exposed to freebase cocaine ("crack") smoking by adults. Children should be protected from environments in which airborne toxins exist (for a discussion of passive second-hand tobacco smoke, see Chapter 46).

The only sure way to prevent poisoning is to remove toxic agents; this means placing containers out of the infant's reach or contact. Because crawling infants soon become climbing toddlers, it is best to keep all toxic agents, especially drugs, in a locked cabinet. Special plastic hooks can be attached to the inside of cabinet doors to keep them securely closed (Fig. 36-13). Firm thumb pressure is required to unlatch the hook, and small children are usually unable to manipulate them. Locks are best, but for frequently used cleaning agents, such as those often kept under a kitchen sink, hooks are a practical alternative.

With several hundred toxic substances in each house, locking up all potentially toxic substances can present a problem; however, careful planning can help. A large surplus of cleaning agents, furniture polishes, laundry additives, paints, insecticides, and solvents should be avoided. Used poison containers should be promptly discarded and not used to store another poison without adequately marking the package. Potentially hazardous substances should not be stored in any type of food container. A popular container used to store toxic liquids is a soda or pop, bottle. A child unaware of the dangerous contents is vulnerable to poisoning. Parents should know the location of local poison control centers and call one in the event of a suspected poisoning. Emergency measures for poisoning are discussed in Chapter 47.

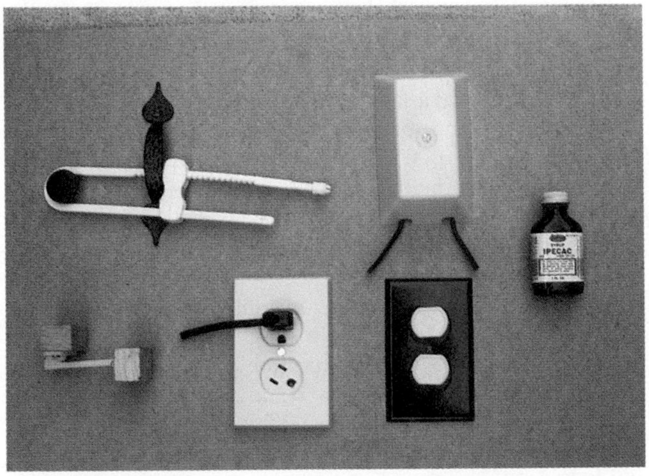

FIG. 36-13 • Safety demonstration board. Clockwise from lower left; two types of cabinet latches; a shock guard for an electrical outlet in use: syrup of ipecac; and two types of outlet covers (the one with the white cover has passive devices that automatically cover the outlet when a plug is removed).

Burns. Scalding from water that is too hot; excessive sunburn; and burns from house fires, electrical wires, sockets, and heating elements such as radiators, registers, and floor furnaces cause a significant number of deaths and many more injuries in infants. The infant's skin is particularly sensitive to irritation, and the mechanisms for temperature perception are not completely developed. As a general precaution, all homes should have smoke alarms installed near the bedroom areas and on each level of the building.

Scald burns from *hot tap water* can be prevented by lowering the water heater to a safe temperature of 49° C (120° F). In addition, the bathwater should be checked before the infant is immersed. Scalds can also occur from bathing infants in the kitchen sink when the garbage disposal, occluded with debris, causes the draining dishwasher effluent to back up into the sink. The temperature of the effluent from a dishwasher is typically that of the maximum water temperature of the household water heater, but many dishwashers are equipped with heating elements that heat water to a temperature that is even higher (Sheridan, Sheridan, and Tompkins, 1993). As a precaution, instruct caregivers to avoid bathing small children in the kitchen sink while the dishwasher is running.

If formula or food is warmed in a *microwave oven,* it must be checked before feeding because the container may remain cool while the contents are hot. Another danger is explosion of the container from the buildup of steam. Because of these dangers, microwaving infant formula or food should be avoided or done using the guidelines in the Home Care box on p. 847. The handles of cooking utensils should be turned toward the back of the stove. When the infant is underfoot, pouring hot liquids and cooking with hot oil are avoided. Hanging tablecloths are also placed out of the infant's reach to prevent pulling hot items off the table.

Sunburn can be a source of a first- or second-degree burn. Exposure to direct sunlight should be avoided for the first 6 months. When infants are in the sun, the body, especially the face and head, should be covered. Sunscreen can be used on older infants, but should be used on small areas of the body and only sparingly in infants under 6 months (American Academy of Pediatrics, 1999b) (see Sunburn, Chapter 53). Although infants burn less readily, their thin skin can become sunburned and needs protection.

Electrical outlets should be covered with protective plastic caps that prevent the child from sucking on the outlet or putting objects such as hairpins into it (see Fig. 36-13). Live wires are placed out of reach so that curious infants cannot chew on them and break the rubber coating (Fig. 36-14). Infants should not be allowed to play near television sets, stereo units, or other appliances.

Any *heat-producing element* should have a guard placed in front of it. Fireplaces should be well screened because they are very appealing and within easy access. Small, portable heaters should be placed on a high surface. Floor furnaces should have barrier gates to prevent children from crawling or walking over them. Burning cigarettes, candles, and incense should be kept out of reach, and infants should not be held by a smoking adult because falling ashes are a hazard, especially to the eyes. Heated-

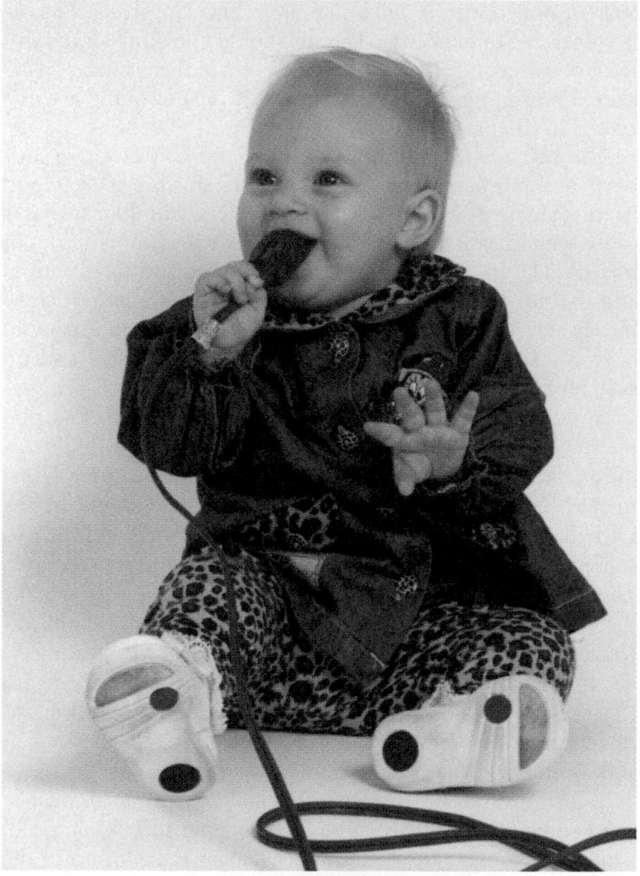

FIG. 36-14 • Infants can find hazardous electrical wires. (Photo by Paul Vincent Kuntz, Texas Children's Hospital.)

mist vaporizers are a source of burns and should not be used. If humidity is needed, only cool-mist vaporizers are safe.

By law, all infant sleepwear must be flame retardant. Unfortunately, this does not apply to all *infant clothing.* Flame-retardant fabric must never be viewed as the ultimate protection against burns. Repeated washing reduces the flame-retardant properties, and the use of soap or bleach destroys the protection. If sleepwear is home sewn, parents are advised to look for specially treated, flame-retardant fabric.

Another type of thermal injury occurs when children are exposed to excessive heat during confinement in poorly ventilated *vehicles.* The practice of leaving the windows open a couple of inches is not protective. The nurse should caution parents never to leave children in parked cars, especially when the automobile is in direct sunlight.

Children can also be burned by overheated metal hardware and vinyl seats in cars parked in the sun. As a precaution, the surface heat of car restraints should be determined before placing children in them. Covering the restraints and hardware (such as metal latches on seat belts) may be necessary to prevent skin burns. An additional safeguard is buying a light-colored restraint, which absorbs less heat.

Drowning. Drowning in this age group can occur in just inches of water. Consequently, infants should always be supervised in a bathtub, hot rub, or near a source of water such as a swimming pool, lake, toilet, or bucket. Organized swimming instruction is not recommended for children under 4 years of age, because it may lead to a false sense of security. No infant can be expected to learn the elements of water safety or to react appropriately in an emergency. Therefore all young children need to be considered at risk when near water (American Academy of Pediatrics, 2000c). Infants and toddlers are also at increased risk of infection and seizures from swallowing large amounts of water.

Bodily Damage. Injuries can occur in numerous ways. Sharp, jagged-edged objects can cause wounds in the skin. Long-pointed articles, such as the common toothpick or fork, can be poked into the eye or ear, causing serious damage. Such articles should be safely stored away from the infant's reach; forks are best avoided for self-feeding until the child has mastered the spoon, usually by age 18 months.

In addition to hazards such as aspiration, small articles can be placed in the ear or nose, and excessive noise from toys can result in sensorineural hearing loss. Although toys with the highest noise levels are model airplanes, air guns, and toy cap guns, even common squeaking toys used by young children may be harmful if placed close to the ear.

Even clothes and hair can present dangers to infants who cannot call attention to the problem. For example, constriction injuries can occur from excessively tight bands on socks, as well as fibers of hair or thread wrapped tightly around appendages, usually toes or fingers.

Another commonly unrecognized danger to infants is animal attacks. As newcomers to the home, helpless infants can provoke jealousy in animals, especially dogs and cats. Parents must be constantly vigilant to protect the child from household pets and farm animals (see Animal Bites, Chapter 53).

Nurse's Role in Injury Prevention. The task of injury prevention begins to be appreciated only when the potential environmental dangers to which infants are vulnerable are considered. Nurses must be aware of the possible causes of injury in each age group in order for anticipatory preventive teaching to occur. For example, the guidelines for injury prevention during infancy presented in Table 36-10 should be discussed before the child reaches the susceptible age group. Preventive teaching ideally occurs during pregnancy. Two thirds of all injuries to children occur in the home, and therefore the importance of safety cannot be overemphasized. The Home Care box summarizes a home safety checklist that can be presented to parents to increase their awareness of danger areas in the home and assist them in implementing safety devices and practices before their absence can inflict injury on infants. In addition, displays such as a safety demonstration board can be helpful in familiarizing parents with inexpensive commercial devices that can be used in the home to prevent injuries. To help parents appreciate the dangers present in their home to young children, suggest that they get eye level with the floor to survey the environment from a child's view.

Injury prevention requires protection of the child and education of the caregiver. Nurses in ambulatory care settings, health maintenance centers, or visiting nurse agencies are in a favorable position for injury education. This does not exclude nurses in inpatient facilities, who could use visiting times as an excellent opportunity for discussing this topic.

One approach to teaching injury prevention is to relate why children in various age groups are prone to specific types of injuries. Stressing prevention is just as important as emphasizing the why of the injury. However, injury prevention must also be practical. Asking parents for their ideas leads to realistic suggestions that can be followed. For instance, bathroom cleaning agents, cosmetics, and personal care items can be placed on a

Home Care

CHILD SAFETY HOME CHECKLIST

Safety: Fire, Electrical, Burns

- ☐ Guards in front of or around any heating appliance, fireplace, or furnace (including floor furnace)*
- ☐ Electrical wires hidden or out of reach*
- ☐ No frayed or broken wires; no overloaded sockets
- ☐ Plastic guards or caps over electrical outlets, furniture in front of outlets*
- ☐ Hanging tablecloths out of reach, away from open fires*
- ☐ Smoke detectors tested and operating properly
- ☐ Kitchen matches stored out of child's reach*
- ☐ Large, deep ashtrays throughout house (if used)
- ☐ Small stoves, heaters, and other hot objects (cigarettes, candles, coffee pots, slow cookers) placed where they cannot be tipped over or reached by children
- ☐ Hot water heater set at 49° C (120° F) or lower
- ☐ Pot handles turned toward back of stove, center of table
- ☐ No loose clothing worn near stove
- ☐ No cooking or eating hot foods or liquids with child standing nearby or sitting in lap
- ☐ All small appliances, such as iron, turned off, disconnected, and placed out of reach when not in use
- ☐ Cool, not hot, mist vaporizer used
- ☐ Fire extinguisher available on each floor and checked periodically
- ☐ Electrical fuse box and gas shutoff accessible
- ☐ Family escape plan in case of a fire practiced periodically; fire escape ladder available on upper-level floors
- ☐ Telephone number of fire or rescue squad and address of home with nearest cross street posted near phone

Safety: Suffocation and Aspiration

- ☐ Small objects stored out of reach*
- ☐ Toys inspected for small removeable parts or long strings*
- ☐ Hanging crib toys and mobiles placed out of reach
- ☐ Plastic bags stored away from young child's reach, large plastic garment bags discarded after tying in knots*
- ☐ Mattress or pillow not covered with plastic or in manner accessible to child*
- ☐ Crib design according to federal regulations (crib slats less than 2⅜ inches [6 cm] apart) with snug-fitting mattress*†
- ☐ Crib positioned away from other furniture or windows*
- ☐ Portable playpen gates up at all times while in use*
- ☐ Accordion-style gates not used*
- ☐ Bathroom doors kept closed and toilet seats down*
- ☐ Faucets turned off firmly*
- ☐ Pool fenced with locked gate
- ☐ Proper safety equipment at poolside
- ☐ Electric garage door openers stored safely and garage door adjusted to rise when door strikes object
- ☐ Doors of ovens, trunks, dishwashers, refrigerators, and front-loading clothes washers and dryers kept closed*
- ☐ Unused appliance, such as a refrigerator, securely closed with lock or doors removed*
- ☐ Food served in small, noncylindric pieces*
- ☐ Toy chests without lids or with lids that securely lock in open position*
- ☐ Buckets and wading pools kept empty when not in use*
- ☐ Clothesline above head level
- ☐ At least one member of household trained in basic life support (CPR) including first aid for choking‡

Safety: Poisoning

- ☐ Toxic substances, including batteries, placed on a high shelf, preferably in locked cabinet
- ☐ Toxic plants hung or placed out of reach*
- ☐ Excess quantities of cleaning fluid, paints, pesticides, drugs, and other toxic substances not stored in home
- ☐ Used containers of poisonous substances discarded where child cannot obtain access
- ☐ Telephone number of local poison control center and address of home with nearest cross street posted near phone
- ☐ Syrup of ipecac in home containing two doses per child
- ☐ Medicines clearly labeled in childproof containers and stored out of reach
- ☐ Household cleaners, disinfectants, and insecticides kept in their original containers, separate from food and out of reach
- ☐ Smoking in areas away from children

Safety: Falls

- ☐ Nonskid mats, strips, or surfaces in tubs and showers
- ☐ Exits, halls, and passageways in rooms kept clear of toys, furniture, boxes, or other items that could be obstructive
- ☐ Stairs and halls well lighted, with switches at both top and bottom
- ☐ Sturdy handrails for all steps and stairways
- ☐ Nothing stored on stairways
- ☐ Treads, risers, and carpeting in good repair
- ☐ Glass doors and walls marked with decals
- ☐ Safety glass used in doors, windows, and walls
- ☐ Gates on top and bottom of staircases and elevated areas, such as porch, fire escape*
- ☐ Guardrails on upstairs windows with locks that limit height of window opening and access to areas such as fire escape*
- ☐ Crib side rails raised to full height; mattress lowered as child grows*
- ☐ Restraints used in high chairs, walkers, or other baby furniture; preferably walkers not used*
- ☐ Scatter rugs secured in place or used with nonskid backing
- ☐ Walks, patios, and driveways in good repair

Safety: Bodily Injury

- ☐ Knives, power tools, and unloaded firearms stored safely or placed in locked cabinet
- ☐ Garden tools returned to storage racks after use
- ☐ Pets properly restrained and immunized for rabies
- ☐ Swings, slides, and other outdoor play equipment kept in safe condition
- ☐ Yard free of broken glass, nail-studded boards, other litter
- ☐ Cement birdbaths placed where young child cannot tip them over*

*Safety measures are specific for homes with young children. All safety measures should be implemented in homes where children reside and visit frequently, such as those of grandparents or baby-sitters.
†Federal regulations are available from U.S. Consumer Product Safety Commission; 1-800-638-CPSC; website: www.cpsc.gov.
‡Community and home care instructions for infant cardiopulmonary resuscitation and infant/child choking are available in Wong DL, Hess CS: ***Wong and Whaley's clinical manual of pediatric nursing,*** ed 5, St Louis, 2000, Mosby.

top shelf in the linen closet, and towels or sheets can be stored on the lower shelves and floor.

If an injury has occurred, the nurse should not be too quick to admonish the parent: injuries do not always indicate neglect. It is a difficult task to watch children carefully without overprotecting or unnecessarily confining them. Small falls help children learn the dangers of heights. Touching a hot object once can emphasize to the child the pain of a burn. Allowing children to explore while maintaining consistent, age-appropriate limits is sound advice.

Parents need to remember that infants and young children cannot anticipate danger or understand when it is or is not present. A dead electrical wire may present no actual harm; but if the child is allowed to play with it, a poor behavior is enforced and will be practiced when the child encounters a live wire. Although it is always wise to explain why something is dangerous, it must be remembered that small children need to be physically removed from the situation.

It is not easy to teach safety, supervise closely, and refrain from saying "no" a hundred times a day. Parents become acutely aware of this dilemma as soon as the infant learns to crawl. Preventing injuries to children is usually the first reason for limit setting and discipline, but limits are also set to prevent danger to valuable household objects. When small children are in the home, dangerous objects must be removed or guarded and valuable articles placed out of reach.

When children are taught the meaning of "no," they should also be taught what "yes" means. Children should be praised for playing with suitable toys, their efforts at behaving or listening should be reinforced, and innovative and creative recreational toys should be provided for them. Infants love to tear paper and avidly pursue books, magazines, or newspapers left on the floor. Instead of always scolding them for destroying a valued book, child-safe books (such as those constructed of fabric) can be kept available for them to play with. If they enjoy pots and pans, a cabinet can be arranged with safe utensils for them to explore.

One additional factor must be stressed concerning injury prevention and education. Children are imitators; they copy what they see and hear. *Practicing safety teaches safety.* This applies to parents and their children and to nurses and their patients. Saying one thing but doing another confuses children and can lead to difficulties as the child grows older.

Anticipatory Guidance—Care of Families

Childrearing is no easy task; it presents challenges to both new and "seasoned" parents. With society's changing roles and mores, combined with a highly mobile population, there is little stability for additional role models and time-honored methods of raising children. As a result, parents look to professionals for guidance. Nurses are in an advantageous position to render assistance and offer suggestions. Every phase of a child's life has its particular traumas—toilet training for toddlers, unexplained fears for preschoolers, and identity crises for adolescents. For parents of an infant, some challenges center around dependency, discipline, increased mobility, and safety. Major areas for parental guidance during the first year are listed in the Home Care box.

Special Health Problems

FEEDING DIFFICULTIES

Regurgitation and "Spitting Up"

The return of small amounts of food after a feeding is a common occurrence during infancy. It should not be confused with actual vomiting, which can be associated with a number of disturbances that may be insignificant or serious. It is usually benign, although persistent regurgitation necessitates medical evaluation to rule out gastroesophageal reflux. For clarification the following terms are defined:

Regurgitation—Return of undigested food from the stomach, usually accompanied by burping

Spitting up—Dribbling of unswallowed formula from the infant's mouth immediately after a feeding

The normal occurrence of regurgitation or spitting up should be explained to parents, especially to those who are unduly concerned about it. Regurgitation can be reduced by some simple measures, such as frequent burping during and after feeding, minimum handling during and after feeding, and positioning the child on the right side with the head slightly elevated after feeding. The inconvenience of spitting up can be managed with the use of absorbent bibs on the infant and protective cloths on the parent.

Home Care

GUIDANCE DURING INFANT'S FIRST YEAR

First 6 Months

- Teach car safety with use of federally approved restraint, facing rearward, in the middle of the back seat—not in a seat with an air bag.
- Understand each parent's adjustment to newborn, especially mother's postpartal emotional needs.
- Teach care of infant and help parents to understand his or her individual needs and temperament and that the infant expresses wants through crying.
- Reassure parents that infant cannot be spoiled by too much attention during the first 4 to 6 months.
- Encourage parents to establish a schedule that meets needs of child and themselves.
- Help parents understand infant's need for stimulation in environment.
- Support parents' pleasure in seeing child's growing friendliness and social response, especially smiling.
- Plan anticipatory guidance for safety.
- Stress need for immunization
- Prepare for introduction of solid foods.

Second 6 Months

- Prepare parents for child's "stranger anxiety."
- Encourage parents to allow child to cling to them and avoid long separation from either.
- Guide parents concerning discipline because of infant's increasing mobility.
- Encourage use of negative voice and eye contact rather than physical punishment as a means of discipline.
- Encourage showing most attention when infant is behaving well, rather than when infant is crying.
- Teach injury prevention because of child's advancing motor skills and curiosity.
- Encourage parents to leave child with suitable caregiver to allow some free time.
- Discuss readiness for weaning.
- Explore parents' feelings regarding infant's sleep patterns.

Sometimes frequent dribbling of formula causes excoriation of the corners of the mouth, the chin, and the neck. Keeping the area dry promotes healing but can be difficult to maintain. Helpful suggestions include applying a thin film of petrolatum or A&D Ointment to the affected areas after cleansing; and using absorbent, nonplastic-lined terry cloth bibs, which are changed often.

Paroxysmal Abdominal Pain (Colic)

Colic is generally described as paroxysmal abdominal pain or cramping that is manifested by loud crying and drawing the legs up to the abdomen. Other definitions include variables, such as duration of cry greater than 3 hours a day occurring more than 3 days per week; and parental dissatisfaction with the child's behavior. Some studies report an increase in symptoms (e.g., fussiness and crying) in the late afternoon or evening; however, in some infants the onset of symptoms occurs at another time. Colic is more common in infants under the age of 3 months than in older infants, and infants with "difficult" temperaments are more likely to be colicky. Despite the obvious behavioral indications of pain, the child tolerates the formula well, gains weight, and usually thrives.

Among the theories that have been investigated as potential causes are too rapid feeding, overeating, swallowing excessive air, improper feeding technique (especially in positioning and burping), and emotional stress or tension between parent and child. Although all of these may occur, there is no evidence that one factor is consistently present. In some infants colic may be a sign of cow's milk allergy or intolerance, and eliminating cow's milk products from the infant's diet and the diet of lactating mothers can reduce the symptoms. Parental smoking has also been associated with colic.

Therapeutic Management. Management of colic should begin with an investigation of diagnosable causes, such as cow's milk allergy. If a sensitivity to cow's milk is strongly suspected, a trial substitution of another formula such as a casein hydrolysate (e.g., Nutramigen, Alimentum, and Pregestimil) is warranted. Soy formulas are avoided because of the possibility of sensitivity to soy protein as well.

The use of drugs, including sedatives, antispasmodics, antihistamines, and antiflatulents, is sometimes recommended. The most commonly used sedatives are phenobarbitol, hydroxyzine hydrochloride (Atarax), and chloral hydrate. Simethicone (Mylicon) may also help allay the symptoms of colic. However, in most controlled studies none of these drugs completely reduce the symptoms of colic (Balon, 1997).

Nursing Considerations. The initial step in managing colic is to take a thorough, detailed history of the usual daily events. Areas that should be stressed include: (1) the infant's diet; (2) the diet of the breastfeeding mother; (3) the time of day when crying occurs; (4) the relationship of the crying to feeding time; (5) the presence of specific family members during the crying and habits of family members, such as smoking; (6) activity of the mother or usual caregiver before, during, and after the crying; (7) characteristics of the cry (e.g., duration, intensity); (8) measures used to relieve the crying and their effectiveness; and (9) the infant's stooling, voiding, and sleeping patterns. Of special emphasis is a careful assessment of the feeding process via demonstration by the parent.

If milk sensitivity is suspected, breastfeeding mothers should follow a milk-free diet for a minimum of 3 to 5 days in an attempt to reduce symptoms in the infant. Mothers need to be cautioned that some nondairy creamers may contain calcium caseinate, a cow's milk protein. If a milk-free diet is helpful, lactating mothers may need calcium supplements to meet the body's requirement. Bottle-fed infants may improve with the same dietary modifications as for the child with cow's milk allergy.

When no cause can be identified, helping parents understand the infant's crying behavior and modifying parent interventions to promptly attend to the infant's needs can decrease the length of fussiness and crying (Dihigo, 1998). Other approaches for relieving colic are listed in the Home Care box. Parents are encouraged to try as many of these approaches as possible, because not all are effective for every infant (Critical Thinking box).

Failure to Thrive (FTT)

FTT is a sign of inadequate growth resulting from inability to obtain and/or use calories required for growth. FTT has no universal definition, although one of the more common parameters is a weight (and sometimes height) that falls below the 5th percentile for the child's age. Growth measurements alone are not used to diagnose children with FTT; rather, the finding of a

Home Care

RELIEVING COLIC

- Place infant prone over a covered hot-water bottle, heated towel, or covered heating pad.
- Massage infant's abdomen.
- Respond immediately to the crying.
- Change infant's position frequently; walk with child's face down and with body across parent's arm, with parent's hand under infant's abdomen, applying gentle pressure (Fig. 36-15).
- Use a front carrier for transporting infant.
- Swaddle infant tightly with a soft, stretchy blanket.
- Place infant in a wind-up swing.
- Take infant for car rides or outside for a change in environment.
- Use bottles that minimize air swallowing (curved bottle and/or inner collapsible bag).
- Use a commercial device* in the crib that stimulates the vibration and sound of a car ride or plays soothing "noise," in utero sounds, or music.†
- Provide smaller, frequent feedings; burp infant during and after feedings using the shoulder position or sitting upright, and place infant in an upright seat after feedings.
- Introduce a pacifier for added sucking.
- In breastfed infants, mother should avoid all milk products for a trial period.
- If household members smoke, avoid smoking near infant; preferably confine smoking activity to outside of home.
- Give appropriate dose of acetaminophen elixir or suppository if suggested by health professional; not recommended for daily use.
- If nothing reduces the crying, place infant in crib and allow to cry; periodically hold and comfort child and put down again.

*Sweet Dreems, Inc., Sleep Tight Order Department, 4710 E. Walnut St., Westerville, OH 43081; 1-800-NO COLIC, 1-800-662-6542.
†Suggested infant relaxation music: "Heartbeat Lullabies" by Terry Woodford. Available from Baby-Go-To-Sleep Center, Audio Therapy Innovations, Inc., P.O. Box 550, Colorado Springs, CO 80901; 1-800-537-7748; website: www.babygotosleep.com.

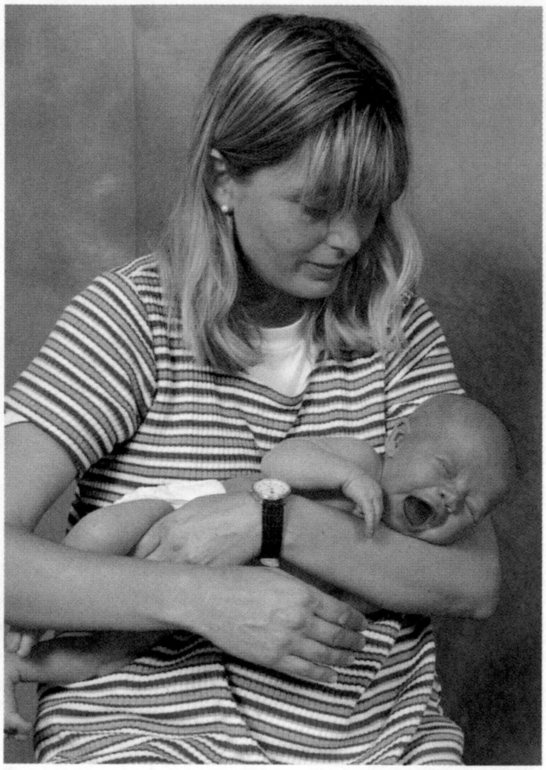

FIG. 36-15 • The "colic carry" may be comforting to an infant with colic. (Photo by Paul Vincent Kuntz, Texas Children's Hospital.)

Critical Thinking

COLIC

During a routine clinic visit you notice that the mother of a 2-month-old infant appears very tired, gets easily confused answering simple questions, and mentions that the infant cries much more than her first child did and for no apparent reason. You direct the focus of the interview on the infant's behavior preceding the crying spells; feeding habits, including dietary history; and patterns of sleep. The mother suspects that the infant has colic. What would be the best response to this mother?

First, Think About It . . .

- **What is the purpose of your thinking?**
- **What would the consequences be if you put your thoughts into actions?**

1. **"Are you concerned that maybe you have done something wrong with this child?"**
2. **"You must feel a little frustrated about this situation; can you tell me more about your concerns and how you are managing?"**
3. **"Colic is a complex problem for which there are few solutions other than giving the child medications and tolerating the crying the best way possible."**
4. **"We have some pamphlets on colic in the lobby; after you see the doctor, be sure to pick one up and read it at home."**

The best response is 2. The purpose is to allow the mother time to express her feelings about the colicky infant, as well as her own fears, and open the door for a discussion of some solutions to the problem. Options 3 and 4 end the discussion and are inappropriate nursing actions. Option 1 is too direct a question at this point in the interview and may suggest a concern the mother never had or may intensify any guilt.

persistent deviation from an established growth curve is cause for concern.

Three general categories of failure to thrive are the following:

1. **Organic failure to thrive** (OFTT)—Result of a physical cause, such as congenital heart defects, neurologic lesions, microencephaly, chronic renal failure, gastroesophageal reflux, malabsorption syndrome, endocrine dysfunction, cystic fibrosis, or acquired immunodeficiency syndrome (AIDS).
2. **Nonorganic failure to thrive** (NFTT)—Has a definable cause that is unrelated to disease. NFTT is most often the result of psychosocial factors, such as inadequate nutritional information by the parent; deficiency in maternal care or a disturbance in maternal-child attachment; or a disturbance in the child's ability to separate from the parent, leading to food refusal to maintain attention.
3. **Idiopathic failure to thrive**—Unexplained by the usual organic and environmental etiologies but may also be classified as NFTT. Both categories of NFTT account for the majority of cases of FTT.

Traditionally the category of NFTT has implied a disturbance in the parent-child interaction; however, this is not always the case. Many other factors can lead to inadequate feeding of the infant, such as the following:

Poverty—Lack of finds to buy sufficient food; may dilute formula to extend available supply

Health and/or childrearing beliefs—Use of fad diets; excessive concern with preventing conditions (e.g., obesity, hypercholesterolemia, or nursing caries); strict use of scheduled feedings

Inadequate nutritional knowledge—Confusion of newly arrived immigrants who are unaware of appropriate food selections in American markets; parents with cognitive impairment

Family stress—Involvement with another chronically ill child; any number of other stresses (e.g., financial, marital, excessive parenting and employment responsibilities, depression, chemical abuse, acute grief)

Feeding resistance—Result of nonoral nutritional therapy early in life

Insufficient breast milk—Result of a number of different causes (e.g., fatigue, illness, poor release of milk, insufficient glandular tissue, lack of maternal confidence)

In these instances parent education and provision of necessary supports (e.g., financial or psychosocial) are successful in correcting the reason for the malnutrition. Dealing with families in which a child has NFTT because of a parent-child disturbance is much more difficult and is the focus of the nursing care discussion.

Diagnostic Evaluation. Diagnosis is initially made from evidence of growth retardation. If FTT is recent, the weight, but not the height, is below accepted standards (usually the 5th percentile); if FTT is long-standing, both weight and height are depressed, indicating chronic malnutrition. Additional diagnostic procedures include a complete health and dietary history, physical examination for evidence of organic causes, developmental assessment, and a family assessment. Other tests are selected only as indicated to rule out organic problems. To prevent the overuse of diagnostic procedures, NFTT should be considered early in the differential diagnosis.

To avoid the social stigma of NFTT during the early investigative phase, many health care workers use the term *growth delay* (or *failure*) until the actual cause is established.

Therapeutic Management. Regardless of the cause of FTT, the treatment is directed at reversing the malnutrition. The goal is to provide sufficient calories to support "catch-up" growth—a rate of growth greater than the expected rate for age. Any coexisting medical problems are treated.

In most cases of NFTT a multidisciplinary team consisting of a physician, nurse, dietitian, child-life specialist, and social worker or mental health professional is needed to deal with the multiple psychologic problems. Efforts are made to relieve any additional stresses on the family, such as referrals to welfare agencies or supplemental food programs.

Prognosis. The prognosis for NFTT is related to the cause. If the parents have simply been ignorant of the infant's needs, teaching may remedy the child's limited caloric intake and permanently reverse the growth failure. Inadequate or decreased feeding periods by the infant's primary caretaker are often observed to be the cause of NFTT in conjunction with family disorganization. When the family dysfunction is extensive, the prognosis is uncertain. Factors related to poor prognosis are severe feeding resistance, lack of awareness in and cooperation from the parent(s), low family income, low maternal educational level, and early age of onset of NFTT.

Nursing Care Management

➤ Assessment

Nurses play a critical role in the diagnosis of NFTT through their assessment of the child, parents, and family interaction. Knowledge of the characteristics of children with NFTT and their families is essential in helping identify these children and hastening the confirmation of a correct diagnosis (Box 36-1). Accurate assessment of initial weight and height and daily weight, as well as recording of all food intake, is mandatory. The feeding behavior of the child is documented, as well as the parent-child interaction during feeding, other caregiving activities, and play.

A 25-item observational scale, the *Feeding Checklist,* was developed specifically for the purpose of observing mother-infant dyads with NFTT. The checklist has helped nurses and other health care professionals in the objective assessment of key aspects of infant and toddler feeding situations related to NFTT (MacPhee and Schneider, 1996).

A feature of many children with NFTT is their irregularity (low rhythmicity) in activities of daily living. Some of these children typify the "difficult" temperament pattern. However, another type is the passive, sleepy, lethargic infant who does not wake up for feedings. Parents who have been advised of "demand feeding schedules" may be unsure of whether to wake the child or let the child sleep. Because of their inexperience and lack of guidance, parents may develop a pattern of infrequent feeding that is inadequate to meet the infant's nutritional needs. Such a pattern is particularly detrimental with the breastfeeding infant, in whom frequent nursing is essential to an adequate milk supply.

Some parents are at increased risk for attachment problems because of (1) isolation and social crisis, (2) inadequate support systems, such as teenage and single mothers, and (3) poor parenting role models as a child. Other factors that should be considered are lack of education; physical and mental health problems such as physical and sexual abuse, depression, or drug dependence; immaturity, especially in adolescent parents; and lack of commitment to parenting, such as giving priority to other ventures such as entertainment or employment. Often these parents and their families are under stress and in multiple chronic emotional, social, and financial crises.

Box 36-1

Clinical Manifestations of Nonorganic Failure to Thrive

Growth failure—below 5th percentile in weight only or weight and height
Developmental retardation—social, motor, adaptive, language
Apathy
Poor hygiene
Withdrawn behavior
Feeding or eating disorders, such as vomiting, anorexia, pica, rumination
No fear of strangers (at age when stranger anxiety is normal)
Avoidance of eye contact
Wide-eyed gaze and continual scan of the environment ("radar gaze")
Stiff and unyielding or flaccid and unresponsive
Minimal smiling

➤ Nursing Diagnoses

A number of nursing diagnoses are prominent in the nursing care of the child with NFTT. The most common nursing diagnoses are as follows:

- Altered nutrition: less than body requirements related to:
  —Deprivation of necessities
  —Emotional deprivation
- Altered growth and development related to:
  —Socially restricted environment (infant deprivation)
  —Physical neglect
- Altered parenting related to:
  —(Specify, e.g., knowledge deficit, poverty)

If an organic cause is found, additional nursing diagnoses may be related to care specific for that disorder, such as heart disease.

➤ Plan of Care and Implementation

Planning needs to begin as soon as possible on admission. The highest-priority nursing goal is providing the infant with sufficient nutrients for growth. More specific nursing care depends on the identified cause of FTT. If an organic cause is confirmed, care is related primarily to management of the disorder. If the problem is one of inadequate knowledge regarding child feeding, parental education is required. When serious psychosocial factors are involved, hospitalization is needed and additional interventions are required to meet the needs of both the child and the family. The following are goals for the hospitalized child with NFTT and the family:

1. The child will experience weight gain.
2. The child will demonstrate positive response to developmental stimulation.
3. The family will demonstrate ability to provide appropriate care to the child.
4. The family will receive adequate support and home services.

Because part of the difficulty between parent and child is dissatisfaction and frustration, the child should have a primary core of nurses (Fig. 36-16). The nurses caring for the child can learn to perceive the child's cues and reverse the cycle of dissatisfaction, especially in the area of feeding. Because these children are not ill with any physical disorder but are debilitated from general malnutrition, they should be placed in a room with noninfectious children of a similar age. Depending on the cause of NFTT, children may be treated on an outpatient basis.

Because many of these children are responding to stimuli that have led to the negative feeding patterns, the first goal is to structure the feeding environment to encourage eating. General guidelines for the feeding process are outlined in the Guidelines box.

Four primary goals in the nutritional management of growth failure (FTT) are: (1) correct nutritional deficiencies and achieve ideal weight for height; (2) allow for catch-up growth; (3) restore optimum body composition; and (4) educate the parents or primary caregivers regarding the child's nutritional requirements and appropriate feeding methods (Maggioni and Lifshitz, 1995). To increase caloric intake in formula-fed infants, supplements such as Polycose or medium-chain triglycerides (MCTs) may be added slowly (Corrales and Utter, 1999). Other carbohydrate additives include rice cereal and vegetable oil. Because vitamin and mineral deficiencies may occur, multivitamin supplementation, including zinc and iron, is recommended. Usually only in extreme cases of malnourishment are tube feedings or intravenous therapy required.

Besides attending to the physical needs of the child, the interdisciplinary team must plan care for appropriate developmental stimulation. Once an approximate developmental age is established, a planned program of play is begun. Ideally a child-life specialist is involved to implement and supervise the stimulation program. Every effort is made to teach the parent how to play and interact with the child.

Nursing care of these children involves a "family systems" approach.

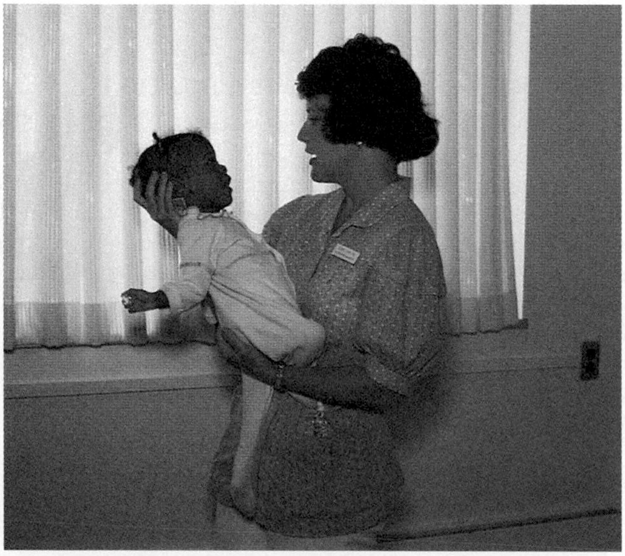

FIG. 36-16 • Consistent nursing contact is important in developing trust in infants with nonorganic failure to thrive.

Teaching infant care techniques to the parents is begun through *example* and *demonstration,* not by lecturing. As the nurse perceives the infant's cues, these are emphasized to the parents. For example, during a feeding the nurse might comment that the infant is still hungry because the child sucks vigorously and looks at the nurse. When the infant is satisfied, the nurse points out that the infant is signaling this by releasing the strong suck, closing the eyes, and breathing deeply and more slowly. By example, the child is gently placed in the crib for a nap.

Plans are made to implement these interventions at home. A home health referral is made, and if a foster grandparent was included, this person should also visit the family. Social agencies that can provide financial or housing assistance to lessen the stress of everyday life are also contacted.

➤ Evaluation

The effectiveness of nursing interventions is determined by continual reassessment and evaluation of care, based on the following observational guidelines and expected outcomes:

1. Record weight and caloric intake daily: document child's reaction to feeding environment: review notes to see

Guidelines

FEEDING CHILDREN WITH NONORGANIC FAILURE TO THRIVE

Provide a primary core of staff to feed the child. The same nurses are able to learn the child's cues and respond consistently.

Provide a quiet, unstimulating atmosphere. A number of these children are very distractable, and their attention is diverted with minimal stimuli. Older children do well at a feeding table; younger children should always be held.

Maintain a calm, even temperament throughout the meal. Negative outbursts may be commonplace in this child's habit formation. Limits on eating behavior definitely need to be provided, but they should be stated in a firm, calm tone. If the nurse is hurried or anxious, the feeding process will not be optimized.

Talk to the child by giving directions about eating. "Take a bite, Lisa" is appropriate and directive. The more distractible the child, the more directive the nurse should be to refocus attention on feeding. Positive comments about feeding are actively given.

Be persistent. This is perhaps one of the most important guidelines. Parents often give up when the child begins negative feeding behavior. Calm perseverance through 10 to 15 minutes of food refusal will eventually diminish negative behavior. Although forced feeding is avoided, "strictly encouraged" feeding is essential.

Maintain a face-to-face posture with the child when possible. Encourage eye contact and remain with the child throughout the meal.

Introduce new foods slowly. Often these children have been exclusively bottle-fed. If acceptance of solids is a problem, begin with pureed food and, once accepted, advance to junior and regular solid foods.

Follow the child's rhythm of feeding. The child will set a rhythm when the previous conditions are met.

Develop a structured routine. Disruption in their other activities of daily living has great impact on feeding responses, so bathing, sleeping, dressing, and playing, as well as feeding, are structured. The nurse should feed the child in the same way and place as often as possible. The length of the feeding should also be established (usually 30 minutes).

whether changes were made as necessary to improve eating and whether consistent group of nurses fed the child.
2. Perform developmental screening tests as needed.
3. Document parents' relationship with the child, staff and other supportive individuals. Note length of time parents visit, appointments kept with referral services, and any requests for help.
4. Keep a record of all patient teaching and note whether outcome behaviors were met.

Expected outcomes include the following:
1. Child gains weight (specify; usually a minimum of 1 to 2 oz/day).
2. Child displays a positive response to interventions (e.g., social smile).
3. Family demonstrates ability to provide appropriate care to child.
4. Family experiences reduction of anxiety and follows through on programs and activities. (See also the Nursing Care Plan "The Child with Nonorganic Failure to Thrive".*)

DISORDERS OF UNKNOWN ETIOLOGY

Sudden Infant Death Syndrome (SIDS)

SIDS is defined as the sudden death of an infant under 1 year of age that remains unexplained after a complete post-mortem examination, including an investigation of the death scene and a review of the case history. In the United States mortality from SIDS declined 38% between 1992 and 1996 (Willinger et al, 1998). The dramatic decrease is attributed to the "Back to Sleep" campaign† (see following section). SIDS is the third leading cause of death in children between the ages of 1 month and 1 year, and claimed the lives of almost 2500 infants in 1998 (Guyer et al, 1999). Table 36-11 summarizes the major epidemiologic characteristics of SIDS.

Etiology. Numerous theories have been proposed regarding the etiology of SIDS; however, the cause remains unknown. The most compelling hypothesis is that SIDS is related to a brainstem abnormality in the neurologic regulation of cardiorespiratory control. Abnormalities include prolonged sleep apnea, increased frequency of brief inspiratory pauses, excessive periodic breathing, and impaired arousal responsiveness to increased carbon dioxide or decreased oxygen. However, sleep apnea is not the cause of SIDS. The vast majority of infants with apnea do not die, and only a minority of SIDS victims have documented *apparent life-threatening events (ALTEs)* (see Apnea of Infancy, p. 874). A theory that has been disproved associated SIDS with diphtheria, tetanus, and pertussis vaccines.

Maternal smoking, both prenatally and postnatally, has been proposed as a possible cause of SIDS, as has poor prenatal care and low maternal age (Leach et al, 1999). Co-sleeping, or bed sharing, has been reported to have a possible association with SIDS, especially in cases of maternal smoking. The American Academy of Pediatrics (1997) recommends that adults follow the same safeguards in the bed as in the crib. In addition, the bed sharer should not smoke or use substances such as alcohol or drugs that may impair arousal. Unlike cribs, which are designed to meet safety standards for infants, adult beds are not so designed and may carry a risk of accidental entrapment and suffocation. Suffocation hazards included wedging between a mattress or bed and wall and oronasal obstruction by a plastic bag (Drago and Dannenberg, 1999).

The most compelling data come from studies that link sleep habits with an increased risk of SIDS. Sleeping in the prone position may cause oropharyngeal obstruction or affect the thermal balance or arousal state.

The American Academy of Pediatrics (1996) recommends that healthy infants be placed to sleep in the supine (on the back) position. There is an increased risk of SIDS in infants placed in the side-lying position, primarily due to their ability to turn to a prone position. Soft bedding such as pillows or quilts should not be used under the infant for bedding. Bedding items such as stuffed animals or towels should be removed from the crib while the infant is asleep to prevent possible asphyxia.

Infants with gastroesophageal reflux and other upper airway anomalies that predispose to airway obstruction may be placed in a prone sleeping position. Most preterm infants being discharged from the hospital should be placed in the supine sleep position unless there are factors that predispose to airway obstruction.

TABLE 36-11
Epidemiology of SIDS

Factors	Occurrence
Incidence	0.6:1000 live births (1998)
Peak age	2 to 4 months; 95% occur by 6 months
Sex	Higher percentage of males affected
Time of death	During sleep
Time of year	Increased incidence in winter
Racial	Greater incidence in Native Americans, African-Americans, and Hispanics
Socioeconomic	Increased occurrence in lower socioeconomic class
Birth	Higher incidence in: Premature infants, especially infants of low birth weight Multiple births* Neonates with low Apgar scores Infants with central nervous system disturbances and respiratory disorders such as bronchopulmonary dysplasia Increasing birth order (subsequent siblings as opposed to firstborn child) Infants with a recent history of illness
Sleep habits	Prone position; use of soft bedding; overheating (thermal stress); co-sleeping with adult, especially on sofa
Feeding habits	Lower incidence in breastfed infants
Siblings	May have greater incidence
Maternal	Young age; cigarette smoking, especially during pregnancy; poor prenatal care; substance abuse (heroin, methadone, cocaine)

*Although a rare event, simultaneous death of twins from SIDS can occur.

*In Wong DL, Hess CS: ***Wong and Whaley's clinical manual of pediatric nursing,*** ed 5, St Louis, 2000, Mosby.
†"Back to Sleep" materials may be ordered by calling 1-800-505-CRIB; fax (301) 496-7101; or write NICHD/Back to Sleep, 31 Center Drive, Room 2A32, Bethesda, MD 20892-2425.

NURSE ALERT • Research findings have important implications for practices that may reduce the risk of SIDS, such as avoiding smoking during pregnancy and near the infant; encouraging the supine sleeping position; avoiding soft moldable mattresses, blankets, and pillows; discouraging bed sharing; encouraging breastfeeding; and avoiding overheating during sleep. The infant's head position should be varied to prevent flattening of the skull *(positioning plagiocephaly).*

Although the etiology is unknown, autopsies reveal consistent pathologic findings such as pulmonary edema and intrathoracic hemorrhages that confirm the diagnosis of SIDS. Consequently, autopsies should be performed on all infants suspected of dying of SIDS, and the findings should be shared with the parents as soon as possible after the death.

Whether subsequent siblings of one SIDS infant are at increased risk for SIDS is unclear. Even if the increased risk is correct, families have a 99% chance that their subsequent child will *not* die of SIDS. Home monitoring is not recommended for this group of children, but it is often used by practitioners and may even be requested by parents. Monitoring is best initiated on an individual basis.

Nursing Considerations. Loss of a child from SIDS presents several crises with which the parents must cope. In addition to grief and mourning for the death of their child, the parents must face a tragedy that was sudden, unexpected, and unexplained. The psychologic intervention for the family must deal with these additional variables. This discussion focuses primarily on the objectives of care for families experiencing SIDS, rather than on the process of grief and mourning, which is explored in Chapter 41.

Finding the Infant. Usually it is the mother who finds the child dead in the crib. Typically the child is in a disheveled bed, with blankets over the head, and huddled in a corner. Frothy, blood-tinged fluid fills the mouth and nostrils, and the infant may be lying face down in the secretions, suggesting that he or she bled to death. The diaper is wet and full of stool, which is consistent with a cataclysmic type of death. The hands may be clutching the sheets, as if the child were in distress before death. The initial appearance of the child, combined with the shock of such an unexpected event, adds to the horror that the parents must face.

Often the mother is alone and must deal with her initial shock, panic, grief, questions of the other siblings, and the decision of where to find help. The first persons to arrive may be the police and ambulance attendants. Hopefully they will handle the situation by asking few questions; giving no indication of wrongdoing, abuse, or neglect; making sensitive judgments concerning any resuscitation efforts for the child; and comforting the members of the family as much as possible. These individuals should be properly informed about SIDS in order to recognize its characteristic signs and tell parents that their child probably died of a disease called sudden infant death syndrome, which cannot be predicted or prevented. A compassionate, sensitive approach to the family during the very first few minutes can help spare them some of the overwhelming guilt and anguish that commonly follow this type of death.

Arriving at the Emergency Department. The first contact that nurses typically have with these families is in the emergency department, when the infant is seen by a physician in order to be pronounced dead. Usually there is no attempt at resuscitation. During the time in the emergency department several aspects warrant special consideration. Parents are asked only factual questions, such as when they found the infant, how he or she looked, and whom they called for help. Any remarks that may suggest responsibility, such as why didn't they go in earlier, didn't they hear the infant cry out, was the head buried in a blanket, or were the other siblings jealous of this child, are avoided.

If statements were made that were misguided, such as "This looks like suffocation," they can be corrected before parents harbor them in their minds as indications of their guilt. The discussion of an autopsy should be presented at this time, emphasizing that a diagnosis cannot be confirmed until the postmortem examination is completed. If the mother was breastfeeding, she needs information about abrupt discontinuation of lactation.

Another important aspect of compassionate care for these parents is allowing them to say good-bye to their child. Because the parents leave the hospital without their infant, it is helpful to accompany them to the car or arrange for someone else to take them home. A debriefing session may help health care workers who dealt with the family and deceased infant to deal with feelings that are often engendered when a SIDS victim is brought into the acute care facility.

Returning Home. When the parents return home, they should be visited by a competent, qualified professional as soon after the death as possible. Printed material that contains excellent information about SIDS (available from the national organizations*) should be provided.

Ideally the number of visits and plans for subsequent intervention need to be flexible. For example, the siblings may initially appear accepting of the explanation and well-adjusted, but may later refuse to go to sleep or ask questions about graves or funerals, indicating their need for further help in dealing with the death. Parents facing the question of a subsequent child will need support. Both the birth of a subsequent child and the survival of that child, especially past the age of death of the previous child, are important transitional stages for parents.

Because the mourning process continues *for at least a year,* and because most health plans do not cover periodic visits to the family to evaluate their progress, referrals to other parents who have lost a child to SIDS should be considered.

Apnea of Infancy (AOI)

AOI generally refers to pathologic apnea in infants of more than 37 weeks' gestation. The clinical presentation of AOI is an *apparent life-threatening event (ALTE)* (previously referred to by the inaccurate and misleading expression, "near-miss SIDS") that is described as:

- Frightening to the observer, who fears the child died or would have died without vigorous intervention

*Sudden Infant Death Syndrome Clearinghouse, 8201 Greensboro Dr., Suite 600, McLean, VA 22102; (703) 821-8955; American Sudden Infant Death Syndrome (SIDS) Institute, 6065 Roswell Rd., Suite 876, Atlanta, GA 30328; 1-800-232-SIDS (in Georgia, 1-800-847-SIDS); website: www.sids.org; The Sudden Infant Death Syndrome Alliance, 1314 Bedford Ave., Suite 210, Baltimore, MD 21208; 1-800-221-SIDS.

- Some combination of:
  - **Apnea**—Cessation of breathing for 20 seconds or more
  - **Color change**—Cyanosis or pallor, but sometimes plethora
  - **Marked change in muscle tone**—Usually marked hypotonia
  - **Choking or gagging**

AOI can be a symptom of many disorders, including sepsis, seizures, upper airway abnormalities, gastroesophageal reflux, hypoglycemia or other metabolic problems, impaired regulation of breathing during sleep or feeding, or a result of intentional poisoning by a caregiver. Abnormal physical properties of pulmonary surfactant have been identified in some children with recurrent ALTE (Silvestri and Weese-Mayer, 1996). However, in about half the cases no cause is identified. Infants with a history of ALTEs are at increased risk for SIDS, but these children constitute less than 7% of all SIDS victims. A diagnosis of AOI is made when no identifiable cause for the ALTE is found.

Diagnostic Evaluation. The most widely used test is continuous recording of cardiorespiratory patterns (cardiopneumogram or pneumocardiogram). Four-channel (or multichannel pneumogram) pneumocardiograms monitor heart rate, respirations (chest impedance), nasal airflow, and oxygen saturation. A more sophisticated test, polysomnography ("sleep study"), also records brain waves, eye and body movements, esophageal manometry, and end-tidal carbon dioxide measurements. However, none of these tests can predict risk. Some children with normal results may still have subsequent apneic episodes.

Therapeutic Management. Treatment usually involves continuous home monitoring of cardiorespiratory rhythms and/or the use of methylxanthines (respiratory stimulant drugs such as theophylline or caffeine). Therapeutic levels are typically 6 to 10 or 13 (g/ml of theophylline and 10 to 20 (g/ml of caffeine. The criteria for discontinuing the monitoring is based on the infant's clinical condition. A general guideline for discontinuation is when infants with ALTEs have gone 2 or 3 months without significant numbers of episodes requiring intervention.

NURSE ALERT • The concentration of theophylline required for apnea is less than that required for bronchodilation.

Nursing Considerations. The diagnosis of AOI engenders great anxiety and concern in parents, and the institution of home monitoring presents additional physical and emotional burdens. If monitoring is required, the nurse can be a major source of support to the family in terms of education about the equipment; observation of the infant's status; and immediate intervention during apneic episodes, including cardiorespiratory resuscitation (CPR) (see Critical Thinking box). To help the family cope with the numerous procedures they must learn, adequate preparation before discharge and written instructions are essential.*

Several types of home monitors are available, and most hospitals select the model that the infant will use at home. Nurses, especially those involved in the care at home, must become familiar with the equipment, including its advantages and disadvantages. Safety is a major concern because monitors can cause electrical burns and electrocution. The following precautions are recommended:

- Remove leads from infant when not attached to monitor.
- Unplug power cord from electrical outlet when cord is not plugged into monitor.
- Use safety covers on electrical outlets to discourage children from inserting objects into a socket.

Siblings should also be supervised when near the infant and taught that the monitor is not a toy. Other safety practices include informing local utility and rescue squads of the home monitoring in case of an emergency. Telephone numbers for these services should be posted near all telephones in the home.

Caregivers need detailed information regarding proper attachment of the electrodes to the infant's chest with impedance monitors that detect chest movement. The electrodes are placed in the midaxillary line, at a space one or two fingerbreadths below the nipple (Fig. 36-17). Adhesive electrodes are attached directly to the skin. For home use, electrodes attached to a belt that is placed around the child's trunk are preferred. The belt is positioned so that the electrodes contact the skin in the same area as shown in Fig. 36-17. Monitors may have memory chips that allow for event recording, which can be an effective tool in evaluating the use of the monitor and reported frequency of alarms.

Monitors are effective only if they are used. They do not prevent death but alert the caregiver to the ALTE in time to inter-

Critical Thinking

HOME APNEA MONITORING

A family has just brought their newborn home on an apnea monitor. The diagnosis is apnea of infancy. You are the nurse making the first home visit. Which of the following should you not expect to find?

First, Think About It . . .

- **What is the purpose of your thinking?**
- **How are you interpreting the information?**

1. **The parent appears knowledgeable about monitor use, responses to alarms, and CPR.**
2. **The infant's respiratory status is stable and color is good.**
3. **The monitor is plugged into an extension cord**
4. **The family appears anxious.**

The best response is 3. The purpose of your thinking may focus on safety, and medical equipment should not be plugged into extension cords. If necessary, furniture and equipment should be rearranged so that an appropriate outlet can be used. Regarding the other answers, parents should be well trained in caring for the child on an apnea monitor before being sent home. You may interpret the information to indicate that the nurse usually only needs to review procedures. However, if parents do not have the necessary information and skills, training should be a priority on the first home visit. Anxiety is common for the first 4 to 8 weeks of home apnea monitoring. An infant with a diagnosis of apnea of prematurity should appear healthy and should not evidence respiratory distress. Signs to the contrary necessitate immediate contact with the family's practitioner.

---

*Community and home care instructions for apnea monitoring and CPR are available in Wong DL, Hess CS: *Wong and Whaley's clinical manual of pediatric nursing,* ed 5, St Louis, 2000, Mosby. Educational materials may also be obtained from the American SIDS Institute, 6065 Roswell Rd., Suite 876, Atlanta, GA 30328.

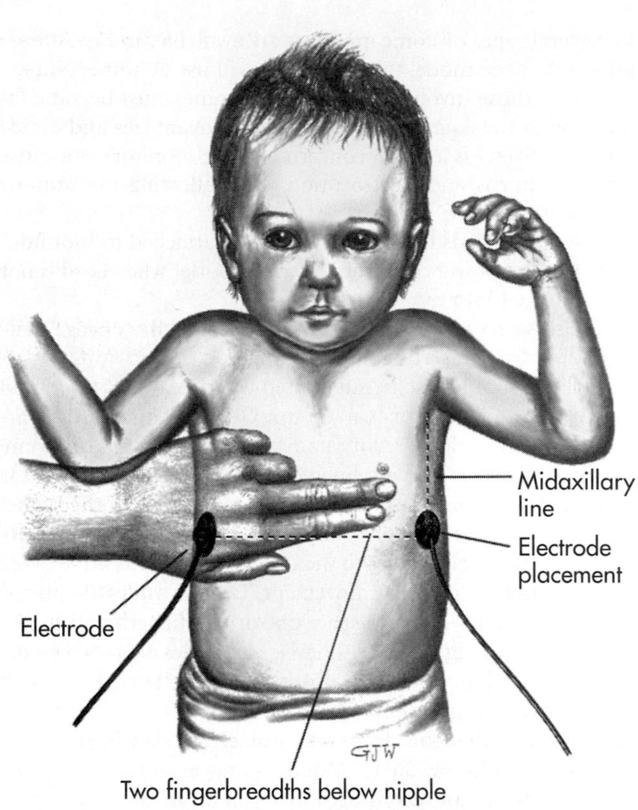

FIG. 36-17 • Electrode placement for apnea monitoring. In small infants one fingerbreadth may be used.

vene. The need to use the monitor and to respond appropriately to alarms must be stressed. Noncompliance can result in the infant's death.

NURSE ALERT • If the infant is apneic, gently stimulate the trunk by patting or rubbing it. If the infant is prone, turn to the back and flick the feet. If there is still no response, begin CPR. Never vigorously shake the child. No more than 15 to 20 seconds are spent on stimulation before implementing CPR.

Family Support. Although AOI is not a chronic illness, many of the stresses observed during the monitoring period are characteristic of those of families with chronically ill children. Parents report increased stress, including concern for the child's survival, fear of incompetency in assuming home responsibility, inadequate respite care, social isolation, constant work, and fatigue. Siblings are impacted as well as the affected child, who may be characterized as "spoiled" and have developmental delays. To deal with these potential effects, nurses need to use the same interventions as those discussed for children with chronic illness (see Chapter 41) and be aware of the need for referral when difficulties are suspected.

To lessen the continuous responsibility of monitoring, other family members such as grandparents should be taught how to manipulate the equipment, read and interpret the signals, and administer CPR. They are encouraged to stay with the infant for regular periods to allow parents respite. Support groups of other families who have successfully completed monitoring can also be of benefit. Because baby-sitters are difficult to locate, support group members or nursing students may be potential sources of qualified caregivers.

Autism

Autism is a complex developmental disorder of brain function accompanied by a broad range and severity of intellectual and behavioral deficits. It is manifested during infancy and early childhood primarily from 18 to 30 months of age. It occurs in 1 in 2500 children; is about 4 times more common in males than in females (although females are more severely affected); and is not related to socioeconomic level, race, or parenting style.

Etiology. The etiology of autism is an unknown. However, considerable evidence supports multiple biologic causes. Individuals with autism may have abnormal electroencephalograms, epileptic seizures, delayed development of hand dominance, persistence of primitive reflexes, metabolic abnormalities (elevated blood serotonin), and cerebellar vermal hypoplasia (part of the brain involved in regulating motion and some aspects of memory).

There is also strong evidence for a genetic basis that in twins is consistent with an autosomal-recessive pattern of inheritance. Twin studies demonstrate a very high concordance (96%) for monozygotic (identical) twins and a 24% concordance for dizygotic (nonidentical) twins. In addition, between 5% and 16% of males with autism are positive for the fragile X chromosome (see Fragile X Syndrome, Chapter 42).

There is a 3% to 8% risk of recurrence of autism in families with one affected child. Although the serotonin-transporter gene has been suggested as a possible causative factor in autism, no specific gene for the disorder has been identified (Rapin, 1997).

Clinical Manifestations and Diagnostic Evaluation. Children with autism demonstrate several peculiar and often seemingly bizarre characteristics, primarily in social interactions, communication, and behavior. Other clinical manifestations typically seen in children with autism are described in Box 36-2. There is a range in severity of clinical manifestations from mild forms, requiring minimal supervision; to severe forms, in which self-abusive behavior is common. The majority of children with autism have some degree of moderate to severe mental retardation. Despite their relatively moderate to severe disability, some children with autism (known as *savants*) excel in particular areas such as art, music, memory, mathematics, or perceptual skills such as puzzle building.

The therapeutic management of autism with the hormone secretin is controversial. One recent study failed to demonstrate significant improvement when autistic children were given one dose of synthetic human secretion (Sandler et al, 1999).*

Prognosis. Autism is usually a severely disabling condition. However, there are reports of children improving with acquisition of language skills and communication with others (Rapin, 1997). Some ultimately achieve independence, but most require lifelong adult supervision. Aggravation of psychiatric symptoms occurs in about half of the children during adolescence, with girls having a tendency for continued deterioration.

*Additional information on secretin may be found at the website: www.autism.org/secretin.html.

Box 36-2
Clinical Manifestations of Autism

SOCIAL RELATIONS AND BEHAVIOR
Extreme interpersonal isolation
Intense, abnormal concern for preservation of sameness
Unyielding to cuddling and holding
Do not respond to verbal stimulation
Bizarre attachment to mechanical objects
Odd repetitive behaviors, such as flicking a light switch on and off
Difficult to manage; passive or irritable
Frequent temper tantrums and/or self-destructive behavior

DEVELOPMENT
Mental retardation, usually severe
May have advanced gross motor skills
Normal to hyperactive
May have exceptional ability (e.g., memory)
Poor suck and feeding responses

LANGUAGE
Echolalia or parrot speech (automatic repetition of words spoken to them)
Pronominal reversal (tendency to use "you" for "I")
Literal, concrete use of words (e.g., "in" to mean "door")

SENSORY/PERCEPTUAL PROCESSES
Sensory deficits even though vision and hearing intact
Act as if deaf, yet may be overly sensitive to sound
Hyposensitive or hypersensitive to pain
Have aversion to touch

Early recognition of behaviors associated with autism is critical in order to implement appropriate interventions and family involvement. The prognosis is most favorable for children with communicative speech development by age 6 years and an intelligence quotient above 50 at the time of diagnosis.

Nursing Considerations. Therapeutic intervention for the child with autism is a specialized area involving professionals with advanced training. Although there is no cure for autism, numerous therapies have been used. The most promising results have been through highly structured and intensive behavior-modification programs. In general, the objective in treatment is to promote positive reinforcement, increase social awareness of others, teach verbal communication skills, and decrease unacceptable behavior. Providing a structured routine for the child to follow is a key in the management of autism.

When these children are hospitalized, the parents are essential to planning care and ideally should stay with the child as much as possible. Nurses should recognize that not all children with autism are the same, and that they will require individual assessment and treatment. Decreasing stimulation by using a private room, avoiding extraneous auditory and visual distraction, and encouraging the parents to bring in possessions the child is attached to may lessen the disruptiveness of hospitalization. Because physical contact often upsets these children, minimum holding and eye contact may be necessary to avoid behavioral outbursts. Care must be taken when performing procedures on, administering medicine to, or feeding these children, because they are either fussy eaters who may willfully starve themselves or gag to prevent eating; or indiscriminate hoarders, swallowing any available edible or inedible items, such as a thermometer.

They need to be introduced slowly to new situations, with visits with staff caregivers kept short whenever possible. Because these children have difficulty organizing their behavior and redirecting their energy, they need to be told directly what to do. Communication should be at the child's developmental level, brief, and concrete. Only one request is given at a time, such as "sit on bed."

Family Support. Parents need expert counseling early in the course of the disorder and should be referred to the Autism Society of America (ASA).* ASA provides information about education, treatment programs and techniques, and facilities such as camps and group homes. There is also a siblings group called SHARE (Siblings Helping Persons with Autism Through Resources and Energy). Other helpful resources are the local and state departments of mental health and developmental disabilities; these organizations provide important programs for autistic children and in-school programs throughout the United States. As the child approaches adulthood and parents become older, the family may require assistance in locating a long-term placement facility (see also Chapter 41).

*7910 Woodmont Ave., Suite 300, Bethesda, MD 20814; 1-800-3-AUTISM, ext. 150; (301) 657-0881; website: www.autism-society.org.

Key Points

- Biologic development of the child encompasses proportional changes; sensory changes, including binocularity, depth perception, and visual preference; maturation of biologic systems; fine motor development; and gross motor development.
- Erikson's theory of psychosocial development (birth to 1 year) is concerned with acquiring a sense of trust while overcoming a sense of mistrust.
- Piaget's theory of cognitive development, as it applies to the infant, focuses on the sensorimotor phase, which includes the use of reflexes, primary circular reactions, secondary circular reactions, and coordination or secondary schemata and their application to new situations.
- Development of body image begins in infancy; by 1 year of age infants recognize that they are distinct from their parents.
- Social development of the infant is guided by attachment, language development, personal-social behavior, and participation in play.
- Temperament influences the type of interaction that occurs between the child and parents and siblings.
- Parents are faced with many concerns, including infant fears, day care, limit setting and discipline, thumb-sucking and pacifier use, teething, and choice of infant shoes.
- Breast milk or formula is the most desirable food for the infant during the first 6 months, followed by gradual introduction of solid food during the second 6 months. Whole milk is not recommended until after 12 months.

- Common sleep problems that develop during infancy—and that are easily prevented—are associated with night crying and feeding. Nurses should instruct the parents, after careful assessment, in strategies to deal with the specific problem.
- Cleaning the teeth regularly and appropriate dietary intake promote good dental health.
- Recommended routine immunizations include those for hepatitis B virus, hepatitis A (in some states), diphtheria, tetanus, pertussis, polio, measles, mumps, rubella, pneumoccoccal, chickenpox, and *Haemophilus influenzae* type b.
- Recommended immunizations for selected groups of children are influenza virus, Lyme, hepatitis A, pneumococcal, and meningococcal vaccines.
- Because injuries are a major cause of death during infancy, parents should be alerted to aspiration of foreign objects, suffocation, falls, poisoning, burns, motor vehicle injuries, and bodily damage, as well as preventive actions needed to make the environment safe for infants.
- Treatment of colic may involve change in feeding practices, correction of a stressful environment, behavior modification, and support of the parent.
- Failure to thrive may be classified as organic, resulting from some physical cause; or nonorganic, resulting from psychosocial factors involving the child and caregiver (e.g., maternal deprivation), environmental causes (e.g., inadequate parental knowledge of child feeding), or unexplained causes.
- Sudden infant death syndrome is the third leading cause of death in children between the ages of 1 month and 1 year.
- Evidence linking SIDS to the prone sleeping position has led to the recommendation that healthy infants sleep supine.
- The primary nursing responsibility in care associated with sudden infant death and other conditions of unknown etiology is emotional support of the family.
- Children with apnea of infancy receive home monitoring to alert the family to an apparent life-threatening event.
- Autism is a disabling, permanent condition characterized by a broad range and severity of deficits in social interaction, communication, and behavior.

References

Advisory Committee on Immunization Practices: Revised recommendations for routine poliomyelitis vaccination, *MMWR Morb Mortal Wkly Rep* 48(27):590, 1999.

American Academy of Pediatrics, Committee on Environmental Health: Ultraviolet light: a hazard to children, *Pediatrics* 104(2):328-333, 1999b.

American Academy of Pediatrics, Committee on Infectious Diseases, Pickering L, editor: *2000 Red Book: report of the Committee on Infectious Diseases,* ed 25, Elk Grove Village, IL, 2000a, The Academy.

American Academy of Pediatrics, Committee on Infectious Diseases: Age for routine administration of the second dose of measles-mumps-rubella vaccine, *Pediatrics* 101(1):129-135, 1998a.

American Academy of Pediatrics, Committee on Infectious Diseases: Poliomyelitis prevention: revised recommendations for use of inactivated and live oral poliovirus vaccines, *Pediatrics* 103(1):171-173, 1999a.

American Academy of Pediatrics, Committee on Infectious Diseases: Recommended childhood immunization schedule—United States, January-December, 2000, *Pediatrics* 105(1): 148-151, 2000b.

American Academy of Pediatrics, Committee on Injury and Poison Prevention: Injuries associated with infant walkers, *Pediatrics* 95(5):778-780, 1995.

American Academy of Pediatrics, Committee on Nutrition: *Pediatric nutrition handbook,* ed 4, Elk Grove Village, IL, 1998b, The Academy.

American Academy of Pediatrics, Committee on Sports Medicine: Infant exercise programs, *Pediatrics* 82(5):800, 1988.

American Academy of Pediatrics, Committee on Sports Medicine and Committee on Injury and Poison Prevention: Swimming programs for infants and toddlers, *Pediatrics* 105(4, part 1 of 2):868-869, 2000c.

American Academy of Pediatrics, Task Force on Infant Positioning and SIDS: Does bed sharing affect the risk of SIDS? *Pediatrics* 109(2):272-273, 1997.

American Academy of Pediatrics, Task Force on Infant Positioning: Positioning and sudden infant death syndrome (SIDS): update, *Pediatrics* 98(6):1218-1220, 1996.

Balon AJ: Management of infantile colic, *Am Fam Physician* 55(1):235-242, 1997.

Biancuzzo M: *Breastfeeding the newborn: clinical strategies for nurses,* St Louis, 1999, Mosby.

Bocar DL: Combining breastfeeding and employment: increasing success, *J Perinat Neonat Nurs* 11(2):23-43, 1997.

Carey WB, McDevitt SC: Revision of the infant temperament questionnaire, *Pediatrics* 61(5):735-739, 1978.

Corbett-Dick P, Bezek SK: Breastfeeding promotion for the employed mother, *J Pediatric Health Care* 11(1):12-19, 1997.

Corrales KM, Utter SL: Failure to thrive. In Samoor PQ, Helm KKI, Lang CE, editors: *Handbook of pediatric nutrition,* ed 2, Gaithersburg, MD, 1999, Aspen Publications.

Dennison BA, Rockwell HL, Baker SL: Excess fruit juice consumption by preschool-aged children is associated with short stature and obesity, *Pediatrics* 99(1):15-22, 1997.

Dewey KG et al: Breastfed infants are leaner than formula-fed infants at 1 year of age: the DARLING study, *Am J Clin Nutr* 57(2):140-145, 1993.

Dihigo SK: New strategies for the treatment of colic: modifying the parent/infant interaction, *J Pediatr Health Care* 12(5):256-262, 1998.

Drago DA, Dannenberg AL: Infant mechanical suffocating deaths in the United States, 1980-1997, *Pediatrics* 103(5):e59, 1999.

Ferber R, Kryger M: *Principles and practice of sleep medicine in the child,* Philadelphia, 1995, WB Saunders.

Guyer B et al: Annual summary of vital statistics—1998, *Pediatrics* 104(6):1229-1246, 1999.

Holida DL: Latex balloons: they can take your breath away, *Pediatr Nurs* 19(1):39-43, 1993.

Horn MI, McCarthy AM: Children's responses to sequential versus simultaneous immunization injections, *J Pediatr Health Care* 13(1):18-23, 1999.

Johns RM, Miller L, Hochstetler I: Mother and baby dental care, *Mother Baby J* 3(3):15-22, 1998.

Jones L, Heermann J: Parental division of infant care: contextual influences and infant characteristics, *Nurs Res* (4):228-234, 1992.

Leach CEA et al: Epidemiology of SIDS and explained sudden infant deaths, *Pediatrics* 104(4):e43, 1999.

MacPhee M, Schneider J: A clinical tool for nonorganic failure-to-thrive feeding interactions, *J Pediatr Nurs* 11(1):29-39, 1996.

Maggioni A, Lifshitz F: Nutritional management of failure to thrive, *Pediatr Clin North Am* 42(4):791-810, 1995.

Medoff-Cooper B: Infant temperament: implications for parenting from birth through 1 year, *J Pediatr Nurs* 10(3):141-145, 1995.

Medoff-Cooper B, Carey WB, McDevitt SC: The early infancy temperament questionnaire, *J Dev Behav Pediatr* 14(4): 230-235, 1993.

Murphy JM: Pediatric occupant car safety: clinical implications, based on recent literature, *Pediatr Nurs* 25(2):137-148, 1999.

Niemela M, Uhari M, Mottonen M: A pacifier increases the risk of recurrent acute otitis media in children in day care centers, *Pediatrics* 96(5, pt 1):884-888, 1995.

Nowak AJ: What pediatricians can do to promote oral health, *Contemp Pediatr* 10(4):90-106, 1993.

Overturf, GD: American Academy of Pediatrics Committee on Infectious Diseases technical report: prevention of pneumococcal infections, including the use of pneumococcal conjugate and polysaccharide vaccines and antibiotic prophylaxis, *Pediatrics* 106(2 Pt 1):367-376, 2000.

Pickler R, Frankel H: The effect of non-nutritive sucking on preterm infants' behavioral organization and feeding performance, *Neonatal Network* 14(2):83, 1995.

Prevention of hepatitis A through active or passive immunization: recommendations of the advisory committee on immunization practices (ACIP), *MMWR* 48(RR12):1-37, Oct. 1, 1999.

Rapin I: Autism, *N Engl J Med* 337(2):97-103, 1997.

Sandler AD et al: Lack of benefit of a single dose of synthetic human secretin in the treatment of autism and pervasive developmental disorder, *N Engl J Med* 341(24):1801-1806, 1999.

Sheridan R, Sheridan M, Tompkins R: Dishwasher effluent burns in infants, *Pediatrics* 91(1):142-143, 1993.

Silvestri JM, Weese-Mayer DE: Respiratory control disorders in infancy and childhood, *Curr Opin Pediatr* 8(3):216-220, 1996.

Skinner JD et al: Fruit juice is not related to children's growth, *Pediatrics* 103(1):58-64, 1999.

Smith MM, Lifshitz F: Excess fruit juice consumption as a contributing factor in nonorganic failure to thrive, *Pediatrics* 93(3):438-443, 1994.

Willinger M et al: Factors associated with the transition to nonprone sleeping positions of infants in the United States: The National Infant Sleep Position study, *JAMA* 280(4):329-335, 1998.

Zuckerman JN, Cockcroft A, Zuckerman AJ: Site of injection for vaccination, *BMJ* 305(6862):1158, 1992.

CHAPTER 37

The Toddler and Family

http://www.harcourthealth.com/MERLIN/Wong/maternal/

Learning Objectives

On completion of this chapter the reader will be able to:

- Identify the major biologic, psychosocial, cognitive, and social developments during the toddler years.
- Relate separation anxiety and negativism to developmental tasks.
- Recognize readiness for toilet training and offer parents guidelines.
- Prepare toddlers for the birth of a sibling.
- Provide parents with guidelines for handling temper tantrums.
- Provide parents with feeding recommendations.
- Outline a preventive dental hygiene plan for toddlers.
- Provide anticipatory guidance to parents regarding injury prevention based on the toddler's developmental achievements.

PROMOTING OPTIMUM GROWTH AND DEVELOPMENT

The term *terrible twos* has often been used to describe the toddler years, the period from 12 to 36 months of age. It is a time of intense exploration of the environment as children attempt to find out how things work and how to control others through temper tantrums, negativism, and obstinacy. Although this can be a challenging time for parents and child as each learns to know the other better, it is an extremely important period for developmental achievement and intellectual growth.

Biologic Development

Proportional Changes. Growth slows considerably during toddlerhood. The average *weight* gain is 1.8 to 2.7 kg (4 to 6 pounds). The birth weight is quadrupled by 2½ years of age. The rate of increase in height also slows. The usual increment is an addition of 7.5 cm (3 inches) per year and occurs mainly in elongation of the legs rather than the trunk. The average *height* of a 2-year-old is 86.6 cm (34 inches). In general, adult height is about twice the 2-year-old child's height. Accurate measurement of height and weight during the toddler years should reveal a steady growth curve that is *steplike* in nature rather than linear (straight), which is characteristic of the growth spurts during the early childhood years.*

The rate of increase in *head circumference* slows somewhat by the end of infancy, and head circumference is usually equal to chest circumference by 1 to 2 years of age. The usual total increase in head circumference during the second year is 2.5 cm (1 inch). Then the rate of increase slows until at age 5 years the increase is less than 1.25 cm (½ inch) per year. The anterior fontanel closes between 12 and 18 months of age.

Chest circumference continues to increase in size and exceeds head circumference during the toddler years. Its shape also changes as the transverse, or lateral diameter exceeds the anteroposterior diameter. After the second year the chest circumference exceeds the abdominal measurement; this, in addition to the growth of the lower extremities, gives the child a taller, leaner appearance. However, the toddler retains a squat, "potbellied" appearance because of the less well developed abdominal musculature and short legs. The legs retain a slightly bowed or curved appearance during the second year from the weight of the relatively large trunk.

Sensory Changes. *Visual acuity* of 20/40 is considered acceptable during the toddler years. Full binocular vision is well developed, and any evidence of persistent strabismus requires professional attention as early as possible to prevent amblyopia. Depth perception continues to develop but, because of the child's lack of motor coordination, falls from heights continue to be a persistent danger.

The senses of *hearing, smell, taste,* and *touch* become increasingly well developed, coordinated with each other, and associated with other experiences. All of the senses are used to explore the environment. Toddlers will visually inspect an object

*For additional information, please view "Growth and Development" in *Whaley and Wong's Pediatric Nursing Video Series,* St Louis, 1996, Mosby; phone 1-800-426-4545; website: www.mosby.com.

by turning it over; they may taste it, smell, it, and touch it several times before they are satisfied with their investigation. They will shake it to see if it makes noise, and vigorously test its durability.

Another example of the integrated function of the senses is the toddler's development of specific *taste preferences.* The child is much less likely than infants to try a new food because of its appearance or smell, not just its taste.

Maturation of Systems. Most of the physiologic systems are relatively mature by the end of toddlerhood. Volume of the *respiratory tract* and growth of associated structures continue to increase during early childhood, lessening some of the factors that predisposed the child to frequent and serious infections during infancy. The internal structures of the ear and throat continue to be short and straight, and the lymphoid tissue of the tonsils and adenoids continues to be large. As a result, otitis media, tonsillitis, and upper respiratory tract infections are common. The respiratory and heart rates slow, and the blood pressure increases (see Appendix J). Respirations continue to be abdominal.

Under conditions of moderate variation in temperature, the toddler rarely has the difficulties of the young infant in maintaining *body temperature.* The mature functioning of the renal systems serves to conserve fluid under times of stress, decreasing the risk of dehydration.

The *digestive processes* are fairly complete by the beginning of toddlerhood. The acidity of the gastric contents continues to increase and has a protective function, since it is capable of destroying many types of bacteria. Stomach capacity increases to allow for the usual schedule of three meals a day.

One of the more prominent changes of the gastrointestinal system is the voluntary control of elimination. With complete myelination of the spinal cord, control of the anal and urethral sphincters is gradually achieved. The physiologic ability to control the sphincters probably occurs somewhere between ages 18 and 24 months. Bladder capacity also increases considerably, and by 14 to 18 months of age the child is able to retain urine for up to 2 hours or longer.

The *defense mechanisms* of the skin and blood, particularly phagocytosis, are much more efficient in toddlers than in infants. The production of antibodies is well established. However, many young children demonstrate a sudden increase in colds and minor infections when they enter preschool or other group situations, such as day care, because of their exposure to pathogens.

Gross and Fine Motor Development. The major *gross motor skill* during the toddler years is the development of locomotion. By 12 to 13 months of age toddlers walk alone using a wide stance for extra balance and by 18 months they try to run but fall easily (Fig. 37-1). Between 2 and 3 years of age, refinement of the upright, biped position is evident in improved coordination and equilibrium. At age 2 years, toddlers can walk up and down stairs; by age 2½ years they can jump using both feet, stand on one foot for a second or two, and manage a few steps on tiptoe. By the end of the second year they can stand on one foot, walk on tiptoe, and climb stairs with alternate footing.

Fine motor development is demonstrated in increasingly skillful manual dexterity. For example, by age 12 months toddlers are able to grasp a very small object but are unable to release it at will. At 15 months they can drop a pellet into a narrow-necked bottle. Casting or throwing objects and retrieving them become almost obsessive activities at about 15 months. By 18 months of age toddlers can throw a ball overhand without losing their balance.

Mastery of gross and fine motor skills is evident in all phases of the child's activity, such as play, dressing, language comprehension, response to discipline, social interaction, and propensity for injuries. Activities occur less in isolation and more in conjunction with other physical and mental abilities to produce a purposeful result. For example, the toddler walks to reach a new location, releases a toy to pick it up or to choose a new one, and scribbles to look at the image produced. The possibilities of the exploration, investigation, and manipulation of the environment—and its hazards—are endless.

Psychosocial Development

Toddlers are faced with the mastery of several important tasks. If the need for basic trust has been satisfied, they are ready to give up dependence for control, independence, and autonomy. Some of the specific tasks to be dealt with include:

- Differentiation of self from others, particularly the mother
- Toleration of separation from parent
- Ability to withstand delayed gratification
- Control over bodily functions
- Acquisition of socially acceptable behavior
- Verbal means of communication
- Ability to interact with others in a less egocentric manner

Mastery of these goals is only begun during late infancy and the toddler years, and such tasks as developing interpersonal relationships with others may not be completed until adolescence. However, crucial foundations for successful completion

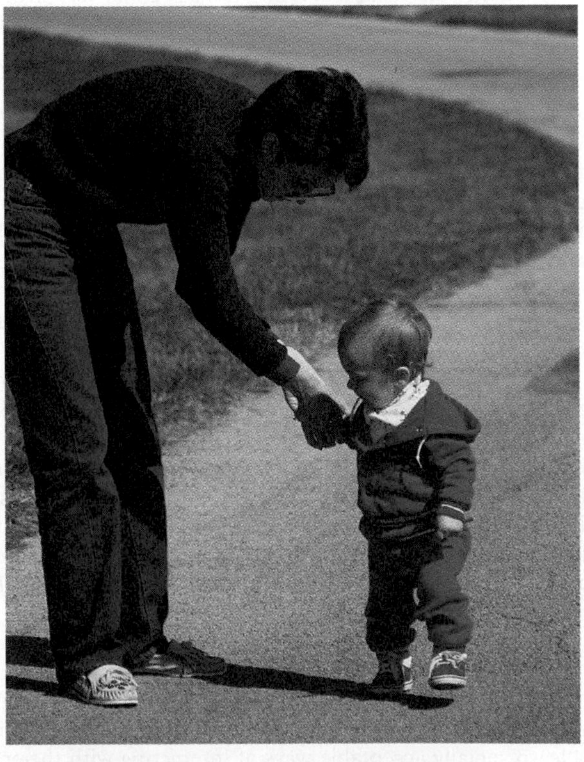

FIG. 37-1 • Typical toddling gait.

of such developmental tasks are laid during these early formative years.

Developing a Sense of Autonomy (Erikson). According to Erikson, the developmental task of toddlerhood is acquiring a sense of *autonomy* while overcoming a sense of *doubt* and *shame.* As infants gain trust in the predictability and reliability of their parents, environment, and interaction with others, they begin to discover that their behavior is their own and that it has a predictable, reliable effect on others. However, although they realize their will and control over others, they are confronted with the conflict of exerting autonomy and relinquishing the much-enjoyed dependence on others. Exerting their will has definite negative consequences, whereas retaining dependent, submissive behavior is generally rewarded with affection and approval. However, continued dependency creates a sense of doubt regarding their potential capacity to control their actions. This doubt is compounded by a sense of shame for feeling this urge to revolt against others' will and a fear that they will exceed their own capacity for manipulating the environment.

Just as the infant has the social modalities of grasping and biting, the toddler has the newly gained modality of holding on and letting go. To hold on and let go is evident with the use of the hands, mouth, eyes, and eventually the sphincters, when toilet training is begun. These social modalities are expressed constantly in the child's play activities, such as casting or throwing objects; taking objects out of boxes, drawers, or cabinets; holding on tighter when someone says, "No, don't touch"; and spitting out food as taste preferences become very strong.

Several characteristics, especially negativism and ritualism, are typical of toddlers in their quest for autonomy. As toddlers attempt to express their will, they often act with *negativism,* the persistent negative response to requests. The words "no" or "me do" can be the sole vocabulary. Emotions become very strongly expressed, usually in rapid mood swings. One minute, toddlers can be engrossed in an activity, and the next minute they might be violently angry because they are unable to manipulate a toy or open a door. If scolded for doing something wrong, they can have a temper tantrum and almost instantaneously pull at the parent's legs to be picked up and comforted. Understanding and coping with these swift changes is often difficult for parents. Many parents find the negativism exasperating and, instead of dealing constructively with it, give in to it, which further threatens children in their search for learning acceptable methods of interacting with others (see Temper Tantrums and Negativism, p. 890).

In contrast to negativism, which often disrupts the environment, *ritualism,* the need to maintain sameness and reliability, provides a sense of comfort. Toddlers can venture out with security when they know that familiar people, places, and routines still exist. One can easily understand why change such as hospitalization represents such a threat to these children. Without the comfortable rituals, there is little opportunity to exert autonomy. Consequently, dependency and regression occur (see Regression, p. 890).

Erikson focuses on the development of the *ego,* which may be thought of as reason or common sense, during this phase of psychosocial development. There is a struggle as the child deals with the impulses of the *id* and attempts to tolerate frustration and learn socially acceptable ways of interacting with the environment. The *ego* is evident as the child is able to tolerate delayed gratification.

There is also a rudimentary beginning of the *superego,* or conscience, which is the incorporation of the morals of society and the process of acculturation. With the development of the ego, children further differentiate themselves from others and expand their sense of trust within themselves. But as they begin to develop awareness of their own will and capacity to achieve, they also become aware of their ability to fail. This ever-present awareness of potential failure creates doubt and shame. Successful mastery of the task of autonomy necessitates opportunities for self-mastery while withstanding the frustration of necessary limit setting and delayed gratification. Opportunities for self-mastery are present in appropriate play activities, toilet training, the crisis of sibling rivalry, and successful interactions with significant others.

Cognitive Development

Sensorimotor and Preconceptual Phase (Piaget). The period from 12 to 24 months of age is a continuation of the final two stages of the sensorimotor phase. During this time the cognitive processes develop rapidly and at times seem similar to those of mature thinking. However, reasoning skills are still quite primitive and need to be understood to effectively deal with the typical behaviors of a child of this age.

Tertiary Circular Reactions. In the fifth stage of the sensorimotor phase (13 to 18 months of age), the child uses active experimentation to achieve previously unattainable goals. Newly acquired physical skills are increasingly important for the function they serve rather than for the acts themselves. The child incorporates the old learning of secondary circular reactions with new skills and applies the combined knowledge to new situations, with emphasis on the results of the experimentation. In this way there is the beginning of rational judgment and intellectual reasoning. During this stage there is further differentiation of oneself from objects. This is evident in the child's increasing ability to venture away from the parent and to tolerate longer periods of separation.

Awareness of a causal relationship between two events is apparent. After flipping a light switch, toddlers are aware that a reciprocal response occurs. However, they are not able to transfer that knowledge to new situations. Therefore, every time they see what appears to be a light switch, they must reinvestigate its function. Such behavior demonstrates the beginning of categorizing data into distinct classes and subclasses. There are innumerable examples of this type of behavior as toddlers continuously explore the same object each time it appears in a new place.

Because classification of objects is still rudimentary, the appearance of an object denotes its function. For example, if the child's toys are stored in a paper bag or large container, that toy receptacle is no different from the garbage pail or laundry basket. If allowed to turn over the toy receptacle, the child will just as quickly do the same to other similar containers because, in the child's mind, there is no difference. Expecting the child to judge which receptacles are permissible to explore and which are not is inappropriate for this age group. Instead, the forbidden object, such as the garbage pail, should be placed out of reach.

The discovery of objects as objects leads to the awareness of their spatial relationships. Children are able to recognize different shapes and their relationship to each other. For example, they can fit slightly smaller boxes into each other (nesting) and can place a round object into a hole, even if the board is turned around, upside down, or reversed. Children are also aware of space and the relationship of their body to dimensions such as height. They will stretch, stand on a low stair or stool, and pull a string to reach an object.

Object permanence has also advanced. Although they still cannot find an object that has been invisibly displaced or moved from under one pillow to another without their seeing the change, toddlers are increasingly aware of the existence of objects behind closed doors, in drawers, and under tables. Parents are usually acutely aware of this developmental achievement and find high places and locked cabinets the only places inaccessible to toddlers.

Invention of New Means Through Mental Combinations. From ages 19 to 24 months the child is in the final sensorimotor stage. During this stage the child completes the more primitive, autistic thought processes of infancy and is prepared for the more complex mental operations that occur during the phase of preoperational thought. One of the most dramatic achievements of this stage is in the area of object permanence. Children will now actively search for an object in several potential hiding places. In addition, they can infer a cause when only experiencing the effect. They can infer that an object was hidden in any number of places even if they only saw the original hiding place.

Imitation displays deeper meaning and understanding. There is greater symbolization to imitation. The child is acutely aware of others' actions and attempts to copy them in gestures and in words. *Domestic mimicry* (imitating household activities) and sex-role behavior become increasingly common during this period and during the second year. Identification with the parent of the same sex becomes apparent by the second year and represents the child's intellectual ability to differentiate different models of behavior and to imitate them appropriately (Fig. 37-2).

The conception of time is still embryonic, but children have some sense of timing in terms of anticipation, memory, and the limited ability to wait. They may listen to the command, "Just a minute," and behave appropriately. However, their sense of timing is exaggerated—1 minute can seem like an hour. Toddlers' limited attention spans also indicate their sense of immediacy and concern for the present.

Preconceptual Phase. At approximately 2 years of age the child enters the preconceptual phase of cognitive development, which lasts until about age 4 years. The preconceptual phase is a subdivision of the preoperational phase, which spans ages 2 to 7 years. The preconceptual phase is primarily one of transition that bridges the purely self-satisfying behavior of infancy and the rudimentary socialized behavior of latency. *Preoperational thought* implies that children cannot think in terms of *operations*—the ability to manipulate objects in relation to each other in a logical fashion. Rather, toddlers think primarily on the basis of their perception of an event. Problem solving is based on what they see or hear directly rather than on what they recall about objects and events. Several characteristics are unique to preoperational thought (Box 37-1).

Within the second year the child increasingly uses language symbolically and is concerned with the "why" and "how" of things. For example, a pencil is "something to write with," and food is "something to eat." However, such mental symbolization is closely associated with prelogical reasoning. For instance, a needle is "something that hurts." Such painful experiences take on new significance because memory is associated with the specific event, and fears are likely to develop, such as resistance to people who wear white uniforms or rooms that look like the practitioner's office. Because of the vulnerability of these early years, it is essential to prepare children for any new experience, whether it is a new baby-sitter or a visit to the dentist.

Spiritual Development

Toddlers have only a vague idea of God and religious teachings because of their immature cognitive processes. However, routines such as saying prayers before meals or at bedtime can be very important and comforting. Near the end of toddlerhood, when children use preoperational thought, there is some advancement of their understanding of God. Religious teachings, such as reward or fear of punishment (heaven or hell) and moral development (see Chapter 32), may influence their behavior (Fina, 1995).

Development of Body Image

As in infancy, the development of body image closely parallels cognitive development. With increasing motor ability, toddlers recognize the usefulness of body parts and gradually learn their respective names. They also learn that certain parts of the body have various meanings; for example, during toilet training the

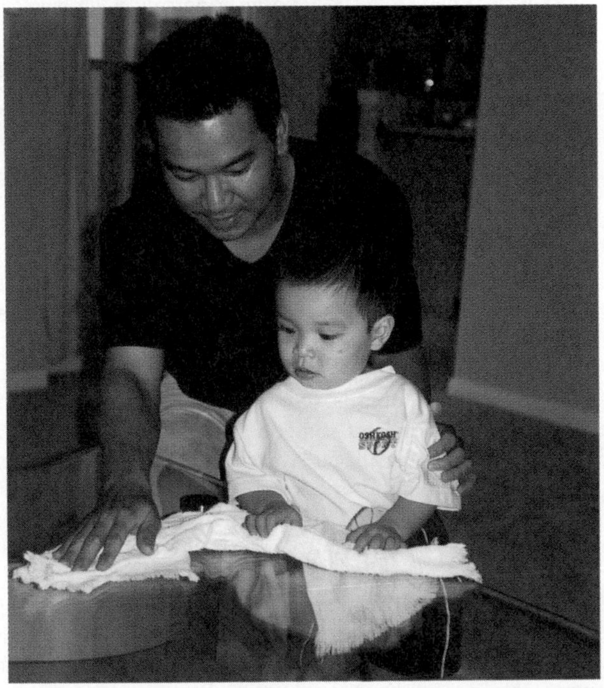

FIG. 37-2 • Domestic mimicry and sex-role behavior are common during toddlerhood.

Box 37-1

Characteristics of Preoperational Thought

Egocentrism—Inability to envision situations from perspectives other than one's own

Example: If a person is positioned between the toddler and another child, the toddler, who is facing the person, will explain that both children can see the middle person's face. The young child is unable to realize that the other person views the middle person from a different perspective, the back.

Implication: Avoid moralizing about "why" something is wrong if it requires an understanding of someone else's feelings or opinion. Telling a child to stop hitting because hitting hurts the other person is often ineffective because, to the aggressor, it feels good to hit someone else. Instead, emphasize that hitting is not allowed.

Transductive—Reasoning from the particular to the particular

Example: Child refuses to eat a food because something previously eaten did not taste good.

Implication: Accept child's reasoning; offer refused food at different time.

Global organization—Reasoning that changing any one part of the whole changes the entire whole

Example: Child refuses to sleep in room because location of bed is changed.

Implication: Accept child's reasoning; use same bed position or introduce change slowly.

Centration—Focusing on one aspect rather than considering all possible alternatives

Example: Child refuses to eat a food because of its color, even though its taste and smell are acceptable.

Implication: Accept child's reasoning.

Animism—Attributing lifelike qualities to inanimate objects

Example: Child scolds stairs for making child fall down.

Implication: Join child in the "scolding." Keep frightening objects out of view.

Irreversibility—Inability to undo or reverse the actions initiated physically

Example: When told to stop doing something, such as talking, child is unable to think of positive activity.

Implication: State requests or instructions *positively* (e.g., "Be quiet.)"

Magical—Believing that thoughts are all-powerful and can cause events

Example: Child wishes someone died; then if the person dies, child feels at fault because of the "bad" thought that made the death happen.

Calling children "bad" because they did something wrong makes children feel as if they are bad.

Implication: Clarify that thoughts do not make things happen and that child is not responsible.

Use "I" messages rather than "you" messages to communicate thoughts, feelings, expectations, or beliefs without imposing blame or criticism. Emphasize that the act is bad, not the child.

Inability to conserve—Inability to understand the idea that a mass can be changed in size, shape, volume, or length without losing or adding to the original mass (instead, children judge what they see by the immediate perceptual clues given to them)

Example: If two lines of equal length are presented in such a way that one appears longer than the other, child will state that one line is longer even if child measures both lines with a ruler or yardstick and finds that each has the same length.

Implication: Change the most obvious perceptual clue to reorient child's view of what is seen. For example, give medicine in a small medicine cup, rather than a large cup, since child will imagine that the large vessel contains more liquid. If child refuses the medicine in the small cup, pour it into a large cup, because the liquid will appear to be less in a tall, wide container.

Give a large, flat cookie rather than a thick, small one, or do the reverse with meat or cheese; child will usually eat larger size of favorite food and smaller size of less favorite food.

genitals become significant and cleanliness is emphasized. By 2 years of age there is recognition of sexual differences and reference to self by name and then by pronoun.

Once they begin preoperational thought, toddlers can use symbols to represent objects, but their thinking may lead to inaccuracies. For example, if someone who is pregnant is called "fat," they will describe all "fat" women as having babies. There is a beginning recognition of words used to describe physical appearance, such as "pretty," "handsome," or "big boy." Such expressions eventually influence how children view their own bodies.

Although there has been little research done on body-image development in young children, it is evident that body integrity is poorly understood and that intrusive experiences are threatening (Colson and Dworkin, 1997). For example, toddlers forcefully resist procedures such as examining the ear or mouth and taking a rectal temperature. Toddlers also have unclear body boundaries and may associate nonviable parts, such as feces, with essential body parts. This can be seen in a toddler who is upset by flushing the toilet and watching the stool disappear.

Nurses can assist parents in fostering a positive body image in their child by encouraging them to avoid negative labels, such as "skinny arms" or "chubby legs"—self-perceptions that can last a lifetime. Body parts, especially those related to elimination and reproduction, should be called by their correct names. Respect for the body should be practiced.

Development of Sexuality

Just as toddlers explore their environment, they also explore their bodies and find that touching certain body parts is pleasurable. Genital fondling (masturbation) can occur and involves manual stimulation, as well as posturing movements (especially in young girls) such as tightening of the thighs or mechanical pressure applied to the pubic or suprapubic area (Lidster and Horsburgh, 1994). Other demonstrations of sensual activities include rocking, swinging, and hugging people and toys. Parental reactions to toddlers' sexual behavior will influence the children's own attitudes and should be accepting rather than critical (Finan, 1997).

Children in this age group are learning vocabulary associated with anatomy, elimination, and reproduction. Certain associations between words and functions become significant and can influence future sexual attitudes. For example, if parents refer to the genitals as dirty, especially in the context of elimination, this association between "genitals" and "dirty" may be transferred to sexual functions.

Sex-role differences become obvious to children and are evident in much of their imitative play. Early attitudes are formed about affectional behaviors between adults from observing parental and other adult sexual/sensual activities. (See also Sex Education, Chapter 38.)

Social Development

A major task of the toddler period is differentiation of self from significant others, usually the mother. The differentiation process consists of two phases: *separation,* the child's emergence from a symbiotic fusion with the mother; and *individuation,* those achievements that mark the child's assumptions of his or her individual characteristics in the environment. Although the process begins during the latter half of infancy, the major achievements occur during the toddler years.

Toddlers have an increased understanding and awareness of object permanence and some ability to withstand delayed gratification and tolerate moderate frustration. As a result, toddlers react differently to strangers than do infants. The appearance of unfamiliar persons does not represent such a significant threat to their attachment to mother. They have learned from experience that parents still exist when physically absent. Repetition of events such as going to bed without the parents, but waking to find them there again reinforces the reliability of such brief separations. Consequently, toddlers are able to venture away from their parents for brief periods of time because of the security of knowing that the parents will be there when they return.

Transitional objects, such as a favorite blanket or toy, provide security for children, especially when they are separated from parents, dealing with a new stress, or just fatigued (Fig. 37-3). Security objects often become so important to toddlers that they refuse to have them taken away. Such behavior is normal; there is no need to discourage this tendency. During separations such as day care, hospitalization, or even staying overnight with a relative, transitional objects should be provided to minimize any feelings of fear or loneliness.

Learning to tolerate and master brief periods of separation is an important developmental task of children in this age group. In addition, it is a necessary component of parenting, since brief periods of separation allow parents to recuperate their energy and patience and to minimize directing their irritations and frustrations at the children.

Language. The most striking characteristic of language development during early childhood is the increasing level of comprehension. Although the number of words acquired—from about 4 at 1 year of age to approximately 300 at age 2 years—is notable, *the ability to comprehend and understand speech is much greater than the number of words the child can say.* This is particularly evident in bilingual families, where the vocabulary may be delayed but comprehension in either language is appropriate (Chiocca, 1998).

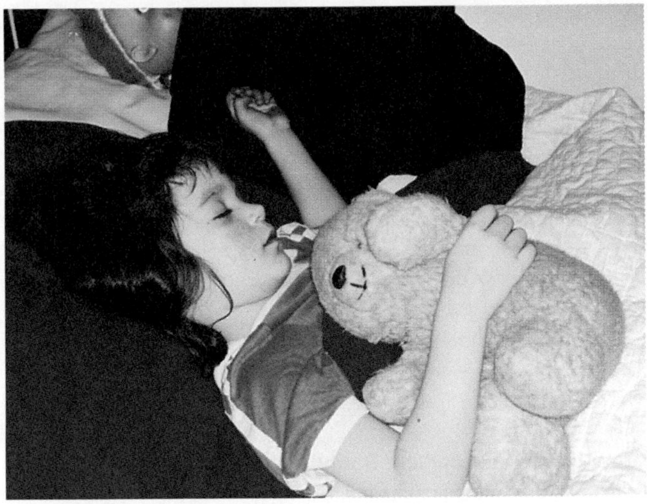

FIG. 37-3 • Transitional objects, such as a fuzzy stuffed animal, are sources of security to a toddler.

At age 1 year the child uses one-word sentences or holophrases. The word "up" can mean "pick me up" or "look up there." For the child, the one word conveys the meaning of a sentence, but to others it may mean many things or nothing. At this age about 25% of the vocalizations are intelligible. By the age of 2 years the child uses multiword sentences by stringing together two or three words, such as the phrases, "mama go bye-bye" or "all gone," and approximately 65% of the speech is understandable.

Personal-Social Behavior. One of the most dramatic aspects of development in the toddler is personal-social interaction. Parents often wonder why their manageable, docile, lovable infant has turned into a determined, strong-willed, volatile-tempered little tyrant. In addition, the tyrant of the terrible twos can swiftly and unpredictably revert back to the adorable infant. All of this is part of "growing up" and is evident in such areas as dressing, feeding, playing, and establishing self-control.

Toddlers are developing skills of independence, and these are evident in all areas of behavior. By 15 months children feed themselves, drink well from a covered cup, and manage a spoon with considerable spilling. By 24 months they use a spoon well and by 36 months may be using a fork. Between ages 2 and 3 years they eat with the family and like to help with chores such as setting the table or removing dishes from the dishwasher; but they lack table manners, and may find it difficult to sit through the family's entire meal.

In dressing, toddlers also demonstrate strides in independence. The 15-month-old child helps by putting the arm or foot out for dressing and pulls shoes and socks off. The 18-month-old child removes gloves, helps with pullover shirts, and may be able to unzip. By age 2 years the toddler removes most articles of clothing and puts on socks, shoes, and pants without regard for right or left and back or front. Help is still needed to fasten clothes.

Play. Play magnifies the toddler's physical and psychosocial development. Interaction with people becomes increasingly important. The solitary play of infancy progresses to *parallel play*—the toddler plays alongside, not with, other children. Although sensorimotor play is still prominent, there is much less emphasis on the exclusive use of one sensory modality. The toddler inspects the toy, talks to the toy, tests it strength and durability, and invents several uses for it. Imitation is one of the most distinguishing characteristics of play and enriches the child's opportunity to engage in fantasy. With less emphasis on sex-stereotyped toys, play objects such as dolls, carriages, dollhouses, dishes, cooking utensils, child-sized furniture, trucks, and dress-up clothes (Fig. 37-4) are suitable for both sexes, although boys will display more gender-specific preferences than girls (Martin, Eisenbud, and Rose, 1995).

Increased locomotive skills make push-pull toys, straddle trucks or cycles, a small gym and slide, balls of various sizes, and rocking horses appropriate for the energetic toddler. Finger paints, thick crayons, chalk, blackboard, paper, and puzzles with large, simple pieces use the child's developing fine motor skills. Interlocking blocks in various sizes and shapes provide hours of fun and, during later years, are useful objects for creative and imaginative play.

Talking is a form of play for the toddler, who enjoys musical toys such as age-appropriate cassette tape players, "talking" dolls

TABLE 37-1
Growth and Development During Toddler Years

Age (Months)	Physical	Gross Motor	Fine Motor
15	Steady growth in height and weight Head circumference 48 cm (19 inches) Weight 11 kg (24 pounds) Height 78.7 cm (31 inches)	Walks without help (usually since age 13 months) Creeps up stairs Kneels without support Cannot walk around corners or stop suddenly without losing balance Assumes standing position without support Cannot throw ball without falling	Constantly casting objects to floor Builds tower of two cubes Holds two cubes in one hand Releases a pellet into a narrow-necked bottle Scribbles spontaneously Uses cup well but rotates spoon
18	Physiologic anorexia from decreased growth needs Anterior fontanel closed Physiologically able to control sphincters	Runs clumsily; falls often Walks up stairs with one hand held Pulls and pushes toys Jumps in place with both feet Seats self on chair Throws ball overhand without falling	Builds tower of three or four cubes Release, prehension, and reach well developed Turns pages in a book two or three at a time In drawing, makes stroke imitatively Manages spoon without rotation
24	Head circumference 49-50 cm (19.5-20 inches) Chest circumference exceeds head circumference Lateral diameter of chest exceeds anteroposterior diameter Usual weight gain of 1.8-2.7 kg (4-6 pounds) Usual gain in height of 10-12.5 cm (4-5 inches) Adult height approximately double height at 2 years of age May have achieved readiness for beginning daytime control of bowel and bladder Primary dentition of 16 teeth	Goes up and down stairs alone with two feet on each step Runs fairly well, with wide stance Picks up object without falling Kicks ball forward without overbalancing	Builds tower of six or seven cubes Aligns two or more cubes like a train Turns pages of book one at a time In drawing, imitates vertical and circular strokes Turns doorknob; unscrews lid
30	Birth weight quadrupled Primary dentition (20 teeth) completed May have daytime bowel and bladder control	Jumps with both feet Jumps from chair or step Stands on one foot momentarily Takes a few steps on tiptoe	Builds tower of eight cubes Adds chimney to train of cubes Good hand-finger coordination; holds crayon with fingers rather than fist Moves fingers independently In drawing, imitates vertical and horizontal strokes; makes two or more strokes for cross

and animals, and toy telephones. Appropriate children's television programs are excellent for children in this age group, who learn to associate words with visual images. Toddlers also enjoy "reading" stories from a picture book and imitating the sounds of animals.

Tactile play is also important for the exploring toddler. Water toys, a sandbox with pail and shovel, finger paints, soap bubbles, and clay provide excellent opportunities for creative and manipulative recreation. Adults sometimes forget the fascination of feeling slippery cream, such as whipped cream or pudding; catching airy bubbles; squeezing and reshaping clay; or smearing paints. These types of unstructured activities are as important as educational play to allow children freedom of expression.

Selection of appropriate toys must involve safety factors, especially in relation to size and sturdiness. The oral activity of toddlers puts them at risk for aspirating small objects or for ingesting toxic substances. Parents need to be especially vigilant of toys of older siblings, or those played with in other children's homes. Toys are a potential source of serious bodily damage to toddlers, who may have the physical strength to manipulate them but not the knowledge to appreciate their danger (see the Home Care box on p. 751).

The major features of growth and development for the age groups of 15, 18, 24, and 30 months are summarized in Table 37-1.

Sensory	Language	Socialization
Able to identify geometric forms; places round object into appropriate hole Binocular vision well developed Displays an intense and prolonged interest in pictures	Uses expressive jargon Says four to six words, including names "Asks" for objects by pointing Understands simple commands May use head-shaking gesture to denote "no" Uses "no" even while agreeing to the request	Tolerates some separation from parent Less likely to fear strangers Beginning to imitate parents, such as cleaning house (sweeping, dusting), folding clothes May discard bottle Manages spoon but rotates it near mouth Kisses and hugs parents; may kiss pictures in a book Expresses emotions; has temper tantrums
	Says 10 or more words Points to a common object, such as a shoe or ball, and to two or three body parts	Great imitator (domestic mimicry) Takes off gloves, socks, and shoes and unzips Temper tantrums may be more evident Beginning awareness of ownership ("my toy") May develop dependency on transitional objects, such as "security blanket"
Accommodation well developed In geometric discrimination, able to insert square block into oblong space	Has vocabulary of approximately 300 words Uses two- or three-word phrases Uses pronouns "I," "me," "you" Understands directional commands Gives first name; refers to self by name Verbalizes need for toileting, food, or drink Talks incessantly	Stage of parallel play Has sustained attention span Temper tantrums decreasing Pulls people to show them something Increased independence from parent Dresses self in simple clothing
	Gives first and last name Refers to self by appropriate pronoun Uses plurals Names one color	Separates more easily from parent In play, helps put things away; can carry breakable objects; pushes with good steering Begins to notice sex differences; knows own sex May attend to toilet needs without help except for wiping

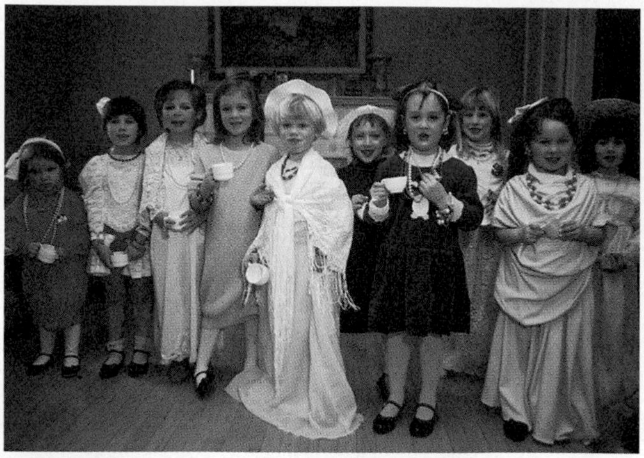

FIG. 37-4 • Young children enjoy dressing up.

Coping with Concerns Related to Normal Growth and Development

Toilet Training. One of the major tasks of toddlerhood is toilet training. Voluntary control of the anal and urethral sphincters is achieved sometime after the child is walking, probably between ages 18 and 24 months. However, complex psychophysiologic factors are required for readiness. The child must be able to recognize the urge to let go and hold on and be able to communicate this sensation to the parent. In addition, there is probably some necessary motivation in the desire to please the parent by holding on, rather than pleasing oneself by letting go.

Usually, physiologic and psychologic readiness for toilet training is not complete until 18 to 24 months of age (Brazelton et al, 1999). By this time, the child has mastered the majority of essential gross motor skills, can communicate intelligibly, is less in conflict with self-assertion and negativism, and is aware of the ability to control the body and please the parent. One of the most important responsibilities of nurses is to help parents identify the readiness signs in their child (Guidelines box).*

Bowel training is usually accomplished before bladder training because of its greater regularity and predictability. There is a stronger sensation for defecation than for urination, and the sensation of defecation can be brought to the child's attention. In fact, nighttime bladder training may not be completed until 4 or 5 years of age, and even later training is normal (Michel, 1999).

A number of techniques can be helpful when initiating training. One is the selection of a potty chair and/or use of the toilet. A freestanding potty chair allows children a feeling of security. Planting the feet firmly on the floor also facilitates defecation. Another option is a portable seat attached to the regular toilet, which may ease the transition from potty chair to regular toilet. Placing a small bench under the feet helps to stabilize the child's position. It is probably best to keep the potty chair in the bathroom and to let the child observe the excreta being flushed down the toilet to associate these activities with usual practices. If a potty chair seat is not available, having the child sit facing the toilet tank provides added support. Boys may begin toilet training in the stand-up position or by sitting on a potty chair or toilet (Fig. 37-5). Imitating one's father is a powerful motivating force during the preschool years.

*The helpful brochure *Toilet Training: A Parent's Guide,* is available from the American Academy of Pediatrics, 141 Northwest Point Blvd., P.O. Box 927, Elk Grove Village, IL 60007; phone (888) 227-1770; fax (847) 228-1281; website: www.aap.org.

Guidelines

ASSESSING TOILET TRAINING READINESS

Physical Readiness

- Voluntary control of anal and urethral sphincters, usually by 18 to 24 months of age
- Ability to stay dry for 2 hours; decreased number of wet diapers; waking dry from nap
- Regular bowel movements
- Gross motor skills of sitting, walking, and squatting
- Fine motor skills to remove clothing

Mental Readiness

- Recognizes urge to defecate or urinate
- Verbal or nonverbal communicative skills to indicate when wet or has urge to defecate or urinate
- Cognitive skills to imitate appropriate behavior and follow directions

Psychologic Readiness

- Expresses willingness to please parent
- Able to sit on toilet for 5 to 10 minutes without fussing or getting off
- Curiosity about adults' or older sibling's toilet habits
- Impatience with soiled or wet diapers; desire to be changed immediately

Parental Readiness

- Recognizes child's level of readiness
- Willing to invest the time required for toilet training
- Absence of family stress or change, such as a divorce, moving, new sibling, or imminent vacation

Practice sessions should be limited to 5 or 10 minutes; a parent should stay with the child, and sanitary habits should be employed after every session. Children should be praised for cooperative behavior and/or successful evacuation. Dressing children in easily removed clothing; using training pants, "pull-on" diapers, or panties; and encouraging imitation by watching others are other helpful suggestions. Forcing children to sit on the potty chair or toilet for long periods, spanking them for having accidents, and other methods of negative control are to be avoided (Taubman, 1997). Daytime accidents are common, particularly during periods of intense activity. Young children become so engrossed in play activity that if they are not reminded, they will wait until it is too late to reach the bathroom. Therefore frequent reminders and trips to the toilet are necessary.

Sibling Rivalry. The natural jealousy and resentment of children to a new child in the family is referred to as *sibling rivalry.* The arrival of a new infant represents a crisis for even the best-prepared toddlers. It is not the infant that toddlers hate or resent but the changes that this additional sibling produces, especially the separation from mother during the birth. The parents now share their love and attention with someone else, the usual routine is disrupted, and toddlers may lose their crib and/or room—all at a time when they thought they were in control of their world. Sibling rivalry tends to be most

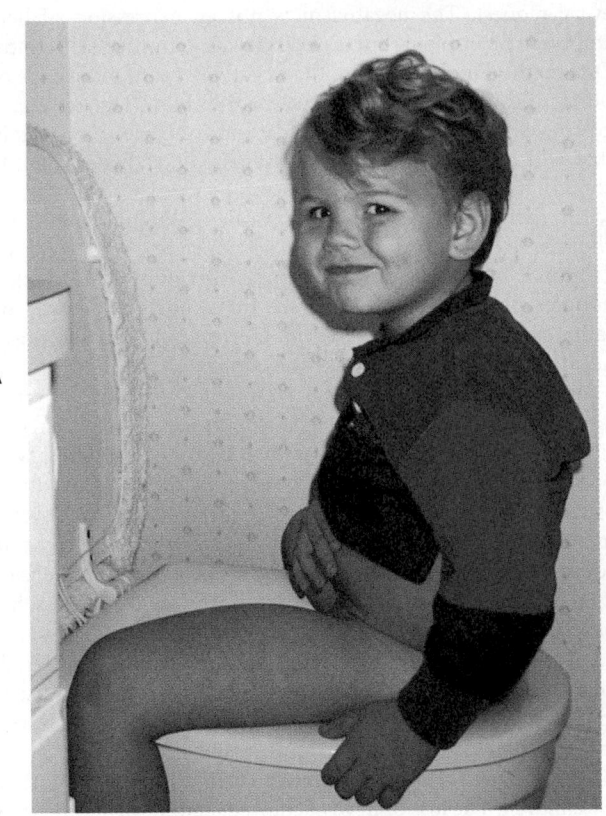

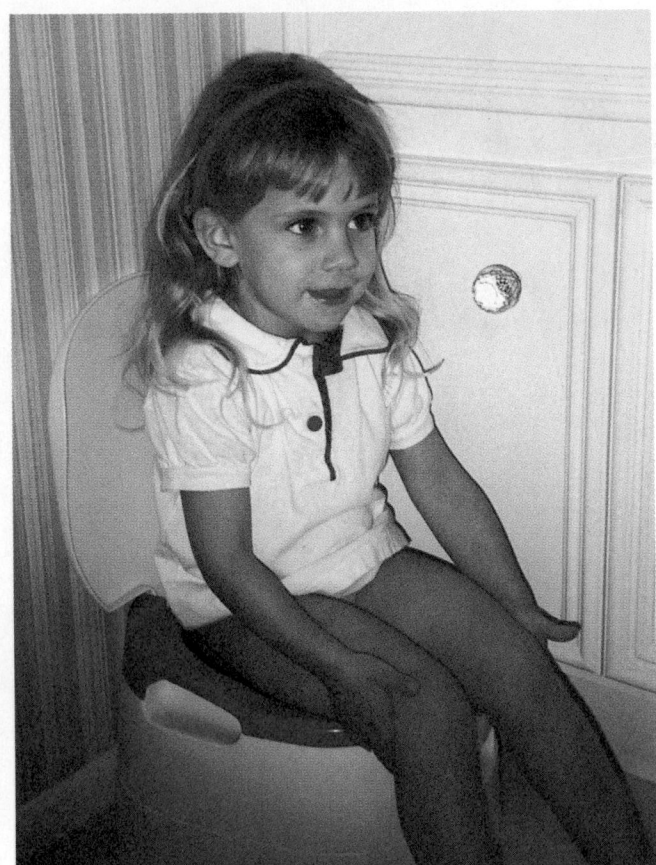

FIG. 37-5 • **A,** Sitting in reverse fashion on a regular toilet provides additional security to a young child. **B,** Children may begin toilet training sitting on a small toilet.

pronounced in the firstborn, who experiences *dethronement* (i.e., loss of sole parental attention). It also seems to be most difficult for young children, particularly in terms of mother-child interaction.

Preparation of children for the birth of a sibling is quite individual, but age dictates some important considerations. Time for toddlers is a vague concept. Tomorrow could be yesterday or next week, and a month from now could be never. Preparing children too soon for the birth may lessen their interest by the time the event occurs. A good time to start talking about the new baby is when toddlers become aware of the pregnancy and the changes taking place in the home in anticipation of the new member.

Toddlers need to have a realistic idea of what the newborn will be like. Telling them that a new playmate will come home soon sets up unrealistic expectations. Rather, parents should stress the activities that will take place when the baby arrives home, such as diapering, bottle- or breastfeeding, bathing, and dressing. At the same time, parents should emphasize which routines will stay the same, such as reading stories or going to the park. If toddlers have had no contact with an infant, it is a good idea to introduce them to one, if feasible. Providing a doll on which toddlers can imitate parental behaviors is another excellent strategy. They can tend to the doll's needs (e.g., diapering and feeding) at the same time the parent is performing similar activities for the infant.

A new sibling in the home is stressful, so any additional stresses for the toddler should be avoided or minimized. For example, moving the toddler to a regular bed or to a different room should be done well in advance of the infant's arrival.

Pregnancy is an abstraction for toddlers. They need concrete illustrations of how the baby is growing inside the mother. It is an excellent opportunity for introducing aspects of reproduction and sexuality. Seeing simple pictures of the uterus and fetus and feeling the fetus move help the child feel involved in the experience (see Fig. 11-2). Children also benefit from classes for siblings that may be part of prenatal sessions (see Fig. 11-3) (Kramer, 1996).

When the new baby arrives, toddlers keenly feel the changed focus of attention. Visitors may initiate problems when they inadvertently shower the infant with attention and presents while neglecting the older child. Parents can minimize this by alerting visitors to the toddler's needs, by having small presents on hand for the toddler, and by including the child in the visits as much as possible. The toddler can also help with the care of the newborn by getting diapers and doing other small tasks (Fig. 37-6).

How children exhibit jealousy is complex. Some will overtly hit the infant, push the child off the mother's lap, or pull the bottle or breast from the infant's mouth. More often the expressions of hostility and resentment are more subtle and covert. Toddlers may verbally express a wish that the infant "go back inside mommy," or they will revert to more infantile forms of be-

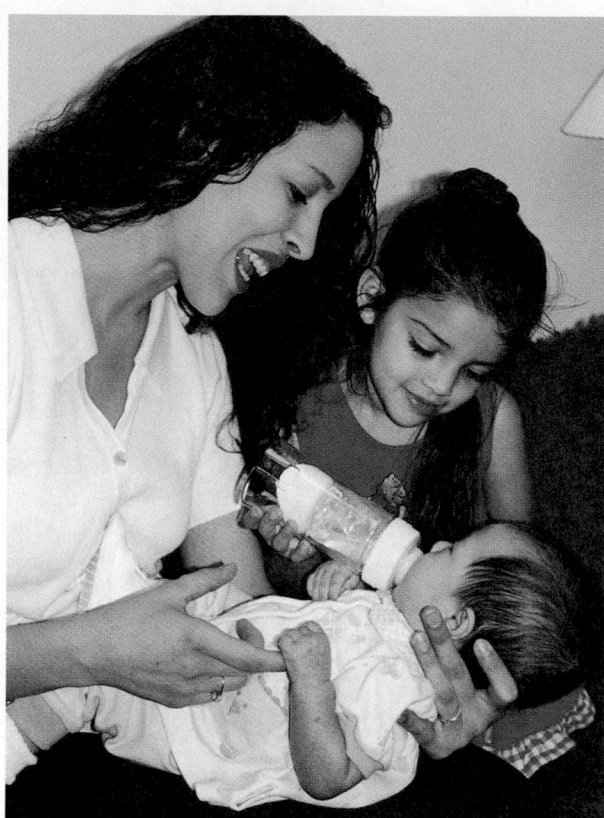

FIG. 37-6 • To minimize sibling rivalry, parents should include the toddler during caregiving activities.

havior, such as demanding a bottle, soiling their underpants, clinging for attention, using baby talk, or aggressively acting out toward others. For this reason, infants must be protected by parental supervision of the interaction between the siblings.

Temper Tantrums. Toddlers may assert their independence by violently objecting to discipline. They may lie down on the floor, kick their feet, and scream at the top of their lungs. Some have learned the effectiveness of holding their breath until the parent relents. Although holding one's breath may cause fainting from lack of oxygen, the accumulation of carbon dioxide will stimulate the respiratory control center, resulting in no physical harm.

The best approach toward extinguishing such attention-seeking behavior is to ignore it, provided the behavior is not injuring the child (e.g., violently banging the head on the floor). However, the parent should remain close by. When the tantrum has subsided, the child needs to feel some control and security. At this time a toy or a favorite activity can be substituted for the ungranted request. (See also Limit Setting and Discipline, Chapter 31.)

Often temper tantrums can be avoided by giving the child advance warning of a request. For example, a popular time for tantrums is before bed. Active toddlers often have trouble slowing down and, when placed in bed, resist staying there. One approach is to establish limited rituals that signal readiness for bed, such as a bath or story. Parents can reinforce the pattern by stating, "After this story it is bedtime," and consistently carrying out the routine.

Negativism. One of the more difficult aspects of rearing children in this age group is their persistent "no" response to every request. The negativism is not an expression of being stubborn or insolent, but a necessary assertion of self-control. One method of dealing with the negativism is to reduce the opportunities for a "no" answer. Asking the child, "Do you want to go to sleep now?" is an almost certain example of a question that will be answered with an emphatic "no." Instead, tell the child that it is time to go to sleep and proceed accordingly.

In their attempt to exert control, children like to make choices. When confronted with appropriate choices, such as "You may have a peanut-butter-and-jelly sandwich or chicken-noodle soup for lunch," they are more likely to choose one rather than automatically say no. However, if their response is negative, parents should make the choice for the child.

Regression. The retreat from one's present pattern of functioning to past levels of behavior is referred to as regression. It usually occurs in instances of discomfort or stress when one attempts to conserve psychic energy by reverting to patterns of behavior that were successful in earlier stages of development. Regression is common in toddlers, because almost any additional stress hinders their ability to master present developmental tasks. Any threat to their autonomy, such as illness, hospitalization, separation, or adjustment to a sibling, represents a need to revert to earlier forms of behavior, such as increased dependency; refusal to use the potty chair; temper tantrums; demand for the bottle, stroller, or crib; and loss of newly learned motor, language, social, and cognitive skills.

At first, such regression appears acceptable and comfortable for children. The loss of newly acquired achievements is actually frightening and threatening, because children are aware of their helplessness. Parents become concerned about regressive behavior and often, in their efforts to deal with it, force the child to cope with an additional source of stress—the pressure to live up to expected standards. Brazelton (1993) suggests that these predictable times of regression, or *touchpoints,* are an opportunity to prepare parents for the next step in their child's development.

When regression does occur, the best approach is to ignore it while praising existing patterns of appropriate behavior. Regression is a child's way of saying, "I can't cope with this present stress and perfect this skill as well, but I will if given patience and understanding." For this reason, it is advisable not to attempt new areas of learning when an additional crisis is present or expected, such as beginning toilet training shortly before a sibling is born or attempting new areas of learning during a brief period of hospitalization.

PROMOTING OPTIMUM HEALTH DURING TODDLERHOOD

Nutrition

During the period from 12 to 18 months of age, the growth rate slows, decreasing the child's need for calories, protein, and fluid. However, the protein (1.2 g/kg) and caloric (102 kcal/kg) requirements are still relatively high to meet the demands for muscle tissue growth and high activity level (Forgac, 1995). The need for minerals such as iron, calcium, and phosphorus is still high, particularly when one considers the poor food habits of children in this age group and the increased mineralization within bones.

At approximately 18 months of age, most toddlers manifest this decreased nutritional need with a decrease appetite, a phenomenon known as *physiologic anorexia.* They become picky, fussy eaters with strong taste preferences. They may eat large amounts one day and almost nothing the next. They are increasingly aware of the nonnutritive function of food: the pleasure of eating, the social aspect of mealtime, and the control of refusing food. They are influenced by factors other than taste when choosing food. If a family member refuses to eat something, toddlers are likely to imitate that response. If the plate is overfilled, they are likely to push it away, overwhelmed by its size. If food does not appear or smell appetizing, they will probably not agree to try it. In essence, mealtime is more closely associated with psychologic components than with nutritional ones.

Developmentally, by 12 months of age most children are eating the same food prepared for the rest of the family. Some may have mastered using a cup with occasional spilling, although most cannot adeptly use a spoon until 18 months of age or later, and generally prefer using their fingers.

Nutritional Counseling. Eating habits established in the first 2 or 3 years of life tend to have lasting effects on subsequent years. If food is used as a reward or sign of approval, a child may overeat for nonnutritive reasons. If food is forced and mealtime is consistently unpleasant, the usual pleasure associated with eating may not develop. Mealtimes should be enjoyable rather than times for discipline or family arguments. The social aspect of mealtime may be distracting for young children; therefore an earlier feeding hour may be appropriate. Young children are unable to sit through a long meal and become restless and disruptive. This is particularly common when children are brought to the table just after active play. Calling them in from play 15 minutes before mealtime allows them ample opportunity to get ready for eating while settling down their active minds and bodies.

The method of serving food also takes on more importance during this period. Toddlers need to have a sense of control and achievement in their abilities. Giving them large, adult-size portions can overwhelm them. In general, what is eaten is much more significant than how much is consumed. Small amounts of meat and vegetables supply greater food value than a large consumption of bread or potato. Serving sizes need to be appropriate for age (Box 37-2). Young children tend to like less spicy, bland food, although this is a culturally determined preference.

Substitutions can be provided for foods that they do not enjoy, although this practice should not cater to all of their desires. Frequent nutritious snacks can replace a meal. "Grazing"—nibbling and snacking—is a good way to ensure proper nutrition, provided that appropriate foods are offered.

NURSE ALERT • Serving Size for Young Children

- A general guide to the serving size of food is 1 tablespoon of solid food per year of age or one fourth to one third of the adult portion size.
- Use the tablespoon guide for easily measured foods such as vegetables or rice.
- Use the fraction guide for bread or milk.

The ritualism of this age also dictates certain principles in feeding practices. Toddlers like the same dish, cup, or spoon every time they eat. They may reject a favorite food simply because it is served in a different utensil. If one food touches another, they often refuse to eat it. Mixed foods, such as stews or casseroles, are rarely favorites. Since toddlers are unpredictable in their table manners, it is best to use plastic dishes and cups, for both economy and safety. For some children a regular mealtime schedule also helps satisfy their desire and need for predictability and ritualism.

Most children by 12 months of age are eating the same food prepared for the rest of the family. However, appetite and food preferences are sporadic. Often the interest in food parallels a growth spurt, so that periods of good eating are interspersed with phases of poor eating. Food "jags" are common.

Such food fads do not ensure a well-balanced diet, but attempts to alter them are usually unsuccessful. It is preferable to accept such extremes and offer other foods in small portions. Introducing at least three items from the different food groups at each meal helps develop a variety of taste preferences and well-balanced eating habits.

Box 37-2

Sample Menu for Toddlers Based on Food Guide Pyramid*

Breakfast	½ cup dry, unsweetened cereal
	½ cup orange juice
	4 oz low-fat milk†
Snack	½-1 whole banana
Lunch	1 tbsp peanut butter
	2 tsp all-fruit preserves
	1 slice whole-wheat bread
	2 tbsp peas
	4 oz low-fat milk†
Snack	2 graham crackers
	4 oz low-fat milk†
Dinner	1 chicken leg, roasted without skin
	¼-½ cup macaroni and cheese
	2 tbsp green beans, cooked
	2 tbsp carrots, cooked
	4-6 oz low-fat milk†
Snack	½ cup frozen yogurt

TOTAL SERVINGS	
Bread, cereal, rice, pasta	6-7
Vegetable	3
Fruit	3-4
Milk, yogurt, cheese	2-3
Meat, poultry, fish, dried beans, eggs, nuts	2

*Use fats, oils, and sweets sparingly. Increase fluids with servings of water. Serving sizes are minimums for nutritional adequacy. Many children eat more.
†Substitute whole milk if child is younger than 24 months.

Sleep and Activity

Total sleep decreases only slightly during the second year and averages about 12 hours a day. Most children take one nap a day, and by the end of the second or third year many relinquish this habit. The activity level is high, and there is rarely a problem with too little physical exercise, provided inappropriate restrictions are not instituted. With increasing numbers of young children being cared for outside the home, attention to the kinds of activity provided is important. For example, children with high activity levels may benefit from an environment in which outdoor play is encouraged.

Sleep problems are common, especially going to bed and falling asleep, and are probably related to fears of separation. Bedtime rituals (e.g., same hour of sleep, snack, and quiet activity) are helpful; and transitional objects, such as a favorite stuffed animal or blanket, can help ease the child's insecurity at bedtime (see Figure 37-3).

Dental Health

Regular Dental Examinations. Ideally, the child should see a dentist (or *pedodontist,* a pediatric dentist) soon after the first teeth erupt and no later than age 2½ years, when primary dentition is completed (Creighton, 1998). Initial visits to the dentist should be nontraumatizing. Since toddlers react negatively to new and potentially frightening experiences, the initial visit can center around meeting the dentist, seeing the equipment, and sitting in the chair. If the child is cooperative, the dentist may just look at the teeth but reserve a more thorough examination for another visit. Modeling, in which the child observes procedures performed on the parent or a cooperative sibling, can also be effective.

Removal of Plaque. The objective of oral hygiene is removal of *plaque,* soft bacterial deposits that adhere to the teeth and cause *dental caries* (*decay* or *cavities*) and *periodontal (gum) disease.* The most effective methods for plaque removal are brushing and flossing. Several brushing techniques exist, although there is no universal agreement regarding the best method. One that is suitable for cleaning the primary teeth is the scrub method. The tips of the bristles are placed firmly at a 45-degree angle against the teeth and gums and moved back and forth in a vibratory motion. The ends of the bristles should be wiggling but not moving forcefully back and forth, which can damage the gums and enamel. All the surfaces of the teeth are cleaned in this manner except the lingual (inner) surfaces of the anterior teeth. To clean these surfaces, the toothbrush is placed vertical to the teeth and moved up and down. Only a few teeth are brushed at one time, using six to eight strokes for each section. A systematic approach is used so that all surfaces are thoroughly cleaned (Fig. 37-7).

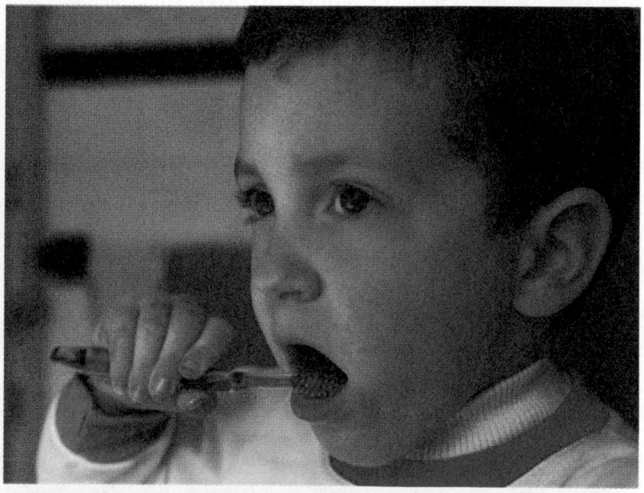

FIG. 37-7 • Young children can participate in toothbrushing, but parents need to brush all the child's teeth thoroughly.

For young children the most effective cleaning is done by parents (Fig. 37-8). Several positions can be used that facilitate access to the mouth and help stabilize the head for comfort:

- Stand with child's back toward adult. (When done in front of a bathroom mirror, both child and adult can see what is being done in the mirror.)
- Sit on a couch or bed with child's head resting in adult's lap.
- Sit on the floor or a stool with child's head resting between adult's thighs.

With all positions, use one hand to cup the chin and the other to brush the teeth. For easier access to back teeth, hold the mouth partially open.

For effective cleaning, a small toothbrush with soft, rounded, multitufted nylon bristles that are short and uniform in length is recommended. Nylon bristles dry more rapidly after use and retain their shape better than natural bristles. Toothbrushes are replaced as soon as the bristles are frayed or bent. With young children, brushing may be more easily accomplished using only water, since many children dislike the foam from toothpaste and the foam interferes with visibility. There is also the danger of swallowing fluoridated toothpaste (see following discussion un-

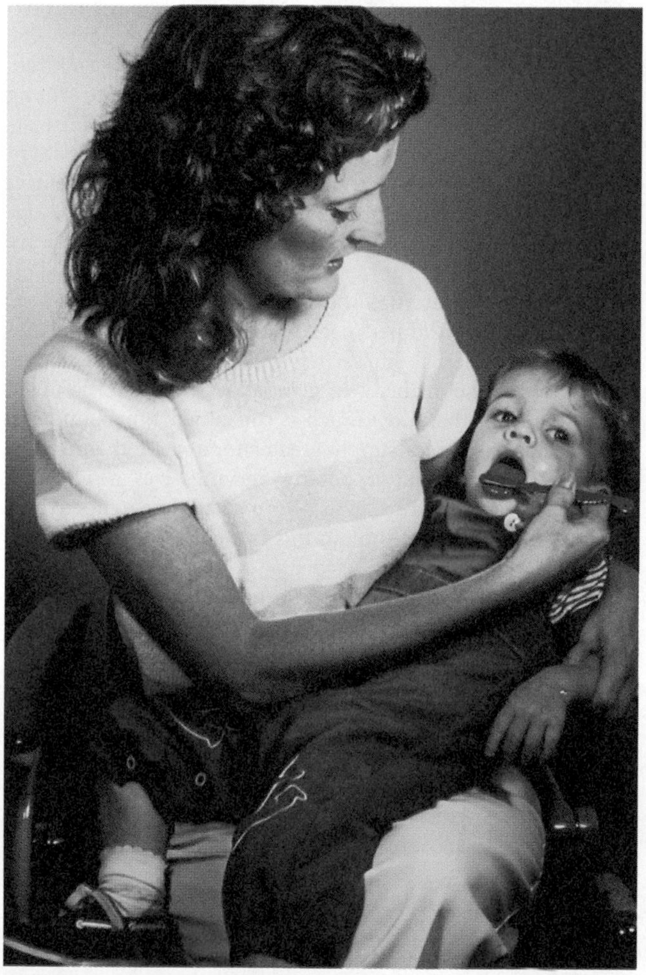

FIG. 37-8 • The most effective cleaning of the teeth is done by parents.

der Fluoride). When using toothpaste, children should select the flavor they like to encourage the brushing habit.

After the teeth have been cleaned, flossing with dental floss is done to remove plaque and debris from between the teeth and below the gum margin, where brushing is ineffective. Since young children do not have the dexterity to manipulate the floss, parents are taught the procedure.

A disclosing agent is helpful in identifying those areas of the teeth where plaque accumulates. It also helps motivate children to clean their teeth because plaque is difficult to see. After cleaning, the mouth is inspected to ensure that all traces of plaque have been removed. Where plaque remains, the teeth are rebrushed.

Ideally, the teeth should be cleaned after each meal and especially before bedtime, and the child should be given nothing to eat or drink after the night brushing except water. At those times when brushing is impractical, the "swish-and-swallow" method of cleaning the mouth is taught: with a mouthful of water the child rinses the mouth and swallows, repeating the procedure three or four times.

Fluoride. Fluoride, a mineral, is found in water, foods, or drinks in which fluoridated water was used as part of the processing system. Because the water fluoridation process and manufacturing of fluoride toothpaste are almost impossible to standardize in the United States, the dosage of fluoride supplements has been lowered to reduce the incidence of fluorosis (Table 37-2). Increased fluoride ingestion leads to enamel protein retention, hypomineralization of the enamel and dentin, and disturbance of crystal formation. The effects caused by this change range from barely discernible white fiberlike lines or spots to gray-brown stains or pitted areas.

Nurses have a responsibility to ensure an optimal fluoride regimen for children and to counsel families regarding correct use of supplements. The nurse should have a knowledge of the fluoride content of the community water supply and provide instruction to parents regarding correct administration of fluoride drops or tablets. Supplements should remain in the mouth for 30 seconds before swallowing and be taken on an empty stomach. Afterward the child should not drink or eat for 30 minutes. All fluoride products (toothpaste, supplements, and rinse) need to be stored away from young children to prevent poisoning. If the water supply is fluoridated, parents are encouraged to use water to prepare drinks and foods.

Low-Cariogenic Diet. Diet is critical to developing good teeth because the carious depends primarily on fermentable sugars, especially sucrose. Refined table sugar, honey, molasses, corn syrup, and dried fruits such as raisins are highly cariogenic.

Ideally, such foods should be eliminated. However, since this is impractical, some suggestions can be helpful. First, *the frequency with which sugar is consumed is more important than the total amount eaten.* Therefore, when sweets are eaten, they are less damaging if consumed immediately after a meal rather than as a snack between meals. When sweets are served as the dessert, the teeth can be cleaned afterward, decreasing the amount of time the sugar is in the mouth.

Second, the form of sugar is important. The more cariogenic foods are those that are sticky or hard, since they remain in the mouth longer. Consequently, sucking on lollipops is more cariogenic than eating a chocolate bar. Sometimes the source of the sugar is "hidden," such as in numerous prescription and nonprescription drugs and in many popular cereals, including the "all-natural" variety. Reading food labels is essential in eliminating sources of sucrose.

A special form of tooth decay in children between 18 months and 3 years of age is *nursing caries* (also called *nursing bottle caries* or *bottle-mouth caries*); this occurs when the child is routinely given a bottle of milk or juice at nap or bedtime or uses the bottle as a pacifier while awake. Frequent nocturnal breastfeeding for prolonged periods also leads to extensive destruction of the teeth (Creighton, 1998). The practice of coating pacifiers in honey can also contribute to caries and may be a potential source of botulism poisoning. As the sweet liquid pools in the mouth, the teeth are bathed for several hours in this cariogenic environment. The maxillary (upper) incisors and molars are affected most, since the mandibular (lower) incisors are protected by the lower lip, tongue, and saliva (Fig. 37-9). Severely decayed teeth may require the application of stainless steel bands to preserve the spacing until the permanent teeth erupt.

Prevention involves eliminating the bedtime bottle completely, feeding the last bottle before bedtime, substituting a bottle of water for milk or juice, not using the bottle as a pacifier, and never coating pacifiers in sweet substances. Putting juice in bottles, especially commercially available ready-to-use bottles, is discouraged: the beverage is especially damaging be-

TABLE 37-2
Fluoride Supplementation*

Age	Water Fluoride Content (in ppm)† <0.3	0.3-0.6	>0.6
Birth-6 months	0	0	0
6 months-3 years	0.25	0	0
3-6 years	0.50	0.25	0
6-16 years	1.00	0.50	0

From American Academy of Pediatrics, Committee on Nutrition: Fluoride supplementation for children, *Pediatrics* 95(5):777, 1995.
*Fluoride daily doses are given in milligrams.
†Parts per million (ppm).

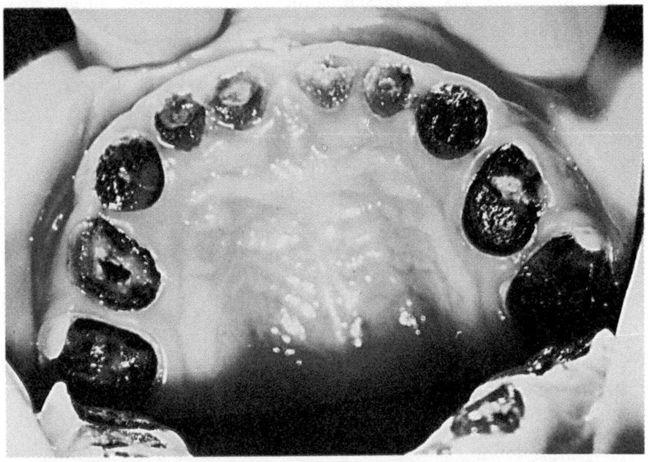

FIG. 37-9 • Nursing caries. Note extensive carious involvement of maxillary primary incisors. (Courtesy Bruce Carter, DDS, Texas Children's Hospital, Houston, Texas.)

TABLE 37-3
Injury Prevention During Early Childhood

Developmental Abilities Related to Risk of Injury	Injury Prevention
Walks, runs, and climbs	***Motor vehicles***
Able to open doors and gates	Use federally approved car restraint; if restraint is not available, use lap belt
Can ride tricycle	Supervise child while playing outside
Can throw ball and other objects	Do not allow child to play on curb or behind a parked car
	Do not permit child to play in pile of leaves, snow, or large cardboard container in trafficked area
	Supervise tricycle riding
	Lock fences and doors if not directly supervising children
	Teach child to obey pedestrian safety rules
	Obey traffic regulations; cross only at crosswalks and only when traffic signal indicates it is safe
	Stand back a step from the curb until it's time to cross
	Look left, right, and left again and check for turning cars before crossing street
	Use sidewalks; when there is no sidewalk, walk on the left, facing traffic
	Wear light colors at night and attach fluorescent material to clothing
Able to explore if left unsupervised	***Drowning***
Has great curiosity	Supervise closely when near any source of water, including buckets
Helpless in water; unaware of its danger; depth of water has no significance	Keep bathroom doors closed and lid down on toilet
	Have fence around swimming pool and lock gate
	Teach swimming and water safety
Able to reach heights by climbing, stretching, and standing on toes	***Burns***
Pulls objects	Turn pot handles toward back of stove
Explores any holes or opening	Place electric appliances, such as coffee maker and popcorn machine, toward back of counter
Can open drawers and closets	Place guardrails in front of radiators, fireplaces, or other heating elements
Unaware of potential sources of heat or fire	Store matches and cigarette lighters in locked or inaccessible area; discard carefully
Plays with mechanical objects	Place burning candles, incense, hot foods, and cigarettes out of reach
	Do not let tablecloth hang within child's reach
	Do not let electric cord from iron or other appliance hang within child's reach
	Cover electrical outlets with protective plastic caps
	Keep electrical wires hidden or out of reach
	Do not allow child to play with electrical appliance, wires, or lighters
	Stress danger of open flames; teach what "hot" means
	Always check bathwater temperature; adjust water heater temperature to 120° F (48.9° C) or lower; do not allow children to play with faucets
	Apply a sunscreen when child is exposed to sunlight
Explores by putting objects in mouth	***Poisoning***
Can open drawers, closets, and most containers	Place all potentially toxic agents out of reach or in a locked cabinet
Climbs	Caution against eating nonedible items, such as plants
Cannot read labels	Replace medications or poisons immediately; replace child-guard caps properly
Does not know safe dose or amount	Administer medications as a drug, not as a candy
	Do not store large surplus of toxic agents
	Promptly discard empty poison containers; never reuse to store a food item or other poison
	Teach child not to play in trash containers
	Never remove labels from containers of toxic substances
	Have syrup of ipecac in home; use only if advised
	Know number and location of nearest poison control center (usually listed in front of telephone directory)
Able to open doors and some windows	***Falls***
Goes up and down stairs	Keep screen in window, nail securely, and use guardrail
Depth perception unrefined	Place gates at top and bottom of stairs
	Keep doors locked or use child-proof doorknob covers at entry to stairs, high porch, or other elevated area, including laundry chute
	Remove unsecured or scatter rugs
	Apply nonskid decals in bathtub or shower
	Keep crib rails fully raised and mattress at lowest level
	Place carpeting under crib and in bathroom

TABLE 37-3—cont'd
Injury Prevention During Early Childhood

Developmental Abilities Related to Risk of Injury	Injury Prevention
	Falls—cont'd
	Keep large toys and bumper pads out of crib or playpen (child can use these as "stairs" to climb out), then move to youth bed when child is able to climb out of crib
	Avoid using walkers, especially near stairs
	Dress in safe clothing (soles that do not "catch" on floor, tied shoelaces, pant legs that do not touch floor)
	Keep child restrained in vehicles; never leave unattended in shopping cart
	Supervise at playgrounds; select play areas with soft ground cover and safe equipment
Puts things in mouth	***Choking and suffocation***
May swallow hard or nonedible pieces of food	Avoid large, round chunks of meat, such as whole hot dogs (slice lengthwise into short pieces)
	Avoid fruit with pits, fish with bones, dried beans, hard candy, chewing gum, nuts, popcorn, grapes, marshmallows
	Choose large, sturdy toys without sharp edges or small removeable parts
	Discard old refrigerators, ovens, and so on; if storing an old appliance, remove the door
	Keep automatic garage door transmitter in inaccessible place
	Select safe toy boxes or chests without heavy, hinged lids
	Keep venetian blind cords out of child's reach
	Remove drawstrings from clothing
	Bodily damage
Still clumsy in many skills	Avoid giving sharp or pointed objects—such as knives, scissors, or toothpicks—especially when walking or running
Easily distracted from tasks	Do not allow lollipops or similar objects in mouth when walking or running
Unaware of potential danger from strangers or other people	Teach safety precautions (e.g., to carry knife or scissors with pointed end away from face)
	Store all dangerous tools, garden equipment, and firearms in locked cabinet
	Be alert to danger of supervised animals and household pets
	Use safety glass and decals on large glassed areas, such as sliding glass doors
	Teach child name, address, and phone number and to ask to help from appropriate people (cashier, security guard, policeman) if lost; have identification on child (sewn in clothes, inside shoe)
	Teach stranger safety
	Avoid personalized clothing in public places
	Never go with a stranger
	Tell parents if anyone makes child feel uncomfortable in any way
	Always listen to child's concerns regarding others' behavior
	Teach child to say "no" when confronted with uncomfortable situations

cause the sugar is more readily converted to acid. Juice should always be offered in a cup to avoid prolonging the bottle-feeding habit. Nurses are in an excellent position to counsel parents regarding the dangers of this habit and other aspects of dental care.*

*Sources of information about nursing caries and other aspects of child dental health include the National Institute of Dental Research, Building 31, 31 Center Dr., MFC-2290, Bethesda, MD 20892-2290; (301) 496-4261; website: www.nidr.nih.gov; Academy of Pediatric Dentistry, 211 E. Chicago Ave., Suite 700, Chicago, IL 60611; (312) 337-2169 or 1-800-544-2174 (outside Illinois); website: www.aapd.org; American Dental Association, 211 E. Chicago Ave., Chicago, IL 60611; (312) 440-2593 or 1-800-621-8099 (outside Illinois); website: www.ada.org; and Canadian Dental Association, 1815 Alta Vista Dr., Ottawa, Ontario K1G 3Y6; (613) 523-1770. Guidelines for children's dental care are available in Wong DL, Hess CS: *Wong and Whaley's clinical manual of pediatric nursing*, ed 5, St Louis, 2000, Mosby.

Injury Prevention

Injuries cause more deaths in children between the ages of 1 to 4 years than in any other childhood age group except adolescence. The injury death rate has remained relatively unchanged during the past decade; however, the corresponding rates from all other causes of death combined have declined significantly. The prominence of injury as the leading cause of death among toddlers and preschoolers underscores the need to emphasize safety awareness among parents and other caregivers (Kopjar and Wickizer, 1996). Child protection and parent education are key determinants in injury prevention.

A major factor in the critical increase of injuries during early childhood is the unrestricted freedom achieved through locomotion combined with an unawareness of danger within the environment. Specific categories of injuries and appropriate prevention are best understood by associating them with the major developmental achievements of young children (Table 37-3).

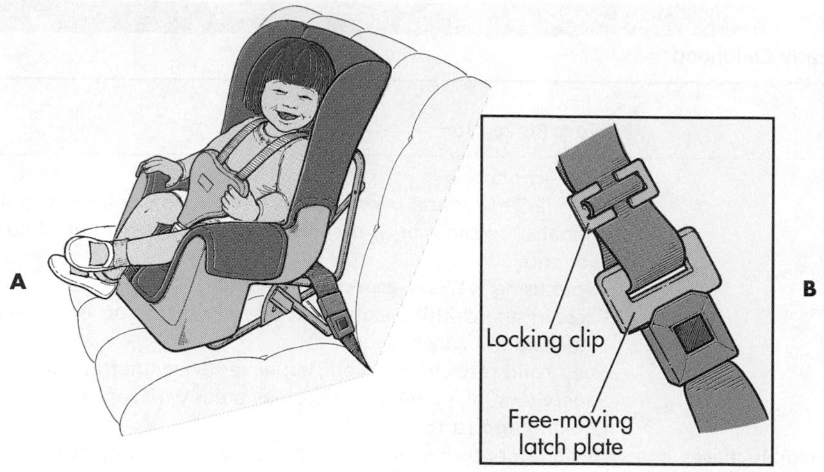

FIG. 37-10 • **A,** Convertible seat in forward-facing position for older infants and children. **B,** Use of locking clip.

The discussions of injuries in Chapters 29 and 36 are also relevant to safety concerns at this age.

Motor Vehicle Injuries. Motor vehicle injuries cause more accidental deaths in all pediatric age groups after age 1 year than any other type of injury or disease, and are responsible for almost one half of all accidental deaths among children ages 1 to 4 years. Many of the deaths are caused by injuries within the car when restraints have not been used or have been used improperly. Approved restraints properly installed and applied can reduce the majority of fatalities and injuries (Murphy, 1999).

Nurses have a responsibility for educating parents regarding the importance of car restraints and their proper use. Five types of restraints are available (1) infant-only devices, (2) convertible models for both infants and toddlers, (3) boosters, (4) safety belts, and (5) devices for children with special needs (see Chapter 41). The infant-type restraints are discussed in Chapter 36; the convertible restraints and boosters are included here.

The *convertible restraint* is suitable for infants in the rearward-facing position and for toddlers in the forward-facing position (Fig. 37-10). The transition point for switching to the forward-facing position is defined by the manufacturer but is generally at a body weight of at least 9 kg (20 pounds) and 1 year of age (Murphy, 1999). Convertible safety seats should be used until the child weighs at least 40 pounds. The restraint consists of a molded hard plastic or metal frame with energy-absorbing padding and a special harness system designed to hold the child firmly in the seat and distribute the forces to body areas that can withstand the impact.

Boosters are not restraint systems like the convertible devices, because they depend on the vehicle belts to hold the child and booster in place. Boosters are of two types: a *low-shield model* that primarily uses a lap belt (Fig. 37-11); and a *belt-positioning model* that uses a lap/shoulder belt. The combination lap/shoulder belt is preferred to the shield (lap belt) model.

Some older model restraints require the use of a top anchor (tether) strap to prevent the child from pitching forward in a crash. If the tether strap is not used, up to 90% of the restraint's protection is lost. Instructions for proper installation of the tether strap and permanent bracket are included with the car restraint. Cars with free-sliding latchplates on the lap/shoulder belt require the use of a metal locking clip to keep the belt in a tight-holding position. The locking clip is threaded onto the belt above the latchplate (see Fig. 37-10, *inset*). If parents have newer cars with automatic lap/shoulder belts, they need to use the lap belts installed to properly secure the infant.

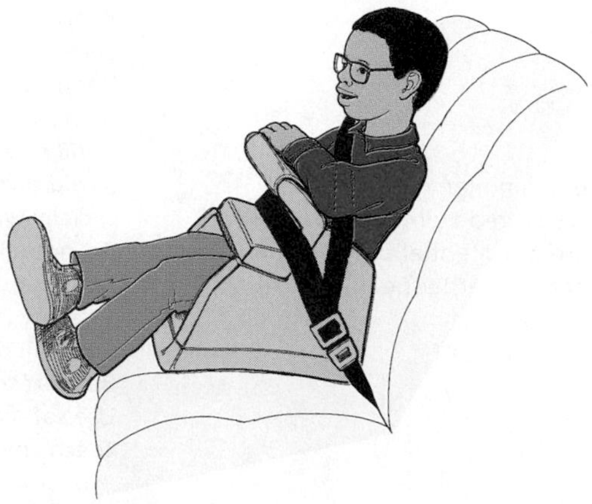

FIG. 37-11 • Automobile booster seat. Note placement of shoulder strap (away from neck or face).

NURSE ALERT • A universal child safety seat system (UCSSS) was implemented as a requirement starting in the fall of 1999 for all new automobiles and child safety seats. This system provides a uniform anchorage consisting of two lower anchorages and one upper anchorage in the rear seat of the vehicle. New child safety seats will have a hook, buckle, strap, or other connector that attaches to the anchorage (Fig. 37-12). Seat belts will no longer be used to anchor child safety seats in newer vehicles. The first phase requires all new cars to have an upper anchorage. By fall of 2002, all new cars must have the entire UCSSS.*

*U.S. Department of Transportation, National Highway Traffic Safety Administration, 400 Seventh St. SW, Washington, DC 20590; 1-800-424-9393; website: www.nhtsa.dot.gov.

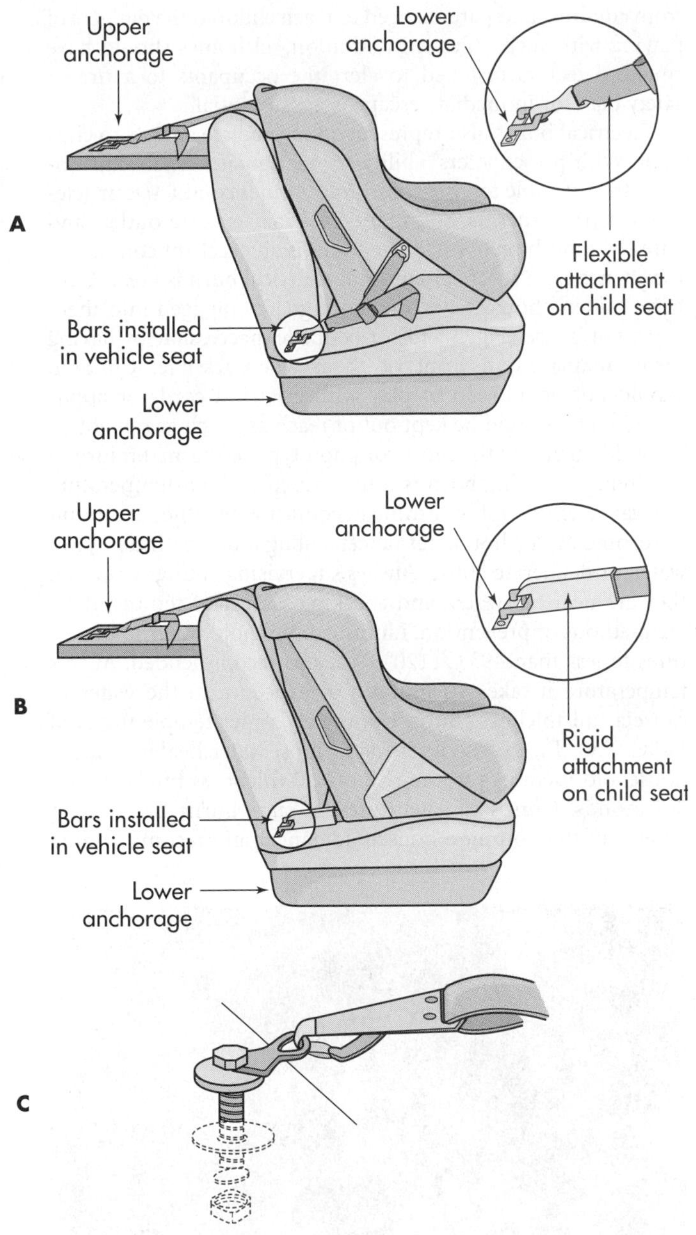

FIG. 37-12 • Universal child safety seat system (UCSSS). **A,** Flexible 2-point attachment with top tether. **B,** Rigid 2-point attachment with top tether. **C,** Top tether. (U.S. Dept. of Transportation, National Highway Traffic Safety Administration.)

Children should use specially designed car restraints until they weigh at least 60 pounds or are 8 years old (Murphy, 1999). Children who outgrow the convertible restraint may still be able to ride safely in a booster seat until the midpoint of the head is higher than the vehicle seat back. If a car safety seat is not available, the lap belt provides more protection than no restraint (except for infants, where there is no safe alternative to approved restraint devices). Shoulder-only automatic belts are designed to protect adults. Children should use the manual shoulder belts in the rear seat. Air bags do not take the place of child safety seats or seat belts and can be lethal to young children. The safest area of the car for children is the back seat. Children who must ride in the passenger side of the front seat with an air bag should be positioned as far back as possible.

Home Care

USING CAR SAFETY SEATS

Read manufacturer's directions and follow them exactly.

Anchor safety seat securely to car's seat and apply harness snugly to child.

Do not start the car until everyone is properly restrained.

***Always* use the restraint, even for short trips.**

If child begins to climb out or undo the harness, firmly say, "No." It may be necessary to stop the car to reinforce the expected behavior. Use rewards, such as stars or stickers, to encourage cooperative behavior.

Encourage child to help attach buckles, straps, and shields, but always double-check fastenings.

Decrease boredom on long trips. Keep soft toys in the car for quiet play; talk to child; point out objects and teach child about them. Stop periodically. If child wishes to sleep, make sure child stays in the restraint.

Insist that others who transport children also follow these safety rules.

NURSE ALERT • Safety belts should be worn low on the hips, snug, and not on the abdominal area. Children should be taught to sit up straight to allow for proper fit. The shoulder belt is used *only* if it does not cross the child's neck or face.

For any restraint to be effective, it must be used consistently and properly. Examples of misuse include misrouting the vehicle seat belt through the restraint; failing to use the vehicle seat belt to secure the restraint; failing to use a tether strap; failing to use the restraint's harness system; and incorrectly positioning the child, especially facing infants forward instead of rearward. To address these issues, nurses must stress correct use of car restraints and rules that ensure compliance (Home Care box). Children riding in car safety seats are generally much better behaved than children left unrestrained, which can be a major benefit to parents and should be emphasized as an additional advantage of restraints.*

Injuries may also occur during sudden stops when objects are left unrestrained. On sudden impact, a loose ball becomes a projectile missile. Therefore all items should be secured or stored in the trunk.

Children over 3 years of age are often involved in pedestrian traffic injuries. Because of their gross motor skills of walking, running, and climbing, and their fine motor skills of opening doors and fence gates, they are likely to be in hazardous areas when unsupervised. Unaware of danger and unable to approximate the speed of a car, they are often hit by moving vehicles. Running after a ball, riding a tricycle, and playing behind a parked car are common activities that may result in a vehicular tragedy. A precaution when children are playing in driveways is attaching to the tricycle a pole with a bright flag that is high enough to be visible through an automobile's back window. An-

*American Academy of Pediatrics, 141 Northwest Point Blvd., P.O. Box 927, Elk Grove Village, IL 60007; (847) 228-5005; website: www.aap.org; and local division of traffic safety or U.S. Department of Transportation, National Highway Traffic Safety Administration, 400 Seventh St. SW, Washington, DC 20590; 1-800-424-9393; website: www.nhtsa.dot.gov. Guidelines for car seat safety are available in Wong DL, Hess CS: *Wong and Whaley's clinical manual of pediatric nursing,* ed 5, St Louis, 2000, Mosby.

other safeguard is the use of a device that beeps when the vehicle is driven in reverse to alert children to the oncoming car, van, or truck.

Preventing vehicular injuries involves protecting and educating children about the danger of moving or parked vehicles. Although preschool children are too young to be trusted to always obey, the parent should emphasize looking for moving vehicles before crossing the street, recognizing the stop and go colors of traffic lights, and following traffic officers' signals. Most important, what is preached must be practiced. Children learn through imitation, and consistency reinforces learning.

Drowning. Drowning, not including drowning from water transportation, ranks second among boys and third among girls ages 1 to 4 years as a cause of accidental death. With well-developed skills of locomotion, toddlers are able to reach potentially dangerous areas, such as bathtubs, toilets, buckets, swimming pools, hot tubs, and lakes. Their intense drive for exploration and investigation, combined with an unawareness of the danger of water and their helplessness in water, makes drowning always a viable threat. It is also one category of injuries that results in death within minutes, diminishing the chance for rescue and survival. Supervising children when near any source of water is essential; teaching swimming and water safety can be helpful but cannot be regarded as sufficient protection.

Burns. Burns rank second among girls and third among boys in this age group as a cause of accidental death. Toddlers' ability to climb, stretch, and reach objects above their heads makes any hot surface a potential source of danger. Scalds from children pulling pots on top of themselves are a major source of burns. As a precaution, pot handles should be turned toward the back of the stove. Ideally, the knobs for controlling the range burners should be out of reach, not on the front panel where nimble fingers can turn them on and accidentally touch the hot burner. Oven doors should be closed whenever the oven is turned on or when it is cooling. The outside of doors of automatic self-cleaning ovens may become hot and, if touched, could cause a burn. Microwave ovens present much less of a burn hazard to toddlers because the outside remains cool, and they are often inaccessible, although foods heated in microwaves can scald children (Dixon, Burd, and Roberts, 1997; Nahlieli et al, 1999).

Other sources of heat, such as radiators, fireplaces, accessible furnaces, kerosene heaters, or wood-burning stoves, should have a guard placed in front of them. The tops of some of these heaters are designed to become hot enough to boil water to provide humidity: they are hazardous if touched or if the pan of water is spilled. Portable electric heaters must be placed in a high area, well out of reach of climbing young children.

Hot objects such as candles, incense, cigarettes, pots of tea or coffee, or irons must be placed away from children. The flame of a candle and the smoke of a cigarette invite investigation. Ashtrays with a center well are preferred to prevent the cigarette from falling off the rim, and adults should try not to smoke, cook, or drink hot liquids when children are physically close. If tablecloths are used, the edges should be placed out of reach to prevent injuries from both burns and falling objects.

Flame burns represent one of the most fatal types of burns and commonly occur when children play with matches and accidentally set themselves (and the home) on fire. To prevent flame burns, matches and lighters must be stored safely away from children, and parents need to teach children the dangers of playing with such objects. In addition, all homes should have smoke detectors installed to alert the occupants to a fire. A safety plan for immediate escape is also essential.

Electrical burns also represent an immediate danger to children. With preschoolers' ability to manipulate small, thin objects, they are able to insert hairpins or other conductive articles into electrical sockets. Young toddlers may explore outlets and wires by mouthing them. Since water is an excellent conductor, the chance for a severe circumoral electrical burn is great. Electrical outlets should have protective guards plugged into them when not in use (Fig. 37-13) or be made inaccessible by having furniture placed in front of them when feasible. Children should not be allowed to play with electrical cords or appliances, which should be kept out of reach as much as possible.

Scald burns are the most common type of thermal injury in children. A scalding burn is often caused by high-temperature tap water, which children come in contact with either as a result of turning on the hot-water faucet, falling into a bathtub of hot water, or deliberate abuse. Always supervising youngsters when they are near tap water, and checking bathwater temperatures are methods of prevention. Limiting household water temperatures to less than 49° C (120° F) is also recommended. At this temperature it takes 10 minutes of exposure to the water to cause a full-thickness burn. Conversely, water temperatures of 54° C (130° F), the usual setting of most water heaters, expose household members to the risk of full-thickness burns within 30 seconds. Nurses can help prevent such burns by advising parents of this common household danger and recommending

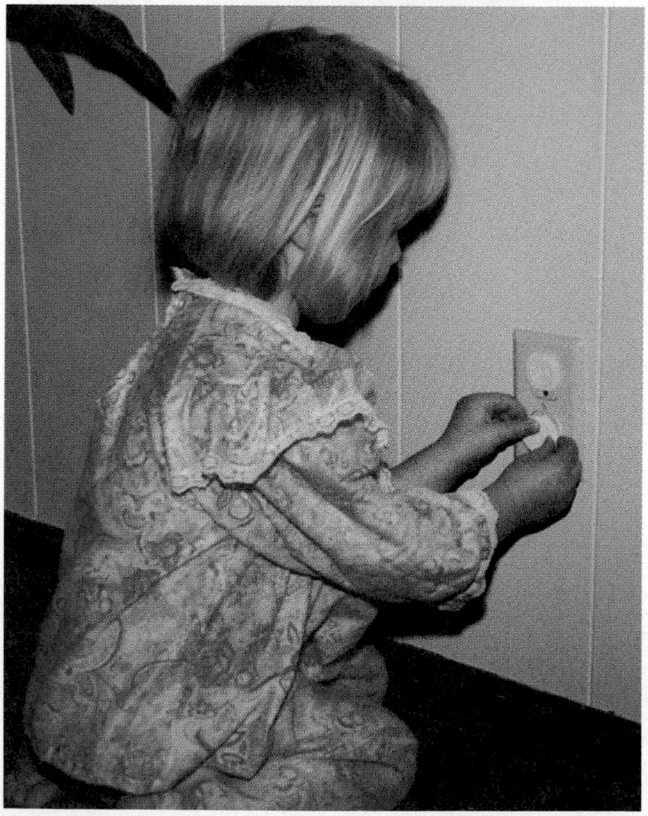

FIG. 37-13 • Special plastic caps in electrical sockets prevent young fingers from exploring dangerous areas.

that they readjust the water heater to a safe temperature. A meat or candy thermometer is a convenient way to measure water temperature. An easy-to-read hot water gauge that changes color to show water temperatures between 120° and 150° F is also available; it shows a "hot," "cool," or "OK" water temperature. A special device can also be added to the faucet that reduces the water flow once the set temperature is reached. Scalding also often occurs when a curious child tries to sip a parent's coffee or tea and spills the boiling liquid down the chin and chest.

Poisoning. Ingestion of toxic agents is common during early childhood. The highest incidence occurs in children in the 2-year-old age group. Although in many instances poisoning does not result in mortality, it may cause significant morbidity, such as esophageal stricture from lye ingestion. Mouthing activity continues to be prevalent after 1 year of age, and exploring objects by tasting them is part of the child's curious investigation. Almost every nonfood substance is potentially harmful, including many house plants (Lamminpaa and Kinos, 1996), and by 2 years of age toddlers are able to climb most heights, open most drawers or closets, and unscrew most lids. By trial and error, younger children also manage to undo tops of bottles, plastic containers, aerosol cans, and jars (including those with child-resistant lids). In addition, pharmacists often transfer drugs to regular containers for the elderly, who may have difficulty with child-resistant lids. Newer forms of drugs, such as transdermal patches and cough-suppressant lozenges, have created additional dangers since they are not packaged with safety caps and the lozenges look like candy.

The major reason for poisoning is improper storage (Fig. 37-14). The guidelines suggested in Chapter 36 apply to children in this age group as well. However, unlike the infant, who was confined to certain heights and unable to unlatch inventive locks, young children manage to find access to many high-level, tight-security places. For this age group only a locked cabinet is safe.

Emergency and preventive measures for accidental poisoning are discussed in Chapter 36. Parents should have ready access to the telephone number for the poison control center and be prepared to act on the advice of the center.

Falls. Falls are still a hazard to children in this age group, although by the later part of early childhood, gross and fine motor skills are well developed, decreasing the incidence of falls down stairs or from chairs. However, playground injuries are common. Children need to be taught safety at play areas, such as no horseplay on high slides or jungle gyms, *sitting* on swings, and staying away from moving swings (McEvoy, Montana, and Panettieri, 1996). Passive prevention includes placement of grass, sand, or wood chips under play equipment. Swing seats should be made of plastic, canvas, or rubber and have smooth or rounded edges. Slides should not exceed an incline of 30 degrees, and should have evenly spaced rungs for climbing and protective "tunnels."

The climbing and running of the typical toddler are complicated by the child's total neglect for and lack of appreciation of danger. Gates must be placed at both ends of stairs. Accessible windows that are left open during warm weather must be screened or guarded with a rail. Falling from open windows is a major cause of accidental death in children from urban, lower socioeconomic groups. Doors leading to stairwells or porches must be locked since preschoolers can easily open them. A convenient type of lock is a sliding bar or hook that can be attached to the door and frame at a level higher than the child can reach.

Cribs and vehicles are other sources of falls. To avoid injury, crib rails should be fully raised, the mattress should be kept at the lowest position, and toys or bumper pads that may be used as steps to climb out should be removed. Ideally, the floor should be carpeted. Once children reach a height of 89 cm (35 inches), they should sleep in a bed rather than a crib. If a bunk bed is selected, parents should be aware of possible dangers such as falls and head entrapment between the mattress and guardrail or between the supporting mattress slats. If the beds are constructed of tubular metal, parents should check for breaks or cracks in the metal and welds that may lead to collapse and injury. Children who sleep on the top bunk should be 6 years or older.

Children who are unrestrained can fall from high chairs, shopping carts, carriages, and car seats (Smith et al, 1996); therefore proper restraint and adequate supervision are essential.

Clothing can also increase the chance of falling. Simple safety measures, such as checking clothing and shoes and keeping shoelaces tied with double knots or using self-adhering closures, can prevent accidents.

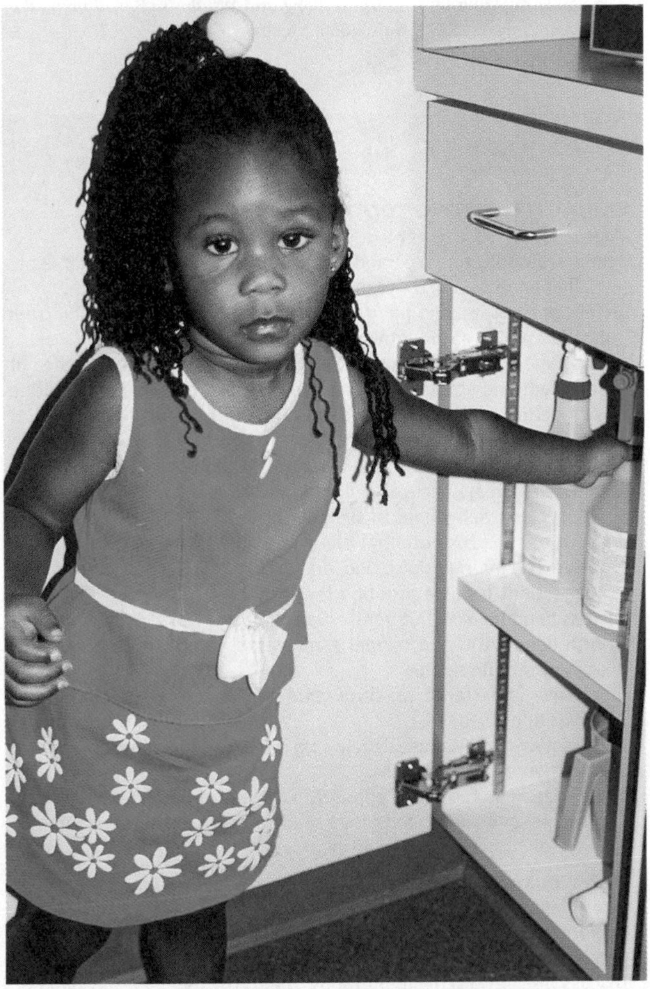

FIG. 37-14 • Children are most likely to ingest substances that are on their level, such as cleaning agents stored under sinks, rat poison, plants, or diaper pail deodorants.

Aspiration and Suffocation. Usually by 1 year of age children chew well, but they may have difficulty with large pieces of food, such as meat and whole hot dogs; and with hard foods, such as nuts or dried beans. Young children cannot discard pits from fruit or bones from fish. It takes practice to learn how to chew gum without swallowing it. Therefore the same precautions as discussed for infants regarding food selection must be implemented (see Chapter 36).

Play objects for toddlers must still be chosen with an awareness of danger from small parts. Large, sturdy toys without sharp edges or removeable parts are safest. Coins, paper clips, pins, bells, button batteries, pull-tabs on cans, thumbtacks, nails, screws, jewelry (especially pierced earrings), and all types of pins are common household objects that can cause significant harm if swallowed or aspirated. Because of the danger of aspiration, parents should be taught emergency procedures for choking (see Airway Obstruction, Chapter 46).*

Another cause of death by traumatic asphyxiation is from electrically operated garage doors. Young children playing in the garage may become trapped under the door. Although the automatic doors should reverse when striking an object, they may not do so when hitting a flexible object or one that is very close to the ground. Precautions include placing controls where they are inaccessible to children, such as high on a wall and in a locked car; and instructing children that the transmitter is not a toy. The door should be checked periodically to ensure that it returns after striking an object.

Suffocation from causes seen during infancy is less common, but old refrigerators, ovens, and other large appliances are an ever-present threat. Toddlers can climb inside these appliances and, if they close the door behind them, can be trapped inside. Discarding old appliances or removing all doors during storage prevents such tragic deaths. Toddlers may also suffocate when unsafe toy box lids accidentally close on their head or neck. Parents should be advised of this danger and encouraged to buy storage chests with lightweight, removeable covers.

Bodily Damage. Toddlers are still clumsy in many of their skills and can seriously harm themselves by walking while holding a sharp or pointed object or by having food or objects such as spoons in their mouths. Preventing such occurrences is the best approach with toddlers. With preschoolers, teaching safety is most important. The child should be taught that when walking with a pointed object such as a knife or scissors, the pointed end is held away from the face. Dangerous garden or workshop equipment and all firearms should be stored in a locked cabinet (Denno et al, 1996). Power lawnmowers are es-

*Community and home care instructions on caring for the choking child are available in Wong DL, Hess CS: *Wong and Whaley's clinical manual of pediatric nursing,* ed 5, St Louis, 2000, Mosby.

Home Care

GUIDANCE DURING TODDLER YEARS

Ages 12 to 18 Months

- Prepare parents for expected behavioral changes of toddler, especially negativism and ritualism.
- Assess present feeding habits and encourage gradual weaning from bottle and increased intake of solid foods.
- Stress expected feeling changes of physiologic anorexia, presence of food fads and strong taste preferences, need for scheduled routine at mealtimes, inability to sit through an entire meal, and lack of table manners.
- Assess sleep patterns at night, particularly habit of a bedtime bottle, which is a major cause of dental caries, and procrastination behaviors that delay hour of sleep.
- Prepare parents for potential dangers of the home, particularly motor vehicle injuries, poisoning, and falling injuries; give appropriate suggestions for safe proofing the home.
- Discuss need for firm but gentle discipline and ways in which to deal with negativism and temper tantrums; stress positive benefits of appropriate discipline.
- Emphasize importance for both child and parents of brief, periodic separations.
- Discuss new toys that use developing gross and fine motor, language, cognitive, and social skills.
- Emphasize need for dental supervision, types of basic dental hygiene at home, and food habits that predispose to caries; stress importance of supplemental fluoride.

Ages 18 to 24 Months

- Stress importance of peer companionship in play.
- Explore need for preparation for additional sibling; stress importance of preparing child for new experiences.
- Discuss present discipline methods, their effectiveness, and parents' feelings about child's negativism; stress that negativism is important aspect of developing self-assertion and independence and is not a sign of spoiling.
- Discuss signs of readiness for toilet training; emphasize importance of waiting for physical and psychologic readiness.
- Discuss development of fears, such as darkness or loud noises, and of habits, such as security blanket or thumb sucking; stress normalcy of these transient behaviors.
- Prepare parents for signs of regression in time of stress.
- Assess child's ability to separate easily from parents for brief periods of separation under familiar circumstances.
- Allow parents opportunity to express their feelings of weariness, frustration, and exasperation; be aware that it is often difficult to love toddlers at times when they are not asleep!
- Point out some of the expected changes of the next year, such as longer attention span, somewhat less negativism, and increased concern for pleasing others.

Ages 24 to 36 Months

- Discuss importance of imitation and domestic mimicry and need to include child in activities.
- Discuss approaches toward toilet training, particularly realistic expectations and attitude toward accidents.
- Stress uniqueness of toddlers' thought processes, especially through their use of language, poor understanding of time, causal relationships in terms of proximity of events, and inability to see events from another's perspective.
- Stress that discipline still must be quite structured and concrete and that relying soley on verbal reasoning and explanation leads to injuries, confusion, and misunderstanding.
- Discuss investigation of preschool or day care center toward completion of second year.

pecially dangerous, and young children should not be allowed in an area where a mower is being used; nor should they be taken for a ride on a mower or allowed to operate that device (Alonso and Sanchez, 1995). Safety education should include respect for firearms and their proper and appropriate use, including nonpowder guns, such as air guns and rifles, which cause serious penetrating injuries (Lie et al, 1994). In addition, the child should be warned of and protected against potential danger from animals (see Animal Bites, Chapter 53).

Toys can be a source of danger, and safety must be a prime consideration when selecting toys (see Home Care box, p. 751). Most toys have age ranges written on them to designate their safety but this information must be used with knowledge of the specific child's readiness.

Household safety should be practiced and includes the usual precautions recommended for any age group (see Home Care box, p. 867). An additional safeguard for young children is the use of safety glass in doors, windows, and tabletops; and the application of decals on glassed areas to lessen the likelihood of running through glass. Also, children should not be allowed to run, jump, wrestle, or play ball near glass structures.

Anticipatory Guidance—Care of Families

Understanding toddlers is fundamental to successful child-rearing. Nurses, particularly those in ambulatory or child health centers, are in a favorable position to assist parents in meeting the tasks and needs of children in this age group. Prevention yields better results than treatment. Anticipatory guidance is paramount if one wishes to prevent future problems (Home Care box). Advice is sometimes not the sole answer. Actual assistance, such as being available for home visits or telephone consulting, should be part of the nurse's flexible repertoire of interventions. Whether parents are experiencing the rearing dilemmas of a first or a subsequent child, they benefit from sharing their feelings, frustrations, and satisfactions. They need adult companionship, freedom from childrearing responsibilities, and periodic separations from their children. Part of a nurse's responsibility is to provide opportunities for parents to express their feelings and to meet their physical, mental, and spiritual needs.

Key Points

- The toddler stage, extending from 12 to 36 months, is a period of intense exploration of the environment.
- Biologic development during the toddler years is characterized by the acquisition of fine and gross motor skills that allow children to master a wide range of activities.
- Although most of the physiologic systems are mature by the end of toddlerhood, development of certain areas of the brain is still occurring, allowing for greater intellectual capacity.
- Locomotion is the major gross motor skill acquired during toddlerhood, followed by increased eye-hand coordination.
- Specific tasks in the psychosocial development of a toddler include differentiating self from others, tolerating separation from parent, coping with delayed gratification, controlling bodily functions, acquiring socially acceptable behavior, communicating verbally, and interacting with others in a less egocentric manner.
- According to Erikson the major developmental task of toddlerhood is acquiring a sense of autonomy while overcoming a sense of doubt and shame.
- In Piaget's sensorimotor and preconceptual phases of development, the toddler experiments by incorporating the old learning of secondary circular reactions with new skills and applies this knowledge to new situations. There is the beginning of rational judgment, an understanding of causal relationships, and discovery of objects as objects.
- Preconceptual thought is characterized by egocentricism, centration, global organization of thought processes, animism, and irreversibility.
- Language is the major cognitive achievement in toddlerhood.
- The most striking characteristic of language development during early childhood is the increasing level of comprehension.
- Development of body image occurs with increasing motor ability, at which point toddlers recognize the importance and capacity of body parts.
- The two phases of differentiation of self from significant others are separation and individuation.
- Parental concerns during the toddler years include toilet training; coping with sibling rivalry; limit setting and discipline; and dealing with temper tantrums, negativism, and regression.
- Effective discipline techniques for toddlers include reward, ignoring or extinction, and time-out.
- Nutrition is important at this stage because eating habits established in toddlerhood tend to have lasting effects in subsequent years.
- Regular dental examinations, fluoride supplementation, removal of plaque, and provision of a low-cariogenic diet promote optimum dental health.
- Because of increased locomotion, toddlers are at high risk for sustaining injuries. Fatal injuries are primarily a result of motor vehicle accidents, drownings, and burns.

References

Alonso JE, Sanchez FL: Lawn mower injuries in children: a preventable impairment, *J Pediatr Orthop* 15(1):83-89, 1995.

Brazelton TB et al: Instruction, timeliness, and medical influences affecting toilet training, *Pediatrics* 103(6):1353-1358, 1999.

Brazelton TB: *Touchpoints*, London, 1993, Viking.

Chiocca EM: Language development in bilingual children, *Pediatr Nurs* 24(1):43-47, 1998.

Colson ER, Dworkin PH: Toddler development, *Pediatr Rev* 18(8):255-259, 1997.

Creighton PR: Common pediatric dental problems, *Pediatr Clin North Am* 45(6):1579-1600, 1998.

Denno DM et al: Safe storage of handguns, *Arch Pediatr Adolesc* 150:927-931, 1996.

Dixon JJ, Burd DA, Roberts DG: Severe burns resulting from an exploding teat on a bottle of infant formula milk heated in a microwave oven, *Burns* 23(3):268-269, 1997.

Fina DK: The spiritual needs of pediatric patients and their families, *AORN* J 64(4):556-564, 1995.

Finan SL: Promoting healthy sexuality: guidelines for infancy through preschool, *Nurse Pract* 22(10):79-80, 83-86, 88, 1997.

Forgac MT: Timely statement of the American Dietetic Association: dietary guidance for healthy children, *J Am Diet Assoc* 95(3):370, 1995.

Kopjar B, Wickizer T: How safe are day care centers: day care versus home injuries among children in Norway, *Pediatrics* 97(1):43-47, 1996.

Kramer L: What's really in children's fantasy play? Fantasy play across transition to becoming a sibling, *J Child Psychiatry* 37(3):327-337, 1996.

Lamminpaa A, Kinos M: Plant poisoning in children, *Hum Exp Toxical* 15(3):245-249, 1996.

Lidster CA, Horsburgh ME: Masturbation: beyond myth and taboo, *Nurs Forum* 29(3):18-27, 1994.

Lie L et al: American Public Health Association/American Academy of Pediatrics Injury Prevention Standards, *Pediatrics* 94(6part2):1046-1048, 1994.

Martin CL, Eisenbud L, Rose H: Children's gender-based reasoning about toys, *Child Dev* 66:1453-1471, 1995.

McEvoy M, Montana B, Panettieri M: A nursing intervention to ensure a safe playground environment, *J Pediatr Health Care* 10(5):209-216, 1996.

Michel RS: Toilet training, *Pediatrics in Review* 20(7):240-245, 1999.

Murphy JM: Pediatric occupant car safety: clinical implications based on recent literature, *Pediatr Nurs* 25(2):137-148, 1999.

Nahlieli O et al: Central palatal burns associated with the eating of microwaved pizzas, *Burns* 25(5):465-466, 1999.

Smith GA et al: Injuries to children related to shopping carts, *Pediatrics* 97(2):161-165, 1996.

Taubman B: Toilet training and toileting refusal for stool only: a perspective study, *Pediatrics* 99(1):54-58, 1997.

CHAPTER 38

The Preschooler and Family

http://www.harcourthealth.com/MERLIN/Wong/maternal/

Learning Objectives

On completion of this chapter the reader will be able to:

- Identify the major biologic, psychosocial, cognitive, moral, spiritual, and social developments that occur during the preschool years.
- List the benefits of imaginary playmates.
- Prepare preschoolers for preschool or day care experience.
- Provide parents with guidelines for sex education.
- Provide parents with guidelines for dealing with a child's fears, stresses, aggression, and sleep problems.
- Recognize the causes of stuttering during the preschool years.
- Offer parents suggestions for preventing speech problems.
- Recognize feeding patterns of preschoolers.
- Provide anticipatory guidance to parents regarding injury prevention based on the preschooler's developmental achievements.
- State three factors thought to be associated with child abuse.
- State four areas of the history that should arouse suspicion of abuse.
- Describe the nursing care of the abused child.

PROMOTING OPTIMUM GROWTH AND DEVELOPMENT

The combined biologic, psychosocial, cognitive, moral, spiritual, and social achievements during the preschool period (3 to 5 years of age) prepare preschoolers for their most significant change in lifestyle—entrance into school. Their control of bodily functions, experience of brief and prolonged periods of separation, ability to interact cooperatively with other children and adults, use of language for mental symbolization, and increased attention span and memory ready them for the next major period—the school years. Successful achievement of previous levels of growth and development is essential for preschoolers to refine many of the tasks that were mastered during the toddler years.

Biologic Development

The rate of physical growth slows and stabilizes during the preschool years. The average weight at 3 years is 14.6 kg (32 pounds), at 4 years is 16.7 kg (36¾ pounds), and at 5 years is 18.7 kg (41¼ pounds). The average weight gain per year remains about 2.3 kg (5 pounds).

Growth in height also remains steady at a yearly increase of 6.75 to 7.5 cm (2½ to 3 inches) and generally occurs in elongation of the legs rather than of the trunk. The average height at 3 years is 95 cm (37¼ inches), at 4 years is 103 cm (40½ inches), and at 5 years is 110 cm (43¼ inches).

Physical proportions no longer resemble those of the squat, potbellied toddler. The preschooler is slender but sturdy, graceful, agile, and posturally erect. There is little difference in physical characteristics according to sex, except as dictated by such factors as dress and hairstyle.

Most bodily systems are mature and stable and can adjust to moderate stress and change. During this period most children are toilet trained. Motor development consists for the most part of increases in strength and refinement of previously learned skills, such as walking, running, and jumping. However, muscle development and bone growth are still far from mature. Excessive activity and overexertion can injure delicate tissues. Good posture, appropriate exercise, and adequate nutrition and rest are essential for optimum development of the musculoskeletal system.

Gross and Fine Motor Behavior. Walking, running, climbing, and jumping are well established by age 36 months. Refinement in eye-hand and muscle coordination is evident in several areas. At age 3 the preschooler rides a tricycle, walks on tiptoe, balances on one foot for a few seconds, and broad jumps. By age 4 the child skips and hops proficiently on one foot (Fig. 38-1) and catches a ball reliably. By age 5 the child skips on alternate feet, jumps rope, and begins to skate and swim.

Fine motor development is evident in the child's increasingly skillful manipulation, such as drawing and dressing. These skills provide readiness for learning and independence for entry into school (Lewit and Baker, 1995).

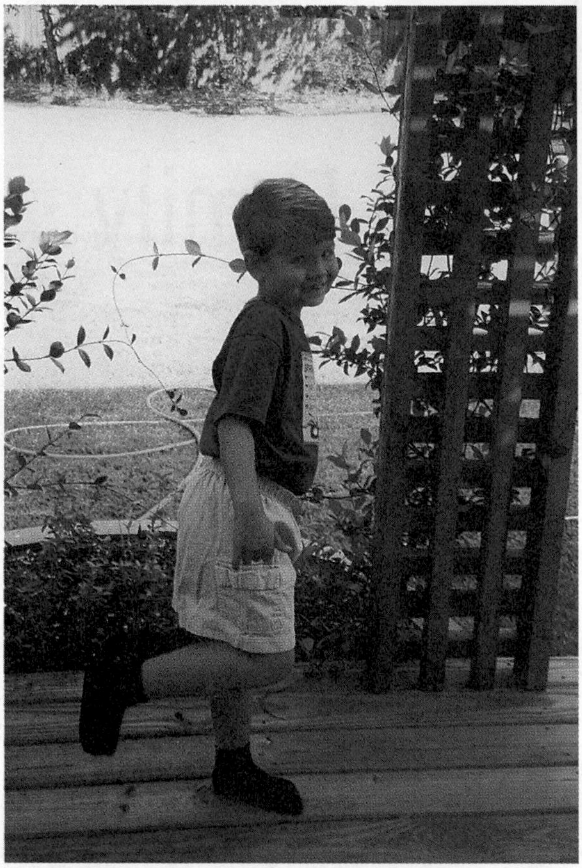

FIG. 38-1 • A 4-year-old child has sufficient balance to walk or hop on one foot.

Psychosocial Development

Developing a Sense of Initiative (Erikson). If preschoolers have mastered the tasks of the toddler period, they are ready to face the developmental endeavors of this stage. The chief psychosocial task of the preschool period is acquiring a sense of *initiative.* Children are in a stage of energetic learning. They play, work, and live to the fullest and feel a real sense of accomplishment and satisfaction in their activities. Conflict arises when children overstep the limits of their ability and inquiry and experience a sense of *guilt* for not having behaved or acted appropriately. Feelings of guilt, anxiety, and fear may also result from thoughts that differ from expected behavior.

A particularly stressful thought is wishing one's parent dead. As a sense of rivalry or competition develops between the child and same-sex parent, the child may think of ways to get rid of the interfering parent. In most situations this rivalry is resolved by strongly identifying with the same-sex parent and peers during the school years. However, if that parent dies before the identification process is completed, the preschooler can be overwhelmed with feelings of guilt for having wished and therefore "caused" the death. Clarifying for children that wishes cannot and do not make events occur is essential in helping them overcome their guilt and anxiety.

Development of the *superego,* or conscience, has its beginnings toward the end of the toddler years and is a major task for preschoolers (Cultural Considerations box). Learning right from wrong and good from bad is the beginning of morality (see Moral Development, p. 905).

Cultural Considerations

LEARNING SOCIOCULTURAL MORES

Developing a conscience implies learning the sociocultural mores of the family's heritage. Depending on the type of attitudes conveyed, children will learn not only appropriate behaviors, but also tolerant, biased, or prejudicial values concerning their ethnic, religious, and social background and those of other groups. Much of this influence may remain dormant until they associate with children or adults of a different heritage. Then, depending on the particular group, they may be accepted or ostracized for their attitudes.

Cognitive Development

One of the tasks related to the preschool period is readiness for school and scholastic learning. Many of the thought processes of this period are crucial for achieving such readiness, and it is intentional that the child begins school between ages 5 and 6 rather than at an earlier age.

Preoperational Phase (Piaget). Piaget's cognitive theory actually does not include a period specifically for children 3 to 5 years old. The *preoperational phase* comprises the age span from 2 to 7 years and is divided into two stages: the *preconceptual phase,* ages 2 to 4; and the *phase of intuitive thought,* ages 4 to 7. One of the main transitions during these two phases is the shift from totally egocentric thought to social awareness and the ability to consider other viewpoints. However, egocentricity is still evident. (For a review of the characteristics of preoperational thought, see Chapter 37.)

Language continues to develop during the preschool period. Speech remains primarily a vehicle of egocentric communication. Preschoolers assume that everyone thinks as they do and that a brief explanation of their thinking makes the entire thought understood by others. Because of their self-referenced, egocentric verbal communication, it is often necessary to explore and understand the young child's thinking through other nonverbal approaches. For children in this age group, the most enlightening and effective method is *play,* which becomes the child's way of understanding, adjusting to, and working out life's experiences.

Preschoolers increasingly use language without comprehending the meaning of words, particularly concepts of right and left, causality, and time. Children may use the concepts correctly, but only in the circumstances in which they have learned them. For example, they may know how to put on shoes by remembering that the buckle is always on the outside of the foot. However, if different shoes have no buckles, they cannot reason which shoe fits which foot. In other words, they do not understand the concept of *right and left.*

Superficially, *causality* resembles logical thought. Preschoolers explain a concept as they heard it described by others, but their understanding is limited. An example is the concept of time. Since *time* is still incompletely understood, the child interprets it according to his or her own frame of reference, such as "A long time means until Christmas." Consequently, time is best explained in relationship to an event, such as "Your mother will visit you after you finish your lunch." Avoiding words such as "yesterday," "tomorrow," "next week," or "Tuesday" to express when an event is expected to occur and associating time with usual expected daily occurrences help children learn about temporal relationships while increasing their trust in others' predictions.

Preschoolers' thinking is often described as *magical thinking.* Because of their egocentrism and transductive reasoning, they believe that thoughts are all-powerful. Such thinking places them in the vulnerable position of feeling guilty and responsible for bad thoughts, which may coincide with the occurrence of a wished event. Their inability to logically reason the cause and effect of illness or an injury makes it especially difficult for them to understand such events.

Moral Development

Preconventional or Premoral Level (Kohlberg). Young children's development of moral judgment is at the most basic level. There is little, if any, concern for why something is wrong. They behave because of the freedom or restriction that is placed on actions. In the *punishment and obedience orientation,* children (ages about 2 to 4 years) judge whether an action is good or bad depending on whether it results in reward or punishment. If children are punished for it, the action is bad. If they are not punished, the action is good, regardless of the meaning of the act. For example, if parents allow hitting, the child will perceive that hitting is good because it is not associated with punishment.

From approximately 4 to 7 years of age children are in the stage of *naïve instrumental orientation,* in which actions are directed toward satisfying their needs and less frequently toward the needs of others. They have a very concrete sense of justice. Reciprocity or fairness involves the philosophy of "You scratch my back, and I'll scratch yours," with no thought of loyalty or gratitude (Thomas, 1996).

Spiritual Development

Children's knowledge of faith and religion is learned from significant others in their environment, usually from the parents and their religious practices (Kenny, 1999). However, young children's understanding of spirituality is influenced by their cognitive level. Preschoolers have a concrete conception of a God with physical characteristics, who is often like an imaginary friend. They understand simple Bible stories and memorize short prayers, but their understanding of the meaning of these rituals is limited. They benefit from concrete representations of religious practices, such as Bible picture books; and small statues, such as those of the Nativity scene.

Development of the conscience is strongly linked to spiritual development. At this age children are learning right from wrong and behave correctly to avoid punishment. Wrongdoing provokes feelings of guilt, and preschoolers often misinterpret illness as a punishment for real or imagined transgressions. It is important that children view God as one who bestows unconditional love, rather than as a judge of good or bad behavior. Praying to God and observing religious traditions (e.g., prayers before meals or bedtime) can help children through stressful periods, such as hospitalization (Fina, 1995).

Development of Body Image

The preschool years play a significant role in the development of body image. With increasing comprehension of language, preschoolers recognize that individuals have undesirable and desirable appearances. They recognize differences in skin color and racial identity, and are vulnerable to learning prejudices and biases. They are aware of the meaning of words such as "pretty" or "ugly," and they reflect the opinions of others regarding their own appearance. By 5 years of age children compare their size with their peers' and can be conscious of being large or short, especially if others refer to them as "so big" or "so little" for their age.

Despite their advances in body-image development, preschoolers have poorly defined body boundaries and little knowledge of their internal anatomy. Intrusive experiences are frightening, especially those that disrupt the integrity of the skin, such as injections and surgery. There is a fear that if the skin is "broken," all of their blood and "insides" can leak out. Therefore bandages are critical to "keeping everything from coming out."

Development of Sexuality

Sexual development during these years is a very important phase of a person's overall sexual identity and beliefs. Preschoolers are forming strong attachments to the opposite-sex parent while identifying with the same-sex parent.

As sexual identity is developing beyond gender recognition, modesty may become a concern, as well as fears of mutilation. There is sex-role imitation, and "dressing up like Mommy (or Daddy)" is an important activity. Attitudes and responses of others to role-playing can condition the child to views of self or others. For example, comments such as "Boys shouldn't play with dolls" can influence a boy's self-concept of masculinity (Finan, 1997).

Sexual exploration may be more pronounced now than ever before, particularly in terms of exploring and manipulating the genitals. Questions about sexual reproduction may come to the forefront in the preschooler's search for understanding (see Sex Education, p. 911 ; and Chapters 39 and 40).

Social Development

During the preschool period the *individuation-separation process* is completed. Preschoolers have overcome much of the anxiety associated with strangers and the fear of separation of earlier years. They relate to unfamiliar people easily and tolerate brief separations from parents with little or no protest. However, they still need parental security, reassurance, guidance, and approval, especially when entering preschool or elementary school. Prolonged separation, such as that imposed by illness and hospitalization, is difficult, but preschoolers respond very well to anticipatory preparation and concrete explanation. They can cope with changes in daily routine much better than toddlers can; however, they may develop more imaginary fears. They gain security and comfort from familiar objects, such as toys, dolls, or photographs of family members. They are able to work through many of their unresolved fears, fantasies, and anxieties through play, especially if guided with appropriate play objects (e.g., dolls or puppets) that represent family members, medical and nursing staff, and other children.

Language. Compared with that of toddlerhood, language during the preschool years is more sophisticated and complex. Both cognitive ability and environment (in particular, consistent role models) influence vocabulary, speech, and comprehension (Huttenlocher, 1998). Language becomes a major mode of communication and social interaction. Vocabulary increases dramatically, from 300 words at age 2 to more than 2100 words at the end of 5 years. Sentence structure, grammatical usage, and intelligibility also advance to a more adult level.

Children between the ages of 3 and 4 form sentences of about three to four words and include only the most essential words to convey a meaning. Such speech is often termed *telegraphic* for its brevity. Three-year-old children ask many questions and use plurals, correct pronouns, and the past tense of verbs. They name familiar objects, such as animals; parts of the body; and relatives and friends. They can give and follow simple commands. They talk incessantly, regardless of whether anyone is listening or answering them. They enjoy musical or talking toys or dolls and imitate near words proficiently.

From ages 4 to 5 years, preschoolers use longer sentences of four to five words and use more words to convey a message, such as prepositions, adjectives, and a variety of verbs. They follow simple directional commands, such as "Put the ball on the chair," but can carry out only one request at a time. They answer questions such as "What do you do when you are hungry?" by describing the appropriate action. The pattern of asking questions is at its peak, and children usually repeat the question until they receive an answer.

By the end of age 5 years, children can use all parts of speech correctly, except for deviations from the rule. They can define simple things by describing their use, shape, or general category of classification, rather than simply describing their outward appearance. For example, they define a ball as "round, something you bounce, or a toy," rather than by its color. They can give some opposites, such as "If Mommy is a woman, Daddy is a man." By the time they are 6 years old, they can describe an object according to its composition, such as "A spoon is made of metal."

Personal-Social Behavior. The pervasive ritualism and negativism of toddlerhood gradually diminish during the preschool years. Although self-assertion is still a major theme, preschoolers demonstrate their sense of autonomy differently. They are able to verbalize their request for independence and perform independently because of their much-refined physical and cognitive development. By 4 or 5 years of age they need little if any assistance with dressing, eating, or toileting (Fig. 38-2). They can also be trusted to obey warnings of danger, although 3- or 4-year-old children may exceed their boundaries at times.

They are also much more sociable and willing to please. They have internalized many of the standards and values of the family and culture. However, by the end of early childhood they begin to question parental values and compare them with those of their peer group and other authority figures; as a result, they may be less willing to abide by the family's code of conduct. Preschoolers become increasingly aware of their position and role within the family. Although this is a more secure age for experiencing the addition of another sibling, relinquishing the position of first or youngest is still difficult and requires appropriate preparation (Sawicki, 1997) (see Sibling Rivalry, Chapter 37).

Play. Various types of play are typical of this period, but preschoolers especially enjoy *associative play*—group play in similar or identical activities but without rigid organization or rules. Play should provide for physical, social, and mental development.

Play activities for physical growth and refinement of motor skills include jumping, running, and climbing. Tricycles, scooter trucks, wagons, gym and sports equipment, sandboxes, wading

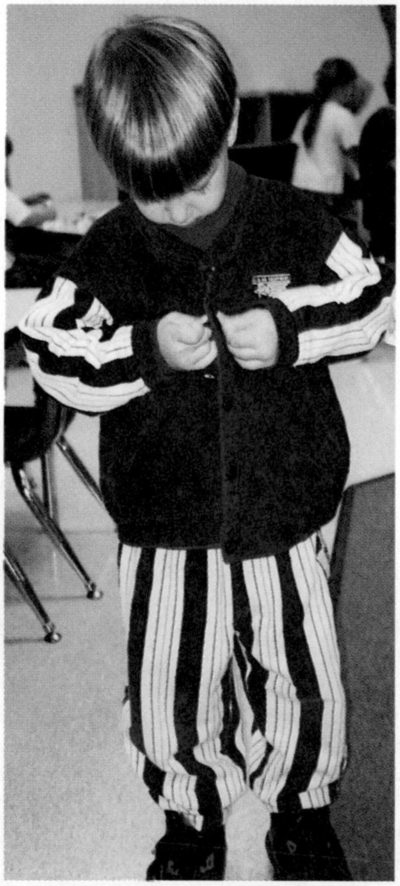

FIG. 38-2 • Most preschoolers are able to dress themselves but need help with more difficult items of clothing.

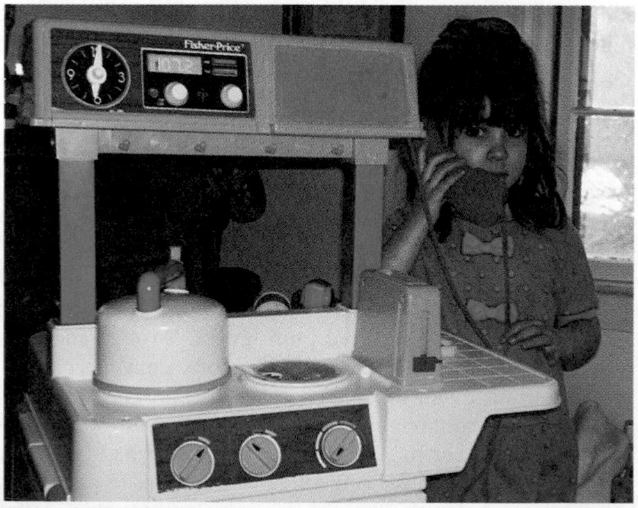

FIG. 38-3 • Imaginative and dramatic play is typical of preschoolers, who enjoy fantasy.

pools, and winter sleds can help develop muscles and coordination. Activities such as swimming, skating, and skiing teach safety as well as muscle development and coordination.

Manipulative, constructive, creative, and educational toys provide for quiet activities, fine motor development, and self-expression. Easy construction sets, large blocks of various sizes and shapes, a counting frame, alphabet or number flash cards, paints, crayons, simple carpentry tools, musical toys, illustrated books, simple sewing or handicraft sets, large puzzles, and clay are suitable toys. Electronic games and educational computer programs are especially valuable in helping children learn basic skills, such as recognizing letters and simple words.

Probably the most characteristic and pervasive preschool activity is *imitative, imaginative,* and *dramatic play.* Dress-up clothes, dolls, housekeeping toys, dollhouses, telephones, farm animals and equipment, village sets, trains, trucks, cars, planes, hand puppets, and doctor and nurse kits provide hours of self-expression (Fig. 38-3). Probably at no other time is the reproduction of adult behavior so faithful and absorbing as in 4- and 5-year-old children (Critical Thinking box). Toward the end of the preschool period, children are less satisfied with make-believe or pretend objects and enjoy actually doing the activity, such as cooking and carpentry.

Television and videotapes also have their places in children's play, although each should be only one part of children's total repertoire of social and recreational activities. Parents and other caregivers should supervise selection of programs, preview programs for appropriateness, and schedule hours for television viewing (Vessey, Yim-Chiplis, and MacKenzie, 1998). (See discussion on television, including Parent Guidelines, in Chapter 33.)

Critical Thinking

IMITATIVE PLAY

In her bedroom 4-year-old Juanita is playing with her dolls. She pretends one doll is "Mommy" and is talking on the telephone: "Be quiet! Can't you see that I am busy? This is an important call. Go away." She hangs up the phone and chooses another doll, pokes it, and cries, "You're bad. Mommy doesn't like you."

Juanita's mother, Mrs. Ortiz, hears this play conversation and realizes she says similar things to Juanita when she is on the telephone. What advice would you give Mrs. Ortiz?

First, Think About It . . .

- **What concepts or ideas are central to your thinking?**
- **How are you interpreting the information?**

1. **Reassure her that imitation is a normal and healthy activity in 4-year-olds.**
2. **Suggest that she use a telephone recorder to return calls at more convenient times.**
3. **Inquire about her reactions to the play conversation and discuss possible ways to avoid the situation.**
4. **Refer the child to a psychologist for further assessment of the apparent child-mother conflict.**

The best response is 3. You want to capitalize on the mother's awareness of the possible messages the child's play has revealed. Your goal is also to empower the parent to find reasonable options that accommodate her lifestyle, which is an important concept in parenting.

Although a telephone recorder is one option, it may not be the best one. Also, you may interpret this play behavior as typical of preschoolers, but premature reassurance will not address the issue or solutions. More assessment is needed before suggesting a referral.

Play is so much a part of the young child's life that reality and fantasy become blurred. The make-believe is reality during play and only becomes fantasy when the toys are put away or the dress-up clothes are removed. It is no wonder that *imaginary playmates* are so much a part of this age period.

The appearance of imaginary companions usually occurs between the ages of 2½ to 3 years, and for the most part such playmates are relinquished when the child enters school. There seems to be a relationship between the level of intelligence and the presence of the imaginary companion. More intelligent children tend to have more vivid and complex pretend playmates.

Imaginary companions serve many purposes: they become friends in times of loneliness, they accomplish what the child is still attempting, and they experience what the child wants to forget or remember. It is not unusual for the "friend" to have a myriad of vices and to be blamed for wrongdoing. Sometimes the child hopes to escape punishment by saying, "My friend George broke the glass." At other times the child may fantasize that the companion misbehaved, and play the role of parent. This becomes a way of assuming control and authority in a safe situation.

Parents often worry about the imaginary playmates, not realizing how normal and useful they are. They need to be reassured that children's fantasy is a sign of health that helps them differentiate between pretend and reality. Parents can acknowledge the presence of the imaginary companion by calling him or her by name and even agreeing to simple requests such as setting an extra place at the table; but they should not allow the child to use the playmate to avoid punishment or responsibility. For example, if the child blames the companion for messing up a room, parents need to state clearly that the child is the only one they see and therefore the child is responsible for cleaning up (Critical Thinking box).

Table 38-1 summarizes the major developmental achievements for children 3, 4, and 5 years old.

Critical Thinking

IMAGINARY PLAYMATES

Mrs. Petner tells you, the nurse, that her 2½-year-old daughter, Kimberly, has an imaginary playmate named Alison. She was not very concerned about this until Kimberly started putting a plate on the table for Alison at mealtimes. What is the best reply?

First, Think About It . . .

- **What is the purpose of your thinking?**
- **What are you taking for granted, and what assumptions are you making?**

1. **"This is highly unusual behavior for children this age and indicates giftedness."**
2. **"This is normal for children this age, and it is fine to allow her to set a place for her imaginary playmate."**
3. **It is best not to allow Kimberly to include her imaginary playmate in activities such as mealtimes."**
4. **"It is important that Kimberly separate reality from fantasy, and a referral to a mental health professional is indicated."**

The best response is 2. Imaginary playmates are normal at this age and serve many purposes. The purpose of our thinking may be to educate parents that they can acknowledge the presence of an imaginary companion as long as the child does not use the playmate to avoid punishment or responsibility. A referral is not necessary. Although the assumption may be that the child is gifted, this one behavior does not indicate that this is true.

TABLE 38-1
Growth and Development During Preschool Years

Age (Years)	Physical	Gross Motor	Fine Motor	Language
3	Usual weight gain of 1.8-2.7 g (4-6 pounds) per year Average weight of 14.6 kg (32 pounds) Usual gain in height of 7.5 cm (3 inches) per year Average height of 95 cm (37¼ inches) May have achieved nighttime control of bowel and bladder	Rides tricycle Jumps off bottom step Stands on one foot for a few seconds Goes up stairs using alternate feet; may still come down using both feet on step Broad jumps May try to dance, but balance may not be adequate	Builds tower of 9 or 10 cubes Builds bridge with three cubes Adeptly places small pellets in narrow-necked bottle In drawing, copies a circle, imitates a cross, names what has been drawn, cannot draw stick figure but may make circle with facial features	Has vocabulary of about 900 words Uses primarily "telegraphic" speech Uses complete sentences of three or four words Talks incessantly regardless of whether anyone is paying attention Repeats sentence of six syllables Asks many questions
4	Pulse and respiration rates decrease slightly Growth rate is similar to that of previous year Average weight of 16.7 kg (36¾ pounds) Average height of 103 cm (40½ inches) Length at birth is doubled Maximum potential for development of amblyopia	Skips and hops on one foot Catches ball reliably Throws ball overhand Walks downstairs using alternate footing	Uses scissors successfully to cut out picture following outline Can lace shoes but may not be able to tie bow In drawing, copies a square, traces a cross and diamond, adds three parts to stick figure	Has vocabulary of 1500 words or more Uses sentences of four or five words Questioning is at peak Tells exaggerated stories Knows simple songs May be mildly profane if associates with older children Obeys four prepositional phrases, such as "under," "on top of," "beside," "in back of," or "in front of" Names one or more colors Comprehends analogies, such as, "If ice is cold, fire is ______"
5	Pulse and respiration rates decrease slightly Average weight of 18.7 kg (41¼ pounds) Average height of 110 cm (43¼ inches) Eruption of permanent dentition may begin Handedness is established (about 90% are right-handed)	Skips and hops on alternate feet Throws and catches ball well Jumps rope Skates with good balance Walks backward with heel to toe Jumps from height of 12 inches and lands on toes Balances on alternate feet with eyes closed	Ties shoelaces Uses scissors, simple tools, or pencil very well In drawing, copies a diamond and triangle; adds seven to nine parts to stick figure; prints a few letters, numbers, or words, such as first name	Has vocabulary of about 2100 words Uses sentences of six to eight words, with all parts of speech Names coins (e.g., nickel, dime) Names four or more colors Describes drawing or pictures with much comment and enumeration Knows names of days of week, months, and other time-associated words Knows composition of articles, such as "A shoe is made of ______" Can follow three commands in succession

Socialization	Cognition	Family Relationships
Dresses self almost completely if helped with back buttons and told which shoe is right or left Pulls on shoes Has increased attention span Feeds self completely Can prepare simple meals, such as cold cereal and milk Can help to set table; can dry dishes without breaking any May have fears, especially of dark and going to bed Knows own sex and sex of others Play is parallel and associative; begins to learn simple games but often follows own rules; begins to share	Is in preconceptual phase Is egocentric in thought and behavior Has beginning understanding of time; uses many time-oriented expressions, talks about past and future as much as about present, pretends to tell time Has improved concept of space, as demonstrated by understanding of prepositions and ability to follow directional command Has beginning ability to view concepts from another perspective	Attempts to please parents and conform to their expectations Is less jealous of younger sibling; may be opportune time for birth of additional sibling Is aware of family relationships and sex-role functions Boys tend to identify more with father or other male figure Has increased ability to separate easily and comfortably from parents for short periods
Very independent Tends to be selfish and impatient Aggressive physically as well as verbally Takes pride in accomplishments Has mood swings Shows off dramatically, enjoys entertaining others Tells family tales to others with no restraint Still has many fears Play is associative Imaginary playmates are common Uses dramatic, imaginative, and imitative devices Sexual exploration and curiosity demonstrated through play, such as being "doctor" or "nurse"	Is in phase of intuitive thought Causality is still related to proximity of events Understands time better, especially in terms of sequence of daily events Unable to conserve matter Judges everything according to one dimension, such as height, width, or order Immediate perceptual clues dominate judgment Is beginning to develop less egocentrism and more social awareness May count correctly but has poor mathematic concept of numbers Obeys because parents have set limits, not because of understanding of right or wrong	Rebels if parents expect too much, such as impeccable table manners Takes aggression and frustration out on parents or siblings Do's and dont's become important May have rivalry with older or younger siblings; may resent older sibling's privileges and younger sibling's invasion of privacy and possessions May "run away" from home Identifies strongly with parent of opposite sex
Less rebellious and quarrelsome than at age 4 years More settled and eager to get down to business Not as open and accessible in thoughts and behavior as in earlier years Independent but trustworthy; not foolhardy; more responsible Has fewer fears; relies on outer authority to control world Eager to do things right and to please; tries to "live by the rules" Has better manners Cares for self totally, occasionally needing supervision in dress or hygiene Not ready for concentrated close work or small print because of slight farsightedness and still unrefined eye-hand coordination Play is associative; tries to follow rules but may cheat to avoid losing	Begins to question what parents think by comparing them with age-mates and other adults May notice prejudice and bias in outside world Is more able to view other's perspective, but tolerates differences rather than understanding them May begin to show understanding of conservation of numbers through counting objects regardless of arrangement Uses time-oriented words with increased understanding Very curious about factual information regarding world	Gets along well with parents May seek out parent more often than at age 4 years for reassurance and security, especially when entering school Begins to question parents' thinking and principles Strongly identifies with parent of same sex, especially boys with their fathers Enjoys activities such as sports, cooking, and shopping with parent of same sex

Coping with Concerns Related to Normal Growth and Development

Preschool and Kindergarten Experience. During the preschool years many children attend some type of early childhood program, usually preschool or a day care center. Group care has become commonplace with the large number of mothers presently employed outside the home (see Alternate Child Care Arrangements, Chapter 36). The effects of early education and stimulation on children have increasingly gained recognition and importance. (For a discussion of the effects of day care on children, see Working Mothers, Chapter 31.) Since social development widens to include age-mates and other significant adults, preschool provides an excellent vehicle for expanding children's experiences with others. It also is an excellent preparation for entrance into elementary school.

In preschool or day care centers, children are exposed to opportunities for learning group cooperation; adjusting to various sociocultural differences; and coping with frustration, dissatisfaction, and anger. If activities are tailored to provide mastery and achievement, children increasingly have feelings of success, self-confidence, and personal competence. Whether or not structured learning is imposed is less important than the social climate, type of guidance, and attitude toward the children that is fostered by the teacher or leader. With a teacher who is aware of preschoolers' developmental abilities and needs, children will learn from the activity that is provided. Most programs incorporate a daily schedule of quiet play, active outdoor activity, group activities such as games and projects, creative or free play, and snack and rest periods. Preschool is particularly beneficial for children who lack a peer-group experience, such as an only child; and for children from impoverished homes. It also is an excellent preparation for kindergarten.

One of the issues that parents face is the child's readiness for preschool or kindergarten. There are no absolute indicators for school readiness, but children's social maturation, especially attention span, is as important as their academic readiness. Using a developmental screening tool that addresses cognitive (especially language), social, and physical milestones can identify children who may benefit from diagnostic testing (Boucher, Doescher, and Sugawara, 1993).

Nurses can be helpful in guiding parents to locate suitable facilities with well-qualified staffs. State licensing agencies can help parents identify day care centers that accept children of specific age groups and that are conveniently located. State-licensed programs are supposed to abide by established standards, which represent the minimum requirements and safeguards; however, enforcement of the standards is sometimes inadequate. Early childhood programs may also belong to a voluntary accreditation system, the National Academy of Early Childhood Programs, which serves as a model for *optimum* care.* References from other parents are also helpful, provided that they have investigated the center carefully.

Other areas for parents to evaluate are the center's daily program, teacher qualifications, student-staff ratio, discipline policy, environmental safety precautions, provision of meals, sanitary conditions, adequate indoor/outdoor space per child, and fee schedule. In terms of an overall evaluation, *there is no substitute for a personal observation of the facility.* Parents should arrange to meet the director and some of the employees, especially those who would be caring for the child. Developing a checklist may be helpful to evaluate the center systematically and make comparisons with other facilities.

One of the areas that is increasingly important in selecting child care centers is the agency's health practices. Substantial evidence shows that children in day care centers, especially those under 3 years of age, have more illnesses (especially diarrhea, hepatitis A, meningitis, otitis media, respiratory tract infections, and cytomegalovirus) than children not in day care centers (Rovers et al, 1999).

Nurses play an important role in infection control. Not only can they advise parents regarding the evaluation of a center's sanitary practices, but they can also take an active part in educating staff in measures to minimize transmission of infection (Lafontaine and Bedard, 1997). For example, in centers caring for children who are not toilet trained, reducing environmental contamination with urine and feces is an important infection control issue (Fig. 38-4).

Children need preparation for the preschool or kindergarten experience.* For young children it represents a change from their usual home environment and prolonged separation from parents.

Before the child begins the school experience, the parents should present the idea as exciting and pleasurable. Talking to the child about activities such as painting, building with blocks, or enjoying swings and other outdoor equipment allows the child to fantasize about the forthcoming event in a positive manner. When the first day of school arrives, the parents should behave confidently. Such behavior requires parents to have resolved their own feelings regarding the experience.

Parents should introduce their child to the teacher and the facility. In some instances it is helpful to remain for at least

*Information about the accreditation criteria and procedures of the National Academy of Early Childhood Programs is available from the National Association for the Education of Young Children, 1834 Connecticut Ave. NW, Washington, DC 20009; (202) 232-8777 or 1-800-424-2460. These criteria are excellent guidelines for evaluating preschools or day care centers.

*Recommended books for preparing young children for day care or school include *Going to Day Care* and *When Your Child Goes to School* by Fred Rogers (GP Putnam's Sons).

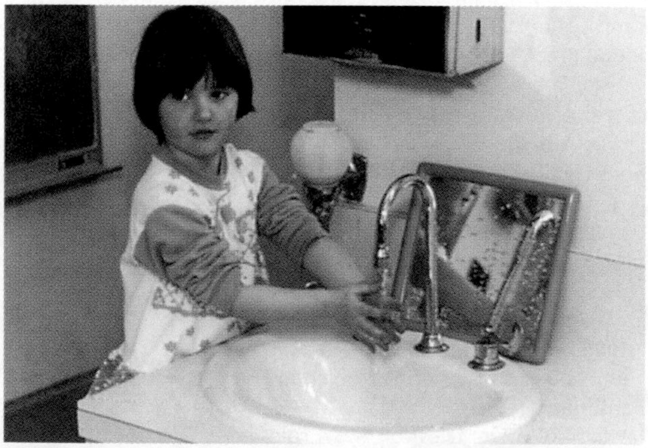

FIG. 38-4 • Thorough handwashing is the single most effective method of preventing infection.

some part of the first day until the child is comfortable and at ease. Other specific actions that can help lessen separation anxiety include providing the school with detailed information about the child's home environment, such as familiar routines, favorite activities, food preferences, names of siblings or pets, and personal habits. Such information helps the child feel familiar in the strange surroundings. When schools automatically request this information, the parent has a valuable clue to evaluating the quality of the program, since the request represents the staff's awareness of each child's needs. Transitional objects, such as a favorite toy, may also help the child bridge the gap from home to school.

Sex Education. Preschoolers have experienced a tremendous amount of information during their short lifetimes. Although their thinking may not be mature, they search constantly for explanations and reasons that are logical and reasonable to them. The word "why" seems to supplant the word "no," which was common in toddlerhood. It is only natural that as they learn about "me," they will also want to know "why me" and "how me." Questions such as "Where do babies come from?" are as casual as "What makes it rain," or "Who is that?" It is the way in which questions about procreation are answered that conditions children, even the youngest, to separate these questions from others about their world.

Two rules govern answering sensitive questions about topics such as sex. The first is to *find out what children know and think.* By investigating the theories children have produced as a reasonable explanation, parents can not only give correct information, but also help children understand why their explanation is inaccurate. Another reason for ascertaining what the child thinks before offering any information is that the "unasked for" answer may be given. For example, 4-year-old Sally asked her father, "Where did I come from?" Both parents quickly took this inquiry as a clue for offering sex education. After the explanation, Sally exclaimed, "I don't know about all that! All I know is Mary came from New York and I want to know where I was born."

The second rule for giving information is to *be honest.* It is true that much of the correct information will be forgotten or misunderstood by the preschooler, but what is more important is that the correct information can be restated until the child absorbs and comprehends the facts. Even though the correct anatomic words may be hard to pronounce or even more difficult to remember, they become foundational content for explaining other concepts later on.

Honesty does not imply imparting to children every fact of life or allowing excessive permissiveness in sexual curiosity. When children ask one question, they are looking for one answer. When they are ready, they will ask about the other "unfinished" parts of the story. Sooner or later they will wonder how the "sperm meets the egg" and "how the baby gets out," but it is best to wait until they ask.

Regardless of whether children are given sex education, they will engage in games of sexual curiosity and exploration. At about 3 years of age children are aware of the anatomic differences between the sexes and are very concerned with how the other "works." This is not really "sexual" curiosity, because many children are still unaware of the reproductive function of the genitals. Their curiosity is for the eliminative function of the anatomy. Little boys wonder how girls can urinate without a penis, so they watch girls go to the bathroom. Since they cannot see anything but the stream of water coming out, they want to observe further for what makes it come out. "Doctor play" is often a game invented for just such investigation. Little girls are no less curious about boys' anatomy. It is very intriguing to have a closer inspection of this "thing" that girls do not have.

One question that parents often have is how to handle such sexual curiosity. A positive approach is to neither condone nor condemn the sexual curiosity but to express that if children have questions, they should ask the parents; then the parents should encourage them to engage in some other activity. In this way children can be helped to understand that there are ways that their sexual curiosity can be satisfied other than through playing investigative games. This in no way condemns the act but stresses alternate methods to seek solutions and answers. Allowing children unrestricted permissiveness only intensifies their anxiety and concern, since exploring and searching usually yield little evidence to satisfy their curiosity.

Many excellent books on sex education are available for preschool children at public libraries, and the Sexuality Information and Education Council of the United States (SIECUS),* local chapters of the Planned Parenthood Federation of America,† and the American Academy of Pediatrics‡ have bibliographies of suggested reading material. Parents should read the book themselves *before* giving or reading it to a child.

Another concern for some parents is *masturbation,* or self-stimulation of the genitals. This occurs at any age for a variety of reasons and, if not excessive, is normal and healthy. It is most common at 4 years of age and during adolescence (Leung and Robson, 1993). For preschoolers it is a part of sexual curiosity and exploration. If parents are concerned about masturbation in their children, it is essential for nurses to investigate the circumstances associated with the activity because it may be an expression of anxiety, boredom, or unresolved conflicts. For example, a boy who repeatedly touches his penis is not masturbating for pleasure but may be reassuring himself that it is intact. Also, children who openly and publicly masturbate are inviting a reaction such as discipline, punishment, or criticism. They may be overwhelmed by their sexual feelings and asking others to help them channel them into more constructive outlets. Since masturbation, like other forms of sex play, is a private act, parents should emphasize this to children as part of teaching them socially acceptable behavior.

Fears. The greatest number and variety of real and imagined fears are present during the preschool years and include fear of the dark, being left alone (especially at bedtime), animals (particularly large dogs and snakes), ghosts, sexual matters (castration), and objects or persons associated with pain (Muris, Merckelbach, and Collaris, 1997). Parents often become perplexed about handling the fears because no amount of logical persuasion, coercion, or ridicule will send away the ghosts, bogeymen, monsters, and devils.

The best way to help children overcome their fears is by actively involving them in finding practical methods to deal with the frightening experience. This may be as simple as keeping a

*130 W. 42nd St., Suite 350, New York, NY 10036; (212) 819-9770; website: www.siecus.org.

†National office: 810 Seventh Ave., New York, NY 10019; (212) 541-7800 or 1-800-829-7732; website: www.plannedparenthood.org.

‡141 Northwest Point Blvd., Elk Grove Village, IL 60007; (888) 227-1770; fax (847) 228-1281; website: aap.org.

night-light on in the child's bedroom for reassurance that no monsters lurk in the dark. Exposing children to the feared object in a safe situation also provides a type of conditioning, or *desensitization.* For instance, children who are afraid of dogs should never be forced to approach or touch one, but they may be gradually introduced to the experience by watching other children play with the animal. This type of modeling, demonstrating fearlessness in others, can be very effective if the child is allowed to progress at his or her own rate (Muris et al, 1996).

Usually by 5 or 6 years of age children relinquish these old fears. Explaining the developmental sequence of fears and their gradual disappearance may help parents feel more secure in handling preschoolers' fears. Sometimes fears do not subside with simple measures or developmental maturation. When children experience severe fears that disrupt family life, professional help is required.

Stress. Although for parents the preschool years generally are less troublesome than toddlerhood, this period of life presents children with many unique stresses. Some, such as fears, are innate and stem from preschoolers' unique understanding of the world; others, such as beginning school, are imposed. Although minimum amounts of stress are beneficial during the early years to help children develop effective coping skills, excessive stress is harmful. Young children are especially vulnerable because of their limited capacity to cope.

To help parents deal with stress in their child's life, they must be aware of signs of stress (see Stress in Childhood, Chapter 33) and be helped to identify the source. In addition, any number of other stresses may be present, such as the birth of a sibling, marital discord, relocation, or illness. The best approach to dealing with stress is prevention—monitoring the amount of stress in children's lives so that levels exceeding their coping ability do not occur. In many instances structuring children's schedules to allow rest and preparing them for change, such as entering school, are sufficient measures.

Aggression. The term *aggression* refers to behavior that attempts to hurt a person or destroy property. Aggression differs from anger, which is a temporary emotional state, but anger may be expressed through aggression. Aggression is influenced by a complex set of biologic, sociocultural, and familial variables. Factors that tend to increase aggressive behavior are gender, frustration, modeling, and reinforcement.

Evidence exists that males are more overtly aggressive than females (Crick, Casas, and Mosher, 1997). *Frustration,* or the continual thwarting of self-satisfaction by disapproval, humiliation, punishment, and insults, can lead children to act out against others. Especially if they fear parents, children will displace anger toward parents to anger toward others. This type of aggression often applies to the child who is well behaved at home but a discipline problem at school.

Modeling, or imitating the behavior of significant others, is a powerful influencing force in preschoolers. Children who see their parents as verbally or physically abusive are observing behavior that they come to know as acceptable (Hart et al, 1998). Another aspect of modeling is the "double standard" for acceptable conduct. For example, in some families, aggression is synonymous with masculinity, and boys are encouraged to defend themselves.

Reinforcement can also shape aggressive behavior. Sometimes the reward for aggression is negative (e.g., punishment) yet reinforcing because it brings attention. For example, children who are ignored by a parent until they hit a sibling learn that this act garners attention.

When extreme behaviors such as aggression are present in children, parents are concerned about the need for professional help. Generally the difference between "normal" and "problematic" behavior is not the behavior itself but its *quantity* (number of occurrences), *severity* (interference with functioning), *distribution* (different manifestations), *onset* (sudden change in behavior), and *duration* (at least 4 weeks).

Speech Problems. The most critical period for speech development occurs between 2 and 4 years of age. During this period children are using their rapidly growing vocabulary faster than they can produce the words. This failure to master sensorimotor integrations results in *stuttering* or *stammering* as children try to say the word they are already thinking about. This dysfluency in speech pattern is a normal characteristic of language development (Castiglia, 1993).

However, when parents or other significant persons place undue emphasis or stress on this pattern of dysfluency, an abnormal speech pattern may result. Chances for reversal of stuttering are good until about 5 years of age; therefore, prevention must begin early.

The nurse should discuss with parents the normal dysfluencies in their child's speech. If excessive concern on the part of the parent, or frustration and struggling by the child is noted, or if a family history of stuttering exists, the child is referred for language and speech evaluation (Ambrose, Yairi, and Cox, 1993).

Children who are pressured into producing sounds ahead of their developmental level may develop *dyslalia* (articulation problems) or revert to using infantile speech. Prevention involves discussing with parents the usual achievement of speech production during childhood. The *Denver Articulation Screening Examination (DASE)* is an excellent tool for assessing articulation skills in the child and for explaining to parents the expected progression of sounds (see Appendix D).

PROMOTING OPTIMUM HEALTH DURING THE PRESCHOOL YEARS*

Nutrition

Nutritional requirements for preschoolers are fairly similar to those for toddlers (U.S. Department of Agriculture, 1999). The requirement for calories per unit of body weight continues to decrease slightly to 90 kcal/kg, for an average daily intake of 1800 calories. Fluid requirements may also decrease slightly to about 100 ml/kg daily but depend on the activity level, climatic conditions, and state of health. The protein requirements are 1.2 g/kg, for an average daily consumption of 24 g (Food and Nutrition Board, 1989). A diet that is moderately reduced in fat may be recommended for healthy preschool children (Williams et al, 1998); however, it is important that the diet not be deficient in nutrients such as calcium (Shea et al, 1993).

Some preschoolers still have food habits that are typical of toddlers, such as food fads and strong taste preferences. When children reach 4 years of age, they seem to enter another period

*For a more comprehensive understanding, the reader is urged to review the material presented in Chapter 37 under Promoting Optimum Health During Toddlerhood.

of finicky eating, which is generally characteristic of the more rebellious and rowdy behavior of children in this age group. By age 5 years children are more agreeable to trying new foods, especially if they are encouraged by an adult who allows them to help with food preparation or experiment with a new taste or different dish (Fig. 38-5). Mealtimes can become battlegrounds if parents expect perfect table manners. Usually the 5-year-old child is ready for the "social" side of eating, but the 3- or 4-year-old child still has difficulty sitting quietly through a long family meal.

The amount and variety of foods consumed by young children vary greatly from day to day (Dennison, Rockwell, and Baker, 1998). Consequently, parents sometimes worry about the quantity of food preschoolers consume. In general, the quality is much more important than the quantity, a fact that should be stressed during nutritional counseling. Some evidence suggests that children self-regulate their caloric intake. If they eat less at one meal, they will compensate at another meal or will snack.

One approach toward lessening this parental concern is advising parents to keep a weekly record of everything the child eats. In particular, the need for measuring the amount of food (e.g., setting aside ½ cup of vegetables, and serving the child from this premeasured amount) is stressed to provide a more accurate estimate of food intake at each meal. Usually by the end of the week, when they look at the food chart, parents are amazed at how much the child has consumed. In general, preschoolers consume only slightly more than toddlers do, or about half an adult's portion.

Sleep and Activity

Sleep patterns vary widely, but the average preschooler sleeps about 12 hours a night and infrequently takes daytime naps. Activity levels continue to be high, although quiet activities, such as watching television, are increasingly appealing and can become an unhealthy substitute for active play. Preschoolers' increased gross motor abilities and coordination provide them with the opportunity to engage in many sports, if only at a novice level. Whether young children should begin formalized training in an activity at this early age is controversial. Children's readiness to participate in organized sports should be determined individually The decision should be based on the child's (not the parent's) motivation and enjoyment. The American Academy of Pediatrics (1992) encourages free play, a variety of physical activities, a noncompetitive atmosphere, and emphasis on fun and safety.

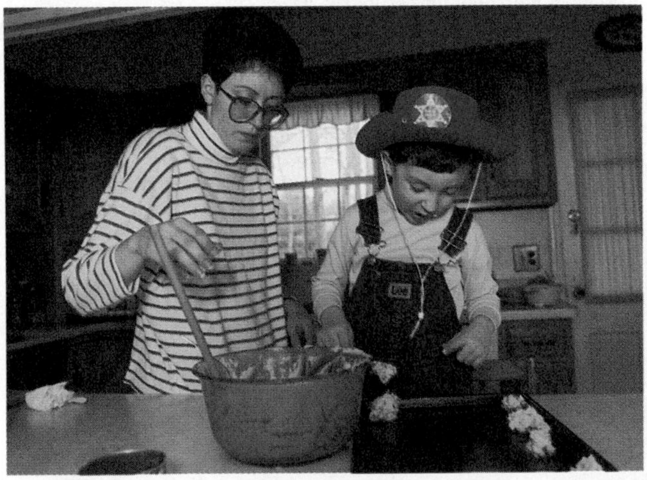

FIG. 38-5 • Preschool-age children enjoy helping adults and are more likely to try new foods if they can assist in their preparation.

Sleep Problems.* The preschool years are a prime time for sleep problems (Kerr and Jowett, 1994). Young children sometimes have trouble going to sleep, especially after so much activity and stimulation during the day. Others may develop bedtime fears, wake during the night, or have nightmares or sleep terrors. Still others may prolong the inevitable through elaborate rituals. Children with reported sleep problems may be more likely to have a difficult temperament than those without sleep disturbances (Atkinson et al, 1995).

Recommendations for sleep disturbance are offered only *after* a thorough assessment of the problem has been completed. Cultural traditions may dictate sleep practices that are contrary to certain well-accepted professional recommendations. Therefore parents may not perceive a particular sleep practice as a problem (Cultural Considerations box).

Interventions can differ greatly; for example, *nightmares* (i.e., frightening dreams that are followed by full waking) and *sleep terrors* (i.e., partial arousal from deep, nondreaming sleep) require very different approaches. Although sleep terrors require no intervention (the best approach is to remain uninvolved so that the child remains asleep), nightmares respond best to the following interventions:

- Accept dream as real fear
- Sit with child; offer comfort, assurance, and sense of protection
- Lie down with child or take to own bed only if child is not calmed by other measures and understands this is a special occasion
- Consider professional counseling for recurrent nightmares unresponsive to the above approaches

For children who delay going to bed, a recommended approach involves counseling parents about the importance of a

*Guidelines for helping parents deal with sleep problems are available in Wong DL, Hess CS: *Wong and Whaley's clinical manual of pediatric nursing,* ed 5, St Louis, 2000, Mosby.

Cultural Considerations

CO-SLEEPING

Although many experts recommend that infants and children be trained to sleep always in their own crib or bed, co-sleeping, or the "family bed" (in which parents allow the children to sleep with them or the siblings to sleep together in one bed), is a relatively common and accepted cultural practice, especially among African-American, Hispanic, and Asian-American families, such as the Japanese.* Other groups that are adopting co-sleeping include (1) single parents, whose need for company may encourage this practice; (2) working parents, who desire the closeness at night that was lost during the day; and (3) parents who have had an issue about sleep or separation in their own past.

*Latz S, Wolf AW, Lozoff B: Co-sleeping in context: sleep practices and problems in young children in Japan and the United States, *Arch Pediatr Adolesc Med* 153(4):339-346, 1999.

consistent bedtime ritual. Attention-seeking behavior is ignored, and the child is not taken into the parents' bed or allowed to stay up past a reasonable hour. Other measures that may be helpful include keeping a light on in the room, providing transitional objects such as a favorite toy, or leaving a drink of water by the bed.

Helping children slow down *before* bedtime also contributes to less resistance to going to bed. One approach is to establish limited rituals that signal readiness for bed, such as a bath or story. Parents can reinforce the pattern by stating, "After this story it is bedtime," and consistently carrying out the routine. If extra stimulation, such as having visitors arrive at bedtime, is disruptive to children's routine, it is advisable to settle children in bed beforehand.

Dental Health

By the beginning of the preschool period the eruption of the deciduous teeth is complete. Dental care is essential to preserve these temporary teeth and to teach good dental habits (see Chapter 37). Although preschoolers' fine motor control is improved, they still require assistance and supervision with brushing, and flossing should be done by parents (American Academy of Pediatric Dentistry, 1996). Professional care and prophylaxis, especially fluoride supplements, should be continued. For children cared for away from home, parents are encouraged to monitor the dental care provided by others, including keeping cariogenic foods to a minimum in the diet.

Injury Prevention

Because of improved gross and fine motor skills, coordination, and balance, preschoolers are less prone to falls than are toddlers. They tend to be less reckless, listen more to parental rules, and are aware of potential dangers, such as hot objects, sharp instruments, and dangerous heights. Putting objects in the mouth as part of exploration has all but ceased, although poisoning is still a danger. Pedestrian motor vehicle injuries increase because of activities such as playing in the street, riding tricycles, running after balls, or forgetting safety regulations when crossing streets.

In general the guidelines suggested for injury prevention in Table 37-3 apply to children in this age group as well. However, emphasis is now on *education* for safety and potential hazards, in addition to appropriate protection. Since preschoolers are great imitators, it is especially essential that parents set a good example by "practicing what they preach." Children quickly observe discrepancies in what they are told to do and what they see others do. Establishing habits at this time, such as wearing bicycle helmets, can create long-term safety behaviors.

Anticipatory Guidance—Care of Families

The preschool years present fewer childrearing difficulties than earlier years, and this stage of development is facilitated by appropriate anticipatory guidance in the areas already discussed (Home Care box). There is a shift in child-rearing practices from protection to education. Whereas injury prevention previously focused on safeguarding the immediate environment, with less emphasis on reasoning, now the protective guardrails or electrical outlet caps may be substituted with verbal explanations of why danger exists and how to avoid it with appropriate judgment and understanding.

During this period an emotional transition between parent and child is also occurring. Although children are still attached to their parents and accepting of all parental values and beliefs,

Home Care

GUIDANCE DURING PRESCHOOL YEARS

Age 3 Years

Prepare parents for child's increasing interest in widening relationships.
Encourage enrollment in preschool.
Emphasize importance of setting limits.
Prepare parents to expect exaggerated tension reduction behaviors, such as need for "security blanket."
Encourage parents to offer child choices when child vacillates.
Prepare parents to expect marked changes at 3½ years, when child becomes less coordinated (motor and emotional), becomes insecure, and exhibits emotional extremes.
Prepare parents for normal dysfluency in speech and advise them to avoid focusing on the pattern.
Prepare parents to expect extra demands on their attention as a reflection of child's emotional insecurity and fear of loss of love.
Warn parents that equilibrium of 3-year-old will change to aggressive, out-of-bounds behavior of 4-year-old.
Inform parents to anticipate more stable appetite with more food selections.
Stress need for protection and education of child to prevent injury (see Injury Prevention, Chapter 37).

Age 4 Years

Prepare parents for more aggressive behavior, including motor activity and offensive language.
Prepare parents to expect resistance to parental authority.
Explore parental feelings regarding child's behavior.
Suggest some kind of respite for primary caregivers, such as placing child in preschool for part of the day.
Prepare parents for child's increasing sexual curiosity.
Emphasize importance of realistic limit setting on behavior and appropriate discipline techniques.
Prepare parents for highly imaginative 4-year-old who indulges in "tall tales" (to be differentiated from lies) and for child's imaginary playmates.
Prepare parents to expect nightmares or an increase in them and suggest that parents make sure child is fully awakened from a frightening dream.
Provide reassurance that a period of calm begins at 5 years of age.

Age 5 Years

Inform parents to expect tranquil period at 5 years.
Help parents to prepare child for entrance into school environment.
Make sure immunizations are up to date before entering school.
Suggest that nonemployed mothers (or fathers if appropriate) consider own activities when child begins school.
Suggest swimming lessons for child.

they are nearing the period of life when they will question previous teachings and prefer the companionship of peers. Entry into school marks a separation from home for parents as well as for children. Parents need help in adjusting to this change, particularly if the mother has focused her daily activity primarily on home responsibilities. As preschoolers begin preschool or elementary school, mothers may need to seek activities beyond the family, such as community involvement or pursuing a career. In this way all family members are adjusting to change, which is part of the process of growth and development.

SPECIAL HEALTH PROBLEMS

Communicable Diseases

The incidence of childhood communicable diseases has declined greatly since the advent of immunizations. Serious complications resulting from such infections have been further reduced with the use of antibiotics and antitoxins. However, infectious diseases do occur, and nurses must be familiar with infectious agents in order to recognize the disease and institute appropriate interventions (Table 38-2). (See also Chapter 53 for a discussion of nursing care for dermatologic conditions.)

Nursing Care Management

➤ Assessment

Identification of the infectious agent is of primary importance to prevent exposure to susceptible individuals. Nurses in ambulatory care settings, child care centers, and schools are often the first persons to see signs of a communicable disease, such as a rash or sore throat. The nurse must operate under a high index of suspicion for common childhood diseases in order to identify potentially infectious cases and to recognize diseases that require medical intervention. An example is the common complaint of sore throat. Although most often a symptom of a minor viral infection, it can signal diphtheria or a streptococcal infection such as scarlet fever. Each of these bacterial conditions requires appropriate medical treatment to prevent serious sequelae.

Assessment of the following is helpful in identifying potentially communicable diseases: (1) recent exposure to a known case; (2) *prodromal symptoms* (symptoms that occur between early manifestations of the disease and its overt clinical syndrome) or evidence of constitutional symptoms, such as a fever or rash (see Table 38-2); (3) immunization history; and (4) history of having the disease. Because immunizations are available for several of the diseases, and since in almost each case an attack confers lifelong immunity, the possibility of many infectious agents can be eliminated based on these two criteria.

➤ Nursing Diagnoses

A number of nursing diagnoses are prominent in the nursing care of the child with a communicable disease, and others specific to individual cases become evident. The most common nursing diagnoses are presented in the Nursing Care Plan on p. 926.

➤ Plan of Care and Implementation

The principal nursing goals, in addition to identification of the communicable disease (see Assessment), are as follows:

- Child will not spread the infection to others.
- Child will not experience complications.
- Child will have minimal discomfort.
- Child and family will receive adequate emotional support.

Prevent Spread. Prevention consists of two components: prevention of the disease and control of its spread to others. Primary prevention rests almost exclusively on immunization. (The nurse's role in immunization of children is discussed in Chapter 36.)

Control measures to prevent spread of the disease include appropriate techniques to reduce risk of cross-transmission of infectious organisms between patients and to protect health care workers from organisms harbored by patients. If the child is hospitalized, the facility's policies for infection control are followed (see Chapter 45). The most important procedure to stress is handwashing. Persons directly caring for the child or handling contaminated articles must wash their hands before beginning care of another patient. The child is instructed to practice good handwashing technique after toileting and before eating. For those diseases spread by droplets, the nurse instructs parents in measures aimed at reducing airborne transmission. The child who is old enough should use a tissue to cover the face during coughing or sneezing; otherwise the parent should cover the child's mouth with a tissue and then discard it. The usual hygiene measures of not sharing eating and drinking utensils are stressed to the family.

NURSE ALERT • If a child is admitted to the hospital with an undiagnosed exanthema, strict isolation is instituted until a diagnosis is confirmed. Childhood communicable diseases requiring strict isolation include diphtheria and chickenpox.

Prevent Complications. Although most youngsters recover without any difficulty, certain groups of children are at risk for serious, even fatal, complications from communicable diseases, especially the viral diseases of chickenpox and erythema infectiosum (EI). Children with an immunodeficiency (e.g., those receiving steroid or other immunosuppressive therapy, those with a generalized malignancy such as leukemia or lymphoma, or those with an immunologic disorder) are at risk for viremia from replication of the *varicella-zoster virus (VZV)** in the blood. VZV is so named because it causes two distinct diseases: *varicella (chickenpox)* and *zoster (herpes zoster or shingles)*. Varicella occurs primarily in children under 15 years of age; however, it leaves the threat of herpes zoster, an intensely painful varicella that is localized to a single dermatome (body area innervated by a particular segment of the spinal cord) (Kakourou et al, 1998). Patients who are immunocompromised and healthy infants under 1 year of age (who also have reduced immunity) are at a higher risk for reactivation of VZV, causing herpes zoster, probably as a result of a deficiency in cellular immunity (Bilgrami et al, 1999).

Children with hemolytic disease, such as sickle cell disease, are at risk for aplastic anemia from EI. The *human parvovirus (HPV)* infects and lyses red blood cell precursors, thus inter-

Text continued on p. 924

*Educational materials for health care providers and families may be obtained from the Varicella Zoster Virus Research Foundation, 40 East 72nd St., New York, NY 10021; or Glaxo-Wellcome, Inc., 3030 Cornwallis Rd., Research Triangle Park, NC 27709; (919) 248-3000 or (888) 825-5249; website: www.glaxowellcome.com.

TABLE 38-2
Communicable Diseases of Childhood

Disease

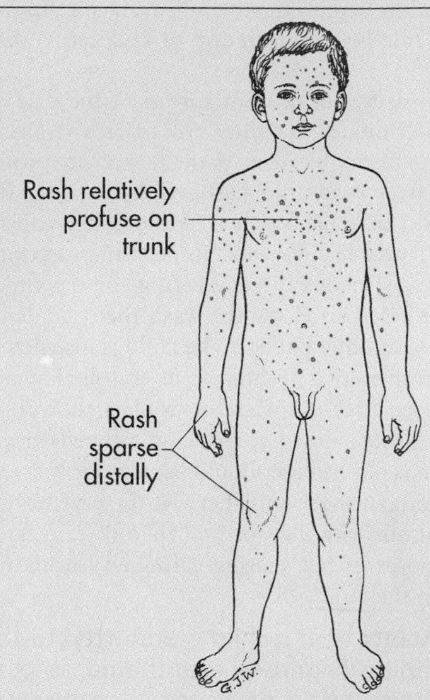

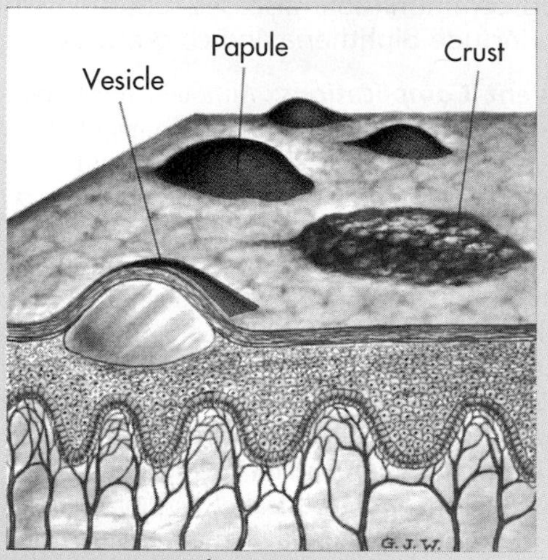

Simultaneous stages of lesions in chickenpox

CHICKENPOX (VARICELLA) (Fig. 38-6)
Agent: Varicella-zoster virus (VZV)
Source: Primary secretions of respiratory tract of infected persons; to a lesser degree, skin lesions (scabs not infectious)
Transmission: Direct contact, droplet (airborne) spread, and contaminated objects
Incubation period: 2-3 weeks, usually 14-16 days
Period of communicability: Probably 1 day before eruption of lesions (prodromal period) to 6 days after first crop of vesicles when crusts have formed

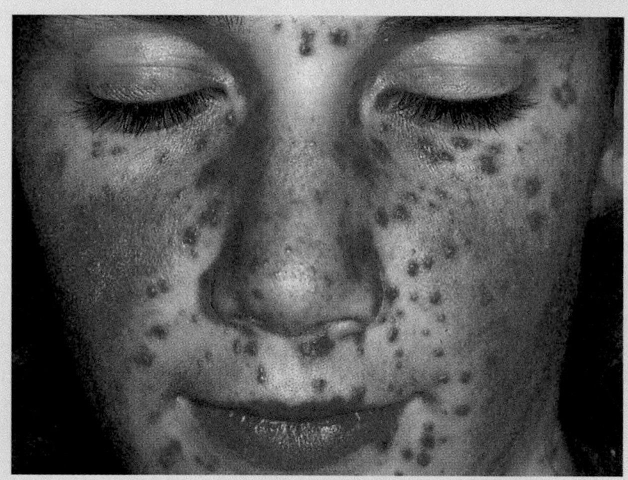

FIG. 38-6 • Chickenpox (varicella). (Clinical view from Habif TP: *Clinical dermatology: a color guide to diagnosis and therapy*, ed 3, St Louis, 1996, Mosby.)

DIPHTHERIA
Agent: *Corynebacterium diphtheriae*
Source: Discharge from mucous membranes of nose and nasopharynx, skin, and other lesions of infected person
Transmission: Direct contact with infected person, a carrier, or contaminated articles
Incubation period: Usually 2-5 days, possibly longer
Period of communicability: Variable; until virulent bacilli are no longer present (identified by three negative cultures); usually 2 weeks but as long as 4 weeks

Clinical Manifestations	Therapeutic Management/ Complications	Nursing Considerations
Prodromal stage: Slight fever, malaise, and anorexia for first 24 hours; rash highly pruritic; begins as macule, rapidly progresses to papule and then vesicle (surrounded by erythematous base, becomes umbilical and cloudy, breaks easily and forms crusts); all three stages (papule, vesicle, crust) present in varying degrees at one time **Distribution:** Centripetal, spreading to face and proximal extremities but sparse on distal limbs and less on areas not exposed to heat (e.g., from clothing or sun) **Constitutional signs and symptoms:** Elevated temperature from lymphadenopathy, irritability from pruritus	**Specific:** Antiviral agent acyclovir (Zovirax); varicella-zoster immune globulin (VZIG) after exposure in high-risk children **Supportive:** Diphenhydramine hydrochloride or antihistamines to relieve itching; skin care to prevent secondary bacterial infection **Complications:** Secondary bacterial infections (abscesses, cellulitis, necrotizing fasciitis, pneumonia, sepsis) Encephalitis Varicella pneumonia (rare in normal children) Hemorrhagic varicella (tiny hemorrhages in vesicles and numerous petechiae in skin) Chronic or transient thrombocytopenia	Maintain strict isolation in hospital Isolate child in home until vesicles have dried (usually 1 week after onset of disease), and isolate high-risk children from infected children Administer skin care; give bath and change clothes and linens daily; administer topical calamine lotion; keep child's fingernails short and clean; apply mittens if child scratches Keep child cool (may decrease number of lesions) Lessen pruritis; keep child occupied Remove loose crusts that rub and irritate skin Tech child to apply pressure to pruritic area rather than scratching it If older child, reason with child regarding danger of scar formation from scratching Avoid use of aspirin; use of acetaminophen controversial
Vary according to anatomic location of pseudomembrane **Nasal:** Resembles common cold, serosanguineous mucopurulent nasal discharge without constitutional symptoms; may be frank epistaxis **Tonsillar/pharyngeal:** Malaise; anorexia; sore throat; low-grade fever; pulse increased above expected for temperature within 24 hours; smooth, adherent, white or gray membrane; lymphadenitis possibly pronounced ("bull's neck"); in severe cases, toxemia, septic shock, and death within 6-10 days **Laryngeal:** Fever, hoarseness, cough, with or without previous signs listed; potential airway obstruction, apprehensive, dyspneic retractions, cyanosis	Antitoxin (usually intravenously); preceded by skin or conjunctival test to rule out sensitivity to horse serum Antibiotics (penicillin or erythromycin) Complete bed rest (prevention of myocarditis) Tracheostomy for airway obstruction Treatment of infected contacts and carriers **Complications:** Myocarditis (second week) Neuritis	Maintain strict isolation in hospital Participate in sensitivity testing; have epinephrine available Administer antibiotics; observe for signs of sensitivity to penicillin Administer complete care to maintain bed rest Use suctioning as needed Observe respiration for signs of obstruction Administer humidified oxygen if prescribed

Continued

TABLE 38-2—cont'd
Communicable Diseases of Childhood

Disease

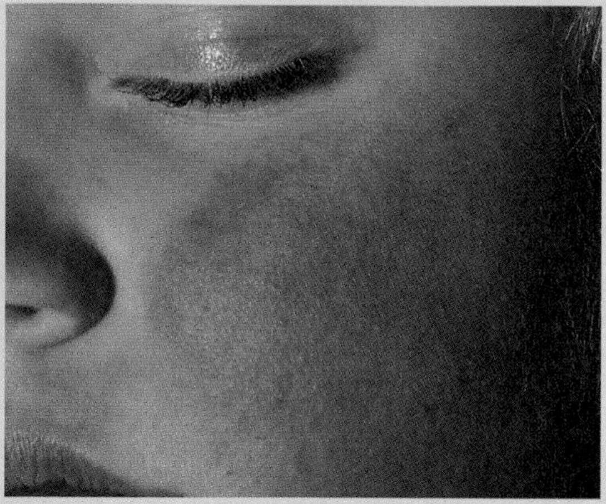

FIG. 38-7 • Erythema infectiosum. (From Habif TP: *Clinical dermatology: a color guide to diagnosis and therapy,* ed 3, St Louis, 1996, Mosby.)

ERYTHEMA INFECTIOSUM (FIFTH DISEASE) (Fig. 38-7)
Agent: Human parvovirus B19 (HPV)
Source: Infected persons
Transmission: Unknown; possibly respiratory secretions and blood
Incubation period: 4-14 days, may be as long as 21 days
Period of communicability: Uncertain but before onset of symptoms in most children; also for about 1 week after onset of symptoms in children with aplastic crisis

EXANTHEMA SUBITUM (ROSEOLA) (Fig. 38-8)
Agent: Human herpesvirus type 6 (HHV-6)
Source: Unknown
Transmission: Unknown (virtually limited to children between 6 months and 3 years of age)
Incubation period: Usually 5-15 days
Period of communicability: Unknown

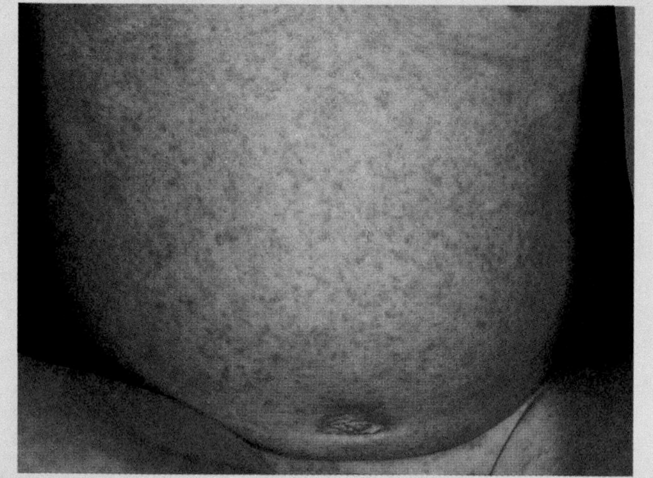

FIG. 38-8 • Roseola infantum. (From Habif TP: *Clinical dermatology: a color guide to diagnosis and therapy,* ed 3, St. Louis, 1996, Mosby.)

Clinical Manifestations	Therapeutic Management/ Complications	Nursing Considerations
Rash appears in three stages: I—Erythema on face, chiefly on cheeks, "slapped face" appearance; disappears by 1-4 days II—About 1 day after rash appears on face, maculopapular red spots appear, symmetrically distributed on upper and lower extremities; rash progresses from proximal to distal surfaces and may last 1 week or more III—Rash subsides but reappears if skin is irritated or traumatized (sun, heat, cold, friction) In children with aplastic crisis, rash is usually absent and prodromal illness includes fever, myalgia, lethargy, nausea, vomiting, and abdominal pain	**Symptomatic and supportive:** Antipyretics, analgesics, antiinflammatory drugs Possible blood transfusion for transient aplastic anemia **Complications:** Self-limited arthritis and arthralgia (arthritis may become chronic)* May result in fetal death if mother infected during pregnancy (documented maternal infection in the first half of pregnancy leads to 10% risk of fetal death, with less risk in second half of pregnancy), but no evidence of congenital anomalies† Aplastic crisis in children with hemolytic disease or immunodeficiency Myocarditis (rare)	Isolation of child not necessary, except hospitalized child (immunosuppressed or with aplastic crises) suspected of HPV infection is placed on respiratory isolation and Standard Precautions Pregnant women: need not be excluded from workplace where HPV infection is present; should not care for patients with aplastic crises; explain low risk of fetal death to those in contact with affected children
Persistent high fever for 3-4 days in child who appears well Precipitous drop in fever to normal with appearance of rash **Rash:** Discrete rose-pink macules or maculopapules appearing first on trunk, then spreading to neck, face, and extremities; nonpruritic, fades on pressure, lasts 1-2 days **Associated signs and symptoms:** Cervical/postauricular lymphadenopathy, inflamed pharynx, cough, coryza	Nonspecific Antipyretics to control fever **Complications:** Recurrent febrile seizures (possibly from latent infection of central nervous system that is reactivated by fever) Encephalitis (rare)	Teach parents measure for lowering temperature (antipyretic drugs) If child is prone to seizures, discuss appropriate precautions, possibility of recurrent febrile seizures

*Nocton JJ et al: Human parvovirus-associated arthritis in children, *J Pediatr* 122(2):186-190, 1993.
†American Academy of Pediatrics, Committee on Infectious Diseases, Pickering L, editor: *2000 Red Book: report of the Committee on Infectious Diseases,* ed 24, Elk Grove Village, IL, 2000, The Academy.

Continued

TABLE 38-2—cont'd
Communicable Diseases of Childhood

	Disease

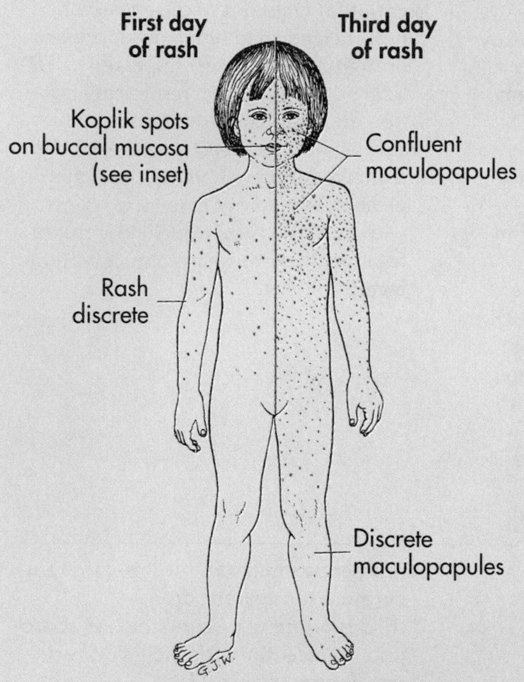

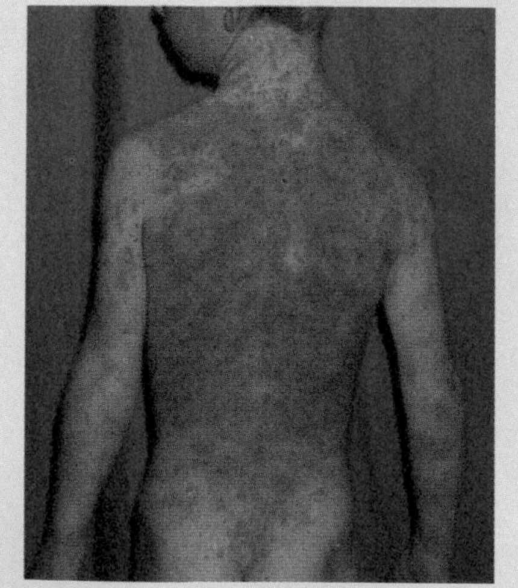

FIG. 38-9 • Measles (rubeola). (Clinical view from Seidel HM et al: *Mosby's guide to physical examination,* ed 4, St Louis, 1999, Mosby; Koplik spots from Zitelli BJ, Davis HW: *Atlas of pediatric physical diagnosis,* ed 3, St Louis, 1997, Mosby.)

MEASLES (RUBEOLA) (Fig. 38-9)
Agent: Virus
Source: Respiratory tract secretions, blood, and urine of infected person
Transmission: Usually by direct contact with droplets of infected person
Incubation period: 10-20 days
Period of communicability: From 4 days before to 5 days after rash appears but mainly during prodromal (catarrhal) stage

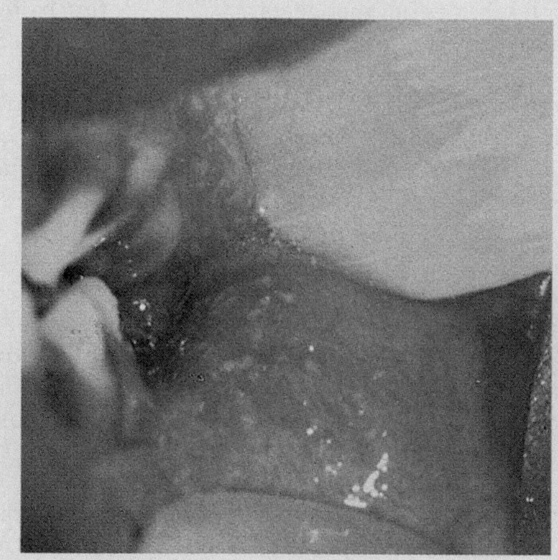

Koplik spots

MUMPS
Agent: Paramyxovirus
Source: Saliva of infected persons
Transmission: Direct contact with or droplet spread from an infected person
Incubation period: 14-21 days
Period of communicability: Most communicable immediately before and after swelling begins

PERTUSSIS (WHOOPING COUGH)
Agent: *Bordetella pertussis*
Source: Discharge from respiratory tract of infected persons

Clinical Manifestations	Therapeutic Management/ Complications	Nursing Considerations
Prodromal (catarrhal) stage: Fever and malaise, followed in 24 hours by coryza, cough, conjunctivitis, Koplik spots (small, irregular red spots with a minute, bluish white center first seen on buccal mucosa opposite molars 2 days before rash); symptoms gradually increase in severity until second day after rash appears, when they begin to subside **Rash:** Appears 3-4 days after onset of prodromal stage; begins as erythematous maculopapular eruption on face and gradually spreads downward; more severe in earlier sites (appears confluent) and less intense in later sites (appears discrete); after 3-4 days assumes brownish appearance, and fine desquamation occurs over areas of extensive involvement **Constitutional signs and symptoms:** Anorexia, malaise, generalized lymphadenopathy	Vitamin A supplementation (see p. 924) **Supportive:** Bed rest during febrile period; antipyretics Antibiotics to prevent secondary bacterial infection in high-risk children **Complications:** Otitis media Pneumonia Bronchiolitis Obstructive laryngitis and laryngotracheitis Encephalitis	Isolation until fifth day of rash; if hospitalized, institute respiratory precautions Maintain bed rest during prodromal stage; provide quiet activity **Fever:** Instruct parents to administer antipyretics; avoid chilling; if child is prone to seizures, institute appropriate precautions (fever spikes to 40° C [104° F] between fourth and fifth days) **Eye care:** Dim lights if photophobia present; clean eyelids with warm saline solution to remove secretions or crusts; keep child from rubbing eyes; examine cornea for signs of ulceration **Coryza/cough:** Use cool-mist vaporizer; protect skin around nares with layer of petrolatum; encourage fluids and soft, bland foods **Skin care:** Keep skin clean; use tepid baths as necessary
Prodromal stage: Fever, headache, malaise, and anorexia for 24 hours, followed by "earache" that is aggravated by chewing **Parotitis:** By third day, parotid gland(s) (either unilateral or bilateral) enlarges and reaches maximum size in 1-3 days; accompanied by pain and tenderness **Other manifestations:** Submaxillary and sublingual infection, orchitis, and meningoencephalitis	**Symptomatic and supportive:** Analgesics for pain and antipyretics for fever Intravenous fluid may be necessary for child who refuses to drink or vomits because of meningoencephalitis **Complications:** Sensorineural deafness Postinfectious encephalitis Myocarditis Arthritis Hepatitis Epididymo-orchitis Sterility (extremely rare in adult males)	Isolation during period of communicability; institute respiratory precautions during hospitalization Maintain bed rest during prodromal phase until swelling subsides Give analgesics for pain; if child is unwilling to chew medication, use elixir form Encourage fluids and soft, bland foods; avoid foods requiring chewing Apply hot or cold compresses to neck, whichever is more comforting To relieve orchitis, provide warmth and local support with tight-fitting underpants (stretch bathing suit works well)
Catarrhal stage: Begins with symptoms of upper respiratory tract infection, such as coryza, sneezing, lacrimation, cough, and low-grade fever; symptoms continue for 1-2 weeks, when dry, hacking cough becomes more severe	Antimicrobial therapy (e.g., erythromycin) Administration of pertussis immune globulin	Isolation during catarrhal stage; if hospitalized, institute respiratory precautions Maintain bed rest as long as fever present

Continued

TABLE 38-2—cont'd
Communicable Diseases of Childhood

	Disease
	PERTUSSIS (WHOOPING COUGH)—cont'd **Transmission:** Direct contact or droplet spread from infected person; indirect contact with freshly contaminated articles **Incubation period:** 6-20 days, usually 7-10 days **Period of communicability:** Greatest during catarrhal stage before onset of paroxysms and may extend to fourth week after onset of paroxysms
	POLIOMYELITIS **Agent:** Enteroviruses, three types: type 1—most common cause of paralysis, both epidemic and endemic; type 2—least commonly associated with paralysis; type 3—second most commonly associated with paralysis **Source:** Feces and oropharyngeal secretions of infected persons, especially young children **Transmission:** Direct contact with persons with apparent or inapparent active infection; spread is via fecal-oral and pharyngeal-oropharyngeal routes **Incubation period:** Usually 7-14 days, with range of 5-35 days **Period of communicability:** Not exactly known; virus is present in throat and feces shortly after infection and persists for about 1 week in throat and 4-6 weeks in feces
	RUBELLA (GERMAN MEASLES) (Fig. 38-10) **Agent:** Rubella virus **Source:** Primarily nasopharyngeal secretions of person with apparent or inapparent infection; virus also present in blood, stool, and urine **Transmission:** Direct contact and spread via infected person; indirectly via articles freshly contaminated with nasopharyngeal secretions, feces, or urine **Incubation period:** 14-21 days **Period of communicability:** 7 days before to about 5 days after appearance of rash

A

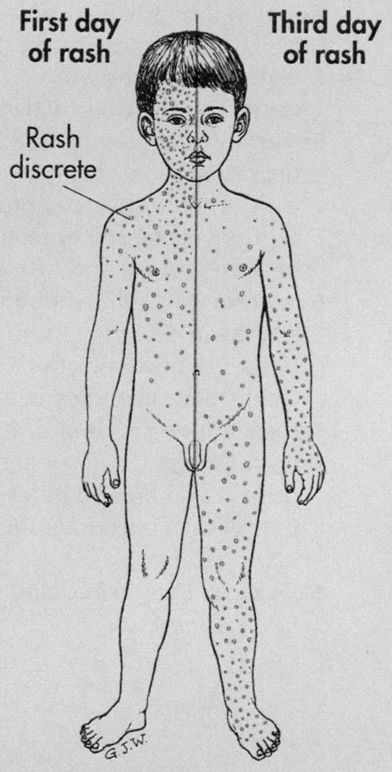

B

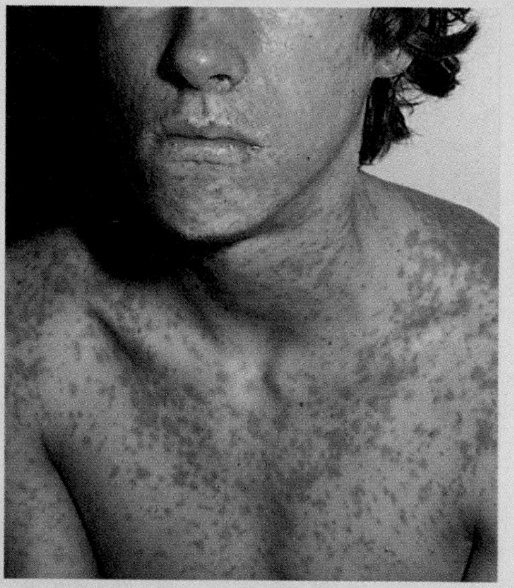

FIG. 38-10 • Rubella (German measles). **A,** Progression of rash. **B,** Clinical view. (Courtesy Dr. Michael Sherlock; in Zitelli BJ, Davis HW: *Atlas of pediatric physical diagnosis,* ed 3, St Louis, 1997, Mosby.)

Clinical Manifestations	Therapeutic Management/ Complications	Nursing Considerations
Paroxysmal stage: Cough most often occurs at night and consists of short, rapid coughs followed by sudden inspiration associated with a high-pitched crowing sound or "whoop"; during paroxysms, cheeks become flushed or cyanotic, eyes bulge, and tongue protrudes; paroxysm may continue until thick mucus plug is dislodged; vomiting commonly follows attack; stage generally lasts 4-6 weeks, followed by convalescent stage	**Supportive treatment:** Hospitalization required for infants, children who are dehydrated, or those who have complications Bed rest Increased oxygen intake and humidity Adequate fluids Intubation possibly necessary **Complications:** Pneumonia (usual cause of death) Atelectasis Otitis media Seizures Hemorrhage (subarachnoid, subconjunctival, epistaxis) Weight loss and dehydration Hernia Prolapsed rectum	Keep child occupied during day (interest in play associated with fewer paroxysms) Reassure parents during frightening episodes of whooping cough Provide restful environment and reduce factors that promote paroxysms (dust, smoke, sudden change in temperature, chilling, activity, excitement); keep room well ventilated Encourage fluids; offer small amount of fluids frequently; refeed child after vomiting Provide high humidity (humidifier or tent); suction gently but often to prevent choking on secretions Observe for signs of airway obstruction (increased restlessness, apprehension, retractions, cyanosis) Involve public health nurse if child cared for at home
May be manifested in three different forms: **Abortive or inapparent**—Fever, uneasiness, sore throat, headache, anorexia, vomiting, abdominal pain; lasts a few hours to a few days **Nonparalytic**—Same manifestations as abortive form but more severe, with pain and stiffness in neck, back, and legs **Paralytic**—Initial course similar to nonparalytic type, followed by recovery and then signs of central nervous system paralysis	No specific treatment, including antimicrobials or gamma globulin Complete bed rest during acute phase Assisted respiratory ventilation in case of respiratory paralysis Physical therapy for muscles following acute stage **Complications:** Permanent paralysis Respiratory arrest Hypertension Kidney stones from demineralization of bone during prolonged immobility	Maintain complete bed rest Administer mild sedatives as necessary to relieve anxiety and promote rest Participate in physiotherapy procedures (use of moist hot packs and range-of-motion exercises) Position child to maintain body alignment and prevent contractures or decubiti; use footboard Encourage child to move; administer analgesics for maximum comfort during physical activity Observe for respiratory paralysis (difficulty in talking, ineffective cough, inability to hold breath, shallow and rapid respirations); report such signs and symptoms to practitioner; have tracheostomy tray at bedside
Prodromal stage: Absent in children, present in adults and adolescents; consists of low-grade fever, headache, malaise, anorexia, mild conjunctivitis, coryza, sore throat, cough, and lymphadenopathy; lasts 1-5 days, subsides 1 day after appearance of rash **Rash:** First appears on face and rapidly spreads downward to neck, arms, trunk, and legs; by end of first day, body is covered with discrete, pinkish red maculopapular exanthema; disappears in same order as it began and is usually gone by third day	No treatment necessary other than antipyretics for low-grade fever and analgesics for discomfort **Complications:** Rare (arthritis, encephalitis, or purpura); most benign of all childhood communicable diseases; greatest danger is teratogenic effect on fetus	Reassure parents of benign nature of illness in affected child Use comfort measures as necessary Isolate child from pregnant women

Continued

TABLE 38-2—cont'd
Communicable Diseases of Childhood

Disease

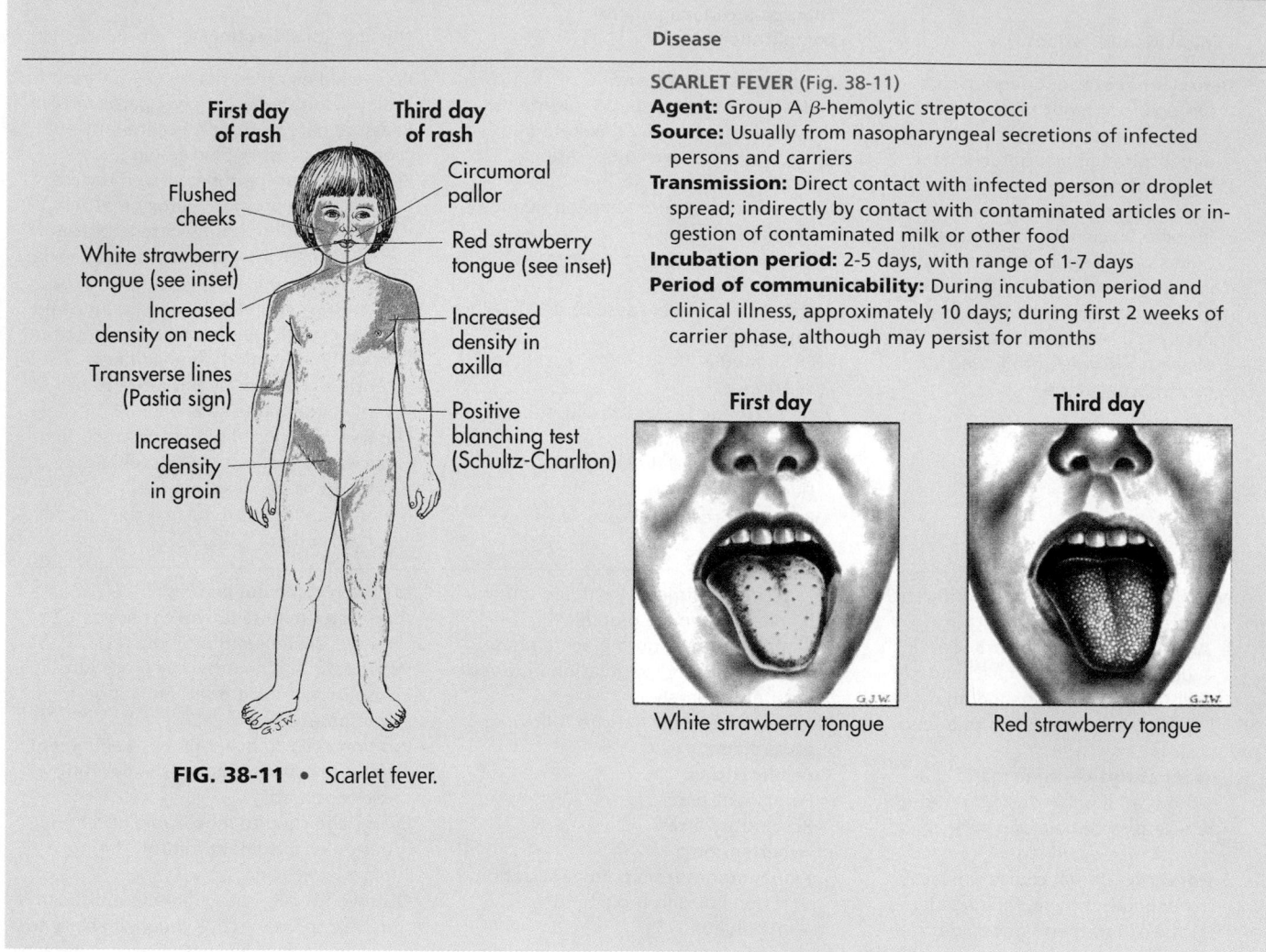

SCARLET FEVER (Fig. 38-11)
Agent: Group A β-hemolytic streptococci
Source: Usually from nasopharyngeal secretions of infected persons and carriers
Transmission: Direct contact with infected person or droplet spread; indirectly by contact with contaminated articles or ingestion of contaminated milk or other food
Incubation period: 2-5 days, with range of 1-7 days
Period of communicability: During incubation period and clinical illness, approximately 10 days; during first 2 weeks of carrier phase, although may persist for months

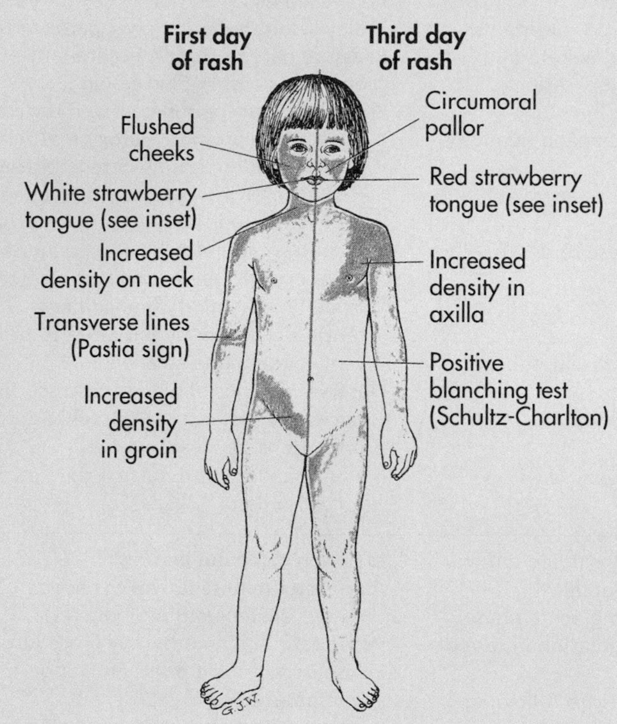

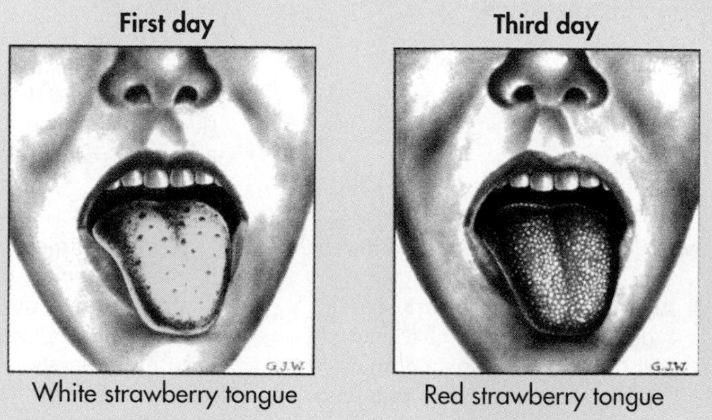

FIG. 38-11 • Scarlet fever.

Text continued from p. 915

rupting the production of red blood cells. Therefore, in patients who need increased red blood cell production to maintain normal red blood cell volumes, the virus may precipitate a severe aplastic crisis. Because the fetus depends on a high rate of red blood cell production and has an immature immune system, the fetus may develop severe anemia as a result of HPV infection in the mother.

NURSE ALERT • High risk children who have signs of these communicable diseases are referred to the practitioner immediately. School nurses are responsible for warning parents about recent outbreaks of these communicable diseases in order to prevent susceptible children's exposure to known cases. In most instances high risk children are kept out of school until the outbreak is over.

Prevention of complications from diseases such as diphtheria and scarlet fever necessitates compliance with antibiotic therapy. With oral preparations the need to complete the entire course of therapy is stressed (see Compliance, Chapter 45). Varicella-zoster immune globulin may be given to high risk children after exposure to chickenpox to prevent the development of varicella. The antiviral agent acyclovir (Zovirax) may be used to treat varicella infections; it is effective in decreasing the number of lesions, shortening the duration of fever, and decreasing itching, lethargy, and anorexia. Acyclovir should be considered for otherwise healthy, nonpregnant individuals over 12 years of age; children with chronic cutaneous or pulmonary conditions; those receiving chronic salicylate therapy; and those receiving short, intermittent, or aerosolized courses of corticosteroids (American Academy of Pediatrics, 2000). Immunocompromised children should receive acyclovir by intravenous infusion (American Academy of Pediatrics, 2000).

Recent evidence suggests that vitamin A supplementation reduces both morbidity and mortality in measles and that all children with severe measles should be given vitamin A supplements (Semba, 1999). A single oral dose of 200,000 IU for

Clinical Manifestations	Therapeutic Management/ Complications	Nursing Considerations
Constitutional signs and symptoms: Occasionally low-grade fever, headache, malaise, and lymphadenopathy **Prodromal stage:** Abrupt high fever, pulse increased out of proportion to fever, vomiting, headache, chills, malaise, abdominal pain **Enanthema:** Tonsils enlarged, edematous, reddened, and covered with patches of exudate; in severe cases appearance resembles membrane seen in diphtheria; pharynx is edematous and beefy red; during first 1-2 days tongue is coated and papillae become red and swollen (white strawberry tongue); by fourth or fifth day white coat sloughs off, leaving prominent papillae (red strawberry tongue); palate is covered with erythematous punctate lesions **Exanthema:** Rash appears within 12 hours after prodromal signs; red pinhead-sized punctate lesions rapidly become generalized but are absent on face, which becomes flushed with striking circumoral pallor; rash is more intense in folds of joints; by end of first week desquamation begins (fine, sandpaper-like on torso; sheetlike sloughing on palms and soles), which may be complete by 3 weeks or longer	Treatment of choice is full course of penicillin (or erythromycin in penicillin-sensitive children); fever should subside 24 hours after beginning therapy Antibiotic therapy for newly diagnosed carriers (nose or throat cultures positive for streptococci) **Supportive measures:** Bed rest during febrile phase, analgesics for sore throat **Complications:** Otitis media Peritonsillar and retropharyngeal abscess Sinusitis Glomerulonephritis Carditis, polyarthritis (uncommon)	Institute respiratory precautions until 24 hours after initiation of treatment Ensure compliance with oral antibiotic therapy (intramuscular benzathine penicillin G [Bicillin] may be given if parents' reliability in giving oral drugs is questionable) Maintain bed rest during febrile phase; provide quiet activity during convalescent period Relieve discomfort of sore throat with analgesics, gargles, lozenges, antiseptic throat sprays (Chloraseptic), and inhalation of cool mist Encourage fluids during febrile phase; avoid irritating liquids (citrus juices) or rough foods; when child is able to eat, begin with soft diet Advise parents to consult practitioner if fever persists after beginning therapy Discuss procedure for preventing spread of infection

children at least 1 year old (half that dose for children 6 to 12 months of age) is recommended. The higher dose may be associated with vomiting and headache for a few hours. The dose should be repeated the next day and at 4 weeks for children with ophthalmologic evidence of vitamin A deficiency (American Academy of Pediatrics, 2000).

NURSE ALERT • Although the risk of vitamin A toxicity from these doses (they are 100 to 200 times the recommended dietary allowance) is very low, nurses should instruct parents on safe storage of the drug. Ideally, vitamin A should be dispensed in the age-appropriate unit dose to prevent excessive administration and possible toxicity.

Provide Comfort. Many of the communicable diseases cause skin manifestations that are bothersome to the child. The chief discomfort from most of the rashes is itching, and measures such as cool baths (usually without soap) and lotions (e.g., calamine) are helpful.

NURSE ALERT • When lotions with active ingredients such as diphenhydramine (in Caladryl) are used, they are applied sparingly, especially over open lesions, where excessive absorption can lead to drug toxicity; and in children simultaneously receiving oral diphenhydramine.

To avoid overheating, which increases itching, children should wear lightweight, loose, nonirritating clothing and keep out of the sun. If the child persists in scratching, the nails are kept short and smooth; mittens and clothes with long sleeves or legs may be needed. For severe itching, antipruritic medication such as diphenhydramine (Benadryl) or hydroxyzine (Atarax) may be required, especially when the child desires to sleep.

An elevated temperature is common, and both antipyretic medicine (acetaminophen or Children's Motrin) and environmental manipulation are implemented (see Controlling Elevated Temperature, Chapter 45). The acetaminophen is effective in lowering the fever but does not significantly reduce the

Nursing Care Plan THE CHILD WITH A COMMUNICABLE DISEASE

NURSING DIAGNOSIS Risk for infection related to susceptible host and infectious agents

EXPECTED OUTCOME Infection remains confined to original source.

Nursing Interventions/*Rationales*

Institute appropriate infection control practices as recommended by the Centers for Disease Control and Prevention (see Chapter 45) *to prevent spread of microorganisms.* **(Scrupulous handwashing by all who have contact with the infected child is critical in control of the disease.)**

Work with family and public health nurse *to ensure adherence to infection control practices and therapeutic regimens if individual is treated in the home.*

Report disease to health department *to monitor outbreak.*

Identify susceptible individuals in community (e.g., high-risk children, close contacts of infected child) who may require prophylactic treatment or need to practice careful avoidance and close monitoring practices *to prevent contracting the disease.*

Promote public education and service programs (e.g., immunization, food handling, animal control, screening) *that aim at prevention/spread of communicable disease on community level.*

NURSING DIAGNOSIS Risk for injury related to disease complications, trauma to skin from scratching

EXPECTED OUTCOME Patient will show no evidence of complications; skin remains intact.

Nursing Interventions/*Rationales*

Involve child and parents in planning and carrying out therapeutic regimen (e.g., bed rest, hydration, feeding, prescribed medications) *to increase compliance.*

Monitor vital signs and appropriate laboratory values and make ongoing assessments of appropriate systems *to detect early signs of potential complications (ear, eye, respiratory infections; seizures, central nervous system involvement; myocarditis, arthritis, hepatitis).* Observe skin *to detect signs of scratching, trauma, infection.*

Institute seizure precautions *if febrile convulsions are a possible complication.*

Maintain good body hygiene; use antipruritics, lotions as needed; keep child's fingernails trimmed, use mittens or restraints, cover affected areas; keep skin cool *to prevent scratching, relieve itching,* and *reduce risk of trauma and secondary infection of lesions.*

Offer small frequent sips of child's favorite liquids and water *to ensure hydration* and frequent small feedings of favorite soft, bland foods (soups, ice cream, pudding, gelatin) *to reduce anorexia, nausea and vomiting.*

NURSING DIAGNOSIS Pain related to skin lesions, malaise

EXPECTED OUTCOME Patient will exhibit minimum signs of discomfort.

Nursing Interventions/*Rationales*

Use comfort measures such as vaporizer, gargles, and lozenges *to keep membranes moist;* petrolatum *for chapped lips;* saline *to cleanse crusted eyes;* cool moist cloths, tepid baths, and lotion *to relieve itching skin.*

Use nonpharmacologic techniques (e.g., distraction, relaxation, guided imagery, positive self-talk, thought stopping) *for pain reduction.*

Administer analgesics, antipyretics, and antipruritics per physician order *to relieve pain, fever, itching.* **(Do not use salicylates because of possible risk of Reye syndrome.)**

NURSING DIAGNOSIS Social isolation related to environmentally imposed constraints secondary to communicable disease

EXPECTED OUTCOME Patient will interact in socially acceptable and developmentally appropriate manner and participate in meaningful diversional activity.

Nursing Interventions/*Rationales*

Explain reasons for confinement *to enhance child's understanding.*

Enlist child's assistance with enforcing restrictions *to provide increased sense of control.*

Allow child to examine and play with any needed isolation supplies (e.g., gown, gloves, mask) *to relieve fears, increase sense of control.*

Have staff identify themselves to child before donning any required protective clothing *to increase child's trust in caregivers.*

Encourage parents to remain with child during hospitalization *to decrease separation and feelings of isolation.*

Encourage contact with peers and siblings by telephone *to maintain social interaction and reduce sense of isolation.*

Plan specific periods of developmentally appropriate diversional activity suited to child's physical condition and energy level *to decrease feelings of boredom and negative self-absorption.*

symptoms of itching, anorexia, abdominal pain, fussiness, or vomiting.

A sore throat, another common symptom, is managed with lozenges, saline rinses (if the child is old enough to cooperate), and analgesics. Since most children are anorectic during an illness, bland foods and increased liquids are usually preferred. During the early stages of the disease, children voluntarily curtail their activity, and although bed rest is beneficial, it should not be imposed unless specifically indicated (e.g., with pertussis). During periods of irritability, quiet activity (e.g., reading, music, television, videos, puzzles, or coloring) helps distract children from the discomfort.

Support Child and Family. Most communicable diseases are benign, but they produce considerable concern and anxiety for some parents. Often the occurrence of a disease such as chickenpox is the first time the child is acutely uncomfortable. Parents need assistance to cope effectively with manifestations of the illness, such as intense itching. Sometimes a visiting nurse may be beneficial to help the family develop a plan of care and encourage compliance with any treatments.

The family and child need reassurance that recovery from the disease is generally rapid. However, visible signs of the dermatosis may be present for some time after the child is well enough to resume usual activities. When the disease involves noticeable signs, such as the crusts of chickenpox, the child may benefit from preparation before returning to school. For example, the parent can discuss the child's physical appearance with the teacher and/or school nurse and request that they explain the child's condition to classmates.

NURSE ALERT • The occurrence of a communicable disease provides the opportunity to ask parents about the child's immunization status and reinforce the benefits of vaccines for children.

➤ Evaluation

The effectiveness of nursing interventions is determined by continual reassessment and evaluation of care based on the following observational guidelines and expected outcomes:

1. Observe or inquire about family members' use of control measures; observe for signs of disease in household contacts.
2. Monitor vital signs, especially temperature; inquire about the identification of high risk contacts and appropriate isolation of the contact; observe or inquire about compliance with antibiotic or antiviral therapy.
3. Inquire about effectiveness of comfort measures.
4. Interview family and child regarding their feelings and concerns, especially when child returns to school.

The expected outcomes are described in the Nursing Care Plan.

CHILD MALTREATMENT

The broad term *child maltreatment* includes intentional physical abuse or neglect, emotional abuse or neglect, and sexual abuse of children, usually by adults. It is one of the most significant social problems affecting children. In 1997, Child Protective Service (CPS) agencies in the United States confirmed that more than one million children were victims of child maltreatment. Of the confirmed cases, 22% suffered physical abuse, 8% sexual abuse, 54% neglect, 4% emotional abuse, and 12% other forms of maltreatment. In 1996, estimates indicated that 1185 children died as a result of child abuse and neglect (Wang and Daro, 1998). Reported statistics only partially represent the actual incidence of child maltreatment, because many cases are believed to go unreported.*

Child Neglect

Child neglect is the most common form of maltreatment. About one half of all reported cases are associated with deprivation of necessities, and more than one third of deaths from maltreatment are in this group. Neglect is generally defined as the failure of a parent or other person legally responsible for the child's welfare to provide for the child's basic needs and an adequate level of care.

Little is known about the etiology of neglect, although it appears that many of the risk factors identified in physical abuse apply to neglect as well (see following discussion). Ignorance of the child's needs and a lack of resources are important contributing factors. For example, neglectful parents often demonstrate poor parenting skills; they may be unaware that an infant needs to be fed every 3 to 4 hours, may not know what to feed the child, and may have insufficient funds to buy food. The most serious lack of knowledge is failure to recognize emotional nurturing as an essential need of children. (See also Failure to Thrive, Chapter 36.)

Types of Neglect. Neglect takes many forms and can be classified broadly as physical or emotional maltreatment. *Physical neglect* involves the deprivation of necessities such as food, clothing, shelter, supervision, medical care, and education. *Emotional neglect* generally refers to failure to meet the child's needs for affection, attention, and emotional nurturance. It may also include lack of intervention for or fostering of maladaptive behavior, such as delinquency or substance abuse. *Emotional abuse,* an even more difficult aspect of maltreatment to define, refers to the deliberate attempt to destroy or significantly impair a child's self-esteem or competence. Emotional abuse may take the following forms: rejecting, isolating, terrorizing, ignoring, corrupting, verbally assaulting, and overpressuring the child (Brodeur and Monteleone, 1994).

Physical Abuse

The deliberate infliction of physical injury on a child, usually by the child's caregiver, is termed *physical abuse.* Minor physical injury is responsible for more reported cases of maltreatment than major physical injury, but major physical abuse causes more deaths. Despite the importance of the problem, a universally accepted definition of what constitutes minor and major physical abuse does not exist. Rather, each state in the United States defines abuse according to its individual reporting laws.

Munchausen Syndrome by Proxy (MSP). One of the more unusual and perplexing types of abuse, usually physical, is MSP, which refers to illness that one person fabricates or induces in another person (Wright, 1997). In children it is usu-

*Additional information is available from the Clearinghouse on Child Abuse and Neglect Information, P.O. Box 1182, Washington, DC 20013-1182; (703) 385-7565 or 1-800-FYI-3366.

ally the mother who fabricates signs and symptoms of illness in her child, the proxy, to gain attention from the medical staff. MSP can take many forms, such as adding maternal blood to the child's urine to simulate hematuria; presenting a fictitious medical history; chronic poisoning of the child; or suffocating the child to cause apnea and seizures. Alleging that the child has been sexually abused by someone else to gain recognition as the child's protector is another form of MSP.

Such cases are often very difficult to confirm and require a high index of suspicion to protect the children. Warning signs of MSP include:

- Unexplained, prolonged, recurrent, or extremely rare illness
- Discrepancies between clinical findings and history
- Illness unresponsive to treatment
- Signs and symptoms occurring only in parent's presence
- Parent knowledgeable about illness, procedures, and treatments
- Parent very interested in interacting with health team members
- Parent very attentive toward child (e.g., refuses to leave hospital)
- Family members with similar symptoms

Consequences for children with MSP can be serious. They often undergo needless and painful medical procedures and treatments. The parent's actions may induce a serious illness in children—one that is fatal in almost 10% of the cases (Souid, Keith, and Cunningham, 1998). Children may develop chronic invalidism, accepting the illness story and believing themselves to be ill. Finally, they may develop MSP as an adult. Even when some of these children are removed from the home, they continue to suffer severe psychologic trauma. Other siblings remaining in the home may become substitute victims.

Factors Predisposing to Physical Abuse. The exact cause of child abuse is not known, although three factors—parental characteristics, characteristics of the child, and environmental characteristics—influence the potential for abuse. However, no one factor or group of factors is predictive of abuse. Rather, the interaction of these factors is thought to increase the risk of abuse occurring in a particular family.

Parental Characteristics. Extensive research has focused on parental characteristics that distinguish abusive parents from nonabusive parents. Unfortunately, the findings from most of these studies provide conflicting evidence. For example, it is commonly believed that abusive parents were abused as children (Brodeur and Monteleone, 1994). Although physical punishment tends to have occurred in the childhoods of abusive parents, most of the parents were not physically abused as children. However, abusive parents who report that they were severely punished as children are much more likely to injure their own children. If the abuse was not overt physical violence, abusive parents typically recall their punishment as unfair and severe, and they characterize their relationship with their parents as negative. Abusive parents tend to have difficulty coping with stress and in controlling anger expression (Burrell, Thompson, and Sexton, 1994; Rodriguez and Green, 1997). Also, spouse-abusing parents have an increased risk of abusing their children (Ross, 1996).

Another finding is that abusive families are often more socially isolated and have fewer supportive relationships than nonabusive parents. Children of teenage mothers are more at risk of abuse than those of older mothers (McCullough and Scherman, 1998). With little or no available support system and the presence of concurrent stresses imposed by the child or environment, these parents are extremely vulnerable to additional crises of any nature and literally strike out at the child as a method of releasing their increasing frustration and anxiety.

Other factors identified in abusive parents include low self-esteem and less adequate maternal functioning. Although inadequate knowledge of childrearing is often cited as a characteristic of abusive parents, research findings do not consistently support this belief. However, this does not mean that these parents cannot benefit from learning more constructive ways of rearing their children, especially nonviolent discipline methods.

Characteristics of the Child. The child also unintentionally contributes to the abusive situation. In families of two or more children, usually only one child is the victim of abuse. This child's temperament, position in the family, additional physical needs if ill or disabled, activity level, or degree of sensitivity to parental needs all contribute to the potential for physical abuse. For example, one child may not be abused if he or she fits into the "easy-child pattern," whereas another sibling with a difficult temperament may add to the parent's stress sufficiently to precipitate an abusive act. However, temperament alone is not the critical factor; rather, it is the "fit" or compatibility between the child's temperament and the parent's ability to deal with that behavioral style.

Occasionally the abused child is illegitimate, unwanted, brain damaged (especially in situations where the parents cannot accept the retardation), hyperactive, or physically disabled. Sometimes children are abused because they remind the parent of someone the parent dislikes, such as a younger brother or sister who received all of the attention from their own parents. Premature infants may be at risk for maltreatment because of the failure of parent-child bonding during early infancy. Often a difficult pregnancy, labor, or delivery is a predisposing factor in abuse, especially when the infant is born prematurely or with congenital anomalies.

Although one child is usually the victim in an abusive family, removing that child from the home often places the other siblings at risk for abuse. Child maltreatment usually is not confined to one child because of a disturbed parent-child relationship but is a result of a family in distress. Therefore no child is safe if left in the abusive environment unless the parents can be helped to learn new parenting skills and to meet their needs and release their frustration through alternatives other than attacking their children.

Environmental Characteristics. The environment is a significant part of the potential abusive situation. Typically the environment is one of chronic stress, including problems of divorce, poverty, unemployment, poor housing, frequent relocation, alcoholism, and drug addiction. Increased exposure between children and parents, such as that which occurs in crowded living conditions, also increases the likelihood of abuse.

Although most reporting of abuse has been from lower socioeconomic populations, child abuse is by no means a problem of any one societal group (Schowengert, 1996). It spans all educational, social, and economic levels. Certainly, stresses imposed by poverty predispose lower socioeconomic families to abusive situations, and abuse in these groups is more apt to be reported. However, concealed crises can also be present in upper-class families. For example, a wealthy family experiencing major life changes, such as rehousing, the birth of an additional child, or marital discord, may have sufficient environmental stressors imposed on them to produce a potentially abusive situation. Wealthy families may be so overinvolved with commitments outside the home that abuse may be inflicted by substitute caregivers. Nurses need to be aware of such factors to identify the less obvious examples of child abuse and neglect.

Sexual Abuse

Sexual abuse is one of the most devastating types of child maltreatment, and current estimates indicate that it has increased significantly during the past decade. However, the increased rate of reporting may not reflect a true increase in prevalence of sexual abuse and rather may be a result of changes in legislation (Wang and Daro, 1998).

As with all forms of child maltreatment, no universal definition for sexual abuse exists. The Child Abuse and Prevention Act (Public Law 100-235) defines *sexual abuse* as "the use, persuasion, or coercion of any child to engage in sexually explicit conduct (or any simulation of such conduct) for producing any visual depiction of such conduct, or rape, molestation, prostitution, or incest with children."

Sexual abuse includes the following types of sexual maltreatment:

Incest—Any physical sexual activity between family members; blood relationship is not required (abusers can include stepparents, nonrelated siblings, grandparents, uncles, and aunts); does not include sexual relations between legally sanctioned partners, such as spouses

Molestation—A vague term that includes "indecent liberties" such as touching, fondling, kissing, single or mutual masturbation, or oral-genital contact

Exhibitionism—Indecent exposure, usually exposure of the genitals by an adult male to children or female adults

Child pornography—Arranging and photographing, in any media, sexual acts involving children, alone or with adults or animals, regardless of consent by the child's legal guardian; also may denote distribution of such material in any form with or without profit

Child prostitution—Involving children in sex acts for profit and usually with changing partners

Pedophilia—Literally means "love of child" and does not denote a type of sexual activity but the preference of an adult for prepubertal children as the means achieving sexual excitement

Characteristics of Abusers and Victims. Anyone, including siblings and mothers, can be sexual abusers, but the typical abuser is a male whom the victim knows. Offenders come from all levels of society. Some are prominent persons in the community; others, especially in the case of pedophiles (also called "child molesters"), are in positions where they work closely with children, such as teaching or coaching.

Pornography and prostitution may involve strangers, as well as the children's own parents. There are no typical characteristics of these offenders, although the abused children tend to be runaways—young adolescents who engage in these activities to obtain money for food, shelter, drugs, and alcohol. Incestuous relationships between father or stepfather and daughter are generally prolonged, and the victims are usually reluctant to report the situation because of fear of retaliation and fear that they will not be believed. Typically, incestuous relationships begin later than other forms of child abuse. The eldest daughter is usually abused, but in her absence another sister is substituted. Sibling incest may also occur (Adler and Schutz, 1995). Sexual abuse by relatives with a strong emotional bond with the victim is the most devastating to the child (Fischer and McDonald, 1998).

Boys are also victims of both intrafamilial and extrafamilial abuse. Male victims are much less likely to report abuse, and they may suffer much greater emotional harm from incestuous relationships, especially between mother and son, than female victims (Moody, 1999). Boys are likely to be subjected to anal penetration and oral-genital contact; to have subtle physical findings; and to be abused by a father, stepfather, or mother's boyfriend.

Initiation and Perpetuation of Sexual Abuse. The cycle of sexual abuse often starts innocently unless it involves an isolated attack, such as rape. Often offenders spend time with the victims to gain their trust before initiating any sexual contact. Most victims are then pressured into being an accessory to the sexual activity through various means (Box 38-1) and may be unaware that sexual activity is part of the offer. Children may not reveal the truth for fear that their parents would not believe them if they told, especially if the offender is a trusted member of the family. Some fear that they will be blamed for the situation, and many young children with limited vocabulary have difficulty describing the activity when they do have the courage or opportunity to reveal the abuse.

Seductiveness by the child does not initiate incest. Most young girls experiment in seduction, especially during the preschool years, but the father's response normally differentiates this playfulness from overt sexual invitation. Although the reasons for incest are complicated and can occur in various family types, it does not occur in healthy families. Most incestuous relationships are directly tied to sexual maladjustment and estrangement between husband and wife. Most begin following the cessation of sexual relationships with the usual partner. Most fathers experience little guilt, and many wives at some level are aware of the incestuous affair. The wife may react by tolerating the situation or may resort to use of denial; some remain unaware of the activity. Consequently, the home offers little protection to young victims, since abusers have easy access to

Box 38-1

Methods Used to Pressure Children into Sexual Activity

- The child is offered gifts or privileges.
- The adult misrepresents moral standards by telling the child that it is "OK to do."
- Isolated and emotionally and socially impoverished children are enticed by adults who meet their needs for warmth and human contact.
- The successful sex offender pressures the victim into secrecy regarding the activity by describing it as a "secret between us" that other people may take away if they find out.
- The offender plays on the child's fears, including fear of punishment by the offender, fear of repercussions if the child tells, and fear of abandonment or rejection by the family.

their victims and the children feel they cannot reveal their secret to other family members. However, not all incestuous relationships follow this pattern of silence. Currently, reports of father-daughter incest during child custody conflicts have become more common and have raised serious concerns regarding the possibility of false accusation. Rather than tolerating or denying the child's sexual abuse, the other parent (usually the mother) is typically the chief accuser.

Nursing Care of the Maltreated Child

➤ Assessment

One of the most critical responsibilities of all health professionals is identifying abusive situations as early as possible. The characteristics that may predispose members of some families to commit abuse can serve as a framework for assessing vulnerability but are never predictive of actual abuse. Rather, a thorough physical examination and a careful, detailed history are the diagnostic tools needed to identify abuse. Nurses have a very special role because they may be the first person to see the child and parent and are the consistent caregivers if the child is hospitalized (Guidelines box).

NURSE ALERT • Nurses must be aware of their biases regarding child abuse. Studies show that nurses are less likely to report abuse when the child is female and from a middle-income, as opposed to lower-income, family (Pillitteri et al, 1992); are significantly less comfortable dealing with sexual abuse, abuse of infants, and fathers as the abusers (Seidl et al, 1993); and experience greater discomfort when dealing with abusers of children with disabilities than with abusers of children without disabilities (Stanton et al, 1994).

Evidence of Maltreatment. Recognition of abuse or neglect necessitates a familiarity with both physical and behavioral signs that suggest maltreatment (Box 38-2). No one indicator can diagnose maltreatment; rather, it is a pattern or combination of indicators that should arouse suspicion and further investigation. In addition, signs of possible abuse must be coupled with an understanding of diseases, such as bleeding disorders, osteogenesis imperfecta, or sudden infant death syndrome (SIDS); and cultural practices, such as cupping or coin rubbing (see Health Practices, Chapter 32), that may mimic physical abuse. Unintentional injuries may also be wrongly diagnosed as abuse, such as burns from metal buckles on car seats, lacerations from seat belts, or retinal hemorrhage after cardiopulmonary resuscitation. Normal variants, such as mongolian spots and congenital anomalies of genitalia, can be mistaken for abuse.

Not all forms of physical abuse demonstrate obvious signs. Violent shaking of children *(shaken baby syndrome [SBS])* can cause fatal intracranial trauma without signs of external head injury (American Academy of Pediatrics, 1993). Nurses should suspect SBS in infants less than 1 year of age who present with subdural and/or retinal hemorrhages in the absence of external signs of trauma (Chiocca, 1995).

NURSE ALERT • Stress to parents the dangers of shaking infants (shaking can cause SBS). Advise against shaking as a method of burping or waking infant; tossing infant in air; or shaking infant when feeling angry or tense.

If abuse is suspected, nurses play an important role in monitoring the parent's activities to identify instances of causing the children's symptoms. Using a hidden video camera to document the parent's behavior is becoming a more common diagnostic procedure, but the parent's right of privacy must be considered (Wilde and Pedroni, 1993).

Neglect and Emotional Abuse. Neglect from deprivation of necessities is easier to identify than emotional neglect or abuse because physical signs are usually evident. Emotional maltreatment may be readily suspected, but it is very difficult to substantiate. Physical signs are often nonspecific, and nurses must rely on behavioral indicators, which range from depression to acting-out behavior, to help identify a possibly abusive situation. Any persistent and unexplained change in the child's behavior is an important clue to possible emotional abuse.

Guidelines

TALKING WITH CHILDREN WHO REVEAL ABUSE

- Provide a private time and place to talk.
- Do not promise not to tell; tell them that you are required by law to report the abuse.
- Do not express shock or criticize their family.
- Use their vocabulary to discuss body parts.
- Avoid using any leading statements that can distort their report.
- Reassure them that they have done the right thing by telling.
- Tell them that the abuse is not their fault, that they are not bad or to blame.
- Determine their immediate need for safety.
- Let them know what will happen when you report.

Box 38-2

Warning Signs of Abuse

- Physical evidence of abuse and/or neglect, including previous injuries
- Conflicting stories about the "accident" or injury from the parents or others
- Cause of injury blamed on sibling or other party
- An injury inconsistent with the history, such as a concussion and broken arm from falling off a bed
- History inconsistent with child's developmental level, such as a 6-month-old turning on the hot water
- A complaint other than the one associated with signs of abuse (e.g., a chief complaint of a cold when there is evidence of first- and second-degree burns)
- Inappropriate response of caregiver, such as an exaggerated or absent emotional response; refusal to sign for additional tests or agree to necessary treatment; excessive delay in seeking treatment; absence of the parents for questioning
- Inappropriate response of child, such as little or no response to pain; fear of being touched; excessive or lack of separation anxiety; indiscriminate friendliness to strangers
- Child's report of physical or sexual abuse
- Previous reports of abuse in the family
- Repeated visits to emergency facilities with injuries

Sexual Abuse. Identifying instances of sexual abuse is particularly difficult because often few if any obvious physical indications of the activity may exist. Also, many individuals are hesitant to believe children and are unwilling to report incidents. Even health professionals are sometimes at fault when they perform cursory physical examinations of the genitalia and ignore behavior or verbal comments that suggest abuse. When sexual abuse is suspected, other children in the family should also be evaluated, since multiple victims are not uncommon.

Unfortunately, there is no typical profile of the victim, and there must be a high index of suspicion to identify these children. Physical signs vary and may include any of those listed for sexual abuse in Box 38-2. The victim may exhibit various behavioral manifestations. Unfortunately, none of these behaviors is diagnostic of sexual abuse. When abused children exhibit these behaviors, the signs may be incorrectly attributed to the normal stresses of childhood, especially in older school-age children or adolescents. Even those signs considered most predictive of sexual abuse, such as certain genital findings, sexually inappropriate behavior for age, enactment of adult sexual activity, and intense focus on sexual activity (e.g., masturbation), do not always indicate that sexual abuse has occurred. Conversely, abused children may not demonstrate more knowledge of sexual activity than non-abused children. However, one difference in the abused children's explanation of sexual activity may be unusual affective responses. For example, abused children may have an increased incidence of sleep disorders, temper tantrums, and depression (Calam et al, 1998).

History Pertaining to the Incident. In addition to observable evidence of abuse, the type of history revealed by the parents or other caregiver, such as the baby-sitter or mother's boyfriend, is a significant factor. Areas of the history that should arouse suspicion of abuse are summarized in Box 38-3.

NURSE ALERT • Incompatibility between the history and the injury is probably the most important criterion on which to base the decision to report suspected abuse.

An important point to remember when taking a history is that maltreated children rarely betray their parents by admitting to the abuse they received. If questioned, they will repeat the same story as the parents and try to defend their parents' actions. If the interviewer directly accuses the parents of abuse, the child may accept responsibility for the act in an attempt to vindicate the parents. Whether children respond in this way out of fear is uncertain; however, children do fear losing whatever security and love they have. Between abusive acts, children may receive some measure of attention and love from the parents. If they betray the parents, they may lose this and be uncertain or fearful of the consequences, such as foster care. Preserving the present situation may be less frightening than the unknown future.

The *disclosure of sexual abuse* can occur in a variety of ways: the act is observed by others, resulting in a direct confrontation; the child tells someone, such as a parent of a friend; visible clues of the relationship are observed, such as an accumulation of coins, gifts, or candy; more obvious clues are seen, such as a child coming home disheveled or becoming pregnant; or physical or behavioral signs and symptoms are observed. Children usually describe the experience in terms of whether it was unpleasant or hurt or was pleasurable (usually a response to hand-genital contact); some indicate no reaction. Young children often feel no guilt or shame because the act is pleasurable and they are unaware of its inappropriateness.

NURSE ALERT • When children report potentially sexually abusive experiences, their reports need to be taken seriously, but also cautiously to avoid alarming the child or falsely accusing someone.

Children's reports of sexual abuse may vary from contradictory stories to unwavering versions of the experience. Stories that sound contradictory may reflect the child's experiences in several instances of abuse. Also, children who repeatedly tell identical facts may have been prompted to do so. Increasing evidence suggests that the types of interrogation children are exposed to following reports of sexual abuse shape their thinking. As a result of the use of leading questions, closed questions (those requiring "yes" or "no" answers), intimidation, prodding, or selective reinforcement for certain answers, children may begin to tell stories that never occurred (Ceci and Bruck, 1995). The Family Focus box discusses false allegations of abuse.

Family Focus

FALSE ALLEGATIONS OF ABUSE

Although health professionals are primarily concerned with detecting child abuse early and protecting the child from further abuse, prevention of abuse must also include prevention of false allegations of abuse. Although some degree of overreporting is expected because the law requires the reporting of suspected maltreatment, the degree of overreporting is considered unreasonably high. Under the present child abuse laws, child protective services have the authority to remove a child from the home solely on the basis of allegations made to an abuse hotline.*

Despite more than half of all reports being unfounded, little attention has been directed to the problem of false accusations and their devastating consequences, such as removal of the child from the home, termination of parental rights, public ridicule of the family, loss of employment, and excessive legal fees to regain custody of the child. Nurses play a critical role in carefully documenting all evidence of abuse, giving alleged offenders the opportunity to present their account of the incident, and recognizing diseases or cultural practices that may be confused with abuse.† In the unfortunate event that a family is wrongly accused of abuse, they may benefit from the services of the National Association of State VOCAL (Victims of Child Abuse Legislation) Organizations,‡ a support group for persons who have experienced false accusations. Another organization that may be helpful to family members who have been accused of sexual abuse by their adult children is the False Memory Syndrome (FMS) Foundation.§ The research and educational institution is dedicated to understanding and preventing allegations of abuse based on "false" memories. In recent years adult children, primarily women, have claimed to suddenly remember childhood sexual abuse, usually by fathers. The abuse is said to have been repressed for many years, but the memory is recovered with the help of a therapist.||

*Radko K: Child abuse: guilty until proven innocent or legalized governmental child abuse, *Issues Child Abuse Accus* 5(2):96-101, 1993.
†Brodeur AE, Monteleone JA: *Child maltreatment, a clinical guide and reference,* St Louis, 1994, Mosby; Hansen KK: Folk remedies and child abuse: a review with emphasis on caida de mollera and its relationship to shaken baby syndrome, *Child Abuse Negl* 22(2):117-127, 1998.
‡11625 E. Old Spanish Trail, Tucson, AZ 85703; (520) 772-1968; hotline: 1-800-745-8778.
§3401 Market St., Suite 130, Philadelphia, PA 19104; 1-800-568-8882; website: www.FMSFonline.org.
||Loftus E: Remembering dangerously, *Skeptical Inquirer* 19(2):20-29, 1995.

Box 38-3

Clinical Manifestations of Potential Child Maltreatment

PHYSICAL NEGLECT

Suggestive Physical Findings

Failure to thrive
Signs of malnutrition, such as thin extremities, abdominal distention, lack of subcutaneous fat
Poor personal hygiene, especially of teeth
Unclean and/or inappropriate dress
Evidence of poor health care, such as nonimmunized status, untreated infections, frequent colds
Frequent injuries from lack of supervision

Suggestive Behaviors

Dull and inactive; excessively passive or sleepy
Self-stimulatory behaviors, such as finger sucking or rocking
Begging or stealing food; Absenteeism from school; Drug or alcohol addiction; Vandalism or shoplifting } in older child

EMOTIONAL ABUSE AND NEGLECT

Suggestive Physical Findings

Failure to thrive
Feeding disorders, such as rumination
Enuresis
Sleep disorders

Suggestive Behaviors

Self-stimulatory behaviors, such as biting, rocking, sucking
During infancy, lack of social smile and stranger anxiety
Withdrawal
Unusual fearfulness
Antisocial behavior, such as destructiveness, stealing, cruelty
Extremes of behavior, such as overcompliant and passive, or aggressive and demanding
Lags in emotional and intellectual development, especially language
Suicide attempts

PHYSICAL ABUSE

Suggestive Physical Findings

Bruises and welts
- On face, lips, mouth, back, buttocks, thighs, or areas of torso
- Regular patterns descriptive of object used, such as belt buckle, hand, wire hanger, chain, wooden spoon, squeeze or pinch marks
- May be present in various stages of healing

Burns
- On soles of feet, palms of hands, back, or buttocks
- Patterns descriptive of object used, such as round cigar or cigarette burns; "glovelike" sharply demarcated areas from immersion in scalding water; rope burns on wrists or ankles from being bound; burns in the shape of an iron, radiator, or electric stove burner
- Absence of "splash" marks and presence of symmetric burns
- Stun gun injury: lesions circular, fairly uniform (up to 0.5 cm), and paired about 5 cm (2 inches) apart*
- Fractures and dislocations
- Skull, nose, or facial structures
- Injury may denote type of abuse, such as spiral fracture or dislocation from twisting of an extremity or whiplash from shaking the child
- Multiple new or old fractures in various stages of healing

Lacerations and abrasions
- On backs of arms, legs, torso, face, or external genitalia
- Unusual symptoms, such as abdominal swelling, pain, and vomiting from punching
- Descriptive marks such as from human bites or pulling hair out

Chemical
- Unexplained repeated poisoning, especially drug overdose
- Unexplained sudden illness, such as hypoglycemia from insulin administration

Suggestive Behaviors

Wary of physical contact with adults
Apparent fear of parents or going home
Lying very still while surveying environment
Inappropriate reaction to injury, such as failure to cry from pain
Lack of reaction to frightening events
Apprehensive when hearing other children cry
Indiscriminate friendliness and displays of affection
Superficial relationships
Acting-out behavior, such as aggression, to seek attention
Withdrawal behavior

SEXUAL ABUSE

Suggestive Physical Findings

Bruises, bleeding, lacerations, or irritation of external genitalia, anus, mouth, or throat
Torn, stained, or bloody underclothing
Pain on urination or pain, swelling, and itching of genital area
Penile discharge
Sexually transmitted disease, nonspecific vaginitis, or venereal warts
Difficulty in walking or sitting
Unusual odor in the genital area
Recurrent urinary tract infections
Presence of sperm
Pregnancy in young adolescent

Suggestive Behaviors

Sudden emergence of sexually related problems, including excessive or public masturbation, age-inappropriate sexual play, promiscuity, or overtly seductive behavior
Withdrawn, excessive daydreaming
Preoccupied with fantasies, especially in play
Poor relationships with peers
Sudden changes, such as anxiety, loss or gain of weight, clinging behavior
In incestuous relationships, excessive anger at mother for not protecting daughter
Regressive behavior, such as bed-wetting or thumb sucking
Sudden onset of phobias or fears, particularly fears of the dark, men, strangers, or particular settings or situations (e.g., undue fear of leaving the house or staying at the day care center or the baby-sitter's house)
Running away from home
Substance abuse, particularly of alcohol or mood-elevating drugs
Profound and rapid personality changes, especially extreme depression, hostility, and aggression (often accompanied by social withdrawal)
Rapidly declining school performance
Suicidal attempts or ideation

*Frechette A, Rimsza ME: Stun gun injury: a new presentation of the battered child syndrome, *Pediatrics* 89(5):898-901, 1992.

Parental Behaviors. Certain behavioral responses of the parents to their child and to the interviewer should alert the nurse to the possibility of maltreatment. Although no one pattern of behaviors is characteristic of these parents, some responses include the following. Abusive parents have difficulty in showing concern toward their child. They are unable to comfort the child and give no indication of realizing how the child may feel, physically or emotionally. Instead, they are critical of and angry with the child for being injured. They maintain that the child is responsible for the injury, and if asked any question regarding their responsibility for protecting or supervising the child, they become hostile and aggressive. They act as if the child's injury is an assault on them. Their entire perception of the incident is in terms of how it affects them, not the child, which is an indication of their preoccupation with their own needs and of their inability to give any support to others.

During the child's hospitalization they may not become involved in the child's care and may show little concern for his or her progress, eventual discharge, or need for follow-up care. However, if they are pressured during interrogation, they immediately demand to take the child home, regardless of the child's readiness for discharge.

Families respond to sexual abuse with a variety of emotional reactions, ranging from not believing the child to being very supportive. Parents and other family members may display the same type of emotional responses as the victim, such as inability to eat or sleep; and somatic complaints, such as headache. In the acute emotional phase, parents have a need to blame someone. The three common targets are the offender, the child, and themselves. The parents often express anger at the child for "stupid" behavior and may even restrict the child's privileges as punishment. When the victim is a girl, the parents may question her sexual provocation of the event. Self-blaming parents assume full responsibility, believing that they have been inadequate parents or should not have allowed the child to go out. When a baby-sitter or trusted relative is involved in the assault, and the child's complaint has not been believed until gross evidence is presented, the parents are often devastated by guilt.

Child Behaviors. Abused children's responses to their parents or the injury may also support the suspicion of abuse. Although no one pattern is typical, extremes of behavior may be observed. Children may be very unresponsive to the parent or excessively clinging and intolerant of separation. They may be overattached to the abusive parent, possibly in the hope of preventing any upset that may precipitate anger and another attack. During care of the injury, children may be passive and accepting of the discomfort or uncooperative and fearful of any physical contact. Some children maintain a wary watchfulness of all strangers; some shy away from strangers as if frightened; others are unusually affectionate and outgoing.

➤ Nursing Diagnoses

A number of nursing diagnoses are prominent in the nursing care of the maltreated child and family, and others specific to individual cases become evident. The most common nursing diagnoses are outlined in the Nursing Care Plan on p. 936.

➤ Plan of Care and Implementation

The main nursing goals related to child maltreatment are as follows:

1. Child will be protected from further abuse.
2. Child and family will receive adequate support.
3. Hospitalized child and family, including foster parents if appropriate, will be prepared for discharge.
4. Child will not experience any maltreatment.

Protect Child from Further Abuse. Initially, identification of instances of suspected abuse or neglect is essential. The nurse may come in contact with abused children in an emergency department, practitioner's office, home, day care center, or school.

NURSE ALERT • The priority is to remove the child from the abusive situation to prevent further injury.

All states and provinces in North America have laws for mandatory reporting of child maltreatment. Suspected child abuse is reported to the local authorities.* Referrals usually come to the state child welfare department and are assigned to a caseworker in an agency such as Child Protective Services (CPS). Once a referral has been made, a caseworker is assigned to investigate the report. Based on the findings, the child is left in the home or temporarily removed.

A court proceeding may be necessary before the child can be placed outside the home or when parental rights are to be terminated. When the courts are involved, they usually require firsthand testimony by the referring parties. Nurses may be subpoenaed to appear in court, or their notes may be introduced as evidence in court hearings. Accurate and factual documentation is essential. A suggested outline for recording pertinent assessment is presented in the Guidelines box. Behaviors are described, not interpreted, and are recorded daily to establish a

*Telephone numbers are usually listed under "Child Abuse" in the business white pages of the local telephone directory; or call the emergency child abuse hotline: 1-800-422-4453 (1-800-4-A-CHILD).

Guidelines

RECORDING ASSESSMENT DATA IN SUSPECTED ABUSE

History of Injury

1. Date, time, and place of occurrence
2. Sequence of events with recorded times
3. Presence of witnesses, especially person caring for child at time of incident
4. Time lapse between occurrence of injury and initiation of treatment
5. Interview with child when appropriate, including verbal quotations and information from drawing or other play activities
6. Interview with parent, witnesses, or other significant persons, including verbal quotations
7. Description of parent-child interactions (verbal interactions, eye contact, touching, parental concern)
8. Name, age, and condition of other children in home (if possible)

Physical Examination

1. Location, size, shape, and color of bruises; approximate location, size, and shape on drawing of body outline
2. Distinguishing characteristics, such as a bruise in the shape of a hand; round burn (possibly caused by cigarette)
3. Symmetry or asymmetry of injury; presence of other injuries
4. Degree of pain; any bone tenderness
5. Evidence of past injuries; general state of health and hygiene
6. Developmental level of child; perform screening test (see Developmental Assessment, Chapter 35)

progress record. Conversations among the nurse, child, and parent are recorded verbatim as much as possible.

Support Child. Often children suspected of abuse are hospitalized for medical management of their injuries. The type of care needed by the sexually abused child depends on the circumstances of the abuse. It varies from reassurance and support when the abuse involves exhibitionism, to long-term counseling in incestuous situations. In interviewing these children, the nurse must be very careful to avoid biasing the child's retelling of the events. Some experts suggest that health professionals limit the interview to the child's physical and mental health concerns and leave topics of the family's social, legal, or other problems to the police or CPS personnel (Hymel and Jenny, 1996). When the sexually abused child has been physically harmed, the care is consistent with that provided to a rape victim. Regardless of the type of abuse, their needs are the same as those of any hospitalized child. The child should be treated as a child with the usual physical needs, developmental tasks, and play interests, not as a dramatic victim of abuse. The nurse is the child's advocate in this goal. The nurse also encourages the child's relationship with the parents.

The nurse does not become a substitute parent to the exclusion of the child's natural parents. Such an intent only intensifies the parents' feelings of inadequacy, worthlessness, and isolation. It does not help them understand their child or promote their trust in health professionals. The goal of the consistent nurse-child relationship is to provide a role model for the parents in helping them to relate positively and constructively to their child and to foster a therapeutic environment for the child in his or her reprieve from the abusing situation.

Support Family. One of the most difficult, yet essential, components of success with abusive parents is the quality of the *therapeutic relationship.* It must be one of genuine concern and treatment, not one of accusation and punishment. Nurses must examine their personal feelings toward these parents, particularly when sexual abuse is present. A therapeutic approach is to view the parent as the patient and the child as the victim of abuse. Unless the nurse's attitude is positive, abusive parents will not be motivated to change, since they will not be working with a trusting person who demonstrates the kind of behavior that is being asked of them.

When parental ignorance of childrearing practices has played a part in the abuse, the nurse can educate the parent regarding children's physical and emotional needs. Because of the parents' own childrearing, they may not be aware of nonviolent methods of discipline, such as time-out or consequences. They may also need help in dealing with their frustration so that they do not vent anger on the child. Since these parents may be sensitive to criticism or domination and already possess a very low self-esteem, teaching is implemented through demonstration and example rather than through lecturing. Any competent parenting abilities they demonstrate are praised to promote their sense of parental adequacy.

Care of the family also depends on the circumstances of the *sexual abuse.* With a nonparent offender, the family may be more able to support the child than if parental incest were involved. Family members are encouraged to express their feelings of anger, guilt, shame, and/or embarrassment, but are also cautioned to avoid displacing such feelings on the child. For example, it is easy for parents to admonish the child with a statement such as "We told you never to go with strangers," which makes the child feel responsible.

Family members are advised to encourage the child to resume normal activities and observe the child for signs of distress (see Postraumatic Stress Disorder, Chapter 39). Children express their feelings primarily through behavior. Parents should be alert for changes in behavior that indicate distress resulting from the incident, such as remaining in the house, refusing to go to school, changes in sleeping patterns, and frequent dreams and nightmares. Children are encouraged to talk about these feelings and nightmares, since the more they can talk about the experience, the more they are able to gain control over it.

Referral to appropriate agencies is also essential. Most abusive parents tend to live in poverty, and the daily stresses imposed by their lifestyle are overwhelming. Resources for financial aid, improved housing, and child care should be sought. Self-help groups also provide important services. Such groups as Parents Anonymous* (a group for parents who have abused or fear that they may abuse their child, but only in terms of physical abuse, not sexual abuse) and Parents United International, Inc.† (a group devoted to helping sexually abused families) are very accepting and nonjudgmental, because everyone has been in the same position.

There is no way to predict which families will be successfully rehabilitated. With father-daughter incest, however, the best results occur when the father accepts full responsibility for the act, the mother acknowledges her role in failing to protect the child, and the child is able to understand and forgive the parents and develop a positive self-image despite the traumatic experience.

Plan for Discharge. Discharge planning should begin as soon as the legal disposition for placement has been decided, which may be temporary foster home placement, return to the parents, or permanent termination of parental rights. The latter is the most drastic solution, but it is necessary in situations of repeated, life-threatening abuse. Whenever children are sent to a foster home or juvenile institution, they must be allowed an opportunity to express their feelings. No matter how severe the abuse, they usually mourn the loss of their parents. They need help to understand why they must not return home, and that this new home is in no way a punishment. Whenever possible, foster parents are encouraged to visit in the hospital, and the nurse should take an active role in helping these new parents understand the child. It is unfortunate that some abused children live in torment as they are sent from one foster home to another, sometimes enduring worse circumstances than those that existed in their original home. Only through constant evaluation of the placement residence and the child's adjustment to a new environment can the vicious circle of abuse, abandonment, and neglect be stopped.

Prevent Abuse. Prevention of child maltreatment has been an extremely difficult goal. Programs aimed at identifying potential abusers and instituting supportive intervention before the occurrence of an abusive act have met with variable success (Flournoy, 1996). However, nurses have played an important role in such programs. For example, prenatal and infancy home visiting by nurses to primiparas who were either teenagers, un-

---

*675 W. Foothill Blvd., Suite 220, Claremont, CA 91711; (909) 621-6181; website: www.parentsanonymous/natl.org.

†P.O. Box 952, San Jose, CA 95108; (408) 453-7616.

married, or of low socioeconomic status resulted in significantly fewer reports of child abuse during the first 2 years but had a less favorable impact on child abuse during the next 2 years (Olds, Henderson, and Kitzman, 1994). The nurses provided information on normal child growth and development and routine health care needs, served as informal support persons, and referred families to appropriate services when a need for assistance was identified.

Such programs provide models that can be used to reduce factors known to increase the risk of abuse. However, nurses in a variety of settings can implement similar activities. Nurses in prenatal clinics can prepare expectant families for the adjustment of parenthood. Nursery and postpartum nurses can foster the attachment process by encouraging parents to hold and look at their infant. Nurses in neonatal intensive care units can minimize the effects of separation by encouraging parents to visit, and can help them become comfortable in the child's care. Those in ambulatory settings can teach parents appropriate methods of bathing, feeding, toileting, disciplining, and preventing injuries, while stressing the normal needs and developmental characteristics of children. Nurses need to be sensitive to the parents' needs for attention, reassurance, and reinforcement. Nurses need to know what kinds of community services are available, including self-help groups, and make timely referrals.

Unlike preventive efforts for neglect and physical abuse, which have been aimed at the potential offender, *prevention of child sexual abuse* has centered on education of children to protect themselves. Currently, much controversy surrounds the effectiveness of these programs. The main issue is whether young children should be expected to participate in their own protection. Some experts suggest that in the struggle between sexual offender and potential child victim, most factors favor the adult, who has superior knowledge, strength, and skill to overcome most children's efforts at self-protection (Conte, Wolf, and Smith, 1989). Clearly, sexual abuse prevention is more than teaching children to say "no" or to recognize their right not to be touched in "private places." It is equally important to teach children safety in terms of potential risk situations. Several suggestions for parents regarding protecting and educating children against possible molestation are presented in the Home Care box.

The nurse is often in a position to discuss this topic with parents as part of health maintenance and to provide guidelines. Books are available for parents that describe sexual abuse and its prevention.* Supporting parental qualities of respect, affection, empathy, and ability to set boundaries; and providing quality child care and education constitute the true preventive approach to sexual abuse (Flournoy, 1996). Helpful games such as "What if the baby-sitter wants to wrestle and hug but tells you to keep it a secret?" can be used to explore dangerous situations in advance and help children learn the importance of saying "no."

They need reassurance that no matter what the other person says or does, the parents want to know about it and will not punish them. Even if children do participate in the activity before telling the parents, they must be reassured that it was not their fault.

In addition, parents need to be made aware that "nice" people, including friends and relatives, can be offenders. Parents should carefully observe how others act toward the child. A sudden change in the child's behavior, and a response such as "I don't like Uncle anymore," are clues to investigate the relationship. In the event of any doubt, further solitary encounters with this person and the child should be prevented. It is sometimes to the child's great misfortune that parents do not take certain comments seriously, such as "He hugs me too tight" or "I don't want to go with him." Casual parental statements such as "He just loves you" or "You do whatever adults tell you to do" can place children in jeopardy. Health professionals can alert par-

Home Care

PREVENTING OR DEALING WITH SEXUAL ABUSE OF CHILDREN

Sexual assault of children is much more common than most people realize. It may be preventable if children have good preparation. *To provide protection and preparation:*

- Pay careful attention to who is around children. (Unwanted touch *may* come from someone liked and trusted.)
- Back up a child's right to say "no."
- Encourage communication by taking seriously what children say.
- Take a second look at signals of potential danger.
- Refuse to leave children in the company of those not trusted.
- Include information about sexual assault when teaching about safety.
- Provide specific definitions and examples of sexual assault.
- Remind children that even "nice" people sometimes do mean things.
- Urge children to tell about *anybody* who causes them to be uncomfortable.
- Prepare children to deal with bribes and threats, as well as possible physical force.
- Virtually eliminate secrets between children and parents.
- Teach children how to say "no," ask for help, and control who touches them and how.
- Model self-protective and limit-setting behavior for children.

Should it ever become necessary *to help a child recover from a sexual assault:*

- Listen carefully to understand the child.
- Support the child for telling through praise, belief, sympathy, and lack of blame.
- Know local resources and choose help carefully.
- Provide opportunities to talk about the assault.
- Provide opportunities for the entire family to go through a recovery process.

Sexual assault affects everyone. *To help deal with this social problem:*

- Provide sympathetic care and support to those who have been victimized.
- Recognize that offenders do not change without intervention.
- Organize neighborhood programs to support each other's efforts to protect children.
- Encourage schools to provide information about sexual assault as a problem of health and safety.
- Organize community groups to support educational treatment and law enforcement programs.

Modified from Adams C, Fay J: *No more secrets: protecting your child from sexual assault,* San Luis Obispo, CA, 1981, Impact.

*Sources of information include Prevent Child Abuse America, Publishing Department, 200 S. Michigan Ave., Suite 1700, Chicago, IL 60604-4357; (312) 663-3520 or 1-800-CHILDREN; website: www.preventchildabuse.org; Kempe Children's Center, 1825 Marion St., Denver, CO 80218; (303) 864-5250; website: www.kempecenter.org; American Association for Protecting Children, American Humane Association, 63 Inverness Dr. E., Englewood, CO 80112; 1-800-227-4645 (outside Colorado) or (303) 792-9900; and National Clearing House on Child Abuse and Neglect Information, 330 C St. SW, Washington, DC 20447; 1-800-394-3366; website: www.calib.com/nccanch.

ents to such dangers and guide them toward an appreciation of the problem, providing concrete guidelines toward child education and protection.

➤ Evaluation

The effectiveness of nursing interventions is determined by continual reassessment and evaluation of care based on the following observational guidelines:

1. Observe child for additional physical and behavioral evidence of abuse; observe child's reactions to health professionals; if child is hospitalized, check staffing patterns for schedule of consistent group of nurses caring for child.
2. Interview parents regarding their knowledge of children's physical and development needs.
3. Interview child regarding feelings about returning home or placement outside the home.
4. Investigate community programs aimed at preventing child maltreatment.

The expected outcomes are described in the Nursing Care Plan.

Nursing Care Plan THE CHILD WHO IS MALTREATED

NURSING DIAGNOSIS Risk for trauma related to characteristics of environment, child, caregiver(s)

EXPECTED OUTCOME Patient will exhibit no evidence of further injury or neglect.

Nursing Interventions/*Rationales*

Identify children at risk for potential abuse *to initiate preventive measures.*

Identify signs of maltreatment and implement measures *to prevent further maltreatment* (e.g., report suspicions to appropriate authorities; assist in removing child from unsafe environment and establishing in a safe environment; institute strict supervision if child is hospitalized).

Keep factual records (e.g., child's physical condition, behavioral responses; family responses; description of environment) *for documentation of maltreatment.*

Help child to recognize situations that place child at risk for sexual abuse and teach assertive responses *to discourage abuse.*

Refer family to appropriate social agencies for assistance with finances, food, shelter, clothing, health care *to help prevent neglect.*

Participate in multidisciplinary team efforts *to assess for continued abuse or neglect and make decisions about removal from and return to the environment.*

NURSING DIAGNOSIS Fear/anxiety related to repeated maltreatment, powerlessness, potential loss of parents

EXPECTED OUTCOME Patient will exhibit decreasing evidence of distress.

Nursing Interventions/*Rationales*

Provide consistent caregivers and therapeutic environment during hospitalization *to build trust and relieve stress.*

Provide support to child (e.g., treat child as someone with the usual age-appropriate physical, developmental, and social needs; avoid interrogation; ask permission to touch child; show attention to praise child's abilities and appropriate behaviors; give child opportunity to talk and ask questions without pressure to do so; use play to promote self-expression) *to decrease anxieties and increase confidence.*

NURSING DIAGNOSIS Altered parenting related to child, caregiver, or situational characteristics that precipitate abusive behavior

EXPECTED OUTCOME Patient will exhibit evidence of changing parenting behaviors.

Nursing Interventions/*Rationales*

Provide support to family (e.g., interactions with parents that reflect care and concern rather than accusation and punishment; encourage parent-child relationship; do not usurp parental role but rather provide a role model for constructive interaction with the child) *to establish trust and provide motivation for change.* Assess parent-childrearing beliefs and practices *to establish baseline for teaching.*

Teach realistic expectations of child behavior and capabilities, emphasizing alternative methods of discipline such as reward, time out *to give parents alternatives to verbal or physical abusive behavior.*

Identify appropriate developmental issues (e.g., toilet training, toddler negativism, independence seeking) that may trigger abuse and help parents work out specific methods for management of the issue *to provide concrete approaches to timely issues.*

Use demonstration, role-modeling approaches rather than lecture or authoritarian approach *to overcome lack of self-esteem and sensitivity to criticism and establish trust.*

Praise competent parenting behaviors *to increase confidence in parenting abilities.*

Refer parent(s) to appropriate sources for classes on how to parent; counseling to explore abuse patterns; support groups *to decrease chances of repeat abuse.*

Key Points

- The preschool years comprise the period from 3 to 5 years of age, a time that is considered critical for emotional and psychologic development.
- Biologic development in the preschool period is characterized by mature body systems and refinement in gross and fine motor behavior, as evidenced by participation in activities such as running, riding a bicycle, and drawing.
- According to Erikson, acquiring a sense of initiative is the chief psychosocial task of the preschooler. Development of the superego occurs during this period, and conscience begins to emerge.
- According to Piaget, the preschool age is characterized by intuitive or prelogical thinking and a move toward logical thought processes through advanced, complex learning, language, and understanding of causality.
- The seeds of moral development are planted during the preschool period. According to Kohlberg, children are in the stage of naïve instrumental orientation, in which they are concerned with satisfying their own needs and less often the needs of others.
- Social development includes further individuation-separation; more sophisticated language; greater independence; and more complex, imaginative forms of play.
- Areas of special concern to parents during the preschool period are preschool and kindergarten experience, sex education, fears, stress, and speech problems.
- In selecting a school or day care, parents should inquire about daily programs, teacher qualifications, accreditation, student-staff ratio, safety, meals, fees, and health practices.
- Two rules that govern answering questions about sex and other sensitive issues are to find out what the child thinks and to be honest.
- Fears constitute a great part of the preschool period; objects, potential annihilation, and parent-induced fears are common sources.
- Preschool aggression may result from frustration, modeling behavior, and reinforcement.
- Hesitancy or dysfluency in speech patterns is a normal characteristic of language development. Speech problems can occur when parents express excessive concern over this pattern.
- Health promotion continues to be directed toward proper nutrition, adequate sleep, proper dental care, and injury prevention.
- Child maltreatment may take the form of physical abuse or neglect, emotional abuse or neglect, or sexual abuse.
- Parental, child, and environmental characteristics are criteria that may predispose children to maltreatment.
- Identification of abuse entails securing evidence of maltreatment, taking a history pertaining to the incident, and assessing parental and child behaviors.
- The reported incidence of sexual abuse has increased in the last decade; common forms are incest, molestation, rape, exhibitionism, child pornography, child prostitution, and pedophilia.

References

Adler NA, Schutz J: Sibling incest offenders, *Child Abuse Negl* 19(7):811-819, 1995.

Ambrose NG, Yairi E, Cox N: Genetic aspects of early childhood stuttering, *J Speech Hear Res* 36(4):701-706, 1993.

American Academy of Pediatrics, Committee on Sports Medicine and Fitness: Fitness, activity and sports participation in the preschool child, *Pediatrics* 90(6):1002-1004, 1992.

American Academy of Pediatrics, Committee on Child Abuse and Neglect: Shaken baby syndrome: inflicted cerebral trauma, *Pediatrics* 92(6):872-875, 1993.

American Academy of Pediatrics, Committee on Infectious Diseases, Pickering L, editor: *2000 Red Book: report of the Committee on Infectious Diseases,* ed 25, Elk Grove Village, IL, 2000, The Academy.

American Academy of Pediatric Dentistry: Reference manual 1996-1997, *Pediatr Dent* 18(6):24-77, 1996.

Atkinson E et al: Sleep disruption in young children, *Child Care Health Dev* 21(4):233-246, 1995.

Bilgrami S et al: Varicella zoster virus infection associated with high-dose chemotherapy and autologous stem-cell rescue, *Bone Marrow Transplant* 23(5):469-474, 1999.

Boucher BH, Doescher SM, Sugawara AI: Preschool children's motor development and self-concept, *Percept Mot Skills* 76(1):11-17, 1993.

Brodeur AE, Monteleone JA: *Child maltreatment, a clinical guide and reference,* St Louis, 1994, Mosby.

Burrell B, Thompson B, Sexton D: Predicting child abuse potential across family types, *Child Abuse Negl* 18(12):1039-1049, 1994.

Calam R et al: Psychological disturbances and child sexual abuse: a follow-up study, *Child Abuse Negl* 22(9):901-913, 1998.

Castiglia PT: Stuttering, *J Pediatr Health Care* 7(6):275-277, 1993.

Ceci SJ, Bruck M: *Jeopardy in the courtroom: a scientific analysis of children's testimony,* Washington, DC, 1995, American Psychological Association Publishing.

Chiocca EM: Shaken baby syndrome: a nursing perspective, *Pediatr Nurs* 21(1):33-38, 1995.

Conte J, Wolf S, Smith T: What sexual offenders tell us about prevention strategies, *Child Abuse Negl* 13:293-301, 1989.

Crick NR, Casas JF, Mosher M: Relational and overt aggression in preschool, *Dev Psychol* 33(4):579-588, 1997.

Dennison BA, Rockwell HL, Baker SL: Fruit and vegetable intake in young children, *J Am Coll Nutr* 17(4):371-378, 1998.

Fina DK: The spiritual needs of pediatric patients and their families, *AORN J* 64(4):556-564, 1995.

Finan SL: Promoting healthy sexuality: guidelines for infancy through preschool, *Nurse Pract* 22(10):79-80, 83-86, 88, 1997.

Fischer DG, McDonald WL: Characteristics of intrafamilial and extrafamilial child sexual abuse, *Child Abuse Negl* 22(9):915-929, 1998.

Flournoy J: Incest prevention: the role of the pediatric nurse practitioner, *J Pediatr Health Care* 10(6):246-254, 1996.

Food and Nutrition Board, National Research Council: *Recommended dietary allowances,* ed 10, Washington, DC, 1989, National Academy Press.

Hart CH et al: Overt and relational aggression in Russian nursery-school-aged children: parenting style and marital linkages, *Dev Psychol* 34(4):687-697, 1998.

Huttenlocher J: Language input and language growth, *Prev Med* 27(2):195-199, 1998.

Hymel KP, Jenny C: Child sexual abuse, *Pediatr Rev* 17(7): 236-249, 1996.

Kakourou T et al: Herpes zoster in children, *J Am Acad Dermatol* 39(2, pt 1):207-210, 1998.

Kenny G: Assessing children's spirituality: what is the way forward? *Br J Nurs* 8(1):28, 30-32, 1999.

Kerr S, Jowett S: Sleep problems in pre-school children: a review of the literature, *Child Care Health Dev* 20(6):379-381, 1994.

Lafontaine G, Bedard L: The prevention of infections in child daycare centers: potential influential factors, *Can J Public Health* 88(4):250-254, 1997.

Leung A, Robson W: Childhood masturbation, *Clin Pediatr* 32(4):238-241, 1993.

Lewit EM, Baker LS: School readiness, *Future Child* 5(2): 128-139, 1995.

McCullough M, Scherman A: Family-of-origin interaction and adolescent mothers' potential for child abuse, *Adolescence* 33(130):375-384, 1998.

Moody CW: Male child sexual abuse, *J Pediatr Health Care* 13(3):112-119, 1999.

Muris P, Merckelbach H, Collaris R: Common childhood fears and their origins, *Behav Res Ther* 35(10):929-937, 1997.

Muris P et al: The role of parental fearfulness and modeling children's fears, *Behav Res Ther* 34(3):265-268, 1996.

Olds DL, Henderson CR Jr, Kitzman H: Does parental and infancy nurse home visitation have enduring effects on qualities of parental caregiving and child health at 25 to 50 months of life? *Pediatrics* 93(1):89-98, 1994.

Pillitteri A et al: Parent gender, victim gender, and family socioeconomic level influences on the potential reporting by nurses of physical child abuse, *Issues Compr Pediatr Nurs* 15(4):239-247, 1992.

Rodriguez CM, Green AJ: Parenting stress and anger expression as predictors of child abuse potential, *Child Abuse Negl* 21(4):367-377, 1997.

Ross S: Risk of physical abuse to children of spouse abusing parents, *Child Abuse Negl* 20(7):589-598, 1996.

Rovers MM et al: Day-care and otitis media in young children: a critical review, *Eur J Pediatr* 158(1):1-6, 1999.

Sawicki JA: Sibling rivalry and the new baby: anticipatory guidance and management strategies, *Pediatr Nurs* 23(3):298-302, 1997.

Schowengert RK: The relationship between parental socioeconomic levels and potential for child abuse, *Nurs Pract* 21(3):144-146, 1996.

Seidl AH et al: Nurses' attitudes toward child victims and the perpetrators of emotional, physical, and sexual abuse, *Issues Child Abuse Accus* 5(1):28-38, 1993.

Semba RD: Vitamin A as "anti-infective" therapy, 1920-1940, *J Nutr* 129(4):783-791, 1999.

Shea S et al: Is there a relationship between dietary fat and stature or growth in children three to five years of age? *Pediatrics* 92:579-586, 1993.

Souid AD, Keith DV, Cunningham AS: Munchausen syndrome by proxy, *Clin Pediatr* 37(8):497-503, 1998.

Stanton M et al: Nurses' attitudes toward emotional, sexual, and physical abusers of children with disabilities, *Rehab Nurs* 19(4):214-218, 1994.

Thomas RM: *Comparing theories of child development,* ed 4, Pacific Grove, CA, 1996, Brooks-Cole.

U.S. Department of Agriculture, Center for Nutrition Policy and Promotion: *Tips for using the Food Guide Pyramid for young children 2 to 6 years old,* Program Aid 1647, March 1999, www.usda.gov/cnpp.

Vessey JA, Yim-Chiplis PK, MacKenzie NR: Effects of television viewing on children's development, *Pediatr Nurs* 23(5): 483-486, 1998.

Wang CT, Daro D: *Current trends in child abuse reporting and fatalities: the results of the 1997 annual fifty state survey,* Chicago, 1998, Prevent Child Abuse America.

Wilde JA, Pedroni AT Jr: Privacy rights in Munchausen syndrome, *Contemp Pediatr* 10(1):83-91, 1993.

Williams CL et al: Healthy Start: a comprehensive health education program for preschool children, *Prev Med* 27(2): 216-223, 1998.

Wright JE: Munchausen syndrome by proxy or medical child abuse, *J Rare Dis* 3(3):5-10, 1997.

CHAPTER 39

The School-Age Child and Family

http://www.harcourthealth.com/MERLIN/Wong/maternal/

Learning Objectives

On completion of this chapter the reader will be able to:

- Describe the physical, cognitive, and moral changes that take place during the middle childhood years.
- Describe ways to help a child develop a sense of accomplishment.
- Demonstrate an understanding of the changing interpersonal relationships of school-age children.
- Discuss the role of the peer group in the socialization of the school-age child.
- Discuss the role of schools in the development and socialization of the school-age child.
- Demonstrate an understanding of the types, causes, and prevention of sports injuries in middle childhood.
- Describe the most common causes of growth and maturation failure in later childhood.
- Discuss the manifestations and nursing management of selected emotional and behavioral problems.
- Outline an appropriate health teaching plan for the school-age child.
- Plan a sex education session for a group of school-age children.
- Identify the causes and discuss the preventive aspects of injury in middle childhood.

PROMOTING OPTIMUM GROWTH AND DEVELOPMENT

The segment of the life span that extends from age 6 to approximately age 12 has a variety of labels, each of which describes an important characteristic of the period. These middle years are most often referred to as *school-age* or the *school years.* This period begins with entrance into the school environment, which has a significant impact on development and relationships. Children affiliate with age-mates, learn the culture of childhood, and establish themselves with peer groups, the first close relationships outside the family group.

Physiologically the middle years begin with the shedding of the first deciduous tooth and end at puberty with the acquisition of the final permanent teeth (with the exception of the wisdom teeth). During the preceding 5 to 6 years children have progressed from helpless infants to sturdy, complicated individuals with the capacity to communicate, conceptualize in a limited way, and become involved in complex social and motor behavior. Physical growth has been equally rapid. In contrast, the period of middle childhood, between the rapid growth of early childhood and the prepubescent growth spurt, is a time of gradual growth and development with more even progress in both physical and emotional aspects.

Biologic Development

During middle childhood, growth in height and weight assumes a slower but steady pace as compared with the earlier years. Between ages 6 and 12, children will grow an average of 5 cm (2 inches) per year to gain 30 to 60 cm (1 to 2 feet) in height and will almost double their weight, increasing 2 to 3 kg (4½ to 6½ pounds) per year. The average 6-year-old child is about 116 cm (45 inches) tall and weighs about 21 kg (46 pounds); the average 12-year-old child stands about 150 cm (59 inches) tall and weighs approximately 40 kg (88 pounds). During this age period, girls and boys differ very little in size, although boys tend to be slightly taller and somewhat heavier than girls. Toward the end of the school-age years, both boys and girls begin to increase in size, although most girls begin to surpass boys in both height and weight, to the acute discomfort of both girls and boys.

Proportional Changes. School-age children are more graceful than they were as preschoolers, and they are steadier on

---

For additional information, please view "Growth and Development" in *Whaley and Wong's Pediatric Nursing Video Series,* St Louis, 1996, Mosby; 1-800-426-4545; website: www.mosby.com.

their feet. Their body proportions take on a slimmer look, with longer legs, varying body proportions, and a lower center of gravity. Posture improves over that of the preschool period to facilitate locomotion and efficiency in using the arms and trunk. These proportions make climbing, bicycle riding, and other activities much easier. Fat gradually diminishes, and its distribution patterns change, contributing to the thinner appearance of the child during the middle years.

Accompanying the skeletal lengthening and fat diminution is an increase in the percentage of body weight represented by muscle tissue. By the end of this age period, both boys and girls will double their strength and physical capabilities, and their steady and relatively consistent acquisition of refined coordination will increase their poise and skill. However, this increased strength can be misleading. Although strength increases, muscles are still functionally immature when compared with those of the adolescent, and they are more readily damaged by muscular injury caused by overuse.

The most pronounced changes, and those that seem to best indicate increasing maturity in children, are a decrease in head circumference in relation to standing height, a decrease in waist circumference in relation to height, and an increase in leg length related to height. These observations often provide a clue to a child's degree of physical maturity that has proved useful in predicting readiness for meeting the demands of school. There appears to be a correlation between physical indications of maturity and success in school.

Facial Changes. Certain physiologic and anatomic characteristics are typical of children in middle childhood. Facial proportions change as the face grows faster in relation to the remainder of the cranium. The skull and brain grow very slowly during this period and increase little in size thereafter. Since all of the primary (deciduous) teeth are lost during this age span, middle childhood is sometimes known as the *age of the loose tooth* (Fig. 39-1) and the early years of middle childhood as the *ugly duckling stage,* when the new secondary (permanent) teeth appear to be much too large for the face.

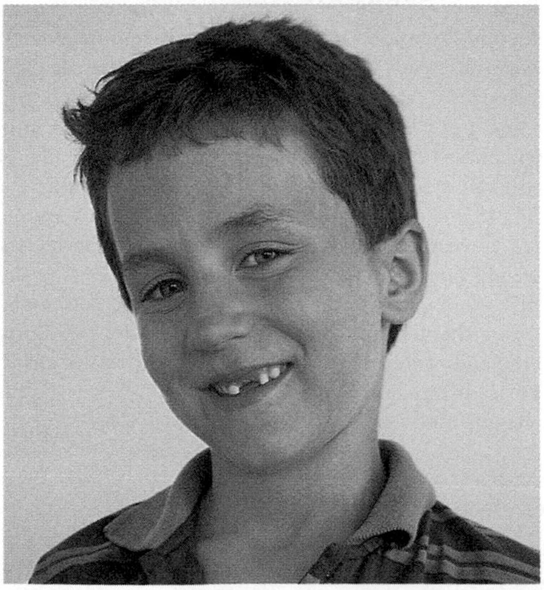

FIG. 39-1 • Middle childhood is the stage of development when deciduous teeth are shed.

Maturation of Systems. Maturity of the gastrointestinal system is reflected in fewer stomach upsets; better maintenance of blood glucose levels; and an increased stomach capacity, which permits retention of food for longer periods. The school-age child does not need to be fed as carefully, as promptly, or as often as before. Caloric needs are less than they were in the preschool years.

Physical maturation is evidenced in other body tissues and organs. *Bladder capacity,* although differing widely among individual children, is generally greater in girls than in boys. The *heart* grows more slowly during the middle years and is smaller in relation to the rest of the body than at any other period of life. Heart and respiratory rates steadily decrease and blood pressure increases during ages 6 to 12 (see Appendix J).

The *immune system* becomes more competent in its ability to localize infections and produce an antibody-antigen response (Wilson, Lewis, and Penix, 1996).

Bones continue to ossify throughout childhood but yield to pressure and muscle pull more than mature bones. Children should have ample opportunity to move around, but they should observe appropriate caution in carrying heavy loads. For example, they should shift books and/or tote bags from one arm to the other. Back packs distribute weight more evenly than tote bags.

Wider differences between children are observed at the end of middle childhood than at the beginning; such differences are sometimes striking. These differences become increasingly apparent and, if extreme or unique, may create emotional problems. The associated characteristics of height and weight relationships, rapid or slow growth, and other important features of development should be explained to children and their families. Physical maturity is not necessarily correlated with emotional and social maturity. Seven-year-old children who look like 10-year-old children will, in fact, think and act like 7-year-old children. To expect behavior appropriate for 10-year-old children from them is unrealistic and can be detrimental to their development of competence and self-esteem. Conversely, to treat 10-year-old children as though they were 7 years old is an equal disservice to them.

Prepubescence. *Preadolescence* is the period that begins toward the end of middle childhood and ends with the thirteenth birthday. Since puberty signals the beginning of the development of secondary sex characteristics, *prepubescence,* the 2-year period that precedes puberty, typically occurs during preadolescence.

Toward the end of middle childhood the discrepancies in growth and maturation between boys and girls become apparent. On the average, there is a difference of approximately 2 years between girls and boys in the age of onset of pubescence. This is a period of rapid growth in height and weight, especially for girls.

There is no universal age at which children assume the characteristics of prepubescence. The first physiologic signs appear at about 9 years of age (particularly in girls) and are usually clearly evident in 11- to 12-year-old children. Although preadolescent children do not want to be different, variability in physical growth and physiologic changes between children of the same sex and between the two sexes is often striking at this time. This variability, especially in relation to the onset of secondary sexual characteristics, is of utmost concern to the preadolescent. Either early or late appearance of these characteristics is a source of embarrassment and uneasiness to both sexes.

Preadolescence is a time when considerable overlapping of developmental characteristics occurs, with elements of both middle childhood and early adolescence. However, there are sufficient unique characteristics to set this apart as an age category. Generally, the earliest age at which puberty begins is 10 years in girls and 12 years in boys, although there has been an increase in the number of girls reaching puberty at age 9. The average age of puberty is 12 years in girls and 14 years in boys. Boys experience little visible sexual maturation during preadolescence.

Psychosocial Development

Middle childhood is the period of psychosexual development that Freud described as *latency period,* a time of tranquility between the Oedipal phase of early childhood and the eroticism of adolescence. During this time children experience relationships with same-sex peers following the indifference of earlier years and preceding the heterosexual fascination that accompanies puberty.

Developing a Sense of Industry (Erikson). Successful mastery of Erikson's first three stages of psychosocial development is probably the most important accomplishment in terms of development of a healthy personality (Erikson, 1963). Successful completion of these stages requires a loving environment within a stable family unit that has prepared the child to engage in experiences and relationships beyond this intimate group.

It has been suggested that the individual's fundamental attitude toward work is established during middle childhood. A *sense of industry,* or a *stage of accomplishment,* is achieved somewhere between age 6 and adolescence. School-age children are eager to develop skills and participate in meaningful and socially useful work. They acquire a sense of personal and interpersonal competence, receive the systematic instruction prescribed by their individual cultures, and develop the skills needed to become useful, contributing members of their social communities.

Interests expand in the middle years, and with a growing sense of independence, children want to engage in tasks that can be carried through to completion (Fig. 39-2). They gain great satisfaction from independent behavior in exploring and manipulating their environment and from interaction with peers. Often the acquisition of skills is a means for achieving success in social activities. Reinforcement in the form of grades, material rewards, additional privileges, and recognition provides encouragement and stimulation.

A sense of accomplishment also involves the ability to cooperate, to compete with others, and to cope effectively with people. Middle childhood is the time when children learn the value of doing things with others and the benefits derived from division of labor in the accomplishment of goals. Peer approval is a strong motivating power.

The danger inherent in this period of personality development is the occurrence of situations that might result in a sense of *inferiority.* This may happen if the previous stages have not been successfully achieved or if the child is incapable of or unprepared to assume the responsibilities associated with developing a sense of accomplishment. Feelings of inferiority or lack of worth can be derived from children themselves or from the social environment. Children with physical or mental limitations may be at a disadvantage for acquisition of certain skills and at risk for feeling inferior. However, no child is able to do well in everything, and children must learn that they will not be able to master each skill that they attempt. All children, even children who usually have positive attitudes toward work and their own capabilities, will feel some degree of inferiority in regard to a specific skill that they cannot master.

Children need and want real achievement. When they have access to tasks that need to be done, that they are able to do well despite individual differences in their innate capacities and emotional development, and for which they are suitably rewarded, children achieve a sense of industry and accomplishment.

Cognitive Development (Piaget). When children enter the school years, they begin to acquire the ability to relate a series of events to mental representations that can be expressed both verbally and symbolically. This is the stage that Piaget describes as *concrete operations,* when children are able to use thought processes to experience events and actions. The rigid, egocentric outlook of the preschool years is replaced by thought processes that allow children to see things from another's point of view.

During this stage, children develop an understanding of relationships between things and ideas. They progress from making judgments based on what they see *(perceptual thinking)* to making judgments based on what they reason *(conceptual thinking).* They are increasingly able to master symbols and to use their memory store of past experiences to evaluate and interpret the present.

One of the major cognitive tasks of school-age children is mastering the concept of *conservation* (Fig. 39-3). At an early age (about 5 to 7 years) they grasp the concept of reversibility of numbers as a basis for simple mathematics problems (e.g., $2 + 4 = 6$ and $6 - 4 = 2$). They learn that certain properties of the environment are not changed simply by altering their arrangement in space, and they become able to resist perceptual cues that suggest such alterations in the physical state of an object. For example, they recognize that changing the shape of a

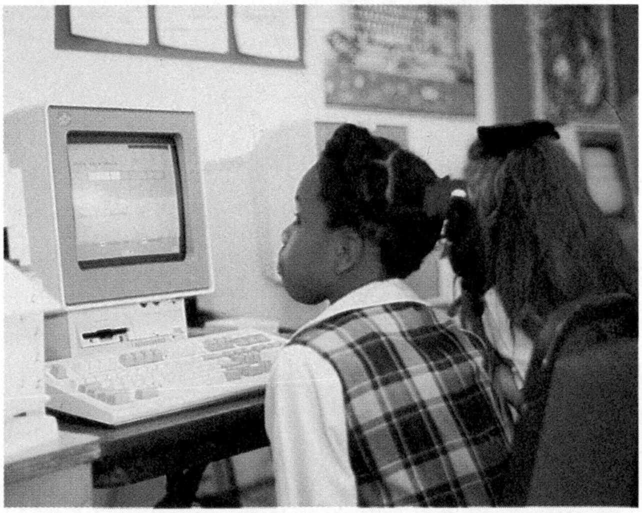

FIG. 39-2 • School-age children are motivated to complete tasks working alone.

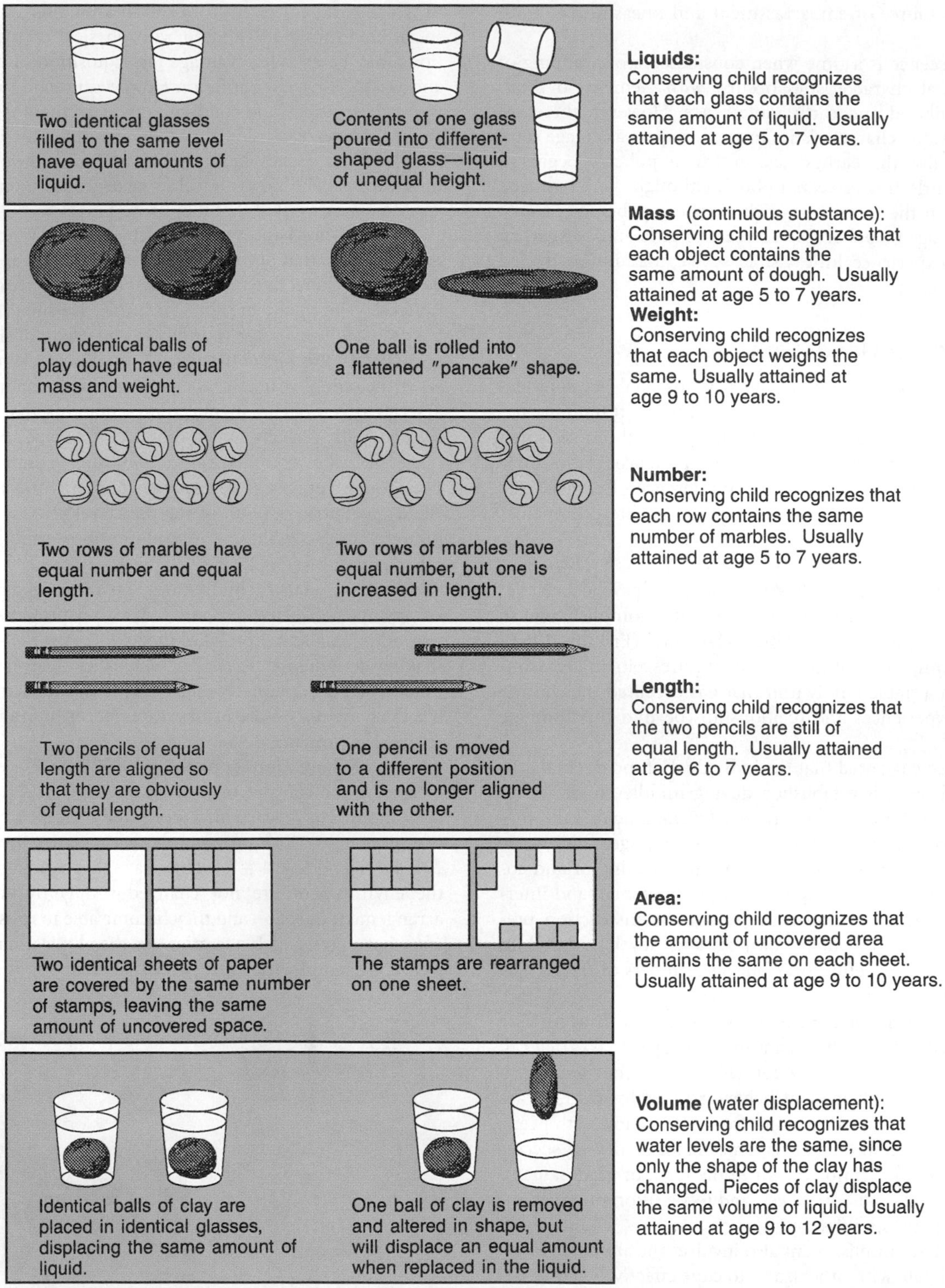

Two identical glasses filled to the same level have equal amounts of liquid.
Contents of one glass poured into different-shaped glass—liquid of unequal height.
Liquids:
Conserving child recognizes that each glass contains the same amount of liquid. Usually attained at age 5 to 7 years.
Two identical balls of play dough have equal mass and weight.
One ball is rolled into a flattened "pancake" shape.
Mass (continuous substance):
Conserving child recognizes that each object contains the same amount of dough. Usually attained at age 5 to 7 years.
Weight:
Conserving child recognizes that each object weighs the same. Usually attained at age 9 to 10 years.
Two rows of marbles have equal number and equal length.
Two rows of marbles have equal number, but one is increased in length.
Number:
Conserving child recognizes that each row contains the same number of marbles. Usually attained at age 5 to 7 years.
Two pencils of equal length are aligned so that they are obviously of equal length.
One pencil is moved to a different position and is no longer aligned with the other.
Length:
Conserving child recognizes that the two pencils are still of equal length. Usually attained at age 6 to 7 years.
Two identical sheets of paper are covered by the same number of stamps, leaving the same amount of uncovered space.
The stamps are rearranged on one sheet.
Area:
Conserving child recognizes that the amount of uncovered area remains the same on each sheet. Usually attained at age 9 to 10 years.
Identical balls of clay are placed in identical glasses, displacing the same amount of liquid.
One ball of clay is removed and altered in shape, but will displace an equal amount when replaced in the liquid.
Volume (water displacement):
Conserving child recognizes that water levels are the same, since only the shape of the clay has changed. Pieces of clay displace the same volume of liquid. Usually attained at age 9 to 12 years.

FIG. 39-3 • Common examples that demonstrate the child's ability to conserve (ages are only approximate).

substance such as a lump of clay does not alter its total mass. They no longer perceive a tall, thin glass of water as containing a greater volume than a short, wide glass; they can distinguish between the weight of items regardless of their size. They recognize that size is not necessarily related to weight or volume. There appears to be a developmental sequence in children's capacity to conserve matter. Conservation of mass usually is accomplished earliest, weight some time later, and volume last.

School-age children also develop *classification* skills. They can group and sort objects according to the attributes that they share; place things in a sensible and logical order; and, in doing so, hold a concept in mind while making decisions based on that concept. It is characteristic of middle childhood that children derive enjoyment from classifying and ordering their environment. They become occupied with numerous and varied collections of objects, such as stickers, stamps, shells, dolls, cars, stones, and anything that is classifiable. They even begin to order friends and relationships (e.g., first best friend, second best friend).

They develop the ability to understand relational terms and concepts, such as bigger and smaller; darker and paler; heavier and lighter; to the right of and to the left of; first, last, and intermediate relationships (fourth, second, and so on); and more than and less than. They can see family relationships in terms of reciprocal roles (e.g., in order to be a brother, one must have a sibling).

School-age children learn the alphabet and the ever-widening world of symbols called words that can be arranged in terms of structure and their relationship to the alphabet. They learn to tell time, to see the relationship of events in time (history) and places in space (geography), and to combine time and space relationships (geology and astronomy).

The most significant skill, the *ability to read,* is acquired during the school years and becomes the most valuable tool for independent inquiry. Children's capacity for exploration, imagination, and expansion of knowledge is enhanced by the ability to read as they progress from the repetition and confusion of early efforts to increasing comprehension.

Moral Development (Kohlberg)

As children move from egocentrism to more logical patterns of thought, they also move through stages in development of conscience and moral standards. Young children do not believe that standards of behavior come from within themselves but rather that rules are established and set down by others. During the preschool years children adopt and internalize the moral values of their parents. They learn the standards for acceptable behavior, act according to these standards, and feel guilty when they violate the standards.

Although children of 6 or 7 years of age know the rules and behaviors expected of them, they do not understand the reasons behind them. Rewards and punishments guide their judgment; a "bad act" is one that breaks a rule or does harm. Young children may believe that what other people tell them to do is right and that what they themselves think is wrong. Consequently, children 6 or 7 years old are more likely to interpret accidents and misfortunes as punishment for misdeeds or "bad" acts.

Older school-age children are able to judge an act by the intentions that prompted it rather than just by the consequences. Rules and judgments become less absolute and authoritarian and begin to be founded more on the needs and desires of others. For older children a rule violation is apt to be viewed in relation to the total context in which it appears; reactions are influenced by the situation as well as by the morality of the rule itself. Although younger children can judge an act only according to whether it is right or wrong, older children take into account a different point of view to make a judgment. They are able to understand and accept the concept of treating others as they would like to be treated.

Cultural Considerations

RELIGIOUS ORIENTATION

Many schools and communities have a Judeo-Christian orientation toward prayer, holidays, and values. This may result in conflict and discomfort for children of other religious/ethnic groups. Sensitivity must be exercised so as not to offend and confuse children from other religious backgrounds, such as the Buddhist, Hindu, and Muslim faiths.

Spiritual Development

Children at this age think in very concrete terms but are avid learners and have a great desire to learn about their God. They picture God as human and use adjectives such as "loving" and "helping" to describe their deity. They are fascinated by the concepts of hell and heaven, and with a developing conscience and concern about rules, they fear going to hell for misbehavior. School-age children want and expect to be punished for misbehavior and, if given the option, tend to choose a punishment that "fits the crime." Often they view illness or injury as a punishment for a real or imagined misdeed. The beliefs and ideals of family and religious personages are more influential than those of their peers in matters of faith.

School-age children begin to learn the difference between the natural and the supernatural but have difficulty understanding symbols. Consequently religious concepts must be presented to them in concrete terms. They are comforted by prayer or other religious rituals, and if these activities are a part of their daily lives, they can help them cope with threatening situations. Their petitions to their God in prayers tend to be for very tangible rewards. Although younger children expect their prayers to be answered, as they get older they begin to recognize that this does not always occur and become less concerned when prayers are not answered. They are able to discuss their feelings about their faith and how it relates to their lives (Cultural Considerations box).

Social Development

One of the most important socializing agents in the life of the school-age child is the peer group. In addition to parents and the schools, the peer group conveys a substantial amount of material to its members. Children have a culture all their own, with secrets, mores, and codes of ethics with which they promote feelings of group solidarity and detachment from adults. Through peer relationships children learn ways in which to deal with dominance and hostility, relate to persons in positions of leadership and authority, and explore ideas and the physical environment.

Identification with peers is a strong influence in the child's gaining independence from parents. The aid and support of the group provide the child with enough security to risk the moderate parental rejection brought about by each small victory in the development of independence.

Much of the child's concept of the appropriate sex role is acquired through relationships with peers. During the early school years there is little difference relative to gender in play experiences of children. Games and many other activities are shared by both girls and boys. However, in the later school years the differences become marked.

Social Relationships and Cooperation. Daily relationships with peers provide the most important social interactions for school-age children. For the first rime, children are able to join in group activities with unrestrained enthusiasm and steady participation. Previous interactions were limited to short periods under considerable adult supervision. With increased skills and wider opportunities, children become involved with one or several peer groups in which they can gain status as respected members.

Valuable lessons are learned from daily interaction with age-mates. First, children learn to appreciate the numerous and varied points of view that are represented in the peer group. As children interact with peers who see the world in ways that are somewhat different from their own, they become aware of the limits of their own point of view. Because age-mates are peers and are not forced to accept each other's ideas as they are expected to accept those of adults, other children have a significant influence on decreasing the egocentric outlook of the child. Consequently, children learn to argue, persuade, bargain, cooperate, and compromise in order to maintain friendships.

Second, children become increasingly sensitive to the social norms and pressures of the peer group. The peer group establishes standards for acceptance and rejection, and children may be willing to modify their behavior to be accepted by the group. The need for peer approval becomes a powerful influence toward conformity. Children learn to dress, talk, and behave in a manner acceptable to the group. A variety of roles, such as class joker or class hero, may be assumed by individual children to gain approval from the group.

Third, the interaction among peers leads to the formation of intimate friendship between same-sex peers. The school-age period is the time when children have "best friends" with whom they share secrets, private jokes, and adventures; they come to one another's aid in times of trouble. In the course of these friendships children also fight, threaten each other, break up, and reunite. These dyadic relationships, in which the child experiences love and closeness for a peer, seem to be important as a foundation for heterosexual relationships in adulthood (Fig. 39-4).

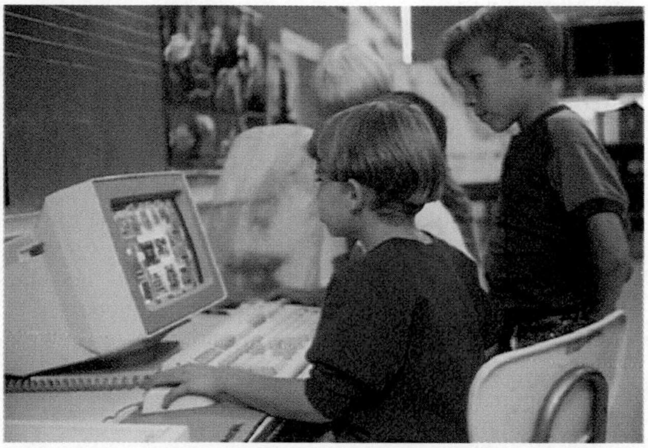

FIG. 39-4 • School-age children enjoy engaging in activities with a "best friend."

Clubs and Peer Groups. One of the outstanding characteristics of middle childhood is the formation of formalized groups, or clubs. A prominent feature of many of these groups is the rigid rules imposed on the members. There is an exclusiveness in the selection of persons who have the privilege of joining. Acceptance in the group is often determined on a pass-fail basis according to social or behavioral criteria. Conformity is the core of the group structure. There are often secret codes, shared interests, and special modes of dress, and each child must abide by a standard of behavior established by the members. Conforming to the rules provides children with feelings of security and relieves them of the responsibility of making decisions. By merging their identities with those of their peers, children are able to move from the family group to an outside group as a step toward seeking further independence. They substitute conformity to a peer-group pattern for conformity to a family pattern at a time when they are still too shaky and insecure to function independently.

During the early school years, groups are rather small and loosely organized, with changing membership and little formal structure. The more prolonged cohesiveness characteristic of groups or cliques in later school years is not obvious. As a rule, girls' groups are less formalized than boys', and although there may be a mixture of both sexes in the earlier school years, the groups of later school years are composed predominantly of children of the same sex. Common interests are a common basis around which a group is structured.

Peer-group identification and association are essential to a child's socialization. Poor relationships with peers and a lack of group identification can contribute to bullying. Bullying occurs when one or more children inflict physical, verbal, or emotional abuse on another child. *Bullying* occurs often in school-age children who lack academic or social skills, and often represents an attempt to act out anger and resentment about peer relationships. Bullying has a negative effect on children who experience this behavior and may increase childhood symptoms such as headache, stomachache, and sleep disturbances (Williams et al, 1996).

There can also be inherent dangers in strong peer-group attachments. Peer pressures may force children into taking risks, even against their better judgment. Peer-group activities that result in unacceptable, unlawful, or criminal *gang violence* are increasing in the United States and represent a significant challenge for health professionals and teachers who work with children.

Relationships with Families. Although the peer group is influential and necessary to normal child development, parents are the primary influence in shaping children's personality, setting standards for behavior, and establishing value systems. Family values usually predominate when parental and peer value systems come into conflict. Although children may appear to reject parental values while testing the new values of the peer group, ultimately they will retain and incorporate into their own value systems the parental values they have found to be of worth. Peer associations seem to remain within the social class systems, and there may be discrimination in membership on the basis of ethnic or racial origin.

Children want to spend more time in the company of peers and may seem eager to leave the house; they often prefer activities of the peer group to family activities. This can be very disturbing to parents. Children become intolerant and critical of parents and their ways when they deviate from those of the group. They discover that parents can be wrong, and they begin to question the knowledge and authority of parents, who previously were considered to be all-knowing and all-powerful.

Although increased independence is the goal of middle childhood, children are not ready to abandon parental control. They need and want restrictions placed on their behavior; they are not yet prepared to cope with all of the problems of their expanding environment. They feel more secure knowing that there is an authority greater than themselves to implement controls and restrictions. Children may complain loudly about the restrictions and try their best to break down parental barriers, but they are uneasy if they succeed in doing so. They respect the adults on whom they can rely to prevent them from acting on each and every urge. Children sense in this behavior an expression of love and concern for their welfare.

Children also need their parents as adults, not as pals. Sometimes parents, hurt at their children's rejection, attempt to maintain their love and gratitude by assuming the role of "pals." Children need the stable, secure strength provided by mature adults to whom they can turn during troubled relationships with peers or stressful changes in their world. During a disruption in their lives, such as times of failure, periods of illness, or a move that separates them from the security of friends, children need the firm, secure anchor of parental interest and concern. With a secure base in a loving family, children are able to develop the self-confidence and maturity needed to break loose from the group and stand independently.

Play. As children enter the school years, their play takes on new dimensions that reflect a new stage of development. Not only does play involve increased physical skill, intellectual ability, and fantasy, but as children form groups and cliques, they begin to develop a sense of belonging to a team or club. To belong to a group is of vital importance; clubs, secret societies, and organizations such as Scouts are part of the culture of childhood.

Rules and Rituals. The need for conformity in middle childhood is strongly manifested in the activities and games so important in the life of school-age children. Up to this point, they have played games they have either invented themselves or have played in the company of a friend or an adult, and the rules more or less evolved with the game. Now they begin to see the need for rules, and the games they play have fixed and unvarying rules that may be bizarre and extraordinarily rigid (especially those made up by the group).

Conformity and ritual permeate the play of school-age children. Not only are they present in games, but they are also evident in much of the children's behavior and language. Childhood is full of chants and taunts, such as "Eeeny, meeny, miney, mo," "Last one is a rotten egg," and "Step on a crack, break your mother's back." Children derive a sense of pleasure and power from such sayings, which have been handed down with few changes through generations.

Team Play. A more complex form of play that evolves from the need for peer interaction is the team game and sports that are part of the early school years. The rules of such games may require the presence of a referee, umpire, or person of authority so that the rules can be followed more accurately. Team play teaches children to modify or exchange personal goals for goals of the group, and that the concept of division of labor is an effective strategy for attaining a goal. They learn about the nature of competition and the importance of winning—an attribute highly valued in the United States.

Team play can also contribute to children's social, intellectual, and skill growth. Children will work hard to develop the skills needed to become team members, to improve their contribution to the group effort, and to anticipate the consequences of their behavior for the group. Team play helps stimulate cognitive growth as children are called on to learn many complex rules, make judgments about those rules, plan strategies, and assess the strengths and weaknesses of members of their own team and members of the opposing team.

Quiet Games and Activities. Although the play of school-age children is highly active, they also enjoy many quiet and solitary activities. The middle years are the time for collections, which constitute another ritual. Young school-age children's collections are an odd assortment of unrelated objects in messy, disorganized piles. Collections of later years are more orderly and selective, and they are organized neatly in scrapbooks, on shelves, or in boxes.

School-age children become fascinated with increasingly complex board or card games, such as Monopoly or rummy, that they can play with a best friend or a group. As in all games, adherence to rules is fanatic. There is usually much discussion and argument, but the disagreement is easily resolved through reading the appropriate rules of the game.

The newly acquired skill of reading becomes increasingly satisfying as school-age children begin to expand their knowledge of the world through books (Fig. 39-5). School-age children never tire of stories, and like preschool children they love to have stories read aloud. Sewing, cooking, carpentry, gardening, and creative activities such as painting are other activities enjoyed. Many creative skills, such as music and art, as well as athletic skills, such as swimming, horseback riding, dancing, and skating, are learned and continue to be enjoyed into adolescence and adulthood (Fig. 39-6).

Ego Mastery. Play also affords children the means to acquire representational mastery over themselves, their environment, and others. Through play they can feel as big, as power-

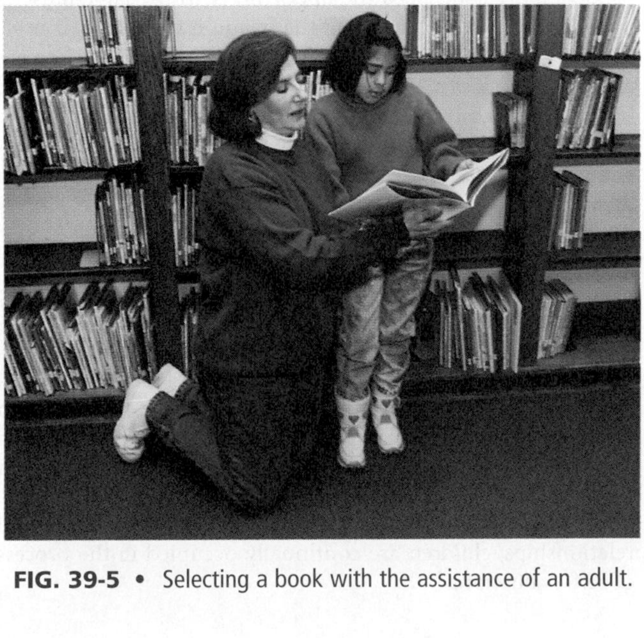

FIG. 39-5 • Selecting a book with the assistance of an adult.

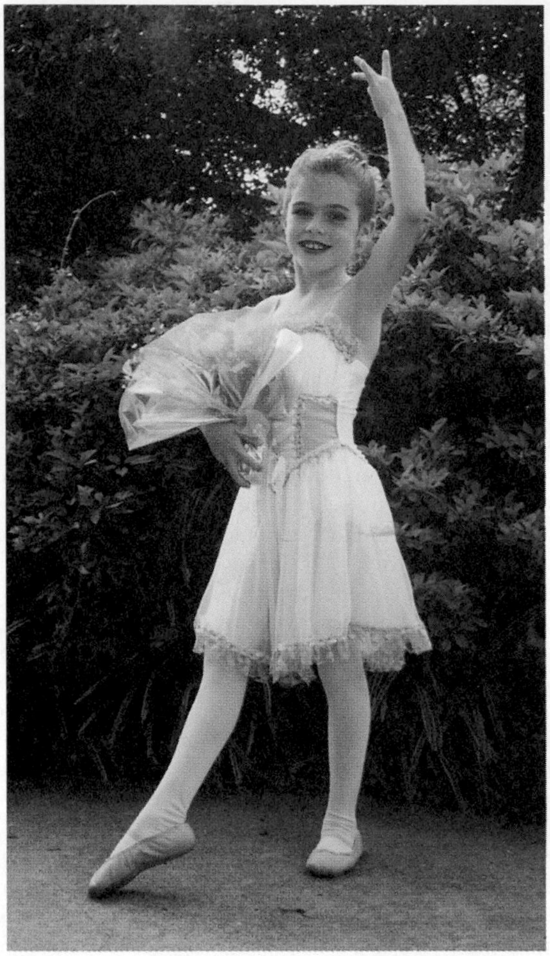

FIG. 39-6 • School-age children take pride in learning new skills.

ful, and as skillful as their imaginations will allow, and they can attain vicarious mastery and power over whomever and whatever they choose. They need to feel in control in their play. Schoolchildren still need the opportunity to use large muscles in exuberant outdoor play and the freedom to exert their new-found autonomy and initiative. They need space in which to exercise large muscles and to work off tensions, frustrations, and hostility. Physical skills practiced and mastered in play help them develop a feeling of personal competence, which contributes to a sense of accomplishment and helps provide a place of status in the peer group.

Developing a Self-Concept

The term *self-concept* refers to a conscious awareness of a variety of self-perceptions, such as one's physical characteristics, abilities, values, self-ideals and expectancy, and idea of self in relation to others. It also includes one's body image, sexuality, and self-esteem. Although primary caregivers continue to impart a great influence on children's self-evaluation, the opinions of peers and teachers provide further input during middle childhood. With the emphasis on skill building and broadened social relationships, children are continually occupied in the process of self-evaluation.

Significant adults in children's lives can often manage to unobtrusively manipulate the environment so that children meet with success. Each small success increases a child's self-image. The more positive children feel about themselves, the more confident they feel in trying again for success. All children profit from feeling that they are in some way special to a significant adult. A positive self-concept makes children feel likable, worthwhile, and capable of valuable contributions. Such feelings lead to self-respect, self-confidence, and a general feeling of happiness. Negative feelings lead to self-doubt.

Developing a Body Image. School-age children have a relatively accurate and positive perception of their physical selves, but in general they like their physical selves less as they grow older. The head appears to be the most important part of the school-age child's perceived image of self, with hair and eye color the characteristics used most commonly to describe the physical self.

Body image is influenced, but not solely determined, by significant others. The number of significant others influencing perception of physical self increases with age. Children are acutely aware of their own body, the bodies of their peers, and those of adults. They are also aware of deviations from the norm. It is important that children know bodily functions and that adults correct misinformation children may have about the body.

Physical impairments (e.g., hearing or visual defects), ears that "stick out," or birthmarks assume great importance. Increasing awareness of these differences, especially when accompanied by unkind comments and taunts from other children, may cause a child to feel inferior and less desirable. This is especially true if the defect interferes with the child's ability to participate in childhood games and activities. When children are teased or criticized about being different, the effect can be lasting.

Table 39-1 summarizes the major developmental achievements of the school-age years.

Coping with Concerns Related to Normal Growth and Development

School Experience. The school serves as the agent for transmitting the values of the society to each succeeding generation of children and as the setting for many relationships with peers. As a socializing agent second only to the family, schools exert a profound influence on the social development of children.

School entrance causes a sharp break in the structure of the child's world. For many children it is their first experience in conforming to a group pattern imposed by an adult who is not a parent and who has responsibility for too many children to be constantly aware of each child as an individual. Children want to go to school, and usually adapt to the new conditions with little difficulty. Successful adjustment is directly related to the physical and emotional maturity of the child and to the parent's readiness to accept the separation associated with school entrance. Unfortunately, some parents express their unconscious attempts to delay the child's maturity by clinging behavior, particularly with their youngest child.

By the time they enter school, most children have a fairly realistic concept of what school involves. They receive information regarding the role of pupil from parents, siblings, playmates, and the media. In addition, most children have had experience with

TABLE 39-1
Growth and Development During School-Age Years

Age (Years)	Physical and Motor	Mental	Adaptive	Personal-Social
6	Height and weight gain continues slowly Weight: 16-23.6 kg (35½-58 pounds); height: 106.6-123.5 cm (42-48 inches) Central mandibular incisors erupt Loses first tooth Gradual increase in dexterity Active age; constant activity Often returns to finger feeding More aware of hand as a tool Likes to draw, print, color Vision reaches maturity	Develops concept of numbers Counts 13 pennies Knows whether it is morning or afternoon Defines common objects such as fork and chair in terms of their use Obeys triple commands in succession Knows right and left hands Says which is pretty and which is ugly of a series of drawings of faces Describes the objects in a picture rather than simply enumerating them Attends first grade	At table, uses knife to spread butter or jam on bread At play, cuts, folds, pastes paper toys; sews crudely if needle is threaded Takes bath without supervision; performs bedtime activities alone Reads from memory; enjoys oral spelling game Likes table games, checkers, simple card games Giggles a lot Sometimes steals money or attractive items Has difficulty owning up to misdeeds Tries out own abilities	Can share and cooperate better Has great need for children of own age Will cheat to win Often engages in rough play Often jealous of younger brother or sister Does what adults are seen doing May have occasional temper tantrums Is a boaster Is more independent, probably influence of school Has own way of doing things Increases socialization
7	Begins to gain at least 5 cm (2 inches) in height per year Weight: 17.7-30 kg (39-66½ pounds); height: 111.8-129.7 cm (44-51 inches) Maxillary central incisors and lateral mandibular incisors erupt More cautious in approaches to new performances Repeats performances to master them Jaw begins to expand to accommodate permanent teeth	Notices that certain parts are missing from pictures Can copy a diamond Repeats three numbers backward Develops concept of time; reads clock or watch correctly to nearest quarter hour; uses clock for practical purposes Attends second grade More mechanical in reading; often does not stop at the end of a sentence, skips words such as "it," "the," and "he"	Uses table knife for cutting meat; may need help with tough or difficult pieces Brushes and combs hair acceptably without help May steal Likes to help and have a choice Is less resistant and stubborn	Is becoming a real member of the family group Takes part in group play Boys prefer playing with boys; girls prefer playing with girls Spends a lot of time alone; does not require a lot of companionship
8-9	Continues to gain 5 cm (2 inches) in height per year Weight: 19.6-39.6 kg (43-87 pounds); height: 117-141.8 cm (46-56 inches) Lateral incisors (maxillary) and mandibular cuspids erupt Movement fluid; often graceful and poised Always on the go; jumps, chases, skips Increased smoothness and speed in fine motor control; uses cursive writing Dresses self completely Likely to overdo; hard to quiet down after recess More limber; bones grow faster than ligaments	Gives similarities and differences between two things from memory Counts backward from 20 to 1; understands concept of reversibility Repeats days of the week and months in order; knows the date Describes common objects in detail, not merely their use Makes change out of a quarter Attends third and fourth grades Reads more; may plan to wake up early just to read	Makes use of common tools such as hammer, saw, screwdriver Uses household and sewing utensils Helps with routine household tasks such as dusting, sweeping Assumes responsibility for share of household chores Looks after all of own needs at table Buys useful articles; exercises some choice in making purchases Runs useful errands Likes pictorial magazines Likes school; wants to answer all the questions	Is easy to get along with at home Likes the reward system Dramatizes Is more sociable Is better behaved Is interested in boy-girl relationships but will not admit it Goes about home and community freely, alone or with friends Likes to compete and play games Shows preference in friends and groups Plays mostly with groups of own sex but is beginning to mix Develops modesty

Continued

TABLE 39-1—cont'd
Growth and Development During School-Age Years

Age (Years)	Physical and Motor	Mental	Adaptive	Personal-Social
8-9—cont'd		Reads classic books, but also enjoys comics More aware of time; can be relied on to get to school on time Can grasp concepts of parts and whole (fractions) Understands concepts of space, cause and effect, nesting (puzzles), conservation (permanence of mass and volume) Classifies objects by more than one quality; has collections Produces simple paintings or drawings	Is afraid of failing a grade; is ashamed of bad grades Is more critical of self Takes music and sport lessons	Compares self with others Enjoys Scouts, group sports
10-12	***Boys:*** Slow growth in height and rapid weight gain; may become obese in this period Weight: 24.3-58 kg (54-128 pounds); height: 127.5-162.3 cm (50-64 inches) Posture is more similar to an adult's; will overcome lordosis ***Girls:*** Pubescent changes may begin to appear; body lines soften and round out Remainder of teeth will erupt and tend toward full development (except wisdom teeth)	Writes brief stories Attends fifth to seventh grades Writes occasional short letters to friends or relatives on own initiative Uses telephone for practical purposes Responds to magazine, radio, or other advertising Reads for practical information or own enjoyment—stores or library books of adventure or romance, animal stories	Makes useful articles or does easy repair work Cooks or sews in small way Raises pets Washes and dries own hair Is responsible for a thorough job of cleaning hair, but may need reminding to do so Is sometimes left alone at home for an hour or so Is successful in looking after own needs or those of other children left in his or her care	Loves friends; talks about them constantly Chooses friends more selectively; may have a "best friend" Enjoys conversation Develops beginning interest in opposite sex Is more diplomatic Likes family; family really has meaning Likes mother and wants to please her in many ways Demonstrates affection Likes father, who is admired and may be idolized Respects parents

day care, preschool, and kindergarten. Middle-class children have fewer adjustments to make and less to learn about expected behavior, since the school tends to reflect dominant middle-class customs and values. If the child has attended a preschool program, the emphasis of the program significantly affects the child's adjustment. Some provide custodial care only; others emphasize emotional, social, and intellectual development.

Classmates have a significant impact on the socialization of individual children. School is usually the first time that most children become members of a large group of individuals their own age. Peer relationships become increasingly important and influential as children proceed through school. The kind of influence exerted by the peer group depends on the background, interests, and abilities of the individual child.

Teachers. To facilitate the transition from home to school, teachers should have personality characteristics that allow them to deal with the needs of young children. Children respond best to teachers with attributes that they would find in a warm, loving parent. Teachers in the early grades perform many of the activities formerly assumed by the parent, such as recognizing children's personal needs (e.g., a need to go to the bathroom or for help with clothing) and helping to develop their social behavior (e.g., manners).

Teachers, like parents, are concerned about the psychologic and emotional welfare of the child. Although the functions of teachers and parents differ, both place constraints on behavior and both are in a position to enforce standards of conduct. However, the teacher's primary responsibility involves stimulating and guiding children's intellectual development, as opposed to providing for their physical welfare beyond the school setting. Teachers share the parental influence in determining the child's attitudes and values.

Teachers serve as models with whom children identify and whom they try to emulate. Teacher approval is sought; teacher disapproval is avoided. The teacher is a very significant person in the life of the early schoolchild, and hero worship of a teacher

Home Care

HELPING CHILDREN IN SCHOOL

General Guidelines

Be supportive—through companionship, share ideas and thoughts.
Be positive—every child should experience some success each day.
Share an interest in reading—use the library; discuss books they are reading.
Support and encourage activity rather than passivity.
Encourage originality—help children make their own projects from discarded articles or other available materials.
Foster the development of hobbies and collections.
Encourage children to wonder and reflect during free time.
Encourage family experiences and trips to places of interest.
Encourage questions—help children discover sources for information or places to explore and investigate.
Stimulate creative thinking and problem solving—help children try out new solutions to problems without fear of making mistakes.
Use rewards rather than punishment.

Specific Guidelines

Meet the teacher at the beginning of school and plan to visit the school to see what is taught and expected.
Send the child to school every day—teachers are concerned when parents make other plans for their children; it conveys the impression that school is unimportant.
Demonstrate an interest in what the child is learning.
Demonstrate an interest in content and growth more than in grades.
Make it clear to the child that schoolwork is between the child and the teacher; teacher and child should set goals for better school performance to allow the child to feel responsible for school successes and failures.
Take advantage of situations that support and reinforce school learning.
Share information with teachers that will help them understand the child better.
Communicate with the teacher if there appears to be a problem—avoid waiting for a scheduled conference.
Provide a quiet, well-lighted area for study that is safe from interruption; do not allow television or radio.
Avoid dictating a study time, but do enforce rules, such as no television until homework is done; accept the child's word that work is complete.
Help with homework should focus on explaining the question, not giving the answer.
Teach the child to break large tasks (e.g., a report) into smaller, manageable tasks spread over the allotted time rather than attempt the entire project the night before it is to be completed.
Limit home tutoring to special circumstances, such as when the teacher requests parental assistance after a child's prolonged absence.
Request special help for children with learning problems.
Support the school staff by showing respect for both the school system and the teacher, at least in the child's presence.

may extend into late childhood and preadolescence. Teachers who make supportive statements that reassure or commend children, use accepting and clarifying statements that help children refine ideas and feelings, and provide assistance that aids children with their own problem solving contribute to the expansion and development of a positive self-concept in the school-age child.

Parents. Parents share responsibility for helping children achieve their maximum potential. There are numerous ways in which parents can supplement the school (Home Care box). Cultivating responsibility is the goal of parental assistance. Being responsible for schoolwork helps children learn to keep promises, meet deadlines, and succeed in their jobs as adults. Responsible children may occasionally ask for help (e.g., with a spelling list), but usually they prefer to think through their work by themselves. Excessive pressure or lack of encouragement from parents may inhibit the development of these desirable traits.

Latchkey Children. The term *latchkey children* is used to describe children in elementary school who are left to care for themselves before or after school without the supervision of an adult. The increasing numbers of single-parent families and working mothers, together with the lack of available child care, have created a stress-provoking situation for many schoolchildren. Some of these children may have a chronic illness as well.

Inadequate adult supervision after school leaves children at greater risk for injury and delinquent behavior. In some instances outside activities are curtailed and relationships with peers may be significantly diminished. Latchkey children feel more lonely, isolated, and fearful than children who have someone to care for them. To cope with their fears and anxieties while alone, these children may devise strategies such as hiding, playing the television at loud volume, or using pets as a comfort.

Many communities and persons concerned about their welfare are trying to help children and their parents deal with this potentially serious problem. School-age care programs have been implemented by some communities and employers. It is important to teach self-help skills to these children and provide telephone check-in and reassurance programs.

Limit Setting and Discipline. Numerous factors influence the amount and manner of discipline and limit setting imposed on school-age children: the psychosocial maturity of the parents, the childhood and childrearing experiences of the parents, the temperament of the children, the context of the children's misconduct, and the response of the children to rewards and punishments. As children are increasingly able to see a situation from the point of view of another, they are able to understand the effects of their reactions on others and themselves.

Disciplinary techniques should help children control their own behavior. Reasoning is an effective technique for this age group. With advancing cognitive skills they are able to benefit from more complex types of disciplinary strategies. For example, withholding privileges, requiring compensation, imposing penalties, and contracting can be used with great success. Problem solving is the best approach to limit setting, and children themselves can be included in the process of determining appropriate disciplinary measures.

Dishonest Behavior. During middle childhood children may engage in what is considered to be antisocial behavior. Lying, stealing, and cheating may become manifest in previously well-behaved children. It is especially disturbing to parents, who may have difficulty coping with this behavior.

Lying can occur for a number of reasons. Preschool children often have difficulty distinguishing between fact and fantasy. By the time they reach school age, they still "tell stories" but can distinguish between what is real and what is make-believe. If not, they need to be taught to distinguish between fantasy and reality. Often children will exaggerate a story or situation as a means of impressing their family or friends.

Young children will lie to escape punishment or to get out of some difficulty even when the evidence of their misbehavior is before their eyes. Older children may lie to meet expectations set by others to which they have been unable to measure up. However, most children are very concerned with the wrongness of lying and cheating—especially in their friends. They are quick to tell on others when they detect cheating.

Parents need to be reassured that all children lie sometimes and that they often have difficulty separating fantasy from reality. Parents should be helped to understand the importance of their own behavior as role models and of being truthful in their relationships with children.

Cheating is most common in young children 5 to 6 years of age. They find it difficult to lose at a game or contest, and so they cheat to win. They have not yet acquired the full realization of the wrongness of this behavior and do it almost automatically. It usually disappears as they mature. However, because children model observed behaviors, parents need to be aware of their own behavior. When parents set examples of honesty, children are more likely to conform to these standards.

As with other ethically related behavior, *stealing* is not an unexpected event in the younger child. Between 5 and 8 years of age, children's sense of property rights is limited; they tend to take something simply because they are attracted to it, or take money for what it will buy. They are equally likely to give away something valuable that belongs to them. When young children are caught and punished, they are penitent—they "didn't mean to" and "promise never to do it again"—but it is quite likely that they will repeat the performance the following day. Often they not only steal but will lie about it as well or attempt to justify the act with excuses. It is seldom helpful to trap children into admission by asking directly if they committed the offense. Children do not take on such responsibility until nearer the end of middle childhood.

There are several reasons why children steal: a lack of a sense of property rights, an attempt to acquire the means with which to bribe favors from other children, a strong desire to own the coveted item, or a means for revenge to "get back at someone" (usually a parent) for what they consider to be unfair treatment. Older children may steal to supplement an inadequate income from other sources. Sometimes stealing is an indication that something is seriously wrong or lacking in the child's life. For example, children may steal to make up for love or another satisfaction that they feel is lacking.

In most situations it is best not to attempt to find a hidden or deep meaning to the stealing. An admonition, together with an appropriate and reasonable punishment, such as having the older child pay back the money or return the stolen items, will ordinarily take care of most cases. Most children can be taught to respect the property rights of others with little difficulty despite the temptations and opportunities presented to them. If children's personal rights are respected, they are more likely to respect the rights of others. Some children simply need more time to learn the importance of the culture's rules regarding private property.

Stress and Fear. Children today face more stresses than children in previous generations. Many children are stressed by conflict within the home and have constant anxiety regarding the separation that these disruptions can cause. The school environment is another stressful experience for some children. Competing with classmates for grades and teacher recognition and being labeled as "stupid" or "learning disabled" can result in emotional discomfort. Increasing *violence* within the family, the school, and the community also serves as a major stressor for children.

To help children cope with the stresses in their lives, the parent, teacher, or health care provider must recognize signs that indicate a child is undergoing stress and identify the source promptly.

NURSE ALERT • The nurse who observes the following signs of stress in a child should explore the situation further:

- Stomach pains or headache
- Sleep problems
- Bed-wetting
- Changes in eating habits
- Aggressive or stubborn behavior
- Reluctance to participate
- Regression to earlier behaviors (e.g., thumb-sucking)

Children need to be taught to recognize signs of stress in themselves, such as a pounding heart, rapid breathing, or "butterflies" in the stomach. Once they are able to recognize that they are stressed, they can employ techniques for managing their stress. Probably the most useful technique is to help them plan a means for dealing with any stress through problem solving.

A variety of anxiety symptoms, including fear of the dark, excessive worry about past behavior, self-consciousness, social withdrawal, and an excessive need for reassurance, are considered normal developmental events for children. School-age children are less fearful of body safety than they were as preschoolers, although they still fear being hurt, kidnapped, or having to undergo surgery. They also fear death and are fascinated by all the aspects of death and dying. The fears of noises, darkness, storms, and dogs lessen. Most of the new fears that trouble school-age children are related to school and family.

PROMOTING OPTIMUM HEALTH DURING THE SCHOOL YEARS

When school-age children enter school, they leave the relatively protected environment of home and neighborhood and experience interpersonal contacts with a larger number of children. Many childhood illnesses can be prevented or lessened by careful health supervision. The body's natural defenses against illness can be supported through careful attention to diet, rest, exercise, and protection from extreme mental and physical stress.

Nutrition

Although caloric needs are diminished in relation to body size during middle childhood, resources are being laid down for the increased growth needs of the adolescent period. It is important to impress on children and their parents the value of a balanced diet to promote growth. Because children usually eat as their families do, the quality of their diet depends to a large extent on the family's pattern of eating.

Likes and dislikes established at an early age continue in middle childhood, although the propensity for single food preferences begins to end and children acquire a taste for an increasing variety of foods. However, with the easy availability of fast-food restaurants, the influence of the mass media, and the temptation of an immense variety of "junk food," it is all too easy for children to fill up on empty calories—foods that do not promote growth, such as sugars, starches, and excess fats. The easy availability of high-calorie foods, combined with the tendency toward more sedentary activities, is contributing to an increasing prevalence of childhood obesity. This problem is discussed further in Chapter 40.

Parents do not know what their children eat when they are away from home. A parent may pack a lunch to be eaten at school but be unaware of how much is eaten, traded, sold, or thrown away. Nutrition education can and should be integrated with other classroom learning throughout the child's school years. In school the Food Guide Pyramid (see Fig. 12-4) and the elements of a wholesome diet are learned, as well as how food products are grown, processed, and prepared. The school nurse can take an active role in nutrition education by working with teachers to plan and implement units on nutrition instruction and by working with parents and children to give nutritional guidance.

Sleep and Rest

The amount of sleep and rest required during middle childhood is highly individualized. There is no specific amount needed by a child at any given age. Rather, the amount depends on the child's age, the activity level, and other factors, such as state of health. The growth rate has slowed; therefore less energy is expended in growth than was expended during the preceding periods.

During the school-age years children usually do not require a nap, but they sleep approximately 9½ hours (Blum, Ditmar, and Charney, 1997). Although fewer bedtime problems occur during these years, occasional difficulties are still associated with the necessary bedtime ritual. Usually there is little problem for children 6 or 7 years old, and the task of going to bed can be facilitated by encouraging quiet activity before bedtime, such as coloring or reading. However, most children in middle childhood must be reminded often to go to bed; children 8- to 11-years-old are particularly resistant. Often children are unaware that they are tired; if allowed to remain up later than usual, they are fatigued the following day. Sometimes bedtime resistance can be resolved by allowing a later bedtime in deference to the child's advancing age. Twelve-year-old children usually offer no difficulty in relation to bedtime. Some even retire early in order to enjoy slow preparations for bed, to read, or to listen to music.

Exercise and Activity

The improved capabilities and adaptability of the school-age child permit greater speed and effort in motor activities; larger, stronger muscles permit longer and increasingly strenuous play without exhaustion. During middle childhood, youngsters acquire the coordination, timing, and concentration that are required to participate in adult-type activities, even though they may lack the strength, stamina, and control of the adolescent and adult. Consequently, a greater amount of physical activity should be expected and encouraged during the school years. However, it must be kept in mind that although school-age children are large and appear to be strong, they may not be ready for strenuous competitive athletics.

All growing children need regular exercise and should be afforded opportunities that provide satisfying experiences to meet individual likes and dislikes. Appropriate activities that promote coordination and development during the school-age years include running, jumping rope, swimming, roller-skating, in-line skating, ice-skating, and bicycle riding. Positive reinforcement achieved by experiencing increasingly smooth, rhythmic, and efficient use of the body conditions the child toward regular physical activity.

Exercise is essential for developmental progress in a number of areas, including muscle development and tone, refinement of balance and coordination, increased strength and endurance, and stimulation of body functions and metabolic processes. Children need ample space in which to run, jump, skip, and climb; and safe facilities and equipment to use both indoors and outdoors. Most children need little encouragement to engage in physical activity. They have so much energy that they seldom know when to stop.

Children with disabling conditions or those who hesitate to become involved in active play, such as obese children, require special assessment and help so that activities that appeal to them, are compatible with their limitations, and meet their developmental needs can be determined.

Sports. Much controversy has surrounded the trend toward earlier participation in competitive athletics and the amount and type of competitive sports that are appropriate for children in the elementary grades. The current view is that virtually every child is suited for some sport, and authorities do not discourage participation if children are matched to the type of sport appropriate to their abilities and to their physical and emotional constitution. School-age children enjoy competition, and when those involved with children in this age group understand children's physical limitations and teach them the proper techniques and safety measures necessary to avoid injury to developing bones and muscles, a safe and appropriate sport can be found for even the most unskilled and noncompetitive child (Fig. 39-7).

Various acceptable sports activities available to school-age children include baseball, soccer, gymnastics, and swimming. Equipment should be maintained in safe condition, and protective apparatus should be worn to prevent serious injury (see Traumatic Injury, Chapter 54).

During the school-age years girls have the same basic body structure as boys and thus have a similar response to systematic exercise training. At puberty, when boys become larger and have more muscle mass, it is usually recommended that girls compete only against other girls. Before puberty there is no essential difference in strength and size between girls and boys, making these precautions unnecessary.

Preadolescence is a time to teach fundamental motor skills; develop fitness in a practical, safe, and gradual manner; and promote desired attitudes and values. Activities should include both practice sessions and unstructured play; the actual game or event should be managed in a manner that stresses mastery of the sport and enhancement of self-image rather than winning or pleasing others. All children should have an opportunity to participate, and special ceremonies should recognize all participants rather than individuals.

Acquisition of Skills. School-age children also demonstrate increasing capacities in fine motor facility and complex artistic skills. Handedness is well established by the beginning of the school years, and children make great strides in writing and drawing during this age period. It is a time of energetic and vibrant creative productivity. With the tools of language and

A

B

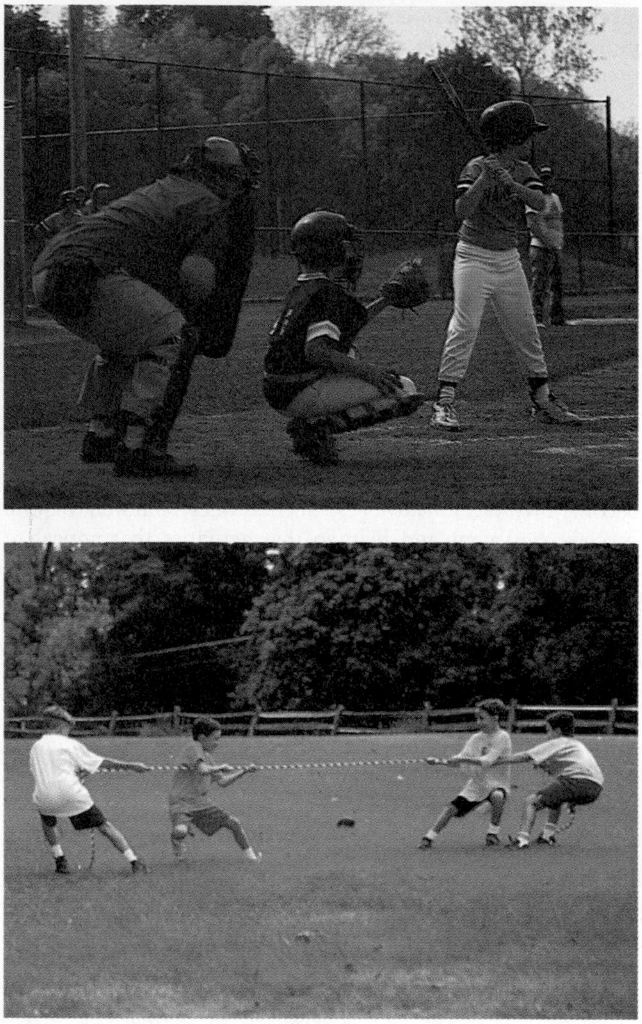

FIG. 39-7 • The activities engaged in by school-age children vary according to interest and opportunity. **A,** Little League competitors. **B,** Playing tug-of-war.

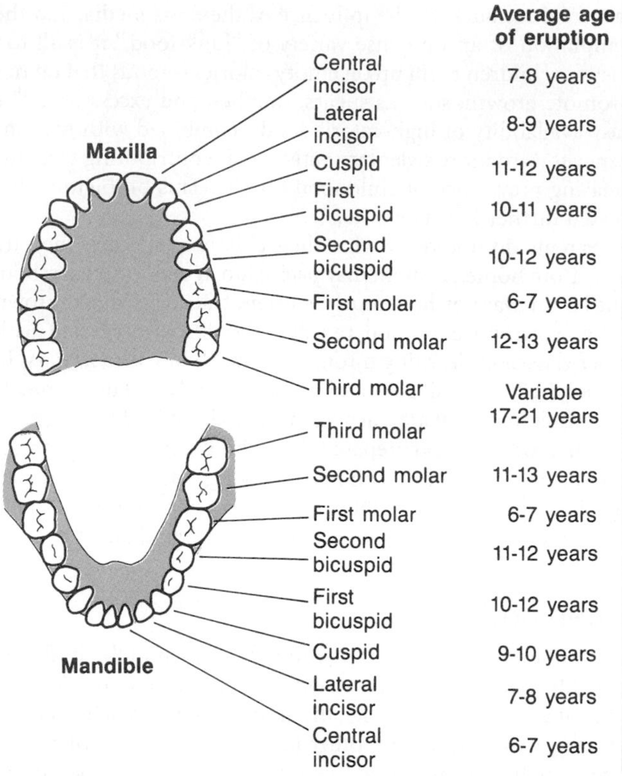

FIG. 39-8 • Sequence of eruption of secondary teeth. (Data from McDonald RE, Avery DR: *Dentistry for the child and adolescent,* ed 6, St Louis, 1994, Mosby.)

reading, children can create poems, stories, and plays. With more advanced fine motor skills, they are able to master an unlimited variety of handicrafts, such as ceramics, needlework, wood carving, and beadwork. They avidly pursue these skills in solitude, with a friend, or in programs offered through organized groups such as boys' or girls' clubs; Scouting; or special interest groups that use crafts or other activities as a means to occupy, entertain, and educate children.

School-age children are capable of assuming responsibility for their own needs, although their distaste for soap and water and "dress" clothes is legendary. School-age children can and want to assume their share of household tasks, which usually are related to the male and female roles that have been defined by their culture. Many also assume responsibility for tasks outside the home, such as baby-sitting, mowing lawns, or paper routes.

Dental Health

The first permanent (secondary) teeth erupt at about 6 years of age, beginning with the 6-year molar, which erupts posterior to the deciduous molars. The others appear in approximately the same order as eruption of the primary teeth (see Teething, Chapter 36) and follow shedding of the deciduous teeth (Fig. 39-8). With the appearance of the second permanent (12-year) molar, most of the permanent teeth are present. Permanent dentition is somewhat more advanced in girls than it is in boys.

Because the permanent teeth erupt during the school-age years, good dental hygiene and regular attention to dental caries are vital parts of health supervision during this period (see Dental Health, Chapter 36). Correct brushing techniques should be taught or reinforced, and the role that fermentable carbohydrates play in production of dental caries should be emphasized. It is important to be alert to possible malocclusion problems that may result from irregular eruption of permanent teeth and that may impair function. Regular dental supervision and continued fluoride supplementation are essential parts of the health maintenance program.

The most effective means of preventing dental caries is proper oral hygiene. Children should be taught to carry out their own dental care with the supervision and guidance of the parents. Parents should learn the brushing technique along with their children, and they should inspect their children's efforts until the children can assume full responsibility.

Teeth should be brushed after meals, after snacks, and at bedtime. Children who brush their teeth often and become accustomed to the feel of a clean mouth at an early age usually maintain the habit throughout life. For the school-age child with mixed and permanent dentition, the best toothbrush is one with soft nylon bristles and an overall length of about 21 cm (6 inches). Numerous methods of brushing have been described and recommended for children, but no conclusive evidence indicates that one method is superior. The thoroughness of the cleaning is more important than the specific technique used. The dentist will assess all factors, such as manipulative skills and special needs of the child, and suggest the most appropriate brushing technique and regimen. Flossing follows brushing. Parents do the flossing until children acquire the manual dexterity needed. Most children are not able to floss properly until about 8 or 9 years of age.

Dental Problems. Limited or inadequate dental care results in the most prevalent of all childhood health problems: dental caries, malocclusion, and periodontal disease. Trauma, especially tooth evulsion, is also an important problem. All of these conditions benefit from early intervention to prevent tooth loss.

Dental caries (cavities) is one of the most common chronic diseases that affect individuals at all ages; it is the principal oral problem in children and adolescents. Reducing the incidence and consequences of the disorder is of primary importance in childhood because dental caries, if untreated, results in total destruction of involved teeth. The ages of greatest vulnerability are 4 to 8 years for the primary dentition and 12 to 18 years for the secondary, or permanent dentition.

Dental caries is a multifactorial disease; it involves susceptible teeth, cariogenic microflora, and an appropriate oral environment. The incidence of lesions and the likelihood of progressive invasion vary considerably and depend on a number of factors being present in the right combination. Oral inspection is an integral part of the nursing assessment of the child. If there is any evidence of dental caries or other unhealthy state, the child is referred for dental services. An alarming number of children do not receive regular dental supervision, and a significant number reach adulthood without having been examined or treated by a dentist.

Periodontal disease, an inflammatory and degenerative condition involving the gums and tissues supporting the teeth, often begins in childhood and accounts for a significant amount of tooth loss in adulthood. The more common periodontal problems are *gingivitis* (simple inflammation of the gums) and *periodontitis* (inflammation of the gums and loss of connective tissue and bone in the supporting structures of the teeth).

The most prevalent periodontal disease, gingivitis, is a reversible inflammatory disease that begins very early in many children and is most often associated with the buildup of plaque on the teeth. Changes take place in the plaque bacteria, in both the type and number of organisms, causing them to release a variety of destructive exotoxins, enzymes, and other noxious agents. They act to produce an inflammatory reaction in the gingival tissues, causing the gums to become red, edematous, tender, and subject to bleeding at the slightest irritation. Management is directed toward prevention by conscientious brushing and flossing, including the use of fluoride. The child should see the dentist at any signs of inflammation or irritation.

Malocclusion occurs when teeth of the upper and lower dental arches do not approximate in the proper relationships; the physiologic function of chewing is less effective and the cosmetic effect is less pleasing. Teeth that are uneven, crowded, or overlapping or are otherwise unable to meet their counterparts in the opposite jaw in the appropriate relationships may be predisposed to disease in later years.

Orthodontic treatment is usually most successful when it is started in the later school-age years or the early teenage years, after the last primary teeth have been shed and before growth ceases. However, referral should be made as soon as malocclusion is evident, since some deformities can be corrected at an earlier age.

Dental injury may occur in childhood and includes fractures of varying degrees of severity, chipping, dislocation, or evulsion. All tooth injuries require prompt treatment by a competent dentist to prevent permanent displacement or loss. Delayed examination and diagnosis of tooth damage can result in infection or pulp involvement. Because it can affect the remaining teeth, replacement of the lost tooth is needed to maintain normal alignment and position of the other teeth.

A tooth that is *evulsed* (i.e., avulsed, exarticulated, or "knocked out") should be replanted by the child, parent, or nurse and stabilized as soon as possible so that the blood supply to the tooth can be reestablished and the tooth kept alive (Emergency box). If the tooth is replaced within 30 minutes, there is a 70% chance that it will become reattached and roots will not resorb or the crown exfoliate. Evulsed primary teeth are usually not reimplanted.

As with all mouth trauma, an evulsed tooth causes a large amount of bleeding, which is frightening to children and their families. Therefore the nurse or anyone faced with dental trauma should be prepared to cope with the emotionality that accompanies tooth evulsion. Using a calm approach and providing gentle reassurance to the child is often successful in reducing anxiety.

> *Emergency*
>
> **EVULSED TOOTH**
>
> Recover tooth.
> Hold tooth by crown; avoid touching root area.
> If tooth is dirty, rinse it gently under running water or saline; be sure to insert stopper in sink or basin (to avoid tooth loss).
> Insert tooth into socket.
> Have child maintain tooth in place.
> Transport child to dentist immediately.
> Avoid sudden stops or sharp turns to prevent dislodging tooth.
>
> **If Child Is Reluctant to Reimplant Tooth:**
>
> Place evulsed tooth in suitable medium for transport:
> a. Cold milk
> b. Saliva—under child's or parent's tongue
> If child is holding tooth in the mouth, avoid sudden stops to prevent swallowing tooth.
> DON'T FORGET TO TAKE TOOTH.

Sex Education

Many children experience some form of sex play during or before preadolescence as a response to normal curiosity, not as a result of love or sexual urge. Children are experimentalists by nature, and this play is incidental and transitory. Any adverse emotional consequences or guilt feelings depend on how the behavior is managed by the parents, if it is discovered; and whether children view their actions as wrong in the eyes of significant persons, particularly the parents.

The child's attitude toward sex is acquired indirectly at a very early age. Initial curiosity about differences in body structure between boys and girls and between children and adults arises in the preschool years. Middle childhood is an ideal time for formal sex education, and many authorities believe that the topic is best presented from a life-span approach. Information about sexual maturation and the process of reproduction helps to minimize the child's uncertainty, embarrassment, and feelings of isolation that often accompany puberty.

An important component of ongoing sex education is effective communication with parents. If parents either repress the child's sexual curiosity or avoid dealing with it, the sexual information that the child receives may be acquired almost entirely from peers. When peers are the primary source of sexual information, it is transmitted and exchanged in secret conversation and contains a large amount of misinformation.

Nurse's Role in Sex Education. No matter where nurses practice, they can provide information on human sexuality to both parents and children. To discuss the topic adequately, nurses must have an understanding of the physiologic aspects of sexuality; a knowledge of cultural and societal values; and an awareness of their own attitudes, feelings, and biases about sexuality.

When sexual information is presented to school-age children, sex should be treated as a normal part of growth and development. Questions should be answered honestly, matter-of-factly, and to the same extent as questions about other topics. Answers should be at the child's level of understanding. There may be times when boys and girls should be taught content separately.

Children need help to differentiate sex and sexuality. Exercises on clarifying values, identifying role models, engaging in problem-solving skills, and practicing responsibility are important to prepare children for early adolescence and puberty. In addition, children need to have sexual information that is provided via the media or jokes explained and defused. Information concerning human immunodeficiency virus (HIV) infection should be presented in simple, accurate terms and should focus on how HIV is transmitted.

Preadolescents need precise and concrete information that will allow them to answer questions such as "What if I start my period in the middle of class?" or "How can I keep people from telling I have an erection?" It is important to tell them what they want to know and what they can expect to happen as they become mature sexually.

During encounters with parents, nurses can be open and available for questions and discussion. They can set an example by the language they use in discussing body parts and their function, and by the way in which they deal with problems that have emotional overtones, such as exploratory sex play and masturbation. Parents need to be helped to understand normal behaviors and to view sexual curiosity in their children as a part of the developmental process. Assessing the parents' level of knowledge and understanding of sexuality provides cues to their need for supplemental information that will better prepare them for the increasingly complex explanations that will be needed as their children grow older.

School Health

Child health maintenance is ultimately the responsibility of the parents; however, the public schools and health departments in the United States have contributed to the improvement of child health by providing a healthful school environment, health services, and health education that emphasizes sound health practices. Most of these functions constitute major components of community health services and involve large amounts of public funds and large numbers of health professionals, including nurses.

A school health program is involved in ongoing health maintenance through assessment, screening, and referral activities. Routine health services provided by most schools include health appraisal, emergency care, safety education, communicable disease control, counseling, and follow-up care. Health education of schoolchildren is directed toward providing knowledge of health and toward influencing habits, attitudes, and conduct in relation to health and injury prevention.

Traditionally, school nurses have been viewed from a limited perspective that placed them in the role of disease detector, applier of bandages, and official caregiver in cases of illness and injury. Although these are still important functions, this traditional role has acquired much broader dimensions. School nurses provide primary health care on a broader scale that includes assessment of physical, psychomedical, psychoeducational, behavioral, and learning disorder problems and comprehensive well-child care. In many settings, school health services have been enlarged to meet the needs of not only schoolchildren, but also their families and the community. School nurse practitioners play an essential role in these school-based centers.

The passage of Public Laws 94-142 and 99-457 required the integration of children with chronic illness or disability into regular classrooms. School nurses are responsible for the medical and nursing needs of these children in the school setting. School nurses also develop, implement, and evaluate the health care plans for these children. Unfortunately, not all schools have a school nurse, and the use of unlicensed assistive personnel (UAP) is increasing. School nurses are faced with the delegation to and supervision of UAP (National Association of School Nurse Consultants, 1995; Rhodes, 1997). School nurses must use nursing assessment and professional judgment in deciding which procedures may be delegated to UAP.

Injury Prevention

Because school-age children have developed more refined muscular coordination and control, and can apply their cognitive capacities to a more judicious course of action, the incidence of injury is diminished in children in this age group as compared with the incidence in early childhood.

The most common cause of severe injury and death in school-age children is motor vehicle accidents—either as pedestrian or passenger. It is imperative that nurses continue to emphasize the importance of three automobile safety measures that have been found to reduce the severity of injuries: effective restraint systems, door-lock mechanisms, and appropriate passenger-seating locations in the motor vehicle. In particular, the American Academy of Pediatrics (1996) recommends that children under the age of 12 years not ride in the front passenger seat of cars with air bags.*

The school-age child's desire for riding bicycles increases the risk of injury on streets and byways. Other serious injuries include accidents on skateboards, roller skates, in-line skates, skis, and other sports equipment. All-terrain vehicles (ATVs), popular with children under 16 years of age, are unstable, difficult to handle, and responsible for an increasing number of childhood

*Guidelines for car seat safety are also available in Wong DL, Hess CS: ***Wong and Whaley's clinical manual of pediatric nursing,*** ed 5, St Louis, 2000, Mosby.

injuries. The American Academy of Pediatrics (1994) views ATVs as a major health hazard for children and opposes their use by children less than 16 years of age.

Most injuries occur in or near the home or school. The most effective means of prevention is education of the child and family regarding the hazards of risk taking and improper use of the equipment. Safety helmets, protective eye and mouth shields, and protective padding are strongly recommended for children engaging in active sports, even though they may not be required equipment. For example, falls from bicycles, ATVs, and skating devices are the cause of a significant number of head injuries in school-age children. Because head injury is the major cause of bicycle-related fatalities, the most important aspect of bicycle safety is to encourage the rider to wear a protective helmet (Fig. 39-9) (American Academy of Pediatrics, 1995). Physically active school-age children are highly susceptible to cuts and abrasions, and the incidence of childhood fractures, strains, and sprains is noteworthy. Trampoline injuries are highest in children 5 through 14 years, and account for numerous fractures, sprains, and head injuries. The American Academy of Pediatrics (1999) recommends against the use of trampolines in the home environment, in routine physical education classes, or in outdoor playgrounds. Injuries of a serious nature are discussed elsewhere in the book: burns (Chapter 53), eye trauma (Chapter 42), near-drowning (Chapter 51), and head injuries (Chapter 51). The prevalence of injuries depends on the dangers present in the environment, the protection offered by adults, and the behavior patterns of the children. Table 39-2 lists the major developmental accomplishments and suggestions for injury prevention, and the Home Care boxes provide guidelines for bicycle, skateboard, and in-line skate safety.

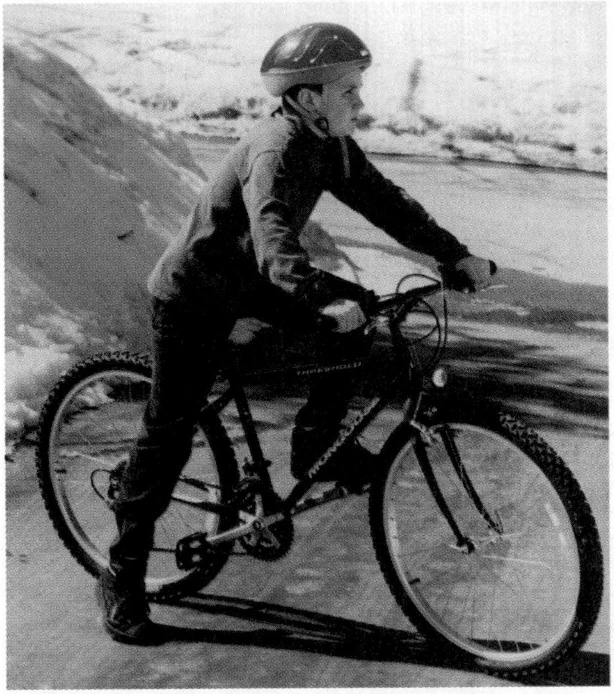

FIG. 39-9 • The right-size bike is important; child should be able to sit on the bike and place balls of both feet on ground. Foot should comfortably reach and manipulate the pedal in the down position. Wearing a protective helmet is mandatory. Helmet should sit on top of head in a level position and should not rock back and forth or from side to side. Strap should always be fastened securely under the chin.

Anticipatory Guidance—Care of Families

Parents of the school-age child find themselves in the position of sharing their child's time with the increasingly important

Home Care

BICYCLE SAFETY

- Always wear properly fitted bicycle helmet that is approved by Snell or the American National Standards Institute (ANSI); replace damaged helmet.
- Ride bicycles with traffic and away from parked cars.
- Ride single file.
- Walk bicycles through busy intersections only at crosswalks.
- Give hand signals well in advance of turning or stopping.
- Keep as close to the curb as practical.
- Watch for drain grates, potholes, soft shoulders, and loose dirt or gravel.
- Keep both hands on handlebars, except with signaling.
- Never ride double on a bicycle.
- Do not carry packages that interfere with vision or control; do not drag objects behind bike.
- Watch for and yield to pedestrians.
- Watch for cars backing up or pulling out of driveways; be especially careful at intersections.
- Look left, right, then left again before turning into traffic or roadway.
- Never hitch a ride on a truck or other vehicle.
- Learn rules of the road and respect for traffic officers.
- Obey all local ordinances.
- Wear shoes that fit securely while riding.
- Wear light colors at night and attach fluorescent material to clothing and bicycle.
- Be certain the bicycle is the correct size for rider.
- Equip bicycle with proper lights and reflectors.
- Have bicycle inspected to ensure good mechanical condition.
- Children riding as passengers must wear appropriate-size helmets in specially designed protective seats.

From American Academy of Pediatrics, Committee on Injury and Poison Prevention: Bicycle helmets, *Pediatrics* 95(4):609-610, 1995.

Home Care

SKATEBOARD AND IN-LINE SKATE SAFETY

- Children younger than 5 years of age should not use skateboard or in-line skates. They are not developmentally prepared to protect themselves from injury.
- Children who use skateboards or in-line skates should wear helmets and other protective equipment, especially on knees, wrists, and elbows, to prevent injury.
- Skateboards and in-line skates should never be used near traffic. Their use should be prohibited on streets and highways. Activities that bring skateboards and vehicles together (e.g., "catching a ride") are especially dangerous.
- Some types of use, such as riding homemade ramps on hard surfaces, may be particularly hazardous.

Modified from American Academy of Pediatrics, Committee on Injury and Poison Prevention: Skateboard injuries, *Pediatrics* 95(4):611-612, 1995.

TABLE 39-2
Injury Prevention during School-Age Years

Developmental Abilities Related to Risk of Injury	Injury Prevention
Is increasingly involved in activities away from home Is excited by speed and motion Is easily distracted by environment Can be reasoned with	***Motor vehicle accidents*** Educate child regarding proper use of seat belts while a passenger in a vehicle Maintain discipline while a passenger in a vehicle (e.g., keep arms inside, do not lean against doors or interfere with driver) Remind parents and children that no one should ride in the bed of a pickup truck Emphasize safe pedestrian behavior Insist on wearing safety apparel (e.g., helmet) when applicable, such as riding bicycle, motorcycle, mo-ped, or all-terrain vehicle (see Home Care box, p. 955)
Is apt to overdo May work hard to perfect a skill Has cautious, but not fearful, gross motor actions Likes swimming	***Drowning*** Teach child to swim Teach basic rules of water safety Select safe and supervised places to swim Check sufficient water depth for diving Swim with a companion Use an approved flotation device in water or boat Advocate for legislation requiring fencing around pools Learn cardiopulmonary resuscitation (CPR)
Has increasing independence Is adventuresome Enjoys trying new things	***Burns*** Make sure smoke detectors are in homes Set water heaters to 48.9° C (120° F) to prevent scald burns Instruct child in behavior in areas involving contact with potential burn hazards (e.g., gasoline, matches, bonfires or barbecues, lighter fluid, firecrackers, cigarette lighters, cooking utensils, chemistry sets); avoid climbing or flying kite around high-tension wires Instruct child in proper behavior in the event of fire (e.g., fire drills at home and school) Teach child safe cooking (use low heat; avoid any frying; be careful of steam burns, scalds, or exploding foods, especially from microwaving)
Adheres to group rules May be easily influenced by peers Has strong allegiance to friends	***Poisoning*** Educate child regarding hazards of taking nonprescription drugs and chemicals, including aspirin and alcohol Teach child to say "no" if offered illegal or dangerous drugs or alcohol Keep potentially dangerous products in properly labeled receptacles, preferably out of reach
Has increased physical skills Needs strenuous physical activity Is interested in acquiring new skills and perfecting attained skills Is daring and adventurous, especially with peers Frequently plays in hazardous places Confidence often exceeds physical capacity Desires group loyalty and has strong need for friends' approval Attempts hazardous feats Accompanies friends to potentially hazardous facilities Delights in physical activity Is likely to overdo Growth in height exceeds muscular growth and coordination	***Bodily damage*** Help provide facilities for supervised activities Encourage playing in safe places Keep firearms safely locked up except during adult supervision Teach proper care of, use of, and respect for devices with potential danger (e.g., power tools, firecrackers) Teach children not to tease or surprise dogs, invade their territory, take dogs' toys, or interfere with dogs' feeding Stress eye, ear, or mouth protection when using potentially hazardous sports Do not permit use of trampolines except as part of supervised training Teach safety regarding use of corrective devices (glasses); if child wears contact lenses, monitor duration of wear to prevent corneal damage Stress careful selection, use, and maintenance of sports and recreation equipment, such as skateboards and in-line skates (see Home Care box, p. 955) Emphasize proper conditioning, safe practices, and use of safety equipment for sports or recreational activities Caution against engaging in hazardous sports, such as those involving trampolines

TABLE 39-2—cont'd
Injury Prevention during School-Age Years

Developmental Abilities Related to Risk of Injury	Injury Prevention
	Bodily damage—cont'd Use safety glass and decals on large glassed areas, such as sliding glass doors Use window guards to prevent falls Teach name, address, and phone number and emphasize that child should ask for help from appropriate people (e.g., cashier, security guard, police) if lost; have identification on child (e.g., sewn in clothes, inside shoe) Teach stranger safety: Avoid personalized clothing in public places Caution child to never go with a stranger Have child tell parents if anyone makes child feel uncomfortable in any way Always listen to child's concerns regarding others' behavior Teach child to say "no" when confronted with uncomfortable situations

Home Care

GUIDANCE DURING SCHOOL YEARS

Age 6 Years

Prepare parents to expect strong food preferences and frequent refusal of specific food items.
Prepare parents to expect increasingly ravenous appetite.
Prepare parents for emotionality as child experiences erratic mood changes.
Help parents anticipate continued susceptibility to illness.
Teach injury prevention and safety, especially bicycle safety.
Encourage parents to respect child's need for privacy and to provide a separate bedroom for child, if possible.
Prepare parents for child's increasing interests outside the home.
Help parents understand the need to encourage child's interactions with peers.

Ages 7 to 10 Years

Prepare parents to expect improvement in health with fewer illnesses, but warn them that allergies may increase or become apparent.
Prepare parents to expect an increase in minor injuries.
Emphasize caution in selecting and maintaining sports equipment and re-emphasize safety.
Prepare parents to expect increased involvement with peers and interest in activities outside the home.
Emphasize the need to encourage independence while maintaining limit setting and discipline.
Prepare mothers to expect more demands at 8 years.
Prepare fathers to expect increasing admiration at 10 years; encourage father-child activities.
Prepare parents for prepubescent changes in girls.

Ages 11 to 12 Years

Help parents prepare child for body changes of pubescence.
Prepare parents to expect a growth spurt in girls.
Make certain child's sex education is adequate with accurate information.
Prepare parents to expect energetic but stormy behavior at 11 years to become more even-tempered at 12 years.
Encourage parents to support child's desire to "grow up" but to allow regressive behavior when needed.
Prepare parents to expect an increase in masturbation.
Instruct parents that the amount of rest the child needs may increase.
Help parents educate child regarding experimentation with potentially harmful activities.

Health Guidance

Help parents understand the importance of regular health and dental care for the child.
Encourage parents to teach and model sound health practices, including diet, rest, activity, and exercise.
Stress the need to encourage children to engage in appropriate physical activities.
Emphasize providing a safe physical and emotional environment.
Encourage parents to teach and model safety practices.

peer group. It is through early peer relationships that children begin to prepare for moving from narrow, sheltered family relationships to a broader world of relationships and increased independence. Parents must learn to provide support as unobtrusively as possible without feeling rejected, hurt, or angry. The nurse can help parents of the school-age child by providing anticipatory guidance and reassurance throughout this period of child development and maturation (Home Care box).

HEALTH PROBLEMS RELATED TO SPORTS PARTICIPATION

Every sport has some potential for injury to the participant, whether the youngster engages in serious competition or participates for enjoyment. Serious injury can occur during rough contact sports or to persons who are not physically prepared for the activity. The risk of injury is greater if the youngster's body build is not suited to the sport, if the muscles and support systems (respiratory and cardiovascular) are insufficiently conditioned to withstand the rigors of the physical stress, or if the youngster lacks the insight and judgment to recognize when an activity is beyond his or her capabilities. More injuries occur during recreational sports participation than during organized athletic competition.

Not only does the activity itself pose a hazard of greater or lesser degree (Fig. 39-10), but the environment and the sports or recreational equipment present additional risks. Children participate in physical activity in a variety of environments: both indoors and outdoors, on floors, on the ground, on snow, on or beneath water surfaces, and sometimes in free air space. These activities often involve equipment that intensifies the risk factor.

Acute overload injuries are those that occur suddenly during an activity and that produce immediate symptoms. They can be caused by a blow or by overstretching, twisting, or sudden stress to tissues. For descriptions and management of traumatic injuries, see Chapter 54.

Overuse Syndromes

To excel in sports, the young athlete is forced to train longer, harder, and earlier in life than previously. The rewards are an increased level of fitness, better performances, faster times, and the satisfaction of attaining a personal goal. However, the risk of overuse injury is always present and can be related to several factors: training errors, muscle-tendon imbalance, anatomic malalignment, incorrect footwear or playing surface, an associated disease state, and growth.

The common feature in overuse injuries is the repetitive microtrauma that occurs to a particular anatomic structure when the same movements are performed over a long period of time; the end result is inflammation of the involved structure with complaints of pain, tenderness, swelling, and disability. Examples of overuse syndromes include "Little League elbow" (tendinitis and osteochondritis from repetitive throwing), "tennis elbow" (lateral epicondylitis from repetitive elbow strain), and Osgood-Schlatter disease (traction apophysitis of the tibial tubercle).

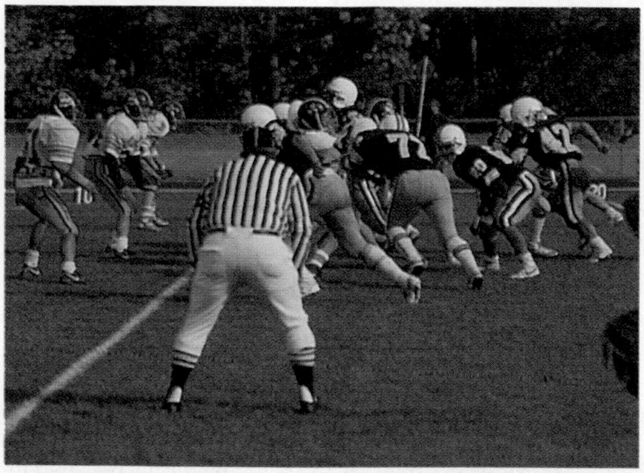

FIG. 39-10 • Football is an example of a strenuous contact sport.

Stress Fractures. Stress fractures occur as a result of repeated muscle contraction and are seen most often in repetitive weight-bearing sports such as running, gymnastics, and basketball. They occur less often in swimmers. The most common symptoms are a sharp, persistent, progressive pain or a deep, persistent, dull ache located over the bone. Sometimes there is pain on impact (heel strike), but the most important clinical sign is pain over the involved bony surface. Diagnosis is established on the basis of clinical observation; occasionally a bone scan may be needed.

Therapeutic Management. Development of inflammation is common to all overuse syndromes; therefore the management is directed toward rest or alteration of activities, physical therapy, and medication. Rest is the primary therapy and is usually interpreted as reduced activity and the use of alternative exercise—*not* bed rest or immobilization with casting. The primary purpose is to alleviate the repetitive stress that initiated the symptoms. It is important to keep the youngster mobile. Training can be continued with alternative exercise that maintains conditioning without aggravating the injury. For example, pool running (treading water in the deep end of a pool) can use the same movements as running but without the weight bearing.

Other modalities include cryotherapy and cold whirlpools. Sometimes taping, bracing, splinting, and other orthotics are employed (treatment is very specific to the injury). Medications such as nonsteroidal antiinflammatory drugs are prescribed for discomfort. Topical medications are of questionable value.

Nurse's Role in Sports for Children and Adolescents

Nurses may become involved in sports activities in the areas of preparation and evaluation for activities, prevention of injury, treatment of injuries, and rehabilitation after injury. Selecting an appropriate sport for both recreation and competition is a joint effort of youngsters, parents, and health professionals. The best approach to counseling children and parents regarding sports participation is to encourage activities that are most likely to provide pleasure and physical benefits throughout childhood and into adulthood. Exposure to a variety of sports activities is probably better for young children than limiting them to one sport. In order that children have ample time for other activities and associations, parents should be cautioned against overprogramming them.

When children sustain athletic injuries, nurses are often responsible for instructing the children and their parents regarding care. Instructions (e.g., schedule for appointments, application of ice, and any restrictions in activity) should be made clear and preferably be accompanied by written directions. The importance of taking medications as prescribed is emphasized, because they may be needed for an extended time and compliance may be difficult.

Prevention of sports injuries is probably the most important aspect of any athletic program. Children should be suited to the activity, and the environment and equipment should be safe for physical activity. Children should be adequately prepared for the sport, especially if it requires strenuous and/or continuous physical exertion. A comprehensive preseason medical examination to identify any conditions that may be exacerbated by athletic activities is recommended (Hergenroeder, 1998).

Nurses, coaches and athletic trainers should collaborate to ensure that safety measures are carried out. Stretching exercises, warm-up and cool-down activities, and an appropriate training program are important for safe participation. Protective measures such as pads, taping, and wrapping are important for areas at risk for injury. Adequate hydration during activities is essential, and requiring sufficient medical coverage at all athletic events is important to ensure prompt treatment for injuries (Hergenroeder, 1998).

ALTERED GROWTH AND MATURATION

The absence of physical and/or sexual maturation at a time when other children are experiencing positive evidence of sexual development and its associated spurt in growth and physical strength is a matter of concern to both the parents and their affected child. Fortunately, in most instances the delay in development is a simple physiologic or *constitutional delay* that merely represents one end of the normal genetically influenced variation of pubertal growth. These children will go through a delayed but normal puberty to finally catch up, in their late teens, with their more rapidly developing age-mates. Less benign causes of delayed development may be of endocrine origin or chromosomal aberrations. In other situations delayed development may be a result of chronic diseases (e.g., malabsorption or chronic asthma) that are serious enough to retard the developmental process; or environmental factors (e.g., stress or poor nutrition).

The rate of maturation is important during the school years, but at puberty it assumes gigantic proportions to youngsters and their parents as well. Girls or boys who lag behind their peers in physical maturation are painfully aware of their shortcomings. Adolescent girls with delayed maturation feel out of place among companions whose hips and breasts are developing, feel cheated if they have not yet menstruated, and may not be a part of the giggling and boy talk of friends. Adolescent boys with delayed maturation feel weak and small compared with more muscular companions with whom they can no longer compete. Slow-maturing youngsters need support and reassurance that they are not abnormal and that they, too, will develop the characteristics for which they yearn.

Serial measurements of growth are plotted periodically on standard growth charts to determine the pattern of growth and to compare the individual child with the norm for that particular age group. When assessing children in the extremes of height ranges, it is important to compare their height with the height of their parents and siblings.

Tall or Short Stature

Tall Stature. Despite the fact that the average height of both boys and girls is steadily increasing, there is a small group of children who, because of some organic disorder or a familial tendency, are excessively tall when compared with their peers. To some, especially boys, it may be a source of pride; to others, especially girls, it may be a source of intense anxiety and a severe social handicap.

When the rate of height change before puberty suggests the probability of excessive adult height, treatment with hormones may be considered, although there is a great deal of controversy regarding their use for this purpose. The use of estrogens has proved effective in controlling height when therapy is initiated before menarche and before the end of the adolescent growth spurt that normally precedes menarche. The selection of children for hormonal therapy is made on the basis of a careful evaluation of physical, psychologic, and social factors.

Short Stature. Short stature is a nonspecific finding that may be the first manifestation of a serious disorder, or it may be of no consequence medically. From a worldwide point of view, the most common cause of short stature and/or delayed development is probably inadequate nutrition; however, the major disorders that produce delayed development are chronic diseases, endocrine dysfunction, and syndromes of primary gonadal failure.

Chronic diseases can interfere with growth; but unless the illness is unduly prolonged, catch-up growth will occur. Diseases and disorders that usually cause some degree of growth delay include asthma, cystic fibrosis, gastrointestinal diseases (e.g., parasitic infections), malabsorption syndromes, cardiac anomalies, and chronic renal disturbances. The duration of the illness is more significant than the intensity in terms of the effect on growth, although the precise length of time necessary to affect growth permanently has not been determined.

Skeletal disorders that affect growth in stature are principally those described as dwarfism. Most are caused by a variety of congenital defects and disorders (e.g., achondroplasia) and by some of the inborn errors of metabolism (e.g., Hurler or Hunter syndrome).

Psychosocial, or *deprivation dwarfism* is a stress-induced growth failure that appears to be more common than previously thought. It is defined as growth retardation in children over 2 years of age caused by environmental (emotional) stress. It is associated with a marked delay in physical growth, delayed developmental skills, and immature behavior. When these children are removed from the deprived environment, their growth proceeds at a normal or increased rate. (See also Failure to Thrive, Chapter 36, and Child Maltreatment, Chapter 38.)

Management consists of continued medical observation, attention to general health and nutrition, and psychologic support. Where growth delay is accompanied by poor self-esteem, many authorities recommend hormonal therapy. Testosterone in carefully regulated doses has proved effective in some cases. Growth hormone is capable of increasing height and is used to treat growth hormone deficiency (see Hypopituitarism, Chapter 52). Its use with children who have constitutional delay is highly controversial.

Nursing Care Management. Deviation from the normal course of puberty is always of concern to the affected adolescent, and to some the concern assumes monumental proportions. Most of the problems of delayed development are those caused by simple constitutional delay of puberty, and in this situation the child can be assured that the normal course of events will eventually take place.

One of the difficulties related to a size that is incongruent with chronologic and mental age is the manner in which others, especially adults, relate to the child. People quite naturally respond to children with short stature as though they are younger than their age. Consequently, these children often react with babyish or juvenile behavior, thus setting in motion a circular pattern of behavior and response. Conversely, children who are tall or physically advanced for their age are commonly treated as though they are more advanced than their years. They are often considered to be retarded or behaviorally immature when they actually perform according to the normal behavioral expectations for their age.

Listening to distressed adolescents and conveying to them interest and concern are prerequisite to any successful intervention. Counseling and therapy are individualized to meet the needs of each youngster. Encouraging these children to accentuate the positive aspects of their bodies and personalities with sound health practices and good grooming helps foster a more positive self-image.

Sex Chromosome Abnormalities

Compared with most hereditary disorders, sex chromosome abnormalities are encountered with relatively high frequency, Most are caused by an alteration in sex chromosome number, some of which are listed in Table 39-3. The more common of these are Turner and Klinefelter syndromes. The following are some general characteristics of sex chromosome abnormalities:

- There is a direct relationship between the male or female body type and the presence or absence of a Y chromosome. It appears that the Y chromosome is essential for development of male characteristics.
- The severity of defects is not related to the number of extra X chromosomes, except for mental retardation, which increases proportionately with each X chromosome.
- The presence of more than one Y chromosome appears to have variable but as yet not well-defined effects on an individual.
- The majority of these conditions are due to nondisjunction.

Turner Syndrome. Turner syndrome is caused by absence of one of the X chromosomes; as a result, the number of chromosomes in these girls is 45: 44 pairs of autosomes and 1 X chromosome (45,X). The incidence of the condition in the population has been estimated at 1 in 2500 female births. Although this disorder is often recognized at birth by the signs of a webbed neck, low posterior hairline, widely spaced nipples, and edema of the hands and feet, it is diagnosed most commonly at puberty because of three outstanding features: short stature, sexual infantilism, and amenorrhea.

Girls with Turner syndrome will always be sterile. They have been found to have difficulty with peer relationships and understanding social cues. They exhibit more behavioral problems, especially in relation to immature, socially isolated behavior. Definitive diagnosis is confirmed on the basis of a negative sex chromatin test; chromosome analysis is rarely necessary.

Therapy is always individualized for these girls and consists primarily of hormone treatment and psychologic counseling for both child and parents. Linear growth often can be increased by the administration of growth hormone, provided that therapy is begun early. Estrogen therapy is initiated during the usual time for puberty to promote the development of secondary sex characteristics. Responses to estrogen therapy vary from girl to girl, but gradual feminization is accomplished to some degree in most individuals.

Klinefelter Syndrome. The most common of all chromosomal abnormalities, Klinefelter syndrome is caused by the presence of one or more additional X chromosomes. The majority of males with this syndrome have a chromosome complement of 47,XXY. In young boys this disorder is seldom diag-

TABLE 39-3
Common Sex Chromosome Abnormalities

Syndrome	Chromosomal Nomenclature	Phenotype	Incidence (Live Births)	Clinical Manifestations
Turner	45,X or 45XO	Female	1:2500 female births*	Short stature; webbed neck; low posterior hairline; shield-shaped chest with widely spaced nipples; sterile; no development of secondary sex characteristics
Triple X, or superfemale	47,XXX (can also be 48,XXXX or 49,XXXXX)	Female	1:850-1250 female births	Normal female characteristics; usually tall; variable mental capacity and behavior; at risk for impaired learning; fertile
XYY male	47,XYY (can also be 48,XYYY or mosaic)	Male	1:900 male births*	Usually normal sexual development; tendency to be tall with long head; poor coordination; may demonstrate aberrant behavior
Klinefelter	47,XXY (48,XXYY, 48,XXXY, 49,XXXXY, and so on, mosaics)	Male	1:850 male births*	Tall with long legs; hypogenitalism; sterile; male secondary sex characteristics may be deficient; may demonstrate aberrant behavior; learning disabled; possible gynecomastia
Fragile X (see also Chapter 42)	46,XY or 46,XX	Predominantly male	Not established	Normocephaly or macrocephaly; prominent mandible; large ears; macro-orchidism; mental retardation

*Data from Nora JJ, Fraser FC: *Medical genetics: principles and practice*, ed 3, Philadelphia, 1989, Lea & Febiger.

nosed before puberty, at which time varying degrees of failure of adolescent virilization occur. Some males are not detected until they appear for evaluation for infertility. All have absence of sperm in the semen (azoospermia), small testes, and defective development of secondary sex characteristics. The incidence of Klinefelter syndrome is estimated to be approximately 1 in 850 live male births. In 80% of these boys there is a chromatin-positive buccal smear, and the extra chromosome is apparent on chromosome analysis.

Cognitive impairment of varying degrees is a common finding and appears to have a direct relationship to the number of X chromosomes in the cells. Boys with Klinefelter syndrome may also have gross motor skill difficulties, developmental language delay, poor verbal skills, and reduced auditory memory. Shyness, passivity, behavioral problems, and school difficulties are often associated with the disorder, but this may be related to the difference in body build and delayed development.

The major effort in medical treatment is directed toward enhancing the masculine characteristics through the administration of male hormones, principally testosterone. Cosmetic surgery will eliminate embarrassment for the boy with gynecomastia.

Nursing Care Management. The nursing care of children with Turner or Klinefelter syndrome is primarily supportive. Nurses assist in diagnosis, explain tests and therapies to children and families, and provide support and encouragement. Since both disorders render the individual unable to reproduce, psychologic counseling, as well as modification of sex education, will be an important aspect of care. Marriage and sexual relationships are still possible, and alternative reproductive options, such as artificial insemination and adoption, should be discussed.

BEHAVIORAL DISORDERS

Attention Deficit Hyperactivity Disorder (ADHD) and Learning Disability (LD)

ADHD refers to developmentally inappropriate degrees of inattention, impulsiveness, and hyperactivity. To be diagnosed as ADHD, the symptoms must have been present before the age of 7 years and must be present in at least two settings. In addition, the persistence of developmentally inappropriate and marked inattention must not be a symptom of another disorder (American Academy of Pediatrics, 2000). An LD refers to a heterogeneous group of disorders manifested by significant difficulties in acquisition and use of listening, speaking, reading, writing, reasoning, mathematics abilities, or social skills.

ADHD and LD conditions affect every aspect of the child's life but are most obvious in the classroom. Early identification of affected children is needed, since the characteristics of the disorder significantly interfere with the normal course of emotional and psychologic development. Many children develop maladaptive behavior patterns that impede psychosocial adjustment while they try to cope with cognitive dysfunction. Their behavior evokes negative responses from others, and repeated exposure to negative feedback adversely affects their self-concept. Research has documented decreased self-perception and increased problems in scholastic competence, social acceptance, and behavioral conduct in children with ADHD (Dumas and Pelletier, 1999).

Diagnostic Evaluations. The behaviors exhibited by the child with ADHD are not unusual aspects of child behavior. The difference lies in the quality of motor activity and developmentally inappropriate inattention, impulsivity, and hyperactivity that the child displays. The manifestations may be numerous or few, mild or severe, and will vary with the developmental level of the child. Any given child will not have every manifestation that is characteristic of the syndrome. The diagnostic criteria established by the American Psychiatric Association (1994) for identifying the child with ADHD are outlined in Box 39-1.

A comprehensive battery of tests is needed to confirm a learning disability. These include intelligence tests (these children tend to have normal or above-average IQs), hand-eye coordination tests, and measurements of auditory and visual perception, comprehension, and memory. Often there is a wide gap between verbal and performance scores on IQ tests.

Therapeutic Management. Management of the child with ADHD usually involves multiple approaches that include family education and counseling, medication, proper classroom placement, environmental manipulation, and sometimes behavioral and/or psychotherapy for the child. Interventions for children with LD are primarily educational.

Medication. Many drugs have been advocated for management of symptoms of ADHD. The most commonly prescribed medications are dextroamphetamine sulfate (Dexedrine) or methylphenidate hydrochloride (Ritalin); however, not all children benefit from medications. Children taking stimulant medication may have symptoms that include nervousness, insomnia, increased blood pressure, and decreased appetite with subsequent weight loss. Long-term use of dextroamphetamine may result in suppression of growth (Critical Thinking box).

Environmental Manipulation. In ADHD the child's environment is simplified by decreasing external stimuli and distractions, reducing alternatives, increasing consistency in routines, and encouraging desired patterns of behavior. Parents need to develop firm but reasonable limits and provide a stable and predictable environment with regular routines of sleeping, eating, working, and playing.

Classroom Education. Special activities are designed to address deficits in visual perception, auditory perception, and other areas involving integration and coordination. The purpose of programs for children with special learning disabilities is to assist them toward more successful achievement, personal adjustment, and eventual retention in the regular classroom. However, according to Public Law 94-142, the Education for All Handicapped Children's Act, children with ADHD or LD must receive free public education in the least restrictive environment (see Chapters 29 and 41).

Prognosis. In the majority of affected children, the disorder is relatively stable through early adolescence. Some children experience decreased symptoms during late adolescence and adulthood, but two thirds of children carry the symptoms into middle adulthood (O'Connell, 1996).

Children with LD grow up to be adults with LD. The goal is to help them identify and compensate for their areas of weakness.

Nursing Care Management. Nurses are active participants in all aspects of management of the child with ADHD or LD. Nurses in the community setting work with families in the home and with school personnel on a long-term basis to help plan and implement therapeutic regimens and to evaluate the effectiveness of therapy. They should explain that children tak-

Box 39-1

Diagnostic Criteria for Attention Deficit Hyperactivity Disorder

A. Either (1) or (2):
   (1) Six (or more) of the following symptoms of ***inattention*** have persisted for at least 6 months to a degree that is maladaptive and inconsistent with developmental level:
   Inattention
   (a) Often fails to give close attention to details or makes mistakes in schoolwork, or other activities
   (b) Often has difficulty sustaining attention in tasks or play activities
   (c) Often does not seem to listen when spoken to directly
   (d) Often does not follow through on instructions and fails to finish schoolwork, chores, or duties in the workplace (not because of oppositional behavior or failure to understand instructions)
   (e) Often has difficulty organizing tasks and activities
   (f) Often avoids, dislikes, or is reluctant to engage in tasks that require sustained mental effort (such as schoolwork or homework)
   (g) Often loses things necessary for tasks or activities (e.g., toys, school assignments, pencils, books, or tools)
   (h) Is often easily distracted by extraneous stimuli
   (i) Is often forgetful in daily activities
   (2) Six (or more) of the following symptoms of ***hyperactivity-impulsivity*** have persisted for at least 6 months to a degree that is maladaptive and inconsistent with developmental level:
   Hyperactivity
   (a) Often fidgets with hands or feet or squirms in seat
   (b) Often leaves seat in classroom or in other situations in which remaining seated is expected
   (c) Often runs about or climbs excessively in situations in which it is inappropriate (in adolescents or adults, may be limited to subjective feelings of restlessness)
   (d) Often has difficulty playing or engaging in leisure activities quietly
   (e) Is often "on the go" or often acts as if "driven by a motor"
   (f) Often talks excessively
   Impulsivity
   (g) Often blurts out answers before questions have been completed
   (h) Often has difficulty awaiting turn
   (i) Often interrupts or intrudes on others (e.g., butts into conversations or games)

B. Some hyperactive-impulsive or inattentive symptoms that caused impairment were present before age 7 years.
C. Some impairment from the symptoms is present in two or more settings (e.g., at school, work, and at home).
D. There must be clear evidence of clinical significant impairment in social, academic, or occupational functioning.
E. The symptoms do not occur exclusively during the course of or are not accounted for by another mental disorder.

From American Psychiatric Association: *Diagnostic and statistical manual of mental disorders,* ed 4 (DSM-IV), Washington, DC, 1994, The Association.

ing stimulant medication need to have it administered in the morning to maximize its effectiveness in the classroom and to decrease its insomnia-producing potential. Parents benefit from practical, specific strategies for helping children with ADHD, such as the need for structure and consistency in dressing, meals, sleep, and discipline.

Nurses must understand which type of LD a child has in order to provide direction for the child, parents, and teachers. Children with an auditory perceptual deficit appear unable to follow directions or to comprehend large amounts of verbal teaching. These children need to be taught with diagrams, pictures, demonstration, and written lists. Children with a visual perceptual deficit may have difficulty reading, lining up numbers for mathematics operations, or judging distance. These children may have dyslexia (letter reversals) and do better with demonstration and a verbal approach. Children with an integrative deficit may have difficulty sequencing data or storing and retrieving sensory data. Multisensory techniques should be used, and comprehension should be checked often throughout instruction. Children with dysgraphia (loss of the ability to write) may need to use computers in the classroom, since their handwriting will *not* improve. They may need to find alternatives to physical competition that requires coordination of movement (Selekman and Snyder, 1996).

Enuresis

Enuresis (bed-wetting) is a common and troublesome disorder that is defined as intentional or involuntary passage of urine into bed (usually at night) or into clothes during the day in children who are beyond the age when voluntary bladder control should normally have been acquired. For the disorder to be diagnosed as enuresis, the chronologic or developmental age of the child must be at least 5 years and the voiding of urine must occur at least twice a week for at least 3 months. The predominant symptom is urgency that is immediate and accompanied by acute discomfort, restlessness, and sometimes urinary frequency.

Enuresis is more common in boys than in girls. It is primarily an alteration of neuromuscular bladder functioning and is often benign and self-limiting. Nocturnal bed-wetting usually ceases between 6 and 8 years of age, although it sometimes continues into adolescence (Cultural Considerations box).

Organic causes that may be related to enuresis should be ruled out before psychogenic factors are considered. These include structural disorders of the urinary tract; urinary tract infection; neurologic deficits; disorders that increase the normal output of urine, such as diabetes; and disorders that impair the concentrating ability of the kidneys, such as chronic renal failure or sickle cell disease. A bladder volume of 300 to 350 ml is

Critical Thinking

ATTENTION DEFICIT HYPERACTIVITY DISORDER

Johnnie, age 8 years, is a third-grader who was diagnosed with attention deficit hyperactivity disorder (ADHD) 1 year ago. Johnnie has been taking the drug methylphenidate (Ritalin) for the past year. Which of the following behaviors indicates that Johnnie may need to have the administration times of his medications changed?

First Think About It . . .

- **What concepts or ideas are central to your thinking?**
- **What precise questions are you trying to answer?**

1. **For the past week, Johnnie has not eaten his lunch. He states that he is not hungry.**
2. **During this school year Johnnie's math grade has increased from a letter grade of D to a grade of B.**
3. **Johnnie's mother told the school nurse that Johnnie has been sleeping very well at night.**
4. **During the past year, Johnnie's teacher has noted that Johnnie has been socializing more with his classmates and that he now has a "best friend."**

The best response is 1. Children taking stimulant medications often experience positive effects such as improvement in schoolwork and increasing self-confidence in social skills. However, there are also negative side effects for some of the drugs used to treat ADHD. For example, side effects for methylphenidate include nervousness, decreased appetite, and insomnia. Recalling these side effects helps you to answer the question precisely. The absorption rate of methylphenidate is increased when this drug is taken with meals; therefore side effects such as decreased appetite may become more pronounced when the medication is taken with meals. Side effects can be alleviated by changing the times that the drug is administered or by switching to a sustained time-release form of the drug that can be given once a day in the morning. When evaluating a child's response to the medication, it is important to obtain reports from the child's teacher, the school nurse, and the parents. Information concerning the child's behavior in at least two settings should be obtained before adjustments are made in the medication dosage or scheduling.

sufficient to hold a night's urine. (To determine a child's bladder capacity, have the child void in a measuring cup after holding urine for as long as possible. Normal bladder capacity [in ounces] is the child's age plus 2 [e.g., a 6-year-old's normal capacity is 8 ounces].) In other cases the enuresis is influenced by emotional factors, although it is doubtful that they are causative factors. Parents report that these children sleep more soundly than other children; however, the depth of sleep has not been identified as the cause of nocturnal anuresis. Enuresis has a strong familiar tendency.

Various therapeutic techniques are employed in the management of enuresis. These include drugs, bladder training, restriction or elimination of fluids after the evening meal, interruption of sleep to void, and some type of electrical device designed to establish a conditioned reflex response to waken the child at the initiation of voiding.

The tricyclic antidepressant drug imipramine (Tofranil) is used to inhibit urination. Another anticholinergic drug, oxybutynin, reduces uninhibited bladder contractions and may be helpful for children with daytime urinary frequency. Desmopressin (DDAVP) nasal spray, an analog of vasopressin, reduces nighttime urine output to a volume less than functional bladder capacity.

Cultural Considerations

ENURESIS

The age at which children attain urinary continence varies widely. For example, Caucasian children in the United States tend to achieve continence earlier than African-American children. In addition, children in Great Britain and Sweden appear to attain continence slightly earlier than children in the United States, and in the extreme, the East African Digos often achieve bladder control by the age of 12 months. Therefore practitioners must be sensitive to the differences among groups before labeling a child enuretic.*

*Rappaport LA: Enuresis. In Levine M et al: *Developmental-behavioral pediatrics,* ed 2, Philadelphia, 1992, WB Saunders.

Nursing Care Management. No matter what techniques are employed, the nurse can help both children and parents to understand the problem of enuresis, the treatment plan, and the difficulties they may encounter in the process. More importantly, the nurse can provide consistent support and encouragement to help sustain them through the inconsistent and unpredictable treatment process. Children need to believe that they are helping themselves, and they need to sustain feelings of confidence and hope.

Encopresis

Encopresis is the repeated voluntary or involuntary passage of feces of normal or near-normal consistency into places not appropriate for that purpose according to the individual's own sociocultural setting. To be diagnosed as encopresis, the fecal incontinence must not be caused by any physiologic effect, such as a laxative; or a general medical condition. The fecal incontinence may be related to emotional problems. The disorder is less common than enuresis, but the two may coexist.

Primary encopresis is identified by age 4 when the child has not achieved fecal continence. Secondary encopresis is fecal incontinence occurring in a child over 4 years of age after a period of established fecal continence. Predisposing factors may be inconsistent toilet training; and psychosocial stress, such as entering school or the birth of a sibling. The disorder is more common in boys than in girls. Incontinence commonly occurs secondary to constipation, painful impaction, or retention of feces with subsequent overflow. It is not unusual for soiling to take place after bathing because of reflex stimulation.

School performance and attendance are affected as the child's offensive odor becomes a target for scorn and ridicule from classmates. This causes further withdrawal and other behavioral manifestations. Therapeutic management consists of determining the cause of the soiling and using appropriate interventions to correct the problem. Interventions may involve dietary changes, relief of a fecal impaction, and/or behavioral therapy. Often psychotherapeutic intervention with the child and the family may be necessary (Vogt and Schaffner, 1996).

Nursing Care Management. The nursing care of the child with encopresis involves education and support of the family as well as treatment of existing constipation. Education regarding the physiology of normal defecation, toilet training as a developmental process, and the treatment outlined for the particular family is essential. Family counseling is directed toward reassurance that most problems resolve successfully, although relapses during periods of stress are possible (Family Focus box).

Posttraumatic Stress Disorder (PTSD)

PTSD refers to the development of characteristic symptoms following exposure to an extremely traumatic experience or catastrophic event. An accident, assault, a natural disaster, sexual abuse, or witnessing violence can lead to PTSD.

Children with PTSD tend to relive or visualize traumatic experiences for years and retain some fear specific to the event. They continue to function as always, but have a feeling of foreboding regarding the future. The way in which children react depends on what resources the individual child brings to the situation (e.g., the coping strategies used, defense mechanisms summoned, and the child's social environment). Although studies indicate that children do not outgrow the trauma, they can be helped to overcome their sense of hopelessness.

The response to the event takes place in three stages. The *initial response* to the stressor is intense arousal, which usually lasts for a few minutes to 1 or 2 hours. The stress hormones are at the maximum as the individual prepares for "fight" or "flight." A prolonged arousal phase may indicate psychosis.

The *second phase,* which lasts approximately 2 weeks, is one in which defense mechanisms are mobilized. It is a period of quiescence in which the event appears to have produced no impression. The victims feel numb, and stress hormone secretion is absent. The reaction is outside their awareness, not well controlled, and involves some type of behavioral pattern. Defense mechanisms are less adaptive to specific situations and may not be what the situation demands. Denial that anything is wrong is a commonly observed defense mechanism.

The *third phase* is one of coping, which normally extends over 2 to 3 months. It is one of consciously directed inquiry. The victims want to know what happened and appear to be getting worse, when actually they are getting better. Numerous psychologic symptoms may be apparent, such as depression, repetitive phenomenon, phobic symptoms, anxiety symptoms, and conversion reactions. Children often display repetitive actions. They play out the situation over and over again in an attempt to come to terms with their fear. Flashbacks are common. This phase can be self-perpetuating, and a prolonged reaction can develop into an obsession with the traumatic event. Some traumatic effects remain indefinitely.

Nursing Care Management. Children need to deal with any traumatic event; much depends on the intensity of the event and their reaction to it. They usually react in much the same manner as their caregivers (contagious pathology); therefore it is important to be aware of these reactions. In the second, or defense phase of the PTSD, the appropriateness of the defense mechanism must be assessed, and children must be assisted in application of their defense. If children do not engage in some catharsis, or if their defense phase is prolonged, they may need referral for special psychologic help.

Coping is a learned response, and children in the third phase can be helped to use their coping strategies to deal with their fear. Children usually are willing to accept reasoning. Those who are assisted in their catharsis and allowed expression will survive without serious lasting effects. It is important for children to be reassured regarding the randomness of an event such as a school shooting, rape, attack, or natural disaster (e.g., hurricane or earthquake). They should be encouraged to play out the stress and/or discuss their feelings about the event. If they are unable to do this, they may become obsessed with the traumatic event and need professional help. Conversion reactions are common obsessive behaviors in children.

Children need professional help if any of the phases of PTSD are prolonged. Boys, more than girls, tend to have a prolonged defense phase. Occasionally the event will be unrecognized, and the affected child will engage in what is considered to be unusual behavior. Children exhibiting any sudden change in behavior need to be assessed for a traumatic event—"Did something happen?" When the change in behavior is traced to a traumatic event, treatment can be implemented.

School Phobia

Children, other than beginning students, who resist going to school or who demonstrate extreme reluctance to attend school for a sustained period of time as a result of severe anxiety or fear of school-related experiences are said to have school phobia. The terms *school refusal* and *school avoidance* are also used to describe this behavior. School phobia occurs in children of all ages but is more common in children 10 years of age and older.

Physical symptoms are prominent and may affect any part of the body (e.g., anorexia, nausea, vomiting, diarrhea, dizziness, headache, leg pains, abdominal pains, or even a low-grade fever). A striking feature of school phobia is the prompt subsiding of symptoms when it is evident that the child can remain at home. Another significant observation is absence of symptoms on weekends and holidays unless they are related to other places such as Sunday school or parties. Occasional mild reluctance is not uncommon among schoolchildren, but if the fear continues for longer than a few days it must be considered a serious problem—a warning of an important personality problem.

Nursing Care Management. Treatment for school phobia depends on the cause. The primary goal is to return the child to school. The longer a child is permitted to stay out of school, the more difficult it is for the child to reenter. Parents must be counseled gently but firmly that *immediate* return is essential and that it is their responsibility to insist on school attendance.

Family Focus

HELPING FAMILIES UNDERSTAND ENCOPRESIS

The prevailing attitude of nurses toward the family of a child with encopresis should be one of no-fault, thus relieving the guilt of both parents and child. Since parents and children are often reluctant to volunteer information, direct questioning about the soiling is more successful. Parents are usually relieved to know that other parents share this problem and are surprised to know that functional changes that take place as the condition develops make control of seepage impossible. Many parents complain that their children soil because they do not take time from play for a bowel movement. Actually, the children may be unaware of a prior sensation and unable to control the urge once it begins. They may be so accustomed to bowel accidents that they are unable to smell or feel it and even deny soiling when it occurs.

A school reentry protocol may be necessary for the child with severe symptoms. In reentry programs, the child role-plays routines involved in getting ready for school and that occur at school. Relaxation techniques are also used. The child usually goes to school initially for a half day and progresses to a full day. Often the school nurse is asked to provide support to the parents and the teacher during the reentry process. If the problem persists, professional help is recommended.

Recurrent Abdominal Pain (RAP)

RAP is a complaint of childhood that is often attributed to a psychogenic etiology, although it can be a symptom of either psychosomatic or organic disease. Children with RAP have real pain that is usually located in the periumbilical and/or epigastric area. On palpation the pain is more likely to be experienced in the epigastric area or in the lower right or left quadrant and is accompanied by vague tenderness without muscle guarding. The pain is irregular in time, duration, and intensity and is associated with either loose or pellet-formed stools. Other symptoms that may accompany the abdominal pain are headache, pallor, dizziness, dysuria, flushing, vomiting, diarrhea, and fatigue.

Support for the psychologic aspects of this disorder is based on observations of aggravation of symptoms during times of tension or stress. Children with RAP tend to be highly sensitive, have a poor self-image, and be uncomfortable with expressions of anger or argument, especially in those persons who are significant in their life. School attendance is adversely affected, and these children may exhibit poor learning performance. It is not uncommon for symptoms to be aggravated during school days.

Treatment involves providing reassurance and reducing or eliminating the symptoms (Hyams and Hyman, 1998). Hospitalization may be necessary, and the child commonly shows improvement in the hospital environment. Initial efforts are directed toward ruling out organic causes of the pain, relieving discomfort, and attempting to determine the situations that precipitate attacks. A high-fiber diet, psyllium bulk agents, lubricants such as mineral oil, and bowel training are emphasized. When simple measures are ineffective, an antispasmodic drug such as propantheline bromide may be prescribed to relieve the muscle spasm.

Nursing Care Management. Once the diagnosis has been established, the parents and the child need an explanation of the pain, which can be compared to a skeletal muscle cramp or "charley horse" for easier comprehension. Reassurance that the symptoms are not unique to their child and that the pain can be expected to subside is helpful in relieving parental fears and anxieties. When parents are reassured that there is no organic cause of the pain, they will need some guidance regarding what they can do during a painful episode. All too often they feel helpless and anxious, which tends to compound the child's distress.

The simple expedient of having the child rest in a peaceful, quiet environment and providing comfort will often relieve the symptoms in a short time. A heating pad may also help ease the discomfort. Teaching the child relaxation techniques and imaging can be helpful (see Nonpharmacologic Pain Management, Chapter 44). If pain is not relieved by these simple measures, the parents are taught how to administer antispasmodics, if prescribed. For example, if pain is precipitated by meals, having the child take the medication 20 to 30 minutes before mealtime may prevent an episode.

The most valuable measures that the nurse can provide are support and reassurance to the family. When open communication is established and families are able to see a relationship between stress-provoking situations and the child's symptoms, the chance for remedial action is enhanced. Follow-up care and continued support are essential, because the symptoms tend to remit and exacerbate; therefore the availability of a supportive health professional can be a source of comfort to the child and family.

Conversion Reaction

Conversion reaction, also known as *hysteria, hysterical conversion reaction,* and *childhood hysteria,* is a psychophysiologic disorder with a sudden onset that can usually be traced to a precipitating environmental event. Once considered rare in childhood, the diagnosis of conversion reaction occurs more commonly than has generally been acknowledged. In childhood the disorder is observed with equal frequency in both sexes, but girls outnumber boys during adolescence.

The manifestations involve primarily the voluntary musculature and special senses and include abdominal pain, fainting, pseudoseizures, paralysis, headaches, and visual field restriction. The most commonly observed symptom is seizure activity, which can be differentiated from symptoms of neurogenic origin by formal tests, the most useful of which is the finding of a normal electroencephalogram.

It has been observed that many children with conversion reaction have experienced a major family crisis before the onset of symptoms, such as loss of a parent or other significant person through death, divorce, or moving.

Nursing Care Management. Nursing care is similar to that for the child with recurrent abdominal pain.

Childhood Depression

Depression in childhood is often difficult to detect. Children may be unable to express their feelings and tend to act out their problems and concerns. Some states of depression are of a temporary nature (e.g., acute depression precipitated by a traumatic event). This might include a period of hospitalization, loss of a parent through death or separation, or loss of a significant relationship with something (a pet), someone (a friend or family member), or a place (move from a familiar home, neighborhood, or city). The characteristics of children with depression are outlined in Box 39-2. The child tends to spend more time in solitary activities, especially television viewing; and schoolwork is impaired. Some children become more dependent and clinging; others become more aggressive and disruptive. The manifestations may last a few days or weeks, usually resolving spontaneously.

More serious and less common are depressive responses to more chronic stress and loss; these are often observed in children with chronic illness or disability when other family members have denial depression. There is usually no apparent precipitating event, but there is often a history of frequent disruptions in important relationships or overwhelming demands (often self-imposed) placed on the youngster. Manifestations are as varied as those observed in acute depression but occur more often and extend over a longer time.

Box 39-2

Characteristics of Children with Depression

BEHAVIOR

Predominantly sad facial expression with absence or diminished range of affective response
Solitary play or work; tendency to be alone; disinterest in play
Withdrawal from previously enjoyed activities and relationships
Lowered grades in school; lack of interest in doing homework or achieving in school
Diminished motor activity; tiredness
Tearfulness or crying
Dependent and clinging or aggressive and disruptive

INTERNAL STATES

Utterance of statements reflecting lowered self-esteem, sense of hopelessness, or guilt
Suicidal ideations

PHYSIOLOGY

Constipation
Nonspecific complaints of not feeling well
Change in appetite resulting in weight loss or gain
Alterations in sleeping pattern, sleeplessness, or hypersomnia

Nursing Care Management. Depressed children are managed by a health team especially prepared in the care of children with mental disorders. Treatment is highly individualized and undertaken in the least restrictive environment. Pharmacotherapy may involve tricyclic antidepressants or serotonin reuptake inhibitors (SRIs) such as fluoxetine (Prozac) and paroxetine (Paxil). Nurses should be aware that depression is a problem that can easily be overlooked in the child and one that can interrupt normal growth and development. Recognizing depression and suicidal tendencies in depressed adolescents and making appropriate referrals is an important nursing function. Identification of the depressed child requires a careful history (health, growth and development, social, and family health), interviews with the child, and observations by the nurse, parents, and teachers (see also Suicide, Ch. 40).

Childhood Schizophrenia

Childhood schizophrenia refers to severe deviations in ego functioning and is generally reserved for psychotic disorders that appear after the first 4 or 5 years of life. Schizophrenia in adults occurs with relative frequency, and although childhood psychosis is not as common, it is by no means rare.

Childhood schizophrenia is characterized by a gradual onset of neurotic symptoms that show wide variation according to each affected child's developmental level, the age of onset, the nature of early childhood experiences, and the type of defense mechanisms used. However, the basic core disturbance is a lack of contact with reality and the subsequent development of a world of the child's own. Secondary characteristics represent impairment in a wide number of areas of development, including cognition, perception, emotion, language, and physical motor control. The most common manifestations involve language disturbances, impaired interpersonal relationships, and inappropriate affect (outward expression of emotion). Treatment has been more successful since newer antipsychotic medications such as risperidone have been used.

Nursing Care Management. Nursing of psychotic children is a highly specialized area, but since these problems are being recognized with increasing frequency, nurses should be alert to the possibility that schizophrenia can occur in children. A child who consistently demonstrates abnormal behavior should be referred for evaluation.

Key Points

- Middle childhood, also known as the school years, is a comfortable period of life that extends from 6 to 12 years of age.
- Although slower than previous years, there is a steady gain in height and weight with maturation of body systems; primary teeth are lost and replaced by permanent teeth.
- School-age children develop what Erikson terms a sense of industry or accomplishment.
- School-age children, although having a limited capacity for abstract thought, can use their thought processes to solve more complex problems, make judgments based on reasoning, and see a situation from the point of view of another.
- The school-age child develops a conscience and is able to understand and adhere to rules and standards set by others.
- Entertaining different points of view, becoming sensitive to social norms, and forming peer friendships are the most important features of social development during the school years.
- Cooperative play, team activities, and acquisition of skills are prime elements of play during the school years; rules and rituals assume greater importance.
- School-age children became proficient at many types of activities.
- Typical parental concerns during middle childhood are beginning separation from the family unit, dishonest behavior, and scholastic achievement.
- Optimum nutrition is often hampered by an affinity for and availability of junk foods, irregular family meals, and schedules of working parents.
- Dental care continues to be important; dental problems include caries, periodontal disease, malocclusion, and tooth evulsion.
- Increased socialization, earlier pubertal development, and constant media exposure make the school years an ideal time for sex education.
- School health ideally offers programs that include health appraisal, emergency care, safety education, communicable disease control, counseling, guidance, and health education with adjustment to individual student needs.
- Injury prevention is directed toward safety education, provision of safe play areas and equipment, and well-supervised sports activities.

- Participation in sports predisposes children and adolescents to both acute injuries and overuse syndromes.
- Alterations in growth and maturation may be manifest in short or tall stature, precocious puberty, and delayed sexual development.
- Tools for assessment of growth include a family history, previous growth patterns, physical examination, bone age determination, and endocrine studies.
- Effective therapies for attention deficit hyperactivity disorder and learning disabilities usually involve a multiple approach: family education and counseling, medication, remedial education, environmental manipulation, and psychotherapy.
- Behavior problems in middle childhood can result from attention deficit hyperactivity disorder, enuresis, encopresis, posttraumatic stress disorder, school phobia, recurrent abdominal pain, childhood depression, conversion reaction, and childhood schizophrenia.

References

American Academy of Pediatrics, Committee on Injury and Poison Prevention: Bicycle helmets, *Pediatrics* 95(4):609-610, 1995.

American Academy of Pediatrics, Committee on Injury and Poison Prevention: Office-based counseling for injury prevention, *Pediatrics* 94:566-567, 1994.

American Academy of Pediatrics, Committee on Injury and Poison Prevention: Selecting and using the most appropriate car safety seats for growing children: guidelines for counseling parents, *Pediatrics* 97:761-763, 1996.

American Academy of Pediatrics, Committee on Injury and Poison Prevention and Committee on Sports Medicine and Fitness: Trampolines at home, school, and recreational centers, *Pediatrics* 103(5, part 1):1053-1056, 1999.

American Academy of Pediatrics, Committee on Quality Improvement, Subcommittee on Attention-Deficit/Hyperactivity Disorder: Clinical practice guideline: diagnosis and evaluation of the child with attention-deficit/hyperactivity disorder, *Pediatrics* 105(5):1158-1170, 2000.

American Psychiatric Association: *Diagnostic and statistical manual of mental disorders,* ed 4 (DSM-IV), Washington, DC, 1994, The Association.

Blum NJ, Ditmar MF, Charney EB: Behavior and development. In Polin RA, Ditmar MF, editors: *Pediatric secrets,* ed 2, St Louis, 1997, Mosby.

Dumas D, Pelletier L: Perception in hyperactive children, *MCN* 24(1):12-19, 1999.

Erikson EH: *Childhood and society,* ed 2, New York, 1963, Norton.

Hergenroeder AC: Prevention of sports injuries, *Pediatrics* 101:1057-1063, 1998.

Hyams JS, Hyman PE: Recurrent abdominal pain and the biopsychosocial model of medical practice, *J Pediatr* 133(4):473-478, 1998.

National Association of State School Nurse Consultants: Delegation of school health services to unlicensed assistive personnel: a position paper, *J Sch Nurs* 11(4):13-16, 1995.

O'Connell KL: Attention deficit hyperactivity disorder, *Pediatr Nurs* 22:30-33, 1996.

Rhodes AM: Liability for unlicensed assistive personnel, part I, *MCN* 22:269, 1997.

Selekman J, Snyder M: Primary care of the child with a learning disability. In Jackson P, Vessey J, editors: *Primary care of children with chronic conditions,* ed 2, St Louis, 1996, Mosby.

Vogt MA, Schaffner B: Pediatric management problems: what is your assessment? Constipation with encopresis, *Pediatr Nurs* 22(5):444-445, 1996.

Williams K et al: Association of common health symptoms with bullying in primary school children, *BMJ* 313:17-19, 1996.

Wilson CB, Lewis DB, Penix LA: Immunodeficiency of immaturity. In Stiehm R, editor: *Immunologic disorders in infants and children,* ed 4, Philadelphia, 1996, WB Saunders.

CHAPTER

40

The Adolescent and Family

http://www.harcourthealth.com/MERLIN/Wong/maternal/

Learning Objectives

On completion of this chapter the reader will be able to:

- Describe the physical changes that occur at puberty.
- Discuss the reactions of the adolescent to physical changes that take place at puberty.
- Demonstrate an understanding of the process by which the adolescent develops a sense of identity.
- Discuss the significance of the changing interpersonal relationships and the role of the peer group during adolescence.
- Outline a health teaching plan for adolescents.
- Identify the causes and discuss the preventive aspects of injuries during adolescence.
- Demonstrate an understanding of common disorders of the male and female reproductive systems.
- Demonstrate an understanding of health problems related to sexuality.
- Outline a plan of care for the child or adolescent with an eating disorder.
- Discuss the manifestations and nursing management of selected emotional and/or behavioral problems.

PROMOTING OPTIMUM GROWTH AND DEVELOPMENT

Adolescence is a period of transition between childhood and adulthood—a time of rapid physical, cognitive, social, and emotional maturing as the boy prepares for manhood and the girl prepares for womanhood (Cultural Considerations box). The precise boundaries of adolescence are difficult to define, but this period is customarily viewed as beginning with the gradual appearance of secondary sex characteristics at about 11 or 12 years of age and ending with cessation of body growth at 18 to 20 years.

Several terms are commonly used in reference to this particular stage of growth and development. *Puberty* primarily refers to the maturational, hormonal, and growth processes that occurs when the reproductive organs begin to function and the secondary sex characteristics develop. This process is sometimes divided into three stages: *prepubescence,* the period of about 2 years immediately before puberty when the child is developing preliminary physical changes that herald sexual maturity; *puberty,* the point at which sexual maturity is achieved, marked by the first menstrual flow in girls but by less obvious indications in boys; and *postpubescence,* a 1- to 2-year period following puberty during which skeletal growth is completed and reproductive functions become fairly well established. *Adolescence,* which literally means "to grow into maturity," is generally regarded as the psychologic, social, and maturational processes initiated by the pubertal changes. It involves three distinct subphases: *early adolescence* (ages 11 to 14), *middle adolescence* (ages 15 to 17), and *late adolescence* (ages 18 to 20). Adolescence tends to begin and end earlier in girls than in boys. The term *teenage years* is used synonymously with *adolescence* to describe ages 13 through 19.

Biologic Development

The physical changes of puberty are primarily the result of hormonal activity under the influence of the central nervous system, although all aspects of physiologic functioning are mutually interacting. The very obvious physical changes are noted in increased physical growth and in the appearance and development of secondary sex characteristics; less obvious are physiologic alterations and neurogonadal maturity, accompanied by the ability to procreate. Physical distinction between the sexes is determined on the basis of distinguishing characteristics: *primary sex characteristics* are the external and internal organs that carry out the reproductive functions (e.g., ovaries, uterus, breasts, and penis); *secondary sex characteristics* are the changes that occur throughout the body as a result of the hormonal change (e.g., voice alterations, development of

---

For additional information, please view "Growth and Development" in ***Whaley and Wong's Pediatric Nursing Video Series,*** St Louis, 1996, Mosby; 1-800-426-4545; website: www.mosby.com.

Cultural Considerations

THE ADOLESCENT YEARS

Other societies in which adolescence is seen as part of the life cycle may have ideas very different from American culture about how the adolescent years are to be spent. For example, some societies discourage contact between adolescent males and females. Sexual experimentation is outlawed, and all grown children, males and females, remain in the home of their parents until they wed. In America we tend to believe that the way our culture is organized is the way all cultures are or should be organized, but of course this is not so. Each society is unique. The way we describe adolescence, the way we experience it, and the predisposition of our adolescents toward violence are peculiar to our American culture.

Modified from Prothrow-Stith D: *Deadly consequences: how violence is destroying our teenage population and a plan to begin solving the problem,* New York, 1993, HarperCollins.

Box 40-1

Usual Sequence of Maturational Changes

GIRLS	BOYS
Breast changes	Enlargement of testicles
Rapid increase in height and weight	Growth of pubic hair, axillary hair, hair on upper lip, hair on face and elsewhere on body (facial hair usually appears about 2 years after appearance of pubic hair)
Growth of pubic hair	Rapid increase in height
Appearance of axillary hair	Changes in the larynx and consequently the voice (usually take place along with growth of penis)
Menstruation (usually begins 2 years after first signs)	Nocturnal emissions
Abrupt deceleration of linear growth	Abrupt deceleration of linear growth

facial and pubertal hair, and fat deposits) but play no direct part in reproduction.

Hormonal Changes of Puberty. It is generally accepted that the events of puberty are caused by hormonal influences and controlled by the anterior pituitary (adenohypophysis) in response to a stimulus from the hypothalamus. Stimulation of the gonads has a dual function: (1) production and release of gametes (i.e., production of sperm in the male and maturation and release of ova in the female) and (2) secretion of sex-appropriate hormones (i.e., estrogen and progesterone from the ovaries [female] and testosterone from the testes [male]).

Sex Hormones. Sex hormones are secreted by the ovaries, testes, and adrenals; they are produced in varying amounts by both sexes throughout the life span. The adrenal cortex is responsible for the small amounts secreted before the pubescent years, but the sex hormone production that accompanies maturation of the gonads is responsible for the variety of biologic changes observed during puberty.

Estrogen, the feminizing hormone, is found in low quantities during childhood; it is secreted in slowly increasing amounts until about age 11 years. In males this gradual increase continues through maturation. In females the onset of estrogen production in the ovaries causes a pronounced increase that continues until about 3 years after the onset of menstruation, at which time it reaches a maximum level that continues throughout the reproductive life of the female.

Androgens, the masculinizing hormones, are also secreted in small and gradually increasing amounts up to about 7 or 9 years of age, at which time there is a more rapid increase in both sexes, especially boys, until about age 15 years. These hormones appear to be responsible for most of the rapid growth changes of early adolescence. With the onset of testicular function, the level of androgens (principally testosterone) in males increases over that in females and continues to increase until a maximum is attained at maturity.

Sexual Maturation. The visible evidence of sexual maturation is achieved in orderly sequence, and the state of maturity can be estimated on the basis of the appearance of these external manifestations. The age at which these changes are observed, and the time required to progress from one stage to another, may vary considerably among children. The time from the appearance of breast buds to full maturity may be 1½ to 6 years for adolescent girls; it may take 2 to 5 years for male genitalia to reach adult size. The stages of the development of secondary sex characteristics and genital development have been defined as a guide for estimating sexual maturity and are often referred to as the *Tanner stages.* The usual sequence of appearance of maturational changes is presented in Box 40-1).

Sexual Maturation in Girls. In most girls the initial indication of puberty is the appearance of breast buds, an event known as *thelarche,* which occurs between 9 and 13½ years of age (Fig. 40-1). This is followed in approximately 2 to 6 months by growth of pubic hair on the mons pubis, known as adrenarche (Fig. 40-2). In a minority of normally developing girls, however, pubic hair may precede breast development.

The initial appearance of menstruation, or *menarche,* occurs about 2 years after the appearance of the first pubescent changes, approximately 9 months after attainment of peak height velocity and 3 months after attainment of peak weight velocity. Menarche has been related to a critical gain in body fat content (i.e., more fat content, earlier menarche), although this is controversial. The normal age range of menarche is usually 10½ to 15 years, with the average age being 12 years 9½ months for North American girls. Initial menstrual periods are usually scanty, irregular, and anovulatory. Ovulation and regular menstrual periods usually occur 6 to 14 months after menarche. Girls may be considered to have *pubertal delay* if breast development has not occurred by age 13 or if menarche has not occurred within 4 years of the onset of breast development.

Sexual Maturation in Boys. The first pubescent changes in boys are testicular enlargement accompanied by thinning, reddening, and increased looseness of the scrotum (Fig. 40-3). These events usually occur between 9½ and 14 years of age. Early puberty is also characterized by the initial appearance of pubic hair. Penile enlargement begins, and testicular enlargement and pubic hair growth continue throughout midpuberty. During this period there is also increasing muscularity, early voice changes, and development of early facial hair. Temporary breast enlargement and tenderness, or *gynecomastia,* is

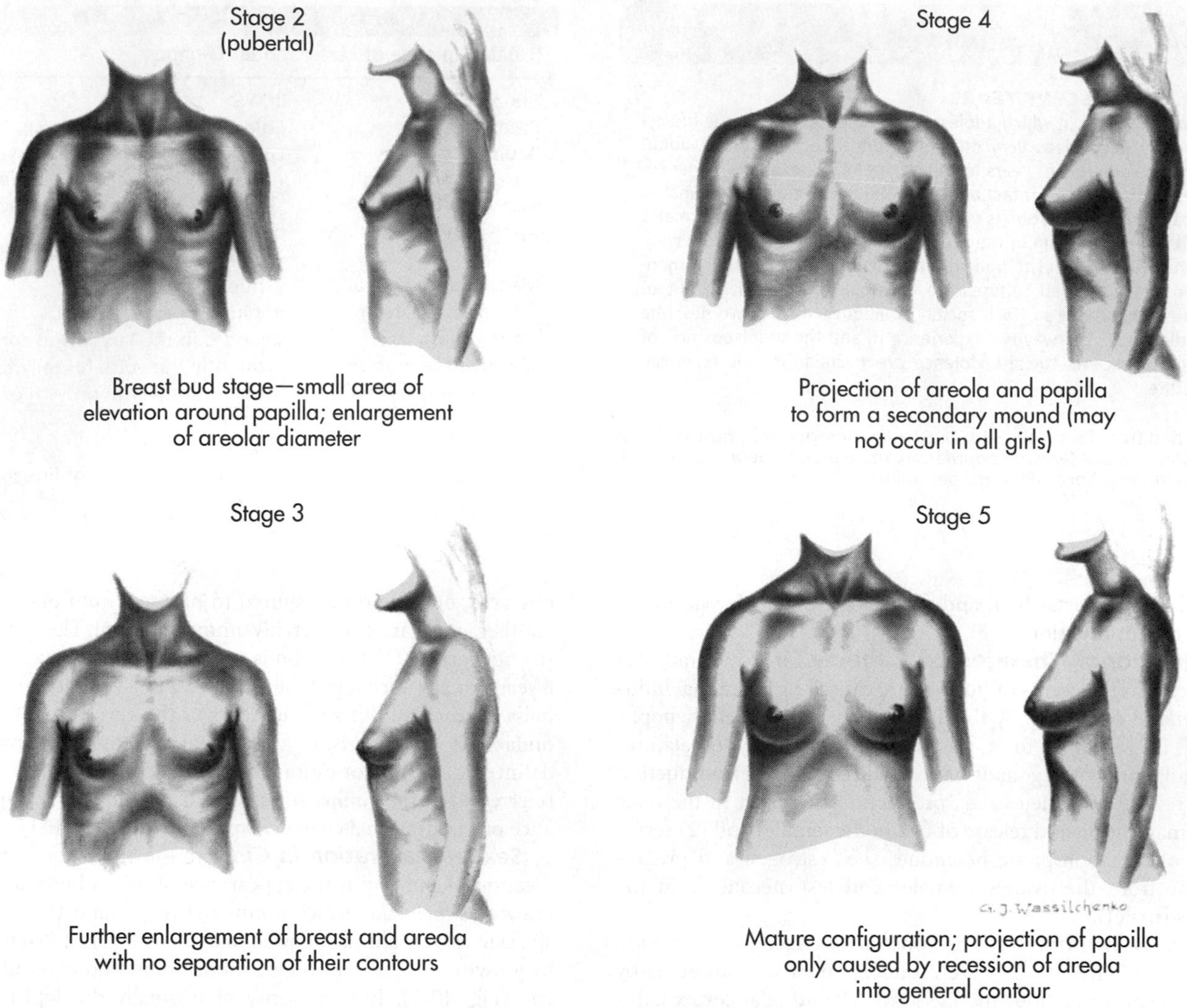

Stage 2
(pubertal)
Breast bud stage—small area of elevation around papilla; enlargement of areolar diameter
Stage 4
Projection of areola and papilla to form a secondary mound (may not occur in all girls)
Stage 3
Further enlargement of breast and areola with no separation of their contours
Stage 5
Mature configuration; projection of papilla only caused by recession of areola into general contour

FIG. 40-1 • Development of the breast in girls—average age span, 11 to 13 years. Stage I (prepubertal—elevation of papilla only) is not shown. (Modified from Marshall WA, Tanner JM: Variations in pattern of pubertal changes in girls, *Arch Dis Child* 44[235]:291-303, 1969; and Daniel WA, Paulshock BZ: A physician's guide to sexual maturity, *Patient Care,* May 13, 1979, pp 122-124.)

common during midpuberty, occurring in up to one third of boys. The spurts in height and weight occur concurrently toward the end of midpuberty. For most boys, breast enlargement disappears within 2 years. By late puberty there is a definite increase in the length and width of the penis, testicular enlargement continues, and first ejaculation occurs. Axillary hair develops, and facial hair extends to cover the anterior neck. Final voice changes occur secondary to the growth of the larynx. Concerns about *pubertal delay* should be considered for boys who exhibit no enlargement of the testes or scrotal changes by 13½ to 14 years of age, or if genital growth is not complete 4 years after the testicles begin to enlarge.

Physical Growth. A constant phenomenon associated with sexual maturation is a dramatic increase in growth. The final 20% to 25% of height is achieved during puberty, and most of this growth occurs during a 24- to 36-month period known as the adolescent *growth spurt.* This accelerated growth occurs in all children but, as in other areas of development, is highly variable in age of onset, duration, and extent. The growth spurt begins earlier in girls, usually between ages 9½ and 14½ years; on the average it begins between ages 10½ and 16 years in boys. During this period the average boy will gain 10 to 30 cm (4 to 12 inches) in height and 7 to 30 kg (15 to 65 pounds) in weight; the average girl, in whom the growth spurt is slower and less extensive, will gain 5 to 20 cm (2 to 8 inches) in height and 7 to 25 kg (15 to 55 pounds) in weight. Growth in height typically ceases 2 to 2½ years after menarche in girls and at age 18 to 20 years in boys.

This increase in size is acquired in a characteristic sequence of changes. Growth in length of the extremities and neck precedes growth in other areas, and because these parts are first to reach adult length, the hands and feet appear larger than normal during adolescence. Increases in hip and chest breadth take place in a few months, followed several months later by an increase in shoulder width. These changes are followed by increases in length of the trunk and depth of the chest. This sequence of changes is responsible for the characteristic long-legged, gawky appearance of the early adolescent child.

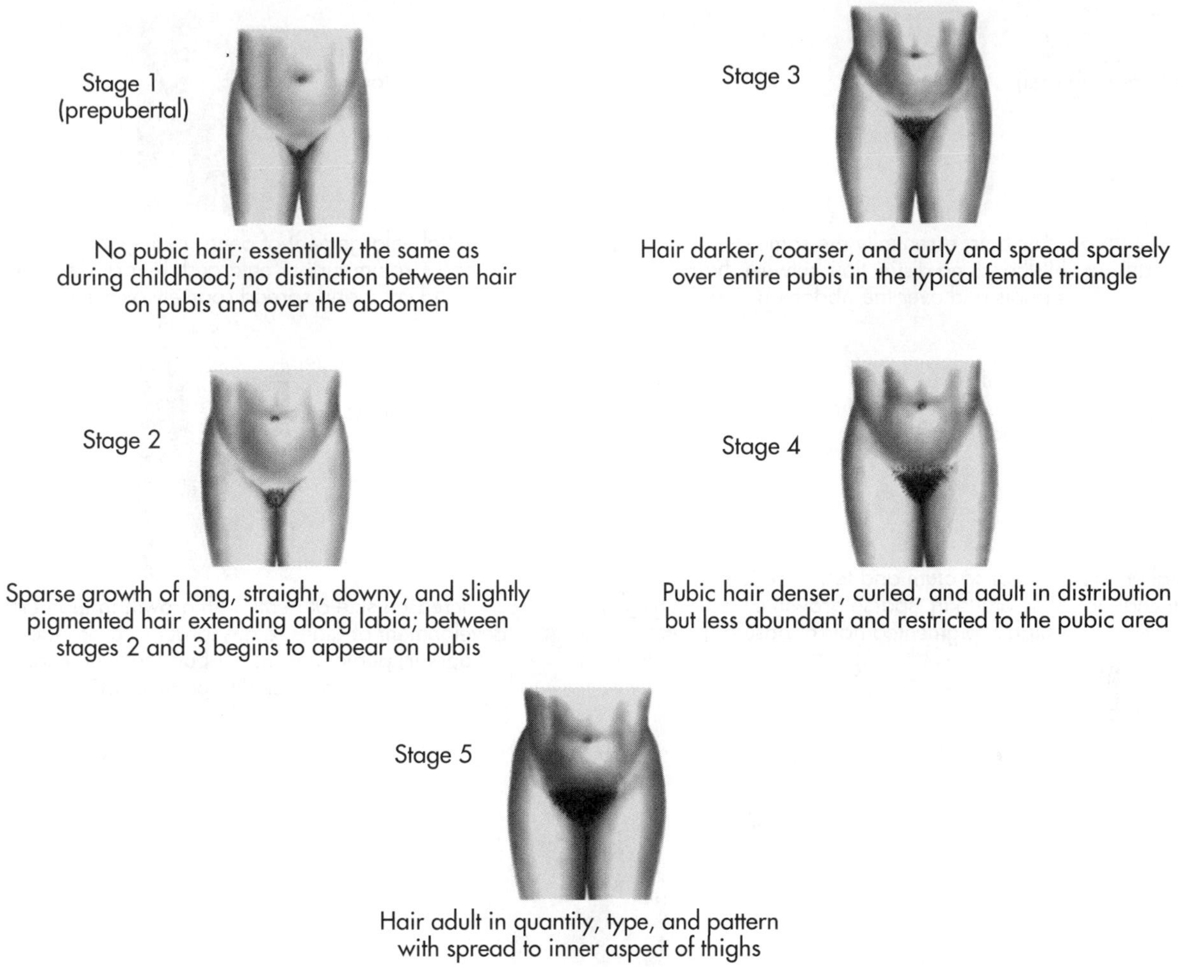
Stage 1
(prepubertal)
No pubic hair; essentially the same as during childhood; no distinction between hair on pubis and over the abdomen
Stage 3
Hair darker, coarser, and curly and spread sparsely over entire pubis in the typical female triangle
Stage 2
Sparse growth of long, straight, downy, and slightly pigmented hair extending along labia; between stages 2 and 3 begins to appear on pubis
Stage 4
Pubic hair denser, curled, and adult in distribution but less abundant and restricted to the pubic area
Stage 5
Hair adult in quantity, type, and pattern with spread to inner aspect of thighs

FIG. 40-2 • Growth in pubic hair in girls—average age span for stages 2 through 5, 11 to 14 years. (Modified from Marshall WA, Tanner JM: Variations in pattern of pubertal changes in girls, *Arch Dis Child* 44[235]:291-303, 1969; and Daniel WA, Paulshock BZ: A physician's guide to sexual maturity, *Patient Care,* May 13, 1979, pp 122-124.)

Sex Differences in General Growth Patterns. Sex differences in general growth and distribution patterns are apparent in skeletal growth, muscle mass, adipose tissue, and skin. Skeletal growth differences between boys and girls are apparently a function of hormonal effects at puberty and are evident primarily in limb length. The earlier cessation of growth in girls is caused by epiphyseal unity under the potent effect of estrogen secretion, and the hormonal effect on female bone growth is much stronger than the similar effect of testosterone in boys. In boys the prolonged growth period before puberty and the less rapid epiphyseal closure are reflected in their greater overall height and longer arms and legs. Other skeletal differences are increased shoulder width in boys and broader hip development in girls.

Hypertrophy of the laryngeal mucosa and enlargement of the larynx and vocal cords occur to produce voice changes in both boys and girls. Girls' voices become slightly deeper and considerably fuller, but the effect in boys is striking. The change in voice of adolescent boys occurs between Tanner stages 3 and 4, with the voice often shifting uncontrollably from deep to high tones in the middle of a sentence. The change is associated with not only a lengthening of the vocal cords, but also an increase in the structure and mass of the vocal folds (Harries et al, 1998).

Growth of lean body mass, principally muscle, which tends to occur after the bone growth spurt, takes place steadily during adolescence. Lean body mass is both quantitatively and qualitatively greater in boys than in girls at comparable stages of pubertal development. Muscle development, under the influence of androgenic hormones, increases steadily. Muscles become remarkably well developed in boys, whereas in girls, muscle mass increase is proportionate to general tissue growth.

Nonlean body mass, primarily fat, is also increased but follows a less orderly pattern. There may be a transient increase in subcutaneous fat just before the skeletal growth spurt, especially in boys. This is followed 1 to 2 years later by a modest to marked decrease, which is again more marked in boys. Later, variable amounts of fat are deposited to fill out and contour the mature physique in patterns characteristic of the adolescent's sex, particularly in the regions over the thighs, hips, and buttocks and around the breast tissue. It should be noted, however, that pediatric obesity is steadily on the increase in the United States, and obesity can change the timing of puberty. In girls, obesity is as-

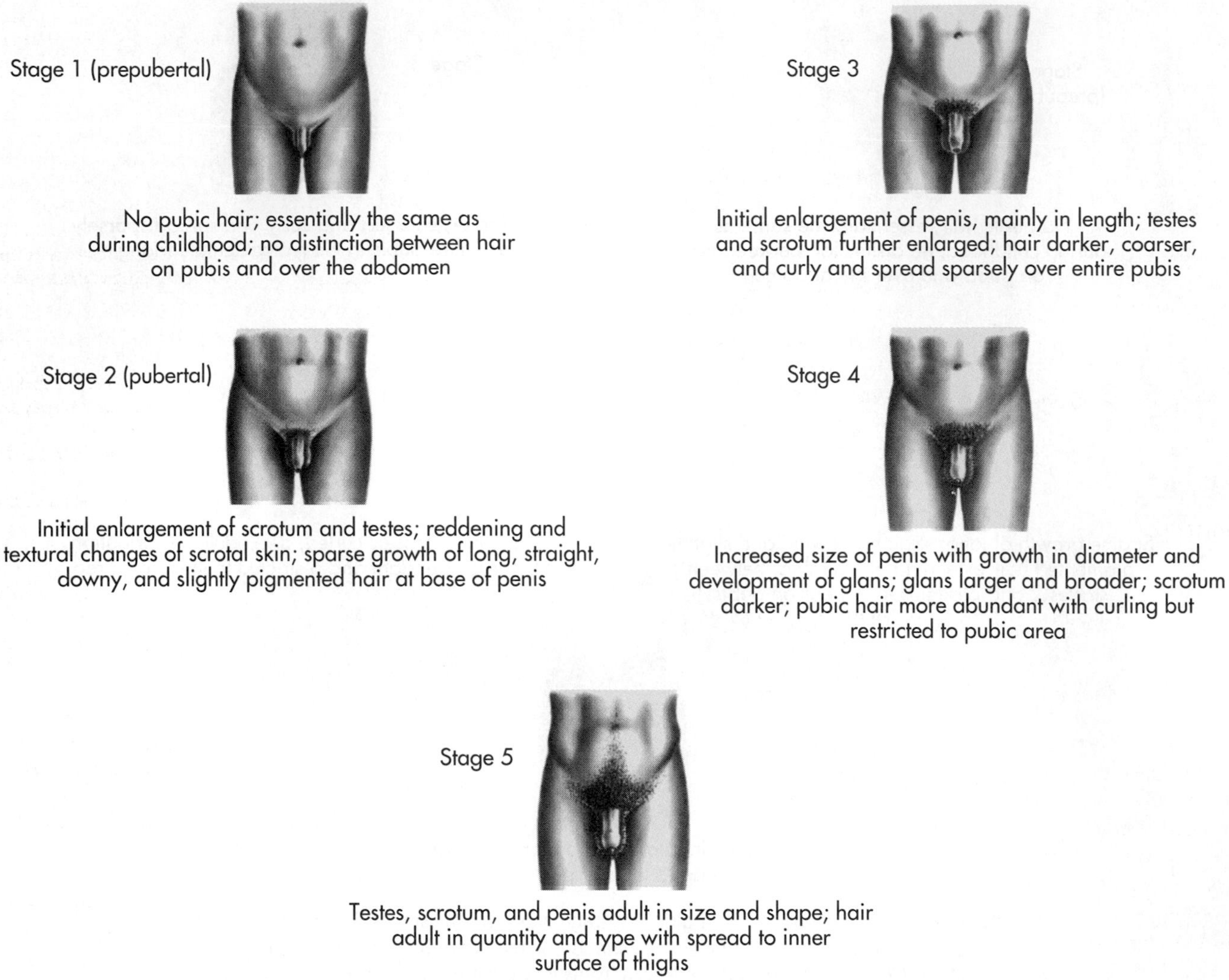
Stage 1 (prepubertal)
No pubic hair; essentially the same as during childhood; no distinction between hair on pubis and over the abdomen
Stage 2 (pubertal)
Initial enlargement of scrotum and testes; reddening and textural changes of scrotal skin; sparse growth of long, straight, downy, and slightly pigmented hair at base of penis
Stage 3
Initial enlargement of penis, mainly in length; testes and scrotum further enlarged; hair darker, coarser, and curly and spread sparsely over entire pubis
Stage 4
Increased size of penis with growth in diameter and development of glans; glans larger and broader; scrotum darker; pubic hair more abundant with curling but restricted to pubic area
Stage 5
Testes, scrotum, and penis adult in size and shape; hair adult in quantity and type with spread to inner surface of thighs

FIG. 40-3 • Developmental stages of secondary sex characteristics and genital development in boys—average age span, 12 to 16 years. (Modified from Marshall WA, Tanner JM: Variations in pattern of pubertal changes in girls, *Arch Dis Child* 44[235]:291-303, 1969; and Daniel WA, Paulshock BZ: A physician's guide to sexual maturity, *Patient Care,* May 13, 1979, pp 122-124.)

sociated with an early onset of puberty and early menarche. In boys, the effects of obesity are less predictable and may result in either early or delayed puberty.

Hormonal influences during puberty cause an acceleration in growth and maturation of the skin and its structural appendages. Sebaceous glands become extremely active at this time, especially those on the genitals and in the "flush areas" of the body (i.e., face, neck, shoulders, upper back, and chest). This increased activity and the structural nature of the glands are extremely important in the pathogenesis of a common problem of puberty: acne (see Chapter 53). The eccrine sweat glands, present almost everywhere on the human skin, become fully functional and respond to emotional as well as thermal stimulation. Heavy sweating appears to be more pronounced in boys than in girls. The apocrine sweat glands, nonfunctional in childhood, reach secretory capacity during puberty. Unlike the eccrine sweat glands, the apocrine glands are limited in distribution and grow in conjunction with hair follicles in the axillae, around the areola of the breast, around the umbilicus, on the external auditory canal, and in the genital and anal regions. Apocrine glands secrete a thick substance as a result of emotional stimulation that, when acted on by surface bacteria, becomes highly odoriferous.

Body hair assumes very characteristic distribution patterns and changes texture during puberty. Under the influence of gonadal and adrenal androgens, hair coarsens, darkens, and lengthens at sites related to secondary sex characteristics. Pubic and axillary hair appears in both sexes, although pubic hair is more extensive in males than in females. Beard, mustache, and body hair on the chest, upward along the linea alba, and sometimes on other areas (e.g., back and shoulders) appears in males and is androgen dependent. Extremity hair appears in varying amounts in both males and females but is also more prolific in the male.

Physiologic Changes. A number of physiologic functions are altered in response to some of the pubertal changes. The size and strength of the heart, blood volume, and systolic blood pressure increase, whereas the pulse rate and basal heat production decrease (see Appendix J). Blood volume, which has increased steadily during childhood, reaches a higher value in boys than in girls, a fact that may be related to the increased muscle mass in pubertal boys. Adult values are reached for all formed elements of the blood. Respiratory rate and basal metabolic rate, decreasing steadily throughout childhood, reach the adult rate in adolescence. Respiratory volume and vital capacity are increased, and to a far greater extent in males than in females. During this period, physiologic responses to exercise change drastically: performance improves, especially in boys, and the body is able to make the physiologic adjustments needed for normal functioning after exercise is completed. These capabilities are a result of the increased size and strength of muscles and the increased level of cardiac, respiratory, and metabolic functioning.

Psychosocial Development

Developing a Sense of Identity (Erikson).

Traditional psychosocial theory holds that the developmental crisis of adolescence leads to the formation of a sense of identity (Erikson, 1963). Throughout childhood, individuals have been going through the process of identification as they concentrate on various parts of the body at specific times. During infancy children identify themselves as being separate from the mother; during early childhood they establish a gender-role identification with the appropriate-sex parent; and in later childhood they establish who they are in relation to others. In adolescence they come to see themselves as distinct individuals, somehow unique and separate from every other individual.

The early period of adolescence begins with the onset of puberty and extends to relative physical and emotional stability at or near graduation from high school. During this time the adolescent is faced with the crisis of *group identity vs. alienation.* In the period that follows, the individual hopes to attain autonomy from the family and develop a sense of *personal identity* as opposed to *role diffusion.* A sense of group identity appears to be essential as a prelude to a sense of personal identity. Young adolescents must resolve questions concerning relationships with a peer group before they are able to resolve questions about who they are in relation to family and society.

Group Identity. During the early stage of adolescence the pressure to belong to a group is intensified. Teenagers find it essential to have a group to which they feel they can belong and that provides them with status. Belonging to a crowd helps adolescents to define the differences between themselves and their parents. They dress as the group dresses and wear makeup and hairstyles according to group criteria, all of which are different from those of the parental generation. Language, music, and dancing reflect a culture that is exclusive to the adolescent. When adults begin to emulate these fashions and interests, the style changes immediately. The evidence of adolescent conformity to the peer group and nonconformity to the adult group provides teenagers with a frame of reference in which they can display their own self-assertion while they reject the identity of their parents' generation. To be different is to be unaccepted and alienated from the group.

Individual Identity. The quest for personal identity is part of the ongoing identification process. As youngsters establish identity within a group, they are also attempting to incorporate multiple body changes into a concept of the self. Body awareness is part of self-awareness, and for some time the adolescent will engage in assimilating the self that is represented by this dimension. In this search for identity, adolescents consider the relationships that have developed between themselves and others in the past, as well as the directions they hope to be able to take in the future.

Significant others hold certain expectations for the behavior of the adolescent. Often these expectations or demands are persistent enough to result in certain decisions that might be made differently or not at all if the individual could be solely responsible for identity formation. It is all too easy to slip into the roles that are expected by these external influences without incorporating personal goals or questioning these decisions in relation to the developing personality. Thus individuals may become what parents or others wish them to be, based on these premature decisions. Young persons might form a negative identity when society or their culture provides them with a self-image that is contrary to the values of the community. Labels such as "juvenile delinquent," "hoodlum," or "failure" are applied to certain adolescents, who then accept and live up to these labels with behaviors that validate and strengthen them.

The process of evolving a personal identity is time-consuming and fraught with periods of confusion, depression, and discouragement. Determining an identity and a place in the world is a critical and perilous feature of adolescence (Critical Thinking box); however, as the pieces are gradually shifted and settled

Critical Thinking

DISCUSSING THE FUTURE

Jeremy, age 17, will be graduating from high school in the spring. His mother, a single parent, tells you that she is concerned because graduation is quickly approaching and Jeremy has made no plans for what he will do with his life after graduation. Whenever Jeremy mentions the topic, his mother tells him, "This is what you must do," and begins to outline the steps he must take. Jeremy just walks away. She asks, "What should I do?" Which of the following would be your must appropriate advice to Jeremy's mother?

First Think About It...

- **From what point of view are you thinking?**
- **What conclusions are you reaching?**

1. **"Think about Jeremy's interests and what he has been successful doing in the past. Arrange for him to speak to someone whose career builds on those interests."**
2. **"Continue to tell him what he must do. Eventually you will get through to him, and he will listen."**
3. **"Be open and available to him. Tell him what you think, but not what to do."**
4. **"You are wise to be concerned. We need to arrange some counseling for Jeremy."**

The best response at this stage is 3. Most adolescents want adult guidance and help, and messages are more likely to be heard if they are presented in an open-ended, nonjudgmental, nondictatorial fashion. Teenagers are unlikely to discuss their concerns on a timetable, and it is important to respect their point of view. Parents create the time and space and then wait. Parents who are available and willing to listen generally find that their adolescents are eager to talk. Answer 1 could be a good second step if Jeremy and his mother explore his interests together. Answer 2 is disrespectful of Jeremy, has not worked in the past, and likely will not work in the future. Answer 4 may be necessary at a later time if other strategies fail.

into place, a positive identity eventually emerges from the confusion. Role diffusion results when the individual is unable to formulate a satisfactory identity from the multiplicity of aspirations, roles, and identifications.

Sex-role Identity. Adolescence is the time for consolidation of a sex-role identity. During early adolescence the peer group begins to communicate some expectations regarding heterosexual relationships, and as development progresses, adolescents encounter expectations for mature sex-role behavior from both peers and adults. Expectations such as these vary from culture to culture, among geographic areas, and among socioeconomic groups.

Emotionality. Adolescents vacillate in their emotional states and between considerable maturity and child-like behavior. One minute they are exuberant and enthusiastic; the next minute they are depressed and withdrawn. Unpredictable but essentially normal outbursts of primitive behavior appear as the teenager loses control over instinctual drives. As the tension is relieved, emotion is brought under control and individuals retreat to review what has happened, to attempt to master their anger, and to grow in their ability to control their emotions and gain from the new experience. Because of these mood swings, adolescents are often labeled as unstable, inconsistent, and unpredictable. Little things can cause an emotional upheaval and, depending on the teenager's interpretation, can mean a great deal.

Teenagers are better able to control their emotions in later adolescence. They can approach problems more calmly and rationally and, although they are still subject to periods of depression, their feelings are less vulnerable and they begin to demonstrate the more mature emotions of later adolescence. Whereas early adolescents react immediately and emotionally, older adolescents can control their emotions until socially acceptable times and places for expression present themselves. They are still subject to heightened emotion; when it is expressed, their behavior reflects feelings of insecurity, tension, and indecision.

Cognitive Development (Piaget)

Cognitive thinking culminates with the capacity for *abstract thinking.* This stage, the period of *formal operations,* is Piaget's fourth and last stage. Adolescents are no longer restricted to the real and actual, which was typical of the period of concrete thought; they are also concerned with the possible. They now think beyond the present. Without having to center attention on the immediate situation, they can imagine a sequence of events that might occur, such as college and occupational possibilities; how things might change in the future, such as relationships with parents; and the consequences of their actions, such as dropping out of school. At this time their thoughts can be influenced by logical principles rather than just their own perceptions and experiences. They now become increasingly capable of scientific reasoning and formal logic.

Adolescents are capable of mentally manipulating more than two categories of variables at the same time. For example, they can consider the relationship between speed, distance, and time in planning a trip. They can detect logical consistency or inconsistency in a set of statements, and evaluate a system or set of values in a more analytic manner. For instance, they question the parent who insists on honesty in the youngster but at the same time cheats on an income tax report or expense account.

Young people are now able to think about both their own thinking and the thinking of others. They wonder what opinion others have of them, and they are increasingly able to imagine the thoughts of others. With this capacity comes the ability to differentiate between others' thoughts and their own, and to interpret the thoughts of others more accurately. Thus they are able to understand that few concepts are absolute or independent of other influencing factors. As they come to know that other cultures and communities have different norms and standards from their own, it becomes easier to accept members of these other cultures, and the decision to behave in their own culture in an accepted manner becomes a more conscious commitment to that culture.

Moral Development (Kohlberg)

Whereas younger children merely accept the decisions or point of view of adults, adolescents, to gain autonomy from adults, must substitute their own set of morals and values. When old principles are challenged but new and independent values have not yet emerged to take their place, young people search for a moral code that preserves their personal integrity and guides their behavior, especially in the face of strong pressure to violate the old beliefs. Their decisions involving moral dilemmas must be based on an *internalized set of moral principles* that provides them with the resources to evaluate the demands of the situation and to plan a course of action that is consistent with their ideals.

Late adolescence is characterized by a serious questioning of existing moral values and their relevance to society and the individual. They understand duty and obligation based on reciprocal rights of others, as well as the concept of justice that is founded on making amends for misdeeds and repairing or replacing what has been spoiled by wrongdoing. However, they seriously question established moral codes, often as a result of observing that adults verbally ascribe to a code but do not adhere to it.

Spiritual Development

As youngsters move toward independence from parents and other authorities, some begin to question the values and ideals of their families. Others cling to these values as a stable element in their lives as they struggle with the conflicts of this turbulent period. Adolescents need to work out these conflicts for themselves, but they also need support from authority figures and/or peers for their resolution. Often the peer group is more influential than parents, although values acquired during the formative years are usually maintained.

Adolescents are capable of understanding abstract concepts and of interpreting analogies and symbols. They are able to empathize, philosophize, and think logically. Most are searching for ideals, and speculate about illogical statements and conflicting ideologies. Their tendency toward introspection and emotional intensity at this age often makes it difficult for others to know what they are thinking. They tend to keep their thoughts private, fearing that no one will understand these feelings, which they perceive to be unique and special; however, they may reveal deep spiritual concerns. They need support and encouragement in their struggle for understanding, and the freedom to question without censure.

Young people may reject formal worship services but engage in individual worship in the privacy of their room. They may need to explore the concept of the existence of God. Comparing their religion with that of others may result in their questioning their own beliefs, but ultimately results in formulating and solidifying their spirituality.

Social Development

To achieve full maturity, adolescents must free themselves from family domination and define an identity independent of parental authority. However, this process is fraught with ambivalence on the part of both teenagers and their parents. Adolescents want to grow up and to be free of parental restraints, but they are fearful as they try to comprehend the responsibilities that are linked with independence. Feelings of immortality and exemption from the consequences of risk-taking behavior, although viewed as negative, can serve an important developmental function at this time. These feelings can give adolescents the courage to separate from their parents and become independent. Part of this emancipation involves developing social relationships outside the family that help teenagers identify their role in society. Adolescence is a time of intense sociability and is often a time of equally intense loneliness. Acceptance by peers, a few close friends, and the secure love of a supportive family are requisites for the interpersonal maturation process.

Relationships with Parents. During adolescence the parent-child relationship changes from one of protection-dependency to one of *mutual affection and equality.* The process of achieving independence often involves turmoil and ambiguity as both parent and adolescent learn to play new roles and work toward this end while, at the same time, resolving the often painful series of rifts essential to establishing the ultimate relationship.

Most of the behavior observed in the adolescent is related to the struggle for independence and the external restrictions and checks that are placed on this spontaneous maturation process. On the one hand, adolescents are accepted as maturing preadults: they are allowed privileges heretofore denied, and are provided with increasing responsibilities. On the other hand, because of their unpredictability and insecurity in evaluating situations and making sound judgments, they must conform to regulations and restrictions set by adults. This state of affairs is exemplified by the struggle between parents and adolescents concerning the nightly curfew.

As teenagers assert their rights for grown-up privileges, they often create tensions within the home. They resist parental control, and conflicts can arise from almost any situation or any subject. Some of the favorite topics of dispute include use of the telephone, manners, dress, chores and duties, homework, disrespectful behavior, friendships, dating, money, automobiles, drinking and/or drugs, and time schedules. Present in these areas of conflict are the overriding argument that "Everyone else has one" or is allowed the desired item or privilege and the ever-present assertions that "You don't understand me or trust me" and "You always treat me like a baby." Spoken or unspoken, parents' reactions consist of "Is this all the thanks I get for what I have done, or am doing, for you?"

The teenager's earliest attempts to achieve emancipation from parental controls are manifested in a period of rejection of the parents. Adolescents are critical, argumentative, and generally remote with both parents. They absent themselves from home and family activities and spend an increasing amount of time with the peer group. They confide less in their parents. Rejection is not consistent, however, and varies with mood changes. Parents continue to play an important role in the personal and health-related decision making of many adolescents.

With advancing adolescence, teenagers become more competent, and with this competence comes a need for more autonomy. Although they may be psychologically prepared for independence, they are often thwarted in their efforts by lack of money or other parental barriers. Conflict arises in relation to the teenager's outside activities and the elements of privacy and trust. Parental supervision remains important throughout adolescence and may have a direct influence on adolescent sexual and substance use behavior. Parents should be guided toward an authoritative style of parenting in which authority is used to guide the adolescent while allowing developmentally appropriate levels of freedom and providing clear, consistent messages regarding expectations (Baker et al, 1999). However, to gain the trust of adolescents, parents must respect their youngster's privacy, as well as show an honest and sincere interest in what the adolescent believes and feels (Family Focus box).

Recent trends of society in terms of equality and relaxation of previous moral standards have made the adjustments of teenagers and parents very difficult. The so-called generation gap is widening in relation to a number of attitudes, values, and beliefs. Parents can no longer find guidance from their own experiences in understanding the needs of today's teenagers.

Relationships with Peers. Although parents remain the primary influence in their lives, for the majority of teenagers, peers assume a more significant role in adolescence than they did during childhood. The peer group serves as a strong support to teenagers. Individually and collectively providing them with a sense of belonging and a feeling of strength

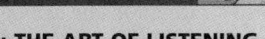

Family Focus

COMMUNICATION WITH TEENS: THE ART OF LISTENING

Conflicts between parents and their adolescents are often a result of a very natural characteristic of parenthood: the desire to protect one's offspring—from harm or from simply doing something "stupid" or embarrassing or something they may later regret. Teenagers sometimes "bounce" their thoughts and ideas off adults. At times they really want some feedback; at other times they simply want to elicit a reaction.

I found it easy to listen openly, thoughtfully, and without interrupting when my teenagers' friends discussed troublesome topics. However, one day, when one of my own teenagers had a similar conversation with me, the parent part kicked in. I felt responsible and spoke my piece on the spot. This brought communication to a halt and resulted in defensiveness. It was a long time before my child tried to talk to me about anything controversial again.

The next time one of my teenagers started a similar conversation, I decided to try to trick myself. Throughout the entire conversation, I told myself over and over again to act as if this were not my teenager, but rather someone else's child. I found this actually worked quite well, and I was able to listen without interrupting. I continued to use the system, sometimes with more success than at other times.

Mother of four

and power, it forms that transitional world between dependence and autonomy.

Peer Group. Adolescents are usually social, gregarious, and group minded. Thus the peer group has an intense influence on adolescents' self-evaluation and behavior. To gain acceptance by a group, younger teenagers tend to conform completely in such things as mode of dress, hairstyle, taste in music, and vocabulary, often at the expense of individuality and self-assertion. The teenager's entire being is measured by the reactions of his or her peers.

The school is psychologically important to adolescents as a focus of social life. Teenagers usually distribute themselves into a relatively predictable social hierarchy. They know to which groups they and others belong. A sense of school connectedness has been found to predict decreased risk-taking behaviors in adolescents (Resnick et al, 1997).

Within the larger groups are smaller, distinct, and rather exclusive crowds or cliques of selected close friends who are emotionally attached to each other. The selection is based on common tastes, interests, and background. Although cliques may become formalized, most remain informal and small. However, each has an identifying feature that proclaims its difference from others and its solidarity within itself, in much the same manner as the adolescent generation as a whole sets itself apart from the adult generation. Cliques are usually made up of one sex, and girls tend to be more cliquish than boys and to have a greater need for close friendships (Fig. 40-4). Within the intimacy of the group, adolescents gain support in learning about themselves, consideration for the feelings of others, and increased ego development and self-reliance.

To belong is of utmost importance; thus adolescents behave in a way that will ensure their establishment in a group. Adolescents are highly susceptible to social approval, acceptance, and demands. To be ignored or criticized by peers creates feelings of inferiority, inadequacy, and incompetence.

Heterosexual Relationships. During adolescence, relationships with members of the opposite sex take on new importance (Fig. 40-5). Although there seems to be a trend toward earlier dating, on the *average* dating activities begin in the seventh and eighth grades, and are usually "crowd" dates at organized school functions. For example, a group of girls just happen to be around a certain group of boys at most activities. During high school, crowd dates are still popular, but now there is more pairing off as couples. Double-dating and then single-pair dating follow group dating. Most adolescents are dating to some degree by the time they leave high school.

The type and degree of seriousness of heterosexual relationships vary. The initial stage is usually noncommittal, extremely mobile, and seldom characterized by any deep romantic attachments. Crushes, those strong feelings of attachment to an important or well-liked adult who embodies the qualities considered most valuable by the adolescent, are common in early adolescence and constitute one of the earliest "love" attachments. In a large sample of early to middle adolescents, boys fell in love earlier and more often than girls. However, both boys and girls had a narrow range for what qualified as being "in love" (Montgomery and Sorrell, 1998).

Middle adolescence is the time when teenagers begin to develop romantic relationships and when most teenagers begin sexual experimentation. Early and middle adolescents choose their partners based on physical and personality characteristics that are acceptable to their peer group. Through these relationships and experimentation, early and middle adolescents begin to explore and understand romantic feelings and experiences. As teenagers move into late adolescence, the partner choice is more likely to be based on individual characteristics and interests.

Sexual Activity. Sexuality and sexual activity is an area that should be addressed with each adolescent in a confidential

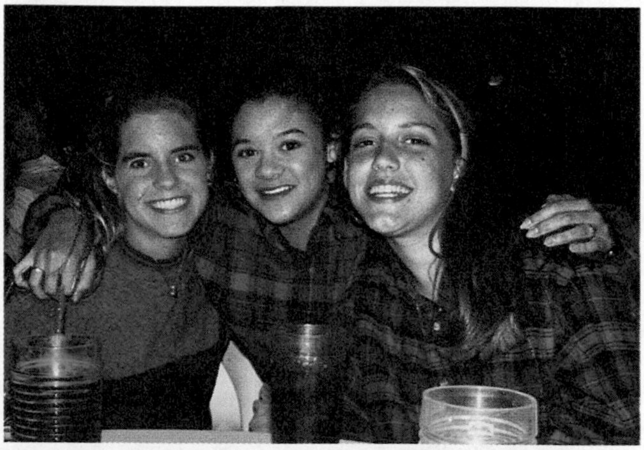

FIG. 40-4 • Teenagers like to gather in small groups.

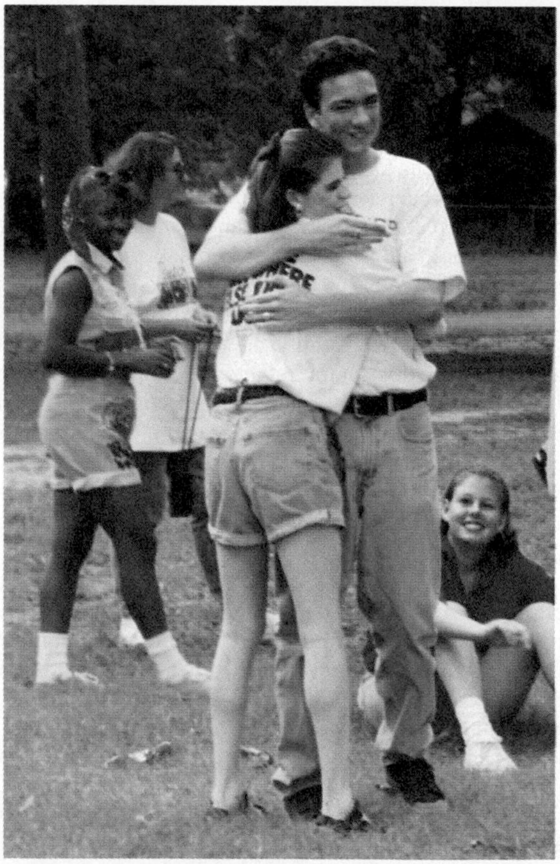

FIG. 40-5 • Heterosexual relationships are an important part of adolescence.

manner. The incidence of sexual activity among teenagers is high and increases with age. Most teenagers younger than 15 years have not had sex; 8 in 10 girls and 7 in 10 boys are still virgins at age 15 years. Among teenagers who have initiated sexual intercourse at an age younger than 14 years, the incidence of sexual abuse is very high. However, by 17 years of age, more than 50% of teenagers have had volitional sexual intercourse (Alan Guttmacher Institute, 1998).

There is a full range of sexual exploration among teenagers, extending from individual masturbation; to petting and mutual masturbation; and to sexual intercourse. In a study of adolescent virgins, 29% reported having engaged in heterosexual masturbation of a partner, and a smaller percentage had engaged in oral sex (Schuster, Bell, and Kanouse, 1996). A careful sexual history helps to determine areas of risk on which the nurse can focus risk reduction messages.

Adolescents become involved in sexual relationships for a variety of reasons: to obtain pleasurable sensations, to satisfy sexual drives, to satisfy curiosity, as a conquest, as an expression of affection, or because they are not able to withstand pressures to conform. Often the urge to belong to and gain reassurance from a group and the wish to really belong to someone provoke a series of increasingly intimate physical contacts with a favored boyfriend or girlfriend.

Girls report less partner pressure for sexual intercourse than boys; however, girls report more disapproval from parents (DeGaston, Weed, and Jensen, 1996). Sex education programs for teenagers need to be sensitive to these gender differences, as well as to the developmental level of the adolescent.

Critical Thinking

DISCUSSING SEXUAL ORIENTATION WITH ADOLESCENTS

John, a 17-year-old adolescent, comes into the school-based clinic and tells the nurse practitioner that he thinks he is homosexual. Which of the following is the most appropriate response for the practitioner to make?

First, Think About It...

- What is the purpose of your thinking?
- What would the consequences be if you put your thoughts into action?

1. "Have you ever tried to have an intimate relationship with a member of the opposite sex?"
2. "How do you know you are not heterosexual?"
3. "Don't worry. This is probably just a phase that you will outgrow."
4. "Tell me more about how you came to this conclusion."

The best response is 4. This response gives John permission to discuss his feelings about this topic. John has come to the nurse practitioner to discuss this matter, and he probably feels comfortable sharing this information with her. The nurse practitioner needs to be open and nonjudgmental in her discussion with John, which is the purpose of her thinking at this point. Above all, John needs to know that she will appreciate his feelings and remain sensitive to his need to talk about this topic. All of the other responses seem to imply that heterosexual relationships are the most appropriate, and that the nurse practitioner assumes that every adolescent will be heterosexual. These responses could end the discussion or convince John that the nurse practitioner is uncomfortable discussing this issue, which could have negative consequences.

Homosexuality in Adolescents. During adolescence, youths develop a sexual identity. This process becomes incredibly complicated when the sexual identity is not heterosexual. Retrospective studies of gay men and lesbians indicate that adolescence is when individuals become aware of same-sex attraction. Gay men become aware of this same-sex attraction at a younger mean age than do gay women. Homosexual and bisexual youths face tremendous challenges to growing up and becoming mentally and physically healthy when confronted with antihomosexual attitudes and values. These adolescents are at increased risk for health-damaging behaviors, not because of the sexual behavior itself, but because of society's reaction to the behavior (Saewyc et al, 1998). Behaviors that place homosexual and bisexual youths at risk for poor health outcomes include early initiation of sexual activity (usually heterosexual), suicide and suicidal ideation, running away from home, and engaging in behaviors that result in sexually transmitted diseases. Nurses who interact with adolescents who are dealing with sexual identity issues must be open to an exploration of these concerns and provide a nonthreatening environment in which teenagers can discuss their problems and ask questions (Wells. 1999) (Critical Thinking box).

Interests and Activities. Adolescents spend a large amount of time engaging in leisure-time activities. As teenagers progress through the developmental stages of adolescence, these leisure-time activities move from being family centered to being peer centered. In addition to providing teenagers with fun and enjoyment, leisure-time activities assist in the development of social, physical, and cognitive skills. Leisure-time activities also allow teenagers the opportunity to learn to set priorities and structure their time (Fig. 40-6).

Today, many adolescents must learn to juggle their time between school, leisure-time activities, and the responsibilities of a job. Adolescent work experiences provide many benefits, including time management, teamwork skills, and increased in-

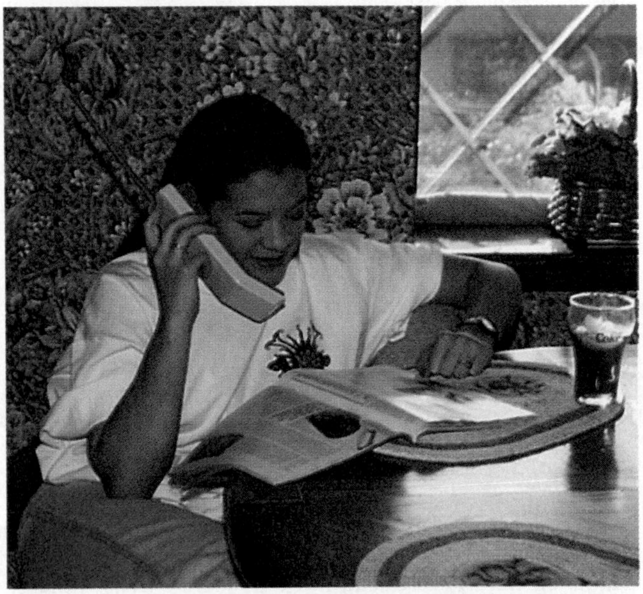

FIG. 40-6 • The telephone, especially the portable phone, provides teenagers with hours of conversation with same-sex and opposite-sex friends.

TABLE 40-1
Growth and Development During Adolescence

Early Adolescence (11-14 Years)	Middle Adolescence (15-17 Years)	Late Adolescence (18-20 Years)
GROWTH		
Rapidly accelerating growth Growth reaches peak velocity Secondary sex characteristics appear	Growth decelerating in girls Stature reaches 95% of adult height Secondary sex characteristics well advanced	Physically mature Structure and reproductive growth almost complete
COGNITION		
Explores newfound ability for limited abstract thought Clumsy groping for new values and energies Comparison of "normality" with peers of same sex	Developing capacity for abstract thinking Enjoys intellectual powers, often in idealistic terms Concern with philosophic, political, and social problems	Established abstract thought Can perceive and act on long-range options Able to view problems comprehensively Intellectual and functional identity established
IDENTITY		
Preoccupied with rapid body changes Trying out of various roles Measurement of attractiveness by acceptance or rejection of peers Conformity to group norms	Modifies body image Very self-centered; increased narcissism Tendency toward inner experience and self-discovery Has a rich fantasy life Idealistic Able to perceive future implications of current behavior and decisions; variable application	Body image and gender-role definition nearly secured Mature sexual identity Phase of consolidation of identity Stability of self-esteem Comfortable with physical growth Social roles defined and articulated
RELATIONSHIPS WITH PARENTS		
Defining independence-dependence boundaries Strong desire to remain dependent on parents while trying to detach No major conflicts over parental control	Major conflicts over independence and control Low point in parent-child relationship Greatest push for emancipation; disengagement Final and irreversible emotional detachment from parents; mourning	Emotional and physical separation from parents completed Independence from family with less conflict Emancipation nearly secured
RELATIONSHIPS WITH PEERS		
Seeks peer affiliations to counter instability generated by rapid change Upsurge of close, idealized friendships with members of the same sex Struggle for mastery takes place within peer group	Strong need for identity to affirm self-image Behavioral standards set by peer group Acceptance by peers extremely important—fear of rejection Exploration of ability to attract opposite sex	Peer group recedes in importance in favor of individual friendship Testing of male-female relationships against possibility of permanent alliance Relationships characterized by giving and sharing
SEXUALITY		
Self-exploration and evaluation Limited dating, usually group Limited intimacy	Multiple plural relationships Decisive turn toward heterosexuality (if homosexual, knows by this time) Exploration of "sex appeal" Feeling of "being in love" Tentative establishment of relationships	Forms stable relationships and attachment to another Growing capacity for mutuality and reciprocity Dating as a male-female pair Intimacy involves commitment rather than exploration and romanticism
PSYCHOLOGIC HEALTH		
Wide mood swings Intense daydreaming Anger outwardly expressed with moodiness, temper outbursts, and verbal insults and name-calling	Tendency toward inner experiences; more introspective Tendency to withdraw when upset or feelings are hurt Vacillation of emotions in time and range Feelings of inadequacy common; difficulty in asking for help	More constancy of emotion Anger more apt to be concealed

come; however, many jobs available to teenagers do not provide opportunities to apply the skills they learn in school, and jobs often have high demands for quick work with low rewards. Very few apprentice opportunities are available for teenagers. It is generally recommended that adolescents limit their work week to no more than 20 hours during the school year.

Development of Self-Concept and Body Image

The sudden growth that takes place in early adolescence creates feelings of confusion for adolescents. They have lost the security of a familiar body and feel a strangeness about their altered body. Consequently, they may try to either hide their body or advertise it, or they may alternate between the two extremes. Teenagers are acutely aware of their appearance as they begin to acquire images of themselves as adults, but they see discrepancies between their ideal and actual skills and abilities.

Adolescents are continually comparing themselves with their peers and making judgments about their own normality based on these observations. Pubertal children feel most comfortable when they are just like their friends and age-mates. Perceived defects or deviations from the group average are threatening to their idealized image. Any blemish is likely to be magnified out of proportion, and any delay of the visible evidence of maturity is cause for worry. Unfortunately, this is also the time when the hormonal effect of the sebaceous glands produces acne, which creates problems for many youngsters. To the adolescent, even the most insignificant pimple may be viewed as a gross disfigurement; every blemish is a major catastrophe. The advent of chronic disease or a permanent physical disability has very special significance during adolescence and creates additional stresses for both the youngster with the condition and health care providers.

It has been determined that the body image established during adolescence is the one that individuals retain throughout life. Much of the adolescent's search for identity takes place before a mirror as they try to read from the reflected features just who they are and what they look like to other people. Adolescents practice facial expressions and postures, try out hair arrangements, worry about a pimple, and in other ways attempt to assess the best means to achieve a maximum effect—to reveal the "true self."

The self-concept becomes more differentiated as adolescents acquire a more complex picture of themselves, one that takes situational factors into account. The self-concept gradually becomes more individualized and more distinct from the concepts of others. Although younger teenagers describe themselves in terms of similarities with peers, as adolescence advances, young people describe themselves in terms of their own special characteristics.

Responses to Puberty. The response to the physical changes of pubertal growth and development is manifested differently depending on the stage of development. During early adolescence, young adolescents become preoccupied with the rapid changes in their body, and they are very interested in the anatomy, physiology, and function of their sexual organs. Boys must also confront the sexual feelings and tensions that accompany puberty, and the appearance of nocturnal emissions may be puzzling, troublesome, or embarrassing events. Unless the boy has been prepared in advance, he may find it difficult to discuss his feelings with his parents and may run to his friends for information and guidance. Many girls also find the rapid changes in their body to be sources of concern. Some girls perceive the increase in weight and associated fat deposition as evidence of obesity and may indulge in fad diets. Although many girls look forward to menstruation and take this event in stride, others may find the first menstrual period a distressing and frightening event. All teenagers, regardless of gender, are very concerned with the question "Am I normal?" To answer this question, they compare their body with the bodies of their peers and with images in the media. This leads to a great deal of uncertainty about their own appearance and attractiveness.

If an adolescent does not enter puberty at the same time as his or her peers, considerable inner conflict may occur. Early-maturing girls and boys, as well as late-maturing boys, have higher rates of risk-taking behaviors than their on-time peers (Graber et al, 1997; Hayward et al, 1997). Nurses who work with adolescents must provide teaching and health care interventions that are appropriate for the chronologic and cognitive development of the adolescent rather than for the physical maturation.

As growth and development proceed through middle adolescence, the rapid body changes diminish, and the adolescent has time to try to make the body more attractive. Adolescents strive to achieve the perfect body within their own cultural norms. The "right" clothes and hairstyle become very important. By late adolescence the heightened concern with body image has ended and is replaced with a general comfort with the body.

The changes that occur during the early, middle, and late phases of adolescence are summarized in Table 40-1.

PROMOTING OPTIMUM HEALTH DURING ADOLESCENCE

The major causes of morbidity and mortality in adolescence are not diseases, but health-damaging behaviors. New sources of morbidity in adolescence include injury, depression, violence, sexually transmitted infections, and pregnancy. Health promotion for this age group consists mainly of teaching and guidance to avoid risk-taking activities and health-damaging behaviors. Adolescence provides an opportunity for teenagers to incorporate healthy lifestyle behaviors that will benefit them not only during the teenage years but also throughout the life span.

Effective health education for adolescents should incorporate a developmentally appropriate, multifaceted approach, but education alone is not enough to change behavior. Effective programs must include opportunities for skill building and must be comprehensive rather than problem focused and include a community-wide approach (Hamburg, 1997).

As teenagers progress through adolescence, they are able to assume additional responsibility for their own health, including maintaining health practices, taking prescribed medications, keeping appointments, and performing procedures when necessary. Health professionals who work with adolescents should consider the adolescent's increasing independence and responsibility while maintaining privacy and ensuring confidentiality (Guidelines and Critical Thinking boxes). Parents should also respect their teenager's independence and move toward the role of consultant about health issues while also maintaining some level of parental involvement throughout adolescence.

Guidelines

INTERVIEWING ADOLESCENTS

Ensure confidentiality and privacy; interview adolescent without parents.

Show concern for adolescent's perspective: "First, I'd like to talk about your main concerns" and "I'd like to know what you think is happening."

Offer a nonthreatening explanation for the questions you ask: "I'm going to ask a number of questions to help me better understand your health."

Maintain objectivity; avoid assumptions, judgments, and lectures.

Ask open-ended questions when possible; move to more directive questions if necessary.

Begin with less sensitive issues and proceed to more sensitive ones.

Use language that both the adolescent and you understand. Clarify terms, such as "having sex."

Use gender neutral terms, such as partner rather than boyfriend or girlfriend.

Restate: reflect back to adolescents what they have said, along with feelings that may be associated with their descriptions.

Critical Thinking

RESPECTING PRIVACY

Jamie S, a 17-year-old girl, arrives with her mother for a routine history and physical examination for college entrance. As you are taking Jamie to an examination room, her mother whispers to you, "I need to speak with you in private." What would be your most appropriate response?

First Think About It...

- What concepts or ideas are central to your thinking?
- What precise question are you trying to answer?

1. Ask Jamie to undress to prepare for the examination while you take her mother to another room to find out what's on her mind.
2. Say to Jamie's mother in Jamie's presence, "Mrs. S, whatever you have to say to me, you need to say in front of Jamie."
3. Say to Jamie and her mother, "I would like to begin by speaking with both of you together, then spend some time just with you, Mrs. S, then just with you, Jamie."
4. Say to Jamie and her mother, "I would like to begin by speaking with both of you together, then spend some time just with you, Jamie, then just with you, Mrs. S."

The best response is 4. Jamie and her mother need to know ahead of time that they will each have an opportunity to express their concerns in private. Since Jamie is your patient, she should be first, which is a central concept in your thinking. Knowing that her mother will also have an opportunity to express concerns, Jamie will likely be more open and may even say, "I know what my mother will tell you," and address the issue herself. Option 1 is disrespectful of Jamie, and option 2 is disrespectful of Jamie's mother and her concerns. Option 1 is poor for two reasons. First, an explanation of what will occur and the interview should precede getting undressed for an examination. Second, Jamie likely will be aware that you are speaking with her mother, feel that her privacy is being violated, and become defensive and distrustful of both you and her mother. Although response 3 gives both mother and daughter an opportunity to express concerns, if Mrs. S goes first, Jamie is likely to spend time trying to draw from you what her mother said and/or become defensive.

In response to changes in adolescent morbidity and mortality, the American Medical Association developed the *Guidelines for Adolescent Preventive Services (GAPS),* which provides a framework for health care providers to use in their clinical practice (Allensworth and Bradley, 1996). The following discussion provides information on specific GAPS topics and recommendations related to screening, guidance, and immunizations.

Immunizations

An immunization update is an important part of adolescent preventive care. Obtaining a record of the teenager's prior immunizations is important. Adolescents should receive a tetanus-diphtheria (Td) vaccine at the age of 11 to 12 years and no later than 16 years if a period of at least 5 years has elapsed since the last dose of diphtheria-tetanus-pertussis or acellular pertussis, or diphtheria-tetanus (DTP, DTaP, or DT) vaccine. Subsequent routine Td boosters are recommended every 10 years. With the exception of pregnant teenagers, all adolescents should receive a second measles-mumps-rubella (MMR) vaccine unless they have documentation of two MMR vaccinations during childhood but not before 12 months of age. All adolescents who have not previously received three doses of hepatitis B vaccine should be vaccinated against hepatitis B virus. All adolescents should also be assessed for previous history of varicella infection or vaccination. Vaccination with the varicella vaccine is recommended for those with no previous history. For adolescents over age 13 years, the varicella vaccine is given in two doses 4 or more weeks apart. Hepatitis A vaccine should be given to adolescents living in communities with high rates of hepatitis A or those with risk factors for hepatitis A such as illicit injectable drug use or high risk sexual activity (American Academy of Pediatrics, 2000). (See also Immunizations, Chapter 36.)

Nutrition

The rapid and extensive increase in height, weight, muscle mass, and sexual maturity of adolescence is accompanied by greater nutritional requirements. Because nutritional needs are closely related to the increase in body mass, the peak requirements occur in the years of maximum growth, during which the body mass almost doubles. The caloric and protein requirements during this time are higher than at almost any other time of life. As a result of increased anabolic need, the adolescent is highly sensitive to caloric restrictions.

The nutritional needs of adolescents are difficult to determine because of meager nutritional information on members of this age group. This difficulty is further complicated by the influence of emotional and other stress factors affecting nutrient utilization and the psychologic factors that influence eating habits. In addition, the wide variations in growth rates during adolescence—and the equally wide variations in ages at which these changes take place—complicate attempts to set minimum dietary standards.

Adolescents usually have sufficient intake of protein to meet their needs, except those who limit their food intake because of economic problems or in an attempt to lose weight. There is a substantial increase in the need for the minerals, calcium, iron, and zinc during periods of rapid growth: calcium for skeletal growth, iron for expansion of muscle mass and blood volume, and zinc for the generation of both skeletal and bone tissue.

Girls with very heavy or frequent menses may be especially susceptible to iron deficiency due to blood loss. Calcium intake from food sources is essential during adolescence to assist in the prevention of osteoporosis. Eventual bone mass is a balance between the amount of bone laid down during adolescence and the amount later lost with aging. Overall, osteoporosis is a result of genetic and environmental factors such as nutrition and exercise (Ralston, 1997). Dietary intervention should promote the regular consumption of breakfast and a balanced intake of a variety of foods.

Eating Habits and Behavior. Eating and attitudes toward food are primarily family centered during early and middle childhood, and food habits are largely related to cultural and individual family preferences and patterns. With adolescence and the move toward independence, family influences on the child change. Children's interests, attitudes, and routines are altered as an increasing number of meals are eaten away from home. These changes are largely a result of the high value that teenagers place on peer acceptability and sociability; therefore their eating habits are easily influenced by their associates.

Pressure for time and commitments to activities adversely affect the teenager's eating habits. Omitting breakfast or eating a breakfast that is nutritionally poor in quality is often a problem. Snacks, usually selected on the basis of accessibility rather than nutritional merit, become more and more a part of the habitual eating pattern during adolescence (Fig. 40-7). Adolescents often eat an insufficient amount of fresh fruits and vegetables, especially those that are rich in ascorbic acid. Milk is usually passed over in favor of soft drinks.

Overeating or undereating during adolescence presents special problems. When they experience the normal increase in weight and fat deposition of the growth spurt, teenage girls often resort to dieting. The desire for a slim figure and a fear of becoming "fat" prompt teenage girls to embark on nutritionally inadequate reducing regimens that drain their energy and deprive their growing bodies of essential nutrients. They resort to diets on their own or with peers in an effort to conform. Many adopt the current fad diets and are victims of food misinformation. Boys are less inclined to undereat; they are more concerned about gaining size and strength. However, they tend to eat foods high in calories but low in other essential nutrients.

Obesity is increasing among both children and adolescents in the United States. The obesity currently seen is not a result of metabolic disturbances, but of poor dietary habits and increased sedentary lifestyles. Childhood obesity often results in obesity in adulthood. However, lifestyle changes necessary for adolescents to lose weight require the involvement of family members who provide support and encourage active participation (Strauss, 1999).

Nursing Care Management. Healthy dietary habits should be discussed with all adolescents. Adolescents need to learn about the Food Guide Pyramid (see Fig. 12-4); the relationships among dietary fat, weight status, and health; and food sources of fat, salt, and fiber (Seidell, 1999). Their food habits must be considered when planning nutritional education and guidance because they reflect many influences and conditions.

To help teenagers select a nutritious diet, it is best to begin with their present diet and actively involve them in the process. Teenagers do not respond well to judgmental attitudes and dislike lectures, but they do respond when their independence is respected and they are given the opportunity to make their own decisions regarding food choices.

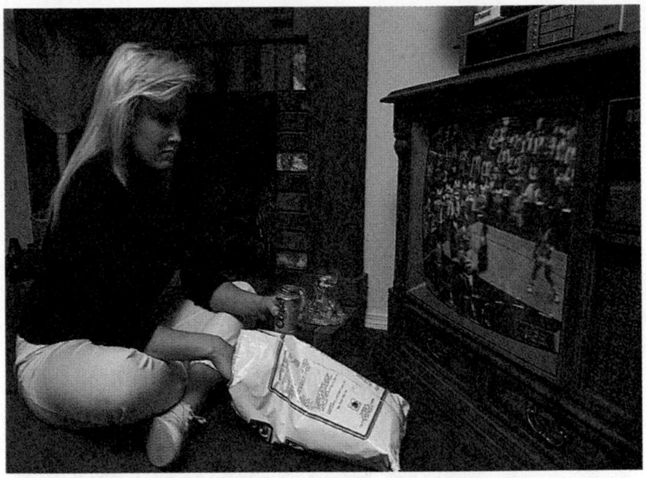

FIG. 40-7 • Snacking on empty calories is common among adolescents, especially during inactivity.

In general, adolescents are body conscious and concerned about their appearance. Concrete messages about the relationship between an attractive appearance and the benefits of a healthy lifestyle are most effective. However, helping young persons arrive at a decision for change is more difficult than providing information. They respond best when the counselor provides straightforward information, uses instructional methods that actively involve them, talks with them and not at them, and listens to what they have to say.

Sleep and Rest

Teenagers vary in their need for sleep and rest. Rapid physical growth, the tendency toward overexertion, and the overall increased activity of this age contribute to fatigue in adolescents. During growth spurts the need for sleep is increased. Their propensity for staying up late makes it very difficult to arise in the morning, and they may sleep late at every opportunity. Adequate sleep and rest at this time are important to a total health regimen.

Exercise and Activity

Although today's youth are less fit than children 20 years ago, adolescents probably spend more time and energy practicing and participating in sports activities than members of any other age group. Many adolescents participate in sports within school settings (Fig. 40-8). School-based, health-oriented physical education may provide both immediate effects of the activity and sustained effects through encouragement of lifelong activity patterns. Although daily physical education classes have decreased in schools in the last 10 years, the physical education classes that are held include more time spent in actual physical activity (Francis, 1999).

The practice of sports, games, and even dancing contributes significantly to growth and development, the education process, and better health. These activities provide exercise for growing

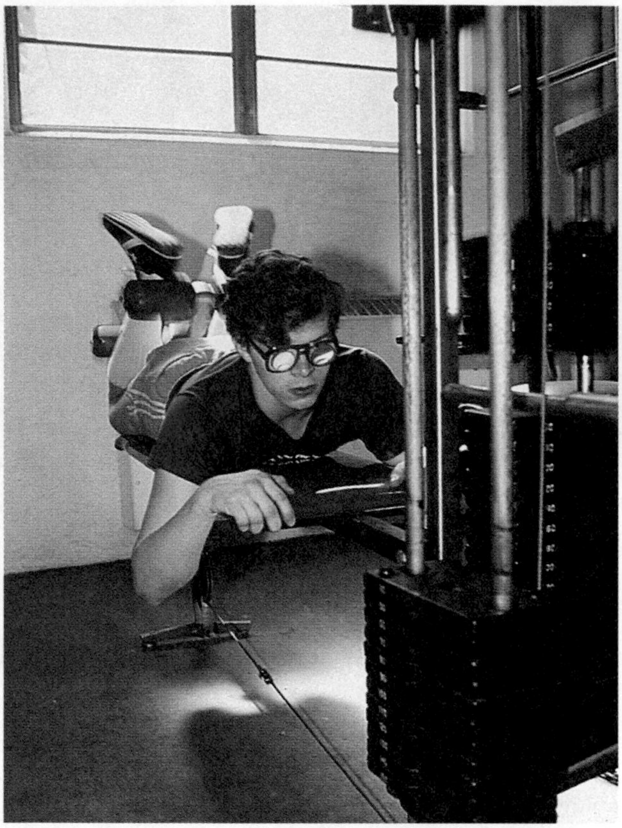

FIG. 40-8 • Adolescents should be encouraged to participate in activities that contribute to lifelong physical fitness.

muscles, interactions with peers, and a socially acceptable means of enjoying stimulation and conflict. In addition, competitive activities help the teenager in the process of self-appraisal, development of self-respect, and concern for others. Because physical fitness appears to be a major influence on one's lifelong health status, children should be encouraged to participate in activities that contribute to lifelong physical fitness. Nurses can encourage participation as a way to promote health and build self-esteem; however, youngsters should not be encouraged to engage in physical activities that are beyond their physical or emotional capacity (see Health Problems Related to Sports Participation, Chapter 39).

Dental Health

Dental health should not be neglected during adolescence, although the rate of caries formation is not as great as in childhood. Early adolescence is usually when corrective orthodontic appliances are worn, and these are often a source of embarrassment and concern to the youngster. Reassurance regarding the temporary nature of the annoyance and anticipation of an improved appearance help to make the inconvenience tolerable. It is also important to reinforce the orthodontist's directions regarding use and care of the appliances, and to emphasize careful attention to toothbrushing during this time (see also Chapters 37 and 39).

Personal Care

The body-conscious teenager is highly amenable to discussion and counseling about personal care and hygiene. Body changes associated with puberty bring with them special needs for cleanliness. The hyperactive sebaceous glands and newly functioning apocrine glands make frequent bathing or showering a necessity, and underarm deodorants assume an important place in personal care. The adolescent will find that hair requires more frequent shampooing, and girls will have questions about hair removal, use of cosmetics, and menstrual hygiene. Many group discussions center around the advantages of particular products or methods. Adolescents are continually bombarded with messages from the media regarding the best way to enhance their popularity and attractiveness. Nurses are in a position to help them evaluate the relative merits of commercial products.

Vision. Regular vision testing is an important part of health care and supervision during adolescence. During adolescence, visual refractive difficulties reach a peak that is not exceeded until the fifth decade of life. The increased demands of schoolwork make adequate vision essential for academic success. Consequently, teenagers are more likely to be referred for visual evaluation. The need for corrective lenses can create psychologic problems for teenagers if they believe that glasses spoil their appearance or do not fit their body image. For those who can afford them, contact lenses are a preferred solution. For some, the impact of a visual defect, no matter how slight, may be stressful.

Hearing. Considerable concern has focused on current teenage practices that cause hearing damage. Cochlear damage from relatively continuous exposure to the loud sound levels of rock music has been documented. The popularity of portable radios, stereo cassettes, and compact disc (CD) players with lightweight earphones are of particular concern to health care professionals. When these units are used for extended periods, permanent hearing loss can occur. Although appeals for more judicious use are not always successful, teenagers should be informed of the risk. Efforts directed toward legislating legal limits to the noise exposure that can be achieved through the sets may be another possible solution. (See Chapter 42 for a discussion of noise-related hearing loss.)

Posture. Many adolescents demonstrate altered posture. Rapid skeletal growth is often associated with slower muscular growth, and as a result, some teenagers may appear awkward or slump, and fail to stand or sit upright. However, some postural defects of adolescence require early medical intervention. Scoliosis is a defect of the spine that occurs commonly in adolescence and is more common in girls than in boys (see Scoliosis, Chapter 54). The majority of the cases are idiopathic, and the defect presents as a painless curvature of the spine. Fortunately, most of these spinal curvatures will not require treatment. However, because there is no way to predict which curvatures will progress, all curvatures of the spine should be referred for further evaluation.

Body Piercing. The popular trend of piercing the ear, nose, nipple, navel, penis, or tongue may sometimes create a health problem in the uninformed teenager. It is a nursing responsibility to caution girls and boys against the practice of having piercing performed by friends, mothers, or themselves. Although in most cases there are few if any serious side effects,

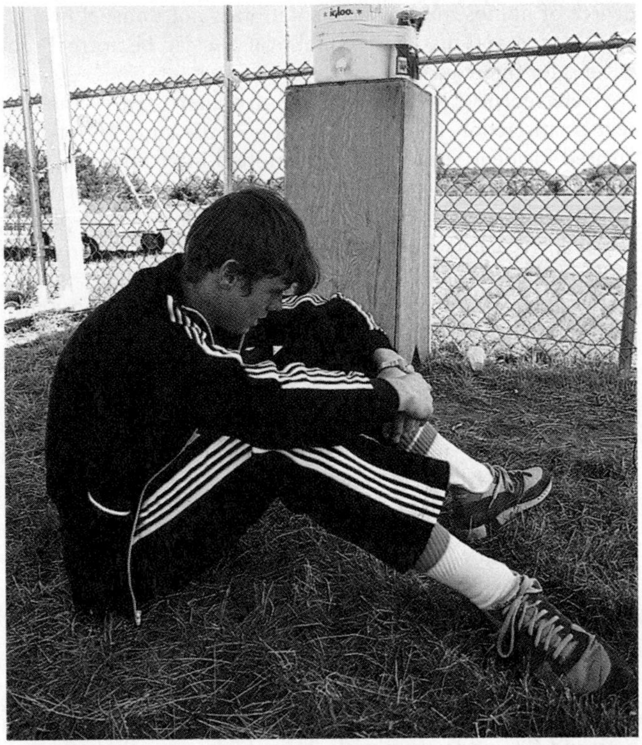

FIG. 40-9 • Adolescents use being alone as a method of coping with stress.

there is always a danger of complications such as infection, cyst or keloid formation, bleeding, dermatitis, or metal allergy. Using the same unsterilized needle to pierce body parts of multiple teenagers presents the same risk of human immunodeficiency virus (HIV) and hepatitis B virus transmission as occurs with other needle-sharing activities.

The procedure should be performed by a qualified operator using proper sterile technique. This is especially important if a youngster has a history of diabetes, allergies, or skin disorders. Adolescents should be informed about the approximate time for healing after body piercing, and the care of the pierced area during and after healing. Some body sites need extra precautions. For example, genital piercing requires special care with condoms, pierced nipples require care not to catch on clothing, and navels take longer to heal because they are covered (Muldoon, 1997).

Suntanning. The quest for an attractive appearance leads many teenagers to excessive sunbathing and artificial means for suntanning. However, this practice has serious long-term risks, and the adolescent should be educated regarding the detrimental effects of sunlight on the skin (see Sunburn, Chapter 53). Long-term effects include premature aging of the skin; increased risk of skin cancer; and, in susceptible individuals, phototoxic reactions.

The increasing popularity of artificial suntanning has prompted concern from health professionals regarding the use of sunlamps and suntanning machines. The long-term effects of tanning machines are similar to those of the sun; dermatologists do not recommend suntanning by this means. Those who insist on using suntanning equipment should be warned that goggles must be worn in tanning booths to prevent serious corneal burning. Education on the use of sunscreens, including hypoallergenic products, with a sun protective factor (SPF) of at least 15 and a nonalcohol base without lanolin, parobens, or fragrance is important (Starr, 1999). Targeting health education messages to adolescents and incorporating educational components relating to sun protection behaviors in school health curricula are also essential (Hoffmann, Rodrique, and Johnson, 1999).

Box 40-2

Areas of Stress in Adolescence

- Body image
- Sexuality conflicts
- Scholastic pressures
- Competitive pressures
- Relationships with parents
- Relationships with siblings
- Relationships with peers
- Finances
- Decisions about present and future roles
- Career planning
- Ideologic conflicts

Stress Reduction

The multiple changes occurring in adolescence can result in great stress (Fig. 40-9 and Box 40-2). Adolescents are faced with pressures from peers that often involve flaunting adult authority and taking serious health risks. Health risks include pressures for sexual experimentation and use of drugs, alcohol, and cigarettes, as well as potentially dangerous physical activities.

Early maturing girls and late-maturing children are especially sensitive to the stresses of being different from their peers. Many feel intense anxiety over their identity. Both early- and late-maturing children feel out of place among their classmates, but slow-maturing children appear to suffer the most pronounced inner turmoil and may be hesitant to voice their concerns. Slow-maturing youngsters need support and reassurance that they are not abnormal and need only be patient until the time comes when they, too, will develop the characteristics for which they yearn.

Sexuality Education and Guidance

Contemporary adolescents are constantly exposed to sexual symbolism and erotic stimulation from the mass media. At the same time, the development of primary and secondary sex characteristics and the increased sensitivity of the genitals produce thoughts and fantasies about sexual relationships. Sexual aspects of interpersonal relationships become particularly important. Societal expectations push adolescents toward dating, and their own inner sex drive urges them toward exploration.

Many adolescents are not prepared for the impact of puberty. A large portion of their knowledge relating to sex is acquired from their peers, television, the movies, and magazines. In addition, some information obtained from their parents may be inaccurate. As a result, the information they accumulate may be incomplete, inaccurate, riddled with cultural and moral judgments, and not very helpful.

The responsibility for providing sexuality education has been assumed by parents, schools, churches, community agencies such as Planned Parenthood Federation of America, Inc.,* and health professionals, especially nurses. Many adolescents perceive nurses, especially school nurses, as individuals who possess important information and who are willing to discuss sex with them. To be able to discuss the topic adequately, nurses must have not only an understanding of the physiologic aspects of sexuality and a knowledge of cultural and societal values, but also an awareness of their own attitudes, feelings, and biases about sexuality.

Comprehensive information about sexuality education is offered by the Sexuality Information and Education Council of the United States (SIECUS)† and the Sex Information and Education Council of Canada (SIEC-CAN).‡ SIECUS maintains that every sexuality education program should present the topic from six aspects: biologic, social, health, personal adjustments and attitudes, interpersonal associations, and the establishment of values.

Whether nurses counsel young people on an individual basis, in mixed groups, or in groups segregated by gender makes little difference. Ideally, boys and girls should be able to discuss sexuality objectively with one another and in groups, but this is not always possible. The differences in the rate of maturation between boys and girls and between different members of the same sex often make it desirable to discuss certain aspects of sexuality in segregated groups. As a general rule, the need for separate discussion groups diminishes as young people progress toward maturity.

Sexuality education should consist of instruction concerning normal body functions and should be presented in a straightforward manner using correct terminology. When discussing sex and sexual activities, nurses should use simple but correct language, not street language, highly scientific terminology, or evasive jargon. Once the meanings of biologic terms such as uterus, testicles, and vagina are understood, most teenagers prefer to use them in their discussions.

Many girls arrive at menarche with ambivalent attitudes, myths, and illogical beliefs. Even girls adequately prepared for menstruation do not always understand its relationship to the total process of reproduction. Many are under the incorrect impression that the "safe" time for sexual intercourse is midway between menstrual periods.

Teenagers' curiosity and desire for information extend beyond the need for anatomic and physiologic knowledge. They need to know more than the mechanics of conception, pregnancy, and birth. Adolescents, girls in particular, want answers to questions such as "What is it like?" "Does it hurt?" "What happens when . . . ?" and "Is it all right if you . . ." Boys are often concerned about the fallacy that a relationship exists between penis size and sexual function. They need reassurance that masturbation is a normal and common practice, that some degree of homosexual experimentation is not unusual in early adolescence, and that oral-genital relations can be normal substitutes for intercourse.

Teenagers need to discuss intercourse, alternative methods of sexual satisfaction, and how to resist peer pressure. With the increased incidence of sexually transmitted infections, especially HIV infection, the topic of "safe sex" (especially abstinence or the use of condoms and abstinence) is essential. Role-playing can help teenagers learn effective approaches to dealing with difficult situations. Sex and sexuality cannot be taught without discussions of mature decision making, sexual responsibility, and values clarification.

Adolescents need role models and life experiences with delayed gratification. Most important, they need problem-solving experience and decision-making skills so that they can anticipate the positive and negative outcomes of a decision. With these types of assistance, teenagers can become sexually responsible young adults.

Injury Prevention

Physical injuries are the greatest single cause of death in the adolescent age group and claim more lives than all other causes combined. The most vulnerable ages are the years 15 to 24, when accidental injuries account for about 60% of deaths in boys and 40% of deaths in girls. These figures remain fairly constant from year to year and are significant because almost all fatal injuries are preventable.

During adolescence, peak physical, sensory, and psychomotor functions give teenagers a feeling of strength and confidence that they have never experienced before, and the physiologic changes of puberty give impetus to many basic instinctual forces. One manifestation of this is an increase in energy that simply must be discharged through action, often at the expense of logical thinking and other control mechanisms. Their propensity for risk-taking behavior, plus feelings of indestructibility, make adolescents especially prone to injuries. Some of the developmental characteristics of teenagers and the common injuries associated with this age group are outlined in Table 40-2.

Vehicle-Related Injuries. The adolescent's newly acquired ability to drive, and the normal developmental need for independence and freedom, make the automobile an attractive part of an adolescent's life. Motor vehicle crashes are the single greatest cause of serious and fatal injuries in adolescents (Cohen and Potter, 1999). Many of these fatal injuries involve alcohol or other substances (Neinstein, 1996). Because there is a significant increase in the number of accidents when adolescents drive at night, many states have effectively enacted driving curfews to curtail this risk. Nurses should educate teenagers and their parents about the risk of driving while drinking alcohol or when intoxicated, or of riding in an automobile with a drunk driver. Many families have developed a plan to arrange a no-questions-asked ride home to prevent an adolescent from riding with a drunk driver. Families should also require adolescents to log several hours of supervised practice driving before taking the car out alone.

Nonautomotive Vehicle Injuries. The increasing use of motorized bicycles, all-terrain vehicles (ATVs), jet skis, and snowmobiles has caused an increase in injuries among youngsters below the legal age for driving automobiles. Many adoles-

*810 Seventh Ave., New York, NY 10019; (212) 541-7800 or 1-800-829-7732; website: www.plannedparenthood.org.

†130 W. 42nd St., Suite 350, New York, NY 10036; (212) 819-9770; website: www.siecus.org.

‡850 Coxwell Ave., EastYork, Ontario M4C 5R1; (416) 466-5304.

TABLE 40-2
Injury Prevention During Adolescence

Developmental Abilities Related to Risk of Injury	Injury Prevention
Need for independence and freedom Testing independence Age permitted to drive a motor vehicle (varies) Inclination for risk taking Feeling of indestructibility Need for discharging energy, often at expense of logical thinking and other control mechanisms Strong need for peer approval May attempt hazardous feats Peak incidence for practice and participation in sports Access to more complex tools, objects, and locations Can assume responsibility for own actions	***Motor/nonmotor vehicles*** ***Pedestrian***—Emphasize and encourage safe pedestrian behavior At night, walk with a friend If someone is following you, go to nearest place with people Do not walk in secluded areas; take well-traveled walkways ***Passenger***—Promote appropriate behavior while riding in a motor vehicle ***Driver***—Provide competent driver education; encourage judicious use of vehicle; discourage drag racing, "playing chicken"; maintain vehicle in proper condition (brakes, tires, etc.) Teach and promote safety and maintenance of two-wheeled vehicles Promote and encourage wearing of safety apparel such as helmet, long trousers, sturdy shoes Reinforce the dangers of drugs, including alcohol, when operating a motor vehicle ***Drowning*** Teach nonswimmer to swim Teach basic rules of water safety Judicious selection of place to swim Sufficient water depth for diving Swimming with companion Review risk of combining use of alcohol with water activities ***Burns*** Reinforce proper behavior in areas involving contact with burn hazards (e.g., gasoline, electric wires, fires) Advise regarding excessive exposure to natural or artificial sunlight (ultraviolet burn) Discourage smoking Encourage use of sunscreen ***Poisoning*** Educate in hazards of drug use, including alcohol ***Falls*** Teach and encourage general safety measures in all activities ***Bodily damage*** Promote acquisition of proper instruction in sports and use of sports equipment Instruct in safe use of and respect for firearms and other devices with potential danger (e.g., power tools, firecrackers) Provide and encourage use of protective equipment when using potentially hazardous devices Promote access to and/or provision of safe sports and recreational facilities Be alert for signs of depression (potential suicide) Discourage use of and/or availability of hazardous sports equipment (e.g., trampoline, surfboards) Instruct regarding proper use of corrective devices (e.g., glasses, contact lenses, hearing aids) Encourage and foster judicious application of safety principles and prevention

cents ride bicycles without helmets and without lights at night, and the overwhelming majority of deaths from bicycle injuries (primarily head injuries) involve teenagers.

Firearms. Firearms are the major cause of intentional fatal injuries in the United States. Adolescence is the peak age for being either a victim or an offender in an injury involving a firearm. Gun carrying among adolescents is on the rise and is not limited to the stereotypic inner-city youth. The rates of gun carrying among Caucasian suburban adolescents have increased more than 130% within the past 10 years (Hayes and Hemenway, 1999). Having a gun in the home increases the risk of adolescent suicide and homicide. All families should be assessed for the presence of a gun in the home and informed of the increased risk for suicide and homicide. When guns are present in the home, families must take preventive action to be sure that the guns are never loaded, that they are locked up in a safe place, and that ammunition is stored and locked up separately in a location where only appropriate adults have access to it.

Nonpowder Firearms. Nonpowder guns (e.g., air rifles and BB guns), although viewed as toys by many, account for almost as many injuries as powder guns. The regulations regarding nonpowder guns are relaxed; they can be purchased legally by youngsters and are labeled as suitable for children as young as 8 years of age. Few states regulate their use. Nurses should act as child advocates and urge passage of laws to regulate the sale of these potentially dangerous "toys."

Sports Injuries. Because the degree of physical maturation, size, coordination, and endurance varies greatly among adolescents of the same age, sports competition between young people who differ greatly in strength and agility is unfair and hazardous. Matching candidates for sports should be done relative to physical maturity, height, weight, and physical fitness and skills, particularly in a sport involving rigorous body contact. Age is a less important consideration.

Every sport has some potential for injury, whether one participates in serious competition or is actively engaged in the activity for pure enjoyment. A large number of severe or fatal injuries occur to persons who are not physically prepared for the activity. The increase in strength and vigor in adolescence may tempt youngsters to overextend themselves, especially boys who are urged on by teammates or are stimulated by the admiration of female observers. The range of injuries sustained in sports or recreational activities can involve any part of the body and extend from relatively minor cuts, bruises, and abrasions to totally incapacitating central nervous system injuries or death. The leading cause of serious sports injuries among boys is participation in football, whereas most girls are injured while participating in gymnastics.

Nursing Care Management. Injury prevention is an ongoing part of nursing responsibility throughout the childhood years. Anticipatory guidance to parents and children regarding the expected problems and hazards related to growth and development does not end as children approach maturity. They need education in basic safety precautions, as well as instruction in skills required in performance of activities such as sports, instruction in handling motor vehicles, and instruction in proper maintenance of equipment. During adolescence, however, health and safety education and guidance are more effective when the young people are directly involved; parents and health professionals can emphasize the importance of safety during performance of activities and the proper conditioning and preparation for sports.

Prevention can occur on a variety of levels. Safety advocacy, changing public policy, and legislation can curtail injuries. Examples of such approaches are laws that mandate wearing seat belts, mandatory helmet use while driving moving vehicles other than automobiles, keeping the legal drinking age at 21 years, and instituting curfews for teen drivers. In addition to improving the environment, health education for teenagers and significant adults is essential. Helping adolescents understand their need for engaging in risky behavior, exploring possible negative outcomes, and weighing possible alternatives are critical components of injury prevention.

Anticipatory Guidance—Care of Families

The parents of the adolescent are often as confused and perplexed about the changes and behavior of this stage of development as the youngster is. Parents need support and guidance to help them through this trying time. They need to understand the changes taking place, to accept the expected behaviors that accompany the process of detachment, to be prepared to "let go," and to promote the changed relationship from one of dependence to one of mutuality. The Home Care box lists suggestions for anticipatory guidance of parents with an adolescent.

Home Care

GUIDANCE DURING ADOLESCENCE

Encourage Parents To:

- Accept adolescent as a unique individual.
- Respect adolescent's ideas, likes and dislikes, and wishes.
- Be involved with school functions and attend adolescent's performances, whether it be a sporting event or a school play.
- Listen and try to be open to teenager's views, even when they disagree with parental views.
- Avoid criticism about no-win topics.
- Provide opportunity for choosing options and accept natural consequences of these choices.
- Allow young person to learn by doing, even when choices and methods differ from those of adults.
- Provide adolescent with clear, reasonable limits.
- Clarify house rules and consequences for breaking them.
- Let society's rules and consequences teach responsibility outside the home.
- Allow increasing independence within limitations of safety and well-being.
- Be available but avoid pressing teenager too far.
- Respect adolescent's privacy.
- Try to share adolescent's feelings of joy or sorrow.
- Respond to feelings, as well as words.
- Be available to answer questions, give information, and provide companionship.
- Try to make communication clear.
- Avoid comparisons with siblings.
- Assist adolescent in selecting appropriate career goals and preparing for adult role.
- Welcome adolescent's friends into the home, and treat them with respect.
- Provide unconditional love.
- Be willing to apologize when mistaken.

Be Aware That Adolescents:

- Are subject to turbulent, unpredictable behavior.
- Are struggling for independence.
- Are extremely sensitive to feelings and behavior that affect them.
- May receive a different message than what was sent.
- Consider friends extremely important.
- Have a strong need "to belong."

Special Health Problems

DISORDERS RELATED TO THE REPRODUCTIVE SYSTEM

Amenorrhea

Menarche, or the first menstrual period, occurs relatively late in female pubertal development. Although there is variation among girls in the onset and rate of progression of pubertal development, the sequence and tempo should be the same. When an adolescent presents with a complaint of absence of menses, a careful history of the timing of her pubertal development will help to determine if there is a need for further evaluation or if reassurance is all that is necessary.

Primary amenorrhea is an absence of secondary sex characteristics and no uterine bleeding by 14 to 15 years of age, or absence of uterine bleeding with secondary sex characteristics by 16 to 16.5 years of age. No uterine bleeding after attaining sexual maturity rating 5 (SMR 5) for 1 year, or after breast development for 4 years, is also considered primary amenorrhea (Neinstein, 1996). The etiology of primary amenorrhea may be anatomic, hormonal, genetic, or idiopathic. A thorough history and physical examination will provide clues to the etiology.

Secondary amenorrhea is defined as the absence of menses for 6 months or at least three cycles after menstruation was previously established. Irregular menstrual cycles are common within the first year or two after menarche. As many as 50% to 80% of young girls have anovulatory cycles resulting in irregular or absent bleeding (Prose, Ford, and Lovely, 1998). Girls with a later onset of menarche will take longer to establish regular ovulatory cycles. Pregnancy is the most common cause of secondary amenorrhea and should be ruled out in both types of amenorrhea, even if the adolescent denies sexual activity. When pregnancy has been ruled out, the history should be evaluated for evidence of stress, changes in environment, weight changes, and eating disorders because these are the next most common causes of a missed period in adolescents (Emans, Laufer, and Goldstein, 1998).

Dysmenorrhea

A certain amount of discomfort during the first day or two of the menstrual flow is extremely common. Most girls experience cramping, abdominal pain, backache, and leg ache, but in a few the pain is intolerable and incapacitating. *Primary dysmenorrhea* is painful menses not related to any pelvic disease. When the discomfort can be attributed to endometriosis, infection, adhesions from peritonitis, or other pelvic disease, the complaint is termed *secondary dysmenorrhea.*

Primary dysmenorrhea is directly related to the occurrence of prior ovulation. There is also a relationship between uterine contractility and the secretion of prostaglandins. Psychogenic factors such as sexual abuse, familial conditioning, sex-role confusion, and school avoidance may also contribute to dysmenorrhea.

A thorough gynecologic examination is carried out to exclude any pelvic abnormalities, and a careful history is taken regarding the type and duration of pain, its relationship to menstrual flow, and any associated symptoms. These questions not only provide information to the examiner, but also provide the girl with evidence that her problem is being taken seriously. An explanation of the physiology of menstruation is reassuring.

Therapeutic Management. First-line treatment for adolescents with dysmenorrhea is the administration of nonsteroidal antiinflammatory drugs that block the formation of prostaglandins for 2 to 3 days of the menstrual cycle. The girl should be instructed to begin the medication at the first sign of cramping or bleeding. Some girls benefit from beginning the medication 1 to 2 days before the onset of their menses. The medications should be taken with food.

Cyclic estrogen therapy and oral contraceptives are also effective. Simple exercises such as pelvic rocking, assuming the knee-chest position, and breathing exercises may be beneficial. Encouraging adequate personal hygiene, participation in regular activities, and methods to decrease stress should also be discussed with the adolescent.

A balanced diet and specific dietary changes that may be helpful include the elimination of caffeine from the diet and the addition of herbal teas. Dietary supplementation with omega-3 fatty acids has been shown to reduce the symptoms of dysmenorrhea in adolescents (Harel et al, 1996).

Nursing Care Management. All adolescent girls need reassurance that menstruation is a normal function. When nurses are asked for advice regarding menstrual problems, they have a valuable opportunity to engage in health teaching concerning menstrual physiology and hygiene, as well as the importance of a well-balanced diet, exercise, and general health maintenance. Health teaching can dispel any myths in relation to menstruation and femininity. When assessment indicates a potential problem and the need for evaluation, referral to an appropriate practitioner, health service, or clinic may be necessary.

One of the most difficult experiences facing the adolescent girl is the gynecologic examination. Whether it is her first experience or not, she is often filled with apprehension. Almost all adolescents are extremely self-conscious about their bodies and the changes taking place. They need continuing support in the form of anticipatory guidance regarding what to expect and suggestions of what to do to help relax during the procedure. Usually the stressful experience of being placed in stirrups for the pelvic examination can be avoided. The adolescent girl who is relaxed may be examined in the supine position with hips and knees flexed and legs abducted. If a female nurse is not the examiner, it is essential for her to remain with the patient during the examination to offer support and guidance.

Vaginitis

Vaginitis can be caused by physical, chemical, or infectious agents. Physical causes may include a forgotten tampon or contraceptive sponge; chemical irritants include bubble bath, douching, deodorant pads, and tampons. Removal of the offending material or discontinuing use of the irritating substance is usually all that is necessary to treat physical or chemical vaginitis. Infectious vaginitis can be caused by *Candida* fungi (yeast), *Trichomonas* protozoa parasites, or bacteria. Diagnosis is confirmed with microscopic evaluation of vaginal secretions. Treatment varies depending on the infectious agent.

Health teaching is important in the prevention and management of all types of vaginitis. Adolescent girls need to be reassured that increased vaginal mucus can occur at the time of ovulation, before menstruation, or with sexual excitement. Many teenage girls mistake these variations as signs of infection. Girls should be taught to wipe from front to back after toileting and to realize that vaginitis can result from irritation, foreign objects, and sexual activity. Nurses need to stress the importance of an evaluation to determine the exact cause.

Disorders of the Male Reproductive System

Most obvious anomalies, such as hypospadias, hydrocele, phimosis, and cryptorchidism, have been identified, and corrective measures have been instituted during early childhood. The most common problems related to the reproductive organs in later childhood are (1) infections, such as urethritis (see Urinary Tract Infection, Chapter 50); (2) hematuria; (3) penile problems, such as nonretractable foreskin in uncircumcised males, carcinoma, and trauma; (4) scrotal conditions, such as varicocele (elongation, dilation, and tortuosity of the veins superior to the testicle); and (5) testicular torsion (a condition in which the testicle hangs free from its vascular structures, which can result in partial or complete venous occlusion with rotation). Tumors of the testes are not common, but when manifested in adolescence, they are generally malignant and demand immediate evaluation.

The usual presenting symptom for testicular cancer is a heavy, hard, painless mass (either smooth or nodular) that is palpated on the testis. Treatment involves surgical removal of the affected testicle (orchiectomy) and possibly chemotherapy and radiation if metastasis has occurred.

Nursing Care Management. The adolescent boy is extremely self-conscious about his changing body and needs preparation for a genital examination. The most successful approach is to assume a matter-of-fact attitude toward the examination, explain precisely what will take place, and maintain a continuous commentary about what is being done and the findings at each phase of the examination.

The routine health assessment of every adolescent boy should include teaching about testicular cancer and how to perform a testicular self-examination every 6 months. This rare malignancy is curable if detected early. Although there is concern that teaching testicular self-examination may cause an unwarranted increase in anxiety (Morris, 1996), nurses are in an ideal role to teach testicular self-examination in a manner that is respectful of the adolescent boy's anxieties, and to promote early treatment (Critical Thinking box).*

The normal testicle is a firm organ with a smooth, egg-shaped contour; the epididymis is palpated as a raised swelling on the superior aspect of the testicle and should not be confused as an abnormality.

Critical Thinking

TESTICULAR SELF-EXAMINATION

At a recent faculty meeting, the school nurse presented plans for a class on testicular self-examination (TSE) to be delivered to the sophomore boys. Several faculty members questioned the value of providing such a class when there is limited time to deliver content relating to "routine academic subjects." Which of the following responses could the nurse use to justify including the TSE class in the curriculum?

First Think About It . . .

- **What assumptions are you making?**
- **What is the purpose of your thinking?**

1. **TSE provides an opportunity for adolescent boys to discover early cases of epididymis, a common infection in this age group.**
2. **TSE allows adolescent boys to determine if they have an asymptomatic sexually transmitted disease.**
3. **TSE permits detection of any tumors of the testes, which are not common in adolescence, but which are often malignant and demand immediate attention whey they occur.**
4. **TSE allows easy identification of malignant testicular tumors, which occur in 5% of adolescent males.**

The best response is 3. TSE is an easily learned technique that allows the adolescent boy to become familiar with his own anatomy and to determine any abnormalities. Although testicular tumors are not common in adolescence, when they do occur, they are often malignant and early detection is essential, which is an important assumption. Although TSE is easily learned by adolescents, the method does not allow the adolescent boy to determine if he has a sexually transmitted disease or epididymitis.

Gynecomastia

The male breast, although not strictly part of the male reproductive system, responds to hormonal changes. Some degree of bilateral or unilateral breast enlargement commonly occurs in boys during puberty. It is estimated that approximately half of adolescent boys have transient gynecomastia (usually lasting less than 1 year) that subsides spontaneously with achievement of male development. A careful assessment of the pubertal stage at the onset of gynecomastia; medication history, including anabolic steroids; and the exclusion of renal, liver, thyroid, and endocrine disorders or dysfunction allow the examiner to reassure the adolescent that the changes are pubertal gynecomastia. No further assessment is indicated for pubertal gynecomastia (Neuman, 1997).

If the condition persists or is extensive enough to cause embarrassment or to produce doubts about gender identity in the young boy, plastic surgery may be indicated for cosmetic and psychologic considerations. Administration of testosterone has no effect on breast development or regression and may aggravate the condition.

Nursing Care Management. Treatment usually consists of assurance to the adolescent and his parents that this is a benign and temporary situation. Adolescents who are distressed about physical integrity and masculinity may benefit from the knowledge that it occurs in more than 50% of all adolescent boys.

EATING DISORDERS

Obesity

Few health problems in childhood and adolescence are so obvious to others, so difficult to treat, and have such long-term effects on psychologic and physical health status as obesity. Several different definitions have been proposed for obesity and overweight. *Obesity* has been defined as an increase in body weight resulting from an excessive accumulation of body fat relative to lean body mass (Keller and Stevens, 1996). *Overweight* refers to the state of weighing more than average for height and

*For information on testicular cancer, contact the Jason A. Struble Memorial Cancer Fund, Inc., 624 Kehrs Mill Rd., Ballwin, MO 63011.

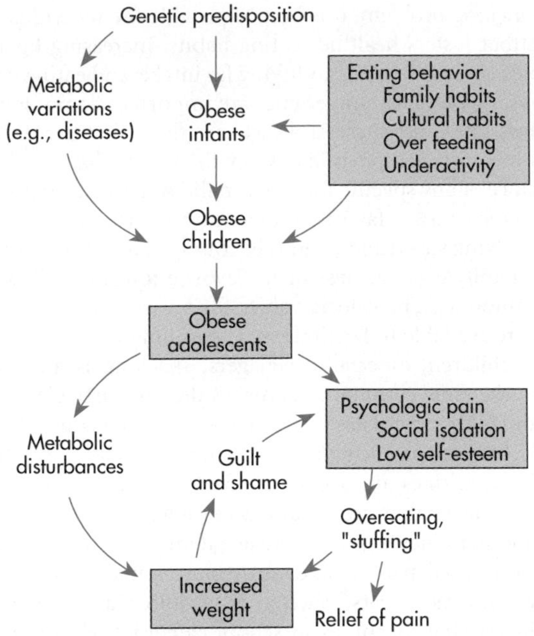

FIG. 40-10 • Complex relationships in adolescent obesity.

body build. Any child whose weight falls in the 95th percentile for age, gender, and height on the NCHS growth chart is considered overweight (Kuczmarski et al, 2000).

BMI-for-age also can be used to identify those at risk for being overweight (≥85th and (95th percentile).

Regardless of the definition used, the number of overweight children in the United States is increasing. Data from the NHANES III survey done from 1988 until 1994 indicated that children ages 12 to 19 years had a 12% increase in obesity from previous survey data (Troiano et al, 1995). Current prevalence of childhood obesity in the United States is estimated to be 25% to 30% (Moran, 1999). These figures translate into poor health outcomes for children who are obese. Recently there has been an increase in type 2 diabetes mellitus among adolescents who are obese, and there is considerable evidence that obese children become obese adults. Obese adults experience several health problems, including hypertension, hyperlipidemia, cardiovascular disease, orthopedic problems, obstructive sleep apnea, colon cancer, and poorer outcomes for the delivery of a healthy infant.

Etiology/Pathophysiology. Obesity is a complex condition and may involve a variety of influences, including metabolic, hypothalamic, hereditary, social, cultural, and psychologic factors (Fig. 40-10). Less than 5% of childhood obesity can be attributed to an underlying disease such as hypothyroidism, adrenal hypercorticoidism, hyperinsulinism, and dysfunction of or damage to the central nervous system.

The metabolism of glucose plays an important role in the regulation of fat deposition, and several theories have been proposed to explain individual variability in metabolism. One theory proposes an increase in metabolic efficiency in obese persons that facilitates fat storage and retention.

Heredity is an important factor in the development of obesity. For example, identical twins reared apart tend to resemble their natural parents to a greater extent than they do their adoptive parents. Obesity can develop in infancy, during childhood, at the onset of puberty, or during adolescence. It is impossible to distinguish between hereditary and environmental factors, because both may be operating in any situation when other family members are obese.

Box 40-3

Clinical Manifestations of Obesity

Overweight appearance
Weight over established standards
Skinfold thickness greater than established standards
Body fat increased above established standards
Body mass index above established standards

Children who are obese are less active than lean children, although it is uncertain whether the inactivity creates the obesity or whether the obesity is responsible for the inactivity. Many people who are obese also demonstrate an overwhelming appetite and overeat when they are not hungry. They eat more rapidly and tend to ingest more calories at one meal rather than over a period of time. Adolescents who are obese are characteristically night eaters and often skip meals, particularly breakfast.

Theories that attempt to explain the development of obesity include:

Adipose cell theory—The number of cells in adipose tissue is increased, the size of the fat cells is increased, or a combination of these. Children who are obese have larger cells that stay the same size once they reach a maximum, and their fat cells appear to increase in number during childhood.

Set point theory—Individuals have a predetermined level for body weight that remains relatively stable during adulthood. With increased caloric intake the metabolic rate increases to burn the excess; when intake is reduced, metabolism decreases to conserve energy.

Sociocultural factors also play a role in weight gain. Patterns of eating are culturally and socially based, and the food preferences of the culture contribute to the development of obesity. Many cultures consider plumpness a sign of health, view obesity as evidence of well-being, and foster weight gain as a desirable feature.

Psychologic factors may provide a basis for eating patterns in childhood. In infancy the child first experiences relief from discomfort through feeding and learns to associate eating with feelings of well-being, security, and the comforting presence of the nurturing person. Soon, eating is associated with the feeling of being loved. Many parents use food, such as candy and other "treats," as a positive reinforcer for desired behavior. This practice may acquire symbolic significance, and the child may use food as a reward, a comfort, and a means for dealing with feelings of depression, hostility, boredom, or loneliness.

Diagnostic Evaluation. Several tests can be employed to assess obesity (Box 40-3). Skinfold measurements; body mass index calculations; plotting of height and weight on standardized growth charts; and body fat measurements as determined by bioelectric impedance, computed tomography, or magnetic resonance imaging measurements may be used for additional data. Appropriate diagnostic tests rule out suspected metabolic and endocrine disorders.

Nursing Care Management

➤ Assessment

The presence of obesity is obvious from appearance alone, and a gross determination can be made by a rough comparison of height and weight with standard growth charts. Currently the body mass index (BMI) measurement has become a very useful tool for assessment of obesity. The BMI is expressed as the child's body weight in kilograms divided by the square of the child's height in meters (kg/m^2). Children with a BMI greater than or equal to the 95th percentile for age and sex should receive an in-depth medical assessment. Children with a BMI in the 85th to 95th percentile range should be evaluated for secondary complications such as hypertension and hyperlipidemia (Barlow and Dietz, 1998; Kuczmarski et al, 2000). Evaluation should also include the height and weight history of the parents and siblings; as well as eating habits, appetite and hunger patterns, and physical activities in which the child is engaged. In addition, a psychosocial history is helpful to understand the impact that this condition has on the child's life.

➤ Nursing Diagnoses

Based on a thorough assessment of the child or adolescent who is obese, nursing diagnoses become apparent. Although the diagnoses vary according to the needs of the individual child, some of the more prominent ones are outlined in Box 40-4.

➤ Plan of Care and Implementation

The goals of a weight loss program include:

1. Child will follow a diet that provides loss of fat content without interfering with growth, normal activity, and psychologic well-being.
2. Child will engage in a regular exercise program.
3. Child will modify eating behavior.
4. Child and family will receive psychologic support.

Motivation to lose weight is the key to success. The reasons children and adolescents desire to lose weight need to be explored, but success is rarely achieved unless youngsters are motivated to lose weight and take personal responsibility for their dietary habits and exercise program. Children who are forced by parents to seek help are seldom sufficiently motivated, become rebellious of parental nagging, and are unwilling to control dietary intake. An approach that focuses on healthy eating habits and enjoyable exercise for all members of the family is more likely to be successful.

Diet. The ideal diet for children and adolescents should meet the criteria outlined in Box 40-5. Because obesity is usually a lifelong problem, it is best to provide the individual with a diet that fosters healthier eating habits. Increasing fiber and complex carbohydrates, modifying fat intake, and eating only in response to physical hunger cues are important components of any diet. The most successful diets are those that use ordinary foods in controlled portions rather than diets that require the avoidance of any specific food. The child or adolescent is taught how to incorporate favorite foods into the diet and how to select satisfying substitutes, and is encouraged to eat what the rest of the family eats, but less of it. Favorite foods are allowed in small amounts. The caloric values for a variety of commercial foods are available to facilitate meal planning.

For children, especially teenagers, snacking is an integral part of the daily routine. This makes dieting particularly difficult for children who are obese. They have little concept of the caloric content of even the most commonplace snack foods. Vending machines are usually stocked with high-calorie, low-nutrient snacks that are readily accessible, and children often have pocket money to purchase these items. Following pressures from concerned parents and nutritionists, many schools provide wholesome "treats," such as fruit, juices, and raw vegetables, in vending machines in school cafeterias. However, fast-food establishments, which are often located near large schools, present problems for children and adolescents who are attempting to lose weight.*

Children and adolescents should not be encouraged to initiate a reduction diet without health assessment and counseling. Significant caloric restriction for children and adolescents who are still growing is usually not recommended. Restriction of calories and nutrients can cause delayed or stunted growth and is effective for only short periods. It is also important to emphasize the undesirable nature of fad diets and crash programs that continually appear in the media. Exotic diets have not been successful, and their unbalanced nature makes them potentially dangerous for growing children or adolescents. To be successful, a dietary program should be nutritionally sound with sufficient satiety value, produce the desired weight loss, and be accompanied by nutrition education and continued support. Long-term weight reduction requires lifestyle changes, modification of eating habits, and adoption of a more active lifestyle.

Exercise. Because weight loss will occur only when caloric expenditure is greater than caloric intake, physical activity in

*Information on the nutrient value of name-brand foods, including menu items from fast-food restaurants, is available from the Nutrition Coordinating Center, 1300 S. Second St., Suite 300, Minneapolis, MN 55414; (612) 626-9450; e-mail: webmaster@keystone.ncc.umn.edu; website: www.ncc.umn.edu.

Box 40-4

Nursing Diagnoses: The Child Who is Obese

- Altered nutrition: more than body requirements related to dysfunctional eating patterns, hereditary factors
- Activity intolerance related to sedentary lifestyle, physical bulk
- Ineffective individual coping related to little or no exercise, poor nutrition, personal vulnerability
- Self-esteem disturbance related to perception of physical appearance, internalization of negative feedback
- Altered family processes related to management of child who is obese

Box 40-5

Essentials of an Ideal Weight Management Program

- Weight maintenance or steady, slow weight loss
- Nutrient, energy, and growth needs met
- Feelings of hunger avoided
- Preservation of lean body mass
- Increased physical activity
- Absence of metabolic complications
- Absence of psychiatric reactions

the form of regularly scheduled exercise, progressively increased over the child's usual activity, is an integral part of a weight-reduction program. Activities should be those that stress self-improvement rather than competition, and teenagers need continued psychologic support and encouragement to participate in physical activities and healthy exercise.

Behavioral Therapy. The most successful method for treating obesity combines diet and exercise with behavior modification, which emphasizes identification and elimination of inappropriate eating habits, as well as problem-solving techniques to identify solutions to use in situations that encourage overeating. Attention is focused not on food but on the social and behavioral aspects surrounding food consumption.

Group Involvement. Some persons on weight-reduction programs find that support and mutual reinforcement provided by a group of persons with a similar problem help them to adjust to the changes needed to accomplish their goals, including weight loss. Commercial groups such as Weight Watchers, TOPS, or diet workshops are composed primarily of adults and may be helpful to a few teenagers; however, a group composed of persons their own age is more effective. Groups for youngsters who are obese include summer camps designed and conducted by health professionals; school groups organized and led by the school nurse; and groups associated with special clinics.

These groups are concerned not only with weight loss but also with the development of a positive self-image. Nutrition education, diet planning, and discussions centered around better grooming and improvement of social skills are essential components of successful groups. Improvement is measured by positive changes in all aspects of behavior.

Medical Therapies. The use of appetite-suppressant drugs is not supported by most practitioners. These drugs are no more effective than diet and exercise in maintaining weight loss, and there is concern that the use of such drugs may become habit forming. Surgical techniques that cause food to bypass a substantial portion of the intestine or that occlude a large segment of the stomach to produce weight loss are hazardous and can cause many metabolic complications.

Prevention. Weight loss programs do not enjoy the success rate that therapeutic interventions for most other disorders do; the failure rate is dismally high. The most successful treatment of preadolescent obesity (which often leads to adult obesity) is to treat preschool obesity with programs that include frequent visits, and with early dietary counseling.

➤ Evaluation

The effectiveness of nursing interventions is determined by continual reassessment based on the following observational guidelines and expected outcomes:

1. Assess weight at regular intervals (usually weekly); discuss with child his or her feelings, reactions, and concerns; analyze daily recordings (log) of activities (e.g., eating, behavior, and exercise) and feelings.
2. Review exercise program with child or teenager.
3. Review log of eating behaviors; discuss observations with child or teenager.
4. Interview child or teenager about the plan of care and progress toward short-term and long-term goals.

Expected outcomes include the following:

1. Eating patterns lead to weight loss; child or teenager expresses feelings and concerns regarding problems
2. Child or teenager engages in preferred exercise and activities regularly
3. Child or teenager demonstrates an understanding of eating patterns
4. Child or teenager evidences a steady weight loss (or weight maintenance in a growing child)

(See also Nursing Care Plan: The Child Who Is Obese.*)

Anorexia Nervosa (AN)

AN is an eating disorder characterized by a refusal to maintain a minimally normal body weight and by severe weight loss in the absence of obvious physical causes. It occurs predominantly in adolescent or young adult females, and the incidence is increasing.

The onset of AN generally takes place at or near menarche. The mean age of onset is 13.75 years, but the age range is from 10 to 25 years (Mackenzie and Neinstein, 1996). Young people who have this disorder are most commonly from the upper or middle socioeconomic groups; are often described as "good children"; are academically high achievers, conforming, and conscientious; and have a high energy level, even with marked emaciation. These adolescents are usually strongly dependent on their parents, and often an ambivalent mother-daughter relationship is present for females. Sexual abuse may be a factor in some cases of AN.

Etiology/Pathology. The etiology of the disorder remains unclear. There is a distinct psychologic component, and the diagnosis is based primarily on psychologic and behavioral criteria. Nevertheless, the physical manifestations of anorexia lend support to possible organic factors in the etiology.

Dominating the psychologic aspects of anorexia nervosa are a relentless pursuit of thinness and a fear of fatness, usually preceded by a period of a year or two of mood disturbances and behavior changes. The weight loss is usually triggered by a typical adolescent crisis (e.g., the onset of menstruation or traumatic interpersonal incidents) that precipitates serious dieting that continues out of control.

Often there is an exaggerated misinterpretation of the normal fat deposition characteristic of the early adolescent period, or someone may comment that the adolescent girl is putting on weight. The weight loss may be a response to teasing or to changing schools or going to college. Youngsters entering the growth phase of puberty, when biologic fat accumulation is normal, are particularly vulnerable. The current emphasis on slimness is a very significant factor: the standard for beauty is exemplified in all forms of media by tall, thin, small-breasted models.

In some situations the adolescent is experiencing severe family stress, such as parental separation or divorce. In these and other circumstances in which the youngster perceives a lack of personal control, the decision to eat or not to eat becomes one area where individual control can be exercised.

Diagnostic Evaluation. Diagnosis is made on the basis of clinical manifestations (Box 40-6) and conformity to the criteria established by the American Psychiatric Association (1994) (Box 40-7).

---

*In Wong DL, Hess CS: ***Wong and Whaley's clinical manual of pediatric nursing,*** ed 5, St. Louis, 2000, Mosby.

Box 40-6
Clinical Manifestations of Anorexia Nervosa

Severe and profound weight loss
Signs of altered metabolic activity:
- Secondary amenorrhea (if menarche not attained)
- Primary amenorrhea (if menarche not attained)
- Bradycardia
- Lowered body temperature
- Decreased blood pressure
- Cold intolerance
- Dry skin and brittle nails
- Appearance of lanugo hair

Box 40-7
Diagnostic Criteria for Anorexia Nervosa

A. Refusal to maintain body weight over a minimal normal weight for age and height (e.g., weight loss leading to maintenance of body weight less than 85% of that expected); or failure to make expected weight gain during period of growth, leading to body weight less than 85% of that expected
B. Intense fear of gaining weight or becoming fat, even though underweight
C. Disturbance in the way in which one's body weight, size, or shape is experienced (e.g., the person claims to "feel fat" even when emaciated, believes that one area of the body is "too fat" even when obviously underweight)
D. In females, absence of at least three consecutive menstrual cycles when otherwise expected to occur (primary or secondary amenorrhea) (a woman is considered to have amenorrhea if her periods occur only following hormone [e.g., estrogen] administration)

From American Psychiatric Association: *Diagnostic and statistical manual of mental disorders,* ed 4 (DSM-IV), Washington, DC, 1994, The Association.

Therapeutic Management. The initial goal is to treat the life-threatening malnutrition with strict adherence to dietary requirements, which sometimes necessitates intravenous (IV) and tube feedings (these methods are usually reserved for severe situations). Rapid weight gain should be avoided because it can be medically unsafe and often overwhelms the patient. Deaths associated with AN occur during rehabilitation as a result of cardiovascular overload. Restoration of body weight to a target weight within 10% of the patient's ideal body weight is often the main goal of nutritional rehabilitation (Fisher, 1997).

One treatment approach that has met with varied degrees of success is behavior modification. This requires team involvement with the following essential aspects:

- The health team determines an approach with the patient and adheres to it consistently.
- All team members are involved.
- There is continuity of caregivers (team members).
- There is clear communication among team members and with the patient so that the patient understands precisely what is expected.
- The patient is supported in his or her efforts (e.g., positive feedback for accomplishments).

Critical Thinking

ANOREXIA NERVOSA

Jane is a 13-year-old whose grades have been excellent and whom the teachers describe as a "model student." Recently some of Jane's friends have expressed concern to the school nurse practitioner that Jane has begun to "jog" at lunch time and seldom eats with them. Jane has told her friends that she gained weight over the winter months and that she is "jogging" because she wants to qualify for the track team this spring. In addition to severe weight loss, which of the following symptoms of anorexia nervosa (AN) is the school nurse practitioner likely to observe when she interviews Jane and performs a sports physical?

First, Think About It . . .

- **What conclusions are you reaching?**
- **If you accept the conclusions, what are the implications?**

1. **Decreased body temperature**
2. **History of dysmenorrhea**
3. **Tachycardia**
4. **Heat intolerance**

The best response is 1. A correct conclusion is that AN is a condition in which several alterations in metabolic activity can occur following excessive weight loss. Also, you may conclude that these alterations include lowered body temperature, bradycardia, secondary amenorrhea, decreased blood pressure, and cold intolerance. When the nutritional status improves and normal body weight has been restored, these metabolic changes are usually reversed.

Individuals whose disorder can be clearly related to a dysfunctional family situation will need intensive family therapy. Many of those whose therapy plan is implemented in the hospital need a continued behavior modification program after discharge to maintain the desired weight.

Family therapy is effective when begun soon after the onset of illness, but it is less successful when the condition has existed for some time. Therapy is directed toward disengagement and redirection of malfunctioning processes in the family. Individual psychotherapy is aimed at helping the young person resolve the adolescent identity crisis, particularly as it relates to a distorted body image.

Nursing Care Management. The management of AN is directed toward correction of the severe state of malnutrition and resolution of the psychologic dynamics. Because of the psychogenic nature of the disorder, treatment is difficult and lengthy. Individuals involved in therapy must consider the adolescent's distorted sense of body image and self-awareness; and the feelings of self-doubt, ineffectiveness, and helplessness that prompt self-damaging behavior in order to feel in control.

Nurses need to adopt and maintain a kind, supportive, yet firm manner in managing the care of a teenager with AN. The child requires sustained support and reassurance to cope with ambivalent feelings related to the body concept and the desire to see oneself as a cooperative and reliable person worthy of receiving kindness. Encouraging education and activities that strengthen self-esteem facilitates the resocialization process and promotes social acceptance among peers.

It is important for nurses to be aware of the physical side effects of AN. Patients with AN may experience urinary tract problems. For example, ketones and protein may be detected in the urine as a result of breakdown of fat and protein. Vital sign instability can be severe (including orthostatic hypotension). The pulse becomes irregular, and the rate decreases markedly. Bradycardia and hypothermia can result in cardiac arrest (Critical Thinking box).

Health professionals, patients, and families can find assistance and information through any of the following organizations: The National Eating Disorders Organization,* the National Association of Anorexia Nervosa and Associated Disorders, Inc.,† and the American Anorexia/Bulimia Association, Inc.‡

(See also Nursing Care Plan: The Adolescent with Anorexia Nervosa.§)

Bulimia

Bulimia is an eating disorder characterized by binge eating. The binge behavior consists of secretive, frenzied consumption of large amounts of high-calorie (or "forbidden") foods during a brief period of time (usually less than 2 hours). The binge is counteracted by a variety of weight control methods (purging), including self-induced vomiting, diuretic and laxative abuse, and rigorous exercise. The frequency of bingeing can be anywhere from once a week to seven or eight times a day. These binge/purge cycles are followed by self-deprecating thoughts, a depressed mood, and an awareness that the eating pattern is abnormal.

The disorder is observed more commonly in older adolescent girls and young women. Characteristically, affected persons have been unsuccessful dieters, have low impulse control, and may have been self-conscious about being overweight in childhood. They fall into two categories: (1) those who purge and (2) those who do not purge. Some are of normal weight or (more often) are slightly above normal weight; others—with *bulimarexia*—become as underweight as anorectic individuals.

Diagnostic Evaluation. The diagnosis may be first suspected from the presence of complications, including fluid and electrolyte disturbances from gastrointestinal losses, abdominal complaints from laxative abuse, erosion of tooth enamel and increased dental caries from vomited gastric acid, and throat complaints. The diagnosis is established on the basis of criteria established by the American Psychiatric Association (1994) (Box 40-8).

Therapeutic Management. Therapy is similar to management of anorexia nervosa. Hospitalization may be required, especially for complications such as potassium depletion and esophageal damage. IV fluids and potassium replacement are essential elements of care, and cardiac monitoring is indicated; behavior therapy may also be used.

Nursing Care Management. Nursing care is similar to care of the patient with AN. Acute care also involves careful monitoring of fluid and electrolyte alterations and observation for signs of cardiac complications.

*6655 S. Yale Ave., Tulsa, OK 74136; (918) 481-4044; website: www.laureate.com.

†Box 7, Highland Park, IL 60035; (847) 831-3438; e-mail: ANAD20@aol.com

‡165 W. 46th St., Suite 1108, New York, NY 10036; (212) 575-6200; e-mail: info@aaba.inc; website: www.aabainc.org.

§In Wong DL, Hess CS: ***Wong and Whaley's clinical manual of pediatric nursing,*** ed 5, St Louis, 2000, Mosby.

Box 40-8

Diagnostic Criteria for Bulimia

A. Recurrent episodes of binge eating (rapid consumption of a large amount of food in a discrete period of time)
B. A feeling of lack of control over eating behavior during the eating binges
C. The person regularly engages in either self-induced vomiting, use of laxatives, or diuretics, strict dieting or fasting or vigorous exercise in order to prevent weight gain
D. A minimum average of two binge eating episodes a week for at least 3 months
E. Persistent overconcern with body shape and weight

From American Psychiatric Association: *Diagnostic and statistical manual of mental disorders,* ed 4 (DSM-IV), Washington, DC, 1994, The Association.

SERIOUS HEALTH PROBLEMS WITH A BEHAVIORAL COMPONENT

Smoking

An alarming number of children and teenagers smoke. A recent analysis of the 1997 Youth Risk Behavior Survey indicated that the prevalence of current cigarette smoking among U.S. high school students increased from 27.5% in 1991 to 36.4% in 1997, and 42.7% of students used cigarettes, smokeless tobacco, or cigars during the 30 days preceding the survey (Centers for Disease Control and Prevention, 1998c). In 1997 there were also increasing trends among all racial and ethnic subgroups. Current smoking increased 80% among African-American students, 34% among Hispanic students, and 28% among Caucasian students (Centers for Disease Control and Prevention, 1998c).

The hazards of smoking at any age are undisputed; however, a preventive approach to teenage smoking is especially important. Smoking almost immediately brings about reduced lung function, "smoker's" cough, and other respiratory difficulties. Most harmful of all is the likelihood of lifelong addiction, because the earlier a person starts smoking, the more difficult it is to later quit. Approximately 90% of all tobacco use begins when children and teenagers are under 18 years of age (Office of Smoking and Health, 1996), and about 23.69% of persons 15 to 24 years of age who try cigarettes move quickly through the continuum of smoking behavior to the stage of nicotine dependence (Centers for Disease Control and Prevention, 1998a). In addition, research findings indicate a clear association between the use of tobacco, the use of alcohol and other drugs, and high risk behaviors (Willard and Schoenborn, 1995).

Etiology. Teenagers begin smoking for a variety of reasons, such as imitation of adult behavior, peer pressure, and emulation of traits popularly attributed to smokers. Teenagers least likely to smoke are those whose families and friends do not smoke; those who are interested in academics or athletics (particularly high-performance sports such as basketball, swimming, and track); and those who plan to go on to college (Family Focus box).

Smokeless Tobacco. Tobacco products that are placed in the mouth but not ignited (e.g., snuff and chewing tobacco) are referred to as smokeless tobacco. This increasingly popular substitute for cigarettes is now posing a serious hazard to children and adolescents, as well as young adults. These products

Family Focus

EARLY SEXUAL MATURATION, ALCOHOL, AND CIGARETTES

Cigarette smoking and the drinking of alcohol among adolescents are complex behaviors that cannot be explained by any single causative factor. However, theorists and investigators have looked at the relationship between biologic maturation and these behaviors. A young girl who is sexually mature at the age of 12 years may be attracted to a group of 14- to 16-year-old girls and boys who smoke and drink. If these teens have not been in any motor vehicle accidents while drinking, the young girl reasons that she, too, will be safe if she smokes and drinks or is in an automobile with friends who are drinking.

Although parents and nurses cannot influence the time of biologic maturation, they can identify young girls who are at risk for the initiation of smoking and drinking because of early puberty. Parents need to understand that an early maturing daughter might be uncomfortable with her body, and they should take advantage of all opportunities to build her self-esteem. Parental sensitivity to the importance of peer-group acceptance is crucial. Parents need to be very supportive of a teenage daughter who feels left out or different. School nurses are in an excellent position to provide anticipatory guidance to girls who enter puberty early and to help them role play responses they can use to cope with situations that involve offers to smoke and drink. In addition, school nurses can provide information on the bodily changes that accompany puberty and emphasize the fact that not all teenagers enter puberty at the same time.

Teachers, coaches, and church leaders can provide opportunities for these girls to "fit in" with their same-age peers through activities that stress mutual goals. For example, an early maturing girl is typically taller than her age-mates and can be an asset in sports such as basketball and track-and-field events.

have been shown to be carcinogenic, and regular use can cause foul-smelling breath, periodontal disease, and tooth erosion or loss. Smokeless tobacco is also associated with lesions in oral soft tissue and can lead to cigarette smoking.

Nursing Care Management. Prevention of regular smoking in teenagers is the most effective way to reduce the overall incidence of smoking. A variety of methods have been employed to deal with the problem. Smoking prevention programs that focus on negative long-term effects of smoking on health have been ineffective. The most effective programs are community-wide programs that involve parents, peers, mass media, and community organizations. Because smoking and smoking-related behavior functions as a key social symbol, antismoking campaigns must be addressed to the norms of the potential smokers without ridicule or threat to the social norms of the group.

Two areas of focus for antismoking programs are (1) peer-led programming emphasizing social consequences of smoking; and (2) use of media, such as videotapes and films, in smoking prevention. If a significant number of influential peers "sell" their classmates on the idea that smoking is not popular, the followers will imitate their behavior. Short-term rather than long-term consequences are emphasized (e.g., the effects of smoking on personal appearance, such as the unattractive stains on teeth and hands and the unpleasant odor that smoking gives to the breath and clothing). Several additional strategies and resources are recommended for health professionals (Community Focus box).

Community Focus

NONSMOKING STRATEGIES

Nurses who work in schools, hospitals, managed care organizations, and other community agencies can take advantage of all opportunities to provide education concerning the dangers of smoking, to discourage smoking initiation by children and adolescents, to encourage smoking cessation, and to promote smoke-free community environments. In particular, school nurses need to be alert to the vulnerability of young preteens when they enter junior high school. These nurses are in an ideal position to assess the degree of stress, personal conflict, concerns about weight, peer pressures, and other factors that place these preteens at risk for smoking initiation. Nurses can also serve as consultants and counselors to student, teacher, and parent groups and as advocates for antismoking legislative efforts. Several additional strategies are recommended*:

- Provide only a cursory mention of long-term health consequences (e.g., cardiovascular and cancer risks).
- Discuss immediate physiologic consequences in some detail (e.g., changes in heart rate and blood pressure, minor respiratory symptoms, and blood carbon monoxide concentrations).
- Mention alternatives to smoking for establishing a self-image that appears tough, independent, mature, or sophisticated (e.g., establishing a weight-lifting regimen, jogging, dancing, joining a Boys Club or a Girls Club, engaging in volunteer work for a hospital or political or religious group).
- Mention the negative effects of smoking (e.g., earlier wrinkling of skin, yellow stains on teeth and fingers, tobacco odor on breath and clothing).
- Mention the increasing ostracism of smokers by nonsmokers, both legal and informal, in the workplace and in public places.
- Mention the increasing evidence that second-hand smoke is injurious to the health of nonsmokers who are regularly exposed, especially small children.
- Acknowledge that many adults once believed that important social benefits were associated with smoking, but point out that the vast majority of adult smokers would now quit smoking if they could.
- Arm the cooperative adolescent with arguments for dealing with peer pressure (e.g., by not smoking, a teenager demonstrates independence and nonconformity—traits normally prized by youth).
- Request posters and pamphlets from local voluntary agencies (e.g., American Cancer Society, American Heart Association, and American Lung Association) to display prominently.

*For information on smoking cessation, nurses can contact the Nursing Center for Tobacco Intervention, 1585 Neil Ave., Columbus, Ohio 43210-1216; (614) 292-0653; fax (614) 292-7976; website: www.con.ohio-state.edu/tobacco/. Information can also be obtained from Stop Teenage Addiction to Tobacco (STAT), a national organization devoted to educating the public and professionals, at 511 E. Columbus Ave., Springfield, MA 01105; (413) 732-STAT; e-mail: stat@exit3.com.

Schools are ideal settings for tobacco use prevention programs. The majority of states have mandated that schools incorporate education that identifies the adverse effects of smoking. Such programs should begin in elementary school and continue through twelfth grade with intensive instruction for students in grades six through eight. Smoking bans in schools also discourage students from starting to smoke, reinforce knowledge of the health hazards of cigarette smoking and exposure to environmental tobacco smoke, and promote a smoke-free environment as the norm. States must also enforce the legal age for buying cigarettes.

Substance Abuse

The use of other substances (primarily drugs) by adolescents to produce an altered state of consciousness is believed to reflect the changes taking place in their lives and the stresses engendered by these changes. Although there is a steady increase in the incidence of adolescents using alcohol and marijuana, teenagers do not become high risk users. Experimentation is limited to 1 adolescent in 5 for stimulants and inhalants; and fewer than 1 in 10 for hallucinogens, sedatives, and "crack" cocaine. Adolescents at greatest risk are the 1% to 2% who use hard drugs regularly (Johnston, O'Malley, and Bachman, 1996).

Drug abuse is the regular use of drugs for other than the accepted medical purposes and to the extent that it results in physical or psychologic harm to the user and/or is detrimental to society. *Drug abuse, misuse,* and *addiction* are culturally defined and are voluntary behaviors. *Drug tolerance* and *physical dependence* are involuntary physiologic responses to the pharmacologic characteristics of drugs. Consequently, an individual can be addicted to a narcotic with or without being physically dependent, and a person may be physically dependent on a narcotic without being addicted (e.g., patients who use opioids to control pain) (see Pain Assessment, Chapter 44).

Most drugs that young people use induce changes in perception, feelings of well-being, a sense of closeness, and a feeling of happiness. In the majority of cases drug use begins with experimentation. The individual may try a drug only once, may use it occasionally, or may make it an integral part of a drug-centered lifestyle.

Motivation. Many factors influence the use of drugs. Adolescents try drugs out of curiosity. For many young people, drugs produce a dreamy state of altered consciousness or a feeling of power, excitement, heightened acuity, or confidence. Others seek visual hallucinatory experiences and sexual sensation. Many youngsters use drugs not only for the perceptual and sensory experiences, but also for the social aspects. They use drugs because their peers use them, and because they want to "belong." Teenagers are highly influenced by society's fads and fashions, and they are, developmentally, sensation-hungry risk takers. Adolescents are also trying to find a means to cope with the stress of the adult world, its social and technologic concerns, and their powerlessness to change it. Many teenagers seek to escape from reality, to achieve a sense of closeness and intimacy with other people, to escape from distress or decision making, or to feel a sense of insight into the mysteries of life and death.

Types of Drugs Abused. Any drug can be abused, and most are potentially harmful to youngsters still going through formative life experiences. Although rarely conceived of as drugs by society, the chemically active substances most often abused are caffeine and theobromines contained in chocolate, tea, coffee, and colas. Ethyl alcohol and nicotine are other substances that, although recognized as drugs, are sanctioned by society. These drugs can produce mild to moderate euphoric and/or stimulant effects and can lead to physical and psychic dependence. Many hazards associated with drug use are also related to adolescents driving a car while under the influence of drugs.

Drugs with mind-altering capacity that are available on the black market and that are of medical and legal concern are the hallucinogenic, narcotic, hypnotic, and stimulant drugs. In addition, health professionals are concerned about the use of alcohol; and various volatile substances such as gasoline, antifreeze, plastic model airplane cement, typewriter correction fluid, and organic solvents, which are inhaled to achieve altered sensation. Drugs available on the street are often mixed with other compounds and fillers so that the purity of the drug, its strength, and the nature of additives are highly variable.

Alcohol. Acute or chronic abuse of ethanol, a socially accepted depressant, is responsible for many acts of violence, suicide, accidental injury, and death. It is the most widely accepted drug, can be purchased legally by adults, is relatively inexpensive, is often used as part of a meal (e.g., wine and beer), and is approved by adults throughout the world when used in moderation. Youngsters may be afraid of hard drugs but feel comfortable with alcohol.

The most noticeable effects of alcohol are on the central nervous system—lack of coordination, marked mood changes, impaired judgment, impaired memory, and impaired perception. Young alcoholics often drink alone and cannot predictably control their use of alcohol. They often rely on alcohol as a defense against depression, anxiety, fear, or anger. Not all of these characteristics are observed, but if several signs are evident, the youngsters should be considered at risk and detoxification therapy initiated to ensure safe and complete withdrawal from the drug. Information about alcohol and answers to questions can be obtained by calling the Alcohol Hotline.*

Cocaine. Although cocaine is not pharmacologically considered a narcotic, it is legally categorized as such. Cocaine is available in two forms: water-soluble cocaine hydrochloride administered by "snorting" or IV injection; and a nonsoluble alkyloid (freebase) used primarily for smoking. "Crack" is a purer and more menacing form of the drug; it can be produced cheaply and smoked in either water pipes or mentholated cigarettes. The increased use of cocaine is related to its availability, affordability, the false perception that it is safe, its association with persons in glamorous occupations, its snob appeal, its reputation as a sexually enhancing drug, and peer pressure.

Cocaine creates a sense of euphoria, or an indefinable high. Withdrawal does not produce the dramatic symptoms observed in withdrawal from other substances. The effects are those more commonly seen in depression, including lack of energy and motivation, irritability, appetite changes, psychomotor retardation, and irregular sleep patterns. More serious symptoms include cardiovascular manifestations and seizures. Physical withdrawal is not to be confused with the so-called crash after a cocaine high, which consists of a long period of sleep. Answers to questions about the health risks of cocaine can be obtained by calling the National Cocaine Hotline,† which also provides referrals to support groups and treatment centers.

Narcotics. Narcotic drugs include opiates such as heroin, morphine, meperidine hydrochloride (Demerol), fentanyl, hydromorphone (Dilaudid), and codeine. These drugs produce a state of euphoria by removing painful feelings and creating a pleasurable experience and a sense of success accompanied by clouding of consciousness and a dreamlike state. Physical signs of narcotic abuse include constricted pupils, respiratory depression and, often, cyanosis. Needle marks may be visible on the arms or legs in chronic users. Withdrawal from opiates is extremely unpleasant unless controlled with supervised substitution of methadone.

---

*1-800-ALCOHOL
†1-800-COCAINE

Perhaps more important are the indirect consequences related to the illegal status of narcotic use and the problems associated with securing the drug (e.g., time-consuming searches and often illegal methods used to meet the high cost). Heath problems result from self-neglect of physical needs (e.g., nutrition, cleanliness, and dental care); overdose; contamination, and infection, including HIV infection and hepatitis B.

Central Nervous System Depressants. A variety of hypnotic drugs that produce physical dependence and withdrawal symptoms on abrupt discontinuation may be used by adolescents. These drugs create a feeling of relaxation and sleepiness but impair general functioning. Drugs in this category include barbiturates, nonbarbiturates (such as methaqualone [Quaalude]), and alcohol. Barbiturates combined with alcohol produce a profound depressant effect.

Central Nervous System Stimulants. Amphetamines and cocaine do not produce strong physical dependence and can be withdrawn without much danger; however, psychologic dependence is strong, and acute intoxication can lead to violent aggressive behavior or psychotic episodes characterized by paranoia, uncontrollable agitation, and restlessness. When combined with barbiturates, the euphoric effects are particularly addictive.

Methamphetamine can be snorted, injected, swallowed, or smoked. It produces a burst of energy in its users, along with intense, alternating attacks of boldness and paranoia. It provokes excitement far more intense than that caused by crack and cocaine. The drug, with the street names "crank," "meth," and "crystal," is inexpensive and has a longer period of action than cocaine. Instead of a short (i.e., a few minutes) high, as achieved with crack, a user can remain "up" for hours on a similar dose of crank.

Mind-Altering Drugs. Hallucinogens (i.e., psychedelic, psychotomimetic, psychotropic, or illusionogenic drugs) produce vivid hallucinations and euphoria. These drugs do not produce physical dependence, and they can be abruptly withdrawn without ill effect. However, acute and long-term effects are variable, and in some individuals the dissociative behavior may be unduly prolonged. This category includes cannabis (e.g., marijuana and hashish) and lysergic acid diethylamide (LSD).

Inhalants. "Sniffing" or "huffing," the inhalation of plastic cement or other volatile substances that youngsters breathe or place in paper or plastic bags to rebreathe the fumes, produces euphoria and altered consciousness. These substances are extremely hazardous to the individual and can cause rapid loss of consciousness and respiratory arrest. Many persons taking these drugs do not have time to remove the bag from their heads and quickly become asphyxiated. An important addition to the list of "sniffing" substances is air dusters, or cans of pressurized gas used to blow dust from such surfaces as computers and camera lenses. The dusters contain chemical solvents and usually a form of freon, which can cause fatal cardiac arrhythmia.

Nursing Care Management. Nurses in almost every setting are likely to have contact with young drug abusers or to be in a position to serve as educator and patient advocate. The nurse most often encounters young drug abusers when they are (1) experiencing overdose symptoms, (2) experiencing withdrawal symptoms, (3) manifesting bizarre behavior or confusion secondary to drug ingestion, (4) worried that they are becoming or will become addicted, or (5) worried about a friend or family member who is addicted.

Nurses who care for hospitalized adolescents need to know if these youths use drugs compulsively. Withdrawal phenomena can seriously complicate other illnesses. Nurses should be alert for physical or behavioral clues that indicate the onset of withdrawal or the effects of drugs. Obstetric and nursery nurses may encounter drug dependence and withdrawal in newborn infants or compulsive drug-using mothers. School nurses and nurses who work in the community also play an essential role in identifying families with substance abuse problems. Early identification of families with substance abuse problems is critical to the prevention of substance abuse among children and adolescents (Werner, Joffe, and Graham, 1999).

Acute Care. Adolescents experiencing toxic drug effects or withdrawal symptoms are often seen in the emergency department. Experienced emergency department personnel are familiar with the management of acute drug toxicosis; the signs, symptoms, and behavioral characteristics of a variety of substances; and differences and similarities among them. Observation of or description of the behavior is often of more value than a report by patients or their friends as to the chemical agent taken.

The treatment for drug toxicity or withdrawal varies according to the drug and the method used. Every effort is made to determine the type and amount of drug taken, the time it was taken, the mode of administration, and factors related to the onset of presenting symptoms. It is helpful to know the individual's pattern of use. For example, if two types of drugs are involved, they may require different treatments. Gastric lavage may be employed when the drug has been ingested recently and the cough reflex is intact, but it is of little value when the drug has been administered by the IV ("mainlined") or intranasal ("sniffed") route. Because the actual content of most street drugs is highly questionable, other pharmaceutical agents are administered with caution, except perhaps naloxone (Narcan) or flumazenil (Romazicon) in cases of suspected opiate or benzodiazepine overdose, respectively. It is also necessary to assess for possible trauma sustained while the patient was under the influence of the drug.

Long-Term Management. A major factor in the treatment and rehabilitation of young drug users is careful assessment, in the nonacute stage, to determine the function that the drug plays in the youngster's life. Adolescents need help to identify the problem that motivated them to use drugs—and to recognize their own role in self-destructive, inappropriate drug abuse behavior—before they can embark on a rehabilitation program.

Rehabilitation begins when youngsters decide that they can and are willing to change. Rehabilitation involves fostering healthy interdependent relationships with caring and supportive adults and exploring alternate mechanisms for problem solving while simultaneously reducing or eliminating drug use. Persons working with troubled youth must be prepared for recidivism, or the tendency to relapse, and maintain a plan for reentry into the treatment process.

Family Support. Organizations that have achieved success in helping others cope with problems of drug abuse are excellent sources for both youngsters and their families. The philosophy of Tough Love* is based on the conviction that parents have the right and responsibility to be the policymakers in the

*P.O. Box 1069, Doylestown, PA 18901; (215) 348-7090; website: www.toughlove.org.

family, to set limits on the behavior of their children, and to take control of the household from out-of-control youngsters. The premise is that allowing teenagers to experience the negative consequences of their behavior will bring them closer to accepting help and/or changing their behavior.

Another group that provides support and counseling for families experiencing crises with their children is Parents Anonymous,* which maintains crisis counseling on a 24-hour basis. Al-Anon, Ala-Teen, and Ala-Tot are support groups for children and families who have an alcoholic family member. Information can be obtained from Alcoholics Anonymous listings in local telephone directories.

Prevention. Substance abuse in adolescence is both an individual and a community problem, and nurses play an important role in education and legislation, as well as in individual observation, assessment, and therapy. In this drug-oriented society, patterns of drug use may be established through parental models and the influence of the media as an effective means to make the user "feel better." Impressionable youth need to be educated regarding appropriate use of chemicals. More important, those associated with adolescents should listen to what they are saying, determine what is bothering them, and try to help them meet their needs through alternative methods before they resort to drugs.

Peer pressure is a powerful tool and can be used effectively in prevention. A group that has had some success in reducing injury from drunk driving is Students Against Driving Drunk (SADD),† an organization designed to help eliminate teenage drunk driving. Techniques used by this group include peer counseling, parental guidelines for teenage parties, and community awareness. Nurses can encourage the formation of chapters of SADD in the high schools in their communities.

The most effective substance abuse prevention strategies are part of a broader, generic prevention effort to promote health and success. Health-compromising behaviors are interconnected and often have common antecedents. Prevention efforts that focus on changing only one behavior (e.g., alcohol and other drug use) are less likely to be successful.

Suicide

Suicide is the third leading cause of death during the teenage years, surpassed only by death from injury and homicide (see Chapter 29). From 1972 to 1992 the suicide rate in the United States for children 10 to 14 years of age more than doubled, and for teenagers 15 to 19 years of age the rate increased 30% (Centers for Disease Control and Prevention, 1995). Specific racial groups have also experienced increases in suicide. From 1980 to 1995 the suicide rate for African-American youths increased 114%; this increase was particularly obvious for African-American youths in the South (Centers for Disease Control and Prevention, 1998b).

Most experts distinguish between suicidal ideation, suicide attempt (or parasuicide), and suicide. *Suicidal ideation* involves a preoccupation with thoughts about committing suicide and may be a precursor to suicide. Although it is not uncommon for adolescents to experience occasional suicidal thoughts, expressions of preoccupation with suicide should be taken seriously, and an assessment should be conducted for appropriate referral. A *suicide attempt* is intended to cause injury or death. The term *parasuicide* is used to refer to all behaviors ranging from gestures to serious attempts to kill oneself; the term does not include intent or motivation. For many adolescents the motivation for a suicidal gesture or attempt may be obscure, complex, and difficult to articulate; however, all parasuicidal activity should be taken seriously.

NURSE ALERT • A history of a previous suicide attempt is a serious indicator for possible suicide completion in the future. Studies of adolescent suicides have found that as many as half of the adolescents had made previous attempts.

Etiology. Adolescence has always been characterized by turmoil, heightened emotionality, and wide variations in mood. With limited capacities for problem solving and with fewer and less sophisticated resources for resolving difficulties, some teenagers have difficulty coping with critical events, especially a situation that is forced on them, such as the death of a friend, parent, or sibling. Impulsive behavior, characteristic of younger children, places children and adolescents at high risk for suicide.

Individual, family, and social/environmental factors have been implicated in suicide. The single most important individual factor is the presence of an active psychiatric disorder (e.g., depression, bipolar disorder, psychosis, substance abuse, or conduct disorder). Gay and lesbian adolescents are at particularly high risk for suicide completion, especially if they are denied support systems (Remafedi et al, 1998) (Community Focus box). Family factors include parental loss; family disruption; a family history of suicide, depression, substance abuse, or emotional disturbance; child abuse or neglect; unavailable parents; poor communication and isolation within the family; family conflict; and unrealistically high parental expectations or parental indifference with low expectations. Social/environmental factors include incarceration, isolation, acute loss of a boyfriend or girlfriend, lack of future options, and increased availability of firearms in the home.

Methods. The outcome of suicidal behavior is influenced by the method used. Violent methods of destruction used by adults, such as jumping from heights or in front of trains, are less commonly employed by youths. Firearms are the most commonly used instruments in completed suicides among males and females. The most common method of suicide attempt is overdose or ingestion of toxic substances such as drugs. Drugs used include medications prescribed for parents (e.g., barbiturates and antidepressants), those intended for household use (e.g., aspirin or acetaminophen), or solvents. Ingestion of medications and strangulation are the second and third methods favored by females; males use hanging and overdose.

NURSE ALERT • Given what is known about youth suicide, nurses should ask parents, especially those with at-risk teenagers, if firearms are available in the house and if so, recommend their removal. Parents must ensure that their children—especially those who are depressed, have poor problem-solving skills, or use drugs or alcohol—do not have access to firearms. Parents must also be educated on the warning signs of suicide (Box 40-9).

*22330 Hawthorne Blvd., No. 208, Torrance, CA 90505; 1-800-352-0386; another source of information is the National Clearinghouse for Alcohol and Drug Information, P.O. Box 2345, Rockville, MD 20847; 1-800-729-6686; website: www.health.org.

†P.O. Box 800, Marlboro, MA 01752; (508) 481-3568 or (877) SADDINC.

Community Focus

SUICIDE, SEXUAL IDENTITY, AND SEXUAL ORIENTATION

A significant number of teenage suicides occur among homosexual youths. Gay or lesbian adolescents who live in families or communities that do not accept homosexuality are likely to suffer low self-esteem, self-loathing, depression, and hopelessness as a result of lack of acceptance from their family or community. Such internalization, without treatment and support, can lead to substance abuse and, eventually, suicide. Youths most at risk are those who struggle with gender identity issues such as gay identity formation at a young age, intrapersonal conflict regarding sexuality, and nondisclosure of orientation to others (Remafedi et al, 1998).

Supportive parents, friends, or relationships serve as protective factors against suicide. However, many gay, lesbian, and bisexual adolescents do not feel supported, understood, or accepted by their friends, parents, and families. Nurses who interact with adolescents must be aware of the association between suicide and adolescent homosexuality and gender nonconformity. School nurses may be the first individuals to discuss issues of sexual identity and orientation with adolescents and/or their families. In their professional capacity, nurses can also serve as support persons for these adolescents and provide the supportive relationship so important to them. Nurses can also provide guidance and resources to families so that they know and understand how best to nurture and support their child.

Nurses must also capitalize on opportunities or experiences that promote the healthy development of self-esteem in youths who choose nontraditional sexual orientation. Educational programs to raise the level of consciousness about the risk factors for and warning signs of suicide are one example. Another possibility could be programs conducted in or outside of school that are designed to foster peer relationships and competency in social skills among high-risk adolescents and young adults, such as support groups and social organizations for these young people.

Box 40-9

Warning Signs of Suicide

- Preoccupation with themes of death—focuses on morbid thoughts
- Wants to give away cherished possessions
- Talks of own death, desire to die
- Loss of energy—loss of interest, listlessness
- Exhaustion without obvious cause
- Changes in sleep patterns—too much or too little
- Increased irritability, argumentativeness, or stubbornness
- Physical complaints—recurrent stomachaches, headaches
- Repeated visits to physician, nurse practitioner, or emergency department for treatment of injuries
- Reckless behavior
- Antisocial behavior—engages in drinking, uses drugs, fights, commits acts of vandalism, runs away from home, becomes sexually promiscuous
- Sudden change in school performance—lowered grades, cutting classes, dropping out of activities
- Resists or refuses to go to school
- Remains distant, sad, remote—flat affect, frozen facial expression
- Describes self as worthless
- Sudden cheerfulness following deep depression
- Social withdrawal from friends, activities, interests that were previously enjoyed
- Impaired concentration
- Dramatic change in appetite

Motivation. Many youngsters cannot identify a cause for their suicidal ideas. Ambivalence about life and death and hopelessness are common feelings. Most suicidal gestures are impulsive acts committed to force parents or other significant persons to pay attention to the youngster's need for help. The attempt usually is the culmination of a behavioral pattern. These youngsters often have a history of attention-getting behaviors that range from minor acts to increasingly dramatic ones. With the ultimate act of attempted suicide, youngsters finally make themselves heard. They seldom actually plan a suicidal act because they really want to die; successful suicides are committed either impulsively or accidentally.

Suicidal ideation is not uncommon in adolescents. It represents numerous fantasies, such as relief from suffering, a means of gaining comfort and sympathy, or a means of revenge against those who have hurt them. Adolescents have the erroneous perception that the act of suicide will evoke remorse and pity and that they will be able to return and witness the grief. Some children and younger adolescents desire to punish others who will be grieved by their death. Angry children who are unable to punish directly those who have injured or insulted them will take revenge on those who love them through self-destruction ("They'll be sorry when they find me dead"; "They'll be sorry they were mean to me").

Occasionally there are adolescents who are so severely depressed that suicide seems to be the only release from their despair. These youngsters rarely give evidence of their intent, concealing their suicidal thoughts for fear of outside intervention. Most adolescents tell their peers of their suicidal thoughts or plans but avoid telling adults. Sometimes this self-destructive behavior on the part of adolescents is a desire to punish themselves for guilt-filled actions or thoughts. Peer pressure also has convinced many young persons that there is something wrong with them if they feel lonely or depressed; therefore they direct these feelings inward to avoid the risk of rejection. Social isolation is the most significant factor in distinguishing adolescents who will kill themselves from those who will not. It is also more characteristic of those who complete suicide than of those who make attempts or threats.

The frequency of contagion, or "copycat" suicides (i.e., an increase in youth suicide that occurs after the suicide of one teenager is publicized) may indicate that suicide is perceived as "glamorous" by teenagers. In addition, young people may not realize the finality of suicide, because they have become desensitized from constantly viewing violence and death on television.

Diagnostic Evaluation. Depression is a symptom common to adolescents who attempt suicide. Depression is characterized by both subjective symptoms and objective signs that reflect the adolescent's grief. Adolescents describe feelings of sadness, despair, helplessness, hopelessness, boredom, loss of interest, and isolation. They may also feel self-reproach, self-deprecation, and guilt. Subjective symptoms of depression or specific changes in behavior place an adolescent at risk for suicide (see Box 40-9).

Therapeutic Management. *Threats of suicide must be taken very seriously.* There has been a tendency to dismiss a suicide attempt as an impulsive act resulting from a temporary crisis or depression. If this attempt to gain attention fails to draw attention to their problems or makes them worse, adolescents may conclude that suicide is the only answer to their unbearable problems.

Children need to know that someone cares, and they must be provided with swift and efficient crisis intervention. Although an acute depressive reaction can be managed without difficulty by ordinary practitioners, the youngster who has made a serious attempt or has made a plan for suicide should receive immediate attention and competent psychiatric care.

NURSE ALERT • Adolescents who express suicidal feelings and have a specific plan should be monitored at all times. They should not have access to firearms, prescription or over-the-counter drugs, belts, scarves, shoestrings, sharp objects, matches, or lighters. If they are intoxicated, they may need to be restrained or placed in a protective environment until they can be assessed by a psychiatrist or psychologist.

Nursing Care Management. Nursing care of the suicidal youngster includes early recognition, management, and prevention. Probably the most important aspect of management is the recognition of warning signs that indicate a youngster is troubled and might attempt suicide. Health professionals need to be alert to the signs of depression, and anyone who exhibits such behavior, subtle or overt, should be referred for thorough psychologic assessment. Depression can be manifested in several ways: young people who feel depressed may talk about suicide and feelings of worthlessness, or they may build themselves a solid defense against such intolerable feelings of depression with behavioral or psychosomatic disturbances.

NURSE ALERT • No threat of suicide should be ignored or challenged in any way. It is a symptom that must be taken seriously. Too often suicidal threats or minor attempts are confused with bids for attention. It is also a mistake to be lulled into a false sense of security when the adolescent's depression is apparently relieved. The improvement in attitude may very well mean that the youngster has made the decision to carry out the threat.

Peers or other confidants are excellent sources of information and valuable observers. They may not be able to diagnose depression, but they are able to sense when a friend has undergone a marked personality change. It is important to emphasize that the peer who detects any changes in a friend is a potential rescuer and should not remain silent about the observations. Friendship does not imply collusion. A peer who believes that a friend may be suicidal should alert someone who is in a position to help—a parent, teacher, guidance counselor, school nurse, or other person.

Routine health assessments of adolescents should include questions that determine the presence of suicidal thought or intent. Information should be gathered to evaluate whether a child or adolescent is depressed, the need for therapy, and the probability of a suicide attempt. Clues to a youth's feelings may be elicited by the following questions (Greydanus and Pratt, 1995):

- Do you consider yourself more a happy person, an unhappy person, or somewhere in the middle?
- Have you ever been so unhappy or upset that you felt like being dead?
- Have you ever thought about hurting yourself?
- Have you ever developed a plan to hurt yourself or kill yourself?
- Have you ever attempted to kill yourself?

If a child or adolescent has expressed suicidal intent, they should be asked to give their written word that they will not attempt suicide during an agreed-on period of time (a week, a day, maybe even just 5 minutes) and that they will contact help immediately if they feel that they cannot keep their contract. The length of time a youngster suggests provides valuable information regarding the seriousness of the threat. Furthermore, most teenagers attach significance to signing their name to a document, and if they sign a no-suicide contract, they will usually honor it. Contracts can be extended when the time limit expires.

Because a suicide attempt is often an outgrowth of family distress, it is essential to deal with the family as well. The most effective approach is recognition of susceptible youngsters during the early stages of intrafamily distress so that family counseling can be started. This emphasizes the importance of parent-child relationships and the role of the nurse in assessing family interactions and recognizing disturbed relationships. Prevention efforts must be directed toward improving child-rearing practices through support and education of parents and changing societal conditions that generate defeat, despair, and maladaptive behavior.

Follow-up care is essential. Although confidentiality is the usual approach with adolescent counseling, in the case of self-destructive behaviors this cannot be honored. Suicidal behavior is reported to the family and other professionals, and youngsters are informed that this will be done. Such action conveys an important message to the youth—that the professionals understand and care.

Many schools have instituted suicide prevention programs designed for high school-age youth, and other schools are attempting to reach elementary school-age children as well. Some school programs include services such as drop-in counseling and a peer-counseling telephone line. Information can also be obtained from the American Association of Suicidology.*

(See also Nursing Care Plan: The Child Who is Suicidal.†)

---

*4201 Connecticut Ave. NW, Suite 408, Washington, DC 20008; phone (202) 237-2280; e-mail: berm101m@ix.netcom.com; website: www.suicidology.org.

†In Wong DL, Hess CS: ***Wong and Whaley's clinical manual of pediatric nursing,*** ed 5, St Louis, 2000, Mosby.

Key Points

- The pubescent growth spurt that begins around age 10 years in girls and age 12 years in boys signals the beginning of adolescence.
- Biologic development during puberty is characterized by increased activity of the pituitary gland, which results in sexual maturity and the appearance of secondary sex characteristics.
- According to Erikson, the major developmental crisis of adolescence is establishing a sense of identity.

- Spiritual development is characterized by the questioning of family values and ideals, a move to more philosophical thinking, and emphasis on personal religion.
- Adolescent relationships with parents may be strained, whereas the influence of the peer group increases and heterosexual relationships assume importance.
- Teenagers demonstrate a variety of interests, and their increased physical and cognitive skills allow them to engage in increasingly difficult and complex activities.
- Adolescents' emotions fluctuate.
- Nutritional needs, especially for calcium, zinc, and iron, may not be met by teenagers' eating habits, such as snacking and irregular mealtimes.
- Motor vehicle injuries are the primary cause of death from injury in the adolescent years.
- The rapid changes, growth, and stress accompanying the transition to adulthood may predispose youngsters to faulty problem solving.
- Cognitive development in adolescence includes abstract thought, thinking beyond the present, logical reasoning, and a sense of idealism.
- Development of body image is closely tied to body changes and social interactions.
- According to Kohlberg's theory of moral development, adolescents begin to question existing moral values and learn to make choices.
- The most common health problems related to the female reproductive system involve menstrual dysfunction.
- Eating disorders observed in middle and late childhood are obesity, anorexia nervosa, and bulimia.
- Smoking is a widespread problem among teenagers: reasons for smoking include social pressure, mass media influence, and a need to develop a self-concept.
- The substances abused by children and adolescents are alcohol, marijuana, narcotics, central nervous system depressants, central nervous system stimulants, hydrocarbons and fluorocarbons, and mind-altering drugs.
- Suicide, the deliberate act of self-injury with the intent to kill, may occur because of difficulties coping with stress, disturbed family environment, chemical dependency, or psychoses.
- No threat of suicide by an adolescent should be ignored or challenged.

References

Alan Guttmacher Institute: *Facts in brief, teen sex, and pregnancy,* New York, 1998, The Institute.

Allensworth DD, Bradley B: Guidelines for adolescent preventive services: a role for the school nurse, *J Sch Health* 66(8):281-285, 1996.

American Academy of Pediatrics, Committee on Infectious Diseases: Recommended childhood immunization schedule—United States, January-December 2000, *Pediatrics* 105(1):148, 2000.

American Psychiatric Association: *Diagnostic and statistical manual of mental disorders,* ed 4 (DSM-IV), Washington, DC, 1994, The Association.

Baker JG et al: Relationship between perceived parental monitoring and young adolescent girls' sexual and substance abuse behaviors, *J Pediatr Adolesc Gynecol* 12(1):17-22, 1999.

Barlow SE, Dietz WH: Obesity evaluation and treatment: expert committee recommendations, *Pediatrics* 102(3):e29, 1998.

Centers for Disease Control and Prevention: Selected cigarette smoking initiation and quitting behaviors among high school students—United States, 1997, *MMWR* 27(19):386-389, 1998a.

Centers for Disease Control and Prevention: *Suicide in the United States 1980-1992,* Atlanta, 1995, National Center for Injury Prevention and Control.

Centers for Disease Control and Prevention: Suicide among black youths—United States, 1980-1995, *MMWR* 47(10): 193-206, 1998b.

Centers for Disease Control and Prevention: Tobacco use among high school students—United States, 1997, *MMWR* 47(12): 229-233, 1998c.

Cohen LR, Potter LB: Injuries and violence: risk factors and opportunities for prevention during adolescence, *Adolesc Med* 10(1):125-135, 1999.

DeGaston JF, Weed S, Jensen L: Understanding the gender differences in adolescent sexuality, *Adolescence* 31(121):217-231, 1996.

Emans SJ, Laufer MR, Goldstein DP: *Pediatric and adolescent gynecology,* ed 4, Philadelphia, 1998, Lippincott-Raven.

Erikson EH: *Childhood and society,* ed 2, New York, 1963, WW Norton.

Fisher M: Anorexia and bulimia nervosa. In Hoekelman RA, editor: *Primary pediatric care,* ed 3, St Louis, 1997, Mosby.

Francis KT: Status of the year 2000 health goals for physical activity and fitness, *Phys Ther* 79(4):405-414, 1999.

Graber JA et al: Is psychopathology associated with the timing of pubertal development? *J Am Acad Child Adolesc Psychiatry* 36:1768-1775, 1997.

Greydanus DE, Pratt HD: Emotional and behavioral disorders of adolescence, part 2, *Adolesc Health Update* 8(1):1-8, 1995.

Hamburg DA: Toward a strategy for healthy adolescent development, *Am J Psychiatry* 154(6):7-12, 1997.

Harel Z et al: Supplementation with omega-3 polyunsaturated fatty acids in the management of dysmenorrhea in adolescents, *Am J Obstet Gynecol* 174:1335-1338, 1996.

Harries M et al: Changes in the male voice at puberty: vocal fold length and its relationship to the fundamental frequency of the voice, *J Laryngeal Otol* 112(5):451-454, 1998.

Hayes DN, Hemenway D: Age within school class and adolescent gun-carrying, *Pediatrics* 103(5):1-6, 1999.

Hayward C et al: Psychiatric risk associated with early puberty in adolescent girls, *J Am Acad Child Psychiatry* 36:255-262, 1997.

Hoffmann RG, Rodrique JR, Johnson JH: Effectiveness of a school-based program to enhance knowledge of sun exposure: attitudes toward sun exposure and sunscreen use among children, *Child Health Care* 28(1):69-86, 1999.

Johnston LD, O'Malley PM, Bachman JG: *Monitoring the future study,* Ann Arbor, Dec 19, 1996, News and Information Services of the University of Michigan.

Keller C, Stevens KR: Childhood obesity: measurement and risk assessment, *Pediatr Nurs* 22(6):494-499, 1996.

Kuczmarski RJ et al: *CDC growth charts: United States. Advance data from vital statistics,* No. 314. Hyattsville, MD: National Center for Health Statistics, June 8, 2000.

Mackenzie R, Neinstein LS: Anorexia nervosa and bulimia. In Neinstein LS, editor: *Adolescent health care,* ed 3, Baltimore, 1996, Williams & Wilkins.

Montgomery MJ, Sorrell GT: Love and dating experience in early and middle adolescence: grade and gender comparisons, *J Adolesc* 21(6):677-689, 1998.

Moran R: Evaluation and treatment of childhood obesity, *Am Fam Physician* 59(4):861-868, 1999.

Morris J: Health promotion, the case against TSE, *Nurs Times* 33:41-42, 1996.

Muldoon KA: Body piercing in adolescence, *J Pediatr Health Care* 11(6):293-301, 1997.

Neinstein LS: *Adolescent health care: a practical guide,* ed 3, Baltimore, 1996, Williams & Wilkins.

Neuman JF: Evaluation and treatment of gynecomastia, *Am Fam Physician* 55:1849-1850, 1997.

Office of Smoking and Health, Division of Adolescent and School Health, National Center for Chronic Disease Prevention and Health Promotion: Tobacco use and usual source of cigarettes among high school students—United States, 1995, *J Sch Health* 66(6):222-224, 1996.

Prose CC, Ford CA, Lovely LP: Evaluating amenorrhea: the pediatrician's role, *Contemp Pediatr* 15:83-110, 1998.

Ralston SH: What determines peak bone mass and bone loss, *Baillieres Clin Rheumatol* 11(3):479-494, 1997.

Remafedi G et al: The relationship between suicide risk and sexual orientation: results of a population-based study, *Am J Public Health* 88(1):57-60, 1998.

Resnick MD et al: Protecting adolescents from harm: findings from the National Longitudianl Study on Adolescent Health, *JAMA* 278:823-832, 1997.

Saewyc EM et al: Gender differences in health and risk behaviors among bisexual and homosexual adolescents, *J Adolesc Health Care* 23:181-188, 1998.

Schuster MA, Bell RM, Kanouse DE: The sexual practices of adolescent virgins: genital sexual activities of high school students who have never had vaginal intercourse, *Am J Public Health* 86(11):1570-1576, 1996.

Seidell JC: Obesity: a growing problem, *Acta Paediatr* 88(428, suppl):46-50, 1999.

Starr NB: Sun smarts: the essentials of sun protection, *J Pediatr Health Care* 13:136-138, 1999.

Strauss R: Childhood obesity, *Curr Probl Pediatr* 29(1):1-29, 1999.

Troiano R et al: Overweight prevalence and trends for children and adolescents, *Arch Pediatr Adolesc Med* 149(10): 1085-1091, 1995.

Wells SW: The health beliefs, values and practices of gay adolescents, *Clin Nurs Spec* 13(2):69-73, 1999.

Werner MJ, Joffe A, Graham AV: Screening, early identification and office-based intervention with children and youth living in substance-abusing families, Pediatrics 103:1099-1112, 1999.

Willard JC, Schoenborn CA: *Relationship between cigarette smoking and other unhealthy behaviors among our nation's youth: United States, 1992,* Advance Data, No. 263, April 24, 1995, Centers for Disease Control and Prevention.

CHAPTER

41

Chronic Illness, Disability, and Death

http://www.harcourthealth.com/MERLIN/Wong/maternal/

Learning Objectives

On completion of this chapter the reader will be able to:

- Identify the scope of and changing trends in care of children with special needs.
- Identify the major reactions of and effects on the family with a child with special needs.
- Define the stages of adjustment to the diagnosis of a chronic condition.
- Recognize the impact of the illness or disability on the developmental stages of childhood.
- Outline nursing interventions that promote the family's optimum adjustment to the child's chronic disorder.
- Outline nursing interventions that support the family at the time of death.
- Define the usual symptoms of normal grief.

PERSPECTIVES ON THE CARE OF CHILDREN WITH SPECIAL NEEDS

Scope of the Problem

A number of terms and defining characteristics have been used to describe chronic illnesses and disability in children (Box 41-1). In recent years there have been continuing efforts to develop a definition that better identifies the numbers of children living with chronic conditions, as well as the impact on health and social services. Currently children with special health care needs are defined as (Newacheck et al, 1998):

> . . . children who have or are at increased risk for a chronic physical, developmental, behavioral, or emotional condition and who also require health and related services of a type or amount beyond that generally required by children.

Ongoing progress in medical and technologic disease management has contributed to the growing number of children with special health care needs. For example, in 1996, as a result of the development of new drugs, death rates for children with human immunodeficiency virus (HIV) infection decreased by 28.8% (Peters, Kochanek, and Murphy, 1998). Technologic advances have substantially increased the survival of extremely- and very-low birth-weight infants. The result of such progress is that an estimated 18% (12.6 million) of children in the United States live with a chronic illness or disability and require specialized health care of a type or amount beyond that generally required by children (Newacheck et al, 1998).

The most commonly occurring conditions causing disability are diseases of the respiratory tract, as well as impairments of speech and intelligence. Mental and nervous system disorders account for about one sixth of all childhood disability (Newacheck and Halfon, 1998).

The impact of chronic illness and disability in children is wide ranging. A child's activity level and development opportunities can be affected. Days can be lost from school. Children with chronic illness or disability may be at increased risk for behavior or emotional problems. Parents may lose days from work, experience financial strain, and be challenged both emotionally and physically as they cope with care of the child. Siblings are affected, as can be extended family members.

Trends in Care

Developmental Focus. Focusing on the child's *developmental level* rather than chronologic age or diagnosis emphasizes the child's abilities and strengths rather than disabilities. Attention focuses on normalizing experiences, adapting the environment, and promoting coping skills. Nurses often are in vital positions to redirect attention from the pathologic model with its focus on weaknesses and problems to the developmental model to meet the unique needs of the child and family.

A developmental focus also considers family development. The life cycle of the family unit reflects changing ages and needs of family members, as well as changing external demands. A

Box 41-1

Common Terms Regarding Children with Special Needs

Chronic illness—A condition that interferes with daily functioning for more than 3 months in a year, causes hospitalization of more than 1 month in a year, or (at time of diagnosis) is likely to do either of these

Congenital disability—A disability that has existed since birth but is not necessarily hereditary

Developmental delay—A maturational lag; an abnormal, slower rate of development in which a child demonstrates a functioning level below that observed in normal children of the same age

Developmental disability—Any mental and/or physical disability that is manifested before age 22 years and is likely to continue indefinitely

Disability—A functional limitation that interferes with a person's ability, for example, to walk, lift, hear, or learn

Handicap—A condition or barrier imposed by society, the environment, or one's own self; not a synonym for disability

Impairment—A loss or abnormality of structure or function

Technology-dependent child—A child between the ages of birth to 21 years with a chronic disability that requires the routine use of a medical device to compensate for the loss of a life-sustaining body function; daily ongoing care and/or monitoring is required by trained personnel

Sources: Childhood-disability definition created, *AAP News* 11(7):4, 1995; Hobbs N, Perrin J, editors: *Issues in the care of children with chronic illness,* San Francisco, 1985, Jossey-Bass; Report to Congress and the Secretary by the Task Force on Technology-Dependent Children: *Fostering home and community-based care for technology-dependent children,* vol 2, Health Care Financing Administration, HCFA Pub. No. 88-02171, Washington, DC, 1988, U.S. DHHS; and Research and Training Center on Independent Living: *Guidelines for reporting and writing about people with disabilities,* ed 3, Lawrence, KS, 1990, The Center.

family member's serious illness or disability can cause significant stress or crisis at any stage of the family life cycle. Just as with individual development, family development may be interrupted or even regress to an earlier level of functioning. Nurses can use the concept of family development to plan meaningful interventions and evaluate care (see Developmental Theory, Chapter 33).

Family-Centered Care. The importance of family-centered care—a philosophy that considers the family as the constant in the child's life—is especially evident in the care of children with special needs (see also Family-Centered Care, Chapter 29). As parents learn about the youngster's health care needs, they often become experts in delivering care. Health care providers, including nurses, are adjuncts to the child's care and need to form partnerships with parents. Collaboration is essential to forming trusting and effective partnerships and has the goal of finding the best ways to meet the needs of the child and family. Collaborative relationships are characterized by communication, dialogue, active listening, awareness, and acceptance of differences (Bishop, Woll, and Arango, 1993).

Communicating with Families. Families whose child is ill react along what health care providers may view as a continuum from the "good" to the "difficult" family stereotype. Nurses readily form relationships with the "good" family, who perceives staff as having power or control and accepts this hierarchy (Satariano and Briggs, 1989). However, this is often not the case with the "difficult" family, who is characterized as being underinvolved or overinvolved in the child's care.

Nurses should respect families' varying styles of interacting with health care providers and can base strategies for working with families on understanding a family's style (Table 41-1). Care conferences, especially multidisciplinary meetings that include the family and key health professionals, provide an opportunity for joint sharing of ideas and expression of feelings or concerns. Individual discussions, especially with the case manager, primary nurse, clinical nurse specialist, or advanced nurse

TABLE 41-1

Strategies for Facilitating Parent-Nurse Interaction

Parent Characteristics	Strategies
SILENT IN CARE	
Have trust and mistrust May not accompany child; prefer to wait outside Are very uncertain, quiet Use little verbal communication Visit on limited or irregular basis	Do not force participation Avoid authoritarian stance Use simple terms and demystify surroundings Explain what will happen Point out how their presence helps child
RECIPIENT OF CARE	
Have total trust Want nurse to make decisions Offer numerous positive comments Are easily impressed with information Are prone to misunderstandings Comply with rules Focus on child while visiting	Offer/provide information; elicit feedback to ensure their understanding Allow unlimited contact with child Engage them in gaining child's cooperation
MONITOR OF CARE	
Have high levels of mistrust Have attitude that "mistakes can happen" Monitor everyone's performance Involved in all decisions Want high levels of information Know agency's hierarchy Seek care from nurses Ask for rule changes	Believe that you can build trust Negotiate, negotiate, negotiate! Be flexible regarding rules Avoid issues of control Ask their opinion and use their suggestions
MANAGER OF CARE	
Are similar to monitors, but less angry Achieve complex coordination of child's chronic care	Recognize them as experts about their child Recognize need for respite

Developed by Donna M. Dixon, Memorial Medical Center, Springfield, IL, 1993. Used with permission. Modified from Knafl KA, Cavallari KA, Dixon DM: *Pediatric hospitalization: family and nurse perspectives,* Glenview, IL, 1988, Scott, Foresman.

practitioner, help establish a consistent and flexible plan of care that can prevent conflicts or deal with them before they become major issues. In family-centered care the goal is to maintain the integrity of the family, empower family members to assume a leadership role, and support the family during stressful times (Baker, 1994).

Issues of culture, ethnicity, and race affect access to services, utilization, and follow-through with referrals and recommendations (Huber, Holditch-Davis, and Brandon, 1993; Newacheck, Stoddard, and McManus, 1993). For some ethnic and minority populations, cultural understandings of illness and disability, the structure of family life, social roles for individuals who are disabled, and other factors related to the perception of children may differ from those of "mainstream" American culture (Groce and Zola, 1993). These factors may affect family needs and family choices regarding the care of their child with special needs.

Although culture cannot completely explain how an individual will think and act, understanding cultural perspectives can help the nurse anticipate and understand why families may make certain decisions (Groce and Zola, 1993; Kelly, 1996; Yoos et al, 1995). Cultural attributes such as values and beliefs regarding illness or disability and its causation, social roles for the ill or disabled, family structure, the role of children, childrearing practices, self vs. group orientation, spirituality, and time orientation also affect a family's response to illness or disability in a child. Developing a plan of care in conjunction with the family while considering their preferences and priorities is an important first step in formulating a plan of care that best meets the family's needs, regardless of their cultural background (Ahmann, 1994).

Normalization. Through application of the principles of normalization, daily routines for the child with illness or disability should be fitted to the family's schedule, rather than vice versa (see also Guidelines box, p. 1017). Age-appropriate expectations for the child's behavior should be applied. As necessary, the environment should be structured to encourage the child's engagement in age-appropriate activities. Thus consequences of the illness are minimized, and the child and family live as normal a life as possible given the disability.

A trend that facilitates normalization is the earlier discharge of children from acute- or chronic-care facilities to the family and community. *Home care* represents the return to a system and set of priorities in which family values are as important in the care of a child with a chronic health problem as they are in the care of other children. Home care seeks to achieve goals that are consistent with the developmental model (Stein, 1985):

- Normalize the life of a child with special needs, including those with technologically complex care, in a family and community context and setting.
- Minimize the disruptive impact of the child's condition on the family.
- Foster the child's maximum growth and development.

With appropriate training and support, families provide complex procedures and treatments in the home. Parents are challenged to retain a homelike setting among monitors, ventilators, and other sophisticated equipment. Throughout the text, home care is discussed as appropriate for specific conditions. The process of transition from hospital to home is elaborated in Chapters 43 and 44.

Paralleling normalization and home care is the process of *mainstreaming,* or integrating children with special needs into regular classrooms. Just as the home is the natural environment for children, so school must also be included as an essential component of their overall physical, intellectual, and social development. Children who attend school have the advantages of learning and socializing with a wide group of peers. There is an increased focus on individualization as the academic needs of these children are planned along with those of the rest of the students.

A variety of supplemental programs have been designed in the school system to accommodate special needs, both at school age and younger, through early intervention, which consists of any sustained and systematic effort to assist children from birth to age 3 years who are young, disabled, and developmentally vulnerable. This change and increasing opportunities for normalization for children with special needs in large part have resulted from the passage of Public Law 94-142 (the Education of All Handicapped Children Act of 1975) and its 1990 amendments (Public Law 101-47b), which changed the name of the act to the Individuals with Disabilities Education Act (IDEA); Public Law 99-457 (the Education of the Handicapped Act Amendments of 1986, which directs states to develop and implement statewide comprehensive, coordinated, multidisciplinary interagency programs of early intervention services for infants and toddlers with disabilities, as well as support services for their families); and the Americans with Disabilities Act (ADA) of 1990 (see also Chapter 29). Nurses can provide parents with information about these laws* and in some cases may participate in the development of individualized educational programs (IEPs) or individualized family service plans (IFSPs) for children with special needs.

Managed Care. Managed care programs have become the major form of health care provision in the United States. The transition to this model of care both offers opportunities and presents challenges with respect to the care of children with special health care needs. Managed care may benefit continuity and coordination of care. At the same time, some research has shown decreased access to pediatric specialists and health-related services in managed care environments.

Managing care for chronically ill children differs greatly from managing care for chronically ill adults in three major ways. First, the large number of rare disorders and low prevalence of children with such disorders make it difficult to monitor the overall quality of care for the total population of chronically ill children. Second, the influence of the child's growth and development on aspects of onset, impact, treatment, and outcomes of chronic conditions varies with the different developmental stages. Third, children rely on adults for access to health care and follow-up with treatment regimens, making it necessary to manage the child's care in the context of the family (American Academy of Pediatrics, 1998; Kuhlthau et al, 1998).

THE FAMILY OF THE CHILD WITH SPECIAL NEEDS

A major goal in working with the family of a child with special needs is to support the family's coping and promote their optimum functioning throughout the child's life. Long-term, comprehensive, family-centered approaches extend beyond sup-

*The NICHCY New Digest, vol 1, No. 1, 1991, was entirely devoted to the topic "The Education of Children and Youth with Special Needs: What Do the Laws Say?" (NICHCY, P.O. Box 1492, Washington, DC 20013.)

porting the child and family during the critical periods of diagnosis and hospitalization. Comprehensive care involves forming parent-professional partnerships that can support a family's adaptation to the many changes that may be necessary in day-to-day life, determine expectations of and for the child, and provide a long-term perspective.

The impact of a child's medical or developmental condition is often experienced as a crisis at the time of diagnosis, which may be at the time of birth, after a long period of physical and/or psychologic testing, or immediately after a tragic injury. It may also begin before the diagnosis is made, when parents are aware that something is wrong with their child but before medical confirmation (Cohen, 1995).

The time of diagnosis is a critical time for parents. Several factors can make it particularly difficult, including a long duration of uncertainty in the diagnostic process and negative perceptions of chronic illness or disability (Cohen, 1995; Garwick et al, 1995). Planning the setting for informing parents, assessing the family's background knowledge and experience, choosing strategies that fit the family's situation, and evaluating the family's understanding of the information will encourage optimum support at the time of diagnosis (Garwick et al, 1995).

Box 41-2

Anticipated Parental Stress Points

Diagnosis of the condition—Requires considerable learning, as well as dealing with emotional response

Developmental milestones—Times that children normally achieve walking, talking, and self-care are delayed or impossible for the child

Start of schooling—Particularly stressful are situations in which appropriate schooling will not be in a regular class placement

Reaching the ultimate attainment—Situations, such as realizing that ambulation will be impossible or that the child will not learn to read, must be handled

Adolescence—Issues such as sexuality and independence become prominent

Future placement—Decisions about placement must be made when the child becomes an adult or when the parents can no longer care for the child

Death of the child

Impact of the Child's Chronic Illness or Disability

Each family who has a child with special needs is affected by the experience. The effects on the parents and their responses are so critical that they directly influence the other members' reactions and the child's own coping.

Parents. Besides grieving for the loss of a perfect child, parents may or may not receive positive feedback from transactions with their child. Many parents feel satisfaction and fulfillment from the parenting role. For others, parenting may be a series of unrewarding experiences, which contributes to parental feelings of inadequacy and failure (Box 41-2). These responses may be most evident in parents who are responsible for the child's care. For example, parents may become preoccupied with their ability to carry out certain procedures, overlooking the child's personal comfort and satisfaction or failing to offer praise for anything less than perfect cooperation or performance. They may pursue a frustrating activity until they achieve "success"—long after the child has become irritable and uncooperative. As a result, parents can become caught in a pattern of interaction that is mutually unrewarding and minimally productive. For these parents, several strategies may be helpful: education regarding what can reasonably be expected of their child, assistance in identifying the child's strengths, praise for a parental job well done, and respite care so that parents can renew their energies.

Parental Roles. Enormous demands may be placed on parental time, energy, and financial resources. Depending on the roles assumed by each partner, these responsibilities may be shared or shifted more heavily to one member. In a shared approach parents often divide tasks in a very specific way, according to their skills or level of comfort. For example, the parent with patience for waiting may be the logical person to take the child for tests, examinations, and procedures. The parent who deals best with the sickness and side effects of treatment can ready the environment for the child's return home. It is important for nurses to realize that the absence of one parent from the hospital or clinic does not necessarily indicate that the shared-parent pattern is not in effect (Clements, Copeland, and Loftus, 1990). On the other hand, making efforts to involve both parents in decision making and in learning how to care for the child's special needs can reduce some of the burden of care often placed on mothers.

In other families, changing sex roles mean added responsibilities for one parent. For example, the working mother may feel the need to continue employment to help defray expenses, but she also incurs the added burden of additional child and home responsibilities. The result can be marital conflict if one partner views his or her share as unequal.

In addition, the partner who is not included in the caregiving activities may feel neglected, because all of the attention is directed toward the child, and resentful that he or she is not sufficiently informed to be competent in the care. Without active participation in the child's care, the parent has little appreciation of the time and energy involved in performing those activities. When this partner does attempt to participate, the other parent often criticizes the less skillful efforts. As a result, communication and support for each other may be adversely affected.

Although marital stress often increases, divorce rates in these families are not substantially higher than those for the general population. Research suggests that families of children with chronic conditions who adjust poorly are those who had problems before the illness. A couple's marital functioning before the birth or diagnosis of a child with special needs may well be the best predictor of long-term marital adjustment. Factors contributing to marital stress include decreased time spent in recreational activities, increased caregiving responsibilities, and fewer exchanges of affection (Quittner et al, 1998).

The nurse can assist the family in avoiding conflicts by providing anticipatory guidance early on. Guidance can address the stressors often cited as having an impact on the marriage: (1) the home care program with the burden of care assumed by primarily one parent, (2) the financial burden, (3) fear of the child dying, (4) pressure from relatives, (5) the hereditary nature of the disease (if applicable), and (6) fear of pregnancy.

Other causes of tension may center on the inconveniences associated with care, such as long waits for appointments, lack of parking near care facilities, or lack of overnight accommodations. Certainly, these last stressors are within health professionals' domain to minimize if not eliminate.

Mother/Father Differences. Mothers and fathers in the same family often adjust and cope differently as parents of a child with special needs. Some mothers experience a peaks-and-valleys periodic crisis pattern, whereas most fathers tend to experience a steady, gradual recovery. Some research suggests that mothers of children with certain conditions may be more susceptible to psychologic distress and feeling worn out than fathers. Mothers are more likely to have to deal with forfeiting or delaying personal goals. Mothers often have greater needs for social support and positive reappraisal of the situation, whereas fathers are more likely to use self-controlling behaviors to cope (Heaman, 1995; Mastroyannopoulou et al, 1997).

The father of a child with special needs struggles with issues that may be quite distinct from those of the mother. He may feel that his role of protector is challenged because he does not know how to help and cannot protect the family from the seemingly overwhelming recurring problems. Dreams of lineage, ego fulfillment, and athletic and vocational achievement are threatened and in turn may threaten the father's self-esteem. Because the traditional paternal role, particularly with sons, emphasizes joint recreation over caregiving, fathers seem to have more difficulty adjusting to a son with special needs than to a daughter with special needs. With today's increased emphasis on fathers' involvement in the lives of their children, this loss is felt more profoundly than in the past. The extensive stresses in the family can leave the father feeling depressed, weak, guilty, powerless, isolated, embarrassed, and very angry. Fearful that he will lose control or be viewed as weak or ineffectual, however, the father will often hide his feelings and display an outward confidence that may lead others to believe that everything is fine. Feelings are further exacerbated by a health care system that often excludes and disregards men. Too often the father feels like an afterthought in the care of his child (May, 1996).

Fathers worry about what the future holds for their children and about their ability to manage the increasing financial burden. Some fathers escape in their work as a means of dulling the pain. Common coping strategies are problem oriented and include praying, getting information, looking at options, and weighing choices (Cayse, 1994), in addition to withdrawing and being practical (Mastroyannopoulou et al, 1997).

Single-Parent Families. Single-parent families are of special concern. The absence of a parent may result from divorce or death, or the parents may never have married. As the only parent of a child who may require extensive, sophisticated, and lifelong care, the single parent may feel an enormous burden. Available financial and emotional resources may already be stretched to the limit. Nurses must recognize that external sources of support and personal inner strength are particularly crucial for single parents to enable them to care for their child (Clements, Copeland, and Loftus, 1990). A special effort should be made to assist the single parent in finding financial and support services that can ease the burden of care. Nurses can also assist the single parent in identifying helping roles that may be acceptable to relatives and friends.

Siblings. Results of studies on how siblings are affected by having a brother or sister with special needs are inconsistent. Some confirm that brothers and sisters of children with chronic or disabling conditions are at high risk for maladjustment; others report that siblings of chronically ill children experience both positive and negative feelings toward their ill sibling (Derouin and Jessee, 1996). However, most investigators do agree that brothers and sisters of children with special needs are no more at risk for *severe* psychiatric problems than are siblings of children without chronic or disabling conditions.

Some difficulties for siblings arise from the demands of the child's condition. For example, at diagnosis the child with special needs by necessity becomes the focus of parental attention and concern. Frequent hospitalizations or trips to the physician or clinic disrupt the family routine. Siblings are pushed to the background, often staying at the homes of family and friends. The child's condition may interfere with holiday celebrations, vacations, and other special events. Siblings may resent these intrusions, which commonly demand self-sacrifice. Their parents may be unable to attend their school functions, ball games, or other activities and at times may be physically and emotionally unavailable for them. The family's financial and emotional resources may be directed toward the child with special needs. When this occurs, there is often not only a decrease in normal family activities but also a decrease in personal items for the other children as well.

Many of the difficulties that siblings encounter are a result of the nature of the sibling relationship itself (see Chapter 31). It is within the sibling relationship that children learn to share, compete, and compromise with others close to them in status. The equality of this relationship is often lost when a brother or sister has special needs. The child with special needs is suddenly "out of tune," unable to contribute to the family or the sibling relationship in his or her usual way. Because identification is another characteristic of sibling relationships, some siblings believe that they too will "catch" the condition, a reasonable assumption in light of experiences with contagious diseases such as chickenpox. Identification, combined with a young child's egocentric thinking, may lead a sibling to feel responsible for a brother's or sister's condition. For example, siblings may believe that playing rough with their brother or sister or even thinking bad thoughts about the sibling caused the condition.

Most brothers and sisters experience mixed and sometimes contradictory feelings. They may feel left out of new family developments and changing roles, guilty that they escaped getting the condition, or sad when their brother or sister is unable to participate in a particular activity or event. Some siblings feel embarrassed and ashamed; having a child in the family who is ill, disfigured, or disabled marks the family as "different." Some siblings worry about the health of the affected child (Faulkner, 1996). Siblings may actually experience a *courtesy stigma*—a spoiled identity because of a close relationship with someone who is devalued and avoided because he or she is different. These painful feelings may lead to isolation and loneliness.

When parents give the child with special needs preferential treatment, siblings may feel resentful and jealous—feelings that are often distorted by the sibling's own sense of loss and concern. Older siblings in particular may resent stepping in as surrogate parents for their younger brothers and sisters. Siblings may be angry at parents for being unable to protect their brother or sister from getting the condition or angry at insensitive friends and classmates. Some siblings must also deal with anger from the child with special needs who resents them for escaping the experience.

Some siblings develop adjustment or behavior problems, especially younger male or older female siblings. Younger children having difficulty tend to become withdrawn and irritable, whereas older siblings tend to act out. Some typical problems include bed-wetting, headaches and other physical symptoms, changes in school performance, school phobia, sleep problems, proneness to injury, depression, and severe separation anxiety.

Often overlooked is the positive caring between children with special needs and their brothers and sisters. Siblings can experience pride and satisfaction in their own contributions to the family, joy and excitement in their brother's or sister's accomplishments, and genuine love. Parents may report an increased closeness among the siblings or an increase in their home responsibilities (Ferrell et al, 1994). Ultimately, most brothers and sisters seem to adapt well, and many demonstrate high levels of self-confidence, independence, maturity, altruism, and tolerance.

Certain factors (e.g., family size, age between children) seem to influence sibling adjustment. However, the most important factors appear to be parental feelings, perceptions, and reactions. Siblings are more at risk for adjustment problems when parents are unaccepting of the child with special needs. Also, certain times seem to be more difficult for siblings (Box 41-3).

How siblings react will have an important impact on the child's overall adjustment. When siblings act in a normal fashion, a secure, stable training ground is provided for social relationships for the child with special needs.

Extended Family Members and Society. In addition to parents and siblings, significant nonnuclear family members or friends may experience the effects of a child's chronic illness or disability. Although extended family relationships are often helpful to parents in rearing a child with special needs, they may also be sources of stress. For example, grandparents or other well-meaning relatives may attempt to reassure the parents that the child "will grow out of" his or her slowness at a time when parents are struggling to accept reality.

Most grandparents experience some ambivalence: they love their grandchild and yet feel personal disappointment. They often experience a double grief, both for their grandchild and for their child, the parent. The future is now unpredictable not only for the grandchild but also for the child's parents. Grandparents do not often acknowledge these emotions and are left to adapt on their own. Support groups for grandparents, although uncommon, can be beneficial (Burns and Madian, 1992).

Considerable stress can also arise from nonfamilial sources, such as friends, neighbors, or strangers. Inability to cope with comments about the disorder or curious stares by others may foster the tendency to isolate and protect the child within the home. The family needs guidance in preparing for these inevitable experiences. Encouraging parents to dress the child like other children as much as possible is one approach. Good grooming is very important in minimizing differences in appearance. Through role-playing, parents can practice responses to comments such as "Is your child retarded?" or "Has he always been crippled?" Through parent groups, family members can share experiences and learn from each other about dealing with probing questions or unkind remarks. Such interventions should include the siblings and the affected child, who also must face and deal with these events.

Parents have to decide how much and what to tell relatives, friends, baby-sitters, and teachers. Concerns about discrimination are very real for parents (Turner-Henson et al, 1994) and must be balanced with the need to share information so that the child receives appropriate care. The nurse can raise the issue by asking parents whether they have concerns about how to inform others of the child's condition. Nurses may be able to offer advice regarding essential safety teaching for others who will care for the child.

Box 41-3

Anticipated Sibling Stress Points

Birth of another child—May be the sibling with special needs or the subsequent birth of another child
Diagnosis of condition—In certain illnesses, times of remission and exacerbations are difficult
When the child is hospitalized—Parental time and attention are focused on the child with special needs
Start of schooling—Particularly stressful if friends reject the child with special needs
Adolescence—When dating begins, may be embarrassed to bring dates home
Future placement—May worry about responsibility for the sibling with special needs, especially if the parents are ill or die
Death of the child

Coping with Ongoing Stress and Periodic Crises

Professionals can help families cope with stress by providing anticipatory guidance, providing emotional support, assisting the family in assessing and identifying specific stressors, aiding the family in developing coping mechanisms and problem-solving strategies, and working collaboratively with parents so that they become empowered in the process.

Concurrent Stresses within the Family. The ability to deal with the overwhelming stresses of a lifelong disability or illness is challenged further when additional stresses are present. Stressors may be situational or developmental. They may be related to marital difficulties, sibling needs, homelessness, or social isolation. Some families may simultaneously be struggling with a family member's alcohol or other drug problem. Even the more minor stresses, such as arranging care for other children, managing the home, and traveling to distant treatment centers, can challenge a family's ability to cope successfully.

For most families, regardless of their income or insurance coverage, financial concerns exist. The costs of caring for a child with special needs can be overwhelming. Nurses and social workers can help a family review various options for financial assistance, including insurance, managed care, or health maintenance organization (HMO) policies, Medicaid, Supplemental Security Income (SSI), WIC (Woman, Infants, and Children program), the state Program for Children with Special Health Needs, disease-related associations, and local philanthropic organizations (Scher and Ahmann, 1996).

Coping Mechanisms. Coping mechanisms are behaviors aimed at reducing the tension caused by a crisis. *Approach* *behaviors* are coping mechanisms that result in movement toward adjustment and resolution of the crisis. *Avoidance behaviors* result in movement away from adjustment or maladaptation to the crisis. Each behavior must be viewed in the context of all of the variables affecting the family. For example, the observation of several avoidance behaviors in an emotionally healthy family may denote significantly less risk to the successful resolution of the crisis than an equal number of avoidance behaviors in an individual who has few available supports.

Parental Empowerment. Empowerment can be seen as a process of recognizing, promoting, and enhancing competence (Gibson, 1995). For parents of children with chronic conditions, empowerment may occur gradually as strength and capabilities are drawn on to master the child's care, manage family life, and plan for the future. Advocating for the child and developing parent-professional partnerships are part of taking charge (Gibson, 1995).

Assisting Family Members in Managing Their Feelings

Although some previous research has postulated stages of adaptation to a chronic illness or disability, there is in fact a great deal of individual variation in responses to the diagnosis, adjustments made, and time frames for coming to terms with a diagnosis. It is important that professionals recognize and respect a wide range of reactions and coping mechanisms. In fact, members of the family of a child with a chronic illness or disability may experience a number of difficult emotions, including fear, guilt, anger, resentment, and anxiety. Learning to manage these emotions promotes adaptive coping (see Guidelines box on p. 1016). Support from professionals, other family members, and friends can assist family members in managing their feelings. The following discussion examines some common phases of adjustment and emotional reactions.

Shock and Denial. The initial diagnosis of a chronic illness or disability is often met with intense emotion and is characterized by shock, disbelief, and sometimes denial, especially if the disorder is not obvious, such as in chronic illness. Denial as a defense mechanism is a necessary cushion to prevent disintegration and is a normal response to grieving for any type of loss. Probably all family members experience various degrees of adaptive denial as they learn of the impact that the diagnosis has on their lives.

Shock and denial can last from days to months, sometimes even longer. Examples of denial that may be exhibited at the time of diagnosis include (1) physician shopping; (2) attributing the symptoms of the actual illness to a minor condition; (3) refusal to believe the diagnostic tests; (4) delay in agreeing to treatment; (5) acting very happy and optimistic despite the revealed diagnosis; (6) refusing to tell or talk to anyone about the condition; (7) insisting that no one is telling the truth, regardless of others' attempts to do so; (8) denying the reason for admission; and (9) asking no questions about the diagnosis, treatment, or prognosis. Generally, these mechanisms should be respected as short-term responses that allow individuals to distance themselves from the onslaught of a tremendous emotional impact and to collect and mobilize their energies toward goal-directed, problem-solving behaviors.

In some instances, various indicators of denial can actually be adaptive behaviors. Searching for another professional option may mean that parents cannot obtain answers to their questions or that they are looking for a different approach to treatment that better meets the needs of their child and family. Sometimes a delay in making decisions or a failure to ask questions simply reflects a lack of information.

In children, the importance of denial has repeatedly been demonstrated as a factor in their positive coping with the diagnosis. Denial allows the child to maintain hope in the face of overwhelming odds and to function adaptively and productively. Like hope, denial may be an adaptive mechanism for dealing with loss that persists until a family or patient is ready or needs other responses.

Denial is probably the least understood and most poorly dealt with reaction. Health professionals typically label denial as "maladaptive" and act inappropriately by attempting to strip it away by repeated and sometimes blunt explanations of the prognosis. However, denial becomes maladaptive only when it prevents recognition of treatment or rehabilitative goals necessary for the child's optimum survival or development.

Adjustment. For most families, adjustment gradually follows shock and is usually characterized by an open admission that the condition exists. This stage may be accompanied by several responses, which are quite normal parts of the adaptation process. Probably the most universal of these feelings are *guilt* and *self-accusation.* Guilt is often greatest when the cause of the disorder is directly traceable to the parent, such as in genetic diseases or from accidental injury. However, it can occur even without any scientific or realistic basis for parental responsibility. Often the guilt stems from a false assumption that the disability is a result of personal failing or wrongdoing, such as not doing something correctly during pregnancy or while giving birth. Guilt may also be associated with cultural or religious beliefs. Some parents are convinced that they are being punished for some previous misdeed. Others may see the disorder as a sacrifice sent by God to test their religious strength and faith. With correct information, support, and time, most parents master guilt and self-accusation. The ability to overcome resentful and self-accusatory feelings of having "caused" the child's disorder is a crucial factor in determining the parents' acceptance of their child.

Children also may interpret their serious illness as retribution for past misbehavior. The nurse should be particularly sensitive to the child who passively accepts all painful procedures. This child may believe that such acts are inflicted as deserved punishment. It is vital that parents and health care professionals reassure children that their illness is not their fault.

Other common and normal reactions to a diagnosis are *bitterness* and *anger.* Anger directed inward may be evident as self-reproaching or punitive behavior, such as neglecting one's health and verbally degrading oneself. Anger directed outward may be manifested in either open arguments or withdrawal from communication and may be evident in the person's relationship with any number of individuals, such as the spouse, the child, and siblings. Passive anger toward the ill child may be evident in decreased visiting, refusal to believe how sick the child is, or inability to provide comfort. Among the most common targets for parental anger are members of the staff. Parents may complain about the nursing care, the insufficient time physicians spend with them, or the lack of skill of those who draw blood or start intravenous infusions.

Children are likely to respond with anger, and this includes the affected child as well as siblings. Children are aware of the loss engendered by their illness or disability and may react angrily to the restrictions imposed or the feelings of being different. Siblings may also feel anger and resentment toward the ill child and parents for the loss of routine and parental attention. It is difficult for older children and almost impossible for younger children to comprehend the plight of the affected child. Their perception is that their brother or sister has the undivided attention of their parents, is showered with cards and gifts, and is the focus of everyone's concern.

During the period of adjustment, four types of parental reactions to the child influence the child's eventual response to the disorder: *overprotection,* in which the parents fear letting the child achieve any new skill, avoid all discipline, and cater to every desire to prevent frustration; *rejection,* in which the parents detach themselves emotionally from the child but usually provide adequate physical care or constantly nag and scold the child; *denial,* in which parents act as if the disorder does not exist or attempt to have the child overcompensate for it; and *gradual acceptance,* in which parents place necessary and realistic restrictions on the child, encourage self-care activities, and promote reasonable physical and social abilities.

Reintegration and Acknowledgment. For many families the adjustment process culminates in the development of realistic expectations for the child and reintegration of family life with the illness or disability in a manageable perspective. Because a large portion of this phase is one of grief for a loss, total resolution is not possible until the child dies or leaves home as an independent adult. Therefore one can regard adjustment as "increased comfort" with everyday living rather than a complete resolution.

This adjustment phase also involves social reintegration in which the family broadens its activities to include relationships outside of the home, with the child as an acceptable and participating member of the group. This last criterion often differentiates the reaction of gradual acceptance during the adjustment period from total acceptance, or perhaps is more descriptive of the acknowledgment process.

Many parents of children with chronic illnesses experience *chronic sorrow,* feelings of sorrow and loss that recur in waves over time. As the child's condition progresses, parents experience repeated losses that present further decline and new caregiving demands. Consequently, families must be assessed on an ongoing basis and offered appropriate support and resources as the needs of the family change over time (Gravelle, 1997).

Establishing a Support System

The diagnosis of a child with a serious health problem or disability is a major situational crisis that affects the entire family system. However, families can experience positive outcomes as they successfully deal with the many challenges that accompany a child with chronic illness or disability. One nursing goal is to assess which families are at greater or lesser risk for succumbing to the effects of the crisis. Several variables—available support system, perception of the event, coping mechanisms, reactions to the child, available resources, and concurrent stresses within the family—influence the resolution of a crisis. Although most families cope well, the needs of families at risk are great. If they receive emotional support and guidance early, there is an increased likelihood that they will also cope successfully.

Although it is easy to assume that families of children with the most severe illnesses or disabilities would have the poorest adjustment, the severity of the condition reflects only one part of the overall picture. The level of adjustment is significantly influenced by the *functional burden* on the individual family (Stein, 1985). This concept considers the issues related to caring for and living with the child in relation to the family's resources and ability to cope. The family of a child with multiple disabilities demanding complex care—yet having many resources and coping skills—may adjust more successfully to the child's situation than the family of a child with a less serious condition and few resources to counter the balance.

Intrafamilial resources, social support from friends and relatives, parent-to-parent support, parent-professional partnerships, and community resources interweave to provide a flexible web of support for the family of a child with a chronic condition.

THE CHILD WITH SPECIAL NEEDS

Impact of Chronic Illness or Disability on the Child

The child's reaction to chronic illness or disability depends to a great extent on his or her developmental level, temperament, and available coping mechanisms; on the reactions of family members or significant others; and to a lesser extent on the condition itself. A child's conceptual understanding of his or her own illness is based not only on age and developmental level but also on the duration and type of experience accumulated with the disease (Yoos, 1994). Knowledge of these variables is essential in providing the kind of information and support needed by these children to cope with a sometimes overwhelming situation.

Developmental Aspects. The impact of a chronic illness or disability is influenced by the age at onset. Chronic illness affects children of all ages, but the developmental aspects of each age group dictate particular stresses and risks for the child. The nurse must also recognize that children need to redefine their condition and its implication as they develop and grow. Children's developmental concepts of illness are discussed in Chapter 44. An understanding of these developmental factors facilitates planning care to support the child and minimize the risks.

Infant. During infancy the child is engaged in the task of developing trust through an intimate, satisfying, consistent relationship with his or her parents. When illness or disability occurs, this relationship is potentially affected. For example, a visible defect can delay parent bonding as the parent mourns the loss of the perfect child. In addition, prolonged illness may impose separations that prevent the child and parent from normal attachment and deprive the infant of a nurturing relationship.

The illness itself affects the infant, especially because sensorimotor experiences are critical at this age. Illness, disability, or both often impair the child's motor abilities by confining the child to a crib and lessening contact with the environment. The messages transmitted to infants about their bodies are influenced by the amount of pain and discomfort they experience. Associating touch with pain can compromise the infant's ability to give and receive affection. Lack of pleasurable sensations can lead to an irritable and unhappy child. Consequently, parents may interpret the behaviors as evidence that they are not adequately meeting the child's physical and emotional needs, which further affects the parent-child relationship and the acquisition of trust. Nursing intervention can be important in helping parents work with the irritable child in a way that encourages understanding and caring.

Nurses should advocate for policies and practices that will best meet the needs of the infant and family. Twenty-four-hour visitation in the neonatal intensive care unit and other infant units is of primary importance. Showing parents how to touch and hold the infant will promote their confidence and competence. "Kangaroo care" has been shown to be both safe and beneficial to the infant. Mothers who choose to breastfeed can be encouraged, with a private space provided for them to nurse or pump and storage facilities made available for breast milk. Sibling visitation can be facilitated.

Toddler. The toddler is in the stage of autonomy; the need for mastery of locomotor and language skills is paramount. The child learning to walk and talk progresses toward becoming a separate person, both physically and psychologically. However, illness or disability can hinder mobility and deprive a child of mastery. In addition, overprotective parents can magnify the problem by setting limits on the child's exploration and experimentation for fear of injury or exertion. Even the most basic self-help skills, such as feeding and dressing, may be done for the child. Age-appropriate tasks such as toilet training may be delayed. Within the constraints of illness or disability, maximum opportunities should be provided for independence in these and other areas.

Illness can impose separations that are detrimental to the toddler. As with the infant, separation is the most anxiety-producing event. A chronic illness or disability can necessitate repeated hospitalizations and painful procedures. If the need to preserve the parent-child relationship is not appreciated, the child may become depressed and eventually detach from the parent. Children seem to have a tremendous capacity to withstand stress, provided that their attachment to the parent is maintained. Parents of toddlers may begin to look for respite care or day care, which is often difficult to find for the child with special needs.* The Americans with Disabilities Act (ADA) requires day care providers to make "reasonable modifications" for equal access to program participation (Siegel, 1995).

Preschooler. The preschooler is in the stage of initiative; numerous tasks are achieved during this age that can be hampered by chronic illness and disability. Impairment can limit the preschooler's learning about the environment, especially in terms of social development. The chronically ill preschooler confined to the home may be slow to develop social skills useful in group or school settings.

One of the major tasks of this period is establishing sexual identity, and one of the principal methods is through imitation of gender-related activities. However, the child with special needs may have fewer opportunities to engage in such activity and may view the parent predominantly in the caregiving role because this may be the focus of their relationship. Some families expect the mother to assume the care of the child while the father provides the financial base by working outside the home. This can limit the child's identification with the male role.

In addition to sexual identity, the child's body image is forming. Children's knowledge of their bodies is limited to what they see, feel, and use. If the child is chronically ill, body awareness is focused on personal pain and the anxiety it causes. The young child may lose control over newly acquired bowel and bladder function and feel embarrassed and inferior. The child with a disability may have difficulty forming a mental image of impaired body parts, such as paralyzed extremities. This poorly developed sense of body integrity makes children especially fearful of intrusive or mutilating experiences, which can be common during prolonged illness.

One of the more critical influences of chronic illness or disability on preschoolers is the feeling of guilt that they "caused" the condition by a real or imagined misdeed. This is probably less a factor if the child is born with the disorder than if it occurs during the preschool years. Such guilt can greatly affect the child's developing but fragile self-esteem. Unlike the child with a temporary physical impairment who has additional opportunities for achieving mastery and thus overcoming feelings of guilt and inferiority, the child with a chronic illness or disability experiences continual insults. Unless situations are structured for success, life can become a series of failures—of never being strong enough or good enough to compete with peers.

School-Age Child. The child of school age is striving to achieve a sense of accomplishment while overcoming a sense of inferiority. Successful mastery of this task depends on the child's ability to cooperate and compete with others. Consequently, physical impairments can greatly affect the ability to achieve and compete. For example, physical disability may hinder participation in sports, and repeated absences from school caused by illness can place the child at an academic disadvantage. If the child must repeat a grade, he or she may have feelings of shame, inadequacy, and inferiority. However, the decision to remain in the same grade can also enhance feelings of success because the work requirements may be easier and new classmates provide a second chance for forming friendships.

During this age there is a transition from relationships with family members to strong identification with peers. Peers increasingly influence school-age children's views of themselves and their self-esteem. Anything that labels children as "different" can affect their sense of belonging to the group. Nurses can help families promote social competence in their children (Breitmayer et al, 1992). For example, if children are helped to deal with their feelings of not being "normal and perfect" and to recognize their unique abilities, they can cope very well. It is to be expected that not all children are able to master every task and that they will feel some degree of disappointment. If this is stressed to children with physical impairment, the burden to achieve is lessened.

Peer interaction is especially important in relation to cognitive development, social development, and maturation. Cognitive development is facilitated by interaction—by exploration of personal, social, and ethical values with peers, parents, and teachers. As school-age children identify more with the peer group and authority figures outside the home, there is a concurrent striving for independence from the family. However, the ill child may be forced into an extended period of dependency either from the disorder or from parental overprotectiveness. Attempts to demonstrate independence may be manifested as

*Access to Respite Care and Help (ARCH) is a national information center on respite programs: ARCH, c/o Chapel Hill Training Outreach Project, 800 Eastowne Dr., Chapel Hill, NC 27514; (919) 490-5577 or 1-800-473-1727 ext. 243; fax (919) 490-4905; website: www.chtop.com (look for ARCH icon).

resentment toward the parents, refusal to comply with treatment, or risk-taking behavior, such as cheating on a special diet. If parents can understand that these behaviors represent a normal phase of development, they may be more tolerant and able to find appropriate outlets for independence (e.g., increasing the child's responsibility for home care or increasing the child's control in non–disease-related activities).

Adolescent. The impact of illness or disability can be most difficult during adolescence. The major task of the adolescent is to establish a personal identity. Pubertal changes must be integrated into the self-image while the teenager is gaining control and mastery over increased physical capabilities and sexuality. During early adolescence this takes place primarily within the peer group. Illness or injury at this time interferes with teenagers' sense of mastery and control over their changing bodies. They are different at a stage of the development when being different is unacceptable to the peer group, which may view a disability in one member as a threat to the established uniformity by which all are measured. At no time of life is an individual so vulnerable to the emotional stress of biologic impairment. In fact, adolescents with physical differences tend to blame most of their problems on the fact that they have something wrong with them. Appearance, skills, and abilities are highly valued by peers (Fig. 41-1); a teenager who is limited in any of these qualities is subject to rejection. This is especially marked when a physical disability interferes with sexual attractiveness.

The subject of sexuality related to the effects of the disorder is a prominent concern of adolescents, but they rarely initiate a discussion of this sensitive topic. Any probable interference in sexual function because of the disability should be discussed openly and candidly with the teenager (Lock, 1998).

Teenagers with special needs are faced with the task of incorporating their disabilities into the changing self-concept. The youngster who becomes ill or acquires a disability during the crucial adolescent years has more difficulty accomplishing this task than the teenager who has been affected since childhood. It appears that the earlier the onset of a limiting condition, the better the individual is able to adapt to it. The youngster with a newly acquired disorder will have the additional task of grieving for lost "perfection" while adjusting to the changes taking place as a natural course of events. He or she often feels rejected because of personal appearance or an inability to engage in activities expected of a healthy adolescent. The threat is greatest during middle adolescence, when the teenager has less available energy to cope with illness because emotional resources are being used to meet the normal demands of this developmental phase.

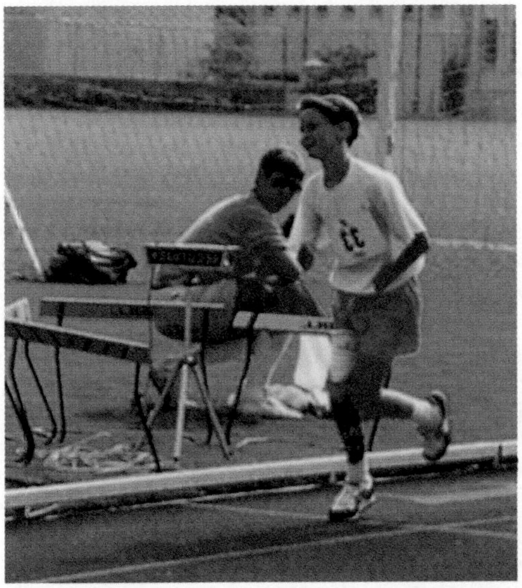

FIG. 41-1 • Children with any type of impairment should have the opportunity to develop their skills. (Courtesy Poyo-Hinton Photography.)

Adolescence is a time for achieving independence from the family and planning for future goals and responsibilities. Adolescents with long-term chronic illness may be less future directed and less independent than healthy peers. Enforced dependency caused by physical impairment can exacerbate the parent-child conflicts surrounding independence. Lack of understanding from both parties can result in bitter feelings and intrafamilial turmoil. The tendency toward rebellion may be directed at the disorder and reflected in decreased compliance with treatment; denial of the disorder to preserve a sense of normalcy with peers; and risk-taking behavior that can place the teenager in jeopardy, such as driving a car despite a disorder that increases the chance of injury. Such behaviors can further strain an already tense parent-child relationship. On the other hand, parents can promote independence by giving the adolescent a greater role in his or her own treatment regimen, encouraging the adolescent to develop a relationship with the health care team that is not mediated by parents, and promoting normalization principles.

Coping Mechanisms. Children's innate and learned coping mechanisms are very important in terms of their ability to deal with their disorder. Individual characteristics and the social support afforded the child are critically important influences on the child's ability to cope with stress. The better the family copes, the better the child is able to deal with the stressors imposed by the illness or disability. Individual characteristics associated with positive coping are female sex, early infancy or age older than 4 years, active or easy temperament, high self-esteem, above-average intelligence, and strong social skills (Garmezy, 1991).

Children with chronic conditions tend to use five distinct patterns of coping (Box 41-4). Children with more positive and accepting attitudes about their chronic illness use a more adaptive coping style characterized by optimism, competence, and compliance. They show fewer behavior problems at home and at school. The two maladaptive coping patterns—"Feels different and withdraws" and "Is irritable and moody and acts out"—are associated with poorer adaptation; children using these strategies have poorer self-concepts, more negative attitudes about their conditions, and more behavior problems at home and at school (Austin, Patterson, and Huberty, 1991).

Well-adapted children gradually learn to accept their physical limitations but find achievement in a variety of compensatory motor and intellectual pursuits. They function well at home, at school, and with peers. They have an understanding of their disorder that allows them to accept their limitations, assume responsibility for care, and assist in treatment and rehabilitation regimens. They express appropriate emotions, such as sadness, anxiety, and anger, at times of exacerbations but ex-

Box 41-4

Coping Patterns Used by Children with Special Needs

Develops competence and optimism. Accentuates the positive aspects of the situation and concentrates more on what he or she has or can do than on what is missing or on what he or she cannot do; is as independent as possible.

Feels different and withdrawn. Sees self as being different from other children because of the chronic health condition; views being different as negative; sees self as less worthy than others; focuses on things he or she cannot do and sometimes overrestricts activities needlessly.

Is irritable, moody, and acts out. Uses proactive and self-initiated coping behaviors, although usually counterproductive in that the behaviors are not ego enhancing or socially responsible and do not result in desired outcomes; acts out irritability, which may or may not be associated with condition's symptoms.

Complies with treatment. Takes necessary medications, treatments; adheres to activity restrictions; also uses behaviors that indicate developing independence (e.g., assumes responsibility for taking medication).

Seeks support. Talks with adults, children, physicians, and nurses; develops plans to handle problems as they occur; uses downward comparison (i.e., realizes that others have it worse).

Modified from Austin J, Patterson J, Huberty T: Development of the Coping Health Inventory for Children, *J Pediatr Nurs* 6(3):166-174, 1991.

press confidence and guarded optimism during periods of clinical stability. They are able to identify with other similarly affected individuals, promoting positive self-images and displaying pride and self-confidence in their ability to master a productive, successful life despite the disability.

Hopefulness. Children, particularly adolescents, are sensitive to the presence or absence of hope. Hopefulness is an internal quality that mobilizes human beings into goal-directed action that may be satisfying and life sustaining. A sense of hopefulness can produce increased participation in health-seeking behaviors and an improved sense of well-being.

Responses to Parental Behavior. The parents' behavior toward the child, especially in terms of childrearing, is one of the most important influencing factors in the child's adjustment. For example, children whose parents are overprotective tend to have marked dependency (especially on the mother), fearfulness, inactivity, and lack of outside interests. Children who are raised by overly solicitous and guilt-ridden parents are often overly independent, defiant, and risk takers. Children who are reared by parents who emphasize their deficits and tend to "hide" or isolate them appear as shy and lonely individuals who harbor resentful and hostile attitudes toward unaffected persons. In contrast, children who are reared by parents who establish reasonable limits tend to develop age-appropriate independence and achievement commensurate with their limitations. In addition, family organization and illness-related support and involvement of parents influence the child's adjustment to chronic illness (Savinetti-Rose, 1994). They often display pride and confidence in their ability to cope successfully with the challenges imposed by their disorder. Anticipatory guidance by the nurse and encouragement of normalizing practices may assist parents in facilitating positive adjustment in their children.

Type of Illness or Disability. The type of illness or disability also influences the child's emotional response. Interestingly, children with more severe disorders often cope better than those with milder conditions. However, the presence of multiple conditions may place a child at risk for more behavioral problems (Newacheck, McManus, and Fox, 1991). Considering children's cognitive ability and their delay in achieving abstract thinking until adolescence, it is likely that an obvious condition is easier to accept because its limitations are concrete. For example, children who are blind or physically disabled are constantly reminded of their inability to run. However, children with cardiac defects not only live by rules they do not understand but also only vaguely and occasionally sense their illness, such as when they try to run and experience dyspnea and fatigue. Therefore some chronic illnesses pose special threats to children.

The onset of a disabling condition may generate a state of confusion for children, who may have trouble differentiating between actual bodily functions and their image of their bodies. They may also experience problems identifying themselves and those extensions of self (e.g., wheelchairs, braces, crutches, or other mechanical or prosthetic devices) and may have difficulty accepting functional aids.

NURSING CARE OF THE FAMILY AND CHILD WITH SPECIAL NEEDS

Assessment

Because the nurse may meet a family during any phase of the adjustment process, several assessment areas are important. Knowledge of the family's available support system is essential and may include the marital relationship, nonmarital partners, extended family, colleagues and co-workers, friends, and health professionals. The family's perception of the illness or disability is also an area that influences family adjustment. Assessment questions should focus on members' general knowledge of the condition even before the child's diagnosis was made, the influence of religion on their thinking, imagined causes of the condition, and the effects of the child's disorder on the family.

Because the family's ability to cope with previous stresses influences the current situation, answers to questions about their usual coping skills are enlightening. Knowledge of concurrent stresses—financial, marital or nonmarital, career, or unemployment—helps identify families who may have fewer resources to cope with the child's needs.

NURSE ALERT • Be aware that many families do not have a telephone, a service most practitioners consider essential for families of children with special needs. Other families may have telephones but may be reluctant to reveal the telephone number. To overcome these difficulties, use the following strategies:

- Help family identify telephone access close to home (e.g., neighbor's home, nearby store).
- Explore methods to obtain telephone service for family (e.g., social service agencies, and charitable organizations).

TABLE 41-2
Assessment of Factors Affecting Family Adjustment

Factors Affecting Adjustment	Assessment Questions
Available support system	
Status of marital relationship	Whom do you talk to when you have something on your mind? (If answer is not the spouse, ask for the reason.)
Alternate support systems	When something is worrying you, what do you do? What helps you most when you are upset?
Ability to communicate	Does talking seem to help when you feel upset?
Perception of the illness/disability	
Previous knowledge of disorder	Have you ever heard the word (name of diagnosis) before? Tell me about it (if answer is yes).
Influence of religion	Has your religion or faith been of help to you? Tell me how (if answer is yes).
Imagined cause of disorder	What are your thoughts about the causes of the disorder?
Effects of illness or disability on family	How has your child's illness or disability affected you and your family? How has your lifestyle changed?
Coping mechanisms	
Reactions to previous crises	Tell me one time you've had another crisis (problem, bad time) in your family. How did you solve that problem?
Reactions to the child Childrearing practices Attitudes	Do you find yourself being a little more cautious with this child than with your other children? Do you feel as comfortable disciplining this child compared with your other children? How is this child different from the siblings or other children of similar age? Describe your child's personality. Is it easy, difficult, or in-between? When you think of your child's future, what thoughts come to mind?
Available resources	What parts of your child's care are causing the most difficulty for you and/or your family? What services are available to help? What services do you need that presently are not available?
Concurrent stresses	What other problems are you facing now? (Be specific; ask about financial, marital, sibling, and extended family/friends concerns.)

- Be sensitive to family's concern for privacy when asking for a telephone number; explain reason for needing number and to whom it will be given.

Finally, awareness of the family members' reactions to the child and the illness or disability is important. Sample questions that the nurse and family can use to evaluate the support system, perception of the illness, coping mechanisms, resources, and concurrent stresses are listed in Table 41-2. Because factors affecting the family's response may change at any point during the illness, assessment must be a continuous process.

Special challenges exist in assessing the child's feelings about having a disability. Chapter 34 presents several approaches to encourage a child to discuss feelings about the condition. The nurse should use a variety of communication techniques, such as drawing and play, as assessment tools rather than relying solely on parental reports. Often children are neglected partners in their care, and their unique needs are not identified.

The needs of working parents and siblings also should be assessed, a goal that requires flexibility in scheduling appointments to include these important family members. When working parents know that their input is valuable, they will often change their work schedule to meet with a health professional. Because siblings can be of any age, the use of appropriate communication strategies for assessment must be considered. Nonverbal techniques such as those discussed in Chapter 34 should be considered for these children. Several instruments can be used to assist the family in assessing their overall functioning and support system (see Chapter 34).

➤ Nursing Diagnoses

A number of nursing diagnoses are prominent in the nursing care of the family and child with special needs. Others specific to individual cases become evident, especially when the child's actual disorder is considered.

➤ Plan of Care and Implementation

The nursing plan depends to a large extent on the child's actual illness or disability. However, the following are basic goals for all families and children with special needs:

1. Child and family will receive support at the time of diagnosis.
2. Family's emotional reactions will be accepted.
3. Child and family will cope with stresses of the situation.
4. Child and family will receive appropriate information about the condition.
5. Family will establish an environment of normalization for the child.
6. Family will establish realistic future goals.

The main objective in working with the family is to help them to cope effectively with those stresses imposed by the child's special needs. To achieve this goal, the entire family should be considered in every aspect of the implementation process (Family Focus box).

Provide Support at the Time of Diagnosis. The time of diagnosis may be experienced as a crisis by some families. The impact of the crisis may occur at the time of birth, after a long period of physical and/or psychologic testing, or immediately after a tragic injury. The impact may begin before the diagnosis is made, when parents are aware that something is wrong with their child but before medical confirmation (Cohen, 1995). It is a critical time for parents. Although they may not hear or remember all that is said to them, they often sense a certain attitude of acceptance, rejection, hope, or despair that may influence their ability to absorb the shock and begin adapting to the family's altered future.

Parents should be encouraged to be together when they are informed of their child's condition, thus avoiding the problem of one parent having to interpret complex findings and deal with the initial emotional reaction of the other. The informing session should take place in a private, comfortable setting free of distractions and interruptions, in an atmosphere in which the parents feel free to express their emotions (Fig. 41-2). If their feelings can be expressed and acknowledged, the parents can be helped to deal openly with them. Their emotional needs are acknowledged by showing acceptance of such expressions as crying, sadness, anger, and disappointment. Emotional support is offered by having tissues available if a family member cries and demonstrating through facial and body language that indeed this is a difficult and painful period. Although touching is a powerful expression of empathy, it must be used wisely. For example, it can prematurely terminate free expression of feelings, especially when combined with statements such as "Everything will be all right." Nurses should also be aware of cultural issues regarding touching (see Chapter 32).

Parents should receive the kind of information they desire. Most parents want a clear, simple explanation of the diagnosis, a prediction of possible futures for the child, advice on what to do next, an opportunity to ask questions, a warm and sympathetic listener, and most important, time. Clarification of explanations is elicited with such questions as "Do you see what I mean?" or "Is this clear to you?" Technical terms are used with simple definitions. If the parents are unaware of the term, they are given written literature or at least a written summary of the diagnosis.

Finally, the informing conference should not end with the presentation of devastating news. Instead, the child's strengths, appealing behaviors, and potential for development are stressed, as well as available rehabilitation efforts or treatment. Parents can be encouraged to view their experiences as a series of challenges that they are capable of handling, particularly with available professional feedback. The parents are assured that the nurse will be available to answer questions and to provide further assistance as needed.

The preceding discussion relates primarily to the initial informing interview. However, because of the need for long-term follow-up, it is only one in a series of continuing discussions. In all interactions the family's input is solicited and incorporated into the plan of care. Some situations require consideration of special problems (Guidelines box).

Accept Family's Emotional Reactions. One of the most supportive interventions is to accept the family's emotional reactions to the child's condition in as nonjudgmental a manner as possible. Although all families respond differently and in varying degrees of intensity, three responses are so common and often so poorly handled that they deserve special consideration.

Denial. The nurse's response to denial is a critical component of the individual's continuing need for this defense mechanism. The most effective method of support is active listening. Silence neither reinforces nor rejects denial (or any other emotional reaction) but implies a willingness and acceptance of the person's need for this behavior. However, silence alone can be misinterpreted. For example, if the person demonstrates denial, such as by saying, "I am sure the doctors made a mistake," and the nurse responds silently and leaves, the person may infer disapproval, agreement, avoidance, or rejection from this behavior.

To be effective, silence and listening must be accompanied by physical and mental concentration and use of body language to communicate interest and concern. Direct eye contact, touch, physical closeness, and body posture, such as sitting and leaning slightly forward, demonstrate silent but effective communication. (See also Communication Techniques, Chapter 34.)

Guilt. Because guilt is such a common response and can cause family members tremendous anxiety, they should be told directly that there is no known cause of the disorder (when appropriate) and that they are not to be blamed. Using the third-person technique is valuable in eliciting thoughts of guilt. For example, with children an appropriate statement may be, "When people get sick, they often wonder whether they did

Family Focus

IDENTIFYING FAMILY NEEDS

To ensure an effective plan of care, attention to *family-identified needs and priorities* is essential. For example, a family may have difficulty focusing on treatment issues if their current priority is obtaining enough food to feed their children.

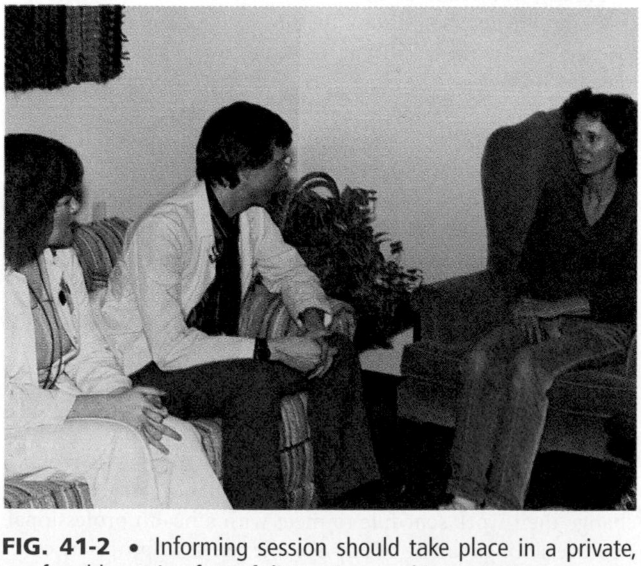

FIG. 41-2 • Informing session should take place in a private, comfortable setting free of distractions and interruptions.

anything to make themselves sick." This allows children an opportunity to explore any feelings of responsibility they harbor.

If family members are expressing feelings of guilt, it is important to allow them to talk about their feelings rather than quickly trying to dispel them with long "scientific" explanations. Statements such as "If you believe you are responsible for Johnny's condition, then no wonder you feel so bad" acknowledge the family member's feelings. This step is often appreciated and necessary before the facts can be presented and absorbed. An effective method in lessening guilt is to *encourage the irrationality of thought.* For example, one mother stated that her son probably developed cancer by sitting too close to the television, which she could have prevented by being more strict. By following her reasoning and talking about how *many* children sit close to the television and how *few* of them ever have cancer, the nurse was able to help the mother realize that this activity was not a cause.

Anger. Anger is one of the more difficult reactions to accept and deal with therapeutically. The responses to anger may be reciprocal anger, fear, acceptance, and/or encouragement. The first two reactions impede communication and express disapproval and rejection of the person. They most commonly occur when the listener views the anger as a personal assault. The last two responses allow the individual to express his or her feelings in an atmosphere of nonjudgmental acceptance. Two basic rules for dealing with the angry person are to avoid losing one's temper and to encourage the person to talk (Guidelines box). One essential element in the successful implementation of this process is to wait for the person to respond to a statement before proceeding to the next step. Because the objective of each

Guidelines

SITUATIONS REQUIRING SPECIAL CONSIDERATION

Congenital anomaly. Tension in the delivery room conveys the sense that something is seriously wrong. Communication is often delayed while the physician is involved with the mother's care. The manner in which the infant is presented may well set the tone for the early parent-child relationship.

- Clarify role with physician in regard to revealing information, to enable immediate parental support.
- Explain to parents briefly in simple language what the defect is and something concerning the immediate prognosis before showing them the infant, when they are more apt to "hear" what is said.
- Be aware of nonverbal communication. Parents watch facial expressions of others for signs of revulsion or rejection.
- Present infant as something precious.
- Emphasize well-formed aspects of infant's body.
- Allow time and opportunity for parents to express their initial response.
- Encourage parents to ask questions, and provide honest, straightforward answers without undue optimism or pessimism.

Cognitive impairment. Unless cognitive impairment (mental retardation) is associated with other physical problems, it is often easy for parents to miss clues to its presence or to make defensive excuses regarding the diagnosis.

- Plan situations that help parents become aware of the problem.
- Encourage parents to discuss their observations of child, but withhold diagnostic opinions.
- Focus on what child can do and appropriate interventions to promote progress (e.g., infant stimulation programs) to involve parents in their child's care while helping them gain an awareness of child's disability.

Physical disability. If loss of motor or sensory ability occurs during childhood, the diagnosis is readily apparent. The challenge lies in helping the child and parents over the period of shock and grief and toward the phase of acceptance and reintegration.

- Institute early rehabilitation (e.g., using a prosthetic limb, learning to read braille, learning to read lips).
- Be aware that physical rehabilitation usually precedes psychologic adjustment.
- When the cause of the disability is accidental, avoid implying that parents or child was responsible for the injury, yet allow them the opportunity to discuss feelings of blame.
- Encourage expression of feelings (see Communication Techniques, Chapter 34).

Chronic illness. Realization of the true impact may take months or years. Conflict over parent's vs. child's concerns may result in serious problems. When condition is inherited, parents may blame themselves, and/or child may blame parents.

- Help each family member gain an appreciation of the other's concerns.
- Discuss hereditary aspect of condition with parents at time of diagnosis to lessen guilt and accusatory feelings.
- Encourage child to express feelings by using third-person technique (e.g., "Sometimes when a person has an illness that was passed on by the parents, that person feels angry or bitter toward them").

Multiple disabilities. The child or parent may require additional time for the shock phase and may be able to attend to only one diagnosis before hearing significant information regarding other disorders.

- Acknowledge parents' understanding and acceptance of all diagnoses, especially when an obvious and more hidden disability co-exists.
- Appreciate the devastating consequences of more than one disability for a child, especially if they interfere with expressive-receptive abilities.

Terminal illness. Parents require much support to deal with their own feelings and guidance in how to tell the child the diagnosis. They may want to conceal the diagnosis from the child. They may believe that the child is too young to know, will not be able to cope with the information, or will lose hope and the will to live.

- Approach the subject of disclosure in a positive way by asking, "How will you tell your child about the diagnosis?"
- Help parents understand the disadvantages of not telling children (e.g., deprives them of the opportunity to discuss their feelings openly and ask questions, incurs the risk of them learning the truth from outside and sometimes less tactful sources, may lessen children's trust and confidence in their parents once they learn the truth).
- Guide parents to see the potential problems involved in fostering a conspiracy.
- Offer parents guidelines for how and what to tell children about their disease or the possibility of death. Explanations should be tailored to child's cognitive ability, be based on knowledge child already has, and be honest. Honesty must be tempered with concern for child's feelings.
- Assure parents that telling a child the name of the illness and the reason for treatment instills hope, provides support from others, and serves as a foundation for explaining and understanding subsequent events.
- Acknowledge that being honest is not always easy because the truth may prompt children to ask other distressing questions, such as "Am I going to die?" However, even this difficult question must be answered.

statement is for the person to speak freely, the responses should avoid yes or no types of answers.

Support Family's Coping Methods. For the family to meet the stresses of optimally adjusting to the child's condition, each member must be individually supported so that the family system is strong. Although the family can indefinitely support a member who is in need of assistance, its greatest strength lies in all members supporting one another. The nurse should bear in mind that the family member in greatest need is not necessarily the affected child but may be a parent or sibling who is dealing with stresses that require intervention.

Parents. The nurse can provide support by being attentive to families' responses to their children. Mothers and fathers need to experience success, joy, and pride in their children to give the support they need. Children also require support for their interactions, adjustments, and efforts. They must be given reinforcement for attempts to get to know their care providers and to communicate their needs to them.

Nurses must examine their attitudes to determine their ability to engage in parent-professional partnerships. An essential characteristic is the belief that parents are equal to professionals and that parents are experts regarding their child (Guidelines box).

Because most mothers and fathers of children with special needs have little or no experience with children who have chronic or disabling conditions, the nurse can serve as a role model for appropriate interactions with the child. Above all, the nurse should ensure that the parents and siblings learn to perceive the child as a child first, with unique and individual needs. The nurse needs to convey a humanistic, accepting approach to the child to enable the parents to observe this acceptance. This attitude of liking, being concerned for, and accepting the child should begin in early infancy and continue throughout the child's life.

Communication among all family members is encouraged. Parent group sessions can help parents to verbalize thoughts and feelings to each other but often do not take into account siblings' or the child's viewpoint. Therefore the nurse may need to set up a family session, such as during a home or clinic visit. Although the ideal situation is to have all of the members present at one time, this is often not possible. However, inviting members to participate at various visits is an appropriate alternative.

Parents can be encouraged to discuss their feelings toward the child, the impact of this event on their marriage, and associated stresses such as financial burdens. For most families, regardless of their income or insurance coverage, financial concerns exist. The costs of caring for a child with special needs can be overwhelming. In addition, the family wage earner may have to sacrifice job opportunities to remain close to a medical facility or to avoid losing insurance benefits.*

The nurse should regard fathers as able, effective parents, competent and capable of coping with the challenges they face. Every effort is made to include the father in visits, such as to the nursery, clinic, special school, and stimulation programs. The father should be included in the assessment process, with specific emphasis on having him describe the child's strengths and difficulties. It is not unusual to find two parents who have differing views of the child's abilities, especially in the area of developmental disabilities.

Numerous volunteer and community resources are available that provide assistance, rehabilitation, equipment, and funding for a variety of health problems.† National and local disease-oriented organizations may provide needed assistance and support to families who qualify. Many of these are discussed in the text under the diagnosis. State and federal departments of health, mental health, social service, and labor may be able to help locate appropriate regional resources. For example, state Programs for Children with Special Health Needs (formerly Crippled Children's Services) provide financial assistance for children with many disabling conditions. Local and national sources of respite care and medical day care may be useful to families. Nurses should become acquainted with those in their communities and with vocational programs for special groups.

Although community resources may exist, it is often very difficult for parents to locate suitable services, and coordination among several agencies may be lacking. Fragmented care is one

---

*Information regarding financial issues is available from the Federation for Children with Special Needs, 95 Berkeley St., Suite 104, Boston, MA 02116; (617) 482-2915.

†General sources of information are the Clearinghouse for Disability Information, Room 3132, Switzer Building, C St. SW, Washington, DC 20202-2524; National Information Center for Children and Youth with Disabilities, P.O. Box 1492, Washington, DC 20013; (202) 884-8200 or 1-800-695-0285; website: www.nichcy.org; and National Center for Children with Chronic Illness and Disability, Box 721-UMHC, Harvard St. at E. River Rd., Minneapolis, MN 55455; (612) 626-2820. A comprehensive list of books and pamphlets for parents and teachers is available from the Easter Seals National Headquarters, 230 W. Monroe St., Suite 1800, Chicago, IL 60606, (312) 726-6200; website: www.easter-seals.org. In Canada these materials are available from the Council of Canadians with Disabilities, Suite 926, 294 Portage Ave., Winnipeg, Manitoba R3C 0B9; (204) 947-0303; website: www.pcs.mb.ca/ccd.

Guidelines

ENCOURAGING EXPRESSION OF EMOTION

Describe the behavior: "You seem angry at everyone."
Give evidence of understanding: "Being angry is only natural."
Give evidence of caring: "It must be difficult to endure so many painful procedures."
Help focus on feelings: "Maybe you wonder why this happened to your child."

Guidelines

DEVELOPING SUCCESSFUL PARENT-PROFESSIONAL PARTNERSHIPS

Promote primary nursing, in nonhospital settings designate a case manager.
Acknowledge parents' overall competence and their unique expertise with their child.
Respect parents' time as having value equal to that of other members of child's health care team.
Explain or define any medical, technical, or disciplinary-specific terms.
Tell families, "I am not sure" or "I don't know," when appropriate.
Facilitate family's effectiveness in team meetings (e.g., provide parents with same information as other participants).

of the chief complaints from families. Consequently, community networking for improved services is essential. Although this topic is beyond the scope of the present discussion, nurses can become key figures in coordinating services.

Parent-to-Parent Support. The support a parent receives from another parent is unique and unobtainable from any other source. A growing number of hospitals and clinics now have a parent on staff. The services these parents provide are particularly valuable for parents of children with special needs who are likely to experience frequent and lengthy hospitalizations as well as numerous routine clinic visits.

Just being with another parent who has shared similar experiences is helpful. A parent of a child with the same diagnosis is not always necessary, because parents in the process of adjusting to a child with special needs—or finding respite services, educational or rehabilitative services, special equipment vendors, and financial counseling—tread a common path. If the agency does not have a parent staff position, the nurse can contact parent groups, which will often send a representative. Another strategy is ask another parent to talk to the parents. The nurse should seek out a parent who is a good listener, has a nonjudgmental approach to differences in families, and possesses good advocacy and problem-solving skills.

The parent self-help group is another way to promote parent-to-parent support.* Group members feel less alone and have the opportunity to observe both coping and mastery role modeling from other members. Parent groups are rich resources for information. Even if parents are unable to attend meetings, they can still benefit from group newsletters and other literature that often accompanies membership. The nurse can foster parent participation in self-help groups by serving as a referral agent, a group advisory board member, a resource person, a group member, or an assistant in founding a group. Sometimes all that is required in starting a group is identifying one or two parents as leaders; sharing with them the names, telephone numbers, and addresses of other families who have expressed both an interest and a willingness to release their phone number and address; and guiding them in how to initiate a first meeting.†

Advocate for Empowerment. Nurses can advocate for methods that foster opportunities for parent empowerment. For example, nurses can suggest reimbursement for travel and child care plus stipends to enable parents' voices to be heard at meetings and conferences. They can encourage parent membership on staff, committees, and boards. They can keep parents informed of pending legislation on child health issues or take action when parents inform them.

The Child. Through ongoing contacts with the child, the nurse (1) observes the child's responses to the disorder, ability to function, and adaptive behavior within the environment and with significant others; (2) explores the child's own understanding of the nature of his or her illness or condition; and (3) provides support while the child learns to cope with his or her feelings. Children are encouraged to express their concerns rather than allowing others to express them for them, because open discussions may reduce anxiety.

Parents sometimes convey concern because children cannot express their anxieties. If children cannot or will not talk, they may have to play out their feelings. They can be provided with toys to express threatening or stressful emotions. The nurse may find that children respond best to drawing pictures or telling stories (see Chapter 34). Puppets can also be used. By demonstrating to parents how useful these techniques are, the nurse also helps them learn new ways of communicating with their child. For youngsters with extremely serious handicaps and/or persistent maladjustment, psychiatric evaluation and management may be needed.

One of the most important interventions is alleviating the child's feeling of being different and normalizing his or her life as much as possible (Guidelines box). Whenever possible, the nurse should assist the family in assessing the child's daily routine for indications of normalizing practices. For example, the child who remains in a bedroom all day is in need of a restructured daily routine to provide activities in different parts of the house, such as eating in the kitchen or dining room with the family. Such children may also be deprived of social, recreational, and academic activities that can be recognized by applying normalization practices. For example, home and out-of-home health-related treatments should be planned at times that least interfere with normal daily activities.

Children who are concerned that their condition detracts from their physical attractiveness need attention focused on the normal aspects of appearance and capabilities. Health professionals must help strengthen and consolidate the self-image by emphasizing the normal, while at the same time allowing children to express anger, isolation, fear of rejection, feelings of sadness, and loneliness. They need positive reinforcement for compliance and any evidence of improvement. Anything that might

Guidelines

PROMOTING NORMALIZATION

Preparation. Prepare child in advance for changes that may occur from the illness or disability; for example, the child is told in advance of the possible side effects of drug therapy.

Participation. Include child in as many decisions as possible, especially those relating to his or her care regimen; for example, the child is responsible for taking medications or scheduling home treatments.

Sharing. Allow both family members and child's peers to be a part of the care regimen whenever possible; for example, the child is given his or her medication when the other siblings receive their vitamins; the parent cooks the same menu for the whole family; and if the child is invited to another's home, the parent advises the family of the child's dietary restrictions.

Control. Identify areas where child can be in control so that feelings of uncertainty, passivity, and helplessness are decreased; for example, the child identifies activities that are appropriate to his or her energy level and chooses to rest when fatigued.

Expectation. Apply the same family rules to the child with a chronic illness or disability as to the well siblings or peers; for example, the child is disciplined, expected to fulfill household responsibilities, and attends school in accordance with abilities.

---

*Information about self-help groups and books and pamphlets are available from the National Self-Help Clearinghouse, 365 5th Ave., Suite 3300, New York, NY 10016-4309; (212) 817-1822; website: www.selfhelpweb.org.

† The following resource is recommended: *The self-help sourcebook: finding and forming mutual aid self-help groups*, by E.J. Madara and A. Meese, available from the New Jersey Self-Help Clearinghouse, 100 E. Hanover Ave., 2nd Floor, Cedar Knolls, NJ 07297; 1-800-367-6274; website: www.njgroups.org.

improve attractiveness and contribute to a positive self-image is employed, such as makeup for a teenager with a scar, clothing that disguises a prosthesis, or a hairstyle or wig to cover a deformity or lost hair.

Siblings. The presence of a child with special needs in a family may result in parents paying less attention to the other children. Siblings may respond by developing negative attitudes toward the child or by expressing anger in different forms. The nurse can help by using "anticipatory guidance," questioning the parents about what they believe is the best way to have siblings respond to the child and guiding them through ways to meet their other children's needs for attention. This questioning should take place before serious negative effects occur.

Siblings may also experience embarrassment associated with courtesy stigma. Parents are then faced with the difficulty of responding to this embarrassment in an understanding and appropriate manner without punishing the siblings for how they feel. Parents should talk with the siblings about how they view their affected sibling. For example, siblings of a child who is retarded may express fears about their ability to bear normal children. Adolescents in particular may not be able to discuss these vital issues with their parents and may prefer to consult with the nurse. Many siblings benefit from sharing their concerns* with other young people who are experiencing a similar situation. Support groups for siblings can help decrease isolation, promote expression of feelings, and provide examples of effective coping skills.

*For information on the Sibling Information Network, contact the Information Network, CUAP, 991 Main St., Suite 3A, East Hartford, CT 06108.

Many parents express concern about when and how to inform the other children in the family about a sibling's disability. The answer depends on each child's level of sophistication and understanding. However, it is usually best to inform the siblings before a neighbor or other nonfamily member does so. Uninformed siblings may fantasize or develop apprehensions that are out of proportion to the child's actual condition. Furthermore, if parents choose to be silent or deceptive about the issue, they are setting a negative precedent for the siblings to follow, rather than encouraging the siblings to cope with the experience in a healthy and nurturing way.

The nurse must be sensitive to the reactions of siblings and whenever possible intervene to promote more positive adjustment. For example, siblings often mention that they are expected to take on additional responsibilities to help the parents care for the child. It is not unusual for them to express a positive reaction to assuming the extra duties but a negative response to feeling unappreciated for doing so. Such feelings can often be minimized by encouraging siblings to discuss this with the parents and by suggesting to parents ways of showing gratitude, such as an increase in allowance, special privileges, and most significantly, verbal praise (Family Focus box).

Extended Family Members and Community. The nurse must also be sensitive to the family's cues regarding

Family Focus

SUPPORTING SIBLINGS

Promote Healthy Sibling Relationships

Value each child individually and avoid comparisons. Remind each child of his or her positive qualities and contribution to other family members.

Help siblings see the differences and similarities between themselves and a child with special needs. Create a climate in which children can achieve successes without feeling guilty.

Teach siblings ways to interact with the child.

Seek to be fair in terms of discipline, attention, and resources; require the affected child to do as much for himself or herself as possible.

Let siblings settle their own differences; intervene only to prevent siblings from hurting one another.

Legitimize reasonable anger. Even children with special needs behave badly sometimes.

Respect a sibling's reluctance to be with or to include the child with special needs in activities.

Help Siblings Cope

Listen to siblings to let them know that their thoughts and suggestions are valued.

Praise siblings when they have been patient, have sacrificed, or have been particularly helpful. Do not expect siblings to always act in this manner.

Acknowledge the personal strengths of siblings and their ability to cope with stress successfully.

Provide age-appropriate information about the child's condition, and update when appropriate.

Let teachers know what is happening so that they can be understanding and helpful.

Recognize special stress times for siblings and plan to minimize negative effects.

Schedule special time with siblings; have a friend or family member substitute when parent is unavailable.

Encourage sibling to join or help establish a sibling support group.

Use the services of professionals when needed. If parent feels that such a service is necessary, it should be provided in as vigorous a manner as a service for the child with special needs.

Involve Siblings

Seek out ways to include siblings realistically in the care and treatment of the child with special needs.

Limit caregiving responsibilities, and give recognition when siblings perform them.

Develop a library of children's books on special needs.

Invite siblings to attend meetings to develop plans for the child with special needs.

Discuss future plans with them.

Solicit their ideas on treatment and service needs.

Have them visit professionals who work with the child.

Help them develop competencies to teach the child new skills.

Provide opportunities for siblings to advocate for the child.

Allow siblings to set their own pace for learning and involvement.

Modified from Powell T, Ogle P: *Brothers and sisters—a special part of exceptional families,* Baltimore, 1985, Brookes; Spokane, Washington, Deaconess Medical Center Pediatric Oncology Unit: Tips for dealing with siblings, *Candlelighters Childhood Cancer Foundation Quarterly Newsletter* 11(3, 4):7, 1987; and Carlson J, Leviton A, Mueller M: Services to siblings: an important component of family-centered practice, *ACCH Advocate* 1(1):53-56, 1993.

sources of stress from extended members, such as grandparents. For example, the nurse may encourage the parents to invite the grandparents to be present during one of the child's visits to a clinic, during the diagnostic workup, or during a parent conference or to provide appropriate literature. Including grandparents in a discussion in which they can share their concerns may help them deal with their feelings, thus reducing stress on the entire family. Grandparents' feelings of blame and anger, as well as any "cure fantasies" they harbor, can be brought out in the open and discussed if necessary. Grandparents can be helped to understand the effects of their behavior on the family with an appropriate statement such as "Your daughter is currently experiencing a great deal of pain and anguish. We realize that this is difficult for you as well as your daughter; however, you can be of tremendous help by being supportive toward her."

Educate About the Disorder and General Health Care. Educating the family about the disorder is actually an extension of revealing the diagnosis.* Education involves not only supplying technical information but also discussing how the condition will affect the child. Parents may be able to digest only so much information at a time. It may be helpful to provide essential information and then follow by asking, "What else would you like to know about your child's condition?" Responding to parents' questions and concerns ensures that information needs are met.

Activities of Daily Living. Parents also need guidance in how the condition may interfere with or alter activities of daily living, such as eating, dressing, sleeping, and toileting. One area commonly affected is nutrition. Common problems are undernutrition, resulting from food being inappropriately restricted, loss of appetite, vomiting, or motor deficits that interfere with feeding, and overnutrition, usually caused by a caloric intake in excess of energy expenditure or boredom and lack of stimulation in other areas. Although the child requires the same basic nutrients as other children, the daily requirements may differ. Special nutritional considerations are discussed as appropriate throughout the text.

Safe Transportation. Modifications may also be needed regarding car safety. Children with conditions such as low birth weight or orthopedic, neuromuscular, or respiratory problems often cannot safely use conventional car restraints. For example, children with hip spica casts cannot sit properly in child safety seats (see Congenital Hip Dysplasia, Chapter 54). Modifications can be made to some commercial models, and for older children a special vest is available that secures the child to the backseat in a lying-down position.†

If a child requires a wheelchair, the family should consult the wheelchair manufacturer for specific instructions regarding safe car transportation. Considerations for wheelchairs used for vehicle transportation must address securing both the wheelchair and the occupant in the wheelchair. Wheelchairs should be secured facing forward with tie downs at four points. The tie-down system should be dynamically crash tested, as should the occupant-securement system that secures the child in the wheelchair. For example, use of trays would not be recommended for transportation. For children who must travel with additional medical equipment, this equipment (i.e., oxygen, monitors, and ventilators) should be anchored to the floor or underneath the vehicle seat or wheelchair. Soft padding should be added around the equipment to reduce movement. A second adult should be present to monitor the condition of a medically fragile child while traveling.

Primary Health Care. Children with special needs require all the usual health care recommended for any child. Attention to injury prevention, immunizations, dental health, and regular physical examinations is essential. Nurses can play an important role in reminding parents of these aspects of care that are so often neglected when the concern is focused on the child's specific illness or disability. Specific discussions of nutrition, sleep and activity, dental health, and injury prevention are presented in the chapters on health promotion for specific age groups. Immunizations are discussed in Chapter 36.

Parents also need to be aware of the importance of communicating the child's condition in the event of a medical emergency. Young children are unable to give information about their disorder, and although older children may be reliable sources, after an accident they may be physically unable to speak. Therefore all children with any type of chronic condition that may affect medical care should wear some type of identification, such as a MedicAlert bracelet,* or carry a card in their wallet that lists the medical condition and a phone number for emergency medical records and other personal information.

Children need information about their condition, the therapeutic plan, and how the disease or the therapy might affect their particular situation. Children nearing puberty also need to understand the maturation process and how their disability may alter this event. Information should not be given all at once but should be timed appropriately to meet the changing needs of the youngsters, and it should be described and repeated as often as the situation demands. The subject of sexuality related to the effects of the disorder is a prominent concern of adolescents, but they rarely initiate a discussion of this sensitive topic. Any probable interference in sexual function because of the disability should be discussed openly and candidly with the teenager.

Promote Normal Development. Aside from knowledge of the condition and its effect on the child's abilities, the family must be guided toward fostering appropriate development in their child. Although each stage may take longer to achieve, parents are guided toward helping the child to fully realize his or her potential in preparation for the next developmental stage. Table 41-3 outlines developmental aspects of chronic illness or disability and supportive interventions. With appropriate planning and knowledge of strategies to improve the child's functional abilities, most children can live fulfilling and productive lives.

One important aspect of promoting normal development is to encourage the child's self-care abilities in both activities of daily living and the medical regimen. An assessment of the child's age and physical, emotional, and mental capacities, as

*Community and home care instructions sheets, which may be copied and given to families, are available in Wong DL, Hess CS: ***Wong and Whaley's clinical manual of pediatric nursing,*** ed 5, St Louis, 2000, Mosby.

†Information on car safety restraints for children with special needs is available from the Automotive Safety for Children Program, Riley Hospital for Children, 575 West Dr., Room 004, Indianapolis, IN 46202; (317) 274-2977 or 1-800-KID-N-CAR (in Indiana); website: www.preventinjury.org.

*P.O. Box 1009, Turlock, CA 95381-1009; 1-800-ID-ALERT; website: https://www.medicalert.org

TABLE 41-3

Developmental Aspects of Chronic Illness or Disability on Children

Developmental Tasks	Potential Effects of Chronic Illness or Disability	Supportive Interventions
INFANCY		
Develop a sense of trust	Multiple caregivers and frequent separations, especially if hospitalized Deprived of consistent nurturing	Encourage consistent caregivers in hospital or other care settings
Bond/attach to parent	Delayed because of separation, parental grief for loss of "dream" child, parental inability to accept the condition, especially a visible defect	Encourage parental presence, "rooming in" during hospitalization, and participation in care Emphasize healthy, perfect qualities of infant Help parents learn special care needs of infant for them to feel competent
Learn through sensorimotor experiences	Increased exposure to painful experiences over pleasurable ones Limited contact with environment from restricted movement or confinement	Expose infant to pleasurable experiences through all senses (touch, hearing, sight, taste, movement) Encourage age-appropriate developmental skills (e.g., holding bottle, finger feeding, crawling)
Begin to develop a sense of separateness from parent	Increased dependency on parent for care Overinvolvement of parent in care	Encourage all family members to participate in care to prevent overinvolvement of one member Encourage periodic respite from demands of care responsibilities
TODDLERHOOD		
Develop autonomy	Increased dependency on parent	Encourage independence in as many areas as possible (e.g., toileting, dressing, feeding)
Master locomotor and language skills	Limited opportunity to test own abilities and limits	Provide gross motor skill activity and modification of toys or equipment, such as modified swing or rocking horse
Learn through sensorimotor experience; beginning preoperational thought	Increased exposure to painful experiences	Give choices to allow simple feeling of control (e.g., choice of what book to look at or what kind of sandwich to eat) Institute age-appropriate discipline and limit setting Recognize that negative and ritualistic behaviors are normal Provide sensory experiences (e.g., water play, sandbox play, finger painting)
PRESCHOOL		
Develop initiative and purpose Master self-care skills	Limited opportunities for success in accomplishing simple tasks or mastering self-care skills	Encourage mastery of self-help skills Provide devices that make task easier (e.g., self-dressing)
Begin to develop peer relationships	Limited opportunities for socialization with peers; may appear "like a baby" to age-mates Protection within tolerant and secure family may cause child to fear criticism and withdraw	Encourage socialization (e.g., inviting friends to play, day care experience, trips to park) Provide age-appropriate play, especially associative play opportunities Emphasize child's abilities; dress appropriately to enhance desirable appearance
Develop sense of body image and sexual identification	Awareness of body may center on pain, anxiety, and failure Sex-role identification focused primarily on mothering skills	Encourage relationships with same-sex and opposite-sex peers and adults Help child deal with criticisms; realize that too much protection prevents child from realities of world
Learn through preoperational thought (magical thinking)	Guilt (thinking he or she caused the illness/disability or is being punished for wrongdoing)	Clarify that cause of child's illness or disability is not his or her fault or a punishment
SCHOOL AGE		
Develop a sense of accomplishment	Limited opportunities to achieve and compete (e.g., many school absences or inability to join regular athletic activities)	Encourage school attendance; schedule medical visits at times other than school; encourage child to make up missed work

TABLE 41-3—cont'd

Developmental Aspects of Chronic Illness or Disability on Children

Developmental Tasks	Potential Effects of Chronic Illness or Disability	Supportive Interventions
SCHOOL AGE—cont'd		
Form peer relationships	Limited opportunities for socialization	Educate teachers and classmates about child's condition, abilities, and special needs
Learn through concrete operations	Incomplete comprehension of the imposed physical limitations or treatment of the disorder	Encourage sports activities (e.g., Special Olympics)
		Encourage socialization (e.g., Girl Scouts, Campfire, Boy Scouts, 4-H Club; having a best friend or club membership)
		Provide child with knowledge about his or her condition
		Encourage creative activities (e.g., Very Special Arts)
ADOLESCENCE		
Develop personal and sexual identity	Increased sense of feeling different from peers and less able to compete with peers in appearance, abilities, special skills	Realize that many of the difficulties the teenager is experiencing are part of normal adolescence (rebelliousness, risk taking, lack of cooperation, hostility toward authority)
Achieve independence from family	Increased dependency on family; limited job/career opportunities	Provide instruction on interpersonal and coping skills
Form heterosexual relationships	Limited opportunities for heterosexual friendships; less opportunity to discuss sexual concerns with peers	Encourage socialization with peers, including peers with special needs and those without special needs
Learn through abstract thinking	Increased concern with issues such as why did he or she get the disorder, can he or she marry and have a family	Provide instruction on decision making, assertiveness, and other skills necessary to manage personal plans
	Decreased opportunity for earlier stages of cognition may impede achieving level of abstract thinking	Encourage increased responsibility for care and management of the disease or condition (e.g., assuming responsibility for making and keeping appointment [ideally alone], sharing assessment and planning stages of health care delivery, contacting resources)
		Encourage activities appropriate for age (e.g., attending mixed-sex parties, sports activities, driving a car)
		Be alert to cues that signal readiness for information regarding implications of condition on sexuality and reproduction
		Emphasize good appearance and wearing stylish clothes, use of makeup
		Understand that adolescent has same sexual needs and concerns as any other teenager
		Discuss planning for future and how condition can affect choices

well as the support and structure provided by the family, should be considered in determining the appropriate level of self-care in the medical regimen (Savinetti-Rose, 1994). Even toddlers can be involved in their own care by holding supplies for the parent during a procedure. Over time, children should be encouraged toward greater autonomy in the self-care arena.

Early childhood. During infancy the child is achieving basic trust through a satisfying, intimate, consistent relationship with his or her parents. However, the affected child's early existence may be stressful, chaotic, and unsatisfying. Consequently, he or she may need more parental support and expressions of affection to achieve trust. Likewise, the parents require assistance in finding ways to meet the infant's needs, such as how to hold a rigid or flaccid infant, how to feed a child with tongue thrust or episodes of dyspnea, and how to stimulate a child who seems incapable of achieving any skills. If hospitalizations are frequent or prolonged, every effort is made to preserve the parent-child relationship (see also Chapter 44). Hospital policies should promote visitation by and involvement of families.

During early childhood the goal is to achieve separation from parents, autonomy, and initiative. However, the natural parental response to having a sick child is overprotection. Parents need help in realizing the importance of brief separations of the child from them and from others involved in the child's care and of providing social experiences outside the home whenever possible. Respite care, which provides temporary relief for family members, can be essential in allowing caregivers time away from daily burdens.

Young children also need the opportunity to develop independence. Commonly the child is able to learn self-help skills, such as holding a bottle, finger feeding, and removing simple articles of clothing, but the parent continues to perform the act. The nurse can guide parents to the usual milestones expected for the child.

When a young child has a disability that interferes with motor development, intervention must be based on providing activities that allow maximum motor development. Also, the activity must take into account the child's need for social interaction, sense of control over the body, feeling of competence and achievement, and an outlet for aggression.

When a child is unable to perform a skill independently, functional aids should be used. With innovation, many adaptations can be implemented in children's environments to increase their mobility and independence and allow them to play like other children their age. For example, with slight modifications, a child with physical limitations may be able to ride a tricycle (Fig. 41-3).

Another critical component for normal child development is discipline. Discipline and guidance serve several purposes, such as providing children with boundaries on which to test out their behavior and teaching them socially acceptable behavior. Resentment and hostility can arise among siblings if different standards are applied to each child. The nurse's responsibility is to help parents learn successful methods of managing a child's behaviors before they become problems (see Chapter 31).

School Age. For school-age children the major tasks are entry into school and achieving a sense of *industry.* Although the importance of school in the life of all children is well known, school absences are significantly higher among children with chronic illness than among their healthy peers. The more school absences the child experiences, the more difficult it is to resume attendance, and "school phobia" may result. The child should return to school as soon as possible after diagnosis or treatments.

Preparation for entry into or resumption of school is best accomplished through a team approach with the parents, child, schoolteacher, school nurse, and primary nurse in the hospital. Ideally this planning should begin before hospital discharge, provided that the child is well enough to resume usual activities. A structured plan should be developed, with attention to those aspects of care that must be continued during school hours, such as administration of medication or other treatments.

Children also need preparation before entering or resuming school. Having a tutor in the hospital or home as soon as children are physically able helps them realize that school will continue and gives them time to consider this prospect (Fig. 41-4). They need to investigate possible answers to the many questions others will ask. One method of anticipatory preparation is to role-play, with the child as the "returned pupil" and the nurse or parent as "other schoolmates." If the child returns to school with some obvious physical change, such as hair loss, amputation, or a visible scar, the nurse might also ask questions about these alterations to prompt preparatory responses from the child.

Classroom peers also need preparation, and a joint plan of the schoolteacher, nurse, and child is best. At a minimum, the classmates should be given a description of the child's condition, prepared for any visible changes in the child, and allowed an opportunity to ask questions. The child should have the op-

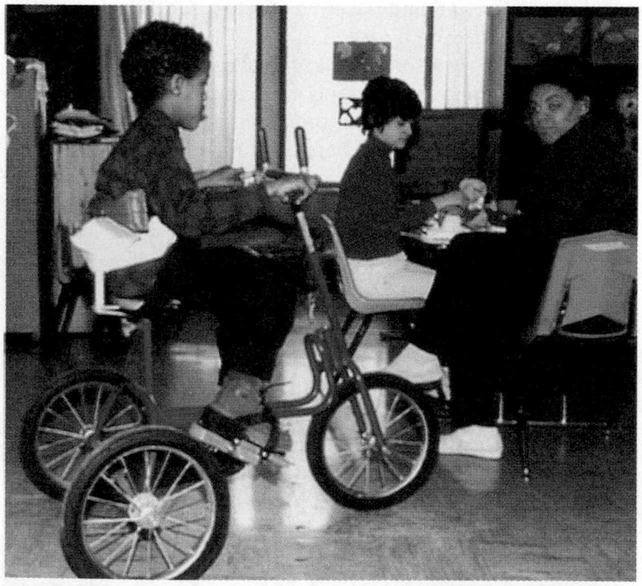

FIG. 41-3 • A modified tricycle with block pedals, self-adhesive straps for support, and modified seat and handle bars can help a child with disabilities gain mobility.

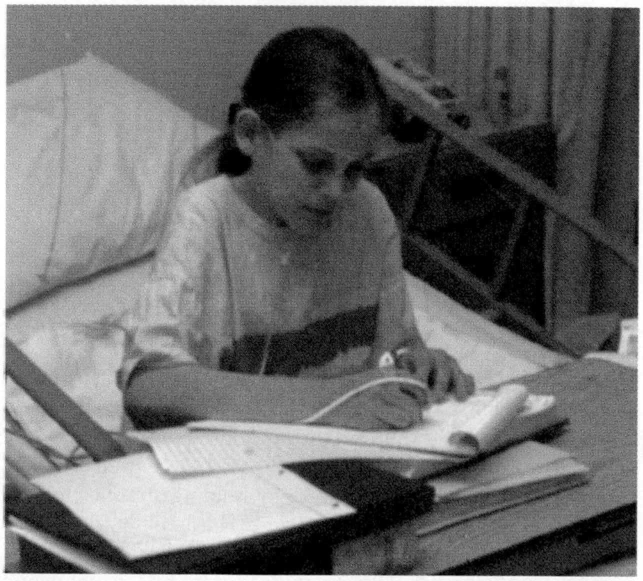

FIG. 41-4 • Children with special needs should continue their schooling as soon as their condition permits.

tion of attending this session. As the child's condition changes, particularly if the illness is potentially fatal, school personnel, including the students, need periodic appraisal of the child's status and preparation for what to expect.

Children with special needs are encouraged to maintain or reestablish relationships with peers and to participate according to their capabilities in any age-appropriate activities. Alternative activities may be substitutes for those that are impossible or that place a strain on the child's condition. Programs such as the Special Olympics* offer children an opportunity to compete with their peers and to achieve athletic skill. Summer camps† allow children to associate with peers and develop a variety of skills. Children with special needs can derive enormous benefits from expressive activities, such as art, music, poetry, dance, and drama. With adaptive equipment and imagination, children can participate in a variety of activities. Organizations such as VSA arts (formerly, Very Special Arts) offer children an opportunity to celebrate and share their accomplishments.‡ Children need the opportunity to interact with healthy peers, as well as to engage in activities with groups or clubs composed of similarly affected age-mates. Such organizations as ostomy clubs, diabetes clubs, and cerebral palsy groups share information and provide support related to the special problems the members face.

Adolescence. Adolescence can be a particularly difficult period for the teenager and family. All of the needs discussed before apply to this age group as well. Developing independence or autonomy, however, is a major task for the adolescent as planning for the future becomes a prominent concern. Although the emphasis in the past has been on achieving independence from physical assistance, recent developments in the fields of special education, adolescent development, and family systems suggest redefining autonomy in terms of individuals' capacities to take responsibility for their own behavior, to make decisions regarding their own lives, and to maintain supportive social relationships. Given this understanding, even individuals with severe impairment can be viewed as autonomous if they perceive their own needs and take responsibility for meeting them, either directly or by engaging the assistance of others. As adolescents become more autonomous, the nurse can help them articulate needs, participate in developing their own plan of care, and discover and express how others can be of greatest assistance.

Physical symptoms are high on the teenager's list of health-related concerns. Because adolescence is a time of enormous physical and emotional changes, it is important for the nurse to make a distinction between body changes that are related to disability and those that are a result of normal body development. It can be a great comfort for teenagers with disabling conditions to know that many of the changes they experience are normal developmental outcomes.

A sense of feeling different from peers can lead to loneliness, isolation, and depression. Participation in groups of teenagers with chronic conditions or disabilities can alleviate feelings of isolation and smooth the transition to a meaningful relationship with one person in adulthood.

Establish Realistic Future Goals. One of the most difficult adjustments is setting realistic future goals for the child and for those involved in his or her continued care. Sometimes the impact of this decision does not surface until the child finishes school or the parents approach retirement, when a crisis can arise because all of the family roles and relationships that maintained stability are now disrupted.

Planning for the future should be a gradual process. All along, the parents should cultivate realistic vocations for the child. For example, if children have physical disabilities, they are directed to intellectual, artistic, or musical pursuits. Children with developmental disabilities are taught manual skills. In this way, the child's development proceeds in the direction of self-support through gainful employment.

With prolonged survival, young persons with chronic illnesses must deal with new decisions and problems, such as marriage, employment, and insurance coverage. With appropriate guidance, gainful employment, marriage, and a family are attainable goals. For those whose conditions are genetic, counseling is needed regarding future offspring. Prospective spouses often benefit from an opportunity to discuss their feelings regarding marriage with an individual with continued health needs and possibly a limited life span. Health insurance coverage is a critical issue because some private carriers may no longer insure a young person who leaves home or may be unwilling to reinsure the person who is independent. Life insurance is another dilemma, especially when children have serious defects such as congenital heart anomalies.

Unfortunately, vocational pursuits and completely independent living are not realistic goals for all persons. Persons with multiple or severe disabilities may require lifelong care and assistance. In these situations parents must look to the time when they will no longer be able to care for their child. Residential placement may be very difficult unless the family mutually participates in the decision-making and planning process. Placement outside the home should not be viewed as abandonment. Not uncommonly it is the only way to preserve the family unit. The nurse should help the family investigate suitable placements, discuss their feelings regarding this decision, and help the family explore measures to maintain meaningful communication between family members.

➤ Evaluation

The effectiveness of nursing interventions is determined by continual reassessment and evaluation of care based on the following observational guidelines:

1. Observe family members' responses to the diagnosis and the types of questions or concerns they have.
2. Interview family regarding their knowledge and understanding of the child's condition; observe whether they have instituted suggestions, such as use of identification devices for children with certain conditions.

---

*1350 New York Ave. NW, Suite 500, Washington, DC 20005-1581; (202) 628-3630. Several pamphlets on sports and recreation for children with disabilities are available from the Easter Seals National Headquarters, 230 W. Monroe St., Suite 1800, Chicago, IL 60606; (312) 726-6200; website: www.easter_seals.org; and the American Alliance for Health, Physical Education, Recreation and Dance (AAHPERD), 1900 Association Dr., Reston, VA 20191; (703) 476-3400; website www.aahperd.org.

†A directory of camps for children with a variety of chronic illnesses or general physical disabilities is available for a fee from the American Camping Association, Publications Service, 5000 State Rd., 67 N., Martinsville, IN 46151; 1-800-428-CAMP.

‡VSA arts has affiliate chapters in all 50 states and in selected sites internationally; yearly festivals are held throughout the world. Information is available from VSA arts, Education Office, John F. Kennedy Center for the Performing Arts, Washington, DC 20566; (202) 628-2800; website: www.vsarts.org.

3. Observe responses of professionals to reactions such as denial, guilt, and anger and whether supportive interventions are used with the family.
4. Observe family's communication patterns with each other and their ability to discuss feelings about issues such as the impact of the child's condition on the marriage or additional care responsibilities; investigate family's use of services, such as self-help groups or other community resources.
5. Perform a developmental screening test in young children and compare results with expected milestones for the child's abilities; investigate use of functional aids to assist children in developing to their potential; question family about the child's attendance at school and interaction with peers.
6. Interview family to determine whether their self-identified needs and concerns have been adequately addressed.

➤ Expected Outcomes

Expected outcomes are listed in the Nursing Care Plan.

PERSPECTIVES ON THE CARE OF CHILDREN AT THE END OF LIFE

Although most childhood illnesses and many injuries and other trauma respond favorably to treatment, some do not. When a child and family face a prolonged and possibly terminal illness, health professionals are faced with the challenge of providing the best possible care to meet the physical, psychologic, spiritual, and emotional needs of the child and family during the uncertain course of the illness and at the time of death. When death is sudden and unexpected, nurses are challenged to respond to a family's grief and shock and provide comfort and support in the absence of a prior relationship.

A child with a life-threatening illness or who has experienced serious, life-threatening trauma needs medical diagnosis and intervention, as well as nursing assessment and care—sometimes for a short time and sometimes over a lengthy period. When cure is no longer possible and life-prolonging measures are resulting in pain and distress to the child, parents need information about care options that are available to assist them in deciding how they want the remaining time with their child to be managed by the health care team. It is important that families be reassured that although their child cannot be cured, active care will continue to be provided to maintain the child's comfort. Support must be provided to assist the child and family during the dying process. As a result, nurses may care for children and families who are making the difficult transition from curative or restorative treatments to palliative care.

Principles of Palliative Care

Palliative care involves a multidisciplinary approach to the management of a terminal illness or the dying process that focuses on symptom control and support rather than on cure or life prolongation in the absence of the possibility of a cure (Billings, 1998). The World Health Organization (1990) defines *palliative care* as the "active total care of patients whose disease is not responsive to curative treatment." Palliative care interventions do not serve to hasten death; rather, they provide pain and symptom management, attention to issues faced by the child and family with regard to death and dying, and promotion of optimal functioning and quality of life during the time the child has remaining. Several principles are the hallmarks of palliative care.

A multidisciplinary team of health care professionals consisting of social workers, chaplains, nurses, personal care aids, and physicians skilled in caring for dying patients assists the family by focusing care on the complex interactions between physical, emotional, social, and spiritual issues.

Palliative care seeks to create a therapeutic environment that is as homelike as possible, if not in the child's own home. Through education and support of family members, an atmosphere of open communication is provided regarding the child's dying process and its impact on all members of the family.

Decision Making at the End of Life

Discussions concerning the possibility that a child's illness or condition is not curable and that death is an inevitable outcome cause everyone involved a great deal of stress. Physicians, other members of the health care team, and families must consider all information regarding the child's situation and make decisions that all parties agree to and that will have a profound impact on the child and family.

Ethical Considerations in End-of-Life Decision Making. A number of ethical concerns arise when parents and health care professionals are deciding the best course of care for the dying child. Many parents and health care providers are concerned that not offering treatment that would cause potential pain and suffering, but might extend life, would be considered euthanasia or assisted suicide. To eliminate such concerns, it is necessary to understand the various terms. *Euthanasia* involves an action carried out by a person other than the patient to end of the life of the patient with a terminal condition. The intent of this action is based on the belief that the act is "putting the person out of his or her misery," and this action has also been called *mercy killing. Assisted suicide* occurs when someone provides the patient with the means to end his or her life and the patient uses that means to do so. The important distinction between these two actions involves who is actually acting to end the person's life.

The American Nurses Association (ANA) (1994) does not support the active intent on the part of a nurse to end a person's life. However, it does permit the nurse to provide interventions to relieve symptoms in the dying patient even when the interventions involve substantial risks of hastening of death. When the prognosis for a patient is poor and death is the expected outcome, it is ethically acceptable to withhold or withdraw treatments that may cause pain and suffering and provide interventions that promote comfort and quality of life. Therefore providing palliative care for patients is the ethically correct choice in such a circumstance.

Parental Decision Making. Rarely are families prepared to cope with the numerous decisions that must be made when a child is dying. When the death is unexpected, as in the case of an accident or trauma, the confusion of emergency services and possibly an intensive care setting presents challenges to parents as they are asked to make very difficult choices. If the child has either experienced a life-threatening illness such as cancer or lived with a chronic illness that has now reached its terminal phase, parents are often unprepared for the reality of

Nursing Care Plan THE CHILD WITH CHRONIC ILLNESS OR DISABILITY

NURSING DIAGNOSIS Altered growth and development related to chronic illness, disability, parent overbenevolence, repeated hospitalization

EXPECTED OUTCOME Patient will exhibit appropriate physical, psychosocial, and cognitive development for age and abilities.

Nursing Interventions/*Rationales*

See Table 41-3.

NURSING DIAGNOSIS Altered family processes related to situational crises (child with chronic disease/disability)

EXPECTED OUTCOME Family will exhibit adaptation of usual roles and will function to accommodate special needs of child; family will exhibit growth-promoting behaviors.

Nursing Interventions/*Rationales*

Provide opportunity for family to absorb and adjust to diagnosis (e.g., repeat information *to allow time for family to hear and understand;* encourage expression of concerns, fears, and feelings about diagnosis and potential impact *to facilitate adjustment;* and identify support systems *to provide resources for coping*).

Assist family to understand expected treatment, rationale, and implications *to provide a sound basis for decision making.*

Explore family reaction to the child; assist them to achieve a realistic view of child's abilities and limitations; encourage family in attempts to promote child growth and development; have family emphasize what child can do; and explore ways for family to include child in family activities *to help family increase abilities to cope with and incorporate child into family structure.*

Arrange for and participate in family conferences *to provide forum for communication, mutual goal setting, and effective strategizing.*

Have parents spend special time with siblings *so that they don't feel neglected or left out.*

Identify additional resource systems (e.g., relatives, friends, church, health care services, community programs) and strategize with family about making good use of these systems *to develop broad base of support.*

Provide a system of ongoing follow-up and evaluation *to ensure long-term adaptation to challenges presented to family functioning by a child with chronic disease/disability.*

NURSING DIAGNOSIS Risk for injury related to physical/developmental limitations

EXPECTED OUTCOME Child will remain free of injury and will exhibit appropriate adaptation to limitations.

Nursing Interventions/*Rationales*

Survey environment for hazards; institute needed safety measures *to decrease risk of injury.*

Encourage use of necessary assistive devices *to enhance safety.*

Help child and parents to identify activities that are appropriate for child's abilities and limitations and encourage participation *to maximize abilities and limit injury.*

Explore limits and rationale for them with child; encourage older child to take responsibility for own safety *to promote involvement of child in care.*

Confer with school nurse, teacher, coach, counselor as needed about special needs *to ensure safe school environment.*

NURSING DIAGNOSIS Impaired social interaction related to repeated hospitalizations, confinement, activity intolerance

EXPECTED OUTCOME Child will engage in appropriate family and peer interactions.

Nursing Interventions/*Rationales*

Encourage regular school attendance and promote peer contacts *to provide opportunity to develop and maintain peer relationships.*

Encourage selection of play activities and recreational outlets *that encourage interaction;* restrict time spent in solo activities *that promote social isolation.*

Encourage contact with peers and siblings by telephone or visit when hospitalized or confined *to maintain social interaction and reduce sense of isolation.*

Plan in specific periods of developmentally appropriate diversional activity suited to child's physical condition and energy level *to decrease feelings of boredom and negative self-absorption.*

NURSING DIAGNOSIS Self-care deficit related to illness/disability

EXPECTED OUTCOME Child will engage in self-care activities commensurate with capabilities.

Nursing Interventions/*Rationales*

Encourage child to assist in self-care activities as age and capabilities permit, and discourage parents form doing it for the child *to foster independence and confidence in abilities.*

Modify environment, introduce use of assistive devices and specialized equipment, and devise alternative methods of completing tasks as needed *to facilitate maximum functioning.*

Use therapeutic play and adapted toys *to increase developmental and functional abilities and encourage cooperation of child.*

Emphasize child's abilities, praise effort and accomplishments, and promote and reinforce successful endeavors *to foster a sense of self-esteem and competence.*

Continued

Nursing Care Plan THE CHILD WITH CHRONIC ILLNESS OR DISABILITY—cont'd

NURSING DIAGNOSIS Body image/self-esteem disturbances related to perception of illness/disability, feeling of being different

EXPECTED OUTCOME Child will demonstrate acceptance of self, physical appearance, and physical and developmental abilities.

Nursing Interventions/*Rationales*

Relate to child on appropriate cognitive level, conveying an attitude of caring and acceptance *to encourage positive feelings about self;* serve as role model for others *to foster positive attitudes of acceptance toward child.*

Encourage child to verbalize feelings and perceptions about the disease/disability (e.g., repeated treatments and hospitalizations, feelings of being different, implications of functional limits, difficulty in making friends, views of self) *to facilitate coping and open expression of problems, fears, wants, wishes, and needs.*

Have child identify strengths, assets, and things he or she likes about self *to increase positive feelings about self and abilities.*

Support positive coping behaviors.

Introduce child to other children who have similar disabilities, and arrange for support groups for child and parents *to increase coping skills.*

Refer child for counseling if needed *to enhance adaptation.*

Encourage use of regular hygiene and grooming practices *to promote positive appearance.*

Family Focus

THE FAMILY OF THE DYING CHILD

No matter whether you have a PhD or many children, when your child dies, it is a new experience and nothing can prepare you for it. Like so many things in life, experience is the best teacher.

Three of our children have died, and by the time the third was dying, we handled many things differently. We learned a lot about dignity and the rights of the child and family. For example, at first, we didn't know that we had a right to have our child die at home. We also didn't understand pain medications and that if children are taking these medicines and are still in agony, they have not overdosed on the medication.

We learned a lot about case management. With our first two children, lots of different people were making decisions and disagreeing about what was best and what should be done. No one had primary authority. With our third child, one doctor took a primary role. Any questions and problems were handled by one person. I could call him 24 hours a day. It made a lot of difference, and I felt our concerns and needs were better heard and respected.

The nurses caring for our third child at home enabled me to step back and just be his mommy. When I could do this, I realized that we were fighting so hard for his life that we weren't really letting him die. His nurses had worked with him for a long time and really loved him. It was hard for them when we decided to let him die. In his last several days we wanted a lot of family time with our son, and I think the nurses felt left out. Something about their reaction to our increased time with him in the last few days made us feel guilty. If we had all been able to communicate a little more openly, I would have understood that they needed more time with him at the end, too. Everyone's needs could have been met.

Jeni Stepanek
Mother
Upper Marlboro, MD

their child's impending death (Family Focus box). Numerous studies have found that families facing the impending death of a child depend on information provided to them by the health care team, particularly an honest appraisal of the child's prognosis, to make difficult decisions regarding care options for their child (Hinds et al, 1997; James and Johnson, 1997; Kirschbaum, 1996).

As the group of health professionals who are most involved with families, nurses are in an excellent position to ensure that families are presented with the options available to them. The nurse's first responsibility is to explore the family's wishes. This is best done in concert with the physician but at times may need to be initiated by the nurse. Statements such as "Tell me about your thought for the type of care you want your child to receive when he is dying" or "Have you considered the types of interventions you would like us to use when your child is near death?" can begin discussion of this sensitive but critical aspect of terminal care.

The Dying Child. Children need honest and accurate information about their illness, treatments, and prognosis; this information needs to be given in clear, simple language. In most situations this best occurs as a gradual process over time, characterized by increasingly open dialogue between parents, professionals, and the child (Lipson, 1993). Providing an atmosphere of open communication early in the course of an illness facilitates answering difficult questions as the child's condition worsens. Providing appropriate literature about the disease, as well as the experience of illness and possible death, is also helpful.

Exactly how and when to involve children in decisions regarding care during their dying process and death is a very individual matter. The age or developmental level of the child is an important consideration in the process (Table 41-4). In general, parents should be asked how they would like their child to be told of his or her prognosis, and should be included in the child's care. Some parents may request that their child not be told that he or she is dying, even if the child asks. This often places health care providers in a difficult situation. Children, even at a young age, are very perceptive. Despite not being told outright that they are dying, they realize that there is something seriously wrong and that it involves them. Often, helping parents understand that honesty and shared decision making between them and their child at this time is very important to the child's emotional health, as well as the emotional health of the family, will encourage parents to allow discussion of dying with

TABLE 41-4
Children's Understanding of and Reactions to Death

Concepts of Death	Reactions to Death	Interventions
INFANTS AND TODDLERS		
Death has least significance to children younger than 6 months of age After parent-child attachment and the development of trust are established, the loss, even if temporary, of the significant person is profound Prolonged separation during the first several years is thought to be more significant in terms of future physical, social, and emotional growth than at any subsequent age Toddlers are egocentric and can only think about events in terms of their own frame of reference—living Their egocentricity and vague separation of fact and fantasy make it impossible for them to comprehend absence of life Instead of understanding death, this age group is affected more by any change in lifestyle	With the death of someone else, they may continue to act as though the person is alive As children grow older, they will be increasingly able and willing to let go of the dead person Ritualism is important; a change in lifestyle could be anxiety producing This age group reacts more to the pain and discomfort of a serious illness than to the probable fatal prognosis This age group also reacts to parental anxiety and sadness	Help parents deal with their feelings, allowing them more emotional reserve to meet the needs of their children Encourage parents to remain as near to child as possible, yet be sensitive to parents' needs Maintain as normal an environment as possible to retain ritualism If a parent has died, encourage having consistent caregiver for child Promote primary nursing
PRESCHOOL CHILDREN		
Believe their thoughts are sufficient to cause death; the consequence is the burden of guilt, shame, and punishment Their egocentricity implies a tremendous sense of self-power and omnipotence Usually have some connotation of its meaning Death is seen as a departure, a kind of sleep May recognize the fact of physical death but do not separate it from living abilities Death is seen as temporary and gradual; life and death can change places with one another No understanding of the universality and inevitability of death	If they become seriously ill, they conceive of the illness as a punishment for their thoughts or actions May feel guilty and responsible for the death of a sibling Greatest fear concerning death is separation from parents May engage in activities that seem strange or abnormal to adults Because of their fewer defense mechanisms to deal with loss, young children may react to a less significant loss with more outward grief than to the loss of a very significant person The loss is so deep, painful, and threatening that the child must deny it for the present in order to survive its overwhelming impact Behavior reactions such as giggling, joking, attracting attention, or regressing to earlier developmental skills indicate children's need to distance themselves from tremendous loss	Help parents deal with their feelings, allowing them more emotional reserve to meet the needs of their children Help parents to understand behavioral reactions of their children Encourage parents to remain near the child as much as possible, to minimize the child's great fear of separation from parents If a parent has died, encourage having a consistent caregiver for child Promote primary nursing
SCHOOL-AGE CHILDREN		
Still associate misdeeds or bad thoughts with causing death and feel intense guilt and responsibility for the event Because of their higher cognitive abilities, they respond well to logical explanations and comprehend the figurative meaning of words	Because of their increased ability to comprehend, they may have more fears, for example: The reason for the illness Communicability of the disease to themselves or others Consequences of the disease The process of dying and death itself	Help parents deal with their feelings, allowing them more emotional reserve to meet the needs of their children Encourage parents to remain near child as much as possible, yet be sensitive to parents' needs

Continued

TABLE 41-4—cont'd
Children's Understanding of and Reactions to Death

Concepts of Death	Reactions to Death	Interventions
SCHOOL-AGE CHILDREN—cont'd		
Have a deeper understanding of death in a concrete sense Particularly fear the mutilation and punishment they associate with death Personify death as the devil, a monster, or the bogeyman May have naturalistic/physiologic explanations of death By age 9 or 10, children have an adult concept of death, realizing that it is inevitable, universal, and irreversible	Their fear of the unknown is greater than their fear of the known The realization of impending death is a tremendous threat to their sense of security and ego strength Likely to exhibit fear through verbal uncooperativeness rather than actual physical aggression Very interested in postdeath services May be inquisitive about what happens to the body	Because of children's fear of the unknown, anticipatory preparation is very important Since the developmental task of this age is industry, interventions of helping children maintain control over their bodies and increasing their understanding allow them to achieve independence, self-worth, and self-esteem and avoid a sense of inferiority Encourage children to talk about their feelings and provide aggressive outlets Encourage parents to honestly answer questions about dying rather than avoiding or fabricating euphemisms Encourage parents to share their moments of sorrow with their children Provide preparation for postdeath services
ADOLESCENTS		
Have a mature understanding of death Still very much influenced by "remnants" of magical thinking and are subject to guilt and shame Likely to see deviations from accepted behavior as reasons for their illness	Straddle transition from childhood to adulthood Have the most difficulty in coping with death Least likely to accept cessation of life, particularly if it is their own Concern is for the present much more than for the past or the future May consider themselves alienated from their peers and unable to communicate with their parents for emotional support, feeling alone in their struggle Adolescents' orientation to the present compels them to worry about physical changes even more than the prognosis Because of their idealistic view of the world, they may criticize funeral rites as barbaric, money making, and unnecessary	Help parents deal with their feelings, allowing them more emotional reserve to meet the needs of their children Avoid alliances with either parent or child Structure hospital admission to allow for maximum self-control and independence Answer adolescents' questions honestly, treating them as mature individuals and respecting their needs for privacy, solitude, and personal expressions of emotions Help parents understand their child's reactions to death/dying, especially that concern for present crises, such as loss of hair, may be much greater than for future ones, including possible death.

their child. Parents may require professional support and guidance in this process from a nurse, social worker, or child life specialist who has a good relationship with the child and family.

If given the opportunity, children will tell others how much they want to know. Asking questions such as "If the disease came back, would you want to know?"; "Do you want others to tell you everything, even if the news isn't good?"; or "If someone were not getting better (or more directly, 'were dying'), do you think he would want to know?" helps children set the limits of how much truth they can accept and cope with. Children need time to process many feelings and much information so that they can assimilate and hopefully accept the inevitable fact of mortality.

Treatment Options for Terminally Ill Children. On the basis of the outcome of the decision by the child and family regarding their wishes for care, there are several options for care that the family may choose.

Hospital. Families may choose to remain in the hospital to receive care if the child's illness or condition is unstable and home care is not an option or if the family is uncomfortable with providing care at home. If a family chooses to remain at the hospital for terminal care, the setting should be made as homelike as possible. Families should be encouraged to bring familiar items from the child's room at home. In addition, there should be a consistent and coordinated plan of care for the child's and family's comfort.

Home Care. Some families may prefer to take their child home and receive services from a home care agency. Generally these services entail periodic nursing visits to administer a treatment or provide medications, equipment, or supplies. The child's care continues to be directed by the primary physician. Home care is often the option chosen by physicians and families because of the traditional view that a child must be considered to have a life expectancy of less than 6 months to be referred to hospice care. Fortunately a number of hospice organizations are expanding their services to children based on the presence of a life-limiting disease process for which cure is not possible, rather than on the sole criteria of a limited 6-month prognosis.

Hospice Care. During the final phases of an illness, parents should be offered the option of caring for their child at home with the assistance of a hospice organization. Hospice is a community health care organization that specializes in the care of dying patients by combining the hospice philosophy with the principles of palliative care. Hospice philosophy regards dying as a natural process and care of dying patients as including management of the physical, psychologic, social, and spiritual needs of the patient and family.* Collaboration between the child's primary treatment team and the hospice care team is essential to the success of hospice care. Families may continue to see their primary care physicians as they choose.

Hospice care is based on a number of important concepts that significantly set it apart from hospital care. First, family members are the principal caregivers and are supported by a team of professional and volunteer staff. Second, the priority of care is comfort. The child's physical, psychologic, social, and spiritual needs are considered. Pain and symptom control are primary concerns, and no extraordinary efforts are used to attempt a cure or prolong life. Third, the needs of the family are considered to be as important as those of the patient. Fourth, hospice is concerned with the family's postdeath adjustment, and care may continue for a year or more.

The goal of hospice care is for children to live life to the fullest without pain, with choices and dignity, in the familiar environment of their home, and with the support of their family. Hospice care is covered under state Medicaid programs, as well as by most insurance plans. Medications, medical equipment, and any necessary medical supplies are provided by the hospice organization providing care.

For children the home has been the more common environment for implementing the hospice concept; it benefits the family in a variety of ways. Children who are dying are allowed the opportunity to remain with those they love and with whom they feel secure. Many children who were thought to be in imminent danger of death have gone home and lived longer than expected. Siblings can feel more involved in the care and often have more positive perceptions of the death. Parental adaptation is often more favorable, as is shown by their perceptions of how the experience at home affected their marriage, social reorientation, religious beliefs, and views on the meaning of life and death.

*National Hospice and Palliative Care Organization, 1700 Diagonal Rd., Suite 300, Arlington, VA 22314; (703) 243-5900; fax (703) 525-5762; website: www.no.org; and Children's Hospice International, Alexandra, VA 22301; (703) 684-0330 or 1-800-24-CHILD; fax (703) 684-0226; website: www.chionline.org.

NURSING CARE OF THE CHILD AND FAMILY AT THE END OF LIFE

Regardless of where the child is cared for during the terminal stage of illness, both the child and the family usually experience the following fears: (1) fear of pain and suffering, (2) fear of dying alone (child) or of not being present when the child dies (parent), and (3) fear of actual death. Nurses can assist families by lessening their fears through attention to the care needs of the child and family (Nursing Care Plan).

Fear of Pain and Suffering

Pain/Symptom Management. Pain control for children in the terminal stages of illness or injury must be given the highest priority. Despite ongoing efforts to educate physicians and nurses on pain management strategies in children, studies have reported that children continue to be undermedicated for their pain (Wolfe et al, 2000). Nearly all children experience some amount of pain in the terminal phase of their illness. The current standard for treating children's pain is according to the World Health Organization's analgesic stepladder (1990). This approach promotes tailoring the pain interventions to the child's level of reported pain. Children's pain should be assessed often, and medications adjusted as necessary. Pain medications should be given on a regular schedule, and extra doses for "breakthrough pain" should be available to maintain comfort. Opioid drugs such as morphine should be given for severe pain, and the dose should be increased as necessary to maintain optimum pain relief. Techniques such as distraction, relaxation techniques, and guided imagery (Lambert, 1999) should be combined with drug therapy to provide the child and family with strategies to control pain (see Chapter 44 for further discussion of pain management strategies).

In addition to pain, children experience a variety of additional symptoms during their terminal course as a result of their disease process or as a side effect of medicines used to manage pain or other symptoms. These symptoms include fatigue, nausea and vomiting, constipation, anorexia, dyspnea, congestion, seizures, anxiety, depression, restlessness, agitation, and confusion (Wolfe et al, 2000). Each of these symptoms should be managed aggressively with appropriate medications or treatments, as well as with interventions such as repositioning, relaxation, massage, and other measures to maintain the child's comfort and quality of life.

Occasionally children require very high doses of opioids to control pain. There are several reasons this occurs. The child receiving long-term opioid pain management can become *tolerant* of the drug, meaning that it is necessary to give more drug to maintain the same level of pain relief. This should not be confused with *addiction,* which is a psychologic dependence on the side effects of opioids. Addiction is not a factor in managing terminal pain in children. Other obvious reasons for requiring increased doses of opioids include progression of disease and other physiologic experiences of pain. It is important to understand that there is no maximum dose that can be given to con-

Nursing Care Plan THE CHILD WHO IS TERMINALLY ILL OR DYING

NURSING DIAGNOSIS Anticipatory grieving related to terminal illness/impending death

EXPECTED OUTCOME Child will participate in age-appropriate constructive anticipatory grief work and will exhibit free expression of feelings.

Nursing Interventions/*Rationales*

Encourage children to express feelings in own way through play, drawing, or verbalization *to promote free expression in accordance with their specific cognitive and emotional abilities.*

Provide a safe, acceptable outlet for expressions of feelings (e.g., crying, sadness, anger, aggression) *as this is needed part of grieving process.*

Structure the care experience to allow child choices and participation in process within constraints of physical condition *to help child maintain a sense of control and self-esteem.*

Encourage family to remain near child and to stay engaged with child *to provide support and to allay child's fear of being abandoned or no longer being loved.*

NURSING DIAGNOSIS Pain related to terminal stage of illness

EXPECTED OUTCOME Child will exhibit minimal signs of physical discomfort.

Nursing Interventions/*Rationales*

Provide and encourage family to provide the child's favorite comfort measures (e.g., rocking, stroking, storytelling, singing); move and turn carefully; avoid excessive noise or light; use noninvasive care monitoring when possible; limit care to essentials *to minimize discomfort and promote comfort.*

Administer treatments as prescribed (e.g., oxygen *for respiratory distress,* anticonvulsants *for seizures,* analgesics *for pain,* anticholinergics *to decrease secretions*) that can cause unpleasant manifestations.

Talk with child in clear, distinct voice *to offer calm reassurance;* avoid whispering or talking about child *to reduce anxiety;* phrase questions to require "yes" or "no" responses *to conserve energy.*

NURSING DIAGNOSIS Anticipatory grieving related to impending loss of a child

EXPECTED OUTCOME Family will exhibit evidence of constructive grief process (verbalization/expression of feelings, maintenance of interpersonal relationships, use of support systems and coping mechanisms).

Nursing Interventions/*Rationales*

Spend time with family to listen, answer questions, provide information *as a way to establish trust, demonstrate support and caring.*

Provide opportunities for family to express their emotions and deal with their feelings *as a part of the grieving process.*

Help family to understand the grief process and to accept feelings being experienced (denial, sadness, guilt, anger, relief) as normal part of the process *to enhance understanding and ability to cope.*

Encourage expression and discussion of perceptions of loss and the impact on life of the family *to provide ventilation and reinforcement of reality.*

Keep family informed of child's status, help them interpret child's responses, and encourage their participation in child's care *to allay fears and anxiety and promote involvement.*

Encourage parents to face child's fears and questions about death openly and honestly *to facilitate grief work by child and parents.*

Explore family religious and cultural beliefs related to death (e.g., prayers, rites, rituals) and arrange for appropriate spiritual care if appropriate.

Emphasize family's identified strengths and provide encouragement for decisions that demonstrate effective coping skills *to help reinforce ability to cope.*

When death is imminent, allow the family privacy and time to be with and hold, touch, and/or talk to the child *to facilitate saying goodbye.*

At death, allow family to remain with child's body for as long as they wish, to rock, hold, bathe or talk with child *to facilitate grieving.*

Be physically present with the family, offer nonverbal comfort, touch if appropriate; help them move through the process of leaving the facility (e.g., gathering belongings, checking out) *to provide supportive presence and guidance in next steps.*

Determine support sources (e.g., relatives, friends, church, community) and how they can help with disruptions that occur in lifestyle (e.g., arrangements, activities of daily living, finances, transportation) *to bolster coping and provide needed support during crisis.*

Refer family to grief counseling if indicated *to aid in coping and to prevent dysfunctional grieving.*

Initiate and maintain contact, attend the funeral, visitation, or memorial service if there was a special closeness with family *to facilitate grief process and termination of therapeutic relationship with caregiver.*

trol pain. However, nurses often express concern that administering doses of opioids that exceed what they are familiar with will hasten the child's death. The principle of double effect addresses such concerns. It provides an ethical standard that supports the use of interventions that have the intention of relieving pain and suffering even though there is a foreseeable possibility that death may be hastened (Siever, 1994). However, in cases where the child is terminally ill and in severe pain, use of large doses of opioids and sedatives to manage pain is justified when no other treatment options are available that would re-

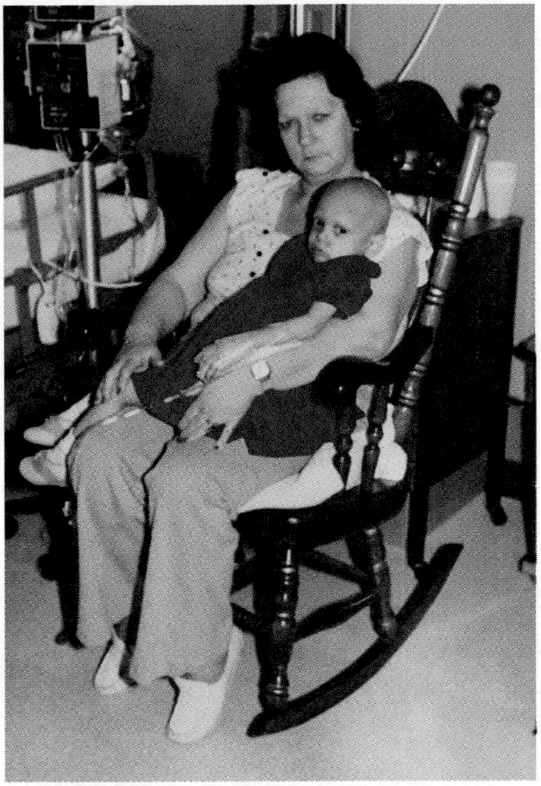

FIG. 41-5 • For the dying child there is no greater comfort than the security and closeness of a parent.

lieve the pain but make the risk of death less likely (Fleischman, 1998). See Chapter 44 for an extensive discussion of pain assessment and management.

Fear of Dying Alone or of Not Being Present When the Child Dies

When a child is being cared for at home, the burden of care experienced by parents and family members can be great. Often, as the child's condition declines, family members begin a "death vigil." Rarely is a child left alone for any length of time. This can be very exhausting for family members, and nurses can help the family by arranging "shifts" so that friends or family members can be present with the child and allow others to rest. If the family has limited resources, community organizations such as hospice or churches often have volunteers who are willing to visit and sit with children. It is important that whoever is sitting with the child be aware of when the parents would like to be notified to return to the child's bedside (Fig. 41-5, Box 41-5).

When a child is dying in the hospital, parents should be given full access to the child at all times. If parents need to leave, they should be provided with a pager or other means of immediate communication and alerted if staff members note any change in the child's condition that may indicate imminent death. Nurses should advocate for the parents' presence in the intensive care and emergency departments and attend to the parents' needs for food, drinks, comfortable chairs, blankets, and pillows.

Box 41-5

Physical Signs of Approaching Death

- Loss of sensation and movement in the lower extremities, progressing toward the upper body
- Sensation of heat, although body feels cool
- Loss of senses:
  - Tactile sensation decreases
  - Sensitive to light
  - Hearing is last sense to fail
- Confusion, loss of consciousness, slurred speech
- Muscle weakness
- Loss of bowel and bladder control
- Decreased appetite/thirst
- Difficulty swallowing
- Change in respiratory pattern:
  - Cheyne-Stokes respirations (waxing and waning of depth of breathing with regular periods of apnea)
  - "Death rattle" (noisy chest sounds from accumulation of pulmonary and pharyngeal secretions)
- Weak, slow pulse; decreased blood pressure

Grief and Mourning

The crisis of loss does not end with the child's death. In many ways it only begins. Unfortunately the child's death often marks the close of the family's contacts with health professionals involved in the care. Consequently many of these families never receive the support and guidance that could assist them in resolving the loss. Fortunately, hospice programs recognize this need and provide regular follow-up after the death.

When death is the expected or possible outcome of a disorder, the child and family members experience the behavioral reactions of anticipatory grief. Anticipatory grief may be manifested in varying behaviors and intensities and may include denial, anger, depression, and other psychologic and somatic symptoms.

When death occurs—whether expected or unexpected—acute grief develops within hours to days. Acute grief is a definite syndrome with psychologic and somatic symptoms that cause intense distress. Anticipatory guidance may assist grieving family members. Health professionals should emphasize that grief reactions such as hearing the dead person's voice, feeling distant from others, or seeking reassurance that they did everything possible for the lost person are normal, necessary, and expected. They in no way signify poor coping, insanity, or an approaching mental breakdown. On the contrary, such behaviors signify that the survivor is working through the acute grief. They are a necessary part of satisfactory resolution of the loss. These reactions are part of the process of resuming or restructuring a meaningful role in the social environment.

After the death, the lengthy process of grief work or mourning begins and extends into a period of adjustment to the loss, with eventual attachment to new persons and the development of new interests. Contrary to the common belief that mourning is completed in a year, research indicates that resolution of grief may take years and that there may be an *intensification* of grief during the early years. The time since a child's death is not necessarily a factor in reducing the intensity of grief for families (Davis and Eng, 1998). Anticipatory guidance regarding the mourning process may be helpful to families so that they can recognize the normalcy of their experiences.

It is important to recognize that some family members may experience "complicated" grief. Complicated grief reactions (more than a year after the loss) include such symptoms as intense intrusive thoughts, pangs of severe emotion, distressing yearnings, feeling excessively alone and empty, unusual sleep disturbance, and maladaptive levels of loss of interest in personal activities (Horowitz et al, 1997). Bereaved persons experiencing such prolonged and complicated grief should be referred to an expert in grief and bereavement counseling.

A child's death can also challenge the marital relationship in several ways. Maternal and paternal reactions often differ (Birenbaum et al, 1996; Moriarty et al, 1996; Vance et al, 1995). Different grieving styles between the couple may hinder communication and support for each other. Differing needs and expectations can place a strain on the marriage.

At times family members may need assistance in their grieving. Mothers in particular often feel a great sense of loneliness and emptiness, and part of their resolving the grief is finding a substitute role that is fulfilling and rewarding. Nurses can be instrumental in this process by (1) preparing the mother for anticipating the *normal* feelings of emptiness, loneliness, and sometimes even failure; (2) helping her reevaluate her role as parent and spouse, stressing that giving up the lost child must occur before she can reestablish emotional relationships; (3) encouraging her to explore fulfilling activities that utilize her special interests, talents, and qualifications; and (4) supporting her as her role changes, particularly assisting with communication between affected family members.

Nurses should also be aware of behaviors that indicate siblings' difficulty with resolving their grief, such as persistent blame and guilt, patterns of overactivity with aggressive and destructive outbursts, compulsive caregiving, persistent anxieties (e.g., fear of another family death or of their own), excessive clinging to the parent, difficulty with forming new relationships, problems at school, or delinquency (e.g., stealing). Providing anticipatory guidance to parents regarding behaviors to watch for may be helpful. Even siblings as young as 2 years of age can experience survivor guilt (Gibbons, 1992). In these situations professional assistance may be required, and the nurse can provide appropriate referral.

Communication with the bereaved family is essential, but often there is a feeling of not knowing what to say and of helplessness in offering words of comfort. The most supportive approach is to avoid judging the family's reactions or offering advice or rationalizations and to focus on feelings. Perhaps the most valuable supportive measure the nurse can perform for families is to listen. Families understand that no words will relieve their pain; all they want is acceptance, understanding, and respect for their grief. A plan for regular follow-up with bereaved families can be beneficial.

It is important for families to understand that mourning takes a long time. Whereas acute grief may last only weeks or months, resolving the loss is measured in years. Holidays and anniversaries can be particularly difficult, and persons who previously had been supportive may now expect the family to have "adjusted." Consequently, prolonged mourning is often silent and lonely.

Many families never receive the support and guidance that could help them resolve the loss. At a minimum, one follow-up phone call or meeting with the family should be arranged. Families can also be referred to self-help groups. When such groups are not available, nurses can be instrumental in networking families or facilitating parent and sibling groups. Formal bereavement programs or bereavement counseling can be helpful as well.

For more information on end-of-life care, visit these websites:

Americans for Better Care of the Dying
www.abcd_caring.com
City of Hope Pain/Palliative Care Resources Center
mayday.coh.org
End-of-Life Physician Education Resource Center
www.eperc.mcw.edu
Growth House
www.growthhouse.org
Last Acts
www.lastacts.org

Key Points

- Trends in the treatment of children with chronic illness or disability have focused on developmental age, the child's strengths and uniqueness, family-centered care, establishment of normalization, early discharge, home care, mainstreaming, and early intervention.
- In response to the child with chronic illness or disability, parents may be affected by feelings of inadequacy and failure; excessive demands on time, energy, and financial resources; and strain on the marital relationship.
- Families' reactions to disability or chronic illness are manifested in the following stages: shock and denial, adjustment, reintegration, and acknowledgment.
- The child's reaction to illness or disability depends on the child's developmental level, coping mechanisms, others' reactions, and the illness itself.
- Assessment of the family's adjustment to a child's chronic illness, disability, or death includes the availability of a support system, their perception of the event, their coping mechanisms, concurrent stressors, and their response to the child.
- To help parents cope with their child's chronic illness or disability, nurses must offer attentiveness, humanistic support, solicitation of suggestions for care, facilitation of communication, verbalization of feelings, and referral to volunteer and community agencies.
- Supporting the child involves encouraging self-expression, alleviating feelings of being different, and strengthening the child's self-image.
- Children's concept of death is determined by their cognitive ability and their experience with life-threatening illness.
- Young children see death as temporary and reversible and mainly fear separation.
- School-age children view death as irreversible but not necessarily inevitable and may fear mutilation.
- Children older than 9 to 10 years realize that death is irreversible, universal, and inevitable but may resist the thought of their own death.

- Siblings have special needs, including the need for information, reassurance about their own health status, assurance that they are not responsible for the illness or death, and support for their own grieving process.
- Special needs of the family facing the unexpected death of a child include support while awaiting news of the child's status; a sensitive pronouncement of death; acknowledgment of feelings of denial, guilt, and anger; an opportunity to view the body; closure; and referrals for support.
- Special decisions at the time of dying and death may involve hospital or hospice care, the child's right to die, visualization of the body, tissue donation and autopsy, and siblings' attendance at the funeral.
- Acute grief is a syndrome with intense and distressing psychologic and somatic symptoms that appear at the time of death.
- Mourning is a prolonged, painful process that consists of four phases: shock and disbelief, expression of grief, disorganization and despair, and reorganization.
- In dealing with stress related to the dying patient, the nurse can cope successfully through self-awareness, consciousness raising, knowledge and practice, an available support system, and maintenance of general good health, and by focusing on the positive rewards of involvement with dying children and their families.

References

Ahmann E: "Chunky stew": appreciating cultural diversity while providing health care for children, *Pediatr Nurs* 20(3):320-324, 1994.

American Academy of Pediatrics, Committee on Children with Disabilities: Managed care and children with special health care needs: a subject review, *Pediatrics* 102(3):657-660, 1998.

American Nurses Association: *Position statement: assisted suicide* (on-line). Available at www.ana.org/readroom/position/ehtics/etscuic.htm.

Austin J, Patterson J, Huberty T: Development of the Coping Health Inventory for Children, *J Pediatr Nurs* 6(3):166-174, 1991.

Baker NA: Avoiding collisions with challenging families, *MCN* 19:97-101, 1994.

Billings JA: What is palliative care? *J Palliat Med* 1(1):73-81, 1998.

Birenbaum LK et al: Health status of bereaved parents, *Nurs Res* 45(2):105-109, 1996.

Bishop KK, Woll J, Arango P: *Family/professional collaboration for children with special health care needs,* Burlington, 1993, Department of Social Work, University of Vermont.

Breitmayer BJ et al: Social competence of school age children with chronic illnesses, *J Pediatr Nurs* 17(3):181-188, 1992.

Burns CE, Madian N: Experiences with a upport group for grandparents of children with disabilities, *Pedatr Nurs* 18(1):17, 1992.

Cayse LN: Fathers of children with cancer: a descriptive study of their stressors and coping strategies, *J Pediatr Oncol Nurs* 11(3):102-108, 1994.

Clements D, Copeland L, Loftus M: Critical times for families with a chronically ill child, *Pediatr Nurs* 16(2):157-161, 224, 1990.

Cohen MH: The stages of the prediagnostic period in chronic life-threatening childhood illness: a process analysis, *Res Nurs Health* 18(1):39-48, 1995.

Davis B, Eng B: Special issues in bereavement and staff support. In Doyle D, Hanks GWC, MacDonald N, editors: *Oxford textbook of palliative medicine,* ed 2, Oxford, 1998, Oxford.

Derouin D, Jessee PO: Impact of chronic illness in childhood: siblings' perceptions, *Issues Compr Pediatr Nurs* 19(2):135-147, 1996.

Faulkner MS: Family responses to children with diabetes and their influence on self-care, *J Pediatr Nurs* 11(2):82-93, 1996.

Ferrell BR et al: The experience of pediatric cancer pain. I. Impact of pain on the family, *J Pediatr Nurs* 9(6):368-379, 1994.

Fleischman AR: Commentary: ethical issues in pediatric pain management and terminal sedation, *J Pain Symptom Manage* 15(4):260-261, 1998.

Garmezy N: Resilience in children's adaptation to negative life events and stressed environments, *Pediatr Ann* 20(9):459-466, 1991.

Garwick AW et al: Breaking the news: how families first learn about their child's chronic condition, *Arch Pediatr Adolesc Med* 149(9):991-997, 1995.

Gibbons MB: A child dies, a child survives: the impact of sibling loss, *J Pediatr Health Care* 6(2):65-72, 1992.

Gibson CH: The process of empowerment in mothers of chronically ill children, *J Adv Nurs* 21(6):1201-1210, 1995.

Gravelle AM: Caring for a child with a progressive illness during the complex chronic phase: parents' experience of facing adversity, *J Adv Nurs* 25:738-745, 1997.

Groce NE, Zola IK: Multiculturalism, chronic illness, and disability, *Pediatrics* 91(5):1048-1055, 1993.

Heaman DJ: Perceived stressors and coping strategies of parents who have children with disabilities: a comparison of mothers with fathers, *J Pediatr Nurs* 10(5):311-320, 1995.

Hinds PS et al: Decision making by parents and healthcare professionals when considering continued care for pediatric patients with cancer, *Oncol Nurs Forum* 24(9):1523-1528, 1997.

Horowitz et al: Diagnostic criteria for complicated grief disorder, *Am J Psychiatry* 154(7):904-910, 1997.

Huber C, Holditch-Davis D, Brandon D: High risk preterm infants at 3 years of age: parental response to the presence of developmental problems, *Child Health Care* 22(2):107, 124, 1993.

James L, Johnson B: The needs of parents of pediatric oncology patients during the palliative care phase, *J Pediatr Oncol Nurs* 14(2):83-95, 1997.

Kelly BR: Cultural considerations in Cambodian childrearing, *J Pediatr Health Care* 10(1):2-9, 1996.

Kirschbaum MS: Advances in nursing science, *Adv Nurs Sci* 19(1):51-71, 1996.

Kuhlthau K et al: Assessing managed care for children with chronic conditions, *Health Aff* 17(4):42-52, 1998.

Lambert S: Distraction, imagery, and hypnosis techniques for management of children's pain, *J Child Fam Nurs* 2(1):5-15, 1999.

Lipson M: What do you say to a child with AIDS? *Hastings Cent Rep* 23(2):6-12, 1993.

Lock J: Psychosexual development in adolescents with chronic medical illness, *Psychosomatics* 39(4):340-349, 1998.

Mastroyannopoulou K et al: The impact of childhood nonmalignant life threatening illness on parents: gender differences and predictors of parental adjustment, *J Child Psychol Psychiatry* 38(7):823-829, 1997.

May J: Fathers: the forgotten parent, *Pediatr Nurs* 22(3):243-246, 271, 1996.

Moriarty H et al: Differences in bereavement reactions within couples following the death of a child, *Res Nurs Health* 19: 461-469, 1996.

Newacheck PW, Halfon N: Prevalence and impact of disabling chronic conditions in childhood, *Am J Public Health* 88(4):610-617, 1998.

Newacheck PW, McManus MA, Fox HB: Prevalence and impact of chronic illness among adolescents, *Am J Dis Child* 145(12):1367-1373, 1991.

Newacheck PW, Stoddard JJ, McManus M: Ethnocultural variations in the prevalence and impact of childhood chronic conditions, *Pediatrics* 91(5):1031-1039, 1993.

Newacheck PW et al: An epidemiologic profile of children with special health care needs, *Pediatrics* 102(1):117-123, 1998.

Peters KD, Kochanek KD, Murphy SL: Deaths: final data for 1996, *National Vital Statistics Report* 47(9):1-100, 1998.

Quittner AL et al: Role strain in couples with and without a child with a chronic illness: associations with marital satisfaction, intimacy, and daily mood, *Health Psychol* 17(2):112-124, 1998.

Satariano HJ, Briggs NJ: The good family syndrome, *Pediatr Nurs* 15(3):285-286, 1989.

Savinetti-Rose B: Developmental issues in managing children with diabetes, *Pediatr Nurs* 20(1):11-15, 1994.

Scher A, Ahmann E: Community resources for the family. In Ahmann E, editor: *Home care for the high risk infant: a family centered approach,* Gaithersburg, MD, 1996, Aspen.

Siegel RD: Child care and the ADA, *Except Parent* 25(2):34, 1995.

Siever BA: Pain management and potentially life-shortening analgesia in the terminally ill child: the ethical implications for pediatric nurses, *J Pediatr Nurs* 9(5):307-312, 1994.

Stein REK: Home care: a challenging opportunity, *Child Health Care* 14(2):90-95, 1985.

Turner-Henson A et al: The experiences of discrimination challenges for chronically ill children, *Pediatr Nurs* 20(6):571-577, 1994.

Vance JC et al: Psychological changes in parents eight months after the loss of an infant from stillbirth, neonatal death, or sudden infant death syndrome—a longitudinal study, *Pediatrics* 96(5):933-938, 1995.

Wolfe J et al: Symptoms and suffering at the end of life in children with cancer, *N Engl J Med* 342(5):326-333, 2000.

World Health Organization: *Cancer pain relief and palliative care: report of a WHO expert committee,* Geneva, Switzerland, 1990, WHO.

Yoos HL: Children's illness concepts: old and new paradigms, *Pediatr Nurs* 20(2):134-140, 1994.

Yoos HL et al: Child rearing beliefs in the African-American community: implications for culturally-competent pediatric care, *J Pediatr Nurs* 10(8):343-353, 1995.

*Resources on Death for Children**

Armstrong-Dailey A: *Hospice for children,* New York, 1996, Oxford University Press.

Bowden VR: Children's literature: the death experience, *Pediatr Nurs* 19(1):17-21, 32-33, 1993.

Delisle R, McNamee A: Children's perceptions of death: a look at the appropriateness of selected picture books, *Death Educ* 5:1-13, 1981.

Fitzgerald H: *The grieving child: a parent's guide,* New York, 1992, Simon & Schuster.

Seibert D, Drolet JO: Death themes in literature for children ages 3-8, *J Sch Health* 63(2):86-90, 1993.

Wass H: Books for children, *Issues Compr Pediatr Nurs* 8(1-6): 373-376, 1985.

Wass H, Corr C, editors: *Helping children cope with death: guidelines and resources,* ed 2, Washington, DC, 1984, Hemisphere.

FOR VERY YOUNG CHILDREN

Anderson JS: *The key into winter,* illustrated by D. Soman, Morton Grove, IL, 1994, Albert Whitman Prairie Books.

Bahr M: *The memory box,* illustrated by D. Cunningham, Morton Grove, IL, 1992, Albert Whitman Prairie Books.

Brown LK, Brown M: *When dinosaurs die: a guide to understanding death,* Boston, 1996, Little, Brown.

Buscaglia L: *The fall of Freddie the Leaf,* Thorofare, NJ, 1982, Slack.

Leighton AO: *A window of time,* illustrated by R. Kyrias, Lake Forest, CA, 1995, Nadja Publishing.

Mellonie B, Ingpen R: *Lifetimes: the beautiful way to explain death to children,* New York, 1993, Bantam Books.

Viorst J: *The tenth good thing about Barney,* illustrated by E. Blevgard, New York, 1971, Aladdin Paperbacks.

Whitbold M: Mending Peter's heart, illustrated by L. Salk, Santa Monica, CA, 1995, Portunus Publishing.

FOR OLDER CHILDREN

Beckleman L: *Grief,* New York, 1995, Crestwood House (A Hotline Book).

Durant PR: *When heroes die,* New York, 1992, Atheneum.

Hipp E: *Help for the hard times: getting through loss,* illustrated by L.K. Hanson, Center City, MN, 1995, Hazelden.

Kuklin S: *After a suicide: young people speak up,* New York, 1994, GP Putnam's Sons.

Liss-Levinson N: *When a grandparent dies: a kid's own workbook for remembering Shiva and the year beyond,* Woodstock, NY, 1995, Jewish Lights Publishing.

*Other sources of publications on life-threatening illness and death are The Compassionate Friends, P.O. Box 3696, Oak Brook, IL 60522-3696; (630) 990-0010; e-mail: TCF_National@progidy.com; Centering Corporation, 1531 N. Saddle Creek Rd., Omaha, NE 68104; (402) 533-1200; website: www.centering.org; Children's Hospice International, 2202 Mt. Vernon Ave., Suite 3-C, Alexandria, VA 22314; 1-800-24-CHILD; e-mail: chiorg@aol.com; website: www.chionline.org; and National Cancer Institute, Cancer Information Service, Building 21, Room 10A29, Bethesda, MD 20892-2580; 1-800-422-6237.

CHAPTER 42

Cognitive and Sensory Impairment

http://www.harcourthealth.com/MERLIN/Wong/maternal/

Learning Objectives

On completion of this chapter the reader will be able to:

- Define the classifications of mental retardation.
- Outline nursing interventions for the child with cognitive impairment that promote optimum development, including during hospitalization.
- Identify the major biologic and cognitive characteristics of the child with Down syndrome.
- Outline nursing interventions for the child with Down syndrome.
- Identify the major characteristics associated with fragile X syndrome.
- List the general classifications of hearing impairment and the effect on speech.
- Outline nursing interventions for the child with hearing impairment, including during hospitalization.
- List the common types of visual disorders in children.
- Outline nursing interventions for the child with visual impairment, including during hospitalization.
- Outline nursing interventions for the child with retinoblastoma.

COGNITIVE IMPAIRMENT

General Concepts

Cognitive impairment is a general term that encompasses any type of mental difficulty or deficiency. In this chapter the term is used synonymously with *mental retardation (MR).* Although the needs and concerns of the family are a primary focus throughout the chapter, the reader is encouraged to review Chapter 41, which details the family's adjustment to disabilities in general.

The definition of MR in children is made up of three components that assess intellectual functioning, functional strengths and weaknesses, and age at time of diagnosis (e.g., less than 18 years of age). Intellectual functioning is measured by the intelligence quotient (IQ), which is found to be 70 to 75 or below. Deficits in functional behaviors are defined by strengths and weaknesses in 10 different adaptive skill areas: communication, self-care, home living, social skills, leisure, health and safety, self-direction, functional academics, community use, and work (Fredericks and Williams, 1998; Schalock et al, 1994). Defining MR in this way has led to the development of a classification system by the American Association of Mental Retardation (AAMR) that allows for identification of the individual's specific needs in each of four established dimensions of care. These dimensions are found in Box 42-1. Careful evaluation to identify the needs of individuals with MR is focused on promoting habilitation for each person. It is anticipated that the functional capabilities of children with MR will improve over time when support is provided.

Diagnosis and Classification. The diagnosis of MR is usually made after a period of suspicion, by professionals and/or the family, that the child's developmental progress is delayed. In some cases it is confirmed at birth because of recognition of distinct syndromes, such as Down syndrome. At the other extreme, the diagnosis is made after the child begins school, when problems such as speech delays arouse concern. In all cases a high index of suspicion for developmental delay and behavioral signs (Box 42-2) is necessary for early diagnosis, and routine developmental screening (see Chapter 35) can assist in early identification. Delays are typically seen in gross and fine motor and speech development, although the latter is most predictive.

Results of standardized tests are used in making the diagnosis of MR. The most commonly used IQ tests include the Stanford-Benet Test and Wechsler Intelligence Scale for Children—Revised (WISC-R). Tests for assessing adaptive behavior include the Vineland Social Maturity Scale and the AAMR Adaptive Behavior Scale. Informal appraisal of adaptive behavior may be made by those fully acquainted with the child

Box 42-1

Dimensions of Care for Mental Retardation

Dimension I	Intellectual functioning and adaptive skills
Dimension II	Psychologic/emotional considerations
Dimension III	Physical/health/etiology considerations
Dimension IV	Environmental considerations

Box 42-2

Early Behavioral Signs Suggestive of Cognitive Impairment

Nonresponsiveness to contact
Poor eye contact during feeding
Diminished spontaneous activity
Decreased alertness to voice or movement
Irritability
Slow feeding

From Crocker A, Nelson R: Mental retardation. In Levine M et al, editors: *Developmental-behavioral pediatrics,* Philadelphia, 1983, WB Saunders.

TABLE 42-1
Classifications of Mental Retardation

Level (IQ)*	Preschool (Birth-5 Years)—Maturation and Development	School Age (6-21 Years)—Training and Education	Adult (21 Years and Older)—Social and Vocational Adequacy
Mild: 50-55 to approximately 70	Often not noticed as retarded by casual observer but is slower to walk, feed self, and talk than most children; follows same sequence in development as normal children	Can acquire practical skills and useful reading and arithmetic to a third- to sixth-grade level with special education; can be guided toward social conformity; achieves mental age of 8-12 years	Can usually achieve social and vocational skills adequate to self-maintenance; may need occasional guidance and support when under unusual social or economic stress; can adjust to marriage but not childrearing
Moderate: 35-40 to 50-55	Noticeable delays in motor development, especially in speech; responds to training in various self-help activities	Can learn simple communication, elementary health and safety habits, and simple manual skills; does not progress in functional reading or arithmetic; achieves mental age of 3-7 years	Can perform simple tasks under sheltered conditions; participates in simple recreation; travels alone in familiar places; usually incapable of self-maintenance
Severe: 20-25 to 35-40	Marked delay in motor development; little or no communication skills; may respond to training in elementary self-care (e.g., self-feeding)	Usually walks, barring specific disability; has some understanding of speech and some response; can profit from systematic habit training; achieves mental age of toddler	Can conform to daily routines and repetitive activities; needs continuing direction and supervision in protective environment
Profound: less than 20-25	Gross retardation; minimum capacity for functioning in sensorimotor areas; needs total care	Obvious delays in all areas of development; shows basic emotional responses; may respond to skillful training in use of legs, hands, and jaws; needs close supervision; achieves mental age of young infant	May walk; needs complete custodial care; has primitive speech; usually benefits from regular physical activity

*Data from American Psychiatric Association: *Diagnostic and statistical manual of mental disorders,* ed 4 (DSM-IV), Washington, DC, 1994, The Association.

(e.g., teachers, parents, or other care providers). Often these observations lead parents to seek evaluation of the child's development.

A more useful approach for clinical application is classification based on educational potential or symptom severity. For educational purposes the terms *educable mentally retarded (EMR)* or *trainable mentally retarded (TMR)* may be used. EMR corresponds to the mildly retarded group, which constitutes about 85% of all people with MR. TMR generally applies to children with moderate levels of cognitive impairment and accounts for about 10% of the MR population (American Psychiatric Association, 1994) (Table 42-1). Although nurses may be familiar with the approximate range of IQ for classifying severity, they should refrain from using numbers as the criterion for assessing or evaluating the child's abilities, because numbers are of little value in counseling parents or training these children.

Etiology. The causes of severe MR are primarily genetic, biochemical, and infectious. Although the etiology is unknown in the majority of cases, familial, social, and environmental causes may predominate. Recent advances suggest that organic etiologies should not be prematurely ruled out (Palmer and Capute, 1994). General categories of events that may lead to retardation include (Camp et al, 1998; Gurrieri et al, 1999):

- Infection and intoxication, such as congenital rubella, syphilis, maternal drug consumption (e.g., excessive alcohol), chronic lead ingestion, or kernicterus
- Trauma or physical agent (i.e., injury to the brain suffered during the prenatal, perinatal, or postnatal period)
- Inadequate nutrition and metabolic disorders, such as phenylketonuria
- Gross postnatal brain disease, such as neurofibromatosis and tuberous sclerosis
- Unknown prenatal influence, including cerebral and cranial malformations, such as microcephaly and hydrocephalus
- Gestational disorders, including prematurity, low birth weight, and postmaturity
- Psychiatric disorders that have their onset during the child's developmental period up to age 18 years, such as autism
- Environmental influences, including evidence of a deprived environment associated with a history of MR among parents and siblings
- Chromosomal abnormalities, such as Down syndrome and fragile X syndrome

NURSING CARE OF CHILDREN WITH COGNITIVE IMPAIRMENT

➤ Assessment

Nurses play a major role in identifying children with cognitive impairment. In the newborn and early infancy period, few signs are present, with the exception of Down syndrome (p. 1041). After this age, however, delayed developmental milestones are the major clues to MR. In addition, nurses must have a high index of suspicion for early behavior patterns that may suggest cognitive impairment (see Box 42-2) and be aware of stereotypes that may delay diagnosis, such as "retarded children have to look dumb." Parental concerns, such as delayed development compared with siblings, need to be taken seriously. All children should receive regular developmental assessment, and the nurse is often the person responsible for performing such assessments (see Chapter 35). When delays are found, the nurse must use sensitivity and discretion in revealing this finding to parents.

➤ Nursing Diagnoses

A number of nursing diagnoses are prominent in the nursing care of the child with cognitive impairment and the child's family; other diagnoses specific to individual cases become evident. The most common nursing diagnoses are outlined in the Nursing Care Plan on p. 1042.

➤ Plan of Care and Implementation

The goals of nursing care for the child with MR and family are as follows:

1. Child will be educated using effective teaching strategies.
2. Child's optimum development will be promoted.
3. Child will learn self-care skills.
4. Family will plan for future care.
5. Child will be cared for appropriately during hospitalization.

Educate Child and Family. To teach children with cognitive impairment, it is necessary to investigate their learning abilities and deficits. This is important for the nurse who may be involved in a home care type of program or who may be caring for the child in a health care setting. The nurse who understands how these children learn can effectively teach them basic skills or prepare them for various health-related procedures.

Children with cognitive impairment have a marked deficit in their ability to discriminate between two or more stimuli because of difficulty in recognizing the relevance of specific cues. However, these children can learn to discriminate if the cues are presented in an exaggerated, concrete form and if all extraneous stimuli are eliminated. For example, the use of colors to emphasize visual cues or the use of singing or rhymes to stress auditory cues can help them learn. Their deficit in discrimination also implies that concrete ideas are learned much more effectively than abstract ideas. Therefore demonstration is preferable to verbal explanation, and learning should be directed toward mastering a skill rather than understanding the scientific principles underlying a procedure.

Another cognitive deficit is in short-term memory. Whereas children of average intelligence can remember several words, numbers, or directions at one time, these children are less able to do so. Therefore they need simple, one-step directions. Learning through a step-by-step process requires a *task analysis,* in which each task is separated into its necessary components and each step is taught completely before proceeding to the next activity.

One critical area of learning that has had a tremendous impact on education for cognitively impaired individuals is *motivation.* Programs based on the motivational principles of behavior modification (i.e., employing positive reinforcement for specific tasks or behaviors) have demonstrated marked improvement in children's ability to learn. Advances in technology have greatly aided in providing reinforcement, especially in children who are severely retarded and who may have physical disabilities that limit their range of capabilities. For example, with the use of specially designed switches, children are given control of some event in the environment, such as turning on the television. The television picture becomes reinforcement for activating the switch. Repetitive use of these switches provides an early, simplistic association with a technical device that may progress to increasingly more complex aids.

Early intervention programs have been widely promoted for children with developmental disabilities, and there is considerable evidence that these programs are valuable for cognitively impaired children. Nurses working with these families need to be aware of the types of programs in their community. Under Public Law 101-476, the Individuals with Disabilities Education Act of 1990, states are encouraged to provide full early intervention services and are required to provide educational opportunities for all children with disabilities from birth to 21 years of age. Services may be provided under state Programs for Children with Special Health Needs (formerly Crippled Children's Program) or Head Start, or by private organizations such as Easter Seals* or the Association of Retarded Citizens of the

*230 W. Monroe, Suite 1800, Chicago, IL 60606-4802; 1-800-221-6827; TTY: (312) 726-4258; fax (312) 726-1494; e-mail: info@easterseals.org; website: www.easter.seals.com.

United States.* Parents should inquire about these programs by contacting the appropriate agencies. The child's education should begin as soon as possible, not at 5 or 6 years of age. As children grow older, their education should be directed toward vocational training that prepares them for as independent a lifestyle as possible within their scope of abilities.

Teach Child Self-Care Skills. When a child with cognitive impairment is born, parents need assistance in promoting normal developmental skills that are almost automatically learned by other children. These include self-care skills such as feeding, toileting, dressing, and grooming. Teaching these skills requires a basic knowledge of the developmental sequence in learning the skills demonstrated by children of average intelligence. For example, children with subaverage intelligence would not be expected to dress themselves as early as unaffected youngsters.

Teaching self-care skills also necessitates a working knowledge of the individual steps needed to master a skill. For example, before beginning a self-feeding program, a task analysis is performed. After a task analysis, the child is observed in a particular situation, such as eating, to determine what skills are possessed and the child's developmental readiness to learn the task. Family members are included in this process because their readiness is as important as the child's is. Numerous self-help aids are available to facilitate independence and can be most helpful in eliminating some of the difficulties of learning, such as using a plate with suction cups to prevent accidental spills (Fig. 42-1).

Promote Child's Optimum Development. Optimum development involves more than achieving independence. It requires appropriate guidance for establishing acceptable social behavior and personal feelings of self-esteem, worth, and security. These attributes are not simply learned through a stimulation program; rather, they must arise from the genuine love and caring that exists among family members. However, families need guidance in providing an environment that fosters optimum development. Often it is the nurse who can provide assistance in these areas of childrearing.

Another important area for promoting optimum development and self-esteem is ensuring the child's physical well-being. Any congenital defects, such as cardiac, gastrointestinal, or orthopedic anomalies, should be repaired. Plastic surgery may be considered when the child's appearance may be substantially improved. Dental health is very significant, and orthodontic and restorative procedures can immensely improve facial appearance.

Play/Exercise. Children who are cognitively impaired have the same needs for recreation and exercise as other children. However, because of the child's slower development, parents may be less aware of the need to provide such activities. Therefore the nurse guides parents toward selection of suitable play and exercise activities. Because play has been discussed for children in each age group in earlier chapters, only the exceptions are presented here.

The type of play is based on the child's developmental age, although the need for sensorimotor play may be prolonged for several years. Parents should use every opportunity to expose the child to as many different sounds, sights, and sensations as possible. Appropriate play includes musical mobiles, stuffed toys, water play, floating toys, a rocking chair or horse, a swing, bells, and rattles. The child should be taken on outings, such as trips to the grocery store or shopping center; other people should be encouraged to visit in the home; and the child should be related to directly, such as by cuddling, holding, rocking, talking to the child in the *en face* (face-to-face) position, and giving "rides" on the parents' shoulders.

Toys are selected for their recreational and educational value. For example, a large inflatable beach ball is a good water toy; it encourages interactive play and can be used to learn motor skills, such as balance, rocking, kicking, and throwing. A doll with removable clothes and different types of closures can help the child learn dressing skills. Musical toys that mimic animal sounds or respond with social phrases are an excellent way of encouraging speech. Toys should be simple in design so that the child can learn to manipulate them without help. For children

*1010 Wayne Ave., Suite 650, Silver Spring, MD 20910 (301) 565-3842; fax (301) 565-5342; e-mail: Info@thearc.org; website: www.thearc.org. Information on early intervention programs in each state is available from the National Down Syndrome Society, 666 Broadway, Eighth Floor, New York, NY 10012-2317; 1-800-221-4602; fax (212) 979-2873; e-mail: info@ndss.org; website: www.ndss.org.

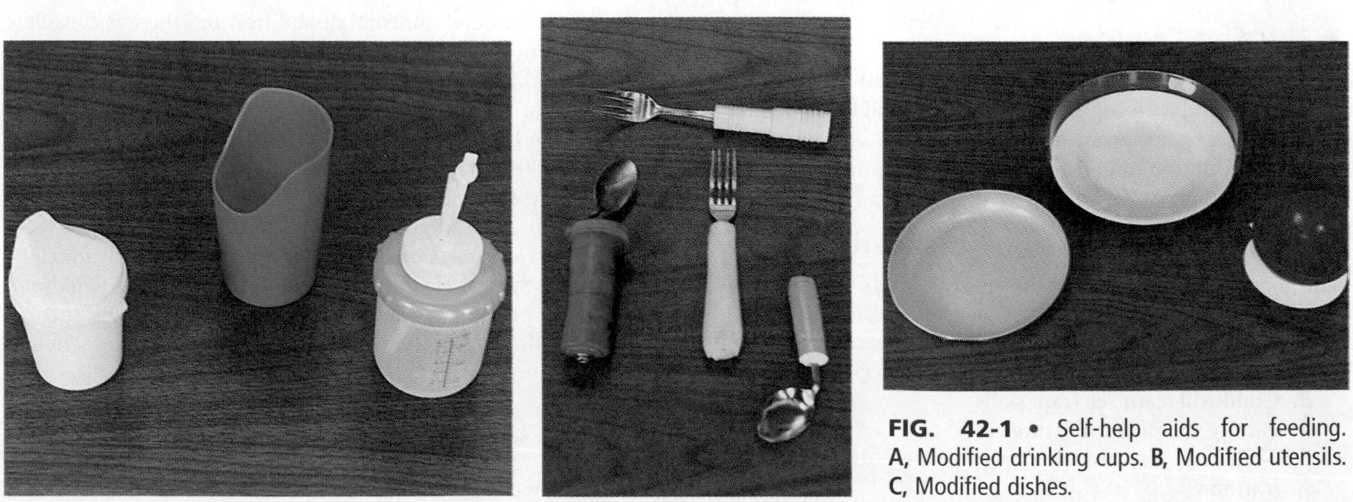

FIG. 42-1 • Self-help aids for feeding. **A,** Modified drinking cups. **B,** Modified utensils. **C,** Modified dishes.

with severe cognitive and physical impairment, electronic switches can be used to allow them to operate toys (Fig. 42-2).

Suitable activities for physical activity are based on the child's size, coordination, physical fitness and maturity, motivation, and health (Fig. 42-3). Some children may have physical problems, such as atlantoaxial instability in children with Down syndrome (p. 1041), that prevent certain sports. These children often have greater success in individual and dual sports than in team sports and enjoy themselves most with children of the same developmental level. The Special Olympics, Inc.* provides these children with a unique competitive opportunity.

Safety is a major consideration in selecting recreational and exercise activities. For example, toys that may be appropriate developmentally may present dangers to a child who is strong enough to break them or to use them incorrectly.

Communication. Verbal skills are typically delayed more than other physical skills. Speech requires hearing and interpretation *(receptive skills)* and facial muscle coordination *(expressive skills)*. Because both types of skills may be impaired, these children need frequent audiometric testing and should be fitted with hearing aids if this is indicated. In addition, they may need help in learning to control their facial muscles. For example, some children may need tongue exercises to correct the tongue thrust or gentle reminders to keep the lips closed.

Nonverbal communication may be appropriate for some of these children, and various devices are available. For the child without associated physical disabilities, a talking picture board is helpful. For children with physical limitations, several adaptations or types of communication devices are available to facilitate selection of the appropriate picture of word (Fig. 42-4). Some children may be taught sign language or *Blissymbols*—a highly stylized system of graphic symbols that represent words, ideas, and concepts. Although they require education to learn their meaning, no reading skill is needed. The symbols are usually arranged on a board, and the person points or uses some type of selector to convey a message.

Discipline. Discipline must begin early. Limit-setting measures need to be simple, consistently applied, and appropriate for the child's mental age. Control measures are based primarily on teaching a specific behavior rather than on understanding the

*1325 G Street NW, Suite 500, Washington, DC 20005; 1-800-700-8585 or (202) 628-3630; fax (202) 824-0200; website: www.specialolympics.org. (Website includes listing of state offices.) In Canada: Canadian Special Olympics, 40 St. Clair Ave. W, Suite 209, Toronto, Ontario M4V 1M2; (416) 927-9050; fax (416) 927-8475; e-mail: solympic@inforamp.net; website: www.cso.on.ca.

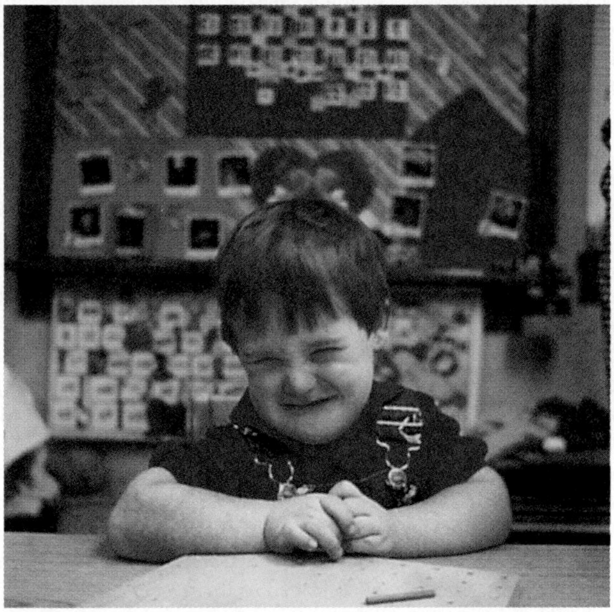

FIG. 42-3 • Play activities for children with cognitive impairments need to be appropriate for their abilities.

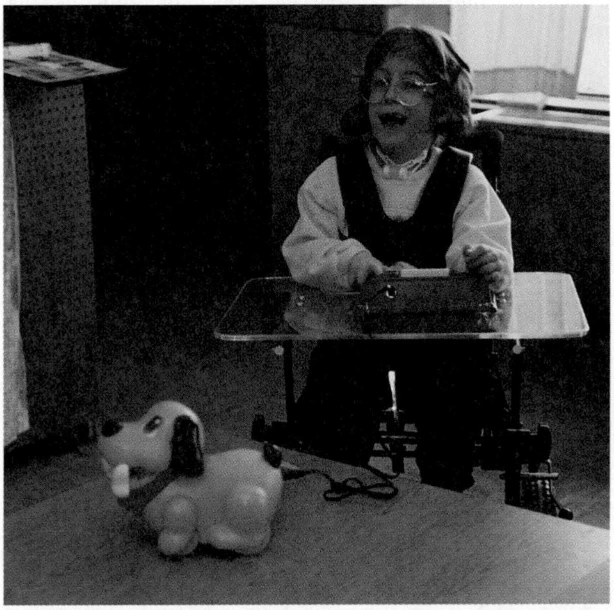

FIG. 42-2 • A manual switch allows a child with cognitive impairment to play with a battery-operated toy.

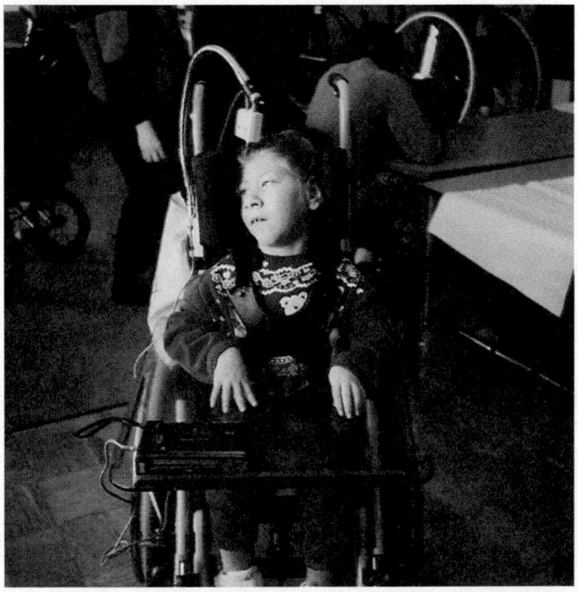

FIG. 42-4 • A child with cognitive and physical impairments can play a tape recorder by moving a device near her head.

reasons behind it. Stressing moral lessons is of little value to a child who lacks the cognitive skills to learn from self-criticism or from a lesson based on previous wrong-doing. Behavior modification, especially reinforcement of desired actions; and time-out are appropriate forms of behavior control.

Socialization. Acquiring social skills is a complex task, as is learning self-care procedures. Active rehearsal, with role-playing and practice sessions, and positive reinforcement for desired behavior have been the most successful approaches. Parents should be encouraged early to teach their child socially acceptable behavior: waving good-bye, saying "hello" and "thank you," responding to his or her name, greeting visitors but not being overly affectionate, and sitting modestly. The teaching of socially acceptable sexual behavior is especially important to minimize sexual exploitation. Parents also need to expose the child to strangers so that he or she can practice manners, because there is no automatic transfer of learning from one situation to another.

Dressing and grooming are also important aspects of socialization. A child who is dressed in age-appropriate clothing and is well groomed is much more likely to be accepted and to develop good self-esteem. Clothes should be clean, up-to-date, and well fitted. Many attractive outfits can be adapted with self-adhering fasteners and elastic openings to facilitate self-dressing.

Children of all ages need peer relationships, and these children are no exception. As soon as possible, parents should enroll the child in appropriate preschool programs. Not only do these programs provide education and training, but they also offer an opportunity for social experiences among the children. As children grow older, they should have peer experiences similar to those of other children, including group outings; sports; and organized activities such as Boy Scouts, Girl Scouts, or Special Olympics. They are encouraged to form a close relationship with a best friend.

Sexuality. Adolescence may be a particularly difficult time for the family, especially in terms of the child's sexual behavior, possibility of pregnancy, future plans to marry, and ability to be independent. Commonly, little anticipatory guidance has been offered parents to prepare the child for physical and sexual maturation. The nurse can help in this area by providing parents with information about sexuality education that is geared to the child's developmental level. For example, the adolescent female needs a *simple* explanation of menstruation and instructions on personal hygiene during the menstrual cycle.

These adolescents also need practical sexual information regarding anatomy, physical development, and conception.* Because of their easy persuasion and lack of judgment, they need a well-defined, concrete code of conduct. The subtleties of social sexual behavior are less beneficial than specific instructions for handling certain situations. For example, a girl should be firmly told never to go alone anywhere with any person she does not know well. A boy should be warned about intimate advances from other males. To protect him or her from abusive sexual activities, parents must closely observe their teenager's activities and associates.

The question of contraceptive protection for these female adolescents is often a parental concern. Permanent contraception through sterilization is a special dilemma because of moral and ethical questions, as well as the psychologic effects on the adolescent. State laws vary: some allow no sterilization, and others permit review of sterilization requests.

Parents of these adolescents are often very concerned about the advisability of marriage between two individuals with significant cognitive impairment. There is no conclusive answer: each situation must be judged individually. In some instances marriage is possible, but parenthood is usually not desirable because of the complexity of childrearing and the potential problem of perpetuating mental deficiency. The nurse should discuss this topic with parents and with the prospective couple, stressing suitable living accommodations and contraceptive methods to prevent pregnancy. If children are conceived, these parents require specialized assistance in learning to meet the needs of their offspring (Shaughnessy et al, 1996).

Help Family Adjust to Future Care. Not all families are able to cope with home care of their affected child, especially one who is severely or profoundly retarded and/or multidisabled. Older parents may not be able to assume care responsibilities once they reach retirement or old age. For these parents, the decision regarding residential placement is a difficult one, and the availability of such facilities varies widely. The nurse working with a family should help them investigate and evaluate various programs, in addition to assisting them in their adjustment to the decision for placement.

Care for Child During Hospitalization. Caring for the child during hospitalization can be a special challenge. Often, nurses are unfamiliar with children who are cognitively impaired, and they may cope with their feelings of insecurity and fear by ignoring or isolating the child. Not only is this approach nonsupportive, it may also be destructive for the child's sense of self-esteem and optimum development, and may hamper the parents' ability to cope with the stress of the experience. One method that successfully avoids this nontherapeutic approach is the use of the mutual participation model in planning the child's care. Parents are encouraged to room with their child but should not be made to feel as if the responsibility is totally theirs.

When the child is admitted, a detailed history is taken (see Chapter 35), especially in terms of all self-care activity. During the interview the child's development age is assessed. It is best to avoid directly asking about IQ levels, because this may make the parents uncomfortable and often tells little about the child's actual abilities. Questions are approached positively. For example, rather than asking, "Is your child toilet trained yet?" the nurse may state, "Tell me about your child's toileting habits." The assessment should also focus on any special devices the child uses, effective measures of limit setting, unusual or favorite routines, and any behaviors that may require intervention. For example, if the parent states that the child engages in self-stimulatory activities, the nurse inquires about events that precipitate them and techniques that the parents use to manage them.

The child's functional level of eating and playing; ability to express needs verbally; progress in toilet training; and relationship with objects, toys, and other children are also assessed. The child is encouraged to be as independent as possible in the hospital.

Realizing that the child may be lonely in the hospital, the nurse makes certain that toys and other activities are provided. The child is placed in a room with other children of approxi-

---

*Sources of information on sexuality and conception are the Association for Retarded Citizens of the United States (see footnote, p. 1038) and the Planned Parenthood Federation of America, 810 Seventh Ave., New York, NY 10019; (212) 541-7800 or 1-800-230-7526; fax (212) 245-1845; e-mail: communication@ppfa.org; website:plannedparenthood.org.

mate developmental age (preferably a room with two beds) to avoid overstimulation. The nurse discusses with the other parents the child's abilities, and introduces the parents and children to each other. By the nurse's example of treating the child with dignity and respect, others who may be fearful of what they do not understand are encouraged to accept the child.

Procedures are explained to the child through methods of communication that are at the appropriate cognitive level. Generally, explanations should be simple, short, and concrete, emphasizing what the child will experience *physically.* Demonstration either through actual practice or with visual aids is always preferable to verbal explanation. The nurse repeats instructions often and evaluates the child's understanding by asking questions such as "What will it feel like?" "What will the doctor look like?" "Show me how you must lie," or "Where will the dressing be?" Parents are included in preprocedural teaching for their own learning and to help the nurse learn effective methods of communicating with the child.

During hospitalization the nurse should also focus on growth-promoting experiences for the child. For example, hospitalization may be an excellent opportunity to emphasize to parents abilities that the child does have but has not had the opportunity to practice, such as self-dressing. It may also be an opportunity for social experiences with peers, group play, or new educational and recreational activities. For example, one child who had the habit of screaming and kicking demonstrated a definite decrease in those behaviors after he learned to pound pegs and use a punching bag. Through social services the parents may become aware of specialized programs for the child. Hospitalization may also offer parents a respite from everyday care responsibilities and an opportunity to discuss their feelings with a concerned professional.

Assist in Measures to Prevent Retardation. Besides having a responsibility to families with a child with MR, nurses also need to be involved in programs aimed at preventing MR. Many of the familial, social, and environmental factors known to cause mild retardation are preventable. Counseling and education can reduce or eliminate such factors (e.g., poor nutrition, cigarette smoking, and chemical abuse), which increase the risk of prematurity and intrauterine growth retardation. Consequently, the major interventions are directed at improving maternal health and educating women regarding the dangers of chemicals, including alcohol during pregnancy and lead during childhood. Other preventive strategies that play an important role include adequate prenatal care; optimum medical care of high risk newborns; rubella immunization; genetic counseling and prenatal screening, especially in terms of Down or fragile X syndromes; use of folic acid supplements during the childbearing years and during pregnancy to prevent neural tube defects; newborn screening for treatable inborn errors of metabolism, such as congenital hypothyroidism, phenylketonuria, and galactosemia; and early appropriate therapies and rehabilitation services for children with developmental disabilities.

➤ Evaluation

The effectiveness of nursing interventions is determined by continual reassessment and evaluation of care based on the following observational guidelines:

1. Observe techniques used to teach child and child's success in ability to learn; inquire if child is enrolled in early stimulation program.
2. Interview family regarding provision of appropriate socialization, discipline, and play for child; observe child's ability to communicate with others; if possible, interview child regarding feelings of self-worth.
3. Observe those activities of daily living that child can completely or partially perform.
4. Interview family regarding any plans for future care and their awareness of community services.
5. Check patient record for evidence of nursing admission history, especially for self-help activities; observe parent's involvement in child's care; observe social interaction of child and family with other patients.
6. Investigate community programs aimed at preventing retardation and inquire as to nursing involvement in these efforts.

The *expected outcomes* are described in the Nursing Care Plan.

Down Syndrome

Down syndrome is the most common chromosomal abnormality of a generalized syndrome, occurring in 1.66 per 1000 live births (Stoll et al, 1998). It occurs slightly more often in Caucasians than in African-Americans, although the incidence in both groups is the same in some socioeconomic classes.

Etiology. The cause of Down syndrome is not known, but evidence from cytogenetic and epidemiologic studies supports the concept of multiple causality. Approximately 95% of all cases of Down syndrome are attributable to an extra chromosome 21 (group G), thus the name *trisomy 21.* Although children with trisomy 21 are born to parents of all ages, there is a statistically greater risk in older women, particularly those over 35 years of age. For example, in women 30 years of age the incidence of Down syndrome is about 1 in 1500 live births, but in women aged 40 it is about 1 in 100. However, the majority (about 80%) of infants with Down syndrome are born to women under age 35. In less than 5% of cases, paternal age is a factor, especially in men 55 years of age or older (Hixon et al, 1998).

About 3% to 4% of the cases may be caused by *translocation* of chromosomes 15 and 21 or 22. This type of genetic aberration is usually hereditary and is not associated with advanced parental age. From 1% to 2% of affected persons demonstrate *mosaicism,* which refers to the presence of cells with both normal and abnormal chromosomes. The degree of physical and cognitive impairment is related to the percentage of cells with the abnormal chromosome makeup.

Diagnostic Evaluation. Down syndrome can usually be diagnosed by the clinical manifestations alone (Box 42-3, Fig. 42-5), but a chromosome analysis should be done to confirm the genetic abnormality.

Several physical problems are associated with Down syndrome. Many of these children have congenital heart malformations, the most common being septal defects. Respiratory tract infections are very prevalent and, when combined with cardiac anomalies, are the chief cause of death, particularly during the first year of life. Hypotonicity of chest and abdominal muscles and dysfunction of the immune system probably predispose to the development of respiratory tract infection. Other physical problems include thyroid dysfunction, especially congenital hypothyroidism; and an increased incidence of leukemia.

Nursing Care Plan THE CHILD WITH MENTAL RETARDATION

NURSING DIAGNOSIS Altered growth and development related to impaired cognitive functioning

EXPECTED OUTCOME Child exhibits evidence of appropriate growth and development behaviors for age and abilities.

Nursing Interventions/*Rationales*

Involve child and family in early developmental stimulation and intervention (refer to available programs) *to maximize developmental potential.*

Assess child's developmental progress at regular intervals and note changes in functional abilities *to revise intervention as needed.*

Help family to set realistic goals and determine child's readiness for specific developmental tasks; encourage and reinforce learning of self-care skills *to facilitate development.*

Emphasize to family that this child has needs that are the same as other children (e.g., play, discipline, interaction, approval), and encourage interventions that help child to meet these needs at appropriate times and in appropriate ways (e.g., teaching socially acceptable behavior; encouraging appropriate grooming, hygiene, and dress; providing opportunities for peer interactions such as school, afterschool activities, special events; reinforcing positive behaviors and setting limits) *to optimize development and socialization.*

As child matures, counsel child and parents on issues such as sexuality, sexual behavior, birth control, marriage and family, and vocational interests and opportunities *to assist in management of ongoing developmental issues.*

NURSING DIAGNOSIS Altered family processes related to having a child with mental retardation

EXPECTED OUTCOME Family members demonstrate acceptance of child.

Nursing Interventions/*Rationales*

Inform family of infant problem as soon as possible after birth *to decrease anxiety of unknown.*

Provide opportunity for family to absorb and adjust to diagnosis (e.g., repeat information *to allow time for family to hear and understand;* encourage expression of concerns, fears, and feelings about diagnosis and potential impact *to facilitate adjustment;* identify support systems *to provide resources for coping).*

Provide family with written materials about child's condition *for long-term reference;* introduce family to other families with similarly affected children *to enhance support mechanisms.*

Demonstrate acceptance of child through own behavior *to serve as role model for family;* encourage family to participate in care *to form emotional attachments.*

Explore family reaction to the child; assist them to achieve a realistic view of child's abilities and limitations; encourage family in attempts to promote child growth and development; have family emphasize what child can do; explore ways for family to include child in family activities *to help family increase abilities to cope with and incorporate child into family structure.*

Arrange for and participate in family conferences *to provide forum for communication, mutual goal setting, and effective strategizing.*

Assess family resources and coping abilities when discussing care options on discharge *so that family can make realistic choices on the basis of their specific circumstances.*

If family opts for home care, assist them in developing a plan of care for the child, and teach them the skills needed in carrying out that plan *to provide optimum care in which the entire family is involved.*

Identify additional resource systems (e.g., relatives, friends, church, health care services, community programs), and strategize with family about making good use of these systems *to develop broad base of support.*

Provide a system of ongoing follow-up and evaluation *to ensure long-term adaptation to challenges presented to family functioning by a child with mental retardation.*

As child ages, help parents explore decisions about future care options that assist in dealing with behavioral management problems, parent debility, or retirement issues *to facilitate long-term care.*

Make referrals to appropriate social agencies *for needed assistance, support, and continuity of care.*

Therapeutic Management. Although no cure exists for Down syndrome, a number of therapies are advocated, such as surgery to correct serious congenital anomalies and possibly the physical stigmata, although the latter is controversial. These children also benefit from regular medical care. Evaluation of sight and hearing is essential, and treatment of otitis media is required to prevent auditory loss, which can influence cognitive function. Periodic testing of thyroid function is recommended, especially if growth is severely delayed. Children participating in sports that may involve stress on the head and neck (e.g., gymnastics, diving, butterfly stroke in swimming, high jump, and soccer) should be evaluated radiologically for *atlantoaxial* instability. Symptoms of the disorder include neck pain, weakness, and torticollis. Affected children are at risk for spinal cord compression.

NURSE ALERT • Report immediately any child with the following signs of spinal cord compression:

- Persistent neck pain
- Loss of established motor skills and bladder or bowel control
- Changes in sensation

Prognosis. Life expectancy for those with Down syndrome has improved in recent years but remains lower than for the general population. More than 80% survive to age 30 years and

Box 42-3

Clinical Manifestations of Down Syndrome

HEAD
*Separated sagittal suture
Brachycephaly
Skull rounded and small
Flat occiput
Enlarged anterior fontanel
Sparse hair (variable)

FACE
Flat profile

EYES
*Oblique palpebral fissures (upward, outward slant)
Inner epicanthal folds
Speckling of iris (Brushfield spots)
Short, sparse eyelashes
Blepharitis

NOSE
*Small
*Depressed nasal bridge (saddle nose)

EARS
Small
Short pinna (vertical ear length)
Overlapping upper helices
Narrow canals

MOUTH
*High, arched, narrow palate
Small osseous orbit
Protruding tongue; may be fissured at lip and furrowed on surface
Hypoplastic mandible
Downward curve (especially noted when crying)
Mouth kept open

TEETH
Delayed eruption
Alignment abnormalities common
Microdontia
Periodontal disease

CHEST
Shortened rib cage
Twelfth rib anomalies
Pectus excavatum/carinatum

NECK
*Skin excess and lax
Short and broad

ABDOMEN
Protruding
Muscles lax and flabby
  Diastasis recti
  Umbilical hernia

GENITALIA
Small penis
Cryptorchidism
Bulbous vulva

HANDS
Broad, short
Stubby fingers
Incurved little finger (clinodactyly)
Transverse palmar crease
Characteristic dermal ridge patterns
  Distally located axial triradius
  Increased ulnar loops on fingers

FEET
*Wide space between big and second toes
*Plantar crease between big and second toes
Broad, stubby, short

MUSCULOSKELETON
*Hyperflexibility
*Muscle weakness
Hypotonia
Atlantoaxial instability

SKIN
Dry, cracked, and frequent fissuring
Cutis marmorata (mottling)

OTHER
Reduced birth weight

*Most common findings. Pueschel SM: The Child with Down Syndrome. In Levine MD et al, editors: *Developmental-behavioral pediatrics,* ed 2, Philadelphia, 1992, WB Saunders.

beyond. As the prognosis continues to improve for these individuals, it will be important to provide for their long-term health care, social, and leisure needs (Carr, 1994).

Nursing Care Management

Support Family at Time of Diagnosis. Because of the unique physical characteristics, the infant with Down syndrome is usually diagnosed at birth, and parents should be informed of the diagnosis at this time. Parents usually prefer that both of them be present during the informing interview so that they can support one another emotionally. They appreciate receiving reading material about the syndrome* and being referred to

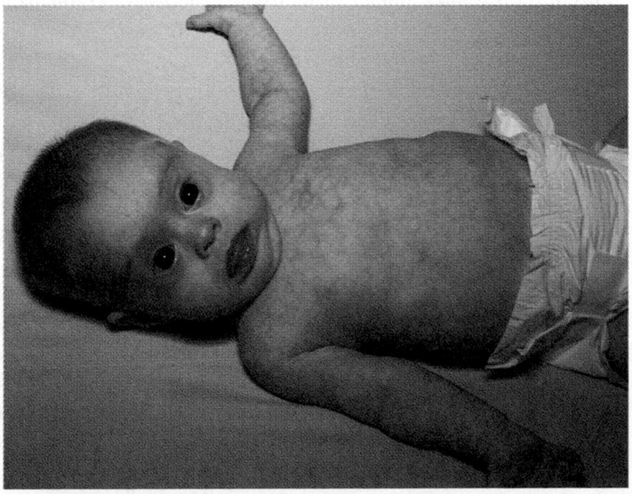

FIG. 42-5 • Down syndrome in infant. Note small, square head with upward slant to the eyes, flat nasal bridge, protruding tongue, mottled skin, and hypotonia.

*Sources of information include the Association for Retarded Citizens of the United States (see footnote, p. 1038); the American Association on Mental Retardation, 444 N. Capitol St. NW, Suite 846, Washington, DC 20001-1512; 1-800-424-3688 or (202) 387-1968; fax (202) 387-2193; website: www.aamr.org; the National Down Syndrome Society, 666 Broadway, Eighth Floor, New York, NY 10012-2317; 1-800-221-4602; fax (212) 979-2873; e-mail: info@ndss.org; website: www.ndss.org; and the National Down Syndrome Congress, 7000 Peachtree-Dunwoody Rd. NE, Lake Ridge 400 Office Park Building 5, Suite 100, Atlanta, GA 30328; 1-800-232-6372 or (770) 604-9500; website: www.ndscenter.org.

others for help or advice, such as parent groups or professional counseling.

Once parents are aware of the diagnosis, they are confronted with the crisis of losing their perfect or dream child and grieving for and accepting their reality child. Consequently, the parents' responses to the child may greatly influence decisions regarding future care. Whereas some families willingly want to take the child home, others consider immediate residential placement. The nurse must carefully answer questions regarding developmental potential. Institutionalization is no longer an option. For families unable or unready to choose taking the newborn home, specialized foster care or adoption are other options (Critical Thinking box).

Assist Family in Preventing Physical Problems. Many of the physical characteristics of Down syndrome present nursing problems. The hypotonicity of muscles and hyperextensibility of joints complicate positioning. The limp, flaccid extremities resemble the posture of a rag doll; as a result, holding the infant is difficult and cumbersome. Sometimes parents perceive this lack of molding to their bodies as evidence of inadequate parenting. The extended body position promotes heat loss because more surface area is exposed to the environment. Parents are encouraged to swaddle or wrap the infant tightly in a blanket before picking up the child to provide security and warmth. The nurse also discusses with parents their feelings concerning attachment to the child, emphasizing that the child's lack of clinging or molding is a physical characteristic, not a sign of detachment or rejection.

Decreased muscle tone compromises respiratory expansion. In addition, the underdeveloped nasal bone causes a chronic problem of inadequate drainage of mucus. The constant stuffy nose forces the child to breathe by mouth, which dries the oropharyngeal membranes, increasing the susceptibility to upper respiratory tract infections. Measures to lessen these problems include clearing the nose with a bulb-type syringe,* rinsing the mouth with water after feedings, using a cool-mist vaporizer to keep the mucous membranes moist and the secretions liquefied, changing the child's position often and performing postural drainage and percussion if necessary, practicing good handwashing, and properly disposing of soiled articles such as tissues. If antibiotics are ordered, the importance of completing the full course of therapy for successful eradication of the infection and prevention of growth of resistant organisms is stressed.

Inadequate drainage resulting in pooling of mucus in the nose also interferes with feeding. Because the child breathes by mouth, sucking for any length of time is difficult. When eating solids, the child may gag on the food because of mucus in the oropharynx. Parents are advised to clear the nose before each feeding; to give small, frequent feedings; and to allow opportunities for rest at mealtime.

The protruding tongue also interferes with feeding, especially of solid foods. Parents need to know that the tongue thrust is not an indication of refusal to feed, but a physiologic response. Parents are advised to use small but long, straight-handled spoon to push the food toward the back and side of the mouth. If food is thrust out, it is refed.

Critical Thinking

DIAGNOSIS OF DOWN SYNDROME

The parents of Melissa, a newborn diagnosed as having Down syndrome, ask you, "What are we supposed to do with her?" They further state that they already have three other children at home. How should you respond?

First, Think About It . . .

- **Within what point of view are you thinking?**
- **What are you taking for granted, and what assumptions are you making?**

1. **Encourage the parents to consider placement arrangements.**
2. **Actively listen to the parents' concerns.**
3. **Refer the parents to their pediatrician.**
4. **Ask the social worker to see the parents.**

The best response is 2. The general point of view is that the parents of a newborn with Down syndrome need time to process information given to them. The best choice for the nurse is not to take anything for granted and to listen. Then the nurse will be able to guide them to appropriate resources, not simply to give them suggestions that would affect their family's future. Options 3 and 4 are appropriate interventions but should not replace the nurse's role with the family.

Dietary intake needs supervision. Decreased muscle tone affects gastric motility, predisposing the child to constipation. Dietary measures such as increased fiber and fluid promote evacuation. The child's eating habits may need careful scrutiny to prevent obesity. Height and weight measurements should be obtained on a serial basis, especially during infancy. Because these children's growth is slower than that of the general pediatric population, special growth charts developed for these children should be used (Toledo et al, 1999).

During infancy the child's skin is pliable and soft; however, it gradually becomes rough and dry and is prone to cracking and infection. Skin care involves the use of minimum soap and the application of lubricants. Lip balm is applied to the lips, especially when the child is outdoors, to prevent excessive chapping.

Assist in Prenatal Diagnosis and Genetic Counseling. Prenatal diagnosis of Down syndrome is possible through chorionic villus sampling and amniocentesis, because chromosome analysis of fetal cells can detect the presence of trisomy or translocation. Testing for low maternal serum alpha-fetoprotein, high chorionic gonadotropin, and low unconjugated estriol levels may identify an affected fetus in women, who can then undergo amniocentesis (American Academy of Pediatrics, 1994; Yankowitz et al, 1998).

The nurse has a role in genetic counseling of women who are of advanced maternal age or who have a family history of the disorder to discuss the possibility of amniocentesis. If the fetus is affected, the nurse must allow the parents to express their feelings concerning elective abortion and support their decision to terminate or proceed with the pregnancy.

(See also Nursing Care Plan: The Child with Down Syndrome.*)

*Community and home care instructions on using a bulb syringe are available in Wong DL, Hess CS: ***Wong and Whaley's clinical manual of pediatric nursing***, ed 5, St Louis, 2000, Mosby.

*In Wong DL, Hess CS: ***Wong and Whaley's clinical manual of pediatric nursing***, ed 5, St Louis, 2000, Mosby.

Fragile X Syndrome

Fragile X syndrome is the most common inherited cause of MR and the second most common genetic cause of MR after Down syndrome. It has been described in all ethnic groups and races; the incidence of affected males is 1 in 1250; the incidence of affected females is 1 in 2500; and the incidence of carrier females is 1 in 259 (Hagerman and Cronister, 1996).

The syndrome is caused by an abnormal gene on the lower end of the long arm of the X chromosome. Chromosome analysis may demonstrate a *fragile site* (a region that fails to condense during mitosis and is characterized by a nonstraining gap or narrowing) in the cells of affected males and females and in carrier females. This fragile site has been determined to be caused by a gene mutation that results in excessive repeats of nucleotide in a specific deoxyribonucleic acid (DNA) segment of the X chromosome. The number of repeats in a normal individual is between 6 and 50. An individual with 50 to 200 base-pair repeats is said to have a *premutation* and is therefore a carrier. When passed from a parent to a child, these base-pair repeats can expand from 200 or more, which is termed a *full mutation.* This expansion occurs only when a carrier mother passes the mutation to her offspring; it does not occur when a carrier father passes the mutation to his daughters.

The inheritance pattern has been termed *X-linked dominant with reduced penetrance.* It is in distinct contrast to the classic X-linked recessive pattern in which all carrier females are normal, all affected males have symptoms of the disorder, and no males are carriers. Consequently, genetic counseling of affected families is more complex than that for families with a classic X-linked disorder, such as hemophilia. Prenatal diagnosis of the fragile X gene mutation is now possible with direct DNA testing in a family with an established history, using amniocentesis or chorionic villus sampling (Murray, 1997). Both affected sexes are fertile and therefore capable of transmitting the fragile X disorder.

Clinical Manifestations. The classic trend of physical findings in adult men with fragile X syndrome consists of a long face with a prominent jaw (prognathism); large, protruding ears; and large testes (macro-orchidism). In prepubertal children, however, these features may be less obvious, and behavioral manifestations may initially suggest the diagnosis (Box 42-4). In carrier females the clinical manifestations are extremely varied.

Therapeutic Management. No cure exists for fragile X syndrome. Medical treatment may include the use of serotonin agents such as carbamazepine (Tegretol) or fluoxetine (Prozac) to control violent temper outbursts, and the use of central nervous system (CNS) stimulants or clonidine (Catapres) to improve attention span and decrease hyperactivity. The use of folic acid, which affects the metabolism of CNS transmitters, is controversial.

All affected children require early speech and language therapy, occupational therapy, and special education assistance. Without appropriate intervention, a progressive decline in IQ can occur.

Prognosis. Individuals with fragile X syndrome are expected to live a normal life span. Their cognitive impairment may be improved by behavioral and educational interventions.

Nursing Care Management. Because cognitive impairment is a fairly consistent finding in individuals with fragile X syndrome, the care given to these families is the same as for any child with MR. Because the disorder is hereditary, genetic counseling is necessary to inform parents and siblings of the risks of transmission. In addition, any male or female with unexplained or nonspecific mental impairment should be referred for genetic testing and, if needed, counseling. Families with a member affected by the disorder should be referred to the National Fragile X Foundation.*

Box 42-4

Clinical Manifestations of Fragile X Syndrome

PHYSICAL FEATURES

- Long, wide, and/or protruding ears
- Long, narrow face with prominent jaw
- In postpubertal males, enlarged testicles
- Long palpebral fissures
- High, arched palate
- Strabismus
- Increased head circumference
- Mitral valve prolapse/aortic root dilation
- Hypotonia
- Hyperextensible finger joints
- Transpalmar crease
- Pes planus (flat feet)

BEHAVIORAL FEATURES

- Mild to severe cognitive impairment (occasionally, normal intelligence with learning disabilities)
- Speech delay; speech may be rapid, with stuttering and repetition of words
- Short attention span, hyperactivity
- Mouthing beyond expected age for behavior
- Hypersensitivity to taste, sounds, touch
- Intolerance to change in routine
- Autistic-like behaviors
- May exhibit aggressive behavior

SENSORY IMPAIRMENT

Hearing Impairment

Hearing impairment is one of the most common disabilities in the United States. An estimated 2 in 1000 infants are born with permanent hearing loss (Applebaum, 1999). For infants admitted to the neonatal intensive care unit, the incidence rises sharply to approximately 2 to 4 per 100 neonates (American Academy of Pediatrics, 1999). There are about 1 million children with hearing impairment ranging in age from birth to 21 years in the United States, and almost a third of these children have other disabilities, such as visual or cognitive deficits.

Definition and Classification. *Hearing impairment* is a general term indicating disability that may range in severity from mild to profound and includes the subsets of deaf and hard-of-hearing. *Deaf* refers to a person whose hearing disability precludes successful processing of linguistic information through audition, with or without a hearing aid. *Hard-of-hearing* refers to a person who, generally with the use of a hearing aid, has residual hearing sufficient to enable successful processing of linguistic information through audition. Other

*P.O. Box 190488, San Francisco, CA 94119; 1-800-688-8765 or (510) 763-6030; fax (510) 763-6223; e-mail: NATLF@sprintmail.com.

terms, such as *deaf and dumb, mute,* or *deaf-mute,* are unacceptable. Persons with hearing impairments are not dumb and, if mute, have no physical speech defect other than that caused by the inability to hear.

Hearing defects may be classified according to etiology, pathology, or symptom severity. Each is important in terms of treatment, possible prevention, and rehabilitation.

Etiology. Hearing loss may be caused by a number of prenatal and postnatal conditions. These include a family history of childhood hearing impairment, anatomic malformations of the head or neck, low birth weight, severe perinatal asphyxia, perinatal infection (e.g., cytomegalovirus, rubella, herpes, syphilis, toxoplasmosis, or bacterial meningitis), chronic ear infection, cerebral palsy, Down syndrome, or administration of ototoxic drugs (Berrettini et al, 1999).

In addition, high risk neonates who are surviving formerly fatal prenatal or perinatal conditions may be susceptible to hearing loss from the disorder or its treatment. For example, sensorineural hearing loss may be a result of continuous humming noises or high noise levels associated with incubators, oxygen hoods, or intensive care units, especially when combined with the use of potentially ototoxic antibiotics.

Environmental noise is a special concern. Sounds loud enough to damage sensitive hair cells of the inner ear can produce irreversible hearing loss. Very loud, brief noise, such as gunfire, can cause immediate, severe, and permanent loss of hearing. Longer exposure to less intense but still hazardous sounds, such as music, can also produce hearing loss (LePage and Murray 1998; Roizen, 1999). The exact sound level that produces hearing loss is unknown.

Pathology. Disorders of hearing are divided according to the location of the defect. *Conductive* or *middle-ear hearing* loss results from interference of transmission of sound to the middle ear. It is the most common of all types of hearing loss and most commonly is a result of recurrent serous otitis media. Conductive hearing impairment involves mainly interference with loudness of sound.

Sensorineural hearing loss, also called *perceptive* or *nerve deafness,* involves damage to the inner ear structures and/or the auditory nerve. The most common causes are congenital defects of inner ear structures; or consequences of acquired conditions, such as kernicterus, infection, administration of ototoxic drugs, or exposure to excessive noise. Sensorineural hearing loss results in distortion of sound and problems in discrimination. Although the child hears some of everything going on around him or her, the sounds are distorted, severely affecting discrimination and comprehension.

Mixed conductive-sensorineural hearing loss results from interference with transmission of sound in the middle ear and along neural pathways. It often results from recurrent otitis media and its complications.

Central auditory imperception includes all hearing losses that do not demonstrate defects in the conductive or sensorineural structures. They are usually divided into organic or functional losses. In the *organic type* of central auditory imperception, the defect involves the reception of auditory stimuli along the central pathways and the expression of the message into meaningful communication. Examples are *aphasia,* the inability to express ideas in any form, either written or verbally; *agnosia,* the inability to interpret sound correctly; and *dysacusis,* difficulty in processing details or discriminating among sounds.

In the *functional type* of hearing loss, no organic lesion exists to explain a central auditory loss. Examples of functional hearing loss are conversion hysteria (an unconscious withdrawal from hearing to block remembrance of a traumatic event), infantile autism, and childhood schizophrenia.

Symptom Severity. Hearing impairment is expressed in terms of a *decibel (dB),* a unit of loudness (Table 42-2). It is measured at various frequencies, such as 500, 1000, and 2000 cycles/sec, the critical listening speech range. Hearing impairment can be classified according to *hearing threshold level* (the measurement of an individual's hearing threshold by means of an audiometer) and the degree of symptom severity as it affects speech (Table 42-3). These classifications offer only general guidelines regarding the effect of the impairment on any individual child, because children differ greatly in their ability to use residual hearing.

Therapeutic Management

Conductive Hearing Loss. Treatment of hearing loss depends on the cause and type of hearing impairment. Many conductive hearing defects respond to medical or surgical treatment, such as antibiotic therapy for acute otitis media or insertion of tympanostomy tubes for chronic otitis media. When the conductive loss is permanent, hearing can be improved with the use of a hearing aid to amplify sound.

The nurse should be familiar with the types, basic care, and handling of hearing aids, especially when the child is hospitalized.* Types of aids include those worn in or behind the ear, models incorporated into an eyeglass frame, or types worn on the body with a wire connection to the ear (Fig. 42-6). One of the most common problems with a hearing aid is *acoustic feedback,* an annoying whistling sound usually caused by improper fit of the ear mold. Sometimes the whistling may be at a frequency that the child cannot hear but that is annoying to others. In this case, if children are old enough, they are told of the noise and asked to readjust the aid.

NURSE ALERT • To reduce or eliminate whistling from a hearing aid, try reinserting the aid, making

*Information about hearing aids is available from the International Hearing Society, 16880 Middlebelt Rd., Suite 4, Livonia, MI 48152; Hearing Aid Helpline: 1-800-521-5247; fax (734) 522-0200; website: www.hearingihs.org.

TABLE 42-2
Intensity of Sounds Expressed in Decibels

Decibels (dB)	Representative Sound
0	Softest sound normal ear can hear
10	Heartbeat, rustling of leaves
20	Whisper at 1.8 m (5 feet)
30-45	Normal conversation
60	Noise in average restaurant
70-80	Street noises
80	Loud radio in home
90-100	Train
120	Thunder, rock music
140	Jet airplane during departure
>140	Pain threshold

certain that no hair is caught between the ear mold and the canal; cleaning the ear mold or ear; or lowering the volume of the aid.

As children grow older, they may be self-conscious about the device. Every effort is made to make the aid inconspicuous, such as an appropriate hairstyle to cover behind-the-ear or in-the-ear models; attractive frames for glasses; and placement of the on-the-body type where it is not seen, such as under a blouse or sweater. Children are given responsibility for the care of the device as soon as they are able, because fostering independence is a primary goal of rehabilitation.

NURSE ALERT • When parents express concern about their child's hearing and speech development, refer the child for a hearing evaluation. Absence of well-formed syllables ("da," "na," "yaya") by 11 months of age should result in immediate referral (Eilers and Oiler, 1994).

Sensorineural Hearing Loss. Treatment for sensorineural hearing loss is much less satisfactory. Because the defect is not one of intensity of sound, hearing aids are of less value in this type of defect. The use of *cochlear implants** (a surgically implanted prosthetic device) provides a sensation of hearing for individuals who have severe hearing loss or are profoundly deaf (Slattery and Fayad, 1999). Children with sensorineural hearing loss have lost or damaged some or all of their hair cells or auditory nerve fibers. Often these children cannot benefit from conventional hearing aids because they only amplify sound that cannot be processed by a damaged inner ear. A cochlear implant bypasses the hair cells to directly stimulate surviving auditory nerve fibers so that they can send signals to the brain. These signals can be interpreted by the brain to produce sound and sensations.

Multichanneled implants are now available. This more sophisticated device stimulates the auditory nerve at a number of locations with differently processed signals. This type of stimulation gives a person the opportunity to use the pitch information present in speech signals, allowing the person to better understand speech.

*Cochlear Implant Club International, Inc., 5335 Wisconsin Ave. NW, Suite 440, Washington, DC 20015; (202) 895-2781; fax (202) 895-2782; e-mail: pwms.cici@worldnet.att.net; website: www.cici.org; Hearing Enrichment Language Program of the Hough Ear Institute, 3434 N.W. 56th St., Oklahoma City, OK 73112; voice: (405) 945-7186; fax (405) 945-7188; e-mail: h.e.l.p.desk@hotbot.com; website: www.oraldeafed.org/schools/help/index.html; Auditory-Verbal International, Inc. (AVI), 2121 Eisenhower Ave., Ste. 402, Alexandria, VA 22314; voice: (703) 739-1049; TDD: (703) 739-0874; fax (703) 739-0395.

TABLE 42-3

Classifications of Hearing Loss Based on Symptom Severity

Hearing Level (dB)	Effect
Slight: 16-25 (hard of hearing)	Has difficulty hearing faint or distant speech Usually is unaware of hearing difficulty Likely to achieve in school but may have problems No speech defects
Mild: 26-40	At 30 dB loss can miss 25%-40% of speech At 35-40 dB loss can miss 50% of discussions May have speech difficulties
Moderate: 41-55	Understands face-to-face conversational speech at a distance of 3-5 feet Likely to have limited vocabulary, delayed or defective syntax, and imperfect speech production
Moderately severe: 56-70 (hard of hearing)	Unable to understand conversational speech unless loud Considerable difficulty with group or classroom discussion Requires special speech training
Severe: 71-90 (deaf)	May hear a loud voice if nearby May be able to identify loud environmental noises Can distinguish vowels but not most consonants Requires speech training
Profound: >91 (deaf)	May hear only loud sounds Requires extensive speech training

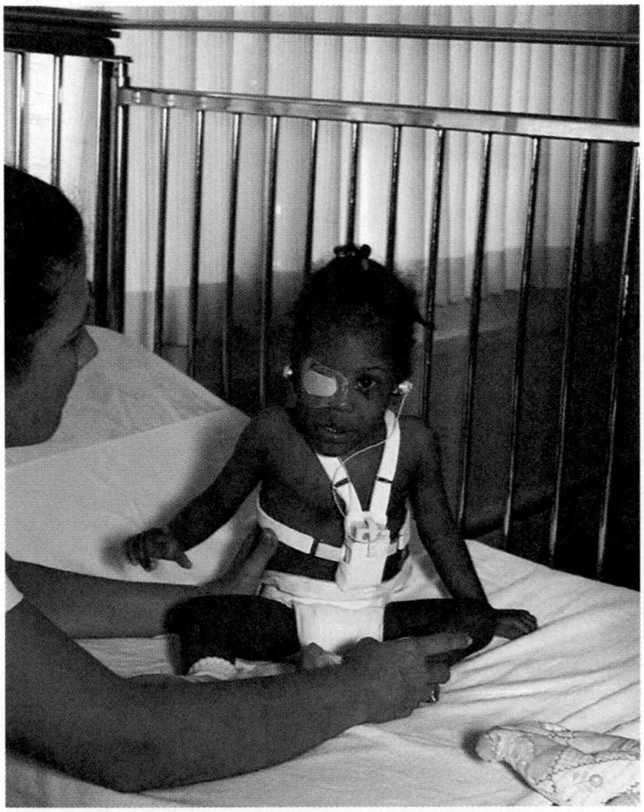

FIG. 42-6 • On-the-body hearing aids are convenient for young children, such as this child with severe bilateral hearing loss. Note eye patching for strabismus.

The trend is toward early use of cochlear implants, usually by 18 months of age, to give the child maximum opportunity to develop listening, language, and speaking skills.

Nursing Care Management

➤ Assessment

Assessment of children for hearing impairment is a critical nursing responsibility. Early detection of hearing loss, preferably within the first 3 to 6 months of life, is essential to improve the language and educational outcomes of those with hearing impairments (Yoshinaga-Itano et al, 1998). To accomplish this goal, the current recommendation is universal newborn hearing screening before discharge from the newborn nursery (American Academy of Pediatrics, 1999). This discussion focuses on developmental and behavioral indexes associated with hearing impairment. Auditory testing is presented in Chapter 35.

Infancy. At birth the nurse can observe the neonate's response to auditory stimuli, as evidenced by the startle reflex, head turning, eye blinking, and cessation of body movement. The infant may vary in the intensity of the response, depending on the state of alertness; however, a consistent absence of a reaction should lead to suspicion of hearing loss. Box 42-5 summarizes other clinical manifestations of hearing impairment in the infant.

Childhood. The child who is profoundly deaf is much more likely to be diagnosed during infancy than the less severely affected one. If the defect is not detected during early childhood, it likely will become evident during entry into school, when the child has difficulty in learning. Unfortunately, some of these children are mistakenly placed in special classes for students with learning disabilities or MR. Therefore it is essential that the nurse suspect a hearing impairment in any child who demonstrates the behaviors listed in Box 42-5.

Of primary importance is the effect of hearing impairment on speech development. A child with a mild conductive hearing loss may speak fairly clearly but in a loud, monotone voice. A child with a sensorineural defect usually has difficulty in articulation. For example, inability to hear higher frequencies may result in the word spoon being pronounced "poon." Children with articulation problems need to have their hearing tested.

NURSE ALERT • Stress to parents the importance of storing batteries for hearing aids in a safe location and teaching children or supervising young children not to remove the battery from the hearing aid. Ingestion of batteries is most often of those from hearing aids, including the child's own aid (Litovitz and Schmitz, 1992).

Box 42-5

Clinical Manifestations of Hearing Impairment

INFANTS

- Lack of startle or blink reflex to a loud sound
- Failure to be awakened by loud environmental noises
- Failure to localize a source of sound by 6 months of age
- Absence of babble or inflections in voice by age 7 months
- General indifference to sound
- Lack of response to the spoken word; failure to follow verbal directions
- Response to loud noises as opposed to the voice

CHILDREN

- Use of gestures rather than verbalization to express desires, especially after age 15 months
- Failure to develop intelligible speech by age 24 months
- Monotone quality, unintelligible speech, lessened laughter
- Vocal play, head banging, or foot stamping for vibratory sensation
- Yelling or screeching to express pleasure, annoyance (tantrums), or need
- Asking to have statements repeated or answering them incorrectly
- Responding more to facial expression and gestures than verbal explanation
- Avoidance of social interaction; often puzzled and unhappy in such situations; prefer to play alone
- Inquiring, sometimes confused facial expression
- Suspicious alertness, sometimes interpreted as paranoia, alternating with cooperation
- Frequently stubborn because of lack of comprehension
- Irritable at not making themselves understood
- Shy, timid, and withdrawn
- Often appear "dreamy," "in a world of their own," or extremely inattentive

➤ Nursing Diagnoses

A number of nursing diagnoses are prominent in the nursing care of the child with hearing impairment and the child's family; other diagnoses specific to individual cases become evident. The most common nursing diagnoses are outlined in the Nursing Care Plan on p. 1052.

➤ Plan of Care and Implementation

The goals of nursing care for the child with hearing impairment and family are as follows:

1. Child will achieve optimum development through enhancement of the communication process and socialization.
2. Child and family will receive support.
3. Child will receive appropriate care during hospitalization.

Promote the Communication Process. The nurse's initial role in rehabilitation is to encourage the family to participate in an auditory training program.* Rehabilitation training consists of learning appropriate methods to improve communication, such as lipreading, sign language, speech language, and therapy.

---

*Home training correspondence programs are sponsored by the John T. Tracy Clinic, 806 W. Adams Blvd., Los Angeles, CA 90007; 1-800-522-4582; TTY: (213) 747-2924; fax (213) 749-1651; website: www.johntracyclinic.org. Other sources of information on several aspects of hearing loss and on the International Parents' Organization are the Alexander Graham Bell Association for the Deaf, 3417 Volta Place NW, Washington, DC 20007; voice: (202) 337-5220; TTY: (202) 337-5221; e-mail: BellChaps@aol.com; website: www.agbell.org; and Canadian Hearing Society, 271 Spadina Rd., Toronto, Ontario M5R 2V3; voice: (416) 964-9595; fax (416) 928-2525; e-mail: info@chs.ca; website: www.chs.ca.

Lipreading. Even though the child may become an expert at lipreading, only about 40% of the spoken word is understood, and less if the speaker has an accent, mustache, or beard. Exaggerating pronunciation or speaking in an altered rhythm further lessens comprehension. Parents can help the child understand the spoken word by using the suggestions in the Guidelines box. The child learns to supplement the spoken word with sensitivity to visual cues, primarily body language and facial expression (e.g., tightening the lips, muscle tension, or eye contact).

Cued Speech. This method of communication is an adjunct to straight lipreading. It uses hand signals to help the child with a hearing impairment distinguish between words that look alike when formed by the lips (e.g., "mat," "bat"). It is most often used by children with hearing impairments who are using speech, rather than those who are nonverbal.

Sign Language. Sign language, such as *American Sign Language (ASL)* or *British Sign Language (BSL),* is a visual gestural language that uses hand signals that roughly correspond to specific words and concepts in the English language. Family members are encouraged to learn signing because using or watching hands requires much less concentration than lipreading or talking. Also, a symbol method enables some children to learn more and to learn faster.

Speech Language Therapy. The most formidable task in the education of a child who is profoundly hearing impaired is learning to speak. Speech is learned through a multisensory approach, using visual, tactile, kinesthetic, and auditory stimulation. Parents are encouraged to participate fully in the learning process.

Additional Aids. Everyday activities present problems for older children with hearing impairment. For example, they may not be able to hear the telephone, doorbell, or alarm clock. Several commercial devices are available to help them adjust to these dilemmas. Flashing lights can be attached to a telephone or doorbell to signal its ringing. Trained hearing ear dogs can provide great assistance because they alert the person to sounds, such as someone approaching, a moving car, a signal to wake up, or a child's cry. Special *teletypewriters* or *telecommunications devices for the deaf (TDD)* help people with impaired hearing communicate with each other over the telephone; the typed message is conveyed via the telephone lines and displayed on a small screen.*

Any audiovisual medium presents dilemmas for these children, who can see the picture but cannot hear the message. However, with *closed captioning* a special decoding device is attached to the television, and the audio portion of a program is translated into subtitles that appear on the screen.†

As children learn to compensate for their lack of hearing, they become extremely perceptive to visual and vibratory changes. Children often know when another person wants to talk to them because the person will walk close by but not pass. They learn to be alert to other people approaching them by seeing their shadows or feeling the vibrations of their footsteps. They are acutely aware of facial expressions and may comprehend the unspoken word more quickly than the spoken word.

Socialization. Because socialization is extremely important to the child's development, the nurse discusses with the family methods of fostering social contact. If children attend a special school for the deaf, they are able to socialize with peers in that setting. Classmates become a potential source of close friendships because they communicate more easily among themselves. Parents are encouraged to promote these relationships whenever possible.

Children with a hearing impairment may need special help with school or social activities. For those children wearing hearing aids, background noise should be kept to a minimum. Because many of these children are able to attend regular classes, the teacher may need assistance in adapting methods of teaching for the child's benefit. The school nurse is often in an optimum position to emphasize methods of facilitated communication, such as lipreading (Guidelines box). Because group projects and audiovisual teaching aids may hinder the child's learning, these educational methods should be carefully evaluated.

In a group setting it is helpful for the other members to sit in a semicircle in front of the child. Because one of the difficulties in following a group discussion is that the child is unaware of who will speak next, someone should point out each speaker. Speakers can also be given numbers, or their names can be written down as each person talks. If one person writes down the main topic of the discussion, the child is able to follow lipreading more closely. Such suggestions can increase the child's ability to participate in sports, organizations such as Boy Scouts or Girl Scouts, and group projects.

Support Child and Family. Once the diagnosis of hearing impairment is made, parents need extensive support to adjust to the shock of learning about their child's disability, and an opportunity to realize the extent of the hearing loss. If the hearing loss occurs during childhood, the child also requires sensitive, supportive care during the long and often difficult adjustment to this sensory loss. Early rehabilitation is one of the best strategies for fostering adjustment. However, progress in learning communication may not always coincide with emotional adjustment. Depression or anger is common, and such feelings are

Guidelines

FACILITATING LIPREADING

- Attract child's attention before speaking; use light touch to signal speaker's presence.
- Stand close to child.
- Face child directly or move to a 45-degree angle.
- Stand still; do not walk back and forth or turn away to point or look elsewhere.
- Establish eye contact and show interest.
- Speak at eye level and with good lighting on speaker's face.
- Be certain nothing interferes with speech patterns, such as chewing food or gum.
- Speak clearly and at a slow and even rate.
- Use facial expression to assist in conveying messages.
- Keep sentences short.
- Rephrase message if child does not understand the words.

*Directory listings stating "TDD only" before a phone number indicate that regular telephone use is not possible; "TDD and voice" indicates that both TDD users and speaking/hearing people can use the telephone number.

†Additional information is available from the National Captioning Institute, Inc., 1900 Gallows Rd., Suite 3000, Vienna, VA 22182; (703) 917-7600; fax (703) 917-9878; website: www.ncicap.org.

a normal part of the grieving process. (See also Chapter 41 for an extensive discussion of the emotional support of the child and family.)

Care for Child During Hospitalization. The needs of the hospitalized child with impaired hearing are the same as those of any other child, but the disability presents special challenges to the nurse (Critical Thinking box). For example, verbal explanations must be supplemented with tactile and visual aids, such as books or actual demonstration and practice. Children's understanding of the explanation needs to be constantly reassessed. If their verbal skills are poorly developed, they can answer questions through drawing, writing, or gesturing. For example, if the nurse is attempting to clarify where a spinal tap is done, the child is asked to point out where the procedure will be done on the body. Because these children often need more time to grasp the full meaning of an explanation, the nurse needs to be patient and allow ample time for understanding.

When communicating with the child, the nurse should use the same principles as those outlined for facilitating lipreading. Ideally, nurses without foreign accents should be assigned to the child. The child's hearing aid is checked to ensure that it is working properly. If it is necessary to awaken the child at night, the nurse gently shakes the child or turns on the hearing aid before arousing the child. The nurse always makes sure that the child can see him or her before any procedures, even routine ones such as changing a diaper or regulating an infusion, are performed. It is important to remember that the child may not be aware of one's presence until alerted through visual or tactile cues.

Ideally, parents are encouraged to room with the child; however, it must be conveyed to them that this is not to serve as a convenience to the nurse but as a benefit to the child. Although the parents' aid can be enlisted in familiarizing the child with the hospital and explaining procedures, the nurse also talks directly to the youngster, encouraging expression of feelings about the experience. If there is difficulty in understanding the child's speech, an effort is made to become familiar with his or her pronunciation of words. Parents often can be helpful by explaining the child's usual speech habits. Nonverbal communication devices that employ pictures or words that the child can point to are also available (see p. 1039). Such boards can also be made by drawing pictures or writing the words of common needs on cardboard, such as *parent, food, water,* or *toilet.*

The nurse has a special role as child advocate with the child and is in a strategic position to alert other health team members and other patients to the child's special needs regarding communication. For example, the nurse should accompany other practitioners on visits to the child's room to ensure that they speak to the child and that the child understands what is said. Caregivers sometimes forget that the child has abilities to perceive and learn despite a hearing loss, and consequently they communicate only with the parents. As a result, the child's needs and feelings remain unrecognized and unmet.

Because children with impaired hearing may have difficulty in forming social relationships with other children, the child is introduced to roommates and encouraged to engage in play activities. The hospital setting can provide growth-promoting opportunities for social relationships. With the assistance of a child-life specialist, the child can learn new recreational activities, experiment with group games, and engage in therapeutic play. The use of puppets, dollhouses, role-playing with dress-up clothes, building with a hammer and nails, finger painting, playing with syringes, and water play can help the child express feelings that previously were suppressed.

Assist in Measures to Prevent Hearing Impairment. A primary nursing role is prevention of hearing loss. Because the most common cause of impaired hearing is chronic otitis media, it is essential that appropriate measures be instituted to treat existing infections and prevent recurrences (see Chapter 46). Children with histories of ear or respiratory infections or any other condition known to increase the risk of hearing impairment should receive periodic auditory testing.

To prevent the causes of hearing loss that begin prenatally and perinatally, pregnant women need counseling regarding the necessity of early prenatal care, including genetic counseling for known familial disorders; avoidance of all ototoxic drugs, especially during the first trimester; tests to rule out syphilis, rubella, or blood incompatibility; medical management of maternal diabetes; strict control of alcohol intake; and adequate dietary intake. The necessity of routine immunization during childhood to eliminate the possibility of acquired sensorineural loss from rubella, mumps, or measles (encephalitis) is stressed.

Exposure to excessive noise pollution is a well-established cause of sensorineural hearing loss. The nurse should routinely assess the possibility of environmental noise pollution and advise children and parents of the potential danger. When individuals engage in activities associated with high-intensity noise, such as flying model airplanes, target shooting, or snowmobil-

Critical Thinking

HEARING IMPAIRMENT

Five-year-old Jason has a severe congenital hearing impairment. You have been assigned to care for him in the outpatient surgery postanesthesia care unit (PACU), where he has just been admitted following a herniorrhaphy. As he emerges from anesthesia, he becomes more and more agitated. The most likely cause for his behavior is which of the following?

First, Think About It . . .

- **What precise question are you trying to answer?**
- **What would the consequences be if you put your thoughts into action?**

1. **This is a normal reaction to anesthesia.**
2. **He is experiencing separation anxiety.**
3. **He is unable to communicate properly.**
4. **He is in pain.**

The best response is 3. Precisely, the focus of the question is on the expected behaviors associated with the emergence from anesthesia. Because Jason became increasingly more agitated as he emerged from anesthesia, his behavior does not suggest the transitory confusion associated with the initial emergence from anesthesia. Rather, it suggests that as he became more aware of his surroundings and tried to communicate with the staff, Jason became increasingly frustrated. Reasons for this might include (a) not having his hearing aid in place; (b) having his arms restrained by intravenous lines, pulse oximetry monitors, and a blood pressure cuff, thus restricting his use of sign language; (c) being unable to read the nurse's lips from a prone position; or (d) not having a nurse who could understand his speech or know or recognize his attempts to use sign language. Although pain is a possibility and needs to be evaluated, regional blocks are typically given during the surgery to keep children comfortable until after they are discharged home. It is unlikely that Jason is having separation anxiety, since this usually occurs in younger children.

ing, they should wear ear protection such as earmuffs or earplugs (not ordinary dry cotton); however, any protection is better than none. Even common household equipment, such as lawn mowers, power vacuum cleaners, and cordless telephones, can be hazardous.

NURSE ALERT • Suspect hazardous noise if the listener experiences (1) difficulty in communication while hearing the sound, (2) ringing in the ears (tinnitus) after exposure to the sound, or (3) muffled hearing after leaving the sound.

➤ Evaluation

The effectiveness of nursing interventions is determined by continual reassessment and evaluation of care based on the following observational guidelines:

1. Observe techniques used to communicate with child; inquire if child is enrolled in an auditory training program; inquire about socialization opportunities for child (e.g., who are child's friends, what are his or her extracurricular activities).
2. Interview family regarding their adjustment to the sensory impairment; observe family members' relationship with child; interview child regarding feelings about the sensory impairment and its effect on activities of daily living (especially important if impairment is recent).
3. Observe types of preparation and communication used to prepare child for hospitalization or procedures; observe parents' involvement in child's care; observe interaction of child and family with other patients.
4. Investigate community programs aimed at preventing or detecting hearing loss and inquire as to nursing involvement in these efforts.

The expected outcomes are described in the Nursing Care Plan.

Visual Impairment

Visual impairment is a common problem during childhood. Globally the prevalence of blindness and serious visual impairment in the pediatric population is estimated at 0.7 per 1000 (Rahi, 1999). In the United States another 100 children per 100,000 have less serious impairment (Davidson, 1992). The nurse's role is clearly one of assessment, prevention, referral, and in some instances, rehabilitation.

Definition and Classification. *Visual impairment* is a general term that refers to visual loss that cannot be corrected with regular prescription lenses. However, more useful definitions for classifying visual impairments include the following. *School vision* (also known as *partially sighted*) refers to visual acuity between 20/70 and 20/200. The child should be able to obtain an education in the usual public school system with the use of normal-sized print. Near vision is almost always better than distance vision. *Legal blindness,* visual acuity of 20/200 or less and/or a visual field of 20 degrees or less in the better eye, is useful only as a legal definition, not as a medical diagnosis. It allows special considerations with regard to taxes, entrance into special schools, eligibility for aid, and other benefits.

Etiology. Visual impairment can be caused by a number of genetic and prenatal or postnatal conditions. These include perinatal infections (e.g., herpes, chlamydia, gonococci, rubella, syphilis, and toxoplasmosis); retinopathy of prematurity; trauma, postnatal infections (meningitis); and disorders such as sickle cell disease, juvenile rheumatoid arthritis, Tay-Sachs disease, albinism, and retinoblastoma. In many instances, such as with refractive errors, the cause of the defect is unknown.

Refractive errors are the most common types of visual disorders in children. The term *refraction* means bending and refers to the bending of light rays as they pass through the lens of the eye. Normally, light rays enter the lens and fall directly on the retina. However, in refractive disorders the light rays either fall in front of the retina *(myopia)* or beyond it *(hyperopia).* Other eye problems, such as strabismus, may or may not include refractive errors, but they are very important because, if untreated, they result in blindness from amblyopia. These, along with other less common visual disorders, are summarized in Box 42-6. In addition to these disorders, other visual problems can be a result of infection or trauma.

Trauma. Trauma is a common cause of blindness in children. Injuries to the eyeball and adnexa (supporting or accessory structures, e.g., eyelids, conjunctiva, and lacrimal glands) can be classified as penetrating or nonpenetrating. *Penetrating wounds* are most often a result of sharp instruments, such as sticks, knives, or scissors; propulsive objects, such as firecrackers, guns, bows, and arrows, or slingshots; or a powerful contusion by a blunt object, which may occur during a fight or from a serious car accident. *Nonpenetrating injuries* may be a result of foreign objects in the eyes, lacerations, a blow from a blunt object such as a ball (baseball, softball, basketball, racquet sports) or fist, or thermal or chemical burns.

Treatment is aimed at preventing further ocular damage and is primarily the responsibility of the ophthalmologist. It involves adequate examination of the injured eye (with the child sedated or anesthetized in severe injuries); appropriate immediate intervention, such as removal of the foreign body or suturing of the laceration; and prevention of complications, such as administration of antibiotics or steroids and complete bed rest to allow the eye to heal and blood to reabsorb (see Emergency box). The prognosis varies according to the type of injury. It is usually guarded in all cases of penetrating wounds because of the high risk of serious complications.

Infections. Infections of the adnexa and structures of the eyeball or globe may occur in children. The most common eye infection is *conjunctivitis* (see Chapter 37). Treatment is usually with ophthalmic antibiotics. Severe infections may require systemic antibiotic therapy. Steroids are used cautiously because they exacerbate viral infections such as herpes simplex, increasing the risk of damage to the involved structures.

Nursing Care Management

➤ Assessment

Assessment of children for visual impairment is a critical nursing responsibility. Discovery of a visual impairment as early as possible is essential to prevent social, physical, and psychological damage to the child. Assessment involves (1) identifying those children who by virtue of their history are at risk, (2) observing for behaviors that indicate a vision loss, and (3) screening all children for visual acuity and signs of other ocular disorders such as strabismus. This discussion focuses on clinical manifestations of various types of visual problems (see Box 42-6). Vision testing is discussed in Chapter 35.

Nursing Care Plan THE CHILD WITH HEARING IMPAIRMENT

NURSING DIAGNOSIS Impaired verbal communication related to conductive and/or sensorineural hearing loss

EXPECTED OUTCOME Child is able to communicate with others in the environment.

Nursing Interventions/*Rationales*

Explore family's knowledge of hearing loss and of the speech development process *to assess baseline for interventions.*

Explain the relationship between the loss of hearing and speech; discuss how speech develops; discuss alternative methods of communication (gestures, drawing, play, sign language, lip reading) *to increase family's understanding of child's speech impairment and how to cope with the loss.*

Encourage family to pursue appropriate communication interventions (e.g., oral speech classes, signing classes) for their child and family members as dictated by the child's degree of hearing loss and the child's developmental level *to promote successful communication.*

Refer family to appropriate community resources such as American Organization for the Education of the Hearing Impaired and family support groups *to aid in coping and adaptation.*

NURSING DIAGNOSIS Sensory/perceptual alterations (auditory) related to conductive and/or sensorineural hearing loss

EXPECTED OUTCOME Child exhibits use of appropriate mechanisms to compensate for hearing loss (e.g., hearing aid, cochlear implants); child is oriented to and displays interest in external environment.

Nursing Interventions/*Rationales*

If appropriate, explore mechanisms *that may enhance hearing abilities* (e.g., hearing aids, visual cues in environment, amplifier devices on telephone, doorbells, cochlear implant surgery).

If hearing aid is used, teach child and family how to use the aid, how to replace batteries, and how to prevent young children from ingesting/aspirating batteries *to promote optimum benefit and safety.*

Use tactile and visual stimuli with child *to enhance sensory stimulation through other modalities.*

Observe child's interaction with and interest in external environment *to assess orientation and function.*

Provide reality orientation *to counteract confusion and disorientation.*

NURSING DIAGNOSIS Risk for altered growth and development related to hearing loss and impaired communication

EXPECTED OUTCOME Child exhibits evidence of appropriate growth and development behaviors for age and abilities.

Nursing Interventions/*Rationales*

If appropriate, explore mechanisms *that may enhance hearing abilities* (e.g., hearing aids, visual cues in environment, amplifier devices on telephone, doorbells, cochlear implant surgery).

Involve child and family in early stimulation and intervention exercises (refer to available programs) *to enhance development of remaining senses and maximize overall development.*

Assess child's developmental progress at regular intervals and note changes in functional abilities *to revise interventions as needed.*

Help family to set realistic goals and determine child's readiness for specific developmental tasks; encourage and reinforce learning of self-care skills *to facilitate development.*

Emphasize to family that this child has needs that are the same as other children (e.g., play, discipline, interaction, approval), and encourage interventions that help child to meet these needs (e.g., selecting toys that maximize visual and tactile resources, using close-captioned television, reinforcing positive behaviors and setting limits, participating in group and peer activities, giving positive feedback for successes and good efforts) *to optimize development and socialization.*

Work with school (teachers, nurse, classmates) *to enhance understanding and ensure meeting of educational needs.*

NURSING DIAGNOSIS Altered family processes related to a diagnosis of deafness of a child

EXPECTED OUTCOME Family members demonstrate acceptance of child.

Nursing Interventions/*Rationales*

Provide opportunity for family to absorb and adjust to diagnosis (e.g., repeat information *to allow time for family to hear and understand;* encourage expression of concerns, fears, and feelings about diagnosis and potential impact *to facilitate adjustment;* identify support systems *to provide resources for coping*).

Provide family written materials about child's condition *for long-term reference;* introduce family to other families with similarly affected children *to enhance support mechanisms.*

Explore family reaction to the child; assist them to achieve a realistic view of child's abilities and limitations; encourage family in attempts to promote child growth and development; have family emphasize what child can do; explore ways for family to include child in family activities; encourage all family members to learn alternative communication measures *to help family increase abilities to cope with and incorporate child into family structure.*

Arrange for and participate in family conferences *to provide forum for communication, mutual goal setting, and effective strategizing.*

Box 42-6

Types of Visual Impairment

REFRACTIVE ERRORS

Myopia

Nearsightedness—Ability to see objects clearly at close range but not at a distance

Pathophysiology

Results from eyeball that is too long, causing image to fall in front of retina

Clinical Manifestations

Rubs eyes excessively
Tilts head or thrusts head forward
Has difficulty in reading or doing other close work
Holds books close to eyes
Writes or colors with head close to table
Clumsy; walks into objects
Blinks more than usual or is irritable when doing close work
Is unable to see objects clearly
Does poorly in school, especially in subjects that require demonstration, such as arithmetic
Dizziness
Headache
Nausea after close work

Treatment

Corrected with biconcave lenses that focus rays on retina
May be corrected with laser surgery

Hyperopia

Farsightedness—Ability to see objects at a distance

Pathophysiology

Results from eyeball that is too short, causing image to focus beyond retina

Clinical Manifestations

Because of accommodative ability, child can usually see objects at all ranges
Most children normally hyperopic until about 7 years of age

Treatment

If correction is required, use convex lenses to focus rays on retina
May be corrected with laser surgery

Astigmatism

Unequal curvatures in refractive apparatus

Pathophysiology

Results from unequal curvatures in cornea or lens that cause light rays to bend in different directions

Clinical Manifestations

Depends on severity of refractive error in each eye
May have clinical manifestations of myopia

Treatment

Corrected with special lenses that compensate for refractive errors
May be corrected with laser surgery

Anisometropia

Different refractive strength in each eye

Pathophysiology

May develop amblyopia or weaker eye is used less

Clinical Manifestations

Depends on severity of refractive error in each eye
May have clinical manifestations of myopia

Treatment

Treated with corrective lenses, preferably contact lenses, to improve vision in each eye so they work as a unit
May be corrected with laser surgery

AMBLYOPIA

Lazy eye—Reduced visual acuity in one eye

Pathophysiology

Results when one eye does not receive sufficient stimulation
Each retina receives different images, resulting in diplopia (double vision)
Brain accommodates by suppressing less intense image
Visual cortex eventually does not respond to visual stimulation, with resultant loss of vision in that eye

Clinical Manifestations

Poor vision in affected eye

Treatment

Preventable if treatment of primary visual defect, such as anisometropia or strabismus, begins before 6 years of age

STRABISMUS

"Squint" or *cross-eye*—Malalignment of eyes
Estropia—Inward deviation of eye
Exotropia—Outward deviation of eye

Pathophysiology

May result from muscle imbalance or paralysis, poor vision, or congenital defect
Since visual axes are not parallel, brain receives two images, and amblyopia can result

Clinical Manifestations

Squints eyelids together or frowns
Has difficulty in focusing from one distance to another
Inaccurate judgment in picking up objects
Unable to see print or moving objects clearly
Closes one eye to see
Tilts head to one side
If combined with refractive errors, may see any of the manifestations listed for refractive errors
Diplopia
Photophobia
Dizziness
Headache
Cross-eye

Continued

Box 42-6

Types of Visual Impairment—cont'd

STRABISMUS—cont'd

Treatment

Treatment depends on cause of strabismus

May involve occlusion therapy (patching stronger eye) or surgery to increase visual stimulation to weaker eye

Early diagnosis is essential to prevent vision loss

CATARACTS

Opacity of crystalline lens

Pathophysiology

Prevents light rays from entering eye and refracting them on retina

Clinical Manifestations

Gradually less able to see objects clearly

May lose peripheral vision

Nystagmus (with complete blindness)

Gray opacities of lens

Strabismus

Absence of red reflex

Treatment

Requires surgery to remove cloudy lens and replace lens (intraocular lens implant, removeable contact lens, prescription glasses)

Must be treated early to prevent blindness from amblyopia

GLAUCOMA

Increased intraocular pressure

Pathophysiology

Congenital type results from defective development of some component related to flow of aqueous humor

Increased pressure on optic nerve causes eventual atrophy and blindness

Clinical Manifestations

Mostly seen in acquired types—loses peripheral vision

May bump into objects not directly in front

Sees halos around objects

May complain of mild pain or discomfort (severe pain, nausea, vomiting, if sudden rise in pressure)

Redness

Excessive tearing (epiphora)

Photophobia

Spasmodic winking (blepharospasm)

Corneal haziness

Enlargement of eyeball (buphthalmos)

Treatment

Requires surgical treatment (goniotomy) to open outflow tracts

May require more than one procedure

Emergency

EYE INJURIES

Foreign Object

Examine eye for presence of a foreign body (evert upper lid to examine upper eye).

Remove a freely moveable object with pointed corner of gauze pad lightly moistened with water.

Do not irrigate eye or attempt to remove a penetrating object (see below).

Caution child against rubbing eye.

Chemical Burns

Irrigate eye copiously with tap water for 20 minutes.

Evert upper lid to flush thoroughly.

Hold child's head with eye under tap of running lukewarm water.

Take to emergency department.

Have child rest with eyes closed.

Keep room darkened.

Ultraviolet Burns

If skin is burned, patch both eyes (make sure lids are completely closed); secure dressing with Kling bandages wrapped around head rather than tape.

Have child rest with eyes closed.

Refer to an ophthalmologist.

Hematoma ("Black Eye")

Use a flashlight to check for gross ***hyphema*** (hemorrhage into anterior chamber; visible fluid meniscus across iris; more easily seen in light-colored than in brown eyes).

Apply ice for first 24 hours to reduce swelling if no hyphema is present.

Refer to an ophthalmologist immediately if hyphema is present.

Have child rest with eyes closed.

Penetrating Injuries

Take child to emergency department.

Never remove an object that has penetrated eye.

Follow strict aseptic technique in examining eye.

Observe for:

- Aqueous or vitreous leaks (fluid leaking from point of penetration)
- Hyphema
- Shape and equality of pupils, reaction to light
- Prolapsed iris (not perfectly circular)

Apply a Fox shield if available (not a regular eye patch) and apply patch over unaffected eye to prevent bilateral movement.

Maintain bed rest with child in 30-degree Fowler position.

Caution child against rubbing eye.

Infancy. At birth the nurse should observe the neonate's response to visual stimuli, such as following a light or object and cessation of body movement. The infant may vary in the intensity of the response, depending on the state of alertness.

Of special importance in detecting visual impairment during infancy are the parents' concerns regarding visual responsiveness in their child. Their concerns, such as lack of eye contact from the infant, must be taken seriously. During infancy the child should be tested for strabismus. Lack of binocularity after

4 months of age is considered abnormal and must be treated to prevent amblyopia.

NURSE ALERT • Suspect blindness if the infant does not react to light, and in any-age child if parents express concern.

Childhood. Because the most common visual impairment during childhood is refractive errors, testing for visual acuity is essential. The school nurse usually assumes major responsibility for vision testing in schoolchildren. Besides refractive errors, the nurse should be aware of signs and symptoms that indicate other ocular problems. If a referral is made to the family requesting further eye testing, the nurse is responsible for follow-up concerning the recommendation.

➤ Nursing Diagnoses

A number of nursing diagnoses are prominent in the nursing care of the child with visual impairment and the child's family; other diagnoses specific to individual cases become evident.

➤ Plan of Care and Implementation

The goals of care for the child with visual impairment and family are as follows:

1. Child and family will receive support and education.
2. Parent-child attachment will develop.
3. Child will achieve optimum development.
4. Child will receive appropriate care during hospitalization.

Support Child and Family. The shock of learning that their child is blind or partially sighted is an immense crisis for families. Of all types of disabilities, many people fear loss of sight the most. Vision is involved in almost every activity of daily living. Parents need support during the initial phase of learning about the diagnosis, and need help to gain a realistic understanding of their child's abilities. The family is encouraged to investigate appropriate stimulation and educational programs for their child as soon as possible. Sources of information include state Commissions for the Blind, local schools for the blind, the American Foundation for the Blind,* National Federation of the Blind,† National Association for Parents of the Visually Impaired, Inc.,‡ National Association for Visually Handicapped,§ and American Council of the Blind.||

When blindness is not congenital but acquired, newly blind children need much support to help them adjust to the disability. They are usually frightened and confused by the sudden or progressive loss of sight, and benefit from an environment that provides security and familiarity.

Promote Parent-Child Attachment. A crucial time in the life of blind infants is when they and their parents are getting acquainted with each other. Pleasurable patterns of interaction between the infant and parents may be lacking if there is not enough reciprocity. For example, if the parent gazes fondly at the infant's face and seeks eye contact, but the infant fails to respond because he or she cannot see the parent, a troubled cycle of responses may occur. The nurse can help parents learn to look for other cues that indicate the infant is responding to them, such as faster or slower breathing, when the parents come near; and whether the infant makes throaty sounds when the parents speak. In time parents learn that the infant has unique ways of relating to them. They are encouraged to show affection using nonvisual methods, such as talking or reading, cuddling, and walking the child.

Promote Child's Optimum Development. Promoting the child's optimum development requires rehabilitation in a number of important areas. These include learning self-help skills and appropriate communication techniques to become independent. Although nurses may not be directly involved in such programs, they can provide direction and guidance to families regarding the availability of programs and the need to promote these activities in their child.

Development and Independence. Motor development depends on sight almost as much as verbal communication depends on hearing. From earliest infancy, parents are encouraged to expose the infant to as many visual-motor experiences as possible, such as sitting supported in an infant seat or swing and being given opportunities for holding up the head, sitting unsupported, reaching for objects, and crawling.

Despite visual impairment, the child can become independent in all aspects of self-care. The same principles used for promoting independence in sighted children apply, with additional emphasis on nonvisual cues. For example, the child may need help in dressing, such as special arrangement of clothing for style coordination and Braille tags to distinguish colors and prints.

The blind child also must learn to become independent in navigational skills. The two main techniques are the *tapping method* (use of a cane to survey the environment for direction and to avoid obstacles); and *guides,* such as a sighted human guide or a Seeing Eye dog. Children who are partially sighted may benefit from ocular aids, such as monocular telescope.

Play and Socialization. Blind children do not learn to play automatically. Because they cannot imitate others or actively explore the environment as sighted children do, they depend much more on others to stimulate and teach them how to play. Parents need help in selecting appropriate play materials, especially those that encourage fine and gross motor development and stimulate the senses of hearing, touch, and smell. Toys with educational value, such as dolls with various clothing closures, are especially useful.

Blind children have the same needs for socialization as sighted children. Because they have little difficulty in learning verbal skills, they are able to communicate with age-mates and participate in suitable activities. The nurse discusses with parents opportunities for socialization outside the home, especially regular preschools. The trend is to include these children with sighted children to help them adjust to the outside world for eventual independence.

---

*11 Penn Plaza, Suite 300, New York, NY 10001; 1-800-232-5463 or (212) 502-7600; TTY: (212) 502-7662; fax (212) 502-7777; e-mail: afbinfo@afbinet; website: www.afb.org.

†1800 Johnson St., Baltimore, MD 21230; (410) 659-9314; website: www.nfb.org.

‡P.O. Box 317, Watertown, MA 02471; 1-800-562-6265; website: www.spedex.com/NAPVI.

§22W. 21st St., New York, NY 10010 (212) 889-3141; fax (212) 727-2931; e-mail: staff@navh.org; website: www.NAVH.org.

||1155 15th St. NW, Suite 1004, Washington, DC 20005, 1-800-424-8666; fax (202) 467-5085; website: www.acb.org.

A source of information in Canada is the Canadian National Institute for the Blind, 1929 Bayview Ave., Toronto, Ontario M4G 3E8; (416) 480-7580; fax (416) 480-7677; website: www.cnib.ca.

To compensate for inadequate stimulation, these children may develop *blindisms* (self-stimulatory activities, e.g., body rocking, finger flicking, arm twirling). Such habits restrict the child's social acceptance and are discouraged. Behavior modification is often successful in reducing or eliminating blindisms.

Education. The main obstacle to learning is the child's total dependence on nonvisual cues. Although the child can learn via verbal lecturing, he or she is unable to read the written word or to write without special education. Therefore the child must rely on *braille,* a system that uses raised dots to represent letters and numbers. The child can then read the braille with the fingers and can write a message using a braille writer. However, unless others read braille, this type of communication is not useful for communicating with others. A more portable system for written communication is the use of a braille slate and stylus (Fig. 42-7) or a microcassette tape recorder. A recorder is especially helpful for leaving messages for others and for note taking during classroom lecturing. For mathematic calculations, portable calculators with voice synthesizers are available.*

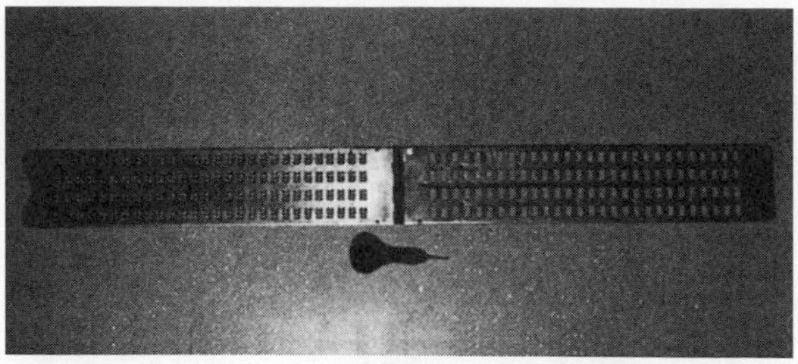

FIG. 42-7 • Braille slate and stylus. The hinged slate consists of a series of open rectangles on one side and standard braille cells on the other. The paper is clamped or sandwiches between these two metal bars, and the appropriate dots are punched with the stylus.

Records and tapes are significant sources of reading material other than braille books, which are large and cumbersome. The Library of Congress† has talking books, braille books, and a special records program, which are available at many local and state libraries and directly from the Library of Congress. The talking book machine and tape player are provided at no cost to families, and there is no postage fee for returning the materials. Recording for the Blind, Inc.,‡ also provides texts and tapes of books, which are very helpful for secondary and college students who are blind.

Learning to use a regular typewriter is another form of writing but has the disadvantage of the blind person's being unable to check the accuracy of the typing. Computers eliminate this drawback; a home computer with a voice synthesizer can be adapted to speak each letter or word that has been typed.

The child with partial sight benefits from specialized visual aids, which produce a magnified retinal image. The basic devices are accommodation (e.g., bringing the object closer), special plus lenses, handheld and stand magnifiers, telescopes, video projection systems, and large print. Special equipment is available to enlarge print. Information about services for the partially sighted is available from the National Association for Visually Handicapped and the American Foundation for the Blind (see footnote on p. 1055). Children with diminished vision often prefer to do close work without their glasses and compensate by bringing the object very near to their eyes. This should be allowed. The exception is the child with vision in only one eye, who should always wear glasses for protection.

Care for Child During Hospitalization. Because nurses are more likely to care for children who are hospitalized for procedures that involve temporary loss of vision than for children who are blind, the following discussion concentrates primarily on the needs of such children. The nursing care objectives in either situation are to (1) reassure the child and family throughout every phase of treatment, (2) orient the child to the surroundings, (3) provide a safe environment, and (4) encourage independence. Whenever possible, the same nurse should care for the child to ensure consistency in the approach. These same principles also apply to the blind child who requires hospitalization.

When sighted children temporarily lose their vision, almost every aspect of the environment becomes bewildering and frightening. They are forced to rely on nonvisual senses for help in adjusting to the blindness without the benefit of any special training. Nurses have a major role in minimizing the effects of temporary loss of vision. They need to talk to the child about everything that is occurring, emphasizing aspects of procedures that are felt or heard. They should approach the child by always identifying themselves as soon as they enter the room. Because unfamiliar sounds are especially frightening, these are explained. Parents are encouraged to room with their child and participate in the care. Familiar objects, such as teddy bear or doll, should be brought from home to help lessen the strangeness of the hospital. As soon as the child is able to be out of bed, he or she is oriented to the immediate surroundings. If the child is able to see on admission, this opportunity is taken to point out significant aspects of the room. The child is encouraged to practice ambulating with the eyes closed to become accustomed to this experience.

The room is arranged with safety in mind. For example, a stool or chair is placed next to the bed to help the child climb in and out of bed. The furniture is always placed in the same position to prevent collisions. Cleaning personnel are reminded of the need to keep the room in order. If the child has difficulty navigating by feeling the walls, a rope can be attached from the bed to the point of destination, such as the bathroom. Attention to details such as well-fitting slippers and robes that do not hang on the floor is important to prevent tripping. Unlike the child who is blind, these children are not familiar with navigating with a cane.

The child is encouraged to be independent in self-care activities, especially if the visual loss may be prolonged or potentially permanent. For example, during bathing the nurse sets up all the equipment and encourages the child to participate. At meal-

*A catalog of numerous products for people with vision problems is available from the American Foundation for the Blind (see footnote p. 1055) and from The Lighthouse, Inc., 1 800-829-0500; website: www.lighthouse.org.

†Division for the Blind and Visually Handicapped, 1291 Taylor St. NW, Washington, DC 20542; 1-800-424-8567; TTY: (202) 707-0744; fax (202) 707-0712; website: www.loc.gov/nls. (A state-by-state listing of libraries for blind and physically handicapped readers, as well as other reference circulars, is available from this office.)

‡20 Roszel Rd., Princeton, NJ 08540; 1-800-221-4792; fax (609) 987-8116; website: www.rfbd.org.

time the nurse explains where each food item is on the tray, opens any special containers, prepares cereal or toast, and encourages the child in self-feeding. Favorite finger foods, such as sandwiches, hamburgers, hot dogs, or pizza, may be good selections. The child is praised for efforts at being cooperative and independent. Any improvements made in self-care, no matter how small, are stressed.

Appropriate recreational activities are provided, and if a child-life specialist is available, such planning is done jointly. Because children with temporary blindness have a wide range of play experiences to draw on, they are encouraged to select activities. For example, if they like to read, they may enjoy being read to. If they prefer manual activity, they may appreciate playing with clay or building blocks or feeling different textures and naming them. If they need an outlet for aggression, activities such as pounding or banging on a drum can be helpful. Simple board and card games can be played with a "seeing partner" or if the opponent helps with the game. They should have familiar toys from home to play with, because familiar items are more easily manipulated than new ones. If parents want to bring presents, they should be objects that stimulate hearing and touch, such as a radio, music box, or stuffed animal.

Occasionally, children who are blind come to the hospital for procedures to restore their vision. Although this is an extremely happy time, it also requires intervention to help them adjust to sight. They need an opportunity to take in all that they see; they should not be bombarded with visual stimuli. They may need to concentrate on people's faces or their own to become accustomed to this experience. They often need to talk about what they see, and to compare the visual images with their mental ones. The child may also go through a period of depression, which must be respected and supported. The nurse or parents should refrain from statements such as "How can you be so sad when you can see again?" Instead the child should be encouraged to discuss how it feels to see, especially in terms of seeing himself or herself.

Newly sighted children also need time to adjust to the ability to engage in activities that were impossible before. For example, they may prefer to use braille to read because of familiarity with the touch system, rather than learning a new "visual" approach. Eventually, as they learn to recognize letters and numbers, they will integrate these new skills into reading and writing. However, parents and teachers must be careful not to push them before they are ready. This applies to social relationships and physical activities as well as learning situations.

Assist in Measures to Prevent Visual Impairment. An essential nursing goal is to prevent visual impairment. This involves many of the same interventions discussed under hearing impairments: (1) prenatal screening for pregnant women at risk, such as those with rubella or syphilis infection and family histories of genetic disorders associated with visual loss; (2) adequate prenatal and perinatal care to prevent prematurity; (3) periodic screening of all children, especially newborns through preschoolers, for congenital blindness and visual impairments caused by refractive errors, strabismus, and other disorders; (4) rubella immunization of all children; and (5) safety counseling regarding the common causes of ocular trauma.

Safety counseling should include safe practices when working with, playing with, or carrying objects such as scissors, knives, and balls.

NURSE ALERT • A helmet with a face mask should be required gear for all children playing football, hockey, baseball, or softball (especially for the catcher, batter, umpire, and base runner).

After detection of eye problems, the nurse has a responsibility to prevent further ocular damage by ensuring that corrective treatment is used. For the child with strabismus, this often necessitates occlusion patching of the stronger eye. Compliance with the procedure is greatest during the early preschool years. It is more difficult to encourage school-age children to wear the occlusive patch because the poor visual acuity of the uncovered weaker eye interferes with school-work and the patch sets them apart from their peers. In school they benefit from being positioned favorably (closer to the chalkboard or other visual media) and allowed extra time to read or complete an assignment. If treatment of the eye disorder requires instillation of ophthalmic medication, the family is taught the correct procedure (see Chapter 45).*

For the child with refractive errors, the nurse helps the child adjust to wearing glasses. Young children, who often pull glasses off, benefit from temporal pieces that wrap around the ears or an elastic strap attached to the frames and around the back of the head to hold the glasses on securely. Once children appreciate the value of clear vision, they are more likely to wear the corrective lenses.

Because trauma is the leading cause of blindness, the nurse has the major responsibility of preventing further eye injury until the specific treatment is instituted. The major principles to follow when caring for an eye injury are outlined in the Emergency box on p. 1054. Because patients with a serious eye injury fear blindness, the nurse should stay with the child and family to provide support and reassurance.

➤ Evaluation

The effectiveness of nursing interventions is determined by continual reassessment and evaluation of care based on the following observational guidelines and expected outcomes:

1. Interview family regarding their adjustments to the sensory impairment; observe family members' relationship with child; interview child regarding feelings about the sensory impairment and its effect on activities of daily living (especially important if a visual loss).
2. Have parents identify those cues that indicate infant is responding to them; observe nonvisual behaviors of parents as they respond to infant.
3. Observe techniques child uses to read and navigate; inquire if child is enrolled in a visual training program; inquire about socialization opportunities for child (e.g., who are child's friends, what are child's extracurricular activities).
4. Observe preparation of the room and self-care activities that provide for safety and independence during hospitalization.

Expected outcomes:

1. Parents express their feelings and concerns regarding loss of sight and demonstrate an understanding of child's disability and its implications.

---

*Community and home care instructions on giving eye medications are available in Wong DL, Hess CS: ***Wong and Whaley's clinical manual of pediatric nursing,*** ed 5, St Louis, 2000, Mosby.

2. Parents demonstrate attachment behaviors.
3. Infant or child engages in appropriate activities for level of development (specify); child demonstrates an attitude of security in the environment.
4. Child and family receive safe and supportive care during hospitalization.

(See also Nursing Care Plan: The Child with Visual Impairment.*)

Deaf-Blind Children

The most traumatic sensory impairment is loss of sight and hearing. Obviously, auditory and visual disabilities have profound effects on the child's development. They interfere with the normal sequence of physical, intellectual, and psychosocial growth. Although such children often achieve the usual motor milestones, their rate of development is slower. These children learn communication only with specialized training. *Finger spelling* is one desirable method often taught to these children. Some deaf-blind children, especially those with residual hearing or sight, can learn to speak. Whenever possible, speech is encouraged, because it allows communication with other individuals.

The future prospects for deaf-blind children are at best unpredictable. Congenital blindness and/or deafness may be accompanied by other physical or neurologic problems, which further lessen the child's learning potential. The most favorable prognosis is for children who have acquired deafness and blindness and have few, if any, associated disabilities. Their learning capacity is greatly potentiated by their developmental progress before the sensory impairments. Although total independence, including gainful vocational training, is the goal, some deaf-blind children are unable to develop to this level. They may require lifelong parental or residential care. The nurse working with such families helps them deal with future goals for the child, including possible alternatives to home care during the parents' advancing years.

Retinoblastoma

Retinoblastoma, which arises from the retina, is the most common congenital malignant intraocular tumor of childhood. Approximately 11 cases per million occur annually, primarily in children under 5 years of age. Of all cases, about 60% are nonhereditary and unilateral, 15% are hereditary and unilateral, and 25% are hereditary and bilateral. Hereditary retinoblastomas are transmitted primarily as an autosomal dominant trait with nearly complete penetrance (Donaldson et al, 1997).

Diagnostic Evaluation. Retinoblastoma has few grossly obvious signs (Box 42-7). Typically it is the parent who first observes a whitish "glow" in the pupil, known as the *cat's eye reflex* (white reflex) or leukokoria. Leukokoria represents visualization of the tumor as the light momentarily falls on the mass (Fig. 42-8).

The first step in diagnosis is carefully listening to and recognizing the significance of reports from family members regarding suspected abnormalities within the eye. Eye abnormalities, including cat's eye reflex, strabismus, decreased vision, and persistent painful erythematous eyes, are referred to an ophthalmologist. Definitive diagnosis is usually based on indirect ophthalmoscopy, which is performed with the patient under general anesthesia with maximum dilation of the pupils.

Therapeutic Management. Treatment of retinoblastoma depends chiefly on the stage of the tumor at the time of diagnosis. *Reese-Ellsworth classification* is the commonly used standard for intraocular disease. In general, early-stage unilateral retinoblastomas are treated with irradiation or other techniques, such as cryotherapy, which freezes the tumor. The aim of therapy is to preserve useful vision in the affected eye and eradicate the tumor.

With advanced tumor growth, especially optic nerve involvement, *enucleation* (removal) of the affected eye is the treatment of choice. The use of chemotherapy in advanced disease is controversial but, if employed, may include vincristine, cyclophosphamide, teniposide, and carboplatin.

With bilateral disease, every attempt is made to preserve useful vision in the least affected eye, with enucleation of the severely diseased eye. When bilateral tumors are found early, radiotherapy or other treatments to both eyes may prevent the need for enucleation.

Prognosis. The overall prognosis for retinoblastoma is very favorable, with a survival rate of nearly 90% for both unilateral and bilateral tumors. Retinoblastoma is one of the tumors that may spontaneously regress.

Of major concern in long-term survivors is the development of secondary tumors, especially osteogenic sarcoma. Children with bilateral disease (hereditary form) are more likely to develop secondary cancers than are children with unilateral dis-

Box 42-7
Clinical Manifestations of Retinoblastoma

Cat's eye reflex (most common sign)
Strabismus (second most common sign)
Red, painful eye, often with glaucoma
Blindness (late sign)

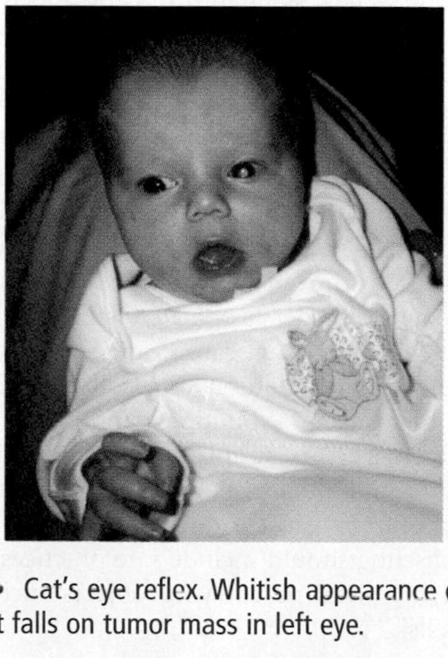

FIG. 42-8 • Cat's eye reflex. Whitish appearance of lens is produced as light falls on tumor mass in left eye.

*In Wong DL, Hess CS: ***Wong and Whaley's clinical manual of pediatric nursing***, ed 5, St Louis, 2000, Mosby.

ease. It is thought that these individuals are predisposed to developing cancer, and radiation increases their risk.

Nursing Care Management. One of the most important nursing goals is to have a high index of suspicion for this rare malignancy. If parents report noticing a strange light in the eye or expression, these concerns must be taken seriously. Families with a history of retinoblastoma require follow-up, and the nurse can be instrumental in reminding parents of appointments.

Because the tumor is usually diagnosed in infants or very young children, most of the preparation for diagnostic tests and treatment involves parents. After indirect ophthalmoscopy, the child may not see very clearly, or the eyes may be sensitive to light because of pupillary dilation. Parents are made aware of these normal reactions before the procedure. They also are informed that a battery of screening tests, such as bone surveys and bone marrow aspiration, may be performed to detect metastasis.

Once the disease is diagnosed, the practitioner confers with the parents regarding treatment. Unless the diagnosis is made very early, an enucleation is performed. Parents are told about the procedure, as well as about the positive benefits of a prosthesis. Showing them pictures of another child with an artificial eye may be very helpful in their adjusting to the thought of disfigurement (Fig. 42-9).

After surgery the parents are prepared for the child's facial appearance. An eye patch is in place, and the child's face may be edematous or ecchymotic. Parents often fear seeing the surgical site because they imagine a cavity in the skull. On the contrary, the lids are usually closed and the area does not appear sunken, because a surgically implanted sphere maintains the shape of the eyeball. The implant is covered with conjunctiva, and when the lids are open, the exposed area resembles the mucosal lining of the mouth. Once the child is fitted for a prosthesis, usually within 3 weeks, the facial appearance returns to normal. Initial instructions for care of the prosthesis are given by the ocularist, who fits and manufactures the device.

Care of the socket is minimal and easily accomplished. The wound itself is clean and has little or no drainage. If an antibiotic ointment is prescribed, it is applied in a thin line on the surface of the tissues of the socket. To cleanse the site, an irrigating solution may be ordered and is instilled daily or more often if necessary, before application of the antibiotic ointment. The dressing consists of an eye pad taped over the surgical site with nonirritating tape; it is changed daily. Once the socket has healed completely, a dressing is no longer necessary, although it is a preventive measure against infection.

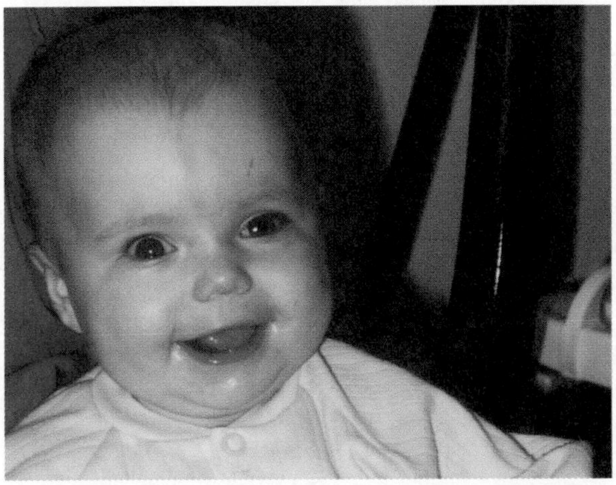

FIG. 42-9 • Infant with left prosthetic eye.

A long-term consideration is the survivor's ability to transmit the defective gene to his or her offspring. Parents are encouraged to seek genetic counseling for themselves and for the child during puberty.

Support Family. Families with a history of the disorder may feel great guilt for transmitting the defect to their offspring. In families with no history of retinoblastoma, the discovery of the diagnosis is a shock, commonly complicated by guilt for not having found it sooner. Because parents often are the first to observe the cat's eye reflex, they may feel angry at themselves or others, especially health professionals, for delaying a more thorough examination. The nurse assesses each of these variables in planning care based on understanding the family's emotional reactions and adjustment (see Chapter 41).

(See also Nursing Care Plan: The Child with Cancer, Chapter 49.)

Key Points

- The definition of mental retardation (MR) is made up of three components that assess intellectual functioning, functional strengths and weaknesses, and age at the time of diagnosis.
- Four dimensions of care for individuals with MR include: intellectual functioning and adaptive skills, psychologic/emotional considerations, physical (health/etiology) considerations, and environmental considerations.
- Causes of severe MR are primarily genetic, biochemical, viral, and developmental. Mild MR is associated primarily with familial, social, and environmental causes, whereas severe MR is more likely to be associated with specific syndromes.
- Education of children with cognitive impairment emphasizes sensory and verbal discrimination, improvement of short-term memory, motivation, and technologic support.
- Promoting optimum development may be achieved through family guidance regarding play, communication, discipline, socialization, and sexuality.
- Prevention efforts regarding MR focus on support for the premature neonate and other high risk newborns, rubella immunization, genetic counseling, and maternal education regarding the risks of chemical use and the importance of adequate nutrition.
- Down syndrome, a chromosomal abnormality, is characterized by retarded intelligence of variable degree, slowed language development, congenital anomalies, sensory problems, and diminished growth and sexual development.
- Fragile X syndrome is characterized by MR and phenotypic findings in affected males. It is considered the second leading chromosomal cause of MR after Down syndrome, and the most common hereditary cause.

- Hearing disorders may be classified according to the location of the defect: conductive, sensorineural, mixed conductive-sensorineural, and central auditory imperception.
- Rehabilitation for hearing loss involves parent education and support, hearing aids, lipreading, sign language, speech therapy, and promotion of socialization.
- Prevention of hearing loss includes treatment of infection, universal newborn screening and child auditory testing, immunization, pregnancy and genetic counseling, and reduction of noise pollution.
- Visual impairments in childhood include refractive errors, amblyopia, strabismus, cataracts, glaucoma, trauma, and infections.
- Nursing goals in visual rehabilitation include helping the family and child adjust to the child's visual impairment, promoting parent-child attachment, fostering optimum development and independence, providing for play and socialization, and being aware of educational facilities.
- For the child undergoing ocular surgery, nursing care is aimed at reassuring the child and family throughout treatment, orienting the child to the surroundings, providing a safe environment, and encouraging independence.
- Prevention of visual impairment focuses on prenatal screening, prenatal and perinatal care, periodic vision screening, immunization, and safety counseling.
- Retinoblastoma is a rare congenital malignant tumor; its most common clinical manifestations are cat's eye reflex (white pupil) and strabismus.

References

American Academy of Pediatrics, Committee on Genetics: Prenatal genetic diagnosis for pediatricians, *Pediatrics* 93(6):1010-1015, 1994.

American Academy of Pediatrics, Task Force on Newborn and Infant Hearing: Newborn and infant hearing loss: detection and intervention, *Pediatrics* 103(2):527-530, 1999.

American Psychiatric Association: *Diagnostic and statistical manual of mental disorders,* ed 4 (DSM-IV), Washington, DC, 1994, The Association.

Applebaum E: Detection of hearing loss in children, *Pediatr Ann* 28(6):351-356, 1999.

Berrettini S et al: Progressive sensorineural hearing loss in childhood, *Pediatr Neurol* 20(2):130-136, 1999.

Camp BW et al: Maternal and neonatal risk factors for mental retardation: defining the "at-risk" child, *Early Hum Dev* 50(2):159-173, 1998.

Carr J: Annotation: long term outcome for people with Down's syndrome, *J Child Psychol Psychiatry* 35(3):425-439, 1994.

Davidson PW: Visual impairment and blindness. In Levine MD, Carey WB, Crocker AC, editors: *Developmental-behavioral pediatrics,* ed 2, Philadelphia, 1992, WB Saunders.

Donaldson S et al: Retinoblastoma. In Pizzo PA, Poplack DG, editors: *Principles and practice of pediatric oncology,* ed 3, Philadelphia, 1997, JB Lippincott.

Eilers RE, Oiler DK: Infant vocalizations and the early diagnosis of severe hearing impairment, *J Pediatr* 124:199-203, 1994.

Fredericks DW, Williams WL: New definition of mental retardation for the American Association of Mental Retardation, *Image J Nurs Sch* 30(1):53-56, 1998.

Gurrieri F et al: Pervasive developmental disorder and epilepsy due to maternally derived duplication of 15q11-q13, *Neurology* 52(8):1694-1697, 1999.

Hagerman RJ, Cronister A: Fragile X syndrome. In Jackson PL, Vessey JA, editors: *Primary care of the child with a chronic condition,* ed 2, St Louis, 1996, Mosby.

Hixon M et al: FISH studies of the sperm of fathers of paternally derived cases of trisomy 21: no evidence for an increase in aneuploidy, *Hum Genet* 103(6):654-657, 1998.

LePage EL, Murray NM: Latent cochlear damage in personal stereo users: a study based on click-evoked otoacoustic emissions, *Med J Aust* 169(11-12):588-592, 1998.

Litovitz T, Schmitz BF: Ingestion of cylindrical and button batteries: an analysis of 2382 cases, *Pediatrics* 89:747-757, 1992.

Murray J et al: Screening for fragile X syndrome, *Health Technol Assess* 1(4):i-iv, 1-71, 1997.

Palmer FB, Capute AJ: Mental retardation, *Pediatr Rev* 15(12):473-479, 1994.

Rahi J: Measuring the burden of childhood blindness, *Br J Ophthalmol* 83:387-388, 1999.

Roizen NJ: Etiology of hearing loss in children: nongenetic causes, *Pediatr Clin North Am* 46(1):49-64, 1999.

Schalock RL et al: The changing conception of mental retardation: implications for the field, *Ment Retard* 32(3):181-193, 1994.

Shaughnessy M et al: *Teaching the mentally retarded parenting skills: international perspectives,* EDRS microfiche report, 1996.

Slattery WH, Fayad JN: Cochlear implants in children with sensorineural inner ear hearing loss, *Pediatr Ann* 28(6):359-363, 1999.

Stoll C et al: Study of Down syndrome in 238,942 consecutive births, *Ann Genet* 41(1):44-51, 1998.

Toledo C et al: Growth curves of children with Down syndrome, *Ann Genet* 42(2):81-90, 1999.

Yankowitz J et al: Prospective evaluation of prenatal maternal serum screening for trisomy 18, *Am J Obstet Gynecol* 178(3):446-450, 1998.

Yoshinaga-Itano C et al: Language of early- and later-identified children with hearing loss, *Pediatrics* 102(5):1161-1171, 1998.

CHAPTER

43

Family-Centered Home Care

http://www.harcourthealth.com/MERLIN/Wong/maternal/

Learning Objectives

On completion of this chapter the reader will be able to:

- Differentiate home care from hospice care.
- List at least three factors contributing to the increasing emphasis on home care services.
- Describe case management/care coordination and its importance in home care.
- List general principles of a family-centered assessment and planning process.
- Identify five key characteristics of collaborative relationships.
- Describe approaches to promoting optimal development, self-care, and education in home care.
- Outline six areas in need of attention for promoting safety in home care.

GENERAL CONCEPTS OF HOME CARE

Definition

Home care is not a new concept in pediatrics. Over time the term has referred to parents caring for mildly ill children at home; to nursing home visits after children are discharged from the hospital; to hospice care; and more recently, to care at home for children with more serious chronic illness and dependence on medical technology. Home care is the fastest growing component of the health care industry.

As discussed in this chapter, *home care* refers to care provided in the family's residence for children with complex health care needs and their families. The purpose of home care services is to promote, maintain, or restore health or to maximize the level of independence while minimizing the effects of disability and illness, including terminal illness. Home care differs from *hospice care,* which is a program of palliative and supportive care services providing physical, psychologic, social, and spiritual care for dying persons, their families, and other loved ones. Hospice services are available in both the home and inpatient settings, and end-of-life planning should be instituted early for any child facing a terminal diagnosis.

Impetus for Home Care

The initial impetus for home care for children with complex medical conditions came from a parental desire to have these children at home and from professionals' willingness to work with families to achieve this goal. Improving the quality of life for both the child and the family was the driving force in the efforts to move technology-dependent children from the hospital to the home setting.

Other factors eventually influenced the shift toward an emphasis on home care for this population, including increasing numbers of children requiring long-term complex medical and nursing care and lower costs for home care as compared with hospital care.

Dramatic advances in medical care over the past several decades have resulted in increased numbers of children requiring long-term complex medical care as a result of (1) improvements in trauma care; (2) increased survival rates for children with leukemia and other cancers, chronic kidney disorders, sickle cell anemia, cystic fibrosis, spina bifida, and cardiac or intestinal malformations; (3) more aggressive care for muscular dystrophy and degenerative neuromuscular disorders; and (4) more children with acquired immunodeficiency syndrome (AIDS).

The cost of care is another critical factor. For third-party payers and the government, the cost of home care is generally less than the cost of hospital care for children dependent on medical technology and requiring substantial and complex care. However, families may absorb many of the costs of home care, including medication, supplies, transportation, shelter, utilities, food, laundry, and housekeeping. Families generally provide at least some portion of the nursing care as well, and some may become unemployed or only partially employed to be able to stay at home. Those out-of-pocket expenses and the loss of income can become a financial burden for the family, and they may need help evaluating options and advocating for the child's needs.

Effectiveness of Home Care

Home care is effective for many children; however, it may not be possible in all circumstances. A number of factors must be considered. First, the child's condition must be medically stable so that care can be managed in the home setting and supported by available home care equipment. Second, the family must want the child at home and must have the motivation and ability to learn to provide the child's care. Families must also be able to live with the intrusion of the child's equipment, care schedule, and nurses and other providers in their daily life. Third, professionals and the community must be prepared to provide the necessary support to make home care successful, including nursing and other therapeutic services, transportation, accessible emergency facilities, case management, and family support. Fourth, financial support, both public and private, is essential.

Even if home care is initially successful for a child and family, alterations in the child's medical condition, the lack of adequate community resources, depletion of the family's financial resources, high levels of family stress and exhaustion, and disagreements between the family members and the health care team can all affect the success of home care. A well-developed system of family support may help avoid a crisis residential placement (Petr, Murdock, and Chapin, 1995); however, short- or long-term residential placement may be a consideration for some families.

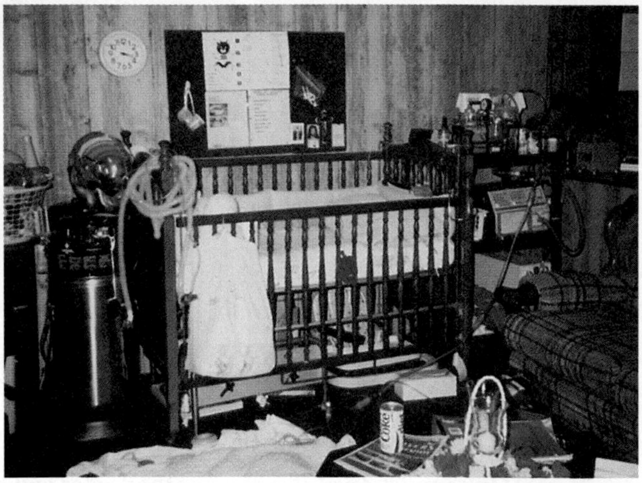

FIG. 43-1 • An essential aspect of preparation for home care is arranging equipment and supplies.

> **Box 43-1**
>
> **Minimum Contents of Written Home Care Instructions**
>
> A schedule of routine care needs
> Correct settings for any equipment required
> A list of signs, symptoms, and parameters (physical and behavioral) that are normal for the individual child
> A list of signs, symptoms, and parameters (physical and behavioral) that indicate a problem for the individual child
> Guidelines for and a list of whom to contact about what problems
> An explanation of pertinent emergency procedures

From Ahmann E: An overview of issues in pediatric high tech home care. In Gorski L: *Best practices in home infusion,* Gaithersburg, MD, 1999, Aspen.

Discharge Planning and Selection of a Home Care Agency

Much of the success of home care for the child who is dependent on medical technology depends on careful planning and preparation. General principles of discharge planning and transition to home care are addressed in Chapter 44. *Discharge planning must begin early, be a multidisciplinary process, and involve the family.* Negotiation with the insurance company or health maintenance organization (HMO) may be necessary. Early involvement of the home care agency promotes continuity of care and a smooth transition from hospital to home. The home care plan for a child with complex care requirements should address the many health and community services that may need to be mobilized. Comprehensive written home care instructions facilitate continuity of care across settings and providers (Box 43-1).* A notebook can be an effective planning and organizing reference for families.

An excellent method of providing home care instructions is with video recordings. Once the family masters the procedures, consider video recording their performance on tape. Visual learning may be most helpful for people who cannot read or who are not fluent in English.

The plans for transition from hospital to home should include at least two family members learning and demonstrating all aspects of the child's care in the hospital. An in-hospital trial period during which parents provide total care for the child is generally beneficial as well. After a successful trial, the family may benefit from taking the child home on a brief pass before making final discharge plans. (This may need to be negotiated with the insurance company.) The home care nurse will play an important role in assessing this experience with the family. Whether or not the child is taken home on a pass, a predischarge home visit offers the home care nurse the opportunity to meet the family, help them assess their preparedness and the preparedness of the home environment, discuss plans for arranging the child's equipment at home (Fig. 43-1), reinforce prior discharge teaching, and implement any additional teaching that may be necessary.

*Numerous community and home care instructions are available in Wong DL, Hess CS: ***Wong and Whaley's clinical manual of pediatric nursing***, ed 5, St Louis, 2000, Mosby.

Case Management

Parents of children with complex care requirements often experience frustration about the fragmentation of services and desire competent case management. Traditional definitions of *case management* generally focus on cost control, attainment of desired clinical outcomes, and monitoring and evaluation of care provided. However, for optimum home care of the child who is technology dependent, case management—or *care coordination*—should be viewed more broadly (see also Chapter 29).

Care coordination has several purposes. Its primary goal is ensuring continuity for the child and family across hospital, home, educational, and other settings. Care should be coordinated among multiple providers to reduce the complexity of care for the child, reduce fragmentation of care, and decrease the burden of care for the family. Care coordination should ensure that the medical, nursing, and health maintenance needs of the child are addressed, as well as the financial issues, psychosocial concerns, and educational issues of the child and family. Assisting families to prepare for the transition at termination of home care is also important (Agazio, 1997).

Care coordination should promote the family's role as primary decision maker and enhance the family's capability to meet the special needs of the child and the family as a whole. Care coordination is most effective if a single person works with the family to accomplish the many tasks and responsibilities involved. These include assessing needs and resources, planning for comprehensive care, coordinating services, and referrals, monitoring and evaluating services, and providing administrative support and advocacy. In 1999 the American Nurses Credentialing Center (ANCC), a subsidiary of the American Nurses Association (ANA), began offering specialty certification in case management.

Role of the Nurse, Training, and Standards of Care

The home care nurse must share a level of technical expertise with the critical care nurse while being able to adapt equipment, procedures, and the nursing process to the home setting. (See Chapter 45 for specific technical skills that may be required in home care practice.) The need for technical expertise must be matched by a knowledge of child development and the ability to work creatively with the child challenged by chronic illness and technology dependence. When practicing in the home, the nurse must be comfortable making independent nursing judgments and problem solving with no immediate assistance. At the same time, the nurse must have excellent interpersonal skills; an ability to work with other professionals and the family; and most importantly, an ability to respect family autonomy. As home care becomes more demanding, specialized educational preparation, credentialing, and advanced practice will become more important.

When working with a home care agency, nurses should expect to receive patient placements appropriate to their expertise. They should also expect orientation in the following areas: to the individual patient's care plan and equipment needs; to the agency's policies and procedures, including procedures for addressing any problems that may occur when care is provided in the home; to documentation procedures (reimbursement-driven documentation in home care differs from documentation practices in the hospital setting); and to legal liability issues. Supervision of practice, including occasional on-site visits by a nursing supervisor, should be provided.

Home care agencies, public or private, that participate in the Medicare or Medicaid programs must be certified by a federally designated, state-certifying body and abide by federal and state regulations. Private agencies that do not participate in the federal programs are not mandated to meet the federal standards, but a variety of organizations can provide some types of credentialing or accreditation for these home health agencies (Gingerich and Ondeck, 1997).

The ANA has developed standards of nursing practice for both community health and home care nurses that should guide practice in the home setting (ANA, 1986a, 1986b). In addition, the ANCC offers both generalist and clinical specialist certification in home health (Wilson, 1996). However, despite some important differences between pediatric and adult care in the home, as of this writing no national standards specific to pediatric home care nursing practice have been developed. Specific texts and articles may provide useful clinical guidelines.

FAMILY-CENTERED HOME CARE

Technology dependence, chronic illness, and complex care requirements cross social, cultural, spiritual, and economic boundaries. Regardless of a family's background, family values must be respected in the provision of home care services. *The home is the family's domain,* and the child is at home because the family's central role is to nurture and raise their child. The nurse must respect the family's central role in the care of the child and must work in collaboration with the family in efforts to care for the child. Family-centered nursing practice is essential in the home setting.

The first of the nine key components of family-centered care (see Chapter 29) provides the philosophic basis for family-centered practice: recognition that the family is the constant in the child's life, whereas the service systems and personnel within those systems fluctuate (Shelton and Stepanek, 1994). Families have the most intimate knowledge of the child's strengths and abilities, the challenges of providing care, and the abilities and needs of other family members. *Believing that no one knows the child better than the family* is critical to the success of any health care plan (Bishop, Woll, Arango, 1993). It is important to recognize the family's central, caring role; their knowledge; and their particular and unique expertise.

Respect for Diversity

Respect for varied family structures and for racial, ethnic, cultural, spiritual, and socioeconomic diversity among families is essential in home care (see also Chapters 31 and 32). Nurses work in close relationship with family members and in the family's own domain. The family's background and their lifestyle choices are respected. Particular attention is given to communication. The meaning of words used and the way they are said may affect various cultural groups in different ways. For example, the words "family support" may be interpreted by some families as an implication that they are weak and in need of help (Patterson and Blum, 1993). Families may also differ in their cultural view of children; in childrearing practices; and in their views of illness, its causes, and its meaning. The views of illness may influence the type or level of investment a family will make in the child's care. Families may have beliefs about health care and healing practices that are foreign to the nurse's background and experience. The home care nurse, aware that value systems drive behavior, needs to learn about the family's culture, ask questions without implying judgment, interpret the mainstream medical culture, and help families design interventions that meet their preferences. Cultural assessment tools and culture-specific teaching materials can be helpful (Narayan, 1997; Spruhan, 1996) (Family Focus box).

Respect for family diversity and awareness of both family developmental stages (see Chapter 31) and the stages of a family's

Family Focus

DEVELOPING A RELATIONSHIP WITH CULTURALLY DIVERSE FAMILIES

I work in the inner city, and my home care patients come from a variety of racial and ethnic backgrounds. I am Caucasian, from Australia. Often, when I first visit a family, there is an initial coolness or apprehension toward me. This is understandable because I am a stranger, and perhaps families think I'll judge them in one way or another. By the end of the first visit, however, there is usually a smile as I leave; by the second visit they often greet me with a smile at the door; and by the third visit we usually have a friendship, a trust, and an ease of communication.

If I'm working on a case for an extended time, I use a holistic nursing approach. This involves being aware of how the illness of the child affects the entire family. As I listen over many weeks to their fears and questions, and often as I share faith perspectives, a bond begins to form. I find it a privilege to share in their joys and their pain, and I feel rewarded by the trust that they invest in me.

Julie Edgerton, RN
Home Care Nurse
Children's National Medical Center
Washington, DC

Critical Thinking

MEDICAL NEGLECT

The home care nurse notes that the family has failed to give a dose of the child's medication. The nurse is responsible for all of the following actions *except* which?

First, Think About It...

- What conclusions are you reaching?
- If you accept your conclusions, what are the implications?

1. Educate and counsel the family about the child's medication requirements and schedule.
2. Report the family for medical neglect.
3. Assess the child's condition.
4. Document the missed dose and any corrective measures taken.

The best answer is 2. It is correct to conclude that some behaviors that might be considered medical neglect may actually result from the family feeling overwhelmed, not being fully educated about the child's care requirements, and/or experiencing denial. The nurse has a responsibility to address these issues with the family. At the same time the nurse should be cognizant that home care providers may have legal liability not only for their own actions but also for those of parents who are "noncompliant" with medical orders. The frequency and severity of "noncompliance" will affect the nurse's responsibility. For example, one missed medication dose may be appropriately handled by documentation and counseling. On the other hand, regularly missed doses or one instance of turning off a ventilator alarm requires a more vigorous response. The point at which these instances cross the line into reportable medical neglect depends in part on the definitions of abuse or neglect in the state in which services are provided.

Modified from Ahmann E: Thinking critically about family-centered home care nursing, *Pediatr Nurs* 20(6):588-590, 1994.

adjustment to illness in a child (see Chapter 41) will assist the home care nurse in recognizing and promoting family strengths and in respecting varied coping mechanisms. Labels such as "dysfunctional," "difficult," and "noncompliant" can reinforce negative expectations and shape behaviors of both parents and professionals (Critical Thinking box). On the other hand, emphasizing, identifying, and building on family strengths and coping mechanisms are strategies that promote a central goal in nursing care of the child and family: family empowerment (see Chapter 29). The nurse working with families should remain flexible and open-minded because new family strengths may emerge over time and coping mechanisms may wax and wane with the stresses of caring for a child with serious or multiple problems.

Parent-Professional Collaboration

Family-centered nursing practice is built on a foundation of parent-professional collaboration, which represents a shift from the traditional unidirectional relationships between health care providers and families. Core competencies for collaboration have been developed (McDaniel and Campbell, 1996). *Collaborative relationships,* essential in the home care setting, are characterized by several features (Bishop, Woll, and Arango, 1993):

Communication—Including complete and unbiased sharing of information with parents about their child's care and prognosis

Dialogue—Exchanging of information and sharing of reactions and ideas

Active listening—Listening beyond the words to hear and understand concerns, including checking to be certain that interpretations are correct

Awareness and acceptance of difference—Willingness to examine one's own cultural biases and to accept that others may think and act out of different value systems

Negotiation—The process of examining different options, priorities, and preferences to best meet the needs of the child and family

Communication with the family should not be invasive. There is no need to collect information from the family that can be obtained from the child's records. The nurse should explain to the family the reason for questions, particularly those that the family may perceive as intrusive, and should inform families of who will have access to the information. The nurse must also assure families that they have a right to expect confidentiality in regard to the data collected. When working in the home, the nurse must respect the privacy of family members' communications with each other that may be overheard.

NURSE ALERT • Home care nurses should restrict their communications with other professionals to clinically relevant information about the family.

Communication with family members should also include sharing with the family, in a supportive manner, complete and unbiased information about all aspects of the child's condition and care, one of the principles of family-centered care (Shelton and Stepanek, 1994). Repeating explanations in simple language may be necessary. Information should be shared with families in a way that will have meaning in their cultural context. Many parents report a preference for interactions with professionals who communicate empathy and concern. Although they want accurate information, many parents prefer that providers moderate the amount of information about possible complications and unfavorable prognoses (Knafl et al, 1992).

Disagreements may arise between parents and nurses over proper procedures for care of the child. In any situation that will not pose danger or risk for the child, nurses should respect parental preferences. Other options to help resolve conflicts include the following (Ahmann and Bond, 1992):

- Work with the family's priorities and reevaluate over time.
- Provide the family with additional information that may affect their perception of priorities.
- Share the nurse's perception of priorities and rationales without judgment.
- Suggest an additional priority goal if the family agrees.

If parents wish to alter a plan of treatment that is part of medical orders, the nurse should ask that they negotiate the change with the practitioner, because the nurse must follow the written medical orders (Klug, 1993).

If disagreements cannot be resolved, the nurse can consult agency policy guidelines, the home care supervisor or case manager, or an ethics committee for guidance.

The Nursing Process

In the home the family is a partner in each step of the nursing process. The use of formal self-report assessment tools can help families identify needs they may have for information, training, services, and support. Assessment should also address family strengths and resources (see Family Assessment, Chapter 34). The principles of communication discussed previously guide data collection. The nurse's observations are shared neutrally, without value judgment, and in a way that preserves the family's own role in decision making (Bond, Phillips, and Rollins, 1994).

All the information gathered as part of the assessment process is shared with the family. The nurse should recognize that the family's perception of their most important need will generally guide their behavior and consume their attention and energy. For this reason, family priorities guide the planning process.

Both short-term and long-term goals should be outlined and agreed on by the child, family, and professionals involved. The plan of care should integrate various disciplines that may be involved with the child in order to minimize duplication and consolidate care requirements. Cross-training of professionals and a transdisciplinary mode of treatment can also be useful when a child has multiple and complex care requirements. For example, certain physical or occupational therapy routines may be incorporated into the child's morning nursing procedures, or speech therapy interventions may be conducted by the parent or nurse around eating times so that the entire day is not occupied by procedures. A written schedule of daily routines should be developed and followed by all caregivers.

Goals of care are supported by intervention strategies that reflect normalization (see Chapter 41) and the interests and abilities of the child and family. Nurses can help families explore a range of alternative strategies, services, and resources so that the family can choose the best match for their situation.

Family participation in evaluating a home care plan can occur on several levels. Families and care providers should regularly review the goals of care and then update the care plan as required. The nurse can also ask the family open-ended questions at regular intervals to assess their opinions on the effectiveness of care. As part of the evaluation process, families should be acknowledged for their successes and accomplishments. Finally, families should be given an opportunity to evaluate individual home care nurses, the home care agency, and other service providers on a periodic basis. The evaluation should address the nurse's knowledge, skills, and respect for the family's choices. It also should address the agency's handling of the schedule, provision of qualified nurses, and problem-solving abilities (Klug, 1993). The evaluations should be used by the agency to improve quality of care (Family Focus box).

Home care nursing encourages a close and rewarding relationship with the family. One of the most important aspects of this relationship is maintaining professional boundaries and a therapeutic role that is supportive but not intrusive (Critical Thinking box).

Technologic trends that may eventually influence the nursing process in home care include the use of laptop computers to document the home visit; and the advent of telemedicine, electronic systems that can transmit physiologic data directly to the clinician via the telephone (Crist, Kaufman, and Crampton, 1996; Warner, 1996).

Family Focus

WHAT I LEARNED ABOUT HOME CARE

I learned many things as a result of having home care for four children over a period of 8 years. Two of the major areas I learned about were communication and families' rights. It took a long time to learn some of these things.

Initially I tried very hard to be sensitive to the professionals and often put my own feelings and needs aside. It took a while to learn that I could stand up for myself and my family and that my child could continue to receive good care. One area that was important to me was to have nurses withhold judgment on our parenting style, even if they might have parented differently.

Communication needs to be open and two-way. Families and nurses ought to tell each other what is going well. For example, "Thanks for keeping the room so neat while you're here" can help a nurse see a family's appreciation. There was so little I could do as just "Mommy" that it really meant a lot to me when nurses would say, "That's such a cute outfit you picked out for him today." Communicating about little things, even inconsequential topics such as favorite TV shows, makes it easier to communicate about more important things and about problems. Communication has to be open about problems, too.

Jeni Stepanek
Mother
Upper Marlboro, MD

Promotion of Optimum Development, Self-Care, and Education

There is little question that living at home offers most children with complex medical problems great social and emotional advantages over living in the hospital or other institutional setting. However, in infancy and throughout the developmental stages, a child's medical condition(s) and the dependence on medical technology can place constraints on and pose challenges to *normal development.* For example, the child may have lengthy and repeated hospitalizations; developmental regression can occur in response to stress; fatigue may be due to underlying pathology, the flare of an illness, or medication side effects; and equipment requirements may impede mobility, exploration, and independence. The challenge of providing support for normal develop-

Critical Thinking

MAINTAINING THERAPEUTIC BOUNDARIES

You are a home care nurse and have been working with a 3-year-old child who is ventilator dependent. You have been visiting the Jones family several days a week for the last 5 months. You notice that the parents are arguing increasingly. Some of the arguments are about whether Mr. Jones helps enough with the child's care. Mrs. Jones approaches you to complain about her husband. Depending on your relationship with the family, you might do any of the following *except* which?

First, think about it...

- **What concepts or ideas are central to your thinking?**
- **If you accent the conclusions, what are the implications?**

1. **Mention that home care can be stressful for a family.**
2. **Indicate that you can provide referrals for counseling should the parents want them.**
3. **Agree with Mrs. Jones that her husband is not contributing enough to the child's care.**
4. **Listen and reflect with Mrs. Jones about her feelings.**

The best response is 3. The concept of therapeutic boundaries supports the idea that they are not rigid and fixed. They must be responsive to the relationship preferred by the family and the style with which the family operates. For this reason, depending on the family, options 1, 2, or 4 (or a combination) might be most appropriate. For any conclusion you may reach, it would be inappropriate to agree with Mrs. Jones that her husband is not helping enough with the child's care. Such an action implies a judgment that is not within the nurse's role to make and undermines rather than supports the family system.

ment in a child who is chronically ill and technology dependent is to optimize opportunities for developmentally appropriate experiences within the constraints posed by the medical condition and the equipment requirements.

Home care plans are designed to promote optimum child development through initial and periodic assessment, planning, and referrals for further assessment or therapeutic services, and by interventions that address normalization issues and self-care. (See Chapter 41 for a discussion of normalization.) General principles for a family-centered assessment and planning process have been addressed earlier in this chapter and are applied in developmental assessment and planning as well.

Some parents may not pursue early developmental intervention because they do not view their child as needing the services. In this case professionals need to explain the child's developmental needs to parents in ways that are meaningful from the parents' own cultural and socioeconomic perspectives. Only then can parents make truly informed decisions. Once parents have been fully informed of the child's condition, likely developmental sequelae, and the expected benefits of intervention, developmental goals outlined by the child and family should guide planning and intervention.

Each family is entitled to an *individual family service plan (IFSP)* to help ensure early intervention. All states in the United States provide agencies that develop IFSPs (American Academy of Pediatrics, 1995).

Several principles underlie appropriate developmental intervention plans for children with complex medical problems. First, nurses should understand the roles of occupational and physical therapists (Pokorni and Sippel, 1997). Second, understanding a child's medical condition ensures that the nurse and family can plan to maximize developmental opportunities at times when the

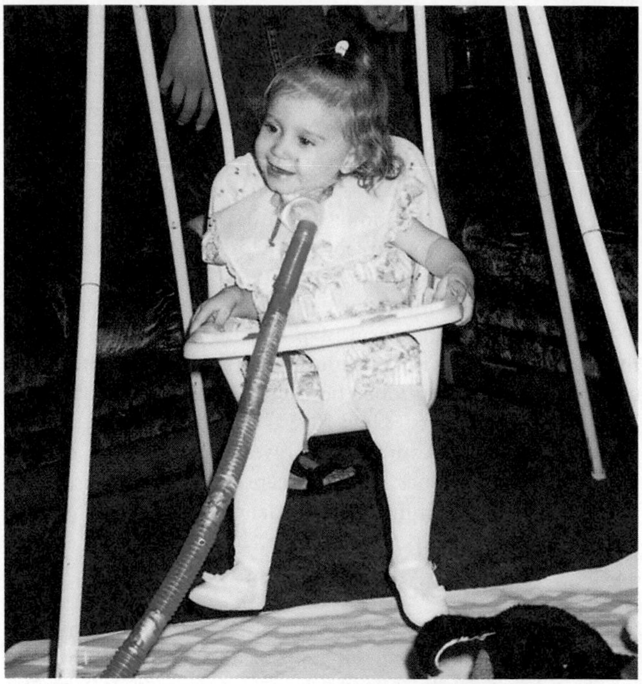

FIG. 43-2 • Use of lengthy tubing facilitates a child's freedom of movement.

child has the most energy and endurance. It also ensures that the stress signals that determine the child's tolerance for type, intensity, and duration of activity will be noticed (Ahmann and Klockenbrink, 1996; Glass and Blinkoff, 1996). Third, plans for developmental support must be flexible and tailored to the individual child's abilities, interests, and needs. Fourth, familiarity with the child's medical equipment will facilitate the planning of creative ways to meet the child's developmental needs. For example, the use of lengthy oxygen tubing allows the active toddler freedom of movement during the day (Fig. 43-2); portable equipment of any type facilitates family outings; and mounting a ventilator to a wheelchair allows the adolescent greater independence.

Many developmental aspects of chronic illness or disability in children are discussed in Chapter 41. Some additional factors apply when children are or have been dependent on medical technology, and these should be considered in developing plans to promote normal development (Ahmann and Lierman, 1992). These special needs may include the following:

- For infants, attention to promoting oral-motor development
- For toddlers, efforts to encourage mobility and exploration and extra assistance with language development
- For preschoolers, assistance in self-care
- For school-age children, provision of games and tasks for mastery and socialization opportunities
- For adolescents, increased independence in managing their own medical care

Promoting coping and capability can buffer stress and contribute to mental health and self-esteem in a child with chronic illness (Patterson and Geber, 1991). The extent to which a child is involved in his or her own care depends on many factors, including the child's developmental age, level of interest, and physical ability, as well as parental comfort and support. *Self-care,* both in activities of daily living and in regard to the medical condition, is important.

The frame of reference for self-care in activities of daily living should be the goal of attaining age-appropriate competence. Some modifications in the environment, in the medical equipment, and/or in the techniques for daily activities may be required to promote and support self-care. Effective teaching for self-care is focused at the child's own level of conceptual understanding and may be augmented by the use of dolls, models and diagrams, simple explanations, and repetition.

For the school-age child or adolescent dependent on medical technology, *educational planning* is important. Despite laws that ensure a "free appropriate public education" to these children, conflict over payment for health care services in the school setting has often been an impediment to mainstreaming children with complex medical problems (Walker, 1991). When a child requiring special medical care is to be placed in an educational setting, the parents, child, school health coordinator, educational evaluation team, and education and administrative staff should meet to determine safe and appropriate placement, as well as necessary services and personnel to enable the child to attend school in the least restrictive environment. Training of educational staff and caregivers is essential to ensuring the child's safety in the educational setting.* Special assistance can also be beneficial in reintegrating previously schooled children, such as those with cancer, into the school setting. Parents may need assistance in developing the skills necessary to advocate effectively for their child in the educational system (DiGregorio-Hixson, Stoff, and White, 1992).

Safety Issues in the Home

Safety is an important consideration in pediatric home care and should be addressed in the home care plan. First, before hospital discharge, emergency preparations must be made. The home should have a telephone. If the family does not have a telephone, arrangements may be made with the telephone company to supply service. Alternatively, one or two nearby neighbors may agree to let the family use their services. In rural areas a local pharmacy or police or ranger station may be willing to receive messages and relay them to the family.

The telephone and electric companies (if use of medical equipment requires electricity) are notified that the family needs to be placed on a priority service list so that the family will learn of any anticipated interruptions in service and receive priority in reinstatement of interrupted services. Prior contact with rescue squad and local emergency facility personnel can help ensure prompt and appropriate interventions if required.

Before hospital discharge, emergency protocols are developed and reviewed with both the parents and the professional caregivers. Cardiopulmonary resuscitation (CPR) guidelines, if appropriate, should be posted near the child's bedside or in another accessible location. A list of emergency telephone numbers can be placed near each home phone and should include those of the rescue squad, emergency room, managing physician(s), nursing agency, and equipment vendor(s).

Another aspect of safety relates to the provision of care by appropriately trained individuals. Family members should receive thorough training in the child's care requirements and have the opportunity to demonstrate knowledge and confidence before hospital discharge. Professional staff caring for the child should have the appropriate background and training for the child's particular care needs. Because of the child's body size, special skill and caution are required both in performing procedures (e.g., gastrostomy feedings and suctioning) and in monitoring the use of equipment (e.g., ventilator settings, intravenous flow rates, total fluid volumes) (see Chapter 45).

The activity level and curiosity of young children raise additional safety considerations in the provision of home care. All medications, needles, syringes, and any contaminated materials are securely stored well out of the reach of curious hands. Special attention is paid to childproofing the control panels for ventilators, pumps, monitors, and other equipment. Use of clear plastic tape, covers, or panels to cover control knobs or buttons reduces the risk of accidental changes in settings. Care must be taken to prevent accidental strangulation on apnea, oximeter, or cardiac monitor wires or lengthy intravenous tubing during sleep. Electrical cords are kept short and out of reach, and safety covers are used on any open outlets. When not in use, equipment is unplugged, and any wires (e.g., lead wires for an apnea monitor) are stored out of reach. Precaution against strangulation includes coiling extra tubing and taping it at the exit site, as well as running wires or tubes out the bottoms of pajamas.

Care at night poses other safety concerns. Parents or other caregivers need to be able to clearly hear monitor, ventilator, or pump alarms at night; an inexpensive intercom system or a baby monitor can be used.

Safe transportation is a vitally important concern. In many cases wheelchairs and other medical equipment must be properly secured to the vehicle, including vans and buses. If necessary, an extra adult should be present to monitor the child while in transit. Additional information on car safety and general health supervision is provided in Chapter 41 (see Educate About the Disorder and General Health Care).

Family-to-Family Support

Family-to-family support networks can be an important source of emotional and instrumental support and empowerment for families of children with chronic health problems. Family-to-family support does not replace professional sources of support but rather is a unique resource promoting family strengths through shared experience (Johnson, Jeppson, and Redburn, 1992). Existing parent support groups may not necessarily meet an individual family's needs; when nurses refer a family to a particular group, they should inform the family of the group's purposes. The value of informal support networks should not be overlooked. Similarly, the support needs of fathers, grandparents, and siblings may be different from those of mothers and should be acknowledged as part of the plan of care. Peer support for school-age children and adolescents with complex care may also be beneficial.

Key Points

- Effective home care depends on many factors, including the child's relative medical stability; the family's willingness, training, and ability to accommodate the child's care requirements; and professional, financial, and community support.

*A thorough discussion of training issues, content, and guidelines for care in the school are provided in Porter S, editor: *Children and youth assisted by medical technology in educational settings: guidelines for care*, ed 2, Baltimore, 1997, Paul H. Brookes.

- Comprehensive, multidisciplinary discharge planning should begin early and should include the family and a home care representative in addition to hospital personnel.
- Thorough training of the family, including a trial of care, a predischarge pass to home, and a predischarge home visit, can ease the transition to home.
- Care coordination ensures continuity of care and reduces fragmentation of services. The family may assume varying degrees of care coordination over time.
- The home care nurse must share a level of technical expertise with the critical care nurse while being able to adapt equipment, procedures, and the nursing process to the home setting. Education and training are increasingly important.
- Federal standards apply to agencies that participate in Medicare or Medicaid; standards of practice by the American Nurses Association can guide nurses in the home setting.
- Specialist and generalist credentialing is available for home care nurses.
- Family-centered nursing practice is applied in the home setting; diversity in family structures, cultural backgrounds, strengths, and coping mechanisms is respected.
- Collaborative relationships are characterized by communication, dialogue, active listening, awareness and acceptance of difference, and negotiation.
- The nursing process is adapted to involve the family in each step and to preserve the family's central role in decision making.
- "House rules" agreed on by the nurse and family allow a family to maintain a feeling of control over their own environment when professionals are present.
- Home care plans are designed to promote optimum development of the child and focus on normalization, on the impact of the child's medical condition and technologic requirements on development, on self-care, and on educational needs.
- Safety in the provision of home care services involves emergency preparations and protocols, appropriate training of family and home care personnel, and safe use and child-proofing of medical equipment.
- Family-to-family support networks can both provide emotional and instrumental support and encourage family empowerment.

References

Agazio JZ: Family transition through the termination of private duty home care nursing. *J Pediatr Nurs* 12(2):74-84, 1997.

Ahmann E, Bond NJ: Promoting normal development in school-age children and adolescents who are technology dependent: a family centered model, *Pediatr Nurs* 18:399-405, 1992.

Ahmann E, Klockenbrink KL: Developmental assessment and intervention in the home. In Ahmann E: *Home care for the high-risk infant: a family-centered approach,* Gaithersburg, MD, 1996, Aspen.

Ahmann E, Lierman C: Promoting normal development in technology-dependent children: an introduction to the issues, *Pediatr Nurs* 18:143-152, 1992.

American Academy of Pediatrics: *The medical home and early interventions,* Elk Grove Village, IL, 1995, The Academy.

American Nurses Association: *Standards of community health nursing practice,* Washington, DC, 1986a, The Association.

American Nurses Association: *Standards of home health nursing practice,* Washington, DC, 1986b, The Association.

Bishop KK, Woll J, Arango P: *Family/professional collaboration,* Burlington, VT, 1993, Department of Social Work, University of Vermont.

Bond N, Phillips P, Rollins JA: Family-centered care at home for families with children who are technology-dependent, *Pediatr Nurs* 20(2):123-130, 1994.

Crist TM, Kaufman SB, Crampton KR: Home telemedicine: a home health agency strategy for maximizing resources, *Home Health Care Manage Pract* 8(4):1-9, 1996.

DiGregorio-Hixson D, Stoff E, White PH: Parents of children with chronic health impairments: a new approach to advocacy training, *Child Health Care* 21(2):111-115, 1992.

Gingerich BS, Ondeck DA: Credentialing and accreditation: what exists for health care provider organizations, *Home Health Care Manage Pract* 9(4):67-68, 1997.

Glass P, Blinkoff R: Overview of developmental issues. In Ahmann E: *Home care for the high-risk infant: a family-centered approach,* Gaithersburg, MD, 1996, Aspen.

Johnson BH, Jeppson ES, Redburn L: *Caring for children and families: guidelines for hospital,* Bethesda, MD, 1992, Association for the Care of Children's Health.

Klug RM: Clarifying roles and expectations in home care, *Pediatr Nurs* 19:374-376, 1993.

Knafl K et al: Parents' view of health care providers: an exploration of the components of a positive working relationship, *Child Health Care* 21(2):90-95, 1992.

McDaniel SH, Campbell TL: Training for collaborative family healthcare, *Fam Systems Health* 14(2):147-150, 1996.

Narayan MC: Cultural assessment in home healthcare, *Home Healthc Nurse* 15(1):663-670, 1997.

Patterson JM, Blum RW: A conference on culture and chronic illness in childhood: conference summary, *Pediatrics* 91:1025-1030, 1993.

Patterson JM, Geber G: Preventing mental health problems in children with chronic illness or disability, *Child Health Care* 20(3):150-161, 1991.

Petr CG, Murdock B, Chapin R: Home care for children dependent on medical technology: the family perspective, *Soc Work Health Care* 21(1):5-22, 1995.

Pokorni JL, Sippel KM: Consultation with physical and occupational therapists to promote the motor development of young children, *Home Healthc Nurse* 15(5):331-339, 1997.

Shelton TL, Stepanek JS: *Family-centered care for children needing specialized health and developmental services,* Bethesda, MD, 1994, Association for the Care of Children's Health.

Spruhan JB: Beyond traditional nursing care: cultural awareness and successful home healthcare nursing, *Home Healthc Nurse* 14(6):445-449, 1996.

Walker P: Where there is a way there is not always a will: technology, public policy, and the social integration of children who are technology-assisted, *Child Health Care* 20(2):68-74, 1991.

Warner I: Introduction to telehealth home care, *Home Healthc Nurs* 14(1):791-796, 1996.

Wilson JS: National certification for home health care nurses: bird by bird, *Home Healthc Nurs* 14(10):817-821, 1996.

CHAPTER

44

Reaction to Illness and Hospitalization

http://www.harcourthealth.com/MERLIN/Wong/maternal/

Learning Objectives

On completion of this chapter the reader will be able to:

- Identify the stressors of illness and hospitalization for children during each developmental stage.
- List the admission procedures for a child on admission to the hospital.
- Outline nursing interventions that prevent or minimize the stress of separation during hospitalization.
- Outline nursing interventions that minimize the stress of loss of control during hospitalization.
- Outline nursing interventions that minimize the fear of bodily injury during hospitalization.
- Describe methods of assessing and managing pain in children.
- Outline nursing interventions that support parents and siblings during a child's illness and hospitalization.
- Describe nursing interventions needed when children are admitted to special units.

STRESSORS OF HOSPITALIZATION

Often illness and hospitalization are the first crises children must face. Children, especially during the early years, are particularly vulnerable to the crises of illness and hospitalization because (1) stress represents a change from the usual state of health and environmental routine, and (2) children have a limited number of coping mechanisms to resolve *stressors* (those events that produce stress). Major stressors of hospitalization include separation, loss of control, bodily injury, and pain. Children's reactions to these crises are influenced by their developmental age; their previous experience with illness, separation, or hospitalization; their innate and acquired coping skills; the seriousness of the diagnosis; and the support system available.

Separation Anxiety

The major stress from middle infancy throughout the preschool years, especially for children aged 6 to 30 months, is separation anxiety, also called *anaclitic depression.* The principal behavioral responses to this stressor during early childhood are summarized in Box 44-1.

During the phase of *protest,* children react aggressively to separation from the parent. They cry and scream for their parents, refuse the attention of anyone else, and are inconsolable in their grief (Fig. 44-1). During the phase of *despair,* the crying stops, and depression is evident. The child is much less active, is uninterested in play or food, and withdraws from others (Fig. 44-2).

The third stage is *detachment,* also called *denial.* Superficially it appears that the child has finally adjusted to the loss. The child becomes more interested in the surroundings, plays with others, and seems to form new relationships. However, this behavior is the result of resignation and is not a sign of contentment. The child detaches from the parent in an effort to escape the emotional pain of desiring the parent's presence and copes by forming shallow relationships with others, becoming increasingly self-centered, and attaching primary importance to material objects. This is the most serious stage in that reversal of the potential adverse effects is less likely to occur once detachment is established. However, in most situations the temporary separations imposed by hospitalization do not cause such prolonged parental absences that the child enters into detachment. In addition, considerable evidence suggests that even with stressors such as separation, children are remarkably adaptable, and permanent ill effects are rare.

Although progression to the stage of detachment is uncommon, the initial stages are commonly observed even with very brief separations from either parent. Unless health team members understand the meaning of each stage of behavior, they may erroneously label the behaviors as positive or negative. For example, they may see the loud crying of the protest phase as

Box 44-1

Manifestations of Separation Anxiety in Young Children

PHASE OF PROTEST

Observed behaviors during later infancy:
- Cries
- Screams
- Searches for parent with eyes
- Clings to parent
- Avoids and rejects contact with strangers

Additional behaviors observed during toddlerhood:
- Verbally attacks strangers (e.g., "Go away")
- Physically attacks strangers (e.g., kicks, bites, hits, pinches)
- Attempts to escape to find parent
- Attempts to physically force parent to stay

Behaviors may last from hours to days

Protest, such as crying, may be continuous, ceasing only with physical exhaustion

Approach of stranger may precipitate increased protest

PHASE OF DESPAIR

Observed behaviors:
- Inactive
- Withdraws from others
- Depressed, sad
- Uninterested in environment
- Uncommunicative
- Regresses to earlier behavior (e.g., thumb-sucking, bed-wetting, use of pacifier, use of bottle)

Behaviors may last for variable length of time

Child's physical condition may deteriorate from refusal to eat, drink, or move

PHASE OF DETACHMENT

Observed behaviors:
- Shows increased interest in surroundings
- Interacts with strangers or familiar caregivers
- Forms new but superficial relationships
- Appears happy

Detachment usually occurs after prolonged separation from parent; rarely seen in hospitalized children

Behaviors represent a superficial adjustment to loss

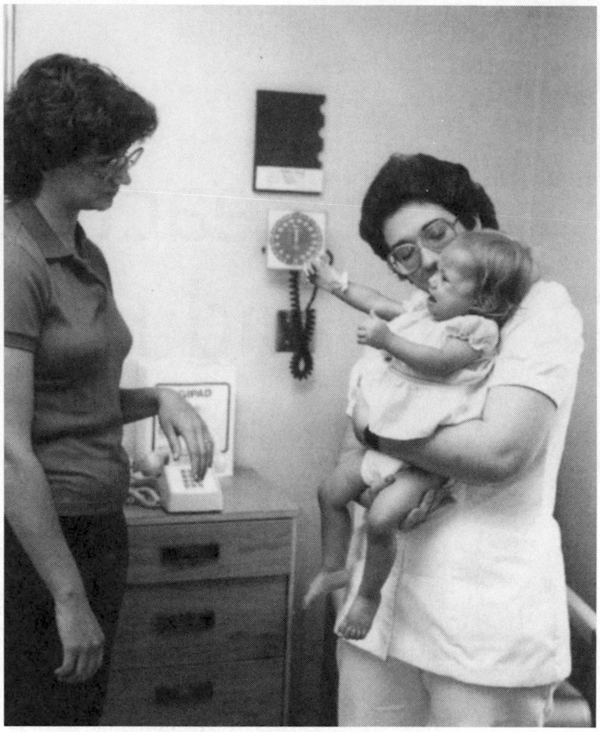

FIG. 44-1 • In the protest phase of separation anxiety, children cry loudly and are inconsolable in their grief for the parent.

"bad" behavior. Because the protesting increases when a stranger approaches the child, they may interpret that reaction as meaning they should stay away. During the quiet, withdrawn phase of despair, health team members may think that the child is finally "settling in" to the new surroundings, and they may see the detachment behaviors as proof of a "good adjustment." The faster this stage is reached, the more likely it is that the child will be regarded as the "ideal patient."

Because children seem to react "negatively" to visits by their parents, uninformed observers feel justified in restricting parental visiting privileges. For example, during the protest stage, children outwardly do not appear happy to see their parents. In fact, they may even cry louder. If they are depressed, they may reject their parents or begin to protest once more. Often they cling to their parents in an effort to ensure their continued presence. Consequently, such reactions may be regarded as "disturbing" the child's adjustment to the new surroundings. If the separation has progressed to the phase of detachment, children will respond no differently to their parents than they would to any other strange or familiar person.

Such reactions are equally distressing to parents who are unaware of their meaning. If parents are regarded as intruders, they will see their absence as "beneficial" to the child's adjustment and recovery. They may respond to the child's behavior by staying for only short periods, visiting less often, or deceiving the child when it is time to leave. The result is a destructive cycle of misunderstanding and unmet needs.

Early Childhood. Separation anxiety is the greatest stress imposed by hospitalization during early childhood. If separation is avoided, young children have a tremendous capacity to withstand any other stress. During this age period the typical reactions previously described are seen. However, children in the toddler stage demonstrate more goal-directed behaviors. For example, they may plead with the parents to stay and physically try to keep the parents with them or try to find parents who have left. They may demonstrate displeasure on the parents' return or departure by having temper tantrums; refusing to comply with the usual routines of mealtime, bedtime, or toileting; or regressing to more primitive levels of development. However, temper tantrums, bed-wetting, or other behaviors may also be expressions of anger or even a physiologic response to stress.

Because preschoolers are more secure interpersonally than toddlers, they can tolerate brief periods of separation from their parents and are more inclined to develop substitute trust in other significant adults. However, the stress of illness usually renders preschoolers less able to cope with separation; as a re-

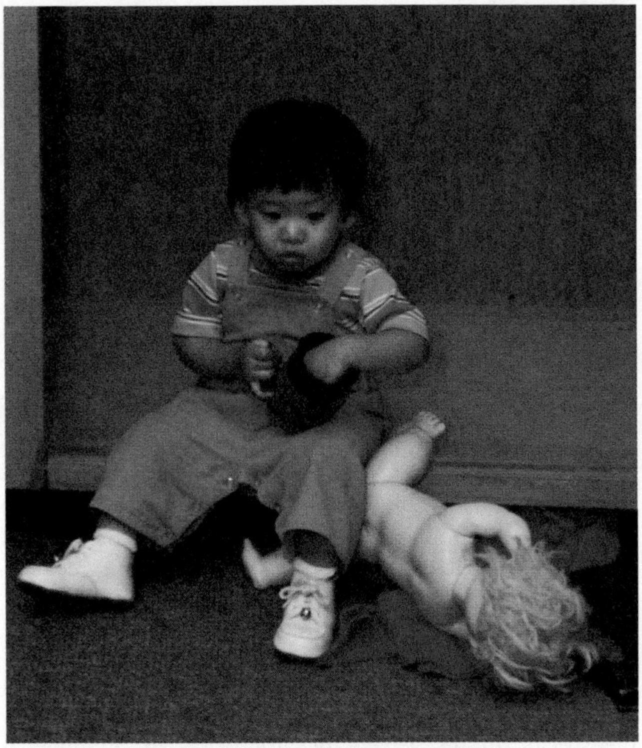

FIG. 44-2 • During the despair phase of separation anxiety, children are sad, lonely, and uninterested in play or food.

sult, they manifest many of the stage behaviors of separation anxiety, although in general the protest behaviors are more subtle and passive than those seen in younger children. Preschoolers may demonstrate separation anxiety by refusing to eat, experiencing difficulty sleeping, crying quietly for their parents, continually asking when the parents will visit, or withdrawing from others. They may express anger indirectly by breaking their toys, hitting other children, or refusing to cooperate during usual self-care activities. Nurses need to be sensitive to these less obvious signs of separation anxiety in order to intervene appropriately.

Later Childhood and Adolescence. Previous research, usually based on adult recollections, indicated that the family does not play as important a role for school-age children as it does during the toddler and preschool years. However, in a recent study that asked children about their fears when hospitalized, children ranked "being away from my family" higher than any other fear associated with hospitalization (Hart and Bossert, 1994; Wilson and Yorker, 1997). Although school-age children are better able to cope with separation in general, the stress and often accompanying regression imposed by illness or hospitalization may increase their need for parental security and guidance. This is particularly true for young school-age children who have only recently left the safety of the home and are struggling with the crisis of school adjustment. Middle and late school-age children may react more to the separation from their usual activities and peers than to the absence of their parents. These children have a high level of physical and mental activity that often finds no suitable outlets in the hospital environment, and even when they dislike school, they admit to missing its routine and worry that they will not be able to compete or "fit in" with their classmates when they return. Feelings of loneliness, boredom, isolation, and depression are common. Such reactions may occur more as a result of separation than from concern over the illness, treatment, or hospital setting.

School-age children may need and desire parental guidance or support from other adult figures but be unable or unwilling to ask for it. Because the goal of attaining independence is so important to them, they are reluctant to seek help directly for fear that they will appear weak, childish, or dependent. Cultural expectations to "act like a man" or to "be brave and strong" bear heavily on these children, especially boys, who tend to react to stress with stoicism, withdrawal, or passive acceptance. Often the need to express hostile, angry, or other negative feelings finds outlets in alternate ways, such as irritability and aggression toward parents, withdrawal from hospital personnel, inability to relate to peers, rejection of siblings, or subsequent behavioral problems in school.

For adolescents, separation from home and parents may be a welcomed and appreciated event. However, loss of peer-group contact may pose a severe emotional threat because of loss of group status, inability to exert group control or leadership, and loss of group acceptance. Deviations within peer groups are poorly tolerated, and although group members may express concern for the adolescent's illness or need for hospitalization, they continue their group activities, quickly filling the gap of the absent member. During the temporary separation from their usual group, ill adolescents may benefit from group associations with other hospitalized age-mates.

Loss of Control

One of the factors influencing the amount of stress imposed by hospitalization is the amount of control that persons perceive themselves as having. Lack of control increases the perception of threat and can affect children's coping skills. Many hospital situations decrease the amount of control a child feels. Although the usual sensory stimulations are lacking, the additional hospital stimuli of sight, sound, and smell may be overwhelming. Without an insight into the type of environment conducive to children's optimum growth, the hospital experience can at best temporarily slow development and at worst permanently restrict it. Because children's needs vary greatly depending on their age, the major areas of loss of control in terms of physical restriction, altered routine or rituals, and dependency are discussed for each age group.

Infants. Infants are developing the most important attribute of a healthy personality—trust. Trust is established through consistent, loving care by a nurturing person. Infants attempt to control their environment through emotional expressions, such as crying or smiling. In the hospital setting, cues may be missed or misinterpreted, and routines may be established to meet the hospital staff's needs instead of the infant's needs. Inconsistent care and deviations from the infant's daily routine may lead to mistrust and a decreased sense of control (Wells et al, 1994).

Toddlers. Toddlers are striving for autonomy, and this goal is evident in most of their behaviors—motor skills, play, interpersonal relationships, activities of daily living, and communication. When their egocentric pleasures meet with obstacles, toddlers react with negativism, especially temper tantrums. Any restriction or limitation of movement, such as the simple act of making toddlers lie down, can cause forceful resistance and noncompliance.

Loss of control also results from altered routines and rituals. Toddlers rely on the consistency and familiarity of daily rituals to provide a measure of stability and control in their complex world of growing and developing. The experience of hospitalization or illness severely limits their sense of expectation and predictability, because practically every detail of the hospital environment differs from that of the home.

Toddlers' main areas for rituals include eating, sleeping, bathing, toileting, and playing. When the routines are disrupted, difficulties can occur in any or all of these areas. The principal reaction to such change is regression. For example, when mealtime and food choices differ from those at home, toddlers often refuse to eat, demand a bottle, or ask others to feed them. Although regression to earlier forms of behavior may seem to increase toddlers' security and comfort, in reality it is very threatening for them to relinquish their most recently acquired achievements.

Enforced dependency is a chief characteristic of the sick role and accounts for the numerous instances of toddler negativism. For example, rigid schedules, different clothes, altered caregiving activities, unfamiliar surroundings, separation from parents, and medical procedures usurp toddlers' control over their world. Although most toddlers initially react negatively and aggressively to such dependency, prolonged loss of autonomy may result in passive withdrawal from interpersonal relationships and regression in all areas of development. Therefore the effects of the sick role are most severe in instances of chronic illnesses or in those families who foster the sick role despite the child's improved state of health.

Preschoolers. Preschoolers also suffer from loss of control caused by physical restriction, altered routines, and enforced dependency. However, their specific cognitive abilities, which make them feel omnipotent, also make them feel out of control. This loss of control in the context of their sense of self-power is a critical influencing factor in their perception of and reaction to separation, pain, illness, and hospitalization.

Preschoolers' egocentric and magical thinking limits their ability to understand events because they view all experiences from their own self-referenced (egocentric) perspective. Without adequate preparation for unfamiliar settings or experiences, preschoolers' fantasy explanations for such events are usually more exaggerated, bizarre, and frightening than the actual facts. One typical fantasy to explain the reason for illness or hospitalization is that it represents punishment for real or imagined misdeeds (Family Focus box). In response to such thinking the child usually feels shame, guilt, and fear.

Preschoolers' preoperational thinking means that explanations are understood only in terms of real events. Purely verbal instructions are often inadequate for them because they are unable to abstract and synthesize beyond what their senses tell them. When combined with their egocentric and magical thinking, this characteristic may lead them to interpret messages according to their particular past experiences. Even with the best preparation for a procedure, they may misconstrue the details.

Because they use transductive reasoning, preschoolers deduct from the particular to the particular, rather than from the specific to the general or vice versa. For example, if preschoolers' concept of nurses is that they inflict pain, preschoolers will think that every nurse (or everyone wearing a similar uniform) will also inflict pain.

School-Age Children. Because of their striving for independence and productivity, school-age children are particularly vulnerable to events that may lessen their feeling of control and power. In particular, altered family roles; physical disability; fears of death, abandonment, or permanent injury; loss of peer acceptance; lack of productivity; and inability to cope with stress according to perceived cultural expectation may result in loss of control.

Because of the nature of the patient role, many routine hospital activities usurp individual power and identity. For school-age children, dependent activities such as enforced bed rest, use of a bedpan, inability to choose a menu, lack of privacy, help with a bed bath, or transport by a wheelchair or stretcher can be a direct threat to their security. Although all of these procedures seem routine and inconsequential, they allow no freedom of choice to children who want to "act grown-up." However, when children are allowed to exert a measure of control, regardless of how limited it may be, they generally respond very well to any procedure. For example, some of the most cooperative, satisfied, and contented patients are school-age children who help make their beds, choose their schedule of activities, assist in procedures, and help the nurses care for younger children. An increased sense of control usually results from a feeling of usefulness and productivity.

In addition to the hospital environment, illness may also cause a feeling of loss of control. One of the most significant problems of children in this age group centers on boredom. When physical or enforced limitations curtail their usual abilities to care for themselves or to engage in favorite activities, school-age children generally respond with depression, hostility, or frustration. Keeping a normally active child on bed rest is no small challenge. However, emphasizing areas of control and

Family Focus

A REFLECTION ON HOSPITALIZATION

Upon my initial hospitalization, determination of an appropriate insulin dosage meant approximately 7 to 10 injections a day for 10 days. While concrete memories of the hospitalization remain sketchy, remnants of my overwhelming feelings of fright persist. In my mind, hospitalization symbolizes the beginning of my diabetic life: daily injections, food restrictions, glucose monitoring, and blood tests administered by my parents, whom I idolized. As children less than age 7 often view illness as a result of human action, I blamed myself for my illness. I considered the daily injections, tests, doctors, and hospitalization "punishment" because I was bad or inferior and thus deserving of these regimens and limitations.

After all, I was "different." During early childhood, I could not eat candy, have birthday cake, choose what and when I wanted to eat, or sleep over at a friend's house without my parents coming to administer my insulin injection. None of my friends, classmates, family members, or siblings had to adhere to such regulations. In my mind, the adversity of these regulations implied wrongdoing and misbehavior on my part and required punishment. Because I continually received the punishment, there was only one conclusion: I was different, I was bad—I was diabetic.

Modified from Levi R: Childhood illness through a child's eyes, *ACCH Advocate* 2(1):43-44, 1995.

capitalizing on quiet activities, particularly hobbies such as building models or collecting specific objects, promote their adjustment to physical restriction. Nursing judgment regarding selection of a roommate is one of the most important contributing factors to their overall adjustment to illness and hospitalization.

Adolescents. Adolescents' struggle for independence, self-assertion, and liberation centers on the quest for personal identity. Anything that interferes with this poses a threat to their sense of identity and results in a loss of control. Illness, which limits one's physical abilities, and hospitalization, which separates one from one's usual support systems, constitute major situational crises.

The patient role fosters dependency and depersonalization. Adolescents may react to dependency with rejection, uncooperativeness, or withdrawal. They may respond to depersonalization with self-assertion, anger, or frustration. Regardless of response, hospital personnel often regard them as difficult, unmanageable patients. Parents may not be a source of help, because these behaviors serve to isolate them further from understanding the adolescent. Although peers may visit, they may not be able to offer the kind of support and guidance needed. Sick adolescents often voluntarily isolate themselves from age-mates until they feel they can compete on an equal basis and meet group expectations. As a result, adolescents may be left with virtually no support system.

Loss of control also occurs for many of the reasons discussed for school-age children. However, adolescents are more sensitive to potential instances of loss of control and dependency than are younger children. For example, both groups seek information about their physical status and rely heavily on anticipatory preparation to decrease fear and anxiety. However, adolescents react not only to the kind of information supplied them but also to the means by which it is conveyed. They may feel very threatened by others who relate facts in a condescending manner. Adolescents want to know that others can relate to them on their own level. This necessitates a careful assessment of their intellectual abilities, previous knowledge, and present needs.

Bodily Injury and Pain

Fears of bodily injury and pain are prevalent among children. The consequences of these fears can be far-reaching; adults who experience more medical fear and pain in childhood are more fearful of pain as adults and tend to avoid medical care (Pate et al, 1996).

In caring for children, nurses must have an appreciation of a child's concerns about bodily harm and the reactions to pain at different developmental periods. Table 44-1 summarizes developmental considerations related to children's understanding of illness and pain. Box 44-2 outlines developmental characteristics of children's reactions to pain.

Infants. Research exploring children's development of illness concepts and how their understanding of illness relates to fears of bodily injury includes no findings for preverbal children. Consequently, the following discussion is limited to infants' reactions to pain.

Infants' responses to pain after the neonatal period are quite similar to earlier reactions, although there is marked variability

TABLE 44-1

Children's Developmental Concepts of Illness and Pain

Concept of Illness*	Concept of Pain†
PREOPERATIONAL THOUGHT (2-7 YEARS)	
Phenomenism: Perceives an external, unrelated, concrete phenomenon as cause of illness (e.g., "being sick because you don't feel well") **Contagion:** Perceives cause of illness as proximity between two events that occurs by "magic" (e.g., "getting a cold because you are near someone who has a cold")	Relates to pain primarily as physical, concrete experience Thinks in terms of magical disappearance of pain May view pain as punishment for wrongdoing Tends to hold someone accountable for own pain and may strike out at person
CONCRETE OPERATIONAL THOUGHT (7-10+ YEARS)	
Contamination: Perceives cause as a person, object, or action external to the child that is "bad" or "harmful" to the body (e.g., "getting a cold because you didn't wear a hat") **Internalization:** Perceives illness as having an external cause but as being located inside the body (e.g., "getting a cold by breathing in air and bacteria")	Relates to pain physically (e.g., headache, stomachache) Is able to perceive of psychologic pain (e.g., someone dying) Fears bodily harm and annihilation (body destruction and death) May view pain as punishment for wrongdoing
FORMAL OPERATIONAL THOUGHT (13 YEARS AND OLDER)	
Physiologic: Perceives cause as malfunctioning or nonfunctioning organ or process; can explain illness in sequence of events **Psychophysiologic:** Realizes that psychologic actions and attitudes affect health and illness	Is able to give reason for pain (e.g., fell and hit nerve) Perceives several types of psychologic pain Has limited life experiences to cope with pain as adult might cope despite mature understanding of pain Fears losing control during painful experience

*From Bibace R, Walsh ME: Development of children's concepts of illness, *Pediatrics* 66(6):912-917, 1980.
†From Hurley A, Whelan EG: Cognitive development and children's perception of pain, *Pediatr Nurs* 14(1):21-24, 1988.

Box 44-2

Developmental Characteristics of Children's Response to Pain

YOUNG INFANT

Generalized body response of rigidity or thrashing, possibly with local reflex withdrawal of stimulated area

Loud crying

Facial expression of pain (brows lowered and drawn together, eyes tightly closed, and mouth open and squarish) (Fig. 44-3)

Demonstrates no association between approaching stimulus and subsequent pain

OLDER INFANT

Localized body response with deliberate withdrawal of stimulated area

Loud crying

Facial expression of pain and/or anger (same facial characteristics as pain but eyes are open)

Physical resistance, especially pushing the stimulus away *after* it is applied

YOUNG CHILD

Loud crying, screaming

Verbal expressions of "Ow," "Ouch," "It hurts"

Thrashing of arms and legs

Attempts to push stimulus away *before* it is applied

Uncooperative; needs physical restraint

Requests termination of procedure

Clings to parent, nurse, or other significant person

Requests emotional support, such as hugs or other forms of physical comfort

May become restless and irritable with continuing pain

All of these behaviors may be seen in anticipation of actual painful procedure

SCHOOL-AGE CHILD

May see all behaviors of young child, especially *during* actual painful procedure but less in anticipatory period

Stalling behavior, such as "Wait a minute" or "I'm not ready"

Muscular rigidity, such as clenched fists, white knuckles, gritted teeth, contracted limbs, body stiffness, closed eyes, wrinkled forehead

ADOLESCENT

Less vocal protest

Less motor activity

More verbal expressions, such as "It hurts" or "You're hurting me"

Increased muscle tension and body control

Data from Craig KD et al: Developmental changes in infant pain expression during immunization injections, *Soc Sci Med* 19(12):1331-1337, 1984; and Katz ER, Kellerman J, Siegel SE: Behavioral distress in children with cancer undergoing medical procedures: developmental considerations, *J Consult Clin Psychol* 48(3):356-365, 1980.

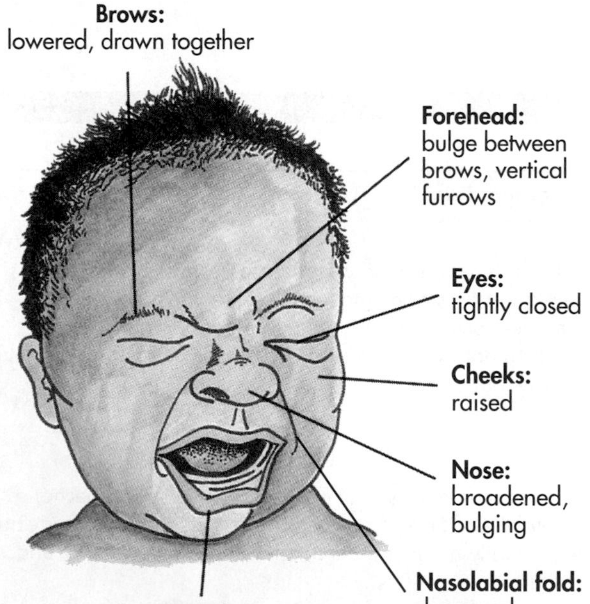

FIG. 44-3 • Facial expression of physical distress is the most consistent behavioral indicator of pain in infants.

in measures of distress, especially the initial cry and heart rate, which may decrease in some infants. The most consistent indicator of distress is a facial expression of discomfort (see Fig. 44-3). Body movements include squirming, writhing, jerking, and flailing (Tamowski and Brown, 1995). Some infants may cry loudly after the procedure, whereas others are easily calmed by a gentle hug. It is important to recognize and respect such early signs of individuality and to realize that children who react less intensely may still be experiencing significant discomfort (Broome et al, 1990).

Infants younger than 6 months seem to have no obvious memory of previous painful experiences and react to a potentially stressful situation with less apprehension and fear than older children. After this time, however, children's response to pain is increasingly influenced by their recall of prior painful experiences and the emotional reaction of parents during the procedure. Older infants react intensely, with physical resistance and uncooperativeness. They may refuse to lie still, attempt to push the person away, or try to escape with whatever motor activity they have achieved. Distraction does little to lessen their immediate reaction to pain, and anticipatory preparation, such as showing them the equipment, can increase their fear and resistance.

Toddlers. Toddlers' concept of body image, particularly the definition of body boundaries, is very poorly developed. Intrusive experiences, such as examining the ears or mouth or checking a rectal temperature, are very anxiety producing. Toddlers may react to such painless procedures as intensely as they do to painful ones.

Toddlers' reactions to pain are similar to those seen during infancy, except that the number of variables influencing the individual response is highly complex and varied. Memory, physical restraint, separation from parents, emotional reactions of others, and lack of preparation partially determine the intensity of the behavioral response. In general, children in this age group continue to react with intense emotional upset and physical resistance to any actual or perceived painful experience. Behaviors indicating pain include grimacing, clenching their teeth and/or lips, opening their eyes wide, rocking, rubbing, and acting aggressively, such as biting, kicking, hitting, or running away. Unlike adults, who usually decrease their activity when in pain, young children typically become restless and overly active; commonly this response is not recognized as a consequence of pain.

By the end of this age period, toddlers usually are able to communicate about their pain. Although they have not developed the ability to describe the type or intensity of the pain, they usually are able to localize it by pointing to a specific area.

Preschoolers. Concepts of illness begin during the preschool period and are influenced by the cognitive abilities of the preoperational stage. Preschoolers differentiate poorly between themselves and the external world. Their thinking is focused on externally perceived events, and causality is based on the proximity of two events. Consequently, children define illness according to what they are told or are given external evidence of, such as "You are sick because you have a fever."

The cause of illness is seen as a concrete action the child does or fails to do, such as "Catching a cold because you go out into cold weather"; consequently, it implies a degree of responsibility and self-blame. Another explanation may be based on contagion, that the proximity of two objects or persons causes the illness; for example, "A person gets a cold when someone else with a cold gets near him."

The psychosexual conflicts of children in this age group make them very vulnerable to threats of bodily injury. Intrusive procedures, whether painful or painless, are threatening to preschoolers, whose concept of body integrity is still poorly developed. Preschoolers may react to an injection with as much concern for withdrawal of the needle as for the actual pain. They fear that the intrusion or puncture will not reclose and that their "insides" will leak out.

Concerns of mutilation are paramount during this age period. Loss of any body part is threatening, but preschool boys' fears of castration complicate their understanding of surgical or medical procedures associated with the genital area, such as circumcision, repair of hypospadias or epispadias, cystoscopy, or catheterization. Their limited comprehension of body functioning also increases their difficulty in understanding how or why body parts are "fixed." For example, telling preschoolers that their tonsils are to be removed may be interpreted as "taking out their voice," or having the penis "fixed"" may be understood as cutting it off. Words such as "dye," "cut off," "take out," or "draw" (e.g., "draw some blood") are understood literally and can lead to confusion and fear (see Communicating with Children, Chapter 34).

Reactions to pain tend to be similar to those seen during toddlerhood, although some differences become apparent. For example, preschoolers respond more favorably than younger children to preparatory interventions, such as explanation and distraction. Physical and verbal aggression are more specific and goal directed. Instead of showing total body resistance, preschoolers may push the offending person away, try to secure the equipment, or attempt to lock themselves in a safe place. Much more thought is evident in their plan of attack or escape.

Verbal expression in particular demonstrates their advanced development in response to stress. They may verbally abuse the nurse by stating, "Get out of here" or "I hate you." They may also use the more cunning approach of trying to persuade the person to give up the intended activity. A common plea is, "Please don't give me a shot; I'll be good." Some statements are not only attempts to avoid the event but also evidence of children's perceptions about the experience.

Preschoolers can locate their pain and can use appropriate pain scales. Children as young as 3 years can use assessment tools that employ facial expressions of pain (see Table 44-2).

School-Age Children. Fears of the physical nature of the illness surface at this time. School-age children may be less concerned with pain than with disability, uncertain recovery, or possible death. Children with chronic illness are more likely to identify intrusive procedures as stressful, whereas children who are acutely ill are more likely to indicate physical symptoms (Bossert, 1994a, 1994b; Boyd and Hunsberger, 1998). Girls tend to express more and stronger fears than boys, and previous hospitalizations may have no effect on the frequency or intensity of these fears. Because of their developing cognitive abilities, school-age children are aware of the significance of different illnesses, the indispensability of certain body parts, potential hazards of treatments, lifelong consequences of permanent injury or loss of function, and the meaning of death. A major concern of school-age children when hospitalized is their fear of being told that something is "wrong" with them (Hart and Bossert, 1994). They generally take a very active interest in their health or illness. Even those children who rarely ask questions usually reveal detailed knowledge of their condition by attentively listening to all that is said around them. They request factual information and quickly perceive lies or half-truths. Seeking information tends to be one way of coping or maintaining a sense of control despite the stress and uncertainty of the condition.

The school-age child defines illness by a set of multiple concrete symptoms, such as signs of a cold, and views the cause as primarily germs or bacteria. Germs have a powerful, almost magical quality, so that in the child's mind, illness can be prevented by avoiding people with germs. There is also the notion of contamination, which is similar to that seen in the younger age group; for example, the illness occurs because of physical contact or because the child engaged in a harmful action and became contaminated. Consequently, feelings of self-blame and guilt may be associated with the reason for becoming ill.

School-age children begin to show concern for the potential beneficial and hazardous effects of procedures. Besides wanting to know whether a procedure will hurt, they want to know what it is for, how it will make them better, and what injury or harm could result. For example, these children may fear the actual procedure of anesthesia. Unlike preschoolers, who fear the mask and the strange surroundings, school-age children fear what may happen while they are asleep, question whether they will wake up, and fear that they may die. Preadolescents also worry about the procedure itself, particularly if it is one that will result in visible changes in body appearance.

Intrusive procedures of a nonsexual nature, such as routine physical examination of the ears, nose, mouth, and throat, are generally well tolerated. However, concerns for privacy become evident and increasingly significant. Although school-age children may cooperate during examination of, or procedures performed on, the genital area, it is usually very stressful for them, especially in the case of preadolescents who are beginning pubertal changes. Nurses who respect children's need for privacy can provide them with much assurance and support.

By 9 or 10 years of age, most school-age children show less fright or overt resistance to pain than younger children. They generally have learned coping methods of dealing with discomfort, such as holding rigidly still, clenching their fists or teeth, or trying to act brave through the "grin-and-bear-it" routine. If they do display signs of overt resistance, such as biting, kicking, pulling away, trying to escape, crying, or plea bargaining, they may deny such reactions later, especially to their peers for fear of embarrassment.

School-age children verbally communicate about their pain with respect to its location, intensity, and description. Unlike younger children, who may have difficulty choosing words to describe pain, children 8 years and older use a wide variety of words and phrases, such as "hurting," "sore," "burning," "stinging," "aching," and "like a sharp knife."

School-age children also use words as a means of controlling their reactions to pain. For example, these children may ask the nurse to talk to them during a procedure. Some prefer to participate in a procedure, whereas others choose to distance themselves by not looking at what is happening. Most appreciate an explanation of the procedure and seem less fearful when they know what to expect. Others try to gain control by attempting to postpone the event. A typical request is, "Give me the shot when I am finished with this." Although the ability to make decisions does increase their sense of control, unlimited procrastination results in heightened anxiety. When choices are allowed, such as selection of the injection site, it is best to structure the number of possible sites and to limit the number of "procrastination" techniques.

Similar to their more passive acceptance of pain is their nondirective request for support or help. School-age children will rarely initiate a conversation about their feelings or request someone to stay with them during a lonely or stressful period. Their visible composure, calmness, and acceptance often mask their inner longing for support. It is especially important to be aware of nonverbal clues, such as a serious facial expression, a half-hearted reply of "I am fine," silence, lack of activity, or social isolation, as signs of the need for help. Usually when someone identifies the unspoken messages and offers support, they readily accept it.

Adolescents. Although the development of body image begins at birth, its relevance is paramount during adolescence. Injury, pain, disability, and death are viewed primarily in terms of how each affects adolescents' views of themselves in the present. Any change that differentiates the adolescent from peers is regarded as a major tragedy. For example, diseases such as diabetes mellitus often present a more difficult adjustment period for children in this age group than for younger children because of the necessary changes in the adolescent's lifestyle. Conversely, serious, even life-threatening illnesses that entail no visible body changes or physical restrictions may have less immediate significance for the adolescent. Therefore the nature of bodily injury may be more important in terms of adolescents' perception of the illness than its actual degree of severity.

Adolescents' rapidly changing body image during pubertal development often makes them feel insecure about their bodies. Illness, medical or surgical intervention, and hospitalization increase their existing concerns for normalcy They may respond to such events by asking numerous questions, withdrawing, rejecting others, or questioning the adequacy of care. Often their fear of loss of control and body-image change is demonstrated as overconfidence, conceit, or a "know-it-all" attitude.

Because of sexual changes, adolescents are very concerned about privacy. Lack of respect for this need can cause greater stress than physical pain. In addition, adolescents look for signs that indicate that they are developing normally and according to acceptable standards. When illness occurs, they fear that growth may be retarded, leaving them behind their peers. Although they may not voice this concern, they may demonstrate it by carefully observing others' reactions to them.

Adolescents typically react to pain with much self-control. Physical resistance and aggression are less likely at this age unless the adolescent is totally unprepared for a procedure. As with older school-age children, adolescents are very concerned with remaining composed and feel embarrassed and ashamed of losing control. They are able to describe their pain experience and to use any of the pain assessment tools developed for adults. However, they may be reluctant to disclose their pain, requiring the nurse to listen closely and observe physical indications, such as limited movement, excessive quiet, or irritability. They may also believe that the nurse knows how they feel; thus they may see no need to ask for analgesia.

Effects of Hospitalization on the Child

Children may react to the stresses of hospitalization before admission, during hospitalization, and after discharge. A child's conception of illness is even more important than age and intellectual maturity in predicting the level of anxiety before hospitalization (Carson, Gravley, and Council, 1992; Clatworthy, Simon, and Tiedeman, 1999). This may or may not be affected by the duration of the condition and/or prior hospitalizations. Therefore nurses should avoid overestimating the illness concepts of children with prior medical experience (Box 44-3).

Individual Risk Factors. A number of risk factors make certain children more vulnerable than others to the stresses of hospitalization (Box 44-4). It has also been noted that rural children exhibit significantly greater degrees of psychologic upset than urban children, possibly because urban children have opportunities to become familiar with a local hospital (Gillis, 1990). Perhaps because separation is such an important issue surrounding hospitalization for young children, children who are active and strong willed tend to fare better when hospitalized than youngsters who are passive. Consequently, nurses should be alert to children who passively accept

Box 44-3

Posthospital Behaviors in Children

YOUNG CHILDREN

Some initial aloofness toward parents; may last from a few minutes (most common) to a few days

Often followed by dependency behaviors:
- Tendency to cling to parents
- Demand parents' attention
- Vigorously oppose any separation (e.g., staying at preschool or with a baby-sitter)

Other negative behaviors include the following:
- New fears (e.g., nightmares)
- Resistance to going to bed, night waking
- Withdrawal and shyness
- Hyperactivity
- Temper tantrums
- Food finickiness
- Attachment to blanket or toy
- Regression in newly learned skills (e.g., self-toileting)

all changes and requests; these children may need more support than the "oppositional" child.

The development of subsequent long-term emotional disturbance may be related to the length and number of hospital admissions and the type of hospital practices. A single hospitalization of 4 weeks or more and repeated hospital admissions have been associated with later disturbances. However, supportive practices, such as frequent family visiting, may lessen the detrimental effects of such admissions. Research also indicates that a child's pain experience determines how the overall hospitalization is experienced (Woodgate and Krisjanson, 1996).

Changes in the Pediatric Population. The pediatric population in hospitals has changed dramatically during the last two decades. Although there is a growing trend toward shortened hospital stays and outpatient surgery, a greater percentage of the children hospitalized today have more serious and complex problems than those hospitalized in the past. Many of these children are fragile newborns and children with severe injuries or disabilities who have survived because of incredible technologic advances, but have been left with chronic or disabling conditions that require frequent and lengthy hospital stays. Research suggests that prior experience and familiarity with medical events related to hospitalization do not reduce fears in children (Hart and Bossert, 1994). Rather, prior experience may simply replace fear of the unknown with fear of the known. The nature of their conditions increases the likelihood that they will experience more invasive and traumatic procedures while they are hospitalized. These factors make them more vulnerable to the emotional consequences of hospitalization and result in their needs being significantly different from those of the short-term patients of the past (see Chapter 41 for further discussion on children with special needs). The majority of these children are infants and toddlers, the age group most vulnerable to the effects of hospitalization.

Concern in recent years has focused on the increasing numbers of these children "growing up in hospitals" (Britton and Johnston, 1993). Discharge is prolonged because of complex medical and nursing care, elusive diagnoses, complicated psychosocial issues, and inconsistent community resources (Wells et al, 1994). Without special attention devoted to meeting the child's psychosocial and developmental needs in the "artificial" hospital environment, the detrimental consequences of prolonged hospitalization may be severe.

Beneficial Effects of Hospitalization. Although hospitalization can be and usually is stressful for children, it can also be beneficial. The most obvious benefit is the recovery from illness, but hospitalization also can present an opportunity for children to master stress and feel competent in their coping abilities. The hospital environment can provide children with new socialization experiences that can broaden their interpersonal relationships. The psychologic benefits need to be considered and maximized during hospitalization. Appropriate nursing strategies to achieve this goal are presented on p. 1110.

STRESSORS AND REACTIONS OF THE FAMILY OF THE CHILD WHO IS HOSPITALIZED

Parental Reactions

The crisis of childhood illness and hospitalization affects every member of the nuclear family. Parents' reactions to illness in their child depend on a variety of influencing factors. Although which factors are most likely to influence their response cannot be predicted, a number of variables have been identified (Box 44-5). (See also Chapter 41.)

Almost all parents respond to their child's illness and hospitalization with remarkably consistent reactions. Initially parents may react with *disbelief,* especially if the illness is sudden and serious. After the realization of illness, parents react with *anger* or *guilt* or both. They may blame themselves for the child's illness or become angry at others for some wrongdoing. Even with the mildest of illnesses, parents question their adequacy as caregivers and review any actions or omissions that could have prevented or caused the illness. When hospitalization is indicated, parental guilt is intensified because the parents feel helpless in alleviating the child's physical and emotional pain.

Fear, anxiety, and *frustration* are common feelings expressed by parents. Fear and anxiety may be related to the seriousness of the illness and the type of medical procedures involved. Often great anxiety is related to the trauma and pain inflicted on the child. Feelings of frustration are often related to lack of information about procedures and treatment, unfamiliarity with hospital rules and regulations, a sense of unwelcomeness from the staff, or fear of asking questions. Much frustration can be alleviated in a pediatric unit when parents are aware of what to expect and what is expected of them, are encouraged to participate in their child's care, and are regarded as the most significant contributors to the child's total health.

Parents eventually may react with some degree of *depression.* The depression usually occurs when the acute crisis is over, such as after hospital discharge or complete recovery. Mothers often comment on their feeling of physical and mental exhaustion af-

Box 44-4

Risk Factors That Increase Children's Vulnerability to the Stresses of Hospitalization

- "Difficult" temperament
- Lack of fit between child and parent
- Age (especially between 6 months and 5 years)
- Male gender
- Below-average intelligence
- Multiple and continuing stresses (e.g., frequent hospitalization)

Box 44-5

Factors Affecting Parents' Reactions to Their Child's Illness

- Seriousness of the threat to the child
- Previous experience with illness or hospitalization
- Medical procedures involved in diagnosis and treatment
- Available support systems
- Personal ego strengths
- Previous coping abilities
- Additional stresses on the family system
- Cultural and religious beliefs
- Communication patterns among family members

ter all of the other family members have adapted to the crisis. Parents may also worry about and miss their other children, who may be left in the care of family, friends, or neighbors. Other reasons for anxiety and depression are related to concerns for the child's future well-being, including negative effects produced by the hospitalization and any financial burden incurred from the hospitalization.

Sibling Reactions

Siblings' reactions to a sister's or brother's illness or hospitalization are discussed in Chapter 41 and differ little when a child becomes temporarily ill. They experience loneliness, fear, and worry, as well as anger, resentment, jealousy, and guilt. Various factors have been identified that influence the effects of the child's hospitalization on siblings. Although these factors are similar to those seen when a child has a chronic illness, Craft (1993) reported that the following factors regarding siblings are related specifically to the hospital experience and have been found to increase the effects on the sibling:

- Younger and experiencing many changes
- Cared for outside the home by care providers who are not relatives
- Received little information about their ill brother or sister
- Perceived their parents to be treating them differently compared with before their sibling's hospitalization

Simon (1993) asked 45 siblings of children who were hospitalized their perceptions of the stress of the hospitalization of a brother or sister. The siblings' perceptions of the stress they experienced were equal to the level of stress of hospitalized children.

Parents are often unaware of the number of effects that siblings experience during the sick child's hospitalization and the benefit of simple interventions to minimize such effects, such as explicit explanations about the illness and provisions for the siblings to remain at home. Sibling visitation is usually beneficial to the patient, sibling, and parent but should be evaluated on an individual basis.

Altered Family Roles

In addition to the effects of separation on family roles, loss of parenting, sibling, and offspring roles may affect each family member differently. One of the most common reactions of parents is specialized and intensified attention toward the sick child. The other children usually regard this as unfair and interpret the parents' attitude toward them as rejection. Although such responses are usually unconscious and unintended, they place unique burdens on ill children. For example, the ill child may feel obligated to play the sick role in order to meet parents' expectations, especially children who have had limited physical ability and regain normal health status, such as after corrective heart surgery. Parents may be unable to perceive the child's recovery and therefore need to continue the pattern of overprotection and indulgent attention.

Ill children may also feel jealousy and resentment from other siblings. Because of their singular position in the family, they may be denied the companionship of their brothers and sisters. Rivalry between siblings tends to be greatest with the sibling who is nearest in age to the ill child. Without an understanding of the interpersonal dynamics between siblings, parents are likely to blame the well children for antisocial behavior. Illness may also result in children's loss of status within either their family or their social group. For example, illness in the oldest child may temporarily terminate special privileges as "big" brother or sister.

NURSING CARE OF THE CHILD WHO IS HOSPITALIZED

Preparation for Hospitalization

The rationale for preparing children for the hospital experience and related procedures is based on the principle that fear of the unknown (fantasy) exceeds fear of the known. Therefore decreasing the elements of the unknown results in less fear. When children do not have paralyzing fear to cope with, they are able to direct their energies toward dealing with the other, unavoidable stresses of hospitalization and to benefit optimally from the growth potential of the experience.

Although preparation for hospitalization is a common practice, no universal standard or program is advocated for all settings. The preparation process may be elaborate, with tours, puppet shows, and playtime with miniature hospital equipment; it may involve the use of books, videos, or films; or it may be limited to a brief description of the major aspects of any hospital stay (Stewart, Algren, and Arnold, 1994). No firm consensus exists on the timing of the event. Some authorities recommend preparing children 4 to 7 years of age about 1 week in advance so that they can assimilate the information and ask questions. For older children the time may be longer. However, for young children, who may begin to fantasize about what they observed, 1 or 2 days before admission is sufficient time for anticipatory preparation. The length of the session should be suited to the children's attention span—the younger the child, the shorter the program. The optimum approach is one that is individualized for each child and family. Regardless of the specific type of program, all children, even those who have been hospitalized before, benefit from an introduction to the environment and routine of the unit.

➤ Assessment

Assessment is the first step in identifying nursing diagnoses and planning care for an individual child. In some instances, such as with elective admission, assessment begins even before the child is hospitalized so that appropriate preadmission preparation can be instituted. At other times, assessment occurs at the time of admission and should be integrated into other admission procedures so that the child's specific needs are recognized *early* in the hospitalization. One critical area is assessment of pain for implementing appropriate relief of discomfort (p. 1085). Although assessment is discussed under nursing care of the child who is hospitalized, a comprehensive approach must involve the child's parents or other caregivers.

The nurse's primary intent is to provide *atraumatic care* (see Chapter 29). Therefore patient assessment should be individualized and include an evaluation of the child's growth and development, psychosocial needs, educational needs, cultural background, and the effects of the illness on the child's family or guardian.

Admission Assessment. A nursing admission history refers to a systematic collection of data about the child and family that allows the nurse to plan individualized care. The nursing admission history presented in Box 44-6 is organized ac-

Box 44-6

Nursing Admission History According to Functional Health Patterns*

HEALTH PERCEPTION–HEALTH MANAGEMENT PATTERN

Why has your child been admitted?
How has your child's general health been?
What does your child know about this hospitalization?
  Ask the child why he or she came to the hospital.
  If the answer is "For an operation or for tests," ask the child to tell you about what will happen before, during, and after the operation or tests.
Has your child ever been in the hospital before?
  How was that hospital experience?
  What things were important to you and your child during that hospitalization? How can we be most helpful now?
What medications does your child take at home?
  Why are they given?
  When are they given?
  How are they given (if a liquid, with a spoon; if a tablet, swallowed with water; or other)?
  Does your child have any trouble taking medication? If so, what helps?
  Is your child allergic to any medications?
What, if any, forms of complementary medicine practices are being used?

NUTRITION-METABOLIC PATTERN

What are the family's usual mealtimes?
Do family members eat together or at separate times?
What are your child's favorite foods, beverages, and snacks?
  Average amounts consumed or usual size of portions
  Special cultural practices, such as family eats only ethnic food
What foods and beverages does your child *dislike?*
What are your child's feeding habits (bottle, cup, spoon, eats by self, needs assistance, any special devices)?
How does your child like the food served (warmed, cold, one item at a time)?
How would you describe your child's usual appetite (hearty eater, picky eater)?
  Has being sick affected your child's appetite? In what ways?
Are there any known or suspected food allergies?
Is your child on a special diet?
Are there any feeding problems (excessive fussiness, spitting up, colic); any dental or gum problems that affect feeding?
What do you do for these problems?

ELIMINATION PATTERN

What are your child's toilet habits (diaper, toilet trained—day only or day and night, use of word to communicate urination or defecation, potty chair, regular toilet, other routines)?
What is your child's usual pattern of elimination (bowel movements)?
Do you have any concerns about elimination (bed-wetting, constipation, diarrhea)?
What do you do for these problems?
Have you ever noticed that your child sweats a lot?

SLEEP-REST PATTERN

What is your child's usual hour of sleep and awakening?
What is your child's schedule for naps; length of naps?
Is there a special routine before sleeping (bottle, drink of water, bedtime story, night light, favorite blanket or toy, prayers)?
Is there a special routine during sleep time, such as waking to go to the bathroom?
What type of bed does your child sleep in?
Does your child have a separate room or share a room; if shares, with whom?
What are the home sleeping arrangements (alone or with others, e.g., sibling, parent, other person)?
What is your child's favorite sleeping position?
Are there any sleeping problems (falling asleep, waking during night, nightmares, sleep walking)?
Are there any problems in awakening and getting ready in the morning?
What do you do for these problems?

ACTIVITY-EXERCISE PATTERN

What is your child's schedule during the day (preschool, day care center, regular school, extracurricular activities)?
What are your child's favorite activities or toys (both active and quiet interests)?
What is your child's usual television-viewing schedule at home?
  What are your child's favorite programs?
  Are there any TV restrictions?
Does your child have any illness or disabilities that limit activity? If so, how?
What are your child's usual habits and schedule for bathing (bath in tub or shower, sponge bath, shampoo)?
What are your child's dental habits (brushing, flossing, fluoride supplements or rinses, favorite toothpaste); schedule of daily dental care?
Does your child need help with dressing or grooming, such as hair combing?
Are there any problems with the above (dislike of or refusal to bathe, shampoo hair, or brush teeth)?
  What do you do for these problems?
Are there special devices that your child requires help in managing (eyeglasses, contact lenses, hearing aid, orthodontic appliances, artificial elimination appliances, orthopedic devices)?
NOTE: Use the following code to assess functional self-care level for feeding, bathing/hygiene, dressing/grooming, toileting:
  0: Full self-care
  I: Requires use of equipment or device
  II: Requires assistance or supervision from another person
  III: Requires assistance or supervision from another person and equipment or device
  IV: Is dependent and does not participate

*The focus of the admission history is the child's psychosocial environment. Most of the questions are worded in terms of parental responses. Depending on the child's age, they should be addressed directly to the child when appropriate.

Continued

Box 44-6

Nursing Admission History According to Functional Health Patterns*—cont'd

COGNITIVE-PERCEPTUAL PATTERN

Does your child have any hearing difficulty?
- Does the child use a hearing aid?
- Have "tubes" been placed in your child's ears?

Does your child have any vision problems?
- Does the child wear glasses or contact lenses?

Does your child have any learning difficulties?
- What is the child's grade in school?

For information on pain, see Box 44-12.

SELF-PERCEPTION–SELF-CONCEPT PATTERN

How would you describe your child (e.g., takes time to adjust, settles in easily, shy, friendly, quiet, talkative, serious, playful, stubborn, easygoing)?

What makes your child angry, annoyed, anxious, or sad? What helps?

How does your child act when annoyed or upset?

What have been your child's experiences with and reactions to temporary separation from you (parent)?

Does your child have any fears (places, objects, animals, people, situations)? How do you handle them?

Do you think your child's illness has changed the way he or she thinks about self (e.g., more shy, embarrassed about appearance, less competitive with friends, stays at home more)?

ROLE-RELATIONSHIP PATTERN

Does your child have a favorite nickname?

What are the names of other family members or others who live in the home (relatives, friends, pets)?

Who usually takes care of your child during the day/night (especially if other than parent, such as baby-sitter, relative)?

What are the parents' occupations and work schedules?

Are there any special family considerations (adoption, foster child, stepparent, divorce, single parent)?

Have any major changes in the family occurred lately (death, divorce, separation, birth of a sibling, loss of a job, financial strain, mother beginning a career, other)? Describe child's reaction.

Who are your child's play companions or social groups (peers, younger or older children, adults, prefers to be alone)?

Do things generally go well for your child in school or with friends?

Does your child have "security" objects at home (pacifier, bottle, blanket, stuffed animal or doll)? Did you bring any of these to the hospital?

How do you handle discipline problems at home? Are these methods always effective?

Does your child have any condition that interferes with communication? If so, what are your suggestions for communicating with your child?

Will your child's hospitalization affect the family's financial support or care of other family members (e.g., other children)?

What concerns do you have about your child's illness and hospitalization?

Who will be staying with your child while hospitalized?

How can we contact you or another close family member outside of the hospital?

SEXUALITY-REPRODUCTIVE PATTERN

(Answer questions that apply to your child's age group.)

Has your child begun puberty (developing physical sexual characteristics, menstruation)? Have you or your child had any concerns?

Does your daughter know how to do breast self-examination?

Does your son know how to do testicular self-examination?

How have you approached topics of sexuality with your child?

Do you feel you might need some help with some topics?

Has your child's illness affected the way he or she feels about being a boy or a girl? If so, how?

Do you have any concerns with behaviors in your child, such as masturbation, asking many questions or talking about sex, not respecting others' privacy, or wanting too much privacy?

Initiate a conversation about an adolescent's sexual concerns with open-ended to more direct questions and using the terms "friends" or "partners" rather than "girlfriend" or "boyfriend":
- Tell me about your social life.
- Who are your closest friends? (If one friend is identified, could ask more about that relationship, such as how much time they spend together, how serious they are about each other, if the relationship is going the way the teenager hoped.)
- Might ask about dating and sexual issues, such as the teenager's views on sexuality education, "going steady," "living together," or premarital sex.
- Which friends would you like to have visit in the hospital?

COPING-STRESS TOLERANCE PATTERN

(Answer questions that apply to your child's age group.)

What does your child do when tired or upset?
- If upset, does your child want a special person or object? If so, explain.

If your child has temper tantrums, what causes them and how do you handle them?

Whom does your child talk to when worried about something?

How does your child usually handle problems or disappointments?

Have there been any big changes or problems in your family recently? If so, how have you handled them?

Has your child ever had a problem with drugs or alcohol or tried to commit suicide?

Do you think your child is "accident prone"? If so, explain.

VALUE-BELIEF PATTERN

What is your religion?

How is religion or faith important in your child's life?

What religious practices would you like continued in the hospital (e.g., prayers before meals/bedtime; visit by minister, priest, or rabbi; prayer group)?

*The focus of the admission history is the child's psychosocial environment. Most of the questions are worded in terms of parental responses. Depending on the child's age, they should be addressed directly to the child when appropriate.

Box 44-7

Complementary Medicine Practices and Examples

Nutrition, diet, and lifestyle/behavioral health changes—Macrobiotics, megavitamins, diets, lifestyle modification, health risk reduction/health education, wellness

Mind/body control therapies—Biofeedback, relaxation, prayer therapy, guided imagery, hypnotherapy, music/sound therapy, aromatherapy, education therapy

Traditional and ethnomedicine therapies—Acupuncture, ayurvedic medicine, herbal medicine, homeopathic medicine, Native-American medicine, natural products, traditional Oriental medicine

Structural manipulation and energetic therapies—Acupressure, chiropractic medicine, massage, reflexology, rolfing, therapeutic touch, QI Gong

Pharmacologic and biologic therapies—Antioxidants, cell treatment, chelation therapy, metabolic therapy, oxidizing agents

Bioelectromagnetic therapies—Diagnostic and therapeutic application of electromagnetic fields (e.g., transcranial electrostimulation, neuromagnetic stimulation, electroacupuncture)

cording to the Functional Health Patterns outlined by Gordon (1994, 1995) (see Nursing Diagnosis, Chapter 29). This assessment framework is a guideline for formulating nursing diagnoses. It would not be practical, however, to include all questions in the nursing admission history.

One of the main purposes of the history is to assess the child's usual health habits at home to promote a more normal environment in the hospital. Therefore questions related to activities of daily living in the nutritional-metabolic, elimination, sleep-rest, and activity-exercise patterns are a major part of the assessment.

The questions found under the health perception–health management pattern are directed toward evaluation of the child's preparation for hospitalization and are key factors in determining whether additional preparation is needed. The questions included in the self-perception–self-concept and role-relationship patterns offer insight into the child's potential reaction to hospitalization, especially in terms of separation.

The nurse should also inquire about the use of any complementary medicine practices (Box 44-7). In a study of children with cancer, 42% had used alternative or complementary therapies simultaneously with or after conventional treatments (Fernandez, Pyesmany, and Stutzer, 1999). Widespread use of complementary medicine is often explored, however, without discussion with the primary care physician or nurse (Moenkhoff et al, 1999; Spiegel, Stroud, and Fyfe, 1998) (Critical Thinking box).

Once the data have been collected, the information must be applied to the nursing process and communicated to other staff. It makes little sense to assess a child's home routine if none of this knowledge is integrated into the plan of care. Most nursing units have provisions for care plans in which specific information about the child's habits and needs is recorded and incorporated into the hospital routine.

Critical Thinking

COMPLEMENTARY MEDICINE PRACTICES

Maria, a 10-year-old Hispanic girl, has had severe nosebleeds. She is admitted to the hospital for a complete workup in an attempt to determine the cause. Her parents and grandparents have gathered around her bed. When you enter her room to begin admitting procedures, you notice an unusual scent. Maria's mother is rubbing the contents from an unfamiliar bottle of liquid on Maria. Meanwhile, the grandmother is rubbing Maria's head. She is startled at your entry and drops something on the floor near your feet. You bend over to pick it up and discover that it is a penny. After introducing yourself and explaining the purpose of your visit, your most appropriate response would be which of the following?

First, Think About It . . .

- **Within what point of view are you thinking?**
- **What would the consequences be if you put your thoughts into action?**

1. **"Here is your penny."**
2. **"I need to take this bottle and have the lab examine its contents."**
3. **"Many families tell me that they use certain medicine practices that are traditional in their families. Can you tell me about yours?"**
4. **"What is going on here?"**

The best response is 3. The third-person technique (see Chapter 34) gives families permission to share information. What you have probably observed is* Santeria, *the African-Caribbean religion that was brought to the New World by slaves from West Africa. It is common among immigrants from Cuba, Puerto Rico, Brazil, and Santo Domingo, and it is believed that a majority of Latin immigrants will have contact with Santeria sometime in their lives. Answer 1 avoids the issue, which could have negative consequences. Although at some point you may need to take action and have the contents of the bottle examined (answer 2), it is an inappropriate initial response. Answer 4 is confrontational and disrespectful.

Besides taking the nursing admission history, nurses should also perform a physical assessment (see Chapter 35) or obtain the information from the medical examination before planning care. At the very least, the nurse's physical assessment of the child should include observation of the body for any bruises, rashes, signs of neglect, deformities, or physical limitations. The nurse should also listen to the heart and lungs to assess overall physical status. For example, it is impossible to evaluate improvement in respiratory function in a child admitted with pulmonary disease unless there are baseline data with which to compare subsequent findings.

➤ Nursing Diagnoses

A number of nursing diagnoses are prominent in the nursing care of children who are ill and/or hospitalized. Other nursing diagnoses specific to individual cases may become evident in addition to those outlined in the Nursing Care Plan on p. 1110.

➤ Plan of Care and Implementation

An effective plan of care for the child who is hospitalized is based on patient- and family-identified needs, as well as those identified by the nurse. Family members and the child should play active roles in developing the plan whenever possible.

The main goals for the child who is ill and/or hospitalized are as follows:

1. Child will be prepared for hospitalization.
2. Child will experience little or no separation.
3. Child will maintain a sense of control.
4. Child will exhibit decreased fear of bodily injury.
5. Child will experience a reduction of pain that is acceptable to child.
6. Child will have opportunities to participate in developmentally appropriate diversional activities.
7. Child will experience maximum benefits from hospitalization.

Preparing Child for Admission. The preparation that children require on the day of admission depends on the kind of prehospital counseling they have received. If they have been prepared in a formalized program, they will usually know what to expect in terms of initial medical procedures, inpatient facilities, and nursing staff. However, prehospital counseling does not preclude the need for support during procedures such as obtaining blood specimens, x-ray tests, or physical examination. For example, undressing young children before they feel comfortable in their new surroundings can be very upsetting to them. Causing needless anxiety and fear during admission may adversely affect the nurse's establishment of trust with these children. Therefore nursing assistance during the admission procedure is vital, regardless of how well prepared any child is for the experience of hospitalization. In addition, spending this time with the child gives the nurse an opportunity to evaluate the child's understanding of subsequent procedures (Fig. 44-4). Ideally, a primary nurse is assigned whenever possible to allow for individualized care and to provide a substitute support person for the child.

When a child is admitted, nurses follow several fairly universal admission procedures, which are outlined in Box 44-8. One particularly important decision is room assignment. The minimum considerations for room assignment are age, sex, and nature of the illness. Ideally, however, room selection should be based on a variety of developmental and psychobiologic needs. Determining compatible roommates, both for the children and for rooming-in parents, greatly influences the growth potential from the hospital experience.

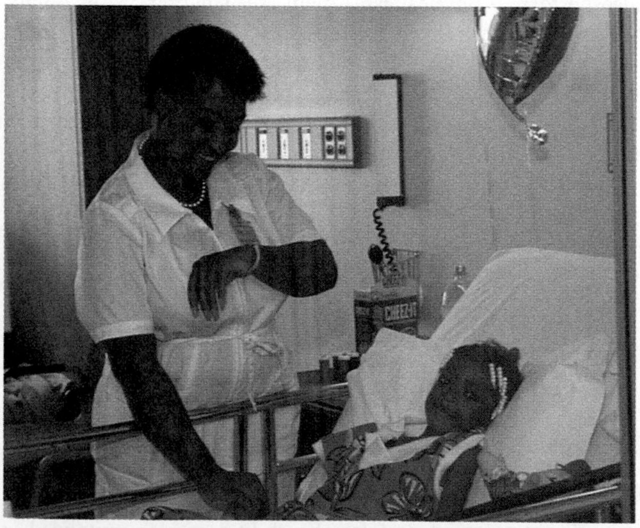

FIG. 44-4 • The initial admission procedures give the nurse an opportunity to get to know the child and to assess the child's understanding of the hospital experience. (Courtesy St Louis Children's Hospital.)

No absolute rules govern room selection, but in general, placing children of the same age group and with similar types of illness in the same room is both psychologically and medically advantageous. However, there are many exceptions. For example, a school-age child may thrive on the responsibility of caring for a younger child. A child in traction may be very therapeutic for another child confined to bed because of a serious illness. A child who is very independent despite physical disabilities may help another child with similar or different limitations, and the parents of the child with disabilities may achieve deeper insight and acceptance of their child's disorder.

Age grouping is especially important for adolescents. Many hospitals make an effort to place teenagers on their own unit or in a separate, designated section of the pediatric or general unit whenever possible.

Preventing or Minimizing Separation. A primary nursing goal is to prevent separation, particularly in children younger than 5 years. Changes in hospitals' policies over recent years reflect a changed attitude toward parents; many hospitals no longer consider parents "visitors" and welcome their presence at all times throughout the child's hospitalization. Many

Box 44-8

Guidelines for Admission

PREADMISSION

Assign a room based on developmental age, seriousness of diagnosis, communicability of illness, and projected length of stay.

Prepare roommate(s) for the arrival of a new patient; when children are too young to benefit from this consideration, prepare parents.

Prepare room for child and family, with admission forms and equipment nearby to eliminate need to leave child.

ADMISSION

Introduce primary nurse to child and family.

Orient child and family to inpatient facilities, especially to assigned room and unit; emphasize positive areas of pediatric unit.

Room: Explain call light, bed controls, television, bathroom, telephone, etc.

Unit: Direct to playroom, desk, dining area, or other areas.

Introduce family to roommate and his or her parents.

Apply identification band to child's wrist, ankle, or both (if not done).

Explain hospital regulations and schedules (e.g., visiting hours, mealtimes, bedtime, limitations [give written information if available]).

Perform nursing admission history (see Box 44-6).

Take vital signs, blood pressure, height, and weight measurements.

Obtain specimens as needed and order needed laboratory work.

Support child and assist practitioner with physical examination (for purposes of nursing assessment).

hospitals have developed a system of family-centered care. This philosophy of care recognizes the integral role of the family in a child's life and emphasizes the importance of providing services that demonstrate the value of collaboration between the health care provider, the child, and the family (see Chapter 29).

At the least, most hospitals welcome parents at any time. Many provide facilities such as a chair or bed for at least one person per child, unit kitchen privileges, and other amenities that create a welcoming atmosphere for parents. However, not all hospitals provide such an invitation, and parents' own schedules may prevent rooming-in. In such instances, strategies to minimize the effects of separation must be implemented.

As previously mentioned, ideally a primary nurse, along with associates, is assigned to meet the child's needs. A thorough, detailed nursing history specifically identifies the child's established daily routine. Usual daily activities, such as food preparation and method of feeding, help establish a complementary schedule of caregiving practices. Incorporating these normal activities also helps the parents feel that they are participating in the child's care, even if through another person. A consistent staff member can be designated to keep the family informed of the child's condition and to support the family's concerns and priorities without being judgmental (Kauffmann et al, 1998; Stepanek and Ahmann, 1995).

Nurses must have an appreciation of the child's separation behaviors. As discussed earlier, the phases of protest and despair are normal. The child is allowed to cry. Even if the child rejects strangers, the nurse provides support through physical presence. *Presence* is defined as spending time being physically close to the child while using a quiet tone of voice, appropriate choice of words, eye contact, and touch in ways that establish rapport and communicate empathy. If behaviors of detachment are evident, the nurse maintains the child's contact with the parents by often talking about them, encouraging the child to remember them, and stressing the significance of their visits, telephone calls, or letters.

Separation may be equally as difficult for parents, especially when they do not understand the behaviors of separation anxiety. To avoid the immediate protest, parents may sneak out or lie to the child about leaving. As a result, the child does not learn that absence is associated with a guaranteed return but that absence means loss of parents. Helping parents recognize that separation behaviors are normal and expected can decrease the parents' anxiety and may ease their fears about leaving without telling the child. Explaining to parents how the child reacts after they leave may also be helpful. Many parents imagine that the child cries for hours after they leave, whereas in reality the child may cry for a few minutes but settle down when comforted by someone else.

Toddlers and preschoolers have a very limited concept of time. The young child's question, "Will my mommy come yesterday?" symbolizes a lack of understanding for usual measurements of time, such as days, hours, and weeks. Time is measured in associations, such as eating dinner "when Daddy comes home." Therefore, when helping parents with their fears of separation, nurses need to suggest ways of explaining leaving and returning. For example, if parents must leave to go to work or to make meals for the other family members, they should tell the child the reason for leaving. They also need to convey the expected time of return in terms of anticipated events. For example, if the parents will return in the morning, they can say to the child, "We'll see you after the sun comes up" or "We'll come back when (a favorite program) is on television."

The young child's ability to tolerate parental absence is very limited. Therefore parental visits should be frequent (e.g., visiting three times a day for short periods rather than once a day for an extended time). This may necessitate that each parent visit at different times to lessen the length of separation. When parents cannot visit, the presence of other significant persons can be most comforting for the child.

If parents leave after the child is asleep, they still need to communicate their absence. The parents of a 5-year-old boy solved this problem by devising a sign; on one side they drew a picture of a telephone, and on the other they drew a hamburger. Before they left, they turned the sign to the appropriate side to tell the child when he awoke that they were out using the telephone or eating.

Older children who know how to tell time may find it helpful to have a clock or watch. However, these children have the same need for honesty from their parents regarding visiting schedules. Because their peer groups are important, adolescents often appreciate planning visiting hours with their parents to ensure that the patient has some private time for friends.

Familiar surroundings also increase the child's adjustment to separation. If parents cannot room-in, they should leave favorite articles from home with the child, such as a blanket, toy, bottle, feeding utensil, or article of clothing. Because young children associate such inanimate objects with significant persons, they gain comfort and reassurance from these possessions. They make the association that if the parents left this, the parents will surely return. Placing an identification band on the toy lessens the chances of its being misplaced and provides a symbol that the toy is experiencing the same needs as the child. Other mementos of home include photographs and audiotape or videocassette recordings of family members reading a story, singing a song, saying prayers before bedtime, relating events at home, or taking a "talking walk" through the home. The tapes can be played at lonely times, such as on awakening or before sleeping. Some units allow pets to visit, which can have therapeutic benefits for a child. Animals should be carefully screened for medical or behavioral problems, and patients should be screened for allergies.

Older children also appreciate familiar articles from home, particularly photographs, a radio, a favorite toy or game, and the usual pajamas. Often the importance of treasured objects to school-age children is overlooked or criticized. However, many school-age children have a special object to which they formed an attachment in early childhood. Therefore such treasured or transitional objects can help even older children feel more comfortable in a strange environment.

The strange sights, smells, and sounds in the hospital that are commonplace for the nurse can be frightening and confusing for children. It is important for the nurse to try to evaluate stimuli in the environment from the child's point of view (considering also what the child may see or hear happening to other patients) and to make every effort to protect the child from frightening and unfamiliar sights, sounds, and equipment. The nurse should offer explanations or prepare the child for those experiences that are unavoidable. Combining familiar or comforting sights with the unfamiliar can relieve much of the harshness of medical equipment.

Helping children maintain their usual nonhome contacts also minimizes the effects of separation imposed by hospitalization. This includes continuing school lessons during the illness and confinement, visiting with friends either directly or through letter writing or telephone calls, and participating in stimulating projects whenever possible (Fig. 44-5). For extended hospitalizations, youngsters enjoy personalizing the hospital room to make it "home" by decorating the walls with posters and cards, rearranging the furniture (when possible), and displaying a collection or hobby.

Minimizing Loss of Control. Feelings of loss of control result from separation, physical restriction, changed routines, enforced dependency, and magical thinking. Although some of these cannot be prevented, most can be minimized through individualized planning of nursing care.

Promoting Freedom of Movement. Younger children react most strenuously to any type of physical restriction or immobilization. Although medical immobilization may be necessary for some interventions such as maintaining an intravenous (IV) line, most physical restriction can be prevented if the nurse gains the child's cooperation.

For young children, particularly infants and toddlers, preserving parent-child contact is the best means of decreasing the need for or stress of restraint. For example, almost the entire physical examination can be done in a parent's lap, with the parent hugging the child for procedures such as otoscopy. For painful procedures the parents' preferences for assisting, observing, or waiting outside the room are assessed.

Environmental factors may also restrict movement. Keeping children in cribs or playpens may not represent immobilization in a concrete sense, but it certainly limits sensory stimulation. Increasing mobility by transporting children in carriages, wheelchairs, carts, or wagons or on stretchers or beds provides them with mechanical freedom.

Maintaining Child's Routine. Altered daily schedules and loss of rituals are particularly stressful for toddlers and early preschoolers and may increase the stress of separation. The nursing admission history provides a baseline for planning care around the child's usual home activities.

A commonly neglected aspect of altered routines is the change in the child's daily activities. A nonhospitalized child's day, especially during the school years, is structured with specific times for eating, dressing, going to school, playing, and sleeping. However, this time structure vanishes when the child is hospitalized. Although the nurses have a set schedule, the child is often unaware of it; new schedules are imposed that may be rigid or flexible. For example, some units have uniform nap times and bedtimes for all children, whereas others allow children to stay up very late. Many children obtain significantly less sleep in the hospital than at home; the primary causes are delay in sleep onset and early termination of sleep because of hospital routines. Not only are sleep hours disrupted, but waking hours are spent in passive activities. For example, few institutions impose any regulation on the amount of time the child spends watching television.

One technique that can minimize the disruption in the child's routine is *time structuring.* This approach is most suitable for the noncritically ill school-age or adolescent child who has mastered the concept of time. It involves scheduling the child's day to include all those activities that are important to the child and nurse, such as treatment procedures, schoolwork, exercise, television, playroom, and hobbies. Together, the nurse, parent, and child plan a daily schedule with times and activities written down (Fig. 44-6). This is left in the child's room, and a clock or watch is available for the child's use. Whenever possible, a calendar is also constructed with special events marked, such as favorite television programs, visits by friends or relatives, events in the playroom, and holidays or birthdays. If specific changes in treatment are expected (e.g., "beginning physical therapy in 2 days"), these are added.

Encouraging Independence. The dependent role of the hospitalized patient imposes tremendous feelings of loss on older children. Principal interventions should focus on respect for individuality and the opportunity for decision making. Although these sound simple, their efficacy lies with nurses who are flexible, tolerant, and personally secure. The last is particularly important because when decision making is geared toward the patient, nurses can feel threatened by a sense of lessened control.

Promoting children's control involves maintaining independence, and the concept of self-care can be most beneficial. *Self-care* refers to the practice of activities that individuals personally initiate and perform on their own behalf in maintaining life, health, and well-being (Orem, 1995). Although self-care is

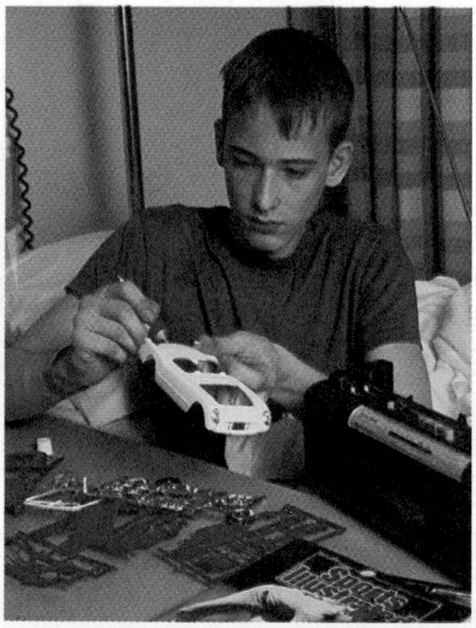

FIG. 44-5 • For extended hospitalizations, children enjoy having projects to occupy time. (Courtesy St Louis Children's Hospital.)

ERIC'S DAILY SCHEDULE:

7:00 AM	– Breakfast, Watch TV, Brush Teeth, Wash up	3:00 PM	– Tutor (M, W, F) Study Time (T, Th)
9:00	– Tub Room, Dressing Change	4:00	– Physical Therapy
		5:00	– Dinner
10:00	– Rest, TV, Snack	6:30	– Dressing Change
11:00	– Physical Therapy	7:00 to 9:00	– TV, Reading, Snack, Friends Visit
12:00 PM	– Lunch		
1:00	– Playroom, Quiet Play, Rest, Friends Visit	9:00	– Brush Teeth, Wash up
		9:15	– Bedtime

FIG. 44-6 • Time structuring is an effective strategy for normalizing the hospital environment and increasing the child's sense of control.

limited by the child's age and physical condition, most children beyond infancy can perform some activities with little or no help. Whenever possible, these activities are encouraged in the hospital. Other approaches include jointly planning care, structuring time, wearing street clothes, making choices in food selections and bedtime, continuing school activities, and rooming with an appropriate age-mate.

Promoting Understanding. Loss of control can occur from feelings of having too little influence on one's destiny, as well as from sensing overwhelming control or power over fate. Although preschoolers' cognitive abilities predispose them most to magical thinking and self-power, all children are vulnerable to misinterpreting causes for stresses such as illness and hospitalization.

Most children feel more in control when they know what to expect because the element of fear is reduced. Anticipatory preparation and providing information help greatly to lessen stress and prevent lack of understanding (see Preparation for Procedures, Chapter 45).

Informing children of their rights while hospitalized fosters greater understanding and may relieve some of the feelings of powerlessness they typically experience. Hospitals providing services to children should have a hospital-wide policy on the rights and responsibilities of these patients and of their parents and/or guardians (Joint Commission on Accreditation of Healthcare Organizations, 1999). An increasing number of hospitals and organizations have developed a "Bill of Rights" that is prominently displayed throughout the hospital or is presented to children and their families on admission (Box 44-9).

Preventing or Minimizing Fear of Bodily Injury. Beyond early infancy all children fear bodily injury from mutilation, bodily intrusion, body-image change, disability, or death. In general, preparation of children for painful procedures decreases their fears. Manipulating procedural techniques for children in each age group also minimizes fear of bodily injury. For example, because toddlers and young preschoolers are traumatized by insertion of a rectal thermometer, axillary temperatures or temperatures taken with electronic or tympanic membrane devices can effectively be substituted. Whenever procedures are performed on young children, the most supportive intervention is to do the procedure as quickly as possible while maintaining parent-child contact.

Because of young children's poorly defined body boundaries, the use of bandages may be particularly helpful. For example, telling children that the bleeding will stop after the needle is removed does little to relieve their fears, whereas applying a small Band-Aid usually provides much reassurance. The size of bandages is also significant to children in this age group; the larger the bandage, the more importance is attached to the wound. Watching their surgical dressings become successively smaller is one way young children can measure healing and improvement. Prematurely removing a dressing may cause these children considerable concern for their well-being.

For children who fear mutilation of body parts, it is essential that the nurse repeatedly stress the reason for a procedure and evaluate the child's understanding. For example, explaining cast removal to preschoolers may seem simple enough, but children's comprehension of the details may vary considerably from the explanation. Asking them to draw a picture of what they think will happen presents substantial evidence of the perceived events.

Children may fear bodily injury from a variety of sources. X-ray machines, use of strange equipment for examination, unfamiliar rooms, or awkward positions can be perceived as potentially hazardous. In addition, thoughts and actions can be imagined sources of bodily damage. For older children, masturbation or sex play may be perceived as powerful weapons of potential destruction. Therefore it is important to investigate imagined reasons, particularly of a sexual nature, for illness. Because children may fear revealing such thoughts, using projective techniques such as drawing or doll play may elicit previously undisclosed misconceptions.

Older children fear bodily injury of both internal and external origins. For example, school-age children are aware of the significance of the heart and may fear the actual operation as much as the pain, the stitches, and the possible scar. Adolescents may express concern about the actual procedure but be much more anxious over the resulting scar. An appreciation of each child's special concerns helps nurses focus on critical areas during preparation for procedures or when giving explanations of the disease processes.

Children can grasp information only if it is presented on or close to their level of cognitive development. This necessitates an awareness of the words used to describe events or processes. For example, young children told that they are going to have a CAT scan may wonder, "Will there be cats or something that scratches?" It is clearer to describe the procedure in simple terms and explain what the letters of the common name stand for.

When children are upset about their illness, their perception can be changed by (1) providing a somewhat different and less negative account of the disease or (2) offering an explanation that is characteristic of the next stage of cognitive development. An example of the first strategy is to reassure a preschooler who has undergone a tonsillectomy that another sore throat does not mean a second operation. Explaining that once tonsils are "fixed" they do not need fixing again can help relieve the fear. An example of the second strategy is to explain that germs made the tonsils sick, and even though germs can cause another sore throat, they cannot cause the tonsils to ever be sick again. This higher level explanation is based on the school-age child's concept of germs as a cause of disease.

Pain Assessment.* Pain assessment is a critical component of the nursing process. Unfortunately, health professionals, including nurses, continue to underestimate and sporadically manage pain in infants and children (Boughton et al, 1998; Broome et al, 1996) (Box 44-10). One of the reasons for inadequate management of pain is a lack of understanding of what

Box 44-9

Bill of Rights for Children and Teens

In this hospital you and your family have the right to:
- Respect and personal dignity
- Care that supports you and your family
- Information you can understand
- Quality health care
- Emotional support
- Care that respects your need to grow, play, and learn
- Make choices and decisions

From Association for the Care of Children's Health: *A pediatric bill of rights,* Bethesda, MD, 1991, The Association.

*For additional information, please view "Pain assessment and management" in ***Whaley and Wong's Pediatric Nursing Video Series,*** St Louis, 1996, Mosby; 1-800-426-4545; website: www.mosby.com.

Box 44-10

Undermedication of Pain in Children

Several studies have examined the pattern of pain medication for children as compared with adults and have found remarkably consistent findings—that children have been undermedicated for pain. Eland and Anderson (1977) investigated the incidence of administration of analgesics to 25 hospitalized children for postoperative pain. Twelve of the children received a total of 24 doses of analgesics; the remaining 13 children were never given any medication for pain relief. In contrast, 18 adults with identical diagnoses received 372 opioid analgesic doses and 299 nonopioid analgesic doses for a total of 671 doses. One of the saddest findings was that more than twice as many children had pain medication ordered as received it. This lack of response to the need for pain medication directly relates to the nurses who failed to administer the analgesic.

Another study investigating analgesic prescriptions given to children and adults after open heart surgery found that all of the adults received medication, for a total of 564 doses, but only three fourths of the children were given medication, for a total of 237 doses during the first 3 postoperative days. This difference was even greater on the fifth postoperative day, when 83% of the adults continued to receive analgesics (a total of 136 doses) but only 12% of the children were medicated (a total of 10 doses) (Beyer et al, 1983).

Another study on postoperative pain found that 75% of the children reported pain on the day of surgery, and if orders for opioid or nonopioid analgesics were written, the nonopioid was given exclusively. In addition, the doses ordered were usually too small and/or too infrequent to be maximally effective. Most orders were written "PRN," which was often interpreted by nursing staff to mean "as little as possible" (Mather and Mackle, 1983).

A review of analgesic use in the emergency department reported significantly low use in children with mild to moderate trauma, including children with painful fractures. Head injury was associated with especially low use of analgesics (Friedland and Kulick, 1994).

Johnston et al (1992) studied 150 randomly selected hospitalized children and found that 87% reported pain, with 19% stating that their pain was severe. Of the 150 children, only 38% had received analgesics during the previous 24 hours.

An even sadder and more disappointing finding is that two decades after Eland's seminal research, some nurses may neither have knowledge about appropriate analgesic medications for children nor appreciate the consequences of undermedication. In the study conducted by Boughton et al (1998), 25% of 36 patients were given no pain medication, and 25% of the patients stated that their pain intervention was only partially effective. *All* patients had PRN orders for analgesics. Clearly, the responsibility for inadequate pain control rested with the nurses.

The situation is even more serious with infants. One analysis of anesthetic practices with newborns undergoing surgical ligation of patent ductus arteriosus found that 76% of the infants received only nitrous oxide and a paralyzing agent. These infants could not move during surgery but could feel all the pain of a thoracotomy (Anand and Aynsley-Green, 1985). In a survey of nurses working in neonatal intensive care units, 79% believed that infants were undermedicated for pain. The same study found that more than half of the medications used for pain relief had no analgesic properties (Franck, 1987). A study comparing premedication for procedures such as arterial line or chest tube placement found that infants in neonatal intensive care units received no premedication much more often than children in pediatric intensive care units (Bauchner, May, and Coates, 1992). In the United States the use of analgesia and anesthesia for newborn circumcision is not routine. A survey of pediatric, obstetric, and family practice residents showed that training in the use of pain reducers during this painful procedure was inadequate (Howard et al, 1998). Unfortunately, the amount of content on pain in nursing curricula also is inadequate, and some of the textbooks contain inaccurate information (Davis, 1998; Ferrell, McCaffery, and Rhiner, 1992).

Much research has been done examining the stress response in premature infants, and the results support the belief that unrelieved pain has detrimental physiologic, anatomic, and behavioral effects (see also Neonatal Pain, Chapter 25). Much less research has been done on the long-term effects of pain on children, from both a psychologic and a physiologic point of view. Stuber et al (1997) examined the psychologic effects on survivors of childhood cancer. Many children reported long-term sequelae that resembled post-traumatic stress syndrome (see Chapter 39). Children's fears were related to their perception of the intensity of treatment, not the illness itself. Symptoms included stomachaches and bad dreams. Another study found that memory of a painful experience may cause anxiety about subsequent procedures. Weisman, Bernstein, and Schechter (1998) showed that children who had a placebo, rather than oral transmucosal fentanyl, before a painful procedure were more anxious than the medicated group for the subsequent procedure *even when the analgesic was given.* Based on their results, the authors argue strongly for aggressive pain control beginning with the first noxious procedure.

On a positive note, Schechter (1997) outlines the growth in research and published literature (33 articles in 1974 to 2966 articles from 1980 to 1991) in pediatric pain management that comprises many topics such as oncology, sickle ceil disease, acute pain, and chronic pain. One outcome of the large number of research studies has been the development of pain teams or pain specialists. Unfortunately, when these services exist, other health care professionals may abandon any responsibility for pain control to the pain experts or neglect to consult the pain team. Although pain teams play a very important role in treating pain adequately (Ferrell et al, 1994), in a survey of 35 pediatric pain services only 17% had written guidelines (Tyc et al, 1998).

Guidelines are available to help practitioners assess and manage pain using methods based on the published scientific literature. In the United States the **Agency for Health Care Policy and Research (AHCPR)** has published guidelines developed by pain experts that focus on the issues of postoperative, procedure-related or trauma, and cancer pain. Other national and international organizations, including the Joint Commission for the Accreditation of Health Care Organizations, have also contributed research-based recommendations that nurses can use to improve pain control.

In your agency, see if these references are readily available to staff. If not, order them, especially the AHCPR publications, and distribute them, stressing that they provide state-of-the-art information. As you practice, carry your copy of the guidelines; mark sections, such as those discussing addiction and listing drug dosages, for quick reference. Compare your pain assessment and management interventions with those in the published guidelines, and make a commitment to increase your knowledge. *Remember: to relieve pain effectively, its management must be based on scientific research, not personal opinion or belief.*

pain is—a personal phenomenon that cannot be experienced by any other individual. Therefore defining pain in terms of another's perceptions is inappropriate and inaccurate. An operational definition that is useful in clinical practice follows: *pain is whatever the experiencing person says it is, existing whenever the person says it does* (McCaffery and Pasero, 1999). This definition implies a very important attitude toward patients—*that that they are believed.* It includes both verbal and nonverbal expressions of pain.

Fallacies and Facts. Children are undertreated for pain for a number of complex and interrelated reasons, including professionals' misconceptions about pain; the complexities of pain assessment, particularly in nonverbal children; and the lack of information regarding currently available pain reduction techniques. A number of fallacies continue to flourish because of incorrect knowledge about pain in infants and children, despite these fallacies having been disproved by current research on pediatric pain (Box 44-11).

Fear of Addiction. A major concern that prevents health professionals from adequately using opioids* to relieve pain is an unwarranted fear of addiction. Studies on addiction rates in patients treated with opioids have found an incidence of less than 1% (McCaffery and Pasero, 1999). The American Society of Addiction Medicine (1997) has defined *physical dependence, tolerance,* and *addiction* as follows:

Physical dependence on an opioid is a physiologic state in which abrupt cessation of the opioid, or administration of an opioid antagonist, results in a withdrawal syndrome. Physical dependency on opioids is an expected occurrence in all individuals in the presence of continuous use of opioids for therapeutic or for nontherapeutic purposes. It does not, in and of itself, imply addiction.

Tolerance is a form of neuroadaptation to the effects of chronically administered opioids (or other medications) that is indicated by the need for increasing or more frequent doses of the medication to achieve the initial effects of the drug. Tolerance may occur both to the analgesic effects of opioids; and to some of the unwanted side effects, such as respiratory depression, sedation, or nausea. The occurrence of tolerance is variable in occurrence, but it does not, in and of itself, imply addiction.

Addiction in the context of pain treatment with opioids is characterized by a persistent pattern of dysfunctional opioid use that may involve any or all of the following:

- Adverse consequences associated with the use of opioids
- Loss of control over the use of opioids
- Preoccupation with obtaining opioids, despite the presence of adequate analgesia

Unfortunately, individuals who have severe, unrelieved pain may become intensely focused on finding relief for their pain. Sometimes behaviors such as "clock watching" make patients appear to others to be preoccupied with obtaining opioids; however, this preoccupation focuses on finding relief of pain, not on using opioids for reasons other than pain control. This

*The term *opioid* refers to natural or synthetic analgesics with morphinelike actions. It is preferred to the term *narcotic,* which in a legal context refers to any substance that causes psychologic dependence, such as cocaine, which is not an opioid. The word *narcotic* also engenders fears of addiction in older children and parents that are unwarranted when opioids are used for pain control.

Box 44-11

Fallacies and Facts about Children and Pain

Fallacy: Infants do not feel pain.

Fact: Infants demonstrate behavioral, especially facial, and physiologic, including hormonal, indicators of pain. Neonates have the neural mechanisms to transmit noxious stimuli by 20 weeks of gestation (Anand and Hickey, 1987; Marshall, 1989; Shapiro, 1989; Stevens, Johnston, and Horton, 1993).

Fallacy: Children tolerate pain better than adults.

Fact: Children's tolerance for pain actually *increases* with age (Haslam, 1969; Lander and Fowler-Kerry, 1991). Younger children tend to rate procedure-related pain higher than older children (Fradet et al, 1990; Humphrey et al, 1992; Wong and Baker, 1988).

Fallacy: Children cannot tell you where they hurt.

Fact: By 4 years of age, children can accurately point to the body area or mark the painful site on a drawing (Savedra et al, 1989, 1993; Van Cleve and Savedra, 1993); children as young as 3 years old can use pain scales, such as faces (Beyer, Denyes, and Villarruel, 1992; Wong and Baker, 1988).

Fallacy: Children always tell the truth about pain.

Fact: Children may not admit having pain to avoid an injection; because of constant pain, they may not realize how much they are hurting; children may believe that others know how they are feeling and not ask for analgesia (Favaloro and Touzel, 1990; Hester, 1989).

Fallacy: Children become accustomed to pain or painful procedures.

Fact: Children often demonstrate *increased* behavioral signs of discomfort with repeated painful procedures (Dolgin et al, 1989; Fitzgerald, Millard, and MacIntosh, 1988; Katz, Kellerman, and Siegel, 1980; Lander and Fowler-Kerry, 1991).

Fallacy: Behavioral manifestations reflect pain intensity.

Fact: Children's developmental level, coping abilities, and temperament, such as activity level and intensity of reaction to pain, influence pain behavior (Beyer, McGrath, and Berde, 1990; Wallace, 1989; Young and Fu, 1988). Children with more active, resisting behaviors may rate pain lower than children with passive, accepting behaviors (Broome et al, 1990).

Fallacy: Narcotics are more dangerous for children than they are for adults.

Fact: Narcotics (opioids) are no more dangerous for children than they are for adults. Addiction to opioids used to treat pain is extremely rare in children (Brozovic et al, 1986; Morrison, 1991; Rogers et al, 1988; Rogers, 1990). Reports of respiratory depression in children are also uncommon (Berde et al, 1991; Billmire, Neale, and Gregory 1985; Dilworth and MacKellar, 1987). By 3 to 6 months of age healthy infants can metabolize opioids similarly to other children (Hertzka et al, 1989; Koren et al, 1985).

phenomenon has been termed *pseudoaddiction* and must not be confused with real addiction.

Nurses must educate older children, parents, and health professionals about the extremely low risk of real addiction (less than 1%) from the use of opioids to treat pain. Infants, young children, and comatose or terminally ill children simply cannot become addicted because they are incapable of a consistent pattern of drug-seeking behaviors such as stealing, drug-dealing, prostitution, and use of family income to obtain opioids for nonanalgesic reasons.

Fear of Respiratory Depression. Although respiratory depression is the most serious side effect of opioids, it is a rare occurrence in children receiving appropriate doses (Graff, Kennedy, and Jaffe, 1996; Jacobson et al, 1997; Mayhew et al, 1995). Evidence suggests that in children older than 3 months, opioids cause no greater respiratory depression than in adults (Kart, Christrup, and Rasmussen, 1997). Respiratory depression is most likely to occur when the opioid is administered with other sedating drugs, such as hydroxyzine (Vistaril), promethazine (Phenergan), chlorpromazine (Thorazine), midazolam (Versed), or diazepam (Valium). Unlike many sedatives, opioids have the advantage of the antidote naloxone (Narcan), which rapidly reverses the respiratory depressant effect. Fortunately, the benzodiazepines, such as diazepam and midazolam, have the drug flumazenil (Romazicon) to treat respiratory depression.

In addition, as tolerance to the analgesic effect of opioids occurs, tolerance to the respiratory depressant effect also occurs. Pain acts as a natural antagonist to the respiratory depressant effect of opioids. With increased pain, a patient can receive increased doses of opioids without necessarily experiencing clinically significant respiratory depression. Respiratory depression is rare in children receiving long-term opioid therapy because tolerance to the respiratory depression develops (Collins, 1997).

Principles of Pain Assessment in Children. Because pain is both a sensory and an emotional experience, several assessment strategies should be used to gather information about pain. One approach to pain assessment in children is QUESTT:

Question the child.
Use a pain rating scale.
Evaluate behavioral and physiologic changes.
Secure parents' involvement.
Take the cause of pain into account.
Take action and evaluate results.

Question the Child. Children's verbal statements and descriptions of pain are the most important factors in assessing pain. However, young children may not know what the word "pain" means and may need help in describing it using familiar language. Therefore using a variety of words to describe pain, such as "owie," "boo-boo," "feel funny," or "hurt," is necessary. The nurse should also use appropriate foreign language words; for example, in Spanish, "pain" is "le le," "duele," "dolor," or "ai ai." Older children benefit from using simple words to describe pain. Asking children to locate the pain is also helpful, and play can provide other means for helping children to reveal discomfort (Fig. 44-7).

When asking children about pain, the nurse must remember that they may deny pain because they fear receiving an injectable analgesic or because they believe they deserve to suffer as punishment for some misdeed. They may also deny pain to a stranger but readily admit it to a parent. This behavior should not be interpreted as seeking attention from the parent, but as a valid indication of pain.

Use a Pain Rating Scale. Pain rating scales (tools) provide a quantitative self-reporting measure of pain. Although various pain scales exist (Table 44-2), not all of them are appropriate for young children. For the most valid and reliable pain intensity rating, a scale is selected that is suitable to the child's age, abilities, and preference. Scales using facial expressions are readily accepted by children and can be used by children as young as 3 years. Some evidence indicates that children may prefer a faces scale to other tools (Keck et al, 1996; West et al, 1994; Wong and Baker, 1988).

It is best to use the same scale with children to avoid confusing them with different instructions and to use the pain measurement scale for pain only. Multiple uses of the scale (e.g., as a general measure of the child's feelings) can cause the child to lose interest in the scale. Ideally, children should be taught to use the scale before pain is expected, such as preoperatively. Familiarizing children with the scale facilitates its use when children are actually in pain.

Evaluate Behavioral and Physiologic Changes. Behavioral changes are common indicators of pain and are especially valuable in assessing pain in nonverbal children. Children's behavioral responses to pain change with age and follow

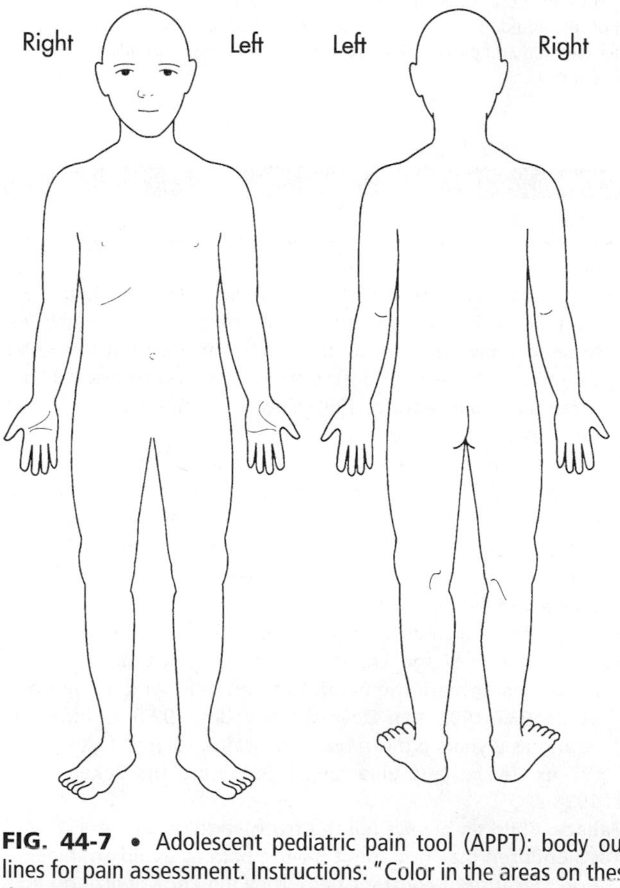

FIG. 44-7 • Adolescent pediatric pain tool (APPT): body outlines for pain assessment. Instructions: "Color in the areas on these drawings to show where you have pain. Make the marks as big or as small as the place where the pain is." (From Savedra MC et al, School of Nursing, University of California-San Francisco, San Francisco, CA. Copyright 1989, 1992.)

TABLE 44-2

Pain Rating Scales for Children

Pain Scale/Description	Instructions	Recommended Age/Comments
FACES PAIN RATING SCALE* (Wong and Baker, 1988, 2000): Consists of six cartoon faces ranging from smiling face for "no pain" to tearful face for "worst pain"	***Original instructions:*** Explain to child that each face is for a person who feels happy because there is no pain (hurt) or sad because there is some or a lot of pain. FACE 0 is very happy because there is no hurt. FACE 1 hurts just a little bit. FACE 2 hurts a little more. Face 3 hurts even more. FACE 4 hurts a whole lot, but FACE 5 hurts as much as you can imagine, although you don't have to be crying to feel this bad. Ask child to choose face that best describes own pain. Record the number under chosen face on pain assessment record. ***Brief word instructions:*** Point to each face using the words to describe the pain intensity. Ask child to choose face that best describes own pain and record the appropriate number.	For children as young as 3 years. Using original instructions without affect words, such as *happy* or *sad,* or brief words resulted in same pain rating, probably reflecting child's rating of pain intensity. For coding purposes, numbers 0, 2, 4, 6, 8, 10 can be substituted for 0-5 system to accommodate 0-10 system. The FACES provides three scales in one: facial expressions, numbers, and words. Use of brief word instructions is recommended.

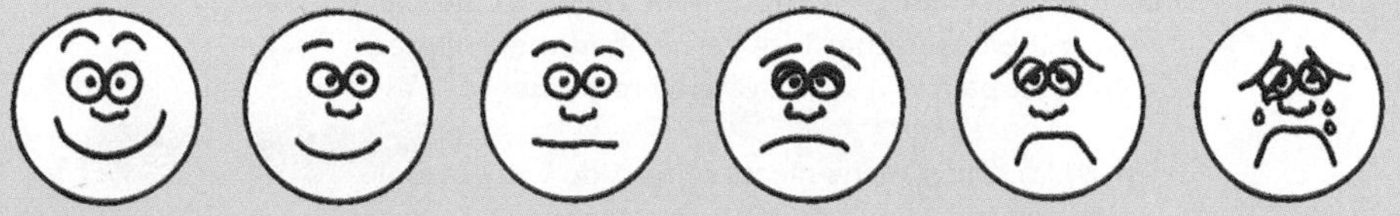

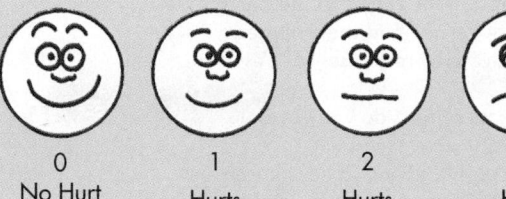

0	1	2	3	4	5
No Hurt	Hurts Little Bit	Hurts Little More	Hurts Even More	Hurts Whole Lot	Hurts Worst

Pain Scale/Description	Instructions	Recommended Age/Comments
OUCHER (Beyer, Denyes, and Villaruel, 1992; Beyer, 1999): Consists of six photographs of child's face representing "no hurt" to "biggest hurt you could ever have"; includes a vertical scale with numbers from 0-100; scales for African-American and Hispanic children have been developed (Villaruel and Denyes, 1991)	**NUMERIC SCALE** Point to each section of scale to explain variations in pain intensity: "0 means no hurt." "This means little hurts" (pointing to lower part of scale, 1-29). "This means middle hurts" (pointing to middle part of scale, 30-69). "This means big hurts" (pointing to upper part of scale, 70-99). "100 means the biggest hurt you could ever have." Score is actual number stated by child. **PHOTOGRAPHIC SCALE** Point to each photograph on Oucher and explain variations in pain intensity using following language: first picture from the bottom is "no hurt," second is "a little hurt," third is "a little more hurt," fourth is "even more hurt than that," fifth is "pretty much or a lot of hurt," and sixth is the "biggest hurt you could ever have." Score pictures from 0-5, with the bottom picture scored as 0. **GENERAL** Practice using Oucher by recalling and rating previous pain experiences (e.g., falling off a bike). Child points to number or photograph that describes pain intensity associated with experience. Obtain current pain score from child by asking, "How much hurt do you have right now?"	For children 3-13 years. Use numeric scale if child can count to 100 by ones and identify larger of any two numbers, or by tens. Determine whether child has cognitive ability to use photographic scale; child should be able to seriate six geometric shapes from largest to smallest. Determine which ethnic version of Oucher to use. Allow child to select a version of Oucher, or use version that most closely matches physical characteristics of child (Jordan-Marsh et al, 1994).

Wong-Baker FACES Pain Rating Scale Reference Manual* describing development and research of the scale is available from the Pain/Palliative Resource Center, City of Hope National Medical Center, 1500 East Duarte Rd., Duarte, CA 91010 (626) 359-8111, ext. 3829; fax (626) 301-894; e-mail: mayday_smtplink.coh.org; website: www.mosby.com/WOW/. A compilation of many pain scales, including the FACES, is available free from Purdue Frederick Company, 100 Connecticut Ave., Norwalk, CT 06850-3950; 1-800-733-1333 or (203) 853-0123, ext. 7378 or 7314; website: www.partnersagainstpain.com. The use of FACES with children is demonstrated in ***Whaley and Wong's Pediatric Nursing Video Series,* "Pain Assessment and Management," narrated by Donna Wong, PhD, RN. Available from Mosby, 11830 Westline Industrial Dr., St. Louis, MO 63146, 1-800-426-4545; fax 1-800-535-9935; website: www.mosby.com.

Continued

TABLE 44-2

Pain Rating Scales for Children—cont'd

Pain Scale/Description	Instructions	Recommended Age/Comments
POKER CHIP TOOL† Uses four red poker chips placed horizontally in front of child (Hester et al, 1998)	Say to child, "I want to talk with you about the hurt you may be having right now." Align the chips horizontally in front of child on bedside table, a clipboard, or other firm surface. Tell child, "These are pieces of hurt." Beginning at the chip nearest child's left side and ending at the one nearest child's right side, point to chips and say, "This [first chip] is a little bit of hurt, and this [fourth chip] is the most hurt you could ever have." For a young child or for any child who may not fully comprehend the instructions, clarify by saying, "That means this [one] is just a little hurt, this [two] is a little more hurt, this [three] is more yet, and this [four] is the most hurt you could ever have." Do not give children an option for zero hurt. Research with the Poker Chip Tool has verified that children without pain will so indicate by responses such as "I don't have any." Ask child, "How many pieces of hurt do you have right now?" After initial use of the Poker Chip Tool, some children internalize the concept "pieces of hurt." If a child gives a response such as "I have one right now," *before* you ask or before you lay out the poker chips, record the number of chips on the Pain Flow Sheet. Clarify child's answer by words such as "Oh, you have a little hurt? Tell me about the hurt."	For children as young as 4 years.
WORD-GRAPHIC RATING SCALE‡ (Tesler et al, 1991): Uses descriptive words (may vary in other scales) to denote varying intensities of pain	Explain to child. "This is a line with words to describe how much pain you may have. This side of the line means no pain, and over here the line means worst possible pain." (Point with your finger where "no pain" is, and run your finger along the line to "worst possible pain," as you say it.) "If you have no pain, you would mark like this." (Show example.) "If you have some pain, you would mark somewhere along the line, depending on how much pain you have." (Show example.) "The more pain you have, the closer to worst pain you would mark. The worst pain possible is marked like this." (Show example.) "Show me how much pain you have right now by marking with a straight, up-and-down line anywhere along the line to show how much pain you have right now." With a millimeter rule, measure from the "no pain" end to the mark and record this measurement as the pain score.	For children 4-17 years.

No pain	Little pain	Medium pain	Large pain	Worst possible pain

†Developed in 1975 by N.O. Hester, University of Colorado Health Sciences Center, School of Nursing, Denver, CO 80262. Also available in Spanish and French.

‡Instructions for Word-Graphic Rating Scale from Acute Pain Management Guideline Panel: *Acute pain management in infants, children, and adolescents; operative and medical procedures; quick reference guide for clinicians.* ACHPR Pub. No. 92-0020, Rockville, MD, 1992. Agency for Health Care Policy and Research, Public Health Service, US Department of Health and Human Services. Word-Graphic Rating Scale is part of the Adolescent Pediatric Pain Tool and is available from Pediatric Pain Study, University of California, School of Nursing, Department of Family Health Care Nursing, 2 Kirkham St., Box 0606, San Francisco, CA 94143-0606; (415) 476-4040; e-mail: savedra@Linex.com.

TABLE 44-2
Pain Rating Scales for Children—cont'd

Pain Scale/Description	Instructions	Recommended Age/Comments
NUMERIC SCALE Uses straight line with end points identified as "no pain" and "worst pain" and sometimes "medium pain" in the middle, divisions along line are marked in units from 0 to 5 or 10 (high number may vary)	Explain to child that at one end of the line is a 0, which means that a person feels no pain (hurt). At the other end is usually a 5 or a 10, which means the person feels the worst pain imaginable. The numbers 1 to 4 or 9 are for a very little pain to a whole lot of pain. Ask child to choose a number that best describes own pain. No pain Worst pain 0 1 2 3 4 5	For children as young as 5 years, as long as they can count and have some concept of numbers and their values in relation to other numbers. Scale may be used horizontally or vertically. Number coding should be same as other scales used in a facility.
VISUAL ANALOGUE SCALE Defined as a vertical or horizontal line that is drawn to a certain length, such as 10 cm, and anchored by items that represent the extremes of the subjective phenomenon, such as pain, that is measured (Cline et al, 1992)	Ask child to place a mark on line that best describes amount of own pain. With a centimeter ruler, measure from the "no pain" end to the mark and record this measurement as the pain score.	For children as young as 4½ years, preferably at least 7 years. Vertical or horizontal scale may be used.
COLOR TOOL Uses crayons or markers for child to construct own scale that is used with body outline (Eland and Banner, 1999)	Present eight crayons or markers to child in random order. Ask child to "pick a crayon with a color that reminds you of the most hurt (or pain) that you could possibly have"; once that crayon is selected, separate it from the others. Next, ask child to select a crayon with a color that "reminds you of pain that is a little less than the pain we just talked about"; once the second crayon is selected, separate it from the group and place it with the first crayon selected. Ask child to select a third crayon with a color "that reminds you of only a little pain"; separate this crayon and move it to the selected group. Finally, ask child to select a crayon with a color that "reminds you of no hurt (or pain)" and separate that fourth color. Show the four crayons selected to the child and arrange them in order of "worst hurt (or pain)" to "no hurt (or pain)" and ask child to show on the body outline "where the hurt is." If child offers any verbal comments, note them.	For children as young as 4 years, provided they know their colors, are not color blind, and are able to construct the scale if in pain.

a developmental trend (see Box 44-2). However, children's responses vary widely, and they may exhibit behaviors at one age that are more typically seen at a different age. Children with more positive moods may appear to be in less pain than they actually are. Children who use passive coping behaviors (offering no resistance, cooperating) may rate pain as more intense than children who use active coping behaviors (resisting, attacking) (Broome et al, 1990). Recent evidence, however, indicates that temperament does not seem to be a useful predictor of response to pain (Broome, Rehwaldt, and Fogg, 1998). Cultural background may also play a role in children's pain responses (Lipson, Dibble, and Minarik, 1996). In addition, cultural and linguistic differences may hinder assessment. Unfortunately, making judgments about pain based solely on behavior may lead to underestimation of severity and inadequate pain management (McCaffery and Pasero, 1999; Tesler, Holzemer, and Savedra, 1998) (Critical Thinking box).

NURSE ALERT • If children's behaviors appear to differ from their rating of pain, believe their pain rating.

Depending on the type and location of pain, children may display behaviors that indicate local body pain, such as pulling the ears for ear pain, rolling the head from side to side for head

Critical Thinking

PAIN ASSESSMENT

Stacy is 14 years old, and this is her second day following abdominal surgery. As you enter her room, she smiles at you and continues to talk and joke with her visitor. Stacy rates her pain as 4 on a scale of 0 to 5, no to worst pain, respectively. Her roommate, Jill, is 12 years old, and this is her third day following scoliosis surgery. She does not smile and is lying very still in bed. Jill rates her pain as 4 on the same scale. Based on your assessment, which of the following would you write in their charts (choose two items).

First, Think About It . . .

- **What information are you using?**
- **How are you interpreting that information?**

1. **Stacy: In no acute distress and appears comfortable, talking and joking with a visitor.**
2. **Jill: Rates her surgical pain as 4 on a 0-to-5 scale and is unable to move because of pain; she appears depressed.**
3. **Stacy: Rates her surgical pain as 4 on a 0-to-5 scale.**
4. **Jill: Rates her surgical pain as 4 on a 0-to-5 scale.**

The best responses are 3 and 4. The best estimate of pain is the person's self-report. Responses 1 and 2 are based on subjective impressions. In response 1 the adolescent's report of pain is totally disregarded. In response 2 there are no assessment data to support that Jill's behavior indicates inability to move or depression.

and ear pain, lying on the side with legs flexed for abdominal pain, limping for leg or foot pain, and refusing to move a body part. Children who experience chronic or repeated pain often develop effective behavioral coping strategies, such as squeezing a hand, talking, counting, relaxing, or thinking about pleasant events. Once these coping skills are identified, the child is encouraged to use them in future experiences with pain.

Physiologic responses indicating pain include flushing of the skin; increases in sweating, blood pressure, pulse, and respiration; restlessness; and dilation of the pupils. However, these signs vary considerably—for example, heart rate may actually decrease—and they may be produced by emotions such as fear, anger, or anxiety. They occur primarily in acute pain from stimulation of the sympathetic nervous system. If pain persists, the body begins to adapt and these responses decrease or stabilize. Consequently, if nurses rely primarily on observing these physiologic indications or expecting "pain" behaviors before believing that pain exists, many instances of pain will go unrecognized (Van Cleve, Johnson, and Pothier, 1996).

One of the most valuable clues to pain is a change in behavior and vital signs after administration of an analgesic. Behaviors such as showing less irritability or ceasing to cry, as well as decreased pulse, respirations, and blood pressure, provide important evidence for pain existing before treatment. Often the change in vital signs is attributed to the depressant effect of opioids, when in reality the return to more normal physiologic functioning is due to pain relief.

Secure Parents' Involvement. Parents should play a key role in the assessment of their child's pain. They know their child, are sensitive to changes in their child's behavior, and typically want to be involved in their child's pain relief. Parents' ability to recognize pain in their children varies. Some parents may never have seen their child in severe pain and may not equate certain responses, such as irritability or withdrawal, with discomfort. Others are aware that certain behaviors signal pain because the child has acted similarly during previous painful events. Parents usually know what comforts their child, such as rocking, stroking, or talking. They are the persons most consistently caring for the child. Encouraging their participation gives them control and a sense of helping.

To better assess the child's pain, the nurse can interview the parents about their child's previous pain experiences. Ideally, this questioning should occur before the child is in pain, such as on admission to the hospital. Parents need to realize that their knowledge of their child is important in providing care. Parents sometimes leave the assessment of pain up to the nurse because "nurses are more experienced," and they expect the nurse to know when their child is in pain (Woodgate and Krisjanson, 1996). Consequently, parents do not report pain. Parents need to be taught nonverbal pain behaviors in children and encouraged to inform the staff when they think their child is in pain.

Take the Cause of Pain into Account. When children exhibit behaviors or other clues that suggest pain, reasons for discomfort should be investigated. The pathologic condition may give clues to the expected intensity and type of pain. For example, pain associated with vaso-occlusive crises in sickle cell disease is severe. Pain caused by bone marrow puncture is typically greater than the discomfort associated with a venipuncture. However, it is a mistake to believe that certain conditions or procedures always produce a standard amount of pain. For example, sore throat pain may be mild or severe—only the child knows the intensity.

NURSE ALERT • A golden rule to follow in pain assessment is this: Whatever is painful to an adult is painful to an infant or child unless proved otherwise.

Take Action and Evaluate Results. The reason for assessing pain is to relieve it (p. 1085). Total pain relief, with the combined use of pharmacologic and nonpharmacologic interventions, should be the goal. However, complete relief may not be possible. When children are able, they can tell the nurse what level of pain is acceptable to them and if that amount of pain allows them to function in terms of sleeping, eating, moving, and resting.

Regardless of the type of pain intervention, *evaluation of the results is essential.* No one pain reduction technique is effective for all children. Therefore a pain assessment record is used to monitor the effectiveness of the interventions (Fig. 44-8). With nonverbal children, behavioral and physiologic signs are evaluated for evidence of pain relief. With verbal children, their statements about pain relief and pain ratings are also recorded. Changes in the medication regimen are made as needed to provide the maximum pain relief with the minimum side effects. Family members are often excellent partners for keeping a pain assessment record for the nurse.

NURSE ALERT • Presenting practitioners with objective documentation of pain, rather than opinion, is more likely to lead to a favorable change in analgesic orders (Walker and Wong, 1991).

Pain Management. Relief of pain is a basic need and right of all children. Effective pain management requires that

Pain Assessment Record

Directions for each column:
1. Record date and time of assessment and analgesic administration; assess analgesic effect ________ minutes later and then ________
2. Use a pain rating scale if child understands its use.
   Name of scale: ________
   Ratings: No pain = _____ Worst pain = _____ Comfort/function goals* _____
3. Record analgesic, dose, and route
4. Record possible indications or effects of pain, such as shallow breathing due to incisional pain, parental request for pain relief; record indications or effects of pain relief, such as "moves easily, playing"
5. Record any other side effects (e.g., nausea, itching)
6. Record LOS (see inset) R (respiratory function); record breaths per minute and/or other observations of respiratory status (e.g., depth of respiration, change in color of skin)
7. Signature or initials of person recording information

Level of Sedation (LOS) Scale†

S = Sleeping, easily aroused
Requires no action
1 = Awake and alert
Requires no action
2 = Occasionally drowsy, easy to arouse
Requires no action
3 = Frequently drowsy, arousable, drifts off to sleep during conversation
Notify practitioner and decrease dose
4 = Somnolent, minimal or no response to stimuli
Notify practitioner and stop opioid

1 Date/time	2 Pain rating	3 Analgesic	4 Possible effects/indications of pain or relief of pain	5 Side effects	6 LOS/R	7 Signature

*Ask the child what pain rating would be acceptable in terms of usual function (e.g., activities of daily living, playing, and attending school). From McCaffery M, Pasero C, editors: *Pain: a clinical manual,* ed 2, St Louis, 1999, Mosby.

†From Pasero C, McCaffery M: Providing epidural analgesia: how to maintain a delicate balance, *Nurs99* 29(8):34-39, 1999.

FIG. 44-8 • Pain assessment record.

health professionals be willing to try a number of interventions to achieve optimum results. Basically, pain-reducing methods can be grouped into two categories: nonpharmacologic and pharmacologic. Whenever possible, both should be used; however, nonpharmacologic measures are not substitutes for analgesics.

Nonpharmacologic Management. Pain is often associated with fears, anxiety, and stress. A number of nonpharmacologic techniques, such as distraction, relaxation, guided imagery, and cutaneous stimulation (Guidelines box), provide coping strategies that may help reduce pain perception, make pain more tolerable, decrease anxiety, and enhance the effectiveness of analgesics (Vessey and Carlson, 1996). Although there is inconclusive research on the effectiveness of many of these interventions, the strategies are safe, noninvasive, and inexpensive, and most are independent nursing functions. Experimentation with several strategies that are appropriate for the child's age, pain intensity, interest, and abilities is often necessary to determine the most effective approach.

NURSE ALERT • Most specific nonpharmacologic strategies require children's understanding and cooperation. Therefore try to match the strategy with the pain severity. Children in severe pain may not be able to expend the effort necessary to learn the technique, and those with very mild symptoms may not be motivated to learn. Therefore these strategies may be most useful with midrange pain.

In the selection of a nonpharmacologic intervention, it is best to use a technique familiar to the child or to describe several strategies and let the child select the most appealing one. Parents should be involved in the selection process; they may be familiar with the child's usual coping skills and can help identify potentially successful strategies. Involving parents also encourages their participation in learning the skill with the child and acting as coach. If the parent cannot assist the child, other appropriate persons may include a grandparent, older sibling, nurse, or child-life specialist.

Guidelines

NONPHARMACOLOGIC STRATEGIES FOR PAIN MANAGEMENT

General Strategies

Use nonpharmacologic interventions to supplement, not replace, pharmacologic interventions and use for mild pain and pain that is reasonably well controlled with analgesics.

Form a trusting relationship with child and family.

- Express concern regarding their reports of pain and intervene appropriately.
- Take an active role in seeking effective pain management strategies.

Use general guidelines to prepare child for procedure (see Chapter 45).

Prepare child before potentially painful procedures but avoid "planting" the idea of pain. For example, instead of saying, "This is going to (or may) hurt," say, "Sometimes this feels like pushing, sticking, or pinching, and sometimes it doesn't bother people. Tell me what it feels like to you."

Use "nonpain" descriptors when possible (e.g., "It feels like heat" rather than "It's a burning pain"). This allows for variation in sensory perception, avoids suggesting pain, and gives child control in describing reactions.

Avoid evaluative statements or descriptions (e.g., "This is a terrible procedure" or "It really will hurt a lot").

Stay with child during a painful procedure.

- Allow parents to stay with child if child and parent desire; encourage parent to talk softly to child and to remain near child's head.
- Involve parents in learning specific nonpharmacologic strategies and in assisting child with their use.

Educate child about the pain, especially when explanation may lessen anxiety (e.g., that pain may occur after surgery and does not indicate something is wrong); reassure that child is not responsible for the pain.

For long-term pain control, give child a doll, which represents "the patient," and allow child to do everything to the doll that is done to the child; pain control can be emphasized through the doll by stating, "Dolly feels better after the medicine." Teach procedures to child and family for later use.

Specific Strategies

Distraction

Involve parent and child in identifying strong distractors.

Involve child in play; use radio, tape recorder, CD player, or computer game; have child sing or use rhythmic breathing.

Have child take a deep breath and blow it out until told to stop (French, Painter, and Coury, 1994).

Have child blow bubbles to "blow the hurt away."

Have child concentrate on yelling or saying "ouch" by focusing on "yelling as loud or soft as you feel it hurt; that way I know what's happening."

Have child look through kaleidoscope (type with glitter suspended in fluid-filled tube) and encourage to concentrate by asking, "Do you see the different designs?" (Vessey, Carlson, and McGill, 1994).

Use humor, such as watching cartoons, telling jokes or funny stories, or acting silly with child.

Have child read, play games, or visit with friends.

Relaxation

With an infant or young child:

- Hold in a comfortable, well-supported position, such as vertically against the chest and shoulder.
- Rock in a wide, rhythmic arc in a rocking chair or sway back and forth, rather than bouncing child.
- Repeat one or two words softly, such as "Mommy's here."

With a slightly older child:

- Ask child to take a deep breath and "go limp as a rag doll" while exhaling slowly; then as child to yawn (demonstrate if needed).
- Help child assume a comfortable position (e.g., pillow under neck and knees).

Begin progressive relaxation: starting with the toes, systematically instruct child to let each body part "go limp" or "feel heavy"; if child has difficulty with relaxing, instruct child to tense or tighten each body part and then relax it.

Allow child to keep eyes open, since children may respond better if eyes are open rather than closed during relaxation.

Guided Imagery

Have child identify some highly pleasurable real or imaginary experience.

Have child describe details of the event, including as many senses as possible (e.g., "feel the cool breezes," "see the beautiful colors," "hear the pleasant music").

Have child write down or tape record script.

Encourage child to concentrate only on the pleasurable event during the painful time; enhance the image by recalling specific details through reading the script or playing the tape.

Combine with relaxation and rhythmic breathing.

Positive Self-Talk

Teach child positive statements to say when in pain (e.g., "I will be feeling better soon," "When I go home, I will feel better, and we will eat ice cream").

Thought Stopping

Identify positive facts about the painful event (e.g., "It does not last long").

Identify reassuring information (e.g., "If I think about something else, it does not hurt as much").

Condense positive and reassuring facts into a set of brief statements and have child memorize them (e.g., "Short procedure, good veins, little hurt, nice nurse, go home").

Have child repeat the memorized statements whenever thinking about or experiencing the painful event.

Cutaneous Stimulation

Includes simple rhythmic rubbing; use of pressure or electric vibrator; massage with hand lotion, powder, or menthol cream; application of heat or cold, such as vapocoolant spray on the site before giving injection or application of ice to the site opposite the painful area (e.g., if right knee hurts, place ice on left knee).

A more sophisticated method is ***transcutaneous electrical nerve stimulation (TENS)*** (use of controlled low-voltage electricity to the body via electrodes placed on the skin).

Another method is the use of ***Pain Relief Therapeutic Electro-Membrane (P.R.E.M.),*** a high-technology membrane electron reservoir fabricated from a nonwoven, nonallergenic dressing that when placed in contact with the skin, releases the stored electrons in the form of microcurrent impulses.*

Behavioral Contracting

Informal—May be used with children as young as 4 or 5 years of age:

- Use stars or tokens as rewards.
- Give uncooperative or procrastinating children (during a procedure) a limited time (measured by a visible timer) to complete the procedure.
- Proceed as needed if child is unable to comply.
- Reinforce cooperation with a reward if the procedure is accomplished within specified time.

Formal—Use written contract, which includes:

- Realistic (seems possible) goal or desired behavior
- Measurable behavior (e.g., agrees not to hit anyone during procedures)
- Contract written, dated, and signed by all persons involved in any of the agreements
- Identified rewards or consequences that are reinforcing
- Goals that can be evaluated
- Commitment and compromise requirements for both parties (e.g., while timer is used, nurse will not nag or prod child to complete procedure)

*For more information contact Helio Medical Supplies, Inc., 606 Charcot Ave., San Jose, CA 95131; (888)-PAINTEM (724 6836); e-mail: eileen @heliomed.com.

Children should learn a specific strategy *before* pain occurs or before it becomes severe. To reduce the child's effort, instructions for a strategy, such as distraction or relaxation, can be audiotaped and played during a period of discomfort.

Pharmacologic Management. Using pharmacologic methods to control pain requires attention to four "rights": right drug, right dose, right route, and right time. In addition, observing for side effects is an essential nursing intervention. Although nurses may not prescribe the medication, knowledge of these essential principles assists in optimally implementing analgesic orders and discussing with other practitioners possible strategies to improve pain control.

Right Drug. Nonopioids, including acetaminophen (Tylenol, paracelamol) and nonsteroidal antiinflammatory drugs (NSAIDs), are suitable for mild to moderate pain; opioids are needed for moderate to severe pain. A combination of the two analgesics attacks pain on two levels: nonopioids primarily at the peripheral nervous system (PNS) and opioids primarily at the central nervous system (CNS). This approach provides increased analgesia without increased side effects. Several commercially available combinations, such as Tylenol with Codeine, may have increasing doses of the opioid but a constant dose of the nonopioid (Box 44-12). Therefore, before the opioid is increased, it may be preferable to increase the nonopioid component (e.g., adding 300 mg of plain Tylenol to Tylenol with Codeine No. 3 before advancing to Tylenol with Codeine No. 4). However, if this approach is not successful, the pain most likely requires a stronger opioid.

Actions of various opioids differ. Morphine is considered the gold standard for the management of severe pain. When morphine is not a suitable opioid, drugs such as oxycodone, hydromorphone (Dilaudid), and fentanyl (Sublimaze) are effective substitutes. Although fentanyl is used as an anesthetic in the operating room, it is classified as an analgesic. It can be safely administered by nurses as a continuous infusion (Algren and Algren, 1998).

Meperidine (Demerol, pethidine) is not recommended as a first-line opioid analgesic for the management of any kind of pain (American Pain Society, 1999; McCaffery and Pasero, 1999). A major drawback in the use of meperidine is its metabolite, normeperidine. Normeperidine is a CNS stimulant that can produce restlessness, irritability, twitching, jerking, agitation, tremors, and seizures (American Pain Society, 1999). The CNS side effects caused by normeperidine are not reversed with naloxone (Reisine and Pasternak, 1996). Research shows that meperidine is more likely than other opioids to cause delirium in postoperative patients (Marcantonio et al, 1994). These symptoms occur in children as well as adults (Kussman and

Box 44-12

Selected Combination Opioid and Nonopioid Oral Analgesics—Nonaspirin Products*

Fioricet with Codeine	30 mg codeine 325 mg acetaminophen 50 mg butalbital 40 mg caffeine
Hydrocet	5 mg hydrocodone 500 mg acetaminophen
Lorcet-HD	5 mg hydrocodone 500 mg acetaminophen
Lorcet Plus	7.5 mg hydrocodone 650 mg acetaminophen
Lorcet 10/650	10 mg hydrocodone 650 mg acetaminophen
Lortab 2.5/500	2.5 mg hydrocodone 500 mg acetaminophen
Lortab 5/500	5 mg hydrocodone 500 mg acetaminophen
Lortab 10/500	10 mg hydrocodone 500 mg acetaminophen
Lortab Elixir (each 15 ml)	7.5 mg hydrocodone 500 mg acetaminophen
Percocet 2.5/325†	2.5 mg oxycodone 325 mg acetaminophen
Percocet-5/325	5 mg oxycodone HCl 325 mg acetaminophen
Percocet 7.5/500	7.5 mg oxycodone 500 mg acetaminophen
Percocet 10/650	10 mg oxycodone 650 mg acetaminophen
Tylenol with Codeine No. 1	7.5 mg codeine 300 mg acetaminophen
Tylenol with Codeine No. 2	15 mg codeine 300 mg acetaminophen
Tylenol with Codeine No. 3	30 mg codeine 300 mg acetaminophen
Tylenol with Codeine No. 4	60 mg codeine 300 mg acetaminophen
Tylenol and Codeine Elixir (each 5 ml)	12 mg codeine 120 mg acetaminophen 7% alcohol
Tylox†	5 mg oxycodone HCl 500 mg acetaminophen
Vicodin	5 mg hydrocodone 500 mg acetaminophen
Vicodin ES	7.5 mg hydrocodone 750 mg acetaminophen
Vicodin HP	10 mg hydrocodone 650 mg acetaminophen
Vicoprofen	7.5 mg hydrocodone 200 mg ibuprofen

*Aspirin is not recommended for children, because of its possible association with Reye syndrome. Analgesic compounds with aspirin include Darvon Compound, Darvon with A.S.A., Percodan, and Percodan-Demi, Darvon or Darvocet (propoxyphene) is not recommended; its analgesic effect is no greater than that from aspirin, acetaminophen, or other NSAIDs. Propoxyphene, an opioid, can depress respirations, and its major metabolite is cardiotoxic and is a central nervous system (CNS) stimulant that can produce seizures (Dahl JL, 1998; Yaster et al, 1997).

†All medications require a prescription, but these are classified as schedule II drugs (like morphine), and each filling requires a written prescription that includes the patient's name and address, the practitioner's DEA (Drug Enforcement Agency) number, and the date. In case of emergency, verbal prescriptions for schedule II substances may be filled; however, the practitioner must provide a signed prescription within 72 hours. Schedule II prescriptions cannot be refilled but require a new prescription.

Sethna, 1998). Another disadvantage of meperidine is the long half-life of its metabolite. Normeperidine has a half-life of 15 to 20 hours, compared with meperidine's half-life of 3 hours.

NURSE ALERT • By any route of administration, the use of meperidine for any type of pain management in children should be questioned because other less toxic, more effective opioid drugs are available. Meperidine should be used only for short-term (48 hours) pain management in healthy patients who have demonstrated an unusual reaction or allergic response during treatment with other opioids. When meperidine is administered, assess the child often for signs of toxicity such as tremors of the outstretched hands, twitching or jerking, or increased agitation. If toxicity is suspected, discontinue the meperidine, maintain the IV infusion, and notify the practitioner immediately. An adverse drug reaction should also be reported.*

Opioids are often combined with other drugs that are considered "potentiators." However, little evidence indicates that any drug potentiates the analgesic effect of opioids; rather, drugs that produce sedation are erroneously equated with producing analgesia. One common drug combination—*meperidine (Demerol [pethidine]), promethazine (Phenergan),* and *chlorpromazine (Thorazine),* known as *DPT* or *lytic cocktail*—has commonly been used to sedate children for procedures (see Preoperative Care, Chapter 45). Meperidine, a short-acting analgesic, provides pain relief for 2 to 3 hours but is irritating to the tissues when given intramuscularly. Promethazine has antianalgesic properties, produces excessive sedation, and can cause extrapyramidal reactions (spasms of neck, face, tongue, and back; fixed eyeballs). Besides producing prolonged deep sedation, all of these drugs can cause respiratory depression and lower the seizure threshold, a particular risk to those with a seizure disorder. In addition, the "cocktail" is usually administered intramuscularly, causing additional pain. *For these reasons, DPT is not recommended for general use* (Acute Pain Management, 1992). Appropriate drugs for sedation are listed in Box 44-13).

Several drugs, known as *adjuvant analgesics* or *coanalgesics,* may be used alone or with opioids to control pain symptoms. Commonly used drugs to relieve anxiety, cause sedation, and provide amnesia are diazepam (Valium) and midazolam (Versed); however, they are not analgesics. Other adjuvants include tricyclic antidepressants (i.e., amitriptyline, imipramine) and epileptics for neuropathic pain (brief, lancinating pain); steroids for inflammation and bone pain; and dextroamphetamine and caffeine for increased analgesia and decreased sedation (McCaffery and Pasero, 1999).

At times, health professionals question whether pain really exists and administer *placebos* to "see if the pain is real." This practice is unjustified and unethical; a positive response to a placebo, such as a saline injection, is common in patients who have a documented, organic basis for pain. Therefore the deceptive use of placebos does not provide useful information about the presence or severity of pain. In addition, the use of placebos can cause side effects similar to those of opioids, can destroy the patient's trust in the health care staff, and raises serious ethical and legal questions (Pasero, 1995). The position of the American Society of Pain Management Nurses (ASPMN, 1998) is that placebos should not be used by any route in the assessment or management of pain in any patient regardless of age or diagnosis.

*The FDA Medical Products Reporting Program, Food and Drug Administration, 5600 Fishers Lane, Rockville, MD 20852-9787; 1-800-FDA-1088; fax 1-800-FDA-0178; website: www.fda.gov/medwatch.

Box 44-13

Suggested Medications for Sedation

OPIOIDS*

Morphine sulfate, 0.05 to 0.1 mg/kg IV over 1 to 2 minutes given 5 minutes before procedure

Fentanyl, 1 to 2 μg/kg (0.001 to 0.002 mg/kg) IV 3 minutes before procedure

Fentanyl Oralet, 5 to 15 μg/kg, maximum to 400 μg, orally 20 to 40 minutes before procedure†

Hydromorphone (Dilaudid), 0.015 to 0.02 mg/kg IV over 1 to 2 minutes given 5 minutes before procedure

Meperidine (if morphine sulfate or fentanyl is not available), 0.5 to 1 mg/kg IV over 1 to 2 minutes given 2 to 5 minutes before procedure or 1.5 mg/kg orally 45 to 60 minutes before procedure

SEDATIVES‡

Midazolam (Versed), 0.25 to 0.5 mg/kg (children 6 months to younger than 6 years old and less cooperative children may require a higher dose of up to 1 mg/kg), maximum to 20 mg, using oral preparation, 10 to 20 minutes, or 0.05 mg/kg IV 3 minutes before procedure

Diazepam (Valium), 0.2 to 0.3 mg/kg, maximum to 10 mg, orally 45 to 60 minutes before procedure

Pentobarbital (Nembutal), 1 to 3 mg/kg IV boluses to maximum of 100 mg until asleep

Chloral hydrate, 50 to 75 mg/kg, to maximum of 100 mg/kg or 2.5 g, orally or rectally 60 minutes before procedure

Modified from Zeltzer LK et al: Report of the subcommittee on the management of pain associated with procedures in children with cancer, *Pediatrics* 86(suppl):826-831, 1990; Coté CJ: Sedation for the pediatric patient, *Pediatr Clin North Am* 41(1):31-58, 1994; and Yaster M et al: *Pediatric pain management and sedation handbook,* St Louis, 1997, Mosby.

*Provide analgesia and sedation.

†Not recommended for children less than 15 kg. Lozenge should be sucked, not chewed and swallowed. If chewed, drug is less effective because part of it is metabolized by liver before entering bloodstream. Swallowing drug rapidly does not increase risk of respiratory depression during first 15 to 30 minutes, period of greatest risk for decreased respiration.

‡Provide sedation but no analgesia.

Right Dosage. The optimum dosage is one that controls pain without causing severe side effects. This usually requires *titration,* the gradual adjustment of drug dosage (usually by increasing or decreasing the dose) until optimum pain relief without excessive sedation is achieved. Dosage recommendations, such as those in Tables 44-3 and 44-4, are only safe initial dosages, not optimum dosages. Children (except infants younger than about 3 to 6 months of age) metabolize drugs more rapidly than adults; younger children may require higher doses of opioids to achieve the same analgesic effect. Therefore the therapeutic effect and duration of analgesia vary. Children's dosages are usually calcu-

TABLE 44-3

Nonsteroidal Antiinflammatory Drugs (NSAIDs) Approved for Children*

Drug (Trade Name)	Dose	Comments
Acetaminophen (Tylenol and other brands)†	10-15 mg/kg/dose every 4-6 hours not to exceed 5 doses in 24 hours or 75 mg/kg/day, orally	Available in numerous preparations Nonprescription Higher dosage range may provide increased analgesia
Choline magnesium trisalicylate (Trilisate)	Children 37 kg or less: 50 mg/kg/day divided into 2 doses Children over 37 kg: 500 mg-1.5 g 2-3 times/day	Available in suspension 500 mg/5 ml Prescription
Ibuprofen† Children's Motrin Children's Advil	Children 6 months and older: 5-10 mg/kg/dose every 6-8 hours not to exceed 40 mg/kg/day	Available in numerous preparations Available in suspension 100 mg/5 ml and drops 100 mg/2.5 ml Nonprescription
Naproxen (Naprosyn)	Children older than 2 years: 10 mg/kg/day divided into 2 doses	Available in suspension 125 mg/5 ml and several different dosages for tablets Prescription
Tolmetin (Tolectin)	Children older than 2 years: 20 mg/kg/day divided into 3 or 4 doses	Available in 200 mg, 400 mg, and 600 mg tablets Prescription

Data from Olin BR et al: *Drug facts and comparisons,* St Louis, 2000, Facts and Comparisons.

NOTE: Newer formulations of NSAIDs, such as celecoxib (Celebrex) or rofecoxib (Vioxx), selectively inhibit one of the enzymes of cyclo-oxygenase (COX-2, which is responsible for pain transmission), but do not inhibit the other (COX-1). Inhibition of COX-1 decreases prostaglandin production, which is necessary for normal organ function. For example, prostaglandins help maintain gastric mucosal blood flow and barrier protection, regulate blood flow to the liver and kidneys, and facilitate platelet aggregation and clot formation. Theoretically, the COX-2 NSAIDs provide similar analgesic and antiinflammatory benefits with fewer side effects than the nonselective agents. Celebrex and Vioxx are approved for use in patients older than 18 years.

*All NSAIDs in the table (except acetaminophen) have significant antiinflammatory, antipyretic, and analgesic actions. Acetaminophen has a weak antiinflammatory action, and its classification as an NSAID is controversial. Patients respond differently to various NSAIDs; therefore, changing from one drug to another may be necessary for maximum benefit.

Acetylsalicylic acid (aspirin) is also an NSAID but is not recommended for children because of its possible association with Reye syndrome. The NSAIDs in the table have no known association with Reye syndrome. However, caution should be exercised in prescribing any salicylate-containing drug (e.g., Trilisate) for children with known or suspected viral infection.

Side effects of ibuprofen, naproxen, and tolmetin include nausea, vomiting, diarrhea, constipation, gastric ulceration, bleeding, nephritis, and fluid retention. Acetaminophen and choline magnesium trisalicylate are well tolerated in the gastrointestinal tract and do not interfere with platelet function. NSAIDs (except acetaminophen) should not be given to patients with allergic reactions to salicylates. All the NSAIDs should be used cautiously in patients with renal impairment.

†For dosage recommendations for specific formulations of acetaminophen and ibuprofen, see Table 45-1.

lated according to body weight, except in children who weigh 50 kg (110 pounds) or more, when the weight formula may exceed the average adult dose. In this case the adult dose is used.

A reasonable starting dose of opioid for infants younger than 6 months who are not mechanically ventilated is one fourth to one third of the recommended starting dose for older children. The infant is monitored very closely for signs of pain relief and respiratory depression. The dose is titrated to effect. Because tolerance can develop rapidly, very large opioid doses may be needed for continued severe pain (American Pain Society, 1999).

If pain relief is inadequate, the initial dosage is increased (usually by 25% to 50% and sometimes more to provide greater analgesic effectiveness). Decreasing the interval between doses may also provide more continuous pain relief. A major difference between opioids and nonopioids is that nonopioids have a *ceiling effect,* which means that doses higher than recommended will not produce greater pain relief. Opioids do not have a ceiling effect other than that imposed by side effects; therefore larger dosages can be given safely for increasing severity of pain (see Critical Thinking box, p. 1102).

NURSE ALERT • A common error in attempts to improve pain control is to change to another analgesic. If an opioid such as morphine, hydromorphone, or fentanyl, is used, rarely is the problem one of drug choice. Rather, the problem is usually one of inadequate dosage. If changing to another analgesic is warranted because of adverse side effects, the new drug should be slightly less potent than or equally potent to the original analgesic.

Parenteral and oral dosages of opioids are not the same. Because of the *first-pass effect,* an oral opioid is rapidly absorbed from the gastrointestinal tract and enters the portal circulation, where it is partially metabolized before reaching the central circulation. Therefore oral dosages must be larger to compensate for the partial loss of analgesic potency to achieve *equianalgesia* (equianalgesic effect). Conversion factors for selected opioids, when a change is made from intramuscular (IM) or IV to oral, are listed in Tables 44-5 and 44-6. Immediate conversion from IM or IV to the suggested equianalgesic oral dose may result in a substantial error in the individual child. For example, the dose

TABLE 44-4
Dosage of Selected Opioids for Children

Drug	Approximate Equianalgesic Oral Dose	Approximate Equianalgesic Parenteral Dose	Recommended Starting Dose (Children Less than 50 kg Body Weight)[a]	
			Oral	Parenteral[b]
Morphine[c]	30 mg every 3-4 hours (around-the-clock dosing)	10 mg every 3-4 hours	0.2-0.4 mg/kg every 3-4 hours 0.3-0.6 mg/kg time released every 12 hours	0.1-0.2 mg/kg IM every 3-4 hours 0.02-0.1 mg/kg IV bolus every 2 hours 0.015 mg/kg every 8 minutes PCA 0.01-0.02 mg/kg/hr IV infusion (neonates) 0.01-0.06 mg/kg/hr IV infusion (child)
Fentanyl (Sublimaze) (oral mucosal form—Fentanyl Oralet)[d]	Not available	0.1 mg IV	5-15 μg/kg; maximum dose 400 μg	0.5-1.5 μg/kg IV bolus every ½ hour 1-2 μg/hr IV infusion
Codeine[e]	200 mg every 3-4 hours	130 mg every 3-4 hours	0.5-1 mg/kg every 3-4 hours	Not recommended
Hydromorphone (Dilaudid)	7.5 mg every 3-4 hours	1.5 mg every 3-4 hours	0.06 mg/kg every 3-4 hours	0.015 mg/kg IV bolus every 2 hours
Hydrocodone (in Lorcet, Lortab, Vicodin, others)	30 mg every 3-4 hours	Not available	0.2 mg/kg every 3-4 hours[g]	Not available
Levorphanol (Levo-Dromoran)	4 mg every 6-8 hours	2 mg every 6-8 hours	0.04 mg/kg every 6-8 hours	0.02 mg/kg every 6-8 hours
Meperidine (Demerol)[f]	300 mg every 2-3 hours	100 mg every 3 hours	Not recommended	0.75 mg/kg every 2-3 hours
Methadone (Dolophine, others)	20 mg every 6-8 hours	10 mg every 6-8 hours	0.2 mg/kg every 6-8 hours	0.1 mg/kg every 6-8 hours
Oxycodone (Roxicodone, Oxycontin; also in Percocet, Percodan, Tylox, others)	20-30 mg every 3-4 hours	Not available	0.2 mg/kg every 3-4 hours[g]	Not available

Data from Acute Pain Management Guideline Panel: *Acute pain management; operative or medical procedures and trauma; clinical practice guideline,* AHCPR Pub. No. 92-0032, Rockville, MD, 1992, Agency for Health Care Policy and Research, Public Health Service, US Department of Health and Human Services; World Health Organization: *Cancer pain relief and palliative care in children,* Geneva, Switzerland, 1998, The Organization; and Yaster et al: *Pediatric pain management and sedation handbook,* St Louis, 1997, Mosby.
IV, Intravenous; *IM,* intramuscular; *PCA,* patient-controlled analgesia.
NOTE: Published tables vary in the suggested doses that are equianalgesic to morphine. Clinical response is the criterion that must be applied for each patient; titration to clinical response is necessary. Because there is not complete cross-tolerance among these drugs, it is usually necessary to use a lower than equianalgesic dose when changing drugs and to retitrate to response. CAUTION: Recommended doses do not apply to patients with renal or hepatic insufficiency or other conditions affecting drug metabolism and kinetics.
[a]CAUTION: Doses listed for patients with body weight less than 50 kg should not be used as initial starting doses in infants younger than 6 months of age. For nonventilated infants younger than 6 months of age, the initial opioid dose should be about one fourth to one third of the dose recommended for older infants and children. For children with body weight greater than 50 kg, the usual adult dose should be used.
[b]IM injections should not be used.
[c]For morphine, hydromorphone, and oxymorphone, rectal administration is an alternate route for patients unable to take oral medications, but equianalgesic doses may differ from oral and parenteral doses because of pharmacokinetic differences.
[d]Fentanyl Oralet is indicated for use in a hospital setting only (1) as an anesthetic premedication in the operating room setting or (2) to induce conscious sedation before a diagnostic or therapeutic procedure in other monitored anesthesia care settings in hospital; is contraindicated in children who weigh less than 15 kg (33 pounds).
[e]CAUTION: Codeine doses greater than 65 mg often are not appropriate because of diminishing incremental analgesia with increasing doses but continually increasing constipation and other side effects.
[f]Meperidine is not recommended for continuous pain control (e.g., postoperatively) because of risk of normeperidine toxicity.
[g]CAUTION: Doses of aspirin and acetaminophen in combination with opioid/NSAID preparations must also be adjusted to patient's body weight.

TABLE 44-5
Selected Analgesics (Equianalgesia)

Drug*	Equal to Oral Morphine (mg)	Equal to IM/IV Morphine (mg)
Hydromorphone (Dilaudid) 1 mg	4	1.3
Codeine 30 mg	4.5	1.5
Meperidine (Demerol) 50 mg	4.8	1.6
30 mg codeine + 300 mg acetaminophen (Tylenol No. 3)	7.2	2.4
Oxycodone 5 mg + 325 mg acetaminophen (Percocet)	7.2	2.4
Oxycodone 5 mg + 325 mg aspirin (Percodan)	7.2	2.4
Hydrocodone 5 mg + 500 mg acetaminophen (Vicodin, Lortab)	9	3
Oxycodone 5 mg + 500 mg acetaminophen (Tylox)	9	3
Dolophine (Methadone) 10 mg	15	7.5
Acetaminophen (Tylenol) 325 mg	2.7	0.9
Aspirin 325 mg	2.7	0.9
Acetaminophen (Tylenol Extra Strength) 500 mg	4	1.3
60 mg codeine + acetaminophen 300 mg (Tylenol No. 4)	11.7	3.9
Transdermal fentanyl patch (Duragesic) (based on 25 μg/hr patch applied every 3 days = 50 mg oral morphine every 24 hours or divided into 6 doses = 8.3 mg)	8.3	2.77

Courtesy Betty R. Ferrell, PhD, FAAN, 1999. Used with permission.
*Oral medication with exception of fentanyl.
NOTE: When converting to oral oxycodone from oral morphine, an appropriate conservative estimate is 15 to 20 mg of oxycodone per 30 mg of morphine; however, when converting to oral morphine from oral oxycodone, an appropriate conservative estimate is 30 mg of morphine per 30 mg of oxycodone. (From McCaffery M, Pasero C, 1999.)

TABLE 44-6
Suggested Intravenous Patient-Controlled Analgesia Opioid Infusion Orders

Drug	Basal Rate (mg/kg/hr)	Bolus Rate (mg/kg/dose)	Lockout Period (min)	Maximum Dose/Hour (mg/kg)
Morphine	10-30	10-30	6-10	0.1-0.15
Hydromorphone	3-5	3-5	6-10	0.015-0.02
Fentanyl	0.5-1.0	0.5-1.0	6-10	0.002-0.004

From Yaster M et al: *Pediatric pain management and sedation handbook,* St Louis, 1997, Mosby.

may be significantly more or less than what the child requires. Small changes ensure small errors.

Right Route. Several routes of analgesic administration exist (Box 44-14). Children should not have to endure pain, such as from IM injections, to achieve pain relief. Therefore the most effective and least traumatic route of administration should be selected.

A significant advance in the administration of IV, epidural, or subcutaneous (SC) analgesics is the use of *patient-controlled analgesia (PCA)*. As the name implies, the patient controls the amount and frequency of the analgesic, which is typically delivered through a special infusion device. Children as young as 5 years who are physically able to push a button and who can understand the concept of pushing a button to obtain pain relief can use PCA (Yaster et al, 1997). Although it is controversial, parents and nurses have used the PCA system for the child (Riemondy et al, 1991; Webb, Paarlberg, and Sussman, 1991). When used as nurse- or parent-controlled analgesia, the concept of patient control is negated however, and the inherent safety of PCA may be compromised. Nevertheless, recent research reported safe and effective PCA was controlled by the patient, parent, or nurse (Algren et al, 1998).

PCA infusion devices typically allow for the following three methods or modes of drug administration to be used alone or in combination:

1. Patient-administered boluses that can be infused only according to the preset amount and lockout interval (time between doses); more frequent pushing of the button means no drug is delivered, but the patient may need the dose and/or time adjusted for better pain control
2. Nurse-administered boluses that are typically used to give an initial loading dose to increase blood levels rapidly and to relieve breakthrough pain (pain not relieved with the usual programmed dose)
3. Continuous basal or background infusion that delivers a constant amount of analgesic and prevents pain from returning during those times, such as sleep, when the patient cannot control the infusion; may decrease safety of PCA

At present the optimum use of these three modes continues to be investigated. However, as with any type of analgesic management plan, continued assessment of the child's pain relief is essential for the greatest benefit from PCA (Critical Thinking box). Typical uses of PCA are for controlling perioperative pain, sickle cell crisis, trauma, and cancer.

Box 44-14

Routes and Methods of Analgesic Drug Administration

ORAL

Preferred because of convenience, cost, and relatively steady blood levels

Higher dosages of oral form of opioids required for equivalent parenteral analgesia

Peak drug effect occurs after 1½ to 2 hours for most analgesics

- Delay in onset is disadvantage when rapid control of severe pain or of fluctuating pain is desired

SUBLINGUAL/BUCCAL/TRANSMUCOSAL

Tablet or liquid placed between cheek and gum (buccal) or under tongue (sublingual)

Highly desirable because more rapid onset than oral route

- Less first-pass effect through liver than oral route, which normally reduces analgesia from oral opioids (unless sublingual/buccal form swallowed, which occurs often in children)

Few drugs commercially available in this form

- Many drugs can be compounded into a sublingual troche or lozenge*

Fentanyl Oralet—Oral transmucosal fentanyl citrate in hard confection base on a plastic holder; used for preoperative or preprocedural sedation/analgesia

Actia—Same formulation as Fentanyl Oralet; indicated only for management of breakthrough cancer pain in patients with malignancies who are already receiving and are tolerant to opioid therapy

INTRAVENOUS (IV) (BOLUS)

Preferred for rapid control of severe pain

Provides most rapid onset of effect, usually in about 5 minutes

- Advantage for acute pain, procedural pain, and break through pain

Initial bolus dose is controversial; one recommendation is one half of intramuscular (IM) dose

Needs to be repeated hourly for continuous pain control

- Drugs with short half-life (morphine, fentanyl, hydromorphone) are preferred, to avoid toxic accumulation of drug

INTRAVENOUS (CONTINUOUS)

Preferred over bolus and IM routes for maintaining control of pain

Provides steady blood levels

Easy to titrate dosage

Amount of initial dose is controversial; one approach to calculating hourly infusion rate is to divide IM dose by drug's expected duration for IM route

Peak effect is delayed; for rapid pain relief, begin with initial IV bolus dose (see preceding section)

SUBCUTANEOUS (SC) (CONTINUOUS)

Used when oral and IV routes not available

Provides equivalent blood levels to continuous IV infusion

Suggested initial bolus dose to equal 2-hour IV dose; total 24-hour dose usually equal to total IV or IM 24-hour dose

PATIENT-CONTROLLED ANALGESIA (PCA)

Generally refers to self-administration of drugs, regardless of route

Typically uses programmable infusion pump (IV, epidural, or SC) that permits self-administration of boluses of medication at preset dose and time interval (*lockout interval* is time between doses)

PCA bolus administration may be combined with initial bolus and continuous (basal or background) infusion of opioid

Optimum lockout interval not known, but must be at least as long as time needed for onset of drug

- Should effectively control pain during movement or procedures
- Longer lockout requires larger dose

FAMILY-CONTROLLED ANALGESIA

One family member (usually a parent) or significant other is designated child's primary pain manager and has responsibility of pressing PCA button

Guidelines for selecting a primary pain manager for family-controlled analgesia:

- Spends a significant amount of time with the patient
- Is willing to assume responsibility of being primary pain manager
- Is willing to accept and respect patient's reports of pain (if able to provide) as best indicator of how much pain the patient is experiencing; knows how to use and interpret a pain rating scale
- Understands the purpose and goals of patient's pain management plan
- Understands concept of maintaining a steady analgesic blood level
- Recognizes signs of pain and side effects and adverse reactions to opioid

NURSE-ACTIVATED DOSING

Child's primary nurse is designated primary pain manager and is only person who presses PCA button during that nurse's shift

Guidelines for selecting primary pain manager for family-controlled analgesia apply to nurse-activated dosing

May be used in addition to a basal rate to treat breakthrough pain with bolus doses; patients are assessed q 30 min for the need for a bolus dose

May be used without a basal rate as a means of maintaining analgesia with around-the-clock (ATC) bolus doses

INTRAMUSCULAR (IM)

NOT RECOMMENDED FOR PAIN CONTROL

Painful administration (hated by children)

Some drugs (e.g., meperidine) can cause tissue damage

Wide fluctuation in absorption of drug from muscle

Faster absorption from deltoid than from gluteal sites

Shorter duration and more expensive than oral drugs

Time consuming for staff

Data primarily from American Pain Society: *Principles of analgesic use in the treatment of acute pain or cancer pain,* ed 4, Glenview, IL, 1999, The Society; and McCaffery M, Pasero C: *Pain: a clinical manual,* ed 2, St Louis, 1999, Mosby.

*For further information about compounding drugs in troche or suppository form, contact: Technical Staff, Professional Compounding Centers of America (PCCA), P.O. Box 368, Sugar Land, TX 77487; 1-800-331-2498; website: www.thecompounders.com.

Box 44-14

Routes and Methods of Analgesic Drug Administration—cont'd

INTRANASAL

Midazolam (Versed) has been used as nasal spray

Although effective, route may be traumatic for children

Available commercially as Stadol NS (butorphanol); approved for those older than 18 years of age; should not be used in patient receiving morphinelike drugs because butorphanol is partial antagonist

INTRADERMAL

Used primarily for skin anesthesia (e.g., before lumbar puncture, bone marrow aspiration, arterial puncture, skin biopsy)

Local anesthetics (such as lidocaine) cause stinging, burning sensation

Duration of stinging may depend on type of "caine" used

To avoid stinging sensation associated with lidocaine:

Buffer the solution by adding 1 part sodium bicarbonate (1 mEq/ml) to 10 parts 1% or 2% lidocaine (see Guidelines box, p. 1103)

TOPICAL/TRANSDERMAL

EMLA (eutectic mixture of local anesthetics [lidocaine/prilocaine]) cream and Anesthetic Disc

Eliminates or reduces pain from most procedures involving skin puncture

Must be placed over puncture site and covered by occlusive dressing or applied as anesthetic disc for 1 hour or more before procedure (see Guidelines box, p. 1103)

LAT (lidocaine/adrenaline/tetracaine) or tetracaine/phenylephrine (tetraphen)

Provides skin anesthesia about 15 minutes after application

Gel (preferable) or liquid placed on wounds for suturing (nonintact skin)

Cocaine should no longer be used because of the risk of systemic absorption and toxicity

Adrenalin must not be used on end arterioles (fingers, toes, tip of nose, penis, earlobes) because of vasoconstriction

Numby Stuff

Uses iontophoresis to transport lidocaine 2% and epinephrine 1:100,000 ***(Iontocaine)*** into the skin

A small battery-powered device delivers current via an electrode with Iontocaine and a ground electrode

Produces local dermal anesthesia in about 10 minutes to a depth of approximately 10 mm at maximum setting

May be frightening to young children when they see the device and feel the mild current

Child should be observed during iontophoresis

Transdermal fentanyl (Duragesic)

Available as "patch" for continuous cancer pain control

Safety and efficacy not established in children under 12 years

Not appropriate for initial relief of acute pain because of long interval to peak effect (from 12 to 24 hours); for rapid onset of pain relief, an immediate-release opioid must be given

Orders for "rescue doses" of an immediate-release opioid should be available for ***breakthrough pain,*** a flare of severe pain that "breaks through" the medication being administered at regular intervals for persistent pain

Has duration of up to 72 hours for prolonged pain relief

If respiratory depression occurs, several doses of naloxone may be needed

Vapocoolant

Use of spray coolant, such as fluori-methane or ethyl chloride; placed on the skin immediately before the needle puncture

Some children dislike the cold; spraying the coolant on a cotton ball and then applying this to the skin may be less uncomfortable

Application of ice to the skin for 30 seconds has been found ineffective

RECTAL

Alternative to oral or parenteral routes

Variable absorption rate

Generally disliked by children

Many drugs can be compounded into rectal suppositories*

REGIONAL NERVE BLOCK

Use of long-acting anesthetic (bupivacaine or ropivacaine) injected into nerves to block pain at site

Provides prolonged analgesia postoperatively, such as after inguinal herniorrhaphy

May be used to provide local anesthesia for surgery, such as dorsal penile nerve block for circumcision or for reduction of fractures

INHALATION

Use of anesthetics, such as nitrous oxide or halothane, to produce partial or complete analgesia for painful procedures

Occupational exposure to high levels of nitrous oxide may cause side effects

EPIDURAL/INTRATHECAL

Involves catheter placed into epidural, caudal, or intrathecal space for continuous infusion or single or intermittent administration of opioid with or without a long-acting anesthetic (e.g., bupivacaine or ropivacaine)

Analgesia primarily from drug's direct effect on opioid receptors in spinal cord

Respiratory depression is rare but may have slow and delayed onset; can be prevented by checking level of sedation and respiratory rate and depth hourly for initial 24 hours and decreasing dose when excessive sedation is detected

Nausea, itching, and urinary retention are common dose related side effects from the epidural opioid

Mild hypotension, urinary retention, and temporary motor and/or sensory deficits are common unwanted effects of epidural local anesthetic

*For further information about compounding drugs in troche or suppository form, contact: Technical Staff, Professional Compounding Centers of America (PCCA), P.O. Box 368, Sugar Land, TX 77487; 1-800-331-2498; website: www.thecompounders.com

Critical Thinking

PAIN MANAGEMENT—PATIENT-CONTROLLED ANALGESIA

Juan, 9 years old, is hospitalized for a fractured pelvis and multiple other trauma as a result of a motor vehicle injury. Since admission, he has been receiving patient-controlled analgesia (PCA) ordered as "morphine, 1.0 to 1.5 mg/hr, lockout 10 minutes; bolus dose 1.5 mg, not to exceed one dose per hour." In assessing his pain, you note that he rates the pain as 4 on a scale of 0 to 5, no pain to worst pain, respectively, and he has been pushing the PCA button an average of 15 times an hour.

What should be the first action you take?

First, think about it. . .

- What assumptions are you making?
- What conclusions are you coming to?

1. Tell Juan that he is pushing the button too often; he should wait 10 minutes before using the PCA machine.
2. Administer the bolus dose of morphine and reassess pain in 10 minutes.
3. Increase the hourly dose of morphine from 1.0 to 1.5 mg and reassess pain in 1 hour.
4. Contact the surgeon about Juan's inadequate pain management.

The best response is 2. The conclusion that Juan's pain is being inadequately treated is correct, and your first intervention is to give the ordered bolus dose. If the bolus dose relieves the pain to an acceptable level for Juan, the next step is to increase the hourly dose of 1.5 mg. Since the PCA order allows titrating (adjusting) the dosage upward, this action precedes calling the surgeon. It is absolutely inappropriate to tell Juan to push the PCA button less often; this response disregards his need for improved pain control and eliminates a valuable assessment parameter, the number of PCA uses.

Morphine is the drug of choice for PCA and is usually prepared at a concentration of 1 mg/ml. Other options are hydromorphone and fentanyl. Because PCA is typically used for continuous and extended pain control, meperidine should not be administered (p. 1095). Another risk for using meperidine is confusion between its concentration (10 mg/ml) and that of morphine when the PCA pump is programmed, which can result in undermedication or overmedication.

Another advance is the use of *epidural analgesia,* primarily after the operation or in selected cases of terminal care. A catheter is placed into the epidural space of the spinal column. An opioid (usually fentanyl hydromorphone or preservative-free morphine), often with a long-acting local anesthetic (usually bupivacaine or ropivacaine), is administered via single or intermittent boluses, continuous infusion, or patient-controlled infusion. Analgesia results from the opioid's direct effect on receptors in the dorsal horn of the spinal cord, which block transmission of pain impulses to the brain (Rasmussen, 1996). Respiratory depression is rare, but if it occurs, it develops slowly and is evident several hours after the infusion begins.

NURSE ALERT • When the epidural route is used, check the child's level of sedation and respiratory rate and depth hourly for the first 24 hours to detect delayed-onset respiratory depression (Pasero, 1999).

Other routes that have benefited from new products for pain control are the *oral transmucosal* and *transdermal routes.* Oral transmucosal *fentanyl* (Fentanyl Oralet) provides atraumatic preoperative oral sedation and analgesia. Fentanyl is also available as a transdermal patch (Duragesic). It may be used for older children and adolescents who have chronic cancer pain.

One of the most significant improvements in the ability to provide atraumatic care to children is the anesthetic cream *EMLA,* a eutectic mixture of local anesthetics (lidocaine 2.5% and prilocaine 2.5%). The eutectic mixture, with a melting point that is lower than that of the two anesthetics alone, permits effective concentrations of the drug to penetrate intact skin. A thick layer of cream under an occlusive transparent dressing or a "peel-and-stick" Anesthetic Disc is applied for 1 hour or more before procedures such as lumbar, venous, arterial, finger, heel, or earlobe punctures; implanted port access; insertion of peripherally inserted central catheter (PICC) lines; superficial biopsy; skin graft; laser treatment of port-wine stains; removal of epicardial (pacing) wires, chest tubes, or hair (electrolysis); bone marrow examination; allergy testing; and IM or SC injections. For deeper pain, such as IM injections, the application time should be extended up to 2½ hours (Guidelines box). The duration of anesthesia is up to 4 hours (Pasero, 1995).

EMLA is approved for children 37 weeks of gestational age and older. It should be used cautiously in infants between 1 and 12 months of age who are receiving treatment with methemoglobin-inducing agents, such as sulfonamides, phenytoin (Dilantin), and acetaminophen (Tylenol). However, the use of these drugs is not a contraindication for applying EMLA, and there are no published reports of methemoglobinemia caused by EMLA when an infant received acetaminophen. Because of their diminished levels of erythrocyte-methemoglobin reductase, infants younger than 3 months are more susceptible to prilocaine-induced *methemoglobinemia,* a very rare and reversible side effect. *Methemoglobin* is a dysfunctional form of hemoglobin that reduces the oxygen-carrying capacity of the blood, causing cyanosis and hypoxemia. The use of IV methylene blue promptly eliminates the methemoglobinemia (McCaffery and Pasero, 1999). Other side effects are very mild and include pallor, erythema, or edema at the application site.

Another intradermal option is *Numby Stuff,* which uses iontophoresis (mild electrical current) to actively push the drug into the skin. This preparation of Iontocaine (lidocaine HCl 2% with epinephrine 1:100,000 topical solution) provides dermal anesthesia to a depth of 10 mm in approximately 10 minutes. It can be used for IV line placement, insertion of PICC lines, lumbar punctures, implantable port needle insertion, and pulsed dye laser therapy (IOMED, 1996). It is important to provide explanations and let the child become familiar with the equipment. Some children may be frightened by the tingling sensation as the drug is administered (McCaffery and Pasero, 1999).

In some situations where there is not ample time for preparations like EMLA to take effect, refrigerant sprays such as ethyl chloride and fluorimethane can be used (Cohen Reis and Holbkov, 1997). When sprayed on the skin, these sprays vaporize, rapidly cool the area, and provide superficial anesthesia.

The *intradermal route* is often used to inject a local anesthetic, typically lidocaine (Zylocaine), into the skin to reduce the pain from a lumbar puncture, bone marrow aspiration, or venous or arterial access. One problem with the use of lidocaine

Guidelines

USING EMLA (EUTECTIC MIXTURE OF LOCAL ANESTHETICS—LIDOCAINE 2.5% AND PRILOCAINE 2.5%)

Explain to child that EMLA is like a "magic cream that takes hurt away." Tap or lightly scratch site of procedure to show child that "skin is now awake."

Apply the "peel-and-stick" Anesthetic Disc or a thick layer (dollop) of EMLA cream over normal intact skin to anesthetize site (about one half of a 5-g tube; can use one third of tube if puncture site is localized and superficial (e.g., intradermal injection or heel/finger puncture).

For venous access, apply to two sites; place enough cream on antecubital fossa to cover medial and lateral veins. Do not rub the cream.

If using the cream, place transparent adhesive dressing (e.g., Tegaderm) over EMLA. Make sure cream remains in a dollop or mound. A piece of plastic film (e.g., Saran Wrap) can be used, with tape to seal the edges. Use only as much adhesive as needed to prevent leakage.

To make the dressing less accessible, cover it loosely with a self-adhering ACE-type bandage (such as Coban) or an IV protector (such as I.V. House*). Label the dressing with "EMLA applied" and the date and time to distinguish it from other types of dressings. Instruct older children not to disturb the dressing. (Covering the dressing with an opaque material may reduce the attraction and discourage "fingering.") Supervise younger or cognitively compromised children throughout the application time.

Leave EMLA on skin for at least 60 minutes for superficial puncture and 2½ hours for deep penetration (e.g., IM injection, biopsy). EMLA may be applied at home† and may need to be kept on longer in persons with dark and/or thicker skin. Anesthesia may last up to 4 hours after EMLA is removed.

Remove Anesthetic Disc or dressing before procedure and wipe cream from skin. For transparent dressing, grasp opposite sides, and while holding dressing *parallel* to skin, pull sides away from each other to stretch and loosen. An adhesive remover may be used.

Observe skin reaction (e.g., either blanched or reddened). If there is no obvious skin reaction, EMLA may not have penetrated adequately. Test skin sensitivity and reapply if needed.

Repeat tapping or lightly scratching on skin to show child that "skin is asleep" and that it cannot feel a needle.

After procedure, assess behavioral response. If child was upset, use pain scale (e.g., FACES) to help child distinguish between pain and fear. (See FACES Pain Rating Scale in Table 44-2.)

In the United States, EMLA is approved for use in infants born at 37 weeks of gestation and older. It should not be used in those rare patients with congenital or idiopathic methemoglobinemia and in infants under the age of 12 months who are receiving treatment with methemoglobin-inducing agents such as sulfonamides, phenytoin (Dilantin), phenobarbital, and acetaminophen (Tylenol). Methemoglobin, a dysfunctional form of hemoglobin, reduces the blood's oxygen-carrying capacity, causing cyanosis and hypoxemia. The use of IV methylene blue promptly eliminates the methemoglobinemia.

NOTE: Although the package insert lists under "Warnings" that patients taking drugs associated with drug-induced methemoglobinemia, such as acetaminophen, are at greater risk for developing methemoglobinemia, there have been no reported cases of this complication occurring in children taking acetaminophen and using EMLA.

Follow the manufacturer's guidelines for MAXIMUM RECOMMENDED APPLICATION AREA TO INTACT SKIN FOR INFANTS AND CHILDREN:

Age and body weight requirements	Maximum total dose of EMLA	Maximum application area
1 to 3 months or <5 kg	1 g	10 cm² (1.25 × 125 in)
4 to 12 months and >5 kg	2 g	20 cm² (1.75 × 1.75 in)
1 to 6 years and >10 kg	10 g	100 cm² (4 × 4 in)
7 to 12 years and >20 kg	20 g	200 cm² (5.5 × 5.5 in)

NOTE: If a patient older than 3 months does not meet the minimum weight requirement, the maximum total dose of EMLA should be restricted to that which corresponds to the patient's weight.

*For more information, contact I.V. House, 7400 Foxmont Dr., Hazelwood, MO 63042-2198; 1-800-530-0400; fax (314) 831-3683; e-mail: ivhouse@ivhouse.com; website: www.ivhouse.com.

†Community and home care instructions on applying EMLA are available in Wong DL, Hess CS: ***Wong and Whaley's clinical manual of pediatric nursing,*** ed 5, St Louis, 2000, Mosby.

is the stinging and burning that initially occur. However, the use of *buffered lidocaine* reduces the stinging sensation (Wong and Pasero, 1997) (Guidelines box). Warming the lidocaine to 37° C (98.6° F) may also accomplish the same effect (Mader, Playe, and Garb, 1994).

Right Time. The right timing for administering analgesics depends on the type of pain. For continuous pain control, such as for postoperative or cancer pain, a preventive schedule of medication *around the clock* (ATC) is effective. The ATC schedule avoids low plasma concentrations that permit breakthrough pain. If analgesics are administered only when pain returns (a typical use of the PRN, or "as needed," order), pain relief may take several hours. This may require higher doses, leading to a cycle of undermedication of pain alternating with periods of overmedication and drug toxicity. This cycle of erratic pain control also promotes "clock watching," which may be erroneously equated with "addiction." Nurses can effectively use PRN orders by giving the drug at regular intervals, because "as needed" can be interpreted to mean "as needed to prevent return of pain."

Preventive pain control is best provided through continuous IV infusion rather than intermittent boluses. If intermittent boluses are given, the intervals between doses should not exceed the drug's expected duration of effectiveness. For extended pain control with fewer administration times, drugs that provide longer duration of action (e.g., some NSAIDs, time-released morphine or oxycodone, methadone, levorphanol) can be used.

Guidelines

USING BUFFERED LIDOCAINE

Supplies: 8.4% sodium bicarbonate (1 mEq/ml), 1% to 2% lidocaine with or without epinephrine, syringe with removeable needle, and a 30-gauge needle

Instructions:

- Use 1 part sodium bicarbonate to 10 parts lidocaine (e.g., draw up 1 ml of lidocaine and 0.1 ml of sodium bicarbonate).
- Change needle used to withdraw buffered lidocaine (BL) to 30-gauge needle for intradermal injection.
- For venipuncture or port access, inject 0.1 ml or less BL intradermally directly over intended puncture site; anesthesia occurs almost immediately.
- Suggested maximum dose of lidocaine for local anesthesia is 4.5 mg/kg.
- If buffering lidocaine vial (e.g., 20 ml lidocaine with 2 ml sodium bicarbonate), solution may be used for 7 days if unrefrigerated or 14 days if refrigerated.

NURSE ALERT • Because breakthrough pain can occur even with optimum ATC scheduling, there should be an order for PRN "rescue" doses of an analgesic.

Continuous analgesia is not always appropriate because not all pain is continuous. Commonly, temporary pain control is needed to provide analgesia before a scheduled procedure. When pain can be predicted, the drug's peak effect should be timed to coincide with the painful event. For example, with opioids the peak effect is only a few minutes for the IV route; with nonopioids the peak effect occurs about 2 hours after oral administration. For rapid onset and peak of action, opioids that quickly penetrate the blood-brain barrier (e.g., IV fentanyl) provide excellent pain control.

Observe for Side Effects. Both NSAIDs and opioids have side effects, although the major concern is with those from opioids (Box 44-15). Respiratory depression is the most serious complication and is most likely to occur in sedated patients. The respiratory rate may decrease gradually or may cease abruptly; lower limits of normal are not established for children, but any significant change from a previous rate calls for increased vigilance. A slower respiratory rate does not necessarily reflect decreased arterial oxygenation; an increased depth of ventilation may compensate for the altered rate (McCaffery and Pasero, 1999). If respiratory depression or arrest occurs, the nurse must be prepared to intervene quickly (Guidelines box).

Although respiratory depression is the most feared side effect, constipation is a common and sometimes serious side effect of opioids, which decrease peristaltic activity and increase anal sphincter tone. Prevention with stool softeners and laxatives is more effective than treatment once constipation occurs. Dietary treatment, such as increased fiber, is usually not sufficient to promote regular bowel evacuation. However, dietary measures, such as increased fluid, fruit, and bran intake, and especially activity, are encouraged.

Pruritus from epidural or IV infusion can be treated with low doses of naloxone infused slowly or with IV nalbuphine. Pruritus from IV infusion usually responds to oral antihistamines. Nausea, vomiting, and sedation usually subside after 2 days of opioid administration, although intravenous, oral, or rectal antiemetics may be necessary.

Both tolerance and physical dependence can occur with prolonged use of opioids. Treatment of tolerance involves increasing the dose or decreasing the duration between doses. Treatment of physical dependence involves gradually reducing the dose over several days to prevent occurrence of withdrawal symptoms (similar to tapering of steroid dosages after chronic

Box 44-15
Side Effects of Opioids

GENERAL

- Constipation (possibly severe)
- Respiratory depression
- Sedation
- Nausea and vomiting
- Agitation, euphoria
- Mental clouding
- Hallucinations
- Orthostatic hypotension
- Pruritus
- Urticaria
- Sweating
- Miosis (may be sign of toxicity)
- Anaphylaxis (rare)

SIGNS OF TOLERANCE

- Decreasing pain relief
- Decreasing duration of pain relief

SIGNS OF WITHDRAWAL SYNDROME IN PATIENTS WITH PHYSICAL DEPENDENCE

Initial signs of withdrawal:
- Lacrimation
- Rhinorrhea
- Yawning
- Sweating

Later signs:
- Restlessness
- Irritability
- Tremors
- Anorexia
- Dilated pupils
- Gooseflesh
- Nausea/vomiting

Guidelines

MANAGING OPIOID-INDUCED RESPIRATORY DEPRESSION

If respirations are depressed:

- Assess sedation level (see Fig. 44-8 for sedation scale).
- Reduce infusion by 25% when possible.
- Stimulate patient (shake gently, call by name, ask to breathe).

If patient cannot be aroused or is apneic (American Pain Society, 1999):

Administer naloxone (Narcan):

- For children less than 40 kg, dilute 0.1 mg of naloxone in 10 ml of sterile saline to make 10 μg/ml solution and give 0.5 μg/kg.
- For children over 40 kg, dilute 0.4-mg ampule in 10 ml of sterile saline and give 0.5 ml.
- Administer bolus slow IV push every 2 minutes until effect is obtained.

Closely monitor patient. Naloxone's duration of antagonist action may be shorter than that of opioid, requiring repeated doses of naloxone.

NOTE: Respiratory depression caused by benzodiazepines (e.g., diazepam [Valium] or midazolam [Versed]) can be reversed with flumazenil (Romazicon). Pediatric dosing experience suggests 0.01 mg/kg (0.1 ml/kg); if no (or inadequate) response after 1 to 2 minutes, administer same dose and repeat as needed at 60-second intervals for maximum dose of 1 mg (10 ml) (Yaster et al, 1997).

steroid therapy). The following are suggested guidelines for treating physical dependence (American Pain Society, 1999):

- Gradually reduce dose (similar to tapering of steroids): Give one half of previous daily dose in q6h doses for first 2 days; then reduce dose by 25% every 2 days.
- Continue this schedule until a total daily dose of 0.6 mg/kg/day of morphine (or equivalent) is reached.
- After 2 days on this dose, discontinue opioid.
- May also switch to oral methadone, using one fourth of equianalgesic dose as initial weaning dose and proceeding as described above.

Use Supportive Statements When Administering Analgesics. The effectiveness of analgesics can be enhanced by a supportive attitude toward the child. By reinforcing the cause and effect of the medication and analgesia, the nurse can condition the child to expect pain relief, provided that the regimen is likely to be effective. Although IM injections should *not* be given, when they are, children need to understand that the "little hurt from the needle will take away the bigger hurt for a long time."

Parents and older children may have concerns about the use of opioids because of fear of addiction. These concerns should be addressed with assurance that any such risk is extremely low. It may be helpful to ask the question, "If you did not have this pain, would you want to take this medicine?" The answer is invariably no, which reinforces the solely therapeutic nature of the drug. It is also important to avoid making statements to the family such as "We don't want you to get used to this medicine" or "By now you shouldn't need this medicine," which may reinforce the fear of becoming addicted.

Providing Developmentally Appropriate Activities. A primary goal of nursing care for the child who is hospitalized is to minimize threats to the child's development. Many strategies (e.g., minimizing separation) have been discussed and may be all that the short-term patient requires. However, children who experience prolonged or repeated hospitalization are at greater risk for developmental delays or regression. The nurse who provides opportunities for the child to participate in developmentally appropriate activities further normalizes the child's environment and helps reduce interference with the child's ongoing development (see Normalization, Chapter 41).

Play is the "work" of children of all ages and assumes a critical role in their development. Because of its other important purposes in the hospital setting, play is the focus of a separate discussion.

Perhaps at no other age is the concept of interference with normal development more crucial than when it is applied to the rapidly developing infant and toddler. The nurse plays a primary role in identifying children at risk and helping to plan, implement, and evaluate developmental intervention (see Chapters 36 and 38).

School is an integral part of the school-age child's and adolescent's development. Accreditation standards for hospitals serving children consider access to appropriate educational services a key factor in the accreditation decision process when a child's treatment requires a significant absence from school (Joint Commission on Accreditation for Healthcare Organizations, 1999). The nurse can encourage children to resume schoolwork as quickly as their condition permits, help them schedule and protect a selected time for studies, and help the family coordinate hospital educational services with their children's schools. Children should have the opportunity to "keep up" with art and music classes, as well as their academic subjects.

To meet the unique developmental needs of adolescents, special units have been developed that provide privacy, increased socialization, and appropriate activities for these young persons. Typically these units are set apart from the general pediatric facility so that the teenagers do not share space with younger children, who are often perceived as a threat to their maturity.

These units also provide more flexible routines and activities, such as more group activity, wearing of street clothes, provisions to leave the adolescent unit temporarily, and access to the items so critical to teenagers—telephones, compact disc and tape players, videocassette recorders (VCRs), computers, and televisions. Because adolescents' food habits are rarely limited to the three traditional meals a day, a ready supply of snacks should be available. However, the most important benefit of these units is increased socialization with peers. In addition, staff members usually enjoy working with this age group and are well suited to establishing the trust so essential for communication.

Providing Opportunities for Play/Expressive Activities. Play is one of the most important aspects of a child's life and one of the most effective tools for managing stress. Because illness and hospitalization constitute crises in a child's life and because these situations are often fraught with overwhelming stresses, children need to play out their fears and anxieties as a means of coping with these stresses.

Play is essential to children's mental, emotional, and social well-being. As with their developmental needs, the need for play does not stop when children are ill or in the hospital. On the contrary, play in the hospital serves many functions (Box 44-16).

> Box 44-16
>
> **Functions of Play in the Hospital**
>
> Provides diversion and brings about relaxation
> Helps the child feel more secure in a strange environment
> Helps to lessen the stress of separation and the feeling of homesickness
> Provides a means for release of tension and expression of feelings
> Encourages interaction and development of positive attitudes toward others
> Provides an expressive outlet for creative ideas and interests
> Provides a means for accomplishing therapeutic goals (see Use of Play in Procedures, Chapter 45)
> Places child in active role and provides opportunity to make choices and be in control

Engaging in such activities puts children in charge, removing them for a time from the usual passive role of recipients of a constant stream of "things" being done to them. In the hospital environment, most decisions are made for the child; play and other expressive activities offer the child much-needed opportunities to make choices. Even if a child chooses not to participate in a particular activity, the nurse has offered the child a choice, perhaps one of but a few real choices the child has had that day.

Of all hospital facilities, probably no room does more to alleviate the stressors of hospitalization than the playroom or activity room. In this room children temporarily distance themselves from the fears of separation, loss of control, and bodily injury. They can work through their feelings in a nonthreatening, comfortable atmosphere and in the manner that is most natural for them. They also know that the boundaries of this room are safe from intrusive or painful procedures and probing questions (Critical Thinking box).

Diversional Activities. Almost any form of play can be used for diversion and recreation, but the activity should be selected on the basis of the child's age, interests, and limitations (Fig. 44-9). Children do not necessarily need special direction for using play materials. All they require is the raw materials with which to work and adult approval and supervision to help keep their natural enthusiasm or expression of feelings from getting out of control. Young children enjoy a variety of small, colorful toys that they can play with in bed or in their room, or more elaborate play equipment, such as playhouses, sandboxes, rhythm instruments, or large boxes and blocks, that may be a part of the hospital playroom.

Games that can be played alone or with another child or an adult are popular with older children, as are puzzles; reading material; quiet, individual activities, such as sewing, stringing beads, and weaving; and Lego blocks and other building materials. Assembling models is an excellent pastime, but one should make certain that all pieces and necessary materials are included in the package so that the child is not disappointed and frustrated.

Well-selected books are of infinite value to the child. Children never tire of stories; having someone read aloud gives them endless hours of pleasure and is of special value to the child who has limited energy to expend in play. A radio, VCR, electronic games, and television, included among most hospital room equipment, are useful tools for entertaining a child. Computers with access to the Internet can provide diversion, educational opportunities, and virtual support groups.

When supervising play for ill or convalescent children, nurses should select activities that are simpler than would normally be chosen according to the specific developmental level of the child. These children usually do not have the energy to cope with more challenging activities. Other limitations also influence the type of activities. Special consideration must be given to the child who is confined in terms of movement, has a restricted extremity, or is isolated. Toys for isolated children may need to be disinfected before and/or after use.

Toys. Parents of hospitalized children often ask nurses about the types of toys that would be best to bring for their child. It is wise to assure the parents that although it is natural to want to provide new toys for their child, it is often better to wait awhile to bring new things, especially in the case of younger children. Small children need the comfort and reassurance of familiar things, such as the stuffed animal the child hugs for comfort and takes to bed at night. These familiar items are a link with home and the world outside the hospital.

Large numbers of toys often confuse and frustrate a small child. A few small, well-chosen toys are usually preferred to one large, expensive one. Children who are hospitalized for an extended time benefit from changes. Rather than a confusing accumulation of toys, older toys should be replaced periodically as interest wanes.

Children love putting things in and taking them out of a larger container. Many simple items, such as a small magnifying glass, a magnet, grooming aids, a small mirror, crayons and

Critical Thinking

THE PLAYROOM

You are watching 7-year-old Hannah playing Candyland with her brother, sister, and several other children in the playroom. A laboratory technician enters the playroom and says, "Hannah, I need to take some blood. I can see that you are playing a game, so I'll just do it while you play. It will just take a minute." Your most appropriate response would be which of the following?

First, Think About It . . .

- **What is the purpose of your thinking?**
- **If you accept the conclusions, what are the implications?**

1. **"Go right ahead. It's silly to have to interrupt her game."**
2. **"Let me help you so that you can finish sooner."**
3. **"Hannah, is this OK with you?"**
4. **"We don't allow any procedures in the playroom."**

The best response is 4. The playroom should be considered a safe place—a sanctuary—and therefore off-limits for procedures. In many hospitals the child's bed is accorded the same status; children are taken to a treatment room for such procedures. Even if you accept the conclusion that it is "OK" with Hannah (number 3), it is important to consider the possible negative implications for the other children in the room, who may be confused about even a simple procedure (e.g., checking blood pressure) or the sanctuary status of the playroom for themselves.

An exception is sometimes made when all of the children present are older and the procedure is a quick, painless one (e.g., checking blood pressure or giving oral medication) that all the children present have experienced. In such cases the patient and the other children are asked if it is OK and give permission before the procedure is undertaken.

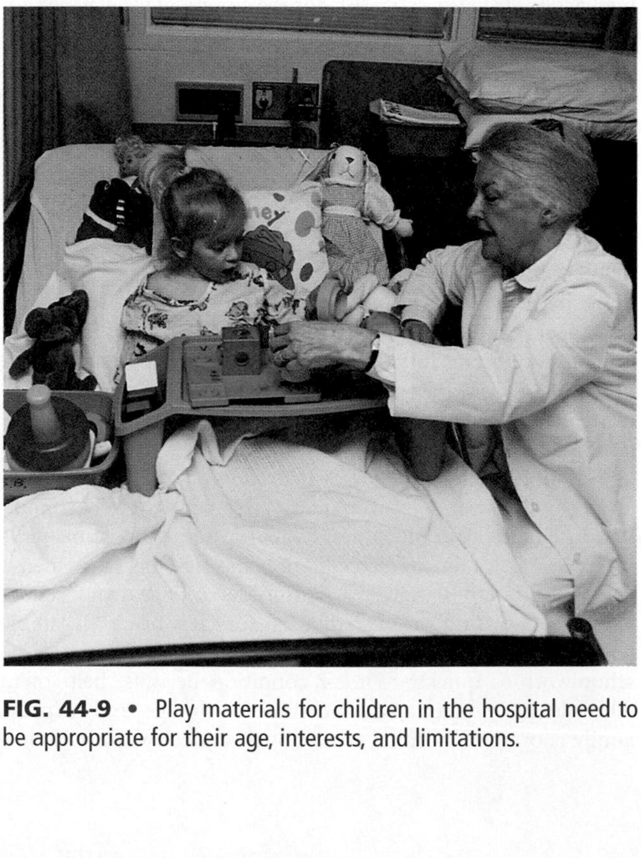

FIG. 44-9 • Play materials for children in the hospital need to be appropriate for their age, interests, and limitations.

drawing paper, colorful paper with scissors and paste, a magic slate, small dolls or toy soldiers, small cars, and beads to string, afford endless hours of amusement. It is the nurse's responsibility to assess the safety of the toys brought to the child.

A highly successful diversion for a child who is hospitalized for a length of time and whose parents are unable to visit often is having the parents bring a box with seven small, inexpensive, brightly wrapped items with a different day of the week printed on the outside of each package. The child will eagerly anticipate the time for opening each one. When the parents know when their next visit will be, they can provide the number of packages that corresponds to the days between visits. In this way the child knows that the diminishing packages also represent the anticipated visit from the parent.

Expressive Activities. Play and other expressive activities provide one of the best opportunities for encouraging emotional expression, including the safe release of anger and hostility. Nondirective play that allows children freedom for expression can be tremendously therapeutic. Therapeutic play, however, should not be confused with *play therapy,* a psychologic technique reserved for use by trained and qualified therapists as an interpretative method with emotionally disturbed children. *Therapeutic play,* on the other hand, is a very effective, nondirective modality for helping children deal with their concerns and fears, and at the same time it often helps the nurse to gain insights into children's needs and feelings.

Tension release can be facilitated through almost any activity, and with younger ambulatory children, large-muscle activity such as use of tricycles and wagons is especially beneficial. Much aggression can be safely directed into pounding and throwing games and activities. Beanbags are often thrown at a target or open receptacle with surprising vigor and hostility. A pounding board is used with enthusiasm by young children; clay and play dough are marvelous media for use at any age.

Creative Expression. Although all children derive physical, social, emotional, and cognitive benefits from engaging in art or other creative activities, children's need for such activities is intensified when they are hospitalized. Children are more at ease expressing their thoughts and feelings through art, because human beings first think in images and later learn to translate these images into words. A child's drawing before surgery, for example, will often reveal unvoiced concerns about mutilation, body changes, and loss of self-control (Clatworthy, Simon, and Tiedeman, 1999). Drawing and painting are excellent media for expression. The child needs only to be supplied with the raw materials, such as crayons and paper; pots of bright poster color, large brushes, and an ample supply of newsprint supported on easels; or materials for finger painting (Fig. 44-10). Children can work individually or collaborate on a group project, such as a mural painted on a long piece of paper. For children confined to bed, an old sheet (acquired from the laundry) spread over the bed and a large gown that extends down over the bedclothes to cover the child's own gown provide protection for clean linen.

Although interpretation of children's drawing requires special training, observing changes in a series of the child's drawings over time can be helpful in assessing psychosocial adjustment and coping (Clatworthy, Simon, and Tiedeman, 1999). The nurse can use children's drawings, stories, poetry, and other products of creative expression as a springboard for discussion of thoughts, fears, and understanding of concepts or events (see Communication Techniques, Chapter 34).

Nurses can incorporate opportunities for musical expression into routine nursing care. For example, simple musical instruments, such as bracelets with bells, can be placed on infants' legs for them to shake to accompany mealtime music or dressing changes. Dance and movement suggestions may encourage a child to ambulate.

Holidays provide stimulus and direction for unlimited creative projects. Children can participate in decorating the pediatric unit, and making pictures and decorations for their rooms gives the children a sense of pride and accomplishment. This is especially beneficial for children who are immobilized and isolated. Making gifts for someone at home helps to maintain interpersonal ties.

Dramatic Play. Dramatic play is a well-recognized technique for emotional release, allowing children to reenact frightening or puzzling hospital experiences. Through use of puppets, replicas of hospital equipment, or some actual hospital equipment, children can play out the situations that are a part of their hospital experience. Dramatic play enables children to learn about procedures and events that will concern them and to assume the roles of the adults in the hospital environment.

Puppets are universally effective for communicating with children. Most children see them as peers and readily communicate with them. Children will relate to the puppet feelings that they hesitate to express to adults. Puppets can share children's own experiences and help them to find solutions to their problems. Puppets dressed to represent figures in the child's environment—for example, a physician, nurse, child patient, therapist, and members of the child's own family—are especially useful (Fig. 44-11). Small, appropriately attired dolls are equally effective in encouraging the child to play out

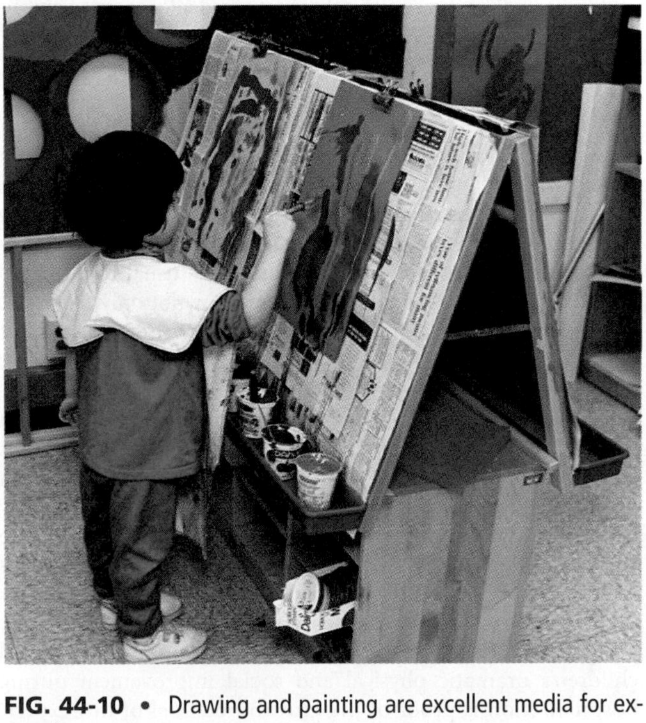

FIG. 44-10 • Drawing and painting are excellent media for expression.

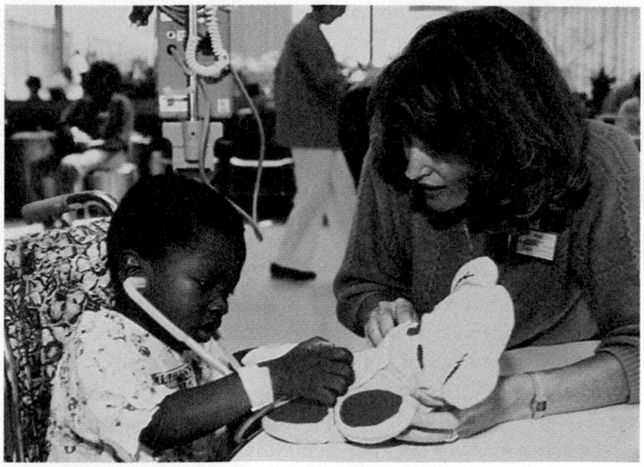

FIG. 44-11 • Playing with stuffed animals allows children to safely explore feelings and concerns. (Courtesy St Louis Children's Hospital.)

situations, although puppets are usually best for direct conversation.

Play must consider medical needs, but at times a procedure can be postponed for a short time to allow the child to complete a special activity (Critical Thinking box). Play must consider any limitations imposed by the child's condition. For example, small children may eat paste and other creative media; therefore a child who is allergic to wheat should not be given finger paint made from wallpaper paste or play dough made with flour. A child whose salt intake is restricted should not play with modeling dough because salt is one of its major constituents. At home the play program can be planned around the therapy regimen. However, play can be satisfactorily incorporated into the child's care if the nurse and others involved allow some flexibility and use creativity in planning for play.

Maximizing Potential Benefits of Hospitalization

Fostering Parent-Child Relationships. The crisis of illness and/or hospitalization can mobilize parents into more acute awareness of the needs of their children. For example, hospitalization provides opportunities for parents to learn more about their children's growth and development. When parents are helped to understand children's usual reactions to stress, such as regression or aggression, they not only are better able to support the child through the hospital experience but also may extend their insights into childrearing practices after discharge.

Difficulties in parent-child relationships that may result in feeding problems, negative behavior, and sleep disturbances may decrease during hospitalization. The temporary cessation of such problems sometimes alerts parents to the role they may be playing in propagating the negative behavior. With assistance from health professionals, parents can restructure ways of relating to their children to foster more positive behavior.

Hospitalization may also represent a temporary reprieve or refuge from a disturbed home. Typically, abused or neglected children's dramatic physical and social improvement during hospitalization is proof of the growth potential of this experience. Hospitalized children temporarily are able to seek support, reassurance, and security from new relationships, particularly with nurses and hospitalized peers.

Critical Thinking

SCHEDULING PROCEDURES

Robert, 5 years old, is recovering from abdominal surgery. You enter his room to check his dressing. His mother is reading him a story. Your most appropriate response would be which of the following?

First, Think About It . . .

- **What concepts or ideas are central to your thinking? What conclusions are you coming to?**

1. **To Robert's mother: "I need to check Robert's dressing."**
2. **"Robert, I need to check your dressing, but I can see that you are in the middle of a story right now. I'll check back in about 10 minutes and do it then."**
3. **"It's time to check your dressing, Robert. Let's get started."**
4. **"Robert, I need to check your dressing. It should take about 5 minutes. Would you like me to check it now, or to come back in about 10 minutes when you have finished hearing the story?"**

The best response is 4, although 2 would also be acceptable. The ideas presented in number 4 not only indicate that you value and respect the activity Robert is engaged in, but also offer him an opportunity to make a choice: to interrupt the story and complete the procedure, or to finish the story and wait for your return. If, because of your own schedule, you conclude that you are unable to offer such choices, express your desire to come back later, but explain that this time it is impossible. Response 1 ignores Robert's presence; number 3 fosters a passive role.

Providing Educational Opportunities. Illness and hospitalization represent excellent opportunities for children and other family members to learn more about their bodies, each other, and the health professions. For example, during a hospital admission for a diabetic crisis, the child may learn about the disease; the parents may learn about the child's needs for independence, normalcy, and appropriate limits; and each of them may find a new support system in the hospital staff.

The special tutoring that children may receive during extended hospitalizations can help them advance their studies and concentrate on subjects that were difficult. The child's relationship with a tutor can foster a more positive attitude toward school and learning.

Illness or hospitalization can also help older children in choosing a vocation. Often children have impressions of physicians or nurses that are disproportionately glorified or horrified. Actual experience with different health professionals can influence their attitude about health professionals and even a decision regarding a health career.

Promoting Self-Mastery. The experience of facing a crisis such as illness or hospitalization, coping successfully with it, and maturing as a result of it constitutes an opportunity for self-mastery. Younger children have the chance to test fantasy vs. reality fears. They realize that they were not abandoned, mutilated, castrated, or punished. In fact, they were loved, cared for, and treated with respect for their individual concerns. It is not unusual for children who have undergone hospitalization or surgery to tell others that "it was nothing" or to display proudly their scars or bandages. For older children, hospitalization may

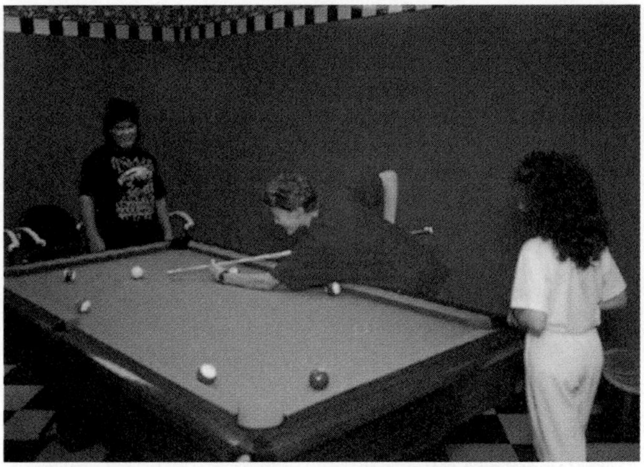

FIG. 44-12 • The hospital environment can present an opportunity for forming new friendships and an accepting peer group for children.

represent an opportunity for decision making, independence, and self-reliance. They are proud of having survived the experience and may feel genuine self-respect for their achievements. Nurses can facilitate such feelings of self-mastery by emphasizing aspects of personal competence in the child and not focusing on uncooperative or negative behavior.

Providing Socialization. Hospitalization may offer children a special opportunity for social acceptance. Lonely, asocial, sometimes delinquent children find a sympathetic environment in the hospital. Children who are physically deformed or in some other way "different" from their agemates may find an accepting social peer group (Fig. 44-12). Although this does not always spontaneously occur, nurses can structure the environment to foster a supportive child group. For example, selection of a compatible roommate can help children gain a new friend and learn more about themselves. Forming relationships with significant members of the health care team, such as the physician, nurse, child-life specialist, or minister, can greatly enhance children's adjustment in many areas of life.

Parents may also encounter a new social group in other parents who have similar problems. The waiting room or hallway "self-help" groups are inherent to every institution. Nurses can capitalize on this informal gathering by encouraging parents to discuss collectively their concerns and feelings. Nurses can also refer parents to organized parent groups or can use the help and support of recovered hospitalized patients.

➤ Evaluation

The effectiveness of nursing interventions is determined by continual reassessment and evaluation of care bared on the following observational guidelines:

1. Interview child and parents regarding the type of preparation for hospitalization the child received.
2. Review the medical record for evidence of parental visitation; interview parents and child regarding strategies used to minimize separation.
3. Observe child's hospital schedule and compare it with the schedule the child typically follows at home; interview child and family for examples of when they were allowed choices in the child's care.
4. Review the medical record for evidence of pain assessment and administration of analgesics or nonpharmacologic pain reducers. Compare child's behavior and pain scores before and after administration of pain reducers for evidence of pain relief.
5. Interview child regarding the types of play and other activities that were introduced by the nurses or child-life specialist and the times the child visited the playroom. For preverbal child, observe child's use of play materials.
6. Interview child and parents regarding their perception of any beneficial aspects of the hospitalization. Observe behaviors that indicate benefits, such as the formation of new friendships.

The expected outcomes are described in the Nursing Care Plan.

NURSING CARE OF THE FAMILY

➤ Assessment

Assessment involves those factors that are most likely to influence the family's responses to the child's illness and/or hospitalization. Although it is not possible to predict exactly which factors are most likely to have an effect on the family's reactions, the areas discussed in Table 41-2 should be included in the assessment process. Other important variables are (1) the seriousness of the child's illness, (2) the family's previous experience with hospitalization, and (3) the medical procedures involved in the diagnosis and treatment. Important information is also obtained in the nursing admission history (see Box 44-6).

Discharge Assessment. Throughout the hospitalization the nurse should be aware of the need for discharge planning and those assessment factors that affect the family's ability to provide home care. Discharge planning must begin early in the hospital admission to permit sufficient time to assess the family's ability to perform care at home and to institute needed teaching. With the current concern for cost containment and recognition of children's emotional needs, home care for children with technologically complex care, such as youngsters on ventilators, has become increasingly common.

In terms of home care for children with complex care, a thorough assessment of the family and home environment should be performed to ensure that the family's emotional and physical resources are sufficient to manage the tasks of home care. (For a discussion of family and home assessment strategies, see Chapter 34; see also Chapter 43 on home care.) In addition to adequate family resources, an investigation of community services, including respite care, is needed to ensure that appropriate support agencies are available, such as emergency facilities, home health agencies, and equipment vendors. Financial resources are also a consideration. To coordinate the immense task of assessment and to plan implementation, a care coordinator or manager should be appointed early in the discharge program.

Discharge planning is also concerned with those skills that parents or children are expected to continue at home. Assessment for planning appropriate teaching includes knowledge of (1) the actual and perceived complexity of the skill, (2) the parents' or child's ability to learn the skill, and (3) the parents' or child's previous or present experience with such procedures.

Nursing Care Plan THE CHILD IN THE HOSPITAL

NURSING DIAGNOSIS Anxiety/fear related to disruption of familiar routine, unfamiliar environment, distressing events and procedures

EXPECTED OUTCOME Patient will exhibit minimal signs of emotional or physical distress (i.e., is calm, relaxed, cooperative; engages in nonnutritive sucking, appropriate play).

Nursing Interventions/*Rationales*

Acknowledge child's fear and help child *to identify sources of that fear to facilitate identification and use of coping strategies.*
Orient the child to hospital sights and sounds; provide child with accurate information about condition, procedures, and treatments; spend time with child *to promote trust and dispel fear.*
Encourage frequent family visitation with active participation in care *to prevent distress from separation.*
Use frequent touch, holding, and talking as appropriate *to provide comfort.*
Provide diversion and sensory stimulation appropriate to the child's developmental level and physical condition.
Instruct family in importance of comfort measures and in their active participation in care *to ease child's fears.*
Prepare child for procedures using developmentally appropriate approaches (therapeutic play) *to reduce fear and promote cooperation.*
Allow child choices when possible *to give some measure of control.*
Work with parents to create a routine similar to the child's usual routine at home *to increase comfort with environment.*

NURSING DIAGNOSIS Diversional activity deficit related to illness and confinement to hospital

EXPECTED OUTCOME Child will engage in activities that are developmentally appropriate and within physical and environmental limitations.

Nursing Interventions/*Rationales*

Schedule therapies and rest periods *to allow time for play activities.*
Time play periods when child may be feeling particularly vulnerable or alone *to provide needed distraction.*
Arrange for social interactions with others *to promote socialization.*
Interview parents and child to discover the child's favorite activities and games; adapt these activities to the child's physical limitations *to provide optimum diversions.*
Have parents bring in treasured toys or objects, decorate room with familiar pictures and drawings *to familiarize an unfamiliar environment.*

NURSING DIAGNOSIS Activity intolerance related to illness and generalized weakness

EXPECTED OUTCOME Patient's vital signs will remain within prescribed limits during activity, and child will tolerate increasing levels of activity.

Nursing Interventions/*Rationales*

Monitor child's vital signs *to assess level of physical tolerance;* monitor child's behavior and look for signs of irritability, shortened attention span, fussiness *that are indicators of a need for rest.*
Balance rest and activity, match play activities with tolerance levels *to conserve energy and prevent intolerance.*
Administer analgesics and sedatives per physician order *to decrease pain and restlessness.*
Remove stimulation and provide a quiet and calm environment during rest periods *to enhance rest and sleep.*

NURSING DIAGNOSIS Risk for injury related to unfamiliar environment, therapies, hazardous equipment

EXPECTED OUTCOME Patient will exhibit no evidence of injury.

Nursing Interventions/*Rationales*

Employ environmental safety measures (e.g., use of side rails; bed in low position; avoidance of hazards; keeping small, sharp and breakable items out of reach) *to prevent injury.*
Transport children using age-appropriate equipment and use of locks and safety belts *to minimize risk of injury.*
Maintain vigilance during trips to bathroom, use of bathtub or shower, performance of procedures *to minimize risk of injury.*
Identify specific motor/sensory deficits and provide appropriate assistive devices *to promote function and enhance safety.*
Instruct family in standard safety practices *to promote safety.*

NURSING DIAGNOSIS Self-care deficit; toileting, bathing/hygiene, dressing/grooming, feeding related to illness, physical restrictions, emotional regression

EXPECTED OUTCOME Patient will exhibit self-care activities within current physical and psychologic capacities.

Nursing Interventions/*Rationales*

Teach parents that some regression is expected when a child is ill *so behavior can be anticipated and viewed as normal part of disease process.*
Identify the level of regression and use developmental strategies appropriate to that level *to facilitate care.*
Involve child in planning and initiating daily routines as appropriate *to foster a sense of control.*
Assist child in performing activities of daily living as indicated, *allowing needed dependency and provision of support.*
Encourage child to perform activities within abilities *to promote self-confidence and independence.*

➤ Nursing Diagnoses

A number of nursing diagnoses are prominent in the nursing care of the family of the hospitalized child, and other specific to individual cases become evident. The most common nursing diagnoses are outlined in the Nursing Care Plan on p. 1110.

➤ Plan of Care and Implementation

The main goals for the family are as follows:

1. Family will participate in child's care to the extent they desire.
2. Family will receive support.
3. Family will be informed of child's care.
4. Family will be prepared for discharge and home care.

Encouraging Parent Participation. Preventing or minimizing separation is a key nursing goal with the child who is hospitalized, but maintaining parent-child contact is also beneficial for the family. One of the best approaches is encouraging parents to stay with their child and to participate in the care whenever possible. Although some health facilities provide special accommodations for parents, the concept of "rooming-in" can be instituted anywhere. The first requirement is the staff's positive attitude toward parents. A negative attitude toward parent participation can create barriers to collaborative working relationships (Johnson and Lindschau, 1996). Although nurses often express explicit support for the concept of family-centered care, some of their practices and beliefs suggest otherwise (Bruce and Ritchie, 1997).

When hospital staff genuinely appreciate the importance of continued parent-child attachment, they foster an environment that encourages parents to stay. When parents are included in the care planning and understand that they are a contributing factor to the child's recovery, they are more inclined to remain with their child and have more emotional reserves to support themselves and the child through the crisis. An empowerment model of helping allows the nurse to focus on parents' strengths and to seek ways to promote growth and family functioning so that the parents become empowered in caring for their child (Fig. 44-13).

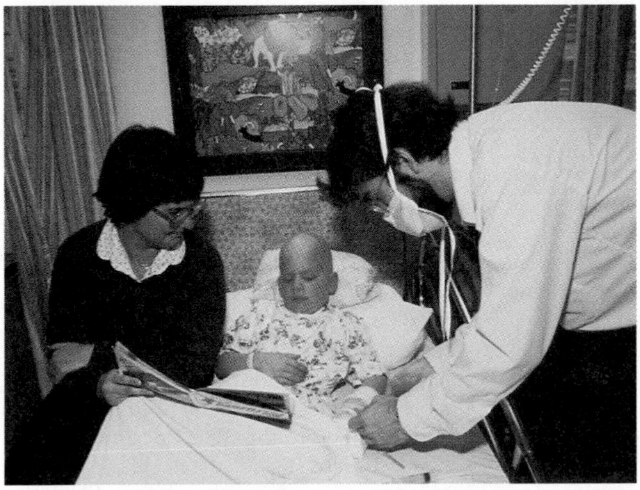

FIG. 44-13 • Parental presence during hospitalization, including during procedures, provides emotional support for the child and increases the parent's sense of empowerment in the caregiver role. (Courtesy St Louis Children's Hospital.)

Because the mother tends to be the usual family caregiver, she typically spends more time in the hospital than the father. However, not all mothers (or fathers) feel equally comfortable in assuming responsibility for their child's care. Some may be under such great emotional stress that they need a temporary reprieve from total participation in caregiving activities (Remmel, 1997). Others may feel insecure in participating in specialized areas of care, such as bathing the child after surgery. On the other hand, some mothers may feel a great need to have control of their child's care. This seems particularly true of young mothers, who have more recently established their role as a parent; mothers of children too young to verbalize their needs; and ethnic minority mothers when the hospital setting is predominantly staffed by nonminority personnel (Schepp, 1992). Individual assessment of each parent's preferred involvement is necessary to prevent the effects of separation while also supporting parents in their needs.

With lifestyles and sex roles changing, fathers may assume all or some of the usual "mothering" roles in the household. In this case it may be the father-child relationship that requires preservation. Fathers need to be included in the plan of care and respected for their parental role. For some fathers the child's hospitalization may represent an opportunity to alter their usual caregiving role and increase their involvement. In single-parent families the caregiver may not be a parent but an extended family member, such as a grandparent or aunt.

One of the potential problems with continuous parent involvement is neglect of the parent's need for sleep, nutrition, and relaxation (Family Focus box). Often the sleeping accommodations are limited to a chair, and sleep is disrupted by nursing procedures. Encouraging the parents to leave for brief periods, arranging for sleeping quarters on the unit but outside the child's room, and planning a schedule of alternating visiting with another family member can minimize the stresses for the parent.

Family Focus

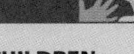

PARENTS' RELUCTANCE TO LEAVE THEIR CHILDREN UNATTENDED

Parents are often very reluctant to leave their children or to ask the nurse to watch their children while they take a break. In his research on the experiences of nurses and parents when parents room-in, Darbyshire (1994) found that many parents did not eat properly or, in some cases, at all. The following are two mothers' experiences:

I just about starved to death the first couple of days . . . just. . . . I mean, it was my own fault really, 'cos I wouldn't leave the wee one. There was always going to be something else happening and I thought . . . if he gets upset I'd better be there when it finishes.

There was one day I couldn't get any of the visitors to look after the wee chap so I could go for something to eat and it was about six o'clock at night and nurse said, "You look awful, are you OK?" and I said, "No, actually I feel awful and I think I'm going to pass out," and she said, "Oh, you've just gone a funny colour," and I said, "What time is it?" and I said, "It's OK, it's just because I haven't eaten all day"—because none of my family had come to take the child from me, and I didn't think to say to a nurse, "Could you watch him till I go for something to eat?"

Data from Darbyshire P: *Living with a sick child in hospital,* London, 1994, Chapman & Hall.

All too often, nurses respond to parent participation by abandoning their patient responsibilities. Nurses need to restructure their roles to complement and augment the caregiving functions of parents. Even in units structured to provide care by parents, parents often feel anxiety in their caregiving responsibilities; those more involved in direct care may feel more anxiety than those less involved in direct care. Therefore 24-hour responsibility may be too much for some parents. Assistance and relief by nursing personnel should always be available to these families, and nurses must often work diligently to establish the strong bond of trust that some parents need in order to take advantage of these opportunities.

Supporting Family Members. Support involves the willingness to stay and listen to parents' verbal and nonverbal messages. Sometimes the nurse does not give this support directly. For example, the nurse may offer to stay with the child to allow the parents time alone or may discuss with other family members the parents' need for extra relief. Often relatives and friends want to help but do not know how. Suggesting ways, such as baby-sitting, preparing meals, tending the garden or home, doing laundry, or transporting the siblings to school, can prompt others to help lessen the responsibilities that burden parents. An ongoing parent support group held on the pediatric unit during the children's traditional nap time has also proved effective in helping parents share emotions and concerns related to hospitalization (Bracht et al, 1998; Santelli, Turnbull, and Higgins, 1997).

Support may also be provided through the clergy. Parents with deep religious beliefs may appreciate the counsel of a clergy member, but because of their stress, they may not have sufficient energy to initiate the contact. Nurses can be supportive by arranging for clergy to visit, upholding parents' religious beliefs, and respecting the individual meaning and significance of those beliefs.

Support involves an acceptance of cultural, socioeconomic, and ethnic values. For example, health and illness are defined differently by various ethnic groups. For some, a disorder that has few outward manifestations of illness, such as diabetes, hypertension, or cardiac problems, is not a sickness. Consequently, following a prescribed treatment may be seen as unnecessary. Nurses who appreciate the influences of culture are more likely to intervene therapeutically. (See also Chapter 32 for an extensive discussion of cultural and religious influences on health care.)

Parents need help in accepting their own feelings toward the ill child. If given the opportunity, parents often disclose their feelings of loss of control, anger, and guilt. They often resist admitting to such feelings because they expect others to disapprove of behavior that is less than perfect. Unfortunately, health personnel, including nurses, sometimes do exercise little tolerance for deviation from the expected norm. This only increases the psychologic impact of a child's illness on family members. Helping parents identify the specific reason for such feelings and emphasizing that each is a normal, expected, and healthy response to stress provides the parents with an opportunity to lessen their emotional burden.

Family-centered care also addresses the needs of siblings. Support may involve preparing siblings for hospital visits, assessing their adjustment, and providing appropriate interventions or referrals when needed. The Home Care box suggests ways that parents can support siblings during hospitalization.

Home Care

SUPPORTING SIBLINGS DURING HOSPITALIZATION

- **Trade off staying at the hospital with spouse or have a parent surrogate who knows the siblings well stay in the home.**
- **Offer information about the child's condition to young siblings as well as older siblings; respect the sibling who avoids information as a means of coping with the situation.**
- **Arrange for children to visit their brother or sister in the hospital if possible.**
- **Encourage phone visits and mail between brothers and sisters; provide children with phone numbers, writing supplies, and stamps.**
- **Help each sibling identify an extended family member or friend to be their support person and provide extra attention during parental absence.**
- **Make or buy inexpensive toys or trinkets for siblings, one gift for each day the child will be hospitalized.**
  - **Wrap each gift separately and place in a basket, box, or other container at each child's bedside.**
  - **Instruct siblings to open one gift each night at bedtime and to remember that he or she is in the parent's thoughts.**
- **If the child's condition is stable and distance is not prohibitive, plan a special time at home with the siblings or have spouse or another relative or friend bring the children to meet parent(s) at a restaurant or other location near the hospital.**
  - **Have extended family members or friends schedule a visit to the child in the hospital during parental absence.**
  - **Arrange a pass for the child to leave the hospital to join the family if the child's condition permits.**

Modified from Craft M, Craft J: Perceived changes in siblings of hospitalized children: a comparison of sibling and parent reports, *Child Health Care* 18(1):42-48, 1989; and Rollins J: *Brothers and sisters: a discussion guide for families,* Landover, MD, 1992, Epilepsy Foundation of America.

Providing Information. One of the most important nursing interventions is providing information about (1) the disease, its treatment, prognosis, and home care; (2) the child's emotional and physical reactions to illness and hospitalization; and (3) the probable emotional reactions of family members to the crisis.

For many families the child's illness is the first contact they have with the hospital experience. Often parents are not prepared for the child's behavioral reactions to hospitalization, such as separation behaviors, regression, aggression, and hostility. Providing the parents with information about these normal and expected behavioral responses can lessen the parents' anxiety during the hospital admission. The family is equally unfamiliar with hospital rules, which often adds to feelings of confusion and anxiety. Therefore the family needs clear explanations about what to expect and what is expected of them.

Parents also need to be aware of the effects of illness on the family and strategies that prevent negative changes. Specifically, parents should keep the family well informed and communicating as much as possible. They should treat all of the children as equally and as normally as before the illness occurred. Discipline, which initially may be lessened for the ill child, should be continued to provide a measure of security and predictability. When ill children know that their parents expect certain standards of conduct from them, they feel certain that they will recover. Conversely, when all limits are removed, they fear that something catastrophic will happen.

Nurses should help parents understand and accept the meaning of posthospitalization behaviors so that the parents can tolerate and support such behaviors. Consequently, parents should be forewarned of the usual continuance of such reactions after discharge (see Box 44-3). Parents who do not expect such reactions may misinterpret them as evidence of the child's "being spoiled" and demand perfect behavior at a time when the child is still reacting to the stress of illness and hospitalization. If the behaviors, especially the demand for attention, are dealt with in a supportive manner, most children are able to relinquish them and assume precrisis levels of functioning.

Nurses should also forewarn parents of the reactions of siblings, particularly anger, jealousy, and resentment. Older siblings may deny such reactions because they provoke feelings of guilt. However, everyone needs outlets for emotions, and the repressed feelings may surface as problems in school or with agemates, as psychosomatic illnesses, or as delinquent behavior.

Probably one of the most neglected areas involves giving information to siblings. Often age becomes the only factor that leads to an awareness of this problem, because older children may begin to ask questions or request explanations. Even in this situation, however, the information may be seriously inadequate. Children in every age group deserve some explanation of the sibling's illness or hospitalization. Although the exact wording may differ, the explanation should focus on the following concerns: (1) "Will I get sick and have to go to the hospital?"; (2) "Did I cause the illness?" (for actual or imagined reasons); and (3) "Will my parents abandon me if my brother or sister doesn't recover?" If parents or nurses address the explanations to these three questions, the siblings' own fears of illness, guilt, and abandonment are minimized (Melnyk and Alpert-Gillis, 1998).

Preparing for Discharge and Home Care. Most hospitalizations necessitate some type of discharge preparation. Often this involves education of the family for continued care and follow-up in the home. Depending on the diagnosis, this may be relatively simple or highly complex. Preparing the family for home care demands a high degree of competence in planning and implementing discharge instructions. This usually is best accomplished using an interdisciplinary team approach, which is a shift from the multidisciplinary team approach used during hospitalization (Hornick, 1996).

Nurses often are responsible for all or some of the teaching as well. The teaching plan incorporates levels of learning, such as observing, participating with assistance, and finally, acting without help or guidance. The skill is divided into discrete steps, and each step is taught to the family member until it is learned. Return demonstration of the skill is requested before new skills are introduced. A record of teaching and performance provides an efficient checklist for evaluation. All families need to receive detailed written instructions about home care,* with telephone numbers for assistance, before they leave the hospital (Critical Thinking box).

Videocassette recordings offer another excellent vehicle for home teaching. The actual teaching session in the hospital can be recorded and played for the family as often as needed. If the family has a VCR at home, the filmed instructions serve as a refresher when parents have questions about the procedure.

Once the family is competent in performing the skill, they are given responsibility for the care. Whenever possible, the family should have a transition or trial period to assume care with minimum supervision. This may be arranged on the unit, during a home pass, or in a facility, such as a motel, near the hospital. Such transitions provide a safe practice period for the family, with assistance readily available when needed, and are especially valuable when the family lives far from the treating center.

In many instances parents need only simple instructions and understanding of follow-up care. However, the often over-

Critical Thinking

DISCHARGE PLANNING AND HOME CARE

Two-year-old Rhonda comes from a rural home 150 miles from the medical center. Last month she suffered a severe case of meningitis that left her profoundly cognitively impaired. During her hospitalization her parents have called infrequently and have never visited because they do not have a telephone or car as a result of their low income. Rhonda is now ready to be discharged from the tertiary care center. As the nurse who is responsible for Rhonda's discharge planning, which of the following activities would you initiate?

First, Think About It . . .

- **What are you taking for granted, what assumptions are you making?**
- **What would the consequences be if you put your thoughts into action?**

1. **Arrange for Rhonda to be institutionalized because her family will be unable to care for her.**
2. **Give to the transport team a list of local services with an encouraging note about the importance of arranging follow-up care to give to her parents.**
3. **Call and arrange for the public health nurse from Rhonda's district to make a home visit shortly after her return.**
4. **Arrange for a multidisciplinary care conference to discuss Rhonda's discharge.**

The best response is 4. Making the arrangements for a multidisciplinary care conference, including the parents, will require some planning. Transportation assistance may be necessary for the parents to attend the care conference. The public health department can be asked to either escort Rhonda's parents to the medical center or arrange for them to participate over a speaker phone. Also, the action taken by the public health nurse from Rhonda's district will include advising the team of the services available in Rhonda's community. Since Rhonda will need care from a variety of professionals, this conference will help ensure that there are no gaps or overlaps in services.

Providing Rhonda's parents with a list of agencies is inappropriate. First, they do not own their own phone. Second, the parents are not in the position of knowing what services they will need. Third, dealing with professional agencies is often an arduous task and one that parents should not be expected to do while adjusting to the child's disability. Although contacting the local public health nurse regarding home visits is a good idea, this should be done well in advance of discharge. This way the nurse could perform a home assessment to help arrange for appropriate services. Institutionalization of children with mental retardation is considered a last resort. All other options should be explored first.

*Community and home care instructions for a wide range of technical skills are available in Wong DL, Hess CS: ***Wong and Whaley's clinical manual of pediatric nursing***, ed 5, St Louis, 2000, Mosby.

whelming care assumed by some families, coupled with other stressors they may be experiencing, necessitates continued professional support after discharge. A follow-up home visit or telephone call gives the nurse a better opportunity to individualize care and provide information in perhaps a less stressful learning environment than the hospital (Snowdon and Kane, 1995). Appropriate referrals and resources may include visiting nurse or home health agencies, private nurse services, the school system, a physical therapist, a mental health counselor, a social worker, and any number of community agencies. Sharing the important issues surrounding the child's and family's needs is essential. Referral summaries should be concise, specific, and factual. When numerous support services are involved, periodic collaboration among the professionals involved and the family is an excellent strategy to ensure efficient usage and comprehensive delivery of services.

➤ Evaluation

The effectiveness of nursing interventions is determined by continual reassessment and evaluation of care based on the following observational guidelines:

1. Observe schedule of parental presence and amount of participation in child's care; observe parents' willingness and ability to take care of their own needs, such as regular breaks to eat, sleep, and care for the family's needs at home.
2. Interview family regarding their concerns; observe support offered by others, such as relatives, friends, and clergy; observe whether special cultural practices (if applicable) are respected in the hospital.
3. Interview family regarding their knowledge of child's illness, child's expected reactions to the hospitalization experience, and the emotional needs of the other family members, especially siblings; observe frequency of siblings' visits and interview siblings regarding their understanding of the ill child's condition.
4. Observe family's performance of skills and determine their understanding of other aspects of home care before discharge; interview family and/or resource persons regarding the family's use of appropriate referral services.

The expected outcomes are described in the Nursing Care Plan.

CARE OF THE CHILD AND FAMILY IN SPECIAL HOSPITAL SITUATIONS

Ambulatory/Outpatient Setting

The ambulatory or outpatient setting provides needed medical services for the child while eliminating the necessity of overnight admission. Among the benefits of ambulatory care are (1) minimization of the stressors of hospitalization, espe-

Nursing Care Plan — THE FAMILY OF THE ILL/HOSPITALIZED CHILD

NURSING DIAGNOSIS Altered family processes and/or ineffective family coping related to situational crisis, threat to role functioning, change in environment

EXPECTED OUTCOME Family will exhibit use of appropriate coping mechanisms, and stress levels are reduced.

Nursing Interventions/*Rationales*

Explore family background, structure, normal roles, and functions, usual coping mechanisms *to identify family strengths and weaknesses and assist in meeting needs.*

Help family arrange a schedule that balances needs of hospitalized child with functions of home and work *to help family manage stress and adapt to the situation.*

Help family prioritize needs, explore options, make decisions *to reduce stress and increase coping.*

Encourage use of available support systems (e.g., extended family, friends, church, community) and make referrals to appropriate social service agencies *to increase support and enhance available resources.*

Keep family informed about child's condition, procedures, and treatments *to reduce anxiety about the unknown.*

Give family members specific suggestions as to what each can contribute to help the child during the hospital stay and recovery *to provide for concrete family contributions and involvement.*

Provide a ready outlet for family to vent feelings, fears, and frustrations *to promote coping.*

Encourage family to take care of their own needs for rest, nutrition, relaxation, and respite *to promote coping.*

NURSING DIAGNOSIS Powerlessness related to health care environment

EXPECTED OUTCOME Family will exhibit a sense of control within the environment.

Nursing Interventions/*Rationales*

Encourage family to identify feelings about having a child in the hospital *to enhance trust, communication, and ventilation.*

Help family identify specific modifications and adjustments that can be made within the environment (e.g., participation in child's care, decision making, scheduling; rearranging and personalizing environmental space; provision of privacy, ready access to specifically identified personnel) *to enhance feelings of control.*

Incorporate family suggestions, needs into plan of care *to enhance sense of contribution and control.*

Keep family informed about child's condition, progress; educate about treatments and procedures *to enhance knowledge.*

cially separation from the family; (2) reduced chance of infection; and (3) cost savings. Admission to the ambulatory or outpatient hospital setting usually is for surgical or diagnostic procedures, such as insertion of tympanostomy tubes, hernia repair, adenoidectomy, tonsillectomy, cystoscopy, or bronchoscopy.

In the ambulatory/outpatient setting, adequate preparation is particularly challenging (Stewart, Algren, and Arnold, 1994). Ideally the child and parents should receive preadmission preparation, including a tour of the facility and a review of the day's events (Brewer and Lambert, 1997). Parents need information to help prepare the child and themselves for surgery and enable them to care for the child at home after the procedure. Parents also appreciate suggestions of items to bring to the hospital (security objects such as blankets or stuffed animals). When preadmission preparation is not possible, time should be allowed on the day of the procedure for children to become acquainted with their surroundings and for nurses to assess, plan, and implement appropriate teaching.

Waiting is usually inevitable in ambulatory settings. Families often report waiting to be the most stressful part of the experience. Providing a pager is one way to allow the family (and at times the child) to leave the area and then be paged to return when needed (Ashenberg et al, 1996). Parents need guidelines on when to call their practitioner regarding a change in the child's condition. A follow-up telephone call system allows for nurses to check on the child's progress within 48 to 72 hours after discharge. It also provides an opportunity for the nurse to review discharge information and answer questions.

Isolation

Admission to an isolation room increases all of the stressors typically associated with hospitalization. There is further separation from familiar persons, additional loss of control, and added environmental changes, such as sensory deprivation and the strange appearance of visitors. Orientation to time and place is affected. These stressors are compounded by children's limited understanding of isolation. Preschool children have difficulty understanding the rationale for isolation because they cannot comprehend the cause-and-effect relationship between germs and illness. They are likely to view isolation as punishment. Older children understand the causality better but still require information to decrease fantasizing or misinterpretation.

When a child is placed in isolation, preparation is essential for the child to feel in control. With young children the best approach is a simple explanation, such as "You need to be in this room to help you get better. This is a special place to make all the germs go away. The germs made you sick, and you could not help that."

All children, but especially younger ones, need preparation in terms of what they will see, hear, or feel in isolation. Therefore they are shown the mask, gloves, and gown and are encouraged to "dress up" in them. Playing with the strange apparel lessens the fear of seeing "ghostlike" people walk into the room. Before entering the room, nurses and other health personnel should introduce themselves and let the child see their face before donning a mask. In this way the child associates them with significant experiences and gains a sense of familiarity in an otherwise strange and lonely environment.

When the child's condition improves, appropriate play activities are provided to minimize boredom, stimulate the senses, provide a real or perceived sense of movement, orient the child to time and place, provide social interaction, and reduce depersonalization. For example, the environment can be manipulated to increase sensory freedom by moving the bed toward the door or window. Opening window shades; providing musical, visual, or tactile toys; and increasing interpersonal contact can substitute mental mobility for the limitations of physical movement. Rather than dwelling on the negative aspects of isolation, the child can be encouraged to view this experience as challenging and positive. For example, the nurse can help the child look at isolation as a method of keeping others out and letting only special persons in. Children often think of intriguing signs for their doors, such as "Enter at your own risk." These signs also encourage people "on the outside" to talk with the child about the ominous greeting.

Emergency Admission

One of the most traumatic hospital experiences for the child and parents is an emergency admission. The sudden onset of an illness or the occurrence of an injury leaves little time for preparation and explanation. Sometimes the emergency admission is compounded by admission to an intensive care unit or the need for immediate surgery. However, even in those instances requiring only outpatient treatment, the child is exposed to a strange, frightening environment and to health professionals who often inflict pain. Thus every medical emergency requires psychologic intervention to reduce the fear and anxiety often associated with the experience.

Lengthy preparatory admission procedures are often inappropriate for emergency situations. In such instances, nurses must focus their nursing interventions on the essential components of admission counseling (Box 44-17) and complete the process as soon as the child's condition is stabilized.

Unless an emergency is life threatening, children need to participate in their care to maintain a sense of control. Because emergency departments are often hectic, there is a tendency to rush through procedures to save time. However, the extra few minutes needed to allow children to participate may save many more minutes of useless resistance and uncooperativeness during subsequent procedures. Other supportive measures include ensuring privacy, accepting various emotional responses to fear or pain, preserving parent-child contact, explaining all events before or as they occur, and remaining calm.

At times, because of the child's physical condition, little or no preparatory counseling for emergency hospitalization can be done. In such situations the implementation of *postvention*, or counseling subsequent to the event, has therapeutic value. The process of postvention involves evaluating children's thoughts regarding admission and related procedures. It is similar to precounseling techniques; however, instead of supplying information, the nurse listens to the explanations offered by the child. Projective techniques such as drawing, doll play, or storytelling are especially effective. The nurse then bases additional information on what has already been revealed.

Intensive Care Unit (ICU)

Admission to an ICU can be a particularly traumatic event for both the child and the parents. The nature and severity of the

Box 44-17

Guidelines for Special Hospital Admission

EMERGENCY ADMISSION

Lengthy preparatory admission procedures are often impossible and inappropriate for emergency situations.

Focus assessment on airway, breathing, and circulation; weigh child whenever possible for calculation of drug dosages.

Unless an emergency is life threatening, children need to participate in their care to maintain a sense of control.

Focus on essential components of admission counseling, including:

- Appropriate introduction to the family
- Use of child's name, not terms such as "honey" or "dear"
- Determination of child's age and some judgment about developmental age (if the child is of school age, asking about the grade level will offer some evidence for concurrent intellectual ability)

Information about child's general state of health, any problems that may interfere with medical treatment (e.g., allergies), and previous experience with hospital facilities

Information about the chief complaint from both the parents and the child

ADMISSION TO INTENSIVE CARE UNIT (ICU)

Prepare child and parents for elective ICU admission, such as for postoperative care after cardiac surgery.

Prepare child and parents for unanticipated ICU admission by focusing primarily on the sensory aspects of the experience and on usual family concerns (e.g., persons in charge of child's care, schedule for visiting, area where family can stay).

Prepare parents regarding child's appearance and behavior when they first visit child in ICU.

Accompany family to bedside to provide emotional support and answer questions.

Prepare siblings for their visit; plan length of time for sibling visitation; monitor siblings' reactions during visit to prevent them from becoming overwhelmed.

Encourage parents to stay with their child:

- If visiting hours are limited, allow flexibility in schedule to accommodate parental needs.
- Give family members a written schedule of visiting times.
- If visiting hours are liberal, be aware of family members' needs and suggest periodic respites.
- Assure family they can call the unit at any time.

Prepare parents for expected role changes and identify ways for parents to participate in child's care without overwhelming them with responsibilities:

- Help with bath or feeding.
- Touch and talk to child.
- Help with procedures.

Provide information about child's condition in understandable language:

- Repeat information often.
- Seek clarification of understanding.
- During bedside conferences, interpret information for family members and child or, if appropriate, conduct report outside room.

Prepare child for procedures, even if this involves explanation while procedure is performed.

Assess and manage pain; recognize that a child who cannot talk, such as an infant or child in a coma or on a ventilator, can be in pain.

Establish a routine that maintains some similarity to daily events in child's life whenever possible:

- Organize care during normal waking hours.
- Keep regular bedtime schedules, including quiet times when television or radio is lowered or turned off.
- Provide uninterrupted sleep cycles (60 minutes for infant, 90 minutes for older child).
- Close and open drapes and dim lights to allow for day/night.
- Place curtain around bed for privacy.
- Orient child to day and time; have clocks or calendars in easy view for older children.

Schedule a time when child is left undisturbed (e.g., during naps, visit with family, playtime, or favorite program).

- Provide opportunities for play.

Reduce stimulation in environment:

Refrain from loud talking or laughing.

Keep equipment noise to a minimum:

- Turn alarms as low as safely possible.
- Perform treatments requiring equipment at one time.
- Turn off bedside equipment that is not in use, such as suction and oxygen.
- Avoid loud, abrupt noises, such as clattering bedpans or toilets flushing.

illness and the circumstances surrounding the admission are major factors, especially for parents. Parents experience significantly more stress when the admission is unexpected rather than expected. Stressors for the child and parent are described in Box 44-18. Although several studies have described what parents perceive as most stressful, the most effective strategy may be to simply ask parents what is stressful and implement interventions that will enhance coping outcomes (Melnyk and Alpert-Gillis, 1998). Assessment should be repeated periodically to account for changes in perceptions over time.

The emotional needs of the family are paramount when a child is admitted to an ICU. Although the same interventions discussed earlier for the stressors of separation, loss of control, and bodily injury and pain apply here, additional interventions may also benefit the family and child (see Box 44-17). Critical care must be centered on the family. Visiting hours should be liberal and flexible enough to accommodate parental needs (Hazinski, 1999).

Critically ill children become the focus of the parents' lives, and parents' most pressing need is for information (Scott, 1998). They want to know whether their child will live and, if so, whether the child will be the same as before. They need to know why various interventions are being done for the child, that the child is being treated for pain and/or is comfortable, and that the child may be able to hear them even though not awake.

Despite the stresses normally associated with ICU admission, a special security develops from being carefully monitored

Box 44-18

Neonatal/Pediatric ICU Stressors for the Child and Family

PHYSICAL STRESSORS

Pain and discomfort (e.g., injections, intubation, suctioning, dressing changes, other invasive procedures)
Immobility (e.g., use of restraints, bed rest)
Sleep deprivation
Inability to eat or drink
Changes in elimination habits

ENVIRONMENTAL STRESSORS

Unfamiliar surroundings (e.g., crowding)
Unfamiliar sounds
- Equipment noise (e.g., monitors, telephone, suctioning, computer printout)
- Human sounds (e.g., talking, laughing, crying, coughing, moaning, retching, walking)

Unfamiliar people (e.g., health care professionals, patients, visitors)
Unfamiliar and unpleasant smells (e.g., alcohol, adhesive remover, body odors)
Constant lights (disturb day/night rhythms)
Activity related to other patients
Sense of urgency among staff
Unkind or thoughtless comments from staff

PSYCHOLOGIC STRESSORS

Lack of privacy
Inability to communicate (if intubated)
Inadequate knowledge and understanding of situation
Severity of illness
Parental behavior (expression of concern)

SOCIAL STRESSORS

Disrupted relationships (especially with family and friends)
Concern with missing school or work
Play deprivation

Data primarily from Tichy AM et al: Stressors in pediatric intensive care units, *Pediatr Nurs* 14(1):40-42, 1988.

and receiving individualized care. Therefore planning for transition to the regular unit is essential and should include (1) assignment of a primary nurse on the regular unit, who visits before the transfer; (2) continued visits by the ICU staff to assess the child's and parents' adjustment and to act as a temporary liaison with the nursing staff; (3) explanation of the differences between the two units and the rationale for the change to less intense monitoring of the child's physical condition; and (4) selection of an appropriate room, such as one that is close to the nursing station, and a compatible roommate.

Key Points

- Children are particularly vulnerable to the stressors of illness and hospitalization because stress represents a change from the usual state of health and routine and because they possess limited coping mechanisms.
- The three phases of separation anxiety are protest, despair, and detachment.
- Feelings of loss of control are caused by unfamiliar environmental stimuli, physical restriction, altered routine, and dependency.
- Fear of bodily pain may be manifested in the following ways: infants—facial expressions, body movements: toddlers-intense emotional upset, physical resistance; preschoolers—aggression, verbal expression, dependency; school-age children—precise verbalization of pain, passive requests for support or help, procrastination technique; adolescents—self-control, limited movement.
- Because of their separation from significant persons, children who are hospitalized may lack the opportunity to form new attachments in the strange environment of the hospital and exhibit negative behaviors after discharge.
- Nursing care of the child in the hospital is aimed at preventing or minimizing separation, decreasing loss of control, minimizing fear of bodily injury, assessing and managing pain, promoting normal development, using play/expressive activities to lessen stress, and maximizing the potential benefits of hospitalization.
- Pain assessment includes questioning the child, using pain rating scales, evaluating behavior, securing parents' involvement, taking the cause of the pain into account, and taking action. Pain management should incorporate both pharmacologic and nonpharmacologic methods.
- The nurse can maximize potential benefits of hospitalization by fostering parent-child relations, providing educational opportunities, promoting self-mastery, and encouraging socialization.
- Family reactions are influenced by the seriousness of the illness, experience with illness or hospitalization and diagnostic or therapeutic procedures, available support systems, personal ego strengths, coping abilities, presence of additional stressors, cultural and religious beliefs, and family communication patterns.
- Fear of contracting illness, their younger age, a close relationship with the ill sibling, substitute child care, minimum explanation of the illness, and perceived changes in parenting all increase the deleterious effects of a brother's or sister's illness and hospitalization on siblings.
- Nursing care of the family involves listening to parents' verbal and nonverbal messages; providing clergy support; accepting cultural, socioeconomic, and ethnic values; giving information to families and siblings; and preparing for discharge and home care.
- Admission to an outpatient setting, emergency department isolation room, or intensive care unit requires additional intervention strategies to meet the child's and family's needs.

References

Acute Pain Management Guideline Panel: *Acute pain management in infants, children and adolescents,* AHCPR Pub. No. 92-0019, Rockville, MD, 1992, Agency for Health Care Policy and Research, Public Health Service, US Department of Health and Human Services.

Algren JT, Algren CL: Management of procedural and perioperative pain in children. In Weiner R, editor: *Pain management: a practical guide for clinicians,* Boca Raton, FL, 1998, St Lucie Press.

Algren JT et al: Efficacy and safety of morphine administered by patient-, parent-, or nurse-controlled analgesia in children, *Anesthesiology* 89:A1003, 1998 (abstract).

American Pain Society: *Principles of analgesic use in the treatment of acute pain and chronic cancer pain,* ed 4, Skokie, IL, 1999, The Society.

American Society of Addiction Medicine: *Public policy statement on the rights and responsibilities of physicians in the use of opioids for the treatment of pain,* April 16, 1997.

American Society of Pain Management Nurses: ASPMN position statement: use of placebos for pain management, *Ostomy Wound Manage* 44(2):56-57, 1998.

Ashenberg MD et al: Easing the wait: development of a pager program for families, *Pediatr Nurs* 22(2):103-107, 1996.

Bossert E: Factors influencing the coping of hospitalized school-age children, *J Pediatr Nurs* 9(5):299-306, 1994a.

Bossert E: Stress appraisals of hospitalized school-age children, *Child Health Care* 23(1):33-49, 1994b.

Boughton K et al: Impact of research on pediatric pain assessment and outcomes, *Pediatr Nurs* 24(1):31-35, 62, 1998.

Boyd J, Hunsberger M: Chronically ill children coping with repeated hospitalizations: their perceptions and suggested interventions, *J Pediatr Nurs* 13(6):330-342, 1998.

Bracht M et al: Initiation and maintenance of a hospital-based parent group for parents of premature infants: key factors for success, *Neonatal Network* 17(3):33-37, 1998.

Brewer S, Lambert C: Preparing children for same day surgery: innovative approaches, *J Pediatr Nurs* 12(4):257-259, 1997.

Britton LJ, Johnston JD: Dependent on technology: a child grows up hospitalized, *Pediatr Nurs* 19(6):579-584, 1993.

Broome M, Rehwaldt M, Fogg L: Relationships between cognitive behavioral techniques, temperament, observed distress, and pain reports in children and adolescents during lumbar puncture, *J Pediatr Nurs* 13:48-54, 1998.

Broome M et al: Children's medical fears, coping behaviors, and pain perceptions during a lumbar puncture, *Oncol Nurs Forum* 17(3):361-367, 1990.

Broome M et al: Pediatric pain practices: a national survey of health professionals, *J Pain Symptom Manage* 11(5):312-320, 1996.

Bruce B, Ritchie J: Nurses' practices and perceptions of family centered care, *J Pediatr Nurs* 12(4):214-222, 1997.

Carson D, Gravley J, Council J: Children's pre-hospitalization conceptions of illness, cognitive development, and personal adjustment, *Child Health Care* 21(2):103-110, 1992.

Clatworthy S, Simon K, Tiedeman ME: Child drawing: hospital—an instrument designed to measure the emotional status of hospitalized school-aged children, *J Pediatr Nurs* 14(1):2-9, 1999.

Cohen Reis E, Holubkov R: Vapocoolant spray is equally effective as EMLA cream in reducing immunization pain in school-aged children, *Pediatrics* 100(6):E5, 1997.

Collins J: Intractable cancer pain in children, *Child Adolesc Psychiatr Clin* 6(4):879-888, 1997.

Craft MJ: Siblings of hospitalized children: assessment and intervention, *J Pediatr Nurs* 8(5):289-297, 1993.

Fernandez C, Pyesmany A, Stutzer C: Alternative therapies in childhood cancer, *N Engl J Med* 340(7):569-570, 1999.

Gillis A: Hospital preparation: the children's story, *Child Health Care* 19(1):19-27, 1990.

Gordon M: *Nursing diagnosis: process and application,* ed 3, St Louis, 1994, Mosby.

Gordon M: *Manual of nursing diagnosis: 1995-1996,* St Louis, 1995, Mosby.

Graff KJ, Kennedy RM, Jaffe DM: Conscious sedation for pediatric orthopaedic emergencies, *Pediatr Emerg Care* 12(1):31-35, 1996.

Hart D, Bossert E: Self-reported fears of hospitalized school-age children, *J Pediatr Nurs* 9(2):83-90, 1994.

Hazinski MF: *Manual of pediatric critical care,* St Louis, 1999, Mosby.

Hornick R: Discharge teams. In Gunter K, Manago R, editors: *Beyond discharge: interdisciplinary perspectives for transitioning children with complex medical needs from hospital to home,* Bethesda, MD, 1996, Association for the Care of Children's Health.

IOMED, Inc: *Iontocaine package insert,* Salt Lake City, UT, 1996, IOMED, Inc.

Jacobson SJ et al: Randomised trial of oral morphine for painful episodes of sickle-cell disease in children, *Lancet* 350(9088):1358-1361, 1997.

Johnson A, Lindschau A: Staff attitudes toward parent participation in the care of children who are hospitalized, *Pediatr Nurs* 22(2):99-102,1996.

Joint Commission on Accreditation of Healthcare Organizations: *AMH92 accreditation manual for hospitals,* Chicago, 1999, The Commission.

Kart T, Christrup LL, Rasmussen M: Recommended use of morphine in neonates, infants and children based on a literature review. I. Pharmacokinetics, *Paediatr Anesth* 7(1):5-11, 1997.

Kauffmann E et al: Stress-point intervention for parents of children hospitalized with chronic conditions, *Pediatr Nurs* 24(4):362-366, 1998.

Keck J et al: Reliability and validity of the FACES and Word Descriptor scales to measure procedural pain, *J Pediatr Nurs* 11(6):368-374, 1996.

Kussman BD, Sethna NF: Pethidine-associated seizure in a healthy adolescent receiving pethidine for postoperative pain control, *Paediatr Anaesth* 8:349-352, 1998.

Lipson J, Dibble S, Minarik P: *Culture and nursing care: a pocket guide,* San Francisco, 1996, UCSF Nursing Press.

Mader TJ, Playe SJ, Garb JL: Reducing the pain of local anesthetic infiltration: warming and buffering have a synergistic effect, *Ann Emerg Med* 23(3):550-554, 1994.

Marcantonio ER et al: The relationship of postoperative delirium with psychoactive medications, *JAMA* 272(19):1518-1522, 1994.

Mayhew JF et al: Low-dose caudal morphine for postoperative analgesia in infants and children: a report of 500 cases, *J Clin Anesth* 7(8):640-642, 1995.

McCaffery M, Pasero C: *Pain: a clinical manual,* ed 2, St Louis, 1999, Mosby.

Melnyk B, Alpert-Gillis L: The COPE Program: a strategy to improve outcomes of critically ill young children and their parents, *Pediatr Nurs* 24(6):521-527, 1998.

Moenkhoff M et al: Parental attitude towards alternative medicine in the paediatric intensive care unit, *Eur J Pediatr* 158(1):12-17, 1999.

Orem D: *Nursing concepts of practice,* ed 5, New York, 1995, Mosby.

Pasero C: Epidural analgesia in children, *Am J Nurs* 99(5):20, 1999.

Pasero C: Pain control: reality check on placebos, *Am J Nurs* 95(8):20, 1995.

Pate J et al: Childhood medical experience and temperament as predictors of adult functioning in medical situations, *Child Health Care* 25(4):281-298, 1996.

Rasmussen G: Epidural and spinal anesthesia and analgesia. In Deshpande J, Tobias J, editors: *Pediatric pain handbook,* St Louis, 1996, Mosby.

Reisine T, Pasternak G: Opioid analgesics and antagonists. In Hardman G, Limbird LM, editors: *Goodman and Gilman's the pharmacological basis of therapeutics,* ed 9, New York, 1996, McGraw-Hill.

Remmel M: Don't assume all parents want to be involved, *RN* 60(9):9, 1997 (letter).

Riemondy S et al: Nurse controlled analgesia: a new method of pediatric pain control, *J Pain Symptom Manage* 6(3):160, 1991 (abstract).

Santelli B, Turnbull A, Higgins C: Parent to parent support and health care, *Pediatr Nurs* 23(3):303-306, 1997.

Schepp K: Correlates of mothers who prefer control over their hospitalized child's care, *J Pediatr Nurs* 7(2):83-89, 1992.

Scott LD: Perceived needs of parents of critically ill children, *J Soc Pediatr Nurses* 3(1):4-12, 1998.

Simon K: Perceived stress of nonhospitalized children during the hospitalization of a sibling, *J Pediatr Nurs* 8(5):298-304, 1993.

Snowdon A, Kane D: Parental needs following the discharge of a hospitalized child, *Pediatr Nurs* 21(5):425-428, 1995.

Spiegel D, Stroud P, Fyfe A: Complementary medicine, *West J Med* 168(4)241-247, 1998.

Stepanek JS, Ahmann E: Parent-professional collaboration when hospital visits are infrequent, *Pediatr Nurs* 21(5):466-468, 1995.

Stewart E, Algren C, Arnold S: Preparing children for a surgical experience, *Todays OR Nurse* 16(2):9-14, 1994.

Stuber M et al: Predictors of posttraumatic stress symptoms in childhood cancer survivors, *Pediatrics* 100(6):958-964, 1997.

Tamowski K, Brown R: Pediatric pain. In Ammerman R, Hersen M, editors: *Handbook of child behavior therapy in the psychiatric setting,* New York, 1995, John Wiley & Sons.

Tesler M, Holzemer W, Savedra M: Pain behaviors: postsurgical responses of children and adolescents, *J Pediatr Nurs* 13(1):41-47, 1998.

Van Cleve L, Johnson L, Pothier P: Pain responses of hospitalized infants and children to venipuncture and intravenous cannulation, *J Pediatr Nurs* 11:161-168, 1996.

Vessey J, Carlson K: Nonpharmacological interventions to use with children in pain, *Issues Compr Pediatr Nurs* 19:169-182, 1996.

Walker M, Wong DL: A battle plan for patients in pain, *Am J Nurs* 91(5):32-36, 1991.

Webb C, Paarlberg J, Sussman M: The use of a PCA device by parents or nurses for postoperative pain in children with cerebral palsy, *J Pain Symptom Manage* 6(3):160, 1991 (abstract).

Wells PW et al: Growing up in the hospital. I. Let's focus on the child, *Pediatr Nurs* 9(2):66-73, 1994.

West N et al: Measuring pain in pediatric oncology ICU patients, *J Pediatr Oncol Nurs* 1(2):64-68, 1994.

Wilson A, Yorker B: Fears of medical events among school-age children with emotional disorders, parents and health care providers, *Issues Ment Health Nurs* 18:57-71, 1997.

Wong DL, Baker C: Pain in children: comparison of assessment scales, *Pediatr Nurs* 14(1):9-17, 1988.

Wong DL, Pasero CL: Pain control: reducing the pain of lidocaine, *Am J Nurs* 97:17-18, 1997.

Woodgate R, Krisjanson L: "Getting better from my hurts": toward a model of the young child's pain experience, *J Pediatr Nurs* 11(4):233-242, 1996.

Yaster M et al: *Pediatric pain management and sedation handbook,* St Louis, 1997, Mosby.

CHAPTER

45

Pediatric Variations of Nursing Interventions

http://www.harcourthealth.com/MERLIN/Wong/maternal/

Learning Objectives

On completion of this chapter the reader will be able to:

- Identify those instances in which informed consent is required and those in which minors may be considered emancipated.
- Formulate general guidelines for preparing children for procedures, including surgery.
- Implement play in therapeutic procedures.
- List general strategies for enhancing compliance in children and families.
- Outline general hygiene and care procedures for hospitalized children.
- Implement feeding techniques that encourage food and fluid intake.
- Describe methods of reducing the temperature of the child with fever or hyperthermia.
- Describe systems that can be used for infection control.
- Describe safe methods of administering oral, parenteral, rectal, optic, otic, and nasal medications to children.
- Identify nursing responsibilities in maintaining fluid balance.
- Demonstrate correct procedures for postural drainage and tracheostomy care.
- Describe the procedures involved in providing nutrition via gavage, gastrostomy, and parenteral routes.
- Describe the procedures involved in administering an enema and ostomy care to children.

GENERAL CONCEPTS RELATED TO PEDIATRIC PROCEDURES

Informed Consent

Informed consent refers to the legal and ethical requirement that the patient clearly, fully, and completely understand the proposed medical treatment to be performed, including significant risks associated with the treatment. The patient must also be informed of alternative treatments that could be offered, including their benefits and risks; and the risks of nontreatment, before giving informed consent. To obtain valid informed consent, the following three conditions must be met:

1. The person must be capable of giving consent; he or she must be over the age of majority (usually age 18) and must be considered competent (i.e., possess the mental capacity to make choices and to understand their consequences).
2. The person must receive the information needed to make an intelligent decision.
3. The person must act voluntarily when exercising freedom of choice without force, fraud, deceit, duress, or other forms of constraint or coercion.

Because of the numerous variations of the laws and institutional policies within the United States, the following discussion of informed consent is presented in general terms and is not to be interpreted as legal advice. Although informing patients of the risks, benefits, and alternatives of a procedure is the physician's responsibility, nurses commonly are responsible for securing the person's signature on a written consent form. In caring for children, special dilemmas may arise regarding who may sign the consent for treatment when parental consent is not available. *The age of majority* is especially important when caring for adolescents, and *competence* is a key issue in decisions involving minors who are retarded or otherwise mentally incapacitated. Also, the judicial system may intervene in cases where the parents' views and the child's best interests conflict. Consequently, nurses need to be familiar with the issues involved in this highly significant and complex subject and must keep current on legal aspects of practice within their community.

Requirements for Obtaining Informed Consent

Written informed consent of the parent or legal guardian is usually required for medical or surgical treatment, including many diagnostic procedures. One blanket consent is not sufficient. Separate informed permissions must be obtained for each surgical or diagnostic procedure, including:

- Major surgery
- Minor surgery (e.g., cutdown, biopsy, dental extraction, suturing a laceration [especially one that may have a cosmetic effect], removal of a cyst, and closed reduction of a fracture)
- Diagnostic tests with an element of risk (e.g., bronchoscopy, needle biopsy, angiography, electroencephalogram, lumbar puncture, cardiac catheterization, ventriculography, and bone marrow aspiration)
- Medical treatments with an element of risk (e.g., blood transfusion, thoracentesis or paracentesis, radiation therapy, and shock therapies)

Situations such as the following are not directly related to medical treatment but also require parental consent:

- Taking photographs for medical, educational, or other public use
- Removal of the child from the health care institution against the advice of the physician
- Postmortem examinations, except in unexplained deaths, such as sudden infant death, violent death, or suspected suicide
- Examination of medical records by unauthorized persons, such as attorneys or insurance representatives (family members have a legal right to medical records)

The need for informed consent is also an issue with proposed treatments or research involving children with a mental age of 7 years or older. *Assent* (usually verbal agreement) requires that the child be informed about the proposed treatment or research and agree or concur with the decisions made by the person(s) who can give informed consent. Multiple methods should be used to explain the study, including age-appropriate methods (e.g., videotapes, peer discussion, diagrams, and written materials). An assent form should be provided to each child to sign, and the child should keep a copy (Broome, 1999). By including children in the decision-making process and gaining their acceptance, children are treated with respect. Assent is not a legal requirement but is an ethical one to protect the rights of children. The nurse, whether acting as a researcher, assisting in research, or caring for the child, must ultimately have the best interest of the child in mind (Algren and Schwartz, 1998).

Eligibility for Giving Informed Consent. In most situations the parent or legal guardian gives informed consent; however, problems may arise when parents are not available to give informed consent, the child is a borderline or emancipated minor, or the parents neglect or refuse care for their minor children. Consent from either divorced parent is sufficient; the consent of both parents is generally not required (Bernardo and Lesniak, 1998).

Informed Consent of Parents or Legal Guardians. Parents have full responsibility for the care and rearing of their minor children, including legal control over them. Therefore as long as children are minors, their parents or legal guardians are required to give informed consent before medical treatment is rendered or any procedure is performed on them. Parents also have a right to withdraw consent later.

Evidence of Consent. A signed consent form is only evidence that the process of informed consent has occurred; it is not legally required, although it may be an institutional policy. Verbal consent is also evidence of the process (Cushing, 1991). For example, when parents are unavailable to sign consent forms, verbal consent may be obtained via telephone. Verbal consent may also be obtained from parents who are unable to sign (e.g., because of injury). It is good risk management to have a witness to a parent's or guardian's verbal consent. Another nurse may be present or listening on a telephone extension. Both nurses record that informed consent was given and the name, address, and relationship of the person giving consent, together with their signatures indicating that they witnessed the consent.

Informed Consent of Mature and Emancipated Minors. State laws differ with regard to the so-called age of majority. Although some variation still exists, children become adults on their eighteenth birthday in most states. Competent adults can give informed consent on their own behalf. Nonetheless, some courts have permitted minors to consent to their treatment based on the *mature minors' doctrine,* which permits minors to give consent even though they are not technically adults as long as they understand the consequences of their decisions. The age for mature minors varies between 14 and 18 years among the states (Sullivan, 1993). For example, statutes in many states permit minors to give consent on their own behalf to certain treatments, such as for sexually transmitted infections, contraceptive services, pregnancy, or drug or alcohol abuse.

An *emancipated minor* is one who is legally under the age of majority but is recognized as having the legal capacity of an adult under circumstances prescribed by state law, such as pregnancy, marriage, high school graduation, living independently, or military service.

Consent to abortion is more complex. The issue of parental notification before or after an abortion is still undecided, although several states have enacted laws stating that minors seeking abortions must involve their parents or obtain court permission (Johannsen, 1995). A woman's right to abortion is an extremely controversial legal and moral issue in the United States.

Treatment without Parental Consent. Exceptions to requiring parental consent before treating minor children occur in situations in which children need prompt medical or surgical treatment and a parent is either not readily available to give consent or refuses to give consent. In the absence of parents or legal guardians, some providers permit persons in charge of the child to give informed consent for treatment. In emergencies, consent is not needed; it is implied according to the law (Sullivan, 1993). Emergencies include danger to life or the possibility of permanent injury.

Refusal to give consent can occur when the treatment, such as blood transfusions, conflicts with the parents' religious beliefs. All states recognize such exceptions and have statutory procedures to permit treatment if the life or health of such a minor is in jeopardy or if delayed treatment would create a risk to the minor's health. The state is also able to intervene in situations that jeopardize the health and welfare of children, as in cases in which parents neglect or impose excessive or improper punishment on a child. Most communities have procedures by which custody of the child can be transferred to a governmental or a private agency when parental neglect or abuse can be proved.

Preparation for Procedures

For most procedures, no special physical preparation is needed, and the focus of care is psychologic preparation of the child and family (see next section). However, some procedures require physical preparation before the procedure, such as cleansing and shaving of the skin before surgery. One area of special concern is the administration of appropriate sedation and/or analgesia before stressful procedures (see p. 1129). The drug is given before the procedure to allow time for the medication to reach its peak effect. Whenever possible, the intravenous (IV) (through an existing infusion), oral, or rectal route is used rather than the intramuscular route because children dislike injections. Some institutions are using short-acting anesthetics (e.g., ketamine or propofol) or potent analgesics (e.g., fentanyl) to eliminate the pain and trauma associated with treatments such as bone marrow tests, lumbar punctures, burn débridement, and suturing. (See also Pain Management, Chapter 44.)

Psychologic Preparation. Preparing children for procedures decreases their anxiety, promotes their cooperation, supports their coping skills and may teach them new ones, and facilitates a feeling of mastery in experiencing a potentially stressful event. Many institutions have developed preadmission teaching programs designed to educate the pediatric patient and family by offering hands-on experience with hospital equipment, the procedure preformed, and departments they will visit (Algren, Ireland, and Stewart, 1998). Preparatory methods may be formal, such as group preparation for hospitalization. Most preparation strategies used by nurses are informal, focus on providing information about the experience, and are directed at stressful and/or painful procedures. In general, young children respond better to play materials, and older youngsters benefit more from viewing peer-modeling films (Bates and Broome, 1986). Especially for painful procedures, the most effective preparation includes the provision of sensory-procedural information and helping the child develop coping skills, such as imagery, distraction, or relaxation (Broome, Rehwaldt, and Fogg, 1998).

General guidelines for preparing children for procedures are described in Box 45-1, and age-specific guidelines that consider children's developmental needs and cognitive abilities are presented in Box 45-2. In addition to these suggestions, nurses should consider the child's temperament, existing coping strategies, and previous experiences in individualizing the preparatory process. Children who are distractible and highly active, as well as those who are "slow to warm up," may need individualized sessions that are shorter for the active child but more slowly paced for the shy child. Youngsters who tend to cope well may need more emphasis on using their present skills, whereas those who appear to cope less adequately can benefit from more time devoted to simple coping strategies such as relaxing, breathing, counting, squeezing a hand, or singing.

Children also are different in their "information-seeking dimension"; some want and actively solicit information about the intended procedure, whereas others characteristically avoid information.

Box 45-1

General Guidelines for Preparing Children for Procedures

Determine details of exact procedure to be performed.
Review parents' and child's present level of understanding.
Plan actual teaching based on child's developmental age and existing level of knowledge.
Incorporate parents in the teaching if they desire, especially if they plan to participate in care.
Inform parents of their role during procedure, such as standing near child's head or in child's line of vision and talking softly to child.
While preparing child and family, allow for ample discussion to prevent information overload and ensure adequate feedback.
Use concrete, not abstract, terms and visual aids to describe procedure. For example, use a simple line drawing of a boy or girl (Fig. 45-1), and mark the body part that will be involved in the procedure. Use nonthreatening but realistic models.*
Emphasize that no other body part will be involved.
If the body part is associated with a specific function, stress the change or noninvolvement of that ability (e.g., following tonsillectomy, child can still speak).
Use words appropriate to child's level of understanding (a rule of thumb for number of words is age in years plus 1).
Avoid words and phrases with dual meanings (see Guidelines box, p. 1125) unless child understands such words.
Clarify all unfamiliar words (e.g., "Anesthesia is a *special* sleep").
Emphasize sensory aspects of procedure—what child will feel, see, smell, and touch and what child can do during procedure (e.g., lie still, count out loud, squeeze a hand, hug a doll).
Allow child to practice those procedures that will require cooperation (e.g., turning, deep breathing, using an incentive spirometer or mask).
Introduce anxiety-laden information last (e.g., starting an intravenous line).
Be honest with child about unpleasant aspects of a procedure but avoid creating undue concern. When discussing that a procedure may be uncomfortable, state that it feels differently to different people and have child describe how it felt.
Emphasize end of procedure and any pleasurable events afterward (e.g., going home, seeing parents).
Stress positive benefits of procedure (e.g., "After your tonsils are fixed, you won't have as many sore throats").

*Soft-sculptured dolls and customized adapters and overlays for preparing children and families about procedures and as teaching models for technical care are available from Legacy Products, Inc., P.O. Box 267, Cambridge City, IN 47327; 1-800-238-7951; e-mail: legacyez2b@aol.com; website: www.legacyproductsinc.com.

The exact timing of the preparation for a procedure varies with the child's age and the type of procedure. There are no exact guidelines to govern timing, but in general the younger the child, the closer the explanation should be to the actual procedure to prevent undue fantasizing and worrying. With complex procedures, more time may be needed for assimilation of information, especially with older children. For example, the explanation for an injection can immediately precede the procedure

Box 45-2

Age-Specific Guidelines for Preparing Children for Procedures Based on Developmental Characteristics

INFANT: DEVELOPING A SENSE OF TRUST AND SENSORIMOTOR THOUGHT

Attachment to Parent

*Involve parent in procedure if desired.
Keep parent in infant's line of vision.
If parent is unable to be with infant, place familiar object with infant (e.g., stuffed toy).

Stranger Anxiety

*Have usual caregivers perform or assist with procedure.
Make advances slowly and in nonthreatening manner.
*Limit number of strangers entering room during procedure.

Sensorimotor Phase of Learning

During procedure use sensory soothing measures (e.g., stroking skin, talking softly, giving pacifier).
*Use analgesics (e.g., local anesthetic, intravenous opioid) to control discomfort.
Cuddle and hug child after stressful procedure; encourage parent to comfort child.

Increased Muscle Control

Expect older infants to resist.
Restrain adequately.
Keep harmful objects out of reach.

Memory for Past Experiences

Realize that older infants may associate objects, places, or persons with prior painful experiences and will cry and resist at the sight of them.
*Keep frightening objects out of view.
*Perform painful procedures in a separate room, not in crib (or bed).
*Use nonintrusive procedures whenever possible (e.g., axillary or tympanic temperatures, oral medications).

Imitation of Gestures

Model desired behavior (e.g., opening mouth).

TODDLER: DEVELOPING A SENSE OF AUTONOMY AND SENSORIMOTOR TO PREOPERATIONAL THOUGHT

Use same approaches as for infant in addition to the following:

Egocentric Thought

Explain procedure in relation to what child will see, hear, taste, smell, and feel.
Emphasize those aspects of procedure that require cooperation (e.g., lying still).
Tell child it's OK to cry, yell, or use other means to express discomfort verbally.

Negative Behavior

Expect treatments to be resisted; child may try to run away.
Use firm, direct approach.
Ignore temper tantrums.
Use distraction techniques (e.g., singing a song *with* a child).
Restrain adequately.

Animism

Keep frightening objects out of view (young children believe objects have lifelike qualities and can harm them).

Limited Language Skills

Communicate using behaviors.
Use a few, simple terms familiar to child.
Give one direction at a time (e.g., "Lie down," then "Hold my hand").
Use small replicas of equipment; allow child to handle equipment.
Use play; demonstrate on doll but avoid child's favorite doll, since child may think doll is really "feeling" procedure.
Prepare parents separately to avoid child's misinterpreting words.

Limited Concept of Time

Prepare child shortly or immediately before procedure.
Keep teaching sessions short (about 5 to 10 minutes).
Have preparations completed before involving child in procedure.
Have extra equipment nearby (e.g., alcohol swabs, new needle, adhesive bandages) to avoid delays.
Tell child when procedure is completed.

Striving for Independence

Allow choices whenever possible but realize that child may still be resistant and negative.
Allow child to participate in care and to help whenever possible (e.g., drink medicine from a cup, hold a dressing).

PRESCHOOLER: DEVELOPING A SENSE OF INITIATIVE AND PREOPERATIONAL THOUGHT

Egocentric

Explain procedure in simple terms and in relation to how it affects child (as with toddler, stress sensory aspects).
Demonstrate use of equipment.
Allow child to play with miniature or actual equipment.
Encourage "playing out" experience on a doll both before and after procedure to clarify misconceptions.
Use neutral words to describe the procedure (see Guidelines box, p. 1125).

Increased Language Skills

Use verbal explanation but avoid overestimating child's comprehension of words.
Encourage child to verbalize ideas and feelings.

Concept of Time and Frustration Tolerance Still Limited

Implement same approaches as for toddler but may plan longer teaching session (10 to 15 minutes); may divide information into more than one session.

Illness and Hospitalization May Be Viewed as Punishment

Clarify why each procedure is performed; a child will find it difficult to understand how medicine can make him or her feel better and can taste bad at the same time.

*Applies to any age.

Continued

Box 45-2

Age-Specific Guidelines for Preparing Children for Procedures Based on Developmental Characteristics—cont'd

Ask child thoughts regarding why a procedure is performed.
State directly that procedures are never a form of punishment.

Animism

Keep equipment out of sight, except when shown to or used on child.

Fears of Bodily Harm, Intrusion, and Castration

Point out on drawing, doll, or child where procedure is performed.
Emphasize that no other body part will be involved.
Use nonintrusive procedures whenever possible (e.g., axillary temperatures, oral medication).
Apply an adhesive bandage over puncture site.
Encourage parental presence.
Realize that procedures involving genitalia provoke anxiety.
Allow child to wear underpants with gown.
Explain unfamiliar situations, especially noises or lights.

Striving for Initiative

Involve child in care whenever possible (e.g., hold equipment, remove dressing).
Give choices whenever possible but avoid excessive delays.
Praise child for helping and attempting to cooperate; never shame child for lack of cooperation.

SCHOOL-AGE CHILD: DEVELOPING A SENSE OF INDUSTRY AND CONCRETE THOUGHT

Increased Language Skills; Interest in Acquiring Knowledge

Explain procedures using correct scientific/medical terminology.
Explain reason for procedure using simple diagrams of anatomy and physiology.
Explain function and operation of equipment in concrete terms.
Allow child to manipulate equipment; use doll or another person as model to practice using equipment whenever possible (doll play may be considered "childish" by older school-age child).
Allow time before and after procedure for questions and discussion.

Improved Concept of Time

Plan for longer teaching sessions (about 20 minutes).
Prepare in advance of procedure.

Increased Self-Control

Gain child's cooperation.
Tell child what is expected.
Suggest ways of maintaining control (e.g., deep breathing, relaxation, counting).

Striving for Industry

Allow responsibility for simple tasks (e.g., collecting specimens).
Include child in decision making (e.g., time of day to perform procedure, preferred site).
Encourage active participation (e.g., removing dressings, handling equipment, opening packages).

Developing Relationships with Peers

May prepare two or more children for same procedure or encourage one to help prepare another peer.
Provide privacy from peers during procedure to maintain self-esteem.

ADOLESCENT: DEVELOPING A SENSE OF IDENTITY AND ABSTRACT THOUGHT

Increasingly Capable of Abstract Thought and Reasoning

Supplement explanations with reasons why procedure is necessary or beneficial.
Explain long-term consequences of procedures.
Realize that adolescent may fear death, disability, or other potential risks.
Encourage questioning regarding fears, options, and alternatives.

Conscious of Appearance

Provide privacy.
Discuss how procedure may affect appearance (e.g., scar) and what can be done to minimize it.
Emphasize any physical benefits of procedure.

Concerned More with Present Than with Future

Realize that immediate effects of procedure are more significant than future benefits.

Striving for Independence

Involve in decision making and planning (e.g., choice of time; place; individuals present during procedure, such as parents; clothing to wear).
Impose as few restrictions as possible.
Suggest methods of maintaining control.
Accept regression to more childish methods of coping.
Realize that adolescent may have difficulty in accepting new authority figures and may resist complying with procedures.

Developing Peer Relationships and Group Identity

Same as for school-age child but assumes even greater significance.
Allow adolescents to talk with other adolescents who have had the same procedure.

for all ages, but preparation for surgery may begin the day before for young children and a few days before for older children, although older children's preferences should be elicited (see Preparation for Hospitalization, Chapter 44).

Establish Trust and Provide Support. The nurse who has spent time with and who has established a positive relationship with a child will usually find it easier to gain the child's cooperation. If the relationship is based on trust, the child will associate the nurse with caregiving activities that give comfort and pleasure most of the time and not regard the nurse as someone who brings discomfort and stress. If the nurse does not know the child, it is best that the nurse be introduced by another staff person whom the child trusts. The first visit with the child should not include any painful procedure and ideally should focus on

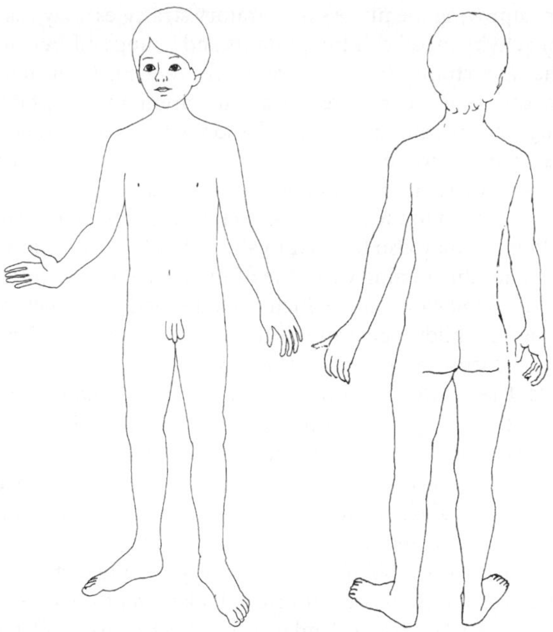

FIG. 45-1 • Examples of line drawings to be used in preparing child for procedures.

Guidelines

SELECTING NONTHREATENING WORDS OR PHRASES

Words/phrases to avoid	Suggested substitutions
Shot, bee sting, stick	Medicine under the skin
Organ	Special place in body
Test	See how (specify body part) is working
Incision	Special opening
Edema	Puffiness
Stretcher, gurney	Rolling bed
Stool	Child's usual term
Dye	Special medicine
Pain	Hurt, discomfort, "owie," "boo-boo"
Deaden	Numb, make sleepy
Cut, fix	Make better
Take (as in "take your temperature" and "take your blood pressure")	See how warm you are Check your pressure; hug your arm
Put to sleep, anesthesia	Special sleep
Catheter	Tube
Monitor	TV screen
Electrodes	Stickers, ticklers
Specimen	Sample

the child first, then on the explanation of the procedure. When talking with the child, the nurse uses the same guidelines for communicating with children that are discussed in Chapter 34.

Parental Support. Children need support during procedures, and for young children the greatest source of comfort is the parents. However, controversy exists regarding the role parents should assume during the procedure, especially if discomfort is involved. Nurses need to consider the issues in deciding whether parental presence is beneficial. The parents' preferences for assisting, observing, or waiting outside the room should be assessed, as well as the child's preference for parental presence. The child's choice should be respected. Parents who want to stay should be educated, because they do not automatically know what to do, where to be, and what to say to help their child through the procedure (Acute Pain Management Guideline Panel, 1992). Simple instructions such as clarifying where parents can stay in the room and positioning them where they have eye contact with the child provide support and lessen anxiety. Parents who do not want to be present or participate are supported in their decision and encouraged to remain close by so that they can be available to console the child immediately after the procedure. Parents should also know that someone will be with their child to provide support. Ideally, this person should inform the parents after the procedure about how the child did.

Provide an Explanation. Children need an explanation for anything that involves them directly. Before performing a procedure, the nurse explains to children what is to be done and what is expected of them. The explanation should be short, simple, and appropriate to the child's level of comprehension. Long explanations are not necessary and may only increase anxiety in a small child. This is especially true regarding painful procedures. When explaining the procedure to parents with the child present, the nurse uses language appropriate to the child because unfamiliar words can be misunderstood (Guidelines box). If the parents need additional preparation, this is done in an area away from the child. Teaching sessions are planned at times most conducive to the child's learning (e.g., after a rest period) and for the usual span of attention.

Special equipment is not necessary for preparing a child, but for young children who cannot yet think in concepts, using objects to supplement verbal explanation is important. Allowing children to handle actual items that will be used in their care, such as a stethoscope, sphygmomanometer, or oxygen mask, helps them to develop familiarity with these items and to reduce the threat often associated with their use. Miniature versions of hospital items such as gurneys and x-ray and intravenous equipment can be used to explain what the children can expect and permit them to safely experience situations that are unfamiliar and potentially frightening. Written and illustrated materials are also valuable aids to preparation.*

Performance of the Procedure. Supportive care continues during the procedure and can be a major factor in a child's ability to cooperate and achieve mastery. Before the procedure is begun, all equipment is assembled and the room is readied to prevent unnecessary delays and interruptions that only serve to increase the child's anxiety.

If at all possible, procedures are performed in a special treatment room rather than the child's hospital room. Traumatic procedures should never be performed in "safe" areas such as the playroom. If the procedure is lengthy, conversation that could be misinterpreted by the child is avoided. As the proce-

*Sources of preparatory materials include *Going to the Hospital* and *Going to the Doctor,* available from Family Communications, Inc., 4802 Fifth Ave., Pittsburgh, PA 15213; (412) 687-2990; *Hospital Friends,* available from the Centering Corporation, 1531 N. Saddle Creek Rd., Omaha, NE 68104; (402) 553-1200; and *Health, Illness, and Disability: A Guide to Books for Children and Young Adults,* available from Pediatric Projects, Inc., P.O. Box 571555, Tarzana, CA 91357-1555; 1-800-947-0947. Other resources include *Berenstein Bears Go to the Doctor* and *Berenstein Bears Visit the Dentist* (Random House), available in most bookstores.

dure is nearing completion, the nurse should inform the child that it is almost over in language that the child understands.

Expect Success. Nurses who approach children with confidence and who convey the impression that they expect to be successful are less likely to encounter difficulty. It is best to approach children as though cooperation is expected. Children sense anxiety in another and may respond to a perceived threat by striking out or with active resistance. Although some children will still exhibit such behavior, a firm approach with a positive attitude on the part of the nurse tends to convey a feeling of security to most children.

Involve the Child. As in any other aspect of care, involving children helps to gain their cooperation. Permitting them to make choices gives them some measure of control. However, a choice is given only in situations in which one is available. Asking children, "Do you want to take your medicine now?" or "I'm going to give you an injection now, okay?" leads them to believe that there is an option and provides them with the opportunity to legitimately refuse or delay the medication. This places the nurse in an awkward, if not impossible, position. It is much better to state firmly, "It's time to drink your medicine now." Children usually like to make choices, but the choice must be one that they may have (e.g., "It's time for your medicine. Do you want to drink it plain or with a little water?").

Many children respond to tactics that appeal to their maturity or courage. This approach also gives them a sense of participation and achievement. For example, preschool children will be proud that they can hold the dressing during the procedure or remove the tape. The same is true for the school-age child, who often cooperates with minimal resistance.

Provide Distraction. When children are occupied with some activity that interests them, they are less likely to focus on the procedure. For example, when an injection is given, it is helpful to give the child something to do or something on which to focus attention. For example, asking the child to point the toes inward and wiggle them not only helps relax the gluteal muscles, but also provides a diversion. Other strategies for diverting attention are to have the child tightly squeeze the hands of a parent or an assistant, count aloud, sing a familiar song such as a nursery rhyme, or verbally express discomfort. It can be helpful to have the child select and practice a coping technique before the procedure. Consider having the parent or some other supportive person, such as a child-life specialist, "coach" the child in learning and using the coping skill. For other interventions that may lessen discomfort, see Pain Management, Chapter 44.

Allow Expression of Feelings. The child is allowed to express feelings of anger, anxiety, fear, frustration, or any other emotion. It is natural for children to strike out in frustration or to try to avoid stress-provoking situations. The child needs to know that it is all right to cry. Behavior is the primary means of communication and coping for children and should be permitted unless it inflicts harm on them or those caring for them.

Postprocedural Support. After the procedure the child continues to need reassurance that he or she performed well and is accepted and loved. If the parents did not participate, the child is united with them as soon as possible so that they can provide comfort.

Encourage Expression of Feelings. Planned activity after the procedure is helpful in encouraging constructive expression of feelings. For verbal children, reviewing the details of the procedure can help clarify misconceptions and provide feedback for improving the nurse's preparatory strategies. Play is an excellent activity for all children. Infants and young children are given the opportunity for gross motor movement. Even older children can vent their anger and frustration in acceptable pounding or throwing activities. Play dough is a remarkably versatile medium for pounding and shaping. Dramatic play provides an outlet for anger and places the child in a position of control, in contrast to the position of helplessness in the real situation. Puppets may also be used to allow the child to communicate in a nonthreatening way. One of the most effective interventions is *therapeutic play,* which includes activities such as permitting the child to give an injection to a doll or stuffed toy to reduce the stress of injections (Fig. 45-2).

Praise the Child. Children need to hear from adults that they know the youngsters did the best they could in the situation, no matter how they behaved. It is important for children to know that their worth is not being judged on the basis of their behavior in a stressful situation. Reward systems, such as earning stars or tokens or saving the empty medicine cup as evidence of achievement, are often helpful. Children who require distasteful medications or injections over time can look with pride on a series of stars or stickers on a calendar, especially if an accumulated number represents a special privilege or reward.

Returning to the child a short while after the procedure helps the nurse to strengthen a supportive relationship. Relating with the child during a relaxed and nonstressful period allows him or her to see the nurse not only as someone associated with stressful situations but also as someone with whom to share pleasurable experiences.

Use of Play in Procedures. The use of play is an integral part of relationships with children. As such, its value in specific situations is discussed throughout this book, such as in Chapter 44, in relation to hospitalization. Nurses can easily include play activities as part of nursing care. Play can be used in teaching, for expression of feelings, or as a method to achieve a therapeutic goal. Consequently, it should be included in preparing children for and encouraging their cooperation during procedures. Play sessions after procedures can be structured, such as directed toward playing with syringes; or general, with a variety of equipment available for children to play with. Suggestions for incorporating play into nursing procedures and activities for the hospitalized child that facilitate learning and adjustment to a new situation are described in Box 45-3. Play

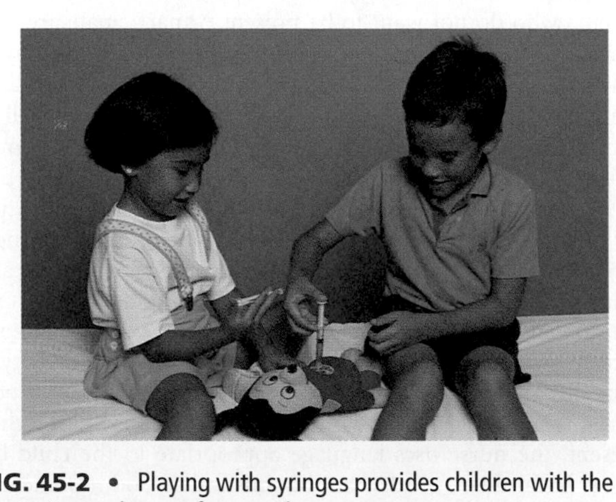

FIG. 45-2 • Playing with syringes provides children with the opportunity to play out fears and concerns.

Box 45-3
Play Activities for Specific Procedures

FLUID INTAKE
Make ice pops using child's favorite juice.
Cut gelatin into fun shapes.
Make a game out of taking a sip when turning page of a book or in games such as Simon Says.
Use small medicine cups; decorate the cups.
Color water with food coloring or powdered drink mix.
Have a tea party; pour at a small table.
Let child fill a syringe and squirt it into mouth or use it to fill small decorated cups.
Cut straws in half and place in a small container (much easier for child to suck liquid).
Decorate a straw: cut out small design with two holes and pass straw through; place small sticker on straw.
Use a "crazy" straw.
Make a "progress poster"; give rewards for drinking a predetermined quantity.

DEEP BREATHING
Blow bubbles with a bubble blower.
Blow bubbles with a straw (no soap).
Blow on a pinwheel, feather, whistle, harmonica, balloon, toy horn, party blower.
Practice band instruments.
Have blowing contest using balloons,* boats, cotton balls, feathers, marbles, Ping-Pong balls, pieces of paper; blow such objects on a table top over a goal line, over water, through an obstacle course, up in the air, against an opponent, or up and down a string.
Use blow bottles with colored water to transfer water from one side to the other.
Dramatize stories such as "I'll huff and puff and blow your house down" from the Three Little Pigs.
Do straw-blowing painting.
Take a deep breath and "blow out the candles" on a birthday cake.
Use a little paint brush to "paint" nails with water and blow nails dry.

RANGE OF MOTION AND USE OF EXTREMITIES
Throw beanbags at a fixed or moveable target or throw wadded-up paper into a wastebasket.
Touch or kick Mylar balloons held or hung in different positions (if child is in traction, hang balloon from a trapeze).
Play "tickle toes"; wiggle them on request.
Play Twister game or Simon Says.
Play pretend and guess games (e.g., imitate a bird, butterfly, or horse).
Have tricycle or wheelchair races in safe area.
Play kickball or throw ball with a soft foam ball in a safe area.
Position bed so that child must turn to view television or doorway.
Climb wall like a "spider."
Pretend to teach "aerobic" dancing or exercises; encourage parents to participate.
Encourage swimming if feasible.
Play video games or pinball (fine motor movement).
Play "hide and seek": hide toy somewhere in bed (or room if ambulatory) and have child find it using specified hand or foot.
Provide clay to mold with fingers.
Paint or draw on large sheets of paper placed on floor or wall.
Encourage combing own hair; play "beauty shop" with "customer" in different positions.

SOAKS
Play with small toys or objects (cups, syringes, soap dishes) in water.
Wash dolls or toys.
Bubbles may be added to bathwater if permissible; move bubbles to create shapes or "monsters."
Pick up marbles or pennies* from bottom of bath container.
Make designs with coins on bottom of container.
Pretend a boat is a submarine by keeping it immersed.
Read to child during soaks, sing with child, or play game, such as cards, checkers, or other board game (if both hands are immersed, move board pieces for child).
Sitz bath: give child something to listen to (music, stories) or look at (Viewmaster, book).
Punch holes in bottom of plastic cup, fill with water, and let it "rain" on child.

INJECTIONS
Let child handle syringe, vial, and alcohol swab, and give an injection to doll or stuffed animal.
Use syringes to decorate cookies with frosting, squirt paint, or target shoot into a container.
Draw a "magic circle" on area before injection; draw smiling face in circle after injection, but avoid drawing on puncture site.
Allow child to have a "collection" of syringes (without needles); make "wild" creative objects with syringes.
If multiple injections or venipunctures, make a "progress poster"; give rewards for predetermined number of injections.
Have child count to 10 or 15 during injection.

AMBULATION
Give child something to push.
  Toddler: push-pull toy
  School-age child: wagon or decorated IV stand
  Adolescent: a baby in a stroller or wheelchair
Have a parade; make hats, drums, etc.

EXTENDING ENVIRONMENT (E.G., FOR PATIENTS IN TRACTION)
Make bed into a pirate ship or airplane with decorations.
Put up mirrors so patient can see around room.
Move patient's bed frequently, especially to playroom, hallway, or outside.

*Small objects such as marbles or coins, as well as gloves or balloons, are unsafe for young children because of possible aspiration. Latex products also carry the risk of an allergic reaction.

can also be spontaneous at the bedside and does not always require many supplies or much nursing time. Small items such as finger puppets or a small bottle of bubbles can be kept in the nurse's pocket for immediate use.

Surgical Procedures

Preoperative Care. Children experiencing surgical procedures require both psychologic and physical preparation. In general, psychologic preparation is similar to that discussed for any procedure and may employ many of the same techniques used in preparing a child for hospitalization, such as films, books, play, and tours. However, some important differences exist. Even though children are asleep for the actual surgical intervention, they are subjected to numerous preoperative and postoperative procedures. Stress points before and after surgery include the admission, the blood test, injection of preoperative medication (if prescribed), the period before and during transport to the operating room, and the return from the postanesthesia care unit (PACU).

Psychologic intervention consisting of systematic preparation, rehearsal of the forthcoming events, and supportive care during times of stress (e.g., admission) has been shown to be more effective than a single-session preparation or consistent supportive care without systematic preparation and rehearsal. Play is always an effective strategy in preparing children, and increased familiarity with medical procedures decreases anxiety.

Although fear of anesthesia is thought to be a major concern among children, little evidence for this exists. One study of school-age children found that the most feared events were the injection and the mask on the face.

Parental presence during induction is becoming a more common practice, although few institutions endorse the policy (Fig. 45-3). Reports from parents who attend the induction are very favorable. Even though some may become anxious, most parents can control their anxiety, do not disrupt the induction, and support the child (Hall et al, 1995; LaRosa-Nash et al, 1995). Some concern surrounds the appropriateness of this practice for all parents.

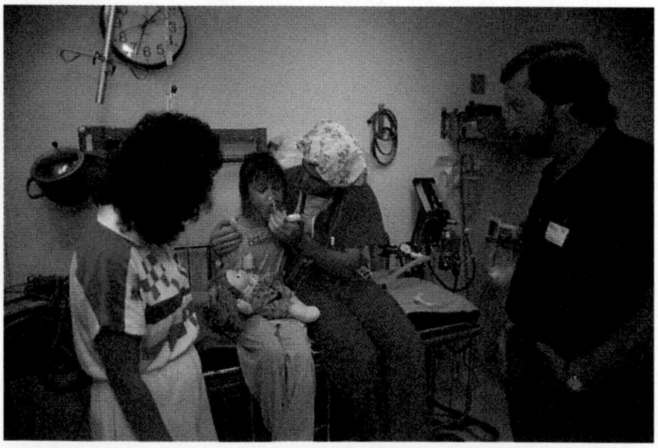

FIG. 45-3 • Parental presence during induction of anesthesia can minimize the child's and parents' anxiety during the preoperative period.

However, based on the parents' favorable response to the practice and most children's desire to have parents with them during any stressful procedure, a policy of offering parents the option of attending the induction, combined with a program that prepares them for what to expect and what is expected of them, is recommended. When parents choose not to or are not allowed to attend this induction, leaving a favorite possession with the child and uniting the child and parents as soon as possible after surgery (preferably in the PACU) are important interventions. During surgery the family should have a designated place to wait and should be kept informed of the child's progress. Family members also should know where and when they can visit the child after surgery.

Aside from possibly being separated from the parents before and after surgery, children may be cared for by a number of unfamiliar practitioners. Although the same supportive nurse should remain with the child through as many of the procedures as possible, the child may have other nurses, especially if the patient returns to a special care unit postoperatively. Many hospitals have surgical tours for children and parents to familiarize them with the strange environment and to introduce them to other individuals who will be involved in their care.

In addition to psychologic preparation, children usually require various types of physical care before surgery, such as those listed in the Nursing Care Plan on p. 1130 and in the preoperative checklist (Guidelines box). An important concern is restriction of food and fluids before surgery to avoid aspiration during anesthesia. Before fluids are restricted, children are encouraged to drink to promote hydration and minimize the dryness and thirst they experience. Infants require special attention to fluid needs;

Guidelines

PREOPERATIVE CHECKLIST

- ☐ Signed informed consent on chart and properly witnessed.
- ☐ Child NPO (nothing by mouth) for appropriate length of time (see Box 45-4).
- ☐ Child's medication orders changed as needed because of NPO status.
- ☐ Results of laboratory tests and vital signs reviewed for abnormal findings, such as elevated temperature, and reported to practitioner.
- ☐ Any specific physical preparation of surgical area, such as shaving or administration of enemas, performed.
- ☐ Child appropriately attired and any personal items (e.g., underwear, favorite toy) labeled.
- ☐ Dental appliances (e.g., retainers) contact lenses, prosthesis, hearing aid, nail polish, and makeup removed.
- ☐ Loose teeth and appliances remaining with child noted on chart.
- ☐ Child voided before preoperative sedation administered.
- ☐ Child wearing correct patient identification.
- ☐ Child's identification charge card on chart.
- ☐ Child and family adequately prepared for surgery experience (e.g., where family can wait for surgeon's report; whether parents can accompany the child to perioperative suite, induction area, or postanesthesia care unit [PACU]).
- ☐ Any special circumstances, such as allergies, skin problems, respiratory or cardiac conditions, paralysis, or family history of malignant hyperthermia, clearly displayed on front of chart.
- ☐ History and physical examination, including child's weight and laboratory test results, indicated on chart.

to avoid glycogen depletion and dehydration they should not be without oral fluids for an extended period preoperatively. Current preoperative fasting guidelines are found in Box 45-4.

Although most preoperative care procedures are routine, nurses should keep in mind that they can be anxiety provoking for children and parents. For example, having to wear a loose-fitting hospital gown without the security of underpants or pajama bottoms can be traumatic for young children. Therefore these articles of clothing should be allowed.

The most upsetting event for children is generally the preoperative injection. Unfortunately, little research has been done on the value of this practice. If children have no preoperative pain, are well prepared psychologically for surgery, and have their parents nearby, preanesthetic medication may be unnecessary. When drugs are used, they should be administered atraumatically by using oral, existing IV, or rectal routes.

Numerous preanesthetic drug regimens are used with children, and no consensus exists on the optimum method (see Pain Management, Chapter 44). Drugs used should achieve five goals (American Academy of Pediatrics, 1992): (1) guard the patient's safety and welfare; (2) minimize physical discomfort or pain; (3) minimize negative psychologic responses to treatment by providing analgesia, and maximize the potential for amnesia; (4) control behavior; and (5) return the patient to a state in which safe discharge, as determined by recognized criteria, is possible.

The use of sedating drugs for procedures has serious associated risks, such as hypoventilation, apnea, airway obstruction, and cardiopulmonary impairment. It is recommended that sedation be viewed as a continuum, ranging from conscious to deep sedation. *Conscious sedation* is a medically controlled state of depressed consciousness that (1) allows protective reflexes to be maintained, (2) retains the patient's ability to maintain a patent airway independently, and (3) permits appropriate response by the patient to physical stimulation or verbal command (e.g., "Open your eyes"). *Deep sedation* is a medically controlled state of depressed consciousness or unconsciousness from which the patient is not easily aroused. This state may be accompanied by (1) partial or complete loss of protective reflexes, (2) loss of the ability to maintain an independent patent airway, and (3) loss of the ability to respond to physical stimulation or verbal command. The loss of these capabilities may progress to general anesthesia (Algren and Algren, 1997).

The American Academy of Pediatrics (1992) has developed policies that provide guidelines for conscious sedation. These guidelines include provision of emergency equipment, such as a positive-pressure oxygen delivery system, airway management and breathing equipment, and an emergency cart. The patient's level of consciousness and responsiveness, heart rate, blood pressure, respiratory rate, and oxygen saturation (via pulse oximetry) must be monitored during the procedure by an individual present for this purpose. In all cases the patient's condition after the procedure is also documented.

Children may also fear induction of anesthesia by mask. Practices that can minimize anxiety related to inhalation anesthesia include (1) disguising the unpleasant odor of anesthetic gases by applying a pleasant-smelling substance on the mask; (2) using a transparent plastic mask rather than an opaque black mask and gradually bringing it toward the face; (3) directing a stream of gas toward the child's face from the bare tube until the child becomes drowsy, then using the mask; (4) allowing the child to sit up rather than lie down for anesthesia induction; and (5) allowing preoperative play with a mask and a doll or mannikin.

Postoperative Care. After surgical procedures, various psychologic and physical interventions and observations are required to prevent or minimize possible untoward effects from anesthesia and the surgical procedure (Nursing Care Plan and Guidelines box). Although most of these interventions are prescribed by physicians, it is the nurse's responsibility to exercise judgment in their implementation. For example, vital signs are taken as often as necessary until they are stable. Simply recording temperature, pulse, respiration, and blood pressure without comparing the present readings with previous ones is a useless technical function. Each vital sign is evaluated in terms of side effects from anesthesia and signs of impending shock, respiratory compromise, or pain. The nurse should also be alert for the development of *malignant hyperthermia,* a potentially lethal genetic myopathy. In susceptible children, certain anesthetic agents trigger the disorder, producing elevated temperature, muscle rigidity, hypermetabolism, and muscle cell destruction. The symptoms may or may not occur during surgery; therefore alert observation in the PACU and regular care unit is essential. Early signs of the disorder include tachycardia, rising blood pressure, tachypnea, mottled skin, and muscle rigidity. An elevated temperature is considered by many to be a late sign of the disorder (Dunn, 1997).

NURSE ALERT • When taking the preoperative history, ask the family if any relatives have had anesthetic difficulties suggesting malignant hyperthermia; report findings immediately.

Providing comfort is a major nursing responsibility after surgery. Pain is assessed, and analgesics are administered to provide comfort and to facilitate the child's cooperation with post-

Box 45-4

Summary of Fasting Recommendations to Reduce the Risk of Pulmonary Aspiration*

Ingested Material	Minimum Fasting Period (Hours)†
Clear liquids‡	2
Breast milk	4
Infant formula	6
Nonhuman milk§	6
Light meal‖	6

From American Society of Anesthesiologists: Practice guidelines for preoperative fasting and the use of pharmacologic agents to reduce the risk of pulmonary aspiration: application to healthy patients undergoing elective procedures, *Anesthesiology* 90(3):896–905, 1999 (www.ASAhq.org/practice/NPO/NPOguide.html).

*These recommendations apply to healthy patients who are undergoing elective procedures. They are not intended for women in labor. Following the guidelines does not guarantee a complete gastric emptying has occurred.

†The fasting periods noted above apply to all ages.

‡Examples of clear liquids include water, fruit juices without pulp, carbonated beverages, clear tea, and black coffee.

§Since nonhuman milk is similar to solids in gastric emptying time, the amount ingested must be considered when determining an appropriate fasting period.

‖A light meal typically consists of toast and clear liquids. Meals that include fried or fatty foods or meat may prolong gastric emptying time. Both the amount and type of foods ingested must be considered when determining an appropriate fasting period.

Nursing Care Plan THE CHILD UNDERGOING SURGERY

NURSING DIAGNOSIS Risk for injury related to surgical procedure, anesthesia

EXPECTED OUTCOME Child shows no evidence of injury.

Nursing Interventions/*Rationales*

Carry out preoperative preparations such as: NPO, anticholinergic medications as ordered *to prevent aspiration;* bathing, cleansing of operative site, antibiotics as ordered *to prevent infection;* emptying of bowel and bladder, insertion of catheter as ordered, cleansing enemas as ordered *to prevent distention and incontinence;* checking vital signs, laboratory values for systematic abnormality *that may complicate surgery* (e.g., elevated temperature, white blood cells [WBCs] *for signs of infection,* hemoglobin [Hb] and hematocrit [Hct] *for anemia,* platelets, clotting times *for bleeding tendencies*): clearly delineate allergies *to prevent reactions or complications;* removal of jewelry, prosthetic devices *to prevent injury;* removal of makeup, nail polish *to improve monitoring for cyanosis;* start IV per order *to provide route for fluids and medications;* dress in attire for operating room (OR) *to provide easy access to surgical site.*

Transport to surgical holding area using safety belt and side rails on stretcher *to prevent falls;* check identification and chart with surgical personnel *to ensure correct identity and completion of all preoperative preparations.*

Carry out intraoperative preparations such as: transfer and proper securing to surgical table *to prevent falls;* check identification *to ensure correct identity;* check chart *to ensure correct surgical procedure at correct site;* talk/play with child before anesthesia administered *to keep anxiety, fear minimal;* after child is anesthetized, careful alignment and positioning *to prevent injury to joints or pressure spots to skin;* apply restraints *to prevent falls;* place on warming blanket per order *to prevent hypothermia;* place grounding plate if electrocautery is to be used *to prevent injury;* cleanse and drape surgical site *to prevent infection;* check expiration dates on all sterile packages before use *to maintain integrity of sterile field;* monitor sterile field and institute immediate corrective measures for technique breaks *to prevent contamination of wound;* ensure correct instrument and sponge count *to prevent loss of foreign substances in wound;* dress surgical site *to prevent infection;* transfer to recovery bed, raise side rails, and transport to recovery room *for postoperative monitoring.*

Carry out recovery room procedures such as: monitor vital signs frequently *to assess for signs of infection, hemorrhage, aspiration;* suction as needed *to prevent aspiration, infection;* monitor neurologic status, gag and swallow reflex, cough *to assess recovery from anesthesia;* monitor intake and output, skin tone and turgor *to assess hydration status;* monitor for signs of sensory overload; orient frequently as child is waking *to prevent overload and confusion;* monitor incision site *for hemorrhage.*

Carry out postoperative procedures such as: employ careful wound care and good handwashing techniques *to prevent infection;* monitor vital signs *to assess for signs of infection, hemorrhage, aspiration;* turn, cough, and deep breathe *to prevent respiratory infection;* encourage graduated nutritious oral intake after bowel sounds heard *to prevent intestinal complications and promote wound healing;* ambulate per physician order *to decrease complications of immobility;* monitor intake and output, skin turgor *to assess hydration status;* monitor and maintain bedside equipment (e.g., IVs, IV pumps, nasogastric [NG] tubes, suction machines, wound drains, chest tubes, catheters) *to ensure function and safe operation.*

NURSING DIAGNOSIS Anxiety/fear related to surgery, separation from support system

EXPECTED OUTCOME Child exhibits reduced signs of fear and anxiety.

Nursing Interventions/*Rationales*

Preoperatively: teach child (using developmentally appropriate approach) what to expect before, during, and after surgery; explain where parents will be during surgery *to reduce fear of unknown;* administer preoperative medications as ordered *to provide relaxation and sleep;* encourage parents to stay with child as long as possible and to touch or hold child until asleep *to reduce fear and feelings of abandonment;* allow child to take a favorite toy to the surgical holding area *to establish a sense of security.*

Postoperatively: orient child as he or she awakes, explain what is happening as it happens, be calm and reassuring *to reduce anxieties;* encourage parental presence as soon as feasible *to decrease separation anxiety.*

NURSING DIAGNOSIS Pain related to surgical incision

EXPECTED OUTCOME Child exhibits minimal evidence of pain.

Nursing Interventions/*Rationales*

Administer postoperative pain medications as ordered before expression of pain *to prevent pain from occurring.*

Splint operative site when coughing or deep breathing: turn and position gently; avoid palpation of surgical site unless necessary *to reduce pain.*

Insert rectal tube as needed *to relieve discomfort from gas.*

Monitor bladder for fullness and encourage voiding *to prevent pain from bladder distention.*

Administer comfort measures (e.g., mouth care, lubrication of eyes if irritated, lubrication of nostril if NG tube present, massage of back) *to reduce discomfort.*

Nursing Care Plan THE CHILD UNDERGOING SURGERY—cont'd

Coordinate nursing activities and procedures with administration of analgesia *to decrease pain and increase effectiveness of activity.*

Administer analgesics, antiemetics per physician order and monitor effectiveness of medications in pain and nausea relief.

NURSING DIAGNOSIS Risk for fluid volume deficit related to NPO status, operative losses, vomiting, loss of appetite

EXPECTED OUTCOME Child exhibits no signs of dehydration.

Nursing Interventions/*Rationales*

Monitor intake and output, IV infusion rate and patency, skin turgor, mucous membranes *to evaluate hydration status.*

Offer oral fluids as ordered and tolerated; use favorite fluids *to establish oral intake after surgery.*

NURSING DIAGNOSIS Risk for infection related to break in skin integrity, anesthesia, immobility, presence of pathogens in environment

EXPECTED OUTCOME Lungs remain clear; surgical incision site is clean.

Nursing Interventions/*Rationales*

Turn, cough, deep breathe, use incentive spirometer or blow bottle *to promote movement and clearing of lung secretions.*

Suction secretions as needed *to keep airway clear.*

Monitor respirations, auscultate breath sounds *to assess respiratory status.*

Ambulate as early as permitted *to promote increased circulation and improved gas exchange.*

Keep surgical site dressed, using careful wound care and handwashing techniques *to prevent infection.*

Monitor temperature; inspect wound for redness, swelling, pus *indicative of infection.*

NURSING DIAGNOSIS Altered family process related to surgical procedure

EXPECTED OUTCOME Family demonstrates understanding of surgery and related processes; family complies with directives.

Nursing Interventions/*Rationales*

Teach family about surgical procedure and related tests and procedures; outline the preoperative, operative, and postoperative processes *to provide understanding of what will happen and prepare family for what is to occur;* allow time for questions; get feedback *to evaluate level of understanding.*

Be available to family *to provide support;* explore family's feelings *to offer needed emotional support.*

Let family know where to wait and whom to talk to while surgery occurring; give them an expected time frame for the procedure; let them know when they can see child after surgery *to provide support.*

Explain child's expected appearance, equipment, and attached apparatus after surgery *to prepare family and reduce fear.*

Explain care after surgery; encourage family to participate in child's care as they feel able *to facilitate a sense of control and ability to cope.*

See also Nursing Care Plan: The Family of the Ill/Hospitalized Child, p. 1114.

operative procedures such as ambulating and deep breathing. Routinely scheduled IV analgesics and the use of patient-controlled analgesia (PCA), rather than PRN (as necessary) orders, afford more satisfactory pain control (see Pain Management, Chapter 44). Mouth care is another important aspect of care because most children are allowed nothing orally until bowel sounds return (see Oral Hygiene, p. 1135).

Because respiratory infections are a potential complication, every effort is taken to aerate the lungs and remove secretions. The lungs are auscultated regularly to identify abnormal sounds or any areas of diminished or absent breath sounds. To prevent hypostatic pneumonia, respiratory movement can be encouraged with incentive spirometers or other motivating activities (see Box 45-3). If these measures are presented as games, the child is more likely to comply. The child's position is changed every 2 hours, and deep breathing is encouraged. Because deep breathing is usually painful after surgery, premedicate the child for pain and have the child splint the operative site (depending on its location) by hugging a small pillow or a favorite stuffed animal.

NURSE ALERT • Early signs of respiratory involvement are abnormal rate, shallow depth, and cough. These findings are reported immediately.

During the recovery period, some time should be spent with children to assess their perception of surgery. Play, drawing, and storytelling are excellent methods of discovering their thoughts. With such information the nurse can support or correct their perceptions and assist children in feeling a sense of mastery for having gone through a stressful procedure.

Compliance

The extent to which the patient's behavior in terms of taking medication, following diets, or executing other lifestyle changes coincides with the prescribed regimen is known as *compliance*

Guidelines

POSTOPERATIVE CARE

- Ensure that preparations are made to receive child.
  - Bed or crib is ready.
  - Intravenous equipment, such as pumps, and any other relevant equipment, such as suction apparatus, oxygen flow meter, or Gomco suction, is at bedside.
- Obtain baseline information:
  - Take vital signs, including blood pressure (BP); keep BP cuff in place and deflated to lessen amount of disturbance to child.
  - Take and record vital signs more frequently if any value fluctuates.
  - Inspect operative area.
    - Check dressing if present.
    - Outline any bleeding area on dressing or cast with pen.
    - Reinforce, but do not remove, loose dressing.
    - Observe areas below surgical site for blood that may have drained toward bed.
    - Assess for bleeding and other symptoms in areas not covered with a dressing, such as throat after tonsillectomy.
  - Assess skin color and characteristics.
  - Assess level of consciousness and activity.
- Notify physician of any irregularities in child's condition.
- Assess for evidence of pain (see Pain Assessment, Chapter 44).
- Review surgeon's orders after completing initial assessment, and check that any preoperative orders, such as seizure or cardiac medications, have been reordered and can be given by available routes (oral preparations may be contraindicated).
- Monitor vital signs as ordered and more often if indicated.
- Check dressings for bleeding or other abnormalities.
- Check bowel sounds.
- Observe for signs of shock, abdominal distention, and bleeding.
- Assess for bladder distention.
- Observe for signs of dehydration.
- Detect presence of infection:
  - Take vital signs every 2 to 4 hours, as ordered.
  - Collect or request needed specimens.
  - Inspect wound for signs of infection—redness, swelling, heat, pain, and purulent drainage.

(or *adherence*). Reviews of compliance rates in children and adolescents with chronic diseases estimate that the rate of noncompliance ranges from 36% to more than 80% (Pidgeon, 1989). Because nurses are commonly responsible for teaching families about treatment protocols, they must have knowledge of factors that influence compliance, methods to measure compliance, and strategies to enhance adherence to prescribed treatment.

Assessment of Compliance. In developing strategies to provide compliance, the nurse must first assess factors that influence compliance in the patient. Because many children are too young to assume partial or total responsibility for their care, parents are usually the primary caregivers in terms of home management. Confusion caused by the transfer of responsibility from parents to the adolescent can play a major role in noncompliance (Tebbi, 1993). Consequently, the nurse needs to assess their ability to carry out instructions. The first approach to assessment is knowledge of those factors that influence compliance, and the second is to apply methods to assess compliance more objectively.

Several factors influence compliance (Box 45-5), although no typical characteristics of noncompliers exist, and even education is not correlated with compliance (Rosenstock, 1988).

Box 45-5

Factors that Positively Influence Compliance

INDIVIDUAL/FAMILY FACTORS
- High self-esteem
- Positive body image
- High degree of autonomy (increased locus of control)
- Supportive and well-adjusted family
- Effective family communication
- Family expectation for successful completion of therapy

CARE-SETTING FACTORS
- Perceived satisfaction with care
- Positive interactions with practitioners
- Continuity of care
- Individualized care
- Minimum waiting time for appointments
- Convenient care-setting

TREATMENT FACTORS
- Simple regimen
- Minimum disruption in usual lifestyle
- Short duration
- Inexpensive
- Visible benefits
- Tolerable side effects

Basically, any aspect of the health care environment that increases the family's satisfaction with the care they are receiving positively influences adherence to the treatment regimen. However, the more complex, expensive, inconvenient, and disruptive the treatment protocol, the less likely the family is to comply. During long-term conditions that involve multiple treatments and considerable rearrangement of lifestyle, compliance is severely affected.

Although it is helpful to know those factors that influence compliance, assessment must include more direct measurement techniques. A number of methods exist, but no one method is totally reliable. The most successful approach combines at least two of the following methods:

Clinical judgment—The nurse judges family compliance. This is a very poor method that is subject to bias and inaccuracy unless the nurse carefully evaluates the criteria used in evaluation.

Self-reporting—The family is asked about their ability to carry out the prescribed treatments, although most people overestimate their compliance by about 20% even when they admit to lapses in treatment.

Direct observation—The nurse directly observes the patient or family performing the treatment. This method is difficult to employ outside the health care setting, and the family's awareness of being observed often affects their performance.

Monitoring appointments—The family's attendance at scheduled appointments is recorded, although this method only indirectly indicates compliance with the prescribed care.

Monitoring therapeutic response—The child's response in terms of benefit from treatment is monitored and preferably recorded on a graph or chart. Unfortunately, few treatments yield directly measurable results (e.g., decreased blood pressure, weight loss).

Pill counts—The nurse counts the number of pills remaining in the original container and compares the amount missing with the number of days the medication should have been taken. Although this is a simple method, families may forget to bring the container or may deliberately alter the number of pills to avoid detection. This method is also poorly suited to liquid medication, which is often prescribed in pediatrics. Another strategy is to call the pharmacy and check on the number of refills for long-term prescriptions.

Chemical assay—For certain drugs, such as digoxin and phenytoin, measurement of plasma drug levels provides information on the amount of drug recently ingested. However, this method is expensive, indicates only short-term compliance, and requires precise timing of the assay for accurate results.

Strategies to Enhance Compliance. *Organizational strategies* refer to those interventions that involve the care setting and the therapeutic plan. They include employing the factors known to positively affect compliance (see Box 45-5). Depending on the individual situation, this may involve increasing the frequency of appointments, designating a primary practitioner, reducing the cost of medication by purchasing generic brands, reducing the treatment's disruption of the family's lifestyle, and using "cues" to minimize forgetting. Numerous devices are available commercially or can be improvised for cueing, such as pill dispensers; watches with alarms; charts to record completed therapy; reminders, such as messages on the refrigerator or morning coffee pot; and treatment schedules that incorporate the treatment plan into the daily routine, such as physical therapy after the evening bath.

Educational strategies are concerned with instructing the family about the treatment plan. Although education is an important component in enhancing compliance and patients who are more knowledgeable about their condition are more likely to comply, education alone does not ensure compliant behavior. Also, for education to be effective, it must incorporate teaching principles known to enhance understanding and retention of material (Guidelines box). Written materials are essential, especially in any regimen requiring multiple or complex treatments, and need to be understandable to the average individual, who reads at about the fourth-grade level. Involvement of the immediate and extended family (e.g., grandparents) in education sessions may enhance compliance (Liptak, 1996).

Guidelines

EFFECTIVE TEACHING OF FAMILY MEMBERS

- Establish rapport; reduce anxiety and fear.
- Assess what family members know and expect to learn, especially if they have concerns, and address their concerns before beginning teaching.
- Assess family's learning style; ask if they prefer to have everything explained in detail or if they prefer knowing only the major facts.
- Use a variety of teaching materials (lecture, demonstration, video or slide presentation, written material).
- Speak family's language, avoid jargon, and clarify all terms.
- Be specific when giving information.
- Divide the information into small steps.
- Keep information short, simple, and concrete.
- Introduce most important information first.
- Use "verbal" headings to organize information, such as "There are two things you need to learn: how to give the medicine and what side effects to look for. First, how to give. . . . Second, what side effects. . . ."
- Stress how important the instructions are and the expected benefits; explain the detrimental effects of inadequate treatment but avoid fear tactics.
- Evaluate the teaching by eliciting feedback to ensure that family members understand the information.
- Repeat information as needed.
- Reward family for learning through verbal praise.
- Use "teachable moments"—times when family members are most likely to accept new information (e.g., when a member asks a question or when symptoms are present).
- Use "hands on" demonstration and return demonstration to encourage mastery of skills and retention of information.

Treatment strategies are related to the child's refusal or inability to take the prescribed medication. The family may also have difficulty following a prescribed treatment regimen. They may remember and understand the instructions but may not be able to give the medicine as prescribed. It is essential to assess the reason for refusal. For example, the child may not be able to swallow pills. In this case, perhaps they can be crushed or a liquid medication substituted. The opposite also may occur; the child may have difficulty drinking a liquid medication but may be able to swallow pills.

Also assess the treatment and medication schedule to determine if it is reasonable for a home situation. Although an every-6-hour or every-8-hour schedule is reasonable for hospitals, a parent would have difficulty awakening one or two times at night when a medication could be given during the day at times that would be easy to remember.

Behavioral strategies encompass those interventions designed to modify behavior directly. Several strategies exist that are effective in encouraging the desired behavior and are very useful with children. Also, positive reinforcement may be employed to strengthen the behavior; this may consist of earning stars or tokens, which gain the child a special privilege or gift. At times, however, techniques such as time-out for young children or withholding privileges for older children may be needed to reduce noncompliance (see Limit Setting and Discipline, Chapter 31).

GENERAL HYGIENE AND CARE

Maintaining Healthy Skin

Skin, the largest organ of the body, is not merely a covering but also a complex structure that serves many functions, the most important of which is to protect the tissues that it encloses and to protect itself. Many routine nursing activities—maintaining an IV line, removing a dressing, positioning a child in bed, changing a diaper, using electrode patches, or maintaining restraints—have the potential to contribute to skin injury. Skin care must go beyond the daily bath and become a part of each nursing intervention. General guidelines for skin care are listed in the Guidelines box.

Assessment of the skin is most easily accomplished during the bath, but often the nurse is not the one who bathes the child. In this case the nurse needs to plan a time to observe the child's

Guidelines

SKIN CARE

Cleanse skin with gentle soap (e.g., Dove) or lotion (e.g., Cetaphil). Rinse well with plain warm water.

Provide daily cleansing of eyes, oral and diaper or perianal areas, and any areas of skin breakdown.

Apply moisturizing agents after cleansing to retain moisture and rehydrate skin; however, cleanse skin of any old cream before adding a new layer.

Use minimum amount tape or adhesive. On very sensitive skin, use a protective, pectin-based or hydrocolloid skin barrier between skin and tape or adhesives.

Use water or possibly adhesive remover (if skin is not fragile) when removing tape or adhesives.

Place pectin-based or hydrocolloid skin barriers directly over excoriated skin. Leave barrier undisturbed until it begins to peel off. With wet, oozing excoriations, place a small amount of stoma powder (as used in ostomy care) on site, remove excess powder, and apply skin barrier. Hold barrier in place for several minutes to allow barrier to soften and mold to skin surface.

Alternate electrode placement and thoroughly assess skin underneath electrodes at least every 24 hours.

Be certain fingers or toes are visible whenever extremity is used for intravenous (IV) or arterial line.

Reduce friction by keeping skin dry (may apply absorbent powder, e.g., cornstarch) and using soft, smooth bed linen and clothes.

Use a draw sheet to move a child in bed or onto a gurney to reduce friction and shearing injuries; do not drag the child from under the arms.

Identify children who are at risk for skin breakdown before it occurs. Employ measures, such as pressure-reducing or pressure-relieving devices, to prevent breakdown.

Do not massage reddened bony prominences because it can cause deep tissue damage; provide pressure relief to those areas instead.

Keep skin free of excess moisture (e.g., urine or fecal incontinence, wound drainage, excessive perspiration).

Routinely assess the child's nutritional status. A child who is NPO (nothing by mouth) for several days and is only receiving IV fluid is nutritionally at risk, which can also affect the skin's ability to maintain its integrity. Hyperalimentation should be considered for these children before they are at risk.

skin and to request feedback from the caregiver. The skin is examined for any early signs of injury, especially for the child who is at risk. Risk factors include impaired mobility, protein malnutrition, edema, incontinence, sensory loss, anemia, and infection. Identification of risk factors helps to determine those children who need a more thorough skin assessment.

When capillary blood flow is interrupted by pressure, the blood flows back into the tissue when the pressure is relieved. As the body attempts to reoxygenate the area, a bright red flush appears. This *reactive hyperemia,* or flush, may be present for one-half to three-fourths as long as the time the pressure occluded the blood flow to the area.

NURSE ALERT • If the redness persists, this may be the first sign of skin breakdown, including the possibility of more extensive damage below the skin.

Staging of pressure ulcers is used to classify the amount of tissue damage that has occurred. The tissue in the wound must be visible to be staged; it is difficult to assess a wound that is covered with necrotic tissue or a scab. Accurate documentation

Critical Thinking

RISK OF SKIN BREAKDOWN

You work on a pediatric surgical unit. In a recent continuous quality improvement report, it was noted that 10% of the patients developed some type of skin breakdown, most often stage II wounds. Which of the following variables identified about this patient population should be investigated further?

First, Think About It . . .

- What precise questions are you trying to answer?
- How are you interpreting the information?

1. Average age of the child is 6 years, and gender is more often male.
2. Major reason for surgery is orthopedic repair, especially as a result of trauma.
3. Average length of surgery is 4 hours, and average duration until appearance of wound is 24 to 48 hours.
4. All children receive adequate pain medication.

The best response is 3. Precisely, the questions are, how prolonged was the surgery and was the patient placed on an adequately padded surface? The excessive pressure on bony prominences causes redness and deeper tissue damage that may not be apparent until hours or days later. An accurate interpretation of the information reveals the fact that these children are most likely to need orthopedic surgery (members of this age group and gender are at risk for injuries), and impaired mobility may also be a risk factor. However, with good pain control, these children should be able to move quite easily. If pressure ulcers develop postoperatively from immobility, they are most likely to develop later than during the first 2 days.

of redness or of obvious skin breakdown is essential. Color, size (diameter and depth), location, presence of sinus tracts, odor, exudate, and response to treatment are observed and recorded at least daily (Critical Thinking box). (For treatment of wounds, see Chapter 53.)

The nurse must also have an understanding of the types of mechanical damage that can occur, such as pressure, friction, shearing, and epidermal stripping. When a combination of risk factors and mechanical injury is present, skin breakdown can occur (Hagelgans, 1993).

When a child is identified as being at risk for skin breakdown, nursing interventions are directed toward prevention of mechanical injury. Wounds caused by pressure can be prevented by using current technology and resources. *Pressure ulcers* can develop when the pressure on the skin and underlying tissues is greater than the capillary closing pressure, causing capillary occlusion. If the pressure remains unrelieved, vessels can collapse, resulting in tissue anoxia and cellular death. Pressure ulcers most often occur over bony prominences. These lesions are usually very deep (stage IV), extending into subcutaneous tissue or even deeper into muscle, tendon, or bone. Prevention of pressure ulcers includes measures that reduce or relieve pressure (Laurent, 1999).

A *pressure-reduction device* reduces pressure by redistributing the pressure. These products do not prevent pressure from causing capillary closing; therefore turning and repositioning are always included when using these devices. Most of these items are overlays that are placed on top of the regular mattress. A pressure-relief device maintains pressure below that which would cause capillary closing. These devices are usually high-technology beds that are used for patients who have multiple problems and cannot be turned effectively.

NURSE ALERT • Use of a polyurethane foam mattress overlay compared with a standard hospital mattress showed a 46% to 52% reduction of soft tissue pressure (Reynolds and Suarez, 1994).

Friction and shear both contribute to pressure ulcers. *Friction* occurs when the surface of the skin rubs against another surface, such as the sheets on the bed. The skin may have the appearance of an abrasion. The skin damage is usually limited to the epidermal and upper layers, and most often occurs over the elbows or heels. Prevention of friction injury includes the use of protective sheepskin over the elbows or heels; moisturizing agents; transparent dressings over susceptible areas; and soft, smooth bed linen and clothing. Friction alone does not cause tissue necrosis, but when friction acts with gravity, it results in shear injury.

Shear is the result of the force of gravity pushing down on the body and friction of the body against a surface, such as the bed or chair. For example, when a patient is in the semi-Fowler position and begins to slide to the foot of the bed, the skin over the sacral area remains in the same place because of the resistance of the bed surface. The blood vessels in the area are stretched and may cause small-vessel thrombosis and tissue death (Bryant and Doughty, 2000). The same type of damage can occur when a patient is pulled up in the bed if the skin does not move with the patient. Prevention of shear injury includes using "lift sheets" when repositioning a patient, elevating the bed no more than 30 degrees for short periods, and using the knee gatch to interrupt the pull of gravity on the body toward the foot of the bed.

Epidermal stripping results when the epidermis is unintentionally removed with tape removal. These lesions are usually shallow and irregularly shaped. Prevention of epidermal stripping includes recognizing fragile skin, such as in neonates; using minimum tape; using solid-wafer skin barriers, transparent dressings, or laced binders to secure dressings (Montgomery straps) on areas where tape must be changed often; using skin sealants under adhesives unless skin is fragile; and using porous tapes. Tape is placed so that there is no tension, traction, or wrinkles on the skin. To remove tape, the nurse slowly peels the tape away while stabilizing the underlying skin. Adhesive remover may be used to break the adhesive bond, but may be drying to the skin; adhesive removers should be avoided in preterm neonates, because absorption rates vary and toxicity may occur. The adhesive is removed with water to prevent absorption and irritation. Wetting the tape with water may facilitate removal.

Chemical factors can also lead to skin damage. Fecal incontinence, especially when mixed with urine; wound drainage; or gastric drainage around gastrostomy tubes can erode epidermis. The skin can very quickly progress from redness to denudement if exposure continues. Moisture barriers, gentle cleansing as soon after exposure as possible, and skin barriers can be used to prevent damage caused by chemical factors (see also Diaper Dermatitis, Chapter 53).

Bathing

Unless contraindicated, most infants and children can be bathed in a tub at the bedside or on the bed; or in a standard bathtub or shower located on the unit, which is often conveniently adapted for pediatric use. For infants and young children confined to bed, the towel method can be used. Two towels are immersed in a dilute soap solution and wrung damp. With the child lying supine on a dry towel, one damp towel is placed on top of the child and used to gently clean the body. This towel is discarded, and the child is dried and turned prone. The procedure is repeated using the second damp towel.

Infants and small children are never left unattended in a bathtub, and infants who are unable to sit alone are securely held with one hand during the bath. The infant's head is supported securely with one hand, or the farther arm is firmly grasped in the nurse's hand while the head rests comfortably on the nurse's wrist or arm. This hold provides secure control of the infant while the other hand is free to wash the infant's body (Fig. 45-4). Infants or children who are able to sit without assistance need only close supervision and a pad placed in the bottom of the tub to prevent slipping and loss of balance, which could result in a bumped head or submersion of the face.

Older children may enjoy a shower if it is available. School-age children may be reluctant to bathe, and many are not accustomed to a daily bath. However, most children who feel well require little encouragement to participate in their daily care. Nurses need to use judgment regarding the amount of supervision the child requires. Some can be trusted to assume this responsibility unaided, whereas others will need someone in constant attendance. Children with mental or physical limitations, and suicidal or psychotic children (who may commit bodily harm) require close supervision.

Areas that require special attention during bed baths and for children performing their own care are the ears, between skinfolds, the neck, the back, and the genital area. The genital area should be carefully cleansed and dried with particular care to skinfolds. In uncircumcised boys, usually those over 3 years of age, the foreskin should be gently retracted and the exposed surfaces cleansed and then the foreskin replaced. Do not attempt to retract the foreskin in newborns. If the condition of the glans indicates inadequate cleaning, such as accumulated smegma, inflammation, phimosis, or foreskin adhesions, teaching proper hygiene is indicated. In the Vietnamese and Cambodian cultures the foreskin is traditionally not retracted until adulthood (Krueger and Osborn, 1986). Older children have the tendency to avoid these areas; therefore they may need a gentle reminder.

Children who are ill or debilitated need more extensive assistance with bathing and other aspects of hygienic care, but they should be encouraged to perform as much as they can without overtaxing their energies. Increasing involvement can be expected with improved strength and endurance. Children with limited capacity for self-care but no other contraindications benefit greatly from tub baths. They can be transported to the tub and, with the aid of lifting devices and/or an appropriate number of persons to assist, gain the advantages of a tub bath.

Oral Hygeine

Mouth care is an integral part of daily hygiene and should be continued in the hospital. Infants and debilitated children require the nurse to perform mouth care. Although young children can manage a toothbrush and should be encouraged to use it, most will need assistance to perform a satisfactory job. Older children, although capable of brushing and flossing without assistance, sometimes need to be reminded that this is a part of their hygienic care. Most hospitals have equipment available for

A

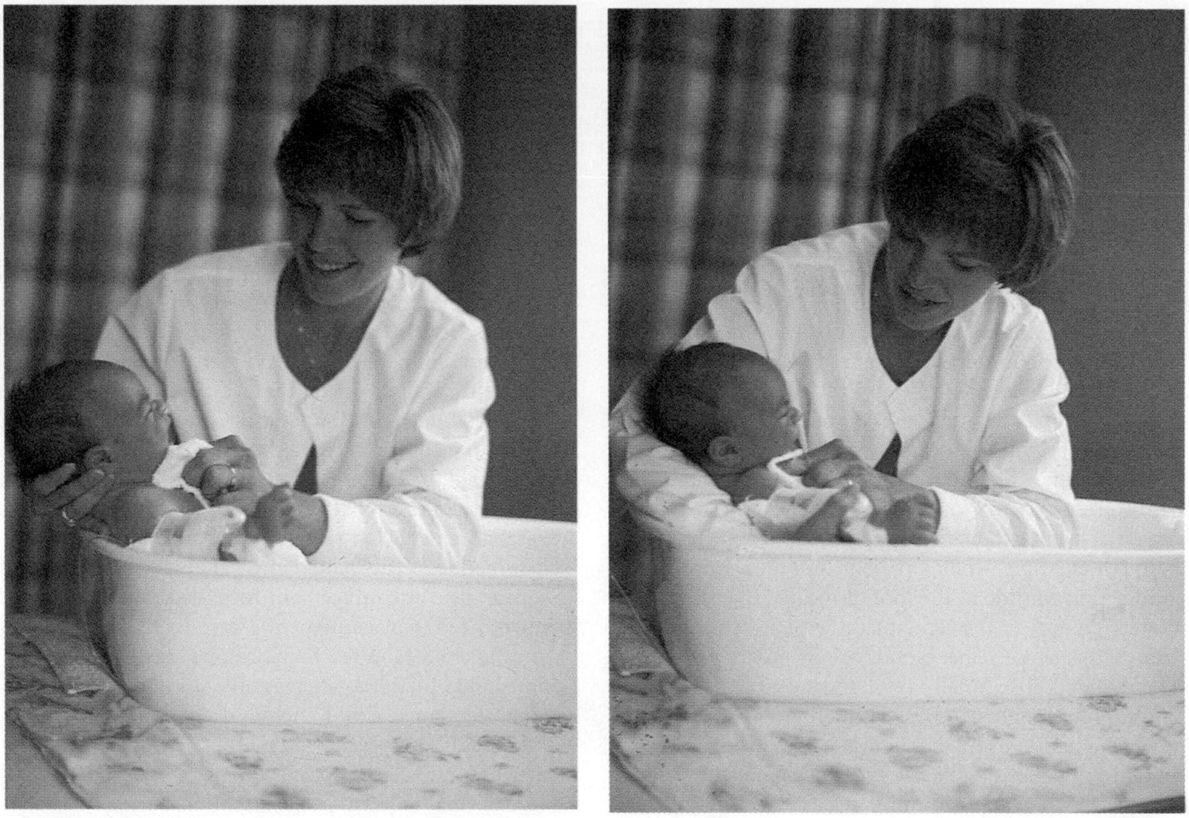

B

FIG. 45-4 • Two methods of supporting infant during tub bath. **A,** Using hand to support neck and head. **B,** Using arm to support neck and head.

those children who do not have a toothbrush or toothpaste of their own. (See Dental Health, Chapters 36 and 37, for specific oral hygiene techniques; mouth care of children with mucosal ulcers is discussed under nursing care of the child with leukemia in Chapter 49.)

Hair Care

Brushing and combing hair are a part of the daily care for all persons in the hospital, including infants and children. If the child does not have a brush or comb, many hospitals provide one as part of the usual admission kit. If not, the parents should be asked to bring hair care equipment for the child's use. Both boys and girls should be helped to comb or brush their hair, or it should be done for them, at least once daily. The hair is styled for comfort and in a manner pleasing to the child and parents. A satisfactory style for girls with longer hair is French braiding, which is done by starting with three equal portions of hair from the top of the scalp; as the hair is braided, segments of hair are added at successive intervals until all the hair has been incorporated into one or more neat, head-hugging braids. The ends are firmly anchored with a coated elastic band or barrette. The hair should not be cut without parental permission, although shaving hair to provide access to a scalp vein for IV needle insertion may be necessary.

If children are hospitalized for more than a few days, the hair may need shampooing. With infants the hair may be washed during the daily bath or less often. For most children, washing the hair and scalp once or twice weekly is sufficient unless there is an indication to wash it more often, such as following a high fever and profuse sweating. Some hospitals have shampoo basins, but almost any child can be conveniently transported by a gurney to an accessible sink or washbasin for shampooing. Those who are unable to be transported can receive a shampoo in their beds with adequate protection and/or specially adapted equipment or positioning. A convenient method involves positioning the child near the edge of the bed, placing towels under the shoulders, and draping a large plastic garbage bag at the edge of the bed with one open side under the shoulders and the other side opened away from the head so that the hair is placed inside the opening. Water can be transported in a basin or placed in a clean enema bag. The nurse should fill a clean enema bag with warm water, hang the bag from an IV pole, and use the clamp on the bag's tubing to adjust the flow of water.

Teenagers, with their normally increased oily sebaceous secretions, are particularly in need of hair care and usually require more frequent shampoos. Commercial no-rinse products also may prove useful on a short-term basis.

African-American children require special hair care, and this need is commonly neglected or inadequately managed. Most standard combs are inadequate and may cause hair breakage and discomfort to the child. If a special comb with widely spaced teeth is not available on the unit, the parent can be reminded to bring a comb from home for the child's use. It is also much easier to comb the hair after shampooing when it is wet.

Guidelines

FEEDING THE SICK CHILD

Take a dietary history (see Chapter 34) and use information to make eating time as much like home as possible.
Encourage parents or other family members to feed child or to be present at mealtimes.
Have children eat at tables in groups; bring nonambulatory children to eating area in wheelchairs, beds, strollers, gurneys, or wagons.
Use familiar eating utensils, such as a favorite plate, cup, or bottle (for small children).
Make mealtimes pleasant; avoid any procedures immediately before or after eating; make sure child is rested and pain free.
Have a nurse present at mealtimes to offer assistance, prevent disruptions, and praise children for their eating.
Serve small, frequent meals rather than three large meals or serve three meals and nutritious between-meal snacks.
Bring in foods from home, especially if food preparation is very different from hospital's; consider cultural differences.
Provide finger foods for young children.
Involve children in food selection and preparation whenever possible.
Serve small portions, and serve each course separately, such as soup first; followed by meat, potatoes, and vegetables; and ending with dessert. With young children, camouflage size of food by cutting meat thicker so that less appears on plate or by folding a cheese slice in half. Offer second helpings. Ensure a variety of foods, textures, and colors.
Provide food selections that are favorites of most children, such as peanut butter-and-jelly sandwiches, hot dogs, hamburgers, macaroni and cheese, pizza, spaghetti, tacos, fried chicken, corn on the cob, and fruit yogurt.
Avoid foods that are highly seasoned, have strong odors, are served hot, or are all mixed together, unless typical of cultural practices.
Provide fluid selections that are favorites of most children, such as fruit punch, cola, ginger ale, sweetened tea, flavored ice pops, sherbet, ice cream, milk and milkshakes, eggnog, pudding, gelatin, clear broth, or creamed soups (see also Box 45-3).
Offer nutritious snacks, such as frozen yogurt or pudding, ice cream, oatmeal or peanut butter cookies, hot cocoa, cheese slices or "kisses," pieces of raw vegetable or fruit, and dried fruit or cereal.
Make food attractive and different; for example:
- Serve a "picnic lunch" in a paper bag.
- Pack food in a Chinese-food container; decorate container.
- Put a "face" or a "flower" on a hamburger or sandwich with pieces of vegetable.
- Use a cookie cutter to shape a sandwich.
- Serve pudding, yogurt, or juice frozen as an ice pop.
- Make slurpies or snow cones by pouring flavored syrup on crushed ice.
- Add food coloring to water or milk.
- Serve fluids through brightly colored or unusually shaped straws.
- Make "bowtie" sandwiches by cutting them in triangles and placing two points together.
- Slice sandwiches into "fingers."
- Grate mounds of cheese.
- Cut apples horizontally to make circles.
- Put a banana on a hot dog bun and spread with peanut butter.
- Break uncooked spaghetti into toothpick lengths and skewer cheese, cold meat, vegetables, or fruit chunks.

Praise children for what they do eat.
Do not punish children for not eating by removing their dessert or putting them to bed.

This type of hair also requires a special hair dressing or pomade, which usually has a coconut oil base. The preparation is rubbed on the hands and then transferred to the hair to make it more pliable and manageable. The child's parents should be consulted regarding the preparation they want to be used on their child's hair, and they should be asked if they can provide some for use during the child's hospitalization. Petroleum jelly should not be used. If braiding or plaiting the hair is desired, the hair should be damp and loosely woven. The hair tightens as it dries, which could result in tension folliculitis (Jackson, 1998).

Feeding the Sick Child

Loss of appetite is a symptom common to most childhood illnesses and is often the initial evidence of illness, preceding fever and other overt signs of infection. In most cases children can be permitted to determine their own need for food. Because an acute illness is usually short, the nutritional state is seldom compromised. In fact, urging foods on the sick child may precipitate nausea and vomiting and in some cases even cause an aversion to the feeding situation that can extend into the convalescent period and beyond.

Refusing to eat may also be one way children can exert power and control in an otherwise helpless situation. For young children, loss of appetite may be related to the depression of separation from their parents and their natural tendency toward negativism. Parents' concern with eating can intensify the problem. Forcing a child to eat only meets with rebellion and reinforces the behavior as a control mechanism. Parents are encouraged to relax any pressure during the period of acute illness. Although it is best to encourage high-quality nutritious foods, the child may desire foods and liquids that contain mostly empty or nonnutritional calories. Some well-tolerated foods include gelatin, clear soups, carbonated drinks, flavored ice pops, dry toast, crackers, and hard candy. Even though these substances are not nutritious, they can provide necessary fluid and calories.

Dehydration is always a hazard when children are febrile or anorexic, especially when this is accompanied by vomiting or diarrhea. An adequate fluid intake is encouraged by offering small amounts of favored fluids at frequent intervals and by offering salty foods (that increase thirst) if allowed. If diarrhea is present, high-carbohydrate liquids (e.g., carbonated beverages, gelatin, flavored ice pops) are avoided because they may aggravate the diarrhea by an osmotic effect. Also, replacing abnormal losses with plain water or undiluted broth, which may worsen the electrolyte imbalance, is not advocated. Fluids should not be forced, and the child should not be wakened from rest to take fluids. Forcing fluids may create the same difficulties as urging unwanted food. Gentle persuasion with preferred beverages will usually meet with success. Using play techniques can also be very effective (Guidelines box).

When children are placed on special diets, such as clear liquids after surgery or during episodes of diarrhea, assessment of

TABLE 45-1
Dosage Recommendations for Ibuprofen* (Children's Motrin)

			Oral Drops 50 mg/1.25 ml			Suspension 100 mg/5 ml		
			Rx		OTC	Rx		OTC
Weight			Fever under 39.2°C (102.5°F)	JRA,† Pain, and Fever ≥39.2°C (102.5°F)		Fever under 39.2°C (102.5°F)	JRA,† Pain, and Fever ≥39.2°C (102.5°F)	
lb	kg	Age (Years)	Droppers (5 mg/kg)	Droppers (10 mg/kg)	Droppers (7.5 mg/kg)	Teaspoons (5 mg/kg)	Teaspoons (10 mg/kg)	Teaspoons (7.5 mg/kg)
12-17	5.4-7.7	6-11 mo	½	1		¼	½	
18-23	8.2-10.4	12-13 mo	1	2		½	1	
24-35	10.9-15.9	2-3	1½	3	2	¾	1½	1
36-47	16.3-21.3	4-5				1	2	1½
48-59	21.8-26.8	6-8				1¼	2½	2
60-71	27.2-32.9	9-10				1½	3	2½
72-95	32.7-43.1	11				2	4	3

Modified from McNeil Consumer Products, Fort Washington, PA, June 1997.
*Doses should be administered every 6 to 8 hours. Another form of nonprescription ibuprofen is Children's Advil.
†The recommended maximum daily dose for JRA is 30 to 40 mg/kg.
Rx, Prescription needed; *OTC,* over the counter; *JRA,* juvenile rheumatoid arthritis.

their intake and readiness to advance to more complex foods is essential.

NURSE ALERT • Evidence of lack of readiness to advance the diet includes the following:
- Vomiting or diarrhea
- Decrease in appetite
- Abdominal cramping or distention
- Absence of bowel sounds
- Dehydration or weight loss

Once the child is feeling better, the appetite usually begins to improve. It is best to take advantage of any hungry period by serving high-quality foods and snacks. If the child still refuses to eat, nutritious fluids, such as prepared breakfast drinks, should be encouraged. Parents can be very helpful by bringing in favorite food items from home, especially if the family's cultural eating habits differ from the hospital's food services.

In general, hot dogs, hamburgers, peanut butter-and-jelly sandwiches, fruit yogurt, milkshakes, spaghetti, tacos, macaroni and cheese, and pizza are favorite foods of most children. Although alone they may not typify well-balanced diets, they can be adjusted to include sufficient amounts from the different food groups. It is better to work with preferred food choices than with selections that children rarely eat. A number of creative approaches to food preparation can increase the child's interest in eating (Guidelines box).

Regardless of the type of diet, charting of the amount consumed is an important nursing responsibility. Descriptions need to be detailed and accurate, such as "4 ounces of orange juice, one pancake, no bacon, and 8 ounces of milk." Comments such as "ate well" or "ate poorly" are inadequate. Charting the percentage of the meal eaten is also inadequate unless food is measured before serving.

NURSE ALERT • Ask the parent if the child ate all of the food from the tray. Occasionally a parent may eat something from the tray because the child did not eat or want it. If a family member has eaten some of the food, this makes a marked difference in the report of how much the child ate.

If parents are involved in the child's care, they are encouraged to keep a list of everything eaten. Using a premeasured cup for fluids ensures a more accurate estimate of intake. A comparison of the intake at each meal can isolate food deficiencies, such as insufficient intake of meat or vegetables. Behaviors associated with mealtime also identify possible factors influencing appetite. For example, the observation that "Child eats well when with other children but plays with food if left alone in room" helps the nurse plan mealtime activities that stimulate the appetite.

Controlling Elevated Temperatures

An elevated temperature, most commonly from fever but occasionally caused by hyperthermia, is one of the most common symptoms of illness in children. This manifestation is often misunderstood and of great, but often unnecessary, concern to parents. To facilitate an understanding of fever, the following terms are defined:

Set point—The temperature around which body temperature is regulated by a thermostat-like mechanism in the hypothalamus

Fever—An elevation in set point such that body temperature is regulated at a higher level; may be arbitrarily defined as temperature above 38° C (100° F)

Hyperthermia—A situation in which body temperature exceeds the set point, which usually results from the body or external conditions creating more heat than the body can

Chewable Tablets 50 mg			Chewable Tablets 100 mg			Caplets 100 mg		
Rx		OTC	Rx		OTC	Rx		OTC
Fever under 39.2°C (102.5°F)	JRA†, Pain, and Fever ≥39.2°C (102.5°F)		Fever under 39.2°C (102.5°F)	JRA,† Pain, and Fever ≥39.2°C (102.5°F)		Fever under 39.2°C (102.5°F)	JRA,† Pain, and Fever ≥39.2°C (102.5°F)	
Tablets (5 mg/kg)	Tablets (10 mg/kg)	Tablets (7.5 mg/kg)	Tablets (5 mg/kg)	Tablets (10 mg/kg)	Tablets (7.5 mg/kg)	Caplets (5 mg/kg)	Caplets (10 mg/kg)	Caplets (7.5 mg/kg)
1	2		½	1				
1½	3	2	¾	1½				
2	4	3	1	2		1	2	
2½	5		1¼	2½	2	1¼	2½	2
3	6		1½	3	2½	1½	3	2½
4	8		2	4	3	2	4	3

eliminate, such as in heatstroke, aspirin toxicity, seizures, or hyperthyroidism

Body temperature is regulated by a thermostat-like mechanism in the hypothalamus. This mechanism receives input from centrally and peripherally located receptors. When temperature changes occur, these receptors relay the information to the thermostat, which either increases or decreases heat production to maintain a constant set point temperature. During an infection, however, pyrogenic substances cause an increase in the body's normal set point, a process that is mediated by prostaglandins. Consequently, the hypothalamus increases heat production until the core (internal) temperature reaches the new set point (Connell, 1997).

Most fevers in children are of viral origin, are of relatively brief duration, and have limited consequences. In addition, fever probably plays a role in enhancing the development of both specific and nonspecific immunity and in aiding recovery and survival from infection. Contrary to popular belief, neither the rise in temperature nor its response to antipyretics indicates the severity or etiology of infection, which casts doubt on the value of using fever as a diagnostic or prognostic indicator.

Measures to Reduce Elevated Temperature. Treatment of elevated temperature depends on whether it is caused by a fever or hyperthermia. Because the set point is normal in hyperthermia but increased in fever, different approaches must be used to lower body temperature successfully.

Fever. The principal reason for treating fever is the relief of discomfort; there is no specific degree of fever that requires treatment. Relief measures include pharmacologic and/or environmental intervention. The most effective intervention is the use of antipyretics to lower the set point.

Antipyretic drugs include acetaminophen, aspirin, and nonsteroidal antiinflammatory drugs (NSAIDs). Acetaminophen is the preferred drug; aspirin should not be given to children because of the association between aspirin use in children with influenza virus or chickenpox and Reye syndrome. One nonprescription NSAID, ibuprofen (Children's Motrin or Children's Advil), is approved for fever reduction in children as young as 6 months of age (Table 45-1). Dosage is based on the initial temperature level: 5 mg/kg of body weight for temperatures less than 39.1° C (102.5° F) or 10 mg/kg for temperatures greater than 39.1° C. The recommended dosage for pain is 10 mg/kg every 6 to 8 hours, and the recommended maximum daily dose for pain and fever is 40 mg/kg. Nonprescription ibuprofen (e.g., Advil, Nuprin, Motrin IB, and Medipren) is not approved for use in children under 12 years of age, and should not be used unless discussed with the primary care provider. Table 45-2 lists the recommended dosages of acetaminophen. It may be given every 4 hours but no more than five times in 24 hours. Because body temperature normally decreases at night, three or four doses in 24 hours are usually sufficient to control most fevers. The temperature is usually retaken 30 minutes after the antipyretic is given to assess its effect but should not be repeatedly measured; the child's level of discomfort is the best indication for continued treatment.

NURSE ALERT • Acetaminophen is an effective antipyretic and analgesic when administered as recommended. However, it is important to recognize its full toxic potential in both acute overdose and excessive therapeutic administration. Several cases of acetaminophen hepatotoxicity have been reported in children who received overdoses of the drug as part of therapeutic administration (Kearns, Leeder, and Wasserman, 1998).

Environmental measures to reduce fever may be used if tolerated by the child and if they do not induce shivering. Shivering is the body's way of maintaining the elevated set point by producing heat. Compensatory shivering greatly increases metabolic requirements above those already caused by the fever.

TABLE 45-2
Dosage Recommendations for Acetaminophen (Tylenol)*

Weight lb	Weight kg	Age (Years)	Infants' Concentrated Drops 80 mg/0.8 ml (Droppers)	Children's Suspension Liquid and Elixir 160 mg/5 ml (Teaspoons)	Children's Chewable Tablets 80 mg (Tablets)	Junior-Strength Chewable Tablets/Caplets 160 mg (Tablets/Caplets)	Suppositories† (not Tylenol) Number (mg)
6-11	2.7-5	0.3 mo	½				½ (80)
12-17	5.4-7.7	4-11 mo	1	½			1 (80)
18-23	8.2-10.4	12-23 mo	1½	¾			1 (120)
24-35	10.9-15.9	2-3	2	1	2		1 (120)
36-47	16.3-21.3	4-5		1½	3		2 (120)
48-59	21.8-26.8	6-8		2	4	2	1 (325)
60-71	27.2-32.2	9-10		2½	5	2½	1 (325)
72-95	32.7-43.1	11		3	6	3	1½ (325)
96	43.5	12				4	2 (325)

Modified from McNeil Consumer Products, Fort Washington, PA, 1997.
*Doses should be administered four or five times daily but should not exceed five doses or 75 mg/kg in 24 hours. Many other brands of acetaminophen are available (e.g., Panadol, Tempra, Liquiprin, St. Joseph Aspirin-Free Chewable, and Feverall suppositories).
†Cut suppository in half *lengthwise.*

NURSE ALERT • Treatment of shivering is directed at modifying or interfering with the rate of heat loss by warming the body with increased clothing (especially on the extremities), higher environmental temperature, and warm baths (Holtzclaw, 1990).

Traditional cooling measures, such as wearing minimum clothing, exposing the skin to the air, reducing room temperature, increasing air circulation, and applying cool, moist compresses to the skin (e.g., the forehead), are effective if employed approximately 1 hour after an antipyretic is given so that the set point is lowered. Cooling procedures such as sponging or tepid baths are ineffective in treating febrile children either when used alone or in combination with antipyretics, and they cause considerable discomfort (Sharber, 1997).

Seizures associated with a fever occur in 3% to 4% of all children, usually those 3 months to 5 years of age. Although most children never have febrile seizures after the first occurrence, a younger age at onset and a family history of febrile seizures are associated with recurring episodes. For children who have febrile seizures, administration of antipyretics does not prevent recurrences.

Hyperthermia. Unlike with fever, antipyretics are of no value in hyperthermia because the set point is already normal. Consequently, cooling measures are used. Cool applications to the skin help to reduce the core temperature. Cooled blood from the skin surface is conducted to inner organs and tissues, and warm blood is circulated to the surface, where it is cooled and recirculated. The surface blood vessels dilate as the body attempts to dissipate heat to the environment and facilitate this cooling process.

Commercial cooling devices, such as cooling blankets or mattresses, are available to reduce body temperature. They are placed on the bed and covered with a sheet or lightweight blanket. Frequent temperature monitoring is essential to prevent excessive cooling of the body.

Traditionally, cool compresses have been used to decrease high temperature; however, no particular temperature of water is agreed on as optimum. For tepid tub baths it is usually best to start with warm water and gradually add cool water until the desired water temperature of 37° C (98.6° F) is reached to accustom the child to the lower water temperature. Generally, the temperature of the water only has to be 1° to 2° (usually a warm temperature) less than the child's temperature to be effective (Kinmonth, Fulton, and Campbell, 1992). The child is placed directly in the tub of tepid water for 20 to 30 minutes while water is gently squeezed from a washcloth over the back and chest or gently sprayed over the body from a sprayer. In the bed or crib, cool washcloths or towels are used, exposing only one area of the body at a time. The sponging is continued for approximately 30 minutes.

After the tub or sponge bath, the child is dried and dressed in lightweight pajamas, a nightgown, or a diaper and placed in a dry bed. The temperature is retaken 30 minutes after the tub bath or sponge bath. The child is dried by gently rubbing the skin surface with a towel to stimulate circulation. The tub or sponge bath should not be continued if the child feels chilled or restarted until the skin surface is warm. Chilling causes vasoconstriction, which defeats the purpose of the cool applications. In this condition, little blood is carried to the skin surface; the blood remains primarily in the viscera to become heated.

Whether a temperature elevation in the critically ill child is caused by fever or hyperthermia, it should be treated more aggressively. The metabolic rate increases 10% for every 1° C increase in temperature, and increases three to five times during shivering; this increases oxygen, fluid, and caloric requirements. If the child's cardiovascular or neurologic system is already compromised, these increased needs are especially hazardous (Bruce and Grove, 1992). In all children with elevated temperature, attention to adequate hydration is essential. Most children's needs can be met through additional oral fluids.

Family Teaching and Home Care

Nurses have a unique opportunity for teaching the family about health care practices while the child is hospitalized. Although most children have learned self-care and hygiene in the home or at school, many have not. For some young children, this is their first introduction to the use of a toothbrush. Much health teaching can be accomplished even when the child is hospitalized for only a short time. The daily bath, handwashing before meals and after bowel and bladder evacuation, and conscientious dental hygiene are taught by example during routine care. Clean hair, nails, and clothing, as well as good grooming, are emphasized as being essential to a pleasing appearance. Positive reinforcement of good hygiene practices helps to create a positive body image, promote the development of self-esteem, and prevent health problems (e.g., teaching girls to wipe the genital area from front to back after toileting).

Although sick children's appetites may be poor and not characteristic of their home eating habits, the hospital stay provides numerous opportunities for nurses to assess the family's knowledge of good nutrition and to implement teaching as needed to improve nutritional intake.

Parental education about elevated temperatures is essential because many parents are unaware of what constitutes a fever, have unrealistic fears about the dangers of fever, and are apt to overmedicate or undermedicate the febrile child. However, when parents' report a fever, research has shown that parents' assessment is quite accurate (Hooker et al, 1996). Parents also need to know that sponging is indicated for elevated temperatures from hyperthermia rather than fever, and that ice water and alcohol are inappropriate, potentially dangerous, solutions. Parents should know how to take the child's temperature and read the thermometer accurately, and should have guidelines for seeking professional care (Home Care box).* Some of the newer temperature-measuring devices, such as tympanic membrane sensors, plastic strips, or digital thermometers, may be better suited for home use because many parents are unable to read a mercury thermometer (see Temperature, Chapter 35).

If the use of acetaminophen and ibuprofen is indicated, the parents need instruction in administering the drug.* It is important to emphasize accuracy in both the amount of drug given and the time intervals at which the drug is administered. Because many forms of acetaminophen are available, the nurse must be certain of the type being used in the home when discussing dosage. For example, the chewable tablets come in two strengths (80 and 160 mg), and the specially coated, swallowable tablets for older children are 160 mg. The nurse should alert the parents to this because the tablets for older children may contain twice the amount of drug as the lower-dose chewable ones. If parents switch from the infant drops to the elixir, they are cautioned against using the dropper to measure the elixir, which is much less concentrated than the drops. Also, as children grow, the dosage needs to be recalculated.

SAFETY

Safety is an essential component of any patient's care, but children have special characteristics that require an even greater concern for safety. Because small children are separated from their usual environment and do not possess the capacity for abstract thinking and reasoning, it is the responsibility of everyone who comes in contact with them to maintain protective measures throughout their hospital stay. Nurses need to understand the age level at which each child is operating and plan for safety accordingly.

Name bands, a part of hospital safety practices, are particularly important for children in the pediatric age group. Infants and unconscious patients are unable to tell or respond to their names. Toddlers may answer to any name or to a nickname only. Older children may exchange places, give an erroneous name, or choose not to respond to their own names as a form of joke, unaware of the hazards of such practices.

Home Care

THE CHILD WITH FEVER

Call Our Office Immediately If:

Your child is less than 3 months old.
The fever is over 40.6°C (105°F).
Your child looks or acts very sick.

Call Within 24 Hours If:

Your child is 3 to 6 months old (unless the fever is due to a diphtheria-pertussis-tetanus [DPT] shot).
The fever is between 40° and 40.6°C (104° and 105°F), especially if your child is less than 2 years old.
Your child has had a fever for more than 24 hours without an obvious cause or location of infection.
Your child has had a fever for more than 3 days.
The fever went away for more than 24 hours and then returned.
You have other concerns or questions.

Modified from Schmitt BD: *Instructions for pediatric patients,* ed 2, Philadelphia, 1999, WB Saunders.

Infection Control

The use of medical asepsis and appropriate barrier precautions to reduce the risk of *nosocomial* (hospital-acquired) infections is essential in caring for children. Children are commonly infected with organisms such as varicella (chickenpox) that are transmissible and may be dangerous to others, especially immunocompromised patients. In addition, children may not have developed good hygiene habits, such as handwashing after toileting. Young children are especially at risk for infection because of their high oral activity. Children in diapers present infection risks if caregivers do not practice meticulous cleaning and disposal techniques.

To assist hospitals in maintaining up-to-date isolation practices, the Centers for Disease Control and Prevention (CDC) and the Hospital Infection Control Practices Advisory Committee (HICPAC) have revised the "CDC Guideline for Isolation Precautions in Hospitals," which was published in 1983. The guideline was revised to meet the following objectives: (1) to be epidemiologically sound; (2) to recognize the importance of all body fluids, secretions, and excretions in the transmission of nosocomial pathogens; (3) to contain adequate precautions for infections transmitted by the airborne, droplet, and contact routes of transmission; (4) to be as simple and user friendly as possible; and (5) to use new terms to avoid confusion with existing infection control and isolation systems (Garner, 1997).

The revised guideline contains two levels of precautions. In the first, and most important, level are those precautions designed for the care of all patients in hospitals regardless of their

*Community and home care instructions on measuring temperature and giving medications are available in Wong DL, Hess CS: ***Wong and Whaley's clinical manual of pediatric nursing***, ed 5, St Louis, 2000, Mosby.

diagnosis or presumed infection status. Implementation of these "standard precautions" is the primary strategy for successful nosocomial infection control. In the second level are precautions designed only for the care of specified patients. These additional "transmission-based precautions" are used for patients known or suspected to be infected or colonized with epidemiologically important pathogens that can be transmitted by airborne or droplet transmission or by contact with dry skin or contaminated surfaces.

Standard Precautions synthesize the major features of Universal (blood and body fluid) Precautions (UP) (designed to reduce the risk of transmission of blood-borne pathogens) and body substance isolation (BSI) (designed to reduce the risk of transmission of pathogens from moist body substances). Standard Precautions involve the use of *barrier protection,* such as gloves, goggles, gown, and/or mask, to prevent contamination from (1) blood; (2) all body fluids, secretions, and excretions *except sweat,* regardless of whether or not they contain visible blood; (3) non-intact skin; and (4) mucous membranes. Standard Precautions are designed to reduce the risk of transmission of microorganisms from both recognized and unrecognized sources of infection in hospitals.

Transmission-based precautions are designed for patients documented or suspected to be infected or colonized with highly transmissible or epidemiologically important pathogens for which additional precautions beyond Standard Precautions are needed to interrupt transmission in hospitals. There are three types of transmission-based precautions: airborne precautions, droplet precautions, and contact precautions. They may be combined for diseases that have multiple routes of transmission (Box 45-6). When used either singularly or in combination, they are to be used in addition to Standard Precautions.

Airborne precautions are designed to reduce the risk of airborne transmission of infectious agents. Airborne transmission occurs by dissemination of either airborne droplet nuclei (i.e., small-particle residue [5 μm or smaller in size] of evaporated droplets that may remain suspended in the air for long periods) or dust particles containing the infectious agent. Microorganisms carried in this manner can be dispersed widely by air currents and may become inhaled by or deposited on a susceptible host within the same room or over a longer distance from the source patient, depending on environmental factors; therefore *special air handling* and *ventilation* are required to prevent airborne transmission. Airborne precautions apply to patients known or suspected to be infected with epidemiologically important pathogens that can be transmitted by the airborne route. Examples of such illnesses include measles, varicella (chickenpox), and tuberculosis.

Droplet precautions are designed to reduce the risk of droplet transmission of infectious agents. Droplet transmission involves contact of the conjunctivae or the mucous membranes of the nose or mouth of a susceptible person with large-particle droplets (larger than 5-m in size) containing microorganisms generated from a person who has a clinical disease or who is a carrier of the microorganism. Droplets are generated from the source person primarily during coughing, sneezing, or talking

Box 45-6

Summary of Types of Precautions and Patients Requiring Them

STANDARD PRECAUTIONS

Use Standard Precautions for the care of all patients.

AIRBORNE PRECAUTIONS

In addition to Standard Precautions, use airborne precautions for patients known or suspected to have serious illnesses transmitted by airborne droplet nuclei. Examples of such illnesses include measles, varicella (including disseminated zoster), tuberculosis.

DROPLET PRECAUTIONS

In addition to Standard Precautions, use droplet precautions for patients known or suspected to have serious illnesses transmitted by large particle droplets. Examples of such illnesses include the following:

- Invasive *Haemophilus influenzae* type b disease, including meningitis, pneumonia, epiglottitis, and sepsis
- Invasive *Neisseria meningitidis* disease, including meningitis, pneumonia, and sepsis
- Other serious bacterial respiratory infections spread by droplet transmission, including diphtheria (pharyngeal), mycoplasmal pneumonia, pertussis, pneumonic plague, streptococcal pharyngitis, pneumonia, or scarlet fever in infants and young children
- Serious viral infections spread by droplet transmission, including adenovirus, influenza, mumps, parvovirus B19, rubella

CONTACT PRECAUTIONS

In addition to Standard Precautions, use contact precautions for patients known or suspected to have serious illnesses easily transmitted by direct patient contact or by contact with items in the patient's environment. Examples of such illnesses include the following:

- Gastrointestinal, respiratory, skin, or wound infections or colonization with multidrug-resistant bacteria judged by the infection control program, based on current state, regional, or national recommendations, to be of special clinical and epidemiologic significance
- Enteric infections with a low infectious dose or prolonged environmental survival, including *Clostridium difficile.* For diapered or incontinent patients: enterohemorrhagic *Escherichia coli* O157:H7, *Shigella,* hepatitis A, or rotavirus
- Respiratory syncytial virus, parainfluenza virus, or enteroviral infections in infants and young children.
- Skin infections that are highly contagious or that may occur on dry skin, including diphtheria (cutaneous), herpes simplex virus (neonatal or mucocutaneous), impetigo, major (noncontained) abscesses, cellulitis or decubiti, pediculosis, scabies, staphylococcal furunculosis in infants and young children, zoster (disseminated or in the immunocompromised host)
- Viral/hemorrhagic conjunctivitis
- Viral hemorrhagic infections (Ebola, Lassa, or Marburg)

From Garner JS. Guidelines for isolation precautions in hospitals, *Infect Control Hosp Epidemiol* 17(1):66, 1996.

and during the performance of certain procedures such as suctioning and bronchoscopy. Transmission via large-particle droplets requires close contact between source and recipient persons, because droplets do not remain suspended in the air and generally travel only short distances, usually 3 feet or less, through the air. Because droplets do not remain suspended in the air, special air handling and ventilation are not required to prevent droplet transmission. Droplet precautions apply to any patient known or suspected to be infected with epidemiologically important pathogens that can be transmitted by infectious droplets (see Box 45-6).

Contact precautions are designed to reduce the risk of transmission of epidemiologically important microorganisms by direct or indirect contact. *Direct-contact transmission* involves a direct body surface-to-body surface contact and physical transfer of microorganisms to a susceptible host from an infected or colonized person, such as occurs when personnel turn patients, bathe patients, or perform other patient care activities that require physical contact. Direct-contact transmission also can occur between two patients (e.g., by hand contact), with one serving as the source of infectious microorganisms and the other as a susceptible host. *Indirect-contact transmission* involves contact of a susceptible host with a contaminated intermediate object, usually inanimate, in the patient's environment (e.g., a contaminated instrument or contaminated hands that are not washed and gloves that are not changed between patients). Contact precautions apply to specified patients known or suspected to be infected or colonized (presence of microorganism in or on the patient but without clinical signs and symptoms of infection) with epidemiologically important microorganisms that can be transmitted by direct or indirect contact.

NURSE ALERT • The most common piece of medical equipment, the stethoscope, can be a potent source of harmful microorganisms and nosocomial infections. One study found that 80% of 200 stethoscopes were contaminated with at least one microbe (Eckler, 1997).

Nurses caring for young children are often in contact with body substances, especially urine, feces, and vomitus. Nurses need to exercise judgment for those situations when gloves, gowns, or masks are necessary. For example, gloves and possibly gowns should be worn for changing diapers when there are loose or explosive stools. Otherwise, the plastic lining of disposable diapers provides a sufficient barrier between the hands and body substances. The type of diaper may be an important aspect of infection control. Superabsorbent disposable diapers with elastic legs contain urine and feces better than cloth diapering systems, and their use can reduce fecal contamination in the environment (Kubiak et al, 1993).

NURSE ALERT • Handwashing is the most critical infection control practice.

During feedings, gowns should be worn if the child is likely to vomit or spit up, which often occurs during burping. If aprons with minimal shoulder protection are worn, the child should be sitting on the nurse's lap, not upright against the shoulder, when the child is bubbled. When gloves are worn, the hands are washed thoroughly after removing the gloves, because both latex and vinyl gloves fail to provide complete protection. The absence of visible leaks does not indicate that gloves are intact. In addition, glove leaks occur more often with vinyl than with latex gloves (Olsen et al, 1993).

Another essential practice of infection control is that all needles (uncapped and unbroken) are disposed of in a rigid, puncture-resistant container located near the site of use. Consequently, these containers are installed in patients' rooms. Because children are naturally curious, extra attention is needed in selecting a suitable type of container and a location that discourages access to the disposed needles (Fig. 45-5). The use of needleless systems allows secure syringe or IV tubing attachment to vascular access devices without the risk of needle-stick injury to the child or nurse.

Environmental Factors

All of the environmental safety measures in operation for the protection of adults apply to children as well. These measures include good illumination, floors clear of fluid or objects that might contribute to falls, and nonskid surfaces in showers and tubs. Electrical equipment should be maintained in good working order; be operated only by personnel familiar with its use; and not placed in contact with moisture or near tubs, where it could prove to be a shock hazard. Beds of ambulatory patients are locked in place and at a height that allows easy access to the

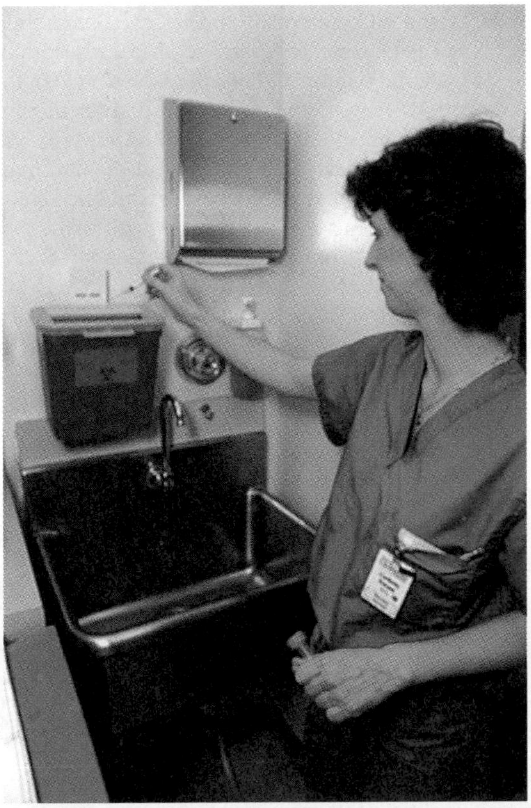

FIG. 45-5 • To prevent needle stick injuries, used needles (and other sharp instruments) are not capped or broken and are disposed of in a rigid, puncture-resistant container located near the site of use. Note placement of the container to prevent children's access to the contents.

floor. A special hazard for children is the danger of entrapment under an electronically controlled bed when it is activated to descend. Staff members should practice proper care and disposal of breakable items such as thermometers and bottles and small items such as syringe caps or needle covers. A well-organized fire plan should be known to all staff members.

All windows should be securely screened, and elevators and stairways made safe. Ideally, electrical outlets should be provided with covers to prevent burns in small children, whose exploratory activities may extend to inserting objects into the small openings. Bathwater is carefully checked before placing the child in it, and children must never be left alone in a bathtub. Infants are helpless in water, and small children (and some older ones) may turn on the hot water faucet and be severely burned.

Furniture is safest when it is scaled to the child's proportions, is sturdy, and is well balanced to prevent its being easily tipped over. Infants and small children must be securely strapped into infant seats, feeding chairs, and strollers. Baby walkers should be discouraged because they provide access to hazards, resulting in burns, falls, and poisonings. Infants; young children; and those who are weak, paralyzed, agitated, confused, sedated, or cognitively impaired are never left unattended on treatment tables, on scales, or in treatment areas. Even premature infants are capable of surprising mobility; therefore portholes in incubators must be securely fastened when not in use. Beds of ambulatory patients should remain locked in place and at a height that allows easy access to the floor.

Crib sides should be elevated and fastened securely unless an adult is at the bedside. It is safer to leave crib sides up, regardless of the child's ability to get out and even when the crib is unoccupied, to remove the child's temptation to climb in. Anyone attending an infant or small child in a crib with the sides down should never turn away without maintaining hand contact with the child; that is, one hand should be kept on the child's back or abdomen to prevent the child from rolling, crawling, or jumping from the open crib (Fig. 45-6). A child who is apt to or has demonstrated the inclination to climb over the sides of the crib is safest when placed in a specially constructed crib with a cover or one that has a safety net placed over the top. If the net is used, it must be tied to the frame in such a manner that there is ready access to the child in case of emergency. Nets are never tied to the movable crib sides, and the knots should be tied in a manner that permits quick release. Cribs are not placed within reach of heating units, appliances, dangling cords, or other objects that can be grabbed by curious hands, and toys are not tied to or across crib rails once children are old enough to reach them.

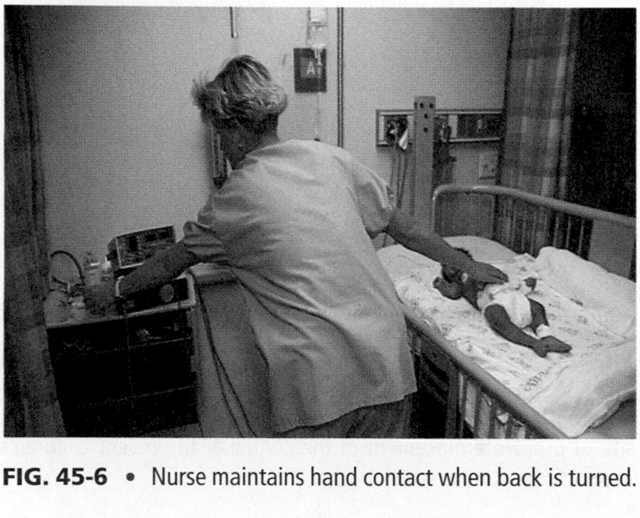

FIG. 45-6 • Nurse maintains hand contact when back is turned.

Toys. Toys play a vital role in the everyday life of children, and they are no less important in the hospital setting. However, nurses are responsible for assessing the safety of toys brought to the hospital by well-meaning parents and friends. Toys and gifts should be appropriate to the child's age, condition, and treatment. For example, if the child is in an oxygen tent, electrical or friction toys cannot be placed in the tent. Toys are inspected to make certain that they are nonallergenic, washable, and unbreakable and that they have no small, removeable parts that can be aspirated or swallowed or that can in other ways inflict injury to a child.

NURSE ALERT • Plants and flowers harbor gram-negative bacteria and molds that may be a risk to the immunocompromised child. These items may also pose the danger of poisoning to curious toddlers.

Limit Setting

Setting limits is essential to a child's safety. Children must understand where they are permitted to go and what they are permitted to do in the hospital. These limitations should be made clear to them, consistently enforced, and repeated as often as necessary to make certain that they are understood. The nurse is responsible for a child's whereabouts at all times. Children can easily wander off unnoticed, and their access to tubs, laundry chutes, medication rooms and carts, and elevators must be prevented. Normally active older children often become restless when their activity is restricted and may resort to pillow fights, water fights, and other rough play that might endanger the safety of the involved children or other children, staff, or visitors. Children in the hospital require supervision, and appropriate tension-reducing activities can be planned and supervised by nurses and/or by the play therapist. A useful discipline technique is time-out (see Limit Setting and Discipline, Chapter 31).

Transporting Infants and Children

In the course of a hospital stay, infants and children usually need to be transported within the unit and to areas outside the pediatric unit. Infants and small children can be carried for short distances within the unit, but for more extended trips the child should be securely transported in a suitable conveyance.

Small infants can be held or carried in the horizontal position with the back supported and the thigh grasped firmly by the carrying arm (Fig. 45-7, *A*). In the football hold, the infant is carried on the nurse's arm with the head supported by the hand and the body held securely between the nurse's body and elbow (Fig. 45-7, *B*). Both of these holds leave the nurse's other arm free for activity. The infant can be held in the upright position with the buttocks on the nurse's forearm and the front of the body resting against the nurse's chest. The infant's head and shoulders are supported by the nurse's other arm to allow for any sudden movement by the infant (Fig. 45-7, *C*). Older infants are able to hold their heads erect but can still make sudden movements.

Infants can be transported to other areas, such as the radiography department, in their bassinets or cribs. Baby carriages are sometimes used for infants who are not likely to stand up. Strollers and wheeled feeding chairs or tables are also convenient transporters in some situations, such as trips to the playroom or nurse's station.

The method of transporting children is determined by their age, condition, and destination. Most older children are safe in wheelchairs or on gurneys. A younger child can be transported in a crib, on a gurney, in a wagon with raised sides, or in a wheelchair with a safety belt. Gurneys should be equipped with high sides and a safety belt, both of which are secured during transport.

Restraining Methods and Therapeutic Hugging

Restraining methods and therapeutic hugging are common practices in nursing to ensure a child's safety or comfort, facilitate examination, and aid in performing diagnostic tests and therapeutic procedures. *Therapeutic hugging* is the use of a secure, comfortable, temporary holding position that provides close physical contact with the parent or other trusted caregiver (see Fig. 45-10).

Nurses need to assess whether or not restraints are needed. Restraints can often be avoided with adequate preparation of the child; parental or staff supervision of the child; and adequate protection of a vulnerable site, such as an infusion device. The nurse needs to take into account the child's development, mental status, potential threat to others or self, and safety. The Joint Commission on Accreditation of Healthcare Organizations (JCAHO) points to the need for a physician's order before application of restraint. However, alternative approaches to restraint must be attempted before seeking a physician's order for restraint (Selekman and Snyder, 1996). Therefore alternative measures to using restraints should be a careful consideration of the nurse. Creative approaches may make physical restraint unnecessary.

When a child must be restrained, it is important to explain to the child the reason for the restraint. This information should be repeated as often as needed to gain cooperation. Have the child verbalize understanding of the need for restraint. Explain how the child can help (e.g., "Your job is to keep your arm as still as a tree"). Most important, reassure the child that the restraint is not a punishment.

Parents need to know the purpose of restraints, how to remove and reapply them, and the signs of complications from their use. Document parental consent for restraints. Sometime parents are upset when their child must be restrained and need to understand how they can help. Explain ways in which they can help to ensure maximal benefit and minimal stress (e.g., have the parent emotionally support the child by staying near the child). Position the parent at the head of the bed (provide a chair for the parent) so that the parent can soothe or calm the child by talking softly, singing, or stroking the child's skin.

After the decision is made that some restraint is necessary, it must be determined what type of restraint should be applied. For example, arm boards are less restrictive than four-point extremity restraints. Using less restrictive restraints is often possible by gaining the cooperation of the child and parents. It is the nurse's responsibility to select the most appropriate and least restrictive type of restraint.

Restraining devices are not without risk and must be checked and documented every 1 to 2 hours to ensure that they are accomplishing their purpose; that they are applied correctly;

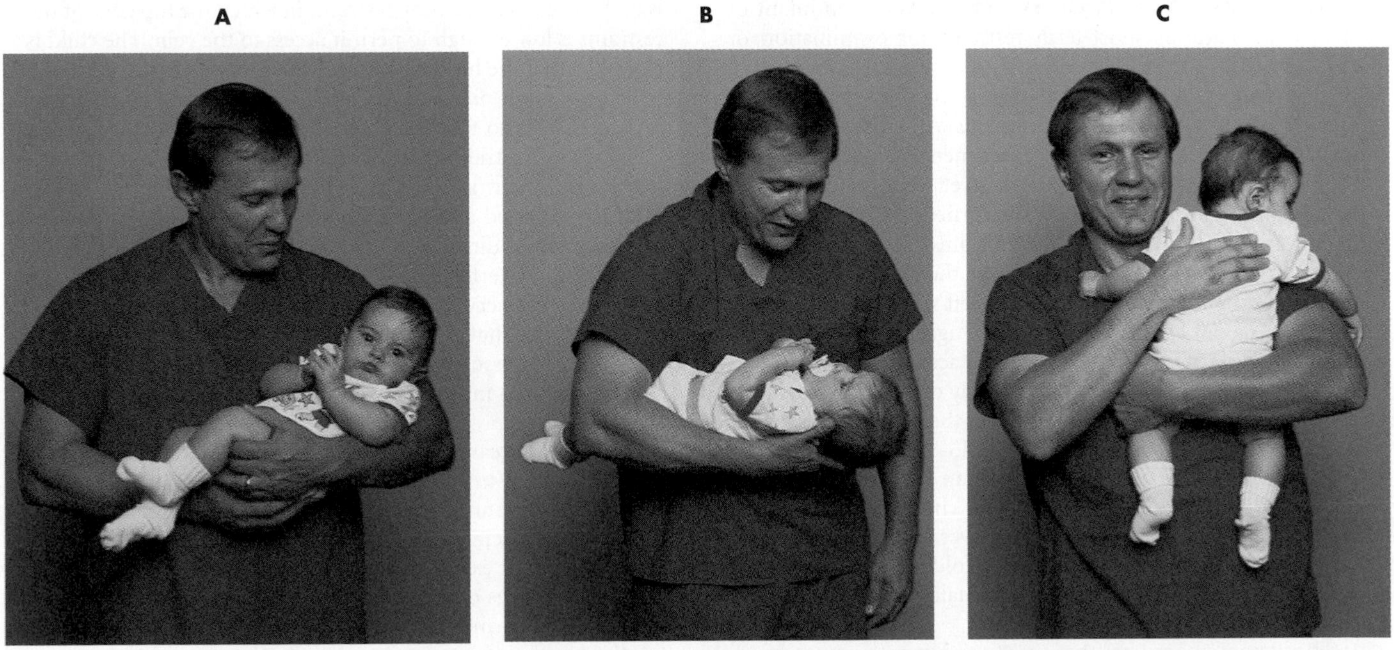

FIG. 45-7 • Transporting infants. **A,** Infant's thigh firmly grasped in nurse's hand. **B,** Football hold. **C,** Back supported.

and that they do not impair circulation, sensation, or skin integrity. Restraints with ties must be secured to the bed or crib frame, not the siderails.

Selekman and Snyder (1997) recommend appropriate nursing interventions for the child who is restrained. Parental participation is always encouraged. These include, but are not limited to, the following:

- Remove and reapply restraints periodically.
- Offer comfort measures; use "therapeutic hugging" rather than mechanical restraint.
- Raise head of bed 30 degrees unless contraindicated.
- Provide range of motion as appropriate.
- Offer food, fluids, and toileting as appropriate; give pacifier.
- Discuss criteria for removal of restraint.
- Administer analgesics and sedatives if ordered, or request if needed.
- Avoid psychologic upset to other patients.
- Provide distraction (e.g., read a book) and touch.
- Maintain child's dignity.
- Provide ongoing nursing assessment.
- Document use of restraints.

Nurses play an important role in the practice of using physical restraints on children. Until more research is available, nurses need to carefully assess the children in their care and apply the nursing process in the use of restraints.

Jacket Restraint. A jacket restraint is sometimes used as an alternative to the crib net to prevent the child from climbing out of the crib or to keep the child safe in various chairs. The jacket is put on the child with the ties in back so that the child is unable to manipulate them. The long tapes, secured to the understructure of the crib, keep the child inside the crib. The jacket restraint is also useful as a means of maintaining the child in a desired horizontal position. A Posey belt scaled to fit the child is an alternative device. The jacket-type restraint has been associated with accidental strangulation deaths in elderly persons.

Mummy Restraint or Swaddle. When an infant or small child requires short-term restraint for examination or treatment that involves the head and neck, such as venipuncture, throat examination, and gavage feeding, the mummy device effectively controls the child's movements. A blanket or sheet is opened on the bed or crib with one corner folded to the center. The infant is placed on the blanket with shoulders at the fold and feet toward the opposite corner (Fig. 45-8, *A*). With the infant's right arm straight down against the body, the right side of the blanket is pulled firmly across the infant's right shoulder and chest and secured beneath the left side of the body (Fig. 45-8, *B*). The left arm is placed straight against the child's side, and the left side of the blanket is brought across the shoulder and chest and locked beneath the child's body on the right side. The lower corner is folded and brought over the body and tucked or fastened securely with safety pins (Fig. 45-8, *C*). Safety pins can be used to fasten the blanket in place at any step in the process.

To modify the mummy restraint for chest examination, the folded edge of the blanket is brought over each arm and under the back, after which the loose edge is folded over and secured at a point below the chest to allow visualization and access to the chest (Fig. 45-8, *D*).

The papoose board has the same function as the mummy restraint. It is a solid board with straps attached that secure the infant or small child to the board, similar to a mummy restraint. For maximum comfort the board should be padded.

Arm and Leg Restraints. Arm and leg restraints are sometimes used to immobilize one or more extremities for treatment or procedures, or to facilitate healing. Several commercial restraining devices are available, including disposable wrist and ankle restraints, or a restraint can be fashioned from gauze tape, muslin strips, or a length of narrow stockinette. When this type of restraint is used, it must be appropriate to the size of the child; it must be padded to prevent undue pressure, constriction, or tissue injury; and the extremity must be observed often for signs of irritation and/or impairment of circulation. The ends of the restraints are never tied to the crib rails, because lowering the rail will disturb the extremity, often with a jerk that may hurt or injure the child.

The *clove hitch restraint* is fashioned from a length of gauze or muslin tape. When properly applied, the restraint should provide a snug fit with minimum danger of pulling too tightly. Fig. 45-9 illustrates the method of tying and applying a clove hitch restraint.

Elbow Restraint. Sometimes it is important to prevent the child from bending an elbow or reaching the head or face (e.g., after lip surgery, when a scalp vein infusion is in place, or to prevent scratching in skin disorders). For this purpose, elbow restraints fashioned from a variety of materials function very well. The most common form of elbow restraint consists of a piece of muslin long enough to reach comfortably from just below the axilla to the wrist with a number of vertical pockets into which tongue depressors are inserted. The restraint is wrapped around the arm and secured with tapes or pins. It may be necessary to pin the top of the restraint to the undershirt sleeve to prevent the restraint from slipping. Similar restraints can be made from commonly available products.

Jugular Venipuncture. The large, superficial external jugular vein may be used to obtain blood specimens from infants and young children. For easy access to the vein, the child is first placed in a mummy restraint in which the top edge of the restraint is low enough to permit access to the vein. The child is placed so that the head and shoulders extend over the edge of a table or a small pillow, with the neck extended and the head turned sharply to the side. One alternate method (therapeutic hugging) for restraining arms and legs is with the parent holding the child's arms and legs at the same time that the child's head is restrained and positioned (Fig. 45-10). It is important for the nurse holding the child to maintain control of the child's head without interfering with the practitioner's approach to the vein. The child's crying during the procedure increases IV pressure, which facilitates visualization of the vein. After venipuncture, digital pressure is applied to the site with a dry gauze square for 3 to 5 minutes or until bleeding stops. Care must be taken not to apply excessive pressure that might compromise circulation or breathing during or after the procedure.

Femoral Venipuncture. Other commonly used sites for venipuncture are the large femoral veins. The nurse restrains the infant by placing the child supine with the legs in a frog position to provide extensive exposure of the groin area. Both the arms and the legs of the infant can be effectively controlled by the nurse's forearms and hands (Fig. 45-11). Only the side used for the venipuncture is uncovered, so the practitioner is protected should the child urinate during the procedure. Pressure

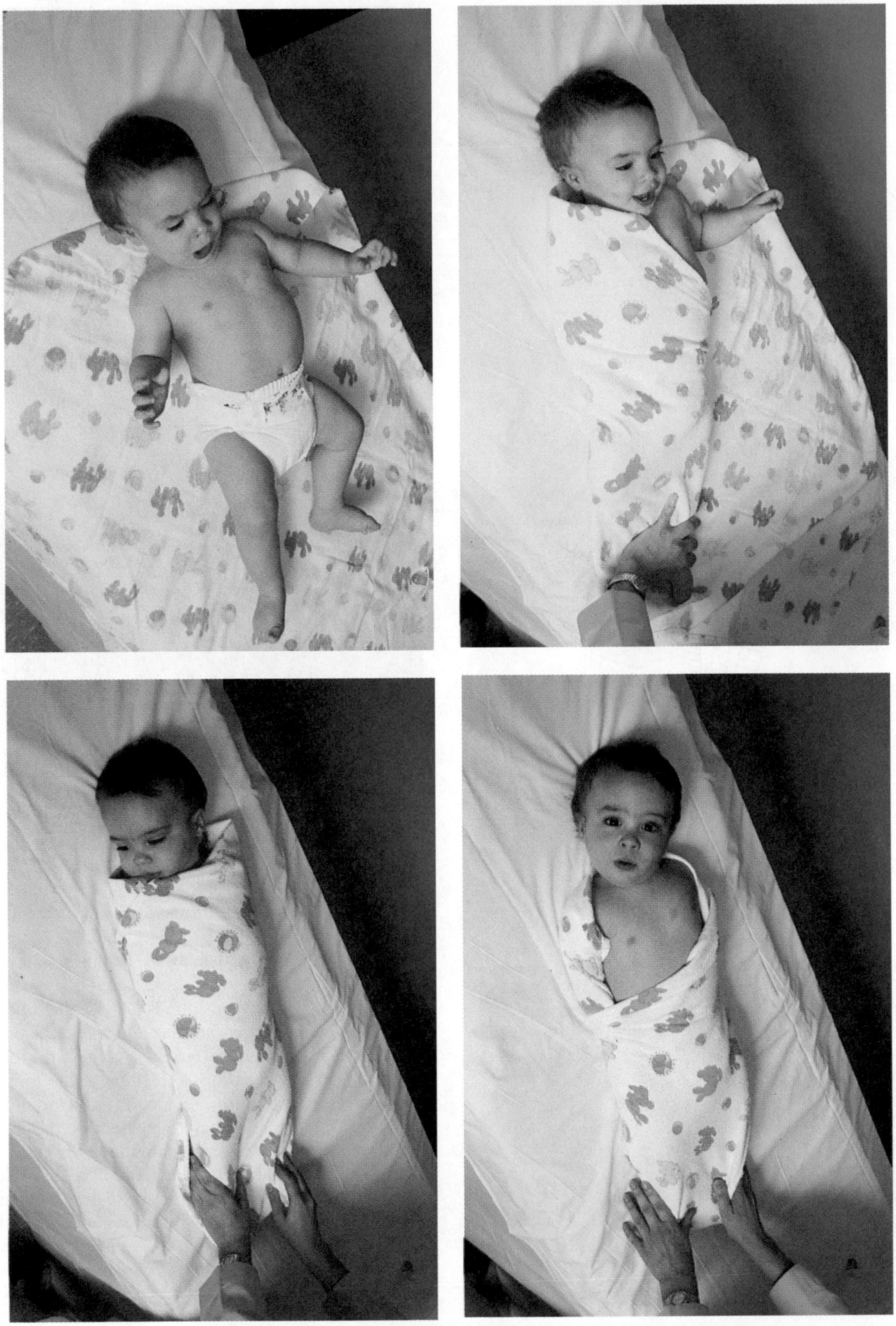

A B C D

FIG. 45-8 • Application of mummy restraint. **A,** Infant placed on folded corner of blanket. **B,** One corner of blanket brought across body and secured beneath body. **C,** Second corner brought across body and secured, and lower corner folded and tucked or pinned in place. **D,** Modified mummy restraint with chest uncovered.

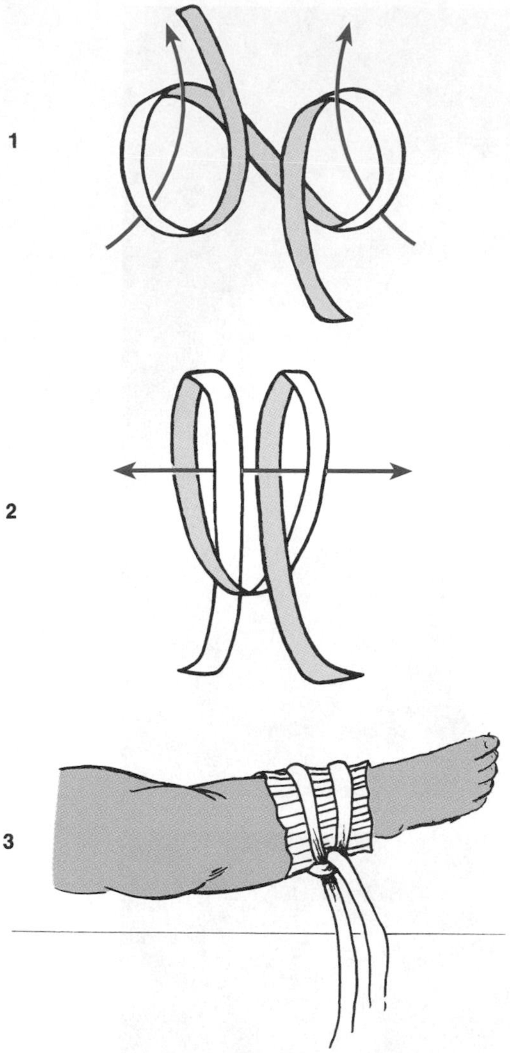

FIG. 45-9 • Clove hitch restraint.

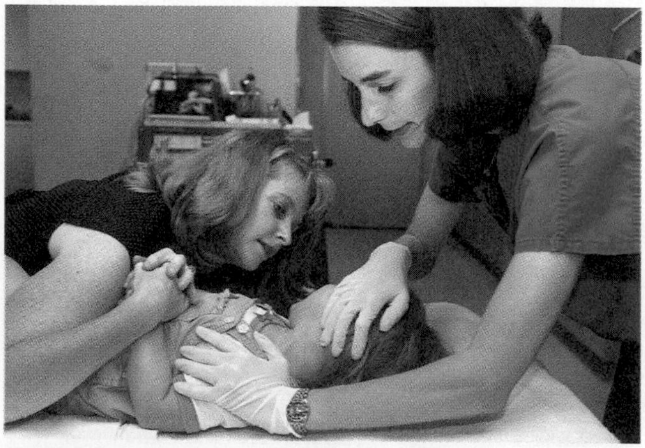

FIG. 45-10 • "Therapeutic hugging" of child for jugular vein puncture with parental assistance.

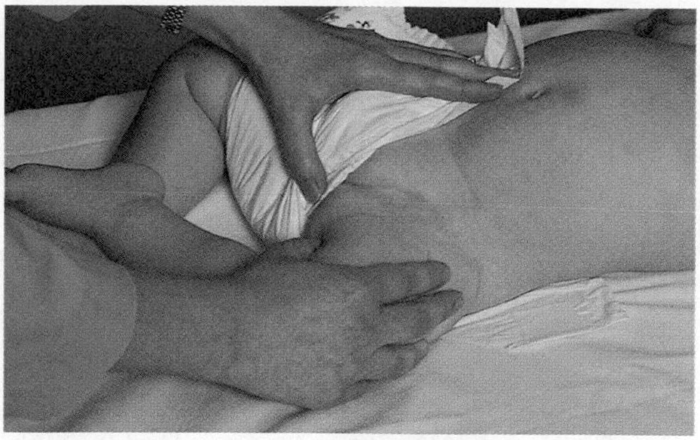

FIG. 45-11 • Restraining infant for femoral vein puncture.

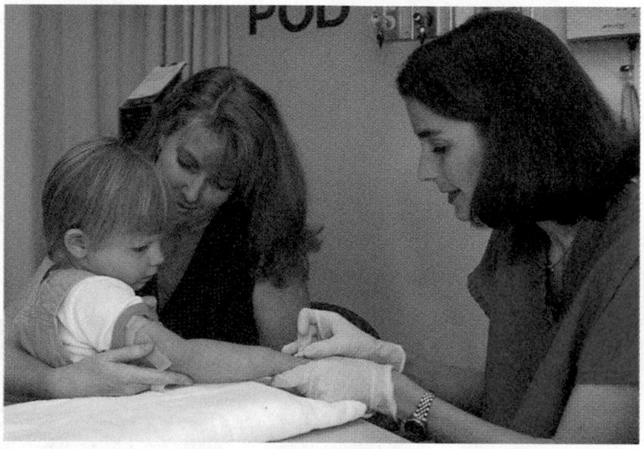

FIG. 45-12 • "Therapeutic hugging" of child for extremity vein puncture with parental assistance.

is applied to the site after the withdrawal of blood to prevent oozing from the site.

Extremity Venipuncture. The most common sites of venipuncture are the veins of the extremities, especially the arm and hand. A convenient position is to place the child in the parent's (or assistant's) lap, with the child facing the parent and in the straddle position. Next, place the child's arm for venipuncture on a firm surface, such as a treatment table, for support and on top of a soft cloth or towel. Have an assistant immobilize the arm for venipuncture, or have the parent do this if an assistant is not available. Then have the parent hug the child around the body to hold the child's free arm, and place the child's legs between the parent's legs (Fig. 45-12). If the child must remain supine, have the parent (or assistant) on one side of the bed and lean over the child's upper body to apply restraint, using the hand to hold the arm for the venipuncture. Have the operator stand on the other side of the bed for access to the arm for venipuncture.

Lumbar Puncture (LP). The technique for LP in infants and children is similar to that in the adult, although modifications are suggested in neonates, who have less distress in a side-lying position with modified neck extension than in flexion or a sitting position (Fig. 45-13, *A*). Neonates tend to have more

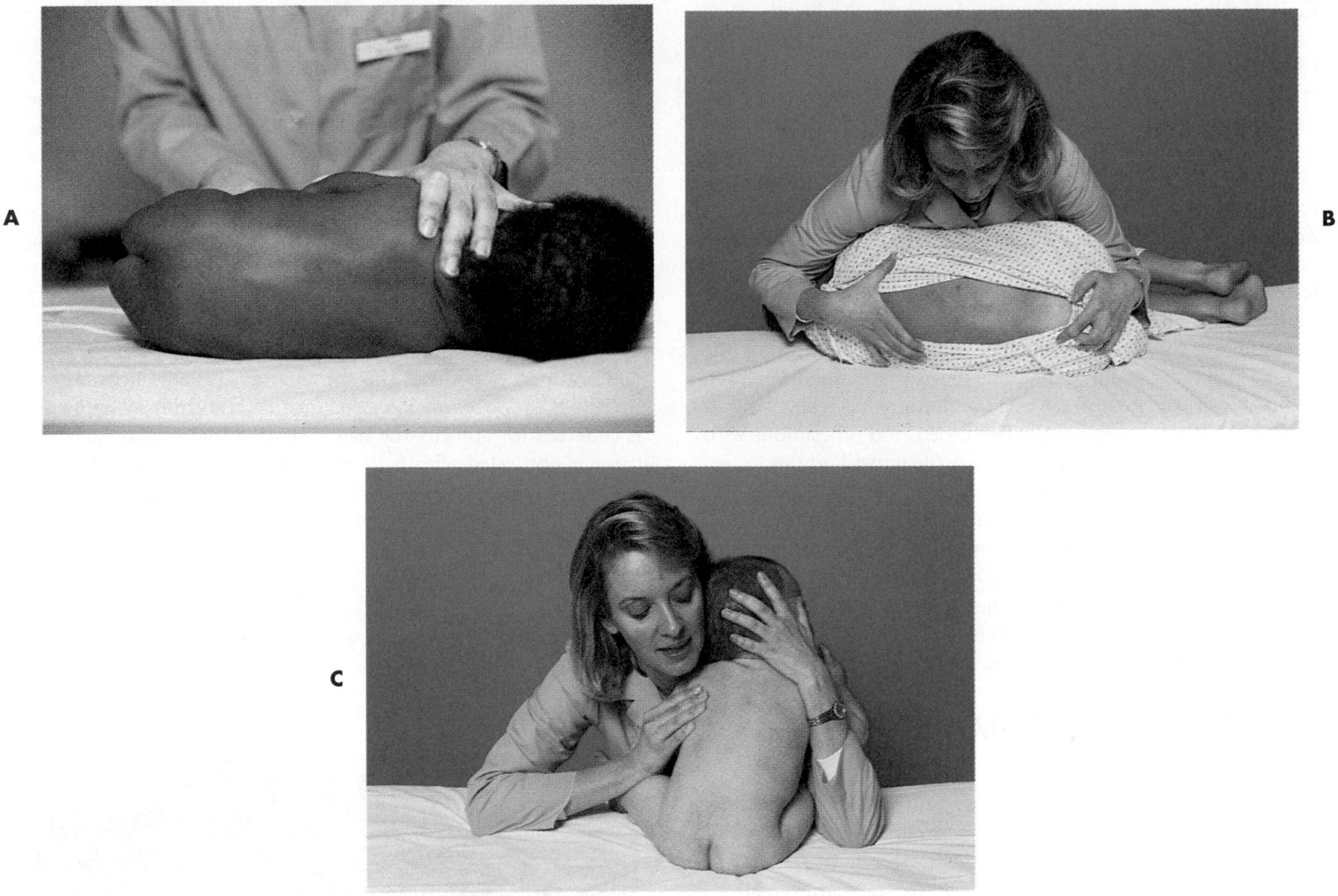

FIG. 45-13 • **A,** Modified side-lying position for lumbar puncture. **B,** Older child in side-lying position. **C,** Infant sitting position allows for flexion of lumbar spine.

cardiorespiratory changes during an LP than older infants regardless of positioning; therefore oximetry and heart rate monitoring are advisable (Lehmann et al, 1990). Pediatric LP sets contain smaller spinal needles, but sometimes the practitioner will specify a particular size or type of needle that the nurse should make certain is placed on the tray.

Children should receive adequate analgesia or anesthesia to relieve pain. EMLA, a mixture of a local and topical anesthetic in a cream form, should be applied before the LP.

Children are usually controlled best in the side-lying position, with the head flexed and the knees drawn up toward the chest. Even cooperative children need to be restrained to prevent possible trauma from unexpected, involuntary movement. They can be reassured that although they are trusted, the holding will serve as a reminder to maintain the desired position. It also provides a measure of support and reassurance to them.

The child is placed on the side with the back close to the edge of the examining table on the side from which the practitioner is working. The nurse maintains the child's spine in a flexed position by holding the child with one arm behind the neck and the other behind the thighs (Fig. 45-13, *B*). The flexed position enlarges the spaces between the lumbar vertebral spines and facilitates access to the spinal fluid space. It is helpful to wrap the legs before positioning to decrease leg movement.

An alternate position used with small infants and some older children is the sitting position. The child is placed with the buttocks at the edge of the table and with the neck flexed so that the chin rests on the chest or the nurse's arm. The infant's arms and legs are immobilized by the nurse's hands (Fig. 45-13, *C*).

NURSE ALERT • The sitting position may interfere with chest expansion and diaphragm excursion, and in infants the soft, pliable trachea may collapse. Therefore observe the child for difficulty with breathing.

Another position that employs close and comforting contact for the child involves holding the child upright against the nurse's (or parent's) chest with the child's legs wrapped around the adult's waist. The adult's arms are used to hug and restrain the child. For ease of the examiner, the adult should be standing. A small pillow is placed between the child's abdomen and the adult to help arch the child's back. If the pillow proves unsuccessful, a third person can place an arm in this space to achieve the desired position. Care should be taken that excessive pressure does not compromise circulation or breathing and that the nose and mouth are not covered by the restrainer's body.

Specimens and spinal fluid pressure are obtained, measured, and sent for analysis in the same manner as for the adult patient. Vital signs are taken as ordered, and the child is observed for any changes in level of consciousness, motor activity, or other neurologic signs. Post-LP headache may occur and is related to postural changes; this is less severe when the child lies flat. Headache is seen much less often in young children than in adolescents.

Bone Marrow Aspiration or Biopsy. Positioning for a bone marrow aspiration or biopsy depends on the location of the chosen site. In children the posterior or anterior iliac crest is most commonly used, although in infants the tibia may be selected because of easy access to the site and holding of the child.

If the posterior iliac crest is used, the child is positioned prone. Sometimes a small pillow or folded blanket is placed under the hips to facilitate obtaining the bone marrow specimen. Children should receive adequate analgesia or anesthesia to relieve pain. If the child awakens, holding may be needed, and is best done with two people—one person to immobilize the upper body and a second person to immobilize the lower extremities.

Other Procedures. For subdural puncture through a fontanel or burr hole, the infant is wrapped in a mummy restraint and placed in the supine position with the head accessible to the examiner. To control the head, the nurse uses a firm hold on each side of it. Procedures for immobilizing the head for examining the ears, nose, or throat are discussed in Chapter 35.

COLLECTION OF SPECIMENS

Urine Specimens

When children are admitted to the hospital or are seen in a clinic or office, a urine specimen may be needed. Older children and adolescents can use a bedpan or urinal or can be trusted to follow directions for collection in the bathroom. However, attention to their special needs and concerns is warranted. School-age children are cooperative but curious. They are likely to ask questions regarding the disposition of their specimen and what one expects to discover from it. Self-conscious adolescents may be reluctant to carry a specimen bottle through a hallway or waiting room and appreciate a paper bag or other means for disguising the container. The presence of menses is sometimes an embarrassment or a concern to teenage girls; therefore it is a good idea to ask if they are menstruating and to make adjustments as necessary. The specimen can be delayed, or a notation made on the laboratory slip to explain the presence of red blood cells.

Preschoolers and toddlers are usually unable to void on request. It is often best to offer them water or other liquids that they enjoy and wait about 30 minutes until they are ready to void voluntarily or to set a timer to alert them that they need to void shortly. The child will better understand what is expected if the nurse uses familiar terms, such as "pee-pee," "wee-wee," "tee-tee," or "tinkle." Some children will have difficulty voiding in an unfamiliar receptacle. Potty chairs or a potty hat placed on the toilet will usually prove satisfactory. Toddlers who have recently acquired bladder control may be especially reluctant, because they undoubtedly have been admonished for "going" in places other than those approved by parents. A useful approach is to enlist the help of parents; they are likely to be successful, and this helps them feel a part of the child's care.

For infants and toddlers who are not toilet trained, special urine collection devices may be used. These devices are clear, plastic, single-use bags with self-adhering material around the opening at the point of attachment. To prepare the infant, the genitalia, perineum, and surrounding skin are washed and dried thoroughly because the adhesive will not stick to a moist, powdered, or oily skin surface. The collection bag is easiest to apply if attached first to the perineum and then progressing to the symphysis (Fig. 45-14). With little girls the perineum is stretched taut during application to that area to ensure a leakproof fit. With small boys the penis and scrotum are placed inside the bag. The adhesive portion of the bag must be firmly applied to the skin all around the genital area to avoid possible leakage. For low-birth-weight infants, small bags with adhesive that is gentle to the skin are available.* Anatomically correct urine collection bags are also available.†

The diaper is carefully replaced. The bag is checked often and removed as soon as the specimen is available because the moist bag may become loosened on an active child. When urine is collected for culture, the bag is removed immediately. If the urine is not tested within 30 minutes, the specimen is refrigerated or placed in a sterile container with a preservative.

*Available from Hollister, Inc., 2000 Hollister Dr., Libertyville, IL 60048; 1-800-323-4060; website: www.hollister.com.

†Available from ConvaTec, CN 5254, Princeton, NJ 08543-5254; 1-800-422-8811; website: www.convatec.com.

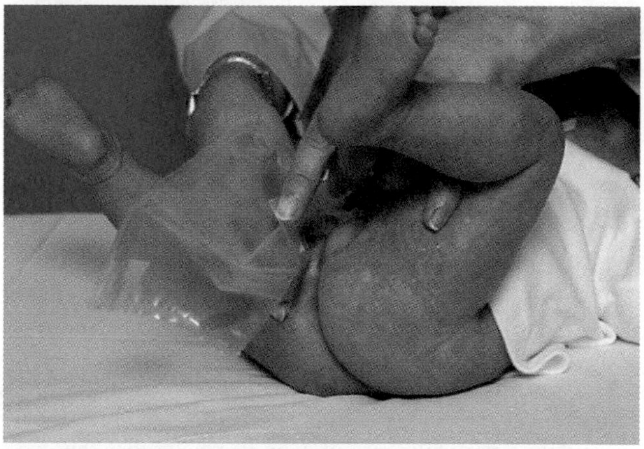

A

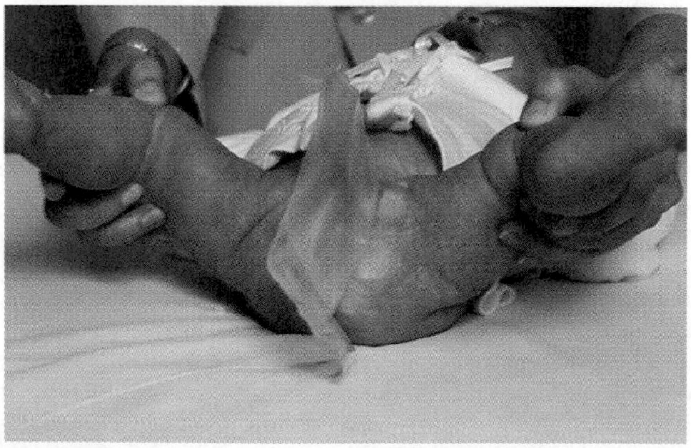

B

FIG. 45-14 • Application of urine collection bag. **A,** On female infant, adhesive portion is applied to exposed and dried perineum first. **B,** Bag adheres firmly around perineal area to prevent urine leakage.

Urine obtained from disposable diapers can be tested accurately for glucose, ketones, protein, blood, bilirubin, urobilinogen, nitrates, potassium, creatinine, and urea. In one study, urine obtained from a disposable diaper provided a valid sample for diagnosing urinary tract infections (Cohen et al, 1997). Erythrocyte and leukocyte counts may be low. Superabsorbent disposable diapers may produce a false crystalluria. Specific gravity measurements are accurate for up to 4 hours provided that the disposable diapers are kept folded. The accuracy of these tests performed on urine obtained from cloth diapers is unknown (Wong et al, 1992). Urine samples collected by the cotton ball method were accurate for pH and specific gravity and were atraumatic to the skin of newborns (Burke, 1995). Traditionally, specific gravity refractometers have been used on nursing units to measure specific gravity. One study showed strong agreement between the use of a refractometer and regeant strip to test urine specific gravity (Barton and Holmes, 1998). However, current regulations have limited the refractometer's use to the laboratory. Urine dipsticks can be used on the nursing unit with reasonable accuracy.

At times parents may be requested to bring a child's urine sample to a health care facility for examination, especially when infants are unable to void during an outpatient visit. In this instance parents need instruction on applying the collection device and storage of the specimen.* Ideally, the specimen should be brought to the designated place as soon as possible; if there is a delay, the sample is refrigerated and the lapsed time reported to the examiner.

Clean-Catch Specimens. The term *clean-catch specimen* traditionally refers to a urine sample obtained for culture after the urethral meatus is cleaned and the first few milliliters of urine are voided before the urine is collected *(midstream specimen)*. The procedure consists of cleaning the perineum or tip of the penis with a soap- or antiseptic-soaked sterile pad and of wiping from front to back only once with each pad in females. This is repeated at least two times. The area may be wiped with sterile water to prevent accidental contamination of the urine with a solution that may destroy the pathogens, although minute amounts of antiseptic such as iodine do not alter bacterial counts.

Although this traditional cleansing procedure is often practiced, studies have found that it does not significantly reduce contamination rates in infants, circumcised or uncircumcised males, or toilet-trained prepubertal children. Also, midstream collection does not significantly reduce contamination rates over nonmidstream specimens (Prandoni et al, 1996).

Twenty-Four–Hour Collection. Collection of urine voided over a 24-hour period creates a special challenge in infants and children. Collection bags are required to collect specimens from infants and small children. Older children require special instruction about notifying someone when they need to void or have a bowel movement so that urine can be collected separately and not discarded. Some older school-age children and adolescents can be trusted to take responsibility for collection of their own 24-hour specimens. They can keep output records and transfer each voiding to the 24-hour collection container if this is permitted.

As in any 24-hour urine collection, the collection period always starts and ends with an empty bladder. At the time the collection begins, the child is instructed to void and the specimen is discarded. All urine voided in the subsequent 24 hours is saved in a container with a preservative or is refrigerated or placed on ice. Twenty-four hours from the time the precollection specimen was discarded, the child is again instructed to void, the specimen is added to the container, and the entire collection is taken to the laboratory for examination.

Infants and small children who need a 24-hour urine collection require a special collection bag; frequent removal and replacement of adhesive collection devices can produce skin irritation. A thin coating of sealant, such as Skin-Prep, applied to the skin helps to protect it and aids adhesion, unless its use is contraindicated, such as in a premature infant or a child with irritated skin. Plastic collection bags with collection tubes attached are ideal when the container must be left in place for a time. These can be connected to a collecting device or emptied periodically by aspiration with a syringe. When such devices are not available, a regular bag with a feeding tube inserted through a puncture hole at the top of the bag serves as a satisfactory substitute. However, care must be taken to empty the bag as soon as the infant urinates to prevent leakage and loss of contents. An indwelling catheter may also be placed for the collection period.

Bladder Catheterization and Other Techniques. Bladder catheterization or *suprapubic aspiration* is employed when a specimen is urgently needed or when the child is unable to void or otherwise provide an adequate specimen. Catheterization is used to obtain a sterile urine specimen and when urethral obstruction or anuria caused by renal failure is believed to be the cause of the child's failure to void. Suprapubic aspiration is useful in clarifying the diagnosis of suspected urinary tract infection in acutely ill infants.

The anxiety, fear, and discomfort experienced during catheterization can be significantly alleviated by adequate preparation of the child and parents, by selection of the correct catheter, and by the appropriate technique of insertion. Specifically, generous lubrication of the urethra before catheterization and use of a lubricant containing 2% lidocaine (Xylocaine) may significantly reduce or eliminate the burning and discomfort often associated with this invasive procedure.

NURSE ALERT • Identify patients who have allergies to povidone-iodine or latex before using these items in catheterization.

Suprapubic aspiration, which is performed by a practitioner skilled in the procedure, involves aspirating bladder contents by inserting a 20- or 21-gauge needle in the midline approximately 1 cm above the symphysis pubis and directed vertically downward. The skin is prepared as for any needle insertion, and the bladder should contain an adequate volume of urine. This can be assumed if the infant has not voided for at least 1 hour or the bladder can be palpated above the symphysis pubis. This technique is useful for obtaining sterile specimens from young infants, because the bladder is an abdominal organ and is easily accessed. Suprapubic aspiration is painful, and therefore pain management during the procedure is important (Atraumatic Care box).

*Community and home care instructions on obtaining a urine sample are available in Wong DL, Hess CS: ***Wong and Whaley's clinical manual of pediatric nursing***, ed 5, St Louis, 2000, Mosby.

Atraumatic Care

BLADDER CATHETERIZATION OR SUPRAPUBIC ASPIRATION

Use distraction to help the child relax (blowing bubbles, deep breathing, singing a song).

Use lidocaine jelly to anesthetize the area before insertion of catheter. EMLA cream may lessen an infant's discomfort as the needle passes through the skin for suprapubic aspiration, but care should be taken that the site is thoroughly cleaned and prepped before the procedure.

Have the parent sit in a chair or on an examining table with a back support. Next, place the child leaning back in the parent's lap with the parent's arms hugging the child's upper body. Then place the child's legs in the frog position with the parent's legs over the child's to stabilize them. In this comfortable position the perineum or lower abdomen is exposed for the procedure.

Children often become agitated at being restrained for either procedure. Use comfort measures through touch and voice, both during and after the procedure, to help reduce the child's distress.

Stool Specimens

Stool specimens are commonly collected in children to identify parasites and other organisms that cause diarrhea, to assess gastrointestinal function, and to check for occult (hidden) blood. Ideally, stool should be collected without contamination with urine, but in children wearing diapers this is difficult unless a urine bag is applied. Children who are toilet trained should urinate first; flush the toilet; then defecate in the toilet, a bedpan (preferably one that is placed on the toilet to avoid embarrassment), or a commercial potty hat.

Stool specimens should be large enough to obtain an ample sampling, not merely a fecal fragment. Specimens are placed in an appropriate container, which is covered and labeled. If several specimens are needed, the containers are marked with the date and time and kept in a specimen refrigerator. Special care is exercised in handling the specimen because of the risk of contamination.

Blood Specimens

Although most blood specimens are obtained by the laboratory staff, nurses are increasingly responsible for specimen collection, especially if the child has an arterial or venous device. However, whether the specimen is collected by the nurse or others, the nurse is responsible for making certain that specimens, such as serial examinations and fasting specimens, are collected on time and that the proper equipment is available, such as correct collection tubes and ice for blood gas samples. Collecting, transporting, and storing of specimens can have a major impact on laboratory results (Frizzell, 1998).

Venous blood samples can be obtained by venipuncture or by aspiration from a peripheral or central access device. Withdrawing blood specimens through peripheral lock devices in small peripheral veins has met with varying degrees of success. Although it avoids an additional venipuncture for the child, attempting to aspirate blood from the peripheral lock may shorten the life of the device. When using an IV infusion site for specimen collection, it is important to consider the type of fluid being infused. For example, a specimen collected for glucose determination would be inaccurate if removed from a catheter through which glucose-containing solution were being administered.

A blood specimen can be obtained from a central venous line or peripheral lock when the infusion solution may interfere with test results by first aspirating a quantity of blood equal to the volume of fluid in the catheter and discarding it; then the blood sample is aspirated.

For a blood culture the first sample of blood is used because organisms are most likely to collect within the catheter itself.

NURSE ALERT • On small or anemic children, keep track of the amount drawn and discarded over time. Frequent taking of blood specimens can rapidly decrease a child's blood volume. Coordinate blood samples and ask the laboratory to save blood as much as possible to reduce the frequency of blood draws.

Arterial blood samples are sometimes needed for blood gas measurement, although noninvasive techniques, such as transcutaneous oxygen/carbon dioxide monitoring and pulse oximetry, are commonly used. Arterial samples may be obtained by arteriopuncture using the radial, brachial, or femoral arteries; by deep heel puncture; or from indwelling arterial catheters (Harrison et al, 1997). Adequate circulation should be assessed before arterial puncture by observing capillary refill or performing the *Allen test,* a procedure that assesses the circulation of the radial, ulnar, or brachial arteries. Because unclotted blood is required, only heparinized collection tubes are used. In addition, no air bubbles should enter the tube, because they can alter blood gas concentration. Crying, fear, and agitation also affect blood gas values; therefore every effort is made to comfort the child. The blood samples are packed in ice to reduce blood cell metabolism and are taken to the laboratory for immediate analysis.

Capillary blood samples are taken from children by a finger or earlobe stick, just as in the adult patient. A common method for taking peripheral blood samples from infants is by a heel stick. Before the blood sample is taken, the heel is warmed with warm, moist compresses for 5 to 10 minutes to dilate the vessels in the area. Although this is a well-accepted practice, one study questioned its effectiveness. In a study of healthy full-term infants, warming the heel with a warm gel pack (40° C [104° F]) for 10 minutes before capillary blood sampling with an automated device (Autolet) did not significantly decrease the sampling time required (Barker et al, 1996).

The area is cleansed with alcohol, and with the infant's foot firmly restrained with the free hand, the heel is punctured with a blade or an automatic lancet device. An automatic device, such as Tenderfoot* or Autolet, delivers a more precise puncture depth and is a less painful puncture than that achieved with a blade or lance (McIntosh, van Veen, and Brameyer, 1994). Although obtaining capillary blood gases is a common practice, some practitioners believe that these measures may not accurately reflect arterial values.

The most serious complication of infant heel puncture is necrotizing osteochondritis from lancet penetration of the un-

*Available from International Technidyne Corporation, 8 Olsen Ave., Edison, NJ 08820; (732) 548-5700 or 1-800-631-5945; website: www.itemed.com.

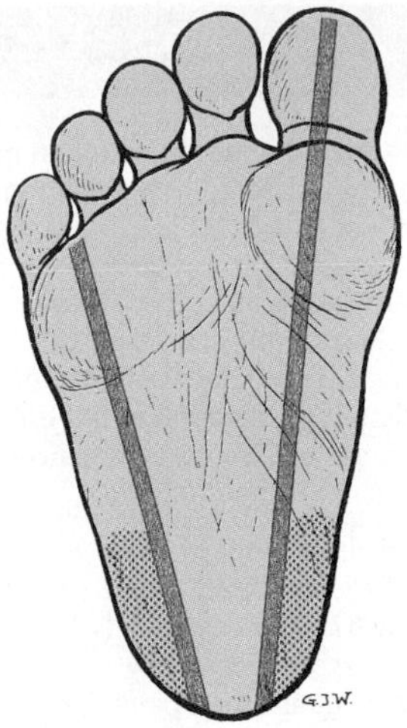

FIG. 45-15 • Puncture site *(colored stippled area)* on sole of infant's foot.

derlying calcaneus bone. To avoid this, the puncture should be no deeper than 2.4 mm and should be made at the outer aspect of the heel. The boundaries of the calcaneus can be marked by an imaginary line extending posteriorly from a point between the fourth and fifth toes and running parallel to the lateral aspect of the heel and another line extending posteriorly from the middle of the great toe and running parallel to the medial aspect of the heel (Fig. 45-15).

The needed specimens are collected quickly, and then pressure is applied to the puncture site with a dry gauze square until bleeding stops. The arm is kept extended, not flexed, while pressure is applied for a few minutes after venipuncture in the antecubital fossa to reduce bruising. The site is then covered with an adhesive bandage. In young children, adhesive bandages pose an aspiration hazard; their use should be avoided or the adhesive bandage should be removed as soon as the bleeding stops. Applying warm compresses to ecchymotic areas increases circulation, helps remove extravasated blood, and decreases pain.

No matter how or by whom the specimen is collected, children, even some older ones, fear the loss of their blood. This is particularly true for children whose condition requires frequent blood specimens. They mistakenly believe that blood removed from their bodies is a threat to their lives. Explaining to them that their blood is continually being produced by their bodies provides them with a measure of reassurance regarding this aspect of the stress-provoking procedure. When the blood is drawn, a simple comment, such as "Just look how red it is. You're really making a lot of nice red blood," confirms this information and affords them an opportunity to express their concern. Covering the puncture site with an adhesive bandage strip gives them added assurance that the vital fluids will not leak out.

Children also dislike the discomfort associated with venous, arterial, or capillary punctures. In fact, children have identified these procedures as the ones most often causing pain during hospitalization, and arterial punctures as being one of the most painful of all procedures experienced (Wong and Baker, 1988). Consequently, nurses need to institute pain reduction techniques to lessen the discomfort of these procedures (Atraumatic Care box). Younger children are more distressed by venipuncture than are older children.

Respiratory Secretions and Throat Specimens

Collection of sputum or nasal discharge is sometimes required for diagnosis of respiratory infections, especially tuberculosis and respiratory syncytial virus (RSV). Older children and adolescents are able to cough as directed and supply sputum specimens when given proper directions. It must be made clear to them that a coughed specimen is needed, not mucus that is cleared from the throat. It is helpful to demonstrate a deep cough so that communication is clear. Infants and small children are unable to follow directions to cough and will swallow any sputum produced; therefore *gastric washings (lavage)* may be used to collect a sputum specimen. Sometimes it is possible to obtain a satisfactory specimen by using a suction device such as a mucus trap if the catheter is inserted into the trachea and the cough reflex is elicited. A catheter that is inserted into the back of the throat is not sufficient. For children with a tracheostomy, a specimen is easily aspirated from the trachea or major bronchi by attaching a collecting device to the suction apparatus.

Nasal washings are usually obtained to diagnose an infection of RSV. The child is placed supine, and 1 to 3 ml of sterile normal saline is instilled with a sterile syringe (without needle) into one nostril. The contents are aspirated using a small, sterile bulb syringe and are placed in a sterile container. To prevent any additional discomfort to the child, all of the equipment should be ready before the procedure is begun.

Other respiratory secretion collection methods include nasopharyngeal swabs to diagnose *Bordetella pertussis* and throat cultures. The nurse swabs both the tonsils and the posterior pharynx when obtaining a throat culture. The swab stick is inserted into the culture tube. Some culture kits require squeezing an ampule to release the culture medium.

NURSE ALERT • Do not attempt to obtain a throat culture if acute epiglottitis is suspected. The trauma from the swab may increase edema, possibly occluding the airway.

ADMINISTRATION OF MEDICATION

Preparation for Safe Administration

The safe administration of medication to children presents a number of problems that are not encountered when giving medication to adult patients. Children vary widely in age; weight; body surface area; and the ability to absorb, metabolize, and excrete medications. Nurses must be particularly alert when computing and administering drugs to infants and children.

Determination of Drug Dosage. It is the physician's responsibility to prescribe drugs in the correct dosage to achieve the desired effect without endangering the health of the child. However, nurses must have an understanding of the safe dosage of medications they administer to children, as well as the expected action, possible side effects, and signs of toxicity (Kennedy, 1996). Unlike with adult medications, there are few standardized pediatric dosage ranges, and with a few exceptions, drugs are prepared and packaged in average adult-dosage strengths.

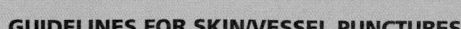

Atraumatic Care

GUIDELINES FOR SKIN/VESSEL PUNCTURES

To Reduce the Pain Associated with Heel, Finger, Venous, or Arterial Punctures:

Apply EMLA topically over the site if time permits (at least 60 minutes). To remove the Tegaderm dressing atraumatically, grasp opposite sides of the film and pull the sides away from each other to stretch and loosen the film. After the film begins to loosen, grasp the other two sides of the film and pull. Use iontophoresis (Numby Stuff) over the site if time permits (8 to 20 minutes, depending on the amount of current), a vapocoolant spray, or buffered lidocaine (injected intradermally near the vein with a 30-gauge needle) to numb the skin.

Use nonpharmacologic methods of pain and anxiety control (e.g., ask child to take a deep breath when the needle is inserted and again when the needle is withdrawn, have child exhale a large breath or blow bubbles to "blow hurt away"; ask child to count slowly and then faster and louder if pain is felt).

Keep all equipment out of sight until used.

Enlist parents' presence and/or assistance if they wish to participate.

Restrain child *only* as needed to perform the procedure safely; use therapeutic hugging (p. 1145).

Allow the skin preparation to dry completely before penetrating the skin.

Use the smallest-gauge needle (e.g., 25 gauge) that permits free flow of blood; a 27-gauge needle can be used for obtaining 1 to 1.5 ml of blood and for prominent veins (needle length is only ½ inch).

Avoid putting an intravenous (IV) line in the dominant hand or the hand the child uses to suck the thumb.

Use an automatic lancet device for precise puncture depth of the finger or heel; press the device lightly against the skin and avoid steadying the finger against a hard surface.

Emphasize that blood entering the syringe or tube does not hurt and reassure young children that you did not "take their blood" away and that they have a lot more inside.

Place a small bandage over the puncture site to make removal easy and less painful and to reassure young children that "their blood will not leak out."*

Have a "two-try" only policy to reduce excessive insertion attempts—two operators each have two insertion attempts; if insertion is not successful after four punctures, consider alternative venous access, such as a peripherally inserted central catheter (PICC); have a policy for identifying children with difficult access and appropriate interventions (e.g., most experienced operator for the first attempt).†

For Multiple Blood Samples:

Use an intermittent infusion device ("saline or heparin lock") to collect additional samples from an existing IV line; consider PICC lines early, not as a last resort. Preferably, use a saline flush for a catheter larger than 24 gauge (less painful, compatible with drugs, and less costly).

Coordinate care to allow several tests to be performed on one blood sample using micromethods of testing.

Anticipate tests (e.g., drug levels, chemistry, immunoglobulin levels) and ask the laboratory to save blood for additional testing.

For Heel Lancing in Newborns:

Heel lancing has been shown to be more painful than venipuncture‡; consider venipuncture when the amount of blood from the heel would require much squeezing (e.g., genetic screening tests).

The effectiveness of EMLA is controversial, although application of 0.5 g for 30 minutes four times a day in preterm infants was found to be safe§.

Place diapered newborn against mother's bare chest in skin-to-skin contact 10 to 15 minutes before and during heel lance.¶

During the procedure, allow newborn to suck a pacifier coated with a slurry of sugar and water: to make an approximate 24% sucrose solution, add 1 teaspoon of table sugar to 4 teaspoons of sterile water. Use this solution to coat the pacifier or administer 2 ml to the tongue 2 minutes before the procedure||.

*Contrary to popular belief, a study of children ages 3 to 6 years found that asking them not to look at the finger stick to avoid the sight of blood, or applying a decorated bandage, did not lessen their rating or pain intensity (Johnston CC, Stevens B, Arbess G: The effect of the sight of blood and use of decorative adhesive bandage on pain intensity ratings by preschool children, *J Pediatr Nurs* 8(3):147-151, 1993).

†For an example of one hospital's guidelines for reducing excessive IV insertion attempts, see Catudal R: Pediatric IV therapy: actual practice, *J Vasc Access Devices* 4(2):27-29, 1999.

‡Larsson BA et al: Alleviation of the pain of venipuncture in neonates, *Acta Paediatr* 87(7):774-779, 1998.

§Essink-Tebbes et al: Safety of lidocaine-prilocaine cream application four times a day in premature neonates: a pilot study, *Eur J Pediatr* 158(5):421-423, 1999.

¶Gray L, Watt L, Blass EM: Skin-to-skin contact is analgesic in healthy newborns, *Pediatrics* 105(1)110-111, 2000; www.pediatrics.org/cgi/content/full/105/1/E14.

||Blass EM, Watt L: Suckling- and sucrose-induced analgesia in human newborns, *Pain* 83(3):611-623, 1999.

Factors related to growth and maturation significantly alter an individual's capacity to metabolize and excrete drugs, and deficiencies associated with immaturity become more important with decreasing age. Immaturity or defects in any or all of the important processes of absorption, distribution, biotransformation, or excretion can significantly alter the effects of a drug. Newborn and premature infants with immature enzyme systems in the liver (where most drugs are broken down and detoxified), lower plasma concentrations of protein for binding with drugs, and immaturely functioning kidneys (where most drugs are excreted) are particularly vulnerable to the harmful effects of drugs. Beyond the newborn period, many drugs are metabolized more rapidly by the liver, necessitating larger doses or more frequent administration. This is particularly important in pain control, when the dosage may need to be increased or the interval between administering analgesics may need to be decreased.

Various formulas involving age, weight, and body surface area as the basis for calculations have been devised to determine children's drug dosage from a standard adult dose. Because the administration of medication is a nursing responsibility, nurses need not only a knowledge of drug action and patient responses, but also some resources for estimating safe dosages for children. The method most often used to determine children's dosage is based on a specific dose per kilogram of body weight, such as 0.1 mg/kg.

The most reliable method for determining children's dosage is to calculate the proportional amount of *body surface area (BSA)* to body weight. The ratio of BSA to weight varies inversely with length; therefore the infant who is shorter and weighs less than an older child or adult has relatively more surface area than would be expected from the weight. The usual determination of BSA requires the use of the *West nomogram* (Fig. 45-16). The BSA is estimated from the height and weight of the child.

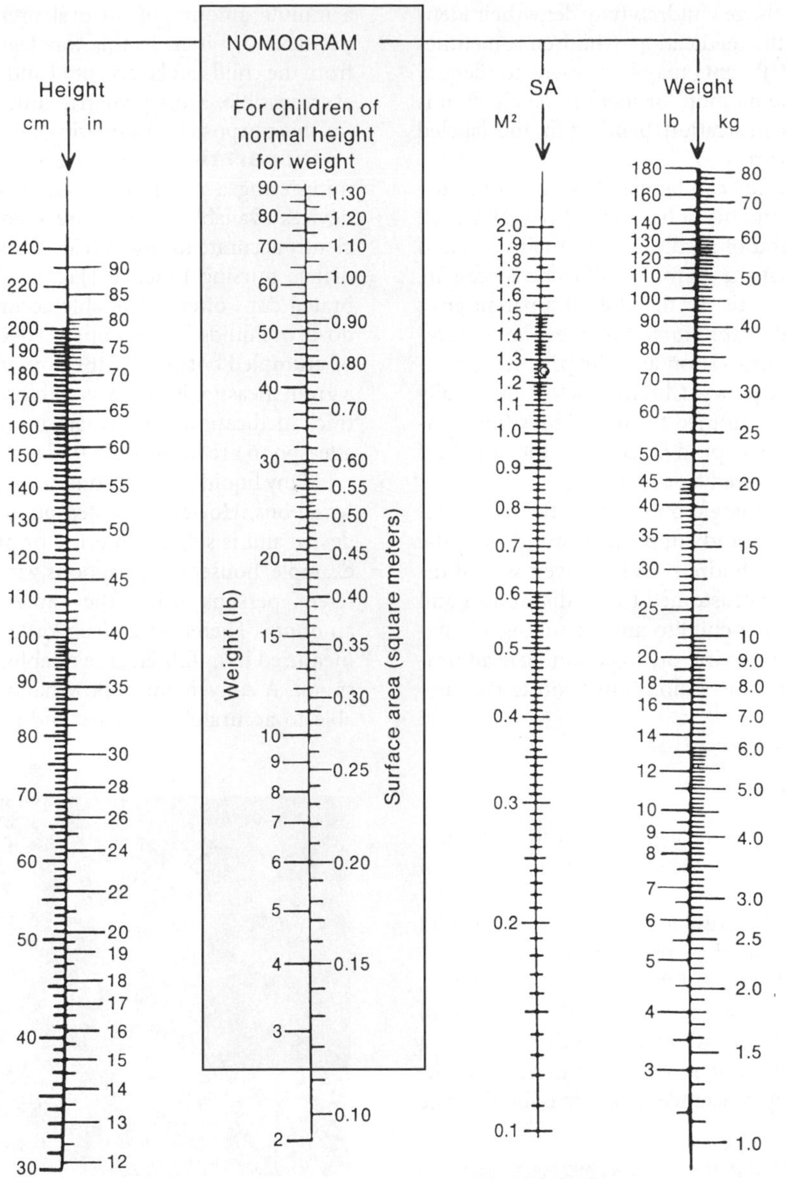

FIG. 45-16 • West nomogram for estimation of surface areas. Surface area is indicated where a straight line connecting height and weight intersects surface area (*SA*) column or, if patient is approximately of normal proportion, from weight alone *(yellow area)*. (Nomogram modified from data of E. Boyd by C.D. West; from Behrman RE, Vaughan VC, editors: *Nelson textbook of pediatrics,* ed 14, Philadelphia, 1992, WB Saunders.)

Checking Dosage. Administering the correct dosage of a drug is a shared responsibility between the practitioner who orders the drug and the nurse who carries out that order. Children react with unexpected severity to some drugs, and ill children are especially sensitive to drugs. Therefore checking the dose if any doubt exists about its accuracy is a professional duty. When a dose is ordered that is outside the usual range, or if there is some question regarding the preparation or the route of administration, the nurse should always check with the prescribing practitioner before proceeding with the administration, because the nurse is legally liable for any drug administered.

Administering some medications requires added safeguards. Even when it has been determined that the dosage is correct for a particular child, many drugs are potentially hazardous or lethal. Most hospital units or other facilities where medications are given to children have regulations requiring that specified drugs be double-checked by another nurse before they are given to the child. Among drugs that require such safeguards are digoxin, heparin, chemotherapeutic agents, and insulin. Others commonly included are epinephrine, opioids, and sedatives. Even if this precaution is not mandatory, nurses are wise to take such precautions for their own sense of security. Errors in decimal point placement may easily occur and may result in a tenfold or more dosage error.

Identification. Before the administration of any medication, the child must be correctly identified, because children are not totally reliable in giving correct names on request. Infants are unable to give their name, a toddler or preschooler may admit to any name, and school-age children may deny their identity in an attempt to avoid the medication. Children sometimes exchange beds during play. Parents may be present to identify their child, but the only safe method for identifying children is to check their hospital identification band with the labeled medication or medication card.

Family Aspects. Parents can be useful sources of information regarding the child and his or her capabilities. Nearly all parents have given some kind of medication to their child and can describe approaches that they have found to be successful. In some cases it is less traumatic for the child if a parent gives the medication, provided that the nurse prepares the medication and supervises its administration and the practice is consistent with hospital or unit policy. Children being given daily medications at home are accustomed to the parent's functioning in this capacity and are less apt to object than they would if the medication were administered by a stranger.

Every child requires psychologic preparation for parenteral administration of medication and supportive care during the procedure (p. 1122). Even if children have received several injections, they rarely become accustomed to the discomfort and have as much right as any other child to understanding and patience from those involved in giving the injection. Safe administration of any drug requires meticulous attention to the safeguards discussed here.

Oral Administration

The oral route is preferred for administering medications to children whenever possible. Because of the ease of administration of oral medications, most are dissolved or suspended in liquid preparations. Although some children are able to swallow or chew solid medications at an early age, solid preparations are not recommended for young children because of the danger of aspiration.

Most pediatric medications come in palatable and colorful preparations for added ease of administration. Some have a slightly unpleasant aftertaste, but most children will swallow these liquids with little if any resistance. The nurse should taste a minute amount of an oral preparation to ascertain if it is palatable or bitter. In this way legitimate complaints of dislike from the child can be accepted and the taste camouflaged whenever possible. Most pediatric units have preparations available for this purpose (Atraumatic Care box).

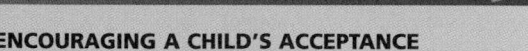

Preparation. Selecting a vehicle for measuring and administering a medication requires careful consideration. The devices available to measure medicines are not always sufficiently accurate for measuring the small amounts needed in pediatric nursing practice (Fig. 45-17). Disposable plastic calibrated cups offer reasonable accuracy in measuring moderate doses of liquids (paper cups are likely to have irregularly shaped or crumpled bottoms). However, the personal interpretation of a given measure is highly variable, and considerable amounts of thick medication may remain in the cup. Measures of less than a teaspoon are impossible to determine accurately with a cup.

Many liquid preparations are prescribed in measurements of teaspoons. However, the teaspoon is an inaccurate measuring device and is subject to error from a number of variables. For example, household teaspoons vary greatly in capacity, and different persons using the same spoon will pour different amounts. Therefore a drug ordered in teaspoons should be measured in milliliters; the established standard is 5 ml per teaspoon. A convenient hollow-handled medicine spoon is available to accurately measure and administer the drug (see Fig.

Atraumatic Care

ENCOURAGING A CHILD'S ACCEPTANCE OF ORAL MEDICATION

Give child a flavored ice pop or small ice cube to suck to numb the tongue before giving the drug.

Mix the drug with a small amount (about 1 teaspoon) of sweet-tasting substance, such as honey (except in infants because of the risk of botulism), flavored syrups, jam, fruit purees, sherbet, or ice cream; avoid essential food items, because the child may later refuse to eat them.

Give a "chaser" of water, juice, soft drink, or ice pop or frozen juice bar after the drug.

If nausea is a problem, give a carbonated beverage poured over finely crushed ice before or immediately after the medication.

When medication has an unpleasant taste, have child pinch the nose and drink the medicine through a straw. Much of what we taste is associated with smell.

Another alternative is to have the pharmacist prepare the drug in a flavored, chewable troche or lozenge.*

*For information about compounding drugs in troches, contact Technical Staff, Professional Compounding Centers of America (PCCA), P.O. Box 368, Sugar Land, TX 77487; 1-800-331-2498; website: www.thecompounders.com.

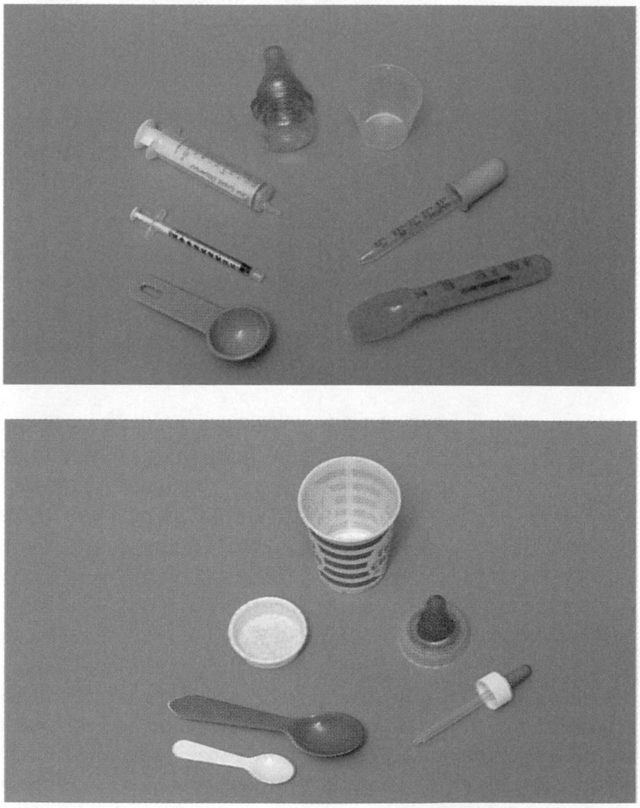

A

B

FIG. 45-17 • **A,** Acceptable devices for measuring and administering oral medication to children *(clockwise from left)*: measuring spoon, plastic syringes, calibrated nipple, plastic medicine cup, calibrated dropper, hollow-handled medicine spoon. **B,** Acceptable devices only for administering premeasured oral medication *(clockwise from left)*: household teaspoons, paper cups, nipple, uncalibrated dropper.

45-17). Household *measuring* spoons can also be used when other devices are not available.

Another unreliable device for measuring liquids is the dropper, which varies to a greater extent than the teaspoon or measuring cup. Droppers are available in numerous sizes, but even with the standard USP dropper, the volume of a drop will vary according to the viscosity of the liquid measured; viscid fluids produce much larger drops than thin liquids. Many medications are supplied with caps or droppers designed for measuring each specific preparation. These are accurate when used to measure that specific medication but are not reliable for measuring other liquids. Emptying dropper contents into a medicine cup invites additional error. Because some of the liquid clings to the sides of the cup, a significant amount of the drug can be lost.

NURSE ALERT • Many pediatric medications are given by drops or dropper. A misunderstanding of these terms by parents can result in a potential overdose. In addition, many droppers that come with medications are marked in tenths of cubic centimeters. If a parent were to use a syringe instead of the dropper, 0.4 cc may be thought to be the same as 4 cc. Provide education to parents on correct methods for giving medication. Demonstrate the technique.

The most accurate means for measuring small amounts of medication is the plastic disposable (never glass) syringe, especially the tuberculin syringe for volumes less than 1 ml. Not only does the syringe provide a reliable measure, but it also serves as a convenient means for transporting and administering the medication. The medication can be placed directly into the child's mouth from the syringe. For added safety, a short length of flexible tubing can be placed on the tip of the syringe to prevent injury to the mouth, although the tubing must be completely emptied of medication.

Young children and some older children as well have difficulty swallowing tablets or pills. Because a number of drugs are not available in pediatric preparations, the tablet needs to be crushed before it can be given to these children. Commercial devices* are available, or simple methods can be employed for crushing tablets. Not all drugs can be crushed (e.g., medication with an enteric or protective coating or those formulated for slow release).

Children who must take oral medication for an extended period can be taught to swallow tablets or capsules. Training sessions include using verbal instruction, demonstration, reinforcement of progressively swallowing larger candy/capsules, no attention for inappropriate behavior, and gradual withdrawal of guidance once children can swallow their medication (Babbitt et al, 1991).

Because pediatric doses often require dividing adult preparations of medication, the nurse may be faced with the dilemma of accurate dosage. With tablets, only those that are scored can be halved or quartered accurately. If the medication is soluble, the tablet or contents of a capsule can be mixed in a small, premeasured amount of liquid and the appropriate portion given. If half a dose is required, the tablet is dissolved in 5 ml of water or flavored liquid and 2.5 ml is given.

Administration. Although administering liquids to infants is relatively easy, the nurse must be careful to prevent aspiration. With the infant held in a semireclining position, the medication is placed in the mouth from a spoon, plastic cup, plastic dropper, or plastic syringe (without needle). The dropper or syringe is best placed along the side of the infant's tongue, with the contents administered slowly in small amounts, allowing the child to swallow between deposits.

In infants up to 11 months of age and children with neurologic impairments, blowing a small puff of air in the face often elicits a swallow reflex.

Medicine cups can be used effectively for older infants who are able to drink from a cup. Because of the natural outward tongue thrust in infancy, medications may need to be retrieved from the lips or chin and refed. Other convenient methods for giving liquid medications to infants are allowing the infant to suck medication that has been placed in an empty nipple; or inserting the syringe or dropper into the side of the mouth, parallel to the nipple, while the infant nurses. Medication is not added to the infant's formula feeding. Dispose of any plastic covers that may be on the ends of syringes: these covers are small enough to be aspirated by young children.

The young child who refuses to cooperate or who resists consistently despite explanation and encouragement may require mild physical coercion. If so, it is carried out quickly and carefully. Every effort is made to determine why the child resists, and the reasons for the coercion are explained to the child in such a way that the child will know that it is being carried out for his or her well-being and is not a form of punishment. There is always a risk in using even mild forceful techniques. A crying child can aspirate a medication, particularly when lying on the back. If the nurse holds the child in the lap with the child's right arm behind the nurse, the left hand firmly grasped by the nurse's left hand, and the head securely restrained between the nurse's arm and body, the medication can be slowly poured into the mouth (Fig. 45-18).

Intramuscular (IM) Administration

Selecting the Syringe and Needle. The volume of medication prescribed for small children and the small amount of tissue for injection require that a syringe be selected that can measure very small amounts of solution. For volumes of less than 1 ml, the tuberculin syringe, calibrated in one-hundredth increments, is appropriate. Very minute doses may require the use of a 0.5-ml, low-dose syringe. These syringes with specially constructed needles minimize the possibility of inadvertently administering incorrect amounts of a drug because of *dead space,* which allows fluid to remain in the syringe and needle after the plunger is pushed completely forward. A minimum of 0.2 ml of solution remains in a standard needle hub; therefore, when very small amounts of two drugs are combined in the syringe, such as mixtures of insulin, the ratio of the two drugs can be altered significantly. Measures that minimize the effect of dead space include the following: (1) when two drugs are combined in the syringe, always draw them up in the same order to maintain a consistent ratio between the drugs; (2) use the same brand of syringe (dead space may vary between brands); and (3) use one-piece syringe units (with needle permanently attached to the syringe).

Dead space is also an important factor to consider when injecting medication, because flushing the syringe with an air bubble or parenteral fluid adds an additional amount of medication to the prescribed dose. This can be hazardous when very small amounts of a drug are given. For example, a tuberculin syringe

*Trademark Medical manufactures a pill crusher and has compiled a list of more than 190 medications that should not be crushed or chewed. Both are available from Trademark Medical, 1053 Headquarters Park, Fenton, MO 63026-2033; 1-800-325-9044; website: www.trademarkmedical.com.

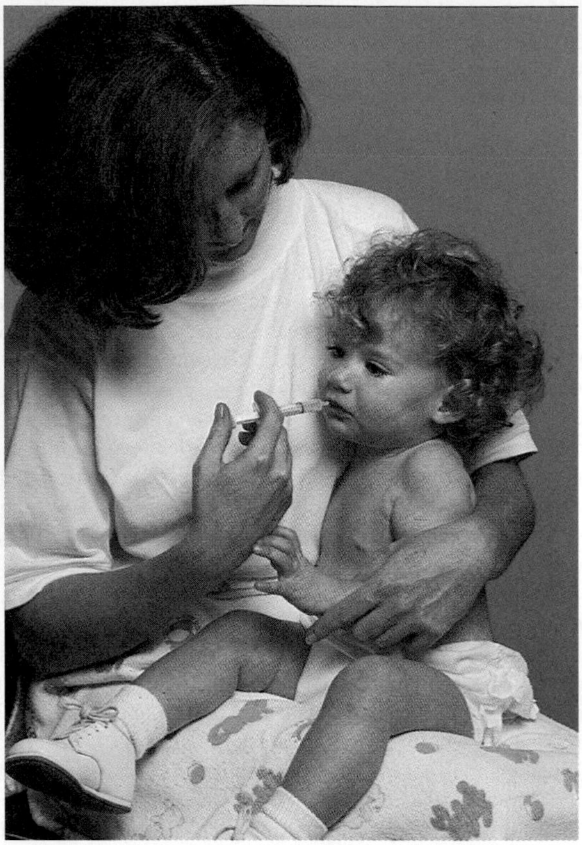

FIG. 45-18 • Nurse partially restrains child for easy and comfortable administration of oral medication.

filled to the 0.05-ml mark can deliver *more than twice* the calculated dose of medication when it is flushed with parenteral fluid from an IV line. Consequently, flushing is not advisable, especially when less than 1 ml of medication is given. Syringes are calibrated to deliver a prescribed drug dose, and the amount of medication left in the hub and needle is not part of the syringe barrel calibrations. However, the air-bubble technique (drawing up about 0.2 ml of air into the syringe after withdrawing the medication) may be beneficial with certain drugs, such as iron dextran and diphtheria and tetanus toxoid, to avoid tracking the drug through the tissue. Other techniques to minimize tracking include changing the needle after withdrawing the fluid from the vial (not always effective); and using the Z-track method.

The *needle length* must be sufficient to penetrate the subcutaneous tissue and deposit the medication in the body of the muscle. Although research is limited on adequate needle length for children, one study found that a 1-inch needle is necessary to adequately penetrate the vastus lateralis muscle in 4-month-old infants, and probably is needed for 2-month-old infants (Hicks et al, 1989).

Based on ultrasonography, two injection techniques have been studied to determine the best needle length for the deltoid and vastus lateralis sites. If the muscle is grasped or bunched, a needle length of 25 mm (1 inch) is recommended. If the muscle is stretched or flattened, a needle length of 16 mm (5/8 inch) is adequate (Groswasser et al, 1997). Unfortunately, the conclusions of the study fail to address whether these lengths apply to both muscles. From the data, it appears more likely that the recommendations apply to the thigh muscle only. Other recommendations for needle size and volume of fluid are based on traditional practice and have not been verified by research.

To estimate the needle length for IM injection, first grasp the lateralis or deltoid muscle and choose a needle length that is approximately half the distance between the thumb and the index finger. With the ventrogluteal or dorsogluteal site, only subcutaneous tissue is grasped, so choose a needle length that is slightly more than half the distance. Choose a final needle length that allows for a small portion of the needle to be exposed at the skin surface as a precaution if the needle should break off from the hub.

The needle gauge should be as small as possible to deliver fluid safely. Smaller-diameter (i.e., 25- to 30-gauge) needles cause the least discomfort, but larger diameters are needed for viscous medication and prevention of accidental bending of longer needles.

Determining the Site. Factors that are considered when selecting a site for an IM injection on an infant or child include:

- The amount and character of the medication to be injected
- The amount and general condition of the muscle mass
- The frequency or number of injections to be given during the course of treatment
- The type of medication being given
- Factors that may impede access to or cause contamination of the site
- The child's ability to assume the required position safely

Older children and adolescents usually pose few problems in selecting a suitable site for IM injections, but infants, with their small and underdeveloped muscles, have fewer available sites. It is sometimes difficult to assess the amount of fluid that can be safely injected into a single site. Usually 1 ml is the maximum volume that should be administered in a single site to small children and older infants. The muscles of small infants may not tolerate more than 0.5 ml. As the child approaches adult size, volumes approaching those given to adults may be used. However, the larger the amount of solution, the larger the muscle must be into which it is injected.

Injections must be placed in muscles large enough to accommodate the medication; however, major nerves and blood vessels must be avoided. There is no universal agreement regarding the best IM injection site for children. The preferred site for infants is the vastus lateralis (the rectus femoris is not an acceptable site). A general recommendation for using the dorsogluteal site is to wait until after the child has been walking (length of suggested time varies but is usually a minimum of 1 year after walking) because the muscle develops with locomotion. Unfortunately, this recommendation is often applied to the ventrogluteal muscle site as well. However, significant differences exist between these two sites. The ventrogluteal site is relatively free of major nerves and blood vessels, is a relatively large muscle with less subcutaneous tissue than the dorsal site, has well-defined landmarks for safe site location, is less painful than the vastus lateralis, and is easily accessible in several positions (Beecroft and Redick, 1990). These advantages make it a preferred site over the dorsogluteal muscle and challenge the recommendation that the ventrogluteal site not be used until children have been walking. Although there are published recommendations regarding age, in clinical practice the ventrogluteal site has been used in children as young as newborns. Table 45-3 summarizes the four major injection sites

TABLE 45-3

Intramuscular Injection Sites in Children

Site	Discussion
VASTUS LATERALIS 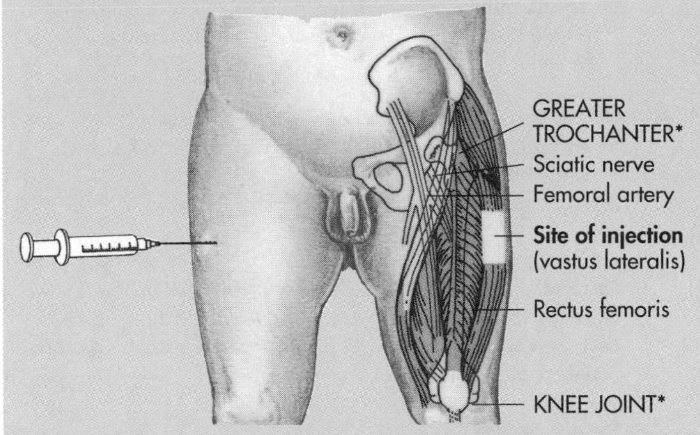	**Location*** Palpate to find greater trochanter and knee joints; divide vertical distance between these two landmarks into thirds; inject into middle third **Needle insertion and size** Insert needle perpendicular to knee in infants and young children or perpendicular to thigh or slightly angled toward anterior thigh 22 to 25 gauge, ⅝ to 1 inch† **Advantages** Large, well-developed muscle that can tolerate larger quantities of fluid (0.5 ml [infant] to 2 ml [child]) Easily accessible if child is supine, side lying, or sitting **Disadvantages** Thrombosis of femoral artery from injection in midthigh area Sciatic nerve damage from long needle injected posteriorly and medially into small extremity More painful than deltoid or gluteal site.
VENTROGLUTEAL 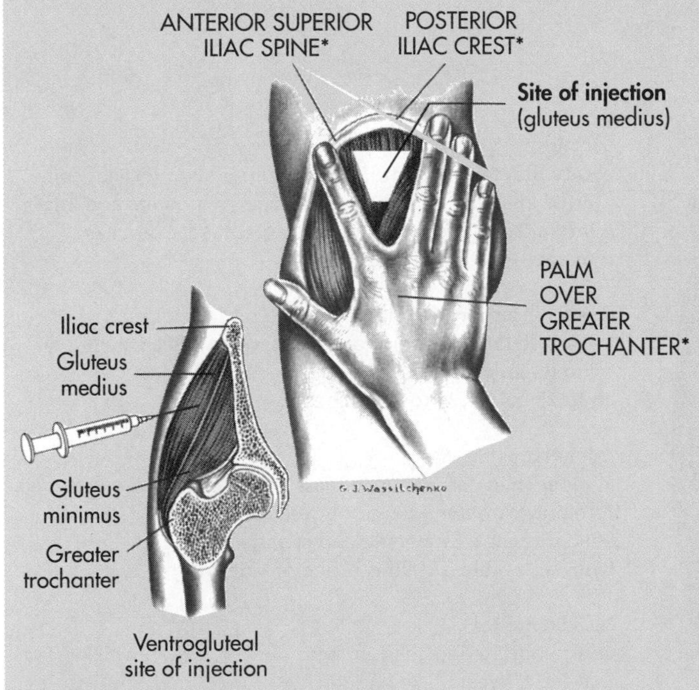	**Location*** Palpate to locate greater trochanter, anterior superior iliac tubercle (found by flexing thigh at hip and measuring up to 1 to 2 cm above crease formed in groin), and posterior iliac crest; place palm of hand over greater trochanter, index finger over anterior superior iliac tubercle, and middle finger along crest of ilium posteriorly as far as possible; inject into center of "V" formed by fingers **Needle insertion and size** Insert needle perpendicular to site but angled slightly toward iliac crest 22 to 25 gauge, ⅝ to 1 inch‡ **Advantages** Free of important nerves and vascular structures Easily identified by prominent bony landmarks Thinner layer of subcutaneous tissue than in dorsogluteal site, thus less chance of depositing drug subcutaneously rather than intramuscularly Can accommodate larger quantities of fluid (0.5 ml [infant] to 2 ml [child]) Easily accessible if child is supine, prone, or side lying Less painful than vastus lateralis **Disadvantages** Health professionals' unfamiliarity with site

*Locations are indicated by asterisks on illustrations.

†Research has shown that a 1-inch needle is needed for adequate muscle penetration in infants 4 months old and possibly in infants as young as 2 months (Hicks et al, 1989).

‡*A Guide for Managing the Pediatric Patient, Reducing the Anxiety and Pain of Injections* (1998) is available from Becton Dickinson & Co., 1 Becton Dr., Franklin Lakes, NJ 07417; (888) 237-2762; fax (201) 847-4682; website: www.bd.com. In Canada: Becton Dickinson Canada, Inc., 2464 S. Sheridan Way, Mississauga, Ontario L5J 2M8; 1-800-268-5430 (Ontario and Quebec) or 1-800-268-5450 (other areas).

Continued

TABLE 45-3
Intramuscular Injection Sites in Children—cont'd

Site	Discussion
DELTOID 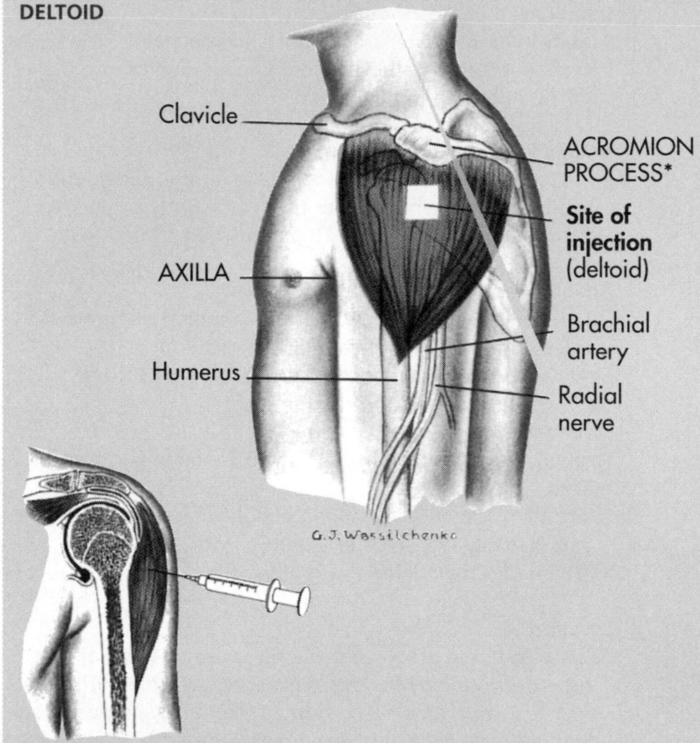 	**Location*** Locate acromion process; inject only into upper third of muscle that begins about 2 fingerbreadths below acromion **Needle insertion and size** Insert needle perpendicular to site but angled slightly toward shoulder 22 to 25 gauge, $\frac{5}{8}$ to 1 inch **Advantages** Faster absorption rates than gluteal sites Easily accessible with minimal removal of clothing Less pain and fewer local side effects from vaccines as compared with vastus lateralis **Disadvantages** Small muscle mass; only limited amounts of drug can be injected (0.5 to 1 ml) Small margins of safety with possible damage to radial and axillary nerves (not shown, lies under deltoid at head of humerus)
DORSOGLUTEAL 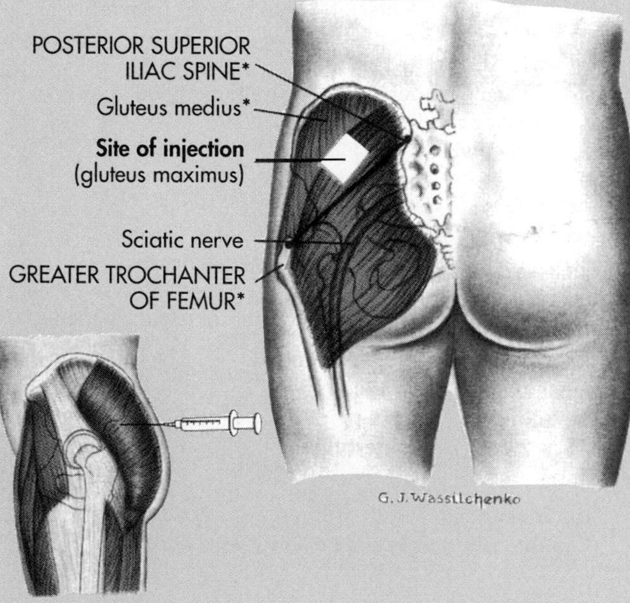 	**Location*** Locate greater trochanter and posterior superior iliac spine; draw imaginary line between these two points and inject lateral and superior to line into gluteus maximus or medius muscle **Needle insertion and size** Insert needle perpendicular to surface on which child is lying when prone 20 to 25 gauge, $\frac{1}{2}$ to $1\frac{1}{2}$ inches **Advantages** In older child, large muscle mass; well-developed muscle can tolerate greater volume of fluid (up to 2 ml) Child does not see needle and syringe Easily accessible if child is prone or side lying **Disadvantages** Contraindicated in children who have not been walking for at least 1 year Danger of injury to sciatic nerve Thick, subcutaneous fat, predisposing to deposition of drug subcutaneously rather than intramuscularly Not suitable for use of a tourniquet Inaccessible if child is supine Exposure of site may cause embarrassment in older child USE ONLY IF NO OTHER SITE EXISTS

*Locations are indicated by asterisks on illustrations.

and illustrates the location of the preferred IM injection sites for children.

Administration. Although injections that are executed with care seldom cause trauma to the child, there have been reports of serious disability related to IM injections in children. Repeated use of a single site has been associated with fibrosis of the muscle with subsequent muscle contracture. Injections close to large nerves, such as the sciatic nerve, have been responsible for permanent disability, especially when potentially neurotoxic drugs are administered. There are several reports of tissue damage from penicillin. One of the difficulties in administering the opaque preparations, such as Bicillin, is that aspirated blood cannot be detected at the bottom of the syringe, thus increasing the risk of injecting into a blood vessel. When such drugs are injected, great care must be used in locating the correct site. When aspirating, the nurse should look for blood at the top of the syringe near the plunger because blood may be drawn up through the column of penicillin. One study of IM injection techniques revealed that the straighter the path of needle insertion (e.g., 90-degree angle), the less displacement there is, causing less discomfort (Katsma and Smith, 1997).

A reported potential hazard with medication in glass ampules is the presence of glass particles in the ampule after the container is broken. When the medication is withdrawn into the syringe, the glass particles may also be withdrawn and subsequently injected into the patient. As a precaution, medication from glass ampules should be drawn up only through a needle with a filter or injected intravenously through a site in the tubing that is distal to an IV filter. Other precautions related to needle use and disposal are on p. 1143.

Children may be unpredictable and cannot be expected to cooperate totally when receiving an injection. Even children who appear to be relaxed and constrained can lose control under the stress of the procedure. It is advisable to have someone available to help hold the child if needed. Because children often jerk or pull away unexpectedly, the nurse should carry an extra needle to exchange for a contaminated one so that the delay is minimal. The child, even a small one, is told that he or she is receiving an injection (preferably using a phrase such as "putting medicine under the skin"), and then the procedure is carried out as quickly and skillfully as possible to avoid prolonging the stressful experience. Delay caused by lengthy explanations, attempts to hide the syringe from sight, or efforts to soothe the child only increase the anxiety. It must be kept in mind that intrusive procedures such as injections are especially anxiety provoking in preschool children and that small children usually associate any assault to the buttocks area with punishment. Most children hate intramuscular injections; studies show that getting an injection is one of the most feared procedures (Huth, 1999). Because injections are painful, the nurse should employ excellent injection technique and effective pain reduction measures to reduce discomfort (Guidelines box).

Small infants offer little resistance to injections. Although they squirm and may be difficult to hold in position, they can usually be restrained without assistance. The body of a larger infant can be securely held between the nurse's arm and body (Fig. 45-19). To inject into the body of the muscle, the muscle mass is firmly grasped between the thumb and fingers to isolate and stabilize the site. In obese children, however, it is preferable first to spread the skin with the thumb and index finger to displace subcutaneous tissue, and then grasp the muscle deeply on each side. For an injection into the arm, place the child in the parent's (or assistant's) lap, with the child facing sideward. Next, place the child's arm that is closest to the parent under the parent's arm and wrap toward the back. Then have the parent hold the arm for the injection against the child's body.

If the medication is given around the clock, the nurse should not try to administer an injection to a sleeping child, even though it may seem to be easier than waking the youngster. This practice can cause the child to fear going to sleep. When awakened first, the child knows that nothing will be done unless he or she is forewarned.

Subcutaneous and Intradermal Administration

Subcutaneous and intradermal injections are commonly administered to children, but the technique differs little from the method used with adults. Examples of *subcutaneous injections* include insulin, hormone replacement, allergy desensitization, and some vaccines. Tuberculin (TB) testing, local anesthesia, and allergy testing are examples of commonly administered *intradermal injections.*

Techniques to minimize the pain associated with these injections include changing the needle if it pierced a rubber stopper on a vial, using 26- to 30-gauge needles (only to inject the solution), and injecting small volumes (up to 0.5 ml). The angle of the needle for the subcutaneous injection is typically 90 degrees. In children with little subcutaneous tissue, some practitioners insert the needle at a 45-degree angle. However, the benefit of using the 45-degree angle rather than the 90-degree angle remains controversial.

Although subcutaneous injections can be given anywhere there is subcutaneous tissue, common sites include the center third of the lateral aspect of the upper arm, the abdomen, and the center third of the anterior thigh. Some practitioners believe it is not necessary to aspirate before injecting subcutaneously. For example, not aspirating is an accepted practice in the administration of insulin. Automatic injector devices do not aspirate before injecting.

When giving an intradermal injection into the volar surface of the forearm, the nurse should avoid the medial side of the arm, where the skin is more sensitive.

Families often need to learn subcutaneous injection technique to administer medications, such as insulin, at home.* Begin teaching as early as possible to allow the family the maximum amount of practice time possible.

Intravenous (IV) Administration

The IV route for administering medications is commonly used in pediatric therapy. For some important drugs it is the only effective route of administration. This method is used for giving drugs to children who have poor absorption as a result of diarrhea, dehydration, or peripheral vascular collapse; children who need a high serum concentration of a drug; children who have resistant infections that require parenteral medication over an

*Community and home care instructions on giving subcutaneous and intramuscular injections are available in Wong DL, Hess CS: ***Wong and Whaley's clinical manual of pediatric nursing***, ed 5, St Louis, 2000, Mosby.

Guidelines

INTRAMUSCULAR ADMINISTRATION OF MEDICATION

Use safety precautions in administering medication (e.g., check child's identification).
Apply EMLA topically over site if time permits (at least 60 minutes, preferably 2 to 2½ hours for (intramuscular [IM] injection) (see Pain Management, Chapter 44).
Prepare medication.
- Select needle and syringe appropriate to the following:
  - Amount of fluid to be administered (syringe size)
  - Viscosity of fluid to be administered (needle gauge)
  - Amount of tissue to be penetrated (needle length)
- Maximum volume to be administered in a single site is 1 ml for older infants and small children.

Determine site of injection (see Table 45-3), make certain that muscle is large enough to accommodate volume and type of medication.
- Older children: select site as with adult patient; allow child some choice of site, if feasible.
- Following are acceptable sites for infants and small or debilitated children:
  - Vastus lateralis muscle
  - Ventrogluteal muscle
- Dorsogluteal muscle is insufficiently developed to be a safe site for infants and small children.

Administer medication.
- Provide for sufficient help in restraining child; children are often uncooperative, and their behavior is usually unpredictable.
- Explain briefly what is to be done and, if appropriate, what child can do to help.
- Expose injection area for unobstructed view of landmarks.
- Select a site where skin is free of irritation and danger of infection; palpate for and avoid sensitive or hardened areas.
  - With multiple injections, rotate sites.
- Place child in a lying or sitting position; child is not allowed to stand because:
  - Landmarks are more difficult to assess.
  - Restraint is more difficult.
  - Child may faint and fall.
- Use a new, sharp needle with smallest diameter that permits free flow of the medication.
- Grasp muscle firmly between thumb and fingers to isolate and stabilize muscle for deposition of drug in its deepest part; in obese children, spread skin with thumb and index finger to displace subcutaneous tissue and grasp muscle deeply on each side.
- Allow skin preparation to dry completely before skin is penetrated.
- Have medication at room temperature.

Decrease perception of pain.
- Distract child with conversation.
- Give child something on which to concentrate (e.g., squeezing a hand or side rail, pinching own nose, humming, counting, yelling "Ouch!").
- Spray vapocoolant (e.g., ethyl chloride or fluori-methane) on site 11 to 15 seconds before injection or place a cold compress or wrapped ice cube on site about 1 minute before injection, or apply cold to contralateral site.
- Say to child, "If you feel this, tell me to take it out, please."
- Have child hold a small adhesive bandage and place it on puncture site after IM injection is given.

Insert needle quickly, using a dartlike motion at a 90-degree angle unless contraindicated.
- Use new needle, not one that has pierced rubber stopper on vial.

Avoid tracking any medication through superficial tissues:
- Replace needle after withdrawing medication, or wipe medication from needle with sterile gauze.
- If withdrawing medication from an ampule, use a needle equipped with a filter that removes glass particles; then use a new, nonfilter needle for injection.
- Use the Z-track and/or air-bubble technique as indicated.
- Avoid any depression of the plunger during insertion of the needle.

Aspirate for blood.
- If blood is found, remove syringe from site, change needle, and reinsert into new location.
- If no blood is found, inject into a relaxed muscle:
  - **Dorsogluteal**—Place child on abdomen with legs and toes rotated inward.
  - **Ventrogluteal**—Place child on side with upper leg flexed and placed in front of lower leg.
- Inject medication slowly.
- Remove needle quickly; hold gauze sponge firmly against skin near needle when removing it to avoid pulling on tissue.
- Apply firm pressure to site after injection; massage site to hasten absorption unless contraindicated, as with irritating drugs.
- Place a small adhesive bandage on puncture site; with young children decorate it by drawing a smiling face or other symbol of acceptance.
- Hold and cuddle young child and encourage parents to comfort child; praise older child.
- Allow expression of feelings.

Discard syringe and uncapped, uncut needle in puncture-resistant container located near site of use.
Record time of injection, drug, dose, and injection site.

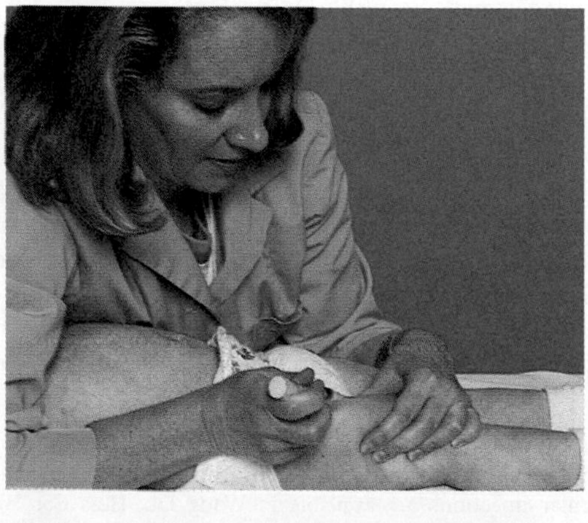

FIG. 45-19 • Holding small child for intramuscular injection. Note how nurse isolates and stabilizes muscle.

extended time; children who need continuous pain relief; and children who require emergency treatment.

Insertion sites and observation of the IV infusion are discussed on p. 1168; however, several factors need to be considered in relation to IV medication. When a drug is administered intravenously, the effect is almost instantaneous and further control is limited. Most drugs for IV administration require a specified minimum dilution and/or rate of flow, and many are highly irritating or toxic to tissues outside the vascular system. In addition to the precautions and nursing observations related to IV therapy, factors to consider when preparing and administering drugs to infants and children by the IV route include the following:

- Amount of drug to be administered
- Minimum dilution of drug and whether child is fluid restricted
- Type of solution in which drug can be diluted
- Length of time over which drug can be safely administered

- Rate of infusion that child and vessels can tolerate safely
- IV tubing volume capacity
- Time that this or another drug is to be administered
- Compatibility of all drugs that child is receiving intravenously

Before any IV infusion, the site of insertion is checked for patency. Medications are never administered with blood products. Only one antibiotic should be administered at a time.

IV infusion is suitable for children who can tolerate the necessary infusion rate and the extra fluid needed to administer the medication. For the very small infant or the fluid-restricted child who is not able to tolerate the increased rate of fluids, special delivery systems such as syringe pumps are used. Regardless of the technique used, the nurse must know the minimum dilutions for safe administration of IV medications to infants and children. The package insert often includes this information, but if there is any doubt regarding the amount of dilution, the pharmacist should be contacted.

Peripheral Venous Access Devices (VADs). The *peripheral lock,* also known as an *intermittent infusion device* or *saline* or *heparin lock,* is used as an alternative for a keep-open infusion when extended access to a vein is required without the need for continuous fluid. It is most commonly employed for intermittent infusion of medication into a peripheral venous route. A short, flexible catheter is used as the lock device, and a site is selected where there will be minimum movement, such as the forearm. The catheter device is inserted and secured in the same manner as for any IV infusion device, but the hub is occluded with a stopper.

The type of device used may vary, and the care and use of the peripheral intermittent infusion device (PIID) are carried out according to the specific protocol of the institution or unit; however, the general concept is the same. The catheter remains in place and is flushed with saline or heparin (usually 1:10 units/ml) after infusion of the medication. The flush solution prevents blood from clotting in the device between infusions. Because heparin is incompatible with many drugs, the peripheral lock must also be flushed with saline before and after administering medication. Many studies have shown that normal saline alone is as effective as heparin in maintaining IV patency, especially in catheters larger than 24 gauge (Beecroft et al, 1997; Heilskov et al, 1998; Kotter, 1996; Paisley et al, 1997). Two factors that may account for the difference in small-gauge catheters is frequency of flush and use of the positive-pressure technique. This technique involves instilling the final flush solution as the clamp is closed. Theoretically the procedure is thought to prevent backflow of blood into the catheter, preventing a small clot from forming.

Children may be discharged with a PIID in place in order to continue receiving medications without hospitalization; this is usually reserved for children who require medications on a short-term basis and who are referred to a home-based infusion company. Those with chronic illnesses who require repeated blood sampling or medications, long-term chemotherapy, or frequent hyperalimentation or antibiotic therapy are best managed with a central venous catheter or a peripherally inserted central catheter.*

*Community and home care instructions on caring for a peripheral intermittent infusion device and central venous catheter are available in Wong DL, Hess CS: ***Wong and Whaley's clinical manual of pediatric nursing,*** ed 5, St Louis, 2000, Mosby.

Central Venous Access Devices (VADs). Central VADs have several different characteristics. The practitioner has to consider the best type of catheter for the individual patient's needs. Factors that can influence the decision include the reason for placement of the catheter (diagnosis), length of therapy, risk to the patient in placement of the catheter, and availability of resources to assist the family in maintaining the catheter (Baranowski, 1993; Freedman and Bosserman, 1993).

Short-term or *nontunneled catheters* are used in acute care, emergency, and intensive care units. These catheters are made of polyurethane and are placed in large veins such as the subclavian, femoral, or jugular. Insertion is by surgical incision or large percutaneous threading. A chest x-ray film should be taken to verify placement of the catheter tip before administration of fluids or medications.

Peripherally inserted central catheters (PICCs) can be used for short-term to moderate-length therapy. Researchers have shown catheter longevity ranging to over 200 days (Donaldson et al, 1995; Frey, 1995). These catheters consist of silicone or polymer material and are placed by specially trained nurses, physicians, or interventional radiologists (Goodwin and Carlson, 1993). The most common insertion site is above the antecubital area using the median, cephalic, or basilic vein. The catheter is threaded either with or without a guidewire into the superior vena cava. PICCs can be trimmed before insertion, and the decision can be made to insert the catheter "midline," which is considered between the insertion site and the head of the clavicle (Kravitz, 1993). If the catheter is threaded midline, total parenteral nutrition (TPN) or any other drug known to irritate a peripheral vein (e.g., chemotherapy drugs), should not be administered. The high concentration of glucose in TPN makes it irritating to the vessel; thus it should be infused through a central catheter.

The decision to insert a PICC needs to be made before there are several unsuccessful attempts at IV lines or blood sampling by phlebotomy. Once the antecubital veins have been punctured repeatedly, they are not considered to be a candidate for this type of catheter. Because this catheter is the least costly and has less chance of complications than other central VADs, it is an excellent choice for many pediatric patients. This catheter is also usually inserted either at the child's bedside or, more appropriately when available, in the unit's treatment room.

NURSE ALERT • Most PICC lines are not sutured into place, so care needs to be maintained when changing the dressing.

Long-term central VADs include tunneled and implanted infusion ports (Table 45-4). They may have single, double, or triple lumens. Several lumens (multilumen catheters) allow more than one therapy to be administered at the same time. Reasons to use multilumen catheters include repeated blood sampling, TPN, administration of blood products or infusion of large quantities and/or concentrations of fluids, ability to administer incompatible drugs or fluids at the same time (through different lumens), and central venous pressure (CVP) monitoring.

With any of the central venous catheters, instilling medication through the injection cap is easily accomplished. With the implanted device the port must be palpated for placement and stabilized; the overlying skin cleansed; and only special noncoring Huber needles used to pierce the port's diaphragm on the top or side, depending on the style. To avoid repeated skin punctures, a special infusion set with a Huber needle and extension

TABLE 45-4
Comparison of Long-term Central Venous Access Devices

Description	Benefits	Care Considerations
TUNNELED CATHETER (E.G., HICKMAN/BROVIAC CATHETER)		
Silicone, radiopaque, flexible catheter with open ends One or two Dacron cuffs or Vitacuffs (biosynthetic material impregnated with silver ions) on catheter(s) enhances tissue ingrowth May have more than one lumen	Reduced risk of bacterial migration after tissue adheres to Dacron cuff or Vitacuff Easy to use for self-administered infusions Removal requires pulling catheter from site (nonsurgical procedure)	Requires daily heparin flushes Must be clamped or have clamp nearby at all times Must keep exit site dry Heavy activity restricted until tissue adheres to cuff Water sports may be restricted (risk of infection) Risk of infection still present Protrudes outside body; susceptible to damage from sharp instruments and may be pulled out; may affect body image More difficult to repair Patient/family must learn catheter care
GROSHONG CATHETER		
Clear, flexible, silicone, radiopaque catheter with closed tip and two-way valve at proximal end Dacron cuff or Vitacuff on catheter enhances tissue ingrowth May have more than one lumen	Reduced time and cost for maintenance care; no heparin flushes needed Reduced catheter damage; no clamping needed because of two-way valve Increased patient safety because of minimum potential for blood backflow or air embolism Reduced risk of bacterial migration after tissue adheres to Dacron cuff or Vitacuff Easily repaired Easy to use for self-administered IV infusions	Requires weekly irrigation with normal saline Must keep exit site dry Heavy activity restricted until tissue adheres to cuff Water sports may be restricted (risk of infection) Risk of infection still present Protrudes outside body; susceptible to damage from sharp instruments and may be pulled out; can affect body image Patient/family must learn catheter care
IMPLANTED PORTS (PORT-A-CATH, INFUS-A-PORT, MEDIPORT, NORPORT, GROSHONG PORT)		
Totally implantable metal or plastic device that consists of self-sealing injection port with top or side access with preconnected or attachable silicon catheter that is placed in large blood vessel	Reduced risk of infection Placed completely under the skin; therefore much less likely to be pulled out or damaged No maintenance care and reduced cost for family Heparinized monthly and after each infusion to maintain patency (Groshong port only requires saline) No limit on regular physical activity, including swimming Dressing only needed when port accessed with Huber needle that is not removed No or only slight change in body appearance (slight bulge on chest)	Must pierce skin for access; pain with insertion of needle; can use local anesthetic (EMLA) or intradermal buffered lidocaine before accessing port Special noncoring needle (Huber) with straight or angled design must be used to inject into port Skin preparation needed before injection Difficult to manipulate for self-administered infusions Catheter may dislodge from port, especially if child "plays" with port site (twiddler syndrome) Vigorous contact sports generally not allowed Removal requires surgical procedure

tubing with a Luer connection can be used (Fig. 45-20). With this attached, the injection procedure is the same as for an intermittent infusion device or a central venous catheter. To prevent infection, meticulous aseptic technique must be used any time the devices are entered, including instillation of heparin or saline to prevent clotting (Long et al, 1996). There should be a protocol stating that the Huber needle needs to be changed at established intervals, usually 5 to 7 days (Baranowski, 1993).

The children and parents are taught the procedure for care of the VAD before discharge from the hospital, including prepa-

A
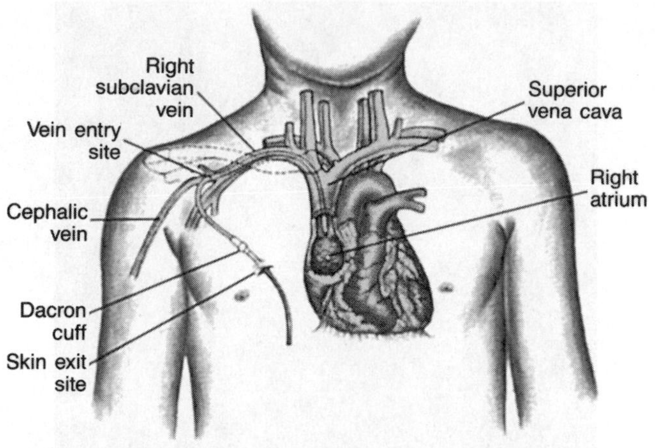

B
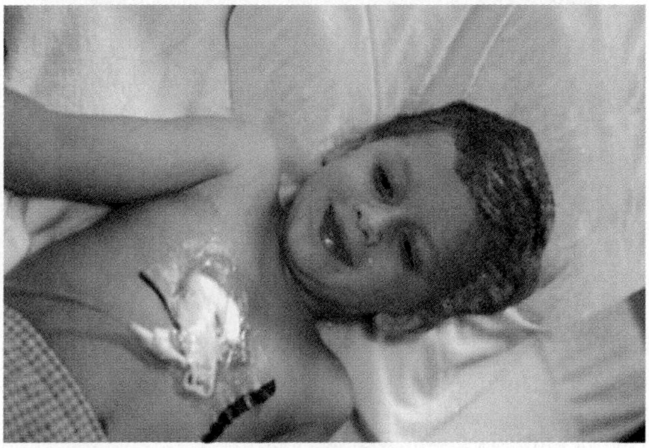

FIG. 45-20 • Venous access devices (VADs). **A,** Central venous catheter insertion and exit site. **B,** Child receiving medication by way of an implantable port. Note needle and extension tubing inserted into port and secured with gauze dressings and a transparent dressing.

ration and injection of the prescribed medication, the flush, and dressing changes. A protective device may be recommended for some active children to prevent their accidentally dislodging the needle. Many children take responsibility for preparing and administering medications. Both verbal and written step-by-step instructions* are provided for the learners.

The use of a spandex-nylon bodysuit on active toddlers has successfully maintained central lines. One study showed that the suit could not be removed by the toddler and fit snugly over the catheter, its exit site, and its connections. The cost of two bodysuits per child, one for wearing while the other is being cleaned, is less than the costs and the risks of repeated central line insertions (Janik, Wayne, and Janik, 1995). A pocket sewn on the inside of a T-shirt provides a place in which to coil the catheter line while the child is at play if a dressing is not used. A commercial elastic vest is also available.†

*Community and home care instructions for caring for a peripheral or central infusion device are available in Wong DL, Hess CS: ***Wong and Whaley's clinical manual of pediatric nursing,*** ed 5, St Louis, 2000, Mosby.

†Available from Advanced Patient Devices, 3564 Sabaka Trail, Verona, WI 53593; 1-800-547-6412; fax: (608) 833-6694.

Infection and an occluded catheter are two of the most common complications of central venous catheters. Although neither is an emergency, both require treatment with antibiotics for infection; and a fibrinolytic agent, such as alteplase, for clots (Reed and Phillip, 1996). Uncapping can be prevented by taping the cap securely to the catheter and the clamped line to the dressing. Leaks can be prevented by using a smooth-edged clamp only. Parents are cautioned to keep scissors away from the child to prevent accidental cutting of the catheter. If the catheter leaks, they are instructed to tape it above the leak and then clamp the catheter at the taped site. The child should be taken to the practitioner as soon as possible to prevent infection or clotting after a catheter leak.

NURSE ALERT • If a central venous catheter is accidentally removed, apply pressure to the entry site to the vein, not the exit site on the skin (Marcoux, Fisher, and Wong, 1990).

Nasogastric, Orogastric, or Gastrostomy Administration

When a child has an indwelling feeding tube or a gastrostomy, oral medications are usually given via that route. An advantage of this method is the ability to administer oral medications around the clock without disturbing the child. A disadvantage is the risk of occluding or "clogging" the tube, especially when giving viscous solutions through small-bore feeding tubes. The most important preventive measure is adequate flushing after the medication is instilled. Guidelines for administration are presented in the Guidelines box.

NURSE ALERT • Sprinkle-type medication should be avoided in a feeding tube. However, if there is no other option and the tube is a large gauge (18 French or greater but usually not a Foley catheter), it may be given by mixing the sprinkles with a small amount of pureed fruit and thinning with water. The fruit keeps the sprinkles suspended so that they do not float to the top. Flush well. This procedure is not recommended for skin-level gastrostomy devices.

Rectal Administration

The rectal route for administration is less reliable but is sometimes used when the oral route is difficult or contraindicated. Some of the drugs available in suppository form are acetaminophen, sedatives, analgesics (morphine), and antiemetics. The difficulty in using the rectal route is that unless the rectum is empty at the time of insertion, the absorption of the drug may be delayed, diminished, or prevented by the presence of feces. Sometimes the drug is later evacuated, securely surrounded by stool. However, the rectal route is used most often in children who are unable to take anything by mouth and are unlikely to have large amounts of stool. It is also used when oral preparations are unsuitable for controlling vomiting.

To insert a suppository, the wrapper is removed and the suppository lubricated with water-soluble jelly or warm water. A gloved finger is used to quickly but gently insert the suppository into the rectum, beyond both of the rectal sphincters. The buttocks are then held or taped together firmly to relieve pressure

Guidelines

NASOGASTRIC, OROGASTRIC, OR GASTROSTOMY MEDICATION ADMINISTRATION IN CHILDREN

Use elixir or suspension (rather than tablet) preparations of medication whenever possible.
Dilute viscous medication or syrup with a small amount of water if possible.
If administering tablets, crush tablet to a very fine powder, and dissolve drug in a small amount of warm water.
- Never crush enteric-coated or sustained-release tablets or capsules.

Avoid oily medications because they tend to cling to side of tube.
Do not mix medication with enteral formula unless fluid is restricted. If adding a drug:
- Check with pharmacist for compatibility.
- Shake formula well and observe for any physical reaction (e.g., separation, precipitation).
- Label formula container with name of medication, dosage, date, and time infusion started.

Have medication at room temperature.
Measure medication in a calibrated cup or syringe.
Check for correct placement of nasogastric or orogastric tube (see Guidelines box, p. 1180).
Attach syringe (with adaptable tip but without plunger) to tube.
Pour medication into syringe.
Unclamp tube and allow medication to flow by gravity.
Adjust height of container to achieve desired flow rate (e.g., increase height for faster flow).
As soon as syringe is empty, pour in water to flush tubing.
- Amount of water depends on length and gauge of tubing.
- Determine amount before administering any medication by using a syringe to fill completely an unused nasogastric or orogastric tube with water. Amount of flush solution is usually 1½ times this volume.
- With certain drug preparations (e.g., suspensions) more fluid may be needed.

If administering more than one drug at the same time, flush tube between each medication with clear water.
Clamp tube after flushing, unless tube is left open.

on the anal sphincter until the urge to expel the suppository has passed—5 to 10 minutes. Sometimes the amount of drug ordered is less than the dosage available. The irregular shape of most suppositories makes the process of dividing them into a desired dose difficult if not dangerous. If the suppository must be halved, it should be cut lengthwise. However, there is no guarantee that the drug is evenly dispersed throughout the petrolatum base.*

Rectal suppositories are usually inserted with the apex (pointed end) foremost. One study demonstrated easier insertion and a lower expulsion rate when the suppository was inserted with the base (blunt end) first (Abd-El-Maeboud et al, 1991).

If medication is administered via a retention enema, the same procedure is used. Drugs given by enema are diluted in the smallest amount of solution possible to minimize the likelihood of being evacuated.

*Information about compounding drugs in suppositories is available from Professional Compounding Centers of America (PCCA), P.O. Box 368, Sugar Land TX 77487; 1-800-331-2498: website: www.thecompounders.com.

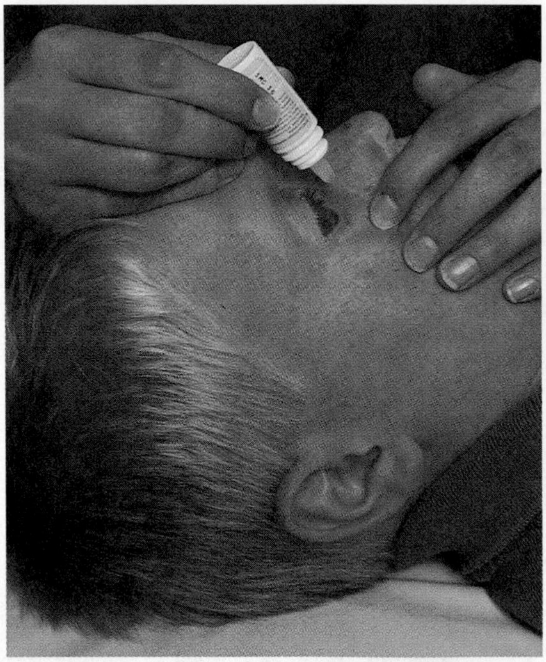

FIG. 45-21 • Administering eye drops.

Optic, Otic, and Nasal Administration

There are few differences in administering eye, ear, and nose medication to children or to adults. The major difficulty is in gaining children's cooperation. The infant's or young child's head is immobilized in the same manner as described in Fig. 35-17. Older children need only explanation and direction. Although the administration of optic, otic, and nasal medication is not painful, these drugs can cause unpleasant sensations that can be eliminated with various techniques. Parental involvement is an important component during administration. A parent's presence can decrease levels of anxiety in the child. To reduce unpleasant sensations, perform the following:

- **Eye**—Apply finger pressure to the lacrimal punctum at the inner aspect of the lid for 1 minute to prevent drainage of medication to the nasopharynx and the unpleasant "tasting" of the drug.
- **Ear**—Allow medications stored in the refrigerator to warm to room temperature before instillation.
- **Nose**—Position the child with the head hyperextended to prevent strangling sensations caused by medication trickling into the throat rather than up into the nasal passages.

To instill eye medication, the child is placed supine or sitting with the head extended, and the child is asked to look up. One hand is used to pull the lower lid downward; the hand that holds the dropper rests on the head so that it may move synchronously with the child's head, thus reducing the possibility of trauma to a struggling child or of dropping medication on the face (Fig. 45-21). As the lower lid is pulled down, a small conjunctival sac is formed; the solution or ointment is applied to this area, never directly on the eyeball. Another effective technique is to pull the lower lid down and out to form a cup, into which the medication is dropped. The lids are gently closed to prevent expression of the medication, and the child is asked to look in all directions to enhance even distribution of the preparation. Excess medication is wiped from the inner canthus outward to prevent contamination to the contralateral eye.

Instilling eye drops in infants can be most difficult, because they often clench the lids tightly closed. One approach is to place the drops in the nasal corner where the lids meet. The medication pools in this area, and when the child opens the lids, the medication flows onto the conjunctiva. For young children, playing a game can be helpful, such as instructing the child to keep the eyes closed until the count of 3 and then open them, at which time the drops are quickly instilled. Ointment can be applied by gently pulling down the lower lid and placing the ointment in the lower conjunctival sac.

NURSE ALERT • If both eye ointment and drops are ordered, give drops first, wait 3 minutes, and then apply the ointment to allow each drug to work. When possible, administer eye ointments before bedtime or naptime, because the child's vision will be blurred temporarily.

Ear drops are instilled with the child in the prone or supine position and the head turned to the appropriate side. For children younger than 3 years of age, the external auditory canal is straightened by gently pulling the pinna downward and straight back. The pinna is pulled upward and back in children older than 3 years of age (see Fig. 35-20). To place the drops deep in the ear canal without contaminating the tip of the dropper, place a disposable ear speculum in the canal and administer the drops through the speculum. After instillation, the child should remain lying on the unaffected side for a few minutes. Gentle massage of the area immediately anterior to the ear facilitates the entry of drops into the ear canal. The use of cotton pledgets prevents medication from flowing out of the external canal; however, the pledgets should be loose enough to allow any discharge to exit from the ear. Premoistening the cotton with a few drops of medication prevents the wicking action from absorbing the medication instilled in the ear.

Nose drops are instilled in the same manner as in the adult patient. Unpleasant sensations associated with medicated nose drops are minimized when care is taken to position the child with the head extended well over the edge of the bed or a pillow (Fig. 45-22). Depending on size, the infant can be positioned in the football hold (see Fig. 45-7, *B*); in the nurse's arm with the head extended and stabilized between the nurse's body and elbow, and the arms and hands immobilized with the nurse's hands; or as in Fig. 45-22. After instillation of the drops, the child should remain in position for 1 minute to allow the drops to come in contact with the nasal surfaces.

Nasal spray dispensers are inserted into the naris vertically and then angled nasally to avoid trauma to the septum and to direct medication toward the inferior turbinate.

Family Teaching and Home Care

The nurse usually assumes the responsibility for preparing families to administer medications at home. The family should have an understanding of why the child is receiving the medication and the effects that might be expected, as well as the amount, frequency, and length of time the drug is to be administered. Instruction should be carried out in an unhurried, relaxed manner, preferably in an area away from busy ward or office routine, following the same guidelines for teaching as outlined in the Guidelines box on p. 1133.

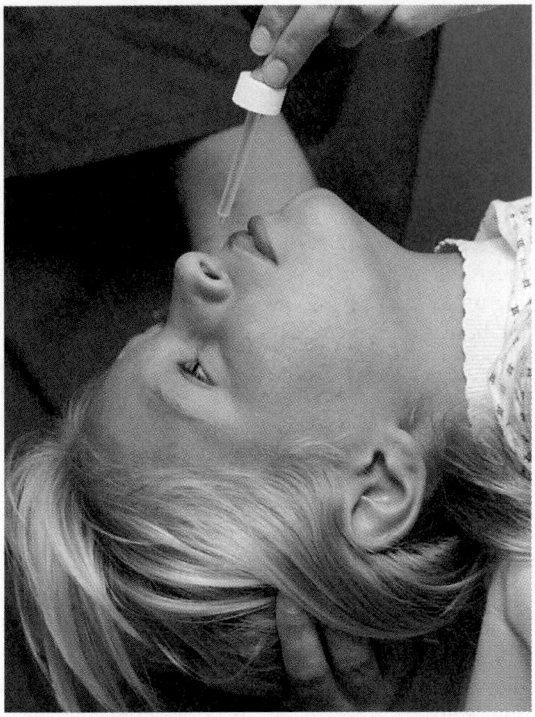

FIG. 45-22 • Proper position for instilling nose drops.

The caregiver is carefully instructed regarding the correct dosage, and the nurse is responsible for preparing parents for the specifics of the task. Some persons have difficulty understanding or interpreting terminology from the pharmacy, and just because they nod or otherwise indicate an understanding, it cannot be assumed that the message is clear. It is important to ascertain their interpretation of a teaspoon, for example, and to be certain they have acceptable devices for measuring the drug. If the drug is packaged with a dropper, syringe, or plastic cup, the nurse should show and/or mark the point on the device that indicates the prescribed dose and demonstrate how the dose is drawn up into a dropper or syringe and measured, and how any bubbles are eliminated. Also, the nurse must be certain that families understand that a prescription ordered in drops means single drops, not dropperfuls, a potential source of administration error (see Nurse Alert, p. 1157). If the nurse has any doubts about the parent's ability to administer the correct dose, the parent should be asked to give a return demonstration. This verification is especially important when the drug has potentially serious consequences from incorrect dosage (e.g., insulin or digoxin) or when more complex administration is required (e.g., parenteral injections). When teaching a parent to give an injection, adequate time for instruction and practice must be allotted.

Home modifications are often necessary because the availability of equipment or assistance can differ from that of the hospital setting. For example, the parent may need guidance in devising methods that allow for one person to hold the child and safely give the drug. One successful method is the following procedure:

- Place child supine on flat surface (bed, couch, floor).
- Sit facing child so that his or her head is between operator's thighs and his or her arms are under operator's legs.

- Place lower legs over child's legs to restrain lower body, if necessary.
- To administer oral medication, place small pillow under child's head to reduce risk of aspiration.
- To administer nasal medication, place small pillow under child's shoulders to aid flow of liquid through nasal passages.

The time that the drug is to be administered is clarified with the parent. For instance, when a drug is prescribed in association with meals, the number of meals that the family is accustomed to eating influences the amount of drug the child receives. Does the child have meals twice a day or five times a day? When a drug is to be given several times during the day, the nurse and parents can together work out a schedule that accommodates the family's routine. This is particularly significant if the drug must be given at equal intervals throughout a 24-hour period. For example, telling parents that the child needs 1 teaspoon of medicine four times a day is subject to misinterpretation, because parents may routinely schedule the doses at incorrect times. Instead, a preplanned schedule based on 6-hour intervals should be set up with the number of days required for therapeutic dosage listed. Modification should also be made to accommodate sleep schedules. For example, at nighttime a 6-hour interval may be extended to 8 hours (e.g., 11 PM, 7 AM, noon, and 6 PM). Written instruction should accompany all drug prescriptions.* If parents have difficulty reading or understanding English, use colors to convey instructions. For example, mark each drug with a color and place the appropriate color on a calendar chart or on a drawing of a clock to identify when the drug needs to be given. If a liquid medication and syringe are used, also mark the syringe at the place the plunger needs to be with color-coded tape.

PROCEDURES RELATED TO MAINTAINING FLUID BALANCE

Measurement of Intake and Output (I&O)

One of the most important roles of the nurse in maintaining fluid balance is accurate measurement of fluid intake and output. Accurate measurements are essential to the assessment of fluid balance. Measurements from all sources—including both gastrointestinal and parenteral I&O from urine, stools, vomitus, fistulas, nasogastric suction, sweat, and drainage from wounds—must be taken and considered. Although the practitioner usually indicates when I&O measurements are to be recorded, it is a nursing responsibility to keep an accurate I&O record on patients in the following situations:

- After major surgery
- IV, diuretic, or corticosteroid therapy
- Severe thermal burns or injuries
- Renal disease or damage
- Congestive heart failure
- Dehydration (vomiting and diarrhea)
- Diabetes mellitus
- Oliguria
- Two years of age or younger
- Respiratory distress

Infants or small children who are unable to use a bedpan or those who have bowel movements with every voiding require the application of a collecting device (p. 1150). If collecting bags are not used, wet diapers or pads are carefully weighed to ascertain the amount of fluid lost. This includes liquid stool, vomitus, and other losses. The volume of fluid in milliliters is equivalent to the weight of the fluid measured in grams. The specific gravity as a measure of osmolality is determined with a refractometer or urine dipsticks and assists in assessing the degree of hydration.

The weighed-diaper method of fluid measurement has disadvantages, including (1) inability to differentiate one type of loss from another because of admixture, (2) loss of urine or liquid stool from leakage or evaporation (especially if the infant is under a radiant warmer), and (3) additional fluid in the diaper (superabsorbent disposable type) from absorption of atmospheric moisture (from high-humidity incubators). However, when several types of diapers, including cloth, conventional disposable, and superabsorbent disposable, were compared for accuracy in terms of evaporative effects, closed superabsorbent disposable diapers followed by open superabsorbent disposable diapers were affected the least (Fox, 1992). To avoid the problem of evaporative losses and leakage of excreta, diapers should be weighed as soon as possible after becoming soiled.

Special Needs When the Child is NPO. Infants or children who are unable or not permitted to take fluids by mouth (NPO) have special needs. To ensure that they do not receive fluids, a sign can be placed in some obvious place, such as over their beds or on their shirts, to alert others to the NPO status. To prevent the temptation to drink, fluids should not be left at the bedside.

Oral hygiene, a part of routine hygienic care, is especially important when fluids are restricted or withheld (p. 1135). For the young child who cannot brush the teeth or rinse the mouth without swallowing fluid, the nurse can institute oral hygiene by wiping the teeth, gums, and tongue with a cloth moistened with saline. To keep the mouth feeling moist when the child is NPO, give ice chips (if this is permitted by the practitioner) or spray the mouth with a fine mist of cool water.

To keep the lips moist and prevent cracking, petrolatum (Vaseline) or some other commercial lip aid is applied. Lemon-glycerin swabs are avoided because they dry the skin, irritate open lesions, and can decay the teeth. To meet the need to suck, the infant is provided with a safe commercial pacifier.

The child who is fluid restricted presents an equal challenge. Limiting fluids is often more difficult for the child than NPO, especially when IV fluids are also eliminated. To make certain the child does not drink the entire amount allowed early in the day, the daily allotment is calculated to provide fluids at periodic intervals throughout the child's waking hours. Serving the fluids in small containers gives the illusion of larger servings. No extra liquid is left at the bedside if compliance is a problem.

Parenteral Fluid Therapy

Site and Equipment. The site selected for IV infusion depends on accessibility and convenience. Although it is possible to use any accessible vein in older children, attention must be directed toward the child's developmental, cognitive, and mobility needs when selecting a site. Ideally in older children, the superficial veins of the forearm should be used, leaving the

*Community and home care instructions on giving medications to children are available in Wong DL, Hess CS: ***Wong and Whaley's clinical manual of pediatric nursing***, ed 5, St Louis, 2000, Mosby.

hands free. An older child can help select the site and thereby maintain some measure of control. For veins in the extremities it is best to start with the most distal site and avoid the child's favored hand in order to reduce the disability related to the procedure. A site is chosen that restricts the child's movements as little as possible—a site over a joint in an extremity, such as the antecubital space, is avoided. In small infants a superficial vein of the hand, wrist, forearm, foot, or ankle is usually most convenient and most easily stabilized (Fig. 45-23). Foot veins should be avoided in children learning to walk and in children already walking. Superficial veins of the scalp have no valves, insertion is easy, and they can be used in infants up to about 9 months of age; but they should be used only when other site attempts have failed.

Selection of a scalp vein as the venipuncture site requires shaving the area around the site to visualize the vein better and to provide a smooth surface on which to tape the catheter hub and tubing. A rubber band slipped onto the head from brow to occiput will usually suffice as a tourniquet. Shaving off a portion of the infant's hair is very upsetting to parents; therefore they should be told what to expect and reassured that the hair will grow in again rapidly (save the hair because parents often wish to keep it). Remove as little as possible, directly over the insertion site and taping surface.

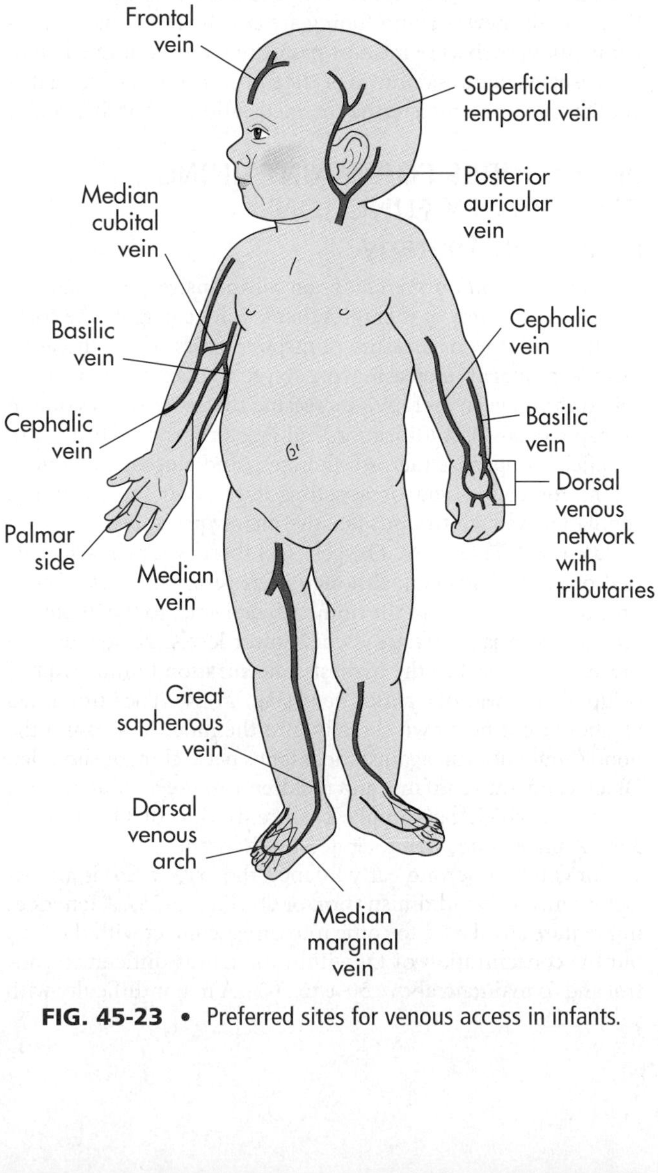

FIG. 45-23 • Preferred sites for venous access in infants.

Situations may occur in which rapid establishment of a systemic access is vital, and venous access may be hampered by peripheral circulatory collapse, hypovolemic shock (secondary to vomiting or diarrhea, burns, or trauma), cardiopulmonary arrest, or other conditions (Banerjee et al, 1994). *Intraosseous infusion* provides a rapid, safe and lifesaving alternate route for administration of fluids and medications until intravascular access can be attained, especially in children who are 6 years of age and younger. A large-bore needle, such as a bone marrow aspiration needle (e.g., Jamshidi) or an intraosseous needle (e.g., Cook), is inserted into the medullary cavity of a long bone, most often the proximal tibia. This procedure is usually reserved for children who are unconscious or for those who are receiving analgesia, because the procedure is painful. Local anesthesia should be used for a semiconscious patient.

For most IV infusions in children, an over-the-needle 22- to 24-gauge catheter may be used if therapy is expected to last less than 5 days. The smallest-gauge and shortest-length catheter that will accommodate the prescribed therapy should be chosen when evaluating the placement of a peripheral IV line. The length of the catheter may be directly related to infection and/or embolus formation—the shorter the catheter, the fewer the complications (Maki, 1994). The gauge of the catheter should maintain adequate flow of the infusate into the cannulated vein while allowing adequate blood flow around the catheter walls to promote proper hemodilution of the infusate. Because stainless steel needles tend to dislodge and infiltrate more often than catheters, the use of these should be limited to short-term or single-dose administration (Intravenous Nurses Society, 1998).

The goal of IV therapy is to deliver the prescribed fluids or medications without complications. Determining the best catheter for the patient early in the therapy provides the best chance of avoiding catheter-related complications (Moureau, 1999). As the length of therapy increases, decisions regarding the type of infusion device (e.g., short peripheral, midline, peripherally inserted central catheter, or central venous catheter) should be explored. Guidelines such as flow charts or algorithms are available to help in these decisions (Catudal, 1999).

Special Care Considerations. To maintain the integrity of the IV line, adequate protection of the site is required. The catheter hub is firmly secured at the puncture site with a transparent dressing or clear, nonallergenic tape. Transparent dressings are ideal because the insertion site is easily observed. Minimal tape should be used at the puncture site and on about 1 to 2 inches of skin beyond the site to avoid obscuring the insertion site for early detection of infiltration.

A protective cover is applied directly over the catheter insertion site to protect the infusion site. Easy access to the IV site for frequent (i.e., 1- to 2-hour) assessments must be considered. Improvised plastic cups that are cut in half with the ridged edges covered with tape should not be used, because they have caused injury to patients (Morris v Children's Medical Center, 1992). A commercial site protector, *I.V. House,** is available in different sizes. Its ventilation holes prevent moisture from accumulating under the dome (Lee and Vallino, 1996). This device is designed to protect the IV site; allow for visibility of the site;

*Available from I.V. House, 7400 Foxmont Dr., Hazelwood, MO 63042; 1-800-530-0400; fax (314) 831-3863; e-mail: ivhouse@ivhouse.com; website: www.ivhouse.com.

minimize use of padded boards, splints, or other restraints and tape; and maintain skin integrity. The connector tubing or extension tubing can be looped to make it small enough to fit under the protective cover to prevent accidental snagging of the catheter. It is important to safely secure the IV tubing to prevent infants and children from becoming entangled in the tubing or from accidentally pulling the catheter or needle out. This securement also eliminates movement of the catheter hub at the insertion site (mechanical manipulation). A colorful and interesting sticker can be applied to the protecting device to add a positive note to the procedure.

When it comes time to discontinue an IV infusion, many children are distressed by the thought of catheter removal; therefore they need a careful explanation of the process and suggestions for helping. Encouraging children to remove or help remove the tape from the site provides them with a measure of control and often encourages their cooperation. The procedure consists of turning off any pump apparatus, occluding the IV tubing, removing the tape, pulling the catheter out of the vessel in the opposite direction of insertion, and exerting firm pressure at the site. A dry dressing (e.g., adhesive bandage strip) is placed over the puncture site. The use of adhesive-removal pads can decrease the pain of tape removal, but the skin should be washed after use because it can become irritated. To remove transparent dressings (e.g., Opsite or Tegaderm), pull the opposing edges parallel to the skin to loosen the bond. If a catheter was used for the IV infusion, the tip is inspected to make certain that the catheter is intact and that no portion remains in the vein.

Complications. The same precautions regarding maintenance of asepsis, prevention of infection, and observation for infiltration are carried out with patients of any age. However, infiltration is more difficult to detect in infants and small children than in adults. The increased amount of subcutaneous fat and the amount of tape used to secure the needle often obscure the signs of early infiltration. When the fluid appears to be infusing too slowly or ceases, the usual assessment for obstruction within the apparatus—kinks, screw clamps, shutoff valve, and positioning interference (e.g., a bent elbow)—often locates the difficulty. When these actions fail to detect the problem, it may be necessary to carefully remove some of the tape and other material that obscure a clear view of the venipuncture site. Dependent areas, such as the palm and undersides of the extremity or the occiput and behind the ears, are examined.

Whenever possible, the IV infusion should be placed in an extremity to which the identification band (or bracelet) is not attached. Serious circulatory impairment can result from infiltrated solution distal to the band, which acts as a tourniquet, preventing adequate venous return. To check for return blood flow through the catheter, the tubing is removed from the infusion pump, and the bag is lowered below the level of the infusion site. If the tubing is connected to an infusion pump, it must be removed from the pump before lowering. A good blood return, or lack thereof, is not always an indicator of infiltration in small infants. Flushing the catheter/needle and observing for edema, redness, or streaking along the vein is an appropriate assessment of IV status (Wilson, 1992). Resistance during flushing or aspiration for blood return also indicates that the IV infusion may have infiltrated surrounding tissue.

NURSE ALERT • Prevention of insertion site infection can be decreased by strict adherence to the following guidelines (Pearson, 1996):

- Practice good handwashing before starting an IV infusion.
- Rigorously cleanse the skin with an appropriate antiseptic, including alcohol or povidone-iodine, before catheter insertion.
- When cleansing the insertion site, use a circular motion starting from the center and working outward.
- Allow the antiseptic to dry for 30 to 60 seconds before inserting the catheter.
- Do not palpate the insertion site after the skin has been cleansed with the antiseptic.

Proper education of the patient and family regarding signs and symptoms of an infected site can help prevent infections from going unnoticed (Messner and Pinkerman, 1992). When an IV infusion continues for several days, the tubing and solution are changed at regular intervals according to hospital policy, most often every 72 hours (Pearson, 1995). The dressing, whether transparent dressing or sterile gauze and tape, can be left in place for the duration of the IV infusion (Maki, 1994) unless the integrity has been compromised. To ensure that the equipment is changed regularly, it is labeled with the date and time that the new bag and tubing are attached. Any signs of inflammation, such as redness or pain, are reported immediately. This usually requires removal of the infusion and restarting it at another site or administering the medication by another route.

PROCEDURES FOR MAINTAINING RESPIRATORY FUNCTION

Inhalation Therapy

The term *inhalation therapy* is an all-inclusive term that encompasses a variety of therapies that involve changing the composition, volume, or pressure of inspired gases. These therapies include primarily increasing the oxygen concentration of inspired gas (oxygen therapy), increasing the water vapor content of inspired gas (humidification), adding airborne particles with beneficial properties (aerosol therapy), and employing various means for controlling or assisting respiration (e.g., artificial ventilation and continuous positive airway pressure).

Oxygen Therapy. Oxygen (O_2) therapy is primarily carried out in the hospital, although increasing numbers of children are receiving O_2 in the home. O_2 delivered to the infant via the incubator is satisfactory when lower levels are adequate to prevent cyanosis, but the highest concentration (almost 100%) is supplied by way of a *plastic hood* (Fig. 45-24). The humidified O_2 should not be blown directly into the infant's face, and the hood should not rub against the infant's neck, chin, or shoulder. Older, cooperative infants and children can use a *nasal cannula* or *prongs,* which can supply a concentration of O_2 of about 50%. A mask is not well tolerated by children.

For children beyond early infancy, the *oxygen tent* is a satisfactory means for administration of O_2 (Fig. 45-25). A tent does not require any device to come into direct contact with the face, but the concentration of O_2 within the tent is difficult to control and to maintain above 30% to 50%. A major difficulty with

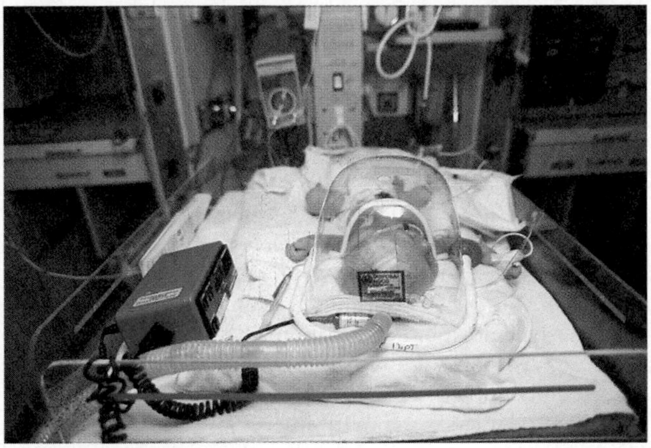

FIG. 45-24 • Oxygen administered to infant by means of a plastic hood. Note oxygen analyzer *(blue machine).*

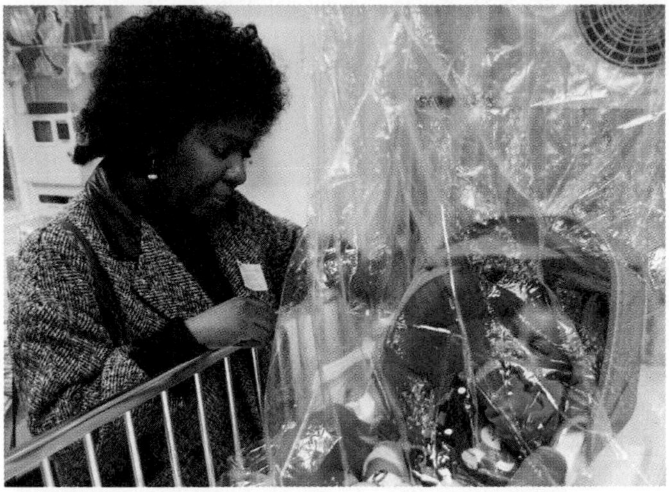

FIG. 45-25 • The tent provides a comfortable method for oxygen administration. (From Wilson SF, Thompson JM: *Respiratory disorders,* St Louis, 1990, Mosby.)

the use of the tent is keeping the tent closed so that the O_2 concentration is maintained.

To reduce O_2 loss, nursing care is planned carefully so that the tent is opened as little as possible. Because O_2 is heavier than air, loss will be greater at the bottom of the tent; therefore the tent is tucked in snugly without open edges. The bottom of the tent should be examined more often when the child is restless and fussy and liable to pull the covers loose. Some tents are even open at the top. Because of the rapid diffusing qualities of carbon dioxide (CO_2), the levels of the gas do not build up within these enclosures.

After the tent has been opened for an extended period, it is flushed with O_2 by increasing the flow meter for a few minutes to quickly raise the O_2 and mist concentration. The flow meter is then reset to the prescribed number of liters.

The enclosed tent becomes very warm; therefore some type of cooling mechanism is provided. The temperature inside the tent must be checked periodically to be certain that it is maintained at the desired level. Although the cool environment can reduce fever and airway inflammation, it can also produce hypothermia and cold stress. It is important to make certain that the child is kept warm and dry. Because O_2 is drying to the tissues, the gas is humidified, which causes moisture to condense on the tent walls.

NURSE ALERT • Keep the child warm and dry by checking the temperature inside the tent and the child's bedding and clothing often. Adjust the temperature and change clothing as often as needed.

The reactions of children to the O_2 tent are variable. Some, especially older children, feel comfortable in the tent and like the cozy, close privacy it affords. Others, more often younger children, may be frightened by the forced enclosure. The plastic walls distort their view of the world and constitute a barrier between them and their source of comfort, their parent. Their distress can be minimized if they are able to see someone nearby and are reassured that they will not be left alone. A favorite toy or object can accompany the child inside the tent; however, all toys should be inspected for safety and suitability. Other familiar items can be placed at the foot of the bed or otherwise in view.

NURSE ALERT • Inspect all toys for safety and suitability (e.g., vinyl or plastic, not stuffed items that absorb moisture and are difficult to keep dry). The high-level O_2 environment makes any source of sparks (e.g., mechanical or electrical toys) a potential fire hazard.

In most instances the child can be removed from the O_2 tent for activities such as feeding and bathing, whereas in other cases the child is placed in the tent only during periods of rest. Still other children may require O_2 continuously and can be removed from the tent or incubator only if an O_2 source is held close to the child's face. Any change in color, increased respiratory effort, or restlessness is an indication to return the child to the O_2 tent.

Oxygen Toxicity. O_2 is essential to life and a valuable therapeutic aid; however, prolonged exposure to high O_2 tensions can be damaging to some body tissues and functions. The organs most vulnerable to the adverse effects of excessive oxygenation are the retina of the premature infant and the lungs of persons at any age.

Oxygen-induced carbon dioxide narcosis is a physiologic hazard of O_2 therapy that may occur in persons with chronic pulmonary disease, such as cystic fibrosis. These children have chronic alveolar hypoventilation with a concomitant chronic CO_2 retention and hypoxemia. In these patients the respiratory center has adapted to the continuously higher arterial carbon dioxide tension ($PaCO_2$) levels, and therefore hypoxia becomes the more powerful stimulus for respiration. When the arterial oxygen tension (PaO_2) level is elevated during O_2 administration, the hypoxic drive is removed, causing progressive hypoventilation and increased $PaCO_2$ levels, and the child rapidly becomes unconscious. CO_2 narcosis can also be induced by the administration of sedation in these patients.

Monitoring Oxygen Therapy. *Pulse oximetry* is a simple, continuous, noninvasive method of determining oxygen saturation (SaO_2) to guide O_2 therapy. A sensor comprising a light-emitting diode (LED) and a photodetector is placed in opposition around a foot, hand, finger, toe, or earlobe, with the LED placed on top of the nail when digits are used (Fig. 45-26). The LED emits red and infrared lights that pass through the skin to the photodetector. The photodetector measures the amount of each type of light absorbed by functional hemoglobins. Hemoglobin saturated with O_2 (oxyhemoglobin) absorbs more infrared light than does hemoglobin not saturated with O_2 (deoxyhemoglobin); therefore pulsatile blood flow is the primary physiologic factor that influences accuracy of the pulse oximeter.

Another noninvasive method is *transcutaneous monitoring (TCM),* which provides continual monitoring of transcutaneous partial pressure of oxygen in arterial blood ($tcPaO_2$), and, with some devices, of carbon dioxide in arterial blood ($tcPaCO_2$). An electrode is attached to the warmed skin to facilitate arterialization of cutaneous capillaries. The site of the electrode must be changed every 3 to 4 hours to prevent burning the skin, and the machine must be calibrated with every site change. TCM is commonly used in neonatal intensive care units, but it may not reflect PaO_2 in infants with impaired local circulation or in older infants whose skin is thicker.

The PaO_2 can be correlated with the SaO_2 by means of the oxyhemoglobin dissociation curve (Fig. 45-27). Most important, changes in PaO_2 do not cause identical changes in SaO_2. Rather, in the steep portion of the curve, small changes in PaO_2 result in large changes in SaO_2. In the flat portion of the curve, large changes in PaO_2 result in only small changes in SaO_2. A quick formula for calculating the correlation of PaO_2 with SaO_2 is the 30-60, 60-90 rule. Assuming a normal pH, $PaCO_2$, and body temperature, this rule can apply: when PaO_2 = 30 mm Hg, SaO_2 = 60%; when PaO_2 = 60 mm, SaO_2 = 90%.

Also, oximetry is insensitive to hyperoxia because hemoglobin approaches 100% saturation for all PaO_2 readings greater than approximately 100 mm Hg, which is a dangerous situation for the premature infant at risk for developing retinopathy of prematurity. Therefore the premature infant being monitored with oximetry should have upper limits identified, such as 90% to 95%, and a protocol established for decreasing O_2 when saturations are high.

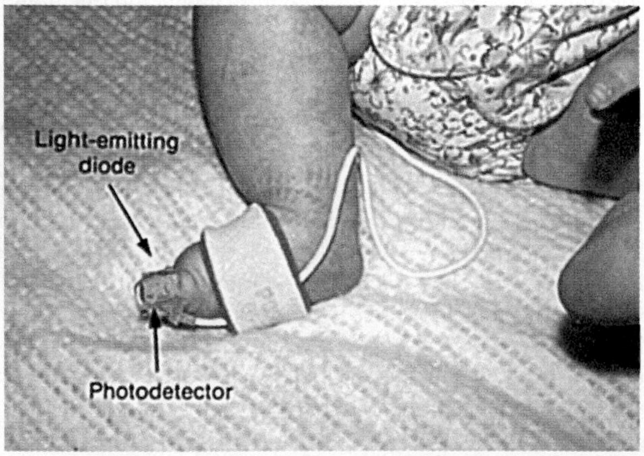

FIG. 45-26 • Oximeter sensor on great toe. Note that sensor is positioned with light-emitting diode opposite photodetector. Cord is secured to foot to minimize movement of sensor.

The degree to which O_2 combines with hemoglobin is affected by several factors. A shift of the curve to the left causes an increased affinity of hemoglobin for O_2, but the O_2 is not easily released to the tissues. This represents an increase in the SaO_2 if it is measured against the same PaO_2 of the normal oxyhemoglobin dissociation curve. This left shift can be caused by an increase in blood pH or a decrease in $PaCO_2$; body temperature; or 2,3-diphosphoglycerate (2,3-DPG), a substance in the red blood cells.

A shift of the curve to the right causes a decreased affinity of hemoglobin for O_2 but improved O_2 release to the tissues. This represents a lower SaO_2 if measured against the same PaO_2 of the normal oxyhemoglobin dissociation curve. This right shift can be caused by a decrease in blood pH or an increase in $PaCO_2$, body temperature, or 2,3-DPG.

Oximetry offers several advantages over TCM. Oximetry (1) does not require heating the skin, thus reducing the risk of burns; (2) eliminates a delay period for transducer equilibration; and (3) maintains an accurate measurement regardless of the patient's age or skin characteristics or the presence of lung disease.

NURSE ALERT • It is important to make certain that sensor connectors and oximeters are compatible. Wiring that is incompatible can generate considerable heat at the tip of the sensor, causing second- and third-degree burns under the sensors. Pressure necrosis can also occur from sensors attached too tightly. Therefore inspect the skin under the sensor often.

Applying the sensor correctly is essential for accurate SaO_2 measurements. Because the sensor must identify every pulse beat to calculate the SaO_2, movement can interfere with sensing. Some devices synchronize the SaO_2 reading with the heartbeat, thereby reducing the interference caused by motion. Sensors are not placed on extremities used for blood pressure monitoring

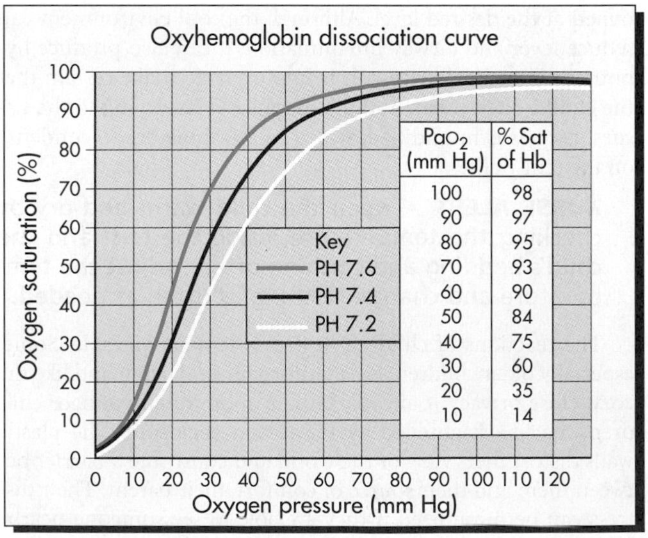

FIG. 45-27 • Oxyhemoglobin dissociation curve. Changes in affinity of hemoglobin for oxygen shift position of curve. Shift to left *(blue line)* indicates increased affinity. Shift to right *(white line)* indicates decreased affinity of hemoglobin for oxygen.

or with indwelling arterial catheters, because pulsatile blood flow can be affected. The following are general guidelines for placing sensors on infants and children:

- **Infant**—Tape the sensor securely to the great toe and tape the wire to the sole of the foot (or use a commercial holder that fastens with a self-adhering closure). Place a snugly fitting sock over the foot.
- **Child**—Tape the sensor securely to the index finger and tape the wire to the back of the hand. Use self-adhering Ace-type wrap (e.g., Coban) around the finger and/or hand to further secure the sensor and wire.

Ambient light from ceiling lights and phototherapy, as well as high-intensity heat and light from radiant warmers, can interfere with readings. Therefore the sensor should be covered to block these light sources. IV dyes; green, purple, or black nail polish; nonopaque synthetic nails; and possibly ink used for footprinting can also cause inaccurate SaO_2 measurements. The dyes should be removed or, in the case of porcelain nails, a different area used for the sensor. Skin color, thickness, and edema do not affect the readings.

Aerosol Therapy. Aerosol therapy can be effective in depositing medication directly into the airway. The value of aerosolized water, or "mist therapy," is controversial. This route of administration can be useful in avoiding the systemic side effects of certain drugs and in reducing the amount of drug necessary to achieve the desired effect. Bronchodilators, steroids, and antibiotics can be suspended in particulate form and then inhaled so that the medication reaches the small airways. The use of aerosol therapy is particularly challenging in children who are too young to cooperate with controlling the rate and depth of breathing. Administration of this therapy requires skill, patience, and creativity.

Medications can be aerosolized or nebulized with air or with O_2-enriched gas. *Handheld nebulizers* are the most commonly used equipment. The medicated "mist" is discharged into a small plastic mask that the child holds over the nose and mouth. To avoid particle deposition in the nose and pharynx, the child is instructed to take slow, deep breaths through an open mouth during the treatment. For home use, an air compressor is necessary to force air through the liquid medication to form the aerosol. Fairly compact, portable units can be rented from health equipment companies. The *metered-dose inhaler (MDI)* is a self-contained, handheld device that allows for intermittent delivery of a specified amount of medication. Many bronchodilators are available in this form and are successfully used by children with asthma. For children under the age of 5 or 6 years, a *spacer device* attached to the MDI can help with coordination of breathing and aerosol delivery. It allows the aerosolized particles to remain in suspension longer. (See also Asthma, Chapter 46.)

A major nursing responsibility during aerosol therapy is to assess the effectiveness of the treatment and the patient's tolerance of the procedure. Assessments of breath sounds and work of breathing should be done before and after treatments. Small children who become upset with having a mask held close to the face may become fatigued with fighting the procedure and may actually appear worse during and immediately after the therapy. Careful assessment is required by the nurse and practitioner to determine if the treatment is worthwhile. It may be necessary to spend a few minutes calming the child after the procedure, and allowing the vital signs to return to baseline to accurately assess changes in breath sounds and work of breathing.

Bronchial (Postural) Drainage

Bronchial drainage is indicated whenever excessive fluid or mucus in the bronchi is not being removed by normal ciliary activity and cough. Positioning the child to take maximum advantage of gravity facilitates removal of secretions. The effect is sometimes dramatic in children with chronic lung disease characterized by thick mucus (e.g., asthma and cystic fibrosis).

Postural drainage is carried out three or four times daily and is more effective when it follows other respiratory therapy, such as bronchodilator and/or nebulization medication. Bronchial drainage is generally performed before meals (or 1 to 1½ hours after meals) to minimize the chance of vomiting and is repeated at bedtime. The length and duration of treatment depend on the child's condition and tolerance level, usually 20 to 30 minutes. There are positions to facilitate drainage from all major lung segments (Fig. 45-28), but all positions are not employed at each session. Children will usually cooperate for four to six positions, but more than six tend to exceed their limits of tolerance. Older children can be expected to tolerate longer periods.

In the hospital an older child can be positioned over an elevated knee rest. Small children and infants can be positioned with pillows or on the therapist's lap and legs (Fig. 45-29). Infants should not be placed in the Trendelenburg position because they do not have an autonomic regulation of blood flow to the head. Special modifications of the techniques are required in children whose conditions contraindicate the standard positioning, such as head injuries, some types of surgical incisions or burns, and casts or traction. At home small children can be positioned on a padded ironing board.* Children who require postural drainage over months or years may benefit from specially constructed tables padded and adjusted to their individual needs. The position used and the frequency and duration of treatment are individualized.

Chest Physiotherapy (CPT)

CPT usually refers to the use of postural drainage in combination with adjunctive techniques that are thought to enhance the clearance of mucus from the airway. These techniques include manual percussion, vibration, and squeezing of the chest; cough; forceful expiration; and breathing exercises; however, the efficacies of these techniques, both individually and combined, are controversial. Postural drainage in combination with forced expiration has been shown to be beneficial, but the benefit of the other techniques has yet to be demonstrated. The results of a study evaluating the effects of noninvasive inspiratory nasal pressure support ventilation (PSV) during CPT showed a significant improvement in respiratory muscle performance and a reduction in O_2 desaturation when used in combination (Fauroux et al, 1999).

The most common technique used in association with postural drainage is manual percussion of the chest wall. Nurses are often responsible for this maneuver if a respiratory therapist is not available, so they should be skilled in the technique. The patient is dressed in a lightweight shirt and placed in a postural

---

*Community and home care instructions on performing postural drainage are available in Wong DL, Hess CS: ***Wong and Whaley's clinical manual of pediatric nursing***, ed 5, St Louis, 2000, Mosby.

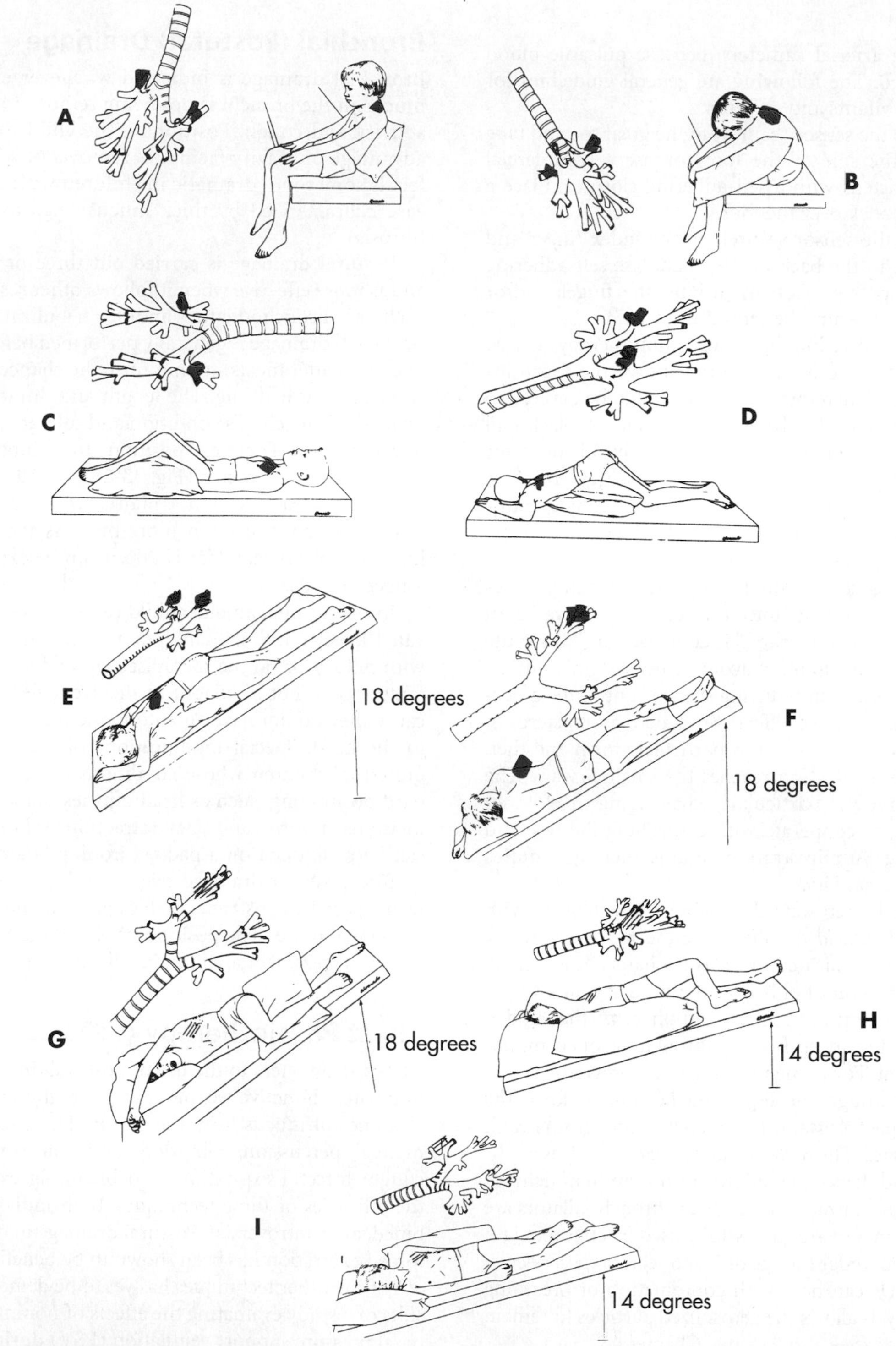

FIG. 45-28 • Bronchial drainage positions for all major segments of child. For each position, model of tracheobronchial tree is projected beside child to show segmental bronchus *(striped)* being drained and pathway *(arrow)* of secretions out of bronchus. Drainage platform is horizontal unless otherwise noted. Striped area on child's chest indicates area to be cupped or vibrated by therapist. **A,** Apical segment of right upper lobe and apical subsegment of apical-posterior segment of left upper lobe. **B,** Posterior segment of right upper lobe and posterior subsegment of apical-posterior segment of left upper lobe. **C,** Anterior segments of both upper lobes; child should be rotated slightly away from side being drained. **D,** Superior segments of both lower lobes. **E,** Posterior basal segments of both lower lobes. **F,** Lateral basal segments of right lower lobe; left lateral basal segment would be drained by mirror image of this position (right side down). **G,** Anterior basal segment of left lower lobe; right anterior basal segment would be drained by mirror image of this position (left side down). **H,** Medial and lateral segments of right middle lobe. **I,** Lingular segments (superior and inferior) of left upper lobe (homologue of right middle lobe). (From Chernick V, editor: *Kendig's disorders of the respiratory tract of children,* ed 5, Philadelphia, 1990, WB Saunders.)

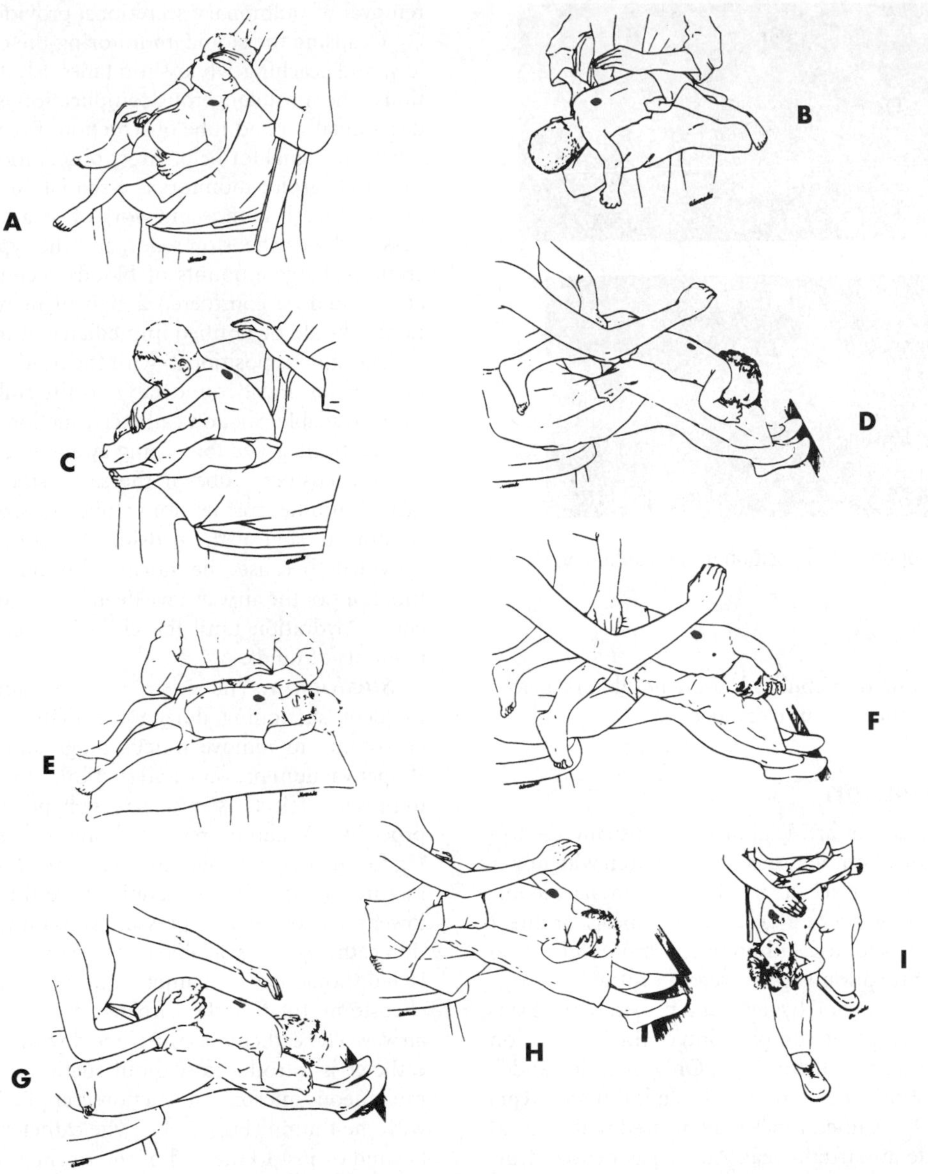

FIG. 45-29 • Bronchial drainage positions for major segments of all lobes in infant. Procedure is most easily carried out in therapist's lap. Therapist's hand on chest indicates area to be cupped or vibrated. **A,** Apical segment of left upper lobe. **B,** Posterior segment of left upper lobe. **C,** Anterior segment of left upper lobe. **D,** Superior segment of right lower lobe. **E,** Posterior basal segment of right lower lobe. **F,** Lateral basal segment of right lower lobe. **G,** Anterior basal segment of right lower lobe. **H,** Medial and lateral segments of right middle lobe. **I,** Lingular segments (superior and inferior) of left upper lobe. (Modified from Cystic Fibrosis Foundation: *Infant segmental bronchial drainage,* Rockville, MD, The Foundation.)

drainage position; then the nurse gently but firmly strikes the chest wall with a cupped hand (Fig. 45-30, *A*). For infants, special devices are available for percussing small areas (Fig. 45-30, *B*). A "popping," hollow sound should be the result, not a slapping sound. The procedure should be done over the rib cage only and should be painless. Percussion can be performed with a soft circular mask (adapted to maintain air trapping) or a percussion cup marketed especially for the purpose of aiding the loosening of secretions.

CPT is contraindicated when patients have pulmonary hemorrhage, pulmonary embolism, end-stage renal disease, increased intracranial pressure, osteogenesis imperfecta, or minimal cardiac reserves.

CPT should be used for patients who have increased sputum production. It is probably of no value to the uncomplicated postoperative patient or the patient with pneumonia. Forced expiration combined with postural drainage is more effective than cough alone, but percussion and vibration have no proven

A

B

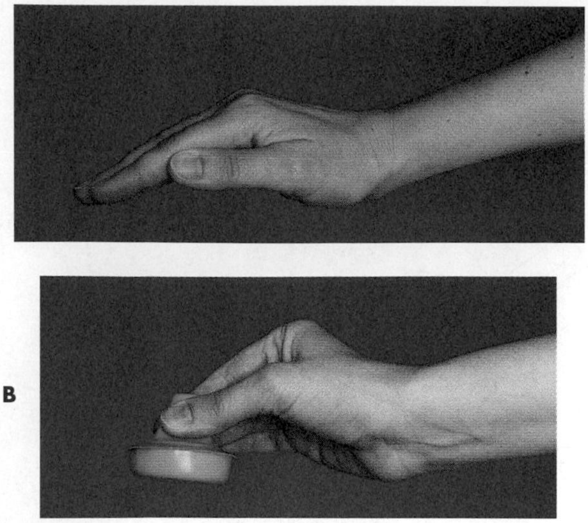

FIG. 45-30 • **A,** Cupped hand position for percussion. **B,** Device for infant percussion.

value. Appropriate use of nebulized bronchodilators before CPT therapy will enhance mucus clearance.

Artificial Ventilation

Artificial Airways. An artificial airway is usually used in association with artificial ventilation and in children with upper airway obstruction. Endotracheal intubation can be accomplished by the nasal (nasotracheal), oral (orotracheal), or direct tracheal (tracheostomy) routes. Although it is more difficult to place, nasotracheal intubation is preferred to orotracheal intubation because it facilitates oral hygiene and provides more stable fixation, which reduces the complication of tracheal erosion and the danger of accidental extubation. Only uncuffed endotracheal (ET) tubes should be used in children less than 8 years of age (Hazinski, 1992). Cuffed tubes may be used with adolescents to help provide an airtight seal. Air or gas delivered directly to the trachea must be humidified as in tracheostomy.

Tracheostomy. A tracheostomy is a surgical opening in the trachea; the procedure may be done on an emergency basis or may be an elective one, and it may be combined with mechanical ventilation.

Pediatric tracheostomy tubes are usually made of plastic or Silastic. The most common types are the Hollinger, Jackson, Aberdeen, and Shiley tubes. These tubes are constructed with a more acute angle than adult tubes; and they soften at body temperature, conforming to the contours of the trachea. Because these materials resist the formation of crusted respiratory secretions, they are made without an inner cannula. Some children require a metal tracheostomy tube (usually made of sterling silver or stainless steel), which contains an inner cannula. The principal advantage of metal tubes is their nonreactivity and decreased chance of causing an allergic reaction.

Children who have undergone a tracheostomy require a hospital stay. During this time the child is closely monitored for the development of complications such as hemorrhage, edema, aspiration, accidental decannulation, tube obstruction, or the entrance of free air into the pleural cavity. The focus of postoperative nursing care is maintaining a patent airway, facilitating the removal of pulmonary secretions, providing humidified air or O_2, cleansing the stoma, monitoring the child's ability to swallow, and teaching while simultaneously preventing complications. The most dangerous complication is related to accidental decannulation and tube obstruction. Because the child may be unable to signal for help, direct observation and use of respiratory and cardiac monitors is essential. Respiratory assessments include breath sounds and work of breathing, vital signs, tightness of the tracheostomy ties, and the type and amount of secretions. Large amounts of bloody secretions are uncommon and should be considered a sign of hemorrhage. The practitioner should be notified immediately if this occurs.

The child is positioned with the head of the bed raised or in the position most comfortable to the child, with the call light easily available. Suction catheters, suction source, gloves, sterile saline, sterile gauze for wiping away secretions, scissors, an extra tracheostomy tube of the same size with ties already attached, another tracheostomy tube one size smaller, and the obturator are kept at the bedside. A source of humidification is provided, because the normal humidification and filtering functions of the airway have been bypassed. IV fluids ensure adequate hydration until the child is able to swallow sufficient amounts of fluids.

Suctioning. The airway must remain patent and requires frequent suctioning during the first few hours after a tracheostomy to remove mucus plugs and excessive secretions. Proper vacuum pressure and suction catheter size are important to prevent atelectasis and decrease hypoxia from the suctioning procedure. Vacuum pressure should range from 60 to 100 mm Hg for infants and children and from 40 to 60 mm Hg for premature infants. Unless secretions are thick and tenacious, the lower range of negative pressure is recommended. Tracheal suction catheters are available in a variety of sizes. The catheter selected should have a diameter one-half the diameter of the tracheostomy tube. If the catheter is too large, it can block the airway. The catheter is constructed with a side port so that the catheter is introduced without suction and removed while simultaneous intermittent suction is applied by covering the port with the thumb (Fig. 45-31). The catheter is inserted to 0.5 cm beyond or just to the end of the tracheostomy tube. Traditionally, a small amount of sterile isotonic saline (usually 1 to 2 ml, depending on the child's size) has been injected into the tube to loosen secretions and crusts for easier aspiration, although the value of this practice is unproved (Blackwood, 1999). Only sterile saline without preservatives can be used.

NURSE ALERT • Suctioning should require no more than 5 seconds (Chandra and Hazinski, 1994).

Counting 1—one thousand, 2—one thousand, 3—one thousand, and so on, is a simple means for monitoring the time while suctioning. Without a safeguard, the airway may be obstructed for too long a period. Hyperventilating the child with 100% O_2 before and after suctioning (using a bag-valve-mask or increasing the fraction of inspired oxygen concentration [FiO_2] ventilator setting) is also performed to prevent hypoxia. Closed tracheal suctioning systems that allow for uninterrupted O_2 delivery may also be used.

The child is allowed to rest for 30 to 60 seconds after each aspiration to allow O_2 tension to return to normal; then the process is repeated until the trachea is clear. Suctioning should be limited to about three aspirations in one period. Oximetry is used to monitor suctioning and prevent hypoxia.

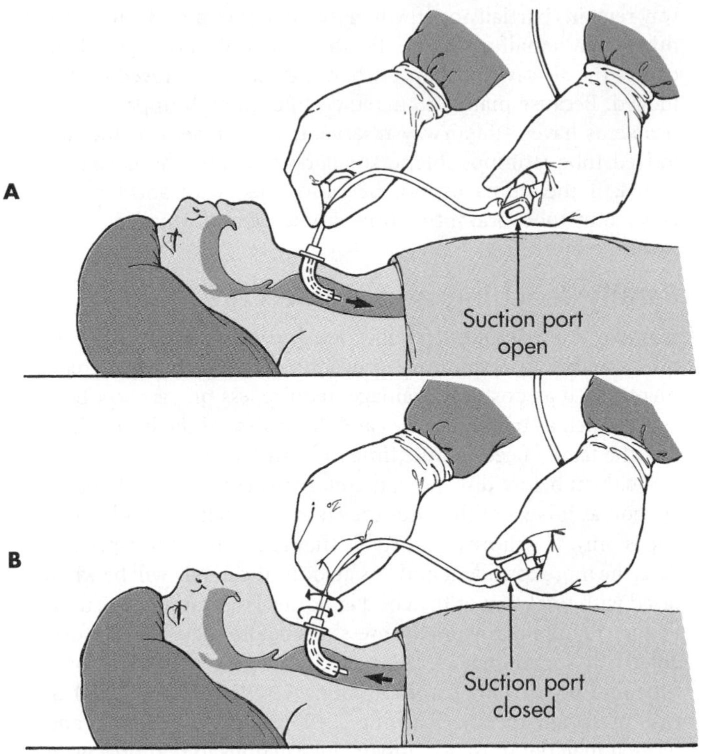

FIG. 45-31 • Tracheostomy suctioning. **A,** Insertion, port open. **B,** Withdrawal, port occluded. Note that catheter is inserted just slightly beyond end of tracheostomy tube.

NURSE ALERT • Suctioning is carried out only as often as needed to keep the tube patent. Signs of mucus partially occluding the airway include an increased heart rate, a rise in respiratory effort, a drop in SaO_2, cyanosis, or an increase in the positive inspiratory pressure (PIP) on the ventilator (Musser, 1992).

In the acute care setting, aseptic technique is used during care of the tracheostomy. Secondary infection is a major concern, because the air entering the lower airway bypasses the natural defenses of the upper airway. Gloves are worn during the aspiration procedure, although a sterile glove is needed only on the hand touching the catheter. A new tube, gloves, and sterile saline solution are used each time (Critical Thinking box).

Routine Care. The tracheostomy stoma requires daily care. Assessments of the stoma area include observations for signs of infection and breakdown of the skin. The skin is kept clean and dry, and secretions around the stoma may be gently removed with half-strength hydrogen peroxide. Hydrogen peroxide should not be used with sterling silver tracheostomy tubes because it tends to pit and stain the silver surface. The nurse should be aware of wet tracheostomy dressings, which can predispose the peristomal area to skin breakdown. Several products are available to prevent or treat excoriation. The Allevyn tracheostomy dressing is a hydrophilic sponge with a polyurethane back that is highly absorptive. Other possible barriers to help maintain skin integrity include the use of hydrocolloid wafers (e.g., Duoderm CGF and Hollister Restore) under the tracheostomy flanges, as well as use of extra-thin hydrocolloid wafers under the chin.

Critical Thinking

PLANNING FOR HOME TRACHEOSTOMY CARE

Jose Munoz, 18 months old, has been ventilator dependent since birth. He is presently hospitalized with pneumonia that has responded well to antibiotic therapy. You are discussing plans for discharge and home care with the family. Jose lives with his mother and her parents. Home nursing support is available only during the day. The family does not want to take Jose home because he is frequently suctioned at night. What should your initial intervention be?

First, Think About It . . .

- **What conclusions are you reaching?**
- **If you accept the conclusions, what are the implications?**

1. **Talk with the night nurses about their suctioning program.**
2. **Design a plan for the family members that allows them to each assume responsibility for night care with scheduled suctioning times.**
3. **Arrange with social services to request additional financial support for the family.**
4. **Suggest that Jose stay in the hospital until he needs less frequent suctioning.**

The best response is 1. If the family managed with daytime nursing assistance before this hospitalization and the pneumonia has resolved, the child should not require intensive suctioning. In talking with the night staff, you find that the nurses suction any time they walk past the room and hear Jose "gurgling." Also, if you accept the conclusion that they do not use premeasured suctioning technique, the implications are that you need to discuss with them a program of premeasured suctioning only as needed to reduce the production of secretion that may be caused from tracheal irritation.

The other three responses assume that the frequent suctioning is needed and are not appropriate initial interventions. Suctioning should be performed not on a set schedule, but only as needed. Requesting additional financial support does not contain costs and does not allow the family members to return to their prehospitalization status. Jose should be discharged as soon as possible to avoid nosocomial infection, promote normalization for a toddler, and contain health care costs. In this case, changing the suctioning regimen decreased the frequency to a minimum of once or twice a night—a level of care the family was able to manage.

The tracheostomy tube is held in place with tracheostomy ties made of a durable, nonfraying material. The ties are changed daily and when soiled. New ties are looped through the flanges and tied snugly in a triple knot at the side of the neck *before* the soiled ties are cut and removed. Some nurses have found that threading the ties through a piece of ¼-inch surgical tubing cushions the ties; others have found the tubing to be irritating to the skin. The ties should be tight enough to allow just a fingertip to be inserted between the ties and the neck (Fig. 45-32). It is easier to ensure a snug fit if the child's head is flexed rather than extended while the ties are being secured. Ties fastened with self-adhering closures are also available. These devices, such as the Dale tracheostomy tube holder, are made of a soft, cushioning, and slightly stretchy material that is very comfortable. They are becoming increasingly popular because of their ease of use and ability to maintain better skin integrity. However, nurses and family members must consider the safety factor and use them only on a child who will not pull and undo the fastener.

Routine tracheostomy tube changes are usually carried out weekly after a tract has been formed to minimize the formation

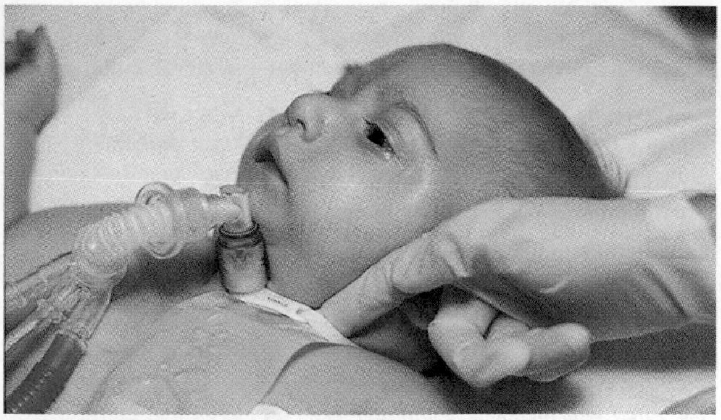

FIG. 45-32 • Tracheostomy ties are snug but allow one finger to be inserted.

of granulation tissue. The first change is usually performed by the surgeon; subsequent changes are performed by the nurse and, if the child is discharged home with the tracheostomy, by either a parent or a visiting nurse. Ideally, two caregivers participate in the procedure to assist with positioning the child.

Changing the tracheostomy tube is accomplished using sterile technique. The new, sterile tube is prepared by inserting the obturator and attaching new ties. The child is suctioned before the procedure to minimize secretions, then restrained and positioned with the neck slightly extended. One caregiver cuts the old ties and removes the tube from the stoma. The new tube is inserted gently into the stoma (using a downward and forward motion that follows the curve of the trachea), the obturator is removed, and the ties are secured. The adequacy of ventilation must be assessed after a tube change because the tube can be inserted into the soft tissue surrounding the trachea; therefore breath sounds and respiratory effort are carefully monitored.

Supplemental O_2 is always delivered with a humidification system to prevent drying of the respiratory mucosa. Humidification of room air for an established tracheostomy can be intermittent if secretions remain thin enough to be coughed or suctioned from the tracheostomy. Direct humidification via a tracheostomy mask can be provided during naps and at night so that the child is able to be up and around unencumbered during much of the day. Room humidifiers are also used successfully.

The inner cannula, if used, should be removed with each suctioning, cleaned with sterile saline and pipe cleaners to remove crusted material, dried thoroughly, and reinserted.

Emergency Care: Tube Occlusion and Accidental Decannulation. Occlusion of the tracheostomy tube is life threatening, and infants and children are at greater risk than adults because of the smaller diameter of the tube. Maintaining patency of the tube is accomplished with suctioning and routine tube changes to prevent the formation of crusts that can occlude the tube.

NURSE ALERT • Life-threatening occlusion is apparent when the child displays signs of respiratory distress and a suction catheter cannot be passed to the end of the tube despite several attempts and instillation of saline. This situation requires an immediate tube change.

Accidental decannulation also requires immediate tube replacement. Some children have a fairly rigid trachea, so the airway remains partially open when the tube is removed. However, others have malformed or flexible tracheal cartilage, which causes the airway to collapse when the tube is removed or dislodged. Because many infants and children with upper airway problems have little airway reserve, if replacement of the dislodged tube is impossible, a smaller-sized tube should be inserted. If the stoma cannot be cannulated with another tracheostomy tube, oral intubation should be performed.

Family Teaching and Home Care

Some of the treatments families need to continue at home are often related to respiratory procedures. Some of these treatments, such as postural drainage, require less preparation than others, such as tracheostomy care. Regardless of the home therapy, the family needs ample time to learn the skills and demonstrate them before discharge; therefore instruction should begin as soon as it is identified that the child will go home with a tracheostomy. The more comfortable they are with all the aspects of care, the more confident and less anxious the family will be when faced with total care of the child at home. For example, the family may require many practice sessions before they feel comfortable with suctioning, cleaning, and changing a tracheostomy tube and performing cardiopulmonary resuscitation (CPR) in case of an emergency. Teaching sessions should be short, and written material must accompany instructions to reinforce what is being taught.* To facilitate the family's adjustment, supplies identical to the ones to which they are accustomed should be available in the home. In the event of substitution, parents need to be reassured that the unfamiliar equipment is safe to use on their child. The home should be properly equipped with all supplies and equipment needed before the child arrives.

A nurse from the public health department or other home care service should be available to the family and should periodically assess the family's ability to carry out the activities needed in care of the child. The parents may find it helpful to talk with parents of other children with similar needs. They also need to know whom to call and where they can get help and support in times of uncertainty or in an emergency.

To prepare for any emergency, the family must be taught infant or child CPR. The local utilities company and local emergency medical services (EMS) should be notified of the child's condition and the equipment used in the home. Prior notification allows for a quicker response if help is needed.

When a child has a tracheostomy, parents are encouraged to provide as normal a life as possible for their child and other family members. Vocalization for the child with a tracheostomy has recently become a reality. Several tracheostomy speaking valves have been created to aid in the development of uninterrupted speech without the necessity of finger occlusion. One valve of several available on the market is the *Passy Muir* valve.† It is a one-way valve that attaches to the hub of all types and sizes of tracheostomies. It can be used in infants and in children who are ventilator assisted (Engleman and Turnage-Carrier, 1997).

---

*Community and home care instructions for tracheostomy care, postural drainage, and CPR are available in Wong DL, Hess CS: ***Wong and Whaley's clinical manual of pediatric nursing,*** ed 5, St Louis, 2000, Mosby.

†Further information can be obtained from Passy & Passy, Inc., 4521 Campus Dr., Suite 273, Irvine, CA 92612; 1-800-634-5397; fax (949) 833-8299; e-mail: info@passy.muir.com; website: www.passy-muir.com.

The child who is physically able (e.g., a child with a tracheostomy without respiratory disability such as recurrent laryngeal polyps) can usually be allowed to engage in most activities that are appropriate for the child's age. The child may play outdoors with a scarf or other protection to loosely cover the tracheostomy stoma. Both child and parents must be cautioned regarding play near any body of water, such as a swimming pool or stream, and informed about safety precautions in the bathtub. The child should not be exposed to noxious fumes (e.g., paint, varnish, hair spray) or talc (baby powder). Young children who may spill food near the stoma should wear a fabric bib (without plastic lining) or other device to prevent dribbled food or crumbs from being aspirated. At all times the family should have a bag with routine and emergency supplies to take with the child.

PROCEDURES RELATED TO ALTERNATIVE FEEDING TECHNIQUES

Some children are unable to take nourishment by mouth because of conditions such as anomalies of the throat, esophagus, or bowel; impaired swallowing capacity; severe debilitation; respiratory distress; or unconsciousness. These children are often fed by way of a tube inserted orally or nasally into the stomach *(orogastric or nasogastric gavage)* or duodenum/jejunum *(enteral gavage)* or by a tube inserted directly into the stomach *(gastrostomy)* or jejunum *(jejunostomy)*. Such feedings may be intermittent or by continuous drip. At times the entire alimentary tract must be bypassed, using IV feeding (total parenteral nutrition [TPN]). Because enteral feedings are used less often than gastric or IV feedings, the following discussion is limited to gastric gavage, gastrostomy, and TPN.

During gavage or gastrostomy (non-oral) feedings, infants are given a pacifier. Nonnutritive sucking has several advantages, such as increased weight gain and decreased crying. However, to prevent the possibility of aspiration, only pacifiers with a safe design may be used. Using improvised pacifiers made from bottle nipples is not a safe practice. (See Injury Prevention: Aspiration in Chapter 36.)

NURSE ALERT • When a child is concurrently receiving continuous-drip gastric or enteral feedings and parenteral (IV) therapy, the potential exists for inadvertent administration of the enteral formula through the circulatory system, especially when the parenteral solution is a fat emulsion, which looks milky. Safeguards to prevent this potentially serious error include (Garvin and Franck, 1989):

- Use a separate, specifically designed enteral feeding pump mounted on a separate pole for continuous-feeding solutions.
- Label all tubing for continuous enteral feeding with brightly colored tape or labels.
- Use specifically designed continuous-feeding bags to contain the solutions instead of parenteral equipment, such as a burette.

Gavage Feeding

Infants and children can be fed simply and safely by a tube passed into the stomach through either the nares or the mouth. The tube can be left in place or inserted and removed with each feeding. In older children it is usually less traumatic to tape the tube securely in place between feedings. When this alternative is used, the tube should be removed and replaced with a new tube according to hospital policy, specific orders, and the type of tube used. Meticulous handwashing is practiced during the procedure to prevent bacterial contamination of the feeding, especially during continuous-drip feedings.

Preparation. The equipment needed for gavage feeding includes:

- A suitable tube selected according to the size of the child and the viscosity of the solution being fed. Feeding tubes are available in silicone rubber, polyurethane, polyethylene, or polyvinylchloride. Polyurethane and silicone rubber tubes are smaller in diameter and more flexible than the others and are often referred to as small-bore tubes.
- A receptacle for the fluid; for small amounts a 10- to 30-ml syringe barrel or Asepto syringe is satisfactory; for larger amounts a 50-ml syringe with a catheter tip is more convenient.
- A syringe to aspirate stomach contents and/or to inject air after the tube has been placed.
- Water or water-soluble lubricant to lubricate the tube; sterile water is used for infants.
- Paper or nonallergenic tape to mark the tube and to attach the tube to the infant's or child's cheek (and nose, if placed through the nares).
- A stethoscope to determine the correct placement in the stomach.
- The solution for feeding.

Not all feeding tubes are the same. Polyethylene and polyvinylchloride types lose their flexibility and need to be replaced often, usually every 3 to 4 days. The polyurethane and silicone rubber tubes are indwelling and remain flexible; thus they can remain in place longer and afford more patient comfort. Use of these small-bore tubes for continuous feeding has greatly reduced the incidence of complications such as pharyngitis, otitis media, and incompetence of the lower esophageal sphincter. Although the increased softness and flexibility of the tubes are advantages, they also result in problems such as difficult insertion (may require a stylet or metal guidewire), collapse of the tube during aspiration of gastric contents when testing for correct placement, dislodgment during forceful coughing, and unsuitability for thick feedings. Traditional methods for verifying placement are less reliable with the small-bore tubes.

Procedure. Infants will be easier to control if they are first wrapped in a mummy restraint (see Fig. 45-8). Even tiny infants with random movements can grasp and dislodge the tube. Premature infants do not ordinarily require restraint, but if they do, a small towel folded across the chest and secured beneath the shoulders is usually sufficient. Care must be taken so that breathing is not compromised.

Whenever possible, the infant should be held during the procedure to associate the comfort of physical contact with the feeding. When this is not possible, gavage feeding is carried out with the infant or child on the back or toward the right side and the head and chest elevated. Feeding the child in a sitting position helps maintain the placement of the tube in the lowest position, thus increasing the likelihood of correct placement in the stomach.

The feeding tube can be passed through either the nose (nasogastric) or the mouth (orogastric). Because most young infants are obligatory nose breathers, insertion through the mouth causes less distress and helps to stimulate sucking. A tube passed through one of the nares in older infants and children is satisfactory once the tube is in place. An indwelling tube is almost always placed through the nose; the tube is alternated between nares with each insertion to minimize irritation, chance of infection, and possible breakdown of mucous membranes from pressure that occurs over time. The procedure for gavage feeding is described in the Guidelines box.

Two standard methods of measuring tube length for insertion are: (1) measuring from the nose to the bottom of the earlobe and then to the end of the xiphoid process; and (2) measuring from the nose to the earlobe and then to a point midway between the xiphoid process and the umbilicus (Fig. 45-33, *A*). However, research on using these methods in infants and children has cast serious doubt on their accuracy (Weibley et al, 1987). Studies have shown that height as a predictor of gastric tube insertion distance may provide a more valid measurement method (Ellett et al, 1992). For very-low-birth-weight infants, daily weight can be used to predict insertion length (Table 45-5).

Unfortunately, "bedside" methods used to verify the placement of the tube have serious shortcomings (see Guidelines box). The most accurate method for testing tube placement is radiography, but this practice is not feasible before each feeding. One method that appears promising is the consideration of aspirate color and pH to determine placement, because respiratory, gastric, and intestinal fluids have a different pH and color. Metheny and colleagues (1998) found that acidic pH values of 4 or less were reasonable indicators of gastric tube placement, whereas respiratory fluid had pH values greater then 6. The color of the gastric fluid aspirated was found to be most often grassy green, off-white to tan, bloody, or brown, whereas the color of pleural fluid was off-white and tinged with mucus and blood. These authors suggest that an aspirate's pH and color can help determine tube placement. Until pH is studied further, especially in children, nurses need to use the traditional methods with an awareness of their limitations. If doubt exists regarding correct placement, the practitioner should be consulted.

Nurses need to take precaution when assessing tube placement. One study reported that out of 201 children, 32 had nasogastric (NG) tube placement errors as viewed by radiography (Ellett, 1998).

Guidelines

NASOGASTRIC TUBE FEEDINGS IN CHILDREN

- Place child supine with head slightly hyperflexed or in a sniffing position (nose pointed toward ceiling).
- Measure the tube for approximate length of insertion and mark the point with a small piece of tape.
- Insert the tube that has been lubricated with sterile water or water-soluble lubricant through either the mouth or one of the nares to the predetermined mark. Since most young infants are obligatory nose breathers, insertion through the mouth causes less distress and helps to stimulate sucking. In older infants and children the tube is passed through the nose and alternated between nostrils. An indwelling tube is almost always placed through the nose.
  - When using the nose, slip the tube along the base of the nose and direct it straight back toward the occiput.
  - When entering through the mouth, direct the tube toward the back of the throat.
  - If the child is able to swallow on command, synchronize passing the tube with swallowing.
- Check the position of the tube by doing *both* of the following:
  - Attach the syringe to the feeding tube and apply negative pressure. Aspiration of stomach contents indicates proper placement, but aspiration of respiratory secretions may be mistaken for stomach contents. However, absence of fluid is not necessarily evidence of improper placement. The stomach may be empty, the tube may not be in contact with stomach contents, or a small-bore flexible tube may collapse. Note the amount and character of any fluid aspirated and return the fluid to the stomach.
  - With the syringe, inject a small amount of air (0.5 to 1 ml in premature or very small infants to 5 ml in larger children) into the tube while simultaneously listening with a stethoscope over the stomach area. Sounds of gurgling or growling will be heard if the tube is properly situated in the stomach, although it is possible to hear the air entering the stomach even when the tube is positioned above the gastroesophageal sphincter.
- Stabilize the tube by holding or taping it to the cheek, not to the forehead, because of possible damage to the nostril. To maintain correct placement, measure and record the amount of tubing extending from the nose or mouth to the distal port when the tube is first positioned. Recheck this measurement before each feeding.
- Warm the formula to room temperature. Do not microwave! Pour formula into the barrel of the syringe attached to the feeding tube. To start the flow, give a gentle push with the plunger, but then remove the plunger and allow the fluid to flow into the stomach by gravity. The rate of flow should not exceed 5 ml every 5 to 10 minutes in premature and very small infants and 10 ml/min in older infants and children to prevent nausea and regurgitation. The rate is determined by the diameter of the tubing and the height of the reservoir containing the feeding and is regulated by adjusting the height of the syringe. A usual feeding may take from 15 to 30 minutes to complete.
- Flush the tube with sterile water (1 or 2 ml for small tubes to 5 to 15 ml or more for large ones), or see discussion of flushing for administering medication through nasogastric tubes in the Guidelines box on p. 1166 to clear it of formula.
- Cap or clamp indwelling tubes to prevent loss of feeding.
  - If the tube is to be removed, first pinch it firmly to prevent escape of fluid as the tube is withdrawn. Withdraw the tube quickly.
- Position the child with the head elevated about 30 degrees and on the right side or abdomen for at least 1 hour in the same manner as following any infant feeding to minimize the possibility of regurgitation and aspiration. If the child's condition permits, bubble the youngster after the feeding.
- Record the feeding, including the type and amount of residual, the type and amount of formula, and how it was tolerated. For most infant feedings, any amount of residual fluid aspirated from the stomach is refed to prevent electrolyte imbalance, and the amount is subtracted from the prescribed amount of feeding. For example, if the infant is to receive 30 ml and 10 ml is aspirated from the stomach before the feeding, the 10 ml of aspirated stomach contents is refed along with 20 ml of feeding. Another method can be used in children. If residual fluid is more than one fourth of the last feeding, return the aspirate and recheck in 30 to 60 minutes. When residual fluid is less than one fourth of the last feeding, give the scheduled feeding. If large amounts of aspirated fluid persist and the child is due for another feeding, notify the practitioner.

Gastrostomy Feeding

Feeding by way of a gastrostomy tube is a variation of tube feeding that is often used for children in whom passage of a tube through the mouth, pharynx, esophagus, and cardiac sphincter of the stomach is contraindicated or impossible. It is also used to avoid the constant irritation of a gastric tube in children who require tube feeding over an extended period. Placement of a gastrostomy tube may be performed with the patient under general anesthesia or percutaneously using an endoscope with the patient sedated and under local anesthesia (percutanous endoscopic gastrostomy [PEG]). The tube is inserted through the abdominal wall into the stomach about midway along the greater curvature and when surgically placed is secured by a purse-string suture. The stomach is anchored to the peritoneum at the operative site. The tube used can be a Foley, wing-tip, or mushroom catheter.

Immediately after surgery the catheter is left open and attached to gravity drainage for 24 hours or more. Postoperative care of the wound site is directed toward prevention of infection and irritation. The area is cleansed with a mild, pH-balanced cleanser such as normal saline. A cotton-tipped applicator is used to remove drainage close to the tube site (O'Brien et al, 1999). After healing takes place, meticulous care is needed to keep the area surrounding the tube clean and dry to prevent excoriation and infection. Daily applications of antibiotic ointment or other preparations may be prescribed to aid in healing and prevention of irritation. Care is exercised to prevent excessive pull on the catheter that might cause widening of the opening and subsequent leakage of highly irritating gastric juices.

For children receiving long-term gastrostomy feeding, a *skin-level device* (e.g., MIC-KEY, Bard Button, or Gastroport) offers several advantages. The small, flexible silicone device protrudes slightly from the abdomen, is cosmetically pleasing in appearance, affords increased comfort and mobility to the child, is easy to care for, and is fully immersible in water. The one-way valve at the proximal end minimizes reflux and eliminates the need for clamping; however, the button requires a well-established gastrostomy site and is more expensive than the conventional tube. In addition, the valve may become clogged. When functioning, the valve prevents air from escaping; therefore the child may require frequent bubbling. With some devices, the child must remain fairly still during feedings because the tubing easily disconnects from the opening. With other devices, extension tubing can be securely attached to the opening (Fig. 45-34). The feeding is instilled at the other end of the tubing in a manner similar to that for a regular gastrostomy. The extension tubing may also have a separate medication port. Both the feeding and the medication ports have plugs attached. Some skin-level devices require a special tube to decompress the stomach (i.e., to check residual or release air).

Feeding of water, formula, or pureed foods is carried out in the same manner and rate as in gavage feeding. A mechanical pump may be used to regulate the volume and rate of feeding. After feedings, in an effort to encourage gastric emptying and reduce potential aspiration, the child is positioned to sleep at a 30-degree angle in bed. Older children are propped up on pillows, whereas the infant can have a small wedge or pillow placed under the head end of the mattress (Holden et al, 1997). It is

TABLE 45-5
Recommended Minimum Insertion Lengths for Orogastric Tubes in Very-low-birth-weight Infants

	Daily Weight (g)			
	<750	750-999	1000-1249	1250-1499
Insertion length (cm)	13	15	16	17

From Gallaher KJ et al: Orogastric tube insertion length in very-low-birth-weight infants (<1500 grams), *J Perinatol* 13(2):128–131, 1993.

A

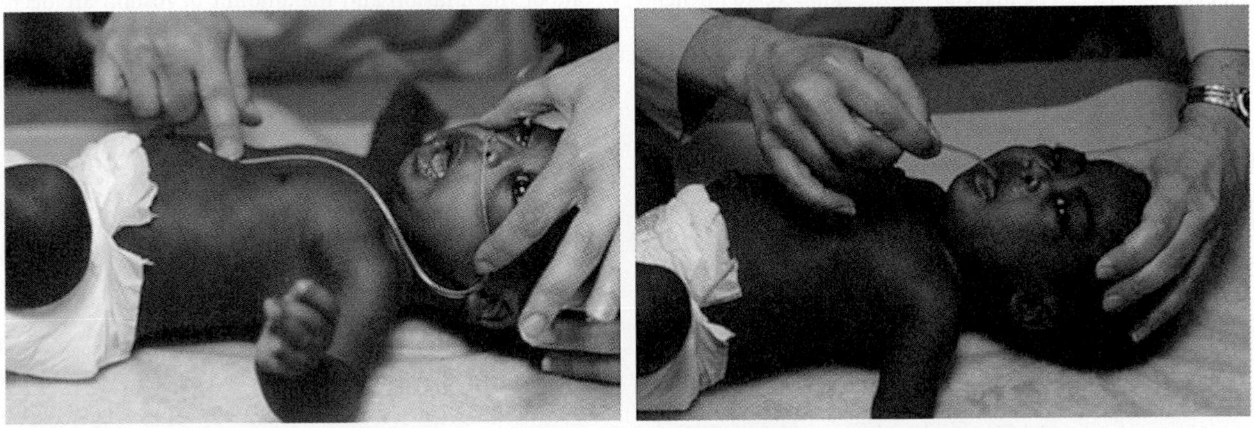

B

FIG. 45-33 • Gavage feeding. **A,** Measuring tube for orogastric feeding from tip of nose to earlobe and to midpoint between end of xiphoid process and umbilicus. **B,** Inserting tube.

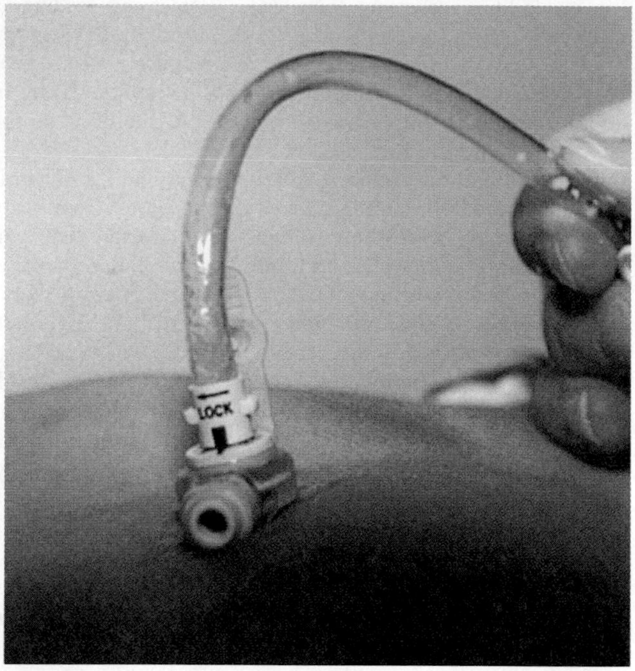

FIG. 45-34 • Child with skin-level gastrostomy device (MIC-KEY), which provides for secure attachment of extension tubing to gastrostomy opening.

also recommended that the infant or child be positioned on the right side. The tube may be clamped, left open, or suspended between feedings, depending on the child's condition. A clamped tube allows more mobility but is appropriate only if the child can tolerate intermittent feedings without vomiting or prolonged backup of feeding into the tube. Sometimes a Y tube is used to allow for simultaneous decompression during feeding. If a Foley catheter is used as the gastrostomy tube, very slight tension is applied. The tube is securely taped to maintain the balloon at the gastrostomy opening to prevent leakage of gastric contents and to prevent the tube's progression toward the pyloric sphincter, where it may occlude the stomach outlet. As a precaution, the length of the tube should be measured postoperatively and then remeasured each shift to be sure it has not slipped. A mark can be made above the skin level to further ensure its placement. When the gastrostomy tube is no longer needed, it is removed; the skin opening usually closes spontaneously by contracture.

Total Parenteral Nutrition (TPN)

TPN, also known as *intravenous alimentation* or *hyperalimentation,* provides for the total nutritional needs of infants or children whose lives are threatened because feeding by way of the gastrointestinal tract is impossible, inadequate, or hazardous.

Hyperalimentation therapy involves IV infusion of highly concentrated solutions of protein, glucose, and other nutrients. The hyperalimentation solution is infused through conventional tubing with a special filter attached to remove particulate matter or microorganisms that may have contaminated the solution. The highly concentrated solutions require infusion into a vessel with sufficient volume and turbulence to allow for rapid dilution. The wide-diameter vessels selected are the superior vena cava and innominate or intrathoracic subclavian veins approached by way of the external or internal jugular veins. The highly irritating nature of concentrated glucose precludes the use of the small peripheral veins in most instances; however, dilute glucose-protein hydrolysates that are appropriate for infusing into peripheral veins are being used with increasing frequency. When peripheral veins are used, intralipid becomes the major calorie source. For long-term alimentation, VADs are usually used (see p. 1163).

The major nursing responsibilities are the same as for any IV therapy: control of sepsis, monitoring of the infusion rate, and assessment of the patient. The TPN solution must be prepared under rigid aseptic conditions best accomplished by specially trained technicians. The solution and tubing are changed and the infusion site redressed by specially trained nurses using meticulous aseptic precautions. In some institutions this may be a nursing responsibility; if so, the procedure is carried out according to hospital protocol.

The infusion is maintained at a constant rate by means of an infusion pump to ensure the proper concentrations of glucose and amino acids. Accurate calculation of the rate is required to deliver a measured amount in a given length of time. Because alterations in flow rate are relatively common, the drip should be checked often to ensure an even, continuous infusion. The hyperalimentation infusion rate should not be increased or decreased without the practitioner being informed, because alterations can cause hyperglycemia or hypoglycemia.

General assessments, such as vital signs, I&O measurements, and checking results of laboratory tests, facilitate early detection of infection or fluid and electrolyte imbalance. Additional amounts of potassium and sodium chloride are often required in hyperalimentation; therefore observation for signs of potassium or sodium deficit or excess is part of nursing care. This is rarely a problem except in children with reduced renal function or metabolic defects. Hyperglycemia may occur during the first day or two as the child adapts to the high-glucose load of the hyperalimentation solution. Although occurring infrequently, insulin may be required to assist the body's adjustment to the hyperglycemia. When this occurs, nursing responsibilities include blood glucose testing. To prevent hypoglycemia at the time the hyperalimentation is disconnected, the rate of the infusion and the amount of insulin are decreased gradually.

In addition to children's physical needs, their developmental needs must also be considered during the often long-term use of TPN. Regular assessment of development should be performed to assess the child's progress, and appropriate interventions should be instituted to encourage expected milestones. Delays in the areas of gross motor and language skills are found most often; therefore special attention should be directed to these areas.

Family Teaching and Home Care

When alternative feedings are needed for an extended period, the family may need to learn how to feed the child with a nasogastric, gastrostomy, or TPN feeding regimen. The same principles discussed earlier in this chapter for compliance, especially in terms of education (p. 1133); and in Chapter 44 for discharge planning and home care, are applied.* Because of the numerous skills the family must learn for home TPN, ample time must be planned for the family to learn and perform the procedures under supervision before assuming full responsibility for the child's care.

The family may be referred to community agencies that provide support and practical assistance. The Oley Foundation† is a nonprofit research and education organization that assists persons receiving enteral nutrition and home TPN.

PROCEDURES RELATED TO ELIMINATION

Enema

The procedure for giving an enema to an infant or child does not differ essentially from that for an adult, except for the type and amount of fluid administered and the distance for inserting the tube into the rectum. Depending on the volume, the nurse uses a syringe with rubber tubing, an enema bottle, or an enema bag (Guidelines box).

NURSE ALERT • Proper insertion of the catheter tip, especially in infants, is essential to prevent rectal damage and perforation (see Fig. 35-7, *B*). If insertion of the enema tip causes discomfort, remove the tip and notify the practitioner.

An isotonic solution is used in children. Plain water is not used because, being hypotonic, it can cause rapid fluid shift and fluid overload. The Fleet enema (pediatric or adult sized) is not advised for children because of the harsh action of its ingredients (sodium biphosphate and sodium phosphate). Commercial enemas can be dangerous to patients with megacolon and to dehydrated or azotemic children. The osmotic effect of the Fleet enema may produce diarrhea, which can lead to metabolic acidosis. Other potential complications are extreme hyperphosphatemia, hypernatremia, and hypocalcemia, which may lead to neuromuscular irritability and coma (McCabe, Sibert, and Routledge, 1991). If prepared saline is not available, it can be made by adding 1 teaspoon of table salt to 500 ml (1 pint) of tap water.

Because infants and young children are unable to retain the solution after it is administered, the buttocks must be held together for a short time to retain the fluid. The enema is administered and expelled while the child is lying with the buttocks over the bedpan and with the head and back supported by pillows. Older children are usually able to hold the solution if they understand what to do and if they are not expected to hold it for too long. The nurse should have the bedpan handy or, for the ambulatory child, ensure that the bathroom is readily available before beginning the procedure. An enema is an intrusive procedure and thus threatening to the preschool child; therefore a careful explanation is especially important to ease possible fear.

A preoperative bowel preparation solution given orally or through a nasogastric tube is increasingly being used instead of an enema. The polyethylene glycol-electrolyte lavage solution (GoLYTELY) mechanically flushes the bowel without significant absorption, thereby avoiding potential fluid and electrolyte imbalances.*

*Community and home care instructions for gavage and gastrostomy feeding are available in Wong DL, Hess CS: ***Wong and Whaley's clinical manual of pediatric nursing***, ed 5, St Louis, 2000, Mosby.

†214 Hun Memorial, A23, Albany Medical Center, Albany, NY 12208; 1-800-776-OLEY; website: web.wizvak.net/oleyfdn/index.html.

Guidelines

ADMINISTRATION OF ENEMAS TO CHILDREN

Age	Amount (ml)	Insertion Distance (cm [inches])
Infant	120–240	2.5 (1 inch)
2–4 years	240–360	5 (2 inches)
4–10 years	360–480	7.5 (3 inches)
11 years	480–720	10 (4 inches)

Ostomies

Children may require stomas for various health problems. The most common causes are necrotizing enterocolitis and imperforate anus in the infant (and, less often, Hirschsprung disease). In the older child the most common causes are inflammatory bowel disease, especially Crohn disease (regional enteritis), and ureterostomies for distal ureter or bladder defects.

Care and management of ostomies in the older child differ little from the care of ostomies in the adult patient. The major emphases in pediatric care are the preparation of the child for the procedure and teaching care of the ostomy to the child and family. The basic principles of preparation are the same as for any procedure (see p. 1122). Simple, straightforward language is most effective, together with the use of illustrations and a replica model (e.g., drawing a picture of a child with a stoma on the abdomen and explaining it as "another opening where bowel movements [or any other term the child uses] will come out"). At another time the nurse can draw a pouch over the opening to demonstrate how the contents are collected. Using a doll to demonstrate the process is an excellent teaching strategy, and special books are available.†

Children with ileostomies are fitted immediately after surgery with an appliance to protect the skin from the proteolytic enzymes in the liquid stool. Parents are usually given a choice of caring for the colostomy with or without an appliance. Pediatric appliances are available in a variety of sizes to ensure an adequate fit.‡

Ostomy equipment consists of a one- or two-piece system with a hypoallergenic skin barrier to maintain peristomal skin integrity. The pouch should be large enough to contain a moderate amount of stool and flatus but not so large as to overwhelm the infant or child. A backing helps minimize the risk of skin breakdown from moisture trapped between the skin and pouch. Small clips or rubber bands should be avoided to prevent choking in the young child. Granulation tissue may grow

*Community and home care instructions for giving an enema are available in Wong DL, Hess CS: ***Wong and Whaley's clinical manual of pediatric nursing***, ed 5, St Louis, 2000, Mosby.

†*Chris Has an Ostomy* is available from United Ostomy Association, Inc., 36 Executive Park, Suite 120, Irvine, CA 92714-6744; 1-800-826-0826.

‡Little Ones Ostomy Products, ConvaTec, CN 5254, Princeton, NJ 08543-5254; 1-800-422-8811; website: www.convatec.com. Parents may find the following pamphlets helpful: *A Parent's Guide to Necrotizing Enterocolitis* or *A Parent's Guide to Ostomy Care for Children*, both available from ConvaTec.

around an ostomy site. This moist, beefy red tissue is not a sign of infection; however, if it continues to grow, the excess moisture can cause irritation of the surrounding skin.

Protection of the peristomal skin is a major aspect of stoma care. Well-fitting appliances are important to prevent leakage of contents. Before the appliance is applied, the skin is prepared with a skin sealant that is allowed to dry. Then stoma paste is applied around the base of the stoma or the back of the wafer. The sealant and paste work together to prevent peristomal breakdown.

In infants with a colostomy left unpouched, skin care is similar to that of any diapered child. However, the peristomal skin is protected with a wafer barrier, such as a hydrocolloid dressing (e.g., Duoderm) or a barrier substance (e.g., zinc oxide ointment [Desitin], karaya products, or a mixture of the zinc oxide ointment and Stoma [Stomahesive*] powder). A gauze dressing may be applied over the stoma and water to absorb stomal drainage. If the skin becomes inflamed, denuded, or infected, the care is similar to the interventions used for diaper dermatitis (see Chapter 53). A product that helps protect healthy skin, heal excoriated skin, and minimize pain associated with skin breakdown is Preshield Plus.* The skin protectant adheres to denuded, weeping skin. It can be applied over topical antifungal and antibacterial agents if infection is present. "No-sting" barrier film† is a skin sealant that has no alcohol base and can be used on open skin without stinging.

With young children, protection of the pouch from being pulled off is also an important consideration. One-piece outfits keep exploring hands from reaching the pouch, and the loose waist prevents any pressure on the appliance. Keeping the child occupied with toys during the pouch change is also helpful. As children mature, their participation in ostomy care is encouraged. Even preschoolers can assist by holding supplies, pulling paper backings from the appliance, and helping clean the stoma area. Toilet training for bladder control needs to begin at the appropriate time as for any other child.

Older children and adolescents should eventually have total responsibility for ostomy care just as they would for usual bowel function. During adolescence, concerns for body image and the ostomy's impact on intimacy and sexuality emerge. The nurse should stress to teenagers that the presence of a stoma need not interfere with their activities. These youngsters can choose which ostomy equipment is best suited to their needs. Attractively designed and decorated pouch covers are well liked by teenagers.

An enterostomal therapy nurse specialist is an important member of the health care team and will have additional suggestions and assistance with skin care information and ostomy pouching options. Further information may be obtained by contacting the Wound, Ostomy, and Continence Nurses Society (WOCN).‡

Family Teaching and Home Care

Because these children are almost always discharged with a functioning colostomy, preparation of the family should begin as early as possible in the hospital. The family is instructed in the application of the device (if used), care of the skin, and instructions regarding appropriate action in case skin problems develop. Early evidence of skin breakdown or stomal complications (e.g., ribbonlike stools, excessive diarrhea, bleeding, prolapse, or failure to pass flatus or stool) is brought to the attention of the physician, the nurse, or the stoma specialist. The same principles are applied as discussed earlier in this chapter for compliance, especially in terms of education (p. 1133), and in Chapter 44 for discharge planning and home care.*

*Healthpoint Medical, 2600 Airport Freeway, Fort Worth, TX 76111; 1-800-441-8227; website: www.healthpoint.com.

†3M, St. Paul, MN; 1-800-228-3957.

‡(888) 224-WOCN: website: www.wocn.org.

*Community and home care instructions on caring for a colostomy are available in Wong DL, Hess CS: ***Wong and Whaley's clinical manual of pediatric nursing***, ed 5, St. Louis, 2000 Mosby.

Key Points

- Informed consent is valid when the person is capable of giving consent (is over the age of majority and is competent), is supplied with information needed to make an intelligent decision, and acts voluntarily when exercising freedom of choice.
- Informed consent is needed for major surgery, minor surgery, and diagnostic tests and medical treatments with an element of risk.
- The major tasks in psychologic preparation of the child for procedures are to establish trust, provide support, and give an explanation in easy-to-understand terms.
- Most parents and children want to be together during stressful procedures and should be offered this opportunity, along with guidance on how the parent can comfort the child.
- In the performance of a procedure the nurse should expect success, involve the child when possible in the procedure, provide distraction, and allow for expression of feelings.
- In giving postprocedural support, the nurse should encourage the child to express feelings and praise the youngster for completion of the procedure.
- Stressful times before and after surgery that produce anxiety in children include admission, blood tests, injection of preoperative medication (if used), transportation to the operating room, and return from the postanesthesia care unit.
- Assessment of compliance entails measuring factors that affect compliance through self-reporting, direct observation, monitoring of appointments and therapeutic response, pill counts, and chemical assay.
- Compliance strategies may be classified as organizational, educational, treatment, and behavioral.
- Knowledge of the sick child's eating habits and favorite foods can help in maintaining adequate nutrition.
- Control of fever may be accomplished by pharmacologic means (administration of antipyretics); hyperthermia is controlled by environmental means (minimum clothing, increased air circulation, cool compresses).

- Infection control is based on two systems: Standard Precautions provide protection when the infected person is undiagnosed; transmission-based precautions add extra interventions for patients diagnosed with or suspected to have an infection.
- Ensuring safety in the hospital setting is a major concern and can be achieved through environmental measures, limit setting, and safe transportation.
- Restraints are used cautiously and typically require a medical order. Therapeutic hugging can avoid the use of restraints.
- Factors that affect drug dosage determination include growth and maturation, difficulty in evaluating drug response, and body surface area.
- Family teaching regarding medication administration includes telling parents why the child is receiving the drug; its possible effects; and the amount, frequency, and length of time the drug is to be administered.
- The preferred sites for intramuscular injection in children are the vastus lateralis and ventrogluteal areas.
- Intermittent venous access is accomplished by a peripheral intermittent infusion device, a peripherally inserted central catheter, a central venous catheter, or an implanted port.
- Several safety catheters and needleless device systems are available to reduce the risk of needle-stick injuries in patients and caregivers.
- Nursing assessment of fluid and electrolyte disturbances entails observation of general appearance, vital signs, and measurement of intake and output.
- Oxygen can be administered by hood, mask, nasal cannula, incubator, or oxygen tent.
- Tracheostomy suctioning involves premeasured insertion of the catheter, application of suction for 5 seconds when withdrawing the catheter, and supplemental oxygen before and after suctioning.
- Alternative forms of feeding include gavage feeding, gastrostomy feeding, and total parenteral nutrition.
- In the care of children with ostomies, nurses play an important role in family support and instruction in care of the stoma site.

References

Abd-El-Maeboud K et al: Rectal suppository: common-sense and mode of insertion, *Lancet* 338(8770):798-800, 1991.

Acute Pain Management Guideline Panel: *Acute pain management: operative or medical procedures and trauma,* Clinical Practice Guideline, AHCPR Pub. No. 92-0032, Rockville, MD, 1992, Agency for Health Care Policy and Research, Public Health Service, US Department of Health and Human Services.

Algren C, Algren J: Pediatric sedation essentials for the perioperative nurse, *Nurs Clin North Am* 32(1):17-30, 1997.

Algren C, Ireland D, Stewart E: Perioperative and perianesthesia care of the child. In Albers AC et al, editors: *Comprehensive care of the pediatric patient: prehospital through rehabilitation,* Park Ridge, IL, 1998, Emergency Nurses Association.

Algren C, Schwartz P: The application of nursing research to the child. In Albers AC et al, editors: *Comprehensive care of the pediatric patient: prehospital through rehabilitation,* Park Ridge, IL, 1998, Emergency Nurses Association.

American Academy of Pediatrics, Committee on Drugs: Guidelines for monitoring and management of pediatric patients during and after sedation for diagnostic and therapeutic procedures, *Pediatrics* 86(6):1110-1115, 1992.

Babbitt RA et al: Teaching developmentally disabled children with chronic illness to swallow prescribed capsules, *J Dev Behav Pediatr* 12(4):229-235, 1991.

Banerjee S et al: The intraosseous route is a suitable alternative to the intravenous route for fluid resuscitation in severely dehydrated children, *Indian Pediatr* 312:1511-1520, 1994.

Baranowski L: Central venous access devices: current technologies, uses and management strategies, *J Intraven Nurs* 16(3):167-194, 1993.

Barker DP et al: Capillary blood sampling: should the heel be warmed? *Arch Dis Child Fetal Neonatal Ed* 74(2):F139-F140, 1996.

Barton S, Holmes S: A comparison of regeant strips and the refractometer for measurement of urine specific gravity in hospitalized children, *Pediatr Nurs* 23(5):480-482, 1998.

Bates T, Broome M: Preparation of children for hospitalization and surgery: a review of the literature, *J Pediatr Nurs* 1(4):230-239, 1986.

Beecroft P, Redick S: Intramuscular injection practices of pediatric nurses: site selection, *Nurse Educ* 15(4):23-28, 1990.

Beecroft PC et al: Intravenous lock patency in children: dilute heparin versus saline, *J Pediatr Pract* 2(4):211-233, 1997.

Bernardo L, Lesniak D: Ethical and legal issues in pediatric nursing. In Albers AC et al, editors: *Comprehensive care of the pediatric patient: prehospital through rehabilitation,* Park Ridge, IL, 1998, Emergency Nurses Association.

Blackwood B: Normal saline instillation with endotracheal suctioning: primum non nocere (first do no harm), *J Adv Nurs* 29(4):928-934, 1999.

Broome M: Consent (assent) for research with pediatric patients, *Semin Oncol Nurs* 15(2):96-103, 1999.

Broome M, Rehwaldt M, Fogg L: Relationship between cognitive behavioral techniques, temperament, observed distress, and pain reports in children and adolescents during lumbar puncture, *J Pediatr Nurs* 13(1):48-54, 1998.

Bruce JL, Grove SK: Fever: pathology and treatment, *Crit Care Nurs* 12(1):40-55, 1992.

Bryant RA, Doughty D, editors: *Acute and chronic wounds: nursing management,* ed 2, St Louis, 2000, Mosby.

Burke N: Alternative methods for newborn urine sample collection, *Pediatr Nurs* 21(6):546-549, 1995.

Catudal R: Pediataric IV therapy: actual practice, *J Vasc Access Devices* 4(2):27-29, 1999.

Chandra NC, Hazinski MF, editors: *Textbook of basic life support for healthcare providers,* Dallas, 1994, American Heart Association.

Cohen HA et al: Urine samples from disposable diapers: an accurate method for urine cultures, *J Fam Pract* 44(3):290-292, 1997.

Connell F: The causes and treatment of fever: a literature review, *Nurs Stand* 12(11):40-43, 1997.

Cushing M: Demystifying informed consent, *Am J Nurs* 91(11):17-19, 1991.

Donaldson JS et al: Peripherally inserted central venous catheters: US-guided vascular access in pediatric patients, *Radiology* 197(2):542-544, 1995.

Dunn D: Malignant hypothermia, *AORN J* 65(4):728-754, 1997.
Eckler J: Combating infection, *Nursing* 27(10):20, 1997.
Ellett ML: Prevalence of feeding tube placement errors and associated risk factors in children, *MCN* 23(5):234-239, 1998.
Ellett ML et al: Predicting the distance for gavage tube placement in children using regression on height, *Pediatr Nurs* 18(2):119-121, 127, 1992.
Engleman SG, Turnage-Carrier C: Tolerance of the Passy-Muir speaking valve in infants and children less than 2 years of age, *Pediatr Nurs* 23:571-573, 1997.
Fauroux B et al: Chest physiotherapy in cystic fibrosis: improved tolerance with nasal pressure support ventilation, *Pediatrics* 103(3):e32, 1999.
Fox MD: Measurement of urine output volume: accuracy of diaper weights in neonatal environments, *Neonatal Network* 11(3):11-18, 1992.
Frey AM: Pediatric peripherally inserted central catheter program report: a summary of 4,536 catheter days, *J Intraven Nurs* 18(6):280-291, 1995.
Freedman SE, Bosserman G: Tunneled catheters: technologic advances and nursing care issues, *Nurs Clin North Am* 28(4):851-858, 1993.
Frizzell J: Avoiding lab test pitfalls, *Am J Nurs* 98(2):34-37, 1998.
Garner JS: What's in a name? The evolution of universal precautions to standard precautions: A guide to the latest recommendations in isolation practices, *Today's Surg Nurse* 19(1):14-21, 1997.
Garvin G, Franck L: Preventing delivery of enteral formula via parenteral route, *Pediatr Nurs* 15(1):17-18, 1989.
Goodwin ML, Carlson I: The peripherally inserted catheter, *J Intraven Nurs* 16(2):92-103, 1993.
Groswasser J et al: Needle length and injection technique for efficient intramuscular vaccine delivery in infants and children evaluated through an ultrasonographic determination of subcutaneous and muscle layer thickness, *Pediatrics* 99(3, pt 1):400-402, 1997.
Hagelgans NA: Pediatric skin care issues for the home care nurse, *Pediatr Nurs* 19(5):499-507, 1993.
Hall PA et al: Parents in the recovery room: survey of parental and staff attitudes, *BMJ* 310(6973):163-164, 1995.
Harrison A et al: Comparison of simultaneously obtained arterial and capillary blood gases in pediatric intensive care unit patients, *Crit Care Med* 25(1):1904-1908, 1997.
Hazinski MF: *Nursing care of the critically ill child,* ed 2, St Louis, 1992, Mosby.
Heilskov J et al: A randomized trial of heparin and saline for maintaining intravenous locks in neonates, *J Soc Pediatr Nurs* 3(3):111-116, 1998.
Hicks JF et al: Optimum needle length for diphtheria-inoculation of infants, *Pediatrics* 84(1):136-137, 1989.
Holden C et al: Enteral nutrition for children, *Nurs Stand* 11(32):49-54, 1997.
Holtzclaw BJ: Control of febrile shivering during amphotericin B therapy, *Oncol Nurs Forum* 17(4):521-524, 1990.
Hooker E et al: Subjective assessment of fever by parents: comparison with measurement by noncontact tympanic thermometer and calibrated rectal glass mercury thermometer, *Ann Emerg Med* 28(3):313-317, 1996.
Huth M: Watch out: the bogeyman is in the hospital closet, *J Child Fam Nurs* 2(2):143-148, 1999.
Intravenous Nurses Society: Revised Intravenous Nursing Standards of Practice, *J Intraven Nurs* 21(1, suppl):S35, S46-S47, S59, 1998.
Jackson F: The ABC's of black hair and skin care, *ABNFJ* 9(5):100-104, 1998.
Janik JP, Wayne ER, Janik JS: Securing central lines in rambunctious toddlers, *Pediatrics* 96(3):523-524, 1995.
Johannsen L: Adolescent abortion and mandated parental involvement, *Pediatr Nurs* 21(1):82-84, 1995.
Katsma D, Smith G: Analysis of needle path during intramuscular injection, *Nurs Res* 46(5):288-292, 1997.
Kearns GL, Leeder SJ, Wasserman GS: Acetaminophen overdose with therapeutic intent, *J Pediatr* 132(1):5-8, 1998.
Kennedy D: Medication "safety checks" in pediatric acute care, *J Intraven Nurs* 19(6):295-302, 1996.
Kinmonth AL, Fulton Y, Campbell MJ: Management of feverish children at home, *BMJ* 305(6862):1134-1136, 1992.
Kotter RW: Heparin vs saline for intermittent intravenous device maintenance in neonates, *Neonatal Network* 15(6):43-47, 1996.
Kravitz GR: Advances in IV delivery, *Hosp Pract* 281(suppl): 21-27, 1993.
Krueger H, Osborn L: Effects of hygiene among the uncircumcised, *J Fam Pract* 22(4):353-355, 1986.
Kubiak M et al: Comparison of stool containment in cloth and single-use diapers using simulated infant feces, *Pediatrics* 91(3):632-636, 1993.
LaRosa-Nash PA et al: Implementing a parent-present induction program, *AORN J* 61(3):526-531, 1995.
Laurent C: And so to beds, *Nurs Times* 95(3):7-8, 1999.
Lee WE, Vallino LM: Intravenous insertion site protection: moisture accumulation in intravenous site protectors, *J Intraven Nurs* 29(4):194-197, 1996.
Lehmann M et al: Upright or lying down: is one better for doing a lumbar puncture (LP)? *Am J Dis Child* 144:427, 1990.
Liptak GS: Enhancing compliance in pediatrics, *Pediatr Rev* 17(4):128-134, 1996.
Long CA et al: Central line associated bacteremia in the pediatric patient, *Pediatr Nurs* 22(3):247-251, 1996.
Maki DG: Infections caused by intravascular devices used for infusion therapy: pathogenesis, prevention, and management. In Bisno AL, Waldvogel FA, editors: *Infections associated with indwelling medical devices,* ed 2, Washington, DC, 1994, American Society for Microbiology.
Marcoux C, Fisher S, Wong D: Central venous access devices in children, *Pediatr Nurs* 16(2):123-133, 1990.
McCabe M, Sibert JR, Routledge PA: Phosphate enemas in childhood: cause for concern, *BMJ* 302(6784):1074, 1991.
McIntosh N, van Veen L, Brameyer H: Alleviation of the pain of heel prick in preterm infants, *Arch Dis Child Fetal Neonatal Ed* 70(3):F177-F181, 1994.
Messner RL, Pinkerman ML: Preventing a peripheral i.v. infection, *Nursing* 92(6):34-41, 1992.
Metheny N et al: pH, color, and feeding tubes, *RN* 61(1):25-27, 1998.
Morris v Children's Hospital Medical Center, 1992.
Moureau N: Practical access, a back-to-basics review of intravenous therapy, *J Vasc Access* Devices 4(2, suppl):1-4, 1999.
Musser V: How do you use shallow-suction technique in children? *Am J Nurs* 92(5):79-83, 1992.
O'Brien B et al: G-tube site care: a practical guide, *RN* 62(2): 52-56, 1999.
Olsen RJ et al: Examination gloves as barriers to hand contamination in clinical practice, *JAMA* 270(3):350-353, 1993.
Paisley MK et al: The use of heparin and normal saline flushes in neonatal intravenous catheters, *Pediatr Nurs* 23(5): 521-527, 1997.

Pearson M: The Hospital Infection Control Practices Advisory Committee: Guidelines for prevention of intravascular-device-related infections, *Infect Control Hosp Epidemiol* 17:438-473, 1995.

Pearson M: Special communication: guidelines for prevention of intravascular device-related infections, parts I and II, *Am J Infect Control* 24(4):262-293, 1996.

Pidgeon V: Compliance with chronic illness regimens: school-aged children and adolescents, *J Pediatr Nurs* 4(1):36-47, 1989.

Prandoni D et al: Assessment of urine collection techniques for microbial culture, *Am J Infect Control* 24(3):219-221, 1996.

Reed T, Phillip S: Management of central venous catheter occlusion and repairs, *J Intraven Nurs* 19(6):289-294, 1996.

Reynolds A, Suarez C: Pressure-reducing capability of Conforma II mattress overlay, *Adv Wound Care* 7(4):36-40, 1994.

Rosenstock IM: Enhancing patient compliance with health recommendations, *J Pediatr Health Care* 2(2):67-72, 1988.

Selekman J, Snyder B: Institutional policies on the use of physical restraints on children, *Pediatr Nurs* 23(5):531-537, 1997.

Selekman J, Snyder B: Uses and alternatives to restraints in pediatric settings, *AACN Clin Issues* 7(4):603-610, 1996.

Sharber J: The efficacy of tepid sponge bathing to reduce fever in young children, *Am J Emerg Med* 15(2):188-192, 1997.

Sullivan D: Minors and emergency medicine, *Emerg Med Clin North Am* 11(4):841-851, 1993.

Swartz ML: NuLYTELY PEG 3350, sodium chloride, sodium bicarbonate, and potassium chloride for oral solution, *Gastroenterol Nurs* 14(4):200-203, 1992.

Tebbi C: Treatment compliance in childhood and adolescence, *Cancer* 71(10):3441-3449, 1993.

Weibley TT et al: Gavage tube insertion in the premature infant, *MCN* 12:24-27, 1987.

Wilson D: Neonatal IVs: practical tips, *Neonatal Network* 11(2):49-53, 1992.

Wong DL, Baker CM: Pain in children: comparison of assessment scales, *Pediatr Nurs* 14(1):9-17, 1988.

Wong DL et al: Diapering choices: a critical review of the issues, *Pediatr Nurs* 18(1):41-54, 1992.

CHAPTER

46 Respiratory Dysfunction

http://www.harcourthealth.com/MERLIN/Wong/maternal/

Learning Objectives

On completion of this chapter the reader will be able to:

- Identify the factors leading to respiratory tract infection in the infant or young child.
- Contrast the effects of various respiratory infections observed in infants and children.
- Describe the postoperative nursing care of the child with a tonsillectomy.
- Outline a nursing care plan for a child with croup.
- Outline a nursing care plan for a child with acute otitis media.
- Demonstrate an understanding of the ways in which inhalation of noninfectious irritants produces pulmonary dysfunction.
- Describe the ways in which the various therapeutic measures relieve the symptoms of asthma.
- Outline a plan for teaching home care for the child with asthma.
- Describe the physiologic effects of cystic fibrosis on the gastrointestinal and pulmonary systems.
- Outline a plan of care for the child with cystic fibrosis.
- List the major signs of respiratory distress in infants and children.

RESPIRATORY INFECTION

General Aspects of Respiratory Infections

Infections of the respiratory tract are described according to the areas of involvement. The *upper respiratory tract*, or *upper airway*, consists primarily of the nose and pharynx. The *lower respiratory tract* consists of the bronchi and bronchioles (the reactive portion of the airway because of their smooth muscle content and ability to constrict) and the alveoli. Authorities disagree about the designation for the structurally stable portion of the airway (including the epiglottis, larynx, and trachea). For this discussion the trachea is considered with lower tract disorders, and infections of the epiglottis and larynx are categorized as croup syndromes. Respiratory infections seldom fall neatly into discrete anatomic areas. Infections often spread from one structure to another because of the contiguous nature of the mucous membrane lining the entire tract. Consequently, infections of the respiratory tract involve several areas rather than a single structure, although the effect on one may predominate in any given illness.

Etiology and Characteristics. Respiratory infections account for the majority of acute illnesses in children. The etiology and course of these infections are influenced by the age of the child, the season, living conditions, and preexisting medical problems.

Infectious Agents. The respiratory tract is subject to a variety of infective organisms, but most infections are caused by viruses, particularly the respiratory syncytial virus (RSV). Other agents involved in primary or secondary invasion include group A β-hemolytic streptococci, staphylococci, *Haemophilus influenzae, Chlamydia trachomatis, Mycoplasma,* and pneumococci.

Age. Infants under age 3 months have a lower infection rate, presumably because of the protective function of maternal antibodies. The infection rate increases from ages 3 to 6 months, the time between the disappearance of maternal antibodies and the infant's own antibody production. The viral infection rate continues to be high during the toddler and preschool years. By the time the child reaches 5 years of age, viral respiratory infections are much less common, but the incidence of *Mycoplasma pneumoniae* and group A β-streptococcal infections increases. The amount of lymphoid tissue increases throughout middle childhood, and repeated exposure to organisms confers increasing immunity as children grow older.

Some viral agents produce a mild illness in older children but cause severe lower respiratory tract illness or croup in infants. For example, whooping cough is a relatively harmless tracheobronchitis in childhood but a serious disease in infancy.

Size. Anatomic differences influence the response to respiratory tract infections. The diameter of the airways is smaller in young children and subject to considerable narrowing from edematous mucous membranes and increased production of secretions. In addition, the distance between structures within the tract is shorter in the young child; therefore organisms move more rapidly down the respiratory tract for more extensive involvement. The relatively short and open eustachian tube in infants and young children allows pathogens easy access to the middle ear.

Resistance. The ability to resist invading organisms depends on several factors. Deficiencies of the immune system place the child at risk for any infectious process. Other conditions that decrease resistance are malnutrition, anemia, fatigue, and chilling of the body. Conditions affecting the respiratory tract that weaken its defenses and predispose to infection include allergies (e.g., allergic rhinitis), asthma, cardiac anomalies that cause pulmonary congestion, and cystic fibrosis. Day care attendance, especially if the caregivers smoke, also increases the likelihood of infection (Blumer, 1998).

Seasonal Variations. The most common respiratory tract pathogens appear in epidemics during the winter and spring months, but mycoplasmal infections occur more often in autumn and early winter. Infection-related asthma (e.g., asthmatic bronchitis) occurs more commonly during cold weather. Winter and spring are typically the "RSV seasons."

Clinical Manifestations. Infants and young children, especially those between 6 months and 3 years of age, react more severely to acute respiratory tract infection than older children. Young children display a number of generalized signs and symptoms—as well as local manifestations—that differ from those seen in older children and adults. Signs and symptoms associated with respiratory illnesses are listed in Box 46-1.

Box 46-1

Signs and Symptoms Associated with Respiratory Infections in Infants and Small Children

FEVER
May be absent in newborn infants
Greatest at ages 6 months to 3 years
  Temperature may reach 39.5° to 40.5° C (103° to 105° F) even with mild infections
Often appears as first sign of infection
May be listless and irritable or somewhat euphoric and more active than normal, temporarily; some children talk with unaccustomed rapidity
Tendency to develop high temperatures with infection in certain families
  May precipitate febrile seizures (see Chapter 51)
  Febrile seizures uncommon after 3 or 4 years of age

MENINGISMUS
Meningeal signs without infection of the meninges
Occurs with abrupt onset of fever
Accompanied by:
  Headache
  Pain and stiffness in the back and neck
  Presence of Kernig and Brudzinski signs
Subsides as the temperature decreases

ANOREXIA
Common with most childhood illnesses
Frequently the initial evidence of illness
Persists to a greater or lesser degree throughout febrile stage of illness; often extends into convalescence

VOMITING
Small children vomit readily with illness
Clue to onset of infection
May precede other signs by several hours
Usually short-lived but may persist during the illness

DIARRHEA
Usually mild, transient diarrhea but may become severe
Often accompanies viral respiratory infections
Frequent cause of dehydration

ABDOMINAL PAIN
Common complaint
Sometimes indistinguishable from pain of appendicitis
Mesenteric lymphadenitis may be cause
Muscle spasms from vomiting may be a factor, especially in nervous, tense child

NASAL BLOCKAGE
Small nasal passages of infants easily blocked by mucosal swelling and exudation
Can interfere with respiration and feeding in infants
May contribute to the development of otitis media and sinusitis

NASAL DISCHARGE
Frequent occurrence
May be thin and watery (rhinorrhea) or thick and purulent
  Depends on the type and/or stage of infection
Associated with itching
May irritate upper lip and skin surrounding the nose

COUGH
Common feature
May be evident only during acute phase
May persist several months after a disease

RESPIRATORY SOUNDS
Sounds associated with respiratory disease:
  Cough
  Hoarseness
  Grunting
  Stridor
  Wheezing
Auscultation:
  Wheezing
  Crackles
  Absence of sound

SORE THROAT
Frequent complaint of older children
Young children (unable to describe symptoms) may not complain even when highly inflamed
  Child will often refuse to take oral fluids or solids

Nursing Care Management

➤ Assessment

Assessment of the respiratory system follows the guidelines described in Chapter 35 (for assessment of the nose, mouth and throat, chest, and lungs). In addition, special attention is given to the observations outlined in Box 46-1 and the components in Box 46-2.

➤ Nursing Diagnoses

After a thorough assessment, several nursing diagnoses may be identified (see Nursing Care Plan, p. 1193). Others may be apparent in individual cases.

➤ Plan of Care and Implementation

The goals for the child with an acute respiratory infection and the family are as follows:

1. Child will exhibit normal respiratory efforts.
2. Child will receive adequate rest.
3. Child will remain comfortable.
4. Child will not spread primary infection to others.
5. Child's temperature will remain within normal limits.
6. Child will maintain normal hydration and adequate nutrition.
7. Child will experience no complications.
8. Child and family will receive information, especially for home care; and support.

Ease Respiratory Efforts. Many acute respiratory infections are mild and cause few symptoms. Although children may feel uncomfortable and have a "stuffy" nose and some mucosal swelling, respiratory distress occurs infrequently. The interventions described in the remainder of the discussion are usually sufficient to relieve minor discomfort and ease respiratory efforts; however, children with croup or epiglottitis may develop sufficient swelling to obstruct the airway. These children may require hospitalization for observation and therapy.

Warm or cool mist has been a common therapeutic measure for symptomatic relief of respiratory discomfort. The moisture soothes inflamed membranes and is beneficial when there is hoarseness or any laryngeal involvement. However, use of steam vaporizers in the home should be discouraged because of the hazards related to their use and limited evidence to support their efficacy. Shallow pans with wide surface areas for evaporation increase humidity but should be placed where they do not pose a safety hazard.

A time-honored method of producing warm mist is the shower. Running a shower of hot water into the empty bathtub or open shower stall with the bathroom door closed produces a quick source of steam. Keeping a child in this environment for 10 to 15 minutes offers the same advantages as the mist tent without the fear and restraint often associated with the confines of a tent. A small child can be held on the lap of a parent or other adult. Older children can sit in the bathroom under the supervision of an adult.

Box 46-2

Components for Assessing Respiratory Function

RESPIRATIONS

The pattern of respirations is observed for rate, depth, ease, and rhythm of breathing:

Rate—Rapid **(tachypnea)**, normal, or slow for the particular child

Depth—Normal, too shallow **(hypopnea)**, too deep **(hyperpnea)**; usually estimated from the amplitude of thoracic and abdominal excursion

Ease—Effortless; labored **(dyspnea)**; **orthopnea** (difficult breathing except in upright position); associated with intercostal and/or substernal retractions (inspiratory "sinking in" of soft tissues in relation to the cartilaginous and bony thorax); **pulsus paradoxus** (blood pressure falls with inspiration and rises with expiration); flaring nares; head bobbing (head of sleeping child with suboccipital area supported on caregiver's forearm bobs forward in synchrony with each inspiration); grunting; wheezing

Labored breathing—Continuous, intermittent, becoming steadily worse, sudden onset, at rest or on exertion, associated with wheezing or grunting, associated with pain

Rhythm—Variation in rate and depth of respirations

OTHER OBSERVATIONS

In addition to respirations, particular attention is addressed to the following:

Evidence of infection—Check for elevated temperature; enlarged cervical lymph nodes; inflamed mucous membranes; and purulent discharges from the nose, ears, or lungs (sputum)

Cough—Observe the characteristics of the cough (if present); under what circumstances the cough is heard (e.g., night only, on arising), nature of the cough (paroxysmal with or without wheeze, "croupy" or "brassy"), frequency of cough, associated with swallowing or other activity, character of the cough (moist and dry), productivity

Wheeze—Expiratory or inspiratory, high-pitched or musical, prolonged, slowly progressive or sudden, associated with labored breathing

Cyanosis—Note distribution (peripheral, perioral, facial, trunk as well as face), degree, duration, associated with activity

Chest pain—May be a complaint of older children. Note location and circumstances: localized or generalized, referred to base of neck or abdomen, dull or sharp, deep or superficial, associated with rapid, shallow respirations or grunting

Sputum—Older children may provide sputum sample by coughing, whereas young children may need use of bulb suction to provide a sample; note volume, color, viscosity, and odor

Bad breath—May be associated with some lung infections

Promote Rest. Children who have an acute febrile illness should be placed on bed rest. This is usually not difficult while the temperature is elevated but may be difficult when children begin to feel better. Often children are more apt to comply if they are allowed to lie quietly on a couch where they can watch television or participate in a quiet activity. If children protest, allowing them to play quietly serves the purpose of rest better than allowing them to cry excessively in bed. Entertainment devices, based on individual interests and developmental stage, can be used to keep children quiet.

Promote Comfort. Older children are usually able to manage nasal secretions with little difficulty. Parents are instructed in the correct administration of nose drops and throat irrigations, if ordered. For very young infants, who normally breathe through their noses, an infant nasal aspirator or a rubber ear syringe is helpful in removing nasal secretions before feeding. This practice, followed by instillation of saline nose drops, may clear nasal passages and promote feeding. Saline nose drops can be prepared at home by dissolving 1 teaspoon of salt in 1 pint of warm water.*

For older infants and children who can better tolerate decongestants, vasoconstrictive nose drops may be administered 15 to 20 minutes before feeding and at bedtime. Two drops are instilled, and because this shrinks only the anterior mucous membranes, 2 more drops are instilled 5 to 10 minutes later. Phenylephrine (Neo-Synephrine) 0.25% and ephedrine 1% may be prescribed. Older cooperative children often prefer nasal sprays. They are taught to compress the plastic container at the moment of inspiration. Spray bottles and bottles of nose drops should be used for one child only and only for one illness, because they become easily contaminated with bacteria. Nose drops or sprays should not be administered for more than 3 days to avoid rebound congestion.

Hot or cold applications sometimes provide relief for other children with painful cervical adenitis. An ice bag or heating pad applied to the neck may decrease the discomfort, but safety precautions must be observed to prevent burns. The ice bag or heating device must be covered, and the heating pad should not be set at high ranges.

Prevent Spread of Infection. Careful handwashing should be carried out when caring for children with respiratory infections. Children and families are taught to throw used tissues into the waste basket immediately after use; to avoid accumulating tissues in a pile; and to avoid sharing cups, washcloths, or towels. They are also taught to use a tissue or their hand to cover their nose and mouth when they cough or sneeze.

NURSE ALERT • To avoid contamination with respiratory viruses, wash hands and do not touch your eyes or nose.

Every endeavor should be made to remove affected children from contact with other children. Parents are encouraged to keep affected children out of school and day care settings to prevent the spread of infection. Ideally, ill children should be isolated in a separate bedroom at the first sign of illness. This is seldom a problem with an only child but is often difficult when living arrangements are crowded and there are several children in the family. An effort should be made to teach well children to stay away from ill children.

Reduce Temperature. If the child has a significantly elevated temperature, controlling the fever becomes important. The parent should know how to take a child's temperature and read the thermometer accurately. Most parents are able to do this, but nurses cannot make this assumption. Those who cannot will require instruction in the use of the thermometer.*

If the practitioner has prescribed acetaminophen or ibuprofen, parents may need help administering the drug. Most parents can read the label and calculate the desired dose, but some may require careful instruction. It is important to emphasize accuracy in both the amount of drug given and the time intervals at which the drug is administered to avoid accumulation effects. Cool liquids are encouraged to reduce the temperature and minimize the chances of dehydration. (See Controlling Elevated Temperatures, Chapter 45.)

Promote Hydration. Dehydration is always a hazard when children are febrile or anorexic, especially when vomiting or diarrhea is also present. Adequate fluid intake should be encouraged by offering small amounts of favorite fluids at frequent intervals. High-calorie liquids, such as colas, fruit juices, water flavored and sweetened with corn syrup, or similar drinks, help prevent catabolism and dehydration but should be avoided if diarrhea is present. Oral rehydration solutions, such as Infalyte or Pedialyte, should then be considered for infants; and sports drinks, such as Gatorade or Exceed, should be considered for older children. Fluids should not be forced, and children should not be awakened to take fluids. Forcing fluids may create the same difficulties as urging unwanted food. Gentle persuasion with preferred beverages is usually successful.

Parents should know how to assess their child's level of hydration (see Chapter 47). They are advised to observe the frequency of voiding and notify the nurse or practitioner if there is insufficient voiding.

Provide Nutrition. Loss of appetite is characteristic of children with acute infections, and in most cases, children can be permitted to determine their own need for food. Many children show no decrease in appetite, and others respond well to foods such as gelatin, soup, and puddings (see Feeding the Sick Child, Chapter 45). Urging foods on anorexic children may precipitate nausea and vomiting, and in some cases even cause an aversion to the feeding situation that can extend into the convalescent period and beyond.

Provide Family Support and Instruction for Home Care. Small children with respiratory infections are irritable and difficult to comfort. Therefore the family needs support, encouragement, and practical suggestions concerning comfort measures and administration of medication.

In addition to antipyretics and nose drops, the child may require antibiotic therapy. Parents of children receiving oral antibiotics need to understand the importance of regular administration and of continuing the drug for the prescribed length of time, regardless of whether the child appears to be ill.

---

*Community and home care instructions for administration of nose drops and nasal aspiration are available in Wong DL, Hess CS: ***Wong and Whaley's clinical manual of pediatric nursing***, ed 5, St Louis, 2000, Mosby.

*Community and home care instructions for measuring temperature and administration of medication are available in Wong DL, Hess CS: ***Wong and Whaley's clinical manual of pediatric nursing***, ed 5, St Louis, 2000, Mosby.

Parents are also cautioned against giving the child any medications that are not approved by the health practitioner. Adverse effects have been noted in children who have received some preparations intended for adults (e.g., some long-acting nose drops [Neo-Synephrine II] and dextromethorphan cough squares [mistaken for candy]). They are also cautioned about giving the child nonprescribed antibiotics left over from a previous illness. Self-medication with nonprescribed antibiotics can produce serious side effects, and the likelihood of adverse reactions is increased when medications are administered to children without consultation with the practitioner. (See Chapter 45 for administration of medications and teaching parents.)

➤ Evaluation

The effectiveness of nursing interventions is determined by continual reassessment and evaluation of care based on the following observational guidelines:

1. Observe child's respiratory effort and movement.
2. Observe signs and symptoms for progress toward health status before illness.
3. Observe child's behavior and activity.
4. Observe other family members and contacts for evidence of infection.
5. Take temperature.
6. Observe for signs of adequate hydration.
7. Observe eating behavior.
8. Assess for complications such as dehydration, weight loss, or spread of infection to other areas of the body.
9. Observe family's behavior and interview members regarding their feelings and concerns.

The expected outcomes are described in the Nursing Care Plan.

UPPER RESPIRATORY TRACT INFECTIONS (URIs)

Nasopharyngitis

Acute nasopharyngitis (the equivalent of the "common cold") is caused by any of a number of different viruses, usually rhinoviruses, RSV, adenovirus, influenza virus, or parainfluenza virus.

Symptoms of nasopharyngitis are more severe in infants and children than in adults. Fever is common, especially in young children. Older children have low-grade fevers, which appear early in the process. Other clinical manifestations are listed in Box 46-3.

Therapeutic Management. Children with nasopharyngitis are managed at home. There is no specific treatment, and effective vaccines are not available. Antipyretics are usually prescribed for mild fever and discomfort (see Chapter 45 for management of fever). Rest is recommended until the child is free of fever for at least 1 day. Decongestants may be prescribed for children and infants over 6 months of age to shrink swollen nasal passages. The decongestants that exert their effect by vasoconstriction are usually less effective when taken orally than when applied topically as nose drops. Because these drugs affect vascular beds, they should be given with caution to children with diabetes.

Cough suppressants containing dextromethorphan may be prescribed for a dry, hacking cough. Some preparations contain up to 22% alcohol; they should not be administered to young children continuously and must be stored securely away from children.

Antihistamines are largely ineffective in treatment of nasopharyngitis. The drugs have a weak atropine-like effect that dries secretions, but they can cause drowsiness or, paradoxically, have a stimulatory effect on children. There is no support for the usefulness of expectorants, and antibiotics are usually not indicated.

Prevention. Nasopharyngitis is so widespread in the general population that it is difficult to prevent. In addition, children are more susceptible because they have not yet developed resistance to many types of viruses. Very young infants are subject to relatively serious complications such as pneumonia; therefore attempts should be made to protect them from exposure.

Nursing Care Management. A cold is often the parents' first introduction to an illness in their infants. Most discomfort of nasopharyngitis is related to the nasal obstruction, especially in small infants. Elevating the head of the bed or crib mattress assists with drainage of secretions; suctioning and vaporization may provide relief. Saline nose drops and gentle suction with a bulb syringe, particularly before feeding, are useful.

Maintaining adequate fluid intake is essential during any infectious process. Although a child's appetite for solid foods is usually diminished for several days, it is important to offer favorite fluids to prevent dehydration. Fluids can be cool or warm, depending on individual preference.

Because nasopharyngitis is spread from secretions, the best means for prevention is avoiding contact with affected persons. This goal is difficult in places where large numbers of people are confined in a small area for a long time, such as classrooms and day care centers. Family members with a cold should try to "keep it to themselves" by carefully disposing of tissues; not sharing towels, glasses, or eating utensils; covering the mouth and nose with tissues when coughing or sneezing; and washing the hands thoroughly after nose blowing or sneezing. The most common carriers of infection are the human hands, which deposit viruses on doorknobs, faucets, and other everyday objects. Therefore children should be taught to wash their hands thoroughly before putting them near their eyes, nose, or mouth.

Family Support. Support and reassurance are important elements of care for families of young children with recurrent URIs. Because URIs are so common in children less than 3 years of age, families may feel they are on an endless roller coaster of illness. They can be reassured that frequent colds are a normal part of childhood and that by 5 years of age, their children will have developed immunity to many viruses. Parents who work outside the home should expect to take time off to care for ill children during the fall and winter months. If children are cared for routinely in day care centers, the infection rate will be higher than if they are cared for in the home. Parents should know the signs of respiratory complications and be counseled to notify a health professional if any signs of complications appear or if the child does not improve within 2 or 3 days (Box 46-4).

Pharyngitis

Group A β-hemolytic streptococci (GABHS) infection of the upper airway *(strep throat)* is not in itself a serious disease, but affected children are at risk for serious sequelae: *acute rheumatic fever (ARF),* an inflammatory disease of the heart, joints, and central nervous system (see Chapter 48); and acute glomeru-

Nursing Care Plan THE CHILD WITH ACUTE RESPIRATORY INFECTION

NURSING DIAGNOSIS Ineffective breathing pattern related to the inflammatory process

EXPECTED OUTCOME Respiration patterns are within normal limits.

Nursing Interventions/*Rationales*

Position and reposition child as needed (e.g., elevate head of bed, tripod or upright sitting position, use of support pillows and wedges) *to maintain open airway, to allow maximum use of accessory muscles,* and *to allow maximum lung and diaphragm expansion for ventilation and comfort.*

Avoid constrictive clothing or bedding *that may interfere with breathing.*

Provide increased humidity and supplemental oxygen per physician order *to aid in oxygenation and breathing.*

Suction airway as needed *to remove secretions.*

Alternate rest and activity cycles *to reduce oxygen demands.*

Administer bronchodilators and other medications as prescribed *to assist with ventilation.*

NURSING DIAGNOSIS Ineffective airway clearance related to inflammation, increased secretions, obstruction

EXPECTED OUTCOME Airway is patent.

Nursing Interventions/*Rationales*

Position child (prone, side lying, sitting) using proper body alignment *for maximum ventilation and prevention of aspiration of secretions.*

Ensure adequate fluid intake *to keep secretions liquid* and provide humidified environment *to keep mucous membranes moist.*

Administer chest physiotherapy (percussion, vibration, postural drainage) *to promote loosening and drainage of lung secretions.*

Assist child to cough and expectorate effectively using suctioning if needed *to clear accumulated secretions.*

Administer expectorants, nebulizer treatments, and bronchodilators as prescribed *to facilitate liquefaction and clearance of secretions.*

Administer prescribed pain medications and provide splinting during coughing *to minimize discomfort and increase effectiveness of coughing.*

NURSING DIAGNOSIS Risk for spread of infection related to presence of infective organisms

EXPECTED OUTCOME Child shows no signs of secondary infection, and there are no signs of infection in others in environment.

Nursing Interventions/*Rationales*

Maintain aseptic environment, use good handwashing techniques, use isolation techniques and universal precautions as needed *to prevent spread of infection and avoid cross contamination and nosocomial infection.*

Administer antibiotics per physician *to treat or prevent infection.*

Instruct child and family in appropriate precautions (e.g., hand washing, tissue disposal) *to prevent spread of infection.*

NURSING DIAGNOSIS Activity intolerance related to inflammatory process, imbalance between oxygen supply and demand

EXPECTED OUTCOME Child shows no signs of increased respiratory distress; child's activity tolerance is appropriate for age and abilities.

Nursing Interventions/*Rationales*

Schedule activities, treatments, visits, and play around child's needs and energy levels *to maximize rest and minimize fatigue.*

Implement measures (quiet, darkened room) *to ensure sleep.*

Encourage frequent rest periods *to balance energy needs.*

Administer pain medications and sedatives per physician order *for restlessness and pain.*

Monitor vital signs *for signs of oxygen lack.*

NURSING DIAGNOSIS Fear/anxiety related to difficulty breathing

EXPECTED OUTCOME Child exhibits reduced signs of fear and anxiety.

NURSING INTERVENTIONS/*RATIONALES*

Acknowledge child's fear and help child identify sources of that fear *to facilitate identification and use of coping strategies.*

Explain respiratory treatments and procedures to child in developmentally appropriate terms *to allay fear of unknown.*

Show child how coughing and deep breathing help aid breathing *to allay fears and give child a measure of control.*

Box 46-3

Clinical Manifestations of Nasopharyngitis and Pharyngitis

NASOPHARYNGITIS

Younger child
- Fever
- Irritability, restlessness
- Sneezing
- Vomiting and/or diarrhea

Older child
- Dryness and irritation of nose and throat
- Sneezing, chilly sensation
- Muscular aches
- Cough, sometimes

Physical Signs
- Edema and vasodilation of mucosa

PHARYNGITIS

Younger child
- Fever
- General malaise
- Anorexia
- Moderate sore throat
- Headache

Older child
- Fever (may reach 40° C [104° F])
- Headache
- Anorexia
- Dysphagia
- Abdominal pain
- Vomiting

Physical Signs

Younger child
- Mild to moderate hyperemia

Older child
- Mild to fiery red, edematous pharynx
- Hyperemia of tonsils and pharynx; may extend to soft palate and uvula
- Often abundant follicular exudate that spreads and coalesces to form pseudomembrane on tonsils
- Cervical glands enlarged and tender

Box 46-4

Early Evidence of Respiratory Complications

Parents are instructed to notify the health professional if any of the following are noted:
- Evidence of earache (see p. 1198)
- Respirations faster than 50 to 60/min
- Fever over 38.3° C (101° F)
- Listlessness
- Increasing irritability with or without fever
- Persistent cough for 2 days or more
- Wheezing
- Crying
- Refusal to eat
- Restlessness and poor sleep patterns

Modified from National Association of Pediatric Nurse Associates and Practitioners (NAPNAP): *Baby's first cold,* New York, 1989, Winthrop Consumer Products. Copies available from NAPNAP, 1101 Kings Hwy. N., No. 206, Cherry Hill, NJ 08034; (609) 667-1773; e-mail: info@napnap.org; website: www.napnap.org

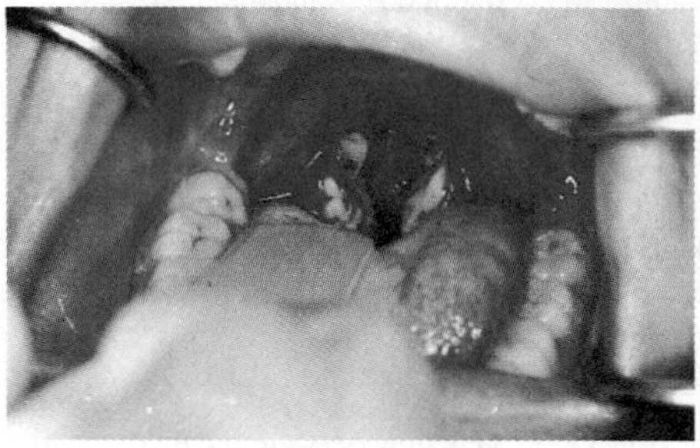

FIG. 46-1 • Tonsillitis and pharyngitis. (Courtesy Dr. Edward L. Applebaum, Head, Department of Otolaryngology, University of Illinois Medical Center, Chicago.)

lonephritis, an acute kidney infection (see Chapter 50). Permanent damage can result from these sequelae, especially ARF.

Clinical Manifestations. GABHS is generally a relatively brief illness that varies in severity from subclinical (i.e., no symptoms) to severe toxicity. The onset is often abrupt and characterized by pharyngitis, headache, fever, and (especially in small children) abdominal pain. The tonsils and pharynx may be inflamed and covered with exudate (Fig. 46-1), which usually appears by the second day of illness. However, streptococcal infections should be suspected in children over 2 years of age who have pharyngitis without exudate (Thuma, 1997). Anterior cervical lymphadenopathy (30% to 50% of cases) usually occurs early, and the nodes are often tender. Pain can be relatively mild to severe enough to make swallowing difficult. Clinical manifestations usually subside in 3 to 5 days unless complicated by sinusitis or parapharyngeal, peritonsillar, or retropharyngeal abscess. Nonsuppurative complications may appear after the onset of GABHS—acute nephritis in about 10 days and ARF in an average of 18 days.

Diagnostic Evaluation. Although 80% to 90% of all cases of acute pharyngitis are viral, a throat culture should be performed to rule out GABHS and (in some cases) *Corynebacterium diphtheriae.* Because some children normally harbor streptococci in their throats, a positive culture is not always conclusive evidence of active disease. Most streptococcal infections are short-term illnesses. Antibody responses appear later than symptoms and are useful only for retrospective diagnosis.

Rapid identification of GABHS is possible with diagnostic test kits, but these kits have problems with sensitivity and should not be considered a substitute for cultures. In addition, the use of some commercial cold medications by the patient can cause false-positive results on rapid strep tests (Armitage, Gross, and Yamauchi, 1999). Therefore a throat culture is recommended for patients who have obvious clinical symptoms and a negative test result with the diagnostic kit (American Academy of Pediatrics, 2000). Practitioners should also consider waiting for culture results before prescribing an antibiotic for otherwise healthy children who have a positive rapid strep test, have few clinical signs of disease, and have been taking a commercial cold medication (Armitage, Gross, and Yamauchi, 1999).

Therapeutic Management. If streptococcal sore throat infection is present, oral penicillin is prescribed in a dose sufficient to control the acute local manifestations and to maintain an adequate level for at least 10 days to eliminate any organisms that might remain to initiate ARF symptoms. Penicillin does not appear to prevent the development of acute glomerulonephritis in susceptible children; however, it may prevent the spread of a nephrogenic strain of GABHS to others in the family. Penicillin usually produces a prompt response within 24 hours. Some patients require retreatment if the organism is not eradicated.

Other antibiotics used to treat GABHS are erythromycin, azithromycin, clarithromycin, cephalosporins such as cefdinir (Omnicef), and amoxicillin (Feder et al, 1999). A combination of penicillin and rifampin is more effective in eradicating GABHS than penicillin alone and is recommended for carriers and persons with GABHS resistant to penicillin.

Nursing Care Management. The nurse often obtains a throat swab for culture and instructs the parents about administering penicillin and analgesics as prescribed. Most children prefer to remain in bed during the acute phase of the illness. Cold or warm compresses to the neck may provide relief. In children old enough to cooperate, warm saline gargles offer some relief of throat discomfort. Pain may interfere with oral intake, and the child should not be forced to eat. Cool liquids or ice chips are usually more acceptable than solids and are encouraged.

Special emphasis is placed on correct administration of oral medication and completing the course of antibiotic therapy (see Administration of Medication; Compliance, Chapter 45). If injections are required, they must be administered deep into a large muscle mass (e.g., vastus lateralis or gluteus muscle). Parents need to be aware of the residual tenderness, which may cause the child to limp for a day or two. Local applications of heat are helpful in relieving discomfort. (For other atraumatic strategies to reduce injection pain, such as application of EMLA over the injection site for 2½ hours, see Administration of Medication: Intramuscular Administration, Chapter 45.)

Nurses also play a key role in preventing the spread of disease. Children are considered noninfectious to others 24 hours after initiation of antibiotic therapy, but they should not return to school or day care until they have been taking antibiotics for a full 24 hours.

NURSE ALERT • When nurses become aware that children have positive throat cultures, they should remind children to discard their toothbrush and replace it with a new one after they have been taking antibiotics for 24 hours.

Tonsillitis

The tonsils are masses of lymphoid tissue located in the pharyngeal cavity. They filter and protect the respiratory and alimentary tracts from invasion by pathogenic organisms and have a role in antibody formation. Although the size of tonsils varies, children generally have much larger tonsils than adolescents or adults. This difference is thought to be a protective mechanism because young children are especially susceptible to URIs.

Pathophysiology. Several pairs of tonsils are part of a mass of lymphoid tissue encircling the nasal and oral pharynx, known as the *Waldeyer tonsillar ring* (Fig. 46-2). The *palatine,* or *faucial tonsils* are located on either side of the oropharynx, behind and below the pillars of the fauces (opening from the mouth). A surface of the palatine tonsils is usually visible during oral examination. The palatine tonsils are those removed during tonsillectomy. The *pharyngeal tonsils,* also known as the *adenoids,* are located above the palatine tonsils on the posterior wall of the nasopharynx. Their proximity to the nares and eustachian tubes causes difficulties in instances of inflammation. The *lingual tonsils* are located at the base of the tongue. The *tubal tonsils,* found near the posterior nasopharyngeal opening of the eustachian tubes, are not part of the Waldeyer tonsillar ring.

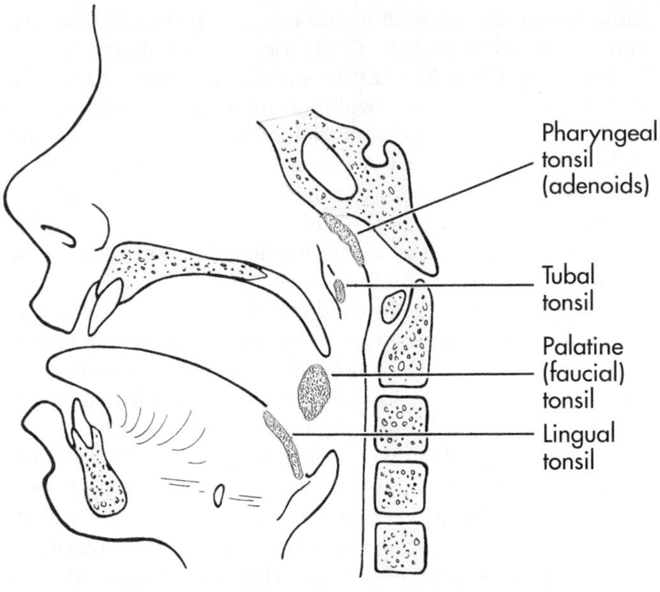

FIG. 46-2 • Location of various tonsillar masses.

Etiology. Tonsillitis often occurs with pharyngitis. Because of the abundant lymphoid tissue and the frequency of URIs, tonsillitis is a common cause of morbidity in young children. The causative agent may be viral or bacterial.

Clinical Manifestations. The manifestations of tonsillitis are caused by inflammation. As the palatine tonsils enlarge from edema, they may meet in the midline (kissing tonsils), obstructing the passage of air or food. The child has difficulty swallowing and breathing. When enlargement of the adenoids occurs, the space behind the posterior nares may become blocked, making it difficult or impossible for air to pass from the nose to the throat. As a result, the child breathes through the mouth.

Therapeutic Management. Because tonsillitis is self-limiting, treatment of viral pharyngitis is symptomatic. Throat cultures positive for GABHS infection warrant antibiotic treatment. It is important to differentiate between viral and streptococcal infection in febrile exudative tonsillitis. Because most infections are of viral origin, early rapid tests can eliminate unnecessary antibiotic administration.

Tonsillectomy (removal of the palatine tonsils) is indicated only in cases of documented recurrent, frequent streptococcal infection; when there is a history of a peritonsillar abscess; or in cases of massive hypertrophy that result in difficulty breathing or eating (Derkay, Darrow, and LeFebvre, 1995). Absolute indications are malignancy and obstruction of the airway. *Adenoidectomy* (removal of the adenoids) is recommended for those children in whom hypertrophied adenoids obstruct nasal breathing. Their removal may be warranted in the child under 3 years of age and should be performed without a tonsillectomy. Contraindications to either tonsillectomy or adenoidectomy are (1) cleft palate, because both tonsils help minimize escape of air during speech; (2) acute infections at the time of surgery, because the locally inflamed tissues increase the risk of bleeding; and (3) uncontrolled systemic diseases or blood dyscrasias.

Nursing Care Management. Nursing care of the child with tonsillitis involves providing comfort and minimizing activities or interventions that precipitate bleeding. A soft to liquid diet is generally preferred. A cool-mist vaporizer helps keep the mucous membranes moist during periods of mouth breathing. Warm salt-water gargles, throat lozenges, and analgesic/antipyretic drugs such as acetaminophen (Tylenol) and codeine are useful to promote comfort.

If surgery is needed, the child requires the same psychologic preparation and physical care as for any other procedure (see Chapters 44 and 45). The following discussion focuses on postoperative nursing care for tonsillectomy and adenoidectomy (T&A), although both procedures may not be performed.

Until they are fully awake, children are placed on the abdomen or side to facilitate drainage of secretions. Suctioning is performed carefully to avoid trauma to the oropharynx. When alert, children may prefer sitting up, although they should remain in bed for the remainder of the day. They are discouraged from coughing frequently, clearing their throat, blowing their nose, or doing any activities that may aggravate the operative site.

Some secretions are common, particularly dried blood from surgery. All secretions and vomitus are inspected for evidence of fresh bleeding (some blood-tinged mucus is expected). Dark brown (old) blood is usually present in the emesis, as well as in the nose and between the teeth. If parents do not expect this, they may be frightened at a time when they need to be calm and reassuring for their children.

The throat is very sore after surgery. An ice collar may provide relief, but many children find it bothersome and refuse to use it. Most children experience significant pain in the first 24 hours after a tonsillectomy, but their parents may be reluctant to give analgesics and may undermedicate their children (Sutters and Miaskowski, 1997). Analgesics may need to be given rectally and should be given in therapeutic doses at regular intervals to lessen pain (see Pain Management, Chapter 44). Local anesthetics such as tetracaine lollipops or ice pops, and transdermal antiemetics such as promethazine (Phenergan) can be made by some pharmacists (see Pain Management, Chapter 44).

Food and fluid are restricted until children are fully alert and there are no signs of hemorrhage. Cool water, crushed ice, flavored ice pops, or dilute fruit juice is given, but fluids with a red or brown color are avoided to distinguish fresh or old blood in emesis from the ingested liquid. Citrus juice may cause discomfort and is usually poorly tolerated. Soft foods, particularly gelatin, cooked fruits, sherbet, soup, and mashed potatoes, are started on the first or second postoperative day or as the child tolerates feeding. The pain from surgery often inhibits intake, reinforcing the need for adequate pain control. Traditionally, milk, ice cream, or pudding have not been offered because milk products coat the mouth and throat, causing the child to clear the throat more often, which may initiate bleeding. However, when children were offered milk or apple juice, more youngsters chose the juice, but over a third also drank the milk. The researchers concluded that children should be given an unrestricted diet postoperatively to increase their food and liquid consumption (Thomas, Moore, and Reilly, 1995).

Postoperative hemorrhage is unusual but can occur; therefore the nurse observes the throat directly for evidence of bleeding, using a good source of light and, if necessary, carefully inserting a tongue depressor. Other signs of hemorrhage are increased pulse (i.e., greater than 120 beats/min), pallor, frequent clearing of the throat or swallowing by a younger child, and vomiting of bright red blood. Restlessness, an indication of hemorrhage, may be difficult to differentiate from general discomfort after surgery. Decreasing blood pressure is a much later sign of shock.

NURSE ALERT • The most obvious early sign of bleeding is the child's continuous swallowing of the trickling blood. While the child is sleeping, note the frequency of swallowing. If continuous bleeding is suspected, notify the surgeon immediately.

Family Support and Home Care. Discharge instructions include (1) avoiding foods that are irritating or highly seasoned, (2) avoiding the use of gargles or vigorous toothbrushing, (3) discouraging the child from coughing or clearing the throat or putting objects in the mouth, (4) using effective analgesics or an ice collar for pain, and (5) limiting activity to decrease the potential for bleeding. Hemorrhage may occur up to 10 days after surgery as a result of tissue sloughing from the healing process. Any sign of bleeding warrants immediate medical attention.

Infectious Mononucleosis

Infectious mononucleosis is an acute, self-limiting infectious disease that is common among young people under 25 years of age. The disease is characterized by an increase in the mononuclear elements of the blood and by general symptoms of an infectious process. The course is usually mild but occasionally can be severe or, rarely, accompanied by serious complications.

Etiology/Pathophysiology. The herpes-like Epstein-Barr virus is the principal cause of infectious mononucleosis. It appears in both sporadic and epidemic forms; the sporadic cases are more common. The mechanism of spread has not been proved, although it is believed to be transmitted by direct intimate contact with oral secretions. It is mildly contagious, and the period of communicability is unknown. The incubation period following exposure is 4 to 6 weeks.

Diagnostic Tests. The onset of symptoms may be acute or insidious. The common presenting symptoms vary greatly in type, severity, and duration (Box 46-5). The leukocyte count may be normal or low, but usually lymphocytic leukocytosis develops. There is also an increase in atypical leukocytes in the peripheral blood smear. The heterophil antibody test determines the extent to which the patient's serum will agglutinate sheep red blood cells. In infectious mononucleosis, a titer of 1:160 is considered diagnostic, although a rising titer during the earlier stages is the best indicator.

The *"spot test" (Monospot),* a slide test of high specificity, is rapid, sensitive, inexpensive, and easy to perform, and has the advantage that it can detect significant agglutinins at lower levels, thus permitting earlier diagnosis. Blood is usually obtained for the test by finger puncture.

Therapeutic Management. There is no specific treatment for infectious mononucleosis. Common symptoms are ordinarily relieved by simple remedies. A mild analgesic is usually sufficient to relieve the bothersome symptoms of headache, fever, and malaise. Bed rest is encouraged for fatigue but is not imposed for any specified period of time. Affected youngsters

Box 46-5
Clinical Manifestations of Infectious Mononucleosis

EARLY SIGNS
Headache
Malaise
Fatigue
Chills
Low-grade fever
Loss of appetite
Puffy eyes

FULL-BLOWN DISEASE
Cardinal Features
Fever
Sore throat
Cervical adenopathy

Common Features
Splenomegaly (may persist for several months)
Palatine petechiae
Macular eruption (especially on trunk)
Exudative pharyngitis/tonsillitis
Hepatic involvement to some degree, often associated with jaundice

are instructed to regulate activities according to their own tolerance unless complicating factors are present. If the spleen is enlarged, activities in which children might receive a blow to the abdomen or chest are avoided.

A short course of oral penicillin is sometimes prescribed for sore throat, especially if β-hemolytic streptococci are present. Administration of ampicillin commonly precipitates a maculopapular rash in affected persons; therefore its use is contraindicated. Sore throat, which can be severe, can be relieved by gargles, hot drinks, anesthetic troches, or analgesics, including opioids. The use of corticosteroids has demonstrated effectiveness in reducing respiratory distress from tonsillar hypertrophy, hemolytic anemia, thrombocytopenia, and neurologic complications; however, the routine use of steroids is not recommended (Barone, Krilov, and Sumaya, 1997).

Prognosis. The course of infectious mononucleosis is self-limiting and usually uncomplicated. Acute symptoms usually disappear within 7 to 10 days, and the persistent fatigue subsides within 2 to 4 weeks. A number of affected youngsters may need to restrict activities for 2 to 3 months; the disease rarely extends for longer periods. Complications are uncommon but can be serious and require appropriate management.

NURSE ALERT • Advise family to seek medical evaluation of the youngster if:
- Breathing becomes difficult.
- Abdominal pain develops.
- Sore throat pain is so severe that the child is unable to eat or drink.

Nursing Care Management. Nursing responsibilities are directed toward providing comfort measures to relieve the symptoms and helping affected youngsters and their families determine appropriate activities according to the stage of the disease and their interests. They may need diet counseling to select foods that contain sufficient calories to meet growth and energy needs but are easy to swallow. Every effort should be made to prevent a secondary infection; therefore the adolescent is counseled to limit exposure to persons outside the family, especially during the acute phase of illness.

The illness and its associated weakness and fatigue can cause depression and resentment on the part of usually vigorous, active teenagers. It is important to spend time with youngsters to listen to their concerns and to allow them to express their feelings and vent their anger. Adolescents need reassurance that the limitations are only temporary, that social activities—so essential at this stage of development—can be resumed after the acute phase, and that they will have sufficient autonomy to determine the extent of their capabilities and the rate of resumption of activities.

Influenza

Influenza, or "flu," is caused by different viruses that may undergo significant changes from time to time. The disease is spread from one individual to another by direct contact (large-droplet infection) or by articles recently contaminated by nasopharyngeal secretions. There is no predilection for a specific age group, but attack rates are highest in young children who have not had previous contact with a strain. It is commonly most severe in infants. During epidemics, infection among school-age children is believed to be a major source of transmission in a community. Influenza is more common during the winter months. The disease has a 1- to 3-day incubation period, and affected persons are most infectious for 24 hours before and after onset of symptoms.

Clinical Manifestations. The manifestations of influenza may be subclinical, mild, moderate, or severe. Most patients have a dry throat and nasal mucosa, a dry cough, and a tendency toward hoarseness. A sudden onset of fever and chills is accompanied by a flushed face, photophobia, myalgia, hyperesthesia, and sometimes prostration. Subglottal croup is common, especially in infants. The symptoms last for 4 to 5 days. Complications include severe viral pneumonia (often hemorrhagic), encephalitis, and secondary bacterial infections such as otitis media, sinusitis, or pneumonia.

Therapeutic Management. Uncomplicated influenza in children usually requires only symptomatic treatment: acetaminophen or ibuprofen for fever, dextromethorphan for cough (if needed), and sufficient fluids to maintain hydration. Amantadine hydrochloride (Symmetrel) has been effective in reducing symptoms associated with type A disease if administered within 24 to 48 hours after onset. It is ineffective against type B or C influenza or other viral diseases. It should not be given to children under 1 year of age but is recommended for unvaccinated high risk children. Children with influenza (or other similar viruses) should not receive aspirin because of its possible link with Reye syndrome.

Prevention. Inactivated influenza viral vaccines are safe and effective for prevention of influenza provided that the antigens in the vaccine correlate with circulating influenza viruses (see Immunizations, Chapter 36). These vaccines are mainly recommended for children with health problems (e.g., heart disease, asthma, human immunodeficiency virus [HIV] infection, cancer, diabetes) that make it risky for them to get the flu (American Academy of Pediatrics, 1998).

Nursing Care Management. Nursing care is the same as for any child with a URI, including helping the family to implement measures to relieve symptoms. The greatest danger to affected children is development of a secondary infection.

NURSE ALERT • Prolonged fever or appearance of fever during early convalescence is a sign of secondary bacterial infection and should be reported to the practitioner for antibiotic therapy.

Otitis Media (OM)

OM is one of the most prevalent diseases of early childhood. The incidence is highest in children ages 6 months to 2 years; it then gradually decreases with age, except for a small increase at age 5 or 6 years, the time of school entry. OM occurs infrequently in children over 7 years of age. Boys are affected more commonly than girls in children less than school age; later the sexes are affected equally. The incidence of acute otitis media (AOM) is highest in the winter months. Children living in households with many members (especially smokers) are more likely to have OM than those living with fewer persons, and children who have siblings or parents with a history of chronic OM have a higher incidence than those who do not.

OM has been defined in a variety of ways. The standard terminology is outlined in Box 46-6.

Etiology. AOM is commonly caused by *Streptococcus pneumoniae* and *Haemophilus influenzae.* The etiology of the noninfectious type is unknown, although it is commonly the result of blocked eustachian tubes from the edema of URIs, allergic rhinitis, or hypertrophic adenoids. Chronic OM is commonly an extension of an acute episode. Passive smoking has been established as a significant factor in the development of OM. Tobacco smoke inhalation may increase the risk of a blocked eustachian tube by impairing mucociliary function, causing congestion of soft nasopharyngeal tissues, or predisposing patients to URI. Day care attendance and living with a smoker are also risk factors for OM (Nafstad et al, 1999).

Infants fed breast milk have a lower incidence of OM compared with formula-fed infants. Breastfeeding may protect infants against respiratory viruses and allergy because breast milk contains secretory immunoglobulin A (IgA) and limits the exposure of the eustachian tube and middle ear mucosa to microbial pathogens and foreign proteins. Reflux of milk up the eustachian tubes is less likely in breastfed infants because of the semivertical positioning during breastfeeding compared with bottle-feeding. There is a definite link between the supine position during feeding and the reflux of fluid into the middle ear (Tully, Bar-Haim, and Bradley, 1995).

Pathophysiology. OM is primarily the result of dysfunctioning eustachian tubes. The eustachian tube, which connects the middle ear to the nasopharynx, is normally closed and flat, preventing organisms from the pharyngeal cavity from entering the middle ear. It opens to allow drainage of secretions produced by the middle ear mucosa and to equalize air pressure between the middle ear and outside environment. Impaired drainage causes retention of secretions in the middle ear. Air, unable to escape through the obstructed tubes, is absorbed into the circulation, causing negative pressure within the middle ear. If the tube opens, this difference in pressure causes bacteria to be swept into the middle ear chamber, where the organisms quickly proliferate and invade the mucosa.

Diagnostic Evaluation. In AOM, otoscopy reveals an intact membrane that appears bright red and bulging, with no visible bony landmarks or light reflex. In OME, otoscopic findings may include a slightly inflamed, dull gray membrane; obscured landmarks; and a visible fluid level or meniscus behind the eardrum if air is present above the fluid. Diagnosis is usually based on clinical manifestations (Box 46-7) and confirmed with *tympanometry,* which measures the change in air pressure in the external auditory canal from movement of the eardrum. The presence of fluid in the middle ear decreases membrane movement or compliance. *Pneumatic otoscopy* also provides an assessment of tympanic membrane mobility. If purulent discharge is present, it should be cultured and a specific antibiotic selected for that organism. Hearing evaluation is recommended for a child who has fluid in both middle ears for a total of 3 months.

Box 46-6

Standard Terminology for Otitis Media

Otitis media (OM)—An inflammation of the middle ear without reference to etiology or pathogenesis

Acute otitis media (AOM)—A rapid and short onset of signs and symptoms lasting approximately 3 weeks

Otitis media with effusion (OME)—An inflammation of the middle ear in which a collection of fluid is present in the middle ear space

Chronic otitis media with effusion—Middle ear effusion that persists beyond 3 months

Box 46-7

Clinical Manifestations of Otitis Media

ACUTE OTITIS MEDIA

Follows an upper respiratory Infection
Otalgia (earache)
Fever
Purulent discharge (otorrhea) may or may not be present

Infant or Very Young Child

Crying
Fussy, restless, irritable
Tendency to rub, hold, or pull affected ear
Rolls head from side to side
Difficulty comforting child
Loss of appetite

Older Child

Crying and/or verbalizes feelings of discomfort
Irritability
Lethargy
Loss of appetite

CHRONIC OTITIS MEDIA

Hearing loss
Difficulty communicating
Feeling of fullness, tinnitus, or vertigo may be present

Therapeutic Management. Because of concerns about penicillin resistance, infectious disease authorities recommend judicious use of antibiotics. Some experts advise that AOM be treated only in children who meet one of the following criteria: more than three ear infections in the past year; a positive respiratory culture; and a high risk for bacterial infections because of immunosuppression, a splenectomy, cystic fibrosis, sickle cell disease, attendance at a day care center, or living with a smoker (Armitage, Gross, and Yamauchi, 1999). When antibiotics are warranted, treatment may involve a 5- or 10-day course of oral antibiotics such as amoxicillin, amoxicillin-clavulanate, sulfonamides, trimethoprim-sulfamethoxazole (Bactrim, Septra), erythromycin-sulfisoxazole (Pediazole), azithromycin, clarithromycin, or cephalosporins (Montville and White, 1998). A single-dose intramuscular (IM) injection of ceftriaxone is also an effective treatment (Barnett et al, 1997). With appropriate therapy, most children improve within 48 to 72 hours.

Myringotomy (surgical incision of the eardrum) may be needed to relieve symptoms in some children, especially if there is severe pain, hearing loss secondary to recurrent and chronic OM, or failure of medical management with prophylactic antibiotics (Williams et al, 1997). Children should be seen after antibiotic therapy to evaluate the effectiveness of the treatment and to identify potential complications, such as effusion or hearing impairment. Analgesic/antipyretic drugs are used to alleviate discomfort and to reduce an elevated temperature.

The major goals in the management of OME are to establish and maintain an aerated middle ear free of fluid with a normal mucosa; and to achieve normal hearing. A course of antibiotics is not recommended as initial treatment for OME but may be indicated for children with persistent effusion for more than 3 months (Dowell et al, 1998).

The use of steroids, decongestants, and antihistamines to shrink the mucous membranes and increase eustachian tube function is not recommended. Surgical treatment involves tympanoplasty or insertion of ventilating tubes. Tympanostomy tubes (pressure-equalizer [PE] tubes or grommets) facilitate continued drainage of fluid and allow ventilation of the middle ear. Myringotomy with or without insertion of PE tubes should not be performed for initial management of OME in an otherwise healthy child. Adenoidectomy is not recommended for treatment of OME in a child 1 to 3 years of age without specific adenoid pathology. Tonsillectomy should not be performed, either alone or with adenoidectomy, for the treatment of OME in a child of any age.

Polyvalent pneumococcal polysaccharide vaccines have reduced the incidence of pneumococcal OM by 50% in children older than 2 years of age (Williams et al 1997). For some high risk infants, an immune globulin containing antibodies against bacterial polysaccharides (BPIG) has resulted in fewer cases of AOM caused by *Streptococcus pneumoniae.*

The Agency for Health Care Planning and Research (AHCPR) has released federal guidelines for the treatment of OME.*

*A parent guide (94-0624) and more detailed Clinical Practice Guidelines (94-0620) are available in English and Spanish from the AHCPR Publications Clearinghouse, OME/AAP, P.O. Box 8547, Silver Spring, MD 20907-8547; 1-800-358-9295; website: www.ahcpr.gov.

Nursing Care Management. Nursing objectives for the child with AOM include: (1) relieving pain, (2) facilitating drainage when possible, (3) preventing complications or recurrence, (4) educating the family in care of the child, and (5) providing emotional support to the child and family.

Analgesics/antipyretics are helpful in reducing the severe earache and fever. The application of heat with a heating pad on low setting and wrapped in a towel may reduce discomfort. Local heat should be placed over the ear with the child lying on the affected side. This position also facilitates drainage of the exudate if the eardrum has ruptured or if myringotomy was performed. An ice compress placed over the affected ear may also provide comfort and reduce edema and pressure. If the child is cooperative, either procedure can be tried to determine which offers maximum relief.

If the ear is draining, the external canal may be cleaned with sterile cotton swabs or pledgets soaked in hydrogen peroxide. If ear wicks or lightly rolled sterile gauze packs are placed in the ear after surgical treatment, they should be loose enough to allow accumulated drainage to flow out of the ear; otherwise the infection may be transferred to the mastoid process. The wicks need to stay dry during shampoos or baths. Occasionally, drainage is so profuse that the auricle and the skin surrounding the ear become excoriated from the exudate. This is prevented by frequent cleansing and application of various moisture barriers (e.g., Aloe Vesta, Proshield Plus) or petrolatum jelly (e.g., Vaseline).

Parents require anticipatory guidance regarding temporary hearing loss that accompanies OM. The nurse should caution parents that the child is not ignoring them but may be unaware of being spoken to. Parents are instructed to speak louder, at closer proximity, and facing the child. Persistent difficulty in hearing beyond the acute stage should be evaluated.

Tympanostomy tubes may allow water to enter the middle ear, but recommendations for earplugs are inconsistent. Research indicates that swimming without earplugs poses no increased risk of infection. However, lake water is contaminated, and wearing earplugs while swimming in a lake will prevent total flooding of the external canal. Bathwater and shampoo water should also be kept out of the ear, if possible, because soap reduces the surface tension of water, facilitating entry through the tube.

Parents should be aware of the appearance of a grommet (usually a tiny, white, plastic spool-shaped tube) so that they can recognize it if it falls out. They are reassured that this is normal and requires no immediate intervention, although they should notify the practitioner.

Prevention of recurrence requires adequate parent education regarding antibiotic therapy. Because the symptoms of pain and fever usually subside within 24 to 48 hours, nurses must emphasize that the infection is not completely eradicated until all of the prescribed medication is taken. Parents should be aware of the potential complications of OM that can occur with inadequate treatment, such as: (1) conductive hearing loss; (2) a perforated and scarred eardrum; (3) *mastoiditis,* an inflammation of the mastoid air cell system; (4) *cholesteatoma,* a cystlike lesion that can invade and destroy surrounding auditory structures; and (5) intracranial infections such as meningitis.

Nurses need to teach parents ways to prevent OM, such as sitting or holding an infant upright during bottle-feeding and breastfeeding. Propping bottles is discouraged to avoid the supine position and to encourage human contact during feeding. Because infants have difficulty expressing themselves verbally, parents should be taught that initial signs of OM may be irritability and ear pulling. Eliminating tobacco smoke and known allergens is also recommended.

(See Nursing Care Plan: The Child with Acute Otitis Media.*)

CROUP SYNDROMES

Croup is a general term applied to a symptom complex characterized by hoarseness, a resonant cough described as "barking" or "brassy" (croupy), varying degrees of inspiratory stridor, and varying degrees of respiratory distress resulting from swelling or obstruction in the region of the larynx. Acute infections of the larynx are of greater importance in infants and small children than they are in older children, because of the increased incidence in children in this age group and the smaller diameter of the airway, which renders it subject to significantly greater narrowing with the same degree of inflammation.

Croup syndromes affect to varying degrees the larynx, trachea, and bronchi; however, laryngeal involvement often dominates the clinical picture because of the severe effects on the voice and breathing. Croup syndromes are usually described according to the primary anatomic area affected (i.e., epiglottitis [or supraglottitis], laryngitis, laryngotracheobronchitis [LTB], and tracheitis). In general, LTB tends to occur in very young children, whereas epiglottitis is more characteristic of older children. A comparison of croup syndromes is provided in Table 46-1.

*In Wong DL, Hess CS: ***Wong and Whaley's clinical manual of pediatric nursing***, ed 5, St Louis, 2000, Mosby.

Acute Epiglottitis

Acute epiglottitis, or *acute supraglottitis,* is a serious obstructive inflammatory process that occurs principally in children between 2 and 5 years of age but can occur from infancy to adulthood. The disorder requires immediate attention. The obstruction is supraglottic as opposed to the subglottic obstruction of laryngitis. The responsible organism is usually *Haemophilus influenzae;* LTB and epiglottitis do not occur together.

Clinical Manifestations. The onset of epiglottitis is abrupt, often preceded by a sore throat, and rapidly progressing to severe respiratory distress. The child usually goes to bed asymptomatic to awaken later, complaining of sore throat and pain on swallowing. The child has a fever; appears sicker than clinical findings suggest; and insists on sitting upright and leaning forward, with the chin thrust out, mouth open, and tongue protruding *(tripod position).* Drooling of saliva is common because of the difficulty or pain on swallowing and excessive secretions.

NURSE ALERT • Three clinical observations that indicate epiglottitis are absence of spontaneous cough, presence of drooling, and agitation.

The child is irritable and extremely restless and has an anxious, apprehensive, and frightened expression. The voice is thick and muffled, with a froglike croaking sound on inspiration. The child is not hoarse. Suprasternal and substernal retractions may be visible. The child seldom struggles to breathe, and slow, quiet breathing provides better air exchange. The sallow color of mild hypoxia may progress to frank cyanosis. The throat is red and inflamed, and a distinctive large, cherry red, edematous epiglottis is visible on careful throat inspection. *Throat inspection should be attempted only when immediate intubation can be performed if needed.*

TABLE 46-1
Comparison of Croup Syndromes

	Acute Epiglottitis (Supraglottitis)	Acute Laryngotracheo-Bronchitis (LTB)	Acute Spasmodic Laryngitis (Spasmodic Group)	Acute Tracheitis
Age group affected	1–8 years	3 months–8 years	3 months-3 years	1 month–6 years
Etiologic agent	Bacterial, usually *Haemophilus influenzae*	Viral	Viral with allergic component	Bacterial, usually *Staphylococcus aureus*
Onset	Rapidly progressive	Slowly progressive	Sudden; at night	Moderately progressive
Major symptoms	Dysphagia Stridor aggravated when supine Drooling High fever Toxic appearance Rapid pulse and respirations	URI Stridor Brassy cough Hoarseness Dyspnea Restlessness Irritability Low-grade fever Nontoxic appearance	URI Croupy cough Stridor Hoarseness Dyspnea Restlessness Symptoms awaken child Symptoms disappear during day Tends to recur	URI Croupy cough Stridor Purulent secretions High fever No response to LTB therapy
Treatment	Antibiotics Airway protection	Humidity Racemic epinephrine	Humidity	Antibiotics

URI, Upper respiratory infection.

Therapeutic Management. The course of epiglottitis may be fulminant, with respiratory obstruction appearing suddenly. Progressive obstruction leads to hypoxia, hypercapnia, and acidosis followed by decreased muscular tone, reduced level of consciousness, and, when obstruction becomes more or less complete, a rather sudden death. A presumptive diagnosis of epiglottitis constitutes an emergency.

The child suspected of having epiglottitis should be examined where facilities are available for coping with this type of emergency. Examination of the throat with a tongue depressor is contraindicated until properly experienced personnel and equipment are at hand to proceed with immediate intubation or tracheostomy in the event that the examination precipitates further or complete obstruction.

If a lateral neck film is indicated, the same experienced personnel should accompany the child to the radiology department. Most practitioners prefer that the child not be transported but remain on the parent's lap in the examination area during portable radiology.

Endotracheal intubation or tracheostomy is usually considered for *H. influenzae* epiglottitis with severe respiratory distress. Intubation, tracheostomy, and any invasive procedure such as starting an intravenous (IV) infusion should be performed in the operating room. Whether or not there is an artificial airway, the child requires intensive observation by experienced personnel. The epiglottal swelling usually decreases after 24 hours of antibiotic therapy, and the epiglottis is near normal by the third day. Intubated children are generally extubated at this time.

Children with suspected bacterial epiglottitis are given antibiotics intravenously, followed by oral administration to complete a 7- to 10-day course. The use of corticosteroids for reducing edema may be beneficial during the early hours of treatment. Most intubated children will have had a course of corticosteroids for 24 hours before extubation.

Prevention. The American Academy of Pediatrics (2000) recommends that all children beginning at 2 months of age receive the *H. influenzae* type B conjugate vaccine (see Immunizations, Chapter 36). Because administration of the vaccine has become a routine part of the regular immunization schedule, a decline in the incidence of epiglottitis has occurred. Patients now tend to be older and have disease caused by other organisms.

Nursing Care Management. Epiglottitis is a serious and frightening disease for the child and family. It is important to act quickly but calmly and provide support without unduly increasing anxiety. The child is allowed to remain in the position that provides the most comfort and security, and parents are reassured that everything possible is being done to obtain relief for their child.

NURSE ALERT • Nurses who suspect epiglottitis should not attempt to visualize the epiglottis directly with a tongue depressor or take a throat culture but should refer the child for medical evaluation immediately (Critical Thinking box).

Acute care of the child is the same as that described for the child with LTB. Continuous monitoring of respiratory status, including pulse oximetry and blood gases, is part of nursing observations, and the IV infusion is maintained as described in Chapter 45.

Acute Laryngitis

Acute infectious laryngitis is a common illness in older children and adolescents. Infants and smaller children experience more generalized involvement (see following section on LTB). Viruses are the usual causative agents, and the principal complaint is hoarseness, which may be accompanied by other upper respiratory symptoms (e.g., coryza, sore throat, and nasal congestion) and systemic manifestations (e.g., fever, headache, myalgia, and malaise). Associated complaints vary with the infecting virus. Adenoviruses and influenza viruses are responsible for more systemic involvement; parainfluenza viruses, rhinoviruses, and RSV cause more mild illness.

Therapeutic Management and Nursing Care Management. The disease is almost always self-limited without long-term sequelae. Treatment is symptomatic with fluids and humidified air (see Nursing Care Plan, p. 1193).

Acute Laryngotracheobronchitis (LTB)

LTB is the most common of the croup syndromes and primarily affects children less than 5 years of age. Organisms responsible for LTB are the parainfluenza virus, RSV, influenza A and B, and *Mycoplasma pneumoniae.* The disease is usually preceded by a URI, which gradually descends to adjacent structures. It is characterized by gradual onset of low-grade fever.

Inflammation of the mucosa lining the larynx and trachea causes a narrowing of the airway. When the airway is significantly narrowed, the child struggles to inhale air past the obstruction and into the lungs, producing the characteristic inspiratory stridor and suprasternal retractions. The typical child with LTB is a toddler who develops the classic barking or seal-like cough and acute stridor after several days of coryza. When the child is unable to inhale a sufficient volume of air, symptoms of hypoxia become evident. Obstruction that is severe enough to prevent adequate exhalation of carbon dioxide causes respiratory acidosis, and eventually the child experiences

Critical Thinking

CROUP SYNDROME

Kim Lee, 4 years old, is admitted to the emergency department with a sore throat, pain on swallowing, drooling, and a fever of 39° C (102.2° F). She looks ill, is agitated, and prefers to sit up and lean over. Which of the following medical orders should you question?

First, Think About It . . .

- **How are you interpreting the information?**
- **What are the consequences if you put your thoughts into action?**

1. **Obtain a complete blood count (CBC) and throat culture immediately.**
2. **Place child on oxygen saturation monitor.**
3. **Start an intravenous line of 5% dextrose in normal saline to run at 30 ml/hr.**
4. **Have a pediatric-sized tracheostomy tray available.**

The best response is 1. Interpreting the information, the nurse should question the order for a throat culture, because the child's symptoms suggest epiglottitis. Negative consequences may result if inappropriate nursing actions are taken, because the action can precipitate obstruction of the airway. The CBC and other interventions are appropriate.

respiratory failure. The progression of symptoms is outlined in Box 46-8.

Therapeutic Management. The major objective in medical management of infectious LTB is maintaining an airway and providing for adequate respiratory exchange. Children with mild croup (no stridor at rest) are managed at home. Parents are taught the signs of respiratory distress so that professional help can be summoned early if needed. Children who progress to stage II respiratory symptoms should receive medical attention.

High humidity with cool mist provides relief for most children. A cool-air vaporizer can be used at home. In the hospital setting, hoods for infants or tents for toddlers may be used to provide increased humidity and supplemental oxygen.

Nebulized epinephrine (racemic epinephrine) is often used in children with more severe disease, stridor at rest, retractions, or difficulty breathing. The α-adrenergic effects cause mucosal vasoconstriction and subsequent decreased subglottic edema. The onset of action is rapid, with detectable clinical improvement within 10 to 15 minutes, although symptoms commonly reappear—typically called "relapse"—within 2 hours. In a significant number of children, however, improvement persists and additional treatments are not necessary.

The use of corticosteroids is beneficial because the anti-inflammatory effects decrease subglottic edema. The onset of action is clinically detectable as early as 6 hours after administration, with continued improvement over 12 to 24 hours.

It is essential to allow children with mild croup to continue to drink beverages they like and to encourage parents to try whatever comforting measures work best with their child (e.g., being held, rocked, walked, or sung to). If the child is unable to take oral fluids, IV fluid therapy might be indicated.

NURSE ALERT • Children with severe respiratory distress (traditionally, infants with a respiratory rate greater than 60 breaths/min) should not be given anything by mouth to prevent aspiration and to decrease the work of breathing.

Nursing Care Management. The most important nursing function in the care of children with LTB is continuous, vigilant observation and accurate assessment of respiratory status. Cardiac, respiratory, and non-invasive blood gas monitoring equipment supplement visual observations. Changes in therapy are commonly based on nurses' observations and assessment of a child's status, response to therapy, and tolerance of procedures. The trend away from early intubation of children with LTB emphasizes the importance of nursing observation and the ability to recognize impending respiratory failure so that intubation can be implemented without delay. Intubation equipment should be readily accessible and taken with the child during transport to other areas (e.g., radiology or operating room).

NURSE ALERT • Early signs of impending airway obstruction include increased pulse and respiratory rate; substernal, suprasternal, and intercostal retractions; flaring nares; and increased restlessness.

To conserve energy, children are given every opportunity to rest. Infants or small children find that being enclosed within a tent, coughing, having laryngeal spasms, and needing IV therapy are additional sources of distress. Infants and small children prefer sitting upright, and most want to be held. Children need the security of the parent's presence. Because crying increases respiratory distress and hypoxia, a child's individual tolerance for these therapies must be assessed. An extremely fussy child may do better when held in the parent's lap with cool mist directed toward the child's face.

The rapid progression of croup, the alarming sound of the cough and stridor, and the child's apprehensive behavior and ill appearance combine to create a very frightening experience for the parents. They need reassurance regarding the child's progress and an explanation of treatments. They may feel guilty for not having suspected the seriousness of the condition sooner. The family should be allowed to remain with their child as much as possible, especially when this decreases the child's distress.

The nurse can provide the parents with an opportunity to express their feelings, thus minimizing any blame or guilt. They need frequent reassurance provided in a calm, quiet manner and education regarding what they can do to make their child more comfortable. Fortunately, as the crisis subsides and the child responds to therapy, breathing becomes easier and recovery is generally prompt. Home care after discharge includes continued humidity, adequate hydration, and nourishment. Parents are encouraged to ask questions about home care and preparation for discharge. Referral to a public health agency for follow-up care may be advisable.

Box 46-8

Progression of Symptoms in Laryngotracheobronchitis

STAGE I
Fear
Hoarseness
Croupy cough
Inspiratory stridor when disturbed

STAGE II
Continuous respiratory stridor
Lower rib retraction
Retraction of soft tissue of neck
Use of accessory muscles of respiration
Labored respiration

STAGE III
Signs of anoxia and carbon dioxide retention
Restlessness
Anxiety
Pallor
Sweating
Rapid respiration

STAGE IV
Intermittent cyanosis
Permanent cyanosis
Cessation of breathing

As described by Forbes. From Krugman S et al: *Infectious diseases of children,* ed 9, St Louis, 1992, Mosby.

Acute Spasmodic Laryngitis

Acute spasmodic laryngitis (*spasmodic croup,* "midnight croup," or "twilight croup") is distinct from laryngitis and LTB and is characterized by paroxysmal attacks of laryngeal obstruction that occur chiefly at night. Signs of inflammation are absent or mild, and there is often a history of previous attacks lasting 2 to 5 days, followed by uneventful recovery. It usually affects children ages 1 to 3 years. Some children appear to be predisposed to the condition; allergy and psychogenic factors are implicated in some cases.

The child goes to bed well or with some very mild respiratory symptoms but awakes suddenly with characteristic barking, metallic cough, hoarseness, noisy inspirations, and restlessness. The child appears anxious, frightened, and prostrated. Dyspnea is aggravated by excitement; but there is no fever, the attack subsides in a few hours, and the child appears well the next day.

Therapeutic Management and Nursing Care Management. Children with spasmodic croup are managed at home. Cool mist is recommended for the child's room. Warm mist provided by steam from hot running water in a closed bathroom may be helpful. Sometimes the spasm is relieved by sudden exposure to cold air (as when the child is taken out into the night air to see the practitioner). Parents are usually advised to have the child sleep in humidified air until the cough has subsided so that subsequent episodes may be prevented. Children with moderately severe symptoms may be hospitalized for observation and therapy with cool mist and racemic epinephrine, as for LTB. Patients may respond to corticosteroid therapy. The disease is usually self-limited.

Bacterial Tracheitis

Bacterial tracheitis, an infection of the mucosa of the upper trachea, is a distinct entity with features of both croup and epiglottitis. The disease is seen in children ages 1 month to 6 years and may be a serious cause of airway obstruction—severe enough to cause respiratory arrest. It is believed to be a complication of LTB, and although *Staphylococcus aureus* is the most common organism responsible, group A β-hemolytic streptococci and *H. influenzae* have also been implicated.

Many of the manifestations of bacterial tracheitis are similar to those of LTB but are unresponsive to LTB therapy. There is a history of previous URI with croupy cough, stridor unaffected by position, toxicity, and high fever. A prominent manifestation is the production of thick, purulent tracheal secretions. Respiratory difficulties are secondary to these copious secretions.

Therapeutic Management and Nursing Care Management. Bacterial tracheitis requires vigorous management. Humidified oxygen, antipyretics, and antibiotics are prescribed. Most children require endotracheal intubation and frequent tracheal suctioning to prevent airway obstruction. The emphasis in this disorder is early recognition to prevent catastrophic airway obstruction.

INFECTIONS OF THE LOWER AIRWAYS

The *reactive portion* of the lower respiratory tract includes the bronchi and bronchioles in children. Cartilaginous support of the large airway is not fully developed until adolescence; consequently, the smooth muscle in these structures represents a major factor in the constriction of the airway, particularly in the bronchioles, that portion that extends from the bronchi to the alveoli. Table 46-2 compares some of the major features of bronchial and bronchiolar infections.

Bronchitis

Bronchitis (sometimes referred to as *tracheobronchitis*) is inflammation of large airways (trachea and bronchi), which is commonly associated with a URI. Viral agents are the primary cause of the disease, although *Mycoplasma pneumoniae* is a com-

TABLE 46-2
Comparison of Conditions Affecting the Bronchi

	Viral-Induced Asthma*	Bronchitis	Bronchiolitis
Description	Exaggerated response of bronchi to infection Bronchospasm, exudation, and edema of bronchi	Usually occurs in association with URI Seldom an isolated entity	More common infectious disease of lower airways Maximum obstructive impact at bronchiolar level
Age group affected	Late infancy and early childhood	Affects children in first 4 years of life	Usually children 2–12 months old; rare after age 2 years Peak incidence at approximately age 6 months
Etiologic agents	Most often viruses but may be any of a variety of URI pathogens	Usually viral Other agents (e.g., bacteria, fungi, allergic disorders, airborne irritants) can trigger symptoms	Viruses, predominantly respiratory syncytial viruses; also adenoviruses, parainfluenza viruses, and *Mycoplasma pneumoniae*
Predominant characteristics	Wheezing, productive cough	Persistent dry, hacking cough (worse at night) becoming productive in 2–3 days	Dyspnea, paroxysmal nonproductive cough, tachypnea with retractions and flaring nares, emphysema; may be wheezing
Treatment	Bronchodilators, corticosteroids	Cough suppressants if needed	Oxygen mist Ribavirin or palivizumab may be used for high-risk populations

*See Asthma, p. 1212.

mon cause in children older than 6 years of age. The condition is characterized by a dry, hacking, and nonproductive cough that is worse at night and becomes productive in 2 to 3 days.

Bronchitis is a mild, self-limiting disease that requires only symptomatic treatment, including analgesics, antipyretics, and humidity. Cough suppressants may be useful to allow rest but can interfere with clearance of secretions. Most patients recover uneventfully in 5 to 10 days.

Respiratory Syncytial Virus (RSV)/Bronchiolitis

Bronchiolitis is an acute viral infection with maximum effect at the bronchiolar level. The infection occurs primarily in winter and spring and is rare in children over 2 years of age. *Respiratory syncytial virus (RSV)* is responsible for at least half of all pediatric hospitalizations for bronchiolitis. Adenoviruses and parainfluenza viruses may also cause acute bronchiolitis. Infection begins in the late fall, reaches a peak during winter, and decreases in spring. It is easily spread from hand to eye, nose, or other mucous membranes.

Pathophysiology. Bronchiole mucosa is swollen, and lumina are filled with mucus and exudate; the walls of the bronchi and bronchioles are infiltrated with inflammatory cells; and peribronchiolar interstitial pneumonitis is usually present. The variable degrees of obstruction produced in small air passages by these changes lead to hyperinflation, obstructive emphysema resulting from partial obstruction, and patchy areas of atelectasis. Dilation of bronchial passages on inspiration allows sufficient space for intake of air, but narrowing of the passages on expiration prevents air from leaving the lungs. Thus air is trapped distal to the obstruction and causes progressive overinflation *(emphysema)*.

Diagnostic Evaluation. Bronchiolitis begins as a URI with serous nasal discharge that may be accompanied by mild fever. Otitis media and conjunctivitis may also be present. The child gradually develops increasing respiratory distress with tachypnea, paroxysmal cough, irritability, wheezing, retractions, crackles, dyspnea, and diminished breath sounds (Box 46-9). Chest radiographs show hyperaeration and areas of consolidation that are difficult to differentiate from bacterial pneumonia.

Apnea may be the first recognized indicator of RSV infection in very young infants. Severe disease may be followed by a rise in arterial carbon dioxide tension ($Paco_2$) (hypercapnia), leading to respiratory acidosis and hypoxemia. Positive identification of RSV is accomplished by enzyme-linked immunosorbent assay (ELISA) or rapid immunofluorescent antibody (IFA) from direct aspiration of nasal secretions or nasopharyngeal washings (see Respiratory Secretion and Throat Specimens, Chapter 45).

Therapeutic Management. Bronchiolitis is treated symptomatically with high humidity, adequate fluid intake, and rest. Most children with bronchiolitis can be managed at home. Hospitalization is usually recommended for children with complicating conditions, such as underlying lung or heart disease; with associated debilitated states; when adequacy of the caregiver is questioned; or when the child is tachypneic, has marked retractions, seems listless, or has a history of poor fluid intake. Mist therapy is generally combined with oxygen by hood or tent in concentrations sufficient to alleviate dyspnea and hypoxia, after which mist alone is continued for mild dyspnea. Fluids by mouth may be contraindicated because of tachypnea, weakness, and fatigue; therefore IV fluids are preferred until the acute crisis of the disease has passed.

Clinical assessments, noninvasive oxygen monitoring, and blood gas values guide therapy. Medical therapy for bronchiolitis is controversial. Bronchodilators, corticosteroids, cough suppressants, and antibiotics have not proved to be effective in uncomplicated disease and are not recommended for routine use. Corticosteroids, theophylline, and furosemide have all been used for intubated and ventilated infants and children.

Prevention of RSV Infection. Two drugs are currently available to use prophylactically to prevent RSV infections. *RSV immune globulin* (*RSV-IGIV* or RespiGam) is an IV preparation of immunoglobulin G that provides neutralizing antibodies against RSV. This drug is given in a monthly IV infusion lasting 3 to 4 hours. However, the volume of fluids administered with this drug may not be well tolerated by pediatric patients whose lung function is already compromised, and it interferes with the measles-mumps-rubella and varicella vaccines. In 1998 the Food and Drug Administration (FDA) approved the *monoclonal antibody, palivizumab (Synagis)*. This drug is preferred for most high risk children because it can be given monthly in an IM injection, it does not interfere with the measles-mumps-rubella vaccine and varicella vaccine, and it has none of the complications associated with IV administration of human immune globulin products (American Academy of Pediatrics, 2000). The main adverse effect of this drug is pain and mild transient erythema at the injection site.

Recommendations by the American Academy of Pediatrics (2000) for the use of palivizumab or RSV-IGIV are as follows:

1. Infants and children younger than 2 years of age with chronic lung disease (CLD) who have received medical therapy for CLD within 6 months before the anticipated RSV season. Patients with more severe CLD may benefit from prophylaxis for 2 RSV seasons.
2. Infants born at 32 weeks of gestation or earlier without CLD also may benefit from RSV prophylaxis. Infants born at 28 weeks' gestation or earlier may benefit from

Box 46-9

Signs and Symptoms of Respiratory Syncytial Virus

INITIAL

Rhinorrhea
Pharyngitis
Coughing/sneezing
Wheezing
Possible ear or eye drainage
Fever

WITH PROGRESSION OF ILLNESS

Increased coughing and wheezing
Air hunger
Tachypnea and retractions
Cyanosis

SEVERE ILLNESS

Tachypnea, greater than 70 breaths/min
Listlessness
Apneic spells
Poor air exchange; poor breath sounds

prophylaxis up to 12 months of age. Infants of 29 to 32 weeks' gestation may benefit most up to 6 months of age. Duration of prophylaxis should be individualized according to the duration of the RSV season.

3. Neither drug is licensed for patients with congenital heart disease (CHD). They are contraindicated for patients with cyanotic CHD; however, patients with CLD, born prematurely, who meet the recommended criteria and who have asymptomatic acyanotic CHD may benefit from prophylaxis.
4. Children with severe immunodeficiencies (e.g., severe combined immunodeficiency or acquired immunodeficiency syndrome) may benefit from prophylaxis.
5. Prophylaxis for RSV should be initiated at the onset of the RSV season and terminated at the end of the season.
6. In hospitalized infants the major means to prevent RSV disease is strict observance of infection control practice and segregation of RSV-infected infants.

Nursing Care Management. Children admitted to the hospital with suspected RSV infection may be assigned separate rooms or grouped with other RSV-infected children. A variety of infection control procedures have been employed over the years, the most important of which is consistent handwashing and not touching the nasal mucosa or conjunctiva. The routine use of gowns and masks has not been shown to be of additional benefit, although gowns may help diminish the potential for fomite spread during close contact when infectious secretions may contaminate clothing. Other isolation procedures of potential benefit are those aimed at diminishing the number of hospital personnel, visitors, and uninfected patients in contact with the child. Another measure includes making patient assignments so that nurses assigned to children with RSV are not taking care of other patients who may be considered high risk.

If patient care warrants opening the tent while the small-particle aerosol generator (SPAG) is running, the nurse should shut the machine off and wait a few moments before opening the tent. Gloves and gowns are not essential, because dermal absorption is negligible. Scavenger devices are commercially available to help decrease the escape of aerosolized ribavirin.

NURSE ALERT • Pregnant health care providers should not care for a child receiving ribavirin.

Children receiving RespiGam should be monitored for symptoms of fluid volume overload during IV administration. Antibodies in RespiGam may interfere with the immune response to live virus vaccines (e.g., mumps, rubella, measles, and chickenpox); therefore these vaccines should be deferred for 9 months after RespiGam infusion (American Academy of Pediatrics, 2000). Atraumatic measures should also be used to alleviate pain associated with IV and IM injections (Atraumatic Care box).

Pneumonias

Pneumonia, inflammation of the pulmonary parenchyma, is common in childhood but occurs more often in infancy and early childhood. Clinically, pneumonia may occur either as a primary disease or as a complication of another illness. Morphologically, pneumonias are recognized as follows:

Lobar pneumonia—All or a large segment of one or more pulmonary lobes is involved. When both lungs are affected, it is known as bilateral or double pneumonia.

Bronchopneumonia—Begins in the terminal bronchioles, which become clogged with mucopurulent exudate to form consolidated patches in nearby lobules; also called lobular pneumonia.

Interstitial pneumonia—The inflammatory process is more or less confined within the alveolar walls (interstitium) and the peribronchial and interlobular tissues.

Pneumonitis is a localized acute inflammation of the lung without the toxemia associated with lobar pneumonia.

The pneumonias are more often classified according to morphology, clinical form, and etiologic agent: viral, atypical (mycoplasmal), bacterial, or aspiration of foreign substances (see Aspiration Pneumonia, p. 1210). Pneumonia may also be caused by histomycosis, coccidioidomycosis, and other fungi. The causative agent is identified from the clinical history, the child's age, the general health history, the physical examination, radiography, and the laboratory examination.

Viral Pneumonia. Viral pneumonias occur more commonly than bacterial pneumonias and are seen in children of all age groups. They are often associated with viral URIs, and RSV accounts for the largest percentage in infants. There are few clinical symptoms to distinguish between the responsible organisms, and differentiations between viruses can be made only by laboratory examination (Box 46-10).

The prognosis is generally good, although viral infections of the respiratory tract render the affected child more susceptible to secondary bacterial invasion, especially when there is denuded bronchial mucosa. Treatment is usually symptomatic and includes measures to promote oxygenation and comfort, such as oxygen administration with cool mist, chest physiother-

Atraumatic Care

INTRAVENOUS RESPIGAM AND INTRAMUSCULAR PALIVIZUMAB

To reduce the pain of monthly intravenous (IV) infusions and intramuscular (IM) injections, apply EMLA cream to at least two possible venous sites (for IV insertion) 60 minutes or to the IM site 2½ hours before the procedure.

Box 46-10

General Signs of Pneumonia

Fever—Usually quite high

Respiratory

- **Cough**—Unproductive to productive with whitish sputum
- Tachypnea
- **Breath sounds**—Rhonchi or fine crackles
- Dullness with percussion
- Chest pain
- Retractions
- Nasal flaring
- Pallor to cyanosis (depends on severity)

Chest x-ray film—Diffuse or patchy infiltration with peribronchial distribution

Behavior—Irritable, restless, lethargic

Gastrointestinal—Anorexia, vomiting, diarrhea, abdominal pain apy and postural drainage, antipyretics for fever management, fluid intake, and family support. Although some authorities recommend antimicrobial therapy in the hope of reducing or preventing secondary bacterial infection, it is usually reserved for children in whom the presence of such infection is demonstrated by appropriate cultures.

Primary Atypical Pneumonia. Infection with *Mycoplasma pneumoniae* is the most common cause of pneumonia in children between ages 5 and 12 years. It occurs in the fall and winter months and is more prevalent where there are crowded living conditions.

Most affected persons recover from acute illness in 7 to 10 days with symptomatic treatment followed by a week of convalescence. Hospitalization is rarely necessary.

Bacterial Pneumonia. In children beyond the neonatal period, bacterial pneumonias display distinct clinical patterns that facilitate their differentiation from other forms of pneumonia, and individual microorganisms produce a distinct clinical picture. Onset is abrupt and is generally preceded by a viral infection that disturbs the natural defense mechanisms of the upper respiratory tract and allows the pathogenic bacteria normally harbored in the upper passages to increase in number.

Children with bacterial pneumonia appear ill and exhibit both general and localized physical findings. Symptoms and signs include fever, malaise, rapid and shallow respirations, cough, and chest pain that is often exaggerated by deep breathing. The pain may be referred to the abdomen and confused with appendicitis. Chills commonly occur, and meningeal symptoms *(meningism)* are also common.

Most older children with pneumococcal pneumonia can be treated at home, especially if the condition is recognized and treatment initiated early. Antibiotic therapy, bed rest, liberal oral intake of fluid, and administration of an antipyretic for fever constitute the principal therapeutic measures. Hospitalization is indicated when pleural effusion or empyema accompanies the disease and is mandatory for children with staphylococcal pneumonia. Pneumonia in the infant or young child is best treated in the hospital, because the course of illness is more variable and complications are more common in very young patients. Fluids are usually given intravenously, and oxygen therapy may be required if the child is in respiratory distress.

At present the classic features and clinical course of pneumonia are rarely seen because of early and vigorous antibiotic and supportive therapy. However, a large number of children, especially infants, with staphylococcal pneumonia develop empyema, pyopneumothorax, or tension pneumothorax. Acute otitis media and pleural effusion are also common in children with pneumococcal pneumonia. A thoracentesis may be performed to remove fluid in the pleural cavity, to obtain a culture of the fluid, and to instill antibiotics directly into the pleural space. Nonpurulent effusions do not require surgical drainage. Continuous closed-chest drainage is instituted when purulent fluid is aspirated, a common finding in staphylococcal infections.

Prognosis. The prognosis for pneumococcal infections is generally good, with rapid recovery when they are recognized and treated early. Streptococcal infections vary in duration but usually resolve spontaneously. The course of staphylococcal pneumonia is generally prolonged. The prognosis varies with the length of illness before treatment is begun, although early recognition and treatment are usually effective. Complications of bacterial pneumonia include pleural effusion, empyema, and tension pneumothorax.

Prevention. Pneumococcal conjugate vaccines are a significant new contribution to the potential control of pneumococcal disease in young children. The American Academy of Pediatrics now recommends that Prevnar be administered to all children at 2, 4, and 6 months of age, with a booster given at 12 to 15 months (see Immunizations, Chapter 36) (Overturf, 2000).

Nursing Care Management. Nursing care of the child with pneumonia is primarily supportive and symptomatic but necessitates thorough respiratory assessment and administration of oxygen and antibiotics. The child's respiratory rate and status, as well as general disposition and level of activity, are frequently assessed. Isolation procedures are instituted according to hospital policy; rest and conservation of energy are encouraged by relief of physical and psychologic stress. The child is disturbed as little as possible by clustering care to encourage the child's regular sleep cycle. If the cough is disturbing, judicious use of antitussives, especially before rest times and meals, is often helpful. To prevent dehydration, fluids are often administered intravenously during the acute phase. Oral fluids, if allowed, are given cautiously to avoid aspiration and to decrease the possibility of aggravating a fatiguing cough.

Children may be placed in a mist tent with oxygen. Cool mist moistens the airways and provides a cool atmosphere that aids in temperature reduction. Children often require frequent clothing and linen changes to prevent chilling in the damp atmosphere. They are usually comfortable in a semierect position but should be allowed to determine the position of comfort. Lying on the affected side (if pneumonia is unilateral) splints the chest on that side and reduces the pleural rubbing that often causes discomfort. Fever is usually controlled by administration of antipyretic drugs as prescribed, and temperature is monitored regularly.

Vital signs and breath sounds are monitored to assess the progress of the disease and to detect early signs of complications. Children with ineffectual cough or those with difficulty handling secretions, especially infants, will require suctioning to maintain a patent airway. A simple bulb syringe is usually sufficient for clearing the nares and nasopharynx of infants, but mechanical suction should be readily available if needed. Older children can usually handle secretions without assistance. Postural drainage and chest physiotherapy are generally prescribed every 4 hours or more often, depending on the child's condition.

The hospitalized child is apprehensive, and the treatments and tests are frightening and stress producing. Reducing anxiety and apprehension reduces psychologic distress in the child, and when the child is more relaxed, the respiratory efforts are lessened. Easing respiratory efforts makes the child less apprehensive, and encouraging the presence of the caregiver provides the child with a customary source of comfort and support.

The family also needs support. The child's dry, hacking cough can be tiring for the parents because it often disturbs the child's and family's sleep. Parents are kept informed of the child's progress and taught appropriate home care, such as use of a nasal aspirator and administration of antibiotics.*

*Community and home care instructions for administration of medication and nasal aspiration are available in Wong DL, Hess CS: ***Wong and Whaley's clinical manual of pediatric nursing***, ed 5, St Louis, 2000, Mosby.

OTHER INFECTIONS OF THE RESPIRATORY TRACT

Pertussis (Whooping Cough)

Pertussis (whooping cough) is an acute respiratory infection caused by *Bordetella pertussis* that occurs chiefly in children younger than 4 years of age who have not been immunized. It is highly contagious and is particularly threatening in young infants, who have a high morbidity and mortality rate. (See Chapter 36 for immunizations.) The incidence is highest in the spring and summer months, and a single attack confers lifetime immunity. Pertussis vaccine is effective, but the immunity diminishes with time after the initial infection or immunization. A small number of immunized adolescents may develop an asymptomatic case of pertussis.

Tuberculosis (TB)

TB is an ancient disease that although controlled in most developed countries, remains a health hazard and the leading cause of death throughout many parts of the world. After decades of steady decline, the incidence of TB in the United States is increasing. Data from 1993 indicate that 38% of all cases of tuberculosis occurred in individuals 25 to 44 years of age (Jackson and McLeod, 1998). The increases are attributed in part to the interaction of foreign-born persons immigrating to the United States, the increase in homelessness, and the HIV epidemic (Hoffman, Kelly, and Futterman, 1996).

TB is caused by *Mycobacterium tuberculosis.* Children are susceptible to both the human *(M. tuberculosis)* and the bovine (*M. bovis*) organisms. In parts of the world where tuberculosis in cattle is not controlled or pasteurization of milk is not practiced, the bovine type is a common source of infection. Although the causative agent is the tubercle bacillus, other factors influence the degree to which the organism is able to produce an altered state in the host, including heredity (resistance to the infection may be genetically transmitted), gender (higher in adolescent girls), age (lower resistance in infants, higher incidence during adolescence), stress (emotional or physical), nutritional state, and intercurrent infection (especially HIV, measles, and pertussis). Multidrug-resistant strains of *M. tuberculosis* have caused outbreaks in hospitals.

The source of infection in children is usually an infected member of the household. It can also be a baby-sitter, domestic worker, or frequent visitor to the household. The lung is the usual portal of entry in humans; the organism *M. bovis* enters less often by ingestion. In the lungs a proliferation of epithelial cells surround and encapsulate the multiplying bacilli in an attempt to wall off the invading organisms, thus forming the typical tubercle. Extension of the primary lesion at the original site causes progressive tissue destruction as it spreads within the lung, discharges material from foci to other areas of the lungs (e.g., bronchi or pleura), or produces pneumonia. Erosion of blood vessels by the primary lesion can cause widespread dissemination of the tubercle bacillus to near and distant sites *(miliary tuberculosis)*. Areas that are commonly affected include lymph nodes, meninges, and bone.

Diagnostic Evaluation. Diagnosis is based on information derived from physical examination, history, reaction to a tuberculin test, radiographic examinations, and organism cultures. In addition, it must be determined whether or not the lesion is in the active, quiescent, or healed stage. Clinical manifestations are listed in Box 46-11.

The *tuberculin test* is the single most important test of whether a child has been infected with the tubercle bacillus. The recommended procedure is the Mantoux test, which uses purified protein derivative (PPD). The standard dose is 5 tuberculin units in 0.1 ml of solution, injected intradermally. Recommendations for TB skin testing of children are listed in Box 46-12. Routine testing of children with no risk factors residing in communities with a low prevalence of TB is not indicated (American Academy of Pediatrics, 2000).

A *positive reaction* indicates that the individual has been infected and has developed a sensitivity to the protein of the tubercle bacillus; however, it does not confirm the presence of active disease. Once individuals react positively, they will always react positively. A previously negative reaction that becomes positive indicates that the person has been infected since the last test. Guidelines for interpreting the Mantoux skin test are listed in Box 46-13.

NURSE ALERT • The American Academy of Pediatrics (2000) recommends that Mantoux skin test results be read by health care professionals.

Therapeutic Management. Medical management of TB lesions in children consists of adequate nutrition, drug therapy, general supportive measures, prevention of unnecessary exposure to other infections that further compromise the body's defenses, prevention of reinfection, and sometimes surgical procedures. Hospitalization is seldom necessary, except for the most serious forms of the disease. Most children with TB receive their nursing care in ambulatory settings, outpatient departments, schools, and public health settings.

Recommended drug therapy for treating tuberculosis usually includes combinations of the following drugs: isoniazid (INH), rifampin, and pyrazinamide (PZA). The American Academy of Pediatrics (2000) recommends a 6-month regimen

Box 46-11

Clinical Manifestations of Tuberculosis

Extremely variable

May be asymptomatic or produce a broad range of symptoms:

- Fever
- Malaise
- Anorexia
- Weight loss
- Cough may or may not be present (progresses slowly over weeks to months)
- Aching pain and tightness in the chest
- Hemoptysis (rare)

With progression:

- Respiratory rate increases
- Poor expansion of lung on the affected side
- Diminished breath sounds and crackles
- Dullness to percussion
- Fever persists
- Generalized symptoms are manifested
- Pallor, anemia, weakness, and weight loss

Box 46-12

Revised Tuberculin Skin Test Recommendations*

CHILDREN FOR WHOM IMMEDIATE SKIN TESTING IS INDICATED

Contacts of persons with confirmed or suspected infectious tuberculosis (TB) (contact investigation); this includes children identified as contacts of family members or associates in jail or prison in the last 5 years.

Children with radiographic or clinical findings suggesting TB.

Children immigrating from endemic countries (e.g., Asia, Middle East, Africa, Latin America).

Children with travel histories to endemic countries and/or significant contact with indigenous persons from such countries.

CHILDREN WHO SHOULD BE TESTED ANNUALLY FOR TB†

Children infected with human immunodeficiency virus (HIV).

Incarcerated adolescents.

CHILDREN WHO SHOULD BE TESTED EVERY 2 TO 3 YEARS†

Children exposed to the following individuals: HIV infected, homeless, residents of nursing homes, institutionalized adolescents or adults, users of illicit drugs, incarcerated adolescents or adults, and migrant farm workers. This would include foster children with exposure to adults in the above high-risk groups.

CHILDREN WHO SHOULD BE CONSIDERED FOR TUBERCULIN SKIN TESTING AT AGES 4 TO 6 AND 11 TO 16 YEARS

Children whose parents immigrated (with unknown tuberculin skin test status) from regions of the world with high prevalence of TB. Continued potential exposure by travel to the endemic areas and/or household contact with persons from the endemic areas (with unknown tuberculin skin test status) should be an indication for repeat tuberculin skin testing.

Children without specific risk factors who reside in high-prevalence areas. In general, a high-risk neighborhood or community does not mean an entire city is at high risk; it is recognized that rates in any area of the city may vary by neighborhood, or even from block to block. Physicians should be aware of these patterns in determining the likelihood of exposure. Public health officials or local TB experts should help clinicians identify areas that have appreciable TB rates.

RISK FOR PROGRESSION TO DISEASE

Children with other medical risk factors, including diabetes mellitus, chronic renal failure, malnutrition, and congenital or acquired immunodeficiencies deserve special consideration; without recent exposure, these persons are not at increased risk of acquiring TB infection. Underlying immune deficiencies associated with these conditions theoretically would enhance the possibility for progression to severe disease. Initial histories of potential exposure to TB should be included for all of these patients. If these histories or local epidemiologic factors suggest a possibility of exposure, immediate and periodic tuberculin skin testing should be considered in these patients. An initial Mantoux TB skin test should be performed before initiation of immunosuppressive therapy in any child with an underlying condition that necessitates immunosuppressive therapy.

From American Academy of Pediatrics, Committee on Infectious Diseases, Pickering L, editor: *2000 Red Book: report of the Committee on Infectious Diseases,* ed 25, Elk Grove Village, IL, 2000, The Academy.
*Bacille Calmette-Guérin (BCG) immunization is not a contraindication to tuberculin skin testing.
†Initial tuberculin skin testing initiated at the time of diagnosis or circumstance.

consisting of INH, rifampin, and PZA given daily for the first 2 months, and INH and rifampin given twice weekly (if administration of the drugs is observed directly) for the remaining 4 months. If a child is suspected of having a multidrug-resistant tuberculosis, either ethambutol or streptomycin (IM injection only) is added. Preventive therapy is intended to keep latent infection from progressing and to prevent initial infection in persons in high risk situations. The most commonly used drug for this is INH for 9 months, or up to 12 months for the HIV-infected child.

Surgical Procedures. Surgery may be required to remove the source of infection in tissues that are inaccessible to drug therapy or that are destroyed by the disease. Orthopedic procedures for correction of bone deformities, bronchoscopy for removal of a tuberculous granulomatous polyp, or resection of a portion of a diseased lung may also be performed.

Prognosis. Most children recover from primary TB infection and are often unaware of its presence. However, very young children have a higher incidence of disseminated disease. It is a serious disease during the first 2 years of life, during adolescence, and in children who are HIV positive. Except in cases of tuberculous meningitis, death seldom occurs in treated children. Antibiotic therapy has decreased the death rate and the hematogenous spread from primary lesions.

Prevention. The only certain means to prevent TB is to avoid contact with the tubercle bacillus. Maintaining an optimum state of health with adequate nutrition and avoiding fatigue and debilitating infections promote natural resistance but do not prevent infection. Pasteurization and routine testing of milk and elimination of diseased cattle have reduced the incidence of bovine tuberculosis.

Limited immunity can be produced by administration of bacille Calmette-Guérin (BCG), vaccine containing bovine bacilli with reduced virulence. The freshly prepared vaccine, injected intradermally, produces a definite although incomplete (about 50%) protection against TB. The distribution of the vaccine is controlled by local or state health departments, but the vaccine is not used extensively, even in areas with a high prevalence of disease.

Nursing Care Management. Most children with pulmonary TB have non-infectious disease; therefore they seldom need to be isolated and can be hospitalized on an open ward if they are receiving drug therapy. Children and adolescents with infectious pulmonary TB should be on isolation precautions until effective drug therapy has been initiated.

Box 46-13

Definition of Positive Mantoux Skin Test (5 TU-PPD) in Children*

INDURATION ≥ 5 MM

Children in close contact with persons who have known or suspected infectious cases of tuberculosis (TB):
- Households with active or previously active cases if (1) treatment cannot be verified as adequate before exposure, (2) treatment was initiated after period of child's contact, or (3) reactivation is suspected

Children suspected to have TB disease:
- Chest x-ray film consistent with active or previously active tuberculosis
- Clinical evidence of TB

Children with immunosuppressive conditions† or human immunodeficiency virus (HIV) infection

INDURATION ≥ 10 MM

Children at increased risk of dissemination from:
- Young age: less than 4 years of age
- Other medical risk factors, including Hodgkin disease, lymphoma, diabetes mellitus, chronic renal failure, and malnutrition

Children with increased environmental exposure:
- Born, or whose parents were born, in regions of the world where TB is highly prevalent
- Frequently exposed to adults who are HIV infected, home less, users of intravenous and other street drugs, residents of nursing homes, incarcerated or institutionalized persons, and migrant farm workers

INDURATION ≥ 15 MM

Children 4 years of age or older without any risk factors

From American Academy of Pediatrics, Committee on Infectious Diseases, Pickering L, editor: *2000 Red Book: report of the Committee on Infectious Diseases*, ed 25, Elk Grove Village, IL, 2000, The Academy.
*These recommendations should apply regardless of whether Bacille Calmette-Guérin (BCG) has been previously administered.
†Including immunosuppressive doses of corticosteroids.

Asymptomatic children are able to lead an essentially unrestricted life. They can and should attend school (or preschool), but older children are restricted from vigorous activities such as competitive games and contact sports during the active stage of primary TB. They should be protected from stresses, including parental anxieties, the tendency toward overprotection, and pressures regarding nutritional intake. The regular immunization schedule should be continued. Care should be taken to maintain an optimum health status with proper diet, adequate rest, and avoidance of infection.

Nurses assume several important roles in management of the disease, including assisting with radiographic examinations, performing skin tests, and obtaining specimens for laboratory examination. Skin tests must be performed correctly and the reaction determined in 48 to 72 hours. Sputum specimens are difficult or impossible to obtain in an infant or young child, because they swallow any mucus coughed from the lower respiratory tract. Therefore the best means for obtaining material for smears or culture is by *gastric washing* (i.e., aspiration of lavaged contents from the fasting stomach). The procedure is carried out and the specimen obtained early in the morning before the customary breakfast time.

Because the success of therapy depends on compliance with the drug regimen, parents are instructed regarding the importance of giving the medication as often and for as long as it is ordered (see Compliance, Chapter 45). Some families may require direct observation to ensure compliance.

PULMONARY DYSFUNCTION CAUSED BY NONINFECTIOUS IRRITANTS

Foreign Body (FB) Aspiration

Small children characteristically explore matter with their mouths and are prone to aspirate an FB into the air passages. Aspiration of an FB can occur at any age but is most common in children under 3 years of age. Severity is determined by the location, type of object aspirated, and extent of obstruction. For example, dry vegetable matter such as a seed, nut, or piece of carrot or popcorn, that does not dissolve and that may swell when wet, creates a particularly difficult problem. The high fat content of potato chips and peanuts may cause the added risk of lipoid pneumonia. "Fun foods" of any kind are among the worst offenders. Offending foods in the order of frequency of aspiration are as follows: hot dog, round candy, peanut or other nut, grape, cookie or biscuit, other meat, carrot, apple, and peanut butter. Round foods are the most common offenders. The first four items together constitute more than 40% of all aspirated food items. A sharp or irritating object produces irritation and edema. A round, pliable object that does not readily break apart is more likely to occlude an airway than an object with a different shape. Latex balloons (uninflated, inflated, or in broken pieces) are especially hazardous. A small object may cause little if any pathologic change, whereas an object of sufficient size to obstruct a passage can produce various changes, including atelectasis, emphysema, inflammation, and abscess.

Diagnostic Evaluation. The diagnosis of FB aspiration is usually suspected on the basis of the history and physical signs. Initially an FB in the air passages produces choking, gagging, wheezing, or coughing. If obstruction progresses, the child's face may become livid, and if the obstruction is total, the child can become unconscious and die of asphyxiation. If obstruction is partial, hours, days, or even weeks may pass without symptoms. Secondary symptoms are related to the anatomic area in which the object is lodged and are usually caused by a persistent respiratory infection distal to the obstruction. An FB is always a possibility in acute or chronic pulmonary lesions. Often, by the time secondary symptoms appear, the parents have forgotten the initial episode of coughing and gagging.

The most common symptoms observed in children brought to medical attention are stridor, wheezing, sternal retraction, and cough. When the object is lodged in the larynx, there is inability to speak or breathe. An object in the bronchi produces cough, decreased airway entry, wheezing, and dyspnea. A nonobstructive, nonirritating object may cause few symptoms; an obstructive object quickly produces pathologic changes; a slight obstruction may be evidenced only by a wheeze.

Radiographic examination reveals opaque FBs but may be of limited use in localizing vegetable matter. Bronchoscopy is required for definitive diagnosis of objects in the larynx and trachea. Fluoroscopic examination is a valuable aid in detecting and localizing FBs in the bronchi.

Therapeutic Management. FB aspiration may result in life-threatening airway obstruction, especially in infants because of the small diameters of their airways. Current recommendations for the emergency treatment of the choking child include the use of abdominal thrusts for children over 1 year of age and back blows and chest thrusts for children less than 1 year of age (see Airway Obstruction, p. 1230).

An FB is rarely coughed up spontaneously; therefore it must be removed instrumentally by direct laryngoscopy or bronchoscopy. This should be carried out as soon as possible, because the progressive local inflammatory process triggered by the foreign material hampers removal; a chemical pneumonia soon develops; and vegetable matter begins to macerate within a few days, causing it to be even more difficult to remove. After removal of the FB, the child is placed in a high-humidity atmosphere, and any secondary infection is treated with appropriate antibiotics.

Nursing Care Management. A major role of nurses caring for the child who has aspirated an FB is to recognize the signs of FB aspiration and implement immediate measures to relieve the obstruction.

All persons working with children should be prepared to deal effectively with aspiration of an FB. Choking on food or other material should not be fatal. Two very simple procedures—back blows and the Heimlich maneuver—can be used by both health professionals and lay persons and can save lives. It is the obligation of nurses to learn these techniques and teach them to parents and other groups.

To aid a child who is choking, nurses need to recognize the signs of distress. Not every child who gags or coughs while eating is truly choking.

NURSE ALERT • The child in distress (1) cannot speak, (2) becomes cyanotic, and (3) collapses. These three signs indicate that the child is truly choking and requires immediate action. The child can die within 4 minutes. Follow-up care after the FB is removed includes chest physiotherapy as indicated, monitoring for respiratory distress, and education of the parents.

Prevention. Small children should not be allowed access to enticing small objects that they might place in their mouth. Rubber balloons are high risk items for children; Mylar balloons are the only safe variety for children. Unlikely items (e.g., foil tabs from soft drink containers, Band-Aids applied to fingers of infants or very small children, plastic tabs from protective coverings on containers and from price tags on clothing) can be hazardous. Peanut butter, a staple in the diet of children, should never be given to a child unless it is spread thinly on bread or a cracker. A spoonful of peanut butter can obstruct the airway and stick to mucous membranes, becoming difficult or impossible for the child to dislodge.

Nurses, as child advocates, are in a position to teach prevention in a variety of settings. They can educate parents singly or in groups about the hazards of FB aspiration in relation to the developmental level of their children, and encourage parents to teach their children safety. Parents teach by example; therefore they should be cautioned about behaviors that their children might imitate (e.g., holding foreign objects such as pins, nails, and toothpicks, in their lips or mouth). Prevention based on the child's age is discussed in Chapters 36 and 37.

Aspiration Pneumonia

Aspiration of fluid or food substances is a particular hazard in the child who has difficulty with swallowing; who is unable to swallow because of paralysis, weakness, debility, congenital anomalies, or absent cough reflex; or who is force-fed, especially while crying or breathing rapidly. In addition to fluids, food, vomitus, and nasopharyngeal secretions, other substances that cause pneumonia are hydrocarbons, lipids, talcum powder, and barium.

Nursing Care Management. Care of the child with aspiration pneumonia is the same as that described for the child with pneumonia from other causes; however, the major thrust of nursing care is aimed at prevention of aspiration. Proper feeding techniques should be carried out for weak, debilitated, and uncooperative children, and preventive measures are used to prevent aspiration of any material that might enter the nasopharynx.

Oily nose drops and oil-based vitamin preparations are not appropriate for infants and small children. Solvents, lighter fluid, and other hydrocarbon substances should be kept away from older infants and small children, who are apt to put anything in their mouths and who may be attracted by the slightly sweet smell. Talcum powder should not be used; if used, careful application (e.g., placing it on the caregiver's hand and then the child's skin) and proper storage are essential.

Infants and debilitated children should be positioned on the right side after feedings to minimize the possibility of aspirating vomitus or regurgitated feeding.

Acute (Adult) Respiratory Distress Syndrome (ARDS)

ARDS poses a major threat to a child recovering from a primary insult. It is a syndrome characterized by respiratory distress and hypoxemia that occur within 72 hours of a serious injury or surgery in a person with previously normal lungs.

The hallmark of ARDS is increased permeability of the alveolar-capillary membrane that results in pulmonary edema. The lungs become stiff, gas diffusion is impaired, and eventually there is bronchiolar mucosal swelling and congestive atelectasis. Surfactant secretion is reduced, and the atelectasis and fluid-filled alveoli provide an excellent medium for bacterial growth. The criteria for diagnosis of ARDS in children are an acute antecedent illness or injury, acute respiratory distress or failure, no evidence of prior cardiopulmonary disease, and diffuse bilateral infiltrates evidenced on chest radiography.

Treatment involves supportive measures, such as prevention of infection, maintenance of vascular pressure and cardiac output, adequate nutrition, comfort measures, positioning to improve functional residual capacity, and psychologic support. Definitive therapy is directed toward improvement of oxygenation. The use of endotracheal intubation and positive end-expiratory pressure (PEEP) may be required to ensure maximum oxygen delivery. Recent developments in the treatment of ARDS include: (1) medications to interrupt the formation or activation of mediators contributing to progression of intrapulmonary shunting and lung injury, such as nonsteroidal antiinflammatory drugs (NSAIDs); (2) immunotherapy with monoclonal antibodies that work against the specific toxins causing the lung injury; and (3) human and artificial surfactant to reduce the severity of and sequelae from RDS.

The prognosis for ARDS varies. Some children recover completely, whereas others are left with varying degrees of pulmonary dysfunction.

Nursing care involves careful monitoring of cardiac output, heart rate, perfusion, capillary filling, and urine output, as well as assessment of respiratory status. Blood gas analysis and pulse oximetry are important evaluation tools. Respiratory distress is a frightening situation for both the child and the parents, and attention to their psychologic needs is a major element in the care of these children.

Inhalation Injury: Smoke and Carbon Dioxide

A number of noxious substances that may be inhaled are toxic to humans. They are primarily products of incomplete combustion and are believed to cause more deaths from fires than flame injuries. The severity of the injury depends on the nature of the substances generated by the material being burned, whether the victim is confined in a closed space, and the duration of contact. Inhaled substances produce injuries (1) locally by irritation, inflammation, and damage to pulmonary tissues or (2) systemically.

Local Injury. A variety of gases may be generated during the combustion of materials such as clothing, furniture, and floor coverings. The synthetic materials are especially toxic. Irritant gases such as nitrous oxide or carbon dioxide combine with water in the lungs to form corrosive acids; aldehydes cause denaturation of proteins, cellular damage, and edema of pulmonary tissues.

Possible inhalation injury is suspected when there is a history of flames in a closed space, whether burns are present or not. Sooty material around the nose or in the sputum; singed nasal hairs; or mucosal burns of the nose, lips, mouth, or throat are all signs that the affected person demands observation for possible pulmonary injury from inhalants. A hoarse voice and cough, inspiratory and expiratory stridor, and signs of respiratory distress are further evidence of airway involvement.

Systemic Injury. Gases that are nontoxic to the airways (e.g., carbon monoxide [CO] and hydrogen cyanide) can cause injury and death by interfering with or inhibiting cellular respiration. CO is responsible for more than half of all fatal inhalation poisonings in the United States. It is a colorless, odorless gas with an affinity for hemoglobin 230 times greater than that of oxygen. When it enters the bloodstream, CO combines readily with hemoglobin to form carboxyhemoglobin (COHb). Because it is released less readily, tissue hypoxia reaches dangerous levels before oxygen is available to meet tissue needs.

NURSE ALERT • In carbon monoxide poisoning, the oxygen saturation ($Sa{O_2}$) obtained by pulse oximetry will be normal because the device measures only oxygenated and deoxygenated hemoglobin; it does not measure dysfunctional hemoglobin, such as COHb.

CO is produced by incomplete combustion of carbon or carbonaceous material such as wood or charcoal. Accidental CO poisoning is most often the result of exposure to fumes from heaters or smoke from structural fires. Poorly ventilated recreational vehicles with improperly operated or maintained gas lamps or stoves, and cooking in underventilated areas with charcoal grills or hibachis are also common causes.

The signs and symptoms of CO poisoning are secondary to tissue hypoxia and vary with the level of COHb. Mild manifestations include headache, visual disturbances, irritability, and nausea; more severe intoxication causes confusion, hallucinations, ataxia, and coma. The bright, cherry red lips and skin often described are less often observed; pallor and cyanosis are seen more commonly.

Therapeutic Management. When smoke inhalation injury is suspected, the patient is given humidified 100% oxygen as quickly as possible, and baseline arterial blood gases and COHb levels are obtained. Surprisingly, arterial oxygen partial pressure ($Pa{O_2}$) may be within normal limits unless there is marked respiratory depression. If CO poisoning is confirmed, 100% oxygen is continued until COHb levels fall to the nontoxic range of about 10%. Artificial ventilation may be implemented in selected cases. Where a hyperbaric oxygen chamber is available, the breakdown of the COHb bond is greatly accelerated.

Respiratory distress may occur early in the course of smoke inhalation as a result of hypoxia, or patients who are breathing well on admission may suddenly develop respiratory distress. Intubation and/or tracheostomy equipment should be available at the bedside. Transient edema of the airways can occur at any level in the tracheobronchial tree. Assessment and localization of the obstruction should be accomplished before severe swelling of the head, neck, or oropharynx occurs. Intubation is often necessary when: (1) severe burns in the area of the nose, mouth, and face increase the likelihood of developing oropharyngeal edema and obstruction; (2) vocal cord edema causes obstruction; (3) the patient has difficulty handling secretions; and (4) progressive respiratory distress requires artificial ventilation. Controversy surrounds tracheostomy, but many prefer this procedure when the obstruction is proximal to the larynx and reserve nasotracheal intubation for lower tract involvement.

Use of corticosteroids, although controversial, may be of value in reducing edema, and bronchodilators are often given intravenously or by nebulizer. Broad-spectrum antibiotics are sometimes administered prophylactically, but this practice is also controversial.

Nursing Care Management. Nursing care of the child with inhalation injury is the same as that for any child with respiratory distress. Vital signs and other respiratory assessments are performed often, and the pulmonary status is carefully observed and maintained. Pulmonary physiotherapy is usually part of the therapeutic program, as is mechanical ventilation, if needed.

In addition to the observation and management of the physical aspects of inhalation injury, the nurse also deals with the psychologic needs of a frightened child and distraught parents. As with any accidental injury, the parents feel overwhelming guilt, even when the injury occurred through no fault of their own. Parents need support, reassurance, and information regarding the child's condition, treatment, and progress.

Passive Smoking

Numerous investigations indicate that parental smoking is an important cause of morbidity in children. Children exposed to environmental tobacco smoke have an increased number of respiratory illnesses and reduced performance on pulmonary function tests. Parental cigarette smoking also increases asthma symptoms, trips to the emergency department and medication use, and impairs recovery after hospitalization for acute asthma (Abulhosm et al, 1997). Maternal cigarette smoking is associated with increased rates of respiratory illnesses (e.g., bronchitis, asthma, and otitis media) decreased fetal growth, increased stillbirths and preterm deliveries, and greater incidence of sudden infant death syndrome (SIDS). Recent studies also indicate that the amount of smoke exposure increases proportionally with the number of smokers in the home (Winkelstein, Tarzian, and Wood, 1997).

Nursing Care Management. Passive smoking during childhood may contribute to the development of chronic lung disease in the adult. Nurses and other health professionals need to include this information in all health assessments of children, especially those with respiratory and allergic illnesses. In families where smokers refuse to quit, house rules should be established for reducing smoke in the child's environment (Home Care box). Nurses should also inform caregivers of the health hazards of children's exposure to tobacco smoke*; set an example for children and families; and become advocates for "no smoking" ordinances in public places, and inclusion of health warnings about secondhand smoke on tobacco products.

LONG-TERM RESPIRATORY DYSFUNCTION

Asthma

Asthma is a chronic inflammatory disorder of the airways in which many cells (e.g., mast cells, eosinophils, and T lymphocytes) may play a role. In susceptible children, inflammation causes recurrent episodes of wheezing, breathlessness, chest tightness, and cough, especially at night or in the early morning. These asthma episodes are associated with airflow limitation or obstruction that is reversible either spontaneously or with treatment. The inflammation also causes an increase in bronchial hyperresponsiveness to a variety of stimuli (National Asthma Education and Prevention Program, 1997).

In 1995 the National Heart, Lung, and Blood Institute developed a classification of asthma based on the symptom indicators of disease severity. This classification includes four categories of asthma: mild intermittent, mild persistent, moderate persistent, and severe persistent. The mild intermittent category has the least number of symptoms; symptoms increase in frequency and/or intensity until the last category of severe persistent asthma (Box 46-14). These categories provide a stepwise approach to the pharmacologic management, environmental control, and educational interventions needed for each category (National Asthma Education and Prevention Program, 1997).

The incidence, severity, and mortality associated with asthma is increasing. These increases may result from increasing air pollution, poor access to medical care, and/or underdiagnosis and undertreatment. Asthma is the most common chronic disease of childhood, is the primary cause of school absences, and is responsible for a major proportion of pediatric admissions to emergency departments and hospitals.

Etiology. Studies of children with asthma indicate that allergy influences both the persistence and severity of the disease. In infants, however, a strong relationship exists between viral

*For a copy of the EPA report *Respiratory Health Effects of Passive Smoking,* contact CERI, U.S. EPA, 26 W. Martin Luther King Dr., Cincinnati, OH 45268; (513) 489-8190 or 1-800-490-9198; fax (513) 489-8695; website: www.epa.gov.

Home Care

HOUSE RULES FOR SMOKING HOUSEHOLDS

Maintain a smoke-free home.
Do not smoke around children.
Restrict smoking to an isolated, outdoor area.
Do not smoke in motor vehicles with children.
Do not smoke in rooms children use.
Do not allow visitors to smoke in the home.

Box 46-14

Asthma Severity Classification in Children 5 Years of Age and Older: Clinical Features*

STEP 4: SEVERE PERSISTENT ASTHMA
Continual symptoms
Frequent exacerbations
Frequent nighttime symptoms
Limited physical activity
Peak expiratory flow (PEF) or forced expiratory volume in 1 second (FEV_1) ≤ 60% of predicted value
PEF variability >30%

STEP 3: MODERATE PERSISTENT ASTHMA
Daily symptoms
Daily use of inhaled short-acting β_2-agonists
Exacerbations affect activity
Exacerbations ≥2 times a week
Exacerbations may last days
Nighttime symptoms >1 time a week
PEF/FEV_1 >60% to <80% of predicted value
PEF variability >30%

STEP 2: MILD PERSISTENT ASTHMA
Symptoms >2 times a week, but <1 time a day
Exacerbations may affect activity
Nighttime symptoms >2 times a month
PEF/FEV_1 ≥80% of predicted value
PEF variability 20% to 30%

STEP 1: MILD INTERMITTENT ASTHMA
Symptoms ≤2 times a week
Exacerbations brief (from a few hours to a few days); intensity may vary
Nighttime symptoms ≤2 times a month
Asymptomatic and normal PEF between exacerbations
PEF or FEV_1 ≥80% of predicted value
PEF variability <20%

From National Asthma Education and Prevention Program: *Expert Panel report II: guidelines for the diagnosis and management of asthma,* Bethesda, MD, 1997, National Heart, Lung, and Blood Institute.
*The presence of one clinical feature of severity is sufficient to place a patient in that category. An individual should be assigned to the most severe grade in which any feature occurs. The characteristics in this table are general and may overlap because asthma is highly variable. An individual's classification may change over time.

infections and asthma. Allergens play a less important role because it takes time for allergic sensitivity to develop. There is also a genetic predisposition for the development of an allergic response to common allergens in the air (National Asthma Education and Prevention Program, 1997). In addition to allergens, other substances and conditions can serve as triggers for asthma episodes (Box 46-15).

Although allergens play an important role in asthma, in some cases no allergic process can be detected. Other theories such as (1) a basic defect in the β-adrenergic receptors on leukocytes, and (2) increased cholinergic activity have been offered. However, most experts agree that asthma involves biochemical, immunologic, infectious, endocrine, and psychologic factors.

Pathophysiology. There is general agreement that inflammation contributes to heightened airway reactivity. The mechanisms responsible for airway inflammation are multiple, and the role that each mechanism plays varies from child to child and during the course of the disease. However, recognition of the importance of inflammation has made the use of antiinflammatory agents a key component of current asthma therapy.

Another important component of asthma is bronchospasm and obstruction. The mechanisms responsible for obstructive symptoms include (Fig. 46-3):

- Inflammation and edema of the mucous membranes
- Accumulation of tenacious secretions from mucous glands
- Spasm of the smooth muscle of the bronchi and bronchioles, which decreases the caliber of the bronchioles.

NURSE ALERT • Airflow is determined by the size of the airway lumen, degree of bronchial wall edema, mucus production, smooth muscle contraction, and muscle hypertrophy.

Box 46-15

Triggers Tending to Precipitate and/or Aggravate Asthmatic Exacerbations

Allergens
- Outdoors: trees, shrubs, weeds, grasses, molds, pollens, air pollution, spores
- Indoors: dust and/or dust mites, mold, cockroach antigen
  - Irritants: tobacco smoke, wood smoke, odors, sprays

Exposure to occupational chemicals
Exercise
Cold air
Changes in weather or temperature
Environmental change: moving to new home, starting new school, etc.
Colds and infections
Animals: cats, dogs, rodents, horses
Medications: aspirin, nonsteroidal antiinflammatory drugs (NSAIDs), antibiotics, beta blockers
Strong emotions: fear, anger, laughing, crying
Conditions: gastroesophageal reflux, tracheoesophageal fistula
Food additives: sulfite preservatives
Foods: nuts, milk/dairy products
Endocrine factors: menses, pregnancy, thyroid disease

Bronchial constriction is a normal reaction to foreign stimuli; but in the child with asthma it is abnormally severe, producing impaired respiratory function. The smooth muscle, arranged in spiral bundles around the airway, causes narrowing and shortening of the airway, which significantly increases airway resistance to airflow. Because the bronchi normally dilate and elongate during inspiration and contract and shorten on expiration, the respiratory difficulty is more pronounced during the expiratory phase of respiration.

Increased resistance in the airway causes forced expiration through the narrowed lumen. The volume of air trapped in the lungs increases as airways are functionally closed at a point between the alveoli and the lobar bronchi. This trapping of gas forces the individual to breathe at higher and higher lung volumes. Consequently, the person with asthma fights to inspire sufficient air. This expenditure of effort for breathing causes fatigue, decreased respiratory effectiveness, and increased oxygen consumption. The inspiration occurring at higher lung volumes hyperinflates the alveoli and reduces the effectiveness of the cough. As the severity of obstruction increases, there is a reduced alveolar ventilation with carbon dioxide retention; hypoxemia; respiratory acidosis; and eventually, respiratory failure.

Diagnostic Evaluation. Children with asthma may experience symptoms that range from acute episodes of shortness of breath, wheezing, and cough followed by a quiet period; to a relatively continuous pattern of chronic symptoms that fluctuate in severity (Box 46-16). An attack may develop gradually or appear abruptly and may be preceded by a URI. The age of the child is often a significant factor, because the first attack in most cases occurs between ages 3 and 8 years. In infancy an attack usually follows a respiratory infection. Some children may experience a prodromal itching at the front of the neck or over the upper part of the back just before an attack.

NURSE ALERT • Shortness of breath with air movement in the chest restricted to the point of absent breath sounds accompanied by a sudden rise in respiratory rate is an ominous sign indicating ventilatory failure and imminent asphyxia.

The diagnosis is determined primarily on the basis of clinical manifestations; history; physical examination; and to a lesser extent, laboratory tests. Radiographic examinations are used primarily to rule out other diseases and to evaluate co-existing

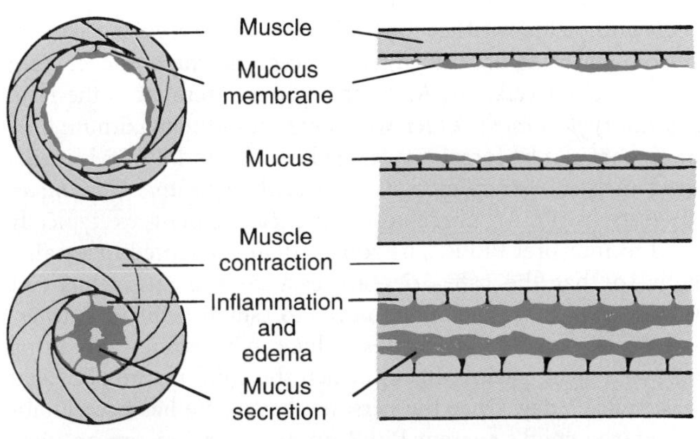

FIG. 46-3 • Mechanisms of obstruction in asthma.

Box 46-16

Clinical Manifestations of Asthma

COUGH

Hacking, paroxysmal, irritative, and nonproductive

Becomes rattling and productive of frothy, clear, gelatinous sputum

RESPIRATORY-RELATED SIGNS

Shortness of breath

Prolonged expiratory phase

Audible wheeze

May have a malar flush and red ears

Lips deep, dark red color

May progress to cyanosis of nail beds and/or circumoral cyanosis

Restlessness

Apprehension

Sweating may be prominent as the attack progresses

Older children may sit upright with shoulders in a hunched-over position, hands on the bed or chair, and arms braced

May speak with short, panting, broken phrases

CHEST

Hyperresonance on percussion

Coarse, loud breath sounds

Wheezes throughout the lung fields

Prolonged expiration

Crackles

Generalized inspiratory and expiratory wheezing; increasingly high pitched

WITH REPEATED EPISODES

Barrel chest

Elevated shoulders

Use of accessory muscles of respiration

Facial appearance: flattened malar bones, circles beneath the eyes, narrow nose, prominent upper teeth

disease. Generally, chronic cough in the absence of infection or diffuse wheezing during the expiratory phase of respiration is sufficient to establish a diagnosis.

Pulmonary function tests (PFTs) provide an objective and reproducible method of evaluating the presence and degree of lung disease, as well as the response to therapy. Spirometry can generally be performed reliably on children by the age of 5 or 6 years and includes either the traditional and simple mechanical spirometer often used in clinics, offices, and the home; or new, computerized versions. Another key measurement is the *peak expiratory flow rate (PEFR),* which measures the maximum flow of air that can be forcefully exhaled in 1 second. PEFR is measured in liters per minute using a *peak expiratory flow meter (PEFM)* (p. 1218). Three zones of measurement are typically used to interpret PEFR. The zone system is adapted to a traffic light so that the categories are easy to use and remember (Guidelines box). Each child needs to establish his or her *personal best value.* A personal best value can be established during a 2- to 3-week period during which the child records PEFR at least twice a day. Once the personal best value has been established, the child's current PEFR on any occasion can be compared with the personal best value.

Guidelines

INTERPRETING PEAK EXPIRATORY FLOW RATES*

- **Green (80% to 100% of personal best) signals all clear. Asthma is under reasonably good control. No symptoms are present, and the routine treatment plan for maintaining control can be followed.**
- **Yellow (50% to 79% of personal best) signals caution. Asthma is not well controlled. An acute exacerbation may be present. Maintenance therapy may need to be increased. Call the practitioner if the child stays in this zone.**
- **Red (below 50% of personal best) signals a medical alert. Severe airway narrowing may be occurring. A short-acting bronchodilator should be administered. Notify the practitioner if the peak expiratory flow rate (PEFR) does not return immediately and stay in yellow or green zones.**

*These zones are guidelines only. Specific zones and management should be individualized for each child.

Atraumatic Care

SKIN TESTING

To help allay children's fears of skin tests, give them a careful and thorough explanation of what is to be done and how many "pricks" are involved (usually series of 8 on each site, for a total of 30 tests). Very young, anxious patients may benefit from one prick on the arm to demonstrate how it feels. The skin is pierced with a stylet rather than a regular needle and syringe; then a drop of allergen is placed on the site. Another helpful strategy is to have the child count off the number of pricks with the nurse as a distraction. For intradermal skin injection, EMLA, a topical anesthetic, reduces or eliminates pain without altering test results.

Skin testing is useful in identifying specific allergens, and those obtained by the puncture technique correlate better than intracutaneous tests with symptoms and measurements of specific immunoglobulin E (IgE) antibody (Atraumatic Care box). *Provocative testing,* direct exposure of the mucous membranes to a suspected antigen in increasing concentrations, helps to identify inhaled allergens. The *radioallergosorbent test (RAST)* helps identify antigens against various foods and is often useful in determining appropriate therapy.

Therapeutic Management. The overall goal of asthma management is to prevent disability and to minimize physical and psychologic morbidity—to help the child live as normal and happy a life as possible. This includes facilitating the child's social adjustments in the family, school, and community and normal participation in recreational activities and sports. To accomplish these goals, efforts are directed toward recognizing acute episodes early, visiting a health care provider regularly and implementing appropriate therapy, identifying and eliminating irritant and allergic factors from the child's environment, educating parents to the long-term nature of the disease and how to manage exacerbations, and helping the child to deal constructively with the disease. Compliance to the prescribed regimen is essential to successful management.

Allergen Control. The goal of nonpharmacologic therapy is prevention and reduction of the child's exposure to airborne

Home Care

"ALLERGY-PROOFING" THE HOME AND ENVIRONMENT

Keep humidity between 30% and 50%; use dehumidifier and/or air conditioner if available; keep air conditioners clean and free of mold; do not use vaporizers or humidifiers.

Encase pillows in zippered allergen-impermeable covers or wash pillows in hot water (at least 54.4°C [130°F]) every week.

Encase mattress and box springs in zippered allergen-impermeable cover.

Use foam rubber mattress and pillows or Dacron pillows and synthetic blankets.

Wash bed linens every 7 to 10 days in hot water (at least 54.4°C).

Encase polyester comforters in allergen-impermeable covers or wash in hot water (at least 54.4°C) every week; if possible, do not use comforters and use cotton blankets.

Do not use a canopy above the bed; children should not sleep on the bottom bunk of a bunk bed.

Store nothing under the bed; keep clothing in a closet with the door shut.

Use washable window shades; avoid heavy curtains; if curtains are used, launder them frequently.

Remove all carpeting if possible; if not possible, vacuum carpet once or twice a week while the child wears a mask; have child remain out of the room while vacuuming occurs and for 30 minutes after vacuuming.

If possible, use a central vacuum cleaner with a collecting bag outside of the home or use cleaner filters (e.g., high-efficiency particulate air [HEPA] filters).

Have air and heating ducts cleaned annually; change or clean filters monthly; cover heating vents with filter material (e.g., cheesecloth) to prevent circulation of dust, especially when heat is turned on after summer.

Remove unnecessary furniture, rugs, stuffed or real animals, toys, books, upholstered furniture, plants, aquariums, and wall hangings from child's room.

Use wipeable furniture (wood, plastic, vinyl, or leather) in place of upholstered furniture; avoid rattan or wicker furniture.

Cover walls with washable paint or wallpaper.

Limit child's exposure to animals (rabbits, gerbils, hamsters) at school; teach child to stay away from zoos, petting farms, and neighbor's pets.

Change child's clothes after playing outdoors; wash child's hair nightly if child is outside and pollen count is high.

Keep child indoors while lawn is being mowed, bushes/trees are being trimmed, or pollen count is high.

Keep windows and doors closed during pollen season; use air conditioner if possible and/or go to places that are air conditioned, such as libraries and shopping malls, when the weather is hot.

Wet-mop bare floors weekly; wet-dust and clean child's room weekly; child should not be present during cleaning activities.

Wash showers and shower curtains with bleach or Lysol at least once a month.

Limit or avoid child's exposure to tobacco and wood smoke; do not allow cigarette smoking in the house or car; select day care centers, play areas, and shopping malls that are smoke free.

Avoid odors or sprays (e.g., perfumes, talcum powder, room deodorizers, chalk dust at school, fresh paint, or cleaning solutions).

Avoid cellar (basement) as a play area if it is damp, and use a dehumidifier in damp basement.

Cover all food, including pet food, and put food away in cabinets.

Store garbage in closed containers.

Use pesticide sprays, roach bait traps, and boric acid powder to kill cockroaches; if living in an apartment or adjacent housing, encourage neighbors to work together to get rid of cockroaches.

Repair leaking or dripping faucets; seal cracks and crevices in cabinets and pantry areas.

allergens and irritants. *House dust mites* and other components of house dust are the agents identified most often in children allergic to inhalants. The most important method to eliminate dust mites is to keep the humidity in the house under 50%, the level below which dust mites do not survive. The *cockroach*, another common household inhabitant, has also been identified as an important allergen in many locations (Rosenstreich et al, 1997). Exterminating live cockroaches, carefully cleaning kitchen floors and cabinets, putting food away after eating, and taking trash out in the evening are essential measures to control cockroaches. Other recommendations for controlling allergens are in the Home Care box.

Specific allergens are identified by skin testing, and steps are taken to eliminate or avoid the offending allergens. Often, simply removing the offending environmental factors (e.g., removal of a dog or cat from the home of a child sensitive to animal dander) will decrease the frequency of asthma episodes. Nonspecific factors that may trigger an episode, such as extremes of temperature, are sometimes controlled by dehumidifiers or air conditioners.

Drug Therapy. The goal of pharmacologic therapy is to prevent and control asthma symptoms, reduce the frequency and severity of asthma exacerbations, and reverse airflow obstruction. A stepwise approach is recommended based on the severity of the child's asthma. Because inflammation is considered an early and persistent feature of asthma, therapy is directed toward long-term suppression of inflammation. Medications are categorized into two general classes: *long-term control medications (preventor medicines)* to achieve and maintain control of inflammation; and *quick-relief medications (rescue medications)* to treat symptoms and exacerbations (National Asthma Education and Prevention Program, 1997).

Many asthma medications are given by inhalation with a nebulizer or *metered-dose inhaler (MDI)*. The MDI may have a spacing unit or reservoir attached, which makes it easier for young children to use. In addition to MDIs, several inhaler devices that do not contain chlorofluorocarbons (CFCs) are now available. Many of these devices use dry powder and are delivered by devices called diskhalers, turbohalers, or rotahalers. These devices are breath activated, and the child needs to inhale as quickly and deeply as possible to use them effectively. Infants and very young children who have difficulty using MDIs or other inhalers can obtain effective relief with *nebulization*. The medication is mixed with saline and then nebulized with compressed air. Children are instructed to breathe normally with the mouth open to provide a direct route to the trachea.

Corticosteroids are antiinflammatory drugs used to treat reversible airflow obstruction and to control symptoms and reduce bronchial hyperreactivity in chronic asthma. Corticosteroids may be administered parenterally, orally, or by aerosol.

Oral medications are metabolized slowly, with an onset of action up to 3 hours after administration and peak effectiveness occurring within 6 to 12 hours. Oral steroids may be given for short periods (i.e., 3- or 10-day "bursts") to gain prompt control of inadequately controlled persistent asthma or to manage severe persistent asthma. These drugs should be given in the lowest effective dose. Long-term use poses the risk of significant adverse effects such as osteoporosis, hypertension, Cushing syndrome, impaired immune mechanisms, and hypothalamic-pituitary-adrenal suppression (National Asthma Education and Prevention Program, 1997).

Inhaled steroids are used for long-term prevention of symptoms, as well as for suppression, control, and reversal of inflammation. These medications have few side effects (e.g., cough and oral thrush), and their use has reduced the need for long-term use of oral steroids (National Asthma Education and Prevention Program, 1997). Recently the FDA ordered that inhaled steroids must carry labels warning that they may slow growth in children. Although the effects of steroids on growth continue to be studied, children receiving inhaled steroids should be seen regularly (at least every 3 to 6 months) by a primary care provider who assesses the systemic effects of these drugs and makes appropriate reductions in dosages and/or changes to other types of asthma therapy (Twarog, 1998).

Cromolyn sodium is an NSAID for asthma. It stabilizes mast cell membranes; inhibits activation and release of mediators from eosinophil and epithelial cells; and inhibits the acute airway narrowing after exposure to exercise, cold dry air, and sulfur dioxide. There is no way to reliably predict whether a child will respond to the drug. Cromolyn sodium has minimal side effects (e.g., occasional coughing on inhalation of the powder formulation) and may be given via nebulizer or MDI. *Nedocromil sodium* is another drug used for maintenance therapy in asthma. This drug has both antiallergic and antiinflammatory properties and few side effects.

β-Adrenergic agonists (primarily *albuterol, metaproterenol,* and *terbutaline*) are used for treatment of acute exacerbations and for the prevention of exercise-induced bronchospasm. They can be given via inhalation or as oral or parenteral preparations. The inhaled drug has a more rapid onset of action than the oral form. Inhalation also reduces troublesome systemic side effects such as irritability, tremor, nervousness, and insomnia.

Inhaled β-adrenergic agents should not be taken more than three or four times daily for acute symptoms. *Salmeterol (Serevent)* is a long-acting bronchodilator that is used twice a day. This drug is added to antiinflammatory therapy and used for long-term prevention of symptoms, especially nighttime symptoms; and exercise-induced bronchospasm.

Methylxanthines, principally *theophylline,* have been used for decades to relieve symptoms and prevent asthma attacks. Theophylline, however, is now considered a third-line agent and unnecessary for treating asthma exacerbations. Theophylline may be taken intravenously, intramuscularly, orally, or rectally (seldom used). The drug is also available in sustained-release oral form. In addition to its bronchodilator effect, theophylline is a central respiratory stimulant and increases respiratory muscle contractility.

When theophylline is used, serum concentrations must be monitored. Monitoring is required for children who fail to exhibit the expected bronchodilator effect, as well as for those who develop an adverse effect with the usual dose. The dosage of theophylline should be adjusted to achieve a serum concentration of 5 to 15 μg/ml (National Asthma Education and Prevention Program, 1997).

There have been reports that theophylline may cause behavior problems and poor school performance, but most research does not support these findings (Milgram and Bender, 1995).

NURSE ALERT • Theophylline toxicity can occur with serum levels greater than 20 μg/ml. Side effects from theophylline include nausea, vomiting, headache, irritability, and insomnia. Early signs of toxicity are nausea, tachycardia, and irritability; seizures and dysrhythmias occur at blood theophylline levels greater than 30 μg/ml.

Leukotriene Modifiers. Leukotrienes are mediators of inflammation that cause increases in airway hyperresponsiveness. Leukotriene modifiers (e.g., zafirlukast, zileuton, and montelukast sodium) block inflammatory and bronchospasm effects. These drugs are given orally in combination with β-agonists and steroids to provide long-term control and prevention of symptoms in mild persistent asthma (Fost and Spahn, 1998).

Exercise. Exercise-induced bronchospasm (EIB) is an acute, reversible, usually self-terminating airway obstruction that develops during or after vigorous activity, reaches its peak 5 to 10 minutes after stopping the activity, and usually stops in another 20 to 30 minutes. Patients with EIB have cough, shortness of breath, chest pain or tightness, wheezing, and endurance problems during exercise; however, an exercise challenge test in a laboratory is necessary to make the diagnosis.

The problem is rare in activities that require short bursts of energy (e.g., baseball, sprints, gymnastics, and skiing) and more common in those that involve endurance exercise (e.g., soccer, basketball, and distance running). Swimming is well tolerated by children with EIB because they are breathing air fully saturated with moisture and because of the type of breathing required in swimming. Exhaling under water is of benefit because it prolongs each expiration and increases the end-expiratory pressure within the respiratory tree (essentially pursed-lip breathing).

Children with asthma are often excluded from exercise by parents, teachers, and practitioners, as well as by the children themselves, because they are reluctant to provoke an attack. This can seriously hamper peer interaction and physical health. Exercise is advantageous for children with asthma, and most children can participate in activities at school and in sports with minimum difficulty provided that the asthma is under control. Participation should be evaluated on an individual basis in terms of tolerance for duration and intensity of effort. Appropriate prophylactic treatment with β-adrenergic agents or cromolyn sodium before exercise will usually permit full participation in strenuous exertion.

Chest Physiotherapy (CPT). CPT includes breathing exercises and physical training. These therapies help produce physical and mental relaxation, improve posture, strengthen respiratory musculature, and develop more efficient patterns of breathing. For the motivated child, breathing exercises and controlled breathing are of value in preventing overinflation and improving efficiency of the cough. However, CPT is not recommended during acute, uncomplicated exacerbations of asthma (National Asthma Education and Prevention Program, 1997).

Hyposensitization. The role of hyposensitization in childhood asthma has become controversial. In the past, immunotherapy has been used for seasonal allergies and when single substances are the offending allergen. It is not recommended for allergens that can be eliminated, such as foods, drugs, and animal dander.

Injection therapy is usually limited to clinically significant allergens. The initial dose of the offending allergen(s), based on the size of the skin reaction, is injected subcutaneously. The amount is increased at weekly intervals until a maximum tolerance is reached, after which a maintenance dose is given at 4-week intervals. This may be extended to 5- or 6-week intervals during the off-season for seasonal allergens. Successful treatment is continued for a minimum of 3 years and then stopped. If no symptoms appear, acquired immunity is said to be retained; if symptoms recur, treatment is reinstituted.

NURSE ALERT • Hyposensitization injections should be administered only with emergency equipment and medications readily available in the event of an anaphylactic reaction.

Prognosis. The outlook for children with asthma varies widely. Many children lose their symptoms at puberty, but up to two thirds of children with asthma continue to have symptoms through puberty and adulthood. The prognosis for control or disappearance of symptoms varies in children, from those who have rare and infrequent attacks to those who are constantly wheezing or are subject to status asthmaticus. In general, when symptoms are severe and numerous, when symptoms have been present for a long time, and when there is a family history of allergy, there is a greater likelihood of a poor prognosis. Many children who outgrow their exacerbations continue to have airway hyperresponsiveness and cough as adults. Furthermore, airway hyperresponsiveness in adults appears to be associated with decreased lung function.

Although death from asthma is rare, the death rate has increased in recent years. The adolescent age group appears to be the most vulnerable, with the greatest increase occurring in ages 10 to 14 years. No reliable data exist to explain this increase. Factors that have been postulated include exposure of atopic persons to more allergens, change in severity of the disease, abuse of drug therapy (toxicity), failure of families and practitioners to recognize the severity of asthma, and psychologic factors such as denial or refusal to accept the disease. Risk factors for asthma deaths appear to be onset at an early age, frequent attacks, difficult-to-manage disease, adolescence, history of respiratory failure, psychologic problems (e.g., refusal to take medications), dependency on or misuse of drugs (high use), presence of physical stigmata (e.g., barrel chest and intercostal retractions), and abnormal pulmonary function tests (Capen and Sherman, 1998).

Status Asthmaticus. Children who continue to display respiratory distress despite vigorous therapeutic measures, especially use of sympathomimetics, are considered to be in status asthmaticus. The condition may develop gradually or rapidly, often coincident with complicating conditions (e.g., pneumonia) that can influence the duration and treatment of the attack. These children are usually seen in the emergency department and may require hospitalization or admission to a pediatric intensive care unit for close observation and continuous cardiorespiratory monitoring.

NURSE ALERT • Status asthmaticus is a medical emergency that can result in respiratory failure and death if untreated. The child who sweats profusely, remains sitting upright, and refuses to lie down is in severe respiratory distress. Also, the child who suddenly becomes agitated, or the agitated child who suddenly becomes quiet, may be seriously hypoxic and requires immediate intervention.

Therapy for status asthmaticus is directed toward improvement of ventilation, correction of dehydration and acidosis, and treatment of any concurrent infection. Bronchospasm is relieved by giving inhaled aerosolized short-acting β_2-agonists (either intermittently or continuously), along with corticosteroids (either orally or intravenously). For the child not responding to either of these therapies, subcutaneous epinephrine (1:1000) at a dose of 0.01 ml/kg, with a maximum dose of 0.3 ml; or subcutaneous terbutaline is administered.

The child is given IV fluids and nothing by mouth except liquids if the condition permits. IV fluids are infused at maintenance rates, and the child is monitored for pulmonary edema.

Correction of dehydration, acidosis, hypoxia, and electrolyte derangements is guided by frequent determination of oxygenation (pulse oximetry), blood gases, and serum electrolytes.

Humidified oxygen is administered by nasal prongs, hood, or face mask to maintain satisfactory oxygenation. Because oxygen is a stimulus for respiration, high levels may significantly depress respirations.

Administration of antibiotics is often advisable in therapy, because infection may be masked or may not always be evident and is always a threatening complication. As the attack subsides, fluids and medication are given orally, and discharge plans are initiated, especially for follow-up care.

Nursing Care Management

➤ Assessment

Physical assessment of asthma involves the same observations and techniques described in the general discussion of assessment of respiratory infection (see Box 46-2) and physical assessment of the chest (see Chapter 35). In addition, some physical characteristics of chronic respiratory involvement are noted and evaluated, including chest configuration, posturing, and type of breathing.

Nurses assist with diagnostic tests, pulmonary function tests, and skin testing, as well as a general health assessment. Nurses also assess how asthma affects the child's everyday activities and self-concept, as well as the child's and family's ability to comply with prescribed therapy. The nurse should determine any cultural or ethnic beliefs or practices that influence self-management and require modifications in educational approaches.

➤ Nursing Diagnoses

Based on a thorough assessment, several nursing diagnoses are identified. The more common diagnoses for the child with asthma are included in the Nursing Care Plan on p. 1221. Others may apply in specific situations.

➤ Plan of Care and Implementation

The goals for the child with asthma and the family include:

1. Child will not experience an asthmatic episode.

2. Child will exhibit improved ventilatory capacity.
3. Child will maintain optimum health.
4. Child will not develop complications.
5. Child will engage in normal activities for age.
6. Child and family will receive appropriate support and education regarding the disease and its management.

Avoid Allergens. One goal of asthma management is avoidance of an exacerbation. Parents need to know how to avoid allergens and/or relieve asthmatic episodes. The nurse assists the parent in modifying the environment to reduce contact with the offending allergen(s) (see Home Care box on p. 1215). Parents are cautioned to avoid exposing a sensitive child to excessive cold, wind, or other extremes of weather; or to smoke, sprays, or other irritants. Foods known to provoke symptoms should be eliminated from the diet.

Home Care

USE OF A PEAK EXPIRATORY FLOW METER

1. Before each use, make sure the sliding marker or arrow on the peak expiratory flow meter (PEFM) points to zero or is at the bottom of the numbered scale.
2. Stand up straight.
3. Remove gum or any food from the mouth.
4. Close your lips tightly around the mouthpiece. Be sure to keep your tongue away from the mouthpiece.
5. Blow out as hard and as quickly as you can, a "fast hard puff."
6. Note the number by the marker on the numbered scale.
7. Repeat entire routine three times; wait 30 seconds between each routine.
8. Record the *highest* of the three readings, not the average.
9. Measure the peak expiratory flow rate (PEFR) close to the same time and same way each day (e.g., morning and evening; before and/or 15 minutes after taking medication).
10. Keep a chart of your PEFRs.

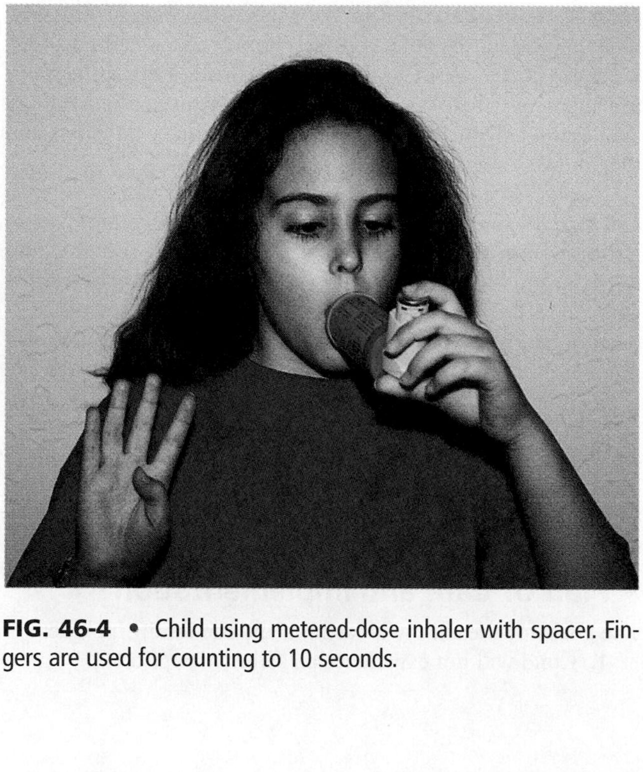

FIG. 46-4 • Child using metered-dose inhaler with spacer. Fingers are used for counting to 10 seconds.

Because approximately 2% to 6% of children with asthma are sensitive to aspirin, acetaminophen is recommended. Those children with aspirin-induced asthma may also be sensitive to salicylate compounds such as Pepto-Bismol, NSAIDs, and tartrazine (yellow dye number 5, a common food coloring).

Relieve Bronchospasm. Parents and older children are taught to recognize early signs and symptoms of an impending attack so that it can be controlled before symptoms become distressing. Most children can recognize prodromal symptoms well before an attack (about 6 hours), and preventive therapy can be implemented. Objective signs that parents may observe include rhinorrhea, cough, low-grade fever, irritability, itching (especially in front of the neck and chest), apathy, anxiety, sleep disturbance, abdominal discomfort, and loss of appetite. A variety of easy-to-use, inexpensive PEFMs are available for use in the home and at school to assess changes in pulmonary function (Home Care box).

Children who use a nebulizer, MDI, diskhaler, or rotahaler to deliver drugs need to learn how to use the device correctly. The MDI device (Fig. 46-4) delivers medication directly to the airways; therefore the child needs to learn to breathe slowly and deeply for better distribution to narrowed airways (Home Care box).

Home Care

USE OF A METERED-DOSE INHALER*

Steps for Checking How Much Medicine is in the Canister

1. If the canister is new, it is full.
2. If the canister has been used repeatedly, it might be empty. (Check product label to see how many inhalations should be in each canister.)
3. To check how much medicine is left in the canister, put the canister (not the mouthpiece) in a cup of water. *Do not use this method with MDIs that contain hydrofluoroalkanes or dry powder.*
   a. If the canister sinks to the bottom, it is full.
   b. If the canister floats sideways on the surface, it is empty.

Steps for Using the Inhaler

1. Remove the cap and hold inhaler upright.
2. Shake the inhaler.
3. Tilt the head back slightly and breathe out.
4. With the inhaler in an upright position, insert the mouthpiece.
   a. About 3 to 4 cm from the mouth or
   b. Into an aerochamber or spacer or
   c. Into the mouth, forming an airtight seal between the lips and the mouthpiece.
5. At the end of a normal expiration, depress the top of the inhaler canister firmly to release the medication (into either the aerochamber or the mouth), and breathe in slowly (about 3 to 5 seconds). Relax the pressure on the top of the canister.
6. Hold the breath for at least 5 to 10 seconds to allow the aerosol medication to reach deeply into the lungs.
7. Remove the inhaler and breathe out slowly through the nose.
8. Wait 1 minute between puffs (if additional one is needed).

Adapted from National Asthma Education and Prevention Program: *Expert Panel Report II: guidelines for the diagnosis and management of asthma.* Pub. No. 97-4051, Bethesda, MD, 1997, National Heart, Lung, and Blood Institute.

*NOTE: Inhaled dry-powder capsules require a different inhalation technique. To use a dry-powder inhaler, it is important to close the mouth tightly around the mouthpiece of the inhaler and inhale rapidly and deeply.

Young children, and those who are unable to manipulate the device or coordinate breathing, should use spacers or holding chambers. These devices allow the parent or child to deliver the medication from the MDI into the spacer, from which the child then inhales the medication (Critical Thinking box). When inhaled steroids are given via an MDI, spacers are also recommended to prevent yeast infections in the mouth.

The child and parents also need to be cautioned about the adverse effects of prescribed drugs and the dangers of overuse of β_2-agonists. They should know that it is important to use them when needed but not indiscriminately or as a substitute for avoiding the symptom-provoking allergen.

NURSE ALERT • Long-acting β-adrenergic inhalers (e.g., salmeterol [Serevent]) should be used only as directed (usually every 12 hours) and not more often. They are not intended to relieve acute asthmatic symptoms.

The family should obtain a PEFM and learn to use this device to monitor their child's asthma. A written asthma action plan that includes the three peak flow meter zones and the child's asthma medications should be obtained from the child's primary care provider. This action plan should be used to make decisions about asthma management at home and at school.

Although foods are an unusual cause of asthma, foods known to provoke symptoms should be eliminated from the diet. Foods most commonly allergenic are eggs, milk, grains, peanuts, and chocolate. Parents are advised to read labels on prepared foods and snacks to determine the presence of allergens. A number of foods contain sodium caseinate or dried-milk products.

The child should be protected from a respiratory infection that can trigger an attack or aggravate the asthmatic state, especially in young children whose airways are mechanically smaller and more reactive. Equipment used for the child, such as nebulizers, must be kept absolutely clean to decrease the chances of contamination with bacteria and fungi.

Breathing exercises and controlled breathing are taught and encouraged for motivated youngsters, and the nurse can provide information concerning activities that promote diaphragmatic breathing, side expansion, and improved mobility of the chest wall.

Self-care is a hallmark of effective asthma management, and self-management programs are important in helping the child and family cope with the disease. The principles conveyed include:

- Asthma is a common disease, and to have asthma is annoying but not disgraceful.
- Persons with asthma are able to live full and active lives.
- It is much easier to prevent than to treat an asthmatic attack.
- Individuals do not become addicted to asthma medication, but they do prefer to breathe more freely whenever possible.

Asthma camps have become popular in recent years as a means of encouraging physical activity in a more homogeneous, controlled, and less competitive environment. Studies indicate that children attending asthma camps have improved attitudes toward asthma and improved self-management skills (Meng, 1997).

Several organizations provide education and services for health professionals and families of children with asthma.* Asthma education and awareness are important aspects of asthma management. Although the principles of self-management are fairly general, specific content must be individualized to meet the special needs of each child and family.

Provide Acute Asthma Care. Children who are admitted to the hospital with acute asthma are ill, anxious, and uncomfortable. In many instances children are admitted on an emergency basis and in acute distress. An IV infusion may be started to provide immediate access; and medications, usually nebulized albuterol and a corticosteroid, are administered to relieve bronchospasm. The child is monitored closely and continuously during therapy for relief of respiratory distress and for signs of side effects.

It is important that the child receive sufficient fluid either orally or intravenously to replace losses through diaphoresis and hyperventilation. Cold liquids may trigger reflex bronchospasm and should be avoided. Nourishment is provided in small, frequent feedings to avoid abdominal distention that might interfere with diaphragmatic excursion.

Older children usually prefer the high-Fowler position, although they may be more comfortable sitting upright or leaning slightly forward. When possible, the nurse communicates in such a way that the child can reply in a few words to avoid fatigue. Shortness of breath makes talking difficult. Oxygen is indicated for relief of dyspnea and cyanosis; however, it is not administered indiscriminately but regulated according to the blood gas analysis; pulse oximetry; and objective observation of color, respiratory effort, and level of consciousness. Associated treatments such as intermittent positive-pressure breathing,

Critical Thinking

ASTHMA

Traditional thinking about the pathophysiology of asthma has changed in recent years. Which one of the following treatments reflects this better understanding of the mechanisms involved in an asthmatic episode?

First, Think About It . . .

- **What precise question are you trying to answer?**
- **What conclusions are you reaching?**

1. **Peak expiratory flow meter (PEFM)**
2. **Metered-dose inhaler (MDI)**
3. **Allergy hyposensitization**
4. **Chest physiotherapy**

The best response is 2. Inflammation of the bronchial airways is now recognized as a critical component in the pathophysiology of asthma. The conclusion that MDIs are used to deliver corticosteroids to decrease the inflammation is correct. The PEFM is an assessment device; the other two choices have been used traditionally.

*Asthma and Allergy Foundation of America (AAFA), 1125 15th St., Washington, DC 20005; (202) 466-7643 or 1-800-7-Asthma; website: www.aafa.org.; American Lung Association, 1740 Broadway, New York, NY 10019; (212) 315-8700 or 1-800-Lung-USA; website: www.lungusa.org; National Heart, Lung, and Blood Institute, Information Center, Code AS-ASHA, P.O. Box 30105, Bethesda, MD 20824-0105; fax (301) 251-1223; website: www.nhlbi.nih.gov/nhlbi.htm.

blood gases, and PFTs may be performed by specialized personnel or may be the nurse's responsibility.

Children with acute asthma are apprehensive and anxious. The calm, efficient presence of a nurse helps to reassure them that they are safe and will be cared for during this stressful period. It is important to assure children that they will not be left alone and that their parents are allowed to remain with them.

Parents need reassurance and want to be informed of their child's condition and therapies. They may feel that they have in some way contributed to the child's condition or could have prevented the episode. Reassurance regarding their efforts expended on the child's behalf and their parenting capabilities can help alleviate their stress. Efforts to reduce parental apprehension will also reduce the child's distress. Anxiety is easily communicated to the child from parents and members of the staff.

Support Child and Family. The nurse working with children with asthma can provide support in a number of ways. Many children voice frustration because their exacerbations interfere with their daily activities and social lives. They need education about their disease, including what to do to prevent an episode and what to do during one. These children need reassurance from the health team and reinforcement of their coping mechanisms.

Both short-term and long-term adaptation of affected children to the disease depends on the family's acceptance of the disorder. The task of living day-to-day with affected children involves the family continually. There are periodic crises and the ever-present threat of a crisis, requiring parental vigilance, sleepless nights, frequent emergency trips to the hospital, and often overwhelming medical expenses. Throughout these stresses, parents are encouraged to promote as normal a life as possible for their children.

➤ Evaluation

The effectiveness of nursing interventions is determined by continual reassessment and evaluation of care based on the following observational guidelines and expected outcomes:

1. Interview family about removal or avoidance of known allergens.
2. Observe child for evidence of respiratory symptoms.
3. Assess child's general health.
4. Observe child and interview family about any infections or other complications.
5. Interview child about daily activities.
6. Determine the degree to which the family and child understand the child's condition and the extent to which the therapies are carried out.

The expected outcomes are described in the Nursing Care Plan.

Cystic Fibrosis (CF)

CF is inherited as an autosomal recessive trait; the affected child inherits the defective gene from both parents, with an overall incidence of 1:4 among carriers of the gene (see Appendix C). The mutated gene responsible for CF is located on the long arm of chromosome 7, along with its protein product, *cystic fibrosis transmembrane regulator (CFTR)*. Although more than 500 mutations from the original sequence of the gene have been reported, the ΔF508 is the most common alteration, found in about 75% of all known mutations (Wilmott, Kaplan, and Perez, 1997).

Pathophysiology. With the discovery of the CFTR gene, research is continuing to determine its multisystemic effects on the body. CF is characterized by several apparently unrelated clinical features: increased viscosity of mucous gland secretions, a striking elevation of sweat electrolytes, an increase in several organic and enzymatic constituents of saliva, and abnormalities in autonomic nervous system function. Although both sodium and chloride are affected, the defect appears to be primarily a result of abnormal chloride movement; the CFTR appears to function as a chloride channel. Further evidence indicates that ΔF508 is closely related to pancreatic insufficiency. The role of CFTR, however, is not definitive.

The primary factor, and the one that is responsible for the multiple clinical manifestations of the disease, is mechanical obstruction caused by the increased viscosity of mucous gland secretions (Fig. 46-5). Instead of forming a thin, freely flowing secretion, the mucous glands produce a thick, inspissated mucoprotein that accumulates and dilates them. Small passages in organs such as the pancreas and bronchioles become obstructed as secretions precipitate or coagulate to form concretions in glands and ducts. The earliest manifestation of CF is *meconium ileus* in the newborn, in which the small intestine is blocked with thick, puttylike, tenacious, mucilaginous meconium.

In the pancreas the thick secretions block the ducts, eventually causing *pancreatic fibrosis*. This blockage prevents essential pancreatic enzymes from reaching the duodenum, which causes marked impairment in the digestion and absorption of nutrients. The disturbed function is reflected in bulky stools that are frothy from undigested fat *(steatorrhea)* and foul smelling from putrefied protein *(azotorrhea)*. The islands of Langerhans may decrease in number as pancreatic fibrosis progresses, and the incidence of diabetes mellitus is becoming a more common finding as children with CF live longer. In the liver, localized biliary obstruction and fibrosis are common and become more extensive with time.

The most common gastrointestinal complication associated with CF is *prolapse of the rectum*, which occurs most often in infancy and childhood. Affected children of all ages are subject to intestinal obstruction from inspissated or impacted feces.

Pulmonary complications are present in almost all children with CF and constitute the most serious threat to life. Most children show evidence of respiratory symptoms before 1 year of age; others may not develop symptoms for weeks, months, or years. Bronchial and bronchiolar obstruction by the abnormally thick, tenacious mucus causes patchy atelectasis with hyperinflation. The child is unable to expectorate the mucus because of its increased viscosity. This retained mucus serves as an excellent medium for bacterial growth. Reduced oxygen-carbon dioxide exchange causes variable degrees of hypoxia, hypercapnia, and acidosis.

Diagnostic Evaluation. An initial evaluation is conducted with overall appraisal in the areas of general activity, physical findings, nutritional status, and findings on chest radiograms (see Box 46-17 for clinical manifestations). The diagnosis of CF is established on the basis of (1) a history of the disease in the family, (2) absence of pancreatic enzymes, (3) increase in electrolyte concentration of sweat, and (4) chronic pulmonary involvement.

Nursing Care Plan THE CHILD WITH ASTHMA

NURSING DIAGNOSIS Risk for suffocation related to interaction of child with allergens

EXPECTED OUTCOME Asthmatic episodes are reduced or eliminated.

Nursing Interventions/*Rationales*

Make an inventory of allergens that trigger reactions or asthmatic episodes *to establish a baseline for prevention.*

Teach child and family how to avoid, limit exposure to, modify or eliminate conditions *that trigger allergy attacks and asthmatic episodes.*

Teach child and family to recognize early signs *so an impending asthmatic episode can be treated early.*

Instruct child and family in correct use of prescribed bronchodilators, antiinflammatants, and other asthma medications *to avoid underuse or overuse of the drugs.*

Instruct child and family in correct use of equipment (e.g., inhalers, nebulizers, peak flow meters) *to ensure correct use and optimum benefit.*

Encourage sound health practices (good nutrition, adequate rest, appropriate exercise, good hygiene) *to support body's natural defenses.*

Encourage child and family to prevent exposure to respiratory infections *since they can serve as triggers for asthma attacks.*

NURSING DIAGNOSIS Ineffective airway clearance related to allergenic response and inflamed bronchial tree

EXPECTED OUTCOME The patient will exhibit evidence of improved ventilatory capacity (i.e., absence of dyspnea, respiration rate and rhythm within normal limits).

Nursing Interventions/*Rationales*

Implement breathing exercises and controlled breathing *to improve chest wall mobility and diaphragmatic expansion.*

Use developmentally appropriate play techniques *to increase expiratory pressure and extend expiratory time.*

Use coughing, percussion, and postural drainage as needed *to clear secretions.*

Supervise use of equipment (e.g., inhalers, nebulizers, peak flow meters) *to evaluate use patterns and optimum benefit.*

Administer medications as ordered *to decrease inflammatory response and improve breathing.*

NURSING DIAGNOSIS Activity intolerance related to imbalance between oxygen supply and demand

EXPECTED OUTCOME The patient's activity level will be within normal limits.

Nursing Interventions/*Rationales*

Balance rest and physical activity, increasing activity levels as tolerated *to regain balance between oxygen supply and demand.*

NURSING DIAGNOSIS Altered family processes related to having a child with chronic health problem

EXPECTED OUTCOME Family exhibits positive adaptive behaviors to child's condition.

Nursing Interventions/*Rationales*

Identify and praise positive coping mechanisms of child and family members *to reinforce long-term use.*

Explore child's and family's understanding of the disease and treatment process *to evaluate family's ability to carry out preventive and emergency intervention.*

Reinforce need for consistent use of preventive measures and need for early response to signs of impending attack *to prevent severe exacerbation.*

Be alert to signs of maladaptation (e.g., parental rejection or overprotection, nonadherence to treatment regimen, lack of alterations in environment or lifestyle, sporadic health care follow-up).

Encourage family to work with school *to develop a consistent plan of care in the school setting.*

Refer family to appropriate support groups and community resources *to provide ongoing support.*

See also the Nursing Care Plan: The Child with Chronic Illness or Disability, Ch. 41.

The consistent finding of abnormally high sodium and chloride concentrations in the sweat is a unique characteristic of CF. Parents commonly observe that their infants taste "salty" when they kiss them. For diagnostic purposes the quantitative *sweat chloride test* is performed on sweat obtained by iontophoresis of pilocarpine. Normally the sweat chloride content is less than 40 mEq/L; a chloride concentration greater than 60 mEq/L is diagnostic of CF.

Chest radiography reveals characteristic patchy atelectasis and obstructive emphysema. PFTs are sensitive indexes of lung function, providing evidence of abnormal function of the small airways in CF. Other diagnostic tools that may aid in diagnosis include stool fat and/or enzyme analysis. Stool analysis requires a 72-hour sample with accurate recording of food intake during that time. Radiographs, including barium enema, are used for diagnosis of meconium ileus.

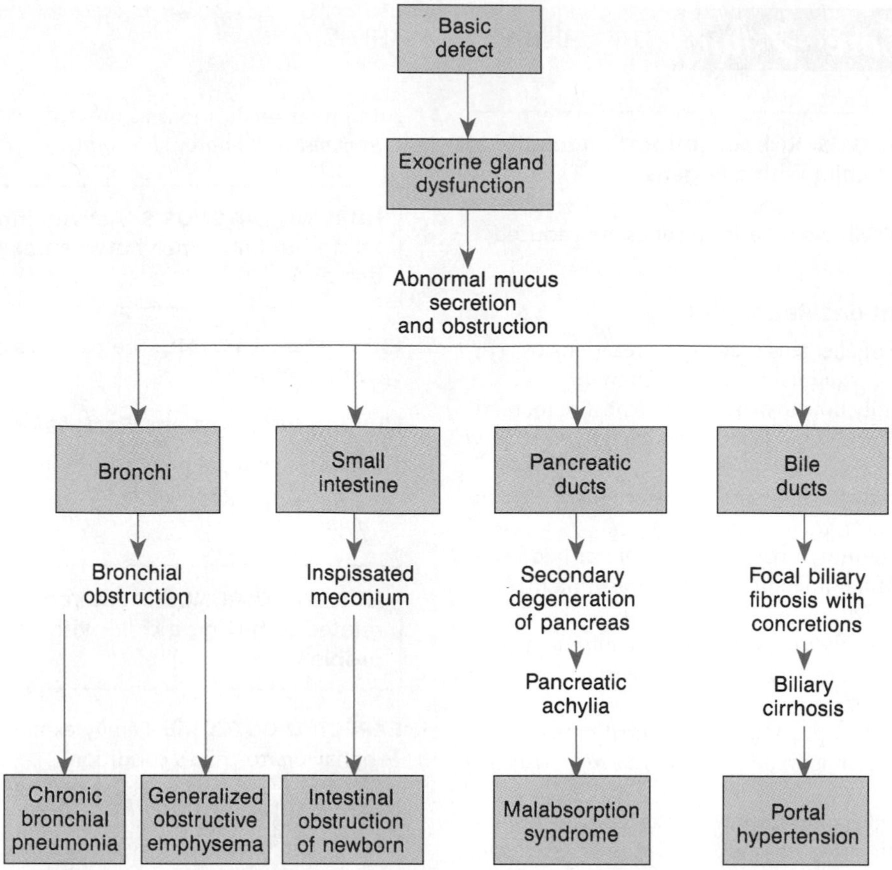

FIG. 46-5 • Various effects of exocrine gland dysfunction in cystic fibrosis (CF).

Box 46-17

Clinical Manifestations of Cystic Fibrosis

MECONIUM ILEUS*
- Abdominal distention
- Vomiting
- Failure to pass stools
- Rapid development of dehydration

GASTROINTESTINAL MANIFESTATIONS
- Large, bulky, loose, frothy, extremely foul-smelling stools
- Voracious appetite (early in disease)
- Loss of appetite (later in disease)
- Weight loss
- Marked tissue wasting
- Failure to grow
- Distended abdomen
- Thin extremities
- Sallow skin
- Evidence of deficiency of fat-soluble vitamins A, D, E, K
- Anemia

PULMONARY MANIFESTATIONS

Initial signs:
- Wheezy respirations
- Dry, nonproductive cough

Eventually:
- Increased dyspnea
- Paroxysmal cough
- Evidence of obstructive emphysema and patchy areas of atelectasis

Progressive involvement:
- Overinflated, barrel-shaped chest
- Cyanosis
- Clubbing of fingers and toes
- Repeated episodes of bronchitis and bronchopneumonia

* In about 10% of cases.

Therapeutic Management. The improved survival rate of patients with CF during the past two decades is attributable largely to antibiotic therapy and improved nutritional management. Goals of therapy are (1) to prevent or minimize pulmonary complications, (2) to ensure adequate nutrition for growth, and (3) to assist the child and family in adapting to a chronic disorder. In attempting to attain these goals, a multisystem approach to treatment modalities is used.

Management of Pulmonary Problems. Management of pulmonary problems is directed toward prevention and treatment of pulmonary infection by improving aeration, removing mucopurulent secretions, and administering antimicrobial agents. Most children develop respiratory symptoms by 3 years of age. Young children normally have small airways and are predisposed to frequent viral infections. The large amounts and viscosity of respiratory secretions in children with CF contribute to the likelihood of infection.

The most common pathogens responsible for pulmonary infections are *Pseudomonas aeruginosa, Burkholderia cepacia, Staphylococcus aureus, Haemophilus influenzae, Escherichia coli,* and *Klebsiella pneumoniae. P. aeruginosa* and *B. cepacia* are particularly pathogenic for children with CF, and infections with these organisms are difficult to clear. In addition, children who are chronically colonized with these organisms have poorer survival rates than children with CF who are not colonized (Wilmott, Kaplan, and Perez, 1997).

Prevention of infection involves a daily routine of CPT to maintain pulmonary hygiene (see Chapter 45). CPT is usually performed twice daily (on rising and in the evening) and more often if needed, especially during pulmonary infection. The *Flutter mucus clearance device** is a small, handheld plastic pipe with a stainless-steel ball on the inside that facilitates removal of mucus. It has the advantage of increasing sputum expectoration and being used without an assistant.

Bronchodilator medication delivered in an aerosol helps open bronchi for easier expectoration and is administered before CPT when the patient exhibits evidence of reactive airway disease and/or wheezing. Another form of aerosolized medication is *recombinant human deoxyribonuclease (rhD-Nase,* known generically as *dornase alfa [Pulmozyme]),* which decreases the viscosity of mucus. It is well tolerated and has no major adverse effects; minor reactions are voice alterations and laryngitis. The drug causes improvement in PFTs and perceptions of well-being, as well as a reduction in the viscosity of sputum.

Physical exercise is an important adjunct to daily CPT. Exercise not only stimulates mucus secretion, it also provides a sense of well-being and increased self-esteem. In some instances, exercise can be substituted for CPT. Any aerobic exercise that is enjoyed by the patient should be encouraged. The ultimate aim of exercise is to establish a good habitual breathing pattern.

Pulmonary infections are treated as soon as they are recognized. Some practitioners prefer to prescribe oral antibiotics prophylactically at the time of diagnosis; others begin therapy when pulmonary symptoms arise. Sputum culture and sensitivity guide the choice of antibiotic. Aerosolized antibiotics such as tobramycin, ticarcillin, and gentamicin have also been beneficial in patients with frequent pulmonary exacerbations (Hagemann, 1996).

IV antibiotics are often administered at home as an alternative to hospitalization. Most children have central venous access devices for home administration of IV medications. When pulmonary function does not improve with outpatient management, hospitalization may be recommended for continued antibiotic therapy and vigorous CPT.

Oxygen administration is usually recommended for children with acute episodes, but because many of these children have chronic carbon dioxide retention, the unsupervised use of oxygen can be harmful (see Oxygen Therapy: Oxygen Toxicity, Chapter 45).

Pneumothorax is most often caused by rupture of subpleural blebs through the visceral pleura and usually occurs in patients with more advanced disease.

NURSE ALERT • Signs of pneumothorax are usually nonspecific and include tachypnea, tachycardia, dyspnea, pallor, and cyanosis.

Management of Gastrointestinal (GI) Problems. The principal treatment for pancreatic insufficiency is replacement of pancreatic enzymes, which are administered with meals and snacks to ensure that digestive enzymes are mixed with food in the duodenum. Enteric-coated products prevent the neutralization of enzymes by gastric acids, thus allowing activation to occur in the alkaline environment of the small bowel. The amount of enzymes depends on the severity of the insufficiency, the response of the child to enzyme replacement, and the philosophy of the practitioner. Usually one to five capsules are administered with a meal, and a smaller amount is taken with snacks. Capsules can be swallowed whole or taken apart and the contents sprinkled on a small amount of food to be taken at the beginning of the meal. The amount of enzyme is adjusted to achieve normal growth and a decrease in the number of stools to one or two per day.

Children with CF require a well-balanced, high-protein, high-caloric diet (because of the impaired intestinal absorption). In fact, they often require up to 150% of the recommended daily allowances to meet their needs for growth. Breast-feeding with enzyme supplementation should be continued whenever possible for parents who prefer this method and, when necessary, supplemented with a higher-calorie-per-ounce formula. For formula-fed infants, commercial cow's milk formulas are usually adequate, although commonly a hydrolysate formula with medium-chain triglycerides (e.g., Pregestimil or Alimentum) may be recommended. Enzymes are mixed into cereal or fruit, such as applesauce. Because the uptake of fat-soluble vitamins is decreased, water-miscible forms of these vitamins (A, D, E, K) are given, along with multivitamins and the enzymes. When high-fat foods are eaten, the child is encouraged to add extra enzymes. Sometimes patients will be placed on supplemental tube feedings or parenteral alimentation in an effort to build up nutritional reserves if there has been a history of inability to maintain weight.

Prognosis. Despite considerable progress and a recent surge in new treatment modalities, CF remains a progressive and incurable disease. The pulmonary involvement ultimately determines the patient's outcome, because pancreatic enzyme deficiency is less of a problem if adequate nutrition is ensured. With advances in technology, parents and adolescents are challenged to set future goals that may include college, careers, social relationships, and marriage. Concurrently, they are faced with increasing morbidity and higher rates of CF complications as they grow older.

Screening. The impact of genetic discoveries on understanding the etiology and treatment of CF is steadily unfolding at the same time that approaches to detection are changing to reflect new technologies. The standard methods of diagnosis rely on either detection of abnormal chloride secretions in sweat or elevated immunoreactive trypsinogen. Carrier screening is available and reliable for siblings and family members of a child with CF.

---

*Manufactured by Scandipharm, Inc., 22 Inverness Center Parkway, Birmingham, AL 35242; (205) 991-8085 or 1-800-950-8085; website: www.scandipharm.com.

Nursing Care Management

➤ Assessment

Assessment of the child with CF involves both pulmonary and GI observations. Pulmonary assessment is the same as that described for asthma (see Box 46-2), with special attention to lung sounds, observation of cough, and evidence or degree of finger clubbing. GI assessment primarily involves observing the frequency and nature of the stools and abdominal distention. The observer is also alert to evidence of failure to thrive (e.g., weight loss, wasting, pallor, and fatigue). Family members are interviewed to determine the child's eating and eliminating habits, to determine salty perspiration, and to confirm a history of frequent respiratory infections or bowel obstruction in infancy.

On initial contact, commonly in the hospital setting, nurses are involved in performing or assisting with diagnostic tests, primarily sweat for laboratory analysis of chloride content and, less often, stool specimens for trypsin and fat.

➤ Nursing Diagnoses

After a careful assessment numerous nursing diagnoses will become evident. The degree of both pulmonary and gastrointestinal involvement varies among affected children; therefore, nursing diagnoses will also vary according to the individual case.

➤ Plan of Care and Implementation

The plan of care for the child with CF involves both the child and the family. Major goals include, but are not limited to, the following:

1. The child will demonstrate signs of adequate gas exchange.
2. The child will expectorate mucus.
3. The child will exhibit signs of adequate digestion.
4. The child will experience few or no complications.
5. The child will demonstrate adequate growth and development.
6. The child and family will receive adequate education about the disease and its management.
7. The child and family will receive adequate support.

Hospital Care. When the child is hospitalized for confirmation of the diagnosis or for pulmonary complications, aerosol therapy is instituted or continued. Respiratory therapy is usually initiated and supervised by a trained respiratory therapist or physiotherapist. In institutions with large support staffs, they may provide all treatments; otherwise it becomes the responsibility of the nurse to perform the prescribed aerosol therapy and CPT and to teach supervised breathing exercises. CPT should not be performed before or immediately after meals. Planning the activity so that it does not coincide with meals is difficult in the hospital situation; however, this is very important and is often overlooked by nursing personnel.

Oxygen is cautiously administered to children in respiratory distress, and the child requires frequent assessment. The hazard of *oxygen narcosis* is a constant threat in children with long-standing disease who receive oxygen (see Chapter 45). The child requires close observation to assist with cough and expectoration.

The diet is implemented for the newly diagnosed child or continued for the child who is hospitalized for pulmonary disease. Children in the early stages of the disease maintain a good appetite, and some will eat excessively. With infection and increased lung involvement, however, the appetite diminishes. Eventually it becomes a challenge to tempt failing appetites. Some younger children may object to the extra fluids that are encouraged to prevent dehydration. Food is considered therapy for these patients. The caloric intake should be increased significantly. Pancreatic enzymes are supplied for each meal or snack, and adequate salt is provided, especially for febrile children. (See Feeding the Sick Child, Chapter 45.)

Frequent skin care is carried out to prevent irritation and skin breakdown over bony prominences. Particular attention is necessary after use of the bedpan or when the diaper is changed. Careful cleansing helps to reduce irritation and odor from offensive stools, and the use of moisture barriers protects the skin. (See Diaper Dermatitis, Chapter 53; and Maintaining Healthy Skin, Chapter 45.)

The child will need support for the many treatments and tests that are a necessary part of the hospital therapy. IV fluids and blood tests are almost always a part of the treatment, and the child soon associates hospitalization with these stress-provoking procedures. Because these children are usually quite thin with little muscle mass, careful selection of injection sites is required.

Providing support to both the child and the family is a vital part of nursing care. The progressive nature of the disease makes each illness requiring hospitalization a potentially life-threatening event. Skilled nursing care and sympathetic attention to the emotional needs of the child and family help them cope with the stresses associated with repeated respiratory infections and hospitalization.

Home Care. After the diagnosis is confirmed and a treatment program determined, preparation for home care is implemented. The plan of care should be flexible enough so that family activities are disrupted as infrequently as possible. Parents will need help in finding the inhalation equipment available for home use that best meets their needs. They will need opportunities to learn how to use the equipment, as well as information about some of the problems they may encounter.

They need to learn about the preferred diet of nutritious meals with tolerated fat, increased protein and carbohydrate, and the administration of pancreatic enzymes. Children usually adjust well to taking pancreatic enzymes. For infants and young children, the enzymes can be mixed with pureed fruit, such as applesauce, and fed with a spoon. Capsules are suitable for older children. It is important to stress to parents that the enzymes, in the amount regulated to the child's needs, should be administered at the beginning of all meals and snacks. They are cautioned about not restricting salt, especially during hot weather; and ensuring an adequate fluid intake, because dehydration aggravates the thick mucus secretions. Oral hygiene is important because of interference with salivation and the increased susceptibility to oral infections.

One of the most important aspects of educating parents for home care is teaching CPT and breathing exercises. The success of a therapy program depends on regular, conscientious performance of these treatments as prescribed. The number of times these therapies are performed each day is determined on an individual basis, and often parents readily learn to adjust the number and intensity of the treatments to the child's needs.

Postural drainage can be achieved with simple activities that are fun, such as hanging by the knees from a bar or low-hanging trapeze that can be easily built in the backyard (or indoors), turning somersaults, or playing "wheelbarrow" with the child suspended head down and propelling with the hands while the adult holds on to the feet. Most children respond to a challenge, such as "How long can you stand on your head?" Small children can "stand on their heads" with their heads on the cushion of a large chair with or without an adult holding on to their feet. Parents soon learn to respond to cues from their children and incorporate spontaneous activities into the treatment regimen.

Another important aspect of home care is the administration of home IV antibiotics. With the use of venous access devices, such as peripherally inserted central catheter (PICC) lines, the parents and child are taught the technique of direct administration into the IV line.* Families also need information about medications and their possible side effects.

Children with CF should receive routine primary care with all recommended routine immunizations. In addition, all patients with CF should be vaccinated yearly for pneumococcus and influenza (American Academy of Pediatrics, 2000).

The nurse can assist the family in contacting resources that provide help to families with affected children. The various special child health services and many local clinics, private agencies, service clubs, and other community groups offer equipment and medications either free or at reduced rates. The Cystic Fibrosis Foundation† has chapters throughout the United States to provide education and services to families and professionals.

Family Support. One of the most important and difficult aspects of providing care for the family of a child with CF is coping with the emotional needs of the child and family. The diagnosis, treatment, and prognosis are fraught with many problems, frustrations, and feelings. The diagnosis, with all its implications, evokes feelings of guilt and self-recrimination in parents. These feelings may be particularly marked if the newly diagnosed child is the second affected child in the family and the parents had been counseled about the 1:4 risk of such an event occurring.

The long-range problems are those encountered in the care of a child with a chronic illness (see Chapter 41). Both the child and the family must make many adjustments, the success of which depends on their ability to cope and also on the quality and quantity of support they receive from outside sources. Combined efforts of a variety of health professionals offer the most comprehensive services to families. It is often the responsibility of the nurse to organize and coordinate these services, to assess the home situation, and to collect the data needed to evaluate the effectiveness of the services in meeting the family's needs.

The persistent need for treatment several times daily also places a strain on the family. Someone must perform the procedures, such as percussion and vibration, even on older children who are able to assume responsibility for their own exercises and respiratory therapy. Children often balk at the treatments, and the parents are placed in the position of insisting on compliance. The stress and anxiety related to this continual routine sometimes generate feelings of resentment, which are commonly focused on one aspect of the regimen, such as the diet or equipment. When possible, occasional trusted respite care should be made available to the parent or parents to allow them the opportunity to leave the situation for short periods without undue anxiety about the child's welfare.

The affected child also may become resentful about the disease, its relentless routine of therapy, and the necessary curtailment it places on activities and relationships. The child's activities are interrupted or built around treatment, medications, and diet, which imposes hardships (e.g., the need to carry medication to school and other places where the child may eat away from home), and the growth retardation associated with most chronic illnesses may be trying. Any of these aspects of the disease may be the cause of ridicule from other children; however, the child should be encouraged to attend school and join age-appropriate groups, such as Scouting, to foster a life that is as normal and productive as possible.

Families affected by CF have psychologic hurdles similar to those of all families coping with a child with a chronic illness. A constant source of anxiety for both parents and child is the ever-present fear of death.

As the disease progresses, family stress should be expected, and the patient may become angry and noncompliant. It is important for the nurse to recognize the changing needs of the family. Families should be made aware of sources for counseling as stressful setbacks occur. Patients need to be guided into activities that enable them to express anger, sorrow, and fear without guilt.

Anticipatory grieving and other aspects related to care of a child with a terminal illness are another important part of nursing care. For example, it is important to prepare family members for end-of-life decisions and care. Families may need information about specific interventions such as hospice, and treatments for pain and dyspnea (see Chapter 41).

It is also important to remember that as life expectancy increases for children with CF, issues related to marriage, childbearing, and career choice become relevant. Men must be informed at some point that they will be unable to produce offspring; however, a distinction should be made between sterility and impotence. Normal sexual relationships can be expected. Female patients may be able to bear children but should be informed of the possible deleterious effects on the respiratory system created by the burden of pregnancy. They also need to know that their children will be carriers of the CF gene.

Life as an independent adult, the goal that most families have for their children, should be encouraged for children with CF. From the time that children can take partial responsibility for their own care (e.g., CPT and taking enzymes), independence and accountability should be fostered. The prognosis for these children has improved, and many children with CF are well adjusted despite numerous hospitalizations and unpleasant complications.

➤ Evaluation

The efficacy of nursing management can be evaluated by application of observational guidelines, which may include the following:

1. Monitor vital signs, especially respiratory parameters.
2. Monitor chest physiotherapy and other procedures to assess the expected outcomes (e.g., expectoration of secretions, increased lung expansion).
3. Monitor meals to ensure that enzymes are taken.
4. Monitor child for evidence of respiratory infection, gastrointestinal dysfunction, and other complications.

---

*Community and home care instructions for giving medications to children are available in Wong DL, Hess CS: ***Wong and Whaley's clinical manual of pediatric nursing***, ed 5, St Louis, 2000, Mosby.

†6931 Arlington Rd., Bethesda, MD 20814-3205; 1-800-FIGHT CF or (301) 951-4422; website: www.eff.org. In Canada: Canadian Cystic Fibrosis Foundation, 586 Eglinton Ave. E., Suite 204, Toronto, Ontario M4P 1P2. Two excellent publications available from the Cystic Fibrosis Foundation are *What Everyone Should Know About Cystic Fibrosis* and *Cystic Fibrosis: A Summary of Symptoms, Diagnosis, and Treatment.* For information about specialized medications, especially Pulmozyme, and equipment for CF and other pulmonary diseases, contact Cystic Fibrosis Pharmacy, Inc., H.H.C.S. Pharmacy Services, 633 E. Colonial Dr., Orlando, FL 32803; 1-800-741-4427.

5. Observe nutritional intake. For the child at home, interview the family regarding the child's intake or have child maintain a log of nutritional intake. Obtain regular measurements of growth, and interview child and family regarding school attendance, interaction with peers, and participation in sports and other activities.
6. Explore family's understanding of the disease and its therapies and the family's ability to carry out the treatment plan.
7. Maintain contact with family (if feasible) at follow-up evaluations and during home care. Interview child and family regarding involvement with agencies and services for children with CF.

Expected outcomes include the following:

1. Child breathes easily and without dyspnea.
2. Child manages secretions with minimum distress.
3. Child takes pancreatic enzymes as prescribed.
4. Child displays no evidence of an infective process.
5. Child is well nourished, exhibits satisfactory weight gain, and engages in appropriate activities.
6. Child and family demonstrate an understanding of the disease and comply with the therapeutic regimen (specify knowledge and method of demonstration).
7. Family maintains contact with health care providers.

(See also the Nursing Care Plan: The Child With Cystic Fibrosis.*)

RESPIRATORY EMERGENCY

Nurses must be prepared to deal effectively with respiratory emergencies. Although the interventions are similar to those used for adults, there are some variations for infants and children.

Respiratory Failure

In general, the term *respiratory insufficiency* is applied to two conditions: (1) children with increased work of breathing but with gas exchange function near normal (ventilatory insufficiency); and (2) children who are unable to maintain normal blood gases and develop hypoxemia and acidosis as a result of carbon dioxide retention.

Respiratory failure is defined as the inability of the respiratory apparatus to maintain adequate oxygenation of the blood, with or without CO_2 retention. *Respiratory arrest* is the cessation of respiration. *Apnea* is the absence of airflow (breathing).

Effective pulmonary gas exchange requires clear airways, normal lungs and chest wall, and adequate pulmonary circulation. Anything that affects these functions or their relationships can compromise respiration.

Diagnostic Evaluation. Respiratory failure that occurs as a result of acute obstruction of a major airway or if cardiac arrest is sudden and readily apparent. Gradual or progressive deterioration of respiratory function is less easily recognized. Therefore nursing observation and judgment are vital to the recognition and early management of respiratory failure. Nurses must be able to assess a situation and initiate appropriate action within moments. Signs of respiratory failure are listed in Box 46-18.

Therapeutic Management. The interventions used in the management of respiratory failure are commonly dramatic, requiring special skills, and are often emergency procedures. Some of the techniques employed to assist ventilation include artificial ventilation, artificial airway, and cardiopulmonary resuscitation (CPR).

Artificial Ventilation. There are a variety of methods for controlling or assisting ventilation. Temporary assistance can be provided by a manual self-inflating ventilation bag with a mask and valve to prevent rebreathing. With the mask placed over the child's nose and mouth (an open airway is established by correct positioning with the chin forward and the neck extended to the "sniffing" position), the bag is rhythmically compressed, forcing the gas from the bag into the child's lungs.

For more prolonged assistance, mechanical ventilation is employed to replace the bellows function of the diaphragm and thoracic wall muscles. The lungs are inflated by the application of either positive or negative pressure. The positive-pressure machine inflates the lung by increasing airway pressure above atmospheric pressure, and a negative-pressure ventilator creates a subatmospheric pressure around the chest wall while airway pressure remains atmospheric. Application of positive pressure by mechanical means usually improves the distribution of gas within the lung and often reinflates partially collapsed lung segments. The overall effect is the improvement of gas exchange.

Box 46-18
Clinical Manifestations of Respiratory Failure

CARDINAL SIGNS
Restlessness
Tachypnea
Tachycardia
Diaphoresis

EARLY BUT LESS OBVIOUS SIGNS
Mood changes, such as euphoria or depression
Headache
Altered depth and pattern of respirations
Hypertension
Exertional dyspnea
Anorexia
Increased cardiac output and renal output
Central nervous system symptoms (decreased efficiency, impaired judgment, anxiety, confusion, restlessness, irritability, depressed level of consciousness)
Flaring nares
Chest wall retractions
Expiratory grunt
Wheezing and/or prolonged expiration

SIGNS OF MORE SEVERE HYPOXIA
Hypotension or hypertension
Dimness of vision
Somnolence
Stupor
Coma
Dyspnea
Depressed respirations
Bradycardia
Cyanosis, peripheral or central

*In Wong DL, Hess CS: ***Wong and Whaley's clinical manual of pediatric nursing***, ed 5, St Louis, 2000, Mosby.

Nursing Care Management. For those families whose child has a respiratory arrest, support focuses on keeping the family informed of the child's status and helping them cope with a near-death experience or an actual death (see Chapter 41). Knowing that their child requires CPR is a frightening and often overwhelming experience for parents. Uncertainty regarding outcome—both mortality and morbidity—is a primary concern. Traditionally, family members are not allowed to be present during resuscitation efforts (Family Focus box). Nurses can serve as the family's advocate by either being present with them or by making sure a support person, such as the clergy, is present. After the child's recovery or death, the family needs continued support and thorough medical information regarding lifesaving measures; the prognosis if the child survives; and the cause of death if the child dies.

Cardiopulmonary Resuscitation (CPR)

Cardiac arrest in the pediatric population is less often of cardiac origin than from prolonged hypoxemia secondary to inadequate oxygenation, ventilation, and circulation (shock). Some causes include injuries, suffocation (e.g., foreign body aspiration), smoke inhalation, SIDS, or infection. Respiratory arrest has been associated with a better survival than cardiac arrest. Once cardiac arrest occurs, the outcome of resuscitative efforts is poor.

Absent respirations, lack of movement, and no response to stimulation signals the need for rapid and vigorous action to prevent cardiac arrest (American Heart Association, 2000). In such situations, nurses must be prepared to initiate action immediately. Neurologically intact survival has occurred only in those children who receive immediate resuscitation and respond promptly. In the hospital, emergency equipment should be readily available in patient care centers, and the status of this resuscitation equipment should be checked at least once daily. Regardless of the cause of the arrest, some basic procedures are carried out and modified somewhat according to the child's size.

NURSE ALERT • Rescuers who have infections that may be transmitted by blood or saliva should not perform mouth-to-mouth resuscitation if the circumstances allow other immediate or effective methods of ventilation.

Outside the hospital situation the first action in an emergency is to assess quickly the extent of any injury and determine whether the child is unconscious. A child who is struggling to breathe but conscious should be transported immediately to an *advanced life support (ALS)* facility, with the child maintaining whatever position affords the most comfort. Attempting to transport a child by automobile wastes valuable time; transport by an *emergency medical service (EMS)* is recommended or preferred. Services in larger communities can institute ALS immediately or en route to a medical facility.

An unconscious child is managed with care to prevent additional trauma if a head or spinal cord injury has been sustained. The circumstances in which the child is found offer clues to a possible injury. For example, a child who has been thrown from a bicycle or fallen from a tree is more likely to sustain trauma than a child who is discovered in bed. The child should be turned as a unit with firm support provided to the head and neck to prevent rolling, twisting, or tilting backward or forward (Chandra and Hazinski, 1997).

Resuscitation Procedure. For effective CPR, the victim is placed on the back on a firm, flat surface, employing appropriate precautions (Fig. 46-6). With loss of consciousness the tongue, which is attached to the lower jaw, relaxes and falls back, obstructing the airway. To open the airway, the head is positioned with either the head tilt/chin lift or jaw thrust maneuver. Health professionals should be able to use both maneuvers. *Head tilt* is accomplished by placing one hand on the victim's forehead and applying firm, backward pressure with the palm to tilt the head back. The fingers of the free hand are placed under the bony portion of the lower jaw near the chin to lift and bring the chin forward *(chin lift)*. This supports the jaw and helps tilt the head back (Fig. 46-7, *A*).

The *jaw thrust* is accomplished by grasping the angles of the victim's lower jaw and lifting with both hands, one on each side, displacing the mandible upward and outward (Fig. 46-7, *B*). In suspected neck injuries the jaw thrust method should be used while the cervical spine is completely immobilized. After restoration of a patent airway by removal of foreign material and secretions (if indicated), and if the child is not breathing, continuation of the airway is maintained and rescue breathing is initiated. To ventilate the lungs in the infant (birth to 1 year of age), the operator's mouth is placed in such a way that both

Family Focus

PARENTAL PRESENCE DURING CARDIOPULMONARY RESUSCITATION

Few acute care facilities allow parents to stay during cardiopulmonary resuscitation (CPR), or a "code." Health professionals' reasons for this decision include believing the experience is too upsetting for the family, fearing the family will need care that will interfere with the staff's resuscitation efforts, experiencing discomfort being "watched" by the family, and fearing increased legal liability if the family knows what has been done or not done.

In reality, when parents do observe their child's CPR, these reasons are not supported. One study found that parents who were given the choice of staying during the code unanimously stated that they would choose this option again. Parents did not interfere with the resuscitation, they were assured that everything was done for their child, and they considered being present one of the most important memories of this difficult experience.

When family members of adult or pediatric patients stayed during CPR, 100% reported that their presence was beneficial for them, the experience caused no negative psychologic effects, and they would do it again. Of the staff, 96% of nurses, 79% of attending physicians, and 19% of residents were satisfied with family presence.* The Emergency Nurses Association† supports the option of family presence during invasive procedures and/or resuscitation efforts.

Based on these findings, we need to question the wisdom of excluding parents during CPR. All may not choose to be present, but shouldn't they be given the opportunity? Whose benefit is served by family exclusion? If the main reason is the staff's own fears and anxieties about being observed and possibly judged on their performance, is depriving the family of their wishes justified? Consider out-of-hospital arrests; emergency medical services personnel routinely perform CPR with family and strangers watching. Why is this public rescue attempt considered acceptable but an in-hospital code considered a private event?

*Meyers TA et al: Family presence during invasive procedures and resuscitation, *Am J Nurs* 100(2):32-42, 2000.
†Emergency Nurses Association: *Position statement: family presence at the bedside during invasive procedures and/or resuscitation,* Park Ridge, IL, 1994, the Association.

	Objectives	ACTIONS		
		Adult (over 8 yr)	Child (1 to 8 yr)	Infant (under 1 yr)
A. AIRWAY	1. Assessment: Determine unresponsiveness.	Tap or gently shake shoulder.		
		Say, "Are you okay?"		Speak loudly.
	2. Get help.	Activate EMS.	Shout for help. If second rescuer available, have person activate EMS.	
	3. Position the victim.	Turn on back as a unit, supporting head and neck if necessary (4-10 seconds).		
	4. Open the airway.	Head-tilt/chin-lift.		
B. BREATHING	5. Assessment: Determine breathlessness.	Maintain open airway. Place ear over mouth, observing chest. Look, listen, feel for breathing (3-5 seconds).*		
	6. Give 2 rescue breaths.	Maintain open airway.		
		Seal mouth to mouth.		Mouth to nose/mouth.
		Give 2 slow breaths. Observe chest rise. Allow lung deflation between breaths.		
		1½ to 2 seconds each	1 to 1½ seconds each	
	7. Option for obstructed airway.	a. Reposition victim's head. Try again to give rescue breaths.		
			b. Activate EMS.	
		c. Give 5 subdiaphragmatic abdominal thrusts (the Heimlich maneuver).		c. Give 5 back blows.
				c. Give 5 chest thrusts.
		d. Tongue-jaw lift and finger sweep.	d. Tongue-jaw lift, but finger sweep only if you see a foreign object.	
		If unsuccessful, repeat a, c, and d until successful.		
C. CIRCULATION	8. Assessment: Determine pulselessness.	Feel for carotid pulse with one hand; maintain head-tilt with the other (5-10 seconds).		Feel for brachial pulse: keep head-tilt.
CPR	Pulse absent: Begin chest compressions: 9. Landmark check.	Run middle finger along bottom edge of rib cage to notch at center (top of sternum).		Imagine a line drawn between the nipples.
	10. Hand position.	Place index finger next to finger on notch:		Place 2-3 fingers on sternum. 1 finger's width below line. Depress ½-1 in.
		Two hands next to index finger. Depress 1½-2 in.	Heel of one hand next to index finger. Depress 1-1½ in.	
	11. Compression rate.	80-100 per minute	100 per minute	At least 100 per minute
	12. Compressions to breaths.	2 breaths to every 15 compressions	1 breath to every 5 compressions	
	13. Number of cycles.	4	20 (approximately 1 minute)	
	14. Reassessment.	Feel for carotid pulse.		Feel for brachial pulse.
		If no pulse, resume CPR, starting with compressions.	If alone, activate EMS. If no pulse, resume CPR, starting with compressions.	
	Pulse present; not breathing: Begin rescue breathing.	1 breath every 5 seconds (12 per minute)	1 breath every 3 seconds (20 per minute)	

*If victim is breathing or resumes effective breathing, place in recovery position: (1) move head, shoulders, and torso simultaneously; (2) turn onto side; (3) leg not in contact with ground may be bent and knee moved forward to stabilize victim; (4) victim should not be moved in any way if trauma is suspected and should not be placed in recovery position if rescue breathing or CPR is required.

FIG. 46-6 • One-rescuer CPR. (Modified from American Heart Association: *Guidelines 2000 for cardiopulmonary resuscitation and emergency cardiovascular care:* International consensus on science, 2000.)

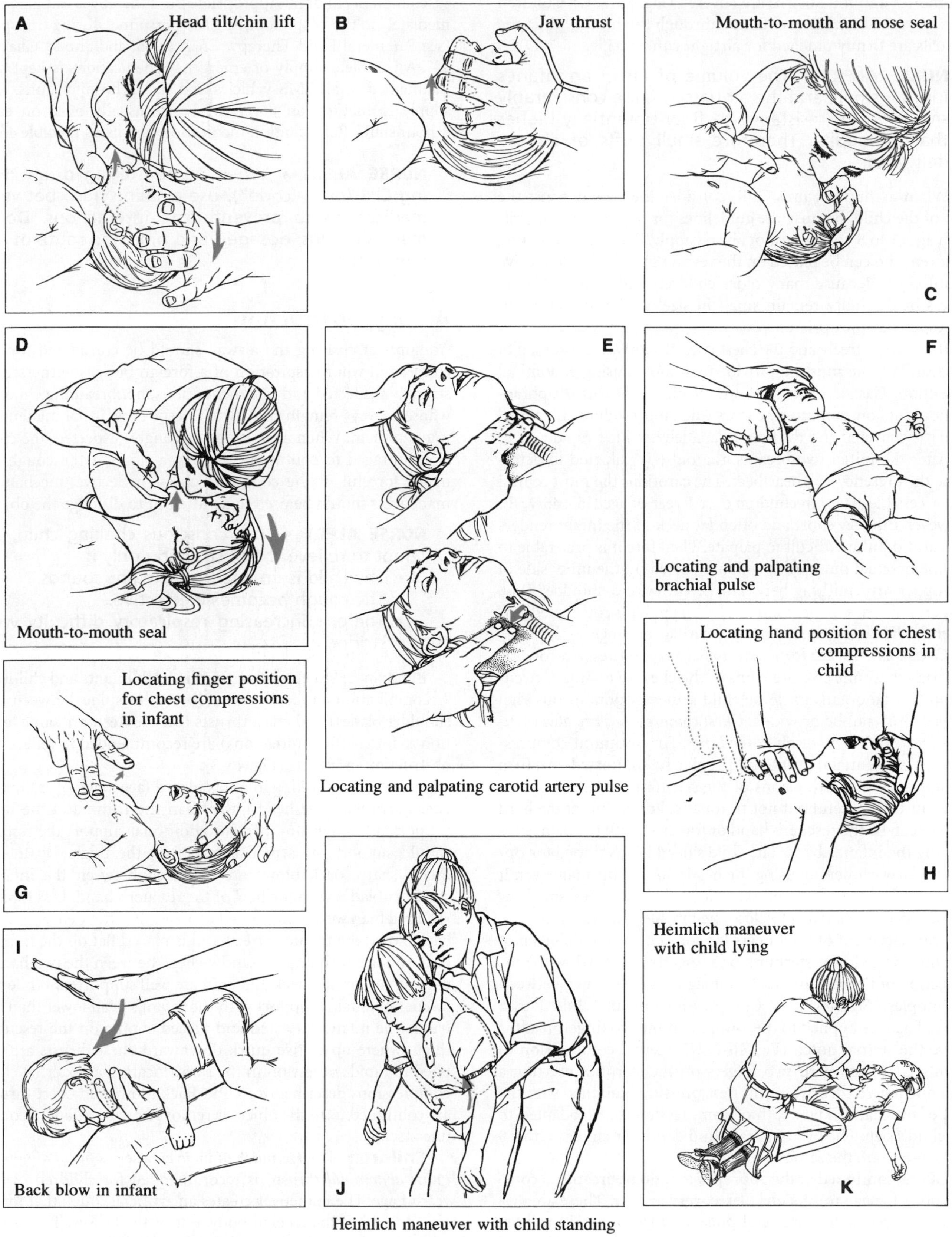

FIG. 46-7 • Procedures for cardiopulmonary resuscitation, **A** to **H**; and airway obstruction, **I** to **K**. (From Chandra NC, Hazinski MF, editors: *Textbook of basic life support for healthcare providers,* Dallas, 1997, American Heart Association.)

the mouth and the nostrils are covered (Fig. 46-7, *C*). Children (over 1 year of age) are ventilated through the mouth while the nostrils are firmly pinched for airtight contact (Fig. 46-7, *D*).

NURSE ALERT • The volume of air in an infant's lungs is small, and the air passages are considerably smaller, with resistance to flow potentially higher than in adults. Therefore small puffs of air are delivered.

When a child requires CPR, consider the size, not just the age, of the child, because the guidelines for infants and for children ages 1 to 8 years may not always apply. For example, young children who can be placed on the rescuer's thigh should receive infant CPR. Because many older children with severe chronic illness or disability remain small in size, pediatric, not adult, CPR may be appropriate.

If air enters freely and the chest rises, the airway is assumed to be clear. Volume must be provided without causing abdominal distention. Gastric distention, which interferes with diaphragmatic excursion, commonly occurs when more volume than necessary is delivered and the breaths are delivered too rapidly.

After the initial two breaths, the pulse is palpated to determine the presence of a heartbeat. The carotid is the most central and accessible artery in children over 1 year of age (Fig. 46-7, *E*). However, the very short and often fat neck of the infant renders the carotid pulse difficult to palpate. Therefore it is preferable to use the brachial pulse in the infant, located on the inner side of the upper arm midway between the elbow and shoulder (Fig. 46-7, *F*). Absence of a carotid or brachial pulse is considered sufficient indication to begin external cardiac massage.

Chest Compression. External chest compression consists of serial, rhythmic compressions of the chest to maintain circulation to vital organs until the child achieves spontaneous vital signs or ALS can be provided. *Chest compressions are always interspersed with ventilation of the lungs.* For optimum compressions, it is essential that the child's spine be supported on a firm surface during compressions of the sternum, and sternal pressure must be forceful but not traumatic. For an infant the hard surface can be the rescuer's hand or forearm, with the palm supporting the infant's back. The child's head is positioned for optimum airway opening using the head tilt/chin lift maneuver. It is essential to prevent over-extension of the head of small infants, because this tends to close the flexible trachea.

The placement of the fingers for compression in infants is at a point on the lower sternum, one fingerbreadth below the intersection of the sternum and an imaginary line drawn between the nipples (Fig. 46-7, *G*). Compressions on the child 1 to 8 years of age are applied to the lower sternum two fingerbreadths above the sternal notch (Fig. 46-7, *H*). Sternal compression to infants is applied with two fingers on the sternum exerting a firm downward thrust; for children, pressure is applied with the heel of one hand. The depth of compression is also adapted to the child's size. The location, rate, and depth for children over 8 years of age are the same as for adults.

CPR is continued at the appropriate ratio of breaths to compressions for age until signs of recovery appear. These are evidenced by palpable peripheral pulses, return of pupils to normal size, the disappearance of mottling and cyanosis, and possibly return of spontaneous respiration.

Medications. Medications are an important adjunct to CPR, especially cardiac arrest, and are used during and after resuscitation in children. Appropriate fluid therapy is initiated immediately in the hospital or by EMS personnel during transport (see Parenteral Fluid Therapy, Chapter 45; and Shock, Chapter 48). A complete supply of emergency medications is kept and maintained in all EMS vehicles and on all hospital units. The supply is checked on a regular basis (usually once on each 8-hour shift). Resuscitation medications are listed in Table 46-3.

NURSE ALERT • When administering drugs during CPR (or a "code"), use a saline flush between medications to prevent drug interactions. Document all drugs, dosages, and time and route of administration.

Airway Obstruction

Attempts at clearing the airway should be considered for (1) children in whom aspiration of a foreign body is witnessed or strongly suspected and (2) unconscious, nonbreathing children whose airways remain obstructed despite the usual maneuvers to open them. When aspiration is strongly suspected, the child is encouraged to continue coughing as long as the cough remains forceful. If the cough becomes ineffective, mechanical maneuvers should be used in an attempt to dislodge the object.

NURSE ALERT • In a conscious choking child, attempt to relieve the obstruction only if:
- The child is unable to make any sounds.
- The cough becomes ineffective.
- There is increasing respiratory difficulty with stridor.

Blind finger sweeps are avoided in both infants and children. A combination of back blows (over the spine between the shoulder blades) and chest thrusts (on the sternum, same location as for chest compressions) are recommended to relieve the obstruction in infants (Fig. 46-8).

Infants. A choking infant is placed face down over the rescuer's arm with the head lower than the trunk and the head supported (see Fig. 46-7, *I*). For additional support the rescuer should support the arm firmly against the thigh. Up to five quick, sharp, back blows are delivered between the infant's shoulder blades with the heel of the rescuer's hand. Less force is required than would be applied to an adult. After delivery of the back blows, the rescuer's free hand is placed flat on the infant's back so that the infant is "sandwiched" between the two hands, making certain the neck and chin are well supported. While the rescuer maintains support with the infant's head lower than the trunk, the infant is turned and placed supine on the rescuer's thigh, where up to five quick downward chest thrusts are applied in rapid succession in the same location as external chest compressions described for CPR. Back blows and chest thrusts are continued until the object is removed or the infant becomes unconscious.

Children. The *Heimlich maneuver,* a series of *subdiaphragmatic abdominal thrusts,* is recommended for children over 1 year of age. The maneuver creates an artificial cough that forces air, and with it the foreign body, out of the airway. The procedure is carried out with the child in a standing, sitting, or lying position (see Fig. 46-7, *J* and *K*). In the conscious choking child, upward thrusts are delivered to the upper abdomen with the fisted hand at a point just below the rib cage (see Fig. 46-7, *J*).

TABLE 46-3

Drugs for Pediatric Cardiopulmonary Resuscitation

Drug/Dose	Action	Implications
Epinephrine HCl IV/IO: 0.01 mg/kg (1:10,000) ET: 0.1 mg/kg (1:1000)	Adrenergic Acts on both alpha- and beta-receptor sites, especially heart and vascular and other smooth muscle	Most useful drug in cardiac arrest Disappears rapidly from bloodstream after injection May produce renal vessel constriction and decreased urine formation
Sodium bicarbonate IV/IO: 1 mEq/kg Newborn: 0.5 mEq/ml 2 mg/kg	Alkalinizer Buffers pH	Infuse slowly and only when ventilation is adequate Don't mix with catecholamines or calcium
Atropine sulfate 0.02 mg/kg/dose Minimum dose: 0.1 mg Maximum single dose: infants and children, 0.5 mg; adolescents, 1 mg	Anticholinergic-parasympatholytic Increases cardiac output, heart rate by blocking vagal stimulation in heart	Used to treat bradycardia after ventilatory assessment Produces pupillary dilation, which constricts with light
Calcium chloride 10% 20 mg/kg 0.2 mg/kg/dose q 10 min	Electrolyte replacement Needed for maintenance of normal cardiac contractility	Used only for hypocalcemia, calcium blocker overdose, hyperkalemia, or hypermagnesemia Administer slowly; very sclerosing; administer in central vein
Lidocaine HCl 1 mg/kg	Antidysrhythmic Inhibits nerve impulses from sensory nerves	Used for ventricular dysrhythmias only
Bretylium 5 mg/kg; may be increased to 10 mg/kg	Antidysrhythmic Inhibits release of norepinephrine in post-ganglionic nerve endings that control ventricular tachycardia	Not a first-line drug for ventricular tachycardia Used if lidocaine is not effective Administer rapidly
Adenosine 0.1 to 0.2 mg/kg Maximum single dose: 12 mg Follow with 2–3 ml normal saline flush	Antidysrhythmic Causes a temporary block through the atrioventricular node and interrupts re-entry circuits	Administer rapidly Very effective Minimal side effects
Naloxone (Narcan) 0.1 mg/kg/dose* May repeat q 2–3 min	Reverses respiratory arrest due to excessive opiate administration	Evaluate level of pain because analgesic effects of opioids are reversed with large dose of naloxone
INFUSIONS		
Epinephrine HCl infusion 0.1–1 μg/kg/min	Adrenergic See above	Titrated to desired hemodynamic effect
Dopamine HCl infusion 2–20 μg/kg/min	Agonist Acts on alpha receptors, causing vasoconstriction Increases cardiac output	Titrated to desired hemodynamic response
Dobutamine HCl infusion 2–20 μg/kg/min	Adrenergic direct-acting β_2 agonist Increases contractility and heart rate	Titrated to desired hemodynamic response Little vasoconstriction, even at high rates
Lidocaine HCl infusion 20–50 μg/kg/min	Antidysrhythmic Increases electrical stimulation threshold of ventricle	See above Lower infusion dose used in shock Used for ventricular tachycardia
Isoproterenol 0.1 to 2 μg/kg/min	Relaxes bronchial smooth muscle, increases cardiac contractility and heart rate	Used for emergency treatment of atropine-resistant bradycardia and shock Increased effects with epinephrine

*Dose of naloxone to reverse respiratory depression without reversing analgesia from opioids is 0.5 μg/kg in children $<$40 kg (American Pain Society, 1999).

IV, Intravenous route; *IO,* intraosseous route; *ET,* endotracheal route.

Signs of life-threatening obstruction

The truly choking child *cannot speak, becomes cyanotic,* and *collapses.*

	Objectives	Actions: Adult (over 8 yr)	Child (1 to 8 yr)	Infant (under 1 yr)
CONSCIOUS VICTIM	1. Assessment: Determine airway obstruction.	Ask, "Are you choking?" Determine if victim can cough or speak.		Observe breathing difficulty, ineffective cough, no strong cry.
	2. Act to relieve obstruction.	Perform up to 5 subdiaphragmatic abdominal thrusts (Heimlich maneuver).		Give 5 back blows. Give 5 chest thrusts.
	Be persistent.	Repeat Step 2 until obstruction is relieved or victim becomes unconscious.		
VICTIM WHO BECOMES UNCONSCIOUS	3. Position the victim: call for help.	Turn on back as a unit, supporting head and neck, face up, arms by sides. Call out, "Help!" Activate EMS. If second rescuer available, have person activate EMS.		
	4. Check for foreign body.	Perform tongue-jaw lift and finger sweep.	Perform tongue-jaw lift. Remove foreign object only if you actually see it.	
	5. Give rescue breaths.	Open the airway with head-tilt/chin-lift. Try to give rescue breaths. If airway is obstructed, reposition head and try to ventilate again.		
	6. Act to relieve obstruction.	Perform up to 5 subdiaphragmatic abdominal thrusts (Heimlich maneuver).		Give 5 back blows. Give 5 chest thrusts.
	7. Be persistent.	Repeat steps 4-6 until obstruction is relieved.		
UNCONSCIOUS VICTIM	1. Assessment: Determine unresponsiveness.	Tap or gently shake shoulder. Shout, "Are you okay?"	Tap or gently shake shoulder.	
		If unresponsive, activate EMS.		
	2. Call for help: position the victim.	Turn on back as a unit, supporting head and neck, face up, arms by sides.		
			Call out for help.	
	3. Open the airway.	Head-tilt/chin-lift.		Head-tilt/chin-lift, but do not tilt too far.
	4. Assessment: Determine breathlessness.	Maintain an open airway. Ear over mouth; observe chest. Look, listen, feel for breathing (3-5 seconds).		
	5. Give rescue breaths.	Make mouth-to-mouth seal.		Make mouth-to-nose-and-mouth seal.
		Try to give rescue breaths.		
	6. If chest is not rising, try again to give rescue breaths.	Reposition head. Try rescue breaths again.		
	7. Activate the EMS system.		If airway obstruction not relieved after about 1 minute, activate EMS as rapidly as possible.	
	8. Act to relieve obstruction.	Perform up to 5 subdiaphragmatic abdominal thrusts (Heimlich maneuver).		Give 5 back blows. Give 5 chest thrusts.
	9. Check for foreign body.	Perform tongue-jaw lift and finger sweep.	Perform tongue-jaw lift. Remove foreign object only if you actually see it.	
	10. Rescue breaths.	Open the airway with head-tilt/chin-lift. Try again to give rescue breaths. If airway is obstructed, reposition head and try to ventilate again.		
	11. Be persistent.	Repeat steps 8-10 until obstruction is relieved.		

FIG. 46-8 • Foreign body airway obstruction management. (Modified from Chandra NC, Hazinski MF, editors: *Textbook of basic life support for healthcare providers,* Dallas, 1997, American Heart Association.)

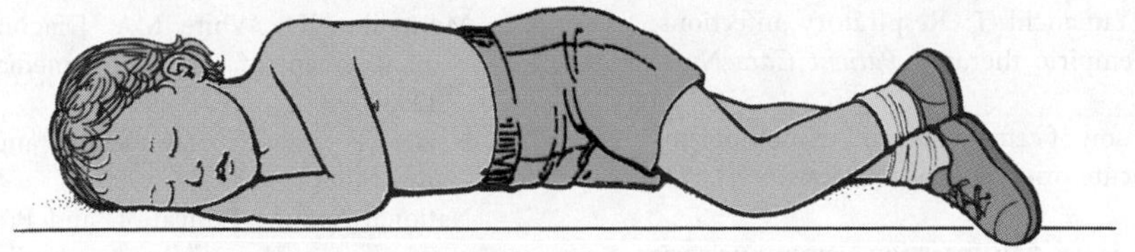

FIG. 46-9 • Recovery position for child after respiratory emergency.

To prevent damage to the internal organs, the rescuer's hands should not touch the xiphoid process of the sternum or the lower margins of the ribs. Five thrusts are repeated in rapid succession until the foreign body is expelled.

It is neither necessary nor desirable to squeeze or compress the arms during the procedure. It is not a punch or a bear hug. The child may vomit after relief of the obstruction and should be positioned to prevent aspiration. After breathing is restored, the child should receive medical attention and be assessed for complications.

The success of the technique is primarily a result of the obstruction occurring at the end of a maximum respiration. The victim is most likely to choke on food during inspiration; therefore the tidal volume plus expiratory reserve volume is present in the lungs. When pressure is exerted on the diaphragm by the maneuver, the food bolus is ejected with considerable force by this trapped air.

NURSE ALERT • If the victim is breathing or resumes effective breathing after emergency interventions, place in the recovery position: move the head, shoulders, and torso simultaneously and turn onto the side. The leg not in contact with the ground may be bent and the knee moved forward to stabilize the victim (Fig. 46-9). The victim should not be moved in any way if trauma is suspected and should not be placed in the recovery position if rescue breathing or CPR is required.

Key Points

- Acute infection of the respiratory tract is the most common cause of illness in infancy and childhood.
- The incidence and severity of respiratory tract infections are influenced by the infectious agents involved, the child's age, and the child's natural defenses.
- Common respiratory tract infections of childhood include nasopharyngitis, pharyngitis (including tonsillitis), influenza, and otitis media.
- Croup syndromes involve acute inflammation and variable degrees of obstruction of the epiglottis, larynx, and/or trachea.
- The primary goals in the care of children with croup are observation for signs of respiratory distress and relief of laryngeal obstruction.
- Common infections of the lower airways are bacterial tracheitis, bronchitis, and respiratory syncytial virus (RSV)/bronchiolitis.
- Pneumonias are classified according to site (lobar, bronchial, or interstitial) or by etiologic agent (viruses, bacteria, mycoplasmas, or associated with aspiration of foreign material).
- In tuberculosis, susceptibility to the bacillus can be influenced by heredity, age, stress, poor nutrition, and intercurrent infection.
- Passive inhalation of cigarette smoke is a major environmental pollutant contributing to respiratory disease in children.
- Asthma is the leading cause of chronic illness in children.
- General therapeutic management of asthma includes allergen control, drug therapy, controlled exercise, physical therapy, and sometimes hyposensitization.
- Support for the family of the child with asthma includes education about the disease and its therapy and facilitation of self-management.
- Cystic fibrosis is the most common inherited disease in children.
- The diagnosis of cystic fibrosis is based on the family history, increased sweat electrolyte content, absent pancreatic enzymes, and chronic pulmonary involvement.
- Choking and respiratory failure are respiratory emergencies that necessitate immediate intervention.
- The Heimlich maneuver is reserved for children in whom foreign body aspiration is witnessed or strongly suspected. A combination of back blows and chest thrusts is used for infants with foreign body aspiration.
- In a conscious choking child, attempts to relieve the obstruction are used only if the child is unable to make any sounds; if the cough becomes ineffective; or if the child has increasing respiratory difficulty with stridor.

References

Abulhosm RS et al: Passive smoke exposure impairs recovery after hospitalization for acute asthma, *Arch Pediatr Adolesc Med* 151:135-139, 1997.

American Academy of Pediatrics: *Influenza guidelines for parents,* Elk Grove Village, IL, 1998, The Academy.

American Academy of Pediatrics, Committee on Infectious Diseases, Pickering L, editor: *2000 Red Book: report of the Committee on Infectious Diseases,* ed 25, Elk Grove Village, IL, 2000, The Academy.

American Heart Association: Guidelines 2000 for cardiopulmonary resuscitation and emergency cardiovascular care: *International consensus on science*, 2000.

Armitage KB, Gross P, Yamauchi T: Respiratory infections: which antibiotics for empiric therapy? *Patient Care Nurse Pract,* Jan 1999, 30-46.

Barnett ED et al: Comparison of ceftriaxone and trimethoprim-sulfamethoxazole for acute otitis media, *Pediatrics* 99(1):23-28, 1997.

Barone SR, Krilov LR, Sumaya CV: Infectious mononucleosis and Epstein-Barr virus infections. In Hoekelman RA et al, editors: *Primary pediatric care,* ed 3, St Louis, 1997, Mosby.

Blumer JL: Traditional management of acute otitis media. In Klein JO, editor: *Otitis media management strategies for the 21st century,* Bala Cynwyd, PA, 1998, Meniscus Educational Institute.

Capen CL, Sherman JM: Fatal asthma in children: a nurse managed model for prevention, *J Pediatr News* 13(6):367-375, 1998.

Chandra NC, Hazinski MF, editors: *Textbook of basic life support for healthcare providers,* Dallas, 1997, American Heart Association.

Derkay CS, Darrow D, LeFebvre S: Pediatric tonsillectomy and adenoidectomy procedures, *AORN J* 62(6):887-904, 1995.

Dowell SF et al: Otitis media: principles of judicious use of antimicrobial agents, *Pediatrics* 101(1, suppl, pt 2):165-171, 1998.

Feder HM et al: Once-daily therapy for streptococcal pharyngitis with amoxicillin, *Pediatrics* 103(1):47-51, 1999.

Fost DA, Spahn JD: The leukotriene modifiers: a new class of asthma medication, *Contemp Pediatr* 15:95-107, 1998.

Hagemann T: Cystic fibrosis—drug therapy, *J Pediatr Health Care* 10(3):127-134, 1996.

Hoffman N, Kelly C, Futterman D: Tuberculosis infection in human immunodeficiency virus-positive adolescents and young adults: a New York City cohort, *Pediatrics* 97(2):198-203, 1996.

Jackson MM, McLeod RP: Tuberculosis in infants, children, and adolescents: an update with case studies, *Pediatr News* 23(5):411-420, 1998.

Meng A: An asthma day camp, *MCN* 22:135-141, 1997.

Milgram H, Bender B: Behavioral side effects of medications used to treat asthma and allergic rhinitis, *Pediatr Rev* 16(9):333-335, 1995.

Montville NH, White MA: Diagnosis and pharmacological management of acute otitis media, *Pediatr Nurs* 23(5):423-429, 1998.

Nafstad P et al: Day care centers and respiratory health, *Pediatrics* 103(4):753-758, 1999.

National Asthma Education and Prevention Program: *Expert Panel report II: guidelines for the diagnosis and management of asthma,* Pub. No. 97-4051, Bethesda, MD, 1997, National Heart, Lung, and Blood Institute, National Institutes of Health.

Overturf GD: The American Academy of Pediatrics, Committee on Infectious Diseases: *Technical report: prevention of pneumococcal infections, including the use of pneumococcal conjugate and polysaccharide vaccines and antibiotic prophylaxis,* June 2000. www.aap.org.

Rosenstreich DL et al: The role of cockroach allergy and exposure to cockroach allergen in causing morbidity among inner-city children with asthma, *N Engl J Med* 336:1356-1363, 1997.

Sutters KA, Miaskowski C: Inadequate pain management and associated morbidity in children at home after tonsillectomy, *J Pediatr Nurs* 12(3):178-186, 1997.

Thomas PC, Moore P, Reilly JS: Child preferences for post-tonsillectomy diet, *Int J Pediatr Otorhinolaryngol* 31:29-33, 1995.

Thuma PE: Pharyngitis and tonsillitis. In Hoekelman RA et al, editors: *Primary pediatric care,* ed 3, St Louis, 1997, Mosby.

Tully SB, Bar-Haim Y, Bradley RL: Abnormal tympanography after supine bottle feeding, *J Pediatr* 126:S105-S111, 1995.

Twarog FJ: Inhaled steroids for asthma—how safe? *Pediatr Alert,* Dec 10, 1998.

Williams RL et al: Use of antibiotics in preventing recurrent otitis media and in treating otitis media with effusion, *JAMA* 270(11):1344-1351, 1997.

Wilmott RW, Kaplan EB, Perez CR: Cystic fibrosis. In Polin RA, Ditmar MF, editors: *Pediatric secrets,* ed 2, St Louis, 1997, Mosby.

Winkelstein ML, Tarzian A, Wood RA: Parental smoking behavior and passive smoke exposure in children with asthma, *Ann Allergy Asthma Immunol* 78(4):419-423, 1997.

CHAPTER

47

Gastrointestinal Dysfunction

http://www.harcourthealth.com/MERLIN/Wong/maternal/

Learning Objectives

On completion of this chapter the reader will be able to:

- Identify children at increased risk of developing nutritional disturbances.
- Outline a nutritional counseling plan for vitamin or mineral deficiency and excess.
- Outline a dietary plan for parents when their infant is sensitive to milk.
- Describe the characteristics of infants that affect their ability to adapt to fluid loss or gain.
- Formulate a plan of care for the infant with acute diarrhea.
- Compare and contrast the inflammatory diseases of the gastrointestinal tract.
- Outline a teaching plan designed to prevent transmission of intestinal parasites.
- Distinguish between aphthous stomatitis and herpetic gingivostomatitis.
- Describe the nursing care of the child with hepatitis.
- Formulate a plan for teaching parents preoperative and postoperative care of the child with a cleft lip and/or palate.
- Formulate a plan of care for the child with an obstructive disorder.
- Identify nutritional therapies for the child with a malabsorption syndrome.
- Identify the principles in the emergency treatment of poisoning.
- Name four sources of lead in the environment.

NUTRITIONAL DISTURBANCES

Vitamin Disturbances

True vitamin deficiencies are rare in the United States, although subclinical deficiencies are commonly seen in population subgroups where dietary intake is imbalanced. A study revealed that only 1 in 5 children ages 2 to 18 years regularly consumed five or more servings of fruit and vegetables per day. In the same group approximately 50% of the children surveyed consumed less than one serving of fruit per day, with boys eating more fruit than girls. The most common vegetable consumed by children and adolescents was French fries (Krebs-Smith et al, 1996).

It has been reported that in children ages 7 to 18 years, approximately one third of the children and two thirds of adolescent girls consume less than the recommended amount of vitamin B_6. Vitamin D-deficiency rickets, once rarely seen because of vitamin D-fortified milk, has increased. Populations at risk include (1) children born of vitamin D-deficient mothers; (2) individuals who are exposed to minimal sunlight because of their particular clothing, religious or cultural beliefs, housing in areas of high pollution, or dark skin pigmentation; (3) those with diets that are low in sources of vitamin D and calcium; and (4) individuals who use milk products not supplemented with vitamin D (e.g., yogurt or raw cow's milk) as the primary source of milk. Children may also be at risk secondary to disorders or their treatment. For example, vitamin deficiencies of the fat-soluble vitamins A and D may occur in malabsorptive disorders. Children receiving high doses of salicylates, such as for rheumatoid arthritis, may have impaired vitamin C storage.

Vitamin A deficiency correlates with increased morbidity and mortality in children with measles. Complications from diarrhea and infections are often increased in infants and children with vitamin A deficiency. The American Academy of Pediatrics (AAP) recommends that vitamin A supplementation be considered in children hospitalized with measles and associated complications (e.g., diarrhea, croup, pneumonia), especially children between the ages of 6 months and 2 years (AAP, 2000).

Of equal, if not greater, concern is the overuse of vitamins, especially as a part of alternative therapies. An excessive dose of a vitamin is generally defined as 10 or more times the recommended dietary allowance, although the fat-soluble vitamins, especially A and D, tend to cause toxic reactions at lower doses. With the addition of vitamins to commercially prepared foods, the potential for hypervitaminosis has increased, especially when combined with the excessive use of vitamin supplements. Hypervitaminosis of A and D presents the greatest problem because these fat-soluble vitamins are stored in the body. Vitamin

D is the most likely of all vitamins to cause toxic reactions in relatively small overdoses. The water-soluble vitamins, primarily niacin, B_6, and C, can also cause toxicity.

One vitamin supplement that is recommended for all women of childbearing age is a daily dose of 0.4 mg of folic acid, the usual recommended dietary allowance (RDA). Folic acid taken before conception and during early pregnancy can reduce the risk of neural tube defects such as spina bifida by at least 50%. Nurses should educate childbearing adolescent females about the need for folic acid to prevent neural tube birth defects. It is easily obtained from a well balanced diet or a daily multivitamin supplement.

Deficiencies and excesses of vitamins A, B complex, C, D, E, and K are summarized in Table 47-1, and the RDAs are listed in Appendix G. General nursing considerations are discussed below, and specific interventions are presented in the table.

Mineral Disturbances

A number of minerals are essential nutrients. The *macrominerals* refer to those with daily requirements greater than 100 mg and include calcium, phosphorus, magnesium, sodium, potassium, chloride, and sulfur. *Microminerals,* or *trace elements,* have daily requirements of less than 100 mg and include several essential minerals and those whose exact role in nutrition is still unclear. The greatest concern with minerals is deficiency, especially iron, calcium, phosphorus, magnesium, and zinc. Low levels of zinc can cause nutritional failure to thrive.

The regulation of mineral balance in the body is a complex process. Dietary extremes of mineral intake can cause a number of mineral-mineral interactions that could result in unexpected deficiencies or excesses. For example, excessive amounts of one mineral, such as zinc, can result in a deficiency of another mineral, such as copper, even if sufficient amounts of copper are ingested.

Deficiencies can also occur when various substances in the diet interact with minerals. For example, iron, zinc, and calcium can form insoluble complexes with *phytates* and/or *oxalates* (substances found in plant proteins), which impair the bioavailability of the mineral. This type of interaction is important in vegetarian diets because plant foods such as soy are high in phytates. Contrary to popular opinion, spinach is not a rich source of iron or calcium because of its high oxylate content. Factors that affect iron absorption are listed in Box 47-1.

Deficiencies and excesses of the essential macrominerals and microminerals are summarized in Table 47-2. General nursing considerations are discussed on p. 1246, and specific interventions are discussed in the table.

Vegetarian Diets

The importance of the relationship between vegetarian diets and potential nutritional deficiencies in children cannot be overemphasized. The stricter the vegetarian diet, the more difficult it becomes to ensure adequate nutrition for infants and children. The major types of vegetarianism are:

Lacto-ovovegetarians, who exclude meat from their diet but consume dairy products and rarely fish

Lactovegetarians, who exclude meat and eggs but drink milk

Pure vegetarians (vegans), who eliminate any food of animal origin, including milk and eggs

Zen macrobiotics, who are even more restrictive than pure vegetarians; small amounts of fruits, vegetables, and legumes are allowed

Semi-vegetarians, who consume a lacto-ovo-vegetarian diet with some fish and poultry; this is an increasingly popular form of vegetarianism and poses little or no nutritional risk to infants unless dietary fat and cholesterol intake is severely restricted.

Many individuals who are concerned about healthy diets subscribe to vegetarian diets that may not be typified by the above categories. Therefore, during nutritional assessment it is necessary to clearly list exactly what the diet includes and excludes (AAP, 1998a).*

The lacto-ovo-vegetarian diet is associated with the least deficiencies, although iron intake needs to be monitored. The major deficiencies in the stricter vegetarian diets are inadequate protein for growth; inadequate calories for energy and growth; poor digestibility, especially for infants, of many of the natural, unprocessed foods; and deficiencies of vitamin B_6, niacin, riboflavin, vitamin D, iron, calcium, and zinc. Strict vegetarian diets also require supplements of vitamin B_{12} and vitamin D. Vitamin D is essential if exposure to sunlight is inadequate (i.e., <5 to 15 minutes per day on the hands, arms and face) or in persons who are dark-skinned or who live in northern latitudes or cloudy or smoky areas (American Dietetic Association, 1997).

Iron deficiency anemia and rickets may also be seen in children on strict vegetarian and macrobiotic diets as a result of consuming plant foods such as unrefined cereals, which impair the absorption of iron, calcium, and zinc (Sanders, 1995).

Nursing Care Management. Identification of nutrient imbalance is the initial nursing goal and requires assessment based on a dietary history and physical examination for signs of deficiency or excess (see Nutritional Assessment, Chapter 34). Once assessment data are collected, this information is evaluated against standard intakes to identify areas of concern. The most widely used standard is the *Recommended Dietary Allowances (RDAs),* developed by the *National Academy of Sciences, Food and Nutrition Board.* The RDAs are not average requirements but recommendations intended to meet the physiologic needs of almost every healthy person. To meet the needs of those with the highest requirements, the RDAs will exceed most people's requirements. Therefore children consuming less than the RDAs are not necessarily consuming an inadequate diet, but they are more likely at risk for deficiency than those who are consuming nutrients in amounts equal to the RDAs.

Several organizations have published dietary advice for the public. The *Dietary Guidelines for Americans* encourage eating a variety of foods; maintaining ideal body weight; consuming adequate starch and fiber; and limiting intake of fat, cholesterol, sugar, salt, and alcohol. The Food Guide Pyramid (FGP) (Fig. 47-1), which replaces the basic four food groups, is used to convey nutrition information to the public and applies to children as young as 2 years of age.

The new FGP includes pictures aimed at younger children. The different food groups and servings are the same, yet the

Text continued on p. 1241

*Further information regarding vegetarian diets may be found at the Vegetarian Resource Group (VRG), (410) 366-VEGE; website: www.vrg.org.

TABLE 47-1
Vitamins and Their Nutritional Significance

Physiologic Functions/Sources	Results of Deficiency or Excess	Nursing Considerations
VITAMIN A (RETINOL)*		
Functions	**Deficiency**	
Necessary component in formation of pigment rhodopsin (visual purple) Formation and maintenance of epithelial tissue Normal bone growth and tooth development Needed for growth and spermatogenesis Involved in thyroxine formation Antioxidant	Night blindness Keratinization (hardening and scaling) of epithelium Xerophthalmia (hardening and scaling of cornea and conjunctiva) Phrynoderma (toad skin) Drying of respiratory, gastrointestinal, and genitourinary tracts Defective tooth enamel Retarded growth Impaired bone formation Decreased thyroxine formation	Encourage foods rich in vitamin A, such as whole cow's milk As milk consumption decreases, encourage foods rich in vitamin A Ensure adequate intake in preterm infants Advise parents of safe use of supplements in child with measles
Sources **Natural form**—Liver, kidney, fish oils, milk and nonskimmed milk products, egg yolk **Provitamin A (carotene)**—Carrots, sweet potatoes, squash, apricots, spinach, collards, broccoli, cabbage, artichokes	**Excess** **Early signs**—Irritability, anorexia, pruritus, fissures at corners of nose and lips **Later signs**—Hepatomegaly, jaundice, retarded growth, poor weight gain, thickening of the cortex of long bones with pain and fragility, hard tender lumps in extremities and occiput of the skull May cause birth defects from excessive maternal intake NOTE: Overdose results from ingestion of large quantities of the vitamin only, not the provitamin; large amounts of carotene (carotenemia) cause yellow or orange discoloration of the skin (not the sclera, urine, or feces as in jaundice), but none of the above symptoms	Emphasize correct use of vitamin supplements and potential hazards of excess Investigate child's dietary habits to calculate approximate intake; if excessive, remove supplemental source (e.g., daily feeding of liver) Advise parents of the benign nature of carotenemia; treatment is avoidance of excess pigmented fruits or vegetables, especially carrots; skin color returns to normal in 2 to 6 weeks
VITAMIN B_1 (THIAMINE)†		
Functions Coenzyme (with phosphorus) in carbohydrate metabolism Needed for healthy nervous system **Sources** Pork, beef, liver, legumes, nuts, whole or enriched grains and cereals, green vegetables, fruits, milk, brown rice	**Deficiency** **Gastrointestinal**—Anorexia, constipation, indigestion **Neurologic**—Apathy, fatigue, emotional instability, polyneuritis, tenderness of calf muscles, partial anesthesia, muscle weakness, paresthesia, hyperesthesia, decreased or absent tendon reflexes, seizures, and coma (in infants) **Cardiovascular**—Palpitations, cardiac failure, peripheral vasodilation, edema **Excess** Headache Irritability Insomnia Rapid pulse Weakness	***Vitamin B complex*** Encourage foods rich in B vitamins Stress proper cooking and storage techniques to preserve potency, such as minimum cooking of vegetables in small amount of liquid; storage of milk in opaque container Explore need for vitamin supplements when dieting or when using goat milk exclusively for infant feeding (deficient in folic acid) or when the breastfeeding mother is a strict vegetarian (vitamin B_{12}) Emphasize correct use of vitamin supplements and potential hazards of excesses

*Fat soluble.
†Water soluble.

Continued

TABLE 47-1—cont'd

Vitamins and Their Nutritional Significance

Physiologic Functions/Sources	Results of Deficiency or Excess	Nursing Considerations
VITAMIN B_2 (RIBOFLAVIN)†		
Functions Coenzyme (with phosphorus) in carbohydrate, protein, and fat metabolism Maintains healthy skin, especially around mouth, nose, and eyes **Sources** Milk and its products, eggs, organ meat (liver, kidney, and heart), enriched cereals, some green leafy vegetables,‡ legumes	**Deficiency** Ariboflavinosis **Lips**—Cheilosis (fissures at corners of lips), perlêche (inflammation at corners of lips) **Tongue**—Glossitis **Nose**—Irritation and cracks at nasal angle **Eyes**—Burning, itching, tearing, photophobia, corneal vascularization, cataracts **Skin**—Seborrheic dermatitis, delayed wound healing and tissue repair **Excess** Paresthesia, pruritus	Same as vitamin B complex
NIACIN (NICOTINIC ACID, NICOTINAMIDE)†		
Functions Coenzyme (with riboflavin) in protein and fat metabolism Needed for healthy nervous system, skin, and normal digestion May lower cholesterol **Sources** Meat, poultry, fish, peanuts, beans, peas, whole or enriched grains except corn and rice Milk and its products are sources of tryptophan (60 mg of tryptophan = 1 mg of niacin)	**Deficiency** Pellagra **Oral**—Stomatitis, glossitis **Cutaneous**—Scaly dermatitis on exposed areas **Gastrointestinal**—Anorexia, weight loss, diarrhea, fatigue **Neurologic**—Apathy, anxiety, confusion, depression, dementia Death **Excess** Release of vasodilator, histamine (flushing, decreased blood pressure, increased cerebral blood flow; aggravates asthma) Dermatologic problems (pruritus, rash, hyperkeratosis, acanthosis nigricans) Increased gastric acidity (aggravates peptic ulcer disease) Hepatotoxicity Increased serum uric acid levels Elevated plasma glucose levels Certain cardiac dysrhythmias	Same as vitamin B complex If used as hypolipidemic agent, stress safe dosage to prevent child's accidental ingestion
VITAMIN B_6 (PYRIDOXINE)†		
Functions Coenzyme in protein and fat metabolism Needed for formation of antibodies, hemoglobin Needed for utilization of copper and iron Aids in conversion of tryptophan to niacin **Sources** Meats, especially liver and kidney, cereal grains (wheat and corn), yeast, soybeans, peanuts, tuna, chicken, salmon	**Deficiency** Scaly dermatitis, weight loss, anemia, retarded growth, irritability, seizures, peripheral neuritis **Excess** Peripheral nervous system toxicity (unsteady gait, numb feet and hands, clumsiness of hands, sometimes perioral numbness) May cause peptic ulcer disease or seizures	Same as vitamin B complex Stress proper cooking and storing techniques to preserve potency Cook food covered in small amount of water Store in light-resistant container

†Water soluble.
‡Green leafy vegetables include spinach, broccoli, kale, turnip greens, mustard greens, collards, dandelion greens, and beet greens.

TABLE 47-1—cont'd
Vitamins and Their Nutritional Significance

Physiologic Functions/Sources	Results of Deficiency or Excess	Nursing Considerations
FOLIC ACID (FOLACIN); REDUCED FORM IS CALLED FOLINIC ACID OR CITROVORUM FACTOR†		
Functions Coenzyme for single-carbon transfer (purines, thymine, hemoglobin) Necessary for formation of red blood cells May prevent neural tube defects (i.e., myelomeningocele) **Sources** Green leafy vegetables,‡ cabbage, asparagus, liver, kidney, nuts, eggs, whole grain cereals, legumes, bananas	**Deficiency** Macrocytic anemia, bone marrow depression, glossitis, intestinal malabsorption **Excess** Rare because megadoses not available over the counter May cause insomnia and irritability	Same as vitamin B complex Stress proper cooking and storing techniques to preserve potency Cook food covered in small amount of water Do not soak food in water Store in light-resistant container Women of childbearing age should receive RDA (0.4 mg/day) to prevent neural tube defects
VITAMIN B_{12} (COBALAMIN)†		
Functions Coenzyme in protein synthesis; indirect effect on formation of red blood cells (particularly on formation of nucleic acids and folic acid metabolism) Needed for normal functioning of nervous tissue **Sources** Meat, liver, kidney, fish, shellfish, poultry, milk, eggs, cheese, nutritional yeast, sea vegetables	**Deficiency** Pernicious anemia (One form of deficiency from absence of intrinsic factor in gastric secretions) General signs of severe anemia Lemon-yellow tinge to skin Spinal cord degeneration Delayed brain growth **Excess** Excess is rare	Same as vitamin B complex
BIOTIN		
Functions Coenzyme in carbohydrate, protein, and fat metabolism Interrelated with functions of other B vitamins **Sources** Liver, kidney, egg yolk, tomatoes, legumes, nuts	**Deficiency** Deficiency is uncommon because synthesized by bacterial flora **Excess** Unknown	Same as vitamin B complex
PANTOTHENIC ACID†		
Functions Coenzyme in carbohydrate, protein, and fat metabolism Synthesis of amino acids, fatty acids, and steroids **Sources** Liver, kidney, heart, salmon, eggs, vegetables, legumes, whole grains	**Deficiency** Deficiency is uncommon because of its multiple food sources and synthesis by bacterial flora **Excess** Minimum toxicity (occasional diarrhea and water retention)	Same as vitamin B complex
VITAMIN C (ASCORBIC ACID)†		
Functions Essential for collagen formation Increases absorption of iron for hemoglobin formation Enhances conversion of folic acid to folinic acid	**Deficiency** *Scurvy* **Skin**—Dry, rough, petechiae, perifollicular hyperkeratotic papules (raised areas around hair follicles)	Encourage foods rich in vitamin C Investigate infant's diet for sources of vitamin, especially when cow's milk is principal source of nutrition

Continued

TABLE 47-1—cont'd
Vitamins and Their Nutritional Significance

Physiologic Functions/Sources	Results of Deficiency or Excess	Nursing Considerations
VITAMIN C (ASCORBIC ACID)†—cont'd		
Functions—cont'd Affects cholesterol synthesis and conversion of proline to hydroxyproline Probably a coenzyme in metabolism of tyrosine and phenylalanine May play role in hydroxylation of adrenal steroids May have stimulating effect on phagocytic activity of leukocytes and formation of antibodies Antioxidant agent (spares other vitamins from oxidation) **Sources** Citrus fruits, strawberries, tomatoes, potatoes, cabbage, broccoli, cauliflower, green peppers, spinach, papaya, mango, cantaloupe, watermelon, enriched fruit juice	**Deficiency—cont'd** **Musculoskeletal**—Bleeding muscles and joints, pseudoparalysis from pain, swelling of joints, costochondral beading (scorbutic rosary) **Gums**—Spongy, friable, swollen, bleed easily, bluish red or black color, teeth loosen and fall out **General disposition**—Irritable, anorexic, apprehensive, in pain, refuses to move, assumes semifroglike position when supine (scorbutic pose) Signs of anemia Decreased wound healing Increased susceptibility to infection **Excess** Diarrhea Increased excretion of uric acid and acidification of urine (may cause urate precipitation and formation of oxalate stones) Hemolysis Impaired leukocytosis activity Damage to beta cells of pancreas and decreased insulin production Reproductive failure "Rebound scurvy" from withdrawal of large amounts	Stress proper cooking and storing techniques to preserve potency Wash vegetables quickly; do not soak in water Cook vegetables in covered pot with minimum water and for short time; avoid copper or cast iron cookware Do not add baking soda to cooking water Use fresh fruits and vegetables as soon as possible; store in refrigerator Store juice in airtight, opaque container Wrap cut fruit or eat soon after exposing to air In caring for child with scurvy: Position for comfort and rest Handle very gently and minimally Administer analgesics as needed Prevent infection Provide good oral care Provide soft, bland diet Emphasize rapid recovery when vitamin is replaced Emphasize correct use of vitamin supplement and potential hazards of excess Identify groups at risk for vitamin C supplements; those with thalassemia; those receiving anticoagulant or aminoglycoside antibiotic therapy
VITAMIN D_2 (ERGOCALCIFEROL) and D_3 (CHOLECALCIFEROL)*		
Functions Absorption of calcium and phosphorus and decreased renal excretion of phosphorus **Sources** Direct sunlight Cod liver oil, herring, mackerel, salmon, tuna, sardines **Enriched food sources**—Milk, milk products, enriched cereals, margarine, breads, many breakfast drinks	**Deficiency** ***Rickets*** **Head**—Craniotabes (softening of cranial bones, prominence of frontal bones), deformed shape (skull flat and depressed toward middle), delayed closure of fontanels **Chest**—Rachitic rosary (enlargement of costochondral junction of ribs) Harrison groove (horizontal depression in lower portion of rib cage), pigeon chest (sharp protrusion of sternum) **Spine**—Kyphosis, scoliosis, lordosis **Abdomen**—Potbelly, constipation **Extremities**—Bowing of arms and legs, knock-knee, saber shins, instability of hip joints, pelvic deformity, enlargement of epiphysis at ends of long bones **Teeth**—Delayed calcification, especially of permanent teeth **Rachitic tetany**—Seizures	Encourage foods rich in vitamin D, especially fortified cow's milk In breastfed infants encourage use of vitamin D supplements if maternal diet inadequate or infant exposed to minimal sunlight In caring for child with rickets: Maintain good body alignment Reposition frequently to prevent decubiti and respiratory infection Handle very gently and minimally Prevent infection Institute seizure precautions Have 10% calcium gluconate available in case of tetany Observe for possibility of overdose from supplements If prescribed, supervise proper use of orthopedic splints or braces Same as vitamin A; may include low-calcium diet during initial therapy

*Fat soluble.
†Water soluble.

TABLE 47-1—cont'd
Vitamins and Their Nutritional Significance

Physiologic Functions/Sources	Results of Deficiency or Excess	Nursing Considerations
VITAMIN D_2—cont'd		
	Excess **Acute**—Vomiting, dehydration, fever, abdominal cramps, bone pain, seizures, and coma **Chronic**—Lassitude, mental slowness, anorexia, failure to thrive, thirst, urinary urgency, polyuria, vomiting, diarrhea, abdominal cramps, bone pain, pathologic fractures **Calcification of soft tissue**—Kidneys, lungs, adrenal glands, vessels (hypertension), heart, gastric lining, tympanic membrane (deafness) Osteoporosis of long bones Elevated serum levels of calcium and phosphorus	
VITAMIN E (TOCOPHEROL)*		
Functions Production of red blood cells and protection from hemolysis Muscle and liver integrity Coenzyme factor in tissue respiration Minimizes oxidation of polyunsaturated fatty acids and vitamins A and C in intestinal tract and tissues Possible role in treatment and prevention of bronchopulmonary dysplasia and retinopathy of prematurity is under investigation	**Deficiency** Hemolytic anemia from hemolysis caused by shortened life of red blood cells, especially in preterm infants, and focal necrosis of tissues Causes infertility in rats, but not in humans (does *not* increase human male virility or potency) **Excess** Little is known: less toxic than other fat-soluble vitamins	Initiate early feeding in preterm infants; may need supplementation
Sources Vegetable oils, wheat germ oil, milk, egg yolk, muscle meats, fish, whole grains, nuts, legumes, spinach, broccoli		
VITAMIN K*		
Functions Catalyst for production of prothrombin and blood-clotting factors II, VII, IX, and X by the liver **Sources** Pork, liver, green leafy vegetables‡ (spinach, kale, cabbage), tomatoes, egg yolk, cheese	**Deficiency** Umbilical cord oozing (or any wounds) and petechiae, hemorrhage **Excess** Hemolytic anemia in individuals who are deficient in glucose-6-phosphate dehydrogenase	Administer prophylactically to all newborns Other indications include intestinal disease, lack of bile, prolonged antibiotic therapy; may be used in management of blood-clotting time when anticoagulants such as warfarin (Coumadin) and dicumarol (bishydroxycoumarin), which are vitamin K antagonists, are used

Text continued from p. 1236

foods are made to appear more realistic than the previous FGP. The names of the groups have also been reduced for children to better understand. The tip of the pyramid emphasizes a decrease in the consumption of fats and sweets.

The number of servings and serving sizes are important components of the Food Guide Pyramid. Suggested serving sizes for the five food groups are listed in Box 47-2. Young children need the same variety of foods as older children but may need less than the 1600 calories provided by the suggested minimum number of servings in each food group. To meet their caloric needs, adjustments are made by using the minimum number of servings and smaller serving sizes; however, it is important that children have the equivalent of at least 2 cups of milk a day. Adolescents, who require increased calories for

Box 47-1

Factors that Affect Iron Absorption

INCREASE

Acidity (low pH)—Administer iron between meals (gastric hydrochloric acid)

Ascorbic acid (vitamin C)—Administer iron with juice, fruit, or multivitamin preparation

Vitamin A

Calcium

Tissue need

Meat, fish, poultry

Cooking in cast iron pots

DECREASE

Alkalinity (high pH)—Avoid any antacid preparation

Phosphates—Milk is unfavorable vehicle for iron administration

Phytates—Found in cereals

Oxalates—Found in many fruits and vegetables (plums, currants, green beans, spinach, sweet potatoes, tomatoes)

Tannins—Found in tea, coffee

Tissue saturation

Malabsorptive disorders

Disturbances that cause diarrhea or steatorrhea

Infection

growth, should have at least 3 cups of milk a day and more fruits, and may require the maximum number of suggested servings. Current recommendations for fat intake for children over 2 years of age are that no more than 30% of calories should come from fat and the remainder of calories should come from carbohydrates and protein (see also Hyperlipidemia [Hypercholesterolemia], Chapter 48).

Because one of the best assurances of nutritional adequacy is eating a variety of foods, families need guidelines for selecting foods that provide essential nutrients without exceeding energy requirements. With a varied diet most children do not need vitamin or mineral supplements. Unfortunately, there are no restrictions on the availability of toxic doses of vitamins or minerals. Nurses need to inquire about alternative therapies that include vitamin or mineral supplements and to inform families of the potential dangers from excess vitamins or minerals. The idea that "more is better" is probably best dispelled by a simple explanation of the body's inability to use more than the needed requirement.

Achieving a nutritionally adequate vegetarian diet requires careful planning and knowledge of nutrient sources. For children the lacto-ovo-vegetarian diet is nutritionally adequate; however, the vegan diet requires supplementation with vitamins D and B_{12} for children ages 2 to 12 years. Infants should be breastfed for the first 6 months and preferably for 1 year, be fed solid foods after about 4 months, and receive iron-fortified cereal for at least 18 months. The American Dietetic Association (1997) recommends iron supplementation in infants exclusively breastfed after 4 to 6 months by vegetarian mothers and no dietary fat restrictions in vegetarian children younger than 2 years. The use of vitamin C juices with foods high in iron will further improve iron absorption; however, breast milk from vegetarian mothers can be deficient in vitamin B_{12}; supplementation of both mother and child is advisable. If cow's or human milk or commercial infant formula is not given, fortified soy milk is recommended. A variety of foods should be introduced during the early years to ensure a more well-balanced intake.

NURSE ALERT • When solid foods are introduced, the safety and digestibility of the selections must be considered. Raw fruits with seeds, vegetables, and nuts are hazardous for infants and young children because of the danger of aspiration. Beans, grain cereals, and vegetables should be served well-cooked and mashed during infancy.

To ensure sufficient protein in the diet, foods with incomplete proteins (i.e., those that do not have all of the essential amino acids) should be eaten with other foods that supply the missing amino acids. The three basic combinations of foods consumed by vegetarians that generally provide the appropriate amounts of essential amino acids are:

1. Grains (cereal, rice, pasta) and legumes (beans, peas, lentils, peanuts)
2. Grains and milk products (milk, cheese, yogurt)
3. Seeds (sesame, sunflower) and legumes

Protein and Energy Malnutrition (PEM)

Malnutrition continues to be a major health problem in the world today, particularly in children under 5 years of age. Lack of food, however, is not always the primary cause for malnutrition. In many developing and underdeveloped nations, *diarrhea* is a major factor. Additional factors are bottle-feeding (in poor sanitary conditions), inadequate knowledge of proper child care practices, parental illiteracy, economic and political factors, and simply the lack of food (David and Lobo, 1995). The most extreme forms of malnutrition, or PEM, are kwashiorkor and marasmus.

In the United States milder forms of PEM are seen, although the classic cases of marasmus and kwashiorkor may also occur. Unlike developing countries, where the main reason for PEM is inadequate food, in the United States PEM occurs despite ample dietary supplies (see Failure to Thrive, p. 869).

Kwashiorkor. Kwashiorkor has been defined in the past as primarily a deficiency of protein with an adequate supply of calories. A diet consisting mainly of starch grains or tubers provides adequate calories in the form of carbohydrates but an inadequate amount of high-quality proteins. There is evidence supporting a multifactorial etiology, including cultural, psychologic, and infective factors that may jointly or singly interact to place the child at risk for kwashiorkor. Taken from the Ga language (Ghana), the word *kwashiorkor* means "the sickness the older child gets when the next baby is born" and aptly describes the syndrome that develops in the first child, usually between 1 and 4 years of age, when weaned from the breast once the second child is born.

The child with kwashiorkor has thin, wasted extremities and a prominent abdomen from edema (ascites). The edema often masks the severe muscular atrophy, making the child appear less debilitated than he or she actually is. The skin is scaly and dry and has areas of depigmentation. Several dermatoses may be evident, partly resulting from the vitamin deficiencies. Permanent blindness often results from the severe lack of vitamin A. Min-

TABLE 47-2
Minerals and Their Nutritional Significance

Physiologic Functions/Sources	Results of Deficiency or Excess	Nursing Considerations
CALCIUM*		
Functions	**Deficiency**	
Bone and tooth development and maintenance (in combination with phosphorus) Muscle contractions, especially the heart Blood clotting Absorption of vitamin B_{12} Enzyme activation Nerve conduction Integrity of intracellular cement substances and various membranes	***Rickets*** Impaired growth, especially of bones and teeth **Excess** Drowsiness, extreme lethargy Impaired absorption of other minerals (iron, zinc, manganese) Calcium deposits in tissues (renal failure)	Encourage foods rich in calcium, especially dairy products Caution that oxalates in leafy vegetables (spinach), oxalates in chocolates, and a high phosphorus intake (especially from carbonated beverages) can decrease calcium absorption Discourage use of whole cow's milk in newborns because the phosphorus-to-calcium ratio favors excretion of calcium Advise against fad diets, especially those that restrict dairy products Emphasize correct use of calcium supplement, especially adequate intake of vitamin D for calcium absorption and the possible interaction between megadoses of calcium and resulting deficiency states of other minerals
Sources Dairy products, egg yolk, sardines, canned salmon with bones, dark green leafy vegetables (except spinach), soybeans, dried beans, and peas		
CHLORIDE*		
Functions	**Deficiency**	
Acid-base and fluid balance Enzyme activation in saliva Component of hydrochloric acid in stomach	Acid-base disturbances (hypochloremic alkalosis, dehydration); occurs mostly in combination with sodium loss **Excess** Acid-base disturbance	Deficiency and excess are unusual; most diets supply adequate chloride (usually in combination with sodium) Disease states such as excessive vomiting can necessitate chloride replacement
Sources Salt, meat, eggs, dairy products, many prepared and preserved foods		
COPPER†		
Functions	**Deficiency**	
Production of hemoglobin Essential component of several enzyme systems	Anemia, leukopenia, neutropenia **Excess** Severe vomiting and diarrhea Hemolytic anemia	Deficiency from inadequate food sources is less likely than from excess intake of other minerals, especially zinc and possibly iron; therefore emphasize the correct use of any vitamin supplement Caution against cooking acid foods in unlined copper pots, which can lead to chronic and toxic accumulation of copper
Sources Organ meats, oysters, nuts, seeds, legumes, corn oil margarine		
FLUORIDE†		
Functions	**Deficiency**	
Formation of caries-resistant teeth Strong bone development	Increased susceptibility to tooth decay **Excess** **Fluorosis** (mottling and/or pitting of enamel) Severe bone deformities	In areas with optimally fluoridated water, encourage sufficient intake to supply recommended amount of fluoride In areas of unfluoridated water or when ready-to-use formula, bottled water, or breast milk is used, stress the importance of fluoride supplements in infants >6 months (see Chapter 37) In areas with excess fluoride in the water, consider the use of bottled water in drinking and possibly cooking to reduce the fluoride intake to safe levels
Sources Fluoridated water and foods or beverages prepared with fluoridated water; fish, tea, commercially prepared chicken for infants		

*Macrominerals—required intake >100 mg/day.
†Microminerals or trace elements—required intake <100 mg/day.

Continued

TABLE 47-2—cont'd
Minerals and Their Nutritional Significance

Physiologic Functions/Sources	Results of Deficiency or Excess	Nursing Considerations
FLUORIDE—cont'd		
		Fluoride has the narrowest range of safe and adequate intake; therefore stress the importance of storing supplements in a safe area
IODINE†		
Functions Production of thyroid hormone Normal reproduction **Sources** Seafood, kelp, iodized salt, sea salt, enriched bread, milk (from dairy processing)	**Deficiency** **Goiter** (enlarged thyroid from decreased thyroxine formation) **Excess** Unknown from food sources; may occur from ingestion of iodine preparations such as saturated solutions of potassium iodide	Encourage use of iodized salt for individuals living far from the sea If iodine preparations are in the home, stress the importance of safe storage
IRON†		
Functions Formation of hemoglobin and myoglobin Essential part of several enzymes and proteins **Sources** Liver, especially pork, followed by calf, beef, and chicken; liverwurst, red meat, poultry, clams, oysters, beans, ham, whole grains, iron-enriched infant formula and cereal, enriched cereals and bread, legumes, nuts, seeds, green leafy vegetables (except spinach), dried fruits, potatoes, molasses, tofu, prune juice	**Deficiency** **Anemia** (see Chapter 49) **Excess** Hemosiderosis (excess iron storage in various tissues of the body, especially the spleen, liver, lymph glands, heart, and pancreas) Hemochromatosis (excess iron storage with cellular damage)	Encourage foods rich in iron Discourage excessive milk consumption, especially more than 1 L per day (milk is a very poor source of iron) If iron supplements are prescribed, teach parents factors that affect absorption (Box 47-1) Stress the importance of storing iron supplements in a safe area To increase consumption of more iron: Make meat loaf by adding up to ½ pound ground liver to 1 pound ground beef; when the seasonings and other ingredients have been added, it is impossible to tell the meat loaf contains liver
MAGNESIUM*		
Functions Bone and tooth formation Production of proteins Nerve conduction to muscles Activation of enzymes needed for carbohydrate and protein metabolism **Sources** Whole grains, nuts, soybeans, meat, green leafy vegetables (uncooked), tea, cocoa, raisins	**Deficiency** Tremors, spasm Irregular heartbeat Muscular weakness Lower extremity cramps Seizures, delirium **Excess** Nervous system disturbances due to imbalance in calcium-to-magnesium ratio	Deficiency and excess are unusual, except in disease states such as prolonged vomiting or diarrhea or kidney dysfunction, where replacement may be needed Death has occurred when megadoses were given to treat constipation (McGuire et al, 2000)
PHOSPHORUS*		
Functions Bone and tooth development (in combination with calcium) Involved in numerous chemical reactions, including protein, carbohydrate, and fat metabolism Acid-base balance	**Deficiency** Weakness, anorexia, malaise, bone pain **Excess** Produces secondary calcium deficiency from disturbed calcium-to-phosphorus ratio	Dietary deficiency is uncommon, although prolonged use of antacids can produce deficiency, in which case supplementation is recommended To preserve calcium-to-phosphorus ratio in newborns, discourage use of whole cow's milk

*Macrominerals—required intake >100 mg/day.
†Microminerals or trace elements—required intake <100 mg/day.

TABLE 47-2—cont'd
Minerals and Their Nutritional Significance

Physiologic Functions/Sources	Results of Deficiency or Excess	Nursing Considerations
PHOSPHORUS*—cont'd **Sources** Dairy products, eggs, meat, poultry, legumes, carbonated beverages		
POTASSIUM* **Functions** Acid-base and fluid balance (major extracellular fluid areas) Nerve conduction Muscular contraction, especially the heart Release of energy **Sources** Bananas, citrus fruit, dried fruits, meat, fish, bran, legumes, peanut butter, potatoes, coffee, tea, cocoa	**Deficiency** Cardiac dysrhythmias Muscular weakness Lethargy Kidney and respiratory failure Heart failure **Excess** Cardiac dysrhythmias Respiratory failure Mental confusion Numbness of extremities	Dietary deficiency and excess are unlikely, although disease states such as prolonged nausea and vomiting or the use of diuretics can result in hypokalemia; In such instances encourage replacement with supplements of rich food sources, such as bananas
SODIUM* **Functions** Acid-base and fluid balance (major extracellular fluid cation) Cell permeability; absorption of glucose Muscle contraction **Sources** Table salt, seafood, meat, poultry, numerous prepared foods	**Deficiency** Dehydration Hypotension Seizures Muscle cramps **Excess** Edema Hypertension Intracranial hemorrhage	Deficiency intake is very rare, although losses secondary to nausea, vomiting, excessive sweating, and use of diuretics can occur and require replacement Encourage parents to limit excessive use of salt in preparing foods and to limit commercial foods with high sodium content, such as smoked meats
ZINC† **Functions** Component of about 100 enzymes Synthesis of nucleic acids and protein in immune system and coagulation Release of vitamin A from liver Improved wound healing with vitamin C **Sources** Seafood (especially oysters), meat, poultry, eggs, wheat, legumes	**Deficiency** Loss of appetite Diminished taste sensation Delayed healing **Skin lesions**—Erythematous, crusted lesions around body orifices Alopecia Diarrhea Growth failure Retarded sexual maturity **Excess** Vomiting and diarrhea Malaise, dizziness Anemia, gastric bleeding Impaired absorption of calcium and copper	Encourage food sources rich in zinc, especially protein Caution that fiber, phytates, oxalates, tannins (in tea or coffee), iron, and calcium adversely affect zinc absorption Recognize groups at risk for zinc deficiency, such as vegetarians and Hispanics, whose diets may have restricted or low meat content and high-fiber, phytate content and patients with malabsorption syndromes Emphasize correct use of zinc supplements and the possible interaction with other minerals

eral deficiencies are common, especially iron, calcium, and zinc. The hair is thin, dry, coarse, and dull. Depigmentation is common, and patchy alopecia may occur.

Diarrhea commonly occurs from a lowered resistance to infection and produces electrolyte imbalance. A large number of fatalities in children with kwashiorkor occurred in those who developed human immunodeficiency virus (HIV) infection, many of whom were breastfed (Brewster, Manary, and Graham, 1997). Behavioral changes are evident as the child grows progressively more irritable, lethargic, withdrawn, and apathetic. Fatal deterioration may be caused by diarrhea and infection or as the result of circulatory failure.

Marasmus. Marasmus results from general malnutrition of both calories and protein. It is a common occurrence in underdeveloped countries during times of drought, especially in cultures where adults eat first; the remaining food is often insufficient in quality and quantity for the children.

Marasmus is usually a syndrome of physical and emotional deprivation and is not confined to geographic areas where food supplies are inadequate. It may be seen in children with failure to thrive in whom the cause is not solely nutritional but primarily emotional. Marasmus may be seen in infants as young as 3 months of age if breastfeeding is not successful and there are no suitable alternatives. *Marasmic-kwashiorkor* is a form of PEM in which clinical findings of both kwashiorkor and marasmus are evident; the child has edema, severe wasting, and stunted growth.

Marasmus is characterized by gradual wasting and atrophy of body tissues, especially of subcutaneous fat. The child appears to be very old, with flabby and wrinkled skin, unlike the child with kwashiorkor, who appears more rounded from the edema. Fat metabolism is less impaired than in kwashiorkor, so that deficiency of fat-soluble vitamins is usually minimal or absent.

The child is fretful, apathetic, withdrawn, and so lethargic that prostration commonly occurs. Intercurrent infection with debilitating diseases such as tuberculosis, parasitosis, and dysentery is common.

Therapeutic Management. The treatment of PEM includes providing a diet with high quality proteins, carbohydrates, vitamins, and minerals. When PEM occurs as a result of diarrhea, three management goals are identified: (1) rehydration with an oral rehydration solution that also replaces electrolytes; (2) medications such as antibiotics and antidiarrheals; and (3) provision of adequate nutrition either by breastfeeding or a proper weaning diet. When the child is too ill to tolerate oral fluids, intravenous administration of fluids and electrolytes will be required to prevent death.

Nursing Care Management. Provision of essential physiologic needs (e.g., protection from infection, rest, and individually tailored activity) is paramount. Because children are usually weak and withdrawn, they depend on others for feeding. Poor skin integrity increases the chance of infections and further skin breakdown. Appropriate developmental stimulation should be provided as appropriate. Tube feedings may be required in infants too weak to breast- or bottle-feed.

A larger problem is the prevention of these conditions through education concerning the importance of proper nutrition, whether breastfeeding or bottle-feeding, when being weaned to semisolid foods. Because children with marasmus may suffer from emotional starvation as well, care should be consistent with care of the child with failure to thrive (p. 869).

Box 47-2

Food Guide Pyramid: Sample Serving Sizes

Grain group—1 slice of bread; 1 ounce of ready-to-eat cereal; ½ cup of cooked cereal, rice, or pasta
Vegetable group—1 cup of raw leafy vegetable; ½ cup of other vegetable, cooked or chopped raw; ¾ cup of vegetable juice
Fruit group—1 medium apple, banana, or orange; ½ cup of chopped, cooked, or canned fruit; ¼ cup of fruit juice
Milk group—2 cups of milk or yogurt; 1½ ounces of natural cheese, 1 ounce of processed cheese
Meat group—2-3 ounces of cooked lean meat, poultry, or fish; ½ cup of cooked dry beans, 1 egg, or 2 tablespoons of peanut butter count as 1 ounce of lean meat

Food Sensitivity

Food sensitivity is a general term that includes any type of adverse reaction to food or food additives. Food sensitivities can be divided into two broad categories:

1. Food allergy or hypersensitivity, which refers to reactions involving immunologic mechanisms, usually immunoglobulin E (IgE); the reactions may be immediate or delayed, and mild or severe (e.g., anaphylactic reaction).
2. Food intolerance, which refers to reactions involving known or unknown nonimmunologic mechanisms; lactose intolerance is an example of a reaction that looks like allergy but is due to deficiency of the enzyme lactase.

However, this classification is not universally accepted; therefore the terms *food sensitivity, hypersensitivity, allergy,* and *intolerance* are often used interchangeably.

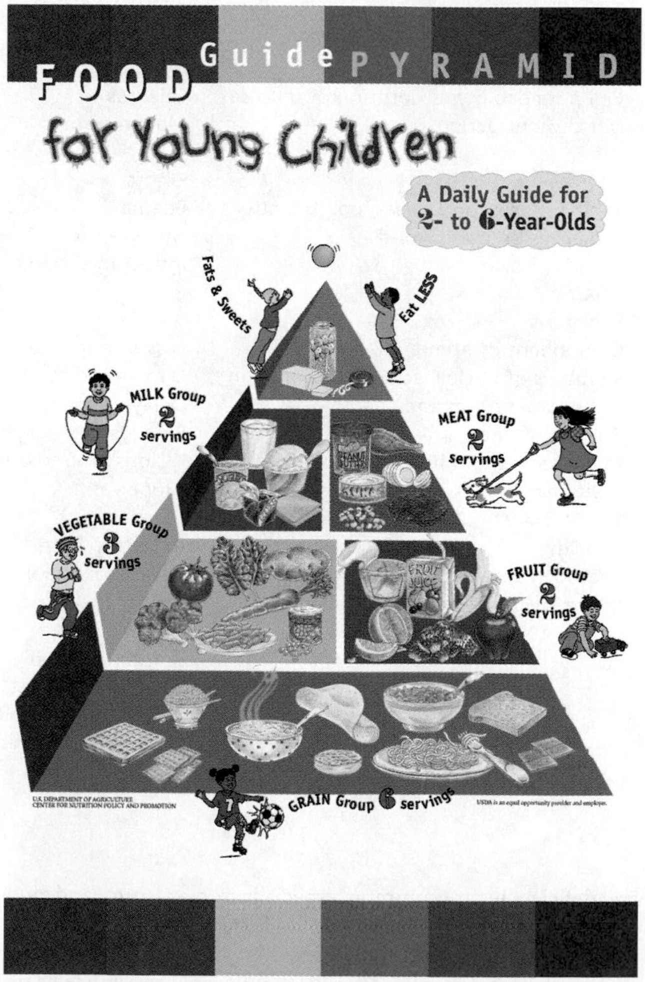

FIG. 47-1 • Food Guide Pyramid for Young Children. (Courtesy U.S. Department of Agriculture Center for Nutrition Policy and Promotion, 1999.)

Food allergy is caused by exposure to *allergens,* usually proteins (but not the smaller amino acids) that are capable of inducing IgE antibody formation ("sensitization") when ingested. *Sensitization* refers to the initial exposure of an individual to an allergen, resulting in an immune response; subsequent exposure induces a much stronger response that is clinically apparent. Consequently, food hypersensitivity typically occurs after the food has been ingested one or more times. In infants an allergic response can occur with the first ingestion because of transplacental sensitization in utero or because of sensitization to the substance passed through breast milk. The most common food allergens are listed in Box 47-3.

Food allergies can occur at any time but are common during infancy because the immature intestinal tract is more permeable to proteins than is the mature intestinal tract, increasing the likelihood of an immune response. Allergies in general demonstrate a genetic component: children who have one parent with allergy have a 50% or greater risk of developing allergy; children who have both parents with allergy have up to a 100% risk of developing allergy. Allergy with a hereditary tendency is referred to as atopy. Some infants with *atopy* can be identified at birth from elevated levels of IgE in cord blood.

Box 47-3

Hyperallergenic Foods/Sources

Milk*—Ice cream, butter, margarine (if it contains dairy products), yogurt, cheese, pudding, baked goods, wieners, bologna, canned creamed soups, instant breakfast drinks, powdered milk drinks, milk chocolate
Eggs*—Mayonnaise, creamy salad dressing, baked goods, egg noodles, some cake icing, meringue, custard, pancakes, French toast, root beer
Wheat*—Almost all baked goods, wieners, bologna, pressed or chopped cold cuts, gravy, pasta, some canned soups
Legumes—Peanuts,* peanut butter or oil, beans, peas, lentils
Nuts*—Some chocolates, candy, baked goods, cherry soda (may be flavored with a nut extract), walnut oil
Fish or shellfish*—Cod liver oil, pizza with anchovies, Caesar salad dressing, any food fried in same oil as fish
Soy*—Soy sauce, teriyaki or worcestershire sauce, tofu, baked goods using soy flour or oil, soy nuts, soy infant formulas or milk, soybean paste, tuna packed in vegetable oil, many margarines
Chocolate—Cola beverages, cocoa, chocolate-flavored drinks
Buckwheat—Some cereals, pancakes
Pork, chicken—Bacon, wieners, sausage, pork fat, chicken broth
Strawberries, melon, pineapple—Gelatin, syrups
Corn—Popcorn, cereal, muffins, cornstarch, corn meal, corn bread, corn tortilla
Citrus fruits—Orange, lemon, lime, grapefruit; any of these in drinks, gelatin, juice, or medicines
Tomatoes—Juice, some vegetable soups, spaghetti, pizza sauce, catsup
Spices—Chili, pepper, vinegar, cinnamon

*Most common allergens.

Deaths have been reported in children who suffered an anaphylactic reaction to food. Onset of the reactions occurred shortly after ingestion (5 to 30 minutes). In most of the children the reactions did not begin with skin signs such as hives, red rash, and flushing, but rather as an acute asthma attack. Parents, teachers, and day care workers should be educated regarding signs and symptoms of food allergies. Those with food sensitivity should avoid unfamiliar foods, as well as restaurants that do not disclose food ingredients. Hidden ingredients in prepared foods have been implicated as a potential source.

NURSE ALERT • Patients with extremely sensitive food allergies should wear medical identification such as a bracelet and have an injectable epinephrine cartridge readily available and know how to use it.

Although the reason is unknown, many children out-grow their food allergies. Children who are allergic to more than one food may develop tolerance to each food at different times. Because of the tendency to lose the hypersensitivity, allergic foods should be reintroduced into the diet after a period of abstinence (usually a year or more) to evaluate if the food can be safely added to the diet. However, foods that are associated with severe anaphylactic reactions, will continue to present a lifelong risk and must be avoided (Anderson, 1997).

Breastfeeding is now considered to be a primary consideration for avoiding atopy in families with known food sensitivities; the breastfeeding mother is encouraged to avoid foods such as peanuts, tree nuts, and fish during the first 6 months of breastfeeding. In addition, supplementation, if required, is best done with hydrolysated, *not soy* formulas (Wood, 1996). The strategies listed in the Guidelines box are those recom-

Guidelines

PREVENTING ATOPY IN CHILDREN

Identify Children at Risk
Family history of allergy
Increased IgE in cord blood and postnatal serum
Dry, flaky skin

Prenatal Precautions (Last Trimester)
Avoid any known food allergens
Avoid milk and other dairy products, peanuts, and eggs
Minimize ingestion of other hyperallergenic foods (see Box 47-3)

Postnatal Precautions
Breast milk or casein/whey hydrolysate formula (e.g., Nutramigen, Pregestimil, Alimentum) exclusively for at least 6 months
No solid food for first 6 months
No cow's milk or soy formula for 12 months
No egg, fish, corn, citrus, peanuts, nuts, or chocolate for 12 months
One new food added at 5-day intervals to identify possible reaction

Environmental Control
Limited exposure to dust mites, molds, furry animals, latex products, and cigarette smoke

Data from Johnstone D: Strategy for intervention of food allergy in infants, *Int Pediatr* 4(4):319–325, 1989; Zeiger R et al: Effectiveness of dietary manipulation in the prevention of food allergy in infants, part 2, *J Allergy Clin Immunol* 78(1, pt 2):224–238, 1986; and Wood RA: Prospects for the prevention of allergy in children, *Curr Opin Pediatr* 8(6):601–605, 1995.

mended by most authorities for infants with a family history of atopy.*

Cow's Milk Allergy. Cow's milk allergy is a multifaceted disorder representing adverse systemic and local gastrointestinal reactions to cow's milk protein. The hypersensitivity may be manifested through a variety of signs and symptoms (Box 47-4) that may appear within 45 minutes of milk ingestion or after a period of several days. The diagnosis may initially be made from the history, although the history alone is not diagnostic; the timing and diversity of clinical manifestations vary greatly. For example, cow's milk allergy may be manifested as colic (see discussion on p. 846) or sleeplessness in an otherwise healthy infant.

Diagnostic Evaluation. A number of diagnostic tests may be performed, including stool analysis for blood (both frank and occult bleeding can occur from the colitis), serum IgE levels, skin-prick or scratch testing; and radioallergosorbent test (RAST), which measures IgE antibodies to specific allergens in serum by radioimmunoassay. Both skin testing and RAST help identify the offending food, but the results are not always conclusive (Wylie, 1996).

The most definitive diagnostic strategy is elimination of milk, followed by challenge testing after improvement of symptoms. Challenge testing involves reintroducing small quantities of milk in the diet to detect resurgence of symptoms; at times challenge testing involves the use of a placebo so that the parent is unaware of or "blind" to the timing of allergen ingestion.

NURSE ALERT • Careful observation of the child is required during a challenge test because of the possibility of anaphylactic reaction.

Therapeutic Management. Treatment of cow's milk allergy is elimination of all dairy products. For infants fed cow's milk formula, this primarily involves changing the formula to a casein hydrolysate milk formula (e.g., Pregestimil, Nutramigen, or Alimentum), in which the protein has been broken down (or "predigested") into its amino acids through enzymatic hydrolysis. Another choice is the amino acid-based formula NEOCATE (Anderson, 1997). Soy-based formula is not recommended because of cross-reactivity to soy (AAP, 1998b). Goat's milk is not an acceptable substitute because it cross-reacts with cow's milk protein, is deficient in folic acid, and is unsuitable as the only source of calories. Infants who are breastfed but have symptoms of cow's milk hypersensitivity are treated by eliminating all dairy products from the lactating mother's diet, although there is evidence that restricting maternal dairy intake is not necessary (Twarog, 1996). If maternal dairy intake is restricted, these women need vitamin D and calcium supplementation to prevent deficiency. Infants are maintained on the dairy-free diet for 1 or 2 years, at which time very small quantities of milk are reintroduced.

Nursing Care Management. The principal nursing objectives are identification of potential milk allergy and appropriate counseling of parents regarding substitute formulas. The protein hydrolysate formulas tend to be less palatable than milk-based formulas. Consequently, reluctance to accept the new formula may be a problem. This can be overcome by introducing the formula gradually over a few days using 1 ounce of new formula to 7 ounces of old formula, then 2:6 ratio, then a 3:4, and as needed. NEOCATE may be made more palatable by adding non-nutritive flavor packets (Ross Laboratories) available in a number of different flavors. Parents also need to be reassured that the infant will receive complete nutrition from the new formula and will suffer no ill effects from the absence of cow's milk. Carnation Good Start, a whey protein hydrolysate, is not appropriate because some children may react to it (Anderson, 1997).

Once solid foods are started, parents need guidance in avoiding all associated milk products (see Box 47-3). Carefully reading all food labels helps avoid ingesting prepared foods containing milk products.

Lactose Intolerance. Lactose intolerance refers to at least three different conditions that involve a deficiency of the enzyme *lactase*, which is needed for the hydrolysis or digestion of lactose in the small intestine; lactose is hydrolyzed into glucose and galactose. *Congenital lactase deficiency* occurs soon after birth once the newborn has consumed lactose-containing milk (human milk or commercial formula). This inborn error of metabolism involves the complete absence or severely reduced presence of lactase; it is rare and requires lifelong lactose-free or extremely reduced lactose diet (McBean and Miller, 1998).

Late-onset lactase deficiency, sometimes referred to as *primary lactase deficiency,* is the most common type of lactose intolerance and is manifested usually around 3 to 7 years of age, although the time of onset is variable. Ethnic groups with a high incidence of lactase deficiency include Orientals, southern Europeans, Arabs, Jews, and African-Americans.

Lactose intolerance *(secondary lactase deficiency)* may occur secondary to damage of the intestinal lumen, which decreases or destroys the enzyme lactase. Cystic fibrosis; sprue; kwashiorkor; or infections such as giardiasis, HIV, or rotavirus may cause a temporary or permanent lactose intolerance.

The primary symptoms of lactose intolerance include abdominal pain, bloating, flatulence, and diarrhea. The onset of symptoms occurs within 30 minutes to several hours of lactose consumption.

Lactose intolerance may be diagnosed on the basis of the history and improvement with a lactose-reduced diet. The breath hydrogen test is used to positively diagnose the condition. Breath samples in lactose-deficient individuals will yield a higher percentage of hydrogen (e.g., 20 ppm or more above baseline).

*Further information for parents of infants with food allergies is available from the American Academy of Allergy, Asthma, and Immunology, 611 E. Wells St., Milwaukee, WI 52202; 1-800-822-2762; website: www.aaaai.org.

Box 47-4

Common Clinical Manifestations of Sensitivity to Cow's Milk

GASTROINTESTINAL	RESPIRATORY	OTHER SIGNS AND SYMPTOMS
Diarrhea	Rhinitis	Eczema
Vomiting	Bronchitis	Excessive crying
Colic	Asthma	Pallor (from anemia secondary to chronic blood loss in gastrointestinal tract)
Abdominal pain	Wheezing	
	Sneezing	
	Coughing	
	Chronic nasal discharge	

Treatment of lactose intolerance is elimination of offending dairy products or the use of enzyme replacement. In infants, soy-based formula can be substituted for cow's milk formula or human milk (AAP, 1998b). Most people are able to tolerate small amounts of lactose (Srinivasan and Minocha, 1998). Milk taken at meals may be better tolerated than when taken alone (Home Care box). Pretreated milk (with microbial-derived lactase) is reported to be effective in improving lactose absorption. Because dairy products are a major source of calcium and vitamin D, supplementation of these nutrients is needed to prevent deficiency. Yogurt contains inactive lactase enzyme, which is activated by the temperature and pH of the duodenum; this lactase activity substitutes for the lack of endogenous lactase. Fresh yogurt may be tolerated better than frozen yogurt.

Nursing Care Management. Nursing care is similar to the interventions discussed for cow's milk allergy: explaining the dietary restrictions to the family; identifying alternate sources of calcium such as yogurt; explaining the importance of supplementation; and discussing sources of lactose, especially hidden sources such as its use as a bulk agent in certain medications, and ways of controlling the symptoms (see Home Care box). Parents are advised to check with the pharmacist regarding this possibility when obtaining medication.

GASTROINTESTINAL (GI) DYSFUNCTION

The extensive surface area of the GI tract and its digestive function represent the major means of exchange between the human organism and the environment. Inflammatory and malabsorptive disorders impair the functional integrity of the GI tract. In addition, because the immune system and mucosal barrier continue to mature after birth, the intestine of infants is extremely vulnerable to infection. Acute infectious diarrhea can cause significant alterations in fluid and electrolyte balance in infants and children.

Numerous general observations provide possible clues to specific GI problems (Box 47-5). In any disorder that involves GI losses (particularly of large amounts of fluid), dehydration poses a serious threat to life and demands immediate attention.

Dehydration

Dehydration is a common body fluid disturbance in infants and children and occurs whenever the total output of fluid exceeds the total intake, regardless of the underlying cause. Dehydration

Home Care

CONTROLLING SYMPTOMS OF LACTOSE INTOLERANCE

- In infants substitute soy-based formula for cow's milk formula or human milk.
- Limit milk consumption to one glass at a time.
- Drink milk with other foods rather than alone.
- Eat hard cheese, cottage cheese, or yogurt instead of drinking milk.
- Use enzyme tablets (Lactaid, Lactrase, Dairy Ease) to predigest the lactose in milk or supplement the body's own lactase (add tablets to milk or sprinkle on dairy products such as ice cream).
- Eat small amounts of dairy foods daily to help colonic bacteria adapt to ingested lactose.

Box 47-5

Clinical Manifestations of Gastrointestinal Dysfunction in Children

Failure to thrive—Deceleration from established growth pattern or consistently below the 5th percentile for height and weight on standard growth charts; sometimes accompanied by developmental delays

Spitting up or **regurgitation**—Passive transfer of gastric contents into the esophagus or mouth

Vomiting—Forceful ejection of gastric contents; involves a complex process under central nervous system control that causes salivation, pallor, sweating, and tachycardia; usually accompanied by nausea

- **Projectile vomiting**—Vomiting accompanied by vigorous peristaltic waves and typically associated with pyloric stenosis or pylorospasm

Nausea—Unpleasant sensation vaguely referred to the throat or abdomen with an inclination to vomit

Constipation—Passage of firm or hard stools or infrequent passage of stool with associated symptoms such as difficulty expelling the stools, blood-streaked stools, and abdominal discomfort

Encopresis—Overflow of incontinent stool causing soiling; often caused by fecal retention or impaction

Diarrhea—Increase in the number of stools with an increased water content as a result of alterations of water and electrolyte transport by the gastrointestinal (GI) tract; may be acute or chronic

Hypoactive, hyperactive, or **absent bowel sounds**—Evidence of intestinal motility problems that may be caused by inflammation or obstruction

Abdominal distention—Protuberant contour of the abdomen that may be caused by delayed gastric emptying, accumulation of gas or stool, inflammation, or obstruction

Abdominal pain—Pain associated with the abdomen that may be localized or diffuse, acute or chronic; often caused by inflammation, obstruction, or hemorrhage

Gastrointestinal bleeding—May be from an upper or lower GI source and may be acute or chronic

- ***Hematemesis***—Vomiting of bright red blood or denatured blood that results from bleeding in the upper GI tract or from swallowed blood from the nose or oropharynx
- ***Hematochezia***—Passage of bright red blood per rectum, usually indicating lower GI tract bleeding
- ***Melena***—Passage of dark-colored, "tarry" stools due to denatured blood, suggesting upper GI tract bleeding or bleeding from the right colon

Jaundice—Yellow coloration of the skin and sclerae associated with liver dysfunction

Dysphagia—Difficulty swallowing caused by abnormalities in the neuromuscular function of the pharynx or upper esophageal sphincter or by disorders of the esophagus

Dysfunctional swallowing—Impaired swallowing caused by central nervous system defects or structural defects of the oral cavity, pharynx, or esophagus; can cause feeding problems or aspiration

Fever—Common manifestation of illness in children with GI disorders; usually associated with dehydration, infection, or inflammation may result from a number of diseases that cause insensible losses through the skin and respiratory tract, through increased renal excretion, and through the GI tract. Although dehydration can result from lack of oral intake (especially in elevated environmental temperatures), more often it is a result of abnormal losses, such as those that occur in vomiting or diarrhea, when oral intake only partially compensates for the abnormal losses. Other significant causes of dehydration are diabetic ketoacidosis and extensive burns.

Water Balance in Infants. Infants and young children have a greater need for water and are therefore more vulnerable to alterations in fluid and electrolyte balance. Compared with older children and adults, they have a greater fluid intake and output relative to size. Water and electrolyte disturbances occur more commonly and more rapidly, and children adjust less promptly to these alterations.

The fluid compartments in the infant vary significantly from those in the adult, primarily because of an expanded extracellular compartment. The *extracellular fluid (ECF)* compartment constitutes more than half the total body water at birth and has a greater relative content of extracellular sodium and chloride. The infant loses a large amount of fluid at birth and still maintains a larger amount of ECF than the adult until about 2 years of age. This contributes to greater and more rapid water loss during this age period.

Fluid losses create compartment deficits that are reflected throughout the duration of dehydration. In general, approximately 60% of fluid is lost from the ECF, and the remaining 40% comes from the *intracellular fluid (ICF)*. The amount of fluid lost from the ECF increases with acute illness and decreases with chronic loss.

Fluid losses are divided into insensible, urinary, and fecal losses and vary with age. Approximately two thirds of *insensible losses* occur through the skin, and the remaining one third is lost through the respiratory tract. Insensible fluid loss is influenced by heat and humidity, body temperature, and respiratory rate. Infants and children have a much greater tendency to become highly febrile than do adults. Fever increases insensible water loss by approximately 7 ml/kg/24 hr for each degree rise in temperature above 37.2° C (99° F). Fever and increased surface area relative to volume are factors that contribute to greater insensible fluid losses in young patients.

Body Surface Area (BSA). The infant's relatively greater BSA allows larger quantities of fluid to be lost in insensible perspiration through the skin. It is estimated that the BSA of the premature neonate is five times as great, and that of the newborn is two to three times as great, as that of the older child or adult. The proportionately longer GI tract in infancy is also a source of relatively greater fluid loss, especially from diarrhea.

Basal Metabolic Rate (BMR). The rate of metabolism in infancy is significantly higher than in adulthood because of the larger BSA in relation to the mass of active tissue. Consequently, there is a greater production of metabolic wastes that must be excreted by the kidneys. Any condition that increases metabolism causes greater heat production, insensible fluid loss, and an increased need for water for excretion. The BMR in infants and children is higher to support growth.

Kidney Function. The kidneys of the infant are functionally immature at birth and are therefore inefficient in excreting waste products of metabolism. Of particular importance for fluid balance is the inability of the infant's kidneys to concentrate or dilute urine, to conserve or excrete sodium, and to acidify urine. The infant is less able to handle large quantities of solute-free water than is the older child and is more apt to become dehydrated when given concentrated formulas or overhydrated when given excessive water or dilute formula.

Fluid Requirements. As a result of these characteristics, infants ingest and excrete a greater amount of fluid per kilogram of body weight than do older children. Because electrolytes are excreted with water and the infant has limited ability for conservation, maintenance requirements include both water and electrolytes. The daily exchange of ECF in the infant is greatly increased over that of older children, which leaves the infant little fluid volume reserve in dehydrated states. Fluid requirements depend on hydration status, size, environmental factors, and underlying disease. Daily maintenance fluid requirements are outlined in Box 47-6.

Types of Dehydration. The pathophysiology of dehydration can best be understood by recognizing that the distribution of water between the ECF and ICF spaces depends on active transport of potassium into and sodium out of cells by energy-requiring processes. Sodium is the chief solute in ECF and thus is the primary determinant of ECF volume. Potassium is primarily intracellular. When ECF volume is reduced in acute dehydration, the total body sodium content is almost always reduced as well, regardless of serum sodium measurements. Replacement of fluid volume should therefore be accompanied by sodium repletion. Sodium depletion in diarrhea occurs in two ways: out of the body in stool, and into the ICF compartment to replace potassium in order to maintain electrical equilibrium.

Dehydration is classified into three categories on the basis of osmolality and depends primarily on the serum sodium concentration: (1) isotonic, (2) hypotonic, and (3) hypertonic.

Isotonic (isosmotic or *isonatremic) dehydration,* the primary form of dehydration in children, occurs in conditions in which the electrolyte and water deficits are present in approximately balanced proportions. Water and salt are lost in approximately equal amounts. The observable fluid losses are not necessarily isotonic, but losses from other avenues make adjustments so that the sum of all losses, or the net loss, is isotonic. There is no osmotic force between the ICF and the ECF, so the major loss is sustained from the ECF compartment. This significantly reduces the plasma volume and also the circulating blood volume, which affects the skin, muscles, and kidneys. Shock is the greatest threat to life, and the child with isotonic dehydration displays symptoms characteristic of hypovolemic shock. Plasma sodium remains within normal limits, between 130 and 150 mEq/L.

Box 47-6

Daily Maintenance Fluid Requirements

1. Calculate weight of child in kilograms:

$$\frac{\text{Weight of child (in pounds)}}{\text{2.2 pounds/kg}} = \text{Weight in kilograms}$$

2. Allow 100 ml/kg for first 10 kg.
3. Allow 50 ml/kg for second 10 kg.
4. Allow 20 ml/kg for remainder of weight in kilograms.
5. Divide total amount by 24 hours to obtain rate in milliliters per hour.

Hypotonic (hyposmotic or *hyponatremic) dehydration* occurs when the electrolyte deficit exceeds the water deficit, leaving the serum hypotonic. Because ICF is more concentrated than ECF in hypotonic dehydration, water moves from the ECF to the ICF to establish osmotic equilibrium. This movement further increases the ECF volume loss, and shock is a common finding. Because there is a greater proportional loss of ECF in hypotonic dehydration, the physical signs tend to be more severe with smaller fluid losses than with isotonic or hypertonic dehydration. Serum sodium concentration is less than 130 mEq/L.

Hypertonic (hyperosmotic or *hypernatremic) dehydration* results from water loss in excess of electrolyte loss and is usually caused by a proportionately larger loss of water and/or a larger intake of electrolytes. This type of dehydration is also the most dangerous, and it requires more specific fluid therapy. Hypertonic dehydration may occur in infants who are given fluids by mouth that contain large amounts of solute, or in children receiving high-protein nasogastric tube feedings that place an excessive solute load on the kidneys. In hypertonic dehydration, fluid shifts from the lesser concentration of the ICF to the ECF. Plasma sodium concentration is greater than 150 mEq/L (Behrman, Kliegman, and Arvin, 2000).

Because the ECF volume is proportionately larger, hypertonic dehydration consists of a greater degree of water loss for the same intensity of physical signs. Shock is less apparent; however, neurologic disturbances (e.g., alterations in consciousness, poor ability to focus attention, lethargy, increased muscle tone with hyperreflexia, and hyperirritability to stimuli) are more likely to occur. Cerebral changes are serious and may result in permanent damage.

Diagnostic Evaluation. Diagnosis of the type and degree of dehydration is necessary to develop an effective plan of therapy. The degree of dehydration has been described as a percentage: 5% (mild), 10% (moderate), or 15% (severe). Water constitutes only 60% to 70% of the infant's weight; however, adipose tissue contains little water and is highly variable in individual infants and children. A more accurate means of describing dehydration is to reflect acute loss (over 48 hours or less) in milliliters per kilogram of body weight. For example, a loss of 50 ml/kg is considered to be a mild fluid loss, whereas a loss of 100 ml/kg produces severe dehydration. Weight is an important determinant of the percent of total body fluid loss in infants and younger children, but other clinical manifestations include a changing level of consciousness (irritability to lethargy), response to stimuli, decreased skin elasticity and turgor, prolonged capillary refill, increased heart rate, and sunken eyes and fontanels (Held, 1995). Any two of the following factors—capillary refill of >2 seconds, absent tears, dry mucous membranes, and an ill general appearance—are predictors of a deficit of at least 5% (Gorelick, Shaw, and Murphy, 1997).

Shock, with tachycardia and very low blood pressure, is a common feature of severe depletion of ECF volume (see Shock, Chapter 48). Clinical signs provide clues to the extent of dehydration (Table 47-3).

Therapeutic Management. (See discussion on therapeutic management of diarrhea, p. 1255.)

Nursing Care Management. Nursing observation and intervention are essential to the detection and therapeutic management of dehydration. A variety of circumstances cause fluid loss in infants, and changes can take place in a very short time. An important nursing responsibility is observation for signs of dehydration. Conditions in which dehydration may develop quickly include diarrhea; vomiting; sweating; fever; disorders such as diabetes, renal disease, and cardiac anomalies; administration of certain drugs, such as diuretics and steroids; and trauma, such as major surgery, burns, and other extensive injury.

Nursing assessment of suspected or potential fluid loss begins with observation of general appearance and proceeds to more specific observations.

Intake and Output. Accurate measurements of fluid intake and output are vital to the assessment of dehydration. This

TABLE 47-3

Evaluating Extent of Dehydration

Level of Dehydration	Mild	Moderate	Severe
Weight loss—infants	5%	10%	15%
Weight loss—children	3%-4%	6%-8%	10%
Pulse	Normal	Slightly increased	Very increased
Blood pressure	Normal	Normal to orthostatic (>10 mm Hg change)	Orthostatic to shock
Behavior	Normal	Irritable, more thirsty	Hyperirritable to lethargic
Thirst	Slight	Moderate	Intense
Mucous membranes*	Normal	Dry	Parched
Tears	Present	Decreased	Absent, sunken eyes
Anterior fontanel	Normal	Normal to sunken	Sunken
External jugular vein	Visible when supine	Not visible except with supraclavicular pressure	Not visible even with supraclavicular pressure
Skin* (less useful in children >2 years)	Capillary refill >2 seconds	Slowed capillary refill (2-4 seconds [decreased turgor])	Very delayed capillary refill (>4 seconds) and tenting; skin cool, acrocyanotic or mottled
Urine specific gravity	>1.020	>1.020; oliguria	Oliguria or anuria

Adapted from Jospe N, Forbes G: Fluids and electrolytes—clinical aspects, *Pediatr Rev* 17(11):395–403, 1996.
*These signs are less prominent in patients who have hypernatremia.

includes oral and parenteral intake and losses from urine, stools, vomiting, fistulas, nasogastric suction, sweat, and wound drainage:

Urine—Frequency, color, consistency, and volume (when weighing diapers, approximately 1 g wet diaper weight equals 1 ml of urine)
Stools—Frequency, volume, and consistency
Vomitus—Volume, frequency, and type
Sweating—Can be only estimated from frequency of clothing and linen changes

In addition to fluid intake and output, the following observations assist in assessment of dehydration:

Vital signs—Temperature (normal, elevated, or lowered depending on degree of dehydration), pulse (tachycardia), respirations (tachypnea), and blood pressure (hypotension)
Skin—Color, temperature, turgor, presence or absence of edema, and capillary refill
Mucous membranes—Moisture, color, and presence of and consistency of secretions
Body weight—Decreased in relation to degree of dehydration
Fontanel (infants)—Sunken, soft, or normal
Sensory alterations—Presence of thirst

For nursing interventions, see discussion under specific disorders.

DISORDERS OF MOTILITY

Diarrhea

Diarrhea is a symptom that results from disorders involving digestive, absorptive, and secretory functions. Diarrhea is caused by abnormal intestinal water and electrolyte transport. Worldwide, approximately 500 million children suffer with diarrhea each year, and 20% of all deaths in children living in developing countries are related to diarrhea and dehydration (Sazawal et al, 1996).

Diarrheal disturbances can involve the stomach and intestines (gastroenteritis), the small intestine (enteritis), the colon (colitis), or the colon and intestines (enterocolitis). Diarrhea is usually classified as acute or chronic.

Acute diarrhea is a leading cause of illness in children younger than 5 years of age. Acute diarrhea is defined as a sudden increase in frequency and a change in consistency of stools, often caused by an infectious agent in the GI tract. It may be associated with upper respiratory or urinary tract infections, antibiotic therapy, or laxative use. Acute diarrhea is usually self-limited (less than 14 days' duration) and subsides without specific treatment if dehydration does not occur. *Acute infectious diarrhea (infectious gastroenteritis)* is caused by a variety of viral, bacterial, and parasitic pathogens (Table 47-4).

Chronic diarrhea is defined as an increase in stool frequency and increased water content with a duration of more than 14 days. It is often caused by chronic conditions such as malabsorption syndromes, inflammatory bowel disease, immune deficiency, food allergy, lactose intolerance, or chronic nonspecific diarrhea; or as a result of inadequate management of acute diarrhea.

Intractable diarrhea of infancy is a syndrome that occurs in the first few months of life, persists for longer than 2 weeks with no recognized pathogens, and is refractory to treatment. The most common cause is acute infectious diarrhea that was not managed adequately.

Chronic nonspecific diarrhea (CNSD), also known as irritable colon of childhood and as toddlers' diarrhea, is a common cause of chronic diarrhea in children 6 to 54 months of age. These children have loose stools, often with undigested food particles, and diarrhea greater than 2 weeks' duration. Children with CNSD grow normally and have no evidence of malnutrition, no blood in their stool, and no enteric infection (Huffman, 1999). Dietary indiscretions and food sensitivities have been linked to chronic diarrhea; in particular, the excessive intake of juices and artificial sweeteners such as sorbitol, found in many commercially prepared beverages and foods, may be a factor.

Etiology. Most pathogens that cause diarrhea are spread by the fecal-oral route through contaminated food or water or are spread from person to person where there is close contact (e.g., day care centers). Lack of clean water, crowding, poor hygiene, nutritional deficiency, and poor sanitation are major risk factors, especially for bacterial or parasitic pathogens. The increased frequency and severity of diarrheal disease in infants is also related to age-specific alterations in susceptibility to pathogens. The immune system of the infant has not previously been exposed to many pathogens and has not acquired protective antibodies.

Rotavirus is the most important cause of dehydrating diarrhea in young children throughout the world. Its symptoms may range from no manifestations to death from dehydration. Rotavirus infection accounts for most hospitalizations for severe diarrhea in young children and is a significant nosocomial (hospital-acquired) pathogen.

Salmonella, Shigella, and *Campylobacter* organisms are the most commonly isolated bacterial pathogens. *Giardia* and *Cryptosporidium* organisms are the parasites that most commonly produce acute, infectious diarrhea (see Table 47-4; see also Intestinal Parasitic Diseases, p. 1264).

Antibiotics are also associated with diarrhea. Antibiotics alter the normal intestinal flora, and the decrease in colonic bacteria results in excessive absorbed carbohydrate and osmotic diarrhea (Behrman, Kliegman, and Arvin, 2000). Antibiotics can also lead to colonization and toxin production by *Clostridium difficile,* which may cause diarrhea and pseudomembranous colitis (Cerquetti et al, 1995; Jobe et al, 1995).

Pathophysiology. Invasion of the GI tract by pathogens produces diarrhea by (1) production of enterotoxins that stimulate secretion of water and electrolytes, (2) direct invasion and destruction of intestinal epithelial cells, and (3) local inflammation and systemic invasion by the organisms. However, the most serious and immediate physiologic disturbances associated with severe diarrheal disease are (1) dehydration, (2) acid-base imbalance with acidosis, and (3) shock that occurs when dehydration progresses to the point that circulatory status is seriously impaired.

Diagnostic Evaluation. The history provides valuable information regarding the duration, severity, associated symptoms, and potential cause of diarrhea. A complete history should include present drugs the child is taking, possible ingestions, family history, and recent travel history (Meyers, 1995). Specific questions include the presence or absence of fever and other symptoms, frequency of vomiting, frequency and character of stools (e.g., watery or bloody), urine output, the child's dietary habits, and recent food and fluid intake.

Extensive laboratory evaluation is not indicated in a child with uncomplicated diarrhea and no evidence of dehydration.

TABLE 47-4
Infectious Causes of Acute Diarrhea

Organism	Pathology	Characteristics	Comments
VIRAL AGENTS			
Rotavirus Incubation period: 1-3 days	Invade epithelium of small bowel mucosa Severely distorted mucosal architecture with atrophic mucosa and severe inflammatory changes Absorption of salt and water decreased	Abrupt onset Fever (38°C [100.4°F] or higher) lasting approximately 48 hours Nausea/vomiting Abdominal pain Associated upper respiratory tract infection Diarrhea may persist for more than 1 week	More infections in winter (90%) with peak incidence (60%) from December through April Affects all age groups (infants 6-12 months of age are most vulnerable, with children older than 3 years rarely symptomatic with severe disease) Usually mild and self-limited Important cause of nosocomial infections in hospitals and gastroenteritis in children attending day care centers
Norwalk-like organisms Incubation period: 1-3 days	Mechanism of effect unknown Blunting of villi and inflammatory changes in lamina propria Reduced enzymes	Fever Loss of appetite Nausea/vomiting Abdominal pain Diarrhea Malaise	Source of infection: drinking water, recreation water, food (including shellfish) Affects all ages Self-limited (2-3 days)
BACTERIAL AGENTS			
Pathogenic *Escherichia coli* Incubation period: highly variable, depends on strain	Usually caused by enterotoxin production (small bowel) Reduces absorption and increases secretion of fluids and electrolytes	Onset gradual or abrupt Variable clinical manifestations Most—green, watery diarrhea with blood and mucus; becomes explosive Vomiting may be present from onset Abdominal distention Diarrhea Fever, appears toxic	Incidence higher in summer Usually interpersonal transmission but may transmit via inanimate objects and undercooked meat, especially chopped beef Cause of nursery epidemics With symptomatic treatment only, may continue for weeks Full breastfeeding has a protective effect Symptoms generally subside in 3-7 days Relapse rate approximately 20%
Salmonella groups (nontyphoidal)—gram negative, nonencapsulated, nonsporulating Incubation period: 6-72 hours for gastroenteritis (usually less than 24); 3-60 days for enteric fever (usually 7-14)	Penetration of lamina propria (small bowel and colon) Local inflammation—no extensive destruction Stimulation of intestinal fluid excretion Systemic invasion of other sites	Rapid onset Variable symptoms—mild to severe Nausea/vomiting and colicky abdominal pain followed by diarrhea, occasionally with blood and mucus Fever Hyperactive peristalsis and mild abdominal tenderness Symptoms usually subside within 5 days May have headache and cerebral manifestations (e.g., drowsiness, confusion, meningismus, seizures) Infants may be afebrile and nontoxic May result in life-threatening septicemia and meningitis Variable in infants	Two thirds of patients are younger than 20 years of age; highest incidence in children younger than age 5 years, especially infants Highest incidence occurs from July through October, lowest from January through April Transmission primarily via contaminated food and drink—most from animal sources, including fowl, mammals, reptiles, and insects Most common sources are poultry and eggs In children—pets (e.g., dogs, cats, hamsters, and especially pet turtles) Communicable as long as organisms are excreted Decreased incidence in last decade

Continued

TABLE 47-4—cont'd
Infectious Causes of Acute Diarrhea

Organism	Pathology	Characteristics	Comments
BACTERIAL AGENTS—cont'd			
S. typhi	Rapid invasion of bloodstream from minor sites of inflammation Marked inflammation and necrosis of intestinal mucosa and lymphatics	Variable in infants Older children—irregular fever, headache, malaise, lethargy Diarrhea occurs in 50% at early stage Cough is common In a few days fever rises and is consistent; fatigue, cough, abdominal pain, anorexia, and weight loss develop; diarrhea begins	Decreased incidence in last decade Acute symptoms may persist for 1 week or more Transmitted by contaminated food or water (primary), infected animals (e.g., pet turtles)
Shigella groups—gram negative, non-motile anaerobic bacilli Incubation period: 1-7 days, usually 2-4	Enterotoxin Stimulates loss of fluids and electrolytes Invasion of epithelium with superficial mucosal ulcerations *S. dysenteriae* forms exotoxin	Onset variable but usually abrupt Fever and cramping abdominal pain initially Fever—may reach 40.5°C (105°F) Seizures in about 10%—usually associated with fever Patient appears sick Headache, nuchal rigidity, delirium Watery diarrhea with mucus and pus starts about 12-48 hours after onset Stools preceded by abdominal cramps; tenesmus and straining follow Symptoms usually subside in 5-10 days	Approximately 60% of cases in children younger than age 9 years with more than one third in children ages 1-4 years Peak incidence in late summer Transmitted directly or indirectly from infected persons Communicable for 1-4 weeks Self-limited Treat with antibiotics Severe dehydration and collapse can affect all patients Acute symptoms may persist for 1 week or more
Yersinia enterocolitica Incubation period: dose dependent, 1-3 weeks		Diarrhea—may be bloody Fever (>38.7°C [102°F]) Abdominal pain in right lower quadrant Vomiting, diarrhea	Seen more frequently in winter Majority in first 3 years of life Transmitted by food and pets Can resemble appendicitis May be relapsing and last for weeks
Campylobacter jejuni Incubation period: 1-7 days or longer	Precise mechanism unclear Jejunum, ileum, and colon involvement Extensive ulceration with hemorrhagic ileitis Broadening and flattening of mucosa	Fever Abdominal pain—often severe, cramping, periumbilical Watery, profuse, foul-smelling diarrhea with blood Vomiting	Person-to-person transmission May be transmitted by pets (e.g., cat, dog, hamster) Food (especially chicken) and water-borne transmission Relapse possible Most patients recover spontaneously Antibiotics may speed recovery Peak incidence in summer
Vibrio cholerae (cholera) groups Incubation period: usually 2-3 days; range from few hours to 5 days	Enterotoxin causes increased secretion of chloride and possibly bicarbonate Intestinal mucosa congested with enlarged lymph foilicles Intact mucosal surface	Sudden onset of profuse watery diarrhea without cramping, tenesmus, or anal irritation, although children may complain of cramping Stools are intermittent at first, then almost continuous Stools are bloody with mucus	Rare in infants younger than 1 year old Mortality high in both treated and untreated infants and small children Transmitted via contaminated food and water Attack confers immunity
Clostridium difficile	Toxin stimulates colonic secretion by damaging epithelium	Diarrhea with blood in stools	May cause pseudomembranous colitis Follows antibiotic therapy

TABLE 47-4—cont'd
Infectious Causes of Acute Diarrhea

Organism	Pathology	Characteristics	Comments
FOOD POISONING			
Staphylococcus Incubation period: 4-6 hours	Produces heat-stable enterotoxin	Severe abdominal cramps Profuse diarrhea Shock may occur in severe cases May be a mild fever	Transferred via contaminated food inadequately cooked or refrigerated (e.g., custards, mayonnaise, cream-filled or cream-topped desserts)
Clostridium perfringens Incubation period: 8-24 hours, usually 8-12	Produces heat-resistant and heat-sensitive toxins	Moderate to severe crampy, midepigastric pain	Self-limited; improvement apparent within 24 hours Excellent prognosis Self-limited
Clostridium botulinum Incubation period: 12-26 hours (range, 6 hours to 8 days)	Highly potent neurotoxin	Nausea, vomiting Diarrhea Central nervous system symptoms with curare-like effect Dry mouth, dysphagia	Transmission by commercial food products, most often meat and poultry Transmitted by contaminated food products Variable severity—mild symptoms to rapidly fatal within a few hours Antitoxin administration

Laboratory tests are indicated when a child is moderately to severely dehydrated. Stool specimens should be obtained in all children with diarrhea that persists for more than a few days. Watery, explosive stools suggest glucose intolerance; foul-smelling, greasy, bulky stools suggest fat malabsorption. Diarrhea that develops after the introduction of cow's milk, fruits, or cereal may be related to an enzyme deficiency or protein intolerance (Leung and Robson, 1996). Neutrophils or red blood cells in the stool indicate bacterial gastroenteritis or inflammatory bowel disease. The presence of eosinophils suggests protein intolerance or parasitic infection.

Cultures of the stool should be performed when blood or mucus is present in the stool, when symptoms are severe, when there is a history of travel to a developing country, and when polymorphonuclear leukocytes are found in the stool. An enzyme-linked immunosorbent assay (ELISA) may be used to confirm the presence of rotavirus or *Giardia.* If there is a history of recent antibiotic use, the stool should be tested for *C. difficile* toxin. The stool should be examined for ova and parasites when bacterial and viral cultures are negative and when diarrhea persists for more than a few days.

A stool pH of less than 6 and the presence of reducing substances may indicate the presence of carbohydrate malabsorption or secondary lactase deficiency. Measurement of stool electrolytes may help identify children with secretory diarrhea.

The urine specific gravity should be determined if dehydration is suspected. A complete blood count (CBC), serum electrolytes, creatinine, and blood urea nitrogen (BUN) should be obtained in the child who requires hospitalization. The hemoglobin, hematocrit, creatinine, and BUN levels are usually elevated in acute diarrhea and should normalize with rehydration.

Therapeutic Management. The major goals in the management of acute diarrhea include (1) assessment of the fluid and electrolyte imbalance, (2) rehydration, (3) maintenance fluid therapy, and (4) reintroduction of an adequate diet. Infants and children with acute diarrhea and dehydration should be treated first with *oral rehydration therapy (ORT).* ORT is one of the major worldwide health care advances of the past decade. It is more effective, safer, less painful, and less costly than intravenous (IV) rehydration. As a result, the AAP, World Health Organization, and Centers for Disease Control and Prevention recommend the use of ORT as the treatment of choice for most cases of dehydration caused by diarrhea (AAP, 1996; Gastanaduy and Begue, 1999; Hugger, Harkless, and Rentschler, 1998; Lasche and Duggan, 1999). Oral rehydration solutions (ORS) enhance and promote the reabsorption of sodium and water, and studies indicate that these solutions greatly reduce vomiting, volume loss from diarrhea, and the duration of the illness. Oral replacement solutions are available in the United States as commercially prepared solutions (e.g., Pedialyte, Infalyte [formerly Ricelyte], and Rehydralyte) and are successful in treating the majority of infants with isotonic, hypotonic, or hypertonic dehydration. Guidelines for rehydration recommended by the AAP are included in Box 47-7.

After rehydration an ORS may be used during maintenance fluid therapy by alternating the solution with a low-sodium fluid such as water, breast milk, lactose-free formula, or half-strength lactose-containing formula. In older children an ORS can be given and a regular diet continued. Ongoing stool losses should be replaced on a 1:1 basis with ORS. If the stool volume is not known, approximately 10 ml/kg (4 to 8 ounces) of ORS should be given for each diarrhea stool.

Solutions for oral hydration are useful in most cases of dehydration, and vomiting is not a contraindication. A child who is vomiting should be given an ORS at common intervals and in small amounts. In young children the fluid may be given with a spoon or small syringe in 5- to 10-ml increments every 1 to 5 minutes by the caregiver. An ORS may also be given via nasogastric or gastrostomy tube infusion. Infants without clinical signs of dehydration do not need ORT; they should, however,

Box 47-7

Model for Rehydration

Rehydration solution should consist of 75 to 90 mEq of sodium (Na^+) per liter.
Give 40 to 50 ml/kg of rehydration solution over 4 hours.
Replacement and maintenance solution should consist of 40 to 60 mEq of Na^+ per liter.
Re-evaluate the need for further rehydration; initiate maintenance therapy using maintenance formulations, with daily volumes not to exceed 150 ml/kg/day.
In children with diarrhea without significant dehydration, the maintenance phase may be initiated without the need for rehydration solution (Acra and Ghishan, 1996).
If additional fluids are needed, use low-salt fluids such as breast milk or water.

Modified from American Academy of Pediatrics, Provisional Committee on Quality Improvement, Subcommittee on Acute Gastroenteritis: Practice parameter: the management of acute gastroenteritis in young children, *Pediatrics* 97(3):424-435, 1996.

receive the same fluids recommended for infants with signs of dehydration in the maintenance phase and for ongoing stool losses.

NURSE ALERT • Diarrhea is not managed by encouraging oral intake of clear fluids, such as fruit juices, carbonated soft drinks, and gelatin. These fluids usually have a high carbohydrate content, a very low electrolyte content, and a high osmolality (Lasche and Duggan, 1999). Caffeinated soda is avoided, because caffeine is a mild diuretic and may lead to increased loss of water and sodium. Chicken or beef broth is not given, because it contains excessive sodium and inadequate carbohydrate. A BRAT diet (i.e., bananas, rice, apples, and toast or tea) is contraindicated for the child and especially for the infant with acute diarrhea, because this diet has little nutritional value (i.e., low in energy and protein), is high in carbohydrates, and is low in electrolytes.

Early reintroduction of nutrients is desirable and is gaining more widespread acceptance. Continued feeding or early reintroduction of a normal diet has no adverse effects and actually lessens the severity and duration of the illness and improves weight gain when compared with the gradual reintroduction of foods (AAP, 1996; Lasche and Duggan, 1999). Infants who are breastfeeding should continue to do so, and an ORS should be used to replace ongoing losses in these infants.

The use of nonhuman milk for infants and children with diarrhea remains controversial. Cow's milk and cow's milk formulas are of concern because poor digestion of lactose can occur in children with infectious diarrhea. However, some studies indicate that well-hydrated infants may resume full-strength nonhuman milk feeding immediately without adverse reactions (Duggan and Nurko, 1997).

Many infants and children can be safely managed with a diet containing cow's milk. Some practitioners advocate the use of a lactose-free formula only if milk or regular formula is not tolerated. In older children a regular diet can generally be offered once rehydration has been achieved. In toddlers there is no contraindication to continuing soft or pureed foods. A diet of easily digestible foods such as cereals, cooked vegetables, and meats is adequate for the older child.

In cases of severe dehydration and shock, IV fluids are initiated whenever the child is unable to ingest sufficient amounts of fluid and electrolytes to (1) meet ongoing daily physiologic losses, (2) replace previous deficits, and (3) replace ongoing abnormal losses. Patients who usually require IV fluids are those with severe dehydration, those with uncontrollable vomiting, those who are unable to drink for any reason (e.g., extreme fatigue or coma), and those with severe gastric distention.

The IV solution is selected on the basis of what is known regarding the probable type and cause of the dehydration—usually a saline solution containing 5% dextrose in water. Sodium bicarbonate may be added because acidosis is usually associated with severe dehydration. Although the initial phase of fluid replacement is rapid in both isotonic and hypotonic dehydration, it is contraindicated in hypertonic dehydration because of the risk of water intoxication, especially in the brain cells.

Once the severe effects of dehydration are under control, specific diagnostic and therapeutic measures are begun to detect and treat the cause of the diarrhea. Enteric infections are generally self-limited conditions. Specific antimicrobial therapy is indicated only for those bacterial or parasitic infections in which therapy can reduce the duration of the illness, severity of symptoms, shedding of organisms, and secondary spread of the organism. Effective antimicrobial therapy is usually not indicated in acute infectious diarrhea and may produce adverse side effects such as worsening of the diarrhea because of slowing of motility or prevention of absorption of medicines or nutrients in the intestine.

Nursing Care Management

➤ Assessment

The nursing assessment of diarrhea begins with observation of the infant's or child's general appearance and behavior. Physical assessment includes all the parameters described for assessment of dehydration, such as decreased urine output; decreased weight; dry mucous membranes; poor skin turgor; sunken fontanel; and pale, cool, dry skin. With more severe dehydration, increased pulse and respiration, decreased blood pressure, and a prolonged capillary refill time (>2 seconds) may indicate impending shock (see Table 47-3).

A history provides valuable information regarding probable etiologic agents, such as introduction of a new food, exposure to infectious agents, travel to an area of high susceptibility, contact with foods that might be contaminated, and contact with pets known to be sources of enteric infections. An allergic, drug, and dietary history may indicate food allergies, use of laxatives or antibiotics, or sources of excess sorbitol and fructose (e.g., apple juice).

➤ Nursing Diagnoses

Several nursing diagnoses become apparent on the basis of a thorough physical assessment. The major diagnoses appropriate for the infant or child are described in the Nursing Care Plan on

p. 1259. Other diagnoses will be evident depending on the age, condition, and etiology of the diarrhea.

➤ Plan of Care and Implementation

The goals for the dehydrated infant or child and for the family are as follows:

1. Infant or child will maintain adequate hydration.
2. Infant or child will maintain appropriate nutrition for age.
3. Infant or child will not spread infection (if etiologic agent) to others.
4. Family will receive appropriate support and education, especially regarding home care.

The management of most cases of acute diarrhea can take place in the home with proper education of the caregiver regarding the cause of the diarrhea, potential complications, and appropriate therapy. Caregivers are taught to monitor for signs of dehydration, especially the number of wet diapers or voidings; to monitor fluids taken by mouth; and to assess the frequency and amount of stool losses. Education relating to ORT, including the administration of maintenance fluids and replacement of ongoing losses, is important (Critical Thinking box). An ORS should be administered in small quantities at frequent intervals. Vomiting is not a contraindication to ORT unless it is severe. Information concerning the introduction of a normal diet is essential. Parents need to know that a slightly higher stool output initially occurs with continuation of a normal diet and with ongoing replacement of stool losses. The potential increase in stool frequency is outweighed by the benefits of a better nutritional outcome with fewer complications and a shorter duration of illness. Parents' concerns should be explored to gain compliance with the treatment plan.

If the child with acute diarrhea and dehydration is hospitalized, an accurate weight must be obtained, as well as careful monitoring of intake and output. The child may be placed on parenteral fluid therapy with nothing by mouth (NPO) for 12 to 48 hours. Monitoring the IV infusion is a primary nursing function, and the nurse must ensure that the correct fluid and electrolyte concentration is infused, the flow rate is adjusted to deliver the desired volume in a given time, and the IV site is maintained.

Accurate measurement of output is essential to determine if renal blood flow is sufficient to permit addition of potassium to the IV fluids. The nurse is responsible for examination of stools and collection of specimens for laboratory examination (see Collection of Specimens, Chapter 45). Care should be exerted in obtaining and transporting stools to prevent possible spread of infection. Stool specimens should be transported to the laboratory in appropriate containers and media according to hospital policy. A clean tongue depressor can be used to obtain specimens for laboratory examination or as an applicator for transfer to a culture medium. Tests for pH, blood, and reducing substance can be done on the nursing unit.

Diarrheal stools are highly irritating to the skin; therefore extra care is needed to protect the skin of the diaper region from becoming excoriated (see Diaper Dermatitis, Chapter 53). Rectal temperatures are avoided because they can stimulate the bowel, increasing passage of stool.

Critical Thinking

DIARRHEA

An 8-month-old infant is evaluated in the primary care clinic because of fever, vomiting, and diarrhea of 12 hours' duration. The caregivers report that the infant had three times as many stools as usual, and the stools are watery in consistency. After the initial examination of the infant, it is apparent that the child is mildly dehydrated because of stool losses secondary to acute infectious diarrhea. Which of the following interventions would be indicated in this situation?

First, Think About It . . .

- **What is the purpose of your thinking?**
- **If you accept the conclusions, what are the implications?**

1. **Recommend that the caregivers offer fruit juice only and delay reintroduction of food for 48 hours.**
2. **Administer antidiarrheal medications.**
3. **Educate the caregivers regarding administration of oral rehydration solution (ORS).**
4. **Administer intravenous (IV) fluids and provide nothing by mouth for several hours.**

The best response is 3. The purpose of your thinking is to establish the goals of management of acute diarrhea, which include assessment of hydration, provision of fluids for rehydration and maintenance, and reintroduction of an adequate diet. In this case, since the infant is mildly dehydrated, oral rehydration therapy (ORT) should be attempted. ORT is effective, safer, less painful, and less costly than IV rehydration. If ORS is administered at frequent intervals, vomiting can be minimized and IV hydration probably avoided.

Early reintroduction of normal nutrients is desirable, and delayed introduction of food may be harmful in terms of nutritional status and duration of illness. Breastfeeding generally should be continued, and most infants who receive cow's milk formulas may resume their usual feedings as soon as they are rehydrated. Occasionally the implications may be that a soy formula is recommended after an episode of acute infectious diarrhea if the infant demonstrates evidence of lactose malabsorption. Use of antidiarrheal medications should not be recommended for acute infectious diarrhea. These drugs may be harmful, because adverse effects such as slowed motility and ileus may occur.

Support for the child and family involves the same care and consideration given all hospitalized children (see Chapter 44). Parents are kept informed of the child's progress and instructed in special care behaviors, such as handwashing and proper disposal of soiled diapers, clothes, and bed linen. Everyone caring for the child must be aware of "clean" areas and "dirty" areas, especially in the hospital, where the sink in the child's room is used for many purposes. Soiled diapers and linen should be discarded in receptacles close to the bedside. To remind caregivers to keep diapers and other soiled articles away from clean areas, place signs identifying "clean" (e.g., bed table) and "dirty" (e.g., sink, bathroom) areas in the room. List on each sign what articles should be stored in each area.

Prevention. The best intervention for diarrhea in infants and children is prevention. Because most infections that cause acute diarrhea are spread by the fecal-oral route, parents need information about preventive measures such as personal hygiene, protecting the water supply from contamination, and careful food preparation.

NURSE ALERT • To reduce the risk of bacteria transmitted via food, encourage parents to:
- Quickly freeze or refrigerate all ground meat and other perishable foods.
- Never thaw food on the counter or let it sit out of the refrigerator for more than 2 hours.
- Wash hands, utensils, and work areas with hot, soapy water after contact with raw meat to keep bacteria from spreading.
- Check ground meat with a fork to make sure no pink is showing before taking a bite.
- Cook all dishes made with ground meat until brown or gray inside or to an internal temperature of 71° C (160° F).

Meticulous attention to perianal hygiene, disposal of soiled diapers, proper handwashing, and isolation of infected persons also minimizes the transmission of infection (see Infection Control, Chapter 45).

Parents also need information about preventing diarrhea while traveling. Recently some medications used by adults to prevent traveler's diarrhea have gained attention, but parents should be cautioned against giving these drugs to their children. Until vaccines or other prophylactic measures are proved to be safe for children, the best measure during travel to areas where water may be contaminated is to allow children to drink only bottled water and carbonated beverages (from the container through a straw supplied from home). Tap water, ice, unpasteurized dairy products, raw vegetables, unpeeled fruits, meats, and seafood should also be avoided.

➤ Evaluation

The effectiveness of nursing interventions is determined by continued reassessment according to the following observational guidelines:

1. Monitor fluid losses with careful intake and output measurements and daily weights.
2. Monitor food intake, especially calories.
3. Observe for evidence of complications from underlying disease (specify) and/or therapy.
4. Observe and interview family to determine extent and effectiveness of care.

The expected outcomes are described in the Nursing Care Plan.

Constipation

Constipation is an alteration in the frequency, consistency, or ease of passing stool. In children, it may be defined as 3 or more days without the passage of stool. It may also be defined as painful bowel movements, which are often blood streaked; or include the retention of stool, with or without soiling, even with a stool frequency of more than three stools per week (Loening-Baucke, 1995). The frequency of bowel movements is not considered a diagnostic criterion, because it varies widely among children. Having extremely long intervals between defecation is termed *obstipation.* Constipation with fecal soiling is referred to as *encopresis.*

Constipation may arise secondary to a variety of organic disorders of the GI tract or in association with a wide range of systemic disorders. Structural disorders of the intestine, such as strictures, ectopic anus, and Hirschsprung disease, may be associated with constipation. Systemic disorders associated with constipation include hypothyroidism, hypercalcemia due to hyperparathyroidism or vitamin D excess, and chronic lead poisoning. Constipation may be associated with drugs such as antacids, diuretics, antiepileptics, antihistamines, opioids, and iron supplementation. Spinal cord lesions may be associated with loss of rectal tone and sensation. Affected children are prone to chronic fecal retention and overflow incontinence.

The majority of children have *idiopathic* or *functional constipation* because no underlying cause can be clearly identified. Chronic constipation may be initiated by environmental or psychosocial factors. Transient illness, withholding and avoidance secondary to painful and/or negative experiences with stooling, and dietary intake with decreased fluid and fiber all play a role in the etiology of constipation.

Newborn Period. Normally the newborn infant passes a first meconium stool within 24 to 36 hours of birth. Any infant who does not do so should be assessed for evidence of intestinal atresia or stenosis, Hirschsprung disease (congenital aganglionic megacolon), hypothyroidism, meconium plugs, or meconium ileus. *Meconium plugs* are caused by meconium that has reduced water content and are usually evacuated following digital examination but may require irrigations of normal saline or the iodinated contrast medium.

Meconium ileus, the initial manifestation of cystic fibrosis, is the luminal obstruction of the distal small intestine by abnormal meconium. Treatment is the same as for a meconium plug. Rarely, surgical intervention may be needed.

Infancy. The onset of constipation commonly occurs during infancy, and medical causes such as Hirschsprung disease, hypothyroidism, and strictures must be ruled out. However, constipation in infancy is often related to dietary practices. It is almost unknown in breastfed infants, who typically have softer stools than bottle-fed infants. Breastfed infants may also have decreased stools because of more complete use of breast milk with little residue. Constipation may occur with the change from human milk or modified cow's milk to whole cow's milk. Simple measures such as adding or increasing the amount of cereal, vegetables, and fruit in the diet of the older infant ordinarily correct the problem. Some bottle-fed infants pass hard stools and develop anal fissures. Stool-withholding behavior may begin at this age in response to pain on defecation (Critical Thinking box).

Childhood. Most constipation in early childhood is due to environmental changes or is related to normal development when a child begins to attain control over bodily functions. Simple constipation may become more severe when stool withholding occurs. A child who has experienced discomfort during bowel movements may deliberately try to withhold stool. The rectum accommodates the accumulation of stool, and the urge to defecate passes. When the bowel contents are ultimately evacuated, the accumulated feces are passed with even greater pain, reinforcing the desire to withhold stool in the future. This pattern may continue for several years and can result in encopresis, which causes additional stress for the child (see Chapter 39).

Constipation in school-age children may also occur as a result of the stress and changes in toileting patterns that accompany going to school for the first time. New-onset constipation may be related to a fear of using the bathrooms at school, the lack of privacy in school bathrooms, and the busy schedules ne-

Nursing Care Plan THE CHILD WITH DIARRHEA (GASTROENTERITIS)

NURSING DIAGNOSIS Fluid volume deficit related to excessive GI losses from diarrhea/emesis

EXPECTED OUTCOME Patient exhibits signs of adequate hydration (i.e., skin—normal turgor, moist mucous membranes; vital signs within normal limits [WNL]; balanced intake and output [I & O]; no thirst; blood—electrolytes, hemoglobin/hematocrit, and osmolality WNL; urine—appearance, specific gravity, and osmolality WNL; clear mental processes).

Nursing Interventions/*Rationales*

Administer prescribed oral rehydration solutions (ORS) and/or intravenous (IV) solutions alternated with small amounts of low-sodium fluids such as water, breast milk, or lactose-reduced formula *for rehydration and replacement.* **(Avoid fluids with high-carbohydrate, low-electrolyte values such as carbonated drinks, fruit juices, and gelatin.)**

Monitor thirst, skin turgor, capillary refill, mucous membranes, mental status, intake and output, vital signs, appropriate blood and urine laboratory results *to assess hydration status.*

Describe all episodes of diarrhea/emesis *to evaluate for continuing fluid loss.*

Instruct family about appropriate administration of fluids, maintenance of I & O records, signs and symptoms of continuing dehydration *to optimize compliance.*

NURSING DIAGNOSIS Altered nutrition: less than body requirements related to diarrheal losses, inadequate intake

EXPECTED OUTCOME Patient exhibits adequate intake of appropriate nourishment and satisfactory gain of any lost weight.

Nursing Interventions/*Rationales*

After rehydration begin refeeding by reintroducing foods from a normal diet as tolerated *to reduce number of stools and weight loss and to shorten the duration of illness.* **(Avoid bananas, rice, apples, and toast or tea [BRAT] diet as it is low in protein, electrolytes, and energy and too high in carbohydrates.)**

Observe and record response to feedings *to assess feeding tolerance.*

Weigh *to monitor weight status.*

Instruct family about appropriate foods *to optimize compliance;* instruct breastfeeding mothers to continue breastfeeding *as it reduces duration and severity of the illness.*

NURSING DIAGNOSIS Risk for transmitting infection related to invasion of the GI tract by microorganisms

EXPECTED OUTCOME Patient shows no evidence of transmission of infection to patient contacts.

Nursing Interventions/*Rationales*

Implement appropriate Standard Precautions, careful handwashing techniques, use of snug-fitting and superabsorbent disposable diapers *to reduce likelihood of fecal transmission.*

Instruct all members in the environment in isolation procedures and handwashing techniques *to optimize compliance and reduce spread of organisms.*

NURSING DIAGNOSIS Impaired skin integrity related to irritation caused by frequent, loose stools

EXPECTED OUTCOME Patient's skin is intact.

Nursing Interventions/*Rationales*

Keep skin clean and dry through frequent diaper changes, use of superabsorbant disposable diapers, and use of gentle nonalkaline soap and water solution *to protect skin from irritation.* **(Avoid commercial baby wipes that contain alcohol as they add to the irritation.)**

Inspect skin for redness and excoriation; expose reddened areas to air *to promote healing;* use a moisture barrier ointment or cream *to protect excoriated areas.*

Inspect perineum and buttocks *for signs of infection such as fungal growth or Candida* and treat with appropriate medication as prescribed.

Instruct family about skin inspection *for early detection of skin problems.*

NURSING DIAGNOSIS Anxiety/fear related to separation from parents, unfamiliar environment, distressing procedures

EXPECTED OUTCOME Patient exhibits minimal signs of emotional or physical distress (e.g., is calm, relaxed, cooperative; engages in nonnutritive sucking, appropriate play).

Nursing Interventions/*Rationales*

Encourage frequent family visitation with active participation in care *to prevent distress from separation.*

Use frequent touch, holding, and talking *to provide comfort;* use pacifier and mouth care for infants who are on nothing by mouth (NPO) status.

Provide diversion and sensory stimulation appropriate to the child's developmental level and physical condition.

Instruct family in importance of comfort measures and in their active participation in care *to ease child's fears.*

Critical Thinking

CONSTIPATION

An 8-month-old infant is seen by the pediatric nurse practitioner. The infant's mother states that the infant usually has one hard stool every 4 to 5 days, which causes discomfort when the stool is passed. The infant has had one episode of diarrhea and two episodes of ribbonlike stools. Abdominal distention and vomiting have not accompanied the constipation, and the infant's growth has been normal. The infant's diet consists of cow's milk formula only. The infant's mother reports that the infrequent passage of hard stools began approximately 6 weeks ago when she stopped breastfeeding. Which of the following interventions should the nurse practitioner include in the initial management of this infant's problem?

First, Think About It . . .

- **What are you taking for granted?**
- **What would the consequences be if you put your thoughts into action?**

1. **Prescribe several medications to be given daily to maintain a loose consistency of stools.**
2. **Tell the infant's mother that she stopped breastfeeding too soon and that if she resumes breastfeeding, the constipation will resolve.**
3. **Reassure the mother that constipation may occur with a change in diet and recommend that the mother slowly introduce cereal and prune juice into the infant's diet.**
4. **Refer the mother to a pediatric gastroenterologist for further evaluation.**

The best responses are 3 and 4. Although functional constipation often occurs in infancy with a change in diet, the episode of diarrhea and the passage of the ribbonlike stools may be manifestations of a medical cause.

The referral is needed to rule out conditions such as Hirschsprung disease. If this infant is determined to have functional constipation, simple measures such as dietary modifications may help to remedy the problem. Often, functional constipation resolves as solid food is introduced into the diet. One or two offerings of fruit juice each day may also help to prevent further constipation. Although breastfed infants may have constipation less frequently than bottle-fed infants, telling the mother to resume breastfeeding may make her feel responsible for her infant's constipation and instill guilt. Medications may be needed if dietary measures fail or if the child is found to have a medical cause for the constipation. However, pharmacologic intervention is not the intervention of choice at this time.

cessitated by school entry. Most schools will liberalize bathroom rules for individual children who have been identified as having toileting problems or who have a parent or school nurse intervene on their behalf.

The management of simple constipation consists of a plan to promote regular bowel movements. Often this is as simple as changing the diet to provide more fiber and fluids (Box 47-8), eliminating any foods known to be constipating, and establishing a bowel routine that allows for regular passage of stool. Stool-softening agents such as docusate or lactulose may also be helpful. If other symptoms such as vomiting, abdominal distention, or pain and evidence of growth failure are associated with the constipation, the condition should be investigated further.

Nursing Care Management. Constipation, unfortunately, tends to be self-perpetuating. A child who has difficulty or discomfort when attempting to evacuate the bowels has a tendency to retain the bowel contents and thus begins a vicious circle. Nursing assessment begins with an accurate history of bowel habits; diet; events that may be associated with the onset of constipation; drugs or other substances that the child may be taking; and the consistency, color, frequency, and other characteristics of the stool. If there is no evidence of a pathologic condition that requires further investigation, the major task of the nurse is to educate the parents regarding normal stool patterns and to participate in the education and treatment of the child.

Dietary modifications are usually essential in preventing constipation. During infancy, simply increasing the carbohydrate in the infant's formula (by adding sugar or corn syrup) will often relieve the problem. During childhood the diet should contain increased amounts of fiber and fluid. Parents benefit from guidance in dietary planning, especially regarding foods that facilitate bowel movements (see Box 47-8). They need reassurance concerning the benign nature of the condition. It is important to discuss with them their attitudes and expectations regarding toilet habits.

Box 47-8

High-fiber Foods

BREAD, GRAINS

Whole-grain bread or rolls
Whole-grain cereals
Bran
Pancakes, waffles, and muffins with fruit or bran
Unrefined (brown) rice

VEGETABLES

Raw vegetables, especially broccoli, cabbage, carrots, cauliflower, celery, lettuce, and spinach
Cooked vegetables, such as those listed above, and asparagus, beans, Brussels sprouts, corn, potatoes, rhubarb, squash, string beans, and turnips

FRUITS

Raw fruits, especially those with skins or seeds, other than ripe banana or avocado
Raisins, prunes, or other dried fruits

MISCELLANEOUS

Nuts, seeds, legumes, popcorn
High-fiber snack bars

Hirschsprung Disease

Hirschsprung disease *(congenital aganglionic megacolon)* is a mechanical obstruction caused by inadequate motility of part of the intestine. It accounts for about one fourth of all cases of neonatal obstruction, although it may not be diagnosed until later in infancy or childhood. It is four times more common in males than in females, follows a familial pattern in a small number of cases, and is considerably more common in children with Down syndrome. The incidence is 1 in 5000 live births. Depending on its presentation, it may be an acute, life-threatening condition or a chronic disorder.

Pathophysiology. The term *congenital aganglionic megacolon* describes the primary defect, which is the absence of

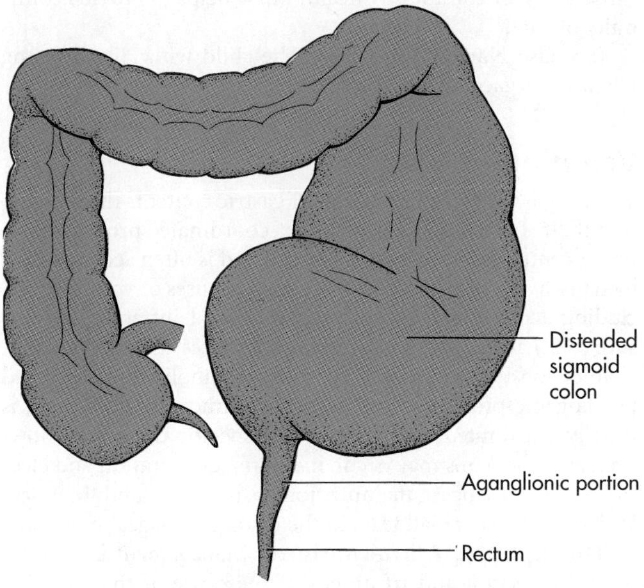

FIG. 47-2 • Hirschsprung disease.

ganglion cells in one or more segments of the colon. The etiology of Hirschsprung disease is not fully understood. The aganglionic segment almost always includes the rectum and a proximal portion of the large intestine. Rarely, "skip segments" or total intestinal aganglionosis may occur. Lack of enervation produces the functional defect that results in absence of propulsive movements (peristalsis) and that causes accumulation of intestinal contents and distention of the bowel proximal to the defect (megacolon). In addition, failure of the internal anal sphincter to relax contributes to the clinical manifestation of obstruction because it prevents evacuation of solids, liquids, and gas (Fig. 47-2). Intestinal distention and ischemia may occur as a result of distention of the bowel wall, which contributes to the development of *enterocolitis* (inflammation of the small bowel and colon), the leading cause of death in children with Hirschsprung disease (Kirschner, 1996).

Diagnostic Evaluation. Clinical manifestations vary according to the age when symptoms are recognized and the presence of complications, such as enterocolitis (Box 47-9). In the neonate, diagnosis is usually made on the basis of clinical signs of intestinal obstruction and failure to pass meconium. Radiographs, barium enema, and anorectal manometric examinations assist in the differential diagnosis, which is confirmed by histologic examination of a full-thickness rectal biopsy demonstrating absence of ganglion cells in the myenteric and submucosal plexus.

Therapeutic Management. Treatment is primarily surgical, to remove the aganglionic portion of the bowel to relieve obstruction and restore normal bowel motility and function of the internal anal sphincter. In most cases this is accomplished in two stages. First, a temporary ostomy is created proximal to the aganglionic segment to relieve obstruction and allow the normally enervated and dilated bowel to return to its normal size. Second, complete corrective surgery is performed, usually when the child weighs approximately 9 kg (20 pounds). There are several surgical procedures that can be performed, including the Swenson, Duhamel, Boley, and Soave procedures.

Box 47-9

Clinical Manifestations of Hirschsprung Disease

NEWBORN PERIOD
- Failure to pass meconium within 24 to 48 hours after birth
- Reluctance to ingest fluids
- Bile-stained vomitus
- Abdominal distention

INFANCY
- Failure to thrive
- Constipation
- Abdominal distention
- Episodes of diarrhea and vomiting
- Ominous signs (often signify the presence of enterocolitis)
  - Explosive, watery diarrhea
  - Fever
  - Severe prostration

CHILDHOOD*
- Constipation
- Ribbonlike, foul-smelling stools
- Abdominal distention
- Visible peristalsis
- Fecal masses easily palpable
- Child usually poorly nourished and anemic

*Symptoms are more chronic.

The Soave endorectal pull-through procedure, one of the most commonly used procedures, consists of pulling the end of the normal bowel through the muscular sleeve of the rectum, from which the aganglionic mucosa has been removed. The ostomy is usually closed at the time of the pull-through procedure.

Prognosis. Most children with Hirschsprung disease require surgery rather than medical therapy. Once the patient is stabilized with fluid and electrolyte replacement, if needed, the temporary colostomy is performed and has a high rate of success. After the later pull-through procedure, anal stricture and incontinence are potential complications that may occur, requiring further therapy, including dilation or bowel-retraining therapy.

Nursing Care Management. The nursing concerns depend on the child's age and the type of treatment. If the disorder is diagnosed during the neonatal period, the main objectives are: (1) to help the parents adjust to a congenital defect in their child, (2) to foster infant-parent bonding, (3) to prepare them for the medical/surgical intervention, and (4) to assist them in colostomy care after discharge.

Preoperative Care. The child's preoperative care depends on the age and clinical condition. A child who is malnourished may not be able to withstand surgery until the physical status improves. Often this involves symptomatic treatment with enemas; a low-fiber, high-calorie, and high-protein diet; and in severe situations, the use of total parenteral nutrition (TPN).

Physical preoperative preparation entails the same measures that are common to any surgery (see Surgical Procedures, Chapter 45). In the newborn, whose bowel is sterile, no additional preparation is necessary; however, in other children, preparation for the pull-through procedure involves emptying the bowel with repeated saline enemas and decreasing bacterial flora with systemic antibiotics and colonic irrigations using antibiotic solution. Oral antibiotics may also be prescribed.

Enterocolitis is the most serious complication of Hirschsprung disease. Emergency preoperative care includes frequent monitoring of vital signs and blood pressure for signs of shock; monitoring fluid and electrolyte replacements, as well as plasma or other blood derivatives; and observing for symptoms of bowel perforation, such as fever, increasing abdominal distention, vomiting, increased tenderness, irritability, dyspnea, and cyanosis.

Because progressive distention of the abdomen is a serious sign, the nurse measures abdominal circumference with a paper tape measure, usually at the level of the umbilicus or at the widest part of the abdomen. The point of measurement is marked with a pen to ensure reliability of subsequent measurements. Abdominal measurement can be performed at the same time that vital signs are taken, and is recorded in serial order so that a change is readily apparent. To reduce stress to the acutely ill child when frequent measurements of abdominal circumference are needed, the tape measure can be left in place beneath the child rather than removed each time.

The child's age dictates the type and extent of psychologic preparation necessary for the child and parents. Because a colostomy is usually performed, the child who is of at least preschool age is told about the procedure in concrete terms, with the use of visual aids (see Chapter 45). It is important to time explanations appropriately to prevent the anxiety and confusion that could result from too much information.

It is important to stress to parents and older children that the colostomy for Hirschsprung disease is temporary, unless so much bowel is involved that a permanent ileostomy must be performed. In most instances the extent of bowel resection is known before surgery, although the nurse should be aware of those instances when doubt exists concerning repair. The nurse should remember that although a temporary colostomy is favorable in terms of future health and adjustment, it requires additional surgery, which may be very stressful to parents and children.

Postoperative Care. Postoperative care is the same as that for any child or infant with abdominal surgery (see Surgical Procedures, Chapter 45). When a colostomy is part of the corrective procedure, stomal care becomes a major nursing task (see Ostomies, Chapter 45). To prevent contamination of the abdominal wound with urine in the infant, the diaper should be pinned below the dressing. Sometimes a Foley catheter is used in the immediate postoperative period to divert the flow of urine away from the abdomen.

Discharge Care. After surgery, parents need instruction concerning colostomy care. Even a preschooler can be included in the care by handing articles to the parent, rolling up the colostomy pouch after it is emptied, or applying barrier preparations to the surrounding skin. Although diagnosis of Hirschsprung disease is less common in school-age children or adolescents, if it is discovered in older children, they should be involved in colostomy care to the point of total responsibility.

Some institutions and communities have enterostomal therapists who provide additional expert assistance in planning home care. If families require financial assistance and additional psychologic support, referral to a social worker, home health care agency, or community health nurse helps to provide continuity of care.*

(See also Nursing Care Plan: The child with Hirschsprung Disease [Megacolon].†)

Vomiting

Vomiting is the forceful ejection of gastric contents through the mouth. It is a well-defined, complex, coordinated process that is under central nervous system control and is often accompanied by nausea and retching. There are many causes of vomiting, including acute infectious diseases, increased intracranial pressure (ICP), toxic ingestions, food intolerances and allergies, mechanical obstruction of the GI tract, metabolic disorders, and psychogenic problems. Vomiting is common in childhood, is usually self-limited, and requires no specific treatment; however, complications may occur, including dehydration and electrolyte disturbances, malnutrition, aspiration, and Mallory-Weiss syndrome (small tears in the distal esophageal mucosa).

Therapeutic Management. Management is directed toward detection and treatment of the cause of the vomiting and prevention of complications from the loss of fluid. Fluids are administered in the same manner and in a similar electrolyte composition to those administered for diarrhea (p. 1256). Although most children respond well to these measures, antiemetic drugs may be needed. The specific antiemetic may block the receptors in the chemoreceptor trigger zone (e.g., ondansetron [Zofran] and trimethobenzamide [Tigan]); enhance gastroduodenal peristalsis (e.g., metoclopramide [Reglan]); or compete for H_1-receptor sites (e.g., promethazine [Phenergan]). For children who are prone to motion sickness, it is often helpful to administer an appropriate dose of dimenhydrinate (Dramamine) before a trip.

Nursing Care Management. The major focus of nursing care of the vomiting infant or child is observation and reporting of vomiting behavior and associated symptoms and the implementation of measures to reduce the vomiting. Accurate assessment of the type of vomiting, the appearance of the vomitus, and the child's behavior in association with the vomiting greatly aids in establishing a diagnosis of disorders that have vomiting as a clinical feature.

Nursing interventions are determined by the cause of the vomiting. When the vomiting is identified as a manifestation of improper feeding methods, establishing proper techniques through teaching and example will usually correct the situation. If the vomiting is assessed as a probable sign of a GI obstruction, food is usually withheld or special feeding techniques are implemented. In situations in which vomiting is related to concurrent infection, dietary indiscretion, or emotional factors, efforts are directed toward maintaining hydration or preventing dehydration.

The thirst mechanism is the most sensitive guide to fluid needs, and ad libitum administration of a glucose-electrolyte solution to an alert child will restore water and electrolytes sat-

*Community and home care instructions on caring for the child with a colostomy are available in Wong DL, Hess CS: ***Wong and Whaley's clinical manual of pediatric nursing***, ed 5, St Louis, 2000, Mosby.

†In Wong DL, Hess CS: ***Wong and Whaley's clinical manual of pediatric nursing***, ed 5, St Louis, 2000, Mosby.

isfactorily. It is important to include carbohydrates to spare body protein and avoid ketosis resulting from exhaustion of glycogen stores. Small, frequent feedings of fluids or foods are preferred. Once vomiting has abated, more liberal amounts of fluids can be offered, followed by gradual resumption of the regular diet.

The vomiting infant or child is positioned on the side or semi-reclining to prevent aspiration, and observed for evidence of dehydration. It is important to emphasize the need for the child to brush the teeth or rinse the mouth after vomiting to dilute hydrochloric acid that comes in contact with the teeth. A flavored mouthwash or brushing also helps freshen the mouth. Careful monitoring of fluid and electrolyte status is important to avoid the possibility of an electrolyte disturbance.

Gastroesophageal Reflux (GER)

GER can best be defined as the transfer of gastric contents into the esophagus. GER occurs in everyone; it is the frequency and persistence that make it abnormal. Approximately 1 in 300 to 1 in 1000 children have a significant problem. It is important to differentiate GER from *gastroesophageal reflux disease (GERD)*. GERD represents symptoms or tissue damage that result from GER; however, GER may occur without reflux disease (GERD), and conversely GERD may occur without regurgitation (Orenstein, 1999). GER becomes disease when complications such as failure to thrive, bleeding, or dysphagia develop. GERD has also been associated with respiratory symptoms including apnea, bronchospasm, laryngospasm, and pneumonia (Zeiter and Hyams, 1999).

The causes of GER are related to dysfunction of the *lower esophageal sphincter (LES)*, delay in gastric emptying, poor clearance of esophageal acid, and the susceptibility of esophageal mucosa to acid injury (Zeiter and Hyams, 1999). In the past, it was thought that GER was the result of decreased LES tone; however, it now appears that *transient relaxation of the lower esophageal sphincter (TRLES)* is the most common mechanism leading to GER. Several factors cause the LES pressure to vary and include gastric distention, increased abdominal pressure caused by coughing, central nervous system (CNS) disease, delayed gastric emptying, hiatal hernia, and gastrostomy placement.

Some infants and children are especially prone to developing GER. These include premature infants; infants with bronchopulmonary dysplasia; and children who have had tracheoesophageal or esophageal atresia repair, neurologic disorders, scoliosis, asthma, cystic fibrosis, or cerebral palsy.

Reflux of stomach contents into the esophagus predisposes the infant or child to aspiration and the development of respiratory symptoms, particularly pneumonia. A particular concern is the association of life-threatening apnea with GER. Repeated irritation of the esophageal lining with gastric acid can lead to esophagitis and subsequent bleeding. Blood loss produces anemia and is seen as hematemesis or melena (blood in stools). Heartburn is also a common symptom in older children who are able to describe it, but it may go unrecognized in infants. A summary of clinical manifestations is provided in Box 47-10.

Diagnostic Evaluation. In addition to the history and physical examination, several tests are available to establish the presence of reflux, including the barium swallow, 24-hour pH probe study, and upper endoscopy. *Scintigraphy* detects radioactive substances in the esophagus after a feeding of the compound and assesses gastric emptying.

Box 47-10

Clinical Manifestations of Gastroesophageal Reflux

INFANTS

Spitting up, regurgitation, vomiting (may be forceful)
Excessive crying, irritability, arching of the back, stiffening
Weight loss, failure to thrive
Respiratory problems (cough, wheeze, stridor, gagging, choking at end of feedings)
Hematemesis
Melena
Anemia

CHILDREN

Heartburn
Abdominal pain
Noncardiac chest pain
Chronic cough
Dysphagia
Nocturnal asthma
Recurrent pneumonia

Adapted from Ault DL, Schmidt D: Diagnosis and management of gastroesophageal reflux in infants and children, *Nurs Pract* 23(6):78, 81-82, 88-89, 1998.

Therapeutic Management. Therapeutic management of GER depends on its severity. No therapy is needed for the infant who is thriving and without respiratory complications. Some children require modification of feeding with small, frequent feedings of thickened formula; and positioning therapy, which may help minimize the symptoms until the child grows and a normal physiologic barrier to reflux develops.

Controversies surround thickened feedings as a treatment for GER. Small, frequent feedings and frequent burping are generally accepted as reasonable strategies to minimize reflux. Constant nasogastric feedings may be necessary for the infant with severe reflux and failure to thrive. Feedings thickened with 1 teaspoon to 1 tablespoon of rice cereal per ounce of formula may be recommended as an initial measure to manage GER. The added calories may benefit the infant with GER.

Several studies have examined the effectiveness of positioning therapy for infants with GER. Traditionally the upright position in an infant seat was recommended for infants with GER; later, a head-elevated prone position was found to be superior. However, another study found no significant differences between the flat prone and head-elevated prone positions, and concluded that the head-elevated prone position is not worth the extra effort required to maintain it. Therefore either the flat prone or the head-elevated prone position after feeding and at night is a reasonable measure for treating infants with GER. The supine position is not used because GER worsens when the infant lies on the back. This is an exception to the recommended supine sleep position for healthy infants to decrease the risk of sudden infant death syndrome (SIDS) (see Chapter 36).

Pharmacologic therapy may be used as an adjunct therapy to treat infants and children with persistent symptoms of GER. H_2 antagonists such as cimetidine (Tagamet), ranitidine (Zantac), or famotidine (Pepcid) have proved effective in reducing the amount of acid present in gastric contents and may prevent esophagitis. Omeprazole (Prilosec) and lansoprazole (Prevacid), proton pump inhibitors, are also effective in blocking acid production. Current investigations are analyzing their effectiveness and potential side effects in infants and children. Metoclopramide (Reglan) has been found to increase resting LES pressure mildly and to increase rates of gastric emptying; however, side effects, including restlessness, drowsiness, and extrapyramidal reaction, may occur, and in some patients, metoclopramide may actually increase the number of reflux episodes.

Cisapride (Propulsid), a drug used to promote gastric emptying, was discontinued in July 2000 because of risk of serious cardiac arrhythmias and death associated with its use; however, the drug will be available through an investigational limited-access program. Bethanechol has been shown to increase LES pressure, but has not been proved to decrease reflux by pH probe studies. Bethanechol also has side effects, including respiratory symptoms such as wheezing.

Surgical management of GER is selected for children with severe complications such as recurrent aspiration pneumonia, apnea, severe esophagitis, or failure to thrive; and for children who have failed to respond to medical therapy. The *Nissen fundoplication* is the most common surgical procedure. This procedure involves a 360-degree wrap of the fundus of the stomach around the distal esophagus.

Unfortunately, complications can occur following fundoplication; therefore the decision to perform this procedure should be carefully considered. Postoperative problems include small bowel obstruction, retching, gas-bloat syndrome, and dumping syndrome. For children with neurologic impairment who are continuously tube fed, a nonsurgical percutaneous gastrojejunostomy and placement of a jejunostomy tube is an alternative to fundoplication with gastrostomy tube placement (Fonkalsrud et al, 1998).

Prognosis. The majority of infants with GER have a mild problem that generally improves by 12 to 18 months of age and requires only conservative lifestyle changes and/or medical therapy. If GER is severe and remains unsuccessfully treated, multiple complications can occur. Esophageal strictures caused by persistent esophagitis with scarring is one of the most significant complications. Recurrent respiratory distress with aspiration pneumonia, another serious complication, is an indication for surgery. Failure to thrive caused by GER can often be managed with medical therapy and nutritional support.

Nursing Care Management. Nursing care is directed at (1) identifying children with symptoms that suggest GER; (2) educating parents regarding home care, including feeding, positioning, and medications when indicated; and (3) if appropriate, providing care for the child undergoing surgical repair (see Surgical Procedures, Chapter 45).

Early in the treatment program, parents should be reassured that most infants and children outgrow GER, and often conservative lifestyle changes are all that will be needed. Parents need support and reassurance to implement these changes effectively. For example, to help parents cope with the inconvenience of dealing with a child who spits up frequently, simple measures such as using bibs and protective cloths during and after feeding are beneficial. When medical management is necessary, it is important to educate parents about the prescribed medications and their potential side effects. Prokinetic medications need to be given before feedings. Medications for acid control need to be given regularly and timed to provide coverage two or three times a day as ordered. Nurses also need to be sensitive to the demands placed on the family.

INTESTINAL PARASITIC DISEASES

Intestinal parasitic diseases, including helminths (worms) and protozoa, constitute the most common infections in the world. In the United States the incidence of intestinal parasitic disease, especially giardiasis, has increased among young children who are attending day care centers. Young children are especially at risk because of typical hand-mouth activity and uncontrolled fecal activity.

Intestinal parasitic diseases in humans are caused by various infecting organisms. This discussion is limited to the two most common parasitic infections among children in the United States: giardiasis and pinworms. Table 47-5 describes the outstanding features of selected helminths that belong to the family of nematodes.

General Nursing Considerations

Nursing responsibilities related to intestinal parasitic infections involve assistance with identification of the parasite, treatment of the infection, and prevention of initial infection or reinfection. Identification of the organism is accomplished by laboratory examination of substances containing the worm, its larvae, or ova. Most are identified by examining fecal smears from the stools of persons suspected of harboring the parasite. Fresh specimens are best for revealing parasites or larvae; therefore collected specimens should be taken directly to the laboratory for examination. If this is not feasible, the specimen is placed in a container with a preservative. Parents need clear instructions on obtaining an adequate sample and on the number of samples required. (See Stool Specimens, Chapter 45.) In most parasitic infections, examination of other family members, especially children, may be carried out to identify those who are similarly affected.

Once the diagnosis is confirmed and an appropriate treatment regimen is planned, parents need further explanation and reinforcement. Compliance in terms of drug therapy, and any other measures, such as thorough handwashing, are essential for eradication of the parasite. The family needs to understand the nature of transmission and that in some cases the medication must be repeated in 2 weeks to 1 month to kill organisms hatched since initial treatment.

The nurse's most important function in relation to these parasites is preventive education of children and families regarding good hygiene and health habits. Thorough handwashing before eating or handling food and after using the toilet is the most important precautionary method. Other preventive practices are listed in the Home Care box.

Giardiasis

Giardiasis is caused by the protozoan *Giardia lamblia* (also called *Giardia intestinalis, Giardia duodenalis,* and *Lamblia intestinalis*). It is the most common intestinal parasitic pathogen in the United States, and its prevalence among children in day

TABLE 47-5
Selected Intestinal Parasites

Clinical Manifestations	Comments
ASCARIASIS—*Ascaris lumbricoides* (Common Roundworm)	
Light infections: asymptomatic Heavy infections: anorexia, irritability, nervousness, enlarged abdomen, weight loss, fever, intestinal colic Severe infections: intestinal obstruction, appendicitis, perforation of intestine with peritonitis, obstructive jaundice, lung involvement—pneumonitis	Transferred to mouth by way of contaminated food, fingers, or toys Largest of the intestinal helminths Affects principally young children 1-4 years of age Prevalent in warm climates
HOOKWORM DISEASE—*Necator americanus*	
Light infections in well-nourished individuals: no problems Heavier infections: mild to severe anemia, malnutrition May be itching and burning ("ground itch") followed by erythema and a papular eruption in areas to which the organism migrates	Transmitted by discharging eggs on the soil, which are picked up, causing infection from direct skin contact with contaminated soil Wearing shoes is recommended, although children playing in contaminated soil expose many skin surfaces
STRONGYLOIDIASIS—*Strongyloides stercoralis* (Threadworm)	
Light infection: asymptomatic Heavy infection: respiratory signs and symptoms; abdominal pain, distention; nausea and vomiting; diarrhea—large, pale stools, often with mucus Threat to life in children with weakened immunologic defenses	Transmission is same as for hookworm except autoinfection common Older children and adults affected more often than young children Severe infections may lead to severe nutritional deficiency
VISCERAL LARVA MIGRANS—*Toxocara canis* (Dogs); Intestinal Toxocariasis—*Toxocara cati* (Cats)	
Depends on reactivity of infected individual May be asymptomatic except for eosinophilia Specific diagnosis difficult	Transmitted by direct contamination of hands from contact with dog, cat, or objects or by ingestion of soil Dogs and cats should be kept away from areas where children play; sandboxes are especially important transmission areas Periodic deworming of diagnosed dogs and cats Control of dog and cat population Continued education and laws to prevent indiscriminate canine and feline defecation
TRICHURIASIS—*Trichuris trichiura* (Whipworm)	
Light infections: asymptomatic Heavy infections: abdominal pain and distention, diarrhea	Transmitted from contaminated soil, vegetables, toys, and other objects Most frequent in warm, moist climates Occurs most often in undernourished children living in unsanitary conditions

care centers may range from 17% to more than 50% during outbreaks (Cody, Sottnek, and O'Leary, 1994). Breastfed infants exposed to *Giardia* develop much less diarrhea but are not protected from becoming infected (Walterspiel et al, 1994).

The potential for transmission is great because the cysts, the nonmotile stage of the protozoa, can survive in the environment for months. Chief modes of transmission are person to person; water, especially mountain lakes, streams, and swimming pools frequented by diapered infants; food; and animals, especially puppies. In children, person-to-person transmission is the most likely cause. Although individuals infected with giardiasis may be asymptomatic, common symptoms include abdominal cramps and diarrhea (Box 47-11).

Diagnosis of giardiasis may be made by microscopic examination of stool specimens or duodenal fluid, or by identification of *G. lamblia* antigens in these specimens by techniques such as enzyme immunoassay (EIA). Because the *Giardia* organisms live in the upper intestine and are excreted in a highly variable pattern, repeated microscopic examination of stool specimens may be required to identify trophozoites (active parasites) or cysts. Duodenal specimens may be obtained by direct aspiration, biopsy, or the *string test.* In the string test, the child swallows a gelatin capsule with a nylon string attached. Several hours later, the string is withdrawn and the contents are sent for laboratory analysis. With the availability of EIA techniques to identify *Giardia* antigens in stool specimens, other tests are being used less often.

Therapeutic Management. The drugs available for treatment of giardiasis are quinacrine (Atabrine), furazolidone (Furoxone), and metronidazole (Flagyl). The drug of choice is furazolidone, unless cost is a factor, in which case quinacrine is substituted. Quinacrine is less than one tenth the cost of fura-

Home Care

PREVENTING INTESTINAL PARASITIC DISEASE

- Always wash hands and fingernails with soap and water before eating and handling food and after toileting.
- Avoid placing fingers in mouth and biting nails.
- Discourage children from scratching bare anal area.
- Use superabsorbent disposable diapers to prevent leakage.
- Change diapers as soon as soiled and dispose of diapers in closed receptable out of children's reach.
- Do not rinse diapers in toilet.
- Disinfect toilet seats and diaper-changing areas; use dilute household bleach (10% solution) or Lysol and wipe clean with paper towels.
- Drink water that is specially treated, especially if camping.
- Wash all raw fruits and vegetables and food that has fallen on the floor.
- Avoid growing foods in soil fertilized with human excreta.
- Teach children to defecate only in a toilet, not on the ground.
- Keep dogs and cats away from playgrounds or sandboxes.
- Avoid swimming in pools frequented by diapered children.
- Wear shoes outside.

Box 47-11

Clinical Manifestations of Giardiasis

- Infants and young children:
  - Diarrhea
  - Vomiting
  - Anorexia
  - Failure to thrive
- Children over 5 years of age:
  - Abdominal cramps
  - Intermittent loose stools
  - Constipation
  - Stools may be malodorous, watery, pale, and greasy
- Most infections resolve spontaneously in 4 to 6 weeks
- Rarely, chronic form occurs:
  - Intermittent loose, foul-smelling stools
  - Possibility of abdominal bloating, flatulence, sulfur-tasting belches, epigastric pain, vomiting, headache, and weight loss

zolidone, and its long-term safety is established over the use of metronidazole. For pregnant women who need treatment, paromomycin may be used first, followed by metronidazole if the initial treatment is unsuccessful (Hill, 1993). Unfortunately, quinacrine has the highest frequency of side effects, especially nausea and vomiting. It also causes temporary yellow staining of the skin, sclera, and urine; and has a very bitter taste.

Nursing Care Management. The most important nursing consideration is prevention of giardiasis, especially among children and staff of day care centers. Attention to meticulous sanitary practices, especially during diaper changes, is essential (Fig. 47-3; see also the Home Care box). Nurses can play an important role in educating day care staff regarding appropriate sanitation practices (see Preschool and Kindergarten Experience, Chapter 38).

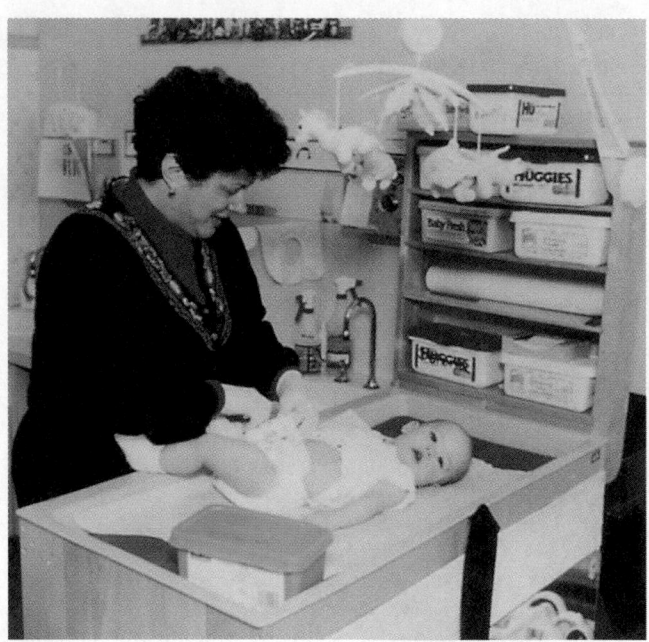

FIG. 47-3 • Prevention of giardiasis, especially in day care centers, requires sanitary practices during diaper changes, such as discarding paper diapers in a covered receptacle, changing paper covers on the diaper-changing surface, and having facilities for handwashing nearby. NOTE: Soiled cloth diapers and clothing should be stored in a plastic bag for transport home.

Once children are infected, family education regarding drug administration is essential. Parents often need suggestions for encouraging the child to take quinacrine. If other household members are infected, the nurse should inquire about their understanding and management of the disease.

To decrease the side effects of quinacrine and increase its palatability:

- Administer the drug with or after meals.
- Crush tablets and mix with a strong flavoring, such as jam or syrup.

Enterobiasis (Pinworms)

Enterobiasis, or pinworms, is caused by the nematode *Enterobius vermicularis.* It is the most common helminthic infection in the United States. It is universally present in temperate climatic zones and may infect more than 30% of all children at any one time. Crowded conditions, such as in classrooms and day care centers, favor transmission.

Infection begins when the eggs are ingested or inhaled (the eggs can be airborne). The eggs hatch in the upper intestine, then mature and migrate through the intestine. After mating, adult females migrate out the anus and lay eggs (AAP, 2000). The movement of the worms on skin and mucous membrane surfaces causes intense itching. As the child scratches, eggs are deposited on the hands and underneath the fingernails. The typical hand-to-mouth activity of youngsters makes them especially prone to reinfection. Pinworm eggs also persist in the indoor environment for 2 to 3 weeks, contaminating anything they contact, such as toilet seats, doorknobs, bed linen, under-

Box 47-12
Clinical Manifestations of Pinworms

Intense perianal itching (principal symptom); evidence of itching in young children includes the following:
- General irritability
- Restlessness
- Poor sleep
- Bed-wetting
- Distractibility
- Short attention span

Perianal dermatitis and excoriation secondary to itching if worms migrate, possible vaginal and urethral infection

wear, and food. Except for the intense rectal itching associated with pinworms, the clinical manifestations (Box 47-12) are nonspecific.

Diagnostic Evaluation. Diagnosis is most commonly made from the tape test (see Nursing Care Management). Repeated tests to collect eggs may be necessary, and if there is a possibility that other family members may be infected, a tape test should be performed on them.

Therapeutic Management. The drugs available for treatment of pinworms include mebendazole (Vermox), pyrantel pamoate (Antiminth), piperazine phosphate (Pripsen), and pyrvinium pamoate (Povan). The drug of choice is mebendazole, which is safe, effective, and convenient, with few side effects. However, it is not recommended for children under 2 years of age. If pyrvinium pamoate is prescribed, parents are advised that the drug stains stool and vomitus bright red, as well as clothing or skin that comes in contact with the drug. Because pinworms are easily transmitted, all household members are treated. The drugs should be repeated in 2 weeks to prevent reinfection.

Nursing Care Management. Nursing care is directed at identifying the parasite, eradicating the organism, and preventing reinfection. Parents need clear, detailed instructions for the *tape test.* A loop of transparent (not "frosted" or "magic") tape, sticky side out, is placed around the end of a tongue depressor, which is then firmly pressed against the child's perianal area. A convenient, commercially prepared tape is also available for this purpose. Pinworm specimens are collected in the morning as soon as the child awakens and *before* the child has a bowel movement or bathes. The procedure may need to be repeated more than once before eggs are collected. Parents are instructed to place the tongue blade in a glass jar or loosely in a plastic bag so that it can be brought in for microscopic examination. For specimens collected in the hospital, practitioner's office, or clinic, the tape is placed smoothly on a glass slide, sticky side down, for examination.

Compliance with the drug regimen is usually excellent because the duration of treatment is typically only one dose. However, the family is reminded of the need to take a second dose in 2 weeks. Posting a reminder on the refrigerator door or bathroom mirror is helpful.

To prevent reinfection, certain cleaning practices, such as washing all clothes and bed linen in hot water and vacuuming the house, may be recommended; however, there is little documentation on their effectiveness because pinworms survive on so many surfaces. Suggestions that are helpful include handwashing after toileting and before eating, keeping the child's fingernails short to minimize the chance of ova collecting under the nails, dressing children in one-piece sleeping outfits, and daily showering rather than tub bathing. Families should be informed that recurrence is common. Repeated infections should be treated in the same manner as the first one.

INFLAMMATORY DISORDERS

Stomatitis

Stomatitis is inflammation of the oral mucosa, which may include the buccal (cheek) and labial (lip) mucosa, tongue, gingiva, palate, and floor of the mouth. It may be infectious or noninfectious and may be caused by local or systemic factors. In children aphthous stomatitis and herpetic stomatitis are typically seen.

Aphthous stomatitis (aphthous ulcer, canker sore) is a benign but painful condition whose cause is unknown. Its onset is usually associated with mild traumatic injury (e.g., biting the check, hitting the mucosa with a toothbrush, or a mouth appliance rubbing on the mucosa), allergy, and emotional stress. The lesions are painful, small, whitish ulcerations surrounded by a red border. They are distinguished from other types of stomatitis by healthy adjacent tissues, absence of vesicles, and no systemic illness. The ulcers persist for 4 to 12 days and heal uneventfully.

Herpetic gingivostomatitis (HGS) is caused by HSV, most often type 1, and may occur as a primary infection or recur in a less severe form known as recurrent herpes labialis (commonly called "cold sores" or "fever blisters"). The primary infection usually begins with a fever; the pharynx becomes edematous and erythematous; and vesicles erupt on the mucosa, causing severe pain. Cervical lymphadenitis often occurs, and the breath has a distinctly foul odor. The disease can last 5 to 14 days with varying degrees of severity.

Therapeutic Management. Treatment for both types of stomatitis is aimed at relief of symptoms, primarily pain. Acetaminophen is usually sufficient for mild cases, but with more severe HGS, stronger analgesics such as codeine may be needed. Topical anesthetics are helpful and include over-the-counter preparations such as Orabase, Anbesol, and Kanka. A mixture of equal parts of diphenhydramine (Benadryl) elixir and Kaopectate, applied topically, provides mild analgesia, anti-inflammatory action, and a protective coating for the lesions. Lidocaine (Xylocaine Viscous) can be prescribed if the child can keep the solution in the mouth for 2 to 3 minutes and then expectorate it. Specific treatment for children with severe cases of HGS is the use of acyclovir (Zovirax) (Olin et al, 2000).

Nursing Care Management. The chief nursing goals for children with stomatitis are relief of pain and prevention of spread of the herpes virus. Analgesics and topical anesthetics are used as needed to provide relief, especially before meals to encourage food and fluid intake. Drinking bland fluids through a straw is helpful in avoiding the painful lesions. Mouth care is encouraged; the use of a very soft bristle toothbrush or disposable foam-tipped toothbrush provides gentle cleaning near ulcerated areas.

Careful handwashing is essential when caring for children with HGS. Because the infection is autoinoculable, children should keep their fingers out of the mouth; contaminated hands also can infect other body parts. Very young children may need elbow restraints to ensure compliance. All articles placed in the mouth are cleaned thoroughly. Newborns and individuals with immunosuppression should not be exposed to infected children.

NURSE ALERT • When examining herpetic lesions, wear gloves. The virus easily enters breaks in the skin and can cause herpetic whitlow of the fingers.

Because herpes infection is often associated with sexual transmission, the nurse should explain to parents and older children that HGS is usually caused by type 1 HSV, the type not associated with sexual activity.

Acute Appendicitis

Appendicitis, or inflammation of the *vermiform appendix* (blind sac at the end of the cecum), is the most common condition requiring abdominal surgery during childhood. Although uncommon in children younger than 2 years of age, it is associated with increased complications and mortality in this age group. Primarily an acute condition, appendicitis rapidly progresses to perforation and peritonitis if it remains undiagnosed. It is a significant pediatric problem because early diagnosis is commonly delayed, the child is often unable to verbalize symptoms, and the clinical signs may be mistaken for other illnesses.

Etiology. The exact cause of appendicitis is poorly understood, but it is almost always a result of obstruction of the lumen of the appendix by hardened fecal material (fecalith), foreign bodies, microorganisms, or parasites. Sometimes a fold of peritoneum causes the appendix to adhere to the cecum, resulting in an obstructive kink. Other causes include lymphoid hyperplasia, fibrous stenosis from an earlier inflammation, and tumors. Dietary habits may play a role. Children with high-fiber diets have a lower incidence of appendicitis than those whose fiber intake is low (Lund and Folkman, 1996). Fiber increases the bulk and softness of the stool—a factor that minimizes the chance of obstruction and promotes evacuation. Pinworms have not been shown to be a cause of appendicitis.

Pathophysiology. With acute obstruction the outflow of mucus secretions is blocked and pressure builds within the lumen, resulting in compression of blood vessels. The resulting ischemia is followed by ulceration of the epithelial lining and bacterial invasion. Subsequent necrosis causes perforation or rupture with fecal and bacterial contamination of the peritoneal cavity. The resulting inflammation spreads rapidly throughout the abdomen *(peritonitis),* especially in young children, who are unable to localize infection. Progressive peritoneal inflammation results in functional intestinal obstruction of the small bowel *(ileus)* because intense GI reflexes severely inhibit bowel motility. Because the peritoneum represents a major portion of total body surface, the loss of ECF to the peritoneal cavity leads to electrolyte imbalance and hypovolemic shock.

Diagnostic Evaluation. Diagnosis is based primarily on the history and physical examination (Box 47-13). Laboratory evaluation includes a white blood cell (WBC) count with a differential that is usually elevated, but seldom higher than 15,000 to 20,000 mm^3, with an elevated percentage of bands (often referred to as "a shift to the left"), indicating an inflammatory process. The diagnostic effectiveness of ultrasonography in the differentiation of pediatric abdominal pain from other causes has essentially replaced abdominal radiographic (x-ray) studies as the most effective method for diagnosing appendicitis (Irish et al, 1998). Findings such as visualization of the appendix and the presence of fluid around the appendix are important sonographic signs.

Box 47-13

Clinical Manifestations of Appendicitis

- Right lower quadrant abdominal pain
- Fever
- Rigid abdomen
- Decreased or absent bowel sounds
- Vomiting (typically follows onset of pain)
- Constipation or diarrhea may be present
- Anorexia
- Tachycardia, rapid shallow breathing
- Pallor
- Lethargy
- Irritability
- Stooped posture

Pain, the cardinal feature, is initially generalized (usually periumbilical); however, it usually descends to the lower right quadrant. The most intense site of pain may be at *McBurney point,* located midway between the anterior superior iliac crest and the umbilicus. Rebound tenderness is not a reliable sign and is extremely painful to the child. Referred pain, elicited by light percussion around the perimeter of the abdomen, indicates the presence of peritoneal irritation. Movement, such as riding over bumps in an automobile or gurney, aggravates the pain. In addition to pain, significant clinical manifestations include a change in behavior, anorexia, and vomiting.

Diagnosis is not always straightforward, and many infectious and inflammatory processes have the same symptoms. Fever, vomiting, abdominal pain, and an elevated blood count are associated with inflammatory bowel disease, pelvic inflammatory disease, gastroenteritis, urinary tract infection, right lower lobe pneumonia, constipation, mesenteric adenitis, Meckel diverticulum, and intussusception. In appendicitis, fever is usually present, varying from 37.5° to 38.5° C (99.5° to 101.5° F). If the temperature is greater than 39° C (102.2° F), a viral illness or perforation is likely. Prolonged symptoms and delayed diagnosis may occur in preschool children because of their inability to verbalize their complaints. Consequently, the risk of perforation is greater.

NURSE ALERT • Signs of peritonitis in addition to fever include sudden relief from pain after perforation, subsequent increase in pain (usually diffuse and accompanied by rigid guarding of the abdomen), progressive abdominal distention, tachycardia, rapid shallow breathing, pallor, chills, and irritability.

Therapeutic Management. Treatment of appendicitis before perforation includes rehydration, antibiotics, and surgical removal of the appendix (appendectomy). Recovery is rapid, and if no complications occur, the hospital stay is short.

Ruptured Appendix. Management of the child diagnosed with peritonitis caused by a ruptured appendix often begins preoperatively with IV administration of fluid and electrolytes, systemic antibiotics, and nasogastric suction. Postoperative management includes IV fluids, continued administration of antibiotics, and nasogastric suction for abdominal decompression until intestinal activity returns. The child with peritonitis is given antibiotics (including ampicillin, gentamicin, and clindamycin) for 7 to 10 days.

In some instances the wound is closed following irrigation of the peritoneal cavity. Many surgeons, however, leave the wound open (delayed closure) to prevent wound infection. A Penrose drain may be used to permit transperitoneal drainage. When delayed closure is used, wound irrigations and wet-to-dry dressings are a routine part of postoperative care.

Prognosis. Complications are uncommon following a simple appendectomy. The mortality rate from perforating appendicitis has improved from nearly certain death a century ago to 1% or less at present (Strahlman, 1997). The most common complications include wound infection and intraabdominal abscess. Early recognition of the illness is essential to prevent complications.

Nursing Care Management

➤ Assessment

Because abdominal pain is the most common childhood complaint with appendicitis, it is important to assess the severity of pain (see Pain Assessment, Chapter 44). One of the most reliable estimates is the degree of change in behavior. For example, a child who stays home from school and voluntarily lies down or refuses to play is much more likely to have considerable discomfort than the child who is absent from school but plays contentedly at home. The younger, nonverbal child will assume a rigid, motionless, side-lying posture with the knees flexed on the abdomen, and there is decreased range of motion of the right hip. Older children may exhibit all of these behaviors while complaining of abdominal pain. They can always indicate a point at which the pain is worse than at any other location.

➤ Nursing Diagnoses

On the basis of a thorough assessment, a number of nursing diagnoses become evident. The more likely diagnoses are listed in Box 47-14. Others will be apparent in specific circumstances.

➤ Plan of Care and Implementation

The goals of care for the child with a simple appendectomy include the following:

1. Child and family will be prepared for surgical intervention.
2. Child will receive postoperative care as described for the child undergoing surgery in Chapter 45.
3. Child with peritonitis will not experience postoperative complications such as spread of infection.
4. Child and family will receive support and education.

➤ Implementation

Physical preparation of the child with appendicitis is the same as that for any child undergoing surgery.

Box 47-14

Nursing Diagnoses: The Child with Appendicitis

Pain related to inflamed appendix
Risk for fluid volume deficit related to decreased intake and losses secondary to loss of appetite, vomiting
Risk for infection related to possibility of rupture
Altered family processes related to illness and hospitalization of a child

NURSE ALERT • In any instance when severe abdominal pain is expected, be aware of the danger of administering laxatives or enemas or applying heat to the area. Such measures stimulate bowel motility and increase the risk of perforation.

Postoperative Care. Postoperative care for the nonperforated appendix is the same as for most abdominal procedures. Care of the child with a ruptured appendix and peritonitis involves more complex care. The course of recovery is considerably longer, usually 7 to 10 days of hospitalization.

The child is maintained on IV fluids, allowed nothing by mouth, and kept on low continuous gastric decompression until there is evidence of intestinal activity. Listening for bowel sounds and observing for other signs of bowel activity (e.g., passage of stool) are part of the routine assessment. Management of IV therapy is the same as for any child receiving fluids and parenteral antibiotics.

A drain is often placed in the wound during surgery, and frequent dressing changes with meticulous skin care are essential to prevent excoriation of the area surrounding the surgical site. Wound care includes irrigation with antibacterial solution.

Management of pain from the incision and repeated dressing changes and irrigations are an essential part of the child's care. Psychologic care of the child and parents is similar to that used in other emergency situations (see Emergency Admission, Chapter 43). Parents and older children need an opportunity to express their feelings and concerns regarding the events surrounding the illness and hospitalization. The nurse can provide important education and psychosocial support to promote adequate coping, with alleviation of anxiety for both the child and the family.

➤ Evaluation

The effectiveness of nursing interventions is determined by continual reassessment and evaluation of care based on the following observational guidelines:

1. Observe child preoperatively for reaction to the situation and compliance with care.
2. Observe for documentation regarding child's emotional and physical needs, especially assessment of pain and administration of analgesics.
3. Monitor child for evidence of infection.
4. Interview and observe child and family for evidence of their understanding of the condition, especially its sudden onset and the need for surgery.

The expected outcomes include the following:

1. Child complies with directives and exhibits evidence of understanding the rationale for care appropriate to his or her age and developmental level (specify).

2. Child is relaxed and exhibits no evidence of distress (specify expected behaviors related to the characteristics of the child).
3. Child exhibits no evidence of dehydration.
4. Child exhibits no evidence of infection at other body sites.
5. Child and family readily express feelings and concerns and appear relaxed within the limitations imposed by the hospitalization (specify behaviors identified for specific case).

(See also the Nursing Care Plan: The Child with Appendicitis.*)

Meckel Diverticulum

Meckel diverticulum is a remnant of the fetal omphalomesenteric duct that connects the yolk sac with the primitive midgut during fetal life. Normally this structure is obliterated by the seventh to eighth week of gestation, when the placenta replaces the yolk sac as the source of nutrition for the fetus. Failure of obliteration may result in an *omphalomesenteric fistula* (a fibrous band connecting the small intestine to the umbilicus, known as Meckel diverticulum).

Meckel diverticulum is a true diverticulum because it arises from the antimesenteric border of the small intestine, and all layers of the intestinal wall are present. The diverticulum is usually found within 100 cm (40 inches) of the ileocecal valve and averages 1 to 10 cm (⅖ to 4 inches) in length.

Meckel diverticulum is the most common congenital malformation of the GI tract and is present in 1% to 3% of the population. It is twice as common in males as in females, and complications are several times more common in males. Most symptomatic cases are seen in childhood.

Pathophysiology. The symptomatic complications of Meckel diverticulum are caused by bleeding, obstruction, or inflammation. Gastric mucosa is the most common ectopic tissue found in Meckel diverticulum. Bleeding, which is the most common problem in children, is caused by peptic ulceration or perforation because of the unbuffered acidic secretion. Several mechanisms may cause obstruction. Intussusception may be led by the diverticulum. Obstruction may also be caused by entanglement of the small intestine around a fibrous cord, trapping of a loop of intestine under the band, incarceration within a hernia sac, or volvulus of the intestinal segment containing the diverticulum. Diverticulitis occurs when peptic ulceration or obstruction leads to inflammation.

Diagnostic Evaluation. Diagnosis is usually based on the history, physical examination, and a specialized radiographic study. The most common clinical presentation of Meckel diverticulum in children includes painless rectal bleeding, abdominal pain, or signs of intestinal obstruction (Box 47-15). Bleeding most commonly appears as dark red or "currant jelly" stools and may be mild or profuse. The Meckel scan, a radionucleotide *scintigraphy,* detects the presence of gastric mucosa with an overall diagnostic accuracy of 90%. Abdominal radiographs, barium enema, and arteriography have not been successful diagnostic tools. Blood studies are part of the general laboratory workup to screen for bleeding disorders and to evaluate the severity of the anemia.

Box 47-15

Clinical Manifestations of Meckel Diverticulum

ABDOMINAL PAIN
Similar to appendicitis
May be vague and recurrent

BLOODY STOOLS*
Painless
Bright or dark red with mucus ("currant jelly" stool)
In infants, bleeding may be accompanied by pain

SOMETIMES
Severe anemia
Shock

*Often a presenting sign.

Therapeutic Management. The standard treatment is surgical removal of the diverticulum. When severe hemorrhage increases the surgical risk, medical intervention to correct hypovolemic shock (e.g., blood replacement, IV fluids, and oxygen) may be necessary. Antibiotics may be used preoperatively to control infection. If intestinal obstruction has occurred, appropriate preoperative measures are used to reverse electrolyte imbalances and to prevent abdominal distention.

Prognosis. If Meckel diverticulum is diagnosed and treated early, full recovery is likely. The mortality rate of untreated Meckel diverticulum has been reported to range from 2.5% to 15%. The complications of untreated Meckel diverticulum include GI hemorrhage and bowel obstruction.

Nursing Care Management. Nursing objectives are the same as for any child undergoing surgery (see Chapter 45). Because the onset is usually rapid, psychologic support is similar to that provided with appendicitis. It is important to remember that the massive intestinal bleeding is traumatic to both the child and the parent and may significantly affect their emotional reaction to hospitalization and surgery.

Specific preoperative considerations when intestinal bleeding is present include (1) frequent monitoring of vital signs and blood pressure for shock, (2) keeping the child on bed rest, and (3) recording the approximate amount of blood lost in stools. In the absence of frank hemorrhage, the nurse tests the stools for occult blood.

Inflammatory Bowel Disease (IBD)

The general term *inflammatory bowel disease* is used for two chronic intestinal disorders: *ulcerative colitis (UC)* and *Crohn disease (CD).* Although UC and CD are grouped under the classification of IBD because they have similar epidemiologic, immunologic, and clinical features, they are two distinct conditions with very important differences (Table 47-6).

In addition to GI symptoms, each of these diseases is characterized by extraintestinal and systemic inflammatory responses. Exacerbations and remissions, without complete resolution, are also characteristic of IBD. In the pediatric population, growth failure is a unique and important problem associated with IBD, especially in CD. CD is often more dis-

*In Wong DL, Hess CS: ***Wong and Whaley's clinical manual of pediatric nursing,*** ed 5, St Louis, 2000, Mosby.

TABLE 47-6
Clinical Manifestations of Inflammatory Bowel Diseases

Characteristics	Ulcerative Colitis	Crohn Disease
Rectal bleeding	Common	Uncommon
Diarrhea	Often severe	Moderate to absent
Pain	Less frequent	Common
Anorexia	Mild or moderate	Can be severe
Weight loss	Moderate	Severe
Growth retardation	Usually mild	Often marked
Anal and perianal lesions	Rare	Common
Fistulas and strictures	Rare	Common
Rashes	Mild	Mild
Joint pain	Mild to moderate	Mild to moderate

abling, it has more serious complications, and medical and surgical treatment is less effective. Theoretically, UC is curable with a colectomy. CD is more common than UC, and the number of affected individuals with CD appears to be rising more than the number of individuals with UC.

Etiology. The exact cause of IBD is unknown, although there is evidence for a multifactorial etiology. It is proposed that IBD is a result of one or more environmental influences (e.g., infectious organisms, dietary habits, and environmental toxins) that promote disease in genetically susceptible individuals. Current research is focused on theories of defective immunoregulation of the inflammatory response to bacteria or viruses in the GI tract in individuals with a genetic predisposition. There appears to be a familial tendency in approximately 20% to 25% of cases. Individuals from higher socioeconomic levels and more Caucasians are affected. The incidence is also higher among Jews living in Europe and North America, and among people living in urban settings. Males and females are affected equally (Leichtner, Jackson, and Grand, 1996). A primary role for psychologic factors has not been supported, although psychologic problems may occur secondary to IBD and may intensify symptoms and influence the course of the disease.

Pathophysiology: Ulcerative Colitis. The inflammation is limited to the colon and rectum, with the distal colon and rectum often the most severely affected. Inflammation affects the mucosa and submucosa and involves continuous segments along the length of the bowel with varying degrees of ulceration, bleeding, and edema. The presentation of UC may be mild, moderate, or severe, depending on the extent of mucosal inflammation and systemic symptoms. Most cases include bloody diarrhea or occult fecal blood, abdominal pain that is most intense during defecation, and varying degrees of systemic manifestations and growth abnormalities (Leichtner, Jackson, and Grand, 1996). Thickening of the bowel wall and fibrosis are unusual, but long-standing disease can result in shortening of the colon and strictures. Extraintestinal manifestations are less common in UC than in CD but may precede colitis.

Pathophysiology: Crohn Disease. The chronic inflammatory process of CD may involve any part of the GI tract from the mouth to the anus but most often affects the terminal ileum. The disease involves all layers of the bowel wall (transmural) in a discontinuous fashion, meaning that between areas of intact mucosa there are areas of affected mucosa (skip lesions). The most common presenting symptoms of CD include abdominal pain with cramps, diarrhea, and weight loss. Other clinical manifestations include fever; anorexia; rectal bleeding; and perineal discomfort, including anal fissures or fistulas. The presence of perianal disease is a strong indication for CD. Mild GI symptoms, poor growth, and extraintestinal manifestations may be present for several years before overt GI symptoms occur. The inflammation may result in ulcerations, fibrosis, adhesions, stiffening of the bowel wall, stricture formation, and fistulas to other loops of bowel, bladder, vagina, or skin. Extraintestinal manifestations are common and include erythema nodosum, large joint arthritis, uveitis, mouth ulcers, liver disease, and renal calculi.

Diagnostic Evaluation. The diagnosis of UC and CD is based on findings from the history, physical examination, laboratory evaluation, and other diagnostic procedures. Laboratory tests include a CBC to evaluate anemia and an erythrocyte sedimentation rate to assess the systemic reaction to the inflammatory process. Levels of total protein, albumin, iron, zinc, magnesium, vitamin B_{12}, and fat-soluble vitamins are measured because they may be low in children with CD. Stools are examined for the presence of blood, leukocytes, and infectious organisms.

An upper GI series with small bowel follow-through is necessary to evaluate small bowel disease in children suspected of having CD. The terminal ileum may be rigid and narrowed with partial obstruction. A computed tomography (CT) scan may be indicated to evaluate abscesses or bowel wall thickening. A barium or air contrast enema is usually performed in children with suspected colitis unless the colitis is severe.

Diagnosis of IBD is confirmed following endoscopy of the upper and lower GI tracts. The bowel is examined for ulcerations or strictures. Mucosal biopsies, obtained during endoscopy, are examined for microscopic changes consistent with inflammation caused by IBD.

Therapeutic Management. The goals of therapy are to (1) control the inflammatory process to reduce or eliminate the symptoms, (2) obtain long-term remission, (3) promote normal growth and development, and (4) allow as normal a lifestyle as possible. Treatment must be individualized and managed according to the type and the severity of the disease, its location, and the response to therapy.

Medical Treatment. Drugs that mediate and control inflammation are the mainstay of IBD treatment. Current medications include 5-aminosalicylic acid (5-ASA) preparations, corticosteroids, azathioprine, 6-mercaptopurine, metronidazole, a variety of antibiotics, and cyclosporine. Corticosteroids are the most effective drugs for treating moderate and severe IBD. High doses of IV steroids are administered for acute episodes and then tapered according to the clinical response. If possible, the steroid dose is decreased or discontinued as soon as possible to minimize side effects such as adrenal suppression, hypertension, osteoporosis, glaucoma, cataracts, hirsutism, diabetes, weight gain, alterations of body composition, and growth retardation.

Sulfasalazine is useful in decreasing the frequency of recurrences in patients with mild cases of IBD. Because IBD interferes with the absorption and utilization of folic acid, daily supplements of folic acid are prescribed. Side effects of sulfasalazine include headache, nausea, vomiting, neutropenia, and oligospermia. Because many of the side effects are caused primarily by the sulfapyridine component of this drug, alternative nonabsorbable salicylate drugs such as olsalazine and mesalamine may be prescribed.

Metronidazole may be used as an adjunctive therapy in children with CD or in children with complications such as perianal disease or small bowel bacterial overgrowth. 6-Mercaptopurine, azathioprine, and cyclosporine are also used to treat IBD; however, these drugs have the major side effect of bone marrow suppression, which can cause leukopenia and opportunistic infections.

Nutritional Support. Nutritional support is a primary component of the treatment of IBD. Growth failure is a common serious complication, especially in CD. Growth failure is characterized by weight loss, alteration in body composition, retarded height, and delayed sexual maturation. Malnutrition causes the growth failure, and the etiology of the malnutrition is multifactorial. Malnutrition occurs as a result of inadequate dietary intake, excessive GI losses, malabsorption, drug-nutrient interaction, and increased nutritional requirements. Inadequate dietary intake occurs with anorexia and episodes of increased disease activity. Excessive loss of nutrients (i.e., protein, blood, electrolytes, and minerals) occurs secondary to intestinal inflammation and diarrhea. Carbohydrate, lactose, fat, vitamin, and mineral malabsorption are common, and vitamin B_{12} and folic acid deficiencies occur with disease episodes, with drug administration, and when the terminal ileum is resected. Finally, nutritional requirements are increased with inflammation, fever, fistulas, and periods of rapid growth (e.g., adolescence).

The goals of nutritional support include (1) correction of specific nutrient deficits and replacement of ongoing losses, (2) provision of adequate energy and protein for healing, and (3) provision of adequate nutrients to promote normal growth. Nutritional support may include both enteral and parenteral nutrition. A well-balanced, high-protein, high-calorie diet is recommended for children whose symptoms do not prohibit an adequate oral intake. There is little evidence that avoiding specific foods influences the severity of the disease. Supplementation with multivitamins, iron, and folic acid is generally recommended.

Special enteral formulas, given either by mouth or by continuous nasogastric infusion (often at night), may be required. Elemental formulas have been used successfully to improve nutritional status, as well as to induce remission in children and adolescents with CD. Elemental formulas are completely absorbed in the small intestine with almost no residue. Several studies have demonstrated that a diet consisting only of elemental formula not only improved nutritional status but also induced disease remission, either without steroids or with a diminished dosage of steroids required. An elemental diet is a safe and potentially effective primary therapy for patients with CD.

TPN has been shown to improve nutritional status in patients with IBD. Short-term remissions have been achieved following TPN, although complete bowel rest has not been proven to reduce inflammation or to add to the benefits of improved nutrition by TPN (Leichtner, Jackson, and Grand, 1996). Nutritional support in patients with UC is less likely to induce a remission than in patients with CD. Improvement of nutritional status is important, however, in preventing deterioration of the patient's health status and in preparing the patient for surgery.

Surgical Treatment. Surgery is indicated for UC when medical and nutritional therapies fail to prevent significant complications. The colectomy is considered to be curative. Surgical options include a *subtotal colectomy* and *ileostomy,* which leaves a rectal stump as a blind pouch. The most commonly used procedure is the colectomy, rectal mucosectomy, and endorectal ileoanal pull-through and anastomosis. A reservoir pouch is created in the configuration of a J or S to help improve continence postoperatively. Eliminating a complete rectal dissection preserves the anorectal sphincter apparatus and parasympathetic innervation to the bladder and genitalia.

Surgery for CD is indicated to drain abscesses, close fistulas, remove short segments of diseased bowel, repair perforations, relieve obstructions, or widen strictures. Surgery is not curative but may be lifesaving or greatly improve the quality of life.

Prognosis. IBD is a chronic disease. Relatively long periods of quiescent disease may follow exacerbations. The outcome of the disease process is influenced by the regions and severity of GI involvement, as well as by appropriate therapeutic management. Malnutrition, growth failure, and GI bleeding are serious complications. The overall prognosis for UC is good.

The development of carcinoma of the colon is a long-term complication of IBD. In UC, removal of the diseased bowel prevents development of carcinoma. In CD, however, surgical removal of the affected bowel does not prevent bowel cancer; therefore routine screening of stool specimens is needed for early detection.

Nursing Care Management. Many nursing considerations relate directly to the therapeutic management of IBD; however, nursing responsibilities extend beyond the immediate period of hospitalization and involve (1) continued guidance of families in terms of dietary management, (2) coping with factors that increase stress and emotional lability, (3) adjusting to a disease of remissions and exacerbations, and (4) when indicated, preparing the child and parents for the possibility of diversionary bowel surgery.

Because nutritional support is an essential part of therapy, encouraging the anorectic child to consume sufficient quantities of food is often a challenge. One approach that is likely to meet with success involves including the child in meal planning; encouraging small, frequent meals or snacks rather than three large meals a day; serving meals around medication schedules, when diarrhea, mouth pain, and intestinal spasm are controlled; and preparing high-protein, high-calorie foods such as eggnog, milkshakes, cream soups, puddings, or custard (if lactose is tolerated) (see Feeding the Sick Child, Chapter 45).

Foods that are known to aggravate the condition are avoided. The routine practice of using bran or a high-fiber diet for IBD is questionable. Bran, even in small amounts, has been shown to worsen the patient's condition. Occasionally the occurrence of aphthous stomatitis further complicates adherence to dietary management. Good mouth care before eating, and the selection of bland foods, help relieve the discomfort of mouth sores.

Nurses play an important role in preparing children and families to administer nasogastric feedings or TPN when indicated. The purpose and the expected outcomes of these therapies should be carefully explained. The child's and family members' anxieties should be acknowledged, and they should be given adequate time to demonstrate the skills necessary to continue the therapy at home if needed* (Critical Thinking box).

*Community and home care instructions on gastrostomy feedings and caring for a central venous catheter (for TPN) are available in Wong DL, Hess CS: ***Wong and Whaley's clinical manual of pediatric nursing***, ed 5, St Louis, 2000, Mosby.

Critical Thinking

INFLAMMATORY BOWEL DISEASE

A 13-year-old girl is admitted to the hospital because of bloody diarrhea, abdominal pain, and weight loss. After a thorough evaluation, including laboratory tests, radiographic studies, and GI endoscopy procedures, the diagnosis of Crohn disease (CD) is made. Medical treatment, including corticosteroid drugs and nutritional support, is initiated in the hospital. Enteral formula administered by continuous nighttime nasogastric (NG) tube infusion and vitamin and mineral supplements will need to be continued at home after the hospitalization. Which of the following interventions would *not* be included as part of important preparations for successful home care?

First, Think About It . . .

- **What information are you using?**
- **How are you interpreting that information?**

1. **Educate the adolescent and family regarding the disease process.**
2. **Educate the adolescent and family regarding medication therapy and administration of NG tube feedings.**
3. **Provide psychosocial support to aid in the adjustment to a chronic disease of remissions and exacerbations.**
4. **Restrict school attendance and extracurricular activities for the duration of home therapy.**

The best response is 4. The information provided in the first sentence indicates the age of the girl, which is an important factor. School absences or inability to compete with peers in some activities may occur during exacerbations of the disease, but self-esteem, positive school performance, and social interactions can be enhanced through support and guidance by the family and health care providers. Once the acute disease exacerbation is under control, the adolescent should resume school attendance and participate with peers in activities of interest. Important nursing responsibilities include educating the adolescent and her family regarding the disease process and therapeutic management and promoting adjustment to the chronic nature of the disease. The importance of continued drug therapy as prescribed despite remission of symptoms should be emphasized. The purpose and expected outcomes of nutritional support therapy should be explained, and the adolescent and her family members should be given adequate time to demonstrate skills relating to NG tube feedings in the hospital environment under supervision before the girl is discharged.

The importance of continued drug therapy despite remission of symptoms must be stressed to the parents and child. Failure to adhere to the pharmacologic regimen can result in exacerbation of the disease process (see Compliance, Chapter 45).

Family Support. Attending to the emotional components of a chronic disease requires a thorough assessment of disease-related stress factors. Commonly the nurse can be instrumental in helping children adjust to the problems of growth retardation, delayed sexual maturation, dietary restrictions, feelings of being "different" or "sickly," inability to compete with peers, and necessary absence from school during exacerbations of the illness (see Chapter 41).

If a permanent colectomy/ileostomy is required, the nurse can help the child and family to accept and adjust to the change by teaching them how to care for the ileostomy; by emphasizing the positive aspects of surgery, particularly accelerated growth and sexual development, permanent recovery, and eliminated risk of colonic cancer in UC; and by stressing the normality of life despite bowel diversion. Introducing the child and parents to other ostomy patients, especially those of the same age, can be effective in fostering eventual acceptance. Whenever possible, the continent ostomies should be offered as options to the child, although they are not performed in all centers throughout the United States.

Because of the chronic and often lifelong nature of the disease, families benefit from many services provided by organizations such as the Crohn's and Colitis Foundation of America, Inc. (CCFA),* which has branches in major communities and provides education regarding the management of IBD. If diversionary bowel surgery is indicated, the United Ostomy Association† and the Wound Ostomy and Continence Nurses Society‡ are available to assist with ileostomy care and provide important psychologic support through their self-help groups. Adolescents often benefit by participating in peer-support groups, which are sponsored in some areas by the CCFA.

(See also Nursing Care Plan: The Child with Inflammatory Bowel Disease.§)

Peptic Ulcer Disease (PUD)

PUD is a chronic condition causing a circumscribed loss of tissue of the mucosal, submucosal, and sometimes muscular layer in parts of the GI tract exposed to acid-pepsin gastric secretions. Ulcers are described as gastric or duodenal and as primary or secondary. A *gastric ulcer* involves the mucosa of the stomach; a *duodenal ulcer* involves the pylorus or duodenum.

Primary ulcers occur in the absence of a predisposing factor. *Secondary ulcers,* or *stress ulcers,* result from the stress of a severe underlying disease or injury (e.g., severe burns, sepsis, intracranial diseases, severe trauma, or multisystem organ failure) or in-

*386 Park Ave. S., 17th Floor, New York, NY 10016; 1-800-932-2423; fax (212) 779-4098; website: www.ccfa.org. In Canada: Crohn's and Colitis Foundation of Canada, 301-21 St. Claire Ave. E, Toronto, Ontario M4T IL9; 1-800-387-1479; fax (416) 929-0365; webite: www.ccfc.ca.

†19772 MacArthur Blvd., Suite 200, Irvine, CA 92612-2405; 1-800-826-0826; website: www.uoa.org.

‡1550 South Coast Highway, Suite 201, Laguna Beach, CA 92651; (888) 224-9626; fax (949) 376-3956; website: www.wocn.org.

§In Wong DL, Hess CS: ***Wong and Whaley's clinical manual of pediatric nursing***, ed 5, St Louis, 2000 Mosby.

gestion of an ulcerogenic drug (e.g., salicylates, nonsteroidal antiinflammatory drugs [NSAIDs], or ferrous sulfate). Stress ulcers occur in all pediatric age groups, including high risk newborns, with critically ill patients at the highest risk. In older children and adolescents the majority of ulcers are primary. The incidence of ulcers in boys is two to three times greater than in girls, although this difference is less in very young children.

Etiology. The exact cause of PUD is unknown, although infectious, genetic, and environmental factors are important. There is an increased familial incidence and increased incidence in persons with blood group O.

There is a significant relationship between the bacterium *Helicobacter pylori* (previously called *Campylobacter pylori*) and ulcers. *H. pylori* is known to colonize the gastric mucosa and has been identified in 90% to 100% of adult patients with PUD. It may cause ulcers by weakening the gastric mucosal barrier and allowing acid to damage the mucosa.

In addition to ulcerogenic drugs, both alcohol and smoking contribute to ulcer formation. There is no conclusive evidence to implicate particular foods, such as caffeine-containing beverages or spicy foods. Polyunsaturated fats and fiber may play a role in ulcer formation.

Psychologic factors may play a role in the development of PUD. Stressful life events, dependency, passiveness, and hostility have all been implicated as contributing factors in PUD.

Pathophysiology. Most likely, the pathogenesis of PUD is caused by an imbalance between destructive factors that promote the formation of peptic ulcers, and protective factors that guard against ulcer formation. The gastroduodenal epithelium secretes a layer of water-insoluble mucus that serves as a protective barrier against hydrogen ions, which are neutralized by the bicarbonate within the mucus. Prostaglandins appear to play a role in mucosal defense because they stimulate both mucus and alkali secretion. When abnormalities in the protective barrier exist, the mucosa is vulnerable to damage by acid and pepsin. Exogenous factors, such as aspirin and NSAIDs, have been shown to cause gastric ulcers by inhibition of prostaglandin synthesis.

Diagnostic Evaluation. Diagnosis is based on the history (pattern of pain) (Box 47-16); physical examination; and diagnostic testing such as radiographs, barium studies, and endoscopy. Upper endoscopy is the most reliable for diagnosing PUD. A biopsy is taken to determine the presence of *H. pylori.* Laboratory studies include a CBC to detect anemia; stool analysis for occult blood; and occasionally, gastric acid measurements (to identify hypersecretion).

Therapeutic Management. The objectives of therapy for children with peptic ulcers are to relieve discomfort, promote healing, prevent complications, and prevent recurrence. The management of ulcers is primarily medical and consists of administration of medications that reduce or neutralize gastric acid secretion. Whenever possible, known stressors are reduced.

Antacids have been beneficial in treating peptic ulcers because these medications neutralize gastric acid; however, to heal the ulcer and eradicate *H. pylori,* antacids are not as effective as medications that inhibit acid secretion (Gormally, Sherman, and Drumm, 1996). The most commonly used antacids are the aluminum or magnesium preparations, which are administered 1 and 3 hours after each meal and at bedtime. The dosage is determined by the size of the child. Common side effects are diarrhea with the magnesium-based products and constipation with the aluminum-based products.

Antisecretory agents that include the *histamine (H_2) receptor antagonists* cimetidine (Tagamet), ranitidine (Zantac), and famotidine (Pepcid) are often prescribed for PUD. These drugs suppress gastric acid production and have few side effects.

Proton pump inhibitors act to block all gastric acid secretion by binding to the hydrogen potassium adenosine-triphosphatase (H^+, K^+, ATPase) enzyme. The binding action blocks movement of H^+ ions out of the parietal cell, thereby inactivating the proton pump and preventing the secretion of hydrochloric acid. These drugs include omeprazole (Prilosec, Losec) and lansoprazole (Prevacid).

Other mucosal protective agents, such as sucralfate and bismuth-containing preparations, may be prescribed. Sucralfate is an aluminum-containing agent that forms a protective barrier over ulcerated mucosa to protect against acid and pepsin. Sucralfate is available in both a pill and a liquid and may be given four times a day for 6 weeks. Because sucralfate blocks the absorption of other medications, it is important that it be given separately from other medications.

Bismuth compounds are sometimes prescribed for the relief of ulcers. The mechanism of their activity is poorly understood, but they do have an effect on inhibiting the growth of microorganisms. Bismuth demonstrates activity against *H. pylori,* and the eradication of *H. pylori* from GI tissue is associated with improved healing of ulcers. Bismuth alone does not eradicate the organism in all cases; however, when bismuth is combined with

Box 47-16

Clinical Manifestations of Peptic Ulcer

NEONATES (USUALLY GASTRIC)
Usually perforation
Often massive hemorrhage
Almost the same as seen in stress ulcers

INFANTS TO 2-YEAR-OLD CHILDREN (GASTRIC OR DUODENAL, PRIMARY OR SECONDARY)
Poor eating, vomiting, crying spells after feeding, abdominal distention, tarry stools, melena
Vague discomfort
Irritability
Usually bleed rather than perforate

2- TO 6-YEAR-OLD CHILDREN (GASTRIC OR DUODENAL)
May have vomiting related to eating, generalized or periumbilical pain, melena, hematemesis
Wake at night or early morning, crying with pain
Perforation more likely in secondary ulcers

6- TO 9-YEAR-OLD CHILDREN (USUALLY DUODENAL AND PRIMARY)
Pain—burning or gnawing sensation in epigastrium related to fasting state, melena, hematemesis, vomiting
Often with obstruction

OVER 9 YEARS (USUALLY DUODENAL)
Same as above
More typical of adult type

an antibiotic, successful long-term eradication is possible. Several combinations of bismuth with one or two antibiotics are used to treat *H. pylori* infection. Antibiotics include ampicillin or amoxicillin, clarithromycin, and metronidazole. Treatment includes a 2-week course of one or two antibiotics combined with bismuth. Bismuth is then continued for an additional 2 to 4 weeks with one of the proton pump inhibitors. The proton pump inhibitor is then continued for another 1 to 2 months. Investigations continue to evaluate which combination of medications and length of treatment is most effective.

The child is provided with a nutritious diet and advised to avoid caffeine. Adolescents are warned about gastric irritation associated with alcohol use and smoking.

A child with an acute ulcer who has developed complications, such as massive hemorrhage, requires emergency care. Administration of IV fluids, blood, or plasma depends on the amount of blood loss. Blood replacement with whole blood or packed cells may be necessary for significant loss.

Surgical intervention may be required in the management of complications of PUD, such as hemorrhage, perforation, or gastric outlet obstruction. Ligation of the source of bleeding or closure of a perforation may be performed. A vagotomy and pyloroplasty may be indicated in children with recurring ulcers despite aggressive medical treatment.

Prognosis. The long-term prognosis for PUD is variable. Many ulcers can be successfully treated with medical therapy; however, primary duodenal peptic ulcers commonly recur. A high incidence of complications such as GI bleeding can occur and extend into adult life. The effect of maintenance drug therapy on long-term morbidity remains to be established with further studies.

Nursing Considerations. The main nursing objective is to promote healing of the ulcer through compliance with the medication regimen. If an analgesic/antipyretic is needed during therapy, acetaminophen, not aspirin or NSAIDs, is used. Critically ill neonates, infants, and children in intensive care units should receive antacids and H_2 blockers to prevent stress ulcers. Critically ill children receiving IV H_2 blockers should have their gastric pH values checked at frequent intervals and buffered with antacid if necessary.

The role of stress in ulcer formation should be considered for nonhospitalized children with chronic illnesses. Many ulcers in children occur secondary to other conditions; the nurse should be aware of family and environmental conditions that may aggravate or precipitate ulcers. Children may also benefit from psychologic counseling and from learning how to cope more constructively with stresses in their lives.

(See also Nursing Care Plan: the Child with Peptic Ulcer Disease.*)

HEPATIC DISORDERS

Acute Hepatitis

Hepatitis, or inflammation of the liver, is a significant health threat and the cause of significant morbidity and mortality in children.

*In Wong DL, Hess CS: ***Wong and Whaley's clinical manual of pediatric nursing***, ed 5, St Louis, 2000, Mosby.

Etiology. Hepatitis in children may be caused by a virus, a chemical or drug reaction, or some other disease process. The majority (90%) of cases of viral hepatitis are caused by six viruses, including:

- Hepatitis A virus (HAV)
- Hepatitis B virus (HBV)
- Hepatitis C virus (HCV)
- Hepatitis D virus (HDV)
- Hepatitis E virus (HEV)
- Hepatitis G virus (HGV)

In the United States, most non-A, non-B hepatitis is caused by HCV (Castiglia, 1996). In addition, cytomegalovirus (CMV), Epstein-Barr virus (EBV), and herpes simplex virus (HSV) may occasionally cause hepatitis. Epidemiologic features and serologic testing are used to differentiate the causes. Table 47-7 compares the characteristics of HAV, HBV, and HCV.

Hepatitis A. HAV infection is usually an acute condition that may be asymptomatic or cause mild illness (e.g., mild nausea, vomiting, and diarrhea). There is no chronic or carrier state. It is a contagious disease that is spread directly or indirectly by the fecal-oral route through ingestion of raw shellfish from polluted waters, direct exposure to infected fecal material, or close contact with an infected person. Infected children who show no symptoms can still spread HAV to others. HAV infection can affect individuals at any age, but the highest incidence occurs among preschool or school-age children under 15 years of age. The incubation period is approximately 3 weeks.

Hepatitis B. HBV infection can occur as an acute and/or chronic infection and may range from being asymptomatic and limited to causing fatal fulminant (rapid and severe) hepatitis. Transmission is usually via the parenteral route through the exchange of blood or any bodily secretion or fluid. Infections from blood transfusion have been reduced as a result of blood product-screening procedures. Transplantation of organs, intimate physical contact, transmission from mother to infant, and the splashing of contaminated fluids into the mouth or eyes are other sources of infection. Adults whose occupations are associated with exposure to blood or blood products (such as health care workers) are at increased risk for infection and should receive HBV vaccination.

Most HBV infection in children is acquired perinatally. Newborns are at risk for hepatitis if the mother is infected with HBV or was a carrier of HBV during pregnancy. Possible routes of maternal-fetal (-infant) transmission include (1) leakage of virus across the placenta late in pregnancy or during labor, (2) ingestion of amniotic fluid or maternal blood, and (3) breastfeeding, especially if the mother has cracked nipples.

HBV infection occurs in children and adolescents in the following high risk groups: (1) individuals with hemophilia and others who have received multiple transfusions, (2) children and adolescents involved in IV drug abuse, (3) institutionalized children and adolescents, (4) preschool-age children in endemic areas, and (5) individuals engaged in heterosexual or homosexual activity with homosexual males. The incubation period of HBV infection varies from 45 to 160 days.

Hepatitis C. HCV infection has been called "non-A, non-B hepatitis" because of the absence of HAV and HBV serologic markers of infection. In the United States, most non-A, non-B hepatitis is caused by the hepatitis C virus (HCV) (Castiglia, 1996). Currently about 0.2% to 0.4% of children under 12 years of age are infected with HCV. The major route of infection in

TABLE 47-7
Comparison of Hepatitis Types A, B, and C

Characteristics	Type A	Type B	Type C
Incubation period	15-50 days, average 25-30 days	45-160 days, average-50 days	6-7 weeks, average 2 weeks-6 months
Period of communicability	Unknown	Variable	Begins before onset of symptoms
	Virus in blood and feces 2-3 weeks before onset of jaundice and for about 1 week after onset of jaundice	Virus in blood or other body fluids during late incubation period and acute stage of disease; may persist in carrier state for years to lifetime	May persist in carrier state for years
Mode of transmission	Principal route—fecal-oral Rarely—parenteral	Principal route—parenteral Less frequent route—oral, sexual, any body fluid Perinatal transfer—transplacental blood (last trimester), at delivery, or during breastfeeding, especially if mother has cracked nipples	Principal route—parenteral Nonparenteral spread possible
Clinical features			
Onset	Usually rapid, acute	More insidious	Usually insidious
Fever	Common and early	Less frequent	Less frequent
Anorexia	Common	Mild to moderate	Mild to moderate
Nausea and vomiting	Common	Sometimes present	Mild to moderate
Rash	Rare	Common	Sometimes present
Arthralgia	Rare	Common	Rare
Pruritus	Rare	Sometimes present	Sometimes present
Jaundice	Present (many cases anicteric)	Present	Present
Immunity	Present after one attack; no crossover to type B or C	Present after one attack; no crossover to type A or C	Present after one attack; no crossover to type A or B
Carrier state	No	Yes	Yes
Chronic infection	No	Yes	Yes
Prophylaxis			
Immune globulin (IG)	Passive immunity Successful, especially in early incubation period and preexposure prophylaxis	Passive immunity Inconsistent benefits: probably of no use	Not currently recommended by Centers for Disease Control and Prevention
HAV vaccine	Two inactivated vaccines are approved for children ages 2-18 years: Havrix and Vaqta; given in a 2-dose schedule (6-12 months between doses)		
HBV immune globulin (HBIG)	No benefit	Postexposure protection possible if given immediately after definite exposure	No benefit
HBV vaccine (see Table 36-4)		Provides active immunity Universal vaccination recommended for all newborns	
Mortality	0.1%-0.2%	0.5%-2% in uncomplicated cases; may be higher in complicated cases	1%-2% in uncomplicated cases; may be higher in complicated cases

children is mother-to-infant transmission (Balistreri, 1999). The second most common route is by percutaneous exposure, which occurs through transfusion of blood or blood products, transplantation of organs or tissues, or through sharing used needles. Transfusion-associated HCV infection is low, but a common cause of infection is injection drug use. The AAP (1998) suggests screening the following groups: (1) all infants born to HCV-infected women, (2) individuals who received blood products before 1992, (3) individuals involved in injection drug use, and (4) individuals who receive hemodialysis. The length of time that maternal antibody is present in infants born to HCV-infected women must be considered, and screening should be done after the infant is 12 months old. However, a routine screening program, such as that for HBV, is not currently recommended.

The clinical course of HCV infection is variable. Incubation averages 6 to 7 weeks, with a range of 2 weeks to 6 months. Some children are asymptomatic, but HCV infection often becomes chronic and can cause cirrhosis and hepatocellular carcinoma. The onset of the disease is often undetected, and progression from the acute phase to cirrhosis and hepatocellular carcinoma usually requires decades or may not occur at all. The severity of the acute illness is also variable. Only a third of affected individuals develop actual symptoms or jaundice; the remainder are anicteric and have subclinical symptoms (Hubbard, 1998).

Current recommendations are to evaluate HCV-infected children at regular intervals to monitor for chronic hepatitis. Most children will be asymptomatic with evidence of chronic hepatitis on liver biopsy. Liver enzyme levels may fluctuate between periods of normal and elevated values (Balistreri, 1999).

Hepatitis D. HDV infection occurs in children already infected with HBV. HDV is a defective ribonucleic acid (RNA) virus that requires the function of HBV. HDV infection occurs primarily in hemophiliac patients and IV drug abusers. The incubation period is 21 to 90 days. Both acute and chronic forms are more severe than HBV infection and can lead to cirrhosis. Testing for HDV infection is recommended in children with chronic HBV infection or severe liver disease, or in children with acute exacerbation of a previously stable liver disease.

Hepatitis E. HEV infection is enterally transmitted non-A, non-B hepatitis. Transmission may occur through the fecal-oral route or from contaminated water. The incubation period is 2 to 9 weeks. This illness is uncommon in children, does not cause chronic liver disease, is not a chronic condition, and has no carrier state. The mortality rate due to submassive hepatic necrosis is low except in pregnant women in their third trimester, in whom mortality reaches 20%.

Hepatitis G. HGV is an RNA virus with a structure similar to that of HCV. HGV is blood-borne. High risk groups include transfusion recipients, IV drug users, and individuals infected with HCV. The virus is responsible for approximately 0.3% of cases of acute viral hepatitis. Individuals with the virus are often asymptomatic, and most infections are chronic.

Diagnostic Evaluation. Diagnosis is based on the history (especially regarding possible exposure to a hepatitis virus), physical examination, and serologic markers for hepatitis A, B, and C. No liver function test is specific for hepatitis. Serum aspartate and alanine aminotransferase (AST, ALT) levels are markedly elevated. Serum bilirubin levels peak 5 to 10 days after clinical jaundice appears.

Histologic evidence from liver biopsy may be required to aid in diagnosis and to assess the severity of liver disease. Serologic markers indicate the antibodies or antigens formed in response to the specific virus and confirm the diagnosis. For example, HAV is diagnosed by the presence of HAV antibody (anti-HAV). During the initial infective period, anti-HAV of the immunoglobulin M (IgM) class is present, but after about 3 to 6 months, this antibody declines and anti-HAV of the IgG class increases. Therefore detection of anti-HAV IgM indicates active infection, and anti-HAV IgG indicates past infection and immunity. Diagnosis of hepatitis B is confirmed by detection of several antigens and antibodies that are produced in response to the virus.

Pathophysiology. The pathologic changes occur primarily in the parenchymal cells of the liver and result in varying degrees of swelling, infiltration of liver cells by mononuclear cells, subsequent degeneration, necrosis, and fibrosis.

Hepatitis can be self-limited, and complete regeneration of liver cells without scarring may occur; however, some forms of hepatitis do not result in complete return of liver function. These include *fulminant hepatitis,* which is characterized by a severe, acute course and massive destruction of the liver that results in liver failure and death in 1 to 2 weeks. *Subacute* or *chronic active hepatitis* is characterized by progressive liver destruction, uncertain regeneration, scarring, and potential cirrhosis.

The initial *anicteric* (absence of jaundice) *phase* usually lasts 5 to 7 days and is often mistaken for influenza. Symptoms include nausea, vomiting, extreme anorexia, malaise, easy fatigability, arthralgia, skin rashes, slight to moderate fever, and epigastric or upper right quadrant abdominal pain.

Symptoms of the *icteric* (jaundice) *phase* include dark urine. Pruritus may accompany jaundice and can be a bothersome symptom; however, many children with acute viral hepatitis do not develop jaundice.

Therapeutic Management. Treatment options for viral hepatitis are limited. The goals of management include early detection, support and monitoring of the disease, recognition of chronic liver disease, and prevention of spread of the disease. There is no specific therapy for acute or chronic hepatitis B or hepatitis C. Special diets are generally of no value. The use of corticosteroids alone or in combination with immunosuppressive drugs is not advocated. Hospitalization may be indicated in the event of coagulopathy or fulminant hepatitis. Currently the immune-modulating agent interferon-α is the only drug approved by the FDA for initial treatment of HCV. Interferon-α has been used with some success in treating chronic hepatitis B and chronic hepatitis C in adults (AAP, 1998; Hubbard, 1998).

Prevention. Proper handwashing and standard isolation precautions can prevent spread of hepatitis. Prophylactic use of standard immune globulin (IG) is effective in preventing HAV infection in situations of preexposure (e.g., anticipated travel to areas where HAV is prevalent) or in situations of postexposure during the early part of the incubation period. Hepatitis B immune globulin (HBIG) is effective in preventing HBV infection after exposure. IGs must be administered less than 2 weeks after exposure.

Active immunizations are not available against the non-A, non-B viruses. Vaccines have been developed to prevent HBV and HAV infection. HBV vaccination is recommended for all newborns and for high risk groups. HAV is also recommended for high risk groups (see Immunizations, Chapter 36).

It is possible to prevent HDV infection by preventing HBV infection.

Prognosis. The prognosis for children with hepatitis is variable and depends on the type of virus causing the disease. HAV usually causes a mild and brief illness with no carrier state. HBV can cause a wide spectrum of acute and chronic illness. Chronic HBV infection leads to cirrhosis in approximately one fourth to one third of the cases. Hepatocellular carcinoma is a potentially fatal complication of HBV infection. HCV infection commonly becomes chronic, and cirrhosis may develop in some patients. Fulminant hepatic failure occurs in a small number of cases of viral hepatitis, regardless of the etiology, and is associated with a high mortality rate.

Nursing Care Management. Nursing objectives depend on the severity of the hepatitis, the medical management, and factors influencing the control and transmission of the disease. Because children with benign viral hepatitis are commonly cared for at home, the responsibility of explaining medical therapies and control measures is commonly left to the clinic or office nurse. When further assistance is needed for parents to comply with such instructions, a public health nursing referral may be necessary.

A well-balanced diet and a realistic schedule of rest and activity adjusted to the child's condition are encouraged. HAV is not infectious within a week or so after the onset of jaundice, and children may feel well enough to resume school. Parents are cautioned about administering any medication to the child, because normal doses of many drugs may become dangerous because of the liver's inability to detoxify and excrete them.

Handwashing is the single most critical measure in reducing risk of hepatitis transmission in any setting. The nurse should explain to parents and children the usual ways in which HAV (oral-fecal route) and HBV (parenteral route) are spread.

Children who are hospitalized are not usually isolated in a separate room unless they are fecally incontinent or their toys and other items might become contaminated with feces. They are discouraged from sharing their toys. (For further discussion, see Infection Control, Chapter 45.)

In young people with HBV infection who have a known or suspected history of illicit drug use, the nurse has the additional responsibility of helping them realize the associated dangers of drug abuse, stressing the parenteral mode of transmission of hepatitis, and encouraging them to seek counseling through a drug program.

(See also Nursing Care Plan: The Child with Acute Hepatitis.*)

Cirrhosis

Cirrhosis occurs at the end stage of many chronic liver diseases, including biliary atresia and chronic hepatitis. Severe damage can be caused by infectious, autoimmune, or toxic factors; and by chronic diseases such as hemophilia and cystic fibrosis. A cirrhotic liver is irreversibly damaged.

Clinical manifestations of cirrhosis develop from features typically seen with all chronic liver disorders. Children with cirrhosis often exhibit jaundice, poor growth, anorexia, muscle weakness, and lethargy. Ascites, edema, GI bleeding, anemia, and abdominal pain may be present in children with impaired intrahepatic blood flow. Pulmonary function may be impaired because of pressure against the diaphragm from hepatosplenomegaly and ascites. Dyspnea and cyanosis may occur, especially on exertion. Intrapulmonary arteriovenous shunts may develop and cause hypoxemia. Spider angiomas and prominent blood vessels are often present on the upper torso.

Therapeutic Management. Therapy is directed toward (1) frequent assessment of liver status with physical examination and liver function tests and (2) management of specific complications. The only successful treatment for end-stage liver disease and liver failure may be liver transplantation, which has improved the prognosis substantially for many children with cirrhosis. Currently, the 1-year survival rate for *liver transplantation* is 85%, and the 5-year survival rate is 75% (United Network for Organ Sharing, 1995).

Prognosis. The succcss of liver transplantation has revolutionized the approach to liver cirrhosis. Liver failure and cirrhosis are currently indications for transplantation. Liver transplantation reflects the failure of other medical and surgical measures to prevent or treat cirrhosis. Careful monitoring of the child's condition and quality of life are necessary to evaluate the need for and timing of transplantation (Family Focus box).

Nursing Care Management. Nursing care of the child with cirrhosis is influenced by several factors, including the cause of the cirrhosis, the severity of complications, and the prognosis. The prognosis for life is often poor unless successful liver transplantation occurs. Therefore nursing care of this child is similar to that for any child with a life-threatening illness (see Chapter 41). Hospitalization is usually required when complications occur.

Biliary Atresia

Biliary atresia, or *extrahepatic biliary atresia (EHBA),* is a progressive inflammatory process that causes both intrahepatic and extrahepatic bile duct fibrosis, resulting in eventual ductal obstruction. The incidence of EHBA is between 1 in 10,000 and 1 in 25,000 live births. There does not seem to be a racial or genetic predilection, although there is a female predominance of 1.4:1 (McEvoy and Suchy, 1996; Whitington, 1996). Associated malformations include polysplenia, intestinal atresia, and malrotation of the intestine. EHBA, if untreated, usually leads to cirrhosis, liver failure, and death in the first 2 years of life.

Etiology/Pathophysiology. The exact cause of biliary atresia is unknown, although immune mechanisms or viral injury may be responsible for the progressive process that results in complete obliteration of the bile ducts. Reports have indicated that biliary atresia is not seen in the fetus, stillborn infant, or newborn infant (Halamek and Stevenson, 1997), suggesting that biliary atresia is acquired late in gestation or in the perinatal period and manifested a few weeks after birth. Inflammation is progressive, causing obstruction and fibrosis of both the intrahepatic and extrahepatic bile ducts. Varying degrees of cholestasis occur, resulting in retention of irritants and toxins that cause severe pruritus. Surgery to obtain effective bile drainage must be achieved within 2 to 3 months after birth to diminish progressive liver damage.

Diagnostic Evaluation. Early diagnosis is the key to the survival of the child with EHBA; the outcome in children surgically treated before 2 months of age is much better than that in patients with delayed treatment. Growth parameters and

Family Focus

END-STAGE LIVER DISEASE

In many cases the child and family must cope with an uncertain progression of the disease. The only hope for long-term survival may be liver transplantation. Transplantation can be very successful, but the waiting period may be long, and there are many more children in need of organs than there are donors. The procedure is very expensive and is performed only at designated medical centers that are often far from the family's home. The nurse should recognize the unique stresses of coping with end-stage liver disease and waiting for transplantation and assist the family in coping with these stressors. The assistance of social workers and support from other parents can be very beneficial.

*In Wong DL, Hess CS: ***Wong and Whaley's clinical manual of pediatric nursing***, ed 5, St Louis, 2000, Mosby.

nutritional status should be assessed because many of these infants and children have nutritional deficiencies and poor growth. The disease is suspected on the basis of clinical signs (Box 47-17). Blood tests, including a CBC, electrolytes, bilirubin, and liver enzymes, are obtained. Additional laboratory analyses, including alpha$_1$-antitrypsin level, TORCHS titers, hepatitis serology, alpha-fetoprotein, urine cytomegalovirus, and a sweat test, may be indicated to rule out other conditions that cause persistent cholestasis and jaundice. Abdominal ultrasonography allows evaluation of the liver and biliary system. Biliary patency can be determined with hepatobiliary scintigraphy. Liver biopsy evaluates hepatic pathology. Definitive diagnosis of EHBA is obtained during an exploratory laparotomy and an intraoperative cholangiogram.

Therapeutic Management. The primary treatment of biliary atresia is *hepatic portoenterostomy (Kasai procedure)*, in which a segment of intestine is anastomosed to the resected porta hepatis to attempt bile drainage. There are several variations of this procedure. In approximately 80% to 90% of infants with EHBA who undergo surgery when younger than 10 weeks of age, bile drainage is achieved (Halamek and Stevenson, 1997); however, progressive cirrhosis still occurs in many children, and up to 80% to 90% will eventually require liver transplantation (Andres, 1996). Prophylactic antibiotics are given following the Kasai procedure to minimize the risk of ascending cholangitis.

Medical management is primarily supportive. It includes nutritional support with infant formulas that contain medium-chain triglycerides and essential fatty acids. Supplementation with fat-soluble vitamins; a multivitamin; and minerals, including iron, zinc, and selenium, is usually required. Aggressive nutritional support in the form of continuous tube feedings or total parenteral nutrition may be indicated for moderate to severe failure to thrive; the enteral solution should be low in sodium. Ursodeoxycholic acid has been used successfully to treat pruritus and hypercholesterolemia in children with liver disease.

Prognosis. Untreated biliary atresia results in progressive cirrhosis and death in most children by 2 years of age. The Kasai procedure does improve the prognosis but is not a cure. Biliary drainage can often be achieved if the surgery is done before the intrahepatic bile ducts are destroyed, usually by 8 weeks of age. Long-term survival has been reported in children who received the Kasai procedure; however, even with successful bile drainage, many children ultimately develop liver failure.

The advances in surgical techniques and the development of immunosuppressive and antifungal drugs have significantly improved the success of transplantation. The major obstacle remains the shortage of donor livers. Success with reduced-sized and split-liver transplantation and retransplantation, as well as increased public awareness, may improve the availability of donor organs for children in the future.

Nursing Care Management. There are important nursing interventions for the child with biliary atresia. Education regarding all aspects of the treatment plan and the rationale for therapy should be provided to the family members. In the immediate postoperative period following a portoenterostomy, nursing care is similar to that following any major abdominal surgery. Teaching includes the proper administration of medications and nutritional therapy, including special formulas, vitamin and mineral supplements, tube feedings, or parenteral nutrition. Pruritus may be a significant problem that can be relieved by drug therapy or comfort measures, including baths and trimming of fingernails.

Children and their families require special psychosocial support. The uncertain prognosis, discomfort, and waiting for transplantation can produce considerable stress. Extended hospitalizations, pharmacologic therapy, and nutritional therapy can impose significant financial burdens on the family. Families of children with liver disease can get help from the Children's Liver Disease Foundation,* an organization that provides educational materials, programs, and support systems to families with liver disease.

Box 47-17

Clinical Manifestations of Extrahepatic Biliary Atresia

- Jaundice
  - Earliest manifestation and most striking feature of disorder
  - First observed in sclera
  - May be present at birth
  - Usually not apparent until age 2 to 3 weeks
- Urine dark and stains diaper
- Stools lighter than expected or white or tan
- Hepatomegaly and abdominal distention common
- Splenomegaly occurs later
- Poor fat metabolism results in:
  - Poor weight gain
  - General failure to thrive
- Pruritus
- Irritability
- Difficult to comfort infant

STRUCTURAL DEFECTS

Cleft Lip (CL) and/or Cleft Palate (CP)

Clefts of the lip and palate are facial malformations that occur during embryonic development, are common to all human populations, and can constitute a severe disability to the affected individual. They may appear separately or, more often, together. CL results from failure of the maxillary and median nasal processes to fuse; CP is a midline fissure of the palate that results from failure of the two sides to fuse. This discussion is concerned primarily with cleft lip and palate (CL/P).

CL may vary from a small notch to a complete cleft extending into the base of the nose (Fig. 47-4). Clefts can be unilateral or bilateral. Deformed dental structures are associated with CL. CP alone occurs in the midline and may involve the soft and hard palates. When associated with CL, the defect may involve the midline and extend into the soft palate on one or both sides.

The incidence of CL with or without CP is approximately 1 in 800 live births. The incidence of CP alone is 1 in 2000 live births. CL with or without CP is more common in males, and CP alone is more common in females. The defect appears more often in Asians and certain tribes of Native Americans than in Caucasians, and less often in African-Americans.

*36 Great Charles St., Birmingham, B33 JY, United Kingdom; (0121) 212-3839; fax (0121) 212-4300; website: www.childliverdisease.org.

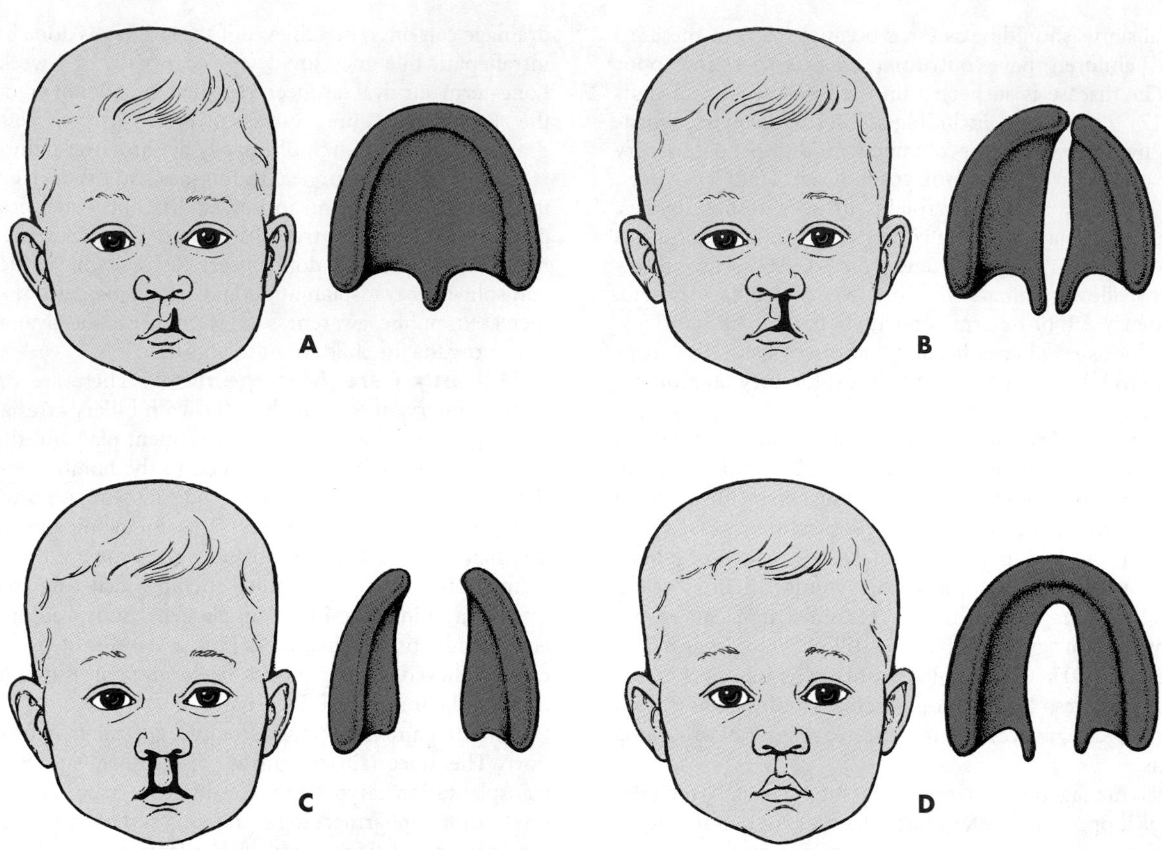

FIG. 47-4 • Variations in clefts of lip and palate at birth. **A,** Notch in vermilion border. **B,** Unilateral cleft lip and palate. **C,** Bilateral cleft lip and palate. **D,** Cleft palate.

Etiology. The majority of cases appear to be consistent with the concept of multifactorial inheritance, as evidenced by an increased incidence in relatives and a higher concordance in monozygotic twins than in dizygotic twins. Many recognized syndromes include these defects as a feature and are the result of chromosomal abnormalities and environmental factors or teratogens that may be responsible for clefts at a critical point in embryonic development. It should be noted that maternal smoking in the first trimester is believed to be the cause of 11% to 12% of all cases of CL and/or CP (Wyszinski, Duffy, and Beatty, 1997).

Pathophysiology. CL/P results from failure of the maxillary and premaxillary processes to come in contact during early embryonic life. Although often appearing together, CL and CP are distinct malformations embryologically, occurring at different times during the developmental process. Merging of the upper lip at the midline is completed between the seventh and eighth weeks of gestation. Fusion of the secondary palate (hard and soft palate) takes place later in development, between the seventh and twelfth weeks of gestation. In the process of migrating to a horizontal position, they are separated by the tongue for a short time. If there is delay in this movement, or if the tongue fails to descend soon enough, the remainder of development proceeds but the palate never fuses.

Diagnostic Evaluation. CL with or without CP is readily apparent at birth and is a defect that elicits severe emotional reactions in parents. CL may be unilateral or bilateral, and the extent of the cleft and degree of nasal deformity are variable. CP may occur as an isolated defect or in association with CL. Less obvious than CL, the defect may not be detected without a thorough assessment of the mouth. The deformity can be identified by placing the examiner's finger directly on the palate. Clefts of the hard palate form a continuous opening between the mouth and the nasal cavity. The severity of the CP has an impact on feeding problems; the infant is unable to generate negative pressure and create suction in the oral cavity. This impairs feeding, even though in most cases the infant's ability to swallow is normal.

Therapeutic Management. Treatment of the child with CL is surgical and usually involves no long-term interventions other than possible scar revision; however, the management of CP involves the cooperative efforts of a multidisciplinary health care team—including pediatrics, plastic surgery, orthodontics, otolaryngology, speech/language pathology, audiology, nursing, and social work—to provide optimum results. Medical management is directed toward closure of the cleft(s), prevention of complications, and facilitation of normal growth and development of the child.

Surgical Correction: CL. Closure of the lip defect precedes that of the palate, usually at 6 to 12 weeks of age. Surgical correction is performed when the infant is free of any oral, respiratory, or systemic infection. The method of repair of the CL involves one of several staggered suture lines (Z-plasty) to minimize notching of the lip from retraction of scar tissue.

Immediately after surgery the suture line is protected from tension and trauma by a thin, arched metal device (the Logan bow) taped to the cheeks; or by a butterfly-type adhesive restraint. The arms are restrained at the elbows to prevent the infant from rubbing the incision with the hands. In the absence of infection or trauma, healing takes place with little scar formation.

Surgical Correction: CP. CP repair is generally postponed until 12 to 18 months of age to take advantage of palatal changes that take place with normal growth. Most surgeons prefer to close the cleft at this time, before the child develops faulty speech habits.

Prognosis. Even with good anatomic closure, the majority of children with CL/P have some degree of speech impairment that requires speech therapy. Physical problems result from inefficient functioning of the muscles of the soft palate and nasopharynx, improper tooth alignment, and varying degrees of hearing loss. Improper drainage of the middle ear, as a result of inefficient function of the eustachian tube, contributes to recurrent otitis media with scarring of the tympanic membrane. This leads to hearing impairment in many children with CP. Upper respiratory infections require immediate and meticulous attention, and extensive orthodontics and prosthodontics may be needed to correct problems of malposition of teeth and maxillary arches.

Some of the more difficult long-term problems are related to social adjustment of the child. The better the physical care, the better is the chance for emotional and social adjustment, although the presence of the defect and the degree of residual disability are not always directly related to a satisfactory adjustment. Physical defects are a threat to the self-image, and abnormal speech quality is an impediment to social expression.

Nursing Care Management

➤ Assessment

Because the lip defect is readily visible at birth, assessment consists of describing the location and extent of the defect. The CP is estimated by visualization during crying. CP without CL is detected by palpating the palate with the finger during the newborn assessment.

The emotional impact of the birth of a child with a cosmetic, as well as a functional, disability is especially traumatic to the family. Consequently, the nursing assessment is concerned with the emotional reaction of the family to the child and to the defect.

➤ Nursing Diagnoses

Based on a thorough physical assessment, a number of nursing diagnoses are evident. These are described in the Nursing Care Plan on p. 1284.

➤ Plan of Care and Implementation

The goals of care for the infant with CL and CP are related to preoperative care, short-term postoperative care, and long-term management. The major goals of care for the infant and family include:

Preoperative care:

1. Family will cope with the impact of an infant with a defect.
2. Infant will receive optimum nutrition.
3. Infant will be prepared for surgery.

Postoperative care:

1. Infant will experience no trauma and minimal or no pain.
2. Infant will receive optimum nutrition.
3. Infant will experience no complications.
4. Infant and family will receive adequate support.
5. Family will be prepared for care at home and long-term needs of a child with CP.

The immediate nursing problems in the care of an infant with CL/P deformities are related to feeding the infant and dealing with the parental reaction to the defect. Facial deformities are particularly disturbing to parents. CL is an especially visible, disfiguring defect that may generate a strong negative response in parents. However, the concept that infants with CL and/or CP are at increased risk for failure of maternal attachment has been challenged by a recent study that indicated that maternal-infant attachment was not negatively affected when measured at 1 year of age (Speltz et al, 1997). During the initial phase after the birth of an infant with CL and/or CP, it is important for the nurse to place emphasis not only on the infant's physical needs, but also on the parents' emotional needs (Speltz et al, 1997). The manner of handling the infant should convey to the parents that the infant is indeed a precious human being. (See Chapter 41 for interventions in assisting parents in accepting a birth defect.)

Throughout the course of therapy, parents need an explanation of the immediate and long-range problems commonly associated with CP. Often they are unaware that more is involved than merely repairing the defect. Whenever possible, they should be referred to a comprehensive CP team.

Feeding. Feeding the infant offers a special challenge to nurses and parents. Growth failure in infants with CL and/or CP has been attributed to preoperative feeding difficulties. Following surgical repair, most infants with isolated CL and/or CP and no associated syndromes gain weight successfully or achieve adequate weight and height for age (Lee, Nunn, and Wright, 1997).

Clefts of the lip or palate reduce the infant's ability to suck, which interferes with compression of the areola and renders breastfeeding and bottle-feeding difficult. Liquid taken into the mouth tends to escape through the nose via the cleft. Feeding is best accomplished with the infant's head in an upright position, either held in the caregiver's hand or cradled in the arm. Normal nipples are unsuitable for these infants, who are unable to generate the suction required; therefore special nipples or other feeding devices are needed. A variety of special "cleft palate" nipples have been devised and used with some success; however, large, soft nipples with large holes; Nursettes; or the long, soft lamb's nipples appear to offer the best means for nipple feeding (Fig. 47-5). The newer "gravity flow" nipple* attached to a squeezable plastic bottle allows formula to be deposited directly into the mouth in much the same manner as with a bulb syringe. Success has also been achieved by the modification of a standard nipple. A single small slit or cross-cut is made in the end of the nipple with a sharp surgical blade or a pair of scissors with sharp, thin blades. The enlarged opening allows the infant to swallow the formula easily, thereby bypassing the suction problem. The size of the slit is adjusted to the infant's needs.

Richard (1991) has developed a feeding technique called ESSR: Enlarge nipple; Stimulate suck reflex; Swallow fluid appropriately; Rest when the infant signals with facial expression. A study of the weights of infants fed with traditional methods

*Ross Laboratories, Columbus, OH 43216.

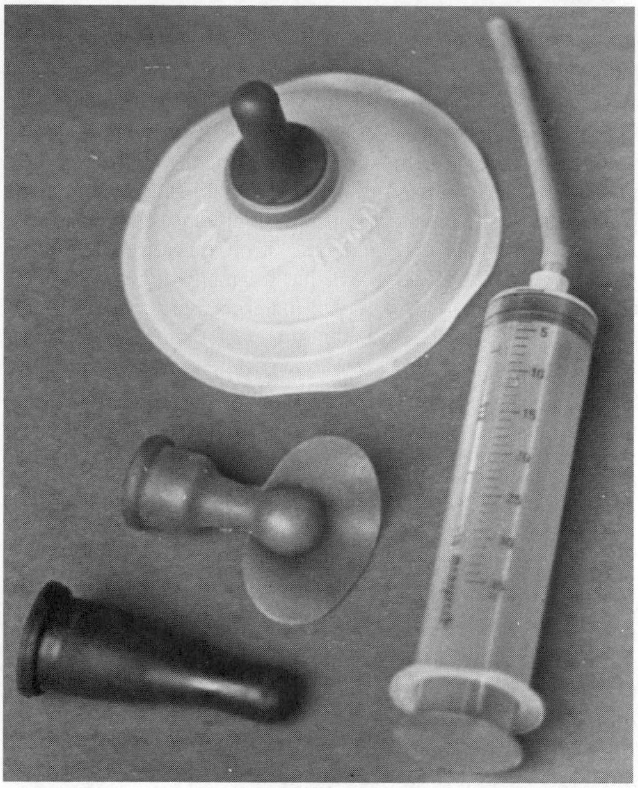

FIG. 47-5 • Some devices used to feed an infant with a cleft lip and palate: (clockwise from left) Lamb's nipple, flanged nipple, special nurser, and syringe with rubber tubing (Breck feeder).

and those fed with the ESSR method revealed a significant increase in mean weight just before surgery in the infants in the ESSR group (Richard, 1994).

Using these types of nipples for feeding also has the advantage of helping to meet the infant's sucking needs. Muscle development is especially important for later development of speech. The nipple is positioned in such a way that it is compressed by the infant's tongue and existing palate. If a single-slit nipple is used, the slit is placed vertically so that the infant will be able to produce and stop a flow of milk by alternately opening and closing the opening. No matter which type of nipple is used, gentle, steady pressure on the base of the bottle reduces the chance of choking or coughing, and the person feeding should resist the temptation to remove the nipple because of the noise the infant makes or for fear that the infant will choke. Because these infants have a tendency to swallow excessive amounts of air, they require frequent burping.

When the infant has trouble with nipple feeding, a rubber-tipped medicine dropper, Asepto syringe, or Breck feeder (a large syringe with soft rubber tubing) often provides an efficient, safe feeding device. The rubber extension should be sufficiently long to extend well back into the mouth to reduce the likelihood of regurgitation through the nose. The formula is deposited on the back of the tongue, and the flow is controlled by bulb or syringe compression that is adjusted to the infant's needs. With some infants, spoon feeding works best, especially if the formula is slightly thickened with cereal. After feeding, the infant is given water to rinse the mouth.

Breastfeeding is also an option. The nipple is positioned and stabilized well back in the oral cavity so that tongue action facilitates milk expression. However, the suction required to stimulate milk may be absent initially; therefore a breast pump may be useful before nursing to stimulate the let-down reflex.

Regardless of the feeding method used, the mother should begin to feed the infant as soon as possible, preferably after the initial nursery feeding. In this way she is able to help determine the method best suited to her and the infant and to become adept in the technique before they are discharged from the hospital.

Preoperative Care. In preparation for surgical repair, the parent is commonly instructed to accustom the infant to the needs of the early postoperative period, particularly if surgery is delayed for several months. It is mandatory for the infant to be positioned on the back or side postoperatively. Most infants tolerate the positions well because they are accustomed to being supine for sleeping. It is also helpful to place the infant or child in arm restraints periodically before admission and, after admission, to feed him or her with a rubber-tipped Asepto syringe or other device in the manner to be used postoperatively.

Postoperative Care: CL. The major efforts in the postoperative period are directed toward protecting the operative site. Following CL repair *(cheiloplasty)*, a metal appliance or adhesive strips are securely taped to the cheeks to relax the surgical site and prevent tension on the suture line caused by crying or other facial movement. Elbow restraints are needed to prevent the infant from rubbing or otherwise disturbing the suture line and are usually applied immediately after surgery. It is advisable to pin the cuff of the restraints to the infant's clothing to keep the restraints in place. The older infant who is able to roll over will require a jacket restraint, in addition to restricting arm movement, to prevent rolling on the abdomen and rubbing the face on the sheet, especially if the repair involves the lip. It is important to remove the restraints periodically to exercise the arms, to provide relief from restrictions, and to observe the skin for signs of irritation. It is advisable to release the restraints one at a time, especially in a very vigorous, active infant. Removing restraints also offers an opportunity for cuddling and body contact. Sitting the infant in an infant seat provides a change of position and a different perspective of the environment. Adequate analgesia is recommended to relieve postoperative pain; sedation is sometimes needed for a very restless, anxious infant.

Clear liquids are offered when the infant has fully recovered from the anesthesia, and feeding is usually resumed when tolerated. The suture site is carefully cleansed of formula or serosanguineous drainage as needed with a cotton-tipped swab dipped in saline. A thin layer of antibiotic ointment may be prescribed for application to the suture line after cleansing. Meticulous care of the suture line is a nursing responsibility because inflammation or infection will interfere with optimum healing and the ultimate cosmetic effect of the surgical repair.

Gentle aspiration of mouth and nasopharyngeal secretions may be necessary to prevent aspiration and respiratory complications. An upright or infant seat position is helpful for the infant in the immediate postoperative period and for one who has difficulty in handling secretions.

Postoperative Care: CP. The child with CP repair *(palatoplasty)* is allowed to lie on the abdomen, especially immediately postoperatively. The child may resume feeding by bottle, breast, or cup shortly after surgery.

NURSE ALERT • Avoid the use of suction or other objects in the mouth, such as tongue depressors, thermometers, spoons, or straws.

Oral packing may be secured to the palate following palatoplasty; this packing is usually removed after 2 to 3 days. Sometimes the infant will have difficulty breathing after surgery, because it is often necessary to alter an established pattern of breathing and adjust to breathing through the nose. This is frustrating but seldom requires more than positioning and support. The elbows may be restrained to keep the child's hand away from the mouth, and parents are instructed to maintain this precaution at home until the palate is healed, usually in 4 to 6 weeks. They are instructed to remove the restraints (usually one at a time) at frequent intervals to allow the child to exercise the arms.

The infant should be assessed for pain postoperatively. Opioids may be prescribed initially, and acetaminophen may be given as needed thereafter.

The older infant may be discharged on a blenderized or soft diet, which parents are instructed to continue until the surgeon directs them otherwise. They are cautioned against allowing the child to eat hard items such as toast, hard cookies, and potato chips, which could damage the newly repaired palate.

Long-term Care. Children with CL/P often require a variety of services during the process of recovery. Families of these children need support and encouragement by health professionals and guidance in activities that facilitate the most normal outcome for their children. In particular, financial stressors are often cited as a difficult issue by parents of a child with a craniofacial anomaly. With the combined efforts of the family and the health team, the majority of these children achieve a satisfactory outcome. Many children with CL/P have surgical correction that creates a near-normal-appearing lip and permits good function. Parents need to understand the function of therapy and the purpose and care of any appliance, as well as the importance of establishing good mouth care and proper brushing habits.

Throughout the child's development, an important goal is the development of a healthy personality and self-esteem. Many local areas have CP parents' groups that offer help and support to families. Several agencies provide services and information for children with CL/P and their families. These include the American Cleft Palate Association and the Cleft Palate Foundation,* the Association of Birth Defect Children (ABDC),† the March of Dimes-Birth Defects Foundation,‡ and state children's medical services.

*1829 Franklin St., Chapel Hill, NC 27514; (412) 418-1376 or 1-800-24-CLEFT; e-mail: cleftline@aol.com.

†827 Irma Ave., Orlando, FL 32803; (407) 245-7035 or 1-800-313-2232; website: www.birthdefects.org.

‡1275 Mamaroneck Ave., White Plains, NY 10605; (914) 428-7100; website: www.modimes.org. In Canada: Aboutface, 99 Crowns Lane, Fourth Floor, Toronto, Ontario M5R3P4; (416) 944-3223 or 1-800-665-3223; website: www.interlog.com/~abtface.

➤ Evaluation

The effectiveness of nursing interventions is determined by continual reassessment and evaluation of care based on the following observational guidelines:

Preoperative care:

1. Observe and interview family members relative to their understanding, feelings, and concerns regarding the defect and anticipated surgery and their interactions with the infant.
2. Observe infant during feeding.
3. Complete preoperative checklist.

Postoperative care:

1. Inspect operative site, including the protective device.
2. Observe for behavioral and physiologic indicators of pain and response to analgesics.
3. Observe infant during feeding, measure intake and output, and weigh infant daily.
4. Observe operative site for evidence of infection, bleeding, sloughing, or irritation.
5. Observe and interview family regarding their understanding and concerns about the infant, including long-term needs.

The expected outcomes are described in the Nursing Care Plan.

Esophageal Atresia with Tracheoesophageal Fistula (TEF)

Congenital atresia of the esophagus and TEF are rare malformations that represent a failure of the esophagus to develop as a continuous passage. These defects may occur as separate entities or in combination (Fig. 47-6) and without early diagnosis and treatment are rapidly fatal.

Etiology. The cause of esophageal atresia and TEF is not known. The incidence has been estimated to be from 1 in 3000 to 1 in 3500 live births. There appears to be an equal sex incidence, but the birth weight of most affected infants is significantly lower than average, and there is an unusually high incidence of prematurity in infants with esophageal atresia. Other congenital anomalies such as VATER or VACTERL syndromes may occur. These syndromes involve a combination of vertebral, anorectal, cardiovascular, tracheoesophageal, renal, and limb abnormalities.

Pathophysiology. In the most commonly encountered form of esophageal atresia and TEF (i.e., 80% to 95% of cases), the proximal esophageal segment terminates in a blind pouch, and the distal segment is connected to the trachea or primary bronchus by a short fistula at or near the bifurcation (Fig. 47-6, *C*). The second most common variety (5% to 8%) consists of a blind pouch at each end, widely separated and with no communication to the trachea (Fig. 47-6, *A*). Less commonly an otherwise normal trachea and esophagus are connected by a common fistula (Fig. 47-6, *E*). Extremely rare anomalies involve a fistula from the trachea to the upper esophageal segment (Fig. 47-6, *B*) or to both the upper and the lower segments (Fig. 47-6, *D*).

Diagnostic Evaluation. The disorder is suspected on the basis of clinical manifestations (Box 47-18). Although the diagnosis is established on the basis of clinical signs and symptoms, the exact type of anomaly is determined by radiographic studies. A radiopaque catheter is inserted into the hypopharynx

Nursing Care Plan THE CHILD WITH CLEFT LIP AND/OR PALATE

NURSING DIAGNOSIS Altered nutrition: less than body requirements, related to physical defect of oral cavity

EXPECTED OUTCOME Patient exhibits signs of adequate nutritional intake (e.g., appropriate weight gain).

Nursing Interventions/*Rationales*

Administer diet appropriate for age and nutritional needs *to ensure adequate nutritional content.*

If infant is breastfeeding, teach mother to stimulate let-down reflex prior to feeding with a breast pump or manually *as required suction from infant may be lacking.*

Have mother position and stabilize nipple well back in infant's oral cavity against existing palate *to facilitate expression of milk.*

Hold child in upright position to feed *to prevent aspiration* and burp frequently as infant takes in excess amounts of air.

If child is unable to maintain adequate suction on a nipple, try using alternative feeding appliances (e.g., Breck feeder, Aesepto syringe) *to facilitate feeding.*

Postoperatively, administer prescribed intravenous fluids *to ensure adequate hydration.*

Maintain feeding records and weigh regularly *to assess adequacy of intake.*

NURSING DIAGNOSIS Potential for altered parenting related to having child with highly visible physical defect

EXPECTED OUTCOME Parents demonstrate acceptance of the infant.

Nursing Interventions/*Rationales*

Allow parents to express feelings, fears *to facilitate coping.*

Convey attitudes and behaviors of acceptance of infant *to serve as a role model for parents.*

Describe results of surgical correction of defect with photos of satisfactory results *to alleviate fears of the unknown and foster hope.*

Arrange for parents to meet with others who have experienced and successfully coped with similar situations *to provide ongoing support.*

NURSING DIAGNOSIS Risk for trauma of surgical site related to position of site

EXPECTED OUTCOME Operative site is undamaged.

Nursing Interventions/*Rationales*

For cleft lip repair, use a lip protective device; position on back or side *to protect suture line.*

For cleft palate repair, prevent sustained crying, placement of objects in mouth *to protect suture line.*

Restrain infant at elbows *to prevent access to operative site;* use jacket restraints on older infants *to prevent rolling onto abdomen and rubbing of suture line on bedding.*

Cleanse suture line after feeding *to reduce presence of foreign materials that may irritate suture line.*

Teach restraint and cleansing techniques to parents *to minimize complications after discharge.*

NURSING DIAGNOSIS Pain related to surgical procedure

EXPECTED OUTCOME Infant is resting comfortably.

Nursing Interventions/*Rationales*

Administer pain medications per physician order *to prevent or minimize pain.*

Remove restraints periodically under careful supervision *to exercise arms and provide relief from restrictions.*

Monitor vital signs and behavior for evidence of pain or discomfort.

See also the Nursing Care Plan: Child Undergoing Surgery, p. 1130.

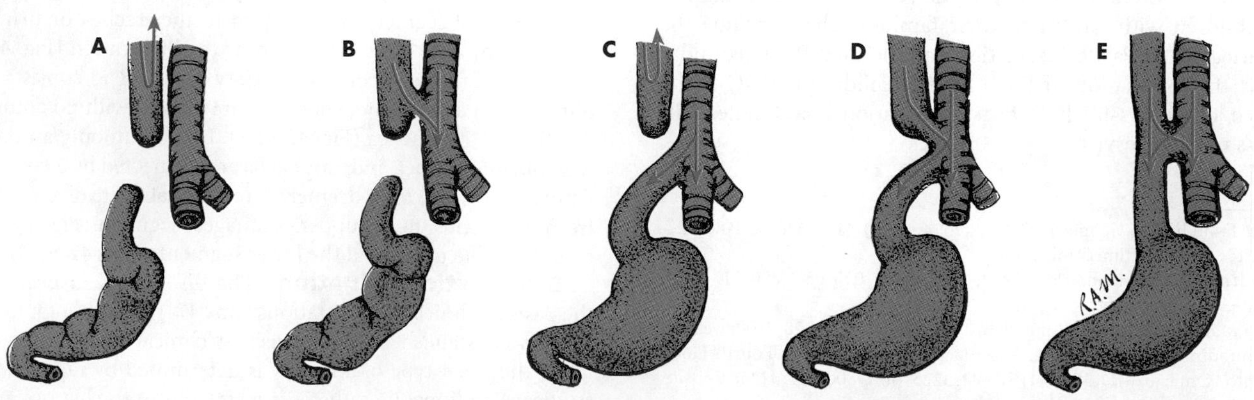

FIG. 47-6 • Five most common types of esophageal atresia and tracheoesophageal fistula.

Box 47-18

Clinical Manifestations of Tracheoesophageal Fistula

Excessive salivation and drooling
Three Cs of tracheoesophageal fistula (TEF)
- Coughing
- Choking
- Cyanosis

Apnea
Increased respiratory distress after feeding
Abdominal distention

and advanced until it encounters an obstruction. Chest films are taken to ascertain esophageal patency or the presence and level of a blind pouch. Sometimes fistulas are not patent, which makes their presence more difficult to diagnose. Complete absence of air in the GI tract indicates esophageal atresia without TEF.

Therapeutic Management. The treatment of esophageal atresia and TEF consists of prevention of pneumonia and surgical repair of the anomaly. When a TEF is suspected, the infant is immediately taken off oral intake, started on IV fluids, and placed in the position least likely to cause aspiration of either mouth or stomach secretions. Removal of secretions from the mouth and upper pouch requires frequent or continuous suction. Because aspiration pneumonia is almost inevitable and appears early, broad-spectrum antibiotic therapy is instituted.

Primary surgical correction consists of a thoracotomy with division and ligation of the TEF and an end-to-end anastomosis of the esophagus. For infants who are premature, have multiple anomalies, or are in very poor condition, a staged procedure is preferred that involves palliative measures including gastrostomy, ligation of the TEF, and provision of constant drainage of the esophageal pouch. A delayed esophageal anastomosis is usually attempted after several weeks when the upper pouch elongates and the lower pouch undergoes hypertrophy. The technique of *bougienage* (the process whereby a blunt metal instrument is used to dilate a fistula or lengthen membranous tissue) of the upper pouch may be performed to elongate this segment. If an esophageal anastomosis still cannot be accomplished, a *cervical esophagostomy* (to allow drainage of saliva) and gastrostomy are performed.

There are rare instances in which a primary anastomosis cannot be accomplished because of insufficient length of the two segments of esophagus. In these cases the defect must be bridged with a colon interposition, gastric tube, or gastric interposition procedure. Endotracheal intubation may be required because many of these infants may also have *tracheomalacia,* a weakness in the tracheal wall that occurs when a dilated proximal pouch compresses the trachea from early in fetal life or when the trachea does not develop normally because of a loss of intratracheal pressure.

Complications of a primary repair include an anastomotic leak, strictures due to tension or ischemia, esophageal motility disorders causing dysphagia, and gastroesophageal reflux. Motility disorders are common following esophageal atresia or TEF repair.

Prognosis. The prognosis for infants with esophageal atresia or TEF is related to the birth weight, associated congenital anomalies, and time of diagnosis. The survival rate is nearly 100% in full-term infants without severe respiratory distress or other anomalies. In premature low-birth-weight infants with associated anomalies, the incidence of complications is high. The overall mortality is 50% (Ryckman, Flake, and Balistreri, 1997).

Nursing Care Management. Nursing responsibility for detection of this serious malformation begins *immediately* after birth. Ideally, the condition is diagnosed before the initial feeding, but often it is not. If fed, the infant swallows normally but suddenly coughs and struggles, and the fluid is aspirated or returns through the nose and mouth. For this reason, it is customary for the nurse to give the infant the first feeding of plain water or to be present when a parent feeds the child in order to observe the infant's response.

NURSE ALERT • Any infant who has an excessive amount of frothy saliva in the mouth or difficulty with secretions and unexplained episodes of cyanosis should be suspected of having a TEF.

Cyanosis is usually a result of laryngospasm caused by overflow of saliva into the larynx from the proximal esophageal pouch, and it normally clears after removal of the secretions from the oropharynx by suctioning. Any suspicion of TEF is reported immediately. The infant is placed in an incubator or under a radiant warmer, and oxygen is administered to help relieve respiratory distress. Positive pressure is contraindicated because it may add to air pressure in the stomach.

The most desirable position for a newborn who is suspected of having a TEF is supine with the head elevated on an inclined plane of at least 30 degrees. This position minimizes the reflux of gastric secretions up the distal esophagus into the trachea and bronchi.

It is imperative that the source of aspiration be removed at once. Oral fluids are withheld, and the infant's fluid needs are met parenterally or via gastrostomy. Until surgery the blind pouch is kept empty by intermittent or continuous suction through an indwelling nasal catheter that extends to the end of the pouch. The catheter needs attention because it has a tendency to become clogged with mucus. It is usually replaced daily by the practitioner. In the event that a staged repair is performed, a gastrostomy tube is inserted and left open so that air entering the stomach through the fistula can escape, thus minimizing the danger that gastric contents will be regurgitated into the trachea. The tube empties by gravity drainage. It is imperative that any secretions that can be a source of aspiration be removed at once.

Postoperative Care. Postoperative care for these infants is essentially the same as the care of any high risk newborn. The infant is returned to the radiant heater, and the gastrostomy tube is returned to gravity drainage until the infant can tolerate feedings, usually by the fifth to seventh postoperative day. At this time the tube is elevated and secured at a point above the level of the stomach. This allows gastric secretions to pass to the duodenum, and swallowed air can escape through the open tube. If tolerated, gastrostomy feedings are continued until the esophageal anastomosis is healed, on about the tenth to fourteenth day, after which oral feedings are initiated.

The initial attempt at oral feeding must be carefully observed to make certain that the infant is able to swallow without choking. Oral feedings are begun with sterile water and followed with frequent, small feedings of formula. Until the infant is able to take a sufficient amount by mouth, oral intake may need to be supplemented by gastrostomy feedings or parenteral nutrition. Ordinarily infants are not discharged until they are taking oral fluids well and the gastrostomy tube has been removed; however, the infant who has undergone palliative surgery will be discharged with the gastrostomy tube in place. The nurse is responsible for making certain that the caregiver is educated and has practiced the care of the gastrostomy (see Chapter 45).*

Special Problems. Upper respiratory complications are a threat to life in both the preoperative and the postoperative period. In addition to pneumonia, there is a constant danger of respiratory distress resulting from atelectasis, pneumothorax, and laryngeal edema. Any persistent respiratory difficulty after removal of secretions is reported to the surgeon immediately. The infant is monitored for anastomotic leaks, as evidenced by purulent chest tube drainage, increased WBC, and temperature instability.

In the infant awaiting esophageal replacement surgery, the catheter is removed and the upper esophageal segment is drained through a cervical esophagostomy. This is a source of annoyance, because the skin may become irritated by moisture from the continual discharge of saliva. Frequent removal of drainage and application of a layer of protective ointment are usually sufficient treatment. Application of a dressing or ostomy appliance may be needed to collect the drainage. An enterostomal therapist may provide helpful guidance in the prevention and/or treatment of skin breakdown.

For the infant who requires esophageal replacement, nonnutritive sucking is provided by a pacifier. Sometimes small amounts of water or formula are given orally, and although the liquid drains from the esophagostomy, this process allows the infant to develop mature sucking patterns. Other appropriate oral stimulation can prevent feeding aversions. Infants who remain NPO for an extended period, or who have not received oral stimulation, often have difficulty with eating by mouth after corrective surgery and may develop oral hypersensitivity and food aversion. After repair they require patient, firm guidance in learning the techniques of taking food into the mouth and swallowing. A referral to a multidisciplinary feeding behavior program may be necessary.

As with any congenital anomaly, parents need support in adjusting to the child's condition (see Chapter 41). One of the difficulties in TEF is the immediate transfer of the sick newborn to the intensive care unit and a sometimes lengthy hospitalization. The attachment process is facilitated by encouraging parents to visit the infant, participate in his or her care when appropriate, and express their feelings regarding the infant's condition. The nurse in the intensive care unit should assume responsibility for ensuring that the parents are kept fully informed of the infant's progress.

(See also Nursing Care Plan: The Child with Esophageal Atresia and Tracheoesophageal Fistula.†)

*Community and home care instructions on giving gastrostomy tube feedings are available in Wong DL, Hess CS: ***Wong and Whaley's clinical manual of pediatric nursing,*** ed 5, St Louis, 2000, Mosby.

†In Wong DL, Hess CS: ***Wong and Whaley's clinical manual of pediatric nursing,*** ed 5, St Louis, 2000, Mosby.

Hernias

A *hernia* is a protrusion of a portion of an organ or organs through an abnormal opening. The danger from herniation arises when the organ protruding through the opening is constricted to the extent that circulation is impaired; or when the protruding organs encroach on and impair the function of other structures. A hernia that cannot be reduced easily is called an *incarcerated hernia.* A *strangulated hernia* is one in which the blood supply to the herniated organ is impaired. The hernias of concern are those that protrude through the diaphragm, the abdominal wall, or the inguinal canal (see also Genitourinary Tract Disorders/Defects, Chapter 50). The other hernias of significance to the pediatric age groups are outlined in Table 47-8.

OBSTRUCTIVE DISORDERS

Obstruction in the GI tract occurs when the passage of nutrients and secretions is impeded by a constricted or occluded lumen or when there is impaired motility *(paralytic ileus).*

Obstructions may be congenital or acquired. Congenital obstructions, such as duodenal, jejunal, or ileal atresia, usually appear in the neonatal period. Malrotation, duodenal web, and Hirschsprung disease often appear after the first few weeks of life. Intestinal obstruction from any cause is characterized by similar signs and symptoms (Box 47-19).

Hypertrophic Pyloric Stenosis (HPS)

HPS occurs when the circular muscle of the pylorus becomes thickened, causing constriction of the pylorus and obstruction of the gastric outlet. This condition usually develops in the first few weeks of life, causing projectile vomiting, dehydration, metabolic alkalosis, and failure to thrive. HPS is more common in firstborn children, and males are affected five times more often than females. HPS is more common in full-term than in premature infants, and it is seen less often in African-American and Asian infants than in Caucasian infants.

The precise etiology is unknown. There is a genetic predisposition, and siblings and offspring of affected persons are at increased risk of developing HPS.

Pathophysiology. The circular muscle of the pylorus is grossly enlarged as a result of both hypertrophy (increased size) and hyperplasia (increased mass). This produces severe narrowing of the pyloric canal between the stomach and the duodenum; consequently, the lumen at this point is partially obstructed. Over time, inflammation and edema further reduce the size of the opening until the partial obstruction may progress to complete obstruction. The muscle is often thickened to as much as twice its usual size (2 to 3 cm), and the hypertrophied pylorus may be palpable as an olive-like mass in the upper abdomen (Fig. 47-7).

Evidence suggests that local innervation is involved in the pathogenesis. In most cases this is an isolated lesion; however, it may be associated with intestinal malrotation, esophageal and duodenal atresia, and anorectal anomalies.

Diagnostic Evaluation. The diagnosis of HPS is often made following the history and physical examination. HPS typically presents when the infant is between 1 and 10 weeks of age. Vomiting usually occurs 30 to 60 minutes after a feeding. Projectile vomiting usually develops within a week and often leads to

TABLE 47-8
Types of Hernias and Their Management

Type	Manifestations/Diagnostic Evaluation	Management
DIAPHRAGMATIC		
Protrusion of abdominal organs through opening in diaphragm	**Symptoms:** Mild to severe respiratory distress within a few hours after birth; tachypnea, cyanosis, dyspnea, absent breath sounds in affected area; impaired cardiac output; possible symptoms of shock, severe acidosis **Diagnosis** suspected on basis of symptoms—confirmed by radiographic study; often diagnosed prenatally as early as 25th week of gestation	**Therapeutic:** Supportive treatment of respiratory distress and correction of acidosis; possible use of endotracheal intubation, gastrointestinal (GI) decompression, and extracorporeal membrane oxygenation (ECMO) Prophylactic antibiotic administration Surgical reduction of hernia and repair of defect **Nursing:** *Preoperative:* Reduce stimulation—environmental/care activities Prompt recognition; resuscitation and stabilization Maintain suction, oxygen, and intravenous (IV) fluids Positioning—head up Administer medications *Postoperative:* Carry out routine postoperative care and observation Relieve pain and provide comfort Support family because this is a critical illness
HIATAL		
Sliding: Protrusion of an abdominal structure (usually stomach) through esophageal hiatus	**Symptoms:** Dysphagia, failure to thrive, vomiting, neck contortions, frequent unexplained respiratory problems, bleeding; usually associated with gastroesophageal reflux (GER); may cause gastric volvulus and obstruction **Diagnosis** made by fluoroscopy	**Therapeutic:** Management of GER symptoms; positioning; pharmacologic treatment; and dietary management Surgical treatment when complications are related to GER despite medical management **Nursing:** Be alert to significant signs and carry out routine postoperative care
ABDOMINAL		
Umbilical: Weakness in abdominal wall around umbilicus; incomplete closure of abdominal wall, allowing intestinal contents to protrude through opening	**Symptoms:** Noted by inspection and palpation of the abdomen High incidence in premature and African-American infants Usually closes spontaneously by 1-2 years of age	**Therapeutic:** No treatment of small defects Operative repair if persists to age 4-6 years or if defect is >1.5-2 cm by age 2 Strangulation requires immediate attention **Nursing:** Discourage use of home remedies (e.g., belly bands, coins) Reassure parents
Omphalocele: Protrusion of intraabdominal viscera into base of umbilical cord; sac is covered with peritoneum without skin **Gastroschisis:** Protrusion of intraabdominal contents through defect in abdominal wall lateral to umbilical ring; there is never a peritoneal sac	**Symptoms:** Obvious on inspection Observe for other malformations	**Therapeutic:** Surgical repair of defect *Preoperative:* Large lesions—gradual reduction of abdominal contents Prophylactic antibiotic administration **Nursing:** (*Preoperative*): Keep sac or viscera moist with saline-soaked pads Use overhead warming unit Carry out routine care of IV line Nasogastric suction NPO

Box 47-19

Clinical Manifestations of Mechanical/paralytic Intestinal Obstruction

Colicky abdominal pain—From peristalsis attempting to overcome the obstruction
Abdominal distention—As a result of accumulation of gas and fluid above the level of the obstruction
Vomiting—Often the earliest sign of a high obstruction; a later sign of lower obstruction (may be bilious or feculent)
Constipation and obstipation—Early signs of low obstructions; later signs of higher obstructions
Dehydration—From losses of large quantities of fluid and electrolytes into the intestine
Rigid and boardlike abdomen—From increased distention
Bowel sounds—Gradually diminish and cease
Respiratory distress—Occurs as the diaphragm is pushed up into the pleural cavity
Shock—Plasma volume diminishes as fluids and electrolytes are lost from the bloodstream into the intestinal lumen
Sepsis—Caused by bacterial proliferation with invasion into the circulation

Box 47-20

Clinical Manifestations of Hypertrophic Pyloric Stenosis

Projectile vomiting
- May be ejected 3 to 4 feet from the child when in a side-lying position, 1 foot or more when in a back-lying position
- Occurs shortly after a feeding (may not occur for several hours)
- May follow each feeding or appear intermittently
- Nonbilious vomitus; may be blood tinged

Infant hungry, avid nurser; eagerly accepts a second feeding after vomiting episode
No evidence of pain or discomfort except that of chronic hunger
Weight loss
Signs of dehydration
Distended upper abdomen
Readily palpable olive-shaped tumor in the epigastrium just to the right of the umbilicus
Visible gastric peristaltic waves that move from left to right across the epigastrium

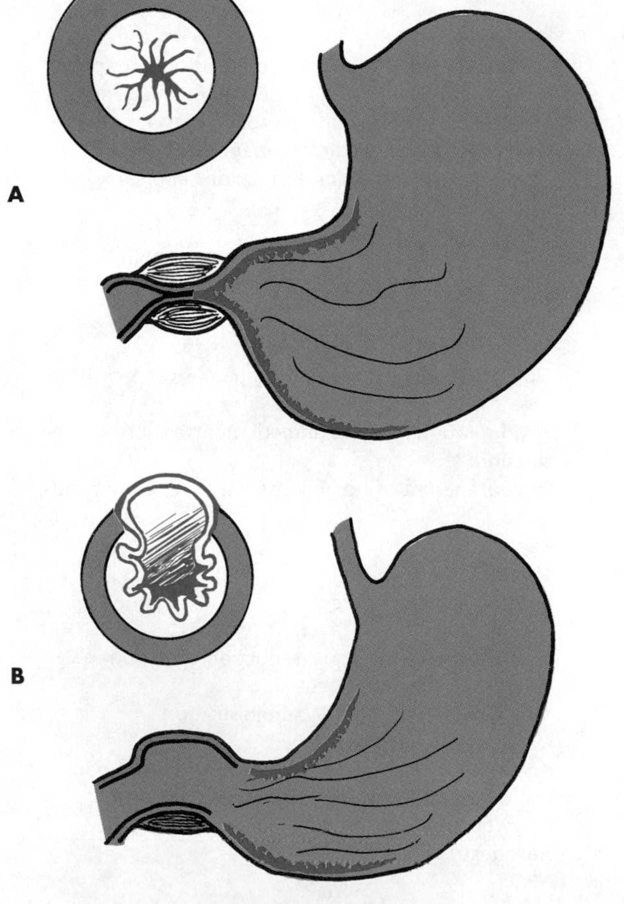

FIG. 47-7 • Hypertrophic pyloric stenosis. **A,** Enlarged muscular tumor nearly obliterates pyloric channel. **B,** Longitudinal surgical division of muscle down to submucosa establishes adequate passageway.

complete obstruction by 4 to 6 weeks of age. Emesis is nonbilious, usually consisting of stale milk. Often these infants become dehydrated and lethargic and appear significantly malnourished.

If the diagnosis is inconclusive from the history and physical signs (Box 47-20), ultrasonography will demonstrate an elongated, sausage-shaped mass with an elongated pyloric channel. If ultrasound fails to demonstrate a hypertrophied pylorus, then upper GI radiography should be done to rule out other causes of vomiting. Laboratory findings reflect the metabolic alterations created by severe depletion of both fluid and electrolytes from extensive and prolonged vomiting. There are decreased serum levels of both sodium and potassium, although these may be masked by the hemoconcentration from ECF depletion. Of greater diagnostic value are a decrease in serum chloride levels; and increases in pH and bicarbonate (carbon dioxide content) characteristic of metabolic alkalosis. The blood urea nitrogen level will be elevated as evidence of dehydration.

Therapeutic Management. Surgical relief of the pyloric obstruction by *pyloromyotomy* (sometimes called *Fredet-Ramstedt procedure*) is the standard treatment for this disorder. The surgical procedure is performed through a right upper quadrant incision (laparotomy) and consists of a longitudinal incision through the circular muscle fibers of the pylorus down to, but not including, the submucosa (Fig. 47-7, *B*). The procedure has a very high success rate when infants receive careful preoperative preparation to correct fluid and electrolyte imbalances.

Feedings are usually begun 4 to 6 hours postoperatively, beginning with small, frequent feedings of glucose water or electrolyte solutions. If clear fluids are retained, about 24 hours after surgery, formula is started in the same stepwise increments, with the amount and interval between feedings gradually increased until a full feeding schedule is reinstated, which usually takes about 48 hours. The infant is ready to be discharged from the hospital by about the second or third postoperative day.

Another procedure, *laparoscopy,* has been found to be safe and successful for infants with HPS (Najmaldin and Tan, 1995). The use of a small incision for the laparoscope may result in a shorter surgical time, more rapid postoperative feeding, and quicker discharge.

Prognosis. Most infants recover completely and rapidly following pyloromyotomy. Postoperative complications include persistent pyloric obstruction and wound dehiscence. Some infants with HPS also have gastroesophageal reflux.

Nursing Care Management

➤ Assessment

HPS should be considered as a possibility in the very young infant who appears alert but fails to gain weight and has a history of vomiting after feedings. Assessment is based on observation of eating behaviors and evidence of other characteristic clinical manifestations.

➤ Nursing Diagnoses

On the basis of a thorough assessment, a number of nursing diagnoses are evident. The most typical are those listed in Box 47-21.

➤ Plan of Care and Implementation

The goals of care for the child with HPS are primarily related to presurgical and postsurgical care of the infant. These include the following:

1. Child will consume sufficient amount of formula.
2. Infant will retain feedings.
3. Child will experience no complications.
4. Family will receive adequate support and education.

Preoperatively the emphasis is placed on restoring hydration and electrolyte balance. Infants with HPS are usually given no oral feedings, and receive IV fluids with glucose and electrolyte replacement based on laboratory serum electrolyte values. Careful monitoring of the IV infusion and diligent attention to intake, output, and urine specific gravity measurements are important to the success of fluid replacement. Any vomiting is observed and recorded accurately, as is the number and character of stools.

Observations include assessment of vital signs, particularly those that might indicate fluid or electrolyte imbalances. These infants are especially prone to metabolic alkalosis from loss of hydrogen ions, and to potassium, sodium, and chloride depletion. The skin and mucous membranes are assessed for alterations in hydration status, and daily weight provides added clues to water gain or loss.

When stomach decompression and gastric lavage are part of preoperative management, the nurse is responsible for ensuring that the tube is patent and functioning properly and for measuring and recording the type and amount of drainage. The infant is usually positioned flat or with the head slightly elevated. The infant who is receiving IV fluids and/or has a nasogastric tube for continuous drainage must be adequately observed to prevent the needle and/or tube from becoming dislodged.

General hygienic care, with particular attention to the skin and mouth in dehydrated infants, is an important part of care. Protection from infection is also important because infants with impaired nutritional status are more susceptible to infection than are normal newborns. Parental involvement is encouraged and promoted.

Postoperative Care. Postoperative vomiting may occur, and most infants, even with successful surgery, exhibit some vomiting during the first 24 to 48 hours. IV fluids are administered until the infant is taking and retaining adequate amounts by mouth. Much of the same care that was instituted before surgery (i.e., observation of physical signs, monitoring of IV fluids, careful observation and recording of intake and output) is continued after surgery. In addition, the infant is observed for responses to the stress of surgery and for evidence of pain. Appropriate analgesics are given. The nasogastric tube may be maintained after surgery for a variable time.

Box 47-21

Nursing Diagnoses: The Infant with Hypertrophic Pyloric Stenosis

High risk for fluid volume deficit related to persistent vomiting
Altered nutrition: less than body requirements related to persistent vomiting
Altered family processes related to hospitalization of infant

Feedings are usually instituted relatively soon, beginning with clear liquids containing glucose and electrolytes. They are offered slowly, in small amounts, and at frequent intervals as ordered by the practitioner. If the infant has been breastfed, breast milk, expressed by the mother, is given by bottle when the infant is able to tolerate feedings, and breastfeeding is resumed as soon as feasible. Observation and recording of feedings and the infant's responses to feedings and feeding techniques are a vital part of postoperative care. Positioning with the head elevated is usually continued postoperatively. Care of the operative site consists of observation for any drainage or signs of inflammation and care of the incision as directed by the surgeon.

As with any child in the hospital, parents are encouraged to remain with their child and become involved in the child's care. Vomiting of a projectile nature is frightening to parents, and they often believe that they may have done something wrong or that surgery was not successful. Most parents need support and reassurance that the condition is caused by a structural problem and is in no way a reflection on their parenting skills and capacities.

➤ Evaluation

The effectiveness of nursing interventions is determined by reassessment based on the following observational guidelines and expected outcomes:

1. Observe feeding behavior, especially vomiting episodes.
2. Weigh infant daily.
3. Observe for evidence of complications.
4. Observe and interview family regarding feelings, understanding, and concerns.

Expected outcomes:

1. Infant will consume a sufficient amount of formula.
2. Infant will take and retain feedings.
3. Infant will recover with no evidence of complications.
4. Family members will express their feelings and concerns, demonstrate an understanding of infant's condition, and be actively involved in infant's care.

(See also the Nursing Care Plan: The Child with Hypertrophic Pyloric Stenosis.*)

*In Wong DL, Hess CS: ***Wong and Whaley's clinical manual of pediatric nursing***, ed 5, St Louis, 2000, Mosby.

Intussusception

Intussusception is one of the most common causes of intestinal obstruction in children and generally occurs between the ages of 3 months and 5 years. Half of the cases occur in children younger than 1 year of age, with a high incidence in children between 3 and 12 months of age. Most other cases occur in children during their second year. Intussusception is twice as common in males as in females and in children with cystic fibrosis. Although specific intestinal lesions can be found in a small percentage of these children, generally the cause is not known. More than 90% of intussusceptions do not have a pathologic lead point such as a polyp, lymphoma, or Meckel diverticulum. The idiopathic cases are most likely a result of hypertrophy of intestinal lymphoid tissue secondary to viral infection.

Pathophysiology. Intussusception is an invagination or telescoping of one portion of the intestine into another. The most common site is the *ileocecal valve* (ileocolic), where the ileum invaginates into the cecum and colon (Fig. 47-8), producing an obstruction to the passage of intestinal contents beyond the defect. In addition, the two walls of the intestine press against each other, causing inflammation, edema, and eventually decreased blood flow. Because fecal material is unable to move beyond the obstruction, the stools contain primarily blood and mucus, resulting in the "currant jelly" stools characteristic of the disorder. Ischemia, perforation, peritonitis, and shock are serious complications of intussusception. If left untreated, this condition is incompatible with life.

NURSE ALERT • A report of severe colicky abdominal pain in a child with vomiting and currant jelly-like stools is a significant clue to intussusception.

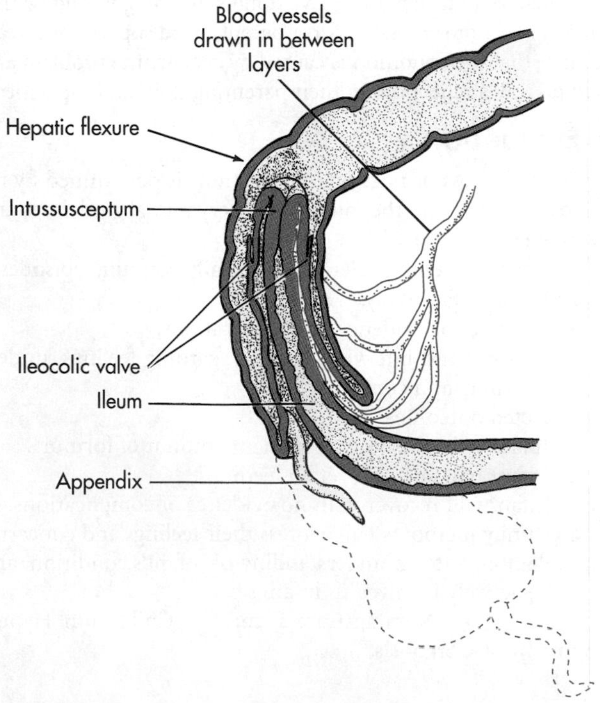

FIG. 47-8 • Ileocolic intussusception.

Diagnostic Evaluation. Commonly the diagnosis can be made on subjective findings alone (Box 47-22). The classic presentation of intussusception is a healthy, thriving child, usually between 3 and 12 months of age, who suddenly develops an episode of acute abdominal pain, vomiting, bloody stool, and a palpable abdominal mass. Definitive diagnosis is based on a barium enema, which clearly demonstrates the obstruction to the flow of barium. Initially, however, an abdominal radiograph is obtained to detect intraperitoneal air from a bowel perforation, which would contraindicate a barium enema. A rectal examination reveals mucus; blood; and occasionally, a low intussusception itself. With atypical cases, lethargy may be the primary presenting symptom (Pearl et al, 1998).

Therapeutic Management. In most cases the initial treatment of choice is nonsurgical hydrostatic reduction by barium enema at the time of diagnostic testing. The force exerted by the flowing barium is usually sufficient to push the invaginated portion of the bowel into its original position, similar to pushing an inverted "finger" out of a glove. Recently, ultrasonography has been advocated for diagnosis and for assistance in hydrostatic reduction of intussusception, because studies have indicated that this procedure is safe and accurate, has a higher success rate than barium enema, and avoids radiation risk (Pearl et al, 1998). Hydrostatic reduction is not recommended if there are clinical signs of shock or perforation. More often, radiologists are using water-soluble contrast and air pressure instead of barium to reduce intussusceptions. The administration of air pressure to reduce intussusception is as successful as barium, is more rapid, and lacks the risk of peritonitis. Fluid resuscitation, nasogastric decompression, and antibiotic therapy may be given before attempts at hydrostatic reduction are made. If these procedures are not successful, the child may require surgical intervention. Surgery involves manually reducing the invagination and, when indicated, resecting any nonviable intestine.

Prognosis. Nonoperative reduction is successful in 80% to 90% of the cases. Surgery is required for patients in whom the contrast enema is unsuccessful. If untreated, approximately 10% of children will have spontaneous reduction or chronic intussusception. The other 90% of untreated children will suffer from complications such as perforation, peritonitis, and sepsis. With early diagnosis and treatment, serious complications and death are very uncommon.

Box 47-22

Clinical Manifestations of Intussusception

- Sudden acute abdominal pain
  - Child screams and draws the knees onto the chest
  - Child appears normal and comfortable during intervals between episodes of pain
- Vomiting
- Lethargy
- Passage of red, currant jelly-like stools (stool mixed with blood and mucus)
- Tender, distended abdomen
- Palpable sausage-shaped mass in upper right quadrant
- Empty lower right quadrant (Dance sign)
- Eventual fever, prostration, and other signs of peritonitis

Nursing Care Management. The nurse can help establish a diagnosis by carefully listening to the parent's description of the child's physical and behavioral symptoms. Parents are astute in detecting that something is wrong with their child, and it is not unusual for parents to express that they felt something was seriously wrong before others shared their concerns. The description of the child's severe colicky abdominal pain combined with vomiting is a significant sign of intussusception.

As soon as a possible diagnosis of intussusception is made, the nurse begins to prepare the parents for the immediate need for hospitalization, the usual nonsurgical technique of hydrostatic reduction, and the possibility of surgery. It is important at this time to explain the basic defect of intussusception. Intussusception is easily demonstrated either by pushing the end of a finger on a rubber glove back into itself or by using the example of a telescoping rod. The principle of reduction by hydrostatic pressure can be simulated by filling the glove with water, which pushes the "finger" into a fully extended position.

Physical care of the child with intussusception differs little from that for any child undergoing abdominal surgery. Even though nonsurgical intervention may be successful, the usual preoperative procedures such as withholding of fluids by mouth, routine laboratory testing (CBC and urinalysis), signed parental consent, and preanesthetic sedation, are carried out. For the child with signs of electrolyte imbalance, hemorrhage, or peritonitis, additional medical preparation such as replacement fluids, whole blood or plasma, and nasogastric suctioning may be performed. Before surgery the nurse monitors all stools.

NURSE ALERT • Passage of a normal brown stool usually indicates that the intussusception has reduced itself. This is immediately reported to the practitioner, who may choose to alter the diagnostic/therapeutic plan of care.

Postprocedural care includes the usual postoperative observations such as vital signs, blood pressure, intact sutures and dressing, and the return of bowel sounds. After hydrostatic reduction or autoreduction, the nurse observes for passage of barium or water-soluble contrast material, and the stool patterns because there may be recurrences of the intussusception. Children may be admitted to the hospital or monitored closely on an outpatient basis. A recurrence of intussusception is usually treated with hydrostatic reduction. A laparotomy is considered for multiple recurrences.

Because this hospitalization may be the child's first separation from the parents, it is especially important to preserve the parent-child relationship by encouraging rooming-in or extended visiting. It may also be the parents' first experience with hospital care for their child, necessitating their preparation for procedures such as IV therapy, frequent vital sign and blood pressure monitoring, dressings, and special orders such as NPO. Because of the rapidity of the onset, diagnosis, and treatment, parents may feel stunned. They may ask few questions; or they may make constant inquiries, sometimes repeating the same ones several times. If the nurse realizes the circumstances surrounding this condition, the parents' reactions are more likely to be understood and accepted.

(See also Nursing Care Plan: The Child with Intussusception.*)

*In Wong DL, Hess CS: ***Wong and Whaley's clinical manual of pediatric nursing***, ed 5, St Louis, 2000, Mosby.

Anorectal Malformations

Anorectal malformations include several forms of imperforate anus, which are often associated with anomalies of the genitourinary and pelvic organs. These malformations are among the more common congenital malformations caused by abnormal development, with an incidence of 1 in 2000 to 5000 live births (Hendren, 1998). *Imperforate anus* encompasses several forms of malformation without an obvious anal opening. Many have a fistula from the distal rectum to the perineum or genitourinary system. Anorectal malformations may occur in isolation or as part of the VACTERL or VATER syndromes.

A persistent cloaca is a complex anorectal malformation in which the rectum, vagina, and urethra drain into a common channel that opens onto the perineum via the usual urethral site. *Cloacal exstrophy* is a rare, severe defect in which there is externalization of the bladder and bowel through the abdominal wall. Often the genitalia are indefinite, and chromosome studies are necessary to determine the child's sex. Gender assignment is almost always female. The exstrophic bladder is separated into two halves by the cecum; other features may include an omphalocele, imperforate anus, and, at times, a neural tube defect. With improved surgical techniques, survival rates for this condition are 88% to 90% in some centers (Smith et al, 1997).

Anorectal anomalies are classified according to sex and abnormal anatomic features, including genitourinary and associated pelvic anomalies. The level of rectal descent is determined by the relationship of the termination of the bowel to the puborectalis sling of the levator ani musculature. The classification of high, intermediate, and low may not always accurately describe the specific anomaly, but the classification is necessary to plan therapy (Table 47-9).

Diagnostic Evaluation. Checking for patency of the anus and rectum is a routine part of the newborn assessment

TABLE 47-9
Classification of Anorectal Malformations

Level	Male	Female
High	Anorectal agenesis With rectoprostatic-urethral fistula Without fistula Rectal atresia	Anorectal agenesis With rectovaginal fistula Without fistula Rectal atresia
Intermediate	Recto-bulbar-urethral fistula Agenesis without fistula	Rectovestibular fistula Rectovaginal fistula Agenesis without fistula
Low	Anocutaneous fistula Anal stenosis	Anovestibular fistula Anocutaneous fistula Anal stenosis
		Cloaca
	Rare malformations	Rare malformations

From Stephens FD et al: *Pediatr Surg Int* 1:200, 1986.

and should include observations regarding the passage of meconium. Inspection of the perineal area reveals absence of the normal anal opening; however, the appearance of the perineum alone does not accurately predict the level of the lesion. Genitourinary and pelvic anomalies associated with anorectal malformations should also be considered.

In the newborn the presence of meconium on the perineum does not always indicate anal patency (particularly in girls) because a fistula may be present and allow evacuation of meconium through the vagina. Fistulas may not be apparent at birth but may become obvious as peristalsis gradually forces the meconium through the fistula. Rectourinary fistulas should be suspected if there is meconium in the urine. Anal stenosis may not be identified until the child is older and presents with a history of difficult defecation, abdominal distention, and ribbon-like stools.

Abdominal ultrasound is performed to further evaluate anatomic malformations. An intravenous pyelogram (IVP) and voiding cystourethrogram are recommended for the infant with a high malformation to identify associated anomalies of the urinary tract. Further examination is also indicated when there is evidence of urinary tract infection or other symptoms. If a syndrome is suspected, cardiac evaluation and spinal films should be obtained to rule out other anomalies.

Therapeutic Management. Successful treatment for anal stenosis is generally accomplished by manual dilations. The procedure, begun by the physician, is repeated on a regular basis by the nurses in the hospital and is continued at home by the parents after they are carefully instructed in the technique. An imperforate anal membrane is excised and followed by daily anal dilations.

Reconstruction of an anus in the proper position is the goal of surgical treatment of other anorectal malformations. Malformations of the lower rectum often can be corrected in the neonatal period by way of simple dilation or a minor perineal procedure. Infants with higher anomalies require a temporary colostomy in the newborn period. Final correction of higher defects is usually postponed for a year, when a pull-through procedure with anorectoplasty is performed.

The long-term prognosis is influenced by the type of defect, the anatomy of the sacrum, and the quality of muscles. In general, if the newborn presents with a deep midline groove, two well-formed buttocks, and an anal dimple, the prognosis for bowel control is better than if the infant has a flat or "rocker" bottom and no midline groove because of associated neurologic problems (Flake and Ryckman, 1997). A functioning interior anal sphincter is important to achieve continence. In its absence, the child may need support with a bowel program to achieve socially acceptable bowel continence. Other potential complications following surgical treatment include strictures, recurrent rectourinary fistula, mucosal prolapse, and constipation.

Nursing Care Management. The first nursing responsibility is identification of undetected anorectal malformations. A poorly developed anal dimple, a genitourinary fistula, or vertebral abnormalities suggest a high lesion. A newborn who does not pass a stool within 24 hours of birth requires further assessment, and meconium that appears at an inappropriate orifice is reported. Preoperative care includes diagnostic evaluation, GI decompression, and IV fluids.

Nursing care following an anorectoplasty is primarily directed toward healing of the surgical site without infection or complications. Special nursing care involves keeping the anal area as clean as possible with scrupulous perineal care. A temporary dressing and drain may be placed initially to manage the continuous passage of stool. Protective ointments (e.g., zinc oxide) and occlusive dressing (e.g., hydrocolloids) will often decrease skin irritation from frequent loose stools. The preferred position is a side-lying prone position with the hips elevated, or a supine position with the legs suspended at a 90-degree angle to the trunk to prevent pressure on perineal sutures.

The infant is given formula when evidence of normal peristalsis is noted. In the meantime, there may be a nasogastric tube for abdominal decompression and IV feedings. Care of the infant with a colostomy involves frequent dressing changes, meticulous skin care, and correct application of a collection device (see Chapter 45).

(See also Nursing Care Plan: The Infant with an Anorectal Malformation.*)

MALABSORPTION SYNDROMES

Malabsorption syndromes are characterized by chronic diarrhea and malabsorption of nutrients. An important complication of malabsorption syndromes in children is failure to thrive. Most are classified according to the location of the supposed anatomic and/or biochemical defect. The term *celiac disease* is often used to describe a symptom complex that has four characteristics in common: (1) steatorrhea (i.e., fatty, foul, frothy, bulky stools), (2) general malnutrition, (3) abdominal distention, and (4) secondary vitamin deficiencies.

Digestive defects are conditions in which the enzymes necessary for digestion are diminished or absent, such as (1) cystic fibrosis, in which pancreatic enzymes are absent; (2) biliary or liver disease, in which bile flow is affected; or (3) lactase deficiency, in which there is congenital or secondary lactose intolerance.

Absorptive defects are conditions in which the intestinal mucosal transport system is impaired. It may be because of a primary defect (e.g., celiac disease) or secondary to inflammatory disease of the bowel (e.g., ulcerative colitis) that results in impaired absorption because bowel motility is accelerated. Obstructive disorders (e.g., Hirschsprung disease) can also cause secondary malabsorption from enterocolitis.

Anatomic defects, such as extensive resection of the bowel or "short-bowel syndrome," affect digestion by decreasing the transit time of substances and affect absorption by severely compromising the absorptive surface.

Celiac Disease (CD)

CD, also known as *gluten-induced enteropathy, gluten-sensitive enteropathy (GSE),* and *celiac sprue,* is a disease of the proximal small intestine characterized by abnormal mucosa and permanent intolerance to gluten. CD is second only to cystic fibrosis as a cause of malabsorption in children. The incidence varies from 1 in 300 to 1 in 4000, and appears to be declining, possibly in relation to environmental factors. It is seen more commonly in Europe than in America and is rarely reported in Asians or African-Americans. The exact cause of CD is not

*In Wong DL, Hess CS: ***Wong and Whaley's clinical manual of pediatric nursing,*** ed 5, St Louis, 2000, Mosby.

known, but there appears to be an inherited predisposition with an influence by environmental factors.

Pathophysiology. The disease is characterized by an intolerance to the protein gluten, found in wheat, barley, rye, and oats. Although the pathologic process is still obscure, susceptible individuals are unable to digest the gliadin component of gluten, resulting in an accumulation of a toxic substance that is damaging to the mucosal cells. Two theories regarding the damaging effect of gluten in CD are that there is a specific enzyme deficiency; or that there is an immunologic abnormality (Walker-Smith, 1996).

Diagnostic Evaluation. Symptoms of CD are usually noted several months after the introduction of gluten-containing grains into the diet, typically between the ages of 1 and 5 years (Box 47-23). The clinical manifestations are usually insidious and chronic. The first evidence of the disease may be failure to thrive and diarrhea.

Currently the diagnosis of celiac disease is based on a biopsy of the small intestine demonstrating the characteristic changes in the mucosa and a positive clinical response to a gluten-free diet. Within a day or two of instituting the diet, most children with CD demonstrate a favorable response, including weight gain and improved appetite. Within a few weeks there is resolution of the diarrhea and steatorrhea.

Serologic testing to detect antibodies to connective tissue (endomysium and reticulin) and to gliadin are available. The presence of antigliadin, antireticulin, and antiendomysial IgG and IgA antibodies (and the disappearance of these antibodies when gluten is removed from the diet), aids in diagnosis (Walker-Smith, 1996). Although these tests may be used as screening tools, they vary in sensitivity and specificity and are often followed by a biopsy (Murray, 1999).

Therapeutic Management. Treatment of chronic CD is primarily dietary management. Although the diet is called "gluten free," it is actually low in gluten because it is impossible to remove every source of this protein. Studies demonstrate that most patients are able to tolerate restricted amounts of gluten. Because gluten is found primarily in the grains of wheat and rye, and also in smaller quantities in barley and oats, these four foods are eliminated. Corn and rice become substitute grain foods.

Children with untreated celiac disease may have associated lactose intolerance related to intestinal mucosal lesions, which usually improve with gluten withdrawal and intestinal healing. Specific nutritional deficiencies are treated with appropriate supplements, including vitamins, iron, and calories.

Prognosis. CD is generally regarded as a chronic disease. The extent of the disease varies among children. The most severe symptoms usually occur in early childhood and again in adult life. Strict dietary avoidance of gluten can prevent symptoms and may minimize the risk of developing lymphoma, one of the most serious complications of the disease.

Nursing Care Management. The main nursing consideration is helping the child adhere to dietary management. Considerable time is involved in explaining to the child and the parents the disease process, the specific role of gluten in aggravating the condition, and those foods that must be restricted. It is especially difficult to maintain a diet indefinitely when the child has no symptoms and temporary transgressions result in no difficulties. However, evidence indicates that the majority of individuals who relax their diet will experience a relapse of their disease and possibly exhibit growth retardation, anemia, or osteomalacia. There is also the risk of developing malignant lymphoma of the small intestine or other GI malignancies.

Although the chief source of gluten is cereal and baked goods, grains are commonly added to processed foods as thickeners or fillers. To add to the difficulty, gluten is added to many foods as "hydrolyzed vegetable protein." The nurse must advise parents to read carefully all ingredients on labels to avoid hidden sources of gluten. Many of the gluten-containing products can be eliminated from the infant's or young child's diet fairly easily, but monitoring the diet of a school-age child or adolescent is much more difficult. Many favorite foods, such as hot dogs, pizza, and spaghetti, are chief offenders. Luncheon preparation away from home is particularly difficult because bread, luncheon meats, and instant soups are not allowed.

In addition to restricting gluten, other dietary alterations may be necessary in the beginning. For example, in some children who have more severe mucosal damage, the digestion of disaccharides is impaired, especially in relation to lactose. Therefore these children often need a temporary lactose-free diet, which necessitates eliminating all milk products.

Generally, management includes a diet high in calories and proteins, with simple carbohydrates, such as fruits and vegetables, but low in fats. Initially the bowel may be inflamed as a result of the pathologic process, so high-fiber foods such as nuts, raisins, raw vegetables, and raw fruits with skin are avoided until inflammation has subsided.

Several resources are available to assist parents in all aspects of coping with CD. The Celiac Sprue Association/United States

Box 47-23

Clinical Manifestations of Celiac Disease

IMPAIRED FAT ABSORPTION
Steatorrhea (excessively large, pale, oily, frothy stools)
Exceedingly foul-smelling stools

IMPAIRED ABSORPTION OF NUTRIENTS
Malnutrition
Muscle wasting (especially prominent in legs and buttocks)
Anemia
Anorexia
Abdominal distention

BEHAVIORAL CHANGES
Irritability
Fretfulness
Uncooperativeness
Apathy

CELIAC CRISIS*
Acute, severe episodes of profuse watery diarrhea and vomiting
May be precipitated by:
- Infections (especially gastrointestinal)
- Prolonged fluid and electrolyte depletion
- Emotional disturbance

*In very young children.

of America* is an organization that provides support and guidance to families and supplies educational materials concerning a gluten-free diet, food sources, recipes, and travel information.†

(See also Nursing Care Plan: The Child with Celiac Disease.‡)

Short-Bowel Syndrome (SBS)

SBS is a malabsorptive disorder that occurs as a result of decreased mucosal surface area, usually as a result of extensive resection of the small intestine. The most common causes of SBS in children include congenital anomalies (e.g., jejunal and ileal atresia, gastroschisis), ischemia (e.g., necrotizing enterocolitis), and trauma or vascular injury (e.g., volvulus [twisting of bowel on itself]). Other causes include bowel resection due to a long-segment Hirschsprung disease and omphalocele. Radiation enteritis can also lead to SBS. The prognosis for infants and children with SBS has dramatically improved in the past 25 years as a result of advances in parenteral nutrition and enteral feeding.

Both the amount and the location of bowel lost are important in determining the severity of the condition. The preservation of the terminal ileum and ileocecal valve influences fluid and nutrient absorption and may avoid problems of bacterial overgrowth by preventing the entrance of bacteria from the colon into the small intestine.

The small intestine has significant capacity for adaptation after resection. During the *adaptation process,* the villus height increases (villus hyperplasia), and the cell number and absorptive surface area are also increased. As villus length and the number of enterocytes available for absorption per centimeter of bowel increase, nutrient absorption increases. Intraluminal enteral feedings stimulate the adaptation process and maintain the structural and functional integrity of the small intestine.

Therapeutic Management. The goals of treatment are (1) to preserve as much length of bowel as possible during surgery; (2) to maintain the child's nutritional status, growth, and development while intestinal adaptation occurs; (3) to stimulate intestinal adaptation with enteral feeding; and (4) to minimize complications related to the disease process and therapy.

Nutritional support becomes the long-term focus of care. The *initial phase* of therapy includes TPN as the primary source of nutrition. Complications associated with SBS and long-term TPN include central venous catheter infection or occlusion, catheter migration, thrombosis or emboli, bacterial overgrowth, metabolic complications, cholestasis, and liver dysfunction.

The *second phase* is the introduction of enteral feeding, which usually begins as soon as possible after surgery. Special elemental formulas containing glucose, sucrose and glucose polymers, hydrolyzed proteins, and medium-chain triglycerides facilitate absorption. Usually these formulas are given by continuous infusion through a nasogastric or gastrostomy tube. As the enteral feedings are advanced, the TPN solution is decreased in terms of calories, amount of fluid, and total hours of infusion per day.

The *final phase* of nutritional support occurs when growth and development are sustained exclusively by enteral feedings. When TPN is discontinued, however, there is a risk of nutritional deficiency secondary to malabsorption of fat-soluble vitamins (A, D, E, K), and trace minerals (iron, selenium, zinc). Serum vitamin and mineral levels should be obtained, and enteral supplementation of vitamins and minerals may be required.

Numerous complications are associated with SBS and long-term TPN. Infectious, metabolic, and technical complications can occur secondary to TPN. Catheter sepsis can occur after improper care of the catheter. The GI tract can also be a source of microbial seeding of the catheter in children with SBS. Bowel atrophy may foster increased intestinal permeability of bacteria. A lack of adequate sites for central lines may become a significant problem for the child in need of long-term TPN. Hepatic dysfunction is also a common complication of TPN. Hepatomegaly with abnormal liver function tests and cholestasis may occur.

Bacterial overgrowth is likely to occur when the ileocecal valve is absent or when stasis exists as a result of a partial obstruction or a dilated segment of bowel with poor motility. Alternating cycles of broad-spectrum antibiotics may be used to reduce bacterial overgrowth. This treatment may also decrease the risk of bacterial translocation and subsequent central venous catheter infections. Other complications of bacterial overgrowth and malabsorption include metabolic acidosis and gastric hypersecretion.

Many surgical interventions, including intestinal valves, tapering enteroplasty or stricturoplasty, intestinal lengthening, and interposed segments have been used to slow intestinal transit, reduce bacterial overgrowth, or increase mucosal surface area. *Intestinal transplantation* has been performed successfully in children; however, the experience is limited, and the long-term results are unknown. Only those children with a permanent dependence on TPN or severe complications of long-term parenteral nutrition are considered candidates for transplantation.

Prognosis. The prognosis for infants with SBS has improved with advances in TPN and with the understanding of the importance of intraluminal nutrition. Improved surgical techniques for the management of therapy-related problems, and the development of more specific immunosuppressive medications for transplantation have all contributed to improved management of SBS. Establishment of the prognosis depends in part on the length of the residual small intestine. An intact ileocecal valve improves the prognosis. Infants and children with SBS usually die of TPN-related problems, such as fulminant sepsis or severe TPN cholestasis. These TPN-related complications can be significant and life-threatening for many of these children.

Nursing Considerations. The most important components of nursing care for children with SBS are administration and monitoring of nutritional therapy. During TPN therapy, care must be taken to minimize the risk of complications related to the central venous access device (e.g., catheter infections, occlusions, dislodgment, or accidental removal). Care of the enteral feeding tubes and monitoring of enteral feeding tolerance are other important ongoing nursing responsibilities.*

When long-term parenteral nutrition is required, preparing the family for home care is a major nursing responsibility that

*P.O. Box 31700, Omaha, NE, 68131-0700; (402) 558-0600; e-mail: celiacusa@aol.com. In Canada: Canadian Celiac Association, Inc., 190 Britannia Rd. E., Unit 11, Mississauga, Ontario, L4Z 1W6; (905) 507-6208; website: www.celiac.ca.

†A booklet, Pointers for Parents: Coping with Celiac Sprue, which provides information on shopping, cooking, and living with an affected child, is available from the Clinical Dietetics Department, Children's Memorial Hospital, 2300 Children's Plaza, Chicago, IL 60614; (773) 880-4793.

‡In Wong DL, Hess CS: ***Wong and Whaley's clinical manual of pediatric nursing,*** ed 5, St Louis, 2000, Mosby.

*Community and home care instructions on caring for a central venous catheter are available in Wong DL, Hess CS: ***Wong and Whaley's clinical manual of pediatric nursing,*** ed 5, St Louis, 2000, Mosby.

should be initiated early to prevent a lengthy hospitalization with subsequent problems such as family dysfunction and developmental delays. Many infants and children can be successfully cared for at home with enteral and parenteral nutrition if the family is thoroughly prepared and provided with adequate support services. Careful follow-up by a multidisciplinary nutritional support service is essential. The nurse can have an active and important role in the success of a home nutrition program. Home infusion companies now provide portable equipment, which enables the child and family to maintain a more normal lifestyle.

When hospitalization is prolonged, the child's developmental and emotional needs must be met. This often requires special planning to promote normal family adjustment and adaptation of the hospital routines. Care of the hospitalized child is discussed in Chapter 44.

INGESTION OF INJURIOUS AGENTS

Since the passage of the Poison Prevention Packaging Act of 1970, which provides that certain potentially hazardous drugs and household products be sold in child-resistant containers, the incidence of poisonings in children has decreased dramatically. However, despite these advances, poisoning remains a significant health concern, with most cases occurring in children under 6 years of age. Although pharmaceuticals such as analgesics, cough and cold preparations, topical preparations, antibiotics, vitamins, gastrointestinal preparations, hormones, and antihistamines are commonly the agents of poisonings, children may be poisoned by a variety of substances. The most commonly ingested poisons include (Litovitz et al, 1997):

1. Cosmetics and personal care products (perfume, cologne, aftershave)*
2. Cleaning products (hypochlorite ["household"] bleach, pine oil disinfectants)
3. Plants (nontoxic gastrointestinal irritants, oxalates; Box 47-24)
4. Foreign bodies, toys, and miscellaneous substances (dessicants, thermometers, bubble-blowing solutions)
5. Hydrocarbons (gasoline)

More than 90% of poisonings occur in the home, although a significant number take place elsewhere, such as in a grandparent's or friend's home, in a school, or in a health care facility.

NURSE ALERT • The following five commonly used and easily available drugs (first four are over-the-counter products) can cause serious or fatal consequences if as little as ¼ teaspoon or ½ tablet is ingested: methyl salicylate, camphor, topical imidazolines (sympathomimetics such as those contained in Visine, Afrin, Otrivin, and Clear Eyes), benzocaine, and diphenoxylate-atropine (e.g., Lomotil). Stress to parents the importance of keeping such drugs away from children. If these agents are ingested, advise parents to seek medical treatment immediately. Emesis is not introduced for significant camphor, topical imidazolines, or Lomotil ingestions (Liebelt and Shannon, 1993).

*The most common substances in each category are in parentheses. Substances ingested are not necessarily most toxic but often represent ready availability.

Box 47-24
Poisonous and Nonpoisonous Plants

Poisonous plants	Toxic parts	Nonpoisonous plants
Apple	Leaves, seeds	African violet
Apricot	Leaves, stem, seed pits	Aluminum plant
Azalea	Foliage and flowers	Asparagus fern
Buttercup	All parts	Begonia
Cherry (wild or cultivated)	Twigs, seeds, foliage	Boston fern
Daffodil	Bulbs	Christmas cactus
Dumb cane, dieffenbachia	All parts	Coleus
Elephant ear	All parts	Gardenia
English ivy	All parts	Grape ivy
Foxglove	Leaves, seeds, flowers	Jade plant
Holly	Berries	Marigolds
Hyacinth	Bulbs	Piggyback begonia
Ivy	Leaves	Piggyback plant
Mistletoe*	Berries, leaves	Poinsettia†
Oak tree	Acorn, foliage	Prayer plant
Philodendron	All parts	Rubber tree
Plum	Pit	Snake plant
Poison ivy, poison oak	Leaves, fruit, stems, smoke from burning plants	Spider plant
Pothos	All parts	Swedish ivy
Rhubarb	Leaves	Wax plant
Tulip	Bulbs	Weeping fig
Water hemlock	All parts	Zebra plant
Wisteria	Seeds, pods	
Yew	All parts	

*Eating one or two berries or leaves is probably nontoxic.
†Mildly toxic if ingested in massive quantities.

The developmental characteristics of young children predispose them to poisoning by ingestion. Infants and toddlers explore their environment through oral experimentation. Because the sense of taste is less discriminatory at this age, many unpalatable substances are ingested. In addition, toddlers and preschoolers are developing autonomy and initiative, which increase their curiosity and noncompliant behavior. Imitation is also a powerful motivator, especially when combined with lack of awareness of danger (Brayden et al, 1993).

This section is primarily concerned with the immediate emergency treatment of ingestion of injurious agents. Specific management of corrosive, hydrocarbon, acetaminophen, salicylate, plant, and iron poisoning is summarized in Box 47-25. Because of the importance of lead poisoning among young children, ingestion of lead is discussed separately. Appropriate suggestions for poison prevention are discussed on p. 1300.

Principles of Emergency Treatment

A poisoning may or may not require emergency intervention, but in every instance medical evaluation is necessary to initiate appropriate action. Parents are advised to call the Poison Control Center (PCC) *before* initiating any intervention. The local PCC telephone number (usually listed in the front of the telephone directory) should be posted near each phone in the

Box 47-25

Common Childhood Poisonings

CORROSIVES (STRONG ACIDS OR ALKALI)

Drain, toilet, or oven cleaners
Electric dishwasher detergent (liquid, because of higher pH, is more hazardous than granular)
Mildew remover
Batteries
Clinitest tablets
Denture cleaners

Clinical Manifestations

Severe burning pain in mouth, throat, and stomach
White, swollen mucous membranes; edema of lips, tongue, and pharynx (respiratory obstruction)
Violent vomiting (hemoptysis)
Drooling and inability to clear secretions
Signs of shock
Anxiety and agitation

Comments

Household bleach is a frequently ingested corrosive but rarely causes serious damage
Liquid preparations cause more damage than granular preparations

Treatment

Inducing emesis is contraindicated (vomiting redamages the mucosa)
Dilute corrosive with water (usually no more than 120 ml [4 ounces]) or milk
Do not neutralize with weak acids or alkalis because reaction produces heat and burns
Provide patent airway if needed
Administer analgesics
Do not allow oral intake
Esophageal stricture may require repeated dilations and/or surgery

HYDROCARBONS

Gasoline
Kerosene
Lamp oil
Mineral seal oil (found in furniture polish)
Lighter fluid
Turpentine
Paint thinner and remover (some types)

Clinical Manifestations

Gagging, choking, and coughing
Nausea
Vomiting
Alterations in sensorium, such as lethargy
Weakness
Respiratory symptoms of pulmonary involvement
- Tachypnea
- Cyanosis
- Retractions
- Grunting

Comments

Immediate danger is aspiration (even small amounts can cause bronchitis and chemical pneumonia)
Gasoline, kerosene, lighter fluid, mineral seal oil, and turpentine cause severe pneumonia

Treatment (Controversial)

Inducing emesis is generally contraindicated
Gastric decontamination and emptying are contraindicated in most hydrocarbon ingestions
Symptomatic treatment of chemical pneumonia includes high humidity, oxygen, hydration, and antibiotics for secondary infection

ACETAMINOPHEN

Clinical Manifestations

Occurs in four stages:
1. Initial period (2 to 4 hours after ingestion)
   - Nausea
   - Vomiting
   - Sweating
   - Pallor
2. Latent period (24 to 36 hours)
   - Patient improves
3. Hepatic involvement (may last up to 7 days and be permanent)
   - Pain in right upper quadrant
   - Jaundice
   - Confusion
   - Stupor
   - Coagulation abnormalities
4. Patients who do not die in hepatic stage gradually recover

Comments

Most common drug poisoning in children
Occurs from acute ingestion
Toxic dose is 150 mg/kg or greater in children
Toxicity from chronic therapeutic use is rare but may occur with ingestion of approximately 150 mg/kg/day, or about double the recommended maximum therapeutic dose (90 mg/kg/day) of acetaminophen, for several days (Douidar, Al-Khalil, and Habersang, 1994); toxicity is more likely in children with hepatic dysfunction or eating disorders (Cheung, Potts, and Meyer, 1994; McDonough, 1998)

Treatment

Activated charcoal
Antidote *N*-acetylcysteine (NAC) (Mucomyst) is given, usually by nasogastric tube because of the antidote's offensive odor (smells like rotten eggs)
Given as 1 loading dose and usually 17 maintenance doses in different dosages
May be given intravenously, but use is investigational

ASPIRIN (ASA)

Clinical Manifestations

Acute poisoning
- Nausea
- Disorientation
- Vomiting
- Dehydration
- Diaphoresis
- Hyperpnea
- Hyperpyrexia

Box 47-25

Common Childhood Poisonings—cont'd

ASPIRIN (ASA)—cont'd

Clinical Manifestations—cont'd

Ollguria
Tinnitus
Coma
Seizures

Chronic poisoning
Same as above but subtle onset (often confused with illness being treated)

Dehydration, coma, and seizures may be more severe
Bleeding tendencies

Comments

May be caused by acute ingestion (severe toxicity occurs with 300 to 500 mg/kg [4 to 7 gr/kg])
May be caused by chronic ingestion (i.e., more than 100 mg/kg/day for 2 or more days); can be more serious than acute ingestion
Time to peak serum salicylate level can vary with enteric aspirin or the presence of concretions (bezoars)

Treatment

Home use of ipecac for moderate toxicity
Hospitalization for severe toxicity
Emesis, lavage, activated charcoal, and/or cathartic
Lavage will not remove concretions of ASA
Activated charcoal is important early in ASA toxicity
Sodium bicarbonate transfusions to correct metabolic acidosis and urinary alkalinization is effective in enhancing elimination
External cooling for hyperpyrexia
Diazepam for seizures
Oxygen and ventilation for respiratory depression
Vitamin K for bleeding
In extreme cases, hemodialysis (not peritoneal dialysis) may be used

IRON

Mineral supplement or vitamin containing iron

Clinical Manifestations

Occurs in five stages:

1. Initial period (½ to 6 hours after ingestion) (if child does not develop gastrointestinal symptoms in 6 hours, toxicity is unlikely)
   Vomiting
   Hematemesis
   Diarrhea
   Hematochezia (bloody stools)
   Gastric pain
2. Latency (2 to 12 hours)
   Patient improves
3. Systemic toxicity (4 to 24 hours after ingestion)
   Metabolic acidosis
   Fever
   Hyperglycemia
   Bleeding
   Shock
   Death (may occur)
4. Hepatic injury (48 to 96 hours)
   Seizures
   Coma
5. Rarely, pyloric stenosis develops at 2 to 5 weeks

Comments

Factors related to frequency of iron poisoning include:
Widespread availability
Packaging of large quantities in individual containers
Lack of parental awareness of iron toxicity
Resemblance of iron tablets to candy (e.g., M&Ms)
Toxic dose is based on the amount of elemental iron in various salts (sulfate, gluconate, fumarate), which ranges from 20% to 33%; ingestions of 60 mg/kg are considered dangerous

Treatment

Emesis or lavage
Lavage for all chewable tablets or liquids if spontaneous vomiting has not occurred
Chelation therapy with deferoxamine in severe intoxication (turns urine a red to orange color)
If intravenous deferoxamine is given too rapidly, hypotension, facial flushing, rash, urticaria, tachycardia, and shock may occur; stop the infusion, maintain the intravenous line with normal saline, and notify the practitioner immediately

PLANTS

See Box 47-24

Clinical Manifestations

Depends on type of plant ingested
May cause local irritation of oropharynx and entire gastrointestinal tract
May cause respiratory, renal, and central nervous system symptoms
Topical contact with plants can cause dermatitis

Comments

Some of most frequently ingested substances
Rarely cause serious problems, although some plant ingestions can be fatal
Can also cause choking and allergic reactions

Treatment

Remove plant parts (emesis)
Wash from skin or eyes
Supportive care as needed

house.* Some evidence indicates that the information given by PCCs is more accurate than instructions given by hospital emergency departments (Wigder et al, 1995) (Critical Thinking box).

Based on the initial telephone assessment, the PCC counsels the parents to begin treatment at home and/or to take the child to an emergency facility. When a call is taken, the name and telephone number of the caller are recorded to reestablish contact if the connection is interrupted. Because most poisonings are managed in the home, expert advice is essential in minimizing adverse effects. When the exact quantity or type of ingested toxin is not known, admission to a hospital for laboratory evaluation and surveillance is critical during the postingestion period.

Assessment. The first and most important principle in dealing with a poisoning is to treat the child first, not the poison. This necessitates an immediate concern for life support; vital signs are taken and respiratory and/or circulatory support instituted as needed. The victim's condition is routinely reevaluated. Because shock is a complication of several types of household poisons (particularly corrosives), measures to reduce the effects of shock, such as elevation of the legs and head to the level of the heart to promote venous drainage and the provision of warmth and rest, are important. Maintenance of respiratory function may require insertion of an airway and/or mechanical ventilation.

The emergency department nurse's responsibility is to be prepared for immediate intervention with any of the necessary equipment. Because time and speed are critical factors in recovery from serious poisonings, anticipation of potential problems and complications may mean the difference between life and death.

Gastric Decontamination. In general, the immediate treatment is to remove the ingested poison by inducing vomiting, adsorbing the toxin with activated charcoal, performing gastric lavage, or increasing bowel motility (catharsis). Because of continuing controversy regarding the use of these methods, each toxic ingestion should be treated individually (Perry and Shannon, 1996). Specific antidotes may be administered for certain poisonings. The preferred method for use at home is to administer *syrup of ipecac,* an emetic that exerts its action by direct stimulation of the vomiting center and through an irritant effect on the gastric mucosa.

NURSE ALERT • Syrup of ipecac is contraindicated in cases of ingestion of corrosive substances and in the child who is comatose or having seizures. In children who have ingested hydrocarbons, ipecac is contraindicated if the risk of aspiration outweighs the benefit of gastric evacuation. Ipecac may cause prolonged vomiting (enduring as long as 12 hours), which makes it relatively contraindicated in ingestions that may cause sedation, coma, or seizures (Perry and Shannon, 1996).

Proper administration of ipecac is essential (Emergency box). Ipecac is available in 30-ml (1-ounce) vials; however, the

*Also available by calling 1-800-555-1212 in any of the United States.

Critical Thinking

POISONING

Mrs. Berry, a neighbor, calls you. She is very upset because her 2-year-old son has eaten several chewable multivitamins with iron. She asks you if she should give syrup of ipecac. What should you advise her to do?

First Think About It...

- **What are you taking for granted, and what assumptions are you making?**
- **How are you interpreting the information?**

1. **First call the Poison Control Center.**
2. **Give the antiemetic.**
3. **Dilute the poison with several glasses of water.**
4. **Wait to see if the child develops symptoms.**

The best response is 1. Regardless of your personal assumptions, the Poison Control Center will advise her of home treatment, such as using ipecac. The goal is to remove the poison, not dilute it, which makes option 3 inappropriate. The correct interpretation of the information presented is that the most toxic ingredient in the multivitamin is iron, which produces symptoms after several hours. Treatment, if needed, should begin long before symptoms appear.

Emergency

POISONING

1. Assess the victim:
   a. Take vital signs; re-evaluate routinely.
   b. Initiate cardiorespiratory support if needed.
   c. Treat other symptoms, such as seizures.
2. Terminate exposure:
   a. Empty mouth of pills, plant parts, or other material.
   b. Flush eyes continuously with normal saline (room-temperature tap water at home) for 15 to 20 minutes.
   c. Flush skin and wash with soap and a soft cloth; remove contaminated clothes, especially if a pesticide, acid, alkali, or hydrocarbon is involved.
   d. Bring victim of an inhalation poisoning into fresh air.
   e. Give one sip of water to dilute ingested poison.
3. Identify the poison:
   a. Question the victim and witnesses.
   b. Look for environmental cues (empty container, nearby spill, odor on breath) and save all evidence of poison (container, vomitus, urine).
   c. Be alert to signs and symptoms of potential poisoning in absence of other evidence, including symptoms of ocular or dermal exposure.
   d. Call Poison Control Center or other competent emergency facility for immediate advice regarding treatment.
4. Remove poison and prevent absorption:
   a. Induce vomiting; administer ipecac if ordered:
      (1) 6 to 12 months: 10 ml; do not repeat.*
      (2) 1 to 12 years: 15 ml; repeat dosage once if vomiting has not occurred within 20 minutes.
      (3) Over 12 years: 30 ml; repeat dosage once if vomiting has not occurred within 20 minutes.
   b. Do not induce vomiting if:
      (1) Victim is comatose, in severe shock, or convulsing, or has lost the gag reflex.
      (2) Poison is a low-viscosity hydrocarbon (unless it contains a more toxic substance [e.g., pesticide or heavy metal] or a strong acid or alkali).
   c. Place child in side-lying, sitting, or kneeling position with head below chest to prevent aspiration.
   d. Administer activated charcoal with cathartic (unless used repeatedly; usual dose 1 g/kg unless amount of toxin is known) 30 to 60 minutes after vomiting from ipecac, if ordered.

*Emesis of children at home is generally contraindicated between ages 6 and 10 months. Ipecac can only be administered safely in a health care facility because of the high risk of aspiration.

label information does not include directions for a second dose if the child fails to vomit after the first dose. Therefore parents need clear instructions for proper use and dosage. As a precaution, parents are advised to have full doses of ipecac for *each child* in the home, to carry the emetic when traveling, and to be certain that other caregivers (e.g., baby-sitters or relatives) have the emetic available. Because children share activities, more than one child may ingest the toxic substance. In an emergency, ipecac can be obtained from an all-night pharmacy, convenience store, emergency squad, or emergency department. Ipecac is also inexpensive.

Although out-of-date ipecac may be used in an emergency, the family is encouraged to replace the expired bottle. Because milk, fluid volume, food, and activity level do not alter ipecac's effectiveness, the common suggestions of forcing fluids and encouraging movement are unnecessary. If liquids are given, clear liquids are preferred for better visualization of pill fragments. For maximum benefit in removing the poison, ipecac should be administered within 1 hour of a toxic ingestion.

If the child is admitted to an emergency facility, *gastric* lavage may also be done to empty the stomach of the toxic agent. Lavage is indicated for the following: young infants in whom ipecac is contraindicated; if the patient is comatose or convulsing, or requires a protected airway; or if the ingested poison is rapidly absorbed (strychnine or cyanide). The use of lavage in petroleum distillate poisoning remains controversial because of the danger of aspiration. When lavage is performed, the largest-diameter tube that can be inserted is used to facilitate passage of gastric contents.

Another method of decontaminating the stomach is the use of *activated charcoal,* an odorless, tasteless, fine black powder that adsorbs many compounds, creating a stable complex. It is mixed with water or a saline cathartic to form a slurry. Slurries are neither gritty nor distasteful but resemble black mud. Potential complications from the use of activated charcoal include aspiration (usually in patients with impaired gag reflexes), constipation, intestinal obstruction, and electrolyte imbalances (Diamont et al, 1994). Cathartics such as sorbitol, sodium, or magnesium may be administered to stimulate evacuation of the bowel, thus decreasing systemic absorption of the poison and aiding in the removal of the charcoal. Many commercial preparations of activated charcoal contain cathartics; however, the use of cathartics is controversial. Cathartics can cause electrolyte imbalances. Sorbitol use in young children has caused excessive fluid losses (Perry and Shannon, 1996). To increase the child's acceptance of activated charcoal, mix it with flavoring or a sweetener and serve it through a straw and in an opaque container with a cover, such as a disposable coffee cup and lid or an ordinary cup covered with aluminum foil or placed inside a small paper bag.

In a minority of poisonings, specific *antidotes* are available to counteract the poison. They are highly effective and should be available in all emergency facilities. The supply of antidotes should be checked routinely and replaced as used or according to expiration dates. Among the more commonly employed antidotes are N-acetylcysteine for acetaminophen poisoning, oxygen for carbon monoxide inhalation, naloxone for opioid overdose, flumazenil (Romazicon) for benzodiazepine (Valium, Versed) overdose, Digibind for digoxin toxicity, and antivenin for certain poisonous bites.

Prevention of Recurrence. The ultimate objective is to prevent poisonings from occurring or recurring. One effective counseling method is first to discuss the difficulties of constantly watching and safeguarding young children (Family Focus box). In this way the challenging task of raising children can lead to a discussion of injury prevention as one part of the parental role. This approach also incorporates other contributory causes for the incident, such as inadequate support systems, marital discord, discipline techniques (especially use of physical punishment), and maternal distress. A visit to the home, especially after a repeat poisoning situation, is recommended as part of the follow-up care to assess hazards (including family factors) and to evaluate appropriate safe-proofing measures. One method of identifying risk areas is to ask specific questions or to have the parent complete a questionnaire designed to isolate factors that predispose children to poisoning. Encourage parents to bend down to the child's eye level and survey the home environment for potential hazards. Having the parents try to open cabinets and reach shelves to access poisons can be helpful.

Passive measures (those that do not require active participation) have been the most successful in preventing poisoning. These include child-resistant closures and limiting the number of tablets in one container. However, these measures alone are not sufficient to prevent poisoning because most toxic agents in the home do not have safety closures. Therefore *active measures* (those that require participation) are essential. Guidelines for preventing the occurrence or recurrence of a poisoning are listed in the Guidelines box.

(See also Nursing Care Plan: The Child with Poisoning.*)

Heavy Metal Poisoning

Heavy metal poisoning in children can occur from the ingestion of a variety of substances, the most common being lead. Other important causes are iron and mercury. *Mercury toxicity,* a rare form of heavy metal poisoning, has occurred in children from a variety of sources, such as broken thermometers or thermostats, broken fluorescent lights, and use of interior latex house paint. Elemental mercury (also called metallic mercury or quicksilver) is nontoxic if ingested and if the gastrointestinal tract is healthy

*In Wong DL, Hess CS: ***Wong and Whaley's clinical manual of pediatric nursing,*** ed 5, St Louis, 2000, Mosby.

Family Focus

POISONING

A poisoning is more than a physical emergency for the child. It usually represents an emotional crisis for the parents, particularly in terms of guilt, self-reproach, and insecurity in the parenting role. The emergency department is no place to admonish the family for negligence, lack of appropriate supervision, or failure to safe-proof the home. Rather, it is a time to calm and support the child and parents while unaccusingly exploring the circumstances of the injury. If the nurse prematurely attempts to discuss ways of preventing such an incident from recurring the parents' anxiety will block out any suggestions or offered guidance. Therefore it is preferable for the nurse to delay the discussion until the child's condition is stabilized or, if the child is discharged immediately after emergency treatment, to make a public health referral or send a packet of information.*

*Woolf AD, Saperstein A, Forjuoh S: Poisoning prevention knowledge and practices of parents after a childhood poisoning incident, *Pediatrics* 90(6):867-870, 1992.

(e.g., has no fistulas). However, mercury is volatile at room temperature and enters the bloodstream after it is inhaled, causing toxicity (e.g., tremors, memory loss, insomnia, gingivitis, diarrhea, anorexia, and weight loss). The classic form of mercury poisoning is called *acrodynia* (or "painful extremities").

Heavy metals have an affinity for certain essential tissue chemicals, which must remain free for adequate cell functioning. When metals are bound to these substances, cellular enzyme systems are inactivated. Treatment involves *chelation,* use of a chemical compound that combines with the metal for rapid and safe excretion.

Lead Poisoning

Poisoning from lead has been a problem throughout history and throughout the world. In the United States the problem facing young children today began in the early 1900s when white lead was added to paints and tetraethyl lead was added to gasoline as an antiknock compound (Berney, 1993). Lead content in paint was decreased in 1950, and in 1978 the use of lead in household paint was banned. The greatest problems remaining are the presence of deteriorating lead-based paint in many older homes and the presence of soil in yards that has a high lead content. Chipping, flaking, and chalking lead-based paint contributes to the environmental dust found in households. Leaded gasoline exhaust contributes to lead hazards in soil (Centers for Disease Control and Prevention [CDC], 1997a, 1997b). Normal hand-to-mouth behavior, coupled with the presence of lead dust in the environment, is the most common method of poisoning (Fisher and Vessey, 1998).

Children 6 years old and under are most vulnerable to the effects of lead. Medicaid recipients are three times as likely to have an elevated blood lead level (U.S. General Accounting Office, 1998). In addition, a disproportionate number of minority children have elevated lead levels (Brody et al, 1994). Any child, however, is at risk for becoming lead poisoned if hazardous conditions for lead are present in their environment.

Causes of Lead Poisoning. Although there are numerous sources of lead (Box 47-26), in most instances of acute childhood lead poisoning the source is nonintact lead-based paint in an older home or lead-contaminated bare soil in the yard. Microparticles of lead gain entryway into a child's body through ingestion or inhalation and, in the case of an exposed pregnant woman, by placental transfer. The blood lead level of an unborn child will be equal to that of the mother (Andrews, Savitz, and Hertz-Picciotto, 1994). Inhalation exposure usually occurs during renovation and remodeling activities in the home, whereas ingestion happens during normal day-to-day play and mouthing activities. Sometimes a child will actually swallow loose chips of lead-based paint because it has a sweet taste. Water and food may also be contaminated with lead.

Guidelines

POISON PREVENTION

- Assess possible contributing factors in occurrence of injury, such as discipline, parent-child relationship, developmental ability, environmental factors, and behavior problems.
- Institute anticipatory guidance for possible future injuries based on child's age and maturational level.
- Refer to visiting nurse agency to evaluate home environment and need for safe-proofing measures.
- Provide assistance with environmental manipulation when necessary, such as lead removal.
- Educate parents regarding safe storage of toxic substances.
- Advise parents to take drugs out of sight of children.
- Advise parents to return all toxic substances *immediately* to safe storage.
- Teach children the hazards of ingesting nonfood items without supervision.
- Advise parents against using plants for teas or medicine.
- Discuss problems of discipline and children's noncompliance and offer strategies for effective discipline (see Limit Setting and Discipline, Chapter 31).
- Instruct parents regarding correct administration of drugs for therapeutic purposes and to discontinue drug if there is evidence of mild toxicity.
- Have syrup of ipecac available—two doses for each child in the family—but to use only if advised to do so by Poison Control Center (PCC) or practitioner.
- Encourage grandparents or other frequent caregivers to keep syrup of ipecac in home.
- Post number of local PCC with emergency phone list by telephone.
- Include by the telephone the home address with nearest cross street in case an ambulance is needed. (In an emergency, family members may not remember the house address, and babysitters may not be aware of the information.)

Box 47-26
Sources of Lead*

- Lead-based paint in deteriorating condition
- Lead solder
- Lead crystal
- Battery casings
- Lead fishing sinkers
- Lead curtain weights
- Lead bullets
- Certain ethnic or cultural products and practices
- Some of the following may contain lead:
  - Ceramic ware
  - Pottery
  - Pewter
  - Dyes
  - Industrial plants
  - Vinyl miniblinds
  - Playground equipment
  - Collectible toys
  - Artists' paints
- Occupations and hobbies involving lead:
  - Battery and aircraft manufacturing
  - Lead smelting
  - Brass foundry work
  - Radiator-repair work
  - Construction work
  - Bridge-repair work
  - Painting
  - Mining
  - Ceramics
  - Stained-glass making
  - Jewelry making

*The U.S. Consumer Product Safety Commission issues alerts an recalls for products that contain lead and that may unexpectedly pose a hazard to young children.

Nurses must be aware of their patients' cultural and ethnic practices and product use. Substances used as natural therapies have been found to contain lead (Cultural Considerations box).

Pathophysiology and Clinical Manifestations. Lead can affect any part of the body, including the renal, hematologic, and neurologic systems (Fig. 47-9). Of most concern for young children is the developing brain and nervous system, which is more vulnerable than that of an older child or adult. Lead in the body moves via an equilibration process between the blood, the soft tissues and organs, and the bones and teeth. At the cellular level it competes with molecules of calcium, interfering with the regulating action of calcium. The inorganic lead found in lead-based paint is not fat soluble and consequently should not cross the blood-brain barrier; however, it does so by impairing the endothelial cells there. Lead interferes with several neurotransmitter mechanisms in the brain. Massive body burdens of lead can lead to cerebral edema and encephalopathy. Fortunately, this is rarely seen today (Finkelstein, Markowitz, and Rosen, 1998).

Lead can also interfere with the binding of iron onto the heme molecule. This sometimes creates a picture of anemia even though the child is not iron deficient. Lead toxicity to the erythrocytes leads to the release of the enzyme erythrocyte protoporphyrin (EP). Because EP is not sensitive to blood lead levels of less than about 16 to 25 μg/dl, it is no longer used as a screening test; however, elevation of the EP level (above 35 μg/dl of whole blood) is a good indicator of toxicity from lead and reflects the length of exposure and body burden of lead in the individual child.

Diagnostic Evaluation. Children with lead poisoning rarely have symptoms, even at levels requiring chelation therapy. A diagnosis of lead poisoning is based only on the lead testing of a venous blood specimen from a venipuncture.

Cultural Considerations

SOURCES OF LEAD

In some cultures the use of traditional ethnic remedies that contain lead may increase children's risk of lead poisoning. These remedies include:

- **Azarcon (Mexico):—For digestive problems; a bright orange powder; usual dose is ¼ to 1 teaspoon, often mixed with oil, milk, or sugar or sometimes given as a tea; sometimes a pinch is added to a baby bottle or tortilla dough for preventive purposes**
- **Greta (Mexico):—A yellow-orange powder, used in the same way as azarcon**
- **Paylooah (Southeast Asia)—Used for rash or fever; an orange-red powder given as ½ teaspoon straight or in a tea**
- **Surma (India)—Black powder applied to the inner lower eyelid that is used as a cosmetic to improve eyesight**
- **Unknown ayurvedic (Tibet)—Small, gray-brown balls used to improve slow development; two balls are given orally three times a day**

Modified from Lead poisoning associated with use of traditional ethnic remedies—California, 1991–1992, *MMWR* 42(27):521–524, 1993.

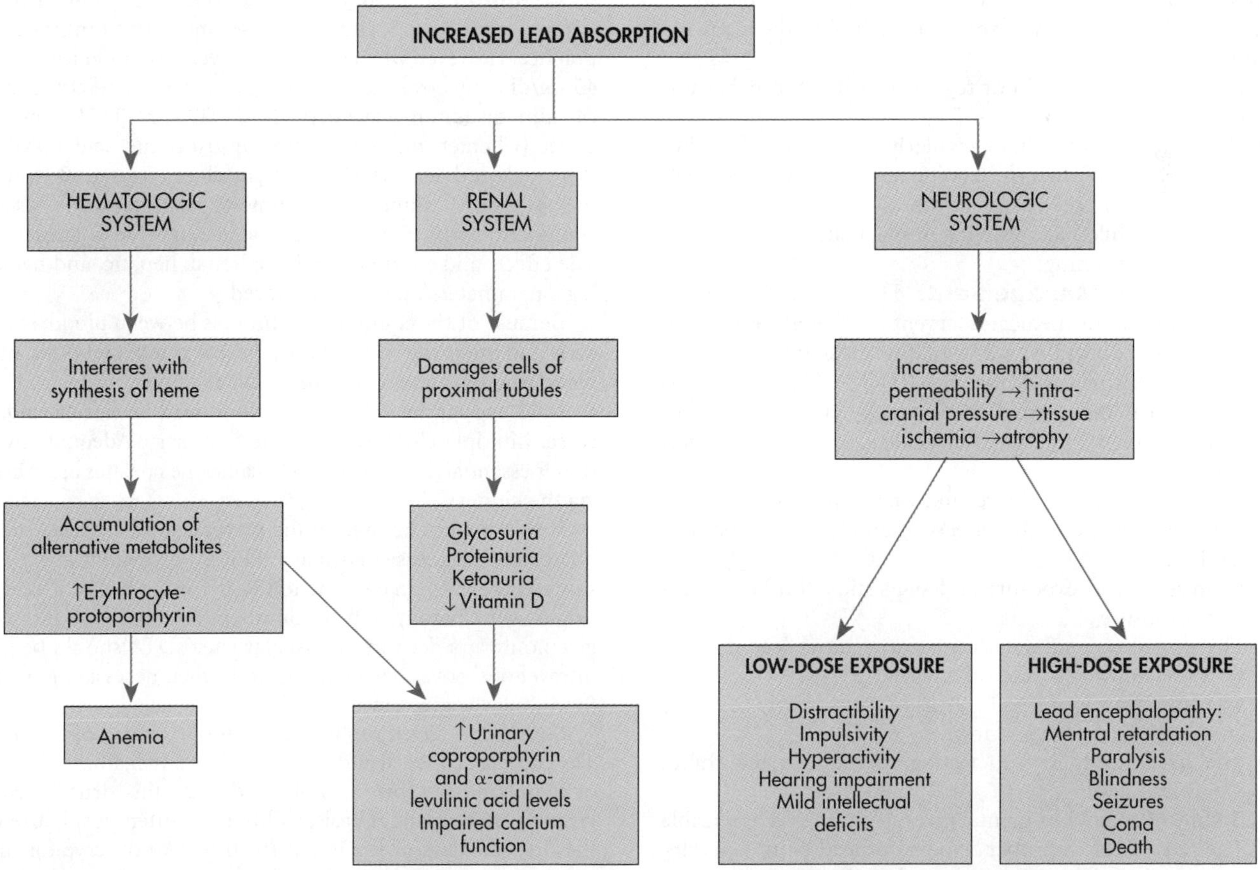

FIG. 47-9 • Main effects of lead on body systems.

The level of concern for an elevated blood lead level has dropped from 80 μg/dl in 1950 to 10 μg/dl today. This is in response to research that has demonstrated lead's harmful effects and to efforts of child health advocates to change lead poisoning prevention policy in the United States (Ryan et al, 1999).

Anticipatory Guidance. Anticipatory guidance lends support to primary prevention efforts. The CDC (1997a) recommends that the following information be made available to families during prenatal care, at 3 to 6 months, and at 1 year of age:

- Hazards of lead-based paint in older housing
- Ways to control lead hazards safely
- Hazards accompanying repainting and renovation of homes built before 1978
- Other exposure sources, such as traditional remedies, that might be relevant for a family

Screening for Lead Poisoning. When primary prevention fails, the secondary prevention effort of screening for elevated blood lead levels can identify children much earlier than in the past. The most recent CDC guidelines (1997a, 1997b) recommend either universal screening or targeted screening, depending on the risk factors and blood lead level surveillance information available for the area.

Universal screening should be done at ages 1 and 2 years. Any child between ages 3 and 6 years who has not been previously screened should also be tested. Any child with risk factors should be screened more often.

Targeted screening is acceptable when an area has been determined by existing data to have less risk. Children should be screened when they live in a high risk geographic area, are members of a group determined to be at risk (e.g., Medicaid recipients), or if their family cannot answer "no" to the following personal risk questions:

- Does your child live in or regularly visit a house that was built before 1950?
- Does your child live in or regularly visit a house built before 1978 with recent or ongoing renovations or remodeling (i.e., within the past 6 months)?
- Does your child have a sibling or playmate who has or did have lead poisoning?

Therapeutic Management. The degree of concern, urgency, and need for medical intervention changes as the lead level increases. Education is one of the most important elements of the treatment process. The CDC (1997a) has identified several areas that should be discussed with the family of every child who has an elevated blood lead level (i.e., 10 μg/dl and above):

- The child's blood lead level and what it means
- Potential adverse health effects of an elevated blood lead level
- Sources of lead exposure and suggestions on how to reduce exposure
- The importance of wet cleaning to remove lead dust on floors, window sills, and other surfaces
- The importance of good nutrition, particularly adequate amounts of calcium and iron
- The need for follow-up testing to monitor the child's blood lead level
- Results of an environmental investigation when applicable
- The hazards of improper removal of lead paint (e.g., dry sanding, scraping, or open-flame burning)

Treatment actions vary depending on the child's blood lead level. Based on a diagnosis from a venous blood lead level test, the CDC (1997a) recommends the following actions:

Blood lead level (μg/dl)	Action
<10	Reassess or rescreen in 1 year. If exposure status changes, do this sooner.
10-14	Provide family with lead poisoning education, follow-up testing, and social service referral if necessary.
15-19	Provide family with lead poisoning education, follow-up testing, and social service referral as needed; if blood lead level persists, initiate actions for blood lead level of 20 to 44 μg/dl.
20-44	Provide coordination of care, clinical management, environmental investigation, and lead hazard control.
45-69	Within 48 hours, provide coordination of care and clinical management, including chelation therapy (medication that removes lead from the blood and, to some extent, in other places in the body), environmental investigation, and lead hazard control. The child must not remain in a lead hazardous environment if resolution is to occur.
≥70	Immediately provide medical treatment and chelation therapy, and begin coordination of care, clinical management, environmental investigation, and lead hazard control.

Chelation Therapy. Medical treatment and chelation therapy for the child with lead poisoning vary from practice to practice. However, when a child has a venous blood lead level of 45 μg/dl and above, two chelating agents are used consistently; calcium disodium edetate ($CaNa_2EDTA$ or EDTA) and succimer (Chemet, meso-2,3 dimercaptosuccinic acid [DMSA]). With a blood lead level of 70 μg/dl or greater, British antilewisite (BAL, dimercaprol, dimercaptopropanol) is used in conjunction with EDTA. All of the agents have potential toxic side effects and contraindications. Renal, hepatic, and hematologic parameters must be monitored.

Because of the equilibration process between blood, soft tissues, and other sites in the body, there is often a rebound of the blood lead level after chelation. Once the body burden of lead is reduced enough to stabilize the blood lead level, rebound will cease. Multiple chelations may be necessary. Adequate hydration is essential during therapy because the chelates are excreted via the kidneys.

BAL must not be used in the presence of a glucose-6-phosphate dehydrogenase deficiency (G6PD) or peanut allergy, nor should it be given in conjunction with iron. It is never used as a single-agent therapy, only in conjunction with EDTA. It must be given only at a deep intramuscular site. EDTA should be given intravenously over several hours and, when necessary to restrict fluids, may be given intramuscularly.

Succimer is given orally over a 19-day course of treatment. The capsule is opened and sprinkled on a small amount of food, or it may be swallowed whole. Although this drug is usually given on an outpatient basis, children are often hospitalized for the first few days of the initial treatment to observe for untoward effects and to plan for discharge to an environment that is

Community Focus

REDUCING BLOOD LEAD LEVELS

Make sure child does not have access to peeling paint or chewable surfaces painted with lead-based paint, especially window sills and wells.

If a house was built before 1960 (possibly before 1980) and has hard-surface floors, wet mop them at least once a week. Wipe other hard surfaces (e.g., window sills, baseboards). If there are loose paint chips in an area, such as a window well, use a wet disposable cloth to pick up and discard them. Do not vacuum hard-surfaced floors or window sills or wells, because this spreads dust. Use vacuum cleaners with agitators to remove dust from rugs rather than vacuum cleaners with suction only. If a rug is known to contain lead dust and cannot be washed, it should be discarded.

Wash and dry child's hands and face frequently, especially before eating.

Wash toys and pacifiers frequently.

If soil around home is or is likely to be contaminated with lead (e.g., if home was built before 1960 or is near a major highway), plant grass or other ground cover; plant bushes around outside of house so that child cannot play there.

During remodeling of older homes, be sure to follow correct procedures. Be certain children and pregnant women are not in the home, day or night, until process is completed. After deleading, thoroughly clean house using cleaning solution to damp mop and dust before inhabitants return.

In areas where lead content of water exceeds the drinking water standard and a particular faucet has not been used for 6 hours or more, "flush" the cold-water pipes by running the water until it becomes as cold as it will get (30 seconds to greater than 2 minutes). The more time water has been sitting in pipes, the more lead it may contain.

Use only cold water for consumption (drinking, cooking, and especially for making infant formula). Hot water dissolves lead more quickly than cold water and thus contains higher levels of lead. May use first-flush water for nonconsumption uses.

Have water tested by a competent laboratory. This action is especially important for apartment dwellers; flushing may not be effective in high-rise buildings or in other buildings with lead-soldered central piping.*

Do not store food in open cans, particularly if cans are imported.

Do not use pottery or ceramic ware that was inadequately fired or is meant for decorative use for food storage or service. Do not store drinks or food in lead crystal.

Avoid folk remedies or cosmetics that contain lead.

Make sure that home exposure is not occurring from parental occupations or hobbies. Household members employed in occupations such as lead smelting should shower and change into clean clothing before leaving work. Construction and lead abatement workers may also bring home lead contaminants.

Make sure child eats regular meals, because more lead is absorbed on an empty stomach.

Make sure child's diet contains sufficient iron and calcium and not excessive fat.

Modified from Centers for Disease Control and Prevention: *Preventing lead poisoning in young children,* Atlanta, 1991, The Centers.

*For more information, contact the county or state department of health or environment for information on local water quality. For general information on lead, call the EPA Safe Drinking Water Hotline, (800) 426-4791; National Lead Information Center (National Safety Council), 1019 19th St. NW, Suite 401, Washington, DC 20036-5105; 1-800-LEAD-FYI; Water Quality Association (WQA), (708) 505-0161, ext. 270; or National Sanitation Foundation (NSF), (213) 769-8010.

safe from lead hazards (Liebelt and Shannon, 1994; Schonfeld and Needham, 1994).

Prognosis. The central nervous system is the focus of the most dramatic effects of lead exposure. Massive amounts of lead are known to cause lead encephalopathy. Seizures, coma, and even death were known to occur in the days before children's exposure to lead was identified early.

Children with smaller amounts of lead poisoning who do not develop encephalopathy are still at risk for neurologic impairment (Needleman, 1992). They are more likely to have a decrease in intellectual functions, to develop learning problems, and to manifest behavior problems than children who have not had lead poisoning (Finkelstein, Markowitz, and Rosen, 1998).

Nursing Care Management. The primary nursing goal in lead poisoning is to prevent the child's initial or further exposure to lead. For children with low-level exposure, this often requires identifying the sources of lead in the environment. Careful history taking is one of the most useful and valuable tools and should concentrate on the personal risk questions (see p. 1302). Suggestions for reducing lead in the child's environment are listed in the Community Focus box.

Children who must undergo chelation therapy are prepared for the injections and allowed to express their pain and anger. Playing with syringes and aggressive play (e.g., pounding clay or throwing beanbags) provides children with an excellent outlet for their frustrations. Children also deserve an explanation of the need for the treatment, particularly that it is not a punishment for eating lead or paint. During home or chelation therapy, parents need to understand the importance of giving the drug as prescribed.

Atraumatic Care

LEAD CHELATION THERAPY

To lessen the pain from intramuscular injection of $CaNa_2EDTA$, the local anesthetic procaine is injected with the drug. Apply EMLA cream over the puncture site 2½ hours before the injection of EDTA and BAL. Administer EDTA intravenously whenever possible.

Chelating agents are administered deeply into a large muscle mass (Atraumatic Care box). To lessen the pain from $CaNa_2EDTA$, the local anesthetic procaine is injected with the drug. Rotation of sites is essential to prevent the formation of painful areas of fibrotic tissue. Because $CaNa_2EDTA$ and lead are toxic to the kidneys, records are kept of intake and output, and the results of urinalysis are assessed to monitor renal functioning. Because of the risk of seizures, appropriate precautions are instituted at the bedside of children with high blood lead levels (BLLs).

NURSE ALERT • $CaNa_2EDTA$ is never given in the absence of an adequate urinary output. Children receiving the drug intramuscularly must be able to maintain adequate oral intake of fluids.

Discharge planning for children with lead poisoning must include thorough education of families regarding safety from lead hazards, clear instructions regarding medication administration and needed follow-up, and confirmation that the child will be discharged to a home without lead hazards. Although caution must be used to avoid alarming parents unnecessarily, it is important that they know the risk implications for their child's behavior and cognitive functions. Nurses are in a position to make observations about the development and behavior of a child who is hospitalized. Concerns that are identified should be more thoroughly evaluated. Referral to a child development or speech and language specialist may be indicated.

As in any situational crisis, parents need support and understanding if their child is treated for lead poisoning. Many of the families at highest risk for lead poisoning have the fewest resources to comply with measures such as relocation or deleading the home. Appropriate referrals are essential in locating assistance for parents. (See also Nursing Care Plan: The Child with Lead Poisoning.*)

*In Wong DL, Hess CS: ***Wong and Whaley's clinical manual of pediatric nursing***, ed 5, St Louis, 2000, Mosby.

Key Points

- Common nutritional disturbances of infancy may result from vitamin and mineral deficiency or excess, some types of vegetarian diets, protein and calorie malnutrition, and food intolerance.
- Food consumption varies among vegetarians; therefore a detailed dietary intake is essential for planning adequate intakes, particularly in children and pregnant and lactating women.
- Protein-energy malnutrition may occur as a complication of underlying disease, lack of parental education about infant nutrition, inappropriate management of food allergy, or incorrect preparation of formula.
- Food intolerance encompasses food allergies and food sensitivities, the most serious of which are cow's milk allergy and lactose intolerance.
- Infants are subject to fluid depletion because of their greater surface area relative to body mass, high rate of metabolism, and immature kidney function.
- Dehydration can be classified as isotonic, hypotonic, and hypertonic.
- Vomiting and diarrhea account for significant fluid depletion, especially in infants and small children.
- The amount, frequency, and characteristics of stool and vomitus are important nursing observations.
- Diarrhea can be caused by an inflammatory process of infectious origin, a toxic reaction to ingestion of poisonous substances, dietary indiscretions, or infections outside the alimentary tract. The primary treatment of diarrhea is the use of oral rehydrating solution.
- Hirschsprung disease requires surgical removal of aganglionic segments of bowel.
- Postoperative care of the child with abdominal surgery involves assessing the abdomen, providing hydration and nutrition, intravenous fluids, proper positioning, wound care, and psychologic support.
- Nursing care of gastrointestinal (GI) reflux is aimed at identifying children with suggestive symptoms, helping parents with home care feeding and positioning, and caring for the child undergoing surgical intervention.
- Common infectious disorders during early childhood include communicable diseases, intestinal parasitic infections, conjunctivitis, and stomatitis.
- Nursing goals in the treatment of a communicable disease are identification, prevention of transmission, provision of comfort, and prevention of complications.
- Intestinal parasitic diseases constitute the most common infections in the world; giardiasis and enterobiasis are the most widespread parasitic infections among children in the United States.
- Although the cause of appendicitis is poorly understood, it is typically a result of obstruction of the lumen, usually by a fecalith. Common signs and symptoms are right lower quadrant abdominal pain, tenderness, and fever.
- Meckel diverticulum is a congenital malformation of the GI tract characterized by bloody stools.
- Inflammatory bowel disease refers to ulcerative colitis and Crohn disease. Chronic diarrhea is the most common feature. It is treated by dietary management and medication, although surgery is needed in some cases.
- Peptic ulcers are poorly understood, but contributing factors include interference with the normal protective mechanisms of the mucosal lining and the presence of *Helicobacter pylori.*
- Viral hepatitis is caused by six types of virus: hepatitis A virus, hepatitis B virus, hepatitis C virus, hepatitis D virus, hepatitis E virus, and hepatitis G virus.
- Hepatitis A virus is spread by the fecal-oral route, whereas hepatitis B and C viruses are transmitted primarily by the parenteral route. The most effective measure in prevention and control of hepatitis in any setting is handwashing.
- Structural disorders of the GI tract include cleft lip, cleft palate, esophageal atresia with tracheoesophageal fistula, anorectal malformations, and biliary atresia.
- Biliary atresia is a serious disorder, often causing progressive liver failure, which is an indication for liver transplantation.
- Cleft lip and palate, the most common facial malformation, may involve nutritional, dental, and speech problems.
- Hernias related to the GI tract can be minor (umbilical) or life threatening (diaphragmatic, gastroschisis, omphalocele).
- General signs of obstruction include colicky abdominal pain, nausea and vomiting, abdominal distention, and decreased stool output.
- Hypertrophic pyloric stenosis is recognized by characteristic projectile vomiting, malnutrition, dehydration, and a palpable mass in the epigastrium; it is relieved by pyloromyotomy.
- Intussusception is one of the most common causes of intestinal obstruction during infancy and is characterized by abdominal pain and blood in stools. Treatment is either non-surgical hydrostatic reduction or surgical reduction.

- Malabsorption syndromes are disorders associated with some degree of impaired digestion and/or absorption. They include digestive defects, absorptive defects, and anatomic defects.
- Celiac disease is characterized by an intolerance to gluten. It is thought to be either an inborn error of metabolism or an immunologic response.
- Short-bowel syndrome is characterized by a loss of intestine resulting in a diminished ability to absorb a regular diet normally. Specialized enteral and parenteral nutrition is a major element of care for these children.
- Although the incidence of poisoning has decreased in the last 30 years as a result of more stringent packaging regulations, childhood poisoning remains a serious health concern.
- The major principles of emergency treatment for poisoning are assessment, supportive measures, gastric decontamination, family support, and prevention of recurrence.
- Ipecac is an effective and safe emetic for home use in poisonings but is contraindicated in situations that increase the risk of aspiration and that involve ingestion of corrosives, in which case vomiting redamages the mucosa.
- Three simple measures that can reduce the severity of a poisoning are knowing the telephone number of the Poison Control Center, having ipecac in the home (two doses per child), and administering it correctly.
- Acetaminophen poisoning is the most common drug poisoning among children and occurs primarily from acute overdose.
- The most important factor contributing to lead poisoning is its availability in the child's environment. Lead-based paint is the most toxic source of lead.
- Because of increasing awareness of the detrimental effects of low levels of lead on the developing nervous system, acceptable blood lead levels have been decreasing and now are at less than 10 μg/dl.

References

American Academy of Pediatrics, Committee on Infectious Diseases, Pickering L, editor: *2000 Red Book: report of the Committee on Infectious Diseases,* ed 25, Elk Grove Village, IL, 2000, The Academy.

American Academy of Pediatrics, Committee on Infectious Diseases: Hepatitis C virus infection, *Pediatrics* 101(3):481-485, 1998.

American Academy of Pediatrics, Committee on Nutrition: *Pediatric nutrition handbook,* ed 4, Elk Grove Village, IL, 1998a, The Academy.

American Academy of Pediatrics, Committee on Nutrition: Soy protein-based formulas: recommendations for its use in infant feeding, *Pediatrics* 101(1):148-153, 1998b.

American Academy of Pediatrics, Provisional Committee on Quality Improvement, Subcommittee on Acute Gastroenteritis: Practice parameter: the management of acute gastroenteritis in young children, *Pediatrics* 97(3):424-435, 1996.

American Dietetic Association: ADA Reports: Position of the American Dietetic Association: vegetarian diets, *J Am Dietetic Assoc* 97(11):1317-1321, 1997.

Anderson JA: Milk, eggs, and peanuts: food allergies in children, *Am Fam Physician* 56(5):1365-1375, 1997.

Andres JM: Neonatal hepatobiliary disorders, *Clin Perinatol* 23(2):321-352, 1996.

Andrews KW, Savitz D, Hertz-Picciotto I: Prenatal lead exposure in relation to gestational age and birth weight: a review of epidemiologic studies, *Am J Ind Med* 26:13-32, 1994.

Balistreri WF: *Hepatitis C—pediatric implications.* Presented at the Thirty-fourth Annual Pediatric Postgraduate Course—Perspectives in Pediatrics, Bal Harbour, FL, Feb 5-11, 1999.

Behrman RE, Kliegman RM, Arvin AM: *Nelson textbook of pediatrics,* ed 16, Philadelphia, 2000, WB Saunders.

Berney B: Round and round it goes: the epidemiology of childhood lead poisoning, 1950-1990, *Milbank Q* 71(1):3-39, 1993.

Brayden RM et al: Behavioral antecedents to pediatric poisonings, *Clin Pediatr* 32(1):30-35, 1993.

Brewster DR, Manary MJ, Graham SM: Case management of kwashiorkor: an intervention project at seven nutrition rehabilitation centres in Malawi, *Eur J Clin Nutr* 51(3):139-147, 1997.

Brody DJ et al: Blood lead levels in the US population: phase I of the Third National Health and Nutrition Examination Survey (NHANES III, 1988-1991), *JAMA* 272:277-283, 1994.

Castiglia PT: Hepatitis in children, *J Pediatr Health Care* 10(6): 286-288, 1996.

Centers for Disease Control and Prevention: *Screening young children for lead poisoning: guidance for state and local public health officials,* Atlanta, 1997a, The Centers.

Centers for Disease Control and Prevention: Update: blood lead levels-United States, 1991-1994, *MMWR* 46(7):141-146, 1997b.

Cerquetti M et al: Role of *Clostridium difficile* in childhood diarrhea, *Pediatr Infect Dis J* 14(7):598-603, 1995.

Cody MM, Sottnek HM, O'Leary VS: Recovery of Giardia lamblia cysts from chairs and tables in child day-care centers, *Pediatrics* 94(6, pt 2):1006-1008, 1994.

David S, Lobo ML: Childhood diarrhea and malnutrition in Pakistan. I. Incidence and prevalence, *J Pediatr Nurs* 10(2):131-137, 1995.

Diamont M et al: Beware the hazards of activated charcoal, *Am J Nurs* 12:10, 1994.

Duggan C, Nurko S: Feeding the gut: the scientific basis for continued enteral nutrition during acute diarrhea, *J Pediatr* 131:801, 1997.

Finkelstein Y, Markowitz ME, Rosen JF: Low-level lead induced neurotoxicity in children: an update on central nervous system effects, *Brain Res Brain Res Rev* 27:168-176, 1998.

Fisher AM, Vessey JA: Preventing lead poisoning and its consequences, *Pediatr Nurs* 24(4):348-350, 1998.

Flake AW, Ryckman FC: Selected anomalies and intestinal obstruction. In Fanaroff AA, Martin RJ, editors: *Neonatal-perinatal medicine: diseases of the fetus and infant,* ed 6, St Louis, 1997, Mosby.

Fonkalsrud EW et al: Surgical treatment of gastroesophageal reflux in children: a combined hospital study of 7467 patients, *Pediatrics* 101(3):419-422, 1998.

Gastanaduy AS, Begue RE: Acute gastroenteritis, *Clin Pediatr* 38(1):1-12, 1999.

Gorelick MH, Shaw KN, Murphy KO: Validity and reliability of clinical signs in the diagnosis of dehydration in children, *Pediatrics* 99(5):e6, 1997.

Gormally S, Sherman PM, Drumm B: Gastritis and peptic ulcer disease. In Walker WA et al, editors: *Pediatric gastrointestinal disease: pathophysiology, diagnosis, management,* ed 2, St Louis, 1996, Mosby.

Halamek LP, Stevenson DK: Neonatal jaundice and liver disease. In Fanaroff AA, Martin RJ, editors: *Neonatal-perinatal medicine: diseases of the fetus and infant,* ed 6, St Louis, 1997, Mosby.

Held JC: Correcting fluid and electrolyte imbalances, *Nursing* 25(4):71, 1995.

Hendren WH: Pediatric rectal and perineal problems, *Pediatr Clin North Am* 45(6):1353-1371, 1998.

Hill DR: Giardiasis: issues in diagnosis and management, *Infect Dis Clin North Am* 7(3):503-525, 1993.

Hubbard P: Hepatitis C, *Am J Nurse Pract* 2(11):17-31, 1998.

Huffman S: Toddler's diarrhea, *J Pediatr Health Care* 13:32-33, 1999.

Hugger J, Harkless G, Rentschler D: Oral rehydration therapy for children with acute diarrhea, *Nurse Pract* 23(12):52-62, 1998.

Irish MS et al: The approach to common abdominal diagnoses in infants and children, *Pediatr Clin North Am* 45(4):729-772, 1998.

Jobe BA et al: *Clostridium difficile* colitis: an increasing hospital-acquired illness, *Am J Surg* 169(5):480-483, 1995.

Kirschner BS: Hirschsprung disease. In Walker WA et al, editors: *Pediatric gastrointestinal disease: pathophysiology, diagnosis, management,* ed 2, St Louis, 1996, Mosby.

Krebs-Smith SM et al: Fruit and vegetable intakes of children and adolescents in the United States, *Arch Pediatr Adolesc Med* 150(1):81-86, 1996.

Lasche J, Duggan C: Managing acute diarrhea: what every pediatrician needs to know, *Contemp Pediatr* 16(2):74-83, 1999.

Lee J, Nunn J, Wright C: Height and weight achievement in cleft lip and palate, *Arch Dis Child* 76(1):70-72, 1997.

Leichtner AM, Jackson WD, Grand RJ: Ulcerative colitis. In Walker WA et al, editors: *Pediatric gastrointestinal disease: pathophysiology, diagnosis, management,* ed 2, St Louis, 1996, Mosby.

Leung AK, Robson WL: Evaluating the child with chronic diarrhea, *Am Fam Physician* 53(2):635-643, 1996.

Liebelt EL, Shannon MW: Small doses, big problems: a selected review of highly toxic common medications, *Pediatr Emerg Care* 9(5):292-297, 1993.

Liebelt EL, Shannon MW: Oral chelators for childhood lead poisoning, *Pediatr Ann* 23:616-626, 1994.

Litovitz T et al: 1996 annual report of the American Association of Poison Control Centers Toxic Exposure Surveillance System, *Am J Emerg Med* 15(5):447-500, 1997.

Loening-Baucke V: Functional constipation, *Semin Pediatr Surg* 4(10):26-34, 1995.

Lund DP, Folkman J: Appendicitis. In Walker WA et al, editors: *Pediatric gastrointestinal disease: pathophysiology, diagnosis, management,* ed 2, St Louis, 1996, Mosby.

McBean LD, Miller GD: Allaying fears and fallacies about lactose intolerance, *J Am Diet Assoc* 98(6):671-676, 1998.

McEvoy CF, Suchy FJ: Biliary tract disease in children, *Pediatr Clin North Am* 43(1):75-98, 1996.

Meyers A: Modern management of acute diarrhea and dehydration in children, *Am Fam Physician* 51(5):1103-1135, 1995.

Murray JA: The widening spectrum of celiac disease, *Am J Clin Nutr* 69:354-365, 1999.

Najmaldin A, Tan HL: Early experience with laparoscopic pyloromyotomy for infantile hypertrophic pyloric stenosis, *J Pediatr Surg* 30(1):37-38, 1995.

Needleman HL: *Human lead exposure,* Boca Raton, 1992, CRC Press.

Olin BR et al: *Drug facts and comparisons,* St Louis, 2000, Facts and Comparisons.

Orenstein SR: Gastroesophageal reflux, *Pediatr Rev* 20(1):24-28, 1999.

Pearl RH et al: The approach to common abdominal diagnoses in infants and children, part II, *Pediatr Clin North Am* 46(6):1287-1326, 1998.

Perry H, Shannon M: Emergency department gastrointestinal decontamination, *Pediatr Ann* 25(1):19-26, 1996.

Richard M: Feeding the newborn with cleft lip and/or palate, the Enlargement, Stimulate, Swallow, Rest (ESSR) method, *J Pediatr Nurs* 6(5):317-321, 1991.

Richard ME: Weight comparisons of infants with complete cleft lip and palate, *Pediatr Nurs* 20(20):191-196, 1994.

Ryan D et al: Protecting children from lead poisoning and building healthy communities, *Am J Public Health* 89(6):822-824, 1999.

Ryckman F, Flake AW, Balistreri WF: Upper gastrointestinal disorders. In Fanaroff AA, Martin RJ, editors: *Neonatal-perinatal medicine: diseases of the fetus and infant,* ed 6, St Louis, 1997, Mosby.

Sanders TAB: Vegetarian diets and children, *Pediatr Clin North Am* 42(4):955-965, 1995.

Sazawal S et al: Zinc supplementation reduces the incidences of persistent diarrhea and dysentery among low socioeconomic children in India, *J Nutr* 126(2):443-450, 1996.

Schonfeld DJ, Needham D: Lead: a practical perspective, *Contemp Pediatr* 11:64-96, 1994.

Smith EA et al: Current urologic management of cloacal exstrophy: experience with 11 patients. *J Pediatr Surg* 32(2):256-262, 1997.

Speltz ML et al: Early predictors of attachment in infants with cleft lip and/or palate, *Child Dev* 68(1):12-25, 1997.

Srinivasan R, Minocha A: When to suspect lactose intolerance: symptomatic, ethnic, and laboratory clues, *Postgrad Med* 104(3):109-123, 1998.

Strahlman RS: Appendicitis. In Hoekelman RA et al, editors: *Primary pediatric care,* ed 3, St Louis, 1997, Mosby.

Twarog F: Another round: do maternal avoidance diets prevent atopy? *Pediatr Alert* 21(24):139-140, 1996.

United Network for Organ Sharing: Update, March 1995.

U.S. General Accounting Office: *Medicaid—elevated blood lead levels in children; Report to the Ranking Minority Member, Committee on Government Reform and Oversight, House of Representatives* (GAO/HEHS-98-78), Washington, DC, 1998.

Walker-Smith J: Celiac disease. In Walker WA et al, editors: *Pediatric gastrointestinal disease: pathophysiology, diagnosis, management,* ed 2, St Louis, 1996, Mosby.

Walterspiel JN et al: Secretory anti-Giardia lamblia antibodies in human milk: protective effect against diarrhea, *Pediatrics* 93(1):28-31, 1994.

Whitington PF: Chronic cholestasis of infancy, *Pediatr Clin North Am* 43(1):1-77, 1996.

Wigder HN et al: Emergency department poison advice telephone calls, *Ann Emerg Med* 25:349-352, 1995.

Wood RA: Prospects for the prevention of allergy in children, *Curr Opin Pediatr* 8(6):601-605, 1996.

Wylie R: Cow's milk protein allergy and hypoallergenic formulas, *Clin Pediatr* 35(10):497-500, 1996.

Wyszinski DF, Duffy DL, Beatty TH: Maternal cigarette smoking and oral clefts: a meta-analysis, *Cleft Palate Craniofac J* 34(3):206-210, 1997.

Zeiter DK, Hyams JS: Gastroesophageal reflux: pathogenesis, diagnosis, and treatment, *Allergy Asthma Proc* 20(1):45-49, 1999.

CHAPTER

48

Cardiovascular Dysfunction

http://www.harcourthealth.com/MERLIN/Wong/maternal/

Learning Objectives

On completion of this chapter the reader will be able to:

- Design a plan for assisting a child during a cardiac diagnostic procedure.
- Demonstrate an understanding of the hemodynamics, distinctive manifestations, and therapeutic management of congenital heart disease.
- Outline a plan of care for an infant or child with congestive heart failure.
- Describe the care for a child who has hypoxia.
- Describe the care for an infant or a child with a congenital heart defect and its surgical repair.
- Discuss the role of the nurse in helping the child and family cope with congenital heart disease.
- Differentiate between rheumatic fever and rheumatic heart disease.
- List the criteria for selected cholesterol screening of children.
- Discuss the assessment and management of hypertension in children and adolescents.
- Outline a plan of care for a child with Kawasaki disease.
- Describe the emergency treatment for shock, including anaphylaxis.

CARDIOVASCULAR DYSFUNCTION

Cardiovascular disorders in children are divided into two major groups: congenital heart disease and acquired heart disorders. *Congenital heart disease* includes primarily anatomic abnormalities present at birth that result in abnormal cardiac function. The clinical consequences of congenital heart defects fall into two broad categories: congestive heart failure and hypoxemia. *Acquired cardiac disorders* refer to disease processes or abnormalities that occur after birth and can be seen in the normal heart or in the presence of congenital heart defects. They result from various factors, including infection, autoimmune responses, environmental factors, and familial tendencies.

Assessment of Cardiac Function

History and Physical Examination. Nursing assessment of children for evidence of cardiac dysfunction begins with a careful history to elicit information regarding possible causes of heart disease: (1) history of heart disease in other family members, such as a parent or sibling; (2) contact with known teratogens, such as rubella, during pregnancy; (3) presence of chromosomal abnormalities, such as Down syndrome; (4) poor weight gain and/or feeding behavior; (5) frequent respiratory infections; (6) prior murmurs; (7) respiratory difficulties, such as tachypnea, dyspnea, and shortness of breath; (8) cyanosis; or (9) recent streptococcal infection in the child. Exercise intolerance and fatigue (e.g., during feeding in the infant) are characteristic features of heart disease.

The physical assessment of suspected heart disease begins with observation of general appearance and then proceeds with more specific observations. The following are supplementary to the general assessment techniques described for physical assessment of the chest and heart in Chapter 35.

Inspection

Nutritional state—Failure to thrive or poor weight gain is associated with heart disease.

Color—Cyanosis is a common feature of congenital heart disease, and pallor is associated with poor perfusion.

Chest deformities—An enlarged heart sometimes distorts the chest configuration.

Unusual pulsations—Visible pulsations of the neck veins are seen in some patients.

Respiratory excursion—This refers to the ease or difficulty of respiration (e.g., tachypnea, dyspnea, presence of expiratory grunt).

Clubbing of fingers—This is associated with cyanosis.

Palpation and Percussion

Chest—These maneuvers help discern heart size and other characteristics (e.g., thrills) associated with heart disease.

Abdomen—Hepatomegaly and/or splenomegaly may be evident.

Peripheral pulses—Rate, regularity, and amplitude (strength) may reveal discrepancies.

Auscultation

Heart rate and rhythm—Listen for fast heart rates (tachycardia), slow heart rates (bradycardia), or irregular rhythms.

Character of heart sounds—Listen for distinct or muffled sounds, murmurs, and additional heart sounds.

Diagnostic Evaluation. A variety of invasive and noninvasive tests may be used in the diagnosis of heart disease (Table 48-1). Cardiac catheterization, an invasive procedure done for both diagnostic and treatment purposes, is discussed in detail.

Cardiac Catheterization

Cardiac catheterization is a diagnostic procedure in which a radiopaque catheter is inserted through a peripheral blood vessel into the heart. The catheter is usually introduced through a cutdown procedure, in which a small incision is made to expose the vessel, or through a percutaneous technique, in which the catheter is threaded through a large-bore needle that is inserted into the vein. The catheter is guided through the heart with the aid of fluoroscopy. Once the tip of the catheter is within a heart chamber, contrast material is injected, and films are taken of the dilution and circulation of the material *(angiography)*. Types of cardiac catheterizations include:

Diagnostic catheterizations—These studies are used to diagnose congenital cardiac detects, particularly in symptomatic infants and before surgical repair. They are divided into right-sided catheterizations, in which the catheter is introduced through a vein (usually the femoral vein) and threaded to the right atrium (most common), and left-sided catheterization, in which the catheter is threaded through an artery into the aorta and into the heart.

Interventional catheterizations (therapeutic catheterizations)—A balloon catheter or other device is used to alter the cardiac anatomy. Examples include dilating stenotic valves or vessels or closing abnormal connections (Table 48-2).

Electrophysiology studies—Catheters with tiny electrodes that record the impulses of the heart directly from the conduction system are used to evaluate dysrhythmias and sometimes destroy accessory pathways that cause some tachydysrhythmias.

Nursing Care Management. Cardiac catheterization has become a routine diagnostic procedure and may be done on an outpatient basis. However, it is not without risks, especially in neonates and seriously ill infants and children. Typical reactions include acute hemorrhage from the entry site (more likely with interventional procedures because larger catheters are

TABLE 48-1

Procedures for Cardiac Diagnosis

Procedure	Description
Chest radiograph (x-ray)	Provides information on heart size and pulmonary blood flow patterns
Electrocardiography (ECG or EKG)	Graphic measure of electrical activity of heart
Holter monitor	24-Hour continuous ECG recording used to assess dysrhythmias
Echocardiography	Use of high-frequency sound waves obtained by a transducer to produce an image of cardiac structures
Transthoracic	Done with transducer on chest
M-mode	One-dimensional graphic view used to estimate ventricular size and function
Two-dimensional (2-D)	Real-time, cross sectional views of heart used to identify cardiac structures and cardiac anatomy
Doppler	Identifies blood flow patterns and pressure gradients across structures
Fetal	Imaging fetal heart in utero
Transesophageal (TEE)	Transducer placed in esophagus behind heart to obtain images of posterior heart structures or in patients with poor images from chest approach
Cardiac catheterization	Imaging study using radiopaque catheters placed in a peripheral blood vessel and advanced into heart to measure pressures and oxygen levels in heart chambers and visualize heart structures and blood flow patterns
Hemodynamics	Measures pressures and oxygen saturations in heart chambers
Angiography	Use of contrast material to illuminate heart structures and blood flow patterns
Biopsy	Use of special catheter to remove tiny samples of heart muscle for microscopic evaluation; used in assessing infection, inflammation, or muscle dysfunction disorders; also to evaluate for rejection after heart transplant
Electrophysiology (EPS)	Special catheters with electrodes used to record electrical activity from within heart; used to diagnose rhythm disturbances
Exercise stress test	Monitoring of heart rate, blood pressure, ECG, and oxygen consumption at rest and during progressive exercise on a treadmill or stationary bicycle
Cardiac magnetic resonance imaging (MRI)	Noninvasive imaging technique; used in evaluation of vascular anatomy outside of heart

used), low-grade fever, nausea, vomiting, loss of pulse in the catheterized extremity (usually transient, resulting from a clot, hematoma, or intimal tear), and transient dysrhythmias (generally catheter induced). Rare risks include stroke, seizures, tamponade, and death.

Preprocedural Care. A complete nursing assessment is necessary to ensure a safe procedure with minimum complications. This assessment should include accurate height (essential to correct catheter selection) and weight. Obtaining a history of allergic reactions is important because some of the contrast agents are iodine based. Specific attention to signs and symptoms of infection is crucial. Severe diaper rash may be a reason to cancel the procedure if femoral access is required. Because assessment of pedal pulses is important after catheterization, the nurse should assess and mark pulses (dorsalis pedis, posterior tibial) before the child goes to the catheterization room. The presence and quality of pulses in both feet are clearly documented. Baseline oxygen saturation using pulse oximetry in children with cyanosis is also recorded.

Preparing the child and family for the procedure is the joint responsibility of the physician and nurse. The cardiologist usually explains the procedure to the parents, but nurses can reinforce and clarify the information. Many parents and older children who undergo both cardiac catheterization and cardiac surgery say, in retrospect, that they were more anxious about cardiac catheterization than about the surgery. Preparation for cardiac catheterization requires the same attention to the principles of preparation for procedures described in Chapter 45.

It is important to describe the catheterization ("cath") room because the x-ray machinery can appear frightening. Other aspects of the procedure that should be explained (using words the child understands) include, specifically, that (1) the groin (or sometimes the antecubital fossa) is cleansed with a special brown solution; (2) the child will receive some medicine (lidocaine) in that area so that the skin will go to sleep; (3) a tube will be placed in a blood vessel, and the child may feel a little pushing at times; (4) when a special "medicine" (referring to the contrast material) is put into the tubing, the child may feel warm for a few seconds; and (5) as soon as the medicine is put in, the lights will go off and a machine will begin to take pictures. The last point is important to stress because younger children may associate the lights going off with "causing" the warm feeling from the contrast agent. As a result, they may become fearful of the dark and the noise from the machines.

Methods of sedation vary among institutions and may include oral or intravenous (IV) medications (Atraumatic Care box). The child's age, heart defect, clinical status, and type of catheterization procedure planned are considered when sedation is determined. General anesthesia may be needed for some interventional procedures. Children are allowed nothing by mouth (NPO) for 4 to 6 hours or more before the procedure according to institutional guidelines. Infants and patients with polycythemia may need IV fluids to prevent dehydration and hypoglycemia.

Postprocedural Care. Essentially the care following cardiac catheterization is the same as general postoperative care. However, because children are not anesthetized during the procedure, they usually return directly to their room. Patients are usually placed on a cardiac monitor and a pulse oximeter for the first few hours of recovery. The most important nursing responsibility is observation of the following for signs of complications:

- Pulses, especially below the catheterization site, for equality and symmetry (pulse distal to the site may be weaker for the first few hours after catheterization but should gradually increase in strength)
- Temperature and color of the affected extremity because coolness or blanching may indicate arterial obstruction
- Vital signs, which are taken as often as every 15 minutes, with special emphasis on heart rate, which is counted for 1 full minute for evidence of dysrhythmias or bradycardia

TABLE 48-2

Current Interventional Cardiac Catheterization Procedures in Children

Intervention	Diagnosis
Balloon atrioseptostomy (BAS) Well established in newborns May also be done under echo guidance	Transposition of great arteries Some complex single-ventricle defects
Balloon dilation Treatment of choice	Valvular pulmonic stenosis Branch pulmonary artery stenosis Congenital valvular aortic stenosis Rheumatic mitral stenosis Recurrent coarctation of aorta Further follow-up required in: Native coarctation of aorta in patients >7 months Congenital mitral stenosis
Coil occlusion Accepted alternative to surgery	Patent ductus arteriosus (<4 mm)
Transcatheter device closure Several devices in clinical trials	Atrial septal defect
Stent placement	Pulmonary artery stenosis Other lesions investigational
Radiofrequency ablation	Some tachydysrhythmias

Data from Allen HD et al: Pediatric therapeutic cardiac catheterization, AHA Scientific Statement, *Circulation* 97:609–625, 1998.

Atraumatic Care

CARDIAC CATHETERIZATION

To reduce the pain of the catheter insertion, apply EMLA topically to the site for 60 minutes or use buffered lidocaine and a 30-gauge needle for intradermal injection (see Pain Management, Chapter 44).

- Blood pressure, especially for hypotension, which may indicate hemorrhage from cardiac perforation or bleeding at the site of initial catheterization
- Dressing, for evidence of bleeding or hematoma formation in the femoral or antecubital area
- Fluid intake, both IV and oral, to ensure adequate hydration (blood loss in the catheterization laboratory, the child's NPO status, and diuretic actions of dyes used during the procedure put children at risk for hypovolemia and dehydration)
- Hypoglycemia, especially in infants who should receive dextrose-containing IV fluids; blood glucose levels should be checked

NURSE ALERT • If bleeding occurs, direct continuous pressure is applied 2.5 cm (1 inch) above the percutaneous skin site to localize pressure over the vessel puncture.

Depending on hospital policy, the child may be kept in bed with the affected extremity maintained straight for 4 to 6 hours after venous catheterization and 6 to 8 hours after arterial catheterization to facilitate healing of the cannulated vessel. If younger children have difficulty complying, they can be held in the parent's lap with the leg maintained in the correct position. The child's usual diet can be resumed as soon as tolerated, beginning with sips of clear liquids and advancing as the condition allows. The child is encouraged to void to clear the contrast material from the blood. Generally there is only slight discomfort at the percutaneous site. To prevent infection, the catheterization area is protected from possible contamination. If the child wears diapers, the dressing can be kept dry by covering it with a piece of plastic film and sealing the edges of the hem to the skin with tape. However, the nurse must be careful to continue to observe the site for any evidence of bleeding (Home Care box and Critical Thinking box).

(See also Nursing Care Plan: The Child Who Undergoes Cardiac Catheterization.*)

*In Wong DL, Hess CS: ***Wong and Whaley's clinical manual of pediatric nursing***, ed 5, St Louis, 2000, Mosby.

Home Care

AFTER CARDIAC CATHETERIZATION

Remove pressure dressing the day after catheterization. Cover site with an adhesive bandage strip for several days.
Keep site clean and dry. Avoid tub baths for several days; may shower.
Observe site for redness, swelling, drainage, and bleeding. Monitor for fever. Notify practitioner if these occur.
Avoid strenuous exercise for several days. May attend school.
Resume regular diet without restrictions.
Use acetaminophen or ibuprofen for pain.
Keep follow-up appointments per practitioner's instruction.

Modified from Children's Hospital (Boston) Cardiovascular Program, 1994.

CONGENITAL HEART DISEASE (CHD)

General Concepts

The incidence of CHD in children is generally believed to be 4 to 10 per 1000 live births and is the major cause of death in the first year (other than prematurity). The sexes are affected differently, depending on the defect. Children with CHD are also more likely to have extracardiac defects, such as tracheoesophageal fistula, renal agenesis, and diaphragmatic hernias.

The etiology of most congenital heart defects is not known. However, several factors are associated with a higher-than-normal incidence of the disease. These include prenatal factors such as (1) maternal rubella during pregnancy, (2) maternal alcoholism, (3) maternal age over 40 years, and (4) maternal type 1 diabetes. Several genetic factors are also implicated, although the influence is multifactorial. For example, there is an increased risk of CHD in the child who (1) has a sibling with a heart defect; (2) has a parent with CHD; (3) has a chromosomal aberration, such as Down syndrome; or (4) is born with other, noncardiac congenital anomalies.

Circulatory Changes at Birth. During fetal life, blood carrying oxygen and nutritive materials from the placenta enters the fetal system through the umbilicus via the large umbilical vein. Oxygenated blood enters the heart by way of the inferior vena cava. Because of the higher pressure of blood entering the right atrium, it is directed posteriorly in a straight pathway across the right atrium and through the *foramen ovale* to the left atrium. In this way the better-oxygenated blood enters the left atrium and ventricle, to be pumped through the aorta to the head and upper extremities. Blood from the head and upper extremities entering the right atrium from the superior vena cava is directed downward through the tricuspid valve into the right ventricle. From here it is pumped through the pulmonary artery, where the major portion is

Critical Thinking

CARDIAC CATHETERIZATION

Tommy, a 4-year-old with tetralogy of Fallot, has just returned from the catheterization laboratory. He has vomited, and his mother calls you to the bedside to tell you that he is bleeding. You arrive to find Tommy crying and sitting up in a puddle of blood. What is the first thing you should do?

First, Think About It . . .

- What concepts are central to your thinking?
- What are the implications?

1. Increase the rate of his IV fluids.
2. Give an antiemetic and keep Tommy NPO (nothing by mouth).
3. Call the cardiologist.
4. Lie Tommy down, remove the dressing, and apply direct pressure above the catheterization site.

The best response is 4. This may be an arterial bleed, and the implications are that Tommy is at risk for losing a large amount of blood in a short time. Your first priority should be to control the bleeding. Pressure is applied above the visible catheterization site where the vessel was entered. Placing the child flat decreases the effect of gravity on the rate of bleeding and is the appropriate position in case of shock. When this is done, you can notify the practitioner and replace fluids and control emesis as ordered.

shunted to the descending aorta via the *ductus arteriosus.* Only a small amount flows to and from the nonfunctioning fetal lungs (Fig. 48-1, *A*).

Before birth the high pulmonary vascular resistance created by the collapsed fetal lung causes greater pressures in the right side of the heart and the pulmonary arteries. At the same time, the free-flowing placental circulation and the ductus arteriosus produce a low vascular resistance in the remainder of the fetal vascular system. With the cessation of placental blood flow from clamping of the umbilical cord and expansion of the lungs at birth, the hemodynamics of the fetal vascular system undergo pronounced and abrupt changes (Fig. 48-1, *B*).

With the first breath, the lungs are expanded, and increased oxygen causes pulmonary vasodilation. Pulmonary pressures start to fall as systemic pressures, given the removal of the placenta, start to rise. Normally the foramen ovale closes as the pressure in the left atrium exceeds the pressure in the right atrium. The ductus arteriosus starts to close in the presence of increased oxygen concentration in the blood and other factors.

Altered Hemodynamics. To appreciate the physiology of heart defects, it is necessary to understand the role of pressure gradients, flow, and resistance within the circulation. As with any fluid, blood flows from an area of high pressure to one of lower pressure and toward the path of least resistance in response to the pumping action of the heart. In general the higher the pressure gradient, the greater the rate of flow; the higher the resistance, the lesser the rate of flow.

Normally the pressure on the right side of the heart is lower than that on the left side, and the resistance in the pulmonary circulation is less than that in the systemic circulation. Vessels entering or exiting these chambers have corresponding pressures. Therefore, if an abnormal connection exists between the heart chambers (such as a septal defect), blood will necessarily flow from an area of higher pressure (left side) to one of lower pressure (right side). Such a flow of blood is termed a *left-to-right shunt.* Anomalies resulting in cyanosis may result from a change in pressure so that the blood is shunted from the right to the left side of the heart *(right-to-left shunt)* because of either increased pulmonary vascular resistance or obstruction to blood flow through the pulmonic valve and artery. Cyanosis may also result from a defect that allows mixing of oxygenated and deoxygenated blood within the heart chambers or great arteries, such as occurs in truncus arteriosus.

Classification of Defects

Congenital heart defects have been divided into two categories. Traditionally cyanosis, a physical characteristic, has been used as the distinguishing feature, dividing the anomalies into *acyanotic defects* and *cyanotic defects.* In clinical practice this system is problematic because children with acyanotic defects may develop cyanosis. Also, more often, those with cyanotic defects may appear pink and have more clinical signs of congestive heart failure (CHF).

A more useful classification system is based on hemodynamic characteristics (blood flow patterns within the heart). These blood flow patterns are (1) *increased pulmonary blood flow,* (2) *decreased pulmonary blood flow,* (3) *obstruction to blood flow* out of the heart, and (4) *mixed blood flow,* in which saturated and desaturated blood mix within the heart or great arteries. As a comparison, both classification systems are outlined in Fig. 48-2.

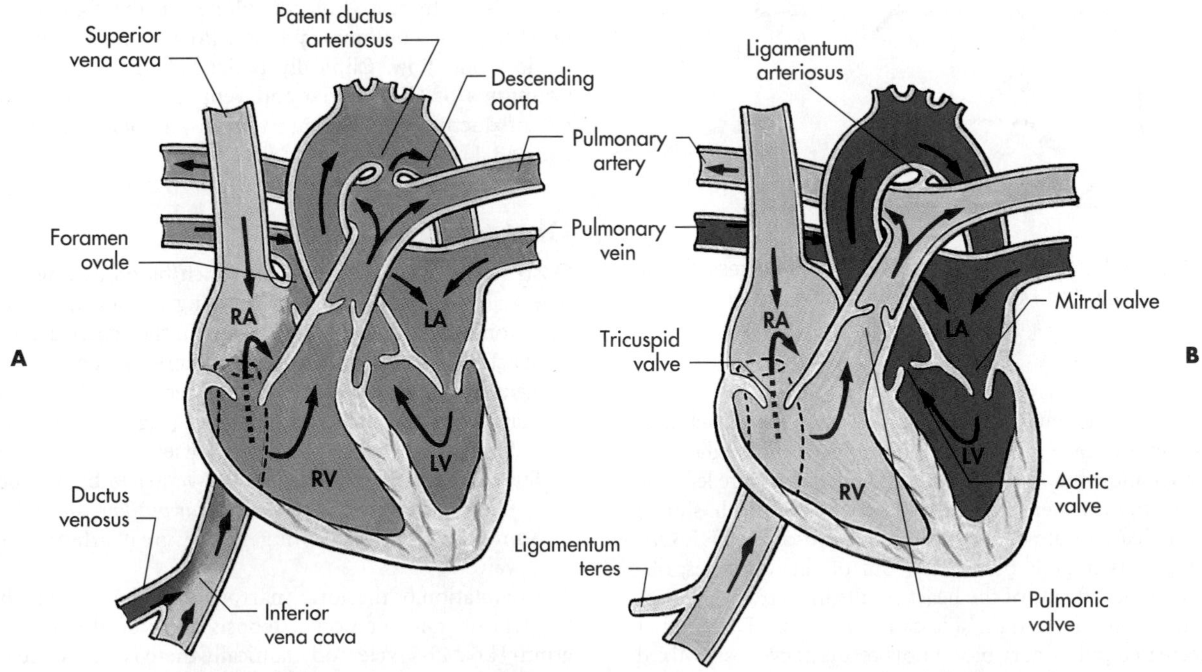

FIG. 48-1 • Changes in circulation at birth. **A,** Prenatal circulation. **B,** Postnatal circulation. Arrows indicate direction of blood flow. Although four pulmonary veins enter the left atrium, for simplicity this diagram shows only two. *RA,* Right atrium; *LA,* left atrium; *RV,* right ventricle; *LV,* left ventricle.

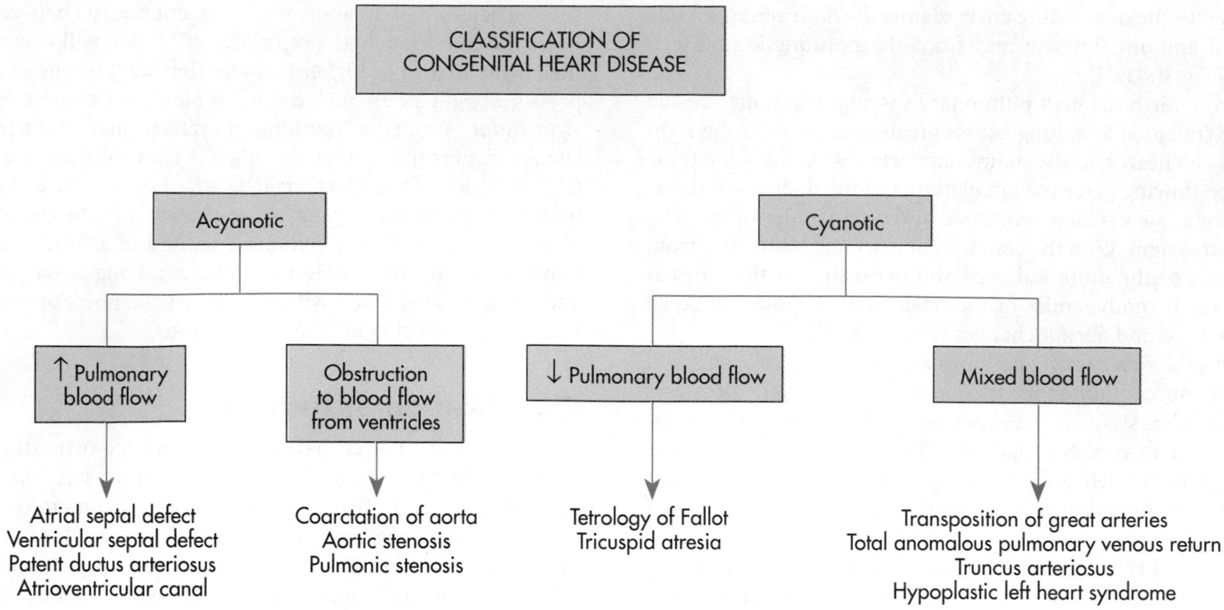

FIG. 48-2 • Comparison of acyanotic-cyanotic and hemodynamic classification systems of congenital heart disease.

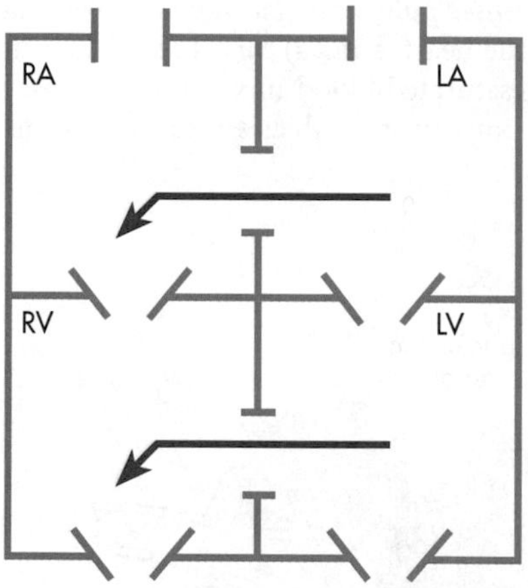

FIG. 48-3 • Hemodynamics in defects with increased pulmonary blood flow. See Fig. 48-1 for abbreviations.

With the hemodynamic classification system, the clinical manifestations of each group are more uniform and predictable. Defects that allow blood flow from the higher-pressure left side of the heart to the lower-pressure right side (left-to-right shunt) result in increased pulmonary blood flow and cause CHF. Obstructive defects impede blood flow out of the ventricles; obstruction on the left side of the heart results in CHF, whereas severe obstruction on the right side causes cyanosis. Defects that cause decreased pulmonary blood flow result in cyanosis. Mixed lesions present a variable clinical picture based on the degree of mixing and amount of pulmonary blood flow; hypoxemia (with or without cyanosis) and CHF usually occur together. This system is used in the following discussion.

Defects with Increased Pulmonary Blood Flow

In this group of cardiac defects, intracardiac communications along the septum or an abnormal connection between the great arteries allows blood to flow from the higher-pressure left side of the heart to the lower-pressure right side of the heart (Fig. 48-3). Increased blood volume on the right side of the heart increases pulmonary blood flow at the expense of systemic blood flow. Clinically patients demonstrate signs and symptoms of CHF. Atrial and ventricular septal defects and patent ductus arteriosus are typical anomalies in this group (Box 48-1).

Obstructive Defects

Obstructive defects are those in which blood exiting the heart meets an area of anatomic narrowing *(stenosis),* causing obstruction to blood flow. The pressure in the ventricle and in the great artery before the obstruction is increased, and the pressure in the area beyond the obstruction is decreased. The location of the narrowing is usually near the valve (Fig. 48-4), as follows:

Valvular—At the site of the valve itself

Subvalvular—Narrowing in the ventricle below the valve (also referred to as the *ventricular outflow tract)*

Supravalvular—Narrowing in the great artery above the valve

Coarctation of the aorta (narrowing of the aortic arch), aortic stenosis, and pulmonic stenosis are typical defects in this group (Box 48-2). Hemodynamically there is a pressure load on the ventricle and decreased cardiac output. Clinically infants and children exhibit signs of CHF. Children with mild obstruction may be asymptomatic. Rarely, as in severe pulmonic stenosis, hypoxemia may be seen.

Box 48-1

Defects With Increased Pulmonary Blood Flow

ATRIAL SEPTAL DEFECT (ASD)

Description: Abnormal opening between the atria, allowing blood from the higher-pressure left atrium to flow into the lower-pressure right atrium. There are three types:

Ostium primum (ASD 1)—Opening at lower end of septum; may be associated with mitral valve abnormalities

Ostium secundum (ASD 2)—Opening near center of septum

Sinus venosus defect—Opening near junction of superior vena cava and right atrium; may be associated with partial anomalous pulmonary venous connection

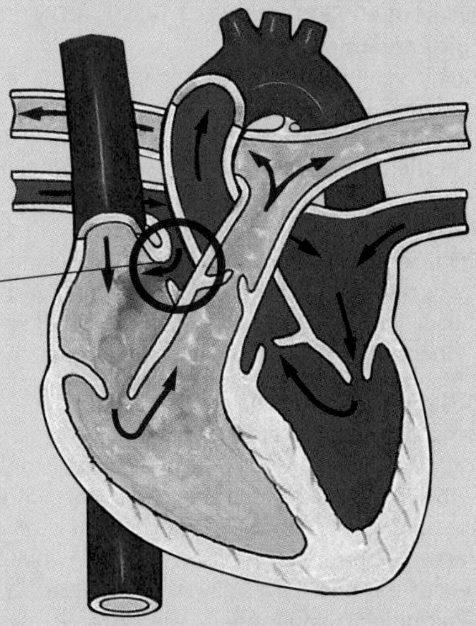

Pathophysiology: Because left atrial pressure slightly exceeds right atrial pressure, blood flows from the left to the right atrium, causing an increased flow of oxygenated blood into the right side of the heart. Despite the low pressure difference, a high rate of flow can still occur because of low pulmonary vascular resistance and the greater distensibility of the right atrium, which further reduces flow resistance. This volume is well tolerated by the right ventricle because it is delivered under much lower pressure than in a ventricular septal defect. Although there is right atrial and ventricular enlargement, cardiac failure is unusual in an uncomplicated ASD. Pulmonary vascular changes usually occur only after several decades if the defect is unrepaired.

Clinical manifestations: Patients may be asymptomatic. They may develop congestive heart failure (CHF). There is a characteristic murmur. Patients are at risk for atrial dysrhythmias (probably caused by atrial enlargement and stretching of conduction fibers) and pulmonary vascular obstructive disease and emboli formation later in life from chronic increased pulmonary blood flow.

Surgical treatment: Surgical Dacron patch closure of moderate to large defects similar to closure of ventricular septal defects. Open repair with cardiopulmonary bypass is usually performed before school age. In addition, the sinus venosus defect requires patch placement, so the anomalous right pulmonary venous return is directed to the left atrium with a baffle. The ASD 1 may require repair or, rarely, replacement of the mitral valve.

Nonsurgical treatment: ASD 2 may also be closed using devices during cardiac catheterization. This technique is in clinical trials in some centers.

Prognosis: Very low operative mortality, less than 1%.

VENTRICULAR SEPTAL DEFECT (VSD)

Description: Abnormal opening between the right and left ventricles. May be classified according to location: membranous (accounting for 80%) or muscular. May vary in size from a small pinhole to absence of the septum, resulting in a common ventricle. Frequently associated with other defects, such as pulmonary stenosis, transposition of the great vessels, patent ductus arteriosus, atrial defects, and coarctation of the aorta. Many VSDs (20% to 60%) are thought to close spontaneously. Spontaneous closure is most likely to occur during the first year of life in children having small or moderate defects. A left-to-right shunt is caused by the flow of blood from the higher-pressure left ventricle to the lower-pressure right ventricle.

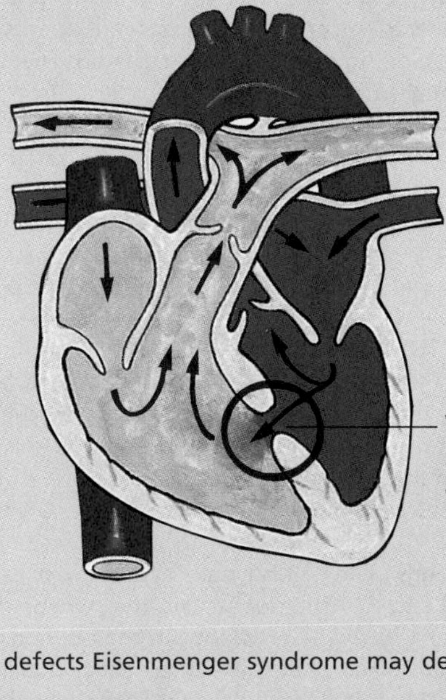

Pathophysiology: Because of the higher pressure within the left ventricle and because the systemic arterial circulation offers more resistance than the pulmonary circulation, blood flows through the defect into the pulmonary artery. The increased blood volume is pumped into the lungs, which may eventually result in increased pulmonary vascular resistance. Increased pressure in the right ventricle as a result of left-to-right shunting and pulmonary resistance causes the muscle to hypertrophy. If the right ventricle is unable to accommodate the increased workload, the right atrium may also enlarge as it attempts to overcome the resistance offered by incomplete right ventricular emptying. In severe defects Eisenmenger syndrome may develop (p. 1330).

Clinical manifestations: CHF is common. There is a characteristic murmur. Patients are at risk for bacterial endocarditis and pulmonary vascular obstructive disease. In severe defects, Eisenmenger syndrome may develop.

Continued

Box 48-1

Defects With Increased Pulmonary Blood Flow—cont'd

VENTRICULAR SEPTAL DEFECT (VSD)—CONT'D

Surgical treatment:

Palliative: Pulmonary artery banding (placing a band around the main pulmonary artery to decrease pulmonary blood flow) in infants in severe CHF was common in the past. It is unusual now as improvements in surgical techniques and postoperative care make complete repair in infancy the preferred approach.

Complete repair (procedure of choice): Small defects are repaired with a purse-string approach. Large defects usually require a knitted Dacron patch sewn over the opening. Both procedures are performed via cardiopulmonary bypass. The repair is generally approached through the right atrium and the tricuspid valve. Postoperative complications include residual VSD and conduction disturbances.

Nonsurgical treatment: Device closure during cardiac catheterization is under clinical trials in some centers for closure of muscular defects that carry a high operative risk.

Prognosis: Risks depend on the location of the defect, number of defects, and other associated cardiac defects. Single membranous defects have a low mortality (less than 5%); multiple muscular defects can have a risk of more than 20%.

ATRIOVENTRICULAR CANAL (AVC) DEFECT

Description: Incomplete fusion of endocardial cushions. Consists of a low atrial septal defect that is continuous with a high ventricular septal defect and clefts of the mitral and tricuspid valves, creating a large central atrioventricular (AV) valve that allows blood to flow between all four chambers of the heart. The directions and pathways of flow are determined by pulmonary and systemic resistance, left and right ventricular pressures, and the compliance of each chamber, although flow is generally from left to right. It is the most common cardiac defect in children with Down syndrome.

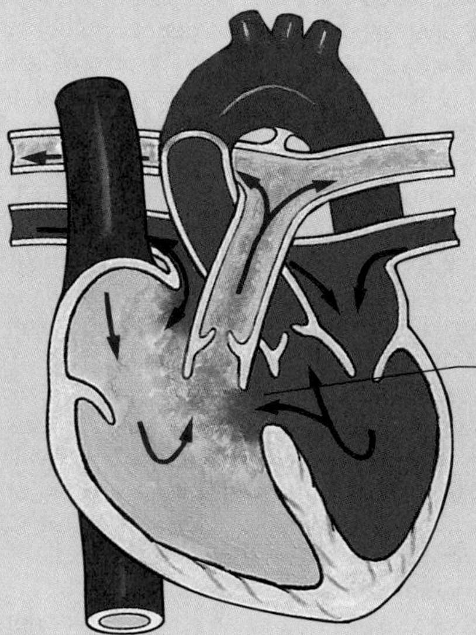

Pathophysiology: The alterations in the hemodynamics depend on the defect's severity and the child's pulmonary vascular resistance. Immediately after birth, while the newborn's pulmonary vascular resistance is high, there is minimum shunting of blood through the defect. Once this resistance falls, left-to-right shunting occurs and pulmonary blood flow increases. The resultant pulmonary vascular engorgement predisposes to development of CHF.

Clinical manifestations: Patients usually have moderate to severe CHF. There is a characteristic murmur. There may be mild cyanosis that increases with crying. Patients are at high risk for developing pulmonary vascular obstructive disease.

Surgical treatment:

Palliative: Pulmonary artery banding for infants with severe symptoms that are caused by increased pulmonary blood flow is performed in some centers. Most centers perform complete repair in infancy.

Complete repair: Surgical repair consists of patch closure of the septal defects and reconstruction of the AV valve tissue (either repair of the mitral valve cleft or fashioning two AV valves). If the mitral valve defect is severe, a valve replacement may be needed. Postoperative complications include heart block, CHF, mitral regurgitation, dysrhythmias, and pulmonary hypertension.

Prognosis: Operative mortality is less than 10%. A potential later problem is mitral regurgitation, which may require valve replacement.

PATENT DUCTUS ARTERIOSUS (PDA)

Description: Failure of the fetal ductus arteriosus (artery connecting the aorta and pulmonary artery) to close within the first weeks of life. The continued patency of this vessel allows blood to flow from the higher-pressure aorta to the lower-pressure pulmonary artery, causing a left-to-right shunt.

Pathophysiology: The hemodynamic consequences of PDA depend on the size of the ductus and the pulmonary vascular resistance. At birth the resistance in the pulmonary and systemic circulations is almost identical, thus equalizing the resistance in the aorta and pulmonary artery. As the systemic pressure exceeds the pulmonary pressure, blood begins to shunt from the aorta, across the duct, to the pulmonary artery (left-to-right shunt). The additional blood is recirculated through the lungs and returned to the left atrium and left ventricle. The effect of this altered circulation is increased workload on the left side of the heart, increased pulmonary vascular congestion and possibly resistance, and potentially increased right ventricular pressure and hypertrophy.

Clinical manifestations: Patients may be asymptomatic or show signs of CHF. There is a characteristic machinery-like murmur. A widened pulse pressure and bounding pulses result from runoff of blood from the aorta to the pulmonary artery. Patients are at risk for bacterial endocarditis and pulmonary vascular obstructive disease in later life from chronic excessive pulmonary blood flow.

Box 48-1
Defects With Increased Pulmonary Blood Flow—cont'd

PATENT DUCTUS ARTERIOSUS (PDA)—CONT'D

Medical management: Administration of indomethacin (prostaglandin inhibitor) has proved successful in closing a patent ductus in premature infants and some newborns.

Surgical treatment: Surgical division or ligation of the patent vessel via a left thoracotomy. A newer technique, visual-assisted thoracoscopic surgery (VATS), uses a thoracoscope and instruments placed through three small incisions on the left side of the chest to place a clip on the ductus. It is used in some centers and eliminates the need for a thoracotomy, thereby speeding postoperative recovery.

Nonsurgical treatment: Use of coils to occlude the PDA in the catheterization laboratory is done in many centers. Small infants (with small-diameter femoral arteries) and those patients with large or unusual PDAs may require surgery.

Prognosis: Both procedures can be done at low risk, with less than 1% mortality.

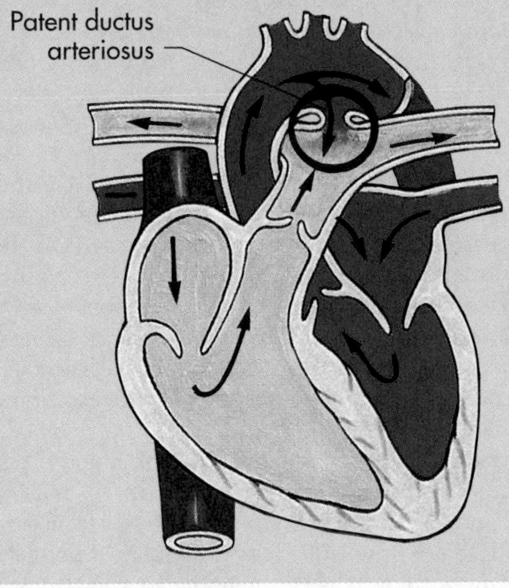

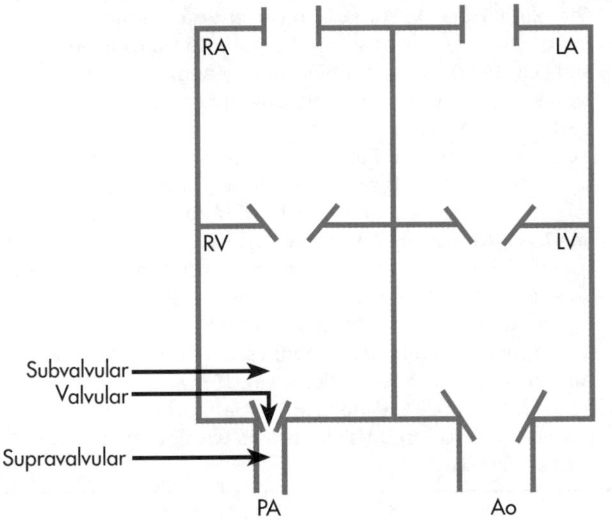

FIG. 48-4 • Obstruction to ventricular ejection can occur at the valvular level (shown), below the valve (subvalvular), or above the valve (supravalvular). Pulmonary stenosis is shown here. See Fig. 48-1 for abbreviations.

Defects with Decreased Pulmonary Blood Flow

In this group of defects, there is obstruction of pulmonary blood flow and an anatomic defect (atrial septal defect [ASD] or ventricular septal defect [VSD]) between the right and left sides of the heart (Fig. 48-5). Because blood has difficulty exiting the right side of the heart via the pulmonary artery, pressure on the right side increases, exceeding left-sided pressure. This allows desaturated blood to shunt right to left, causing desaturation in the left side of the heart and in the systemic circulation. Clinically these patients are hypoxemic and usually appear cyanotic. Tetralogy of Fallot and tricuspid atresia are the more common defects in this group (Box 48-3).

Mixed Defects

Many complex cardiac anomalies are classified together in the *mixed* category (Box 48-4) because survival in the postnatal period depends on mixing of blood from the pulmonary and systemic circulations within the heart chambers. Hemodynamically, fully saturated systemic blood flow mixes with the desaturated pulmonary blood flow, causing a relative desaturation of the systemic blood flow. Pulmonary congestion occurs because the differences in pulmonary artery pressure and aortic pressure favor pulmonary blood flow. Cardiac output decreases because of a volume load on the ventricle. Clinically these patients have a variable picture that combines some degree of desaturation (although cyanosis is not always visible) and signs of CHF. Some defects, such as transposition of the great arteries, cause severe cyanosis in the first days of life and later cause CHF. Others, such as truncus arteriosus, cause severe CHF in the first weeks of life and mild desaturation.

CLINICAL CONSEQUENCES OF CONGENITAL HEART DISEASE

Congestive Heart Failure (CHF)

CHF is the inability of the heart to pump an adequate amount of blood to the systemic circulation at normal filling pressures to meet the metabolic demands of the body. In children CHF most commonly occurs secondary to structural abnormalities (e.g., septal defects) that result in increased blood volume and pressure within the heart. It can also result from myocardial failure in which the contractility of the ventricle is impaired. This can occur with cardiomyopathy, dysrhythmias, or severe electrolyte

Box 48-2

Obstructive Defects

COARCTATION OF THE AORTA (COA)

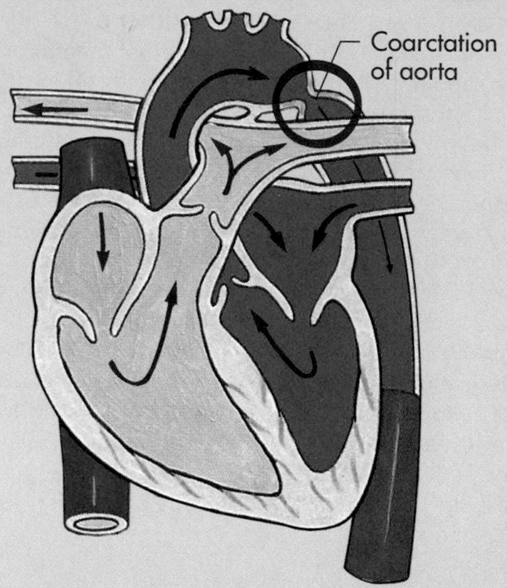

Description: Localized narrowing near the insertion of the ductus arteriosus, resulting in increased pressure proximal to the defect (head and upper extremities) and decreased pressure distal to the obstruction (body and lower extremities).

Pathophysiology: The effect of a narrowing within the aorta is increased pressure proximal to the defect and decreased pressure distal to it. In the preductal type of COA the lower half of the body is supplied with blood by the right ventricle through the ductus arteriosus. In the postductal type, right ventricular outflow cannot maintain blood flow to the descending aorta. Therefore collateral circulation develops during fetal life to maintain flow from the ascending to the descending aorta.

Clinical manifestations: There may be high blood pressure and bounding pulses in arms, weak or absent femoral pulses, and cool lower extremities with lower blood pressure. There are signs of congestive heart failure (CHF) in infants. Often these patients' hemodynamic condition deteriorates rapidly, and they are admitted to the intensive care unit near death, usually severely acidotic and hypotensive. Mechanical ventilation and inotropic support are often necessary before surgery. Older children may experience dizziness, headaches, fainting, and epistaxis resulting from hypertension. Patients are at risk for hypertension, ruptured aorta, aortic aneurysm, or stroke.

Surgical treatment: Either resection of the coarcted portion with an end-to-end anastomosis of the aorta or enlargement of the constricted section using a graft of prosthetic material or a portion of the left subclavian artery. Because this defect is outside the heart and pericardium; cardiopulmonary bypass is not required and a thoracotomy incision is used. Postoperative hypertension (greater than 160 mm Hg) is treated with intravenous sodium nitroprusside or amrinone, followed by oral medications, such as captopril, hydralazine, and/or propranolol. Residual permanent hypertension after repair of COA seems to be related to age and time of repair. To prevent both hypertension at rest and exercise-provoked systemic hypertension after repair, elective surgery for COA is advised within the first 2 years of life. There is a 5% to 10% risk of recurrent narrowing in patients who underwent surgical repair as infants (Hougen and Sell, 1995). Percutaneous balloon angioplasty techniques have proved to be very effective in relieving residual postoperative coarctation gradients.

Nonsurgical treatment: Balloon angioplasty as a primary intervention for COA is being performed in some centers, but concerns about inadequate relief of gradients, risk of aneurysm formation, and restenosis have limited its widespread use. Recent studies have demonstrated that balloon angioplasty is effective in children and that aneurysm formation is rare. The high restenosis rate in infants younger than 7 months old limits its application in this group, and further study is needed (Allen et al, 1998).

Prognosis: Less than 5% mortality in patients with isolated coarctation; increased risk in infants with other complex cardiac defects.

AORTIC STENOSIS (AS)

Description: Narrowing or stricture of the aortic valve, causing resistance to blood flow in the left ventricle, decreased cardiac output, left ventricular hypertrophy, and pulmonary vascular congestion. The prominent anatomic consequence of AS is the hypertrophy of the left ventricular wall, which eventually will lead to increased end-diastolic pressure, resulting in pulmonary venous and pulmonary arterial hypertension. Left ventricular hypertrophy also interferes with coronary artery perfusion and may result in myocardial infarction or scarring of the papillary muscles of the left ventricle, causing mitral insufficiency. ***Valvular stenosis,*** the most common type, is usually caused by malformed cusps resulting in a bicuspid rather than tricuspid valve or fusion of the cusps. ***Subvalvular stenosis*** is a stricture caused by a fibrous ring below a normal valve; ***supravalvular stenosis*** occurs infrequently. Valvular AS is a serious defect for the following reasons: (1) the obstruction tends to be progressive; (2) sudden episodes of myocardial ischemia, or low cardiac output, can result in sudden death; and (3) surgical repair rarely results in a normal valve. This is one of the rare instances in which strenuous physical activity may be curtailed because of the cardiac condition.

Pathophysiology: A stricture in the aortic outflow tract causes resistance to ejection of blood from the left ventricle. The extra workload on the left ventricle causes hypertrophy. If left ventricular failure develops, left atrial pressure will increase; this causes increased pressure in the pulmonary veins, resulting in pulmonary vascular congestion (pulmonary edema).

Clinical manifestations: Infants with severe defects demonstrate signs of decreased cardiac output with faint pulses, hypotension, tachycardia, and poor feeding. Children show signs of exercise intolerance, chest pain, and dizziness when standing for a long period. There is a characteristic murmur. Patients are at risk for bacterial endocarditis, coronary insufficiency, and ventricular dysfunction.

Box 48-2
Obstructive Defects—cont'd

Valvular Aortic Stenosis

Surgical treatment: Aortic valvotomy under inflow occlusion.

Prognosis: Aortic valvotomy in critically ill neonates and infants still carries a mortality of 10% to 20% in major medical centers (Park, 1996). Results of aortic valvotomy in older children are very good, with mortality close to 0%. However, aortic valvotomy remains a palliative procedure, and approximately 25% of patients require additional surgery within 10 years for recurrent stenosis. A valve replacement may be required at the second procedure.

Nonsurgical treatment: Dilating narrowed valve with balloon angioplasty in the catheterization laboratory.

Prognosis: Complications include aortic insufficiency or valvular regurgitation, tearing of the valve leaflets, and loss of pulse in the catheterized limb. Relief of obstruction is similar to that for surgical valvotomy (Justo, 1996).

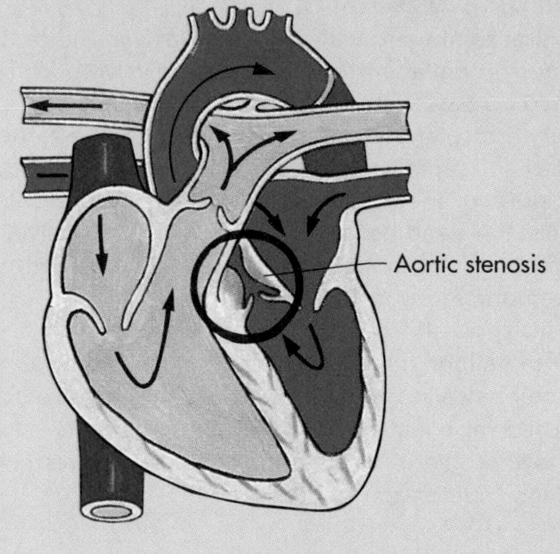

Subvalvular Aortic Stenosis

Surgical treatment: May involve incising a membrane if one exists or cutting the fibromuscular ring. If the obstruction results from narrowing of the left ventricular outflow tract and a small aortic valve annulus, a patch may be required to enlarge the entire left ventricular outflow tract and annulus and replace the aortic valve, an approach known as the ***Konno*** procedure. An aortic homograft with a valve may also be used ***(extended aortic root replacement),*** or the pulmonary valve may be moved to the aortic position and replaced with a homograft valve (***Ross*** procedure).

Prognosis: Mortality from surgical repairs of subvalvular AS is less than 2% in major centers; however, about 10% of these patients develop recurrent subaortic stenosis and require additional surgery (Park, 1996). All operations to replace the aortic root and enlarge the left ventricular outflow tract require further evaluation.

PULMONIC STENOSIS (PS)

Description: Narrowing at the entrance to the pulmonary artery. Resistance to blood flow causes right ventricular hypertrophy and decreased pulmonary blood flow. ***Pulmonary atresia*** is the extreme form of PS in that there is total fusion of the commissures and no blood flows to the lungs. The right ventricle may be hypoplastic.

Pathophysiology: When PS is present, resistance to blood flow causes right ventricular hypertrophy. If right ventricular failure develops, right atrial pressure will increase, and this may result in reopening of the foramen ovale, shunting of unoxygenated blood into the left atrium, and systemic cyanosis. If PS is severe, CHF occurs, and systemic venous engorgement will be noted. An associated defect such as a patent ductus arteriosus (PDA) partially compensates for the obstruction by shunting blood from the aorta to the pulmonary artery and into the lungs.

Clinical manifestations: Patients may be asymptomatic; some have mild cyanosis of CHF. Newborns with severe narrowing will be cyanotic. There is a characteristic murmur. Cardiomegaly is evident on chest x-ray film. Patients are at risk for bacterial endocarditis, with progressive narrowing causing increased symptoms.

Surgical treatment: In infants, transventricular (closed) valvotomy ***(Brock)*** procedure. In children, pulmonary valvotomy with cardiopulmonary bypass. Need for surgical treatment is uncommon with widespread use of balloon angioplasty techniques.

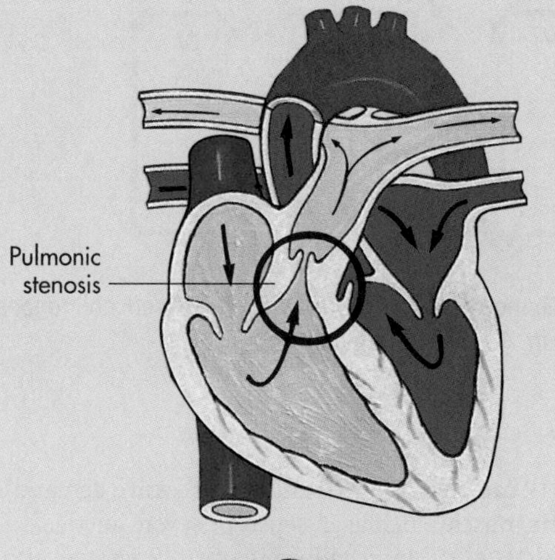

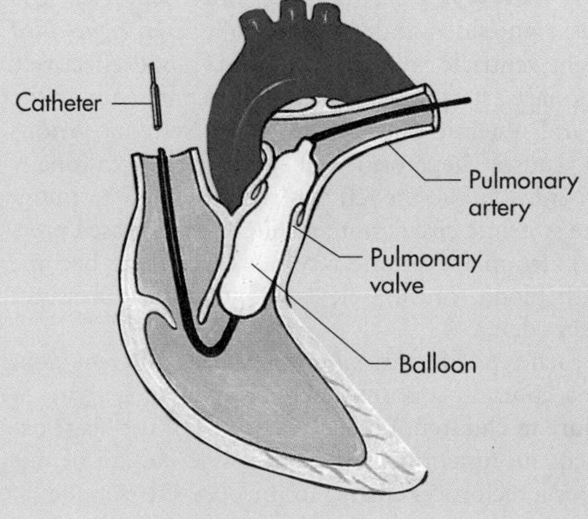

Continued

Box 48-2

Obstructive Defects—cont'd

PULMONIC STENOSIS—cont'd

Nonsurgical treatment: Balloon angioplasty in the cardiac catheterization laboratory to dilate the valve. A catheter is inserted across the stenotic pulmonic valve into the pulmonary artery, and a balloon at the end of the catheter is inflated and rapidly passed through the narrowed opening (see figure, p. 1317). The procedure is associated with few complications and has proved to be highly effective. It is the treatment of choice for discrete PS in most centers and can be done safely in neonates.

Prognosis: Low risk for both procedures; less than 2% mortality. Both balloon dilation and surgical valvotomy leave the pulmonic valve incompetent because they involve opening the fused valve leaflets; however, these patients are clinically asymptomatic. Long-term problems with restenosis or valve incompetence may occur.

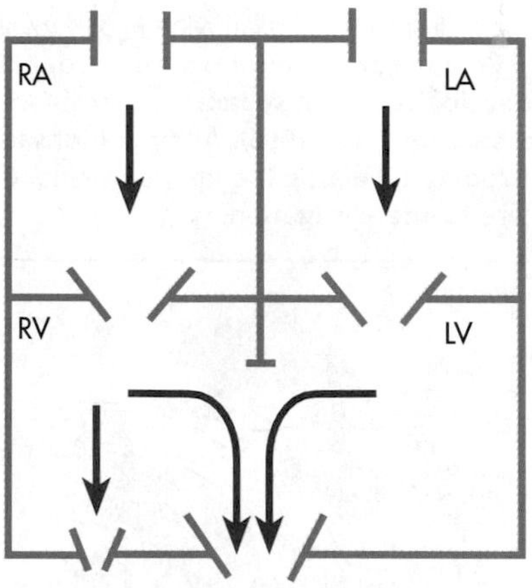

FIG. 48-5 • Hemodynamic defects with decreased pulmonary blood flow. See Fig. 48-1 for abbreviations.

disturbances. CHF can also occur because of excessive demands on a normal heart muscle, such as in sepsis or severe anemia.

Pathophysiology. Heart failure is often separated into two categories: right-sided and left-sided failure. In *right-sided failure* the right ventricle is unable to pump blood effectively into the pulmonary artery, resulting in increased pressure in the right atrium and systemic venous circulation. Systemic venous hypertension causes hepatosplenomegaly and occasionally edema. In *left-sided failure* the left ventricle is unable to pump blood into the systemic circulation, resulting in increased pressure in the left atrium and pulmonary veins. The lungs become congested with blood, causing elevated pulmonary pressures and pulmonary edema.

Although each type of heart failure produces different signs and symptoms, clinically it is unusual to observe solely right- or left-sided failure in children. Because each side of the heart depends on adequate function of the other side, failure of one chamber causes a reciprocal change in the opposite chamber.

If the abnormalities precipitating CHF are not corrected, the heart muscle becomes damaged. Despite compensatory mechanisms, the heart is unable to maintain an adequate cardiac output. Decreased blood flow to the kidneys continues to stimulate sodium and water reabsorption, leading to hypervolemia, increased workload on the heart, and congestion in the pulmonary and systemic circulations (Fig. 48-6).

The signs and symptoms of CHF can be divided into three groups: (1) impaired myocardial function, (2) pulmonary congestion, and (3) systemic venous congestion (Box 48-5). Because these hemodynamic changes occur from different causes and at differing times, the clinical presentation may vary among children.

Diagnostic Evaluation. Diagnosis of CHF is made on the basis of clinical manifestations. A chest x-ray film demonstrates cardiomegaly and increased pulmonary vascular markings caused by increased pulmonary blood flow. Ventricular hypertrophy appears on the electrocardiogram (ECG).

Therapeutic Management. The goals of treatment are to (1) improve cardiac function, (2) remove accumulated fluid, (3) decrease cardiac demands, and (4) improve tissue oxygenation and decrease oxygen consumption.

Improve Cardiac Function. Myocardial efficiency is improved through administration of digitalis glycosides. The beneficial effects are increased cardiac output, decreased heart size, decreased venous pressure, and relief of edema. In pediatrics, *digoxin (Lanoxin)* is used almost exclusively because of its more rapid onset. It is available as an elixir (0.05 mg/ml) for oral administration. For infants the dose is calculated in micrograms (1000 μg = 1 mg).

Treatment consists of a digitalizing dose, given orally or intravenously in divided doses over 24 hours to produce optimum cardiac effects, and a maintenance dose, given orally twice a day to maintain blood levels. During digitalization the child is monitored by means of an ECG to observe for the desired effects (prolonged P-R interval and reduced ventricular rate) and detect side effects, especially dysrhythmias.

NURSE ALERT • Therapeutic serum digoxin levels range from 0.8 to 2.0 μg/L.

Text continued on p. 1325

Box 48-3

Defects With Decreased Pulmonary Blood Flow

TETRALOGY OF FALLOT (TOF)

Description: The classic form includes four defects: (1) ventricular septal defect, (2) pulmonic stenosis, (3) overriding aorta, and (4) right ventricular hypertrophy.

Pathophysiology: The altered hemodynamics vary widely, depending primarily on the degree of pulmonary stenosis, but also on the size of the ventricular septal defect (VSD) and the pulmonary and systemic resistance to flow. Because the VSD is usually large, pressures may be equal in the right and left ventricles. Therefore the shunt direction depends on the difference between pulmonary and systemic vascular resistance. If pulmonary vascular resistance is higher than systemic resistance, the shunt is from right to left. If systemic resistance is higher than pulmonary resistance, the shunt is from left to right. Pulmonic stenosis decreases blood flow to the lungs and, consequently, the amount of oxygenated blood that returns to the left side of the heart. Depending on the position of the aorta, blood from both ventricles may be distributed systemically.

Clinical manifestations:

Infants: Some infants may be acutely cyanotic at birth; others have mild cyanosis that progresses over the first year of life as the pulmonic stenosis worsens. There is a characteristic murmur. There are acute episodes of cyanosis and hypoxia, called *blue spells* or *tet spells* (p. 1330). Anoxic spells occur when the infant's oxygen requirements exceed the blood supply, usually during crying or after feeding.

Children: With increasing cyanosis, there may be clubbing of the fingers, squatting, and poor growth.

Patients are at risk for emboli, cerebrovascular disease, brain abscess, seizures, and loss of consciousness or sudden death following an anoxic spell.

Surgical treatment:

Palliative shunt: In infants who cannot undergo primary repair, a palliative procedure to increase pulmonary blood flow and increase oxygen saturation may be performed. The preferred procedure is the ***Blalock-Taussig*** or ***modified Blalock-Taussig shunt,*** which provides blood flow to the pulmonary arteries from the left or right subclavian artery (see Table 48-4). In general, however, shunts are avoided because they may result in pulmonary artery distortion.

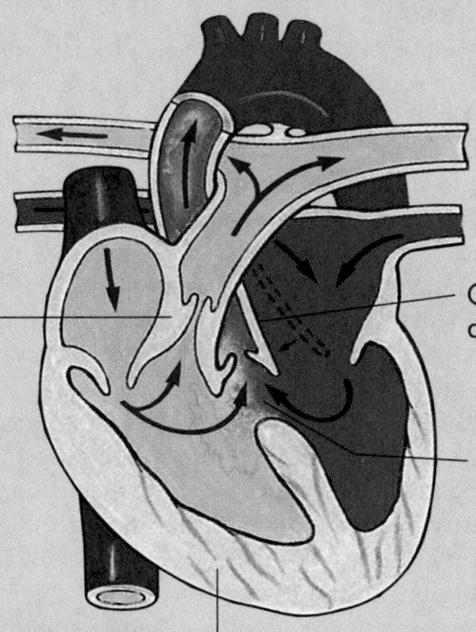

Complete repair: Elective repair is usually performed in the first year of life. Indications for repair include increasing cyanosis and the development of hypercyanotic spells. Complete repair involves closure of the VSD and resection of the infundibular stenosis, with a pericardial patch to enlarge the right ventricular outflow tract. The procedure requires a median sternotomy and the use of cardiopulmonary bypass.

Prognosis: The operative mortality for total correction of TOF is less than 5%. With improved surgical techniques there is a lower incidence of dysrhythmias and sudden death; surgical heart block is rare. Congestive heart failure (CHF) may occur postoperatively.

Continued

Box 48-3

Defects With Decreased Pulmonary Blood Flow—cont'd

TRICUSPID ATRESIA

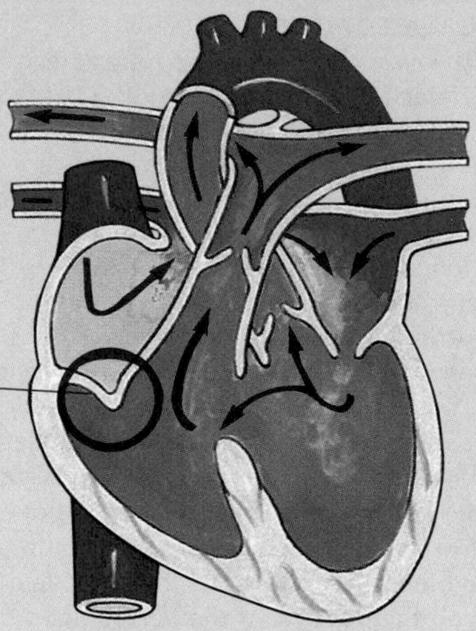

Description: Failure of the tricuspid valve to develop; consequently, there is no communication from the right atrium to the right ventricle. Blood flows through an atrial septal defect (ASD) or a patent foramen ovale to the left side of the heart and through a VSD to the right ventricle and out to the lungs. It is often associated with pulmonic stenosis and transposition of the great arteries. There is complete mixing of unoxygenated and oxygenated blood in the left side of the heart, resulting in systemic desaturation and varying amounts of pulmonary obstruction, causing decreased pulmonary blood flow.

Pathophysiology: At birth the presence of a patent foramen ovale (or other atrial septal opening) is required to permit blood flow across the septum into the left atrium; the patent ductus arteriosus allows blood flow to the pulmonary artery into the lungs for oxygenation. A VSD allows a modest amount of blood to enter the right ventricle and pulmonary artery for oxygenation. Pulmonary blood flow usually is diminished.

Clinical manifestations: Cyanosis is usually seen in the newborn period. There may be tachycardia and dyspnea. Older children have signs of chronic hypoxemia with clubbing. Patients are at risk for bacterial endocarditis, brain abscess, and stroke.

Therapeutic management: For the neonate whose pulmonary blood flow depends on the patency of the ductus arteriosus, a continuous infusion of prostaglandin E_1 is started until surgical intervention can be arranged.

Surgical treatment: ***Palliative*** treatment is the placement of a shunt ***(pulmonary-to-systemic artery anastomosis)*** to increase blood flow to the lungs. If the ASD is small, an atrial septostomy is done during cardiac catheterization. Some children have increased pulmonary blood flow and require ***pulmonary artery banding*** to lessen the volume of blood to the lungs. A ***bidirectional Glenn shunt*** (cavopulmonary anastomosis) may be performed at 6 to 9 months as a second stage.

Modified Fontan procedure: Systemic venous return is directed to the lungs without a ventricular pump through surgical connections between the right atrium and the pulmonary artery. A fenestration (opening) in the right atrial baffle is sometimes done to relieve pressure. The patient must have normal ventricular function and a low pulmonary vascular resistance for the procedure to be successful. The modified Fontan procedure separates oxygenated and unoxygenated blood inside the heart and eliminates the excess volume load on the ventricle but does not restore normal anatomy or hemodynamics.

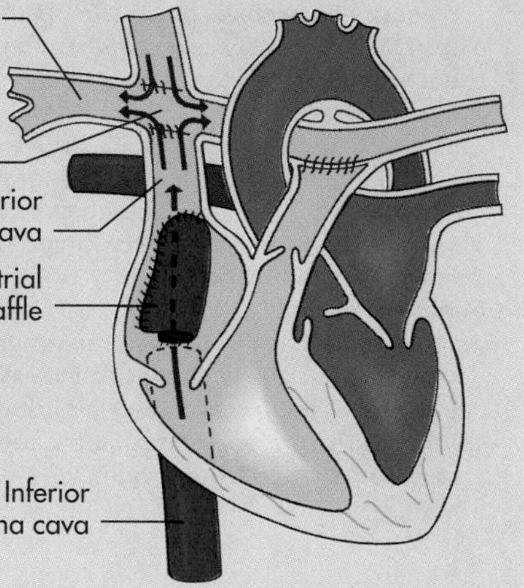

Prognosis: Surgical mortality varies. It is less than 10% in many centers and increases with more complex anatomy and other risk factors. Postoperative complications include dysrhythmias, systemic venous hypertension, pleural and pericardial effusions, and ventricular dysfunction. Although initial results have been encouraging, long-term survival and morbidity must await future studies.

Box 48-4

Mixed Defects

TRANSPOSITION OF THE GREAT ARTERIES (TGA) OR TRANSPOSITION OF THE GREAT VESSELS (TGV)

Description: The pulmonary artery leaves the left ventricle, and the aorta exits from the right ventricle, with no communication between the systemic and pulmonary circulations.

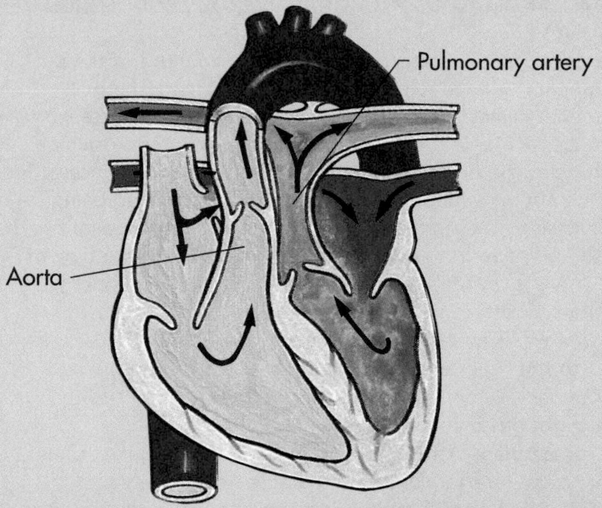

Pathophysiology: Associated defects such as septal defects or patent ductus arteriosus (PDA) must be present to permit blood to enter the systemic circulation and/or the pulmonary circulation for mixing of saturated and desaturated blood. The most common defect associated with TGA is a patent foramen ovale. At birth there is also a PDA, although in most instances this closes after the neonatal period. Another associated anomaly may be a ventricular septal defect (VSD). The presence of these defects increases the risk of congestive heart failure (CHF), since they often produce high pulmonary blood flow under high pressure. For example, a large VSD permits blood to flow from the right to the left ventricle, into the pulmonary artery, and finally to the lungs. However, it also produces high pulmonary blood flow under high pressure, which can result in pulmonary vascular resistance. The same series of events occurs with a large PDA, since blood directly from the aorta flows under high pressure into the pulmonary artery and lungs.

Clinical manifestations: Depend on the type and size of the associated defects. Children with minimum communication are severely cyanotic and depressed at birth. Those with large septal defects or a PDA may be less severely cyanotic but may have symptoms of CHF. Heart sounds vary according to the type of defect present. Cardiomegaly is usually evident a few weeks after birth.

Therapeutic management:

To provide intracardiac mixing: The administration of intravenous prostaglandin E_1 may be initiated to temporarily increase blood mixing if systemic and pulmonary mixing is inadequate to provide an oxygen saturation of 75% or to maintain cardiac output. During cardiac catheterization a balloon atrial septostomy ***(Rashkind procedure)*** may also be performed to increase mixing and maintain cardiac output over a longer period.

Surgical treatment:

Arterial switch procedure: Procedure of choice performed in first weeks of life. Involves transecting the great arteries and anastomosing the main pulmonary artery to the proximal aorta (just above the aortic valve) and anastomosing the ascending aorta to the proximal pulmonary artery. The coronary arteries are switched from the proximal aorta to the proximal pulmonary artery, creating a new aorta. Reimplantation of the coronary arteries is critical to the infant's survival, and they must be reattached without torsion or kinking to provide the heart with its supply of oxygen. The advantage of the arterial switch procedure is the reestablishment of normal circulation, with the left ventricle acting as the systemic pump. Potential complications of the arterial switch include narrowing at the great artery anastomoses or coronary artery insufficiency.

Intraatrial baffle repairs: Intraatrial baffle repairs are rarely performed, although many adolescents and adults survive today with repairs that were done 10 to 25 years ago. An intraatrial baffle is created to divert venous blood to the mitral valve and pulmonary venous blood to the tricuspid valve using the patient's atrial septum ***(Senning procedure)*** or a prosthetic material ***(Mustard procedure).*** They are performed in the first year of life. A disadvantage is the continuing role of the right ventricle as the systemic pump and the late development of right ventricular failure and rhythm disturbances. Other potential postoperative complications include loss of normal sinus rhythm, baffle leaks, and ventricular dysfunction.

Rastelli procedure: Operative choice in infants with TGA, VSD, and severe pulmonic stenosis (PS). It involves closure of the VSD with a baffle, directing left ventricular blood through the VSD into the aorta. The pulmonic valve is then closed, and a conduit is placed from the right ventricle to the pulmonary artery, creating a physiologically normal circulation. Unfortunately, this procedure requires multiple conduit replacements as the child grows.

Prognosis: Operative mortality is about 5% to 10% with all procedures; with atrial level repairs, there is a later risk of dysrhythmias and ventricular dysfunction.

Continued

Box 48-4

Mixed Defects—cont'd

TOTAL ANOMALOUS PULMONARY VENOUS CONNECTION (TAPVC)

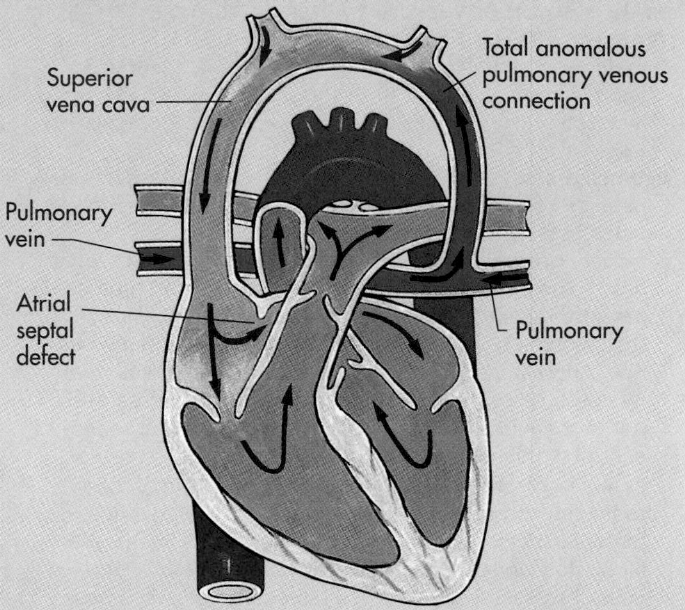

Description: Rare defect characterized by failure of the pulmonary veins to join the left atrium. Instead, the pulmonary veins are abnormally connected to the systemic venous circuit via the right atrium or various veins draining toward the right atrium, such as the superior vena cava. The abnormal attachment results in mixed blood being returned to the right atrium and shunted from the right to the left through an atrial septal defect (ASD). The type of TAPVC is classified according to the pulmonary venous point of attachment as:

Supracardiac—Attachment above the diaphragm, such as to the superior vena cava (most common form)

Cardiac—Direct attachment to the heart, such as to the right atrium or coronary sinus

Infracardiac—Attachment below the diaphragm, such as to the inferior vena cava (most severe form)

TAPVC is also called total anomalous pulmonary venous return (TAPVR) or total anomalous pulmonary venous drainage (TAPVD).

Pathophysiology: The right atrium receives all the blood that normally would flow into the left atrium. As a result, the right side of the heart hypertrophies, whereas the left side, especially the left atrium, may remain small. An associated ASD or patent foramen ovale allows systemic venous blood to shunt from the higher-pressure right atrium to the left atrium and into the left side of the heart. As a result, the oxygen saturation of the blood in both sides of the heart (and ultimately, in the systemic arterial circulation) is the same. If the pulmonary blood flow is large, pulmonary venous return is also large and the amount of saturated blood is relatively high. However, if there is obstruction to pulmonary venous drainage, pulmonary venous return is impeded, pulmonary venous pressure rises, and pulmonary interstitial edema develops and eventually contributes to CHF. Infracardiac TAPVC is often associated with obstruction to pulmonary venous drainage and is a surgical emergency.

Clinical manifestations: Most infants develop cyanosis early in life. The degree of cyanosis is inversely related to the amount of pulmonary blood flow—the more pulmonary blood, the less cyanosis. Children with unobstructed TAPVC may be asymptomatic until pulmonary vascular resistance decreases during infancy, increasing pulmonary blood flow, with resulting signs of CHF. Cyanosis becomes worse with pulmonary vein obstruction; once obstruction occurs, the infant's condition usually deteriorates rapidly. Without intervention, cardiac failure will progress to death.

Surgical treatment: Corrective repair in early infancy. The surgical approach varies with the anatomic defect. In general, however, the common pulmonary vein is anastomosed to the left atrium, the ASD is closed, and the anomalous pulmonary venous connection is ligated. The cardiac type is most easily repaired; the infracardiac type has the highest morbidity and mortality because of the higher incidence of pulmonary vein obstruction. Potential postoperative complications include reobstruction; bleeding; dysrhythmias, particularly heart block; pulmonary artery hypertension; and persistent heart failure.

Prognosis: The cardiac type has a surgical mortality of less than 5%; the incidence of morbidity is greater with the other types and increases with the presence of pulmonary vein obstruction.

TRUNCUS ARTERIOSUS (TA)

Description: Failure of normal septation and division of the embryonic bulbar trunk into the pulmonary artery and the aorta, resulting in a single vessel that overrides both ventricles. Blood from both ventricles mixes in the common great artery, causing desaturation and hypoxemia. Blood ejected from the heart flows preferentially to the lower-pressure pulmonary arteries, causing increased pulmonary blood flow and reduced systemic blood flow. There are three types:

Type I—A single pulmonary trunk arises near the base of the truncus and divides into the left and right pulmonary arteries.

Type II—The left and right pulmonary arteries arise separately but in close proximity and at the same level from the back of the truncus.

Type III—The pulmonary arteries arise independently from the sides of the truncus.

Pathophysiology: Blood ejected from the left and right ventricles enters the common trunk, mixing pulmonary and systemic circulations. Blood flow is distributed to the pulmonary and systemic circulations according to the relative resistances of each system. The amount of pulmonary blood flow depends on the size of the pulmonary arteries and the pulmonary vascular resistance. Generally, resistance to pulmonary blood flow is less than systemic vascular resistance, resulting in preferential blood flow to the lungs. Pulmonary vascular disease develops at an early age in patients with truncus arteriosus.

Clinical manifestations: Most infants are symptomatic with moderate to severe CHF and variable cyanosis, poor growth, and activity intolerance. There is a characteristic murmur. Patients are at risk for brain abscess and bacterial endocarditis.

Box 48-4

Mixed Defects—cont'd

Surgical treatment: Early repair in the first few months of life. Corrective repair is a modified Rastelli procedure. It involves closing the VSD so that the truncus arteriosus receives the outflow from the left ventricle, excising the pulmonary arteries from the aorta, and attaching them to the right ventricle by means of a homograft. Currently, homografts (segments of cadaver aorta and pulmonary artery that are treated with antibiotics and cryopreserved) are preferred over synthetic conduits to establish continuity between the right ventricle and pulmonary artery. Homografts are more flexible and easier to use during the procedure and appear less prone to obstruction. Postoperative complications include persistent heart failure, bleeding, pulmonary artery hypertension, dysrhythmias, and residual VSD. These children require additional procedures to replace the conduit as its size becomes inadequate in relation to the children's growth.

Prognosis: Mortality is greater than 10%; future operations are required to replace the conduits.

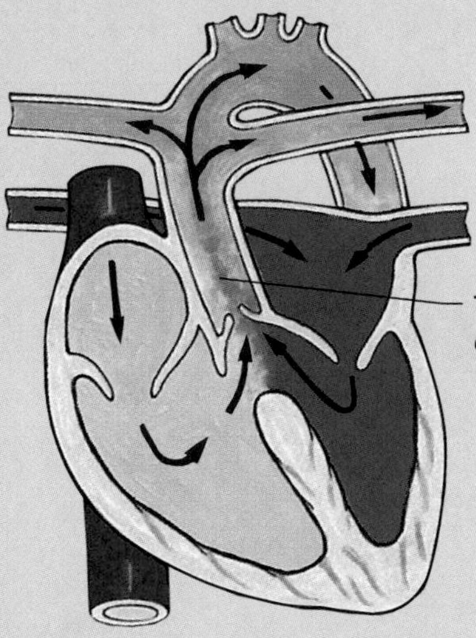

HYPOPLASTIC LEFT HEART SYNDROME (HLHS)

Description: Underdevelopment of the left side of the heart, resulting in a hypoplastic left ventricle and aortic atresia. Most blood from the left atrium flows across the patent foramen ovale to the right atrium, to the right ventricle, and out the pulmonary artery. The descending aorta receives blood from the patent ductus arteriosus supplying systemic blood flow.

Pathophysiology: An ASD or patent foramen ovale allows saturated blood from the left atrium to mix with desaturated blood from the right atrium, and to flow through the right ventricle and out into the pulmonary artery. From the pulmonary artery the blood flows to the lungs, then through the ductus arteriosus into the aorta and out to the body. The amount of blood flow to the pulmonary and systemic circulations depends on the relationship between the pulmonary and systemic vascular resistances. The coronary and cerebral vessels receive blood by retrograde flow through the hypoplastic ascending aorta.

Clinical manifestations: There is mild cyanosis and signs of congestive heart failure until the patent ductus arteriosus closes, then progressive deterioration with cyanosis and decreased cardiac output, leading to cardiovascular collapse. It is usually fatal in the first months of life without intervention.

Therapeutic management: Neonates require stabilization with mechanical ventilation and inotropic support preoperatively. A prostaglandin E_1 infusion is needed to maintain ductal patency, ensuring adequate systemic blood flow.

Surgical treatment: Several-staged approach: First stage is ***Norwood procedure:*** Anastomosis of the main pulmonary artery to the aorta to create a new aorta, shunting to provide pulmonary blood flow, and creation of a large ASD. Postoperative complications include imbalance of systemic and pulmonary blood flow, bleeding, low cardiac output, and persistent heart failure. The second stage is often a ***bidirectional Glenn shunt*** done at 6 to 9 months of age to relieve cyanosis and reduce the volume load on the right ventricle. The final repair is a ***modified Fontan procedure*** (see Tricuspid Atresia in Box 48-3).

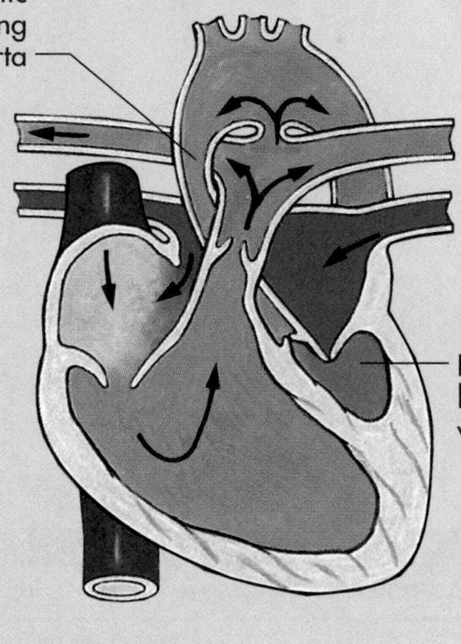

Transplantation: Some programs believe that heart transplantation in the newborn period is the best option for these infants. Problems include the shortage of newborn organ donors, risk of rejection, long-term problems with chronic immunosuppression, and infection (see Heart Transplantation, p. 1350).

Prognosis: Mortality risks of more than 25% with both surgery and transplantation. Results vary widely in different centers. This may improve in the future. Because of the high-risk nature of both surgical palliation and neonatal heart transplantation, some cardiologists continue to recommend no treatment for this defect.

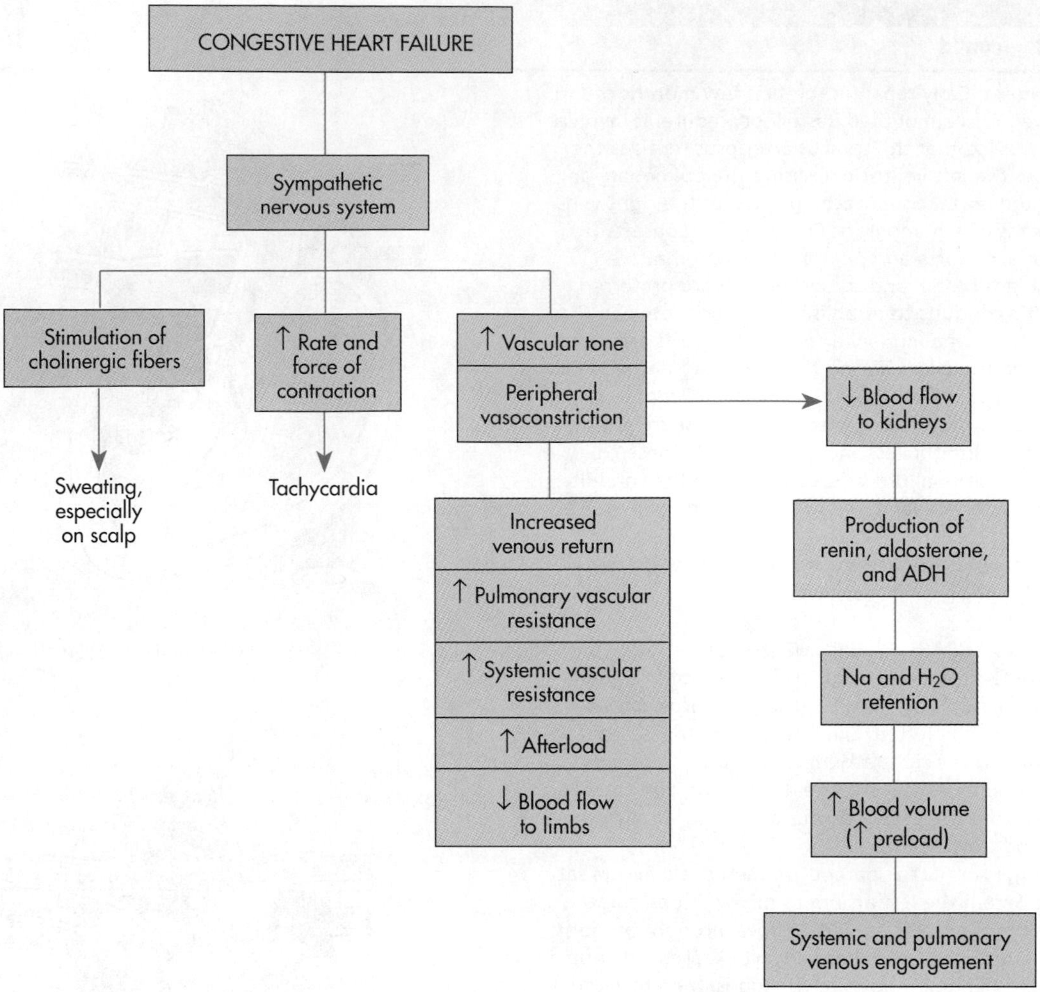

FIG. 48-6 • Pathophysiology of congestive heart failure.

Box 48-5

Clinical Manifestations of Congestive Heart Failure

IMPAIRED MYOCARDIAL FUNCTION

Tachycardia
Sweating (inappropriate)
Decreased urine output
Fatigue
Weakness
Restlessness
Anorexia
Pale, cool extremities
Weak peripheral pulses
Decreased blood pressure
Gallop rhythm
Cardiomegaly

PULMONARY CONGESTION

Tachypnea
Dyspnea
Retractions (infants)
Flaring nares
Exercise intolerance
Orthopnea
Cough, hoarseness
Cyanosis
Wheezing
Grunting

SYSTEMIC VENOUS CONGESTION

Weight gain
Hepatomegaly
Peripheral edema, especially periorbital
Ascites
Neck vein distention (children)

Text continued from p. 1318

A newer group of drugs used in the treatment of CHF are the *angiotensin-converting enzyme (ACE) inhibitors.* As their name implies, these drugs inhibit the normal function of the renin-angiotensin system in the kidney. The ACE inhibitors block the conversion of angiotensin I to angiotensin II so that instead of vasoconstriction, vasodilation occurs. Vasodilation results in decreased pulmonary and systemic vascular resistance, decreased blood pressure, and a reduction in afterload. Two ACE inhibitors are commonly used in pediatrics: *captopril (Capoten),* given three times a day, and *enalapril (Vasotec),* given twice a day. Captopril is used in infants and young children because it can be given in smaller doses; its principal side effects are hypotension, renal dysfunction, and cough.

NURSE ALERT • Because ACE inhibitors also block the action of aldosterone, the addition of potassium supplements or spironolactone (Aldactone) to the drug regimen of patients taking diuretics is usually not needed and may cause hyperkalemia.

Remove Accumulated Fluid. Treatment consists of diuretics, possible fluid restriction, and possible sodium restriction. Diuretics are the mainstays of therapy to eliminate excess water and salt to prevent reaccumulation. The most commonly used agents are *furosemide (Lasix),* the *thiazides (chlorothiazide suspension* or *hydrochlorothiazide tablets),* and *spironolactone (Aldactone)* (Table 48-3). Because furosemide and the thiazides are potassium-losing diuretics, potassium supplements may be prescribed, and rich sources of the electrolyte are encouraged in the diet.

NURSE ALERT • A fall in the serum potassium level enhances the effects of digitalis, increasing the risk of digoxin toxicity. Therefore serum potassium levels must be carefully monitored.

Fluid restriction may be required in the acute states of CHF and must be carefully calculated to avoid dehydrating the child, especially if cyanotic CHD and significant polycythemia are present. Infants rarely need fluid restrictions because CHF makes feeding so difficult that they struggle to take maintenance fluids.

Sodium-restricted diets are used less often in children than in adults to control CHF because of their potential negative effects on appetite. If salt intake is restricted, additional table salt and highly salted foods are avoided.

Decrease Cardiac Demands. The workload on the heart is reduced when metabolic needs are kept to a minimum. This is accomplished by limiting physical activity (bed rest), preserving body temperature, treating any infections, reducing the effort of breathing (semi-Fowler position), and using medication to sedate an irritable child.

TABLE 48-3
Diuretics Used in Congestive Heart Failure

Action	Comments	Nursing Considerations
FUROSEMIDE (LASIX)		
Blocks reabsorption of sodium and water in proximal renal tubule and interferes with reabsorption of sodium	Drug of choice in severe congestive heart failure (CHF) Causes excretion of chloride and potassium (hypokalemia may precipitate digitalis toxicity)	Begin to record output as soon as drug is given Observe for dehydration caused by profound diuresis Observe for side effects (nausea and vomiting, diarrhea, ototoxicity, hypokalemia, dermatitis, postural hypotension) Encourage foods high in potassium and/or give potassium supplements Monitor chloride and acid-base balance with long-term therapy Observe for signs of digoxin toxicity
CHLOROTHIAZIDE (DIURIL)		
Acts directly on distal tubules to decrease sodium, water, potassium, chloride, and bicarbonate absorption	Less commonly used drug Causes hypokalemia, acidosis from large doses May be given on alternate days or for 4 or 5 days and stopped for 2 days to allow for reabsorption of potassium	Observe for side effects (nausea, weakness, dizziness, paresthesia, muscle cramps, skin eruptions, hypokalemia, acidosis) Encourage foods high in potassium and/or give potassium supplements
SPIRONOLACTONE (ALDACTONE)		
Blocks action of aldosterone, which promotes retention of sodium and excretion of potassium	Weak diuretic Has potassium-sparing effect; commonly used with thiazides, furosemide Poorly absorbed from gastrointestinal tract Takes several days to achieve maximum actions	Observe for side effects (skin rash, drowsiness, ataxia, hyperkalemia) Do not administer potassium supplements

Improve Tissue Oxygenation and Decrease Oxygen Consumption. All of the preceding measures serve to increase tissue oxygenation, either by improving myocardial function or by lessening tissue oxygen demands. Supplemental cool, humidified oxygen is usually provided to increase the amount of available oxygen during inspiration. Oxygen is a vasodilator that decreases pulmonary vascular resistance. The amount of cool humidity is carefully regulated to prevent chilling.

NURSE ALERT • Oxygen is a drug and is administered only with an appropriate order. In some uncommon circumstances in patients with complex hemodynamics, oxygen can be detrimental.

Nursing Care Management. The infant or child with CHF is usually admitted to the hospital, where intensive nursing care is available. The child is positioned for optimum ventilation and administered oxygen by the most effective means, IV access is established, and cardiac and respiratory function is monitored continuously using a cardiac monitor and pulse oximeter to monitor oxygen saturation. Urine output and serum electrolytes are evaluated often.

➤ Assessment

Nurses need to be alert to signs of CHF in infants and children with suspected or known congenital defects. Signs of CHF indicate a worsening clinical condition; the earlier they are detected, the sooner treatment can be begun.

NURSE ALERT • The early signs of CHF are the following:

- Tachycardia, especially during rest and slight exertion
- Tachypnea
- Profuse scalp sweating, especially in infants
- Fatigue and irritability
- Sudden weight gain
- Respiratory distress

➤ Nursing Diagnoses

A number of nursing diagnoses are identified after a thorough assessment. Some of these are included in the Nursing Care Plan on p. 1329. Others may become apparent in special circumstances and with children in different age groups.

➤ Plan of Care and Implementation

The goals for the infant or child with CHF and the family are as follows:

1. Child will exhibit improved cardiac output.
2. Child will experience decreased cardiac demands.
3. Child will exhibit improved respiratory function.
4. Child will maintain adequate nutritional status.
5. Child will exhibit no evidence of fluid excess.
6. Child and family will receive adequate support and education.

Although the objectives of nursing care are the same, the interventions differ depending on the child's age. Interventions for infants are quite different from those for older children.

Assist in Measures to Improve Cardiac Function. The nurse's responsibility in administering digoxin includes observing for signs of toxicity, calculating and administering the correct dosage, and instituting parental teaching regarding drug administration at home. The child's apical pulse is always checked before administering digoxin. As a general rule, the drug is not given if the pulse is below 90 to 110 beats/min in infants and young children or below 70 beats/min in older children (the cutoff point for adults is 60 beats/min). However, because the pulse rate varies in children in different age groups, the written drug order should specify at what heart rate the drug is withheld. The nurse should also use judgment in evaluating the pulse rate. If it is significantly lower than the previous recording, the dose should be withheld until the practitioner is notified.

The apical rate is taken because a pulse deficit (radial pulse rate lower than apical) may be present with decreased cardiac output. It is auscultated for 1 full minute to evaluate alterations in rhythm. If the child is monitored by means of an ECG, a rhythm strip is obtained and attached to the chart for rate and rhythm analysis, such as abnormal lengthening of the P-R interval (more than a 50% increase over predigitalization interval) and dysrhythmias.

Digoxin is a potentially dangerous drug because the margin of safety of therapeutic, toxic, and lethal doses is very narrow. Many toxic responses are extensions of its therapeutic effects. Therefore the nurse must maintain a high index of suspicion for signs of toxicity when administering digoxin (Box 48-6).

Because digoxin toxicity can occur from accidental overdose, great care must be taken in properly calculating and measuring the dosage. When converting milligrams to micrograms to milliliters, the nurse carefully checks the placement of the decimal point because an error causes a significant change in dosage. For example, 0.1 mg is 10 times the dosage of 0.01 mg.

NURSE ALERT • Infants rarely receive more than 1 ml (50 μg or 0.05 mg) in one dose; a higher dose is an immediate warning of a dosage error. To ensure safety, ask another staff member to check the calculation before giving the drug.

These same principles are taught to parents in preparation for discharge, although the correct dose in milliliters is usually specified on the container, thus reducing potential errors in calculation. The nurse watches the parent measure the elixir in the dropper and stresses that the level mark is the meniscus of the fluid that is observed at eye level. Other instructions for administering digoxin are listed in the Home Care and the Critical Thinking boxes.

Parents are also advised of the signs of toxicity. According to the practitioner's preference, they may be taught to take the pulse before giving the drug. A return demonstration of the procedure from both parents or other principal caregiver is included as part of the teaching plan. Their level of anxiety in counting the pulse is assessed, because overconcern about the heart rate may result in excessive withholding of the drug.

Box 48-6

Common Signs of Digoxin Toxicity in Children

GASTROINTESTINAL	CARDIAC
Nausea	Bradycardia
Vomiting	Dysrhythmias
Anorexia	

Afterload Reduction. For patients receiving ACE inhibitors for afterload reduction, the nurse should carefully monitor blood pressure before and after dose administration, observe for symptoms of hypotension, and notify the practitioner if blood pressure is low. Numerous medications affecting the kidney can potentiate renal dysfunction, so children taking multiple diuretics along with an ACE inhibitor require careful assessment of serum electrolytes and renal function.

Decrease Cardiac Demands. The infant requires rest and conservation of energy for feeding. Every effort is made to organize nursing activities to allow for uninterrupted periods of sleep. Whenever possible, parents are encouraged to stay with their infant to provide the holding, rocking, and cuddling that help children sleep more soundly. To minimize disturbing the infant, changing of bed linens and complete bathing are done only when necessary. Feeding is planned to accommodate the infant's sleep and wake patterns. The child is fed when hungry, such as when sucking on fists rather than when crying for a bottle, because the stress of crying exhausts the limited energy supply. Because infants with CHF tire easily and may sleep through feedings, smaller feedings every 3 hours may be helpful. Gavage feedings may be instituted to provide adequate nutrition and allow the infant to rest.

Every effort is made to minimize unnecessary stress. Older children need an explanation of what is happening to them to decrease anxiety about their illness and necessary treatments such as cardiac monitoring, oxygen administration, and medications. Outlining a plan for the day, preparing the child for tests and procedures, providing quiet activities, and providing adequate rest periods are all helpful interventions with older children. Some infants and children require sedation during the acute phase of illness to allow them to rest.

Temperature is carefully monitored because hyperthermia or hypothermia increases the need for oxygen. Febrile states are reported to the physician, because infection must be treated promptly. Maintaining body temperature is of special importance in children who are receiving cool, humidified oxygen and in infants who tend to be diaphoretic and lose heat by way of evaporation.

Skin breakdown from edema is prevented with a change of position every 2 hours (from side to side while in semi-Fowler position) and use of a mattress or bed. The skin, especially over the sacrum, is checked for evidence of redness from pressure.

Reduce Respiratory Distress. Careful assessment, positioning, and oxygen administration can reduce respiratory distress. Respirations are counted for 1 full minute during a resting state. Any evidence of increased respiratory distress is reported because this may indicate worsening CHF.

Infants are positioned to encourage maximum chest expansion, with the head of the bed elevated; they should sit up in an infant seat or be held at a 45-degree angle. Children prefer to sleep on several pillows and remain in a semi-Fowler or high-Fowler position during waking hours. Shirts and diapers are pinned loosely to allow maximum chest expansion. Safety restraints, such as those used with infant seats, are applied low on the abdomen and loosely enough to provide both safety and maximum expansion.

The infant or child is often given humidified supplemental oxygen via an oxygen hood or tent, nasal cannula, or mask. The child's response to oxygen therapy is carefully evaluated by noting respiratory rate, ease of respiration, color, and especially oxygen saturations, as measured by oximetry.

Home Care

ADMINISTERING DIGOXIN

Give digoxin at regular intervals, usually every 12 hours, such as 8 AM and 8 PM.

Plan the times so that the drug is given *1 hour before or 2 hours after* feedings.

Use a calendar to mark off each dose that is given, or post a reminder, such as a sign on the refrigerator.

Have the prescription refilled *before* the medication is completely used.

Administer the drug carefully by slowly directing it on the side and back of the mouth.

Do not mix it with other foods or fluids, since refusal to consume these results in inaccurate intake of the drug.

If the child has teeth, give water after administering the drug; whenever possible, brush the teeth to prevent tooth decay from the sweetened liquid.

If a dose is missed and more than 4 hours has elapsed, withhold the dose and give the next dose at the regular time; if less than 4 hours has elapsed, give the missed dose.

If the child vomits, do not give a second dose.

If more than two consecutive doses have been missed, notify the practitioner.

Do not increase or double the dose for missed doses.

If the child becomes ill, notify the practitioner immediately.

Keep digoxin in a safe place, preferably a locked cabinet.

In case of accidental overdose of digoxin, call the nearest Poison Control Center immediately; the number is usually listed in the front of the telephone directory.

Critical Thinking

DIGOXIN TOXICITY

You are visiting a 3-month-old infant at home who began receiving digoxin and Lasix 5 days ago for management of CHF. The infant seems well. The mother mentions that the infant vomited several times yesterday and again this morning. Your assessment reveals an irregular heartbeat at 104 beats/min. What should you do?

First, Think About It . . .

- What conclusions are you reaching?
- What are the implications of your assessment?

1. Give the digoxin and instruct the mother to call the cardiologist in a few days if the vomiting persists.
2. Explain that vomiting and a slow heart rate are common side effects of digoxin.
3. Calm the infant and check the heart rate again.
4. Notify the health care provider of your findings before giving digoxin.

The correct answer is 4. Your assessment reveals a slow, irregular heartbeat and intermittent vomiting. These are common signs of digoxin toxicity in infants. This medication was started only 5 days ago. The practitioner should be notified for further assessment and management. The implications of the assessment are essential because the margin of safety for digoxin blood levels is narrow. Continuing to give the digoxin can cause a fatal toxic reaction.

Respiratory infections can exacerbate CHF and should be appropriately treated and prevented if possible. The child should be protected from persons with respiratory infections and have a noninfectious roommate. With an older child, it is advantageous to choose a roommate who is also confined to bed and relatively quiet in order to promote a restful environment. Good handwashing is practiced before and after caring for any hospitalized child. Antibiotics may be given to combat respiratory infection. The nurse ensures that the drug is given at equally divided times over a 24-hour schedule to maintain high blood levels of the antibiotic.

Maintain Nutritional Status. Meeting the nutritional needs of infants with CHF or serious cardiac defects is a nursing challenge. The metabolic rate of these infants is greater because of poor cardiac function and increased heart and respiratory rates. Their caloric needs are greater than those of the average infant because of their increased metabolic rate; however, their ability to take in adequate calories is hampered by their fatigue. Feeding for a fragile infant with serious CHD is similar to exercise in an adult, and they often do not have the energy or cardiac reserve to do extra work. The nurse seeks measures to enable the infant to feed easily without excess fatigue and to increase the caloric density of the formula.

The infant should be well rested before feeding and fed soon after awakening so as not to expend energy on crying. A 3-hour feeding schedule works well for many infants. (Feeding every 2 hours does not provide enough rest between feedings, and a 4-hour schedule requires an increased volume of feeding, which many infants are unable to take.) The feeding schedule should be individualized to the infant's needs. A soft preemie nipple or a slit in a regular nipple to enlarge the opening decreases the energy expenditure of the infant while sucking. Infants should be well supported and fed in a semiupright position. The infant may need to rest often and may need to have the jaw and cheeks stroked to encourage sucking. Generally, giving an infant about a half hour to complete a feeding is reasonable. Prolonging the feeding time can exhaust the infant and decrease the rest period between feedings.

Infants with feeding difficulties are often gavage fed using a nasogastric tube to supplement their oral intake and ensure adequate calories. If they are very stressed and fatigued, in respiratory distress, or tachypneic to 80 to 100 breaths/min, oral feedings may be withheld and all nutrition given by gavage feedings. Gavage feedings are usually a temporary measure until the infant's medical status improves and nutritional needs can be met through oral feedings. Some infants with severe CHF, neurologic deficits, or significant gastroesophageal reflux may need placement of a gastrostomy tube to allow adequate nutrition.

Increasing the caloric density of formulas by concentration and then adding corn oil, medium-chain triglycerides (MCT oil), or Polycose is commonly done. Infant formulas provide 20 Kcal/oz, and the use of additives can increase the nutritional value to 30 Kcal/oz or more. This allows the infant to obtain more calories despite a smaller-volume intake of formula. The caloric density of the formula needs to be increased slowly (by 2 Kcal/oz per day) to prevent diarrhea or formula intolerance. Breastfeeding mothers are encouraged to provide the infant with alternating feedings of breast milk and high-calorie formulas. Some lactating mothers will prefer to feed the child expressed breast milk that has been fortified with Similac or Enfamil powder, Polycose, or corn oil to increase caloric intake. A supplemental nurser may also be helpful. A diet plan specific to the individual infant's needs is calculated and prescribed by the nutritionist in collaboration with the other health personnel. The nurse needs to reinforce this information with the parents as necessary.

Assist in Measures to Promote Fluid Loss. When diuretics are given, the nurse records fluid intake and output and monitors body weight at the same time each day to evaluate benefit from the drug. Because profound diuresis may cause dehydration and electrolyte imbalance (loss of sodium, potassium, chloride, bicarbonate), the nurse observes for signs indicating either complication, as well as signs and symptoms suggesting reactions to the drugs. Diuretics should be given early in the day to children who are toilet trained to avoid the need to urinate at night. If potassium-losing diuretics are given, the nurse encourages foods high in potassium, such as bananas, oranges, whole grains, legumes, and leafy vegetables, and administers prescribed supplements. Serum potassium levels are checked often.

Fluid restriction is rarely necessary in infants because of their difficulty in feeding. However, if fluids are restricted, the nurse plans fluid intake schedules for a 24-hour period, allowing for most fluids during waking hours. Toddlers and preschoolers should be given small amounts of liquid in small cups so that the containers appear full. Suitable utensils are decorated medicine cups, paper cups, doll-sized teacups, or measuring cups. It is also important to avoid leaving extra fluids at the bedside because older children may help themselves to additional servings. Older children's cooperation is gained by placing them in charge of recording fluid intake.

If sodium intake is limited, the nurse discusses food sources of sodium with the family and discourages their bringing salt-containing treats to the child. At mealtime the child's tray is checked to make sure the appropriate diet is given.

Support Child and Family. CHF is a serious complication of heart disease. Parents and older children are usually acutely aware of the critical nature of the condition. Because stress places additional demands on cardiac function, the nurse should focus on reducing anxiety through anticipatory preparation, frequent communication with the parent regarding the child's progress, and constant reassurance that everything possible is being done.

Home care involves many of the same interventions discussed under Plan for Discharge and Home Care (p. 1337). The nurse teaches the family about the medications that need to be administered and alerts them to the signs of worsening CHF that require medical attention, such as increased sweating, decreased urine output (noted in fewer wet diapers or infrequent use of the toilet), or poor feeding. Compliance is a major issue, and every effort is extended to improve the family's adherence to the medication schedule (see Chapter 45). Written instructions regarding correct administration of digoxin are essential (see Home Care box, p. 1327), including an explanation regarding signs of toxicity.

If CHF is the end stage of a severe heart defect, the nurse cares for this child as for any child who is terminally ill, using the principles discussed in Chapter 41.

➤ Evaluation

The effectiveness of nursing interventions for the family and the child with CHF is determined by continual reassessment and evaluation of care based on the following observational guidelines:

1. Monitor heart rate and quality, respiratory rate and efforts, and color, and observe behaviors that provide clues to expended effort.
2. Observe nutritional intake, feeding behaviors, and weight.
3. Monitor intake, output, and weight.
4. Interview and observe behaviors of family.

The expected outcomes are described in the Nursing Care Plan.

Nursing Care Plan — THE CHILD WITH CONGESTIVE HEART FAILURE

NURSING DIAGNOSIS **Decreased cardiac output related to structural defect, myocardial dysfunction**

EXPECTED OUTCOME Patient exhibits signs of improved cardiac output (i.e., strong, regular pulse with rates within normal limits [WNL]; blood pressure WNL; absence of pallor, adequate capillary refill).

Nursing Interventions/*Rationales*

Administer digoxin (Lanoxin) per physician order *to improve myocardial efficiency:* make certain dosage is within safe limits; count pulse for 1 minute before giving drug and withhold if too slow; monitor for adverse or toxic effects. Ensure adequate intake of potassium and monitor potassium levels, *since decreased levels enhance toxicity of digoxin.*

Administer medications *to decrease afterload as ordered*; monitor for hypotension and electrolyte levels.

Administer oxygen per physician order *to increase supply to myocardium.*

Monitor apical and radial pulses frequently for rate and rhythm *to detect presence of dysrythmias;* monitor skin color, temperature, capillary refill, vital signs *to assess for status of cardiac output.*

Plan child's care and activities to prevent overexertion, *which increases myocardial oxygen demand.*

Administer stool softeners as ordered *to prevent straining at stool and resultant bradycardia.*

NURSING DIAGNOSIS **Ineffective breathing pattern related to pulmonary congestion**

EXPECTED OUTCOME Patient exhibits signs of improved respiratory function (i.e., regular, even respirations with rates WNL; good color; adequate oxygen saturations; decreased restlessness).

Nursing Interventions/*Rationales*

Place in inclined posture of 30 to 45 degrees and avoid constrictive clothing or restraints around abdomen or chest *to encourage maximum chest expansion.*

Administer humidified oxygen as ordered *to reduce hypoxia.*

Monitor respiratory rate, rhythm, ease of breathing, skin color, oxygen saturations by oximetry, breath sounds, restlessness *to assess pulmonary status.*

Suction airway as needed *to remove secretions.*

Plan child's care and activities with adequate rest *to prevent fatigue and reduce oxygen demand.*

NURSING DIAGNOSIS **Fluid volume excess related to pulmonary congestion and fluid accumulation**

EXPECTED OUTCOME Patient exhibits evidence of fluid loss (i.e., increased urine output, weight loss, reduction of edema).

Nursing Interventions/*Rationales*

Administer diuretics as prescribed *to induce diuresis.*

Monitor weight, intake and output, level of edema, urine specific gravity, electrolytes *to assess fluid status;* blood urea nitrogen, creatinine levels *to assess renal function.*

Monitor intravenous and oral intake carefully *to prevent further fluid overload.*

Provide skin care and reposition frequently when edematous *to prevent skin breakdown;* provide oral care *to prevent drying of mucous membranes.*

Monitor skin turgor *to assess for dehydration.*

NURSING DIAGNOSIS **Activity intolerance related to oxygen imbalance**

EXPECTED OUTCOME Patient's activity level is within normal limits.

Nursing Interventions/*Rationales*

Maintain neutral thermal environment *to decrease oxygen demands.*

Feed small volumes at frequent intervals using soft nipple with moderately large opening *to decrease fatigue;* implement gavage feeding if necessary *to prevent fatigue and ensure adequate intake.*

Implement measures to reduce anxiety, crying, signs of distress, *which increase demand for oxygen.*

Perform only necessary functions *to reduce fatigue and energy expenditure.*

Balance rest and physical activity, increasing activity levels as tolerated *to regain balance between oxygen supply and demand.*

See also the Nursing Care Plan: The Family of the Ill/Hospitalized Child, Chapter 44.

Hypoxemia

Hypoxemia refers to an arterial oxygen tension (or pressure, Pa_{O_2}) that is less than normal and can be identified by a decreased arterial saturation or a decreased Pa_{O_2}. *Hypoxia* is a reduction in tissue oxygenation that results from low oxygen saturations and Pa_{O_2} and results in impaired cellular processes. *Cyanosis* is a blue discoloration in the mucous membranes, skin, and nail beds of the child with reduced oxygen saturation. It results from the presence of deoxygenated hemoglobin (hemoglobin not bound to oxygen) in a concentration (5 g/dl of blood). Cyanosis is usually apparent when arterial oxygen saturations are 80% to 85%. Determination of cyanosis is subjective. It can vary depending on skin pigment, quality of light, color of the room, or clothing worn by the child. The presence of cyanosis may not accurately reflect arterial hypoxemia because both oxygen saturation and the amount of circulating hemoglobin are involved. Children with severe anemia may not be cyanotic despite severe hypoxemia because the hemoglobin level may be too low to produce the characteristic blue color. Conversely patients with polycythemia may appear cyanotic despite a near-normal Pa_{O_2}. Heart defects that cause hypoxemia and cyanosis result from desaturated venous blood (blue blood) entering the systemic circulation without passing through the lungs.

Adolescents and young adults may become cyanotic because of unrepaired septal defects in which the increased pulmonary blood flow over many years results in pulmonary vascular changes. *Eisenmenger complex (syndrome)* refers to the clinical situation in which a left-to-right shunt becomes a right-to-left shunt because of a progressive increase in pulmonary vascular resistance. With increasing pulmonary vascular thickening, the resistance in the pulmonary circulation can exceed or equal that in the systemic circulation, causing a reversal of blood flow from the right to the left ventricle.

Clinical Manifestations. Over time, two physiologic changes occur in the body in response to chronic hypoxemia: polycythemia and clubbing. *Polycythemia,* an increased number of red blood cells, increases the oxygen-carrying capacity of the blood. However, anemia may result if iron is not readily available for the formation of hemoglobin. Polycythemia increases the viscosity of the blood and crowds out clotting factors. Clubbing, a thickening and flattening of the tips of the fingers and toes, is thought to occur because of chronic tissue hypoxemia and polycythemia (Fig. 48-7). Infants with mild hypoxemia may be asymptomatic except for cyanosis and exhibit near-normal growth and development. Those with more severe hypoxemia may exhibit fatigue with feeding, poor weight gain, tachypnea, and dyspnea. Severe hypoxemia resulting in tissue hypoxia is manifested by clinical deterioration and signs of poor perfusion.

Squatting, most characteristic of children with tetralogy of Fallot, is seen in toddlers and older children as an unconscious attempt to relieve chronic hypoxia, especially during exercise. Because of early surgical intervention during infancy, squatting is rarely seen.

Hypercyanotic spells, also referred to as *blue spells* or *tet spells* because they are often seen in infants with tetralogy of Fallot, may occur in any child whose heart defect includes obstruction to pulmonary blood flow and communication between the ventricles. The infant becomes acutely cyanotic and hyperpneic because sudden infundibular spasm decreases pulmonary blood flow and increases right-to-left shunting (the proposed mechanism in tetralogy of Fallot). Spells, rarely seen before 2 months of age, occur most commonly in the first year of life. They occur more often in the morning and may be preceded by feeding, crying, defecation, or stressful procedures (Critical Thinking box). Because profound hypoxemia causes cerebral hypoxia, hypercyanotic spells require prompt assessment and treatment to prevent brain damage or possibly death.

Persistent cyanosis as a result of cyanotic heart defects places the child at risk for significant *neurologic complications.* Cerebrovascular accident (CVA, stroke), brain abscess, and develop-

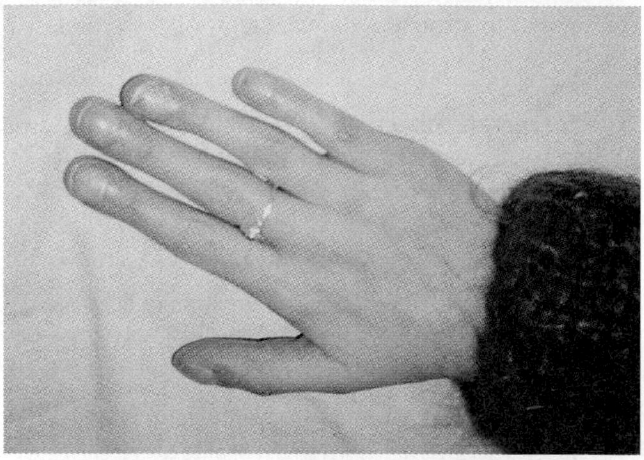

FIG. 48-7 • Clubbing of the fingers.

Critical Thinking

HYPERCYANOTIC SPELL

A 4-month-old infant known to have tetralogy of Fallot is seen in the emergency department because of a 2-day history of diarrhea, low-grade fever, and poor oral intake. When blood tests are done, he becomes acutely cyanotic with rapid shallow respirations. What should you do?

First, Think About It . . .

- **What precise questions are you trying to answer?**
- **If you accept the conclusions, what are the implications?**

1. **Begin cardiopulmonary resuscitation (CPR).**
2. **Calm the infant, place in the knee-chest position and administer blow-by oxygen, and call for assistance.**
3. **Continue the procedure; this is expected for an infant with tetralogy of Fallot.**
4. **Stop the procedure and wait for color to improve before completing the blood test.**

The best response is 2. Precisely, the questions are focused on what symptoms the infant is experiencing, and what the priority nursing action is. The infant is having a hypercyanotic, or "tet," spell, and the first actions should be to calm the infant, place in the knee-chest position, and give supplemental oxygen. A hypercyanotic spell will likely worsen without intervention, so prompt action is needed. CPR is inappropriate at this time because the infant has an adequate heart rate and effective respirations. If you fail to accept the conclusions, negative implications may result, since a severe hypercyanotic spell may require intravenous medications, hydration, and resuscitative measures to stabilize the infant.

mental delays (especially in motor and cognitive development) may result from chronic hypoxia.

Therapeutic Management. Hypercyanotic spells occur suddenly, and prompt recognition and treatment are essential. In the hospital setting, spells are often seen during blood drawing or IV insertion, when the child is highly agitated, or after cardiac catheterization. Treatment of a hypercyanotic spell is outlined in the Guidelines box. Morphine, administered subcutaneously or through an existing IV line, helps to reduce infundibular spasm. A spell indicates the need for prompt surgical treatment if possible. In infants with defects not amenable to surgical repair, a shunt may be created surgically to increase blood flow to the lungs. Currently used types of shunts are described in Table 48-4 and Fig. 48-8.

The cyanotic infant and child are well hydrated to keep the hematocrit and blood viscosity within acceptable limits to reduce the risk of CVAs. Fevers are carefully evaluated because bacteremia can result in bacterial endocarditis. The infant is monitored closely for anemia because of the risk of CVAs and the reduced arterial oxygen-carrying capacity that occurs. Iron supplementation and possibly blood transfusion are used as needed.

Respiratory infections or reduced pulmonary function from any cause can worsen hypoxemia in the cyanotic child. Aggressive pulmonary hygiene, chest physiotherapy, administration of antibiotics, and use of oxygen to improve arterial saturations are important interventions.

Nursing Care Management. The general appearance of infants and children with significant cyanosis poses unique concerns. Blue lips and fingernails are obvious signs of their hidden heart defect. Clubbing and small, thin stature in older children further indicate severe heart disease. Adolescents are especially concerned about their body image; children with cyanosis are often teased about their appearance and singled out as different. Many children, when asked what surgery will do, reply, "Make me pink." Their joy and excitement after surgery are evident when they see their pink fingers. Accentuating the normal and positive and being careful not to call attention to their cyanosis are helpful interventions. Meeting other children in the clinic or hospital who are cyanotic reassures them that they are not the only ones who are blue.

Parents are often fearful of their child's bluish color because cyanosis is usually associated with lack of oxygen and severe illness. They also must deal with comments from relatives, friends, and strangers about their child's abnormal color. They need a simple explanation of hypoxemia and cyanosis and reas-

Guidelines

TREATING HYPERCYANOTIC SPELLS

Place infant in knee-chest position.
Use calm, comforting approach.
Administer 100% oxygen by face mask.
Give morphine subcutaneously or through existing intravenous (IV) line.
Begin IV fluid replacement and volume expansion if needed.
Repeat morphine administration.

TABLE 48-4
Selected Shunt Procedures for Children with Cardiac Defects

Shunt Location	Comments
MODIFIED BLALOCK-TAUSSIG (BT) SHUNT	
Subclavian artery to pulmonary artery using Gore-Tex or Impra tube graft	Shunt flow sometimes excessive, requiring use of diuretics Possibility of thrombosis; antiplatelet therapy may be used postoperatively Easy to ligate at time of definitive correction Shunt size fixed and may become too small as child grows
CENTRAL SHUNT	
Ascending aorta to main pulmonary aorta using Gore-Tex graft	Length of shunt acts to restrict blood flow, limiting symptoms of congestive heart failure (CHF); may require diuretics Uncommon; used when modified BT shunt cannot be done Easy to perform and remove at time of repair
GLENN SHUNT	
Superior vena cava to side of right pulmonary artery, which is ligated from main pulmonary artery Blood flow to right lung only	Used as a second shunt procedure if complete repair is not possible High mortality in infants younger than 6 months Superior vena cava syndrome may occur Pulmonary arteriovenous fistulas may occur many years later Difficult to take down at time of definitive repair
BIDIRECTIONAL GLENN (CAVOPULMONARY ANASTOMOSIS) SHUNT	
Superior vena cava to side of right pulmonary artery Blood flow to both lungs	Done as a second shunt; often as a staging step to a Fontan procedure Can be incorporated into eventual modified Fontan procedure Relieves cyanosis and decreases volume overload on ventricle

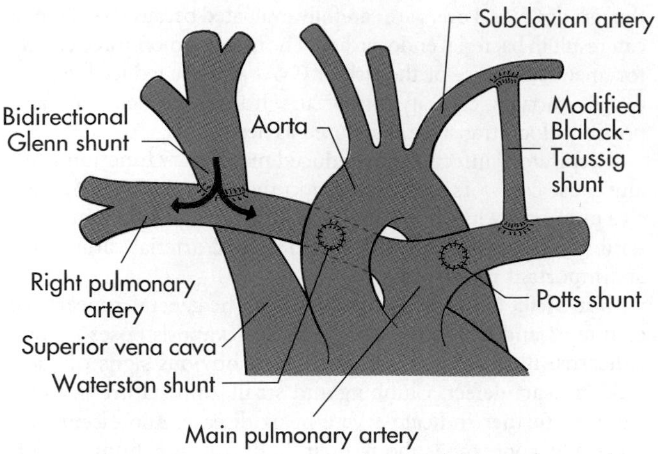

FIG. 48-8 • Schematic diagram of cardiac shunts. NOTE: Two early shunt procedures—Waterston shunt (ascending aorta to right pulmonary artery) and Potts shunt (descending aorta to left pulmonary artery)—are no longer performed because of problems with excessive pulmonary blood flow and distortion of the pulmonary arteries. Adult patients may have had these shunts done as their initial repair.

surance that cyanosis does not imply a lack of oxygen to the brain. Their questions and fears need to be addressed in a calm, supportive manner, and positive aspects of their child's growth and development are emphasized. They are taught the treatment for hypercyanotic spells (see Guidelines box, p. 1331).

Dehydration must be prevented in hypoxemic children because it potentiates the risk of CVAs. Fluid status is carefully monitored, with accurate intake and output and daily weight measurements. Maintenance fluid therapy is the minimum requirement, supplemental fluids should be readily available, and gavage feeding or IV hydration is given to children unable to take adequate oral fluids. Fever, vomiting, and diarrhea can cause dehydration and require prompt treatment. Parents are instructed in the importance of adequate fluid intake and measures to prevent dehydration. An oral electrolyte solution should be available at home in the event that the infant is unable to tolerate the usual formula. The practitioner should be notified of fever, vomiting, diarrhea, or other problems.

Preventive measures and accurate assessment of respiratory infection are important nursing considerations. Any compromise in pulmonary function will increase the infant's hypoxemia. Good handwashing and protection from individuals with an obvious respiratory infection are important. Aggressive pulmonary hygiene, treatment with antibiotics or antiviral agents as indicated, and supplemental oxygen to decrease hypoxemia are necessary measures. Infants may need to be gavage fed or given parenteral hydration if respiratory distress prevents oral feeding.

NURSE ALERT • Intracardiac shunting of blood from the right side (desaturated) to the left side of the heart allows air in the venous system to go directly to the brain, resulting in an air embolism. Therefore all IV lines should have filters in place to prevent air from entering the system, the entire tubing should be checked for air, all connections should be taped securely, and any air should be removed.

NURSING CARE OF THE FAMILY AND CHILD WITH CONGENITAL HEART DISEASE

➤ Assessment

When a child is born with a severe cardiac anomaly, the parents are faced with the immense psychologic and physical tasks of adjusting to the birth of a child with special needs. The reactions and nursing interventions required to support the family are similar to those of other parents whose children have serious chronic conditions and are discussed in Chapter 41.

The following discussion is primarily directed (1) toward the family of an infant who has a serious heart defect and requires home care before definitive repair and (2) toward preparation and care of the child and family when heart surgery is performed. For nursing care related to the child with hypoxemia and CHF, the reader should refer to earlier discussions of these topics.

Nursing care of the child with a congenital heart defect begins as soon as the diagnosis is suspected. Prenatal diagnosis of congenital heart defects is becoming increasingly common. Severe congenital heart defects are usually diagnosed in infancy.

Some children do not display symptoms of heart disease until the child's growth and/or energy expenditure exceeds the heart's ability to supply oxygenated blood to the tissues. The onset of symptoms may be gradual, and the child may curtail activities.

➤ Nursing Diagnoses

Many nursing diagnoses are apparent after a thorough assessment of the child and family. Some of these are developed in the Nursing Care Plan on p. 1338. Others will be evident on the basis of assessment of individual cases.

➤ Plan of Care and Implementation

The goals for the infant with CHD and the family include the following:

1. Family and child (if appropriate) will adjust to the diagnosis.
2. Family will be knowledgeable regarding symptoms of the disease and their management.
3. Family will cope with effects of the disorder.
4. Child (if appropriate) and family will be prepared for surgical repair of a defect.
5. Child undergoing cardiac surgery will receive appropriate care.
6. Family will receive adequate emotional support.
7. Family will be prepared for home care.

Help Family Adjust to the Disorder. Once parents learn of the heart defect, whether it is soon after the child's birth or at a later period in life, they are initially in a period of shock, followed by high anxiety and fear that the child will die. The family needs time to grieve before they can assimilate the meaning of the defect. Unfortunately the demands for medical treatment may not allow this, necessitating that the parents immediately give informed consent for diagnostic/therapeutic procedures. The nurse can be instrumental in supporting parents in their loss, assessing their level of understanding, supplying information as needed, and helping other members of the health care team to understand the parents' reactions (Family Focus box).

Severely distressed newborns usually remain in the hospital. This can seriously affect parent-infant attachment unless

Family Focus

THE DIAGNOSIS OF HEART DISEASE

Remember, we don't have your experience. We don't see children everyday who have heart disease. We would have been upset finding out our child had to have his tonsils out. How could we ever be prepared for this? Please remember, we only know people who have trivial heart murmurs. How could we ever expect this to happen? And to us, this is the worst problem we've ever heard of.

We still fear most what we don't know and understand. Be honest with us. If you don't know either, tell us. But at least don't leave us wondering about what you know and we don't. Not knowing anything really can be worse than knowing something bad. Be honest, but don't strip us of hope. . . .

Please, remember we are trying to learn complex information in a moment of time. And trying to learn it in a context of great pain and emotional investment. This is our lives you're talking about. Please be thorough, but keep it simple. Tell us again, maybe even again and again, when we can hear better.

From Schrey C, Schrey M: A parent's perspective: our needs and our message, *Crit Care Nurs Clin North Am* 6(1):113–119, 1994.

parents are encouraged to hold, touch, and look at their child. Every effort must be made by health personnel to foster attachment.

The effect of a child with a serious heart defect on the family is complex. No member, regardless of the degree of positive adjustment, is unaffected. Mothers commonly feel inadequate in their mothering ability because they gave birth to a child with a defect and are unable to keep the child well. They often feel constantly exhausted from the pressures of caring for these children and the other family members. Fathers and siblings may feel neglected and resentful, a reaction similar to the feelings of family members toward other chronic conditions (see Chapter 41). Often, parents do not feel confident leaving the child in another's care. This often sets up a trap for parents, especially mothers, who become locked into the child's care with no relief. Although the fears are justified, they can be minimized by gradually teaching someone (a reliable relative or neighbor) how to care for the child.

The need to maintain discipline and set consistent limits cannot be overemphasized. Using behavior modification techniques, either in the form of concrete awards (e.g., a favorite activity) or social reinforcement (e.g., approval), can be effective. However, it is most beneficial if used before the child learns to control the family. Therefore it is necessary to guide parents toward the need for discipline while the child is in infancy to prevent later problems. Use of behavior modification techniques also teaches these children how to tolerate frustration and delayed gratification (this ability often is lacking because all their needs are satisfied immediately).

Another issue that may develop within family relationships is the child's overdependency. This is often the result of parental fear that the child may die. The best approach to dealing with this dilemma is prevention. Parents need guidance to recognize the eventual hazards of continuing dependency and protectiveness as the child grows older, and the nurse can assist parents in learning ways to foster optimum development. Unless parents are shown what activities the child can do, they may focus on physical limitations and encourage dependency.

The child also needs opportunities for social development. These children do not need to be prevented from playing with other children because of concern regarding overexertion. Children usually limit their activities if allowed to set their own pace. Such practices foster increased dependency in the home environment. Parents need to be encouraged to seek appropriate social activity, especially before kindergarten.

Having a child with CHD may constitute a long-term family crisis. Commonly the continuing unremitting stresses of care—physical exhaustion, financial costs, emotional upset, fear of death, and concern for the child's future—are not fully appreciated by those caring for the family. Even when the child's condition is stabilized or corrected, the family may need to make new adjustments in their lifestyle. Introducing them to other families with similarly affected children can help them adjust to the daily stresses.*

Educate Family about the Disorder. Once parents are ready to hear about the heart condition, it is essential that they be given a clear explanation based on their level of understanding. Lack of familiarity with the cardiovascular system may be a major reason for lack of parental understanding, and it is usually helpful to review the basic structure and function of the heart before describing the defect. A simple diagram, pictures, or a model of the heart can be most helpful in visualizing the heart and the congenital defect. Parents appreciate receiving written information about the specific condition.† Parents also require information on the treatment options for the cardiac condition and the prognosis.

Another fact to remember is that different health personnel may convey the same information using different diagrams and medical terms. To prevent this from becoming a problem, which often happens when several health team members work with a family, the same type of diagram should be used, and the parents should write down any unclear terms or ask for clarification. Sometimes it is helpful to provide the family with a glossary of commonly used words for reference.

Infants and children with CHD require good nutrition. Providing infants with adequate nutrition is especially difficult because of their high caloric requirements and inability to suck effectively because of fatigue and tachypnea. Instructing parents in feeding methods that decrease the work of the infant and giving high-calorie formula are important interventions. (See p. 1328 for a discussion on feeding the infant with CHF.)

Children with severe cardiac defects are often anorexic. Encouraging them to eat can be a tremendous challenge. Because of the parents' concern over eating, children learn early to manipulate parents through eating, such as making unrealistic demands for foods that are not available. The nurse advises parents of this potential problem because prevention yields greater success than intervention. For example, the child should be given a choice of available high-quality foods. Suggestions for feeding sick children are discussed in Chapter 45.

The family also needs to be knowledgeable regarding the therapeutic management of the disorder, especially in terms of

---

*Some local chapters of the American Heart Association have organized parent groups.

†The booklet *If Your Child Has a Congenital Heart Defect: A Guide for Parents,* as well as other information, is available from the American Heart Association, 7272 Greenville Ave., Dallas, TX 75231; (214) 373-6300 or 1-800-AHA-USA1; website: www.americanheart.org.

the medications that the child is receiving. Parents are taught the correct procedure for giving drugs* and cautioned to keep them in a safe area to prevent accidental ingestion.

Children of various ages have different ideas about their hearts. Children between 4 and 6 years of age have heard about the heart, know its approximate anatomic location in the chest or back, illustrate it as valentine shaped, and characterize it by sounds such as tick-tock and thump. Children 7 to 10 years of age have a clearer concept of the heart, realizing that it is not shaped like a valentine and that it has vital functions, such as "It makes you live." However, their knowledge of its integrated functions to pump blood through a system of vessels to all parts of the body is still hazy. By 10 or 11 years of age, children have a much more involved concept of the heart, with knowledge of veins, valves, pumping action, and circulation. They are beginning to understand why death occurs when the heart stops.

Information given to the child must be tailored to the child's developmental age. As the child matures, the level of information is revised to meet the child's new cognitive level. Preschoolers need basic information about what they will experience more than about what is actually occurring physiologically. School-age children benefit from a concrete explanation of the defect. Preadolescents and adolescents often appreciate a more detailed description of how the defect affects their hearts. Children of all ages need to express their feelings concerning the diagnosis.

Help Family Cope with Effects of the Disorder. Parents should be aware of the symptoms of their child's heart condition (if the child is symptomatic). Parents of children who may develop CHF should be familiar with these symptoms (p. 1324) and know when to contact the practitioner. Parents of children with cyanosis should be informed about fluid management and hypercyanotic spells (p. 1331). Parents should know how to contact their child's cardiologist at all times and know what to do in an emergency.

Another area of parental concern is the child's level of physical activity. Children do not need to restrict activity, and the best approach is to treat the child normally and allow limited activity. Deliberately attempting to prevent crying should be avoided because it can establish a maladaptive parental pattern of relating to the infant. Exceptions to self-determined activity primarily involve strenuous recreational and competitive sports.

NURSE ALERT • Although decisions regarding activity restrictions are made on an individual basis on the cardiologist's advice, children with moderate to severe aortic stenosis or insufficiency are usually not permitted to engage in strenuous activity (Koster, 1994).

Prepare Child and Family for Surgery. Few surgical procedures demand as much planning for preoperative preparation and postoperative care as heart surgery. The reader is urged to review the general principles for preparing for procedures such as surgery, discussed in Chapter 45. This discussion focuses on those measures specific to cardiovascular procedures. Preoperative preparation is often done in the outpatient setting, and children are admitted the day of surgery. Infants and patients with other medical needs are admitted the day before surgery.

Introduce Child and Family to the Environment. Ideally, when the child is admitted, a plan should be made to provide consistent caregivers. In some institutions the nurse who will care for the child postoperatively in the intensive care unit (ICU) is also assigned to the child at admission to facilitate forming a relationship with the family and to share preoperative teaching, such as introduction to the recovery room and ICU. To increase familiarity, all nurses should call the child and parents by name and refer to themselves by name. Wearing a name tag reinforces this point. Postoperatively the family will feel more at ease recognizing familiar names, faces, and voices.

If a visit to the recovery room and/or ICU is planned, it should take place when there is least activity in the area, the parents can accompany the child, and the child is well rested. Usually a day before surgery is ample time to allow the child to ask questions and to prevent undue fantasizing about the experience. If a visit is included in the teaching plan, the nurse can use a book, preferably with pictures or photographs of the actual rooms, to explain the environment to the child.

During the visit to the ICU, the child and parents should experience everything that directly affects the child's care, such as the sounds of ECG monitors, oxygen tents, and placement of the bed. All positive, nonfrightening aspects of the environment are emphasized, such as the play area, visitors' section, pictures or mobiles in the room, or television. If it is a pediatric ICU, the nurse can introduce the family to other children who may be recovering from surgery. The child should be protected from the frightening sights in the unit, and equipment not in view postoperatively, such as equipment located behind or below the bed, needs less attention. The child and parents are encouraged to ask questions or to explore further any equipment in the room, but they should not be pushed to assimilate more information than they appear to be tolerating.

Familiarize Child and Family with Equipment and Procedures. Some of the equipment, such as the stethoscope, blood pressure apparatus, and thermometer, will already be familiar to the child and parents; however, the nurse emphasizes that procedures involving such equipment will be done more often. If monitoring devices, such as blood pressure or oximetry, are used, the child is told about the placement of the sensor on the skin.

Types of equipment new to many families are the oxygen mask, suction device, chest tubes, endotracheal tubes, incentive spirometers, nasogastric tube, and IV tubing. Each of these is shown and demonstrated either on a doll or on the child, if he or she appears ready. With a younger child, miniaturized equipment suitable for use with a doll or puppet is often less anxiety producing than the actual samples. If other children in the unit have an IV infusion or are in oxygen tents, the older child may benefit from seeing them, but this must be planned carefully to avoid frightening the child.

Several IV lines are inserted preoperatively: (1) an ordinary line for infusion of fluids, inserted in a peripheral vein; (2) a venous pressure line, inserted into the right subclavian or jugular vein; and (3) an arterial line for direct measurement of arterial pressure. Younger children need only know the location of each tubing. Older children may appreciate knowing the reason for

*Community and home care instructions on giving medications to children are available in Wong DL, Hess CS: ***Wong and Whaley's clinical manual of pediatric nursing***, ed 5, St Louis, 2000, Mosby.

each infusion. Because the lines are inserted during surgery, they are not painful; they only cause discomfort because movement is restricted.

The type and size of incision the child will have after surgery are discussed and can be shown on a doll. Usually one of two types of incisions is made: a *median sternotomy,* which splits the sternum, or a *lateral thoracotomy,* which extends from the midaxillary line to the scapula. Minimally invasive surgical techniques using a *ministernotomy* (opening the lower half of the sternum) are becoming more widely used to decrease postoperative pain and speed postoperative recovery. Commonly no sutures are visible because subcuticular, absorbable sutures may be used. If this is done, it should be pointed out to the child and parents, who may fear the incision will open.

The child may be told about chest tubes and their purpose in draining fluid from around the heart and lungs. An endotracheal (ET) tube is inserted during surgery and may be left in place for ventilatory assistance and tracheobronchial suctioning. However, it may be best to prepare older children for the ET tube only if prolonged ventilatory support is planned. The ET tube can be presented as a "breathing tube" that is placed in the nose or mouth. The nurse explains that while the tube is in, the child will feel it in the throat and will not be able to talk, but nothing is wrong. The child can express desires by pointing or using a picture communication board. At this point, communicating the amount of discomfort from the surgery can also be discussed, especially using measurement tools such as numbers or faces (see Pain Assessment, Chapter 44). The nurse stresses that the tube will be removed as soon as possible, often during the first postoperative day.

Preoperative physical care differs little, if any, from that for any other surgery and is discussed in Chapter 45. The child should be assured that the parents will be there when he or she wakes up; parents should be allowed to accompany their child as far as possible to the operating suite. After all the equipment and procedures have been explained, it is important to talk about "getting well" and going home. If a doll was used during the preparatory session, the tubes can be removed, and the doll can be dressed in regular clothes in anticipation of discharge.

Provide Postoperative Care. Immediate postoperative care is usually provided by specially trained nurses in ICUs. Many of the procedures, such as arterial pressure and central venous pressure (CVP) monitoring, and the observations related to vital functions require advanced educational training (the reader should refer to critical care texts for further information). However, nurses caring for the child before surgery and during the convalescent period need to be familiar with the major principles of care. Selected complications that may occur postoperatively are described in Box 48-7.

Observe Vital Signs. Vital signs and blood pressure are recorded frequently until stable. Heart rate and respirations are counted for 1 full minute, compared with the ECG monitor, and recorded with activity. The heart rate is normally increased after surgery. The nurse observes cardiac rhythm and notifies the practitioner of any changes in regularity. Dysrhythmias may occur postoperatively secondary to anesthetics, acid-base and electrolyte imbalance, hypoxia, surgical intervention, or trauma to conduction pathways (p. 1342).

At least hourly the lungs are auscultated for breath sounds. Diminished or absent sounds most likely indicate an area of atelectasis, which necessitates further medical assessment.

Box 48-7

Common Complications After Cardiac Surgery and Their Treatment Approaches

CARDIAC

Congestive heart failure: Digoxin, diuretics (p. 1326)

Low cardiac output: Intravenous inotropes (Shock, p. 1346)

Dysrhythmias: Identification, drug treatment, possible pacing, cardioversion (p. 1342)

Tamponade (blood or fluid in the pericardial space constricting the heart): Prompt removal of fluid by pericardiocentesis

RESPIRATORY

Atelectasis: Chest physiotherapy, coughing, deep breathing, ambulation

Pulmonary edema: Diuretics

Pleural effusions: Diuretics, possible chest tube drainage

Pneumothorax: Possible chest tube drainage

NEUROLOGIC

Seizures: Assessment, antiepileptic drugs

Cerebrovascular accident (stroke), cerebral edema, neurologic deficits: Assessment and treatment

INFECTIOUS DISEASE

Infections (especially wound, pneumonia, otitis media, and sepsis): Antibiotics

HEMATOLOGIC

Anemia: Iron supplementation, possible transfusion

Postoperative bleeding: Initially, clotting factors, blood products; may need repeat surgery to locate and ligate source of bleeding

OTHER

Postpericardiotomy syndrome (syndrome of fever, leukocytosis, friction rub, pericardial and pleural effusions, lethargy seen about 7 to 21 days after cardiac surgery; possible viral or autoimmune etiologies): Antipyretics, diuretics, antiinflammatory medications

Temperature changes are typical during the early postoperative period. Hypothermia is expected immediately after surgery from hypothermia procedures, effects of anesthesia, and loss of body heat to the cool environment. During this period the child is kept warm to prevent additional heat loss. Infants may be placed under radiant heat warmers. During the next 24 to 48 hours the body temperature may rise to 37.7° C (100° F) or slightly higher as part of the inflammatory response to tissue trauma. After this period an elevated temperature is most likely a sign of infection and warrants immediate investigation for probable cause.

Maintain Respiratory Status. The child is generally maintained on mechanical ventilation in the immediate postoperative period. Early extubation in the operating room or early postoperative period is becoming more common. When weaning and extubation are completed, humidified oxygen is delivered by mask or hood. The child is kept warm and dry because excessive chilling from wet linens causes an increased metabolic need and consequent increased cardiac demand. The child is encouraged to turn and breathe deeply at least hourly. Every measure is used to enhance ventilation and decrease pain, such as splinting of the operative site and judicious use of analgesics.

Suctioning is performed only as needed and maintained for no more than 5 seconds at a time to prevent depleting the oxygen supply. To prevent hypoxia, supplemental oxygen is administered with a manual resuscitation bag before and after the procedure. Heart rate is monitored after suctioning to detect changes in rhythm or rate, especially bradycardia. The child should be positioned facing the nurse to permit assessment of the child's color and tolerance of the procedure.

NURSE ALERT • During suctioning, observe for signs and symptoms of respiratory distress, such as tachypnea, use of accessory muscles for breathing, restlessness, and changes in oxygen saturation on the pulse oximeter.

Drainage from chest tubes is checked hourly for color and quantity. Immediately after surgery the drainage may be bright red, but afterward it should be serous. The largest volume of drainage occurs in the first 12 to 24 hours and is greater in extensive heart surgery.

NURSE ALERT • Chest tube drainage greater than 3 ml/kg/hr for more than 3 consecutive hours is excessive and may indicate postoperative hemorrhage. The surgeon is notified immediately, because cardiac tamponade can develop rapidly and is life threatening.

Chest tubes are usually removed on the first to third postoperative day. Removal of chest tubes is a painful, frightening experience. Analgesics such as morphine sulfate, often combined with midazolam (Versed), should be given before the procedure. To decrease pain, a topical anesthetic such as EMLA can be placed over the chest tube insertion site for 3 hours before removal (Valenzuela and Rosen, 1999). Older children are forewarned that they will feel a sharp, momentary pain. After the suture is cut, the tubes are quickly pulled out at the end of full inspiration to prevent intake of air into the pleural cavity. A purse-string suture (placed when the tubes were inserted) is pulled tight to close the opening. A petrolatum-covered gauze dressing is immediately applied over the wound and securely taped on all four sides to the skin so that an airtight seal is formed. The dressing is checked for signs of drainage and any evidence of infection.

Monitor Fluids. Intake and output of all fluids must be accurately calculated. Intake is primarily IV fluids; however, a record of fluid used to flush the arterial and CVP lines or to dilute medications is also kept. Output includes hourly recordings of urine (usually a Foley catheter is inserted and attached to a closed collecting device), drainage from chest and nasogastric tubes, and blood drawn for analysis. Urine is analyzed for specific gravity to assess the concentrating ability of the kidneys and to assess approximately the body's degree of hydration. Renal failure is a potential risk from a transient period of low cardiac output.

NURSE ALERT • The signs of renal failure are decreased urine output (less than 1 ml/kg/hr) and elevated levels of blood urea nitrogen and serum creatinine.

Fluids are restricted during the immediate postoperative period to prevent hypervolemia, which places additional demands on the myocardium, predisposing to cardiac failure. To monitor fluid retention, the child is weighed daily, and the same scale is used at approximately the same time each day to avoid errors in measurement. The child is usually designated NPO for the first 24 hours. If an ET tube is inserted, oral fluids are usually withheld until the child is extubated. Fluid restriction may be imposed even when oral fluids are given. The nurse calculates the distribution over a 24-hour period based on the child's preoperative weight and drinking habits. The distribution should allow for most fluid to be given during the child's most wakeful and active periods.

Provide Rest and Progressive Activity. After heart surgery, rest should be provided to decrease the workload of the heart and promote healing. The simplest way to ensure individualized, efficient, high-quality care is to plan at the beginning of the shift the nursing procedures to be done, with periods of rest identified. The schedule should be shared with parents to allow them to sit at the most advantageous times, such as after a rest period when no special treatments are anticipated.

A progressive schedule of ambulation and activity is planned, based on the child's preoperative activity patterns and postoperative cardiovascular and pulmonary function. Ambulation is initiated early, usually by the second postoperative day, when chest tubes, arterial lines, and assisted ventilatory equipment may be removed. Activity progresses from sitting on the edge of the bed and dangling the legs to standing up and to sitting in a chair. Heart rate and respirations are carefully monitored to assess the degree of cardiac demand imposed by each activity. Tachycardia, dyspnea, cyanosis, desaturation, progressive fatigue, or dysrhythmias indicate the need to limit further energy expenditure.

Provide Comfort and Emotional Support. Heart surgery is both painful and frightening for children, and comfort is a primary nursing concern. Continuous IV opioid infusions, particularly morphine and fentanyl, are safe and effective analgesics. Patient-controlled analgesia may be used with children old enough to understand the concept. Nonsteroidal antiinflammatory drugs (NSAIDs) such as ketorolac (Toradol) may be used intravenously. Epidural morphine may be another option because it affords very good pain control when a thoracotomy is performed. Paralyzing agents such as pancuronium (Pavulon) or metocurine (Metubine) may also be used with the analgesics for children who are very agitated or hemodynamically unstable.

Most patients need IV analgesics for pain control during the immediate postoperative period. After extubation and removal of lines and tubes, pain can be satisfactorily controlled with oral medications such as ibuprofen, codeine with acetaminophen (Tylenol), or oxycodone and acetaminophen (Tylox). Acetaminophen alone provides adequate pain relief for most children at discharge. Sternotomy incisions are usually well tolerated, with some discomfort when walking and coughing. Thoracotomy incisions are usually more painful because the incision is through muscle; a more aggressive pain management plan with around-the-clock medications for several days is often necessary to allow for adequate rest, ambulation, and pulmonary hygiene.

In addition to pharmacologic pain control, every effort is made to minimize the discomfort of procedures, such as using a firm pillow or favorite stuffed animal placed against the chest incision during movement and performing treatments after pain medication is given, preferably at a time that coincides with the drug's peak effect. Nonpharmacologic measures are used to lessen the perception of pain, and parents are encouraged to comfort their child as much as possible. (See also Pain Assessment; Pain Management, Chapter 44.)

Children may also be angry and uncooperative after surgery as a response to the physical pain and to the loss of control imposed by the surgery and treatments. They need an opportunity to express feelings, either verbally or through activity. Children also may express feelings of anger or rejection toward parents. The nurse must reassure parents that this is normal and that with continued support the anger will subside.

The nurse can support the parents by being available for information and explaining all the procedures to them. The first few postoperative days are particularly difficult because parents see their child in pain and realize the potential risks from surgery. They often are overwhelmed by the physical environment of the ICU and feel useless because they can do so little for their child. The importance of their presence in making the child feel more secure is stressed, even if they do not provide physical care.

Plan for Discharge and Home Care. Ideally, discharge planning begins on admission for cardiac surgery and includes an assessment of the parents' adjustment to the child's altered state of health. As mentioned earlier, one of the most common parental reactions is overprotection, and the nurse needs to be aware of times when the family may need help in recognizing the child's improved health status. With surgical correction of heart anomalies occurring during infancy, there is less likelihood of this pattern of overdependency developing.

The family will need both verbal and written instructions on medication, nutrition, activity restrictions, subacute bacterial endocarditis, return to school, wound care, and signs and symptoms of infection or complications (Home Care box). Referrals to community agencies may be warranted to assist parents in the transition from hospital to home and to reinforce the teaching.

The parents will also need clear instructions on when to seek medical care, such as for a change in the child's behavior or an unexplained fever. Follow-up with the cardiologist is also arranged before discharge. Appropriate identification, such as a Medic-Alert device, is indicated for children with a pacemaker or a heart transplant and for those receiving anticoagulation therapy or antidysrhythmic medication.

Home Care

TOPICS TO INCLUDE IN DISCHARGE TEACHING AFTER CARDIAC SURGERY

Medication teaching (for digoxin, see Home Care box, p. 1327)
Activity restrictions
Diet and nutrition
Wound care (include dressings if any, suture removal, bathing)
Bacterial endocarditis prophylaxis (see Box 48-9)
Follow-up appointments (cardiologist, primary care provider)
Community agencies as needed (visiting nurse service, early developmental intervention)
When to call practitioner; signs and symptoms of postoperative problems

The nurse also discusses common behavior disturbances that may occur after discharge, such as nightmares, sleep disturbances, separation anxiety, and overdependence. A supportive, consistent response is essential to allow the child to overcome the surgical experience. The child should be encouraged to work out feelings and fears through therapeutic play.

Although surgical correction of heart defects has improved dramatically, it is still not possible to completely repair many of the complex anomalies. For many children, repeat procedures are required to replace conduits or grafts or to manage complications such as restenosis. Consequently the long-term prognosis is uncertain, and full recovery is not always possible. For these families, medical follow-up and continued emotional support are essential. The nurse can often serve as an important primary health professional and as a resource for referrals when needed.

➤ Evaluation

The effectiveness of nursing interventions for the child with CHD and the family is determined by continual reassessment and evaluation of care based on the following observational guidelines and expected outcomes:

1. Interview family and observe their behavior with infant or child.
2. Encourage family to discuss their feelings and concerns; observe their response to education.
3. Interview child and observe his or her behavior and concerns; encourage verbal child to express feelings.
4. Interview family and observe family interactions and relationships.
5. Interview family regarding their understanding of the condition and the proposed surgery.
6. Monitor and observe infant or child and family preoperatively and postoperatively.
7. Observe and interview child and family regarding their understanding of home care needs, ability to carry out care, and compliance with the plan of care.

Also see the Nursing Care Plan.

ACQUIRED CARDIOVASCULAR DISORDERS

Bacterial Endocarditis (BE)

BE, or infective endocarditis (IE), also referred to as *subacute bacterial endocarditis (SBE),* is an infection of the valves and inner lining of the heart. Although it can occur without underlying heart disease, IE most often is a sequela of bacteremia in the child with acquired or congenital anomalies of the heart or great vessels. It especially affects children with valvular abnormalities, prosthetic valves, recent cardiac surgery with invasive lines, and rheumatic heart disease with valve involvement. In addition, a growing problem is endocarditis associated with drug abuse (Dajani and Taubert, 1995). The most common causative agent is *Streptococcus viridans;* other causative agents are *Staphylococcus aureus,* gram-negative bacteria, and fungi such as *Candida albicans.*

Pathophysiology. Organisms may enter the bloodstream from any site of localized infection. The most common portals of entry are oral from dental work *(S. viridans);* the urinary tract, such as from urinary tract infection after catheterization (gram-negative bacilli); the heart, from cardiac surgery, especially if synthetic material is used (valves, patches, conduits); and the bloodstream from long-term indwelling

Nursing Care Plan THE CHILD WITH CONGENITAL HEART DISEASE

NURSING DIAGNOSIS Potential for decreased cardiac output related to structural defect

EXPECTED OUTCOME Patient exhibits signs of adequate cardiac output (i.e., strong, regular pulse with rates within normal limits [WNL]; blood pressure WNL; absence of pallor, adequate capillary refill).

Nursing Interventions/*Rationales*

Administer digoxin per physician order using established precautions *to prevent toxicity* (see pp. 1326-1327); monitor for adverse or toxic effects. Ensure adequate intake of potassium and monitor potassium levels, *as decreased levels enhance toxicity of digoxin.*

Administer diuretics as ordered (see p. 1325).

Administer afterload reduction medications as ordered (see p. 1327).

Monitor apical and radial pulses frequently for rate and rhythm *to detect presence of dysrhythmias;* monitor skin color, temperature, capillary refill, vital signs *to assess for status of cardiac output.*

Plan child's care and activities to prevent overexertion, *which increases myocardial oxygen demand.*

NURSING DIAGNOSIS Activity intolerance related to oxygen imbalance

EXPECTED OUTCOME Patient's activity level is within normal limits for physical condition.

Nursing Interventions/*Rationales*

Prevent temperature extremes, *which can increase oxygen demands.*

Implement measures to reduce anxiety and signs of distress, *which can increase oxygen demands.*

Balance rest and physical activity, increasing activity levels as tolerated *to maintain balance between oxygen supply and demand.* Help child to select activities appropriate to age, physical condition, and capabilities.

NURSING DIAGNOSIS Altered growth and development related to inadequate oxygenation of tissues; social isolation

EXPECTED OUTCOME Patient exhibits height, weight gains that follow growth curve; patient exhibits gross and fine motor abilities, language abilities, and social skills that are WNL for age.

Nursing Interventions/*Rationales*

Provide well-balanced, highly nutritious diet *to promote adequate growth.*

Monitor height and weight using growth charts *to plot growth trends.*

Administer iron supplements as ordered *to correct or prevent anemia.*

Encourage age-appropriate activity *to build gross and fine motor skills.*

Plan regular storytelling or reading sessions *to enhance verbal abilities.*

Encourage interaction with other children *to promote social interaction.*

Test child's developmental level periodically *to evaluate for developmental delay.*

NURSING DIAGNOSIS Potential infection related to debilitated physical status

EXPECTED OUTCOME Patient exhibits no signs of infection.

Nursing Interventions/*Rationales*

Avoid high-exposure social settings such as nursery schools, day care, crowds, *which increase risk of infection.*

Screen visitors and playmates and prevent contact with infected persons *to decrease infection risk.*

Provide for adequate rest and nutrition *to support body's natural defenses.*

Have family and child practice good hygiene and handwashing techniques *to contain germ spread.*

NURSING DIAGNOSIS Potential for injury (complications) related to cardiac status and therapies

EXPECTED OUTCOME Signs of cardiac complications are absent or detected in a timely fashion.

Nursing Interventions/*Rationales*

Teach family to recognize early signs of congestive heart failure (e.g., tachycardia, tachypnea, profuse scalp sweating, fatigue and irritability, sudden weight gain, respiratory distress); hypoxemia (e.g., cyanosis, restlessness); digoxin toxicity (e.g., nausea, vomiting, anorexia, bradycardia, dysrhythmias) *to ensure timely intervention.*

Give family written instructions about what to do and whom to call if any of the signs occurs *to ensure timely intervention.*

NURSING DIAGNOSIS Altered family processes related to having child with heart condition

See the Nursing Care Plan: Child with Chronic Illness or Disability, Chapter 41.

catheters. The microorganisms grow on the endocardium, forming vegetations (verrucae), deposits of fibrin, and platelet thrombi. The lesion may invade adjacent tissues, such as aortic and mitral valves, and may break off and embolize elsewhere, especially in the spleen, kidney, and central nervous system.

Diagnostic Evaluation. The diagnosis of IE is suspected on the basis of clinical manifestations (Box 48-8). Several laboratory findings may suggest IE (e.g., ECG changes [prolonged P-R interval], radiographic evidence of cardiomegaly, anemia, elevated erythrocyte sedimentation rate, leukocytosis, and microscopic hematuria). Vegetations on the valve and abnormal valve function can often be visualized by echocardiography. Definitive diagnosis rests on growth and identification of the causative agent in the blood.

Therapeutic Management. Treatment should be instituted immediately and consists of administration of high doses of appropriate antibiotics intravenously and/or intramuscularly for at least 4 weeks. Blood cultures are taken periodically to evaluate response to antibiotic therapy.

IE in susceptible children is prevented by administering prophylactic antibiotic therapy both before and for a short period after procedures known to increase the risk of entry of organisms, including dental work and any manipulation of the respiratory, genitourinary, or gastrointestinal tract. In female adolescents this includes childbirth (Box 48-9).

Nursing Care Management. Ideally, the objective of nursing care is prevention through counseling parents of high risk children about the need for prophylactic antibiotic therapy before procedures such as dental work. Unless parents are aware of the risk inherent in exposing their child to these procedures, they may not be inclined to seek medical treatment beforehand. As an added precaution and to ensure that preventive treatment is carried out, the family's regular dentist should be advised of existing cardiac problems in the child.

Treatment of IE requires hospitalization for the institution of parenteral drug therapy. In many patients IV antibiotics may be administered at home with nursing supervision to complete the course of treatment. Nursing goals during this period are (1) preparation of the child for continuous IV infusion, possibly for several venipunctures for blood cultures; (2) observation for side effects of antibiotics; and (3) observation for complications, especially from embolism, and the possibility of heart failure. For specific interventions see Nursing Care Plan: The Child with Congestive Heart Failure, p. 1329.

Box 48-8

Clinical Manifestations of Infective Endocarditis

- Onset usually insidious
- Unexplained fever (low grade and intermittent)
- Anorexia
- Malaise
- Weight loss
- Characteristic findings caused by extracardiac emboli formation:
  - Splinter hemorrhages (thin black lines) under the nails
  - Osler nodes (red, painful intradermal nodes found on pads of phalanges)
  - Janeway lesions (painless hemorrhagic areas on palms and soles)
  - Petechiae on oral mucous membranes
- May be present:
  - Congestive heart failure
  - Cardiac dysrhythmias
  - New murmur or change in previously existing one

Rheumatic Fever (RF)

RF, or acute RF, is an inflammatory disease affecting the heart, joints, central nervous system, and subcutaneous tissue. It derives its name from involvement of joints and the presence of fever in the acute stage. The most significant sequela of RF is *rheumatic heart disease,* especially damage to and scarring of the mitral valve. Although the disease has declined during the past 30 years, recent outbreaks have been reported in several areas of the United States, causing concern among health professionals. RF remains a devastating problem in Third World countries.

Etiology. Strong evidence supports a relationship between upper respiratory infection with group A streptococci and subsequent development of RF (usually within 2 to 6 weeks). In almost all cases of RF a previous infection with group A streptococci can be documented by laboratory evidence of rising

Box 48-9

Endocarditis Prophylaxis Recommendations

DENTAL PROCEDURES

- Dental extractions
- Periodontal procedures, including surgery, scaling and root planing, probing, and recall maintenance
- Dental implant placement and reimplantation of avulsed teeth
- Endodontic (root canal) instrumentation or surgery only beyond the apex
- Subgingival placement of antibiotic fibers/strips
- Initial placement of orthodontic bands but not brackets
- Intraligamentary local anesthetic injections
- Prophylactic cleaning of teeth or implants where bleeding is anticipated

OTHER PROCEDURES

Respiratory Tract

- Surgical operations that involve respiratory mucosa
- Bronchoscopy with a rigid bronchoscope
- Tonsillectomy and/or adenoidectomy

Gastrointestinal Tract

- Sclerotherapy for esophageal varices
- Esophageal stricture dilation
- Endoscopic retrograde cholangiography with biliary obstruction
- Biliary tract surgery
- Surgical operations that involve intestinal mucosa

Genitourinary Tract

- Prostatic surgery
- Cystoscopy
- Urethral dilation

From Dajani AS et al: Prevention of bacterial endocarditis: recommendations by the American Heart Association, *JAMA* 277: 1794–1801, 1997.

antibody titers. Prevention or treatment of group A streptococcal infection prevents RF.

Diagnostic Evaluation. Diagnosis is based on a set of guidelines recommended by the American Heart Association. These guidelines, known as *modifications of the Jones criteria,* suggest that the presence of two major manifestations or one major and two minor manifestations, such as fever and arthralgia, with supportive evidence of recent streptococcal infection, indicates a high probability of RF (Guidelines box).

Guidelines

DIAGNOSIS OF INITIAL ATTACK OF RHEUMATIC FEVER (JONES CRITERIA, 1992 UPDATE)*

Major Manifestations

Carditis

Tachycardia out of proportion to degree of fever
Cardiomegaly
New murmurs or change in preexisting murmurs
Muffled heart sounds
Precardial friction rub
Precardial pain
Changes in ECG (especially prolonged P-R interval)

Polyarthritis

Swollen, hot, red, painful joint(s)
After 1 to 2 days affects different joint(s)
Favors large joints—knees, elbows, hips, shoulders, wrists

Erythema Marginatum

Erythematous macules with clear center and wavy, well-demarcated border
Transitory
Nonpruritic
Primarily affects trunk and extremities (inner surfaces)

Chorea (St. Vitus Dance, Sydenham Chorea)

Sudden aimless, irregular movements of extremities
Involuntary facial grimaces
Speech disturbances
Emotional lability
Muscle weakness (can be profound)
Muscle movements exaggerated by anxiety and attempts at fine motor activity; relieved by rest

Subcutaneous Nodes

Nontender swelling
Located over bony prominences
May persist for some time, then gradually resolve

Minor Manifestations

Clinical findings
- Arthralgia
- Fever

Laboratory Findings

Elevated acute-phase reactants
- Erythrocyte sedimentation rate
- C-reactive protein

Supporting Evidence of Antecedent Group A Streptococcal Infection

Positive throat culture or rapid streptococcal antigen test
- Elevated or rising streptococcal antibody titer

From Special Writing Group of the Committee on Rheumatic Fever, Endocarditis, and Kawasaki Disease of the Council on Cardiovascular Disease in the Young of the American Heart Association: Guidelines for the diagnosis of rheumatic fever: Jones criteria, 1992 (update), *JAMA* 268:2069-2073, 1992.

*If supported by evidence of preceding group A streptococcal infection, the presence of two major manifestations or of one major and two minor manifestations indicates a high probability of acute rheumatic fever.

Children suspected of having RF are tested for streptococcal antibodies. The most reliable and best standardized test is an elevated or rising *antistreptolysin-O (ASO* or *ASLO) titer,* which occurs in 80% of children with RF. Others include anti-DNase B and anti-DPNase tests, erythrocyte sedimentation rate, and C-reactive protein. ECGs and radiographs are obtained to detect any evidence of heart involvement.

Therapeutic Management. The goals of medical management are (1) eradication of hemolytic streptococci, (2) prevention of permanent cardiac damage, (3) palliation of other symptoms, and (4) prevention of recurrences of RF. Penicillin is the drug of choice, with erythromycin as a substitute in penicillin-sensitive children. Salicylates are used to control the inflammatory process, especially in the joints, and reduce the fever and discomfort. Bed rest is recommended during the acute febrile phase but need not be strict.

Prophylactic treatment against recurrence of RF is started after the acute therapy and involves monthly intramuscular injections of benzathine penicillin G (1.2 million U), two daily oral doses of penicillin (200,000 U), or one daily dose of sulfadiazine (1 g). The duration of long-term prophylaxis is uncertain. Because of the risk of IE in rheumatic heart disease, the same prophylaxis discussed earlier is implemented. The antibiotic regimens used to prevent recurrences of RF are inadequate for the prevention of IE.

Children who have had acute RF are susceptible to recurrent RF for the rest of their lives and should undergo medical follow-up for at least 5 years. Children and families must be aware of the need for continuing antibiotic prophylaxis for dental work, infection, and invasive procedures.

Nursing Care Management. The objectives of nursing care for the child with RF are to (1) encourage compliance with drug regimens, (2) facilitate recovery from the illness, (3) provide emotional support, and (4) prevent the disease. Because compliance is a major concern in long-term drug therapy, every effort is made to encourage adherence to the therapeutic plan (see Compliance, Chapter 45). When compliance is poor, monthly injections may be substituted for daily oral administration of antibiotics, and children need preparation for this often-dreaded procedure.

Interventions during home care are primarily concerned with providing rest and adequate nutrition. Usually, once the febrile stage is over, children can resume moderate activity, and their appetite improves. If carditis is present, the family must be aware of any activity restrictions and may need help in choosing less strenuous activities for the child.

One of the most disturbing and frustrating manifestations of the disease is *chorea.* The onset is gradual and may occur weeks to months after the illness; it sometimes even occurs in children in whom RF has not been diagnosed. It may be mistaken for nervousness, clumsiness, behavioral changes, inattentiveness, and learning disability. It is usually a source of great frustration to the child because the movements, incoordination, and weakness severely limit physical ability. The child needs an opportunity to verbalize feelings. Of utmost importance is stressing to parents and schoolteachers the involuntary, sudden nature of the movements, that the chorea is transitory, and that all manifestations eventually disappear.

Nurses also have a role in prevention, primarily in screening school-age children for sore throats caused by group A streptococci. This may involve actively participating in throat culture screening programs or in referring children with a possible streptococcal infection for testing.

(See also Nursing Care Plan: The Child with Rheumatic Fever.*)

Hyperlipidemia (Hypercholesterolemia)

Hyperlipidemia is a general term for excessive lipids (fat and fat-like substances); *hypercholesterolemia* refers to excessive cholesterol in the blood. High lipid or cholesterol levels are believed to play an important role in producing atherosclerosis (fatty plaques on the arteries), which eventually can lead to coronary artery disease, a primary cause of morbidity and mortality in the adult population. Current research indicates that a presymptomatic phase of atherosclerosis begins in childhood. Preventive cardiology is focusing on the screening and management of lipid levels in childhood. The goal is to identify those children at high risk and intervene early.

Cholesterol is part of the lipoprotein complex in plasma that is essential for cellular metabolism. Triglycerides, natural fats synthesized from carbohydrates, are used for energy. Both are major lipids transported on *lipoproteins,* a combination of lipids and proteins, which include:

Low-density lipoproteins (LDLs)—Contain low concentrations of triglycerides, high levels of cholesterol, and moderate levels of protein. LDL is the major carrier of cholesterol to the cells. Cells use cholesterol for synthesis of membranes and steroid production. Elevated circulating LDL is a strong risk factor in cardiovascular disease.

High-density lipoproteins (HDLs)—Contain very low concentrations of triglycerides, relatively little cholesterol, and high levels of protein. They transport free cholesterol to the liver for excretion in the bile. High levels of HDL are thought to protect against cardiovascular disease.

Diagnostic Evaluation. Hyperlipidemia is diagnosed on the basis of analysis of blood for a full lipid profile. Two samples drawn in the fasting state (12 hours) should be analyzed, and the average of the values used for diagnosis. Blood samples should be collected after having the child sit for 5 minutes, and the tourniquet should be applied immediately before the needle puncture, because posture and vascular stasis may affect results. Diagnostic values for acceptable, borderline, and high total cholesterol and LDL cholesterol levels are listed in Table 48-5.

Screening children for hypercholesterolemia is a controversial issue, with some authorities advocating universal screening and others proposing selective screening. Current guidelines recommended by the National Cholesterol Education Program (NCEP) (1992) recommend a strategy that combines two complementary approaches: (1) a population approach that aims to lower the average levels of blood cholesterol among all American children through population-wide changes in nutrient intake and eating patterns; and (2) an individualized approach that targets children and adolescents for screening who have a family history of premature cardiovascular disease or at least one parent with high blood cholesterol (240 mg/dl or higher).

*In Wong DL, Hess CS: ***Wong and Whaley's clinical manual of pediatric nursing***, ed 5, St Louis, 2000, Mosby.

TABLE 48-5

Classification of Cholesterol Levels in Children From Families with a History of Heart Disease

Category	Total Cholesterol (mg/dl)	LDL Cholesterol (mg/dl)
Acceptable	<170	<110
Borderline	170-199	110-129
High	≥200	≥130

From National Cholesterol Education Program: Report of the Expert Panel on Blood Cholesterol Levels in children and adolescents, *Pediatrics* 89(3 pt 2):527, 1992.

Therapeutic Management. Treatment of high cholesterol is primarily dietary. The NCEP guidelines recommend a two-step dietary approach that restricts the intake of cholesterol and fat. Children with borderline levels of LDL cholesterol are advised to follow the *step one diet.* It recommends the same nutrient intake as for the general population (i.e., less than 10% of total calories from saturated fatty acids, no more than 30% of calories from total fat, less than 300 mg/day of cholesterol, and adequate calories to support growth and development and to reach or maintain desirable body weight). Children with high LDL cholesterol levels initially are also given this diet. If these dietary modifications fail to achieve satisfactory levels of LDL after 3 months of therapy, the *step two diet* is initiated. These dietary restrictions include a further reduction of saturated fatty acid intake to 7% of calories and of cholesterol intake to less than 200 mg/day.

New research continues to support the benefit of diets low in saturated fats. Current thinking favors a "Mediterranean"-type diet. Whole grains, fruits, and vegetables form the foundation of this diet. In addition, this diet allows the use of monounsaturated fats, such as olive oil and canola oil, which have beneficial effects on HDL cholesterol values. The use of these fats also makes the diet more realistic.

NURSE ALERT • The Report of the Expert Panel on Blood Cholesterol Levels in Children and Adolescents regarding recommendations for fat intake are not intended for infants from birth to 2 years of age, whose fast growth requires a higher percentage of calories from fat. Toddlers 2 to 3 years of age may safely make the transition to the recommended eating pattern as they begin to eat with the family. No treatment recommendations are made for any child younger than 2 years of age.

For children with severe hypercholesterolemia who do not respond to dietary modifications, drug therapy may be necessary. Two drugs recommended for treatment are the bile acid–binding resins or sequestrants *cholestyramine* and *colestipol.* These two drugs act by binding bile acids in the intestinal lumen. Because they are not absorbed by the intestine, they do not produce systemic toxicity and are safe for children. Cholestyramine (Questran) and colestipol (Colestid) are both powders that are mixed with water or juice just before ingestion. Some patients cannot tolerate the medication because of the taste and the side effects, the most significant being constipation, abdominal pain, gastrointestinal bloating, flatulence, and nausea.

Patients should be instructed to take one multivitamin supplement with iron daily, because cholestyramine may interfere with the absorption of fat-soluble vitamins. It may also interfere with the absorption of other medications, which should be given at least 1 hour before or 6 hours after the resin-binding agent is ingested.

Niacin (nicotinic acid), a B vitamin, may be given in therapeutic doses to older children. Although available without a prescription, niacin is treated as a prescription medicine in children. Its use is monitored closely by a health care professional with clinical and laboratory monitoring, especially liver function tests (Colletti et al, 1993).

Nursing Care Management. Nurses play an important role in the screening, education, and support of children with hyperlipidemia and their families. When a child is referred to a lipid clinic, it is essential that the family be adequately prepared for the first visit. Generally the parents will be asked to keep a record of the child's dietary intake before this visit. Sometimes they will need to complete a questionnaire regarding the child's normal dietary habits over the preceding year. Families should be instructed to keep their child fasting for at least 12 hours before screening. Therefore it is important to schedule the blood test early in the morning and to arrange for nourishment immediately thereafter. At the visit, a full family history should be taken, including the health of both parents and all first-degree relatives. Specific questions should be asked regarding early heart disease, hypertension, strokes (CVAs), sudden death, hyperlipidemia, diabetes, and endocrine abnormalities. Nurses may also uncover risk factors when obtaining a health history for other purposes. It is therefore important that nurses be familiar with current screening practices and the availability of resources for children with positive family histories.

Parents and extended families should be informed about cholesterol and hyperlipidemia. This education should include a brief introduction to the different lipoprotein categories, including cholesterol, HDL, LDL, and triglycerides. Also, behavioral risk factors for heart disease, such as smoking and lack of exercise, should be reviewed. For management to be effective, parents need to understand the rationale for dietary and/or pharmacologic intervention. The key is prevention of future cardiovascular disease.

Stringent dietary guidelines may become an issue of control and a source of great stress for many families. Children should not be viewed as having a disease. Rather, the positive aspects of healthful eating, regular exercise, and smoking avoidance should be emphasized. Basic dietary changes should be encouraged for the whole family so that the affected sibling is not singled out. Cultural differences must be considered, and recommendations individualized. Substitution rather than elimination needs to be emphasized. Visual aids are often helpful, especially for the children (e.g., test tubes depicting the amount of fat in a hot dog). Diets should be flexible and individually tailored by a nutritionist experienced in combining recommendations that meet both the nutritional demands of the growing child and the lipid modifications. Parents are encouraged to participate in dietary and educational sessions, ask questions, and share ideas and experiences.

Parents often feel guilty about the hereditary component of hyperlipidemia. Many also believe they have failed if the diet alone is not making a significant difference in their child's lipid profile. They need to be reassured that a dietary approach alone is often not sufficient, especially for children with LDL values greater than 130 mg/dl.

Parents of children who require pharmacologic therapy need to understand the purpose, dosage, and possible side effects of the various drugs. Medication schedules should remain flexible and should not interfere with the child's daily activities. For example, children of elementary school age may have better compliance if they take a resin-binding agent (e.g., cholestyramine, colestipol) twice a day (i.e., before school and at night) rather than the standard three times a day. Follow-up phone calls by the nurse between visits allow parents to discuss their concerns and ask any questions that have arisen.

Cardiac Dysrhythmias

Cardiac dysrhythmias, or abnormal heart rhythms, occur less commonly in children than in adults. However, they are not rare, and the incidence is rising. The survival rate of children undergoing complex cardiac surgical procedures is higher, and conduction system damage may be a complication.

The basic diagnostic procedure is the ECG, including 24-hour Holter monitoring. *Electrophysiologic cardiac catheterization* allows for identification of the conduction disturbance and immediate investigation of drugs that may control the dysrhythmia. Another procedure that may be used is *transesophageal recording.* An electrode catheter is passed to the lower esophagus and, when in position at a point proximal to the heart, is used to stimulate and record dysrhythmias.

Classification. Dysrhythmias can be classified according to various criteria, such as effect on heart rate and rhythm, as follows:

Bradydysrhythmias—Abnormally slow rate
Tachydysrhythmias—Abnormally rapid rate
Conduction disturbances—Irregular heart rate

Before classifying an infant or child with an abnormal rate, nurses must be familiar with the standards of normal heart rate for the particular age group (see inside back cover). Heart rate variations considered normal for a particular child can vary tremendously.

Bradydysrhythmias. The most common bradydysrhythmia in children is *complete atrioventricular block (AV block),* also referred to as *complete heart block.* This can be either congenital or acquired, as seen in postoperative patients after surgery has been performed in the area of the AV valves and ventricular septum.

Sinus bradycardia in children can be caused by the influence of the autonomic nervous system, as with hypervagal tone, or in response to hypoxia and hypotension. *Junctional* or *nodal rhythms* are common in the postoperative patient. The impulse for these rhythms originates further down the conduction system, in the AV node. Identification is marked by absence of P waves on the ECG, and often little change occurs in the heart rate or cardiac output. If there is no significant compromise to the patient's cardiac status, no treatment is necessary.

Tachydysrhythmias. *Sinus tachycardia* caused by fever, anxiety, pain, anemia, dehydration, or any other etiologic factor requiring increased cardiac output should be ruled out before diagnosing an increased heart rate as pathologic. *Supraventricular tachycardia (SVT)* is one of the most common dysrhythmias found in children and refers to a rapid regular heart rate of 200 to 300 beats/min. The onset of SVT is often sudden, and the duration is variable. Infants and young children with SVT may be unable to communicate that they have a rapid heart rate, and the clinical course can progress to CHF. Important signs in the infant and young child are poor feeding, extreme irritability, and pallor.

Conduction Disturbances. Most rhythm disturbances are seen postoperatively in the child undergoing cardiac surgery and are of little significance. AV blocks are most often related to edema around the conduction system and resolve without treatment. Temporary epicardial wires are placed in most patients at surgery; if a rhythm disturbance occurs, temporary pacing can be used. Just before discharge, the health practitioner removes the wires by pulling slowly and deliberately down on them from the site of insertion.

Premature contractions can occur from an atrial, ventricular, or junctional focus. Their significance depends on the degree of compromise and the presence or absence of underlying CHD.

Therapeutic Management. Treatment of dysrhythmias depends on the cause and severity. Whenever possible, the underlying cause is treated. However, in some cases it is necessary to use antidysrhythmic drugs, with the goal being control, not cure. A permanent *pacemaker* may be needed in some children, such as those with postsurgical AV block or, less commonly, congenital AV block. The pacemaker takes over or assists in the conduction function of the heart. The surgical implantation of a pacemaker is usually a low risk procedure. Once the wire has been introduced, a small incision is made, and a pocket is formed under the muscle to house and protect the generator. Continuous ECG monitoring is necessary during the recovery phase to assess pacemaker function. The nurse should be aware of the programmed rate and expected individual generator variations. A baseline ECG strip should be documented for future comparison.

The treatment of SVT depends on the degree of compromise imposed by the dysrhythmia. In some instances, *vagal maneuvers,* such as applying ice to the face, massaging the carotid artery (on one side of the neck only), or having an older child perform a Valsalva maneuver (e.g., exhaling against a closed glottis, blowing on the thumb as if it were a trumpet for 30 to 60 seconds), have reversed the SVT. When vagal maneuvers fail, adenosine may be used to end the episode of SVT by impairing AV node conduction. If the infant or child is minimally symptomatic, digitalization should be undertaken, with careful monitoring of vital signs and patient response to the intervention. If cardiac output is significantly compromised or signs of CHF exist, esophageal overdrive pacing or synchronized cardioversion can be used in the intensive care setting.

Nursing Care Management. An initial nursing responsibility is recognition of an abnormal heartbeat, in either rate or rhythm. When a dysrhythmia is suspected, the apical rate is counted for 1 full minute and compared with the radial rate. Consistently high or low heart rates should be regarded as suspicious. Accurate nursing assessment, especially in regard to cardiac output, is essential.

The onset and diagnosis of a cardiac dysrhythmia are frightening experiences for parents and the older child. Sometimes the dysrhythmia rapidly leads to heart failure and an emergency medical crisis. In this situation parents need much support to express their feelings, understand the diagnosis, and comply with home therapy, such as daily drug administration. Often an unspoken fear of potential death exists even if the dysrhythmia is benign, and repeated explanations are needed to allay the anxiety.

A primary focus of nursing care is education of the family regarding the specific treatment of the dysrhythmia. After the first episode of SVT, parents should be taught to take a pulse for 1 full minute. If medication is prescribed, instructions regarding accurate dosage and the importance of administering the correct dose at specified intervals are stressed.

When a pacemaker is implanted, the education of the parents and child includes an explanation of the device, a description of the component parts and the surgical procedure, and discharge teaching. For example, discharge teaching includes information about the signs and symptoms of infection, general wound care, and any specific limitations to activity. Instructions for telephone transmission of ECG readings are also given. Children with pacemakers should wear a Medic-Alert device, and their parents should have a pacer identification card with specific pacer data in case of an emergency.

VASCULAR DYSFUNCTION

Systemic Hypertension

Hypertension is defined as the consistent elevation of blood pressure (BP) beyond values considered to be the upper limits of normal. The National Heart, Lung, and Blood Institute's report (1996) on BP control in children defines BP categories as follows:

Normal BP—Systolic and diastolic pressure below the 90th percentile for age and sex

Normal high BP—Average systolic and/or average diastolic BP between the 90th and 95th percentiles for age and sex

High BP (hypertension)—Average systolic and/or average diastolic BP at or greater than the 95th percentile for age and sex with measurements obtained on at least three occasions

The two major categories are *essential hypertension* (no identifiable cause) and *secondary hypertension* (subsequent to an identifiable cause). Hypertension is a primary risk for CVAs and a major risk factor for myocardial infarction in adults. In recent years there has been increasing interest in this disorder in adolescents and children, particularly in terms of prevention of later morbidity and mortality.

Routine DP measurements have detected hypertension with surprising frequency in asymptomatic children, especially teenagers. Although the prevalence of the condition in adolescents is difficult to evaluate, evidence is accumulating to indicate that the essential hypertension of adulthood may have its origin in childhood; thus its early detection has significance for prevention and treatment.

Etiology. Most instances of hypertension observed in young children occur secondary to a structural abnormality or an underlying pathologic process, although this is being challenged by screening programs of relatively healthy children. The most common cause of secondary hypertension is renal disease, followed by cardiovascular, endocrine, and some neurologic disorders.

The causes of essential hypertension are undetermined, but evidence indicates that both genetic and environmental factors play a role. The incidence of hypertension has been shown to be higher in children whose parents are hypertensive. African-

Americans have a higher incidence of hypertension than Caucasians, and in these persons it develops earlier, is commonly more severe, and results in mortality at an earlier age. Environmental factors that contribute to the risk of developing hypertension include obesity, excessive salt ingestion, smoking, and stress.

Diagnostic Evaluation. Because of the increasing numbers of hypertensive or potentially hypertensive children and adolescents being identified, a BP determination should be a routine part of annual assessment in children. Although clinical manifestations associated with hypertension depend largely on the underling cause, some observations can provide clues to the examiner that an elevated BP may be a factor (Box 48-10). In infants and very young children who cannot communicate symptoms, observation of behavior provides clues, although gross behavioral changes may not be apparent until complications are present.

No definitive cutoff values are used in the diagnosis of hypertension in the pediatric patient. The suggested classification is given in Table 48-6. *Significant hypertension* is a BP persistently between the 95th and 99th percentiles for age and sex. *Severe hypertension* is a BP persistently at or above the 99th percentile for age and sex. It is important to note that a child who is very tall for his or her age (above the 90th percentile) may have a higher normal BP than a child of average height. Newer BP tables have been developed that adjust for age, sex, and height (see Appendix J). Before a diagnosis is made, BP should be measured on at least three separate occasions.

In children with suspected primary hypertension, initial laboratory data are also obtained. This generally includes a urinalysis, renal function studies such as creatinine and blood urea nitrogen, a lipid profile, complete blood count, and electrolytes. More intensive tests may be indicated for those with probable secondary hypertension.

Therapeutic Management. Therapy for secondary hypertension involves diagnosis and treatment of the underlying cause. In cases amenable to surgical repair, the nature of the condition, the type of surgery, and the age of the child are all important considerations. Children or adolescents with consistently elevated BP readings from no known cause or those with secondary hypertension not amenable to surgical correction may be treated with a combination of nonpharmacologic and pharmacologic interventions. Dietary practices and lifestyle changes are important in the control of hypertension both for children and for adults. Nonpharmacologic measures, such as limitation of dietary salt, weight control, increased exercise, and avoidance of stress and smoking, carry no risk and should be instituted first, except in severe cases. Because the long-term effects of antihypertensive agents on children are not known, drug treatment of asymptomatic children with mild or borderline hypertension is not recommended.

Drug therapy is instituted with caution in children with significant elevations of BP resistant to nonpharmacologic intervention. The treatment should begin with one drug and should add other drugs only if control is not obtained. Compliance with antihypertensive drug regimens is extremely difficult. The oral antihypertensive drugs used most often in children include beta blockers (propranolol), ACE inhibitors, diuretics, and occasionally a vasodilator (hydralazine). The goal is to achieve a normotensive state throughout the day without accompanying drug side effects.

Box 48-10

Clinical Manifestations of Hypertension

ADOLESCENTS AND OLDER CHILDREN

Frequent headaches
Dizziness
Changes in vision

INFANTS OR YOUNG CHILDREN

Irritability
Head-banging or head-rubbing
May wake up screaming in the night

TABLE 48-6

Classification of Hypertension by Age Group

Age Group	Significant Hypertension (mm Hg)	Severe Hypertension (mm Hg)
Newborn (7 days)	Systolic BP ≥96	Systolic BP ≥106
(8–30 days)	Systolic BP ≥104	Systolic BP ≥110
Infant (<2 years)	Systolic BP ≥112	Systolic BP ≥118
	Diastolic BP ≥74	Diastolic BP ≥82
Children (3-5 years)	Systolic BP ≥116	Systolic BP ≥124
	Diastolic BP ≥76	Diastolic BP ≥84
Children (6-9 years)	Systolic BP ≥122	Systolic BP ≥130
	Diastolic BP ≥78	Diastolic BP ≥86
Children (10-12 years)	Systolic BP ≥126	Systolic BP ≥134
	Diastolic BP ≥82	Diastolic BP ≥90
Adolescents (13-15 years)	Systolic BP ≥136	Systolic BP ≥144
	Diastolic BP ≥86	Diastolic BP ≥92
Adolescents (16-18 years)	Systolic BP ≥142	Systolic BP ≥150
	Diastolic BP ≥92	Diastolic BP ≥98

From National Heart, Lung, and Blood Institute: Report of the Second Task Force on Blood Pressure Control in Children, 1987, *Pediatrics* 79(1): 1-25, 1987.

Nursing Care Management. The nurse is active in detection, diagnosis, and therapy in many settings. Nurses are commonly the persons who operate well-child care and follow-up units and are usually the primary contact between health services and the child and family.

BP measurement should always be a part of the routine assessment of infants and children. To avoid false readings caused by excitement, care is taken to quiet the child or relax the adolescent while the measurement is recorded. The chief cause of falsely elevated BP readings is the use of improperly fitting, narrow cuffs. Therefore attention to correct measurement technique is essential (see Blood Pressure, Chapter 35).

Nursing counseling and guidance of affected children are challenges. Education aimed at understanding hypertension and its implication over the life span is essential in promoting patient and family compliance with both nonpharmacologic and pharmacologic therapies (see Compliance, Chapter 45).

Home BP measurements can facilitate surveillance in youngsters with chronic hypertension and can document effectiveness of therapy. A family member can be instructed on how to take and record accurate BP measurements, thus decreasing the number of trips to a health care facility. This individual needs to understand when to contact the practitioner regarding elevated values. The school nurse can often be a valuable resource in monitoring BP.

The nurse plays an important role in assessing individual families and providing targeted information regarding nonpharmacologic modes of intervention, such as diet, weight loss, smoking, and exercise programs. If extensive dietary counseling is required, the child should be referred to a nutritionist with expertise in working with children and adolescents. Exercise regimens should be individualized. School children and young adolescents generally prefer team sports rather than individual training, which they may view as a burden rather than an enjoyable activity. If peers and family members can be encouraged to participate in any of the management strategies, the child's compliance is likely to be greater.

Young hypertensive women should avoid oral contraceptives because of their pressor effects. Other options need to be presented before this form of birth control is discontinued (see Contraception, Chapter 40).

If drug therapy is prescribed, the nurse needs to provide information to the family regarding the reasons for it, how the drug works, and possible side effects. General instructions for antihypertensive drugs include:

- Rise slowly from a horizontal position and avoid sudden position changes.
- Take drug as prescribed.
- Notify practitioner if unpleasant side effects occur, but do not discontinue drug.
- Avoid alcohol and stay on prescribed diet.

The need for follow-up is stressed, especially because antihypertensive therapy can sometimes be safely discontinued if BP remains under control over time.

Kawasaki Disease (KD) (Mucocutaneous Lymph Node Syndrome)

KD is an acute systemic vasculitis. It is seen in every racial group, and about 80% of cases occur in children younger than 5 years, with peak incidence in the toddler age group. The acute disease is self-limited. Without treatment, however, approximately 20% of children with KD develop cardiac sequelae. Infants younger than 1 year are most seriously affected by KD and are at the greatest risk for heart involvement.

The etiology of KD remains a mystery. Although it is not spread by person-to-person contact, several factors support infectious etiologic factors. It is often seen in geographic and seasonal outbreaks, with most cases reported in the late winter and early spring.

Pathophysiology. The principal area of involvement is the cardiovascular system. During the initial stage of the illness, extensive inflammation of the arterioles, venules, and capillaries occurs, which later progresses to the formation of coronary artery aneurysms in some children. When death occurs, it is usually the result of coronary thrombosis or severe scar formation and stenosis of the main coronary artery.

Clinical Manifestations. Because no specific diagnostic test exists for KD, the diagnosis is established on the basis of clinical findings and associated laboratory results (Box 48-11). KD manifests in three phases: acute, subacute, and convalescent. The *acute phase* begins with the abrupt onset of high fever that is unresponsive to antibiotics and antipyretics. The child then develops the remaining diagnostic symptoms. During this stage the child is typically very irritable. The *subacute phase* begins with resolution of the fever and lasts until all clinical signs of KD have disappeared. During this phase the child is at greatest risk for the development of coronary artery aneurysms. Echocardiograms are used to monitor myocardial and coronary artery status. A baseline echocardiogram should be obtained at the time of diagnosis for comparison with future studies. Irritability persists during this phase. In the *convalescent phase,* all the clinical signs of KD have resolved, but the laboratory values have not returned to normal. This phase is complete when all blood values are normal (6 to 8 weeks after onset). At the end of this stage the child has regained his or her usual temperament, energy, and appetite.

Cardiac Involvement. The most serious complication of KD is the potential for myocardial infarction, which generally results from thrombotic occlusion of a coronary aneurysm. The main symptoms of acute myocardial infarction in children are abdominal pain, vomiting, restlessness, inconsolable crying, pallor, and shock.

Box 48-11

Diagnostic Criteria for Kawasaki Disease

The child must exhibit five of the following six criteria, including fever:

1. Fever for 5 or more days (often diagnosed with shorter duration of fever if other symptoms are present)
2. Bilateral conjunctival injection (inflammation) without exudation
3. Changes in the oral mucous membranes, such as erythema, dryness, and fissuring of the lips; oropharyngeal reddening; or "strawberry tongue" (large papillae are exposed)
4. Changes in the extremities, such as peripheral edema, erythema of the palms and soles, and periungual desquamation (peeling) of the hands and feet
5. Polymorphous rash
6. Cervical lymphadenopathy (one lymph node >1.5 cm)

Therapeutic Management. The current treatment of KD includes high-dose IV gamma globulin along with salicylate therapy. Gamma globulin has been demonstrated to be effective at reducing the incidence of coronary artery abnormalities when given within the first 10 days of the illness. A single large infusion of 2 g/kg over 10 to 12 hours is safe and effective in reducing fever and aneurysm formation (American Academy of Pediatrics, 2000).

Aspirin is given initially in an antiinflammatory dose (80 to 100 mg/kg/day in divided doses every 6 hours) to control fever and symptoms of inflammation. Once fever has subsided, aspirin is continued at an antiplatelet dose (3 to 5 mg/kg/day). Low-dose aspirin is continued in patients without echocardiographic evidence of coronary abnormalities until the platelet count has returned to normal (6 to 8 weeks). If the child develops coronary abnormalities, salicylate therapy is continued indefinitely. Additional anticoagulation with Coumadin may be indicated in children with giant aneurysms.

Prognosis. Most children with KD recover fully after treatment. However, when cardiovascular complications occur, serious morbidity may result. Death occurs rarely and almost always results from coronary thrombosis.

Nursing Care Management. In the initial phase the nurse must monitor the child's cardiac status carefully. Intake and output and daily weight measurements are recorded. Although the child may be reluctant to eat and therefore may be partially dehydrated, fluids need to be administered with care because of the usual finding of myocarditis. The child should be assessed often for signs of CHF, including decreased urine output, gallop rhythm (an additional heart sound), tachycardia, and respiratory distress.

Administration of gamma globulin should follow the same guidelines as for any blood product, with frequent monitoring of vital signs. Patients must be watched for allergic reactions (see Table 48-6). Cardiac status must be monitored because of the large volume being administered to patients with myocarditis and diminished left ventricular function.

Most nursing care focuses on symptomatic relief. To minimize skin discomfort, cool cloths, nonscented lotions, and soft, loose clothing are helpful. During the acute phase, mouth care, including lubricating ointment for the lips, is important for the mucosal inflammation. Clear liquids and soft foods can be offered.

Patient irritability is perhaps the most challenging problem. These children need a quiet environment that promotes adequate rest. Their parents need to be supported in their efforts to comfort an often inconsolable child. They may need time away from their child, and nurses can often provide respite care for the family. Parents need to understand that irritability is a hallmark of KD and that they need not feel guilty or embarrassed about their child's behavior.

Discharge Teaching. Parents need accurate information about the progression of KD, including the importance of follow-up monitoring and when they should contact their practitioner. Irritability is likely to persist for up to 2 months after the onset of symptoms. Peeling of the hands and feet is painless and occurs primarily in the second and third weeks. Arthritis, especially of the larger weight-bearing joints, may persist for several weeks. Children are typically most stiff in the mornings, during cold weather, and after naps. Passive range-of-motion exercises in the bathtub are often helpful in increasing flexibility. Any live immunizations (e.g., measles-mumps-rubella) should be deferred for 3 months after the administration of gamma globulin because the body might not produce the appropriate amount of antibodies. The decision to give the varicella (chickenpox) vaccine while the child is receiving aspirin therapy is made individually by the practitioner. Temperature should be recorded after discharge until the child has been afebrile for several days.*

All parents should understand the unlikely but real possibility of myocardial infarction, as well as the signs and symptoms of cardiac ischemia, in a child. At discharge the ultimate cardiac sequela is generally not known because changes occur up to a month after the onset of KD. In addition, the parents of children with known severe coronary artery sequelae may be taught cardiopulmonary resuscitation.*

Shock

Shock, or *circulatory failure,* is a complex clinical syndrome characterized by inadequate tissue perfusion to meet the metabolic demands of the body, resulting in cellular dysfunction and eventual organ failure. Although the causes are different, the physiologic consequences are the same: hypotension, tissue hypoxia, and metabolic acidosis.

Circulatory failure in children is a result of hypovolemia, altered peripheral vascular resistance, or pump failure. Types of shock are listed in Box 48-12.

Pathophysiology. A healthy child's circulatory system is able to transport oxygen and metabolic substrates to body tissues, which require a constant source of these essential needs. The cardiac output and distribution to various body tissues can change rapidly in response to intrinsic (myocardial and intravascular) or extrinsic (neuronal) control mechanisms. In shock states these mechanisms are altered or challenged.

Reduced blood flow, as in hypovolemic shock, causes diminished venous return to the heart, low CVP, low cardiac output, and hypotension. Vasomotor centers in the medulla are signaled, causing a compensatory increase in the force and rate of cardiac contraction and constriction of arterioles and veins, thereby increasing peripheral vascular resistance. Simultaneously the lowered blood volume leads to the release of large amounts of catecholamines, antidiuretic hormone, adrenocorticosteroids, and aldosterone in an effort to conserve body fluids. This causes reduced blood flow to the skin, kidneys, muscles, and viscera in order to shunt the available blood to the brain and heart. Consequently, the skin feels cold and clammy, there is poor capillary filling, and glomerular filtration and urine output are significantly reduced.

As a result of impaired perfusion, oxygen is depleted in the tissue cells, causing them to revert to anaerobic metabolism, producing lactic acidosis. The acidosis places an extra burden on the lungs as they attempt to compensate for the metabolic acidosis by increased respiratory rate to remove excess carbon dioxide. Prolonged vasoconstriction results in fatigue and atony of the peripheral arterioles, which leads to vessel dilation. Venules, less sensitive to vasodilator substances, remain constricted for a time, causing massive pooling in the capillary and venular beds, which further depletes blood volume.

*Community and home care instructions for measuring a child's temperature and for infant and child cardiopulmonary resuscitation are available in Wong DL, Hess CS: ***Wong and Whaley's clinical manual of pediatric nursing***, ed 5, St Louis, 2000, Mosby.

Box 48-12

Types of Shock

HYPOVOLEMIC SHOCK

Characteristics

Reduction in size of vascular compartment
Falling blood pressure
Poor capillary filling
Low central venous pressure

Most Common Causes

Blood loss (hemorrhagic shock)—trauma, gastrointestinal bleeding, intracranial hemorrhage
Plasma loss—increased capillary permeability associated with sepsis and acidosis, hypoproteinemia, burns, peritonitis
Extracellular fluid loss—vomiting, diarrhea, glycosuric diuresis, sunstroke

DISTRIBUTIVE SHOCK

Characteristics

Reduction in peripheral vascular resistance
Profound inadequacies in tissue perfusion
Increased venous capacity and pooling
Acute reduction in return blood flow to the heart
Diminished cardiac output

Most Common Causes

Anaphylaxis (anaphylactic shock)—extreme allergy or hypersensitivity to a foreign substance
Sepsis (septic shock, bacteremic shock, endotoxic shock)—overwhelming sepsis and circulating bacterial toxins
Loss of neuronal control (neurogenic shock)—interruption of neuronal transmission (spinal cord injury)
Myocardial depression and peripheral dilation—exposure to anesthesia or ingestion of barbiturates, tranquilizers, opiolds, antihypertensive agents, or ganglionic blocking agents

CARDIOGENIC SHOCK

Characteristic

Decreased cardiac output

Most Common Causes

After surgery for congenital heart disease
Primary pump failure—myocarditis, myocardial trauma, biochemical derangements, congestive heart failure
Dysrhythmias—paroxysmal atrial tachycardia, atrioventricular block, and ventricular dysrhythmias; secondary to myocarditis or biochemical abnormalities (occasionally)

Complications of shock create further hazards. Central nervous system hypoperfusion may eventually lead to cerebral edema, cortical infarction, or intraventricular hemorrhage. Renal hypoperfusion causes renal ischemia with possible tubular or glomerular necrosis and renal vein thrombosis. Reduced blood flow to the lungs can interfere with surfactant secretion and result in adult respiratory distress syndrome (ARDS), characterized by sudden pulmonary congestion and atelectasis with formation of a hyaline membrane. Gastrointestinal tract bleeding and perforation are always possible after splanchnic ischemia and necrosis of intestinal mucosa. Metabolic complications of shock may include hypoglycemia, hypocalcemia, and other electrolyte disturbances.

Box 48-13

Clinical Manifestations of Shock

COMPENSATED

Apprehensiveness
Irritability
Unexplained tachycardia
Normal blood pressure
Narrowing pulse pressure
Thirst
Pallor
Diminished urine output
Reduced perfusion of extremities

UNCOMPENSATED

Confusion and somnolence
Tachypnea
Moderate metabolic acidosis
Oliguria
Cool, pale extremities
Decreased skin turgor
Poor capillary filling

IRREVERSIBLE

Thready, weak pulse
Hypotension
Periodic breathing or apnea
Anuria
Stupor or coma

Diagnostic Evaluation. The etiology of shock can be discerned from the history and the physical examination. The severity of the shock is determined by measurements of vital signs, including CVP and capillary filling (Box 48-13). Shock can be regarded as a form of compensation for circulatory failure. Because of the progressive nature of shock, it can be divided into the following three stages or phases:

1. *Compensated shock.* Vital organ function is maintained by intrinsic compensatory mechanisms; blood flow is usually normal or increased but generally uneven or maldistributed in the microcirculation.

NURSE ALERT • Unexplained mild tachycardia and a decrease in perfusion of the hands and feet are differentiating features of compensated shock.

2. *Uncompensated shock.* Efficiency of the cardiovascular system gradually diminishes until perfusion in the microcirculation becomes marginal despite compensatory adjustments. The outcomes of circulatory failure that progress beyond the limits of compensation are tissue hypoxia, metabolic acidosis, and eventual dysfunction of all organ systems.

NURSE ALERT • Tachycardia is pronounced; BP is maintained, but pulse pressure (difference between systolic and diastolic BP) becomes narrowed; there is poor capillary filling; and the child in uncompensated shock exhibits decreased responsiveness, confusion, and sleepiness.

3. *Irreversible, or terminal, shock.* Damage to vital organs, such as the heart or brain, is of such magnitude that the entire organism will be disrupted regardless of therapeutic intervention. Death occurs even if cardiovascular measurements return to normal levels with therapy.

At all stages the principal differentiating signs are observed in the (1) degree of tachycardia and perfusion to extremities, (2) level of consciousness, and (3) BP. Additional signs or modifications of these more universal signs may be present depending on the type and cause of the shock. Initially the child's ability to compensate is effective; therefore early signs are subtle. As the shock state advances, signs are more obvious and indicate early decompensation.

Additional signs may be present, depending on the type and etiology of the shock. In early septic shock there are chills, fever, and vasodilation, with increased cardiac output that results in warm, flushed skin (hyperdynamic or "hot" shock). A later and ominous development is disseminated intravascular coagulation (see Chapter 49), the major hematologic complication of septic shock. Anaphylactic shock is commonly accompanied by urticaria and angioneurotic edema, which is life threatening when it involves the respiratory passages (see Anaphylaxis, p. 1349).

Laboratory tests that assist in assessment are blood gas measurements, pH, and sometimes liver function tests. Coagulation tests are evaluated when there is evidence of bleeding, such as oozing from a venipuncture site, bleeding from any orifice, or petechiae. Cultures of blood and other sites are indicated when there is a high suspicion of sepsis. Renal function tests are performed when impaired renal function is evident.

Therapeutic Management. Treatment of shock consists of three major thrusts: (1) ventilation, (2) fluid administration, and (3) improvement of the pumping action of the heart (vasopressor support). The first priority is to establish an airway and administer oxygen. Once the airway is ensured, circulatory stabilization is the major concern.

Ventilatory Support. The lung is the organ most sensitive to shock. Decreased or redistribution of blood flow to respiratory muscles plus the increased work of breathing can rapidly lead to respiratory failure. Critically ill patients are unable to maintain an adequate airway. To place the lung at rest and improve ventilation, tracheal intubation is initiated early with positive-pressure ventilation. Supplemental oxygen is always given as soon as possible. Blood gases and pH are monitored often.

Increased extravascular lung water caused by edema contributes to the development of respiratory complications. Therapy is directed toward maintaining normal arterial blood gas measurements, normal acid-base balance, and circulation. Efforts are made to remove fluid and prevent its accumulation with the use of diuretics.

Cardiovascular Support. In most cases, rapid restoration of blood volume is all that is needed for resuscitation of the child in shock. An isotonic crystalloid solution (normal saline or Ringer's lactate) is the fluid of choice; colloids such as albumin are also used. Successful resuscitation is reflected by an increase in BP and a reduction in heart rate; increased cardiac output will result in improved capillary circulation and skin color. CVP measurements of right atrial pressure help guide fluid therapy, and urine output measurement is an important indicator of adequacy of circulation. Correction of acidosis, hypoxemia, and any metabolic derangements is mandatory.

Temporary pharmacologic support may be required to enhance myocardial contractility to reverse metabolic or respiratory acidosis, and/or to maintain arterial pressure. The principal agents used to improve cardiac output and circulation are the sympathetic amines administered by constant infusion pump. Those given most often are catecholamines, such as dopamine (Intropin), epinephrine (Adrenalin), and isoproterenol (Isuprel). Vasodilators that are sometimes used include nitroprusside (Nipride) and hydralazine (Apresoline).

Acidosis is corrected with adequate ventilatory support, including oxygen, and the administration of sodium bicarbonate. Calcium chloride may be administered to improve cardiac function. Appropriate antibiotics are administered to patients with septic shock. In cases of septic shock caused by gram-negative organisms, corticosteroids are of value. Other complicating disorders are treated appropriately.

Nursing Care Management. When shock is a likely complication, the child is observed carefully for any early signs, which are reported immediately for further medical evaluation.

NURSE ALERT • Early clinical signs include apprehension, irritability, normal BP, narrowing pulse pressure (difference between diastolic and systolic BP), thirst, pallor, diminished urine output, unexplained mild tachycardia, and a decrease in perfusion of the hands and feet.

The child who is in shock requires intensive observation and care. *The initial action is to ensure adequate tissue oxygenation.* The nurse should be prepared to administer oxygen by the appropriate route and to assist with any intubation and ventilatory procedures indicated. Other procedures and activities that require immediate attention are establishing an IV line, weighing the child, obtaining baseline vital signs, placing an indwelling catheter, obtaining blood gas and other measurements, and administering medications as indicated. The child is best positioned flat with the legs elevated.

The nurse's responsibilities are to monitor the IV infusion, intake and output, vital signs (including CVP), and general systems assessments on a routine basis. IV medications are titrated according to patient responses, and vital signs are taken every 15 minutes during the critical periods and thereafter as needed. Urine output is measured hourly; blood gases, hematocrit, pH, and electrolytes are monitored frequently to assess the status of the child and the efficacy of therapy. An apnea and cardiac monitor is attached and monitored continuously. In the initial stages of acute shock, the care of the child often requires the attendance of more than one nurse in order to manage all the necessary activities that must be carried out simultaneously (Emergency box).

Emergency

SHOCK

Ventilation

Establish airway—be prepared for intubation.
Administer oxygen, usually 100% by mask.

Fluid Administration

Restore blood or fluid volume as ordered.

Cardiovascular Support

Administer vasopressors, especially epinephrine in dose of 0.01 mg/kg until maximum dose of 0.5 ml of 1:1000 dilution subcutaneously; may repeat in 30 minutes.

General Support

Keep child flat with legs raised above level of heart.
Keep child warm and calm.

In Addition

Septic shock: Administer broad-spectrum antibiotics intravenously.
Anaphylaxis: Remove allergen if possible; may place tourniquet above site of injection.

Throughout the intense activity the family must not be overlooked. Someone should contact family members at short intervals to inform them about what is being done and whether there is any progress. Ideally someone should remain with the parents to serve as liaison between them and the intensive care team. However, this is not always feasible in such a critical situation. As soon as possible, they should be allowed to see the child. A member of the clergy may be called to help provide comfort and support.

(See also Nursing Care Plan: The Child in Circulatory Failure [Shock].*)

Anaphylaxis

Anaphylaxis is an acute clinical syndrome resulting from the interaction of an allergen and a patient who is hypersensitive. When the antigen enters the circulatory system, a generalized reaction occurs rapidly. Vasoactive amines (principally histamine or a histamine-like substance) are released and cause vasodilation, bronchoconstriction, and increased capillary permeability.

Severe reactions are immediate in onset, are often life threatening, and commonly involve multiple systems, primarily the cardiovascular, respiratory, gastrointestinal, and integumentary systems. Exposure to the antigen can be by ingestion, inhalation, skin contact, or injection. Examples of common allergens associated with anaphylaxis include drugs (e.g., antibiotics, chemotherapeutic agents, and radiologic contrast media), latex, foods, bee or snake venoms, and biologic agents (e.g., antisera, enzymes, hormones, an blood products).

NURSE ALERT • Penicillin allergy is associated with immediate onset (within an hour of administration) or accelerated onset (1 to 72 hours after administration) of skin eruption, especially a urticarial rash, or more serious symptoms such as laryngeal edema or anaphylactic shock.

Clinical Manifestations. The onset of clinic symptoms usually occurs within seconds or minutes of exposure to the antigen, and the rapidity of the reaction is directly related to its intensity: the sooner the onset, the more severe the reaction. The reaction may be preceded by symptoms of uneasiness, restlessness, irritability, severe anxiety, headache, dizziness, paresthesia, and disorientation. The patient may lose consciousness. Cutaneous signs of flushing and urticaria are common early on, followed by angioedema, most notably in the eyelids, lips, tongue, hands, feet, and genitalia.

Bronchiolar constriction may follow, causing narrowing of the airway; pulmonary edema and hemorrhage also may occur. Laryngeal edema with severe acute upper airway obstruction may be life threatening and requires rapid intervention. Shock occurs as a result of mediator-induced vasodilation, which causes capillary permeability and loss of intravascular fluid into the interstitial space. Sudden hypotension and impaired cardiac output with poor perfusion are seen.

Therapeutic Management. Successful outcome of anaphylactic reactions depends on rapid recognition and institution of treatment. The goals of treatment are to provide ventilation, restore adequate circulation, and prevent further exposure by identifying and removing the cause when possible.

A mild reaction with no evidence of respiratory distress or cardiovascular compromise can be managed with subcutaneous administration of antihistamines, such as diphenhydramine (Benadryl) and epinephrine.

Moderate or severe distress presents a potentially life-threatening emergency. As with all shock states, establishing an airway is the first concern. Epinephrine is given subcutaneously or intravenously as an antihistamine and to support the cardiovascular system and increase blood pressure. Other routes for giving epinephrine are intramuscular and via the airway, either nebulized or injected through an ET tube. In severe anaphylaxis, epinephrine by any route is better than none. Fluids are given to restore blood volume. Additional vasopressors may be given to improve cardiac output. Children with serious anaphylaxis should be hospitalized and monitored for at least 24 hours because relapses may occur (Bochner and Lichtenstein, 1991).

Prevention of a reaction is preferable. Preventing exposure is more easily accomplished in children known to be at risk, including those with (1) a history of previous allergic reaction to specific antigen, (2) a history of atopy, (3) a history of severe reactions in immediate family members, and (4) a reaction to a skin test, although skin tests are not available for all allergens. Desensitization may be recommended in certain cases.

Nursing Care Management. The major nursing responsibility in anaphylaxis is anticipating which children are likely to develop a reaction, recognizing the early signs, and intervening appropriately. When an anaphylactic reaction is suspected, both immediate intervention and preparation for medical therapy are nursing responsibilities. Ventilation is ensured by placing the child in a head-elevated position, unless contraindicated by hypotension, to facilitate breathing and administer oxygen. If the child is not breathing, cardiopulmonary resuscitation (CPR) is initiated, and emergency medical services are summoned.

If the cause can be determined, measures are implemented to slow the spread of the offending substance. For example, a tourniquet is applied above the point of entry (e.g., sting, injection), or IV medication or dye infusion is discontinued. An IV infusion is established immediately. Emergency medications are given intravenously whenever possible; however, epinephrine may be given subcutaneously (see Emergency box). Vital signs and urine output are monitored frequently. Medications are administered as prescribed, with regular assessment to monitor effectiveness and to detect signs of side effects of medication and fluid overload.

To prevent an anaphylactic reaction, parents are always asked about possible allergic responses to foods, latex, medications, and environmental conditions. (See Guidelines box, Taking an Allergy History, p. 770). These are displayed prominently on the patient's chart. The specific allergen is noted, as well as the type and severity of the reaction. Parents are excellent historians, especially when the child has displayed a pronounced reaction to a substance. Drugs, including related drugs (e.g., penicillin, nafcillin), and other items, such as latex, that have produced a reaction previously are never used. If the child is allergic to insect venom, the family is instructed to purchase an emergency kit to be kept with the child at all times. Both the family and the child, if the child is old enough, are taught how to use the equipment. Medical identification should be carried by the patient at all times.

*In Wong DL, Hess CS: ***Wong and Whaley's clinical manual of pediatric nursing***, ed 5, St Louis, 2000, Mosby.

Toxic Shock Syndrome (TSS)

TSS is a relatively rare disease that occurs predominantly (but not exclusively) in previously healthy young women during their menstrual periods. The organism implicated is the phage group 1 *S. aureus,* which is believed to produce an epidermal toxin. The disease has been observed primarily in women who use tampons during their menstrual periods. The tampons may carry the organism from the fingers or the vulva into the vagina during insertion; the tampon might traumatize the vaginal wall and provide a focus of infection; or the tampon itself may provide a favorable environment for growth of the organism or elaboration of its toxin.

Diagnostic Evaluation. Diagnosis is established on the basis of the criteria established by the Centers for Disease Control and Prevention's toxic case definition (Box 48-14). A history of tampon use contributes to the diagnosis. Additional laboratory tests include cultures from blood, vagina, cervix, and any discharge. Other laboratory tests are those that facilitate the management of shock.

Therapeutic Management. The management of TSS is the same as management of shock of any etiology and may range from supportive care in mild cases to hospitalization and intensive care in severe cases. Appropriate parenteral antibiotics are usually administered after cultures are obtained.

Nursing Care Management. Nursing care and observation of the acutely ill patient are the same as those described for shock of any etiology. Because the disease is relatively rare, the major efforts of nursing are directed toward prevention. The association between the disease and the use of tampons provides some direction for education. Avoiding the use of tampons offers the most certain preventive measure, although this approach is probably unacceptable to most adolescent girls, who prefer the freedom, comfort, and inconspicuousness that tampons afford.

Adolescent girls who use tampons can be taught general hygiene measures, such as handwashing before insertion of the tampon and not using a tampon that has been dropped or otherwise soiled. Tampons should be inserted carefully to avoid vaginal abrasion. Also, it is wise to modify their use. For example, tampons may be used intermittently during the menstrual cycle, alternating with sanitary napkins—perhaps using the napkins during the night, when at home during the day, and when flow is light. Young girls are advised not to use superabsorbent tampons and not to leave any tampon in the body for more than 4 to 6 hours. Patients who use tampons need to understand that they should remove the tampon and consult their health professional if they develop a sudden high fever, vomiting, diarrhea, muscle pain, dizziness, fainting or near fainting when standing, or a rash that resembles a sunburn.

HEART TRANSPLANTATION

Heart transplantation has become a treatment option for infants and children with worsening heart failure and a limited life expectancy despite maximum medical and surgical management. Indications for heart transplantation in children are cardiomyopathy and end-stage congenital heart disease. It is also an option for patients with some forms of complex congenital heart defects, such as hypoplastic left heart syndrome, for whom conventional surgical approaches have a high mortality.

The heart transplant procedure may be orthotopic or heterotopic. *Orthotopic heart transplantation* refers to removing the recipient's own heart and implanting a new heart from a donor who has been pronounced brain dead but whose heart remains healthy. The donor and recipient are matched by weight and blood type. *Heterotopic heart transplantation* refers to leaving the recipient's own heart in place and implanting a new heart to act as an additional pump or "piggyback" heart; this type of transplant is rarely done in children.

Before transplantation, potential recipients undergo a careful cardiac evaluation to determine whether there are any other medical or surgical options to improve the patient's cardiac status. Other organ systems are assessed to identify problems that might preclude or increase the risk of transplantation. A psychosocial evaluation of the patient and family is done to assess family function, support systems, and the family's ability to comply with the complex medical regimen after the transplant. Support services to help the family successfully care for their child are provided when possible. Parents and older adolescents need extensive education about the risks and benefits of transplantation so that they can make an informed decision. In a study of factors that influenced parent decision making about heart transplantation, family beliefs and values were found to be most important (Higgins and Kayser-Jones, 1996).

Box 48-14

Criteria for Definition of Toxic Shock Syndrome

1. Fever of 38.9° C (102°F) or higher
2. Presence of diffuse macular erythroderma
3. Desquamation, particularly of palms and soles, 1 to 2 weeks after onset of illness
4. Hypotension, defined as a systolic blood pressure of 90 mm Hg or less for adults and below the 5th percentile for children younger than 16 years old; or an orthostatic drop in diastolic blood pressure of 15 mm Hg or more with a change from lying to sitting; or orthostatic syncope; or orthostatic dizziness
5. Involvement of three or more of the following organ systems: gastrointestinal, muscular, mucous membrane, renal, hepatic, hematologic, and central nervous system.

Toxic shock syndrome is probable when four of the five major criteria are fulfilled. In addition, if blood and cerebrospinal fluid cultures are obtained, they must be negative for any organisms other than *Staphylococcus aureus.* Serologic tests for Rocky Mountain spotted fever, leptospirosis, and measles also must be negative.

Modified from American Academy of Pediatrics, Committee on Infectious Diseases, Pickering L, editor: *2000 Red Book: report of the Committee on Infectious Diseases,* ed 25, Elk Grove Village, IL, 2000, The Academy.

Patients are listed on a national computer network organized by the United Network for Organ Sharing (UNOS) to match donors and recipients. Because of the limited donor supply, from 10% to 25% of infants waiting for heart transplants will die before receiving a donor heart. (See also Organ or Tissue Donation/Autopsy, Chapter 41.)

The heart transplant registry sponsored by the International Society of Heart and Lung Transplantation recently reported a subset of pediatric data for patients aged 0 to 18 years (Boucek et al, 1991). The registry includes information on 3800 pediatric heart transplant recipients who underwent transplantation from 1987 to 1997. Worldwide, approximately 360 pediatric heart transplants were performed each year during the 1990s. Most of these were done in the United States (about 250 transplants per year). Infants and young children are the largest group. The actuarial survival rate of all pediatric patients in the registry is 78% at 1 year and 68% at 5 years. Infants have a higher mortality rate in the first year after transplant than older children and adolescents. The ongoing rate of patient loss (as a measure of late mortality) is approximately 2.5% each year during the first 10 years. Survivors have an excellent functional status, with more than 90% reporting no activity limits.

The posttransplant course is complex. Although heart function is greatly improved or normal after transplantation, the risk of rejection is serious. The leading cause of death after heart transplantation is rejection (Shaddy et al, 1996). Rejection of the heart is diagnosed primarily by endomyocardial biopsy in older children. Serial echocardiograms are often used in infants and young children to reduce the need for invasive biopsies. Immunosuppressants must be taken for life and have many systemic side effects. Infection is always a risk. Potential long-term problems that may limit survival include chronic rejection, causing coronary artery disease; renal dysfunction and hypertension resulting from cyclosporine administration; lymphoma; and infection. In the short term, after successful transplantation, children are able to return to full participation in age-appropriate activities and appear to adapt well to their new lifestyle. Transplantation is not a cure because patients must live with the lifetime consequences of chronic immunosuppression. The long-term prognosis is unknown because heart transplantation is a relatively new therapy in the pediatric population, begun in 1985.

Nursing Care Management. Nursing care after transplantation is demanding and complex, and careful attention must be paid to both the physical needs of the child and the emotional needs of the child and family. Successfully caring for a child after heart transplantation requires the expertise and dedication of many members of the health care team. Nurses play vital roles in assessment, coordination of care, psychosocial support, and patient and family education. The heart transplant recipient must be carefully monitored for signs of rejection, infection, and the side effects of the immunosuppressant medications. Care of the immunosuppressed child is reviewed in Chapter 49. Psychosocial concerns and appropriate interventions for the child with a life-threatening disorder are presented in Chapter 41.

The first 6 to 12 months after the transplant are most intense because the risk of complications is greatest and the patient and family are adjusting to a new lifestyle. Patients are monitored closely by the health care team, with frequent visits and laboratory tests. Care is usually shared between local health care providers and the transplant center. Many patients are able to return to school and other age-appropriate activities within 2 to 3 months after the transplant.

Key Points

- Congenital heart disease (CHD) is the most common form of heart disease in children.
- Major categories to investigate in the cardiac history are poor weight gain, poor feeding habits, and fatigue during feeding; frequent respiratory infections and difficulties; and evidence of exercise intolerance.
- The most common tests used in assessing cardiac function are radiography, electrocardiography, echocardiography, and cardiac catheterization.
- Cardiac catheterization procedures can be divided into three groups: (1) diagnostic procedures, including angiography, that measure pressures and saturations to establish cardiac diagnosis; (2) interventional procedures, in which catheters or balloon devices are used to correct cardiac defects; and (3) electrophysiology studies, in which catheters with electrodes are used to evaluate dysrhythmias.
- Diagnostic cardiac catheterization provides important information about oxygen saturation of blood within the chambers and great vessels, pressure changes, changes in cardiac output or stroke volume, and anatomic abnormalities.
- Several prenatal factors may predispose children to CHD: maternal rubella during pregnancy, maternal alcoholism, maternal age above 40 years, and maternal type 1 diabetes.
- Congenital heart defects can be divided into four main groups, as determined by hemodynamic patterns: (1) defects that result in increased pulmonary blood flow, (2) obstructive defects, (3) defects that result in decreased pulmonary blood flow, and (4) mixed defects.
- Clinical consequences of congenital heart defects include congestive heart failure (CHF) and hypoxemia. A child can have both hypoxemia and CHF, although usually they occur independently.
- Clinical manifestations of CHF are impaired myocardial function (tachycardia, cardiomegaly), pulmonary congestion (dyspnea, tachypnea, orthopnea, cyanosis), and systemic congestion (hepatosplenomegaly, edema, distended veins).
- Nursing measures in the care of a child with CHF are to assist in improving cardiac function, decrease cardiac demands, reduce respiratory distress, maintain nutritional status, promote fluid loss, and provide family support.
- Clinical manifestations of hypoxemia are cyanosis, polycythemia, clubbing, and delayed growth and development. The child is at increased risk for hypercyanotic spells, cerebrovascular accidents, brain abscess, and bacterial endocarditis.
- Caring for the child with CHD and the family requires helping them to adjust to the disorder and to cope with the effects of the defect and fostering growth-promoting family relationships.

- Preoperative care of the child with a congenital heart defect involves introducing the child and family to the hospital and preparing them for preoperative and postoperative procedures.
- Providing postoperative care includes observing vital signs and arterial/venous pressures, maintaining respiratory status, allowing maximum rest, providing comfort, monitoring fluids, planning for progressive activities, giving emotional support, observing for complications of surgery, and planning for discharge and home care.
- Acquired cardiovascular disorders include bacterial endocarditis, rheumatic fever, hyperlipidemia (hypercholesterolemia), and cardiac dysrhythmias.
- Prevention of bacterial endocarditis in certain children with CHD involves administration of prophylactic antibiotics when specific procedures are performed.
- Acute rheumatic fever is a systemic inflammatory disease that can damage the cardiac valves and is associated with previous group A streptococcal infection. Its incidence has increased in some areas of the United States.
- Cholesterol screening in children is controversial; currently children with known risk factors for hyperlipidemia are screened and treated as needed. The influence of childhood cholesterol levels on later development of coronary artery disease is under investigation.
- Common dysrhythmias in children include slow rhythms (bradycardias, heart block) and fast rhythms (sinus tachycardia, supraventricular tachycardia).
- Heart transplantation has been extended to infants and children with cardiopulmonary and complex congenital heart defects involving ventricular dysfunction, such as hypoplastic left heart syndrome.
- Education of the child with hypertension and the family focuses on drug therapy, diet control, and appropriate exercise.
- Kawasaki disease is an extensive inflammation of small vessels and capillaries that may progress to involve the coronary arteries, causing aneurysm formation. The administration of gamma globulin is an important aspect of treatment.
- Emergency treatment for shock includes ensuring ventilation; administering vasopressors, fluids/blood, and antibiotics as needed; and providing supportive measures such as correct positioning, warmth, and psychologic reassurance to the child and family.
- Persons at risk for anaphylaxis may be identified by a history of previous allergic reaction, history of atopy, history of severe reactions in the family, and positive skin test response to the allergen.
- Nursing management of the patient with toxic shock syndrome focuses on prevention primarily through education concerning safe tampon use.

References

American Academy of Pediatrics, Committee on Infectious Diseases, Pickering L, editor: *2000 Red Book: report of the Committee on Infectious Diseases,* ed 25, Elk Grove Village, IL, 2000, The Academy.

Bochner BS, Lichtenstein LM: Anaphylaxis, *N Engl J Med* 324(25):1785-1790, 1991.

Boucek MM et al: The registry of the International Society of Heart and Lung Transplantation: second official pediatric report 1998, *J Heart Lung Transplant* 17:1141-1160, 1998.

Colletti RB et al: Niacin treatment of hypercholesterolemia in children, *Pediatrics* 92(1):78-82, 1993.

Dajani AS, Taubert KA: Infective endocarditis. In Emmanouilides GC et al, editors: *Heart disease in infants, children and adolescents,* ed 5, Baltimore, 1995, Williams & Wilkins.

Higgins SS, Kayser-Jones J: Factors influencing parent decision making about pediatric cardiac transplantation, *J Pediatr Nurs* 11(3):152-160, 1996.

Koster NK. Physical activity and congenital heart disease, *Nurs Clin North Am* 29(2):345-356, 1994.

National Cholesterol Education Program: Report of the expert panel on blood cholesterol levels in children and adolescents, *Pediatrics* 89:525-584, 1992.

National Heart, Lung, and Blood Institute: Update on the 1987 Task Force Report on High Blood Pressure in Children and Adolescents: a working group report from the National High Blood Pressure Education Program: National High Blood Pressure Education Program Working Group on Hypertension Control in Children and Adolescents, *Pediatrics* 98(4, pt 1):649-658, 1996.

Shaddy RE et al: Outcome of cardiac transplantation in children: survival in a contemporary multi-institutional pediatric heart transplant study, *Circulation* 94(9, suppl):1169-1173, 1996.

Valenzuela RC, Rosen DA: Topical lidocaine-prilocaine cream (EMLA) for thoracostomy tube removal, *Anesth Analg* 88:1107-1108, 1999.

CHAPTER 49

Hematologic and Immunologic Dysfunction

http://www.harcourthealth.com/MERLIN/Wong/maternal/

Learning Objectives

On completion of this chapter the reader will be able to:

- Distinguish between the various categories of anemia.
- Describe the prevention of and care of the child with iron deficiency anemia.
- Compare sickle cell anemia and β-thalassemia major in relation to pathophysiology and nursing care.
- Describe the mechanisms of inheritance and nursing care of the child with hemophilia.
- Relate the pathophysiology and clinical manifestations of leukemia.
- Demonstrate an understanding of the rationale of therapies for neoplastic disease.
- Outline a plan of care for the child with neoplastic disease and the family.
- Contrast the pathophysiology and management of the immunodeficiency disorders.
- List nursing precautions and responsibilities during blood transfusion.
- Describe the types of bone marrow transplants.

HEMATOLOGIC/IMMUNOLOGIC DYSFUNCTION

Assessment of Hematologic Function

Several tests can be performed to assess hematologic function, including additional procedures to identify the cause of the dysfunction. The following discussion is limited to a description of the most common and one of the most valuable tests, the *complete blood count (CBC)*. Other procedures, such as those related to iron, coagulation, and immune status, are discussed throughout the chapter as appropriate. The nurse should be familiar with the significance of the findings from the CBC (Table 49-1) and aware of normal values for age, which are listed in Appendix F.

As with any disorder, the history and physical examination are essential to identification of hematologic dysfunction, and the nurse is often the first person to suspect a problem based on information from these sources. Comments by the parent regarding the child's lack of energy, food diary of poor sources of iron, frequent infections, and bleeding that is difficult to control offer clues to the more common disorders affecting the blood. A careful physical appraisal, especially of the skin, can reveal findings (e.g., pallor, petechiae, bruising) that may indicate minor or serious hematologic conditions. Nurses need to be aware of the clinical manifestations of blood diseases to assist in recognizing symptoms and establishing a diagnosis.

RED BLOOD CELL (RBC) DISORDERS

Anemia

The term *anemia* describes a condition in which the number of RBCs and/or the hemoglobin (Hgb or Hb) concentration is reduced below normal. As a result of this decrease, the oxygen-carrying capacity of the blood is diminished, causing a reduction in the oxygen available to the tissues. Anemia is the most common hematologic disorder of infancy and childhood and is not a disease itself but an indication or manifestation of an underlying pathologic process.

Classification. Anemias are classified in relation to (1) *etiology* or *physiology,* manifested by erythrocyte and/or Hgb depletion; and (2) *morphology,* the characteristic changes in RBC size, shape, and/or color. Although the morphologic classification is more useful in terms of laboratory evaluation of anemia, the etiologic approach provides direction for planning nursing care. For example, anemia with reduced Hgb concentration may be caused by a dietary depletion of iron, and the principal intervention is replenishing iron stores. Etiologic factors responsible for anemia are described in Box 49-1.

TABLE 49-1

Tests Performed as Part of the Complete Blood Count

Test (Average Value)*	Description/Comments
Red blood cell (RBC) count (4.5-5.5 million/mm^3)	Number of RBCs/mm^3 of blood Indirectly estimates Hgb content of blood Reflects function of bone marrow
Hemoglobin (Hgb) determination (11.5-15.5 g/dl)	Amount of Hgb/dl of whole blood Total blood Hgb primarily depends on number of circulating RBCs, but also on amount of Hgb in each cell
Hematocrit (Hct) (35%-45%)	Percentage or volume of packed RBCs to whole blood Indirectly measures Hgb content Is approximately three times Hgb content
RBC indexes	MCV and MCH depend on accurate counts of RBCs, whereas MCHC does not; therefore MCHC is often more reliable All indexes depend on *average* cell measurements and do not show anisocytosis (individual RBC variations)
Mean corpuscular volume (MCV) (77-95 μm^3)	Average of mean volume (size) of a single RBC MCV values expressed as cubic microns (μm^3) or femtoliters (fl)
Mean corpuscular hemoglobin (MCH) (25-33 pg/cell)	Average or mean quantity (weight) of Hgb in a single RBC MCH values expressed as picograms (pg) or micromicrograms ($\mu\mu g$)
Mean corpuscular hemoglobin concentration (MCHC) (31%-37% Hgb [g]/dl RBC)	Average concentration of Hgb in a single RBC MCHC values expressed as % Hgb (g)/cell or Hgb (g)/dl RBC
RBC volume distribution width (RDW) (13.4% $\pm$ 1.2%)	Average size of RBCs Differentiates some types of anemia
Reticulocyte count (0.5%-1.5% erythrocytes)	% Reticulocytes to RBCs Index of production of mature RBCs by bone marrow Decreased count indicates depressed bone marrow function Increased count indicates erythrogenesis in response to some stimulus When reticulocyte count is extremely high, other forms of immature RBCs (normoblasts, even erythroblasts) may be present Indirectly estimates hypochromic anemia Usually elevated in patients with chronic hemolytic anemia
White blood cell (WBC) count (4.5-13.5 $\times 10^3$ cells/mm^3)	Number of WBCs/mm^3 of blood Total number of WBCs less important than differential count
Differential WBC count	Inspection and quantification of WBC types present in peripheral blood Values are expressed as percentages; to obtain absolute number of any type of WBCs, multiply its respective percentage by total number of WBCs
Neutrophils (polys) (54%-62%) (3-5.8 $\times 10^3$ cells/mm^3)	Primary defense in bacterial infection; capable of phagocytizing and killing bacteria
Bands (3%-5%) (0.15-0.4 $\times 10^3$ cells/mm^3)	Immature neutrophils Increased numbers in bacterial infection Also capable of phagocytosis and killing
Eosinophils (1%-3%) (0.05-0.25 $\times 10^3$ cells/mm^3)	Named for their staining characteristics with eosin dye Increased in allergic disorders, parasitic diseases, certain neoplasms, and other diseases
Basophils (0.075%) (0.015-0.030 cells/mm^3)	Named for their characteristic basophilic stippling Contain histamine, heparin, and serotonin; believed to cause increased blood flow to injured tissues while preventing excessive clotting
Lymphocytes (25%-33%) (1.5-3.0 $\times 10^3$ cells/mm^3)	Involved in development of antibody and delayed hypersensitivity
Monocytes (3%-7%)	Large phagocytic cells that are involved in early stage of inflammatory reaction
Absolute neutrophil count (ANC) (>1000)	% Neutrophils $\times$ WBC count Indicates body's capability to handle bacterial infections
Platelet count (150-400 $\times 10^3$/mm^3)	Number of platelets/mm^3 of blood Cellular fragments that are necessary for clotting to occur
Stained peripheral blood smear	Visual estimation of amount of Hgb in RBCs and overall size, shape, and structure of RBCs Various staining properties of RBC structures may be evidence of immature forms of erythrocytes Shows variation in size and shape of RBCs: microcytic, macrocytic, poikilocytic (variable shapes)

*See Appendix for normal values according to ages.

Box 49-1

Classification of Anemia

ETIOLOGY/PATHOPHYSIOLOGY

Excessive blood loss—From acute or chronic hemorrhage (internal or external); until stores are replaced, there is usually a normocytic (normal size), normochromic (normal color) anemia, provided that there are sufficient iron stores for hemoglobin (Hgb) synthesis

Destruction (hemolysis) of erythrocytes—As a result of an intracorpuscular defect within the red blood cell (RBC) (e.g., sickle cell anemia) or an extracorpuscular factor (e.g., infectious agents, chemicals, immune mechanisms) that causes destruction to outpace production

Decreased or impaired production of erythrocytes or their components—As a result of bone marrow failure (caused by factors such as neoplastic diseases, irradiation, chemicals, or disease) or deficiency of essential nutrients (e.g., iron)

MORPHOLOGY

Size—Cell size; for example, ***normocytes*** (normal), ***microcytes*** (smaller than normal), or ***macrocytes*** (larger than normal)

Shape—Irregularly shaped RBCs; for example, ***poikilocytes*** (irregularly shaped cells), ***spherocytes*** (globular cells), and ***drepanocytes*** (sickle cells)

Staining characteristics or color—Reflects the hemoglobin concentration; for example, ***normochromic*** (sufficient or normal amount) or ***hypochromic*** (reduced amount)

Box 49-2

Clinical Manifestations of Anemia

GENERAL MANIFESTATIONS

Muscle weakness
Easy fatigability
- Frequent resting
- Shortness of breath
- Poor sucking (infants)

Pale skin
- Waxy pallor seen in severe anemia

Pica—eating clay, ice, paste

CENTRAL NERVOUS SYSTEM MANIFESTATIONS

Headache
Dizziness
Light-headedness
Irritability
Slowed thought processes
Decreased attention span
Apathy
Depression

SHOCK (BLOOD LOSS ANEMIA)

Poor peripheral perfusion
Skin moist and cool
Low blood pressure and central venous pressure
Increased heart rate

Consequences of Anemia. The basic physiologic defect caused by anemia is a decrease in the oxygen-carrying capacity of blood and consequently a reduction in the amount of oxygen available to the cells. When the anemia has developed slowly, the child usually adapts to the declining Hgb level.

The effects of anemia on the circulatory system can be profound. Because the viscosity of blood depends almost entirely on the concentration of RBCs, the resulting hemodilution of severe anemia decreases peripheral resistance, causing greater quantities of blood to return to the heart. The increased circulation and turbulence within the heart may produce a murmur. Because the cardiac workload is greatly increased, especially during exercise, infection, or emotional stress, cardiac failure may ensue.

Children seem to have a remarkable ability to function quite well despite low levels of Hgb. *Cyanosis* (the result of the quantity of deoxygenated Hgb in arterial blood) is typically not evident. Growth retardation, resulting from decreased cellular metabolism and coexisting anorexia, is a common finding in chronic severe anemia and is commonly accompanied by delayed sexual maturation in the older child.

Diagnostic Evaluation. In general, anemia may be suspected from findings during the history taking and physical examination, such as lack of energy, easy fatigability, and pallor, but unless the anemia is severe, the first clue to the disorder may be alterations in the CBC, such as decreased RBCs and hematocrit (Hct) levels (Box 49-2). Although anemia is sometimes defined as an Hgb level below 10 or 11 g/dl, this arbitrary cutoff is inappropriate for all children because Hgb levels normally vary with age (see Table 49-1 and Appendix F).

Other tests specific to a particular type of anemia are used to determine the underlying cause of anemia. These are discussed in relation to the particular disorder.

Therapeutic Management. The objective of medical management is to reverse the anemia by treating the underlying cause and to make up for any deficiency of blood, blood component, or substance the blood needs for normal functioning. For example, blood or blood cells are replaced after hemorrhage; in nutritional anemias the specific substance that is deficient is replaced.

In patients with severe anemia, supportive medical care may include oxygen therapy, bed rest, and replacement of intravascular volume with intravenous (IV) fluids. Medical management of selected anemias is outlined in Table 49-2. The prognosis for anemia depends on the correction of the cause.

Nursing Care Management

➤ Assessment

The assessment of anemia includes the basic techniques that are applicable to any condition. The age of the infant or child provides some clues regarding the possible etiology of the anemia. For example, iron deficiency anemia occurs more commonly in infants between 6 and 24 months of age and during the growth spurt of adolescence.

Racial or ethnic background is a significant factor. For example, the anemias related to abnormal Hgb levels are found in Southeast Asians and persons of African or Mediterranean ancestry. These same groups may be genetically deficient in the enzyme lactase after the period of infancy. Affected individuals are unable to tolerate lactose in the diet, with consequent intestinal irritation and chronic blood loss.

Special emphasis is placed on a careful history to elicit any information that might help identify the cause of the anemia. For example, a statement such as "The baby drinks lots of milk"

TABLE 49-2
Description and Management of Selected Anemias

Type of Anemia	Description	Management
Blood loss anemia	Until 20% or more of blood volume is lost with normal vital signs	No therapy needed
	Altered vital signs with losses of 30%-40% of blood volume and signs of shock	Blood replacement Plasma or plasma protein product until blood is available
Iron deficiency anemia	Decreased RBC production	See discussion in text
Anemia of renal disease	Usually not until symptomatic and Hgb is less than 7 to 8 mg/dl	Transfusion of packed RBCs
Hemolytic anemias Spherocytosis Elliptocytosis	Shortened survival of RBCs	Splenectomy
Sickle cell anemia	Shortened survival of RBCs	See discussion in text
Thalassemia	Shortened survival of RBCs	See discussion in text

is a common finding in infants with iron deficiency anemia. An episode of diarrhea may have precipitated a temporary lactose intolerance in infants.

Stool examination for occult (invisible) blood (Hemoccult test) can identify chronic intestinal bleeding that results from a primary or secondary lactase deficiency. It is also important to understand the significance of various blood tests. Blood loss from overt hemorrhage may be manifested as shock.

➤ Nursing Diagnoses

A variety of nursing diagnoses may be evident after the assessment of anemia. Some of the general aspects of nursing management are included in the Nursing Care Plan on p.1357. Others become apparent in specific situations.

➤ Plan of Care and Implementation

The goals of care for the infant or child with anemia depend on the severity of the condition and the cause. Most children tolerate mild anemia well, and a major goal is preparing them for diagnostic tests and possible blood transfusion (p. 1355). Other goals of care are the following:

1. Child and family will receive adequate support and education.
2. Child will exhibit minimal physical or emotional exertion.
3. Child will experience no complications from anemia or its treatment.

Prepare Child and Family for Laboratory Tests. Usually, several blood tests are ordered, but because they are generally done sequentially rather than at one time, the child is subjected to multiple finger or heel punctures and/or venipunctures. Laboratory technicians commonly are not aware of the trauma that repeated punctures represent to a child. However, these invasive procedures need not be painful (see Blood Specimens, Chapter 44). For example, the topical application of *EMLA (eutectic mixture of local anesthetics)* before needle punctures can eliminate any pain (see Pain Management, Chapter 44). Therefore the nurse is responsible for preparing the child and family for the tests by (1) explaining the significance of each test, particularly why the tests are not done at one time; (2) encouraging parents or another supportive person to be with the child during the procedure; and (3) allowing the child to play with the equipment on a doll and/or participate in the actual procedure (e.g., by cleansing the finger with an alcohol swab). Older children may appreciate the opportunity to observe the blood cells under a microscope or in photographs. This experience is an especially important consideration if a serious blood disorder, such as leukemia, is suspected because it serves as a foundation for explaining the pathophysiology of the disorder.

Bone marrow aspiration is not a routine hematologic test but is essential for definitive diagnosis of the leukemias, lymphomas, and certain anemias.

The following are suggested explanations for teaching children about blood components:

- **Red blood cells (RBCs)**—Carry the oxygen you breathe from your lungs to all parts of your body
- **White blood cells (WBCs)**—Help keep germs from causing infection
- **Platelets**—Small parts of cells that help make bleeding stop; platelets help your body stop bleeding by forming a clot (scab) over the hurt area
- **Plasma**—The liquid portion of blood; has clotting factors that help make bleeding stop

Decrease Tissue Oxygen Needs. Because the basic pathology in anemia is a decrease in oxygen-carrying capacity, an important nursing responsibility is to assess the child's energy level and minimize excess demands. The child's level of tolerance for activities of daily living and play is assessed, and adjustments are made to allow as much self-care as possible without undue exertion. During periods of rest the nurse takes vital signs and observes behavior to establish a baseline of nonexertional energy expenditure. During periods of activity the nurse repeats these measurements and observations to compare them with resting values.

NURSE ALERT • Signs of exertion include tachycardia, palpitations, tachypnea, dyspnea, shortness of breath, hyperpnea, breathlessness, dizziness, light-headedness, diaphoresis, and change in skin color. The child looks fatigued (sagging, limp posture; slow, strained movements; inability to tolerate additional activity; difficulty sucking in infants).

Nursing Care Plan THE CHILD WITH ANEMIA

NURSING DIAGNOSIS Anxiety/fear related to diagnostic procedures, transfusions

EXPECTED OUTCOME Child and family will exhibit minimal signs of fear or anxiety.

Nursing Interventions/*Rationales*

Prepare child and family for tests and procedures using a developmentally appropriate approach (e.g., demonstration of procedure using dolls) *to relieve fear of unknown.*

Explain purpose of tests, procedures, and interventions such as transfusions to child and family *to increase understanding and relieve anxiety.*

Remain with child during tests and procedures and provide comfort measures *to provide support.*

Encourage a parent to remain *to minimize separation anxiety.*

Enlist the child's and parent's help during procedure, giving them very specific tasks and a range of choices as appropriate *to provide a measure of control.*

NURSING DIAGNOSIS Activity intolerance related to generalized weakness, diminished oxygen delivery to tissues

EXPECTED OUTCOME Child's activity level is within normal limits for his or her physical condition.

Nursing Interventions/*Rationales*

Observe for signs of physical exertion (e.g., tachycardia, palpitations, tachypnea, shortness of breath, dizziness, sweating, fatigue) *to assess need for rest.*

Balance rest and activity when planning nursing and medical interventions and play *to diminish exertion.*

Provide quiet diversional activities *that promote rest and prevent boredom.*

Administer oxygen as ordered *to increase oxygenation of tissues.*

Administer blood products as ordered *to replace lost blood and stimulate new blood cell formation;* observe child carefully during and after transfusion *for possible side effects and complications.*

NURSING DIAGNOSIS Altered nutrition: less than body requirements related to inadequate iron intake

EXPECTED OUTCOME Child receives minimum daily requirements of iron.

Nursing Interventions/*Rationales*

Teach caregiver what iron does, what the minimum daily requirements of iron are, and what foods are iron-rich *to promote adequate iron intake in child's diet.*

Administer iron preparations as prescribed *to replenish depleted iron stores.*

Instruct family regarding correct administration of iron preparation (e.g., give between meals *for maximum absorption,* give with fruit juice or multivitamin preparation *because vitamin C appears to increase absorption,* do not give with milk or antacids *since they decrease absorption*).

Observe stools *as adequate dosages of oral iron turn stools a tarry green.*

Diversional activities are planned that promote rest but prevent boredom and withdrawal. Because short attention span, irritability, and restlessness are common in anemia and increase stress demands on the body, appropriate activities are planned, such as listening to music; using a tape recorder; watching television; reading or listening to stories or comics; continuing a favorite hobby, such as stamp collecting, coloring, or drawing; playing board and card games; or being wheeled in a carriage or chair. Choosing the appropriate roommate, such as a child of similar age with a diagnosis that also requires restricted activity, is a helpful intervention.

If infants or young children are hospitalized, the importance of preventing separation from parents must be considered. Crying and fretfulness place increased stress demands on the body, which increases oxygen needs. Parents need help in understanding the importance of their presence, even though the child may be less responsive than usual. The nurse also explains the reason for mood changes and the necessity of allowing the child's dependency.

Prevent Complications. Children who are so severely anemic that they are hospitalized may require oxygen to prevent or reduce tissue hypoxia. Because these children are susceptible to infection, every effort is expended to prevent exposure to infectious agents. All the usual precautions are taken to prevent infection, such as practicing thorough handwashing, selecting an appropriate room in a noninfectious area, restricting visitors or hospital personnel with active infection, and maintaining adequate nutrition. The nurse also observes for signs of infection, particularly temperature elevation and leukocytosis.

Support Family. See Nursing Care Plan: The Child with Anemia for other supportive and educative strategies.

➤ Evaluation

The effectiveness of nursing interventions is determined by continual reassessment and evaluation of care based on the following observational guidelines and expected outcomes:

1. Interview the child and family regarding their understanding of diagnostic procedures and the blood disorder, as well as regarding their feelings and concerns.
2. Monitor therapeutic interventions and the child's tolerance for activity.
3. Assess the child for evidence of complications of therapies.

Expected outcomes are listed in the Nursing Care Plan.

Iron Deficiency Anemia

Anemia caused by an inadequate supply of dietary iron is the most prevalent nutritional disorder in the United States and the most common mineral disturbance (Pappas and Cheng, 1998). However, the prevalence has decreased, probably in part because of families' participation in the Women, Infants, and Children (WIC) program, which provides iron-fortified formula for the first year of life. Premature infants are especially at risk because of their reduced fetal iron supply. Adolescents are also at risk because of their rapid growth rate combined with poor eating habits (Pappas and Cheng, 1998).

Pathophysiology. Iron deficiency anemia can be caused by any number of factors that decrease the supply of iron, impair its absorption, increase the body's need for iron, or affect the synthesis of Hgb. Although the clinical manifestations and diagnostic evaluation are quite similar regardless of the cause, the therapeutic and nursing considerations depend on the specific reason for the iron deficiency. The following discussion is limited to iron deficiency anemia resulting from inadequate iron in the diet.

During the last trimester of pregnancy, iron is transferred from mother to fetus. Most of the iron is stored in the circulating erythrocytes of the fetus, with the remainder stored in the fetal liver, spleen, and bone marrow. These iron stores are usually adequate for the first 5 to 6 months in a full-term infant but for only 2 to 3 months in premature infants or multiple births. If dietary iron is not supplied to meet the infant's growth demands once the fetal iron stores are depleted, iron deficiency anemia results. Physiologic anemia should not be confused with iron deficiency anemia resulting from nutritional causes.

Although most infants with iron deficiency anemia are underweight, many are overweight because of excessive milk ingestion (known as *milk babies*). These children become anemic for two reasons: milk, a poor source of iron, is given almost to the exclusion of solid foods, and some infants fed cow's milk have an increased fecal loss of blood.

Therapeutic Management. Once the diagnosis of iron deficiency anemia is made, therapeutic management focuses on increasing the amount of supplemental iron the child receives. This is usually done through dietary counseling and the administration of oral iron supplements.

In formula-fed infants the most convenient and best sources of supplemental iron are iron-fortified commercial formula and iron-fortified infant cereal. Iron-fortified formula provides a relatively constant and predictable amount of iron and is not associated with an increased incidence of gastrointestinal (GI) symptoms, such as colic, diarrhea, or constipation. To decrease the possibility of iron deficiency from GI blood loss occurring from allergy to the milk protein, infants under 12 months of age should *not* be given fresh cow's milk. Dietary addition of iron-rich foods is usually inadequate as the sole treatment of iron deficiency anemia because the iron is poorly absorbed and provides insufficient supplemental quantities of iron.

If dietary sources of iron cannot replace body stores, oral iron supplements are prescribed for approximately 3 months. Ferrous iron, more readily absorbed than ferric iron, results in higher Hgb levels. Ascorbic acid (vitamin C) appears to facilitate absorption of iron and may be prescribed in addition to the iron preparation.

If the Hgb level is very low or if levels fail to rise after 1 month of oral therapy, it is important to assess whether the iron is being administered correctly. Parenteral (IV or intramuscular [IM]) iron administration is painful, expensive, and occasionally associated with regional lymphadenopathy or serious allergic reaction (Miller, 1995). Therefore parenteral iron is reserved for children who have iron malabsorption or chronic hemoglobinuria. Transfusions are indicated for the most severe anemia and in cases of serious infection, cardiac dysfunction, or surgical emergency when anesthesia is required. Packed RBCs (2 to 3 cc/kg), not whole blood, are used to minimize the chance of circulatory overload. Supplemental oxygen is administered when tissue hypoxia is severe.

Prognosis. The prognosis for a child with this condition is very good. However, there is some evidence that if the iron deficiency anemia is severe and long-standing, cognitive, behavioral, and motor impairment may result (Lozoff et al, 2000).

Nursing Care Management. An essential nursing responsibility is instructing parents in the administration of iron. Oral iron should be given as prescribed in two divided doses between meals, when the presence of free hydrochloric acid is greatest, because more iron is absorbed in the acidic environment of the upper GI tract. A citrus fruit or juice taken with the medication aids in absorption.

An adequate dosage of oral iron turns the stools a tarry green color. The nurse advises parents of this normally expected change and inquires about its occurrence on follow-up visits. Absence of the greenish black stool may be a clue to poor administration of iron, either in schedule or in dosage. Vomiting and/or diarrhea can occur with iron therapy. If the parents report these symptoms, the iron can be given with meals and the dosage reduced and then gradually increased until tolerated.

Liquid preparations of iron may temporarily stain the teeth. If possible, the medication should be taken through a straw or given through a syringe or medicine dropper placed toward the back of the mouth. Brushing the teeth after administration of the drug lessens the discoloration.

If parenteral iron preparations are prescribed, iron dextran must be injected deeply into a large muscle mass using the Z-tract method. The injection site is not massaged after injection to minimize skin staining and irritation. Because no more than 1 ml should be given in one site, the IV route should be considered to avoid multiple injections. Careful observation is required because of the risk of adverse reactions, such as anaphylaxis, with IV administration. A test dose is recommended before routine use.

Diet. A primary nursing objective is to prevent nutritional anemia through family education. The nurse discusses with parents the importance of using iron-fortified formula and the introduction of solid foods at the appropriate age. The best solid-food source of iron is commercial infant cereals. It may be difficult at first to teach the infant to accept foods other than milk. The same principles are applied as those for introducing new foods (see Nutrition, Chapter 36), especially feeding the solid food before the milk. Predominantly milk-fed infants rebel against solid foods, and parents are cautioned about this and the need to be firm in not relinquishing control to the child. It may require intense problem solving on the part of both the family and the nurse to overcome the child's resistance.

A difficulty encountered in discouraging the parents from feeding milk to the exclusion of other foods is dispelling the popular myth that milk is a "perfect food." Many parents believe that milk is best for the infant and equate the weight gain with a "healthy child" and "good mothering." They are not concerned about providing other foods as long as the child continues to take milk. The nurse can also stress that overweight is not synonymous with good health.

Diet education of teenagers is especially difficult, especially because teenage girls are particularly prone to following weight-reduction diets. Emphasizing the effect of anemia on appearance (pallor) and energy level (difficulty maintaining popular activities) may be useful.

Sickle Cell Anemia (SCA)

SCA is one of a group of diseases collectively termed *hemoglobinopathies,* in which normal adult hemoglobin (Hgb A [HbA]) is partly or completely replaced by abnormal sickle hemoglobin (HbS). *Sickle cell disease (SCD)* includes all those hereditary disorders whose clinical, hematologic, and pathologic features are related to the presence of HbS. Even though SCD is sometimes used to refer to SCA, this use is incorrect. Other correct terms for SCA are *SS* and *homozygous sickle cell disease.*

The following are the most common forms of SCD in the United States:

Sickle cell anemia, the homozygous form of the disease (HbSS or SS)

Sickle cell-C disease, a heterozygous variant of SCD, including both HbS and HbC (SC)

Sickle cell–hemoglobin E disease, a variant of SCD in which glutamic acid has been substituted for lysine in the number-26 position of the β-chain (SE)

Sickle thalassemia disease, a combination of sickle cell trait and β-thalassemia trait (Sβthal). β^+ refers to the ability to still produce some normal HbA. β^0 indicates that there is no ability to produce HbA.

Of the SCDs, SCA is the most common form in African-Americans, followed by sickle cell–C disease and sickle β-thalassemia.

SCA is found primarily in African-Americans, occasionally in Hispanics, and infrequently in Caucasians (especially those of Mediterranean descent). The incidence of the disease varies in different geographic locations. Among African-Americans the incidence of sickle cell trait is about 8%. In West Africa the incidence is reported to be as high as 40% among the native population. The high incidence of sickle cell trait in West Africans is believed by some to be the result of selective protection afforded trait carriers against one type of malaria.

The gene that determines the production of HbS is situated on an autosome; when present, it is always detectable and therefore dominant. Persons with heterozygous inheritance have both normal HbA and abnormal HbS and are said to have *sickle cell trait.* Persons with homozygous inheritance have predominantly HbS and have *sickle cell anemia.* The inheritance pattern is essentially that of an autosomal recessive disorder (see Appendix C). Therefore, when both parents have the sickle cell trait, each offspring they produce has a 25% chance of having SCA.

Although the defect is inherited, the sickling phenomenon is usually not apparent until later in infancy because of the presence of fetal hemoglobin (HbF). As long as HbF persists, sickling does not occur because there is less HbS. The newborn has from 60% to 80% HbF, but this rapidly decreases during the first year, so the child is at risk for sickle cell–related complications (Lane, 1996).

Pathophysiology. The clinical features of SCA are primarily the result of (1) *obstruction* caused by the sickled RBCs, and (2) increased RBC *destruction* (Fig. 49-1). The entanglement and enmeshing of rigid sickle-shaped cells with one another intermittently block the microcirculation, causing vaso-occlusion. The resultant absence of blood flow to adjacent tissues causes local hypoxia, leading to tissue ischemia and infarction (cellular death). Most of the complications seen in SCA can be traced to this process and its impact on various organs of the body. The effect of sickling and infarction on organ structures occurs in the following sequence (see also consequences in Box 49-3):

1. Stasis with enlargement
2. Infarction with ischemia and destruction
3. Replacement with fibrous tissue (scarring)

Clinical Manifestation. The clinical manifestations of SCA vary greatly in severity and frequency. The most acute symptoms of the disease occur during periods of exacerbation called *crises.* There are several types of episodic crises: vaso-occlusive, acute splenic sequestration, aplastic, hyperhemolytic, cerebrovascular accident (CVA [stroke]), chest syndrome, and infection. The crises may occur individually or concomitantly with one or more other crises. The episode may be a *vaso-occlusive crisis,* preferably called a "painful episode," characterized by distal ischemia and pain; *sequestration crisis,* a pooling of blood in the liver and spleen with decreased blood volume and shock; *aplastic crisis,* diminished RBC production resulting in profound anemia; or *hyperhemolytic crisis,* an accelerated rate of RBC destruction characterized by anemia, jaundice, and reticulocytosis. This complication commonly suggests other co-existing conditions, such as viral illness, or glucose-6-phosphate dehydrogenase (G6PD) deficiency, which is also common in African-Americans.

Another serious complication is *chest syndrome,* which is clinically similar to pneumonia. It is also associated with chest pain, fever, pneumonia-like cough, and associated anemia. A CVA is a sudden and severe complication, often with no related illnesses. Sickled cells block the major blood vessels in the brain, resulting in cerebral infarction, which causes variable degrees of neurologic impairment. Repeat CVAs causing progressively greater brain damage occur in 47% to 93% of children who have already experienced one stroke (Pegelow et al, 1995).

Diagnostic Evaluation. Newborn screening for SCA is mandatory in most of the United States so that infants can be identified before symptoms occur. At birth the infant has up to 80% HbF, which does not carry the defect. During the first months of life the infant begins production of RBCs with HbA and with HbS if the gene is present. At this point the child may become symptomatic. Because levels of HbS are low at birth, Hgb electrophoresis or other tests that measure Hgb concentrations are indicated. Early diagnosis (before 3 months of age) enables initiation of appropriate interventions to minimize complications. The family is taught to administer prophylactic antibiotics and identify early signs of infection in order to seek medical therapy as soon as possible.

If SCA is not diagnosed in early infancy, it is likely to manifest symptoms during the toddler and preschool years. SCA is occasionally first diagnosed during a crisis that follows an acute respiratory or GI infection. Routine hematologic tests are done to evaluate the anemia. Several specific tests detect the presence of the abnormal Hgb in the heterozygote and/or the homozy-

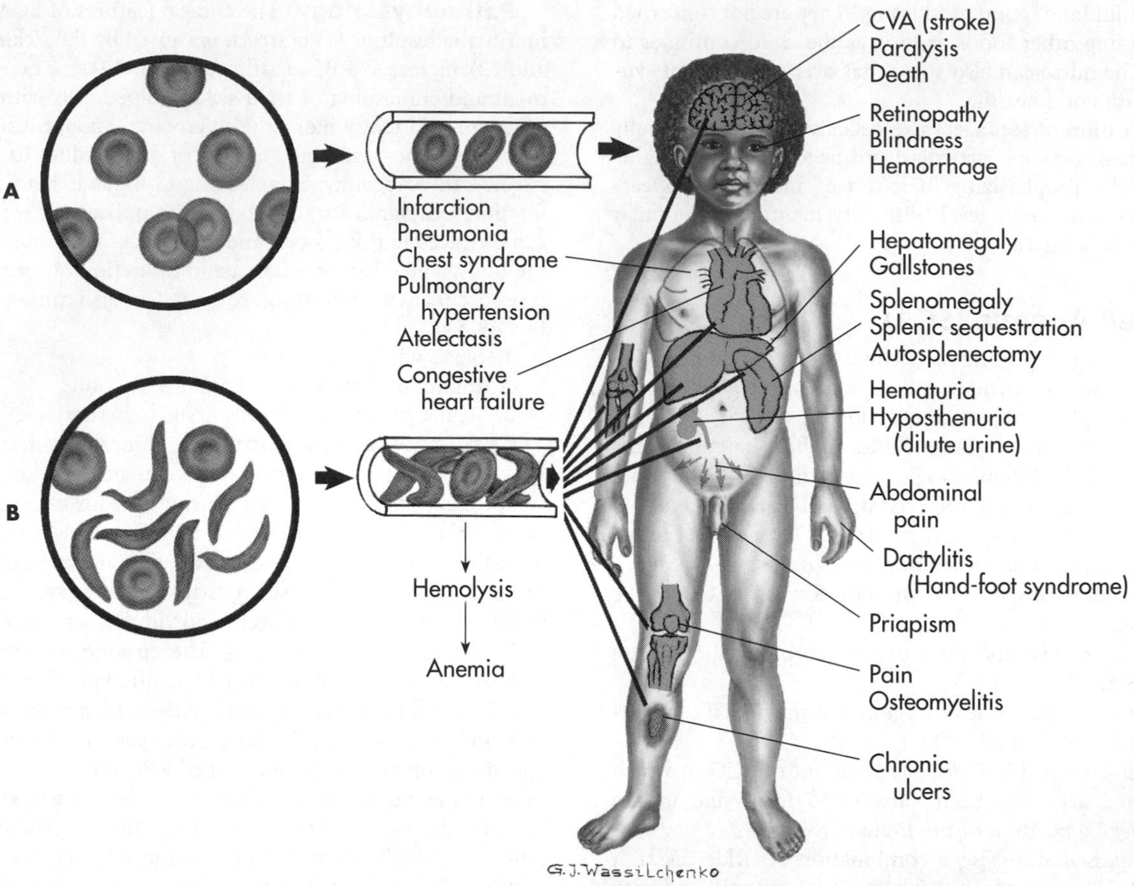

FIG. 49-1 • Differences between effects of **A**, normal, and **B**, sickled RBCs on circulation with selected consequences in a child.

Box 49-3

Clinical Manifestations of Sickle Cell Anemia

GENERAL

Possible growth retardation
Chronic anemia (Hgb 6 to 9 g/dl)
Possible delayed sexual maturation
Marked susceptibility to sepsis

VASO-OCCLUSIVE CRISIS

Pain in area(s) of involvement
Manifestations related to ischemia of involved areas:
- Extremities—painful swelling of hands and feet (sickle cell dactylitis, or "hand-foot syndrome"), painful joints
- Abdomen—severe pain resembling acute surgical condition
- Cerebrum—stroke, visual disturbances
- Chest—symptoms resembling pneumonia, protracted episodes of pulmonary disease
- Liver—obstructive jaundice, hepatic coma
- Kidney—hematuria
- Genital—priapism (painful constant penile erection)

SEQUESTRATION CRISIS

Pooling of large amounts of blood:
- Hepatomegaly
- Splenomegaly
- Circulatory collapse

EFFECTS OF CHRONIC VASO-OCCLUSIVE PHENOMENA

Heart—cardiomegaly, systolic murmurs
Lungs—altered pulmonary function, susceptibility to infections, pulmonary insufficiency
Kidneys—inability to concentrate urine, progressive renal failure, enuresis
Liver—hepatomegaly, cirrhosis, intrahepatic cholestasis
Spleen—splenomegaly, susceptibility to infection, functional reduction in splenic activity progressing to autosplenectomy
Eyes—intraocular abnormalities with visual disturbances, sometimes progressive retinal detachment and blindness
Extremities—skeletal deformities, especially lordosis and kyphosis, chronic leg ulcers, susceptibility to osteomyelitis
Central nervous system—hemiparesis, seizures (acute, not chronic)

gote. For *screening* purposes the *sickle-turbidity test (Sickledex)* is commonly used because it can be performed on blood from a finger stick and yields accurate results in 3 minutes. However, if the test is positive, Hgb electrophoresis is necessary to distinguish between those children with the trait and those with the disease. *Hemoglobin electrophoresis* ("fingerprinting" of the protein) is an accurate, rapid, and specific test for detecting the homozygous and heterozygous forms of the disease, as well as the percentages of the various types of Hgb.

Therapeutic Management. The aims of therapy are (1) to prevent conditions that enhance sickling phenomena, which are responsible for the pathologic sequelae; and (2) to treat the medical emergencies of sickle cell crisis. Prevention consists of maintaining hemodilution. The successful implementation of this goal depends more often on nursing interventions than on medical therapies. Research is investigating hydroxyurea and erythropoietin, which may increase the concentration of Hbf and ultimately reduce complications (Charache et al, 1996; Claster and Vichinsky, 1996; Jayabose et al, 1996; Ware, Steinberg, and Kinney, 1995). A promising area of research is bone marrow transplantation as a possible cure for SCD (Walters, 1999; Walters et al, 2000). Limiting factors include proper patient selection as well as the availability of suitable donors (Mentzer, 2000). This technology raises many ethical issues regarding patient access and availability of therapy (Platt and Guinan, 1996).

Medical management of a crisis is usually directed at supportive and symptomatic treatment. The main objectives are to provide (1) bed rest to minimize energy expenditure and oxygen use; (2) hydration through oral and IV therapy; (3) electrolyte replacement, because hypoxia results in metabolic acidosis, which also promotes sickling; (4) analgesics for the severe pain from vaso-occlusion; (5) blood replacement to treat anemia and to reduce the viscosity of the sickled blood; and (6) antibiotics to treat any existing infection.

Administration of pneumococcal and meningococcal vaccines is recommended for these children because of their susceptibility to infection as a result of a functional asplenia. With the likelihood of transfusion therapy for individuals with SCA, hepatitis B vaccine is recommended for those children who have not received it as part of their routine immunization schedule. (See immunizations, Chapter 36.) Oral penicillin prophylaxis is also recommended by 2 months of age (Sickle Cell Disease Guideline Panel, 1993).

Short-term oxygen therapy may be helpful if a child has symptoms of respiratory difficulty. Severe hypoxia must be prevented because this causes massive systemic sickling that can be fatal. Although oxygen may prevent more sickling, it usually is not effective in reversing sickling, because the oxygen is unable to reach the enmeshed sickled erythrocytes in clogged vessels (Chiocca, 1996). In addition, prolonged administration can depress bone marrow, further aggravating the anemia (Khoury and Grimsley, 1995).

Exchange transfusion, which reduces the number of circulating sickle cells and slows down the vicious circle of hypoxia, thrombosis, tissue ischemia, and injury, has been successful. The procedure is sometimes advocated as a possible preventive technique. However, multiple transfusions carry the risk of transmission of viral infection, hyperviscosity, transfusion reactions, alloimmunization, and hemosiderosis (Lane, 1996). Once a CVA has occurred, blood transfusions are usually given every 4 to 5 weeks to help prevent a repeat stroke. To reduce iron overload, home subcutaneous chelation therapy may be started (see p. 1365).

In children with recurrent life-threatening splenic sequestration, splenectomy may be a lifesaving measure. However, because the spleen usually atrophies on its own through progressive fibrotic changes *(functional asplenia),* routine splenectomy is not recommended because of the risk of overwhelming infection. Any procedure that requires anesthesia has increased risk for these children. *Painful priapism (continual erection)* may be treated by aspiration of the corpora cavernosum. This complication is particularly common in vaso-occlusive crises.

The most common problem for patients with SCA is *vaso-occlusive pain* (Fig. 49-2). The chronic nature of this pain can greatly affect the child's development. A multidisciplinary approach is best for its management. When mild to moderate pain is reported, ibuprofen or acetaminophen is used initially. If these drugs are not effective alone, codeine can be added. The dosages of both drugs are titrated (adjusted) to a therapeutic level. Opioids such as immediate- and sustained-release morphine, oxycodone, hydromorphone (Dilaudid), and methadone are administered intravenously or orally for severe pain and are given around the clock. Patient-controlled analgesia (PCA) has been used successfully for sickle cell–related pain. PCA reinforces the patient's role and responsibility in managing the pain and pro-

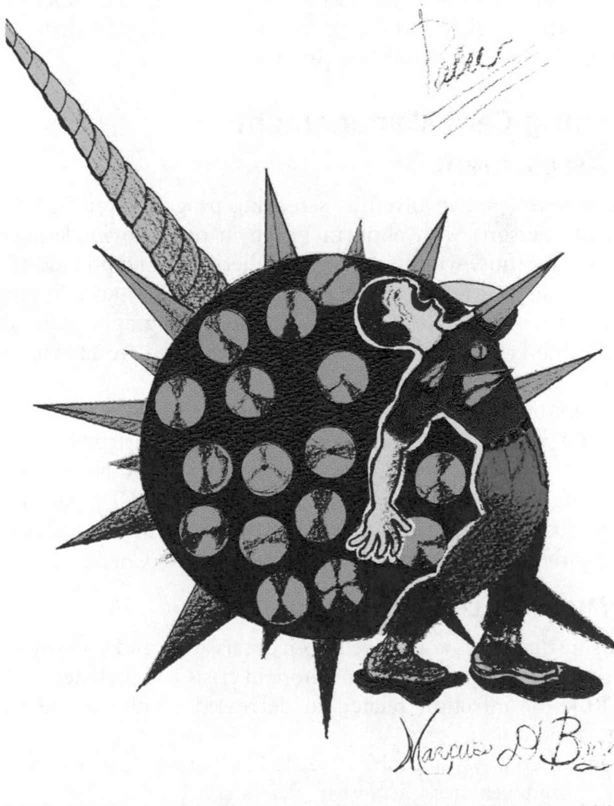

FIG. 49-2 • Drawing of sickle cell pain by a 17-year-old boy. When asked what message he would like to give health professionals about treating pain, he stated, "Tell them to listen to the patient and family. They know about the pain."

vides flexibility in dealing with pain, which may vary in severity over time. The use of high-dose methylprednisolone has decreased the duration of severe pain in children (Griffin, McIntire, and Buchanan, 1994). (See Pain Management, Chapter 44.)

NURSE ALERT • Meperidine (pethidine [Demerol]) is not recommended. Normeperidine, a metabolite of meperidine, is a central nervous system stimulant that produces anxiety, tremors, myoclonus, and generalized seizures when it accumulates with repetitive dosing. Patients with SCD are particularly at risk for normeperidine-induced seizures (American Pain Society, 1999).

Prognosis. The prognosis varies. Most of the time children are without symptoms and participate in normal activities without restrictions. The greatest risk is usually in children younger than 5 years, and the majority of deaths in these children are caused by overwhelming infection. Consequently, SCA is a chronic illness with a potentially terminal outcome.

Individuals with higher levels of HbF are more likely to have fewer complications than those with lower levels (Gribbons, Zahr, and Opas, 1995; Lane, 1996). Research is investigating hydroxyurea and crythropoietin, which may increase the concentration of HbF and ultimately reduce complications (Jayabose et al, 1996).

Physical and sexual maturation are delayed in adolescents with SCA. Although adults achieve normal height, weight, and sexual function, the delay may present problems to the adolescent (Gribbons, Zahr, and Opas, 1995). Bone marrow transplantation offers the hope of a cure for some children, although the mortality related to the procedure is significant (Mentzer, 2000; Walters et al, 2000) (see p. 1390).

Nursing Care Management

➤ Assessment

Many nurses are involved in screening programs for SCA to identify persons with abnormal Hgb in order to implement therapy for those with homozygous inheritance and provide genetic counseling for those with heterozygous inheritance. Young children from families of at-risk racial or geographic origins who exhibit any of the signs previously described are advised to seek medical attention immediately.

Assessment of the child in sickle cell crisis involves all areas and systems that can be affected by circulatory obstruction, including vital signs, neurologic signs, and vision and hearing assessment, as well as assessment of the respiratory, GI, renal, and musculoskeletal systems. It is also important to assess the location and intensity of pain (see Pain Assessment, Chapter 44).

➤ Nursing Diagnoses

Nursing diagnoses are derived from observation and assessment of children with the disease or those in crisis and include:

Risk for infection related to decreased or absent splenic function
Impaired physical mobility related to tissue ischemia, generalized weakness
Altered family processes related to child with a chronic condition
Sickle cell crisis
Pain related to tissue ischemia (sickle cell crisis)
Altered tissue perfusion related to impaired arterial blood flow

➤ Plan of Care and Implementation

The primary goals are as follows:

1. The family and child (when appropriate) will receive education regarding the sickling phenomenon and possible consequences and early recognition of crises and infection.
2. The child will receive supportive therapies during crises.
3. The child and parents will adjust to a lifelong, potentially fatal hereditary disease.
4. Family members will receive genetic counseling.

Educate Family and Child. Family education begins with an explanation of the disease and its consequences. After this explanation, the most important issues to teach the family are to (1) seek early intervention for problems, such as fever of 38.5° C (101.5° F) or greater; (2) give penicillin as ordered; (3) recognize signs and symptoms of splenic sequestration, as well as respiratory problems that can lead to hypoxia; and (4) treat the child normally. The nurse tells the family that the child is healthy but can get sick in ways that other children cannot.

The nurse emphasizes the importance of adequate hydration to prevent sickling and to delay the stasis-thrombosis-ischemia cycle in a crisis. It is not sufficient to advise parents to "force fluids" or "encourage drinking." They need specific instructions on how many daily glasses or bottles of fluid are required. Many foods are also a source of fluid, particularly soups, flavored ice pops, ice cream, sherbet, gelatin, and puddings.

NURSE ALERT • Advise parents to be particularly alert to situations where dehydration may be a possibility, such as during hot weather, and to recognize early signs of reduced intake, such as decreased urine output (e.g., fewer wet diapers) and increased thirst.

Increased fluids combined with impaired kidney function result in the problem of *enuresis.* Parents who are unaware of this fact commonly use the usual measures to discourage bedwetting, such as limiting fluids at night, and may resort to punishment and shame to force bladder control. Enuresis is treated as a complication of the disease, such as joint pain or some other symptom, in order to alleviate parental pressure on the child.

Promote Supportive Therapies During Crises. The success of many of the medical therapies relies heavily on nursing implementation. Management of pain is an especially difficult problem and often involves experimenting with various analgesics, including opioids, and schedules before relief is achieved. Unfortunately, these children tend to be undermedicated, resulting in their "clock watching" and demands for additional doses sooner than might be expected. Often this incorrectly raises suspicions of drug addiction, when in fact the problem is one of improper dosage (Family Focus box). In choosing and scheduling analgesics, the goal should be prevention of pain.

Any pain program should be combined with psychologic support to help the child deal with the depression, anxiety, and fear that may accompany the disease. This includes regular visits with the child to discuss any concerns during the hospitalization and positive reinforcement of coping skills, such as successful methods of dealing with the pain and compliance with treatment prescriptions. To reduce the negative connotation associated with the term "crisis," it is best to say "pain episode."

Family Focus

FEAR OF ADDICTION

Although pain is usually severe and opioids are warranted, many families fear that their child will become addicted to the narcotic. Unfortunately, misinformed health professionals may foster this unfounded fear, resulting in needless suffering. Few, if any, children who receive opioids for severe pain become behaviorally addicted to the drug (Gribbons, Zahr, and Opas, 1995). Families and older children, especially adolescents, need to be reassured that opioids are medically indicated, high doses may be needed, and addiction is rare.

Often, heat to the affected area is soothing. Cold compresses are not applied to the area because this enhances sickling and vasoconstriction. Bed rest is usually well tolerated during a crisis, although actual rest depends greatly on pain alleviation and organized schedules of nursing care. Some activity, particularly passive range-of-motion exercises, is beneficial to promote circulation. Usually the best course of action is to let children dictate their activity tolerance.

If blood transfusions or exchange transfusions are given, the nurse has the responsibility of observing for signs of transfusion reaction. Because hypervolemia from too rapid transfusion can increase the workload of the heart, the nurse also is alert to signs of cardiac failure.

In splenic sequestration the size of the spleen is gently measured by abdominal palpation (see Abdomen, Chapter 35). The nurse should be aware of spleen size because an increasing splenomegaly is an ominous sign. A decreasing spleen size denotes response to therapy. Vital signs and blood pressure are also closely monitored for impending shock. Anemia is typically not a presenting complication in vaso-occlusive crises but is a critical problem in other types of crises. The nurse monitors for evidence of increasing anemia and institutes appropriate nursing intervention (see p. 1356). Oxygen is not beneficial in vaso-occlusive episodes unless hypoxemia is present (Chiocca, 1996). It does not reverse sickled RBCs, and if used in the nonhypoxic patient, it will decrease erythropoiesis (Shapiro, 1993). Because prolonged use of oxygen can aggravate the anemia, signs of lack of therapeutic benefit, such as restlessness, increased pallor, and continued pain, are reported.

Intake, especially of IV fluids, and output are recorded. The child's weight should be taken on admission because it serves as a baseline for evaluating hydration. Because diuresis can result in electrolyte loss, the nurse also observes for signs of hypokalemia and should be familiar with normal serum electrolyte values to report changes.

Recognize Other Complications. Nurses also need to be aware of the signs of chest syndrome and CVA, both potentially fatal complications.

NURSE ALERT • Report signs of the following immediately:

Chest syndrome:

Severe chest pain, sometimes spreading to abdomen

Fever of 38.8° C (102° F) or higher

Very congested cough

Dyspnea, tachypnea

Retractions

Declining oxygen saturation (oximetry)

Cerebrovascular accident:

Jerking or twitching of the face, legs, or arms

Seizures

Strange, abnormal behavior

Inability to move an arm and/or a leg

Stagger or an unsteady walk

Stutter or slurred speech

Weakness in the hands, feet, or legs

Changes in vision

Severe, unrelieved headaches

Severe vomiting

Support Family. Families need the opportunity to discuss their feelings regarding transmitting a potentially fatal, chronic illness to their child. Because of the widely publicized prognosis for children with SCA, many parents express their prevalent fear of the child's death. Because there is no way to predict which child will follow a favorable course, nursing care for the family should be the same as for any family with a child with a life-threatening illness. Particular emphasis is placed on the siblings' reactions, the stress on the marital relationship, and the childrearing attitudes displayed toward the child (see Chapter 41).

Several resources are available to the family with a sickling disorder.*

The nurse advises parents to inform all treating personnel of the child's condition. The use of medical identification, such as a bracelet, is another way of ensuring awareness of the disease.

If family members have the SCD trait and/or SCA, genetic counseling is necessary. A primary goal is informing parents who carry the trait, in language they can understand, that each of their children will have a 1 in 4 chance of having the disease.

*National Association for Sickle Cell Disease, Inc., 3345 Wilshire Blvd., Suite 1106, Los Angeles, CA 90010-1880; (213) 736-5455 or 1-800-421-8453; website: www.sicklecelldisease.org; Center for Sickle Cell Disease, Howard University, 2121 Georgia Ave. NW, Washington, DC 20059; (202) 806-7930; and National Heart, Lung, and Blood Institute, 9000 Rockville Pike, Building 31, Room 4A-21, Bethesda, MD 20892; (301) 496-4236; website: www.nhlbi.nih.gov/nhlbi/nhlbi.htm. The Agency for Health Care Policy and Research (AHCPR) has published three booklets on sickle cell disease: *Sickle Cell Disease: Comprehensive Screening, Diagnosis, Management, and Counseling in Newborns and Infants, Quick Reference Guide for Clinicians No. 6,* Pub. No. AHCPR-0563; and *Sickle Cell Disease in Newborns and Infants: A Guide for Parents,* Pub. No. AHCPR 93-0564. They are available from the AHCPR Publications Clearinghouse, P.O. Box 8547, Silver Spring, MD 20907; 1-800-358-9295; website: www.ahcpr.gov/. *Guideline for the Management of Acute and Chronic Pain in Sickle Cell Disease* is available from American Pain Society, 4700 W. Lake Ave., Glenview, IL 60025-1485; (847) 375-4715; fax (847) 375-6315; e-mail: info@ampainsoc.org; website: www.ampainsoc.org; *Clinical Reference Guide for Health Care Providers; Sickle Cell Related Pain: Assessment and Management—A Guide for Patients and Parents* is available from the New England Regional Genetics Groups (NERGG), No. 28 Clarendon St., Newton, MA 02460; (617) 243-3033; e-mail: maryaten@mediaone.net; website: www.acadia.net/NERGG. A video, *Sickle Cell Disease Is More Than Pain Management,* is available from Maxishare, P.O. Box 2041, Milwaukee, WI 53201; 1-800-444-7747. Information is also available from the Sickle Cell Disease Association of America, Inc., 200 Cooperate Pointe, Suite 495, Culver City, CA 90230-7633.

➤ Evaluation

The effectiveness of nursing interventions is determined by continual reassessment and evaluation of care based on the following observational guidelines and expected outcomes:

1. Interview family regarding their understanding of the disease, the sickling phenomenon, its consequences, and early recognition of complications.
2. Observe child for any evidence of sickling; monitor preventive strategies and therapies, especially pain assessment and management.
3. Interview and observe child and family regarding the way the disease has affected their lives.
4. Interview the family to determine their understanding of the risk of having another child with SCA.
5. Advise family to seek medical attention appropriately.

Expected outcomes include the following:

1. The family demonstrates an understanding of the disease and its consequences and verbalizes symptoms to report (specify knowledge and method of demonstration).
2. The family gives antibiotic on a consistent basis.
3. The child exhibits few episodes of sickling; pain is effectively controlled.
4. The family takes advantage of genetic counseling services and medical care.
5. The child and family express their feelings and concerns regarding the disease.

(See also Nursing Care Plan: The Child with Sickle Cell Disease.*)

β-Thalassemia (Cooley Anemia)

The term *thalassemia,* which is derived from the Greek word *thalassa,* meaning "sea," is applied to a variety of inherited blood disorders characterized by deficiencies in the rate of production of specific globin chains in Hgb. The name appropriately refers to descendants of or those people living near the Mediterranean Sea, who have the highest incidence of the disease, namely, Italians, Greeks, and Syrians. Evidence suggests that the high incidence of the disorders among these groups is a result of selective advantage of the trait to malaria, as is postulated in sickle cell disease. However, the disorder has a wide geographic distribution, probably as a result of genetic migration through intermarriage or possibly as a result of spontaneous mutation.

β-Thalassemia is the most common of the thalassemias and occurs in three forms: a heterozygous form, *thalassemia minor* or *thalassemia trait,* which produces a mild microcytic anemia; *thalassemia intermedia,* which is manifested as splenomegaly and moderate to severe anemia; and a homozygous form, *thalassemia major* (also known as *Cooley anemia*), which results in a severe anemia that would lead to cardiac failure and death in early childhood without transfusion support.

Pathophysiology. Normal postnatal Hgb is composed of two β- and two β-polypeptide chains. In β-thalassemia there is a partial or complete deficiency in the synthesis of the β-chain of the Hgb molecule. Consequently, there is a compensatory increase in the synthesis of β-chains, and β-chain production remains activated, resulting in defective Hgb formation. This unbalanced polypeptide unit is very unstable; when it disintegrates, it damages RBCs, causing severe anemia.

To compensate for the hemolytic process, an overabundance of erythrocytes is formed unless the bone marrow is suppressed by transfusion therapy. Excess iron from hemolysis of supplemental RBCs in transfusions and from the rapid destruction of defective cells is stored in various organs (hemosiderosis).

Diagnostic Evaluation. The onset of thalassemia major may be insidious and not recognized until the latter half of infancy. The clinical effects of thalassemia major are primarily attributable to (1) defective synthesis of HbA, (2) structurally impaired RBCs, and (3) shortened life span of erythrocytes (Box 49-4).

Hematologic studies reveal the characteristic changes in RBCs (i.e., microcytosis, hypochromia, anisocytosis, poikilocytosis, target cells, and basophilic stippling of various stages). Low Hgb and Hct levels are seen in severe anemia, although they are typically lower than the reduction in RBC count because of the proliferation of immature erythrocytes. Hgb electrophoresis confirms the diagnosis, and radiographs of involved bones reveal characteristic findings.

Therapeutic Management. The objective of supportive therapy is to maintain sufficient Hgb levels to prevent bone marrow expansion and the resulting bony deformities, as well as to provide sufficient RBCs to support normal growth and normal physical activity. Transfusions are the foundation of medical management. Recent studies have evaluated the benefits of maintaining the child's Hgb level above 10 g/dl, a goal that may require transfusions as often as every 3 weeks. The advantages

Box 49-4

Clinical Manifestations of β-Thalassemia

ANEMIA (BEFORE DIAGNOSIS)
Unexplained fever
Poor feeding
Greatly enlarged spleen

WITH PROGRESSIVE ANEMIA
Signs of chronic hypoxia
- Headache
- Precordial and bone pain
- Decreased exercise tolerance
- Listlessness
- Anorexia

OTHER FEATURES
Small stature
Delayed sexual maturation
Bronzed, freckled complexion (if not chelated)

BONE CHANGES (OLDER CHILDREN IF UNTREATED)
Enlarged head
Prominent frontal and parietal bosses
Prominent malar eminences
Flat or depressed bridge of the nose
Enlarged maxilla
Protrusion of the lip and upper central incisors and eventual malocclusion
Oriental appearance of eyes

---

*In Wong DL, Hess CS: ***Wong and Whaley's clinical manual of pediatric nursing,*** ed 5, St Louis, 2000, Mosby.

of this therapy include (1) improved physical and psychologic well-being because of the ability to participate in normal activities, (2) decreased cardiomegaly and hepatosplenomegaly, (3) fewer bone changes, (4) normal or near-normal growth and development until puberty, and (5) fewer infections.

One of the potential complications of frequent blood transfusions is iron overload. Because the body has no effective means of eliminating the excess iron, the mineral is deposited in body tissues. To minimize the development of hemosiderosis, *deferoxamine (Desferal),* an iron-chelating agent, is given with small oral supplements of vitamin C. Vitamin C should be used only in patients whose ascorbate levels are depleted and only while deferoxamine is being administered. As ferritin levels decrease toward normal, the role of vitamin C in increasing iron excretion disappears (Benz and Giardina, 1995). Deferoxamine is given intravenously or subcutaneously, often at home using a portable infusion pump, over 8 to 24 hours (usually during sleep) for 5 to 7 days a week. It is also given intravenously over a period of 4 hours at the time of blood transfusion (Benz and Giardina, 1995). Creative strategies such as behavioral contracting have been used to assist the child in complying with the deferoxamine regimen.

In some children with severe splenomegaly who demonstrate increased transfusion requirements, a splenectomy may be necessary to decrease the disabling effects of abdominal pressure and to increase the life span of supplemental RBCs. Over time, the spleen may accelerate the rate of RBC destruction and thus increase transfusion requirements. After a splenectomy, children generally require fewer transfusions, although the basic defect in Hgb synthesis remains unaffected. A major postsplenectomy complication is severe and overwhelming infection. Therefore these children continue to receive prophylactic antibiotics with close medical supervision for many years and should receive the pneumococcal and meningococcal vaccines in addition to the regularly scheduled immunizations (see Immunizations, Chapter 36).

NURSE ALERT • Ensure that the family/patient understands the need to notify the health professional of all fevers of 38.5° C (101.5° F) or greater because of the risk of sepsis in a child with asplenia.

Prognosis. Most children treated with blood transfusion and early chelation therapy survive well into adulthood. The most common cause of death is iron-induced heart disease, followed by infection, liver disease, and malignancy (Benz and Giardina, 1995). A promising treatment for some children is bone marrow transplantation (BMT) (p. 1390). For children with symptomatic disease, BMT is the only curative therapy (Mentzer, 2000).

Nursing Care Management. The objectives of nursing care are to (1) promote compliance with transfusion and chelation therapy, (2) assist the child in coping with the anxiety-provoking treatments and the effects of the illness, (3) foster the child's and family's adjustment to a chronic illness, and (4) observe for complications of multiple blood transfusions. Basic to each of these goals is explaining to parents and older children the defect responsible for the disorder, its effect on RBCs, and the potential effects of untreated iron overload (such as diabetes and heart disease). Because the prevalence of this condition is high among families of Mediterranean descent, the nurse also inquires about the family's previous knowledge about thalassemia. All families with a child with thalassemia should be tested for the trait and referred for genetic counseling.

As with any chronic illness, the needs of the family must be met for optimum adjustment to the stresses imposed by the disorder (see Chapter 41). Sources of information for the family include Cooley's Anemia Foundation* and the Thalassemia Action Group. Genetic counseling for the parents and fertile offspring is mandatory, and both prenatal diagnosis using amniocentesis at 10 weeks of gestation or fetal blood sampling at 20 weeks and screening for thalassemia trait are available.

Aplastic Anemia

Aplastic anemia refers to a condition in which all formed elements of the blood are simultaneously depressed. The peripheral blood smear demonstrates pancytopenia or the triad of profound anemia, leukopenia, and thrombocytopenia. *Hypoplastic anemia* is characterized by a profound depression of RBCs but normal or slightly decreased WBCs and platelets.

Etiology. Aplastic anemia can be *primary* (*congenital,* or present at birth) or *secondary (acquired).* The best-known congenital disorder of which aplastic anemia is an outstanding feature is *Fanconi syndrome,* a rare hereditary disorder characterized by pancytopenia, hypoplasia of the bone marrow, and patchy brown discoloration of the skin due to the deposition of melanin and associated with multiple congenital anomalies of the musculoskeletal and genitourinary systems. The syndrome appears to be inherited as an autosomal recessive trait with varying penetrance; therefore affected siblings may demonstrate several different combinations of defects.

Several factors contribute to the development of acquired hypoplastic anemia. The most common causes of acquired aplastic anemia are listed in Box 49-5. The following discussion focuses on acquired aplastic anemia, which carries a poorer prognosis and follows a more rapidly fatal course than the primary types.

Diagnostic Evaluation. The onset of clinical manifestations, which include anemia, leukopenia, and decreased platelet count, is usually insidious, not unlike that seen in leukemia. Definitive diagnosis is determined from bone mar-

*129-09 26th Ave., Flushing, NY 11354; (718) 321-2873 or 1-800-522-7222; fax (718) 321-3340; website: www.thalassemia.org

Box 49-5

Common Causes of Acquired Aplastic Anemia

- Infection with the human parvovirus (HPV), hepatitis, or overwhelming infection
- Irradiation
- Drugs such as the chemotherapeutic agents and several antibiotics, one of the most notable being chloramphenicol
- Industrial and household chemicals, including benzene and its derivatives, which are found in petroleum products, dyes, paint remover, shellac, and lacquers
- Infiltration and replacement of myeloid elements, such as in leukemia or the lymphomas
- Idiopathic, in which no identifiable precipitating cause can be found

row aspiration, which demonstrates the conversion of red bone marrow to yellow, fatty bone marrow.

Therapeutic Management. The objectives of treatment are based on the recognition that the underlying disease process is failure of the bone marrow to carry out its hematopoietic functions. Therefore therapy is directed at restoring function to the marrow and involves two main approaches: (1) immunosuppressive therapy to remove the presumed immunologic functions that prolong aplasia and/or (2) replacement of the bone marrow through transplantation. BMT is the treatment of choice for severe aplastic anemia when a suitable donor exists (see p. 1390).

Currently, *antilymphocyte globulin (ALG)* or *antithymocyte globulin (ATG)* is the principal drug treatment for aplastic anemia. The rationale for using ATG is based on the theory that aplastic anemia may be a result of autoimmunity. ATG suppresses T-cell–dependent autoimmune responses but does not cause bone marrow suppression. The optimum schedule for ATG administration is still under investigation. It is usually given intravenously over 12 to 16 hours, after a test dose to check for hypersensitivity. Subsequent doses are given depending on the reduction in circulating lymphocytes.

Colony-stimulating factors (CSFs), given parenterally, may be used to enhance bone marrow production. Androgens may be used with ATG to stimulate erythropoiesis, although the exact mechanism of erythropoietic action is unclear. Cyclosporine may also be administered in children who fail to respond to ATG, and success has also been achieved using high-dose methylprednisolone.

Because of the relatively poor prognosis in aplastic anemia treated with drug therapy, BMT should be considered early in the course of the disease if a compatible donor can be found. Transplantation is more successful when performed before multiple transfusions have sensitized the child to leukocyte and human leukocyte antigens (HLAs). BMT is associated with a 69% 15-year survival rate (Doney et al, 1997).

Nursing Care Management. The care of the child with aplastic anemia is similar to that of the child with leukemia (see p. 1380)—specifically, preparing the child and family for the diagnostic and therapeutic procedures, preventing complications from the severe pancytopenia, and emotionally supporting them in terms of a potentially fatal outcome. Because each of these nursing considerations is discussed in the section on leukemia, only the exceptions are presented here.

The drug ATG is usually administered by way of a central vein. If not, vigilant care must be directed to the IV infusion to prevent extravasation. Meticulous care of the venous access is essential because of the child's susceptibility to infection. CSFs are usually given by subcutaneous injection over a period of several days. The anesthetic cream EMLA minimizes the puncture pain.

Testosterone produces several undesirable effects that when combined with the effects of steroid therapy, such as moon face, result in dramatic body image alterations. The virilizing effects of testosterone include deepening of the voice, hirsutism, growth of pubic hair, enlargement of the penis in males, flushing of the skin, and acne. Potentially testosterone can cause muscular and skeletal maturation, resulting in severely retarded height in a young child. Not only are these changes difficult to accept, but they also are especially difficult to explain to children not approaching puberty. Parents may feel embarrassed because they are unprepared for the sexual changes. Information and support are available from the Aplastic Anemia and MDS International Foundation, Inc.*

Because chemotherapeutic agents may be used, many of the reactions, such as nausea and vomiting, alopecia, and painful mucosal ulceration, can be encountered. In addition, extensive ecchymotic areas of the oral mucosa that result from thrombocytopenia require meticulous mouth care to prevent breakdown, bleeding, and infection. Local anesthetics are usually not necessary, but anorexia is still a consequence because of the edematous nature of the lesions. Liquid, bland, and soft diets are usually tolerated best (see Feeding the Sick Child, Chapter 45). Specialized care is required for children who have a bone marrow transplant (see p. 1390).

DEFECTS IN HEMOSTASIS

Hemostasis is the process that stops bleeding when a blood vessel is injured. Vascular and plasma clotting factors, as well as platelets, are required. A complex system of clotting, anticlotting, and clot breakdown *(fibrinolysis)* mechanisms exists in equilibrium to ensure clot formation only in the presence of blood vessel injury and to limit the clotting process to the site of vessel wall injury. Dysfunction in these systems will lead to bleeding or abnormal clotting. Although the coagulation process is complex, clotting depends on three factors: (1) vascular influence, (2) platelet role, and (3) clotting factors.

Hemophilia

The term *hemophilia* refers to a group of bleeding disorders in which there is a deficiency of one of the factors necessary for coagulation of the blood. Although the symptoms are similar regardless of which clotting factor is deficient, the identification of specific factor deficiencies allows definitive treatment with replacement agents.

In about 80% of all cases of hemophilia, the inheritance pattern is demonstrated as X-linked recessive (see Appendix C). The two most common terms of the disorder are *factor VIII deficiency (hemophilia A,* or *classic hemophilia)* and *factor IX deficiency (hemophilia B,* or *Christmas disease). von Willebrand disease (vWD)* is a hereditary bleeding disorder characterized by a deficiency, abnormality, or absence of the protein called *von Willebrand factor (vWF)* and a deficiency of factor VIII. Unlike hemophilia, vWD affects both males and females. The following discussion is primarily concerned with factor VIII deficiency, which accounts for about 75% of all cases.

Pathophysiology. The basic defect of hemophilia A is a deficiency of *factor VIII (antihemophilic factor [AHF])*. AHF is produced by the liver and is necessary for the formation of thromboplastin in phase I of blood coagulation. The less AHF found in the blood, the more severe the disease. Individuals with hemophilia have two of the three factors required for coagulation: vascular influence and platelets. Therefore they may bleed for longer periods, but not at a faster rate.

Bleeding into tissue can occur anywhere, but hemorrhage into joint cavities and muscles is the most common type of in-

*P.O. Box 613, Annapolis, MD 21404; 1-800-747-2820; website: www.aamdj.org.

ternal bleeding. Bony changes and crippling deformities occur after repeated bleeding episodes over several years. Bleeding in the neck, mouth, or thorax is serious because the airway can become obstructed. Intracranial hemorrhage can have fatal consequences and is one of the major causes of death. Hemorrhage anywhere along the GI tract can lead to anemia, and bleeding into the retroperitoneal cavity is especially hazardous because of the large space for blood to accumulate. Hematomas in the spinal cord can cause paralysis.

Diagnostic Evaluation. Overt, prolonged hemorrhage is readily apparent; bleeding into tissues is less apparent (Box 49-6). The diagnosis is usually made from a history of bleeding episodes, evidence of X-linked inheritance (only one third of the cases are new mutations), and laboratory findings. The tests specific for hemophilia plasma depend on specific factors for a reaction to occur, such as the partial thromboplastin time (PTT). Specific determination of factor deficiencies requires assay procedures normally performed in specialized laboratories. Carrier detection is possible in classic hemophilia using DNA testing and is an important consideration in families in which female offspring may have inherited the trait.

Therapeutic Management. The primary therapy for hemophilia is replacement of the missing clotting factor. The products currently available are *factor VIII concentrate* from pooled plasma or a genetically engineered recombinant, to be reconstituted with sterile water immediately before use, and *DDAVP (1-deamino-8-D-arginine vasopressin)*, a synthetic form of vasopressin that is the treatment of choice in mild hemophilia and vWD (except types IIB and III) if the child shows an appropriate response. Vigorous therapy is instituted to prevent chronic crippling effects from joint bleeding.

Other drugs may be included in the therapy plan, depending on the sources of the hemorrhage. Corticosteroids are given for hematuria, acute hemarthrosis, and chronic synovitis. Nonsteroidal antiinflammatory drugs (NSAIDs), such as ibuprofen, are effective in relieving pain caused by synovitis; however, they must be used with caution because they inhibit platelet function (Dragone and Karp, 1996; Hilgartner and Corrigan, 1995). Oral administration and/or local application of epsilon-aminocaproic acid (Amicar) prevents clot destruction; however, its use is limited to mouth or trauma surgery, and a dose of factor concentrate must be given first.

A regular program of exercise and physical therapy is an important aspect of management. Physical activity within reasonable limits strengthens muscles around joints and may decrease the number of spontaneous bleeding episodes.

Box 49-6

Clinical Manifestations of Hemophilia

- Prolonged bleeding anywhere from or in the body
- Hemorrhage from any trauma—loss of deciduous teeth, circumcision, cuts, epistaxis, injections
- Excessive bruising—even from a slight injury, such as a fall
- Subcutaneous and intramuscular hemorrhages
- Hemarthrosis (bleeding into the joint cavities), especially the knees, ankles, and elbows
- Hematomas—pain, swelling, and limited motion
- Spontaneous hematuria

Treatment without delay results in more rapid recovery and a decreased likelihood of complications; therefore most children are treated at home. The family is taught the technique of venipuncture and to administer the AHF to children older than 2 to 3 years. The child learns the procedure for self-administration at 8 to 12 years of age. Home treatment is highly successful, and the rewards, in addition to the immediacy, are less disruption of family life, fewer school or work days missed, and enhancement of the child's self-esteem and independence.

Primary prophylaxis in hemophilia patients has been practiced for many years in European countries (Nilsson et al, 1994; van den Berg et al, 1994) and has proved to be effective in preventing arthropathy. Primary prophylaxis involves the infusion of factor VIII concentrate on a regular basis before the onset of joint damage. In 1994 the Medical and Scientific Advisory Council (MASAC) of the National Hemophilia Foundation recommended that prophylaxis be considered optimum therapy for children with severe hemophilia (MASAC, 1994). Secondary prophylaxis involves the infusion of factor VIII concentrate on a regular basis after the child experiences his first joint bleed. The infusions are given three times a week. Aggressive factor replacement (or "enhanced episodic care") may be a cost-effective alternative to primary prophylaxis. This involves the infusion of a high dose of factor VIII concentrate when a joint bleed occurs, followed by 2 days of more standard doses of factor VIII concentrate (Cross and Koerper, 1997).

Prognosis. Although there is no cure for hemophilia, its symptoms can be controlled and its potentially crippling deformities greatly reduced or even avoided. Today many children with hemophilia function with minimal or no joint damage. They are healthy children with an average life expectancy in every respect but one: they have a tendency to bleed, which is a significant inconvenience but not necessarily a life-threatening event.

Unfortunately, those individuals with hemophilia who were treated before current purification techniques for factor VIII concentrate (between 1979 and 1985) may have been exposed to the human immunodeficiency virus (HIV). It is estimated that over 50% of these patients have seroconverted to HIV-positive status, and 30% have acquired immunodeficiency syndrome (AIDS) (Hilgartner and Corrigan, 1995). As these individuals become sexually active, the issue of sexual transmission of HIV becomes increasingly important. The adolescent must be knowledgeable regarding safe sexual behavior. Individuals with hemophilia diagnosed and treated with factor concentrates since 1985 are at virtually no risk for developing HIV infection from treatment. Current manufacturing techniques have also greatly reduced the risk of hepatitis transmission.

Gene therapy may prove to be a treatment option in the future. This therapy involves introducing a working copy of the factor VIII gene into a patient who has a flawed copy of the gene (Cross and Koerper, 1997).

Nursing Care Management

➤ Assessment

The earlier a bleeding episode is recognized, the more effective it can be treated. Signs that indicate internal bleeding are especially important to recognize. Children are aware of internal bleeding and are very reliable in telling the examiner where an internal bleed is. In addition to the manifestations described (see Box 49-6), the nurse maintains a high level of suspicion when a child with hemophilia demonstrates signs such as headache, slurred speech, loss of consciousness (from cerebral bleeding), and black tarry stools (from GI bleeding).

➤ Nursing Diagnoses

Nursing diagnoses for the child with hemophilia include but are not limited to the following:

Risk for injury (trauma)
Pain related to bleeding into tissues
Impaired physical mobility related to hemorrhaging into joints and other tissues
Altered family processes related to child with a chronic illness

➤ Plan of Care and Implementation

The objectives of care can be divided into immediate needs and long-term goals. The patient and family goals for nursing care include the following:

1. The family and child will receive education regarding hemophilia and early recognition of bleeding episodes.
2. Bleeding episodes will be recognized and controlled, and the child will receive supportive therapy.
3. The child and parents will adjust to a chronic hereditary disease.
4. Family members will receive genetic counseling.

Prevent Bleeding. The goal of prevention of bleeding episodes is directed toward decreasing the risk of injury. Prevention of bleeding episodes is geared mostly toward appropriate exercises to strengthen muscles and joints and to allow age-appropriate activity. During infancy and toddlerhood the normal acquisition of motor skills creates innumerable opportunities for falls, bruises, and minor wounds. Restraining the child from mastering motor development can herald more serious long-term problems than allowing the behavior. However, the environment should be made as safe as possible, with close supervision maintained during playtime, to minimize incidental injuries.

For older children the family usually needs assistance in preparing for school. A nurse who knows the family can be instrumental in discussing the situation with the school nurse and in jointly planning an appropriate schedule of activity. Because almost all persons with hemophilia are boys, the physical limitations in regard to active sports may be a difficult adjustment, and activity restrictions must be tempered with sensitivity to the child's emotional, as well as physical, needs. Use of protective equipment, such as padding and helmets, is particularly important, and noncontact sports, especially swimming, are encouraged (Dragone and Karp, 1996; National Hemophilia Foundation and American Red Cross, 1996).

To prevent oral bleeding, some readjustment in terms of dental hygiene may be needed to minimize trauma to the gums, such as using a water irrigating device, softening the toothbrush in warm water before brushing, or using a sponge-tipped disposable toothbrush. A regular toothbrush should be soft bristled and small.

Because any trauma can lead to a bleeding episode, all persons caring for these children must be aware of their disorder. These children should wear medical identification, and older children should be encouraged to recognize situations in which disclosing their condition is important, such as during dental extraction or injections. Health personnel need to take special precautions to prevent the use of procedures that may cause bleeding, such as IM injections. The subcutaneous route is substituted for IM injections whenever possible. Venipunctures for blood samples are usually preferred for these children. There is usually less bleeding after the venipuncture than after finger or heel punctures. Neither aspirin nor any aspirin-containing compound should be used. Acetaminophen (Tylenol) is a suitable aspirin substitute, especially for use during control of pain at home.

Recognize and Control Bleeding. As noted, the earlier a bleeding episode is recognized, the more effectively it can be treated. Factor replacement therapy should be instituted according to established medical protocol, and supportive measures may be implemented, such as RICE, which is (1) rest, (2) ice, (3) compression, and (4) elevation. When parents and older children are taught such measures beforehand, they can be prepared to initiate immediate treatment. Plastic bags of ice or cold packs should be kept in the freezer for such emergencies. However, such measures do not take the place of factor replacement.

Prevent Crippling Effects of Bleeding. As a result of repeated episodes of hemarthrosis, incompletely absorbed blood in the joints, and limitation of motion, bone and muscle changes occur that result in flexion contractures and joint fixation. During bleeding episodes the joint is elevated and immobilized. Active range-of-motion exercises are usually instituted after the acute episode. This allows the child to control the degree of exercise and discomfort. If an exercise program is instituted in the home, a physical therapist or public health nurse may need to supervise compliance with the regimen. Rarely, orthopedic intervention, such as casting, application of traction, or aspiration of blood, may be necessary to preserve joint function. Diet is also an important consideration because excessive body weight can increase the strain on affected joints, especially the knees, and predispose to hemarthrosis. Consequently, calories need to be supplied in accordance with energy requirements.

Support Family and Prepare for Home Care. Genetic counseling is essential as soon as possible after diagnosis. Unlike many other disorders in which both parents carry the trait, the feeling of responsibility for this condition usually rests with the mother. Without an opportunity to discuss her feelings, the marital relationship can suffer. Technology is now available to identify carriers in approximately 80% of cases and may reduce the anxiety regarding childbearing in females who may be at risk of carrying the defective gene, such as sisters or maternal aunts of an affected male. The discovery of factor concentrates has greatly changed the outlook for these children. Bleeding can be minimized, and the child can live a much more normal, unrestricted life. Children are taught to take responsibility for their disease at an early age. They learn their limitations and other preventive measures, as well as self-administration of the prophylactic AHF.

The needs of families who have children with hemophilia are best met through a comprehensive team approach of physicians (pediatrician, hematologist, orthopedist), nurse practitioner, nurse, social worker, and physical therapist. Parent-group discussions are beneficial in meeting those needs often best met by similarly affected families. For example, with the improved prognosis for these children, parents and adolescents with hemophilia are faced with vocational and financial problems, in addition to concern over future childbearing. Once children reach 21 years of age, many insurance companies will no longer carry them. This can be disastrous in terms of the cost of treatment. The National Hemophilia Foundation* and the Canadian Hemophilia Society† provide numerous services and publications for both health providers and families. Financial support is particularly important. A person with severe hemophilia may require factor replacement therapy and other medical treatments that cost in excess of $70,000 to $90,000 a year.

Children who have become infected with HIV through transfusions and factor replacement products are faced with the consequences of this dreaded disease. Consequently they need the support of health professionals, especially in the areas of safe sexual practices to avoid disease transmission, public education regarding AIDS, and ways to deal with public reactions to persons who have AIDS (see p. 1384).

➤ Evaluation

The effectiveness of nursing interventions is determined by continual reassessment and evaluation of care based on the following observational guidelines and expected outcomes:

1. Interview the child and family regarding preventive measures implemented and any bleeding episodes the child has.
2. Observe the child for evidence of bleeding episodes; monitor preventive strategies and therapies, especially pain management and management.
3. Observe and interview the family regarding treatments and the schedule for prophylactic administration of antihemophilic factor.
4. Interview the family and/or consult the genetic counseling service regarding the carrier status of other members of the family.

Expected outcomes:

1. The child exhibits no evidence of bleeding.
2. The child exhibits no evidence of tissue damage.
3. The child and family discuss their feelings and concerns and demonstrate an understanding of the disease and its therapy (specify knowledge and method of demonstration).
4. The family seeks genetic counseling.

(See also Nursing Care Plan: The Child with Hemophilia.‡)

Idiopathic Thrombocytopenic Purpura (ITP)

ITP is an acquired hemorrhagic disorder characterized by (1) *thrombocytopenia,* excessive destruction of platelets; and (2) *purpura,* a discoloration caused by petechiae beneath the skin. Although the cause is unknown, it is believed to be an autoimmune response to disease-related antigens. It is the most commonly occurring thrombocytopenia of childhood. The greatest frequency of occurrence is between 2 and 8 years of age.

The disease occurs in one of two forms: an acute, self-limiting course or a chronic condition (greater than 6 months' duration). The acute form is most often seen after upper respiratory infections; after the childhood diseases measles, rubella, mumps, and chickenpox; or after infection with parvovirus B19.

Diagnostic Evaluation. The diagnosis is suspected on the basis of clinical manifestations (Box 49-7). In ITP the platelet count is reduced to below 20,000 mm^3; therefore tests that depend on platelet function, such as the tourniquet test, bleeding time, and clot retraction, yield abnormal results. Although there is no definitive test on which to establish a diagnosis of ITP, several are usually performed to rule out other disorders in which thrombocytopenia is a manifestation, such as systemic lupus erythematosus, lymphoma, or leukemia.

Therapeutic Management. Management of ITP is primarily supportive because the course of the disease is self-limited in the majority of cases. Activity is restricted at the onset while the platelet count is low and while active bleeding or progression of lesions is occurring. Treatment for acute presentation is symptomatic and has included prednisone, IV immunoglobulin (IVIG), and anti-D antibody. These are not curative therapies. Some experts suggest that no therapy is necessary for the asymptomatic patient, with no difference in the recovery of platelet counts over time. *Anti-D antibody* is a relatively new therapy for ITP. Infusion of anti-D antibody causes a transient hemolytic anemia in the patient. Along with the clearance of antibody-coated RBCs, there is prolonged survival of platelets due to the blockade of the Fc receptors of the reticuloendothelial cells. The platelet count does not increase until 48 hours after an infusion of anti-D antibody; therefore it is not appropriate therapy for patients who are actively bleeding. The benefits of choosing anti-D antibody therapy over prednisone or IVIG is that anti-D antibody can be given in one dose over a period of 5 to 10 minutes and is significantly less expensive than IVIG. Historically, patients who are treated with prednisone must first undergo a bone marrow examination to rule out leukemia. Therefore the use of anti-D antibody alleviates the need for a bone marrow examination. Premedication with acetaminophen (such as Tylenol) 5 to 10 minutes before infusion is recommended.

Box 49-7

Clinical Manifestations of Idiopathic Thrombocytopenic Purpura

- Easy bruising
  - Petechiae
  - Ecchymoses
  - Most often over bony prominences
- Bleeding from mucous membranes
  - Epistaxis
  - Bleeding gums
  - Internal hemorrhage evidenced by:
    - Hematuria
    - Hematemesis
    - Melena
    - Hemarthrosis
    - Menorrhagia
- Hematomas over lower extremities

---

*110 Green St., Room 303, New York, NY 10012; (212) 431-8541 or 1-800-42HANDI; fax (212) 431-0906; website www.infonhf.org/.

†625 President Kennedy, Suite 1210, Montreal, Quebec H3A 1K2; (514) 848-0503; e-mail: chs@odysee.net

‡In Wong DL, Hess CS: ***Wong and Whaley's clinical manual of pediatric nursing,*** ed 5, St Louis, 2000, Mosby.

NURSE ALERT • After administration of anti-D antibody, observe the child for a minimum of 1 hour and maintain a patent IV line. Obtain baseline vital signs before the infusion and again 5, 20, and 60 minutes after the infusion is begun. Fever, chills, and headache may occur during or shortly after the infusion. If fever, chills, or headache occurs, diphenhydramine (Benadryl) and hydrocortisone sodium succinate (Solu-Cortef) should be given and the patient should be observed for an additional hour.

Splenectomy is reserved for those patients in whom ITP has persisted for 1 year or longer. It is the only treatment associated with long-term remission for 70% to 90% of children. Splenectomy removes the risk of hemorrhage, as well as the need for parents to closely monitor their child's activities (Bussel and Corrigan, 1995). Before considering splenectomy, parents are generally advised to wait until the child is more than 5 years old because of the increased risk of bacterial infection in younger children. Pneumococcal and meningococcal vaccines are recommended before splenectomy. (See Immunization, Chapter 36). The child also receives penicillin prophylaxis after splenectomy. The length of prophylactic therapy is controversial, but in general a minimum of 3 years is recommended.

Prognosis. The majority of children have a self-limited course without major complications. Some children will develop chronic ITP and require ongoing therapy. A splenectomy may modify the disease process, and the child will be asymptomatic.

Nursing Care Management. Nursing care is largely supportive and should include teaching regarding possible side effects of therapy and limitation in activities while the child's platelet count is <50,000 to 100,000/mm^3. Children with ITP should not participate in any contact sports, bike riding, skateboarding, in-line skating, gymnastics, climbing, or running. Parents are encouraged to engage their children in quiet activities and to prevent any injuries to the child's head. The harmful effects of using aspirin and NSAIDs to control pain are critical for these children; therefore salicylate substitutes (such as acetaminophen) are always used. As in any condition with an uncertain outcome, the family needs emotional support.

Disseminated Intravascular Coagulation (DIC)

DIC, also known as *consumption coagulopathy,* is a secondary disorder of coagulation that occurs as a complication of a number of pathologic processes, such as hypoxia, acidosis, shock, and endothelial damage. It can result from many severe systemic diseases, such as congenital heart disease, necrotizing enterocolitis, gram-negative bacterial sepsis, rickettsial infections, and some severe viral infections. The disorder is characterized by inappropriate systemic activation and acceleration of the normal clotting mechanism.

Pathophysiology. DIC occurs when the first stage of the coagulation process is abnormally stimulated. Although no well-defined sequence of events occurs, two distinct phases can be identified. First, when the clotting mechanism is triggered in the circulation, thrombin is generated in greater amounts than can be neutralized by the body. Consequently there is rapid conversion of fibrinogen to fibrin, with aggregation and destruction of platelets. If local and widespread fibrin deposition in blood vessels takes place, obstruction and eventual necrosis of tissues occur. Second, the fibrinolytic mechanism is activated, causing extensive destruction of clotting factors. With a deficiency of clotting factors the child is vulnerable to uncontrollable hemorrhage into vital organs. An additional complication is damage and hemolysis of RBCs (Fig. 49-3).

Diagnostic Evaluation. DIC is suspected when the patient has an increased tendency to bleed (Box 49-8). Hematologic findings include prolonged prothrombin time (PT), partial thromboplastin time (PTT), and thrombin time (TT). There is a profoundly depressed platelet count, fragmented RBCs, and depleted fibrinogen.

Therapeutic Management. Treatment of DIC is directed toward control of the underlying or initiating cause, which in most instances stops the coagulation problem spontaneously. Platelets and fresh-frozen plasma may be needed to replace lost plasma components, especially in the child whose underlying disease remains uncontrolled. The extremely ill newborn infant may require exchange transfusion with fresh blood. The IV administration of heparin to inhibit thrombin formation is most often restricted to patients who have not responded to treatment of the underlying disease or replacement of coagulation factors and platelets.

Nursing Care Management. The goals of nursing care are to be aware of the possibility of DIC in the severely ill

Box 49-8

Clinical Manifestations of Disseminated Intravascular Coagulation

- Petechiae
- Purpura
- Bleeding from openings in the skin
  - Venipuncture site
  - Surgical incision
- Bleeding from umbilicus, trachea (newborn)
- Evidence of gastrointestinal bleeding
- Hypotension
- Organ dysfunction from infarction and ischemia

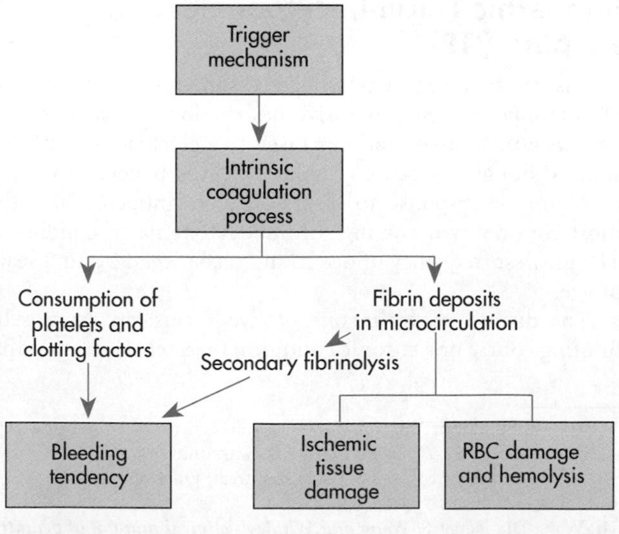

FIG. 49-3 • Effects of disseminated intravascular coagulation.

child and to recognize signs that might indicate its presence. The skills needed to monitor IV infusion and blood transfusions and to administer heparin are the same as for any child receiving these therapies (see p. 1388). (See Chapter 41 for care of the child with a life-threatening illness.)

Epistaxis (Nosebleeding)

Isolated and transient episodes of epistaxis, or nosebleeding, are common in childhood. The nose, especially the septum, is a highly vascular structure, and bleeding usually results from direct trauma, including blows to the nose, foreign bodies, and nose picking, or from mucosal inflammation associated with allergic rhinitis and upper respiratory infections. The bleeding ordinarily stops spontaneously or with minimum pressure and requires no medical evaluation or therapy.

Recurrent epistaxis and severe bleeding may indicate an underlying disease, particularly vascular abnormalities, leukemia, thrombocytopenia, and clotting factor deficiency diseases (e.g., hemophilia and vWD). Nosebleeds are sometimes associated with administration of aspirin, even in normal amounts. Persistent episodes of epistaxis require medical evaluation.

Nursing Care Management. In the event of a nosebleed, an essential intervention is to remain calm. Otherwise, the child will become more agitated, the blood pressure will increase, and the child will not cooperate. Although in most instances a nosebleed is not serious, it can be very upsetting to family members as well. They need reassurance that the loss of blood is not serious and that the bleeding usually stops within 10 to 15 minutes.

To control the bleeding, the child is instructed to sit up and lean forward (not to lie down) to avoid aspiration of blood. Most of the nosebleeding originates in the anterior part of the nasal septum and can be controlled by applying pressure to the soft lower portion of the nose with the thumb and forefinger (Emergency box). During this time the child breathes through the mouth.

In the event that hemorrhage continues, the child should be evaluated by a practitioner, who may pack the nose with epinephrine-soaked gauze. After a nosebleed, petroleum or water-soluble jelly can be inserted into each nostril to prevent crusting of old blood and to lessen the likelihood of the child's picking at the nose and restarting the hemorrhage. If a child has numerous nosebleeds, factors believed to increase the likelihood of bleeds are eliminated, such as discouraging nose picking or altering the household humidity by placing a cool-mist humidifier in the child's room. Repeated bleeding episodes lasting longer than 30 minutes may be an indication to refer the child for evaluation for the possibility of a bleeding disorder.

Emergency

EPISTAXIS

- Have child sit up and lean forward (not lying down).
- Apply continuous pressure to nose with thumb and forefinger for at least 10 minutes.
- Insert cotton or wadded tissue into each nostril, and apply ice or cold cloth to bridge of nose if bleeding persists.
- Keep child calm and quiet.

NEOPLASTIC DISORDERS

Neoplastic disorders are the leading cause of death from disease in children past infancy, and almost half of all childhood cancers involve the blood or blood-forming organs. Leukemias and lymphomas are discussed here. Malignant solid tumors of childhood are discussed elsewhere in relation to the tissues or organs involved.

Leukemias

Leukemia, cancer of the blood-forming tissues, is the most common form of childhood cancer. The annual incidence is 3 to 4 cases per 100,000 Caucasian children younger than 15 years (Margolin and Poplack, 1997). It occurs more commonly in males than in females after 1 year of age, and the peak onset is between 2 and 6 years of age. It is one of the forms of cancer that have demonstrated dramatic improvements in survival rates. Current long-term disease-free survival for children with acute lymphoid leukemia approaches 75% (Friebert and Shurin, 1998), whereas acute nonlymphoid leukemia has a 40% survival rate (Ebb and Weinstein, 1997). (See also Prognosis, p. 1373).

Classification. *Leukemia* is a broad term given to a group of malignant diseases of the bone marrow and lymphatic system. Current research has revealed that it is a complex disease of varying heterogeneity. Consequently, classification has become increasingly complex, sophisticated, and essential because identification of the subtype of leukemia has therapeutic and prognostic implications. The following is a brief overview of the major classification systems currently being used.

Morphology. Two forms are generally recognized in children: *acute lymphoid leukemia (ALL)* and *acute nonlymphoid (myelogenous) leukemia (ANLL* or *AML)*. Synonyms for ALL include lymphatic, lymphocytic, lymphoblastic, and lymphoblastoid leukemia. Usually the terms *stem cell* or *blast cell leukemia* also refer to the lymphoid type of leukemia. Synonyms for the AML type include granulocytic, myelocytic, monocytic, myelog enous, monoblastic, and monomyeloblastic.

Cytochemical Markers. Several chemical stains aid in differentiation between ALL and ANLL. For instance, ALL will stain positive for terminal deoxynucleotidyl transferase (TdT), whereas ANLL is nonreactive (Margolin and Poplack, 1997).

Chromosome Studies. Chromosome analysis has become an important tool in the diagnosis of acute lymphoblastic leukemia. For example, children with trisomy 21 have 20 times the risk of other children for developing ALL. Children with more than 50 chromosomes on the leukemic cells (hyperdiploid) have the best prognosis (Margolin and Poplack, 1997). Translocations of chromosomes also found on the leukemic cells can denote good prognosis, as in the trisomies 4 and 10, or a poor prognosis, as in the t(9:22) or Philadelphia chromosome.

Cell-Surface Immunologic Markers. Cell-surface antigens have permitted differentiation of ALL into three broad classes: non-T, non-B ALL; B-cell ALL; and T-cell ALL. Children with non-T, non-B ALL have the best prognosis, especially if they have the common acute lymphocytic leukemia antigen, known as CALLA positive, on their cell surfaces (Margolin and Poplack, 1997).

Pathophysiology. Leukemia is an unrestricted proliferation of immature WBCs in the blood-forming tissues of the body. Although not a "tumor" as such, the leukemic cells demonstrate the same neoplastic properties as solid cancers. Therefore the resulting pathologic condition and clinical manifestations are caused by infiltration and replacement of any tissue of the body with nonfunctional leukemic cells. Highly vascular organs, such as the spleen and liver, are the most severely affected.

To understand the pathophysiology of the leukemic process, it is important to clarify two common misconceptions. First, although leukemia is an overproduction of WBCs, most often in the acute form the leukocyte count is low (thus the term *leukemia*). Second, these immature cells do not deliberately attack and destroy the normal blood cells or vascular tissues. Cellular destruction takes place by infiltration and subsequent competition for metabolic elements (Table 49-3).

In all types of leukemia the proliferating cells depress the production of formed elements of the blood in bone marrow by competing for and depriving the normal cells of the essential nutrients for metabolism. The most common presenting signs and symptoms of leukemia are a result of infiltration of the bone marrow. The three main consequences are (1) *anemia* from decreased RBCs, (2) *infection* from neutropenia, and (3) *bleeding tendencies* from decreased platelet production. The invasion of the bone marrow with leukemic cells gradually causes a weakening of the bone and a tendency toward fractures. As leukemic cells invade the periosteum, increasing pressure causes severe pain.

The spleen, liver, and lymph glands demonstrate marked infiltration, enlargement, and eventually fibrosis. Hepatosplenomegaly is typically more common than lymphadenopathy. The next most important site of involvement is the central nervous system (CNS) secondary to leukemic infiltration, which may cause increased intracranial pressure (see Box 51-1).

Leukemic cells may also invade the testes, kidneys, prostate, ovaries, GI tract, and lungs. With long-term survivors becoming more common, such sites of leukemia invasion, especially the testes, are becoming more important clinically.

Diagnostic Evaluation. Leukemia is usually suspected by the history, physical manifestations (see Table 49-3), and a peripheral blood smear that contains immature forms of leukocytes, commonly combined with low blood counts. Definitive diagnosis is based on bone marrow aspiration or biopsy. Typically the bone marrow is hypercellular, with primarily blast cells. Once the diagnosis is confirmed, a lumbar puncture is performed to determine whether there is any CNS involvement. A few children will have CNS involvement at diagnosis, although most are asymptomatic.

Therapeutic Management. Treatment of leukemia involves the use of chemotherapeutic agents, with or without cranial irradiation, in four phases: (1) *induction therapy,* which achieves a complete remission or less than 5% leukemic cells in the bone marrow; (2) *CNS prophylactic therapy,* which prevents leukemic cells from invading the CNS; (3) *intensification therapy* (consolidation), which eradicates residual leukemia cells, followed by delayed intensification, which prevents emergence of resistant leukemic clones; and (4) *maintenance therapy,* which serves to maintain the remission phase. Although the combination of drugs and radiation may vary according to institutions, the prognostic or risk characteristics of the patient, and the type of leukemia being treated, the following general principles for each phase are used quite consistently.

Remission Induction. Almost immediately after confirmation of the diagnosis, induction therapy is begun and lasts for 4 to 6 weeks. The principal drugs used for induction in ALL are corticosteroids (especially prednisone), vincristine, and L-asparaginase, with or without doxorubicin. Drug therapy for AML includes doxorubicin or daunorubicin (daunomycin) and cytosine arabinoside; various other drugs may be used.

Because many of the drugs also cause myelosuppression of normal blood elements, the period immediately after a remission can be critical. The body is defenseless against and highly

TABLE 49-3
Pathology and Related Clinical Manifestations of Leukemia

Organ or Tissue	Consequences	Manifestations
Bone marrow dysfunction	Decreased RBCs—anemia	Pallor, fatigue
	Neutropenia—infection	Fever
	Decreased platelets—bleeding tendencies	Hemorrhage (petechiae)
	Invasion of bone marrow—bone weakness; invasion of periosteum	Tendency toward fractures Pain
Liver Spleen Lymph glands	Infiltration, enlargement, eventual fibrosis	Hepatomegaly Splenomegaly Lymphadenopathy
Central nervous system: meninges	Increased intracranial pressure, ventricular enlargement	Severe headache Vomiting Irritability, lethargy Papilledema Eventual coma
	Meningeal irritation	Pain Stiff neck and back
Hypermetabolism	Cell deprivation of nutrients by invading cells	Muscle wasting Weight loss Anorexia Fatigue

susceptible to infection and spontaneous hemorrhage. Consequently, supportive therapy during this time is essential.

CNS Prophylactic Therapy. Treatment of the CNS consists of prophylactic therapy using intrathecal chemotherapy with methotrexate, cytarabine, and hydrocortisone. Sometimes methotrexate, as well as cytarabine, may be given intrathecally as a single agent. Because of the concern regarding late effects of cranial irradiation, this treatment is reserved for high risk patients and those with CNS disease.

Intensification or Consolidation Therapy. Once complete remission is obtained, a period of intensified treatment is begun to eradicate residual leukemic cells; this is followed by delayed intensification to prevent emergence of resistant leukemic clones. Intrathecal along with systemic chemotherapy, including L-asparaginase, high-dose or intermediate-dose methotrexate, cytarabine, vincristine, and mercaptopurine, is administered over a period of several months.

Maintenance Therapy. Maintenance therapy is begun after completion of successful induction and consolidation therapy to preserve the remission and further lessen the number of leukemic cells. Combined drug regimens, including daily mercaptopurine, weekly methotrexate, and periodic intrathecal therapy, are administered over the remaining 2-year period. Also, during maintenance therapy periodic CBCs are taken to evaluate the marrow's response to the drugs.

Reinduction after Relapse. The presence of leukemic cells in the bone marrow, CNS, or testes constitutes a relapse. Therapy for the child with a relapse includes reinduction with prednisone and vincristine, along with a combination of other drugs not previously used. CNS preventive therapy and maintenance therapy follow, as outlined before, once remission occurs.

Bone Marrow Transplantation (BMT). BMT has been used successfully for treating children who have ALL and AML. BMT is not recommended for children with ALL during the first remission because of the excellent results possible with chemotherapy. Because of the poorer prognosis in children with AML, allogeneic BMT may be considered during the first remission (Ebb and Weinstein, 1997). Allogeneic BMT involves obtaining bone marrow from a matched, histocompatible family member, usually a sibling.

Bone marrow used for BMT may be not only from antigen-matched related donors but also from matched unrelated donors or mismatched donors. Peripheral blood stem cells are also used. Peripheral blood stem cell transplants are capable of differentiating into specialized cells of the hematologic system and can be obtained from related or unrelated donors or from umbilical cord blood (see also p. 1390). Regardless of the type of transplant, it is accompanied by significant morbidity and mortality, including graft-vs.-host disease, overwhelming infection, or severe organ damage. Cure after BMT ranges from 30% to 60%; relapse after BMT creates a dismal outlook (Sanders, 1997).

Prognosis. The most important prognostic factors for determining long-term survival for children with ALL (in addition to treatment) are (1) the initial WBC count, (2) the child's age at the time of diagnosis, (3) the type of cell involved, (4) the sex of the child, and (5) karyotype analysis. Children with a normal or low WBC count and who have non-T, non-B ALL and are CALLA positive have a much better prognosis than those with a high count or other cell types. Children whose disease is diagnosed between 2 and 9 years of age have consistently demonstrated a better outlook than those whose disease is diagnosed before 2 or after 10 years of age, and girls appear to have a more favorable prognosis than boys. Children with a DNA index greater than 1.16 (hyperdiploid) and translocation of chromosomes 4 and 10 have a better prognosis (Margolin and Poplack, 1997). In addition, it appears that the more rapid the induction of a remission in AML, the better the chance for an ultimate long-term, continuous remission.

Late Effects of Treatment. Although vigorous treatment of childhood cancers has resulted in dramatically improved survival rates, increasing concern surrounds late effects—adverse changes related to treatment modalities—and recurrence of the disease process. Almost no organ is exempt, and almost every antineoplastic agent, including and especially irradiation, is responsible for some adverse effect.

The most devastating late effect is development of a second malignancy. Children who received cranial irradiation at age 5 years or younger are most susceptible to developing brain tumors (Pui, 1997). Treatment with anthracycline is associated with cardiomyopathy; cranial irradiation and intrathecal chemotherapy are associated with cognitive and neuropsychologic deficits, which are just a few of the long-term sequelae. Consequently, close monitoring for late effects is essential, especially with the advent of additional clinical trials.

Nursing Care Management. Nursing care of the child with leukemia is directly related to the regimen of therapy.

➤ Assessment

The history and physical examination often yield the first clues to the presence of neoplastic disease. Vague symptoms such as fatigue, pain in a limb, night sweating, lack of appetite, headache, and general malaise, may be the earliest clues of leukemia.

➤ Nursing Diagnoses

A number of nursing diagnoses become apparent after an assessment of the child with leukemia and the family. Some are considered in the Nursing Care Plan on pp. 1380-1382. Others will be identified in specific situations.

➤ Plan of Care and Implementation

The goals of nursing care of the child with leukemia and the family include:

1. Child will receive appropriate primary health care.
2. Child and family will be prepared for diagnostic and therapeutic procedures.
3. Child will experience minimal complications of myelosuppression.
4. Problems of radiation and drug toxicity will be managed.
5. Child and family will receive adequate support and education.

Nursing care of the child with leukemia is directly related to the regimen of therapy. Nurses working with families of children with cancer have a significant supportive role in helping them understand the various therapies, preventing or managing expected side effects or toxicities, observing for late effects of treatment, and helping the child and family live as normal a life as possible and cope with the emotional aspects of the disease. Education is a constant feature of the nursing role, especially in terms of clinical trials and home care. Diagnosis of leukemia tends to generate anxiety in families and patients. The nurse is instrumental in providing support and reassurance, as well as accurate explanation regarding diagnostic tests, procedures, and treatment plans.

Prepare Child and Family for Diagnostic and Therapeutic Procedures. From the time before diagnosis to cessation of therapy, children must undergo several tests; the most traumatic are bone marrow aspiration or biopsy and lumbar punctures. Multiple finger sticks and venipunctures for blood analysis and drug infusion are common occurrences. Therefore the child needs an explanation of each procedure and what can be expected. In addition, effective pharmacologic measures, including conscious and unconscious sedation, and nonpharmacologic strategies are used to reduce discomfort associated with these painful procedures.

Relieve Pain. The effective use of analgesia is especially important when the malignant process is uncontrolled and causes acute pain. Dosages of opioids (narcotics) are adjusted or *titrated to the child's needs* and administered *around the clock* for optimum pain control. Nonpharmacologic strategies should be implemented as needed but are not substitutes for pharmacologic management. The reader is encouraged to review the principles of pain assessment and management presented in Chapter 44 and Preparation for Procedures in Chapter 45 when caring for a child with leukemia.

Prevent Complications of Myelosuppression. The leukemic process and most of the chemotherapeutic agents cause myelosuppression. The reduced numbers of blood cells result in secondary problems of infection, bleeding tendencies, and anemia. Supportive care involves both medical and nursing management. Because these are so closely linked, they are discussed together rather than separately.

Infection. A common complication of treatment for childhood cancer is overwhelming infection secondary to neutropenia. The child is most susceptible to overwhelming infection during three phases of the disease: (1) at the time of diagnosis and relapse when the leukemic process has replaced normal leukocytes, (2) during immunosuppressive therapy, and (3) after prolonged antibiotic therapy that predisposes to the growth of resistant organisms. However, the use of granulocyte colony-stimulating factor (GCSF) has reduced the incidence and duration of infection in children receiving treatment for cancer.

The first defense against infection is prevention. When the child is hospitalized, the nurse uses all measures to control transfer of infection. These typically include the use of a private room, restriction of all visitors and health personnel with active infection, and strict handwashing technique with an antiseptic solution. In some research centers, special germ-free environments are available during complete myelosuppression from intensive chemotherapy or for bone marrow transplant.

NURSE ALERT • Because the live viral infections of childhood are particularly dangerous, the child is not immunized against these diseases (measles, rubella, mumps, and polio) until the immune system is capable of responding appropriately to the vaccine. If given when the immune system is depressed, the attenuated virus can result in an overwhelming infection. The child can receive the Salk (inactivated) vaccine.

The child is evaluated for potential sites of infection (e.g., mucosal ulceration; skin abrasion; or skin tear, such as a hangnail) and observed for any elevation in temperature. To identify the source of infection, chest radiographs and blood, stool, urine, and nasopharyngeal cultures are taken. IV antibiotics are administered, and if this therapy is prolonged, a venous access device, such as a peripherally inserted central catheter (PICC), intermittent infusion device (saline lock or PRN adaptor), catheter, or implanted infusion port, is used to maintain IV access.

Prevention of infection continues to be a priority after discharge from the hospital. Ordinarily, the child is allowed to return to school when the WBC count is at a satisfactory level, usually an absolute neutrophil count (ANC) greater than $500/mm^3$ (Guidelines box). At all times, family members are encouraged to practice good handwashing to prevent introducing pathogens into the home. The child may need to be isolated from school contacts in the event of an outbreak of a childhood disease, especially chickenpox.

Nutrition is another important component of infection prevention. An adequate protein-caloric intake provides the child with better host defenses against infection and increased tolerance to chemotherapy and irradiation. However, providing optimum nutrition during periods of anorexia and vomiting from chemotherapy is a tremendous challenge (see Feeding the Sick Child, Chapter 45).

Hemorrhage. Before the use of transfused platelets, hemorrhage was a leading cause of death in patients with leukemia. Now most bleeding episodes can be prevented or controlled with the administration of platelet concentrates or platelet-rich plasma.

Because infection increases the tendency toward hemorrhage and because bleeding sites become more easily infected, skin punctures are avoided whenever possible. When finger sticks, venipunctures, IM injections, and bone marrow aspirations are performed, aseptic technique must be used, as well as continued observation for bleeding. Meticulous mouth care is essential because gingival bleeding with resultant mucositis is a common problem. Because the rectal area is prone to ulceration from various drugs, feces and urine are removed immediately, and the perianal area is washed. Rectal temperatures are avoided to prevent trauma. Children are advised to avoid activities that might cause injury or bleeding, such as riding bicycles or skateboards, climbing trees or playground equipment, and playing contact sports.

Platelet transfusions are generally reserved for active bleeding episodes that do not respond to local treatment and that may occur during induction or relapse therapy. Epistaxis and gingival bleeding are the most common. The nurse teaches parents and older children measures to control nosebleeding (see

Guidelines

CALCULATING THE ABSOLUTE NEUTROPHIL COUNT

Determine the total percent of neutrophils ("polys" or "segs" and "bands").

Multiply white blood cell (WBC) count by percent of neutrophils.

Example:

WBC = 1000, neutrophils = 7%, nonsegmented neutrophils (bands) = 7%

Step 1: 7% + 7% = 14%

Step 2: 0.14 × 1000 = 140 absolute neutrophil count (ANC)

p. 1371). Pressure at the site without disturbing clot formation is the general rule.

During bleeding episodes the parents and child need much emotional support. Often parents will request a platelet transfusion, unaware of the need for trying local measures first. The nurse can be instrumental in allaying anxiety by acknowledging the feelings of the child and family and explaining the reason for delaying a platelet transfusion until absolutely necessary.

Anemia. Initially anemia may be profound because of complete replacement of the bone marrow by leukemic cells. During induction therapy, blood transfusions may be necessary. The usual precautions in caring for the child with anemia are instituted (see p. 1356).

Use Precautions in Administering and Handling Chemotherapeutic Agents. Many chemotherapeutic agents are vesicants (sclerosing agents) that can cause severe cellular damage if even minute amounts of the drug infiltrate surrounding tissue. Only nurses experienced with chemotherapeutic agents should administer vesicants. Guidelines are available* and must be followed exactly to prevent tissue damage to patients. Interventions for extravasation vary, but each nurse should be aware of the institution's policies and implement them at once.

NURSE ALERT • Chemotherapeutic drugs must be given through a free-flowing IV line. The infusion is stopped immediately if any sign of infiltration (pain, stinging, swelling, or redness at the cannulation site) occurs.

In addition to extravasation, a potentially fatal complication is anaphylaxis, especially from L-asparaginase, teniposide (VM-26), etoposide (VP-16), bleomycin, and cisplatin. Nursing responsibilities include prevention of, recognition of, and preparation for serious reactions. Prevention begins with a careful history for known allergy.

NURSE ALERT • When certain chemotherapeutic and immunologic agents are given (see Box 49-9), the child must be observed for 20 minutes after the infusion for signs of anaphylaxis (cyanosis, hypotension, wheezing, severe urticaria). Emergency equipment (especially blood pressure monitor and bag-valve-mask) and emergency drugs (especially oxygen, epinephrine, antihistamine, aminophylline, corticosteroids, and vasopressors) must be available. If a reaction is suspected, the drug is discontinued, the IV line is flushed with saline solution, and the child's vital signs and subsequent responses are monitored.

In addition to the many responsibilities nurses must have in regard to the child and family, they must also use safeguards to protect themselves. Handling chemotherapeutic agents may present risks to handlers and to their offspring, although the exact degree of risk is not known.

Some children have a venous access device, which facilitates administration of IV drugs. During treatment and remission, many drugs are taken orally at home. Compliance with the medication schedule is essential, and nurses play an important role in educating the family about the drugs and encouraging adherence to the plan.*

Manage Problems of Drug Toxicity. Chemotherapy presents several nursing challenges. The complexity of the treatment protocols is often overwhelming to families. In addition, each therapy is associated with a number of predictable side effects. Nurses must be aware of these side effects and use judgment in recognizing actions, as well as toxicities (Box 49-9).

Nausea and Vomiting. The nausea and vomiting that occur shortly after administration of several of the drugs and from cranial or abdominal radiation can be profound. The serotonin-receptor antagonists (e.g., ondansetron [Zofran]) are effective in the control of nausea and vomiting occurring after emetogenic chemotherapy and radiation therapy. When combined with dexamethasone, these agents are the treatment of choice in the prevention of cisplatin-induced emesis (Tonato, Roila, and Del Favero, 1994).

The most beneficial regimen for antiemetic control has been the administration of the antiemetic *before* the chemotherapy begins. The goal is to prevent the child from ever experiencing nausea or vomiting, thus preventing development of anticipatory symptoms (the conditioned response of developing nausea and vomiting before receiving the drug).

Anorexia. Loss of appetite is a direct consequence of the chemotherapy and/or irradiation. It is a major problem for parents because it is the one area they feel responsible for, particularly when so many other facets of care are outside their control. There are no universally successful techniques for encouraging a sick child to eat. However, the guidelines in Chapter 45 can be helpful during the anorexic period and can prevent additional problems during the remission.

Some children still do not eat despite these approaches. When loss of appetite and weight persists, the nurse should investigate the family situation to determine whether any factors (e.g., conditioned aversion to food, environmental stress related to eating, controlling behavior, anger) might be contributing to the problem. Nasogastric tube feedings or total parenteral nutrition may be implemented for children with significant nutritional problems.

Mucosal Ulceration. One of the most distressing side effects of several drugs is GI mucosal cell damage, which can produce ulcers anywhere along the alimentary tract. Oral ulcers greatly compound anorexia because eating is extremely uncomfortable, but the following interventions may be helpful: (1) provide a bland, moist, soft diet appropriate for the child's age and preferences; (2) use a soft sponge toothbrush (Toothettes)† or cotton-tipped applicator; (3) provide frequent mouthwashes with normal saline solution (1 teaspoon of table salt added to 1 pint of water) or sodium bicarbonate mouthrinses (1 teaspoon of baking soda added to 1 quart of water); and (4) use local anesthetics (e.g., Chloraseptic lozenges) or nonprescription preparations without alcohol (e.g., Orabase and Ulcerease). Although local anesthetics are effective in temporarily relieving the pain, many children dislike the taste and numb feeling they produce.

**Cancer Chemotherapy Guidelines* can be obtained from the Oncology Nursing Society, 501 Holiday Dr., Pittsburgh, PA 15220-2749; (412) 921-7373.

*Community and home care instructions on caring for a venous access device and administering medications to children are available in Wong DL, Hess CS: ***Wong and Whaley's clinical manual of pediatric nursing,*** ed 5, St Louis, 2000, Mosby.

†Manufactured by Halbrand, Inc., Willoughby, OH.

Box 49-9

Summary of Selected Chemotherapeutic Agents Used in the Treatment of Childhood Leukemias and Lymphomas*

BLEOMYCIN (BLENOXANE)

Administration

IV, IM, SC

Side Effects and Toxicity

Allergic reaction—fever, chills, hypotension, anaphylaxis
Fever (nonallergic)
N/V (mild)†
Stomatitis
Cumulative dose effects include:
- Skin—rash, hyperpigmentation, thickening, ulceration, peeling, nail changes, alopecia
- Lungs—pneumonitis with infiltrate that can progress to fatal fibrosis

Comments and Specific Nursing Considerations

Should give test dose (SC) before therapeutic dose is administered
Have emergency drugs at bedside
Hypersensitivity occurs with first one to two doses
May give acetaminophen before drug to reduce likelihood of fever
Concentration of drug in skin and lungs accounts for toxic effects

CORTICOSTEROIDS (PREDNISONE)

Administration

PO; IM or IV rarely used

Side Effects and Toxicity, Short-Term

For short-term use, no acute toxicity
Usual side effects are mild: moon face, fluid retention, weight gain, mood changes, increased appetite, gastric irritation, insomnia, susceptibility to infection

Comments and Specific Nursing Considerations

Explain expected effects, especially in terms of body image, increased appetite, and personality changes
Monitor weight gain
Recommend moderate salt restriction
Administer with antacid and early in morning (sometimes given every other day to minimize side effects)
May need to disguise bitter taste (crush tablet and mix with syrup, jam, ice cream, or other highly flavored substance; use ice to numb tongue before administration; place tablet in gelatin capsule if child can swallow it)
Observe for potential infection sites; usual inflammatory response and fever are absent

Side Effects and Toxicity, Long-Term

Long-term effects of chronic steroid administration are mood changes, hirsutism, trunk obesity (buffalo hump), thin extremities, muscle wasting and weakness, osteoporosis, poor wound healing, bruising, potassium loss, gastric bleeding, hypertension, diabetes mellitus, growth retardation

Comments and Specific Nursing Considerations

Same as for short-term use; in addition, encourage foods high in potassium (bananas, raisins, prunes, coffee, chocolate)
Test stools for occult blood
Monitor blood pressure
Test blood for sugar and urine for acetone
Observe for signs of abrupt steroid withdrawal: flulike symptoms, hypotension, hypoglycemia, shock

DAUNORUBICIN (DAUNOMYCIN, RUBIDOMYCIN) AND DOXORUBICIN (ADRIAMYCIN)

Administration

IV

Side Effects and Toxicity

N/V (moderate)†
Stomatitis
BMD (7 to 14 days later)
Fever, chills
Local phlebitis
Alopecia
Cumulative-dose toxicity includes:
- Cardiac abnormalities
- Electrocardiographic changes
- Heart failure

Comments and Specific Nursing Considerations

Vesicant‡ (extravasation may *not* cause pain)
Use only sterile distilled water as a diluent
Observe for any changes in heart rate or rhythm and signs of failure
Cumulative dose must not exceed 400 mg/m^2
Warn parents that drug causes urine to turn red (for up to 12 days after administration); this is normal, not hematuria

L-ASPARAGINASE (ELSPAR)

Administration

IM, IV

Side Effects and Toxicity

Allergic reactions (including anaphylactic shock)
Fever
N/V (mild)†
Anorexia
Weight loss
Arthralgia
Toxicity:
- Liver dysfunction
- Hyperglycemia
- Renal failure
- Pancreatitis

Comments and Specific Nursing Considerations

Have emergency drugs at bedside
Record signs of allergic reaction, such as urticaria, facial edema, hypotension, or abdominal cramps

*Includes principal drugs used in the treatment of childhood leukemias and lymphomas. Several other conventional and investigational chemotherapeutic agents may be used in the treatment regimen.
†*N/V,* Nausea and vomiting. Mild = <20% incidence; moderate = 20% to 70% incidence; severe = >75% incidence.
‡Vesicants (sclerosing agents) can cause severe cellular damage if even minute amounts of the drug infiltrate surrounding tissue.
IV, Intravenous; *IT,* intrathecal; *PO,* by mouth; *IM,* intramuscular; *SC,* subcutaneous; *BMD,* bone marrow depression.

Box 49-9

Summary of Selected Chemotherapeutic Agents Used in the Treatment of Childhood Leukemias and Lymphomas*—cont'd

L-ASPARAGINASE (ELSPAR)—cont'd

Comments and Specific Nursing Considerations—cont'd

Check weight daily

Normally, blood urea nitrogen (BUN) and ammonia levels rise as a result of drug; not evidence of liver damage

Check urine for sugar and blood amylase

MECHLORETHAMINE (NITROGEN MUSTARD, MUSTARGEN)

Administration

IV

Side Effects and Toxicity

N/V (30 minutes to 8 hours later) (severe)†

BMD (2 to 3 weeks later)

Alopecia

Local phlebitis

Comments and Specific Nursing Considerations

Vesicant

MERCAPTOPURINE (6-MP, PURINETHOL)

Administration

PO

Side Effects and Toxicity

N/V (mild)†

Diarrhea

Anorexia

Stomatitis

BMD (4 to 6 weeks later)

Immunosuppression

Dermatitis

Less often may be hepatic dysfunction

Comments and Specific Nursing Considerations

6-MP is an analog of xanthine; therefore allopurinol (Zyloprim) delays its metabolism and increases its potency, necessitating a lower dose (⅓ to ¼) of 6-MP

METHOTREXATE (MTX, AMETHOPTERIN)

Administration

PO, IV, IM, IT

May be given in conventional doses (mg/m^2) or high doses (g/m^2)

Side Effects and Toxicity

N/V (severe at high doses)†

Diarrhea

Mucosal ulceration (2 to 5 days later)

BMD (10 days later)

Immunosuppression

Dermatitis

Photosensitivity

Alopecia (uncommon)

Toxic effects include:

- Hepatitis (fibrosis)
- Osteoporosis
- Nephropathy
- Pneumonitis (fibrosis)

Neurologic toxicity with IT use—pain at injection site, meningismus (signs of meningitis without actual inflammation), especially fever and headache; potential sequelae—transient or permanent hemiparesis, seizures, dementia, death

Comments and Specific Nursing Considerations

Side effects and toxicity are dose related

Potency and toxicity are increased by reduced renal function, salicylates, sulfonamides, and aminobenzoic acid; avoid use of these substances, such as aspirin

Avoid exposure to sun

High-dose therapy:

- Citrovorum Factor (folinic acid or leucovorin) decreases cytotoxic action of MTX; used as an antidote for overdose and to enhance normal cell recovery after high-dose therapy; avoid use of vitamins containing folic acid during MTX therapy unless prescribed by physician

IT therapy:

- Drug *must* be mixed with preservative-free diluent
- Report signs of neurotoxicity immediately

PROCARBAZINE (MATULANE)

Administration

PO

Side Effects and Toxicity

N/V (moderate)†

BMD (3 to 4 weeks later)

Lethargy

Dermatitis

Myalgia

Arthralgia

Less often:

- Stomatitis
- Neuropathy
- Alopecia
- Diarrhea

Comments and Specific Nursing Considerations

Central nervous system (CNS) depressants (phenothiazines, barbiturates) enhance CNS symptoms

Monoamine oxidase (MAO) inhibition sometimes occurs; therefore all other drugs are avoided unless medically approved; red wine, fava beans, and broad bean pods are avoided

VINCRISTINE (ONCOVIN) AND VINBLASTINE (VELBAN)

Administration

IV

Side Effects and Toxicity

Neurotoxicity (less severe with vinblastine)—paresthesia (numbness); ataxia; weakness; footdrop; hyporeflexia; constipation (dynamic ileus); hoarseness (vocal cord paralysis); abdominal, chest, and jaw pain; mental depression

Fever

N/V (mild)†

BMD (minimal; 7 to 14 days later)

Alopecia

Continued

Box 49-9

Summary of Selected Chemotherapeutic Agents Used in the Treatment of Childhood Leukemias and Lymphomas*—cont'd

Comments and Specific Nursing Considerations
Vesicant
Report signs of neurotoxicity because may necessitate cessation of drug
Individuals with underlying neurologic problems may be more prone to neurotoxicity
Monitor stool patterns closely; administer stool softener
Excreted primarily by liver into biliary system; administer cautiously to anyone with biliary disease

CYTOSINE ARABINOSIDE (ARA-C, CYTOSAR, CYTARABINE)
Administration
IV, IM, SC, IT

Side Effects and Toxicity
N/V (mild)†
BMD (7 to 14 days later)
Mucosal ulceration
Immunosuppression
Hepatitis (usually subclinical)

Comments and Specific Nursing Considerations
Crosses blood-brain barrier
Use with caution in patients with hepatic dysfunction

CYCLOPHOSPHAMIDE (CYTOXAN, CTX, NEOSAR)
Administration
PO, IV, IM

Side Effects and Toxicity
N/V (3 to 4 hours later) (severe at high doses)†
BMD (10 to 14 days later)
Alopecia
Hemorrhagic cystitis
Severe immunosuppression
Stomatitis (rare)
Hyperpigmentation
Transverse ridging of nails
Infertility

Comments and Specific Nursing Considerations
BMD has platelet-sparing effect
Give dose early in day to allow adequate fluids afterward
Force fluids before administering drug and for 2 days after to prevent chemical cystitis; encourage frequent voiding even during night
Warn parents to report signs of burning on urination or hematuria to practitioner

DACARBAZINE (DTIC)
Administration
IV

Side Effects and Toxicity
N/V (especially after first dose) (severe)†
BMD (7 to 14 days later)
Alopecia
Flulike syndrome
Burning sensation in vein during infusion (not extravasation)

Comments and Specific Nursing Considerations
Vesicant (less sclerosive)‡
Must be given cautiously in patients with renal dysfunction
Decrease IV rate or use warm, moist towels on IV site to decrease burning

*Includes principal drugs used in the treatment of childhood leukemias and lymphomas. Several other conventional and investigational chemotherapeutic agents may be used in the treatment regimen.
†*N/V,* Nausea and vomiting. Mild = <20% incidence; moderate = 20% to 70% incidence; severe = >75% incidence.
‡Vesicants (sclerosing agents) can cause severe cellular damage if even minute amounts of the drug infiltrate surrounding tissue. *IV,* Intravenous; *IT,* intrathecal; *PO,* by mouth; *IM,* intramuscular; *SC,* subcutaneous; *BMD,* bone marrow depression.

NURSE ALERT • Viscous lidocaine is not recommended for young children; if applied to the pharynx, it may depress the gag reflex, increasing the risk of aspiration. Seizures rarely have been associated with the use of oral viscous lidocaine (Hess and Walson, 1988).

Other preparations that may be used to prevent or treat mucositis include chlorhexidine gluconate (Peridex) because of its dual effectiveness against candidal and bacterial infections, antifungal troches (lozenges) or mouthwash, and lip balm (e.g., Aquaphor) to keep the lips moist. Agents that should not be used include lemon glycerine swabs (irritate eroded tissue and can decay teeth), hydrogen peroxide (delays healing by breaking down protein), and milk of magnesia (dries mucosa).

Stomatitis may cause such difficulty with eating that the child may require hospitalization for hydration, parenteral nutrition, and pain control (often with IV morphine). The child will usually choose the foods that are best tolerated, and the nurse should encourage parents to relax any eating pressures. Because the stomatitis is a temporary condition, the child can resume good food habits once the ulcers heal. Dental hygiene can become a serious problem for children with orthodontic appliances. Sometimes it may be necessary to remove the braces to allow chemotherapy to continue.

Rectal ulcers are managed by meticulous toilet hygiene and use of an occlusive ointment or dressing applied to the ulcerated area to promote epithelialization. Exposing the denuded skin to air, heat, or supplemental oxygen delays healing. (See Maintaining Healthy Skin, Chapter 45, and Process of Wound Healing, Chapter 53). Parents are advised to record bowel movements because the child may voluntarily avoid defecation to prevent discomfort. The use of rectal thermometers and suppositories is contraindicated because insertion may further traumatize the area.

Neuropathy. Vincristine and, to a lesser extent, vinblastine can cause various neurotoxic effects. Nursing interventions for management of these effects include (1) administering stool softeners or laxatives for severe constipation caused by decreased bowel innervation; (2) maintaining good body alignment and, if on bed rest, using a footboard or high-top shoes to minimize or prevent footdrop; (3) carrying out safety measures during ambulation because of weakness and numbing of the extremities, which may cause difficulty in walking or fine hand movement; and (4) providing a soft or liquid diet for severe jaw pain.

Hemorrhagic Cystitis. Sterile hemorrhagic cystitis, a side effect of chemical irritation to the bladder from cyclophosphamide, can be decreased and often prevented by (1) a liberal fluid intake (at least one and a half times the recommended daily fluid requirement); (2) frequent voiding immediately after feeling the urge, before bed, and after arising; (3) administering the drug early in the day to allow for sufficient oral intake and voiding; and (4) administering mesna (an agent that provides protection to the bladder) as ordered. If oral home administration is prescribed, the family needs *specific* instructions regarding exactly how much fluid the child must have.

NURSE ALERT • If signs of cystitis occur, such as burning on urination, prompt medical evaluation is needed.

Alopecia. Hair loss is a common side effect of several chemotherapeutic drugs and cranial irradiation, although not all children lose their hair during drug therapy. It is better to warn children and parents of this side effect than to allow them to think that it is only a remote possibility. A soft cotton cap is the most comfortable head wear for children. Polyester increases perspiration and causes itching. Other options include scarves, hats, or a wig.

The nurse should also inform the family that hair regrows in 3 to 6 months and may be of a different color and texture. Commonly the hair is darker, thicker, and curlier than before. If the child chooses not to wear a wig, attention to some type of head covering, especially in cold climates and during exposure to sun, and scalp hygiene are important. The scalp should be washed like any other body part.

Moon Face. Short-term steroid therapy produces no acute toxicities and produces two beneficial reactions: increased appetite and a sense of well-being. However, it does produce alterations in body image, which although not clinically significant, can be extremely distressing to older children. One of these is moon face, in which the child's face becomes rounded and puffy. It is not unusual for other children to make fun of the child with such remarks as "Miss Piggy," "Porky Pig," or "fat face." It is helpful to reassure children who experience such name-calling that after cessation of the drug the face will return to normal. Unlike hair loss, little can be done to camouflage this obvious change. If the child resumes activity early in the course of treatment, the change may be less noticeable to peers than after a long absence.

Mood Changes. Shortly after beginning steroid therapy, children experience a number of mood changes that range from feelings of well-being and euphoria to depression and irritability. If parents are unaware of these drug-induced changes, they may become unduly concerned. Therefore the nurse should warn them of the reactions and encourage them to discuss the behavioral changes with each other and the child.

Provide Continued Physical Care and Emotional Support. Because of the improved survival of these children, continued monitoring of physical and intellectual growth and development is essential. Nurses should stress the importance of regular follow-up care.

An important aspect of continued emotional support involves the prognosis. Although leukemia is no longer invariably fatal, it must be remembered that survival statistics are only average estimates and apply to those children treated with the latest protocols since diagnosis. For the low-risk child the chances may be better, but for the high risk child they may be significantly poorer. Of those who do survive after discontinuing therapy, some will have a relapse. Therefore, at present, only the passage of time is positive confirmation of the child's being ultimately "cured" of the disease. Remission, even in excess of 5 years, cannot be equated with a cure. With increasing concern regarding late effects of treatment, continued surveillance of the child's health status is needed. The nurse who is working with family members must individualize information regarding the "numbers" and the potential risks. An understanding of each member's emotional needs, as well as competent care of physical ones, is essential to the positive, growth-promoting support of the family. Comprehensive emotional support for the family of the child with a potentially fatal illness is discussed in Chapter 41.

➤ Evaluation

The effectiveness of nursing interventions is determined by continual reassessment and evaluation of care based on the following observational guidelines:

1. Compare number of visits for primary health with recommended schedule of health supervision.
2. Monitor growth, development, and other aspects of regular health assessment; check mouth for adequacy of dental hygiene; review immunization record for age-appropriate vaccines and use of non-live virus preparations.
3. Interview child and family regarding their understanding of treatments and diagnostic tests.
4. Use pain assessment techniques for procedural pain.
5. Make careful observations of physical status.
   a. Take vital signs regularly.
   b. Observe for evidence of bleeding, infection, neuropathy, cystitis, and mucosal ulceration.
   c. Observe and record intake and output.
6. Interview child and family and observe behaviors as a result of complications of therapies.
7. Interview child and family and observe behaviors that provide clues to their response to the disease, its therapy, and nursing interventions.

The expected outcomes are described in the Nursing Care Plan.

Lymphomas

Pediatric lymphomas are the third most common group of malignancies in children and adolescents. The lymphomas, a group of neoplastic diseases that arise from the lymphoid and hemopoietic systems, are divided into Hodgkin disease and non-Hodgkin lymphoma (NHL). These diseases are further subdivided according to tissue type and extent of disease. NHL is more prevalent in children younger than 14 years, whereas Hodgkin disease is prevalent in adolescence and the young adult period, with a striking increase between ages 15 and 19 years.

Nursing Care Plan THE CHILD WITH CANCER

NURSING DIAGNOSIS Risk for injury related to malignant process and treatment

EXPECTED OUTCOME Complications from chemotherapy are minimized, and the child exhibits signs of complete or partial remission.

Nursing Interventions/*Rationales*

Administer chemotherapeutic agents per physician order and monitor IV site closely for signs of infiltration *to prevent severe tissue damage.*

Obtain allergy history *to prevent anaphylaxis.*

Observe child for at least 20 minutes after chemotherapy infusion *for signs of anaphylaxis* (cyanosis, wheezing, hypotension, urticaria); stop infusion and flush IV line *to minimize reaction;* have emergency equipment and drugs readily available *to prevent delay in treatment of anaphylactic reaction.*

NURSING DIAGNOSIS Risk for injury (hemorrhage, hemorrhagic cystitis) related to interference with cell proliferation

EXPECTED OUTCOME The child exhibits no evidence of bleeding or hematuria.

Nursing Interventions/*Rationales*

Monitor platelet counts and administer platelets per physician order *to raise platelet count and minimize bleeding tendencies.*

Avoid aspirin products *as they interfere with platelet function.*

Teach child and family to limit activity when platelet count drops *to minimize chances of accidental injury.*

Use care in the administration of therapy (e.g., avoid grabbing with fingers and friction with clothing and bedclothes when turning; keep skin clean and dry and sheets clean and wrinkle free; use soft sponge for oral care) *to reduce bruising and injury.*

Turn and reposition frequently, use pressure-relieving mattresses *to prevent pressure ulcers.*

Implement only essential skin puncturing procedures; monitor puncture site carefully; apply gentle pressure, ice to bleeding sites *to minimize bleeding.*

Teach child and parents how to manage nosebleeds *to reduce blood loss.*

Administer ordered drugs that are irritating to the bladder mucosa early in day *to allow sufficient fluid intake and voiding for flushing of irritants.*

Ensure increased oral intake as ordered and encourage frequent voiding *to flush metabolites from system and prevent irritation.*

Observe for and report signs of cystitis (burning and pain on urination) *to ensure prompt medical treatment.*

NURSING DIAGNOSIS Risk for infection related to depressed body defenses

EXPECTED OUTCOME The child exhibits no evidence of infection.

Nursing Interventions/*Rationales*

Place child in private room and screen all visitors and staff for signs of infection *to minimize exposure to infective organisms.*

Teach child and family about good hygiene and careful handwashing techniques *to prevent spread of infection.*

Use good handwashing for all contacts with child and scrupulous aseptic technique for all invasive procedures *to minimize exposure to infection.*

Encourage a nutritionally complete diet *to support body's natural defenses.*

Administer antibiotics and GCSF per physician order *to prevent infection.*

Monitor vital signs and observe skin and mucosa *to detect signs of infection.*

Avoid administration of live attenuated virus vaccines (i.e., measles-mumps-rubella, oral polio, varicella zoster) to child with depressed immune system *to prevent overwhelming the system and introducing an infectious disease;* use inactivated virus vaccines as prescribed (i.e., chickenpox, Salk polio, influenza) *to prevent common childhood illnesses.*

NURSING DIAGNOSIS Risk for fluid volume deficit related to chemotherapy-induced nausea and vomiting

EXPECTED OUTCOME The child is adequately hydrated.

Nursing Interventions/*Rationales*

Administer initial dose of antiemetic before starting chemotherapy *to reduce incidence of nausea and vomiting.*

Administer regular doses of antiemetic as ordered for the duration of expected cycle of nausea and vomiting *to decrease or prevent nausea and vomiting episodes.*

Administer IV fluids as ordered *to maintain hydration;* encourage oral fluids and foods in small amounts *to increase toleration.*

Monitor child's response to antiemetic *as reactions are idiosyncratic and adjustments in drugs or dose may be needed.*

Monitor intake and output *to ensure adequate hydration.*

Avoid foods with strong odors *that may induce nausea and vomiting.*

Encourage frequent intake of fluids in small amounts *since small portions are usually better tolerated.*

Nursing Care Plan THE CHILD WITH CANCER—cont'd

NURSING DIAGNOSIS Altered mucous membranes related to administration of chemotherapeutic agents

EXPECTED OUTCOME The child exhibits no evidence of oral mucositis or rectal ulceration.

Nursing Interventions/*Rationales*

Institute meticulous oral hygiene (e.g., soft sponge toothbrush *to avoid trauma;* frequent mouthwashes *to promote healing;* lip balm *to keep lips moist*). **Avoid use of lemon glycerin swabs,** *which irritate eroded tissue and induce tooth decay;* **hydrogen peroxide,** *which delays healing of ulcers;* and **milk of magnesia,** *which dries oral mucosa.*

Inspect oral mucosa daily for ulcers and report immediately *to ensure early treatment.*

Apply local anesthetics as ordered to ulcerated areas before meals *to relieve pain and increase food intake.* **Avoid use of viscous lidocaine in young children** ***as it may depress gag reflex.***

Serve a bland, moist soft diet; avoid juices with ascorbic acid; use a straw for fluids; avoid oral and rectal temperature-taking *to decrease pain and injury to ulcerated areas.*

Administer prescribed antiinfective agents *to prevent or treat mucositis,* analgesics *to control pain.*

Wash perianal area after stools *to lessen irritation.*

Use warm sitz baths *to ease pain and promote healing.*

Expose reddened mucosal areas to air; apply protective skin barriers to perianal area *to protect mucosa and promote healing.*

Use stool softeners, bulk laxatives *to prevent constipation.*

Track frequency and description of bowel movements *to assess for constipation.*

NURSING DIAGNOSIS Altered nutrition: less than body requirements related to chemotherapeutically induced loss of appetite

EXPECTED OUTCOME Nutritional intake is adequate.

Nursing Interventions/*Rationales*

Allow child any food tolerated, fortify foods with supplements, use small frequent feedings, make food appealing, involve child in selection and preparation *to increase intake and tolerance.*

Take family history *to assess any food issues that may require intervention* (e.g., use of food as control mechanism or reward and punishment).

NURSING DIAGNOSIS Impaired skin integrity related to administration of chemotherapy, radiotherapy, immobility

EXPECTED OUTCOME Skin is clean and intact.

Nursing Interventions/*Rationales*

Provide meticulous skin care, turn and reposition frequently *to prevent skin breakdown.*

Inspect skin frequently *to assess for areas of impending breakdown.*

Encourage adequate caloric-protein intake *to prevent negative nitrogen balance.*

NURSING DIAGNOSIS Impaired physical mobility related to neuromuscular impairment (neuropathy)

EXPECTED OUTCOME The child is as mobile as condition permits, and signs of neuropathy are minimal.

Nursing Interventions/*Rationales*

Match activity level to physical condition and abilities *to prevent overexertion and injury.*

If bedridden, have patient perform passive range of motion *to retain full range of motion;* use a footboard or high-top shoes *to prevent footdrop;* position body in correct alignment with adequate support *to prevent pain and contractures.*

NURSING DIAGNOSIS Pain related to cancer and treatments

EXPECTED OUTCOME The child exhibits no signs of discomfort.

Nursing Interventions/*Rationales*

Be judicious in caregiving and handling *to minimize pain.*

Administer analgesics as prescribed on a regular schedule *to prevent start or recurrence of pain.*

Implement appropriate nonpharmacologic pain reduction techniques *as an adjunct to analgesics.*

Monitor child for vital signs, signs of irritability, restlessness *to assess need for and effectiveness of pain management techniques.*

Continued

Nursing Care Plan THE CHILD WITH CANCER—cont'd

NURSING DIAGNOSIS Fear related to diagnosis, prognosis, treatment procedure

EXPECTED OUTCOME The child exhibits signs of reduced fear.

Nursing Interventions/*Rationales*

Acknowledge child's fear and help child to identify sources of that fear *to facilitate identification and use of coping strategies.*

Orient child to hospital sights and sounds; provide child with accurate information about condition, procedures, and treatments; spend time with child *to promote trust and dispel fear.*

Encourage frequent family visitation with active participation in care *to prevent distress from separation.*

Use frequent touch, holding, and talking as appropriate *to provide comfort.*

Provide diversion and sensory stimulation appropriate to the child's developmental level and physical condition.

Instruct family in importance of comfort measures and in their active participation in care *to ease child's fears.*

Prepare child for procedures using developmentally appropriate approaches (therapeutic play) *to reduce fear and promote cooperation.*

Allow child choices when possible *to give child some measure of control.*

Work with parents to create a routine that is similar to the child's usual routine at home *to increase comfort with environment.*

NURSING DIAGNOSIS Altered family processes related to situational crises (child with life-threatening disease), treatment approaches

EXPECTED OUTCOME The family exhibits adaptation of their usual roles, functions to accommodate special needs of child, and exhibits growth-promoting behaviors.

Nursing Interventions/*Rationales*

Provide opportunity for family to absorb and adjust to diagnosis (e.g., repeat information *to allow time for family to hear and understand;* encourage expression of concerns, fears, and feelings about diagnosis and potential impact *to facilitate adjustment;* identify support systems *to provide resources for coping*).

Assist family to understand expected treatment, rationale, and implications *to provide a sound basis for decision making.*

Teach family about expected side effects and toxicities of treatment *to prevent surprises and prepare them for what will happen.*

Explore family reaction to the child; assist them to achieve a realistic view of child's condition; have family emphasize what child can do; explore ways for family to include child in family activities *to help family increase abilities to cope with child's illness and to help child remain a part of the family structure.*

Arrange for and participate in family conferences *to provide forum for communication, mutual goal setting, and effective strategizing.*

Have parents spend special time with siblings *so that they do not feel neglected or left out.*

Identify additional resource systems (e.g., relatives, friends, church, health care services, community programs) and strategize with family about making good use of these systems *to develop broad base of support.*

NURSING DIAGNOSIS Anticipatory grieving related to impending loss of a child

See the Nursing Care Plan: The Child Who Is Terminally Ill or Dying, Chapter 41.

Hodgkin Disease

Hodgkin disease is a neoplastic disease that originates in the lymphoid system and primarily involves the lymph nodes. It predictably metastasizes to nonnodal or extralymphatic sites, especially the spleen, liver, bone marrow, and lungs, although no tissue is exempt from involvement (Fig. 49-4). It is classified according to four histologic types: (1) lymphocytic predominance, (2) nodular sclerosis, (3) mixed cellularity, and (4) lymphocytic depletion. Accurate staging of the extent of disease is the basis for treatment protocols and expected prognoses. The well-established Ann Arbor staging system assigns stage based on the number of sites of lymph node involvement, presence of extranodal disease, and history of any symptoms. Class A includes patients who are asymptomatic and class B includes those who have the following symptoms: temperature of 38° C (100.4° F) or higher for 3 consecutive days, drenching night sweats, or unexplained loss of body weight (10% or more) over the preceding 6 months (Hudson and Donaldson, 1997).

Asymptomatic enlarged cervical or supraclavicular lymphadenopathy is the most common presentation of Hodgkin disease (Box 49-10). Other systemic symptoms, including fever, weight loss, and night sweats, as well as cough, abdominal discomfort, anorexia, nausea, and pruritus, may be manifested. Because multiple organs may be involved, diagnosis is based on the results of several tests and the extent of metastatic disease. Tests include a CBC, erythrocyte sedimentation rate, serum

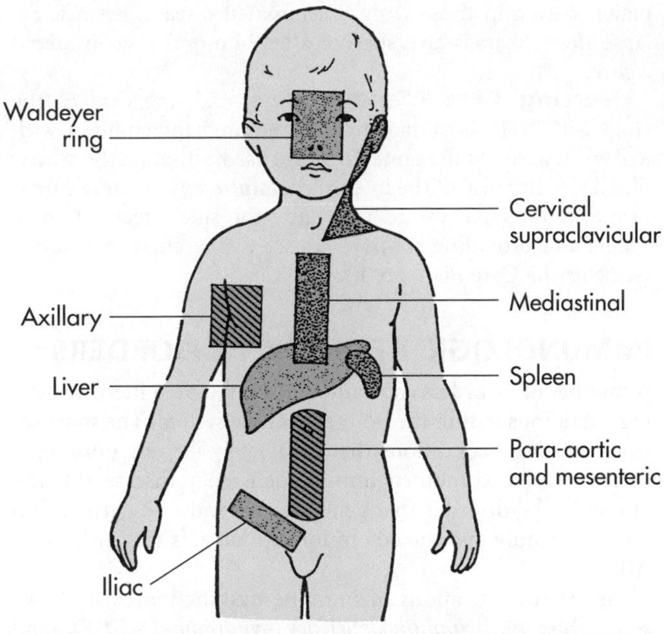

FIG. 49-4 • Main areas of lymphadenopathy and organ involvement in Hodgkin disease.

copper, ferritin level, fibrinogen, immunoglobulins, uric acid level, liver function tests, T-cell function studies, and urinalysis. Radiographic tests include computed tomography (CT) scans of the neck, chest, abdomen, and pelvis; a gallium scan (identifies metastatic/recurrent disease); a chest x-ray film; and if clinically indicated, a bone scan to identify metastatic disease. With the advent of CT and gallium scans, a lymphangiogram may not be needed, although elimination is controversial.

Although used rarely, *lymphangiography* may be performed. This is visualization of the lymphatic circulation of the lower extremities, groin, iliopelvic and abdominal-aortic regions, and thoracic duct by way of a radiopaque medium injected in the feet or hands.

A lymph node biopsy is essential to establish histiologic diagnosis and staging. The presence of Reed-Sternberg cells is characteristic of Hodgkin disease. These large cells, which are multilobed and nucleated with abundant cytoplasm and a typically halolike clear zone around the nucleolus, are often described as having an "owl's eyes" appearance (Hudson and Donaldson, 1997). A bone marrow aspiration or biopsy is performed. With the advent of CT and gallium scans to identify metastatic disease and multiagent chemotherapy to eradicate metastatic disease, a laparotomy is avoided except in a few selected cases.

Therapeutic Management. The primary modalities of therapy are radiation and chemotherapy. Each may be used alone or in combination based on the clinical staging. Radiation may involve only the involved field (IF), an extended field (EF) (involved areas plus adjacent nodes), or total nodal irradiation (TNI), depending on the extent of involvement.

An effective combination of chemotherapy widely used is MOPP (mechlorethamine, vincristine [Oncovin], procarbazine, and prednisone) alternating with ABVD (adriamycin, bleomycin, vinblastine, and dacarbazine) over a period of several months. However, this therapy combination caused severe late effects, especially secondary malignancies. At present, use of ABVD alternating with COPP (cyclophosphamide, vincristine, prednisone, procarbazine) as a substitute for MOPP is being investigated in hopes of minimizing late effects.

Box 49-10

Clinical Manifestations of Hodgkin Disease

Painless enlargement of the lymph nodes:
- Enlarged, firm, nontender, moveable nodes in the cervical area are most common
- "Sentinel" node located near the left clavicle may be first enlarged node
- Axillary and inguinal lymph nodes less frequently

Other signs and symptoms of lymphadenopathy:
- Enlarged mediastinal nodes cause persistent nonproductive cough
- Enlarged retroperitoneal nodes produce unexplained abdominal pain

Systemic symptoms (usually indicate advanced involvement):
- Low-grade and/or intermittent fever
- Anorexia
- Nausea
- Weight loss
- Night sweats
- Pruritus

Follow-up care of children no longer receiving therapy is essential to identify relapse and secondary cancers. In children with splenectomy due to laparotomy, prophylactic antibiotics are administered for an indefinite period. Also, immunizations against pneumococci and meningococci are recommended before the splenectomy.

Prognosis. Long-term survival for all stages of Hodgkin disease is excellent. Early-stage disease can have survival rates greater than 90%, with advanced-stage disease having rates between 65% and 75%.

Nursing Care Management. Nursing care involves the same objectives as for patients with other types of cancer—specifically, (1) preparation for diagnostic and operative procedures, (2) explanation of treatment side effects (see Box 49-9), and (3) child and family support (see Chapter 41). Because this is most often a disease of adolescents and young adults, the nurse must have an appreciation of their psychologic needs and reactions during the diagnostic and treatment phases (see Nursing Care Plan, pp. 1380-1382).

Once the child is hospitalized for suspected Hodgkin disease, a battery of diagnostic tests is ordered. The family needs an explanation of why each test is performed because many of them, such as bone marrow aspiration, are not routine.

The most common side effect of radiation is fatigue, which may last for a year after treatment. This is particularly difficult for active, outgoing school-age children and adolescents because it prevents them from keeping up with their peers. Sometimes adolescents will push themselves to the point of physical exhaustion rather than admit and succumb to the decreased activity tolerance. The nurse cautions parents to observe for behavior such as extreme fatigue at the end of the day, falling asleep at the dinner table, inability to concentrate on homework, or an increased susceptibility to infection. A regular bedtime and scheduled rest periods are important for these children, especially during chemotherapy, when myelosuppression increases the risk of infection and debilitation. Before discharge the nurse should discuss a feasible school schedule with the parents and child.

An area of concern for adolescents is the high risk of sterility from radiation and chemotherapy. Both radiation to the gonads; and drugs, particularly procarbazine and alkylating agents, can lead to infertility. Adolescents should be informed of these side effects early in the course of the diagnosis and treatment. In adolescent boys, sperm banking is now offered at many cancer centers before the initiation of treatment. Sexual function is not altered, although the appearance of secondary sexual characteristics and menstruation may be delayed in the pubescent child. Delayed sexual maturation may be an extremely sensitive and stressful issue for children.

Non-Hodgkin Lymphoma (NHL)

Approximately 60% of pediatric lymphomas are classified as NHL, with an incidence of 7 to 8 cases per million in children younger than 15 years (Shad and Magrath, 1997). Histologic classification of childhood NHL is strikingly different from that of Hodgkin disease, as demonstrated in the following statements:

- The disease is usually diffuse rather than nodular.
- The cell type is either undifferentiated or poorly differentiated.
- Dissemination occurs early, more often, and rapidly.
- Mediastinal involvement and invasion of meninges are common.

NHL exhibits a variety of morphologic, cytochemical, and immunologic features, not unlike the diversity seen in leukemia. Classification is based on the histologic pattern: (1) lymphoblastic, (2) Burkitt or non-Burkitt, or (3) large cell. Immunologically these cells are also classified as T cells; B cells; or non-T, non-B cells (lacking immunologic properties).

The clinical staging system used in Hodgkin disease is of little value in NHL, although it has been modified and other systems have been developed.

Diagnostic Evaluation. Because the clinical presentation of most children with NHL is widespread disseminated disease, thorough pathologic staging is unnecessary. Clinical manifestations depend on the anatomic site and extent of involvement. These manifestations include many of those seen in Hodgkin disease and leukemia, as well as organ symptoms related to pressure from enlargement of adjacent lymph nodes, such as intestinal or airway obstruction, cranial nerve palsies, and spinal paralysis.

Current recommendations for staging include surgical biopsy of an enlarged node, histopathologic confirmation of disease with cytochemical and immunologic evaluation, bone marrow examination, radiographic studies (especially tomograms of the lungs and GI organs), and lumbar puncture.

Therapeutic Management. The present treatment protocols for NHL include aggressive use of radiation and chemotherapy. Similar to leukemic therapy the protocols include induction, consolidation, and maintenance phases, some with intrathecal chemotherapy. Several drug combinations are employed, most of which contain several antineoplastic agents.

Prognosis. The prognosis is excellent for children with localized disease, and long-term remissions are possible in many patients, even in those with disseminated disease. Because relapse after 2 years is rare, survival after 24 months is considered a cure.

Nursing Care Management. Nursing care of the child with NHL is similar to that required for children with leukemia. Many of the same drugs are used, although the schedules differ. Because of the intense chemotherapy, nursing care is primarily directed toward managing the side effects of these agents and providing supportive care to the child and family (see Nursing Care Plan, pp. 1380-1382).

IMMUNOLOGIC DEFICIENCY DISORDERS

A number of disorders can cause profound, often life-threatening alterations within the body's immune system. The most serious are those conditions that completely depress immunity, such as severe combined immunodeficiency disease (SCID). However, the disorder that generates the most anxiety, within both the family and the community at large, is HIV infection/AIDS.

Several classifications of immune dysfunction exist. *AIDS, severe combined immunodeficiency syndrome (SCIDS),* and *Wiskott-Aldrich syndrome* are syndromes wherein the body is unable to mount an immune response. The immune response can also be misdirected. In *autoimmune disorders,* antibodies, macrophages, and lymphocytes attack healthy cells.

Human Immunodeficiency Virus (HIV) Infection and Acquired Immunodeficiency Syndrome (AIDS)

Because the first cases of AIDS were identified in the early 1980s, HIV infection has generated intense medical investigation. Research has led to early diagnosis of and improved medical treatments for HIV infection, changing this disease from a rapidly fatal one to a chronic, but terminal, disease of childhood.

Epidemiology. The World Health Organization estimates reveal that by late 1999, 1.3 million children (aged 0 to 14 years) worldwide had been infected with HIV and had died (UNAIDS, 2000). As of December 1999, 8718 pediatric cases of AIDS had been reported to the Centers for Disease Control and Prevention in the United States (CDC, 1999a). Eighty-eight percent of these children acquired the disease perinatally from their mothers (CDC, 1999b). Fewer children were infected through the transfusion of contaminated blood/blood products before 1985 or through sexual abuse. In contrast, sexual activity and IV drug use are major sources of HIV infection in adolescents. More than 4000 cases of AIDS in adolescents aged 13 to 19 years had been reported through December 1998 (CDC, 1999a).

Etiology. There are different strains of HIV. HIV-2 is prevalent in Africa, whereas HIV-1 is the dominant strain in the United States and elsewhere. *Horizontal transmission* of HIV occurs through intimate sexual contact or parenteral exposure to blood or body fluids containing visible blood. *Perinatal (vertical) transmission* occurs when an HIV-infected pregnant woman passes the infection to her infant. There is no evidence that casual contact between infected and uninfected individuals can spread the virus.

Pathophysiology. The HIV virus primarily infects a specific subset of T lymphocytes, the CD_4^+ T cells. The virus takes over the machinery of the CD_4^+ lymphocyte, using it to replicate itself, rendering the CD_4^+ cell dysfunctional. The CD_4^+ lymphocyte count gradually decreases over time, leading to progressive immune deficiency. The count eventually reaches a critical level below which there is substantial risk of opportunistic illnesses followed by death.

Clinical Manifestations. Common clinical manifestations of HIV infection in children are varied (Box 49-11). The diagnosis of AIDS is based on the occurrence of certain illnesses or conditions (CDC, 1994). The most common AIDS-defining conditions observed among American children are listed in Box 49-12. Other problems in these children may include short stature, malnutrition, and cardiomyopathy. CNS abnormalities due to HIV infection may include neuropsychologic deficits; developmental disabilities; and deficits in motor skills, communication, and behavioral functioning.

Diagnostic Evaluation. For children 18 months of age and older, the HIV enzyme-linked immunosorbent assay (ELISA) and Western blot immunoassay are performed to determine HIV infection. In infants born to HIV-infected mothers, these assays will be positive because of the presence of maternal antibodies derived transplacentally. Maternal antibodies may persist in the infant up to 18 months of age. Therefore other diagnostic tests are used, most commonly the HIV polymerase chain reaction (PCR) for detection of proviral DNA. With this technique, disease can be diagnosed in more than 95% of infected infants by 1 month of age (Luzuriaga and Sullivan, 1998).

The CDC (1994) has developed a classification system to describe the spectrum of HIV disease in children. The system indicates the severity of clinical signs and symptoms and the degree of immunosuppression. Mild signs and symptoms include lymphadenopathy, parotitis, hepatosplenomegaly, and recurrent or persistent sinusitis or otitis media. Moderate signs and symptoms include lymphoid interstitial pneumonitis (LIP) and a variety of organ-specific dysfunctions and/or infections. Severe signs and symptoms include AIDS-defining illnesses with the exception of LIP. Children with LIP have a better prognosis than those with other AIDS-defining illnesses. In children whose HIV infection is not yet confirmed, the letter *E* (vertically exposed) is placed in front of the classification. The immune categories are based on CD_4^+ lymphocyte counts and percentages. Age adjustment of these numbers is necessary because normal counts, which are relatively high in infants, decline steadily until 6 years of age, when they reach adult norms.

Box 49-11

Common Clinical Manifestations of HIV Infection in Children

Lymphadenopathy
Hepatosplenomegaly
Oral candidiasis
Chronic or recurrent diarrhea
Failure to thrive
Developmental delay
Parotitis

Box 49-12

Common AIDS-Defining Conditions in Children

Pneumocystis carinii pneumonia (PCP)
Lymphoid interstitial pneumonitis (LIP)
Recurrent bacterial infections
Wasting syndrome
HIV encephalopathy
Candidal esophagitis
- Cytomegalovirus disease
- *Mycobacterium avium-intracellulare* complex infection
- Severe herpes simplex infection
- Pulmonary candidiasis

Cryptosporidiosis

Therapeutic Management. The goals of therapy for HIV infection include slowing the growth of the virus, preventing and treating opportunistic infections, and providing nutritional support and symptomatic treatment. *Antiretroviral drugs* work at various stages of the HIV life cycle to prevent reproduction of functional new virus particles. Although not a cure, these drugs can suppress viral replication, preventing further deterioration of the immune system, and thus delay disease progression. Classes of antiretroviral agents include nucleoside reverse transcriptase inhibitors (e.g., zidovudine, didanosine, stavudine, lamivudine, abacavir), nonnucleoside reverse transcriptase inhibitors (e.g., nevirapine, delavirine, efavirenz), nucleotide reverse transcriptase inhibitors (e.g., adefovir), protease inhibitors (e.g., indinavir, saquinavir, ritonavir, nelfinavir, amprenavir), and adjunctive antiretrovirals (e.g., hydroxyurea). Combinations of these drugs are used to forestall the emergence of drug resistance. Antiretroviral therapy regimens and guidelines are continually evolving. Therapy is lifelong, making adherence difficult. Laboratory markers (CD_4^+ lymphocyte count, viral load) assist in monitoring both disease progression and response to therapy.

Pneumocystis carinii pneumonia (PCP) is the most common opportunistic infection of children infected with HIV. It occurs most commonly between 3 and 6 months of age. All infants born to HIV-infected women should receive prophylaxis during the first year of life according to guidelines set by the CDC (1995). After 1 year of age, the need for prophylaxis is determined by the presence of severe immunosuppression or a history of PCP (CDC, 1995). Trimethoprim-sulfamethoxazole (TMP-SMZ) is the agent of choice.

Prophylaxis is often used for other opportunistic infections, such as disseminated *Mycobacterium avium-intracellulare* complex (MAC), candidiasis, and herpes simplex. IV immunoglobulin has been helpful in preventing recurrent or serious bacterial infections in some HIV-infected children.

Immunization against common childhood illnesses is recommended for all children exposed to and infected with HIV (American Academy of Pediatrics, 2000). The only changes in the schedule are the avoidance of varicella (chickenpox) vaccine and the use of inactivated poliovirus (IPV) rather than oral poliovirus (OPV) for these children and their close contacts. The pneumococcal and influenza vaccines are recommended. Because antibody production to vaccines may be poor or decrease over time, immediate prophylaxis after exposure to several vaccine-preventable diseases (e.g., measles, varicella) is warranted. As a result of the occurrence of severe measles in some infected children, the measles-mumps-rubella (MMR) vaccine is given if they are not severely immunocompromised. It should be recognized that children receiving IV gamma globulin prophylaxis may not respond to the MMR vaccine (American Academy of Pediatrics, 2000).

HIV infection often leads to marked failure to thrive and multiple nutritional deficiencies. Nutritional management may be difficult because of recurrent illness, diarrhea, and other physical problems. Intensive nutritional interventions should be instituted when the child's growth begins to slow or weight begins to decrease.

Prognosis. Perinatally infected infants generally have more rapid disease progression than children infected at an older age or adults. It has been reported that the risk of dying is higher for children in whom AIDS is diagnosed early in life and in those who develop PCP (Kline et al, 1995; Turner et al, 1995). The mean survival time from birth to death has been reported to be about 9.4 years (Barnhart et al, 1996). Mortality related to HIV infection has decreased 71% since 1995 and is no longer considered one of the 15 leading causes of death (Guyer et al, 1999).

Nursing Care Management. Education concerning transmission and control of infectious diseases, including HIV infection, is essential for children with HIV infection and anyone involved in their care. The basic tenets of standard precautions should be presented in an age-appropriate manner, with careful consideration of the educational levels of the individuals (see Infection Control, Chapter 45). Safety issues, including appropriate storage of special medications and equipment (e.g., needles and syringes), are emphasized. Unfortunately, relatives, friends, and others in the general public may be fearful of contracting HIV infection, and criticism and ostracism of the child and family may occur. In an effort to protect the child, the family may limit the child's activities outside the home. Although certain precautions are justified in limiting exposure to sources of infections, they must be tempered with concern for the child's normal developmental needs. Both the family and the community need ongoing education about HIV to dispel many of the myths that have been perpetuated by uninformed persons.*

Prevention is a key component of HIV education. Educating adolescents about HIV is essential in preventing HIV infection in this age group. Education should include the routes of transmission; the hazards of IV and other recreational drug use, and the value of sexual abstinence and safe sex practices. Such education should be a part of anticipatory guidance provided to all adolescent patients. Nurses can also encourage adolescents at risk to undergo HIV counseling and testing. In addition to identifying infected teenagers and getting them into care, such counseling affords adolescents an opportunity to learn about, and possibly change, their risk behaviors.

The nurse's role in the care of the child with HIV is multifaceted. The nurse serves as educator, direct care provider, case manager, and advocate. As with all persons with chronic illnesses, these children will have much involvement with the health care system. The need for HIV medications is lifelong. Nurses are instrumental in encouraging and empowering these children (and their caretakers) to adhere to their medication regimens. Clinic visits and hospitalizations may become frequent as the disease progresses. The physiologic care of the child is directed at minimum exposure to infections; nutritional support; comfort measures, including pain management; and assessment and recognition of changes in status that may indicate new complications. The scope of nursing care will change with new symptoms, changes in treatment, and disease progression. The unpredictability of the course of pediatric HIV infection is a continual source of stress to these children and their caretakers. Psychologic interventions will vary with the unique circumstances of each child and family.

Common psychosocial concerns include disclosing the diagnosis to the child, making custody plans when the parent is infected, and anticipating the loss of a family member. Other stressors may include financial difficulties, HIV-associated stigma, striving to keep the diagnosis a secret, infection of other family members, and the multiple losses associated with HIV. Many mothers of these children are single mothers who are also HIV infected. As primary caretakers, they often attend to the needs of their child first, neglecting their own health in the process (Family Focus box). The nurse can encourage the mother to receive regular health care.

Children with HIV infection attend day care centers and schools. It is well established that the risk of HIV transmission in these settings is minimal. These institutions are required to follow CDC and Occupational Safety Health Administration (OSHA) guidelines for infection control measures. Standard precautions describing proper management of blood and body fluids should also be followed. It is recommended that school personnel receive current HIV information and include it in the health education curriculum for kindergarten through twelfth grade (American Academy of Pediatrics, 1998). School nurses play a vital role in educating the school staff, students, and parents. They are also invaluable in monitoring the needs of children who are known to be infected.

Confidentiality is a major issue in day care or school attendance. Parents and legal guardians have the right to decide whether they inform these agencies of their child's HIV diagnosis. Unfortunately, myths about HIV infection continue, and the family often wishes to avoid any potential criticism or ostracism of the child.

Nursing care of the child with HIV infection is summarized in the Nursing Care Plan.

Family Focus

CAREGIVERS AND THE INFANT WITH HIV INFECTION

Unlike other fatal pediatric diseases, HIV infection is associated with special family alterations. The infant infected in utero faces multiple physical and parental problems. Because the mother is infected, she may be ill or dying and therefore unable to care for the child. If possible, grandparents or other relatives may assume care. Foster care is often difficult to arrange because of the nature of the disease, especially in relation to the social stigma and the child's multiple medical needs. These children may require frequent hospitalizations with progression of their HIV disease. When children remain in the hospital, the importance of consistent caregivers, especially primary nurses, who attend to the youngsters' physical, developmental, and emotional needs cannot be overemphasized. However, primary nurses may face the risk of overinvolvement and must be aware of the boundaries of a therapeutic relationship.

*Additional information is available from the AIDS Hotline: 1-800-342-2437 (AIDS); and from the National Pediatric HIV Resource Center, 30 Bergen St., ADMC 4, Newark, NJ 07107; (473) 972-0399 or 1-800-362-0071; website: www.pedhivaids.org.

Nursing Care Plan THE CHILD WITH HIV INFECTION

NURSING DIAGNOSIS Risk for infection related to impaired body defenses

EXPECTED OUTCOME The child exhibits no evidence of infection and no evidence of spread of the virus.

Nursing Interventions/*Rationales*

Place child in private room and screen all visitors and staff for signs of infection *to minimize exposure to infective organisms.*

Teach child and family about good hygiene and careful handwashing techniques *to prevent spread of infection.*

Use good handwashing for all contacts with child and scrupulous aeseptic technique for all invasive procedures *to minimize exposure to infection.*

Encourage a nutritionally complete diet *to support body's natural defenses.*

Administer prescribed antibiotics *to prevent infection,* antiretroviral drugs *to increase lymphocyte production,* trimethoprim sulfamethoxazole tablets *to prevent pneumocystis pneumonia,* rifabutin *to prevent Mycobacterium avium.*

Monitor vital signs and observe skin and mucosa, auscultate lungs *to detect signs of infection.*

Avoid administration of live attenuated virus vaccines (i.e., MMR, oral polio, varicella zoster) to child with depressed immune system *to prevent overwhelming the system and introducing an infectious disease;* use inactivated virus vaccines as prescribed (i.e., Salk polio, influenza) *to prevent common childhood illnesses.*

Instruct child and family about protective methods (e.g., handwashing after using bathroom, avoidance of blood and body fluids by others; avoidance of biting, scratching behaviors) *to prevent spread of virus.*

Use appropriate universal precautions when administering care and performing invasive procedures *to prevent spread of HIV virus.*

NURSING DIAGNOSIS Altered nutrition: less than body requirements related to recurrent illness, diarrhea, loss of appetite, oral thrush

EXPECTED OUTCOME The child's nutritional intake is adequate.

Nursing Interventions/*Rationales*

Provide high-calorie, high-protein diet *to meet body requirements for metabolism and growth;* fortify foods with nutritional supplements *to maximize quality of intake.*

Involve child in selection and preparation *to increase intake and tolerance.*

Use creativity to encourage child to eat (see Feeding the Sick Child, Chapter 45).

Monitor height and weight *to assess for slowed growth or weight loss.*

Administer antifungal medications as ordered *to prevent or treat thrush.*

NURSING DIAGNOSIS Impaired social interaction related to recurrent illness, social stigma of HIV

EXPECTED OUTCOME The child is involved in age-appropriate peer group and family activities.

Nursing Interventions/*Rationales*

Assist child to identify personal strengths *to facilitate coping.*

Educate school personnel and classmates about HIV *so child is not unnecessarily isolated.*

Encourage family to plan activities that include child as a participating member *to increase family interaction.*

Encourage child to maintain phone contact with friends during hospitalization *to reduce feelings of isolation.*

Introduce child to other children with HIV *to provide mutual support system.*

NURSING DIAGNOSIS Altered sexuality pattern related to risk of disease transmission

EXPECTED OUTCOME The adolescent displays appropriate sexual behavior and exhibits positive sexual identity.

Nursing Interventions/*Rationales*

Educate adolescent about sexual transmission risks, perinatal infection risks, avoidance of high-risk behavior, abstinence/use of condoms *so adolescent can make informed decisions about safe and healthy expressions of sexuality.*

Encourage adolescent to talk about feelings and concerns related to sexuality *to facilitate coping.*

NURSING DIAGNOSIS Altered family processes related to situational crises (child with life-threatening disease) and treatment approaches

See the Nursing Care Plan: The Child with Cancer, pp. 1380-1382 and the Nursing Care Plan: The Child Who Is Terminally Ill or Dying, p. 1030.

Severe Combined Immunodeficiency Disease (SCID)

SCID is a defect characterized by absence of both humoral and cell-mediated immunity. The terms *Swiss-type lymphopenic agammaglobulinemia* (an autosomal recessive form of the disease) and *X-linked agammaglobulinemia* have been used to describe this disorder, which as the names imply, can follow either mode of inheritance.

Susceptibility to infection occurs early in life, most often during the first month. The child has chronic infection, fails to completely recover from an infection, is often reinfected, and is infected with unusual agents. Failure to thrive is a consequence of the persistent illnesses.

Diagnosis is usually based on a history of recurrent, severe infections from early infancy; a familial history of the disorder; and specific laboratory findings, which include lymphopenia, lack of lymphocyte response to antigens, and absence of plasma cells in the bone marrow. Documentation of immunoglobulin deficiency is difficult during infancy because of the normally delayed response of infants in producing their own immunoglobulins and material transfer of immunoglobulin G (IgG).

Therapeutic Management. The only definitive treatment for SCID is a bone marrow transplant from a histocompatible donor, usually a sibling. If a compatible sibling is not available, a parent's marrow can be used after the T lymphocytes have been depleted. IVIg can be used to augment the humoral immunity until the transplant is performed.

Nursing Care Management. Nursing care focuses on the prevention of infection and support of the child and family. If BMT is attempted, the care is consistent with that needed for BMT for any condition (see p. 1390). Because the prognosis for SCID is very poor if a compatible bone marrow donor is not available, nursing care is directed at supporting the family in caring for a child with a life-threatening illness (see Chapter 41). Genetic counseling is essential because of the modes of transmission in either form of the disorder.

Wiskott-Aldrich Syndrome

Wiskott-Aldrich syndrome is an X-linked recessive disorder characterized by a triad of abnormalities: (1) thrombocytopenia, (2) eczema, and (3) immunodeficiency of selective functions of B lymphocytes and T lymphocytes. At birth the major effect of the disorder is bleeding as a result of the thrombocytopenia. As the child grows older, recurrent infection and eczema become more severe, and the bleeding becomes less frequent.

Eczema is typical of the allergic type and easily becomes superinfected. Chronic infection with herpes simplex is a common problem and may lead to chronic keratitis of the eye with loss of vision. Chronic pulmonary disease, sinusitis, and otitis media result from repeated infections. In those children who survive the bleeding episodes and overwhelming infections, malignancy presents an additional risk to survival.

Specific tests for immunologic function confirm the diagnosis. Medical treatment involves (1) counteracting the bleeding tendencies with platelet transfusions, (2) using IV gamma globulin to provide passive immunity (de Martino et al, 1994; Baehner and Miller, 1995), and (3) administering prophylactic antibiotics to prevent and control infection. Bone marrow transplants have been attempted but, even if successful, do not reverse all the defects of this disorder.

Nursing Care Management. Because of the poor prognosis for these children, the main nursing consideration is supporting the family in the care of a fatally ill child (see Chapter 41). Physical care is directed at controlling the problems imposed by the disorder. The measures used to control bleeding are similar to those for hemophilia and vWD (see earlier discussions). Another major goal is prevention or control of infection. Because eczema is a troublesome problem, nursing measures specific to this condition are especially important (see Chapter 53). The genetic implications of this X-linked recessive disorder differ little from those of any other X-linked disorder.

TECHNOLOGIC MANAGEMENT OF HEMATOLOGIC/IMMUNOLOGIC DISORDERS

Blood Transfusion Therapy

Technologic advances in blood banking and transfusion medicine enable the administration of only the blood component needed by the child, such as packed RBCs in anemia or platelets for bleeding disorders. However, regardless of the blood component infused, all transfusions have some risks. Therefore nurses need to be aware of the possible complications and the appropriate interventions. Table 49-4 summarizes the major hazards of transfusions, the signs and symptoms typically associated with each, and nursing responsibilities. General guidelines that apply to all transfusions include:

- Take vital signs, including blood pressure, before administering blood to establish baseline data for intratransfusion and posttransfusion comparison and then every 15 minutes for 1 hour while blood is infusing.
- Check the identification of the recipient with the donor's blood group and type, regardless of the blood product used.
- Administer the first 50 ml of blood or 20% of the volume (whichever is smaller) slowly and stay with the child.
- Administer with normal saline solution on a piggyback setup or have normal saline solution available.
- Administer blood through an appropriate filter to eliminate particles in the blood and prevent the precipitation of formed elements; gently shake the container often.
- Use blood within 30 minutes of its arrival from the blood bank; if it is not used, return it to the blood bank—do not store in the regular unit refrigerator.
- Infuse a unit of blood (or the specified amount) within 4 hours. If the infusion will exceed this time, the blood should be divided into appropriately sized quantities by the blood bank, and the unused portion refrigerated under controlled conditions.
- If a reaction of any type is suspected, take vital signs, stop the transfusion, maintain a patent IV line with normal saline solution and new tubing, notify the practitioner, and do not restart the transfusion until the child's condition has been medically evaluated.

Although hemolytic reactions are rare, ABO incompatibility remains the most common cause of death from blood transfusion, and human error is usually responsible (administration of the wrong type to the patient or mislabeling of the blood product) (Lubin, 1995). Hemolysis can also cause the release of large quantities of phospholipids, which are capable of stimulating disseminated intravascular coagulation (see p. 1370). Acute kid-

TABLE 49-4
Nursing Care of the Child Receiving Blood Transfusions

Complication	Signs/Symptoms	Precautions/Nursing Responsibilities
IMMEDIATE REACTIONS		
Hemolytic reactions Most severe type, but rare Incompatible blood Incompatibility in multiple transfusions	Chills Shaking Fever Pain at needle site and along venous tract Nausea/vomiting Sensation of tightness in chest Red or black urine Headache Flank pain Progressive signs of shock and/or renal failure	Identify donor and recipient blood types and groups before transfusion is begun; verify with another nurse or practitioner Transfuse blood slowly for first 15-20 minutes and/or initial 20% of blood volume; remain with patient Stop transfusion immediately in event of signs or symptoms, maintain patent intravenous line, and notify practitioner Save donor blood to re-crossmatch with patient's blood Monitor for evidence of shock Insert urinary catheter and monitor hourly outputs Send sample of patient's blood and urine to laboratory for presence of hemoglobin (indicates intravascular hemolysis) Observe for signs of hemorrhage resulting from disseminated intravascular coagulation (DIC) Support medical therapies to reverse shock
Febrile reactions Leukocyte or platelet antibodies Plasma protein antibodies	Fever Chills	May give acetaminophen for prophylaxis Leukocyte poor red blood cells (RBCs) are less likely to cause reaction Stop transfusion immediately; report to practitioner for evaluation
Allergic reactions Recipient reacts to allergens in donor's blood	Urticaria Flushing Asthmatic wheezing Laryngeal edema	Give antihistamines for prophylaxis to children with tendency toward allergic reactions Stop transfusions immediately Administer epinephrine for wheezing or anaphylactic reaction
Circulatory overload Too rapid transfusion (even a small quantity) Excessive quantity of blood transfused (even slowly)	Precordial pain Dyspnea Rales Cyanosis Dry cough Distended neck veins	Transfuse blood slowly Prevent overload by using packed RBCs or administering divided amounts of blood Use infusion pump to regulate and maintain flow rate Stop transfusion immediately if signs of overload Place child upright with feet in dependent position to increase venous resistance
Air emboli May occur when blood is transfused under pressure	Sudden difficulty in breathing Sharp pain in chest Apprehension	Normalize pressure before container is empty when infusing blood under pressure Clear tubing of air by aspirating air with syringe at nearest Y connector if air is observed in tubing; disconnect tubing and allow blood to flow until air has escaped only if a Y connector is not available
Hypothermia	Chills Low temperature Irregular heart rate Possible cardiac arrest	Allow blood to warm at room temperature (less than 1 hour) Use approved mechanical blood warmer or electric warming coil to warm blood rapidly; never use microwave oven Take temperature if patient complains of chills; if subnormal, stop transfusion
Electrolyte disturbances Hyperkalemia (in massive transfusions or in patients with renal problems)	Nausea, diarrhea Muscular weakness Flaccid paralysis Paresthesia of extremities Bradycardia Apprehension Cardiac arrest	Use washed RBCs or fresh blood if patient is at risk

Continued

TABLE 49-4
Nursing Care of the Child Receiving Blood Transfusions—cont'd

Complication	Signs/Symptoms	Precautions/Nursing Responsibilities
DELAYED REACTIONS		
Transmission of infection Hepatitis Human immunodeficiency virus (HIV) Malaria Syphilis Bacteria or viruses Other	Signs of infection (e.g., jaundice) Toxic reaction: high fever, severe headache or substernal pain, hypotension, intense flushing, vomiting/diarrhea	Blood is tested for antibiotics to HIV, hepatitis C virus (HCV), and hepatitis B core antigen (HBcAg); in addition, blood is tested for hepatitis B surface antigen (HBsAg) and alanine aminotransferase (ALT), and a serology test is performed for syphilis; positive units are destroyed; individuals at risk for carrying certain viruses are deferred from donation Report any sign of infection and, if occurring during transfusion, stop transfusion immediately, send sample for culture and sensitivity tests, and notify practitioner
Alloimmunization Antibody formation Occurs in patients receiving multiple transfusions	Increased risk of hemolytic, febrile, and allergic reactions	Use limited number of donors Observe carefully for signs of reactions
Delayed hemolytic reaction	Destruction of RBCs and fever 5-10 days after transfusion	Observe for posttransfusion anemia and decreasing benefit from successive transfusion

ney shutdown and eventual renal failure are a result of renal vasoconstriction from antigen-antibody complexes derived from the RBC surface.

Blood is usually administered to children by infusion pump; therefore the usual precautions and management related to pumps apply. When the blood is started with a standard transfusion set, the filter chamber is filled to allow the total filter to be used. The drip chamber is partially filled with blood to permit counting of the drops. In adjusting the flow rate, it is important to remember that blood administration sets do not use microdrops (60 drops/ml) but regular drops (usually 10 or 15 drops/ml). Therefore this must be considered when calculating the flow rate.

Bone Marrow Transplantation (BMT)

Another approach to the treatment of childhood cancer is BMT. Candidates for transplantation are children who have malignancies that are unlikely to be cured by other means. BMT allows for lethal doses of chemotherapy, often combined with radiation therapy, to be given in order to rid the body of all cancer cells (Abramovitz and Senner, 1995). Once the body is free of malignant cells and the immune system is suppressed to prevent rejection of the transplanted marrow, the donor marrow or stem cells or the cells previously stored from the patient are given to the patient by IV transfusion. The newly transfused marrow or stem cells will begin to produce functioning nonmalignant blood cells. In essence, a new blood-forming organ will be accepted by the recipient.

The selection process of a suitable donor and the potential complications in transplantation are related to the *HLA system complex.* Some of the major HLA antigens are A, B, C, D, and DR. There is wide diversity for each of these HLA loci. More than 20 different HLA-A antigens and more than 40 different HLA-B antigens can be inherited.

The genes are inherited as a single unit or *haplotype.* A child inherits one unit from each parent; thus a child and each parent have one identical and one nonidentical haplotype. Because the possible haplotype combinations among siblings follow the laws of mendelian genetics, there is a 25% chance that two siblings have two identical haplotypes and are perfectly matched at the HLA loci.

The importance of HLA matching is to prevent the serious complication known as *graft-vs.-host disease (GVHD).* Because the child's immune system is essentially rendered nonfunctional, there is little difficulty with bone marrow rejection by the recipient. However, the donor's marrow may contain antigens not matched to the recipient's antigens, which begin attacking body cells. The more closely the HLA systems match, the less likely GVHD is to develop. However, it can occur even with a perfect HLA match because there are as yet unidentified and thus unmatched histocompatibility antigens (Sanders, 1997).

Different types of BMT are now performed in children with cancer. *Allogeneic BMT* involves the matching of a histocompatible donor with the recipient. However, allogeneic BMT is limited by the presence of a suitable marrow donor.

Because of the limited numbers of patients having HLA-identical siblings, other types of allogeneic transplants have evolved. *Umbilical cord blood stem cell transplantation* is a new source of hematopoietic stem cells for use in children with cancer (Wagner et al, 1995). Because stem cells can be found with high frequency in the circulation of newborns, cord blood transplantation has become an alternative for some children (Amos and Gordon, 1995). The benefit of using umbilical cord blood is the blood's relative immunodeficiency at birth, allowing for partially matched unrelated cord blood transplants to be successful, with a lower risk of GVHD-related problems (Varadi et al, 1995).

Autologous BMTs use the patient's own marrow that has been collected from disease-free tissue, frozen, and sometimes treated to remove malignant cells. Children with solid tumors such as neuroblastoma, Hodgkin disease, NHL, rhabdomyosarcoma, Ewing sarcoma, and Wilms tumor have been treated with autologous BMTs.

Peripheral stem cell transplants (PSCTs) are also used in children with cancer. PSCT, a type of autologous transplant, differs in the way stem cells are collected from the patient. Colony-stimulating factor (CSF) is first given to stimulate the production of many stem cells (Bensinger et al, 1995). Once the WBC count is high enough, the stem cells are collected by an "apheresis" machine. This machine filters out peripheral stem cells from whole blood, returning the remainder of the blood cells and plasma to the child. Stem cells have been collected in small children, weighing 20 kg or less, without problems (Takaue et al, 1995). The peripheral stem cells are then frozen until the patient is ready for the PSCT.

Nursing Care Management. The care of children undergoing BMT is similar to that of any child receiving chemotherapy and radiation therapy. The hospitalization is typically 3 to 6 weeks in an isolated environment, during which time the child is subjected to numerous procedures and side effects of therapy. Throughout this long ordeal there is the family's concern for successful engraftment and fear of fatal complications (Family Focus box). Consequently nurses involved with the child and family need to provide sensitive care and maintain a supportive attitude during the many crises that may arise. If the procedure is not successful, the care needed by these families is consistent with that required by the family of any child with a life-threatening disorder (see Chapter 41).

Apheresis

Apheresis is the removal of blood from an individual, separation of the blood into its components, retention of one or more of these components, and reinfusion of the remainder of the blood into the individual. Apheresis is most often used to remove large quantities of platelets from healthy adult donors. These transfusion products have greatly prolonged the survival of patients with hematologic and oncologic diseases.

This technique is used to remove peripheral blood stem cells (PBSCs) from children before they receive bone marrow transplants or high-dose chemotherapy and/or radiation therapy, which is severely toxic to the bone marrow. These PBSCs can then be used to restore the child's bone marrow. Apheresis is also used as a therapeutic modality. The blood component that is diseased or toxic is separated from the blood, and the remainder is returned to the individual. Therapeutic apheresis is considered part of standard therapy for many diseases. Plasma is selectively removed from individuals with hyperviscosity, life-threatening complications of myasthenia gravis, Guillain-Barré syndrome, thrombotic thrombocytopenic purpura, and certain drug overdoses. WBCs are removed from individuals with high-WBC-count leukemia.

Nursing Care Management. Difficult venous access and small blood volume can limit the ability to use this therapy in the infant and young child. Education of the family and child focuses on the purposes of the therapy, as well as the technology.

Specially trained individuals perform the apheresis procedure. Attention focuses on rate of removal, blood component separation, and reinfusion of blood into the child. Vital signs are monitored, and the child is continuously observed for any adverse reactions secondary to the circulatory volume changes and the anticoagulant used.

Family Focus

THE DECISION FOR A BONE MARROW TRANSPLANT

A family's decision for a child to undergo bone marrow transplantation (BMT) may be fraught with challenges. Often the child is facing certain death from the malignancy. The preparation of the child for the transplant also places the patient at great medical risk.

Once the preparatory regimen is begun and the child's immune system is destroyed, there is no turning back. Unlike kidney transplantation, BMT does not have a "rescue" procedure, such as dialysis, for supportive therapy. If the donor is a sibling, the issue of his or her marrow "saving" the brother or sister can be a concern, especially if the transplant fails. Parents often must leave the home to stay at the transplant center and encounter additional stressors such as arranging child care, taking a leave from work, and managing finances. The patient faces the greatest stress—fear of BMT failure or life-threatening complications.

When apheresis components are infused, nursing measures will differ if the product is autologous (blood component from the child) or allogeneic (blood component from another individual). Autologous components are the child's own blood; therefore a major precaution is proper identification to ensure the correct component. The rate of infusion should be adjusted to the child's tolerance. If the product is allogeneic, all precautions for blood transfusions apply.

Key Points

- Anemia is defined as reduction of red blood cell volume or hemoglobin concentration to levels below normal; disorders are classified either by etiology/physiology or by morphology.
- The role of the nurse in treatment of anemia is to assist in establishing a diagnosis, prepare the child for laboratory tests, administer prescribed medications, decrease tissue oxygen needs, implement safety precautions, and observe for complications.
- The main nursing goal in prevention of nutritional anemia is parent education regarding correct feeding practices.
- Sickle cell anemia is a hereditary hemoglobinopathy affecting primarily African-Americans.
- Nursing care of the child with sickle cell anemia is aimed at teaching the family how to prevent and recognize sickling, managing pain during crises, and helping the child and parents adjust to a lifelong, potentially fatal disease.
- Nursing care of the child with thalassemia involves observing for complications of multiple blood transfusions, assisting the child in coping with the effects of illness, and fostering parent-child adjustment to long-term illness.
- Causes of acquired aplastic anemia include irradiation, drugs, industrial and household chemicals, infections, infiltration and replacement of myeloid elements, and idiopathic conditions.
- The human body controls bleeding through three processes: vascular spasm, platelet aggregation, and coagulation and clot formation.

- Nursing care of the child with hemophilia involves preventing bleeding by decreasing the risk of injury, recognizing and managing bleeding with factor replacement, preventing the crippling effects of joint degeneration, and preparing and supporting the child and family for home care.
- Goals in the care of the child with leukemia are to prepare the family for diagnostic and therapeutic procedures, prevent complications of myelosuppression, manage problems of irradiation and drug toxicity, and provide continued emotional support.
- The lymphomas include Hodgkin and non-Hodgkin lymphoma and are disorders involving the lymph glands.
- Immunodeficiency disorders are those that in some way render the affected individual unable to fight infectious organisms.
- HIV infection is primarily acquired in infants from a parent with HIV infection and in adolescents from engaging in high risk behaviors. Blood transfusions are no longer a source of HIV infection but in the past were responsible for HIV infection in children treated with multiple blood transfusions, especially those with hemophilia.
- Blood transfusions supply needed blood components.
- Bone marrow transplantation replaces the diseased or malfunctioning bone marrow with viable blood stem cells.
- Apheresis is the selective removal of a blood component. It can be used to supply cellular elements needed for therapy (i.e., platelets or stem cells) or to remove diseased components.

References

Abramovitz LZ, Senner AM: Pediatric bone marrow transplantation update, *Oncol Nurs Forum* 22(1):107-115, 1995.

American Academy of Pediatrics, Committee on Infectious Diseases, Pickering L, editor: *2000 Red Book: report of the Committee on Infectious Diseases,* ed 25, Elk Grove Village, IL, 2000, The Academy.

American Academy of Pediatrics, Committee on Pediatric AIDS: Human immunodeficiency virus/acquired immunodeficiency syndrome education in schools, *Pediatrics* 101(5):933-935, 1998.

American Pain Society: *Guidelines for the management of acute and chronic pain in sickle-cell disease,* Glenview, IL, 1999, American Pain Society.

Amos TA, Gordon MY: Sources of human hematopoietic stem cells or transplantation—a review, *Cell Transplant* 4(6):547-569, 1995.

Baehner RL, Miller DR: Disorders of granulopoiesis. In Miller DR, Baehner RL, editors: *Blood diseases of infancy and childhood,* ed 7, St Louis, 1995, Mosby.

Barnhart HX et al: Natural history of human immunodeficiency virus disease in perinatally infected children: an analysis from the Pediatric Spectrum of Disease Project, *Pediatrics* 97(5):710-716, 1996.

Bensinger W et al: Factors that influence collection and engraftment of autologous peripheral blood stem cells, *J Clin Oncol* 13(10):2547-2555, 1995.

Benz E, Giardina PV: Thalassemia syndromes. In Miller DR, Baehner RL, editors: *Blood diseases of infancy and childhood,* ed 7, St Louis, 1995, Mosby.

Bussel JB, Corrigan JJ: Platelet and vascular disorders. In Miller DR, Baehner RL, editors: *Blood diseases of infancy and childhood,* ed 7, St Louis, 1995, Mosby.

Centers for Disease Control and Prevention: Pediatric HIV/AIDs Surveillance, 1999a. http://www.cdc.gov/hiv/stats/hasrlink/htm

Centers for Disease Control and Prevention: Pediatric HIV/AIDS Surveillance, Slide series through 1999, 1999b. http://www.cdc.gov/hiv/graphics/surveill.htm

Centers for Disease Control and Prevention: 1994 revised classification system for human immunodeficiency virus infection in children less than 13 years of age, *MMWR* 43(RR-12):1-10, 1994.

Centers for Disease Control and Prevention: 1995 revised guidelines for prophylaxis against *Pneumocystis carinii* pneumonia for children infected with or perinatally exposed to human immunodeficiency virus, *MMWR* 44(RR-4):1-11, 1995.

Charache S et al: Hydroxyurea and sickle cell anemia: clinical utility of a myelosuppressive switching agent, *Medicine* 75(6):300-326, 1996.

Chiocca EM: Sickle cell crisis: severe pain and potential tissue necrosis are the major concerns, *Am J Nurs* 96(9):49, 1996.

Claster S, Vichinsky E: First report of reversal of organ dysfunction in sickle cell anemia by the use of hydroxyurea: splenic regeneration, *Blood* 88(6):1951-1953, 1996.

Cross S, Koerper M: Symposium report: prophylaxis in hemophilia—primary, secondary, and beyond, *Hemaware* 2(2):7-12, 34, 1997.

de Martino M et al: Effects of different intravenous immunoglobulin regimens on hemorrhages, platelet numbers and volume in a child with Wiskott-Aldrich syndrome, *Vox Sang* 67:317-319, 1994.

Doney K et al: Primary treatment of acquired aplastic anemia: outcomes with bone marrow transplantation and immunosuppressive therapy, *Ann Intern Med* 126(2):107-115, 1997.

Dragone MA, Karp S: Bleeding disorders. In Jackson PL, Vessey JA, editors: *Primary care of the child with a chronic condition,* ed 2, St Louis, 1996, Mosby.

Ebb DH, Weinstein HJ: Diagnosis and treatment of childhood acute myelogenous leukemia, *Pediatr Clin North Am* 4(4):847-862, 1997.

Friebert S, Shurin SB: ALL: diagnosis and outlook, *Contemp Pediatr* 15(2):118-136, 1998.

Gribbons D, Zahr LK, Opas SR: Nursing management of children with sickle cell disease: an update, *J Pediatr Nurs* 10(4):232-242, 1995.

Griffin TC, McIntire D, Buchanan GR: High-dose intravenous methylprednisolone therapy for pain in children and adolescents with sickle cell disease, *N Engl J Med* 330(11):733-737, 1994.

Guyer B et al: Annual summary of vital statistics—1998, *Pediatrics* 104(6):1229-1245, 1999.

Hess G, Walson P: Seizures secondary to oral viscous lidocaine, *Ann Emerg Med* 17:725-727, 1988.

Hilgartner MW, Corrigan JJ: Coagulation disorders. In Miller DR, Baehner RL, editors: *Blood diseases of infancy and childhood,* ed 7, St Louis, 1995, Mosby.

Hudson MM, Donaldson SS: Hodgkin's disease, *Pediatr Clin North Am* 44(4):891-904, 1997.

Jayabose S et al: Clinical and hematologic effects of hydroxyurea in children with sickle cell anemia, *J Pediatr* 129(4):559-565, 1996.

Khoury H, Grimsley E: Oxygen inhalation in nonhypoxic sickle cell patients during vaso-occlusive crisis, *Blood* 86(10):3998, 1995.

Kline MW et al: Characteristics of children surviving to 5 years of age or older with vertically acquired HIV infection, *Pediatr AIDS HIV Infect Fetus Adolesc* 6(6):350-353, 1995.

Lane PA: Sickle cell disease, *Pediatr Hematol* 43(3):639-664, 1996.

Lozoff B et al: Poorer behavioral and developmental outcome more than 10 years after treatment for iron deficiency in infancy, *Pediatrics* 105(4; part 1 of 2):852, 2000.

Lubin NLC: Blood groups and blood component transfusion. In Miller DR, Baehner RL, editors: *Blood diseases of infancy and childhood,* ed 7, St Louis, 1995, Mosby.

Luzuriaga K, Sullivan JL: Prevention and treatment of pediatric HIV infection, *JAMA* 280(1):17-18, 1998.

Margolin JF, Poplack DG: Acute lymphoblastic leukemia. In Pizzo PA, Poplack DG: *Principles and practice of pediatric oncology,* ed 3, Philadelphia, 1997, JB Lippincott.

Medical and Scientific Advisory Committee of the National Hemophilia Foundation: *MASAC recommendations concerning prophylaxis,* Medical Bulletin 193, New York, 1994, The Foundation.

Mentzer WD: Bone marrow transplantation for hemoglobinopathies, *Curr Opin Hematol* 7:95-100, 2000.

Miller DR: Erythropoiesis, hypoplastic anemias, and disorders of heme synthesis. In Miller DR, Baehner RL, editors: *Blood diseases of infancy and childhood,* ed 7, St Louis, 1995, Mosby.

National Hemophilia Foundation and American Red Cross: *Hemophilia sports and exercise,* New York, 1996, National Hemophilia Foundation.

Nilsson IM et al: Prophylactic treatment of severe hemophilia A and B can prevent joint disability, *Semin Hematol* 31(2, suppl 12):5-9, 1994.

Pappas DE, Cheng TL: Iron deficiency anemia, *Pediatr Rev* 19(9):321-322, 1998.

Pegelow CH et al: Risk of recurrent stroke in patients with sickle cell disease treated with erythrocyte transfusions, *J Pediatr* 126(6):896-899, 1995.

Platt OS, Guinan EC: Bone Marrow tranplantation in sickle cell anemia: the dilemma of choice, *N Eng J Med* 335(6):426-427, 1996.

Pui C: Acute lymphoblastic leukemia, *Pediatr Clin North Am* 44(4):831-846, 1997.

Sanders TE: Bone marrow transplantation for pediatric malignancies, *Pediatr Clin North Am* 44(4):1005-1018, 1997.

Shad A, Magrath I: Non-Hodgkin's lymphoma, *Pediatr Clin North Am* 44(4):863-890, 1997.

Shapiro BS: Management of painful episodes in sickle cell disease. In Schecter NL, Berde CB, Yaster M, editors: *Pain in infants, children, and adolescents,* Baltimore, 1993, Williams & Wilkins.

Sickle Cell Disease Guideline Panel: *Sickle cell disease: screening, diagnosis, management, and counseling in newborns and infants,* No 93-0562, Rockville, MD, 1993, Agency for Health Care Policy and Research.

Takaue Y et al: Collection and transplantation of peripheral blood stem cells in very small children weighing 20 kg or less, *Blood* 86(1):372-380, 1995.

Tonato M, Roila F, Del Favero A: Are there differences among the serotonin antagonists? *Support Care Cancer* 2(5):293-296, 1994.

Turner BJ et al: A population-based comparison of the clinical course of children and adults with AIDS, *AIDS 1995* 9(1):65-72, 1995.

UNAIDS: *Report on the global HIV/AIDS epidemic,* Geneva, Switzerland, 2000, UNAIDS.

van den Berg HM et al: Hemophilia prophylaxis in the Netherlands, *Semin Hematol* 31(2, suppl 2):13-15, 1994.

Varadi G et al: Human umbilical cord blood for hematopoietic progenitor cells transplantation, *Leuk Lymphoma* 20(12):51-58, 1995.

Wagner JE et al: Allogeneic sibling umbilical-cord-blood transplantation in children with malignant and nonmalignant disease, *Lancet* 346:214-219, 1995.

Walters MC: Bone marrow transplantation for sickle cell disease: Where do we go from here? *J Pediatr Hematol/Oncol* 21(6):467-474, 1999.

Walters MC et al: Impact of bone marrow transplantation for symptomatic sickle cell disease: an interim report, *Blood* 95(6):1918-1924, 2000.

Ware RE, Steinberg MH, Kinney TR: An alternative to transfusion therapy for stroke in sickle cell anemia, *Am J Pediatr Hematol Oncol* 50:140-143, 1995.

CHAPTER 50 Genitourinary Dysfunction

http://www.harcourthealth.com/MERLIN/Wong/maternal/

Learning Objectives

On completion of this chapter the reader will be able to:

- Describe the various factors that contribute to urinary tract infections in infants and children.
- Discuss the preoperative preparation of the child and parents when the child has a structural defect of the genitourinary tract.
- Demonstrate an understanding of the causes and mechanisms of edema formation in nephrotic syndrome.
- Compare the child with minimal-change nephrotic syndrome and the child with acute glomerulonephritis in terms of clinical manifestations and nursing care.
- Contrast the causes, complications, and management of acute and chronic renal failure.
- List the types of renal dialysis.
- Recognize signs of kidney transplant rejection.

GENITOURINARY DYSFUNCTION

Assessment of Renal Function

Assessment of kidney and urinary tract integrity and diagnosis of renal or urinary tract disease are based on several evaluative tools. Physical examination, history taking, and observation of symptoms are the initial procedures. In suspected urinary tract diseases or disorders, further assessment by laboratory, radiologic, and other evaluative methods is carried out.

Clinical Manifestations. As in most disorders of childhood, the incidence and type of kidney or urinary tract dysfunction changes with the age and maturation of the child. In addition, the presenting complaints and the significance of these complaints varies with maturation. For example, a complaint of enuresis has greater significance at 8 years of age than at 4 years of age. In the newborn, urinary tract disorders are associated with a number of obvious malformations of other body systems, including the curious and unexplained but common association between malformed or low-set ears and urinary tract anomalies.

Many of the clinical manifestations of renal disease are common to a variety of childhood disorders, but their presence is an indication to obtain further information from the past history, family history, and laboratory studies as part of a complete physical examination. Suspected renal disease can be further evaluated by means of radiographic studies and renal biopsy (Table 50-1).

Laboratory Tests. Both urine and blood studies contribute vital information for detection of renal problems. The single most important test is probably routine urinalysis. Specific urine and blood tests provide additional information. Because nurses are usually the persons who collect the specimens for examination, and also often perform many of the screening tests, they should be familiar with the test, its function, and the factors that can alter or distort the results of the test. The major urine and blood tests are outlined in Tables 50-2 and 50-3.

Nursing Care Management. Nursing responsibilities in assessment of genitourinary disorders and/or diseases begin with observation of the child for any manifestations that might indicate dysfunction. Many conditions have specific characteristics that distinguish them from other disorders. These are discussed as appropriate throughout the chapter.

The nurse is generally the person who is responsible for preparing infants, children, and parents for tests and for collection of urine and (sometimes) blood specimens for observation and laboratory analysis (see Preparation for Procedures, Chapter 45 and Collection of Specimens, Chapter 45). An important nursing responsibility is to maintain careful *intake and output* and *blood pressure measurements* on children with genitourinary dysfunction and also those who might be at risk for developing renal complications (e.g., children in shock and postoperative patients). For example, any significant degree of renal disease can diminish the glomerular filtration rate, a measure of the amount of plasma from which a given substance is totally cleared in 1 minute. A number of substances can be used, but the most useful clinical estimation of glomerular filtration is the clearance of *creatinine,* an end product of protein metabolism

TABLE 50-1
Radiologic and Other Tests of Urinary System Function

Test	Procedure	Purpose	Comments and Nursing Responsibilities
Intravenous pyelography (IVP) (intravenous urogram; excretory urogram)	Intravenous injection of a contrast medium Medium secreted and concentrated by tubules X-ray films made 5, 10, and 15 minutes after injection; delayed films (30, 60 minutes, etc.) are obtained if obstruction suspected	Defines urinary tract Provides information about integrity of kidneys, ureters, and bladder Retroperitoneal masses visualized when they shift position of ureters	Preparation for test: Infants younger than 2 years old—no solid food, omit one bottle on morning of examination; studies should be performed early to avoid withholding of fluids Children aged 2-14 years—give cathartic evening before examination, nothing orally after midnight,* enema (Fleet [See Nursing Alert, p. 1183] or soapsuds) morning of examination
Retrograde pyelography	Contrast medium injected through ureteral catheter	Visualizes pelvic calyces, ureters, and bladder	Prepare the child for cystoscopy
Renal angiography	Contrast medium injected directly into renal artery via catheter placed in femoral artery (or umbilical artery in newborn) and advanced to renal artery	Visualizes renal vascular system, especially for renal arterial stenosis	Give cathartic if ordered Give preoperative medication if ordered Observe for reaction to contrast medium Monitor vital signs following procedure
Radioisotope imaging studies	Contrast medium injected intravenously; computer analysis to measure uptake or washout (excretion) for analysis of organ function	**DTPA** radioisotope used to measure glomerular filtration rate; estimate of differential renal function and renal washout to determine presence and location of upper urinary tract obstruction **DMSA** radioisotope allows visualization of renal scars and differential renal function; ureters and bladder are not visualized **MAG 3** radioisotope combines features of DTPA (evaluation of upper urinary tract obstruction) with features of DMSA radioisotope (differential renal function)	Insert or assist with insertion of intravenous infusion Monitor intravenous infusion Urethral catheterization may accompany DTPA radioisotope scan; prepare child for catheterization when indicated
Voiding cystourethrography	Contrast medium injected into bladder through urethral catheter until bladder is full; films taken before, during, and after voiding	Visualizes bladder outline and urethra, reveals reflux of urine into ureters, and shows complications of bladder emptying	Prepare child for catheterization
Radionuclide (nuclear) cystogram	Radionuclide-containing fluid injected through urethral catheter until bladder is full; images generated before, during, and after voiding	Alternative to voiding cystourethrography in children with allergy to intravesical contrast material Allows evaluation of reflux, although visualization of anatomic details is relatively poor	Prepare child for catheterization Reassure patient and parents that allergic response to contrast materials is avoided by use of radionuclide

*Current research supports oral intake of clear fluids up to 2 hours before test.

Continued

TABLE 50-1
Radiologic and Other Tests of Urinary System Function—cont'd

Test	Procedure	Purpose	Comments and Nursing Responsibilities
Scout film	Flat plate roentgenogram of abdomen and pelvis for kidney, ureters, bladder (KUB)	Detects and establishes renal outlines, presence of calculi, or opaque foreign bodies in bladder	Prepare as for routine x-ray film
Cystoscopy	Direct visualization of bladder and lower urinary tract through small scope inserted via urethra	Investigation of bladder and lower tract lesions; visualizes ureteral openings, bladder wall, trigone, and urethra	Give nothing orally after midnight* Carry out preoperative preparations
Renal biopsy	Removal of kidney tissue by open or percutaneous technique for study by light, electron, or immunofluorescent microscopy	Yields histologic and microscopic information about glomeruli and tubules; helps to distinguish between types of nephrotic syndromes Distinguishes other renal disorders	Give nothing orally 4-6 hours before test* Premedicate as ordered Prepare setup for procedure Assist with procedure Take vital signs Apply pressure to area with pressure dressing and, if feasible, a sandbag Bed rest for 24 hours Observe for abdominal pain, tenderness Monitor input and output; surgical incision may be required in infants
Renal/bladder ultrasound	Transmission of ultrasonic waves through renal parenchyma, along ureteral course, and over bladder	Allows visualization of renal parenchyma, renal pelvis without exposure to external beam radiation or radioactive isotopes Visualization of dilated ureters and bladder wall also possible	Noninvasive procedure
Testicular (scrotal) ultrasound	Transmission of ultrasonic waves through scrotal contents and testis	Allows visualization of scrotal contents, including testis Testicular ultrasound is used to identify masses, and Doppler-enhanced ultrasound is used to differentiate hyperemia of epididymo-orchitis from ischemia of torsion	Noninvasive procedure
Computed tomography (CT)	Narrow-beam x-rays and computer analysis provide precise reconstruction of area	Visualizes vertical or horizontal cross section of kidney Especially valuable to distinguish tumors and cysts	Noncontrast scan is noninvasive Contrast-enhanced CT scan preparation is similar to intravenous pyelogram (IVP) preparation
Urine culture and sensitivity	Collection of sterile specimen	Determines presence of pathogens and the drugs to which they are sensitive	Does not require specific parental permission Send specimen to laboratory immediately after collection Catherization, clean-catch, or suprapubic specimen

*Current research supports oral intake of clear fluids up to 2 hours before test.

TABLE 50-1
Radiologic and Other Tests of Urinary System Function—cont'd

Test	Procedure	Purpose	Comments and Nursing Responsibilities
Urodynamics	Set of tests designed to measure bladder filling, storage, and evacuation functions **Uroflowmetry** is a test to determine efficiency of urination **Cystometrogram** is a graphic comparison of bladder pressure as a function of volume **Sphincter electromyogram** (EMG) is a test of pelvic muscle function during bladder filling and evacuation **Voiding pressure study** is a comparison of detrusor contraction pressure, sphincter EMG, and urinary flow	Determine characteristics of voiding dysfunction Used to identify type (cause) of incontinence or urinary retention Especially valuable for voiding dysfunction complicated by urinary infection, urinary retention, or neurogenic bladder dysfunction	Prepare child for catheterization Insertion of a rectal tube will produce feelings of rectal fullness or pressure Insertion of needles may be required for sphincter EMG
Whitaker perfusion test	Injection of contrast material through renal pelvis and ureters Pressures are measured in renal pelvis and urinary bladder	Determines presence of obstruction causing upper urinary tract dilation	Prepare child for insertion of a spinal needle or perfusion catheter in renal pelvis (anesthesia often required)

in muscle and a substance that is freely filtered by the glomerulus and secreted by renal tubular cells. The nurse's responsibility in this test is collection of urine, usually a 12- or 24-hour specimen.

GENITOURINARY TRACT DISORDERS/DEFECTS

Urinary Tract Infection (UTI)

Infection of the genitourinary tract is one of the most common conditions of childhood. UTI may involve the urethra; bladder (lower urinary tract); and/or the ureters, renal pelvis, calyces, and renal parenchyma (upper urinary tract). Because it is often impossible to localize the infection, the broad designation UTI is applied to the presence of significant numbers of microorganisms anywhere within the urinary tract, except the distal one third of the urethra, which is usually colonized with bacteria. The peak incidence of UTI not caused by structural anomalies occurs between 2 and 6 years of age, and except for the neonatal period, females have a higher risk for developing UTI. This period coincides with toilet training and establishing voiding habits.

Classification. Infection of the urinary tract may be present with or without clinical symptoms. As a result, the site of infection is often difficult to pinpoint with any degree of accuracy. Various terms used to describe urinary tract disorders include:

Bacteriuria—Presence of bacteria in the urine

Asymptomatic bacteriuria—Significant bacteriuria with no evidence of clinical infection (usually defined as greater than 100,000 colony-forming units [CFUs])

Symptomatic bacteriuria—Bacteriuria accompanied by physical signs of urinary infection (i.e., dysuria, suprapubic discomfort, hematuria, and fever)

Recurrent UTI—Repeated episode of bacteriuria or symptomatic UTI

Persistent UTI—Persistence of bacteriuria despite antibiotic treatment

Febrile UTI—Bacteriuria accompanied by fever and other physical signs of urinary infection; presence of a fever typically implies a pyelonephritis

Cystitis—Inflammation of the bladder

Urethritis—Inflammation of the urethra

Pyelonephritis—Inflammation of the upper urinary tract and kidneys

Urosepsis—Febrile urinary tract infection coexisting with systemic signs of bacterial illness; blood culture reveals presence of urinary pathogen

Etiology. A variety of organisms can be responsible for UTI. *Escherichia coli* (80% of cases) and other gram-negative enteric organisms are most commonly implicated; these organisms are usually found in the anal and perineal region. Other organisms associated with UTI include *Proteus, Pseudomonas, Klebsiella, Staphylococcus aureus, Haemophilus,* and coagulase-negative *Staphylococcus.* Several factors contribute to the development of UTI in childhood.

Anatomic and Physical Factors. The structure of the lower urinary tract is believed to account for the increased incidence of bacteriuria in females. The short urethra, which measures about 2 cm (¾ inch) in young girls and 4 cm (1½ inches) in mature women, provides a ready pathway for invasion of organisms. In addition, the closure of the urethra at the end of

TABLE 50-2
Urine Tests of Renal Function

Test	Normal Range	Deviations	Significance of Deviations
PHYSICAL TESTS			
Volume	Age related	Polyuria	Osmotic factors (urinary glucose level in diabetes mellitus)
		Oliguria	Retention caused by obstructive disease
			Inadequate bladder emptying caused by neurogenic bladder or obstructive disorder
		Anuria	Obstruction of urinary tract; acute renal failure
Specific gravity	With normal fluid intake: 1.016-1.022	High	Dehydration
			Presence of protein or glucose
	Newborn: 1.001-1.020		Presence of radiopaque contrast medium after radiologic examinations
	Others: 1.001-1.030	Low	Excessive fluid intake
			Distal tubular dysfunction
			Insufficient antidiuretic hormone
			Diuresis
Osmolality	Newborn: 50-600 mOsm/L	Fixed at 1.010	Chronic glomerular disease
	Thereafter: 50-1400 mOsm/L	High or low	Same as for specific gravity
			More sensitive index than specific gravity
Appearance	Clear pale yellow to deep gold	Cloudy	Contains sediment
		Cloudy reddish pink to reddish brown	Blood from trauma or disease
			Myoglobin after severe muscle destruction
		Light	Dilute
		Dark	Concentrated
		Red	Trauma
CHEMICAL TESTS			
pH	Newborn: 5-7	Weak acid or neutral	If associated with metabolic acidosis, suggests tubular acidosis
	Thereafter: 4.8-7.8		If associated with metabolic alkalosis, suggests potassium deficiency
	Average: 6		Urinary tract infection
		Alkaline	Metabolic alkalosis
Protein level	Absent	Present	Abnormal glomerular permeability (e.g., glomerular disease, changes in blood pressure)
			Most kidney disease
			Orthostatic in some individuals
Glucose level	Absent	Present	Diabetes mellitus
			Infusion of concentrated glucose-containing fluids
			Glomerulonephritis
			Impaired tubular reabsorption
Ketone levels	Absent	Present	Conditions of acute metabolic demand (stress)
			Diabetic ketoacidosis
Leukocyte esterase	Absent	Present	Can identify both lysed and intact white blood cells via enzyme detection
Nitrites	Absent	Present	Most species of bacteria convert nitrates to nitrites in the urine

TABLE 50-2
Urine Tests of Renal Function—cont'd

Test	Normal Range	Deviations	Significance of Deviations
MICROSCOPIC TESTS			
White blood cell count	Less than 1 or 2	More than 5 polymorphonuclear leukocytes/field	Urinary tract inflammatory process
		Lymphocytes	Allograft rejection Malignancy
Red blood cell count	Less than 1 or 2	4-6/field in centrifuged specimen	Trauma Stones Glomerular injury Infection Neoplasms
Presence of bacteria	Absent to a few	More than 100,000 organisms/ml in centrifuged specimen	Urinary tract infection
Presence of casts	Occasional	Granular casts	Tubular or glomerular disorders Degenerative process in advanced renal disease
		Cellular casts	Pyelonephritis
		White blood cell	Glomerulonephritis
		Red blood cell	Proteinuria; usually transient
		Hyaline casts	

TABLE 50-3
Blood Tests of Renal Function

Test	Normal Range (mg/dl)	Deviations	Significance of Deviations
Blood urea nitrogen (BUN)	Newborn: 4-18 Infant, child: 5-18	Elevated	Renal disease—acute or chronic (the higher the BUN, the more severe the disease) Increased protein catabolism Dehydration Hemorrhage High protein intake Corticosteroid therapy
Uric acid	Child: 2.0-5.5	Increased	Severe renal disease
Creatinine	Infant: 0.2-0.4 Child: 0.3-0.7 Adolescent: 0.5-1.0	Increased	Severe renal impairment

micturition may return contaminated bacteria to the bladder. The longer urethra (as long as 20 cm [8 inches] in an adult) and the antibacterial properties of prostatic secretions inhibit the entry and growth of pathogens in the male.

Considerable evidence suggests there are fewer UTIs among circumcised male infants than among uncircumcised male infants, but the difference is not significant enough to recommend routine circumcision in newborns (American Academy of Pediatrics, 1999).

The single most important host factor influencing the occurrence of UTI is *urinary stasis.* Ordinarily urine is sterile, but at 37° C (98.6° F) it provides an excellent culture medium. Under normal conditions the act of completely and repeatedly emptying the bladder flushes away any organisms before they have an opportunity to multiply and invade surrounding tissue. However, urine that remains in the bladder allows bacteria from the urethra to rapidly become established in the rich medium. Incomplete bladder emptying (stasis) may result from *reflux* (see Vesicoureteral Reflux), anatomic abnormalities (especially those involving the ureters), dysfunction of the voiding mechanism, or extrinsic ureteral or bladder compression that may be caused by constipation. The key to preventing UTI is to maintain adequate blood supply to the bladder wall by avoidance of overdistention and high bladder pressure.

Altered Urine and Bladder Chemistry. Several mechanical and chemical characteristics of the urine and bladder mucosa help maintain urinary sterility. An increased fluid intake promotes flushing of the normal bladder and lowers the concentration of organisms in the infected bladder. Diuresis also seems to enhance the antibacterial properties of the renal medulla.

Most pathogens favor an alkaline medium. Normally, urine is slightly acidic. A urine pH of about 5 hampers bacterial multiplication, although acidification rarely eliminates bacteriuria. Much has been reported about the use of cranberry juice for the prevention of UTI. This mechanism was initially thought to result from increased urine acidity. In a study of elderly women done by Fleet (1994), cranberry juice did not lower the pH of urine when compared with the placebo group; however, later studies found substances in cranberries that prevent adherence of bacteria to the mucosal surfaces of the urinary tract (Kuzminski, 1996). For children unwilling to drink cranberry juice, dried cranberries may be offered.

Diagnostic Evaluation. The clinical manifestations of UTI depend on the age of the child (Box 50-1). Diagnosis of UTI is confirmed by detection of bacteriuria in urine culture, but urine collection is often difficult, especially in infants and very small children. Several factors may alter a urine specimen, and contamination of a specimen by organisms from sources other than the urine, such as perineal and perianal flora in bag specimens, is the most common cause of false-positive results. Unless the specimen is a first morning sample, a recent high fluid intake may indicate a falsely low organism count. Therefore children should not be encouraged to drink large volumes of water in an attempt to obtain a specimen quickly.

Box 50-1

Signs and Symptoms of Urinary Tract Disorders or Disease at Different Ages

NEONATAL PERIOD (BIRTH TO 1 MONTH)
- Poor feeding
- Vomiting
- Failure to gain weight
- Rapid respiration (acidosis)
- Respiratory distress
- Spontaneous pneumothorax or pneumomediastinum
- Frequent urination
- Screaming on urination
- Poor urine stream
- Jaundice
- Seizures
- Dehydration
- Other anomalies or stigmata
- Enlarged kidneys or bladder

INFANCY (1 TO 24 MONTHS)
- Poor feeding
- Vomiting
- Failure to gain weight
- Excessive thirst
- Frequent urination
- Straining or screaming on urination
- Foul-smelling urine
- Pallor
- Fever
- Persistent diaper rash
- Seizures (with or without fever)
- Dehydration
- Enlarged kidneys or bladder

CHILDHOOD (2 TO 14 YEARS)
- Poor appetite
- Vomiting
- Growth failure
- Excessive thirst
- Enuresis, incontinence, frequent urination
- Painful urination
- Swelling of face
- Seizures
- Pallor
- Fatigue
- Blood in urine
- Abdominal or back pain
- Edema
- Hypertension
- Tetany

More accurate estimates of bacterial content are obtained from *suprapubic aspiration* (in children younger than 2 years of age) and properly performed bladder catheterization (as long as the first few milliliters are excluded from collection). The specimen should be taken directly to the laboratory for immediate culture.

Tests to detect bacteriuria are being used with increased frequency in screening for UTI. The dipstick tests that test for leukocyte esterase or nitrite are quick and inexpensive methods for detecting infection before obtaining final culture results.

Localization of the infection site may involve more specific tests, including percutaneous kidney taps and bladder washout procedures. Other tests such as ultrasonography, voiding cystourethrogram (VCUG), intravenous pyelogram (IVP), and DMSA (dimercaptosuccinic acid) scan may be performed after the infection subsides to identify anatomic abnormalities contributing to the development of infection and kidney changes resulting from recurrent infection.

Therapeutic Management. The objectives of treatment of children with UTI are (1) to eliminate current infection, (2) to identify contributing factors to reduce the risk of recurrence, (3) to prevent systemic spread of the infection, and (4) to preserve renal function. Antibiotic therapy should be initiated on the basis of identification of the pathogen, the child's history of antibiotic use, and the location of the infection. A variety of antimicrobial drugs are available for treating UTI, but all of them can occasionally be ineffective because of resistance of organisms. Common antiinfective agents used for UTI include the penicillins, sulfonamide (including trimethoprim and sulfisoxazole in combination), the cephalosporins, and nitrofurantoin.

If anatomic defects such as primary reflux or bladder neck obstruction are present, surgical correction of these abnormalities may be necessary to prevent recurrent infection. Follow-up study is an important component of medical management because the relapse rate is high and infection tends to recur 1 to 2 months after termination of treatment. The aim of therapy and careful follow-up is to reduce the chance of renal scarring; however, recurrent infection of the urinary bladder predisposes the individual to transient episodes of vesicoureteral reflux.

Vesicoureteral Reflux (VUR). VUR refers to the abnormal retrograde flow of bladder urine into the ureters. During voiding, urine is swept up the ureters and then flows back into the empty bladder, where it acts as a reservoir for bacterial growth until the next voiding. *Primary reflux* results from congenitally abnormal insertion of ureters into the bladder; *secondary reflux* occurs as a result of an acquired condition.

It is not clear that reflux necessarily causes infections. What is clear is that reflux is more likely to be associated with recurring kidney infections than with simple bladder infections (cystitis). In the presence of reflux, infected urine (bacteria) from the bladder has access to the kidney, resulting in kidney infections (pyelonephritis). These children are usually very symptomatic with high fevers, vomiting, and chills. Reflux when associated with UTI is the most common cause of renal scarring in children. Renal scarring may occur with the first episode of febrile UTI. Reflux in the presence of sterile urine does not cause renal damage; therefore the most important concept in managing VUR is preventing bacteria from reaching the kidneys. VUR is managed conservatively with daily low-dose antibiotic therapy. A urine culture should be done every 2 to 3 months and any time the child has a fever. This method of management requires a motivated, reliable, and cooperative family. Many children will outgrow the reflux over a period of years. An annual voiding cystourethrogram is done to assess the status of the reflux.

Indications for surgical intervention include significant anatomic abnormality at the ureterovesical junction, recurrent UTIs, severe forms of VUR, noncompliance with medical therapy, intolerance to antibiotics, and VUR after puberty in females.

Prognosis. With prompt and adequate treatment at the time of diagnosis, the long-term prognosis for UTI is usually excellent. However, the hazard of progressive renal injury is greatest when infection occurs in young children (especially under 2 years of age) and is associated with congenital renal malformations and reflux. Therefore early diagnosis of children at risk is particularly important during infancy and toddlerhood.

Nursing Care Management

➤ Assessment

Nurses should instruct parents to observe regularly for clues suggesting UTI. Unfortunately, the signs of UTI are not as evident as those of upper respiratory tract infection. Therefore many cases go undetected because no one thought to investigate this very common problem.

NURSE ALERT • A child who exhibits the following should be evaluated for UTI:
- Incontinence in a toilet-trained child
- Strong-smelling urine
- Frequency and/or urgency

Because infants and young children are unable to express their feelings and sensations verbally, it is difficult to detect discomfort they may be experiencing from dysuria. A careful history regarding voiding habits, stooling pattern, and episodes of unexplained irritability may assist in detecting less obvious cases of UTI. Consequently, parents should be cautioned to observe for specific clues of UTI in suspected cases.

➤ Nursing Diagnoses

A number of nursing diagnoses become evident following a thorough assessment. These diagnoses include but are not limited to the following:
- Risk for injury related to possibility of kidney damage from chronic infection
- Anxiety related to unfamiliar procedures
- Altered family processes related to illness of a child

➤ Plan of Care and Implementation

The goals of care for the child with UTI and the family are as follows:
1. Child and family will be prepared properly for needed tests and procedures.
2. Parents and child will receive appropriate education regarding prevention and treatment of infection.

When infection is suspected, collecting an appropriate specimen is essential. It is the nurse's responsibility to take every precaution to obtain acceptable clean-voided specimens to avoid the use of other collecting procedures except when absolutely indicated. Because of the unreliability of a specimen obtained via a urine collection bag, suprapubic aspiration of urine or sterile catheterization should be done in the infant or young child who presents with fever.

Commonly, additional tests are performed to detect anatomic defects. Children are prepared for these tests as appropriate for their age. This includes an explanation of the procedure, its purpose, and what the children will experience (see Preparation for Procedures, Chapter 45). Sometimes a simple description of the urinary system is helpful. Especially for preschool children, the nurse must clarify that the urinary tract is separate from any sexual function and that the test is for a problem that they did not cause. Children may associate blame for perceived wrongdoing (e.g., masturbation) or unacceptable thoughts with the reason for the illness or the tests. For children under 3 to 4 years of age, the procedure can be explained on a doll. For those who are older, a simple drawing of the bladder, urethra, ureters, and kidneys makes the explanation more understandable.

Handling actual equipment when feasible can be helpful in allaying anxiety in children of all ages. Anticipatory instruction on distraction techniques such as deep breathing, storytelling, and imagery may help the child relax and be more cooperative during the actual procedures. If surgery is indicated, the child will be able to encounter the impending procedure with facts and understanding of the procedure that will help to decrease his or her fear and anxiety concerning more extensive medical-surgical intervention.

Because antibacterial drugs are indicated in UTI, the nurse advises parents of proper dosage and administration. When antiseptics such as nitrofurantoin are used for prolonged therapy to maintain urine sterility, parents need an explanation of the drug's continued necessity when no signs of infection are present.* For all children an adequate or increased fluid intake is encouraged.

Prevention. Prevention is the most important goal in both primary and recurrent infection, and most preventive measures are simple hygienic habits that should be a routine part of daily care (Guidelines box). For example, parents are taught to cleanse their infant's genital areas from front to back to avoid contaminating the urethral area with fecal organisms. Female children are taught to wipe from front to back after voiding or defecating. Children should void as soon as they feel the urge (Critical Thinking box).

Sexually active adolescent females are advised to urinate as soon as possible after they have intercourse to flush out bacteria introduced during the activity. Children who have recurrent UTIs or neurogenic bladder are commonly maintained on daily low-dose antibiotics. The nurse should reinforce the importance of compliance to parents and older children.

➤ Evaluation

The effectiveness of nursing interventions is determined by continual reassessment and evaluation of care on the basis of the following observational guidelines and expected outcomes:
1. Question children and families regarding their understanding of the disease and the diagnostic measures re-

*Community and home care instructions for giving medications to children and collecting a urine sample are available in Wong DL, Hess CS: ***Wong and Whaley's clinical manual of pediatric nursing,*** ed 5, St Louis, 2000, Mosby.

Guidelines

PREVENTION OF URINARY TRACT INFECTION

Factors Predisposing to Development	Measures of Prevention
Short female urethra close to vagina and anus	Perineal hygiene: wipe from front to back. Avoid tight clothing or diapers; wear cotton panties rather than nylon. Check for vaginitis or pinworms, especially if child scratches between legs.
Incomplete emptying (reflux) and overdistention of bladder	Avoid "holding" urine; encourage child to void frequently, especially before long trip or other circumstances where toilet facilities are not available. Empty bladder completely with each void. Have the child "double void" (void, wait a few minutes and void again). Severe cases may require clean, intermittent catheterization or biofeedback instruction. Avoid straining during defecation and avoid constipation.
Concentrated urine	Encourage generous fluid intake.

quired for identifying the presence of infection or physical abnormalities.

2. Observe and interview family and child regarding preventive practices and observe laboratory reports of urinalyses and cultures for evidence of treatment efficacy.

Expected outcomes include the following:

1. Child and family demonstrate an understanding of the illness and diagnostic tests (specify knowledge and means of demonstration).
2. Child and family demonstrate an understanding of preventive practices (specify means of demonstration).

(See Nursing Care Plan: The Child with Urinary Tract Infection.*)

Critical Thinking

URINARY TRACT INFECTION AND CONSTIPATION

During your assessment of Ginger, a 4-year-old admitted to the hospital for a severe urinary tract infection (UTI), her mother tells you that Ginger has bowel movements every third to fourth day. They are usually large, hard-formed stools, and Ginger sometimes has trouble evacuating the stool. What should you do?

First, Think About It . . .

- What assumptions are you making?
- If you accept the conclusions, what are the implications?

1. Explain to the mother that this may be normal for Ginger, because her mother has the same pattern and Ginger will have less trouble as she gets older.
2. Explain to the mother the relationship of diet to constipation as you develop a line of inquiry to elicit the fat content of Ginger's diet.
3. Explain to the mother that the diarrhea associated with the antibiotics Ginger is now receiving should correct the constipation.
4. Explain to the mother the relationship between chronic constipation and UTI as you move into a complete elimination history.

The best response is 4. Although Ginger may have an elimination pattern similar to her mother's, 3 to 4 days is a long interval between stools, even for an adult. In this instance the presence of a large stool mass within the colon is likely to cause pressure on the bladder and urethra and not allow the bladder to empty completely. The implications of stasis of urine within the bladder can then lead to infection. Although a diet and fluid intake history is part of the assessment of children with UTI and constipation, the fat content of Ginger's diet is not the most critical information at this time. Finally, Ginger may or may not develop diarrhea secondary to her antibiotic regimen. However, one bout of diarrhea will not eliminate the constipation, which has been present over a long period of time.

Obstructive Uropathy

Structural or functional abnormalities of the urinary system that obstruct the normal flow of urine can produce renal disorders. When there is interference with urine flow, the backup of urine above the obstruction causes *hydronephrosis* (dilation of the renal pelvis from distention) with eventual pressure destruction leading to renal parenchyma, although the dilating ureters form a reservoir that reduces the effect on the kidneys for a long time.

Obstruction may be congenital or acquired, unilateral or bilateral, complete or incomplete, and the manifestations may be acute or chronic. The obstruction can occur at any level of the upper or lower urinary tract (Fig. 50-1). Partial obstruction may not be symptomatic unless there is a water or solute diuresis. Boys are affected more commonly than girls, and malformations should be suspected when patients have some other congenital defects (e.g., prune belly syndrome, chromosomal anomalies, anorectal malformations, or defects of the pinna of the ear).

Damage to distal nephrons in chronic uropathy alters the ability to concentrate urine, contributing to increased urine flow and metabolic acidosis occurring from decreased excretion of acid secondary to impaired ability of the distal nephron to secrete hydrogen ions. Partial obstruction results in progressive loss of renal function as a result of irreversible damage to the nephrons. Pooled urine serves as a medium for bacterial growth; therefore UTIs further increase the extent of renal damage.

Early diagnosis and surgical correction; or procedures that divert the flow of urine to bypass the obstruction, such as placement of a temporary percutaneous nephrostomy tube or cutaneous ureterostomy, are essential to prevent progressive renal damage. Medical complications of acute or chronic renal failure and/or infection are managed as described for those disorders.

Nursing Care Management. Nursing goals in urinary tract obstruction include helping to identify cases, assisting with diagnostic procedures, and caring for children with complications. Preparing parents and children for procedures is a major nursing responsibility. Preparation for urinary diversion procedures is of special importance (see Preparation for Procedures, Chapter 45).

Parents and children need emotional support and counseling during the lengthy management of these disorders. Many

*In Wong DL, Hess CS: ***Wong and Whaley's clinical manual of pediatric nursing,*** ed 5, St Louis, 2000, Mosby.

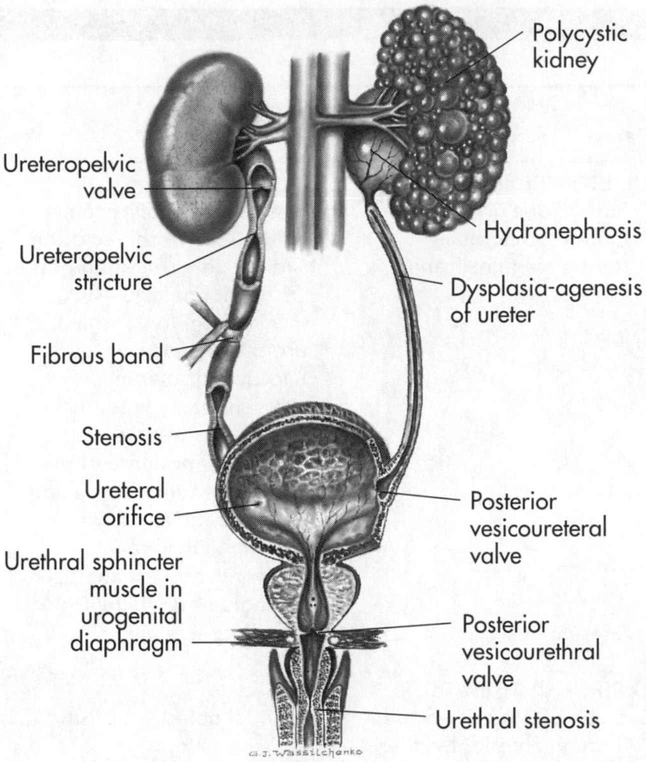

FIG. 50-1 • Major sites of urinary tract obstruction.

children are discharged with ureteral drainage systems in place that must be protected from damage, and the danger of infection is a constant concern. Parents are taught to care for the equipment and to recognize the signs of possible obstruction or infection within the system. Maintaining adequate urine flow is imperative. Fluids should be encouraged. The tube should be observed often for indications of obstruction due to sediment, small blood clots, or kinking. The physician should inspect any drainage from around the tube.

Children with external diversional systems will need psychologic support and guidance, especially as they reach adolescence and body image concerns assume more prominence. Those with progressive renal deterioration may face the prospect of dialysis and/or transplantation and the emotional aspects that accompany these procedures.

External Defects

Defects of the external genitourinary tract are serious conditions primarily because of the psychologic impact on the child. Satisfactory surgical repair is successful for the more common disorders and is carried out or initiated as early as possible. The major anomalies of the lower genitourinary tract, their description, and their management are outlined in Table 50-4.

Psychologic Problems Related to Genital Surgery. Surgery involving sexual organs can be particularly disruptive to children, especially to preschoolers who fear punishment, retaliation, body mutilation, or castration. Some of the problems of hospitalization, separation, and anxiety can be eased by hospital practices that are sensitive to the needs of the child (see Chapter 44).

The body image of a child is largely formed as a result of feedback from the primary caregivers, and parental anxiety regarding an acceptable physical appearance and adequate future sexual competency is readily communicated to the affected child. Therefore children with birth defects are at risk for developing a distorted body image that reflects the caregiver's subtly communicated evaluation of their bodies. The trend toward repair of visible genital defects is based in large part on these psychologic variables. The earlier a repair can be effected, the more likely the possibility that the child will develop a normal body image.

During the years from 3 to 6, the phallic-oedipal period, children show a strong interest and concern about the genital area, sex differences, and genital normality or its lack. It is also a time when children are frightened of what they perceive to be threats to their body and bodily function. They also view any untoward happening as a punishment for real or imagined wrongdoing or unacceptable sexual feelings, such as masturbation, sex play, or erotic feelings. Surgical repair is recommended before these fears and anxieties develop.

After extensive review of the emotional, cognitive, and body-image problems that may occur in children undergoing surgical reconstruction of a genital deformity, it was recommended that surgery be accomplished between the ages of 6 and 15 months to minimize the psychologic effects of surgery and anesthesia (Kass, 1996).

Nursing Care Management. Preparing children and their families for diagnostic and surgical procedures (see Preparation for Procedures, Chapter 45) and for home care are major nursing functions. Most postoperative care involves care of the surgical site. Tub baths are discouraged for 1 week following simple surgeries. The surgical site is kept clean and otherwise protected from infection and is inspected for signs of infection. Dressings, if any, are inspected regularly. More complex surgeries require additional care and observation (e.g., catheter care for urethral reconstruction and care of urinary diversion stomas and collection devices).

Some activities of older children (e.g., pushing, lifting, playing with straddle toys or in sandboxes, swimming, and rough activities) may be restricted for some types of surgical repairs. Precise restrictions depend on the specific type of surgery. Activities of infants and toddlers are not limited.

In most cases the results of surgery are quite satisfactory. However, in some of the more severe defects, such as exstrophy and those that require stomas, additional emotional interventions may be needed. A major concern of parents and children is related to surgery affecting the genitalia. Concerns about penile size, appearance of the genitalia, potential ability to procreate, and rejection by peers (especially the opposite sex) are potential fears that require psychologic adjustment, particularly during adolescence.

GLOMERULAR DISEASE

Nephrotic Syndrome

Nephrotic syndrome is a clinical state that includes massive proteinuria, hypoalbuminemia, hyperlipemia, and edema. The disorder can occur (1) as a primary disease known as *idiopathic nephrosis, childhood nephrosis,* or *minimal-change nephrotic syndrome (MCNS);* (2) as a secondary disorder that occurs as a clinical manifestation after or in association with glomerular

TABLE 50-4
Defects of the Genitourinary Tract

Defect	Therapeutic Management
INGUINAL HERNIA Protrusion of abdominal contents through inguinal canal into scrotum	Detected as painless inguinal swelling of variable size Surgical closure of inguinal defect
HYDROCELE Fluid in scrotum	Surgical repair indicated if spontaneous resolution not accomplished in 1 year
PHIMOSIS Narrowing or stenosis of preputial opening of foreskin	Mild cases: manual retraction of foreskin and proper cleansing of area Severe cases: circumcision or vertical division and transverse suturing of foreskin
HYPOSPADIAS Urethral opening located behind glans penis or anywhere along ventral surface of penile shaft	Objectives of surgical correction: To enable child to void in standing position and direct stream voluntarily in usual manner Improve physical appearance of genitalia Produce a sexually adequate organ
CHORDEE Ventral curvature of penis, often associated with hypospadias	Surgical release of fibrous band causing the deformity
EPISPADIAS Meatal opening located on dorsal surface of penis	Surgical correction, usually including penile and urethral lengthening and bladder neck reconstruction (if necessary)
CRYPTORCHIDISM Failure of one or both testes to descend normally through inguinal canal	Detected by inability to palpate testes within scrotum Medical: administration of human chorionic gonadotropin (older child) Surgical: orchiopexy Objectives of therapy: Prevent damage to undescended testicle Decrease incidence of malignant tumor formation Avoid trauma and torsion Close inguinal canal Prevent cosmetic and psychologic disability from empty scrotum
EXSTROPHY OF BLADDER Eversion of posterior bladder through anterior bladder wall and lower abdominal wall; associated with open pubic arch (a severe defect)	Potential objectives of surgical correction: Preserve renal function Attain urinary control Adequate reconstructive repair Improve sexual function (especially in males)
AMBIGUOUS GENITALIA Types:	Assignment of gender sex
Masculinized female (female pseudohermaphrodite)	Surgical correction if needed; gender assignment—female
Incompletely masculinized male (male pseudohermaphrodite)	Gender assignment—usually female, but controversial
True hermaphrodite (both ovaries and testes)	Gender assignment depends on predominant characteristics
Mixed gonadal dysgenesis	Gender assignment depends on predominant characteristics

damage of known or presumed etiology; or (3) as a congenital form inherited as an autosomal recessive disorder. The disorder is characterized by increased glomerular permeability to plasma protein, which results in massive urinary protein loss. The glomerulus is responsible for the initial step in the formation of urine, and the filtration rate depends on an intact glomerular membrane. This discussion is devoted to MCNS because it constitutes 80% of nephrotic syndrome cases.

Pathophysiology. The onset of MCNS can occur at any age but occurs predominantly in children between 2 and 7 years of age. It is rare in children younger than 6 months of age, uncommon in infants younger than 1 year of age, and unusual after the age of 8. Patients with MCNS are twice as likely to be male.

The pathogenesis of MCNS is not understood. There may be a metabolic, biochemical, physiochemical, or immune-mediated disturbance that causes the basement membrane of the glomeruli to become increasingly permeable to protein, but the cause and mechanisms are only speculative.

The glomerular membrane, normally impermeable to albumin and other proteins, becomes permeable to proteins, especially albumin, which leak through the membrane and are lost in urine *(hyperalbuminemia)*. This reduces the serum albumin level *(hypoalbuminemia)*, decreasing the colloidal osmotic pressure in the capillaries. As a result, the vascular hydrostatic pressure exceeds the pull of the colloidal osmotic pressure, causing fluid to accumulate in the interstitial spaces *(edema)* and body cavities,

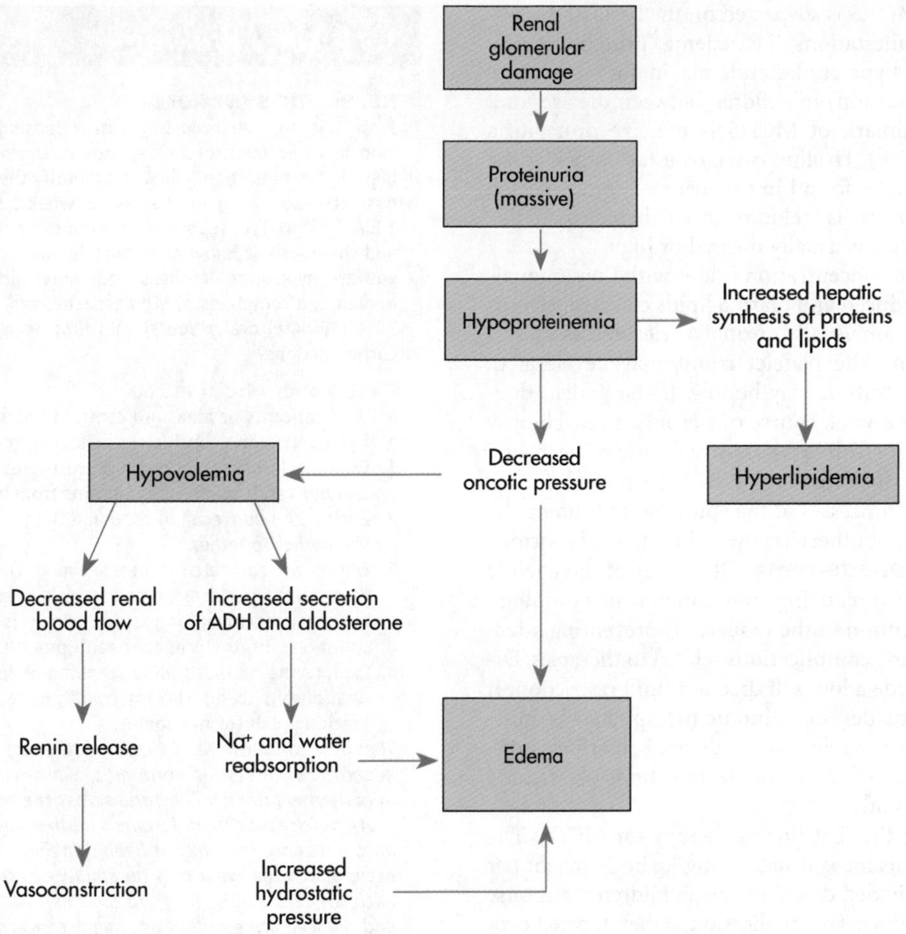

FIG. 50-2 • Sequence of events in nephrotic syndrome.

particularly in the abdominal cavity *(ascites)*. The shift of fluid from the plasma to the interstitial spaces reduces the vascular fluid volume *(hypovolemia)*, which in turn stimulates the renin-angiotensin system and the secretion of antidiuretic hormone and aldosterone. Tubular reabsorption of sodium and water is increased in an attempt to increase intravascular volume. The elevation of serum lipids is unexplained. The sequence of events in nephrotic syndrome is presented in Fig. 50-2.

Diagnostic Evaluation. The disease is suspected on the basis of clinical manifestations (Box 50-2), especially when weight gain in a previously well child increases slowly over days or weeks. The generalized edema may develop rapidly or gradually but eventually prompts the family to seek medical attention. Parents usually give a history of the child being well but steadily gaining weight and then becoming anorexic, irritable, and less active.

NURSE ALERT • A child who exhibits the following should be evaluated for the possibility of nephrotic syndrome:
- Weight gain over that expected based on previous pattern
- Parent observation that the child's clothes fit tightly
- Decreased urine output
- Pallor, fatigue

Box 50-2

Clinical Manifestations of Nephrotic Syndrome

- Weight gain
- Puffiness of face (facial edema):
  - Especially around the eyes
  - Apparent on arising in the morning
  - Subsides during the day
- Abdominal swelling (ascites)
- Pleural effusion
- Labial or scrotal swelling
- Edema of intestinal mucosal may cause:
  - Diarrhea
  - Anorexia
  - Poor intestinal absorption
- Ankle/leg swelling
- Irritability
- Easily fatigued
- Lethargic
- Blood pressure normal or slightly decreased
- Susceptibility to infection
- Urine alterations:
  - Decreased volume
  - Frothy

The diagnosis of MCNS is suspected on the basis of the history and clinical manifestations (i.e., edema, proteinuria, hypoalbuminemia, and hypercholesterolemia in the absence of hematuria and hypertension) in children between the ages of 2 and 8 years. The hallmark of MCNS is massive proteinuria (>3+ on urine dipstick). Hyaline casts, oval fat bodies, and a few red blood cells can be found in the urine of some affected children, although there is seldom gross hematuria. The glomerular filtration rate is usually normal or high.

Total serum protein concentration is low, with the serum albumin significantly reduced and plasma lipids elevated. Hemoglobin and hematocrit are usually normal or elevated as a result of hemoconcentration. The platelet count may be elevated. Serum sodium concentration may be low. If the patient does not respond to a 4- to 8-week course of steroids, a renal biopsy may be needed to distinguish between other types of nephrotic syndrome. The biopsy of children with MCNS is remarkable for effacement of the foot processes of the epithelial cells lining the basement membrane, but otherwise the kidney tissue is normal.

Therapeutic Management. Objectives of therapeutic management include: (1) reducing excretion of urinary protein, (2) reducing fluid retention in the tissues, (3) preventing infection, and (4) minimizing complications related to therapies. Dietary restrictions include a low-salt diet and fluid restriction. If complications of edema develop, diuretic therapy may be initiated to provide temporary relief from edema. Sometimes infusions of 25% albumin are used. Acute infections are treated with appropriate antibiotics.

Corticosteroids are the first line of therapy for MCNS. The starting dose for prednisone is usually 2 mg/kg body weight per day, in one or more divided doses. In most children a response occurs within 7 to 21 days. The medication is then tapered over a period of several weeks and eventually stopped if the child remains asymptomatic. About two thirds of children with MCNS have a relapse, heralded first by increased urine protein. Relapses can be diagnosed early if parents are taught routine home monitoring of urine protein by dipstick. Relapses are treated with a repeated course of high-dose steroid therapy. Side effects of the steroids include weight gain, rounding of the face, and increased appetite. Long-term therapy may result in hirsutism, growth retardation, cataracts, hypertension, gastrointestinal bleeding, bone demineralization, infection, and hyperglycemia. Children who do not respond to steroid therapy, those who have frequent relapses, and those in whom the side effects threaten their growth and general health may be considered for a course of therapy using other immunosuppressant medications (e.g., cyclophosphamide, chlorambucil, or cyclosporine).

MCNS episodes, both the first episode and relapse, often happen in conjunction with a viral or bacterial infection. Relapses can also be triggered by allergies and immunizations. Relapses in children with MCNS may continue over many years.

Complications of nephrotic syndrome include infection, circulatory insufficiency secondary to hypovolemia, and thromboembolism. Infections that may be seen in children with nephrotic syndrome include peritonitis, cellulitis, and pneumonia; these require prompt recognition and vigorous treatment with appropriate antibiotic therapy (Critical Thinking box).

Prognosis. The prognosis for ultimate recovery in most cases is good. It is a self-limiting disease, and in children who respond to steroid therapy the tendency to relapse decreases with time. With early detection and prompt implementation of therapy to eradicate proteinuria, progressive basement membrane damage is minimized, so that when the tendency to exacerbations is past, renal function is usually normal or near normal. It is estimated that approximately 80% of affected children have this favorable prognosis.

Critical Thinking

NEPHROTIC SYNDROME

Jerome is an 8-year-old boy with relapsing nephrotic syndrome who has become steroid dependent. During your initial assessment in the outpatient clinic you identify the following: (1) weight has increased 2 kg in the last 2 weeks; (2) blood pressure is 100/70; (3) mother reports that Jerome is not urinating very much, and she does not know how much he has been drinking; (4) while you are measuring Jerome's abdominal girth, he guards his abdomen and complains of stomachache; and (5) his temperature is 38°C (100.4°F) orally. You should first do which of the following correct actions?

First, Think About It . . .

- **What concepts or ideas are central to your thinking?**
- **If you accept the conclusions, what are the implications?**

1. **Examine Jerome's abdomen more thoroughly while eliciting a 24-hour recall of illness symptoms from his mother.**
2. **Elicit a 24-hour recall of food and fluid intake from Jerome and his mother together.**
3. **Obtain a clean-catch urine specimen. Divide the specimen so that you can perform a dipstick analysis immediately and retain the other specimen for possible urinalysis and culture after consultation with the primary health practitioner.**
4. **Explore the mother's understanding of Jerome's illness and its relationship to his current condition to begin outlining your teaching plan for this family.**

The best response is 1. One of the complications of severe nephrotic syndrome is peritonitis, which can occur secondary to migration of intestinal bacteria across the bowel wall and into the protein-rich acidic fluid. Jerome's mother has already said that she does not know what he has been drinking. Therefore the idea may occur to you that your only possibility of assessing his intake is to elicit the recall while they are together. Although his weight gain and reduced urine output are major concerns, they are secondary to peritonitis. (It should be recognized that children on strict fluid restrictions are prone to obtain fluids from unauthorized sources.) Obtaining a urine specimen for dipstick analysis is part of the initial assessment for Jerome. Also, you may initially conclude that the fever and abdominal pain are the first priority. As with option 3, the fourth choice must be addressed, along with evaluation of the current stress level in the home, after the implications of fever and pain have been addressed.

Nursing Care Management

➤ Assessment

Continuous monitoring of fluid retention or excretion is an important nursing function. Strict intake and output records are essential but may be difficult to obtain from very young children. Application of collection bags is highly irritating to edematous skin that is subject to breakdown. Application of diapers or weighing wet pads may be necessary.

Other methods of monitoring progress include urine examination for albumin, daily weight, and measurement of abdominal girth. Assessment of edema (e.g., increased or decreased swelling around the eyes and dependent areas, the degree of pitting) and the color and texture of skin are part of nursing care. Vital signs are monitored to detect any early signs of complications such as shock or an infective process.

➤ Nursing Diagnoses

Constant reassessment and evaluation reveal a number of nursing diagnoses that are relevant to the care of these children and their families:

Risk for fluid volume deficit
Altered nutrition
Fluid volume excess
Risk for impaired skin integrity
Activity intolerance
Body image disturbance

➤ Plan of Care and Implementation

The goals of nursing care of the child with nephrotic syndrome and the family are as follows:

1. Child will exhibit no evidence of fluid accumulation.
2. Child will exhibit no evidence of skin breakdown or infection.
3. Child will receive optimum nutrition.
4. Child and family will express feelings and concerns.

Children hospitalized with MCNS may be placed on bed rest during the edema phase of the disease. They seldom offer resistance because they are usually lethargic and easily fatigued, and their cumbersome edematous bulk is not conducive to movement.

Reducing the excretion of urinary protein primarily involves the administration of corticosteroids. Nurses must be aware of the problems associated with these drugs and be alert to complications from their use.

Infection is a constant source of danger to edematous children and to those receiving corticosteroid therapy. These children are particularly vulnerable to upper respiratory infection; therefore they must be kept warm and dry; turned frequently; and protected from contact with infected roommates, visitors, and personnel. Vital signs are monitored to detect any early signs of an infective process.

The loss of appetite that accompanies active nephrosis creates a perplexing problem for nurses. During this time the combined efforts of the nurse, dietitian, parents, and child are needed to formulate a nutritionally adequate and attractive diet. Salt is usually restricted (but not eliminated) during the edema phase, and fluid restriction (if prescribed) is limited to short-term use during massive edema. Every effort should be made to serve attractive meals with preferred foods and a minimum of fuss, but it usually requires a considerable amount of ingenuity and enticement to get the child to eat (see Feeding the Sick Child, Chapter 45).

As the edema subsides, children are allowed increased activity. Although easily fatigued, children usually adjust activities according to their tolerance level. However, they may require guidance in selecting play activities. Suitable recreational and diversional activities are an important part of their care. Once edema fluid has been lost, children are allowed to resume their usual activities with discretion. Irritability and mood swings that accompany the inactivity, disease process, and steroid therapy are not unusual; they create an additional challenge to the nurse and the family.

Family Support and Home Care. Continuous support of the child and family is a major nursing consideration. Many children are treated at home during exacerbations. Parents are taught to detect signs of relapse and to call for changes in treatment at the earliest indications. Unless the edema and proteinuria are severe, or the parents, for some reason, are unable to care for the ill child, *home care is preferred*. Parents are instructed in testing urine for albumin, administration of medications, and general care. Parents are also instructed regarding avoiding contact with infected playmates, but the child should attend school.

The prolonged course of the relapsing form of nephrotic syndrome is taxing to both the child and the family. The up-and-down course of remissions and exacerbations—with periodic disruption of family life by hospitalization—places a severe strain, both psychologically and financially, on the child and the family. Reassurance regarding this characteristic of the course of the disease, with emphasis on the importance of long-term care, needs to be provided to parents and children to gain their cooperation. A satisfactory response is more likely when relapses are detected and therapy is instituted early, and remissions are prolonged when instructions are carried out faithfully. Continuous support of the child and family is a major nursing consideration (see Chapter 41).

➤ Evaluation

The effectiveness of nursing interventions is determined by continual reassessment and evaluation of care on the basis of the following observational guidelines and expected outcomes:

1. Measure intake and output and examine urine for albumin.
2. Monitor vital signs and assess the skin for evidence of breakdown or infection.
3. Assess appetite and eating behaviors.
4. Observe and interview child and family regarding their understanding of the disease, therapies, and compliance with the prescribed regimen.

(See Nursing Care Plan: The Child with Nephrotic Syndrome.*)

Acute Glomerulonephritis (AGN)

AGN may be a primary event or a manifestation of a systemic disorder that can range from minimal to severe. Common features include oliguria, edema, hypertension and circulatory congestion, hematuria, and proteinuria. Most cases are postinfectious and have been associated with pneumococcal, streptococcal, and viral infections. *Acute poststreptococcal glomerulonephritis (APSGN)* is the most common of the postinfectious renal diseases in childhood and the one for which a cause can be established in the majority of cases. APSGN can occur at any age but affects primarily early school-age children, with a peak age of onset of 6 to 7 years. It is uncommon in children younger than 2 years of age, and males outnumber females 2:1.

Etiology. APSGN is an immune-complex disease that occurs after an antecedent streptococcal infection with certain strains of the group A ß-hemolytic streptococcus. Most streptococcal infections do not cause APSGN. A latent period of 10 to

*In Wong DL, Hess CS: ***Wong and Whaley's clinical manual of pediatric nursing***, ed 5, St Louis, 2000, Mosby.

21 days occurs between the streptococcal infection and the onset of clinical manifestations. Disease secondary to streptococcal pharyngitis is more common in the winter or spring, but when APSGN is associated with pyoderma (principally *impetigo*), it may be more prevalent in later summer or early fall, especially in warmer climates. Second episodes of AGN are rare.

Pathophysiology. The pathophysiology of APSGN is still uncertain. Immune complexes are deposited in the glomerular basement membrane. The glomeruli become edematous and infiltrated with polymorphonuclear leukocytes, which occlude the capillary lumen. The resulting decrease in plasma filtration results in an excessive accumulation of water and retention of sodium that expands plasma and interstitial fluid volumes, leading to circulatory congestion and edema. The cause of the hypertension associated with AGN cannot be completely explained by fluid retention. Excess renin may also be produced.

Diagnostic Evaluation. Typically, affected children are in good health until they experience the streptococcal infection. In some instances there is a history of only a mild cold or no previous infection at all. The onset of nephritis appears after an average latent period of about 10 days (Box 50-3). Because the child appears to be well during the latest period, the association is not recognized by the parents. The edema is relatively moderate and may not be appreciated by someone unfamiliar with the child's normal appearance.

Urinalysis during the acute phase characteristically shows hematuria and proteinuria. Proteinuria generally parallels the hematuria and may be 3+ or 4+ in the presence of gross hematuria. Gross discoloration of the urine reflects red blood cell and hemoglobin content. Microscopic examination of the sediment shows many red blood cells, leukocytes, epithelial cells, and granular and red blood cell casts. Bacteria are not seen.

Azotemia that results from impaired glomerular filtration is reflected in elevated blood urea nitrogen and creatinine levels in at least 50% of cases. Occasionally proteinuria is excessive and the patient may have nephrotic syndrome (i.e., hypoproteinemia and hyperlipidemia).

Cultures of the pharynx are rarely positive for streptococci because the renal disease occurs weeks after the infection.

NURSE ALERT • A child who exhibits the following should be evaluated for possible AGN:
- Orbital edema, which parents report is worse in the morning
- Loss of appetite
- Decreased output
- Dark-colored urine
- Antecedent streptococcal infection

Some serologic tests are necessary to make the diagnosis of AGN. Circulating serum antibodies to streptococcus indicate the presence of a previous infection. The antistreptolysin O (ASO) titer is the most familiar and readily available test for streptococcal infection. Other antibodies that may aid in diagnosis are elevated antihyaluronidase (AHase), antideoxyribonuclease B (ADNase-B), and streptozyme.

All patients with APSGN have reduced serum complement (C3) activity in the early stages of the disease. Rising C3 levels are used as a guide to indicate improvement of the disease and should be normal in almost all patients 8 weeks after the disease onset.

Studies that may be useful include chest x-ray examination, which generally shows cardiac enlargement, pulmonary congestion, and/or pleural effusion during the edematous phase of acute disease. Renal biopsy for diagnostic purposes is seldom required but may be useful in the diagnosis of atypical cases.

Therapeutic Management. Management consists of general supportive measures and early recognition and treatment of complications. Children who have normal blood pressure and a satisfactory urine output can generally be treated at home. Those with substantial edema, hypertension, gross hematuria, and/or significant oliguria should be hospitalized because of the unpredictability of complications.

Dietary restrictions depend on the stage and severity of the disease, especially the extent of edema. Moderate sodium restriction and even fluid restriction may be instituted for children with hypertension and edema. Foods with substantial amounts of potassium are generally restricted during the period of oliguria.

Regular measurement of vital signs, body weight, and intake and output is essential in order to monitor the progress of the disease and to detect complications that may appear at any time during the course of the disease. *A record of daily weight is the most useful means for assessing fluid balance.* Rarely, children with AGN will develop acute renal failure with oliguria that significantly alters the fluid and electrolyte balance (resulting in hyperkalemia, acidosis, hypocalcemia, and/or hyperphosphatemia). These children require careful management. Peritoneal dialysis or hemodialysis is seldom needed.

Acute hypertension must be anticipated and identified early. Blood pressure measurements are taken every 4 to 6 hours. A variety of antihypertensive medications, as well as diuretics, are used to control hypertension.

Antibiotic therapy is indicated only for those children with evidence of persistent streptococcal infections. It is used to prevent transmission of nephritogenic streptococci to other family members.

Box 50-3

Clinical Manifestations of Acute Poststreptococcal Glomerulonephritis

- Edema:
  - Especially periorbital
  - Facial edema more prominent in the morning
  - Spreads during the day to involve extremities and abdomen
- Anorexia
- Urine:
  - Cloudy, smoky brown (resembles tea or cola)
  - Severely reduced volume
- Pallor
- Irritability
- Lethargy
- Child appears ill
- Child seldom expresses specific complaints
- Older children may complain of:
  - Headaches
  - Abdominal discomfort
  - Dysuria
- Vomiting possible
- Mild to moderately elevated blood pressure

Prognosis. Almost all children correctly diagnosed as having APSGN recover completely, and specific immunity is conferred so that recurrences are uncommon. A few of these children have been reported to develop chronic disease, but most of these cases are now believed to be different glomerular diseases misdiagnosed as poststreptococcal disease.

Nursing Care Management

➤ Assessment

Nursing care of the child with glomerulonephritis involves careful assessment of the disease status with regular monitoring of vital signs (including frequent measurement of blood pressure), fluid balance, and behavior.

Vital signs provide clues to the severity of the disease and early signs of complications. They are carefully measured, and any deviations are reported and recorded. The volume and character of urine is noted, and the child is weighed daily. Children with restricted fluid intake, especially those who are not severely edematous or those who have lost weight, are observed for signs of dehydration.

Assessment of the child's appearance for signs of cerebral complications is an important nursing function because the severity of the acute phase is variable and unpredictable. The child with edema, hypertension, and gross hematuria may be subject to complications, and anticipatory preparations such as seizure precautions and intravenous equipment are included in the nursing care plan.

➤ Nursing Diagnoses

Several nursing diagnoses become obvious on the basis of assessment. Others may be evident in specific situations.

Fluid volume excess related to decreased plasma filtration

Activity intolerance related to fatigue

Altered patterns of urinary elimination related to fluid retention and impaired glomerular filtration

Altered family processes related to the child with a renal disorder

➤ Plan of Care and Implementation

The goals of care for the child with AGN and the family include the following:

1. Child will receive optimum rest.
2. Child will receive sufficient nutrition.
3. Child will exhibit no evidence of complications.
4. Child and family will receive appropriate support and education regarding child's condition.

For most children a regular diet is allowed, but it should contain no added salt. Foods high in sodium and salted treats are eliminated, and parents and friends are advised not to bring items such as potato chips or pretzels. However, the total amount of salt ingested is usually less than prescribed because of the child's poor appetite. Fluid restriction, if prescribed, is more difficult, and the amount permitted should be evenly divided throughout the waking hours. Meal preparation and service require special attention because the child is indifferent to meals during the acute phase. Again, collaboration with parents and the dietitian and special consideration for food preferences facilitate meal planning.

During the acute phase children are generally quite content to lie in bed. As they begin to feel better and their symptoms subside, they will want to be up and about. Activities should be planned to allow for frequent rest periods and avoidance of fatigue. Children who have mild edema and no hypertension, as well as convalescent children who are being treated at home, need follow-up care. Parents are instructed regarding general measures, including diet, and prevention of infection.

Health supervision is continued with weekly, then monthly visits for evaluation and urinalysis. Parent education and support in preparation for discharge and home care includes education in home management and the need for follow-up care and health supervision.

➤ Evaluation

The effectiveness of nursing interventions is determined by continual reassessment and evaluation of care on the basis of the following observational guidelines and expected outcomes:

1. Observe child's behavior.
2. Monitor dietary and fluid intake; interview family regarding child's diet and appetite.
3. Monitor vital signs, intake and output, and observe for signs of complications such as hypertension, increased intracranial pressure, and infection.
4. Observe behaviors and interview child and family regarding reaction to the disease and therapies.

Expected outcomes

1. Child plays and rests quietly.
2. Child consumes a sufficient amount of appropriate foods.
3. Child exhibits no evidence of complications.
4. Child and family demonstrate an understanding of the disease and its therapy (specify learning and methods of demonstration), and they express their feelings and concerns.

(See also Nursing Care Plan: The Child with Acute Poststreptococcal Glomerulonephritis.*)

MISCELLANEOUS RENAL DISORDERS

Hemolytic-Uremic Syndrome (HUS)

HUS is an uncommon, acute renal disease that occurs primarily in infants and small children between the ages of 6 months and 5 years. HUS is the most common cause of acquired acute renal failure in children (Brandt et al, 1994). The clinical features of the disease include acquired hemolytic anemia, thrombocytopenia, renal injury, and central nervous system symptoms. The etiology of HUS is thought to be associated with bacterial toxins, chemicals, and viruses. The appearance of the disease has been associated with *Rickettsia,* viruses (especially coxsackie virus, echovirus, and adenovirus), *Escherichia coli,* pneumococci, *Shigella,* and *Salmonella* and may represent an unusual response to these infections. Multiple cases of HUS caused by enteric infection of the *E. coli* 0157:H7 serotype have been traced to undercooked meat, especially ground beef (Brandt et al, 1994). Other sources are unpasteurized milk or fruit juice (especially apple), alfalfa sprouts, lettuce, and salami; and drinking or swimming in sewage-contaminated water. The clinical presentation is usually a history of a prodromal illness (most often gastroenteritis or an upper respiratory infection) followed by the sudden onset of hemolysis and renal failure.

*In Wong DL, Hess CS: ***Wong and Whaley's clinical manual of pediatric nursing,*** ed 5, St Louis, 2000, Mosby.

Pathophysiology. The primary site of injury appears to be the endothelial lining of the small glomerular arterioles, which become swollen and occluded with deposits of platelets and fibrin clots (intravascular coagulation). Red blood cells are damaged as they attempt to move through the partially occluded blood vessels. These damaged cells are removed by the spleen, causing acute hemolytic anemia. The platelet aggregation within the damaged blood vessels or the damage and removal of platelets produce the characteristic thrombocytopenia.

Diagnostic Evaluation. The triad of anemia, thrombocytopenia, and renal failure is sufficient for diagnosis (Box 50-4). Renal involvement is evidenced by proteinuria, hematuria, and the presence of urinary casts; blood urea nitrogen and serum creatinine levels are elevated. A low hemoglobin and hematocrit and a high reticulocyte count confirm the hemolytic nature of the anemia.

Therapeutic Management. The goals of therapy are early diagnosis and aggressive, supportive care of the acute renal failure and hemolytic anemia. The most consistently effective treatment of HUS is hemodialysis or peritoneal dialysis, which is instituted in any child who has been anuric for 24 hours or who demonstrates oliguria with uremia or hypertension and seizures. Other treatments include use of pharmacologic agents, fresh-frozen plasma, and plasma pheresis. Blood transfusions with fresh, washed packed cells are administered for severe anemia but are used with caution to prevent circulatory overload from added volume.

Prognosis. With prompt treatment the recovery rate is about 95%, but residual renal impairment ranges from 10% to 50% in various areas. Long-term complications include chronic renal failure, hypertension, and central nervous system disorders. Death is usually caused by residual renal impairment or central nervous system injury.

Nursing Care Management. Nursing care is the same as that provided in acute renal failure and, for children with continued impairment, includes management of chronic disease. Because of the sudden and life-threatening nature of the disorder in a previously well child, parents are often ill-prepared for the impact of hospitalization and treatment. Therefore support and understanding are especially important aspects of care.

Box 50-4

Clinical Manifestations of Hemolytic-Uremic Syndrome

- Vomiting
- Irritability
- Lethargy
- Marked pallor
- Hemorrhagic manifestations:
  - Bruising
  - Petechiae
  - Jaundice
  - Bloody diarrhea
- Oliguria or anuria
- Central nervous system involvement:
  - Seizures
  - Stupor/coma
- Signs of acute heart failure (sometimes)

Wilms Tumor

Wilms tumor, or nephroblastoma, is the most common malignant renal and intraabdominal tumor of childhood. Its incidence is estimated to be 8.1 cases per million Caucasian children less than 15 years of age (Green, 1997). Wilms tumor occurs about three times more often in African-Americans than in East Asians in the United States. The peak age at diagnosis is approximately 3 years, and occurrence is slightly more common in boys than in girls. Eighty percent of patients with Wilms tumor are diagnosed at under 5 years of age, with 1% to 2.5% having a familial origin (Petruzzi and Green, 1997). Unfortunately, there is no method of identifying gene carriers at this time.

Etiology. Wilms tumor probably arises from a malignant, undifferentiated cluster of primordial cells capable of initiating the regeneration of an abnormal structure. Its occurrence slightly favors the left kidney, which is advantageous because surgically this kidney is easier to manipulate and remove. In about 10% of cases both kidneys are involved. Studies have shown that development of Wilms tumor involves genetic and somatic mosaicism and is commonly associated with aniridia, hemihypertrophy, Beckwith-Wiedemann syndrome, and genitourinary anomalies (Green et al, 1997).

Diagnostic Evaluation. In a child suspected of having Wilms tumor, special emphasis is placed on the history and physical examination for the presence of congenital anomalies, a family history of cancer, and signs of malignancy (e.g., weight loss, enlarged liver and spleen, indications of anemia, and lymphadenopathy). Most children with Wilms tumor are brought to the practitioner because of abdominal swelling or an abdominal mass (Box 50-5). Specific tests include radiographic studies, including abdominal ultrasound; computed tomography; hematologic studies (polycythemia is sometimes present if the tumor secretes excess erythropoietin); biochemical studies; and urinalysis. Studies to demonstrate the relationship of the tumor to the ipsilateral kidney and the presence of a normal functioning kidney on the contralateral side are essential. If a large tumor is present, an inferior venacavagram is necessary to demonstrate possible tumor involvement adjacent to the vena

Box 50-5

Clinical Manifestations of Wilms Tumor

- Abdominal swelling or mass:
  - Firm
  - Nontender
  - Confined to one side
- Hematuria (less than one fourth of cases)
- Fatigue/malaise
- Hypertension (occasionally)
- Weight loss
- Fever
- Manifestations resulting from compression of tumor mass
- Secondary metabolic alterations from tumor or metastasis
- If metastasis, symptoms of lung involvement:
  - Dyspnea
  - Cough
  - Shortness of breath
  - Chest pain (sometimes)

cava. A bone marrow aspiration may be performed to rule out metastasis, which is rare in children with Wilms tumor.

Therapeutic Management. Combined treatment of surgery and chemotherapy with or without radiation is based on the histologic pattern and clinical stage.

Surgery is scheduled as soon as possible after confirmation of a renal mass, usually within 24 to 48 hours of admission. A large transabdominal incision is performed for optimum visualization of the abdominal cavity. The tumor, affected kidney, and adjacent adrenal gland are removed. Great care is taken to keep the encapsulated tumor intact because rupture can seed cancer cells throughout the abdomen, lymph channel, and bloodstream. The contralateral kidney is carefully inspected for evidence of disease or dysfunction. Regional lymph nodes are inspected, and a biopsy is performed when indicated. Any involved structures, such as part of the colon, diaphragm, or vena cava, are removed. Metal clips are placed around the tumor site for exact marking during radiotherapy.

If both kidneys are involved, the child may be treated with radiation therapy and/or chemotherapy before surgery to decrease the size of the tumor, allowing more conservative surgery. It may be possible to perform a partial nephrectomy on the less affected kidney, with a total nephrectomy on the opposite side. When a transplant is feasible (e.g., from a twin, sibling, or parent), bilateral nephrectomy is considered as a last resort.

Postoperative radiation therapy is indicated for children with large tumors, metastasis, residual postoperative disease, unfavorable histology, or recurrence. Chemotherapy is indicated for all stages. The most effective agents for treating Wilms tumor are actinomycin D (dactinomycin), vincristine, and adriamycin with the addition of cyclophosphamide for unfavorable histology or advanced disease (Green, 1997). The duration of therapy ranges from 6 to 15 months.

Prognosis. Survival rates for Wilms tumor are the highest among all childhood cancers. Children with localized tumor (stages I and II) have a 90% chance of cure with multimodal therapy. Factors that favorably affect the success of further therapy include initial treatment with only vincristine and dactinomycin, relapse to the lungs only, relapse in the abdomen of a patient who received no prior abdominal radiation, and relapse more than 12 months after diagnosis. Wilms tumor may recur, especially in the lungs. Both chemotherapy and radiation therapy can induce second tumors, usually in areas that have been irradiated (Green, 1997).

Nursing Care Management. Nursing care of the child with Wilms tumor is similar to that of children with other cancers treated with surgery, radiation, and chemotherapy; however, there are some significant differences. These differences are discussed for each phase of nursing intervention.

Preoperative Care. The preoperative period is one of swift diagnosis. The nurse is faced with the challenge of preparing the child and parents for all laboratory and operative procedures within 24 to 48 hours of admission. Because the minimal amount of available preparatory time, explanations should be simple, repetitive, and focused on the child's actual experiences. In addition to the usual preoperative observations, blood pressure is monitored because hypertension from excess renin production is a possibility.

There are several special preoperative concerns, the most important of which is that *the tumor is not palpated unless absolutely necessary,* because manipulation of the mass may cause dissemination of cancer cells to adjacent and distant sites.

NURSE ALERT • To reinforce the need for caution, it may be necessary to post a sign on the bed that reads "DO NOT PALPATE ABDOMEN." Careful bathing and handling are also important in preventing trauma to the tumor site.

Because radiation therapy and chemotherapy are usually begun immediately after surgery, parents need an explanation of what to expect (e.g., major benefits and side effects). The timing of the information should be considered to avoid overwhelming the family. Ideally, the nurse should be present during physician-parent conferences to answer questions as they arise. It is usually better to postpone telling the child about these side effects until after surgery. Alopecia, usually of most concern to older children, does not occur until approximately 2 weeks after the initial treatment regimen. Therefore the child can be prepared for the hair loss postoperatively.

Postoperative Care. Despite the extensive surgical intervention necessary in many children with Wilms tumor, the recovery is usually rapid. The major nursing responsibilities are the same as those after any abdominal surgery (see Surgical Procedures, Chapter 45). Because these children are at risk for intestinal obstruction from vincristine-induced adynamic ileus, radiation-induced edema, and postsurgical adhesion formation, gastrointestinal activity (e.g., bowel movements, bowel sounds, distention, vomiting, and pain) is carefully monitored.

The nurse also monitors blood pressure, urine output, and signs of infection, as well as instituting pulmonary hygiene to prevent postoperative pulmonary complications.

NURSE ALERT • Because the child is left with one kidney, certain precautions, such as avoiding contact sports, are recommended to prevent injury to the remaining organ. Prompt detection and treatment of any genitourinary signs or symptoms is mandatory.

Family Support. The postoperative period is commonly difficult for parents. The shock of seeing their child immediately after surgery may be the first realization of the seriousness of the diagnosis. It also marks the confirmation of the stage of the tumor. During this period, the nurse should be with the parents to assure them of the child's recovery after surgery and to assess the parents' understanding of the total experience. They need an opportunity to express their feelings and need to be provided the same emotional care discussed in Chapter 41 for families who have a child with a life-threatening disorder.

Older children need an opportunity to deal with their feelings concerning the many procedures to which they have been subjected in rapid succession. Play therapy with dolls or puppets or through drawing can be extremely beneficial in helping them adjust. It is not unusual for children to feel angry because of the extent of surgery, the need for additional therapy, or the seriousness of the disorder.

RENAL FAILURE

Renal failure is the inability of the kidneys to excrete waste material, concentrate urine, and conserve electrolytes. It can occur suddenly *(acute renal failure)* in response to inadequate perfusion, kidney disease, or urinary tract obstruction; or it can develop slowly *(chronic renal failure)* as a result of long-standing kidney disease or an anomaly.

Azotemia and uremia are terms often used in relation to renal failure. *Azotemia* is the accumulation of nitrogenous waste within the blood. *Uremia* is a more advanced condition in which retention of nitrogenous products produces toxic symptoms. Azotemia is not life threatening, whereas uremia is a serious condition that often involves other body systems.

Acute Renal Failure (ARF)

ARF is said to exist when the kidneys suddenly are unable to regulate the volume and composition of urine appropriately in response to food and fluid intake and the needs of the organism. The principal feature of ARF is oliguria* associated with azotemia, metabolic acidosis, and diverse electrolyte disturbances. ARF is not common in childhood, but the outcome depends on the cause, associated findings, and prompt recognition and treatment.

The pathologic conditions that produce ARF caused by glomerulonephritis and hemolytic-uremic syndrome have been discussed in relation to those disorders. ARF can also develop as a result of a large number of related or unrelated clinical conditions: poor renal perfusion; urinary tract obstruction; acute renal injury; or the final expression of chronic, irreversible renal disease. The most common cause in children is transient renal failure resulting from severe dehydration or other causes of poor perfusion that may respond to restoration of fluid volume.

Pathophysiology. ARF is usually reversible, but the deviations of physiologic function can be extreme, and mortality in the pediatric age group remains high. There is severe reduction in the glomerular filtration rate, an elevated blood urea nitrogen level, and a significant reduction in renal blood flow.

The clinical course is variable and depends on the cause. In reversible ARF there is a period of severe oliguria, or a low-output phase; followed by an abrupt onset of diuresis, or a high-output phase; and then a gradual return to, or toward, normal urine volumes.

Diagnostic Evaluation. In many instances of ARF the infant or child is already critically ill with the precipitating disorder, and the explanation for development of oliguria may or may not be readily apparent (Box 50-6). When a previously well child develops ARF without obvious cause, a careful history is taken to reveal symptoms that may be related to glomerulonephritis, obstructive uropathy, or exposure to nephrotoxic chemicals (e.g., ingestion of heavy metals or inhalation of carbon tetrachloride or other organic solvents or drugs known to be toxic to the kidneys). Significant laboratory measurements during renal shutdown that serve as a guide for therapy are blood urea nitrogen, serum creatinine, pH, sodium, potassium, and calcium.

Therapeutic Management. Treatment of ARF is directed toward (1) treatment of the underlying cause, (2) management of the complications of renal failure, and (3) provision of supportive therapy within the constraints imposed by the renal failure.

*The definition of oliguria varies extensively in the literature, from 1.8 to 4 dl/m²/24 hr.

Box 50-6

Clinical Manifestations of Acute Renal Failure

Specific:
- Oliguria
- Anuria uncommon (except in obstructive disorders)

Nonspecific (may develop):
- Nausea
- Vomiting
- Drowsiness
- Edema
- Hypertension

Manifestations of underlying disorder or pathologic condition

Treatment of poor perfusion resulting from dehydration consists of volume restoration, as described in Chapter 47 in treatment of dehydration. If oliguria persists after restoration of fluid volume, or if the renal failure is caused by intrinsic renal damage, the physiologic and biochemical abnormalities that have resulted from kidney dysfunction must be corrected or controlled. Initially a Foley catheter is inserted to rule out urine retention, to collect available urine for analysis, and to monitor results of diuretic administration. The catheter may or may not be removed during the oliguric phase.

The amount of exogenous water provided should not exceed the amount needed to maintain zero water balance. It is calculated on the basis of estimated endogenous water formation and losses from sensible (primarily gastrointestinal) and insensible sources. No allotment is calculated for urine as long as oliguria persists.

When the output begins to increase, either spontaneously or in response to diuretic therapy, the intake of fluid, potassium, and sodium must be monitored and adequate replacement provided to prevent depletion and its consequences. Some patients pass enormous amounts of electrolyte-rich urine.

Complications. The child with ARF has a tendency to develop water intoxication and hyponatremia, which makes it difficult to provide calories in sufficient amounts to meet the needs of the child and reduce the tissue catabolism, metabolic acidosis, hyperkalemia, and uremia. If the child is able to tolerate oral foods, food sources high in concentrated carbohydrate and fat but low in protein, potassium, and sodium may be provided. However, many children have functional disturbances of the gastrointestinal tract, such as nausea and vomiting; therefore the intravenous (IV) route is generally preferred and usually consists of essential amino acids or a combination of essential and nonessential amino acids administered by the central venous route.

Control of water balance in these patients requires careful monitoring of feedback information, such as accurate intake and output, body weight, and electrolyte measurements. In general, during the oliguric phase, no sodium, chloride, or potassium is given unless there are other large, ongoing losses. Regular measurement of plasma electrolyte, pH, blood urea nitrogen, and creatinine levels is required to assess the adequacy of fluid therapy and to anticipate complications that require specific treatment.

Hyperkalemia is the most immediate threat to the life of the child with ARF. Hyperkalemia can be minimized and sometimes avoided by eliminating potassium from all food and fluid, by reducing tissue catabolism, and by correcting acidosis. Measures employed for the reduction of serum potassium levels are oral or rectal administration of an ion-exchange resin such as sodium polystyrene sulfonate (Kayexalate) and peritoneal dialysis or hemodialysis (p. 1417). The resin produces its effect by exchange of its sodium for the potassium, thus binding potassium for removal from the body. This increased sodium concentration may contribute to fluid overload, hypertension, and cardiac failure. Dialysis removes potassium and other waste products from the serum by diffusion through a semipermeable membrane.

NURSE ALERT • Any of the following signs of hyperkalemia constitute an emergency and are reported immediately:

- Serum potassium concentrations in excess of 7 mEq/L
- Presence of electrocardiographic abnormalities such as prolonged QRS complex, depressed ST segment, high peaked T waves, bradycardia, or heart block

Hypertension is a common and serious complication of ARF, and to detect it early, blood pressure measurements are made every 4 to 6 hours. The most common cause of hypertension in ARF is overexpansion of extracellular fluid and plasma volume together with activation of the renin-angiotensin system. Hypertension is controlled with antihypertensive drugs. Other measures that may be used include limiting fluids and salt.

Anemia is commonly associated with ARF, but transfusion is not recommended unless the hemoglobin drops below 6 g/dl. Transfusions, if used, consist of fresh, packed red blood cells given slowly to reduce the likelihood of increasing blood volume, hypertension, and hyperkalemia.

Seizures occur rather often when renal failure progresses to uremia and are also related to hypertension, hyponatremia, and hypocalcemia. Treatment is directed to the specific cause when known. More obscure causes are managed with antiepileptic drugs.

Cardiac failure with pulmonary edema is almost always associated with hypervolemia. Treatment is directed toward reduction of fluid volume, with water and sodium restriction and administration of diuretics.

Prognosis. The prognosis of ARF depends largely on the nature and severity of the causative factor or precipitating event and the promptness and competence of management. The outcome is least favorable in children with rapidly progressive nephritis and cortical necrosis. Children in whom ARF is a result of hemolytic-uremic syndrome or acute glomerulitis may recover completely, but residual renal impairment or hypertension is more often the rule. Complete recovery is usually expected in children whose renal failure is a result of dehydration, nephrotoxins, or ischemia. ARF following cardiac surgery is less favorable. It is often impossible to assess the extent of recovery for several months.

Nursing Care Management

➤ Assessment

Meticulous attention to fluid intake and output is mandatory and includes all of the physical measurements discussed previously in relation to problems of fluid balance. Monitoring fluid balance and vital signs is a continuous process, and observers are constantly on the alert for signs of complications so that appropriate interventions can be implemented. Because these children require intensive observation (and often, specialized treatment such as dialysis), they are usually admitted to an intensive care unit in which needed equipment and trained personnel are available.

NURSE ALERT • **Diminished urine output and lethargy in a child who is dehydrated, in shock, or recently postoperative should be evaluated for possible acute kidney failure.**

➤ Nursing Diagnoses

A number of nursing diagnoses are evident following a thorough assessment of the child with ARF. Others, including the following, will be noted depending on the age of the child, the cause of the renal failure, and any concomitant complications:

- Fluid volume excess related to failure of or compromised renal regulatory mechanisms
- Risk for injury related to accumulated electrolytes and waste products
- Risk for infection related to lowered body defenses, fluid overload
- Altered family processes related to a child with a serious disorder

➤ Plan of Care and Implementation

The major goals for the child with ARF and the family are as follows:

1. Child will maintain appropriate fluid volume.
2. Child will maintain normal electrolyte levels.
3. Child will maintain blood pressure within acceptable limits.
4. Child will experience minimized risk of infection.
5. Child and family will receive adequate support.

The major nursing task in the care of the infant or child with ARF is monitoring and assessing fluid and electrolyte balance.

Limiting fluid intake requires ingenuity on the part of caregivers to cope with the child who is thirsty. One strategy is to ration the daily intake in small amounts of fluid served in containers that give the impression of larger volumes. Older children who understand the rationale of fluid limits can help determine how their daily ration should be distributed.

Meeting nutritional needs is sometimes a problem; the child may be nauseated, and encouraging concentrated foods without fluids may be difficult. When nourishment is provided by the IV route, careful monitoring is essential to prevent fluid overload. In addition, nursing measures such as maintaining an optimum thermal environment, reducing any elevation of body temperature, and reducing restlessness and anxiety are employed to decrease the rate of tissue catabolism.

The nurse must be continually alert for changes in behavior that indicate the onset of complications. Infection from reduced resistance, anemia, and general morbidity is a constant threat. Fluid overload and electrolyte disturbances can precipitate cardiovascular complications such as hypertension and cardiac failure. Fluid and electrolyte imbalances, acidosis, and accumulation of nitrogenous waste products can produce neurologic involvement manifested by coma, seizures, or alterations in sensorium.

Although children with ARF are usually quite ill and voluntarily diminish their activity, infants may become restless and irritable, and children are often anxious and frightened. There are frequent, painful, and stress-producing treatments and tests that must be performed. The presence of a supportive, empathetic nurse can provide comfort and stability in a threatening and unnatural environment.

Family Support. Providing support and reassurance to parents is among the major nursing responsibilities. The seriousness of ARF and its emergency nature are stressful to parents, and most feel some degree of guilt regarding the child's condition, especially when the illness is a result of either ingestion of a toxic substance, dehydration, or a genetic disease. Parents need reassurance and a sympathetic listener. They also need to be kept informed of the child's progress and provided explanations regarding the therapeutic regimen. The equipment and the child's behavior are sometimes frightening and anxiety provoking. Nurses can do much to help parents comprehend and deal with the stresses of the situation.

➤ Evaluation

The effectiveness of nursing interventions is determined by continual reassessment and evaluation of care on the basis of the following observational guidelines and expected outcomes:

1. Carry out frequent assessment of vital signs and behaviors.
2. Observe eating behaviors and energy expenditure; monitor intake of protein and calories; carefully monitor intake and output; weigh daily or more often as prescribed.
3. Monitor vital signs, sensorium, and other neurologic signs; evaluate laboratory results and observe for signs of electrolyte imbalance.
4. Observe and interview child and family regarding their understanding of the disease and therapies; encourage child and family to express feelings and concerns.

Expected outcomes include the following:

1. Alterations in vital signs and behavior are detected.
2. Child consumes a sufficient amount of appropriate nutrients without evidence of fluid gain or waste product accumulation.
3. Child exhibits no evidence of infection.
4. Evidence of complications is detected early, and appropriate interventions are implemented.
5. Child and family express their feelings and concerns and demonstrate their understanding of the condition and the therapies (specify knowledge and method of demonstration).

(See Nursing Care Plan: The Child with Acute Renal Failure.*)

Chronic Renal Failure (CRF)

The kidneys are able to maintain the chemical composition of fluids within normal limits until more than 50% of functional renal capacity is destroyed by disease or injury. Chronic renal insufficiency or failure begins when the diseased kidneys can no longer maintain the normal chemical structure of body fluids under normal conditions. Progressive deterioration over months or years produces a variety of clinical and biochemical disturbances that eventually culminate in the clinical syndrome known as *uremia.*

A variety of diseases and disorders can result in CRF. The most common causes are congenital renal and urinary tract malformations, vesicoureteral reflux associated with recurrent urinary tract infection, chronic pyelonephritis, hereditary disorders, chronic glomerulonephritis, and glomerulonephropathy associated with systemic diseases such as anaphylactoid purpura and lupus erythematosus.

Pathophysiology. Early in the course of progressive nephrotic destruction, the child remains asymptomatic with only minimal biochemical abnormalities. Unless the presence of CRF is detected in the process of routine assessment, signs and symptoms that indicate advanced renal damage commonly emerge only late in the course of the disease. Midway in the disease process, as increasing numbers of nephrons are totally destroyed and most others are damaged to varying degrees, the few that remain intact are hypertrophied but functional. These few normal nephrons are able to make sufficient adjustments to stresses to maintain reasonable degrees of fluid and electrolyte balance. Definitive biochemical examination at this time will reveal restricted tolerance to excesses or restrictions. As the disease progresses to the end stage, because of a severe reduction in the number of functioning nephrons, the kidneys are no longer able to maintain fluid and electrolyte balance, and the features of uremic syndrome appear.

The accumulation of various biochemical substances in the blood, a result of diminished renal function, produces complications such as the following:

- Retention of waste products, especially the blood urea nitrogen and creatinine
- Water and sodium retention, which contributes to edema and vascular congestion
- Hyperkalemia of dangerous levels
- Metabolic acidosis of a sustained nature because of continual hydrogen ion retention and bicarbonate loss
- Calcium and phosphorus disturbances resulting in altered bone metabolism, which in turn causes growth arrest or retardation, bone pain, and deformities known as *renal osteodystrophy*
- Anemia caused by hematologic dysfunction, including shortened life span of red blood cells, impaired red blood cell production related to decreased production of erythropoietin, prolonged bleeding time, and nutritional anemia
- Growth disturbance, probably caused by such factors as renal osteodystrophy, poor nutrition associated with dietary restrictions and loss of appetite, and biochemical abnormalities

Children with CRF seem to be more susceptible to infection, especially pneumonia, urinary tract infection, and septicemia, although the reason for this is unclear. These children become extraordinarily sensitive to changes in vascular volume that may cause pulmonary overload, central nervous system symptoms, hypertension, and cardiac failure.

Diagnostic Evaluation. The diagnosis of CRF is usually suspected on the basis of any number of clinical manifestations, a history of prior renal disease, and/or biochemical findings. The onset is usually gradual, and the initial signs and symptoms are vague and nonspecific (Box 50-7).

*In Wong DL, Hess CS: ***Wong and Whaley's clinical manual of pediatric nursing,*** ed 5, St Louis, 2000, Mosby.

Laboratory and other diagnostic tools and tests are of value in assessing the extent of renal damage, biochemical disturbances, and related physical dysfunction (see Tables 50-1, 50-2, and 50-3). Often they can help establish the nature of the underlying disease and differentiate between other disease processes and the pathologic consequences of renal dysfunction.

Therapeutic Management. In irreversible renal failure the goals of medical management are (1) to promote maximal renal function, (2) to maintain body fluid and electrolyte balance within safe biochemical limits, (3) to treat systemic complications, and (4) to promote as active and normal a life as possible for the child for as long as possible. The child is allowed unrestricted activity and is allowed to set his or her own limits regarding rest and extent of exertion. School attendance is encouraged as long as the child is able. When the effort is too great, home tutoring is arranged.

Box 50-7

Clinical Manifestations of Chronic Renal Failure

- Early signs:
  - Loss of normal energy
  - Increased fatigue on exertion
  - Pallor, subtle (may not be noticed)
  - Elevated blood pressure (sometimes)
- As the disease progresses:
  - Decreased appetite (especially at breakfast)
  - Less interest in normal activities
  - Increased or decreased urine output with compensatory intake of fluid
  - Pallor more evident
  - Sallow, muddy appearance of skin
- Child may complain of:
  - Headache
  - Muscle cramps
  - Nausea
- Other signs and symptoms:
  - Weight loss
  - Facial edema
  - Malaise
  - Bone or joint pain
  - Growth retardation
  - Dryness or itching of the skin
  - Bruised skin
  - Sensory or motor loss (sometimes)
  - Amenorrhea (common in adolescent girls)
- Uremic syndrome (untreated):
  - Gastrointestinal symptoms
    - Anorexia
    - Nausea and vomiting
  - Bleeding tendencies
    - Bruises
    - Bloody diarrheal stools
    - Stomatitis
    - Bleeding from lips and mouth
  - Intractable itching
  - Uremic frost (deposits of urea crystals on skin)
  - Unpleasant "uremic" breath odor
  - Deep respirations
  - Hypertension
  - Congestive heart failure
  - Pulmonary edema
  - Neurologic involvement
    - Progressive confusion
    - Dulled sensorium
    - Coma (ultimately)
    - Tremors
    - Muscular twitching
    - Seizures

Diet regulation is the most effective means, short of dialysis, for reducing the quantity of materials that require renal excretion. The goal of the diet in renal failure is to provide sufficient calories and protein for growth while limiting the excretory demands made on the kidney, to minimize metabolic bone disease *(osteodystrophy)*, and to minimize fluid and electrolyte disturbances. Dietary protein intake is limited only to the recommended daily allowance (RDA) for the child's age. Restriction of protein intake below the RDA is believed to negatively affect growth and neurodevelopment. Malnutrition may develop in patients with CRF even before they need dialysis (Steiber, 1999).

Sodium and water are not usually limited unless there is evidence of edema or hypertension, and potassium is not usually restricted; however, restrictions of any or all three may be imposed in later stages or at any time that abnormal serum concentrations are evident.

Dietary phosphorus is controlled to prevent or correct the calcium/phosphorus imbalance by the reduction of protein and milk intake. Phosphorus levels can be further reduced by oral administration of calcium carbonate preparations that combine with the phosphorus to decrease gastrointestinal absorption and thus the serum levels of phosphate. At the same time that serum calcium levels are increased from the calcium carbonate, vitamin D therapy is begun to increase calcium absorption.

Metabolic acidosis is alleviated through administration of alkalizing agents such as sodium bicarbonate or a combination of sodium and potassium citrate.

Growth failure is one major consequence of CRF, especially in the preadolescent. These children grow poorly both before and after the initiation of hemodialysis. The use of recombinant human growth hormone to accelerate growth in children with growth retardation secondary to CRF has been successful (Schaefer F, 1999). *Osseous deformities* that result from renal osteodystrophy, especially those related to ambulation, are troublesome and require correction if they occur. *Dental defects* are common in children with CRF, and the earlier the onset of the disease, the more severe are the dental manifestations (e.g., hypoplasia, hypomineralization, tooth discoloration, alteration in size and shape of teeth, malocclusion, and ulcerative stomatitis). Therefore regular dental care is especially important in these children.

Anemia in children with CRF is related to decreased production of erythropoietin. Recombinant human erythropoietin (rHuEPO) is being offered to these children as thrice-weekly or weekly subcutaneous injections and is replacing the need for frequent blood transfusions. The drug corrects the anemia and in turn increases appetite, activity, and general well-being in the children who receive it.

Hypertension of advanced renal disease may be managed initially by cautious use of a low-sodium diet, fluid restriction, and perhaps diuretics such as hydrochlorothiazide or furosemide. Severe hypertension requires the use of antihypertensive agents, singly or in combinations.

Intercurrent infections are treated with appropriate antimicrobials at the first sign of infection; however, any drug eliminated through the kidneys is administered with caution. Other complications are treated symptomatically (e.g., central-acting antiemetics for *nausea,* antiepileptics for *seizures,* and diphenhydramine [Benadryl] for *pruritus*).

Once evidence of end-stage renal disease (ESRD) appears in a child, the disease runs its relentless course and results in death in a few weeks, unless waste products and toxins are removed from body fluids by dialysis and/or kidney transplantation. Because these techniques have been adapted for infants and small children, these alternatives have been implemented in most cases of renal failure once conservative management is no longer effective (see Technologic Management of Renal Failure, p. 1417).

Prognosis. Dialysis and transplantation are the only treatments currently available for children with ESRD. Although children may survive on dialysis, it is not an ideal long-term modality. Complications include infection of access sites, growth failure, and disruption of normal socialization. Many pediatric centers encourage families of children with ESRD to consider renal transplantation. The North American Renal Transplantation in Children Report of the Pediatric Renal Transplant Cooperative Study reports a graft survival of 90% at 1 year and 74% at 6 years for living donor kidneys, and 80% at 1 year and 58% at 6 years for cadaver kidneys (Benfield et al, 1999).

Posttransplant complications include infection, hypertension, steroid toxicity, hyperlipidemia, aseptic necrosis, malignancy, and growth retardation (Suthanthiran and Strom, 1994). Long-term graft survival is not guaranteed, and many children require a second or third transplant. Successful renal transplantation does improve rehabilitation of children with CRF, both educationally and psychologically. Increasing use of primary or preemptive renal transplants is becoming the optimum form of renal replacement therapy, leading to substantial improvement in quality of life (Laine et al, 1998).

Nursing Care Management

➤ Assessment

Assessment of the child with CRF is primarily one of observation for signs of complications and evidence of improvement through therapy. Some of the first changes observed are growth failure, developmental delay, bone disease, and hypertension.

➤ Nursing Diagnoses

A number of nursing diagnoses become evident on assessment of the child. The most relevant in the majority of cases are outlined in the Nursing Care Plan on pp. 1418-1419. Others will be appropriate for individual children and their families.

➤ Plan of Care and Implementation

The goals of care for the child with CRF (especially one in ESRD) and the family are as follows:

1. Child will receive encouragement in his or her normal growth and development, minimizing the impact of the disease process.
2. Child will remain free of complications.
3. Child and family will receive appropriate support, guidance, and education.

The multiple complications of ESRD are managed according to medical protocols prescribed for the care of those specific problems. However, progressive disease places a number of stresses on the child and family, including those of a potentially fatal illness (see Chapter 41). There is a continuing need for repeated examinations that often entail painful procedures, side effects, and frequent hospitalizations. Diet therapy becomes progressively more restricted and intense, and the child is required to take a variety of medications. Ever present in all aspects of the treatment regimen is the agonizing realization that without treatment, death is inevitable.

Some specific stresses related to ESRD and its treatment are predictable. When it first becomes apparent that ESRD is inevitable, both parents and child experience depression and anxiety. Acceptance is particularly difficult if renal failure progresses rapidly after diagnosis. Denial and disbelief are usually pronounced, especially among the parents. Once the kidney failure is established and symptoms become progressively more distressing, the initiation of hemodialysis is usually perceived as a positive experience, and after experiencing initial concerns regarding the treatment, the child begins to feel better and parental anxiety is relieved for a time.

Initiating a hemodialysis regimen is a traumatic and anxiety-provoking experience for most children because it involves surgery for implantation of a graft, fistula, or peritoneal catheter. The initial experience with the hemodialysis procedure is frightening to most children. They need reassurance about the nature of the preparations for hemodialysis and the conduct of the treatment.

Both the graft and the fistula require needle insertions at each dialysis. The goal is to perform pain-free venipuncture. Using buffered lidocaine with a small-gauge needle (30 gauge) to anesthetize the area before venipuncture of the graft/fistula is one method. Using an anesthetizing topical preparation such as EMLA (eutectic mixture of local anesthetics [lidocaine and prilocaine]) 1 hour before venipuncture is another approach (see Pain Management, Chapter 44).

External dual-lumen venous access devices eliminate the need for needles but are more prone to infection and other central line complications.

Adolescents, with their increased need for independence and their urge for rebellion, usually adapt less well. They resent the control and enforced dependence imposed by the rigorous and unrelenting therapy program. They resent being dependent on hemodialysis technology, their parents, and the professional staff. Depression and/or hostility are common in adolescents undergoing hemodialysis.

The availability of home dialysis has offered a greater degree of freedom for persons undergoing long-term dialysis. The nurse is responsible for teaching the family about (1) the disease, its implications, and the therapeutic plan; (2) the possible psychologic effects of the disease and the treatment; and (3) the technical aspects of the procedure. The family learns to manage the various aspects of the dialysis procedure, how to maintain accurate records, and how to observe for signs of complications that need to be reported to the proper persons.

Body changes related to the disease process (e.g., skin color, growth retardation, and lack of sexual maturation) are stress provoking. Dietary restrictions are particularly burdensome for both children and parents. Children feel deprived when they are unable to eat foods previously enjoyed and that are unrestricted for other family members. Consequently, failure to cooperate may occur. Diet restrictions may be interpreted as punishment. Some children, unable to understand fully the purpose of restrictions, will sneak forbidden food items at every opportunity. Allowing children, especially adolescents, maximum participation in and responsibility for their own treatment program is helpful.

After months or years of dialysis, the parents and child feel anxiety associated with the prognosis and continued pressures of the treatment. The relentless need for treatment interferes with family plans. The time spent in transportation to and from the dialysis unit and the time spent undergoing dialysis treatments cut into time for outside activities, including school. Graft and fistula problems, as well as peritoneal catheter exit site infections, may develop and present a common source of aggravation (Family Focus box).

The possibility of renal transplantation often provides hope for relief from the rigors of hemodialysis and peritoneal dialysis. Most children and families respond well to a kidney transplant, and most children can be successfully rehabilitated.

The National Kidney Foundation* and other agencies provide a number of services and information for families of children with renal disease.

➤ Evaluation

The effectiveness of nursing interventions is determined by continual reassessment and evaluation of care based on the following observational guidelines:

1. Observe and interview family regarding their compliance with the medical and dietary regimen.
2. Monitor vital signs, growth measurements, laboratory reports, behavior, and appearance.
3. Observe and interview child and family regarding their feelings, concerns, and fears; observe reactions to therapies and prognosis.

The expected outcomes are described in the Nursing Care Plan.

*30 E. 33rd St., New York, NY 10016; (212) 889-2210 or 1-800-622-9010; website: www.kidney.org. In Canada: Kidney Foundation of Canada, 5160 Boulevard Decarie, Bureau 780, Montreal, Quebec H3X 2H9; (514) 369-4806.

Family Focus

FAMILY PRIORITIES

Families who have children with long-term chronic illnesses, such as end-stage renal disease, spend much time in hospitals, outpatient clinics, and primary health care facilities. When they miss appointments or respond less quickly than anticipated, sometimes they are quickly labeled "noncompliant." It is important to remember that families have to develop priorities for the unit as a whole. Sometimes the family may decide that it is more important for the parent to go to work or to attend a sibling's school performance than to attend an appointment scheduled for them by health care personnel. The chronically ill child cannot and should not always be the number-one priority for the family. The professional staff who works with the family can help the parents prioritize the needs of the ill child within the needs of the family constellation.

Teresa Hall, MS, RN
Hathaway Children's Services
Sylmar, CA

TECHNOLOGIC MANAGEMENT OF RENAL FAILURE

Dialysis

Dialysis is the process of separating colloids and crystalline substances in solution by the difference in their rate of diffusion through a semipermeable membrane. Methods of dialysis currently available for clinical management of renal failure are *peritoneal dialysis,* wherein the abdominal cavity acts as a semipermeable membrane through which water and solutes of small molecular size move by osmosis and diffusion according to their respective concentrations on either side of the membrane; and *hemodialysis,* in which blood is circulated outside the body through artificial membranes that permit a similar passage of water and solutes. A third type of dialysis is *hemofiltration,* in which blood filtrate is circulated outside the body by hydrostatic pressure exerted across a semipermeable membrane with simultaneous infusion of a replacement solution. Types of hemofiltration include *continuous arteriovenous hemofiltration (CAVH), continuous arteriovenous hemodialysis (CAVHD),* and *continuous venovenous hemofiltration (CVVH).* CAVH, CAVHD, and CVVH are used primarily in acute conditions, such as to remove fluid overload, rather than in ESRD.

Peritoneal dialysis is the preferred form of dialysis for children/parents who wish to remain independent, families who live a long distance from the medical center, and children who prefer fewer dietary restrictions and a gentler form of dialysis. Chronic peritoneal dialysis is most often performed at home. The two types of peritoneal dialysis are *continuous ambulatory peritoneal dialysis (CAPD)* and *continuous cycling peritoneal dialysis (CCPD).* In both methods, commercially available sterile dialysate is instilled into the peritoneal cavity through a surgically implanted indwelling catheter tunneled subcutaneously and sutured into place. The warmed solution is allowed to enter the peritoneal cavity by gravity and remains a variable length of time according to the procedure used. The care and management of the procedure are the responsibility of the parents of young children. Use of home health nurses to give parents respite from care has been initiated in some centers (Cascio et al, 1994). Older children and adolescents can carry out the procedure themselves, which provides them with some control and less dependency. This is especially important for adolescents.

NURSE ALERT • Observe for changes in the color of the dialysate draining from the child. The solution should be straw colored. If the color is pink, bright yellow, or brown, or if the solution is cloudy, notify the practitioner immediately.

Hemodialysis requires the creation of a vascular access and the use of special dialysis equipment—the hemodialyzer, or so-called artificial kidney. Vascular access may be one of three types: fistulas, grafts, or external vascular access devices. An *atriovenous fistula* is an access in which a vein and artery are connected surgically. The preferred site is the radial artery and a forearm vein. An alternative is the creation of a subcutaneous (internal) *arteriovenous graft* by anastomosing a segment of a saphenous vein autograft or a bovine arterial xenograft to the brachial artery and brachiocephalic vein, which produces dilation and thickening of the superficial vessels of the forearm to provide easy access for repeated venipuncture. Both the graft and the fistula require needle insertions at each dialysis.

Nursing Care Plan THE CHILD WITH CHRONIC RENAL FAILURE

NURSING DIAGNOSIS Risk for injury related to accumulated electrolytes and waste products

EXPECTED OUTCOME Child exhibits no evidence of accumulation of waste products and no evidence of injury.

Nursing Interventions/*Rationales*

Provide diet low in protein, potassium, sodium, and phosphorous; high in calories and calcium; and supplemented with essential amino acids as ordered *to reduce excretory demand on kidneys.*

Assist and monitor renal or peritoneal dialysis as prescribed *to maintain excretory function.*

Administer potassium-removing resins as prescribed *to reduce potassium levels;* antihypertensives *for hypertension;* diuretics *for edema;* phosphate binders *for hyperphosphatemia;* antiinfectives *for infection;* and antipruritics *for itching.*

Monitor for signs of accumulating waste products (e.g., elevated BUN, creatinine; hyperkalemia, hyperphosphatemia; muscle twitching; muscle cramps; anorexia, nausea, vomiting; hypertension; pruritis; yellowing skin; confusion, lethargy) *to ensure prompt treatment.*

Balance activity and rest and plan appropriate activities *to reduce fatigue and chances of injury.*

Provide meticulous skin care and avoid shearing and frictional forces *to reduce injury to skin.*

NURSING DIAGNOSIS Fluid volume excess related to failure of renal regulatory mechanisms

EXPECTED OUTCOME Child exhibits no evidence of increase in fluid accumulation.

Nursing Interventions/*Rationales*

Instruct child and family about fluid restrictions and strategize ways to maintain those restrictions (e.g., keeping mouth moist with hard candies, gum, ice chips; keeping lips lubricated; divide fluids into small, even quantities throughout day) *to decrease chances of fluid overload.*

Monitor I & O, weight changes, girth measurements *to track fluid accumulation.*

NURSING DIAGNOSIS Altered nutrition: less than body requirements related to restricted diet and loss of appetite

EXPECTED OUTCOME Child exhibits adequate and appropriate food intake.

Nursing Interventions/*Rationales*

Provide dietary instructions for child and family, including allowed foods, recipes, and menus *to increase successful use of restrictive diet and to reduce excretory demand on kidneys.*

NURSING DIAGNOSIS Body image/self-esteem disturbance related to altered appearance, chronic illness, frequent treatments, feelings of being different

EXPECTED OUTCOME Child exhibits signs of acceptance of self and of alteration in appearance; child exhibits signs of coping with disease process.

Nursing Interventions/*Rationales*

Relate to child on appropriate cognitive level, conveying an attitude of caring and acceptance *to encourage positive feelings about self;* serve as role model for others *to foster positive attitudes of acceptance toward child.*

Encourage child to verbalize feelings and perceptions about CRF (e.g., repeated treatments and hospitalizations, feelings of differentness, implications of functional limits, difficulty in making friends, views of self) *to facilitate coping and open expression of problems, fears, wants, wishes, and needs.*

Have child identify strengths, assets, and things he or she likes about self *to increase positive feelings about self and abilities.*

Support positive coping behaviors.

Involve child in care and management of disease *to promote a sense of control, independence, and self-esteem.*

Introduce child to other children who have similar disabilities; arrange for support groups for child and parents *to increase coping skills.*

Refer child for counseling if needed *to enhance adaptation.*

Encourage use of regular hygiene and grooming practices *to promote positive appearance.*

NURSING DIAGNOSIS Impaired social interaction related to repeated hospitalizations, confinement, activity intolerance

EXPECTED OUTCOME Child engages in appropriate family and peer interactions.

Nursing Interventions/*Rationales*

Encourage regular school attendance and promote peer contacts *to provide opportunity to develop and maintain peer relationships.*

Encourage selection of play activities and recreational outlets *that encourage interaction;* restrict time spent in solo activities *that promote social isolation.*

Encourage contact with peers and siblings by telephone or visit when hospitalized or confined *to maintain social interaction and reduce sense of isolation.*

Plan specific periods of developmentally appropriate diversional activity suited to child's physical condition and energy level *to decrease feelings of boredom and negative self-absorption.*

Nursing Care Plan THE CHILD WITH CHRONIC RENAL FAILURE—cont'd

NURSING DIAGNOSIS Altered family processes related to child with chronic illness

EXPECTED OUTCOME Family exhibits adaptation of usual roles and functions to accommodate special needs of child; family exhibits growth-promoting behaviors.

Nursing Interventions/*Rationales*

Provide opportunity for family to absorb and adjust to diagnosis (e.g., repeat information *to allow time for family to hear and understand;* encourage expression of concerns, fears, and feelings about diagnosis and potential impact *to facilitate adjustment;* identify support systems *to provide resources for coping*).

Assist family to understand expected treatment, rationales, and implications *to provide a sound basis for decision making.*

Explore family reaction to the child, assist them to achieve a realistic view of child's abilities and limitations, encourage family in attempts to promote child growth and development, have family emphasize what child can do, and explore ways for family to include child in family activities *to help family increase abilities to cope with and incorporate child into family structure.*

Arrange for and participate in family conferences *to provide forum for communication, mutual goal setting, and effective strategizing.*

Have parents spend special time with siblings *so that they do not feel neglected or left out.*

Identify additional resource systems (e.g., relatives, friends, church, health care services, community programs) and strategize with family about making good use of these systems *to develop broad base of support.*

Provide a system of ongoing follow-up and evaluation *to ensure long-term adaptation to challenges presented to family functioning by a child with chronic disease.*

For external vascular access devices, percutaneous catheters are inserted in the femoral, subclavian, or internal jugular veins, even in very small children. A more permanent form of external access is available via a central catheter inserted surgically into the subclavian vein or internal jugular vein. This catheter has a dual lumen, which allows differentiation between arterial and venous blood. Catheters eliminate the need for skin punctures but require some home care.*

Hemodialysis is best suited to children who do not have someone in the family who is capable of learning to perform home dialysis; and to those children who live close to a dialysis center. The procedure is usually performed three times a week for 4 to 6 hours, depending on the size of the child. Hemodialysis achieves rapid correction of fluid and electrolyte abnormalities but can cause problems in association with this rapid change, such as muscle cramping and hypotension. Disadvantages include school absence during dialysis and strict fluid and dietary restrictions between dialysis sessions. Boredom for the child and family is often a problem during dialysis, and planned quiet activities should be introduced (Fig. 50-3).

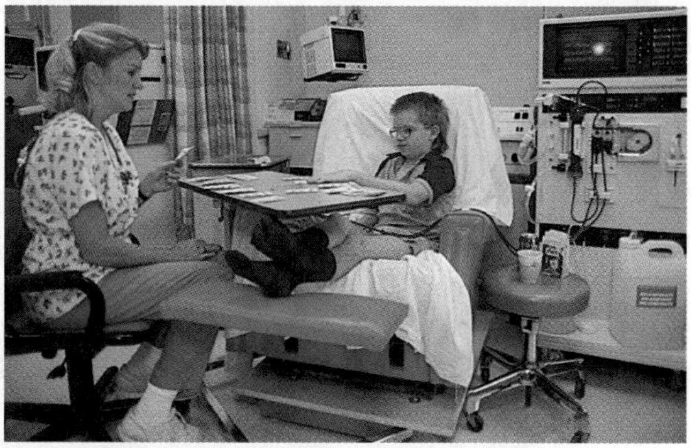

FIG. 50-3 • Diversional activities help lessen the boredom children can experience during hemodialysis.

Most children show rapid clinical improvement with the implementation of dialysis, although it is directly related to the duration of uremia before dialysis and the extent to which dietary regulations are followed. Growth rate and skeletal maturation improve, but recovery of normal growth occurs infrequently. In many cases, sexual development, although delayed, progresses to completion.

Transplantation

Renal transplantation is now an acceptable and effective means of therapy in the pediatric age group. Although peritoneal dialysis and hemodialysis are life preserving, both require major alterations in lifestyle. Transplantation offers the opportunity for a relatively normal life and is the preferred form of treatment for children with CRF. Primary or preemptive transplants maintain the greatest amount of normalcy in the family's life.

Kidneys for transplant are available from two sources: a *living related donor (LRD),* usually a parent or a sibling; or a *cadaver donor (CAD),* wherein the family of a dead or brain-dead patient consents to donation of a healthy kidney. Retransplantation occurs commonly.

The primary goal in transplantation is the long-term survival of grafted tissue by securing tissue that is antigenically similar to that of the recipient and by suppressing the recipient's immune mechanism. The immunosuppressant therapy of choice has been corticosteroids (Prednisone) in conjunction with cyclosporine and azathioprine. Other therapies include antilymphoblast globulin or monoclonal antibodies. New im-

*Community and home care instructions on central venous catheters are available in Wong DL, Hess CS: ***Wong and Whaley's clinical manual of pediatric nursing,*** ed 5, St. Louis, 2000, Mosby.

munosuppressant medications are rapidly coming into clinical trials and into use in large transplant centers. It is important for the nurse to learn about the medications and their side effects used in the antirejection protocol(s). Because the immunosuppressant medications are taken indefinitely, transplant patients experience many side effects of the drugs, including hypertension, growth retardation, cataracts, risk of infection, obesity, characteristics of Cushing syndrome, and hirsutism.

Rejection of the transplanted kidney is the most common cause of transplant failure. Rejection is treated aggressively with immunosuppressant medications and can often be reversed. Some patients do not respond to treatment of acute rejection or develop chronic rejection and must eventually return to dialysis or undergo another kidney transplant.

NURSE ALERT • The child with a recent kidney transplant (i.e., within a few days) or one who was grafted approximately 6 months previously who exhibits any of the following should be evaluated immediately for possible rejection:

Fever
Swelling and tenderness over graft area
Diminished urine output
Elevated blood pressure

Key Points

- Common inflammatory disorders of the genitourinary tract include urinary tract infection, nephrotic syndrome, and acute glomerulonephritis.
- Management of urinary tract infections is directed at eliminating infection, detecting and correcting functional or anatomic abnormalities, preventing recurrences, and preserving renal function.
- Vesicoureteral reflux is the retrograde flow of bladder urine into the ureters.
- Obstructive uropathy is a result of structural or functional abnormalities of the urinary system that obstruct the normal flow of urine.
- The more common defects of the genitourinary tract include phimosis, cryptorchidism, inguinal hernia, hydrocele, and hypospadias.
- Body-image concerns and castration anxiety are particularly intense in children with defects in the genital area.
- Nephrotic syndrome is characterized by increased glomerular permeability to protein, with massive urinary loss of protein resulting in hypoproteinemia and edema.
- Management of nephrotic syndrome is aimed at reducing excretion of protein, reducing or preventing fluid retention by tissues, and preventing infection and other complications.
- Common features of acute glomerulonephritis are oliguria, edema, hypertension, circulatory congestion, hematuria, and proteinuria.
- Therapeutic management of acute glomerulonephritis is maintenance of fluid balance, treatment of hypertension, and antibiotic therapy.
- Management of hemolytic-uremic syndrome is aimed at control of complications and hematologic manifestations of renal failure.
- Wilms tumor is the most common malignant neoplasm of the kidney in infants and children.
- In acute renal failure, management is directed at determining treatment of the underlying cause, management of complications of renal failure, and supportive therapy.
- Abnormalities in chronic renal failure are waste product retention, water and sodium retention, hyperkalemia, acidosis, calcium and phosphorus disturbance, anemia, and growth disturbances.
- The types of dialysis used in end-stage renal disease are peritoneal dialysis and hemodialysis.
- When the child will need home dialysis, the nurse educates the family about the disease, its implications, the therapeutic plan, possible psychologic effects of the disease, and the treatment and technical aspects of the procedure.
- The major concerns in renal transplantation are tissue matching and prevention of rejection, psychologic concerns involve self-image as related to possible body changes as a result of the effects of corticosteroid therapy.

References

American Academy of Pediatrics: Task Force on Circumcision, *Pediatrics* 103(3):686-693, 1999.

Benfield MR et al: The 1997 Annual Renal Transplantation in Children Report of the North American Pediatric Renal Transplant Cooperative Study (NAPRTCS), *Pediatr Transplant* 3(2):152-167, 1999.

Brandt et al: Escherichia coli 0 157:H7-associated hemolytic-uremic syndrome after ingestion of contaminated hamburgers, *J Pediatr* 125(4):519-526, 1994.

Cascio C et al: Use of private duty nurses for daily CCPD and family relief in pediatric PD patients, *Adv Perit Dial* 10:304-306, 1994.

Fleet JC: New support for a folk remedy: cranberry juice reduces bacteriuria and pyuria in elderly women, *Nutr Rev* 52(5):168-170, 1994.

Green D: Wilms tumor. In Pizzo PA, Poplack DP, editors: *Principles and practices of pediatric oncology,* ed 3, Philadelphia, 1997, JB Lippincott.

Kass E: Timing of elective surgery on the genitalia of male children with particular reference to the risks, benefits, and psychological effects of surgery and anesthesia, *Pediatrics* 97(4):590-594, 1996.

Kuzminski LN: Cranberry juice and urinary tract infections: is there a beneficial relationship? *Nutr Rev* 54(11, pt 2):587-590, 1996.

Laine J et al: Pediatric kidney transplantation, *Ann Med* 30(1):45-57, 1998.

Petruzzi MJ, Green DM: Wilms' tumor, *Pediatr Clin North Am* 44(4):939-952, 1997.

Schaefer F: Long-term experience with growth hormone treatment in children with chronic renal failure, *Perit Dial Int* 19(suppl 2):S467-S472, 1999.

Steiber AL: Clinical indicators associated with poor oral intake of patients with chronic renal failure, *J Ren Nutr* 9(2):84-88, 1999.

Suthanthiran M, Strom TB: Renal transplantation, *N Engl J Med* 331(6):365-375, 1994.

CHAPTER 51

Cerebral Dysfunction

http://www.harcourthealth.com/MERLIN/Wong/maternal/

Learning Objectives

On completion of this chapter the reader will be able to:

- Describe the various modalities for assessment of cerebral function.
- Differentiate between the stages of consciousness.
- Formulate a plan of care for the unconscious child.
- Distinguish between the types of head injuries and the serious complications.
- Describe the nursing care of a child with a tumor of the central nervous system.
- Outline a plan of care for the child with bacterial meningitis.
- Differentiate between the various types of seizure disorders.
- Demonstrate an understanding of the manifestations of a seizure disorder and the management of a child with such a disorder.
- Describe the preoperative and postoperative care of a child with hydrocephalus.

CEREBRAL DYSFUNCTION

Assessment of Cerebral Function

Most of the information about the status of the brain is obtained by indirect measurements. Some of these measurements are discussed elsewhere in relation to numerous aspects of child care (e.g., as part of assessments of health [Chapter 35], newborn status [Chapter 36], mental retardation [Chapter 42], hypoxic injury [cerebral palsy, Chapter 55], and attainment of developmental milestones at each stage of development). Because increased intracranial pressure and altered states of consciousness have such prominent places in neurologic dysfunction, they are described here, followed by techniques for neurologic assessment and diagnostic tests.

General Aspects. Children younger than 2 years require special evaluation because they are unable to respond to directions designed to elicit specific neurologic responses. Early neurologic responses in infants are primarily reflexive; these responses are gradually replaced by meaningful movement in the characteristic cephalocaudal direction of development. This evidence of progressive maturation reflects more extensive myelinization and changes in neurochemical and electrophysiologic properties.

Most information about infants and small children is gained by observing their spontaneous and elicited reflex responses as they develop increasingly complex locomotor and fine motor skills and by eliciting progressively sophisticated communicative and adaptive behaviors. Delay or deviation from expected milestones helps identify high risk children. Persistence or reappearance of reflexes that normally disappear indicates a pathologic condition. In evaluating the infant or young child, it is also important to obtain the pregnancy and delivery history to determine the possible effect of intrauterine environmental influences known to affect the orderly maturation of the central nervous system (CNS). These influences include maternal infections, chemicals, trauma, and metabolic insults.

General aspects of assessment that provide clues to the etiology of dysfunction include:

Family history—Sometimes offers clues regarding possible genetic disorders with neurologic manifestations

Health history—May provide valuable clues regarding the cause of dysfunction (e.g., injury, short febrile illness, encounter with an animal or insect, ingestion of neurotoxic substances, inhalation of chemicals, past illness, or known diabetes mellitus)

Physical evaluation of infants—Includes observation of the following:

Size and shape of the head

Spontaneous activity and postural reflex activity

Sensory responses

- Attitude—normal flexed posture, extreme extension, opisthotonos, and hypotonia
- Symmetry in movement of extremities
- Excessive tremulousness or frequent twitching movements
- Altered expiratory cycle:
  - Prolonged apnea
  - Ataxic breathing
  - Paradoxic chest movement
  - Hyperventilation
- Skin and hair texture
- Distinctive facial features
- Presence of a high-pitched, piercing cry
- Abnormal eye movements
- Inability to suck or swallow
- Lip smacking
- Asymmetric contraction of facial muscles
- Yawning (may indicate cranial nerve involvement)
- Muscular activity and coordination
- Level of development

Increased Intracranial Pressure (ICP). The brain, tightly enclosed in the solid bony cranium, is well protected but highly vulnerable to pressure that may accumulate within the enclosure. Its total volume—brain, cerebrospinal fluid (CSF), and blood—must remain approximately the same at all times. A change in the proportional volume of one of these components (e.g., increase or decrease in intracranial blood) must be accompanied by a compensatory change in another. In this way the volume and pressure normally remain constant. Examples of compensatory changes are reduction in blood volume, decrease in CSF production, increase in CSF absorption, or shrinkage of brain mass by displacement of intracellular and extracellular fluid. Children with open fontanels compensate by skull expansion and widened sutures. However, at any age the capacity for spatial compensation is limited. An increase in ICP may be caused by tumors or other space-occupying lesions, accumulation of fluid within the ventricular system, bleeding, or edema of cerebral tissues. Once compensation is exhausted, any further increase in volume will result in a rapid rise in ICP.

Early signs and symptoms of increased ICP are often subtle and assume many patterns (Box 51-1). As pressure increases, signs and symptoms become more pronounced, and the level of consciousness deteriorates.

Box 51-1

Clinical Manifestations of Increased Intracranial Pressure in Infants and Children

INFANTS

Tense, bulging fontanel; lack of normal pulsations
Separated cranial sutures
Macewen sign (cracked-pot sound on percussion)
Irritability
High-pitched cry
Increased occipitofrontal circumference
Distended scalp veins
Changes in feeding
Cries when held or rocked
Setting-sun sign

CHILDREN

Headache
Nausea
Vomiting—often without nausea
Diplopia, blurred vision
Seizures

PERSONALITY AND BEHAVIOR SIGNS

Irritability (toddlers), restlessness
Indifference, drowsiness, or lack of interest
Decline in school performance
Diminished physical activity and motor performance
Increased complaints of fatigue, tiredness; increased time devoted to sleep
Significant weight loss possible from anorexia and vomiting
Memory loss if pressure is markedly increased
Inability to follow simple commands
Progression to lethargy and drowsiness

LATE SIGNS

Lowered level of consciousness
Decreased motor response to command
Decreased sensory response to painful stimuli
Alterations in pupil size and reactivity
Decerebrate or decorticate posturing
Cheyne-Stokes respirations
Papilledema

Altered States of Consciousness. *Consciousness* implies awareness—the ability to respond to sensory stimuli and have subjective experiences. There are two components of consciousness: *alertness,* an arousal-waking state, including the ability to respond to stimuli; and *cognitive power,* including the ability to process stimuli and produce verbal and motor responses.

An altered state of consciousness usually refers to varying states of unconsciousness that may be momentary or may extend for hours, for days, or indefinitely. *Unconsciousness* is depressed cerebral function—the inability to respond to sensory stimuli and have subjective experiences. *Coma* is defined as a state of unconsciousness from which the patient cannot be aroused even with powerful stimuli.

Level of Consciousness (LOC). Assessment of LOC remains the earliest indicator of improvement or deterioration in neurologic status. LOC is determined by observations of the child's responses to the environment. Other diagnostic tests, such as motor activity, reflexes, and vital signs, are more variable and do not necessarily directly parallel the depth of the comatose state. The most consistently used terms are described in Box 51-2.

Coma Assessment. Several scales have been devised in an attempt to standardize the description and interpretation of the degree of depressed consciousness. The most popular of these is the *Glasgow Coma Scale (GCS),* which consists of a three-part assessment: eye opening, verbal response, and motor response (Fig. 51-1). When LOC is being assessed in young children, it is often useful to have a parent present to help elicit a desired response. An infant or child may not respond in an unfamiliar environment or to unfamiliar voices. Children older than 3 years should be able to give their name, although they may not be cognizant of place or time.

Numeric values are assigned to the levels of response in each category, and the sum of these numeric values provides an objective measure of the patient's LOC. The lower the score, the

Box 51-2
Levels of Consciousness

Full consciousness—Awake and alert; oriented to time, place, and person—behavior appropriate for age
Confusion—Impaired decision making
Disorientation—Disorientation to time and place, decreased level of consciousness
Lethargy—Limited spontaneous movement, sluggish speech
Obtundation—Arousable with stimulation
Stupor—Remains in a deep sleep, responsive only to vigorous and repeated stimulation
Coma—No motor or verbal response to noxious (painful) stimuli
Persistent vegetative state (PVS)—The permanently lost function of the cerebral cortex—eyes follow objects only by reflex or when attracted to the direction of loud sounds; all four limbs are spastic but can withdraw from painful stimuli; hands show reflexive grasping and groping; the face can grimace, some food may be swallowed, and the child may groan or cry but utter no words.

Modified from Hazinski MF, editor: *Care of the critically ill child*, ed 2, St Louis, 1992, Mosby.

deeper the coma. A person with an unaltered LOC would score the highest, 15; a score of 7 or below is generally accepted as a definition of coma; the lowest score, 3, indicates deep coma. In cases of irreversible coma, the Task Force for the Determination of Brain Death in Children has established physical examination criteria.

NURSE ALERT • Lack of response to painful stimuli is abnormal and is reported immediately.

Neurologic Examination. The purpose of the neurologic examination is to establish an accurate, objective baseline of neurologic information. It is essential that the neurologic examination be documented in a fashion that can be reproduced by others. Descriptions of behaviors should be simple, objective, and easily interpreted: "Drowsy but awake and conversationally rational/oriented"; "Sleepy but arousable with vigorous physical stimuli. Pressure to nail base of right hand results in upper extremity flexion/lower extremity extension."

Vital Signs. Pulse, respiration, and blood pressure provide information regarding the adequacy of circulation and the possible underlying cause of altered consciousness. Autonomic activity is most intensively disturbed in deep coma and in brainstem lesions.

Body temperature is often elevated, and sometimes the elevation may be extreme. Coma of a toxic origin may produce hypothermia. High temperature is most commonly a sign of an acute infectious process or heat stroke but may be caused by ingestion of some drugs (especially salicylates, alcohol, and barbiturates) or intracranial bleeding, especially subarachnoid hemorrhage. A fever sometimes follows a cerebral seizure.

The *pulse* is variable and may be rapid, slow and bounding, or feeble. *Blood pressure* may be normal, elevated, or at shock levels. The Cushing reflex or pressor response, which causes a slowing of the pulse and an increase in blood pressure, is uncommon in children; when it occurs, it is a very late sign. Vital signs are also affected by medications. For assessment purposes,

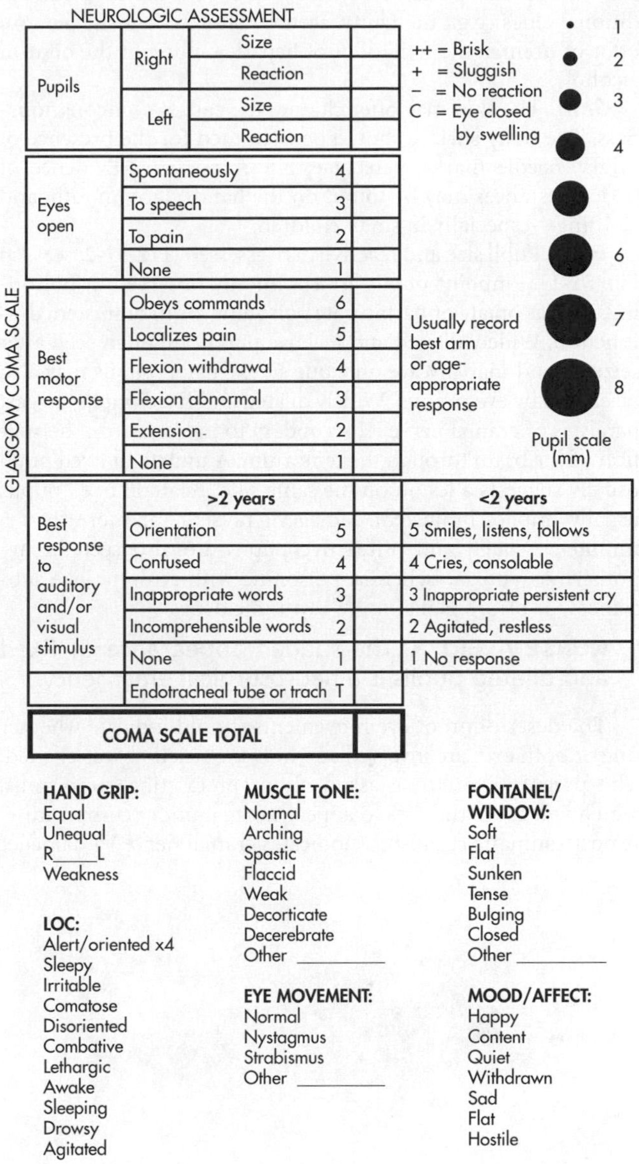

FIG. 51-1 • Pediatric coma scale.

changes in pulse and blood pressure are more important than whether they increase or decrease.

Respirations are often slow, deep, and irregular. Slow, deep breathing is often seen in the heavy sleep caused by sedatives, after seizures, or in cerebral infections. Slow, shallow breathing may result from sedatives or opioids (narcotics). Hyperventilation (deep and rapid respirations) is usually a result of metabolic acidosis or abnormal stimulation of the respiratory center in the medulla caused by salicylate poisoning, hepatic coma, or Reye syndrome.

Breathing patterns have been described with a number of terms (e.g., apneustic, cluster, ataxic, Cheyne-Stokes). However, it is better to describe what is being observed rather than placing a label on it. The terms are often used and interpreted incorrectly. Periodic or irregular breathing is an ominous sign of brainstem (especially medullary) dysfunction that often precedes complete apnea. The *odor* of the breath may provide additional clues (e.g., the fruity, acetone odor of ketosis; the foul odor of uremia; the fetid odor of hepatic failure; or the odor of alcohol).

Skin. The skin may offer clues to the cause of unconsciousness. The body surface should be examined for the presence of injury, needle marks, petechiae, bites, and ticks. Evidence of toxic substances may be found on the hands, face, mouth, and clothing—especially in small children.

Eyes. Pupil size and reactivity are assessed (Fig. 51-2; see also Fig. 51-1). Pinpoint pupils are commonly observed in poisoning, such as opiate or barbiturate poisoning, or in brainstem dysfunction. Widely dilated and reactive pupils are often seen after seizures and may involve only one side. Dilated pupils may also be caused by eye trauma. Widely dilated and fixed pupils suggest paralysis of cranial nerve III secondary to pressure from herniation of the brain through the tentorium. A unilateral fixed pupil usually suggests a lesion on the same side. Bilateral fixed pupils usually implies brainstem damage if present for more than 5 minutes. Dilated and unreactive pupils are also seen in hypothermia, anoxia, ischemia, poisoning with atropine-like substances, or prior instillation of mydriatic drugs.

NURSE ALERT • The sudden appearance of fixed and dilated pupils is a neurosurgical emergency.

The description of eye movements should indicate whether one or both eyes are involved and how the reaction was elicited. The parents should be asked about preexisting strabismus, which will cause the eyes to appear normal under compromise. A posttraumatic strabismus indicates cranial nerve VI damage.

Special tests, usually performed by qualified persons, include the following:

Doll's head maneuver—Elicited by rotating the child's head quickly to one side and then to the other. Conjugate (paired or working together) movement of the eyes in the direction opposite to the head rotation is normal. Absence of this response suggests dysfunction of the brainstem or oculomotor nerve (cranial nerve III).

NURSE ALERT • Any tests that require head movement are not attempted until after cervical spine injury has been ruled out.

Caloric test, or oculovestibular response—Elicited with the child's head up by irrigating the external auditory canal with ice water, which normally causes conjugate movement of the eyes toward the side of stimulation. This is lost when the pontine centers are impaired, thus providing important information in assessment of the comatose patient.

NURSE ALERT • The caloric test is painful and is never performed on a child who is awake or who has a ruptured tympanic membrane.

Funduscopic examination—Reveals additional clues. If papilledema develops at all, it will not be evident early in the course of unconsciousness because it takes 24 to 48 hours for papilledema to develop. The presence of preretinal (subhyaloid) hemorrhages in children is almost invariably a result of acute trauma with intracranial bleeding, usually subarachnoid or subdural hemorrhage.

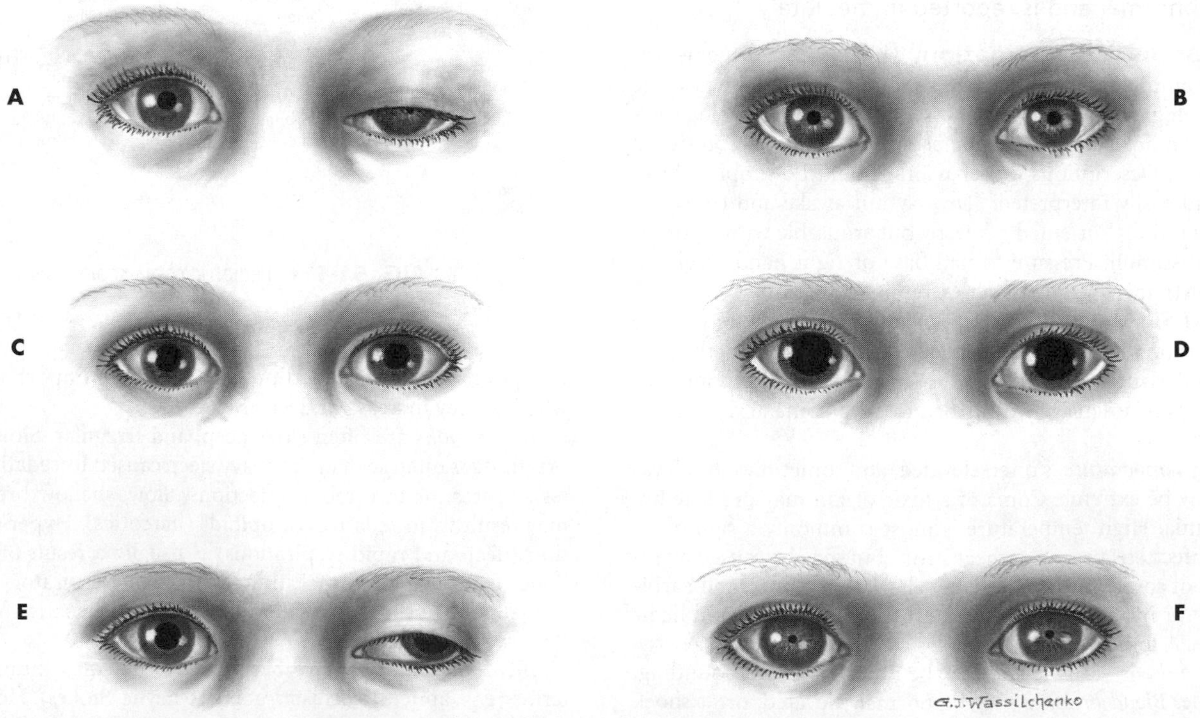

FIG. 51-2 • Variations in pupil size with altered states of consciousness. **A,** Ipsilateral pupillary constriction with slight ptosis. **B,** Bilateral small pupils. **C,** Midposition, light fixed to all stimuli. **D,** Bilateral dilated and fixed pupils. **E,** Dilated pupils, left eye abducted with ptosis. **F,** Pinpoint pupils.

Motor Function. Observing spontaneous activity, posture, and response to painful stimuli provides clues to the location and extent of cerebral dysfunction. Even subtle movements (e.g., the outward rotation of a hip) should be noted, and the child should be observed for other signs. Asymmetric movements of the limbs or absence of movement suggests paralysis. In hemiplegia the affected limb lies in external rotation and will fall uncontrollably when lifted and allowed to drop. These observations should be described rather than labeled.

In the deeper comatose states there is little or no spontaneous movement, and the musculature tends to be flaccid. There is considerable variability in the motor behavior in lesser degrees of coma. For example, the child may be relatively immobile or restless and hyperkinetic; muscle tone may be increased or decreased. Tremors, twitching, and spasms of muscles are common observations. The patient may display purposeless plucking or tossing movements. Combative or negativistic behavior is not uncommon. Hyperactivity is more common in acute febrile and toxic states than in cases of increased ICP. Seizures are common in children and may be present in coma from any cause. Any repetitive or seizure movements should be described.

Posturing. Because cortical control over motor function is lost in brain dysfunction, primitive postural reflexes emerge. These are evident in posturing and motor movements directly related to the area of the brain involved. *Decorticate posturing* (Fig. 51-3, *A*) is seen when there is severe dysfunction of the cerebral cortex. Typical decorticate posturing includes adduction of the arms at the shoulders, flexion of the arms on the chest with the wrists flexed and the hands fisted, and extension and adduction of the lower extremities. *Decerebrate posturing* (Fig. 51-3, *B*), a sign of dysfunction at the level of the midbrain, is characterized by rigid extension and pronation of the arms and legs. The posturing may not be evident when the child is quiet but can usually be elicited by applying painful stimuli, such as a blunt object pressed on the base of the nail.

A

B

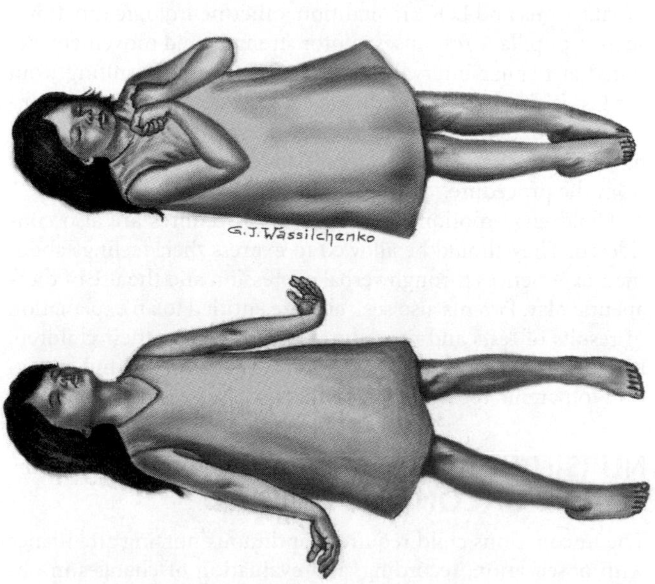

FIG. 51-3 • **A,** Decorticate posturing. **B,** Decerebrate posturing.

Reflexes. Testing of some reflexes may be of limited value. In general, the corneal, pupillary, muscle-stretch, superficial, and plantar reflexes tend to be absent in deep coma. The state of reflexes is variable in lighter grades of unconsciousness and depends on the underlying pathologic process and the location of the lesion. Absence of corneal reflexes and presence of a tonic neck reflex are associated with severe brain damage. The Babinski reflex (see Extremities, Chapter 35) may be of value if it is found to be present consistently in children older than 18 months. A positive Babinski reflex is significant in assessment of pyramidal tract lesions when it is unilateral and associated with other pyramidal signs.

NURSE ALERT • Three key reflexes that demonstrate neurologic health in young infants are the Moro, tonic neck, and withdrawal reflexes.

Special Diagnostic Procedures. Numerous diagnostic procedures are used for assessment of cerebral function. Laboratory tests that may help to determine the cause of unconsciousness include blood glucose, urea nitrogen, and electrolyte (pH, sodium, potassium, chloride, calcium, and bicarbonate) tests; clotting studies, hematocrit, and a complete blood count; liver function tests; blood cultures if there is fever; and sometimes studies to detect lead or other toxic substances, such as drugs.

Highly sophisticated tests are carried out with specialized equipment by skilled personnel. Most of these tests are outlined in Box 51-3. Because such tests can be threatening to children, a child will need preparation for, and support and reassurance during, the tests (see Preparation for Procedures, Chapter 45).

Children who are old enough to understand require careful explanation of the procedure, why it is being done, what they will experience, and how they can help. School-age children usually appreciate a more detailed description of why contrast material is injected. The importance of lying still for tests needs to be stressed. Children unfamiliar with the machines can be shown a picture beforehand. Although radiographic examinations are not painful, the machinery is often so frightening in appearance that the child protests because of anxiety.

Tests such as computed tomography (CT) and magnetic resonance imaging (MRI) require that children be immobilized. Chin and cheek pads are sometimes used to prevent the slightest head movement, and straps are applied to the body to prevent a slight change in body position. The nurse can explain these events to a frightened child by comparing them to an astronaut's preparation for spaceflight. It is very important to emphasize to the child that at no time is the procedure painful.

The nurse should not expect cooperation from a young child. Conscious sedation may be required. Drugs commonly used are intravenous (IV) pentobarbital or oral chloral hydrate. Chloral hydrate may be the drug of choice for children younger than 2 years. The suggested oral dosage is (Barkovich, 1995):

- $<$10 kg: 75 to 100 mg/kg, or
- $>$10 kg: 75 to 100 mg/kg plus 50 mg/kg for each kilogram of weight $<$10 kg (to a maximum dose of 2 g)
- If child is still awake after 20 minutes, supplementary doses may be given up to a total dose of 2 g.
- The drug should be given 35 to 45 minutes before the anticipated imaging time.

It is helpful for nurses to become acquainted with the equipment and the general environment in which the test will take

Box 51-3

Procedures Used in Cerebral Assessment

LUMBAR PUNCTURE (LP)
Diagnostic: measures spinal fluid pressure, obtains cerebrospinal fluid (CSF) for visualization and laboratory analysis

SUBDURAL TAP
Helps rule out subdural effusions
Relieves intracranial pressure (ICP)

ELECTROENCEPHALOGRAPHY (EEG)
Measures electric activity of cerebral cortex
Detects electric abnormalities—diagnosis of seizures
Used to determine brain death

VIDEO EEG
Split-screen simultaneous visualization of whole-body, facial, and EEG recording

COMPUTED TOMOGRAPHY (CT) SCAN
Visualizes horizontal and vertical cross section of brain at any axis
Distinguishes density of various intracranial tissues and structures—congenital abnormalities, hemorrhage, tumors, and demyelinating and inflammatory processes

NUCLEAR BRAIN SCAN
Test material accumulates in areas where blood-brain barrier is defective
Identifies focal brain lesions (e.g., tumors, abscesses)
Positive uptake of material with encephalitis and subdural hematoma
Visualizes CSF pathways

TRANSILLUMINATION
Varying degrees of localized glowing may be seen in abnormal fluid accumulation in various areas of head

ECHOENCEPHALOGRAPHY
Identifies shifts in midline structures from their normal positions as a result of intracranial lesions
May show ventricular dilation

RADIOGRAPHY
Shows fractures, dislocations, spreading suture lines, and craniostenosis
Shows degenerative changes, bone erosion, and calcifications

MAGNETIC RESONANCE IMAGING (MRI)
Permits visualization of morphologic features of target structures
Permits tissue discrimination unavailable with many techniques

POSITRON EMISSION TRANSAXIAL TOMOGRAPHY (PETT) OR POSITRON EMISSION TOMOGRAPHY (PET)
Detects and measures such functions as blood volume and flow in brain, metabolic activity, and biochemical changes within tissues

REAL-TIME ULTRASONOGRAPHY (RTUS)
Allows high-resolution anatomic visualization in variety of imaging planes

DIGITAL SUBTRACTION ANGIOGRAPHY (DSA)
Visualizes vasculature of target tissue
Visualizes finite vascular abnormalities

place so that they can better explain the procedure to children at their level of understanding. Equipment is often strange and ominous to a child and may be perceived as a frightening monster. They need constant reassurance from a trusted companion. Because children are particularly frightened of needles, they need to be informed of any medication or contrast media to be administered intravenously.

Physical preparation may involve administering a sedative or providing IV access for infusion of contrast material. If so, children should be given a local anesthetic (e.g., eutectic mixture of local anesthetic [EMLA]), before the IV line is placed, helped through the preparation and administration, and assured that someone will remain with them (if this is possible). Children will need continual support and reinforcement during procedures in which they remain conscious. Vital signs and physiologic response to the procedure are monitored throughout. Conscious sedation records become part of the child's chart. Many diagnostic procedures performed on an outpatient basis require sedation, and children need recovery time and observation. Written instructions should be reviewed with parents if the child is discharged to home after a procedure (Critical Thinking box).

Children who have undergone a procedure while under general anesthesia require postanesthesia care, including positioning to prevent aspiration of secretions and frequent assessment of vital signs and LOC. In addition, other neurologic functions, such as pupillary responses, motor strength, and movement, are tested at regular intervals. Any surgical wound resulting from the test is checked for bleeding, CSF leakage, and other complications. Children who undergo repeated subdural taps should have their hematocrit measured daily to detect any blood loss from the procedure.

Children's emotional reactions to procedures are also considered. They should be allowed to express their feelings about their experiences through verbal expression and the use of therapeutic play. Parents also seek and are entitled to an explanation of results of tests and procedures performed on their children. Nurses are in a unique position to provide support and education to parents regarding procedures.

NURSING CARE OF THE UNCONSCIOUS CHILD

The unconscious child requires continuous nursing attendance with observation, recording, and evaluation of changes in objective signs. These observations provide valuable information regarding the patient's progress. Often they serve as a guide to

Critical Thinking

CONSCIOUS SEDATION

Brian, 4 weeks old, is returned to his room after a CT scan to evaluate a seizure episode. On examination you find a sleepy infant who is arousable with vigorous stimulation and has pale, dusky skin and mucous membranes. The vital signs are temperature of 35.8°C (96.4°F), pulse of 110, respiratory rate of 20, and blood pressure of 82/40; the oxygen saturation is 89% to 92%. His weight is 5 kg, and he received 500 mg of chloral hydrate (<10 kg: 75-100 mg/kg dosage) as ordered before leaving for the CT. During the report the CT nurse reviews the conscious sedation record, and you note that it does not include the infant's temperature. An additional dosage of 250 mg of chloral hydrate was administered during the CT scan to achieve sleep for Brian. What is the best intervention?

First, Think About It . . .

- **What information are you using?**
- **What conclusions are you reaching?**

1. **Monitor the vital signs and cover the infant.**
2. **Place a radiant warmer over the infant and notify the physician.**
3. **Fill out a medication error report.**
4. **Allow the infant to sleep.**

The best response is 2. The information provided indicates that Brian is experiencing thermoregulation problems compounded by the administration of too much chloral hydrate for conscious sedation. You may appropriately conclude that the maximum dosage of sedation was exceeded for this infant. Conscious sedation flow sheets to record vital signs often do not include temperature measurement, which is an essential observation in infants because of their inability to maintain body temperature.

diagnosis and treatment. Therefore careful and detailed observations are essential for the patient's welfare. In addition, vital functions must be maintained and complications prevented through conscientious and meticulous nursing care. The outcome of unconsciousness may be early complete recovery, death within a few hours or days, persistent and permanent unconsciousness, or recovery with varying degrees of residual mental and/or physical disability. The outcome and recovery of the unconscious child may depend on the level of nursing care and observational skills.

Emergency measures are directed toward ensuring a patent airway, treatment of shock, and reduction of ICP (if present). Delayed treatment often leads to increased damage. As soon as emergency measures have been implemented—in many cases concurrently—therapies for specific causes are begun. Because nursing care is closely related to medical management, both are considered here.

➤ Assessment

Continual observation of LOC, pupillary reaction, and vital signs is essential to management of CNS disorders. Regular assessment of neurologic signs is a vital part of nursing comatose children. Vital signs are taken and recorded regularly. The frequency depends on the cause of coma, the status, and the progression of cerebral involvement. Intervals may be as short as every 15 minutes or as long as every 2 hours. Significant alterations are reported immediately. Temperature is taken every 2 to 4 hours, depending on the patient's condition.

An elevated temperature may occur in children with CNS dysfunction; therefore a light covering is sufficient. Vigorous efforts, such as tepid sponge baths or application of a hypothermia blanket, are needed to prevent brain damage if the child's temperature exceeds 40° C (104° F) rectally.

The LOC is assessed periodically, including size, equality, and reaction of pupils to light, as well as signs of meningeal irritation, such as nuchal rigidity. This also includes response to vocal commands, spontaneous behavior, resistance to care, and response to painful stimuli. Motions of any type, changes in muscle tone or strength, and body position are noted. Seizure activity is described according to the type and length of seizure and body areas involved (see Box 51-13). An antiepileptic drug such as phenytoin (Dilantin) or phenobarbital is ordered for control of seizure activity.

Pain management for the comatose child requires astute nursing observation and management. Signs of pain include changes in behavior (e.g., increased agitation and rigidity and alterations in physiologic parameters); usually increased heart rate, respiratory rate, and blood pressure; and decreased oxygen saturation. Because these findings are not specific for pain, the nurse should observe for their appearance during times of induced or suspected pain and for their disappearance after the inciting procedure or the administration of analgesia. A pain assessment record should be used to document indications of pain and the effectiveness of interventions (see Pain Assessment, Chapter 44).

The use of opioids, such as morphine, to relieve pain is controversial because they may mask signs of altered consciousness or depress respirations. However, unrelieved pain activates the stress response, which can elevate ICP. To block the stress response, some authorities advocate the use of analgesics, sedatives, and in some cases such as head injury, paralyzing agents via continuous IV infusion. A commonly used combination is fentanyl, midazolam (Versed), and vecuronium. If there are concerns about assessing the LOC or respiratory depression, naloxone can be used to reverse the opioid effects. Acetaminophen and codeine may also be effective analgesics for mild to moderate pain. Regardless of which drugs are used, adequate dosage and regular administration are essential to provide optimum pain relief (see Pain Management, Chapter 44).

Other measures to relieve discomfort include providing a quiet, dimly lit environment; limiting the number of visitors; preventing any sudden, jarring movement, such as banging into the bed; and preventing an increase in ICP. The last is most effectively achieved by proper positioning and prevention of straining, such as during coughing, vomiting, or defecating.

NURSE ALERT • When opioids are used, bowel elimination must be closely monitored because of the potential constipating effect. Stool softeners and laxatives should be given as needed to prevent constipation.

➤ Nursing Diagnoses

Based on a thorough assessment, several nursing diagnoses are identified. The more common diagnoses for the unconscious child are included in the Nursing Care Plan on pp. 1433-1434. Others may apply in specific situations.

➤ Plan of Care and Implementation

The goals for the unconscious child and the family include:

1. Child will maintain respiratory integrity.
2. Child will not experience increasing ICP.
3. Child will have basic needs (hygiene, nutrition, hydration, elimination) met.
4. Child will not experience complications of immobility.
5. Family will receive adequate support and education.

Respiratory Management. Respiratory effectiveness is the primary concern in the care of the unconscious child, and establishment of an adequate airway is always the first priority. Carbon dioxide has a potent vasodilating effect and will increase cerebral blood flow (CBF) and ICP. Cerebral hypoxia that lasts longer than 4 minutes nearly always causes irreversible brain damage.

NURSE ALERT • Respiratory obstruction and subsequent compromise lead to cardiac arrest. It is of the utmost importance to maintain an adequate, patent airway.

Children in lighter states of coma may be able to cough and swallow, but those in deeper states are unable to handle secretions, which tend to pool in the throat and pharynx. Dysfunction of cranial nerves IX and X places the child at risk for aspiration and cardiac arrest; therefore the child is positioned to prevent aspiration of secretions, and the stomach is emptied to reduce the likelihood of vomiting. In infants, blockage of air passages from secretions can happen in seconds. In addition, upper airway obstruction from laryngospasm is a common complication in comatose children.

An oral airway can be used for the child with a temporary loss of consciousness, such as after a contusion, seizure, or anesthesia. For children who remain unconscious for a time, a nasotracheal or orotracheal tube is inserted to maintain the open airway and facilitate removal of secretions. A tracheostomy is performed in cases in which laryngoscopy for introduction of an endotracheal tube would be difficult or dangerous. Suctioning is used only as needed to clear the airway, exerting care to prevent increasing ICP. Respiratory status is observed and evaluated regularly. Signs of respiratory embarrassment may be an indication for ventilatory assistance.

When the respiratory center is involved, mechanical ventilation is usually indicated (see Chapter 45). Blood gas analysis is performed regularly, and oxygen is administered when indicated. Moderately severe hypoxia and respiratory acidosis are often present but are not always evident from clinical manifestations. Hyperventilation commonly accompanies unconsciousness and may lead to respiratory alkalosis, or it may represent the body's attempt to compensate for metabolic acidosis. Therefore blood gas and pH determinations are essential guides for electrolyte therapy. Chest physiotherapy is carried out on a regular basis, and the child's position is changed at least every 2 hours to prevent pulmonary complications.

Intracranial Pressure Monitoring. Management of the child with increased ICP is possibly the most formidable task and the most controversial subject in pediatric critical care. It appears that the outcome in pediatric neurologic injury may reflect more the initial cerebral damage than subsequent intracranial hypertension. Of note, ICP gives little indication of the severity of the initial insult (Pople et al, 1995).

When increased ICP is a result of accumulation of CSF from obstruction of CSF flow, a ventricular tap will provide relief quickly and effectively. Evacuation of a hematoma reduces pressure from this source. Indications for inserting an ICP monitor are (1) GCS evaluation of less than 7, (2) GCS evaluation of less than 8 with respiratory assistance, (3) deterioration of condition, and (4) subjective judgment regarding clinical appearance and response.

Four major types of ICP monitors are (1) intraventricular catheter with fiberscopic sensors attached to a monitoring system, (2) subarachnoid bolt (Richmond screw), (3) epidural sensor, and (4) anterior fontanel pressure monitor. Transducers for both ventricular and subarachnoid monitoring should be set up without the use of a flush device. Direct ventricular pressure measurement remains the gold standard of ICP monitoring.

The catheter method involves introduction of a catheter into the lateral ventricle on the nondominant side, if known, or placement in the subdural space. The catheter has the advantage of providing a means of extraventricular (or continuous) drainage to reduce pressure. A drainage bag attached to the system is kept at the level of the ventricles and can be lowered to decrease ICP (Critical Thinking box).

NURSE ALERT • If the external ventricular drain (EVD) is unclamped for CSF drainage, carefully monitor the level of the collection container. If the container is too low, improper CSF decompression could lower ICP too rapidly, causing bleeding and pain.

With the bolt method the end of the bolt is placed into the subarachnoid space. The bolt cannot be adequately secured in a

Critical Thinking

HYDROCEPHALUS

Three-year-old Emma is 5 days postoperative for removal of a posterior fossa tumor. Although an external ventricular drain (EVD) was placed to treat her hydrocephalus, she continues to demonstrate signs of increased ICP, including holding the back of her head, anorexia, crying when moved or when strangers enter the room, and lethargy. On examination, fluid drainage is noted on the mother's clothes, and Emma is experiencing repetitive, rapid eyelid blinking. What is the best intervention?

First, Think About It . . .

- **What precise question are you trying to answer?**
- **What conclusions are you reaching?**

1. **Lower the EVD drain.**
2. **Check the EVD dressing site, perform a neurologic examination, and notify the practitioner.**
3. **Change the dressing to a transparent adhesive.**
4. **Request a CT scan.**

The best response is 2. Precisely, the question is whether the EVD is draining correctly. Your conclusion should be that it is not draining properly but is taking the path of least resistance through the insertion site. Lowering the EVD may cause rapid drainage of the CSF, resulting in subdural complications. The dressing may need to be changed to a clear adhesive so that the site can be observed. A CT scan may be required, but the priority is to stabilize Emma, who is demonstrating signs of increased ICP and cranial neuropathy.

small child's pliant skull, although special modifications have been developed for children younger than 6 years.

NURSE ALERT • The bolt is stabilized with dressings, but these are not changed or disturbed, even to check the site.

The placement of the bolt is not adjusted by anyone except the neurosurgeon who placed the device. The neurosurgeon is notified if a satisfactory waveform is not observed.

An epidural sensor can be placed between the dura and the skull through a burr hole and connected to a stopcock assembly and a transducer, which provides a readout of the pressure. Correlation of pressure readings is less invasive but may be inconsistent. In infants a fontanel transducer can be used to detect impulses from a pressure sensor and convert them to electrical energy. The electrical energy is then converted to visible waves or numeric readings on an oscilloscope. ICP measurement from the anterior fontanel is noninvasive but may prove to be inaccurate if the equipment is poorly placed or inconsistently recalibrated. The intraparenchymal pressure–monitoring device (e.g., Camino) is a result of fiberoptic technology and has a reliable performance.

ICP can be increased by instillation of solutions; therefore antibiotics are administered systemically if a positive CSF culture is obtained. However, IV ICP monitoring rarely causes infection. Because CSF is a body fluid, standard precautions are implemented according to hospital policy (see Infection Control, Chapter 45).

Nurses caring for patients with intracranial monitoring devices must be acquainted with the system, assist with insertion, interpret the monitor readings, and be able to distinguish between danger signals and mechanical dysfunction.

For increased ICP resulting from cerebral edema, several medical measures are available. Osmotic diuretics may provide rapid relief in emergency situations. Although their effect is transient, lasting only about 6 hours, they can be lifesaving in emergencies. These substances are rapidly excreted by the kidneys and carry with them large quantities of sodium and water. Mannitol (or sometimes urea) administered intravenously is the drug most commonly used for rapid reduction. The infusion is generally given slowly but may be pushed rapidly if there is herniation or impending herniation. Because of the profound diuretic effect of the drug, an indwelling catheter is inserted to ensure bladder emptying. Adrenocorticosteroids are not recommended for cerebral edema secondary to head trauma. $Pa{CO_2}$ should be maintained at 25 to 30 mm Hg to produce vasoconstriction, which reduces CBF, thereby decreasing ICP.

Nursing Activities. In cases of high levels of increased ICP, nursing procedures tend to trigger reactive pressure waves in many patients. For example, increased intrathoracic or abdominal pressure will be transmitted to the cranium. Particular care should be taken in positioning these patients to avoid neck vein compression, which may further increase ICP by interfering with venous return.

The child can be propped to one side or the other, and the use of an alternating-pressure mattress reduces the chance of prolonged pressure to vulnerable areas. Frequent clinical assessment of the child cannot be replaced by an ICP-monitoring device.

NURSE ALERT • The head of the bed is elevated 15 to 30 degrees, and the child is positioned so that the head is maintained in the midline to facilitate venous drainage and avoid jugular compression. Turning side to side is contraindicated because of the risk of jugular compression.

It is important to avoid activities that may increase ICP by causing pain or emotional stress. Gentle range-of-motion exercises can be carried out but should not be performed vigorously. Nontherapeutic touch can cause an increase in ICP. Any disturbing procedures to be performed should be scheduled to take advantage of therapies that reduce ICP, such as osmotherapy and sedation. Efforts are taken to minimize or eliminate environmental noise. Assessment and intervention to relieve pain are important nursing functions to decrease ICP. Individualizing nursing activities and minimizing environmental stimuli by decreasing noxious procedures help to control ICP (Vernon-Levett, 1998).

Suctioning. Suctioning and percussion are poorly tolerated and are therefore contraindicated unless there are concurrent respiratory problems. Hypoxia and the Valsalva maneuver associated with cough both acutely elevate ICP. Vibration, which does not increase ICP, accomplishes excellent results and should be tried first if treatment is needed. If suctioning is necessary, it should be brief and preceded by hyperventilation with 100% oxygen, which can be monitored during suctioning with a pulse oxygen sensor reading to determine oxygen saturation.

Nutrition and Hydration. Fluids and calories are supplied initially by the IV route (see Chapter 45). An IV infusion is started early, and the type of fluid administered is determined by the general condition of the patient. Fluid therapy requires careful monitoring and adjustment based on neurologic signs and electrolyte determinations. Often, comatose children are unable to cope with the same amounts of fluid they could tolerate at other times, and overhydration must be avoided to prevent fatal cerebral edema.

Later, nutrition is provided in a balanced formula given by nasogastric or gastrostomy tube. The nasogastric tube is usually taped in place with care to prevent pressure on the nares. Most children have continuous feedings, but if bolus feedings are used, the tube is rinsed with water after each feeding. Tubes are replaced according to unit policy. Nostrils are alternated with each replacement to prevent nasal irritation and pressure. Overfeeding should be avoided to prevent vomiting with its attendant danger of aspiration. Stomach contents are aspirated and measured before feeding to ascertain the amount remaining in the stomach. If the residual volume is excessive (depending on the size of the child), the dietitian and physician should be consulted regarding alteration of the formula composition to provide the needed calories and nutrients in a smaller volume. The aspirated contents should always be refed.

Hydration is maintained in the same manner. When cerebral edema is a threat, fluids may be restricted to reduce the chance of fluid overload. Skin and mucous membranes are examined for signs of dehydration. Observation for signs of altered fluid balance related to abnormal pituitary secretions is a part of nursing care.

Altered Pituitary Secretion. An altered ability to handle fluid loads is attributed in part to the syndrome of inappropriate antidiuretic hormone secretion (SIADH) and diabetes insipidus (DI) resulting from hypothalamic dysfunction (see Chapter 52). SIADH commonly accompanies CNS diseases such as head injury, meningitis, encephalitis, brain abscess, brain tumor, and subarachnoid hemorrhage. In the patient with SIADH, scant quantities of urine are excreted, electrolyte analysis reveals hyponatremia and hyposmolality, and manifestations of overhydration are evident. It is important to evaluate all parameters because the reduced urine output might be erroneously interpreted as a sign of dehydration.

The treatment of SIADH consists of restriction of fluids until serum electrolytes and osmolality return to normal levels. Because SIADH commonly occurs with meningitis in children, fluid restriction is often prescribed. Likewise, DI may occur after intracranial trauma. There is increased urine volume and the accompanying danger of dehydration (Table 51-1 compares fluid changes in SIADH and DI). Adequate replacement of fluids is essential, and observation of electrolyte balance is necessary to detect signs of hypernatremia and hyperosmolality. Exogenous vasopressin may be administered.

Medications. The cause of unconsciousness determines specific drug therapies. Children with infectious processes are given antibiotics appropriate to the disease and the infecting organism, and corticosteroids are prescribed for inflammatory conditions and edema. Cerebral edema is an indication for osmotherapy with osmotic diuretics. Sedatives or antiepileptics are prescribed for seizure activity (see p. 1456). Sedation in the combative child provides amnesic and anxiolytic properties in conjunction with a paralytic agent. The combination decreases ICP and allows treatment of cerebral edema. Usual drugs include morphine, midazolam (Versed), and pancuronium. Midazolam is attractive because of its short half-life.

Deep coma, induced by administration of barbiturates, is controversial in the management of ICP. Barbiturates are currently reserved for the reduction of increased ICP when all else has failed. Barbiturates decrease the cerebral metabolic rate for oxygen and protect the brain during times of reduced cerebral perfusion pressure (CPP). Barbiturate coma requires extensive monitoring, cardiovascular and respiratory support, and ICP monitoring to assess response to therapy. Paralyzing agents such as pancuronium (Pavulon) also may be needed to aid in performing diagnostic tests, improving effectiveness of therapy, and reducing risks of secondary complications. Elevation of ICP and/or heart rate of patients who are being given paralyzing agents or are under sedation may indicate the need for another dose of either or both medications.

Thermoregulation. Hyperthermia often accompanies cerebral dysfunction; if it is present, measures are implemented to reduce the temperature to prevent brain damage and to reduce metabolic demands generated by the increased body temperature. Antipyretics are the method of choice for fever reduction; cooling devices are used for hyperthermia. Laboratory tests and other methods are used in an attempt to determine the cause, if any, of the hyperthermia.

Elimination. A retention catheter is usually inserted in the acute phase, although diapers may be used and weighed to record urine output. The child who formerly had bowel and bladder control is generally incontinent. If the child remains comatose for a long period, the indwelling catheter may be removed and periodic bladder emptying accomplished by intermittent catheterization. Stool softeners are usually sufficient to maintain bowel function, but suppositories or enemas may be needed occasionally for adequate elimination and to prevent an impaction. The passage of liquid stool after a period of no bowel activity is usually a sign of an impaction. To avoid this preventable problem, daily recording of bowel activity is essential.

Hygienic Care. Routine measures for cleansing and maintaining skin integrity are an integral part of nursing care of the unconscious child. Skin folds require special attention to prevent excoriation. The child who is unable to move is prone to developing tissue breakdown and pressure necrosis; therefore the child may be placed on a pressure-reducing or pressure-relieving device to prevent pressure on prominent areas of the body. The goal is prevention by regular change of position and inspection of vulnerable areas, such as the ankle, trochanter, and shoulder. Because unconscious children undergo numerous invasive procedures, these skin sites require special assessment and intervention to promote healing and to prevent infection. Bed linen and any clothing are kept dry and free of wrinkles. If the child requires surgery or radiography, the nurse checks all dressings, bony sites, catheters, and IV access lines (see also Maintaining Healthy Skin, Chapter 45).

Mouth care is performed at least twice daily because the mouth tends to become dry or coated with mucus. The teeth are carefully brushed with a soft toothbrush or cleaned with gauze saturated with saline solution. Commercially prepared cleansing devices, such as Toothettes, are convenient for cleansing the mouth and teeth. Lips are coated with ointment or other preparations to protect them from drying, cracking, or blistering.

The deeply comatose child is also prone to eye irritation. The corneal reflexes are absent; therefore the eyes are easily irritated or damaged by linen, dust, or other substances that may come in contact with them. There is excessive dryness as a result of decreased secretions, especially if the child is undergoing osmotherapy to reduce or prevent brain edema, and incomplete closure of the eyes.

NURSE ALERT • The eyes should be examined regularly and carefully for early signs of irritation or inflammation. Artificial tears (methylcellulose) are placed in the eyes every 1 to 2 hours. Sometimes eye dressings may be needed to protect the eyes from possible damage.

The hair is combed and styled neatly. Long hair is usually braided and secured with rubber bands. The scalp should be kept clean with dry or wet shampoos as needed. The child's head may be shaved for tests or surgical procedures. If so, the hair is saved, if possible, and given to the family.

TABLE 51-1
Effects of Altered Pituitary Secretion

Measurement	DI	SIADH
Urine output	Increased	Decreased
Specific gravity	Decreased	Increased
Serum sodium	Increased (hypernatremia)	Decreased (hyponatremia)

DI, Diabetes insipidus; *SIADH,* syndrome of inappropriate antidiuretic hormone secretion.

Positioning and Exercise. The unconscious child is positioned to prevent aspiration of saliva, nasogastric secretions, and vomitus and to minimize ICP. The head of the bed is elevated, and the child is placed in a side-lying or semiprone position. A small, firm pillow is placed under the head, and the uppermost limbs are flexed and supported with pillows. The weight of the body should not rest on the dependent arm. In the semiprone position the child lies with the dependent arm at the side behind the body, the opposite side supported on pillows, and the uppermost arm and leg flexed and resting on the pillows. This position prevents undue pressure on the dependent extremities. The dependent position of the face encourages drainage of secretions and prevents the flaccid tongue from obstructing the airway.

Normal range-of-motion exercises help to maintain function and prevent contractures of joints. Exercises should be done gently and with full range of motion. A small rolled pad can be placed in the palms to help maintain proper position of fingers; footboards or boots can be used to help prevent footdrop; splinting may be needed to prevent severe contractures of the wrist, knee, or ankle in decerebrate children.

Stimulation. Sensory stimulation is important in the care of the unconscious child, just as it is in the care of the alert child. For the temporarily unconscious or semiconscious child, sensory stimulation helps to arouse the child to the conscious state and orient the child in terms of time and place. Auditory and tactile stimulation are especially valuable. Tactile stimulation is not appropriate for the child in whom it may elicit an undesirable response. However, for other children tactile contact often has a relaxing and calming effect. When the child's condition permits, holding or rocking has a soothing effect and provides the body contact needed by young children.

The auditory sense is often present in a state of coma. Hearing is the last sense to be lost and the first one to be regained; therefore the child should be spoken to as is any other child. Conversation around the child should not include thoughtless or derogatory remarks. A radio playing soft music, a music box, or a record player is commonly used to provide auditory stimulation. Singing the child's favorite songs or reading a favorite story is a tactic used to maintain the child's contact with a familiar world. Having parents tape songs or stories provides a continuous source of familiar stimulation.

Regaining Consciousness. Awakening from a coma is a gradual process; however, sometimes children regain consciousness within a short time. Regaining orientation involves knowing person, place, and time, in that order.

Certain behaviors have been observed when children awaken from the unconscious state. The stress and anxiety they appear to feel in a strange and unfamiliar environment are consistently expressed in silent and withdrawn behavior. Children respond to basic questioning but usually do not display their prehospitalization personality and social behavior until they are transferred from the critical care area.

Family Support. Helping parents of an unconscious child cope with the situation is especially difficult. They may demonstrate all the guilt, fear, hostility, and anxiety of any parent of a seriously ill child (see Chapter 41). In addition, these parents are faced with the uncertain outcome of the cerebral dysfunction. The fear of death, mental retardation, or other permanent disability is present. Nursing intervention with parents depends on the nature of the pathologic condition, the personality of the parents, and the parent-child relationship before the injury or illness.

If there is little or no residual effect, the child will be discharged to home care fairly soon. The parents need the most intensive nursing intervention during the period of crisis and uncertainty. During the recovery phase they are given information, information is clarified, and they are encouraged to become involved in the child's care. Often the child's hospitalization is brief; however, some children require extended hospitalization for intensive therapy and rehabilitation.

The parents of children who die within hours or days require the support and guidance that the parents of any dying child would need in coping with the reality of the death and resolving their grief (see Chapter 41).

Probably the most difficult situations are those that involve children who are unconscious permanently or for an indefinite period. Unlike parents who lose a child through death, the finality is lacking for these parents, often leaving them in a state of suspended grief. The presence of the child renders the parents unable to resolve the loss. Like parents of dying children, parents of the comatose child search for any signs of hope. Well-meaning friends and relatives relate instances of miraculous recoveries. The parents seek confirmation and support for such possibilities and assign erroneous meanings to any sign in the child, such as reflexive muscle contractions, that might be interpreted as evidence of recovery.

At these times nurses need to respond with compassion and gentle honesty. They can acknowledge that miraculous recoveries do occur, but they are rare. The important message is to maintain open communication with the family.

Like parents who lose a child through death, the parents of the child lost to their world attempt to reconstitute a representation of the child. They bring items that belong to the child, such as favorite toys, music, and other objects cherished by the child. This is interpreted as an attempt to provide stimulation for the child in the hope of eliciting a response, to let the hospital staff know the child as the unique individual he or she was so that the parents' distress can be better appreciated, and to reconstitute an image of the child "lost" to them and for whom they mourn. An awareness of these behaviors and coping mechanisms provides nurses with the understanding that helps them support the parents in their grief process.

Along with grieving for the "lost" child, parents may be faced with making difficult decisions. When the child's brain is so severely damaged that vital functions must be maintained by artificial means, the parents must make the final decision to remove life support systems. Because the decision is so difficult for parents, the practitioner is commonly placed in a position of making the decision indirectly. After providing the parents with all of the information, the practitioner will suggest that the child be removed from the life support to test whether the child can live without it. The approach relieves the parents of the decision and can be effective, but it is based on an evaluation of the parents' intellectual level and emotional state. Sometimes parents may even choose to refuse treatment if they believe it to be best for the child and the family (informed dissent). At other times parents request that everything possible be done for the child.

The nurses can be instrumental in providing guidance and clarifying information—a valued but demanding undertaking. It is not unusual for the family to ask the same questions and to compare responses elicited from different staff members. A child's death is an intensely personal issue that deserves direct involvement by the nurse and auxiliary support systems.

When the child has survived the illness or injury that produced the brain damage but is left permanently unconscious, the parents must decide whether to place the child in a chronic care facility or arrange to care for the child at home. The nurse can listen to the parents' discussions regarding alternatives, provide information when appropriate, and support the family in their decision. The nurse can help the family prepare for the transfer of the child and make referrals to persons or agencies that can provide additional assistance.

When the child has survived the cerebral insult and is not comatose, but physical and/or mental capacity is limited either minimally or severely, families must cope with the long and tedious rehabilitation process and uncertain outcome. The drain on financial, emotional, and social resources can be enormous.

For parents who choose to care for their child at home, planning for home care begins early in the process of recovery. The family should become involved with the care of the child as soon as they indicate an interest and ability to do so. They need education and support in learning to care for the child, regular follow-up observation and assessment of the home management, and planning for some respite care of the child. Parents need to understand that it is important to plan for periodic relief from the continual care of the child (see Preparing for Discharge and Home Care, Chapter 44; and Family-Centered Home Care, Chapter 43).

➤ Evaluation

The effectiveness of nursing interventions for the unconscious child is determined by continual reassessment and evaluation of care based on the following observational guidelines:

1. Monitor child's neurologic signs, vital signs, and behavior.
2. Observe child's response to nursing activities, therapies, and diagnostic procedures; monitor ICP.
3. Observe child's color, position, and motor activity; measure fluid and nutritional intake and output.
4. Monitor status of child's respiratory, renal, and gastrointestinal systems and skin.
5. Observe family behaviors and interview members regarding their understandings and their feelings and concerns.

The expected outcomes are described in the Nursing Care Plan.

CEREBRAL TRAUMA

Head Injury

Head injury is a pathologic process involving the scalp, skull, meninges, or brain as a result of mechanical force. According to national statistics and the Safe Kids Campaign,* injuries are the number one health risk for children and the leading cause of death in children older than 1 year. Yearly, 1 in 4 children in the United States will have an injury serious enough to require medical attention. Tragically, 8000 children are killed every year by injuries. It has been estimated that 300 per 100,000 children per year have a traumatic brain injury and that 10 per 100,000 children per year die as a result of the brain injury. Studies indicate that as many as three fourths of the childhood deaths caused by mechanical trauma are the direct result of a brain injury.

Etiology. The three major causes of brain damage in childhood in order of importance are falls, motor vehicle injuries, and bicycle injuries. Neurologic injury accounts for the highest mortality, with boys usually affected twice as often as girls. In motor vehicle accidents children younger than 2 years are almost exclusively injured as passengers, whereas older children may also be injured as pedestrians or cyclists. The majority of deaths from brain trauma caused by bicycle injuries occur between the ages of 5 and 15 years. With the advent of bike helmet laws, this should be a decreasing trend.

The exposed nature of the head renders it particularly vulnerable to external violence, and many of the physical characteristics of children predispose them to craniocerebral trauma. For example, infants are commonly left unattended on beds, in high chairs, and in other places from which they can fall. Because the head of an infant or toddler is large and heavy in relation to other body parts, it is the most likely to be injured. Incomplete motor development contributes to falls at young ages, and the natural curiosity and exuberance of children increase their risk of an injury.

Pathophysiology. The pathology of brain injury is directly related to the force of impact. Intracranial contents (brain, blood, CSF) are damaged because the force is too great to be absorbed by the skull and musculoligamentous support of the head. The elastic, pliable skulls of infants and young children absorb much of the direct energy of physical impact to the head and afford some protection to intracranial structures. Although nervous tissue is delicate, it usually requires a severe blow to cause significant damage.

A child's response to head injury is different from that of adults. The larger head size and insufficient musculoskeletal support render the very young child particularly vulnerable to acceleration-deceleration injuries.

Primary head injuries are those that occur at a time of trauma and include skull fracture, contusions, intracranial hematoma, and diffuse injury. Subsequent complications include hypoxic brain damage, ICP, infection, and cerebral edema. The predominant feature of a child's brain injury is the diffuse amount of swelling that occurs. Hypoxia and hypercapnia threaten the energy requirements of the brain and increase CBF. The added volume across the blood-brain barrier and the loss of autoregulation exacerbate cerebral edema. Pressure inside the skull greater than the arterial pressure results in inadequate perfusion.

Cerebral hyperemia occurs more often in children, and this volume expansion may account for their tendency to develop intracranial hypertension. However, because the cranium of very young children has the ability to expand and the thin skull is more pliant, they may tolerate increases in ICP better than older children and adults. Children have a significantly higher percentage of good outcomes and a lower mortality rate, as well as a lower incidence of surgical mass lesions after severe head trauma. However, their thinner, softer brain may sustain greater long-term damage than previously suggested.

Physical forces act on the head through *acceleration*, *deceleration*, or *deformation*. Acceleration or deceleration is more de-

*SAFE KIDS, 1301 Pennsylvania Ave. NW, Suite 1000, Washington, DC 20004-1707; (202) 662-0600; fax (202) 393-2072; website: www.safekids.org.

Nursing Care Plan THE UNCONSCIOUS CHILD

NURSING DIAGNOSIS Risk for suffocation (aspiration) related to ineffective airway clearance secondary to depressed sensorium, impaired motor function

EXPECTED OUTCOME Patent airway is maintained; no signs of cerebral hypoxia are present.

Nursing Interventions/*Rationales*

Position semiprone or side-lying with neck slightly extended, nose in "sniffing" position *to provide optimal ventilation and prevent aspiration.* **Avoid neck hyperextension, which can block airway.**

Insert oral airway if indicated *to promote ventilation.*

Remove pooled secretions promptly *to prevent aspiration.*

Have emergency equipment available for insertion of endotracheal tube or tracheostomy *to prevent delay in treatment response to blocked airway.*

Administer oxygen, hyperventilate as ordered *to increase oxygenation to tissues.*

Monitor vital signs, blood gases, and pH *for evidence of hypoxia.*

NURSING DIAGNOSIS Risk for infection (respiratory) related to coma, immobility, pooling or respiratory secretions

EXPECTED OUTCOME Patient exhibits no evidence of infection; lungs are clear.

Nursing Interventions/*Rationales*

Place child in private room and screen all visitors and staff for signs of infection *to minimize exposure to infective organisms.*

Teach family about good hygiene and careful handwashing techniques *to prevent spread of infection.*

Observe careful asepsis in all procedures *to prevent spread of infection.*

Remove nasal and oral secretions as they form and provide good oral hygiene *to remove medium for growth of microorganisms.*

Monitor vital signs, auscultate lungs *to detect signs of infection.*

NURSING DIAGNOSIS Risk for injury related to depressed sensorium, intracranial abnormality

EXPECTED OUTCOME Child exhibits no evidence of injury (i.e., no increased ICP, cerebral edema, seizure activity).

Nursing Interventions/*Rationales*

Elevate head of bed 15 to 30 degrees with child's head in midline position *to facilitate venous drainage and prevent jugular compression.*

Prevent constipation, excessive stimuli in environment, painful stimuli, vigorous suctioning, or percussing, *as these activities can lead to increased ICP and seizure activity.*

Use stool softeners as ordered; monitor bowel movements *to prevent constipation and Valsalva maneuver.*

Keep room darkened, quiet; play soothing background music: place earphones over child's ears; use touching and calm, soothing voice to talk with child when performing care *to reduce environmental stimuli.*

Use sedation as ordered *for episodes of agitation or restlessness.*

Observe child for signs of pain (e.g., agitation, increases in pulse, blood pressure), and medicate with analgesic or paralyzing agents as ordered *to reduce pain.*

Arrange painful procedures to occur after sedation or analgesic administration *to decrease chances of increasing ICP.*

Administer antiseizure medication as ordered *to prevent seizure activity.*

Monitor neurologic vital signs *to assess neurosensory status.*

NURSING DIAGNOSIS Ineffective thermoregulation related to intracranial abnormality. CNS dysfunction

EXPECTED OUTCOME Child maintains body temperature at normothermic levels.

Nursing Interventions/*Rationales*

Monitor and record body temperature frequently *to assess status of thermoregulatory system and effectiveness of interventions.*

Administer antipyretics as ordered *for fever.*

Remove blankets, administer tepid sponge bath, use hypothermia blankets *to reduce hyperthermia.*

Maintain adequate hydration *to reduce or prevent fever.*

Use blankets, bed warmers *to reduce hypothermia.*

Prevent shivering, *which can increase ICP and metabolic rate.*

Monitor blood urea nitrogen (BUN), pH, electrolyte, glucose levels, *as they may be affected by thermal instability.*

NURSING DIAGNOSIS Risk for disuse syndrome related to coma, prolonged immobility

EXPECTED OUTCOME Child maintains full range of motion; muscle tone (no contractures, footdrop); skin integrity (no skin redness, irritation, breakdown, decubiti); normal patterns of elimination (no constipation, renal retention, renal calculi); normal circulatory function (no thrombus formation, venous stasis); adequate dietary intake (no weight loss, muscle wasting).

Nursing Interventions/*Rationales*

Turn and reposition every 2 hours *to promote circulation and prevent skin breakdown* (align properly, provide positional supports, use handrolls or splints *to position hands in functional position;* use footboard or hightop tennis shoes *to prevent footdrop*); perform passive range of motion fre-

Continued

Nursing Care Plan THE UNCONSCIOUS CHILD—cont'd

quently *to maintain full range in all joints and prevent contracture formation:* seat in chair *to improve circulation;* place on tilt table *to prevent loss of bone density to long bones.*

Use pressure reduction mattress overlay *to prevent pressure necrosis;* use foam pads on ankles, heels, elbows *to protect bony prominences;* massage skin with lotion regularly *to stimulate circulation and prevent friction and shearing effects;* keep bedclothes clean, dry, and wrinkle-free *to prevent skin irritation;* lubricate lips *to prevent drying and cracking;* lubricate eyes and keep them closed *to prevent drying and corneal irritation;* cleanse skin, mucous membranes of mouth and perianal area regularly *to prevent irritation and breakdown;* keep skin folds clean and dry *to prevent excoriation;* inspect skin, mucous membranes, corneas regularly *to assess for early signs of irritation or breakdown.*

Ensure adequate fluid intake, administer stool softeners *to maintain urinary output, prevent calculi, and aid bowel elimination;* monitor intake and output (I & O), hydration status, electrolytes, BUN, creatinine, urine characteristics *to assess for adequate hydration.*

Apply elastic stockings as indicated *to promote venous return, prevent stasis.*

Provide tube feedings that are adequate *to support the nutritional and metabolic needs of child (e.g., increased fiber, protein, vitamin C; decreased calcium);* monitor weight daily *to assess nutritional adequacy.*

NURSING DIAGNOSIS Altered family processes related to situational crises (child in coma)

EXPECTED OUTCOME Family exhibits adaptation of usual roles and functions to accommodate special needs of child; family exhibits growth-promoting behaviors.

Nursing Interventions/*Rationales*

Provide opportunity for family to absorb and adjust to diagnosis (e.g., repeat information *to allow time for family to hear and understand;* encourage expression of concerns, fears, and feelings about diagnosis and potential impact *to facilitate adjustment;* identify support systems *to provide resources for coping*).

Keep family informed of child's status, assist family to understand expected treatment *to promote trust and provide a sound basis for decision making.*

Explore parents' reaction to the child, involve them in child's daily care routines, have them touch and hold child *to provide some measure of control.*

Have parents spend special time with siblings *so they don't feel neglected or left out.*

Identify additional resource systems (e.g., relatives, friends, church, health care services, community programs) and strategize with family about making good use of these systems *to develop broad base of support.*

Provide a system of ongoing follow-up observation and evaluation *to ensure long-term adaptation to challenges presented to family functioning by a child who is in a long-term comatose state.*

scriptive of the circumstances responsible for most head injuries. When the stationary head receives a blow, the sudden acceleration causes deformation of the skull and mass movement of the brain. Continued movement of the intracranial contents allows the brain to strike parts of the skull (e.g., the sharp edges of the sphenoid or the irregular surface of the anterior fossa) or the edges of the tentorium.

Although the brain volume remains unchanged, significant distortion takes place as the brain changes shape in response to the force of impact to the skull. This movement can cause bruising at the point of impact *(coup)* and/or at a distance as the brain collides with the unyielding surfaces far removed from the point of impact *(contrecoup)* (Fig. 51-4). Thus a blow to the occipital region can cause severe injury to the frontal and temporal areas of the brain. Sudden deceleration, such as takes place during a fall, causes the greatest cerebral injury at the point of impact. Children with an acceleration/deceleration injury demonstrate diffuse generalized cerebral swelling produced by increased blood volume or a redistribution of cerebral blood volume (cerebral hyperemia) rather than by increased water content (edema), as seen in adults.

Another effect of brain movement is shearing stresses, which may tear small arteries and cause subdural hemorrhages. Another source of damage occurs when severe compression of the skull causes the brain to be forced through the tentorial opening. This can produce irreparable damage to the brainstem (Fig. 51-5).

Concussion. The most common head injury is concussion, a transient and reversible neuronal dysfunction, with instantaneous loss of awareness and responsiveness, that results from trauma to the head and persists for a relatively short time, usually minutes or hours. It is generally followed by amnesia for the moment of the injury and a variable period after the injury. The common misconception that loss of consciousness is the hallmark of concussion is not true, especially for children. Concussion is correctly defined as "a traumatically induced alteration in mental status." Confusion and amnesia after head injury are the hallmarks of concussion.

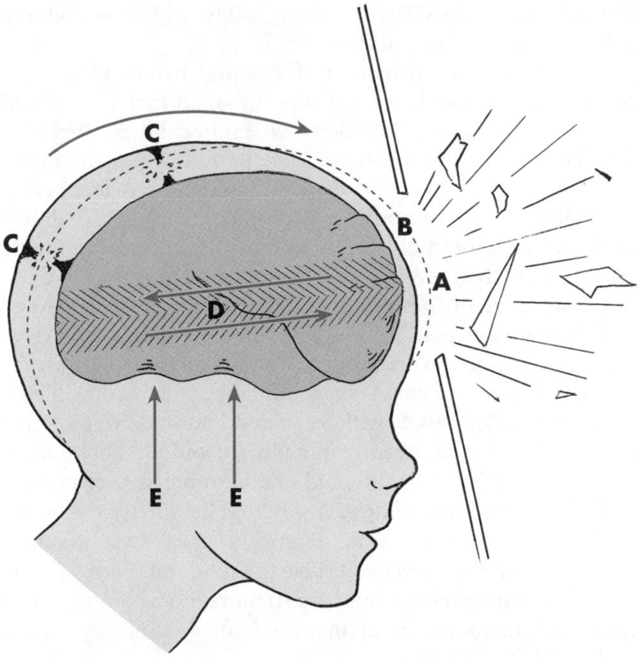

FIG. 51-4 • Mechanical distortion of cranium during closed head injury. **A,** Preinjury contour of skull. **B,** Immediate postinjury contour of skull. **C,** Torn subdural vessels. **D,** Shearing forces. **E,** Trauma from contact with floor of cranium. (Redrawn from Grubb RL, Coxe WS: Central nervous system trauma: cranial. In Eliasson SG, Presky AL, Hardin WB Jr, editors: *Neurological pathophysiology,* New York, 1974, Oxford University Press.)

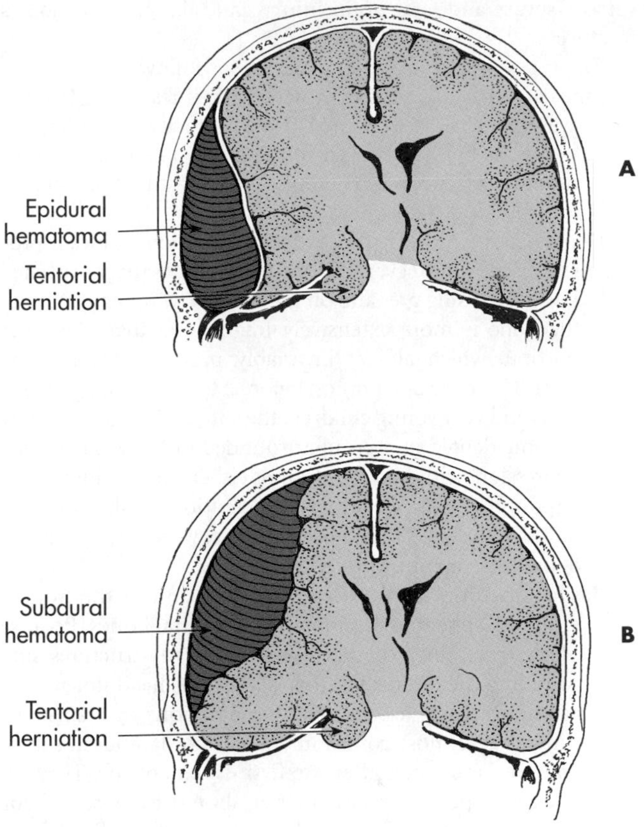

FIG. 51-5 • **A,** Epidural (extradural) hematoma and compression of temporal lobe through tentorial hiatus. **B,** Subdural hematoma.

The pathogenesis of concussion is still unclear but may be a result of shearing forces that cause stretching, compression, and tearing of nerve fibers, particularly in the area of the central brainstem, the seat of the reticular activating system. It has also been suggested that the anatomic alterations of nerve fibers cause the release of large quantities of acetylcholine into the CSF and a reduction in oxygen consumption with increased lactate production.

Contusion and Laceration. The terms *contusion* and *laceration* are used to describe visible bruising and tearing of cerebral tissue. Contusions represent petechial hemorrhages along the superficial aspects of the brain at the site of impact (coup injury) and/or a lesion remote from the site of direct trauma (contrecoup injury). In serious accidents there may be multiple sites of injury.

The major areas of the brain susceptible to contusion or laceration are the occipital, frontal, and temporal lobes. Also, the irregular surfaces of the anterior and middle fossae at the base of the skull are capable of producing bruises or lacerations on forceful impact. Contusions may cause focal disturbances in strength, sensation, or visual awareness. The degree of brain damage in the contused areas varies according to the extent of vascular injury. Signs will vary from mild, transient weakness of a limb to prolonged unconsciousness and paralysis. However, the signs and symptoms may be clinically indistinguishable from those of concussion.

The lower incidence of cerebral contusion in infancy has been attributed to the infant's pliable skull with less convolutional markings of the inner space between brain tissue and bone. Also, the infant's brain tissue has a softer consistency, which also reduces surface injury. However, infants who are roughly shaken (shaken baby syndrome [SBS]) can sustain profound neurologic impairment, seizures, retinal hemorrhages, and intracranial subarachnoid or subdural hemorrhages. In addition to these classic injuries, high cervical spinal cord hemorrhages and contusions can occur.

Cerebral lacerations are generally associated with penetrating or depressed skull fractures. However, they may occur without fracture in small children. When brain tissue is actually torn, with bleeding into and around the tear, more severe and prolonged unconsciousness and paralysis usually occur, leaving permanent scarring and some degree of disability.

Fractures. Because of its flexibility, the immature skull is able to sustain a greater degree of deformation than the adult skull before it incurs a fracture. A great deal of force is required to produce a fracture in the skull of an infant. However, the undersurface of the skull contains grooves in which the meningeal arteries lie. A fracture that runs through one of these grooves may tear the artery and produce severe and damaging hemorrhage. Hypovolemic hypotension can occur in infants with skull fractures. Note that a skull fracture may occur, and the patient may experience little or no brain damage. Conversely, severe and fatal brain injury can take place without a fracture.

The types of fractures that occur are as follows:

Linear fractures are those in which the lines of the fracture are predetermined by the site and velocity of the impact, as well as by the strength of the bone. These are uncommon before 2 to 3 years of age but constitute the majority of childhood skull fractures.

Depressed fractures are those in which the bone is locally broken, usually into several irregular fragments that are pushed inward, causing pressure on the brain. The inner portion of the bone is more extensively fragmented than the outer portion, which almost invariably produces tears in the dura. These are uncommon before 2 to 3 years of age. In infants and very young children, the soft, malleable bone may become dented in a peculiar rounded or "Ping-Pong ball" depression, without laceration of either skin or dura.

Compound fractures consist of laceration of skin that extends to the site of the bony fracture, which can be linear, depressed, or comminuted.

Basilar fractures involve the basilar portion of the frontal, ethmoid, sphenoid, temporal, or occipital bones. Because of the proximity of the fracture line to structures surrounding the brainstem, this is a serious head injury.

Diastatic fractures are traumatic separations of cranial sutures. These most commonly affect the lambdoid suture and are rarely seen after the first 4 years of life. They require no specific treatment but should be observed for "growing fractures" or development of a fluid-filled cyst.

Complications. The major complications of trauma to the head are hemorrhage, infection, edema, and herniation through the tentorium. Infection is always a hazard in open injuries, and edema is related to tissue trauma. Vascular rupture may occur even in minor head injuries, causing hemorrhage between the skull and cerebral surfaces. Compression of the underlying brain produces effects that can be rapidly fatal or insidiously progressive.

NURSE ALERT • Posttraumatic meningitis should be suspected in children with increasing drowsiness and fever who also have basilar skull fractures.

Epidural Hemorrhage. The blood accumulates between the dura and the skull to form a hematoma, which because of the difficulty with which dura is stripped from bone, forces the underlying brain contents downward and inward as the brain expands (see Fig. 51-5, *A*). Because bleeding is generally arterial, brain compression occurs rapidly. Most often the expanding hematoma is located in the parietotemporal region, forcing the medial portion of the temporal lobe under the edge of the tentorium, where it causes pressure on nerves and blood vessels. The lower incidence of epidural hematoma in childhood has been attributed to the fact that the middle meningeal artery is not embedded in the bone surface of the skull until approximately 2 years of age. Therefore a fracture of the temporal bone is less likely to lacerate the artery. Second, the dura closely adheres to the inner table of the skull, especially at the level of the sutures, making separation from bleeding less likely. However, a child's skull can be indented with sufficient force to tear the middle meningeal artery and then rebound intact without causing a fracture. Hemorrhage can also derive from dural veins or the dural sinuses, especially in infants and small children, in whom fracture is less likely to occur. In 20% to 40% of children a skull fracture is not detectable.

The classic clinical picture of epidural hemorrhage (momentary unconsciousness followed by a normal period and then lethargy or coma) is seldom evident in children (Box 51-4 lists the clinical manifestations). The period of impaired consciousness is commonly lacking, and the symptom-free period is atypical because of nonspecific problems such as irritability, headache, and vomiting. The symptom-free period commonly lasts longer than 48 hours. Clinically significant epidural hematomas are uncommon in children younger than 4 years. These differences may be caused by the decreased tendency of the resilient skull to fracture; the ability of blood to escape through widened sutures, an open fontanel, or a fracture; bleeding from smaller vessels with less rapid and massive bleeding; lower systolic blood pressure in children; and possibly the decreased susceptibility of the child's brain to pressure changes.

Subdural Hemorrhage. A subdural hemorrhage is bleeding between the dura and the cerebrum, usually as a result of rupture of cortical veins that bridge the subdural space (see Fig. 51-5, *B*). Subdural hematomas are 10 times more common than epidural hematomas, occurring most often in infancy, with a peak incidence at 6 months.

Unlike epidural hemorrhage, which develops inwardly against the less resistant brain tissue, subdural hemorrhage

Box 51-4

Clinical Manifestations of Acute Head Injury

MINOR INJURY

May or may not lose consciousness
Transient period of confusion
Somnolence
Listlessness
Irritability
Pallor
Vomiting (one or more episodes)

SIGNS OF PROGRESSION

Altered mental status (e.g., difficulty rousing child)
Mounting agitation
Development of focal lateral neurologic signs
Marked changes in vital signs

SEVERE INJURY

Signs of increased ICP (see Box 51-1)
- Increased head size (infant)
- Bulging fontanel (infant)

Retinal hemorrhage
Extraocular palsies (especially cranial nerve VI)
Hemiparesis
Quadriplegia
Elevated temperature
Unsteady gait (older child)
Papilledema (older child)
Retinal hemorrhages

ASSOCIATED SIGNS

Skin injury (to area of head sustaining injury)
Other injuries (e.g., to extremities)

tends to develop more slowly and spreads thinly and widely until it is limited by the dural barriers—the falx and tentorium. Subdural hematoma is fairly common in infants, typically as a result of birth trauma, falls, assaults, or violent shaking. The small subdural space and dura firmly attached to the skull in this area are highly vulnerable to increased ICP.

NURSE ALERT • Children with a subdural hematoma and retinal hemorrhages should be evaluated for the possibility of child abuse, especially SBS.

Repeated subdural taps often provide relief in the infant, as revealed by follow-up CT scans, improved neurologic status, and a flat anterior fontanel. Surgical evacuation of the hematoma is the treatment of choice in the older child and is commonly required in infants.

Cerebral Edema. Some degree of brain edema is expected, especially 24 to 72 hours after craniocerebral trauma. Cerebral edema caused by direct cellular injury or vascular injury induces vascular stasis, anoxia, and further vasodilation. If the progression continues unchecked, ICP exceeds arterial pressure and fatal anoxia ensues, and/or the pressure causes herniation of a portion of the brain over the edge of the tentorium, compressing the brainstem and occluding the posterior cerebral arteries. Diffuse cerebral swelling and changes in CBF are common patterns after head injury in children.

NURSE ALERT • If a child loses consciousness or vomits more than three times, medical attention should be sought.

Diagnostic Evaluation. A detailed history, especially a health history, both past and present, is essential in evaluating the child with a craniocerebral trauma. Certain disorders, such as drug allergies, hemophilia, diabetes mellitus, or epilepsy, may produce similar symptoms. Furthermore, even minor traumatic injury can aggravate a preexisting disease process. Events surrounding the injury often supply significant data. It must be determined whether the infant or child exhibited alterations in consciousness, and any other signs and behaviors exhibited by the child must be noted. Because head injuries are commonly accompanied by injuries in other areas, the examination is performed with care to avoid further damage.

NURSE ALERT • Stabilize a child's spine after head injury until a spinal cord injury is ruled out.

Initial Assessment. Priorities in the initial phase of the care of a child with a head injury include assessment of the ABCs (airway, breathing, circulation); evaluation for shock; neurologic examination, especially LOC; pupillary symmetry and response to light; and seizures. The assessment is carried out quickly in relation to vital signs (Emergency box). Excited and irritable children may have a rapid pulse, hyperventilate, appear pale, and feel clammy shortly after an injury.

NURSE ALERT • Deep, rapid, periodic, or intermittent and gasping respirations; wide fluctuations or noticeable slowing of the pulse; and widening pulse pressure or extreme fluctuations in blood pressure are signs of brainstem involvement. It is important to note that marked hypotension may represent internal injuries.

Ocular signs such as fixed and dilated pupils, fixed and constricted pupils, and pupils that are poorly reactive or unreactive to light and accommodation indicate increased ICP or brainstem involvement. It is important to remain with the child who has fixed and dilated pupils because these are ominous signs and there is a probability of respiratory arrest. Dilated, nonpulsating blood vessels indicate increased ICP before the appearance of papilledema. Retinal hemorrhages are seen in acute head injuries.

NURSE ALERT • Observation of asymmetric pupils or one dilated, unreactive pupil in a comatose child is a neurosurgical emergency.

Less urgent but important additional assessments include examination of the scalp for lacerations and palpation for other abnormalities. However, a significant amount of blood loss can occur from scalp lacerations.

NURSE ALERT • Bleeding from the nose or ears needs further evaluation, and a watery discharge from the nose (rhinorrhea) that is positive for glucose (as tested with Dextrostix) suggests leaking of CSF from a skull fracture.

Emergency

HEAD INJURY

Assess child:
- **A—Airway**
- **B—Breathing**
- **C—Circulation**

Stabilize neck and spine.

Clean any abrasions with soap and water.
- **Apply clean dressing.**
- **If bleeding, apply ice for 1 hour to relieve pain and swelling.**

Give only clear liquids until no vomiting for at least 6 hours.

Assess pain.

Check pupil reaction every 4 hours (including twice during night) for 48 hours.

Awaken twice during night to check level of consciousness.

Seek medical attention if there is any of the following:
- **Injury sustained:**
  - **At high speed (e.g., automobile)**
  - **Fall from a significant distance (e.g., roof, tree)**
  - **From great force (e.g., baseball bat)**
  - **Under suspicious circumstances**
- **Child younger than 12 months old**
- **Loss of consciousness**
- **Discomfort (crying) more than 10 minutes after injury**
- **Headache that is severe, worsening, interferes with sleep**
- **Vomiting three or more times**
- **Swelling in front of or above earlobe or swelling that increases in size**
- **Confused or not behaving normally**
- **Difficult to rouse from sleep**
- **Difficulty with speaking**
- **Blurring of vision or seeing double**
- **Unsteady gait**
- **Difficulty using extremities**
- **Neck pain**
- **Pupils dilated or fixed**
- **Infant with bulging fontanel**
- **Bruising below the eyes ("raccoon eyes")**

An accurate assessment of clinical signs provides baseline information. Serial evaluations, preferably by a single observer, help to detect changes in the neurologic status. Alterations in mental status, evidenced by increased difficulty in rousing the child, mounting agitation, development of focal lateral neurologic signs, or marked changes in vital signs, usually indicate extension or progression of the basic pathologic process.

Special Tests. After a thorough clinical examination, a variety of diagnostic tests are helpful in providing a more definitive diagnosis of the type and extent of the trauma. The severity of a head injury may not be apparent on clinical examination of a child, but it will be detectable on a CT scan. Whenever the child has a history consistent with a serious head injury (unrestrained occupant in a severe motor vehicle accident or a fall from a significant height), it is important that a scan be performed even if the child initially appears alert and oriented. All children with head injuries who have any alteration of consciousness, headache, vomiting, skull fracture, seizure, or a predisposing medical condition should also undergo CT scanning.

MRI and neurobehavioral assessment after early head injury may be useful in documenting cognitive impairment in relation to structural alterations in the young brain. MRI provides details of soft tissues better than any other noninvasive device. Electroencephalography is not particularly helpful for early diagnosis but is useful for defining seizure activity or focal destructive lesions after the acute phase of illness. Lumbar puncture is rarely used in craniocerebral trauma and is contraindicated in the presence of increased ICP. In some centers monitoring ICP is part of the assessment.

Posttraumatic Syndromes. Posttraumatic syndromes can be clinically manifested because of structural complications resulting from a head injury and through the signs and symptoms demonstrated by the child. Structural complications can include hydrocephalus and focal deficits such as optic atrophy, cranial nerve palsies, motor deficits, diabetes insipidus, aphasia, and seizures. Behavioral disturbances include sleep disturbances, phobias, emotional lability, altered school performance, and changes related to aggressiveness or withdrawal. *Postconcussion syndrome* is a common sequela to brain injury and occurs within minutes to an hour after a minimal head injury. The manifestations vary with the age of the child. The syndrome occurs very commonly in children younger than 1 year. The syndrome in adolescents is similar to that in adults. The duration of manifestations can vary from several days to several months. Death from concussion is preventable unless overwhelming secondary brain injury has occurred (Durkin et al, 1998).

Posttraumatic seizures occur often in children who survive a head injury and are more common in children than in adults. Seizures are more likely to occur within the first few days of the head injury (Kaufman and Park, 1997). *Structural complications* (e.g., hydrocephalus) may occur after a head injury. The type of residual effect depends on the location and nature of the disorder. True mental retardation occurs only after severe injuries.

Therapeutic Management. The majority of children with mild to moderate concussion who have not lost consciousness can be cared for and observed at home after careful examination reveals no serious intracranial injury. Nurses should provide parents with clear explanations and instructions and should encourage them to ask questions both before and after leaving the medical facility if clarification is needed (Family Focus box). The parents are instructed to check the child every 2 hours to determine any changes in responsiveness. The sleeping child should be awakened to determine whether he or she can be roused normally. Parents are advised to maintain contact with the health professional, who usually wants to examine the child again in 1 or 2 days. The manifestations of epidural hematoma in children do not generally appear until 24 hours or more after injury.

> ***Family Focus***
>
> **MAINTAINING CONTACT**
>
> **Maintaining contact with parents for continued observation and reevaluation of the child, when indicated, facilitates early diagnosis and treatment of possible complications from head injury, such as hematoma, hydrocephalus, cysts, and posttraumatic seizures. Children are generally hospitalized for 24 to 48 hours' observation if their family lives far from medical facilities or lacks transportation or a telephone that would provide access to immediate help. Other circumstances such as language or other communication barriers, or even emotional trauma, may hinder learning and make it difficult for families to feel confident in caring for their child at home.**

Children with severe injuries, those who have lost consciousness for more than a few minutes, and those with prolonged and continued seizures or other focal or diffuse neurologic signs must be hospitalized until their condition is stable and their neurologic signs have diminished.

The child is given nothing by mouth or is restricted to clear liquids, if able to take fluids by mouth, until it is determined that vomiting will not occur. IV fluids are indicated in the child who is comatose or displays dulled sensorium and/or in the child with persistent vomiting. Fluid balance is closely monitored by daily weights; accurate intake and output measurements; and serum osmolality to detect early signs of water retention, excessive dehydration, and states of hypertonicity or hypotonicity.

The volume of IV fluid is carefully monitored to avoid aggravating any cerebral edema and to minimize the possibility of overhydration in case of SIADH. However, damage to the hypothalamus or pituitary gland may produce diabetes insipidus with its accompanying hypertonicity and dehydration.

If necessary, restlessness can be satisfactorily managed with mild sedation, and headache is usually controlled with acetaminophen (Tylenol). Antiepileptics are used for seizure control and commonly in cases of suspected contusion or laceration. Antibiotics may be administered if there are lacerations, CSF leakage, or excessive cerebral tissue damage. Prophylactic tetanus toxoid is given as appropriate. Cerebral edema is managed as described for the unconscious child. Hyperthermia is controlled with tepid sponges or a hypothermia blanket.

Surgical Therapy. Scalp lacerations are sutured after the underlying bone is carefully examined (Atraumatic Care box). Depressed fractures require surgical reduction and removal of bone fragments. Torn dura is sutured. "Ping-Pong ball" skull fractures in very young infants ordinarily correct themselves within a few weeks and do not require specific treatment, although they can be reduced by pressure against the bone.

Prognosis. The outcome of craniocerebral trauma depends on the extent of injury and complications. However, the outlook is generally more favorable for children than for adults (Ward,

Atraumatic Care

NONINVASIVE LOCAL ANESTHESIA

The use of topical lidocaine, epinephrine, and tetracaine (LET) solution* or lidocaine, adrenaline, and tetracaine (LAT) gel provides noninvasive anesthesia for suturing.† Both of these preparations provide an acceptable alternative to tetracaine, adrenaline, and cocaine (TAC), which is more expensive, is a restricted narcotic, and carries a higher potential for toxicity.‡

*Adler AJ, Dubinsky I, Eisen J: Does the use of topical lidocaine, epinephrine and tetracaine solution provide sufficient anesthesia for laceration repair? *Acad Emerg Med* 5:108-112, 1998.
†Ernst AA et al: Topical lidocaine adenaline tetracaine (LAT gel) versus injectable buffered lidocaine for local anesthesia in laceration repair, *West J Med* 167:79-81, 1997.
‡Keyes PD, Tallon JM, Rizos J: Topical anesthesia, *Can Fam Physician* 44:2152-2156, 1998.

1995). Over 90% of children with concussions or simple linear fractures recover without symptoms after the initial period. The incidence of fatalities and neurologic sequelae is lower in children, even in those with severe head injuries. The prognosis for recovery is primarily related to the duration of coma and the degree of injury. The combination of impaired consciousness and skull fracture carries the highest risk of complication.

The concern regarding outcome is increasingly focused on cognitive, emotional, and/or mental problems. Recent studies indicate that children have a higher frequency of psychologic disturbances after head injury, whereas adults are more prone to physical symptoms.

Children may be more vulnerable than adults to long-term cognitive and behavioral dysfunction after diffuse brain injury. Even with recovery, the effects of brain injury on a child's potential can never be known.

True coma (not obeying commands, eyes closed, and not speaking) usually does not last more than 2 weeks. A child's eventual outcome can range from brain death to a persistent vegetative state to complete recovery. However, even the best recovery may be associated with personality changes, including mood lability and loss of confidence, impaired short-term memory, headaches, and subtle cognitive impairments. Many children are left with significant disabilities after head injury that appear months later as learning difficulties, behavioral changes, or emotional disturbances (Cattelani et al, 1998). Generally, within 6 months to 1 year after the injury, 90% of the long-term neurologic outcome has been achieved.

Nursing Care Management. The hospitalized child requires careful neurologic assessment and evaluation (including vital signs) repeated at frequent intervals to provide information needed to establish a correct diagnosis, to reveal signs and symptoms of increased ICP, to determine clinical management, to prevent many complications, and to provide support to the child and family during the recovery phases.

The child is placed on bed rest, usually with the head of the bed elevated slightly, and appropriate safety measures, such as siderails kept up for older children and seizure precautions for children of all ages, are implemented. For the extremely restless child, hard surfaces may have to be padded and restraint used to prevent the possibility of further injury. Care is individualized according to the specific needs of the child. The unconscious child is managed as described in the previous section, but most childhood head injuries are those causing momentary stunning or temporary unconsciousness. Children may be restless and irritable, but more often their reaction is to fall asleep when left undisturbed. A quiet environment helps reduce the restlessness and irritability. Shining bright lights directly into the child's face is irritating and often makes checking the ocular responses more difficult and more aggravating to the child.

Frequent examinations of vital signs, neurologic signs, and LOC are extremely important nursing observations. When possible, they should be performed by a single observer to better detect subtle changes that may indicate worsening of neurologic status. Pupils are checked for size, equality, reaction to light, and accommodation. After the initial elevations usually seen after injury, the vital signs generally return to normal unless there is brainstem involvement. An axillary measurement of temperature is the safest method because seizures are not uncommon and vomiting is a frequent response in children, especially when the child is disturbed.

The most important nursing observation is assessment of the child's LOC. Alterations in consciousness appear earlier in the progression of an injury than alterations of vital signs or focal neurologic signs. Some expected responses may be misinterpreted as deviations from the norm. Frequent examinations of alertness are fatiguing to the child; therefore the child often wants to fall asleep, which may be confused with depressed consciousness. When left alone, the child promptly dozes. It is not uncommon to observe ocular divergence through the partially closed eyelids.

A key nursing role is to provide sedation and analgesia for the child. The conflict between the need to promote comfort and relieve anxiety in the child vs. the need to be able to assess for neurologic changes presents a dilemma. However, both goals can be achieved with close observation of the child's LOC and response to analgesics, use of a pain assessment record, and effective communication with the practitioner. To differentiate between sedation from an opioid or the injury, naloxone (Narcan) can be given slowly to reverse the opioid's sedative effect. Decreasing restlessness after administration of an analgesic most likely reflects pain control rather than a decreasing LOC.

Observations of position and movement provide additional information. Any abnormal posturing is noted, as well as whether it occurs continuously or intermittently. Are the child's handgrips strong and equal in strength? Are there any signs of decerebrate or decorticate posturing? What is the child's response to stimulation? Is movement purposeful, random, or absent? Are movement and/or sensation equal on both sides or restricted to one side only?

The child may report headache or other discomfort. The child who is too young to describe a headache will be fussy and resist being handled. The child who has vertigo will often assume a position of comfort and vigorously resist efforts to be moved. Forcible movement causes the child to vomit and display spontaneous nystagmus. Seizures, relatively common in children with craniocerebral trauma, may be of any type but are more often generalized, regardless of the type of injury. Any seizure activity should be carefully observed and described in detail. Children in postictal (postseizure) states are more lethargic and have sluggish pupils.

Drainage from any orifice is noted. Bleeding from the ear suggests the possibility of a basal skull fracture. The amount and characteristics of the drainage are observed, and because the auditory canal may be a source of infection, dry, sterile cotton can be placed loosely at the orifice and changed when soiled.

NURSE ALERT • Suctioning through the nares is contraindicated because there is a risk of the catheter entering the brain parenchyma through a fracture in the skull.

Head trauma is commonly accompanied by other undetected injuries; therefore any bruises, lacerations, or evidence of internal injuries or fractures of the extremities is noted and reported. Associated injuries are evaluated and treated appropriately.

The child with normal LOC is usually allowed clear liquids unless fluid is restricted. If the child has an IV infusion, it is maintained as prescribed. The diet is advanced to that appropriate for the child's age as soon as the condition permits. Intake and output are measured and recorded, and any incontinence of bowel or bladder is noted in the child who has been toilet trained.

The child should be observed for any unusual behavior, but behavior should be interpreted in relation to the child's normal behavior. For example, urinary incontinence during sleep would be of no consequence in a child who routinely wets the bed but would be highly significant for one who never does. In addition, a child who has nightmares might cry out and demonstrate agitated behavior at night. Parents are valuable resources. Information obtained from parents at or shortly after admission is helpful in evaluating the child's behavior (e.g., the ease with which the child is roused normally, the usual sleeping position, how much the child sleeps during the day, motor activity the child is capable of [rolling over, sitting up, climbing], hearing and visual acuity, appetite, and manner of eating [spoon, bottle, cup]). There would be less concern about a child who falls asleep several times during the day if this particular type of behavior is consistent with the child's usual behavior.

Family Support. The emotional and educational support of the family of children who have suffered head injury presents a formidable, challenging aspect to nursing care. Witnessing the parents' ordeal of grief and helplessness on seeing their child in an intensive care unit connected to monitoring equipment in an altered state evokes empathy. The nurse can encourage the family to be involved in the child's care, to bring in familiar belongings, or to make a tape recording of familiar voices and sounds. Parents may need a demonstration on how to touch or cuddle their child and may want to talk about their grief. The nurse can listen attentively, reinforce what is being done to assist the child, and direct parents toward signs and symptoms of recovery to instill hope without promises. A common phenomenon is for families to seek information from all health care providers by asking, "What will she be like? What do you know?" as they search for some clue that the child is recovering. Honesty and kindness, along with competent care, distinguish excellent nursing abilities.

When the child is discharged, the parents are advised of probable posttraumatic symptoms that may be expected, such as behavioral changes, sleep disturbances, phobias, and seizures. They should understand observations that need to be made and how to contact the physician, nurse, or health facility in case the child develops any unusual signs or symptoms. The importance of follow-up evaluation should be emphasized. It is often advisable to refer the family to a public health agency for home follow-through to be certain that the child receives posthospital evaluation.

Rehabilitation. The rehabilitation and management of the child with permanent brain injury are essential aspects of care. Rehabilitation of brain-injured children is begun as soon as feasible and usually involves the family and a rehabilitation team. Careful assessment of the child's capabilities, limitations, and probable potential is made as early as possible, and appropriate interventions are implemented to maximize the residual capacities. The Brain Injury Association* "arose from the mutual frustration and sense of hopelessness experienced by families in their search for appropriate facilities and support to return head-injured loved ones to their maximum functioning potential." It provides information and listings of rehabilitation services and support groups throughout the country.

Pediatric trauma rehabilitation is a national concern. Coordinating care and services for early rehabilitation involves identifying the child's and family's responses to the traumatic injury and disability, securing available resources, and recognizing the parental role in the process.

The child with a disability resulting from head trauma requires assessment on a physical, cognitive, emotional, and social level. The child has experienced separation, pain, sensory deprivation and overload, changes in circadian cycle, and fear of the unknown. Recovery and transition require new coping strategies at the same time that regressive and acting-out behavior may start. Parents and children need honest communication for decision making. Rehabilitation is advocated when the child is making progress beyond what can be provided in a hospital setting. The Rancho Los Amigos Scale provides a systematic assessment of the progress a child with a severe head injury may achieve.

Prevention. Tremendous strides have been made in the prevention of cerebral damage after head injury in children. New developments requiring research point to the prevention of cellular injury or the primary insult. However, the greatest benefit lies in prevention of head injuries. Nurses can exert a valuable influence on behalf of children through education. The reason injuries remain preventable is that unnecessary risks go unchecked. Inadequate supervision combined with a child's natural sense of indestructibility and exploration can lead to lethal results. Nurses are in the unique position of influencing caregivers in terms of growth and development. Banning the use of infant walkers is an example. This equipment does not help develop motor skills but places infants at risk for head and neck injuries from falls, especially down steps. Public education, coupled with legislative support, can prevent childhood injuries.

(For extensive discussions of childhood injuries, see the discussions on injury prevention in Chapters 36, 37, 38, 39, and 40. See also Childhood Mortality, Chapter 29; and Nursing Care Plan: The Child with a Head Injury.†)

Near-Drowning

Drowning is the second most common cause of accidental death in children. Most cases of drowning are accidental, usu-

---

*105 North Alfred St., Alexandria, VA 22314; (703) 236-6000; fax (703) 236-6001; website: www.biausa.org.

†In Wong DL, Hess CS: ***Wong and Whaley's clinical manual of pediatric nursing,*** ed 5, St Louis, 2000, Mosby.

ally involving children who are helpless in water, such as inadequately attended children in or near swimming pools or infants in bathtubs; small children who fall into ponds, streams, and flooded excavations, usually near home; occupants of pleasure boats who fail to wear life preservers; children who have diving accidents; and children who are able to swim but overestimate their endurance. Accidental drowning occurs five times more often in boys than in girls; 50% of children younger than 4 years, and 90% of cases occur in private swimming pools (National Center for Injury Prevention and Control, 1999).

Drowning can take place in any body of water, including such unlikely ones as a pail of water. Top-heavy toddlers fall head first into a pail of water, their arms become trapped, and they are unable to free themselves. Hot tubs and whirlpool spas have been implicated in childhood drowning injury. The suction created at the outlet is strong enough to trap even larger children underwater. Drowning as a form of fatal child abuse has also been recognized as a problem. Homicidal drownings are typically unwitnessed, they usually occur in the home, and the victims are often either infants or toddlers.

With expeditious treatment many children can be and are being saved. For purposes of this discussion, two terms need clarification:

Drowning—Death from asphyxia while submerged, regardless of whether fluid has entered the lungs

Near-drowning—Survival at least 24 hours after submersion in a fluid medium

Pathophysiology. The major pulmonary changes that occur in drowning are directly related to the length of submersion (regardless of the type and amount of fluid aspirated), the physiologic response of the victim, and the development and degree of immersion hypothermia. In addition, cerebral recovery depends on the effectiveness of initial resuscitation and subsequent critical care measures to support cerebral salvage.

Physiologic factors that influence the extent of damage from immersion include resistance to asphyxia and anoxia, which shows some individual variation. There is greater resistance with diminishing age; young children can withstand longer periods of submersion. More important is the drowning, or diving reflex. This neurologic response is triggered by immersion of the face in cold water. Blood is shunted away from the periphery, and the flow is predominantly concentrated to the brain and heart.

The problems created by near-drowning are (1) hypoxia and asphyxiation, (2) aspiration, and (3) hypothermia (except near-drowning in hot tubs). Cardiopulmonary arrest is secondary to asphyxia.

Hypoxia is the primary problem because it results in global cell damage, and different cells tolerate variable lengths of anoxia. Neurons, especially cerebral cells, sustain irreversible damage after 4 to 6 minutes of submersion. The heart and lungs can survive up to 30 minutes. Regardless of the amount of water aspirated, there is arterial hypoxemia (resulting from atelectasis with shunting of blood through the nonventilated alveoli) and a combined respiratory acidosis (resulting from retained carbon dioxide) and metabolic acidosis (caused by buildup of acid metabolites from anaerobic metabolism). The pathologic events are directly related to the duration of submersion. The major difficulty is acute ventilatory insufficiency. Approximately 10% of drowning victims die without aspirating fluid but die of acute asphyxia as a result of prolonged reflex laryngospasm.

Aspiration of fluid occurs in the majority of drownings. The aspirated fluid results in pulmonary edema, atelectasis, airway spasm, and pneumonitis, which aggravate the hypoxia. It was previously thought that near-drowning in salt water produced a different physiologic response than near-drowning in fresh water. However, there is no clinically significant difference in the response of human survivors, and the submersion does not alter the therapy or outcome.

Hypothermia occurs rapidly in infants and children, partly because of their large surface area relative to body mass and partly as a result of the cold water itself. Water is an excellent heat conductor, and the contact with the skin is increased by struggling. Hypothermia may make resumption or maintenance of cardiac function possible if body temperature is less than 30° C (86° F). Profound hypothermia is usually evidence of lengthy submersion.

Therapeutic Management. Resuscitative measures should begin at the scene of a drowning, and the victim should be transported to the hospital with maximum ventilatory and circulatory support. Many victims need care for some time after aspiration of fluid. In the hospital, intensive pulmonary care is implemented and continued according to the needs of the patient.

In general, the management of the near-drowning victim is based on the degree of cerebral insult (Box 51-5). The first pri-

Box 51-5

Clinical Manifestations of Near-Drowning*

Category A: Awake (minimum injury)
- Fully conscious
- Mild hypothermia
- Mild chest radiographic changes
- Mild arterial blood gas abnormalities

Category B: Blunted sensorium (moderate injury)
- Obtunded
- Stuporous
- Purposeful response to painful stimuli
- Mild to moderate hypothermia
- Respiratory distress (frequently)
- Chest radiographs abnormal
- Arterial blood gas abnormalities

Category C: Comatose (severe anoxia)
- Unarousable
- Abnormal response to pain
- Abnormal respiratory pattern
- Seizures
- Shock
- Marked arterial blood gas abnormalities
- Abnormal chest radiographs
- Dysrhythmias
- Metabolic acidosis
- Hyperkalemia, hyperglycemia
- Disseminated intravascular coagulation

Also:
- **C1:** Decorticate, Cheyne-Stokes respirations
- **C2:** Decerebrate, central hyperventilation
- **C3:** Flaccid, apneustic, or cluster breathing
- **C4:** Flaccid, apneic, no detectable circulation

*Directly related to the degree of consciousness following rescue and resuscitation.

ority is to restore oxygen delivery to the cells and prevent further hypoxic damage. A spontaneously breathing child will do well in an oxygen-enriched atmosphere; the more severely affected child will require endotracheal intubation and mechanical ventilation. Blood gases and pH are monitored frequently as a guide to oxygen, fluid, and electrolyte therapies.

NURSE ALERT • All children who have a near-drowning experience should be admitted to the hospital for observation. Although many patients do not appear to have had adverse effects from the event, complications (e.g., respiratory compromise, cerebral edema) may occur as long as 24 hours after the incident.

Aspiration pneumonia is a common complication that occurs about 48 to 72 hours after the episode. Bronchospasm, alveolocapillary membrane damage, atelectasis, abscess formation, and acute respiratory distress syndrome are other complications that occur after aspiration of fluid.

Prognosis. Studies report that the best predictors of a good outcome were submersion in non-icy water (>5° C [41° F]) for less than 5 minutes and the presence of sinus rhythm, reactive pupils, and neurologic responsiveness at the scene. The worst prognoses—for death or severe neurologic impairment—were in children submerged for more than 10 minutes and not responding to advanced life support within 25 minutes. All children without spontaneous, purposeful movement and normal brainstem function 24 hours after near-drowning experienced severe neurologic deficits or died (Zuckerman, Gregory, and Santos-Damiani, 1998).

Nursing Care Management. Nursing care depends on the condition of the child. A child who survives may need intensive respiratory nursing care with attention to vital signs, mechanical ventilation and/or tracheostomy, blood gas determination, chest therapy, and IV infusion. Commonly the child is comatose for an indefinite period and requires the same care as an unconscious child.

A difficult aspect in the care of the child victim of near-drowning is helping the parents cope with severe guilt reactions. The magnitude of the event is so great that efforts to provide comfort and support are of only limited success. Parents need to hear that everything possible is being done to treat the child, and this message needs to be repeated often.

The parents of the child who is saved from death are also faced with the anxiety of not knowing what the outcome will be, and sometimes they wish for the death of the child. Because their situation generates such intense feelings of loneliness, it is important for families to know that they are not alone. They need to be reminded often that there are caring persons to assist them both during the crisis and later. Additional sources of support that can be recommended are psychiatric and social work consultants, community services, and religious support. Self-help groups are excellent if these are available in the community.

Nurses often have difficulty relating to the parents if obvious neglect has precipitated the accident and subsequent problems; therefore it is important for those who care for these children and their families to assess their own feelings about the situation, as well as the coping abilities and resources of the family. Caring for near-drowning victims and their families requires nurses to be sensitive to the needs of the child and the family and to recognize their own reactions and emotions.

Prevention. Most drownings, particularly of infants or small children, can be prevented with adequate supervision. Water safety and survival training should be required for all school-age children, and nurses can be active advocates in their communities. Nurses are also in a position to emphasize the importance of adequate adult supervision when children are in the water. Aquatic programs for infants and toddlers do not decrease the risk of drowning; they should never be left unattended when in or near the water (American Academy of Pediatrics, 2000b). Parents with pools should know cardiopulmonary resuscitation (CPR) techniques.* See also Injury Prevention, Chapters 36, 37, 38, 39, and 40.

NERVOUS SYSTEM TUMORS

Brain tumor and neuroblastoma are two major forms of childhood cancer derived from neural tissue. CNS tumors account for approximately 20% of all childhood cancers, with an annual incidence of 2.4 per 100,000 children younger than 5 years (Heideman et al, 1997). Both of these types of tumors are difficult to treat and have not demonstrated the dramatic improvements in survival seen in other forms of childhood cancer.

Brain Tumors

Brain tumors are the most common solid tumors in children and are the second most common childhood cancer. The majority of tumors (about 60%) are *infratentorial* (below the tentorium cerebelli), which means that they occur in the posterior third of the brain, primarily in the cerebellum or brainstem. This anatomic distribution accounts for the frequency of symptoms resulting from increased ICP. The other tumors are *supratentorial,* or within the anterior two thirds of the brain, mainly the cerebrum.

Brain tumors, whether benign or malignant, can arise from any cell within the cranium. Consequently the cranial cells' origin provides a histologic classification for major tumors. For instance, astrocytes (cells that form the supportive tissue for neurons) may form a common glial tumor called an *astrocytoma.* The major infratentorial tumors are medulloblastomas, cerebellar astrocytomas, brainstem gliomas, and ependymomas, and the major supratentorial tumors are astrocytomas, hypothalamic tumors, optic pathway tumors, and craniopharyngiomas.

Diagnostic Evaluation. The signs and symptoms of brain tumors are directly related to their anatomic location and size and, to some extent, the age of the child. In infants, whose cranial sutures are still open, virtually no early detectable symptoms develop. It is not until spinal fluid obstruction causes markedly increased head size that a lesion may be suspected. Even in older children, clinical manifestations are nonspecific. However, the most common symptoms are headache, especially on awakening, and vomiting that is not related to feeding. The common clinical manifestations of brain tumors are presented in Box 51-6.

Diagnosis of a brain tumor is based subjectively on presenting clinical signs and objectively on neurologic tests and histo-

*Community and home care instructions for CPR are available in Wong DL, Hess CS: ***Wong and Whaley's clinical manual of pediatric nursing,*** ed 5, St Louis, 2000, Mosby.

Box 51-6

Clinical Manifestations of Brain Tumors

SIGNS AND SYMPTOMS

Headache

Recurrent and progressive
In frontal or occipital areas
Usually dull and throbbing
Worse on arising, less during day
Intensified by lowering head and straining, such as during bowel movement, coughing, sneezing

Vomiting

With or without nausea or feeding
Progressively more projectile
More severe in morning
Relieved by moving about and changing position

Neuromuscular Changes

Incoordination or clumsiness
Loss of balance (use of wide-based stance, falling, tripping, banging into objects)
Poor fine motor control
Weakness
Hyporeflexia or hyperreflexia
Positive Babinski sign
Spasticity
Paralysis

Behavioral Changes

Irritability
Decreased appetite
Failure to thrive
Fatigue (frequent naps)
Lethargy
Coma
Bizarre behavior (staring, automatic movements)

Cranial Nerve Neuropathy

Cranial nerve involvement varies according to tumor location
Most common signs
- Head tilt
- Visual defects (nystagmus, diplopia, strabismus, episodic "graying out" of vision, visual field defects)

Vital Sign Disturbances

Decreased pulse and respiration
Increased blood pressure
Decreased pulse pressure
Hypothermia or hyperthermia

Other Signs

Seizures
Cranial enlargement*
Tense, bulging fontanel at rest*
Nuchal ridigity
Papilledema (edema of optic nerve)

*Present only in infants and young children.

logic diagnosis via surgery. Because the signs and symptoms are vague and easily overlooked, early diagnosis necessitates a high index of suspicion during history taking. A number of tests may be used in the neurologic evaluation, but the most common diagnostic procedure is MRI, which determines the location and extent of the tumor. Other tests that may be used include CT, angiography, electroencephalography, and lumbar puncture. Lumbar puncture is dangerous in the presence of increased ICP because of the possibility of brainstem herniation after a sudden release of pressure. However, the definitive diagnosis is based on brain tissue specimens obtained during surgery.

Therapeutic Management. Treatment may involve the use of surgery, radiotherapy, and chemotherapy. All three may or may not be used, depending on the type of tumor. The treatment of choice is total removal of the tumor without residual neurologic damage. Patients with the most complete tumor removal have the greatest chance of survival. Radiotherapy is used to treat most tumors and to shrink the size of the tumor before attempting surgical removal. Chemotherapy has emerged in the past decade to delay radiation in children younger than 5 years (Shiminski-Maher and Shields, 1995) and is also used as adjunct therapy for residual tumor, nonresectable tumor, or recurrent tumor. The most commonly used chemotherapy is cisplatin, carboplatin, vincristine, cyclophosphamide, lomustine, carmustine, etoposide, and thiotepa. Surgery (biopsy, resection, laser, or stereotactic), radiotherapy (hyperfractionated, fractionated, or stereotactic), and/or multiagent chemotherapy are all instrumental in the treatment of brain tumors.

Prognosis. The prognosis for the child with a brain tumor depends on the type of brain tumor, the size of the tumor, the extent of the disease, and the age of the child. Problems associated with treatment and a relatively poor prognosis, primarily in infants and young children, are compounded by serious late effects of therapy. A decline in incidence of children with medulloblastoma has been significantly linked with a protective effect of maternal folate, iron, and multivitamin supplementation. Along with the recent advances of surgical instrumentation allowing aggressive surgical intervention, modifications in radiation and use of chemotherapy have increased the long-term survival rates for many children with brain tumors (Shiminski-Maher and Shields, 1995).

Nursing Care Management

➤ Assessment

A child admitted to the hospital with neurologic dysfunction is often suspected of having a brain tumor, although the actual diagnosis is as yet unconfirmed. Establishing a baseline of data on which to compare preoperative and postoperative changes is an essential step toward planning physical care and preventing complications. It also allows the nurse to assess the degree of physical incapacity and the family's emotional reaction to the diagnosis.

Vital signs, including blood pressure and pulse pressure (the difference between systolic and diastolic pressures), are taken routinely and more often when any change is noted. Any sudden variations are reported immediately. It is especially important to note a change in vital signs during or after diagnostic procedures. A routine neurologic assessment is also performed at the same time as vital signs, and head circumference is measured in infants and very young children.

The child is observed for evidence of headache, vomiting, and any seizure activity. The location, severity, and duration of the headache are noted, as well as its relationship to activity and time of day. Behaviors such as lying flat and facing away from light or refusing to engage in play are clues to discomfort in the nonverbal child. The child's gait is observed at least once daily. Head tilt and other changes in posturing are always noted.

➤ Nursing Diagnoses

A number of nursing diagnoses will be evident after a thorough assessment of the child and family. Some of these are outlined in Box 51-7. Others may be determined in individual cases.

➤ Plan of Care and Implementation

The goals of care for the child with a brain tumor are as follows:

1. Child and family will be prepared for diagnostic/operative procedures.
2. Child will experience no postoperative complications.
3. Child and family will receive adequate support.
4. Child will return to normal functioning.

The suspected diagnosis of a brain tumor is always a crisis event. Despite the fact that some tumors are removed with excellent results, the physician can rarely give definitive answers regarding prognosis until after surgery. Therefore parents and older children require much emotional support to face the diagnostic procedures and a craniotomy.

Prepare Child and Family for Diagnostic/Operative Procedures. The child's preparation for the diagnostic tests depends on his or her age and previous experience. Because most of the tests involve x-ray equipment, the child may be familiar with the procedure. By the time most children are late preschoolers, they know that the head and brain are important parts of their bodies. It may be helpful to have them draw their concept of the brain in order to clarify misconceptions and base the explanation on their level of understanding.

Although the temptation is to justify the need for surgery by stating that removing the tumor will take away various symptoms, the nurse should refrain from emphasizing this point too strenuously. Postsurgery headaches and cerebellar symptoms, such as ataxia, may be aggravated rather than improved. Surgery may not improve vision. With optic gliomas the child will be blind in one eye. Finally, surgical removal of the mass may be impossible, and after surgery there may be temporary deterioration of functioning. Being honest before surgery most often makes honesty after the operation easier because no false hopes were created.

However, honesty does not negate instilling hope. A truthful explanation regarding the operation is as follows: "The surgeon will see exactly where the tumor is. If it is small and in one place, it will be removed. If it is large, as much of it as possible will be removed so that some of your symptoms will go away." It is best to deliver information in small amounts to let the child pursue additional answers. For example, some children will ask about what happens when part of the tumor is left in. An honest reply is that after surgery the practitioner will attempt to destroy the remaining tumor with radiation and/or chemotherapy. A further explanation of radiation or chemotherapy should be delayed until a decision regarding these treatments is made.

The hair may be shaved in the operating room just before surgery or in the child's room, usually the night before surgery. When shaving is done with the child awake, the procedure is approached in a sensitive, positive way. If the child's hair is long, it should be braided so that the long swatch can be saved. Showing children how they look at different stages of the process helps them prepare for the final appearance.

Once the hair is clipped very short or shaved, the child can be given a cap or scarf to wear to camouflage the baldness. Every precaution is taken to provide privacy during the procedure and to protect the child from teasing or ridicule by other children before surgery. It is also emphasized that the hair will regrow shortly after surgery. Depending on the child's immediate adjustment to the hair loss, the nurse may introduce the idea of wearing a wig until the hair is grown in, particularly if additional irradiation or chemotherapy is anticipated.

The child is also told about the size of the dressing. Usually the entire scalp is covered to maintain a tight wound closure, even if a small incision is made. Infratentorial head dressings may be attached to the upper back and extend forward on the neck to maintain slight extension and alignment as a precaution against wound rupture. Applying a similar dressing or "special hat" to a doll is often a less traumatic way of demonstrating the physical appearance.

The child also needs a brief explanation of how he or she will feel after surgery and where he or she will be. Ordinarily children will return to a special intensive care unit, which they should visit beforehand. The child should be aware that he or she may be sleepy for some time after surgery and that a headache is likely, although it should last only a few days.

Parents need similar explanations before surgery, especially in terms of special equipment used in the intensive care unit, dressings, and their child's behavior. For example, they should know that it is not unusual for the child to be comatose or lethargic for a few days after surgery. The nurse may wish to encourage less visiting during this period so that parents can rest and be able to provide support when the child awakens.

The nurse should participate in preoperative conferences with the physician and parents. The nurse needs to know what information the parents have been given to be able to give further explanations or emotional support when necessary.

Box 51-7

Nursing Diagnoses: the Child with a Brain Tumor

Sensory/perceptual alterations (visual, auditory, kinesthetic, gustatory, tactile, olfactory related to altered sensory reception, transmission, and/or integration)
Pain related to increased ICP
Altered family processes related to situational crisis (child with a serious illness)
Anxiety related to diagnosis, diagnostic and treatment procedures
Anticipatory grieving related to potential loss of child

Prevent Postoperative Complications. Usually the surgeon will prescribe specific orders for vital signs, neurologic checks, positioning, fluid regulation, and medication. These vary somewhat, depending on the location of the craniotomy. The following are general principles of care for infratentorial or supratentorial surgery. Additional aspects of care that are discussed elsewhere may include care of the child with seizures and care of the unconscious child in terms of neurologic assessment.

Vital signs are taken as often as every 15 to 30 minutes until stable. Temperature measurement is particularly important because of hyperthermia resulting from surgical intervention in the hypothalamus or brainstem and from some types of general anesthesia. To prepare for this reaction, a cooling blanket should be placed on the bed before the child returns to the unit so that it is ready for use when needed. The temperature is monitored carefully when any cooling measures are taken because hypothermia can occur suddenly. Recognizing signs of other complications such as increased ICP, meningitis, and respiratory tract infection is imperative.

NURSE ALERT • When temperature is elevated, an infectious process must always be suspected, particularly if the febrile state occurs 1 to 2 days after surgery.

Neurologic checks are an essential aspect of care and include pupillary reaction to light, LOC, sleep patterns, and response to stimuli. Although children may be comatose for a few days, once they regain consciousness, there should be a steady increase in alertness. Regression to a lethargic, irritable state indicates increasing pressure, possibly caused by meningitis or cerebral edema.

NURSE ALERT • Sluggish, dilated, or unequal pupils are reported immediately because they may indicate increased ICP and potential brainstem herniation, a medical emergency.

Observations for function are not instituted until the child regains consciousness. However, as soon as possible the nurse should begin testing reflexes, handgrip, and functioning of the cranial nerves. Muscle strength is usually diminished as a result of general weakness after surgery but should improve daily. Ataxia may be significantly worse with cerebellar intervention, but it will improve slowly. Edema near the cranial nerves may depress important functions such as the gag, blink, or swallowing reflex.

Dressings are observed for evidence of drainage. If soiled, the dressing is not removed but reinforced with dry sterile gauze. The approximate amount of drainage is estimated and recorded. A drain may be placed in the operative site.

NURSE ALERT • To keep an accurate account of drainage, the soiled area is circled with a pen every hour or so. In this way, continuous bleeding is easily recognized. The presence of colorless drainage is reported immediately, because it most likely is CSF from the incisional area. A foul odor from the dressing may indicate an infection. Such a finding is reported, and a culture is taken.

Once the younger child is alert, the arms may need to be restrained to preserve the dressing. Even a child who has been cooperative before surgery must be closely supervised during the initial stages of regaining consciousness, when disorientation and restlessness are common. Correct positioning after surgery is critical to prevent pressure against the operative site, reduce ICP, and avoid the danger of aspiration. If a large tumor was removed, the child is not placed on the operative site because the brain may suddenly shift to that cavity, causing trauma to the blood vessels, linings, and the brain itself. The nurse confers with the surgeon to be certain of the correct position, including degree of neck flexion. The first 24 to 48 hours after brain surgery are critical. If the child's position is restricted, notice of this is posted above the head of the bed. When the child is turned, every precaution is used to prevent jarring or malalignment in order to prevent undue strain on the sutures. Two nurses, one supporting the head and the other the body, are needed. The use of a turning sheet may facilitate turning a heavy child.

The child with an infratentorial procedure is usually positioned flat and on either side. Pillows should be placed against the child's back, not head, to maintain the desired position. Ordinarily the head and neck are kept in midline with the body and slightly extended. In a supratentorial craniotomy the head is usually elevated above the heart to facilitate CSF drainage and decrease excessive blood flow to the brain to prevent hemorrhage.

NURSE ALERT • The Trendelenburg position is contraindicated in both infratentorial and supratentorial surgeries because it increases ICP and the risk of hemorrhage. If shock is impending, the practitioner is notified immediately, before the head is lowered.

With an infratentorial craniotomy the child is allowed nothing by mouth for at least 24 hours, or longer if the gag and swallowing reflexes are depressed or the child is comatose. With a supratentorial operation, clear fluids may be resumed soon after the child is alert, sometimes within 24 hours. If the child vomits, oral liquids are stopped. Vomiting not only predisposes to aspiration but also increases ICP and the potential for incisional rupture.

The child should be fed to conserve energy and minimize movement. If there is any sign of facial paralysis, the child is fed slowly to prevent choking or aspiration. Sometimes gavage feeding is necessary when bodily functions are too depressed to permit safe oral feedings or when the child refuses to eat or drink. IV fluids are continued until oral fluids are well tolerated. Because of the cerebral edema postoperatively and danger of increased ICP, fluids are carefully monitored.

Headache may be severe and is mainly a result of cerebral edema. Measures to relieve some of the discomfort include providing a quiet, dimly lit environment; restricting visitors; preventing any sudden jarring movement, such as banging into the bed; and preventing an increase in ICP. Avoiding increased ICP is most effectively achieved by proper positioning and prevention of straining, such as during coughing, vomiting, or defecating. The use of opioids, such as morphine, to relieve pain is controversial because it is thought that they may mask signs of altered consciousness or depress respirations. However, they can be given safely because naloxone can be used to reverse opioid effects, such as sedation or respiratory depression. Acetaminophen and codeine are also effective analgesics for mild to moderate pain. Regardless of the drugs used, adequate dosage and regular administration are essential to providing optimum pain relief (see also Pain Assessment; Pain Management, Chapter 44). Placing an ice bag on the forehead may also provide some headache relief, especially if facial edema is severe.

Bowel movements are monitored to prevent constipation. Stool softeners may be given as soon as liquids are tolerated to facilitate easy passage of stool. Saline drops, or artificial tears, may be needed if the eyelids do not close completely, to prevent corneal ulceration.

Support Child and Family. The emotional needs of the family are immense when the diagnosis is a brain tumor, and feelings are influenced by the extent of surgery, any neurologic deficits, the expected prognosis, and additional therapy. Because few definitive answers can be given before surgery, the surgeon's report is a significant finding that can vary from a completely benign, resected neoplasm to a highly malignant, invasive, and only partially removed tumor. Although parents try to prepare themselves for a potentially fatal diagnosis, it is a shock for them.

Ideally a nurse should be with the family when the physician visits with them to discuss with parents the expected prognosis and plan of therapy. Although parents may hear only a fraction of what they are told, they can begin to put the future into perspective. Whereas some children will be cured, those with residual tumor may die within a relatively short period of time or live for several years. Regardless of the future prospects, the parents' thinking must be directed toward helping the child recover and resume a normal life to his or her maximum potential.

It is also a time to encourage parents to verbalize their feelings about the diagnosis. Often they express tremendous guilt for attributing the insidious onset of symptoms, such as ataxia, visual difficulty, or headache, to "minor complaints" by the child. Any comments that insinuate that the parents should have sought medical advice sooner are avoided because such remarks only add to the parents' guilt feelings.

During this period the nurse should also discuss with parents what they plan to tell the child. If the child was prepared honestly, as described previously, the diagnosis can be expressed in a similar manner. During recovery the child will need additional explanation about the treatment, as well as the reason for any residual neurologic effects, such as ataxia or blindness.

Promote Return to Optimum Functioning. The ultimate goal is a cured child who has maximum functioning. As soon as possible, the child should resume usual activities within tolerable limits, especially returning to school.* Until the skull is completely healed, the child may need to wear a helmet when engaging in any active sport. The school nurse and teacher should confer with the parents to discuss activity restrictions, such as physical education and the reactions of schoolmates to the child's appearance. Because children often equate brain surgery with "going crazy," it is important to prepare the child for possible remarks to this effect. As one child told a classmate, "It's your head they should have fixed because you're crazy. Can't you see that I'm all better?"

After discharge, the family needs continuing medical and emotional support from health personnel. Children who are long-term survivors after treatment for a brain tumor may have residual disabilities, such as growth retardation, cranial nerve palsies, sensory defects, motor abnormalities (especially ataxia), intellectual deficits, memory loss, dysphagia, dysgraphia, and behavioral problems. The high frequency of late effects attests to the tremendous need for follow-up care despite successful treatment of the tumor.

➤ Evaluation

The effectiveness of nursing interventions is determined by continual reassessment and evaluation of care based on the following observational guidelines and expected outcomes:

1. Interview child and family regarding their understanding of scheduled tests and procedures; observe child's behavior during procedures.
2. Monitor child's vital signs, neurologic signs, and dressing.
3. Interview child and family and observe their behaviors during hospitalization and recovery.
4. Interview child and family regarding activities and interests.

Expected outcomes include the following:

1. Child is able to demonstrate an understanding of the tests and procedures and copes with a minimum of stress.
2. Child exhibits no evidence of complications.
3. Child and family demonstrate evidence of healthy coping.
4. Family devises and carries out a realistic activity schedule, and child attends school with reasonable regularity (specify).

(See Nursing Care Plan: The Child with Cancer, Chapter 49; and Nursing Care Plan: The Child with a Brain Tumor.*)

Neuroblastoma

Neuroblastomas are the most common malignant extracranial solid tumors of childhood (Black and Atkinson, 1997). They occur in about 1 per 10,000 live births, with a slightly higher incidence in male infants. About half the cases occur in children younger than 2 years, and another fourth occur in children younger than 4 years. These tumors originate from embryonic neural crest cells that normally give rise to the adrenal medulla and the sympathetic ganglia. Consequently the majority of tumors develop in the adrenal gland or the retroperitoneal sympathetic chain. Other sites may be in the head, neck, chest, or pelvis.

Neuroblastoma is a "silent" tumor. In more than 70% of cases, diagnosis is made after metastasis occurs, with the first signs caused by involvement in the nonprimary site, usually the lymph nodes, bone marrow, skeletal system, skin, or liver.

Diagnostic Evaluation. The objective of diagnosis is to locate the primary site and areas of metastasis. The signs and symptoms of neuroblastoma depend on the location and stage of the disease. Most presenting signs are caused by compression of adjacent structures (Box 51-8). Skeletal survey; skull, neck, chest, abdominal, and bone CT scans; and a bone marrow test are used to locate a tumor mass and/or metastasis. An IV pyelogram may provide evidence of renal involvement.

Urinary excretion of catecholamines is detected in approximately 95% of children with adrenal or sympathetic tumors.

---

*Excellent publications, including the pamphlet *When Your Child Is Ready to Return to School,* are available from the American Brain Tumor Association, 2720 River Rd., Des Plaines, IL 60018; 1-800-886-2282; fax (847) 827-9918; e-mail: info@abta.org; website: www.abta.org.

*In Wong DL, Hess CS: ***Wong and Whaley's clinical manual of pediatric nursing,*** ed 5, St Louis, 2000, Mosby.

Box 51-8

Clinical Manifestations of Neuroblastoma

ABDOMINAL TUMORS

Firm, nontender, irregular mass
Crosses the midline
Compression of kidney, ureter, or bladder may cause urinary frequency or retention

DISTANT METASTASIS

Ocular:
- Supraorbital ecchymosis
- Periorbital edema
- Proptosis (exophthalmos) from invasion of retrobulbar soft tissue

Lymphadenopathy, especially cervical and supraclavicular
Skeletal: bone pain may or may not be present
Intracranial: neurologic impairment
Thoracic: respiratory obstruction
Spinal cord: varying degrees of paralysis
Adrenal:
- Increased catecholamine excretion
- Flushing
- Hypertension
- Tachycardia
- Diaphoresis

WIDESPREAD METASTASIS—VAGUE SYMPTOMS

Pallor
Weakness
Irritability
Anorexia
Weight loss

Analyzing the breakdown products excreted in the urine—namely vanillylmandelic acid (VMA), homovanillic acid (HVA), dopamine, and norepinephrine—permits detection of suspected tumor before and after medical/surgical intervention (Heideman et al, 1997). Amplification of *N-myc* gene and chromosomal abnormalities correlates strongly with advanced-stage disease, rapid tumor progression, and a poor prognosis (Black and Atkinson, 1997).

Therapeutic Management. Accurate clinical staging is important for establishing initial treatment. Therefore surgery is used both to remove as much of the tumor as possible and to obtain biopsy specimens. In early stages, complete surgical removal of the tumor is the treatment of choice. If the tumors are large, partial resection is attempted, with a course of irradiation postoperatively to shrink the tumor in the hope of complete removal at a later date. Radiation therapy also offers palliation for metastatic lesions in the bones, lung, liver, or brain. Chemotherapy is the mainstay of therapy for extensive local or disseminated disease.

Prognosis. If all stages are grouped together, the survival rates are 75% for children 1 year of age or younger and less than 50% for children older than 1 year (Brodeur and Castleberry, 1997). Generally the younger the child is at diagnosis (especially if younger than 1 year), the better the survival rate. Neuroblastoma is one of the few tumors that demonstrates spontaneous regression (especially stage IV-s), possibly as a result of maturity of the embryonic cell or the development of an active immune system.

Nursing Care Management. Nursing considerations are similar to those discussed for leukemia and brain tumors, including psychologic and physical preparation for diagnostic and operative procedures; prevention of postoperative complications for abdominal, thoracic, or cranial surgery; and explanation of chemotherapy and radiotherapy and their side effects.

Because this tumor carries a poor prognosis for many children, every consideration must be given the family in terms of coping with a life-threatening illness (see Chapter 41). Because of the high degree of metastasis at the time of diagnosis, many parents may feel guilty for not having recognized signs earlier. Often the guilt is expressed as anger toward practitioners for not diagnosing it sooner. Parents need support in dealing with these feelings and expressing them to the appropriate persons.

INTRACRANIAL INFECTIONS

The nervous system and its coverings are subject to infection by the same organisms that affect other organs of the body. However, the nervous system is limited in the ways in which it responds to injury. Infectious processes share virtually the same clinical and pathologic features. They differ primarily in the growth and virulence of the specific organism. It is generally difficult to distinguish between the various etiologic agents by looking at clinical manifestations. Laboratory studies are needed to identify the causative agent. The inflammatory process can affect the meninges *(meningitis),* the brain *(encephalitis),* or the spinal cord *(myelitis).*

The most common infection of the CNS is meningitis. It can be caused by a variety of organisms, but the three main types are the following:

1. Bacterial, or pyogenic, caused by pus-forming bacteria, especially the meningococcus, pneumococcus, and influenza bacillus
2. Tuberculous, caused by the tubercle bacillus
3. Viral, or aseptic, caused by a variety of viral agents

Bacterial Meningitis

Bacterial meningitis is an acute inflammation of the CNS. The advent of antimicrobial therapy has had a marked effect on the course and prognosis of the illness, although the use of conjugate vaccines against *Haemophilus influenzae* type B (Hib vaccine) since 1990 has led to the most dramatic change in the epidemiology of bacterial meningitis (Feigin and Perlman, 1998). In 1993 the incidence of *H. influenzae* had decreased to 2 cases per 100,000 children younger than 5 years, from 41 per 100,000 in 1987 (Anderson et al, 1994). Today *H. influenzae* type B infection has virtually been eradicated in areas of the world where the vaccine is administered routinely (Kaplan, 1999). However, bacterial meningitis caused by other organisms remains a serious illness in children. It is significant because of the residual damage caused by undiagnosed and untreated or inadequately treated cases. Ninety percent of reported cases occur in children between 1 month and 5 years of age (Feigin and Perlman, 1998).

Bacterial meningitis can be caused by any of a variety of bacterial agents. *Streptococcus pneumoniae* (pneumococcal) and *Neisseria meningitidis* (meningococcal) organisms are responsible for bacterial meningitis in 95% of children older than 2 months. The leading causes of neonatal meningitis are the group B streptococci and *Escherichia coli* organisms. *E. coli* infection is seldom seen beyond infancy. Meningococcal (epidemic cerebrospinal) meningitis occurs in an epidemic form and is the only form readily transmitted to others. It is transmitted by droplet infection from nasopharyngeal secretions. Although it may develop at any age, the risk of meningococcal infection increases with the number of contacts; therefore it occurs predominantly in school-age children and adolescents.

Pathophysiology. Meningitis appears to occur as an extension of a variety of bacterial infections, probably as a result of the lack of acquired resistance to the various causative organisms. The most common route of infection is by vascular dissemination from a focus of infection elsewhere. Organisms also gain entry by direct implantation after penetrating wounds, skull fractures that provide an opening into the skin or sinuses, lumbar puncture or surgical procedures, anatomic abnormalities such as spina bifida, or foreign bodies such as a ventricular shunt. Once implanted, the organisms spread into the CSF, which serves as a conduit for spread of infection throughout the subarachnoid space.

The infective process is that seen in any bacterial infection—inflammation, exudation, white blood cell accumulation, and varying degrees of tissue damage. The brain becomes hyperemic and edematous, and the entire surface of the brain is covered with a layer of purulent exudate. As infection extends to the ventricles, thick pus, fibrin, or adhesions may occlude the narrow passages, obstructing the flow of CSF.

NURSE ALERT • Any child who is ill and develops a purpuric or petechial rash may have overwhelming meningococcemia and must receive medical attention immediately (Box 51-9).

Diagnostic Evaluation. A lumbar puncture is the definitive diagnostic test. The fluid pressure is measured, and samples are obtained for culture, Gram stain, blood cell count, and determination of glucose and protein content. The findings are usually diagnostic. Culture and stain are needed to identify the causative organism. Spinal fluid pressure is usually elevated, but interpretation is often difficult when the child is crying. Sedation with meperidine (Demerol) or fentanyl and midazolam (Versed) can alleviate the child's pain and fear associated with this procedure. EMLA, applied to the skin overlying L3 to L5 1

Box 51-9

Clinical Manifestations of Bacterial Meningitis

CHILDREN AND ADOLESCENTS

Usually abrupt onset
Fever
Chills
Headache
Vomiting
Alterations in sensorium
Seizures (often the initial sign)
Irritability
Agitation
May develop:
- Photophobia
- Delirium
- Hallucinations
- Aggressive behavior
- Drowsiness
- Stupor
- Coma

Nuchal rigidity
- May progress to opisthotonos

Positive Kernig and Brudzinski signs
Hyperactive but variable reflex responses
Signs and symptoms peculiar to individual organisms:
- Petechial or purpuric rashes (meningococcal infection), especially when associated with a shocklike state
- Joint involvement (meningococcal and *H. influenzae* infection)
- Chronically draining ear (pneumococcal meningitis)

INFANTS AND YOUNG CHILDREN

Classic picture (above) rarely seen in children between 3 months and 2 years of age
Fever
Poor feeding
Vomiting
Marked irritability
Frequent seizures (often accompanied by a high-pitched cry)
Bulging fontanel
Nuchal rigidity may or may not be present
Brudzinski and Kernig signs are not helpful in diagnosis
- Difficult to elicit and evaluate in this age group

Subdural empyema (*H. influenzae* infection)

NEONATES: SPECIFIC SIGNS

Extremely difficult to diagnose
Manifestations vague and nonspecific
Well at birth but within a few days begins to look and behave poorly
Refuse feedings
Poor sucking ability
Vomiting or diarrhea
Poor tone
Lack of movement
Weak cry
Full, tense, and bulging fontanel may appear late in course of illness
Neck usually supple

NEONATES: NONSPECIFIC SIGNS THAT MAY BE PRESENT

Hypothermia or fever (depending on the maturity of the infant)
Jaundice
Irritability
Drowsiness
Seizures
Respiratory irregularities or apnea
Cyanosis
Weight loss

hour before lumbar puncture, reduces pain for children undergoing this procedure.

There is generally an elevated white blood cell count, predominantly polymorphonuclear leukocytes, but it may be extremely variable. The glucose level is reduced, generally in proportion to the duration and severity of the infection. The protein concentration is usually increased. A blood culture is advisable for all children suspected of having meningitis and occasionally proves positive when results of CSF culture are negative. Nose and throat cultures may provide helpful information in some cases.

Therapeutic Management. Acute bacterial meningitis is a medical emergency that requires early recognition and immediate institution of therapy to prevent death and avoid residual disabilities. The initial therapeutic management includes:

- Isolation precautions
- Initiation of antimicrobial therapy
- Maintenance of optimum hydration
- Maintenance of ventilation
- Reduction of increased ICP
- Management of bacterial shock
- Control of seizures
- Control of temperature extremes
- Correction of anemia
- Treatment of complications

The child is isolated from other children, usually in an intensive care unit, and observed closely. An IV infusion is started to facilitate the administration of antimicrobial agents, fluids, antiepileptic drugs, and blood if needed. The child is placed on a cardiac monitor.

The choice of antibiotic is based on the known sensitivity of the organism. Except under special circumstances, the drugs are administered intravenously throughout the course of treatment. They are given in large doses, and the period of therapy is determined by CSF findings (normal glucose level and negative culture) and the child's clinical condition. Dexamethasone is currently recommended for the treatment of *H. influenzae* type b meningitis and should be considered for use in other types of bacterial meningitis (American Academy of Pediatrics, 2000a). It should not be used if aseptic or nonbacterial meningitis is suspected (Feigin and Perlman, 1998).

Maintaining hydration is a primary concern, and the decision to administer IV fluids and the type and amount of fluid are determined by the patient's condition. The optimum hydration involves correction of any fluid deficits followed by maintenance hydration at minimum levels to prevent cerebral edema. Cerebral edema and electrolyte disturbances are complications associated with poor neurologic outcomes (Brown and Feigin, 1994). If indicated, measures are taken to reduce ICP as described previously (p. 1429).

Complications are treated appropriately, such as aspiration of subdural effusion in infants and heparin therapy for children who develop disseminated intravascular coagulation syndrome. If shock occurs, it is managed by restoration of blood volume and maintenance of electrolyte balance. Seizures, which occur in many children, are controlled with anticonvulsants.

Lumbar puncture is carried out as needed to determine the effectiveness of therapy. The patient is evaluated neurologically during the convalescent period and at regular intervals during the succeeding year.

Prognosis. The age of the child, the type of organism, the severity of the infection, the duration of the illness before the onset of therapy, and the sensitivity of the organism to antimicrobial drugs are important factors in determining the prognosis. Sequelae are most commonly seen when the disease occurs in the first 2 months of life and least often in children with meningococcal meningitis. The residual deficits in infants are primarily a result of communicating hydrocephalus and the greater effects of cerebritis on the immature brain. In older children the residual effects are related to the inflammatory process itself or result from vasculitis associated with the disease. The mortality rate and incidence of poor neurologic outcome are highest in patients with pneumococcal meningitis (Kaplan, 1997). Evaluation of cranial nerve VIII is needed for at least a 6-month follow-up period to assess for possible hearing loss.

Prevention. Vaccines are available for types A, C, Y, and W-135 meningococci and *H. influenzae* type b. Routine meningococcal vaccination of children is not recommended. However, routine vaccinations for *H. influenzae* type b are recommended for all children beginning at 2 months of age (see Immunizations, Chapter 36). Pneumococcal conjugate vaccine is now recommended for all children beginning at 2 months of age (American Academy of Pediatrics, 2000c).

Nursing Care Management. Nurses should take necessary precautions to protect themselves and others from possible infection. Parents are taught the proper procedures and supervised in their application.

> **NURSE ALERT** • A major priority of nursing care of a child suspected of having meningitis is to administer the antibiotic as soon as it is ordered. The child is also placed on respiratory isolation for at least 24 hours after implementation of antimicrobial therapy.

The room should be kept as quiet as possible, and environmental stimuli are kept at a minimum because most affected children are sensitive to noise, bright lights, and other external stimuli. Most children are more comfortable without a pillow and with the head of the bed slightly elevated. A side-lying position is more often assumed because of nuchal rigidity. The nurse should avoid actions, such as lifting the child's head, that cause pain or increase discomfort. Measures are taken to ensure safety because the child is often restless and subject to seizures.

The nursing care of the child with meningitis is determined by the child's symptoms and treatment. Observation of vital signs, neurologic signs, LOC, urine output, and other pertinent data is carried out at frequent intervals. The unconscious child is managed as described previously (see p. 1426), and all children are observed carefully for signs of the complications just described, especially signs of increased ICP, shock, or respiratory distress. Head circumference is measured in the infant because subdural effusions and obstructive hydrocephalus can develop as a complication of meningitis.

Fluids and nourishment are determined by the child's status. The child with dulled sensorium is usually given nothing by mouth. Other children are allowed clear liquids initially and progress to a diet suitable for their age. Careful monitoring and recording of intake and output are needed to determine deviations that might indicate impending shock or increasing fluid accumulation, such as cerebral edema or subdural effusion.

One of the problems in nursing care of children with meningitis is maintaining the IV infusion for the length of time needed to provide adequate antimicrobial therapy (usually 10 days). Because continuous IV fluids are usually not necessary, an intermittent infusion device is used. In some cases children who are recovering uneventfully are sent home with the device, and parents are taught IV drug administration.*

(See also Nursing Care Plan: The Child with Acute Bacterial Meningitis.†)

Family Support. The sudden nature of the illness makes emotional support of the child and parents extremely important. Parents are very upset and concerned about their child's condition and commonly feel guilty for not having suspected the seriousness of the illness sooner. They need reassurance that the natural onset of meningitis is sudden and that they acted responsibly in seeking medical assistance when they did. The nurse encourages them to openly discuss their feelings to minimize blame and guilt. They also are kept informed of the child's progress and of all procedures and treatments. In the event that the child's condition worsens, they need the same psychologic care as parents facing the possible death of their child (Family Focus box; see also Chapter 41).

Nonbacterial (Aseptic) Meningitis

Aseptic meningitis is caused by a number of agents, principally viruses, and is commonly associated with other diseases, such as measles, mumps, herpes, and leukemia. Enteroviruses and mumps viruses account for many cases.

The onset may be abrupt or gradual. The initial manifestations are headache, fever, malaise, gastrointestinal symptoms, and signs of meningeal irritation that develop a day or two after the onset of illness. Abdominal pain and nausea and vomiting are common; back and leg pain, sore throat, chest pain, photophobia, and generalized muscular aches or pains are found occasionally. There may be a maculopapular rash. These symptoms usually subside spontaneously and rapidly, and the child is well in 3 to 10 days with no residual effects.

Diagnosis is based on clinical features and CSF findings, which include increased lymphocytes, predominantly mononuclear cells. It is important to differentiate this self-limited disorder from the more serious form of meningitis and to diagnose and treat any disease of which it is a manifestation.

*Community and home care instructions for caring for an intermittent infusion device are available in Wong DL, Hess CS: ***Wong and Whaley's clinical manual of pediatric nursing,*** ed 5, St Louis, 2000, Mosby.

†In Wong DL, Hess CS: ***Wong and Whaley's clinical manual of pediatric nursing,*** ed 5, St Louis, 2000, Mosby.

Family Focus

PREVENTING BACTERIAL MENINGITIS

With the change in immunization schedules calling for administration of Hib vaccine to infants at 2 months of age, parents should be encouraged to bring their child to a health facility so that the full series of inoculations is completed. With the high mortality associated with bacterial meningitis, early immunization can prevent families from experiencing the tragic death of a child. Nurses play a significant role in educating families regarding preventive measures, such as early Hib vaccination.

Treatment is primarily symptomatic, such as acetaminophen for headache and muscle pain and positioning for comfort. Antimicrobial agents may be administered and isolation enforced until a definitive diagnosis is made as a precaution against the possibility that the disease might be of bacterial origin.

Nursing care is similar to nursing care of the child with bacterial meningitis.

Encephalitis

Encephalitis is an inflammatory process of the CNS producing altered function of various portions of the brain and spinal cord. Encephalitis can be caused by a variety of organisms, including bacteria, spirochetes, fungi, protozoa, helminths, and viruses. Most infections are associated with viruses, and this discussion is limited to these etiologic agents.

Etiology. Encephalitis can occur as a result of (1) direct invasion of the CNS by a virus, or (2) postinfectious involvement of the CNS after a viral disease. Often the specific type of encephalitis in a particular child may not be identified for some time or at all. The majority of cases of known etiology are associated with the childhood viral diseases. Most other viral infections are those involved with arthropod vectors and those associated with hemorrhagic fevers. The vectors for most agents pathogenic to human beings and detected in the United States are mosquitos and ticks; therefore most cases of encephalitis appear during the hot summer months.

Herpes simplex encephalitis is an uncommon disease, but 30% of cases involve children. The initial clinical findings are nonspecific (fever, altered mental status), but most cases evolve to demonstrate focal neurologic signs and symptoms. Children may experience focal seizures. The CSF is abnormal in most cases. Because of a rise in the number of children with herpes simplex virus encephalitis, suspected cases require prompt attention, especially because the diagnosis can be difficult. The clinical diagnosis can be confirmed by the rapid appearance of IgM antibody to herpes simplex virus type 1 in CSF and serum. The early use of IV acyclovir reduces mortality and morbidity.

Diagnostic Evaluation. The clinical features are similar, regardless of the agent involved. Manifestations can range from a mild, benign form that resembles aseptic meningitis, lasting a few days and followed by rapid and complete recovery, to a fulminating encephalitis with severe CNS involvement (Box 51-10).

Box 51-10

Clinical Manifestations of Encephalitis

ONSET: SUDDEN OR GRADUAL	SEVERE CASES
Malaise	High fever
Fever	Stupor
Headache	Seizures
Dizziness	Disorientation
Apathy	Spasticity
Neck stiffness	Coma (may proceed to death)
Nausea and vomiting	Ocular palsies
Ataxia	Paralysis
Tremors	
Hyperactivity	
Speech difficulties	

The diagnosis is made on the basis of clinical findings, circumstances associated with the disease, and (where possible) identification of the specific virus. A diagnostic evaluation of encephalitis may include a brain biopsy, usually from the temporal lobe area. Arboviruses are rarely detected in the blood or spinal fluid, but viruses of herpes, mumps, and measles and enteroviruses may be found in CSF. Serologic diagnosis may be reached by means of a variety of antibody tests. The first should be drawn as soon after onset as possible, and the second 2 or 3 weeks later. Laboratory detection of herpes simplex virus–DNA in CSF may be used to expedite the diagnosis of herpes simplex encephalitis.

Therapeutic Management. Patients suspected of having encephalitis are hospitalized promptly for skilled nursing care and observation. Treatment is primarily supportive, including conscientious nursing care, control of cerebral manifestations, and adequate nutrition and hydration, with observations and management as for other disorders involving cerebral injury. Follow-up care with periodic reevaluation and rehabilitation are important requisites to survivors with residual effects of the disease.

Prognosis. The prognosis for the child with encephalitis depends on the child's age, the type of organism, and residual neurologic damage. Children younger than 2 years may exhibit increased neurologic disability, including learning difficulties and seizure disorders.

Nursing Considerations. Nursing care of the child with encephalitis is the same as for any unconscious child and the child with meningitis. Neurologic monitoring, administration of medications, and support to the child and parents are the major aspects of care.

Reye Syndrome (RS)

RS is a toxic encephalopathy associated with other characteristic organ involvement. It is characterized by fever, profoundly impaired consciousness, and disordered hepatic function.

The etiology of the disorder is obscure, but most cases of RS follow a common viral illness, most commonly influenza or varicella. The potential association between aspirin therapy for the treatment of fever in children with varicella or influenza and the development of RS precludes its use in these patients (Saez-Llorenz and McCracken, 1997). The use of aspirin and nonsteroidal antiinflammatory drugs (NSAIDs), such as ibuprofen, is not recommended for children with varicella or those suspected of having influenza.

Pathophysiology. RS has been defined by the Centers for Disease Control and Prevention as acute noninflammatory encephalopathy and hepatopathy, with no reasonable explanation for the cerebral and hepatic abnormalities. The pathology of RS is a mitochondrial insult induced by different viruses, drugs, exogenous toxins, and genetic factors.

Diagnostic Evaluation. Elevated ammonia levels tend to correlate with the clinical manifestations and prognosis. Definitive diagnosis is established by liver biopsy (Box 51-11). Children who in the past would have been diagnosed with RS are now assigned other diagnoses, such as metabolic disorders, as a result of improved diagnostic techniques.

Therapeutic Management. The most important aspect of successful management of the child with RS is early diagnosis and aggressive therapy. Rapid progression through coma stages and high peak ammonia concentrations are associated with a more serious prognosis. Cerebral edema with increased ICP represents the most immediate threat to life. Recovery from RS is rapid and usually without sequelae if there has been early diagnosis and implementation of therapy.

Prognosis. Although the incidence of RS is declining, survivors may have subtle neuropsychologic deficits. Generally recovery is good given the gravity of the disease (Quam, 1994).

Nursing Care Management. The child who is acutely ill with RS requires continuous and intensive nursing care. In addition to an appraisal of vital functions and neurologic status, the nurse assists with a lumbar puncture, obtains blood for laboratory examination, and inserts various IV lines such as peripheral, arterial, and central venous pressure. A retention catheter and a nasogastric tube are inserted, and when respirations are compromised, an endotracheal tube is inserted and attached to a respirator for controlled respirations.

Care and observations are implemented as for any child with an altered state of consciousness (p. 1426) and increasing ICP. Accurate and frequent monitoring of intake and output is essential for adjusting fluid volumes to prevent both dehydration and cerebral edema. The child who is paralyzed and in a drug-induced coma is totally dependent on the caregivers, and meticulous vigilance and attention to all biologic needs are mandatory. Because hypovolemic shock is a constant danger in children with controlled fluid intake and osmotic diuresis, vital signs, including central venous pressure and/or cardiac output (Swan-Ganz catheter), are monitored often. Because of related liver dysfunction, the nurse must observe for signs of impaired coagulation such as prolonged bleeding time.

Family Support. Parents of children with RS need a great deal of emotional support. They are usually frightened by the child's appearance, the treatment, and the life-threatening severity and suddenness of the illness. Their distress is increased if they believe that their actions may have contributed to a delay in diagnosis. They need to be kept informed regarding the child's progress, to have diagnostic procedures and therapeutic management explained, and to be given concerned and sympathetic support.

Box 51-11

Staging Criteria for Reye Syndrome

Stage I: Vomiting, lethargy, and drowsiness; liver dysfunction; type I electroencephalogram (EEG); follows commands; pupillary reaction brisk

Stage II: Disorientation, combativeness, delirium, hyperventilation, hyperactive reflexes, appropriate responses to painful stimuli; evidence of liver dysfunction, type I EEG; pupillary reaction sluggish

Stage III: Obtunded, coma, hyperventilation, decorticate rigidity, preservation of pupillary light reaction and oculovestibular reflexes (although sluggish); type II EEG

Stage IV: Deepening coma, decerebrate rigidity, loss of oculocephalic reflexes, large and fixed pupils, loss of doll's eye reflex, loss of corneal reflexes; minimal liver dysfunction; type III or IV EEG; evidence of brainstem dysfunction

Stage V: Seizures, loss of deep tendon reflexes, respiratory arrest, flaccidity; type IV EEG; usually no evidence of liver dysfunction

The National Reye's Syndrome Foundation* was established by the parents of a child who died of this disease. These parents hoped to encourage research of the disease and to educate parents and health professionals.

Human Immunodeficiency Virus (HIV) Encephalopathy

Children with HIV encephalopathy, a complication of acquired immunodeficiency syndrome (AIDS), present a nursing challenge. Progressive encephalopathy occurs in 30% to 50% of infants and children infected with HIV; 82% are younger than 5 years.

Neurologic manifestations in children suggest that progressive encephalopathy is a result of primary and persistent infection of the brain with the virus. Unexplained neurodevelopmental regression and focal seizures are the dominant clinical features of the disorder. Others include progressive motor dysfunction and atypical CNS infections. These manifestations indicate a poor prognosis and, almost invariably, a fatal outcome. However, earlier implementation of therapies for AIDS may allow for slower progression of these neurologic complications.

Appropriate precautions are practiced by nurses when caring for these children. Excellent nursing requires careful handling of these children because they may experience pain, isolation, social stigma, susceptibility to infection, and abandonment resulting in less than minimum sensorimotor stimulation. Nursing assessment and intervention warrant planning time to meet developmental needs, especially holding, rocking, and comforting the child. Pain management is essential and may require use of several drugs to effectively treat the neuropathic pain (see Pain Assessment and Pain Management, Chapter 44). (See Chapter 49 for a more extensive discussion of AIDS.)

Rabies

Rabies is an acute infection of the nervous system caused by a virus that is almost invariably fatal if left untreated. It is transmitted to human beings by the saliva of an infected mammal introduced through a bite or skin abrasion. After entry into a new host, the virus multiplies in muscle cells and is spread through neural pathways without stimulating a protective host immune response.

Approximately 88% of rabies cases come from wild animals, and 12% come from domestic animals. Cats are now the most common domestic animals and should be the target of rabies vaccination programs. Carnivorous wild animals (especially raccoons, skunks, and foxes) and bats are the animals most often infected with rabies and the cause of most indigenous cases of human rabies in the United States (Centers for Disease Control and Prevention, 1998). The likelihood of human exposure to a rabid domestic animal has decreased greatly. The circumstances of a biting incident are important. An unprovoked attack is more likely to indicate a rabid animal than a provoked attack. Bites inflicted on a child attempting to feed or handle an apparently healthy animal can generally be regarded as provoked. Any child bitten by a wild animal is assumed to be exposed to rabies.

NURSE ALERT • Unusual behavior in an animal is cause for suspicion; children should be warned to beware of wild animals that appear friendly.

The disease is uncommon in human beings, but the highest incidence occurs in children younger than 15 years. The incubation period usually ranges from 1 to 3 months but may be as short as 10 days or as long as 8 months. Only 10% to 15% of persons bitten develop the disease, but once symptoms are present, rabies progresses inexorably to a fatal outcome. Diagnosis is made on the basis of the history and clinical features (Box 51-12). Although treatment is of little avail once symptoms appear, the long incubation period allows time for induction of active and passive immunity before the onset of illness.

Therapeutic Management. Two types of immunizing products are available for use in human beings: (1) the *inactivated rabies vaccines*, which induce an active immune response, and (2) the *globulins*, which contain preformed antibodies. The two types of products should be used concurrently for rabies postexposure treatment when prophylaxis is indicated.

The current therapy for a rabid animal bite consists of thorough cleansing of the wound and passive immunization with *human rabies immune globulin (HRIG)* as soon as possible after exposure (Centers for Disease Control and Prevention, 1999).

Postexposure active immunity is conferred by administration of the *human diploid cell rabies vaccine (HDCV)*. The first dose of the vaccine is given at the same time as the immune globulin and followed by intramuscular injections at 3, 7, 14, and 28 days after the first dose. An additional dose in 90 days is recommended by the World Health Organization. Before antirabies prophylaxis is initiated, the local or state health department is consulted.

Nursing Care Management. Both parents and children are frightened by the urgency and seriousness of the situation. They need anticipatory guidance for the therapy, and support and reassurance regarding the efficacy of the preventive measures for this dreaded disease. EMLA cream can be placed

Box 51-12

Clinical Manifestations of Rabies

INITIAL SIGNS
General malaise
Fever
Sore throat

EXCITEMENT PHASE
Hypersensitivity
Increased reaction to external stimuli
Seizures
Maniacal behavior
Choking

SEVERE SPASM OF RESPIRATORY MUSCLES*
Apnea
Cyanosis
Anoxia

*From attempts at swallowing (characteristics from which the term *hydrophobia* was derived).

*P.O. Box 829, Bryan, OH 43506; (419) 636-2679.

on the injection site $2\frac{1}{2}$ hours before the procedure to reduce the pain.

Mass immunization is unnecessary and unlikely to be implemented. Certain circumstances may warrant vaccination, such as when a child is being taken to an area of the world where rabies in stray dogs is still a problem.

SEIZURE DISORDERS

Seizures are brief malfunctions of the brain's electric system resulting from cortical neuronal discharge. The manifestations of seizures are determined by the site of origin and may include unconsciousness or altered consciousness; involuntary movements; and changes in perception, behaviors, sensations, and posture. Seizures are the most commonly observed neurologic dysfunction in children and can occur with a variety of conditions involving the CNS.

Epilepsy

Seizures result from paroxysmal discharges in cortical neurons and are symptoms of abnormal brain function. They are considered to be a symptom of an underlying disease process. Once it is determined that the child has had a seizure, it is important to distinguish whether the episode was an epileptic or a nonepileptic seizure. Seizures are the indispensable characteristic of epilepsy; however, not every seizure is epileptic. Epilepsy is a chronic seizure disorder with recurrent and unprovoked seizures.

Etiology. Seizure disorders have numerous and varied causes (e.g., tumors, infections, neoplasms). Most are *idiopathic.* Although the cause of idiopathic epilepsy is unknown, genetic factors may in some way alter the seizure threshold to influence neuronal discharge. A seizure disorder also can be *acquired* as a result of brain injury during prenatal, perinatal, or postnatal periods. This injury may be caused by trauma, hypoxia, infections, exogenous or endogenous toxins, and a variety of other factors. Biochemical events (e.g., hypoglycemia, hypocalcemia, and certain nutritional deficiencies) produce seizure activity.

The incidence of causative factors associated with childhood seizures is commonly related to the age of the child. Seizures are more common during the first 2 years of life than during any other period of childhood. In very young infants the most common causes are birth injuries, such as intracranial trauma, hemorrhage, or anoxia, and congenital defects of the brain. Acute infections are a common cause of seizures in late infancy and early childhood but become an infrequent cause in middle childhood. In children older than 3 years the most common factor is idiopathic epilepsy.

Seizure activity is believed to be caused by spontaneous electric discharge initiated by a group of hyperexcitable cells referred to as the *epileptogenic focus.* These cells display increased electric excitability in response to any of a variety of physiologic stimuli, such as cellular dehydration, abnormal blood glucose levels, electrolyte imbalance, fatigue, emotional stress, and endocrine changes. When neuronal excitation from the epileptogenic focus spreads to the brainstem, a generalized seizure develops. Seizures are designated as *focal (localized), focal with rapid generalization,* and *generalized,* on the basis of the characteristic neuronal discharges. In a large proportion of children focal seizures spread to other areas, ultimately becoming generalized with loss of consciousness.

Classification. There are many different types of epileptic seizures, and each has unique characteristics. The onset of a seizure is abrupt, paroxysmal, and transitory, and signs are highly variable. The current classification system divides seizures into two major categories: partial and generalized (Box 51-13). Some of these are described in the following section.

Partial seizures are caused by abnormal electric discharges from epileptogenic foci limited to a more or less circumscribed region of the cerebral cortex. Focal seizures may arise from any area of the cerebral cortex, but the frontal, temporal, and parietal lobes are the ones that are most often affected. The area of cerebral involvement is reflected by clinical manifestations. Partial seizures are subdivided into three types. *Simple partial seizures* have elementary or simple symptoms and are accompanied by no alteration of consciousness (also called an *aura*). *Complex partial seizures* involve complex symptoms and impairment of consciousness. These seizures may begin with an *aura,* a simple partial seizure that is usually a sensation or sensory phenomenon that reflects the complicated connections and integrative functions of that area of the brain. The aura is part of the seizure event and is associated with electroencephalogram (EEG) changes (Van Donselaar, Geerts, and Schimscheimer, 1990). *Simple* or *complex seizures secondarily generalized* develop into generalized seizures, usually a tonic-clonic event.

Generalized seizures without a focal onset appear to arise in the reticular formation, and the clinical observations indicate that the initial involvement is from both hemispheres. Commonly loss of consciousness occurs and is the initial clinical manifestation. Unlike partial seizures that become generalized, there is no aura. Episodes occur at any time, day or night, and the interval between episodes may be minutes, hours, weeks, or even years. Most affected persons first experience seizures in childhood, and children whose seizures begin before 4 years of age have mental retardation and behavioral and learning problems more often than those whose seizures begin after 4 years of age.

Diagnostic Evaluation. Establishing a diagnosis is critical. The process of diagnosis in a child with a seizure disorder has two major foci: (1) to ascertain the type of seizure the child has experienced and (2) to attempt to understand the cause of the events. The assessment and diagnosis rely heavily on a thorough history, skilled observation, and use of several diagnostic tests.

During the assessment process it is unusual to observe the child having a seizure; therefore a complete, accurate, and detailed history should be obtained from a reliable and knowledgeable informant. This history involves prenatal, perinatal, and neonatal periods, including any instances of infection, apnea, colic, or poor feeding, and information regarding any previous accidents or serious illnesses.

Another treatment for refractory seizures is the use of the *ketogenic diet,* which severely restricts carbohydrate and protein intake and uses fat as the primary fuel to produce ketosis. A recent review of the effects of the diet indicate that some children have fewer seizures during treatment, but the long-term effects, such as increased blood lipids, are not known (Lefevre and Aronson, 2000).

Seizure history should be equally detailed, including the type of seizure or description of the child's behavior during the

Box 51-13

Classification and Clinical Manifestations of Seizures

PARTIAL SEIZURES

Simple Partial Seizures with Motor Signs

Characterized by:
- Localized motor symptoms
- Somatosensory, psychic, autonomic symptoms
- Combination of these
- Abnormal discharges remain unilateral

Manifestations:
- Aversive seizure (most common motor seizure in children)
  - Eye or eyes and head turn away from the side of the focus
  - Awareness of movement or loss of consciousness
- Rolandic (Sylvan) seizure
  - Tonic-clonic movements involving the face
  - Salivation
  - Arrested speech
  - Most common during sleep
- Jacksonian march (rare in children)
  - Orderly, sequential progression of clonic movements beginning in a foot, hand, or face and moving or "marching" to adjacent body parts

Simple Partial Seizures With Sensory Signs

Characterized by various sensations, including:
- Numbness, tingling, prickling, paresthesia, or pain originating in one area (e.g., face or extremities) and spreading to other parts of the body
- Visual sensations or formed images
- Motor phenomena such as posturing or hypertonia
- Uncommon in children younger than 8 years

Complex Partial Seizures (Psychomotor Seizures)

Observed more often in children from 3 years through adolescence

Characterized by:
- Period of altered behavior
- Amnesia for event (no recollection of behavior)
- Inability to respond to environment
- Impaired consciousness during event
- Drowsiness or sleep usually follows seizure
- Confusion and amnesia may be prolonged
- Complex sensory phenomena (aura)
  - Most frequent sensation—strange feeling in the pit of the stomach that rises toward the throat
  - Often accompanied by:
    - Odd or unpleasant odors or tastes
    - Complex auditory or visual hallucinations
    - Ill-defined feelings of elation or strangeness (e.g., deja vu, a feeling of familiarity in a strange environment)
- May be strong feelings of fear and anxiety, distorted sense of time and self
- Small children may emit a cry or attempt to run for help

Patterns of motor behavior:
- Stereotypic
- Similar with each subsequent seizure
- May suddenly cease activity, appear dazed, stare into space, become confused and apathetic, and become limp or stiff or display some form of posturing
- May be confused
- May perform purposeless, complicated activities in a repetitive manner (automatisms), such as walking, running, kicking, laughing, or speaking incoherently, most often followed by postictal confusion or sleep; may be oropharyngeal activities, such as smacking, chewing, drooling, swallowing, and nausea or abdominal pain followed by stiffness, a fall, and postictal sleep; rarely manifests as rage or temper tantrums; aggressive acts uncommon during seizure

GENERALIZED SEIZURES

Tonic-Clonic Seizures (Formerly Known as Grand Mal)

Most common and most dramatic of all seizure manifestations

Occur without warning

Tonic phase: lasts approximately 10 to 20 seconds

Manifestations:
- Eyes roll upward
- Immediate loss of consciousness
- If standing, falls to floor or ground
- Stiffens in generalized, symmetric tonic contraction of entire body musculature
- Arms usually flexed
- Legs, head, and neck extended
- May utter a peculiar piercing cry
- Apneic, may become cyanotic
- Increased salivation and loss of swallowing reflex

Clonic phase: lasts about 30 seconds but can vary from only a few seconds to a half hour or longer

Manifestations:
- Violent jerking movements as the trunk and extremities undergo rhythmic contraction and relaxation
- May foam at the mouth
- May be incontinent of urine and feces

As event ends, movements become less intense, occur at longer intervals, then cease entirely

Status epilepticus: series of seizures at intervals too brief to allow the child to regain consciousness between the time one event ends and the next begins
- Requires emergency intervention
- Can lead to exhaustion, respiratory failure, and death

Postictal state:
- Appears to relax
- May remain semiconscious and difficult to arouse
- May awaken in a few minutes
- Remains confused for several hours
- Poor coordination
- Mild impairment of fine motor movements
- May have visual and speech difficulties
- May vomit or complain of severe headache
- When left alone, usually sleeps for several hours
- On awakening is fully conscious
- Usually feels tired and complains of sore muscles and headache
- No recollection of entire event

Absence Seizures (Formerly Called Petit Mal or Lapses)

Characterized by:
- Onset usually between 4 and 12 years of age
- More common in girls than in boys
- Usually cease at puberty

Box 51-13

Classification and Clinical Manifestations of Seizures—cont'd

Absence Seizures (Formerly Called Petit Mal or Lapses)—cont'd
- Brief loss of consciousness
- Minimal or no alteration in muscle tone
- May go unrecognized because little change in child's behavior
- Abrupt onset; suddenly develops 20 or more attacks daily
- Event often mistaken for inattentiveness or daydreaming
- Events can be precipitated by hyperventilation, hypoglycemia, stresses (emotional and physiologic), fatigue, or sleeplessness

Manifestations:
- Brief loss of consciousness
- Appear without warning or aura
- Usually last about 5 to 10 seconds
- Slight loss of muscle tone may cause child to drop objects
- Able to maintain postural control; seldom falls
- Minor movements such as lip smacking, twitching of eyelids or face, or slight hand movements
- Not accompanied by incontinence
- Amnesia for episode
- May need to reorient self to previous activity

Atonic and Akinetic Seizures (Also Known As Drop Attacks)

Characterized by:
- Onset usually between 2 and 5 years of age
- Sudden, momentary loss of muscle tone and postural control
- Events recur frequently during the day, particularly in the morning hours and shortly after awakening

Manifestations:
- Loss of tone causes child to fall to the floor violently
  - Unable to break fall by putting out hand
  - May incur a serious injury to the face, head, or shoulder
- Loss of consciousness only momentary

Myoclonic Seizures

A variety of seizure episodes

May be isolated as benign essential myoclonus

May occur in association with other seizure forms

Characterized by:
- Sudden, brief contractures of a muscle or group of muscles
- Occur singly or repetitively
- No postictal state
- May or may not be symmetric
- May or may not be loss of consciousness

Infantile Spasms

Also called: infantile myoclonus, massive spasms, hypsarrhythmia, salaam episodes, or infantile myoclonic spasms

Most commonly occur during the first 6 to 8 months of life

Twice as common in males as in females

Child may have numerous seizures during the day without postictal drowsiness or sleep

Outlook for normal intelligence poor

Manifestations:
- Possible series of sudden, brief, symmetric, muscular contractions
- Head flexed, arms extended, and legs drawn up
- Eyes may roll upward or inward
- May be preceded or followed by a cry or giggling
- May or may not be loss of consciousness
- Sometimes flushing, pallor, or cyanosis

Infants who are able to sit but not stand:
- Sudden dropping forward of the head and neck with trunk flexed forward and knees drawn up—the "salaam" or "jack-knife" seizure

Less often: alternate clinical forms observed
- Extensor spasms rather than flexion of arms, legs, and trunk and head nodding
- Lightning events involving a single, momentary, shocklike contraction of the entire body

event, the age at onset, and the time at which the seizure occurs (e.g., in early morning, before meals, while awake, or during sleep). Any factors that may have precipitated the seizure are important, including fever, infection, falls that may have caused trauma to the head, anxiety, fatigue, activity (e.g., hyperventilation), and environmental events (exposure to strong stimuli such as bright, flashing lights or loud noises). If the child can describe any sensory phenomena, these are recorded. The duration and progression of the seizure (if any) and the *postictal* (period after the seizure) feelings and behavior, such as confusion, inability to speak, amnesia, headache, and sleep, are recorded. The ability to identify seizure types accurately has resulted from the technologic advances in video recording and long-term EEG monitoring.

A complete physical and neurologic examination, including developmental assessment of language, learning, behavior, and motor abilities, often provides clues to neurologic disturbances. A family history can offer clues to paroxysmal disorders such as migraine, breath-holding spells, febrile seizures, or neurologic diseases that may be related to the seizure disorder.

Laboratory studies that may prove to be of value include a complete blood cell count and white blood cell count (for signs of infection). Blood and CSF glucose may give evidence of hypoglycemic episodes or infection, and serum electrolytes, blood urea nitrogen, calcium, and other blood studies might indicate metabolic disturbances. Lumbar puncture can confirm a suspected diagnosis of cerebrospinal infection.

Skull radiographs, CT scans, and other studies help to identify skull abnormalities, separation of sutures, and intracranial calcifications. Focal seizures in children younger than 1 year are indications for MRI to rule out a supratentorial tumor. An EEG is obtained for all children with seizure activity and is the most useful tool for evaluating seizure disorders. The EEG is carried out under varying conditions—with the child asleep, awake, awake with provocative stimulation (flashing lights, noise), and hyperventilating. Stimulation elicits abnormal electric activity, which is recorded on the EEG.

Variations of the EEG are video recordings and simultaneous polygraphs of the patient during waking and/or sleeping. These techniques can be used concurrently and are especially valuable in differentiating epileptic activity from paroxysmal behavior or nonepileptic motor events.

Therapeutic Management. The objectives of treatment of seizure disorders are to (1) control the seizures or reduce their frequency, (2) discover and correct the cause when possible, and (3) help the child who has recurrent seizures to live as normal a life as possible. Seizures of a recurrent nature are treated as soon as the diagnosis is established. If the seizure activity is a manifestation of an infectious, traumatic, or metabolic process, the seizure therapy is instituted as a part of the general therapeutic regimen. Seizure control is considered to prevent secondary brain cell injury from the neuronal discharge and hypoxia.

It is known that persons predisposed to epilepsy have seizures when their basal level of neuronal excitability exceeds a critical point or threshold; no event occurs if the excitability is maintained below this threshold. The administration of antiepileptic drugs serves to raise this threshold and prevent seizures. Consequently, the primary therapy for seizure disorders is the administration of the appropriate antiepileptic drug or combination of drugs in a dosage that provides the desired effect without causing undesirable side effects or toxic reactions.

Numerous drugs are available for control of seizures. The primary drugs prescribed for partial seizures and/or generalized tonic-clonic seizures are carbamazepine (Tegretol), phenytoin (Dilantin), fosphenytoin (Cerebyx), and valproic acid (Depakote or Depakene). The drug of choice for absence seizures is ethosuximide (Zarontin) and valproic acid. The dosage is determined by monitoring serum drug levels. Complete control can be achieved in only 50% to 75% of affected children, however, even with careful attention to details of therapy.

There is increasing evidence that diminishing polypharmacy can bring about a better quality of life; therefore single-drug therapy is recommended. Several new drugs have also increased seizure control for many children. These include gabapentin (Neurontin), lamotrigine (Lamictal), and felbamate (Felbatol). The use of felbamate is controversial because of the side effects of aplastic anemia or hepatic failure.

Once seizures are controlled, the drug or drugs are continued for a prolonged time. However, periodic reevaluation of the drug is important to assess the continued effectiveness and to alter the dosage if indicated. The dosage will need to be increased as the child grows.

Withdrawal of antiepileptic therapy follows a predesigned protocol, usually begun when the child has been seizure free for at least 2 years with a normal EEG. Relapse in children may be related to factors such as neurologic deficit or a positive family history for epilepsy. Recurrence is most likely within the first year after discontinuance of the medication. When a medication is discontinued, the dosage should be reduced gradually over 1 to 2 weeks. Sudden withdrawal of a drug can cause an increase in the number and severity of seizures, often precipitating status epilepticus. If the time for reducing the medication coincides with puberty or, in younger children, occurs during periods when the child is subject to frequent infections, the drug is continued for a longer period. Repeat EEGs are generally obtained every 6 months to 2 years.

When seizure activity is determined to be caused by a hematoma, tumor, or other progressive cerebral lesion, surgical removal is the treatment. Surgery also may be indicated for those who have repetitive, incapacitating seizures that are caused by a focal brain abnormality, if removal of the lesion does not result in significant loss of vital functions, such as speech and movement. The risks of brain surgery cannot be underestimated. Also, the costs of surgical interventions must be taken into consideration, as well as the numerous tests necessary to assess the child before surgery.

Status Epilepticus. Status epilepticus is a continuous seizure that lasts more than 30 minutes or a series of seizures from which the child does not regain a premorbid level of consciousness. The initial treatment is directed toward support and maintenance of vital functions, including maintenance of an adequate airway, administration of oxygen, and hydration, and is followed by IV administration of either diazepam (Valium) or phenobarbital. Rectal diazepam is a simple, effective, and safe treatment for prehospital management (Dieckmann, 1994). Lorazepam (Ativan) may be replacing IV diazepam as the drug of choice. It has a longer duration of action and causes less respiratory distress in children older than 2 years.

> **NURSE ALERT** • Fosphenytoin (Cerebyx) is often used instead of IV phenytoin to treat seizures because of possible complications and drug interactions associated with IV phenytoin. If IV phenytoin is used, it should be administered via slow IV push and at a rate that does not exceed 50 mg/min. Because phenytoin precipitates when mixed with glucose, only normal saline solution is used to flush the tubing or catheter. Fosphenytoin may be given in saline or glucose solutions at a rate of up to 150 mg PE (phenytoin equivalent) per minute, and it may be given intramuscularly if necessary.

The child must be closely monitored during administration to detect early alterations in vital signs that may indicate impending cardiac arrest or respiratory depression. When diazepam is ineffective, phenobarbital, often in extremely high levels that may require respiratory support, is given intravenously as the initial medication. Patients who do not respond to drug therapy may require the use of IV lidocaine, general anesthesia, or a potent skeletal muscle relaxant such as curare. This should be administered by an anesthesiologist.

> **NURSE ALERT** • Status epilepticus is a medical emergency requiring immediate intervention to prevent permanent injury to the brain, respiratory failure, and death.

Prognosis. The course and prognosis for children with seizures depend on the etiology, type of seizure, age at onset, and family and medical histories. In one study of children with epilepsy (excluding those with generalized absence, myoclonus, akinetic, atonic, and infantile seizures), 55% of children "outgrew" the disorder and remained seizure free without medication during an average 7-year follow-up period. At diagnosis the best predictors of remission were age under 12 years at onset, normal intelligence, no prior neonatal seizures, and fewer than 21 seizures before treatment (Camfield and Camfield, 1993).

Risk factors associated with recurrence of epilepsy include being 16 years or older, taking more than one antiepileptic drug, having seizures after starting drug treatment, having a history of primary or secondarily generalized tonic-clonic seizures or an EEG showing myoclonic seizures, and having an abnormal EEG. The risks of seizures recurring decreases with increasing time without seizures (Medical Research Council, 1993).

Box 51-14

Assessment of the Child During a Tonic-Clonic Seizure

OBSERVE SEIZURE

Describe

Order of events
Duration of seizure

Onset

Significant preseizure events—bright lights, noise, excitement, emotional outbursts
Behavior
- Change in facial expression, such as of fear
- Cry or other sound
- Stereotyped or automatous movements
- Random activity

Position of head, body, extremities
- Unilateral or bilateral posturing of one or more extremities
- Body deviation to side

Time of onset

Movement

Change of position, if any
Site of commencement—extremity, generalized
Tonic phase, if present—duration, parts of body involved
Clonic phase—twitching or jerking movements, parts of body involved, sequence of parts involved, generalized, change in character of movements
Absence of movement of any extremity

Face

Color change—pallor, cyanosis, flushing
Diaphoresis
Mouth—position, deviating to one side, teeth clenched, tongue bitten, excessive salivation, bleeding

Eyes

Position—straight ahead, deviation upward, deviation outward, conjugate or divergent gaze
Pupils (if able to assess)—change in size, equality, reaction to light and accommodation

Respiratory Effort

Presence and length of apnea
Presence of stridor

Other

Incontinence of urine or stool

Observe Postictally

State of consciousness—unresponsive, drowsy, confused
Orientation to time, place, persons
Sleeping but arousable
Duration of sleep
Motor ability
- Any change in motor function
- Ability to move all extremities
- Weakness

Speech—changes, peculiarities, difficulties
Sensations
- Discomfort or pain
- Visual or auditory impairment
- Preseizure sensations, warning of event, aura

The prognosis after treatment for status epilepticus is more favorable than previously reported. The majority of children will probably have no intellectual impairment. Children who do have cognitive deficits or who die are likely to have preceding developmental delay, neurologic abnormality, or concurrent serious illness (Verity, Ross, and Golding, 1993).

Nursing Care Management

➤ Assessment

An important nursing function during a seizure is observing the seizure and describing its pertinent features. Any alterations in behavior and characteristics of the seizure, such as sensory-hallucinatory phenomena (e.g., an aura), motor effects (e.g., eye movements, muscular contractions, laterality, and complex activities), alterations in consciousness, and postictal state, are noted and recorded (Box 51-14).

Generalized seizures and others with dramatic manifestations are easily detected, but absence seizures may be more difficult to detect. They are easily misinterpreted as inattention. Any unusual behavior, even seemingly inconsequential behavior such as a momentary interruption of activity, staring, or mental blankness, should be described. The more detailed these descriptions, the more valuable they are for assessment. The nurse notes the time the seizure began and the duration of the seizure.

Box 51-15

Nursing Diagnoses: The Child with Epilepsy

Risk for injury related to sudden and unexpected loss of consciousness
Body image disturbance related to perception of seizure disorder
Altered family processes related to chronic disease of a child

History taking is a vital tool for helping to identify factors that are valuable in establishing a cause of the seizures. Interviewing the child and family helps to elicit problems related to the psychologic impact of the disorder on their lives.

➤ Nursing Diagnoses

Several nursing diagnoses that become apparent after an assessment of the child with a seizure disorder are listed in Box 51-15. Others may be identified in specific cases.

➤ Plan of Care and Implementation

The goals for the child with a seizure disorder and the family include the following:

1. Child will be protected during a seizure.
2. Child will experience as few seizures as possible.

Emergency

SEIZURES

Tonic-Clonic Seizure

During the Seizure

Time seizure episode.
Approach calmly.
If child is standing or seated, ease child down.
Place pillow or folded blanket under child's head. If no bedding is available, place own hands under child's head.
Do not:
- Attempt to restrain child or use force
- Put anything in child's mouth
- Give any food or liquids

Loosen restrictive clothing.
Remove eyeglasses.
Clear area of any hazards or hard objects.
Allow seizure to end without interference.
If vomiting occurs, try to turn child to one side as a unit.

After the Seizure

Time postictal period.
Check for breathing. Check position of head and tongue. Reposition if head is hyperextended. If breathing is not present, give rescue breathing and call emergency medical service (EMS).
Check around mouth for evidence of burns or suspicious substances that might indicate poisoning.
Keep child on side.
Remain with child until full recovery.
Do not give food or liquids until fully alert and swallowing reflex has returned.
Call EMS when necessary.
Look for medical identification and determine what factors occurred before onset of seizure and that may have been triggering factors.
Check head and body for possible injuries and fractures.
Check inside of mouth to see if tongue or lips have been bitten.

Complex Partial Seizure

During the Seizure

Do not restrain unless in danger.
Remove harmful objects from path.
Redirect to safe area.
Do not agitate; instead, talk in calm, reassuring manner.
Do not expect child to follow instructions.
Watch to see if seizure generalizes to tonic-clonic type.

After the Seizure

Stay with child and reassure until fully conscious.

Call EMS if:

Child stops breathing
There is evidence of injury, or youngster is diabetic or pregnant
Seizure lasts for more than 5 minutes (unless duration of seizure is typically longer than 5 minutes by history)
Status epilepticus occurs
Pupils are not equal in size after seizure
Child vomits continuously 30 minutes after seizure has ended (sign of possible acute problem)
Child cannot be awakened and is unresponsive to pain after seizure has ended
Seizure occurs in water (shock and aspiration may be delayed)
This is child's first seizure

Modified from *Seizure recognition and first aid,* Landover, MD, 1989, Epilepsy Foundation of America.

Box 51-16
Seizure Precautions

Extent of precautions depends on type, severity, and frequency of seizures
May include the following:
- Siderails raised when child is sleeping or resting
- Siderails and other hard objects padded
- Waterproof mattress/pad on bed/crib
- Appropriate precautions during potentially hazardous activities:
  - Swimming with a companion
  - Use of protective helmet and padding during bicycle riding, skateboarding, in-line skating
  - Supervision during use of hazardous machinery/equipment

Have child carry or wear medical identification
Alert other caregivers to need for any special precautions
Identify and avoid triggering factors whenever possible

3. Child and family will cope with the challenges associated with the disorder.
4. Child will develop a positive self-image.
5. Child and family will identify triggering factors.

The child must be protected from injury during the seizure (Emergency box). It is impossible to halt a seizure once it has begun, and no attempt should be made to do so. The nurse must remain calm, stay with the child, and prevent the child from sustaining any harm during the seizure. If possible, the child should be isolated from the view of others by closing a door or pulling screens. A seizure can be very upsetting to the child, other visitors, and their families. If other persons are present, they should be assured that everything is being done for the child. After the seizure, they can be given a simple explanation of the event as needed.

NURSE ALERT • Do not move or forcefully restrain the child during a tonic-clonic seizure and do not place a solid object between the teeth.

If the nurse is able to reach the child in time, a child who is standing or is seated in a chair (including a wheelchair) is eased to the floor immediately. During and sometimes after the tonic-clonic seizure, the swallowing reflex is lost, salivation increases, and the tongue is hypotonic. Therefore the child is at risk for aspiration and airway obstruction. Placing the child on the side facilitates drainage and helps to maintain a patent airway. If the child becomes cyanotic, oxygen is administered. After the seizure the child is kept on the side in bed to allow the youngster to sleep. When feasible, the child is reintegrated into the environment as soon as possible. Sending a child with a chronic seizure disorder home from school after a seizure is not necessary, unless the parents request this.

Children who are known to have seizures or who are under observation for seizures will require some precautions. The extent of these measures depends on the type and frequency of the seizure (Box 51-16).

Long-Term Care. Care of the child with a recurrent seizure disorder involves physical care and instruction regarding the importance of the drug therapy and, probably more significant, the problems related to the emotional aspects of the disorder. Few diseases generate as much anxiety among relatives as epilepsy. Fears and misconceptions about the disease and its treatment abound in the layperson's mind. For many it represents the archetype of severe hereditary affliction. Therefore the foci of nursing care are directed toward helping the child and the family to deal with the psychologic and sociologic problems related to the disorder and educating the child, the family, peers, and the public toward a more realistic and liberal view of the disease.

Children subject to seizures are given some type of drug therapy. The nurse can help the parents plan the administration of the medication at convenient times to minimize disruption to the family routine. The most convenient times for administration seem to be with meals or at bedtime. Although antiepileptic drugs are available in liquid extracts or emulsions, the tablet form is preferred by neurologists. The unequal distribution of the drug in the solute and the increased likelihood of inaccurate measurements make liquid medication less desirable. For small children a tablet of the proper dosage can be crushed and administered in syrup, jelly, or other palatable substances.

NURSE ALERT • Children taking phenobarbital and/or phenytoin should receive adequate vitamin D and folic acid because deficiencies of both have been associated with these antiepileptics. Phenytoin should not be taken with milk.

It is important to impress on the family the need to continue the medication regularly without interruption for as long as required. The parents and the child will need to know the common side effects of the drug prescribed and observe for signs that might indicate unfavorable reactions.

Parents need to be warned of possible behavioral changes as the seizures are controlled in children taking primidone, phenobarbital, or phenytoin. Changes in personality, indifference to school activities and family, hyperactivity, or even psychotic behavior may sometimes be observed. The potential effects of antiepileptics on learning and behavior should be considered. Progressive intellectual deterioration in a child with epilepsy requires investigation of present medication plus the role of the underlying cerebral pathology. Parents should notify the health professional if the child has an illness, including vomiting or fever. Vomiting can interfere with drug absorption; fever may increase metabolic requirements; both can precipitate seizure activity.

Rectal preparations of some medications are highly useful and effective when a child is unable to take oral medications because of repeated vomiting, gastrointestinal surgery, or status epilepticus. Administration of rectal drugs can be learned by parents for home treatment during a seizure.* Rectal lorazepam (Ativan) is useful as an adjunctive home treatment for children at risk for prolonged seizures.

The degree to which activities are restricted is individualized for each child and depends on the type, frequency, and severity of the seizures; the child's response to therapy; and the length of time the seizures have been controlled. Normal healthy activities are encouraged for children, and participation in competitive sports is determined on an individual basis. With encouragement most older children can accept the restrictions placed on activities. Only essential restrictions should be placed on children regarding sports and peer activity to reduce the likelihood of needlessly accentuating differences.

Because the child is encouraged to attend school, camp, and other normal activities, the school nurse and the teacher should be made aware of the child's condition and therapy. They can help to ensure regularity of medication and any special care the child might need. Teachers, child care providers, camp counselors, youth organization leaders, coaches, and other adults who assume responsibility for children should be instructed regarding care of the child during a seizure so that they can act in a calm manner for the welfare of the child and to influence the attitude of the child's peers.*

Triggering Factors. Careful and detailed documentation of seizures over a period of time may reveal a pattern. When this occurs, the nurse or responsible adult may intervene to identify the triggering factors and make changes in the environment that may prevent or decrease seizure frequency. Commonly the necessary changes are very simple and cost free but can make an enormous difference in the child's and family's lives (Critical Thinking box).

Critical Thinking

SEIZURES

Since age 2 years, Jane Little has had epilepsy that is well controlled with medication. However, now that she has begun elementary school, her seizures have returned. On the way home Jane usually has a seizure on the bus; however, on weekends and holidays she is seizure free. As the school nurse, what should you advise Jane's parents to do?

First, Think About It . . .

- **What information are you using?**
- **How are you interpreting that information?**

1. **Take her for medical reevaluation.**
2. **Increase her antiepileptic medication.**
3. **Drive her home from school.**
4. **Ride with her on the school bus.**

The best response is 4. Your first priority is to help the family identify triggering events, which would yield pertinent and necessary information. At your suggestion, Mrs. Little rode the school bus home with Jane. As the child began to seize, the mother noted that they had just passed a white picket fence, the triggering factor. Once the child was seated on the other side of the bus, the seizure episodes stopped.

With the consistent pattern and abrupt onset of the seizures, seeking medical reevaluation should be advised only if no triggering event is identified. An accurate interpretation of the information is that it is not within the scope of nursing practice for you to change the dosage of the medication. Even if the child rides home in a car, the seizures may occur if Jane sits in the same position as on the school bus.

*Community and home care instructions for administering oral and rectal medications are available in Wong DL, Hess CS: ***Wong and Whaley's clinical manual of pediatric nursing,*** ed 5, St Louis, 2000, Mosby.

*An excellent resource is *Students with Seizures: A Manual for School Nurses* by N. Santilli, W.E. Dodson, and A.V. Walton (Landover, MD, 1991, Epilepsy Foundation of America).

Factors that may trigger seizures in children include changes in dark-light patterns, such as those that occur with a flash on a camera, automobile headlights, walking by a picket fence, reflections of light on snow or water, or rotating blades on a fan; sudden loud noises; specific voices, songs, or nursery rhymes; startling or sudden movements; extreme or drastic changes in temperature; dehydration; fatigue; hyperventilation; hypoglycemia; caffeine; and insufficient protein in the diet (protein is needed to metabolize some antiepileptic drugs). Although there have been reports of seizures triggered by flashing video games, this relationship has not been confirmed by controlled studies. Seizures may be caused by the length of playing time, which may cause sleep deprivation, fatigue, excitement, or photosensitivity (Ferrie et al, 1994). On the basis of current knowledge, the overwhelming majority of children with seizures can play video games without the risk of seizures.*

If a child is photosensitive, it may be necessary to avoid things such as wallpaper with stripes, a ceiling fan, and blinking lights; view the television screen from a distance of at least 2 yards; and cover one eye.

Family Support. Parental attitudes and management of a child with a seizure disorder are as varied as those of other parents of children with a chronic disorder, and they are subject to the same long-term problems (see Chapter 41). Whether the seizures result from illness, injury, or unknown etiology, the parents may feel guilt, anxiety, and often humiliation. They want to know whether it will affect the child's mental capacities. To many persons, epilepsy is erroneously associated with mental deficiency. Seizures do commonly accompany other manifestations of severe brain damage from disease or injury, but children with seizures, like any population of healthy children, display a wide range of intelligence.

Parents also wonder how the illness will affect the child's future and need reassurance that it will not shorten the life of the child and that the child can attend school, marry, and elect to have children. The child will need vocational guidance, and the parents should become familiar with the laws in their state regarding any limitations that might be imposed on the child because of the disorder. It should be emphasized that seizures can be controlled or greatly reduced in the majority of children and that new studies hold the promise of progress in future treatment. Parents also need reassurance that today less stigma is attached to the disease than there has been in the past.

It is important to encourage a healthy attitude toward the child and the disease and to help the parents feel competent in their ability to meet their responsibilities. The child should be reared as any normal child, with natural concern tempered by the understanding of the need of the child not to be overprotected. Many parents refrain from correcting or punishing the child, especially if they have had the experience of such an emotional stress precipitating a seizure. The child must not be made to feel different in any way. Parents should be encouraged to be honest and open about the disorder with the child and with others. Some parents are tempted to try to conceal the nature of the child's illness because of their belief that the disorder is shameful or a disgrace to the family.

*For more information on video games and epilepsy, contact the Epilepsy Foundation of America, 4351 Garden City Dr., Landover, MD 20785; (301) 459-3700 or 1-800-EFA-1000; website: www.efa.org.

Restrictions on the child's activities will be necessary for safety, but this area can be approached in a positive way in terms of what the child can do rather than what the child cannot do. Sometimes parents curtail the child's activities more than necessary. The child needs to experience the maturing influences of play and work. The Epilepsy Foundation of America* is a national organization that works toward and for the welfare of persons with epilepsy and their families; helps with employment and legal problems; and provides education to patients, families, and communities.

The Child with Epilepsy. The child who is provided the security of a loving family, rewards and punishments no different from those of other children, and support in acquiring self-esteem is more likely to have a positive attitude toward the disease. Children derive their self-concept and self-esteem from observations of others' reactions to them and their own perception of their capabilities. The suddenness and unpredictability of seizures and the reactions of others further influence their feelings. When others consider children to be different, inferior, or objects of ridicule, they come to view themselves as different, inferior, and incapable.

Children with epilepsy need to learn about their disease and the role that the medication plays in contributing to their prolonged well-being. As soon as they are old enough, children should assume responsibility for taking their own medication and be advised to carry medical identification with pertinent information about their condition. Planning activities with children and emphasizing those in which they can engage rather than those in which they cannot participate help them succeed and gain satisfaction in their achievements. They should be offered opportunities and encouraged to exercise judgment in their daily lives.

The adolescent period may prove to be a trying time for the child with epilepsy. Limits imposed on the young person's activities at a time when freedom and independence are desired may bring the disability into sharp focus. For example, some states do not allow persons with epilepsy to obtain a driver's license, even when the disease is controlled; in others there are restrictions on employment insurance.

Epilepsy should not be a severe impairment to most youngsters, and the nurse, by assuming the role of patient advocate, helping to educate the public regarding the disease, working toward making opportunities available to persons with the disorder, and lobbying for legislation that recognizes the needs of the individual with a seizure disorder, can help to erase the stigma that still remains regarding the disease.

➤ Evaluation

The effectiveness of nursing interventions for the child with epilepsy is determined by continual reassessment and evaluation of care based on the following observational guidelines and expected outcomes:

1. Observe child's behavior for evidence of seizure activity and assess the environment for situations that could cause injury to child in the event of a seizure; interview family regarding management of child during a seizure.

*4351 Garden City Dr., Landover, MD 20785; (301) 459-3700 or 1-800-EFA-1000; website: www.efa.org.

2. Interview child and family regarding compliance with the medication regimen and identification of triggering factors.
3. Observe and interview family regarding their feelings and concerns and their understanding of child's condition.
4. Observe child's interactions with others and interview child about any feelings or concerns about own health.

Expected outcomes include the following:

1. Child exhibits no evidence of physical injury.
2. Family complies with instructions; child remains free of seizure activity.
3. Child exhibits no or minimal complications from medication.
4. Child and family identify triggering factors and make adjustments that diminish the frequency of seizure episodes.
5. Child expresses feelings and concerns and has a positive self-image.
6. Child and family demonstrate a healthy view of the disorder and alterations in lifestyle that it imposes.

(See Nursing Care Plan: The Child with Epilepsy.*)

Febrile Seizures

Febrile seizures are transient disorders of childhood that occur in association with a fever. They are one of the most common neurologic disorders of childhood, affecting about 4% of children. Most febrile seizures occur after 6 months of age and usually before 3 years of age, with increased frequency in children younger than 18 months. They are unusual after 5 years of age. Boys are affected about twice as often as girls, and there is an increased susceptibility in families, indicating a possible genetic predisposition. Most febrile seizures are generalized and last less than 5 minutes (Farwell et al, 1994). About 30% to 40% of children will have one recurrence.

The cause of febrile seizures is still uncertain. In most children the height but not the rapidity of the temperature elevation seems to be a factor. The fever usually exceeds 38.8° C (101.8° F) and occurs during the temperature rise rather than after a prolonged elevation. Sometimes it constitutes the dramatic beginning of an illness. Febrile seizures usually accompany an upper respiratory or gastrointestinal infection. Although pertussis vaccine does not cause febrile seizures, this immunization is a precipitating factor in initial episodes of febrile seizures in children prone to having seizures (Cherry et al, 1993).

Most febrile seizures have stopped by the time the child is taken to a medical facility. However, if the seizure continues, treatment consists of controlling the seizure with diazepam (Valium) and reducing the temperature by administration of acetaminophen. In children with simple febrile seizures, prophylactic antiepileptic therapy is not recommended. The most important interventions are parental education and emotional support (American Academy of Pediatrics, 1999). Little risk of neurologic deficit, epilepsy, mental retardation, or altered behavior has been observed as sequelae of febrile seizures.

Parents need reassurance of the benign nature of febrile seizures (almost 95% of children with febrile seizures will not develop epilepsy or any neurologic damage). They should be told that their child is in no danger of dying of a febrile seizure. They also need education regarding protecting the child from harm and observing exactly what happens to the child during the event. Attempts to lower the temperature with acetaminophen or to use diazepam to prevent a seizure are of no benefit in most children (Uhari et al, 1995). Tepid sponge baths are ineffective in significantly lowering the temperature, the shivering effect further increases metabolic output, and cooling causes discomfort in the child.

NURSE ALERT • If a febrile seizure lasts more than 10 minutes, parents should seek medical attention right away. Encourage them to drive carefully; a few extra minutes will not make any significant difference (Camfield and Camfield, 1993).

CEREBRAL MALFORMATIONS

Cranial Deformities

In the healthy newborn the cranial sutures are separated by membranous seams several millimeters wide. For the first few hours to 1 to 2 days after birth, the cranial bones are highly mobile, which allows them to mold and slide over one another, adjusting the circumference of the head to accommodate to the changing shape and character of the birth canal. The principal sutures in the infant's skull are the sagittal, coronal, and lambdoidal sutures, and the major soft areas at the juncture of these sutures are the anterior and posterior fontanels.

After birth, growth of the skull bones occurs *perpendicular* to the line of the suture, and normal closure occurs in a regular and predictable order. Although there are variations in the age at which closure takes place in individual children, normally all sutures and fontanels are ossified by the following ages:

8 weeks: Posterior fontanel closed
6 months: Fibrous union of suture lines and interlocking of serrated edges
18 months: Anterior fontanel closed
12 years: Sutures unable to be separated by increased ICP

Solid union of all sutures is not completed until very late childhood. Closure of a suture before the expected time inhibits the perpendicular growth. Because normal increase in brain volume requires expansion, the skull is forced to grow in a direction *parallel* to the fused suture. This alteration in skull growth always produces a distortion of the head shape when the underlying brain growth is normal. The small head with closed and normal shape is a result of deficient brain growth; the suture closure is secondary to this brain growth failure. Failure of brain growth is not secondary to suture closure.

Various types of cranial deformities are encountered in early infancy. These include the enlarged head with frontal protrusion (bossing; characteristic of hydrocephalus), the parietal bossing that is seen in chronic subdural hematoma, the small head, and a variety of skull deformities (Box 51-17). Some occur during prenatal development; in others, head circumference is usually within normal limits at birth, and the deviation from normal development becomes apparent with advancing age.

Prognosis. The majority of infants presenting with craniosynostosis have normal brain development. The exceptions are those genetic disorders that involve brain pathology.

*In Wong DL, Hess CS: ***Wong and Whaley's clinical manual of pediatric nursing,*** ed 5, St Louis, 2000, Mosby.

Box 51-17

Cranial Deformities

Microcephaly—Head circumference more than 2 standard deviations below average for age, sex, and gestation; caused by failure of brain development
  Management—No treatment available

Craniosynostosis—Premature closure of single or multiple sutures of cranial vault, face, and base of skull
  Scaphocephaly—Premature closure of sagittal suture causes skull to become elongated in an anteroposterior direction with a high cranial vault and a subnormal transverse diameter
  Brachycephaly—Premature closure of coronal sutures causes skull to become shortened in an anteroposterior direction with flattening of occiput and forehead
  Oxycephaly—Premature closure of both coronal and sagittal sutures causes an excessively high and narrow skull that tapers upward on all sides
  Plagiocephaly—Unilateral closure of one coronal or lambdoidal suture causes skull to become asymmetric
  Craniofacial dysostosis (Crouzon disease)—Premature closure of any or all cranial sutures, most frequently the coronal, and a typical facial deformity (widely spaced eyes, hypoplastic maxilla, and beaklike nose; tongue appears large and protruding; frequently with exophthalmos)
    Management—Surgical release of closed sutures; Crouzon disease—surgical correction of major facial deformities

Nursing Care Management. Nursing care of families in which there is a child with a cranial defect involves identifying children with deformities and referring them for evaluation. Because no therapy is available for children with microcephaly, nursing care is directed toward helping parents adjust to rearing a child with brain damage (see Chapter 42).

Caring for infants who benefit from surgery requires special emphasis on observation for signs of decreased hematocrit and hemoglobin because of the large blood loss during surgery (Family Focus box). A cardiac monitor may demonstrate a resting heart rate of 200 beats/min. Nursing care includes observation for signs of hemorrhage, infection, pain, and swelling and parental education for suture care and safety. Surgical sutures should remain dry and intact. Parents need to observe for any signs of redness, drainage, or swelling and report any temperature greater than 38.4° C (101° F).

Early surgical management of craniosynostosis allows proper expansion of the brain and the creation of an acceptable appearance. Parents require special support and education during this time, especially from other parents whose infants have undergone similar operations. (Richard, 1994). The nurse can serve as a liaison for this type of parental support.

Family Focus

BLOOD DONATION

Parents may wish to provide a compatible blood donor for their infant undergoing a planned surgical correction for craniosynostosis. Nurses need to inform and guide parents through this blood bank procedure.

Hydrocephalus

Hydrocephalus is a condition caused by an imbalance in the production and absorption of CSF in the ventricular system. When production is greater than absorption, CSF accumulates within the ventricular system, usually under increased pressure, producing passive dilation of the ventricles.

Pathophysiology. The two mechanisms by which CSF is formed include secretion by the choroid plexuses and lymphatic-like drainage by the extracellular fluid of the brain. CSF circulates throughout the ventricular system and then is absorbed within the subarachnoid spaces by a mechanism that is not entirely clear. Prenatal diagnosis is undoubtedly having an impact on the current prevalence at birth of hydrocephalus. The advent of MRI and CT scanning has provided valuable information about the pathophysiology of various diseases. The causes are diverse; they are either congenital (maldevelopment or intrauterine infection) or acquired (neoplasm, hemorrhage, or infection).

Hydrocephalus is a symptom of an underlying brain disorder resulting in either (1) impaired absorption of CSF within the subarachnoid space (ventricles communicate; *communicating hydrocephalus*), or (2) obstruction to the flow of CSF within the ventricles (ventricles do not communicate; *noncommunicating hydrocephalus*). Any imbalance of secretion and absorption causes an increased accumulation of CSF in the ventricles, which become dilated and compress the brain substance against the surrounding rigid bony cranium. When this occurs before fusion of the cranial sutures, it produces enlargement of the skull, as well as dilation of the ventricles (Fig. 51-6). In children younger than 10 to 12 years, previously closed suture lines, especially the sagittal suture, may become diastatic or opened (Swaiman, 1994).

Most cases of noncommunicating hydrocephalus are a result of developmental malformations. Although the defect usually is apparent in early infancy, it may become evident at any time from the prenatal period to late childhood or early adulthood. Other causes include neoplasms, infections, and trauma. An obstruction to the normal flow can occur at any point in the CSF pathway to produce increased pressure and dilation of the pathways proximal to the site of obstruction.

Developmental defects (e.g., Arnold-Chiari malformations [ACMs], aqueduct stenosis, aqueduct gliosis, and atresia of the foramina of Luschka and Magendie [Dandy-Walker syndrome]) account for most cases of hydrocephalus from birth to 2 years of age. Hydrocephalus is so often associated with myelomeningocele that all such infants should be observed for its development. In the remainder of cases there is a history of intrauterine infection, perinatal hemorrhage, and neonatal meningoencephalitis. In older children hydrocephalus is most often a result of space-occupying lesions, intracranial infections, hemorrhage, or preexisting developmental defects, such as aqueduct stenosis or the *Arnold-Chiari malformation* (a congenital anomaly in which the cerebellum and medulla oblongata extend down through the foramen magnum).

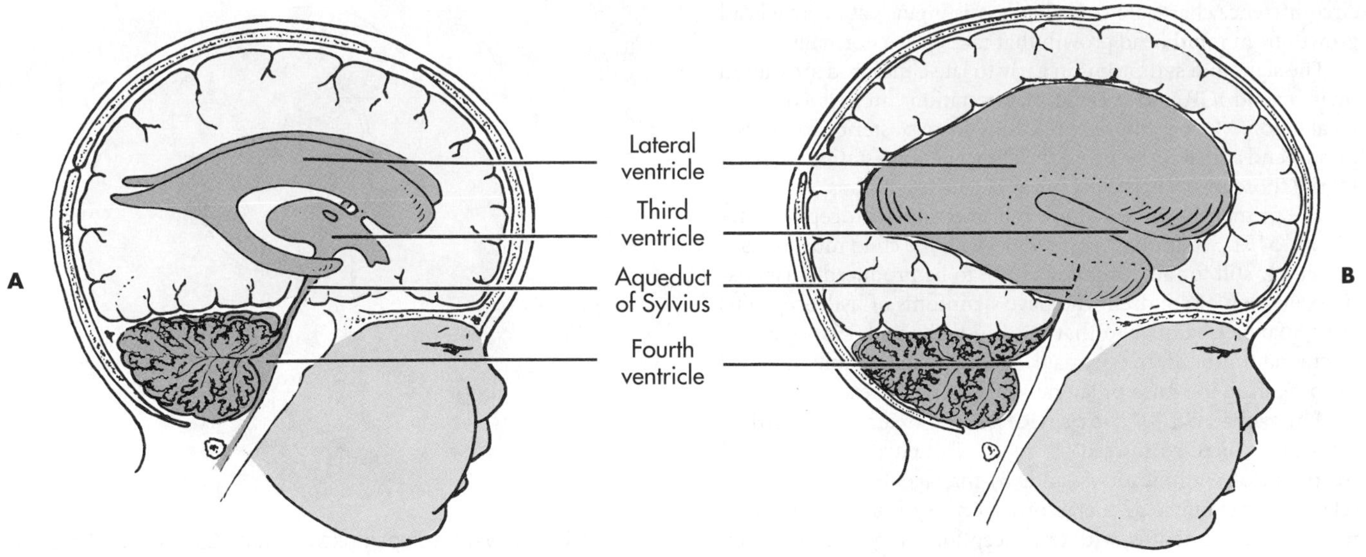

FIG. 51-6 • Hydrocephalus: a block in flow of cerebrospinal fluid. **A,** Patent cerebrospinal fluid circulation. **B,** Enlarged lateral and third ventricles caused by obstruction of circulation—stenosis of aqueduct of Sylvius.

Box 51-18

Clinical Manifestations of Hydrocephalus

INFANCY, EARLY

- Abnormally rapid head growth
- Bulging fontanels (especially anterior) sometimes without head enlargement:
  - Tense
  - Nonpulsatile
- Dilated scalp veins
- Separated sutures
- Macewen sign (cracked-pot sound on percussion)
- Thinning of skull bones

INFANCY, LATER

- Frontal enlargement, or bossing
- Depressed eyes
- Setting sun sign (sclera visible above the iris)
- Pupils sluggish, with unequal response to light

INFANCY, GENERAL

- Irritability
- Lethargy
- Infant cries when picked up or rocked and quiets when allowed to lie still
- Early infantile reflex acts may persist
- Normally expected responses fail to appear
- May display:
  - Change in level of consciousness
  - Opisthotonos (often extreme)
  - Lower extremity spasticity
  - Vomiting
- Advanced cases:
  - Difficulty in sucking and feeding
  - Shrill, brief, high-pitched cry
  - Cardiopulmonary embarrassment

CHILDHOOD

- Headache on awakening; improvement following emesis or upright posture
- Papilledema
- Strabismus
- Extrapyramidal tract signs (e.g., ataxia)
- Irritability
- Lethargy
- Apathy
- Confusion
- Incoherence
- Vomiting

Diagnostic Evaluation. The two factors that influence the clinical picture in hydrocephalus are the time of onset and the presence of preexisting structural lesions. In infancy, before closure of the cranial sutures, head enlargement is the predominant sign, whereas in older infants and children the lesions responsible for hydrocephalus produce other neurologic signs through pressure on adjacent structures before causing CSF obstruction (Box 51-18).

In infancy the diagnosis of hydrocephalus is based on head circumference that crosses one or more grid lines on the measurement chart within a period of 2 to 4 weeks and on associated neurologic signs that are present and progressive. However, other diagnostic studies are needed to localize the site of CSF obstruction. Routine daily head circumference measurements are carried out in infants with myelomeningocele and intracranial infections. In evaluation of a premature infant, specially adapted head circumference charts are consulted to distinguish abnormal head growth from rapid head growth that takes place normally.

The signs and symptoms in early to late childhood are caused by increased ICP, and specific manifestations are related to the focal lesion. Most commonly resulting from posterior fossa neoplasms and aqueduct stenosis, the clinical manifestations are primarily those associated with space-occupying lesions.

The primary diagnostic tools for detecting hydrocephalus are CT and MRI. Sedation is required because the child must remain absolutely still for an accurate picture to be produced. Diagnostic evaluation of children who have symptoms of hydrocephalus after infancy is similar to that used in those with suspected intracranial tumor. In the neonate, echoencephalography is useful in comparing the ratio of lateral ventricle to cortex.

Therapeutic Management. The treatment of hydrocephalus is directed toward (1) relief of the hydrocephalus, (2) treatment of complications, and (3) management of problems related to the effect of the disorder on psychomotor development. The treatment is, with few exceptions, surgical. This is accomplished by direct removal of an obstruction (such as a tumor) or a shunt procedure that provides primary drainage of the CSF from the ventricles to an extracranial compartment, usually the peritoneum *(ventriculoperitoneal [VP] shunt)* (Fig. 51-7).

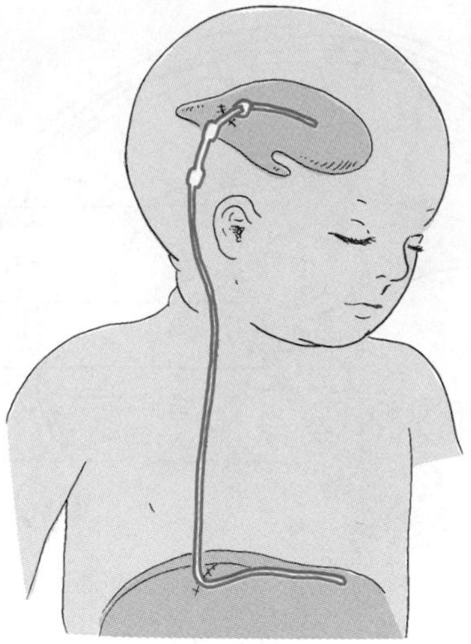

FIG. 51-7 • Ventriculoperitoneal shunt. Catheter is threaded beneath the skin.

Most shunt systems consist of a ventricular catheter, a flush pump, a unidirectional flow valve, and a distal catheter. In all models the valves are designed to open at a predetermined intraventricular pressure and close when the pressure falls below that level, thus preventing backflow of secretions.

The initial shunt is placed when necessary to relieve CSF obstruction, and revisions are needed when there are signs of malfunction. In all mechanisms the initial success rate is relatively high; however, shunts are associated with complications that interfere with continued shunt function or that threaten the life of the child.

The major complications of VP shunts are infection and malfunction. All shunts are subject to mechanical difficulties, such as kinking, plugging, or separation or migration of the tubing. Malfunction is most often caused by mechanical obstruction either within the ventricles from particulate matter (tissue or exudate) or at the distal end from thrombosis or displacement as a result of growth. The child with a shunt obstruction is often first seen in an emergency department with clinical manifestations of increased ICP, commonly accompanied by worsening neurologic status.

The most serious complication, shunt infection, can occur at any time, but the period of greatest risk is 1 to 2 months after placement. The infection is generally a result of intercurrent infections at the time of shunt placement. Infections include septicemia, bacterial endocarditis, wound infection, shunt nephritis, meningitis, and ventriculitis. Meningitis and ventriculitis are of greatest concern because any complicating CNS infection is a significant predictor of intellectual outcome. Infection is treated with massive doses of antibiotics administered by the IV route. A persistent infection requires removal of the shunt until the infection is controlled. External ventricular drainage (EVD) is used until CSF is sterile.

Prognosis. The prognosis of children with treated hydrocephalus depends largely on the rate at which hydrocephalus develops, the duration of raised ICP, the frequency of complications, and the cause of the hydrocephalus. For example, malignant tumors may have a high mortality rate regardless of other complicating factors.

Surgically treated hydrocephalus with continued neurosurgical and medical management has a survival rate of about 80%, with the highest incidence of mortality occurring within the first year of treatment. Of the surviving children, approximately one third are both intellectually and neurologically normal, and one half have neurologic disabilities.

Nursing Care Management

➤ Assessment

Preoperatively the infant with diagnosed or suspected hydrocephalus is observed carefully for signs of increasing ICP. In infants the head is measured daily at the point of largest measurement—the occipitofrontal circumference (OFC) (see Head Circumference, Chapter 35, for technique). Fontanels and suture lines are gently palpated for size, signs of bulging, tenseness, and separation. An infant with normal ICP will display bulging under certain circumstances such as straining or crying; therefore such accompanying behavior should be noted. Irritability, lethargy, or seizure activity, as well as altered vital signs and feeding behavior, may indicate an advancing pathologic condition.

In older children, who are usually admitted to the hospital for elective or emergency shunt revision, the most valuable indicator of increasing ICP is an alteration in the child's LOC and the way in which the child interacts with the environment. Changes are identified by observation and by comparison of present behavior with customary behavior, sleep patterns, developmental capabilities, and habits, all obtained through a detailed history and a baseline assessment. This baseline information serves as a guide for postoperative assessment and evaluation of shunt function.

➤ Nursing Diagnoses

After a thorough assessment, nursing diagnoses become apparent. These include, but are not limited to, those listed in Box 51-18.

➤ Plan of Care and Implementation

The goals of care of the child with hydrocephalus and family include the following:

1. Child will experience no complications of hydrocephalus and/or corrective surgery.
2. The family will receive adequate education and emotional support.

General nursing care of the infant with hydrocephalus may present special problems. Maintaining adequate nutrition often requires flexible feeding schedules to accommodate diagnostic procedures because feeding before or after handling can precipitate an episode of vomiting. Small feedings at shorter intervals are often better tolerated than larger ones spaced farther apart. These infants are often difficult to feed and require extra time and innovation.

The nurse is responsible for preparing the child for diagnostic tests such as tomography and for assisting the practitioner with procedures such as a ventricular tap, which is often performed to relieve excessive pressure during the preoperative period and for CSF examination. Sedation is required because the child must remain absolutely still during diagnostic testing. IV pentobarbital or oral chloral hydrate is commonly used for these procedures. (See Chapter 45 for preparing children for procedures.)

NURSE ALERT • If surgery is anticipated, IV infusions should not be placed in a scalp vein in a child with hydrocephalus.

Fortunately, almost all affected children are recognized, and treatment is begun early. For those children with significant head enlargement, care must be exercised to ensure that the head is well supported when the infant is fed or moved to prevent extra strain on the infant's neck, and measures must be taken to prevent development of pressure areas. As the hydrocephalus progresses, untreated children become increasingly helpless and prone to the multiple problems of immobility (e.g., pressure sores and contracture deformities). Not infrequently, infants with irreversible brain damage or with severe developmental defects such as hydranencephaly, in which both cerebral hemispheres fail to develop and are replaced with a membranous sac filled with CSF, are placed in long-term care facilities.

Postoperative Care. Routine postoperative care and observation are instituted. In addition, the infant or child is positioned carefully on the unoperated side to prevent pressure on the shunt valve and pressure areas. The child is kept flat to help avert complications resulting from too rapid reduction of intracranial fluid. When the ventricular size is reduced too rapidly, the cerebral cortex may pull away from the dura and tear the small interlacing veins, producing a subdural hematoma. This is not a problem in children with elective shunt revision because their intraventricular size and pressure have been normal. The surgeon indicates the position to be maintained and the extent of activity allowed. If there is increased ICP, the surgeon will prescribe elevation of the head of the bed and/or that the child be allowed to sit up to enhance gravity flow through the shunt. Pain management can usually be achieved with acetaminophen with or without codeine for mild to moderate pain and opioids for severe pain (see Pain Management, Chapter 44).

Observation for signs of increased ICP, which indicates obstruction of the shunt, is continued. Neurologic assessment includes evaluation of pupillary dilation (pressure causes compression or stretching of the oculomotor nerve, producing dilation on the same side as the pressure) and blood pressure (hypoxia to the brainstem causes variability in these vital signs).

NURSE ALERT • Arbitrary pumping of the shunt may cause obstruction or other problems and should not be performed unless indicated by the neurosurgeon.

The child is also observed for abdominal distention because CSF may cause peritonitis or a postoperative ileus as a complication of distal catheter placement. In addition, intake and output are carefully monitored. Children may be placed on fluid restriction with nothing by mouth for 24 hours. The IV infusion is closely monitored to prevent fluid overload. Routine feeding is resumed after the prescribed period of no oral intake, but the presence of bowel sounds is determined before feeding children with VP shunts.

Because infection is the greatest hazard of the postoperative period, nurses are continually on the alert for the usual manifestations of CSF infection, which may include elevated vital signs, poor feeding, vomiting, decreased responsiveness, and seizure activity. There may be signs of local inflammation at the operative sites and along the shunt tract. The child's diaper should be kept off the peritoneal dressing site or suture line. Antibiotics are administered by the IV route as ordered, and the nurse may also need to assist the practitioner with intraventricular instillation. The incision site is inspected for leakage, and any suspected drainage is tested for glucose, an indication of CSF.

Meticulous skin care is continued postoperatively, with extra care taken to prevent tissue damage from pressure. A pressure-reducing mattress or overlay pad underneath the child helps prevent pressure on prominent areas. Skin is inspected regularly for any signs of pressure, irritation, or infection.

Family Support. Specific needs and concerns of parents during periods of hospitalization are related to the reason for the child's hospitalization (shunt revision, infection, diagnosis) and the diagnostic and/or surgical procedures to which the child must be subjected. Often parents have very little understanding of anatomy; therefore they need further exploration and reinforcement of information that was given to them by the physician and neurosurgeon, as well as information about what they can expect. They are especially frightened of any procedure that involves the brain, and the fear of retardation or brain damage is very real and pervasive. Nurses can do much to allay their anxiety by explaining the rationale underlying the various nursing and medical activities, such as positioning or testing, and by simply being available and willing to listen to their concerns.

To prepare for the child's discharge and home care, the parents are instructed on how to recognize signs that indicate shunt malfunction or infection and how to pump the shunt, if necessary. Active children may have accidents, such as a fall, that can damage the shunt, and the tubing may pull out of the distal insertion site or become disconnected during normal growth.

Safe transportation is an essential issue to discuss with parents. The tendency for the enlarged head to fall forward and to turn to the side, combined with poor head control, influences the type of child restraint system needed. Small infants can be restrained reclining in an approved car restraint bed.

The management of hydrocephalus in a child is a demanding task for both family and health professionals, and helping a family cope with the child is an important nursing responsibility. It is important to emphasize that hydrocephalus is a lifelong problem and that the child will require evaluation on a regular basis. The overall aim is to establish realistic goals and an appropriate educational program that will help the child to achieve his or her optimum potential.

Anticipatory guidance will prepare parents for possible problems and help them to avoid being overprotective of the child. Few restrictions (mainly contact sports) need be placed on the child's activities, and the child should be encouraged to live as would any other child of the same age and abilities. Parents need support and encouragement in coping with the child and with problems the child may encounter in relationships with peers and others. Reactions of other children when the child has a noticeably enlarged head or requires shaving at the times of revision are stressful situations for both the child and parents. (See Chapter 41 for a discussion on problems and coping with the child with a disability.)

Families can be referred to community agencies for support and guidance. The National Hydrocephalus Foundation (NHF)* provides information on the condition for families and assists interested groups in establishing local organizations. Helpful booklets are available from this and other sources.

➤ Evaluation

The effectiveness of nursing interventions is determined by continual reassessment and evaluation of care based on the following:

Observational guidelines:

1. Monitor child's neurologic status (physical signs and behavior), take temperature, and examine skin at points of pressure.
2. Interview family regarding their feelings and concerns.

Expected outcomes:

1. Child remains free from complications of the disorder and surgical correction.
2. Family discusses their feelings and concerns regarding child's condition.

(See also the Nursing Care Plan: The Child with Hydrocephalus.†)

*12413 Centralia Rd., Lakewood, CA 90715-1623; (562) 402-3523; fax (562) 924-6666; website: www.nhfonline.org.

†In Wong DL, Hess CS: ***Wong and Whaley's clinical manual of pediatric nursing***, ed 5, St Louis, 2000, Mosby.

Key Points

- Level of consciousness (LOC) is the most important indicator of neurologic health; altered levels include full consciousness, confusion, disorientation, lethargy, obtundation, stupor, coma, and persistent vegetative state.
- Complete neurologic examination includes LOC; posture; motor, sensory, cranial nerve, and reflex testing; and vital signs.
- Nursing care of the unconscious child focuses on managing respiratory function, assessing neurologic status, monitoring intracranial pressure (ICP), supplying adequate nutrition and hydration, providing drug therapy, promoting elimination, providing hygienic care, ensuring proper positioning and exercise, providing stimulation, and encouraging family support.
- Fractures resulting from head injuries may be classified as depressed, compound, basilar, and diastatic.
- Primary head injury involves features that occur at the time of trauma, including fractured skull, contusions, intracranial hematoma, and diffuse injury. Secondary complications include hypoxic brain damage, increased ICP, infection, cerebral edema, and posttraumatic syndromes.
- The young child's response to head injury is different because of the following features: larger head size; expandable skull; larger amount of blood volume to the brain; small subdural spaces; and thinner, softer brain tissue.
- Problems resulting from near-drowning include hypoxia and asphyxiation, aspiration, and hypothermia.
- Nursing care of the child with a brain tumor includes observing for signs and symptoms related to the tumor, preparing the child and family for diagnostic tests and operative procedures, preventing postoperative complications, planning for discharge, and promoting a return to optimum health.
- Nursing care of the child with meningitis includes administering antibiotics, instituting isolation precautions, removing environmental stimuli, ensuring correct positioning, monitoring vital signs, providing intravenous therapy, promoting adequate fluid and nutritional status, and providing supportive care of the family.
- Routine immunization of infants against *Haemophilus influenzae* type B infection has reduced the incidence of bacterial meningitis.
- Encephalitis may result from direct invasion of the central nervous system by a virus or from involvement of the central nervous system after viral disease.
- A seizure is a symptom of an underlying pathologic condition and may be manifested by sensory-hallucinatory phenomena, motor effects, sensorimotor effects, and loss of consciousness.
- Partial seizures are categorized as simple (without associated impairment of consciousness) or complex (with impaired consciousness); both types may become generalized.
- Generalized seizures are categorized as tonic-clonic convulsive absence, atonic and akinetic, myoclonic, and infantile spasms.
- Long-term care of the child with recurrent seizure disorders includes physical care and education regarding the importance of drug therapy and problems related to emotional aspects of the disorder.
- Febrile seizures are frightening to parents but are usually benign events that do not require antipyretic or antiepileptic therapy.
- Many cranial deformities are amenable to surgical correction.

- Hydrocephalus is a symptom of underlying brain pathology, demonstrated by impaired absorption of cerebrospinal fluid (CSF) or obstruction to the flow of CSF within the ventricles.
- Therapy for hydrocephalus involves relief of the hydrocephalus, treatment of the underlying brain disorder if possible, prevention and/or treatment of complications, and management of problems related to psychomotor development.

References

American Academy of Pediatrics, Committee on Infectious Diseases, Pickering L, editor: *2000 Red Book: report of the committee on infectious diseases,* ed 25, Elk Grove Village, IL, 2000a, The Academy.

American Academy of Pediatrics: Committee on Quality Improvement, Subcommittee on Febrile Seizures: Practice parameter: long-term treatment of the child with simple febrile seizures, *Pediatrics* 103(6):1307-1309, 1999.

American Academy of Pediatrics: Committee on Sports Medicine and Fitness and Committee on Injury and Poison Prevention: Swimming programs for infants and toddlers, *Pediatrics* 105(4):868-870, 2000b.

American Academy of Pediatrics: Recommendations for the prevention of pneumococcal conjugate vaccine (Prevnar), pneumococcal polysaccharide vaccine, and antibiotic prophylaxis, *Pediatrics* 106:362-366, 2000c.

Anderson G et al: Progress toward elimination of *Haemophilus influenzae* type b disease among infants and children—United States, 1987-1993, *MMWR* 43:144-148, 1994.

Barkovich AJ: Techniques and methods in pediatric imaging. In Barkovich AJ, editor: *Pediatric neuroimaging,* ed 2, New York, 1995, Raven Press.

Black CT, Atkinson JB: Neuroblastoma, *Semin Pediatr Surg* 6(1):2-10, 1997.

Brodeur GM, Castleberry RP: Neuroblastoma. In Pizzo PA, Poplack DG, editors: *Principles and practice of pediatric oncology,* Philadelphia, 1997, JB Lippincott.

Brown LW, Feigin RD: Bacterial meningitis: fluid balance and therapy, *Pediatr Ann* 23(2):93-98, 1994.

Camfield CS, Camfield PE: Febrile seizures: an Rx for parent fears and anxiety, *Contemp Pediatr* 10(4):26-44, 1993.

Cattelani R et al: Traumatic brain injury in childhood: intellectual, behavioural and social outcome into adulthood, *Brain Inj* 12:283-296, 1998.

Centers for Disease Control and Prevention: Human rabies—Texas and New Jersey, 1997, *MMWR* 47:1-5, 1998.

Centers for Disease Control and Prevention: Human rabies prevention—United States, 1999, *MMWR* 48(RR-1):1-21, 1999.

Cherry JD et al: Pertussis immunization and characteristics related to first seizures in infants and children, *J Pediatr* 122(6):900-903, 1993.

Dieckmann RA: Rectal diazepam for prehospital pediatric status epilepticus, *Ann Emerg Med* 23:216-224, 1994.

Durkin MS et al: The epidemiology of urban pediatric neurological trauma: evaluation of, and implications for, injury prevention programs, *Neurosurgery* 42:300-310, 1998.

Farwell JR et al: First febrile seizures: characteristics of the child, the seizure, and the illness, *Clin Pediatr* 33(5):263-267, 1994.

Feigin RD, Perlman E: Bacterial meningitis beyond the neonatal period. In Feigin RD, Cherry JD: *Textbook of pediatric infectious diseases,* ed 4, Philadelphia, 1998, WB Saunders.

Ferrie CD et al: Video-game epilepsy, *Lancet* 344(8938):1710-1711, 1994.

Heideman RL et al: Tumors of the central nervous system. In Pizzo PA, Poplack DG, editors: *Principles and practice of pediatric oncology,* ed 3, Philadelphia, 1997, JB Lippincott.

Kaplan SL: Acute bacterial meningitis beyond the neonatal period. In Long SS, Pickering LS, Prober CG, editors: *Principles and practice of pediatric infectious diseases,* New York, 1997, Churchill Livingstone.

Kaplan SL: Clinical presentations, diagnosis, and prognostic factors of bacterial meningitis, *Infect Dis Clin North Am* 13:579-594, 1999.

Kaufman BA, Park TS: Head injury and intracranial pressure. In Oldham KT, Colombani PM, Foglia RO, editors: *Surgery of infants and children; scientific principles and practice,* Philadelphia, 1997, Lippincott-Raven.

Lefevre F, Aronson N: Ketogenic diet for the treatment of refractory epilepsy in children: a systematic review of efficacy, *Pediatrics* 105(4):e46, 2000, www.pediatrics.org/cgi/content/full/105/4/e46.

Medical Research Council Antiepileptic Drug Withdrawal Study Group: Prognostic index for recurrence of seizures after remission of epilepsy, *BMJ* 306:1374-1378, 1993.

National Center for Injury Prevention and Control: *Unintentional injury: drowning fact sheet,* 1999, www.cdc.gov/ncipc/duip/drown.htm.

Pople IK et al: Results and complications of intracranial pressure monitoring in 303 children, *Pediatr Neurosurg* 23:64-67, 1995.

Quam DA: Recognizing a case of Reye's syndrome, *Am Fam Physician* 15(7):1491-1496, 1994.

Richard ME: Common pediatric craniofacial reconstructions, *Nurs Clin North Am* 29(4):791-799, 1994.

Saez-Llorenz X, McCracken GH: Genesis of fevers and the inflammatory response. In Long SS, Pickering LS, Prober CG, editors: *Principles and practice of pediatric infectious diseases,* New York, 1997, Churchill Livingstone.

Shiminski-Maher T, Shields M: Pediatric brain tumors: diagnosis and management, *J Pediatr Oncol Nurs* 12(4):188-198, 1995.

Swaiman KF: *Pediatric neurology: principles and practice,* ed 2, St Louis, 1994, Mosby.

Uhari M et al: Effect of acetaminophen and of low intermittent doses of diazepam on prevention of recurrences of febrile seizures, *J Pediatr* 126(6):991-995, 1995.

Van Donselaar CA, Geerts AT, Schimscheimer RJ: Usefulness of an aura for classification of a first generalized seizure, *Epilepsia* 31(5):529-535, 1990.

Verity CM, Ross EM, Golding J: Outcome of childhood status epilepticus and lengthy febrile convulsions: findings of national cohort study, *BMJ* 307:225-228, 1993.

Vernon-Levett P: Neurologic system. In Slota MC, editor: *Core curriculum for pediatric critical care nursing,* Philadelphia, 1998, WB Saunders.

Ward JD: Craniocerebral injuries. In Buntain WL, editor: *Management of pediatric trauma,* Philadelphia, 1995, WB Saunders.

Zuckerman GB, Gregory PM, Santos-Damiani SM: Predictors of death and neurologic impairment in pediatric submersion injuries: the pediatric risk of mortality score, *Arch Pediatr Adolesc Med* 152:134-140, 1998.

CHAPTER 52 Endocrine Dysfunction

http://www.harcourthealth.com/MERLIN/Wong/maternal/

Learning Objectives

On completion of this chapter the reader will be able to:

- Differentiate between the disorders caused by hypopituitary and hyperpituitary dysfunction.
- Describe the manifestations of thyroid hypofunction and hyperfunction and the management of children with the disorders.
- Distinguish between the manifestations of adrenal hypofunction and hyperfunction.
- Differentiate among the various categories of diabetes mellitus.
- Discuss the management and nursing care of the child with diabetes mellitus in the acute care setting.
- Distinguish between a hypoglycemic reaction and a hyperglycemic reaction.
- Design a teaching plan for a child with diabetes mellitus.
- Formulate a teaching plan for instructing the parents of a child with diabetes mellitus.

DISORDERS OF PITUITARY FUNCTION

The *pituitary gland,* or *hypophysis,* is often referred to as the *master gland* because of its role in regulating other endocrine glands. Under the influence of secretions from the hypothalamus, the anterior lobe of the pituitary (adenohypophysis) releases or withholds seven hormones (Table 52-1). These hormones control the secretion of hormones from other endocrine glands and influence somatic and sexual development. Because of this relationship, a dysfunction observed in target tissues can be a result of malfunction of the hypothalamus, the pituitary gland, or the target gland. If the tropic hormones are involved, the resulting disorder reflects the altered stimulus to the target gland. For example, if thyroid-stimulating hormone is deficient, thyroid hormone is also deficient, and the child displays the manifestations of hypothyroidism. Overproduction of pituitary hormone is thought to be caused by hyperplasia of the pituitary cells or by a primary hypothalamic defect that results in excess production of the hormone's releasing factor.

Deficiencies of the anterior pituitary hormones may be a result of organic defects or of idiopathic etiology and may occur as a single hormonal problem or in combination with other hormonal deficiencies. The clinical manifestations depend on the hormones involved and the age of onset. This discussion is limited to dysfunction related primarily to the secretion of growth hormone.

NURSE ALERT • Children with panhypopituitarism should wear medical identification such as a bracelet.

Hypopituitarism: Growth Hormone (GH) Deficiency

Hypopituitarism is primarily a disorder associated with deficient secretion of GH (somatotropin). It may be caused by a variety of conditions, including: development defects; destructive lesions such as tumors; trauma, vascular abnormalities, or surgery; certain hereditary disorders; or functional disorders such as anorexia nervosa or psychosocial dwarfism. In more than half of children with hypopituitarism, no lesion is evident and the cause is unknown. This is called *idiopathic hypopituitarism* or *idiopathic pituitary growth failure.*

GH deficiency inhibits somatic growth in all body cells (Fig. 52-1). The primary site of dysfunction in the syndrome appears to be in the hypothalamus. The extent of idiopathic GH deficiency may be complete or partial, but the cause is unknown. It is commonly associated with other pituitary hormone deficiencies and is treated more often in boys than in girls.

Diagnostic Evaluation. Only a small number of children with delayed growth or short stature have hypopituitary dwarfism. In the majority of instances the cause is constitutional delay. Although children with hypopituitarism are normal at birth, they show growth patterns that progressively deviate from the normal growth rate, often beginning in infancy. The chief complaint in most instances is short stature (Box 52-1).

A complete diagnostic evaluation should include a family history, a history of the child's growth patterns and previous health status, physical examination, psychosocial evaluation,

TABLE 52-1
Endocrine Glands and Their Functions

Hormone	Primary Effect
ADENOHYPOPHYSIS (ANTERIOR PITUITARY GLAND)	
Growth hormone (GH)	Promotes growth of bone and soft tissues
Thyroid-stimulating hormone (TSH)	Stimulates thyroid hormone secretion
Adrenocorticotropic hormone (ACTH)	Stimulates adrenal cortex to secrete glucocorticoids and androgens
Gonadotropins Follicle-stimulating hormone (FSH) Luteinizing hormone (LH)	Stimulate gonads to mature and produce sex hormones and germ cells
Prolactin	Stimulates milk secretion
Melanocyte-stimulating hormone (MSH)	Promotes pigmentation of skin
NEUROHYPOPHYSIS (POSTERIOR PITUITARY GLAND)	
Antidiuretic hormone (ADH)	Acts on kidney tubules to reabsorb water
Oxytocin	Stimulates uterine contractions Causes milk ejection reflex
THYROID GLAND	
Thyroid hormones	Regulate metabolic rate Control rate of body cell growth
Thyrocalcitonin	Influences ossification and development of bone
PARATHYROID GLANDS	
Parathyroid hormone (PTH)	Regulates calcium metabolism
ADRENAL CORTEX	
Aldosterone	Regulates sodium retention and excretion
Sex hormones	Influence development of bones, reproductive organs, and secondary sex characteristics
Glucocorticoids	Promote metabolism Mobilize body defenses during stress Suppress inflammatory reaction
ADRENAL MEDULLA	
Catecholamines	Produce a sympathetic response Increase blood pressure and blood glucose levels
ISLETS OF LANGERHANS OF PANCREAS	
Insulin	Promotes utilization of glucose by cells; decreases blood glucose levels
Glucagon	Increases blood glucose levels Accelerates glyconeogenesis
Somatostatin	Inhibits secretion of insulin and glucagon
OVARIES	
Estrogen	Stimulates ripening of ova Produces female secondary sex characteristics Promotes epiphyseal closure of bones
Progesterone	Prepares uterus for fertilization
TESTES	
Testosterone	Stimulates spermatogenesis Produces male secondary sex characteristics Promotes epiphyseal closure of bones

drug intake, parental heights, birth size, nutritional state, review of systems, radiographic surveys, and endocrine studies. Definitive diagnosis is based on radioimmunoassay of plasma GH levels stimulated pharmacologically with two or more agents. GH levels below 10 ng/ml after two provocative tests establish the diagnosis (Shulman and Bercu, 1998).

Radiographic examination of the hand and wrist for centers of ossification is an important procedure in evaluating growth. Endocrine studies to detect tropic hormone deficiencies are also performed if there is evidence of hypothyroidism, hypersecretion of cortisol, or gonadal aplasia.

Therapeutic Management. Treatment of GH deficiency caused by organic lesions is directed toward correction of the underlying disease process (e.g., surgical removal or irradiation of a tumor). The definitive treatment of GH deficiency is replacement of GH. *Biosynthetic GH* prepared by recombinant DNA technology is the therapy of choice. Children with other hormone deficiencies require replacement therapy to correct the specific disorders. This may involve administration of thyroid extract, cortisone, testosterone, or estrogens and progesterone. The sex hormones are usually begun during adolescence to promote normal sexual maturation. Currently, much contro-

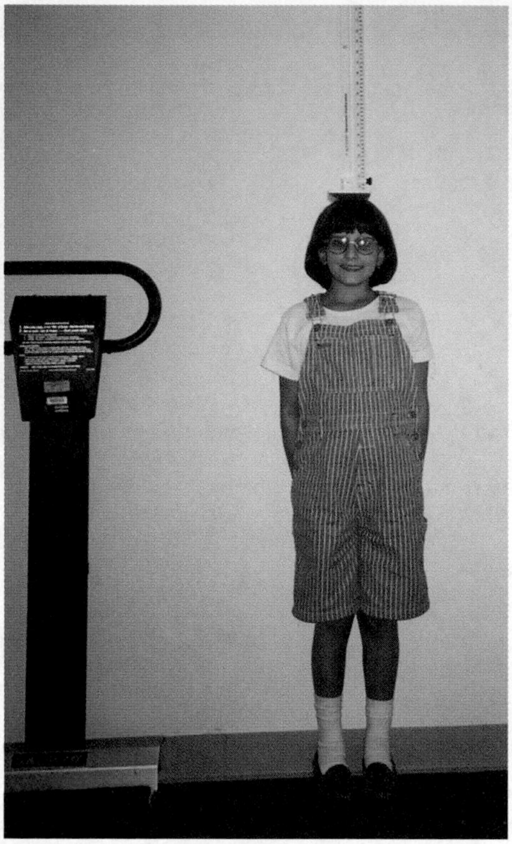

FIG. 52-1 • Thirteen-year-old girl with short stature. Height is 133 cm. Normal height for age is 145 to 168 cm.

versy exists over the use of GH in children who are short but not GH deficient.

Prognosis. GH replacement is successful in 80% of affected children. Children who respond to therapy typically increase their growth rate from 3.5 to 4 cm/year before treatment to 8.7 ± 1.5 cm/year after treatment. Young children, obese children, and severely GH-deficient children respond best. Growth responses to GH will vary depending on age, length of treatment, frequency of administration, dosage, weight, and GH receptor amount (Blethen et al, 1996). Overall studies have noted improved actual or near-final adult height. Early diagnosis and initiation of therapy is important to successful therapy (August, Julius, and Blethen, 1998).

Creutzfeldt-Jakob disease (CJD), a rare neurodegenerative condition, was reported in some patients after administration of cadaver derived human growth hormone (HGH) but does not occur with the use of biosynthetic GH. Circumstances make it likely that HGH contaminated with CJD, a slow-growing, viruslike particle, may have been responsible for fatalities in patients treated with HGH. Blood banks do not accept donation from former HGH recipients because of the inability to test for infection with CJD (Rosenfeld, 1996).

Nursing Care Management. Nursing care is primarily directed toward assisting in establishing the diagnosis and providing emotional support to the child and family (see Chapter 41). Because these children appear younger than their chronologic age, others often relate to them in childish ways.

Box 52-1

Clinical Manifestations of Hypopituitarism

- Presenting complaint—short stature
  - Usually normal growth first year
  - Growth during second year drops below established percentile
  - Growth measurements below 5th percentile
- Premature aging common in later life
- Height may be retarded more than weight
- Appear well nourished
- Skeletal proportions normal
- Tend to be relatively inactive
- Less apt to participate in aggressive, sporting-type activities
- Bone age nearly always retarded but closely related to height age
- Usually primary teeth appear at expected age; eruption of permanent teeth delayed
- Teeth are overcrowded and malpositioned (because of underdeveloped jaw)
- Sexual development usually delayed but normal

Parents and teachers benefit from guidance directed toward realistic expectations of the child based on age and abilities (Zimet et al, 1997).

Children undergoing hormone replacement require additional support, such as preparation for daily subcutaneous injections and education for self-management during the school-age years* (Critical Thinking box).

NURSE ALERT • Injections are given at bedtime to most closely approximately physiologic release of GH.

Even when hormone replacement is successful, these children attain their eventual adult height at a slower rate than that of their peers; thus they need assistance in setting realistic expectations regarding the expected outcome. Professionals and families may find education and support from the Human Growth Foundation.† The treatment is expensive—up to $20,000 to $30,000 per year depending on dosage.

Pituitary Hyperfunction

Excess GH before closure of the epiphyseal shafts results in proportional overgrowth of long bones; the individual can reach a height of 8 feet or more. Vertical growth is accompanied by rapid and increased development of muscles and viscera. Weight is increased but usually is in proportion to height. Proportional enlargement of head circumference also occurs and may result in delayed closure of the fontanels. Children with a pituitary-secreting tumor may also demonstrate signs of increasing intracranial pressure, especially headache.

If hypersecretion of GH occurs after epiphyseal closure, growth is in the transverse direction, producing a condition known as *acromegaly.* Typical facial features include overgrowth

*Community and home care instructions on giving subcutaneous injections are available in Wong DL, Hess CS: ***Wong and Whaley's clinical manual of pediatric nursing,*** ed 5, St Louis, 2000, Mosby.

†1997 Glen Cove Ave., Glen Head, NY 11545; 1-800-451-6434; e-mail: hgfl@hgfound.org; website: www.hgfound.org.

Critical Thinking

GROWTH HORMONE DEFICIENCY

Kevin, an 11-year-old boy, is being treated for growth hormone (GH) deficiency. A workup was initiated after Kevin's mother noticed that his pants size had not changed in 2 years and that his 8-year-old brother was rapidly becoming taller than Kevin. Kevin has become increasingly hostile to his brother and is refusing to attend school on a regular basis. Kevin's mother is administering the daily injections of GH. Which of the following interventions should be initiated first to allow Kevin to regain feelings of mastery and control over his environment?

First, Think About It . . .

- **What concepts or ideas are central to your thinking?**
- **What conclusions are you coming to?**

1. **Preparation for home schooling**
2. **Family counseling related to sibling rivalry**
3. **Education and support related to self-administration of GH**
4. **Encouragement and assurance that the therapy is temporary and will maximize his adult height**

The best response is 3. The idea that children with GH deficiency may develop behaviors related to feelings of inadequacy and loss of control is developmentally sound. Often families, teachers, and peers relate to the child relative to his or her short height rather than his or her chronologic age. Children of 11 years are competent to draw up and administer daily injections of GH, which will allow them increased control over their environment and a feeling that they are responsible for treatment of his growth deficit.

Option 1 is incorrect; these children must remain in regular school. At this point, option 2 is probably not necessary, since increasing Kevin's control may reduce his hostility. Although option 4 is always appropriate, it does not address the principal issue—the conclusion that Kevin should be independently responsible for his therapy.

of the head, lips, nose, tongue, jaw, and paranasal and mastoid sinuses; separation and malocclusion of the teeth in the enlarged jaw; disproportion of the face to the cerebral division of the skull; increased facial hair; and thickened, deeply creased skin.

Diagnostic Evaluation. Diagnosis is based on a history of excessive growth during childhood and evidence of increased levels of GH. Radiologic studies may reveal a tumor in an enlarged sella turcica; normal bone age; enlargement of bones, such as the paranasal sinuses; and evidence of joint changes. Endocrine studies to confirm excess of other hormones, such as cortisol and sex hormones, are also included in the differential diagnosis.

Therapeutic Management. If a lesion is present, surgical treatment, including cryosurgery or hypophysectomy, may be warranted to remove the tumor whenever feasible. Other therapies that destroy pituitary tissue include external radiation and radioactive implants. Depending on the extent of surgical extirpation and the degree of pituitary insufficiency, hormone replacement with thyroid extract, cortisone, and sex hormones may be necessary.

Nursing Care Management. The primary nursing consideration is early identification of children with excessive growth rates. Although medical management does not diminish the height already attained, it can retard further growth. The earlier the treatment is begun, the better the chance to attain a normal adult height.

Children with excessive growth rates require as much emotional support as those with short stature. Girls may suffer from the effects of excessive height much more than boys, who may find their height an asset when pursuing sports such as basketball. A compassionate nurse can be very supportive to these children, especially before adolescence when they are larger than their peers. The nurse can emphasize to a tall girl that boys become taller as they grow older, and she will not always be looking down at them. Because early adolescence is a time of idol worship, the nurse can point out celebrity couples in which the woman is taller than the man to help the girl gain a perspective that not all heterosexual relationships must follow stereotypic models.

Precocious Puberty

Manifestations of sexual development in boys younger than 9 or in girls younger than 8 are considered precocious and should be investigated. Early sexual development can have a number of causes and may result from a disorder of the gonad, the adrenal gland, or the hypothalamic-pituitary gonadal axis. The disorder occurs far more commonly in girls than in boys. No causative factor can be found in 80% to 90% of girls and in 50% of boys with the condition (Rosenfeld, 1996).

True, or *complete precocious puberty* is always isosexual and results from premature activation of the hypothalamic pituitary-gonadal axis, which produces early maturation and development of the gonads with secretion of sex hormones, development of secondary sex characteristics, and sometimes production of mature sperm or ova. Precocious puberty is explained only as an unusually early activation of the maturation process that is regarded as a normal course of events at a later age. There is early acceleration of linear growth with early epiphyseal fusion and ultimate height less than that anticipated with later pubertal onset. *Precocious pseudopuberty,* or *incomplete puberty,* differs from true sexual precocity in that there is no early secretion of gonadotropin. Most cases result from early overproduction of sex hormone, usually caused by a tumor of the ovary or testis, a tumor or hyperplasia of the adrenal gland, or exogenous sources of androgens or estrogens.

Therapeutic Management. Treatment of precocious pseudopuberty is directed toward the specific cause when known. Precocious puberty of central origin is managed with monthly subcutaneous injections of a synthetic analog of *luteinizing hormone-releasing hormone (LHRH; Lupron),* which regulates pituitary secretions. This therapy slows the prepubertal growth in affected children to normal rates. Treatment is discontinued at a chronologically appropriate time, allowing pubertal changes to resume.

Nursing Care Management. Psychologic support and guidance of the child and family are the most important aspects of management. Parents need a detailed explanation and reassurance of the benign nature of the condition. Dress and activities for the physically precocious child should be appropriate to the chronologic age.

Despite the early sexual development, maturation of the gonads and the appearance of secondary sexual characteristics proceed in the usual order. After puberty, physical differences from peers are no longer present. Heterosexual interest is not usually advanced beyond the child's chronological age; however, the nurse should emphasize to parents that the child is fertile.

No form of contraception is necessary, however, unless the child is sexually active.

Children receiving LHRH therapy need preparation for the subcutaneous injections. Both parents and children should be taught the injection procedure.*

Diabetes insipidus (DI)

The principal disorder of posterior pituitary hypofunction is DI, also known as *neurogenic DI.* The disease is a result of hyposecretion of *antidiuretic hormone (ADH),* or *vasopressin,* which produces a state of uncontrolled diuresis. Primary causes are familial or idiopathic; secondary causes include trauma (accidental or surgical), tumors, granulomatous disease, infections (meningitis or encephalitis), or vascular anomalies (aneurysm). The disorder is not to be confused with nephrogenic DI, a rare hereditary disorder caused by unresponsiveness of the renal tubules to the hormone.

Clinical Manifestations. The cardinal signs of DI are polyuria and polydipsia. In the older child excessive urination accompanied by a compensatory insatiable thirst may be so intense that the child does little other than drink fluids and void. Not infrequently, the first sign is enuresis. In the infant the initial symptom is irritability that is relieved with feedings of water but not milk. The infant is also prone to dehydration, electrolyte imbalance, hyperthermia, azotemia, and potential circulatory collapse.

NURSE ALERT • The child with DI complicated by congenital absence of the thirst center must be encouraged to drink sufficient quantities of liquid to prevent electrolyte imbalance.

Diagnostic Evaluation. The simplest test used to diagnose this condition is restriction of oral fluids and observation of consequent changes in urine volume and concentration. In DI, fluid restriction has little or no effect on urine formation but causes weight loss from dehydration. If this test is positive, the child should be given a test dose of injected *aqueous vasopressin (Pitressin),* which should alleviate the polyuria and polydipsia. Unresponsiveness to exogenous vasopressin usually indicates nephrogenic DI.

NURSE ALERT • Small children require close supervision during fluid restriction to prevent them from drinking, even from toilet bowls, plants, or other unlikely sources of fluid.

Therapeutic Management. The usual treatment requires daily hormone replacement of vasopressin. The drug of choice is *desmopressin acetate (DDAVP),* a synthetic analog of vasopressin. DDAVP may also be given orally. Recent studies have found this to be an effective alternative (Boulgourdjian et al, 1997). Nasal DDAVP has widely replaced the use of vasopressin tannate in peanut oil. The injectable form has the advantage of lasting 48 to 72 hours, which affords the child a full night's sleep; however, it has the disadvantages of requiring frequent injections and proper preparation of the drug.

*Community and home care instructions on giving subcutaneous injections are available in Wong DL, Hess CS: ***Wong and Whaley's clinical manual of pediatric nursing,*** ed 5, St Louis, 2000, Mosby.

DDAVP is available and administered intranasally by way of a flexible tube to achieve adequate control. It is usually administered twice daily. The response pattern of the child is variable, with duration ranging from 8 to 20 hours. Children receiving DDAVP need to be observed for a possible overdose of the drug. The signs of overdosage are those of water intoxication and are similar to manifestations of inappropriate antidiuretic hormone secretion.

Nursing Care Management. The initial objective of care is identification of the disorder. After confirmation of the diagnosis, parents need a thorough explanation of the condition, with special emphasis on distinguishing between diabetes insipidus and diabetes mellitus. The parents must realize that treatment is lifelong. If the child is to receive the injectable vasopressin, ideally both parents, as well as children who are over 7 years of age, should be taught the correct procedure for preparation and administration of the drug.* Once children are old enough, they should be encouraged to assume full responsibility for care.

NURSE ALERT • To be effective, vasopressin must be thoroughly resuspended in the oil by being held under warm running water for 10 to 15 minutes and shaken vigorously before being drawn into the syringe. If this is not done, the oil may be injected without ADH. Small brown particles, which indicate drug dispersion, must be seen in the suspension.

For emergency purposes these children should wear medical alert identification. Older children are advised to carry the nasal vasopressin spray with them for temporary relief of symptoms. School personnel should be made aware of the problem so that the child is granted unrestricted use of the lavatory and drinking water. Failure to permit this may result in embarrassing accidents that often lead to the child's unwillingness to attend school.

Syndrome of Inappropriate Antidiuretic Hormone Secretion (SIADH)

Hypersecretion of the posterior pituitary ADH (vasopressin) produces the disorder known as SIADH. SIADH is observed with increased frequency in a variety of conditions, especially those involving infections, tumors, and trauma of the central nervous system.

The manifestations observed are directly related to fluid retention and hypotonicity. Increased secretion of ADH causes the kidneys to reabsorb water, which increases the fluid volume and decreases serum osmolality. When serum sodium levels are lowered to 120 mEq/L, the child displays anorexia, nausea (sometimes vomiting), stomach cramps, irritability, and personality changes. With progressive reduction in sodium, other neurologic signs, stupor, and seizures may be evident. The symptoms disappear when the underlying disorder is corrected. Immediate management consists of restricting fluids.

Nursing Care Management. The first goal of nursing management is recognizing the presence of SIADH from symptoms described in patients at risk. Accurately measuring intake,

*Community and home care instructions on giving intramuscular or subcutaneous injections are available in Wong DL, Hess CS: ***Wong and Whaley's clinical manual of pediatric nursing,*** ed 5, St Louis, 2000, Mosby.

output, and daily weight; and observing for signs of fluid overload are primary nursing functions, especially in the child receiving intravenous (IV) fluids.

NURSE ALERT • Children with SIADH develop an expanded circulatory volume but do not form edema, which is an excess of both water and sodium (Gildea, 1993).

Seizure precautions are implemented, and the child and family need education regarding the rationale for fluid restriction. The rare child with chronic SIADH will be placed on a long-term regimen of ADH-antagonizing medication and will require instructions for its administration.

DISORDERS OF THYROID FUNCTION

The thyroid gland secretes two types of hormones: *thyroid hormone (TH)*, which consists of the hormones *thyroxine* (T_4) and *triiodothyronine* (T_3); and *thyrocalcitonin*. The secretion of thyroid hormones is controlled by *thyroid-stimulating hormone (TSH)* from the anterior pituitary. Hypothyroidism or hyperthyroidism may result from a defect in the target gland or from a disturbance in secretion of TSH or its releasing factor in the hypothalamus.

Because the functions of T_3 and T_4 are qualitatively the same, the term *thyroid hormone (TH)* is used throughout this discussion.

The synthesis of TH depends on available sources of dietary iodine and tyrosine. The thyroid is the only endocrine gland capable of storing excess amounts of hormones for release as needed. The main physiologic action of TH is to regulate the basal metabolic rate and thereby control the processes of growth and tissue differentiation.

Thyrocalcitonin helps maintain blood calcium levels by decreasing the calcium concentration. Its effect is the opposite of parathormone; it inhibits skeletal demineralization and promotes calcium deposition in the bone.

Juvenile Hypothyroidism

Hypothyroidism is one of the most common endocrine problems of childhood. It may be either congenital or acquired and represents a deficiency in secretion of TH. Hypothyroidism from dietary insufficiency of iodine is rare in the United States because iodized salt is a readily available source of the nutrient. This discussion is limited to the juvenile form of hypothyroidism.

Beyond infancy, primary hypothyroidism may be caused by a number of defects. For example, a congenital hypoplastic thyroid gland may provide sufficient amounts of TH during the first year or two but be inadequate when rapid body growth increases demands on the gland. A partial or complete thyroidectomy for cancer or thyrotoxicosis can leave insufficient thyroid tissue to furnish hormones for body requirements. Irradiation for Hodgkin disease or other malignancies or infectious processes may be a cause of hypothyroidism (August et al, 1996). A high risk for thyroid disease, including thyroid cancer and Graves disease, persists for more than 25 years after patients have received radiation therapy (Ron et al, 1995).

Clinical manifestations depend on the extent of dysfunction and the age of the child at the onset (Box 52-2). Because brain growth is nearly complete by 2 to 3 years of age, mental retardation or neurologic sequelae are not associated with juvenile hypothyroidism.

Box 52-2
Clinical Manifestations of Juvenile Hypothyroidism

- Decelerated growth
  - Less when acquired at later age
- Myxedematous skin changes
  - Dry skin
  - Puffiness around eyes
  - Sparse hair
  - Constipation
  - Sleepiness
  - Mental decline

Therapy is oral TH replacement, the same as for hypothyroidism in the infant, although the prompt treatment needed for brain growth in the infant is not required in the child. In children with severe symptoms, the restoration of euthyroidism is achieved more gradually, with administration of increasing amounts of L-thyroxine over 4 to 8 weeks to avoid symptoms of hyperthyroidism that can occur with treatment of chronic hypothyroidism.

Nursing Care Management. Early recognition in the infant is important. Cessation or retardation of growth in a child whose growth has previously been normal should alert the observer to the possibility of hypothyroidism. After diagnosis and implementation of thyroxine therapy, the importance of compliance and periodic monitoring of the response to therapy should be stressed to the parents. Children should learn to take responsibility for their health as soon as they are old enough, at about 9 to 10 years of age.

Goiter

A goiter is an enlargement or hypertrophy of the thyroid gland. It can be congenital or acquired. Congenital disease usually occurs as a result of antithyroid drugs and/or iodides administered to the mother during pregnancy. The acquired disease can result from increased secretion of pituitary thyrotropic hormone in response to decreased circulating levels of TH, neoplastic or inflammatory processes, or dietary iodine deficiency.

Enlargement of the thyroid gland may be mild and noticeable only when there is an increased demand for TH (e.g., during periods of rapid growth). Enlargement of the thyroid at birth can be sufficient to cause severe respiratory distress. TH replacement is necessary to treat the hypothyroidism and reverse the TSH effect on the gland.

Nursing Care Management. Large goiters are identified by their obvious appearance. Smaller nodules may be evident only on palpation. Nurses in ambulatory settings need to be aware of the possibility of neck enlargement from goiters and report such findings.

NURSE ALERT • If an infant is born with a goiter, immediate precautions are instituted for emergency ventilation, such as supplemental oxygen and a tracheostomy set. Positioning the child with the neck hyperextended often facilitates breathing.

Immediate surgery to remove part of the gland may be lifesaving. When thyroid replacement is necessary, parents have the same needs regarding its administration as discussed for the parents of children who have hypothyroidism.

Lymphocytic Thyroiditis

Lymphocytic thyroiditis *(Hashimoto disease, juvenile autoimmune thyroiditis)* is the most common cause of thyroid disease in children and adolescents, and it accounts for the largest percentage of juvenile hypothyroidism. It also accounts for many of the enlarged thyroid glands formerly designated as thyroid hyperplasia of adolescence, or "adolescent goiter." The disease is more common in girls than in boys, and more common in Caucasians than African-Americans. It occurs more often after age 6, reaching a peak incidence in adolescence; there is evidence that the disease is self-limited.

Pathophysiology. There is a strong genetic predisposition to the development of autoimmune thyroiditis, although no mode of inheritance has been delineated and the basic stimulus or autoimmune defect is unknown. The disease is characterized by lymphocytic infiltration of the gland; inflammation; and, in many patients, replacement with fibrous tissue. In the early stages there may be only hyperplasia.

Diagnostic Evaluation. The enlarged thyroid gland may be detected by the practitioner during a routine examination, although it may be noted by parents when the youngster swallows. Most children are euthyroid, but some display symptoms of hypothyroidism. Others have signs that suggest hyperthyroidism (Box 52-3).

Thyroid function tests are usually normal, although TSH levels may be slightly or moderately elevated. With progressive disease the T_4 decreases, followed by a decrease in T_3 levels and an increase in TSH. A variety of abnormalities in radioactive iodine uptake may be noted. The majority of children have serum antibody titers to thyroid antigens, but fewer children have a positive red blood cell hemagglutination test. When both tests are used, almost all children with thyroid autoimmunity are detected.

Therapeutic Management. In many cases the goiter is transient and asymptomatic and regresses spontaneously within a year or two. Therapy of a nontoxic diffuse goiter is usually simple, uncomplicated, and effective. Oral administration of TH depresses TSH, thus decreasing the size of the gland significantly. Surgery is contraindicated in this disorder.

Nursing Care Management. Nursing care consists of identifying the youngster with thyroid enlargement, reassuring the child that the condition is probably only temporary, and reinforcing instructions for thyroid therapy.

Box 52-3

Clinical Manifestations of Lymphocytic Thyroiditis

ENLARGED THYROID GLAND
- Usually symmetric
- Firm
- Freely moveable
- Nontender

TRACHEAL COMPRESSION
- Sense of fullness
- Hoarseness
- Dysphagia

HYPERTHYROIDISM (POSSIBLE)
- Nervousness
- Irritability
- Increased sweating
- Hyperactivity

Hyperthyroidism (Graves Disease)

The largest percentage of hyperthyroidism in childhood is caused by Graves disease, which is usually associated with an enlarged thyroid gland and exophthalmos. The peak incidence of the disease occurs between 12 and 14 years of age, but it may be present at birth in children of thyrotoxic mothers. The incidence is five times higher in girls than in boys. The disease is apparently caused by a serum thyroid-stimulating immunoglobulin, but no specific etiology has been identified. There is definitive evidence for familial association; a large number of persons with the disease possess the histocompatibility antigen HLA-B8.

Diagnostic Evaluation. The development of manifestations is highly variable (Box 52-4). Manifestations develop gradually, with an interval between onset and diagnosis of approximately 6 to 12 months. Diagnosis is established on the basis of increased levels of T_4 and T_3. TSH is suppressed to unmeasurable levels. Other tests are rarely indicated.

Box 52-4

Clinical Manifestations of Hyperthyroidism (Graves Disease)

CARDINAL SIGNS
- Emotional lability
- Physical restlessness, characteristically at rest
- Decelerated school performance
- Voracious appetite with weight loss in 50% of cases
- Fatigue

PHYSICAL SIGNS
- Tachycardia
- Widened pulse pressure
- Dyspnea on exertion
- Exophthalmos (protruding eyeballs)
- Wide-eyed, staring expression with lid lag
- Tremor
- Goiter (hypertrophy and hyperplasia)
- Warm, moist skin
- Accelerated linear growth
- Heat intolerance (may be severe)
- Hair fine and unable to hold a curl
- Systolic murmurs

THYROID STORM
- Acute onset:
  - Severe irritability and restlessness
  - Vomiting
  - Diarrhea
  - Hyperthermia
  - Hypertension
  - Severe tachycardia
  - Prostration
- May progress rapidly to:
  - Delirium
  - Coma
  - Death

Therapeutic Management. Therapy for hyperthyroidism is controversial, but all methods are directed toward retarding the rate of hormone secretion. The three acceptable modes available are (1) the antithyroid drugs (including propylthiouracil [PTU] and methimazole [MTZ, Tapazole]), which interfere with the biosynthesis of TH; (2) subtotal thyroidectomy; and (3) ablation with radioiodine (^{131}I-iodide). When affected children exhibit signs and symptoms of hyperthyroidism, their activity should be limited. Vigorous exercise is restricted until thyroid levels are decreased to normal or near-normal values.

Thyrotoxicosis (thyroid crisis or thyroid storm) may occur from sudden release of the hormone. Although it is unusual in children, a crisis can be life threatening. A crisis may be precipitated by acute infection, surgical emergencies, or discontinuation of antithyroid therapy. Treatment, in addition to antithyroid drugs, is administration of β-adrenergic blocking agents (e.g., propranolol), which provide relief from the disturbing side effects of the reaction.

Nursing Care Management. The initial nursing objective is identification of children with hyperthyroidism. Because the clinical manifestations often appear gradually, the goiter and ophthalmic changes may not be noticed and the excessive activity may be attributed to behavioral problems. Nurses in ambulatory settings, particularly those caring for children in school, need to be alert to signs that suggest this disorder, especially weight loss despite an excellent appetite, academic difficulties resulting from a short attention span and inability to sit still, unexplained fatigue and sleeplessness, and difficulty with fine motor skills (such as writing). Exophthalmos may develop long before the onset of signs and symptoms of hyperthyroidism and may be the only presenting sign (Bartley et al, 1996).

Much of the care during diagnosis and initial medical therapy is related to the physical symptoms. The child needs a quiet, unstimulating environment that is conducive to rest, and sometimes hospitalization is necessary during the immediate treatment phase. A regular routine is beneficial, as are frequent rest periods, minimizing the stress of coping with unexpected demands, and meeting the child's needs promptly. Physical activity is restricted; for example, school physical education classes are discontinued. Despite the excessive activity of these children, they tire easily, experience muscle weakness, and are unable to relax to recoup their strength.

Emotional lability is often manifested by sudden episodes of crying or elation. Such behavior, together with irritability, disrupts interpersonal relationships and creates difficulties within and outside the home. Heat intolerance may produce considerable family conflict: because a cooler environment is preferred, the child is likely to open windows, complain about the heat, wear minimal clothing, and kick off blankets while sleeping. Hygiene should be stressed because of excessive sweating.

Dietary requirements are regulated to meet the child's increased metabolic rate. Although the need for calories is increased, these should be provided in wholesome foods rather than "junk" foods. Vitamin supplements may be needed to meet daily requirements. Rather than three large meals, the child's appetite may be better satisfied by five or six moderate meals throughout the day.

Once therapy is instituted, the nurse explains the drug regimen, emphasizing the importance of observing for side effects of antithyroid drugs. Untoward effects of propylthiouracil and related compounds include skin rash, drug fever, enlargement of the salivary and cervical lymph glands, diminished sense of taste, hepatitis, and edema of the lower extremities (Critical Thinking box).

Parents should also be aware of the signs of hypothyroidism, which can occur from overdose of the drugs. The most common indications are lethargy and somnolence.

Surgical Care. If surgery is anticipated, iodine is usually administered for a few weeks before the procedure. Because oral iodine preparations are unpalatable, they should be mixed with a strong-tasting fruit juice (e.g., grape or punch flavors) and be given through a straw. Compliance with iodine therapy is essential to avoid the danger of thyroid crisis after sudden discontinuation.

NURSE ALERT • Children being treated with propylthiouracil must be carefully monitored for side effects of the drug. Because sore throat and fever accompany the grave complication of leukopenia, these children should be seen by a practitioner if such symptoms occur. Parents and children should be taught to recognize and report symptoms immediately.

Psychologic preparation of children for thyroidectomy is similar to that for any other surgical procedure (see Chapter 45); however, the site of the incision is of special consideration.

Critical Thinking

GRAVES DISEASE

Susie, 15 years old, has noticed a racing pulse, ravenous appetite with continued weight loss, heat intolerance and sensitivity, and eyes that appear to be bulging from their sockets. After a diagnosis of Graves disease, Susie is started on a therapeutic dose of propylthiouracil. Because of tachycardia, Susie is advised to participate in sedentary activities only and to discontinue school physical education classes. Environmental temperature and appropriate dress related to heat sensitivity, as well as dietary adjustments to meet increased metabolic needs, are addressed by the nurse. Susie is shown that exopthalmos can be minimized with artful application of cosmetics. Episodic emotional lability is discussed with Susie and her family. The drug regimen is explained with special emphasis on its side effects. After 6 weeks of treatment Susie presents with a sore throat and fever. Which of the following interventions is most appropriate?

First, Think About It . . .

- **What precise question are you trying to answer?**
- **What conclusions are you coming to?**

1. **Immediate follow-up by the practitioner**
2. **Further instruction related to heat sensitivity**
3. **Instruction related to symptomatic relief of the common cold**
4. **Psychosocial interventions related to somatization of emotional lability**

The best response is 1. Precisely, the question is focused on the complications of propylthiouracil. Therapeutic levels of propylthiouracil can be accompanied by the grave complication of leukocytopenia. Any indication of infection must be promptly evaluated and appropriate therapy instituted. An accurate conclusion is that none of the other options addresses the immediate problem.

The fear of having the throat cut is very real, and in older children is associated with death. The nurse should explain that only the skin, not the throat, is cut to allow for removal of the gland. Showing children a picture of the anatomic location of the thyroid around the trachea is often helpful. Children should be prepared for the dressing around the neck and the possibility of an endotracheal or breathing tube after surgery.

Postoperative care involves positioning with the neck slightly flexed to avoid strain on the sutures and to observe for bleeding and complications. Children are taught to support the neck in this position when they sit up. Damage to the recurrent laryngeal nerve is evidenced by severe stridor and/or hoarseness, although some hoarseness is expected. Observation for signs of hypoparathyroidism, which causes hypocalcemia, should be implemented in the immediate postoperative period.

NURSE ALERT • The earliest indication of hypoparathyroidism may be anxiety and mental depression, followed by paresthesia and evidence of heightened neuromuscular excitability, such as:

- **Chvostek sign**—Facial muscle spasm elicited by tapping the facial nerve in the region of the parotid gland
- **Trousseau sign**—Carpal spasm elicited by pressure applied to nerves of the upper arm
- **Tetany**—Carpopedal spasm (sharp flexion of wrist and ankle joints), muscle twitching, cramps, seizures, and sometimes stridor

DISORDERS OF PARATHYROID FUNCTION

The parathyroid glands secrete *parathormone (PTH),* whose main function, along with vitamin D, is to maintain homeostasis of blood calcium concentrations. PTH exerts its effect by: (1) increasing the release of calcium and phosphate from the bone (bone demineralization); (2) increasing the absorption of calcium and the excretion of phosphate by the kidneys; and (3) promoting calcium absorption in the gastrointestinal tract. The net result of these actions is to increase the plasma calcium concentration while lowering the plasma phosphate concentration.

Hypoparathyroidism

Two classic forms of hypoparathyroidism are observed during childhood. *Autoimmune hypoparathyroidism,* in which there is deficient production of PTH, may occur as a component of multiglandular failure, usually in relation to autoimmune phenomena. *Familial hypoparathyroidism* is inherited as an autosomal recessive trait and has early onset, usually in the first month of life. In *pseudohypoparathyroidism,* production of PTH is increased but end-organ responsiveness to the hormone is deficient. Pseudohypoparathyroidism is also thought to be inherited as an X-linked dominant trait with variable expressivity. Transient hypoparathyroidism may also be observed in infants born to mothers with the disease or in infants fed a milk formula with a high phosphate-to-calcium ratio.

Diagnostic Evaluation. The diagnosis of hypoparathyroidism is made on the basis of clinical manifestations associated with *decreased serum calcium* and *increased serum phosphorus levels* (Box 52-5). Levels of plasma PTH are low in idiopathic hypoparathyroidism but high in pseudohypoparathyroidism. End-organ responsiveness is tested by the administration of PTH with measurement of urinary cyclic adenosine monophosphate (cAMP). Kidney function tests are included in the differential diagnosis to rule out renal insufficiency. Although bone radiographs are usually normal, they may demonstrate increased bone density and suppressed growth.

Box 52-5

Clinical Manifestations of Hypoparathyroidism

PSEUDOHYPOPARATHYROIDISM

Short stature
Round face
Short, thick neck
Short, stubby fingers and toes
Dimpling of skin over knuckles
Subcutaneous soft tissue calcifications
Mental retardation a prominent feature

IDIOPATHIC HYPOPARATHYROIDISM

None of the above physical characteristics observed
Papilledema may be seen
May be mental retardation

BOTH TYPES

- Dry, scaly, coarse skin with eruptions
- Hair often brittle
- Nails thin and brittle with characteristic transverse grooves
- Dental and enamel hypoplasia
- Muscle contractions:
  - Tetany
  - Carpopedal spasm
  - Laryngospasm (laryngeal stridor)
  - Muscle cramps and twitching
  - Positive Chvostek and/or Trousseau signs (see Nurse Alert, p. 1478)
- Paresthesias, tingling
- Neurologic:
  - Headache
  - Seizures (generalized, absence, or focal)
  - Swings of emotion
  - Loss of memory
  - Depression
  - Confusion can occur
- Gastrointestinal:
  - Muscle cramps
  - Diarrhea
  - Vomiting

Therapeutic Management. The objective of treatment is to maintain normal serum calcium and phosphate levels with a minimum of complications. Acute or severe tetany is corrected immediately by IV and oral administration of calcium gluconate and follow-up daily doses to achieve normal levels. When the diagnosis is confirmed, *vitamin D therapy* is begun. Long-term management consists of administration of massive doses of vitamin D; oral calcium supplementation may be useful, although it is not essential.

Nursing Care Management. The initial objective is recognition of hypocalcemia. Unexplained seizures, irritability (especially to external stimuli), gastrointestinal symptoms (e.g., diarrhea, vomiting, and abdominal cramps), and signs of tetany should lead the nurse to suspect this disorder. Much of the initial nursing care is related to the physical manifestations and includes institution of seizure and safety precautions, reduction of environmental stimuli (e.g., sudden noises or movements and bright lights), and observation for signs of laryngospasm.

NURSE ALERT • The signs of laryngospasm are stridor, hoarseness, and a feeling of tightness in the throat. A tracheostomy set and injectable calcium gluconate should be placed near the bedside for emergency use. The IV administration of calcium gluconate requires precautions against extravasation of the drug and resulting tissue destruction.

After initiation of treatment, the nurse discusses with the parents the need for continuous daily administration of calcium salts and vitamin D. Because vitamin D toxicity can be a serious consequence of therapy, parents are advised to watch for signs, which include weakness, fatigue, lassitude, headache, nausea, vomiting, and diarrhea. Early renal impairment is manifested by polyuria, polydipsia, and nocturia.

Hyperparathyroidism

Hyperparathyroidism is rare in childhood but can be primary or secondary. The most common cause of primary hyperparathyroidism is adenoma of the gland. The most common causes of secondary hyperparathyroidism are chronic renal disease, renal osteodystrophy, and congenital anomalies of the urinary tract. The common factor is hypercalcemia. The manifestations of hyperparathyroidism are listed in Box 52-6.

Diagnostic Evaluation. Blood studies to confirm the presence of *elevated calcium* and *lowered phosphorus levels* are routinely performed. Measurement of PTH, as well as several tests to isolate the cause of the hypercalcemia, such as renal function studies, should be included. Other procedures employed to substantiate the physiologic consequences of the disorder include electrocardiography and radiographic bone surveys.

Therapeutic Management. Treatment depends on the cause. The treatment of primary hyperparathyroidism is surgical removal of the tumor or hyperplastic tissue. Treatment of secondary hyperparathyroidism is directed at the underlying contributing cause, thus subsequently restoring the serum calcium balance. However, in some instances the underlying disorder is irreversible, such as in chronic renal failure (see Chapter 50). In this instance treatment is the same as the treatment for renal osteodystrophy.

Nursing Care Management. Because surgical removal is the major treatment modality, nursing care is similar to that discussed for the child with hyperthyroidism (p. 1475). Because hypocalcemia is a potential complication, observation for signs of tetany, institution of seizure precautions, and having calcium gluconate available for emergency use are part of the nursing care.

Box 52-6

Clinical Manifestations of Hyperparathyroidism

GASTROINTESTINAL
Nausea
Vomiting
Abdominal discomfort
Constipation

CENTRAL NERVOUS SYSTEM
Delusions
Confusion
Hallucinations
Impaired memory
Lack of interest and initiative
Depression
Varying levels of consciousness

NEUROMUSCULAR
Weakness
Easy fatigability
Muscle atrophy (especially proximal muscles of lower limbs)
Tongue twitching
Paresthesias in extremities

SKELETAL
Vague bone pain
Subperiosteal resorption of phalanges
Spontaneous fractures
Absence of lamina dura around teeth

RENAL
Polyuria
Polydipsia
Renal colic
Hypertension

DISORDERS OF ADRENAL FUNCTION

The *adrenal cortex* secretes three main groups of hormones collectively called steroids and classified according to their biologic activity: (1) *glucocorticoids* (cortisol, corticosterone); (2) *mineralocorticoids* (aldosterone); and (3) sex steroids (androgens, estrogens, and progestins). Alterations in the levels of these hormones produce significant dysfunction in a variety of body tissues and organs. Because the adrenocortical cells are capable of producing any of the steroids, pathologic conditions may result in a deficiency or an excess of more than one type of hormone. However, these pathologic conditions are rare in children.

The *adrenal medulla* secretes the *catecholamines epinephrine* and *norepinephrine.* Both hormones have essentially the same effects on various organs as those caused by direct sympathetic stimulation, except that the hormonal effects last several times longer. Catecholamine-secreting tumors are the primary cause of adrenal medullary hyperfunction.

Acute Adrenocortical Insufficiency

The acute form of adrenocortical insufficiency *(adrenal crisis)* may result from a number of causes during childhood. Although a rare disorder, some of the more common etiologic factors include hemorrhage into the gland from trauma (which may be caused by a prolonged, difficult labor); fulminating infections such as meningococcemia, that result in hemorrhage and necrosis (Waterhouse-Friderichsen syndrome); abrupt withdrawal of exogenous sources of cortisone or failure to increase exogenous supplies during stress; and congenital adrenogenital hyperplasia of the salt-losing type.

Diagnostic Evaluation. There is no rapid, definitive test for confirmation of acute adrenocortical insufficiency. Routine procedures such as measurement of plasma cortisol levels are too time consuming to be practical. Therefore diagnosis is usually based on clinical symptoms (Box 52-7). Improvement with cortisol therapy confirms the diagnosis.

Therapeutic Management. Treatment involves replacement of cortisol, replacement of body fluids to correct dehydration and hypovolemia, administration of glucose solutions to correct hypoglycemia, and specific antibiotic therapy in the presence of infection. If hemorrhage has been severe, whole blood may be replaced. In the event that these measures do not reverse the circulatory collapse, vasopressors are used for immediate vasoconstriction and elevation of blood pressure. Once the child's condition is stabilized, oral doses of cortisone, fluids, and salt are given, similar to the regimen used for chronic adrenal insufficiency.

Nursing Care Management. Because of the abrupt onset and potentially fatal outcome of this condition, prompt recognition is essential. Vital signs and blood pressure are measured often to monitor the hyperpyrexia and shocklike state. Seizure precautions are instituted because seizures from the elevated temperature are not uncommon. As soon as therapy is instituted, the nurse monitors the child's response to fluid and cortisol replacement, being alert to signs of too rapid administration of fluids and drugs. Overtreatment with cortisol and sodium chloride can precipitate complications such as an ascending flaccid paralysis. The nurse should observe for signs of hypokalemia and should evaluate serum electrolyte levels. The condition is rapidly corrected with IV and oral potassium replacement. Intake and urine output are measured and recorded.

NURSE ALERT • Monitor serum electrolyte levels and observe for signs of hypokalemia or hyperkalemia, (e.g., weakness, poor muscle control, paralysis, cardiac dysrhythmias, and apnea).

The sudden, severe nature of this disorder requires considerable emotional support for the child and family. The child is usually in an intensive care unit, where the surroundings are strange and frightening. Because recovery within 24 hours is often dramatic, the nurse should keep the parents apprised of the child's condition, emphasizing signs of improvement such as a lowered temperature and elevated blood pressure. If paralysis occurs, the nurse should assure them that this condition is temporary and quickly reversed.

Box 52-7

Clinical Manifestations of Acute Adrenocortical Insufficiency

EARLY SYMPTOMS
- Increased irritability
- Headache
- Diffuse abdominal pain
- Weakness
- Nausea and vomiting
- Diarrhea

GENERALIZED HEMORRHAGIC MANIFESTATIONS (WATERHOUSE-FRIDERICHSEN SYNDROME)
- Fever—increases as condition worsens
- Central nervous system signs
  - Nuchal rigidity
  - Seizures
  - Stupor
  - Coma

SHOCKLIKE STATE
- Weak, rapid pulse
- Decreased blood pressure
- Shallow respirations
- Cold, clammy skin
- Cyanosis
- Circulatory collapse (terminal event)

NEWBORN
- Hyperpyrexia
- Tachypnea
- Cyanosis
- Seizures
- Gland may be evident as palpable retroperitoneal mass (hemorrhagic)

Chronic Adrenocortical Insufficiency (Addison Disease)

Chronic adrenocortical insufficiency is rare in children. When it does occur, it is usually caused by a destructive lesion of the adrenal glands, by a neoplasm, or it has an idiopathic cause.

Evidence of this disorder is usually gradual in onset because 90% of adrenal tissue must be nonfunctional before signs of insufficiency are manifested (Box 52-8). However, during periods of stress, when demands for additional cortisol are increased, symptoms of acute insufficiency may appear in a previously well child.

Definitive diagnosis is based on measurements of functional cortisol reserve. The cortisol and urinary 17-hydroxycorticosteroid levels are low and fail to rise, whereas plasma adrenocorticotropic hormone (ACTH) levels are elevated with corticotropin stimulation, the definitive test for the disease.

Therapeutic Management. Treatment involves replacement of *glucocorticoids (cortisol)* and *mineralocorticoids (aldosterone).* Some children are able to be maintained solely on oral supplements of cortisol (cortisone or hydrocortisone preparations) with a liberal intake of salt. Other forms of therapy include monthly injections of desoxycorticosterone acetate or subcutaneous implantation of desoxycorticosterone acetate pellets every 9 to 12 months. During stressful situations such as infection, emotional upset, or surgery, the dosage must be tripled to accommodate the body's increased need for glucocorticoids. Failure to meet this requirement will precipitate an acute crisis. Overdosage produces Cushingoid signs (Fig. 52-2).

Nursing Care Management. Once the disorder is diagnosed, parents need guidance concerning drug therapy. They must be aware of the continuous need for cortisol replacement. Sudden termination of the drug because of inadequate supplies, or inability to ingest the oral form because of vomiting, places the child in danger of an acute adrenal crisis. Ideally, the parents should have a prefilled syringe of hydrocortisone in the home and should be taught the proper technique for intramuscular administration of the drug in case of a crisis.* Unnecessary administration of cortisone will not harm the child but, if needed, may be lifesaving. Any evidence of acute insufficiency is reported immediately to the practitioner.

Because the body cannot supply endogenous sources of cortical hormones during times of stress, the home environment should be stable and relatively unstressful. Parents need to be aware that during periods of emotional or physical crisis the child requires additional hormone replacement. The child should wear medical identification to permit medical personnel to adjust the requirements during emergency care.

*Community and home care instructions on giving intramuscular injections are available in Wong DL, Hess CS: ***Wong and Whaley's clinical manual of pediatric nursing,*** ed 5, St Louis, 2000, Mosby.

Box 52-8

Clinical Manifestations of Chronic Adrenocortical Insufficiency

NEUROLOGIC SYMPTOMS
Muscular weakness
Mental fatigue
Irritability, apathy, and negativism
Increased sleeping, listlessness

PIGMENTARY CHANGES
Previous scars
Palmar creases
Mucous membranes
Hair
Hyperpigmentation over pressure points (elbows, knees, or waist)
Less frequently, vitiligo (loss of pigmentation)

GASTROINTESTINAL SYMPTOMS
Dehydration
Anorexia
Weight loss

CIRCULATORY SYMPTOMS
Hypotension
Small heart size
Dizziness
Syncopal (fainting) attacks

HYPOGLYCEMIA
Headache
Hunger
Weakness
Trembling
Sweating

OTHER SIGNS (SEEN IN SOME CHILDREN)
Recurrent, unexplained seizures
Intense craving for salt
Acute abdominal pain
Electrolyte imbalances

Cushing Syndrome

Cushing syndrome is a characteristic group of manifestations caused by excessive circulating free cortisol. It can result from a variety of etiologies that generally fall into five categories (Box 52-9).

Box 52-9

Etiology of Cushing Syndrome

Pituitary—Cushing syndrome with adrenal hyperplasia, usually attributed to an excess of adrenocorticotropin hormone (ACTH)
Adrenal—Cushing syndrome with hypersecretion of glucocorticoids, generally a result of adrenocortical neoplasms
Ectopic—Cushing syndrome with autonomous secretion of ACTH, most often caused by extrapituitary neoplasms
Iatrogenic—Cushing syndrome, frequently a result of administration of large amounts of exogenous corticosteroids
Food dependent—Inappropriate sensitivity of adrenal glands to normal postprandial increases in secretion of gastric inhibitory polypeptide (Magiakou et al, 1994)

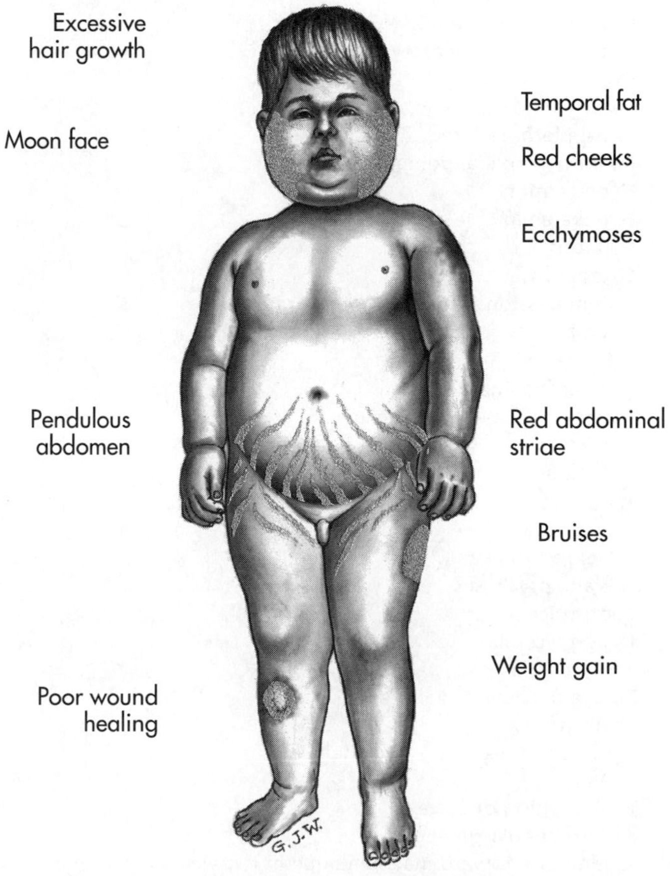

FIG. 52-2 • Characteristics of Cushing syndrome.

Cushing syndrome is uncommon in children. When seen, it is often caused by excessive or prolonged steroid therapy, which produces a Cushingoid appearance (Box 52-10; see also Fig. 52-2). This condition is reversible once steroids are discontinued. Abrupt withdrawal may precipitate acute adrenal insufficiency; gradual withdrawal of exogenous supplies is necessary to allow the anterior pituitary an opportunity to secrete increasing amounts of ACTH to stimulate the adrenals to produce cortisol.

Diagnostic Evaluation. Several tests are helpful in confirming excess cortisol levels. These include fasting blood glucose levels for hyperglycemia, serum electrolyte levels for hypokalemia and alkalosis, 24-hour urinary levels of elevated 17-hydroxycorticoids and 17-ketosteroids, and radiographic studies of bone for evidence of osteoporosis and of the skull for enlargement of the sella turcica. Administration of an exogenous supply of cortisone normally suppresses ACTH production; however, in individuals with Cushing syndrome, cortisol levels remain elevated. This test is helpful in differentiating between children who are obese and those who appear to have Cushingoid features.

Box 52-10
Clinical Manifestations of Cushing Syndrome

- Centripetal fat distribution
  - Truncal obesity
  - Supraclavicular fat pads
  - Fat pads on neck and back ("buffalo hump")
- Rounded or "moon" face
- Muscular wasting
  - Thin extremities
  - Pendulous abdomen
  - Muscle weakness
- Thin skin and subcutaneous tissue
- Poor wound healing
- Increased susceptibility to infection
- Decreased inflammatory response
- Excessive bruising
- Petechial hemorrhages
- Facial plethora ("red cheeks")
- Reddish purple abdominal striae
- Hypertension
- Hypokalemia
- Alkalosis
- Osteoporosis
  - Compression fractures of vertebrae
  - Kyphosis
  - Backache
  - Retarded linear growth
- Hypercalciuria—renal calculi
- Psychoses
  - Irritability
  - Insomnia
  - Euphoria
  - Depression
  - Frank psychoses
- Peptic ulcer
- Hyperglycemia
  - Glycosuria
  - Latent or overt diabetes
- Virilization
  - Hirsutism (excessive body hair)
  - Acne
  - Deepening of voice
  - Clitoral enlargement
  - Tendency toward male physique in female
- Amenorrhea
- Impotence

Therapeutic Management. Treatment depends on the cause. In most cases surgical intervention involves bilateral adrenalectomy and postoperative replacement of the cortical hormones (the therapy for this is the same as that outlined for chronic adrenal insufficiency). If a pituitary tumor is found, surgical extirpation or irradiation may be chosen. In either of these instances treatment of panhypopituitarism with replacement of growth hormone, thyroid extract, antidiuretic hormone, gonadotropins, and steroids may be necessary for an indefinite period.

Nursing Care Management. Nursing care also depends on the cause. When cushingoid features are caused by steroid therapy, the effects may be lessened with administration of the drug early in the morning and on an alternate-day basis. Giving the drug early in the day maintains the normal diurnal pattern of cortisol secretion. If given during the evening, the drug is more likely to produce symptoms because endogenous cortisol levels are already low and the additional supply exerts more pronounced effects. An alternate-day schedule allows the anterior pituitary an opportunity to maintain more normal hypothalamic-pituitary-adrenal control mechanisms.

If an organic cause is found, nursing care is related to the treatment regimen. Although a bilateral adrenalectomy permanently solves one condition, it also produces another syndrome. Before surgery, parents need to be adequately informed of the operative benefits and disadvantages. Postoperative teaching regarding drug replacement is a nursing function.

NURSE ALERT • Postoperative complications of adrenalectomy are related to the sudden withdrawal of cortisol. Observe for signs of a shocklike state, especially hypotension and hyperpyrexia.

Congenital Adrenal Hyperplasia (CAH)

Disorders caused by excessive secretion of androgens by the adrenal cortex are known as a family of inherited disorders causing dysfunction in the production of steroids. Although hyperfunction of the adrenal gland can occur from a number of causes, such as a virilizing adrenal tumor, in children the most common cause is congenital adrenogenital hyperplasia, an inborn deficiency of various enzymes necessary for the biosynthesis of cortisol. CAH is inherited as an autosomal-recessive disorder or may result from a tumor or from maternal ingestion of steroids.

Pathophysiology. Interference in the biosynthesis of cortisol during fetal life results in an increased production of ACTH, which stimulates hyperplasia of the adrenal gland. Depending on the enzymatic defect, increased quantities of cortisol precursors and androgens are secreted. There are six major types of biochemical defects; in each there is excess production of androgens, which causes ambiguous genitalia in females and precocious genital development in males. In both sexes, linear growth is accelerated and epiphyseal closure is premature, ultimately resulting in short stature. Other forms of CAH do not result in excess production of androgens but cause various degrees of hypoaldosteronism or hyperaldosteronism.

The most common biochemical defect is partial or complete *21-hydroxylase deficiency.* With partial deficiency, enough aldosterone is produced to preserve sodium, and adequate cortisol is produced to prevent signs of adrenocortical insufficiency. In the complete or salt-losing form, insufficient amounts of aldosterone and cortisol are produced so that circulatory collapse occurs without immediate replacement of the mineralocorticoids and glucocorticoids.

Diagnostic Evaluation. Clinical diagnosis is initially based on congenital abnormalities that lead to difficulty in assigning sex to the newborn (Box 52-11) and on signs and symptoms of adrenal insufficiency or hypertension. Definitive diagnosis is confirmed by evidence of increased 17-ketosteroid levels in most types of CAH. Blood electrolytes demonstrate loss of sodium and chloride and elevation of potassium. A karyotype for positive sex determination should always be done in any case of ambiguous genitalia.

Ultrasonography can also be used to visualize the presence of pelvic structures. It is especially useful in CAH to identify the absence or presence of female reproductive organs in a newborn or child with ambiguous genitalia. Because it yields immediate results, it has the advantage of determining the child's gender long before the more complex laboratory results for chromosome analysis or steroid levels are available.

Therapeutic Management. The initial medical objective is to confirm the diagnosis and assign a sex to the child, usually according to the genotype. In both sexes cortisone is administered to suppress the abnormally high secretions of ACTH. Cortisone depresses the secretion of ACTH by the adenohypophysis; this in turn inhibits the secretion of adrenocorticosteroids, which stems the progressive virilization. If cortisol is given early enough, the signs and symptoms of masculinization in the female gradually disappear, and excessive early linear growth is slowed. Puberty occurs normally at the appropriate age.

Because these children are unable to produce cortisol in response to stress, the dosage is increased during episodes of infection, fever, or other stresses. Acute emergencies require immediate IV or intramuscular administration. Children with the salt-losing type of CAH require aldosterone replacement and supplementary dietary salt.

Depending on the degree of masculinization in the female, reconstructive surgery may be required to reduce the size of the clitoris, separate the labia, and create a vaginal orifice. This should be done after the infant is physically able to tolerate the procedure and before she is old enough to be aware of the abnormal genitalia. Plastic surgery is generally done in stages and yields excellent cosmetic results. The capacity for orgasm and sexual gratification is not necessarily impaired.

Unfortunately, not all children with CAH are diagnosed at birth and raised in accordance with their genetic sex. Particularly in the case of affected females, masculinization of the external genitalia may have led to sex assignment as a male. In these situations it is advisable to continue rearing the child as a male in accordance with the assigned sex and phenotype. Hormone replacement may be required to permit linear growth and to initiate male pubertal changes. Surgery is usually indicated to remove the female organs and reconstruct the phallus for satisfactory sexual relations. These individuals are not fertile. Diagnosis in males is usually delayed until early childhood, when signs of virilism appear.

Nursing Care Management. The nursing care of the child with CAH and the family is concerned primarily with identifying the condition and providing support and assistance. Of major importance is recognition of ambiguous genitalia in newborns. If there is any question regarding assignment of sex, the parents need to be told immediately in order to prevent the embarrassing situation of informing family members of the child's sex and then having to change the announcement. As with any congenital defect, the parents require an adequate explanation of the condition and some time to grieve for the loss of perfection. Parents need an explanation regarding this disorder that facilitates their explaining it to others. The external genitalia are referred to as sex organs, and the similarity between the penis/clitoris and scrotum/labia during fetal development is emphasized to help parents understand that too much male hormone secretion caused some organs to overdevelop. Using a correct vocabulary allows parents to explain the abnormalities to others in a straightforward manner, just as they would if the defect involved the heart or an extremity. As soon as the sex is determined, parents are informed of the findings and encouraged to choose an appropriate name. The child is identified as a male or female, with no reference to ambiguous sex. If the appearance of the enlarged genitalia in a female child concerns the parents, they are encouraged to discuss their feelings.

Nursing considerations regarding cortisol and aldosterone replacement are the same as those for chronic adrenocortical insufficiency. A follow-up visit by a home health nurse may be desirable to ensure that parents understand and comply with the treatment regimen. Likewise, nurses in well-child facilities

Box 52-11

Clinical Manifestations of Adrenogenital Hyperplasia

Female: Masculinization
- Enlarged clitoris (appears as small phallus)
- Fusion of labia (saclike structure resembling a scrotum)
- Vaginal orifice usually closed by fused labia

Male: Precocious genital development
- Genital enlargement (macrogenitosomia precox)
- Frequent erections

Untreated: Early sexual maturation
- Enlargement of external sexual organs
- Development of axillary, pubic, and facial hair
- Deepening of voice
- Acne
- Marked increase in musculature (changes toward an adult male physique)
- Accelerated linear growth
- Premature epiphyseal closure (short stature by end of puberty)

Female:
- No breast development
- Females remain amenorrheic and infertile

Male:
- Testes remain small

should assume responsibility for guidance and supervision regarding this aspect of care during each visit.

Because these infants are especially prone to dehydration and salt-losing crises, parents need to be aware of the signs of dehydration and the urgency of immediate medical intervention to stabilize the child's condition. Parents, and later the child, need to understand that the medical regimen must be a lifelong commitment; therefore they should be provided with the education and counseling that is most likely to ensure informed and willing compliance. They also need to know that growth retardation that may have occurred before therapy cannot be overcome and that normal stature is not a realistic expectation, even though growth velocity may improve with medication. The parents are also taught to give necessary injections (see Chapter 45).*

NURSE ALERT • The parents should be advised that there is no physical harm in treating for suspected adrenal insufficiency that is not present, whereas the consequence of not treating acute adrenal insufficiency can be fatal (Ruble, 1996).

In the unfortunate situation in which the sex is erroneously assigned and the correct sex determined later, parents need a great deal of help in understanding the reason for the incorrect sex identification and the options for sex reassignment and/or medical/surgical intervention. Because children become aware of their sexual identity by 18 months to 2 years of age, it is believed that any reassignment after this period can cause tremendous psychologic conflicts in the child. Therefore sex rearing should be continued as previously established with medical/surgical intervention as required.

Because the hereditary form of adrenogenital hyperplasia is an autosomal-recessive disorder, parents should be referred for genetic counseling before conceiving another child. Affected offspring also require genetic counseling because both sexes are generally able to reproduce. (See genetic counseling in Appendix C.)

Hyperaldosteronism

Excessive secretion of aldosterone may be caused by an adrenal tumor; also, in some types of adrenogenital syndromes, symptoms are caused by increased sodium levels, water retention, and potassium loss. The clinical diagnosis is suspected when there are findings of hypertension, hypokalemia, and polyuria that fail to respond to antidiuretic hormone administration.

Therapeutic Management. Temporary treatment of the disorder involves replacement of potassium and administration of spironolactone (Aldactone), a diuretic that blocks the effects of aldosterone. Definitive treatment is similar to that for chronic adrenocortical insufficiency.

Nursing Care Management. An important nursing consideration is recognition of the syndrome, particularly in children who demonstrate high blood pressure. After the diagnosis, nursing care is related to the treatment regimen, such as education about the diuretic and potassium supplements (see Nurse Alert, p. 1478). Parents need to be aware of the signs of hypokalemia and hyperkalemia (see Nurse Alert, p. 1478).

*Community and home care instructions for giving injections are available in Wong DL, Hess CS: ***Wong and Whaley's clinical manual of pediatric nursing,*** ed 5, St Louis, 2000, Mosby.

Pheochromocytoma

Pheochromocytoma is an adrenal tumor characterized by secretion of catecholamines. The tumor most commonly arises from the chromaffin cells of the adrenal medulla but may occur wherever these cells are found, such as along the paraganglia of the aorta or thoracolumbar sympathetic chain. In children this type of tumor is most commonly bilateral or multiple and is generally benign. Often there is a familial transmission of the condition as an autosomal-dominant trait that tends to favor males. The clinical manifestations of pheochromocytoma are caused by an increased production of catecholamines, and they mimic those of other disorders, such as hyperthyroidism, diabetes mellitus, or functional hyperventilation (Box 52-12).

Therapeutic Management. Definitive treatment consists of surgical removal of the tumor. In children the tumors may be bilateral, requiring a bilateral adrenalectomy and lifelong glucocorticoid and mineralocorticoid therapy.

Nursing Care Management. An initial nursing objective is identification of children with this disorder. Outstanding clues are hypertension and hypertensive attacks. Preoperative nursing care involves frequent monitoring of vital signs and observing for evidence of hypertensive attacks and congestive heart failure. Urine should be tested at least daily for glucose and ketones. Any signs of hyperglycemia are noted and reported immediately.

NURSE ALERT • DO NOT PALPATE MASS. Preoperative palpation may facilitate release of catecholamines, which can stimulate severe hypertension and tachyarrhythmias.

The environment should be conducive to rest and free of emotional stress. This requires adequate preparation during hospital admission and before surgery. Parents are encouraged to room-in with their child and to participate in the care. Play activities need to be tailored to the child's energy level, but should not be overly strenuous or challenging because these can increase the metabolic rate and promote frustration and anxiety.

After surgery the child is observed for signs of shock from removal of excess catecholamines. If a bilateral adrenalectomy was performed, the nursing interventions are the same as those discussed for chronic adrenocortical insufficiency.

Box 52-12
Clinical Manifestations of Pheochromocytoma

- Hypertension
- Tachycardia
- Headache
- Decreased gastrointestinal activity; resultant constipation
- Anorexia
- Weight loss
- Hyperglycemia
- Polyuria
- Polydipsia
- Hyperventilation
- Nervousness
- Heat intolerance
- Diaphoresis
- Signs of congestive heart failure in severe cases

DISORDERS OF PANCREATIC HORMONE FUNCTION

The islets of Langerhans of the pancreas have three major functioning cells:

1. The *alpha cells* produce *glucagon,* which increases the blood glucose levels by stimulating the liver and other cells to release stored glucose (glycogenolysis).
2. The *beta cells* produce *insulin,* which lowers blood glucose levels by facilitating the entrance of glucose into the cells for metabolism.
3. The *delta cells* produce *somatostatin,* which is believed to regulate the release of insulin and glucagon.

The discussion of disorders of pancreatic hormone secretion is limited to diabetes mellitus.

Diabetes Mellitus (DM)

DM is a disease of metabolism characterized by a total or partial deficiency of the hormone *insulin,* resulting in a metabolic adjustment or physiologic change in almost all areas of the body. It is the most common endocrine disorder of childhood, with the peak incidence reached during early adolescence.

The classification of DM was changed in 1997 to avoid confusion regarding treatment, cause, and nomenclature (American Diabetes Association, 1998). DM can be classified into three major groups:

1. Type 1 diabetes is characterized by destruction of pancreatic beta cells, which produce insulin, usually leading to absolute insulin deficiency. Onset is typically in childhood and adolescence but can be at any age.
2. Type 2 diabetes usually arises because of insulin resistance, in which the body fails to use insulin properly, combined with a relative insulin deficiency. Onset is usually after age 40, and there appears to be considerable heterogeneity; affected persons may or may not require daily insulin injections.
3. Maturity onset diabetes of the young (MODY) is transmitted as an autosomal-dominant disorder in which there is formation of structurally abnormal insulin that has decreased biologic activity. Onset is generally before age 25 years.

Because DM of childhood is, with few exceptions, the type 1 form, the remainder of this discussion is devoted to this important cause of long-term health problems. However, type 2 diabetes is included as is appropriate for comparison throughout. Also, Native American, Hispanic, and African-American children are at increased risk for type 2 diabetes (American Diabetes Association, 1998).

Etiology. The clinical syndrome of DM results from a large variety of etiologic and pathogenic mechanisms. Type 1 DM is now believed to be an autoimmune disease that arises when a person with a genetic predisposition is exposed to a precipitating event, such as a viral infection.

Genetic Factors. Type 1 DM is not inherited, but heredity is a prominent factor in the etiology. A variety of genetic mechanisms have been proposed, but most authorities favor a multifactorial inheritance or a recessive gene somehow linked to the human lymphocyte antigen (HLA). However, the genetic influences in type 1 DM and type 2 DM appear to differ in several ways. Studies of type 2 DM in identical twins demonstrate a 100% concordance throughout the lifespan, whereas studies of type 1 DM in identical twins demonstrate a 30% to 50% concordance rate. The lower rate suggests that environmental and genetic factors are important in the genesis of type 1 DM (Stoffer et al, 1997; Winters, Chihara, and Schatz, 1993).

Autoimmune Mechanisms. An autoimmune process is involved in persons who develop type 1 DM. The current theory is that the presence of the HLA genes causes a defect in the immune system that renders the possessor susceptible to a trigger event, which can be a dietary source (Atkinson and Ellis, 1997), virus, bacterium, or a chemical irritant. The predisposing event initiates an autoimmune process that gradually destroys beta cells. Without beta cells no insulin can be produced. There is also a strong association between type 1 DM and other autoimmune endocrine disorders such as thyroiditis and Addison disease.

Pathophysiology. Insulin is needed to support the metabolism of carbohydrates, fats, and proteins; this is done primarily by facilitating the entry of these substances into the cell, with the exception of nerve cells and vascular tissue. With a deficiency of insulin, glucose is unable to enter the cell, and its concentration in the bloodstream increases *(hyperglycemia).* The increased concentration of glucose produces an osmotic gradient that causes the movement of body fluid from the intracellular space to the extracellular space; from there the body fluid is excreted by the kidneys. When the serum glucose level exceeds the renal threshold (±180 mg/dl), glucose "spills" into the urine *(glycosuria)* along with an osmotic diversion of water *(polyuria),* a cardinal sign of diabetes. The urinary fluid losses cause the excessive thirst *(polydipsia)* observed in diabetes. As might be expected, this water washout results in a depletion of other essential chemicals.

Protein is also wasted during insulin deficiency. Because glucose is unable to enter the cells, protein is broken down and converted to glucose by the liver *(glucogenesis);* this glucose then contributes to the hyperglycemia. Without the use of carbohydrates for energy, fat and protein stores are depleted as the body attempts to meet its energy needs. The hunger mechanism is triggered, but the increased food intake *(polyphagia)* enhances the problem by further elevating the blood glucose.

Ketoacidosis. When insulin is absent, glucose is unavailable for cellular metabolism and the body chooses alternate sources of energy, principally fat. Consequently fats break down into fatty acids, and glycerol in the fat cells and liver is converted to ketone bodies (β-hydroxybutyric acid, acetoacetic acid, and acetone). The ketone bodies can be used as an alternative source of fuel for glucose, but they are used in the cells at a limited rate. Any excess is eliminated in the urine *(ketonuria)* or the lungs (acetone breath). The ketone bodies in the blood *(ketonemia)* are strong acids that lower serum pH, producing *ketoacidosis.* The respiratory system attempts to eliminate the excess carbon dioxide by increased depth and rate (*Kussmaul respirations,* the hyperventilation characteristic of metabolic acidosis).

With cellular death, potassium is released from the cell into the interstitial spaces and then into the bloodstream. It is then excreted by the kidney, where the loss is accelerated by osmotic diuresis. The total-body potassium is then decreased even though the serum potassium level may be elevated as a result of the decreased fluid volume in which it circulates. Alteration in serum and tissue potassium can make cardiac arrest a potential problem.

If these conditions are not reversed by insulin therapy in combination with correction of the fluid deficiency and electrolyte imbalance, progressive deterioration occurs, with dehydration, electrolyte imbalance, acidosis, coma, and death. *Diabetic ketoacidosis (DKA)* is a pediatric emergency and should be diagnosed promptly, with therapy instituted.

Long-term Complications. Long-term complications of diabetes involve the small, as well as larger, blood vessels. The principal microvascular complications are *nephropathy* and *retinopathy.* The process appears to be one of *glycosylation,* wherein proteins from the blood become deposited in the basement membrane of small vessels (e.g., glomeruli, retina), where they become trapped by "sticky" glucose compounds (glycosyl radicals). The buildup of these substances over time causes narrowing of the vessels with subsequent interference with microcirculation to the affected areas. With poor control, vascular changes appear as early as $2\frac{1}{2}$ to 3 years after diagnosis; with good control, changes have been postponed for 20 or more years.

Neuropathy appears to be an identical process, but glycosylation occurs on the sheath of nerves, interrupting neurotransmission of stimuli. Macrovascular disease may develop after 25 years of diabetes and creates the predominant complications in patients with type 2 DM. Intensive insulin therapy appears to delay the onset and slow the progression of clinically important retinopathy (including vision loss), nephropathy, and neuropathy from 35% to more than 70% (Wunderlich et al, 1998).

Maturity-Onset Diabetes of the Young (MODY). Although most childhood diabetes is recognized during the rapid initial deterioration in carbohydrate metabolism, other cases with more benign disease are being identified with increasing frequency. A few are detected accidentally by urinalysis before overt symptoms are observed. MODY is sometimes seen in an obese teenager. It is similar to type 2 DM and can often be controlled with dietary modifications and oral hypoglycemic agents if needed.

NURSE ALERT • Recurrent urinary tract and vaginal infections, especially with *Candida albicans,* are often an early sign of type 1 DM, especially in adolescents.

Diagnostic Evaluation. Three groups of children who should be considered at risk for diabetes are (1) those who have glycosuria, polyuria, and a history of weight loss or failure to gain despite a hearty appetite; (2) those with transient or persistent glycosuria; and (3) those who display manifestations of metabolic acidosis, with or without stupor or coma. Clinical manifestations of type 1 DM are outlined in Box 52-13. Diabetes is a great imitator; influenza, gastroenteritis, and appendicitis are the conditions most often mistaken for it.

Diagnosis is based on *serum glucose levels.* A fasting serum glucose level of >126 mg/dl or a random blood glucose level of ≥200 mg/dl accompanied by classic signs of type 1 DM is almost certain to indicate diabetes (American Diabetes Association, 1998). Postprandial blood glucose determinations and the traditional oral glucose tolerance tests are not usually necessary for establishing a diagnosis. Serum insulin levels may be normal or moderately elevated at the onset of diabetes; delayed insulin response to glucose indicates the presence of impaired glucose tolerance.

Ketoacidosis must be differentiated from other causes of acidosis or coma, including hypoglycemia, uremia, gastroenteritis with metabolic acidosis, salicylate intoxication, encephalitis, and other intracranial lesions. DKA is determined by the presence of hyperglycemia (blood glucose measurement of ≥250 mg/dl), ketonemia (strongly positive), acidosis (pH of <7.20 and bicarbonate of <15 mEq/L), glycosuria, and ketonuria (American Diabetes Association, 1998). Tests used to determine ketonuria are urine test strips such as Ketostex.

Box 52-13

Clinical Manifestations of Type 1 Diabetes Mellitus

- Polyphagia
- Polyuria
- Polydipsia
- Weight loss
- Enuresis or nocturia
- Irritability and "not himself" or "herself"
- Shortened attention span
- Lowered frustration tolerance
- Fatigue
- Dry skin
- Blurred vision
- Poor wound healing
- Flushed skin
- Headache
- Frequent infections
- Hyperglycemia:
  - Elevated blood glucose levels
  - Glucosuria
  - Diabetic ketosis:
    - Ketones, as well as glucose, in urine
    - Dehydration may or may not be present
  - Diabetic ketoacidosis:
    - Dehydration
    - Electrolyte imbalance
    - Acidosis
    - Deep, rapid breathing (Kussmaul)

Therapeutic Management. The management of the child with type 1 DM consists of a multidisciplinary approach involving the family; the child (when appropriate); and professionals, including a pediatric endocrinologist, diabetes nurse educator, and nutritionist, as well as an exercise physiologist. Often psychologic support from a mental health professional is also needed. Communication among the team members is essential and extends to other individuals in the child's life such as teachers, the school nurse, school guidance counselor, and coach.

The definitive treatment is replacement of insulin; however, insulin needs are affected by nutritional intake, activity, emotions, and other life events such as illnesses and puberty. Medical and nutritional guidance are primary, but management also includes continuing diabetes education, family guidance, and emotional support.

Insulin Therapy. Insulin is available in highly purified pork preparations and in human insulin manufactured by biosynthesis. Most clinicians suggest human insulin as the treatment of choice. It is available in rapid-, short-, intermediate-, and long-acting preparations, and all are packaged in the strength of 100 units/ml. (Other dosages are available for situations where extraordinarily large or small dosages are required.)

The precise dose of insulin needed cannot be predicted; therefore a regimen of total dosage and the percentage of rapid- or short- to intermediate-acting insulin is determined for each child. The amount of insulin is based on capillary blood glucose levels, which the child or family member tests by means of a drop of blood on a chemically treated test strip with the aid of a color chart or a glucose monitor.

Daily insulin is administered subcutaneously by twice-daily injections, by multiple-dose injections, or by means of a portable pump. Diabetes can be controlled satisfactorily in most children with a *twice-daily insulin* regimen consisting of a combination of *rapid-acting (lispro)* or *short-acting (regular)* and *intermediate-acting (NPH* or *Lente)* insulin given in the same syringe before breakfast and before the evening meal. The amount of insulin is determined by measurements of the blood glucose level after the peak effect of the insulin has occurred. For example, the amount of regular insulin at breakfast is determined by a pattern of the previous lunchtime blood glucose values. Regular insulin is best given at least 30 minutes before meals to allow sufficient time for absorption. On the other hand, lispro insulin is best given no more than 10 to 15 minutes before the meal. Some children require more frequent administration of insulin. This includes children with difficult-to-control diabetes and children during the adolescent growth spurt. An intensive insulin management program has been shown to reduce microvascular complications in young, healthy patients who have type 1 DM (Diabetes Control and Complications Trial Research Group, 1993).

The *insulin pump* is designed to deliver fixed amounts of regular or lispro insulin continuously, thereby more closely imitating the release of the hormone by the islet cells. The system consists of a syringe to hold the insulin, a plunger, and a computerized mechanism to drive the plunger. The insulin flows from the syringe through a catheter to a needle inserted into subcutaneous tissue (the abdomen or thigh), and the lightweight device is worn on a belt or a shoulder holster. The tubing and catheter are changed every 48 hours by the child or parent, using aseptic technique, and taped in place.

Although the pump provides more even insulin release, it has disadvantages. It should not be removed for more than 1 to 2 hours, which may limit some activities such as bathing and swimming, although some water-safe models are now available. Skin infections are common; and, like any other mechanical device, it is subject to malfunction. However, the pumps are equipped with alarms that signal problems that may arise such as depleted batteries, an occluded needle or tubing, or a microprocessor malfunction.

Researchers are experimenting with *intranasal* and *inhaled insulin administration.* Given nasally or deep into the lungs, the insulin is able to cross the mucosa to increase serum levels. The duration of action is not long enough to be a total replacement for injections but may be of value as insulin supplementation at mealtime.

Islet cell or *whole pancreas transplantation* may offer hope to patients in the future. Viable insulin-producing cells have been injected into the portal vein, where they take root in the liver and eventually produce up to two thirds of the needed insulin. The major use of transplants has been in persons who have serious complications, particularly those whose deteriorating kidneys have required renal transplants and who are receiving immunosuppression therapy. However, islet cell and pancreatic transplants tend not to be sustainable over time despite continuation of therapy. The use of nonhuman islets encapsulated in immunoprotective, semipermeable membranes may have a future in the treatment of type 1 DM (Lanza et al, 1999).

Monitoring. *Self-blood glucose monitoring (SBGM)* has improved diabetes management and is used successfully by children from the onset of their diabetes. By testing their own blood, children and parents are able to change their insulin regimen to maintain their glucose level in the euglycemic (normal) range of 80 to 120 mg/dl. Diabetes management depends to a great extent on SBGM.

Laboratory measurement of *glycosylated hemoglobin (hemoglobin A_{1c})* levels reflects the average blood glucose levels during the previous 2 to 3 months and is of value in assessing glucose control in any person with diabetes. As red blood cells circulate in the bloodstream, glucose molecules gradually attach to the hemoglobin A molecules and remain there for the lifetime of the red blood cell, approximately 120 days. Nondiabetic hemoglobin A_{1c} values are generally between 4% and 6% but can vary by laboratory. Acceptable diabetes control for children is typically a hemoglobin A_{1c} value $<7.5\%$.

Urine testing for glucose is no longer used for diabetes management; there is poor correlation between simultaneous glycosuria and blood glucose concentrations. However, urine testing can be carried out to detect evidence of ketonuria.

NURSE ALERT • It is recommended that urine be tested for ketones every 3 hours during an illness and whenever the blood glucose level is $\geq$240 mg/dl when illness is not present.

Nutrition. The nutritional needs of children with diabetes essentially are no different from those of unaffected children. Children with diabetes require no special foods or supplements. They need sufficient calories to balance daily expenditure for energy and to satisfy the requirement for growth and development. They also need consistent intake and timing of food, especially carbohydrates.

Normally insulin is secreted in response to food intake; however, insulin injected subcutaneously has a relatively predictable time of onset, peak effect, duration of action, and absorption rate, depending on the type of insulin used. Consequently, the timing of food consumption is regulated to correspond to the time and action of the insulin prescribed. Meals and snacks must be eaten at the same times each day, and the total number of calories and proportions of basic nutrients must be consistent from day to day. The distribution of calories, especially carbohydrates, is determined to fit the activity pattern of each child. Alterations in food intake are made so that food, insulin, and exercise are balanced. Extra food is needed for extra activity.

The food intake is based on a balanced diet that incorporates six basic food groups: milk, meat, vegetables, fat, fruit, and bread. The family may follow the exchange system approved by the American Diabetes Association, the carbohydrate counting system, or the point system (based on 75 kcal equaling 1 point). The exchange system indicates the amount (portion size) of each food by volume or weight and is prescribed in terms of the number of exchanges from each food group that constitutes each meal and snack. This ensures day-to-day consistency in total calories, protein, fat, and carbohydrate while allowing a choice from a variety of foods. Fiber is important in dietary planning because of its influence on digestion, absorption, and metabolism of many nutrients; it diminishes the rise in the blood glucose level after meals.

Exercise. Because it lowers blood glucose levels, exercise is encouraged and never restricted unless indicated by other health conditions. It is included as part of diabetes management and is planned around the child's interests and capabilities. However, in most instances children's activities are unplanned, and the resulting decrease in the blood glucose level can be compensated for by providing extra snacks before (and, if prolonged, during) the activity. Besides providing a feeling of well-being, regular exercise aids in the body's use of food and often decreases insulin requirements.

Hypoglycemia. Even a child with well-controlled diabetes may often experience mild symptoms of hypoglycemia; but if the signs and symptoms are recognized early (see Table 52-2) and relieved promptly by appropriate therapy, the child's activity should not be interrupted for more than a few minutes.

NURSE ALERT • Hypoglycemic episodes most commonly occur before meals, or when the insulin effect is peaking.

The most common causes of hypoglycemia, or *insulin reaction,* are bursts of physical activity without additional food; or delayed, omitted, or incompletely consumed meals or snacks. Reglycosalation of muscles and replenishment of liver glycogen may occur over the ensuing 24 hours. Therefore particular vigilance related to hypoglycemia may be necessary during the night after vigorous exertion.

In the majority of cases simple concentrated sugar, such as honey, that can be held in the mouth for a short time will elevate the blood glucose level and alleviate the symptoms. The simpler the carbohydrate, the more rapidly it will be absorbed. For a mild reaction, low-fat milk is a good food to use in children; it supplies lactose or milk sugar, as well as a more prolonged action from the protein and fat. All children with diabetes should carry with them a source of glucose such as glucose tablets, Insta-Glucose, hard candy, or sugar cubes. The rapid-releasing sugar is followed by a complex carbohydrate and protein, such as a slice of bread or a cracker spread with peanut butter.

Glucagon is sometimes prescribed for home treatment of severe hypoglycemia. It is available by prescription as a prefilled syringe and is administered intramuscularly or subcutaneously. Glucagon functions by releasing stored glycogen from the liver; it requires about 10 minutes to elevate the blood glucose level. Once the child is responsive, the lost glycogen stores are replaced by small amounts of sugar-containing fluid administered frequently until the child feels comfortable about trying solid foods.

NURSE ALERT • Vomiting may occur after administration of glucagon; therefore precautions against aspiration must be taken (e.g., placing the child on the side) because the child will be unconscious.

The *Somogyi effect* should be recognized as a response separate from hypoglycemia. This phenomenon occurs when the blood glucose level decreases to the point where stress hormones (e.g., epinephrine, growth hormone, and corticosteroids) are released, causing a rebound hyperglycemia. Prevention consists of increasing the amount of food eaten and/or decreasing the insulin.

Illness Management. Illness alters diabetes management. Maintaining blood glucose control is usually related to the seriousness of the illness. As the illness runs its course, the goal of diabetes management is to maintain some euglycemia while recognizing and treating urinary ketones and preventing dehydration. Some hyperglycemia and ketonuria are expected in most illnesses, even with diminished food intake, and indicate the need for increased insulin. Insulin should never be omitted during an illness, although dosage requirements may increase, decrease, or remain unchanged depending on the severity of the illness and the child's appetite. In addition, supplemental doses of lispro or regular insulin are often used to manage the hyperglycemia associated with illness. Illness management must always include careful attention to fluid balance. Hyperglycemia contributes to dehydration, and the child will require extra oral fluids while ill.

Management of Diabetic Ketoacidosis. DKA, the most complete state of insulin deficiency, is a life-threatening situation. The child is admitted to an intensive care facility for management, which consists of rapid assessment, adequate insulin to reduce the elevated blood glucose level, fluids to overcome dehydration, and electrolyte replacement (especially potassium). The preferred method for administering insulin to the child with ketoacidosis is a continuous IV infusion of low-dose regular insulin.

NURSE ALERT • Because insulin can chemically bind to plastic tubing and in-line filters, thereby reducing the amount of the medication reaching the bloodstream, an insulin mixture is run through the tubing to saturate the insulin binding sites before the infusion is begun.

Current trends suggest cautious fluid resuscitation and blood glucose management to reduce risk of cerebral edema. The fluid deficit is replaced evenly over 24 to 48 hours. Serum potassium levels may be normal on admission, but rapid return of potassium to cells following initiation of fluid and insulin can seriously deplete serum levels, with the attendant risk of cardiac arrhythmias. A cardiac monitor is employed as a guide to therapy and to determine changes that might indicate alterations in potassium concentration.

NURSE ALERT • Potassium must never be given until the serum potassium level is known to be normal or low and voiding of urine is observed. All maintenance IV fluids should include 20 to 40 mEq/L of potassium. Never give potassium as a rapid IV bolus; cardiac arrest may result.

When the critical period is over, the task of regulating insulin dosage to diet and activity is begun. Children should be actively involved in their own care and are given responsibility according to their ability and guidance of the nurse.

Nursing Care Management

➤ Assessment

Daily monitoring of blood glucose levels; periodic urine analysis for ketones; and observation for signs of hypoglycemia, hyperglycemia, or other complications is part of the daily life of the child with diabetes and the family. Diabetes should be suspected in any child who exhibits the manifestations outlined in Box 52-13, and the child should be referred for further assessment and appropriate testing.

The signs and symptoms of hypoglycemia are caused by both increased adrenergic activity and impaired brain function, and it is often difficult to distinguish between hyperglycemia and a hypoglycemic reaction (Table 52-2). Because the symptoms are similar and usually begin with changes in behavior, the simplest way to differentiate between the two is to test the blood glucose level (low in hypoglycemia; elevated in hyperglycemia).

The nurse should also be alert to evidence of complications, although these are usually not manifested until adulthood. Assessment of skin for evidence of breakdown is important in or-

TABLE 52-2

Comparison of Manifestations of Hypoglycemia and Hyperglycemia

Variable	Hypoglycemia	Hyperglycemia
Onset	Rapid (minutes)	Gradual (days)
Mood	Labile, irritable, nervous, weepy	Lethargic
Mental status	Difficulty concentrating, speaking, focusing, coordinating Nightmares	Dulled sensorium Confused
Inward feeling	Shaky feeling, hunger Headache Dizziness	Thirst Weakness Nausea/vomiting Abdominal pain
Skin	Pallor Sweating	Flushed Signs of dehydration
Mucous membranes	Normal	Dry, crusty
Respirations	Shallow, normal	Deep, rapid (Kussmaul)
Pulse	Tachycardia, palpitations	Less rapid, weak
Breath odor	Normal	Fruity, acetone
Neurologic	Tremors Late: hyperflexia, dilated pupils, seizure	Diminished reflexes Paresthesia
Ominous signs	Shock, coma	Acidosis, coma
Blood:		
Glucose	Low: less than 60 mg/dl	High: 250 mg/dl or more
Ketones	Negative	High/large
Osmolarity	Normal	High
pH	Normal	Low (7.25 or less)
Hematocrit	Normal	High
HCO_3	Normal	Less than 20 mEq/L
Urine:		
Output	Normal	Polyuria (early) to oliguria (late) Enuresis, nocturia
Glucose	Negative	High
Ketones	Negative/trace	High
Visual	Diplopia	Blurred vision

der that appropriate care can be implemented to facilitate healing and prevent infection. Because illnesses such as respiratory infections or gastrointestinal upsets complicate diabetes management, they should be detected early.

Education is the cornerstone of diabetes management and the major responsibility in diabetes nursing care. Whether teaching is conducted on an outpatient basis or in a preparatory, in-depth manner on an inpatient basis, the ability and readiness of the individual learner must be accurately assessed. This includes assessment of the educational background and emotional stability of the individual(s) involved; and the use of appropriate measurement tools, such as a pretest or an objective assessment of the learner's educational level and literacy.

➤ Nursing Diagnoses

A number of nursing diagnoses are prominent in the nursing management of type 1 DM, and others specific to individual cases become evident. The most common are outlined in the Nursing Care Plan on p. 1494.

➤ Plan of Care and Implementation

The goals of care for the child with DM and the family are as follows:

1. Child and family will be educated about the disease, assessment techniques, and therapy.
2. Child will experience a minimum of complications of diabetes.
3. Child will develop a positive self-image.
4. Child and family will receive adequate support.

Once the child with diabetes is diagnosed and insulin therapy initiated, the major nursing responsibility is the education of the family and reinforcement of information. The parents must supervise and manage the child's therapeutic program, but the child should assume responsibility for self-management as soon as he or she is capable. Children can assist with blood glucose testing at a relatively young age (4 to 5 years), and most should be able to administer their own insulin with supervision at about 9 years of age. In situations in which the parents are inconsistent and/or unreliable, the child is taught self-care at an earlier age and additional adult support is sought.

The first 3 or 4 days after diagnosis is not an optimum time for learning; therefore the family should be given only essential or survival information first and intense information later. A child learns best when sessions are kept short, no more than 15 to 20 minutes. The parents do best in periods of 45 to 60 minutes, or longer if they are inquisitive. Education should involve all the senses, and although visual aids are valuable tools, participation is the most effective method for learning. For example, to teach blood testing the technique is explained, the procedure is demonstrated, and the learner is allowed to perform the procedure; this is followed by a review of the material by visual aids, and the learning is validated by some testing method that includes feedback. Varying the presentation with a number of audiovisual materials (e.g., videotapes, slide-tape programs, and books) stimulates the senses and helps the individual to learn.

Several organizations are prepared to assist with education and dissemination of knowledge about diabetes. The American Diabetes Association, Inc.,* Canadian Diabetes Association,† Juvenile Diabetes Foundation International,‡ Juvenile Diabetes Foundation—Canada,§ and American Association of Diabetes Educators|| are valuable resources for a wide range of educational materials. The National Diabetes Information Clearinghouse¶ publishes a number of comprehensive annotated bibliographies, including *Educational Materials for and about Young*

---

*1660 Duke St., Alexandria, VA 22314; 1-800-232-3472; website: www.diabetes.org.

†15 Toronto St., Suite 800, Toronto, Ontario M5C 2E3; (416) 363-3373 or 1-800-BANTING; website: www.diabetes.ca.

‡120 Wall St., New York, NY 10005; 1-800-223-1138; website: www.jdf.org.

§89 Granton Dr., Richmond Hill, Ontario L4B 2N5; 1-800-668-0274; website: www.jdfc.ca.

||100 W. Monroe, Suite 400, Chicago, IL 60603; 1-800-338-3633; website:www.aadenet.org.

¶1 Information Way, Bethesda, MD 20892-3560; (301) 654-3327; fax (301) 907-8906; e-mail: ndic@info.niddk.gov; website: www.niddk.nih.gov/health/diabetes/ndic.htm.

People with Diabetes (a compilation of resource materials for children, siblings, parents, teachers, and health professionals) and *Sports and Exercise for People with Diabetes.*

Self-management, the ultimate goal for the child with diabetes, is more likely to occur when the child understands the disorder and the care it requires. Properly educated and with adequate resources, any family should be able to follow a program of regulated control satisfactorily. The following information will allow the family to manage the daily aspects of care.

Identification. One of the first issues to raise with parents is the need for the child to wear medical identification. This essential and immediate information could save the child's life. Identification tags come in a variety of forms including neck chains, bracelets, and tags for shoes.

Nature of Diabetes. The better the parents understand the pathophysiology of diabetes, and the function and action of insulin and glucagon in relation to caloric intake and exercise, the better their understanding of the disease and its effect on the child. Parents need answers to a number of questions (voiced or unvoiced) because those answers will provide them with an increased feeling of security in coping with the disease. Parents initially may worry about what diabetes is, how their child developed diabetes, and if their other children are at risk of developing diabetes. In addition, they will worry about what to tell family, friends, and school personnel. They may have fears about complications and about how they will afford the cost of diabetes care.

Meal Planning. Normal nutrition is a major aspect of the family education program. Diet instruction is usually conducted by the nutritionist, with reinforcement and guidance from the nurse (Fig. 52-3). Learning about foods within specific food groups helps in making choices. Weights and measures of foods, used as eye-training devices in defining portion sizes, should be practiced repeatedly, with gradual conversion to estimating foods. Members of the family are also guided in reading labels for the nutritional value of foods and food contents. Meals and snacks are modified to suit the child and the present food menu, preserving cultural patterns and preferences as much as possible.

Lists of popular fast-food items and items served at the major fast-food chains can be obtained from the American Diabetes Association and help guide food selections. Children are advised to use sugar substitutes with moderation in items such as soft drinks. "Sugar-free" chewing gum and candy made with sorbitol may be used in moderation; however, sorbitol is metabolized to fructose and then to glucose, and large amounts of sorbitol can cause an osmotic diarrhea. Dietetic foods that contain sorbitol are more expensive than regular foods, and often the total carbohydrate content of the food is the same or even greater.

Insulin. Families need to understand the treatment method and the insulin prescribed, including the effective duration, onset, and peak action. They also need to know the characteristics of the various types of insulins and their proper mixing and dilution. Insulin may be kept safely at room temperature or refrigerated, provided the temperature is maintained above freezing and below 30° C (86° F). Insulin, once opened, should be discarded in 1 month (even if refrigerated). Unopened insulin is good until the expiration date on the bottle.

Injection Procedure. Learning to give the insulin injections is a source of anxiety for the family and the child. It is helpful for the learner to know that this important aspect of care will become as routine as brushing the teeth. First, the basic injection technique is taught, using an orange or similar item and saline solution for practice.* To gain the confidence of the child, the nurse demonstrates the technique by giving a skillful injection to the parent, who then returns the demonstration by giving the nurse an injection. With practice, family members soon are able to give the insulin injection to the child. Both parents should participate, and as little time as possible should elapse between instruction and the actual injection, especially with parents and the teenage learner.

Insulin is injected at a 90-degree angle into subcutaneous tissue, where it is slowly absorbed (Fig. 52-4). Newly diagnosed children may have lost adipose tissue, and care should be exercised not to inject into the muscle. The pinch technique is the most effective method for obtaining skin tightness to allow easy entrance of the needle into subcutaneous tissues in children. The site selected will sometimes depend on whether the child or parent administers the insulin. The upper arms, thighs, hips, and abdomen are usual injection sites for insulin. The child can reach the thighs, abdomen, and part of the hip and arm easily but may require help to inject other sites. For example, a parent can pinch a loose fold of skin on the arm while the child injects the insulin.

*Community and home care instructions on subcutaneous injection are available in Wong DL, Hess CS: ***Wong and Whaley's clinical manual of pediatric nursing,*** ed 5, St Louis, 2000, Mosby.

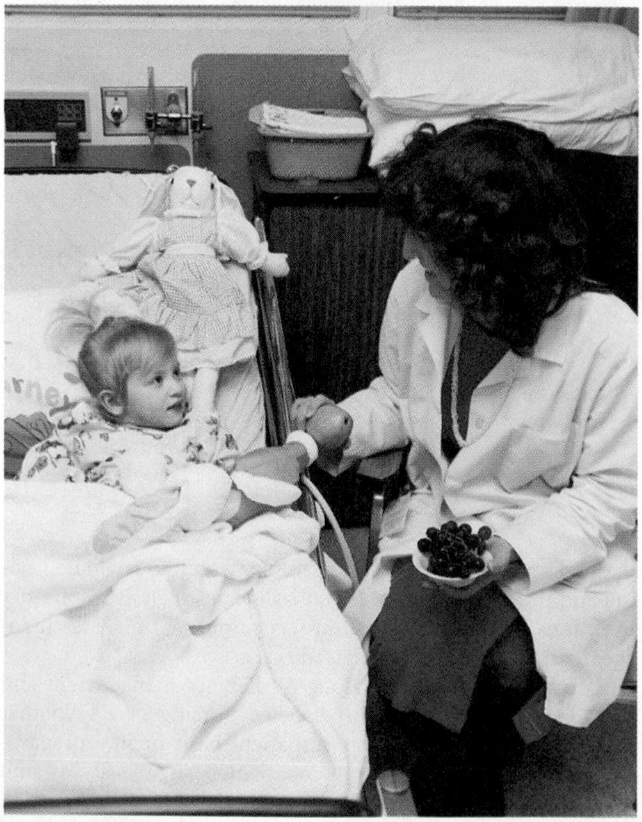

FIG. 52-3 • Nutritionist instructs child, using food to explain food exchanges.

Injections are rotated to various areas of the body to enhance absorption, because insulin absorption is slowed by the fat pads that develop in overused areas of injection. The parents and child are helped to work out a rotation pattern, which involves giving about four to six injections in one area (each injection about 1 inch, or the diameter of the insulin vial, away from the previous injection) and then moving to another area. In this way injection sites for an entire month can be planned in advance on a simple chart or illustration, such as an outline of a body or a teddy bear. It is a good idea for the parents each to give one or two injections a week in the areas that are difficult to reach in order to keep in practice.

It is important to remember that the absorption rate varies in different parts of the body (Table 52-3). Methodically using one anatomic area and then moving to another minimizes variation in absorption rates. New recommendations suggest rotating injections within an anatomic area (Fleming, 1999). An example of this would be using the abdomen for morning injections and the thighs for evening injections. This may assist with obtaining more consistent blood glucose levels. Injecting small doses of insulin also minimizes changes in plasma glucose levels. Absorption is also altered by vigorous exercise, which enhances absorption from exercised muscles. Therefore it is recommended that excess exercise be avoided during the time the insulin is expected to peak.

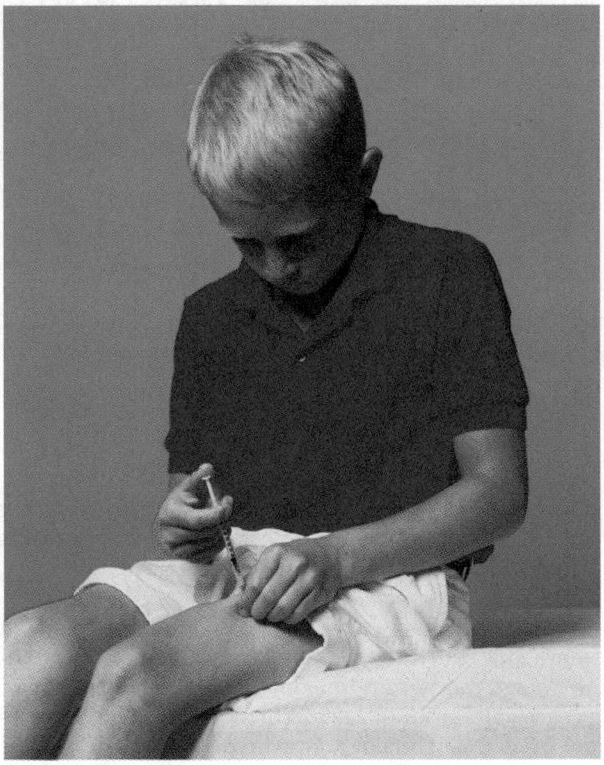

FIG. 52-4 • School-age children are able to administer their own insulin.

Teaching includes the proper way to equalize pressure in the bottle by injecting an amount of air equal to the amount of solution withdrawn and how to remove air bubbles from the syringe. When insulin dosages are small, an air bubble in the syringe can displace a significant amount of medication. Since the introduction of the $\frac{5}{10}$-ml and $\frac{3}{10}$-ml syringes, the risk of incorrect dosage has diminished; however, insulin injections of less than 2 units of U100 have an unacceptably large error. Diluted insulin should be used if the prescribed dose is less than 2 units (Gnanalingham, Newland, and Smith, 1998). Aspiration for blood before injecting the insulin is not routinely done.

Insulin syringes should be compared for accuracy, comfort, and strength. The family and/or child should be able to choose both "their" insulin and "their" syringe from a variety of samples. Use of the same type of syringe (even during hospitalization) is recommended to prevent errors in dosage caused by different markings and varying amounts of dead space among syringes.

When the child's dosage requires the injection of both rapid- or short-acting and intermediate-acting insulin at the same time, most families prefer to mix the two and use a single injection; however, there are some problems associated with this accepted practice, and the family should understand what happens when insulins are mixed. Longer-acting insulins contain ingredients that bind to insulin, allowing for gradual release after injection. Some brands contain extra binding compounds that can bind with rapid- or short-acting insulin, blunting the action of the quicker insulin and altering the effect on blood glucose. The degree of alteration depends on the type of longer-acting insulin, the ratio of rapid- or short-acting insulin to long-acting insulin, and how long the mixture is allowed to stand before injection. The mixture should be injected less than 5 minutes after mixing (before the zinc content of the long-acting insulin affects the action time of the rapid- or short-acting insulin) or longer than 15 minutes after mixing (to allow the insulins to resume long-acting and short-acting properties).

To obtain the maximum benefit from mixing insulins, the recommended practice is to:

1. Inject the measured amount of air (equivalent to the dosage) into the longer-acting insulin (cloudy).

TABLE 52-3
Onset and Duration of Action Related to Insulin Injection Site

	Site of Injection			
	Abdomen	**Arm**	**Leg**	**Buttock**
Rate	Very fast	Fast	Slow	Very slow
Duration	Very short	Short	Long	Very long

From Albisser AM, Sperlich M: Adjusting insulins, *Diabetes Educ* 18(3):211-218, 1992.

2. Inject the measured amount of air into the rapid- or short-acting (clear) insulin and, without removing the needle, withdraw the clear insulin.
3. Insert the needle (already containing the clear insulin) into the longer-acting insulin and withdraw the desired amount.

NURSE ALERT • When mixing types of insulin, always withdraw the clear insulin first, then the longer-acting insulin next to avoid contaminating the clear insulin with the longer-acting insulin.

It has become acceptable practice (though not recommended by all professionals) to reuse disposable needles and syringes. Bacteria counts are unaffected, and there is a considerable cost saving. It is important to stress the importance of vigorous handwashing before handling any equipment, as well as capping the syringe immediately after use. Syringes may be stored at room temperature (American Diabetes Association, 1996). Nurses should also teach proper disposal of equipment after use in the home. Although it is not standard practice in the hospital, the use of a needle clipper is recommended to safely remove and house the used needle. In addition, the syringe plunger can be broken before disposal. An excellent means for syringe disposal is use of an opaque, puncture-resistant container, such as an empty coffee can, bleach bottle, or milk carton that is labeled "bio-hazardous waste" and is discarded with similar material only, not with household refuse. Many pharmacies now carry commercially produced sharps containers.

Other devices are available for insulin injection and may offer advantages to some children. Children who do not wish to give themselves injections can be taught to use a syringe-loaded injector *(Injectease)*. With the device, puncture is always automatic. Adolescents respond well to a self-contained and compact device resembling a fountain pen (e.g., *Novopen*), which eliminates conventional vials and syringes. Preloaded pens may also cause less pain, because the needle is not blunted by piercing the rubber top of the insulin vial (Saudek, 1997).

Some children are considered candidates for continuous subcutaneous insulin infusion with a portable insulin pump. The child and the parents are taught to operate the device, including the mechanics of the pump, battery changes, and alarm systems. They learn how to load the syringe, insert the catheter, adjust the insulin flow for routine needs and for illnesses, and connect and disconnect the catheter. Nurses who work where the pumps are part of the therapeutic regimen should become familiar with the operation of the specific device being used and the protocol of the regimen.

Glucose Monitoring. Nurses should also be prepared to teach and supervise blood glucose monitoring. Blood for testing can be obtained by two different methods: manually or with a spring-loaded puncturing device. The automatic lancet device is recommended because its precise puncture depth produces better blood flow and less pain; however, the child and family should learn to use both methods in the event of mechanical failure. Several lancet devices are available from which to choose, and each provides a means for obtaining enough blood for testing (Fig. 52-5). Many lancet devices may be adjusted for depth of puncture.

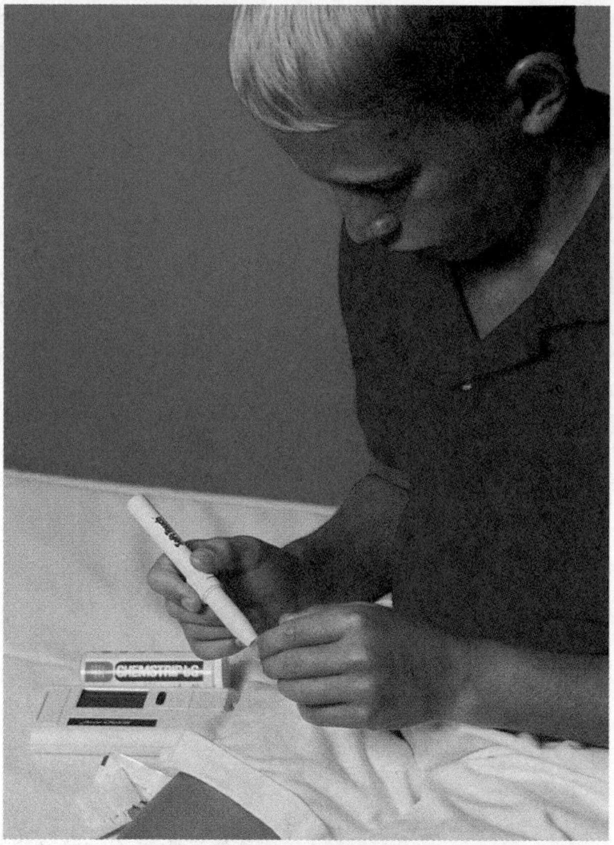

FIG. 52-5 • Child using finger-stick device to obtain blood sample. Blood glucose monitor and reagent strips are nearby.

NURSE ALERT • Caution children not to allow anyone else to use their lancet or lancet device because of the risk of contracting hepatitis B virus or human immunodeficiency virus (HIV) infection.

Repeated finger punctures can be painful, but most children become accustomed to the procedure (Atraumatic Care box). However, persistent signs of redness and soreness at the puncture site should be investigated. It may be evidence of poor technique or poor skin healing relative to poor control.

The least expensive testing method uses a visually read reagent strip to which blood is applied. After blotting, the color change is compared with a color scale for an estimation of the blood glucose level. The strips can be cut in half (although this is not recommended by all professionals) to obtain two readings per strip. This method might be ideal for use at school, where expensive equipment can be lost or broken.

Many types of glucose monitors are available for home use. The family should be shown features of several meters, including advantages and disadvantages, and allowed to choose equipment that best meets their needs. One important consideration is the amount of blood needed. Choosing devices that require small amounts may prevent repunctures.

Urine Testing. Urine ketone testing is easily taught but requires careful attention to technique. The test strip must be

Atraumatic Care

MINIMIZING PAIN OF BLOOD GLUCOSE MONITORING

To enhance blood flow to the finger, hold it under warm water for a few seconds before the puncture.

When obtaining blood samples, use the ring finger or thumb (blood flows more easily to these areas), and puncture the finger just to the side of the finger pad (more blood vessels and fewer nerve endings).

To prevent a deep puncture, press the platform of the lancet device lightly against the skin and avoid steadying the finger against a hard surface.

Use glucose monitors that require very small blood samples to avoid repunctures (e.g., Glucometer Elite).

Apply EMLA to the puncture site, especially when the child is newly diagnosed and the skin is still very sensitive (see Pain Management, Chapter 44).

Emergency

HYPOGLYCEMIA

Mild Reaction: Adrenergic Symptoms

Give child 10 to 15 g of simple carbohydrate (preferably liquid; e.g., 3 to 6 ounces of orange juice).

Follow with starch-protein snack.

Moderate Reaction: Neuroglycopenic Symptoms

Give child 10 to 15 g of simple carbohydrate as above.

Repeat in 10 to 15 minutes if symptoms persist.

Follow with larger snack.

Watch child closely.

Severe Reaction: Unresponsive, Unconscious, and/or Seizures

Administer glucagon as prescribed.

Follow with planned meal or snack when child is able to eat, or add a snack.

Nocturnal Reaction

Give child 10 to 15 g of simple carbohydrate.

Follow with a snack.

used accurately and the test timed precisely. Because the test strip is visually read, there must be adequate lighting available. Testing for ketones is recommended during times of illness or when glucose readings are high. Because moisture will cause changes to take place in both glucose and ketone strips, families are instructed to discard strips that are discolored, that have been open for a specified time, or after an expiration date. Test strips are available for testing both glucose and ketones.

Hyperglycemia and Hypoglycemia. Severe hyperglycemia is most often caused by illness, growth, emotional upset, or inaccurate or missed insulin doses. With careful glucose monitoring, most elevations can be managed by adjustment of insulin or food intake. Parents should understand how to adjust food, activity, and insulin at the time of illness or when the child is treated for an illness with a medication known to raise the blood glucose level (e.g., cough syrup or steroids). The hyperglycemia is managed by increasing insulin soon after the increased glucose is noted.

Hypoglycemia is caused by imbalances of food intake, insulin, and activity. Ideally, hypoglycemia should be prevented, and parents need to be prepared to prevent, recognize, and treat the problem. They should be familiar with the signs of hypoglycemia and instructed in treatment, including care of the child with seizures (see Chapter 51). Hypoglycemia can be managed effectively as outlined in the Emergency box.

Exercise. Exercise should be planned (as may be necessary for the sedentary teenager) or observed (as in most active children). If the child is more active at one time of the day than at another, food and/or insulin can be altered to meet the activity pattern of the individual. Food should be increased in the summer when children tend to be more active. Decreased activity on return to school may require a decrease in food intake. The child who is active in team sports will need additional food intake on the days of activity in the form of a carbohydrate snack about ½ hour before the anticipated activity. Races or other competition may call for a slightly higher food intake than practice times.

Food will usually need to be repeated for prolonged activity periods, often every 45 minutes to 1 hour. Families should be informed that if increased food is not tolerated, decreased insulin is the next course of action. If the blood glucose level is elevated (≥240 mg/dl) and ketone values are positive before planned exercise, the activity should be postponed until the blood glucose is controlled. Moderate to large ketone values should be reported to the practitioner.

Record Keeping. Recording information about food, insulin, blood glucose measurements, and ketonuria is useful to the practitioner as well as to the family. Insulin reactions are noted, including the time, severity, treatment, and response to treatment. Dietary variations are noted so that an increased blood glucose level can be analyzed in relation to the insulin dose, food intake, and activity level. Record keeping should also include identified stresses such as school exams, birthday parties, and injuries.

Self-Management. Self-management is the key to close control. Being able to make changes at the time they are needed rather than waiting until the next contact with health professionals is important for self-management and gives the child and parents the feeling that they have control over the disease. As children grow and assume more and more responsibility for self-management, they develop confidence in their ability to manage their disease and in themselves as persons. Self-management techniques to be mastered are the testing of blood and urine, administration of insulin, and adjustment of insulin and diet with alterations in day-to-day activities and unusual occurrences.

Hygiene. All aspects of personal hygiene are emphasized for the child with diabetes. The child should be cautioned against wearing shoes without socks, wearing sandals, or walking barefoot. The correct method of nail and extremity care instituted for each particular child (with the guidance of a podiatrist) can begin health practices that last a lifetime. Eyes should be checked once a year, unless the child wears glasses, and then as directed by the ophthalmologist. Regular dental care is emphasized, and cuts and scratches should be treated with plain soap and water unless otherwise indicated.

Acute Care. Children with diabetes may be admitted to the hospital at the time of their initial diagnosis, during illness or surgery, or during episodes of DKA—especially in the small number who exhibit a degree of metabolic lability or who have repeated episodes of DKA. Most children with diabetes are able to keep the disease under control with periodic assessment and adjustment of insulin, diet, and activity as needed under health supervision.

The child with DKA requires intensive nursing care. On admission to the hospital, usually an intensive care unit, an IV infusion is started immediately to hydrate the child and to administer insulin, usually as a continuous infusion (see Management of Diabetic Ketoacidosis, p. 1486). The blood glucose level is monitored at regular intervals, and the insulin administered as ordered.

Sodium, potassium, and bicarbonate levels are monitored and replaced as indicated. Because potassium and sodium reenter the cells rapidly after administration of insulin, depletion of these electrolytes can be a serious consequence. The child is attached to a cardiac monitor for continual assessment of cardiac status, especially when potassium levels are markedly altered.

Careful and accurate records are maintained, including vital signs, blood pressure, IV fluids, electrolytes, insulin, blood glucose level, intake and output, and weight. A urine collection device is used to obtain the urine measurements, which include volume, specific gravity, and glucose and ketone values. The volume relative to the glucose content is important, because 5% glucose in a 300-ml sample is a significantly greater amount than a similar reading from a 75-ml sample. A diabetic flow sheet maintained at the bedside provides an ongoing record of the vital signs, urine and blood tests, amount of insulin given, and intake and output of the patient. The level of consciousness is assessed and recorded at frequent intervals. Any change or deterioration in the level of consciousness must be reported to the health care provider. Such changes may indicate an increase in intracranial pressure and must be managed aggressively. The comatose child generally regains consciousness fairly soon after initiation of therapy but until then is managed as is any unconscious child.

Family Support. In any educational program the psychologic needs of the child are just as important as the physical needs. Adjustment to a chronic illness is difficult and follows the grief process (see Chapter 41). A noticeable adjustment cycle occurs during the week-long education course. First, there is interest and perhaps some anger and doubt, followed by denial and accompanied by the overwhelming feeling of "Why me?" There are doubts regarding the ability to absorb so much essential information. Then follows the acceptance and synthesis of material, as the learners realize that they are able to state and demonstrate their understanding of the material.

Young children usually adjust well to problems related to the disease; however, challenges exist, such as providing regular feedings to the sick infant or to the negative toddler. With toddlers and preschoolers insulin injections and glucose testing may be difficult at first. However, they usually accept the procedures when the parents use a matter-of-fact approach without calling attention to a "hurt" and treat the procedure like any other routine part of a child's life. Following the injection time with some special and positive attention, such as reading, talking, or some other pleasant activity, is one way to convert children who initially refuse injections to those who accept them.

School-age children tend to accept their condition more easily than adolescents. School-age children can understand the basic concepts related to their disease and its treatment. They are able to test blood glucose and urine; recognize food groups; give injections; keep records; and distinguish between feelings of fear, excitement, and hypoglycemia. They understand how to recognize, prevent, and treat hypoglycemia. However, they still need considerable parental involvement.

Adolescents appear to have the most difficulty in adjusting. Adolescence is a time when there is much stress toward being "perfect" and being like peers, and no matter what others say, the person with diabetes is different. Some youngsters are more upset about not being able to have a candy bar than about injections, diet, and other aspects of management. If children can accept the difference as a part of life—or in other words, that each person is different in some way—then with adequate family support they should be able to adjust (Family Focus box and Critical Thinking box).

For all families, daily compliance with numerous procedures and structured living schedules is difficult. Maintaining good blood glucose control requires ongoing motivation. Nurses can encourage families to adhere to treatment regimens and lifestyle adjustments by emphasizing the benefits of preventing complications such as hypoglycemia. In some families complications can have a favorable impact. Once parents experience the child's having a severe insulin reaction with a seizure, or the adolescent has one in a public place, the desire to maintain better control is reinforced. They must understand how to prevent problems and how to handle problems calmly if they occur. (See Compliance, Chapter 45.)

Parents develop guilt feelings when they have a child with any chronic disease, especially one with a hereditary component. They cope with these feelings in a number of ways. For example, they may be either overprotective or neglectful. Parents may blame themselves, consciously or subconsciously, for the disease. Nevertheless they must come to realize, through education and counseling, that there was nothing they could have done to delay or prevent the disease and that it was not their fault, because environmental, as well as hereditary, factors may be involved in the development of the disease.

Problems in the parental response provide a challenge for the nurse who must assist through counseling or, if the problems are severe enough, refer the parents to appropriate resources designed to help them alter their behavior. Times should be set aside during the child's health visit or afterward to meet the needs of the parents. Parents should also be included in special sessions to keep them abreast of the child's management, to help them continue to participate in the child's care, and to provide them with an opportunity to express their own feelings concerning their own or their child's adjustment to the disease. The amount of information that they offer at this time can give clues to their level of support of the child and help assist in decisions concerning the therapeutic management of the child.

Camps for children with diabetes and other special groups are very useful. In these special camps children learn that they are not alone. As a result, most children become more independent and resourceful outside the camp setting. Camp time also provides parents a respite from the child's daily regimen. Information about such camps and organizations can be obtained from the American Diabetes Association. A free list of accredited camps specifically for children and teenagers with diabetes is also available.*

*Camp Directory, 1660 Duke St., Alexandria, VA 22314; 1-800-232-3472.

Family Focus

THE ADOLESCENT WITH TYPE 1 DIABETES MELLITUS

As a nurse caring for adolescents with type 1 diabetes mellitus (DM), I am constantly aware of the wide range of adolescent behaviors that affect the course of this disease. Education of the child and the parents can often make the difference between a disease in control of the teenager and a teenager in control of the disease.

I have cared for many adolescent girls who have episodes of hyperglycemia at the time of menstruation that can result in diabetic ketoacidosis (DKA). I have found that education regarding sick-day protocol with sliding-scale rapid-acting insulin instituted at the first sign of hyperglycemia, which may occur 1 to 2 days before onset of menses, can keep the adolescent girl out of the intensive care unit and in control of her diabetes.

Eating disorders, such as bulimia or anorexia nervosa, in the teenager with type 1 DM pose a serious health hazard. Also, insulin manipulation or omission has been identified as a weight loss method used by some adolescents (Barber and Lowes, 1998). Poor disease control may also be used by depressed teens as a method of suicide. Nurses working with these adolescents must be aware of the hazards and openly discuss the risks with the young person. A referral for specialized intervention may be needed.

Another group of adolescents with diabetes who are at risk are those who drink alcohol. I have found that confusion about the effects of alcohol on blood glucose is common. Teenagers may believe that alcohol will increase blood glucose levels, when in fact the opposite occurs. Ingestion of alcohol inhibits the release of glycogen from the liver, therefore resulting in hypoglycemia. Teenagers with diabetes who drink alcohol may become hypoglycemic but be treated as if they were inebriated (drunk). Behaviors may be similar, such as shakiness, combativeness, slurred speech, and loss of consciousness.

Education regarding the effects of alcohol is important and must be included in a teaching plan. If teenagers insist on drinking alcohol, they can be cautioned to use sweetened mixers or eat snacks when consuming alcoholic beverages.

Episodes of hyperglycemia or hypoglycemia may become a serious issue for adolescents who are leaving home for the first time. One teenager confided that her mother always recognized her combative, antisocial behavior as impending hypoglycemia and treated her with the appropriate intervention. The teenager feared that a college roommate might be offended by the behavior and leave her alone with impending hypoglycemia.

One young man realized he could not live alone when he "took a nap because of feeling tired" and woke up 4 days later in the hospital. Fortunately, his family realized he was in a coma and summoned emergency medical service. The fatigue signaled the beginning of a viral infection, which led to a blood glucose level of 410 mg/dl. Nurses need to address these fears openly and facilitate ways in which the teenager can enlist the aid of significant peers who may be available during hyperglycemic or hypoglycemic episodes.

Susan Zekauskas, MSN, RN, PNP

➤ Evaluation

The effectiveness of nursing interventions is determined by continual reassessment and evaluation of care based on the following observational guidelines:

1. Interview family to determine their understanding of the disease; have child and family demonstrate and discuss the needed assessment and therapeutic techniques.
2. Interview family regarding their understanding of tight control; analyze and evaluate management records.
3. Discuss child's disease with him or her.
4. Interview family and child regarding their feelings and concerns about the disease.

The expected outcomes are described in the Nursing Care Plan.

Critical Thinking

TYPE 1 DIABETES MELLITUS

Rebecca, 15 years old, has a 3-year history of type 1 diabetes mellitus and has been admitted to the pediatric intensive care unit for treatment of diabetic ketoacidosis (DKA). This is her fifth hospital admission for DKA in the past year. Rebecca's parents are divorced, and she has four younger siblings, none of whom has diabetes. Rebecca's mother has maintained two jobs for the past 5 years and frequently leaves Rebecca in charge of the household. In anticipation of her discharge, you plan a patient education program for Rebecca and her mother. Areas of diabetes management that must be emphasized are (1) careful dietary management, (2) an appropriate exercise program, (3) conscientious self-testing of blood glucose and appropriate administration of daily insulin, (4) adherence to sliding-scale insulin therapy as prescribed, (5) urine ketone testing when blood glucose levels are elevated, and (6) effective methods of handling emotional stressors. Of the following issues that might be influencing the recurrent episodes of DKA, which one should you address initially?

First, Think About It . . .

- What precise question are you trying to answer?
- What conclusions are you coming to?

1. The responsibility Rebecca feels for the care of her four younger siblings
2. Fluctuation of blood glucose levels around the time of menses with inadequate insulin dosage
3. Stress related to the absence of Rebecca's mother and the loss of the close relationship Rebecca shared with her father
4. Adolescent issues, such as seeking independence, feeling different from her peers, and alcohol use

The best response is 2. The nurse should concentrate first on situations directly related to hyperglycemia. The concept that adolescent girls with diabetes tend to have frequent fluctuation of blood glucose levels, especially increased blood glucose immediately before, during, or after their menses, is correct. Emotional stress related to increased responsibilities, normal developmental tasks of adolescence, and personal loss from divorce can also precipitate a stress response and elevate blood glucose levels. The nurse should address these issues if there is time during teaching or make a referral for special support services, since negative consequences could result if no action is taken.

Nursing Care Plan THE CHILD WITH DIABETES MELLITUS

NURSING DIAGNOSIS Risk for injury related to hypoglycemia or hyperglycemia

EXPECTED OUTCOME Child demonstrates normal blood glucose levels.

Nursing Interventions/*Rationales*

Obtain blood glucose level *to determine appropriate insulin dose and monitor glucose level.*

Administer insulin as ordered *to maintain normal glucose level.*

Make sure nutritional intake is appropriate, timely, and adequate *to maintain blood glucose level.*

Monitor for signs of hypoglycemia (e.g., sweating, shaky nervousness, faintness, fatigue, palpitations, confusion) and hyperglycemia (nausea, urinary frequency, thirst, hunger, tiredness, fruity breath) and correct appropriately (e.g., readily absorbed carbohydrates followed by complex carbohydrate and protein for hypoglycemia; insulin for hyperglycemia) *to maintain glucose balance and prevent long-term complications.*

NURSING DIAGNOSIS Knowledge deficit related to new health condition (diabetes mellitus)

EXPECTED OUTCOME Child and family delineate plan of care for management of diabetes; child and family exhibit evidence of incorporation of care behaviors into daily routine.

Nursing Interventions/*Rationales*

Ascertain family's general knowledge of diabetes *to assess baseline knowledge.* Set up an environment conducive to learning (e.g., teaching methods appropriate to age of child and family; use of written materials, pictures, audiovisuals; use of short repetitive teaching sessions with ongoing reinforcement of information and feedback; encouragement of questions; clarification of misconceptions) *to maximize learning.*

Discuss the pathology and potential sequelae of diabetes, the function and actions of insulin in relation to eating and exercise, the need for careful adherence to the plan of care, and the importance of regular health care *to ensure adequate understanding and promote compliance.*

Help family understand diabetic diet and dietary exchanges and to plan any needed dietary changes within family cultural and food preferences; help with menus, recipes, shopping strategies (refer to dietitian if available) *to promote successful adaptation of dietary practices.*

Teach family the importance of careful blood glucose monitoring *to maintain consistent blood glucose levels and prevent ketoacidosis.*

Teach family about importance of judicious exercise and the need for glucose monitoring after vigorous exercise *to prevent hypoglycemia.*

Teach family about need for careful oral and body hygiene, prompt treatment of cuts and scrapes, careful foot care; regular visits to the dentist, ophthalmologist, and endocrinologist *to prevent or detect early signs of complications.*

Teach family how to use and interpret glucose monitoring equipment; how to store, draw up, and administer insulin; how to rotate injection sites; use of any needed supplies or equipment by using a demonstration—return demonstration technique *to ensure comfort and ability to perform needed procedures and handle equipment.*

Have child wear a medical identification device (bracelet, necklace) at all times *to ensure prompt and proper emergency care if needed.*

Increase child's role in self-management of disease by using age-appropriate guidelines *to move child into a long-term role as independent manager of the disease process and associated treatments.*

NURSING DIAGNOSIS Altered family processes related to situational crises (child with chronic disease/disability)

See the Nursing Care Plan: The Child with Chronic Illness, Disability, Chapter 41.

Key Points

- Pituitary dysfunction is manifested primarily by growth disturbance.
- The main physiologic action of thyroid hormone is to regulate the basal metabolic rate and control the processes of growth and tissue differentiation.
- Disorders of thyroid function include hypothyroidism, autoimmune thyroiditis, goiter, and hyperthyroidism.
- Therapy for hyperthyroidism is directed at retarding the rate of hormone secretion and may include drug therapy, thyroidectomy, or radioiodine therapy.
- Classic forms of hypoparathyroidism in childhood are idiopathic—deficient production of parathyroid hormone (PTH)—and pseudohypoparathyroidism—increased PTH production with end-organ unresponsiveness to PTH.

- The adrenal cortex secretes three important groups of hormones: glucocorticoids, mineralocorticoids, and sex steroids.
- Disorders of adrenal function include acute adrenocortical insufficiency, chronic adrenocortical insufficiency, Cushing syndrome, congenital adrenogenital hyperplasia, and hyperaldosteronism.
- Four categories of Cushing syndrome are pituitary, adrenal, ectopic, and iatrogenic.
- Management of congenital adrenogenital hyperplasia includes assignment of a sex according to genotype, administration of cortisone, and, possibly, reconstructive surgery.
- Diabetes mellitus is categorized as type 1 diabetes, type 2 diabetes, and maturity-onset diabetes of the young.
- The focus of type 1 diabetes management is insulin replacement, diet, and exercise.
- Education of families includes explanation of diabetes, meal planning, administering insulin injection, monitoring, general hygienic practices, promoting exercise, record keeping, and observing for complications.

References

American Diabetes Association: *Complete guide to diabetes,* Alexandria, VA, 1996, American Diabetes Association.

American Diabetes Association: Clinical practice recommendations 1998; report of the Expert Committee on the Diagnosis and Classification of Diabetes Mellitus, *Diabetes Care* 21(suppl 1):S5-S19, 1998.

Atkinson MA, Ellis TM: Infants' diets and insulin-dependent diabetes: evaluating the "cows' milk hypothesis" and a role for antibovine serum albumin immunity, *J Am Coll Nutr* 16(4):334-340, 1997.

August GP, Julius JR, Blethen SL: Adult height in children with growth hormone deficiency who are treated with biosynthetic growth hormone: The National Cooperative Growth Study Experience, *Pediatrics* 102(2):512-516, 1998.

August M et al: Complications associated with therapeutic neck radiation, *J Oral Maxillofac Surg* 54(12):1409-1415, 1996.

Bartley GB et al: Clinical features of Graves' ophthalmopathy in an incidence cohort, *Am J Ophthalmol* 121:284-290, 1996.

Blethen SL et al: Safety of recombinant deoxyribonucleic acid-derived growth hormone, *J Clin Endocrinol Metab* 81(5):1704-1710, 1996.

Boulgourdjian EM et al: Oral desmopressin treatment of central diabetes insipidus in children, *Acta Pediatr* 86:1261-1262, 1997.

Diabetes Control and Complications Trial Research Group: The effect of intensive treatment of diabetes on the development and progression of long-term complications in insulin-dependent diabetes mellitus, *N Engl J Med* 329(14):977-986, 1993.

Fleming DF: Challenging traditional insulin injection practices, *Am J Nurs* 99(2):72-74, 1999.

Gildea J: High and dry—low and wet: the key to DI and SIADH, *Pediatr Nurs* 19(5):478-481, 1993.

Gnanalingham MG, Newland P, Smith CP: Accuracy and reproducibility of low dose insulin administration using pen-injectors and syringes, *Arch Dis Child* 79(1):59-62, 1998.

Lanza RP et al: Xenotransplantation of cells using biodegradable microcapsules, *Transplant* 67(8):1105-1111, 1999.

Ron E et al: Thyroid cancer after exposure to external radiation: a pooled analysis of seven studies, *Radiat Res* 141:259-277, 1995.

Rosenfeld RR: Disorders of growth hormone and insulin-like growth factor secretion and action. In Sperling MA, editor: *Pediatric endocrinology,* Philadelphia, 1996, WB Saunders.

Ruble JA: Congenital adrenal hyperplasia. In Jackson PL, Vessey JA, editors: *Primary care of the child with a chronic condition,* ed 2, St Louis, 1996, Mosby.

Saudek CD: Novel forms of insulin delivery, *Endocrinol Metab Clin North Am* 26(3):599-610, 1997.

Shulman DI, Bercu BB: Growth hormone therapy: an update, *Contemp Pediatr* 15(8):95-108, 1998.

Stoffer DA et al: Early onset type-2 diabetes mellitus (MODY 4) linked to IPFI, *Nat Genet* 117:138-139, 1997.

Winters WE, Chihara T, Schatz D: The genetics of autoimmune 2 diabetes, *Am J Dis Child* 147(12):1282-1290, 1993.

Wunderlich RP et al: Pathophysiology and treatment of painful diabetic neuropathy of the lower extremity, *South Med J* 91(10):894-898, 1998.

Zimet GD et al: Psychosocial outcome of children evaluated for short stature, *Arch Pediatr Adolesc Med* 151(10):1017-1023, 1997.

CHAPTER 53 Integumentary Dysfunction

http://www.harcourthealth.com/MERLIN/Wong/maternal/

Learning Objectives

On completion of this chapter the reader will be able to:

- Describe the distribution and configuration of the various skin lesions.
- List the benefits of a moist environment for wound healing.
- Discuss the nursing care related to therapies for skin disorders.
- Contrast the manifestations of and therapies for bacterial, viral, and fungal infections of the skin.
- Compare the skin manifestations related to age in children.
- Outline a plan of care to prevent and treat diaper dermatitis.
- Outline a plan of care for a child with atopic dermatitis.
- Formulate a teaching plan for an adolescent with acne.
- Describe the methods for assessing a burn wound.
- Discuss the physical and emotional care of a child with a severe burn wound.

INTEGUMENTARY DYSFUNCTION

Skin Lesions

Lesions of the skin can result from a variety of etiologic factors. In general, skin lesions originate from (1) contact with injurious agents (e.g., infective organisms, toxic chemicals, or physical trauma); (2) hereditary factors; (3) an external factor that produces a reaction in the skin (e.g., allergens); or (4) a systemic disease in which lesions are a cutaneous manifestation (e.g., measles, lupus erythematosus, or nutritional deficiency diseases). Responses are highly individualized. An agent that may be harmless to one individual may be damaging to another, and a single agent may produce various types of responses in different individuals.

Another factor involved in the etiology of skin manifestations is the age of the child. For example, infants are subject to "birthmark" malformations and atopic dermatitis that appear early in life; the school-age child is susceptible to ringworm of the scalp; and acne is a characteristic skin disorder of puberty. Contact dermatitis, such as poison ivy, is seen only where the noxious agent is a feature of the area. Similarly, insect bites are associated with life-cycle and seasonal activities. Although less common in children, tension and anxiety may produce, modify, or prolong many skin conditions.

Skin of Younger Children. The major skin layers arise from different embryologic origins. Early in the embryonic period, a single layer of epithelium forms from the ectoderm, while simultaneously the corium develops from the mesenchyme. In the infant and small child the epidermis is still loosely bound to the dermis. This poor adherence causes the layers to separate readily during an inflammatory process to form blisters. This is especially true in preterm infants, who have an even greater propensity to blister formation and separation during careless handling (such as removal of adhesive tape). The skin is thinner than in older children, and the cells of all strata are more compressed.

Several characteristics influence skin responses in infants and young children. Their skin is far more susceptible to superficial bacterial infection. They are more likely to have associated systemic symptoms with some infections and are more apt to react to a primary irritant than to a sensitizing allergen. Infants and young children are more commonly affected by chronic atopic dermatitis (eczema). The infant's skin is much more prone to develop a toxic erythema as a result of skin eruptions or drug reactions and is subject to maceration, infection, and the moisture retention associated with diaper rash.

Pathophysiology of Dermatitis. Over half of dermatologic problems are various forms of dermatitis. This implies a sequence of inflammatory changes in the skin that are grossly and microscopically similar but diverse in course and causation. Acute responses produce intercellular and intracellular edema, the formation of intradermal vesicles, and an initial infiltration of inflammatory cells into the epidermis. In the dermis there is edema, vascular dilation, and early perivascular cellular infiltration. The location and manner of these reactions produce the lesions characteristic of each disorder. The changes are reversible, and the skin ordinarily recovers without blemish and completely intact unless complicating factors are present such as ulceration from the primary irritant, scratching, and infection; or unless underlying vascular disease develops. In chronic conditions permanent effects are seen that vary according to the disorder, the general condition of the affected individual, and available therapy.

Diagnostic Evaluation. Although the history and subjective symptoms are explored first, objective findings are often noted simultaneously. One of the more advantageous aspects of skin lesions is that often the diagnosis is readily established after simple, careful inspection.

History and Subjective Symptoms. Many cutaneous lesions are associated with local symptoms, the most common of which is itching *(pruritus)* that varies in kind and intensity. Pain or tenderness often accompanies some skin lesions, and other sensations may be described as burning, prickling, stinging, or crawling. Alterations in local feeling or sensation include absence of sensation *(anesthesia)*, excessive sensitiveness *(hyperesthesia)*, diminished sensation *(hypesthesia* or *hypoesthesia)*, or abnormal sensation, such as burning or prickling *(paresthesia)*. These symptoms may remain localized or may migrate; may be constant or intermittent; and may be aggravated by a specific activity or circumstance, such as exposure to sunlight.

It is also important to determine whether the child has had an allergic condition such as asthma or hay fever or has had previous skin disease. Atopic dermatitis, often associated with allergies, commonly begins in infancy. It should be determined when the lesion or symptom first became apparent, as well as whether it is related to ingestion of a food or other substance, including any medication the child might be taking. It should be kept in mind that the condition may be related to an activity such as contact with plants, insects, or chemicals.

Objective Findings. Much can be determined by the distribution, size, morphology, and arrangement of the lesions. Extrinsic causes usually result from physical, chemical, or allergic irritants or from an infectious agent such as bacteria, fungi, viruses, or animal parasites. Skin manifestations can be produced by such intrinsic causes as a specific infection (such as measles or chickenpox), drug sensitization, or other allergic phenomena. Other diagnostic tools are subjective symptoms, the history, and medical and laboratory studies.

Lesion. According to the nature of the pathologic process, lesions assume more or less distinct characteristics.

Names that have been applied to these lesions are important for descriptive purposes in the processes of record keeping and communication. Nurses should also become familiar with the more common terms used to describe skin lesions seen in dermatologic conditions:

Erythema—A reddened area caused by increased amounts of oxygenated blood in the dermal vasculature

Ecchymoses (bruises)—Localized red or purple discolorations caused by extravasation of blood into dermis and subcutaneous tissues

Petechiae—Pinpoint, tiny, and sharp circumscribed spots in the superficial layers of the epidermis

Primary lesions—Skin changes produced by some causative factor; common primary lesions in pediatric skin disorders are macules, papules, and vesicles (Fig. 53-1)

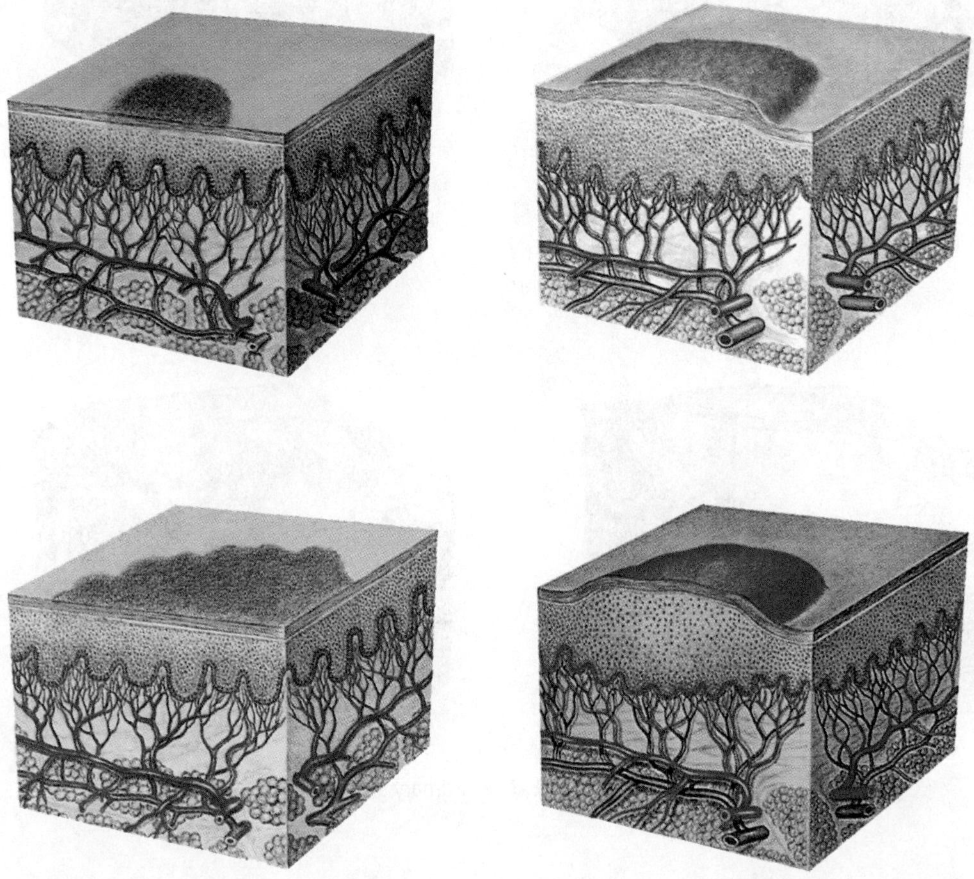

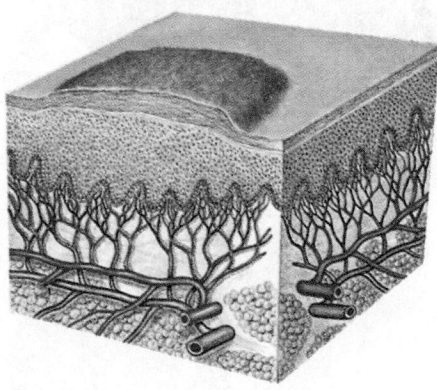

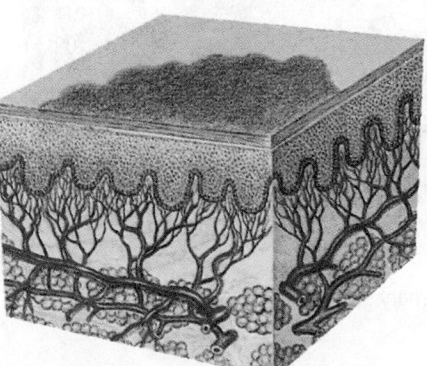

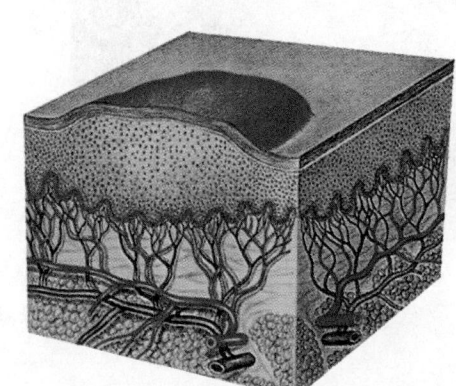

FIG. 53-1 • Primary skin lesions. (From Seidel HM et al: *Mosby's guide to physical examination*, ed 4, St Louis, 1999, Mosby.)

Continued

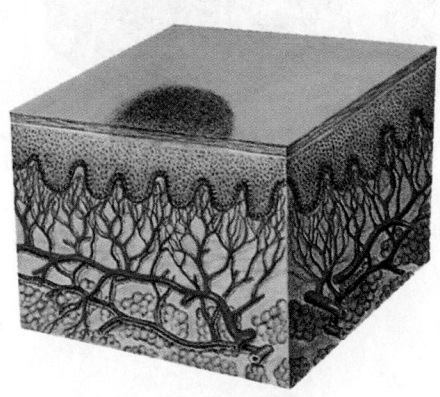

Papule—elevated; palpable; firm; circumscribed; less than 1 cm in diameter; brown, red, pink, tan, or bluish red in color
Examples: Warts; drug-related eruptions; pigmented nevi

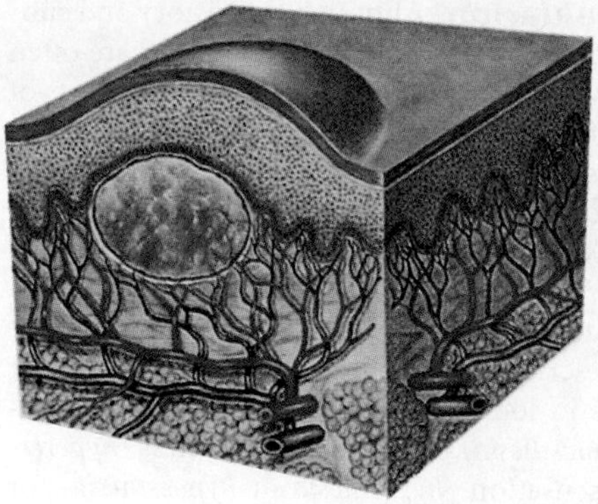

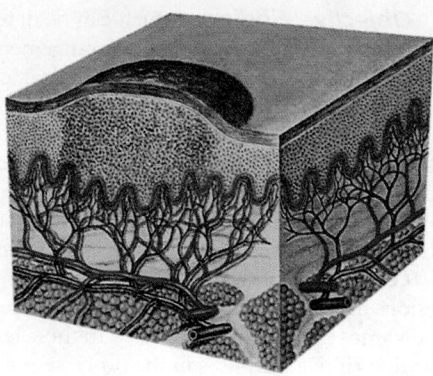

Nodule—elevated; firm; circumscribed; palpable; deeper in dermis than papule; 1 to 2 cm in diameter
Examples: Erythema nodosum; lipomas

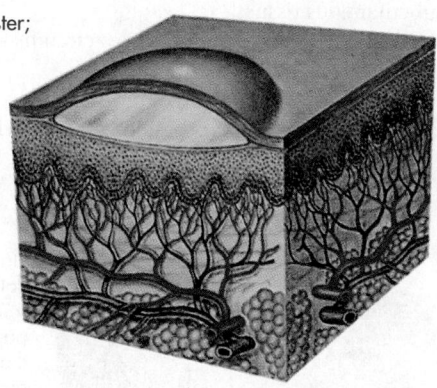

Vesicle—elevated; circumscribed; superficial; filled with serous fluid; less than 1 cm in diameter
Examples: Blister; varicella

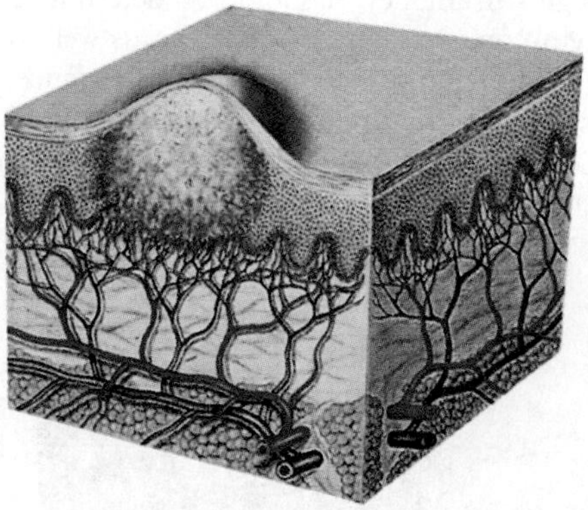

Pustule—elevated; superficial; similar to vesicle but filled with purulent fluid
Examples: Impetigo; acne; variola

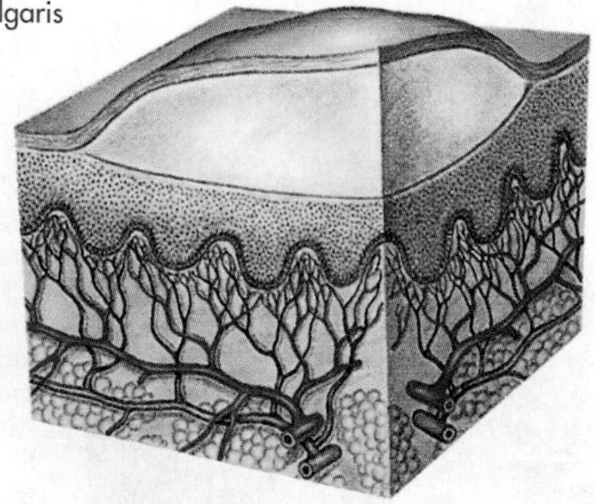

Bulla—vesicle greater than 1 cm in diameter
Examples: Blister; pemphigus vulgaris

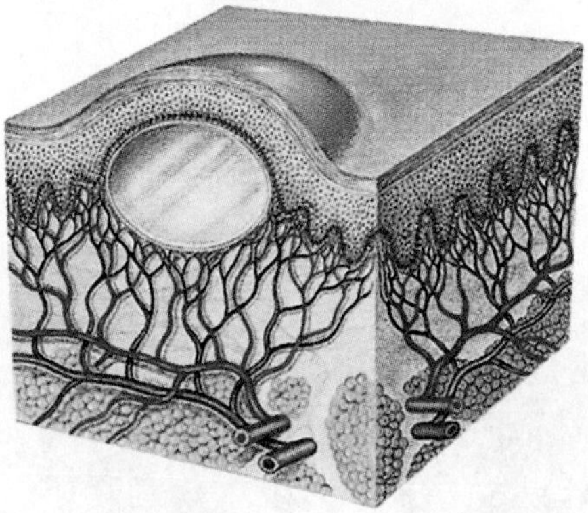

Cyst—elevated; circumscribed; palpable; encapsulated; filled with liquid or semisolid material
Example: Sebaceous cyst

FIG. 53-1, cont'd • Primary skin lesions.

Secondary lesions—Changes that result from alteration in the primary lesions, such as those caused by rubbing, scratching, medication, or involution and healing (Fig. 53-2)

Distribution pattern—The pattern in which lesions are distributed over the body, whether local or generalized, and specific areas associated with the lesions

Configuration and arrangement—The size, shape, and arrangement of a lesion or groups of lesions (e.g., discrete, clustered, diffuse, or confluent)

Laboratory Studies. When it is suspected that a skin problem might be related to a systemic disease, such as one of the collagen diseases or immunodeficiency disease, studies are needed to rule out these possibilities. Diagnostic modalities include microscopic examination, cultures, skin scrapings or biopsy, cytodiagnosis, patch testing, and Wood light examination. Allergic skin testing and various other laboratory tests (e.g., blood count and sedimentation rate) are used when indicated.

Wounds

Wounds are structural or physiologic disruptions of the integument that call for normal or abnormal tissue repair responses. All wounds can be classified as acute or chronic. *Acute wounds* are those that heal uneventfully within the usual time frame. *Chronic wounds* are those that do not heal in the expected time frame or are associated with many complications. In children most wounds are acute and can be prevented from becoming chronic wounds through appropriate nursing care. Wounds are classified in the same manner as burns: partial-thickness, full-thickness, and complex wounds that include muscle and/or bone.

Epidermal Injuries. Abrasions are the most common epidermal wounds of childhood, usually in the form of a skinned knee or elbow. In most injuries the margins of the abraded area are superficial, involving only the outer layers of epidermis, although the central portion may extend into the dermis. Initially the defect is filled by a blood clot and necrotic debris, which subsequently dehydrate to form a scab. Epithelial tissue is composed of *labile cells,* which are constantly destroyed and replaced throughout life. Injury to these tissues results in *regeneration* (i.e., rapid replacement by similar cells).

The epithelial wound heals by migration and proliferation of epithelial cells from the wound margin and from cells surviving in transected skin appendages. This response begins within 24 to 48 hours after the wound is incurred. Cell migration ceases when migrating cells make contact with epithelial cells migrating from all other sites. Fixed basal cells adjacent to the wound edge and in skin appendages begin to divide rapidly to replace the migrated cells. As resurfacing is accomplished, the migrated cells begin to divide and thicken the new epithelial layer.

Epithelial cells advance over the wound surface by "flowing." The first cell advances, anchors, and then moves no more. Instead, a cell from behind advances over it, anchors, and subsequently is overridden by other cells that advance over both the primary cells—similar to a leapfrog movement. Epithelial cells

Crust—dried serum, blood, or purulent exudate; slightly elevated; size varies; brown, red, black, tan, or straw in color
Examples: Scab on abrasion; eczema

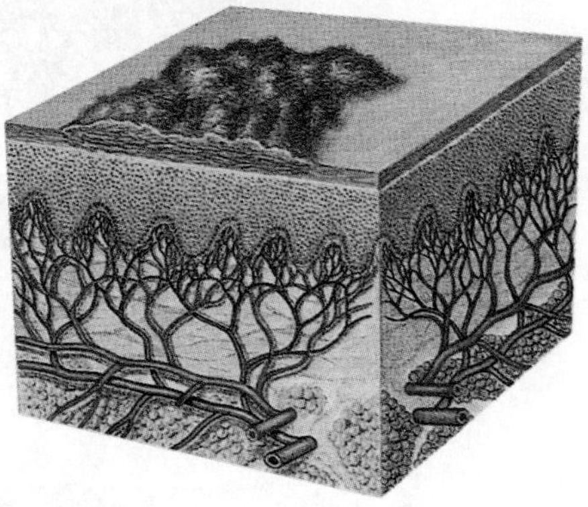

Scale—heaped-up keratinized cells; flaky exfoliation; irregular; thick or thin; dry or oily; varied size; silver, white, or tan in color
Examples: Psoriasis; exfoliative dermatitis

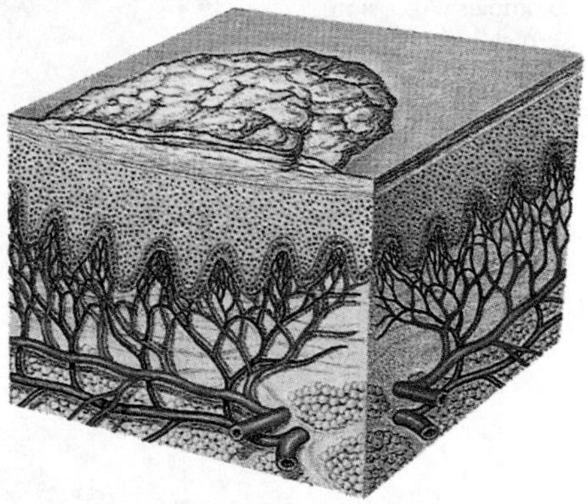

Lichenification—rough, thickened epidermis; accentuated skin markings caused by rubbing or irritation; often involves flexor aspect of extremity
Example: Chronic dermatitis

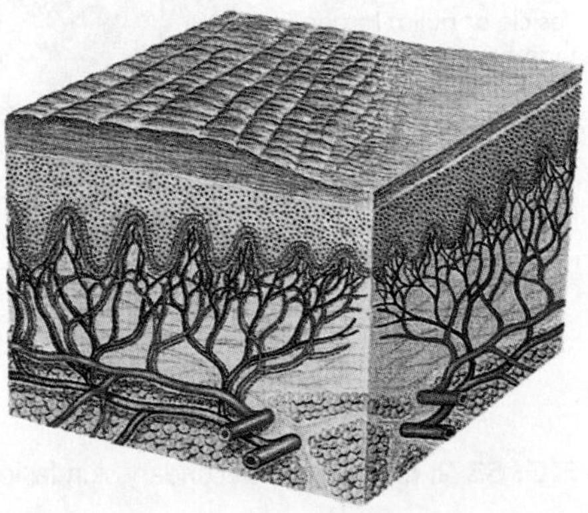

FIG. 53-2 • Secondary skin lesions. (From Seidel HM et al: *Mosby's guide to physical examination,* ed 4, St Louis, 1999, Mosby.) *Continued*

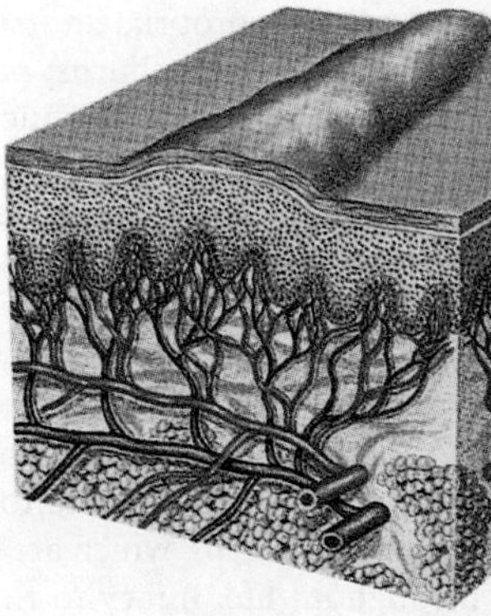

Scar—thin to thick fibrous tissue replacing injured dermis; irregular; pink, red, or white in color; may be atrophic or hypertrophic
Example: Healed wound or surgical incision

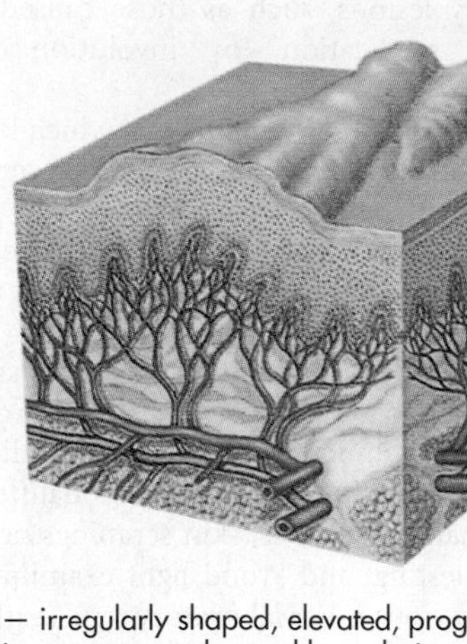

Keloid— irregularly shaped, elevated, progressively enlarging scar; grows beyond boundaries of wound; caused by excessive collagen formation during healing
Example: Keloid from ear piercing or burn scar

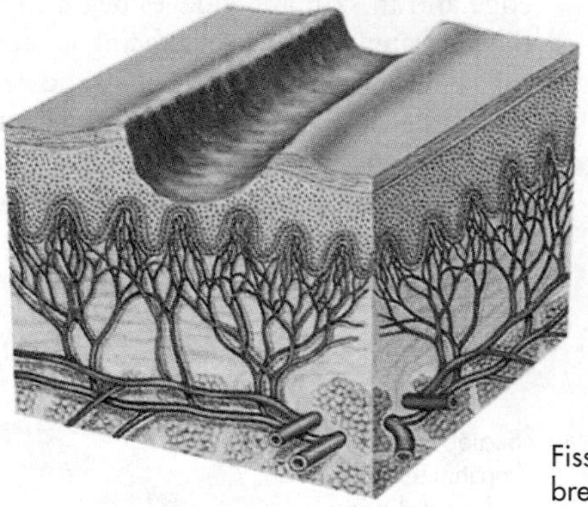

Excoriation—loss of epidermis; linear or hollowed-out crusted area; dermis exposed
Examples: Abrasion; scratch

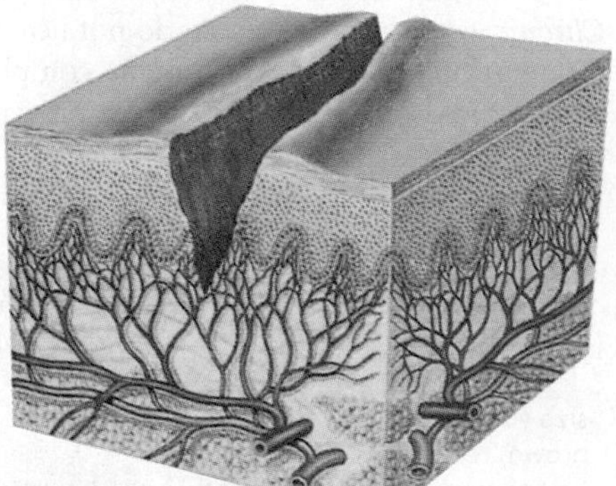

Fissure—linear crack or break from epidermis to dermis; small; deep; red
Examples: Athlete's foot; cheilosis

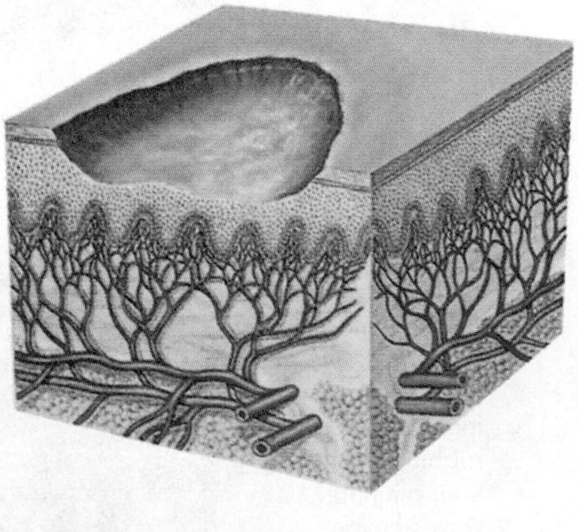

Erosion—loss of all or part of epidermis; depressed; moist; glistening; follows rupture of vesicle or bulla; larger than fissure
Examples: Varicella; variola following rupture

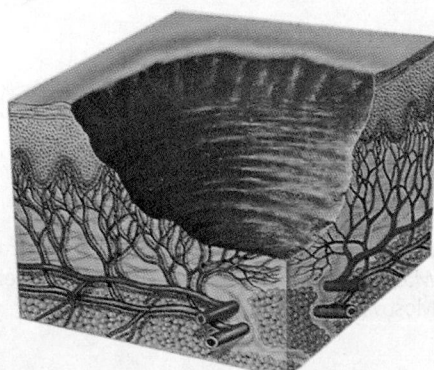

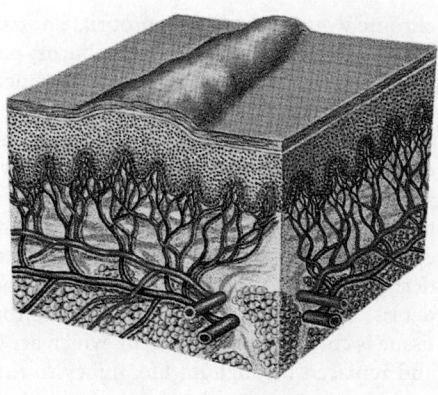

Ulcer—loss of epidermis and dermis; concave; varies in size; exudative; red or reddish blue
Examples: Decubiti; stasis ulcers

FIG. 53-2, cont'd • Secondary skin lesions.

move most rapidly in moist environments, and the rate of epithelization depends on a variety of elements, particularly the amount of oxygen supplied to the wound.

Injury to Deeper Tissues. Tissues composed of *permanent cells,* such as muscle and nerve cells, are unable to regenerate. Therefore these tissues repair themselves by substituting fibrous connective tissue for the injured tissue. This fibrous tissue, or *scar,* serves as a patch to preserve or restore the continuity of the tissue. Wounds involving permanent cells include surgical incisions, lacerations, ulcers, evulsions, and full-thickness burns. Injured cells of glandular organs and bones, composed of *stable* cells, multiply less vigorously and heal more slowly.

Process of Wound Healing. The nonspecific repair mechanism of wound healing with scar formation involves the processes of *inflammation,* fibroplasia, contraction, and scar maturation. The initial response at the site of injury is inflammation, a vascular and cellular response that prepares the tissues for the subsequent repair process. There is a transient constriction of transected blood vessels, lasting 5 to 10 minutes, followed by active vasodilation of all local small vessels and increased blood flow to the area. This is accompanied by increased permeability of small venules, allowing plasma to leak into surrounding tissues *(edema).* A blood clot is formed along wound edges, forming a framework for future growth of capillaries *(angiogenesis)* and epithelial cells.

At the same time, vessel walls become lined with leukocytes, primarily neutrophils, which pass through the walls and concentrate at the injured site, where they ingest bacteria and debris *(phagocytosis).* The presence of neutrophils is superseded by macrophages, which continue phagocytosis, and also by growth factors needed for skin repair and angiogenesis. Fibroblasts attracted to the area from blood vessels deposit fibrin throughout the clot. Adjacent capillaries begin to form buds that stretch across the supporting fibrin threads, and epithelial cells secrete a fibrolytic enzyme that allows their advancement across the wound. This initial phase of wound healing takes place during the first 3 to 5 days after injury. The wound is weakest at this time.

Fibroplasia (granulation or *proliferation),* the second phase of healing, lasts from 5 days to 4 weeks. Fibroblasts, immature connective tissue cells, migrate to the healing site and begin to secrete collagen into the meshwork spaces. Granulation tissue is highly vascular, "beefy" red, and shiny connective tissue that organizes and restructures, forming thicker, stronger fibers arranged in orderly layers. A thin layer of epithelial tissue is regenerated over the surface of the wound, and leukocytes gradually disappear from the area.

During *contraction* and *maturation,* the third and fourth phases of wound healing, collagen continues to be deposited and organized into layers, compressing the new blood vessels and gradually ceasing blood flow across the wound. Fibroblasts disappear as the wound becomes stronger. Fibroblast movement causes contraction of the healing area, helping to bring wound edges closer together. A mature scar is then formed. The maturation process may continue for years, and the extent to which the scar remodels and matures varies among individuals.

Children heal aggressively with abundant scar tissue, especially during growth spurts. The highly elastic quality of children's skin pulls on wounds, which defend against the pull by aggressive scarring. Consequently, the child's skin heals with more scar tissue than the less elastic skin of the adult.

Factors that Influence Healing. During the last two decades, understanding of wound healing has revolutionized the interventions used to promote healing. Emphasis has shifted from interventions directed at maintaining a dry environment that promoted eschar formation to those that promote a moist, crust-free environment that enhances the migration of epithelial cells across the wound and facilitates resurfacing. An acute full-thickness wound kept in a moist environment usually reepithelializes in 12 to 15 days, whereas the same wound when kept open to the air heals in approximately 25 to 30 days.

Numerous factors have been identified that delay healing (Table 53-1). Many traditional practices, such as the use of antiseptics (e.g., hydrogen peroxide and povidone-iodine [Betadine] solutions), thought to prevent infection, actually have a cytotoxic effect on healthy cells and minimal effect on controlling infections. Povidone-iodine may be absorbed through the skin, especially in neonates and young children.

NURSE ALERT • Do not put anything in a wound that you would not put in the eye. The safest solution is normal saline.

General Therapeutic Management

The human body tends to heal; therefore treatment is directed toward eliminating or ameliorating influences that interfere with normal healing processes. Some disorders may demand aggressive therapy, but by and large the major aim of any treatment is to prevent further damage, eliminate the cause, prevent complications, and provide relief from discomfort while tissues undergo healing. Factors that contribute to the dermatitis and prolong the course of the disease must be eliminated when possible. The most common offenders in pediatrics are environmental factors (e.g., soaps, bubble baths, shampoos, rough or tight clothing, wet diapers, blankets, and toys) and the natural elements (e.g., dirt, sand, heat, cold, moisture, and wind). Dermatitis can also be aggravated by home remedies and medications.

Dressings. Dressings serve several useful functions. They (1) provide a moist healing environment, (2) protect the wound from infection and trauma, (3) provide compression in the event of anticipated bleeding or swelling, (4) apply medication, (5) absorb drainage, (6) debride necrotic tissue, (7) reduce pain, and (8) control odor. To provide a moist environment, open wounds are covered with an occlusive ointment or dressing (Table 53-2). No one dressing meets the needs of all types of wounds. The traditional gauze dressing should not be used on open wounds because it allows the wound surface to dry, does little to prevent bacterial invasion, and adheres to the dried scab so that removal disturbs the newly regenerating epithelial cells. In many situations, traditional gauze dressings have been replaced with new "active occlusive" dressings that allow moist wound healing.

Topical Therapy. A variety of agents and methods are available for treatment of dermatologic problems. In selecting a therapeutic program, the practitioner considers (1) a choice of active ingredient, (2) a proper vehicle or base, (3) the cosmetic effect, (4) the cost, and (5) instructions for its use. In addition, several basic concepts are kept in mind. Overtreatment is avoided. For example, when the dermatitis is acute,

TABLE 53-1
Factors that Delay Wound Healing

Factor	Effect on Healing
Dry wound environment	Allows epithelial cells to dry out and die; impairs migration of epithelial cells across wound surface
Nutritional deficiencies	
Vitamin C	Inhibits formation of collagen fibers and capillary development
Protein	Reduces supply of amino acids for tissue repair
Zinc	Impairs epithelialization
Impaired circulation	Reduces supply of nutrients to wound area
	Inhibits inflammatory response and removal of debris from wound area
Stress (pain, poor sleep)	Releases catecholamines that cause vasoconstriction
Antiseptics	
Hydrogen peroxide	Toxic to fibroblasts; can cause subcutaneous gas formation (mimics gas-forming infection)
Povidone-iodine	Toxic to white and red blood cells and fibroblasts
Chlorhexidine	Toxic to white blood cells
Corticosteroids	Impairs phagocytosis
	Inhibits fibroblast proliferation
	Depresses formation of granulation tissue
	Inhibits wound contraction
Foreign bodies	Inhibits wound closure
	Increases inflammatory response
Infection	Increases inflammatory response
	Increases tissue destruction
Mechanical friction	Damages or destroys granulation tissue
Fluid accumulation	Accumulation in area inhibits tissues from approximating
Radiation	Inhibits fibroblastic activity and capillary formation
	May cause tissue necrosis
Diseases	
Diabetes mellitus	Inhibits collagen synthesis
	Impairs circulation and capillary growth
	Hyperglycemia impairs phagocytosis
Anemia	Reduces oxygen supply to tissues

the applications should be mild and bland to avoid further irritation. Broken or inflamed skin, especially in children, is more absorbent than intact skin, and chemicals that are nonirritating to intact skin may be quite irritating to inflamed skin.

Topical applications may be applied to treat the disorder, reduce the itching associated with many diseases, decrease external stimuli, or apply external heat or cold. The emollient action of soaks, baths, and lotions provides a soothing film over the skin surface that reduces external stimuli. Ordinarily lukewarm, tepid, or cool applications offer the greatest relief.

NURSE ALERT • Application of heat tends to aggravate most conditions, and its use is usually reserved for reducing specific inflammatory processes such as folliculitis and cellulitis.

Topical Corticosteroid Therapy. The glucocorticoids are the therapeutic agents used most commonly for skin disorders. Their local antiinflammatory effects are merely palliative, so that the medication must be applied until the disease state undergoes a remission or the causative agent is eliminated. Corticosteroids are applied directly to the affected area and, because they are essentially nonsensitizing and have only minor side effects, can be applied over prolonged periods with continuing effectiveness. As with the use of any steroids, their use in large amounts may mask signs of infection, and symptoms may be exacerbated after termination of the drug. Families are cautioned that the medication cannot be used for all skin disorders. The concentrations available without prescription are not adequate for some stubborn conditions (e.g., psoriasis) and may cause worsening of inflammation caused by fungus or bacteria. It has also been found that users apply too much topical hydrocortisone; they should be counseled that it is both effective and economical to apply only a thin film and massage it into the skin.

Other Topical Therapies. Other topical treatments include chemical cautery (especially useful for warts), cryosurgery, electrodesiccation (chiefly used for warts, granulomas, and nevi), ultraviolet therapy (primarily used in psoriasis and acne), laser therapy (especially for birthmarks), and special acne therapies such as dermabrasion and chemical peels.

Systemic Therapy. Therapeutic agents are often used as an adjunct to topical therapy in dermatologic disorders, and those most commonly used therapeutically are the corticosteroids and the antibiotics. The corticosteroid hormones, with their capacity to inhibit inflammatory and allergic reactions, are valuable in the treatment of severe skin disorders. Dosage is carefully adjusted and gradually tapered to the minimum that is effective and tolerated. In infants and children, dosage is larger than is usually calculated from body weight ratios; however, prolonged use may temporarily suppress growth.

Antibiotics, which interfere with the growth of microorganisms, are used in severe or widespread skin infections; however, because they tend to produce hypersensitivity in the patient, they are used with caution. Antifungal agents are the only means for treating systemic fungal infections.

Nursing Care Management of the Child with a Skin Disorder

To help establish a diagnosis, it is important for nurses to accurately describe any deviation in the character of the skin. Using both inspection and palpation, the color, shape, and distribution of the lesions or wounds are noted. The individual lesions are described according to the accepted terminology and may involve more than one type (e.g., a maculopapular rash). Wounds are assessed for depth of tissue damage, evidence of healing, and signs of infection.

TABLE 53-2

Properties of Commonly Used Occlusive Dressings and Other Products*

Examples	Indications	Advantages	Disadvantages	Considerations
POLYURETHANE FILMS				
Op-Site, Tegaderm, Bioclusive, Blister-film, Acu-derm, Polyskin II, Transorb, Epi View	Protection of partial-thickness red wounds Cover dressing for hydrophilic preparations and hydrogels Autolytic debridement of wounds with dry eschar	Transparent; good adhesion; reduce pain, minimize friction forces to wound; timesaving; easy to store; cost-effective Moisture, vapor, and oxygen transmission Impermeable to water and bacteria	Adhesive injury to intact and new skin; nonabsorbent; some products difficult to apply; variable barrier function; can promote wound infection Unsuitable for electrical stimulation wound healing	Protect wound margins; avoid in wounds with infection, copious drainage, tracts or fragile skin surrounding lesion Change only if dressing leaks
POLYMERIC FOAMS				
Allevyn, Allevyn Adhesive, Allevyn Cavity, Nu-Derm, Lyofoam, PolyMem	Used when a nonadherent dressing is needed Used on burns	Moisture is absorbed into foam; maceration is decreased Removal does not cause reinjury to wound Comfortable, easy to apply; cushion and protect wound	Requires an additional dressing to secure	Do not use on infected wounds
HYDROCOLLOIDS				
DuoDerm CGF, DuoDerm Extra Thin, Comfeel, Restore, Tegasorb, Signa-Dress, Cutinova Hydro, Ultec, Acti-derm, Replicare	Protection of superficial and small, deep red wounds Autolytic debridement of small, noninfected yellow wounds† Partial thickness, stages 2 and 3; shallow full thickness, granulating with minimal to moderate exudate, stage 4	Absorbent; nonadhesive to healing tissue; waterproof; reduce pain; easy to apply; timesaving; easy to store Moldable to area; occlusive; provide insulation; maintain moist wound surface; wet-to-dry adherence	Nontransparent; may soften and lose shape with heat or friction; odor and brown drainage on removal (melted dressing material)	Frequency of changes depend on amount of exudate (change as needed for leakage) DO NOT USE for heavily exudative wounds, sinus tracts, or infected wounds; shape dressing to wound area
HYDROGELS/SHEETS				
Vigilon, Elastogel, Aquasorb, Nu-Gel, Duo-Derm Gel, Second Skin, Hypergel, Intra-Site gel	Protection of superficial and moderately deep red wounds Autolytic debridement of small, noninfected yellow or black wounds† Delivery system for topical antimicrobial creams (increases penetration) Partial and full thickness	Absorbent; nonadhesive; reduce pain; compatible with topicals; good conformity; easy to store Maintain a moist wound surface, have a "cooling" effect	Poor barrier; semitransparent; require cover dressing to secure; can promote growth of *Pseudomonas* and other gram-negative bacteria and yeast Unused portion will dessicate Not for weight-bearing ulcers Expensive; nonadhesive High water content can macerate surrounding skin	Avoid in infected wounds; change every 8 hours or as needed for leakage Cut and shape to wound DO NOT REMOVE poly backing

Modified from Cuzzell JZ: Choosing a wound dressing: a systematic approach, *AACN Clin Issues Crit Care Nurse* 1(3):566–577, 1990; Krasner D, Kane D: *Chronic wound care; a clinical source book for healthcare professionals,* ed 2, Wayne, PA, 1997, Health Management Publications; and McCulloch JM, Kloth LC, Feedar JA: *Wound healing alternatives in management,* Philadelphia, 1995, FA Davis.

*Stephen Jones, MS, RNC, PNP, ET, assisted in the revision of this table.

†NOTE: Users should read package inserts for any contraindications to the use of these products. Some dressings, such as Duoderm CGF, have been approved for application to infected wounds, provided that the wound is cultured and treated for the infection. However, Duoderm CGF should not be used on full-thickness burns.

Continued

TABLE 53-2
Properties of Commonly Used Occlusive Dressings and Other Products*—cont'd

Examples	Indications	Advantages	Disadvantages	Considerations
HYDROCOLLOID ABSORPTION POWDERS, PASTES, BEADS, AND GRANULES				
Bard absorption dressing, Comfeel Ulcus paste, Comfeel Ulcus powder, Multidex powder and gel, Debrisan	Used on uneven and exudating ulcers	Control bacteria Cleanse wound Reduce odor Cost-effective		Cleanse with lukewarm water or saline to remove
ALGINATES				
Sorbsan, Kaltostat, Curasorb, Algi Site	Used for leg ulcers, burns, donor sites, infected traumatic or exudating wounds	Nonallergenic; biodegradable; little to no local tissue reaction Decrease pain at wound site	Expensive; easily displaced by mechanical forces Permeable to bacteria, urine	Change daily after proper cleansing if used on infected wounds

NURSE ALERT • Signs of wound infection are:
- Increased erythema, especially beyond wound margin
- Edema
- Purulent exudate
- Pain
- Increased temperature

To confirm or amplify the findings made by inspection, the skin is gently palpated to detect characteristics such as temperature, moisture, texture, elasticity, and the presence of edema. It should be indicated whether the findings are restricted to the area of the lesion(s) or are generalized.

The child's subjective symptoms provide additional information. Older children are able to describe the condition as painful, itching, or tingling or in other descriptive terms. However, much can be determined by observing the younger child's behavior and the parents' account of these reactions. Does the child scratch? Is the child restless or irritable? Does the child favor or avoid using a body part? A careful history may provide clues. Has the child had access to chemicals or been in the woods or around a woodpile? Has the child eaten a new food? Is the child taking medication? Has the child any known allergy? Do any playmates have a similar lesion? A doubtful diagnosis is commonly confirmed on the basis of history.

Therapeutic programs are usually designed to provide general measures such as rest, protection, and relief of discomfort; and specific treatments such as a definitive medication or physical technique. Because only a few skin diseases are contagious, it is usually not necessary to isolate the affected child unless there is a danger of acquiring a secondary infection (e.g., the child receiving large doses of corticosteroids or other immunosuppressant drugs or the child with an immunologic deficiency disorder). If the skin manifestation is caused by a viral exanthema, such as measles or chickenpox, the child is prevented from exposing other susceptible children.

Wound Care. Small wounds to the skin are managed by the parents at home. The parents are instructed to wash their hands and then wash the wound gently with mild soap and water for several minutes, followed by thorough rinsing. Open wounds are covered with a dressing such as a commercial adhesive bandage, although larger wounds may benefit from the use of occlusive dressings (see Table 53-2). If occlusive dressings are applied, instruct the parents on their correct application and removal. For example, hydrocolloid dressings adhere best if a wide margin is left around the wound and the dressing is pressed against intact skin until it adheres.* The edges of the dressing can be secured to the skin with waterproof tape. They are removed if leakage occurs or after a specific time interval, usually 7 days. Dressings are removed carefully to protect intact skin and prevent damage to the epithelial surface of the wound. To remove transparent or hydrocolloid dressings, raise one edge of the dressing and pull *parallel* to the skin to loosen the adhesive. The longer the dressings are left on, the easier they are to remove.

NURSE ALERT • Advise parents that the yellow gel forming under hydrocolloid dressings may look like pus and has a distinct odor (somewhat fruity) but is normal leakage.

Lacerations present a special challenge. The injured child and family are usually very distressed by the bleeding and are in variable degrees of shock; parental guilt usually accompanies the injury. Because scalp lacerations bleed so profusely, they are especially frightening. The initial nursing intervention is to apply pressure to the area and attempt to calm the child before further examination. Unless there is bleeding from a severed artery, the wound can be cleansed with a forced jet of sterile tepid water or saline (via syringe) and examined for extent, depth, and presence of foreign material such as dirt, glass, or fabric fragments.

NURSE ALERT • Hydrogen peroxide and povidone-iodine are contraindicated for cleaning fresh, open wounds. Hydrogen peroxide can cause formation of subcutaneous gas when applied under pressure.

*Information on the use of the hydrocolloid dressing Duoderm is available from ConvaTec Professional Services, P.O. Box 5254, Princeton, NJ 08543; 1-800-422-8811; fax (908) 281-2405; website: www.convatec.com.

The location of the wound also dictates assessment. For example, wounds over bony areas may contain bone chips, and clear fluid seeping from severe head wounds may indicate leakage of cerebrospinal fluid. A pressure dressing is applied for transfer to medical care; the child in a medical facility is prepared for suturing (Atraumatic Care box).

Puncture wounds that do not require a tetanus booster are soaked in warm water and soap for several minutes. Causing the wound to rebleed may be helpful. An adhesive bandage can be applied if desired. Puncture wounds of the head, chest, or abdomen—and those that could still contain a portion of the puncturing object—must be evaluated.

Parents are cautioned against opening blisters or kissing a wound "to make it better." The wound can easily become contaminated from germs in the human mouth. If scabs form, they are allowed to slough off without assistance; picking or early removal may cause scarring. Parents are advised to seek medical help if there is evidence of infection.

Relief of Symptoms. Most of the therapeutic regimens for skin lesions are directed toward relief of pruritus, the most common subjective complaint. Cooling the affected area; increasing the skin pH with measures such as cool baths or compresses to reduce external stimuli to the area; and alkaline applications (e.g., baking soda baths) to increase skin pH all help to prevent scratching. Clothing and bed linen should be soft and lightweight to decrease the irritation from friction and stimulation.

During any type of treatment, both affected and unaffected skin is protected from damage and secondary infection. Preventing scratching is of primary importance. Older children will usually cooperate, although they may need to be reminded to stop scratching or rubbing. In smaller and uncooperative children, the use of techniques and devices such as mittens (especially during sleep) or special coverings is required. Keeping fingernails short, well trimmed, and clean helps reduce the chance of secondary infection.

Antipruritic medications such as diphenhydramine (Benadryl) or hydroxyzine (Atarax) may be prescribed for severe itching, especially if it disturbs the child's rest. Pain and discomfort are usually managed with nonpharmacologic measures and mild analgesia; severe pain may require more potent medication. Occlusive dressings over wounds reduce pain. For suturing wounds a topical anesthetic or intradermal buffered lidocaine can be used. (See Pain Management, Chapter 44.)

Topical Therapy. Therapy usually involves some type of topical treatment, and the mode of application depends on the nature and location of the lesion being treated. It is especially important to wash the hands before and after application of topical therapies. The skin is assessed before the treatment or application of medication and reassessed after the treatment is completed. Any observed changes are noted and described.

Wet compresses or *dressings* cool the skin by evaporation, relieve itching and inflammation, and cleanse the area by loosening and removing crusts and debris. Any of a variety of ingredients, such as plain water or Burow solution (available without a prescription), can be applied on Kerlix gauze, plain gauze, or (preferably) soft cotton cloths such as freshly laundered handkerchiefs or strips from diapers, sheeting, or pillowcase material.

Dressings immersed in the desired solution are wrung out slightly and applied to the affected area wet but not dripping. They are applied flat and smooth and in such a way that motion is not totally restricted: fingers are wrapped separately, and arms and legs are wrapped so that elbows and knees can bend. Dressings are kept in place by Kerlix or other cotton wrap, tubular stockinette, mittens, and socks (two pairs—one to hold the dressings in place, the other to take up movement) but are left uncovered. When evaporation begins to dry them, the dressings are removed, rewet in the solution, and reapplied to the area using aseptic technique. The solution is not poured or syringed directly over the dressings. As fluid evaporates, the solution becomes increasingly concentrated and thus stronger, which may be damaging to sensitive lesions.

Fresh solution at room temperature is applied at 2-, 3-, or 4-hour intervals and is allowed to remain on the lesion from 30 minutes to 1½ hours. Wet dressings are seldom continued after 48 hours. The child must be guarded against chilling during treatment, and no more than 20% of the body should be covered at one time to avoid the risk of hypothermia. After treatment, the skin is dried thoroughly by patting with a towel. Application of lotion or other medication may be ordered at this time.

When children are uncooperative in the use of wet dressings, *soaks* with the same solution as for wet compresses are often used for removal of crusts and for their mild astringent action. Gaining young children's cooperation for hand or foot soaks is difficult unless the procedure is made attractive to them through play.

Older infants and toddlers delight in playing with brightly colored objects or poker chips scattered over the bottom of the receptacle, and preschoolers can be challenged to hold a floating item beneath the water's surface. These activities require supervision; infants and small children will often place items in their mouths, and children can easily lose control with water play. Washing dishes, cars, dolls, or doll clothes will occupy many children for quite some time.

Although older children are able to cooperate, they may need something to do during the procedure, such as listening to music or a story, or watching television. A single extremity (e.g., a foot or a hand) can be easily soaked by placing the solution and the extremity in a plastic sealable bag. The closure is then zipped snugly around the limb.

Atraumatic Care

PAINLESS SUTURING AND WOUND CLEANSING

A variety of topical anesthetic solutions, such as lidocaine, adrenaline, and tetracaine combined (LAT) and tetracaine-phenylephrine (tetraphen), applied to wounds, especially on the head, scalp, and face, provide anesthesia in 10 to 15 minutes (Smith et al, 1996). Tetracaine, adrenaline, and cocaine combined (TAC) or AC (without tetracaine) should not be used because of the potential for lethal cocaine intoxication. LAT is as effective, is safer, and is much less expensive than TAC. If further anesthesia is required or if the topical preparations are not available, using buffered lidocaine administered with a 30-gauge needle reduces the stinging and burning of the injection (see Pain Management, Chapter 44). The use of a noninvasive tissue adhesive (e.g., Derma Bond*) provides a faster and less painful method of facial laceration repair with cosmetic results comparable to those obtained with suturing (Osmond, Klassen, and Quinn, 1995).

*Manufactured by Closure Medical Corporation, Raleigh, NC.

Baths are especially useful in the treatment of widespread dermatitis because they evenly distribute the soothing antipruritic and antiinflammatory effects of the solution, usually an oatmeal or mineral oil preparation. The solution is added to a tub of lukewarm water. The temperature of the bath is tepid, and the treatment usually lasts 15 to 30 minutes. Therapeutic baths are always more interesting when the child has toy boats or other items for water play.

Topical applications are applied to skin lesions to ease discomfort, prevent further injury, and facilitate healing. Most preparations are placed directly on the skin and left uncovered; others may be applied under an occlusive dressing. A thin application of the ointment or cream is covered with plastic film and anchored with adhesive or covered with a commercial transparent dressing. Occlusive dressings promote moisture retention and nonevaporation of the preparation, increasing the penetration of the medication. Regardless of the type of preparation used, parents need detailed information on how to apply it and how long the preparation should remain on the skin or under an occlusive dressing.

Apply topical applications systematically with the contour of the body surface (not simply up and down). Children love to be "painted": therefore, lotion applications can be fun when applied with an ordinary paintbrush.

NURSE ALERT • Provide written instructions and demonstrate to parents the correct amount of topical medication to apply (e.g., size of a pea, or a thin film to cover). If more than one preparation is applied, mark the containers 1 and 2 for parents to remember the correct order. Stress that more is not necessarily better with some medications, such as steroids.

Home Care and Family Support. Dermatologic conditions always involve the family. Because few situations require hospitalization and children who are hospitalized will complete a therapy program at home, the family must carry out the treatment plan; therefore their cooperation is essential. Regimens that are simple to accomplish in the hospital or office may be frustrating and baffling at home. The family often needs assistance in adapting equipment available in the home to the therapy.

It is important that the child and family be given as detailed an explanation as possible about both the expected and unexpected results of treatment, including any ill effects that might occur. If unexplained reactions do develop, the family is directed to discontinue treatment and report the reactions to the appropriate person(s). The use of over-the-counter medicines is discouraged unless they have first been discussed with the attending practitioner and received approval.

Because the skin is the most visible portion of the body, defects that alter its appearance are sometimes a source of distress to the child and of revulsion and rejection by others. Parents of other children may fear that their children will "catch" the disorder. Occasionally the affected child's own family members will reduce their interaction with him or her (especially close physical contact) or otherwise demonstrate distaste for the condition. The child may interpret this as rejection. This is seldom a difficulty with dermatitis of short duration, but chronic conditions can create problems in development of a positive self-concept (Nursing Care Plan).

INFECTIONS OF THE SKIN

Bacterial Infections

Normally, the skin harbors a variety of bacterial flora, including the major pathogenic varieties of staphylococci and streptococci. The degree of their pathogenicity depends on the invasiveness and toxigenicity of the specific organism, the integrity of the skin, and the immune and cellular defenses of the host. Children with congenital or acquired immunodeficiency disorders (e.g., acquired immunodeficiency syndrome [AIDS]), those in a debilitated condition, those receiving immunosuppressant agents, and those with a generalized malignancy such as leukemia or lymphoma are at risk for developing bacterial infections.

Because of the characteristic "walling-off" process of the inflammatory reaction (abscess formation), staphylococci are more difficult to attack, and the local infected area is associated with an increase in numbers of bacteria all over the skin surface that serve as a source of continuing infection. Staphylococcal infections occur most often in younger children, and the incidence decreases with advancing age. All of these factors emphasize the importance of careful handwashing and cleanliness when caring for infected children and their lesions, both to prevent spread of the infection and as an essential prophylactic measure. Common bacterial skin disorders are outlined in Table 53-3.

Nursing Care Management. The major nursing functions related to bacterial skin infections are to prevent the spread of infection and to prevent complications. Handwashing is mandatory before and after contact with the affected child. Handwashing is also emphasized to both the child and the family, and the child should be provided with towels separate from those of other family members. Impetigo contagiosa is easily spread by self-inoculation; therefore the child must be cautioned against touching the involved area. This is difficult to accomplish; distraction or reminders are useful but are not helpful when the child is alone, such as at bedtime.

Children and parents are often tempted to squeeze follicular lesions. They must be warned that squeezing will not hasten the resolution of the infection and that there are risks of making the lesion worse and of spreading the infection. No attempt should be made to puncture the surface of the pustule with a needle or sharp instrument. A child with a sty may awaken with the eyelids of the affected eye sealed shut with exudate. The child or the parents are instructed to gently wipe the lid from the inner to the outer edge with warm water and a clean washcloth until the exudate has been removed.

The child with limited cellulitis of an extremity is usually managed at home on a regimen of oral antibiotics and warm compresses. The parents are taught the procedures and instructed in administration of the medication. Children with more extensive cellulitis, especially around a joint with lymphadenitis or on the face, are usually admitted to the hospital for parenteral antibiotics with continued treatment at home. Nurses are responsible for teaching the family to administer the medication and apply compresses.

Viral Infections

Viruses are intracellular parasites that produce their effect by using the intracellular substances of the host cells. Composed of

Nursing Care Plan THE CHILD WITH A SKIN DISORDER

NURSING DIAGNOSIS Impaired skin integrity related to environmental agents, somatic factors, immunologic deficit

EXPECTED OUTCOME The child exhibits signs of skin healing, intact skin remains free of irritation or secondary infection, and there is no evidence of recurring lesions.

Nursing Interventions/*Rationales*

Provide moist environment for lesions (dressing ointment) *to provide optimum healing of wounds.*

Administer topical and systemic medications as ordered *to aid healing and prevent infection.*

Keep lesions, surrounding skin, clothing, and linens clean and dry *to promote healing and prevent secondary infection and mechanical trauma.*

Use good handwashing technique before and after administration of care *to prevent infection;* teach child and family about importance of handwashing and hygiene measures *to prevent spread of infection.*

Use methods as appropriate (e.g., short nails, mittens, elbow splints, clothing that covers lesions) *to prevent child from touching or scratching lesions and prevent autoinoculation and secondary infection.*

Teach child and family to recognize and avoid contact with agents/allergens known to precipitate skin reaction *to prevent recurrence of lesions.*

Observe skin frequently for signs of spread, secondary infection, irritation, or breakdown *so appropriate treatment measures can be instituted.*

NURSING DIAGNOSIS Risk for infection related to presence of infective organisms

EXPECTED OUTCOME Infection is confined to primary site.

Nursing Interventions/*Rationales*

Implement universal precautions, use careful handwashing, avoid unnecessary close contact during infective stage *to prevent spread of infection.*

Implement isolation techniques as appropriate, including proper disposal of all items that come in contact with infective lesions *to prevent spread of infection.*

Teach child and family about handwashing and hygiene techniques *to reduce risk of spread of infection.*

NURSING DIAGNOSIS Pain related to itching, trauma of skin lesions

EXPECTED OUTCOME The child exhibits signs of comfort, and there is no evidence of scratching.

Nursing Interventions/*Rationales*

Administer topical and systemic agents as ordered *to reduce pain and itching.*

Implement nonpharmacologic pain reduction techniques as appropriate (e.g., distraction, relaxation, guided imagery, positive self-talk, cutaneous stimulation) *to relieve pain.*

Advocate for child regarding appropriate anesthesia for wound suturing *to prevent unnecessary pain and emotional trauma.*

NURSING DIAGNOSIS Body-image disturbance related to appearance altered by skin lesions

EXPECTED OUTCOME The child demonstrates a positive body image.

Nursing Interventions/*Rationales*

Encourage child to express feelings and ask questions about appearance and perceived reactions of others *to facilitate coping.*

Discuss with child and family the expected progression of the skin lesions and healing process *to provide a sense of hope and control.*

Have child participate in care and maintain usual routine and activities as much as possible *to promote a sense of normalcy and adequacy.*

only a DNA or RNA core enclosed in an antigenic protein shell, viruses are unable to provide for their own metabolic needs or to reproduce themselves. After a virus penetrates the cell of the host organism, it sheds its outer shell and disappears within the cell, where the nucleic acid core stimulates the host cell to form more virus material from its intracellular substance. In a viral infection the epidermal cells react with inflammation and vesiculation (as in herpes simplex) or by proliferating to form growths (as in warts).

Most of the communicable diseases of childhood are associated with rashes, and each rash is characteristic. The type of lesion and the configuration of the viral exanthemas of rubeola, rubella, and chickenpox are described in Table 38-1. Other common viral disorders of the skin are outlined in Table 53-4.

TABLE 53-3
Bacterial Infections

Disorder/Organism	Manifestations	Management	Comments
Impetigo contagiosa (Fig. 53-3)—*Staphylococcus*	Begins as a reddish macule Becomes vesicular Ruptures easily, leaving superficial, moist erosion Tends to spread peripherally in sharply marginated irregular outlines Exudate dries to form heavy, honey-colored crusts Pruritus common Systemic effects: minimal or asymptomatic	Careful removal of undermined skin, crusts, and debris by softening with 1:20 Burow solution compresses Topical application of bactericidal ointment Systemic administration of oral or parenteral antibiotics (penicillin) in severe or extensive lesions	Tends to heal without scarring unless secondary infection Autoinoculable and contagious Very common in toddler, preschooler May be superimposed on eczema
Pyoderma—*Staphylococcus, Streptococcus*	Deeper extension of infection into dermis Tissue reaction more severe Systemic effects: fever, lymphangitis	Soap and water cleansing Wet compresses Bathing with antibacterial soap as prescribed	Autoinoculable and contagious May heal with or without scarring
Folliculitis (pimple), furuncle (boil), carbuncle (multiple boils)—*Staphylococcus aureus*	Folliculitis: infection of hair follicle Furuncle: larger lesion with more redness and swelling at a single follicle Carbuncle: more extensive lesion with widespread inflammation and "pointing" at several follicular orifices Systemic effects: malaise, if severe	Skin cleanliness Local warm, moist compresses Topical application of antibiotic agents Systemic antibiotics in severe cases Incision and drainage of severe lesions, followed by wound irrigations with antibiotics or suitable drain implantation	Autoinoculable and contagious Furuncle and carbuncle tend to heal with scar formation A lesion should *never* be squeezed
Cellulitis—*Streptococcus, Staphylococcus, Haemophilus influenzae* (Fig. 53-4)	Inflammation of skin and subcutaneous tissues with intense redness, swelling, and firm infiltration Lymphangitis "streaking" frequently seen Involvement of regional lymph nodes common May progress to abscess formation Systemic effects: fever, malaise	Oral or parenteral antibiotics Rest and immobilization of both affected area and child Hot moist compresses to area	Hospitalization may be necessary for child with systemic symptoms Otitis media may be associated with facial cellulitis
Staphylococcal scalded skin syndrome—*S. aureus*	Macular erythema with "sandpaper" texture of involved skin Epidermis becomes wrinkled (in 2 days or less), and large bullae appear	Systemic administration of antibiotics Gentle cleansing with saline, Burow solution, or 0.25% silver nitrate compresses	Infant subject to fluid loss; impaired body temperature regulation; and secondary infection, such as pneumonia, cellulitis, and septicemia Heals without scarring

Dermatophytoses (Fungal Infections)

The dermatophytoses (ringworm) are infections caused by a group of closely related filamentous fungi that invade primarily the stratum corneum, hair, and nails. These are superficial infections that live on, not in, the skin. They are confined to the dead keratin layers and are unable to survive in the deeper layers. Because the keratin is being desquamated constantly, the fungus must multiply at a rate that equals the rate of keratin production to maintain itself; otherwise, the infection would be shed with the discarded skin cells. Common dermatophytoses are outlined in Table 53-5.

Dermatophytoses are designated by the Latin word *tinea,* with further designation related to the area of the body where they are found (e.g., tinea capitis [ringworm of the scalp]). Dermatophyte infections are most often transmitted from one person to another or from infected animals to humans. Diagnosis is made from microscopic examination of scrapings taken from the advancing periphery of the lesion, which almost always produces scale.

TABLE 53-4
Viral Infections

Infection	Manifestations	Management	Comments
Verruca (warts) Cause: human papillomavirus (various types)	Small, benign tumors Usually well-circumscribed, gray or brown, elevated, firm papules with a roughened, finely papillomatous texture Occur anywhere, but usually appear on exposed areas such as fingers, hands, face, and soles May be single or multiple Asymptomatic	Not uniformly successful Local destructive therapy, individualized according to location, type, and number—surgical removal, electrocautery, curettage, cryotherapy (liquid nitrogen), caustic solutions (lactic acid and salicylic acid in flexible collodion, retinoic acid, salicylic acid plasters), x-ray treatment, laser Hypnotherapy may be effective	Common in children Tend to disappear spontaneously Course unpredictable Most destructive techniques tend to leave scars Autoinoculable Repeated irritation will cause to enlarge Apply topical anesthetic EMLA
Verruca plantaris (plantar wart)	Located on plantar surface of feet and, because of pressure, are practically flat; may be surrounded by a collar of hyperkeratosis	Apply caustic solution to wart, wear foam insole with hole cut to relieve pressure on wart; soak 20 minutes after 2-3 days; repeat until wart comes out	Destructive techniques tend to leave scars, which may cause problems with walking Apply topical anesthetic EMLA
Herpes simplex virus Type I (cold sore, fever blister) Type II (genital)	Grouped, burning, and itching vesicles on inflammatory base, usually on or near mucocutaneous junctions (lips, nose, genitals, buttocks) Vesicles dry, forming a crust, followed by exfoliation and spontaneous healing in 8-10 days May be accompanied by regional lymphadenopathy	Avoidance of secondary infection Burow solution compresses during weeping stages Topical therapy (penciclovir) can shorten duration of cold sores Oral antiviral (acyclovir) for initial infection or to reduce severity in recurrence Valacyclovir (Valtrex), an oral antiviral used for episodic treatment of recurrent genital herpes, reduces pain, stops viral shedding, and has a more convenient administration schedule than acyclovir	Heal without scarring unless secondary infection Type I cold sores can be prevented by using sunscreens protecting against ultraviolet A (UVA) and ultraviolet B (UVB) light to prevent lip blisters Aggravated by corticosteroids Positive psychologic effect from treatment May be fatal in children with depressed immunity
Varicella zoster virus (herpes zoster; shingles)	Caused by same virus that causes varicella (chickenpox) Virus has affinity for posterior root ganglia, posterior horn of spinal cord, and skin; crops of vesicles usually confined to dermatome following along course of affected nerve Usually preceded by neuralgic pain, hyperesthesias, or itching May be accompanied by constitutional symptoms	Symptomatic Analgesics for pain Mild sedation sometimes helpful Local moist compresses Drying lotions may be helpful Ophthalmic variety: systemic corticotropin (adrenocorticotropic hormone [ACTH]) and/or corticosteroids Acyclovir Lidoderm topical anesthetic	Pain in children usually minimal Postherpetic pain does not occur in children Chickenpox may follow exposure; Isolate affected child from other children in a hospital or school May occur in children with depressed immunity; can be fatal
Molluscum contagiosum Cause: pox virus	Flesh-colored papules with a central caseous plug (umbilicated) Usually asymptomatic	Cases in well children resolve spontaneously in about 18 months Treatment reserved for troublesome cases Apply topical anesthetic EMLA Curettage or cryotherapy	Common in school-age children Spread by skin-to-skin contact, including autoinoculation and fomite-to-skin contact

TABLE 53-5
Dermatophytoses (Fungal Infections)

Disease/Organism	Manifestations	Management	Comments
Tinea capitis—*Trichophyton tonsurans, Microsporum audouini, Microsporum canis* (Fig. 53-5, *A*)	Lesions in scalp but may extend to hairline or neck Characteristic configuration of scaly, circumscribed patches and/or patchy, scaling areas of alopecia Generally asymptomatic, but severe, deep inflammatory reaction may occur that manifests as boggy, encrusted lesions (kerions) Pruritic Microscopic examination of scales is diagnostic	Oral griseofulvin Oral ketoconazole for difficult cases Selenium sulfide shampoos Topical antifungal agents (e.g., clotrimazole, haloprogin, miconazole)	Person-to-person transmission Animal-to-person transmission Rarely, permanent loss of hair *M. audouini* transmitted from one human being to another directly or from personal items; *M. canis* usually contracted from household pets, especially cats Atopic individuals more susceptible
Tinea corporis—*Trichophyton rubrum, Trichophyton mentagrophytes, M. canis, Epidermophyton* (see Fig. 53-5, *B*)	Generally round or oval, erythematous scaling patch that spreads peripherally and clears centrally; may involve nails (tinea unguium) Diagnosis: direct microscopic examination of scales Usually unilateral	Oral griseofulvin Local application of antifungal preparation such as tolnaftate, haloprogin, miconazole, clotrimazole; apply 1 inch beyond periphery of lesion; continual application 1 to 2 weeks after no sign of lesion	Usually of animal origin from infected pets Majority of infections in children caused by *M. canis* and *M. audouini*
Tinea cruris ("jock itch")—*Epidermophyton floccosum, T. rubrum, T. mentagrophytes*	Skin response similar to tinea corporis Localized to medial proximal aspect of thigh and crural fold; may involve scrotum in males Pruritic Diagnosis: same as for tinea corporis	Local application of tolnaftate liquid Wet compresses or sitz baths may be soothing	Rare in preadolescent children Health education regarding personal hygiene
Tinea pedis ("athlete's foot")—*T. rubrum, Trichophyton interdigitale, E. floccosum*	On intertriginous areas between toes or on plantar surface of feet Lesions vary: Maceration and fissuring between toes Patches with pinhead-sized vesicles on plantar surface Pruritic Diagnosis: direct microscopic examination of scrapings	Oral griseofulvin Local applications of tolnaftate liquid and antifungal powder containing tolnaftate Acute infections: compresses or soaks followed by application of glucocorticoid cream Elimination of conditions of heat and perspiration by clean, light socks and well-ventilated shoes; avoidance of occlusive shoes	Most frequent in adolescents and adults; rare in children, but occurrence increases with wearing of plastic shoes Transmission to other individuals rare despite general opinion to contrary Ointments not successful
Candidiasis (monillasis)—*Candida albicans*	Grows in chronically moist areas Inflamed areas with white exudate, peeling, and easy bleeding Pruritic Diagnosis: characteristic appearance	Amphotericin B, nystatin ointment, or other antifungal preparations to affected areas	Common form of diaper dermatitis (see Fig. 53-11) Oral form common in infants Vaginal form in older females May be disseminated in immunosuppressed children

Nursing Care Management. When teaching families regarding the care of children with ringworm, the nurse should emphasize good health and hygiene. Because of the infectious nature of the disease, affected children should not share with other children any grooming items, headgear, scarves, or other articles of apparel that have been in proximity to the infected area. Affected children are provided with their own towels and directed to wear a protective cap at night to avoid transmitting the fungus to bedding, especially if they sleep with another person. Because the infection can be acquired by animal-to-human transmission, all household pets should be examined for the presence of the disorder. Other sources of infection are seats

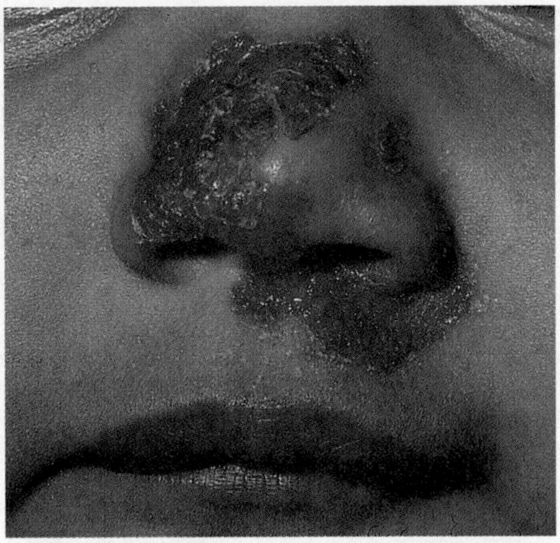

FIG. 53-3 • Impetigo contagiosa. (From Weston WL, Lane AT, Morelli JG: *Color textbook of pediatric dermatology,* ed 2, St Louis, 1996, Mosby.)

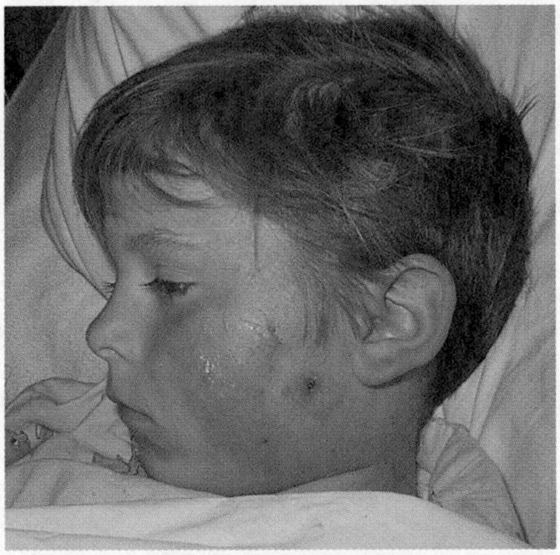

FIG. 53-4 • Cellulitis of cheek from puncture wound. (From Weston WL, Lane AT, Morelli JG: *Color textbook of pediatric dermatology,* ed 2, St Louis, 1996, Mosby.)

A

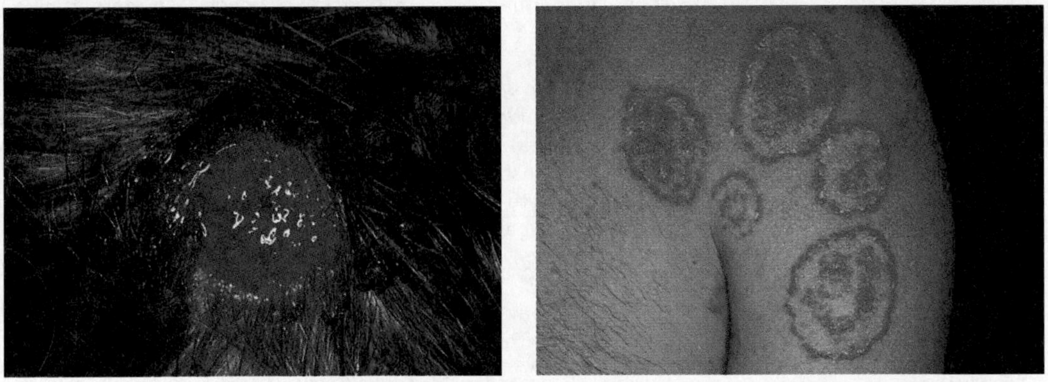

B

FIG. 53-5 • **A,** Tinea capitis. **B,** Tinea corporis. Both infections are caused by *Microsporum canis,* the "kitten" or "puppy" fungus. (From Habif TP: *Clinical dermatology: a color guide to diagnosis and therapy,* ed 3, St Louis, 1996, Mosby.)

with headrests (e.g., theater seats), seats in public transportation, helmets, and gymnasium mats.

Treatment with the drug griseofulvin commonly continues for weeks or months, and because subjective symptoms subside, children or parents may be tempted to decrease or discontinue the drug. The nurse should emphasize to family members the importance of maintaining the prescribed dosage schedule and of taking the medication with high-fat foods for best absorption. They are also instructed regarding the possibility of side effects from the drug (e.g., headache, gastrointestinal upset, fatigue, insomnia, and photosensitivity). For children who take the drug over many months, periodic testing is required to monitor leukopenia and to assess liver and renal function.

Systemic Mycotic (Fungal) Infections

Mycotic (systemic or deep fungal) infections have the capacity to invade the viscera as well as the skin. The best known of these infections are primarily lung diseases, which are usually acquired by inhalation of fungal spores. These fungi produce a variable spectrum of disease, and some are quite common in certain geographic areas. They are not transmitted from person to person but appear to reside in the soil, from which their spores become airborne. The cutaneous lesions caused by deep fungal infections are granulomatous and appear as ulcers, plaques, nodules, fungating masses, and abscesses. The course of deep fungal diseases is chronic with slow progression that favors sensitization (Table 53-6).

SKIN DISORDERS RELATED TO CHEMICAL OR PHYSICAL CONTACTS

Contact Dermatitis

Contact dermatitis is an inflammatory reaction of the skin to chemical substances, natural or synthetic, that evoke a hypersensitivity response; or to those agents that cause direct irritation. The initial reaction occurs in an exposed region, most commonly the face and neck, backs of the hands, forearms, male genitalia, and lower legs. There is characteristically a sharp delineation between inflamed and normal skin early in the reaction

TABLE 53-6
Systemic Mycoses

Disorder/Organism	Skin Manifestations	Systemic Manifestations	Treatment	Comments
North American blastomycosis—*Blastomyces dermatitidis*	Chronic granulomatous lesions and microabscesses in any part of body Initial lesion is a papule; undergoes ulceration and peripheral spread	Pulmonary symptoms, such as cough, chest pain, weakness, and weight loss May have skeletal involvement, with bone destruction and formation of cutaneous abscesses	Intravenous (IV) administration of amphotericin B	Usual portal of entry is lungs Source of infection unknown Noninfectious Pulmonary infections may be mild and self-limiting and require no treatment Progressive disease often fatal
Cryptococcosis—*Cryptococcus neoformans (Torula histolytica)*	Usually on face; acneiform, firm, nodular, painless eruption	Central nervous system (CNS) manifestations: headache, dizziness, stiff neck, and signs of increased intracranial pressure Low-grade fever, mild cough, lung infiltration	IV amphotericin B; may be administered intrathecally for CNS involvement 5-Fluorocytosine for meningitis Excision and drainage of local lesions	Acquired by inhalation of dust but may enter through skin Prognosis serious Noninfectious Increased incidence in persons receiving corticosteroids with lymphoreticular malignancies, or type 2 diabetes
Histoplasmosis—*Histoplasma capsulatum*	Not distinctive or uniform but most appear as punched-out or granulomatous ulcers	General systemic symptoms may include pallor, diarrhea, vomiting, irregular spiking temperature, hepatosplenomegaly, and pulmonary symptoms Any tissue of body may be involved with related symptoms	IV amphotericin B for severe cases Oral ketoconazole	Organism cultured from soil, especially where contaminated with fowl droppings Fungus enters through skin or mucous membranes of mouth and respiratory tract Endemic in Mississippi and Ohio River valleys Disseminated diseases most common in infants and children
Coccidioidomycosis (valley fever)—*Coccidioides immitis*	Erythema nodosum Erythema multiforme Erythematous maculopapular rash	Primary lung disease usually asymptomatic May be sign of acute febrile illness Disseminated disease is very serious	IV amphotericin B IV miconazole (synthetic imidazole) Intraventricular miconazole plus oral ketoconazole for CNS involvement Surgical resection of persistent pulmonary cavities	Inhalation of aerospores from soil Endemic in southwestern United States Usually resolves spontaneously Increased incidence in dark-skinned races (Filipino, African-American, Hispanic, Asian-American)

that ranges from a faint, transient erythema to massive bullae on an erythematous swollen base. Itching is a constant symptom.

The cause may be a primary irritant or a sensitizing agent. A *primary irritant* is one that irritates any skin. A *sensitizing agent* produces an irritation on those who have met the irritant or something chemically related to it, have undergone an immunologic change, and have become sensitized. Prior exposure is not necessarily a factor in the reaction. A sensitizer irritates in relatively low concentrations only persons who are allergic to it. Sometimes with repeated exposure and reactions the skin loses its capacity to return to normal, or secondary factors become predominant to produce a chronic inflammatory process.

The major goal in treatment is to prevent further exposure of the skin to the offending substance. Provided there is no further irritation, the normal recuperative powers of the skin will produce satisfactory results without treatment. The most common offenders are plant and animal irritants, the prototype of which is poison ivy (see following section).

The most common contact dermatitis in infants occurs on the convex surfaces of the diaper area (see Diaper Dermatitis,

p. 1521). Other agents that commonly produce dermatologic responses from contact are animal irritants such as wool, feathers, and furs; vegetable irritants such as oleoresins, oils, and turpentine; and chemicals of all kinds, including synthetic fabrics (e.g., shoe components), dyes, metals, cosmetics, perfumes, and soaps (including bubble baths). The list is endless.

Nursing Care Management. Nurses commonly detect evidence of contact dermatitis during routine physical assessments. Skin manifestations in specific areas suggest limited contact, such as around the eyes (mascara), areas of the body covered by clothing but not protected by undergarments (wool), or areas of the body not covered by clothing (ultraviolet injury). Generalized involvement is more likely to be caused by bubble bath or soap. Often nurses are able to determine the offending agent and counsel families regarding management. However, if the lesions persist, are extensive, or show evidence of infection, medical evaluation is indicated.

Poison Ivy, Oak, and Sumac

Contact with the dry or succulent portions of any of three poisonous plants (i.e., poison ivy, oak, and sumac) produces localized, streaked or spotty, oozing, and painful impetiginous lesions. The offending substance in these plants is urushiol, an extremely potent oil. Sensitivity to urushiol is not inborn but is developed after one or two exposures and may change over a lifetime. All parts of these plants contain the oil, so even dried leaves and stems contain the irritant (Fig. 53-6). Even smoke from burning brush piles can produce a reaction.

Animals do not seem to be affected by the oil; however, dogs or other animals that have run or played in the plants may carry the sap on their fur, and animals who eat the plants can transfer the oil in saliva. Shoes, tools, and toys can transfer the oil. Golf balls that have been in the rough also are sources of contact.

Urushiol takes effect as soon as it touches the skin. It penetrates through the epidermis and bonds with the dermal layer, where it initiates an immune response. The full-blown reaction is evident after about 2 days, with redness, swelling, and itching at the site of contact. Several days later, streaked or spotty blisters oozing serum from damaged cells produce the characteristic impetiginous lesions (Fig. 53-7). The lesions dry and heal spontaneously, and itching stops by 10 to 14 days.

Therapeutic Management. Treatment of the lesions includes calamine lotion, soothing Burow solution compresses, and/or Aveeno baths to relieve discomfort. Topical corticosteroid gel is very effective for prevention or relief of inflammation, especially when applied before blisters form. Oral corticosteroids may be needed for severe reactions, and a sedative such as diphenhydramine (Benadryl) may be ordered.

Nursing Care Management. When it is known that the child has made contact with the plant, the area is flushed with *cold* running water immediately (preferably within 15 minutes) to neutralize the urushiol not yet bonded to the skin. If there is a stream nearby, an effective method is to have the child enter the water (clothes and all) and allow the water to rinse the oil from both skin and clothing. Harsh soap is contraindicated because it removes protective skin oils and dilutes the urushiol, allowing it to spread; hard scrubbing irritates the skin. All clothing that has come in contact with the plant is removed with care and thoroughly laundered in hot water and detergent. Every effort is made to keep the child from scratching the lesions. Although the lesions do not spread by contact with the blister serum or from scratching, they can become secondarily infected (Critical Thinking box).

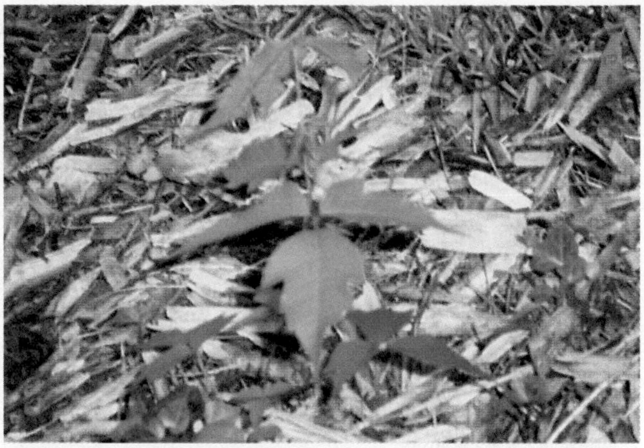

FIG. 53-6 • Poison ivy plants.

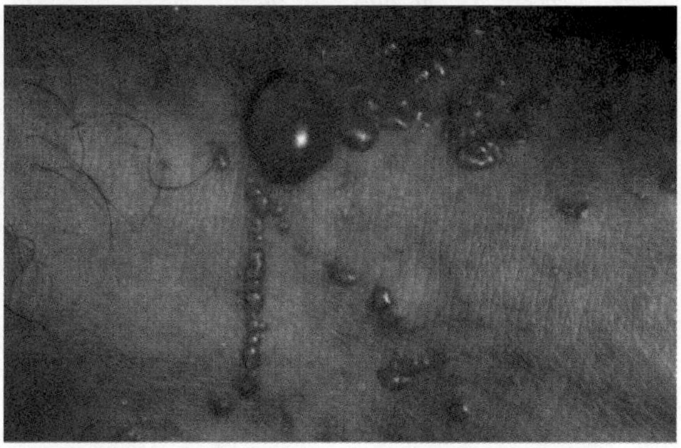

FIG. 53-7 • Poison ivy; note "streaked" blisters surrounding one large blister. (From Habif TP: *Clinical dermatology: a color guide to diagnosis and therapy,* ed 3, St Louis, 1996, Mosby.)

Prevention. Prevention is best accomplished by avoidance of contact and removal of these plants from the environment when feasible. All children, especially those known to be sensitive, should be taught to recognize these plants. Information regarding means for destroying plants can be obtained from the U.S. Department of Agriculture or Forestry Service. An example of a cream that helps protect exposed skin from poison oak and ivy is Stokogard.*

Drug Reactions

Adverse reactions to drugs are seen more often in the skin than in any other organ, although any organ of the body can be affected. The reaction may be a result of toxicity related to drug concentration, individual intolerance to the average dosage of

*Distributed in the United States by Stockhausen, Inc., Greensboro, NC 27406; 1-800-334-0242.

Critical Thinking

POISON IVY

While on an overnight camping trip, Billy, age 9, runs up to the camp nurse with some leaves he has picked on a trail in the woods. The nurse recognizes the leaves as poison ivy. What would be the best intervention for the camp nurse to implement?

First, Think About It . . .
- **What information are you using?**
- **What are you taking for granted, and what assumptions are you making?**

1. **Isolate Billy from his classmates and telephone his parents to pick him up immediately from the camp.**
2. **Scrub Billy's hands vigorously with a strong soap.**
3. **Rinse Billy's hands in the cool water of the nearby stream and apply calamine lotion.**
4. **Throw the poison ivy leaves into the camp fire and examine Billy's hands for any reddened areas.**

The best response is 3. Poison ivy lesions are not contagious, which is important information. Also, children who are exposed to poison ivy do not need to be isolated. However, the leaves of a poison ivy plant do contain an oil called urushiol, which begins to initiate an immune response as soon as the oil touches the human skin. Contact with the leaves should not be taken for granted. An effective way to remove this oil is by rinsing the skin with cold, running water; the cool water of a running stream is ideal. Calamine lotion will relieve the itching and discomfort. Harsh soaps dilute the urushiol and allow the oil to spread; vigorous scrubbing irritates the skin. Burning the leaves is dangerous because contact with the smoke can not only cause a skin reaction, but is dangerous to the lungs if it is inhaled.

the drug, or an allergic or idiosyncratic response. The manifestations may be associated with side effects or secondary effects of a drug, either of which are unrelated to its primary pharmacologic actions.

Although any drug is capable of producing almost any form of reaction in the susceptible individual, some have a tendency to produce a particular reaction consistently, and some are more likely than others to produce an untoward effect. Many are allergenic responses after a prior administration of the drug, even a topical application. Other factors influence a drug response in a particular individual. For example, the incidence increases with the number and amount of drugs given.

Manifestations of drug reactions may be delayed or immediate. A period of 7 days is usually required for a child to develop sensitivity to a drug that has never been administered previously. With prior sensitivity the manifestations appear almost immediately.

Rashes are the most common manifestation of adverse drug reactions in children; however, individual drug reactions may vary from a single lesion to extensive, generalized epidermal necrosis, seen in Stevens-Johnson syndrome (see Table 53-9). Cutaneous manifestations can resemble almost any skin disease and can be seen in almost any degree of severity. With few exceptions, the distribution of a drug eruption is widespread because it results from a circulating agent; appears as an inflammatory response with itching; is sudden in onset; and may be associated with constitutional symptoms such as fever, malaise, gastrointestinal upsets, anemia, or liver and kidney damage.

In most cases treatment for simple cutaneous reactions consists of discontinuing the drug. Sometimes a decision is made to continue the drug (e.g., an antibiotic in an infant or small child) until the cause of the rash is clearly indicated. In urticarial-type eruptions antihistamines may be ordered, and for widespread and severe lesions corticosteroids are beneficial. Severe anaphylactic reactions are a medical emergency (see Anaphylaxis, Chapter 48).

Nursing Care Management. The most effective means of management is prevention. Parents always remember a severe reaction. A careful history will elicit evidence of a previous drug reaction. The history should include the name of the drug, nature of the reaction, drug dose, and how soon after administration the reaction occurred (see Chapter 34).

Nurses who suspect that a rash is caused by a medication should withhold any further dose and report the eruption to the practitioner. Common offenders in drug reactions are penicillin and sulfonamides, and nurses must be alert to this possibility. However, even commonplace drugs, including aspirin, barbiturates, chemical agents in some foods, flavoring agents, and preservatives, are capable of producing an undesired response. Persons who have severe reactions should wear an identification bracelet or pendant to prevent inadvertent administration of the offending drug in an emergency.

Foreign Bodies

Small wooden splinters can be removed by parents with a needle and tweezers that have been sterilized with alcohol or a flame. The area around the sliver is washed with soap and water before removal is attempted. The sliver is exposed with the needle, then grasped firmly by the tweezers and pulled out. Some foreign bodies, such as a fishhook, a piece of glass, a difficult-to-see object, or a deeply embedded object (such as a needle in a foot or near a joint), may need medical evaluation.

Cactus prickles or spines may be removed by the following methods:

- Apply a thin layer of water-soluble household glue and cover with gauze; when the glue dries, peel off the gauze
- Apply hair removal wax or body sugar (Aplon*); let dry and remove
- Place cellophane tape, sticky side down, over the spines and lift off

SKIN DISORDERS RELATED TO INSECT AND ANIMAL CONTACTS

Scabies

Scabies is an endemic infestation caused by the scabies mite, *Sarcoptes scabiei*. Lesions are created as the impregnated female burrows into the stratum corneum of the epidermis (never into living tissue) to deposit her eggs and feces. The inflammatory response and itching occur after the host becomes sensitized to the mite, approximately 30 to 60 days after initial contact.

If the person has been previously sensitized to the mite, the response occurs within 48 hours after exposure. After this time, anywhere the mite has traveled will begin to itch and develop

*Distributed by Corsa, Ltd., 555 N. Lane, Suite 5025, Conshohocker, PA 19428; (610) 834-1555; website: www.corsa.com.

the characteristic eruption (Box 53-1). Consequently, mites will not necessarily be located at all sites of eruption.

There is great variability in the type of lesions. Infants often develop an eczematous eruption; therefore the observer must look for discrete papules, burrows, or vesicles.

Nursing Care Management. The treatment of scabies is the application of a scabicide. Scabicides such as permethrin 5% cream (Elimite) and lindane have been used to treat scabies. Nurses instructing families in the use of scabicides should emphasize the importance of following directions carefully. If lindane lotion is prescribed, it is applied to cool, dry skin over the entire cutaneous surface from the neck down. Lindane is left on for the recommended time, usually 4 to 6 hours; however, permethrin 5% cream is the currently preferred topical treatment for scabies because it is safer, avoids the risk of neurotoxicity, and is more effective than lindane. Permethrin is applied to all skin surfaces (not just the areas with rash, but also between the fingers and toes, the umbilicus, and the cleft of the buttocks). Permethrin cream should remain on the skin for 8 to 14 hours. One liberal application is sufficient, but all persons in the family (including baby-sitters and others who have close contact with the child) should be treated. Families need to know that although the mite will be killed, the rash and the itch will not be eliminated until the stratum corneum is replaced, which takes approximately 2 to 3 weeks. Soothing ointments or lotions can be applied for itching. Antibiotics may be given for secondary infection.

Recently an oral medicine, ivermectin, has been used to treat scabies (Dourmishev, Serafimova, and Dourmishev, 1998; Offidani et al, 1999). This medication is effective, safe, and easy to use, and it seems to be particularly useful in patients with secondary excoriations, for whom the topical scabicides are very irritating and less well tolerated. At the present time, the safety and efficacy of this medication for pediatric patients weighing less than 15 kg (33 pounds) has not been established.

Box 53-1

Clinical Manifestations of Scabies

LESION

Children—minute grayish-brown, threadlike (mite burrows), pruritic
- Black dot at end of burrow (mite)

Infants—eczematous eruption, pruritic

DISTRIBUTION

Generally in intertriginous areas—interdigital, axillary-cubital, popliteal, inguinal

Children over 2 years of age—primarily hands and wrists

Children younger than 2 years—primarily feet and ankles

Box 53-2

Clinical Manifestations of Pediculosis

Pruritus (caused by crawling insect and insect saliva on skin)

Nits observable on hair shaft (see Fig. 53-8)

DISTRIBUTION

Occipital area

Behind ears

Nape of neck

Eyebrows and eyelashes (occasionally) (caused by pubic lice)

Pediculosis Capitis

Pediculosis capitis (head lice) is an infestation of the scalp by *Pediculus humanus capitis,* a very common parasite, especially in school-age children. The adult louse lives only about 48 hours when away from a human host, and the life span of the average female is 1 month. The female lays the majority of the eggs at the junction of a hair shaft and close to the skin because the eggs need a warm environment. The *nits,* or eggs, hatch in approximately 7 to 10 days. Itching is usually the only symptom. Common areas involved are the occipital area, behind the ears, and the nape of the neck (Box 53-2).

Diagnostic Evaluation. Diagnosis is made by observation of the white eggs (nits) firmly attached to the hair shafts (Box 53-2). Because of their brief life span and mobility, adult lice are more difficult to locate. Nits must be differentiated from dandruff, lint, hair spray, and other items of similar size and shape. Scratch marks and/or inflammatory papules, caused by secondary infection, may also be found on the scalp in the vulnerable areas.

Therapeutic Management. Treatment consists of the application of pediculicides and manual removal of nit cases. The drug of choice for infants and children is permethrin 1% creme rinse (Nix), which kills both lice and nits after one application. This product and preparations of pyrethrin with piperonyl butoxide (RID or A-200 Pyrinate) can be obtained without a prescription and are more effective and safer than lindane. Because there are concerns that head lice may be developing increased resistance to chemical shampoos, and that repeated exposure of children to strong chemicals on the scalp may not be wise, research for alternative therapies is ongoing. Recently Robi-Comb, an electronic head lice detector and remover, has been used to kill head lice. When this instrument is used to comb a child's hair, an auditory alert signals the presence of a louse and a small electrical charge passes from one tooth of the comb through the louse to the next tooth (O'Brien, 1998). The louse is killed with no irritation or discomfort to the child. The comb is completely safe, but it does not kill the nits or eggs. To destroy any new lice, the comb should be used at least 5 minutes daily for 2 weeks. When this instrument is used in schools to screen for head lice, however, nurses should be sure that the comb is sanitized with a germicidal spray between children so that there is no chance of transferring lice from one child to another (O'Brien, 1998).

Nursing Care Management. Nurses should be aware of several things to successfully manage or assist parents in coping with pediculosis. It should be emphasized that *anyone* can get pediculosis; it has no respect for age, socioeconomic level, or cleanliness. The louse does not jump or fly, but it can be transmitted from one person to another on personal items. Lice are more apt to infest Caucasian children, those with straight hair, and girls. Children are cautioned against sharing combs, hair ornaments, hats, caps, scarves, coats, and other items used on or near the hair. Children who share lockers are more likely to contract an infestation, and slumber parties place children at risk. Lice are not carried or transmitted by pets.

If a child scratches the head more than usual, nurses or parents should carefully inspect the head for bite marks, redness, and nits. The hair is systematically spread with two flat-sided sticks or tongue depressors, and the scalp is observed for any movement that indicates a louse. Nurses should wear gloves when examining the hair. Lice are small and grayish tan, have no wings, and are visible to the naked eye. The nits, or eggs, appear as tiny whitish oval specks adhering to the hair shaft about ¼ inch from the scalp. The adherent nature of the nits distinguishes them from dandruff, which falls off readily. *Empty nit cases,* indicating hatched lice, are translucent rather than white and are located more than ¼ inch from the scalp (Fig. 53-8).

If evidence of infestation is found, it is important to perform the treatment according to the directions described on the label of the pediculicide. Parents are advised to read the directions carefully before beginning treatment. Instructions on the labels indicate that dead lice and remaining nits are removed with an extra–fine-toothed comb. Most preparations include a comb to dislodge the firmly adhered nits. Commercial products (e.g., Step 2 or Clear) may be used to loosen attached nits for removal; however, if the comb is ineffective in removing the nit cases, they must be removed with tweezers or between the fingernails.

The child is made as comfortable as possible during the application process because the pediculicide must remain on the scalp and hair for several minutes.

Playing "beauty parlor" during the shampoo is a useful strategy. The child lies supine, with the head over a sink or basin, and covers the eyes with a dry towel or washcloth. This prevents the medication, which can cause chemical conjunctivitis, from splashing into the eyes. If eye irritation occurs, the eyes must be flushed well with tepid water.

Lice can survive for up to 48 hours away from the host. Nits are shed into the environment and are capable of hatching in 7 to 10 days. Therefore measures must be taken to prevent further infestation (Community Focus box). Spraying with insecticide is not recommended because of the danger to children and animals. Families should also be advised that the pediculicide is relatively expensive, especially when several members of the household require treatment.

The psychologic effects of lice infestations can be highly stressful to children. They are influenced by the reactions of others, including their parents, and may be made to feel ashamed or guilty. Parents are strongly cautioned against cutting a child's hair or, worse, shaving a child's head. Lice infest short hair as readily as long hair, and these actions only compound the child's distress and serve as a continual reminder to peers, who are always ready to taunt another with something out of the ordinary.

Prevention. The increasing incidence of pediculosis in schoolchildren has become a serious concern for school nurses, parents, and community health agencies. School nurses usually coordinate school-community prevention control programs for pediculosis. The National Pediculosis Association* offers education and advocates a "no nits" policy for treated children's reentry to school.

Arthropod Bites and Stings

Bites and stings account for a significant incidence of mild to moderate discomfort, and most are managed by simple symptomatic measures such as compresses, calamine lotion, and prevention of secondary infection.

Arthropods include insects and arachnids such as mites, ticks, spiders, and scorpions. Major offending creatures, their manifestations, and management are outlined in Table 53-7.

When a hymenopteran (bees in particular) stings, its barbed stinger penetrates into the skin. As long as the stinger remains in the skin, the muscles push the stinger deeper and the venom is pumped into the wound. The best approach is to remove the stinger as quickly as possible and to get away from the vicinity of other insects to prevent further injury. Children who have become sensitized to hymenopteran bites may demonstrate a severe systemic response that can be life threatening. One sting can produce generalized urticaria, respiratory difficulty (from laryngeal edema), hypotension, and death. Intramuscular administration of epinephrine provides immediate relief and must be available for emergency use.

*P.O. Box 6101891, Newton, MA 02161; (617) 449-6487 or 1-800-446-4NPA; fax (781) 449-8129; website: www.headlice.org.

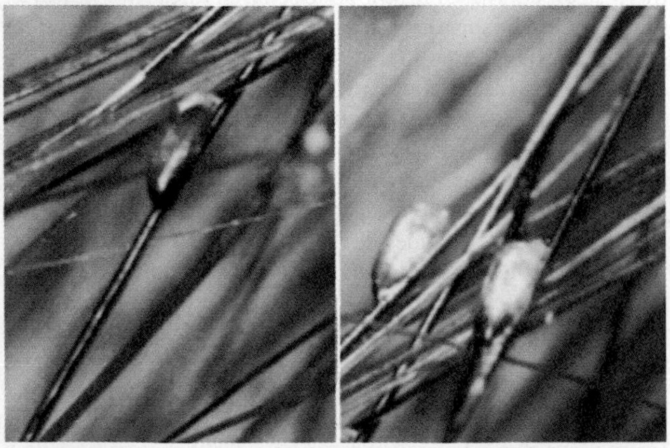

A B

FIG. 53-8 • A, Empty nit case. B, Viable nits. (From *The contemporary approach to the control of head lice in schools and communities,* Pittsburgh, 1991, SmithKline Beecham.)

Community Focus

PREVENTING THE SPREAD AND RECURRENCE OF PEDICULOSIS

Machine wash all washable clothing, towels, and bed linens in hot water, and dry in a hot dryer for at least 20 minutes. Dry-clean nonwashable items.

Thoroughly vacuum carpets, car seats, pillows, stuffed animals, rugs, mattresses, and upholstered furniture.

Seal nonwashable items in plastic bags for 14 days if unable to dry-clean or vacuum.

Soak combs, brushes, and hair accessories in lice-killing products for 1 hour or in boiling water for 10 minutes.

In day care centers, store children's clothing items such as hats and scarves and other headgear in separate cubicles.

Discourage the sharing of items such as hats, scarves, hair accessories, combs, and brushes among children in group settings such as day care centers.

Avoid physical contact with infested individuals and their belongings, especially clothing and bedding.

Inspect children in a group setting regularly for head lice.

Provide educational programs on the transmission of pediculosis, its detection, and treatment.

From Benenson AS, editor: *Control of communicable diseases manual,* Washington, DC, 1995, American Public Health Association.

TABLE 53-7
Skin Lesions Caused by Arthropods

Mechanism/Characteristics	Manifestations	Management
FLIES, GNATS, MOSQUITOES, FLEAS		
Mechanism: Foreign protein in insects' saliva is introduced when skin is penetrated for a blood-sucking meal	Hypersensitivity reaction Papular urticaria Firm papules; may be capped by vesicles or excoriated Little or no reaction in nonsensitized person	Treatment Use antipruritic agents and baths Administer antihistamines Prevent secondary infection Prevention: Avoid contact Remove focus, such as treating furniture, mattresses, carpets, and pets, where insects may live Apply insect repellent when exposure is anticipated
CHIGGERS—HARVEST MITE		
Mechanism: Attach with claws and secrete a digestive substance that liquefies the host's epidermis Manifestations: Erythematous papules Intense itching	Same as insect bites Favor warm areas of body, especially intertriginous areas and areas covered with clothing	Avoid contact, especially in areas of tall grass and underbrush Apply insect repellant when exposure is anticipated; insecticides such as diazinon can also be sprayed in yards May require systemic steroids for extensive bites
HYMENOPTERANS—BEES, WASPS, HORNETS, YELLOW JACKETS, FIRE ANTS		
Mechanism: Injection of venom through stinging apparatus Venom contains histamine, allergenic proteins, and often a spreading factor, hyaluronidase Severe reactions caused by hypersensitivity and/or multiple stings	Local reaction: small red area, wheal, itching, and heat Systemic reactions: may be mild to severe, including generalized edema, pain, nausea and vomiting, confusion, respiratory embarrassment, and shock	Treatment: Carefully scrape off stinger or pull out stinger as quickly as possible Cleanse with soap and water Apply cool compresses Apply common household product (e.g., lemon juice, paste made with aspirin or baking soda) Administer antihistamines Severe reactions: administer epinephrine, corticosteroids; treat for shock Prevention: Teach child to wear shoes; to avoid wearing bright clothing, flowery prints, shiny jewelry, or perfumed grooming products (cologne, scented hairspray), which might attract the insect; and to avoid places where the insect may be contacted Hypersensitive children should wear medical identification to indicate allergy and therapy needed; family should keep emergency medication and be taught its administration
BLACK WIDOW SPIDER		
Mechanism: Venom injected through a claw-like appendage; has neurotoxic action Characteristics: Spider is shiny black, with a body about 1.25 cm (0.5 inches) long and a red or orange hourglass-shaped marking on underside Avoids light and bites in self-defense	Mild sting at time of bite Area becomes swollen, painful, and erythematous Dizziness, weakness, and abdominal pain May produce delirium, paralysis, seizures, and (if large amount of venom absorbed) death	Treatment: Cleanse wound with antiseptic Apply cool compresses Administer antivenin Administer muscle relaxant, such as calcium gluconate; analgesics and/or sedatives; hydrocortisone or diazepam intravenously Prevention: Teach children to avoid places that harbor the spider (e.g., woodpiles)

Continued

TABLE 53-7
Skin Lesions Caused by Arthropods—cont'd

Mechanism/Characteristics	Manifestations	Management
BROWN RECLUSE SPIDER		
Mechanism: Venom injected via fangs Venom contains powerful necrotoxin Characteristics: Spider is slender, with long legs and body length of 1 to 2 cm; color is fawn to dark brown; recognized by fiddle-shaped mark on head Shy; bites only when annoyed or surprised Prefers dark areas where seldom disturbed	Mild sting at time of bite Transient erythema followed by bleb or blister; mild to severe pain in 2-8 hours; purple, star-shaped area in 3-4 days; necrotic ulceration in 7-14 days (Fig. 53-9) Systemic reactions may include fever, malaise, restlessness, nausea, vomiting, and joint pain Generalized petechial eruption Wounds heal with scar formation	Treatment: Apply cool compresses locally Administer antibiotics, corticosteroids Relieve pain Wound may require skin graft Prevention: Teach children to avoid possible nesting sites
SCORPIONS		
Mechanism: Sting by means of a hooked caudal stinger that discharges venom Venom of more venomous species contains hemolysins, endotheliolysins, and neurotoxins Characteristics: Usual habitat is southwestern United States	Intense local pain, erythema, numbness, burning, restlessness, vomiting Ascending motor paralysis with seizures, weakness, rapid pulse, excessive salivation, thirst, dysuria, pulmonary edema, coma, and death Some species produce only local tissue reaction with swelling at puncture site (distinctive) Symptoms subside in a few hours Deaths occur among children younger than 4 years old, usually in first 24 hours	Treatment: Delay absorption of venom by keeping child quiet; place involved area in dependent position Administer antivenin Relieve pain Admit to pediatric intensive care unit for surveillance Prevention: Teach children to avoid possible nesting sites
TICKS		
Mechanism: In process of sucking blood, head and mouth parts are buried in skin Characteristics: Feed on blood of mammals Significant in humans because of pathologic organism carried May be vectors of various infectious diseases, such as Rocky Mountain spotted fever, Q fever, tularemia, relapsing fever, Lyme disease, tick paralysis Must attach and feed for 1-2 hours to transmit disease Usual habitat is very wooded area	Tick usually attached to skin, head embedded Produce firm, discrete, intensely pruritic nodules at site of attachment May cause urticaria or persistent localized edema	Treatment: Grasp tick with tweezers (forceps) as close as possible to point of attachment Pull straight up with steady, even pressure; if bare hands, use a tissue to touch tick during removal; wash hands thoroughly with soap and water Remove any remaining part (e.g., head) with sterile needle Cleanse wounds with soap and disinfectant Prevention: Teach children to avoid areas where prevalent Inspect skin (especially scalp) after being in wooded areas

Hypersensitive children should wear medical identification such as a bracelet. They should also have a kit that contains epinephrine and a hypodermic syringe. Families are reminded to check the expiration date on the kit and to replace an outdated one. They should determine whether a nurse is available at the school, and what the school policy is regarding administration of drugs. If a school nurse is not present, someone at the school should be designated to inject the epinephrine in an emergency.

Most arthropods in the United States, including tarantulas, are relatively harmless. Although all spiders produce venom that is injected via fangs, some are unable to pierce the skin; others produce a venom that is insufficiently toxic to be harmful. Only scorpions and two spiders—the brown recluse and the black widow—inject venom deadly enough to require immediate attention. Children bitten by these arachnids must receive medical attention as soon as possible.

TABLE 53-8
Disorders Transmitted by Arthropods

Disorder/ Organism/Host	Manifestations	Management	Comments
Rocky Mountain spotted fever—*R. rickettsii* Arthropod: tick Transmission: tick Mammal source: wild rodents; dogs	Gradual onset: fever, malaise, anorexia, myalgia Abrupt onset: rapid temperature elevation, chills, vomiting, myalgia, severe headache Maculopapular or petechial rash primarily on extremities (ankles and wrists) but may spread to other areas, characteristically on palms and soles	Control: protection from tick bite by wearing proper apparel, tick repellent Tetracycline or chloramphenicol Vigorous supportive therapy	Usually self-limited in children Onset in children may resemble any infectious disease Severe disease rare in children Children and dogs should be inspected regularly if they play in wooded areas
Epidemic typhus—*R. prowazekii* Arthropod: body louse Transmission: infected feces into broken skin Mammal source: humans	Abrupt onset of chills, fever, diffuse myalgia, headache, malaise Maculopapular rash becomes petechial 4 to 7 days later, spreading from trunk outward	Control: immediate destruction of vectors Tetracycline or chloramphenicol Supportive treatment	Patient should be isolated until deloused See discussion on p. 1515 for management of pediculosis Excreta from infected lice also in dust—disinfect patient's clothing, bedding, and possessions and wash in hot water
Endemic typhus—*R. typhi* Arthropod: rat fleas or body lice Transmission: flea bite; inhaling or ingesting flea excreta Mammal source: rats	Headache, arthralgia, backache followed by fever; may last 9-14 days Maculopapular rash after 1-8 days of fever; begins in trunk and spreads to periphery; rarely involves face, palms, soles	Control: eliminate rat reservoir, insect vectors, or both Tetracycline or chloramphenicol Supportive treatment	Fairly common in United States Shorter duration than epidemic typhus Mild, seldom fatal illness Difficult to distinguish from epidemic typhus
Rickettsialpox—*R. akarl* Arthropod: mouse mite Transmission: mite Mammal source: house mouse	Maculopapular rash following primary lesion; eschar at site of bite; fever, chills, headache	Control: eradication of rodent reservoir and mite vector Tetracycline or chloramphenicol Supportive treatment	Self-limited nonfatal disease Endemic in New York City Found in many cities in United States

Infections Transmitted by Arthropods

The organisms responsible for a number of disorders are transmitted to human beings via arthropods (Table 53-8). Rickettsiae are intracellular parasites, similar in size to bacteria, that inhabit the alimentary tract of a wide range of natural hosts. Mammals become infected only through the bites of infected lice, fleas, ticks, and mites, all of which serve as both infectors and reservoirs. Rickettsial diseases are more common in temperate and tropical climates and in areas where humans live in association with arthropods. Infection in humans is incidental (except epidemic typhus) and not necessary for the survival of the rickettsial species. However, once the organism invades a human, it causes a disease that varies in intensity from a benign, self-limiting illness to a fulminating and commonly fatal one.

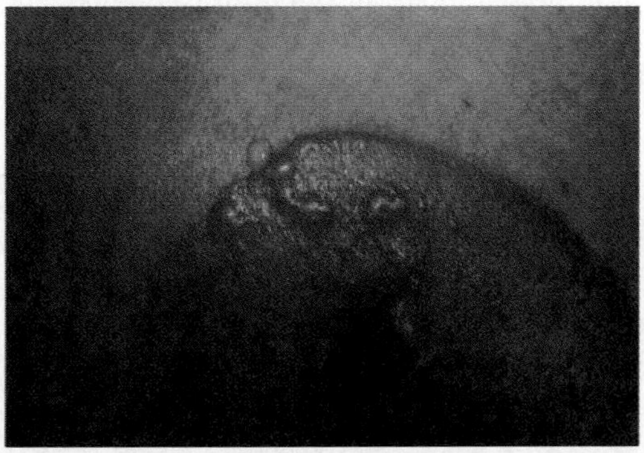

FIG. 53-9 • Brown recluse spider bite; note central necrosis surrounded by purplish area and blisters. (From Weston WL, Lane AT: *Color textbook of pediatric dermatology,* St Louis, 1991, Mosby.)

Lyme Disease (LD)

LD is the most common tick-borne disorder in the United States. It is caused by a spirochete, *Borrelia burgdorferi,* which enters the skin and bloodstream through the saliva and feces of biting ticks, especially the deer tick. The disease may present in any of three stages: (1) the tick bite at the time of inoculation, followed in 3 to 32 days by the development of *erythema chronicum migrans (ECM)* at the site of the bite (Fig. 53-10); (2) the most serious stage of the disease, characterized by systemic involvement of neurologic, cardiac, and musculoskeletal systems that appears several weeks after the cutaneous phase is completed; and (3) development of musculoskeletal pain involving the tendons, bursae, muscles, and synovia. Arthritis may occur, and late neurologic problems include deafness and chronic encephalopathy.

Diagnostic Evaluation. Diagnosis is based on history, observation of lesions, and development of clinical manifestations. Serologic testing may be used to establish the diagnosis in later stages of the disease.

Therapeutic Management. Early and appropriate treatment is essential to prevent complications. Children over 8 years of age are treated with oral doxycycline or amoxicillin; children under 8 years of age are given amoxicillin or penicillin. For patients allergic to penicillin, an alternative drug is cefuroxime axetil (Ceftin). Intramuscular ceftriaxone is used to manage the neurologic, cardiac, and arthritic manifestations.

A vaccine against LD, *LYMErix,* has been licensed by the Food and Drug Administration (FDA). The vaccine is recommended for individuals ages 15 to 70 years at high risk for LD from significant exposure to tick habitats in endemic areas (currently, the northeast and north central United States) and for those who have been infected with LD. It is administered on a 0-, 1-, and 12-month schedule; doses 2 and 3 should be given several weeks before *B. burgdorferi* season, which usually begins in April (American Academy of Pediatrics, 2000.)

Nursing Care Management. The major thrust of nursing care is prevention. Parents should be educated to protect their children from exposure to ticks. Children should avoid tick-infested areas; or when in wooded areas wear light-colored clothing so that ticks can be spotted easily, tuck pant legs into socks, and wear a long-sleeved shirt tucked into pants. Grass and shrubbery where ticks may be lurking should be avoided, and children and adults should walk in the center of trails. Parents and children need to perform regular tick checks when they are in infested areas. After a hike, a bare skin check (with special attention to the scalp, neck, armpits, and groin areas) is important to spot any ticks and remove them. The use of insect repellents containing diethyltoluamide (DEET) and permethrin can protect against ticks, but parents should use these chemicals cautiously because DEET is absorbed through the skin and can cause toxicity in infants and children. Information about Lyme disease can also be obtained from the American Lyme Disease Foundation, Inc.*

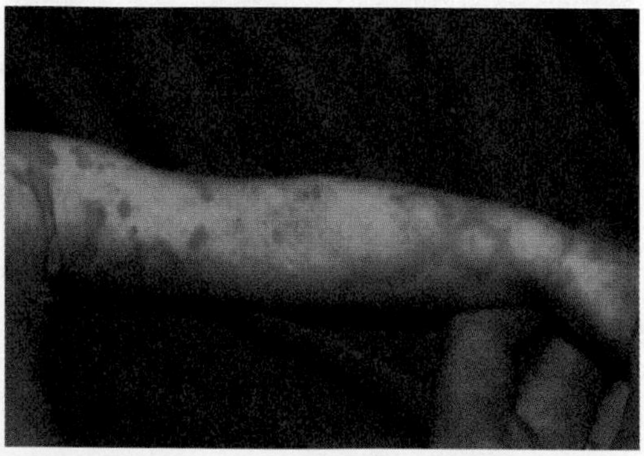

FIG. 53-10 • Lyme disease. Note annular red rings in erythema chronicum migrans. (From Weston WL, Lane At: *Color textbook of pediatric dermatology,* St Louis, 1991, Mosby.)

Animal Bites

Animal bites are common in childhood. Children are bitten more often by animals belonging to the family or to neighbors than by stray animals. More than half the victims of dog bites are less than 4 years of age; boys are bitten more often than girls. Most dog or cat injuries are to the upper extremities. Small children are more likely to be bitten or scratched on the head, face, and neck because they tend to put their heads near the animal's head and flail their arms rather than protecting their heads. The injuries vary from small puncture wounds to complete evulsion of tissue and significant crush injury. Animal bites are potentially serious because of the likelihood of significant infection.

Therapeutic Management. General wound care consists of rinsing the wound with copious amounts of saline or Ringer's lactate under pressure via a large syringe; and of washing the surrounding skin with mild soap. A clean pressure dressing is applied, and the extremity is elevated if the wound is bleeding. Medical evaluation is advised because there is danger of tetanus and rabies, although dogs in most urban areas are required to be immunized against rabies. Bites from wild animals such as squirrels, bats, raccoons, foxes, and skunks are potentially dangerous.

Prophylactic antibiotics are indicated for puncture wounds and wounds in areas that may prove to be cosmetically or functionally impaired if infected. Extensive lacerations are debrided and loosely sutured to allow for drainage in the event of infection. Tetanus toxoid is administered according to standard guidelines (see Immunizations, Chapter 36), and rabies protocol is followed (see Rabies, Chapter 51). Injuries to poorly vascularized areas such as the hands are more likely to become infected than those in more vascularized areas such as the face; puncture wounds are more apt to become infected than lacerations.

Nursing Care Management. The most important aspect related to animal bites is prevention. Children should understand animal behavior and develop a respect for animals. Parents should monitor their children's behavior with dogs and instruct them not to tease or surprise a dog, invade its territory, interfere with its feeding or sleeping, take its toy, or interact with a sick or injured dog or a dog with pups (Humane Society of United States, 1998). Parents who are considering getting a pet, especially a dog, for themselves or their children should select one that is least likely to be a danger to their children. Dogs that are too clumsy, impetuous, or vigorous are not suitable for small children.

Human Bites

Children often acquire lacerations from the teeth of other humans in rough play, during fights, or as victims of child abuse. Many preschool children bite others out of frustration or anger. Because human dental plaque and gingiva harbor pathogenic organisms, all human bites should receive attention. Delayed treatment increases the risk of infection.

*Mill Pond Offices 293, Route 100, Suite 204, Somers, NY 10589; (914) 277-6970 or 1-800-876-LYME; fax (914) 277-6974; website: www.aldf.com.

If the laceration is less than $\frac{1}{4}$ inch in length, the wound can be treated at home. The wound is washed thoroughly with soap and water, and a pressure dressing is applied to stop bleeding. Ice applications minimize discomfort and swelling. Increased pain or redness at the wound site is an indication that the child should receive medical attention for antibiotic therapy. Tetanus toxoid is needed if the child is insufficiently immunized. Larger wounds should receive medical attention.

Cat Scratch Disease (CSD)

CSD is a subacute regional adenitis that follows the scratch or bite of an animal, especially a cat (99% of cases). The disease is usually a benign, self-limiting illness that resolves spontaneously in about 2 to 4 months. Diagnosis is made on the basis of three of the following: (1) contact (usually a kitten) and regional inoculation lesion, (2) lymphadenopathy, (3) positive CSD skin test, and (4) biopsy of a lymph node with histopathology compatible with CSD. The disease may persist for several months before gradual resolution. In some children, especially those who are immunocompromised, the adenitis may progress to suppuration and serious complications. Treatment is primarily supportive.

MISCELLANEOUS SKIN DISORDERS

A number of skin lesions are caused by extrinsic or intrinsic factors. Other skin lesions occur as a result of congenital disorders and are usually inherited as an autosomal-dominant trait (Table 53-9). *Ichthyoses* are a heterogenous group of disorders characterized by scaling; their treatment poses a challenge. These disorders are not discussed in detail because of their variability.

SKIN DISORDERS ASSOCIATED WITH SPECIFIC AGE GROUPS

Several common and important dermatologic conditions are confined primarily to children in specific age groups. These conditions include atopic, seborrheic, and diaper dermatitis and the acne of adolescence. Treatment modalities include those previously described, but some special needs and therapies are involved with these disorders.

Diaper Dermatitis

Diaper dermatitis, one of the most common dermatoses in infants, is one of several acute inflammatory skin disorders caused either directly or indirectly by the wearing of diapers. The peak age of occurrence is 9 to 12 months of age, and the incidence is greater in bottle-fed infants than in breastfed infants.

Pathophysiology and Clinical Manifestations. Diaper dermatitis is caused by prolonged and repetitive contact with an irritant (e.g., urine, feces, soaps, detergents, ointments, and friction). Although the irritant in the majority of incidences is urine and feces, the specific components that contribute to irritation include a combination of factors.

Prolonged contact of the skin with diaper wetness produces higher friction, greater abrasion damage, increased transepidermal permeability, and increased microbial counts. These combine to make healthy skin less resistant to potential irritants.

Although ammonia was once thought to cause diaper rash because of the association between the strong odor on diapers and dermatitis, ammonia alone is not sufficient. The important function of urine is related to an increase in pH from the breakdown of urea in the presence of fecal urease. The increased pH promotes the activity of fecal enzymes, principally proteases and lipases, which act as irritants. Fecal enzymes also increase the permeability of skin to bile salts, another potential irritant in feces.

The eruption of diaper dermatitis can be manifested primarily on convex surfaces or in folds. The lesions can represent a variety of types and configurations. Eruptions involving the skin in most intimate contact with the diaper (e.g., the convex surfaces of buttocks, inner thighs, mons pubis, and scrotum) but sparing the folds are likely to be caused by chemical irritants, especially from urine and feces (Fig. 53-11). Other causes are detergents or soaps from inadequately rinsed cloth diapers, or the chemicals in disposable wipes. Perianal involvement is usually a result of chemical irritation from feces, especially diarrheal stools. *Candida albicans* infection produces perianal inflammation with satellite lesions (Fig. 53-12).

Nursing Care Management. Nursing interventions are aimed at altering the three factors considered to produce dermatitis—wetness, pH, and fecal irritants. The most significant factor amenable to intervention is the moist environment created in the diaper area. Changing the diaper as soon as it becomes wet eliminates a large part of the problem, and removing the diaper to expose healthy skin to air facilitates drying.

NURSE ALERT • A heat lamp, hair dryer, or source of oxygen should not be used on very reddened or denuded skin because these interventions dry the skin and retard healing. Instead, occlusive ointments are applied to provide a moist healing environment.

Diaper construction has a significant impact on the incidence and severity of diaper dermatitis. Superabsorbent disposable paper diapers have been shown to reduce diaper dermatitis. They contain an absorbent gelling material that binds water tightly to decrease skin wetness, maintain pH control by providing a buffering capacity, and decrease skin irritation by preventing mixing of urine and feces in the diaper. Another advance in diapers is the addition of an inner layer or topsheet that is impregnated with petrolatum (e.g., Ultra Pampers with Tender Touch Liner*).

Guidelines for controlling diaper rash are presented in the Home Care box.† A common misconception about using cornstarch on skin is that it promotes the growth of *Candida albicans.* Neither cornstarch nor talc promotes the growth of the fungi under conditions normally found in the diaper area. Cornstarch is also more effective in reducing friction and tends to cake less than talc when the skin is wet. On the basis of these properties, and its safety in terms of inhalation injury, cornstarch is the preferred product.

Atopic Dermatitis (AD) (Eczema)

Eczema or eczematous inflammation of the skin refers to a descriptive category of dermatologic diseases and not to a specific etiology. AD is a type of pruritic eczema that usually begins during infancy and is associated with allergy with a hereditary

*Manufactured by Procter & Gamble Company, Cincinnati, OH 45224; 1-800-285-6064; website: www.pampers.com.

†Pamphlets describing the development and treatment of diaper rash include *Diaper Rash,* available from the American Academy of Pediatrics, 141 Northwest Point Blvd., Elk Grove Village, IL 60009; (888) 227-1770; fax (847) 228-1281; website: www.aap.org.

TABLE 53-9
Miscellaneous Skin Disorders

Disease/Causative Agent	Local Manifestations	Management	Comments
Urticaria—Usually allergic response to drugs or infection	Development of wheals Vary in size and configuration and tend to appear quickly, spread irregularly, and fade within a few hours May be constant or intermittent, sparse or profuse, small or large, discrete or confluent May be acute, chronic, or recurrent in acute attacks	Local soothing and antipruritic applications Antihistamines Epinephrine or ephedrine Cortisone in severe cases Severe upper respiratory involvement may require tracheostomy	Known etiologic agents should be avoided May be accompanied by malaise, fever, lymphadenopathy Severe cases may involve mucous membranes, internal organs, and joints Obstruction to air passages constitutes medical emergency (see Chapter 48)
Intertrigo—Mechanical trauma and aggravating factors of excessive heat, moisture, and sweat retention	Red, inflamed, moist, partially denuded, marginated areas, the shape of which is determined by location Appears where opposing skin surfaces rub together, such as intergluteal folds, groin, neck, and axilla Excessive moisture and obesity are often factors	Affected areas kept clean and dry Skinfolds kept separated with a generous supply of non-medicated powder Expose to air and light Remove excess clothing	A form of diaper irritation Prevent recurrence by keeping susceptible areas clean and dry Frequently associated with overheating from too much clothing
Psoriasis—Unknown; hereditary predisposition; may be triggered by stress	Round, thick, dry, reddish patches covered with coarse, silvery scales over trunk and extremities; first lesions commonly appear in scalp; facial lesions more common in children than in adults Affected cells proliferate at a much more rapid rate than normal cells	Exposure to sunlight, ultraviolet light Topical corticosteroids Tar derivates Keratolytic agents (salicylic acid) Emollients may provide relief	Uncommon in children younger than 6 years old Persons are otherwise healthy individuals Coal tar and psoralin act synergistically with ultraviolet light Keratolytic agents enhance absorption of corticosteroids Humidifiers may help in winter
Alopecia*			
Alopecia areata	Sudden onset of asymptomatic, noninflammatory, round, bald patches in hairy parts of body	Psychologic support Inducement of allergic contact dermatitis to stimulate growth of hair Minoxidil (peripheral vasodilator)	Family history in 10%-26% of cases Some concern regarding drug therapy safety Refer to support groups*
Traumatic alopecia	Traction alopecia around scalp margins from tight hair styles (e.g., braids, pony tails, corn rows)	Counseling regarding hair styling, use of hair cosmetics, hot combs, rollers	More prevalent in African-American children and adolescents Prolonged traction can produce fibrosis of hair root and permanent loss
Trichotillomania	Compulsive hair pulling	Determine and treat cause	Chronic hair pulling may require psychologic therapy
Tinea capitis	See Table 53-5	See Table 53-5	See Table 53-5

*National Alopecia Areata Foundation, 710 C St., Suite 11, San Rafael, CA 94901; (415) 456-4644; fax (415) 456-4274; e-mail: 74301.1642@compuserve.com.

TABLE 53-9
Miscellaneous Skin Disorders—cont'd

Disease/Causative Agent	Local Manifestations	Management	Comments
Erythema multiforme (Stevens-Johnson syndrome)—Unknown; associated with ingestion of some drugs; often follows upper respiratory infection	Erythematous papular rash Lesions enlarge by peripheral expansion; develop central vesicle Involves most skin surfaces except scalp May extend to mucous membranes, especially oral, ocular, and urethral	Symptomatic and supportive Maintain adequate intake of fluids (oral or intravenous), calories, and protein Cutaneous hygiene Appropriate treatment of complications Diligent monitoring of urine volume and specific gravity, hemoglobin and hematocrit, serum electrolyte levels, total body weight	Rash often preceded by fever and malaise Complications include renal failure and severe eye disease Respiratory involvement in a number of cases Self-limiting, but recovery may extend for weeks; skin lesions may subside without scarring; mucous membrane lesions may persist for months Recurrence rate 20%; mortality as high as 10% High mutation rate
Neurofibromatosis—Inherited disorder; autosomal-dominant inheritance pattern	Café-au-lait spots, pigmented nevi, axillary freckling Slow-growing cutaneous and subcutaneous neurofibromas	Symptomatic treatment of associated manifestations (e.g., speech defects, seizures, skeletal defects [scoliosis, kyphosis], learning disabilities) Surgical removal of troublesome tumors	Refer to support groups* Family needs to know about genetic implications

*National Neurofibromatosis Foundation, Inc., 95 Pine St., 16th Floor, New York, NY 10005; 1-800-323-7938 or (212) 344-6633; fax (212) 747-0004; e-mail: nnff@nf.org; website: www.nf.org.

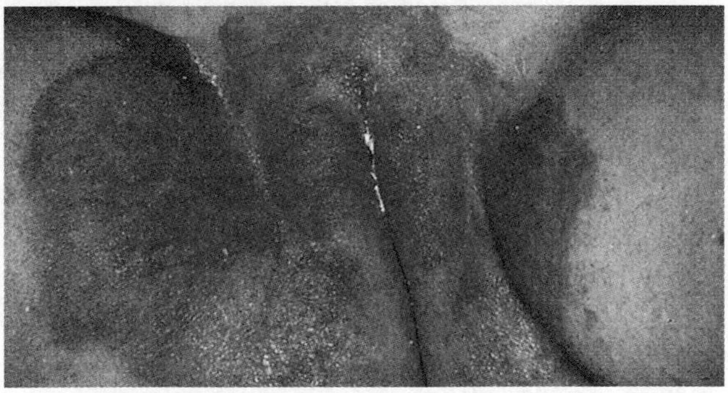

FIG. 53-11 • Irritant diaper dermatitis. Note sharply demarcated edges. (From Habif TP: *Clinical dermatology: a color guide to diagnosis and therapy,* ed 3, St Louis, 1996, Mosby.)

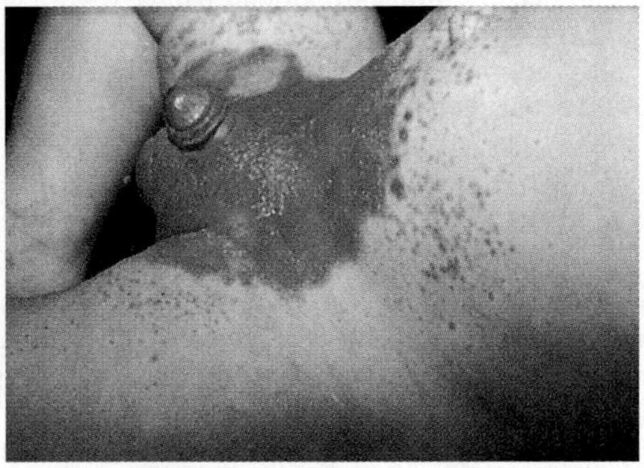

FIG. 53-12 • Candidiasis of diaper area. Note beefy red central erythema with satellite pustules. (From Weston WL, Lane AT, Morelli JG: *Color textbook of pediatric dermatology,* ed 2, St Louis, 1996, Mosby.)

tendency *(atopy)*. AD presents in three forms based on the age of the child and the distribution of lesions:

1. **Infantile (infantile eczema)**—Usually begins at 2 to 6 months of age and generally undergoes spontaneous remission by 3 years of age.
2. **Childhood**—May follow the infantile form; it occurs at 2 to 3 years of age, and 90% of children with AD will manifest the disease by age 5 years.
3. **Preadolescent and adolescent**—Begins at about 12 years of age and may continue into the early adult years or indefinitely.

The diagnosis of AD is based on a combination of history and morphologic findings (Box 53-3). Children with the disease have a lower threshold for cutaneous itching, and many authorities believe the dermatologic manifestations appear subsequent to scratching of the intense pruritus. For example, infants will rub their faces against bed linen, and crawling (a form of scratching) results in irritation of knees and elbows. Lesions will disappear if the scratching is stopped.

The majority of children with infantile AD have a family history of eczema, asthma, food allergies, or allergic rhinitis; this strongly supports a genetic predisposition. The cause is un-

Home Care

CONTROLLING DIAPER RASH

Keep skin dry.
- **Use superabsorbent disposable diapers to reduce skin wetness.**
- **If using cloth diapers, use only overwraps that allow air to circulate; avoid rubber pants.**
- **Change diapers as soon as soiled, especially with stool, whenever possible, preferably once during the night.**
- **Expose healthy or only slightly irritated skin to air, not heat, to dry completely.**

Apply ointment, such as zinc oxide or petrolatum, to protect skin, especially if skin is very red or has moist, open areas.
- **When soiled, wipe off top layer of ointment and reapply.**
- **To completely remove ointment, especially zinc oxide, use mineral oil; do not wash vigorously.**

Avoid overwashing the skin, especially with perfumed soaps or commercial wipes, which may be irritating.
- **May use a moisturizer or nonsoap cleanser, such as cold cream or Cetaphil, to wipe urine from skin.**
- **Gently wipe stool from skin using water and mild soap, such as Dove.**

NOTE: Powder helps keep the skin dry, but talc is very dangerous if breathed into the lungs. Plain cornstarch or cornstarch-based powder is safer. When using any powder product, shake it first into your hand, then apply it to the diaper area. Store the container away from the infant's reach; keep the container closed when not in use.

known but appears to be related to abnormal function of the skin, including alterations in sweating, peripheral vascular function, and heat tolerance. The symptoms improve in humid climates and become worse in fall and winter when homes are heated and environmental humidity is lower. The disorder can be controlled but not cured.

Therapeutic Management. The major goals of management are to (1) relieve pruritus, (2) hydrate the skin, (3) reduce inflammation, and (4) prevent or control secondary infection. Most of the general measures for managing AD serve to reduce pruritus, as well as other aspects of the disease. General management includes avoiding exposure to skin irritants, avoiding overheating, improving skin hydration, and administration of medications such as antihistamines, topical steroids, and (as indicated) mild sedatives.

Differing philosophies regarding cleansing and hydrating the skin of the child with AD focus on two methods—the wet and the dry methods. In the *dry method* baths are infrequent and skin is cleansed with a nonlipid, hydrophilic agent such as Cetaphil. The *wet method* consists of frequent baths (up to four times per day) followed immediately by the application of a lubricant (while the skin is still damp) to trap moisture in the skin. Either no soap or a very mild, nonperfumed soap (e.g., Dove, Lowila, or Neutrogena) is used. Some advocate oil or oilated oatmeal baths with light drying so that a protective, oily film remains on the skin. Showers are acceptable as long as a moisturizer is applied within 3 minutes to prevent drying and damaging the skin.

Enhancing skin hydration can be accomplished by application of preparations that occlude the skin to prevent evaporation and retain moisture in the upper skin layers; and/or by replacement of natural moisturizing substances in the skin. Glycerin-based lubricants are preferred over lanolin-based creams because of the sensitivity of many of these children to wool and wool products (Vernon, 1998). For the majority of patients, lotions applied twice or three times daily maintain satisfactory hydration. The frequency may be increased if greater hydration is required. Creams or ointments provide more occlusion, and those that contain urea or lactic acid improve the binding of water in the skin and prevent evaporation of moisture.

Sometimes colloid baths (e.g., 2 cups of cornstarch added to a tub of warm water) provide temporary relief of itching, and may help the child sleep if given before bedtime. Cool wet compresses are soothing to the skin and provide antiseptic protection.

Moderate or severe pruritus is usually relieved by oral antihistamine drugs such as hydroxyzine (Atarax) or diphenhydramine

Box 53-3
Clinical Manifestations of Atopic Dermatitis

DISTRIBUTION OF LESIONS

Infantile form—generalized, especially checks, scalp, trunk, and extensor surfaces of extremities (Fig. 53-13)

Childhood form—flexural areas (antecubital and popliteal fossae, neck), wrists, ankles, and feet

Preadolescent and adolescent form—face, sides of neck, hands, feet, face, and antecubital and popliteal fossae (to a lesser extent)

APPEARANCE OF LESIONS

Infantile form:
- Erythema
- Vesicles
- Papules
- Weeping
- Oozing
- Crusting
- Scaling
- Often symmetric

Childhood form:
- Symmetric involvement
- Clusters of small erythematous or flesh-colored papules or minimally scaling patches
- Dry and may be hyperpigmented
- Lichenification (thickened skin with accentuation of creases)
- Keratosis pilaris (follicular hyperkeratosis) common

Adolescent/adult form:
- Same as childhood manifestations
- Dry, thick lesions (lichenified plaques) common
- Confluent papules

OTHER PHYSICAL MANIFESTATIONS

Intense itching

Unaffected skin dry and rough

African-American children likely to exhibit more papular and/or follicular lesions than Caucasian children

May exhibit one or more of the following:
- Lymphadenopathy, especially near affected sites
- Increased palmar creases (many cases)
- Atopic pleats (extra line or groove of lower eyelid)
- Prone to cold hands
- Pityriasis alba (small, poorly defined areas of hypopigmentation)
- Facial pallor (especially around nose, mouth, and ears)
- Bluish discoloration beneath eyes ("allergic shiners")
- Increased susceptibility to unusual cutaneous infections (especially viral)

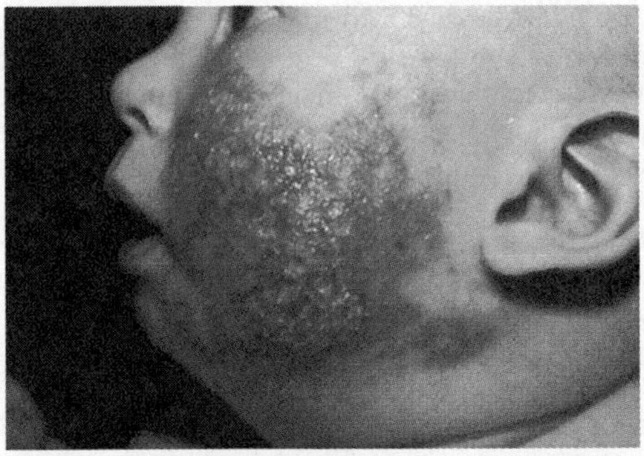

FIG. 53-13 • Infantile atopic dermatitis with oozing and crusting of lesions. (From Weston WL, Lane AT, Morelli JG: *Color textbook of pediatric dermatology,* ed 2, St Louis, 1996, Mosby.)

(Benadryl). Nonsedating antihistamines such as loratadine (Claritin) or fexofenadine (Allegra) may be preferred for daytime.

Occasional flare-ups require the use of topical steroids to diminish inflammation. Low-, moderate-, or high-potency topical corticosteroids are prescribed, depending on the degree of involvement, the area of the body to be treated, the age of the child, and the type of vehicle to be used (e.g., cream, lotion, or ointment).

Alternating corticosteroids with lubricants will reduce the risks associated with prolonged steroid use. Secondary infection is managed with appropriate antibiotic therapy.

Prevention of AD by limiting exposure of the fetus and child to allergens is controversial; however, the precautions in the Guidelines box may be recommended.

Prognosis. Most affected children (90%) "outgrow" AD by adolescence, but some continue to have chronic AD in adulthood.

Nursing Care Management

➤ Assessment

Assessment of the child with AD includes a family history for evidence of atopy, a history of previous involvement, and any environmental or dietary factors associated with the present and previous exacerbations. The skin lesions are examined for type, distribution, and evidence of secondary infection. Parents are interviewed regarding the child's behavior, especially in relation to scratching, irritability, and sleeping patterns. Exploration of the family's feelings and methods of coping should also be included.

➤ Nursing Diagnoses

A number of nursing diagnoses identified for the child with AD are outlined in Box 53-4. Others will be apparent individual cases.

➤ Plan of Care and Implementation

The objectives for nursing care of the child with AD and the family are as follows:

1. Child will experience no or minimal pruritus.
2. Child will receive appropriate treatment for skin hydration.
3. Child will experience no complications.
4. Child and family will receive adequate support.

Guidelines

PREVENTING ATOPY IN CHILDREN

Identify Children at Risk

Family history of allergy
Increased IgE in cord blood and postnatal serum
Dry, flaky skin

PRENATAL PRECAUTIONS (LAST TRIMESTER)

Avoid any known food allergens
Avoid milk and other dairy products, peanuts, and eggs
Minimize ingestion of other hyperallergenic foods

POSTNATAL PRECAUTIONS

Breast milk or casein/whey hydrolysate formula (e.g., Nutramigen, Pregestimil, Alimentum) exclusively for at least 6 months
No solid food for 6 months
No cow's milk or soy formula for 12 months
No egg, fish, corn, citrus, peanuts, nuts, or chocolate for 12 months
One new food added at 5-day intervals to identify possible reaction

ENVIRONMENTAL CONTROL

Limited exposure to dust, molds, animals, and cigarette smoke

Data from Johnstone D: Strategy for intervention of food allergy in infants, *Int Pediatr* 4(4):319-325, 1989; Zeiger R et al: Effectiveness of dietary manipulation in the prevention of food allergy in infants, part II, *J Allergy Clin Immunol* 78(1, pt 2):224-238, 1986; and Wood RA: Prospects for the prevention of allergy in children, *Curr Opin Pediatr* 8(6):601–605, 1995.

Box 53-4

Nursing Diagnoses: The Child with Atopic Dermatitis

Impaired skin integrity related to eczematous lesions
Risk for infection related to risk of secondary infection of primary lesions
Altered family processes related to child's discomfort and lengthy therapy

The child with AD presents a nursing challenge. Controlling the intense pruritus is imperative if the disorder is to be successfully managed, because scratching leads to new lesions and may cause secondary infection. In addition to the medical regimen, other measures can be taken to prevent or minimize the scratching. Fingernails and toenails are cut short, kept clean, and filed often to prevent sharp edges. Gloves or cotton stockings can be placed over the hands and pinned to shirtsleeves. To prevent reaching the affected skin, elbow restraints are sometimes necessary. One-piece outfits with long sleeves and long pants also decrease direct contact with the skin. If gloves or socks are used, the child needs some periods free from such restrictions. An excellent time to remove protective devices is during the bath or after receiving sedative or antipruritic medication.

NURSE ALERT • Do not remove elbow restraints during sleep because of the likelihood that the child will scratch while asleep.

Conditions that increase itching are eliminated when possible. Woolen clothes or blankets, rough fabrics, and furry stuffed animals are removed. Because heat and humidity cause perspiration, which intensifies the itching, proper dress for climatic conditions is essential. Pruritus is often precipitated by exposure to the irritant effects of components of common products such as soaps, detergents, fabric softeners, perfumes, and powders. Most children experience less itching when soft cotton fabrics are worn next to the skin. During cold months, synthetic fabrics (not wool) should be used for overcoats, hats, gloves, and snowsuits. Exposure to latex products such as gloves and balloons should also be avoided.

Clothes and sheets are laundered in a mild detergent and rinsed thoroughly in clear water (without fabric softeners or antistatic chemicals). Putting the clothes through a second complete wash cycle without using detergent reduces the amount of residue remaining in the fabric.

Preventing infection is usually secondary to preventing scratching. Baths are given as prescribed: the water is kept tepid, and soaps (except as indicated) and bubble baths are avoided, as are oils or powders. Skinfolds and diaper areas need frequent cleansing with plain water. A room humidifier or vaporizer may benefit children with extremely dry skin.

NURSE ALERT • If the child is being treated with frequent baths for hydration, it is imperative that the emollient preparation be applied immediately after bathing (while the skin is still slightly moist) to prevent drying.

Soaks and compresses are applied and medications for pruritus or infection are administered as directed. The family is given explicit instructions on the preparation and use of soaks, special baths, and topical medications, including the order of application if more than one is prescribed. It is important to emphasize that one thick application of topical medication is *not* equivalent to several thin applications. Excessive use (particularly of steroids) can be hazardous. If children have difficulty remaining still for a 10- or 15-minute soak, bath, or dressing application, these can be carried out at naptime or when the child is engrossed in television, a story, or playing with tub toys.

Because adequate rest is important for these children, who are usually fretful and irritable, planning meals, baths, medications, and treatments during periods when they are awake is paramount. Sleepy, tired children are normally cranky, and such behavior only intensifies the urge to scratch. During periods of irritability, these children tend to have a poor appetite, which is worsened by restriction of their usual foods.

Diet modification is another source of frustration to parents. When a hypoallergenic diet is prescribed, parents need help in understanding the reason for the diet and the guidelines for following it. Because hypoallergenic diets take time before effects are apparent, parents need reassurance that results may not be seen immediately.

Family Support. Parents are assured that the lesions will not produce scarring (unless secondarily infected) and that the disease is not contagious; however, the child will be subject to repeated exacerbations and remissions.

During acute phases, emotional stress can become intense for the family. They need time to discuss negative feelings and to be reassured that these feelings are normal. Efforts to relieve as much anxiety as possible in both parents and child has a beneficial emotional and physical effect, because stress aggravates the severity of the condition.

➤ Evaluation

The effectiveness of nursing interventions is determined by continual reassessment and evaluation of care based on the following observational guidelines:

1. Observe child's behavior, clothing, and activities.
2. Examine skin for evidence of dryness.
3. Examine skin lesions for evidence of secondary infection.
4. Interview aspects of family and encourage dialogue regarding the child and aspects of care.

Expected outcomes include the following:

1. Child does not scratch and rests or plays quietly.
2. Skin appears well hydrated.
3. There is no evidence of secondary infection.
4. Family members comply with the therapeutic regimen, freely discuss their feelings and concerns, and appear to be coping with the inconveniences imposed by the disorder (specify).

(See also Nursing Care Plan: The Child with Atopic Dermatitis [Eczema].*)

Seborrheic Dermatitis

Seborrheic dermatitis is a chronic, recurrent, inflammatory reaction of the skin. It occurs most commonly on the scalp (cradle cap), but may involve the eyelids (blepharitis), external ear canal (otitis externa), nasolabial folds, and inguinal region. The cause is unknown, although it is more common in early infancy when sebum production is increased. The lesions are characteristically thick, adherent, yellowish, scaly, oily patches that may or may not be mildly pruritic. Unlike atopic dermatitis, seborrheic dermatitis is not associated with a positive family history for allergy and is very common in infants shortly after birth and after puberty. Diagnosis is made primarily by the appearance and location of the crusts or scales.

Nursing Care Management. Cradle cap may be prevented with adequate scalp hygiene. Not infrequently, parents omit shampooing the infant's hair for fear of damaging the "soft spots," or fontanels. It is important to discuss how to shampoo the infant's hair and to emphasize that the fontanel is like skin anywhere else on the body—it does not puncture or tear with mild pressure.

When seborrheic lesions are present, the treatment is directed at removing the crusts. Parents are taught the appropriate procedure to clean the scalp, which may require a demonstration. Shampooing should be done daily with a mild soap or commercial baby shampoo; medicated shampoos are not necessary, but an antiseborrheic shampoo containing sulfur and salicylic acid may be used. Shampoo is applied to the scalp and allowed to remain on until the crusts are softened, and then the scalp is thoroughly rinsed. Using a fine-tooth comb or a soft facial brush after shampooing helps remove the loosened crusts from the strands of hair.

Acne

There is one skin disorder that, although not limited to the adolescent age group, appears predominantly at this time: *acne vul-*

*In Wong DL, Hess CS: ***Wong and Whaley's clinical manual of pediatric nursing,*** ed 5, St Louis, 2000, Mosby.

garis. Acne is an almost universal occurrence during these years and involves anatomic, physiologic, biochemical, genetic, immunologic, and psychologic factors of significant import.

It is estimated that about 85% of the population will have had acne by the end of the teenage years. Although the disorder can appear before this time, the peak incidence is in mid to late adolescence, at age 16 to 17 years in girls and 17 to 18 years in boys. It is more common in males than in females. The degree to which an individual is affected may range from nothing more than a few isolated comedones to a severe inflammatory reaction. Although the disease is self-limited and not life threatening, its significance to the adolescent is great, and it is a mistake to underestimate the impact that it can have on young people.

Numerous factors can affect the development and course of acne. Its distribution in families and a high degree of concordance in identical twins suggest hereditary factors. Premenstrual flares of acne occur in nearly 70% of adolescent girls, suggesting a hormonal cause. Studies do not indicate a clear association between stress and acne, although adolescents commonly cite stress as a cause for acne outbreaks. Cosmetics containing lanolin, petrolatum, vegetable oils, lauryl alcohol, butylstearate, and oleic acid can increase comedome production. Exposure to oils in cooking grease can be a precursor in adolescents who work in fast-food restaurants. There is no known link between dietary intake and the development or worsening of acne.

Pathophysiology. Acne is a disease that involves the *pilosebaceous follicles* (the hair follicle and sebaceous gland complex) of the face, neck, chest, and upper back. Three pathophysiologic factors are involved in the development of acne: excessive sebum production, comedogenesis, and the overgrowth of *Propionibacterium acnes* (Hurwitz, 1995).

Comedogenesis (formation of comedones) results in a *noninflammatory lesion* that may be either an *open comedone* ("blackhead") or a *closed comedone* ("whitehead"). Inflammation occurs with the proliferation of *Propionibacterium acnes,* a benign organism always present on the skin, resulting in papules, pustules, nodules, and cysts (Fig. 53-14).

A

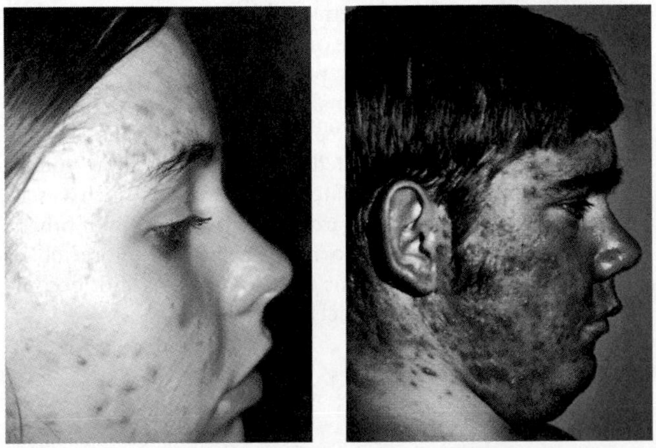

B

FIG. 53-14 • Acne vulgaris. **A,** Comedones with a few inflammatory pustules. **B,** Papulopustular acne. (From Weston WL, Lane AT: *Color textbook of pediatric dermatology,* St Louis, 1991, Mosby.)

Adolescents' concern about their appearance tempts them to pick, finger, squeeze, and otherwise manipulate the lesions; this plays an important role in the perpetuation of acne and possible secondary infection. In addition to the precipitating factors mentioned previously, the application of creams and oils, including heavy makeup bases, may aggravate acne.

Therapeutic Management. Successful management of acne depends on a cooperative effort between the health care provider, the adolescent, and the parents. Unlike many dermatologic conditions, acne lesions resolve slowly, and improvement may not be apparent for at least 6 weeks. Individual comedones may take several weeks to months to resolve, and papules and pustules usually resolve in about 1 week.

The multifactorial causes of acne necessitate a combined approach for successful treatment. Treatment consists of general measures of care and specific treatments determined by the type of lesions involved.

General Measures. Improvement of the adolescent's overall health status is part of the general management. Adequate rest, moderate exercise, a well-balanced diet, reduction of emotional stress, and elimination of any foci of infection are all part of general health promotion.

Medications. The wide range of topical medications available for the treatment of acne has nearly eliminated the need for systemic treatment (Berson and Shalita, 1995). *Tretinoin (Retin-A)* is the only drug that effectively interrupts the abnormal follicular keratinization that produces microcomedones, the invisible precursors of the visible comedones. Tretinoin alone is usually sufficient for management of comedonal acne. Tretinoin is available as a cream, gel, or liquid, but it can be extremely irritating to the skin and requires careful patient education for optimum usage. The patient should be instructed to begin with a pea-sized dot of medication, which is divided into the three main areas of the face and then gently rubbed into each area. The medication should not be applied for at least 20 to 30 minutes after washing to decrease the burning sensation. Avoidance of the sun and the use of daily sunscreen must be emphasized, because sun exposure can result in severe sunburn. Adolescents should be advised to apply the medication at night and to use a sunscreen with a sun protection factor (SPF) of at least 15 in the daytime.

Topical *benzoyl peroxide* kills *P. acnes* organisms, is effective against both inflammatory and noninflammatory acne, and can be used as a single therapy for mild acne. This medication is available as a cream, lotion, gel, or wash. The patient should be informed that the medication may have a bleaching effect on sheets, bedclothes, and towels. Accommodation to the medication can be gained with a gradual increase in the strength and frequency of application.

When inflammatory lesions accompany the comedones, a *topical antibacterial agent* may be prescribed. Clindamycin, erythromycin, metronidazole, azelaic acid, and the combination of either benzoyl peroxide and erythromycin (Benzamycin) or benzoyl peroxide and glycolic acid are all choices for topical antibacterial therapy (Leyden, 1997). Tretinoin improves the penetration of other topical agents, and combination therapy with tretinoin and an antibacterial treatment is the only way to address three of the pathogenic causes of acne: keratinization, *P. acnes,* and inflammation (Berson and Shalita, 1995).

Systemic antibiotic therapy is used when moderate to severe acne does not respond to topical treatments. Oral antibiotics that are considered extremely safe to use to treat acne include tetracycline, erythromycin, minocycline, doxycycline, clindamycin, and trimethoprim-sulfamethoxazole (Leyden, 1997).

Females with mild to moderate acne may respond well to topical treatment and the addition of an *oral contraceptive pill (OCP)*. Oral contraceptive pills reduce the endogenous androgen production and decrease the bioavailability of the circulating androgens. Both of these actions result in decreased acne.

Isotretinoin, 13-cis retinoic acid (Accutane), a very potent and effective oral agent, is reserved for severe cystic acne that has not responded to other treatments. Isotretinoin decreases sebum production, which ultimately results in a decrease in *P. acnes*. However, management of this medication should be done only by a dermatologist. Adolescents with multiple, active, deep dermal or subcutaneous cystic and nodular acne lesions are treated for 20 weeks. Multiple side effects can occur, including dry skin and mucous membranes, nasal irritation, dry eyes, decreased night vision, photosensitivity, arthralgia, headaches, mood changes, depression, and suicidal tendencies. The most significant side effects are the teratogenic effects. The drug is absolutely contraindicated in pregnancy, and practitioners must follow strict guidelines when prescribing the drug for female patients. Before treatment, identify whether or not the adolescent is sexually active. Sexually active young women must use an effective contraceptive method during treatment and for 1 month after treatment. Patients using isotretinoin should also be monitored for elevated cholesterol and triglyceride levels. Significant elevation of these laboratory values may require discontinuation of the medication.

Cleansing. Acne is not caused by dirt or oil on the surface of the skin. Gentle cleansing with a mild cleanser once or twice daily is usually sufficient. Antibacterial soaps are ineffective and may be too drying in combination with topical acne medications. For some adolescents hygiene of the hair and scalp appears to be related to the clinical activity of the acne. Acne on the forehead may be improved by brushing the hair away from the forehead and more frequent shampooing.

Prognosis. Acne will resolve spontaneously over a variable amount of time, depending on the individual.

Nursing Care Management. Because acne is so common and its appearance may seem so mild, the health care provider may underestimate the relative importance of this phenomenon to the adolescent. The nurse should assess the individual adolescent's level of distress, current management, and perceived success of any regimen before initiating a referral. If adolescents do not perceive the acne to be a problem, they will not be motivated to follow the daily routine necessary to treat the acne (Critical Thinking box).

Teenagers need a supportive, caring individual to help them maintain the persistence required to deal with the disorder over such an extended period. The adolescent needs education regarding the disease process and instruction in the prescribed therapy. Instruction should be definite and as specific as practical for each individual youngster. A written instruction sheet that describes the etiology and therapeutic regimen is often helpful, and parents should be cautioned against nagging. Adolescents should assume responsibility for following through on the instructions. They are cautioned against damaging the skin through too vigorous scrubbing. Several points are emphasized as particularly important: using only those preparations prescribed for their particular needs, carrying out associated directions, and not leaving cosmetics on the face overnight. Teenagers are subject to the influence of commercial advertising from a variety of media. Washing with a mild, nonabrasive cleanser, such as Dove (unscented), is adequate for cleansing.

Teenagers should be advised not to expect any visible improvement for 4 to 6 weeks after initiation of therapy. Acne may appear to worsen initially. Medications often cause erythema, peeling, itching, burning, and drying when first applied. The use of comedone extractors to remove blackheads is not recommended because this procedure can cause increased scarring. Females taking oral contraceptive pills and oral antibiotics should be instructed to use an additional form of contraception.

During conversations with teenagers the nurse can dispel the common myths often associated with acne and allow youngsters to discuss any feelings related to the disorder, such as self-consciousness or anxieties regarding relationships with others. Sometimes the nurse can also help teenagers explore job or other after-school interests. The acne lesions need not become an excuse to avoid social contacts and activities.

Critical Thinking

ACNE

Kim, who is 16 years old, recently started "breaking out." During her visit to the nurse practitioner, she was diagnosed as having a mild form of acne and was told to cleanse her face twice a day and apply Retin-A and benzoyl peroxide daily. Which instructions describe the correct skin care schedule?

First, Think About It . . .

- **What precise questions are you trying to answer?**
- **What information are you using?**

1. **Use a mild facial scrub in the morning and apply the Retin-A; at night use an astringent to remove makeup and apply benzoyl peroxide.**
2. **Wash the face with soap in the morning and at night; wait 30 minutes after the night cleansing to apply Retin-A, followed by benzoyl peroxide.**
3. **Wash the face with soap in the morning and apply benzoyl peroxide; wash the face before bedtime and apply Retin-A.**
4. **Wash the face with soap in the morning and apply benzoyl peroxide; wash the face in the evening and apply Retin-A about 30 minutes later.**

The best response is 4. Precisely, the most important aspects of the skin care regimen are to apply the topical preparation at different times of the day, because it is less effective when applications are close together. Also, the face should be completely dry before applying Retin-A to reduce skin irritation. Although either preparation can be used first, it is preferable to suggest applying Retin-A at night, when the teenager has time to wait after cleansing the skin. The information that you need to recall is that facial scrubs and astringents are not used, because they increase skin dryness.

THERMAL INJURY

Burns

Burn injuries are usually attributed to extreme heat sources but may also result from exposure to cold, chemicals, electricity, or radiation. Most burns are relatively minor and do not require definitive medical treatment; however, burns involving a large body surface area, critical body parts, or the geriatric or pediatric population often benefit from treatment in specialized burn centers. The American Burn Association has established criteria to guide decisions regarding the severity of injury and the need for transfer for specialized care. Burn prevention is also discussed in Chapters 36, 37, 39, and 40.

When burns are characterized by patients' age and type of injury, the following pattern arises: (1) toddlers most often sustain hot-water scalds; (2) older children are most likely to have received flame-related burns; (3) 20% of all pediatric admissions can be attributed to child abuse (Herndon et al, 1996); and (4) children playing with matches or lighters account for 1 in 10 house fires.

The extent of tissue destruction is determined by considering the intensity of the heat source, duration of contact or exposure, conductivity of the tissue involved, and rate at which the heat energy is dissipated by the skin. A brief exposure to high-intensity heat from a flame can produce burn injuries similar to those induced by long exposure to less intense heat in hot water.

Characteristics of Burn Injury. The physiologic responses, therapy, prognosis, and disposition of the injured child are all directly related to the *amount of tissue destroyed;* therefore the severity of the burn injury is assessed on the basis of the percentage of surface burned and the depth of the burn. In the school-age group or younger, a burn that is 10% of the *total body surface area (TBSA)* can be life threatening if not treated correctly. Also important in determining the seriousness of the injury are the location of the wounds, the age of the child, the causative agent, the presence of respiratory involvement, the general health of the child, and the presence of any associated injury or condition.

Type of Injury. The majority of burns result from contact with thermal agents such as a flame, hot surfaces, or hot liquids. Electrical injuries caused by household current have the greatest incidence in young children, who insert conductive objects into electrical outlets and bite or suck on connected electrical cords (Herndon et al, 1996). They occur most commonly during the spring and summer months and are also associated with risk-taking behaviors in boys. Direct contact with high- or low-voltage current, as well as lightning strikes, are the most common mechanism of injury. The resistance of the tissue and the path of the electric current are responsible for the damage incurred. Electric current travels through the body on the path of least resistance—tissue, fluid, blood vessels, and nerves. A more localized burn is produced if skin resistance is high at the area of contact, whereas a more systemic pattern of injury is produced if skin resistance is low. Often compared with a crush injury, serious electrical trauma results from current passing through vital organs, muscle compartments, and nerve or vascular pathways. Loss of limbs, cardiac fibrillation, respiratory collapse, and burns are common sequelae after exposure to electrical energy.

Chemical burns are seen in the pediatric population and can cause extensive injury. The severity of injury is related to the chemical agent (e.g., acid, alkali, or organic compound) and the duration of contact. The mechanism of injury differs from other burns in that there is a chemical disruption and alteration of the physical properties of the exposed body area. Noxious agents exist in many cleaning products commonly found in the home. In addition to concern for localized damage, the potential for systemic toxicity must be addressed. Of particular concern is the exposure of the eyes to chemical agents and the ingestion of caustic substances.

Extent of Injury. The extent of a burn is expressed as a percentage of the *TBSA.* This is most accurately estimated by using specially designed age-related charts (Fig. 53-15). It is more efficient to use a chart designed to assign body proportions to children of different ages.

A

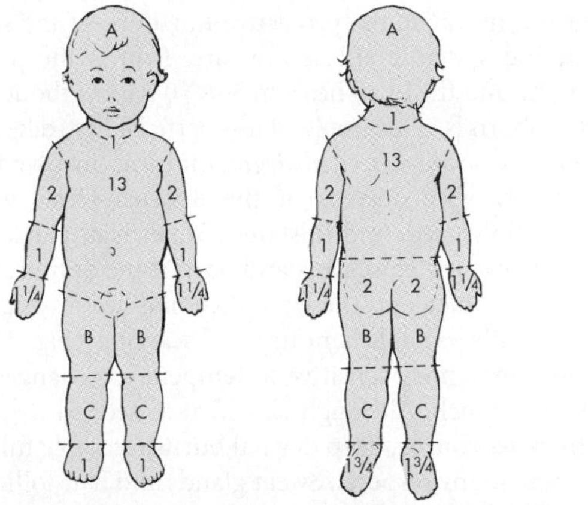

RELATIVE PERCENTAGES OF AREAS AFFECTED BY GROWTH

AREA	BIRTH	AGE 1 YR	AGE 5 YR
A = ½ of head	9½	8½	6½
B = ½ of one thigh	2¾	3¼	4
C = ½ of one leg	2½	2½	2¾

B

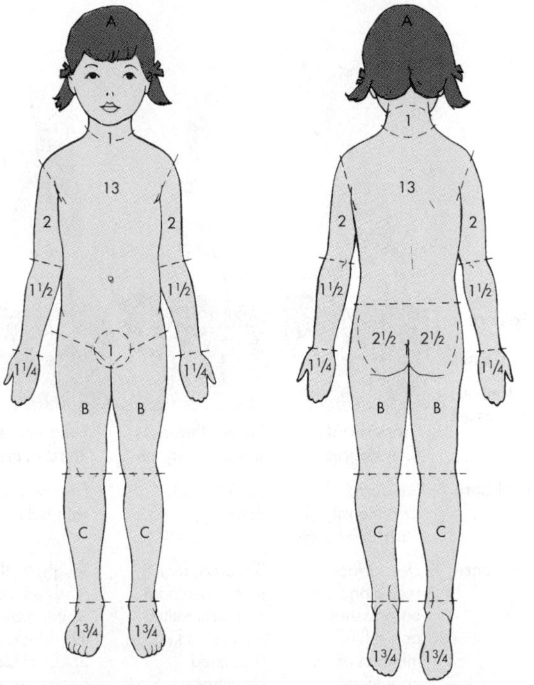

RELATIVE PERCENTAGES OF AREAS AFFECTED BY GROWTH

AREA	AGE 10 YR	AGE 15 YR	ADULT
A = ½ of head	5½	4½	3½
B = ½ of one thigh	4½	4½	4¾
C = ½ of one leg	3	3¼	3½

FIG. 53-15 • Estimation of distribution of burns in children. **A,** Children from birth to age 5 years. **B,** Older children.

Depth of Injury. A thermal injury is a three-dimensional wound and therefore is also assessed in relation to depth of injury. Traditionally the terms *first-*, *second,-* and *third-degree* have been used to describe the depth of tissue injury; however, with the current emphasis on wound healing, these have been replaced by more descriptive terms based on the extent of destruction to the epithelializing elements of the skin (Fig. 53-16).

Superficial (first-degree) burns are usually of minor significance. There is often a latent period followed by erythema. Tissue damage is minimal, the protective functions of the skin remain intact, and systemic effects are rare. Pain is the predominant symptom, and the burn heals in 5 to 10 days without scarring. A mild sunburn is an example of a superficial first-degree burn.

Partial-thickness (second-degree) injuries involve the epidermis and varying degrees of the dermis. These wounds are painful, moist, red, and blistered. Superficial partial-thickness burns involve the epidermis and part of the dermis. Dermal elements are intact, and the wound should heal in approximately 14 days with variable amounts of scarring (Fig. 53-17). The wound is extremely sensitive to temperature changes, exposure to air, and touch. Although classified as second-degree or partial-thickness burns, deep dermal burns resemble full-thickness injuries in many respects. Sweat glands and hair follicles remain intact. The burn may appear mottled, with pink, red, or waxy white areas exhibiting blisters and edema formation. Systemic effects are similar to those encountered with full-thickness burns. Although these wounds heal spontaneously in approximately 30 days, they do so with extensive scarring.

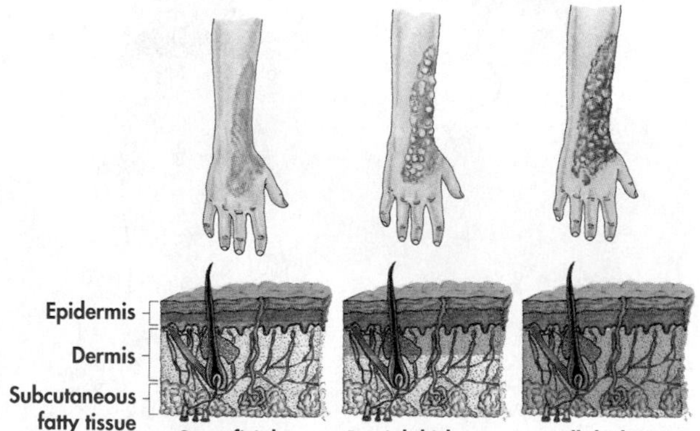

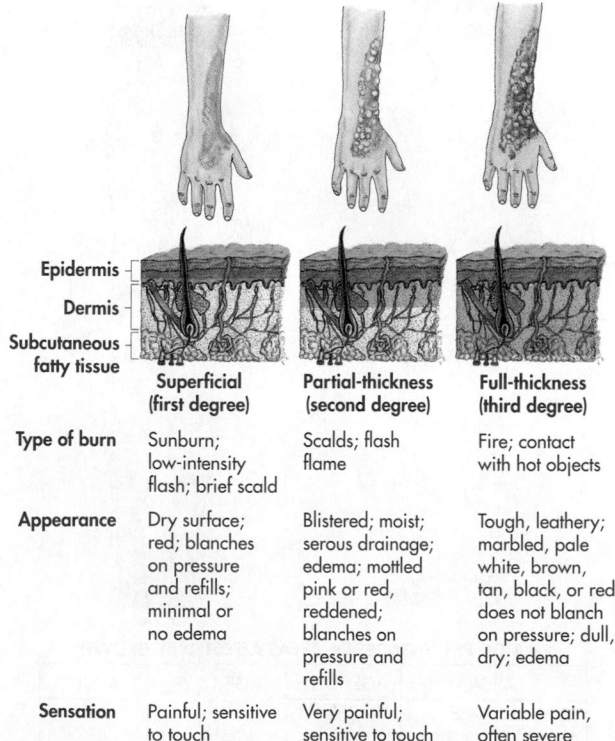

	Superficial (first degree)	Partial-thickness (second degree)	Full-thickness (third degree)
Type of burn	Sunburn; low-intensity flash; brief scald	Scalds; flash flame	Fire; contact with hot objects
Appearance	Dry surface; red; blanches on pressure and refills; minimal or no edema	Blistered; moist; serous drainage; edema; mottled pink or red, reddened; blanches on pressure and refills	Tough, leathery; marbled, pale white, brown, tan, black, or red; does not blanch on pressure; dull, dry; edema
Sensation	Painful; sensitive to touch	Very painful; sensitive to touch	Variable pain, often severe

FIG. 53-16 • Classification of burn depth. (Redrawn from Grant HD, Murray RH: *Emergency care,* ed 7, Upper Saddle River, NJ, 1995, Prentice-Hall.)

Full-thickness (third-degree) burns are serious injuries that involve the entire epidermis and dermis and extend into subcutaneous tissue (see Fig. 53-16). Nerve endings, sweat glands, and hair follicles are destroyed. The burn varies in color from red to tan, waxy white, brown, or black and is distinguished by a dry, leathery appearance (Fig. 53-18). Normally, full-thickness

A

B

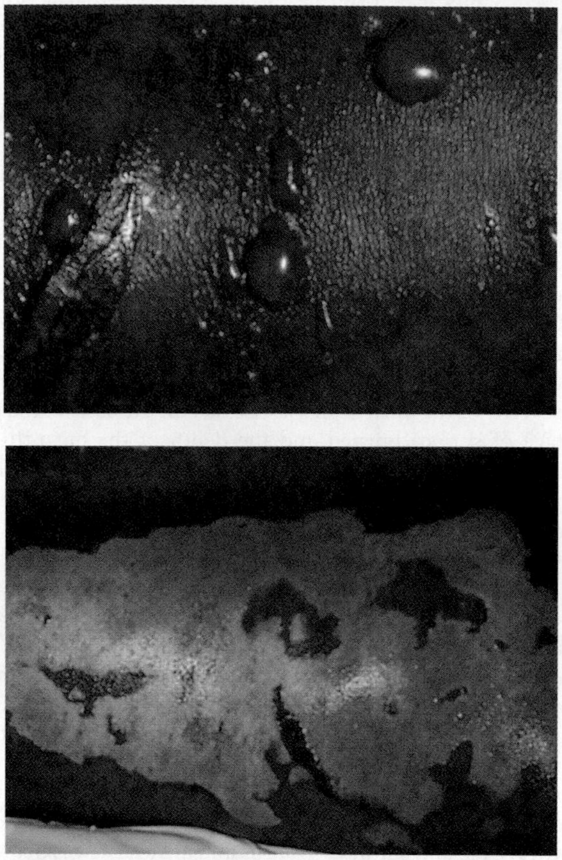

FIG. 53-17 • Superficial partial-thickness burns on an African-American child. **A,** Blisters intact. **B,** Blisters removed. (Courtesy of Hillcrest Medical Center, Tulsa, OK.)

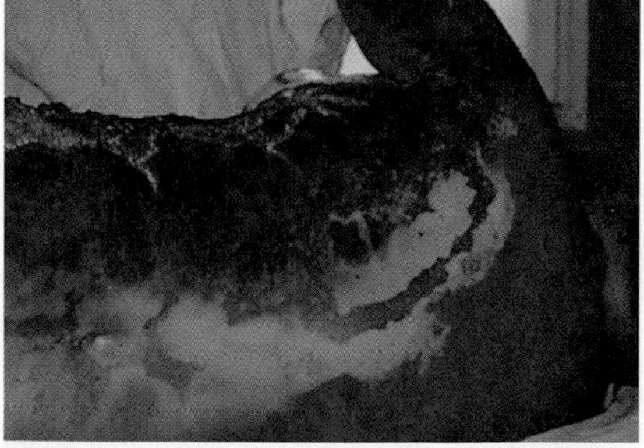

FIG. 53-18 • From bottom to top: Deep partial-thickness burn (red area); full-thickness burn (white area); full-thickness burn with eschar (brown area). (Courtesy Hillcrest Medical Center, Tulsa, OK.)

burns lack sensation in the area of injury because of the destruction of nerve endings; however, most full-thickness burns have superficial and partial-thickness burned areas at the periphery of the burn, where nerve endings are intact and exposed. Excised eschar and donor sites also cause exposed nerve fibers. Finally, as peripheral fibers regenerate, painful sensations return. Consequently, children often experience severe pain related to the size and depth of the burn. Full-thickness wounds are not capable of reepithelialization and require surgical excision and grafting to close the wound.

Fourth-degree burns are full-thickness injuries that involve underlying structures such as muscle, fascia, and bone. The wound appears dull and dry, and ligaments, tendons, and bone may be exposed (Fig. 53-19).

Severity of Injury. Burns are classified as minor, moderate, or major, which is useful in determining the disposition of the patient for treatment. Burn patients can usually be distinguished as (1) those with a *major burn injury,* who require the services and facilities of a specialized burn center; (2) those with a *moderate burn,* who may be treated in a hospital with expertise in burn care; and (3) those with *minor injuries,* who are able to be treated on an outpatient basis. The severity of the injury is determined by the extent and depth of the burn (Table 53-10), the causative agent, the body area involved, the patient's age, and concomitant injuries and illnesses.

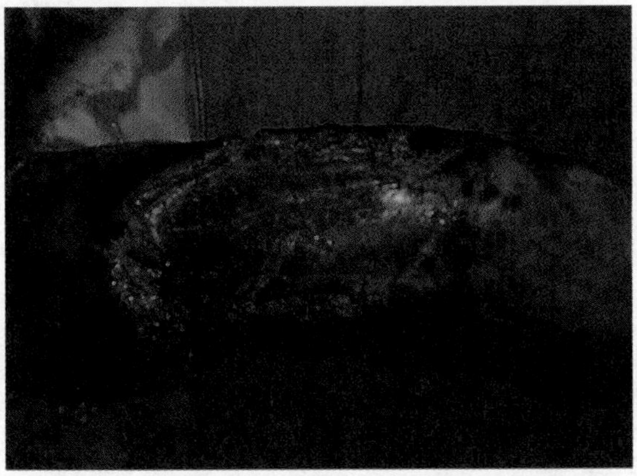

FIG. 53-19 • Full-thickness burn with muscle and fascia involved. (Courtesy Hillcrest Medical Center, Tulsa, OK.)

Because infants' skin is so thin, it is likely to sustain deeper injuries. Children younger than 2 years of age, especially 6 months or younger, have a significantly higher mortality rate than older children with burns of similar magnitude. Acute or chronic illnesses or superimposed injuries also complicate burn care and response to treatment.

Inhalation Injury. Trauma to the tracheobronchial tree often follows inhalation of the heated gases and toxic chemicals produced during combustion. Although direct thermal injury to the upper airway may occur, heat damage below the vocal cords is rare. Inspired heated air is cooled in the upper airway before reaching the trachea. Reflex closure of the cords and laryngeal spasm prevent full inhalation. Evidence of direct thermal injury to the upper airway includes burns of the face and lips, singed nasal hairs, and laryngeal edema. Clinical manifestations may be delayed as long as 24 to 48 hours. Wheezing, increasing secretions, hoarseness, wet rales, and carbonaceous secretions are signs of respiratory tract involvement. Upper airway obstruction is often associated with burn shock and fluid resuscitation. In such situations endotracheal intubation may be necessary to preserve a patent airway.

Inhalation of carbon monoxide is suspected when the fire has occurred in an enclosed space. Respiratory injury is manifested by mucosal erythema and edema, followed by sloughing of the mucosa. A mucopurulent membrane replaces the mucosal lining and seriously compromises respiration and ventilation.

Early in the postburn period the largest percentage of pulmonary infections result from nosocomial exposure, immobility, and abdominal distention. The hematogenous variety occurs later and is related to the septic burn wound or other foci, such as phlebitis at the site of an invasive IV line. A significant increase in mortality has been observed when inhalation injury and pneumonia are both present.

Deep burns, especially those circling the thorax, may cause restriction of chest excursion as a result of edema and inelastic eschar formation. Young children are particularly at risk because of the pliability of the skeletal structure. Hypoxia is relieved by an escharotomy incision, which allows expansion of the chest wall to facilitate ventilation.

Pathophysiology. Thermal injuries produce both local and systemic effects that are related to the extent of tissue destruction. In superficial burns the tissue damage is minimal. In partial-thickness burns there is considerable edema and more severe capillary damage. With a major burn greater than 30% of the TBSA, there is a systemic response involving an increase in

TABLE 53-10

Severity Grading System Adopted by the American Burn Association

	Minor*	Moderate	Major
Partial-thickness burns	<10% of total body surface area (TBSA)	10%-20% of TBSA	>20% of TBSA
Full-thickness burns			All
Treatment	Usually outpatient; may require 1- to 2-day admission	Admission to hospital, preferably one with expertise in burn care	Admission to a burn center

From Vaccaro P, Trofino RB: Care of the patient with minor to moderate burns. In Trofino RB, editor: *Nursing care of the burn-injured patient,* Philadelphia, 1991, FA Davis.

*Minor burns exclude any burn involving the face, hands, feet, perineum, or crossing joints; electrical burns; any injury complicated by the presence of inhalation injury or concomitant trauma; children with psychosocial factors impacting the injury.

capillary permeability, allowing plasma proteins, fluids, and electrolytes to be lost. Maximum edema formation in a small wound occurs about 8 to 12 hours after injury. After a larger injury, hypovolemia, associated with this phenomenon, will slow the rate of edema formation, with maximum effect at 18 to 24 hours.

Another systemic response is anemia, caused by direct heat destruction of red blood cells, hemolysis of injured red blood cells, and trapping of red blood cells in the microvascular thrombi of damaged cells. A long-term decrease in the number of red blood cells may result in diminished red blood cell life span. Initially there is an increased blood flow to the heart, brain, and kidneys, with decreased blood flow to the gastrointestinal tract. There is an increase in metabolism to maintain body heat, providing for the increased energy needs of the body.

Complications. Thermally injured children are subject to a number of serious complications, both from the wound and from systemic alterations resulting from the injury. The immediate threat to life is related to airway compromise and profound shock. During healing, infection—both local and systemic sepsis—is the primary complication. Mortality associated with thermal trauma in children increases with the severity of injury and decreases as age advances. In children older than 3 years, the mortality rate is similar to that of adults. Below this age, the survival rate from burns and their associated complications lessens considerably.

A less apparent respiratory injury is inhalation of carbon monoxide. Carbon monoxide has a greater affinity for hemoglobin than does oxygen, thereby depriving peripheral tissues and oxygen-dependent organs (such as the heart and brain) of the oxygen needed for survival. Treatment is 100% oxygen, which reverses the situation rapidly.

Pulmonary problems are a major cause of fatality in children with either thermal burns or complications in the respiratory tract. Respiratory problems include inhalation injuries, aspiration in unconscious patients, bacterial pneumonia, pulmonary edema, pulmonary embolus, posttraumatic pulmonary insufficiency, and atelectasis. The most common cause of respiratory failure in the pediatric age group is bacterial pneumonia, which requires prolonged intubation and sometimes necessitates a tracheostomy. Tracheostomies increase the incidence of serious complications, and they are performed only in extreme cases.

A less common complication is pulmonary edema resulting from fluid overload or acute respiratory distress syndrome (ARDS) in association with gram-negative sepsis. This syndrome results from pulmonary capillary damage and leakage of fluid into the interstitial spaces of the lung. A loss of compliance and interference with oxygenation are the consequences of pulmonary insufficiency in conjunction with systemic sepsis.

Wound Sepsis. Sepsis is a critical problem in the treatment of burns and an ever-present threat after the shock phase. Initially, burn wounds are relatively pathogen free unless they are contaminated with potentially infectious material such as dirt or polluted water. However, dead tissue and exudate provide a fertile field for bacterial growth. On approximately the third postburn day, early colonization of the wound surface by a preponderance of gram-positive organisms (primarily staphylococci) changes to predominantly gram-negative opportunistic organisms, particularly *Pseudomonas aeruginosa.* By the fifth postburn day, bacterial invasion is well under way beneath the surface of the burn wound. Early surgical excision of eschar, together with placement of autograft, has reduced the incidence of sepsis today.

Therapeutic Management

Emergency Care. The initial management of the burn patient begins at the scene of injury. The first priority is to stop the burning process (Emergency box). The child should then be transported immediately to the nearest medical facility for treatment and evaluation. The child and the family will be extremely frightened and anxious; sensitivity to their emotional state will provide reassurance during the transport process.

Stop the Burning Process. The chief aim of rescue in flame burns is to smother the fire, not fan it. Children tend to panic and run, which spreads the flames and makes assistance more difficult. The injured child should be placed in a horizontal position and rolled in a blanket, rug, or similar article, with care taken not to cover the head and face because of the danger of inhalation of toxic fumes. If nothing is available, the victim should lie down and roll over slowly to extinguish the flames. Remaining in the vertical position may cause the hair to ignite or cause inhalation of flames, heat, or smoke.

Major burns with large amounts of denuded skin should not be cooled. Heat is rapidly lost from burned areas, and additional cooling leads to a drop in core body temperature and potential circulatory collapse. Wet dressings also promote vasoconstriction because of cooling, resulting in impaired circulation to the burned area and increased tissue damage. Chemical burns present special circumstances and require continuous flushing with large amounts of water during transport to a medical facility. The use of neutralizing agents on the skin is contraindicated because a chemical reaction is initiated and further injury may result. If the chemical is in powder form, the addition of water may spread the caustic agent. The powder should be brushed off if possible.

Burned clothing is removed to prevent further damage from smoldering fabric and hot beads of melted synthetic materials. Jewelry is removed to eliminate the transfer of heat from the

Emergency

BURNS

Minor Burns

Stop the burning process:
- Apply cool water to the burn or hold the burned area under cool running water. Do not use ice.

Do not disturb any blisters that form.
Do not apply anything to the wound.
Cover with a clean cloth if risk of damage or contamination.
Remove burned clothing and jewelry.

Major Burns

Stop the burning process:
- Flame burns—smother the fire.
- Place victim in the horizontal position.
- Roll victim in a blanket or similar object; avoid covering the head.

Assess for an adequate airway and breathing.
If not breathing, begin mouth-to-mouth resuscitation.
Remove burned clothing and jewelry.
Cover wound with a clean cloth.
Keep victim warm.
Transport to medical aid.
Begin intravenous and oxygen therapy as prescribed.

metal and constriction resulting from edema formation. This also provides access to the wound and prevents painful removal later on.

Assess the Victim's Condition. As soon as the flames are extinguished, the child is assessed. Airway, breathing, and circulation are the priority concerns. Cardiopulmonary complications may result from exposure to electric current, inhalation of toxic fumes and smoke, hypovolemia, and shock. Emergency measures are instituted as appropriate.

Cover the Burn. The burn wound should be covered with a clean cloth to prevent contamination, decrease pain by eliminating air contact, and prevent hypothermia. No attempt should be made to treat the burn. Application of topical ointments, oils, or other home remedies is contraindicated.

Transport the Child to Medical Aid. The child with an extensive burn is not given anything by mouth to avoid aspiration in the presence of paralytic ileus and upper airway edema and to prevent water intoxication. The child is transported to the nearest medical facility. If this cannot be accomplished within a relatively short period of time, IV access should be established, if possible, with a large-bore catheter. Oxygen is administered, if available, at 100%. A report of the initial assessment and any interventions implemented is given to the medical facility assuming care of the child.

Provide Reassurance. Providing reassurance and psychologic support to both the family and the child helps immeasurably during postinjury crisis. Reducing anxiety conserves energy needed to cope with the physiologic and emotional stress of injury.

Minor Burns. Treatment of burns classified as minor can usually be managed adequately on an outpatient basis when it is determined that the parent can be relied on to carry out instructions for care and observation. Patients with less than optimum circumstances may require close follow-up to ensure compliance with treatment.

The wound is cleansed with a mild soap and tepid water. Debridement of the wound includes removal of any embedded debris, chemicals, and devitalized tissue. Removal of intact blisters remains controversial. Some argue that blisters provide a barrier against infection; others maintain that blister fluid is an effective medium for the growth of microorganisms. Most practitioners favor covering the wound with an antimicrobial ointment to reduce the risk of infection and to provide some form of pain relief. The dressing consists of a fine-mesh gauze placed over the ointment and a light wrap of gauze dressing that avoids interference with movement. This helps to keep the wound clean and protect it from trauma. The caregiver is instructed to wash the wound, reapply the dressing, and return the child to the office or clinic as directed for wound observation. The frequency of dressing changes may vary from every other day to twice a day.

Some practitioners prefer an occlusive dressing, such as a hydrocolloid, which is placed over the wound after cleansing. The dressing is changed once leakage occurs or at regular intervals. This method eliminates the discomfort associated with frequent dressing changes but impairs visualization of the wound surface.

If there is a high probability of infection or other complications, or if there is doubt about the ability to carry out instructions, the caregiver may be directed to bring the patient in daily for dressing changes and inspection, or a nurse may be assigned to make a home visit for that purpose. Frequent removal of the dressing is an effective mode of debridement. Soaking the dressing in tepid water before removal will help loosen the dressing and debris and reduce discomfort. Burns of the face are usually treated by an open method. The wound is washed and debrided in the same manner, and a thin film of antimicrobial ointment is applied.

A tetanus history is obtained on admission. When there is no history of immunization, or more than 5 years have passed since the last immunization, tetanus prophylaxis is administered. Administration of antibiotics for minor burns is controversial. A mild analgesic such as acetaminophen is usually sufficient to relieve discomfort; the antipyretic effect of the drug also alleviates the sensation of heat.

Most minor burns heal without difficulty, but if the wound margin becomes erythematous, if gross purulence is noted, or if the child develops evidence of systemic reaction such as fever or tachycardia, hospitalization is indicated. The child should also be evaluated for functional impairment, and the caregiver should be instructed in the exercise and ambulation program. After wound healing, an evaluation of scar maturation and range of motion will indicate any need for further therapy.

Major Burns. The first priority is airway maintenance. The inhalation of noxious agents or respiratory burns is suggested when there is a history of injury in an enclosed space; edema of the oral and nasal membranes; thermal injury to the face, nares, and upper torso; hyperemia; and blisters or evidence of trauma to the upper respiratory passages. When respiratory involvement is suspected or evident, 100% oxygen is administered and blood gas values, including carbon monoxide levels, are determined.

If the child exhibits changes in sensorium, air hunger, or other signs of respiratory distress, an endotracheal tube is inserted to maintain the airway. When severe edema of the face and neck is anticipated, intubation is performed before swelling makes intubation difficult or impossible. Controlled intubation is preferred to an emergency procedure. Intubation allows for the delivery of humidified oxygen, the removal of secretions from respiratory passages, and the provision of ventilatory support.

When full-thickness burns encircle the chest, constricting eschar may limit chest wall excursion, and the child becomes more difficult to ventilate. Escharotomy of the chest relieves this constriction and improves ventilation.

Fluid Replacement Therapy. The objectives of fluid therapy are to (1) compensate for water and sodium lost to traumatized areas and interstitial spaces, (2) replenish sodium deficits, (3) restore circulating volume, (4) provide adequate perfusion, (5) correct acidosis, and (6) improve renal function.

Fluid replacement is required during the first 24 hours because of fluid shifts that are occurring. Many formulas are used to calculate these needs, and the one adopted depends on practitioner preference. Crystalloid solutions are used during this initial phase of therapy. Adequacy of fluid resuscitation is determined by parameters such as vital signs (especially heart rate), urine output volume, adequacy of capillary filling, and state of sensorium.

After the initial 24-hour period, theoretically there is a capillary seal, and capillary permeability is restored. Colloid solutions such as albumin, Plasma-Lyte, or fresh frozen plasma are useful in maintaining plasma volume; however, children with burn injuries usually require fluids in excess of their calculated maintenance and replacement volume. Reasons for this may include underestimation of burn size (particularly in pediatric patients), pulmonary injury that sequesters resuscitation fluid in the lung, electrical injury with greater tissue destruction than that which is visible, and a delay in the initiation of fluid resuscitation. Irreversible burn shock that persists despite aggressive fluid resuscitation remains a significant cause of death in the immediate postburn period. Fluid balance may continue to be a problem throughout the course of treatment, especially during the periods in which there may be considerable evaporative loss from the wound.

Nutrition. The enhanced metabolic requirements and catabolism in severe burns make nutritional needs of paramount importance and often difficult to provide. The diet must provide sufficient calories to meet the increased metabolic needs and sufficient protein to avoid protein breakdown. Hypoglycemia can result from the stress of the burn injury as the liver glycogen stores are rapidly depleted.

A high-protein, high-calorie diet is encouraged after resolution of paralytic ileus; however, many children have poor appetites and are unable to meet energy requirements solely by oral feeding. Most children with burns in excess of 25% of the TBSA require supplementation with tube feeding. Early and continued nutritional support is an important part of therapy for seriously burned patients. Enteral feeding has been found to directly nourish the gastrointestinal tract and may help to reverse the defective gut barrier that accompanies burn shock (Hansbrough, 1998).

If nutritional requirements cannot be met entirely by the enteral route, parenteral hyperalimentation can be used to supplement intake. However, enteral feeding increases blood flow in the intestinal tract, preserves gastrointestinal function, and minimizes bacterial translocation by decreasing mucosal atrophy of the intestines. This makes enteral feeding the preferred route of nutritional support (Herndon et al, 1996).

To facilitate growth and proliferation of epithelial cells, administration of vitamins A and C is begun early in the postburn period. Zinc is also supplemented because of its important role in wound healing and epithelialization.

Medication. Antibiotics are usually not administered prophylactically. The administration of systemic antibiotics to control wound colonization is not indicated because decreased circulation to the injured area prevents delivery of the medication to areas of deepest injury. Surveillance cultures and monitoring of the clinical course provide the most reliable indicators of developing infection. Appropriate antibiotics can then be instituted to treat the identified organism. Otitis media should not be overlooked as a source of fever in the pediatric population.

Some form of sedation and analgesia is required in the care of burned children. Morphine sulfate is the drug of choice for severe burn injuries. Morphine has extensive distribution but is eliminated rapidly; continuous infusion or frequent administration is needed for pain management in burns. Morphine is administered intravenously and titrated to individual need. The unstable circulatory status and edema formation preclude intramuscular or subcutaneous administration. When combined, midazolam (Versed) and fentanyl (Sublimaze) also provide excellent IV sedation and analgesia to control procedural pain in children with burns (Herndon et al, 1996). The oral form of fentanyl, Fentanyl Oralet, provides effective analgesia in a convenient form that the child sucks. The dose is 5 to 15 μg/kg (maximum 400 μg) (Kahana, 1997). Tolerance to opioids may develop and requires dosage monitoring. IV analgesics are most effective if administered just before the onset of procedural pain.

The use of short-acting anesthetic agents such as propofol and nitrous oxide has proved beneficial in eliminating procedural pain. Pharyngeal reflexes remain intact, thus ensuring a patent airway. Propofol (Diprivan) is an IV sedative hypnotic agent that produces sedation in less than 1 minute and lasts only a few minutes.

Nitrous oxide is a useful short-term analgesic when given in a mixture of gases on a fixed ratio of 50% nitrous oxide and 50% oxygen (Annequin et al, 2000). Initiation of action is approximately 1 minute, with peak effect reached in 3 to 5 minutes. Nitrous oxide is useful to alleviate anxiety and raise the threshold of pain during procedures. The child may self-administer the nitrous oxide mixture with assistance. For any conscious or unconscious sedation, the child is monitored continuously during the procedure. (See Preoperative Care, Chapter 45, and Pain Assessment and Pain Management, Chapter 44.)

Management of the Burn Wound. After the initial period of shock and the restoration of fluid balance, the primary concern is the burn wound. The objectives of wound management include prevention of infection, removal of devitalized tissue, and closure of the wound. The application of dressings and topical antimicrobial therapy reduce pain by minimizing the exposure to air.

Primary excision. In children with large, full-thickness burn wounds, excision is performed as soon as the patient is hemodynamically stable after initial resuscitation. Because the burn wound is precipitating the exaggerated physiologic response, many complications do not resolve until the eschar is excised and the wound is closed. Early excision of deep partial-thickness and full-thickness burns reduces the incidence of infection and the threat of sepsis.

Debridement. Hydrotherapy is employed to cleanse the wound and involves soaking in a tub or showering once or twice a day for no more than 20 minutes. Hydrotherapy helps to cleanse not only the wound but the entire body and aids in maintenance of range of motion.

Partial-thickness wounds require debridement of devitalized tissue to promote healing. Debridement is very painful and requires some type of analgesia before the procedure. The water acts to loosen and remove sloughing tissue, exudate, and topical medications. Mesh gauze serves to entrap the exudative slough and is readily removed during hydrotherapy. Any loose tissue is carefully trimmed away before the wound is redressed.

Topical antimicrobial agents. Methods used for managing the burn wound include:

Exposure—Wounds are left open to air; crust forms on partial-thickness wounds, and eschar forms on full-thickness burns

Open—Topical antimicrobial agent is applied directly to the wound surface, and the wound is left uncovered

Modified—Antimicrobial is applied directly or impregnated into thin gauze and applied to the wound; gauze or net secures the area

Occlusive—Antimicrobial is impregnated in gauze or applied directly to the wound; multiple layers of bulky gauze are placed over the primary layer and secured with gauze or net

All of these methods provide wound coverage and employ some type of topical agent.

Topical agents do not eliminate organisms from the wound but can effectively inhibit bacterial growth. To be effective, a topical application must be nontoxic, capable of diffusing through eschar, harmless to viable tissue, inexpensive, and easy to apply. It should not encourage the development of resistant strains of bacteria and should produce minimum electrolyte derangement. A comparison of commonly used agents is summarized in Table 53-11.

Biologic skin coverings. Permanent coverage of extensive burns is a prolonged process that requires repeated operations for debridement and grafting. Early closure shortens the period of metabolic stress and decreases the likelihood of burn wound sepsis. In the acute phase, biologic dressings cover and protect the wound from contamination, reduce fluid and protein loss, increase the rate of epithelialization, reduce pain, and facilitate movement of joints to retain range of motion.

Allograft (homograft) skin is obtained from human cadavers that are screened for communicable diseases. Homograft is particularly useful in the coverage of surgically excised deep partial-thickness and full-thickness wounds in extensive burns when available donor sites are limited. Severe immunosuppression occurs in massively burned children, and the allograft becomes adherent. The homograft can remain in place until suitable donor sites become available. Typically, rejection is seen approximately 14 days after application. The use of homograft is limited by the availability of tissue banks and a supply of suitable donors.

Xenograft from a variety of species, most notably pigs, is commercially available. In large burns, the porcine xenograft is commonly applied when extensive early debridement is indicated to cover a partial-thickness burn; this allows available autograft to be applied to the full-thickness areas (Still et al, 1996). Pigskin dressings are replaced daily or every 2 to 3 days. They are particularly effective in children with partial-thickness scald burns of the hands and face because they allow relatively pain-free movement, which reduces contracture formation and has the added benefit of improving appetite and morale.

When applied early to a superficial partial-thickness injury, biologic dressings stimulate epithelial growth and faster wound healing; however, biologic dressings must be applied to clean wounds. If the dressing covers areas of heavy microbial contamination, infection occurs beneath the dressing. In the case of partial-thickness burns, such infection may convert the wound to a full-thickness injury.

NURSE ALERT • Observe the wound daily for any sign of an infectious process, such as purulence, erythema, cellulitis around the wound edges, or temperature elevation.

TABLE 53-11
Comparison of Common Topical Preparations

Agent	Dressings	Advantages	Disadvantages
Silver nitrate 0.5% ($AgNO_3$)	Open, modified or occlusive; impedes joint movement; dressings changed twice daily; keep dressing moist, rewet at least every 2 hours	Greatly reduces evaporative losses; does not interfere with wound healing; bacteriostatic action against major burn flora, including *Pseudomonas* and *Staphylococcus;* inexpensive	Does not penetrate eschar; ineffective on established burn wound infections; little effect on *Klebsiella* and *Aerobacter* groups; stains skin, clothing, linens; makes assessment of the wound difficult because of staining; hypotonicity pulls electrolytes from the wound, depleting sodium, potassium, chloride, and magnesium; stings on application
Silver sulfadiazine 1% (AgSD)	Occlusive; motion of joints maintained; applied twice daily; do not use with a history of allergy to sulfa	Little pain on application; bactericidal by altering DNA and cell metabolism; effective against gram-positive and gram-negative bacteria; easy to apply; nontoxic	Transient neutropenia; does not penetrate eschar; forms proteinaceous gel on wound surface that is painful to remove; occasional rashes and pruritus; decreases granulocyte formation
Mafenide acetate 10% (Sulfamylon)	***Cream:*** Usually open; do not apply to face; apply twice daily ***Solution:*** Occlusive; keep dressing moist (rewet at least every 2 hours); protect solution from light	Penetrates eschar and diffuses rapidly into burn wound and underlying tissues; effective in deep flame, electrical, and infected wounds; biostatic against many gram-positive and gram-negative organisms, including *Pseudomonas* and *Clostridium*	Difficult and painful to remove cream; pain on application; metabolic acidosis, hypercapnia, and carbonic anhydrase inhibition; inhibits wound healing; hypersensitivity in some patients
Bacitracin	Open, modified; motion of joints maintained; change dressing twice daily	Bactericidal and bacteriostatic against gram-positive organisms; low toxicity; painless application; ease of application	Limited activity against gram-negative organisms; allergic reaction in sensitive individuals

Synthetic skin coverings are available for the management of partial-thickness burn wounds. Ideally, the dressing should provide the properties of human skin: adherence, elasticity, durability, and hemostasis. Synthetic skin substitutes are readily available, have an indefinite shelf life, and are relatively inexpensive.

Synthetic dressings are composed of a variety of materials and can be used successfully in the management of superficial partial-thickness burns and donor sites. Examples include adherent elastic films, hydroactive materials, or colloidal suspensions that are usually permeable to air, vapor, and fluids. BCG Matrix consists of a film-backed mesh-reinforced hydrocolloid dressing. Biobrane is a flexible silicone-nylon membrane bonded to collagenous peptides of porcine skin. Calcium alginate is another treatment for donor sites. As with biologic dressings, it is important that the wound be free of debris before the dressing is applied. Body temperature elevation or evidence of purulence, erythema, or cellulitis around the wound edges may indicate that the wound has become infected beneath the dressing. Prompt discontinuance of the synthetic dressing is indicated. All synthetic dressings are reputed to hasten wound healing and reduce discomfort.

Permanent skin coverings. Permanent coverage of deep partial-thickness and full-thickness burns is usually accomplished with a split-thickness skin graft. This graft consists of the epidermis and a portion of the dermis removed from an intact area of skin by a special instrument, the dermatome (Fig. 53-20) (Atraumatic Care box).

With extensive burns it is often difficult to find enough viable skin to cover the wounds; therefore available donor sites and special techniques are used. Split-thickness skin grafts may be sheet graft or mesh graft:

Sheet graft—A sheet of skin, removed from the donor site, is placed intact over the recipient site and sutured in place; used in areas where cosmetic results are most visible (Fig. 53-21)

Mesh graft—A sheet of skin is removed from the donor site and passed through a mesher, which produces tiny slits in the skin that allow the skin to cover 1½ to 9 times the area of the sheet graft; results in a less desirable cosmetic and functional outcome (Fig. 53-22)

The donor site is dressed with synthetic wound coverings or fine-mesh gauze until the dressing separates at 10 to 14 days when the wound is healed. Dressings are not changed on donor sites to avoid damage to newly healed, delicate epithelium. Healed donor sites are available for reharvesting in patients with extensive burns and limited undamaged skin, but the quality of skin is decreased when multiple grafts are taken.

Artificial skin. The development of Integra,* a product that allows the dermis to regenerate, has produced significant improvement in burn wound healing and decreased scar forma-

*Integra Life Sciences Corporation, 105 Morgan Lane, Plainsboro, NJ; (609) 275-0500; fax (609) 779-3297.

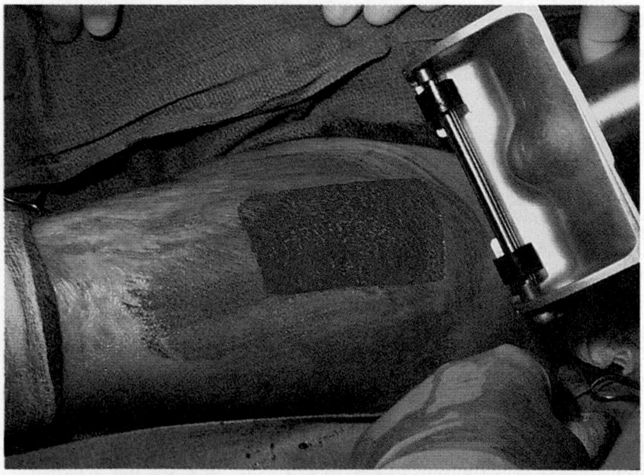

FIG. 53-20 • Removal of split-thickness skin graft with a dermatome.

Atraumatic Care

SKIN GRAFTING

The removal of skin with a dermatome is a very painful procedure. The child should be given unconscious sedation.

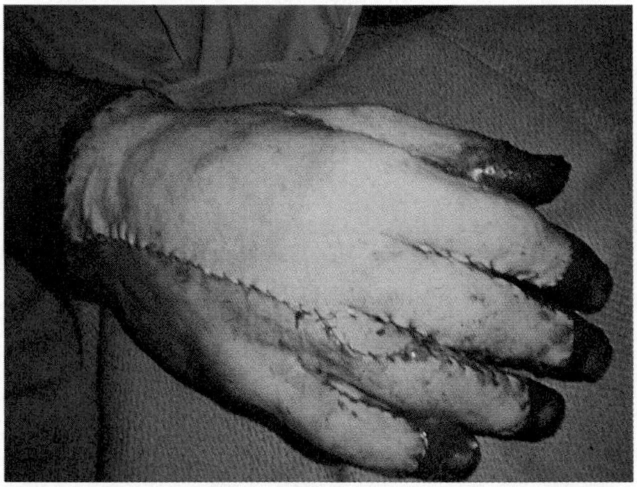

FIG. 53-21 • Sheet graft.

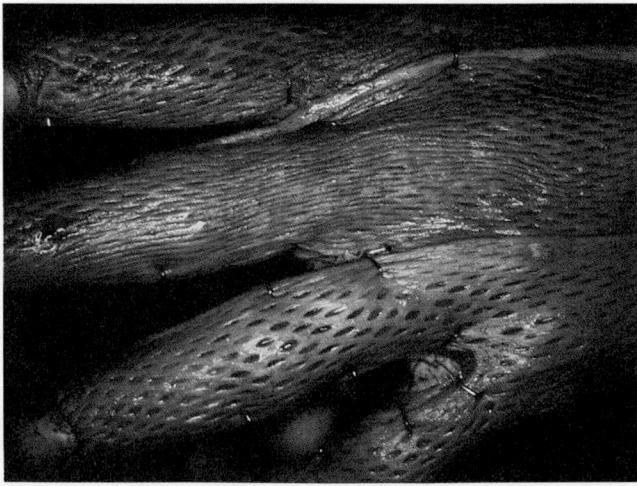

FIG. 53-22 • Mesh graft.

tion. It is applied to partial-thickness and full-thickness burns. The two-layer membrane is made of collagen (a fibrous protein from animal tendons and cartilage) and silicone rubber (i.e., Silastic). The Silastic layer is peeled off after the dermis is formed. The application of artificial skin does not replace the grafting procedure, but it prepares the burn wound to accept an ultrathin autograft. Advantages include faster healing of the burn wound when integrity of the dermis is restored, faster healing of donor sites with the use of ultrathin grafts, and restoration of sweat glands and hair follicles. A disadvantage is its high cost.

Cultured epithelium. When burns are extensive and donor sites for split-thickness skin grafting are limited, it is possible to culture cells from a full-thickness skin biopsy and produce coherent sheets that can be applied to clean, excised full-thickness wounds. Epithelial cell culture grafts offer the possibility of an unlimited source of autografts in patients with extensive burns. Cultured epithelial autografts are effective in early wound closure. The child's own skin is fractionated and cultured in a porcine media to form a thin epithelial layer that is applied to the burn wound. This technique offers an improved rate of survival in patients with extensive burns and limited donor sites.

Prognosis. Children differ from adults in their responses to thermal injury, and the mortality rates in young children are significantly higher than those in older children and adults. Mortality is greatest for children younger than 48 months of age. Many children who do survive have long-term functional and cosmetic impairments.

Nursing Care Management. Because the care of burned children encompasses a broad range of skills, it has been divided into segments that correspond with the major phases of burn treatment. The *acute phase,* also referred to as the emergent or resuscitative phase, involves the first 24 to 48 hours. The *management phase* extends from the completion of adequate resuscitation through wound coverage. The *rehabilitative phase* begins once the majority of the wounds have healed and rehabilitation has become the predominant focus of the plan of care. This phase continues until all reconstructive procedures and corrective measures have been accomplished and often extends over a period of months or years.

Acute Phase. The primary emphasis during the emergent phase is the treatment of burn shock and management of pulmonary status. Monitoring vital signs, output, fluid infusion, and respiratory parameters are ongoing activities in the hours immediately following injury. IV infusion is begun immediately and is regulated to maintain a urine output of at least 1 to 2 ml/kg in children weighing less than 30 kg; an output of 30 to 50 ml/hr is expected in children weighing more than 30 kg. Urine output and specific gravity, vital signs, laboratory data, and objective signs of adequate hydration guide the rate of fluid administration.

Children who are hospitalized with burns require constant observation and assessment for complications. Alterations in electrolyte balance can produce clinical symptoms of confusion, weakness, cardiac irregularities, and seizures. Changes in respiratory function and gas exchange are reflected clinically by restlessness, irritability, increased work of breathing, and alterations in blood gas values. The loss of protective function of the skin exposes burned children to increased risk of hypothermia. Edema formation and circulatory impairment can result in loss of sensation, deep throbbing pain, and loss of sensation in extremities.

NURSE ALERT • Evaluate the extremity and check the pulse every hour. If unable to palpate, use Doppler to ascertain loss of circulation and pulse. If the pulse is lost, escharotomy may be necessary to relieve the edema causing pressure on blood vessels and to restore adequate circulation.

Burn units maintain a pictorial record of the wound to record progress and for legal purposes (if child abuse is suspected). The burn wound is treated according to the protocol of the specific burn facility. Baseline cultures are obtained on admission. The burn team monitors infection control procedures and ensures that staff and visitors comply with established protocols to prevent cross-contamination in the burn unit.

Throughout the acute phase of care, the psychosocial needs of the children and their families should not be overlooked. The child is frightened, uncomfortable, and often confused. Children may be isolated from familiar persons and surroundings; the overwhelming physical needs at this time are the primary focus of the staff and parents. In addition to feeling concern for their child, the family experiences guilt, which has nothing to do with the burn injury. This guilt is related to the fact that the parents did not or could not protect their child. Consistency in the information presented and in the attitude of the staff creates a sense of familiarity and stability during the emergent phase.

Management and Rehabilitative Phases. After the patient's condition is stabilized, the management phase begins. The multidisciplinary team concentrates on preventing wound infections, closing the wound as quickly as possible, and managing the numerous complications. Although the rehabilitative phase begins when permanent wound closure has been achieved, rehabilitation issues are identified on admission and are included in the plan of care throughout the hospital course.

➤ Assessment

Wound assessment and comprehensive assessment of the child's general condition and behaviors are of major importance. The nurse must assess signs of complications, infection, and the need for and effectiveness of pain management.

NURSE ALERT • Disorientation in the burned patient is one of the first signs of overwhelming sepsis and may indicate inadequate hydration. Assessment of the sensorium is another important indicator of the adequacy of hydration. A spiking fever and diminished bowel sounds accompanied by paralytic ileus are noted and progressively increase over 48 to 72 hours, after which the temperature falls to subnormal limits. At this time the wound deteriorates, the white blood cell count is depressed, and septic shock becomes manifest.

➤ Nursing Diagnoses

Nursing diagnoses identified for the child with severe or extensive burns are included in the Nursing Care Plan on p. 1542. Additional diagnoses may be ascertained for individual children.

➤ Plan of Care and Implementation

The goals for the child with a burn injury and the family are as follows:

1. Child will experience reduction of pain.
2. Child will exhibit evidence of wound healing.
3. Child will receive adequate nutrition and will achieve reduction in metabolic losses.
4. Child will not experience complications during acute care.
5. Child will not experience complications during long-term care.
6. Child and family will receive emotional support.

Comfort Management. The severe pain of the wound and resultant therapies, the anxiety generated by these experiences, sleep deprivation, itching related to wound healing, and the conscious and unconscious interpretations of traumatic events contribute to the psychologic behaviors commonly observed in children with burns. It is always difficult to deal with a child in pain, and to inflict pain on a helpless child is contrary to the empathic nature of nursing. Interventions may include medications (including IV morphine or midazolam and short-term anesthetics such as propofol), relaxation techniques, distraction therapy, cutaneous stimulation by touching, and family participation.

Children need age-appropriate explanations before all procedures. When children appear to accept pain with little or no response, psychologic consultation may be needed. Consistency in caregivers is important. If this is not possible, a carefully developed, multidisciplinary plan of care is necessary to provide consistency.

Care of the Burn Wound. The nurse has a major responsibility for cleansing, debriding, and applying topical medications and dressings to the burn wound. Medication should be administered so that the peak effect of the drug coincides with the procedure. Children who have an understanding of the procedure to be performed and some perceived control demonstrate less maladaptive behavior. Children also respond well to participating in decisions (Guidelines box).

Outer dressings are removed. Any dressings that have adhered to the wound can be more easily removed by applying tepid water. Loose or easily detached tissue is debrided during the cleansing process. In dressing the wound, it is important that all areas be clean, that medication be amply applied, and that no two burned surfaces touch each other (e.g., fingers or toes, or ears touching the side of the head). If they are touching, the burned surfaces will heal together, causing deformity and/or dysfunction.

Topical medications may be applied directly to the wound with a clean, gloved hand or impregnated into fine-mesh gauze before application. Dressings are then applied to assist in exudate absorption, wound debridement, and increased patient comfort. All dressings applied circumferentially should be wrapped in a distal-to-proximal manner. The dressing is applied with sufficient tension to remain in place but not so tightly as to impair circulation or limit motion. Elastic bandages are applied over dressings to prevent epithelial breakdown, decrease edema formation, stimulate circulation, and improve mobility. The bandage is applied in a figure-8 to promote optimum circulation. A stable dressing is especially important when the child is ambulatory.

Standard precautions, including the use of protective garb and barrier techniques, should be followed when caring for all patients with thermal injuries. Frequent hand and forearm washing is the single most important element of the infection control program. Strict policies for cleaning the environment and patient care equipment should be implemented to minimize the risk of cross-contamination. All visitors and members of other departments should be oriented to the infection control policies, including the importance of hand and forearm washing and use of protective garb. Visitors should be screened for infection and contagious diseases before patient contact.

Nutrition. Oral feedings are encouraged unless the child is intubated or paralytic ileus persists. Because children often lack an appetite, a great deal of encouragement, help, and patience is required of the nursing staff. Consultation between the caregiver and the dietitian helps to determine food preferences. Children who are old enough to participate should be included in meal planning. In addition, many children prefer an atmosphere more nearly like that provided at home. Therefore, when possible, many children enjoy sitting at a table and interacting with other children at mealtimes. Painful procedures should not be scheduled near mealtimes because most children will be too physically exhausted and emotionally upset to eat.

Children who require enteral supplementation must be monitored for feeding intolerance and tube malposition. The nurse should also monitor and report any abdominal distention, diarrhea, or electrolyte and metabolic deviations.

Prevention of Complications

Acute Care. The maintenance of body temperature is important to the child with burns. Core body temperature is supported when energy is conserved with an environmental temperature of 28° to 33° C (82° to 91° F). Large areas of the body should not be exposed simultaneously during dressing changes. Warmed solutions, linens, occlusive dressings, heat shields, a radiant warmer, and warming blankets assist in preventing hypothermia.

The chief danger during acute care is infection—wound infection, generalized sepsis, or bacterial pneumonia. Accurate and ongoing assessments of all parameters that provide clues to the early diagnosis and treatment of infection are essential. Symptoms of sepsis include a change in the level of consciousness, a rising or falling white blood cell count, hypothermia or hyperthermia, a loss of the progression of wound healing, in-

Guidelines

REDUCING THE STRESS OF BURN CARE PROCEDURES

Have all materials ready before beginning.
Administer appropriate analgesics.
Remind the child of the impending procedure to allow sufficient time to prepare.
Allow the child to test and approve the temperature of the water.
Allow the child to select the area of the body on which to begin.
Allow the child to request a short rest period during the procedure.
Allow the child to remove the dressings if desired.
Provide something constructive for the child to do during the procedure (e.g., holding a package of dressings or a roll of gauze).
Inform the child when the procedure is near completion.
Praise the child for cooperation.

creasing fluid requirements, hypoactive or absent bowel sounds, a rising or falling blood glucose level, tachycardia, tachypnea, and thrombocytopenia.

Children are reluctant to move if movement causes pain, and they are likely to assume a position of comfort. Unfortunately, the most comfortable position often encourages the formation of contractures and loss of function. Ongoing efforts to prevent contractures include maintaining proper body alignment, positioning and splinting of involved extremities in extension, active and passive physical therapy, and encouragement of spontaneous movement when feasible. Frequent position changes are important to improve bronchopulmonary hygiene and capillary perfusion to common pressure areas. Low-air loss beds are beneficial for the morbidly obese or children with posterior grafts. Special attention should be given to areas at risk for increased pressure such as the posterior scalp, heels, and areas exposed to mechanical irritation from splints and dressings.

Long-Term Care. The rehabilitative phase of care begins once wound coverage has been achieved. Scar formation becomes a major problem as burn wounds heal (Fig. 53-23). Contractile properties of the scar tissue can result in disabling contractures, deformity, and disfigurement.

Uniform pressure applied to the scar decreases the blood supply. When pressure is removed, blood supply to the scar is immediately increased; therefore periods without pressure should be brief to avoid nourishment of the hypertrophic tissue. Continuous pressure to areas of scarring can be achieved by elastic bandages or commercially available pressure garments. Because these custom-made garments are often worn for months, revision may be required as the child grows. It is much easier to prevent scarring and contracture of the wound than to resolve an existing problem. Splints and appliances may also be needed until wound maturation is achieved (Fig. 53-24).

Scar tissue has certain significant properties, particularly for growing children. Intense itching occurs in healing burn wounds and scar tissue until the scar is no longer active. Itching is usually treated with hydroxyzine (Atarax) or diphenhydramine (Benadryl) and frequent applications of a moisturizer such as Eucerin, cocoa butter, or Nivea. Massage therapy during the application of moisturizers is also beneficial to stretch scar tissue and aid in contracture prevention. Scar tissue has no sweat glands, and children with extensive scarring may experience difficulty during hot weather. Caregivers should be alerted to this possibility and be prepared to institute alternate methods of cooling when necessary.

Scar tissue does not grow and expand as does normal tissue, which may create difficulties, especially in functional areas such as the hands and over joints. Additional surgery is sometimes required to allow independent functioning in daily activities, to improve cosmetic appearance, or to restore anatomic integrity.

The nursing activities in the rehabilitative phase of treatment focus on the child's and family's adaptation to the burn injury and their ability to reintegrate into the community. The psychologic pain and sequelae of severe burn injury are as intensive as the physical trauma. The impact of severe burns taxes the capabilities at all ages. Very young children, who suffer acutely from separation anxiety; and adolescents, who are developing an identity, are probably the most affected psychologically. Toddlers cannot understand why the parents they love and who have protected them can leave them in such a frightening and unfamiliar place. Adolescents, in the process of achieving independence from the family, find themselves in a dependent role with a damaged body. Being different from others at a time when conformity with peers is so important is difficult to accept.

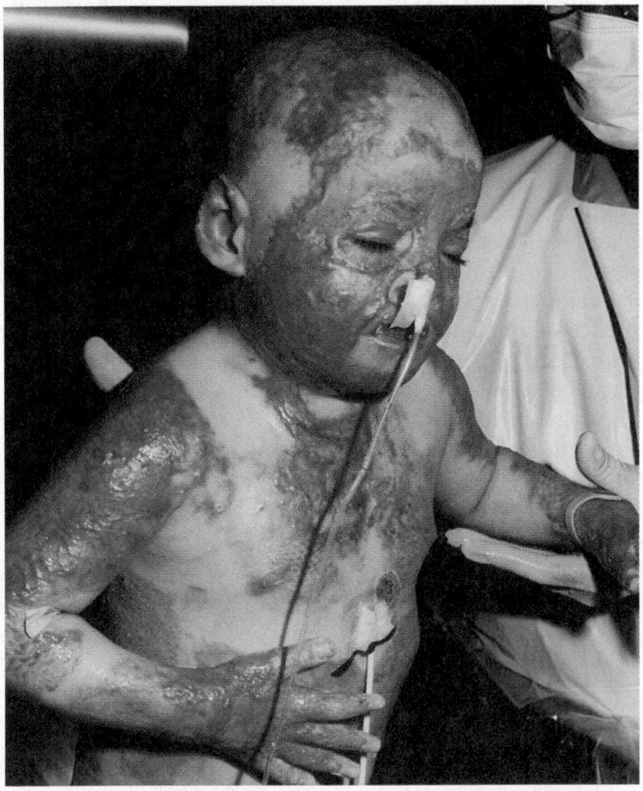

FIG. 53-23 • Extensive scars from flame burn. (Courtesy C.R. Boeckman Regional Burn Center, Akron, OH.)

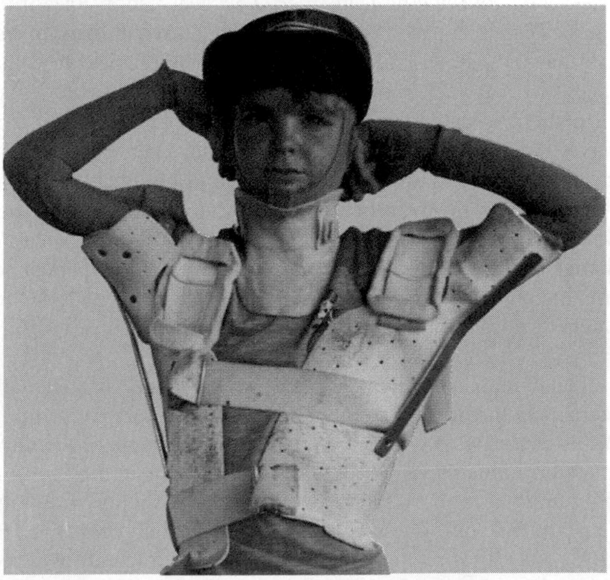

FIG. 53-24 • Child in elasticized (Jobst) garment and "airplane" splints.

Anticipation of the return to school can be overwhelming and frightening. It is essential that health care professionals recognize the importance of preparing teachers and classmates for the child's return. Teachers need to be provided with information to assist the child and family and to promote the child's optimum adjustment. Hospital-sponsored school reentry programs use a variety of methods to provide education and information about the implications of the injury, the garments and appliances, and the need for support and acceptance. Telephone calls, videotapes, information packets, and visits by members of the health care team offer opportunities to help with reintegration into the school environment—a focal point of the child's life.

Psychosocial Support of the Child. Children should begin early to do as much for themselves as possible and to be active participants in their care. Loss of control and perceived helplessness may result in acting-out behaviors. During illness, children regress to a previous developmental level that allows them to deal with stress. As children begin to participate in their care, they gain confidence and self-esteem. Fears and anxieties diminish with accomplishment and self-confidence. If the child demonstrates nonadherence in the rehabilitative phase, a behavior modification program can be initiated to promote or reward the child's accomplishment in care.

Children need to know that their injury and the treatments are not punishment for real or imagined transgressions and that the nurse understands their fear, anger, and discomfort. They also need body contact. This is often difficult to arrange for the child with massive burns; stroking areas of unburned skin is comforting. Even older children enjoy sitting on the parent's lap and being cuddled and hugged. This can be a reward or a comfort in times of stress, but most of all it should be kept in mind that it is a natural part of childhood.

Psychosocial Support of the Family. Recognizing and respecting each family's strengths, differences, and methods of coping allows the nurse to respond to their unique needs by implementing a family-centered approach to care. In the acute phase, all attention is focused on the child, and the parents feel powerless and ineffectual. Most parents feel overwhelming guilt, whether or not the guilt is justified. They feel responsible for the injury. These feelings may impede the child's rehabilitation. Parents may indulge the child and allow nonadherent behaviors that affect physical and emotional recovery. Parents need to be informed of the child's progress and helped to cope with their feelings while providing support to their child. The nurse can help them understand that it is not selfish to look after themselves and their own needs in order to better meet the needs of their child. It is important to recognize the parents' need to grieve the change in the normal appearance of their child as a part of the grieving process. Definitive professional help may be needed for parents whose response to the injury is severe or whose response to stress is manifested in destructive behavior.

The parents are members of the multidisciplinary team and participate in the development of the plan of care. It is important to facilitate their input; to consider all aspects of the physical, emotional, social, and cultural factors impacting the child and family; and to establish a realistic home therapy program. The family's willingness to assume responsibility for care and their ability to implement the therapeutic regimen are assessed. Home, school, and other environmental factors are explored; financial concerns and available community resources are discussed; and a specific plan of care for the child, with an anticipated follow-up program, is developed.

Prevention of Burn Injury. The best intervention is to prevent burns from occurring. Infants and toddlers are most commonly injured by hot liquids in the kitchen and bathroom. Hot liquids should be kept out of reach; tablecloths and dangling appliance cords are often pulled by toddlers, spilling hot grease and liquids on them. Electrical cords and outlets represent a potential risk to small children, who may chew on accessible cords and insert objects into outlets.

In 1974 the Consumer Product Safety Commission recommended a reduction of water heater thermostats to a maximum of 48.9° C (120° F). The "dial-down" recommendation has been suggested by utility companies, burn treatment centers, medical personnel, and others interested in public safety; however, many water heaters remain set at levels well above the safe level. Small children are especially at risk for scald injuries from hot tap water because of their decreased reaction time and agility, their curiosity, and the thermal sensitivity of their skin. Caregivers should be educated never to leave a child unattended in a bath and without adult supervision. Water should always be tested before a child is placed in the tub or shower.

The increased use of microwave ovens has resulted in burn injuries from the extremely hot internal temperatures generated in heated items. Baby formula, jelly-filled pastries, and hot liquids and dishes may result in cutaneous scalds or the ingestion of overheated liquids. Parents should use caution when removing items from the microwave oven and should always test the food before giving it to children.

As children mature, risk-taking behaviors increase. Matches and lighters are very dangerous in the hands of the young. Adults must remember to keep potentially hazardous items out of the reach of children; a lighter, like a match, is a tool for adult use.

Education related to fire safety and survival should begin with the very young. "Stop, drop, and roll" to extinguish a fire can be practiced. The fire escape route, including a safe meeting place away from the home in case of fire, also should be practiced.

Community activities are also very helpful in supporting burn survivors and preventing burns. The Aluminum Cans for Burned Children (ACBC) is an exemplary effort based in the Clifford R. Boeckman, MD, Regional Burn Center, Akron, Ohio.* Activities funded by ACBC include Burn Survivors Support Group, Burn Camp, and meetings of Juvenile Firestoppers (for children with fire-setting behavior). Adult weekend retreats and school and family education sessions are a part of this program. Burn center staff and fire department staff provide the personnel to present programs.

Additional information on burn care and prevention can be obtained from the American Burn Association† and the National Safety Council.‡ The Alisa Ann Ruch Burn Foundation§ provides assistance to burn victims and burn centers. The Shriners Burn Institutes are staffed to treat pediatric patients following acute burn injuries and those requiring rehabilitative and reconstructive services as a result of scarring and functional

*Children's Hospital Medical Center of Akron, 1 Perkins Square, Akron, OH 44308-1062; (330) 379-8224; fax (330) 379-8152; website: www.akronchildrens.org.

†625 North Michigan Ave., Suite 1530, Chicago, IL 60611; (312) 642-9260 or 1-800-548-2876; fax (312) 642-9130; e-mail: aba@ameriburn.org.

‡1121 Spring Lake Dr., Itasca, IL 60143-3201; 1-800-621-7615; website: www.nsc.org.

§20944 Sherman Way, Suite 115, Canoga Park, CA 91303; (818) 883-7700; website: www.aarbf.org.

impairment. Information can be obtained from local Shrine Temples and Shrine Clubs, from Shriners Hospitals, or by contacting the International Shrine Headquarters.* The Alisa Ann Ruch Foundation and Shriners Hospitals for Crippled Children support research to improve burn care and treatment and promote public education in burn prevention.

➤ Evaluation

The effectiveness of nursing interventions is determined by continual reassessment and evaluation of care based on the following observational guidelines:

1. Observe child's behavior during all aspects of care; listen to verbal cues; use a pain assessment record to evaluate the effectiveness of analgesia.
2. Observe the burn wound and child's general condition.
3. Observe child's eating behavior and the amount of food consumed; weigh daily or as indicated.
4. Inspect the burn wound for signs of infection; measure vital signs; observe for evidence of respiratory complications, gastric bleeding, altered hemoglobin level, and neurologic signs.
5. Observe for evidence of healing, scar formation, and contracture; assess effectiveness of physical therapy and appliances (e.g., splints, pressure garments).
6. Observe child's and family's behaviors; interview child and family regarding their feelings and concerns.

The expected outcomes are described in the Nursing Care Plan.

Sunburn

Sunburn is a very common skin injury caused by overexposure to ultraviolet (UV) light waves. The sun emits a continuous spectrum of visible and nonvisible light rays that range in length from very short to very long. The shorter, higher-frequency waves are more damaging than longer wavelengths, but much of the light is filtered out as it travels through the atmosphere. Of the light that does filter through, *ultraviolet A (UVA)* waves are the longest and cause only minimum burning, but they potentiate *ultraviolet B (UVB)* waves. UVB waves are shorter and are responsible for tanning, burning, and most of the harmful effects attributed to sunlight, especially skin cancer.

Numerous factors influence the amount of UVB exposure. Maximum exposure occurs at midday (10 AM to 3 PM), when the sun is highest in the sky. There is more exposure at higher altitudes, and less when the sky is hazy (although the amount of UV radiation that does penetrate is easily underestimated). Window glass effectively screens out UVB but not UVA rays. Fresh snow and water reflect UV rays, especially when the sun is directly overhead; some rays are reflected by sand.

Nursing Care Management. Protection from sunburn is the major goal of medical and nursing management, and the harmful effects of the sun on the delicate skin of infants and children are receiving increased attention. To protect skin exposed to the sun for extended periods, skin should be covered with clothing, and FDA-approved sun protection agents should be applied.

Two types of products are available for protection from the sun: *topical sunscreens,* which partially absorb UV light; and *sun blockers,* which block out UV rays by reflecting sunlight. The most commonly recommended sun blockers are zinc oxide and titanium dioxide ointments. Sunscreens are products containing a *sun protection factor (SPF)* based on evaluation of effectiveness against UV rays. The SPF is indicated by a number, such as 15, which indicates that if individuals normally burn in 10 minutes without a sunscreen, use of a sunscreen with SPF 15 allows them to remain in the sun 15×10, or 150 minutes ($2\frac{1}{2}$ hours) before acquiring the same degree of burn. The most effective sunscreens against UVB are *p-aminobenzoic acid (PABA)* and *PABA-esters.*

Claims such as "broad-spectrum" or "UVA-UVB sunblock" are usually unsubstantiated. One product that affords protection against UVA is *Parsol 1789,* found in Photoplex and UVA Guard.

Sunscreens are applied evenly to all exposed areas, with special attention given to skinfolds and areas that might become exposed as clothing shifts. Parents are directed to read labels of sunscreen products carefully for the SPF and follow the manufacturer's directions for application.

> **NURSE ALERT** • Infants under 6 months of age may have sunscreen applied over small areas of skin such as the face and back of hands that may not be adequately covered by clothing when exposed to the sun (American Academy of Pediatrics, 1999). Infants should be kept out of the sun or kept shaded from it. Fabric with a tight weave, such as cotton, offers good protection.

Individuals in the community who work with children, such as teachers, day care workers, coaches, and youth-group leaders, as well as relatives, should all be made aware of sun safety for children. Sunscreens must be applied *liberally.*

Sunburn is usually an epidermal burn, although severe sunburn can be a partial-thickness burn with blister formation. Treatment involves stopping the burning process, decreasing the inflammatory response, and rehydrating the skin. Local application of cool-tap water soaks, or immersion in a tepid-water bath for 20 minutes or until the skin is cool limits tissue destruction and relieves the discomfort. Moisturizing lotion is then applied. Partial-thickness burns are treated the same as those from any heat source (see earlier discussion on burns).

Cold Injury

Cold injuries are most commonly seen in very cold regions. The nature of the heat-regulating mechanisms of the body are such that the inner portion of the body, or core, produces heat and the periphery, or outer area, conserves or dissipates heat. When the body attempts to conserve heat, the outer tissues are subjected to low temperatures, and local trauma may result.

Chilblain, redness and swelling of the skin, occurs when extremities, usually the hands, are exposed intermittently to temperatures of $-1.1°$ to $15.5°$ C ($30°$ to $60°$ F). The response may vary but is characterized by intense vasodilation that increases the temperature of involved tissues above that of unaffected tissue and produces edematous, reddish blue patches that itch and

*2900 Rocky Point Dr., Tampa, FL 33607; 1-800-237-5055 (in Florida: 1-800-282-9161); International Shrine Headquarters website: www.shrinershq.org; Shriners Burn Institutes website: www.shrinershq.org/Hospitals/BurnInst/.

Nursing Care Plan THE CHILD WITH A FULL-THICKNESS BURN MORE THAN 25% TBSA

NURSING DIAGNOSIS Impaired skin integrity related to thermal injury

EXPECTED OUTCOME The child exhibits signs of wound healing, and skin grafts remain intact.

Nursing Interventions/*Rationales*

Thoroughly cleanse wound and debride devitalized skin *to decrease infection and promote healing.*

Apply topical and systemic bacterial agents to wounds as ordered *to decrease chances of infection.*

Dress wounds as ordered *to protect against infection and fluid loss.*

Monitor serum electrolytes and blood gases *for potential adverse affects of topical agents.*

Monitor wound appearance for signs of infection or healing *to guide ongoing treatment.*

Monitor grafts for evidence of hematoma/fluid collection; aspirate or express fluids *to maintain graft contact with base of site.*

Use appropriate measures (e.g., splints, dressings, restraints) *to prevent child from touching or picking at wound and graft sites.*

Offer high-calorie, high-protein meals and snacks *to meet nutritional requirements caused by increased metabolism and catabolism.*

Administer supplemental vitamins A, B, C, iron, and zinc *to facilitate wound healing and epithelialization.*

NURSING DIAGNOSIS Fluid volume deficit related to active loss of body fluids secondary to thermal injury

EXPECTED OUTCOME The child exhibits signs of adequate fluid volume and electrolyte balance.

Nursing Interventions/*Rationales*

Administer intravenous fluids with sodium as ordered *to prevent burn shock and maintain perfusion.*

Monitor vital signs, skin turgor, mucous membranes *for signs of fluid volume/electrolyte balance.*

Monitor intake and output (including wound drainage, urinary output) *to assess fluid balance and circulatory status.*

Monitor electrolytes, blood gases, specific gravity *to assess hydration, electrolyte balance.*

NURSING DIAGNOSIS Risk for fluid volume excess related to retention of fluids and sodium secondary to intravenous therapy, edema formation

EXPECTED OUTCOME The child exhibits signs of adequate fluid volume and electrolyte balance.

Nursing Interventions/*Rationales*

Discontinue intravenous fluids as ordered when an established rate of urinary output is reached and adequate circulatory volume is restored *to prevent fluid overload.*

Monitor respiratory status *for signs of fluid accumulation in lungs;* tissue pressures *for signs of edema that may cause permanent injury to underlying nerves and muscles.*

NURSING DIAGNOSIS Risk for infection related to denuded or absence of skin, presence of pathogenic organisms, and altered immune response

EXPECTED OUTCOME The child exhibits no evidence of infection.

Nursing Interventions/*Rationales*

Place child in appropriate protective environment (e.g., laminar air flow, isolation, private room) and screen all visitors and staff for signs of infection *to minimize exposure to infective organisms.*

Teach child and family about good hygiene and careful handwashing techniques *to prevent spread of infection.*

Use good handwashing for all contacts with child and scrupulous aseptic technique with gown, cap, mask, and gloves for all wound care procedures *to minimize exposure to infection.*

Cleanse and debride eschar, crust, and blisters *to remove infection reservoir.*

Administer prescribed topical antimicrobials and cover wound with dry dressings per protocol *to provide a barrier to organisms.*

Encourage a nutritionally complete diet (high-calorie, high-protein) *to support body's natural defenses.*

Monitor vital signs, observe wounds, and obtain wound cultures *to detect signs of infection.*

NURSING DIAGNOSIS Anxiety/pain related to trauma from burns and debridement therapy and other treatments

EXPECTED OUTCOME The child exhibits a reduced level of pain and/or anxiety.

Nursing Interventions/*Rationales*

Monitor closely for pain relief needs and administer medications as ordered *to decrease pain;* anticipate need and administer medication before onset of severe pain and at regular intervals *to better manage pain levels;* medicate before procedures such as debridement, hydrotherapy, dressing changes *to better manage pain levels.*

Administer medications as prescribed, apply lotions *for the relief of itching of scar tissue.*

Prepare child and family for procedures and allow the child to make active choices during procedures (e.g., testing

Nursing Care Plan THE CHILD WITH A FULL-THICKNESS BURN MORE THAN 25% TBSA—cont'd

temperature of water for hydrotherapy, selecting which site to start debridement, saying when to stop procedure for a rest, helping with the procedure) *to promote sense of control and cooperation.*

Implement nonpharmacologic pain reduction techniques as appropriate (e.g., distraction, relaxation, guided imagery, positive self-talk, cutaneous stimulation) *to relieve pain.*

NURSING DIAGNOSIS Impaired physical mobility related to pain, scar formation, joint contracture

EXPECTED OUTCOME The child exhibits a reduced level of pain and/or anxiety.

Nursing Interventions/*Rationales*

Implement active/passive range of motion *to prevent contractures, keep joints mobile, minimize pain.*

Use positioning techniques, splinting, conformers, pressure garments *to prevent flexion and scar contractures.*

Ambulate as soon as possible, promote self-help activities, encourage play *to maintain mobility.*

Use lotion and massage healed areas *to soften scars and promote relaxation.*

Administer analgesic before painful activity (e.g., physical therapy) *so that child is more likely to cooperate and be mobile.*

NURSING DIAGNOSIS Ineffective thermoregulation related to loss of skin surface, sweat glands

EXPECTED OUTCOME The child exhibits tolerance to the environment.

Nursing Interventions/*Rationales*

Carefully control and monitor temperature in environment, limit exposure to temperature extremes *to prevent hypothermia or hyperthermia.*

Avoid vigorous physical activity *that may lead to heat prostration.*

Monitor temperature *to assess for hypothermia or hyperthermia.*

NURSING DIAGNOSIS Body-image/self-esteem disturbance related to scar formation, alterations in appearance and function

EXPECTED OUTCOME The child demonstrates an acceptance of self, his or her own physical appearance, and physical abilities.

Nursing Interventions/*Rationales*

Relate to child, conveying an attitude of caring and acceptance *to encourage positive feelings about self;* serve as role model for others *to foster positive attitudes of acceptance toward child.*

Encourage child to verbalize feelings and perceptions about the burn incident, wounds, and scarring (e.g., nightmares, fears of fire, pain of therapy, multiple treatments and prolonged and multiple hospitalizations, feelings of differentness, implications of functional limits, difficulty in making friends, views of self) *to facilitate coping and open expression of problems, fears, wants, wishes, and needs.*

Have child identify strengths, assets, things he or she likes about self *to increase positive feelings about self and abilities.*

Support positive coping behaviors.

Introduce child to other children who have had similar experiences, arrange for support groups for child and parents *to increase coping skills.*

Refer child and family for counseling as needed *to enhance adaptation.*

Encourage use of regular hygiene and grooming practices, use of accessories (e.g., wigs, concealing makeup, concealing clothing) *to promote positive appearance.*

Prepare peers for child's appearance *to encourage acceptance and support.*

NURSING DIAGNOSIS Altered family processes related to situational crises (child with scarring, altered appearance and function)

EXPECTED OUTCOME Family members exhibit adaptation of usual roles and functions to accommodate special needs of the child and exhibit growth-promoting behaviors.

Nursing Interventions/*Rationales*

Provide opportunity for family to absorb and adjust to diagnosis (e.g., repeat information *to allow time for family to hear and understand;* encourage expression of concerns, fears, and feelings about diagnosis and potential impact *to facilitate adjustment;* identify support systems *to provide resources for coping*).

Assist family to understand expected treatment, rationale, and implications *to provide a sound basis for decision making.*

Explore family's reaction to the child; assist them to achieve a realistic view of child's abilities and limitations; encourage family in attempts to promote child's growth and development; have family emphasize what child can do; explore ways for family to include child in family activities *to help family increase abilities to cope with and incorporate child into family structure.*

Arrange for and participate in family conferences *to provide forum for communication, mutual goal setting, and effective strategizing.*

Have parents spend special time with siblings *so they do not feel neglected or left out.*

Identify additional resource systems (e.g., relatives, friends, church, health care services, community programs) and strategize with family about making good use of these systems *to develop broad base of support.*

Provide a system of ongoing follow-up and evaluation *to ensure long-term adaptation to challenges presented in family functioning by a child with severely altered appearance and scarring.*

burn. As warming takes place, the sensations become more intense, but ordinarily they subside in a few days.

Frostbite is the term used to describe tissue damage caused when excessive heat loss to local tissues allows ice crystals to form in tissues. The frostbitten part appears white or blanched, feels solid, and is without sensation. Rapid rewarming produces a flush (sometimes deep purple) and a return of sensation, which is extremely painful. In 24 to 48 hours after rewarming, large blisters appear, which begin to reabsorb within 5 to 10 days, followed by the formation of a hard black eschar. Superficial injury often heals without incident. Rewarming is accomplished by immersing the part in well-agitated water at 37.8° to 42.2° C (100° to 108° F). Discomfort is managed with analgesics and sedatives. Care of blistered skin is similar to that described for burns. It is seldom possible to estimate the extent of tissue loss until new skin layers are revealed after the eschar layer separates.

Key Points

- Therapeutic management of skin disorders includes a variety of methods and agents to cool, soothe, and reduce the irritating effects of external stimuli.
- A moist environment promotes healing of wounds.
- Skin infections can be caused by bacteria, viruses, or fungi.
- Some diseases manifested in the skin are transmitted by arthropod vectors, especially ticks.
- The most common skin infestations of childhood—scabies and pediculosis capitis—can affect children of any age and from any social class.
- Contact dermatitis may involve a primary irritant or a sensitizing agent.
- Adverse reactions to drugs are manifested more often in the skin than in any other body organ.
- The most common skin disorders of infancy are diaper dermatitis, seborrheic dermatitis, and atopic dermatitis.
- Acne, a disorder affecting a large proportion of adolescents, is related to excessive sebum production, the formation of comedones, and the overgrowth of the *Propionibacterium acnes* organism.
- Medication and gentle facial cleansing are the treatments of choice for acne.
- Burns are caused by thermal, chemical, electric, or radioactive agents.
- Burns are assessed on the extent, depth, and severity of the wound.
- Essentials of emergency care of burn injury include stopping the burning process, covering the burn, transporting the injured child to medical aid, and providing reassurance to the child and family.
- Management of minor burns consists of facilitating wound healing, relieving discomfort, and preventing complications.
- Management of major burns consists of facilitating wound healing, relieving discomfort, replacing destroyed skin, preventing and/or treating complications, and providing rehabilitation.
- Sunscreen is recommended for use when the skin is exposed to the damaging effects of the sun's rays.
- Thermal injuries to the skin can result from exposure to extreme cold.

References

American Academy of Pediatrics, Committee on Environmental Health: Ultraviolet light: a hazard to children, *Pediatrics* 104(2):328-333, 1999.

American Academy of Pediatrics, Committee on Infectious Diseases: Prevention of Lyme disease, *Pediatrics* 105(1):142-147, 2000.

Annequin D et al: Fixed 50% nitrous oxide oxygen mixture for painful procedures: a French survey, *Pediatrics* 105(4):e47, 2000, www.pediatrics.org/cgi/content/full/105/4/e47.

Berson DS, Shalita AR: The treatment of acne: the role of combination therapies, *J Am Acad Dermatol* 32:S31-S41, 1995.

Dourmishev A, Serafimova D, Dourmishev L: Efficacy and tolerance of oral ivermectin in scabies, *J Eur Acad Dermatol Venereol* 11(3):247-251, 1998.

Hansbrough JF: Enteral nutritional support in burn patients, *Gastrointest Endosc Clin North Am* 8(3):645-647, 1998.

Herndon DN et al: *Total burn care,* London, 1996, WB Saunders.

Humane Society of the United States: *Preventing and avoiding dog bites,* Washington, DC, 1998, The Society.

Hurwitz S: Acne treatment for the '90s, *Contemp Pediatr* 12: 19-32, 1995.

Kahana M: From theory to practice: Fentanyl Oralet in the pediatric burn unit, *Am J Anesthesiol* 24(1, suppl):17-18, 1997.

Leyden JJ: Therapy for acne vulgaris, *N Engl J Med* 336: 1156-1162, 1997.

O'Brien E: Detection and removal of head lice with an electronic comb: zapping the louse, *J Pediatr Nurs* 13(4):265-266, 1998.

Offidani A et al: Treatment of scabies with ivermectin, *Eur J Dermatol* 9(2):100-101, 1999.

Still JM Jr et al: Decreasing length of hospital stay by early excision and grafting of burns, *South Med J* 89(6):578-582, 1996.

Vernon PL: The "itch that rashes": responding to atopic dermatitis, *Adv Nurse Pract,* pp 36-40, 50, Sept 1998.

CHAPTER

54

Musculoskeletal or Articular Dysfunction

http://www.harcourthealth.com/MERLIN/Wong/maternal/

Learning Objectives

On completion of this chapter the reader will be able to:

- Outline a plan for the care of a child immobilized with an injury or a degenerative disease.
- Formulate a teaching plan for the parents of a child in a cast.
- Explain the functions of the various types of traction.
- Devise a nursing care plan for a child in traction.
- Differentiate among the various congenital skeletal defects.
- Design a teaching plan for the parents of a child with a congenital skeletal deformity.
- Describe the therapies and nursing care of a child with scoliosis.
- Outline a plan of care for a child with osteomyelitis.
- Differentiate between osteosarcoma and Ewing sarcoma.
- Describe the nursing care of a child with juvenile rheumatoid arthritis.
- Demonstrate an understanding of the management of systemic lupus erythematosus.

THE IMMOBILIZED CHILD

Immobilization

Immobilization, or bed rest, was once thought to have a restorative influence on a child's recovery from a variety of illnesses and injuries. It is now well established that immobilization has serious consequences for physical, social, and psychologic health and is prescribed only for the briefest period necessary. Some of the disorders that may impose limited immobilization include fractures of the pelvis and femur, avascular necrosis, osteomyelitis, spinal cord and head injuries, and medical conditions such as congestive heart failure and pulmonary disease.

Physiologic Effects of Immobilization. The stresses a child places on the body and organs through normal activities of daily living help determine functional capacity (Buschbacher, 1996). Disuse from illness, injury, or a sedentary lifestyle can limit function and potentially delay age-appropriate milestones. Most of the pathologic changes that occur during immobilization are primary and produce a direct effect; others seem to be more indirect, or secondary, and affect more than one body system.

The major effects of immobilization are outlined briefly in Table 54-1. They are related directly or indirectly to decreased muscle activity, which produces numerous primary changes in the musculoskeletal system with secondary alterations in the cardiovascular, respiratory, metabolic, and renal systems. The musculoskeletal changes that occur during disuse are a result of alterations in gravity and stress on the muscles, joints, and bones. Clinical studies in adults and animals document significant decrease in muscle weight, growth, contractile force, and velocity within a week of disuse. This results in muscles that are smaller, weaker, and slower to respond (Wedrick et al, 1997). During immobilization a joint contracture begins when the arrangement of collagen, the main structural protein of connective tissues, is altered, resulting in a denser tissue that does not glide as easily. Eventually muscles, tendons, and ligaments can shorten and reduce joint movement, ultimately producing contractures that restrict function. The daily stresses on bone created by motion and weight bearing maintain the balance between bone formation (osteoblastic activity) and bone reabsorption (osteoclastic activity). During immobilization, increased calcium leaves the bone, causing osteopenia (demineralization of the bones), which may predispose bone to pathologic fractures. The major musculoskeletal consequences of immobilization are (1) significant decrease in muscle size, strength, and endurance; (2) bone demineralization leading to osteoporosis; and (3) contractures and decreased joint mobility. The larger the

TABLE 54-1
Summary of Physical Effects of Immobilization*

Primary Effects	Secondary Effects
MUSCULAR SYSTEM	
Decreased muscle strength, tone, and endurance	Decreased venous return and decreased cardiac output Decreased metabolism and need for oxygen Decreased exercise tolerance Bone demineralization
Disuse atrophy and loss of muscle mass	Catabolism Loss of strength
Loss of joint mobility	Contractures, ankylosis of joints
Weak back muscles	Secondary spinal deformities
Weak abdominal muscles	Impaired respiration
SKELETAL SYSTEM	
Bone demineralization—osteoporosis, hypercalcemia	Negative calcium balance Pathologic fractures Calcium deposits Extraosseous bone formation, especially at hip, knee, elbow, and shoulder Renal calculi
Negative calcium balance	Life-threatening electrolyte imbalance
METABOLISM	
Decreased metabolic rate	Slowing of all systems Decreased food intake
Negative nitrogen balance	Decline in nutritional state Impaired healing
Hypercalcemia	Electrolyte imbalance
Decreased production of stress hormones	Decreased physical and emotional coping capacity
CARDIOVASCULAR SYSTEM	
Decreased efficiency of orthostatic neurovascular reflexes	Inability to adapt readily to upright position Pooling of blood in extremities in upright posture
Diminished vasopressor mechanism	Orthostatic hypotension with syncope—hypotension, decreased cerebral blood flow, tachycardia
Altered distribution of blood volume	Decreased cardiac workload Decreased exercise tolerance
Venous stasis	Pulmonary emboli and/or thrombi
Dependent edema	Tissue breakdown and susceptibility to infection
RESPIRATORY SYSTEM	
Decreased need for oxygen	Altered oxygen—carbon dioxide exchange and metabolism
Decreased chest expansion and diminished vital capacity	Diminished oxygen intake Dyspnea and inadequate arterial oxygen saturation; acidosis
Poor abdominal tone and distention	Interference with diaphragmatic excursion
Mechanical or biochemical secretion retention	Hypostatic pneumonia Bacterial and viral pneumonia Atelectasis
Loss of respiratory muscle strength	Poor cough Upper respiratory infection
GASTROINTESTINAL SYSTEM	
Distention caused by poor abdominal muscle tone	Interference with respiratory movements
No specific primary effect	Difficulty in feeding in prone position; gravitation effect on feces through ascending colon, or weakened smooth muscle tone may cause constipation Anorexia
URINARY SYSTEM	
Alteration of gravitational force	Difficulty in voiding in prone position
Impaired ureteral peristalsis	Urinary retention in calyces and bladder Infection Renal calculi
INTEGUMENTARY SYSTEM	
No specific primary effect	Decreased circulation and pressure leading to tissue injury and decreased healing capacity Difficulty with personal hygiene

*Not all problems will apply in every situation.

portion of the body immobilized and the longer the immobilization, the greater the hazards of immobility.

Psychologic Effects of Immobilization. Throughout childhood, physical activity is an integral part of daily life and is essential for physical growth and development. The activity helps children deal with a variety of feelings and impulses and provides a mechanism by which they can exert control over inner tensions. Children respond to anxiety with increased activity. Removal of this power deprives them of necessary input and a natural outlet for their feelings and fantasies.

When children are immobilized by disease or as part of a treatment regimen, they experience diminished environmental stimuli with a loss of tactile input and an altered perception of themselves and their environment. Sudden or gradual immobilization narrows the amount and variety of environmental stimuli children receive by means of all of their senses: touch; sight; hearing; taste; smell; and proprioception, or the feeling of where they are in their environment. This sensory deprivation commonly leads to feelings of isolation and boredom, and of being forgotten, especially by peers.

Physical interference with the activity of infants and young children gives them a feeling of helplessness. Even speech and language skills require sensorimotor activity and experience. Children who are restrained by casts, splints, or straps during the first 3 years of life may have more difficulty with language than children whose activities are unrestricted.

For the toddler, exploration and imitative behaviors are essential to developing a sense of autonomy; the preschooler's expression of initiative is evidenced by the need for vigorous physical activity; the school-age child's development is strongly influenced by physical achievement and competition; and the adolescent relies on mobility to achieve independence. The quest for mastery at every stage of development is related to mobility.

The monotony of immobilization can lead to sluggish intellectual and psychomotor responses, decreased communication skills, increased fantasizing, and even hallucinations and disorientation. Children are likely to become depressed over their loss of ability to function or any marked changes in body image. They may seek the attention of others by reverting to earlier developmental behaviors, such as wanting to be fed, bed-wetting, and baby talk.

Also, limbs in casts or traction transmit less than normal sensory data. Children who have limited ability to feel others touching them not only experience less tactile stimuli in a physical sense, but are also deprived of warm, loving feelings that arise from being touched. The loss of feeling derived from touch can further add to their sense of being isolated and unwanted.

Children may react to immobility by active protest, anger, and aggressive behavior; or they may become quiet, passive, and submissive. Children should be allowed to discharge their anger, but it should be within the limits of safety to their self-esteem and not damaging to the integrity of others. For example, providing an object to attack rather than a person or a valued possession is safe and therapeutic. When children are unable to express anger, aggression is often displayed inappropriately through regressive behavior and outbursts of crying or temper tantrums.

Effect on Families. Brief periods of immobilization have few effects on the family; however, catastrophic illness or disability may severely tax their resources.

The family's needs often must be met by the services of a multidisciplinary team, and nurses play a key role in anticipating the services they will need and in coordinating conferences to plan care. In preparation for discharge, home visits are advisable, and home management is commonly planned weeks in advance of the actual discharge. Such planning includes special considerations for cultural, economic, physical, and psychologic needs. A child with a severe disability is very dependent, and caregivers need rest periods to revitalize themselves. Individual and group counseling is beneficial for preproblem-solving situations and provides an emotional support system. Parent groups are also helpful and often allow nonthreatening social contact. The families of children with permanent disabilities need long-term resources because some of the most difficult problems arise as they try to sustain high-quality care for many years (see Chapter 41).

Nursing Care Management

➤ Assessment

Physical assessment of the child who is immobilized as a result of an injury or a degenerative disease focuses not only on the injured part (e.g., fracture or damaged joint) but also on the functioning of other systems that may be affected secondarily (e.g., the circulatory, renal, respiratory, muscular, and gastrointestinal systems). With long-term immobilization there may also be neurologic impairment and changes in electrolytes (especially calcium), nitrogen balance, and the general metabolic rate. The psychologic impact of immobilization should also be assessed.

➤ Nursing Diagnoses

Nursing diagnoses for the immobilized child are outlined in the Nursing Care Plan on p. 1549. Others will be identified in specific cases.

➤ Plan of Care and Implementation

The general goals of care for the immobilized child and family include the following:

1. Child will experience no physical injury.
2. Child will experience no psychologic complications.
3. Child will engage in appropriate diversional activities.
4. Child and family will receive adequate support.

Frequent position changes help to prevent dependent edema and to stimulate circulation, respiratory function, gastrointestinal motility, and neurologic sensations. The use of antiembolism stockings or Ace wraps may minimize or prevent dependent edema and fluid shifts to third spaces. Metabolism is increased by activity within the limitations of the disability and capabilities of the child. High-protein, high-calorie foods are encouraged for correction of negative nitrogen balance, which may be difficult to correct by diet, especially if there is loss of appetite. Stimulating the appetite with small servings of attractively arranged, preferred foods may be sufficient. Sometimes supplementary nasogastric feedings or hyperalimentation may be needed.*

NURSE ALERT • Lying in a prone position during feeding increases the risk of aspiration. Therefore suction is kept nearby.

Adequate hydration and, when possible, an upright position and remobilization promote bowel and kidney function and help prevent complications in these systems. A sensitive discussion of elimination needs and toileting may help reduce embarrassment and complications of stool holding. Hydration, in ad-

*Community and home care instructions on giving nasogastric tube feedings and gastrostomy tube feedings are available in Wong DL, Hess CS: ***Wong and Whaley's clinical manual of pediatric nursing,*** ed 5, St Louis, 2000, Mosby.

dition to restriction of high-calcium foods, is also a primary measure for managing hypercalcemia.

Children are encouraged to be as active as their condition and restrictive devices allow. This poses few problems for children, whose innate ingenuity and natural inclination toward mobility provide them with the impetus for physical activity. They need the opportunity, the materials or objects to stimulate activity, and the encouragement and participation of others. Those who are unable to move need passive exercise and movement, perhaps in consultation with a physical therapist (PT).

Whenever possible, transporting the child by stretcher, stroller, or wagon outside the confines of the room increases environmental stimuli and provides social contact with others. Hospitalized children benefit from frequent visitors, from using clocks and calendars, and from programs of diversional therapy, all of which help them to function in a more normal way. If available, a play therapist or child-life specialist should be consulted for recreational planning. As soon as possible, hospitalized children should resume school and preinjury hobbies. The use of play (see Chapter 44) and any activity that is tolerated (e.g., turning in bed or changing the location of the bed within the room) help to alter the monotony of immobilization and decrease tension and frustration.

Using dolls to illustrate and explain the restraining method is a valuable tool for small children. Placing a cast, tubing, or other restraining equipment on the doll offers the child a nonthreatening opportunity to express, through the doll, feelings concerning the restrictions and feelings toward the nurse and other health care providers. It also provides a means for anticipatory teaching and explanation of needed restraining devices.

One of the most useful interventions to help children cope with immobility is participation in their own care. Self-care is usually well received by children. They can help plan their daily routine; select their diet (when possible); and choose "street clothes," including innovative adornments such as baseball caps or brightly colored stockings, to express their autonomy and individuality. They are encouraged to do as much as they are able to for themselves in order to keep muscles active and their interest alive. If feasible, they should be placed where they can benefit from the company of other children who are immobilized, which assures them that they are not singled out for this treatment.

It is important for children to understand behavioral limitations or rules, and their questions should be answered. For example, they need to know the reasons for medical and nursing measures as well as occupational and physical therapy, and they need to know that schedules are necessary. In some areas they have a choice; in others they do not. They may or may not be permitted to sleep late, but they can choose their own clothing. Most of children's activity of daily living is play; therefore therapies that incorporate this concept are more apt to gain their cooperation.

Visits from significant persons, such as family members and friends, offer occasions for emotional support and also provide opportunities for learning how to care for the child. Some privacy is needed, particularly by the teenager, and most long-term health care facilities recognize that rooms shared by two to four children, rather than large wards, are better environments for habilitation or rehabilitation. Selecting roommates according to age and companionship gives each child the chance to test out thoughts and feelings safely with others. If a traumatic incident caused the child's disability, guilt feelings may be displayed overtly or masked behind regressive or aggressive behavior. The feeling that "I must have been bad for this to happen" is common, and honest feedback stating, "It just happened—it was an accident," needs to be repeated many times.

For a child with greatly restricted movement (e.g., the quadriplegic child or the child with a large bilateral hip spica cast), nursing care is a challenge. These situations require long-term care either in the hospital or at home; but wherever the care occurs, consistent planning and coordination of activities with professionals and significant others are vital nursing functions.

Family Support and Home Care. The needs of a child with severe disabilities can be very complex, and family members require time to assimilate the teachings and demonstrations needed to understand the child's situation and care. Even the child who is confined on a short-term basis can be a challenge for the family, which is usually unprepared for the problems imposed by the child's special needs. Home modification is usually needed for facilitating care, especially when it involves traction, large casts, or extended confinement. Suitable child care may be needed for times when all family members work.

Just as in the hospital, the child at home is encouraged to be as independent as possible and to follow a schedule that approximates his or her normal lifestyle as nearly as possible, such as continuing school lessons, regular bedtime, and suitable recreational activities.

➤ Evaluation

The effectiveness of nursing interventions is determined by continual reassessment and evaluation of care based on the following observational guidelines and expected outcomes:

1. Observe vital signs, neurologic signs, and respiratory, gastrointestinal, and renal functioning; inspect skin; observe effects of correct functioning of equipment and appliances (e.g., restraints, traction, cast, and braces)
2. Observe child's behavior; engage in dialogue to elicit feelings, concerns, and interests
3. Observe child's activities and interests
4. Interview child and family regarding their feelings and concerns; observe family interaction at home, if possible

Expected outcomes are contained in the Nursing Care Plan.

TRAUMATIC INJURY

Soft Tissue Injury

Injuries to the muscles, ligaments, and tendons are common in children (Fig. 54-1). In young children, soft tissue injury usually results from mishaps during play. In older children and adolescents, participation in sports is the more common cause.

Contusions. A contusion is damage to the soft tissue, subcutaneous structures, and muscle. The tearing of these tissues and small blood vessels and the inflammatory response lead to hemorrhage, edema, and associated pain when the child attempts to move the injured part. The escape of blood into the tissues is observed as *ecchymosis,* a black-and-blue discoloration.

Large contusions cause gross swelling, pain, and disability, and those sustained while the child is participating in sports usually receive immediate attention from health personnel. The less spectacular, smaller injuries may go unnoticed, allowing continued participation; however, they can become disabling after rest be-

Nursing Care Plan THE CHILD WHO IS IMMOBILIZED

NURSING DIAGNOSIS Impaired physical mobility related to mechanical restrictions, physical disability

EXPECTED OUTCOME Child engages in activities appropriate to physical limitations.

Nursing Interventions/*Rationales*

Arrange for appropriate transport (e.g., wheelchair, stretcher, crutches, stroller) *to maintain mobility;* plan trips outside confines of room *to prevent isolation.*

Rearrange furniture in room when child is confined for long term *to break monotony and provide variety.*

Encourage mobility freedom of movement, independence in activities of daily living and play within physical limits *to maintain sense of autonomy and control.*

Encourage child to make choices about daily routine, food, clothing, play within physical limits *to maintain sense of control.*

NURSING DIAGNOSIS Risk for impaired skin integrity related to immobility, therapeutic devices

EXPECTED OUTCOME Skin is clean, dry, and intact.

Nursing Interventions/*Rationales*

Turn and reposition every 2 hours *to promote circulation and prevent skin breakdown* (align properly, provide positional supports; use handrolls or splints *to position hands in functional position;* use footboard or high top tennis shoes *to prevent footdrop*); perform passive range of motion frequently *to maintain full range in all joints and prevent contracture formation;* seat child in chair *to improve circulation;* place on tilt table *to prevent loss of bone density to long bones.*

Use pressure reduction mattress overlay *to prevent pressure necrosis;* use foam pads on ankles, heels, elbows *to protect bony prominences;* massage skin with lotion regularly *to stimulate circulation and prevent friction and shearing effects;* keep bedclothes clean, dry, and wrinkle-free *to prevent skin irritation;* cleanse skin, mucous membranes of mouth, and perianal area regularly *to prevent irritation and breakdown;* keep skinfolds clean and dry *to prevent excoriation;* inspect skin, mucous membranes, corneas regularly *to assess for early signs of irritation or breakdown.*

NURSING DIAGNOSIS Risk for injury related to impaired mobility

EXPECTED OUTCOME Child exhibits no evidence of injury.

Nursing Interventions/*Rationales*

Promote and teach child and family proper transfer techniques, use of mobilizing devices (e.g., wheelchairs, crutches, walkers, braces) *to enhance safety.*

Modify environment as appropriate (e.g., place call bell in easy reach, remove hazards and barriers, clear traffic areas) *to enhance safety.*

NURSING DIAGNOSIS Diversional activity deficit related to mobility impairment and confinement

EXPECTED OUTCOME Child engages in activities that are developmentally appropriate and within physical and environmental limitations.

Nursing Interventions/*Rationales*

Schedule therapies and rest periods *to allow time for play activities.* Time play periods when child may be feeling particularly vulnerable or alone *to provide needed distraction.*

Arrange for social interactions with others *to promote socialization.*

Interview parents and child to discover the child's favorite activities and games; adapt activities to the child's physical limitations *to provide optimal diversions.*

Have parents bring in treasured toys or objects; decorate room with familiar pictures and drawings *to familiarize child with an unfamiliar environment.*

cause of pain and muscle spasm. The young athlete is commonly instructed to work it out or disregard the pain. Unfortunately, this can result in myositis ossificans, which requires a lengthy recovery. Immediate treatment consists of cold application, as in the treatment of sprains described below. Return to participation is allowed when the strength and range of motion of the affected extremity are equal to those of the opposite extremity.

Related to contusions are crush injuries that occur in children when their fingers are compressed (e.g., slammed in doors, or caught in folding chairs or equipment) or hit (e.g., struck while using a hammer). A severe crush injury involves the bone, with swelling and bleeding beneath the nail (subungual) and sometimes laceration of the pulp of the distal phalanx. The subungual hematoma can be released by drilling holes at the proximal end of the nail.

Dislocations. Long bones are held in approximation to one another at the joint by ligaments. A dislocation occurs when the force of stress on the ligament is so great as to displace the normal position of the opposing bone ends or to displace the bone end from its socket. The predominant symptom is pain that increases with attempted passive or active movement of the extremity. In dislocations there may be an obvious deformity and inability to move the joint. Children with naturally lax joints, such as children with Down syndrome, are more prone

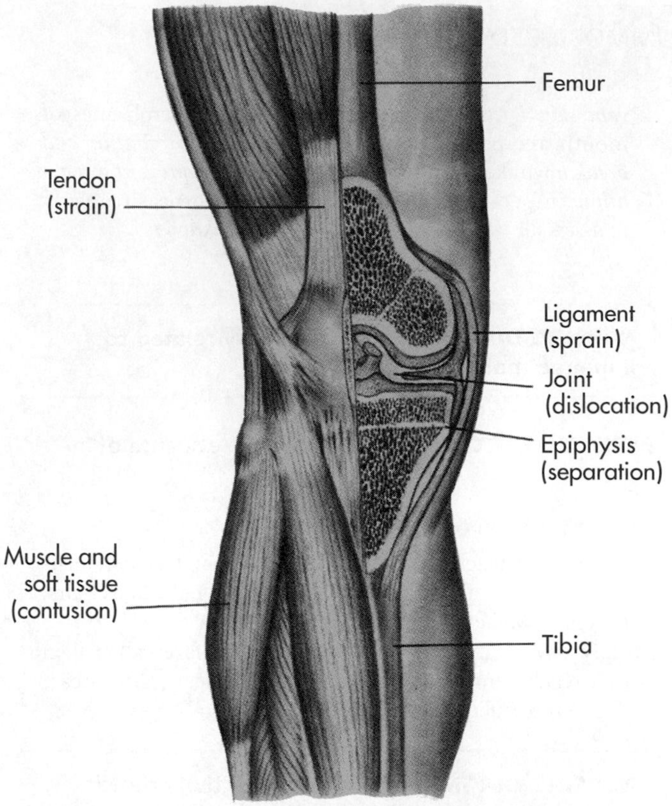

FIG. 54-1 • Sites of injuries to bones, joints, and soft tissues.

to dislocation of joints. Dislocation of the phalanges is the most common type seen in children, followed by elbow dislocation. The most common dislocation of the elbow involves the radial head. Called "pulled elbow" or "nursemaid's elbow," it is most commonly found in children between ages 1 and 5. Realignment of the bony structure can be accomplished by manipulation of the forearm while holding the radial head. Recovery of mobility after the dislocation is related to the length of time the joint remains dislocated.

Hip dislocation in children less than 5 years of age is usually caused by a fall. The greatest risk following this injury is the potential loss of blood supply to the head of the femur. Relocation of the hip within 60 minutes after the injury provides the best chance for prevention of damage to the femoral head.

Shoulder dislocations occur most often in older adolescents and are often sports related. Temporary restriction of the joint, with a sling or bandage that secures the arm to the chest, provides sufficient comfort and immobilization until medical help is received.

Simple dislocations should be reduced as soon as possible with the child under conscious sedation (and often, local anesthesia). Also, the use of anesthetics, such as nitrous oxide, parenteral or oral ketamine, or intravenous (IV) propofol, can be used to produce partial or complete analgesia (Annequin et al, 2000; Kennedy and Luhmann, 1999). An unreduced dislocation will be complicated by increased swelling, making reduction difficult and increasing the risk of neurovascular problems. Reduction is accomplished by simple traction and slight flexion, followed by immobilization in a splint for 10 to 16 days or up to 3 weeks or more for healing of torn ligaments.

Sprains. A sprain occurs when trauma to a joint is so severe that a ligament is partially or completely torn or stretched by the force created as a joint is twisted or wrenched, often accompanied by damage to associated blood vessels, muscles, tendons, and nerves.

The presence of joint laxity is the most valid indicator of the severity of a sprain. In a severe injury the child complains of the joint "feeling loose" or as if "something is coming apart," and may describe hearing a "snap," "pop," or "tearing." Pain is seldom the principal subjective symptom. There is a rapid onset with swelling (often diffuse), accompanied by immediate disability and appreciable reluctance to use the injured joint.

Strains. A strain is a microscopic tear to the musculotendinous unit and has features in common with sprains. The area is painful to touch and swollen. Most strains are incurred over time rather than suddenly, and the rapidity of the appearance provides clues regarding severity. In general, the more rapidly the strain occurs, the more severe the injury. When the strain involves the muscular portion, there is more bleeding, often palpable soon after injury and before edema obscures the hematoma.

Therapeutic Management. The first 6 to 12 hours are the most critical for virtually all soft tissue injuries. Basic principles of managing sprains and other soft tissue injuries are summarized in the acronyms *RICE* and *ICES:*

R—Rest	I—Ice
I—Ice	C—Compression
C—Compression	E—Elevation
E—Elevation	S—Support

Soft tissue injuries should be iced immediately. This is best accomplished with crushed ice wrapped in a towel or encased in a screw-top ice bag or resealable storage bag. A wet elastic wrap, which transfers cold better than dry wrap, is applied to provide compression and to keep the ice pack in place. Ice has a rapid cooling effect on tissues that reduces the pain threshold. However, ice should never be applied for more than 30 minutes at a time.

Elevating the extremity uses gravity to facilitate venous return and to reduce edema formation in the damaged area. The point of injury should be kept several inches above the level of the heart for therapy to be effective. Several pillows can be used effectively for elevation. Allowing the extremity to be dependent causes excessive fluid accumulation in the area of injury, delaying healing and causing painful swelling.

Torn ligaments, especially those in the knee, are usually treated by immobilization with a cast for 3 to 4 weeks or strapping of the joint with adhesive or Elastoplast bandage. Passive leg exercises are begun as soon as sufficient healing has taken place and gradually increased to active exercise. Parents and children are cautioned against using any form of liniment or other heat-producing preparation before examination. If the injury requires casting or splinting, the heat generated in the enclosed space can cause extreme discomfort and may even cause tissue damage.

Fractures

Bone fractures occur when the resistance of bone yields to the stress force being exerted. Fractures are a common injury at any age but are more likely to occur in children and older adults. Because of the characteristics of the child's skeleton, the pattern of fractures, problems of diagnosis, and methods of treatment differ in the child and the adult.

Fracture injuries in children are a result of traumatic incidents at home, at school, in a motor vehicle, or in association with recreational activities. Children's everyday activities include vigorous play that predisposes them to injury from climbing, falling down, running into immovable objects, and receiving blows to any part of their bodies.

Aside from vehicular accidents, true injuries that cause fractures rarely occur in infancy; therefore bone injury in children of that age group warrants further investigation. In any small child, radiographic evidence of fractures at various stages of healing are, with few exceptions, a result of physical abuse. Any investigation of fractures in infants, particularly multiple fractures, should include consideration of osteogenesis imperfecta.

The clavicle is probably the bone most commonly broken in childhood, with approximately half of clavicle fractures occurring in children under 10 years of age. Common mechanisms of injury include a fall with an outstretched hand or direct trauma to the bone.

Fractures in school-age children are often a result of bicycle-automobile or skateboard injuries. Adolescents are vulnerable to multiple and severe trauma because they are mobile on bikes and motorcycles and are active in sports.

Epiphyseal Injuries. The weakest point of long bones is the cartilage growth plate or epiphyseal plate. Consequently, this is a common site of damage during trauma. Detection of epiphyseal injuries is sometimes difficult, but critical. Fractures involving the epiphysis or epiphyseal plate present special problems in determining whether or not bone growth will be affected. Treatment of these fractures may include open reduction and internal fixation to prevent or reduce growth disturbances.

Types of Fractures. A fractured bone consists of fragments—the fragment closer to the midline, or the proximal fragment; and the fragment farther from the midline, or the distal fragment. When fracture fragments are separated, the fracture is *complete;* when fragments remain attached, the fracture is *incomplete.* The fracture line can be any of the following:

Transverse—Crosswise, at right angles to the long axis of the bone

Oblique—Slanting but straight, between a horizontal and a perpendicular direction

Spiral—Slanting and circular, twisting around the bone shaft

The twisting of an extremity while the bone is breaking results in a spiral break. If the fracture does not produce a break in the skin, it is a *simple,* or *closed fracture. Open,* or *compound fractures* are those with an open wound through which the bone is or has protruded. If the bone fragments cause damage to other organs or tissues (such as the lung or bladder), the injury is said to be a *complicated fracture.* When small fragments of bone are broken from the fractured shaft and lie in the surrounding tissue, the injury is a *comminuted fracture.* This type of fracture is rare in children. The types of fractures that are seen most often in children are described in Box 54-1 and in Fig. 54-2.

NURSE ALERT • A spiral fracture in children may indicate child abuse. Further assessment and immediate involvement of interdisciplinary team members, such as a social worker, is necessary.

Box 54-1

Types of Fractures in Children

Bend—Occurs when the bone is bent but not broken. A child's flexible bone can be bent 45 degrees or more before breaking. However, if bent, the bone will straighten slowly, but not completely, to produce some deformity but without the angulation seen when the bone breaks. Bends occur most commonly in the ulna and fibula, often in association with fractures of the radius and tibia.

Buckle, or **torus, fracture**—Produced by compression of the porous bone; appears as a raised or bulging projection at the fracture site. These fractures occur in the most porous portion of the bone near the metaphysis (the portion of the bone shaft adjacent to the epiphysis) and are more common in young children.

Greenstick fracture—Occurs when a bone is angulated beyond the limits of bending. The compressed side bends, and the tension side fails, causing an incomplete fracture similar to the break observed when a green stick is broken.

Complete fracture—Divides the bone fragments. These fragments often remain attached by a periosteal hinge, which can aid or hinder reduction.

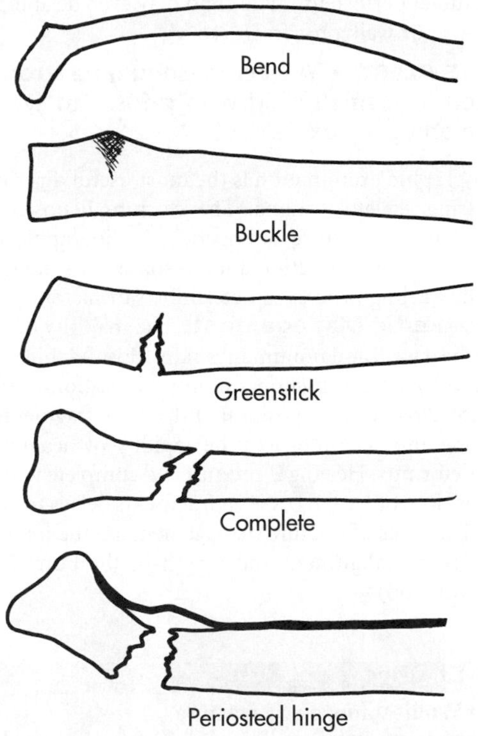

FIG. 54-2 • Types of fractures in children.

Immediately after a fracture occurs, the muscles contract and physiologically splint the injured area. This phenomenon accounts for the muscle tightness observed over a fracture site and the deformity that is produced as the muscles pull the bone ends out of alignment. This muscle response must be overcome by traction or complete muscle relaxation (e.g., with anesthesia) in order to realign the distal bone fragment to the proximal bone fragment.

Bone Healing and Remodeling. Bone healing is characteristically rapid in children because of the thickened periosteum and generous blood supply. When there is a break in the continuity of bone, the osteoblasts are stimulated to maximum activity. New bone cells are formed in immense numbers almost immediately after the injury and, in time, are evidenced by a bulging growth of new bone tissue between the fractured bone fragments. This is followed by deposition of calcium salts to form a *callus.*

Fractures heal in less time in children than in adults. The approximate healing times for a femoral shaft are as follows:

- Neonatal period—2 to 3 weeks
- Early childhood—4 weeks
- Later childhood—6 to 8 weeks
- Adolescence—8 to 12 weeks

Diagnostic Evaluation. A history is often lacking in childhood injuries. Infants are unable to communicate, and older children seldom volunteer information (even under direct questioning) when the injury occurred during forbidden activities. Unless they are witnesses to the injury, parents may misinterpret what the child is trying to say. In cases of child abuse, parents may give false information to protect themselves.

The child may exhibit the same manifestations seen in adults (Box 54-2). However, often a fracture is remarkably stable because of intact periosteum. The child may even be able to use an affected arm or walk on a fractured leg.

NURSE ALERT • A fracture should be strongly suspected in a small child who refuses to walk or to move an upper extremity.

Radiographic examination is the most useful diagnostic tool for assessing skeletal trauma. The calcium deposits in bone make the entire structure radiopaque. Radiographic films are taken after fracture reduction and, in some cases, may be taken during the healing process to determine satisfactory progress.

Therapeutic Management. The majority of children's fractures heal well, and nonunion is rare. Most fractures are readily reduced by simple traction and immobilization until healing takes place. However, the position of the bone fragments in relation to one another influences the rapidity of healing and the residual deformity. Healing is prompt and complete with end-to-end apposition, but a gap between fragments delays (or prevents) healing. The goals of fracture management are the following:

1. To regain alignment and length of the bony fragments (reduction)
2. To retain alignment and length (immobilization)
3. To restore function to the injured parts
4. To prevent further injury

In children the bone fragments are usually realigned and immobilized by traction or by closed manipulation and casting until an adequate callus is formed. Weight bearing on lower extremity fractures and active movement for the purpose of regaining function can begin after the fracture site is stable. The child's natural tendency to be active is usually sufficient to restore normal mobility, and physical therapy is rarely needed. In most cases children's fractures can be managed by closed reduction and plaster immobilization, which is most often provided on an outpatient basis with reevaluation in 7 to 10 days.

Children are most commonly hospitalized for fractures of the femur and the supracondylar area of the distal humerus. If simple reductions cannot be achieved, or if a neurovascular problem is detected after injury, observation in a hospital is indicated. Severe contusions with profound swelling cannot be treated with a cast, which would act as a tourniquet on the extremity. A badly malaligned fracture requires traction for a time before a cast is applied.

The major methods for immobilizing a fracture, casting and traction, are described in the following sections.

Nursing Care Management. Nurses are commonly the persons who make the initial assessment of a child with a suspected fracture (Emergency box). The child and parents are frightened and upset; the child is in pain; and because most fractures are obvious, the parents and (commonly) the child are already convinced of the diagnosis. Therefore, if the child is alert and there is no evidence of hemorrhage, the initial nursing interventions are directed toward calming and reassuring the child and parents so that a more extensive assessment can be more easily accomplished.

While remaining calm and speaking in a quiet voice, the nurse can ask the parents and older child to describe what happened and how they feel about it. Because the child usually ar-

Box 54-2

Clinical Manifestations of a Fracture

Signs of injury:
- Generalized swelling
- Pain or tenderness
- Diminished functional use of affected part

May be:
- Bruising
- Severe muscular rigidity
- Crepitus (grating sensation at fracture site)

Emergency

Emergency

FRACTURE

Assess the extent of injury—5 *P's;*
- **Pain and point of tenderness**
- **Pulse—distal to the fracture site**
- **Pallor**
- **Paresthesia—sensation distal to the fracture site**
- **Paralysis—movement distal to the fracture site**

Determine the mechanism of injury.
Move the injured part as little as possible.
Cover open wounds with a sterile or clean dressing.
Immobilize the limb, including joints above and below the fracture site; do not attempt to reduce the fracture or push protruding bone under the skin.
- **Soft splint (pillow or folded towel)**
- **Rigid splint (rolled newspaper or magazine)**
- **Uninjured leg can serve as a splint for a leg fracture if no splint available**

Reassess neurovascular status.
Apply traction if circulatory compromise is present.
Elevate the injured limb if possible.
Apply cold to the injured area.
Call emergency medical service or transport to medical facility.

rives with the limb supported in some manner, this time does not delay or endanger the treatment. Initially it is best not to touch the child but to ask him or her to point to the painful area and to wiggle the fingers or toes. By this time the child usually feels relatively safe and will allow someone to gently touch the area just enough to feel the pulse and test for sensation. A child's anxiety is greatly influenced by previous experiences with injury and with health personnel; however, he or she needs to be told what will happen and what to do to help. The affected limb need not be palpated, and it should not be moved unless properly splinted. If the child is at home or if the practitioner is not present to examine the child, some type of splint is applied carefully for transport to the medical facility.

The Child in a Cast

The completeness of the fracture, the type of bone involved, and the amount of weight bearing influence how much of the extremity must be included in the cast to immobilize the fracture site completely. In most cases the joints above and below the fracture are immobilized to eliminate the possibility of movement that might cause displacement at the fracture site. Four major categories of casts are used for fractures: *upper extremity* to immobilize the wrist and/or elbow, *lower extremity* to immobilize the ankle and/or knee, *spinal* and *cervical* for immobilization of the spine, and *spica casts* to immobilize the hip and knee.

The Cast. Casts are constructed from gauze strips and bandages impregnated with plaster of paris or, more commonly, from synthetic lighter-weight and water-resistant materials (e.g., fiberglass and polyurethane resin).

Both types of casting produce heat from chemical reaction immediately after application. Plaster casts mold closely to the body part, take 10 to 72 hours to dry, have a smooth exterior, and are inexpensive. Synthetic casting material is lighter, dries in 5 to 30 minutes, and is water-resistant. The disadvantages of synthetic casting include its inability to mold closely to body parts; its rough exterior, which may scratch surfaces; and its increased cost. Synthetic casts have special advantages for children. They come in different colors and with designs (e.g., cartoons and stripes). They are lightweight, durable, easy to clean, and water-resistant. With a special Gore-Tex liner, the cast can be immersed in water. One other drawback—their rough surface is harder to autograph!

Application of a Cast. When a cast is to be applied, the nurse often must set up the cast materials and hold the extremity in alignment. In most instances only the cast material is required; however, special cast tables that hold the child's body are used for applying large hip spica casts. If possible, children should be allowed to play with a doll that has a cast so that they understand what will be done.

Before the cast is applied, the extremities are checked for any abrasions, cuts, or other alterations in the skin surface and for the presence of rings or other items that might cause constriction from swelling; such objects are removed. If hospitalization is anticipated identification bands are placed on a noninjured extremity.

A tube of stockinette is stretched over the area to be casted, and bony prominences are padded with soft cotton sheeting. Some practitioners use a special plastic material or Gore-Tex liner under a spica cast to prevent skin breakdown. Dry rolls of casting material are immersed in a pail of water. The wet rolls are put on in a bandage fashion and molded to the extremity. During application of the cast, the underlying stockinette is pulled over the raw edges of the cast and secured with a layer of wet plaster ½ to 1 inch below the rim to form a smooth, padded edge to protect the skin.

If the operator does not form such a protective edge with a stockinette, the raw edges of the cast can be protected by a "petaled" edge. Small pieces approximately 2 to 3 inches long are cut from 1- or 1½-inch-wide adhesive tape or moleskin. The edges are rounded with scissors, and these "petals" are placed over the edge of the cast, with each petal slightly overlapping the previous petal to form a smooth, neat edge. It is easier to apply the petal to the underside of the cast first and then bring the unadhered edge to the front, pressing firmly so that the edges remain securely attached. Adhesive bandages can be used instead of the tape petals for quicker preparation and a slightly padded cast edge.

Nursing Care Management. The complete evaporation of the water from a hip spica cast can take 24 to 48 hours when plaster is used. Drying occurs within minutes with new, quick-drying substances. The cast must remain uncovered to allow it to dry from the inside out. Turning the child in a plaster body cast at least every 2 hours will help to dry the cast evenly and prevent complications related to immobility. A regular fan or cool-air hair dryer to circulate air may be helpful when the humidity is high.

NURSE ALERT • Heated fans or dryers are not used because they cause the cast to dry on the outside and remain wet beneath. They also can cause burns from heat conduction by way of the cast to the underlying tissue.

A wet cast should be supported by a pillow that is covered with plastic. The cast should be handled by the palms of the hands to prevent indenting the cast, which can create pressure areas. A dry plaster of paris cast produces a hollow sound when it is tapped with the finger. If "hot spots" are felt on the cast surface (usually indicating infection beneath the area), this should be reported so that a window can be made in the cast to observe the site.

During the first few hours after a cast is applied, the chief concern is that the extremity may continue to swell to the extent that the cast becomes a tourniquet, shutting off circulation and producing neurovascular complications. To reduce the likelihood of this problem, the body part can be elevated, thereby increasing venous return. If edema is excessive, casts are bivalved (i.e., cut to make anterior and posterior halves that are held together with an elastic bandage). The cast and the involved extremity are observed frequently for neurovascular integrity and for any signs of compromise. Permanent muscle and tissue damage can occur within 6 to 8 hours.

NURSE ALERT • Observations such as pain, swelling, discoloration (pallor or cyanosis) of the exposed portions, lack of pulsation and warmth, or the inability to move the exposed part(s) are reported immediately.

When an extremity that has sustained an open fracture is casted, a window is often left over the wound area to allow for observation and for dressing of the wound. A surgical reduction is usually casted as for a closed fracture. For the first few hours after surgery, there may be substantial bleeding that will soak through the cast. Periodically the circumscribed blood-stained area should be outlined with a ball-point pen or pencil, and the time indicated to provide a guide for assessing the amount of bleeding.

Usually the child is discharged to home care after a cast is applied in the emergency department or clinic. Parents need instructions on drying and caring for the cast and on checking for signs and symptoms that indicate the cast is too tight (Home Care box). They should also be told to take the child to the health professional for attention if the cast becomes too loose, because a loose cast no longer serves its purpose. A cast is a badge of honor for the child and serves as visible evidence of an otherwise invisible injury.

Nurses can help families adapt the child's home environment to meet the temporary encumbrance of a cast. Home care creates problems of various magnitude, especially for children in large casts (e.g., a hip spica). Commonplace situations become problematic (e.g., returning the child home safely and comfortably). Standard seat belts and car seats may not be readily adapted for use by children in some casts. There are specially designed car seats and restraints available that meet safety requirements* (Fig. 54-3). Alterations to standard car seats to accommodate the cast are not recommended because the structure may be adversely altered.

*For additional information contact the Automotive Safety for Children Program, James Whitcomb Riley Hospital for Children, Indiana University School of Medicine, 575 West Dr., Room 004, Indianapolis, IN 46202; (317) 274-2977 (in Indianapolis 1-800-KID-N-CAR); website: www.preventinjury.org.

Home Care

CAST CARE

- **Keep the casted extremity elevated on pillows or similar support for the first day, or as directed by the health professional.**
- **Avoid indenting the cast while still wet to avoid creating pressure points.**
- **Observe the extremities (fingers or toes) for any evidence of swelling or discoloration (darker or lighter than a comparable extremity), and contact the health professional if noted.**
- **Check movement and sensation of the visible extremities frequently.**
- **Follow health professional's orders regarding any restriction of activities.**
- **Restrict strenuous activities for the first few days.**
  - **Engage in quiet activities but encourage use of muscles.**
  - **Move the joints above and below the cast on the affected extremity.**
- **Encourage frequent rest for a few days, keeping the injured extremity elevated while resting.**
- **Avoid allowing the affected limb to hang down for any length of time.**
  - **Keep an injured upper extremity elevated (e.g., in a sling) while upright.**
  - **Elevate a lower limb when sitting and avoid standing for too long.**
- **Do not allow the child to put anything inside the cast.**
  - **Keep small items that might be placed inside the cast away from small children.**
- **Keep a clear path for ambulation.**
  - **Remove toys, hazardous floor rugs, pets, or other items over which the child might stumble.**
- **Use crutches appropriately if lower limb fracture.**
  - **The crutches should fit properly, have a soft rubber tip to prevent slipping, and be well padded at the axilla.**

Parents are taught the proper care of the cast (or orthotic device) and are helped to devise means for maintaining cleanliness. A superabsorbent disposable diaper (newborn size) is tucked beneath the entire perineal opening of the cast. A larger (toddler size) diaper can be applied and fastened over the small diaper and cast.

For tightly fitting casts, transparent film dressings can be cut into strips as for petaling, and one edge applied to the cast edge and the other directly to the perineum; this forms a continuous, waterproof bridge between the perineum and the cast to prevent leakage. An additional advantage to the use of this transparent dressing is that it keeps both the skin and the cast dry while allowing for observation of skin beneath the dressing.

Older infants and small children may stuff bits of food, small toys, or other items under the cast; parents should be alerted to this possibility so that suitable preventive measures can be initiated.

Feeding the infant in a hip spica cast offers problems in positioning. Very young infants can be fed in the supine position with the head elevated; with the infant's hips and legs supported on a pillow at the side, the parent can cuddle the infant in his or her arms during feeding. A somewhat similar position can be used for breastfeeding (i.e., with the infant supported on pillows or held in a "football" hold facing the mother with the legs behind

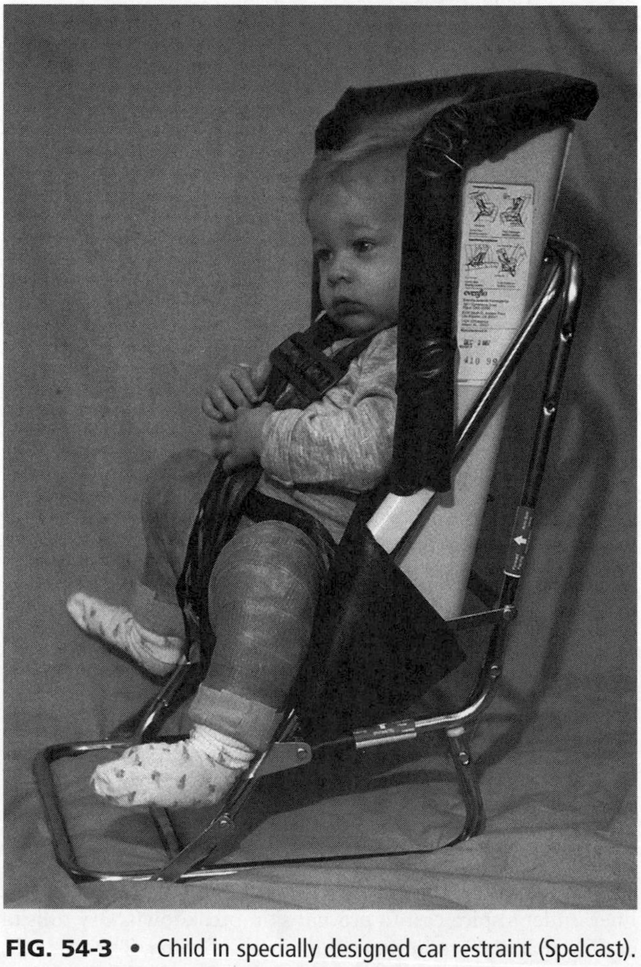

FIG. 54-3 • Child in specially designed car restraint (Spelcast).

her). An alternate position is to hold the infant upright on the caregiver's lap with the legs of the infant astride the adult's leg.

Children in spica casts usually find the prone position easier for self-feeding from a small table placed next to the dining table. The use of a conventional toilet is almost impossible. Small bedpans or other containers offer alternatives for elimination. The nurse may suggest waterproofing methods, using plastic wraps, that can help with elimination and showers. Baths are possible only if the plaster cast is kept out of the water and covered to prevent it from becoming wet from splashes. Synthetic casts can be immersed in water if a special type of cast liner is used.

Cast Removal. Cutting the cast to remove it or to relieve tightness is commonly a frightening experience for children. They fear the sound of the cast cutter and are terrified that their flesh, as well as the cast, will be cut. Because it works by vibration, a cast cutter cuts only the hard surface of the cast. This can be demonstrated on the nurse or person removing the cast. The oscillating blade vibrates very rapidly back and forth and will not cut when placed lightly on the skin. Children have described it as producing a tickling sensation. The vibration also generates heat that may be felt by the child. Both of these feelings should be explained.

Preparation for the procedure will help reduce anxiety, especially if a trusting relationship has been established between the child and the nurse. Many young children come to regard the cast as part of themselves, which intensifies their fear of removal. Using the analogy of having fingernails trimmed or a haircut sometimes helps reduce their anxiety. They need continual reassurance that all is going well and that their behavior is accepted.

After the cast is removed, the skin surface will be caked with desquamated skin and sebaceous secretions. Simple soaking in a bathtub is usually sufficient for their removal, but a several days may be required to eliminate the accumulation completely. Application of olive oil or skin lotion may provide comfort. The parents and child should be instructed not to pull or forcibly remove this material with vigorous scrubbing because it may cause excoriation and bleeding.*

The Child in Traction

Bone fragments that cannot be aligned initially by simple traction and stabilization with a cast require the extended pulling force supplied by continuous traction. Traction may be used for other purposes, including the following:

- To provide rest for an extremity
- To help prevent or improve contracture deformity
- To correct a deformity
- To treat a dislocation
- To allow preoperative or postoperative positioning and alignment
- To provide immobilization of specific areas of the body
- To reduce muscle spasms (rare in children)

Purposes of Traction. The three essential components of traction management are traction, countertraction, and friction (Fig. 54-4). To reduce or realign a fracture site, *traction* (forward force) is produced by attaching weight to the distal bone fragment; body weight provides *countertraction* (backward force); and the patient's contact with the bed constitutes the *frictional* force. These forces are used to align the distal and proximal bone fragments by adjusting the line of pull upward or downward and adducting or abducting the extremity.

To attain equilibrium, the amount of forward force is adjusted by adding weight to or subtracting weight from the traction, and/or countertraction can be increased by elevating the foot of the bed to create a greater gravitational pull to the backward force. A bed board placed under the mattress of heavy children prevents sagging, which might otherwise change the direction of the forces applied to the fracture.

The three primary purposes of traction for reduction of fractures are:

1. To fatigue the involved muscle and reduce muscle spasm so that bones can be realigned
2. To position the distal and proximal bone ends in desired realignment to promote satisfactory bone healing
3. To immobilize the fracture site until realignment has been achieved and sufficient healing has taken place to permit casting or splinting

The *all-or-none law,* characteristic of muscle contractibility, influences the complete relaxation. When muscle is stretched, muscle spasm ceases and permits the realignment of the bone ends. The continuous maintenance of traction is important

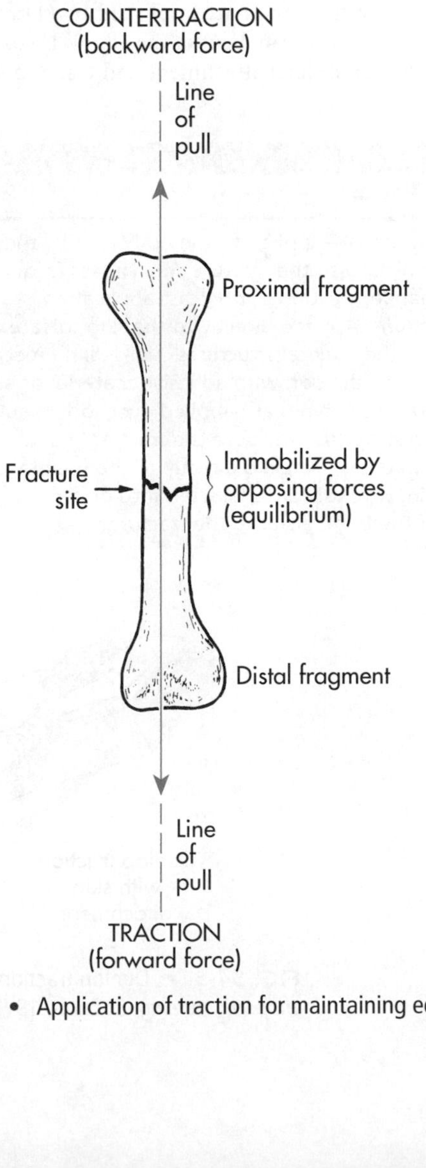

FIG. 54-4 • Application of traction for maintaining equilibrium.

---

*Community and home care instructions for the child in a cast are available in Wong DL, Hess CS: ***Wong and Whaley's clinical manual of pediatric nursing,*** ed 5, St Louis, 2000, Mosby.

during this phase because releasing the traction allows the normal contracting ability of the muscle to again cause a malpositioning of the bone ends.

The realignment of the fragments is a gradual process that is achieved more rapidly in infants, who have limited muscle tone, than in muscular teenagers. The desired line of pull and callus formation are checked periodically by radiographic examination. The traction pull to some degree immobilizes the fracture site; however, adjunctive immobilizing devices such as splints or casts are sometimes used with skeletal traction. In injuries in which there is severe soft tissue swelling or vascular and nerve damage, it is customary to use traction until these complications have been resolved and it is safe to apply a cast. Immobilization with traction will be maintained until the bone ends are in satisfactory realignment, after which a less confining type of immobilization, usually a cast, will be applied.

Types of Traction (General). The pull needed for traction can be applied to the distal bone fragment in several ways (Box 54-3). The type of traction applied is determined primarily by the age of the child, the condition of the soft tissues, and the type and degree of displacement of the fracture. Fractures most commonly treated by application of traction are those involving the humerus, femur, and vertebrae. The major types of traction for specific fractures are discussed in the following sections.

Upper Extremity Traction. Treatment of fractures of the humerus by traction is accomplished by (1) *overhead suspension,* in which the arm, bent at the elbow, is suspended vertically by skin or skeletal attachment and traction is applied to the distal end of the humerus; or (2) *Dunlop traction.* With Dunlop traction (Fig. 54-5), the arm is suspended horizontally, using either skin or skeletal attachment. A skeletal wire placed in the upper arm to allow additional weight may be applied in certain instances, such as a supracondylar fracture. When skin traction is used, straps are placed on the lower and upper arm with the arm flexed to accomplish pull in two directions, one along the longitudinal direction of the upper arm and one to maintain vertical alignment of the lower arm.

Fractures of the humerus, which usually result from a fall with the arm in extension, commonly involve the supracondylar portion. These fractures especially place the patient at risk for nerve damage and angulation deformities; therefore they must be reduced carefully, sometimes with the patient under anesthesia. Because of the danger of complications, children with closed reduction of supracondylar fractures are often hospitalized for observation. In severely malaligned fractures, closed reduction with the patient under anesthesia is followed by application of skeletal traction for 2 to 3 weeks, after which a long arm cast is applied for an additional 2 to 3 weeks.

Lower Extremity Traction. The severity of the fracturing force and the ability of the muscles to hold the fracture out of alignment will determine the fracture type and the amount of overriding of the fragments. The periosteum may remain intact, which helps maintain alignment. A fracture in the middle third of the shaft of the femur results in significant overriding but minimal displacement. In a fracture in the lower one third of the shaft, the pull of the gastrocnemius muscle causes the distal fragment to become downwardly displaced.

Fractures of the femur can often be reduced with immediate application of a hip spica cast in young children. When traction is required, several types may be used, based on the initial assessment.

Bryant traction is a type of running traction in which the pull is only in one direction. Skin traction is applied to the legs, which are flexed at a 90-degree angle at the hips. The child's trunk (buttocks are raised slightly off the bed) provides countertraction.

NURSE ALERT • Bryant traction is not recommended because of the gravitational vascular draining of the elevated extremities; the possible tourniquet effect of the bandages; and the effect of the traction, which can trigger vasospasms and avascular necrosis.

Box 54-3

Types of Traction

Manual traction—Applied to the body part by the hand placed distally to the fracture site. Nurses frequently provide manual traction during cast application.

Skin traction—Applied directly to the skin surface and indirectly to the skeletal structures. The pulling mechanism is attached to the skin with adhesive material or an elastic bandage. Both types are applied over soft, foam-backed traction straps to distribute the traction pull.

Skeletal traction—Applied directly to the skeletal structure by a pin, wire, or tongs inserted into or through the diameter of the bone distal to the fracture.

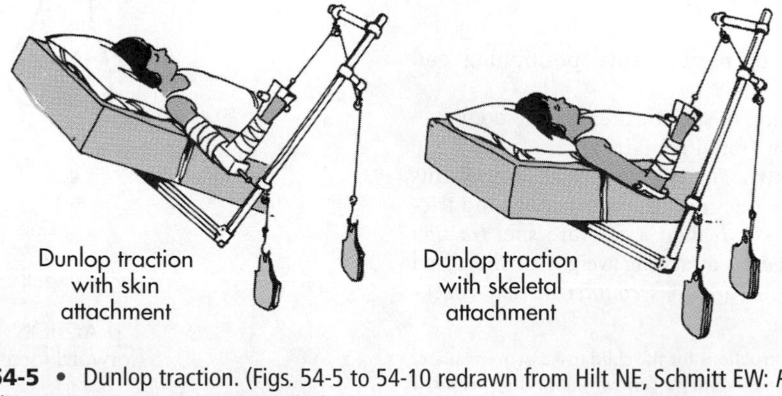

FIG. 54-5 • Dunlop traction. (Figs. 54-5 to 54-10 redrawn from Hilt NE, Schmitt EW: *Pediatric orthopedic nursing,* St Louis, 1975, Mosby.)

Buck extension (Fig. 54-6) is a type of skin traction with the legs in an extended position. Except for fracture cases, turning from side to side is permitted, with care to maintain the involved leg alignment. Buck extension is used primarily for short-term immobilization, preoperatively with dislocated hips, for correcting contractures, or for bone deformities such as Legg-Calvé-Perthes disease.

Russell traction (Fig. 54-7) uses skin traction on the lower leg and a padded sling under the knee. Two lines of pull, one along the longitudinal line of the lower leg and one perpendicular to the leg, are produced. This combination of pulls allows realignment of the lower extremity and immobilizes the hip and knee in a flexed position. The hip flexion must be kept at the prescribed angle to prevent fracture malalignment, because there is no direct support under the fracture and the skin traction may slip. Special nursing measures include carefully checking the position of the traction so that the amount of desired hip flexion is maintained and damage to the common peroneal nerve under the knee does not produce footdrop.

The most common skeletal traction is *90-degree-90-degree* traction (Fig. 54-8). The lower leg is supported by a boot cast or a calf sling, and a skeletal Steinmann pin or Kirschner wire is placed in the distal fragment of the femur, resulting in a 90-degree angle at both the hip and the knee. From a nursing standpoint, this traction facilitates position changes, toileting, and prevention of complications related to traction (Houston, 1996).

Balance suspension traction (Fig. 54-9) may be used with or without skin or skeletal traction. Unless used with another traction, the balanced suspension merely suspends the leg in a desired flexed position to relax the hip and hamstring muscles and does not exert any traction directly on a body part. A *Thomas splint* extends from the groin to midair above the foot, and a *Pearson attachment* supports the lower leg. Towels or pieces of felt covered with stockinette are clipped or pinned to the splints for leg support. When the child is lifted off the bed, the traction lifts with the child without loss of alignment. This traction requires very careful checking of splints and ropes to make certain that no slippage or fraying has occurred. The traction is of great value in an older and heavier child when it is essential to lift the patient for care.

Cervical Traction. The cervical area is a vulnerable site for flexion or extension injuries to muscle, vertebrae, and/or the spinal cord. Cervical muscle trauma without other complications is treated with a cervical soft or hard collar to relieve the weight of the head from the fracture site. Intermittent cervical skin traction might be used with a child halter and weight to decrease muscle spasms (Fig. 54-10). Injuries limited to cervical

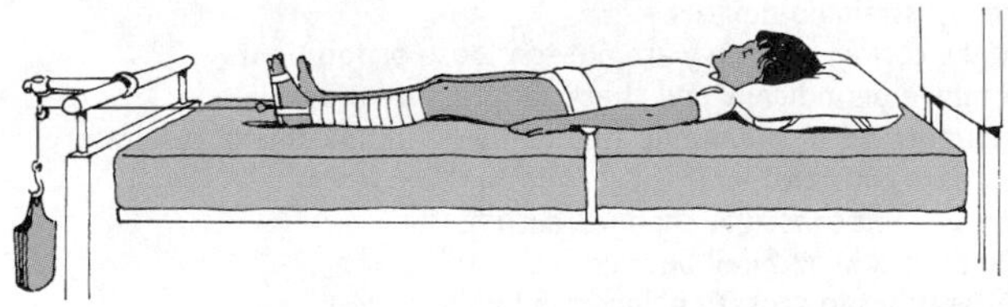

FIG. 54-6 • Buck extension traction.

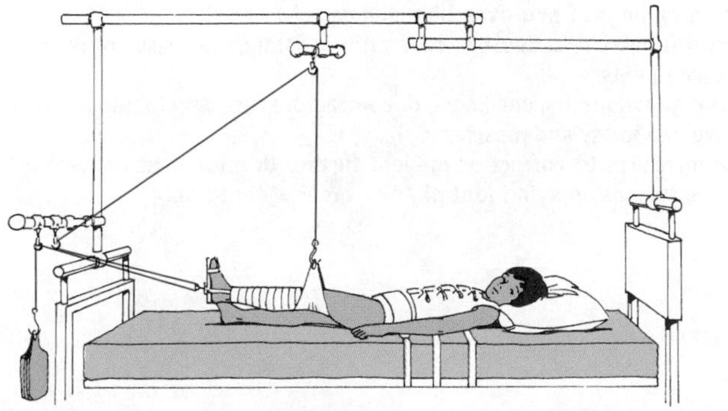

FIG. 54-7 • Russell traction.

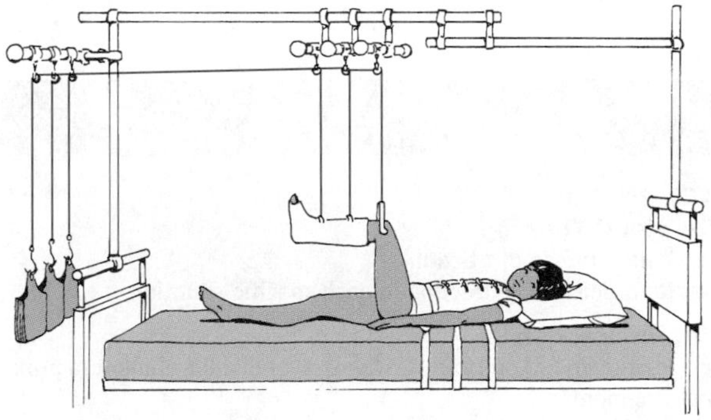

FIG. 54-8 • "Ninety-ninety" traction.

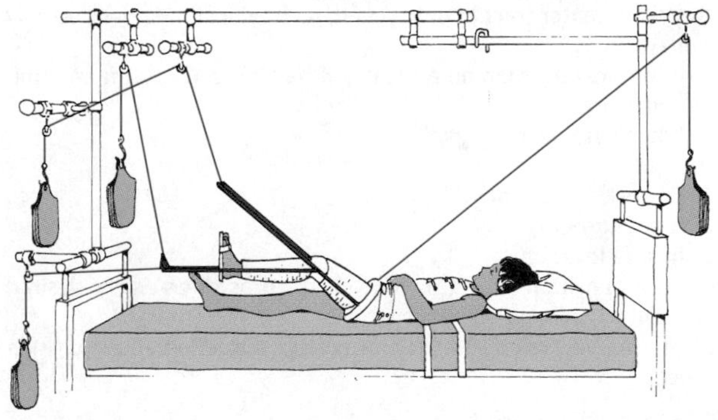

FIG. 54-9 • Balance suspension with Thomas ring splint and Pearson attachment.

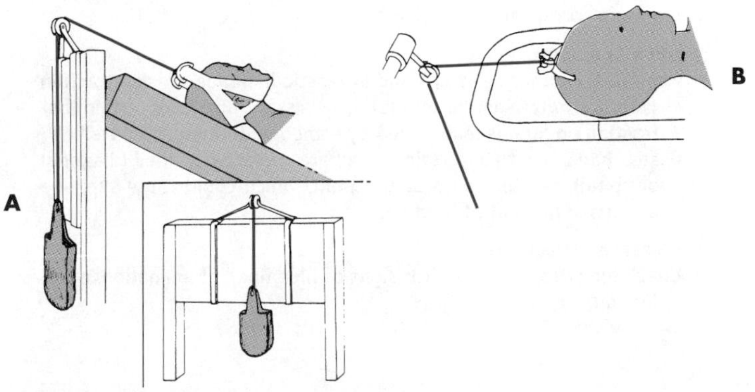

FIG. 54-10 • A, Cervical traction. B, Crutchfield tong traction.

muscles can be very uncomfortable, but with prompt medical care usually resolve with conservative treatment.

When a child displaces or fractures a cervical vertebra, it is necessary to reduce and immobilize the site with cervical skeletal traction. The spinal cord runs through the intravertebral canal, and dislocation or fracture of the vertebrae can also cause spinal cord injury. Nursing assessment of neurologic function is essential to prevent further injury during the application and use of cervical skeletal traction.

Cervical traction is usually accomplished by the insertion of *Crutchfield* or *Barton tongs* through burr holes in the skull and weights attached to the hyperextended head. As the neck muscles fatigue with constant traction pull, the vertebral bodies gradually separate so that the cord is no longer pinched between the vertebrae. Immobilization until fracture healing can occur is an essential goal of cervical traction. If the injury has been limited to a vertebral fracture without neurologic deficit, a halo cast can be applied to permit earlier ambulation.

Nursing Care Management. To assess the child in traction, it is essential to know the purpose for which the traction is applied and to understand the basic principles of traction. Regular assessment of both the child and the traction apparatus is required (Guidelines box). Many of the nursing problems associated with a child in traction are related to immobility.

NURSE ALERT • Skeletal traction is never released by the nurse. This precaution includes not lifting weights (e.g., while moving the child in bed or for repositioning) that are applying traction.

Guidelines

TRACTION CARE

Understand Therapy

Understand purpose of traction.
Understand function of traction in each specific situation.

Maintain Traction

Check desired line of pull and relationship of distal fragment to proximal fragment.
- Check whether fragment is being directed upward, adducted, or abducted.

Check function of each component.
- Position of bandages, frames, splints
- Ropes: In center tract of pulley, taut, no fraying, knots tied securely
- Pulleys:
  - In original position on attachment bar; have not slid from original site
  - Wheels freely moveable
- Weights:
  - Correct amount of weight
  - Hanging freely
  - In safe location

Check bed position—head or foot elevated as directed for desired amount of pull and countertraction.
Do not remove skeletal traction or adhesive traction straps on skin traction.

Maintain Alignment

Observe for correct body alignment with emphasis on alignment of shoulder, hip, and leg.
Check after child has moved.
Apply restraints when indicated.
Maintain correct angles at joints.

Skin Traction

Replace nonadhesive straps and/or elastic bandage on skin traction *when permitted* and/or absolutely necessary, but make certain that traction on limb is maintained by someone during procedure.
Assess bandages to ascertain if they are correctly applied (diagonal or spiral), not too loose or too tight, which could cause slippage and malalignment of traction.

Skeletal Traction

Check pin sites frequently for signs of bleeding, inflammation, or infection.
Cleanse and dress pin sites as ordered.
Apply topical antiseptic or antibiotic daily as ordered.
Cover ends of pins with protective cord or padding to prevent child's being scratched by pin.
Note pull of traction on pin; pull should be even.
Check pin screws to be certain that screws are tight in metal clamp that attaches traction apparatus to pin.

Prevent Skin Breakdown

Provide foam overlay or alternating-pressure mattress underneath hips and back.
Make total-body skin checks for redness or breakdown, especially over areas that receive greatest pressure.
Wash and dry skin at least daily.
Stimulate circulation with gentle massage over pressure areas.
Change position at least every 2 hours to relieve pressure.

Prevent Complications

Check pulse in affected area and compare with pulse in contralateral site.
Assess circular dressings for excessive tightness.
Assess restraining devices.
- Make certain that they are not too loose or too tight.
- Remove periodically and check for pressure areas.

Encourage deep breathing frequently with maximum inspiratory chest expansion.
Note any neurovascular changes, such as:
- Color in skin and nail beds
- Alterations in sensation, increased pain
- Alterations in motor ability

Take immediate action to correct problem or report to practitioner if neurovascular changes are found.
Record findings of neurovascular changes.
Carry out passive, active, or active-with-resistance exercises of uninvolved joints.
Note if any tightness, weakness, or contractures are developing in uninvolved joints and muscles.
Take measures to correct or prevent further development of weakness, such as applying foot plate to prevent footdrop.

When indicated by the attending practitioner, the nurse may remove nonadhesive skin traction. In these cases intermittent traction is periodically released and reapplied as ordered. When skin traction must be constantly maintained, such as in fractures, nurses may occasionally remove and reapply the elastic bandage if this is approved by the attending practitioner, provided that *someone manually maintains the traction during the rewrapping process.* A child may have several types of traction at one time, and each traction must be assessed separately to avoid problems.

In addition to routine skin observation and care, the child in skeletal traction will need special skin care at the pin site according to hospital policy or practitioner preference. A pressure reduction device, such as a foam overlay or an alternating pressure mattress placed beneath the hips and back, reduces the chance of skin breakdown in these vulnerable areas.

When the child is first placed in traction, an increase in discomfort is common as a result of the traction pull fatiguing the muscle. It has been determined that orthopedic conditions are associated with a higher-than-average number of painful events and a higher percentage of bodily symptoms than other common conditions. Analgesics, including opioids, and muscle relaxants help during this phase of care and should be administered liberally.

Children are given an explanation at their level of understanding about what is happening and why they must remain in the device. Children are reassured that someone will be present to aid them in adjusting to the traction and in coping with the problems of immobilization.

The specific nursing responsibilities for the patient in traction are outlined in the Guidelines box.

Distraction

Unlike traction, which helps bones realign and fuse properly, distraction is the process of separating opposing bone to encourage regeneration of new bone in the created space. Distraction can also be used when limbs are of unequal lengths and new bone is needed to elongate the shorter limb.

External Fixation. The *Ilizarov external fixator (IEF)* is the most common external fixation device. The IEF uses a system of wires, rings, and telescoping rods that permits limb lengthening to occur by manual distraction. In addition to lengthening bones, the device can be used to correct angular or rotational defects or to immobilize fractures. The device is attached surgically by securing a series of external full or half rings to the bone with wires. External telescoping rods connect the rings to each other. Manual distraction is accomplished by manipulating the rods to increase the distance between the rings. A percutaneous ostomy is performed when the device is applied to create a "false" growth plate. A special osteotomy or corticotomy involves cutting only the cortex of the bone while preserving its blood supply, bone marrow, endosteum, and periosteum. Capillary blood flow to the transected area is essential for proper bone growth. Cut bone ends typically grow at a rate of 1 cm/month. The IEF can result in up to a 15-cm gain in length (Carlino, 1991).

Nursing Care Management. Success of the IEF depends on the child's and family's cooperation; therefore, before surgery they must be fully informed of the appearance of the device, how it accomplishes bone growth, needed alterations in activities, and home and follow-up care. Children are involved in learning to adjust the device to accomplish distraction. Children, as well as parents, should be instructed in pin care, including observation for infection and loosening of the pins. Cleaning routines for the pin sites vary among practitioners but should not traumatize the skin.

Children who participate actively in their care report less discomfort. Because the device is external, the child and family need to be prepared for the reactions of others and assisted in camouflaging the device with appropriate apparel, such as wide-legged pants that close with self-adhering fasteners around the device (Fig. 54-11). Partial weight bearing is allowed, and the child needs to learn to walk with crutches. Alterations in activity include modifications at school and in physical education. Full weight bearing is not allowed until the distraction is completed and bone consolidation has occurred. Follow-up care is essential to maintaining appropriate distraction until the desired leg length is achieved. The device is removed surgically after the bone has consolidated, and the child may need to use crutches or have a cast for 4 to 6 weeks following removal.

Amputation

A child may be born with the congenital absence of a body part, have a traumatic loss of an extremity, or need a surgical amputation for a pathologic condition such as osteogenic sarcoma. With today's surgical technology and the quick thinking of bystanders who save a traumatically amputated body part, some children have had fingers and arms reattached with variable degrees of functional use regained. A severed part should be wrapped lightly in a clean cloth or gauze saturated with normal saline and sealed in a watertight plastic bag. One should avoid using ice, which might come in contact with the tissue and make implantation impossible. The bag should be labeled with the child's name, the date, and the time and taken to the hospital with the child.

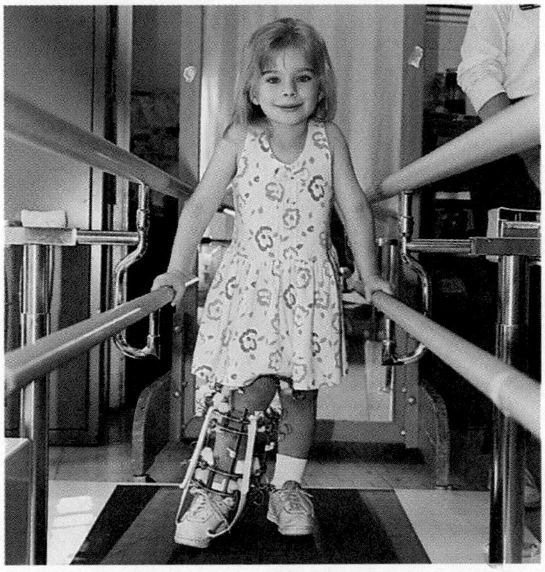

FIG. 54-11 • Children with the Ilizarov external fixator must cope with the visible nature of the device.

Surgical amputation or the surgical repair of a permanently severed limb focuses on constructing an adequately nourished stump. A smooth, healthy, padded stump, free of nerve endings, is important in prosthesis fitting and subsequent ambulation. In some situations in which there is no vascular or neurologic deficit, a cast is applied to the stump immediately after the procedure, and a pylon, metal extension, and artificial foot are attached so that the patient can walk on the temporary prosthesis within a few hours.

Nursing Care Management. Stump shaping is done postoperatively with special elastic bandaging using a figure-8 bandage, which applies pressure in a cone-shaped fashion. This technique decreases stump edema, controls hemorrhage, and aids in developing desired contours so that the child will bear weight on the posterior aspect of the skin flap rather than on the end of the stump. Stump elevation may be used during the first 24 hours, but after this time the extremity should not be left in this position because contractures will develop in the proximal joint and seriously hamper ambulation. Monitoring proper body alignment will further decrease the risk of flexion contractures.

For older children and adolescents, arm exercises and bed pushups (as well as parallel bars, which are used in prosthesis-training programs) help build up the arm muscles necessary for walking with crutches. Full range-of-motion exercises of joints above the amputation must be performed several times daily using active and isotonic exercises. Young children are spontaneously active and require little encouragement.

Depending on the age of the child, children or their parents will need to learn stump hygiene, including careful soap and water washing every day and checking for skin irritation, breakdown, or infection. A tube of stockinette or powder is used to slide the prosthesis on more easily. Skin must be checked carefully every time the prosthesis is removed, and prosthesis tolerance time must be adjusted to prevent skin breakdown.

For children who have had an amputation, *phantom limb sensation* is an expected experience because the nerve-brain connections are still present. Gradually these sensations fade, although in many amputees they persist for years. Preoperative discussion of this phenomenon will aid a child in understanding these "unusual feelings" and in not hiding the experiences from others. Limb pain, especially pain that increases with ambulation, should be evaluated for the possibility of a neuroma at the free nerve endings in the stump, or other problems such as a poorly fitting prosthesis or joint instability.

CONGENITAL DEFECTS

There are numerous skeletal defects that can be diagnosed at or shortly after birth. The alert nurse is commonly the person who detects the defect and refers the family for correction of the condition. The deviation is often difficult to detect without careful inspection. Therefore it is imperative that nurses become acquainted with signs of these defects and understand the principles of therapy in order to direct others in the care and management of these children.

Developmental Dysplasia of the Hip (DDH)

The broad term *developmental dysplasia of the hip* describes a group of disorders related to abnormal development of the hip. A change in terminology from congenital hip dysplasia (CHD) and congenital dislocation of the hip (CDH) to DDH more properly reflects a variety of hip abnormalities in which there is a shallow acetabulum, subluxation, or dislocation.

The incidence of hip instability of some kind is approximately 10 per 1000 live births. The incidence of frank dislocation or a dislocatable hip is 1 per 1000. The left hip is involved in 60% of cases, the right hip in 20%, and both hips in 20%. Sixty percent of the patients are girls. Caucasian children have a higher incidence of DDH than other groups (Maher, Salmond, and Pellino, 1998).

Pathophysiology. Three degrees of DDH can be identified (Fig. 54-12):

Acetabular dysplasia (or preluxation)—The mildest form, in which there is neither subluxation nor dislocation. The dysplasia reflects an apparent delay in acetabular development evidenced by osseous hypoplasia of the acetabular roof that is oblique and shallow, although the cartilaginous roof is comparatively intact. The femoral head remains in the acetabulum.

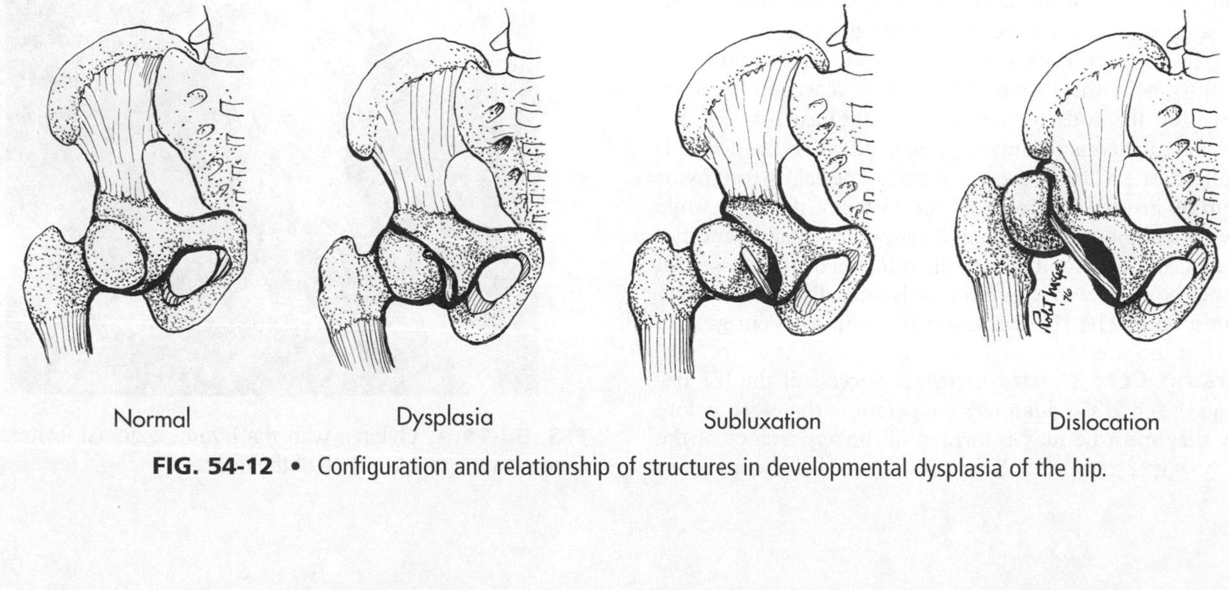

FIG. 54-12 • Configuration and relationship of structures in developmental dysplasia of the hip.

Subluxation—Accounts for the largest percentage of congenital hip dysplasias. Subluxation implies incomplete dislocation of the hip and is sometimes regarded as an intermediate state in the development from primary dysplasia to complete dislocation. The femoral head remains in contact with the acetabulum, but a stretched capsule and ligamentum teres cause the head of the femur to be partially displaced. Pressure on the cartilaginous roof inhibits ossification and produces a flattening of the socket.

Dislocation—In which the femoral head loses contact with the acetabulum and is displaced posteriorly and superiorly over the fibrocartilaginous rim. The ligamentum teres is elongated and taut.

Prenatal factors that influence development of hip abnormalities are maternal hormone secretion and mechanical factors of intrauterine posture. The maternal hormone secretion, principally of estrogen, that produces laxity of the maternal pelvis toward the end of gestation affects the fetal joints as well. Reliable evidence indicates an association between a higher incidence of developmental hip deformities with breech presentations and cesarean section (often necessitated by abnormal intrauterine position). Legs in frank breech position (i.e., with the hips acutely flexed and knees extended) is an important factor. Other prenatal factors that contribute to hip dysplasia include twinning and large infant size. Factors related to infant handling are indicated in the Cultural Considerations box.

Diagnostic Evaluation. The diagnosis of DDH should be made in the newborn period if possible because treatment initiated before 2 months of age is most successful (Box 54-4). In the newborn period dysplasia usually appears as hip joint laxity rather than as outright dislocation (Fig. 54-13). Subluxation and the tendency to dislocate can be demonstrated by the Ortolani or Barlow tests (Fig. 54-13, *B, C,* and *D*). There are cases in which dislocation is not diagnosed by these standard tests, and the disorder may not be apparent at birth. Therefore it is recommended that hip examination be included as part of health supervision until the child begins to walk and the gait is obviously normal.

Radiographic examination in early infancy is not reliable because the bones are largely cartilaginous and difficult to visualize; however, the cartilaginous head can be visualized directly with real-time high-resolution ultrasonography. In infants over the age of 4 months and in children, radiographic examination is useful in confirming the diagnosis. An upward slope in the roof of the acetabulum (the acetabular angle) greater than 40 degrees with upward and outward displacement of the femoral head is a common finding in older children.

Cultural Considerations

DEVELOPMENTAL DYSPLASIA OF THE HIP

A striking relationship exists between the development of the dislocation and methods of handling infants. Among the cultures with the highest incidence of dislocation, newly born infants are tightly wrapped in blankets or other swaddling material or are strapped to cradle boards. In cultures such as the Far East, where mothers traditionally carry infants on their backs or hips in the widely abducted straddle position, the disorder is virtually unknown.

Therapeutic Management. Treatment is begun as soon as the condition is recognized because early intervention is more favorable to the restoration of normal bony architecture and function. The longer treatment is delayed, the more severe the deformity, the more difficult the treatment, and the less favorable the prognosis. The treatment varies with the age of the child and the extent of the dysplasia.

Newborn to Age 6 Months. The hip joint is maintained by splinting with the proximal femur centered in the acetabulum in an attitude of flexion. Of the numerous devices available, the *Pavlik harness* is the most widely used, and with time, motion, and gravity the hip works into a more abducted, reduced position (Fig. 54-14). The harness is worn continuously until the hip is clinically and radiographically stable, usually in about 3 to 6 months.

When adduction contracture is present, other devices such as skin traction are used to slowly and gently stretch the hip to full abduction, after which wide abduction is maintained until stability is attained. When there is difficulty in maintaining stable reduction, a hip spica cast is applied and changed periodically to accommodate the child's growth. After 3 to 6 months, sufficient stability is acquired to allow transfer to a removeable protective abduction brace. The duration of treatment depends on development of the acetabulum but is usually accomplished within the first year.

Ages 6 to 18 Months. In this age group the dislocation is not recognized until the child begins to stand and walk, when attendant shortening of the limb and contractures of hip adductor and flexor muscles become apparent. Gradual reduction by traction is followed by cast immobilization, which is maintained until radiographic examination confirms a stable joint.

Box 54-4

Clinical Manifestations of Developmental Dysplasia of the Hip

INFANT

Shortening of limb on affected side (Galleazzi sign, Allis sign)
Restricted abduction of hip on affected side
Unequal gluteal folds (infant prone)
Positive Ortolani test
Positive Barlow test

OLDER INFANT AND CHILD

Affected leg shorter than the other
Telescoping or piston mobility of joint
- Head of femur can be felt to move up and down in buttock when extended thigh is pushed first toward child's head and then pulled distally

Trendelenburg sign
- When child stands first on one foot and then on the other (holding onto a chair, rail, or someone's hands) bearing weight on affected hip, pelvis tilts downward on normal side instead of upward, as it would with normal stability

Greater trochanter is prominent and appears above a line from anterior superior iliac spine to tuberosity of ischium
Marked lordosis (bilateral dislocations)
Waddling gait (bilateral dislocations)

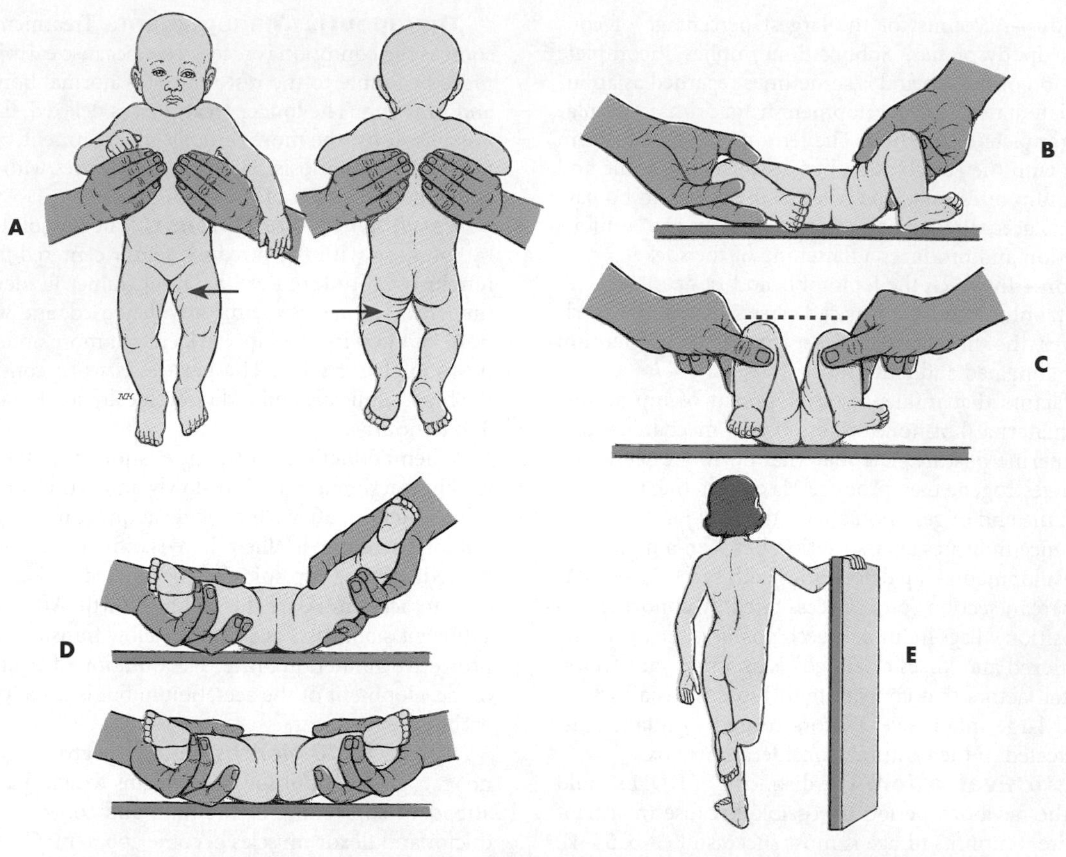

FIG. 54-13 • Signs of developmental dysplasia of the hip. **A,** Asymmetry of gluteal and thigh folds. **B,** Limited hip abduction, as seen in flexion. **C,** Apparent shortening of the femur, as indicated by the level of the knees in flexion. **D,** Ortolani click (if infant is under 4 weeks of age). **E,** Positive Trendelenburg sign or gait (if child is weight bearing).

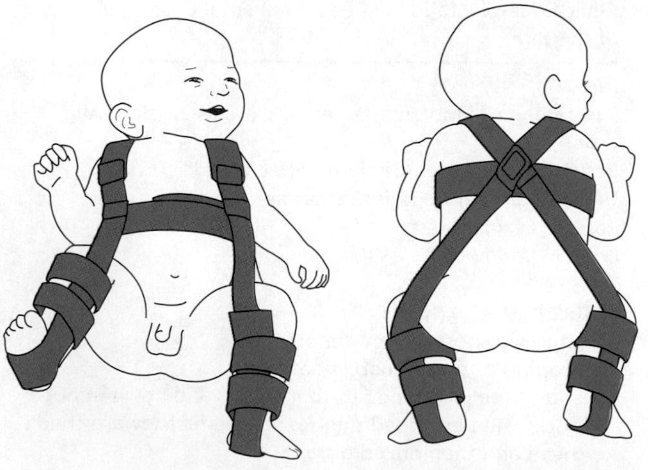

FIG. 54-14 • Child in Pavlik harness. (From Ball JW: *Mosby's pediatric patient teaching guides,* St Louis, 1998, Mosby.)

Often soft tissue may obstruct and complicate reduction and subsequent joint development. In this case open reduction is performed to remove the obstruction, followed by postoperative spica cast immobilization, and later replacement with an abduction splint.

Older Child. Correction of the hip deformity in older children is inherently more difficult than in the preceding age groups because secondary adaptive changes complicate the condition. Operative reduction—which may involve preoperative traction, tenotomy of contracted muscles, and any one of several innominate osteotomy procedures designed to construct an acetabular roof—is usually required. After the cast is removed and before weight bearing is permitted, range-of-motion exercises help restore movement. Next, rehabilitative measures are instituted. Successful reduction and reconstruction become increasingly difficult after the age of 4 years and are usually impossible or inadvisable in children over 6 years of age because of severe shortening and contracture of muscles and deformity of the femoral and acetabular structures.

Nursing Care Management

➤ Assessment

Nurses are in a unique position to detect DDH in the newborn. During the infant assessment process and routine nurturing activities the hips and extremities are inspected for any deviations from normal. Usually only nurses specially trained in the technique are permitted to perform Ortolani and Barlow tests, but any nurse can be alert to other signs of DDH. These observations are reported to the attending practitioner, and the ambulatory child who displays a limp or an unusual gait should be referred for evaluation. This may indicate an orthopedic or neurologic problem. Nonambulatory children with cerebral palsy should also be assessed for evidence of dislocation.

➤ Nursing Diagnoses

Nursing diagnoses identified for the child with congenital hip dysplasia are:

Impaired physical mobility related to correction device
Risk for impaired skin integrity related to presence of correction device
Altered family processes related to care of a child in a corrective device

➤ Plan of Care and Implementation

The goals of care for the child in a mechanical device for correction of DDH are as follows:

1. Child will maintain correct position of hip in acetabulum.
2. Child will experience no complications related to wearing corrective device.
3. Family will adapt routine nurturing activities to accommodate corrective device.

NURSE ALERT • Observations during routine care such as diapering provide an excellent opportunity to observe the infant for limited movement and a wide perineum, which is an indication to assess for leg shortening, unequal gluteal folds, and limited abduction.

The major nursing problems in the care of an infant or child in a cast or other device are related to maintenance of the device and adaptation of nurturing activities to meet the needs of the infant or child. Generally, treatment and follow-up care of these children is carried out in a clinic, practitioner's office, or outpatient unit. Hospitalization may be necessary for cast application or brace fitting but seldom exceeds 24 to 48 hours. Longer hospitalization is required for open reduction.

The primary nursing goal is teaching parents to apply and maintain the reduction device. The Pavlik harness allows for easy handling of the infant and usually produces less apprehension in the parent than heavy braces and casts. It is important that parents understand the correct use of the appliance, which may or may not allow for its removal during bathing. When the infant has a harness that is not removed, a sponge bath is recommended, and the skin beneath the harness is assessed daily for irritation. Powders and lotions are not used because they tend to cake or "ball" underneath straps or clothing.

To prevent skin irritation from the straps, long socks and a shirt are worn under the device. Extensions on the shirt that snap at the crotch help keep the shirt in place. Unbuckling or removal of the harness is determined individually on the basis of the family's level of understanding and the degree of deformity in the hip. In general, parents should not adjust the harness without supervision. The child should be examined by the practitioner before any adjustment is attempted to make certain the hips are in correct placement before the harness is resecured.

Casts and orthotics devices (braces) offer more challenging nursing problems because they cannot be removed for routine care, although sometimes a brace may be removed for bathing. Care of an infant or small child with a cast requires nursing innovation to reduce irritation and to maintain cleanliness of both the child and the cast, particularly in the diaper area. (See p. 1553 for care of the child in a cast.)

It is important for nurses, parents, and other caregivers to understand that children in corrective devices need to be involved in all the activities of any child in the same age group. Toys are chosen that can be used in a prone position on the floor or in the seats devised for feeding and other activities. Confinement in a cast or appliance should not exclude children from family (or unit) activities. They can be held astride the lap for comfort and transported to areas of activity. The child may be allowed to walk in a cast or orthotic device. An adapted wheelchair, stroller, or scooter can offer mobility to the older infant or child.

➤ Evaluation

The effectiveness of nursing interventions is determined by continual assessment and evaluation of care based on the following observational guidelines and expected outcomes:

1. Inspect corrective device regularly.
2. Inspect child's skin and circulation regularly.
3. Observe family's behavior with child and interview them regarding identified problems and solutions.

Expected outcomes include the following:

1. Hip remains in desired position; corrective device is positioned properly.
2. Skin remains free of irritation; circulation is unimpaired.
3. Family adjusts nurturing activities to accommodate corrective device.

Congenital Clubfoot

The general term *clubfoot* is used to describe a common deformity in which the foot is twisted out of its normal shape or position. Any foot deformity involving the ankle is called *talipes,* derived from *talus,* meaning ankle; and *pes,* meaning foot. Deformities of the foot and ankle are described according to the position of the ankle and foot. The more common positions involve the following variations:

Talipes varus—An inversion or a bending inward
Talipes valgus—An eversion or bending outward
Talipes equinus—Plantar flexion in which the toes are lower than the heel
Talipes calcaneus—Dorsiflexion, in which the toes are higher than the heel

Most cases of clubfoot are a combination of these positions, and the most commonly occurring type of clubfoot (approximately 95%) is the composite deformity *talipes equinovarus (TEV),* in which the foot is pointed downward and inward in varying degrees of severity (Fig. 54-15). Unilateral clubfoot is somewhat more common than bilateral clubfoot and may occur as an isolated defect or in association with other disorders or syndromes, such as chromosomal aberrations, arthrogryposis (a generalized immobility of the joints), cerebral palsy, or spina bifida.

The incidence of clubfoot in the general population is 1 per 700 to 1 per 1000 live births, with boys affected twice as often as girls. The precise cause of clubfoot is unknown. Some authorities attribute the defect to abnormal positioning and restricted movement in utero, although the evidence is not conclusive. Other experts implicate arrested or abnormal embryonic development. Arrested development during this early stage tends to result in a rigid deformity, whereas mechanical pressures from intrauterine positioning are likely causes of more flexible deformities.

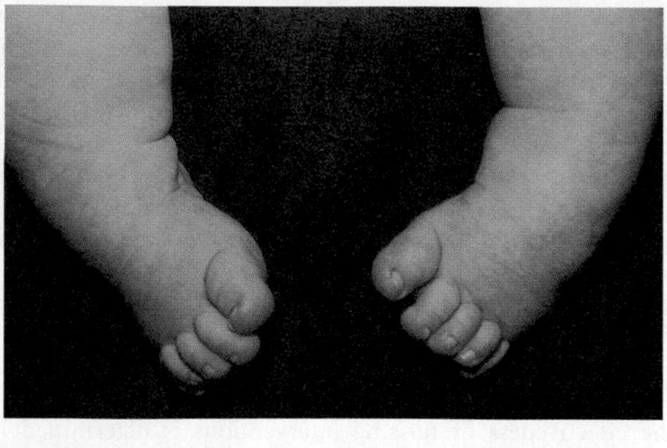

FIG. 54-15 • Bilateral congenital talipes equinovarus (congenital clubfoot) in 2-month-old infant. (From Zitelli BJ, Davis HW: *Atlas of pediatric physical diagnosis,* ed 3, St Louis, 1997, Mosby.)

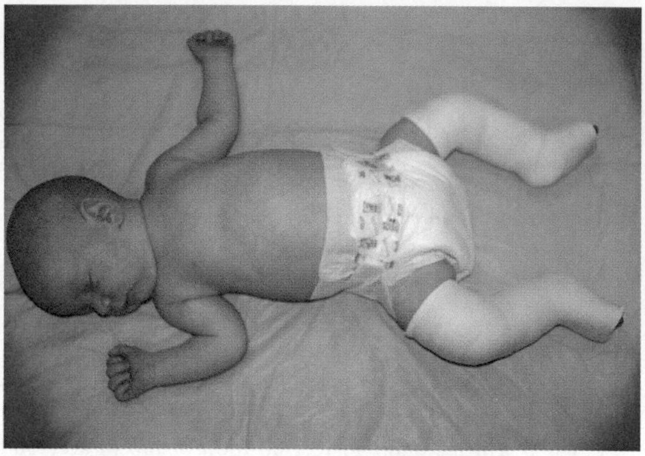

FIG. 54-16 • Feet casted for correction of bilateral congenital talipes equinovarus.

Classification. Medical literature describes three major categories of clubfoot: mild, tetralogic, and idiopathic. The mild, or postural, clubfoot may correct spontaneously or may require passive exercise or serial casting. There is no bony abnormality, but there may be tightness and shortening of the soft tissues medially and posteriorly. The tetralogic clubfoot is associated with other congenital anomalies such as myelodysplasia or arthrogryposis. These feet usually require surgical correction and have a high incidence of recurrence. The congenital idiopathic clubfoot, or "true clubfoot," almost always requires surgical intervention because there is bony abnormality.

Diagnostic Evaluation. The deformity is readily apparent and easily detected prenatally through ultrasonography or at birth. However, it must be differentiated from some positional deformities that can be passively corrected or overcorrected. The true clubfoot is fixed. Paralytic changes in the lower extremity of children with neuromuscular involvement often produce equinovarus deformity.

Therapeutic Management. Treatment of clubfoot involves three stages: (1) correction of the deformity, (2) maintenance of the correction until normal muscle balance is regained, and (3) follow-up observation to avert possible recurrence of the deformity. Some feet respond to treatment readily; some respond only to prolonged, vigorous, and sustained efforts; and the improvement in others remains disappointing even with maximum effort on the part of all concerned.

Serial casting is begun immediately or shortly after birth. Successive casts allow for gradual stretching of skin and tight structures on the medial side of the foot (Fig. 54-16). Manipulation and casting are repeated often (i.e., every few days for 1 to 2 weeks, then at 1- to 2-week intervals) to accommodate the rapid growth of early infancy. The extremity or extremities are casted until maximum correction is achieved, usually within 8 to 12 weeks. A radiograph is then taken to see the relationship of the bones to each other. Failure to achieve normal alignment indicates the need for surgical intervention. The optimum age for surgery is generally acknowledged to be between 4 months and 1 year.

Nursing Care Management. Nursing care of the child with clubfoot is the same as for any child who has a cast (see p. 1553). Because the child will spend considerable time in a corrective device, nursing care plans include both long-term and short-term goals. Conscientious observation of the skin and circulation is particularly important in young infants because of their normally rapid growth rate. Because treatment and follow-up care are handled in the orthopedist's office, clinic, or outpatient department, parent education and support are important in nursing care of these children.

Parents need to understand the overall treatment program, the importance of regular cast changes, and the role they play in the long-term effectiveness of the therapy. Reinforcing and clarifying the orthopedist's explanations and instructions, teaching parents about care of the cast or appliance (including vigilant observation for potential problems), and encouraging parents to facilitate normal development within the limitations imposed by the deformity or therapy are all part of nursing responsibilities.

Metatarsus Adductus (Varus)

Metatarsus adductus, or metatarsus varus, is probably the most common congenital foot deformity. In most instances it is a result of abnormal intrauterine positioning and is usually detected at birth. The deformity is characterized by medial adduction of the toes and forefoot, commonly in association with inversion, and by convexity of the lateral border of the foot. Unlike TEV, with which it is often confused, the angulation occurs at the tarsometatarsal joint, whereas the heel and ankle remain in a neutral position. This deformity often causes a pigeon-toed gait in the child.

Management depends on the rigidity of the deformity. Correction can usually be accomplished by gentle manipulation and passive stretching of the foot, which the parent is taught to perform. Repeated and consistent stretching is continued for the first 6 weeks, after which the treatment is based on the flexibility of the foot. Those feet that do not respond to the manipulation require orthopedic therapy. If the child is able to actively overcorrect the deformity voluntarily on stimulation, continued stretching is generally sufficient. If the foot cannot be actively or passively overcorrected, the feet are stretched and manipulated and held with casts and/or orthoses.

Nursing Care Management. The nursing role primarily involves identifying the defect so that early therapy and instruction of the parents can be initiated. The nurse teaches the parents how to hold the heel firmly and to stretch only the forefoot; otherwise, undue force on the heel may produce a valgus deformity. If casting is needed, the nurse instructs the parents in cast care and observation (see p. 1553).

Skeletal Limb Deficiency

Congenital limb deficiencies, or reduction malformations, are manifested by a variety of degrees of loss of functional capacity. They are characterized by underdevelopment of skeletal elements of the extremities. The range of malformation can extend from minor defects of the digits to serious abnormalities such as *amelia,* absence of an entire extremity; or *meromelia,* partial absence of an extremity that includes *phocomelia* (seal limbs), interposed deficiency of long bones with relatively good development of hands and feet attached at or near the shoulder or the hips. Most reduction defects are primary defects of development of the limb, but prenatal destruction of the limb can occur, such as the amputation of a limb in utero from constriction of an amniotic band.

Pathophysiology. Limb deficiencies can be attributed to both hereditary and environment and can originate at any stage of limb development. Formation of limbs may be suppressed at the time of limb bud formation, or there may be interference in later stages of differentiation and growth. Heredity appears to play a prominent role, and prenatal environmental insults have been implicated in a number of cases. The latter includes the well-publicized thalidomide tragedy of the 1950s and early 1960s, which demonstrated a clear relationship between the time of exposure of the pregnant woman to the antiemetic drug and the presence and type of limb deformity in the newborn.

Therapeutic Management. Children with congenital limb deficiencies should be fitted with prosthetic devices whenever possible, and the devices should be applied at the earliest possible stage of development in an attempt to match the motor readiness of the infant. This favors natural progression of prosthetic use. For example, a young infant with an upper extremity deficiency is fitted with a simple passive device, such as a mitten prosthesis, to encourage limb exploration, sitting (with the extremities needed for support), and bilateral hand activities.

Lower limb prostheses are applied when the infant is ready to pull to a standing position. In preparation for prosthetic devices, surgical modification is often necessary to ensure the most favorable use of the device because severe deformity can interfere with its effective use. Phocomelic digits are preserved for controlling switches of externally powered appliances in upper extremities. Digits (in both upper and lower extremities) provide the child with surfaces for tactile exploration and stimulation. Prostheses are replaced to accommodate growth and increasing capabilities of the child.

Nursing Care Management. Prosthetic application training and habilitation are most successfully carried out in a center that specializes in meeting the special needs of these children, especially very young children and those with multiple amputations. It involves a team of health professionals and the parents, who must encourage the child in making age-commensurate adjustments to the environment. Although these children need assistance, excessive overprotection may produce overdependency, with later maladjustment to school and other situations.

Box 54-5

Classification of Osteogenesis Imperfecta

Type		Characteristics
I*	A	Mild bone fragility; blue sclerae; normal teeth, presenile deafness (occurs between ages 20 and 30 years); autosomal-dominant inheritance
	B	Same as A except dentinogenesis imperfecta instead of normal teeth
	C	Same as B; no bone fragility
II		Lethal; stillborn or die in early infancy; severe bone fragility, multiple fractures at birth; 10% of cases of osteogenesis imperfecta (OI), autosomal recessive inheritance
III		Severe bone fragility leads to severe progressive deformities; normal sclerae; marked growth failure; most autosomal-recessive inheritance; few autosomal-dominant inheritance
IV	A	Mild to moderate bone fragility; normal sclerae; short stature; variable deformity; autosomal-dominant inheritance
	B	Same as A except dentinogenesis imperfecta instead of normal teeth, approximately 6% of cases of OI

*Two thirds of cases are type I.

Osteogenesis Imperfecta (OI)

OI refers to a group of heterogeneous inherited disorders of connective tissue characterized by excessive fragility of and resultant bone defects. The inheritance pattern is autosomal dominant in the majority of cases, although the most severe form demonstrates autosomal-recessive inheritance (Box 54-5).

Genetic mutation is the cause of OI, and occurs in one of two ways: either by decreased synthesis of normal type I procollagen; or by structural aberrations of type I procollagen (Bender, 1991).

At present, OI is believed to consist of four different types (see Box 54-5). Type II, the most severe form of OI, is characterized by multiple intrauterine or perinatal fractures resulting in severe deformity and, commonly, early death. The brittle bones easily fracture from the slightest trauma. OI types I, III, and IV run a milder course. The tendency to fracture may appear later in childhood and disappear after puberty.

During childhood the shafts of long bones are slender, with reduced cortical thickness resulting from defective periosteal bone formation. In addition to the features already described, the child with OI has thin skin, hyperextensibility of ligaments, a tendency toward recurrent epistaxis, excess diaphoresis, a tendency to bruise easily, and mild hyperpyrexia. The disease shows variable expressivity; that is, the number and extent of pathologic features appear in any individual range, from severe to minimal involvement. The incidence of fractures decreases at puberty, when the body's production of hormones helps strengthen bones.

Therapeutic Management. The treatment is primarily supportive. Several drugs have been tried but appear to be of limited benefit. Lightweight braces and splints help support limbs, prevent fractures, and aid in ambulation. Physical therapy helps prevent disuse osteoporosis and strengthens muscles, which in turn improves bone density.

Surgical techniques are used to correct deformities that interfere with bracing, standing, or walking. For the child with recurrent fractures, inserting an intermedullary rod provides stability to bones. Two types of rods are used. Telescoping rods will not need to be replaced but have complications such as failure to expand, bending from falls, and penetration of the ends of the bones. Nontelescoping rods are safer but have to be replaced as the child grows; otherwise, fractures may occur through the unprotected portion of the bone.

Nursing Care Management. Infants and children with this disorder require careful handling to prevent fractures. They must be supported when they are being turned, positioned, moved, and fondled. Even changing a diaper may cause a fracture in severely affected infants. These children should never be held by the ankles when being diapered but should be gently lifted by the buttocks or supported with pillows.

Both parents and the affected child need education regarding the child's limitations and guidelines in planning suitable activities that promote optimum development while protecting the child from harm. Realistic occupational planning and genetic counseling are part of the long-term goals of care. Educational materials and information can be obtained from the Osteogenesis Imperfecta Foundation, Inc,* which also has a network that can put a family in contact with other families with a similar problem.

OI is a differential diagnosis that must be ruled out in the event of multiple fractures that may be attributed to nonaccidental injury. A detailed history, no evidence of associated soft tissue injury, and the presence of other symptoms related to OI help to determine the diagnosis.

NURSE ALERT • Children with OI have an increased risk of dehydration from excessive loss of fluid through the skin. During surgery and the perioperative period there is also potential for hyperthermia and diuresis. Careful monitoring of temperature and hydration is critical.

ACQUIRED DEFECTS

Legg-Calvé-Perthes Disease

Legg-Calvé-Perthes disease is a self-limited juvenile idiopathic avascular necrosis of the femoral head. The disease affects children ages 3 to 12 but most commonly boys between 4 and 8 years of age. Bilateral hip involvement is present in 10% to 15% of cases; most of the affected children have delayed bone age. Recurrent disease is rare (Martinez and Weinstein, 1991).

Pathophysiology. The cause of the disease is unknown, but there is a disturbance of circulation to the femoral capital epiphysis that produces an ischemic aseptic necrosis of the femoral head. During middle childhood, circulation to the femoral epiphysis is more tenuous than at other ages and can become obstructed by trauma, inflammation, coagulation defects, and a variety of other causes (Burg et al, 1995). The pathologic events seem to take place in four stages (Box 54-6). The entire process may encompass as little as 18 months or continue for several years. The reformed femoral head may be severely altered or appear entirely normal.

Clinical Manifestations and Diagnostic Evaluation. The onset is insidious, and the history may reveal only intermittent appearance of a limp on the affected side or a symptom complex including hip soreness, ache, or stiffness that can be constant or intermittent. The pain may be experienced in the hip, along the entire thigh, or in the vicinity of the knee joint. The pain and limp are usually most evident on arising and at the end of a long day of activities. The pain is usually accompanied by joint dysfunction and limited range of motion. There may be a vague history of trauma. The diagnosis is established by radiographic examination.

Therapeutic Management. Because deformity occurs early in the disease process, the aim of treatment is to keep the head of the femur contained in the acetabulum, which serves as a mold to preserve the spherical shape of the head and to maintain a full range of motion. However, there is no agreement regarding the best treatment in terms of conservative vs. surgical approaches (Poussa et al, 1993). Often, treatment approaches vary with the severity of presentation (Rang, 1996). Activity causes microfractures of the soft, ischemic epiphysis, which tend to induce synovitis, stiffness, and adductor contractures (Burg et al, 1995). The initial therapy is rest and non-weight bearing, which helps to reduce inflammation and restore motion. Later, active motion is encouraged. In some cases traction is applied to stretch tight adductor muscles.

Containment can be accomplished in several ways. One method is the use of nonweight-bearing devices (e.g., an abduction brace, leg casts, or a leather harness sling) that prevent weight bearing on the affected limb. Another method includes the use of various weight-bearing appliances, such as abduction-ambulation braces or casts after a period of bed rest and traction. A third method consists of surgical reconstruction and containment procedures. Conservative therapy must be continued for 2 to 4 years, although braces constructed from lightweight materials allow the child to maintain a nearly normal ac-

Box 54-6

Stages of Legg-Calvé-Perthes Disease

Stage I: Aseptic necrosis or infarction of the femoral capital epiphysis with degenerative changes producing flattening of the upper surface of the femoral head—the **avascular stage**

Stage II: Capital bone absorption and revascularization with fragmentation (vascular resorption of the epiphysis) that gives a mottled appearance on radiographs—the **fragmentation,** or **revascularization, stage**

Stage III: New bone formation, which is represented on radiographs as calcification and ossification or increased density in the areas of radiolucency; this filling-in process appears to take place from the periphery of the head centrally—the **reparative stage**

Stage IV: Gradual reformation of the head of the femur without radiolucency and, it is hoped, to a spherical form—the **regenerative stage**

*804 W. Diamond Ave., Suite 210, Gaithersburg, MD 20878; 1-800-981-2663; e-mail: bonelink@oif.org.

tivity level. Surgical correction, although subjecting the child to additional risks (e.g., from anesthesia, infection, and blood transfusion), returns the child to normal activities in 3 to 4 months. The use of home traction has been explored (Stevens et al, 1995).

Prognosis. The disease is self-limited, but the ultimate outcome of therapy depends on early and efficient treatment and the age of the child at onset of the disorder. Younger children, whose epiphyses are more cartilaginous, have the best prognosis for complete recovery. The later the diagnosis is made, the more femoral damage has occurred before treatment is implemented. In most cases, with good patient compliance, the prognosis is excellent.

Nursing Care Management. Nurses are often the first health professionals to identify affected children and to refer them for medical evaluation. They are also persons on whom the child and the family can rely to help them understand and adjust to the therapeutic measures. Because most of the child's care is conducted on an outpatient basis, the major emphasis of nursing care is teaching the family the care and management of the corrective appliance selected for therapy. The family needs to learn the purpose, function, application, and care of the corrective device and the importance of compliance in order to achieve the desired outcome.

One of the most difficult aspects associated with the disorder is coping with a normally active child who feels well but who must remain relatively inactive. Suitable activities must be devised to meet the needs of the child in the process of developing a sense of initiative or industry. Activities that meet the creative urges are well received. This is also an opportune time to encourage the child to begin a hobby such as starting a collection, model building, or crafts.

Slipped Femoral Capital Epiphysis (SFCE)

SFCE refers to the slipping of the proximal femoral epiphysis in a posterior and inferior direction. It is the most common hip disorder in adolescence and occurs during the growth spurt. The average age of affected girls is 12 years, and the average age of boys is 13.5 years. Bilateral involvement occurs in up to 40% of cases (Loder, 1998).

Pathophysiology. Most cases of SFCE are idiopathic, although it can be associated with endocrine disorders, growth hormone therapy, renal osteodystrophy, and radiation therapy. The cause of idiopathic SFCE is multifactorial and includes obesity, physeal architecture and orientation, and puberty hormone changes that affect physeal strength. Although obesity stresses the physeal plate, SFCE can also occur in children who are not obese (Loder, 1998). Radiographs show medial displacement of the epiphysis and uncovered upper portion of the femoral neck adjacent to the physis. There is a widened growth plate and irregular metaphysis. The capital femoral epiphysis remains in the acetabulum, but the femoral neck slips, deforming the femoral head and stretching blood vessels to the epiphysis.

Diagnostic Evaluation. The disorder is suspected when an adolescent or preadolescent youngster displays clinical signs or complains of pain (Box 54-7). The diagnosis is confirmed by radiographic examination.

Therapeutic Management. Treatment goals include avoiding avascular necrosis, avoiding chondrolysis, preventing further slip, and correcting the deformity (Aronsson and Loder, 1996). Surgical treatment varies with the degree of displacement; methods include presurgery bed rest/traction followed by a single pin, multiple pins and screws, and/or osteotomy for deformity correction if needed. Postsurgery care includes non-weight-bearing with crutch ambulation until acceptable, painless range of motion is achieved (Aronsson and Loder, 1996). SFCE is an emergency and requirements early diagnosis and treatment to increase the likelihood of a satisfactory cure.

Nursing Care Management. Nursing care is the same as that for a child in a cast or a child in traction, as discussed earlier in this chapter.

Kyphosis and Lordosis

The spine, consisting of numerous segments, can acquire deformity curves of three types: kyphosis, lordosis, and scoliosis (Fig. 54-17). *Kyphosis* is an abnormally increased convex angulation in the curvature of the thoracic spine (Fig. 54-17, *B*). It can occur secondary to disease processes such as tuberculosis, chronic arthritis, osteodystrophy; or to compression fractures of the thoracic spine. The most common form of kyphosis is "postural." Children, especially during the time when skeletal growth outpaces growth of muscle, are prone to exaggeration of a normal kyphosis. They assume abnormal sitting and standing positions. This is particularly common in self-conscious adolescent girls who assume a round-shouldered, slouching posture in an attempt to hide their developing breasts.

Postural kyphosis is almost always accompanied by a compensatory postural lordosis, an abnormally exaggerated concave lumbar curvature. Treatment consists of postural exercises to strengthen shoulder and abdominal muscles, and may include bracing for more marked deformity. Unfortunately, treatment is difficult; the normal rebellious tendencies of the adolescent, together with continual parental nagging to "stand up straight," often interfere with compliance to a therapeutic regimen. The best approach is to emphasize the cosmetic value of corrective therapy and to place the responsibility on the adolescent for carrying out an exercise program at home with regular visits to and assessments by a therapist. Most adolescents respond well to selected sports as a supplement to regular exercise. Boys prefer weight lifting (preferably performed from a prone or supine position on a bench) and track sports. Girls respond well to dancing classes (ballet or modern dancing). Swimming is excellent and has the added advantages of exercising all muscles, eliminating much of the effects of gravity, and teaching breath

Box 54-7

Clinical Manifestations of Slipped Femoral Capital Epiphysis

- May be obese
- Limp on affected side
- Pain in hip
  - Continuous or intermittent
  - Frequently referred to groin, anteromedial aspect of thigh, or knee
- Restricted internal rotation on adduction with external rotation deformity
- Loss of abduction and internal rotation as severity increases
- Shortening of lower extremity

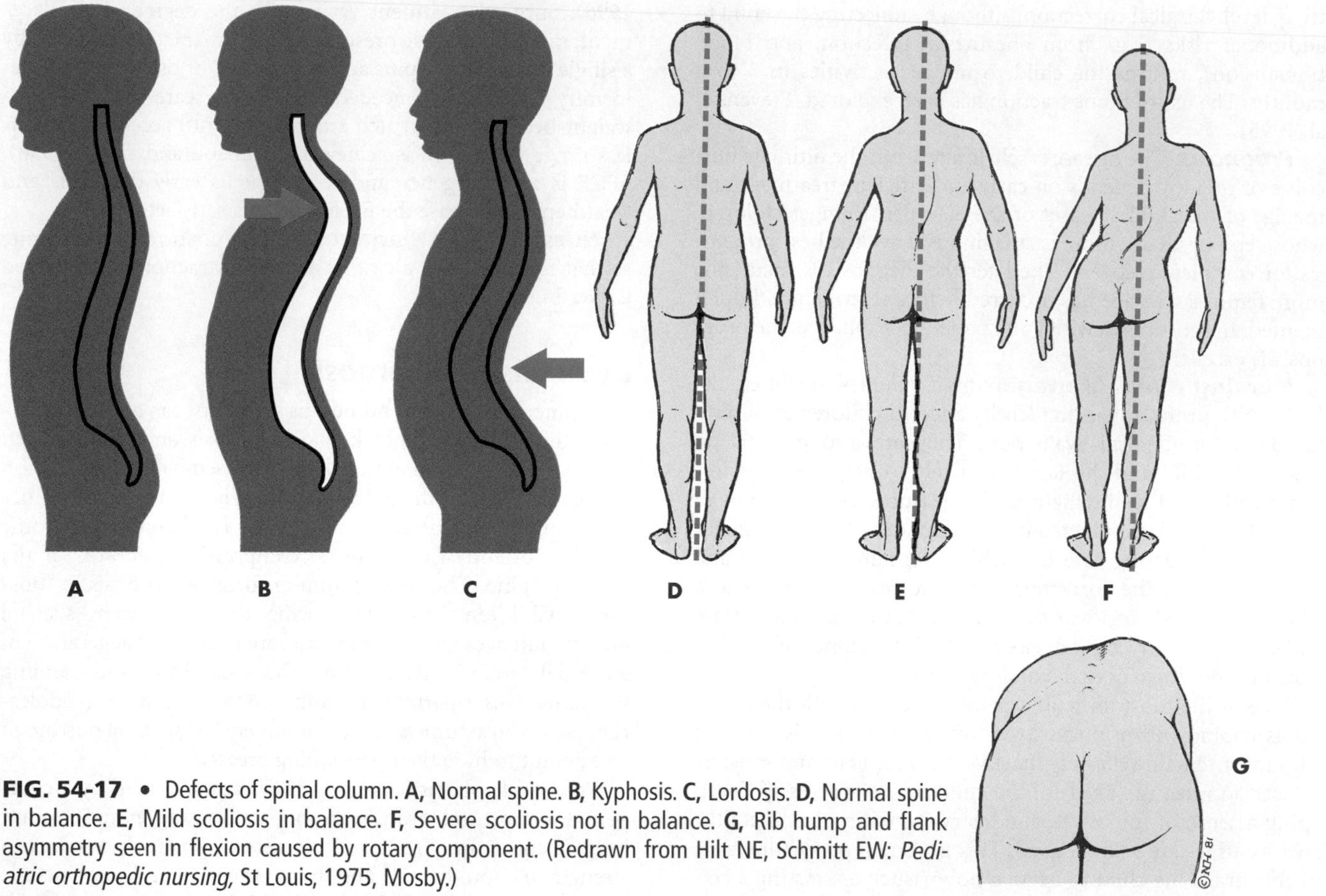

FIG. 54-17 • Defects of spinal column. **A,** Normal spine. **B,** Kyphosis. **C,** Lordosis. **D,** Normal spine in balance. **E,** Mild scoliosis in balance. **F,** Severe scoliosis not in balance. **G,** Rib hump and flank asymmetry seen in flexion caused by rotary component. (Redrawn from Hilt NE, Schmitt EW: *Pediatric orthopedic nursing,* St Louis, 1975, Mosby.)

control. Treatment with a brace may be indicated until skeletal maturity, and surgical fusion may be considered for severe, painful, or progressive kyphotic curves.

Lordosis is an accentuation of the cervical or lumbar curvature beyond physiologic limits (see Fig. 54-17, *C*). It may be a secondary complication of a disease process, a result of trauma, or idiopathic. It is often seen in association with flexion contractures of the hip, obesity, congenital dislocated hip, and slipped femoral capital epiphysis. During the pubertal growth spurt, lordosis of varying degrees is observed in teenagers, especially girls. In obese children the weight of the abdominal fat alters the center of gravity, causing a compensatory lordosis. Unlike kyphosis, severe lordosis is usually accompanied by pain.

Treatment involves management of the predisposing cause when possible, such as weight loss and correction of deformities. Postural exercises and/or support garments are helpful in relieving symptoms in some cases; however, these do not usually effect a permanent cure.

Scoliosis

Scoliosis is a complex spinal deformity in three planes, usually involving lateral curvature, spinal rotation causing rib asymmetry, and thoracic hypokyphosis. It is the most common spinal deformity. It can be congenital, or it can develop during infancy or childhood; but it is most common during the growth spurt of early adolescence. Scoliosis can be caused by a number of conditions and may occur alone or in association with other diseases, particularly neuromuscular conditions. In most cases, however, there is no apparent cause, and it is called idiopathic scoliosis. There is evidence that it may be genetic.

Idiopathic scoliosis is most noticeable during the preadolescent growth spurt. Parents commonly bring a child for follow-up on an abnormal school scoliosis screening or because of "ill-fitting" clothes, such as uneven hems. School screening remains controversial because there are no controlled studies to demonstrate improved outcomes (Screening, 1993).

Diagnostic Evaluation. Diagnosis is made by observation of standing radiographs, which establish the degree of curvature. Observation is performed behind an undressed, standing child, noting asymmetry of shoulder height, scapular or flank shape, or hip height. When the child bends forward at the waist with hanging arms, asymmetry of the ribs and flanks may be appreciated. Often a primary curve and a compensatory curve will place the head in alignment with the gluteal cleft. However, in the uncompensated curve the head and hips are not aligned (see Fig. 54-17, *E* and *F*). (See Spine, Chapter 35, for additional information.)

Therapeutic Management. A thorough assessment of the child, including history and examination, is carried out to evaluate the status of the deformity, factors contributing to the defect, and factors that may influence the outcome of therapy. Treatment is best carried out in a center in which a team is available that specializes in management of scoliosis. Current

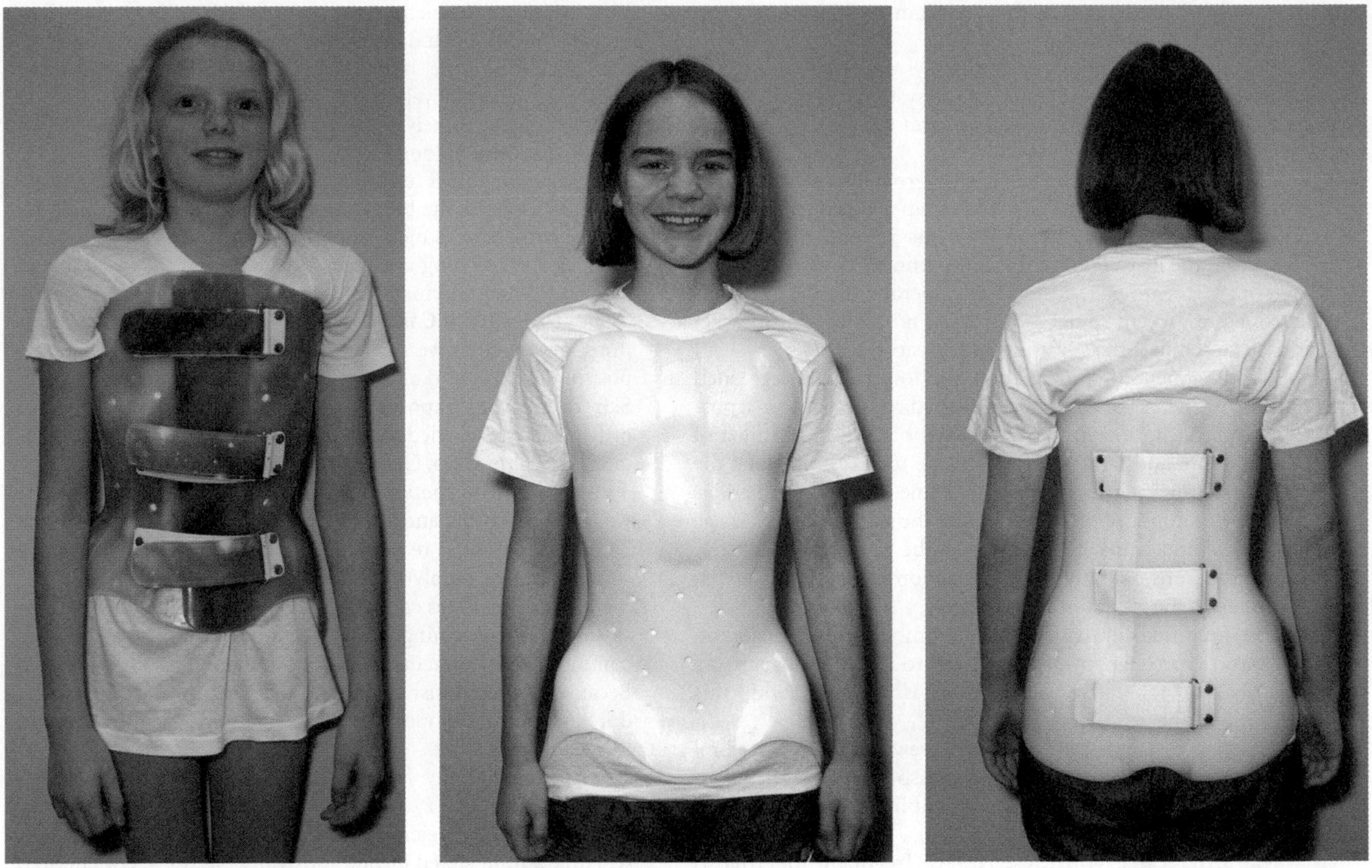

A B C

FIG. 54-18 • A, Standard TLSO brace for idiopathic scoliosis. Note the color and design incorporated into the brace to make it more acceptable to children and adolescents. **B,** Variation of a standard TLSO that fastens in the back, **C,** to provide needed support for the spine curvature.

management options include observation with regular clinical and radiographic evaluation, orthotic intervention (bracing), and surgical spinal fusion. Treatment decisions are based on the magnitude, location, and type of curve; the age and skeletal maturity of the child; and any underlying or contributing disease process.

Bracing and Exercise. For many curves in the growing child and adolescent, bracing may be the treatment of choice. It is important to realize that bracing is not curative, but that it may slow the progression of the curvature to allow skeletal growth and maturity. The two most common types of bracing are (1) the *Boston brace,* an underarm orthosis customized from prefabricated plastic shells, with corrective forces for each patient using lateral pads and decreasing lumbar lordosis; and (2) a *TLSO (thoracolumbosacral orthotic),* which is an underarm orthosis fabricated out of plastic that is custom molded to the body and then shaped to correct or hold the deformity (Fig. 54-18). The Milwaukee brace, which is an individually adapted brace that includes a neck ring, is rarely used in scoliosis but is sometimes used in the treatment of kyphosis.

External electrical stimulation of spinal muscles, transmitted by pads on the back during sleep, was not found to be an effective alternative to orthotic treatment (Weinstein, 1994). Exercises are of benefit when used in conjunction with bracing to maintain and strengthen spinal and abdominal muscles during treatment; but exercises alone are rarely of value in managing scoliosis.

Surgical Management. Surgical intervention may be required for correction of severe curves. The degree of curvature and its cause determine the decision for surgery. Bracing and exercise have been universally disappointing in curves greater than 40 degrees, and paralytic and congenital curves, which will eventually progress, are best treated with early surgical stabilization if the health status of the child will allow major surgery. The age of the child and location of the curvature influence the decision for surgery, and any progressive or severe curve that does not respond to more conservative orthotic measures requires surgical correction. Difficulties with balance or seating, respiratory excursion, and pain are also considered.

The surgical technique consists of realignment and straightening with internal fixation and instrumentation combined with bony fusion *(arthrodesis)* of the realigned spine. The goals of surgical intervention are to correct the curvatures on the sagittal and coronal planes and to have a solid, pain-free fusion in a well-balanced torso, with maximum mobility of the remaining spinal segments.

There are several instrumentation systems that are used to facilitate spinal fusion. Selection of the system is individualized according to the needs of the patient and the preference of the surgeon.

The Harrington system, the first internal spinal instrumentation device, consists of distraction and compression rods, hooks, and nuts. The posterior elements are decorticated, and bone from the iliac crest and/or donor bone is placed across the vertebrae to provide fusion. Postoperatively the child is logrolled to prevent spinal motion, and a molded plastic jacket is used to stabilize the spine until the fusion is solid.

L-rod segmental spinal instrumentation provides segmental stability by the use of wires and L-shaped rods. By way of a posterior approach, the wires are threaded beneath the lamina of each vertebra and tightened around the rods resting along the transverse processes to stabilize the spine. Bone from the iliac crest and/or donor bone is used to fuse the spine. The advantage of this method is that the patient can be mobile within a few days and no postoperative immobilization is required. The disadvantage is the risk of nerve damage.

The multihook instrumentation combines the Harrington and L-rod approaches by using bilateral rods and hooks at many sites. No postoperative stabilization is required with this method.

Anterior instrumentation using screws into the vertebral bodies connected by a cable or rod is also available. These systems provide better correction but require immobilization of the spine postoperatively.

Nursing Care Management. Treatment for scoliosis extends over a significant portion of the affected child's period of growth. In adolescents this period is the one in which their identity, physical and psychologic, is formed. The identification of scoliosis as a "deformity," in combination with unattractive appliances and a significant surgical procedure, can have a negative effect on the already-fragile adolescent body image (Noonan et al, 1997). Although these adolescents are encouraged to participate in most peer activities, necessary therapeutic modifications are likely to make them feel different and apart.

When a child first faces the prospect of a prolonged period in a brace, cast, or other device, the therapy program and the nature of the device must be explained thoroughly to both the child and the parents so that they will have an understanding of the anticipated results, how the appliance corrects the defect, the freedoms and constraints imposed by the device, and what they can do to help achieve the desired goal. The management involves the skills and services of a team of specialists, including the orthopedist, physical therapist, orthotist (a specialist in fitting orthopedic braces), nurse, social worker, and sometimes a pulmonary specialist.

It is difficult for a child to be restricted at any phase of development, but the teenager needs continual positive reinforcement, encouragement, and as much independence as can be safely assumed during this time. Adolescents appreciate guidance and assistance regarding anticipated problems, such as selection of clothing and participation in social activities. Socialization with peers is encouraged, and every effort is expended to help the adolescent feel attractive and worthwhile.

Preoperative Care. The preoperative workup usually involves a radiographic series, including bending and traction films; pulmonary function studies; arterial blood gases; and laboratory studies, including prothrombin and partial thromboplastin clotting time, blood count, electrolytes, urinalysis and urine culture, and levels of any medications. Autologous blood donations are routinely obtained from the youngster before the surgery to replace blood loss during the operation.

Surgery for spinal fusion is quite complex, and often adolescents who require the procedure because of idiopathic scoliosis are not familiar with medical terms, procedures, or experiences. Preoperative teaching is critical for the adolescent to be able to cooperate and participate in his or her treatment and recovery.

Postoperative Care. Following surgery, patients are monitored in an intensive care unit and logrolled when changing position to prevent damage to the fusion and instrumentation. Skin care is very important, and pressure-relieving mattresses or beds may be needed to prevent pressure wounds (see Maintaining Healthy Skin, Chapter 45).

In addition to the usual postoperative assessments (i.e., of wound, circulation, and vital signs), the neurologic status of the patient's extremities requires special attention. There is usually some degree of paralytic ileus following the procedure; therefore nursing includes care of the nasogastric intubation and assessment for returning bowel function. Urinary retention is common and often requires insertion of an indwelling catheter. Because of the extensive blood loss during the surgical procedure and renal hypoperfusion, observation of urine output is especially important.

The child usually has considerable pain for the first few days following surgery and requires frequent administration of pain medication, preferably opioids administered on a regular schedule administered intravenously or epidurally. For children able to understand the concept, patient-controlled analgesia (PCA) is a recommended alternative (see Pain Assessment; Pain Management, Chapter 44).

All patients are started on physiotherapy as soon as they are able, beginning with range-of-motion exercises and many of the activities of daily living. Self-care, such as washing and eating, is always encouraged. Some simple physical therapy may be begun during this acute stage. Throughout the hospitalization diversional activities and contact with family and friends are important parts of nursing care and planning.

The family is encouraged to become involved with the patient's care to facilitate the transition from hospital to home management. Family members learn to apply and care for the brace or learn cast care. An organization that provides education and services to both families and professionals is the National Scoliosis Foundation, Inc.* The Scoliosis Research Society,† an organization of physicians and scientists, has published an excellent book, *Scoliosis,* and has educational information available on its website.

(See also Nursing Care Plan: The Child with Structural Scoliosis.‡)

---

*5 Cabot Place, Stoughton, MA 02072; (617) 341-6333 or 1-800-673-6922; e-mail: scoliosis@aol.com.

†6300 N. River Rd., Suite 727, Rosemont, IL 60018-4226; (847) 698-1627; fax (847) 823-0536; website: www.srs.org.

‡In Wong DL, Hess CS: ***Wong and Whaley's clinical manual of pediatric nursing,*** ed 5, St Louis, 2000, Mosby.

INFECTIONS OF BONES AND JOINTS

Osteomyelitis

Osteomyelitis is an infectious process of bone that can occur at any age but that occurs most commonly between 5 and 14 years of age. It is twice as common in boys as in girls.

Pathophysiology. Osteomyelitis can be acquired from exogenous or hematogenous sources. *Exogenous osteomyelitis* is acquired by invasion of the bone by direct extension from the outside as a result of a penetrating wound, open fracture, contamination during surgery, or secondary extension from an overlying abscess or burn. *Hematogenous osteomyelitis* occurs from spread of organisms from preexisting infectious foci, including furuncles, skin abrasions, impetigo, upper respiratory tract infections, acute otitis media, tonsillitis, abscessed teeth, pyelonephritis, or infected burns.

Any organism can cause osteomyelitis, and there is some relationship between the age of the child and the type of organism responsible. *Staphylococcus aureus* is the most common organism in children more than 5 years of age. *Haemophilus influenzae* predominates in the younger child. In children with sickle cell anemia, *Salmonella* organisms are commonly the responsible agents. Other factors that predispose to development of osteomyelitis are poor physical condition, inadequate nutrition, and surroundings that are not hygienic.

Infective emboli from the focus of infection travel to the small end arteries in the bone metaphysis, where they set up an infectious process that leads to local bone destruction and abscess formation.

Diagnostic Evaluation. The signs and symptoms of *acute hematogenous osteomyelitis* begin abruptly and build up to a maximum intensity during the first few days of the disease, usually less than 1 week (Box 54-8). Symptoms often resemble those observed in other disorders involving bones (e.g., leukemia and arthritis). There is marked leukocytosis and an elevated erythrocyte sedimentation rate. Blood cultures may be positive, but patients already receiving antibiotics are likely to have negative cultures. Bone cultures from biopsy or aspirate may yield positive cultures in patients with negative blood cultures. Early plain radiographs are often normal. Technetium-labeled bone scans are more sensitive in early disease (Karwowska et al, 1998).

Box 54-8

Clinical Manefestations of Acute Osteomyelitis

GENERAL MANIFESTATIONS

History of trauma to affected bone (frequent)
Child appears very ill
Irritability
Restlessness
Elevated temperature
Rapid pulse
Dehydration

LOCAL MANIFESTATIONS

Tenderness
Increased warmth
Diffuse swelling over involved bone
Involved extremity painful, especially on movement
Involved extremity held in semiflexion
Surrounding muscles tense and resist passive movement

Most cases involve the femur or tibia, and to a lesser extent, the humerus and hip. In infants the diagnosis is more difficult because of a lack of systemic symptoms, and the disease may involve multiple bones or joints because of the difficulty in confining an infectious process in children in this age group.

In *subacute hematogenous osteomyelitis,* symptoms have been present for a longer period of time, and the child sometimes has been treated with antibiotics, often for another infection, which modifies the clinical symptoms. In some instances the infection may produce a walled-off abscess rather than a spreading infection.

Therapeutic Management. As soon as blood cultures have been drawn, prompt and vigorous IV antibiotic therapy is initiated. The choice of antibiotic is influenced by age, and the dosage determined is sufficient to ensure high blood and tissue levels. The appropriate antibiotic is usually continued for at least 3 to 4 weeks, but the length of therapy is determined by the duration of symptoms, the initial response to treatment, and the sensitivity of the specific organism. In select cases oral antibiotics may follow a shorter intensive IV course with good results (Karwowska et al, 1998). Because of prolonged high-dose therapy, it is important to monitor hematologic, renal, hepatic, and other organ systems that might be adversely affected by the drugs (e.g., those that are ototoxic).

Antibiotic therapy is accompanied by local treatment. The child is placed on complete bed rest. Immobilization of the affected extremity, which may require a splint or bivalved cast, is continued throughout therapy to limit the spread of infection and, when it is a complication of a fracture, to maintain alignment of bone fragments.

Opinions differ regarding surgical intervention, but many advocate sequestrectomy (removal of dead bone) and surgical drainage to prevent abscess formation. When surgical drainage is carried out, polyethylene tubes are placed in the wound—one tube instills an antibiotic solution directly into the infected area by gravity; the other, connected to a suction apparatus, provides drainage.

Nursing Care Management. During the acute phase of illness any movement of the affected limb will cause discomfort; therefore the child is positioned comfortably with the affected limb supported. Moving and turning are carried out carefully and gently to minimize pain. Pain medication is administered to provide comfort. Vital signs are taken and recorded frequently, and measures are implemented to reduce a significant temperature elevation.

Antibiotic therapy requires careful observation and monitoring of the IV equipment and site. Because more than one antibiotic is usually administered, the compatibility of the drugs is determined and care is taken to avoid mixing noncompatible drugs. For long-term antibiotic therapy, an intermittent infusion device or peripherally inserted central catheter (PICC) is used (see Peripheral Venous Access Devices, Chapter 45). Antibiotic therapy is often continued at home.*

The child with an open wound may be placed on contact isolation. The wound is managed as prescribed. Antibiotic solution administered directly into the wound is most efficiently accom-

*Community and home care instructions on caring for an intermittent infusion device or a central venous catheter are available in Wong DL, Hess CS: ***Wong and Whaley's clinical manual of pediatric nursing,*** ed 5, St Louis, 2000, Mosby.

plished with a regular IV infusion setup that is prepared and regulated in the same manner as any other. The drainage tubes are connected to low Gomco or wall suction for continuous removal. Intake and output are measured and recorded, and the character of the wound drainage is noted. The amount and character of drainage on the wound dressing are also noted.

Casts are sometimes used for immobilization, and if so, routine cast care is carried out. The extremity is examined for sensation, circulation, and pain, and the area over the inflammation is usually left open for observation. The affected area, casted or uncasted, is assessed for color, swelling, heat, and tenderness.

The child usually has a poor appetite at first. Nourishment in the form of high-calorie liquids, such as fruit juices, gelatin, and flavored ice pops, is encouraged until the child begins to feel better. The appetite returns as the acute symptoms subside. During convalescence adequate nutrition must be maintained to aid healing and formation of new bone.

When the acute stage subsides, the child begins to feel better, the appetite improves, and the child becomes interested in the surroundings and relationships and may move about in bed. However, weight bearing on the affected limb is not permitted until healing is well under way in order to avoid pathologic fractures. Diversional and constructive activities become important nursing interventions. The child is usually confined to bed for some time after the acute phase but may be allowed to move about in a wheelchair when isolation and bed rest are no longer necessary. As the infection subsides, physical therapy is instituted to ensure restoration of optimum function.

Septic (Suppurative, Pyogenic, Purulent) Arthritis

Infections of the joints, like those of bone, usually develop through hematogenous dissemination from another focus; occasionally they result from direct extension of a soft tissue infection. Joint infections occur predominantly in males, especially in the adolescent age group. In infancy, however, the incidence in boys and girls is nearly equal. Any joint may be involved, but the hip, knee, shoulder, and other large joints are most commonly affected. Usually only one joint is involved.

Therapeutic Management and Nursing Care Management. Treatment consists of open surgical drainage of infections of the hip and shoulder joints, and repeated needle aspirations of the joint space in other joints. The goals are (1) to cleanse the joint to avoid destruction of articular cartilage; (2) to decompress the joint to avoid interference with the blood supply to the epiphysis; (3) to eradicate the infection with adequate antibiotic therapy; and (4) to prevent secondary bone infection and hematogenous spread. Therapy is similar to that for osteomyelitis: IV antibiotic therapy, relief of pain, immobilization of the joint, and prohibition of weight bearing until healing is complete. Nursing care is the same as that for osteomyelitis.

Tuberculosis

Tubercular infection of bones and joints is acquired by hematogenous dissemination of pulmonary tuberculosis. The joint infection is typically spread from adjoining osteomyelitis. Common sites are digits of the upper and lower extremities, resulting in tuberculous dactylitis. Tuberculosis of the spine can involve one or more vertebrae, eroding the bone and destroying the disk space and resulting in Pott disease. Clinical manifestations are not specific; this, combined with a child who may not have verbal skills, can make diagnosis difficult. There may be pain over the affected area, pain with motion, posture change to a position of comfort, a limp, or localized swelling over the affected area. The diagnosis should be considered in a child with a family or environmental exposure to tuberculosis and a positive purified protein derivative (PPD) test. Treatment involves immobilization, surgical debridement, and oral antituberculosis chemotherapy for 1 year (Wang et al, 1999). The prognosis for recovery is excellent.

Nursing Care Management. The nursing responsibilities are similar to those for other types of osteomyelitis and septic arthritis, but include monitoring tuberculosis drug therapy and identifying positive family or environmental active disease contacts.

BONE AND SOFT TISSUE TUMORS

General Concepts: Bone Tumors

Neoplastic disease can arise from any tissues involved in bone growth. In children the two types that account for 85% of all primary malignant bone tumors are osteogenic sarcoma (osteosarcoma) and Ewing sarcoma.

The peak childhood ages for these sarcomas are 15 to 19 years. The sexes are affected equally until puberty, at which time the ratio approaches 2:1 in favor of males. This propensity for males, with a peak incidence during adolescence, is thought to be related to the accelerated growth rate of osseous tissue. These two bone tumors have several characteristics in common, and these are discussed in the following sections. Specific information related to each tumor is also presented.

Diagnostic Evaluation. A primary objective in diagnosis of bone neoplasm is to rule out causes such as trauma or infection. A history and careful questioning regarding pain help determine the duration and rate of tumor growth (Box 54-9). Physical assessment focuses on the functional status of the affected area, signs of inflammation, size of the mass, involvement of regional lymph nodes, and any systemic indication of generalized malignancy.

Definitive diagnosis is based on radiologic studies, particularly computed tomography (CT) scans, radioisotope bone scans, and either needle or surgical bone biopsy to determine the histologic type. Radiologic findings are characteristic for each type of tumor. In osteogenic sarcoma the needlelike bone projections present a "sunburst" appearance, whereas the layers of

Box 54-9
Clinical Manifestations of Bone Tumors

- Pain localized at affected site
  - May be severe or dull
  - Often relieved by position of flexion
  - Frequently brought to attention when child:
    - Limps
    - Curtails own physical activity
    - Is unable to hold heavy objects

new bone in Ewing sarcoma will have an "onionskin" or "hair-on-end" appearance (Himelstein and Dormans, 1996). MRI provides information regarding neurovascular structures, intramedullary bone involvement, and soft tissue extension; this information is useful particularly in limb-salvage procedures.

At present there is no reliable biochemical test for bone cancers, although elevated alkaline phosphatase levels may occur in osteoid tumors. Several tests may be performed to rule out metastatic disease from other neoplasms. Lung tomography is usually a standard procedure, because pulmonary metastasis is the most common complication of primary bone tumors. Bone marrow aspiration is helpful in diagnosing Ewing sarcoma in the rare event that the child has bone marrow metastasis.

Osteogenic Sarcoma

Osteogenic sarcoma is the most commonly encountered malignant bone cancer in children, with a peak incidence between 10 and 25 years of age (Link and Eilber, 1997). Most primary tumor sites are in the metaphysis of long bones (i.e., the wider part of the shaft, next to epiphyseal growth plate), especially in the lower extremities. More than half occur in the femur, particularly the distal portion, with the rest involving the humerus, tibia, pelvis, jaw, and phalanges.

Therapeutic Management. Optimum treatment of osteosarcoma is controversial. The traditional approach has consisted of radical surgical resection or amputation of the affected area. Depending on the tumor site, surgery consists of amputation of the affected extremity at least 7.5 cm (3 inches) above the proximal tumor margin or above the joint proximal to the involved bone (Link and Eilber, 1997). With tumors of the distal femur, preservation of the hip joint may be possible. Other procedures include an above-the-knee amputation for tumors of the tibia or fibula, a hemipelvectomy for tumors of the innominate (hip) bone, and a forequarter amputation (i.e., removal of the arm, the scapula, and a portion of the clavicle on the affected side) for tumors of the upper humerus. *Limb-salvage procedures* entail en bloc resection of tumor-bearing bone with prosthetic replacement of the involved bone. Partial limb salvage by a *rotationplasty procedure* involves resection of the tumor, including the knee joint, with the lower part of the leg rotated 180 degrees and retransplanted to the thigh, creating a shortened leg with the ankle joint at the position of the former knee joint (Kotz, 1997).

Antineoplastic drugs such as high-dose methotrexate with citrovorum rescue, Adriamycin, actinomycin D, cyclophosphamide, ifosfamide, and cisplatin may be administered in combination or singly both before and after surgery.

Prognosis. Surgical procedures (e.g., limb-salvage procedures, amputation, and thoracotomy) accompanied by multiagent chemotherapy have significantly improved survival rates in patients with osteosarcoma. Approximately 65% to 75% of patients with osteosarcoma can expect long-term survival (Pearson, 1998). To improve long-term survival, a compound known as muramyl tripeptide phosphatidylethanolamine (MTP-PE) is being studied. MTP-PE is designed to stimulate macrophages to kill tumor cells, consequently reducing the risk of recurrence in patients with osteosarcoma (Meyers and Gorlick, 1997).

Nursing Care Management. Nursing care depends on the type of surgical approach, and in either instance preparation of the child and family is crucial. Obviously, the family may have more difficulty adjusting to an amputation than a limb-salvage procedure. Straightforward honesty is essential to gain the cooperation and trust of the child. The diagnosis of cancer should not be disguised with falsehoods such as "infection." To accept the need for radical surgery, the child must be aware of the lack of alternatives for treatment. Although the task of informing the child is the responsibility of the physician, the nurse should be present for the discussion or be aware of exactly what is said to the child. The child should be told a few days before surgery, so that he or she has time to think about the diagnosis and consequent treatment and to ask questions.

Sometimes children have many questions about the prosthesis, the limitations on physical ability, and their prognosis in terms of cure. At other times they react with silence or with a calm manner that masks their concern and fear. Either response is part of the grieving process that accompanies a loss and must be accepted. Children should not be overwhelmed with information. A supportive approach is to answer their questions without offering additional information and to express a willingness to talk. The nurse should not push the topic unless the child initiates the discussion. Silence does not always mean nonacceptance.

The child is also informed of the need for chemotherapy and its side effects before surgery. Caution must be exercised in offering too much information at one time. It is wise to discuss hair loss with emphasis on positive aspects, such as wearing a wig or baseball cap. Because bone tumors affect adolescents and young adults, it is not unusual for them to become angry over all of the radical body alterations.

If an amputation is performed, the child may be fitted with a temporary prosthesis immediately after surgery; this permits early functioning and fosters psychologic adjustment. If this is not done, the child requires stump care, which is the same as for any amputee. A permanent prosthesis is usually fitted within 6 to 8 weeks. During hospitalization the child begins physical therapy to become proficient in the use and care of the device.

In rotationplasty, a prosthesis is fitted over the newly created knee joint; however, the appearance of a foot placed backward on the leg to create a substitute knee is a major change in body image. Children often need help in dealing with their own feelings and other people's reactions to the leg.

Phantom limb pain may develop following amputation. This symptom is characterized by pain, tingling, itching, burning, and/or cramping in the area of the amputated leg. The child and family need to know that the sensations are real, not imagined. Amitriptyline (Elavil) has been used successfully in children to decrease the pain (Olsson, 1999).

Discharge planning must begin early during the postoperative period. Every effort is made to promote normality and gradual resumption of realistic preamputation activities.* Role-playing in anticipation of such experiences is very beneficial in preparing the child for the inevitable confrontation by others.

*Information about special programs for children with amputations, such as "Sunshine Skiers," is available from the Candlelighters Childhood Cancer Foundation, 1901 Pennsylvania Ave. NW, Suite 1001, Washington, DC 20006; website: www.candlelighters.org. Information about prostheses can be obtained from the National Amputation Foundation, Inc., 3840 Church St., Malverne, NY 11565; (516) 887-3600. In Canada: War Amputations of Canada, 2827 Riverside Dr., Ottawa, Ontario KlV 0C4; (613) 731-3821; www.waramps.ca.

Environmental barriers, such as stairs, are assessed in terms of the accessibility of the school and/or home, especially because the child may need to use crutches or a wheelchair before complete healing and prosthetic competency are achieved.

The family and child need a great deal of support in adjusting not only to a life-threatening diagnosis, but also to alteration in body image and function. Because loss of a limb requires a grieving process, those caring for the child need to recognize that anger and depression are normal and necessary reactions. Often parents view the anger as a direct affront to them for allowing the amputation, or they view the depression as rejection. These are not personal attacks but the child's attempts to cope with the loss.

(See also Nursing Care Plan: The Child with Cancer [Chapter 49] and Nursing Care Plan: The Child with a Bone Tumor.*)

Ewing Sarcoma (Primitive Neuroectodermal Tumor)

Ewing sarcoma, a primitive neuroectodermal tumor, is the second most common malignant bone tumor (after osteogenic sarcoma) in children and adolescents (Grier, 1997). It arises in the marrow spaces of the bones such as the femur, tibia, fibula, ulna, humerus, vertebrae, pelvis, scapula, ribs, and skull. The disease occurs almost exclusively in individuals under age 30, with most occurrences in individuals between 4 and 25 years of age.

Therapeutic Management. Surgical amputation is not routinely recommended but may be considered when the results of radiotherapy render the extremity useless or deformed (such as from retarded growth in young children) or when the tumor appears resectable. The treatment of choice is intensive radiation therapy of the involved bone combined with chemotherapy. A widely used drug regimen includes vincristine, actinomycin D, and cyclophosphamide; or ifosfamide, VP-16, and Adriamycin.

Prognosis. The prognosis is best for children who do not have metastasis at the time of diagnosis. Children with massive tumors or lung and bone marrow metastasis have a much poorer prognosis. Children with distal lesions have the best chance for cure.

Nursing Care Management. The psychologic adjustment to Ewing sarcoma is typically less traumatic than to osteogenic sarcoma because of the preservation of the affected limb. Many families accept the diagnosis with a sense of relief in knowing that this type of bone cancer does not necessitate amputation, and initially they may not be aware of the deleterious effects on the irradiated site, especially severely affected growth, function, and appearance. Consequently, they need preparation for the various diagnostic tests, including bone marrow aspiration and surgical biopsy, and adequate explanation of the treatment regimen.

High-dose radiation therapy often causes a skin reaction of dry or moist desquamation followed by hyperpigmentation. The nurse advises the child to wear loose-fitting clothes over the radiated area to minimize additional skin irritation. Because of increased sensitivity, the radiated skin is protected from sunlight and from sudden changes in temperature, such as those caused by the use of heating pads or ice packs. The child is encouraged to use the extremity as tolerated. Occasionally an active exercise program may be planned by the physical therapist to preserve maximum function.

The child needs the same considerations as any other patient with cancer in adjusting to the effects of chemotherapy, such as hair loss, severe nausea and vomiting, peripheral neuropathy, and possibly cardiotoxicity. Every effort should be made to outline a treatment plan that allows the child maximum resumption of a normal lifestyle and activities.

(See also Nursing Care Plan: The Child with Cancer in Chapter 49.)

Rhabdomyosarcoma

Soft tissue sarcomas are the fourth most common type of solid tumor in children. These malignant neoplasms originate from undifferentiated mesenchymal cells in muscles, tendons, bursae, and fascia; or from such cells in fibrous, connective, lymphatic, or vascular tissue. These disorders derive their name from the specific tissue(s) of origin, such as *myosarcoma (myo=muscle)* or *rhabdomyosarcoma (rhabdo=striated)*. Because striated (skeletal) muscle is found almost anywhere in the body, these tumors occur in many sites, the most common of which are the head (especially the orbit) and neck. The disease occurs most commonly in children younger than 5 years.

Diagnostic Evaluation. The initial signs and symptoms are related to the site of the tumor and compression of adjacent organs (Box 54-10). Some tumor locations, particularly the orbit, produce symptoms early in the course of the illness and contribute to rapid diagnosis and improved prognosis. Other tumors, such as those of the retroperitoneal area, produce no symptoms until they are large, invasive, and widely metastasized. Unfortunately, many of the signs and symptoms attributable to rhabdomyosarcoma are vague and commonly suggest a common childhood illness, such as "earache" or "runny nose." In some instances a primary tumor site is never identified.

Diagnosis begins with a careful examination of the head and neck area, particularly palpation of a nontender, firm, hard mass. The nasopharynx and oropharynx are inspected for any evidence of a visible mass. Radiographic studies are performed to isolate a tumor site; accompanied by chest radiographic examinations, chest CT scans, bone surveys, and bone marrow aspiration to rule out metastasis. A lumbar puncture is indicated for head and neck tumors. An excisional biopsy is performed to confirm the histologic type.

Therapeutic Management. Because this tumor is highly malignant, with metastasis commonly occurring at the time of diagnosis, aggressive multimodal therapy is recommended. Complete removal of the primary tumor is advocated whenever possible. However, biopsy is performed only in certain tumor locations, such as those of the orbit when followed by radiation and chemotherapy. This avoids the devastating effects of enucleation, amputation, or pelvic exenteration.

High-dose radiation to the primary tumor is recommended for most tumors. Radiation usually begins after several chemotherapy courses have been given to shrink the tumor. Drugs that are cytotoxic for rhabdomyosarcoma are vincristine, actinomycin D, and cyclophosphamide, with or without Adri-

---

*In Wong DL, Hess CS: ***Wong and Whaley's: clinical manual of pediatric nursing,*** ed 5, St Louis, 2000, Mosby.

Box 54-10

Clinical Manifestations of Rhabdomyosarcoma According to Tumor Site

ORBIT
Rapidly developing unilateral proptosis
Ecchymosis of conjunctiva
Loss of extraocular movements (strabismus)

NASOPHARYNX
Stuffy nose (earliest sign)
Nasal obstruction—dysphagia, nasal voice (obstruction of posterior nasal conchae), serous otitis media (obstruction of eustachian tube)
Pain (sore throat and ear)
Epistaxis
Palpable neck nodes
Visible mass in oropharynx (late sign)

PARANASAL SINUSES
Nasal obstruction
Local pain
Discharge
Sinusitis
Swelling

MIDDLE EAR
Signs of chronic serous otitis media
Pain
Sanguinopurulent drainage
Facial nerve palsy

RETROPERITONEAL AREA
Usually a "silent" tumor
Abdominal mass
Pain
Signs of intestinal or genitourinary obstruction

PERINEUM
Visible superficial mass
Bowel or bladder dysfunction (from tumor compression)

amycin; as well as ifosfamide, cisplatin, etoposide, and carboplatin. These may be given for 1 to 2 years.

Prognosis. With current treatment protocols, survival rates have increased considerably for children with tumors detected at all clinical stages. Data suggest that children who remain disease free for 2 years are probably cured; however, if relapse occurs, the prognosis for long-term survival is extremely poor (Wexler and Helman, 1997).

Nursing Care Management. The nursing responsibilities are similar to those for other types of cancer, especially the solid tumors when surgery is used. Specific objectives include (1) careful assessment for signs of the tumor, especially during well-child examinations; (2) preparation of the child and family for the multiple diagnostic tests; and (3) supportive care during each stage of multimodal therapy. The reader is urged to review Nursing Care Management under Leukemias in Chapter 49 for physical care of the child, and Chapter 41 for emotional support of the family in the event of a poor prognosis.

DISORDERS OF JOINTS

Juvenile Rheumatoid Arthritis (JRA)

JRA, also known as juvenile chronic arthritis (JCA) or idiopathic arthritis of childhood (IAC), is an inflammatory disease with an unknown cause. Possible causes include infection, autoimmunity, and trauma. There are two peak ages of onset: between 1 and 3 years of age and between 8 and 10 years of age. Twice as many girls as boys have JRA. Although the exact incidence is not known, because many cases remain undiagnosed, studies suggest a minimum incidence of 4.08 per 100,000 children (Malleson, Fung, and Rosenberg, 1996).

JRA is not a single disease, but a heterogeneous group of diseases. Three major types include pauciarticular onset, polyarticular onset, and systemic onset. *Pauciarticular onset,* which involves arthritis in four or fewer joints, accounts for 50% of all cases. *Polyarticular onset,* which involves five or more joints, accounts for 40% of all cases. *Systemic onset* has variable arthritis with systemic features of high fevers with late-evening spikes, transient maculopapular rash, hepatosplenomegaly, pericarditis, pleuritis, and lymphadenopathy. Systemic onset represents 10% of all cases. Although JRA and adult disease both involve arthritis, the diseases are distinct. In contrast to adult disease, JRA occurs in children younger than 16 years; children have a negative rheumatoid factor in 90% of cases, systemic features in 10% of cases, and the associated complication of eye disease (iridocyclitis) in 8% to 20% of cases. A large portion of JRA cases tend to "burn out" and become inactive.

Pathophysiology. The rheumatic process is characterized by chronic inflammation of the synovium with joint effusion and eventual erosion, destruction, and fibrosis of the articular cartilage. Adhesion between joint surfaces and ankylosis of joints occurs with disease progression.

Clinical Manifestations. Whether a single joint or multiple joints are involved, stiffness, swelling, and loss of motion develop in the affected joints. They are swollen and warm to touch but seldom red. The swelling results from joint effusion and synovial thickening. The affected joints may be tender and painful to touch or relatively painless. The limited motion early in the disease is a result of muscle spasm and joint inflammation; later it is caused by ankylosis or soft tissue contractures. Morning stiffness, or "gelling," of the joint(s), is characteristic and present on arising in the morning or after inactivity. Infections, injuries, or surgical procedures often precipitate a flare of the arthritis; therefore prompt recognition and treatment of infections is necessary.

In severe, long-standing cases growth is significantly retarded. Corticosteroid therapy is also a contributing factor. There may be growth disturbances, either overgrowth or undergrowth, adjacent to the inflamed joints (e.g., altered leg length after knee involvement) and micrognathia (receding chin) from temporomandibular arthritis.

Diagnostic Evaluation. JRA is a clinical diagnosis; there are no definitive tests. The diagnosis is based on the criteria, established by the American College of Rheumatology, of (1) age of onset younger than 16 years, (2) arthritis in one or more joints, (3) duration of arthritis for 6 weeks or longer, and (4) exclusion of other forms of arthritis (Cassidy and Petty, 1995). Laboratory tests may provide supporting evidence of disease. An elevated sedimentation rate may or may not be present. Leukocytosis is commonly present during flares of systemic disease. Rheumatoid factor (RF) is positive in only 10% of children with JRA. Antinuclear antibodies are more common in JRA, but they are not specific for JRA. They do, however, help identify children (particularly young girls) with pauciarticular disease, who are at greater risk for uveitis.

Therapeutic Management. There is no specific cure for JRA. The major goals of therapy are to preserve joint function, prevent physical deformities, and relieve symptoms without iatrogenic harm. The child is treated at home under the supervision of the health team, and intermittent treatment by qualified professionals is administered. Hospitalization may be needed during severe exacerbations or when intercurrent illness warrants. *Iridocyclitis,* also known as *uveitis* (inflammation of the iris and ciliary body), is a serious disorder unique to JRA that requires the attention of an ophthalmologist.

Drugs. Several drugs, given alone or in combination, are effective in suppressing the inflammatory process and relieving pain:

Nonsteroidal antiinflammatory drugs (NSAIDs) were the first drugs used. Historically aspirin was the drug of choice; however, most treatment centers now initiate therapy with ibuprofen, naproxen, or Tolectin sodium because they have fewer side effects, are easier to administer, and are very effective (Cassidy and Petty, 1995). Newer formulations of NSAIDs, such a celecoxib (Celebrex) and rofecoxib (Vioxx), are being prescribed for some children. These drugs selectively inhibit one of the enzymes (COX-2) of cyclooxygenase, which is responsible for pain transmission; but do not inhibit the enzyme COX-1, which is necessary for production of prostaglandins that help maintain gastric mucosal blood flow and barrier protection, regulate blood flow to the liver and kidneys, and facilitate platelet aggregation and clot formation. Theoretically the COX-2 NSAIDs provide similar analgesic and antiinflammatory benefits with fewer gastrointestinal and blood-clotting side effects than the nonselective agents (Schuna and Megeff, 2000).

Slow-acting antirheumatic drugs (SAARDs) may require months to be effective and typically work in combination with NSAIDs. SAARDs include hydroxychloroquine, sulfasalazine, gold, and D-penicillamine.

Cytotoxic drugs are used in children with severe arthritis who have failed treatment with NSAIDs. Low-dose methotrexate is an established therapy for polyarticular JRA and commonly supersedes use of SAARDs (Wallace, 1998). Potential bone marrow suppression and liver toxicity require weekly blood monitoring initially and monthly blood monitoring thereafter (Kremer et al, 1994). Treatment with other cytotoxic agents (e.g., azathioprine, cyclosporine, and cyclophosphamide) is largely anecdotal and used only in children who are severely debilitated and nonresponsive to other medications (Cassidy and Petty, 1995).

Corticosteroids are potent immunosuppressives used for life-threatening disease, incapacitating arthritis, and iridocyclitis. They are administered in the lowest effective dose for the briefest period of time and discontinued on a tapering schedule. High-dose "pulse" IV steroids are occasionally administered to patients with severe, disabling disease. A single intraarticular corticosteroid injection may provide effective relief for children with pauciarticular disease nonresponsive to NSAIDs (Padeh and Passwell, 1998). Prolonged use of systemic steroids is associated with significant side effects, including Cushing syndrome, osteoporosis, increased infection risk, glucose intolerance, cataracts, and growth suppression. Despite these risks, corticosteroids may be necessary in the treatment of severe disease (Cassidy and Petty, 1995).

Immunologic modulators are aimed at altering the immune response to decrease inflammation, because children with JRA have known immunologic abnormalities. Tumor necrosis factor-α is an immune mediator that plays a major role in the inflammatory response. Early trials of etanercept (recombinant human tumor necrosis factor receptor) have shown improvement in children who have failed other therapy (Lovell et al, 1998).

Physical Management. Programs of physical management are individualized for each child and designed to reach the ultimate goal: preserving function and/or preventing deformity. Physical therapy is directed toward specific joints, focusing on strengthening muscles, mobilizing restricted joint motion, and preventing or correcting deformities. Occupational therapy assumes responsibility for generalized mobility and performance of activities of daily living.

General treatment or maintenance programs vary; physiotherapists may be involved several times weekly to monthly in management of a home program; or their visits may be limited to infrequent review of the home program for compliance, effectiveness, and need. Normal activities of daily living and the child's natural tendency to be active are usually sufficient to maintain muscle strength and joint mobility.

Exercising in a pool is excellent therapy because it allows freedom of movement with support and minimal gravitational pull. If there is pain on motion, a hot pack or warm bath before therapy may help.

Practitioners may recommend nighttime splinting to help minimize pain and prevent or reduce flexion deformity. Joints most commonly splinted are the knees, wrists, and hands. Positioning during rest is also important. The child rests on a firm mattress with no pillow or a very low one and has no support under the knee. Loss of extension in the knee, hip, and wrist causes special problems and requires vigilance to detect the earliest signs of involvement and vigorous attention to prevent deformity with specialized passive stretching, positioning, and resting splints.

Prognosis. The course of JRA is highly variable. Thirty percent to 40% of patients have active disease 10 years after the diagnosis, have substantial disability as adults, and require long-term drug therapy. The prognosis is best for children with pauciarticular JRA and worst for children with chronic, polyarticular disease, especially those positive for RF (Wallace and Levinson, 1991).

Nursing Care Management

➤ Assessment

Nursing the child with JRA involves assessment of the child's general health, the status of involved joints, and the child's emotional response to all ramifications of the disease (e.g., discomfort, physical restrictions, therapies, and self-concept).

➤ Nursing Diagnoses

Nursing diagnoses and management identified for the child with JRA include the following:

Chronic pain related to joint inflammation

Impaired physical mobility related to joint discomfort and stiffness

Bathing/hygiene, dressing/grooming, feeding, or toileting self-care deficit related to impaired joint mobility

Altered family processes related to a situational crisis (child with a chronic illness)

➤ Plan of Care and Implementation

Goals for the child with JRA and family include the following:

1. Child will experience reduction of pain to level acceptable to child.
2. Child will remain healthy.
3. Child will exhibit signs of adequate joint function.
4. Child will perform activities of daily living.
5. Child and family will receive adequate support.

The effects of JRA are manifested in every aspect of the child's life, physical activities, social experiences, and personality development. Although children with severe disease may have more physical barriers to overcome, studies show that emotional and behavioral functioning is most closely linked with maternal depression and parental distress, not with physical disability (Frank et al, 1998). Nursing interventions to support the parents may foster a successful adaptation for the entire family. Parental concerns about the disease prognosis, financial and insurance issues, spouse/sibling relationships, and job and schedule conflicts must all be addressed. Referral to social workers, counselors, or support groups may be needed.

Relieve Pain. The pain of JRA is related to several aspects of the disease—disease severity, functional status, individual pain threshold, family variables, and psychologic adjustment. The aim is to provide as much relief as possible with medication and other therapies to help children tolerate the pain and cope as effectively as possible. At present, opioid administration is not a routine therapy for the chronic pain. Nonpharmacologic modalities have proved effective in modifying pain perception (see Pain Management, Chapter 44) and activities that aggravate pain. Behavioral and cognitive therapy, such as relaxation techniques, may be useful tools in treating arthritis pain in children (Schanberg et al, 1997).

Promote General Health. The general health of the child must be considered. A well-balanced diet with sufficient calories to maintain growth is essential. If the child is relatively inactive, caloric intake needs to match energy needs to avoid excessive weight gain, which places additional stress on affected joints. Sleep and rest are essential for children with JRA. Some children will require rest during the day; however, daytime napping that interferes with nighttime sleepiness should be avoided. A bedtime routine that involves comfort measures can help induce sleep. A firm mattress, heated water bed, electric blanket, or sleeping bag help provide warmth, comfort, and rest. Nighttime splints needed to maintain range of motion might initially be a source of bedtime conflict. The family needs instruction on how to use the splint appropriately so that it does not cause pain or impede sleep. Behavior modification programs that reward splint and exercise compliance may be helpful in reducing compliance barriers. Well-child care to assess growth and development as well as immunization requirements needs to be coordinated between the primary care provider and the rheumatologist. Common childhood illnesses such as upper respiratory infections may cause arthritis to worsen; consequently, medical attention must be sought quickly for relatively minor illness to prevent flares. Effective communication between the family, the primary care provider, and the rheumatology team is essential for care coordination.

Children are encouraged to attend school, even on days when there may be some pain or discomfort. The aid of the school nurse is enlisted so that a child is permitted to take the prescribed medication at school and to arrange for rest in the nurse's office during the day. Split days or half days may help a child remain involved in school. Permitting the child to come to school late allows time to gain joint movement and reduces the time at school to avoid exhaustion. It is important that the child attend school to learn skills and engage in social interaction, especially if the JRA continues to limit physical skills. Arranging for two sets of textbooks eliminates the need to carry heavy or numerous books to and from school, thus reducing discomfort and difficulty ambulating. A formal school hearing may be necessary to obtain an individualized education plan, ensured by public law, which includes intensive school modifications (Bartholomew et al, 1994).

Facilitate Compliance. The child and family are involved in the therapeutic plan. They need to know the purpose and correct use of any splints and appliances and the medication regimen. The family is instructed regarding administration of medications, as well as the value of a regular schedule of administration to maintain a satisfactory drug level in the body. They need to know that NSAIDs should not be given on an empty stomach and to be alert for signs of medication toxicity. If evidence of drug toxicity is noted, the family is instructed to notify the health professional and follow that person's instructions.

Encourage Heat and Exercise. Heat has been shown to be beneficial to children with arthritis. Moist heat is best for relieving pain and stiffness, and the most efficient and practical method is in the bathtub with warm water. Sometimes a daily whirlpool bath, paraffin bath, or hot packs may be used as needed for temporary relief of acute swelling and pain. Hot packs are easily applied using a bath towel wrung out after being immersed in hot water or heated in a microwave oven; covered with plastic, it is applied to the area for 20 minutes. Commercial pads that warm in only a few minutes in the microwave are also available. Painful hands or feet can be immersed in a pan of water for 10 minutes two or three times daily in addition to tub baths.

Pool therapy is the easiest method for exercising a large number of joints. Swimming activities strengthen muscles and maintain mobility in larger joints. Very small children who are frightened of the water can carry out their exercises in the bathtub. Small children love to splash, kick, and throw things in the water. Remember, adult supervision is necessary for all water activities.

Activities of daily living provide satisfactory exercise for older children to maintain maximum mobility with minimum pain. These children are encouraged in their efforts to be independent and patiently allowed to dress and groom themselves, to assume daily tasks, and to care for their belongings. It is often difficult for children to manipulate buttons, to comb or brush hair, and to operate faucets; but unless there is an acute flare, parents and other caregivers should not offer assistance. In addition, children should learn and understand why others do not help them. Many helpful devices, such as self-adhering fasteners, tongs for manipulating difficult items, and grab bars installed in bathrooms for safety, can be used to facilitate tasks. A raised toilet seat often makes the difference between dependent and independent toileting because weak quadriceps muscles and sore knees inhibit the ability to raise the body from a low sitting position.

A child's natural affinity for play offers many opportunities for incorporating therapeutic exercises. Throwing or kicking a ball and riding a tricycle (with the seat raised to achieve maximum leg extension) are excellent moving and stretching exercises for a very young child whose daily living activities are physically limited.

An effective approach to beginning the day's activities is to awaken children early to give them their medication and then to allow them to sleep for an hour. On arising, children take a hot bath (or shower) and perform a simple ritual of limbering-up exercises, after which they commence the activities of the day, such as going to school. Exercise, heat, and rest are spaced throughout the remainder of the day according to the child's individual needs and schedules. Parents are instructed in exercises that meet the needs of the child.

The Arthritis Foundation* and the American Juvenile Arthritis Foundation* provide services for both parents and professionals, and nurses should refer families to these agencies as an added resource.

Support Child and Family. JRA affects every aspect of life for the child and family. Physical limitations may interfere with self-care, school participation, and recreational activities. The intensive treatment plan, including multiple medications, physical therapy, comfort measures, and medical appointments, is intrusive and very disruptive to the parents' work schedule and the family's routine. To prevent isolation and encourage independence, the family is encouraged to pursue their normal activities. Unfortunately, the adaptations necessary to make that happen take resourcefulness and commitment from all family members. At diagnosis and throughout the span of JRA, it is essential to recognize signs of stress and counterproductive coping and provide the necessary support to maximize adaptation. The problems and needs of the family with a chronic illness like JRA are discussed in Chapter 41, and the reader is directed to that chapter for guidance in planning care.

➤ Evaluation

The effectiveness of nursing interventions is determined by continual reassessment and evaluation of care based on the following observational guidelines:

1. Observe child's behavior and use pain assessment techniques.
2. Conduct routine assessment of child's general health.
3. Observe child during planned and unplanned activities, assess mobility of joints, and observe the use of prescribed appliances.
4. Observe child's ability to perform activities of daily living.
5. Observe and interview child and family regarding feelings and concerns.

Expected outcomes include the following:

1. Child is able to move with minimum or no discomfort.
2. Child attains and maintains optimal health status (specify).
3. Child engages in activities suitable to interests, capabilities, and developmental level; joints are mobile, flexible, and free of deformity.
4. Child is involved in self-care activities to maximum capabilities.
5. Child and family demonstrate an understanding of the child's disease and therapies; they verbalize their feelings and concerns.

(See also the Nursing Care Plan: The Child with Juvenile Rheumatoid Arthritis.*)

Systemic Lupus Erythematosus (SLE)

SLE is a chronic, multisystem, autoimmune disease of the connective tissues and blood vessels characterized by inflammation in potentially any body tissue. Its course and symptoms are variable and unpredictable, with mild to life-threatening complications. In addition to SLE, there are other forms of lupus, such as neonatal lupus, which occurs when maternal autoantibodies cross the placenta and cause transient lupuslike symptoms in the newborn with the potential serious complication of heart block. This discussion focuses on SLE.

The estimated minimum incidence of SLE is 0.28 per 100,000 children younger than 16 years (Malleson, Fung, and Rosenberg, 1996). SLE is more common in girls, with an approximate 5:1 female-to-male ratio; and typically occurs between the ages of 10 and 19 years. There is a familial tendency, although many newly diagnosed patients are unaware of other affected family members. SLE has been reported in all cultures, but within the United States there has been a disproportionately higher report in African-American, Asian, and Hispanic children.

The cause of SLE is unknown. Potential triggers include hormonal imbalance; immune abnormalities; and environmental exposures, including drugs, infection, sun exposure, stress, and chemical agents.

Clinical Manifestations and Diagnostic Evaluation. The child with SLE may have any clinical manifestation (Box 54-11) with mild to life-threatening severity. The diagnosis is established when 4 of the 11 diagnostic criteria are met (Box 54-12). Kidney involvement heralds progressive disease and the need for rigorous therapeutic management.

Therapeutic Management. The goal of treatment is to ensure the health of the child by balancing the medications necessary to avoid exacerbation and complications while preventing or minimizing treatment-associated morbidity. Therapy in-

*1314 Spring St. NW, Atlanta, GA 30309; (404) 872-7100 or 1-800-283-7800; website: www.arthritis.org. In Canada: the Arthritis Society, 250 Bloor St. E., Suite 401, Toronto, Ontario M4W 3P2; (416) 979-7228.

*In Wong DL, Hess CS: ***Wong and Whaley's clinical manual of pediatric nursing,*** ed 5, St Louis, 2000, Mosby.

Box 54-11

Clinical Manifestations of Systemic Lupus Erythematosus Related to Tissues Involved

Cutaneous lesions—Erythematous blush or scaly erythematous patches over bridge of nose and extending to each check symmetrically ("butterfly rash"); may extend to scalp, neck, chest, and extremities; sometimes pruritic resemble severe sunburn or hives or may become bullous
Musculoskeletal system—Generalized weakness, usually accompanied by arthritis, myalgia, joint swelling, and stiffness; usually not severe enough to cause deformity; pain may cause temporary disability
Central nervous system—Varies from forgetfulness, excitability, and headache to seizures and frank psychosis; seizures may be early sign; any cranial nerves can be affected; paralysis (spinal cord involvement)
Heart and lungs—Serous linings may be inflamed; pleurisy (lungs), pericarditis (heart); usually reversible with rest
Kidneys—Glomerulus is usual site of destruction; proteinuria; kidney failure
Blood—Anemia from decreased erythrocytes is common; amenorrhea secondary to anemia; platelets and plasma proteins may be affected
Lymphoid system—Spleen and cervical, axillary, and inguinal lymph nodes are enlarged (sometimes); hepatitis may develop
Gastrointestinal tract—Nausea, vomiting, diarrhea, and abdominal pain are possible

Box 54-12

Criteria for Diagnosis of Systemic Lupus Erythematosus

Butterfly rash
Discoid rash
Photosensitivity
Oral ulcers
Arthritis
Serositis
Renal disorder
Neurologic disorder(s) (psychosis, coma, seizures, paresis)
Hematologic disorder(s) (anemia, thrombocytopenia, leukopenia)
Immunologic disorder(s) (anti-DNA, anti-SM, STS, antiphospholipid antibodies)
Antinuclear antibody (ANA)

volves the use of specific medications and general supportive care. The drugs used to control inflammation are corticosteroids administered in doses sufficient to control inflammation, then tapered to the lowest suppressive dose. Other drugs include antimalarial preparations, which are useful for rash and arthritis; NSAIDs, which relieve muscle and joint inflammation; and immunosuppressive agents, such as cyclophosphamide, for renal and central nervous system disease. Antihypertensives, aspirin, and antibiotics are just a few of the additional drugs that may be necessary to treat or avoid complications.

General supportive care includes sufficient nutrition, sleep and rest, and exercise. Exposure to the sun and ultraviolet B (UVB) light is limited because of its association with SLE exacerbation (Rihner and McGrath, 1992).

Nursing Care Management. The principal nursing goal is to help the child and family positively adjust to the disease and therapy. The child and family must learn to recognize subtle signs of disease flare and potential complications of medication therapy, and to communicate these concerns to their care provider. Consequently, patient/family education is an ongoing process initiated at diagnosis and tailored to the patient's individual needs. Referral to a social worker, psychologist, or support group may help the child and family make a successful adjustment. Support groups are associated with the Lupus Foundation of America, Inc.,* and the Arthritis Foundation (p. 1578).†

Key issues include therapy compliance; body-image problems associated with rash, hair loss, and steroid therapy; school attendance; vocational activities; social relationships; sexual activity; and pregnancy. (See Chapter 41 for a discussion on adjusting to a chronic illness.) Specific instructions for avoiding exposure to the sun and UVB light, such as sunscreens, sun-resistant clothing, and altering outdoor activities, must be provided with great sensitivity to ensure compliance while minimizing the associated feeling of being different from peers (see Sunburn, Chapter 53). Patients need to be instructed to maintain regular medical supervision and seek attention quickly during illness or before elective surgical procedures, such as dental extraction, because of potential needs for increased steroids or prophylactic antibiotics. People with SLE should carry medical identification for their disease and steroid dependence.

*4 Research Place, Suite 180, Rockville, MD 20850; (301) 670-9292 or 1-800-558-0121; website: www.lupus.org.
†A recommended booklet available from the Arthritis Foundation is *Meeting the Challenge: A Young Person's Guide to Living with Lupus.*

Key Points

- Immobility has a profound effect on all aspects of growth and development.
- The major physical consequences of immobilization are loss of muscle strength, endurance, and muscle mass; bone demineralization; loss of joint mobility; and contractures.
- Features of children's fractures not observed in the adult include presence of growth plate, thicker and stronger periosteum, bone porosity, more rapid healing, and less joint stiffness.
- The goals of fracture management are to regain alignment and length of bony fragments, retain alignment and length, and restore function to injured parts.
- The method of fracture reduction is determined by the age of the child, degree of displacement, amount of overriding, amount of edema, condition of the skin and soft tissues, sensation, and circulation distal to the fracture.
- The primary purposes of traction are to fatigue involved muscles and reduce muscle spasm, position bone ends in desired realignment, and immobilize

the fracture site until realignment has been achieved to permit casting or splinting.

- The development of developmental dysplasia of the hip appears to be related to intrauterine, genetic, and cultural factors.
- Treatment of clubfoot consists of manipulation and casting to correct the deformity, maintenance of the correction, and prevention of possible recurrence of the deformity.
- Acquired hip deformities are managed with non-weight-bearing devices (Legg-Calvé-Perthes disease) or surgical stabilization (slipped femoral capital epiphysis).
- Observation for scoliosis is an important part of a routine physical assessment.
- Scoliosis is managed by bracing and exercise, or surgical correction.
- Bone infections are managed with vigorous antibiotic therapy, immobilization of the affected part, and (sometimes) surgical drainage.
- Osteosarcoma is a neoplasm of bone-forming tissues; Ewing sarcoma is a neoplasm that arises from bone marrow spaces.
- Rhabdomyosarcoma may occur almost anywhere in the body, but the most common sites are the head and neck.
- Nursing care of the child with juvenile arthritis consists of promoting general health, relieving discomfort, preventing deformity, and preserving function.
- Lupus erythematosus is a chronic autoimmune disorder that affects the collagen tissues of the body.

References

Annequin D et al: Fixed 50% nitrous oxide oxygen mixture for painful procedures: a French survey, *Pediatrics* 105(4):c47, 2000; www.pediatrics.org/cgi/content/full/105/4/c47.

Aronsson DD, Loder RT: Treatment of the unstable (acute) slipped capital femoral epiphysis, *Clin Orthop* 322:99-110, 1996.

Bartholomew LK et al: An educational needs assessment of children with chronic juvenile rheumatoid arthritis, *Arthritis Care Res* 7(3):136-143, 1994.

Bender LH: Osteogenesis imperfecta, *Orthop Nurs* 10(4):23-32, 1991.

Burg FD et al: *Gillis and Kagan's current pediatric therapy,* ed 15, Philadelphia, 1995, WB Saunders.

Buschbacher RM: Deconditioning, conditioning, and the benefits of exercise. In Braddom RL, editor: *Physical medicine and rehabilitation,* ed 1, Philadelphia, 1996, WB Saunders.

Carlino HY: The child with an Ilizarov external fixator, *Pediatr Nurs* 17(4):355-358, 1991.

Cassidy J, Petty R: *Textbook of pediatric rheumatology,* ed 3, Philadelphia, 1995, WB Saunders.

Frank RG et al: Disease and family contributors to adaptation in juvenile rheumatoid arthritis and juvenile diabetes, *Arthritis Care Res* 11(3):166-176, 1998.

Grier H: The Ewing family of tumors: Ewing's tumors, *Pediatr Clin North Am* 44(4):991-1004, 1997.

Himelstein BP, Dormans JP: Malignant bone tumors of childhood, *Pediatr Clin North Am* 43(4):967-983, 1996.

Houston MS: Care of the school-aged child in 90/90 traction, *Orthop Nurs* 15(2):57-64, 1996.

Karwowska A et al: Epidemiology and outcomes of osteomyelitis in the era of sequential intravenous-oral therapy, *Pediatr Infect Dis J* 17:1021-1026, 1998.

Kennedy RM, Luhmann JD: The "ouchless emergency department": getting closer: advances in decreasing distress during painful procedures in the emergency department, *Pediatr Clin North Am* 46(6):1215-1247, 1999.

Kotz R: Rotationplasty, *Semin Surg Oncol* 13(1):34-40, 1997.

Kremer JM et al: Methotrexate for rheumatoid arthritis: suggested guidelines for monitoring liver toxicity, *Arthritis Rheum* 37:316-328, 1994.

Link MP, Eilber F: Osteosarcoma. In Pizzo PA, Poplack DG, editors: *Principles and practice of pediatric oncology,* ed 3, Philadelphia, 1997, JB Lippincott.

Loder RT: Slipped capital femoral epiphysis, *Am Fam Physician* 59(9):2135-2142, 1998.

Lovell DJ et al: Safety and efficacy of tumor necrosis factor receptor P75 FC fusion protein (TNFR: FC: Enbrel) in polyarticular course juvenile rheumatoid arthritis, *Arthritis Rheum* 41 (suppl 9):S130, 1998 (abstract).

Maher AB, Salmond SW, Pellino TA: *Orthopedic nursing,* ed 2, Philadelphia, 1998, WB Saunders.

Malleson P, Fung M, Rosenberg A: The incidence of pediatric rheumatic diseases: results from the Canadian Ped Rheumatology Association Disease Registry, *J Rheumatol* 23(11): 1981-1987, 1996.

Martinez AG, Weinstein SL: Recurrent Legg-Calve-Perthes disease, *J Bone Joint Surg* 73A(7):1081-1085, 1991.

Meyers PA, Gorlick R: Osteosarcoma, *Pediatr Clin North Am* 44(4):973-989, 1997.

Noonan KJ et al: Long term psychosocial characteristics of patients treated for idiopathic scoliosis, *J Pediatr Orthop* 17: 712-717, 1997.

Olsson GL: Neuropathic pain in children. In McGrath PJ, Finley GA, editors: *Chronic and recurrent pain in children and adolescents,* Seattle, 1999, IASP Press.

Padeh S, Passwell P: Intraarticular corticosteroid injection in the management of children with chronic arthritis, *Arthritis Rheum* 41(7):1210-1214, 1998.

Pearson M: Historical perspective of the treatment of osteosarcoma: an interview with Dr. Norman Jaffe, *J Pediatr Oncol Nurs* 15(2):90-94, 1998.

Poussa M et al: Conservative vs. operative treatment of Perthes' disease, *Clin Orthop* 297:82-86, 1993.

Rang M: Musculoskeletal O & A: management of Legg-Calvé-Perthes disease varies with severity, *J Musculoskel Med* 12(4):10-11, 1996.

Rihner M, McGrath H Jr.: Fluorescent light photosensitivity in patients with systemic lupus erythematosus, *Arthritis Rheum* 35:949, 1992.

Schanberg LE et al: Pain coping and the pain experience in children with juvenile chronic arthritis, *Pain* 73(2):181-189, 1997.

Screening for adolescent idiopathic scoliosis: policy statement, US Preventive Services Task Force, *JAMA* 269(20):2664-2666, 1993.

Schuna AA, Megeff C: New drugs for the treatment of rheumatoid arthritis, *Am J Health Syst Pharm* 57(3):225-234, 2000.

Stevens B et al: Evaluation of a home-based traction program for children with congenital dislocated hips and Legg Perthes disease, *Can J Nurs Res* 27(40):133-150, 1995.

Wallace CA: The use of methotrexate in childhood rheumatic disease, *Arthritis Rheum* 41:381-391, 1998.

Wallace CA, Levinson JE: Juvenile rheumatoid arthritis: outcome and treatment for the 1990s, *Rheum Dis Clin North Am* 17(4):891-905, 1991.

Wang M et al: Tuberculous osteomyelitis in young children, *J Pediatr Orthop* 19:151-155, 1999.

Wedrick JJ et al: Effect of 17 days of bed rest on peak isometric force and unloaded velocity of human soleus fibers, *Am J Physiol* (Cell Physiol 43):1690-1699, 1997.

Weinstein SL: *The pediatric spine: principles and practice,* New York, 1994, Raven Press.

Wexler LH, Helman LJ: Rhabdomyosarcoma and the undifferentiated sarcoma. In Pizzo PA, Poplack DG, editors: *Principles and practice of pediatric oncology,* ed 3, Philadelphia, 1997, JB Lippincott.

CHAPTER 55

Neuromuscular or Muscular Dysfunction

http://www.harcourthealth.com/MERLIN/Wong/maternal/

Learning Objectives

On completion of this chapter the reader will be able to:

- Discuss the nursing role in helping parents cope with a child with cerebral palsy.
- Formulate a nursing care plan for the preoperative and postoperative care of a child with myelomeningocele.
- Outline a plan of care for a child with Duchenne muscular dystrophy.
- Discuss the prevention and treatment of tetanus.
- Identify the causes of botulism in infants and children.
- List three causes of spinal cord injury in children.

CONGENITAL NEUROMUSCULAR OR MUSCULAR DISORDERS

Cerebral Palsy (CP)

CP is a nonspecific term applied to disorders characterized by early onset of impaired movement and posture. It is nonprogressive and may be accompanied by perceptual problems, language deficits, and intellectual impairment. The etiology, clinical features, and course are variable and are characterized by abnormal muscle tone and coordination as the primary disturbances. CP is the most common permanent physical disability of childhood, and the incidence is reported as 1.5 to 3 in every 1000 live births (Dabney, Lipton, and Miller, 1997).

A variety of prenatal, perinatal, and postnatal factors contribute to the etiology of CP singly or multifactorially. Although the prevalent hypothesis has been that CP results from perinatal problems, especially birth asphyxia, it is now known that CP results more often from existing *prenatal* brain abnormalities. Premature delivery continues to be the single most important risk factor for CP; however, in approximately 24% of cases, no cause is determined (Paneth, 1993).

Pathophysiology. It is difficult to establish a precise location of neurologic lesions based on etiology or clinical signs because no characteristic pathologic pattern exists. Some patients have gross malformations of the brain; others may have evidence of vascular occlusion, atrophy, loss of neurons, and degeneration. Anoxia plays the most significant role in the pathologic state of brain damage, which is commonly caused by other mechanisms.

CP has been classified in several ways, but the most useful classification is based on the nature and distribution of neuromuscular dysfunction (Box 55-1).

Diagnostic Evaluation. Neurologic examination and history are the primary modalities for diagnosis of CP. A thorough knowledge of normal variations of motor development is required for detecting abnormal progress, and a careful history is elicited to detect possible etiologic factors. The alert observer may be suspicious when a child demonstrates some of the manifestations outlined in Box 55-2. The child's spontaneous movements and behavior are observed, including posture; attitude; and muscle size, function, and tone. Persistence of primitive reflexes may be of value, and two of these aid in diagnosis: asymmetric tonic neck reflex and crossed extensor reflex (Nehring and Steele, 1996).

Supplemental diagnostic tests may be used, such as electroencephalography, tomography, screening for metabolic defects, and serum electrolyte values. The possibility that the manifestations are those of slowly progressive degenerative disease or early-onset, slowly growing brain tumors must be ruled out.

Therapeutic Management. The goals of therapy for children with CP are early recognition and promotion of optimum development to enable affected children to attain their potential within the limits of their brain dysfunction. The dis-

Box 55-1

Clinical Classification of Cerebral Palsy

Spastic—May involve one or both sides
- Hypertonicity with poor control of posture, balance, and coordinated motion
- Impairment of fine and gross motor skills
- Active attempts at motion increase abnormal postures and overflow of movement to other parts of the body

Dyskinetic/athetoid—Abnormal involuntary movement
- Athetosis, characterized by slow, wormlike, writhing movements that usually involve the extremities, trunk, neck, facial muscles, and tongue
- Involvement of the pharyngeal, laryngeal, and oral muscles causes drooling and dysarthria (imperfect speech articulation)
- Involuntary movements may take on choreoid (involuntary, irregular, jerking movements) and dystonic (disordered muscle tone) manifestations that increase in intensity with emotional stress and around adolescence

Ataxic
- Wide-based gait
- Rapid, repetitive movements performed poorly
- Disintegration of movements of the upper extremities when the child reaches for objects

Mixed type/dystonic—Combination of spasticity and athetosis

order is permanent, and therapy is chiefly symptomatic and preventive.

The broad aims of therapy are (1) to establish locomotion, communication, and self-help; (2) to gain optimum appearance and integration of motor functions; (3) to correct associated defects as effectively as possible; (4) to provide educational opportunities adapted to the individual child's needs and capabilities; and (5) to promote socialization experiences with other affected and unaffected children. Each child is evaluated and managed on an individual basis. The plan of therapy may involve a variety of settings, facilities, and specially trained persons, including the parents.

Ankle-foot orthoses (AFOs, braces) are worn by many of these children and are used to help prevent or reduce deformity, increase the energy efficiency of gait, and control alignment. Other mobilization devices include wheeled scooter boards that allow children to propel themselves while on the abdomen, wheeled go-carts that provide sitting balance and serve as early "wheelchair" experience for young children, and special devices that leave the upper extremities free (Figs. 55-1 and 55-2).

NURSE ALERT • The use of infant walkers is discouraged. They pose a risk of injury to healthy children and are especially hazardous for children with CP. Also, jumping seats, such as those that hang in doorways, should not be used.

Orthopedic surgery may be required to correct contracture or spastic deformities, to provide stability for an uncontrollable joint, and to provide balanced muscle power. This includes tendon-lengthening procedures (especially heel-cord lengthening), release of spastic wrist flexor muscles, and correction of hip and adductor muscle spasticity or contracture to improve locomotion. A neurosurgical intervention, *selective dorsal rhizotomy*, is used selectively in some children with CP. The procedure involves selectively cutting dorsal column sensory rootlets that have an abnormal response to electrical stimulation. Achieving the benefits from the surgery requires intensive physical therapy and family commitment. Because the procedure results in flaccid muscles, the child must be retaught to sit, stand, and walk.

Box 55-2

Clinical Manifestations of Cerebral Palsy

DELAYED GROSS MOTOR DEVELOPMENT
- A universal manifestation
- Delay in all motor accomplishments
- Increases as growth advances
- Delays more obvious as growth advances

ABNORMAL MOTOR PERFORMANCE
- Very early preferential unilateral hand use
- Abnormal and asymmetric crawl
- Standing or walking on toes
- Uncoordinated or involuntary movements
- Poor sucking
- Feeding difficulties
- Persistent tongue thrust

ALTERATIONS OF MUSCLE TONE
- Increased or decreased resistance to passive movements
- Opisthotonic postures (exaggerated arching of back)
- Feels stiff on handling or dressing
- Difficulty in diapering
- Rigid and unbending at the hip and knee joints when pulled to sitting position (an early sign)

ABNORMAL POSTURES
- Maintains hips higher than trunk in prone position with legs and arms flexed or drawn under the body
- Scissoring and extension of legs, with the feet plantar flexed in supine position
- Persistent infantile resting and sleeping posture:
  - Arms abducted at shoulders
  - Elbows flexed
  - Hands fisted

REFLEX ABNORMALITIES
- Persistence of primitive infantile reflexes:
  - Obligatory tonic neck reflex at any age
  - Nonpersistence beyond 6 months of age
- Persistence or hyperactivity of the Moro, plantar, and palmar grasp reflexes
- Hyperreflexia, ankle clonus, and stretch reflexes elicited in many muscle groups on fast, passive movements

ASSOCIATED DISABILITIES*
- Subnormal learning and reasoning (mental retardation in about two thirds of individuals)
- Seizures
- Impaired behavioral and interpersonal relationships
- Sensory impairment (vision, hearing)

*May or may not be present.

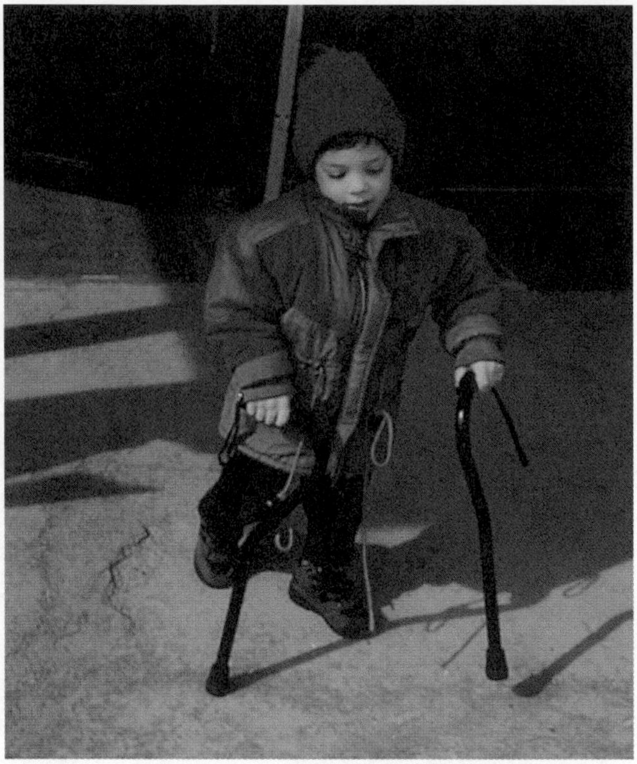

FIG. 55-1 • Mobilization device for child.

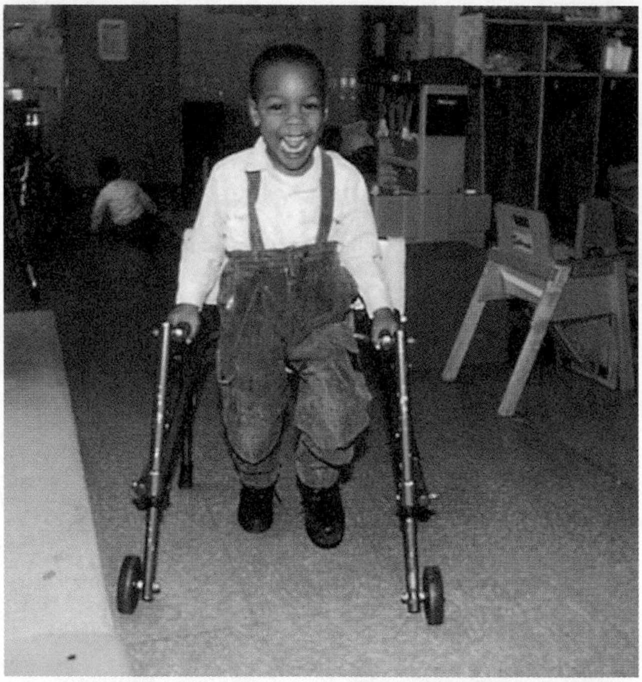

FIG. 55-2 • Child ambulating with use of assistive device.

Surgical intervention is usually reserved for the child who does not respond to the more conservative measures, but it is also indicated for the child whose spasticity causes progressive deformities. Surgery is primarily used to improve function rather than for cosmetic purposes and is followed by physical therapy.

Pharmacologic agents given orally have had little effectiveness in improving overall function in children with CP. Antianxiety agents have been used to some extent to relieve excessive motion and tension, particularly in the child with athetosis. Skeletal muscle relaxants, such as dantrolene (Dantrium), baclofen (Lioresal), and methocarbamol (Robaxin) may be used on a short-term basis for older children and adolescents. Diazepam (Valium) is used commonly but should be restricted to older children and adolescents. A local nerve block to motor points of a muscle with a neurolytic agent such as phenol solution reduces spasticity temporarily. Botulinum toxin (Botox) is also being used to paralyze specific muscles (Dabney, Lipton, and Miller, 1997).

The neurosurgical and pharmacologic approach to managing the spasticity associated with CP involves the implantation of a pump to infuse baclofen directly into the intrathecal space surrounding the spinal cord to provide relief of spasticity. High doses of oral baclofen are associated with significant side effects, including drowsiness and confusion, but are often unable to provide adequate relief of spasticity. Direct infusion of baclofen into the intrathecal space provides relief without the associated side effects (Albright, 1996; Armstrong et al, 1997).

Patients are screened before pump placement by the infusion of a "test dose" of intrathecal baclofen delivered via a lumbar puncture. Close monitoring for side effects and relief of spasticity occurs for several hours after the infusion. If a positive effect is noted, the patient is considered a candidate for pump placement. The implantation procedure is done in the operating room by a neurosurgeon. The pump is placed in the subcutaneous space of the midabdomen. An intrathecal catheter is tunneled from the lumbar area to the abdomen and connected to the pump. The pump is filled with baclofen and programmed to provide a set dose using a telemetry wand and a computer. The patient remains hospitalized for 3 to 7 days to adjust the dose and ensure proper healing. Outpatient visits to refill the pump and make dosage adjustments occur about every 4 to 6 weeks, depending on the patient's response to the treatment. This procedure is most suited for a multidisciplinary setting where rehabilitation specialists are readily available and consistently involved in the patient's ongoing care (Rawlins, 1995).

Antiepileptic medications, especially phenobarbital and phenytoin, are prescribed routinely for children who have seizures, and hyperactive, dyskinetic children perform better when given dextroamphetamine or other drugs used for the child with attention deficit hyperactivity disorder. Care of visual and auditory deficits requires the attention of appropriate specialists, and speech therapy involves the services of a speech therapist. Dental care is especially important. Regular visits to the dentist and prophylaxis, including brushing, using fluoride, and flossing, should be instituted as soon as the teeth erupt. This is especially important for children being given phenytoin, who often develop gum hyperplasia.

A wide range of technical aids are available to improve the functioning of children with CP. These include electromechanical toys that use biofeedback and operate from a head unit. The toy is manipulated only when the head and trunk are in correct alignment. Eye-hand coordination can also be enhanced by appropriately designed toys and games. Microcomputers combined with voice synthesizers help children with speech difficulties "speak." These and others print messages onto screen monitors and paper. These devices have made it apparent that some children have been erroneously considered to be mentally retarded.

Many other electronic devices allow independent functioning. Sensors can be activated and deactivated by using a head-stick, tongue, or other voluntary muscle movement over which the child has control. The application of this technology makes it possible for persons with CP to function in their own residences, and use of these devices can be extended into the workplace.

Physical therapy is one of the most commonly used conservative treatment modalities. It requires the specialized skills of a qualified therapist with an extensive repertoire of exercise methods who can design a program to stimulate each child to achieve his or her functional goals.

An active therapy program involves the family, the physical therapist, and often other members of the health team, especially the nurse. The major approach uses traditional types of therapeutic exercises that consist of stretching, passive, active, and resisted movements applied to specific muscle groups or joints to maintain or increase range of motion, strength, or endurance.

Prognosis. Survival rates of children with moderate disability from CP are about the same as those of unaffected children for the first 20 years of life. Children with severe disability have about a 50% probability of surviving 20 or more years (Hutton, Cook, and Pharaoh, 1994).

Nursing Care Management

➤ Assessment

Early recognition of CP is often a result of alert observation by the nurse. Detection begins at birth, and the nurse should be especially observant for signs in an infant who has a history that includes any of the prenatal or perinatal conditions that predispose to brain damage. Unusual manifestations in a newborn can be signs of a variety of conditions, but an infant who displays poor feeding, rigidity, tenseness, or hypotonia merits closer scrutiny. A history of these unexplained signs is cause for repeated assessment. The disorder is not readily identifiable in the early months of life; often evidence is not apparent until the child begins to walk. Delayed attainment of developmental milestones is one of the most valuable clues to recognizing CP; therefore slow development in a child offers one of the earliest indications of neurologic impairment (Box 55-3).

➤ Nursing Diagnoses

Based on a thorough assessment, several nursing diagnoses identified for the child with CP are primarily related to self-help and to facilitating mobility (see Nursing Care Plan, p. 1588. Other diagnoses may apply in specific cases.

➤ Plan of Care and Implementation

The goals of nursing care for the child with CP and the family are as follows:

1. Child will acquire mobility within personal capabilities.
2. Child will acquire communication skills or use appropriate assistive devices.
3. Child will engage in self-help activities.
4. Child will receive appropriate education.
5. Child will develop a positive self-image.
6. Family will receive appropriate education and support in their efforts to meet the child's needs.
7. Child will receive appropriate care if hospitalized.

Because children are being treated at an earlier age, parents are participating earlier in treatment programs for their disabled child. They are taught the proper handling and home care of young children with CP and need a carefully planned program so that their change of role from parent to therapist can be melded into the already-established relationship. Nurses reinforce the therapeutic plan and assist the family in devising and modifying equipment and activities to continue the therapy program in the home.

Therapeutic interventions are those that are most appropriate for the specific problem and that best suit the needs of the individual child at any given time. Passive range-of-motion exercises, stretching, and elongation exercises are valuable at any age, even at early ages when the child is unable to cooperate. They are of particular value for postural abnormalities around various joints.

Training in manual skills and activities of daily living proceeds along developmental lines and according to the child's functional level. Sitting, balancing, crawling, and walking are encouraged at appropriate ages, accompanied by stimulation of protective extension and equilibrium reactions. Hand activities are begun early to improve motor function and provide the child with sensory experiences and information about the environment. As the child progresses from simple feeding and self-care activities, training is extended to include other tasks, such as cooking or typing, that are within the child's developmental and functional capabilities.

Incorporating play into the therapeutic program often requires great ingenuity and inventiveness from those involved in the child's care. Objects and toys are chosen to provide needed sensory input, using a variety of shapes, forms, and textures. Nurses can help parents integrate therapy into play activities in natural ways.

The child may need considerable help (and patience) in learning to feed, dress, and care for personal hygiene needs.

Box 55-3
Warning Signs of Cerebral Palsy

PHYSICAL SIGNS
Poor head control after 3 months of age
Stiff or rigid arms or legs
Pushing away or arching back
Floppy or limp body posture
Cannot sit up without support by 8 months
Uses only one side of the body, or only the arms to crawl

BEHAVIORAL SIGNS
Extreme irritability or crying
Failure to smile by 3 months
Feeding difficulties
- Persistent gagging or choking when fed
- After 6 months of age, tongue pushes soft food out of the mouth

Data from Pathways Awareness Foundation: *Parents . . . if you see any of these warning signs . . . don't delay,* Chicago, 1991, The Foundation.

Children should be fed in the normal eating position. When they have difficulty with sucking and swallowing, it is tempting to hold them in a semireclining posture to make use of gravity flow. This method does not promote active swallowing, however, and the neck hyperextension may even interfere with swallowing. A more flexed sitting position with arms brought forward to decrease the tendency toward back and neck extension is more natural during bottle- or spoon-feeding and encourages active swallowing (Suresh-Babu et al, 1998).

Because jaw control is compromised, more normal control can be achieved if the feeder provides stability of the oral mechanism from the side or front of the face. When directed from the front, the middle finger of the nonfeeding hand is placed posterior to the body portion of the chin, the thumb is placed below the bottom lip, and the index finger is placed parallel to the child's mandible (Fig. 55-3). Manual jaw control from the side assists with head control, correction of neck and trunk hyperextension, and jaw stabilization. The middle finger of the nonfeeding hand is placed posterior to the bony portion of the chin, the index finger is placed on the chin below the lower lip, and the thumb is placed obliquely across the cheek to provide lateral jaw stability (Fig. 55-4).

Speech training under the supervision of a speech therapist is begun early, before the child learns poor habits of communication. Parents and others can help by following the directions of the speech therapist and by talking slowly to the child and using pictures or handling objects about which the adult is speaking. Feeding techniques that force the child to use the lips and tongue in eating help to facilitate speech (e.g., placing food at the side of the tongue, first one side and then the other; making the child use the lips to take food from a spoon rather than placing it directly on the tongue; and avoiding using the teeth to remove the food from the utensil). If severe dysarthria prevents articulate speech and the child has reasonable intelligence, nonverbal communication, such as sign language, is taught.

As in all aspects of care, educational requirements are determined by the child's needs and potential. Children with mild to moderate involvement are generally able to participate, for varying amounts of time, in regular classes. Resource rooms are available in most schools to provide more individualized attention to a child's particular needs. Integration of these children into regular classrooms should be the initial goal. For those who are unable to benefit from formal education, a training program may be appropriate. At adolescence, prevocational and vocational counseling and guidance are arranged. At any phase or in any setting, education is geared toward the child's assets.

Recreational outlets and after-school activities should be considered for the child who is unable to participate in the regular athletic programs and other peer activities. Some children can compete in athletic and artistic endeavors, and many games and pastimes are suited to their capabilities. Competitive sports are also becoming increasingly available to children with disabilities and offer an added dimension to physical activities. Information on training programs and competition on local, state, regional, and national levels can be obtained from the National Association of Sports for Cerebral Palsy through United Cerebral Palsy Associations.*

Recreational activities serve to stimulate children's interest and curiosity, help them adjust to their disability, improve their functional abilities, and build self-esteem. Any accomplishment that helps children approach a "normal" way of life enhances their self-concept.

Family Support. Probably the nursing interventions most valuable to the family are support and help in coping with the emotional aspects of the disorder, many of which are discussed in relation to the child with a disability (see Chapter 41). Initially the parents need supportive counseling directed toward understanding the implications of the diagnosis and all of the feelings that it engenders. Later they need clarification regarding what they can expect from the child and from health pro-

*1660 L St. NW, Suite 700, Washington, DC 20036; 1-800-872-5827; voice/TDD: (202) 776-0406; fax (202) 776-0414; e-mail: ucpntl.org; website: www.ucpa.org. In Canada: Ontario Federation of Cerebral Palsy, 1630 Lawrence Ave. W, Suite 104, Toronto, Ontario M6L 1C5; (416) 244-9686.

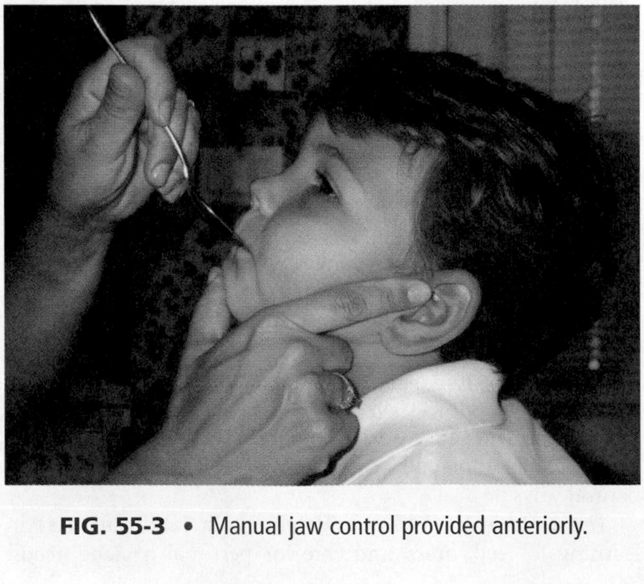

FIG. 55-3 • Manual jaw control provided anteriorly.

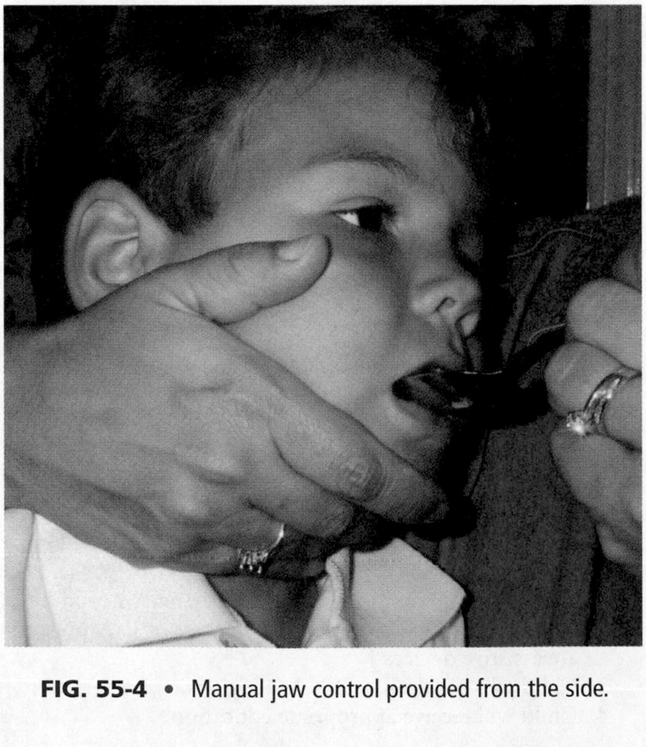

FIG. 55-4 • Manual jaw control provided from the side.

fessionals. Having a child with CP creates numerous challenges of daily management and changes in family life.

The nurse needs to support the parents in their frustration, their problem solving, their concerns, their approaches to helping the child, and their lack of gratification, as well as the positive approaches they use. All of these aspects must be explored and discussed. Parents, as well as other members of the family, require support and counseling. Siblings of a child with a disability are affected and may respond to the presence of the child with overt or less evident behavioral problems. The family needs a relationship with nurses who can provide continued contact, support, and encouragement through the long process of habilitation.

Parents can also find help and solace from parent support groups. They can share problems and concerns with, and derive comfort and practical information from others. Parent groups are most helpful through sharing experiences and accomplishments. For example, parents can understand from others what it is like to have a child with CP, which is generally not possible from professionals (Family Focus box). The national organization United Cerebral Palsy Associations has branches in most communities. The address of the nearest branch can be obtained by consulting a local telephone directory, local agency directory, or a local health department or by writing to the national headquarters. The association provides a variety of services for children and families. A number of excellent books also are available to serve as guides for parents and nurses who work with the child with CP.

The Hospitalized Child. CP is not a disorder that requires hospitalization; therefore, when children with CP are hospitalized, they are usually admitted for another reason or for corrective surgery. Consequently, many nurses are not accustomed to handling these children. Nurses who have never been associated with a child with CP may react in a variety of ways, including fear, revulsion, or overwhelming pity. The basic concept to keep in mind when caring for these children is that they are, first of all, children, who happen to have a disorder that limits their capacities in performing some activities of daily living and, for some, in communicating with others.

Children with CP should be approached and treated the same as any children in the hospital. The nurse's actions should convey acceptance, affection, and friendliness and promote a feeling of trust and dependability in the child. This is especially true with older children who have normal intelligence but who may have communication problems. Speech impairment is common in children with CP. All too often, nurses tend to "talk down" to these children and do things for them that they are perfectly capable of doing for themselves, although not as adeptly. This is especially humiliating to teenagers, who value their independence and self-esteem.

To facilitate the care and management of these children, the therapy program should be continued, insofar as their condition allows, during the time they are hospitalized. This should be incorporated into the nursing care plans and every effort should be made to ensure that the ground that has been so laboriously gained is not lost. Encouraging the parent to room-in and actively participate in the child's care facilitates a continuation of the home therapy program and helps the child adjust to an unfamiliar environment. However, it is equally important to remember that a hospitalization may be the first time a parent can defer care to a nurse and not be the primary caregiver. This respite may be crucial to the parent's well-being.

➤ Evaluation

The effectiveness of nursing interventions is determined by continual reassessment and evaluation of care based on the following observational guidelines:

1. Observe child's movements and use of mobilization devices.
2. Observe child's speech and ability to use communication devices.
3. Observe child's activities, especially those related to self-care.
4. Interview family regarding child's activities and school attendance.
5. Observe child's interactions with others and choice of activities; interview child regarding feelings and concerns.
6. Interview family regarding their feelings and concerns and observe family members' interaction with the child.
7. Observe child's behavior and responses during hospitalization.

The expected outcomes are described in the Nursing Care Plan.

Family Focus

THE REALITY OF ACCEPTANCE OF CEREBRAL PALSY

Acceptance is rarely achieved in the length of time implied in the literature.

In the first place, what is it? To me, it is the end of comparing my son with every other child I see. I focus on *his* gains, not society's expectations.

It is also being able to laugh periodically *at* his "clumsiness." It is "gallows humor" as he achieves adulthood; jokes about CP can be funny now.

The bitterness is gone; I am now happy for people who have children without CP.

I no longer feel sorry for my son, but rather for the people who cannot see him for the great person he is; the CP does *not* come first.

He is now a young man of 25 years and I am learning to accept his independence.

It is a "never-ending story."

Elaine A. Dunham, RN
Shriner's Hospital
Springfield, MA

Spina Bifida (Myelomeningocele)

Abnormalities that are derived from the embryonic neural tube *(neural tube defects [NTDs])* constitute the largest group of congenital anomalies that is consistent with multifactorial inheritance. Normally the spinal cord and cauda equina are encased in a protective sheath of bone and meninges (Fig. 55-5, *A*). Failure of neural tube closure produces defects of varying degrees (Box 55-4). They may involve the entire length of the neural tube or may be restricted to a small area.

In the United States, rates of NTDs have declined from 1.3 per 1000 births in 1970 to 0.32 per 1000 births in 1996 (Lary and Edmonds, 1996). A partial explanation is the increased use

Nursing Care Plan THE CHILD WITH CEREBRAL PALSY

NURSING DIAGNOSIS Impaired physical mobility related to neuromuscular impairment

EXPECTED OUTCOME Child engages in activities appropriate to physical limitations.

Nursing Interventions/*Rationales*

Encourage gross and fine motor activities (e.g., sitting, crawling, walking, grasping, throwing) at appropriate ages *to facilitate optimum motor development.*

Refer to therapeutic modalities (physical therapy) that strengthen muscles, relax increased muscle tone, and improve control and balance *to facilitate optimum motor development.*

Balance rest and activity *to provide optimum energy for motor trials.*

Use aids such as parallel bars, crutches, and orthoses (braces) *to facilitate locomotion.*

Use passive and active range of motion and stretching exercises *to facilitate muscle development, prevent flexion contractures, and maintain joint flexibility.*

NURSING DIAGNOSIS Self-care deficit related to physical disability

EXPECTED OUTCOME Child engages in self-care activities commensurate with capabilities.

Nursing Interventions/*Rationales*

Encourage child to assist in self-care activities as age and capabilities permit, discourage parents from doing them for the child *to foster independence and confidence in abilities.*

Modify environment, introduce use of assistive devices and specialized equipment, devise alternative methods of completing tasks as needed *to facilitate maximum functioning.*

Use therapeutic play and adapted toys *to increase developmental and functional abilities and encourage cooperation of child.*

Emphasize child's abilities, praise effort and accomplishments, promote and reinforce successful endeavors *to foster a sense of self-esteem and competence.*

Refer to therapeutic modalities (e.g., physical therapy [PT], speech therapy, and occupational therapy [OT]) for strengthening of oral motor muscles, development of swallowing control, evaluation and work with adaptive devices *to enhance functional ADLs.*

NURSING DIAGNOSIS Risk for injury related to physical, perceptual impairment

EXPECTED OUTCOME Child exhibits no evidence of injury.

Nursing Interventions/*Rationales*

Promote and teach child and family proper use of adaptive and protective devices (e.g., crutches, walkers, braces, helmets, large-handled utensils) *to enhance safety.*

Modify environment as appropriate (e.g., pad furniture: avoid throw rugs, polished floors, deep carpets; put side rails on bed; remove hazards and barriers, clear traffic areas) *to enhance safety.*

Provide adequate rest *to prevent fatigue, which increases injury risk.*

Use feeding techniques and assistive devices (feed in upright position, stroke throat to aid swallowing), which encourage intake and proper swallowing *to minimize choking and aspiration.*

Use restraints in car and when seated *to enhance safety.*

Institute seizure precautions if appropriate and administer seizure medications as ordered *to prevent seizure activity and possible injury.*

NURSING DIAGNOSIS Impairment verbal communication related to physical, perceptual impairment

EXPECTED OUTCOME Child demonstrates ability to communicate needs and wants to caregivers.

Nursing Interventions/*Rationales*

Refer to therapeutic modalities (OT, speech therapy) for strengthening of oral motor muscles, evaluation of oral motor abilities, exercises that promote vocalizations/verbalizations, development of verbal and nonverbal communication modalities *to enhance communication.*

Teach caregivers (family, schoolteachers, therapists, nurses) how to use various verbal and nonverbal communication methods and adaptive communications equipment (e.g., communication boards, sign language, computer aids, voice synthesizers) *to enhance communication with others in environment.*

NURSING DIAGNOSIS Fatigue related to increased energy expenditure

EXPECTED OUTCOME Child exhibits signs of adequate rest and optimum nutritional intake.

Nursing Interventions/*Rationales*

Balance activity with frequent rest periods: monitor for any signs of tiredness *to reduce fatigue.*

Provide high-calorie, high-protein diet *to meet increased energy expenditure needs.*

Monitor weight *to evaluate adequacy of intake.*

Carry out a regular schedule of health promotion and maintenance (regular checkups with physician, dentist; immunizations; avoidance of people with infections) *to enhance general state of health.*

Nursing Care Plan THE CHILD WITH CEREBRAL PALSY—cont'd

NURSING DIAGNOSIS Body image/self-esteem disturbances related to perception of disability, feeling different

EXPECTED OUTCOME Child demonstrates acceptance of self, physical appearance, and physical and developmental abilities

Nursing Interventions/*Rationales*

Relate to child on appropriate cognitive level, conveying an attitude of caring and acceptance *to encourage positive feelings about self;* serve as role model for others *to foster positive attitudes of acceptance toward child.*

Encourage child to communicate feelings about the disability (e.g., feelings of differentness, implications of functional limit, difficulty in making friends, views of self) *to facilitate coping.*

Have child identify strengths, assets, things he or she likes about self *to increase positive feelings about self.*

Support positive coping behaviors.

Introduce child to other children who have similar disabilities, arrange for support groups for child and parents *to increase coping skills.*

Refer child for counseling if needed *to enhance adaptation.*

Encourage use of good grooming and age-appropriate dress *to enhance appearance.*

NURSING DIAGNOSIS Altered family processes related to situational crises (child with lifelong disability)

EXPECTED OUTCOME Family will exhibit adaptation of usual roles and functions to accommodate special needs of child, and they will exhibit growth-promoting behaviors.

Nursing Interventions/*Rationales*

Provide opportunity for family to absorb and adjust to diagnosis (e.g., repeat information *to allow time for family to hear and understand;* encourage expression of concerns, fears, and feelings about diagnosis and potential impact *to facilitate adjustment;* identify support systems *to provide resources for coping*).

Assist family to understand expected treatment, rationale, and implications *to provide a sound basis for decision making.*

Explore family reaction to the child; assist them to achieve a realistic view of child's abilities and limitations; encourage family in attempts to promote child growth and development; have family emphasize what child can do; explore ways for family to include child in family activities *to help family increase abilities to cope with and incorporate child into family structure.*

Identify additional resource systems (e.g., relatives, friends, church, health care services, community programs) and strategize with family about making good use of these systems *to develop broad base of support.*

Provide a system of ongoing follow-up and evaluation *to ensure long-term adaptation to challenges presented to family functioning by a child with a chronic disability.*

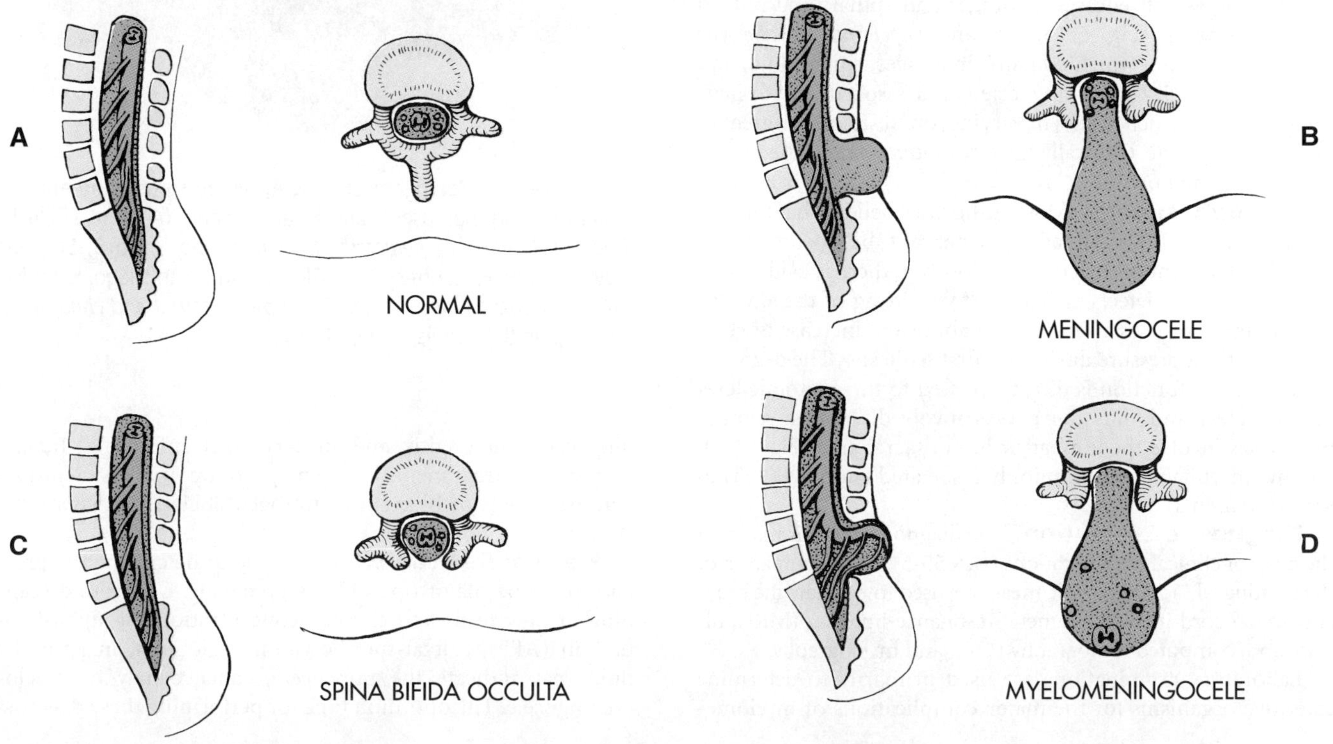

FIG. 55-5 • Midline defects of osseous spine with varying degrees of neural herniations.

Box 55-4

Significant Neural Tube Defects

Cranioschisis—A skull defect through which various tissues protrude
Exancephaly—Brain totally exposed or extruded through an associated skull defect; fetus usually aborted
Anencephaly—If fetus with exancephaly survives, degeneration of the brain to a spongioform mass with no bony covering; incompatible with life usually beyond a few days
Encephalocele—Herniation of brain and meninges through a defect in the skull producing a fluid-filled sac
Rachischisis or **spina bifida**—Fissure in the spinal column that leaves the meninges and spinal cord exposed
Meningocele—Hernial protrusion of a saclike cyst of meninges filled with spinal fluid (Fig. 55-5, *C*)
Myelomeningocele (meningomyelocele)—Hernial protrusion of a saclike cyst containing meninges, spinal fluid, and a portion of the spinal cord with its nerves (Fig. 55-5, *D*)

of prenatal diagnostic techniques and termination of pregnancies. (See also Prevention, p. 1592.)

Myelodysplasia refers broadly to any malformation of the spinal canal and cord. Midline defects involving failure of the osseous (bony) spine to close are called *spina bifida (SB),* the most common defect of the central nervous system. SB is categorized into two types: spina bifida occulta and spina bifida cystica.

Spina bifida occulta refers to a defect that is not visible externally. It occurs most commonly in the lumbosacral area (L5 and S1) (Fig. 55-5, *B*). SB occulta may not be apparent unless there are associated cutaneous manifestations or neuromuscular disturbances.

Spina bifida cystica refers to a visible defect with an external saclike protrusion. The two major forms of SB cystica are *meningocele,* which encases meninges and spinal fluid but no neural elements (Fig. 55-5, *C*), and *myelomeningocele* (or *meningomyelocele*), which contains meninges, spinal fluid, and nerves (Fig. 55-5, *D*). Meningocele is not associated with neurologic deficit, which occurs in varying, often serious, degrees in myelomeningocele. Clinically the term *spina bifida* is used to refer to myelomeningocele.

Pathophysiology. Most authorities believe that the primary defect in NTDs is a failure of neural tube closure during early development of the embryo. However, there is evidence to indicate that the defects are caused by splitting of the already-closed neural tube as a result of an abnormal increase in cerebrospinal fluid pressure during the first trimester. The degree of neurologic dysfunction is directly related to the anatomic level of the defect and thus the nerves involved. Most myelomeningoceles involve the lumbar or lumbosacral area (Fig. 55-6), and hydrocephalus is a commonly associated anomaly (90% to 95% of patients).

Diagnostic Evaluation. The diagnosis of SB is made on the basis of clinical manifestations (Box 55-5) and examination of the meningeal sac. Diagnostic measures used to evaluate the brain and spinal cord include magnetic resonance imaging (MRI), ultrasound, computed tomography (CT), and myelography.

Laboratory examinations are used primarily to determine causative organisms for the major complications of myelomeningocele—meningitis and urinary tract infections. Infants with urinary tract incontinence may require urinalysis, culture, and evaluation of blood urea nitrogen (BUN) and creatinine clearance.

A

B

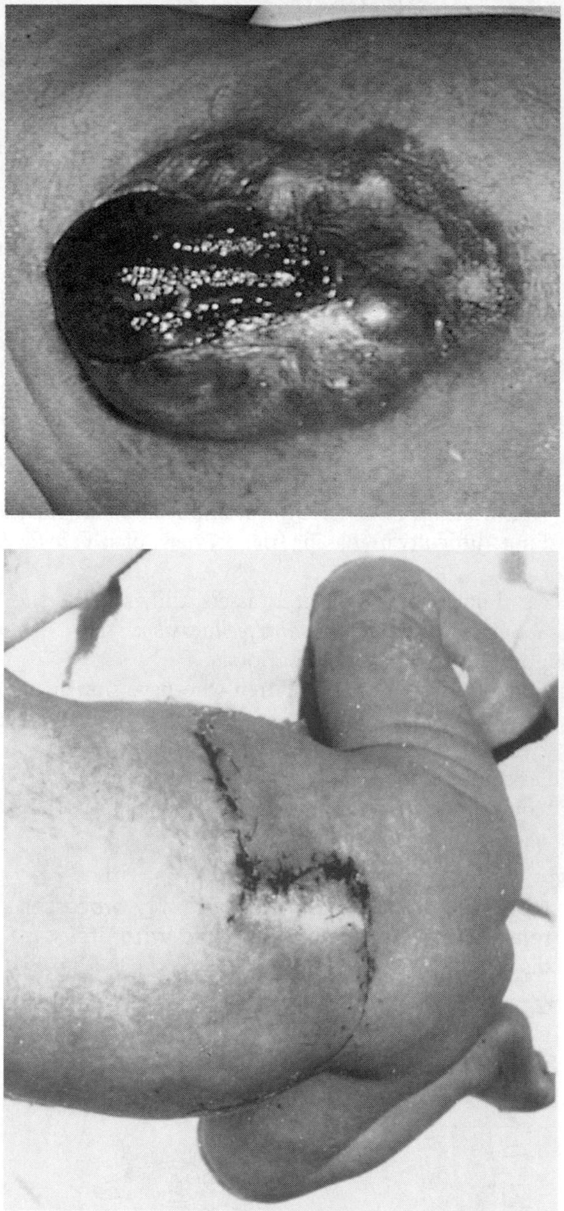

FIG. 55-6 • Meningomyelocele. **A,** before surgery (an antibacterial dressing was used); and **B,** after repair. (A, from Zitelli BJ, Davis HW: *Atlas of pediatric physical diagnosis,* ed 3, St Louis, 1997, Mosby; B, Courtesy M.C. Gleason, MD, San Diego. From Novak JC, Broom BL: *Ingalls and Salerno's maternal and child health nursing,* ed 8, St Louis, 1995, Mosby.)

Prenatal Detection. It is possible to determine the presence of some major open NTDs prenatally. Ultrasound scanning of the uterus and elevated concentrations of alpha-fetoprotein (AFP), a fetal-specific gamma$_1$-globulin, in amniotic fluid may indicate the presence of anencephaly or myelomeningocele. The optimum time for performing these diagnos-

Box 55-5

Clinical Manifestations of Spina Bifida

SPINA BIFIDA CYSTICA

Sensory disturbances usually parallel motor dysfunction
- Below second lumbar vertebra:
  - Flaccid, partial paralysis of lower extremities
  - Varying degrees of sensory deficit
  - Overflow incontinence with constant dribbling of urine
  - Lack of bowel control
  - Rectal prolapse (sometimes)
- Below third sacral vertebra:
  - No motor impairment
  - May be saddle anesthesia with bladder and anal sphincter paralysis

Joint deformities (sometimes produced in utero):
- Talipes valgus or varus contractures
- Kyphosis
- Lumbosacral scoliosis
- Hip dislocations

SPINA BIFIDA OCCULTA

Often no observable manifestations

May be associated with one or more cutaneous manifestations:
- Skin depression or dimple
- Port-wine angiomatous nevi
- Dark tufts of hair
- Soft, subcutaneous lipomas

May be neuromuscular disturbances:
- Progressive disturbance of gait with foot weakness
- Bowel and bladder sphincter disturbances

tic tests is between 16 and 18 weeks of gestation, before AFP concentrations normally diminish and in sufficient time to permit a therapeutic abortion. Chorionic villus sampling (CVS) is also a measure for prenatal diagnosis of NTDs. It is recommended that such diagnostic procedures be considered for all mothers who have borne an affected child, and testing is offered to all pregnant women. In addition, elective prelabor cesarean birth may result in less motor dysfunction.

Therapeutic Management. Management of the child who has a myelomeningocele requires a multidisciplinary approach involving the specialties of neurology, neurosurgery, pediatrics, urology, orthopedics, rehabilitation, and physical therapy, as well as intensive nursing care in a variety of specialty areas. The collaborative efforts of these specialists are focused on (1) the myelomeningocele and the problems associated with the defect—hydrocephalus, paralysis, orthopedic deformities, and genitourinary abnormalities; (2) possible acquired problems that may or may not be associated, such as meningitis, hypoxia, and hemorrhage; and (3) other abnormalities, such as cardiac or gastrointestinal malformations.

Infancy. Initial care of the newborn involves prevention of infection; neurologic assessment, including observation for associated anomalies; and dealing with the impact of the anomaly on the family. Although meningoceles are repaired early, especially if there is danger of rupture of the sac, the philosophy regarding skin closure of myelomeningocele varies. Most authorities believe that early closure, within the first 24 to 72 hours, offers the most favorable outcome. Early closure, preferably in the first 12 to 18 hours, not only prevents local infection and trauma to the exposed tissues but also avoids stretching of other nerve roots, which may occur as the meningeal sac expands during the first hours after birth, thus preventing further motor impairment.

Associated problems are assessed and managed by appropriate surgical and supportive measures. Shunt procedures provide relief from imminent or progressive hydrocephalus (see Chapter 51). Meningitis, urinary tract infection, and pneumonia are treated with vigorous antibiotic therapy and supportive measures. Surgical intervention for Arnold-Chiari malformation (a downward herniation of the brain into the brainstem) or for tethered cord (scar tissue binding the spinal cord) is indicated only when the child is symptomatic.

Improved surgical techniques do not alter the major physical disability, spinal defect, or chronic urinary tract and pulmonary infections that affect the quality of life for these children. Superimposed on the physical problems are the effects that the disorder has on family life and finances, including the need for specialized school and hospital services.

Orthopedic Considerations. According to most orthopedists, musculoskeletal problems that will affect later locomotion should be evaluated early, and treatment, where indicated, should be instituted without delay. Neurologic assessment will determine the neurosegmental level of the lesion, recognition of spasticity and progressive paralysis, potential for deformity, and functional expectations. Orthopedic management includes preventing joint contractures, correcting the deformity, preventing skin breakdown, and obtaining the best possible locomotor function. The status of the neurologic deficit remains the most important factor in determining the child's ultimate functional abilities.

A variety of devices are available to provide mobility to children with spinal cord lesions, including lightweight braces, special "walking" devices, and custom-built wheelchairs (see also Chapter 42). Corrective procedures, when indicated, are best initiated at an early age so that the child will not lag significantly behind age-mates in developmental progress. Where there is little hope for lower extremity functioning, surgery is seldom recommended unless it will improve sitting position in a wheelchair and function for activities of daily living and mobility.

Management of Genitourinary Function. Myelomeningocele is one of the most common causes of *neuropathic (neurogenic) bladder dysfunction* in children. In infants the goal of treatment is to preserve renal function. In older children the goal is to preserve renal function and achieve optimum urinary continence. Urinary incontinence, a chronic, often debilitating problem, typically arises from the dysfunctional bladder. In addition, neuropathic bladder dysfunction may predispose the child to *urinary system distress* (e.g., infection, ureterohydronephrosis, and vesicoureteral reflux). The characteristics of bladder dysfunction in children vary according to the level of the lesion and the influence of bony growth and development on the spine. Therefore urodynamic testing during infancy and early childhood is important because bladder function changes. The presence of hydrocephalus has the potential to affect bladder function, although spinal influences are predominant.

Treatment of renal problems includes (1) regular urologic care with prompt and vigorous treatment of infections; (2) some type of regular emptying of the bladder, such as clean intermittent catheterization (CIC) taught to and performed by parents and self-catheterization taught to children; (3) medications to improve bladder storage and continence, such as oxybutynin chloride (Ditropan), propantheline (Pro-Banthine), and tolterodine (Detrol); and (4) surgical procedures such as *vesicostomy* (stoma created on the abdominal wall for urinary drainage) and *augmentation enterocystoplasty* (increases bladder capacity and reduces high bladder pressures).

Rarely children with myelodysplasia may develop severe dysfunction of the bladder that compromises renal function or produces debilitating urinary incontinence that is intractable to other means. *Urinary diversion,* typically using a continent neobladder constructed from bowel or stomach, may be required. Whenever feasible, the neobladder is constructed in a way that allows continence, and CIC is used to regularly evacuate urine.

Bowel Control. Some degree of fecal continence can usually be achieved in most children with myelomeningocele with diet modification, regular toilet habits, and prevention of constipation and impaction. It is commonly a lengthy process. Fiber supplements, laxatives, suppositories, and/or enemas aid in producing regular evacuation.

Prognosis. The early prognosis for the child with myelomeningocele depends on the neurologic deficit present at birth, including motor ability and bladder innervation and the presence of associated cerebral anomalies. Early surgical repair of the spinal defect, antibiotic therapy to reduce the incidence of meningitis and ventriculitis, prevention of urinary system dysfunction, and early detection and correction of hydrocephalus have significantly increased the survival rate of such children. Based on current medical knowledge and ethical considerations, aggressive management is favored for the child with myelomeningocele.

Prevention. The widespread use of folic acid among women of childbearing age is expected to significantly decrease the incidence of SB. It has been estimated that a daily intake of 0.4 mg of folic acid in women of childbearing age will prevent 50% to 70% of all cases of neural tube defects (Centers for Disease Control and Prevention [CDC], 1999). For women who have had a previous pregnancy affected by NTDs, this intake is increased to 4 mg under supervision of a practitioner beginning 1 month before a planned pregnancy and continuing during the first trimester. Supplementation of 4 mg of folate should not be given in multivitamin preparations because of the risk of overdose of other vitamins. However, despite the recommendations of several health care and public agencies (Institute of Medicine, 1998) for the daily intake of 0.4 folic acid in the periconceptual period, a recent survey revealed that only a small percentage of women of childbearing age actually follow these guidelines (CDC, 1999). Awareness of the benefits of folic acid for the prevention of birth defects was lowest in women aged 18 to 24 years and in women with less than a high school education. These results indicate that nurses and other health care workers have an important task in disseminating information that may decrease the incidence of birth defects in children by promoting maternal consumption of folic acid.* To ensure adequate daily intake of the recommended amount of folic acid, women must take a folic acid supplement, eat a fortified breakfast cereal containing 100% of the Recommended Dietary Allowance (RDA) of folic acid (Kellogg's Product 19 and General Mills Total and Multi-Grain Cheerios Plus), or increase their consumption of fortified foods (cereal, bread, rice, grits, pasta), and foods naturally rich in folate (green leafy vegetables and citrus fruits).

NURSE ALERT • Because approximately one half of all pregnancies in the United States are unplanned (Henshaw, 1998), adolescent girls and women of childbearing age need to be educated about the necessity of folic acid to prevent neural tube defects. The daily dose of 0.4 mg (400 μg) is most easily obtained from a multivitamin supplement.

Nursing Care Management. At birth an examination is performed to assess the intactness of the membranous cyst. During transport to the nursery, every effort is made to prevent trauma to this protective covering. In addition to the routine assessment of the newborn, the infant is assessed for the level of neurologic involvement. Movement of extremities or skin response, especially an anal reflex, that might provide clues to the degree of motor or sensory impairment is noted. It is important to observe the infant's behavior in conjunction with the stimulus because limb movements can be induced in response to spinal cord reflex activity that has no connection with the higher centers. Observation of urine output, especially if a diaper remains dry, may indicate urinary retention. Abdominal assessment revealing bladder distention, even with a wet diaper, may indicate urinary overflow in a retentive bladder. The head circumference is measured daily (see Chapter 35), and the fontanels are examined for signs of tension or bulging.

NURSE ALERT • Avoid measuring rectal temperatures in infants with SB. Because bowel sphincter function is commonly affected, the thermometer can cause irritation and rectal prolapse.

Care of the Myelomeningocele Sac. The infant is usually placed in an incubator or warmer so that temperature can be maintained without clothing or covers that might irritate the delicate lesion. When an overhead warmer is used, the dressings over the defect require more frequent moistening because of the dehydrating effect of the radiant heat.

Before surgical closure the myelomeningocele is prevented from drying by the application of a sterile, moist, nonadherent dressing over the defect. The moistening solution is usually sterile normal saline solution. Dressings are changed frequently (every 2 to 4 hours), and the sac is closely inspected for leaks, abrasions, irritation, or any signs of infection. The sac must be carefully cleansed if it becomes soiled or contaminated. Sometimes the sac ruptures during delivery or transport, and any opening in the sac greatly increases the risk of infection to the central nervous system.

NURSE ALERT • Observe for early signs of infection, such as elevated temperature (axillary), irritability, and lethargy, and for signs of increased intracranial pressure (ICP), which might indicate developing hydrocephalus.

*Information is available from the Centers for Disease Control and Prevention, "Flo" CDC, NCEH, BDPG, MS F-45 4770 Buford Highway NE, Atlanta, GA 30341; (888) 232-6789; e-mail: Flo@cdc.gov; website: www.cdc.gov/nceh/folicacid; and March of Dimes Resource Center, 1275 Mamaroneck Ave., White Plains, NY 10605; (888) MODIMES; website: www.modimes.org.

One of the most difficult, important, and challenging aspects in the early care of the infant with myelomeningocele is positioning. Before surgery the infant is kept in the prone position to minimize tension on the sac and the risk of trauma. The prone position allows for optimum positioning of the legs, especially in cases of associated hip dysplasia. The infant is placed flat with the hips only slightly flexed to reduce tension on the defect. The legs are maintained in abduction with a pad between the knees to counteract hip subluxation, and a small roll is placed under the ankles to maintain a neutral foot position. A variety of aids, including diaper rolls, pads, small sandbags, or specially designed frames and appliances can be used to maintain the desired position.

Prevent Complications. The prone position affects other aspects of the infant's care. For example, in this position the infant is more difficult to keep clean, pressure areas are a constant threat, and feeding becomes a problem. The infant's head is turned to one side for feeding. Fortunately, most defects are repaired early, and the infant can be held for feeding soon after surgery. Special care must be taken to avoid pressure on the operative site.

Diapering the infant may be contraindicated until the defect has been repaired and healing is well advanced or epithelialization has taken place. The padding beneath the diaper area is changed as needed to keep the skin dry and free of irritation. When urinary retention is detected, CIC is used.* Because the bowel sphincter is commonly affected, there is continual passage of stool, often misinterpreted as diarrhea, which is a constant irritant to the skin and a source of infection to the spinal lesion.

Areas of sensory and motor impairment are subject to skin breakdown and therefore require meticulous care. Placing the infant on a special mattress or mattress overlay reduces pressure on the knees and ankles. Periodic cleansing, application of lotion, and gentle massage aid circulation.

Gentle range-of-motion exercises are sometimes carried out to prevent contractures, and stretching of contractures is performed when indicated. However, these exercises may be restricted to the foot, ankle, and knee joint. Where the hip joints are unstable, stretching against tight hip flexors or adductor muscles, which act much like bowstrings, may aggravate a tendency toward subluxation. Consultation with a physical therapist is an important aspect of the short- and long-term management of infants with myelomeningocele.

Some infants with unrepaired myelomeningocele are unable to be held in the arms and cuddled as unaffected infants are, so their need for tactile stimulation is met by caressing, stroking, and other comfort measures. To facilitate handling and to reduce parental anxiety, the infant can recline on a pillow placed in the parent's lap. Individualized developmental care with age-appropriate stimulation is provided.

Provide Postoperative Care. Postoperative care of the infant with myelomeningocele involves the same basic care as that of any postsurgical infant: monitoring vital signs, monitoring intake and output, providing nourishment, observing for signs of infection, and managing pain as needed. Care of the operative site is carried out under the direction of the surgeon and includes close observation for signs of leakage of cerebrospinal fluid. General care is continued as preoperatively.

The prone position is maintained after surgical closure, although many neurosurgeons allow a side-lying or partial side-lying position unless it aggravates a coexisting hip dysplasia or permits undesirable hip flexion. This offers an opportunity for position changes, which reduce the risk of pressure sores and facilitate feeding. If permitted, the infant can be held upright against the body, with care taken to avoid pressure on the operative site. Once the effects of anesthesia have subsided and the infant is alert, feedings may be resumed unless there are other anomalies or associated complications.

Because children who have SB are prone to develop an allergy to latex, reducing exposure to latex from birth on is hoped to decrease the chance of allergy development. Parent education must emphasize preventive measures to avoid latex sensitization. The establishment of a latex-safe environment is being accomplished in many health care facilities where patients (and health care workers) are at high risk (see Latex Allergy, below).

Support Family and Educate About Home Care. As soon as the parents are able to cope with the infant's condition, they are encouraged to become involved in care. They need to learn how to continue at home the care that has been initiated in the hospital—positioning, feeding, skin care, and range-of-motion exercises when appropriate. They are taught CIC technique when it is prescribed. They need to know the signs of complications and how to obtain assistance when needed. When the defect has not been repaired, they are taught to care for the lesion.

The long-range planning with and support of the parents and child begin in the hospital and extend throughout childhood and even beyond. Long-term care of these children is of uncertain length, although the life expectancy is of average length, well into adulthood. Nurses assume an important role as a central member of the health team. As a coordinator, the nurse reviews information with the family, takes responsibility for family teaching, and acts as a liaison between inpatient and outpatient services. The child may need numerous hospitalizations over the years, and each one will be a source of stress, to which the younger child is especially vulnerable. (See Chapter 41 for a discussion of care of the child with a disability.)

Habilitation involves not only solving problems of self-help and locomotion but also solving the distressing problem of incontinence, which threatens the child's social acceptability. Assistance with preparing the child and the school regarding the special needs of the child helps provide a better initial adjustment to this broader social experience. The Spina Bifida Association of America* is organized to provide services and support for families of children with spinal lesions.

(See also Nursing Care Plan: The Infant with Myelomeningocele.†)

Latex Allergy. Latex allergy was identified as being a serious health hazard when a report linked intraoperative anaphylaxis with latex in children with SB. These children are at

*Community and home care instructions on performing clean intermittent self-catheterization (CIC) are available in Wong DL, Hess CS: ***Wong and Whaley's clinical manual of pediatric nursing,*** ed 5, St Louis, 2000, Mosby.

*4590 MacArthur NW, Suite 250, Washington, DC 20007-4226; (202) 944-3285 or 1-800-621-3141; website: www.sbaa.org.

†In Wong DL, Hess CS: ***Wong and Whaley's clinical manual of pediatric nursing,*** ed 5, St Louis, 2000, Mosby.

high risk for developing latex allergy because of repeated exposure to latex products during surgery and from numerous bladder catheterizations (Carroll, 1999). Allergic reactions range from urticaria, wheezing, watery eyes, and rashes to anaphylactic shock. More severe reactions tend to occur when latex comes in contact with mucous membranes, wet skin, the bloodstream, or an airway. There also can be cross-reactions to a number of foods (e.g., banana, avocado, kiwi, chestnut). In addition to patients with SB, high risk populations include patients with urogenital anomalies or multiple surgeries, as well as health care workers. Box 55-6 lists the medical conditions associated with SB. The incidence of latex allergy in children with SB ranges from an estimated 18% to 67% (Carroll, 1999; Kellett, 1997).

The most important goals are prevention of latex allergy and identification of children with a known hypersensitivity (Guidelines box). High risk and latex-allergic individuals must be managed in a *latex-safe* environment. Care must be taken so that they do not come in direct or secondary contact with products or equipment containing latex at any time during medical treatment. Allergy testing has been used with varying success to identify latex allergy. Skin prick testing and provocation testing carry the risk of allergic reaction or anaphylaxis. The radioallergosorbent test (RAST) has been used to measure the serum level of latex-specific IgE. The RAST has been shown to be 90% to 95% sensitive (Kellett, 1997). Pretreatment with antihistamines and steroids (dexamethasone) before and after surgery to reduce the possibility of a serious reaction remains controversial because it may interfere with healing.

Latex, a natural product derived from the rubber tree, is used in combination with other chemicals to give elasticity, strength, and durability to many products. There are published lists of products, such as vinyl gloves, that may be substituted for latex.* In the health care arena it is important to use products with the lowest potential risk of sensitizing patients and staff members. User labeling for latex-containing devices that come into contact directly or indirectly with live human tissue was instituted by the Food and Drug Administration (FDA) in 1998.

The American Nurses Association (ANA) (1997), National Institute for Occupational Safety and Health (NIOSH) (1997), and Occupational Safety and Health Administration (OSHA) (1999) have issued statements on latex allergies emphasizing that all health care institutions should abandon the unnecessary use of latex gloves and provide low-allergen, powder-free latex gloves in other settings. Procedures for the identification and treatment of latex-sensitive patients, provision of latex-free medical products, and reporting of allergic events related to latex medical devices to the FDA MedWatch Program are also strongly advocated by the ANA.† In addition, the ANA recommends that each health care facility have a multidisciplinary task force to develop occupational health guidelines to ensure a safe environment for health care workers to minimize latex exposure, identify those at risk for reaction to latex, and accommodate the needs of latex-sensitive employees.

The identification of those sensitive to latex is best accomplished through careful screening of *all* patients. (See Guidelines box for questions related to latex allergy.)

NURSE ALERT • **During the health interview ask all patients, not only those at risk, about allergic reactions to latex. Be sure that this is a routine part of all preoperative and preprocedural histories. Stress the importance of the allergy history to all personnel (e.g., phlebotomists).**

Children with latex allergy should carry or wear some form of medical identification. Education programs regarding latex hypersensitivity are aimed at those who care for high risk groups, such as children with SB, and may include relatives, school nurses, teachers, child care workers, and baby-sitters. In addition to educating caregivers about the child's exposure to medical products that contain latex, nurses need to inform them of common nonmedical latex objects. Items brought to

Box 55-6

Medical Conditions Associated with Risk of Latex Allergy

Spina bifida
Urogenital anomalies
Imperforate anus
Tracheoesophageal fistula
VATER association (*v*ertebral defects, imperforate *a*nus, *t*racheoesophageal fistula, and *r*adial and renal dysplasia)
Preterm infants
Ventriculoperitoneal shunt
Mental retardation
Cerebral palsy
Quadriplegia
Multiple surgeries
Atopy

Guidelines

IDENTIFYING LATEX ALLERGY

Does your child have any symptoms, such as sneezing, coughing, rashes, or wheezing, when handling rubber products (e.g., balloons, tennis or Koosh balls, adhesive bandage strips), or when in contact with rubber hospital products (e.g., gloves, catheters)?
Has your child ever had an allergic reaction during surgery?
Does your child have a history of rashes, asthma, or allergic reactions to medication or foods, especially milk, kiwi, bananas, or chestnuts?
How would you identify or recognize an allergic reaction in your child?
What would you do if an allergic reaction occurred?
Has anyone ever discussed latex or rubber allergy or sensitivity with you?
Has your child had any allergy testing?
When did your child last come in contact with any type of rubber product? Were you present?

Modified from Romanczuk A: Latex use with infants and children: it can cause problems, *MCN* 18(4):208–212, 1993.

*For an updated list of latex-free items (medical and community) and alternative products, contact the Spina Bifida Association of America, 4590 MacArthur Blvd. NW, Suite 250, Washington, DC 20007-4226; (202) 944-3285 or 1-800-621-3141; website: www.sbaa.org. Additional information regarding latex allergy may be found at the following website: www.latexallergyhelp.com.

†The FDA Medical Products Reporting Program, Food and Drug Administration, 5600 Fishers Lane, Rockville, MD 20852-9787; 1-800-FDA-1088; fax 1-800-FDA-0178; website: www.fda.gov/medwatch.

the hospital, such as floral bouquets, are also screened for latex toys or balloons. Parents should also be given literature explaining signs and symptoms of latex hypersensitivity and appropriate emergency treatment (see Anaphylaxis, Chapter 48).

Progressive Infantile Spinal Muscular Atrophy (Werdnig-Hoffmann Disease)

Progressive infantile spinal muscular atrophy (Werdnig-Hoffmann disease) is characterized by progressive weakness and wasting of skeletal muscles. It is inherited as an autosomal-recessive trait and is the most common paralytic form of the *floppy infant syndrome (congenital hypotonia).* The degeneration occurs in the anterior horn cells of the spinal cord and the motor nuclei of the brainstem, with the primary result being atrophy of skeletal muscles. The age of onset is variable, but the earlier the onset, the more disseminated and severe the motor weakness (Iannaccone, 1998).

Therapeutic Management. The diagnosis is suspected on the basis of clinical manifestations (Box 55-7). It is established by electromyography demonstrating a denervation pattern and is confirmed by muscle biopsy. Treatment is symptomatic and preventive, primarily preventing infection and treating orthopedic problems, the most serious of which is scoliosis. Many children benefit from powered chairs, lifts, special mattresses, and accessible environmental controls. Vigorous antibiotic therapy and chest physiotherapy are implemented during upper respiratory infections.

Prognosis. Prognosis varies according to age of onset or group as described in Box 55-7. However, recent observations suggest that the classification is not valid. Individuals with group 1 manifestations had a life span of 4 months to 31 years. Also, some affected persons did not demonstrate progressive loss of strength and function (Russman, 1996).

Nursing Care Management. The infant or small child with extensive paralysis requires frequent change of position to prevent physical injury and complications, especially pneumonia. The pharynx requires suctioning to remove secretions, and feeding must be carried out slowly and carefully to prevent aspiration. Because these children are intellectually normal, verbal, tactile, and auditory stimulation are important aspects of care. Supporting them so that they can see the activities around them and transporting them in appropriate conveyances (i.e., carriage, wagon, wheelchair) for a change of environment provide stimulation and a broader scope of contacts.

Children who are able to sit require proper support and attention to alignment to prevent deformities and other complications. Children who survive beyond infancy will need attention to educational needs and opportunities for social interaction with other children. The parents of a child who is chronically or potentially fatally ill require support and encouragement (see Chapter 41). The parents of a child with a genetically transmitted disorder also need to be encouraged to seek genetic counseling, especially if they are planning to have other children.

Box 55-7

Clinical Manifestations of Spinal Muscular Atrophy

GROUP 1 (WERDNIG-HOFFMANN DISEASE)

Disease acquired in utero or during first 2 months of life
Inactivity is most prominent feature
Infant lies in the frog position with legs externally rotated, abducted, and flexed at knees
Weakness
Limited movements of shoulder and arm muscles
Active movement is usually limited to fingers and toes
Diaphragmatic breathing with sternal retractions
Weak cry and cough
Secretions tend to pool in pharynx
Alert facies
Normal sensation and intellect
Affected infants do not progress to sit alone, roll over, or walk
Early death (usually by 4 years of age) from respiratory failure or infection

GROUP 2 (INTERMEDIATE SMA)

Disease manifested between 2 and 12 months of age
Early—weakness confined to arms and legs
Later—becomes generalized
Legs usually involved to greater extent than arms
Prominent pectus excavatum
Movements absent during complete relaxation or sleep
Some infants able to sit if placed in position
Life span varies from 7 months to 7 years

GROUP 3 (KUGELBERG-WELANDER SYNDROME)

Onset of symptoms in first year of life
Normal head control and can sit unassisted by 6 to 8 months of age
Thigh and hip muscles weak
In those who manage to walk:
- Lumbar lordosis
- Waddling gait
- Genu recurvatum
- Protuberant abdomen
- Ambulation becomes increasingly difficult
- Confined to a wheelchair by second decade

Deep tendon reflexes may be present early but disappear

NOTE: These classifications are general, but some research suggests there may be variations in life span and other characteristics (Russman et al, 1992; Russman, 1996).

Juvenile Spinal Muscular Atrophy (Kugelberg-Welander Disease)

Juvenile spinal muscular atrophy (Kugelberg-Welander disease, juvenile proximal hereditary muscular atrophy) is also a result of anterior horn cell and motor nerve degeneration. The disease is characterized by a pattern of muscular weakness similar to that of infantile spinal muscular atrophy (see Box 55-7). Several modes of inheritance have been reported for the disease: autosomal-recessive, autosomal-dominant, and X-linked recessive.

The onset occurs from less than 1 year of age into adulthood, with symptoms resembling those of group 3 infantile spinal muscular atrophy; proximal muscle weakness (especially of the lower limbs) and muscular atrophy are the predominant features. The disease runs a slowly progressive course. Some children lose the ability to walk 8 to 9 years after the onset of symptoms, but many can still walk after 30 years or more. Many affected persons have a normal life expectancy (Iannaccone, 1998).

Therapeutic Management and Nursing Care Management. The management is primarily symptomatic and supportive and is related to maintaining mobility as long as possible, preventing complications, and providing support to the child and family.

Muscular Dystrophies (MDs)

MDs constitute the largest and most important single group of muscle diseases of childhood. They all have a genetic origin in which there is gradual degeneration of muscle fibers, and they are characterized by progressive weakness and wasting of symmetric groups of skeletal muscles, with increasing disability and deformity. In all forms of MD there is insidious loss of strength, but each type differs in regard to muscle groups affected (Fig. 55-7), age of onset, rate of progression, and inheritance patterns. Although the etiology of MD is unknown, it appears to be related to a metabolic disturbance unrelated to the nervous system. Serum creatinine phosphokinase is consistently elevated in affected individuals, which assists in diagnosis and early detection (Voit, 1998). The most common form, *Duchenne muscular dystrophy,* is considered separately in the next section.

Facioscapulohumeral (Landouzy-Déjérine) muscular dystrophy is inherited as an autosomal-dominant disorder with onset in early adolescence. It is characterized by difficulty in raising the arms over the head, lack of facial mobility, and a forward slope of the shoulders. The progression is slow, and the life span is usually unaffected.

Limb-girdle muscular dystrophy is an autosomal-recessive disease of later childhood or adolescence with variable but usually slow progression; it is characterized by weakness of proximal muscles of the pelvic and shoulder girdles.

Treatment of the MDs consists mainly of supportive measures, including physical therapy, orthopedic procedures to minimize deformity, and assistance for the affected child in meeting the demands of daily living.

Pseudohypertrophic (Duchenne) Muscular Dystrophy (DMD)

DMD is the most severe and the most common MD of childhood. An X-linked inheritance pattern is identified in most patients; about one third of all cases represent fresh mutations. As in all X-linked disorders, males are affected almost exclusively. At the genetic level, DMD results from mutation of the gene that encodes *dystrophin,* a protein product in skeletal muscle. The incidence is approximately 1:3500 male births (Multicenter Study Group, 1992). Box 55-8 describes the characteristics of DMD.

Evidence of muscle weakness usually appears during the third year, although there may have been a history of delay in motor development, particularly walking. Difficulties in running, riding a bicycle, and climbing stairs are usually the first symptoms noted. Later, abnormal gait on a level surface be-

Box 55-8

Characteristics of Duchenne Muscular Dystrophy

- Early onset, usually between 3 and 5 years of age
- Progressive muscular weakness, wasting, and contractures
- Calf muscle hypertrophy in most patients
- Loss of independent ambulation by 9 to 11 years of age
- Slowly progressive, generalized weakness during teenage years
- Relentless progression until death from respiratory or cardiac failure

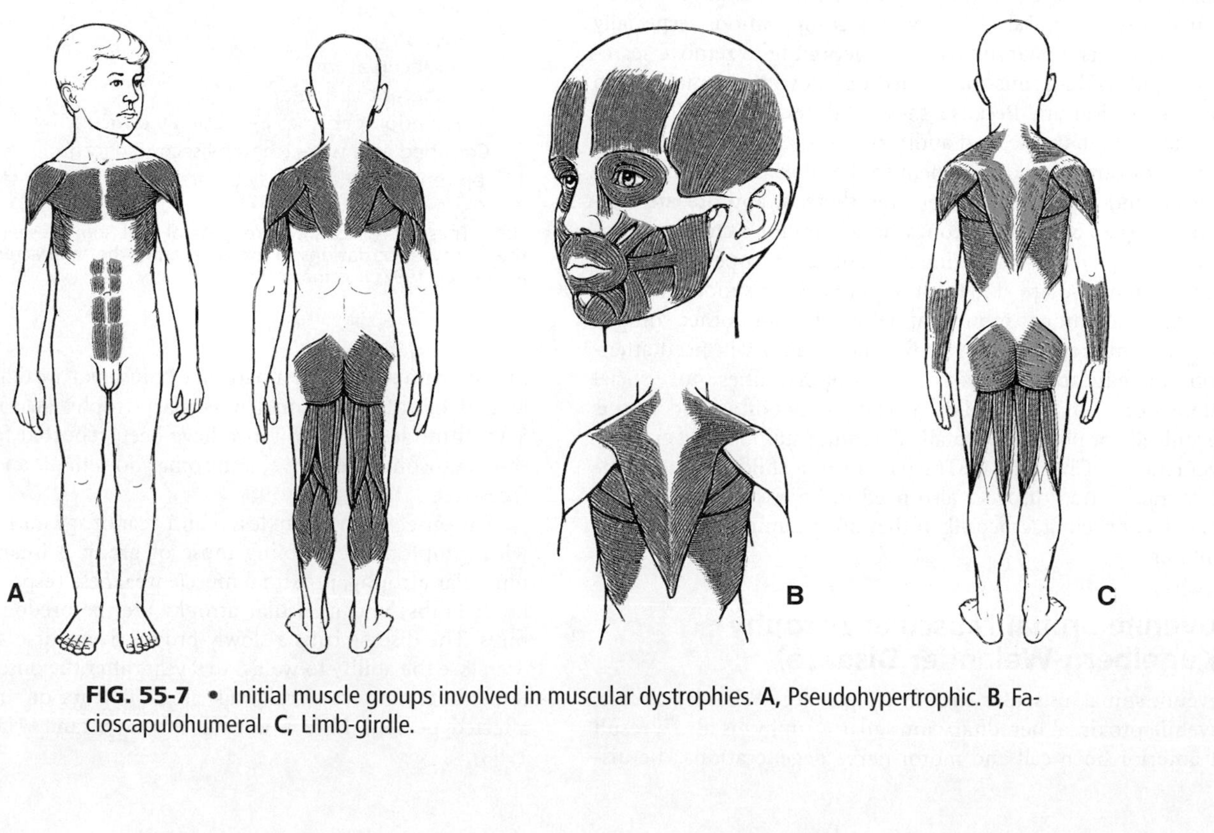

FIG. 55-7 • Initial muscle groups involved in muscular dystrophies. **A,** Pseudohypertrophic. **B,** Facioscapulohumeral. **C,** Limb-girdle.

comes apparent. In the early years rapid developmental gains may mask the progression of the disease. Questioning the parents may reveal that the child has difficulty in rising from a sitting or supine position. Occasionally the parents notice enlarged calves.

The term *pseudohypertrophy* is derived from muscular enlargement caused by fatty infiltration. Profound muscular atrophy occurs in later stages, and as the disease progresses, contractures and deformities involving large and small joints are common complications. Ambulation usually becomes impossible by 12 years of age. Facial, oropharyngeal, and respiratory muscles are spared until the terminal stages of the disease. Ultimately the disease process involves the diaphragm and auxiliary muscles of respiration, and cardiomegaly is common. Mild mental delay is commonly associated with MD (Voit, 1998). The cause of death is usually respiratory tract infection or cardiac failure.

Diagnostic Evaluation. The disease is suspected on the basis of clinical manifestations (Box 55-9) and confirmed by serum enzyme measurement, muscle biopsy, and electromyography (EMG). The serum creatine phosphokinase, aldolase, and serum glutamic-oxaloacetic transaminase (SGOT) (more recent term, aspartate aminotransferase [AST]) levels are extremely high in the first 2 years of life before the onset of clinical weakness. They diminish with muscle deterioration but do not reach normal levels until severe muscle wasting and incapacitation have occurred. Muscle biopsy reveals degeneration of muscle fibers, with fibrosis and fatty tissue replacement. EMG readings show a decrease in amplitude and duration of motor unit potentials.

Therapeutic Management. No effective treatment exists for childhood MD. Increased muscle bulk and muscle power have been reported after a course of corticosteroids; however, this therapy requires further evaluation before it becomes routine management. Maintaining function in unaffected muscles for as long as possible is the primary goal. It has been found that children who remain as active as possible are able to avoid wheelchair confinement for a longer time. Early recourse to a wheelchair accelerates deconditioning and promotes the development of lower extremity contractures. Maintenance of function often includes range-of-motion exercises, surgery to release contracture deformities, bracing, and performance of activities of daily living. Genetic counseling is recommended for parents, female siblings, and maternal aunts and their female offspring (Voit, 1998).

Nursing Care Management. The major emphasis of nursing care is to help the child and family cope with the progressive, incapacitating, and fatal nature of the disease; to help design a program that will allow a greater degree of independence and reduce the predictable and preventable disabilities associated with the disorder; and to help the child and family deal constructively with the limitations the disease imposes on their daily lives.

Working closely with other team members, nurses assist the family in developing the child's self-help skills to give the child the satisfaction of being as independent as possible for as long as possible. This requires continual evaluation of the child's capabilities, which are often difficult to assess. It is not always possible to know when children seek parental assistance because they want a little extra attention, when parents are being overprotective, or when the muscles are overtired. Fortunately, most children with MD instinctively recognize the need to become as independent as possible and strive to do so.

Practical difficulties faced by families are physical limitations of housing and mobility. Parents also need assistance in buying and modifying clothing for their child. It is difficult to find clothing and footwear to wear comfortably in a wheelchair, to fit over contracted limbs, and to fit hypertrophied muscles. The parent's social activities are also restricted, and the family's activities must be continually modified to meet the needs of the affected child.

When the child becomes increasingly helpless, the family may consider a skilled nursing facility or respite care to provide the care needed. Nurses can assist with decision making and support the family in the decision.

No matter how successful the program or how well the family adapts to the disorder, superimposed on the physical and emotional problems associated with a child with a long-term disability is the constant presence of the ultimate outcome of the disease. All of the manifestations seen in the child with a chronic fatal illness are encountered in these families (see Chapter 41). The guilt feelings of the mother may be particularly pronounced with this disorder because of the mother-to-son transmission of the defective gene.

Nurses are especially valuable health professionals as they come to know the family and the family's problems. Nurses can be alert to the problems and needs of the families and make necessary referrals when supplementary services are indicated. The Muscular Dystrophy Association of America, Inc.,* has branches in most communities to provide assistance to families in which there is a member with MD.

Box 55-9

Clinical Manifestations of Duchenne Muscular Dystrophy

- Waddling gait
- Lordosis
- Frequent falls
- Gower sign (child turns onto side or abdomen, flexes knees to assume a kneeling position, then with knees extended gradually pushes torso to an upright position by "walking" the hands up the legs)
- Enlarged muscles (especially thighs and upper arms)
  - Feel unusually firm or woody on palpation
- Later stages: profound muscular atrophy
- Mental deficiency (common)
  - Mild (about 20 IQ points below normal)
  - Frank mental deficit present in 25% of patients
- Complications:
  - Contracture deformities of hips, knees, and ankles
  - Disuse atrophy
  - Obesity

*3300 E. Sunrise Dr., Tucson, AZ 85718; 1-800-572-1717; fax (520) 529-5300; e-mail: mda@mdausa.org; website: www.mdausa.org. In Canada: Muscular Dystrophy Association of Canada, 2345 Yonge St., Suite 900, Toronto, Ontario M4P 2E5; (416) 488-0030 or 1-800-567-2873 (Canada only); fax (416) 488-7523; website: www.mdac.ca.

ACQUIRED NEUROMUSCULAR DISORDERS

Guillain-Barré Syndrome (GBS) (Infectious Polyneuritis)

GBS, also known as infectious polyneuritis, is an uncommon acute demyelinating polyneuropathy with a progressive, usually ascending flaccid paralysis. Children are less often affected than adults, with children between 4 and 10 years of age having higher susceptibility. Both sexes are affected with equal frequency (Jones, 1996).

Pathophysiology. GBS is an immune-mediated disease often associated with a number of viral or bacterial infections or the administration of vaccines. It has been associated with infectious mononucleosis, measles, mumps, *Borrelia burgdorferi* (Lyme disease), *Helicobacter pylori,* and *Mycoplasma* and *Pneumocystis* infections. Pathologic changes in spinal and cranial nerves consist of inflammation and edema with rapid, segmented demyelination and compression of nerve roots within the dural sheath. Nerve conduction is impaired, producing ascending partial or complete paralysis of muscles innervated by the involved nerves.

Diagnostic Evaluation. Diagnosis of GBS is based on the paralytic manifestations (Box 55-10) and/or EMG findings. Cerebrospinal fluid analysis reveals an increased protein concentration, but other laboratory studies are noncontributory. The symmetric nature of the paralysis helps differentiate this disorder from spinal paralytic poliomyelitis, which usually affects sporadic muscles.

Therapeutic Management. Treatment of GBS is symptomatic. In some reports, corticosteroid therapy has been of benefit in the early stages. Respiratory and pharyngeal involvement requires assisted ventilation, commonly with tracheostomy. Plasma exchange (plasmapheresis) may be beneficial both in shortening the length of illness and in lessening the long-term disability; intravenous (IV) immunoglobulin is also advocated in the acute stages (Vasjar et al, 1994).

Course and Prognosis. Better outcomes are associated with younger age, no requirement for respiratory assistance, slower progression of disease, normal peripheral nerve function on EMG, and treatment by plasmapheresis (Graf et al, 1999).

Almost all deaths are caused by respiratory failure; therefore early diagnosis and access to respiratory support are especially important. Muscle function begins to return 2 days to 2 weeks after the onset of symptoms, and recovery is complete in most patients. The rate of recovery is usually related to the degree of involvement, which may extend from a few weeks to months. The greater the degree of paralysis, the longer the recovery phase.

Nursing Care Management. Nursing care is essentially supportive and is the same as that required for quadriplegia from any cause. The emphasis of care is on close observation to assess the extent of paralysis and on prevention of complications.

During the acute phase of GBS the child's condition should be carefully observed for possible difficulty in swallowing and respiratory involvement. The child's cardiorespiratory function is monitored, and a ventilator, suction apparatus, tracheostomy tray, and vasoconstrictor drugs are kept available at the bedside. Vital signs and level of consciousness are monitored frequently. For the child who develops respiratory dysfunction, the care is the same as that for any child with respiratory distress requiring mechanical ventilation.

Throughout the recovery phase, special emphasis is placed on prevention of complications, including proper postural alignment, frequent change of position, and passive range-of-motion exercises. Children with oral and pharyngeal involvement are usually fed via a nasogastric tube to ensure adequate feeding. Bowel and bladder care is needed to avoid constipation and urine retention. Sensory impairment makes the child susceptible to burns and trophic ulcers.

Physical therapy is limited to passive range-of-motion exercises during the evolving phase of the disease. Later, as the disease stabilizes and recovery begins, an active physical therapy program is implemented to prevent contracture deformities and facilitate muscle recovery. This may include active exercise, gait training, and bracing.

Throughout the course of the illness, support of the child and parents is paramount. The usual rapidity of the paralysis and the long period of recovery greatly tax the emotional reserves of all family members. The parents and child benefit from repeated reassurance that recovery is occurring and from realistic information regarding the possibility of permanent disability. In the event of a residual disability, the family needs assistance in accepting and adjusting to the loss of function (see Chapter 41). The Guillain-Barré Syndrome Foundation International* is a nonprofit organization devoted to support, education, and research. It provides support to families from recovered persons, publishes informational literature and a newsletter, and maintains a list of practitioners experienced with the disease.

Box 55-10

Clinical Manifestations of Guillain-Barré Syndrome

INITIAL SYMPTOMS

Muscle tenderness
Paresthesia and cramps (sometimes)
Proximal symmetric muscle weakness

PARALYSIS

Ascends from lower extremities
Frequently involves muscles of trunk, upper extremities, and those supplied by cranial nerves (especially facial)
Flaccid paralysis with loss of reflexes
May involve facial, extraocular, labial, lingual, pharyngeal, and laryngeal muscles
Intercostal and phrenic nerves:
- Breathlessness in vocalizations
- Shallow, irregular respirations

OTHER MANIFESTATIONS

Tendon reflexes depressed or absent
Variable degrees of sensory impairment
Muscle tenderness or sensitivity to slight pressure
Urinary incontinence or retention and constipation (frequently)

Tetanus

Tetanus, or *lockjaw,* is an acute, preventable, and often fatal disease caused by an exotoxin produced by the anaerobic, spore-

*P.O. Box 262, Wynnewood, PA 19096; (610) 667-0131.

forming, gram-positive bacillus *Clostridium tetani.* The disorder is characterized by painful muscular rigidity primarily involving the masseter and neck muscles. There are four requirements for the development of tetanus: (1) presence of tetanus spores or vegetative forms of the bacillus, (2) injury to the tissues, (3) wound conditions that encourage multiplication of the organism, and (4) a susceptible host.

Tetanus spores are found in soil, dust, and the intestinal tracts of human beings and animals, especially herbivorous animals. The organisms are more prevalent in rural areas but are readily carried to urban areas by the wind. The organisms are not invasive but enter the body by way of wounds, particularly a puncture wound, burn, or crushed area. They may enter through a very minor, unnoticed break in the skin, such as a thorn or needle prick, bee sting, or scratch. In the newborn, infection may occur through the umbilical cord, usually in situations in which infants are delivered in severely contaminated surroundings. The disease has the greatest incidence in months when persons are more involved in outdoor activities. Substance abusers are especially susceptible from poor injection technique and the use of street heroin, which is often mixed with quinine, a protoplasmic poison that favors the growth of the organism (American Academy of Pediatrics, 2000).

Pathophysiology. When conditions are favorable, the organisms proliferate and excrete a potent exotoxin that affects the central nervous system to produce the clinical manifestations of the disease. The ideal conditions for growth of the organisms are devitalized tissues without access to air, such as wounds that have not been washed or kept clean and those that have crusted over, trapping pus beneath. The exotoxin appears to reach the central nervous system by way of either the neuron axons or the vascular system. The toxin becomes fixed on nerve cells of the anterior horn of the spinal cord and the brainstem. The toxin acts at the myoneural junction to produce muscular stiffness and lower the threshold for reflex excitability.

Several forms of the disease exist, but the generalized form is the most common and most dangerous. The incubation period for tetanus varies from 3 days to 3 weeks but generally averages 8 days. The traditional belief that the more extensive the injury, the shorter the incubation period and the more severe the symptoms, has not been confirmed in the United States.

The manner of onset varies, but the initial symptoms are usually a progressive stiffness and tenderness of the muscles in the neck and jaw. Eventually all voluntary muscles are affected (Box 55-11). As the child recovers from the disease, the paroxysms become less frequent and gradually subside. Survival beyond 4 days usually indicates recovery, but complete recovery may require weeks.

The mortality rate is about 30%, but the disease is almost invariably fatal in the newborn. The incubation period is short, with the appearance of symptoms 3 to 10 days after exposure. The first symptom is difficulty sucking, which progresses to total inability to suck, excessive crying, irritability, and nuchal rigidity (American Academy of Pediatrics, 2000).

Therapeutic Management. Preventive measures are based on the immune status of the affected child and the nature of the injury. Specific prophylactic therapy after trauma is administration of either *tetanus toxoid* or *tetanus antitoxin* (see Immunizations, Chapter 36).

The unprotected or inadequately immunized child who sustains a "tetanus-prone" wound (such as, but not limited to, wounds contaminated with dirt, feces, soil, and saliva; puncture wounds; avulsions; and wounds resulting from missiles, crushing, burns, and frostbite) should receive *tetanus immune globulin (TIG).* Concurrent administration of both TIG and tetanus toxoid at separate sites is recommended both to provide protection and to initiate the active immune process. Completion of active immunization is carried out according to the usual pattern (American Academy of Pediatrics, 2000).

The affected child is best treated in an intensive care facility where close and constant observation and equipment for monitoring and respiratory support are readily available. A quiet environment is preferred to reduce external stimuli. Neonates are placed in an open warmer unit or incubator to maintain a constant environmental temperature.

General supportive care, including maintenance of adequate fluid and electrolyte balance and caloric intake, is indicated. Indwelling oral or nasogastric feedings are used whenever possible, but severe laryngospasm may necessitate IV parenteral nutrition or gastrostomy feeding. Recurrent laryngospasm or excessive accumulation of secretions may require endotracheal intubation.

TIG therapy to neutralize toxins is the most specific therapy for tetanus. Antibiotics are administered to control the proliferation of the vegetative forms of the organism at the site of infection. Local care of the wound by surgical debridement and cleansing helps reduce the numbers of proliferating organisms

Box 55-11

Clinical Manifestations of Tetanus

INITIAL SYMPTOMS

Progressive stiffness and tenderness of muscles in neck and jaw
Characteristic difficulty in opening the mouth (trismus)
Risus sardonicus (sardonic smile) caused by facial muscle spasm

PROGRESSIVE INVOLVEMENT

Opisthotonos
Boardlike rigidity of abdominal and limb muscles
Difficulty swallowing
High sensitivity to external stimuli (slight noise, gentle touch, or bright light):
- Trigger paroxysmal muscular contractions that last seconds to minutes
- Contractions recur with increased frequency until almost continuous

Laryngospasm and tetany of respiratory muscles:
- Accumulated secretions
- Respiratory arrest
- Atelectasis
- Pneumonia

OTHER ASPECTS

Mentation unaffected; patient alert
Pain and distress are reflected in:
- Rapid pulse
- Sweating
- Anxious expression

Fever usually absent or only mild

at the site of injury. The cleansing should be repeated several times during the first 48 hours, and deep, infected lacerations are usually exposed and debrided.

Sedatives or muscle relaxants are administered to help reduce muscle spasm and prevent seizures. The most widely used is diazepam (Valium), but phenobarbital, chloral hydrate, the phenothiazines, and paraldehyde may be used. Patients with severe tetanus and those who do not respond to other sedatives require the administration of a neuromuscular blocking agent, usually pancuronium bromide (Pavulon) or vecuronium. Because of their paralytic effect on respiratory muscles, use of these drugs requires mechanical ventilation with endotracheal intubation or tracheostomy and constant attendance by trained personnel until muscle spasms are controlled. Endotracheal tube insertion or tracheostomy is often indicated and should be performed before severe respiratory distress develops. Administration of corticosteroids has met with success in some instances.

Nursing Care Management. In caring for the child with tetanus, every effort is made to control or eliminate stimulation from sound, light, and touch. Although a darkened room is ideal, sufficient light is essential so that the child can be carefully observed; light appears to be less irritating than vibratory or auditory stimuli. The infant or child is handled as little as possible, and sudden and/or loud noise is avoided.

Medications are administered as prescribed, and vital signs are observed and recorded at frequent intervals. The location and extent of muscle spasms and assessment of their severity are important nursing observations. Respiratory status is carefully evaluated for any signs of distress, and appropriate emergency equipment is kept available at all times. Muscle relaxants and sedatives that may be prescribed can also cause respiratory depression; therefore the child must be assessed for excessive central nervous system depression. Oxygen saturation is monitored, and when needed, blood gases are obtained frequently to evaluate respiratory status. Attention to hydration and nutrition may involve monitoring an IV infusion, monitoring nasogastric or gastrostomy feedings, and suctioning oropharyngeal secretions when indicated.

If a potent muscle relaxant such as pancuronium bromide is used, the total paralysis makes oral communication impossible. Therefore all the child's needs must be anticipated and procedures carefully explained beforehand. As the dose of medication is decreased, the child regains movement of the eyelids and facial muscles, which gives the child some opportunity to express emotions and indicate choices through a signal system (e.g., blinking the lids to indicate yes or no).

Because their mental status is clear, children with tetanus are aware of what is happening to them and are often in a state of terror. They should not be left alone, and all efforts should be made to reduce anxiety, which can contribute to muscular spasms. A calm and reassuring manner and sympathetic understanding can assist immeasurably in helping a child through this crisis situation. Parents are encouraged to stay with the child to offer security and support.

Botulism

Botulism is a serious food poisoning that results from ingestion of the preformed toxin produced by the anaerobic bacillus *Clostridium botulinum*. The most common source of the toxin is improperly sterilized home-canned foods. Central nervous system symptoms appear abruptly about 12 to 36 hours after ingestion of contaminated food and may not have been preceded by acute digestive disturbance (Box 55-12).

Treatment consists of IV administration of botulism antitoxin and general supportive measures, primarily respiratory and nutritional. Toxins vary in protein-binding capacity. Some have a relatively short half-life and do not bind to tissues firmly; therefore therapy is continued until paralysis abates. Other toxins appear to bind irreversibly to nerve endings and are therefore not amenable to neutralization. Respiratory support is often needed and should be available at the bedside, ready for use if indicated (Ferrari and Weisse, 1995).

Infant Botulism. Infant botulism, unlike the disease in older persons, is caused by ingestion of spores or vegetative cells of *C. botulinum* and the subsequent release of the toxin from organisms colonizing the gastrointestinal tract. There appears to be no common food or drug source of the organisms; however, the *C. botulinum* organisms have been found in honey and light or dark corn syrup fed to affected infants (American Academy of Pediatrics, 2000).

There is wide variation in the severity of the disease, from mild constipation to progressive sequential loss of neurologic function and respiratory failure (see Box 55-12). The affected infant is usually well before the onset of symptoms. Constipation is a common presenting symptom, and almost all infants exhibit generalized weakness and a decrease in spontaneous movements. Deep tendon reflexes are usually diminished or absent; cranial nerve deficits are common, as evidenced by loss of head control, difficulty in feeding, weak cry, and reduced gag reflex. The most commonly recognized form of the disease is consistent with the hypotonic infant. Botulism toxin exerts its effect by inhibiting the release of acetylcholine at the myoneural junction, thereby impairing motor activity of muscles innervated by affected nerves.

Diagnosis is made on the basis of the history, physical examination, and laboratory detection of the organism in the patient or the implicated food. Treatment consists of supportive meas-

Box 55-12

Clinical Manifestations of Botulism

GENERAL SIGNS
- Weakness
- Dizziness
- Headache
- Difficulty talking and speaking
- Diplopia
- Vomiting
- Progressive, life-threatening respiratory paralysis

INFANT BOTULISM
- Constipation (a common symptom)
- Generalized weakness
- Decrease in spontaneous movements
- Diminished or absent deep tendon reflexes
- Loss of head control
- Difficulty feeding
- Weak cry
- Reduced gag reflex
- Progressive respiratory paralysis

ures, primarily respiratory and nutritional. Botulism antitoxin, used in adults and older children, is not administered to infants. Evidence indicates that infants recover without the antitoxin and that its efficacy is lacking.

The prognosis is generally good if the patient is adequately supported, although recovery may be very slow, requiring weeks to months after severe illness. An infant who is recovering from botulism must avoid contact with other infants for about 3 months or until excretion of the organisms has ceased (Glatman-Freedman, 1996).

Nursing Care Management. Nursing responsibilities include observing for and reporting signs of muscle impairment and providing intensive nursing care when the infant is hospitalized. Parental support and reassurance are important. Most infants recover when the disorder is recognized and therapy is implemented. Parents should be aware that during recovery, patients tire easily when muscular action is sustained. This has important implications for timing the resumption of feedings, because of the risk of aspiration. Parents should also be advised that normal bowel action may not return for several weeks; therefore a stool softener can be beneficial. Cathartics and enemas are not advised.

Spinal Cord Injuries

Spinal cord injuries with major neurologic involvement are not a common cause of physical disability in childhood. However, a sufficient number of children with these injuries are admitted to major medical centers, and because of the increased survival rate as a result of improved management, nurses are more likely to become involved with such children.

Mechanisms of Injury. In motor vehicle accidents (MVAs) most spinal cord injuries in children are a result of indirect trauma caused by sudden hyperflexion or hyperextension of the neck, often combined with a rotational force. Trauma to the spinal cord without evidence of vertebral fracture or dislocation is particularly likely to occur in an MVA when proper restraints are not used. An unrestrained child becomes a projectile during sudden deceleration and is subject to injury from contact with a variety of objects inside and outside the vehicle. Individuals who use only a lap seat belt restraint are at greater risk of spinal cord injury than those who use a combination lap and shoulder restraint.

Falling from heights occurs less often in children than in adults, but vertebral compression from blows to the head or buttocks can occur in water sports (diving and surfing), falls from horses, or other athletic activities. Birth injuries may occur in breech deliveries from traction force on the spinal cord during delivery of the head and shoulders. An increasing number of teenagers receive spinal cord injuries from gunshot wounds or violent inflicted injury.

The injury sustained can affect any of the spinal nerves, and the higher the injury, the more extensive the damage. The child can be left with complete or partial paralysis of the lower extremities *(paraplegia)* or with damage at a higher level and without functional use of any of the four extremities *(quadriplegia)*. A high cervical cord injury that affects the phrenic nerve paralyzes the diaphragm and leaves the child dependent on a ventilator.

A mild but equally frightening form of cord trauma is *spinal cord compression,* a temporary neural dysfunction without visible damage to the cord. Complete quadriplegia can result but initially may not be differentiated from serious cord injury (Menezes and Osenbach, 1994).

Therapeutic Management. The management of the child with spinal cord injury is complex and controversial. Initial care begins at the scene of the accident; therefore education and training of rescue personnel in stabilization and transfer techniques to prevent or reduce the severity of injury are critically important. Because of the complexity and relative infrequency of these injuries, it is usually recommended that these persons be transferred to a spinal injury center for care by specially trained personnel (Lang and Bernardo, 1993).

Nursing Care Management. The nursing care of the paraplegic or quadriplegic child is complex and challenging. As a member of the acute care and rehabilitation teams, the nurse is involved in all aspects of care. Ideally, initial care takes place in a special intensive care unit with personnel trained to handle spinal cord injuries. Nursing management is concerned primarily with prevention of complications and maintenance of function.

Once the acute period is over, the lesion is usually static and nonprogressive, regardless of whether the paralysis is secondary to trauma, a congenital defect, infection, a treated tumor, or surgery. The nurse is a member of a team of specialists, including physicians from a number of specialty areas, physical and occupational therapists, psychologists, social workers, teachers, and vocational counselors. Each team member makes a unique contribution, and specific areas of responsibility and evaluation of progress are mutually agreed on during regularly scheduled team conferences.

Key Points

- Clinical manifestations of cerebral palsy include delayed gross motor development; abnormal motor performance; alterations of muscle tone; abnormal postures; reflex abnormalities; and associated disabilities such as mental retardation, seizures, attention deficit hyperactivity disorder, and sensory impairment.
- Therapy for cerebral palsy takes into account the nature of the physical disability, defects associated with the disorder, and interpersonal and social influences encountered by the affected child.
- Care of the infant and child with myelomeningocele is directed toward protecting the meningeal sac, preventing infection and skin breakdown, and observing for signs of complications.
- Werdnig-Hoffmann disease is characterized by progressive weakness and wasting of skeletal muscles caused by degeneration of anterior horn cells of the spinal cord.
- Muscular dystrophies are the greatest and most important cause of muscular dysfunction of childhood.
- Major complications of Duchenne muscular dystrophy include joint contractures, disuse atrophy, infections, obesity, and cardiopulmonary problems.
- Nursing care of the child with Guillain-Barré syndrome consists of monitoring vital signs, ensuring alignment and positioning, providing physical therapy, and providing support to the child and family.

- Tetanus occurs when tetanus spores or vegetative bacilli enter a wound and multiply in a susceptible host.
- Infant botulism results from the release of toxins from *Clostridium botulinum* colonizing the gastrointestinal tract.
- Therapeutic management of spinal cord injury is directed toward preventing further neuronal damage, avoiding complications, and maintaining vital functions.

References

Albright AL: Baclofen in the treatment of cerebral palsy, *J Child Neurol* 11(2):773-776, 1996.

American Academy of Pediatrics, Committee on Infectious Diseases, Pickering L, editor: *2000 Red Book: report of the Committee on Infectious Diseases,* ed 25, Elk Grove Village, IL, 2000, The Academy.

American Nurses Association: Position statement on latex allergy, *Okla Nurse* 42(4):32-33, 1997.

Armstrong RW et al: Intrathecally administered baclofen for treatment of children with spasticity of cerebral origin, *J Neurosurg* 87(3):409-414, 1997.

Carroll P: Latex allergy: what you need to know, *RN* 62(9):41-45, 1999.

Centers for Disease Control and Prevention: *Preventing neural tube defects with folic acid: working together for healthier babies,* NCEH Pub. No. 99-0082, 1999.

Dabney KW, Lipton GE, Miller F: Cerebral palsy, *Curr Opin Pediatr* 9(1):81-88, 1997.

Ferrari ND, Weisse ME: Botulism, *Adv Pediatr Infect Dis* 10:81-91, 1995.

Glatman-Freedman A: Infant botulism, *Pediatr Rev* 17(5):185-186, 1996.

Graf WD et al: Outcome in severe pediatric Guillain-Barré syndrome after immunotherapy or supportive care, *Neurology* 52(7):1494-1497, 1999.

Henshaw SK: Unintended pregnancy in the United States, *Fam Plann Perspect* 30:24-29, 1998.

Hutton JL, Cook T, Pharaoh P: Life expectancy in children with cerebral palsy, *BMJ* 309(6952):431-435, 1994.

Iannaccone ST: Spinal muscular atrophy, *Semin Neurol* 18(1): 19-26, 1998.

Institute of Medicine: *Dietary reference intake: folate, other B vitamins, and choline,* Washington, DC, 1998, National Academy Press.

Jones HR: Childhood Guillian-Barré syndrome: clinical presentation, diagnosis and therapy, *J Child Neurol* 11(1):4-12, 1996.

Kellett PB: Latex allergy: a review, *J Emerg Nurs* 23(1):27-36, 1997.

Lang SM, Bernardo CM: SCIWORA syndrome: nursing assessment . . . spinal cord injury without radiographic abnormality, *Dimens Crit Care Nurs* 12(5):247-254, 1993.

Lary JM, Edmonds LD: Prevalence of spina bifida at birth—United States 1983-1990: a comparison of two surveillance systems, *MMWR CDC Surveill Summ* 45(2):15-26, 1996.

Menezes AH, Osenbach RK: Spinal cord injury. In Cheek WR, editor: *Pediatric neurosurgery,* ed 3, Philadelphia, 1994, WB Saunders.

Multicenter Study Group: Diagnosis of Duchenne and Becker muscular dystrophies by polymerase chain reaction, *JAMA* 276(19):2609-2615, 1992.

National Institute for Occupational Safety and Health: *NIOSH alert: preventing allergic reactions to natural rubber latex in the workplace,* DHHS Pub. No. 97-135, Washington, DC, 1997, NIH.

Nehring WM, Steele S: Cerebral palsy. In Jackson PL, Vessey JA, editors: *Primary care of the child with a chronic illness,* ed 2, St Louis, 1996, Mosby.

Occupational Safety and Health Administration: *Technical information bulletin—potential for allergy to natural rubber latex gloves and other natural rubber products,* Washington, DC, April 12, 1999, U.S. Department of Labor.

Paneth N: The causes of cerebral palsy: recent evidence, *Clin Invest Med* 16(2):95-102, 1993.

Rawlins P: Intrathecal baclofen for spasticity of cerebral palsy: project coordination and nursing care, *J Neurosci Nurs* 27(2):157-163, 1995.

Russman BS: Function changes in spinal muscular atrophy II and III: the DCN/SMA group, *Neurology* 47(4):973-976, 1996.

Suresh-Babu MV et al: Nutrition in children with cerebral palsy, *J Pediatr Gastroenterol Nutr* 26(4):484-485, 1998.

Vasjar J et al: Plasmapheresis vs intravenous immunoglobulin treatment in childhood Guillain-Barré syndrome, *Arch Pediatr Adolesc Med* 148(11):1210-1211, 1994.

Voit T: Congenital muscular dystrophies: 1997 update, *Brain Dev* 20(2):65-74, 1998.

APPENDIX

A Relationship of Drugs to Breast Milk and Effect on Infant

http://www.harcourthealth.com/MERLIN/Wong/maternal/

The drugs listed in this appendix have been categorized by their major use. The ratings given are those published by the American Academy of Pediatrics (AAP) Committee on Drugs. These ratings label drugs that transfer into human milk. Not every drug in the list has an AAP rating. The ratings are described as follows:

1. Drugs that are contraindicated during breastfeeding
2. Drugs of abuse that are contraindicated during breastfeeding
3. Radioactive compounds that require temporary cessation of breastfeeding
4. Drugs with unknown effects on breastfeeding but which may be of concern
5. Drugs that have been associated with significant effects on some breastfeeding infants and that should be given to breastfeeding mothers with caution
6. Maternal medication usually compatible with breastfeeding
7. Food and environmental agents: effect on breastfeeding

Drug	Excreted in Milk	% Adult Dose in Milk	AAP Rating	Comments
ANALGESICS AND ANTIINFLAMMATORY DRUGS (NONNARCOTIC)				
Acetaminophen (Datril, Tylenol)	Yes	0.04 to 1.85	6	Detoxified in liver. Avoid in immediate postbirth period; otherwise no problems with therapeutic dose.
Aspirin (e.g., Bayer, Anacin, Bufferin, Excedrin)	Yes	10.55 ± 10.45	6	Long history of experience shows complications rare. Can cause interference with platelet aggregation and diminished factor XII (Hageman factor) at birth. When mother requires high, continuing level of medication for arthritis, aspirin is drug of choice. Observe infant for bruisability. Platelet aggregation can be evaluated. Salicylism seen only in maternal overdosing. Mother should increase vitamin C and vitamin K intake.
Ibuprofen (e.g., Advil, Nuprin, Motrin)	Yes	<0.8	6	No apparent effects in therapeutic doses.
Indomethacin (Indocin)	Yes	0.11 to 0.98	6	Convulsions in breastfed neonate (case report). Used to close patent ductus arteriosus. Insufficient data as to effect on other vessels. May be nephrotoxic.
Mefenamic acid (Ponstel)	Yes	0.036 to 0.8	6	No apparent effect on infant at therapeutic doses; infant able to excrete via urine.
Naproxen (Naproxyn, Anaprox, Naprosyn, Aleve)	Yes	1.1		Less toxic in adults than some other organic derivatives.
Propoxyphene (Darvon)	Yes	Trace amounts	6	Only symptoms detectable would be failure to feed and drowsiness. On daily, around-the-clock dosage, infant could consume 1 mg/day.

Compiled from Lawrence R. *Breastfeeding: A guide for the medical profession,* ed 5, St Louis, 1999, Mosby; and The Committee on Drugs, American Academy of Pediatrics: The transfer of drugs and other chemicals into human breast milk, *Pediatrics* 93(1):137-150, 1994.

Continued

Drug	Excreted in Milk	% Adult Dose in Milk	AAP Rating	Comments
ANTIINFECTIVES (May change intestinal flora of infant and sensitize for later allergic reaction)				
Acyclovir (Zovirax)	Yes	5.6 ± 4.4	6	Minimal absorption through maternal skin.
Ampicillin (Polycillin, Amcill, Omnipen, Penbritin)	Yes	0.05 to 0.04		Sensitivity resulting from repeated exposure; diarrhea or secondary candidiasis.
Carbenicillin (Pyopen, Geopen)	Yes	0.001		Levels not significant. Drug is given to neonate. Not well absorbed from gastrointestinal (GI) tract.
Cefazolin (Ancef, Kefzol)	Yes	0.075	6	Probably not significant. Detected in milk if given intravenously (IV).
Cephalexin (Keflex)	Yes	0.86 ± 0.35		Completely gone by 8 hours; absorption less in first few months.
Cephalothin (Keflin)	Yes	0.4		Negligible.
Chloramphenicol (Chloromycetin)	Yes	1.6	4	Gray syndrome. Infant does not excrete drug well, and small amounts may accumulate. Contraindicated. May be tolerated in older infant with mature glycuronide system.
Colistin (Colymycin)	Yes	0.07		Not absorbed orally.
Demeclocycline (Declomycin)	Yes	Trace		Not significant in therapeutic doses. Can be given to infants. Drug remains in milk 3 days after dose.
Erythromycin (Ilosone, E-Mycin, Erythrocin)	Yes	0.1 to 2.1	6	Higher concentrations have been reported in milk than in plasma. Should not be given under 1 month of age because of risk of jaundice. Dose in milk higher when given IV to mother.
Gentamicin	Yes			Not absorbed from GI tract, may change gut flora. Drug is given to newborns directly.
Isoniazid (Nydrazid)	Yes	2.3		Infant at risk for toxicity, but need for breast milk may outweigh risk.
Kanamycin (Kantrex)	Yes	0.95	6	Infant absorbs little from GI tract. Infants can be given drug.
Metronidazole (Flagyl)	Yes	0.13 to 36	4	Caution should be exercised because of its high milk concentrations. Contraindicated when infant under 6 months; may cause neurologic disorders and blood dyscrasia. AAP says to discard milk for 12 hours if mother takes 2-g dose.
Nitrofurantoin (Furadantin, Macrodantin)	Yes	0.6	6	No significant effect in therapeutic doses except in infant with G-6-PD deficiency.
Novobiocin (Albamycin, Cathomycin)	Yes	0.15		Infant can be given drug directly.
Nystatin (Mycostatin)	No	Not absorbed orally		Can be given to infant directly.
Oxacillin (Prostaphlin)	No	Trace		
Penicillin G, benzathine (Bicillin)	Yes	0.8		Clinical need should supersede possible allergic responses.
Penicillin G, potassium	Yes	0.8		Infant can be given penicillin directly. Parents should be told to inform physician that infant has been exposed to penicillin because of potential sensitivity.
Streptomycin	Yes	0.5	6	Not to be given more than 2 weeks. Ototoxic and nephrotoxic with long use. Is given to infants directly.
Sulfisoxazole (Gantrisin)	Yes	0.45	6	To be avoided during first month after birth; may cause kernicterus.
Tetracycline HCl (Achromycin, Panmycin, Sumycin)	Yes	0.3 to 4.8	6	Not enough to treat an infection in an infant. May cause discoloration of the teeth in the infant; the antibiotic, however, may be largely bound to the milk calcium. Do not give longer than 10 days or repeatedly.

Compiled from Lawrence R. *Breastfeeding: a guide for the medical profession,* ed 5, St Louis, 1999, Mosby; and The Committee on Drugs, American Academy of Pediatrics: The transfer of drugs and other chemicals into human breast milk, *Pediatrics* 93(1):137-150, 1994.

Drug	Excreted in Milk	% Adult Dose in Milk	AAP Rating	Comments
ANTICOAGULANTS				
Coumarin derivatives Dicumarol (bishydroxy-coumarin), warfarin (Panwarfin)	Yes	6.5	6	Monitor prothrombin time. Give vitamin K to infant. Discontinue if surgery or trauma occurs. Drug of choice if mother to continue breastfeeding. May cause bleeding.
Heparin	No			Heparin ineffective orally.
ANTICONVULSANTS AND SEDATIVES (Barbiturates may pass into milk but do not sedate infant)				
Magnesium sulfate	Yes	0.5	6	May produce sedation in infant.
Pentobarbital (Nembutal)	Yes	Traces		Depends on liver for detoxification so may accumulate in first week of life until infant is able to detoxify. No problem for older infant in usual doses.
Phenytoin (Dilantin)	Yes	1.4 to 7.2	6	No problem if mother's dose is in therapeutic range.
Phenobarbital (Luminal)	Yes	1.5		Sleepiness and decreased sucking possible. On usual analeptic doses, infants alert and feed well. On hypnotic doses, infants depressed and difficult to rouse.
Sodium bromide (Bromo-Seltzer and OTC sleeping aids)	Yes	6.7		Drowsy, decreased crying, rash, decreased feeding. No longer available in the United States.
ANTIHISTAMINES (May suppress lactation; administer after breastfeeding; all pass into breast milk)				
Brompheniramine (Dimetane)	Yes	Unknown		Drugs used in neonates. May cause sedation or decreased feeding, or may produce stimulation and tachycardia. Should avoid long-acting preparations, which may accumulate in infant.
Diphenhydramine (Benadryl)	Yes	Unknown		When combined with decongestants, may cause decrease in milk.
Promethazine (Phenergan)	Yes	Unknown	6	Passage into breast is expected; increases serum prolactin levels.
AUTONOMIC DRUGS				
Atrophine sulfate*	Yes	Traces	6	Hyperthermia, atropine toxicity, infants especially sensitive; also inhibits lactation. Infant dose 0.01 mg/kg.
Ergotamine	Yes	Unknown	1	May inhibit lactation.
Neostigmine	No	No known harm to infant		
Propantheline bromide (Pro-Banthine)	No	Uncontrolled data indicate no measurable levels		Drug rapidly metabolized in maternal system to inactive metabolite; however, mother should avoid long-acting preparations.
CARDIOVASCULAR DRUGS				
Diazoxide (Hyperstat)				Arteriolar dilators and antihypertensive, given only IV, not active orally.
Digoxin	Yes	0.07 to 14	6	Not detected in infant's plasma.
Hydralazine (Apresoline)	Yes	0.8	6	Jaundice, thrombocytopenia, electrolyte disturbances possible.
Methyldopa (Aldomet)	Yes	0.02 to 0.09		Galactorrhea. No specific data except as affects mother's milk production.
Propranolol (Inderal)	Yes	Traces		Risk of effect almost nonexistent.
Quinidine	Yes	4.1	6	Arrhythmia may occur.

*An ingredient in many prescription and nonprescription drugs.

Continued

Drug	Excreted in Milk	% Adult Dose in Milk	AAP Rating	Comments
CATHARTICS				
Cascara	Yes	Low	6	Causes colic and diarrhea in infant.
Milk of magnesia	No	None	6	No effect.
Mineral oil	No	None	6	No effect.
Phenolphthalein	Unknown	Unknown	6	Reported to cause symptoms in some.
Rhubarb	Unknown	None	6	None in syrup form. Fresh rhubarb may give symptoms of colic and diarrhea.
Saline cathartics	No	None	6	No effect.
Senna	No	None	6	No effect.
Stool softeners and bulk-forming laxatives	No	None	6	No effect.
Suppositories (for constipation)	No	None	6	Not absorbed.
DIURETICS				
Furosemide (sulfamoylanthranilic acid) (Lasix)	Possible	Not found in all samples		Drug is given to children under medical management.
Spironolactone (Aldactone)	Yes	Canrenone, a metabolite, appears	6	Acts as antagonist of aldosterone; causes sodium excretion and potassium retention. The metabolite apparently has some activity.
Thiazides (Diuril, Enduron, Esidrix, HydroDiuril, Oretic, Thiuretic tablets)	Yes	0.25 to 0.43	6	Risk of dehydration and electrolyte imbalance, especially sodium loss, which would require monitoring. Watch weight and wet diapers and take an occasional specific gravity reading of urine and serum sodium to indicate status of infant. Risk, however, is extremely low. May suppress lactation because of dehydration in mother.
HORMONES AND CONTRACEPTIVES				
Contraceptives (oral) Ethinyl estradiol, mestranol, 19-nortestosterone, norethindrone (Norlutin)	Yes	0.16 ± 0.14	6	May diminish milk supply. May decrease vitamins, protein, and fat in milk. Most significant concern is long-range influence of hormone on young infant, which is not certain. Reports of feminization of infant.
Corticotropin	Yes	1.1	6	May decrease quantity and quality of milk.
Cortisone	Yes	Significant amounts		May affect infant in therapeutic doses.
Epinephrine (Adrenalin)	Yes			Destroyed in GI tract of infant.
Estrogen	Yes	0.1	6	Risks as with oral contraceptives. May alter quality and quantity of milk.
Insulin	No			Destroyed in intestinal tract.
Medroxyprogesterone acetate (Provera)	Yes	0.86 to 5	6	6-month injection may affect milk supply; 3-month injection should not decrease supply.
Prednisone	Yes	0.06 to 3.6	6	Minimum amount not likely to cause effect on infant in short course.
Tolbutamide (Orinase)	Yes	18	6	Watch for jaundice.
NARCOTICS				
Cocaine	Yes	Significant levels in milk	1, 2	No metabolites or drug found in milk after 36 hours or in infant's urine after 60 hours.
Codeine	Yes	5 ± 2	6	No effect in therapeutic level and transient use. Can accumulate. Individual variation. Watch for neonatal depression. Asians metabolize drug less rapidly than Caucasians do.
Heroin	Yes		2	Level in milk enough to cause addiction in infant.

Compiled from Lawrence R. *Breastfeeding: a guide for the medical profession,* ed 5, St Louis, 1999, Mosby; and The Committee on Drugs, American Academy of Pediatrics: The transfer of drugs and other chemicals into human breast milk, *Pediatrics* 93(1):137-150, 1994.

Drug	Excreted in Milk	% Adult Dose in Milk	AAP Rating	Comments
NARCOTICS—cont'd				
Marijuana (*Cannabis sativa* L.)	Yes		2	Shown in laboratory animals to produce structural changes in nursling's brain cells; impairs DNA and RNA formation. Infant at risk of inhaling smoke during feeding or when held by person who is smoking.
Meperidine (Demerol)	Yes	Trace		Trace amounts may accumulate if drug taken around the clock when infant is neonate. Watch for drowsiness and poor feeding.
Methadone	Yes	2.2	6	When dosage not excessive, infant can be breastfed if monitored for evidence of depression and failure to thrive. Suggest mother take daily dose after evening feeding and supplement formula at next feeding.
Morphine	Yes	0.8 to 1.2	6	Single doses have minimum effect. Potential for accumulation. May be addicting to neonate. Amounts in breast milk too variable to consider breastfeeding as means of treating withdrawal symptoms.
Percodan (oxycodone [derived from opiate thebaine], aspirin, phenacetin, caffeine)	Yes	Unknown		Consider for its component parts. In neonatal period, sleepiness and failure to feed, which increase maternal engorgement and neonatal weight loss, have been observed, probably caused by oxycodone.
PSYCHOTROPIC AND MOOD-CHANGING DRUGS				
Alcohol (Ethanol)	Yes	1 to 19.5	6	Milk may smell like alcohol. Ethanol in doses of 1 to 2 g/kg to mother causes depression of milk-ejection reflex (dose dependent). No acetaldehyde found because infant cannot metabolize ethanol.
Amphetamine	Yes	6.1 ± 0.1	2	Has caused stimulation in infants with jitteriness, irritability, sleeplessness. Long-acting preparations cumulative.
Benzodiazepines* Chlordiazepoxide (Librium)	Yes			Not sufficient to affect infant first week when glucuronyl system needed for detoxification. May accumulate. May cause jaundice. Older infant has no apparent problem.
Diazepam (Valium)	Yes	2 to 4.7	4	Detoxified in glucuronyl system. In first weeks of life may contribute to jaundice. Metabolite active. Effect on infant: hypoventilation, drowsiness, lethargy, weight loss. Single doses over 10 mg contraindicated during breastfeeding. Accumulation in infant possible.
Haloperidol (Haldol)	Yes	0.15 to 2	4	An antipsychotic: animal studies in nurslings show behavior abnormalities.
Lithium carbonate (Eskalith, Lithane, Lithonate)	Yes	1.8		Measurable lithium in infant's serum. Infant kidney can clear lithium; however, lithium inhibits adenosine 3′,5′-cyclic monophosphate, significant for brain growth. Also affects amine metabolism. Report of cyanosis and poor muscle tone and ECG changes in breastfeeding infant.
Meprobamate (Miltown, Equanil)	Yes	2 to 4 times maternal plasma level		If therapy continued, infant should be followed closely.
Phencyclidine (PCP)	Yes		1	Animal studies show PCP in milk even after drug has been discontinued for 40 days.

*Alcohol enhances the effects of these drugs.

Continued

Drug	Excreted in Milk	% Adult Dose in Milk	AAP Rating	Comments
PSYCHOTROPIC AND MOOD-CHANGING DRUGS—cont'd				
Phenothiazines				
Chlorpromazine (Thorazine)	Yes	0.07 to 0.2		Drowsiness and lethargy in infants.
Thioridazine (Mellaril)	Yes	No information		Thioridazine is less potent in general than other phenothiazines. Probably safe.
Trifluoperazine (Stelazine)	Yes	Minimum		
Tricyclic antidepressants				Apparently no accumulation. No infants who have been observed showed symptoms.
Amitriptyline (Elavil)	Yes	0.8 ± 0.2	4	Watch for depression or failure to feed; increases maternal prolactin secretion.
Desipramine (Norpramin, Pertofrane)		1	4	
Imipramine (Tofranil)	Yes	0.1	4	
STIMULANTS				
Caffeine	Yes	0.66 to 10	6	Accumulates when intake moderate and continual. Causes jitteriness, wakefulness, and irritability. Caffeine present in many hot and cold drinks. Consider if infant very wakeful.
Theobromine	Yes	20	7	No adverse symptoms observed in the infants. Chocolate the most common cause of exposure.
Theophylline	Yes	<1 to 15	6	Irritability, fretfulness.
THYROID AND ANTITHYROID MEDICATIONS				
Thiouracil	Yes	0.3 to 2.6	6	Get baseline levels of T_3, T_4, and TSH before and 6 weeks after mother starts medication.
Thyroid and thyroxine	Yes	0.3 to 2.6	6	Does not produce adverse symptoms on long-range follow-up study. Noted to improve milk supply of hypothyroid mothers. No contraindication.
MISCELLANEOUS				
DPT	Yes	Minimum		Does not interfere with immunization schedule.
Methotrexate	Yes	0.93	1	Antimetabolite. Infant would receive 0.26 g/dl, which researchers consider nontoxic for infant.
Nicotine	Yes		2	Decreases milk production. Smoking may interfere with let-down reflex if smoking started before onset of a feeding. Smoke exposure may be a concern.
Poliovirus vaccine	No			Live vaccine taken orally. Not necessary to withhold breastfeeding 30 minutes before and after dose. Provide booster after infant no longer breastfeeding.
Rh antibodies	Yes			Destroyed in GI tract; not effective orally.
Rubella virus vaccine	Yes	Minimum		Will not confer passive immunity. Mother should not be given vaccine when at risk for pregnancy.
Tuberculin test	No			Tuberculin-sensitive mothers can adaptively immunize their infants through breast milk, and that immunity may last several years.
Chest x-rays				No effect.

Compiled from Lawrence R. *Breastfeeding: a guide for the medical profession,* ed 5, St Louis, 1999, Mosby, and The Committee on Drugs, American Academy of Pediatrics: The transfer of drugs and other chemicals into human breast milk, *Pediatrics* 93(1):137-150, 1994.

APPENDIX

B Family Assessment

Family APGAR Questionnaire

PART I

The following questions have been designed to help us better understand you and your family. You should feel free to ask questions about any item in the questionnaire.

The space for comments should be used when you wish to give additional information or if you wish to discuss the way the question is applied to your family. Please try to answer all questions.

Family is defined as the individual(s) with whom you usually live. If you live alone, your "family" consists of persons with whom you now have the strongest emotional ties.*

For each question, check only one box

	Almost always	Some of the time	Hardly ever
I am satisfied that I can turn to my family for help when something is troubling me. Comments: ______	☐	☐	☐
I am satisfied with the way my family talks over things with me and shares problems with me. Comments: ______	☐	☐	☐
I am satisfied that my family accepts and supports my wishes to take on new activities or directions. Comments: ______	☐	☐	☐
I am satisfied with the way my family expresses affection and responds to my emotions, such as anger, sorrow, and love. Comments: ______	☐	☐	☐
I am satisfied with the way my family and I share time together. Comments: ______	☐	☐	☐

*According to which member of the family is being interviewed the interviewer may substitute for the word 'family' either spouse, significant other, parents, or children.

A

FIG. B-1 • Family APGAR questionnaire; may be photocopied for clinical use. (Modified from Smilkstein G, Ashworth C, Montano D: Validity and reliability of the family APGAR as a test of family function. *J Fam Pract* 15(2):303-311, 1982. **A,** Part I.

Continued

Family APGAR Questionnaire

PART II

Who lives in your home?* List by relationship (e.g., spouse, significant other,†child, or friend).

Please check below the column that best describes how you now get along with each member of the family listed.

Relationship	Age	Sex	Well	Fairly	Poorly
____________	__	__	☐	☐	☐
____________	__	__	☐	☐	☐
____________	__	__	☐	☐	☐
____________	__	__	☐	☐	☐
____________	__	__	☐	☐	☐
____________	__	__	☐	☐	☐

B

If you don't live with your own family, please list below the individuals to whom you turn for help most frequently. List by relationship, (e.g., family member, friend, associate at work, or neighbor).

Please check below the column that best describes how you now get along with each person listed.

Relationship	Age	Sex	Well	Fairly	Poorly
____________	__	__	☐	☐	☐
____________	__	__	☐	☐	☐
____________	__	__	☐	☐	☐
____________	__	__	☐	☐	☐
____________	__	__	☐	☐	☐
____________	__	__	☐	☐	☐

*If you have established your own family, consider home to be the place where you live with your spouse, children, or significant other; otherwise, consider home as your place of origin, e.g., the place where your parents or those who raise you live.

†"Significant other" is the partner you live with in a physically and emotionally nurturing relationship, but to whom you are not married.

FIG. B-1, cont'd • **B,** Part II.

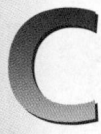

APPENDIX

C Patterns of Inheritance

http://www.harcourthealth.com/MERLIN/Wong/maternal/

GLOSSARY

congenital The condition is present at birth. The disorder may be brought about by genetic causes, nongenetic causes, or a combination of these.

familial A disorder that "runs in families" or is present in more members of a family than would be expected by chance.

genetic The disorder is caused by a single harmful gene, by several genes, or by a deviation in chromosome number or structure. It may or may not be apparent at birth.

genotype The genetic constitution that determines the physical and chemical characteristics of an individual.

heterozygous Having dissimilar genes at a given position (locus) on a pair of chromosomes.

homozygous Having the same genes at a given position (locus) on a pair of chromosomes.

inherited (heritable, hereditary) Synonymous with genetic, although in the past often used to describe a disorder that appeared in parent and offspring over several generations.

mutation Structural or chemical alteration in genetic material that, when changed, remains changed and is transmitted to future generations. Mutations usually occur naturally *(spontaneous);* or can be *induced* by a variety of external agents, or *mutagens* (e.g., temperature, certain chemicals, and radiation).

phenotype The physical or chemical characteristics of an individual, produced by the interaction of the environment with the genotype.

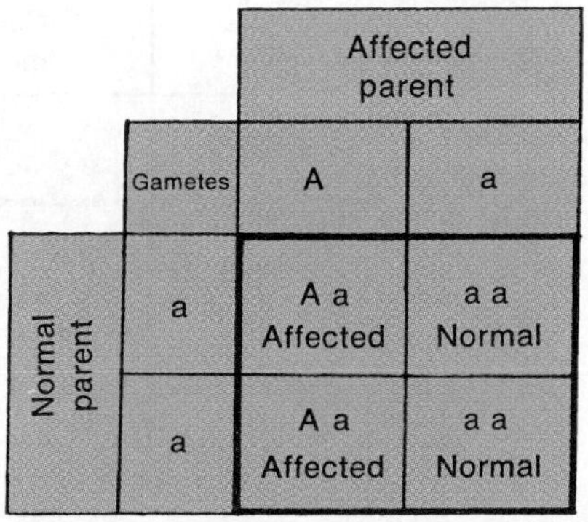

Affected parent
Gametes
A
a
Normal parent
a
A a Affected
a a Normal
a
A a Affected
a a Normal

FIG. C-1 • Possible offspring of mating between normal parent, aa, and parent with an autosomal-dominant trait, Aa.

MODIFICATIONS OF BASIC INHERITANCE PATTERNS

heterogeneity The same or similar manifestations that result from (1) different mutant genes at the same location on a chromosome or (2) mutant genes at different locations on a chromosome (e.g., the hemophilias, which produce defects in coagulation; and the muscular dystrophies, which produce muscular weakness), but that exhibit different inheritance patterns.

linkage Some genes are located too close together on a chromosome, so they segregate and migrate together during cell division; therefore, the characteristics they produce always appear together in the phenotype.

penetrance The regularity with which an inherited trait is manifested in the person who carries the gene. When a gene produces its effect on the phenotype each time it is present in the genotype, it is said to be *fully penetrant* or to exhibit *complete penetrance.* For example, achondroplasia (a form of dwarfism) is always evident whenever the gene is present. If a trait is not recognized in a person who carries the responsible gene, it is said to be *nonpenetrant* in that individual. This phenomenon accounts for what appears to be skipped generations.

pleiotropy The multiple, different, and seemingly unrelated effects associated with a particular disorder; the varied clinical features that constitute a syndrome. For example, Marfan syndrome, a disorder of the elastic fibers of connective tissue, may be manifested in an individial by any or all of the symptoms associated with it—aortic aneurysm, dislocation of the optic lens, or any of a number of skeletal deformities.

variable expressivity The degree of severity of, or the variability in, the manifestations seen in persons of a particular genotype. For instance, polydactyly can be expressed as any number of extra digits, or the extra digits may be fingers in one generation and toes in another. The severity of a disorder may be so mild as to be almost undetected or so severe that the affected individual is totally incapacited.

Autosomal Dominant Inheritance

Characteristics of a condition caused by a dominant gene on an autosome include the following (Fig. C-1):

1. Males and females are affected with equal frequency.
2. Affected individuals have an affected parent (unless the condition is caused by a fresh mutation).
3. Half the children of a heterozygous affected parent will possess the defective gene, although it may be nonpenetrant.
4. Unaffected children of affected parents will have unaffected children (unless the gene is nonpenetrant).

Autosomal Recessive Inheritance

Characteristics of a condition caused by a recessive gene on an autosome include the following (Fig. C-2):

1. Males and females are affected with equal frequency.
2. Affected individuals have unaffected parents who are heterozygous for the trait.
3. There is a one in four chance that any child of two unaffected heterozygous parents will be affected.
4. Two affected parents will have affected children exclusively.
5. Affected individuals married to unaffected individuals will have normal children, all of whom will be carriers.
6. There is usually no evidence of the trait in previous generations—a negative family history.

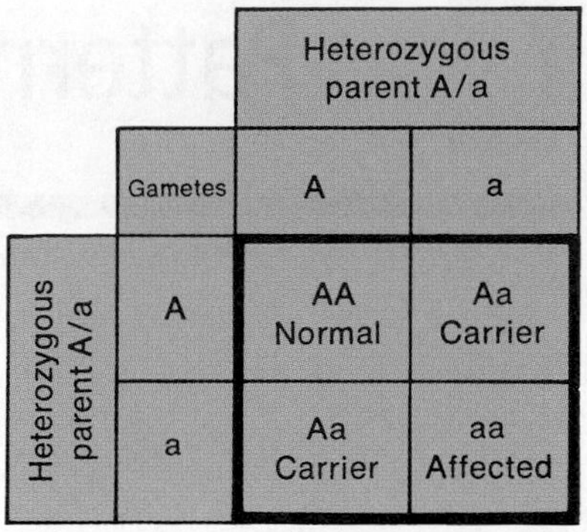

FIG. C-2 • Possible offspring of mating between two parents with a recessive gene, a, on an autosome.

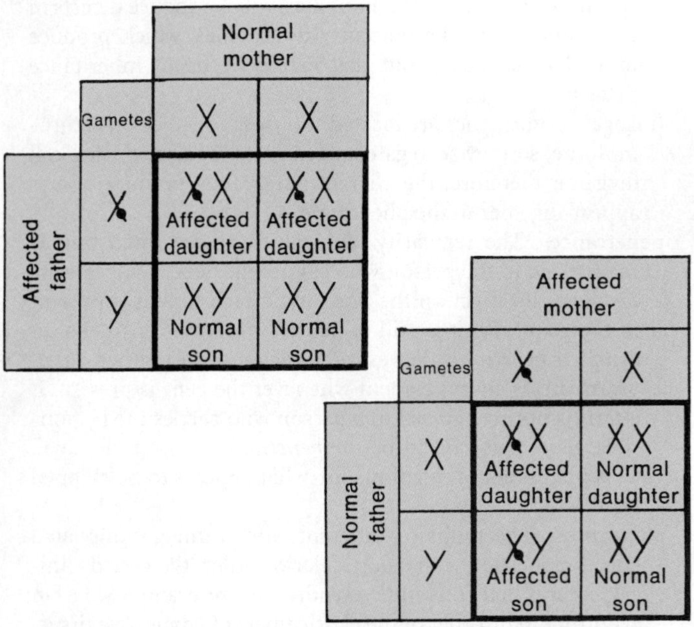

FIG. C-3 • Sex differences in offspring ratios in X-linked dominant inheritance. ●, Dominant allele on X chromosome.

X-Linked Dominant Inheritance

Characteristics of a condition caused by a dominant gene on an X chromosome include the following (Fig. C-3):

1. Affected individuals have an affected parent.
2. All the daughters but none of the sons of an affected male will be affected.
3. Half the sons and half the daughters of an affected female will be affected.
4. Normal children of an affected parent will have normal offspring.
5. There are no carriers.
6. The inheritance pattern shows a positive family history.

X-Linked Recessive Inheritance

Characteristics of a disorder caused by a recessive gene on the X chromosome include the following (Fig. C-4):

1. Affected individuals are principally males.
2. Affected individuals have unaffected parents (except in the rare possibility that the father is affected and the mother is a carrier).
3. Half of the female siblings of an affected male will be carriers of the trait.
4. Unaffected male siblings of an affected male cannot transmit the disorder.
5. Sons of an affected male are unaffected.
6. Daughters of an affected male are carriers.
7. The unaffected male children of a carrier female do not transmit the disorder.

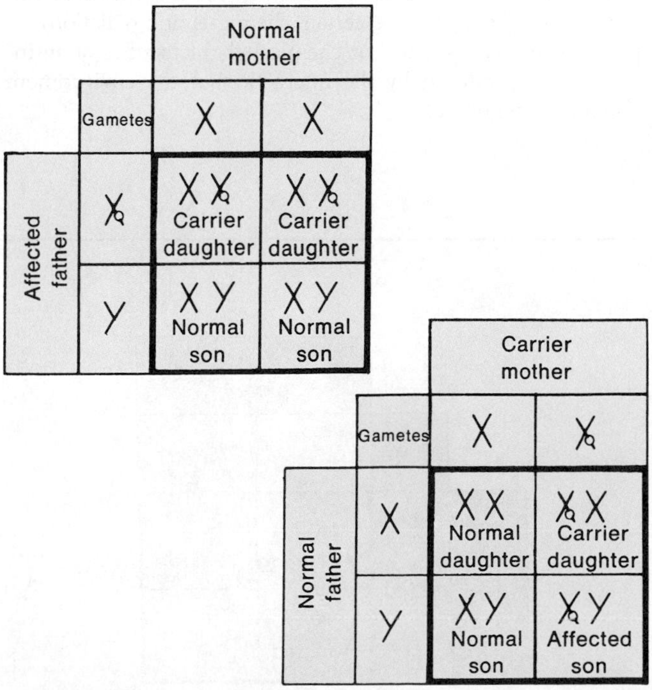

FIG. C-4 • Differences in offspring ratios in X-linked recessive inheritance. O, Recessive allele on X chromosome.

APPENDIX

D Developmental/Sensory Assessment

http://www.harcourthealth.com/MERLIN/Wong/maternal/

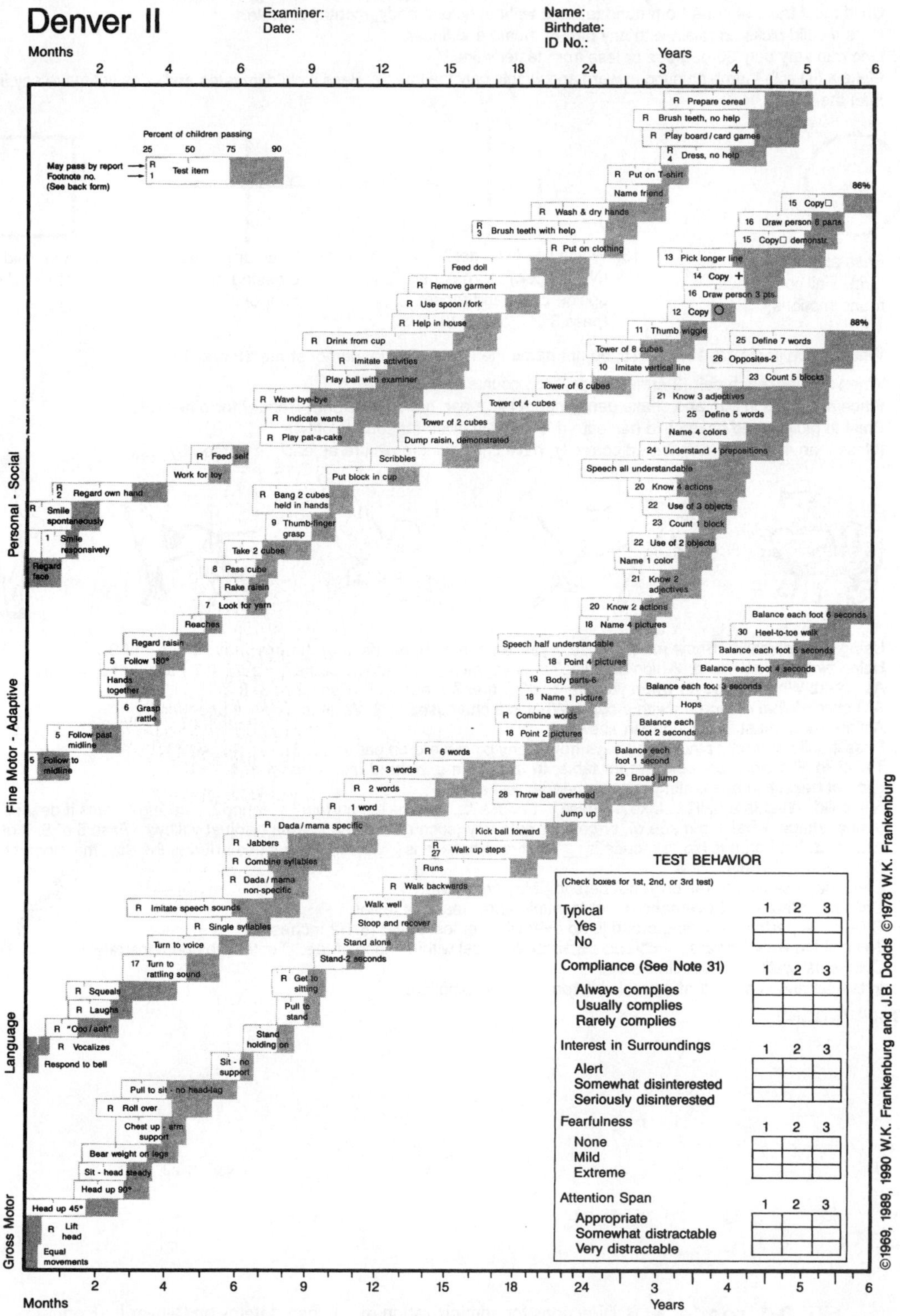

A

FIG. D-1 • **A,** Denver II. (From W.K. Frankenburg and J.B. Dodds, 1990.) *Continued*

DIRECTIONS FOR ADMINISTRATION

1. Try to get child to smile by smiling, talking or waving. Do not touch him/her.
2. Child must stare at hand several seconds.
3. Parent may help guide toothbrush and put toothpaste on brush.
4. Child does not have to be able to tie shoes or button/zip in the back.
5. Move yarn slowly in an arc from one side to the other, about 8" above child's face.
6. Pass if child grasps rattle when it is touched to the backs or tips of fingers.
7. Pass if child tries to see where yarn went. Yarn should be dropped quickly from sight from tester's hand without arm movement.
8. Child must transfer cube from hand to hand without help of body, mouth, or table.
9. Pass if child picks up raisin with any part of thumb and finger.
10. Line can vary only 30 degrees or less from tester's line.
11. Make a fist with thumb pointing upward and wiggle only the thumb. Pass if child imitates and does not move any fingers other than the thumb.

12. Pass any enclosed form. Fail continuous round motions.

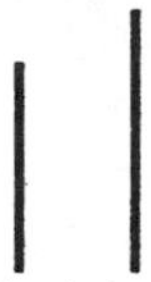

13. Which line is longer? (Not bigger.) Turn paper upside down and repeat. (pass 3 of 3 or 5 of 6)

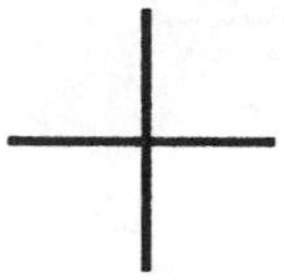

14. Pass any lines crossing near midpoint.

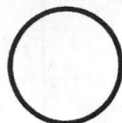

15. Have child copy first. If failed, demonstrate.

When giving items 12, 14, and 15, do not name the forms. Do not demonstrate 12 and 14.

16. When scoring, each pair (2 arms, 2 legs, etc.) counts as one part.

B

17. Place one cube in cup and shake gently near child's ear, but out of sight. Repeat for other ear.
18. Point to picture and have child name it. (No credit is given for sounds only.) If less than 4 pictures are named correctly, have child point to picture as each is named by tester.

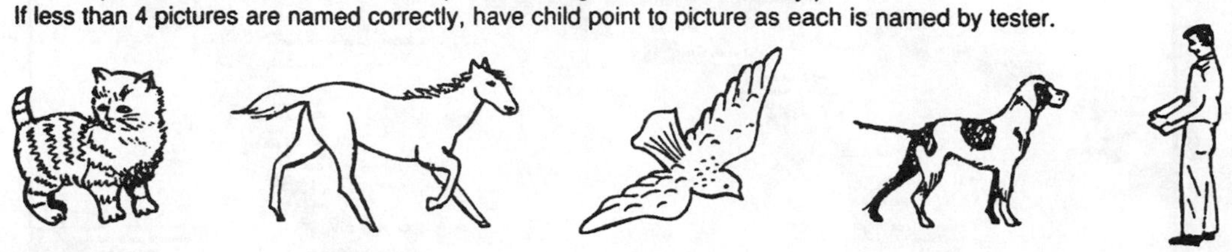

19. Using doll, tell child: Show me the nose, eyes, ears, mouth, hands, feet, tummy, hair. Pass 6 of 8.
20. Using pictures, ask child: Which one flies?... says meow?... talks?... barks?... gallops? Pass 2 of 5, 4 of 5.
21. Ask child: What do you do when you are cold?... tired?... hungry? Pass 2 of 3, 3 of 3.
22. Ask child: What do you do with a cup? What is a chair used for? What is a pencil used for? Action words must be included in answers.
23. Pass if child correctly places <u>and</u> says how many blocks are on paper. (1, 5).
24. Tell child: Put block **on** table; **under** table; **in front of** me, **behind** me. Pass 4 of 4. (Do not help child by pointing, moving head or eyes.)
25. Ask child: What is a ball?... lake?... desk?... house?... banana?... curtain?... fence?... ceiling? Pass if defined in terms of use, shape, what it is made of, or general category (such as banana is fruit, not just yellow). Pass 5 of 8, 7 of 8.
26. Ask child: If a horse is big, a mouse is __? If fire is hot, ice is __? If the sun shines during the day, the moon shines during the __? Pass 2 of 3.
27. Child may use wall or rail only, not person. May not crawl.
28. Child must throw ball overhand 3 feet to within arm's reach of tester.
29. Child must perform standing broad jump over width of test sheet (8 1/2 inches).
30. Tell child to walk forward, heel within 1 inch of toe. Tester may demonstrate. Child must walk 4 consecutive steps.
31. In the second year, half of normal children are non-compliant.

OBSERVATIONS:

FIG. D-1, cont'd • B, Directions for administration of numbered items on Denver II. (From W.K. Frankenburg and J.B. Dodds, 1990.)

DENVER ARTICULATION SCREENING EXAM
for children 2½ to 6 years of age

Name:

Instructions: Have child repeat each word after you. Circle the underlined sounds that he pronounces correctly. Total correct sounds is the Raw Score. Use charts on reverse side to score results.

Hosp. No.:

Address: ______________________

____

Date: __________ Child's age: __________ Examiner: __________ Raw score: ____
Percentile: ______ Intelligibility: __________ Result: __________

1. table	6. zipper	11. sock	16. wagon	21. leaf
2. shirt	7. grapes	12. vacuum	17. gum	22. carrot
3. door	8. flag	13. yarn	18. house	
4. trunk	9. thumb	14. mother	19. pencil	
5. jumping	10. toothbrush	15. twinkle	20. fish	

Intelligibility: (circle one)
1. Easy to understand
2. Understandable ½ the time
3. Not understandable
4. Can't evaluate

Comments:

Date: __________ Child's age: __________ Examiner: __________ Raw score: ____
Percentile: ______ Intelligibility: __________ Result: __________

1. table	6. zipper	11. sock	16. wagon	21. leaf
2. shirt	7. grapes	12. vacuum	17. gum	22. carrot
3. door	8. flag	13. yarn	18. house	
4. trunk	9. thumb	14. mother	19. pencil	
5. jumping	10. toothbrush	15. twinkle	20. fish	

Intelligibility: (circle one)
1. Easy to understand
2. Understandable ½ the time
3. Not understandable
4. Can't evaluate

Comments:

A

Date: __________ Child's age: __________ Examiner: __________ Raw score ____
Percentile: ______ Intelligibility: __________ Result: __________

1. table	6. zipper	11. sock	16. wagon	21. leaf
2. shirt	7. grapes	12. vacuum	17. gum	22. carrot
3. door	8. flag	13. yarn	18. house	
4. trunk	9. thumb	14. mother	19. pencil	
5. jumping	10. toothbrush	15. twinkle	20. fish	

Intelligibility: (circle one)
1. Easy to understand
2. Understandable ½ the time
3. Not understandable
4. Can't evaluate

FIG. D-2 • **A,** Denver Articulation Screening Examination (DASE) for children $2^1/_2$ to 6 years of age. (From A.F. Drumwright, University of Colorado Medical Center, 1971.) *Continued*

To score DASE words: Note raw score for child's performance. Match raw score line (extreme left of chart) with column representing child's age (to the closest previous age group). Where raw score line and age column meet number in that square denotes percentile rank of child's performance when compared to other children that age. Percentiles above heavy line are ABNORMAL percentiles, below heavy line are NORMAL.

PERCENTILE RANK

B

Raw Score	2.5 yr.	3.0	3.5	4.0	4.5	5.0	5.5	6 years
2	1							
3	2							
4	5							
5	9							
6	16							
7	23							
8	31	2						
9	37	4	1					
10	42	6	2					
11	48	7	4					
12	54	9	6	1	1			
13	58	12	9	2	3	1	1	
14	62	17	11	5	4	2	2	
15	68	23	15	9	5	3	2	
16	75	31	19	12	5	4	3	
17	79	38	25	15	6	6	4	
18	83	46	31	19	8	7	4	
19	86	51	38	24	10	9	5	1
20	89	58	45	30	12	11	7	3
21	92	65	52	36	15	15	9	4
22	94	72	58	43	18	19	12	5
23	96	77	63	50	22	24	15	7
24	97	82	70	58	29	29	20	15
25	99	87	78	66	36	34	26	17
26	99	91	84	75	46	43	34	24
27		94	89	82	57	54	44	34
28		96	94	88	70	68	59	47
29		98	98	94	84	84	77	68
30		100	100	100	100	100	100	100

To score intelligibility:

	NORMAL	ABNORMAL
2½ years	Understandable ½ the time, or, "easy"	Not understandable
3 years and older	Easy to understand	Understandable ½ time Not understandable

Test result: 1. NORMAL on DASE and Intelligibility = NORMAL

2. ABNORMAL on DASE and/or Intelligibility = ABNORMAL

*If abnormal on initial screening, rescreen within 2 weeks.
If abnormal again, child should be referred for complete speech evaluation.

FIG. D-2, cont'd • **B,** Percentile rank. (From A.F. Drumwright, University of Colorado Medical Center, 1971.)

DENVER EYE SCREENING TEST

Name:
Hospital No.:
Ward:
Address:

	1ST SCREENING: DATE:						RESCREENING: DATE:					
	Right Eye			Left Eye			Right Eye			Left Eye		
Vision Tests	Normal	Abnormal	Untestable	Normal	Abnormal	Untestable	Normal	Abnormal	Untestable	Normal	Abnormal	Untestable
1. "E" (3 years and above—3 to 5 trials)	3P	3F	U	3P	3F	U	3P	3F	U	3P	3F	U
2. Picture card (2 1/2 - 2 11/12 yrs.—3 to 5 trials)	3P	3F	U	3P	3F	U	3P	3F	U	3P	3F	U
3. Fixation (6 months - 2 5/12 years)	P	F	U	P	F	U	P	F	U	P	F	U
4. Squinting		yes			yes			yes			yes	
Tests for Non-Straight Eyes	Normal		Abnormal			Untestable	Normal		Abnormal			Untestable
1. Do your child's eyes turn in or out, or are they ever not straight?	NO		YES			U	NO		YES			U
2. Cover Test	P		F			U	P		F			U
3. Pupillary Light Reflex	P		F			U	P		F			U
Total Test Rating (Both Eyes)												
Normal (passed vision test plus no squint, plus passed 2/3 tests for non-straight eyes)	Normal						Normal					
Abnormal (abnormal on any vision test, squinting or 2 of 3 procedures for non-straight eyes)	Abnormal						Abnormal					
Untestable (untestable on any vision test or untestable on 2/3 tests for non-straight eyes)	Untestable						Untestable					
Future Rescreening Appointment for Total Test Rating (Abnormal or Untestable)	Date:						Date:					

FIG. D-3 • Denver Eye Screening Test. (From W.K. Frankenburg and J.B. Dodds, University of Colorado Medical Center, 1969.)

SNELLEN SCREENING*

Preparation

1. Hang the Snellen chart on a light-colored wall so that the 20- to 30-foot lines are at eye level when children 6 to 12 years old are tested in the standing position.
2. Secure the chart to the wall with double-stick tape on the back side of all four corners. If the chart must be reversed for use of letter or E chart, secure it at the top and bottom with tacks. Make sure that the chart does not swing when in place.
3. The illumination intensity on the chart should be 10 to 30 foot candles, without any glare from windows or light fixtures. The illumination should be checked with a light meter.
4. Mark an exact 20-foot distance from the chart. Mark the floor with a piece of tape or "footprints" positioned so that the heels touch the 20-foot-line.

Procedure

1. Place the child at the 20-foot mark, with the heel edging the line if the child is standing or with the back of the chair placed at the marker if the child is seated.
2. If the E chart is used, accustom the child to identifying which direction the "legs of the E" are pointing. Use a demonstration E card for this purpose.
3. Teach the child to use the occluder to cover one eye. Instruct the child to keep both eyes open during the test. Provide a clean cover card for each child and then discard after use.
4. If the child wears glasses, test only with glasses on.
5. Test both eyes together, then the right eye, then the left eye.
6. Begin with the 40- or 30-foot line and proceed with the test to include the 20-foot line.
7. With a child suspected of low vision, begin with the 200-foot line, and proceed until child can no longer correctly read three out of four or four out of six symbols on a line.
8. Use covers on the Snellen chart to expose only one symbol or one line at a time. When screening kindergarten or older children, expose one line but use a pointer to point to one symbol at a time.

*Modified from recommendations of the **National Society to Prevent Blindness:** *Guide to testing distance visual acuity,* Schaumburg, IL, 1988, The Society.

Recording and Referral

1. Record the last line the child read correctly (three out of four or four out of six symbols).
2. Record visual acuity as a fraction. The numerator represents the distance from the chart, and the denominator represents the last line read correctly. For example, 20/30 means that the child read the 30-foot line at a 20-foot distance.
3. Observe the child's eyes during testing and record any evidence of squinting, head tilting, thrusting the head forward, excessive blinking, tearing, or redness.
4. Only make referrals after a second screening has been made on children who are potential candidates for referral.
5. The following children should be referred for a complete eye examination:
   a. Three-year-old children with vision in either eye of 20/50 or less (inability to correctly identify one more than half the symbols on the 40-foot line) *or* a two-line difference in visual acuity between the eyes in the passing range (e.g., 20/20 in one eye and 20/40 in the other)
   b. All other ages and grades with vision in either eye of 20/40 or less (inability to correctly identify one or more than half the symbols on the 30-foot line)
   c. All children who consistently show any of the signs of possible visual disturbances, regardless of visual acuity

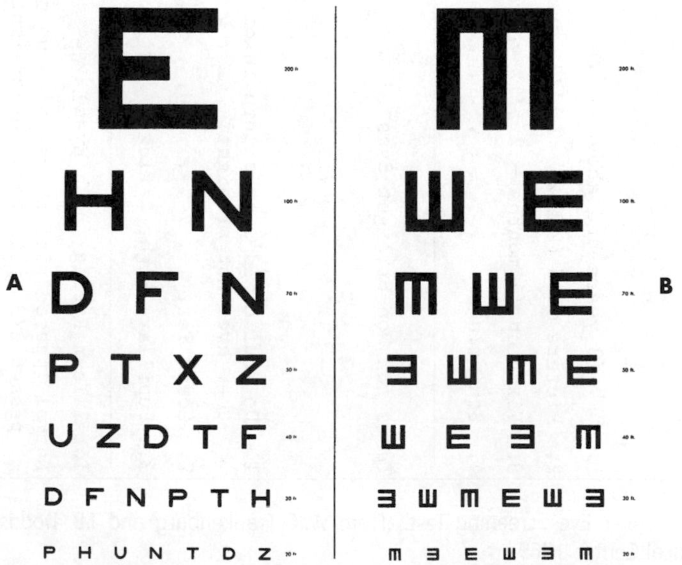

FIG. D-4 • Snellen chart. **A,** Letter (alphabet) chart. **B,** Symbol E chart. (From National Society to Prevent Blindness, Inc., Schaumburg, IL.)

APPENDIX

E Growth Measurements

http://www.harcourthealth.com/MERLIN/Wong/maternal/

Height and Weight Measurements for Boys

	Height by Percentiles						Weight by Percentiles					
	5		50		95		5		50		95	
Age*	cm	inches	cm	inches	cm	inches	kg	lb	kg	lb	kg	lb
Birth	46.4	18¼	50.5	20	54.4	21½	2.54	5½	3.27	7¼	4.15	9¼
3 months	56.7	22¼	61.1	24	65.4	25¾	4.43	9¾	5.98	13¼	7.37	16¼
6 months	63.4	25	67.8	26¾	72.3	28½	6.20	13¾	7.85	17¼	9.46	20¾
9 months	68.0	26¾	72.3	28½	77.1	30¼	7.52	16½	9.18	20¼	10.93	24
1	71.7	28¼	76.1	30	81.2	32	8.43	18½	10.15	22½	11.99	26½
1½	77.5	30½	82.4	32½	88.1	34¾	9.59	21¼	11.47	25¼	13.44	29½
2†	82.5	32½	86.8	34¼	94.4	37¼	10.49	23¼	12.34	27¼	15.50	34¼
2½†	85.4	33½	90.4	35½	97.8	38½	11.27	24¾	13.52	29¾	16.61	36½
3	89.0	35	94.9	37¼	102.0	40¼	12.05	26½	14.62	32¼	17.77	39¼
3½	92.5	36½	99.1	39	106.1	41¾	12.84	28¼	15.68	34½	18.98	41¾
4	95.8	37¾	102.9	40½	109.9	43¼	13.64	30	16.69	36¾	20.27	44¾
4½	98.9	39	106.6	42	113.5	44¾	14.45	31¾	17.69	39	21.63	47¾
5	102.0	40¼	109.9	43¼	117.0	46	15.27	33¾	18.67	41¼	23.09	51
6	107.7	42½	116.1	45¾	123.5	48½	16.93	37¼	20.69	45½	26.34	58
7	113.0	44½	121.7	48	129.7	51	18.64	41	22.85	50¼	30.12	66½
8	118.1	46½	127.0	50	135.7	53½	20.40	45	25.30	55¾	34.51	76
9	122.9	48½	132.2	52	141.8	55¾	22.25	49	28.13	62	39.58	87¼
10	127.7	50¼	137.5	54¼	148.1	58¼	24.33	53¾	31.44	69¼	45.27	99¾
11	132.6	52¼	143.3	56½	154.9	61	26.80	59	35.30	77¾	51.47	113½
12	137.6	54¼	149.7	59	162.3	64	29.85	65¾	39.78	87¾	58.09	128
13	142.9	56¼	156.5	61½	169.8	66¾	33.64	74¼	44.95	99	65.02	143¼
14	148.8	58½	163.1	64¼	176.7	69½	38.22	84¼	50.77	112	72.13	159
15	155.2	61	169.0	66½	181.9	71½	43.11	95	56.71	125	79.12	174½
16	161.1	63½	173.5	68¼	185.4	73	47.74	105¼	62.10	137	85.62	188¾
17	164.9	65	176.2	69¼	187.3	73¾	51.50	113½	66.31	146¼	91.31	201¼
18	165.7	65¼	176.8	69½	187.6	73¾	53.97	119	68.88	151¾	95.76	211

Modified from National Center for Health Statistics (NCHS), Health Resources Administration, Department of Health, Education and Welfare, Hyattsville, MD. Conversion of metric data to approximate inches and pounds by Ross Laboratories.
*Years unless otherwise indicated.
†Height data include some recumbent length measurements, which make values slightly higher than if all measurements had been of stature (standing height).

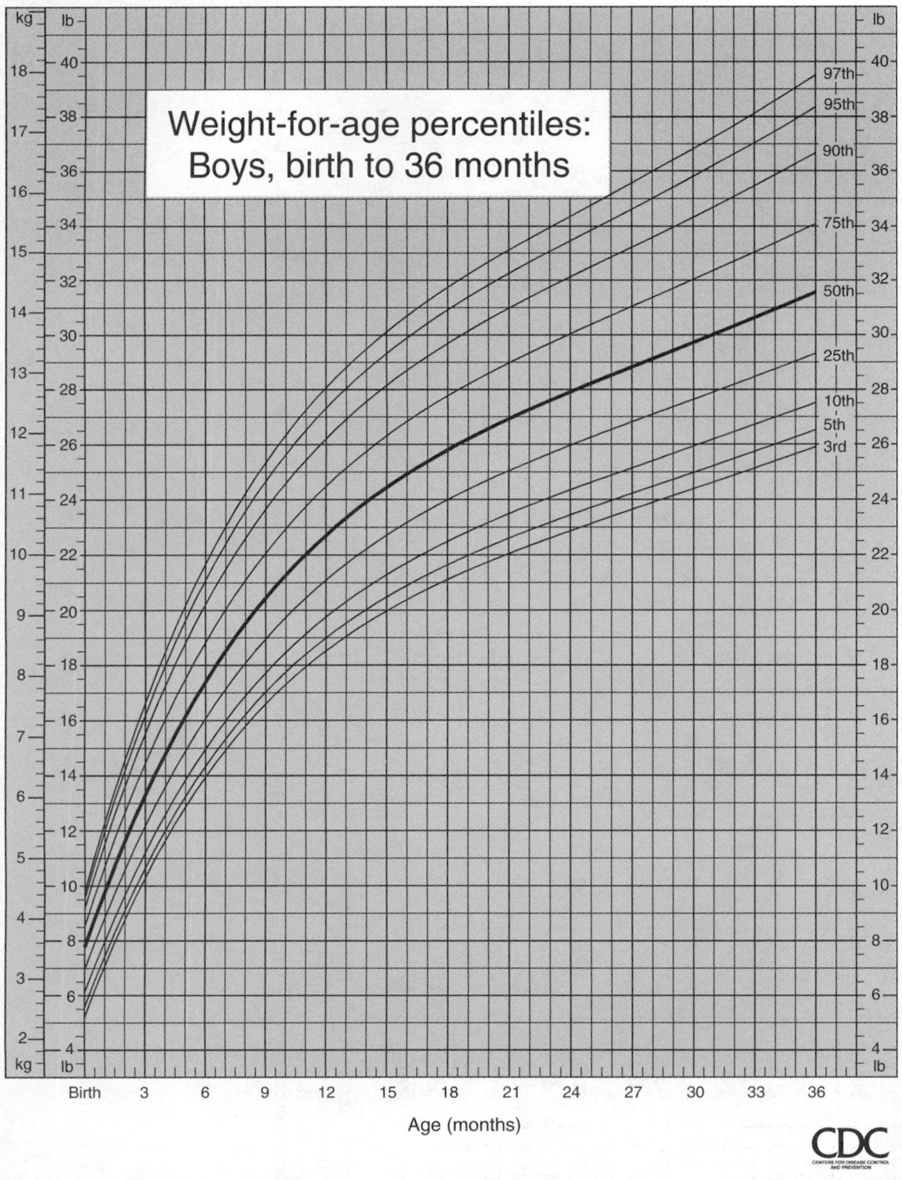

FIG. E-1 • Weight-for-age percentiles, boys, birth to 36 months, CDC growth charts: United States. (Developed by the National Center for Health Statistics in collaboration with the National Center for Chronic Disease Prevention and Health Promotion [2000].)

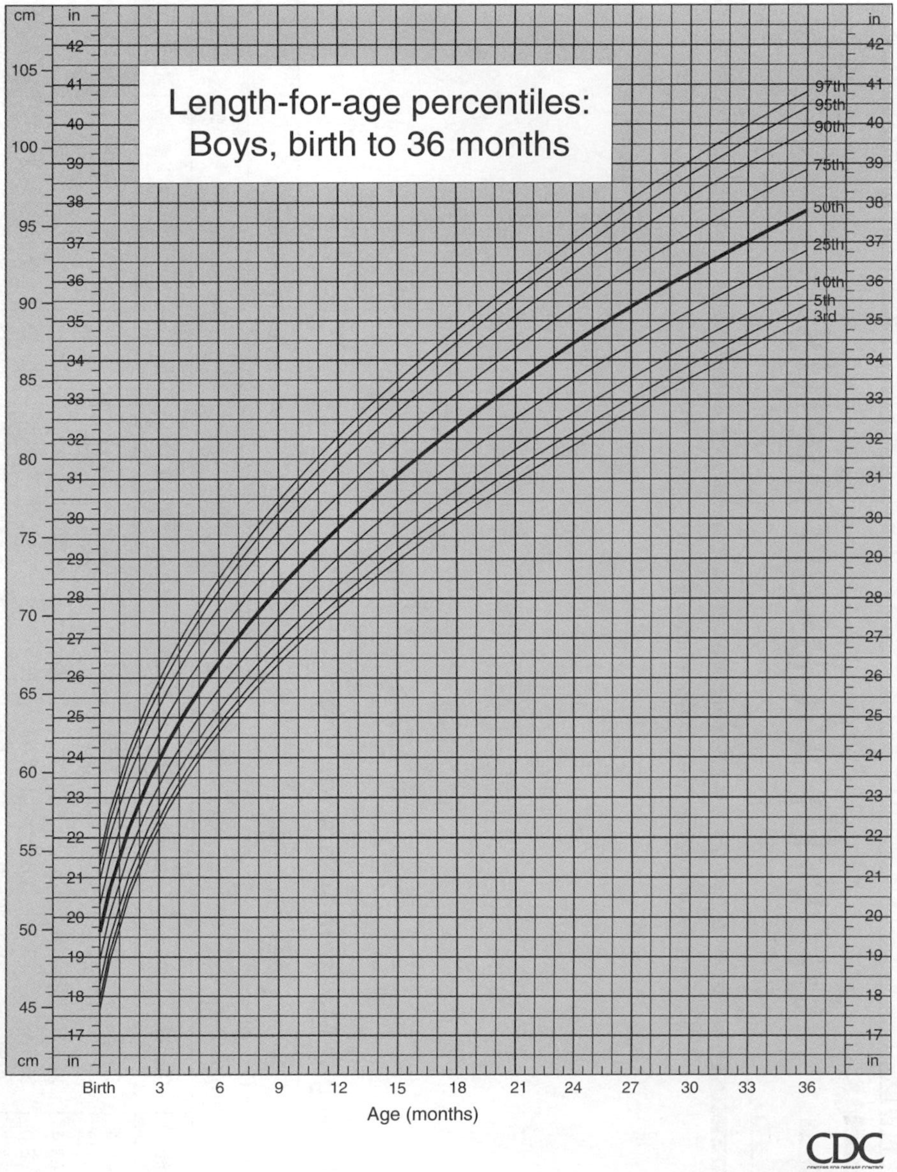

FIG. E-2 • Length-for-age percentiles, boys, birth to 36 months, CDC growth charts: United States. (Developed by the National Center for Health Statistics in collaboration with the National Center for Chronic Disease Prevention and Health Promotion [2000].)

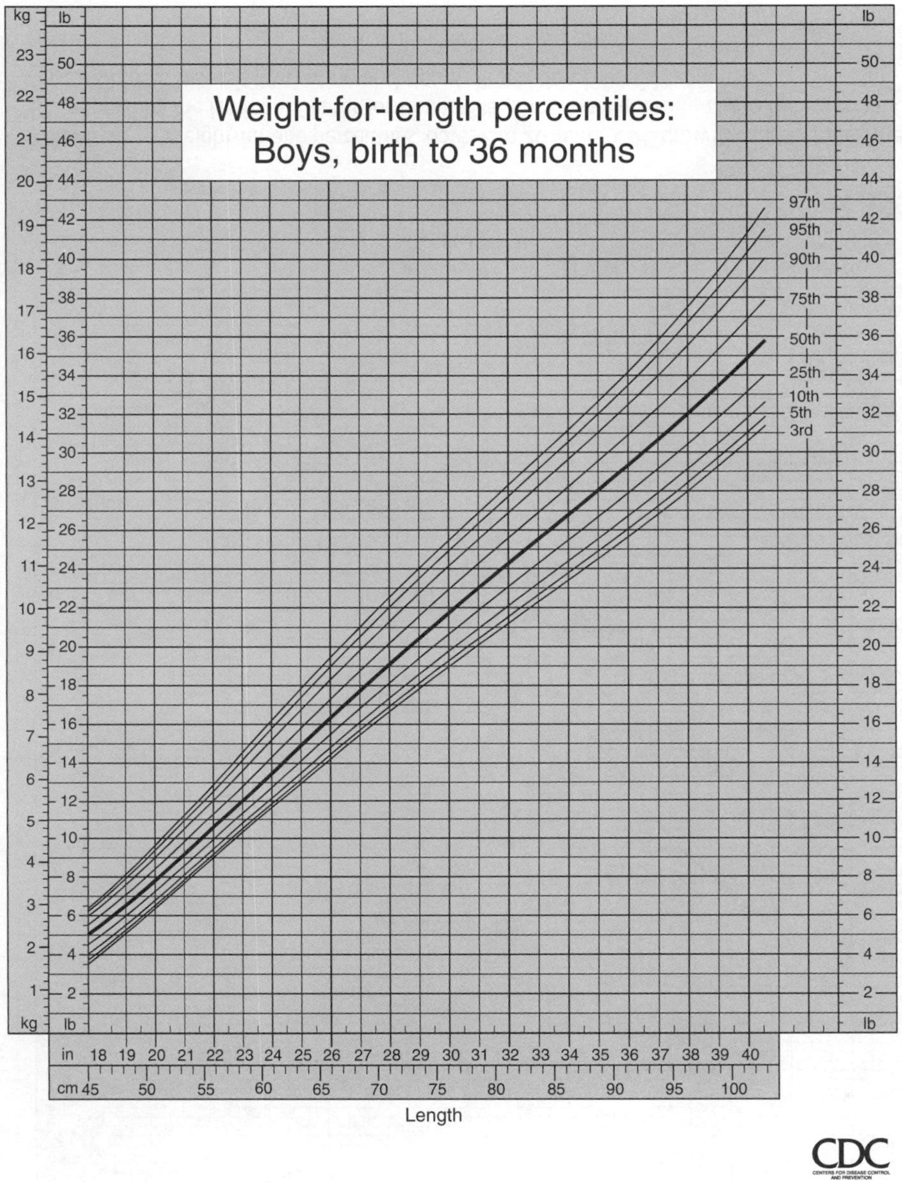

FIG. E-3 • Weight-for-length percentiles, boys, birth to 36 months, CDC growth charts: United States. (Developed by the National Center for Health Statistics in callaboration with the National Center for Chronic Disease Prevention and Health Promotion [2000].)

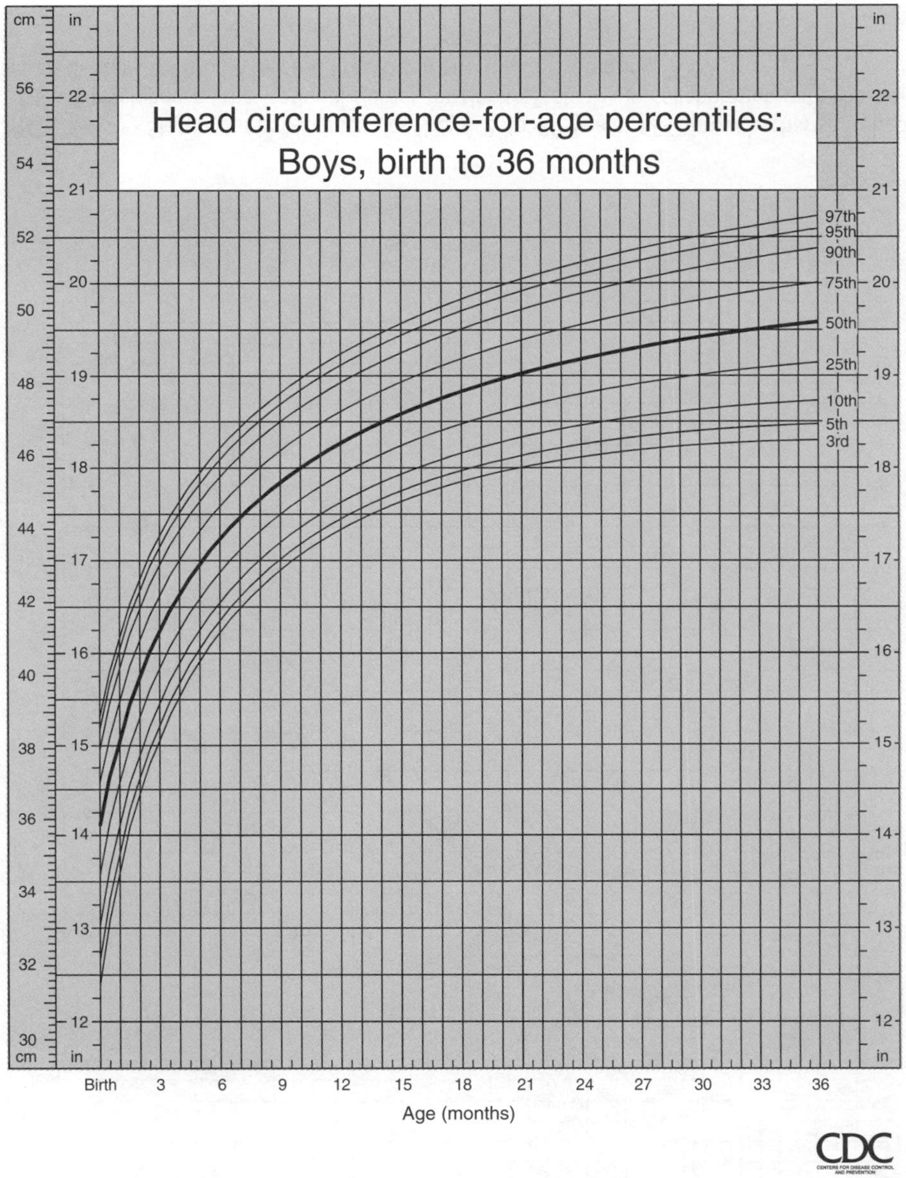

FIG. E-4 • Head circumference-for age percentiles, boys, birth to 36 months, CDC growth charts: United States. (Developed by the National Center for Health Statistics in collaboration with the National Center for Chronic Disease Prevention and Health Promotion [2000].)

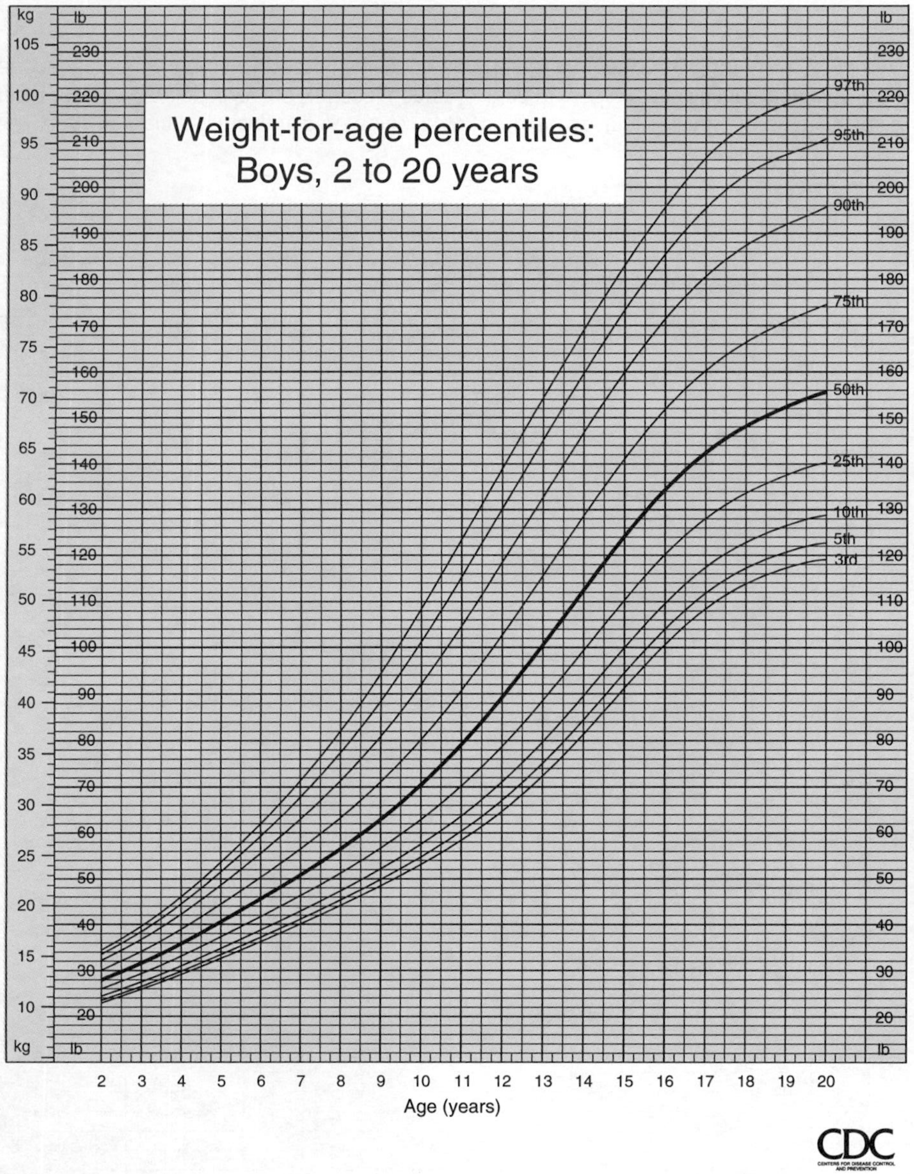

FIG. E-5 • Weight-for-age percentiles, boys, 2 to 20 years, CDC growth charts: United States. (Developed by the National Center for Health Statistics in collaboration with the National Center for Chronic Disease Prevention and Health Promotion [2000].)

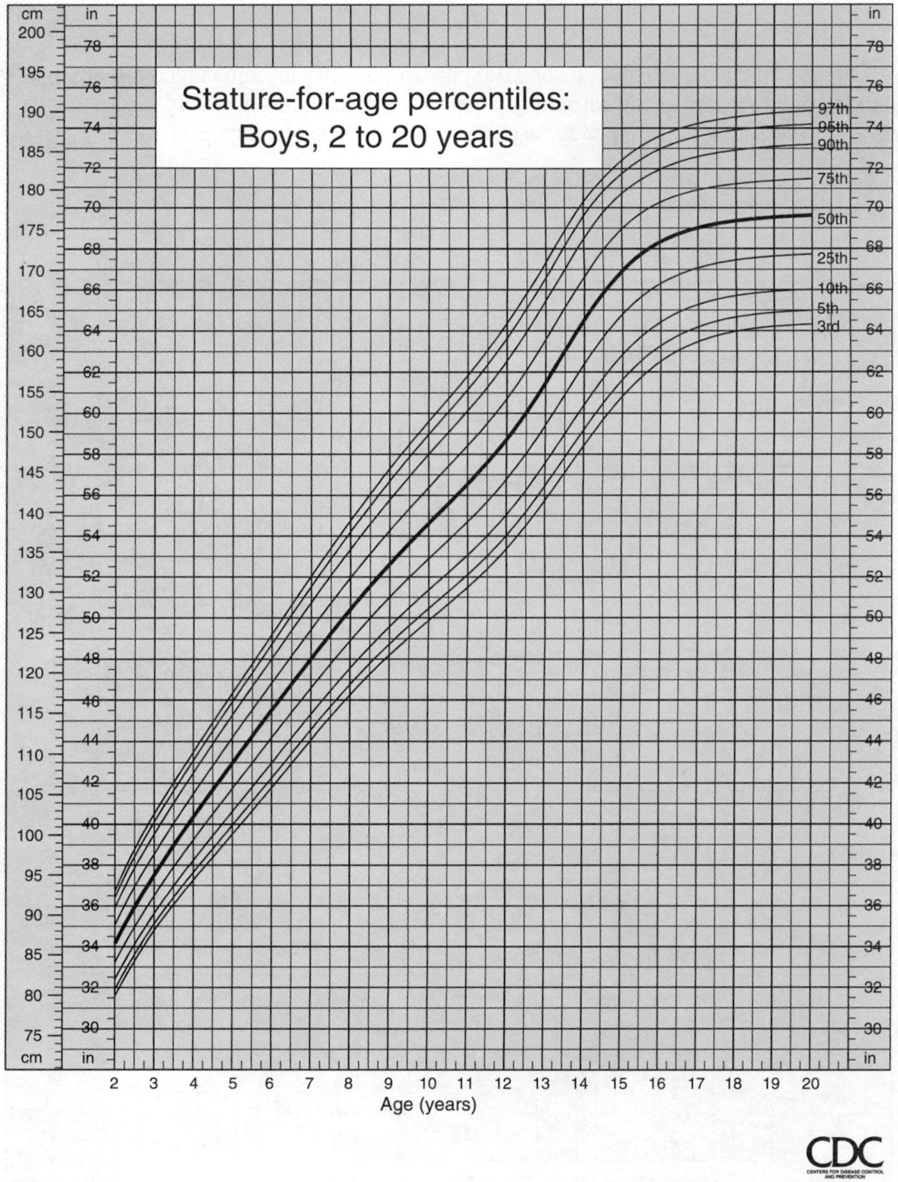

FIG. E-6 • Stature-for-age percentiles, boys, 2 to 20 years, CDC growth charts: United States. (Developed by the National Center for Health Statistics in collaboration with the National Center for Chronic Disease Prevention and Health Promotion [2000].)

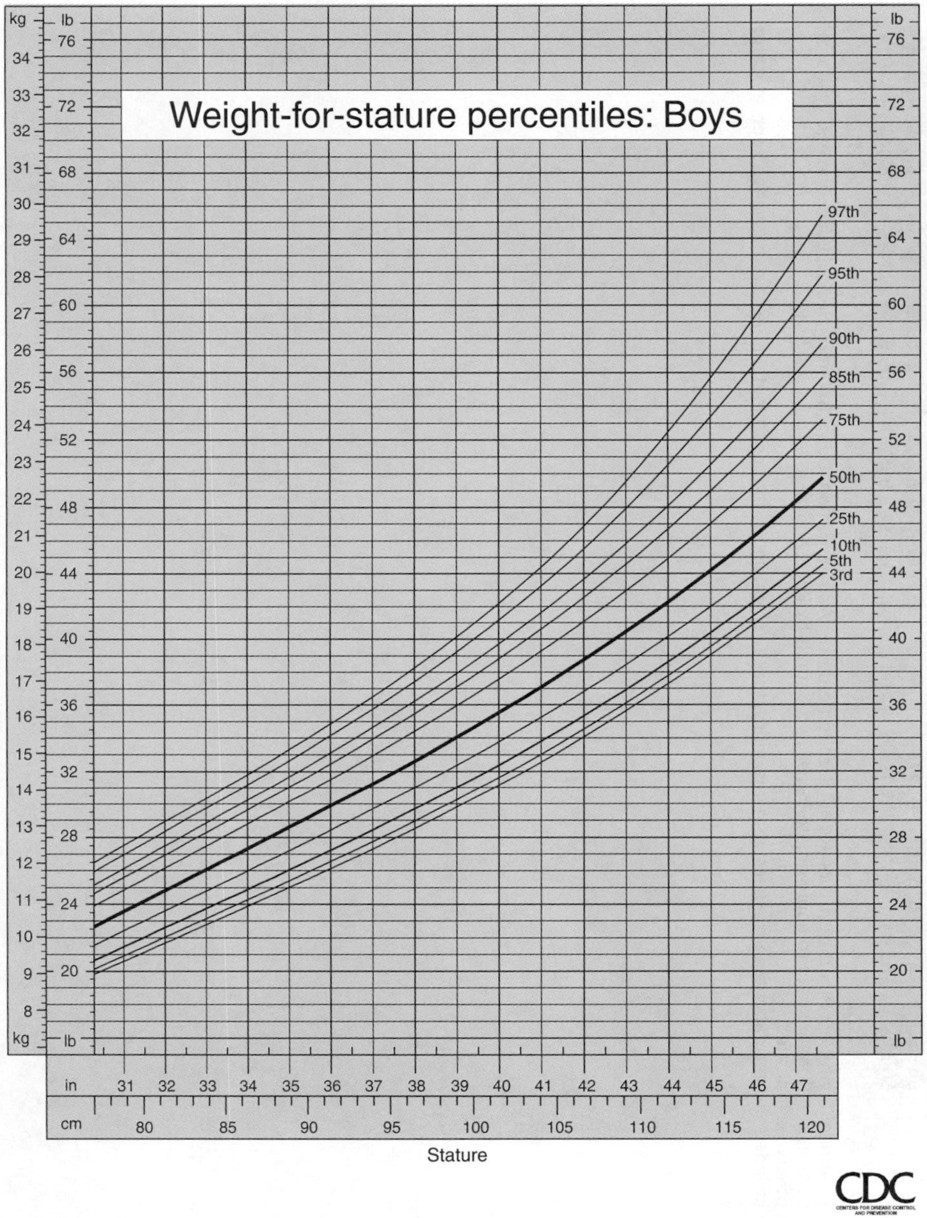

FIG. E-7 • Weight-for stature percentiles, boys, CDC growth charts: United States. (Developed by the National Center for Health Statistics in collaboration with the National Center for Chronic Disease Prevention and Health Promotion [2000].)

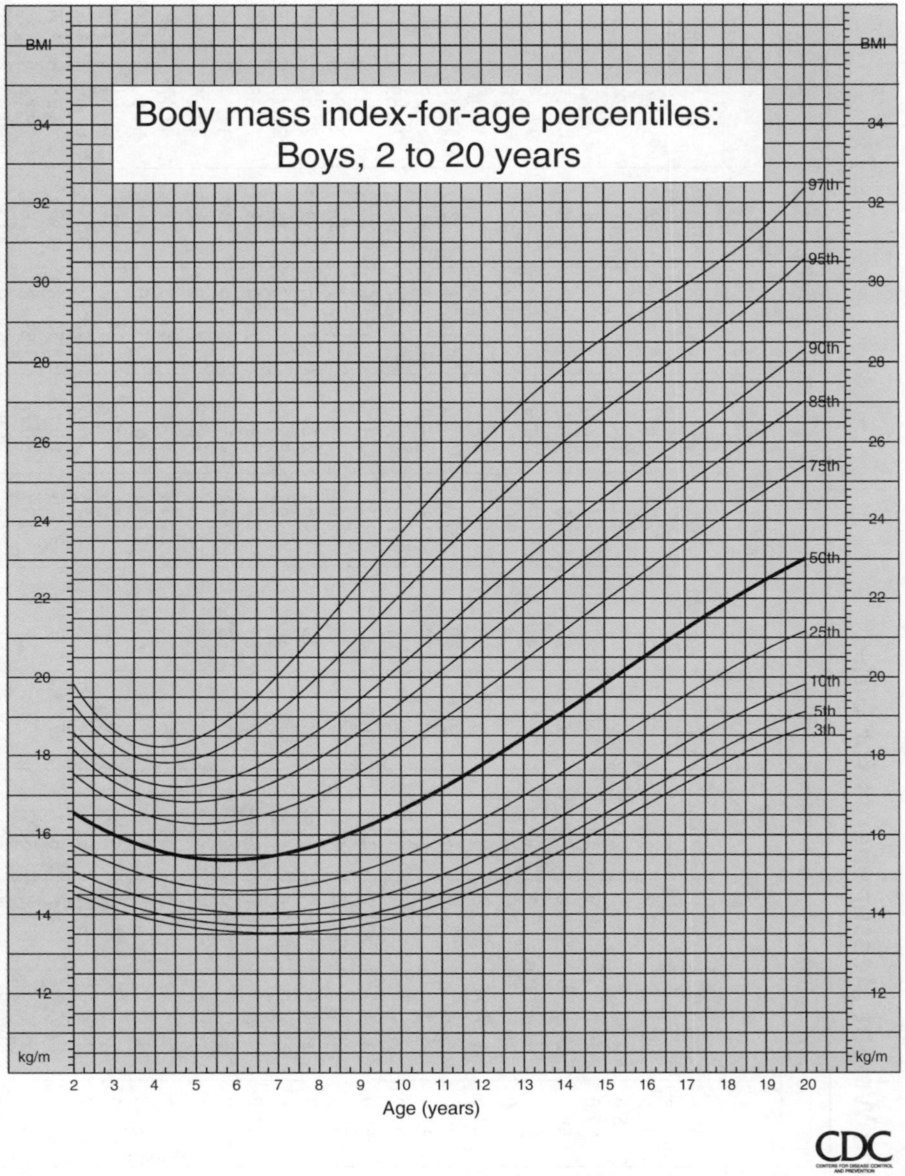

FIG. E-8 • Body mass index-for-age percentiles, boys, 2 to 20 years, CDC growth charts: United States. (Developed by the National Center for Health Statistics in collaboration with the National Center for Chronic Disease Prevention and Health Promotion [2000].)

Height and Weight Measurements for Girls

	Height by Percentiles						Weight by Percentiles					
	5		50		95		5		50		95	
Age*	cm	inches	cm	inches	cm	inches	kg	lb	kg	lb	kg	lb
Birth	45.4	$17^{3}/_{4}$	49.9	$19^{3}/_{4}$	52.9	$20^{3}/_{4}$	2.36	$5^{1}/_{4}$	3.23	7	3.81	$8^{1}/_{2}$
3 months	55.4	$21^{3}/_{4}$	59.5	$23^{1}/_{2}$	63.4	25	4.18	$9^{1}/_{4}$	5.4	12	6.74	$14^{3}/_{4}$
6 months	61.8	$24^{1}/_{4}$	65.9	26	70.2	$27^{3}/_{4}$	5.79	$12^{3}/_{4}$	7.21	16	8.73	$19^{1}/_{4}$
9 months	66.1	26	70.4	$27^{3}/_{4}$	75.0	$29^{1}/_{2}$	7.0	$15^{1}/_{2}$	8.56	$18^{3}/_{4}$	10.17	$22^{1}/_{2}$
1	69.8	$27^{1}/_{2}$	74.3	$29^{1}/_{4}$	79.1	$31^{1}/_{4}$	7.84	$17^{1}/_{4}$	9.53	21	11.24	$24^{3}/_{4}$
$1^{1}/_{2}$	76.0	30	80.9	$31^{3}/_{4}$	86.1	34	8.92	$19^{3}/_{4}$	10.82	$23^{3}/_{4}$	12.76	$28^{1}/_{4}$
2†	81.6	$32^{1}/_{4}$	86.8	$34^{1}/_{4}$	93.6	$36^{1}/_{4}$	9.95	22	11.8	26	14.15	$31^{1}/_{4}$
$2^{1}/_{2}$†	84.6	$33^{1}/_{4}$	90.0	$35^{1}/_{2}$	96.6	38	10.8	$23^{3}/_{4}$	13.03	$28^{3}/_{4}$	15.76	$34^{3}/_{4}$
3	88.3	$34^{3}/_{4}$	94.1	37	100.6	$39^{1}/_{2}$	11.61	$25^{1}/_{2}$	14.1	31	17.22	38
$3^{1}/_{2}$	91.7	36	97.9	$38^{1}/_{2}$	104.5	$41^{1}/_{4}$	12.37	$27^{1}/_{4}$	15.07	$33^{1}/_{4}$	18.59	41
4	95.0	$37^{1}/_{2}$	101.6	40	108.3	$42^{3}/_{4}$	13.11	29	15.96	$35^{1}/_{4}$	19.91	44
$4^{1}/_{2}$	98.1	$38^{1}/_{2}$	105.0	$41^{1}/_{4}$	112.0	44	13.83	$30^{1}/_{2}$	16.81	37	21.24	$46^{3}/_{4}$
5	101.1	$39^{3}/_{4}$	108.4	$42^{3}/_{4}$	115.6	$45^{1}/_{2}$	14.55	32	17.66	39	22.62	$49^{3}/_{4}$
6	106.6	42	114.6	45	122.7	$48^{1}/_{4}$	16.05	$35^{1}/_{2}$	19.52	43	25.75	$56^{3}/_{4}$
7	111.8	44	120.6	$47^{1}/_{2}$	129.5	51	17.71	39	21.84	$48^{1}/_{4}$	29.68	$65^{1}/_{2}$
8	116.9	46	126.4	$49^{3}/_{4}$	136.2	$53^{1}/_{2}$	19.62	$43^{1}/_{4}$	24.84	$54^{3}/_{4}$	34.71	$76^{1}/_{2}$
9	122.1	48	132.2	52	142.9	$56^{1}/_{4}$	21.82	48	28.46	$62^{3}/_{4}$	40.64	$89^{1}/_{2}$
10	127.5	$50^{1}/_{4}$	138.3	$54^{1}/_{2}$	149.5	$58^{3}/_{4}$	24.36	$53^{3}/_{4}$	32.55	$71^{3}/_{4}$	47.17	104
11	133.5	$52^{1}/_{2}$	144.8	57	156.2	$61^{1}/_{2}$	27.24	60	36.95	$81^{1}/_{2}$	54.0	119
12	139.8	55	151.5	$59^{3}/_{4}$	162.7	64	30.52	$67^{1}/_{4}$	41.53	$91^{1}/_{2}$	60.81	134
13	145.2	$57^{1}/_{4}$	157.1	$61^{3}/_{4}$	168.1	$66^{1}/_{4}$	34.14	$75^{1}/_{4}$	46.1	$101^{3}/_{4}$	67.3	$148^{1}/_{4}$
14	148.7	$58^{1}/_{2}$	160.4	$63^{1}/_{4}$	171.3	$67^{1}/_{2}$	37.76	$83^{1}/_{4}$	50.28	$110^{3}/_{4}$	73.08	161
15	150.5	$59^{1}/_{4}$	161.8	$63^{3}/_{4}$	172.8	68	40.99	$90^{1}/_{4}$	53.68	$118^{1}/_{4}$	77.78	$171^{1}/_{2}$
16	151.6	$59^{3}/_{4}$	162.4	64	173.3	$68^{1}/_{4}$	43.41	$95^{3}/_{4}$	55.89	$123^{1}/_{4}$	80.99	$178^{1}/_{2}$
17	152.7	60	163.1	$64^{1}/_{4}$	173.5	$68^{1}/_{4}$	44.74	$98^{3}/_{4}$	56.69	125	82.46	$181^{3}/_{4}$
18	153.6	$60^{1}/_{2}$	163.7	$64^{1}/_{2}$	173.6	$68^{1}/_{4}$	45.26	$99^{3}/_{4}$	56.62	$124^{3}/_{4}$	82.47	$181^{3}/_{4}$

Modified from National Center for Health Statistics (NCHS), Health Resources Administration, Department of Health, Education and Welfare, Hyattsville, MD. Conversion of metric data to approximate inches and pounds by Ross Laboratories.
*Years unless otherwise indicated.
†Height data include some recumbent length measurements, which make values slightly higher than if all measurements had been of stature.

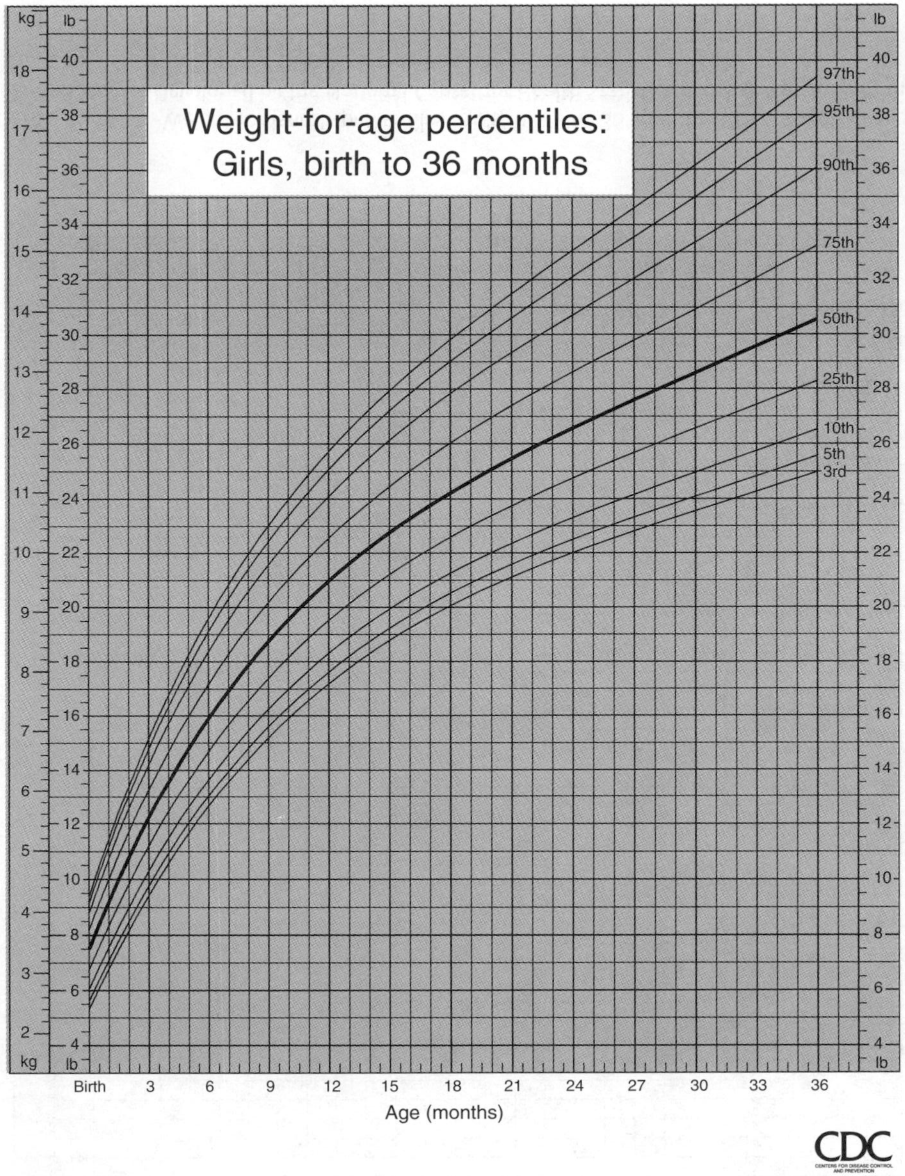

FIG. E-9 • Weight-for-age percentiles, girls, birth to 36 months, CDC growth charts: United States. (Developed by the National Center for Health Statistics in collaboration with the National Center for Chronic Disease Prevention and Health Promotion [2000].)

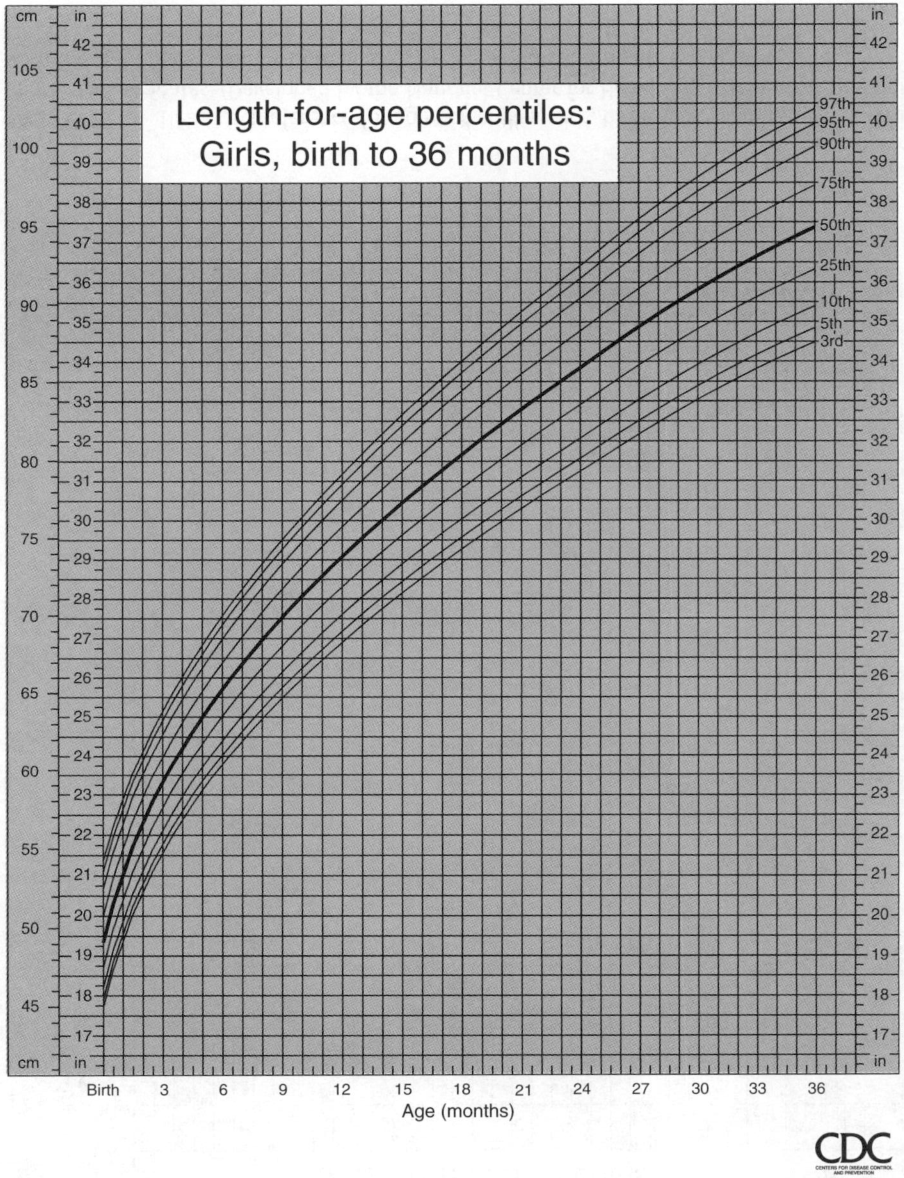

FIG. E-10 • Length-for-age percentiles, girls, birth to 36 months, CDC growth charts: United States. (Developed by the National Center for Health Statistics in collaboration with the National Center for Chronic Disease Prevention and Health Promotion [2000].)

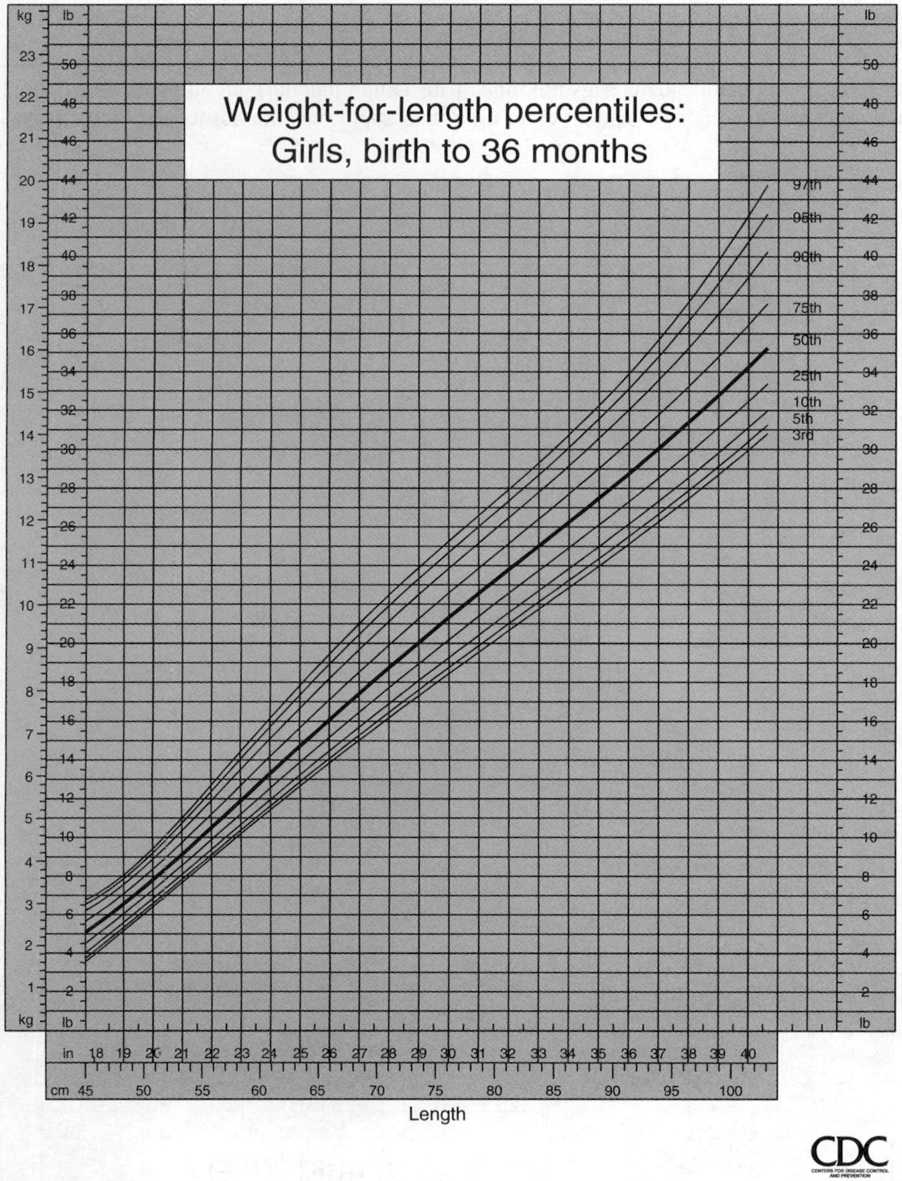

FIG. E-11 • Weight-for-length percentiles, girls, birth to 36 months, CDC growth charts: United States. (Developed by the National Center for Health Statistics in collaboration with the National Center for Chronic Disease Prevention and Health Promotion [2000].)

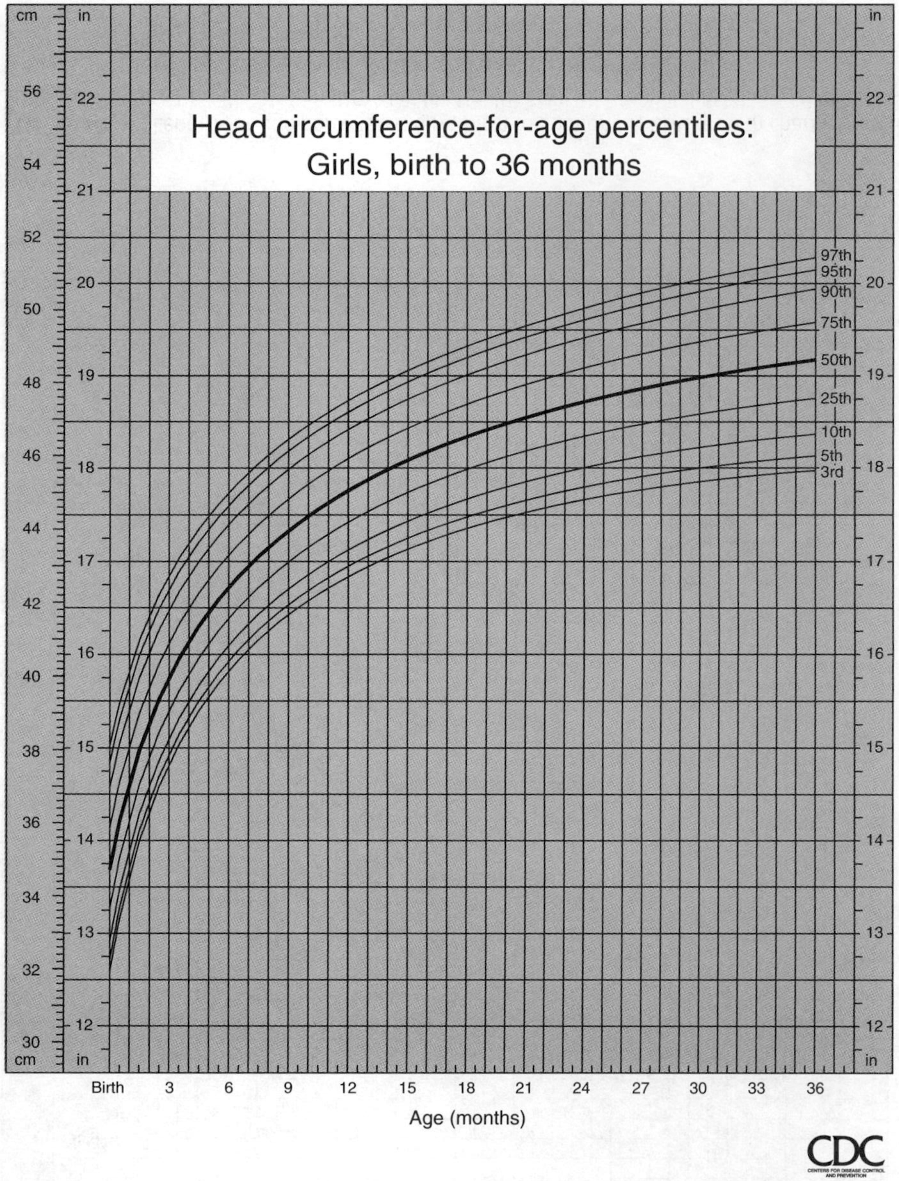

FIG. E-12 • Head circumference-for-age percentiles, girls, birth to 36 months, CDC growth charts: United States. (Developed by the National Center for Health Statistics in collaboration with the National Center for Chronic Disease Prevention and Health Promotion [2000].)

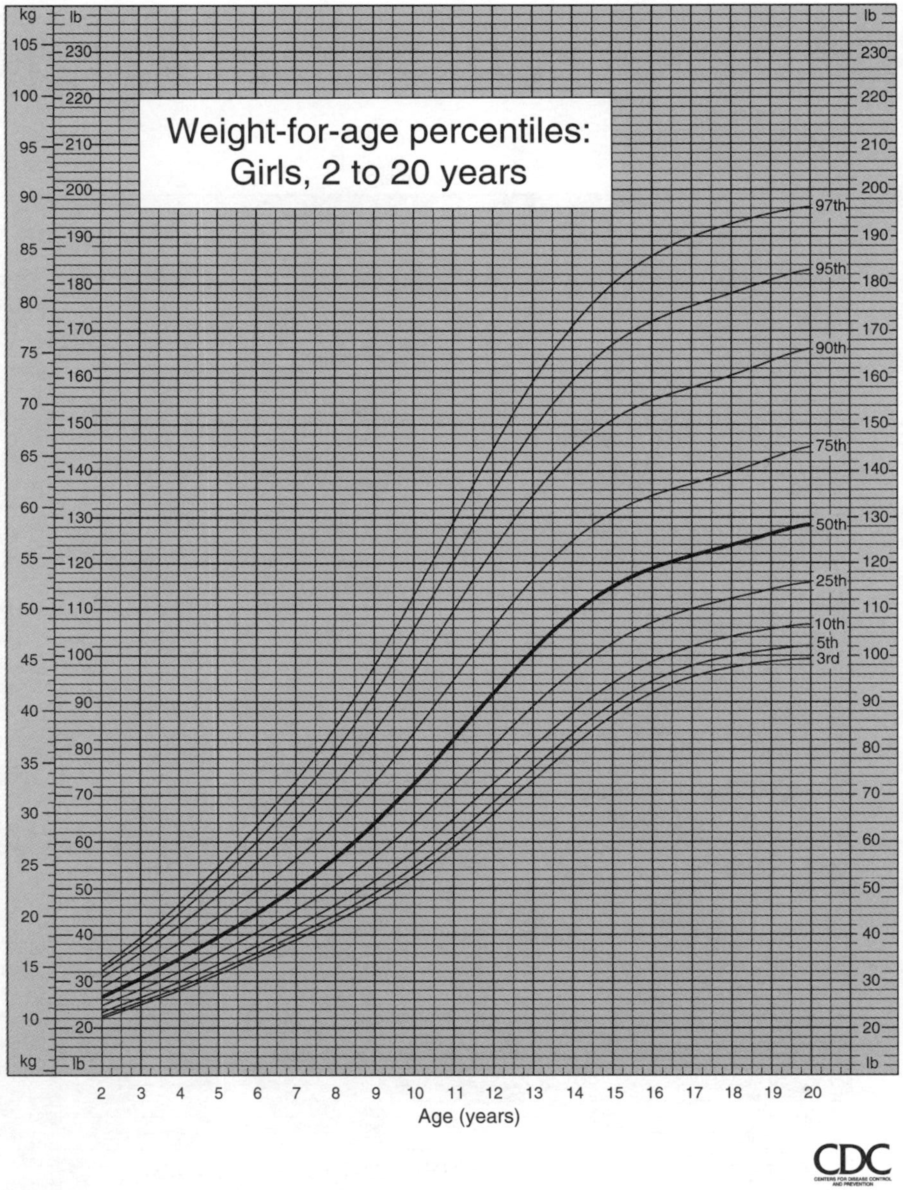

FIG. E-13 • Weight-for-age percentiles, girls, 2 to 20 years, CDC growth charts: United States. (Developed by the National Center for Health Statistics in collaboration with the National Center for Chronic Disease Prevention and Health Promotion [2000].)

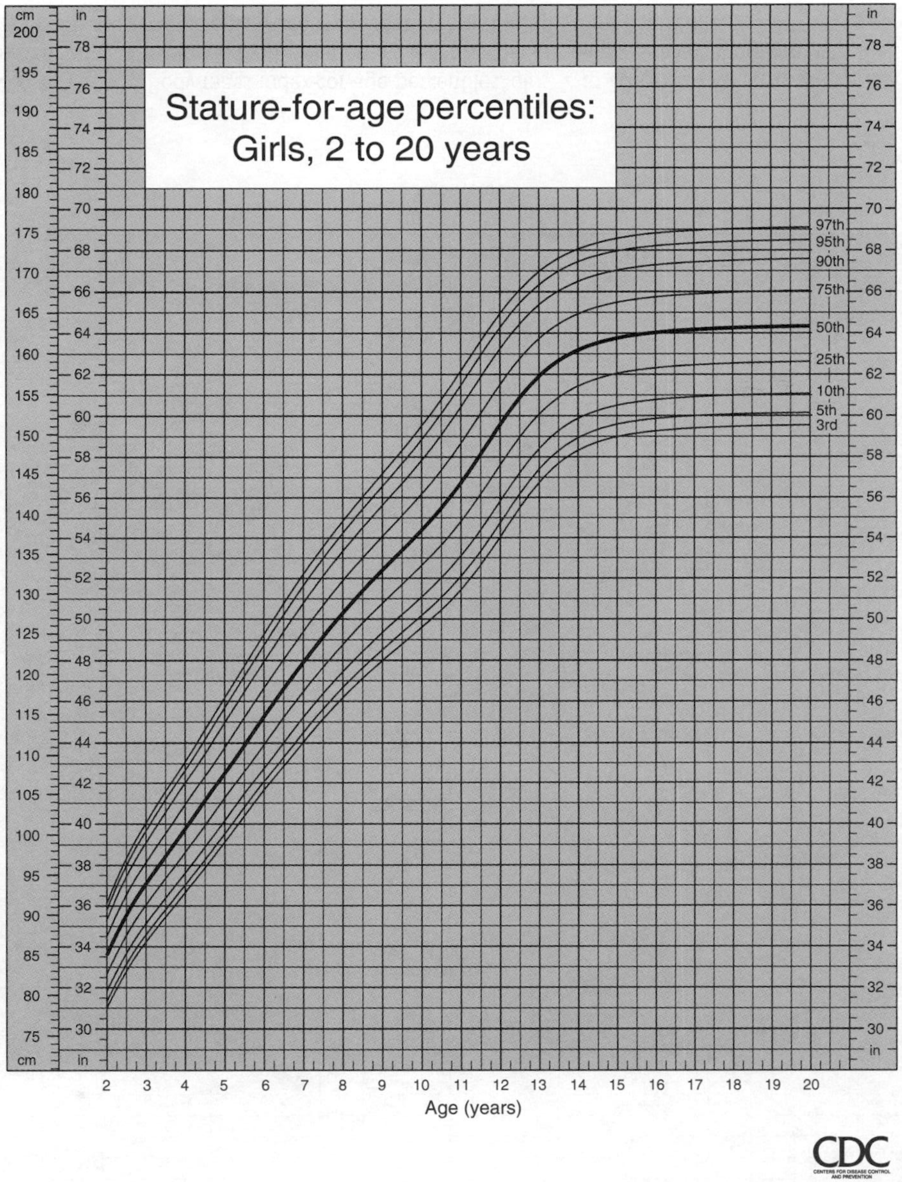

FIG. E-14 • Stature-for-age percentiles, girls, 2 to 20 years, CDC growth charts: United States. (Developed by the National Center for Health Statistics in collaboration with the National Center for Chronic Disease Prevention and Health Promotion [2000].)

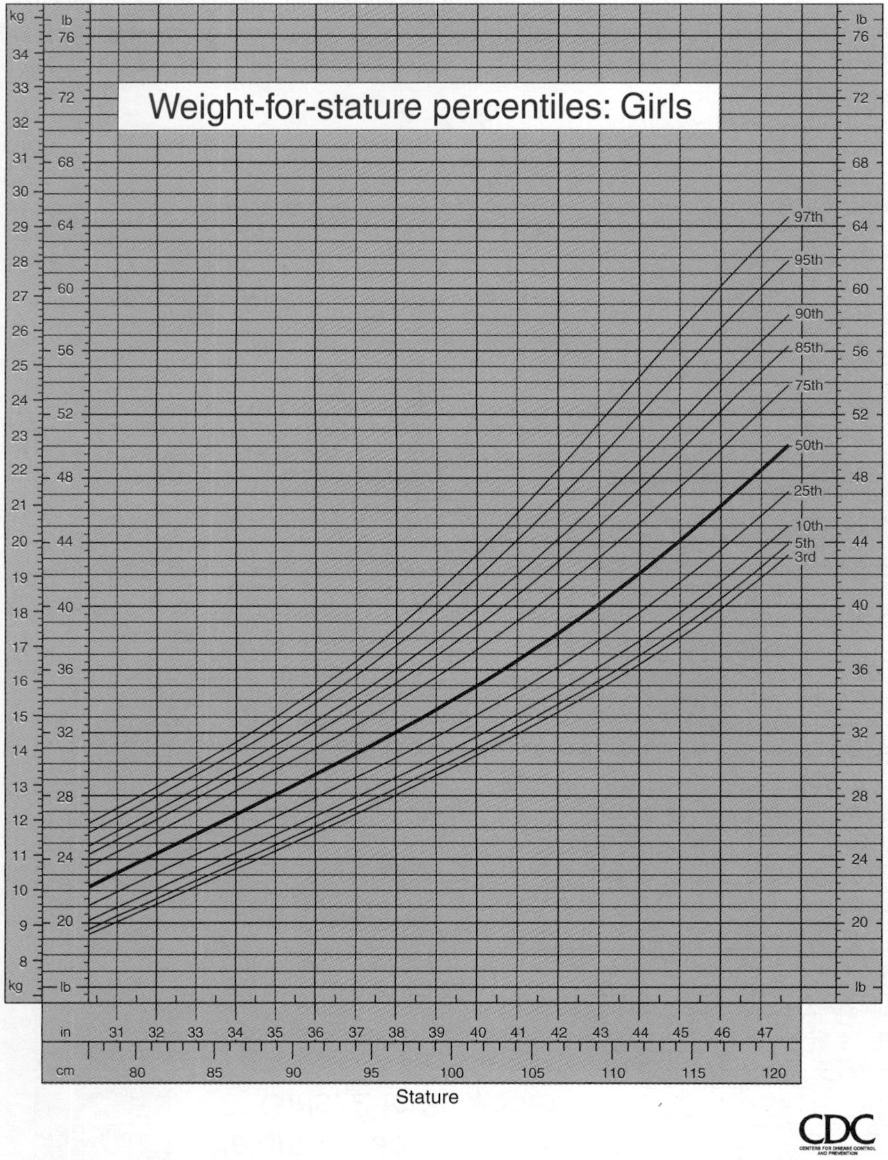

FIG. E-15 • Weight-for-stature percentiles, gorls, CDC growth charts: United States. (Developed by the National Center for Health Statistics in collaboration with the National Center for Chronic Disease Prevention and Health Promotion [2000].)

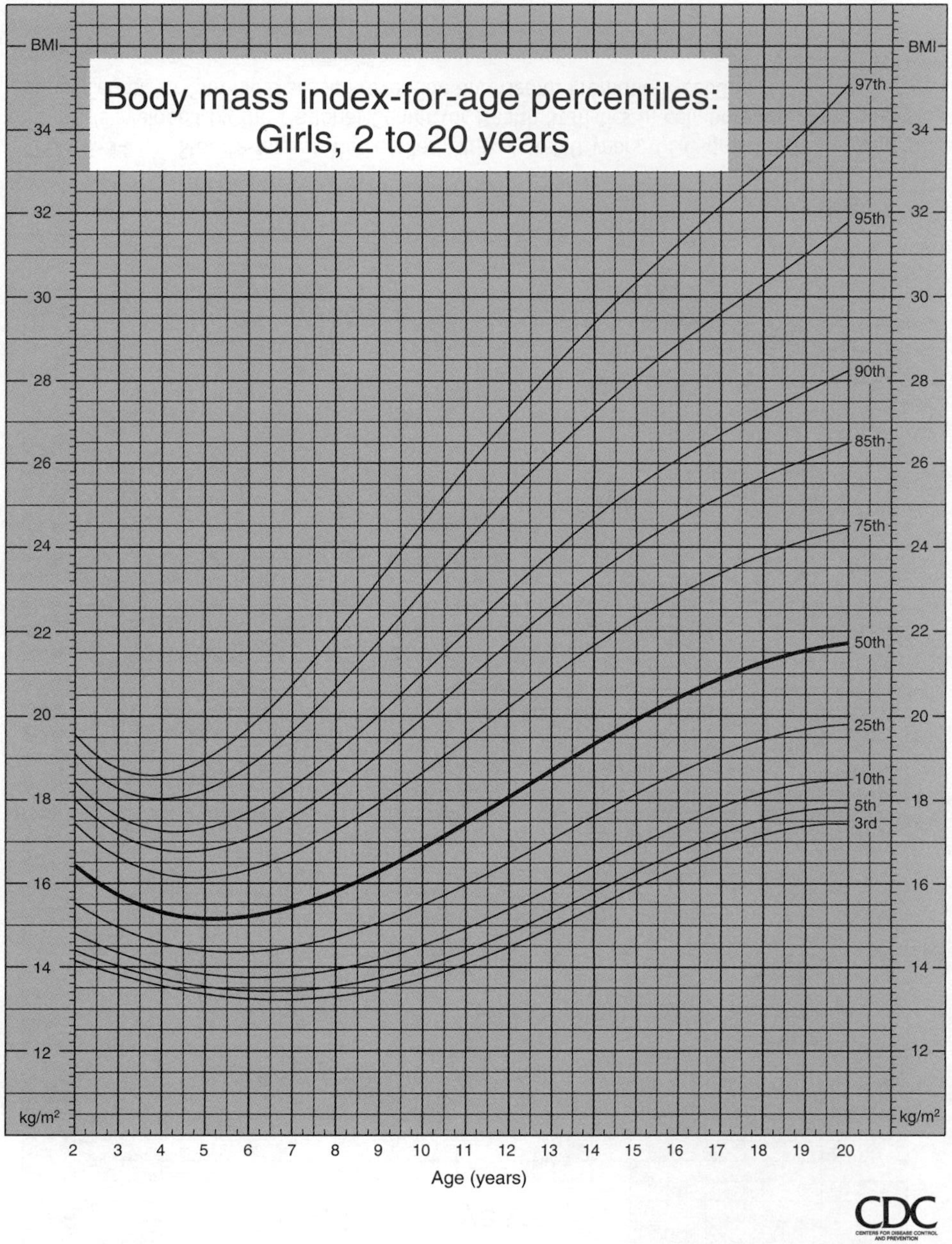

FIG. E-16 • SBody mass index-for-age percentiles, girls, 2 to 20 years, CDC growth charts: United States. (Developed by the National Center for Health Statistics in collaboration with the National Center for Chronic Disease Prevention and Health Promotion [2000].)

Growth Standards of Healthy Chinese Children

Age (Months or Years)	Weight (kg)		Height (cm)		Head Circumference	
	Boys	Girls	Boys	Girls	Boys	Girls
Birth	3.27	3.17	50.6	50.0	34.3	33.7
1 month	4.97	4.64	56.5	55.5	38.1	37.3
2 months	5.95	5.49	59.6	58.4	39.7	38.7
3 months	6.73	6.23	62.3	60.9	41.0	40.0
4 months	7.32	6.69	64.4	62.9	42.0	41.0
5 months	7.70	7.19	65.9	64.5	42.9	41.9
6 months	8.22	7.62	68.1	66.7	43.9	42.8
8 months	8.71	8.14	70.6	69.0	44.9	43.7
10 months	9.14	8.57	72.9	71.4	45.7	44.5
12 months	9.56	9.04	75.6	74.1	46.3	45.2
15 months	10.15	9.54	78.3	76.9	46.8	45.6
18 months	10.67	10.08	80.7	79.4	47.3	46.2
21 months	11.18	10.56	83.0	81.7	47.8	46.7
24 months	11.95	11.37	86.5	85.3	48.2	47.1
2.5 years	12.84	12.28	90.4	89.3	48.8	47.7
3 years	13.63	13.16	93.8	92.8	49.1	48.1
3.5 years	14.45	14.00	97.2	96.3	49.4	48.5
4 years	15.26	14.89	100.8	100.1	49.7	48.9
4.5 years	16.07	15.63	103.9	103.1	50.0	49.1
5 years	16.88	16.46	107.2	106.5	50.2	49.4
5.5 years	17.65	17.18	110.1	109.2	50.5	49.6
6 years	19.25	18.67	114.7	113.9	50.8	50.0
7 years	21.01	20.35	120.6	119.3	51.1	50.2
8 years	23.08	22.43	125.3	124.6	51.4	50.6
9 years	25.33	24.57	130.6	129.5	51.7	50.9
10 years	27.15	27.05	134.4	134.8	51.9	51.3
11 years	30.13	30.51	139.2	140.6	52.3	51.7
12 years	33.05	34.74	144.2	146.6	52.7	52.3
13 years	36.90	38.52	149.8	150.7	53.0	52.8

Data from Bejing Children's Hospital, 1987, China.

HEAD CIRCUMFERENCE CHARTS

A

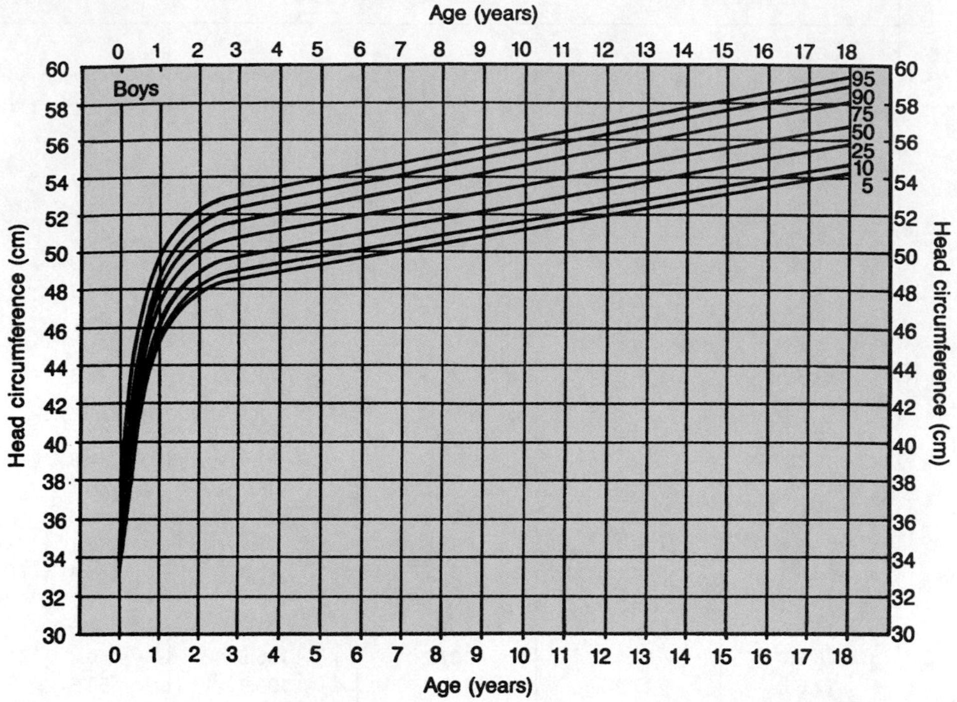

B

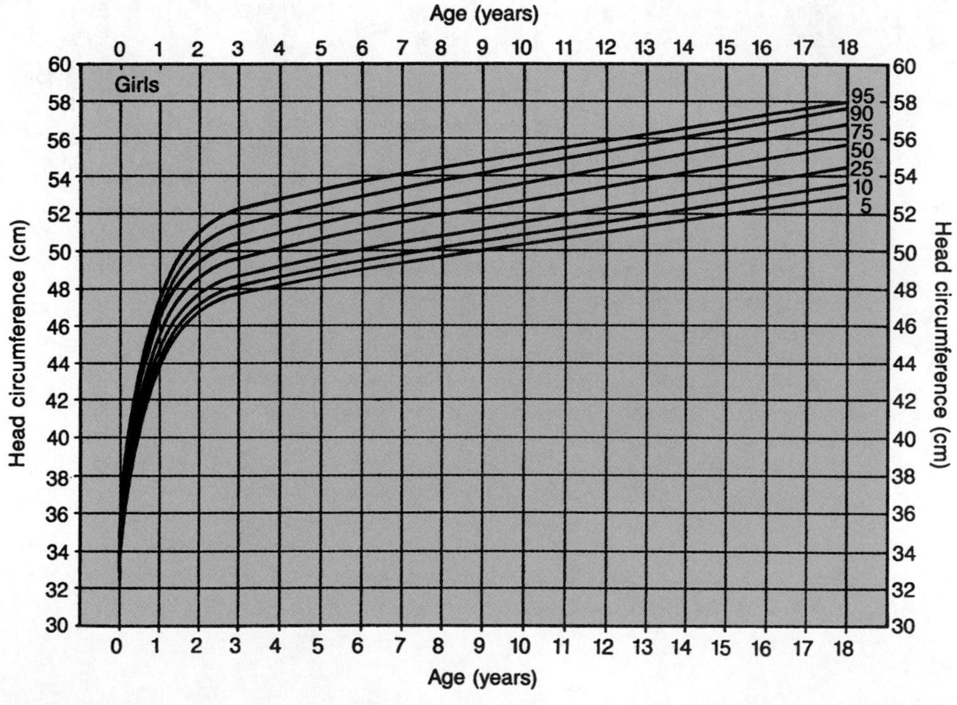

FIG. E-17 • Selected percentiles for smoothed head circumference values of children from birth to 18 years. **A,** Boys. **B,** Girls. (From Roche AF et al: Head circumference reference data: birth to 18 years, *Pediatrics* 79(5):706-712, 1987.)

Percentiles for Triceps Skinfold

	Triceps Skinfold Percentiles (mm)									
	Males					Females				
Age-Group (Years)	5	25	50	75	95	5	25	50	75	95
1-1.9	6	8	10	12	16	6	8	10	12	16
2-2.9	6	8	10	12	15	6	9	10	12	16
3-3.9	6	8	10	11	15	7	9	11	12	15
4-4.9	6	8	9	11	14	7	8	10	12	16
5-5.9	6	8	9	11	15	6	8	10	12	18
6-6.9	5	7	8	10	16	6	8	10	12	16
7-7.9	5	7	9	12	17	6	9	11	13	18
8-8.9	5	7	8	10	16	6	9	12	15	24
9-9.9	6	7	10	13	18	8	10	13	16	22
10-10.9	6	8	10	14	21	7	10	12	17	27
11-11.9	6	8	11	16	24	7	10	13	18	28
12-12.9	6	8	11	14	28	8	11	14	18	27
13-13.9	5	7	10	14	26	8	12	15	21	30
14-14.9	4	7	9	14	24	9	13	16	21	28
15-15.9	4	6	8	11	24	8	12	17	21	32
16-16.9	4	6	8	12	22	10	15	18	22	31
17-17.9	5	6	8	12	19	10	13	19	24	37
18-18.9	4	6	9	13	24	10	15	18	22	30
19-24.9	4	7	10	15	22	10	14	18	24	34

From Frisancho A: New norms of upper limb fat and muscle areas for assessment of nutritional status, *Am J Clin Nutr* 34:2540-2545, 1981.

Percentiles of Upper Arm Circumference

	Arm Circumference Percentiles (mm)									
	Males					Females				
Age-Group (Years)	5	25	50	75	95	5	25	50	75	95
1-1.9	142	150	159	170	183	138	148	156	164	177
2-2.9	141	153	162	170	185	142	152	160	167	184
3-3.9	150	160	167	175	190	143	158	167	175	189
4-4.9	149	162	171	180	192	149	160	169	177	191
5-5.9	153	167	175	185	204	153	165	175	185	211
6-6.9	155	167	179	188	228	156	170	176	187	211
7-7.9	162	177	187	201	230	164	174	183	199	231
8-8.9	162	177	190	202	245	168	183	195	214	261
9-9.9	175	187	200	217	257	178	194	211	224	260
10-10.9	181	196	210	231	274	174	193	210	228	265
11-11.9	186	202	223	244	280	185	208	224	248	303
12-12.9	193	214	232	254	303	194	216	237	256	294
13-13.9	194	228	247	263	301	202	223	243	271	338
14-14.9	220	237	253	283	322	214	237	252	272	322
15-15.9	222	244	264	284	320	208	239	254	279	322
16-16.9	244	262	278	303	343	218	241	258	283	334
17-17.9	246	267	285	308	347	220	241	264	295	350
18-18.9	245	276	297	321	379	222	241	258	281	325
19-24.9	262	288	308	331	372	221	247	265	290	345

From Frisancho A: New norms of upper limb fat and muscle areas for assessment of nutritional status, *Am J Clin Nutr* 34:2540-2545, 1981.

APPENDIX

F Common Laboratory Tests*

http://www.harcourthealth.com/MERLIN/Wong/maternal/

		Conventional Units		International Units (SI)	
Test/Specimen	**Age/Sex/Reference**	**Normal Ranges**			
Acetaminophen					
Serum or plasma	Therap. conc.	10-30 μg/ml		66-200 μmol/L	
Ammonia nitrogen	Toxic conc.	>200 μg/ml		>1300 μmol/L	
Plasma or serum	Newborn	90-150 μg/dl		64-107 μmol/L	
	0-2 wk	79-129 μg/dl		56-92 μmol/L	
	>1 mo	29-70 μg/dl		21-50 μmol/L	
	Thereafter	0-50 μg/dl		0-35.7 μmol/L	
Urine, 24 hr		500-1200 mg N/d		36-86 μmmol/d	
Antistreptolysin O titer (ASO)					
Serum	2-4 yr	<160 Todd units			
	School-age children	170-330 Todd units			
Base excess					
Whole blood	Newborn	(−10)-(−2) mEq/L		(−10)-(−2) mmol/L	
	Infant	(−7)-(−1) mEq/L		(−7)-(−1) mmol/L	
	Child	(−4)-(+2) mEq/L		(−4)-(+2) mmol/L	
	Thereafter	(−3)-(+3) mEq/L		(−3)-(+3) mmol/L	
Bicarbonate (HCO_3)					
Serum	Arterial	21-28 mEq/L		21-28 mmol/L	
	Venous	22-29 mEq/L		22-29 mmol/L	
		Premature (mg/dl)	**Full term (mg/dl)**	**Premature (μmol/L)**	**Full term (μmol/L)**
Bilirubin, total					
Serum	Cord	<2.0	<2.0	<34	<34
	0-1 d	<8.0	<6.0	<137	<103
	1-2 d	<12.0	<8.0	<205	<137
	2-5 d	<16.0	<12.0	<274	<205
	Thereafter	<20.0	<10.0	<340	<171
Bilirubin, direct (conjugated)					
Serum		0.0-0.2 mg/dl		0-3.4 μmol/L	
Bleeding time					
Blood from skin puncture					
Ivy	Normal	2-7 min		2-7 min	
	Borderline	7-11 min		7-11 min	
Simplate (G-D)		2.75-8 min		2.75-8 min	
Blood volume					
Whole blood	Male	52-83 ml/kg		0.052-0.083 L/kg	
	Female	50-75 ml/kg		0.050-0.075 L/kg	
C-reactive protein (CRP)					
Serum	Cord	52-1330 ng/ml		52-1330 μg/L	
	2-12 y	67-1800 ng/ml		67-1800 μg/L	
Calcium, ionized					
Serum, plasma, or whole blood	Cord	5.0-6.0 mg/dl		1.25-1.50 mmol/L	
	Newborn, 3-24 hr	4.3-5.1 mg/dl		1.07-1.27 mmol/L	
	24-48 hr	4.0-4.7 mg/dl		1.00-1.17 mmol/L	

Modified from Behrman RE et al, editors: *Nelson textbook of pediatrics,* ed 16, Philadelphia, 2000, WB Saunders; and Mc Millan A et al, editors: *Oski's pediatrics—principles and practice,* ed 3, Philadelphia, 1999, Lippincott-Williams-Wilkins.

*For a description of abbreviations see p. 1641.

Test/Specimen	Age/Sex/Reference	Conventional Units	International Units (SI)
		Normal Ranges	
Calcium, ionized—cont'd			
Serum, plasma, or whole blood—cont'd	Thereafter	4.8-4.92 mg/dl or 2.24-2.46 mEq/L	1.12-1.23 mmol/L
Calcium, total			
Serum	Cord	9.0-11.5 mg/dl	2.25-2.88 mmol/L
	Newborn, 3-24 hr	9.0-10.6 mg/dl	2.3-2.65 mmol/L
	24-48 hr	7.0-12.0 mg/dl	1.75-3.0 mmol/L
	4-7 d	9.0-10.9 mg/dl	2.25-2.73 mmol/L
	Child	8.8-10.8 mg/dl	2.2-2.70 mmol/l
	Thereafter	8.4-10.2 mg/dl	2.1-2.55 mmol/L
Carbon dioxide, partial pressure (Pco_2)			
Whole blood, arterial	Newborn	27-40 mm Hg	3.6-5.3 kPa
	Infant	27-41 mm Hg	3.6-5.5 kPa
	Thereafter: Male	35-48 mm Hg	4.7-6.4 kPa
	Female	32-45 mm Hg	4.3-6.0 kPa
Carbon dioxide, total (tCO_2)			
Serum or plasma	Cord	14-22 mEq/L	14-22 mmol/L
	Premature (1 wk)	14-27 mEq/L	14-27 mmol/L
	Newborn	13-22 mEq/L	13-22 mmol/L
	Infant, child	20-28 mEq/L	20-28 mmol/L
	Thereafter	23-30 mEq/L	23-30 mmol/L
Cerebrospinal fluid (CSF)			
Pressure		70-180 mm water	70-180 mm water
Volume	Child	60-100 ml	0.06-0.10 L
	Adult	100-160 ml	0.10-0.16 L
Chloride			
Serum or plasma	Cord	96-104 mEq/L	96-104 mmol/L
	Newborn	97-110 mEq/L	97-110 mmol/L
	Thereafter	98-106 mEq/L	98-106 mmol/L
Sweat	Normal (homozygote)	<40 mEq/L	<40 mmol/L
	Marginal (e.g., asthma, Addison disease, malnutrition)	45-60 mEq/L	45-60 mmol/L
	Cystic fibrosis	>60 mmol/L	>60 mmol/L
Cholesterol, total			
Serum or plasma*	Acceptable	<170 mg/dl	<4.4 mmol/L
	Borderline	170-199 mg/dl	4.4-5.1 mmol/L
	High	≥200 mg/dl	≥5.2 mmol/L
Clotting time (Lee-White)			
Whole blood		5-8 min (glass tubes)	5-8 min
		5-15 min (room temp)	5-15 min
		30 min (silicone tube)	30 min
Creatine kinase (CK, CPK)			
Serum	Cord blood	70-380 U/L	70-380 U/L
	5-8 hr	214-1175 U/L	214-1175 U/L
	24-33 hr	130-1200 U/L	130-1200 U/L
	72-100 hr	87-725 U/L	87-725 U/L
	Adult	5-130 U/L	5-130 U/L
Creatinine			
Serum	Cord	0.6-1.2 mg/dl	53-106 μmol/L
	Newborn	0.3-1.0 mg/dl	27-88 μmol/L
	Infant	0.2-0.4 mg/dl	18-35 μmol/L
	Child	0.3-0.7 mg/dl	27-62 μmol/L
	Adolescent	0.5-1.0 mg/dl	44-88 μmol/L
	Adult: Male	0.6-1.2 mg/dl	53-106 μmol/L
	Female	0.5-1.1 mg/dl	44-97 μmol/L

*From National Cholesterol Education Program: Report of the expert panel on blood cholesterol levels in children and adolescents, *Pediatrics* 89 (3, pt 2):527, 1992.

Continued

Test/Specimen	Age/Sex/Reference	Conventional Units (Normal Ranges)	International Units (SI) (Normal Ranges)
Creatinine—cont'd			
Urine, 24 hr	Premature	8.1-15.0 mg/kg/24 hr	72-133 μmol/kg/24 hr
	Full term	10.4-19.7 mg/kg/24 hr	92-174 μmol/kg/24 hr
	1.5-7 yr	10-15 mg/kg/24 hr	88-133 μmol/kg/24 hr
	7-15 yr	5.2-41 mg/kg/24 hr	46-362 μmol/kg/24 hr
Creatinine clearance (endogenous)			
Serum or plasma and urine	Newborn	40-65 ml/min/1.73 m^2	
	<40 yr: Male	97-137 ml/min/1.73 m^2	
	Female	88-128 ml/min/1.73 m^2	
Digoxin			
Serum, plasma; collect at least 12 hr after dose	Therap. conc.		
	CHF	0.8-1.5 ng/ml	1.0-1.9 nmol/L
	Arrhythmias	1.5-2.0 ng/ml	1.9-2.6 nmol/L
	Toxic conc.		
	Child	>2.5 ng/ml	>3.2 nmol/L
	Adult	>3.0 ng/ml	>3.8 nmol/L
Eosinophil count			
Whole blood, capillary blood		50-250 cells/mm^3 (μl)	50-250 × 10^6 cells/L
Erythrocyte (RBC) count			
Whole blood			
	Cord	3.9-5.5 million/mm^3	3.9-5.5 × 10^{12} cells/L
	1-3 d	4.0-6.6 million/mm^3	4.0-6.6 × 10^{12} cells/L
	1 wk	3.9-6.3 million/mm^3	3.9-6.3 × 10^{12} cells/L
	2 wk	3.6-6.2 million/mm^3	3.6-6.2 × 10^{12} cells/L
	1 mo	3.0-5.4 million/mm^3	3.0-5.4 × 10^{12} cells/L
	2 mo	2.7-4.9 million/mm^3	2.7-4.9 × 10^{12} cells/L
	3-6 mo	3.1-4.5 million/mm^3	3.1-4.5 × 10^{12} cells/L
	0.5-2 yr	3.7-5.3 million/mm^3	3.7-5.3 × 10^{12} cells/L
	2-6 yr	3.9-5.3 million/mm^3	3.9-5.3 × 10^{12} cells/L
	6-12 yr	4.0-5.2 million/mm^3	4.0-5.2 × 10^{12} cells/L
	12-18 yr: Male	4.5-5.3 million/mm^3	4.5-5.3 × 10^{12} cells/L
	Female	4.1-5.1 million/mm^3	4.1-5.1 × 10^{12} cells/L
Erythrocyte sedimentation rate (ESR)			
Whole blood			
Westergren (modified)	Child	0-10 mm/hr	0-10 mm/hr
	<50 yr: Male	0-15 mm/hr	0-15 mm/hr
	Female	0-20 mm/hr	0-20 mm/hr
Wintrobe	Child	0-13 mm/hr	0-13 mm/hr
	Adult: Male	0-9 mm/hr	0-9 mm/hr
	Female	0-20 mm/hr	0-20 mm/hr
Fibrinogen			
Plasma	Newborn	125-300 mg/dl	1.25-3.00 g/L
	Thereafter	200-400 mg/dl	2.00-4.00 g/L
Galactose			
Serum	Newborn	0-20 mg/dl	0-1.11 mmol/L
	Thereafter	<5 mg/dl	<0.28 mmol/L
Urine	Newborn	≤60 mg/dl	≤3.33 mmol/L
	Thereafter	<14 mg/24 hr	<0.08 mmol/d
Glucose			
Serum	Cord	45-96 mg/dl	2.5-5.3 mmol/L
	Newborn, 1 d	40-60 mg/dl	2.2-3.3 mmol/L
	Newborn, >1 d	50-90 mg/dl	2.8-5.0 mmol/L
	Child	60-100 mg/dl	3.3-5.5 mmol/L
	Thereafter	70-105 mg/dl	3.9-5.8 mmol/L
Whole blood	Adult	65-95 mg/dl	3.6-5.3 mmol/L

Test/Specimen	Age/Sex/Reference	Conventional Units (Normal Ranges)		International Units (SI) (Normal Ranges)	
Glucose—cont'd					
CSF	Adult	40-70 mg/dl		2.2-3.9 mmol/L	
Urine (quantitative)		<0.5 g/d		<2.8 mmol/d	
(Qualitative)		Negative		Negative	
Glucose tolerance test (GTT), oral					
Serum					
Dosages		**Normal**	**Diabetic**	**Normal**	**Diabetic**
Adult: 75 g	Fasting	70-105 mg/dl	≥126 mg/dl	3.9-5.8 mmol/L	≥7.0 mmol/L
Child: 1.75 g/kg of ideal weight up to maximum of 75 g	60 min	120-170 mg/dl	≥200 mg/dl	6.7-9.4 mmol/L	≥11 mmol/L
	90 min	100-140 mg/dl	≥200 mg/dl	5.6-7.8 mmol/L	≥11 mmol/L
	120 min	70-120 mg/dl	≥200 mg/dl	3.9-6.7 mmol/L	≥11 mmol/L
Growth hormone (hGH, somatotropin)					
Plasma	1 d	5-53 ng/ml		5-53 μg/L	
	1 wk	5-27 ng/ml		5-27 μg/L	
	1-12 mo	2-10 ng/ml		2-10 μg/L	
	Fasting child/adult	<0.7-6.0 ng/ml		<0.7-6.0 μg/L	
Hematocrit (HCT, Hct)					
Whole blood	1 d (cap)	48%-69%		0.48-0.69 vol. fraction	
	2 d	48%-75%		0.48-0.75 vol. fraction	
	3 d	44%-72%		0.44-0.72 vol. fraction	
	2 mo	28%-42%		0.28-0.42 vol. fraction	
	6-12 yr	35%-45%		0.35-0.45 vol. fraction	
	12-18 yr: Male	37%-49%		0.37-0.49 vol. fraction	
	Female	36%-46%		0.36-0.46 vol. fraction	
Hemoglobin (Hb)					
Whole blood	1-3 d (cap)	14.5-22.5 g/dl		2.25-3.49 mmol/L	
	2 mo	9.0-14.0 g/dl		1.40-2.17 mmol/L	
	6-12 yr	11.5-15.5 g/dl		1.78-2.40 mmol/L	
	12-18 yr: Male	13.0-16.0 g/dl		2.02-2.48 mmol/L	
	Female	12.0-16.0 g/dl		1.86-2.48 mmol/L	
Hemoglobin A					
Whole blood		>95% of total		>0.95 fraction of Hb	
Hemoglobin F					
Whole blood	1 d	63%-92% HbF		0.62-0.92 mass fraction HbF	
	5 d	65%-88% HbF		0.65-0.88 mass fraction HbF	
	3 wk	55%-85% HbF		0.55-0.85 mass fraction HbF	
	6-9 wk	31%-75% HbF		0.31-0.75 mass fraction HbF	
	3-4 mo	<2%-59% HbF		<0.02-0.59 mass fraction HbF	
	6 mo	<2%-9% HbF		<0.02-0.09 mass fraction HbF	
	Adult	<2.0% HbF		<0.02 mass fraction HbF	
Immunoglobulin A (IgA)					
Serum	Cord blood	1.4-3.6 mg/dl		14-36 mg/L	
	1-3 mo	1.3-53 mg/dl		13-530 mg/L	
	4-6 mo	4.4-84 mg/dl		44-840 mg/L	
	7 mo-1 yr	11-106 mg/dl		110-1060 mg/L	
	2-5 yr	14-159 mg/dl		140-1590 mg/L	
	6-10 yr	33-236 mg/dl		330-2360 mg/L	
	Adult	70-312 mg/dl		700-3120 mg/L	
Immunoglobulin D (IgD)					
Serum	Newborn	None detected		None detected	
	Thereafter	0-8 mg/dl		0-80 mg/L	
Immunoglobulin E (IgE)					
Serum	M	0-230 IU/ml		0-230 kIU/L	
	F	0-170 IU/ml		0-170 kIU/L	

Continued

Test/Specimen	Age/Sex/Reference	Conventional Units	International Units (SI)
		Normal Ranges	
Immunoglobulin G (IgG)			
Serum	Cord blood	636-1606 mg/dl	6.36-16.06 g/L
	1 mo	251-906 mg/dl	2.51-9.06 g/L
	2-4 mo	176-601 mg/dl	1.76-6.01 g/L
	5-12 mo	172-1069 mg/dl	1.72-10.69 g/L
	1-5 yr	345-1236 mg/dl	3.45-12.36 g/L
	6-10 yr	608-1572 mg/dl	6.08-15.72 g/L
	Adult	639-1349 mg/dl	6.39-13.49 g/L
Immunoglobulin M (IgM)			
Serum	Cord blood	6.3-25 mg/dl	63-250 mg/L
	1 mo-4 mo	17-105 mg/dl	170-1050 mg/L
	5 mo-9 mo	33-126 mg/dl	330-1260 mg/L
	10 mo-1 yr	41-173 mg/dl	410-1730 mg/L
	2-8 yr	43-207 mg/dl	430-2070 mg/L
	9-10 yr	52-242 mg/dl	520-2420 mg/L
	Adult	56-352 mg/dl	560-3520 mg/L
Iron			
Serum	Newborn	100-250 μg/dl	18-45 μmol/L
	Infant	40-100 μg/dl	7-18 μmol/L
	Child	50-120 μg/dl	9-22 μmol/L
	Thereafter: Male	65-170 μg/dl	12-30 μmol/L
	Female	50-170 μg/dl	9-30 μmol/L
	Intoxicated child	280-2550 μg/dl	50.12-456.5 μmol/L
	Fatally poisoned child	>1800 μg/dl	>322.2 μmol/L
Iron-binding capacity, total (TIBC)			
Serum	Infant	100-400 μg/dl	17.90-71.60 μmol/L
	Thereafter	250-400 μg/dl	44.75-71.60 μmol/L
Lead			
Whole blood	Child	<10 μg/dL	<0.48 μmol/L
Urine, 24 hr		<80 μg/L	<0.39 μmol/L
Leukocyte count (WBC count)		**× 1000 cells/mm³ (μl)**	**× 10^9 cells/L**
Whole blood	Birth	9.0-30.0	9.0-30.0
	24 hr	9.4-34.0	9.4-34.0
	1 mo	5.0-19.5	5.0-19.5
	1-3 yr	6.0-17.5	6.0-17.5
	4-7 yr	5.5-15.5	5.5-15.5
	8-13 yr	4.5-13.5	4.5-13.5
	Adult	4.5-11.0	4.5-11.0
		× 1000 cells/mm³ (μl)	**× 10^6 cells/L**
CSF	Premature	0-25 mononuclear	0-25
		0-10 polymorphonuclear	0-10
		0-1000 RBC	0-1000
	Newborn	0-20 mononuclear	0-20
		0-10 polymorphonuclear	0-10
		0-800 RBC	0-800
	Neonate	0-5 mononuclear	0-5
		0-10 polymorphonuclear	0-10
		0-50 RBC	0-50
	Thereafter	0-5 mononuclear	0-5

Test/Specimen	Age/Sex/Reference	Conventional Units (Normal Ranges)		International Units (SI) (Normal Ranges)
Leukocyte differential count				
Whole blood	Myelocytes	0%	0 cells/mm^3 (μl)	Number fraction 0
	Neutrophils—"bands"	3%-5%	150-400 cells/mm^3 (μl)	Number fraction 0.03-0.05
	Neutrophils—"segs"	54%-62%	3000-5800 cells/mm^3 (μl)	Number fraction 0.54-0.62
	Lymphocytes	25%-33%	1500-3000 cells/mm^3 (μl)	Number fraction 0.25-0.33
	Monocytes	3%-7%	285-500 cells/mm^3 (μl)	Number fraction 0.03-0.07
	Eosinophils	1%-3%	50-250 cells/mm^3 (μl)	Number fraction 0.01-0.03
	Basophils	0%-0.75%	15-50 cells/mm^3 (μl)	Number fraction 0-0.0075
Mean corpuscular hemoglobin (MCH)				
Whole blood	Birth	31-37 pg/cell		0.48-0.57 fmol/cell
	1-3 d (cap)	31-37 pg/cell		0.48-0.57 fmol/cell
	1 wk-1 mo	28-40 pg/cell		0.43-0.62 fmol/cell
	2 mo	26-34 pg/cell		0.40-0.53 fmol/cell
	3-6 mo	25-35 pg/cell		0.39-0.54 fmol/cell
	0.5-2 yr	23-31 pg/cell		0.36-0.48 fmol/cell
	2-6 yr	24-30 pg/cell		0.37-0.47 fmol/cell
	6-12 yr	25-33 pg/cell		0.39-0.51 fmol/cell
	12-18 yr	25-35 pg/cell		0.39-0.54 fmol/cell
	18-49 yr	26-34 pg/cell		0.40-0.53 fmol/cell
Mean corpuscular hemoglobin concentration (MCHC)				
Whole blood	Birth	30%-36% Hb/cell or g Hb/dl RBC		4.65-5.58 mmol Hb/L RBC
	1-3 d (cap)	29%-37% Hb/cell or g Hb/dl RBC		4.50-5.74 mmol Hb/L RBC
	1-2 wk	28%-38% Hb/cell or g Hb/dl RBC		4.34-5.89 mmol Hb/L RBC
	1-2 mo	29%-37% Hb/cell or g Hb/dl RBC		4.50-5.74 mmol Hb/L RBC
	3 mo-2 yr	30%-36% Hb/cell or g Hb/dl RBC		4.65-5.58 mmol Hb/L RBC
	2-18 yr	31%-37% Hb/cell or g Hb/dl RBC		4.81-5.74 mmol Hb/L RBC
	>18 yr	31%-37% Hb/cell or g Hb/dl RBC		4.81-5.74 mmol Hb/L RBC
Mean corpuscular volume (MCV)				
Whole blood	1-3 d (cap)	95-121 μm^3		95-121 fl
	0.5-2 yr	70-86 μm^3		70-86 fl
	6-12 yr	77-95 μm^3		77-95 fl
	12-18 yr: Male	78-98 μm^3		78-98 fl
	Female	78-102 μm^3		78-102 fl
Osmolality				
Serum	Child, adult	275-295 mOsmol/kg H_2O		
Urine, random		50-1400 mOsmol/kg H_2O, depending on fluid intake After 12-hr fluid restriction: >850 mOsmol/kg H_2O		
Urine, 24 hr		≈300-900 mOsmol/kg H_2O		
Oxygen, partial pressure (Po_2)				
Whole blood, arterial	Birth	8-24 mm Hg		1.1-3.2 kPa
	5-10 min	33-75 mm Hg		4.4-10.0 kPa
	30 min	31-85 mm Hg		4.1-11.3 kPa
	>1 hr	55-80 mm Hg		7.3-10.6 kPa
	1 d	54-95 mm Hg		7.2-12.6 kPa
	Thereafter (decreased with age)	83-108 mm Hg		11-14.4 kPa

Continued

Test/Specimen	Age/Sex/Reference	Conventional Units	International Units (SI)
		Normal Ranges	
Oxygen saturation (Sao_2)			
Whole blood, arterial	Newborn	85%-90%	Fraction saturated 0.85-0.90
	Thereafter	95%-99%	Fraction saturated 0.95-0.99
Partial thromboplastin time (PTT)			
Whole blood (Na citrate)			
Nonactivated		60-85 s (Platelin)	60-85 s
Activated		25-35 s (differs with method)	25-35 s
pH			H^+ concentration
Whole blood, arterial	Premature (48 hr)	7.35-7.50	31-44 nmol/L
	Birth, full term	7.11-7.36	43-77 nmol/L
	5-10 min	7.09-7.30	50-81 nmol/L
	30 min	7.21-7.38	41-61 nmol/L
	>1 hr	7.26-7.49	32-54 nmol/L
	1 d	7.29-7.45	35-51 nmol/L
	Thereafter	7.35-7.45	35-44 nmol/L
	Must be corrected for body temperature		
Urine, random	Newborn/neonate	5-7	0.1-10 μmol/L
	Thereafter	4.5-8 (average ≈6)	0.01-32 μmol/L (average ≈ 1.0 μmol/L)
Stool		7.0-7.5	31-100 nmol/L
Phenylalanine			
Serum	Premature	2.0-7.5 mg/dl	120-450 μmol/L
	Newborn	1.2-3.4 mg/dl	70-210 μmol/L
	Thereafter	0.8-1.8 mg/dl	50-110 μmol/L
Urine, 24 hr	10 d-2 wk	1-2 mg/d	6-12 μmol/d
	3-12 yr	4-18 mg/d	24-110 μmol/d
Plasma volume	Thereafter	trace-17 mg/d	trace-103 μmol/d
Plasma	Male	25-43 ml/kg	0.025-0.043 L/kg
Platelet count (thrombocyte count)	Female	28-45 ml/kg	0.028-0.045 L/kg
Whole blood (EDTA)	Newborn (After 1 wk, same as adult)	84-478 × 10^3/mm^3 (μl)	84-478 × 10^9/L
Potassium	Adult	150-400 × 10^3/mm^3 (μl)	150-400 × 10^9/L
Serum	Newborn	3.0-6.0 mEq/L	3.0-6.0 mmol/L
Plasma (heparin)	Thereafter	3.5-5.0 mEq/L	3.5-5.0 mmol/L
Urine, 24 hr		3.4-4.5 mEq/L	3.4-4.5 mmol/L
Protein		2.5-125 mEq/d varies with diet	2.5-125 mmol/L
Serum, total	Premature	4.3-7.6 g/dl	43-76 g/L
	Newborn	4.6-7.4 g/dl	46-74 g/L
	1-7 yr	6.1-7.9 g/dl	61-79 g/L
	8-12 yr	6.4-8.1 g/dl	64-81 g/L
	13-19 yr	6.6-8.2 g/dl	66-82 g/L
Total			
Urine, 24 hr		1-14 mg/dl	10-140 mg/L
		50-80 mg/d (at rest)	50-80 mg/d
		<250 mg/d after intense exercise	<250 mg/d after intense exercise
Total			
CSF		Lumbar: 8-32 mg/dl	80-320 mg/L
Prothrombin time (PT)			
One-stage (Quick)			
Whole blood (Na citrate)	In general	11-15 s (varies with type of thromboplastin)	11-15 sec
	Newborn	Prolonged by 2-3 sec	Prolonged by 2-3 sec
Two-stage modified (Ware and Seegers)			
Whole blood (Na citrate)		18-22 sec	18-22 sec

Test/Specimen	Age/Sex/Reference	Conventional Units	International Units (SI)
		Normal Ranges	
RBC count, see erythrocyte count			
Red blood cell volume			
Whole blood	Male	20-36 ml/kg	0.020-0.036 L/kg
Reticulocyte count	Female	19-31 ml/kg	0.019-0.031 L/kg
Whole blood	Adults	0.5%-1.5% of erythrocytes or 25,000-75,000/mm^3 (μl)	0.005-0.015 (number fraction) or: 25,000-75,000 $\times 10^6$/L
Capillary	1 d	0.4%-6.0%	0.004-0.060 (number fraction)
	7 d	<0.1%-1.3%	<0.001-0.013 (number fraction)
	1-4 wk	<0.1%-1.2%	<0.001-0.012 (number fraction)
	5-6 wk	<0.1%-2.4%	<0.001-0.024 (number fraction)
	7-8 wk	0.1%-2.9%	0.001-0.029 (number fraction)
	9-10 wk	<0.1%-2.6%	<0.001-0.026 (number fraction)
	11-12 wk	0.1%-1.3%	0.001-0.013 (number fraction)
Salicylates			
Serum, plasma	Therap. conc.	15-30 mg/dl	1.1-2.2 mmol/L
	Toxic conc.	>30 mg/dl	>18.5 mmol/L
Sedimentation rate: see erythrocyte sedimentation rate			
Sodium			
Serum or plasma	Newborn	134-146 mEq/L	134-146 mmol/L
	Infant	139-146 mEq/L	139-146 mmol/L
	Child	138-145 mEq/L	138-145 mmol/L
	Thereafter	136-146 mEq/L	136-146 mmol/L
Urine, 24 hr		40-220 mEq/L (diet dependent)	40-220 mmol/L
Sweat	Normal	<40 mEq/L	<40 mmol/L
	Indeterminate	45-60 mEq/L	45-60 mmol/L
	Cystic fibrosis	>60 mEq/L	>60 mmol/L
Specific, gravity			
Urine, random	Adult	1.002-1.030	1.002-1.030
	After 12 hr fluid restriction	>1.025	>1.025
Urine, 24 hr		1.015-1.025	
Theophylline			
Serum, plasma	Therap. conc.		
	Bronchodilator	10-20 μg/ml	56-110 μmol/L
	Premature apnea	5-10 μg/ml	28-56 μmol/L
	Toxic conc.	>20 μg/ml	>110 μmol/L
Thrombin time			
Whole blood (Na citrate)		Control time ± 2 sec when control is 9-13 sec	Control time ± 2 sec when control is 9-13 sec
Thyroxine, total (T_3)			
Serum	Cord	8-13 μg/dL	103-168 nmol/L
	Newborn	11.5-24 (lower in low-birth-weight infants)	148-310 nmol/L
	Neonate	9-18 μg/dL	116-232 nmol/L
	Infant	7-15 μg/dL	90-194 nmol/L
	1-5 yr	7.3-15 μg/dL	94-194 nmol/L
	5-10 yr	6.4-13.3 μdL	83-172 nmol/L
	Thereafter	5-12 μg/dL	65-155 nmol/L
	Newborn screen (filter paper)	6.2-22 μg/dL	80-284 nmol/L

Continued

Test/Specimen	Age/Sex/Reference	Conventional Units		International Units (SI)	
		Normal Ranges			
Triglycerides (TG)					
Serum, after ≥12 hr fast		mg/dl		g/L	
		M	F	M	F
	Cord blood	10-98	10-98	0.10-0.98	0.10-0.98
	0-5 yr	30-86	32-99	0.30-0.86	0.32-0.99
	6-11 yr	31-108	35-114	0.31-1.08	0.35-1.14
	12-15 yr	36-138	41-138	0.36-1.38	0.41-1.38
	16-19 yr	40-163	40-128	0.40-1.63	0.40-1.28
Triiodothyronine, free					
Serum	Cord	20-240 pg/dl		0.3-3.7 pmol/L	
	1-3 d	200-610 pg/dl		3.1-9.4 pmol/L	
	6 wk	240-560 pg/dl		3.7-8.6 pmol/L	
	Adults (20-50 yr)	230-660 pg/dl		3.5-10.0 pmol/L	
Triiodothyronine, total (T_3-RIA)					
Serum	Cord	30-70 ng/dl		0.46-1.08 nmol/L	
	Newborn	72-260 ng/dl		1.16-4.00 nmol/L	
	1-5 yr	100-260 ng/dl		1.54-4.00 nmol/L	
	5-10 yr	90-240 ng/dl		1.39-3.70 nmol/L	
	10-15 yr	80-210 ng/dl		1.23-3.23 nmol/L	
	Thereafter	115-190 ng/dl		1.77-2.93 nmol/L	
Urea nitrogen					
Serum or plasma	Cord	21-40 mg/dl		7.5-14.3 mmol urea/L	
	Premature (1 wk)	3-25 mg/dl		1.1-9 mmol urea/L	
	Newborn	3-12 mg/dl		1.1-4.3 mmol urea/L	
	Infant/child	5-18 mg/dl		1.8-6.4 mmol urea/L	
	Thereafter	7-18 mg/dl		2.5-6.4 mmol urea/L	
Urine volume					
Urine, 24 hr	Newborn	50-300 ml/d		0.050-0.300 L/d	
	Infant	350-550 ml/d		0.350-0.500 L/d	
	Child	500-1000 ml/d		0.500-1.000 L/d	
	Adolescent	700-1400 ml/d		0.700-1.400 L/d	
	Thereafter: Male	800-1800 ml/d		0.800-1.800 L/d	
	Female	600-1600 ml/d (varies with intake and other factors)		0.600-1.600 L/d	
WBC, see leukocyte					

ABBREVIATIONS USED IN LABORATORY TESTS

Abbreviation	Term
cap	capillary
CHF	congestive heart failure
conc.	concentration
CSF	cerebrospinal fluid
d	day; diem
EDTA	ethylenediaminetetraacetate
g	gram
m	meter
hr	hour
L, l	liter
mEq	milliequivalent
min	minute
mm	millimeter
mm^3	cubic millimeter
mo	month
mol	mole
mOsmol	milliosmole
s	second
SI	International system of units
Therap.	therapeutic
U	International unit of enzyme activity
vol	volume
wk	week
yr	year
$>$	greater than
$\geq$	greater than or equal to
$<$	less than
$\leq$	less than or equal to
$\pm$	plus/minus
$\simeq$	approximately equal to

PREFIXES DENOTING DECIMAL FACTORS

Prefix	Symbol	Amount
deci	d	one tenth (10^{-1})
centi	c	one hundredth (10^{-2})
milli	m	one thousandth (10^{-3})
micro	μ	one millionth (10^{-6})
nano	n	one billionth (10^{-9})
pico	p	one trillionth (10^{-12})
femto	f	one quadrillionth (10^{-15})

APPENDIX

G Recommended Daily Dietary Allowances

http://www.harcourthealth.com/MERLIN/Wong/maternal/

Recommended Dietary Allowances[a] Designed for the Maintenance of Good Nutrition of Practically All Healthy People in the United States

		Weight[b]		Height[b]			Fat-Soluble Vitamins			
Category	Age (Years) or Condition	(kg)	(lb)	(cm)	(in)	Protein (g)	Vitamin A (μ RE)[c]	Vitamin D (μg)[d]	Vitamin E (mg/α-TE)[e]	Vitamin K (μg)
Infants	0.0-0.5	6	13	60	24	13	375	7.5	3	5
	0.5-1.0	9	20	71	28	14	375	10	4	10
Children	1-3	13	29	90	35	16	400	10	6	15
	4-6	20	44	112	44	24	500	10	7	20
	7-10	28	62	132	52	28	700	10	7	30
Males	11-14	45	99	157	62	45	1000	10	10	45
	15-18	66	145	176	69	59	1000	10	10	65
	19-24	72	160	177	70	58	1000	10	10	70
	25-50	79	174	176	70	63	1000	5	10	80
	51+	77	170	173	68	63	1000	5	10	80
Females	11-14	46	101	157	62	46	800	10	8	45
	15-18	55	120	163	64	44	800	10	8	55
	19-24	58	128	164	65	46	800	10	8	60
	25-50	63	138	163	64	50	800	5	8	65
	51+	65	143	160	63	50	800	5	8	65
Pregnant						60	800	10	10	65
Lactating	1st 6 months					65	1300	10	12	65
	2nd 6 months					62	1200	10	11	65

From Food and Nutrition Board, National Research Council: *Recommended dietary allowances,* ed 10, Washington, DC, 1989, National Academy of Sciences.

[a]The allowances, expressed as average daily intakes over time, are intended to provide for individual variations among most normal persons as they live in the United States under environmental stresses. Diets should be based on a variety of common foods in order to provide other nutrients for which human requirements have been less well defined.

[b]Weights and heights of reference adults are actual medians for the U.S. population of the designated age, as reported by National Health and Nutrition Examination Survey (NHANES) II. The median weights and heights of those under 19 years of age were taken from Hamill PV and others: Physical growth: National Center for Health Statistics percentiles, *Am J Clin Nutr* 32:607-629, 1979. The use of these figures does not imply that the height-to-weight ratios are ideal.

[c]Retinol equivalent. 1 retinol equivalent = 1 μg retinol or 6 μ β-carotene.

[d]As cholecalciferol. 10 μg cholecalciferol = 400 IU vitamin D.

[e]α-Tocopherol equivalents. 1 mg *d-a*-tocopherol = 1 α-TE.

[f]1 NE (niacin equivalent) is equal to 1 mg of niacin or 60 mg of dietary tryptophan.

Water-Soluble Vitamins							Minerals						
Vitamin C (mg)	Thiamine (mg)	Riboflavin (mg)	Niacin (mg NE)[f]	Vitamin B_6 (mg)	Folate (μg)	Vitamin B_{12} (μg)	Calcium (mg)	Phosphorus (mg)	Magnesium (mg)	Iron (mg)	Zinc (mg)	Iodine (μg)	Selenium (μg)
30	0.3	0.4	5	0.3	25	0.3	400	300	40	6	5	40	10
35	0.4	0.5	6	0.6	35	0.5	600	500	60	10	5	50	15
40	0.7	0.8	9	1.0	50	0.7	800	800	80	10	10	70	20
45	0.9	1.1	12	1.1	75	1.0	800	800	120	10	10	90	20
45	1.0	1.2	13	1.4	100	1.4	800	800	170	10	10	120	30
50	1.3	1.5	17	17	150	2.0	1200	1200	270	12	15	150	40
60	1.5	1.8	20	2.0	200	2.0	1200	1200	400	12	15	150	50
60	1.5	1.7	19	2.0	200	2.0	1200	1200	350	10	15	150	70
60	1.5	1.7	19	2.0	200	2.0	800	800	350	10	15	150	70
60	1.2	1.4	15	2.0	200	2.0	800	800	350	10	15	150	70
50	1.1	1.3	15	1.4	150	2.0	1200	1200	280	15	12	150	45
60	1.1	1.3	15	1.5	180	2.0	1200	1200	300	15	12	150	50
60	1.1	1.3	15	1.6	180	2.0	1200	1200	280	15	12	150	55
60	1.1	1.3	15	1.6	180	2.0	800	800	280	15	12	150	55
60	1.0	1.2	13	1.6	180	2.0	800	800	280	10	12	150	55
70	1.5	1.6	17	2.2	400	2.2	1200	1200	320	30	15	175	65
95	1.6	1.8	20	2.1	280	2.6	1200	1200	355	15	19	200	75
90	1.6	1.7	20	2.1	260	2.6	1200	1200	340	15	16	200	75

Estimated Safe and Adequate Daily Dietary Intakes of Selected Vitamins and Minerals[a]

		Vitamins	
Category	Age (Years)	Biotin (μg)	Pantothenic Acid (mg)
Infants	0-0.5	10	2
	0.5-1	15	3
Children and adolescents	1-3	20	3
	4-6	25	3-4
	7-10	30	4-5
	11+	30-100	4-7
Adults		30-100	4-7

From Food and Nutrition Board, National Research Council: *Recommended dietary allowances,* ed 10, Washington, DC, 1989, National Academy of Sciences.
[a]Because there is less information on which to base allowances, these figures are not given in the main table of RDAs and are provided here in the form of ranges of recommended intakes.
[b]Since the toxic levels for many trace elements may be only several times usual intakes, the upper levels for the trace elements given in this table should not be habitually exceeded.

Estimated Sodium, Chloride, and Potassium Minimum Requirements of Healthy Persons[a]

Age	Weight (kg)[a]	Sodium (mg)[a,b]	Chloride (mg)[a,b]	Potassium (mg)[c]
Months				
0-5	4.5	120	180	500
6-11	8.9	200	300	700
Years				
1	11.0	225	350	1000
2-5	16.0	300	500	1400
6-9	25.0	400	600	1600
10-18	50.0	500	750	2000
>18[d]	70.0	500	750	2000

From Food and Nutrition Board, National Research Council: *Recommended dietary allowances,* ed 10, Washington, DC, 1989, National Academy of Sciences.
[a]No allowance has been included for large, prolonged losses from the skin through sweat.
[b]There is no evidence that higher intakes confer any health benefit.
[c]Desirable intakes of potassium may considerably exceed these values (~3500 mg for adults).
[d]No allowance included for growth. Values for those younger than 18 years of age assume a growth rate at the 50th percentile reported by the National Center for Health Statistics and averaged for males and females.

Trace Elements[b]				
Copper (mg)	Manganese (mg)	Fluoride (mg)	Chromium (μg)	Molybdenum (μg)
0.4-0.6	0.3-0.6	0.1-0.5	10-40	15-30
0.6-0.7	0.6-1.0	0.2-1.0	20-60	20-40
0.7-1.0	1.0-1.5	0.5-1.5	20-80	25-50
1.0-1.5	1.5-2.0	1.0-2.5	30-120	30-75
1.0-2.0	2.0-3.0	1.5-2.5	50-200	50-150
1.5-2.5	2.0-5.0	1.5-2.5	50-200	75-250
1.5-3.0	2.0-5.0	1.5-4.0	50-200	75-250

Median Heights and Weights and Recommended Energy Intake

		Weight		Height			Average Energy Allowance (kcal)[b]		
Category	Age (Year) or Condition	(kg)	(lb)	(cm)	(in)	REE[a] (kcal/day)	Multiples of REE	Per kg	Per Day[c]
Infants	0.0-0.5	6	13	60	24	320		108	650
	0.5-1.0	9	20	71	28	500		98	850
Children	1-3	13	29	90	35	740		102	1300
	4-6	20	44	112	44	950		90	1800
	7-10	28	62	132	52	1130		70	2000
Males	11-14	45	99	157	62	1440	1.70	55	2500
	15-18	66	145	176	69	1760	1.67	45	3000
	19-24	72	160	177	70	1780	1.67	40	2900
	25-50	79	174	176	70	1800	1.60	37	2900
	51+	77	170	173	68	1530	1.50	30	2300
Females	11-14	46	101	157	62	1310	1.67	47	2200
	15-18	55	120	163	64	1370	1.60	40	2200
	19-24	58	128	164	65	1350	1.60	38	2200
	25-50	63	138	163	64	1380	1.55	36	2200
	51+	65	143	160	63	1280	1.50	30	1900
Pregnant	1st trimester								+0
	2nd trimester								+300
	3rd trimester								+300
Lactating	1st 6 months								+500
	2nd 6 months								+500

From Food and Nutrition Board, National Research Council: *Recommended dietary allowances,* ed 10, Washington, DC, 1989, National Academy of Sciences.
[a]Resting energy expenditure.
[b]In the range of light to moderate activity, the coefficient of variation is ±20%
[c]Figure is rounded.
The data in this table have been assembled from the observed median heights and weights of children together with desirable weights for adults for the mean heights of men (70 inches) and women (64 inches) between the ages of 18 and 34 years as surveyed in the United States population (HEW/NCHS data). The energy allowances for the young adults are for men and women doing light work. The allowances for the two older age-groups represent mean energy needs over these age spans, allowing for a 2% decrease in basal (resting) metabolic rate per decade and a reduction in activity of 200 kcal/day for men and women between 51 and 75 years of age, 500 kcal for men over 75, and 400 kcal for women over 75. The customary range of daily energy output is shown for adults in parentheses and is based on a variation in energy needs of ±400 kcal at any one age, emphasizing the wide range of energy intakes appropriate for any age group of people. Energy allowances for children through age 18 are based on medium energy intakes of children these ages followed in longitudinal growth studies.

APPENDIX

H NANDA-Approved Nursing Diagnoses 2001-2002

http://www.harcourthealth.com/MERLIN/Wong/maternal/

- Activity intolerance
- Activity intolerance, risk for
- Adjustment, impaired
- Airway clearance, ineffective
- Anxiety
- Anxiety, death
- Aspiration, risk for
- Body image, disturbed
- Body temperature, imbalanced, risk for
- Bowel incontinence
- Breastfeeding, effective
- Breastfeeding, ineffective
- Breastfeeding, interrupted
- Breathing pattern, ineffective
- Cardiac output, decreased
- Caregiver role strain
- Caregiver role strain, risk for
- Comfort, impaired
- Communication, impaired verbal
- Confusion, acute
- Confusion, chronic
- Constipation
- Constipation, perceived
- Constipation, risk for
- Coping, defensive
- Coping, ineffective community
- Coping, family, compromised
- Coping, family, disabled
- Coping, ineffective
- Coping, readiness for enhanced community
- Coping, readiness for enhanced family
- Decisional conflict
- Denial, ineffective
- Dentition, impaired
- Development, delayed, risk for
- Diarrhea
- Disuse syndrome, risk for
- Diversional activity, deficient
- Dysreflexia, autonomic
- Dysreflexia, autonomic, risk for
- Energy field, disturbed
- Environmental interpretation syndrome, impaired
- Failure to thrive, adult
- Falls, risk for
- Family processes, interrupted
- Family processes, dysfunctional: alcoholism
- Fatigue
- Fear
- Fluid volume, deficient
- Fluid volume, deficient, risk for
- Fluid volume excess
- Fluid volume imbalance, risk for
- Gas exchange, impaired
- Grieving
- Grieving, anticipatory
- Grieving, dysfunctional
- Growth, disproportionate, risk for
- Growth and development, delayed
- Health maintenance, ineffective
- Health-seeking behaviors
- Home maintenance, impaired
- Hopelessness
- Hyperthermia
- Hypothermia
- Incontinence, urinary, functional
- Incontinence, urinary, reflex
- Incontinence, urinary, stress
- Incontinence, urinary, total
- Incontinence, urinary urge
- Incontinence, urinary urge, risk for
- Infant behavior, disorganized
- Infant behavior, disorganized: risk for
- Infant behavior, organized: readiness for enhanced
- Infant feeding pattern, ineffective
- Infection, risk for
- Injury, perioperative positioning: risk for
- Injury, risk for
- Intracranial adaptive capacity, decreased
- Knowledge, deficient
- Latex allergy response
- Latex allergy response, risk for
- Loneliness, risk for
- Memory, impaired
- Mobility, impaired bed
- Mobility, impaired physical
- Mobility, impaired wheelchair
- Nausea
- Noncompliance
- Nutrition, imbalanced: less than body requirements
- Nutrition, imbalanced: more than body requirements
- Nutrition, imbalanced: risk for more than body requirements
- Oral mucous membrane, impaired
- Pain, acute
- Pain, chronic
- Parent/infant/child attachment, impaired: risk for
- Parental role conflict
- Parenting, impaired
- Parenting, impaired, risk for
- Peripheral neurovascular dysfunction, risk for
- Personal identity, disturbed
- Poisoning, risk for
- Post trauma syndrome
- Post trauma syndrome, risk for
- Powerlessness
- Powerlessness, risk for
- Protection, ineffective
- Rape-trauma syndrome
- Rape-trauma syndrome: compound reaction
- Rape-trauma syndrome: silent reaction
- Relocation stress syndrome
- Relocation stress syndrome, risk for
- Role performance, ineffective
- Self-care deficit, bathing/hygiene
- Self-care deficit, dressing/grooming
- Self-care deficit, feeding
- Self-care deficit, toileting
- Self-esteem, chronic low
- Self-esteem, situational low
- Self-esteem, situational low: risk for
- Self-mutilation
- Self-mutilation, risk for
- Sensory perception, disturbed
- Sexual dysfunction
- Sexuality patterns, ineffective
- Skin integrity, impaired
- Skin integrity, impaired, risk for
- Sleep deprivation
- Sleep pattern disturbed
- Social interaction, impaired
- Social isolation
- Sorrow, chronic
- Spiritual distress
- Spiritual distress, risk for
- Spiritual well-being, readiness for enhanced

North American Nursing Diagnosis Association: *Nursing diagnoses: definitions and classification* 2001-2002, Philadelphia, 2001, NANDA.

- Suffocation, risk for
- Suicide, risk for
- Surgical recovery, delayed
- Swallowing, impaired
- Therapeutic regimen management, community: ineffective
- Therapeutic regimen management, family: ineffective
- Therapeutic regimen management, effective
- Therapeutic regimen management; ineffective
- Thermoregulation, ineffective
- Thought processes, disturbed
- Tissue integrity, impaired
- Tissue perfusion, ineffective
- Transfer ability, impaired
- Trauma, risk for
- Unilateral neglect
- Urinary elimination, impaired
- Urinary retention
- Ventilation, impaired spontaneous
- Ventilatory weaning response, dysfunctional
- Violence, risk for: other-directed
- Violence, risk for: self-directed
- Walking, impaired
- Wandering

APPENDIX

I Translations of Faces Pain Rating Scale*

http://www.harcourthealth.com/MERLIN/Wong/maternal/

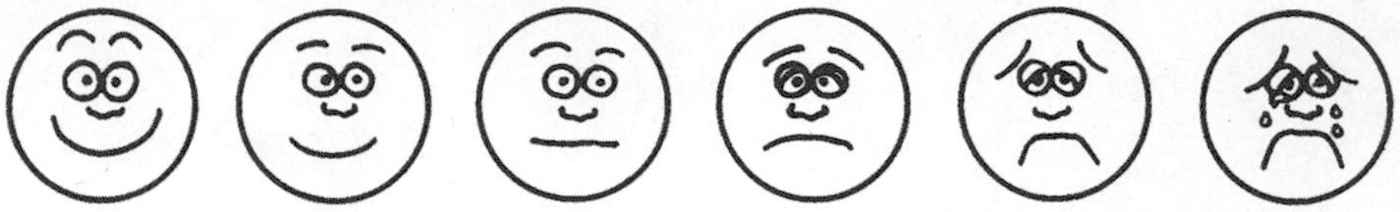

0–5 coding	0	1	2	3	4	5
0-10 coding	0	2	4	6	8	10

ENGLISH	No Hurt	Hurts Little Bit	Hurts Little More	Hurts Even More	Hurts Whole Lot	Hurts Worst
SPANISH	No duele	Duele un poco	Duele un poco más	Duele mucho	Duele mucho más	Duele el máximo
FRENCH	Ne fait pas mal	Fait mal un petit peu	Fait mal un petit plus	Fait mal encore plus	Fait beaucoup mal	Fait très, très mal
ITALIAN	Non fa male	Fa male un poco	Fa male un po di piu	Fa male ancora di piu	Fa molto male	Fa maggior-mente male
PORTUGUESE	Não doi	Doi um pouco	Doi um pouco mais	Doi muito	Doi muito mais	Doi o máximo
BOSNIAN	Ne boli	Boli samo malo	Boli malo više	Boli još više	Boli puno	Boli najviše
GREEK	Δεν Πονaï	Πονaï Λιγο	Πονaï Λιγο Πιο Πολν	Πονaï Πολν	Πονaï Πιο Πολν	Πονaï Παρa Πολν

BRIEF WORD INSTRUCTIONS (ABOVE):

Point to each face using the words to describe the pain intensity. Ask the child to choose face that best describes own pain and record the appropriate number. NOTE: Use of these instructions is recommended. Rating scale can be used with people 3 years and older.

ORIGINAL INSTRUCTIONS:

English

Explain to the person that each face is for a person who feels happy because he has no pain (hurt) or sad because he has some or a lot of pain. Face 0 is very happy because he doesn't hurt at all. Face 1 hurts just a little bit. Face 2 hurts a little more. Face 3 hurts even more. Face 4 hurts a whole lot. Face 5 hurts as much as you can imagine, although you don't have to be crying to feel this bad. Ask the person to choose the face that best describes how much hurt he has.

Rating scale is recommended for persons age 3 years and older.

---

*Wong-Baker FACES Pain Rating Scale: Available at no charge from The Purdue Frederick Company, 100 Connecticut Ave., Norwalk, CT 06850-3590; (230) 853-0123, ext. 7378 or 7314. Spanish and Portuguese translations by Ellen Johnsen; French translation by Thomas Angelo; Italian translation by Madeline Mitchko; Romanian translation by Bogdan R. Dinu; Bosnian translation by Barbara Bogomolor; Vietnamese translation by Yen B. Isle; Greek translation by Nicholas Mamalis; Chinese translation by Hung-Shen Lin; Japanese translation from *After the announcement of cancer,* Tokyo, 1993, Iwanami Shoten, Pub; German translation from Wong DL: *Pediatric quick reference,* Berlin, Wiesbaden, 1997, Ullstein Mosby.

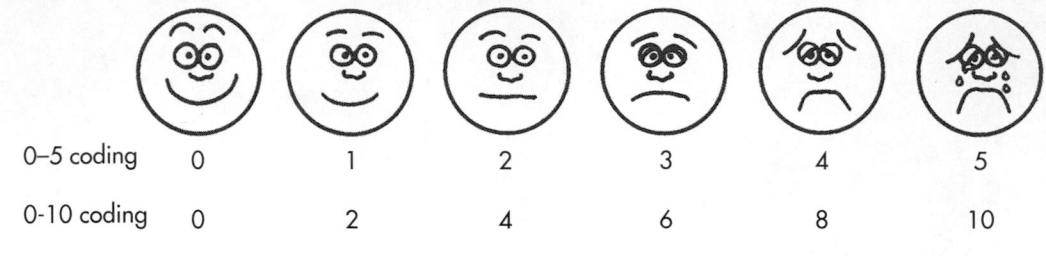

Spanish

Expliquele a la persona que cada cara representa una persona que se siente feliz porque no tiene dolor o triste porque siente un poco a mucho dolor. **Cara 0** se siente muy feliz porque no tiene dolor. **Cara 1** tiene un poco de dolor. **Cara 2** tiene un poquito más de dolor. Cara 3 tiene más dolor. **Cara 4** tiene mucho dolor. **Cara 5** tiene el dolor más fuerte que usted pueda imaginar, aunque usted no tiene que estar llorando para sentirse asi de mal. Pidale a la persona que escoja la cara que mejor describe su proprio dolor.

Esta escala se puede usar con personas de tres años de edad o más.

French

Expliquez á la personne que chaque visage représent un personne qui est heureux parce qu'elle n'a pas point du mal ou triste parce qu'il a un peu ou beaucoup du mal. **Visage 0** est trés heureux parce qu'elle n'a pas point du mal. **Visage 1** a un point peu de mal. **Visage 2** a plus du mal. **Visage 3** a encore plus du mal. **Visage 4** a beaucoup du mal. **Visage 5** a autant mal que vous pouvez imaginer, bien que ces mauvals sentiments ne finissent pas nécessairement a vous faire pleurer. Demandez à la personne de choisir le visage qui convient le mieux avec ses sentiments.

Ces evaluations sont recommendé pour des personnes de trois ans et davantage.

Italian

Spiegare a la persona che ogni facien è per una persona che si sente felice perchè non tiene dolore oppure triste penchè ha poco o molto dolore. **Faccia 0** è molto felice perchè non tiene dolore. **Faccia 1** tiene poco dolore. **Faccia 2** tiene un po più di dolore. **Faccia 3** tiene più dolore. **Faccia 4** tiene molto dolore. **Faccia 5** tiene molto dolore che non puoi immaginare però non devi piangere per tenere dolore. Domandi ala persona di scegliere quale faccia meglio descrive come si sente.

Grado scale è raccomandata a la persona di tre anni in sù.

Portuguese

Explique a pessoa que cada face representa uma pessoa que está feliz porque não têm dor, ou triste por ter um pouco ou muita dor. **Face 0** está muito feliz porque não têm nenhuma dor. **Face 1** tem apenas um pouco de dor. **Face 2** têm um pouco mais de dor. **Face 3** têm aioda mais dor. **Face 4** têm muita dor. **Face 5** têm uma dor máxima, apesar de que nem sempre provoca o choro. Peça a pessoa que escolhe a face que melhor descreve como ele se sente.

Esta escala é aplicável a pessoas de tres anos de idade ou mais.

Bosnian

Objasnite osobi da je svako lice namjenjeno za osobu koja se osjeća sretnom jer ne osjeća bol ili tužnom jer osjeća malo ili puno boli. Lice 0 je sretno jer ne osjeća nikakvu bol. Lice 1 osjeća samo malu bol. Lice 2 osjeća malo više boli. Lice 3 osjeća jos vecúbol. Lice 4 osjeća puno boli. Lice 5 osjeća onoliku bol koju je moguće zamisliti, što ne znaći da osoba koja osjeća tu bol mora plakati. Upitajte osobu da izabere lice koje najbolje opisuju kako se osjeća. Skala procijene bola se preporućuje za osobe starosti 3 godine ili više.

Upirati prstom na svako lice objašnjavajući riječima intensitet boli. Pitajte dijere da izabere lice koje najbolje opisuje njihovu bol i zabiljezue odgovarajući broj.

Vietnamese

Xin cắt nghỉa cho mổi người, từng khuôn mặt của một người cãm thấy vui vẽ tại vì không có sự đau đớn hoặc, buồn vì có chút ít hay rất nhiều sự đau đớn.

Cái **mặt** với **số 0** thì rất là vui tại vì mặt ấy không có sự đau đớn. **Mặt số 1** chỉ đau một chút thôi. **Mặt số 2** hơi đau hơn một chút nữa. **Mặt số 3** đau hơn chút nữa. **Mặt số 4** đau thật nhiều. **Mặt số 5** đau không thể tưởng tượng, mặc dù người ta không cần phải khóc mới cảm thấy được sự buồn khổ như thế.

Bạn hỏi từng người tự chọn khuôn mặt nào diển tả được sự đau đớn của chính mình.

Chinese

解釋給人聽用每張臉譜來代表著一個人的感覺是因爲沒有疼痛〔傷痛〕而感快樂或是因爲些許疼痛或者是許多疼痛而感傷心。第零張臉是很快樂的因爲他一點也不覺得疼痛。第一張臉只痛一丁點兒。第二張臉又痛多了一些。第三張臉痛得更多了。第四張臉是非常痛了。第五張臉是爲人們所能想像到的劇痛既使感到這樣難過，卻不一定哭出來。請這人選擇出最能代表他現在感覺的一張臉譜。此量表適用於三歲以上的人。

Japanese

3歳以上の患者に望ましい。それぞれの顔は、患者の痛み(pain, hurt)がないのでご機嫌な感じ、または、ある程度の痛み・沢山の痛みがあるので悲しい感じを表現していることを説明して下さい。0＝痛みがまったくないから、とても幸せな顔をしている、1＝ほんの少し痛い、2＝もう少し痛い、3＝もっと痛い、4＝とっても痛い、5＝痛くて涙を流す必要はないけれども、これ以上の痛みは考えられないほど痛い。今、どのように感じているか最もよく表わしている顔を選ぶよう、患者に求めて下さい。

Romanian

Explică persoanei că fiecare faţă este specifică diferitelor stări fizice; o persoană este ferioita pentru că nu are nici o durere ori tristă pentru că suferă puţin sau mai mult. **Faţa 0** este foarte ferioită pentru că nu are absolut nici o durere. **Faţa 1** are un pic de durere. **Faţa 2** are ceva mai mult. **Faţa 3** suferă şi mai mult. **Faţa 4** suferă foarte mult. **Faţa 5** este greu de imaginat cât de mult suferă, căci nu trebuie neapărat să plângi, oricat de tare te-ar dureă. Intreabă persoana să indice figura care-i desorie cel mai bine starea fizică.

Acest **grad de durere** este racomandat pentru persoanele de la 3 ani în sus.

German

Erläutern Sie dem Kind, daβ jedes Gesicht zu einer Person gehört, die froh darüber ist, keine Schmerzen zu haben, oder die sehr traurig ist, weil sie mäβige bis starke Schmerzen hat. **Gesicht 0** ist sehr froh, weil es keine Schmerzen hat. **Gesicht 1** sagt, es tut ein biβchen weh. **Gesicht 2** hat ein biβchen mehr Schmerzen. **Gesicht 3** sagt, es tut noch mehr weh, und **Gesicht 4**, es tut ziemlich weh. **Geisicht 5** leidet unter so starken Schmerzen, wie Du Dir nur vorstellen kannst, auch wenn dabei nicht unbedingt Tränen flieβen müssen. Bitten Sie das Kind, das Gesicht auszuwählen, das seinem Empfinden am besten entspricht. Empfohlen für Kinder ab 3 Jahren.

APPENDIX

J Pediatric Vital Signs and Parameters

http://www.harcourthealth.com/MERLIN/Wong/maternal/

Normal Temperatures in Children

Age	°F—Temperature—°C	
3 months	99.4	37.5
6 months	99.5	37.5
1 year	99.7	37.7
3 years	99.0	37.2
5 years	98.6	37.0
7 years	98.3	36.8
9 years	98.1	36.7
11 years	98.0	36.7
13 years	97.8	36.6

Modified from Lowrey GH: *Growth and development of children,* ed 8, St Louis, 1986, Mosby.

Centigrade to Fahrenheit Temperature Conversions

°C	°F	°C	°F	°C	°F
35.0	**95.0**	**37.0**	**98.6**	**39.0**	**102.2**
35.2	95.4	37.2	99.0	39.2	102.6
35.4	95.7	37.4	99.3	39.4	102.9
35.6	96.1	37.6	99.7	39.6	103.3
35.8	96.4	37.8	100.0	39.8	103.6
36.0	96.8	38.0	100.4	40.0	104.0
36.2	**97.2**	**38.2**	**100.8**	**40.2**	**104.4**
36.4	97.5	38.4	101.1	40.4	104.7
36.6	97.9	38.6	101.5	40.6	105.1
36.8	98.2	38.8	101.8	40.8	105.4
				41.0	**105.8**

CONVERSION FORMULAS
°F = (°C × $^9/_5$) + 32 or (°C × 1.8) + 32
°C = (°F − 32) × $^5/_9$ or (°F − 32) × 0.55

Normal Heart Rates for Infants and Children

Age	Rate (Beats/Min)		
	Resting (Awake)	Resting (Sleeping)	Exercise (Fever)
Newborn	100-180	80-160	Up to 220
1 week to 3 months	100-220	80-200	Up to 220
3 months to 2 years	80-150	70-120	Up to 200
2 years to 10 years	70-110	60-90	Up to 200
10 years to adult	55-90	50-90	Up to 200

From Gillette PC: Dysrhythmias. In Adams FH, Emmanoulides GC, Riemenschneider TA, editors: *Moss, heart disease in infants, children, and adolescents,* ed 4, Baltimore, 1989, Williams & Wilkins.

Normal Respiratory Rates for Children

Age	Rate (Breaths/Min)
Newborn	35
1 to 11 months	30
2 years	25
4 years	23
6 years	21
8 years	20
10 years	19
12 years	19
14 years	18
16 years	17
18 years	16-18

Normal Blood Pressure Readings for Children—Girls

		Systolic BP (mm Hg)							Diastolic BP (mm Hg)						
Age	Height Percentiles*→ BP† ↓	5%	10%	25%	50%	75%	90%	95%	5%	10%	25%	50%	75%	90%	95%
1	90th	97	98	99	100	102	103	104	53	53	53	54	55	56	56
	95th	101	102	103	104	105	107	107	57	57	57	58	59	60	60
2	90th	99	99	100	102	103	104	105	57	57	58	58	59	60	61
	95th	102	103	104	105	107	108	109	61	61	62	62	63	64	65
3	90th	100	100	102	103	104	105	106	61	61	61	62	63	63	64
	95th	104	104	105	107	108	109	110	65	65	65	66	67	67	68
4	90th	101	102	103	104	106	107	108	63	63	64	65	65	66	67
	95th	105	106	107	108	109	111	111	67	67	68	69	69	70	71
5	90th	103	103	104	106	107	108	109	65	66	66	67	68	68	69
	95th	107	107	108	110	111	112	113	69	70	70	71	72	72	73
6	90th	104	105	106	107	109	110	111	67	67	68	69	69	70	71
	95ty	108	109	110	111	112	114	114	71	71	72	73	73	74	75
7	90th	106	107	108	109	110	112	112	69	69	69	70	71	72	72
	95th	110	110	112	113	114	115	116	73	73	73	74	75	76	76
8	90th	108	109	110	111	112	113	114	70	70	71	71	72	73	74
	95th	112	112	113	115	116	117	118	74	74	75	75	76	77	78
9	90th	110	110	112	113	114	115	116	71	72	72	73	74	74	75
	95th	114	114	115	117	118	119	120	75	76	76	77	78	78	79
10	90th	112	112	114	115	116	117	118	73	73	73	74	75	76	76
	95th	116	116	117	119	120	121	122	77	77	77	78	79	80	80
11	90th	114	114	116	117	118	119	120	74	74	75	75	76	77	77
	95th	118	118	119	121	122	123	124	78	78	79	79	80	81	81
12	90th	116	116	118	119	120	121	122	75	75	76	76	77	78	78
	95th	120	120	121	123	124	125	126	79	79	80	80	81	82	82
13	90th	118	118	119	121	122	123	124	76	76	77	78	78	79	80
	95th	121	122	123	125	126	127	128	80	80	81	82	82	83	84
14	90th	119	120	121	122	124	125	126	77	77	78	79	79	80	81
	95th	123	124	125	126	128	129	130	81	81	82	83	83	84	85
15	90th	121	121	122	124	125	126	127	78	78	79	79	80	81	82
	95th	124	125	126	128	129	130	131	82	82	83	83	84	85	86
16	90th	122	122	123	125	126	127	128	79	79	79	80	81	82	82
	95th	125	126	127	128	130	131	132	83	83	83	84	85	86	86
17	90th	122	123	124	125	126	128	128	79	79	79	80	81	82	82
	95th	126	126	127	129	130	131	132	83	83	83	84	85	86	86

From the update on the Task Force Report (1987) on High Blood Pressure in Children and Adolescents: A Working Group Report from the National High Blood Pressure Education Program. NIH Pub. No. 96-3790, September 1996, National Heart, Lung and Blood Institute, Bethesda, MD.
*Height percentile determined by standard growth curves.
†Blood pressure percentile determined by a single measurement.

Normal Blood Pressure Readings for Children—Boys

		Systolic BP (MM Hg)							Diastolic BP (MM Hg)						
Age	Height Percentiles*→ BP† ↓	5%	10%	25%	50%	75%	90%	95%	5%	10%	25%	50%	75%	90%	95%
1	90th	94	95	97	98	100	102	102	50	51	52	53	54	54	55
	95th	98	99	101	102	104	106	106	55	55	56	57	58	59	59
2	90th	98	99	100	102	104	105	106	55	55	56	57	58	59	59
	95th	101	102	104	106	108	109	110	59	59	60	61	62	63	63
3	90th	100	101	103	105	107	108	109	59	59	60	61	62	63	63
	95th	104	105	107	109	111	112	113	63	63	64	65	66	67	67
4	90th	102	103	105	107	109	110	111	62	62	63	64	65	66	66
	95th	106	107	109	111	113	114	115	66	67	67	68	69	70	71
5	90th	104	105	106	108	110	112	112	65	65	66	67	68	69	69
	95th	108	109	110	112	114	115	116	69	70	70	71	72	73	74
6	90th	105	106	108	110	111	113	114	67	68	69	70	70	71	72
	95th	109	110	112	114	115	117	117	72	72	73	74	75	76	76
7	90th	106	107	109	111	113	114	115	69	70	71	72	72	73	74
	95th	110	111	113	115	116	118	119	74	74	75	76	77	78	78
8	90th	107	108	110	112	114	115	116	71	71	72	73	74	75	75
	95th	111	112	114	116	118	119	120	75	76	76	77	78	79	80
9	90th	109	110	112	113	115	117	117	72	73	73	74	75	76	77
	95th	113	114	116	117	119	121	121	76	77	78	79	80	80	81
10	90th	110	112	113	115	117	118	119	73	74	74	75	76	77	78
	95th	114	115	117	119	121	122	123	77	78	79	80	80	81	82
11	90th	112	113	115	117	119	120	121	74	74	75	76	77	78	78
	95th	116	117	119	121	123	124	125	78	79	79	80	81	82	83
12	90th	115	116	117	119	121	123	123	75	75	76	77	78	78	79
	95th	119	120	121	123	125	126	127	79	79	80	81	82	83	83
13	90th	117	118	120	122	124	125	126	75	76	76	77	78	79	80
	95th	121	122	124	126	128	129	130	79	80	81	82	83	83	84
14	90th	120	121	123	125	126	128	128	76	76	77	78	79	80	80
	95th	124	125	127	128	130	132	132	80	81	81	82	83	84	85
15	90th	123	124	125	127	129	131	131	77	77	78	79	80	81	81
	95th	127	128	129	131	133	134	135	81	82	83	83	84	85	86
16	90th	125	126	128	130	132	133	134	79	79	80	81	82	82	83
	95th	129	130	132	134	136	137	138	83	83	84	85	86	87	87
17	90th	128	129	131	133	134	136	136	81	81	82	83	84	85	85
	95th	132	133	135	136	138	140	140	85	85	86	87	88	89	89

From the update on the Task Force Report (1987) on High Blood Pressure in Children and Adolescents: A Working Group Report from the National High Blood Pressure Education Program. NIH Pub. No.96-3790, September 1996, National Heart, Lung and Blood Insitute, Bethesda, MD.
*Height percentile determined by standard growth curves.
†Blood pressure percentile determined by a single measurement.

Index

Page numbers followed by *b* indicate boxes; *f* indicates figures; *t* indicates tables.

C

H

J

P

S

Critical Thinking

MATERNITY

PEDIATRICS

Community Focus

MATERNITY

PEDIATRICS